MANUAL OF Molecular AND Clinical Laboratory Immunology

7TH EDITION

MANUAL OF Molecular AND Clinical Laboratory Immunology

7TH EDITION

EDITORS

Barbara Detrick
Johns Hopkins University, School of Medicine
Baltimore, MD

Robert G. Hamilton
Johns Hopkins University, School of Medicine
Baltimore, MD

James D. Folds
University of North Carolina, School of Medicine
University of North Carolina Hospitals
Chapel Hill, NC

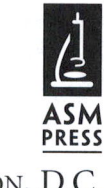

ASM PRESS

WASHINGTON, D.C.

Library of Congress Cataloging-in-Publication Data

Manual of molecular and clinical laboratory immunology / editors, Barbara Detrick, Robert G. Hamilton, and James D. Folds.—7th ed.
    p. ; cm.
  Rev. ed. of: Manual of clinical laboratory immunology. 6th ed. c2002.
  Includes bibliographical references and index.
  ISBN-13: 978-1-55581-364-2
  ISBN-10: 1-55581-364-X
    1. Immunodiagnosis—Handbooks, manuals, etc. 2. Immunology—Handbooks, manuals, etc.
3. Molecular immunology—Handbooks, manuals, etc.
  [DNLM: 1. Immunologic Techniques—Laboratory Manuals. 2. Immunologic
Tests—methods—Laboratory Manuals. QW 525 M2925 2006] I. Detrick, Barbara. II. Hamilton,
Robert G. III. Folds, James D. IV. Manual of clinical laboratory immunology.
RB46.5.M36 2006
616.07′56—dc22

                      2005037941

10 9 8 7 6 5 4 3 2 1

Address editorial correspondence to: ASM Press, 1752 N St., N.W., Washington, DC 20036-2904, U.S.A.

Send orders to: ASM Press, P.O. Box 605, Herndon, VA 20172, U.S.A.
Phone: 800-546-2416; 703-661-1593
Fax: 703-661-1501
Email: Books@asmusa.org
Online: estore.asm.org

Contents

Editorial Board

Contributors

JOSEPH W. ADELSBERGER
Clinical Services Program, NCI-Frederick, SAIC Frederick, Inc., P.O. Box B, Frederick, MD 21702-1201

JOHN ALTMAN
Emory Vaccine Center, 954 Gatewood Rd., Atlanta, GA 30329

BURT E. ANDERSON
Dept. of Medical Microbiology and Immunology, University of South Florida College of Medicine, MDC Box 10, 12901 Bruce B. Downs Blvd., Tampa, FL 33612

GRANT J. ANHALT
Dept. of Dermatology, Johns Hopkins School of Medicine, Ross Research Bldg., Room 771, 720 Rutland Ave., Baltimore, MD 21205

AFTAB A. ANSARI
Dept. of Pathology and Laboratory Medicine, Emory University School of Medicine, Atlanta, GA 30322

MARY D. ARI
Meningitis and Special Pathogens Branch, Division of Bacterial and Mycotic Diseases, National Center for Infectious Diseases, Centers for Disease Control and Prevention, Atlanta, GA 30333

WILLIAM M. BALDWIN, III
Transplantation Laboratory, Dept. of Pathology, Johns Hopkins School of Medicine, Ross Research Bldg., Room 659B, 720 Rutland Ave., Baltimore, MD 21205-2196

MICHAEL W. BASELER
Applied and Developmental Research Program, SAIC-Frederick, Inc., P.O. Box B, Bldg. 469-6, NCI-FCRDC, Frederick, MD 21701

LEE ANN BAXTER-LOWE
Immunogenetics & Transplantation Laboratory, University of California, San Francisco, Box 0508, San Francisco, CA 94143-0508

MAURO BENDINELLI
Dept. of Experimental Pathology and Retrovirus Center, University of Pisa, 37, Via San Zeno, I-56127 Pisa, Italy

DEBORAH L. BIRX
U.S. Military HIV Research Program, Walter Reed Army Institute of Research, 13 Taft Court, Rockville, MD 20850

GUY BOIVIN
Centre de Recherche en Infectiologie, Centre Hospitalier Universitaire de Québec, and Dept. of Medical Biology, Laval University, Québec City, Quebec G1V 4G2, Canada

GRAHAM H. BOTHAMLEY
NE London TB Network, Homerton University Hospital, Homerton Row, London E9 6SR, United Kingdom

ARTHUR R. BRADWELL
Dept. of Immunology, The Medical School, University of Birmingham, Vincent Drive, Birmingham B15 2TJ, United Kingdom

RICHARD A. BRONSON
Dept. of Obstetrics and Gynecology and Dept. of Pathology, Health Science Center, State University of New York, Stony Brook, NY 11794-8091

MARY B. BROWN
Dept. of Pathobiology, College of Veterinary Medicine, University of Florida, Gainesville, FL 32611-0880

C. LYNNE BUREK
Dept. of Pathology, Johns Hopkins University School of Medicine, 648 Ross Research Building, 720 Rutland Ave., Baltimore, MD 21205

ANDREW W. O. BURGESS
Dept. of Medical Microbiology and Immunology, University of South Florida College of Medicine, MDC Box 10, 12901 Bruce B. Downs Blvd., Tampa, FL 33612

RUFUS W. BURLINGAME
INOVA Diagnostics, Inc., San Diego, CA 92131-1638

LEE ANN CAMPBELL
Dept. of Pathobiology, Box 357238, Room F-161F, Health Sciences Bldg., 1959 N.E. Pacific St., University of Washington, Seattle, WA 98195

KAI CAO
CW Bill Young Marrow Donor Recruitment and Research Program and Dept. of Oncology, Georgetown University Medical Center, E404 Research Bldg., 3970 Reservoir Rd., NW, Washington, DC 20057

MARY CARRINGTON
Laboratory of Genomic Diversity, SAIC-Frederick, Inc., National Cancer Institute, Frederick, MD 21702

CHI-CHAO CHAN
Immunopathology Section, Laboratory of Immunology, National Eye Institute, National Institutes of Health, Building 10-Room 10N103, Bethesda, MD 20892

DANIEL W. CHAN
Dept. of Pathology, Division of Clinical Chemistry, Johns Hopkins University School of Medicine, 600 North Wolfe St., Meyer B-121, Baltimore, MD 21287-7065

EDWARD K. L. CHAN
Dept. of Oral Biology, University of Florida, P.O. Box 100424, Gainesville, FL 32610-0424

CHUNG-CHE (JEFF) CHANG
Dept. of Pathology, Methodist Hospital/Baylor College of Medicine, 6565 Fannin, MS 205, Houston, TX 77030

STEPHEN J. CHANOCK
Pediatric Oncology Branch and Advanced Technology Center, National Cancer Institute, 8717 Grovemont Circle, Bethesda, MD 20892-4605

KEVIN CHESTERTON
Immunogenetics Laboratory, Dept. of Medicine, Johns Hopkins University School of Medicine, 2041 E. Monument St., Baltimore, MD 21205-2222

MARIAN S. CHIN
Immunology & Virology Section, Laboratory of Immunology, National Eye Institute, National Institutes of Health, Building 10-Room 10N248, Bethesda, MD 20892

IAN CHIN-YEE
The London Health Sciences Centre, London, Ontario N6A 4G5, Canada

A. BERNARD COLLINS
Dept. of Pathology, Massachusetts General Hospital and Harvard Medical School, 32 Fruit St., Boston, MA 02114

ROBERT B. COLVIN
Dept. of Pathology, Massachusetts General Hospital and Harvard Medical School, 32 Fruit St., Boston, MA 02114

MARY ELLEN CONLEY
Dept. of Pediatrics, University of Tennessee College of Medicine, and Dept. of Immunology, St. Jude Children's Research Hospital, 332 N. Lauderdale, Memphis, TN 38105

LINDA COOK
Molecular Virology Laboratory, Seattle Cancer Care Alliance, Fred Hutchinson Cancer Research Center, Seattle, WA 98109

ROSS L. COPPEL
Dept. of Microbiology, Monash University, Clayton, Victoria, Australia

JOSEPHINE H. COX
U.S. Military HIV Research Program, Henry M. Jackson Foundation for the Advancement of Military Medicine, 13 Taft Court, Rockville, MD 20850

NANCY J. COX
Influenza Branch, Division of Viral and Rickettsial Diseases, National Center for Infectious Diseases, Centers for Disease Control and Prevention, 1600 Clifton Rd., Mail Stop G16, Atlanta, GA 30333

LETA K. CRAWFORD-MIKSZA
Food and Drug Laboratory Branch, California Dept. of Health Services, 850 Marina Bay Parkway, Richmond, CA 94804

JOHN T. CURNUTTE
Schering-Plough Biopharma, 901 California Ave., Palo Alto, CA 94304-1104

JEFFREY R. CURRIER
Henry M. Jackson Foundation, 13 Taft Ct., Suite 200, Rockville, MD 20850

DARSHANA DADHANIA
Division of Nephrology, Dept. of Medicine, Weill Medical College of Cornell University, and Dept. of Transplantation Medicine and Extracorporeal Therapy, New York-Presbyterian Hospital, New York, NY 10021

M. R. DAHA
Dept. of Nephrology, C3P-29, Leiden University Medical Center, Albinusdreef 2, 2333 ZA Leiden, The Netherlands

DEREK A. DAMIN
Private Practice, Kentuckiana Allergy, PSC, Louisville, KY 40222

INGER K. DAMON
Poxvirus Program, Division of Viral and Rickettsial Diseases, Centers for Disease Control and Prevention, 1600 Clifton Rd., Mail Stop G-43, Atlanta, GA 30333

RICHARD T. DAVEY, JR.
Office of Clinical Research, National Institute of Allergy and Infectious Diseases, National Institutes of Health, Bethesda, MD 20892

STEPHEN DEALLER
Pathology Dept., Royal Lancaster Infirmary and University of Lancaster, Lancaster LA1 4RP, United Kingdom

MARK DESOUZA
U.S. Military HIV Research Program, Armed Forces Research Institute of Medical Sciences, 315/6 Rajvithi Rd., Bangkok 10400, Thailand

BARBARA DETRICK
Immunology Laboratory, Dept. of Pathology/Meyer B125, Johns Hopkins University School of Medicine, 600 N. Wolfe St., Baltimore, MD 21205

NICOLETTE C. DEVORE
Center for Biologics Evaluation and Research, U.S. Food and Drug Administration, 29 Lincoln Dr., Bethesda, MD 20892

ROBIN L. DEWAR
Clinical Services Program, NCI-Frederick, SAIC Frederick, Inc., P.O. Box B, Frederick, MD 21702-1201

STEVEN D. DOUGLAS
Division of Allergy-Immunology, Clinical Immunology Laboratories, The Children's Hospital of Philadelphia, Dept. of Pediatrics, University of Pennsylvania School of Medicine, 3615 Civic Center Blvd., Abramson Bldg., Rm 1208, Philadelphia, PA 19104-4318

BRUCE E. DUNN
Dept. of Pathology, Medical College of Wisconsin, 8700 W. Wisconsin Ave., Milwaukee, WI 53226, and Veterans Integrated Service Network 12, Clement J. Zablocki VA Medical Center, 5000 W. National Ave., Milwaukee, WI 53295-1000

PAUL H. EDELSTEIN
Dept. of Pathology and Laboratory Medicine and Dept. of Medicine, University of Pennsylvania School of Medicine, Philadelphia, PA 19104-4283

TAREK ELBEIK
Dept. of Laboratory Medicine, University of California, San Francisco, and San Francisco General Hospital, Bldg. NH, Room 2M35, 1001 Potrero Ave., San Francisco, CA 94110

MELISSA E. ELDER
Division of Immunology, Rheumatology, and Infectious Diseases, Dept. of Pediatrics, University of Florida Health Sciences Center, 1600 SW Archer Rd., R1-118, Gainesville, FL 32610-0296

ANDREW L. FELDMAN
Laboratory of Pathology, Center for Cancer Research, National Cancer Institute, and FDA-NCI Clinical Proteomics Program, Bethesda, MD 20892

HEINZ FELDMANN
Special Pathogens Program, National Microbiology Laboratory, Public Health Agency of Canada, and Dept. of Medical Microbiology, University of Manitoba, Winnipeg, Manitoba R3E 3R2, Canada

NINGGUO FENG
Division of Gastroenterology and Hepatology, Stanford University School of Medicine, 300 Pasteur Dr., Stanford, CA 94305-5187

GUIDO FERRARI
Dept. of Surgery, P.O. Box 2926, Duke University Medical Center, Durham, NC 27710-2996

BOURKE L. FIRFER
Dept. of Pathology, Stroger Hospital of Cook County, Rosalind Franklin University of Medicine and Science, Chicago, Illinois

DAVID M. FLEISCHER
Dept. of Pediatric Allergy and Immunology, Johns Hopkins Hospital, CMSC 1102, 600 N. Wolfe St., Baltimore, MD 21287

THOMAS A. FLEISHER
Dept. of Laboratory Medicine, Clinical Center, National Institutes of Health, Bethesda, MD 20892-1508

CARL E. FRASCH
Laboratory of Bacterial Polysaccharides, Center for Biologics Evaluation and Research, Mailstop HFM-428, 1401 Rockville Pike, Rockville, MD 20852

GIULIA FREER
Dept. of Experimental Pathology and Retrovirus Center, University of Pisa, 37, Via San Zeno, I-56127 Pisa, Italy

MARVIN J. FRITZLER
Dept. of Biochemistry and Molecular Biology, University of Calgary, HRB 410B, 3330 Hospital Dr. NW, Calgary, Alberta T2N 4N1, Canada

MIHAELA GADJEVA
New Research Building, Brigham and Women's Hospital, 77 Louis Pasteur, Room 652, Boston, MA 02115

DENNIS GALANAKIS
Dept. of Pathology, State University of New York at Stony Brook, Stony Brook, NY 11794

CHARLOTTE A. GAYDOS
Division of Infectious Diseases, School of Medicine, Johns Hopkins University, Baltimore, MD 21205

M. ERIC GERSHWIN
Division of Rheumatology/Allergy and Clinical Immunology, School of Medicine, University of California at Davis, Davis, CA 95616

SMITA A. GHANEKAR
BD Biosciences Immunocytometry Systems, 2350 Qume Dr., San Jose, CA 95131

PATRICIA C. GICLAS
Clinical Reference Laboratories, Complement Laboratory, Dept. of Pediatrics, Division of Allergy and Immunology, National Jewish Medical and Research Center, 1400 N. Jackson, Denver, CO 80206-2761

JAMES A. GOEKEN
Dept. of Pathology, University of Iowa Healthcare, 5231-G RCP, 200 Hawkins Dr., Iowa City, IA 52242-1009

JUDITH A. GOODSHIP
Institute of Human Genetics, University of Newcastle upon Tyne, Newcastle upon Tyne NE1 3BZ, United Kingdom

TIMOTHY H. J. GOODSHIP
Institute of Human Genetics, International Centre for Life, University of Newcastle upon Tyne, Central Parkway, Newcastle upon Tyne NE1 3BZ, United Kingdom

PETER D. GOREVIC
Division of Rheumatology, The Mount Sinai Medical Center, Annenberg Building, Room 5-207M, Box 1244, 1425 Madison Ave., New York, NY 10029-6574

JAN GRATAMA
Dept. of Medical Oncology, Erasmus MC - Daniel den Hoed Cancer Center, Rotterdam, The Netherlands

ALLEN GROLLA
Special Pathogens Program, National Microbiology Laboratory, Public Health Agency of Canada, Winnipeg, Manitoba, Canada

PAULETTE HAHN
Division of Rheumatology & Clinical Immunology, University of Florida, P.O. Box 100221, Gainesville, FL 32610-0221

SCOTT A. HALPERIN
Dept. of Pediatrics and Dept. of Microbiology & Immunology, Dalhousie University and the IWK Health Centre, 5850/5980 University Ave., Halifax, Nova Scotia, Canada B3K 6R8

ROBERT G. HAMILTON
Johns Hopkins University School of Medicine, Johns Hopkins Asthma & Allergy Center, DACI Reference Laboratory, 5501 Hopkins Bayview Circle/Room 1A20, Baltimore, MD 21224-6801

RONALD J. HARBECK
Dept. of Medicine and Immunology, Clinical Laboratories, National Jewish Medical and Research Center, 1400 Jackson St., Denver, CO 80206

CHOLI HARTONO
Division of Nephrology, Dept. of Medicine, Weill Medical College of Cornell University, and Dept. of Transplantation Medicine and Extracorporeal Therapy, New York-Presbyterian Hospital, New York, NY 10021

KARIM E. HECHEMY
Division of Infectious Disease, Wadsworth Center, New York State Dept. of Health, 120 New Scotland Ave., Albany, NY 12208

RICHARD L. HENGEL
Infectious Disease Solutions, 35 Collier Rd., Suite M245, Atlanta, GA 30309

PAUL G. HEYWORTH
Schering-Plough Biopharma, 901 California Ave., Palo Alto, CA 94304-1104

JEANETTE HIGGINS
Clinical Services Program, NCI-Frederick, SAIC Frederick, Inc., P.O. Box B, Frederick, MD 21702-1201

HELENE C. HIGHBARGER
Clinical Services Program, NCI-Frederick, SAIC-Frederick, Inc., P.O. Box B, Frederick, MD 21702-1201

BRIAN HJELLE
Depts. of Pathology, Molecular Genetics & Microbiology, and Biology, University of New Mexico School of Medicine, MSCO8 4640, 1 University of New Mexico, Albuquerque, NM 87131

RICHARD L. HODINKA
Dept. of Pediatrics and Dept. of Pathology, Clinical Virology Laboratory, Children's Hospital of Philadelphia, and University of Pennsylvania School of Medicine, Abramson Research Center, Rm 716D, 3615 Civic Center Blvd., Philadelphia, PA 19104-4399

ALEX R. HOFFMASTER
Meningitis and Special Pathogens Branch, National Center for Infectious Diseases, Centers for Disease Control and Prevention, 1600 Clifton Rd., MS G34, Atlanta, GA 30333

AKI HOJI
Dept. of Infectious Diseases and Microbiology, University of Pittsburgh Graduate School of Public Health, Pittsburgh, PA 15261

STEVEN M. HOLLAND
Laboratory of Clinical Infectious Diseases, National Institute of Allergy and Infectious Diseases, National Institutes of Health, Bldg. 10, CRC B3-4141, MSC 1684, 10 Center Dr., Bethesda, MD 20892-1684

JOHN J. HOOKS
Immunology & Virology Section, Laboratory of Immunology, National Eye Institute, National Institutes of Health, Bldg. 10, Room 10N248, Bethesda, MD 20892

D. CRAIG HOOPER
Center for Neurovirology, Dept. of Microbiology and Immunology, Thomas Jefferson University, 1020 Locust St., Room 454, Philadelphia, PA 19107-6799

GLEN L. HORTIN
Dept. of Laboratory Medicine, Warren G. Magnusson Clinical Center, National Institutes of Health, 10 Center Dr., MSC 1508, Bethesda, MD 20892-1508

JULIE A. HOUP
Immunogenetics Laboratory, Dept. of Medicine, Johns Hopkins University School of Medicine, 2041 E. Monument St., Baltimore, MD 21205-2222

C. ALAN HOWARD
National Marrow Donor Program, Minneapolis, MN 55413

ERIC D. HSI
Depts. of Anatomic and Clinical Pathology, Cleveland Clinic Foundation, L-11, 9500 Euclid Ave., Cleveland, OH 44195

PATRICIA A. HUGHES
Dept. of Pediatrics, Section of Infectious Disease, Albany Medical Center, Room A-615, MC 88, 47 New Scotland Ave., Albany, NY 12208

RICHARD G. HUGHES
The Binding Site Ltd., P.O. Box 11712, Birmingham B14 4ZB, United Kingdom

LANCE HULTIN
Dept. of Medicine, Cellular Immunology and Cytometry, University of California, Los Angeles, 12-236 Factor Bldg., 10833 Le Conte Ave., Los Angeles, CA 90095-1745

PATRICIA HULTIN
Dept. of Medicine, Cellular Immunology and Cytometry, University of California, Los Angeles, 12-236 Factor Bldg., 10833 Le Conte Ave., Los Angeles, CA 90095-1745

RICHARD L. HUMPHREY
Johns Hopkins Hospital, Meyer B121C, 600 N. Wolfe St., Baltimore, MD 21287-7021

CAROLYN KATOVICH HURLEY
CW Bill Young Marrow Donor Recruitment and Research Program and Dept. of Oncology, Georgetown University Medical Center, E404 Research Bldg., 3970 Reservoir Rd., NW, Washington, DC 20057

HIROMI IMAMICHI
Clinical Services Program, NCI-Frederick, SAIC-Frederick, Inc., P.O. Box B, Frederick, MD 21702-1201

TOMOZUMI IMAMICHI
Clinical Services Program, NCI-Frederick, SAIC-Frederick, Inc., P.O. Box B, Frederick, MD 21702-1201

ELAINE S. JAFFE
Hematopathology Section, Laboratory of Pathology, National Cancer Institute, 10 Center Dr., Bldg. 10, Room 2N110, MSC-1500, Bethesda, MD 20892-1500

PETER B. JAHRLING
U.S. Army Medical Research Institute of Infectious Diseases, Fort Detrick, Frederick, MD 21702

HAL B. JENSON
Baystate Health and Tufts University School of Medicine, Western Campus, Springfield, MA 01199

BARBARA J. B. JOHNSON
Div. of Vector-Borne Infectious Diseases, National Center for Infectious Diseases, Centers for Disease Control and Prevention, Fort Collins, CO 80522

ANDRÉ A. KAJDACSY-BALLA
Dept. of Pathology, University of Illinois Medical Center at Chicago, 1819 West Polk St., Room 446, Chicago, IL 60612-7335

EDWARD KAPLAN
Dept. of Pediatrics, University of Minnesota Medical School, World Health Organization Collaborating Center for Reference and Research on Streptococci, 420 Delaware St., S.E., Minneapolis, MN 55455

KEVIN L. KAREM
Poxvirus Program, Division of Viral and Rickettsial Diseases, Centers for Disease Control and Prevention, 1600 Clifton Rd., Mail Stop G-43, Atlanta, GA 30333

A. R. KARIM
Dept. of Neuroimmunology, The Medical School, Edgbaston, Birmingham, United Kingdom

JACQUELINE M. KATZ
Influenza Branch, Division of Viral and Rickettsial Diseases, National Center for Infectious Diseases, Centers for Disease Control and Prevention, 1600 Clifton Rd., Mail Stop G16, Atlanta, GA 30333

JERRY A. KATZMANN
Protein Immunology Laboratory, Mayo Clinic College of Medicine, 210F Hilton Bldg., 200 First St. SW, Rochester, MN 55905

MICHAEL KEENEY
The London Health Sciences Centre, London, Ontario N6A 4G5, Canada

DAVID F. KEREN
Warde Medical Laboratory, 300 West Textile Rd., Ann Arbor, MI 48108-9548

THOMAS S. KICKLER
Dept. of Pathology, Johns Hopkins University School of Medicine, Weinberg Bldg. Room 2337, 600 N. Wolfe St., Baltimore, MD 21205

THOMAS J. KIPPS
Dept. of Medicine, Division of Hematology/Oncology, Moores Cancer Center, University of California-San Diego School of Medicine, 9500 Gilman Dr., La Jolla, CA 94093-0663

ALEXANDER I. KLIMOV
Influenza Branch, Division of Viral and Rickettsial Diseases, National Center for Infectious Diseases, Centers for Disease Control and Prevention, 1600 Clifton Rd., Mail Stop G16, Atlanta, GA 30333

AMY D. KLION
Laboratory of Parasitic Diseases, Bldg. 4, Room 126, National Institute of Allergy and Infectious Diseases, National Institutes of Health, 4 Center Dr., Bethesda, MD 20892-0425

MEGHAVI KOSBOTH
Division of Rheumatology & Clinical Immunology, University of Florida, P.O. Box 100221, Gainesville, FL 32610-0221

PAUL KROGSTAD
David Geffen School of Medicine at UCLA, Dept. of Pediatrics and Dept. of Molecular and Medical Pharmacology, University of California, Los Angeles, 10833 Le Conte Ave., Room 22-442 MDCC, Los Angeles, CA 90095

NIELS KRUSE
Institute for Multiple Sclerosis Research, Medical Faculty, University of Göttingen, and Gemeinnützige Hertie-Stiftung, Waldweg 33, D 37073 Göttingen, Germany

JIACHUN X. KUNG
Dept. of Clinical Pathology, Cleveland Clinic Foundation L-11, 9500 Euclid Ave., Cleveland, OH 44195

CHO-CHOU KUO
Dept. of Pathobiology, Box 357238, Room F-161A, Health Sciences Bldg., 1959 N.E. Pacific St., University of Washington, Seattle, WA 98195

ROBERT A. KYLE
Mayo Clinic College of Medicine, 628 Stabile Bldg., 200 First St. SW, Rochester, MN 55905

ROBERT S. LANCIOTTI
Arboviral Diseases Branch, Division of Vector-Borne Infectious Diseases, National Center for Infectious Diseases, Centers for Disease Control and Prevention, P.O. Box 2087, Fort Collins, CO 80522-2087

MARIE LOUISE LANDRY
Dept. of Laboratory Medicine, Yale University School of Medicine, P.O. Box 208035, New Haven, CT 06520-8035

ANA M. LAZARO
CW Bill Young Marrow Donor Recruitment and Research Program and Dept. of Oncology, Georgetown University Medical Center, E404 Research Bldg., 3970 Reservoir Rd., NW, Washington, DC 20057

HOWARD M. LEDERMAN
Division of Pediatric Allergy & Immunology, Johns Hopkins Hospital - CMSC 1102, 600 N. Wolfe St., Baltimore, MD 21287-3923

MARY S. LEFFELL
Immunogenetics Laboratory, Dept. of Medicine, School of Medicine, Johns Hopkins University, 2041 E. Monument St., Baltimore, MD 21205

DIANE S. LELAND
Dept. of Pathology and Laboratory Medicine, Indiana University School of Medicine, Riley Hospital, Room 0969, 702 Barnhill Dr., Indianapolis, IN 46202

RICHARD A. LEMPICKI
Clinical Services Program, NCI-Frederick, SAIC Frederick, Inc., P.O. Box B, Frederick, MD 21702-1201

MARTHA L. LEPOW
Dept. of Pediatrics, Section of Infectious Disease, Albany Medical Center, Room A-615, MC 88, 47 New Scotland Ave., Albany, NY 12208

PATRICK S. C. LEUNG
Division of Rheumatology/Allergy and Clinical Immunology, School of Medicine, University of California at Davis, Davis, CA 95616

PAUL N. LEVETT
Provincial Laboratory, Saskatchewan Health, 3200 Albert St., Regina, Saskatchewan, Canada S4S 5W6

MYRON M. LEVINE
Center for Vaccine Development, Dept. of Medicine and Dept. of Pediatrics, University of Maryland School of Medicine, 685 W. Baltimore St., Rm 480, Baltimore, MD 21201

MARK D. LINDSLEY
Mycotic Diseases Branch, Division of Bacterial and Mycotic Diseases, National Center for Infectious Diseases, Centers for Disease Control and Prevention, 1600 Clifton Rd., N.E., Mailstop G-11, Atlanta, GA 30333

STEPHEN E. LINDSTROM
Influenza Branch, Division of Viral and Rickettsial Diseases, National Center for Infectious Diseases, Centers for Disease Control and Prevention, 1600 Clifton Rd., Mail Stop G16, Atlanta, GA 30333

LANCE A. LIOTTA
Center for Applied Proteomics and Molecular Medicine, George Mason University, Manassas, VA 20110

VLADIMIR N. LOPAREV
Centers for Disease Control and Prevention, 1600 Clifton Rd., MS G-18, Atlanta, GA 30333

ROBIN G. LORENZ
University of Alabama at Birmingham, Birmingham, AL 35294

THOMAS P. LOUGHRAN
Penn State Cancer Institute, Pennsylvania State University College of Medicine, Hershey, PA 17033

MARK LOWENTHAL
Laboratory of Pathology, Center for Cancer Research, National Cancer Institute, and FDA-NCI Clinical Proteomics Program, Bethesda, MD 20892

JULIA LUBORSKY
Endocrine Immunology, Dept. of Pharmacology and Dept. of Obstetrics and Gynecology, Rush University Medical Center, Chicago, IL 60612

DONNA P. LUCAS
Immunogenetics Laboratory, Dept. of Medicine, Johns Hopkins University School of Medicine, 2041 E. Monument St., Baltimore, MD 21205-2222

ANDREW D. LUSTER
Center for Immunology and Inflammatory Diseases, Division of Rheumatology, Allergy and Immunology, Massachusetts General Hospital, CNY 8301, 149 13th St., Charlestown, MA 02129

ROBERT LYONS
Division of Rheumatology and Clinical Immunology, Dept. of Medicine, University of Florida, P.O. Box 100221, 1600 S.W. Archer Rd., ARB R3-110, Gainesville, FL 32610-0221

KEVIN MACALUSO
Dept. of Pathobiological Sciences, School of Veterinary Medicine, Louisiana State University, Skip Berman Dr. #3213, Baton Rouge, LA 70803

HOLDEN T. MAECKER
BD Biosciences Immunocytometry Systems, 2350 Qume Dr., San Jose, CA 95131

FABRIZIO MAGGI
Dept. of Experimental Pathology and Retrovirus Center, University of Pisa, 37, Via San Zeno, I-56127 Pisa, Italy

JAMES B. MAHONY
Dept. of Pathology and Molecular Medicine, McMaster University, and the Regional Virology & Chlamydiology Laboratory, St. Joseph's Hospital, 50 Charlton Ave. E., Hamilton, Ontario L8N 4A6, Canada

VERNON C. MAINO
BD Biosciences Immunocytometry Systems, 2350 Qume Dr., San Jose, CA 95131

EUGENE O. MAJOR
Molecular Medicine and Virology Section, Laboratory of Molecular Medicine and Neuroscience, National Institute of Neurological Disorders and Stroke, Bldg 36, Room 5W21, 36 Convent Dr., MSC 4164, Bethesda, MD 20892-4164

MICHAEL P. MANNS
Dept. of Gastroenterology and Hepatology, Zentrum Innere Medizin, Medizinische Hochschule Hannover, Hannover, Germany

SUZANNE M. MATSUI
Gastroenterology Section (111-GI), VA Palo Alto Health Care System, 3801 Miranda Ave., Palo Alto, CA 94304, and Division of Gastroenterology and Hepatology, Stanford University School of Medicine, 300 Pasteur Dr., Stanford, CA 94305-5187

THOMAS W. McCLOSKEY
The Institute for Medical Research, North Shore University Hospital / New York University School of Medicine, 350 Community Dr., Manhasset, NY 11030

THERON McCORMICK
Baylor College of Medicine and Pediatric Allergy and Immunology Service, Texas Children's Hospital, 6621 Fannin St., FC330.01, Houston, TX 77030-2399

BENJAMIN D. MEDOFF
Center for Immunology and Inflammatory Diseases, Division of Rheumatology, Allergy and Immunology, and Pulmonary and Critical Care Unit, Massachusetts General Hospital, Harvard Medical School, Boston, MA 02114

JULIA A. METCALF
Office of Clinical Research, National Institute of Allergy and Infectious Diseases, National Institutes of Health, Bethesda, MD 20892

STEPHEN A. MIGUELES
Laboratory of Immunoregulation, National Institute of Allergy and Infectious Diseases, National Institutes of Health, Bethesda, MD 20892

CHRISTINE J. MORRISON
Mycotic Diseases Branch, Division of Bacterial and Mycotic Diseases, National Center for Infectious Diseases, Centers for Disease Control and Prevention, 1600 Clifton Rd., N.E., Mailstop G-11, Atlanta, GA 30333

MOON H. NAHM
University of Alabama at Birmingham, 845 19th St. South (BBRB-614), Birmingham, AL 35294

STANLEY J. NAIDES
Division of Rheumatology, H038, BMR C5840, Milton S. Hershey Medical Center, Pennsylvania State University College of Medicine, 500 University Dr., Hershey, PA 17033-0850

SONALI NARAIN
Division of Rheumatology and Clinical Immunology, Dept. of Medicine, University of Florida, P.O. Box 100221, 1600 S.W. Archer Rd., ARB R3-110, Gainesville, FL 32610-0221

SONALI NARAIN
Division of Rheumatology & Clinical Immunology, University of Florida, P.O. Box 100221, Gainesville, FL 32610-0221

VEN NATARAJAN
Clinical Services Program, NCI-Frederick, SAIC-Frederick, Inc., P.O. Box B, Frederick, MD 21702-1201

JAMES P. NATARO
Center for Vaccine Development, Dept. of Pediatrics, University of Maryland School of Medicine, 685 W. Baltimore St., Rm 480, Baltimore, MD 21201

JENNIFER NG
CW Bill Young Marrow Donor Recruitment and Research Program and Dept. of Pediatrics, Georgetown University Medical Center, Washington, DC 20057

CODY NICHOLS
Division of Rheumatology and Clinical Immunology, Dept. of Medicine, University of Florida, P.O. Box 100221, 1600 S.W. Archer Rd., ARB R3-110, Gainesville, FL 32610-0221

DOUGLAS F. NIXON
Gladstone Institute of Virology and Immunology and University of California, San Francisco, 1650 Owens St., San Francisco, CA 94158

CARLOS H. NOUSARI
Institute for Immunofluorescence, DermPath Diagnostics South Florida, and Dept. of Dermatology, University of Miami, Miami, FL 33069

THOMAS NUTMAN
Helminth Immunology Section and Clinical Parasitology Unit, Laboratory of Parasitic Diseases, Bldg. 4, Rm B1-03, National Institutes of Health, Bethesda, MD 20892-0425

SUSAN B. NYLAND
Penn State Cancer Institute, Pennsylvania State University College of Medicine, Hershey, PA 17033

MAURICE R. G. O'GORMAN
Dept. of Pathology, Childrens Memorial Hospital, 2300 Children's Plaza, Chicago, IL 60614-3394

ANDREW R. PACHNER
Dept. of Neurosciences, UMDNJ-New Jersey Medical School, 185 S. Orange Ave., Newark, NJ 07103

SAVITA PAHWA
Dept. of Microbiology and Immunology, University of Miami School of Medicine, 1580 NW 10th Ave., BCRI-712, Miami, FL 33136

ELISABETH PAIETTA
Our Lady of Mercy Cancer Center, New York Medical College, 600 East 233rd St., Bronx, NY 10466

MARCELA F. PASETTI
Center for Vaccine Development, Dept. of Pediatrics, University of Maryland School of Medicine, 685 W. Baltimore St., Rm 480, Baltimore, MD 21201

BRUCE K. PATTERSON
Dept. of Pathology and Medicine, Division of Infectious and Geographic Medicine, Stanford University School of Medicine, 300 Pasteur Dr., Rm H1537J, Stanford, CA 94305-5629

R. STOKES PEEBLES, JR.
Division of Allergy, Pulmonary, and Critical Care Medicine, Vanderbilt University School of Medicine, Center for Lung Research, T-1217 MCN, Vanderbilt University Medical Center, Nashville, TN 37232-2650

SUHAS PHADNIS
Dept. of Pathology, Medical College of Wisconsin, 8700 W. Wisconsin Ave., Milwaukee, WI 53226, and Clement J. Zablocki VA Medical Center, 5000 W. National Ave., Milwaukee, WI 53295-1000

BARBARA N. PHENIX
The Institute for Medical Research, North Shore University Hospital / New York University School of Medicine, 350 Community Dr., Manhasset, NY 11030

PEDRO A. PIEDRA
Dept. of Molecular Virology and Microbiology and Dept. of Pediatrics, Baylor College of Medicine, Room 248E, One Baylor Plaza, Houston, TX 77030

DAVID S. PISETSKY
Division of Rheumatology, Duke University Medical Center, Durham, NC 27710, and Durham VA Medical Center, Box 151G, 508 Fulton St., Durham, NC 27705

MAURO PISTELLO
Dept. of Experimental Pathology and Retrovirus Center, University of Pisa, 37, Via San Zeno, I-56127 Pisa, Italy

RAYMOND P. PODZORSKI
Dept. of Pathology, Waukesha Memorial Hospital, 725 American Ave., Waukesha, WI 53188

VICTORIA POPE
National Center for HIV, STD, and TB Prevention, Centers for Disease Control and Prevention, 1600 Clifton Rd., N.E., Atlanta, GA 30333 [retired]

TANJA POPOVIC
Office of the Chief Science Officer, Centers for Disease Control and Prevention, 1600 Clifton Rd., MS D50, Atlanta, GA 30333

HARRY PRINCE
Focus Diagnostics, Inc., 5785 Corporate Ave., Cypress, CA 90630

MARK RAFFELD
Hematopathology Section, Laboratory of Pathology, National Cancer Institute, 10 Center Dr., Bldg. 10, Room 2N110, MSC-1500, Bethesda, MD 20892-1500

ALEX J. RAI
Dept. of Pathology, Division of Clinical Chemistry, Johns Hopkins University School of Medicine, 600 North Wolfe St., Meyer B-121, Baltimore, MD 21287

SILVIA RATTO-KIM
U.S. Military HIV Research Program, Armed Forces Research Institute of Medical Sciences, 315/6 Rajvithi Rd., Bangkok 10400, Thailand

WESTLEY H. REEVES
Division of Rheumatology and Clinical Immunology, Dept. of Medicine, University of Florida, P.O. Box 100221, 1600 S.W. Archer Rd., ARB R3-110, Gainesville, FL 32610-0221

NANCY L. REINSMOEN
Dept. of Pathology, Duke University Medical Center, Box 3712 DUMC, Research Park Bldg., 111 Research Dr., Durham, NC 27710

ALAN T. REMALEY
Dept. of Laboratory Medicine, Warren G. Magnusson Clinical Center, National Institutes of Health, 10 Center Dr., MSC 1508, Bethesda, MD 20892-1508

DANIEL G. REMICK
Dept. of Pathology, University of Michigan Medical School, M2210 Medical Science I, 1301 Catherine Rd., Ann Arbor, MI 48109-0602

PETER RIECKMANN
Dept. of Neurology, Clinical Research Unit for Multiple Sclerosis and Neuroimmunology, Julius Maximilians University, Josef-Schneider-Str. 11, D 97080 Würzburg, Germany

YASUKO RIKIHISA
Dept. of Veterinary Biosciences, College of Veterinary Medicine, The Ohio State University, 1925 Coffey Rd., Columbus, OH 43210

CHARLES R. RINALDO, JR.
Dept. of Infectious Diseases and Microbiology, University of Pittsburgh Graduate School of Public Health, Pittsburgh, PA 15261, and Dept. of Pathology, Clinical Virology Laboratory, University of Pittsburgh Medical Center, Pittsburgh, PA 15213

PATRICK C. ROCHE
Ventana Medical Systems, Inc., 1910 Innovation Park Dr., Tucson, AZ 85737

JOHN T. ROEHRIG
Arboviral Diseases Branch, Division of Vector-Borne
Infectious Diseases, National Center for Infectious Diseases,
Centers for Disease Control and Prevention, P.O. Box 2087,
Fort Collins, CO 80522-2087

CHAIM M. ROIFMAN
Division of Immunology and Allergy and Program of Infection,
Immunity, Injury and Repair, The Hospital for Sick Children
and The University of Toronto, Toronto, Ontario M5G 1X8,
Canada

A. ROOS
Dept. of Nephrology, C3P-29, Leiden University Medical
Center, Albinusdreef 2, 2333 ZA Leiden, The Netherlands

NOEL R. ROSE
Dept. of Pathology, Johns Hopkins University School of
Medicine, Baltimore, MD 21205

SARBJIT SAINI
Johns Hopkins Asthma and Allergy Center, 5501 Hopkins
Bayview Circle, Room 1A38A, Baltimore, MD 21224

MINORU SATOH
Division of Rheumatology and Clinical Immunology, Dept. of
Medicine, University of Florida, P.O. Box 100221, 1600 S.W.
Archer Rd., ARB R3-110, Gainesville, FL 32610-0221

PETER M. SCHANTZ
Division of Parasitic Diseases, National Center for Infectious
Diseases, Centers for Disease Control and Prevention, MS F-
36, 4770 Buford Hwy., Atlanta, GA 30341-3724

D. SCOTT SCHMID
Herpesvirus Team, Centers for Disease Control and
Prevention, 1600 Clifton Rd., Bldg. 7, Room 230, MS G-18,
Atlanta, GA 30333

JOHN L. SCHMITZ
Dept. of Pathology & Laboratory Medicine, University of
North Carolina, Chapel Hill, Room 1035 East Wing, UNC
Hospitals, Chapel Hill, NC 27514

DAVID SCHNURR
Viral and Rickettsial Disease Laboratory, California Dept. of
Health Services, 850 Marina Bay Parkway, Richmond, CA 94804

MARTIN E. SCHRIEFER
Bacterial Zoonoses Branch, Division of Vector-Borne
Infectious Diseases, National Center for Infectious Diseases,
Centers for Disease Control and Prevention, Ft. Collins, CO
80522

JOHN T. SCHROEDER
Johns Hopkins Asthma and Allergy Center, 5501 Hopkins
Bayview Circle, Baltimore, MD 21224

M. A. SEELEN
Dept. of Internal Medicine, Division of Nephrology, University
Medical Center Groningen, Hanzeplein 1, 9713 GZ
Groningen, The Netherlands

SUMAN SETTY
Dept. of Pathology (M/C 847), University of Illinois Medical
Center at Chicago, 1819 West Polk St., Room 446, Chicago,
IL 60612-7335

BARBARA L. SHACKLETT
Dept. of Medical Microbiology and Immunology, School of
Medicine, University of California at Davis, 3327 Tupper Hall,
1 Shields Ave., Davis, CA 95616

KEERTI V. SHAH
Dept. of Molecular Microbiology and Immunology, Johns
Hopkins University, Blooomberg School of Public Health, 615
N. Wolfe St., Baltimore, MD 21205

WILLIAM T. SHEARER
Baylor College of Medicine and Allergy and Immunology
Service, Texas Children's Hospital, 6621 Fannin St., FC330.01,
Houston, TX 77030-2399

ANITA SHET
Aaron Diamond AIDS Research Center, Rockefeller
University, 455 First Ave., New York, NY 10016

VINOD B. SHIDHAM
Dept. of Pathology, Medical College of Wisconsin, 9200 W.
Wisconsin Ave., Milwaukee, WI 53226

JERRY W. SIMECKA
Dept. of Molecular Biology and Immunology, University of
North Texas Health Science Center, 3500 Camp Bowie Blvd.,
Fort Worth, TX 76107

JAY E. SLATER
Center for Biologics Evaluation and Research, U.S. Food and
Drug Administration, 29 Lincoln Dr., Bethesda, MD 20892

THOMAS F. SMITH
Dept. of Laboratory Medicine and Pathology, Division of
Clinical Microbiology, Mayo Clinic and Foundation, 200 First
St. SW, Rochester, MN 55905

STEVEN C. SPECTER
Office of Student Affairs (MDC 4), University of South
Florida COM, 12901 Bruce B. Downs Blvd., Tampa,
FL 33612-4799

KIRSTEN ST. GEORGE
Clinical Virology Program, New York State Dept. of Health,
Wadsworth Center - Griffin Laboratories, Slingerlands,
NY 12159

NORIKO STEINER
CW Bill Young Marrow Donor Recruitment and Research
Program and Dept. of Oncology, Georgetown University
Medical Center, E404 Research Bldg., 3970 Reservoir Rd.,
NW, Washington, DC 20057

RANDY A. STEVENS
Clinical Services Program, NCI-Frederick, SAIC Frederick,
Inc., P.O. Box B, Frederick, MD 21702-1201

LISA STRAIN
Institute of Human Genetics, University of Newcastle upon
Tyne, Newcastle upon Tyne NE1 3BZ, United Kingdom

JAMES E. STRONG
Special Pathogens Program, National Microbiology Laboratory,
Public Health Agency of Canada, and Childrens Hospital,
Health Sciences Centre, University of Manitoba, Winnipeg,
Manitoba, Canada

J. BRUCE SUNDSTROM
Dept. of Pathology and Laboratory Medicine, Emory
University School of Medicine, 2309 WMB, 101 Woodruff
Circle, Atlanta, GA 30322

MANIKKAM SUTHANTHIRAN
Division of Nephrology, Dept. of Medicine, Weill Medical
College of Cornell University, and Dept. of Transplantation
Medicine and Extracorporeal Therapy, New York-Presbyterian
Hospital, New York, NY 10021

D. ROBERT SUTHERLAND
Princess Margaret Hospital, The University Health Network, Room 4-107, 610 University Ave., Toronto, Ontario M5G 2M9, Canada

TING TANG
CW Bill Young Marrow Donor Recruitment and Research Program and Dept. of Pediatrics, Georgetown University Medical Center, Washington, DC 20057

STEFFEN THIEL
Dept. of Medical Microbiology and Immunology, Bartholin Building, University of Aarhus, Aarhus DK8000, Denmark

HERBERT A. THOMPSON
Viral and Rickettsial Zoonosis Branch, National Center for Infectious Diseases, Centers for Disease Control and Prevention, MS G-13, 1600 Clifton Rd., N.E., Atlanta, GA 30333

RUSSELL H. TOMAR
Dept. of Pathology, LL850, Stroger Hospital of Cook County, 1901 West Harrison St., Chicago, IL 60612

TRINH T. TRAN
Division of Rheumatology, Duke University Medical Center, Durham, NC 27710

KENNETH S. K. TUNG
Dept. of Pathology and Dept. of Microbiology, University of Virginia Health Sciences Center, Box 214, Old Medical School, 4th Flr., Rm. 4888, Charlottesville, VA 22908-0001

DOLLY B. TYAN
HLA & Immunogenetics Laboratory, SSB-197, Medical Genetics Institute, Cedars-Sinai Medical Center, 8723 Alden Dr., Los Angeles, CA 90048

KENNETH E. UGEN
Dept. of Medical Microbiology and Immunology and Center for Molecular Delivery, University of South Florida College of Medicine, MDC 10, 12901 Bruce B. Downs Blvd., Tampa, FL 33612

MARIALINDA VATTERONI
Dept. of Experimental Pathology and Retrovirus Center, University of Pisa, 37, Via San Zeno, I-56127 Pisa, Italy

RENATO VEGA
Immunogenetics Laboratory, Dept. of Medicine, Johns Hopkins University School of Medicine, 2041 E. Monument St., Baltimore, MD 21205-2222

KEN B. WAITES
Dept. of Pathology, University of Alabama at Birmingham, Birmingham, AL 35233

DAVID W. WARNOCK
Mycotic Diseases Branch, Division of Bacterial and Mycotic Diseases, National Center for Infectious Diseases, Centers for Disease Control and Prevention, 1600 Clifton Rd., N.E., Mailstop G-11, Atlanta, GA 30333

JEFFREY S. WARREN
Division of Clinical Pathology, Dept. of Pathology, University of Michigan Medical School, Medical Science I Bldg., M5242, 1301 Catherine Rd., Ann Arbor, MI 48109-0602

ADRIANA WEINBERG
Dept. of Pediatrics and Medicine, University of Colorado Health Sciences Center, 4200 East 9th Ave., Campus Box C227, Denver, CO 80262

KENT J. WEINHOLD
Dept. of Surgery, P.O. Box 2926, Duke University Medical Center, Durham, NC 27710-2996

THERESA L. WHITESIDE
Depts. of Pathology, Immunology, and Otolaryngology, University of Pittsburgh School of Medicine and University of Pittsburgh Cancer Institute, Pittsburgh, PA 15213

J. WIESLANDER
Wieslab IDEON, Lund, Sweden

ALLAN WIIK
Autoimmunology, Statens Seruminstitut, Artillerivej 5, 2300 Copenhagen S., Denmark

HUGH J. WILLISON
Division of Clinical Neurosciences, University of Glasgow, Southern General Hospital, Glasgow G51 4TF, Scotland

MARIANNA WILSON
Division of Parasitic Diseases, National Center for Infectious Diseases, Centers for Disease Control and Prevention, MS F-36, 4770 Buford Hwy., Atlanta, GA 30341-3724

MARY E. WINTERS
Laboratory of Pathology, Center for Cancer Research, National Cancer Institute, and FDA-NCI Clinical Proteomics Program, Bethesda, MD 20892

BRENT LEE WOOD
Dept. of Laboratory Medicine, #357110, University of Washington Medical Center, 1959 NE Pacific St., Seattle, WA 98195

ROBERT A. WOOD
Dept. of Pediatric Allergy and Immunology, Johns Hopkins Hospital, CMSC 1102, 600 N. Wolfe St., Baltimore, MD 21287

STEPHEN A. YOUNG
Microbiology/Virology, TriCore Reference Laboratories, Albuquerque, NM 87102, and Dept. of Molecular Genetics & Microbiology, University of New Mexico School of Medicine, MSCO8 4660, 1 University of New Mexico, Albuquerque, NM 87131

ANDREA A. ZACHARY
Immunogenetics Laboratory, Dept. of Medicine, Johns Hopkins University School of Medicine, 2041 E. Monument St., Baltimore, MD 21205-2222

ADRIANA ZEEVI
Dept. of Pathology, University of Pittsburgh Medical Center, Pittsburgh, PA 15261

CHENGSHENG ZHANG
Dept. of Pathology and Molecular Medicine, McMaster University, and the Regional Virology & Chlamydiology Laboratory, St. Joseph's Hospital, 50 Charlton Ave. E., Hamilton, Ontario, L8N 4A6, Canada

Preface

Over the past several decades, dramatic progress has taken place in the field of immunology. As a consequence, significant advances have been realized not only in the research realm but also in the diagnostic and clinical arena.

Clinical immunology, a dynamic and ever-evolving discipline, has witnessed remarkable advances. Exciting discoveries in molecular biology, recombinant DNA and proteins, cytokine biology, and human genetics have enhanced our understanding of immune-mediated diseases and have led the way for novel therapeutics for many immunologic disorders. With these advances, clinical immunology has matured and its applications have increased extensively. Furthermore, the scope of clinical immunology, which extends to a wide and diverse group of human diseases, has become integrated into nearly every medical specialty. This widespread feature of clinical immunology may be seen in, but not limited to, disciplines such as hematology, transplantation, rheumatology, oncology, dermatology, infectious disease, allergy, and neurology. Thus, it is the clinical laboratory immunologist who serves as the interface for communication among these various disciplines, while providing leadership and knowledge for the best laboratory approaches to evaluate patients with immune-mediated diseases.

Given their strategic position in the hospital setting, it is imperative that clinical and diagnostic immunology laboratories have a blueprint to follow with regard to sound and appropriate laboratory procedures. As the field of immunology continues to explode with new discoveries and applications, the laboratory director is the key person who can harness basic immunologic research findings and translate them into useful and reliable laboratory applications. Furthermore, the immunology laboratory director serves as a consultant to the clinician regarding the interpretation of laboratory testing and as the facilitator for the exchange of basic and new concepts in immunology.

This Manual has traditionally served to assist and guide the laboratory director in immunology. For six editions, the *Manual of Clinical Laboratory Immunology* has fulfilled this mission under the excellent guidance of Noel R. Rose, editor-in-chief. In fact, for nearly 30 years, this Manual has served as the primary reference manual for clinical immunology laboratories around the world, providing up-to-date methodologies for diagnosis and monitoring of immune-mediated disorders. We now offer the 7th edition of the Manual, with the goal of following the renowned reputation of the past six editions. The 7th edition continues to provide a concise review of the basic principles underlying each procedure, detailed descriptions of the methodology, and special focus on interpretation of the laboratory findings.

In an effort to capture the exciting new dimensions in the field of immunology and to reflect the continuous evolution of clinical immunology, significant changes have been introduced into this edition. First, the name of the Manual has been modified. The new title, *Manual of Molecular and Clinical Laboratory Immunology*, reflects the tremendous impact of molecular biology on the discipline. Molecular immunology has emerged as a significant development in the field, and numerous applications are quickly moving into the clinical and diagnostic laboratories. The first section of the book delineates the varied and timely molecular applications that the immunology laboratory will be implementing in the laboratory environment. The chapter on general methods introduces this new information and the theme is continued in several other sections throughout the book.

Second, each chapter in the Manual has been substantially revised and updated to present the most current information on that topic. Just as in the previous editions, experts once again have contributed to the various chapters and included important additions to provide the most contemporary procedures. Moreover, the Manual features not only timely and current long-standing laboratory procedures but also several chapters dedicated to cutting-edge topics that may shortly be implemented in the clinical immunology laboratory. Some of these ground-breaking areas can be seen in the sections pertaining to transplantation, monitoring of cytokines and chemokines, multiple applications of flow cytometry, allergic diseases, and cancer.

Noel Rose's insightful goal for this Manual was that it must not only serve the needs of today's clinical immunology laboratory but also look to the future, where even more dramatic progress in diagnosis and treatment can be anticipated. I share that vision with him and hope that this edition will follow in that outstanding tradition.

The publication of this Manual is the joint effort of many dedicated individuals. I wish to acknowledge the tremendous support and outstanding commitment of our volume editors, section editors, and chapter authors, who as experts in their areas have contributed their extraordinary experience, energy, and generous time to the success of this edition. In addition, I wish to express special appreciation to the editorial and production staff at ASM Press for their excellent work. In particular, I would like to thank Ellie Tupper, our senior editor, for her guidance, patience, nudging, and incredible support through the many phases of this production.

I would also like to acknowledge the valuable assistance of Jeff J. Holtmeier, Director, ASM Press, and the creative endeavors of Jennifer Adelman, Marketing Director.

BARBARA DETRICK, PH.D.
EDITOR-IN-CHIEF

GENERAL METHODS

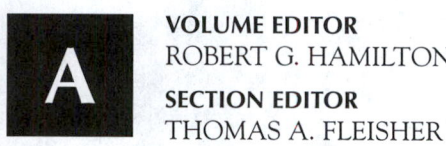

VOLUME EDITOR
ROBERT G. HAMILTON
SECTION EDITOR
THOMAS A. FLEISHER

Proteomics and Genomics Methodology in the Clinical Immunology Laboratory

THOMAS A. FLEISHER

1

Major advances in proteomics and genomics have occurred since the last edition of this book, and these are further impacting the field of diagnostic and clinical immunology. The completion of the Human Genome Project has fueled the field of genomics and provided the critical database from which to expand genomic studies. This has been complemented by recognition that proteins, the products of the genome, are highly evolved and varied to carry out the work of the cell. A vast array of proteins provide a wide range of functional elements in the immune system. Expanded evaluation of these critical products should provide new insights into the biology of the immune system and pathology of immunologic disorders. The future will depend on linking genomic and proteomic studies as partners in understanding the immune response and characterizing the underlying basis of immunologic diseases.

The laboratory methods available to evaluate proteins and nucleic acids form the substance of the following four chapters. These are developed in the setting of a recognition that our current approaches leave the vast majority of the world of human proteins untouched and the reality that specific and reliable biomarkers of human disease remain an unfulfilled promise. In light of this, new strategies to expand the range of evaluating the proteome are introduced by Remaley and Hortin in chapters 2 and 3 that include multiplex immunoassays, two-dimensional gel electrophoresis, and mass spectrometry. It is likely that these and additional technologies will provide the means to measure new markers for early specific disease detection and monitoring the effectiveness of therapy. Parallel developments in the field of genomics also impact on the field of diagnostic and clinical immunology. In chapter 5 by Podzorski, a general survey is provided of methods available in the field of molecular biology. Many of these techniques have already found their way into the diagnostic laboratory, and it is likely that this trend will continue at an even faster pace. In chapter 4, by Chanock, the emerging technology of microarray analysis is summarized, an approach that has already resulted in an approved assay system for clinical laboratory use.

The information garnered by the expanding range of analytes and technologies available to evaluate the proteome and genome is fueling a new vision of scientific discovery referred to as systems biology (1). This integrated proteomic and genomic approach should afford far better understanding of the perturbations that lead to human disease. Furthermore, such a multiparametric approach applied in the evaluation of a patient should allow for the identification of disease-specific therapies and the real possibility of strategies that will ultimately prevent disease.

REFERENCE

1. **Hood, L., J. R. Heath, M. E. Phelps, and B. Lin.** 2004. Systems biology and new technologies enable predictive and preventative medicine. *Science* **306:**640–643.

Introduction to Protein Analysis

GLEN L. HORTIN AND ALAN T. REMALEY

2

PROTEIN DIVERSITY AND ITS DIAGNOSTIC SIGNIFICANCE

Proteome Complexity

The complete set of human proteins in an individual, what was first termed the proteome by Wilkins in 1994, represents even greater complexity than the genome. In the stepwise flow of genetic information from approximately 25,000 genes comprising the human genome (7) to mRNAs to proteins, there is likely to be a progressive increase in complexity (Fig. 1). Alternative splicing of RNA leads to the possibility of producing several mRNAs from each gene.

There are multiple sources of variation in individual proteins and in the proteome, as outlined in Table 1. Posttranslational modifications of the primary translation products of mRNAs potentially lead to large numbers of structural variants of individual gene products. A total of more than 200 types of posttranslational modifications have been described (11, 12), including biosynthetic modifications such as glycosylation, phosphorylation, acetylation, sulfation, proteolysis, and chemical modification by reactants in the environment such as sugars, aldehydes, reactive oxygen species, and free radicals. Thus, the complete human proteome derived from typical somatic cells is likely to contain more than 1,000,000 different structures, although current technologies are able to detect only a small subset of the expected protein diversity (1–3, 9).

As proteins undergo extracellular and intracellular degradation, a complex array of peptides is generated, quite possibly even more complex than the original set of proteins. Analysis of ultrafiltrates of plasma has identified thousands of peptides (10), which are likely a small sampling of the total. Currently, there is little understanding of the complete range of peptides generated, the peptidome, although some subsets of the peptidome, such as the diverse range of peptides generated for antigen presentation on histocompatibility antigens, have been investigated and are recognized to have a critical role in directing immune responses (4, 5). Peptide splicing has recently been identified as another mechanism that may increase peptide diversity (6).

Somatic recombination and mutation of selected genes in immune cells, such as those encoding immunoglobulins, add further to the genetic and polypeptide complexity (8). Different cells within an individual encode millions of variants of immunoglobulin genes, which are expressed as even larger numbers of variant mRNAs and proteins. In practice, the complex mixtures of proteins comprising immunoglobulins usually are analyzed as a class, such as immunoglobulin G. The exception is in cases of multiple myeloma, where there is massive expansion of a clonal line expressing a single defined polypeptide sequence. Subsets of immunoglobulin molecules often are defined for diagnostic purposes by their antigen-binding specificity, although these sets generally also consist of a complex mixture of variant protein structures with subtle variations in binding specificity.

Bacteria, viruses, fungi, dietary components, therapeutic agents, and other environmental exposures contribute a diverse range of other potential protein and peptide components that may occur within the body. These components represent important immunogens, allergens, toxins, therapeutic agents, and targets for diagnostic applications.

Challenges of Proteome Analysis

Analysis of the proteome is a supremely complex and difficult problem (1–3, 9). For reasons outlined in Table 1, analysis of the proteome is substantially more complicated than analysis of genetic variation. Genes are a relatively fixed linear combination of only four nucleotides. Proteins have a primary linear structure of 20 primary amino acids that may undergo multiple modifications and form branched or cross-linked structures joined by disulfides or other cross-links. The peptide chain folds into local secondary structures, such as alpha helices and beta sheets, and then, in many cases, into globular domains that comprise the tertiary structure. Multiple polypeptide chains may come together, forming the quaternary structure of proteins with multiple subunits, and there may be multiple associations with other inorganic ions, cofactors, and ligands. Many proteins participate in complex interaction networks or assemble further into supramolecular structures, such as organelles, membranes, ribosomes, and filaments. Analysis of protein interaction networks is a challenging aspect of proteome analysis. Furthermore, proteins are distributed into all cellular and extracellular compartments, whereas the genetic material is restricted to the nucleus. In order to understand many pathophysiological processes, such as prion diseases, amyloidosis, hemoglobinopathies, and apoptotic processes, simple primary sequence analysis of proteins

Increasing Complexity Through Steps in Expression of Genetic Information

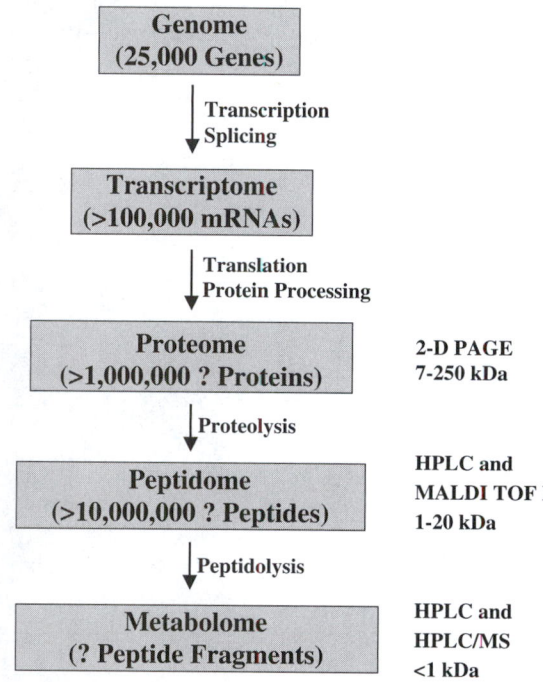

FIGURE 1 Molecular diversity: increasing complexity through steps in expression of genetic information and common methods of analysis. 2-D PAGE, two-dimensional polyacrylamide gel electrophoresis; HPLC, high-performance liquid chromatography; MALDI TOF MS, matrix-assisted laser desorption ionization–time of flight mass spectrometry.

TABLE 1 Elements of protein diversity

Type of variation
Structural
Primary structure (amino acid sequence)
Genetic variation
RNA splicing variants
Biosynthetic modifications
Chemical modification by reactants
Secondary structure (helix and sheet formation)
Tertiary structure (folding into domains)
Quaternary structure (combination of subunits)
Formation of supramolecular structures (protein interactions): organelles, ribosomes, filaments, membranes, lipoproteins
Association with ligands: inorganic ions, cofactors, ligands
Quantitative
Changes in abundance over time
Localization
Distribution among subcellular, cellular, and tissue compartments

such as two-dimensional gel electrophoresis, have the capability of resolving only up to a few thousand components in a single analysis. Therefore, current analytical technologies permit analysis of only a small subset of the human proteome, usually only a survey of the most abundant components.

is inadequate. Often it is essential to identify not only the primary structural variation of proteins but also variation in their folding, aggregation, or abnormal localization within or outside of cells.

Two additional challenges to protein analysis that are nearly as great as structural diversity are (i) the dynamic nature of protein concentration and (ii) the wide range of protein concentrations. Unlike genes, which occur in most cells at a constant two copies per cell except during cell division, the concentrations of individual proteins change continually as an ongoing balance between synthesis and export or degradation. Since the proteome changes from moment to moment, the time of specimen collection is an important variable, and it is often necessary to perform repeated analysis to examine changing patterns of proteins during pathophysiological processes. Not only are concentrations of proteins undergoing constant change, but also the concentrations of proteins in blood vary over a huge range—from millimolar concentrations of albumin and hemoglobin down to concentrations far below any current methods for detection. Assuming that some proteins may present at concentrations as low as a few molecules per liter, the range of concentrations is more than 10^{20}-fold. Unlike the case for nucleic acids, there is no simple method for amplification of the concentration of proteins. Most methods for protein analysis have a practical analytical concentration range of only about 100- to 10,000-fold, and the highest-resolution separation methods for protein analysis,

REFERENCES

1. **Anderson, N. L., and N. G. Anderson.** 2002. The human plasma proteome: history, character, and diagnostic prospects. *Mol. Cell. Proteomics* **1:**845–867.
2. **Anderson, N. L., M. Polanski, R. Pieper, T. Gatlin, R. S. Tirumalai, T. P. Conrads, T. D. Veenstra, J. N. Adkins, J. G. Pounds, R. Fagan, and A. Lobley.** 2004. The human plasma proteome: a nonredundant list developed by combination of four separate sources. *Mol. Cell. Proteomics* **3:**311–326.
3. **De Hoog, C. L., and M. Mann.** 2004. Proteomics. *Annu. Rev. Genomics Hum. Genet.* **5:**267–293.
4. **Engelhard, V. H.** 1994. Structure of peptides associated with class I and class II molecules. *Annu. Rev. Immunol.* **12:**181–207.
5. **Engelhard, V. H., A. G. Brickner, and A. L. Zarling.** 2002. Insights into antigen processing gained by direct analysis of the naturally processed class I MHC associated peptide repertoire. *Mol. Immunol.* **39:**127–137.
6. **Hanada, K., J. W. Yewdell, and J. C. Yang.** 2004. Immune recognition of a human renal cancer antigen through post-translational protein splicing. *Nature* **427:**252–256.
7. **International Human Genome Sequencing Consortium.** 2004. Finishing the euchromatic sequence of the human genome. *Nature* **431:**931–945.
8. **Li, Z., C. J. Woo, M. D. Iglesias-Ussel, D. Ronai, and M. D. Scharff.** 2004. The generation of antibody diversity through somatic hypermutation and class switch recombination. *Genes Dev.* **18:**1–11.
9. **Pieper, R., C. L. Gatlin, A. J. Makusky, P. S. Russo, C. R. Schatz, S. S. Miller, Q. Su, A. M. McGrath, M. A. Estock, P. P. Parmar, M. Zhao, S. T. Huang, J. Zhou, F. Wang, R. Esquer-Blasco, N. L. Anderson, J. Taylor, and S. Steiner.** 2003. The human serum proteome: display of nearly 3700 chromatographically separated protein spots on two-dimensional electrophoresis gels and identification of 325 distinct proteins. *Proteomics* **3:**1345–1364.

10. **Rudolf, R., P. Schulz-Knappe, M. Schrader, L. Standker, M. Jurgens, H. Tammen, and W.-G. Forssmann.** 1999. Composition of the peptide fraction in human blood plasma: database of circulating human peptides. *J. Chromatogr. B* **726:**25–35.

11. **Seo, J., and K. J. Lee.** 2004. Post-translational modifications and their biological functions: proteomic analysis and systematic approaches. *J. Biochem. Mol. Biol.* **37:**35–44.

12. **Veenstra, T. D.** 2003. Proteome analysis of posttranslational modifications. *Adv. Prot. Chem.* **65:**161–194.

Protein Analysis for Diagnostic Applications

ALAN T. REMALEY AND GLEN L. HORTIN

3

CLINICAL LABORATORY ANALYSIS OF COMPONENTS OF THE PROTEOME

In the context of the amazingly diverse and dynamic array of proteins in the human proteome, a relatively tiny set of proteins representing a few hundred gene products are analyzed for diagnostic purposes. This represents only about 2% of all gene products and leaves the huge realm of the other 98% of gene products remaining to be evaluated as potentially useful diagnostic markers. In most cases, current diagnostic analyses of proteins analyze a single gene product at a time and measure the sum total of many posttranslationally modified forms of an individual gene product. Until very recently, the arrays of hundreds of thousands of variant protein structures from posttranslational processing or of perhaps an even larger number of peptide fragments of proteins derived from degradation of proteins have been, for the most part, untapped universes for diagnostic analysis.

Recent refinements in methods for protein separations have led to methods for simultaneous analyses of hundreds of plasma proteins (1, 2, 12, 58). Applications of mass spectrometry to analysis of plasma peptide components over the last few years suggest that there are a large number of potential diagnostic markers among these components (10, 55, 64, 72). Mass spectrometric analyses of peptides are applicable to a variety of fluids and even to direct tissue analysis (9). Recent approaches for profiling hundreds of peptide components in a single analysis show promise for rapid discovery of potential new markers of disease and for direct diagnostic application (9, 10, 55, 64, 72). It appears that many peptide components circulate in blood bound to larger carrier proteins so that they are not cleared rapidly by filtration in the kidneys (48). Further description of analysis of proteins by two-dimensional electrophoresis and peptides by mass spectrometry are in the final section of this chapter, which describes research and potential future clinical laboratory methods.

PREANALYTICAL VARIABLES IN ANALYSIS OF PROTEINS

Approaches to Sampling of Proteins for Diagnostic Purposes

Considering that proteins are differentially distributed among cellular compartments, types of cells, tissues, and different body compartments, the sites and methods of sample collection are critical factors in what types of diagnostic information can be obtained. Potential types of diagnostic specimens are summarized in Table 1. Due to ease of access and analysis, biological fluids are the most common diagnostic specimens. Biological fluids often have both liquid and cellular components. Usually, different approaches are required for analysis of soluble components, e.g., by immunoassay, while analysis of proteins in cellular components requires either a solubilization step or methods for cellular analysis such as flow cytometry, immunohistochemistry, or tests of cellular function. Analysis of proteins in solution is useful for providing information about the concentration within a particular compartment, such as the blood circulation, and may allow analysis of structural variants of proteins. Analysis of proteins in cellular elements provides additional information about protein distribution and localization within cells and assists with classification of cells. Assays of cellular function, such as cellular adhesion, response to antigens, or metabolic responses to stimuli, simultaneously assess the function of many protein components along signaling and functional pathways. These may serve as useful screening methods to identify pathways with dysfunctional or deficient protein components.

Direct tissue sampling by biopsy provides additional information about the distribution and spatial organization of proteins within cells and about cellular abnormalities based on protein expression. Analysis of proteins in these types of specimens depends on immunohistochemistry or sampling of proteins from microdissection specimens or other extraction methods.

Functional and spatial analysis of proteins noninvasively in the intact body would offer the ideal analysis. Skin testing for allergens and a variety of other immunogens for many years has been applied as an approach for in vivo evaluation of specific protein-directed pathways (see section M of this book). A variety of endocrinological stimulation and challenge tests similarly quantitatively evaluate a number of complex protein responses in vivo. Recent progress in molecular imaging has yielded information about the function and distribution of specific proteins within the body (24, 60). These techniques offer the prospects of noninvasively evaluating the concentration and localization of specific proteins across the entire human body—or at least the compartments accessible to the molecular probes—rather than from a limited tissue or fluid sampling.

TABLE 1 Types of specimens for diagnostic evaluation of proteins

Type of specimen
Proteins in solution
Plasma or serum (from blood)
Urine
Cerebrospinal fluid
Other fluids—pleural, peritoneal, pericardial, joint, nasal, ocular, and abscess fluids and saliva
Stool extracts or suspensions
Cells in suspension
Blood
Urine
Cerebrospinal fluid
Other fluids—pleural, peritoneal, pericardial, joint, and abscess fluids
Tissue aspirates
Tissues
Needle biopsy samples
Excisional biopsy samples
In vivo analysis
Skin testing
Physiological tests
Molecular imaging

Variables in Specimen Collection and Processing

Many preanalytical variables can impact efforts to sample the diverse range of proteins for diagnostic purposes. Considering the highly dynamic nature of the concentration and distribution of proteins, timing of sampling can be a major variable in the analysis of circulating proteins. Some components undergo diurnal rhythms or respond to recent dietary intake. Physiological stresses such as exercise, psychological trauma, or physical pain can evoke complex physiological responses. For many diagnostic tests, efforts are made to collect specimens in a fasting state in order to minimize postprandial changes in components such as lipoproteins and to avoid turbidity of specimens from lipemia. Recent posture of the person undergoing sampling—recumbent, sitting, or standing—can introduce some redistribution of fluids within the body and changes in protein concentrations in the vascular compartment. Transfusions, intravenous fluids, and medications may directly or indirectly alter the composition and distribution of protein and cellular elements in the circulation. The tissue distribution and the number of circulating white blood cells and platelets may change acutely in response to a variety of stimuli, such as infection, medication, or thrombosis.

Timing of sampling in relation to ongoing disease or physiological processes can be critical. Collection of several specimens over a day is important for identifying a diagnostic pattern associated with acute injury such as myocardial infarction, whereas collection of specimens over several weeks may be required to assess a serological response to an infection.

Blood represents the most common specimen collected for protein analysis. Since blood circulates throughout the body and contacts diverse tissues, it provides a sampling of most proteins secreted by tissues or released by cellular death or injury throughout the body. Specimens usually are collected from peripheral veins, but occasionally, selected venous or arterial sampling is applied to identify local gradients of a protein such as renin or insulin to localize the site of production.

Blood commonly is fractionated into cellular and serum or plasma fractions for analysis. Cellular elements within the blood allow in situ analysis of protein components within a number of cell types, by techniques such as flow cytometry. For analysis of the components of the serum or plasma fraction, blood usually either is drawn into a collection tube and allowed to clot or is collected in syringes or tubes containing inhibitors of coagulation such as citrate, EDTA, or heparin. Following centrifugation, these procedures, respectively, yield serum or anticoagulated plasma. During the clotting process to form serum, a number of components, such as fibrinogen and clotting factors, are consumed or bound into the clot, decreasing the total protein content by about 5%. Additional peptide and protein components, such as activation peptides of coagulation factors and platelet proteins, are released into serum during clotting. Collection of blood in chelating agents such as EDTA avoids the activation of calcium-dependent proteases in the coagulation cascade and inhibits other proteases and peptidases that require metal cofactors. Use of chelating agents such as EDTA, together with rapid chilling and centrifugation of specimens, is necessary to achieve high recovery of some highly protease-sensitive proteins and peptides. Heparin serves as an alternative anticoagulant for plasma. Heparin acts by accelerating the inhibition of coagulation factors by endogenous inhibitors rather than by chelation of calcium. Plasma contains a diverse range of endo- and exopeptidases that can cleave polypeptides. Although chelating agents inhibit some of these, there is no collection procedure that will universally block protease activities.

Multiple factors in the collection process, as listed in Table 2, may affect the serum or plasma collected. The collection technique affects whether other tissue components are added from local tissue trauma and cells are ruptured by

TABLE 2 Factors affecting specimen collection

Factor
Time of collection related to physiological processes
Time of day—diurnal rhythms
Physiological stresses
Recent dietary intake
Posture
Disease processes
Treatments
Transfusions or infusions
Medications
Intravenous fluids
Collection process
Site of collection
Tourniquet time
Collection technique
Collection materials
Rate of collection
Type of collection tube
Tube additives—clot activators, surfactants, and clot inhibitors
Specimen processing
Time delay before processing
Storage temperature before processing
Centrifugation force
Centrifugation time and temperature
Rotor type—swinging bucket vs fixed angle
Specimen storage

high shear rates while flowing through collection needles. Any component contacting blood may activate clotting, adsorb selected components, or shed contaminating compounds into blood. Blood collection tubes are not simply inert containers for blood but have several constituents, including a surface coating to prevent binding of cells to tube walls, lubricants for stoppers, a reduced internal pressure to draw in blood, and, in some cases, polymeric gels to serve as a barrier between cells and serum after centrifugation (6). Either clot activators or inhibitors are added, depending on whether the device is for collection of serum or plasma. The materials of stoppers and tube walls are selected to serve as either a clot activator or an inert surface. Recent studies have found that polymeric components are released by many types of collection tubes (16) and that quantitative immunoassays in some cases can be affected unpredictably by components released from blood collection tubes (6).

Processing steps introduce additional variables. The time delay and temperature of the specimen before centrifugation influence the extent of clot formation, contraction, cross-linking, and fibrinolysis. Centrifugation time and speed influence the efficiency of separation of cells, particularly for plasma, where centrifugation speed and time affect the number of platelets remaining in specimens. The duration and conditions of storage of specimens waiting for analysis can affect the recovery of particular proteins and peptides. Freezing of specimens generally slows protein degradation, but cycles of freezing and thawing of proteins also can lead to denaturation, aggregation, and loss of function of some proteins. Selected plasma proteins may form a cryoprecipitate in samples that are frozen and thawed or stored under refrigeration, resulting in selective loss of components. Frozen specimens may require warming and extensive mixing to dissolve all components, and there may be some physical changes in components such as lipoprotein particles.

DIAGNOSTIC GOALS IN PROTEIN ANALYSIS

There are a variety of different types of diagnostic questions that are addressed by protein analysis. The simplest is the qualitative question of whether a protein serving as a physiological marker is present or absent in a particular specimen. The goal of such a test may be to identify previous exposure to or infection with an infectious agent, such as cytomegalovirus or human immunodeficiency virus, or to determine whether a woman is pregnant or to identify the presence of a specific autoantibody. These qualitative assays may be interpreted by visual inspection, and in most cases, there is little need for highly precise quantitative measurements due to the large difference between positive and negative responses.

A second qualitative question is whether there is structural variation of a protein. The diagnostic issue may be whether there is a genetic variant of a protein, change in isoenzyme distribution, or variation in posttranslational modification. Addressing these issues often requires physical separation techniques such as electrophoresis, chromatography, or mass spectrometry. Some examples of these types of analyses are analyses of genetic variants of hemoglobin and transthyretin, analysis of serum proteins by electrophoresis and immunofixation for detection of abundant monoclonal immunoglobulins rather than the usual polyclonal pattern, analysis of creatine kinase isoenzymes and isoforms as markers for myocardial infarction, analysis of glycoforms of transferrin as markers for alcohol abuse, and analysis of glycoforms of α-fetoprotein as markers for hepatic carcinoma.

More commonly, diagnostic analyses of proteins involve questions of quantitative analysis, e.g., how does the concentration of a protein component compare to a reference range or to previous values for the same patient? In these cases, reference ranges for the appropriate population and the precision of the quantitative measurements become significant issues in the interpretation of whether the values represent physiological abnormality or a change versus a previous value for the same subject. Measurements of changes for an individual patient rely on having specimens collected at the appropriate times, such as acute- and convalescent-phase specimens for serological analysis.

METHODS OF PROTEIN ANALYSIS

Functional Assays

Measurements of protein function can serve as a means to specifically measure the quantity of a single protein or of entire pathways, as in the example of complement activation assays (see section C of this book) or coagulation assays. In general, the methods for performing functional assays are relatively specific for the protein or pathway of interest.

Functional assays can serve as rapid screens for either quantitative deficiencies of a protein or functionally defective variants that may be present in normal quantities. The high specificity of many enzymes for particular substrates allows relatively simple and selective measurement of the activity of some proteins by monitoring of absorbance in reactions. Analysis of selected intracellular enzymes in serum offers a common diagnostic tool for detecting cellular injury and leakage of intracellular products from specific tissues. Activity of enzyme inhibitors, such as C1 inhibitor, can be measured indirectly through loss of activity of their target enzymes.

Binding assays represent the broadest range of functional assays for proteins in the clinical laboratory. These are used most often for identifying or quantifying subsets of immunoglobulins that recognize specific antigens. These types of assays, including serological assays, are covered below.

Immunoassay Methods

Immunoassays are among the most versatile and widely used methods for the analysis of proteins, peptides, and other molecules in the clinical laboratory. Qualitative immunoassays developed by Landsteiner and Witt for identifying red cell antigens and antibodies served as the foundation for practice of transfusion medicine (42). The first report of a quantitative immunoassay was over 70 years ago by Heidelberger and Kendall (27), who used antibodies to measure capsular polysaccharides from streptococci. Immunoassays began to be widely applied as quantitative methods following the development by Yalow and Berson of the radioimmunoassay (RIA) (79). Although myriad types of immunoassays have been developed over the years, each with their own advantages and disadvantages and sometimes cryptic acronyms, all immunoassays depend upon a few basic principles which are summarized here.

Antibodies as Immunoassay Reagents

A fundamental prerequisite for any immunoassay is to have a reagent that specifically recognizes and binds the analyte of interest. Antibodies, due to their high versatility and specificity in molecular recognition, are ideally suited as recognition elements in immunoassays. Antibodies offer high specificity and affinity, the most important features of the recognition element, that often are sufficient to allow the measurement of low-abundance molecules in complex mixtures such as serum without any prior purification step. Other molecules, such as receptors, binding proteins, lectins, and oligonucleotide aptamers, occasionally have been substituted for antibodies as recognition elements in assays, but generally these alternatives offer more limited variation in binding specificity and lower binding affinity.

Immunoglobulins offer great diversity in binding specificities due to the millions of amino acid sequence permutations within their antigen binding domains (44). These variations result from recombination events during the differentiation of B lymphocytes between the various immunoglobulin gene segments and from somatic mutation that by clonal selection allows further affinity maturation.

Each plasma cell produces antibodies with a single antigen binding domain and, therefore, epitope specificity. During the immune response to large, complex antigens such as proteins, however, many different clones of plasma cells are stimulated to produce antibodies to different epitopes. Polyclonal antibodies from immunization of animals with a protein, therefore, represent a heterogeneous mixture of antibodies that react to many different epitopes on a protein antigen with widely different affinities. Antisera collected from animals or humans therefore represent very complex mixtures that change in antigen specificity, affinity, and titer from one batch to the next. Only a small proportion of the antibodies recognize the specific antigen of interest. To improve the specificity of antisera, adsorption procedures may be applied to remove unwanted antigen specificities or affinity purification may be applied to select antibodies with only the desired specificities.

Small molecules, such as peptides, often have low immunogenicity. Development of strong immune responses may require conjugation to an immunogenic carrier protein or chemical synthesis of peptides as branched, polyvalent structures. Development of peptide-specific antisera offers one approach for developing reagents of greater specificity for a particular segment of a protein.

Monoclonal antibodies, in contrast to polyclonal antibodies, are derived from a single plasma cell clone and, therefore, express a single antigen-binding specificity. Monoclonal antibodies are produced by fusing a single plasma cell, usually isolated from the spleen of an immunized mouse, with an immortalized B-cell myeloma cell line to produce an immortalized hybridoma cell line (40). A monoclonal antibody represents a single discrete reagent that should have a constant binding specificity for each batch of antibody produced. Monoclonal antibodies also allow the selection of an antibody directed against a single epitope; this potentially provides improved specificity of an immunoassay. Monoclonal antibodies have allowed a detailed analysis of the nature of epitopes in proteins (20, 71). Continuous sequence epitopes are defined by peptide sequences of about 3 to 7 residues in length. Conformational or discontinuous sequence epitopes depend on the folding and conformation of a protein. Some continuous epitopes may be inaccessible or masked in the native folded structure of proteins and may become accessible as the protein is unfolded or denatured, while at the same time, conformational epitopes may be lost. Some proteins may become denatured during purification, storage, freezing and thawing of solutions, or immobilization on surfaces; this introduces a complicating factor in selecting antibodies that will recognize the native protein. Screening assays for assessing antibody binding should use a form of the protein similar to that occurring in specimens.

Deciding on whether to use polyclonal or monoclonal antibodies depends on a variety of factors. Polyclonal antibodies often have overall higher affinity than individual monoclonal antibodies, and this may assist in assays of low-abundance components. Polyclonal antibodies are easier to produce, but they have substantial lot-to-lot variability. In immunoassay formats relying on aggregate formation such as radial immunodiffusion (RID), immunofixation, turbidimetry, and nephelometry, polyclonal antiserum promotes the formation of cross-linked aggregates more efficiently. Monoclonal antibodies may allow better targeting of molecular specificity. This may be advantageous where the goal is to bind only a specific molecular form of a protein, but it can be a disadvantage if the goal is to recognize the sum total of all molecular forms of a protein. Depending on the particular immunoassay application and format, either polyclonal or monoclonal antibodies or a combination of antibodies may be most favorable.

Antigen-Antibody Interaction

The interaction between an antigen and its antibody can be described by the following reaction and the equation related to it:

$$Ag + Ab \underset{K_d}{\overset{K_a}{\rightleftharpoons}} Ag - Ab$$

$$K_{eq} = K_a/K_d = (Ag - Ab)/(Ab)(Ag)$$

K_{eq}, which is the ratio of the association constant (K_a) over the dissociation constant (K_d), is called the equilibrium binding constant of the antigen (Ag)-antibody (Ab) reaction and provides an overall index of the strength of the interaction between an antigen and antibody. The equilibrium binding constant can be determined from the slope of a Scatchard plot, which is the plot of the ratio of the concentration of antibody-bound antigen to free antigen against the concentration of the antibody-bound antigen. Alternatively, application of new methods, such as surface plasmon resonance measurements, permits the continuous monitoring of antibody-antigen binding and dissociation reactions to determine the association constants (62).

The term "affinity" is formally used to refer to the binding constant for a single antigen binding domain, and the term "avidity" is used to describe the overall interaction of an antibody with its antigen, which takes into account the number of antigen binding sites, as well as the valency or number of epitopes on the antigen. For example, the avidity of immunoglobulin M (IgM) for antigens is much higher than the affinity of its individual antigen binding sites, because it forms pentamers and has a total of 10 binding sites per complex. The avidity of an antibody that is necessary for developing an immunoassay depends on the assay design and on the concentration of the antigen being measured. In general, the equilibrium binding constant for most antibodies used in immunoassays ranges between 10^8 and 10^{12} liters/mol.

Because antibodies are bivalent molecules, the molecular configuration of the antigen-antibody complex is dependent upon the molar ratio of antigen to antibody. The different types of antigen-antibody complexes that form can be broadly classified into three configurations based on the three zones of the immunoprecipitin curve (Fig. 1). When there is a vast molar excess of antibody to antigen, most of the antigen-antibody complexes will exist as a single antibody bound to a single antigen. Conversely, when there is much more antigen

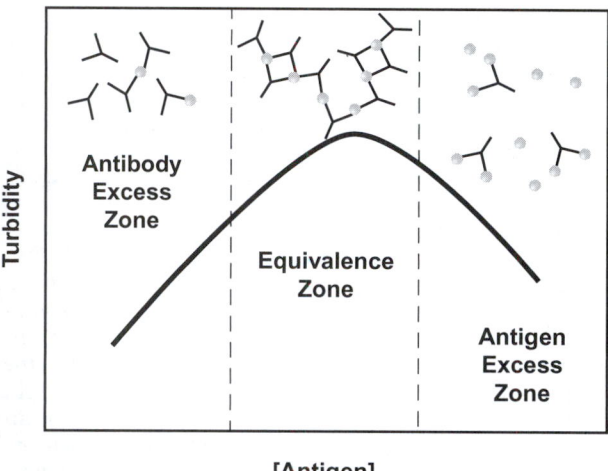

FIGURE 1 Immunoprecipitin curve. At a fixed concentration of antibody, the type of antigen-antibody complex that forms is dependent upon the antigen concentration.

than antibody, the complexes that form will mostly be single antibodies that are fully saturated with two antigens. At the point of equivalence, which is usually at a molar ratio of antibody to antigen of approximately 2 to 3, large insoluble lattice-like complexes form between the antigen and antibody. This occurs because of the ability of polyclonal antibodies to bind to multiple epitopes on each protein molecule and then to form cross-linked structures bridged by antibody molecules with proteins bound at both antigen binding sites (Fig. 1). Monoclonal antibodies, because of their specificity for a single epitope, do not form large antigen-antibody complexes, unless the antigen is multivalent. The antigen-antibody complexes that form at the point of equivalence are as large as 100 nm in diameter and will increase the turbidity of a solution because of their ability to reflect light. In addition, these large immune complexes, when present in a semisolid support such as agarose gels, will self-aggregate and form visible precipitin lines. If a constant amount of antibody is used, the precipitation reactions will vary depending on the antigen concentration, and monitoring of the aggregation reaction, e.g., by turbidimetry, nephelometry, or RID, can provide a quantitative measure of antigen concentration.

Immunoassay Formats

A wide variety of different immunoassay formats have been described that vary in the formats for antigen binding and signal generation (23, 78). However, it is possible to classify the many immunoassay formats based on the immunoprecipitin curve into antigen excess, antibody excess, and antigen-antibody equivalence assays (Table 3). A further differentiation can be made between homogeneous assays, where all components are present and measurements are performed in a homogeneous mixture, and heterogeneous assays, which require physical separation of bound and free components before signal analysis is performed.

Antigen excess assays are competitive assays in which the antibody is in limiting amounts with respect to the concentration of the analyte. These types of assays are often used to measure small molecules, such as peptides, drugs, and steroid hormones, which exist in the micromolar to nanomolar concentration range. These types of assays can be further subdivided based on the type of signal detection system used

TABLE 3 Immunoassay formats

Format
Antigen excess assays
Heterogeneous methods
RIA
FIA
EIA
Chemiluminoimmunoassay
Homogeneous methods
FPIA
EMIT
CEDIA
Antigen-antibody equivalence assays
Passive gel diffusion
RID
Double immunodiffusion
Active gel diffusion (electroimmunoassay)
Agglutination method (latex agglutination)
Photometric methods
Turbidimetry
Nephelometry
Antibody excess assays
One-site methods
Immunoblotting (Western blotting)
Immunohistochemistry
Immunofluorescence
Two-site methods
IRMA
Immunofluorimetric assay
Immunochemiluminometric assay
Immunoenzymetric assay

and whether the free analyte has to first be separated (heterogeneous) or not (homogeneous) from the antibody-bound analyte before signal measurement.

In antibody excess-type assays, the antibody is in molar excess relative to the concentration of the antigen. These are noncompetitive assays and usually involve the use of either one (one-site) or two different (two-site) antibodies for binding to the analyte. These assays are best suited for large antigens, such as proteins, with multiple epitopes. Antibody excess-type assays can achieve high sensitivity, with detection of low-abundance analytes in the picomolar to femtomolar concentration range.

By convention, antigen excess assays are usually named based on the signal detection system used followed by the word immunoassay, as in fluoroimmunoassay (FIA), which uses a fluorescent tag for detection. Antibody excess assays are in general termed immunometric assays, and the individual types of assays are identified by inserting the word for the signal detection system in the middle of the name. For example, the immunofluorometric assay is an immunometric assay that utilizes fluorescence for quantification. The enzyme-linked immunosorbent assay (ELISA) is a generic name for all enzyme-labeled assays that are performed on a microtiter plate and can be either an antibody excess or antigen excess assay. The surfaces of microtiter plates nonspecifically adsorb substances in a noncovalent-type interaction and are used as a solid support for binding either the antibody or antigen.

Antigen-Antibody Equivalence Assays

Antigen-antibody equivalence assays were the first type of immunoassays developed, because they do not require labeling of either the antigen or antibody or a sophisticated detection system. The antigen-antibody reaction can be interpreted visually by the formation of an aggregate or agglutination of particles such as red cells. For most of these assays to work, antigen and antibody need to be approximately at the equivalence point. If either is in large excess, a visible reaction may not occur.

Heterogeneous assay formats for antigen-antibody equivalence assays rely on a separation process to achieve the equivalence point between antigen and antibody. Gel diffusion-based assays use a transparent semisolid support, such as agar or agarose, as a diffusion medium for antibody and antigen. At the distance within the support where antigen and antibody achieve equivalence, a precipitin line is formed. There are many different variations of gel diffusion assays. One of the first to be developed and the simplest is the RID assay. In this method, a test solution containing the antigen is put in the well of a gel, and its corresponding antibody is incorporated into the gel matrix. As the antigen passively diffuses away from the well and into the gel, its concentration decreases progressively, and it forms a circular precipitin line at a distance from the well where it reaches the equivalence point with antibody in the gel. The greater the radius of the circular precipitin line, the greater the concentration of the antigen in the original test solution. Double-immunodiffusion-type assays involve the diffusion of both the antigen and antibody from separate wells in a gel in what are commonly termed Ouchterlony plates. This technique allows one to compare the antigen or antibody concentrations in two or more solutions and to test for cross-reactivity between samples.

The diffusion of antibody and or antigen in a gel can be accelerated by electroimmunoassay, in which electrophoresis drives the migration of an antigen from the sample well in one direction. The migrating antigen forms a rocket-shaped precipitin line with antibody in the gel, and the height of the rocket is related to the concentration of the antigen. Compared to other immunoassay formats, gel diffusion assays are relatively insensitive (0.1 μg/ml to 10 mg/ml), are only semiquantitative, and are also slow and cumbersome to perform. For these reasons, clinical use of these methods has declined.

Homogeneous forms of antigen-antibody equivalence assays are commonly performed as qualitative agglutination assays or as quantitative assays of aggregate formation. Agglutination assays also involve measurement of the antigen-antibody complex, but the size of the complex is enhanced by attaching either the antigen or antibody to a small particle, such as a latex bead or red blood cell. These assays can be used for measuring either antigen or antibody in a competitive or noncompetitive format. The testing for endogenous blood group antigens on red blood cells by this technique, termed the "direct hemagglutination test," is still widely used in blood banks. The attachment of antigen or antibody to a particle increases its valency, thus facilitating antigen-antibody complex formation, and the particles assist visualization of the immune complexes. The detection limits of these types of assays can be as low as 1 μg/ml. Latex agglutination tests have been used to develop simple screening tests on slides, such as for pregnancy testing (detection of urinary human chorionic gonadotropin [hCG]), although more sensitive and easier-to-use immunochromatographic lateral-flow tests (54) are replacing most agglutination tests.

Some agglutination tests have persisted, however, as screening tests for infectious agents and transfusion medicine.

Quantitative applications of antigen-antibody equivalence assays use instrumentation to measure the absorbance or light scattering of solutions during the antigen-antibody reaction by turbidimetry or nephelometry (8, 75). These tests depend upon the formation of large antigen-antibody immune complexes in the presence of a fixed concentration of excess antibody. The specimen is diluted to achieve an antigen concentration near the equivalence point with antibody. Measurement of either the rate or final endpoint change of light absorbance or scattering relates to the antigen concentration. Turbidimetry relies on spectrophotometric measurements of changes in absorbance during the antigen-antibody reaction. Nephelometry measures light scattered to the side by aggregates formed in the antigen-antibody reaction. Nephelometry generally measures a larger proportional change in signal than does turbidimetry, because the amount of scattered light at the start of a reaction is small unless the specimen is lipemic or contains particles. Therefore, nephelometry usually allows detection of lower antigen concentrations than does turbidimetry. Sample turbidity due to lipemia or other causes can serve as an interference with either type of assay.

The attachment of antibodies and antigens to particles, such as latex beads, and/or the addition of polymers, such as polyethylene glycol, promotes the formation of the immune complexes and can enhance the sensitivity of turbidimetry and nephelometry approximately 10- to 100-fold (8, 26, 27, 75). Attachment of small antigens, such as peptides or drugs, to particles also increases their size and valency to allow the application of these techniques for analysis of small molecules. Competitive assay formats, in which antigen in solution competes with particle-bound antigen for antibody binding and inhibits aggregation of particles, offer another variation in this technique (8).

Turbidimetric and nephelometric methods are readily automated because all components are in solution, no separation step is required, and simple photometric detection is used. Most automated turbidimetric and nephelometric assays perform checks for antigen excess to ensure that an acceptable ratio of antibody to antigen is achieved. Relatively abundant proteins that exist in serum or plasma in concentrations greater than 1 to 10 mg/liter, such as apolipoproteins, complement factors, fibrinogen, and immunoglobulins, are all commonly measured by clinical laboratories by automated nephelometric or turbidimetric analyzers. Turbidimetric assays are available on the routine test menus of many general chemistry analyzers.

Antigen Excess Assays

RIA (Fig. 2), as first described in the 1950s (79), is the prototypical antigen excess assay. Its development represented a major milestone in the history of quantitative immunoassays. RIA and other antigen excess assays usually are competitive assays (Fig. 2). A relatively small amount of radiolabeled antigen, the tracer, competes with unlabeled antigen in the specimen for a fixed and limited amount of antibody. The more antigen that is in the sample, the less tracer that is bound to the antibody. The amount of tracer bound to the antibody is measured after bound tracer is separated from the unbound tracer. Radioactive counts from the bound tracer are inversely related to the antigen concentration in the original sample. The detection limits of an RIA depend upon the avidity of its antibody for antigen and the specific activity of the radiolabeled tracer.

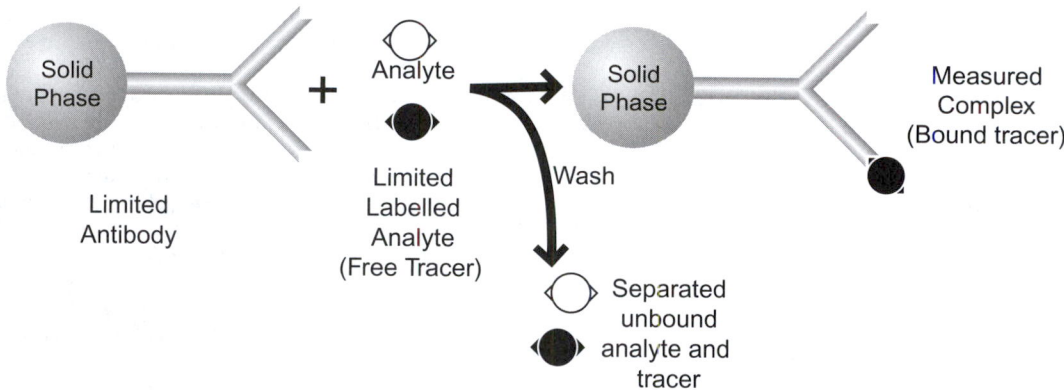

FIGURE 2 Diagram of an antigen excess-type assay using a solid support to immobilize the antibody.

Free and bound tracers have been separated by many different techniques, such as charcoal adsorption, gel filtration, polymer or salt precipitation, and secondary antibody precipitation. The most convenient and widely used separation method involves attaching the antibody or antigen to a solid support, such as beads or the reaction tube itself. The analyte bound to the antibody can then be separated from the unbound free analyte by a simple washing step (Fig. 2). Microparticles a few micrometers in diameter are often used as a solid support; their large surface area and small size promote rapid reaction. Superparamagnetic microparticles are used in many assay formats to allow retention of particles during washing steps.

As an alternative to the method shown in Fig. 2, one can also perform an RIA by radiolabeling the antibody and immobilizing a limited amount of antigen to the solid support. The more antigen in the test sample, the less radiolabeled antibody will be bound to the antigen immobilized to the solid support. The choice of RIA format depends in part on whether the antigen or antibody is more suitable for labeling.

Many types of radioisotopes have been used to label the tracer for RIAs, but ^{125}I and ^{3}H (tritium) have been the most frequently used isotopic labels. Whatever radioisotope or labeling procedure is used, it is critical to determine that the chemical modification during labeling does not significantly alter the antigen-antibody interaction. A standard curve or calibration curve is typically performed with each RIA run to control for decay of the tracer and other variables. A variety of mathematical approaches have been applied for mathematical fitting of calibration curves and calculation of results (19). Because the accuracy of the final result depends upon the accuracy of assigning concentrations to calibrators, their concentrations must be carefully established, and ideally, the calibrators should be in a matrix similar to the sample. For many routine diagnostic tests, calibrator concentrations are related to certified reference materials, which are available from various government and international organizations, such as the National Institute of Standards and Technology or the World Health Organization, and contain an assigned antigen concentration.

Nonisotopic labels have largely replaced radioisotopic labels for routine use in competitive assays in the clinical laboratory (23, 78). Nonisotopic labels are more amenable to automation, are more stable, and reduce safety concerns and regulatory requirements related to the use of radioisotopes. Use of fluorescent labels to develop FIAs offers a sensitive and versatile approach for labeling tracer molecules. High background signals from endogenous fluorescent compounds are one limiting factor in the sensitivity of common fluorescent dyes such as fluorescein. Organic chelates of the rare-earth lanthanide europium serve as improved fluorescent labels due to their relatively long fluorescent lifetime and a large Stokes' shift, the difference between the excitation and emission fluorescent wavelengths (28, 34). Use of time-resolved fluorescence measurements with europium labels provides a large enhancement of signal versus background fluorescence that has been employed for what has been termed dissociation-enhanced lanthanide fluorescence immunoassay (DELFIA), with substantial enhancement in the sensitivity of detection.

Chemiluminoimmunoassays are the chemiluminescent assay equivalent of an RIA. Chemiluminescent molecules emit light after activation in a chemical reaction, usually an oxidation reaction. Chemiluminescent labels usually offer greater sensitivity than fluorescent labels, because chemiluminescence uses no light excitation source that can produce scattered light and because background signal from specimens is very low. Chemiluminescent labels, such as isoluminol, and acridinium esters have been widely applied in automated immunoassays (23, 78).

In enzyme immunoassays (EIAs), the antibody or antigen is labeled by covalently coupling it with an enzyme, which generates a signal through the catalytic action of the enzyme. Enzymes can be directly conjugated to an antibody or antigen, using various chemical cross-linkers, or can be attached to a reagent, such as a secondary antibody or streptavidin, which recognizes the primary antibody modified by biotinylation (14). A wide variety of enzymes have been used as enzyme labels, but peroxidase and alkaline phosphatase are the most common because they are relatively stable, have a very high catalytic rate, and have readily available chromogenic substrates (23, 78). EIAs are quantified by measuring the activity of the enzyme with either a chromogenic, fluorogenic, or chemiluminescent substrate. Several enzyme cascade-type reactions have also been used to further amplify the signal (67). In these reactions, the product of the covalently attached enzyme is utilized by two or more coupled reactions that continuously recycle the original product, and with each cycle more signal is generated.

A number of homogeneous formats for antigen excess assays have been developed (Table 3). Elimination of a separation step makes these assays easier and more rapid to perform, but generally they have lower sensitivity than heterogeneous assays. Fluorescence polarization immunoassay

(FPIA) was one of the first homogeneous assays developed and became widely available in the Abbott TDx analyzer (11). FPIA depends on the change in rotational movement of a small fluorescence-labeled antigen when it binds to antibody. When the fluorescent label is excited with plane polarized light, the decreased rotational movement of the bound tracer results in a greater polarization of the emitted fluorescent light. FPIAs are competitive-type assays in which the antigen in the test sample competes with the fluorescently labeled antigen for binding to a limited amount of antibody. FPIAs have been developed for many different therapeutic drugs and other small molecules and are sensitive down to the micromolar to nanomolar concentration range.

Two other homogeneous competitive immunoassays that are also commonly used to measure small antigens, such as drugs, are the enzyme multiplied immunoassay technique (EMIT) (65) and the cloned enzyme donor immunoassay (CEDIA) (29). In EMIT assays, the target antigen is covalently attached to an enzyme and when an antibody specific to the drug binds to the drug-enzyme complex, the activity of the enzyme is decreased by steric blockade of the active site. Addition of antigen in a specimen competes for antibody binding and frees up labeled enzyme molecules to have increased enzyme activity.

In CEDIA, one of two recombinant fragments of beta-galactosidase is conjugated to the antigen being measured. The two enzyme fragments normally spontaneously assemble in solution to create an active enzyme complex. However, this assembly is prevented if the reagent antibody binds to the antigen-enzyme fragment. Antigen in the test sample competes for antibody binding and frees up the antigen-labeled fragment to form active enzyme. Important practical advantages of the EMIT and CEDIA are that they require simple absorbance measurements and no separation step.

Antibody Excess Assays

Antibody excess assays, unlike competitive RIAs, employ an excess of antibody or binding reagent in a noncompetitive assay format. Although not frequently considered classic immunoassays, immunoblotting, immunohistochemistry, direct immunofluorescence, and flow cytometry, which are used to detect antigens in gel membranes, tissue sections, cell lines, and cells in suspension, respectively, are simple reactions generally with excess antibody relative to antigen.

Immunoradiometric assays (IRMAs) (29, 50, 77) are the antibody excess assay equivalent of RIAs. Generally, IRMAs use an excess of two or more antibodies (23, 78) that recognize different epitopes on the analyte and are called two-site or sandwich-type assays (Fig. 3). Unlike in competitive assays, the signal from the assay is directly proportional to the concentration of the analyte. These assays are well-suited for large protein antigens that have multiple epitopes. Reliance on the binding of antibodies to two different epitopes helps improve the specificity of these assays. Frequently, at least one of the two antibodies is a monoclonal antibody to ensure that the two antibodies recognize different epitopes and do not compete with each other. The two antibodies can be incubated with the antigen simultaneously (one-step assay) or sequentially (two-step assay), with a wash step between the two antibody steps. Typically, one of the antibodies is attached to some type of solid support and is called the capture antibody, whereas the other antibody is labeled to generate the signal and is called the signal or detector antibody. The sandwich-type complex that is formed between the two antibodies and the antigen is then separated from excess free labeled antibody by a wash step before measurement of bound signal (Fig. 3).

Like for antigen excess assays, both isotopic and nonisotopic signal detection systems can be used in these types of assays, and the name of the signal detection system is usually incorporated into the assay name (Table 3). Two-site immunometric assays are typically more sensitive than competitive-type assays and can routinely detect analytes down to the femtomolar concentration range. These assays are also usually significantly faster than competitive-type assays, because the use of excess antibody increases the rate of the reaction between the antibody and antigen. Disadvantages of the immunometric assays are the requirement for the target antigen to be large enough to have two separate epitopes without steric hindrance of simultaneous antibody binding and use of larger amounts of antibody reagent. Use of excess labeled antibody also potentially increases the background from nonspecific binding, which often becomes the major factor limiting the sensitivity of these assays. Blocking proteins,

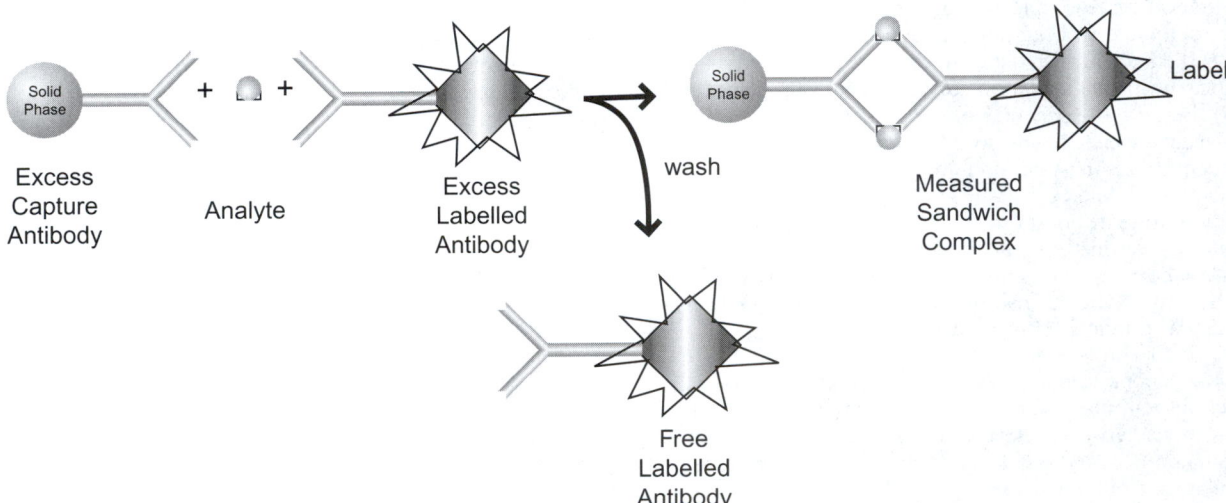

FIGURE 3 Diagram of a two-site antibody excess-type immunometric (labeled-antibody) assay.

such as albumin, and mild detergents are frequently added to the reaction buffer and wash solutions to reduce the background from nonspecific binding.

By reversing the assay format to use antigen as a capture reagent, many serological assays to detect antibodies with particular binding specificities can be performed in reagent excess formats. Describing these assay formats as antibody excess is somewhat of a misnomer in that excess antigen replaces antibody as the capture reagent, and it would be more accurate to term these assays as reagent excess rather than antibody excess. One example of this type of assay is the radioallergosorbent test, in which allergen-specific IgE antibodies are detected by incubating the sample with a solid support coated with an excess of a specific allergen (25). After a wash step, any bound IgE is then measured after detection with a labeled secondary antibody that is specific to human IgE. Antibodies to antigens of many infectious agents, such as hepatitis viruses, human immunodeficiency virus, and many other pathogens, can be assessed by measuring binding of selected classes of immunoglobulins to immobilized antigens of the pathogen.

Automation of Immunoassays

Except for turbidimetric and nephelometric tests, which were first automated in the late 1960s (63), automated analyzers for performing most immunoassays were relatively slow to evolve compared to other kinds of laboratory testing. The discovery of nonisotopic labels and homogeneous assays in the 1970s heralded the development of fully automated immunoassay analyzers in the early 1980s for drugs and other small molecules (11). The emergence of dedicated analyzers in the early 1990s that could use a solid support for separating bound and free analytes made it possible also to automate heterogeneous immunoassays for low-abundance proteins, such as peptide hormones. Currently, there are over two dozen different types of automated immunoassay analyzers (74), and like for the rest of the clinical laboratory, automation has greatly improved both the consistency and efficiency of immunoassay testing.

Automated assays are now available for almost all common diagnostic immunoassays and have largely replaced manual testing (4, 74). Manual RIA and ELISA are primarily limited to esoteric testing and research assays. Many automated immunoassay analyzers can perform over 50 different types of tests, with a throughput over 200 tests per hour. Manual immunoassays often take several hours to a day to perform; the antigen-antibody reaction is often allowed to approach equilibrium in order to maximize the signal and to reduce any variability from subtle differences in the timing of the various steps. In contrast, analysis time for most automated immunoassays is less than 1 h; these assays are performed under nonequilibrium conditions. This is possible because automated immunoassays use sensitive signal detection systems, such as fluorescence and chemiluminescence, that generate enough signal even with short reaction times, and automation enables very precise timing of all steps in assays. As a consequence, the intra-assay and interassay variabilities of automated immunoassays are also usually much better than for manual tests.

The menu for automated immunoassay analyzers has steadily increased and has now expanded to include a wide spectrum of tests, such as drug assays, protein hormones, steroids, tumor markers, and even serological tests, which in the past may have been done by different parts of the clinical laboratory. Automated immunoassays have, therefore, improved the efficiency of clinical laboratories by facilitating consolidation. Currently, there is also great interest and effort in developing immunoassay analyzers that can be integrated with other automated systems, such as general chemistry analyzers, to allow even greater lab integration and efficiency from full laboratory automation.

Because of the wide variety of automated immunoassay analyzers that are currently available, it is sometimes difficult to identify the best instrument for any given laboratory (4). Besides the analytical quality of the lab tests that are available on any given analyzer, there are many other factors to consider when choosing the best immunoassay platform (Table 4). The characteristics of the laboratory and how any new analyzer will fit with the operation and goals of the laboratory must be considered.

TABLE 4 Factors in selection of an immunoassay

Factor
Analytical
Sensitivity
Precision
Accuracy/test standardization
Linearity
Interferences
Carryover effects
Calibration stability
Economic
Purchase cost
Lease options
Maintenance costs
Reagent costs
Operator time and costs
Disposable costs
Instrument
Maintenance requirements
Automation compatibility
Space requirements
Utility requirements
Autodilution ability
Tube handling capability
Reliability
Information system compatibility
Clot error detection
Manufacturer
Future product plans
Reputation
Technical support
Menu expansion plans
Operational
Test menu
Test mode capability
Throughput
Reagent capacity
Reagent stability
Onboard reagent stability
STAT capability
Reflex testing capability
Reagent kit size
Training requirements
Operating complexity
Waste requirements
Reagent storage requirements
Downtime plans

Rapid, Point-of-Care Immunoassays

Small point-of-care devices represent one of the fastest-growing forms of immunoassay testing. These types of tests allow rapid pregnancy or ovulation testing in a home or clinic setting. The menu of tests that can be performed with simple point-of-care devices includes a wide variety of tests, such as assays for rapid detection of influenza virus or streptococcal antigens, serum markers for myocardial infarction or congestive heart failure, drugs of abuse in urine, and antibodies to human immunodeficiency virus.

Point-of-care devices rely on the same basic principles as other immunoassays, but the methods for physical separation of bound and unbound components and for signal generation differ somewhat from most other applications of immunoassay methods. Most of the current generation of point-of-care immunoassays employ single-use lateral-flow devices (7, 26). A specimen is applied to a membrane strip and the specimen flows along the strip by capillary action. An early zone of the membrane contains small colored particles derivatized with a specific antibody or antigen which interacts with the specimen. As the mixture of particles and specimen continues to flow along the membrane, they pass over a zone of immobilized antibody or antigen. If the specimen contains a large antigen, such as hCG, that is targeted in the assay, it forms a sandwich between antibody-coated particles and immobilized antibodies on the membrane. This creates a visible colored line on the membrane that can be detected visually or with a photometer. If no antigen is present, the particles are not retained by the immobilized antibody and they are swept away by continued flow of the specimen, which serves as a washing and separation step. The situation described represents a typical antibody excess reaction. Some lateral-flow assays, for example, for molecules (such as drugs of abuse) that are too small to serve as bridges in sandwich-type assays, represent competitive or antigen excess formats in which a positive result is represented by a decrease in binding of particles to the zone of recognition.

Visually interpreted assays are best suited for qualitative interpretations such as positive or negative results for pregnancy or influenza virus antigen detection. However, progressive miniaturization of photometers and other components of analyzers makes it possible to perform virtually any immunoassay method with a small portable analyzer. Analysis of parathyroid hormone (PTH) by portable analyzers in operating rooms serves as one example of the feasibility of performing virtually any quantitative assay with small portable analyzers (69).

Methods for Analyzing Structural Variation in Proteins

Clinical laboratories have applied a variety of electrophoretic, chromatographic, and other separation techniques to analysis of proteins. These techniques are useful for qualitative analysis of the size, charge, associations, and other physical properties of proteins that may not be distinguished by quantitative methods such as immunoassays or functional assays.

Fractionation by Precipitation or Flotation

Centrifugation represents one of the simplest methods for separating proteins into two or more fractions, usually a precipitate and a soluble fraction. Prior to centrifugation the specimen may be incubated in the cold to allow cryoprecipitate formation, or the composition of the specimen may be adjusted with additives to change ionic strength, pH, or other properties of the solution. These simple separations have been applied to a variety of clinical applications: analysis of cryoprecipitates, identification of antibody-bound versus free proteins, separating protein-bound from free components, separating various lipoproteins by density or differential precipitation, and preparative cell and subcellular fractionations. Because these techniques generally do not have an associated method for detection other than by visual inspection, these separation techniques commonly are used as preparative steps to generate a soluble precipitate fraction that is subjected to another analytical technique.

Electrophoretic Methods

There are a large number of different electrophoretic techniques based on variation in electrolyte composition, support or separation medium, and detection method. Separations are based on the differential migration of proteins in an electric field due to variation in protein charge or size. Clinical laboratory analyses of proteins in biological fluids such as serum, cerebrospinal fluid, and urine provide quantitative analysis of specific components and qualitative identification of unusual components, such as abundant monoclonal immunoglobulins. Tiselius originally described electrophoretic separations of proteins in open columns (70). Subsequently, many variations of this technique using different support and separation media, such as paper, nitrocellulose membranes, agarose gels, and polyacrylamide gels, were described (37), and recently electrophoresis in open columns has returned as a common clinical technique in the form of capillary electrophoresis (5). These low-resolution analyses separate components into prealbumin, albumin, and one or more α, β, and γ fractions. Protein stains such as amido black visualize the distribution of all protein components. In capillary electrophoresis, all proteins are detected without staining by measurement of absorbance in the UV region as proteins migrate through an absorbance detector. Other staining procedures such as immunofixation followed by staining, use of lipid stains, or addition of enzyme substrates allow selective detection of different components. Immunofixation analysis is commonly applied to evaluate monoclonal immunoglobulins.

Isoelectric focusing is an equilibrium method in which a pH gradient is formed by the electrolyte or support medium and proteins migrate until they reach their isoelectric point (pH at which the protein has no net charge). This method provides higher resolution than the typical methods for serum protein analysis, and it is applied in the clinical laboratory to achieve higher-resolution separations of immunoglobulins for evaluation of oligoclonal bands in cerebrospinal fluid. Isoelectric focusing also is commonly applied as a first-dimension separation in two-dimensional electrophoresis, which is discussed later in this chapter.

Electrophoretic separations based primarily on protein size can be performed by using gels with a gradient of decreasing pore size or by analysis of proteins in a denaturant, such as sodium dodecyl sulfate (SDS), that dissociates proteins into individual peptide chains. These techniques have been applied clinically to analysis of the size distribution of urinary proteins and lipoproteins (45, 47). The technique described by Laemmli (41) for SDS-polyacrylamide gel electrophoresis also has been applied frequently as a research tool due to its relatively high resolution and size-based separation of polypeptides.

Chromatographic Methods

Chromatographic methods allow the separation of proteins and peptides based on size, charge, or adsorption to a variety of hydrophobic or affinity matrices. Size separation of proteins and peptides by gel filtration or size exclusion chromatography is best suited for separating molecules or complexes that have a relatively large difference in size (76). It has been applied to analysis of a variety of antibody-antigen complexes such as macroenzymes formed by binding of an enzyme to cognate autoantibodies or by binding of a small hormone, such as insulin, to a cognate autoantibody. Gel filtration allows rapid separation of bound and free antigens in these cases based on the much smaller size of the free antigen.

Ion-exchange chromatography allows separation of proteins and peptides primarily based on differences in net charge that result in differential binding to a solid phase bearing groups with an opposite charge. An example of an application in clinical laboratories is the analysis of glycated hemoglobin (21). This technique can be used as a preparative technique such as for the preparation of a partially purified immunoglobulin fraction from serum or as part of a multistep purification of virtually any protein or peptide.

Most peptides and proteins have some affinity for hydrophobic stationary phases such as octyl (C_8) or octadecyl (C_{18}) silica (32). Differential elution of peptides and proteins can be achieved using a gradient of progressively increasing hydrophobicity such as aqueous solution with an increasing concentration of acetonitrile. This technique of reverse-phase chromatography has been of greatest utility for separations of peptides. Separations of proteins generally are less efficient due to lesser variability in their absorption characteristics and denaturation of proteins in the organic solvents.

Many different types of adsorptive phases have been used for affinity chromatography (30). Immobilized antibodies provide a highly selective phase for rapid purification of selected antigen molecules that might be eluted for analysis of molecular variation by a technique such as mass spectrometry. Lectins, streptavidin, or a variety of other affinity matrices can be used for separations of classes of molecules interacting with the affinity matrix. Binding of glycated hemoglobin to phenylboronate groups has been applied by clinical laboratories to determine the fraction of hemoglobin occurring as a glycated form.

QUALITY ASSURANCE OF TESTING

General Quality Assurance Measures

The goal of quality assurance activities is to make sure that the complete testing process is performed reliably and reported in a manner most appropriate for clinical interpretation. Usually, the central components of a quality assurance program are considered to be quality control (QC) and proficiency testing (PT) programs. However, QC and PT serve as checks only for the analytical process, and there are many other critical steps in the testing process. Some other measures that generally are necessary to monitor and ensure proper performance of the testing process include thorough evaluation of new tests, identification of any test limitations or interferences, determination of reference ranges, development of procedures and appropriate materials for patient preparation and specimen collection and processing, development of information sources and ordering procedures that help direct accurate and appropriate ordering of tests, ensuring appropriate staff qualifications and training, programs for equipment maintenance, criteria for repeat testing in the case of questionable or critical results, monitoring of turnaround times, and review of information systems and reporting processes.

QC programs evaluate testing for repeated analysis of pooled material and are designed primarily to identify systematic changes in an analytical process, such as from deterioration of a reagent over time. Consistent values for QC materials determine that a test has stable performance but do not necessarily ensure that test results are accurate. Federal regulations in the United States mandate that at least two levels of QC material be analyzed daily for each test that is performed. For qualitative tests, these would be materials representing positive and negative specimens, and for quantitative tests, these should represent high and low results. QC materials should be selected to have values that ensure appropriate performance near important clinical decision values, so for some tests, more than two levels of QC material may be desirable. The stability of test systems needs to be evaluated to determine whether QC testing should be performed daily or at more frequent intervals. Some point-of-care devices have internal procedural controls that check on the performance of each test or have electronic simulators that may check performance of an analyzer. The degree to which these measures substitute for analysis of QC materials is controversial, and laboratories need to review the extent to which regulations allow these substitutions. Another alternative process for QC of procedures is to perform statistical evaluation of patient results. This may help detect gradual shifts in testing processes or changes in the preanalytical process such as changes in patient preparation, collection devices, or specimen processing that are not monitored by traditional QC.

PT compares the analysis of the same pooled specimens by different laboratories. PT serves as a measure of test accuracy and variation in performance between laboratories. Target values for a specific test may be established by statistical analysis of all participating laboratories or, for selected tests, by analysis of specimens by reference methods.

QC and PT serve as indicators of systematic changes in a testing process, but they are not effective measures for detecting sporadic errors due to problems such as specimen dilution with intravenous fluid, hemolysis of specimens, or specimen clots or bubbles which interfere with sampling. Checks of the specimen for potential interferences such as hemoglobin or lipemia and criteria for repeat analyses based on extreme values or changes from previous values (delta checks) may identify some specimen collection problems or sporadic errors.

Troubleshooting Immunoassay

Immunoassays have several limitations which are important to recognize, particularly when interpreting unexpected or discordant test results (39, 66). One important inherent limitation of immunoassays is that they sometimes lack sufficient specificity and either endogenous or exogenous substances can affect the accuracy of the result (51). For example, many protein hormones can exist in a large variety of different structural forms, not all of which are biologically active. The biologically active form of PTH has 84 amino acids, but several inactive carboxyl-terminal proteolytic fragments of PTH can accumulate in patients to variable degrees, depending on renal function (15). The particular forms of PTH that are detected by any given assays are dependent upon which epitopes or regions of the PTH molecule the antibodies are directed against. Similarly, in the case of drug immunoassays, depending on the antibody used in an assay, an inactive catabolite of the drug, as well as the active drug, may be detected. Many parent drugs are also similar in structure and hence will often cross-react in immunoassays. Some protein analytes may also be highly polymorphic in their primary amino acid sequence and/or in posttranslational modifications. Some of these variant forms may therefore not be detected, particularly when highly specific monoclonal antibodies are used in assays (57). The ability of an antibody to react with a protein antigen can also be affected by whether the protein is bound to another protein or other subunit, which may mask an epitope on the protein antigen and interfere with binding to an antibody. Also, some molecules seemingly unrelated in terms of overall structure may cross-react or interfere with an immunoassay, because they may still share a relatively small region or epitope. Depending on the assay design, cross-reactive substances can result in either a positive or a negative bias.

Depending on the assay design, unusually high concentrations of an analyte may paradoxically cause a falsely low result by a phenomenon called a hook or prozone effect. Those analytes that have a wide concentration range, such as hCG and tumor markers, are most likely to be affected by this problem. Two-site immunometric assays are particularly prone to hook problems when the antigen concentration is sufficiently high that different antigen molecules are bound to the capture and labeled antibodies. When this occurs a sandwich complex is not formed (Fig. 3), which results in a falsely low value. This problem can be ameliorated by performing the assay on a diluted sample or making sure that there is sufficient excess antibody even for those samples with unusually high levels of the analyte. Two-step immunometric assays that are performed in a sequential manner so that only one antibody is used per step and with a wash step between antibodies also reduce the likelihood of hook effect problems.

Heteroantibodies are another important cause of immunoassay problems (39, 43, 66). Heteroantibodies are nonreagent antibodies that come from the test sample and, depending on the assay design, can cause a positive or negative bias, by reacting with the antibody reagents or the analyte. For example, autoantibodies, such as rheumatoid factor, which binds IgG, can interfere with immunoassays by blocking the reagent antibody from reacting with the analyte or by cross-linking the reagent antibody. Autoantibodies that are induced as a consequence of the administration of a therapeutic recombinant protein may also interfere with the immunoassay of that protein by competing with the reagent antibody. Heterophile antibodies, which are a group of poorly defined antibodies that react with a wide range of antigens, are the most common source of heteroantibody problems. Human anti-mouse antibodies are heterophile antibodies that react with mouse immunoglobulins, and they frequently interfere with immunoassays by binding to mouse monoclonal antibody reagents. Heterophile antibodies may develop due to environmental exposure to different animal immunoglobulins, but they may also develop in patients after the intravenous administration of a therapeutic or diagnostic mouse monoclonal antibody. In order to reduce interference from heterophile antibodies, immunoassay reagents frequently contain mouse and other animal serum or excess nonimmune animal immunoglobulins to compete for the binding of heterophile antibodies.

Various preanalytical factors can also affect immunoassays. Similar to other laboratory tests, hemolysis, lipemia, and bilirubinemia often adversely affect immunoassays. Radioisotopes and fluorescent contrast material given to patients for various radiological imaging procedures can also create problems, depending on the immunoassay label. Some immunoassays are also incompatible with the various blood collection tube additives. For example, EDTA in plasma collection tubes will often interfere with assays that use alkaline phosphatase, because it will chelate Zn from the reaction mixture, which is a necessary cofactor for the enzyme. Many protein analytes are labile and are prone to proteolysis and must, therefore, be processed quickly and properly stored to get accurate results. Finally, in the case of drugs and those analytes that show a large diurnal variation, the specimen must be collected at the appropriate time in order to properly interpret the result.

As with all diagnostic assays, it is critical that the clinical laboratory assess the analytical performance of its immunoassays with a QC program. Immunoassays are particularly prone to drift between lots of reagents because of subtle differences in the binding properties of the antibody reagents. It is also required for clinical laboratories to participate in an external PT program, such as the one offered by the College of American Pathologists. An overall quality assurance program should also be implemented to ensure that the immunoassays are meeting the medical needs of the ordering physicians. Because of the complexity in interpreting many immunoassays, it is especially important for the laboratory to monitor, in conjunction with the ordering physicians, that their immunoassay results are being interpreted and utilized correctly.

RESEARCH APPLICATIONS AND FUTURE DEVELOPMENTS FOR PROTEIN ANALYSIS

Advances in Immunoassay Technologies

There has been ongoing progress in immunoassay methods since their inception over 70 years ago. These provide incremental improvements in sensitivity down to attomolar (10^{-18} M) or zeptomolar (10^{-21} M) limits of detection and progressive miniaturization and acceleration of analyses. Some more fundamental potential changes in immunoassay techniques are (i) the application of new specificity elements such as single-chain antibodies, imprinted polymers (38), or RNA aptamers (36) which may provide chemically defined recognition elements with a different range of specificities and (ii) applications of nanotechnology that offer potential dramatic miniaturization of assays (35) and new detection technologies with high sensitivity such as immuno-PCR, which uses PCR as the reporter system for an immunoassay (52).

Multiplex Immunoassays

Another fundamental change in immunoassay technology is presented by multiplex immunoassays, which measure many components in a single assay rather than one component at a time. Small panels of tests in a single lateral-flow immunoassay device are in common use for applications such as detection of markers for myocardial infarction or for screening for a panel of drugs of abuse (7). However, technological advances in multiplex assays offer the possibility of analyzing a much larger number of components in a single analysis. At present, multiplex assays are in two basic forms—surface based and particle based. In surface-based multiplex assays, an array of spots of different antigens or antibodies is prepared on a surface such as a silica chip, a glass slide, or the well of a microtiter plate (13). Binding of components in a specimen to each spot is analyzed as a separate reaction, using a labeled antigen or antibody component applied after the specimen. Particle-based assays rely on the ability to distinguish particles based on size, color, or other properties (17). This allows the simultaneous analysis of addressable beads derivatized with different antigens or antibodies. Following incubation with specimen and a labeled detection reagent, the signal attached to beads can be analyzed by flow cytometry. Multiplex immunoassays offer the advantages of being able to measure a large number of components simultaneously and to perform replicate analyses of individual components as an internal quality assurance measure. However, there are major challenges in ensuring reproducibility of multiplex assays, in optimizing assays for each of multiple components, and in analyzing the large amount of data generated. As the number of results from a multiplex assay grows, the interpretation of results may need to rely increasingly on sophisticated informatics tools.

Two-Dimensional Gel Electrophoresis and Chromatography

Sequentially combining two separation technologies with different principles of separation allows separation of many more components than either technique alone. The most widely used approaches have been variations of the technique described by O'Farrell (53), which employs isoelectric focusing in the first dimension in the presence of denaturants and nonionic detergents and SDS-polyacrylamide gel electrophoresis in the second dimension. This technique can provide resolution of more than 1,000 components in a single analysis. Two-dimensional electrophoresis has served as a valuable research tool, but clinical use has been limited by low throughput, labor-intensiveness, and complexity in standardization and interpretation of data. Completion of sequencing of the human genome and improvement in mass spectrometric methods for peptide analysis have greatly advanced the ability to identify components separated in two-dimensional gels. The number of plasma components that can be analyzed by two-dimensional gels also has been increased by recent applications of immunosubtraction methods to remove the most abundant plasma components such as albumin, transferrin, and immunoglobulins, which otherwise overload the capacity of the method and limit detection of low-abundance components (22, 59). Considering the large number of potential protein components in plasma, even the highest-resolution methods for two-dimensional gel analysis probably evaluate only a small subset of the most abundant components in plasma.

Two-dimensional gel electrophoresis will fail to detect proteins and peptides that are more basic or acidic than the pH range of the isoelectric focusing analysis and that are smaller than about 7,000 Da. Two-dimensional chromatography offers a separation technology for components that may not be observed by two-dimensional gel electrophoresis, such as small peptides. Two-dimensional or multidimensional chromatography combines complementary separation methods such as chromatofocusing or ion-exchange chromatography with reverse-phase chromatography (73). The first dimension is run in a series of steps that are collected as fractions that are each analyzed by the second mode of separation. This technique has been coupled to detection by tandem mass spectrometry to allow sequence analysis of a thousand or more peptide components in a single run.

Mass Spectrometric Methods

The Nobel Prize in Chemistry was awarded in 2002 to Fenn and Tanaka for the development of two major advances—electrospray ionization and matrix-assisted laser desorption/ionization–time of flight (MALDI-TOF)—in mass spectrometric analysis of proteins (18, 46). These methods have provided new tools for the analysis and identification of proteins and peptides. In the technique of electrospray ionization, a solution containing proteins or peptides is sprayed into fine droplets which, after solvent evaporation, yield individual multiply charged protein molecules. The protein ions are analyzed in a vacuum by a mass spectrometer. This technique uses a liquid specimen so that it can be linked directly to the outflow from liquid chromatography. A single protein tends to generate a number of peaks due to different forms of the protein. Thus, it is difficult to analyze complex mixtures of proteins by this technique. Usually, it is applied to samples enriched for a single protein or to mixtures of peptides that are analyzed by liquid chromatography linked to electrospray ionization mass spectrometry. A recent example is the analysis of molecular variants of transthyretin that are related to hereditary amyloidosis (3).

MALDI-TOF mass spectrometry uses a laser to vaporize a small amount of solid specimen that consists of protein specimens dried with a light-absorbing compound that then serves as the sample matrix. Vaporization of the sample by the laser tends to release predominantly intact polypeptide molecules with a single charge. The charged polypeptides are analyzed in a vacuum by accelerating them in an electric field and measuring how long it takes them to reach a detector (time of flight). Lighter peptides reach a higher speed; analysis of the time of flight allows accurate determination of polypeptide mass. MALDI-TOF mass spectrometry is complementary to electrophoretic methods in that it has highest resolution and detection sensitivity for small peptides. It is possible to analyze large proteins as well, although there is progressive loss of resolution and detection sensitivity as protein size increases. MALDI-TOF mass spectrometry also allows the analysis of profiles of complex mixtures of peptides such as those occurring in biological fluids, resolving up to hundreds of different peaks. It serves as a relatively rapid and simple method of analysis that could find clinical applications. Some processing or fractionation of specimens prior to analysis is required to avoid suppressive effects of salts and abundant protein components. A variation of this technique in which fractionation of the specimen is performed using specimen target plates with a modified surface has been termed surface-enhanced laser desorption/ionization–time-of-flight mass spectrometry (33, 49). In this method, the target surface serves as a selective capture surface that is analyzed by MALDI-TOF mass spectrometry. This technique has generated both excitement as a discovery tool for potential markers of disease (10, 56) and controversy with regard to how to analyze complex sets of data (61) and to achieve acceptable reproducibility for clinical use (31, 68). It is not clear yet whether mass spectrometry will find common clinical laboratory use as a diagnostic tool or whether it will be used primarily as a discovery tool for potential new markers that will then be analyzed by methods such as immunoassay.

REFERENCES

1. **Anderson, N. L., and N. G. Anderson.** 2002. The human plasma proteome: history, character, and diagnostic prospects. *Mol. Cell. Proteomics* **1:**845–867.
2. **Anderson, N. L., M. Polanski, R. Pieper, T. Gatlin, R. S. Tirumalai, T. P. Conrads, T. D. Veenstra, J. N. Adkins, J. G. Pounds, R. Fagan, and A. Lobley.** 2004. The human plasma proteome: a nonredundant list developed by combination of four separate sources. *Mol. Cell. Proteomics* **3:**311–326.
3. **Bergen, H. R., III, S. R. Zeldenrust, M. L. Butz, D. S. Snow, P. J. Dyck, C. J. Klein, J. F. O'Brien, S. N. Thibodeau, and D. C. Muddiman.** 2004. Identification of

transthyretin variants by sequential proteomic and genomic analysis. *Clin. Chem.* **50**:1544–1552.

4. **Blick, K. E.** 1996. Specifications for the selection of automated immunoassay systems. *J. Clin. Immunol.* **19**:220–228.

5. **Bossuyt, X.** 2004. Interferences in clinical capillary zone electrophoresis of serum proteins. *Electrophoresis* **25**:1485–1487.

6. **Bowen, R. A. R., Y. Chan, J. Cohen, N. N. Rehak, G. L. Hortin, G. Csako, and A. T. Remaley.** 2005. Effect of blood collection tubes on total triiodothyronine and other laboratory assays. *Clin. Chem.* **51**:424–433.

7. **Buechler, K. F., S. Moi, B. Noar, D. McGrath, J. Villela, M. Clancy, A. Shenhav, A. Colleymore, G. Valkirs, T. Lee, et al.** 1992. Simultaneous detection of seven drugs of abuse by the Triage panel for drugs of abuse. *Clin. Chem.* **38**:1678–1684.

8. **Cambiasco, C. L., H. A. Riccomi, P. L. Mason, and J. F. Hermans.** 1974. Automated nephelometric immunoassay: its application to the determination of hapten. *J. Immunol. Methods* **5**:293–302.

9. **Chaurand, P., M. E. Sanders, R. A. Jensen, and R. M. Caprioli.** 2004. Proteomics in diagnostic pathology: profiling and imaging proteins directly in tissue sections. *Am. J. Pathol.* **165**:1057–1068.

10. **Clarke, W., Z. Zhang, and D. W. Chan.** 2003. The application of clinical proteomics to cancer and other diseases. *Clin. Chem. Lab. Med.* **41**:1562–1570.

11. **Dandliker, W. B., R. J. Kelly, J. Dandliker, J. Farquahar, and J. Levin.** 1973. Fluorescence polarization immunoassay. Theory and experimental method. *Immunochemistry* **10**:219–227.

12. **De Hoog, C. L., and M. Mann.** 2004. Proteomics. *Annu. Rev. Genomics Hum. Genet.* **5**:267–293.

13. **Delehanty, J. B., and F. S. Ligler.** 2002. A microarray immunoassay for simultaneous detection of proteins and bacteria. *Anal. Chem.* **74**:5681–5687.

14. **Diamandis, E. P., and T. K. Christopoulos.** 1991. The biotin-(strept)avidin system: principles and applications in biotechnology. *Clin. Chem.* **37**:625–636.

15. **Dilena, B. A., and G. H. White.** 1989. Interference with measurement of intact parathyrin in serum from renal dialysis patients. *Clin. Chem.* **35**:1543–1544.

16. **Drake, S. K., R. A. R. Bowen, A. T. Remaley, and G. L. Hortin.** 2004. Potential interferences from blood collection tubes in mass spectrometric analyses of serum polypeptides. *Clin. Chem.* **50**:2398–2401.

17. **Dunbar, S. A., C. A. Vander Zee, K. G. Oliver, K. L. Karem, and J. W. Jacobson.** 2003. Quantitative, multiplexed detection of bacterial pathogens: DNA and protein applications of the Luminex LabMAP system. *J. Microbiol. Methods* **53**:245–252.

18. **Fenn, J. B., M. Mann, D. K. Meng, S. F. Wong, and C. M. Whitehouse.** 1989. Electrospray ionization for mass spectrometry of large biomolecules. *Science* **246**:64–71.

19. **Gerlach, R. W., R. J. White, S. N. Deming, J. A. Palasota, and J. M. van Emon.** 1993. An evaluation of five commercial immunoassay data analysis software systems. *Anal. Biochem.* **212**:185–193.

20. **Geysen, H. M., T. J. Mason, and S. J. Rodda.** 1988. Cognitive features of continuous antigenic epitopes. *J. Mol. Recognit.* **1**:32–41.

21. **Goldstein, D. E., R. R. Little, H. M. Wiedmeyer, J. D. England, and E. M. McKenzie.** 1986. Glycated hemoglobin. Methodologies and clinical applications. *Clin. Chem.* **32**(Suppl.):B64–B70.

22. **Gorg, A., W. Weiss, and M. J. Dunn.** 2004. Current two-dimensional electrophoresis technology for proteomics. *Proteomics* **4**:3665–3685.

23. **Gosling, J. P.** 2000. *Immunoassays: a Practical Approach.* Oxford University Press, Oxford, United Kingdom.

24. **Gross, S., and D. Piwnica-Worms.** 2005. Spying on cancer: molecular imaging in vivo with genetically encoded reporters. *Cancer Cell* **7**:5–15.

25. **Hamilton, R. G., and N. F. Adkinson, Jr.** 2003. Clinical laboratory assessment of IgE-dependent hypersensitivity. *J. Allergy Clin. Immunol.* **111**:S687–S701.

26. **Harvey, M. A., C. A. Audette, and R. McDonogh.** 1996. The use of microporous polymer membranes in immunoassays. *IVD Technol.* **2**:34–39.

27. **Heidelberger, M., and F. W. Kendall.** 1929. A quantitative study of the precipitin reaction between type III pneumococcus polysaccharide and purified homologous antibody. *J. Exp. Med.* **50**:809–823.

28. **Hemmila, I., S. Dakubu, V. M. Mukkala, H. Siitari, and T. Lovgren.** 1984. Europium as a label in time-resolved immunofluorometric assays. *Anal. Biochem.* **137**:335–343.

29. **Henderson, D. R., S. B. Friedman, J. D. Harris, W. B. Manning, and M. A. Zoccoli.** 1986. CEDIA, a new homogeneous immunoassay system. *Clin. Chem.* **32**:1637–1641.

30. **Hermanson, G. T., A. K. Mallia, and P. K. Smith.** 1992. *Immobilized Affinity Ligand Techniques.* Academic Press, San Diego, Calif.

31. **Hortin, G. L.** 2005. Can mass spectrometric protein profiling meet desired standards of clinical laboratory practice? *Clin. Chem.* **51**:3–5.

32. **Issaq, H. J., T. P. Conrads, G. M. Janini, and T. D. Veenstra.** 2002. Methods for fractionation, separation and profiling of proteins and peptides. *Electrophoresis* **23**:3048–3061.

33. **Issaq, H. J., T. D. Veenstra, T. P. Conrads, and D. Felschow.** 2002. The SELDI-TOF MS approach to proteomics: protein profiling and biomarker identification. *Biochem. Biophys. Res. Commun.* **292**:587–592.

34. **Jackson, T. M., and R. P. Ekins.** 1986. Theoretical limitations on immunoassay sensitivity. Current practice and potential advantages of fluorescent Eu3+ chelates as nonradioisotopic tracers. *J. Immunol. Methods* **87**:13–20.

35. **Jain, K. K.** 2003. Nanodiagnostics: applications of nanotechnology in molecular diagnostics. *Expert Rev. Mol. Diagn.* **3**:153–161.

36. **Jayasena, S. D.** 1999. Aptamers: an emerging class of molecules that rival antibodies in diagnostics. *Clin. Chem.* **45**:1628–1650.

37. **Jeppson, J.-O., C.-B. Laurell, and B. Franzen.** 1979. Agarose gel electrophoresis. *Clin. Chem.* **25**:629–638.

38. **Kitade, T., K. Kitamura, T. Konishi, S. Takegami, T. Okuno, M. Ishikawa, M. Wakabayashi, K. Nishikawa, and Y. Muramatsu.** 2004. Potentiometric immunosensor using artificial antibody based on molecularly imprinted polymers. *Anal. Chem.* **76**:6802–6807.

39. **Klee, G. G.** 2004. Interferences in hormone immunoassays. *Clin. Lab. Med.* **24**:1–18.

40. **Kohler, G., and C. Milstein.** 1975. Continuous culture of fused cells secreting specific antibody of predicted specificity. *Nature* **256**:495–497.

41. **Laemmli, U. K.** 1970. Cleavage of structural proteins during the assembly of the head of bacteriophage T4. *Nature* **227**:680–685.

42. **Landsteiner, K., and D. H. Witt.** 1926. Observations on the human blood groups. Irregular reactions. Iso-agglutinin in sera of group 4. The factor A1. *J. Immunol.* **2**:221–229.

43. **Levinson, S. S., and J. J. Miller.** 2002. Towards a better understanding of heterophile (and the like) antibody interference with modern immunoassays. *Clin. Chim. Acta* **325**:1–15.

44. **Li, Z., C. J. Woo, M. D. Iglesias-Ussel, D. Ronai, and M. D. Scharff.** 2004. The generation of antibody diversity through somatic hypermutation and class switch recombination. *Genes Dev.* **18**:1–11.

45. **Maachi, M., S. Fellahi, A. Regeniter, M. E. Diop, J. Capeau, J. Rossert, and J. P. Bastard.** 2004. Patterns

of proteinuria: urinary sodium dodecyl sulfate electrophoresis versus immunonephelometric protein marker measurement followed by interpretation with the knowledge-based system MDI-LabLink. *Clin. Chem.* **50**:1834–1837.

46. **Marvin, L. F., M. A. Roberts, and L. B. Fay.** 2003. Matrix-assisted laser desorption/ionization time-of-flight mass spectrometry in clinical chemistry. *Clin. Chim. Acta* **337**:11–21.

47. **McNamara, J., H. Campos, J. Ordovas, J. Peterson, P. Wilson, and E. Schaefer.** 1987. Effect of gender, age, and lipid status on low-density lipoprotein subfraction distribution: results of the Framingham Offspring Study. *Arteriosclerosis* **7**:483–490.

48. **Mehta, A. I., S. Ross, M. S. Lowenthal, V. Fusaro, D. A. Fishman, E. F. Petricoin III, and L. A. Liotta.** 2003. Biomarker amplification by serum carrier protein binding. *Dis. Markers* **19**:1–10.

49. **Merchant, M., and S. R. Weinberger.** 2000. Recent advancements in surface-enhanced laser desorption/ionization-time of flight-mass spectrometry. *Electrophoresis* **21**:1164–1167.

50. **Miles, L. E., and C. N. Hales.** 1968. Labelled antibodies and immunological assay systems. *Nature* **219**:186–189.

51. **Miller, J. J., and R. Valdes.** 1991. Approaches to minimizing interference by cross-reacting molecules in immunoassays. *Clin. Chem.* **37**:144–153.

52. **Niemeyer, C. M., M. Adler, and R. Wacker.** 2005. Immuno-PCR: high sensitivity detection of proteins by nucleic acid amplification. *Trends Biotechnol.* **23**:208–216.

53. **O'Farrell, P. H.** 1975. High resolution two-dimensional electrophoresis of proteins. *J. Biol. Chem.* **250**:4007–4021.

54. **Paek, S. H., S. H. Lee, J. H. Cho, and Y. S. Kim.** 2000. Development of rapid one-step immunochromatographic assay. *Methods* **22**:53–60.

55. **Petricoin, E. F., A. M. Ardekani, B. A. Hitt, P. J. Levine, V. A. Fusaro, S. M. Steinberg, G. B. Mills, C. Simone, D. A. Fishman, E. C. Kohn, and L. A. Liotta.** 2002. Use of proteomic patterns in serum to identify ovarian cancer. *Lancet* **359**:572–577.

56. **Petricoin, E. F., J. Wulfkuhle, V. Espina, and L. A. Liotta.** 2004. Clinical proteomics: revolutionizing disease detection and patient tailoring therapy. *J. Proteome Res.* **3**:209–217.

57. **Pettersson, K., Y.-Q. Ding, and I. Huhtaniemi.** 1991. Monoclonal antibody-based discrepancies between two-site immunometric tests for lutropin. *Clin. Chem.* **37**:1745–1748.

58. **Pieper, R., C. L. Gatlin, A. J. Makusky, P. S. Russo, C. R. Schatz, S. S. Miller, Q. Su, A. M. McGrath, M. A. Estock, P. P. Parmar, M. Zhao, S. T. Huang, J. Zhou, F. Wang, R. Esquer-Blasco, N. L. Anderson, J. Taylor, and S. Steiner.** 2003. The human serum proteome: display of nearly 3700 chromatographically separated protein spots on two-dimensional electrophoresis gels and identification of 325 distinct proteins. *Proteomics* **3**:1345–1364.

59. **Pieper, R., Q. Su, C. L. Gatlin, S. T. Huang, N. L. Anderson, and S. Steiner.** 2003. Multi-component immunoaffinity subtraction chromatography: an innovative step towards a comprehensive survey of the human plasma proteome. *Proteomics* **3**:422–432.

60. **Piwnica-Worms, D., D. P. Schuster, and J. R. Garbow.** 2004. Molecular imaging of host-pathogen interactions in intact small animals. *Cell. Microbiol.* **6**:319–331.

61. **Ransohoff, D. F.** 2005. Lessons from controversy: ovarian cancer screening and serum proteomics. *J. Natl. Cancer Inst.* **97**:315–319.

62. **Rich, R. L., and D. G. Myszka.** 2000. Advances in surface plasmon resonance biosensor analysis. *Curr. Opin. Biotechnol.* **11**:54–61.

63. **Ritchie, R. F., C. A. Alper, and J. A. Graves.** 1969. Experience with a fully automated system for immunoassay of specific serum proteins. *Arthritis Rheum.* **12**:693–699.

64. **Rosenblatt, K. P., P. Bryant-Greenwood, J. K. Killian, A. Mehta, D. Geho, V. Espina, E. F. Petricoin III, and L. A. Liotta.** 2004. Serum proteomics in cancer diagnosis and management. *Annu. Rev. Med.* **55**:97–112.

65. **Rubenstein, K. E., R. S. Schneider, and E. F. Ullman.** 1972. "Homogeneous" enzyme immunoassay. A new immunochemical technique. *Biochem. Biophys. Res. Commun.* **47**:846–851.

66. **Selby, C.** 1999. Interference in immunoassay. *Ann. Clin. Biochem.* **36**:704–721.

67. **Self, C. H.** 1985. Enzyme amplification—a general method applied to provide an immunoassisted assay for placental alkaline phosphatase. *J. Immunol. Methods* **76**:389–393.

68. **Semmes, O. J., Z. Feng, B.-L. Adam, L. L. Banez, D. Campos, L. H. Cazares, D. W. Chan, W. E. Grizzle, E. Izbicka, J. Kagan, G. Malik, D. McLerran, J. W. Moul, A. Partin, P. Prasanna, J. Rosenzweig, L. J. Sokoll, S. Srivastava, S. Srivastava, I. Thompson, M. J. Welsh, N. White, M. Winget, Y. Yasui, Z. Zhang, and L. Zhu.** 2005. Evaluation of serum protein profiling by surface-enhanced laser desorption/ionization time-of-flight mass spectrometry for the detection of prostate cancer. I. Assessment of platform reproducibility. *Clin. Chem.* **51**:102–112.

69. **Sokoll, L. J., F. H. Wians, Jr., and A. T. Remaley.** 2004. Rapid intraoperative immunoassay of parathyroid hormone and other hormones: a new paradigm for point-of-care testing. *Clin. Chem.* **50**:1126–1135.

70. **Tiselius, A.** 1937. A new apparatus for electrophoresis: analysis of colloidal mixtures. *Trans. Faraday Soc.* **33**:524–529.

71. **Tribbick, G.** 2002. Multipin peptide libraries for antibody and receptor epitope screening and characterization. *J. Immunol. Methods* **267**:27–35.

72. **Villanueva, J., J. Philip, D. Entenberg, C. A. Chaparro, M. K. Tanwar, E. C. Holland, and P. Tempst.** 2004. Serum peptide profiling by magnetic particle-assisted, automated sample processing and MALDI-TOF mass spectrometry. *Anal. Chem.* **76**:1560–1570.

73. **Wang, H., and S. Hanash.** 2003. Multi-dimensional liquid phase separations in proteomics. *J. Chromatogr. B* **787**:11–18.

74. **Wheeler, M. J.** 2001. Automated immunoassay analysers. *Ann. Clin. Biochem.* **38**:217–229.

75. **Whicher, J. T., C. P. Price, and K. Spencer.** 1983. Immunonephelometric and immunoturbidimetric assays for proteins. *Crit. Rev. Clin. Lab. Sci.* **18**:213–260.

76. **Winzor, D. J.** 2003. Analytical exclusion chromatography. *J. Biochem. Biophys. Methods* **30**:15–52.

77. **Woodhead, J. S., G. M. Addison, and C. N. Hales.** 1974. Radioimmunoassay and saturation analysis. The immunoradiometric assay and related techniques. *Br. Med. Bull.* **30**:44–49.

78. **Wu, J. T.** 2000. *Quantitative Immunoassays: a Practical Guide for Assay Establishment, Troubleshooting, and Clinical Application.* AACC Press, Washington, D.C.

79. **Yalow, R. S., and S. A. Berson.** 1959. Assay of plasma insulin in human subjects by immunological methods. *Nature* **184**:1648–1649.

Genomics and Chip Technology

STEPHEN J. CHANOCK

4

The genomics revolution has ushered in a new age in scientific research which has notably expanded the paradigm of scientific investigation. Until recently, genetic studies examined individual gene expression by Northern blotting or single polymorphisms by gel-based restriction fragment length polymorphism analysis, but with new high-throughput technologies, it is possible to survey the expression of all transcripts in a cell in parallel or analyze thousands of sequence variants at once. This shift towards examining expression patterns in a single genome has been possible because of the technical advances in microchips and bead arrays. Incidentally, the same technologies can interrogate thousands of genetic variants in one individual genome.

The genomic age has tremendous potential to explore the interactions between a host and either its environment or pathogens. The genomic paradigm becomes more complex as the analysis incorporates genomic observations derived from both host and pathogen. Still, the near future promises to see the realization of patterns of genes integral to disease susceptibility and outcomes, which can be used to develop new drug targets or preventive strategies (7). Already, we have seen examples in pharmacogenomics, such as the association of drug efficacy in lung cancer patients receiving the targeted therapy gefitinib in subjects with a particular type of somatic mutation in the tumor (16).

As a consequence of the high-throughput analytical platforms, there has been an explosion in the generation of data, particularly in public databases (17). Accordingly, analytical capabilities for these ambitious large-scale studies have lagged behind the generation of genomic data. The creation of common databases replete with search tools has made this staggering amount of data available to many investigators, some of whom will undoubtedly continue to forge novel analytical approaches. In turn, validation can easily be based on analysis of existing data and the robustness of a new approach can be judged against current standard practices and previous publications. In a short period, the genomics age has shifted a substantial proportion of study to the search for patterns or profiles of expression or genetic variants in specific diseases. Eventually, it will be necessary to refine the paradigm so that the transition from research observation can seamlessly move into clinical practice under standards agreed upon by all.

DNA MICROARRAY EXPRESSION

There are two different techniques for spotting known DNA sequences in microarray expression analyses; either cDNA clones or synthesized oligonucleotides (notably, the length of oligonucleotides has increased over the past decade) are spotted as DNA probes on a solid support, such as a glass microscope slide. All genes expressed in an organism or cell type can be spotted onto a surface using robotics and an informatic grid that locates the precise position of each DNA probe. Annotated double-stranded cDNA clones, usually presequenced for validation, are PCR amplified, purified, and spotted in a predetermined array pattern. Oligonucleotides can be synthesized as short (25 bp) or long (50 to 75 bp) and directly printed on a glass surface or synthesized onto the glass or silicon surface. Photolithography technology has emerged as a standard technology for spotting oligonucleotides on array surfaces, which, incidentally, is the same technology as used for computer microchips (15).

Microarray analysis interrogates total RNA or mRNA purified from cell or tissue sources. If a sufficient quantity of RNA is available, reverse transcription can be performed directly, but if there is limited RNA, protocols for amplification of the cDNA can faithfully represent the target RNA with a modicum of variance (24). cDNA is labeled with either dUTP-biotin or a conjugated fluorescent dye, such as Cy3 or Cy5, which is easily detected with a fluorescent scanner. Depending on the study design, the labeled probes are singly or in combination hybridized to the microarray slides prior to scanning for digital imaging. The coordinates for each spot and known duplicates guide the collection of data and permit facile determination of individual gene expression profiles.

The prospect of developing more accurate diagnostic profiles of diseases represents a major goal of microarray technology applied to gene expression. In one experiment, one can assess the relative differences in expression of all transcripts in a cell type or tissue, providing a snapshot of what is turned on and off. Harvest of total RNA or mRNA is critical; technical problems or degradation fatally undermines the interpretation of expression data. Hence, the timely extraction of RNA from fresh or carefully frozen tissue is a requirement for performing expression array analysis.

Naturally, the quality control steps for ensuring that RNA is not degraded must be established, and in circumstances in which insufficient RNA is available, careful amplification of RNA can be performed during the generation of cDNA (24). It is notable that expression studies do not establish the absolute expression level but, instead, when conducted carefully, an accurate assessment of the differential expression of all genes in a particular cell type.

Global analysis of gene expression using microarrays can be applied to many research questions. Distinct expression profiles can be used as molecular signatures of diseases (12, 14). In some cases, this approach in population-based studies can identify profiles of genes that subtype a disease, such as breast cancer or non-Hodgkin's lymphoma (1, 8). Moreover, the clustering of specific genes in breast cancer portends outcome and is beginning to be used in studies to determine therapeutic intervention (8, 19, 21). Certainly, additional prospective studies are needed to fully address these critical issues. Intense effort has been directed at applying expression profiles to therapeutic response (e.g., pharmacogenomics); in some cases, studies have sought to identify signature expression patterns that correlate with response or toxicity. Conversely, microarray studies have identified suitable genes or pathways for development of novel drug targets. In this regard, sequence analysis of genes altered in expression in breast cancer have led to the characterization of a new tumor suppressor gene, GATA3 (22).

Once the hybridization steps are completed, sophisticated scanning technology is required to capture images of differences in signal. The immense collection of raw data can be mined according to distinct analytical algorithms. With so many data points, the standard visualization tool is a pseudo-color coding of the ratio between the expression of two samples hybridizing to the same DNA sequence. Background noise can be reduced by filtering raw data prior to visualization steps.

An analytical plan seeks to reduce the complexity of ratios and seek patterns or profiles of gene expression which, in turn, reflect biologically significant observations. Some investigators choose not to supervise the analysis and thus with no prior knowledge define relationships between samples. Many investigators utilize a supervised analysis in which a training set is validated in an independent data set; the purpose of this approach is to discover markers that are specific to each group. Furthermore, some have stated that to navigate immensely dense data sets, an artificial intelligence program can provide sophisticated analyses. For instance, each of the following has been successfully used to classify biologically confirmed sets: artificial neural networks, advanced clustering, and support vector machines (3). Alternatively, others choose to conduct standard statistical tests, such as t tests, and classify on the basis of classical statistics. The classification of data includes determination of gene ontogeny, which is usually drawn from one of several public databases, and the clustering of data is intended to visualize the data. Both dendrograms and multidimensional scaling are used to visualize the relationship between expression patterns in a graphic representation that reflects a presumed biological relationship between sets of samples that differentiates two or more subsets.

Recently, the microarray platform has been used to perform comparative genomic hybridization to identify regions of allelic loss or amplification. Instead of using cDNA generated from harvested RNA, DNA extracted from tissue, including archived material, is hybridized to DNA chips. Currently, most studies have used cDNA or oligonucleotide-based arrays to identify regions of loss of heterozygosity or gene amplifications (2, 6).

MICROARRAY ANALYSIS OF SEQUENCE VARIATION

There are several substantive differences between the analyses of gene expression patterns and germ line genetic variants. Unlike the study of expressed transcripts, which utilizes a technique that captures all known transcripts by priming with the poly(A) tail, common and rare genetic variants have to be interrogated base by base. Since there is no common handle to capture sequence variants, analysis has to specifically examine unique regions by PCR amplification. This requires detailed knowledge of flanking sequence and amplification conditions for each region of interest. Therefore, for large-scale analysis, large-scale multiplex analysis has been developed and has several limitations: single-nucleotide polymorphisms (SNPs) in close proximity are difficult to assay; selected regions, often high in GC content, do not faithfully amplify both alleles; and random drop-out of assays occurs, though, with optimization, at a tolerable level that does not significantly undermine the ability to estimate haplotype structure from unphased genotype data (18). There are probably over 10 million common SNPs in the human genome (with a mean allele frequency of more than 5% in at least one studied population). Furthermore, SNP frequencies can vary substantially by population.

Chip technology was initially applied to single-base pair mutation detection, using a similar hybridization technology but with genomic DNA as a template. Modifications of laying SNPs on microchips quickly progressed from a single-SNP analysis to analysis of thousands of SNPs (11). Currently, there are four commercial technologies available for large-scale, high-throughput genotype analysis (Table 1). For each technology, substantial effort and cost must be expended to optimize the panel of SNPs, which are fixed prior to analysis. As the International HapMap Consortium completes its first phase of genotype analysis, it will be possible to analyze the structure of genetic variation across the genome in a more comprehensive manner (13). This strategy, known as whole-genome scanning, is based on the observation that there is linkage disequilibrium across any gene or region and estimates the haplotype structure of a region. Since SNPs are inherited in units, haplotype blocks can vary in size according to the region of the genome and the population under study (10). These blocks can decrease the complexity and permit analysis of a subset of SNPs, known as

TABLE 1 Current high-throughput genotype technologies

Technology
Affymetrix: simplification of the genome by restriction digestion, and addition of universal adapting linkers, which are amplified prior to fragmentation and labeling. SNPs are assayed on a microchip using an address system.
ParAllele: allele-specific primer extension followed by ligation and amplification prior to reading on a bead or microarray platform
Illumina: allele-specific gap fill followed by ligation and amplification prior to readout on a microarray or microchip system
Perlegen: a PCR-based sample preparation that targets amplification across the genome. High-density oligonucleotide arrays consisting of short DNA probes are synthesized on a glass surface and used to determine genotypes with great redundancy. The technology is vendor based and not exportable to academic or government labs.

haplotype tagging SNPs, which captures a high proportion of ancestral haplotypes. These facts underscore the dynamic history of selection and adaptation of genetic variation in response to differential challenges, such as diet, pathogens, and climate. In some regions of the genome, there is little linkage disequilibrium, requiring an alternative analysis plan with a more dense collection of neighboring SNPs.

With these new technologies, the search for genetic contributions to disease susceptibility and outcomes can systematically evaluate all genes as well as the intergenic regions of the genome. Because most SNPs are silent and have no apparent functional consequence, the challenge is to identify the set of informative SNPs that are "causal."

Laboratory analyses (e.g., in vitro or animal work) will be necessary to investigate the basic mechanism of an SNP or haplotype, which alters either expression or function. The laboratory component continues to be outpaced by the advances in technical capabilities in genomics. For instance, we can now consider analyzing a large set of common SNPs across the genome, chosen on the basis of haplotype structure in the search for germ line genetic risk factors for disease or outcome (including toxicity or efficacy associated with therapeutic intervention) (9).

The new technologies for SNP detection will enable studies to look at genetic variation across all genes of a pathway or biological process as well as across the entire genome (which comes at a formidable cost). Similar to the analytical challenges of the microarray expression studies, analytical approaches will continue to evolve in SNP research (4). Since SNPs are low penetrance and impact risk, the challenge of finding the informative SNPs for a disease or outcome is daunting. Innovative strategies coupled with sufficiently large population-based studies will minimize false positives and improve the probability of obtaining findings that can be replicated, a central requirement for SNP studies (5, 23).

FUTURE DIRECTIONS IN SEQUENCE TECHNOLOGIES

One of the major goals of the coming decade is the development of high-throughput sequence technologies. Sequence analysis across a region or gene captures all of the common and rare variants. Since neighboring SNPs can undermine the fidelity of a genotype SNP assay, large-scale sequence analysis should be more accurate. When sequencing platforms are cost-effective, perhaps an entire genome can be sequenced for a reasonable cost—the so-called "$1,000 genome." At this point, it will be possible to examine common and uncommon genetic variants in large population-based studies. However, these developments are not imminent, so there is adequate time to begin to consider the analytical challenges ahead, namely, identifying rare variants that lead to significant phenotypes (20). Since most rare variants are probably not causal, interpretation of rare genetic variants will require corollary functional data or detailed family pedigree analysis to establish a critical relationship with disease outcome.

REFERENCES

1. Alizadeh, A. A., M. B. Eisen, R. E. Davis, C. Ma, I. S. Lossos, A. Rosenwald, J. C. Boldrick, H. Sabet, T. Tran, X. Yu, J. I. Powell, L. Yang, G. E. Marti, T. Moore, J. Hudson, Jr., L. Lu, D. B. Lewis, R. Tibshirani, G. Sherlock, W. C. Chan, T. C. Greiner, D. D. Weisenburger, J. O. Armitage, R. Warnke, R. Levy, W. Wilson, M. R. Grever, J. C. Byrd, D. Botstein, P. O. Brown, and L. M. Staudt. 2000. Distinct types of diffuse large B-cell lymphoma identified by gene expression profiling. *Nature* **403**:503–511.
2. Barrett, M. T., A. Scheffer, A. Ben-Dor, N. Sampas, D. Lipson, R. Kincaid, P. Tsang, B. Curry, K. Baird, P. S. Meltzer, Z. Yakhini, L. Bruhn, and S. Laderman. 2004. Comparative genomic hybridization using oligonucleotide microarrays and total genomic DNA. *Proc. Natl. Acad. Sci. USA* **101**:17765–17770.
3. Bishop, C. M. 1995. *Neural Networks for Pattern Recognition.* Clarendon Press, Oxford, United Kingdom.
4. Botstein, D., and N. Risch. 2003. Discovering genotypes underlying human phenotypes: past successes for Mendelian disease, future approaches for complex disease. *Nat. Genet.* **33**:228–237.
5. Chanock, S., and S. Wacholder. 2002. One gene and one outcome? No way. *Trends Mol. Med.* **8**:266–269.
6. Chen, Q. R., S. Bilke, J. S. Wei, C. C. Whiteford, N. Cenacchi, A. L. Krasnoselsky, B. T. Greer, C. G. Son, F. Westermann, F. Berthold, M. Schwab, D. Catchpoole, and J. Khan. 2004. cDNA array-CGH profiling identifies genomic alterations specific to stage and MYCN-amplification in neuroblastoma. *BMC Genomics* **5**:70.
7. Collins, F. S., E. D. Green, A. E. Guttmacher, M. S. Guyer, and the U.S. National Human Genome Research Institute. 2003. A vision for the future of genomics research. *Nature* **422**:835–847.
8. Dave, S. S., G. Wright, B. Tan, A. Rosenwald, R. D. Gascoyne, W. C. Chan, R. I. Fisher, R. M. Braziel, L. M. Rimsza, T. M. Grogan, T. P. Miller, M. LeBlanc, T. C. Greiner, D. D. Weisenburger, J. C. Lynch, J. Vose, J. O. Armitage, E. B. Smeland, S. Kvaloy, H. Holte, J. Delabie, J. M. Connors, P. M. Lansdorp, Q. Ouyang, T. A. Lister, A. J. Davies, A. J. Norton, H. K. Muller-Hermelink, G. Ott, E. Campo, E. Montserrat, W. H. Wilson, E. S. Jaffe, R. Simon, L. Yang, J. Powell, H. Zhao, N. Goldschmidt, M. Chiorazzi, and L. M. Staudt. 2004. Prediction of survival in follicular lymphoma based on molecular features of tumor-infiltrating immune cells. *N. Engl. J. Med.* **351**:2159–2169.
9. Evans, W. E., and M. V. Relling. 2004. Moving towards individualized medicine with pharmacogenomics. *Nature* **429**:464–468.
10. Gabriel, S. B., S. F. Schaffner, H. Nguyen, J. M. Moore, J. Roy, B. Blumenstiel, J. Higgins, M. DeFelice, A. Lochner, M. Faggart, S. N. Liu-Cordero, C. Rotimi, A. Adeyemo, R. Cooper, R. Ward, E. S. Lander, M. J. Daly, and D. Altshuler. 2002. The structure of haplotype blocks in the human genome. *Science* **296**:2225–2229.
11. Gilles, P. N., D. J. Wu, C. B. Foster, P. J. Dillon, and S. J. Chanock. 1999. Single nucleotide polymorphic discrimination by an electronic dot blot assay on semiconductor microchips. *Nat. Biotechnol.* **17**:365–370.
12. Golub, T. R., D. K. Slonim, P. Tamayo, C. Huard, M. Gaasenbeek, J. P. Mesirov, H. Coller, M. L. Loh, J. R. Downing, M. A. Caligiuri, C. D. Bloomfield, and E. S. Lander. 1999. Molecular classification of cancer: class discovery and class prediction by gene expression monitoring. *Science* **286**:531–537.
13. International HapMap Consortium. 2003. The International HapMap project. *Nature* **426**:789–796.
14. Khan, J., J. S. Wei, M. Ringner, L. H. Saal, M. Ladanyi, F. Westermann, F. Berthold, M. Schwab, C. R. Antonescu, C. Peterson, and P. S. Meltzer. 2001. Classification and diagnostic prediction of cancers using gene expression profiling and artificial neural networks. *Nat. Med.* **7**:673–679.
15. Lipshutz, R. J., S. P. Fodor, T. R. Gingeras, and D. J. Lockhart. 1999. High density synthetic oligonucleotide arrays. *Nat. Genet.* **21**:20–24.

16. Lynch, T. J., D. W. Bell, R. Sordella, S. Gurubhagavatula, R. A. Okimoto, B. W. Brannigan, P. L. Harris, S. M. Haserlat, J. G. Supko, F. G. Haluska, D. N. Louis, D. C. Christiani, J. Settleman, and D. A. Haber. 2004. Activating mutations in the epidermal growth factor receptor underlying responsiveness of non-small-cell lung cancer to gefitinib. *N. Engl. J. Med.* **350:**2129–2139.

17. Marth, G., R. Yeh, M. Minton, R. Donaldson, Q. Li, S. Duan, R. Davenport, R. D. Miller, and P. Y. Kwok. 2001. Single-nucleotide polymorphisms in the public domain: how useful are they? *Nat. Genet.* **27:**371–372.

18. Packer, B. R., M. Yeager, B. Staats, R. Welch, A. Crenshaw, M. Kiley, A. Eckert, M. Beerman, E. Miller, A. Bergen, N. Rothman, R. Strausberg, and S. J. Chanock. SNP500Cancer: a public resource for sequence validation and assay development for genetic variation in candidate genes. *Nucleic Acids Res.* **32**(Database issue)**:**D528–532.

19. Paik, S., S. Shak, G. Tang, C. Kim, J. Baker, M. Cronin, F. L. Baehner, M. G. Walker, D. Watson, T. Park, W. Hiller, E. R. Fisher, D. L. Wickerham, J. Bryant, and N. Wolmark. 2004. A multigene assay to predict recurrence of tamoxifen-treated, node-negative breast cancer. *N. Engl. J. Med.* **351:**2817–2826.

20. Pritchard, J. K. 2001. Are rare variants responsible for susceptibility to complex diseases? *Am. J. Hum. Genet.* **69:**124–137.

21. Sorlie, T., R. Tibshirani, J. Parker, T. Hastie, J. S. Marron, A. Nobel, S. Deng, H. Johnsen, R. Pesich, S. Geisler, J. Demeter, C. M. Perou, P. E. Lonning, P. O. Brown, A. L. Borresen-Dale, and D. Botstein. 2003. Repeated observation of breast tumor subtypes in independent gene expression data sets. *Proc. Natl. Acad. Sci. USA* **100:**8418–8423.

22. Usary, J., V. Llaca, G. Karaca, S. Presswala, M. Karaca, X. He, A. Langerod, R. Karesen, D. S. Oh, L. G. Dressler, P. E. Lonning, R. L. Strausberg, S. Chanock, A. L. Borresen-Dale, and C. M. Perou. 2004. Mutation of GATA3 in human breast tumors. *Oncogene* **23:**7669–7678.

23. Wacholder, S., S. J. Chanock, M. Garcia-Closas, L. El Ghormli, and N. Rothman. 2004. Assessing the probability that a positive report is false: an approach for molecular epidemiology studies. *J. Natl. Cancer Inst.* **96:**434–442.

24. Wang, E., L. D. Miller, G. A. Ohnmacht, E. T. Liu, and F. M. Marincola. 2000. High-fidelity mRNA amplification for gene profiling. *Nat. Biotechnol.* **18:**457–459.

Introduction to Molecular Methodology

RAYMOND P. PODZORSKI

5

The genomics revolution involving chip technology is overviewed in chapter 4. This chapter is intended to provide a more detailed discussion of the molecular techniques and equipment that are available, or under development, for use in the clinical laboratory. While sufficient detail is provided to understand the design and strengths and weaknesses of the various techniques, this chapter is not intended to provide complete step-by-step instructions for each molecular diagnostic procedure. The reader is encouraged to investigate other chapters of this manual or other sources for more detailed descriptions of these procedures and their applications (see references).

MOLECULAR SPECIMENS

Prior to performing a molecular assay on a specimen, DNA or RNA of interest must be available and in a functional form for testing. The specimen processing component of a molecular assay involves liberating the nucleic acid from the target of interest to remove or inactivate potential inhibitors of nucleic acid amplification or hybridization and concentrate the nucleic acid prior to analysis. In many instances, the most labor-intensive portion of a molecular assay is specimen processing. The labor costs alone associated with specimen processing can determine whether a particular molecular assay is worth being run in-house.

The actual amount of manipulation that will be required prior to placing an aliquot of the specimen into a molecular assay depends upon a number of factors. These include the specimen type, or types, the sensitivity required, and the volume of specimen anticipated. Types of specimens differ considerably in terms of the difficulty in isolating functional nucleic acids. Specimens such as cerebrospinal fluid, whole blood, serum, or plasma are typically more amenable to relatively uncomplicated specimen processing protocols compared to specimens such as tissue, bone, sputum, or stool. In addition, it is well known that microorganisms differ in terms of the relative ease of nucleic acid extraction. For example, mycobacteria and many fungi are relatively difficult to process, while viruses are typically far easier to process for a nucleic acid sample.

When contemplating bringing molecular diagnostics in-house, it is a common concern that the assays will be so labor-intensive, complicated, and procedurally foreign to the technologists that it will be difficult to maintain a high level of competency with the assays. Fortunately for those in the market for molecular testing, the days of having to make all your nucleic acid extraction reagents are effectively over. Because of the tremendous growth in the number of specimen processing reagents, kits, and instruments available today, it is beyond the scope of this chapter to present any meaningful evaluation or comparison of these products. However, it would be very prudent for those pondering bringing molecular assays into their laboratories to give considerable thought to their specimen processing requirements. In certain instances there may be little flexibility in terms of how specimen processing can be done. For example, molecular-assay-based kits that have been approved by the U.S. Food and Drug Administration (FDA) typically come with specimen processing reagents and/or procedures designating which specimen types the kit is designed for, how the specimens must be processed, and what reagents should be used. However, when developing and using homebrew molecular assays, or assays using an analyte-specific reagent (ASR), individualized specimen processing protocols may provide considerable latitude in terms of protocol options.

A particularly important point to note is that for some molecular assays, complex processing procedures are not required. Some nucleic acid amplification-based assays require only "boil-and-go" processing. This type of processing involves heating a small aliquot of the specimen at 100°C for a short period, cooling and spinning the aliquot at 10,000 to 15,000 $\times g$ for 2 to 3 min to pellet any insoluble material, and taking the supernatant and using it directly in the assay. Specimens that are less likely to contain strong inhibitors of nucleic acid amplification tests and are known to consistently contain a certain amount of the target nucleic acid are good candidates for boil-and-go processing. When more elaborate specimen processing procedures are required, relatively recent advances in semiautomated and automated specimen processing instruments are changing the landscape of nucleic acid extraction in the clinical laboratory. The use of specimen processing instruments, coupled with real-time amplification technology discussed below, and the availability of FDA-approved kits, or ASRs, for molecular assays have markedly reduced the complexity of many molecular procedures. While the first automated specimen processing instruments that came onto the market were large and expensive, a number of new, smaller, and less costly specimen processing instruments have been introduced recently and initial evaluations of these instruments have been encouraging. These instruments automate many, or all, of the steps involved in nucleic acid isolation, minimizing the demands of manual processing procedures that were common a few years ago. Semiautomated or automated specimen processing instruments are now within reach of most clinical laboratories and allow the laboratory to more easily maintain a level of quality, proficiency, and competency in their nucleic acid extractions over a range of specimen types and instrument users. However, the performance of automated specimen processors has been reported to vary. Some users have found that additional up-front steps are required with some specimens to reach the same DNA extraction efficiency seen with manual procedures. Discussing the performance of an automated processing instrument of interest with an experienced user, or doing an in-house evaluation of the instrument, before purchasing it is strongly suggested.

CLASSICAL MOLECULAR DIAGNOSTIC TESTING

Molecular testing in the clinical laboratory consists of two major areas: (i) the use of DNA probes to directly detect or characterize a specific target and (ii) the use of nucleic acid amplification technologies to detect or characterize a specific target DNA or RNA. The use of DNA probe technology is discussed first; nucleic acid amplification technology and nucleic acid sequencing are discussed later, followed by molecular arrays, a more elaborate application of probe technology. The procedures for use of DNA probes are now well standardized and frequently simpler than those for nucleic acid target or probe amplification assays. However, the sensitivity that can be attained with many probes is still lower than that of nucleic acid amplification procedures, and this remains the main drawback of more widespread use of probe technology directly on patient specimens (79). Classical molecular techniques that are DNA probe based can be divided into three general categories: solid-phase hybridization, solution-phase hybridization, and in situ hybridization. Each type of probe hybridization assay is discussed individually, as are probe amplification procedures.

Solid-Phase Hybridization

In the slot or dot blot DNA probe hybridization procedure, intact cells are lysed and the DNA is denatured, brought into direct contact with a nylon membrane by vacuum aspiration in a dot or slot configuration, and then fixed onto the membrane (9, 22). Nucleic acids bound to solid supports such as nylon membranes are still available to participate in hybridization reactions. The membrane is immersed in a hybridization solution containing the DNA reporter probe and allowed to hybridize. In solid-phase assays the hybridization reaction is very slow and typically requires an overnight incubation to complete. Following hybridization, the unbound reporter probes are washed away and the bound probe is detected by one of several methods. Dot or slot blots are especially useful for the processing of multiple specimens at one time, since numerous specimens can be screened on a single filter. A variation on the dot or slot blot utilizes sandwich or capture hybridization (70, 85, 118). This procedure utilizes two probes that bind to different sites on the target nucleic acid. One probe is attached to the membrane and serves to capture the target nucleic acid in the sample. The second probe is labeled and serves as the detector. This system was developed to circumvent the direct binding of target DNA to the membrane. In some cases, sandwich hybridization has been found to be more sensitive than standard membrane hybridization.

The Southern blot is a solid-phase hybridization assay that allows size determination of DNA fragments bound by the reporter probe (8, 22, 99). The Northern blot, a variation on the Southern blot, is a molecular assay to detect RNA instead of DNA (10, 88). These procedures generally require purified DNA or RNA. In the Southern blot, sample DNA is isolated and digested with a restriction endonuclease, and the fragments are separated by size using agarose gel electrophoresis. In the Northern blot, total sample RNA is isolated and separated by size using denaturing agarose gel electrophoresis. In both types of blots the nucleic acids are then transferred to a nylon membrane for hybridization with a specific probe. These assays typically require 2 to 3 days to complete because the transfer of the nucleic acid to the membrane is usually done overnight and the probing of the membrane is also done overnight. A very well-known molecular assay that involves Southern blot analysis is testing for T-cell receptor gene rearrangements.

Solution-Phase Hybridization

Some commercially available DNA probe kits for use in the clinical laboratory are based on solution-phase hybridization, or some variant, in which both the target nucleic acid and the probe are free to interact in an aqueous reaction mixture (7, 59, 114, 115). The free target-probe interaction in the aqueous environment has very rapid hybridization kinetics, typically requiring just 1 h or less to complete, a considerably shorter time than the overnight hybridization frequently required in a solid-phase hybridization reaction. The key to solution-phase hybridization is that the nucleic probe must be single stranded and not hybridize with itself.

In the clinical laboratory, one popular method for detecting probe hybridization in solution is a bacterial and fungal culture confirmation procedure that utilizes the hybridization protection assay (HPA) (3, 67). In HPA, an acridinium ester-labeled DNA probe is hybridized to target rRNA. After 15 min the hybridization reaction mixture is treated with alkali. After an additional 15 min, the reaction mixture is placed in a luminometer, peroxides are added, and the acridinium ester emits detectable light. In HPA, hybridization of the acridinium ester-labeled DNA probe protects the acridinium ester from alkaline hydrolysis, and upon addition of peroxides, the acridinium ester will emit detectable light. However, if the acridinium ester-labeled DNA probe is not hybridized, the acridinium ester is not protected from alkali and is hydrolyzed to a form that does not emit light; thus, the quantity of light emitted is a reflection of the degree of hybridization. HPA can be performed in a few hours and does not require removal of excess unbound acridinium ester-labeled DNA probe. Because HPA is proprietary technology of Gen-Probe, it has seen little use outside of various kits offered by Gen-Probe.

Another solution-phase hybridization method suited for use in the clinical laboratory is a reverse hybridization assay using free detection probes and tethered (but with considerable mobility) capture probes. Following sample extraction the DNA is denatured, mixed with free biotinylated detection probes, and placed in a microtiter plate with capture oligonucleotide probes tethered to the wells. The solution is incubated for about 1 h. The capture probes bind to areas of the target DNA that are unique from those sites bound by the detection probes. Following hybridization, unbound material is washed away and an alkaline phosphatase-conjugated antibiotin antibody is added. After the appropriate incubation, the wells are washed again and the substrate is added. The bound alkaline phosphatase can be detected using either a colorimetric or chemiluminescent substrate (51, 82).

In Situ Hybridization

In situ hybridization assays involve the same general principles as solid- and solution-phase hybridizations. However, in situ hybridization occurs within the morphological context of individual cells or a tissue sample (31, 101). When considered in conjunction with tissue morphology and host response, the results of these assays confirm that specific DNA or RNA targets are present in the specimen under study and provide additional information regarding distribution and abundance. In clinical settings, formalin-fixed paraffin-embedded tissue sections frequently form the starting material for in situ hybridization assays. In situ hybridization requires that target nucleic acid be made accessible for hybridization while the cellular morphology is preserved for subsequent interpretation and analysis. Therefore, the tissue processing must be delicate enough to preserve the cellular structure while denaturing the nucleic acids in the cell to make them accessible to the DNA probe. The sensitivity of in situ hybridization is limited by the accessibility of target nucleic acids within the cell. Because of the accessibility limitations associated with mammalian cells, it has been found that relatively small probes (500 bases or less) are optimal to favor tissue penetration (104).

Signal Amplification Schemes

Several ingenious signal amplification schemes have been developed in recent years to increase the sensitivity of probe-based assays (24, 45, 91, 117). Unlike nucleic acid target amplification or probe amplification procedures, signal amplification procedures are designed to increase the signal generated by the probe hybridized to a specific sequence of target DNA or RNA. The fact that signal amplification procedures do not involve nucleic acid target or probe amplification is a theoretical advantage, because it makes these amplification procedures less prone to the contamination problems that are of concern in enzyme-catalyzed amplification procedures. However, a relative lack of sensitivity compared to nucleic acid amplification procedures is still a drawback to some of these procedures. While some assays have sensitivities to below 100 nucleic acid targets per ml (16), other signal amplification procedures require a minimum of 10^3 to 10^5 nucleic acid targets (depending upon specimen processing) (44), which is well below the sensitivity of highly optimized nucleic acid target or probe amplification procedures. The chief limitation of some signal amplification systems is the background noise due to nonspecific binding of reporter probes. Problems with high backgrounds have led to modifications such as incorporating gray zones into the interpretation of the assay when the result is close to the positive cutoff and procedural modifications, such as the use of target capture probes and isonucleotides, to reduce the background noise levels associated with some signal amplification procedures (16, 37).

bDNA

One of the most well-known signal amplification systems is the branched DNA (bDNA) probe system (Bayer Corporation), which utilizes multiple probes together with multiple reporters (16, 95, 109). This system utilizes a specific target capture step for isolation of the nucleic acid sequence of interest followed by hybridization with unlabeled label extender and preamplifier probes (Fig. 1). One

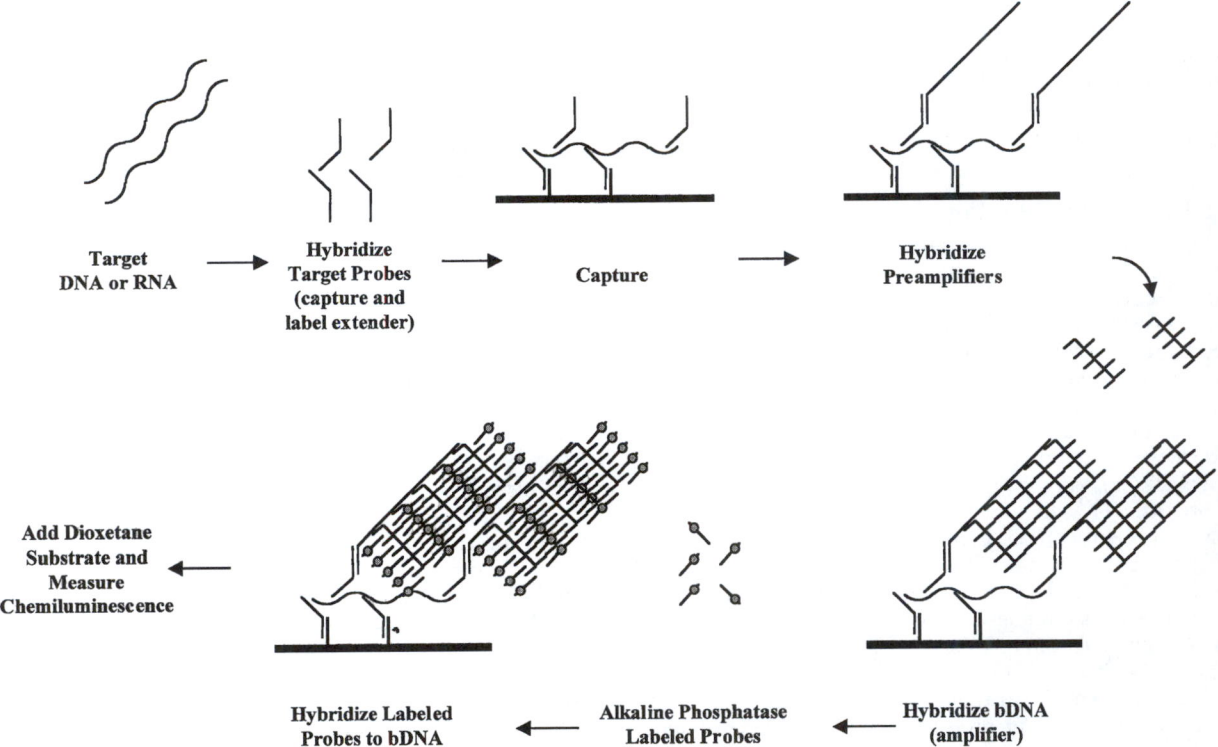

FIGURE 1 bDNA-based signal amplification. Target nucleic acid is released by cell disruption and captured to a solid surface via multiple contiguous capture extender probes. Label extender probes hybridize with adjacent target sequences and contain additional sequences homologous to the preamplifier probes. Preamplifier probes bind multiple bDNA (amplifier) probes. Enzyme-labeled oligonucleotides bind to the bDNA by homologous base pairing, and the enzyme-probe complex is measured by detection of chemiluminescence.

region of the label extender is complementary to the target nucleic acid, and another part of the label extender is capable of hybridizing with the preamplifier. The preamplifier and bDNA amplifier are the keys to the amplifying power of this technique. The bDNA amplifier is chemically synthesized with a comb-like backbone made from a branching nucleoside analog that is incorporated at regular intervals along the oligonucleotide. The bDNA binds many labeled probes, providing a significant boost in signal. Depending upon the specific version of bDNA kit used, over 10,000 reporter molecules can be incorporated onto each target sequence. The most recent bDNA probe system has high specificity because both capture and target probes must bind before the signal amplification can take place, and the use of nonnatural bases, isocytidine and isoguanosine, decreases nonspecific hybridization. In this bDNA probe system, nonspecific hybridization rarely results in hybridization of both capture and target probes to the same nontarget sequence. Because bDNA probe systems provide quantitative detection over a range of several orders of magnitude, such assays are very useful for monitoring therapeutic responses during disease therapy. The determination of responses to therapy has been demonstrated to be useful in assessing the need for further therapy or for adjusting doses of therapeutic agents for certain infectious diseases (human immunodeficiency virus type 1 and hepatitis C virus [HCV]).

Hybrid Capture

The most commonly used technology for human papillomavirus (HPV) testing of cervical specimens is Digene's hybrid capture (4, 26, 35, 38, 102). This is a signal amplification system that is based upon the binding of multiple alkaline phosphatase-conjugated antibodies that are specific

for DNA-RNA hybrids (Fig. 2). Isolated target DNA is denatured and hybridized to a complementary RNA probe at 65°C for 1 h. The DNA-RNA hybrids are transferred to a capture microtiter plate with wells that are coated with polyclonal antibodies that are specific for DNA-RNA hybrids and incubated at room temperature for 1 h with rotary shaking. The hybridization solution is discarded, and alkaline phosphatase-conjugated antibodies specific for DNA-RNA hybrids are added to the capture plate and incubated at room temperature for 30 to 45 min. These antibodies have the same specificity as the capture antibodies on the plate and bind to open epitopes on the captured DNA-RNA hybrids. The plate is rigorously washed, and a chemiluminescent substrate is added to the plate, which is incubated in the dark for 15 to 30 min at room temperature and then read in a luminometer.

The sensitivity of hybrid capture for HPV is reported by the company to be 1.08 pg/ml (product insert). Based upon a genome size of about 8,000 bp for HPV, this translates to approximately 134,000 DNA copies/ml of specimen. This sensitivity closely compares to what Digene has reported for this technology in a quantitative HBV assay that is under development (142,000 copies/ml of blood) (44). However, up-front ultracentrifugation of specimens for HBV testing by hybrid capture increases the sensitivity to approximately 4,700 DNA copies/ml. This sensitivity is below what would be expected for a target amplification assay such as PCR. Use of a signal amplification assay raises a concern about the signal-to-noise ratio on samples with a low target DNA copy number. For the HPV assay, Digene defines a gray zone for weakly positive specimens because the signal amplification specificity is suspect for samples with signals just above the positive breakpoint. A new version of the assay that is under

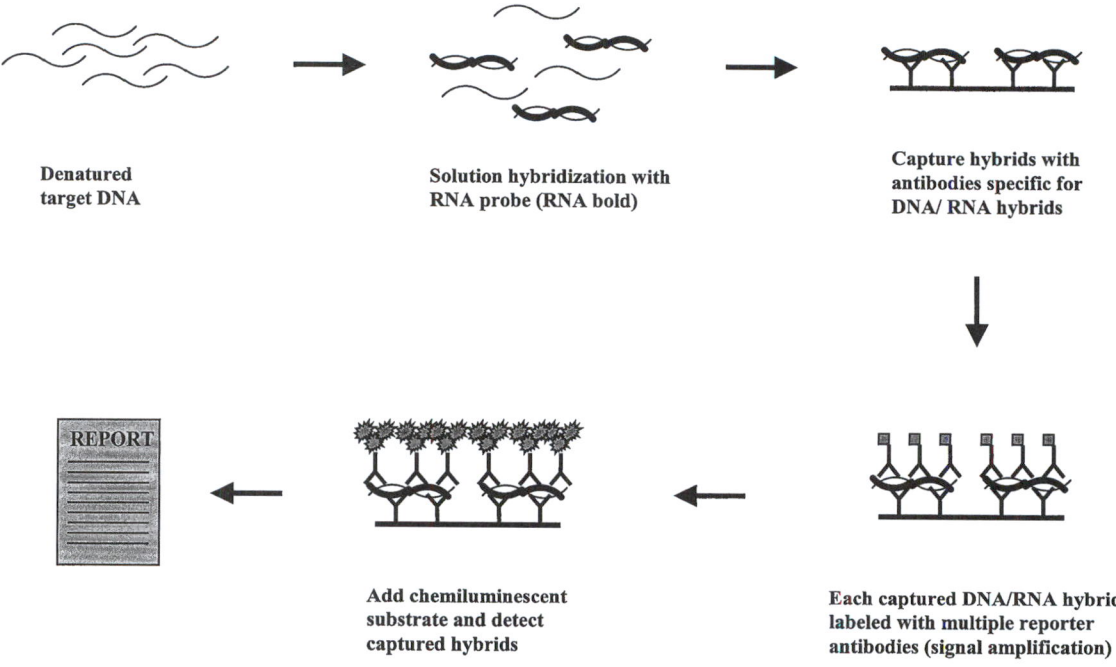

Denatured target DNA

Solution hybridization with RNA probe (RNA bold)

Capture hybrids with antibodies specific for DNA/RNA hybrids

Add chemiluminescent substrate and detect captured hybrids

Each captured DNA/RNA hybrid labeled with multiple reporter antibodies (signal amplification)

REPORT

FIGURE 2 Hybrid capture. Target DNA is released by cell disruption, denatured, and allowed to hybridize to specific RNA probes. Double-stranded DNA-RNA hybrids are captured to a solid surface via antibodies specific for the hybrids. Multiple reporter antibodies specific for the hybrids bind each captured DNA-RNA hybrid, setting the stage for signal amplification. A chemiluminescent substrate is added and the reporter antibody-hybrid complex is measured by detection of chemiluminescence.

development attempts to improve the specificity of the assay by incorporating avidin-coated wells which bind to specific single-stranded biotinylated oligonucleotide capture probes (11). The single-stranded capture probes capture the desired DNA-RNA hybrids in a sequence-specific fashion. This modification lowers the possibility of nonspecific DNA-RNA hybrids being captured by the polyclonal anti-DNA-RNA antibodies. Digene is looking to use hybrid capture as a basic platform for a number of assays. In addition to the HPV test, a number of additional assays are available or under development (quantitative cytomegalovirus, HBV, chlamydia, and *Neisseria gonorrhoeae* tests).

Invader

Invader technology (Third Wave Technologies, Inc., Madison, Wis.) is a signal amplification procedure that generates large numbers of reporter probes from a single target-bound DNA probe (45, 91). This procedure is isothermal and done in a microtiter format, and the results are read on a fluorescence plate reader. The assay utilizes two major components: (i) a cleavase enzyme that specifically cuts a bound probe and (ii) three oligonucleotide probes, i.e., a primary probe, an "invader" probe, and a reporter probe. The primary probe and invader probe are designed so the Invader assay will interrogate one specific base in the target nucleic acid (Fig. 3). In the primary reaction, the invader oligonucleotide probe and primary probe bind together to the target nucleic acid sequence, creating a structure with a 1-bp overlap and a nonhybridized flap on the 5' end of the primary probe. The cleavase enzyme recognizes this overlapping structure and cleaves the 5' flap off the primary probe. Each time the correct structure forms, the cleavase enzyme cuts the 5' flap off the primary probe. The reactions are deliberately carried out at temperatures near the denaturation temperature of the primary probe. This results in a dynamic hybridization reaction allowing multiple uncleaved primary probes to bind to the same nucleic acid without temperature cycling, and in linear signal amplification because 1,000 to 10,000 5' flaps are

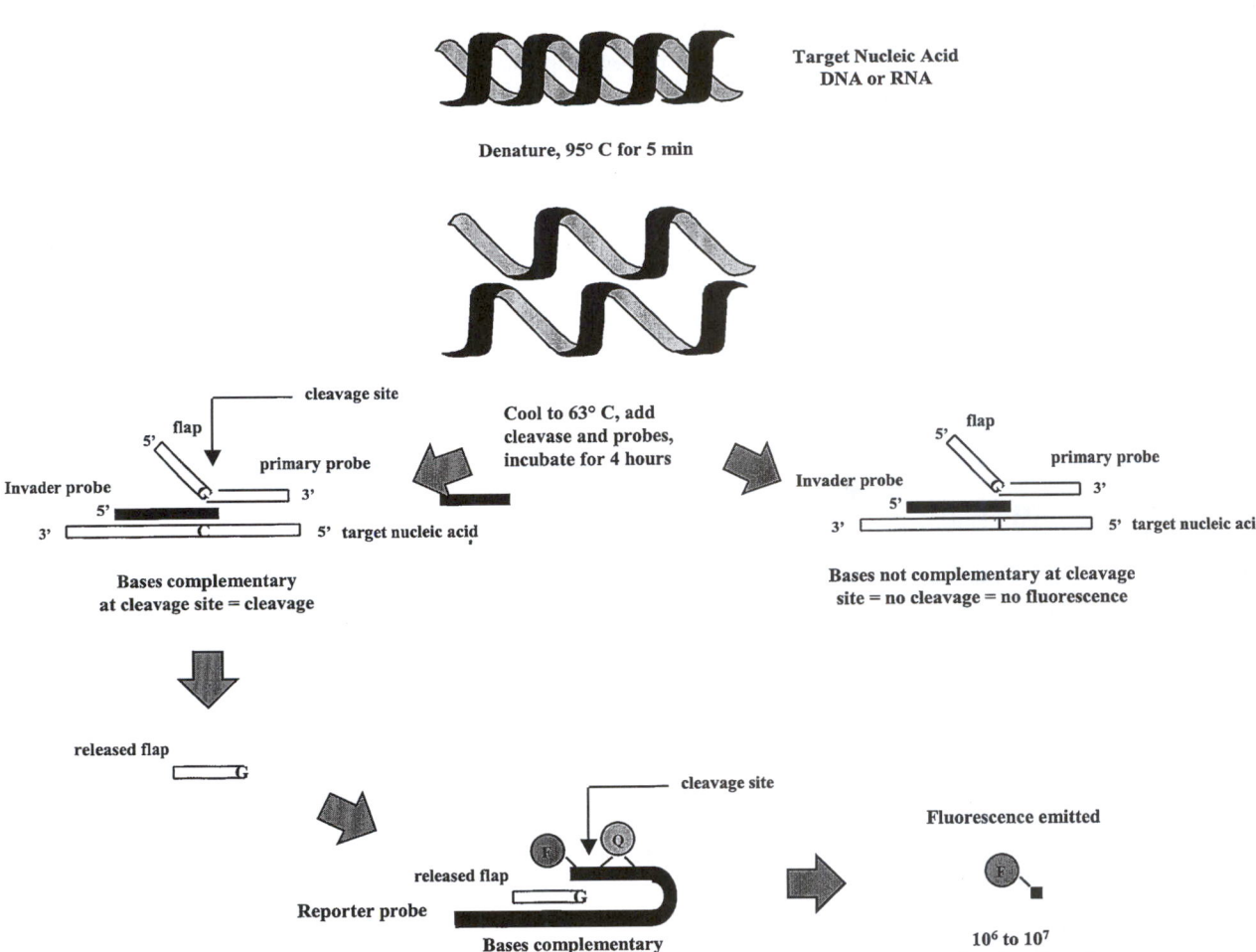

FIGURE 3 Invader. A primary probe, with a 5' flap, and an invader probe bind to the target nucleic acid and form a 1-bp overlap. Cleavase recognizes this substrate and cleaves the 5' flap from the primary probe. The free 5' flap acts as secondary invader probe with the reporter probe. Cleavase cleaves the fluorescein (F) from the 5' end of the reporter probe, separating it from the quencher dye (Q), allowing a fluorescent signal that can be detected. If the target region of the primary probe and the invader probe do not match perfectly with the target DNA, the proper substrate is not formed and the cleavase will not cleave the 5' flap from the primary probe (right panel).

being cleaved from primary probes per hour for each target molecule in the reaction. When the primary probe and the target nucleotide do not complement each other perfectly, the correct overlapping structure does not form and the cleavase enzyme will not cut the primary probe.

The accumulating 5′ flaps released from the cleaved probes participate in the secondary detection reaction. The free 5′ flaps are designed to act as secondary invader probes, and the reporter probe acts as both the secondary probe and the target. Each reporter probe, regardless of the target in the primary reaction, has the identical sequence and is designed to fold over on itself to mimic a probe hybridized to a target and make a 5′ flap. The principle of the reporter probe used in the Invader assay is fluorescent energy transfer. The reporter probe contains a fluorescein at the 5′ end and a quencher dye attached nearby in the sequence. When the two dyes are proximal to each other, no fluorescence is produced. Once a free 5′ flap binds to the reporter probe, the two form the overlapping structure recognized and cut by the cleavase enzyme. When the cleavase enzyme cuts the fluorescein off the 5′ end of the reporter probe, the dyes are separated and a fluorescent signal can be detected. Under the conditions of the assay, 5′ flaps readily cycle on and off the reporter probes. Every time a 5′ flap and uncleaved reporter probe form the correct overlapping structure, the cleavase cuts the 5′ fluorescein off the reporter probe. Each free 5′ flap can cause the cleavage of 1,000 to 10,000 reporter probes in 1 h. As a result, the primary and secondary reactions work together to produce a 1 million- to 10-million-fold linear amplification of the signal from a single target gene. Because of its linear signal amplification, Invader technology is inherently quantitative and can be employed in quantitative and qualitative assays. Currently the maker of Invader assays has a number of hemostasis testing ASRs available; these include tests for Factor V Leiden, Factor II, and MTHFR, as well as many others (49). Invader reagents for infectious disease testing are relatively few, with ASRs for HCV genotyping and an HPV assay available.

NUCLEIC ACID AMPLIFICATION TECHNIQUES

The primary objective of nucleic acid amplification techniques is to improve the sensitivity of assays based on nucleic acids and to eventually simplify these assays by development of automated assay formats such as real-time detection. The technology behind nucleic acid amplification methods is highly diverse and constantly changing. Because of this complexity, it is useful to assign such methods to one of three general categories: (i) target amplification systems such as PCR, nucleic acid sequence-based amplification (NASBA), transcription-mediated amplification (TMA), and strand displacement amplification (SDA); (ii) probe amplification systems, which include the ligase chain reaction; and (iii) signal amplification systems (described above), in which the signal generated from each probe molecule is increased by using compound probes or branched probes, or by generation of large numbers of reporter probes. Ligase chain reaction is not discussed in this edition of this manual; readers are referred to the previous edition for an in-depth discussion of this technology.

PCR

PCR is based upon the ability of DNA polymerase to copy a strand of DNA by elongation of complementary strands initiated from a pair of closely spaced oligonucleotide primers

(64, 65, 66). Theoretically, each cycle of the reaction will double the amount of target DNA, resulting in millionfold levels of amplification.

PCR can be used on all types of specimens (2, 5, 23, 60, 74, 79, 80, 93, 98, 110, 116). As with all the nucleic acid target amplification procedures, some knowledge of the target sequence must be available in order to design the two single-stranded DNA oligonucleotide primers that will be used to amplify target DNA (Fig. 4). These PCR primers, each about 20 to 25 nucleotides long, can be synthesized by using an automated DNA synthesizer or ordered from a commercial supplier. PCR has high sequence specificity because the two unique primers must hybridize in relatively close proximity to each other on the target DNA sequence under stringent temperature and reaction conditions before exponential amplification can occur.

A commonly used set of cycling temperatures includes denaturation of double-stranded DNA at 94°C for 10 to 30 s, hybridization of oligonucleotide primers at 52°C for 10 to 30 s, and extension (polymerase-mediated complementary strand synthesis) from the primers at 72°C for 15 s to 1.5 min (Fig. 4) (93). These three steps are repeated for 25 to 45 cycles. In the early cycles of the reaction, the initially synthesized strands of new DNA are variable in length depending upon the processivity of the DNA polymerase. However, after a few cycles the primers begin to use the newly synthesized strands of DNA as templates, and the predominant product of PCR becomes a double-stranded DNA sequence, the length of which is the sum of the lengths of the two primers plus the intervening target DNA. PCR is an exponential amplification reaction such that after n cycles there is $(1 + x)^n$ times as much target as was present initially, where x is the mean efficiency of the reaction for each cycle. Theoretically, as few as 20 cycles would yield approximately 1 million times the amount of target DNA initially present. In practice, however, the theoretical maxima are never reached, and more cycles are necessary to achieve such a level of amplification.

NASBA

The first non-PCR nucleic acid amplification technique was a transcription-based amplification system (TAS) developed in 1989 by Kwoh et al. (46). In TAS, amplification of RNA is based upon a repeated two-cycle reaction of cDNA synthesis followed by transcription of the cDNA template into multiple copies of RNA. A major drawback to TAS was that heat was needed to denature the RNA-DNA intermediate formed during each cycle of the reaction. Heating inactivated the enzymes used in TAS, requiring their replenishment at the end of each cycle. During the development of TAS, it was discovered that the addition of *Escherichia coli* RNase H to the reaction resulted in degradation of the RNA template within the double-stranded RNA-DNA intermediates, allowing the cycling reaction to proceed under isothermal conditions (29). One variation of this nucleic acid amplification reaction is known as NASBA (also called 3SR for self-sustained sequence replication) and has been patented by Organon Teknika (17, 89).

NASBA utilizes the collective activities of three enzymes (avian myeloblastosis virus reverse transcriptase, RNase H, and bacteriophage T7 DNA-dependent RNA polymerase) to isothermally amplify an RNA target (Fig. 5). The initial steps in the reaction involve the formation of cDNAs from the target RNA using specific oligonucleotide primers; one of the primers contains a T7 RNA polymerase binding site at its 5′ end. The RNase H in the reaction

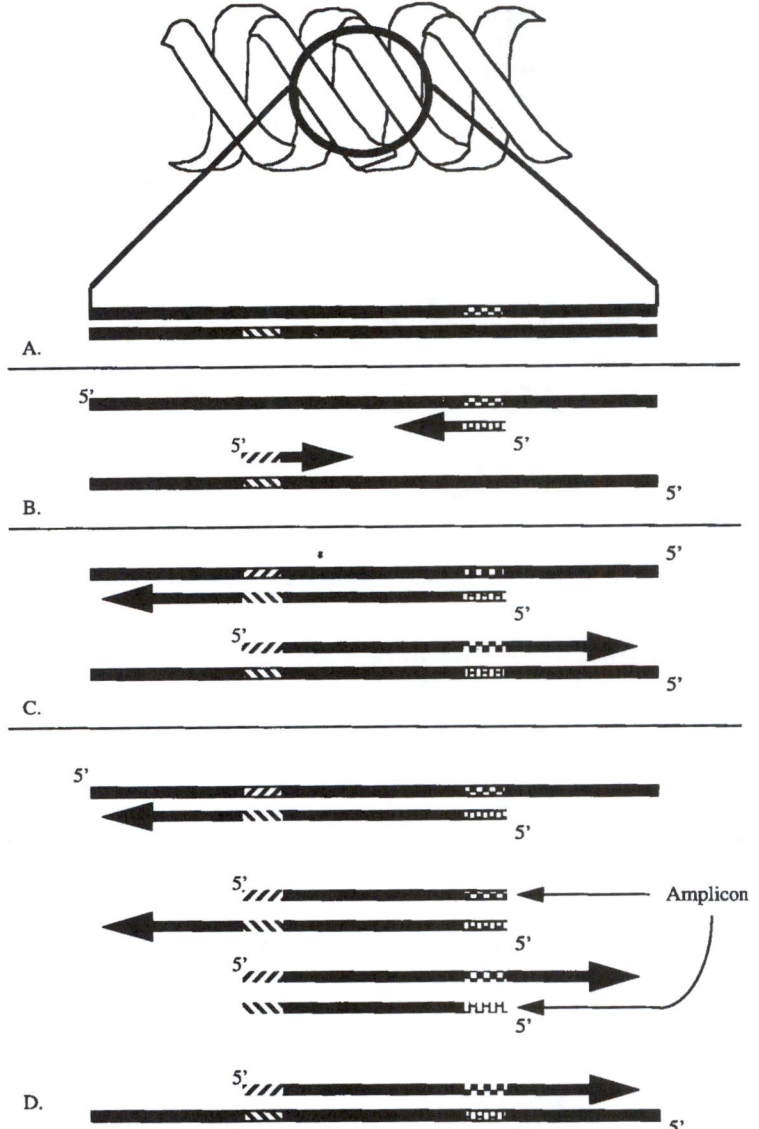

FIGURE 4 PCR. (A) In the first cycle, a double-stranded DNA target sequence is used as template, with the primer binding sites indicated by the hatched lines. (B) The two DNA strands are separated by heat denaturation, and two synthetic oligonucleotide primers (complementary cross-hatched lines) anneal to their recognition sites in the 5' to 3' orientation when the reaction cools. Note that the 3' ends of the primers (arrowheads) are facing each other. (C) *Taq* DNA polymerase initiates synthesis at the 3' end of each primer. Extension of the primer via DNA polymerization (synthesis) results in new primer binding sites. The net result after one round of polymerization is one copy of each (two total) strand of the original target DNA of unspecified length. (D) In the second cycle, each of the four DNA strands shown in panel C anneals to primers (present in excess) to initiate a new round of DNA polymerization. Of the eight single-stranded products, two are of a length defined by the distance between and including the primer annealing site. This amplification product (amplicon) accumulates exponentially in subsequent cycles.

degrades the initial strands of target RNA in the RNA-DNA hybrids after they have served as templates for the first primer. The second primer binds to the newly formed cDNA and is extended, resulting in the formation of double-stranded cDNAs with one strand capable of serving as a transcription template for T7 RNA polymerase. It is reported that approximately 10 million-fold amplification occurs after a 1- to 2-h incubation, with an initial rate of

amplification of 10-fold every 2.5 min for the first 10 min. Organon Teknika has developed an electrochemiluminescence-based solid-phase sandwich hybridization system to automate the detection of the amplified product from NASBA. This is a generic detection system so it can be used to detect the amplified product from Organon Teknika-supplied kits or can be used to detect the product from in-house-developed NASBA assays.

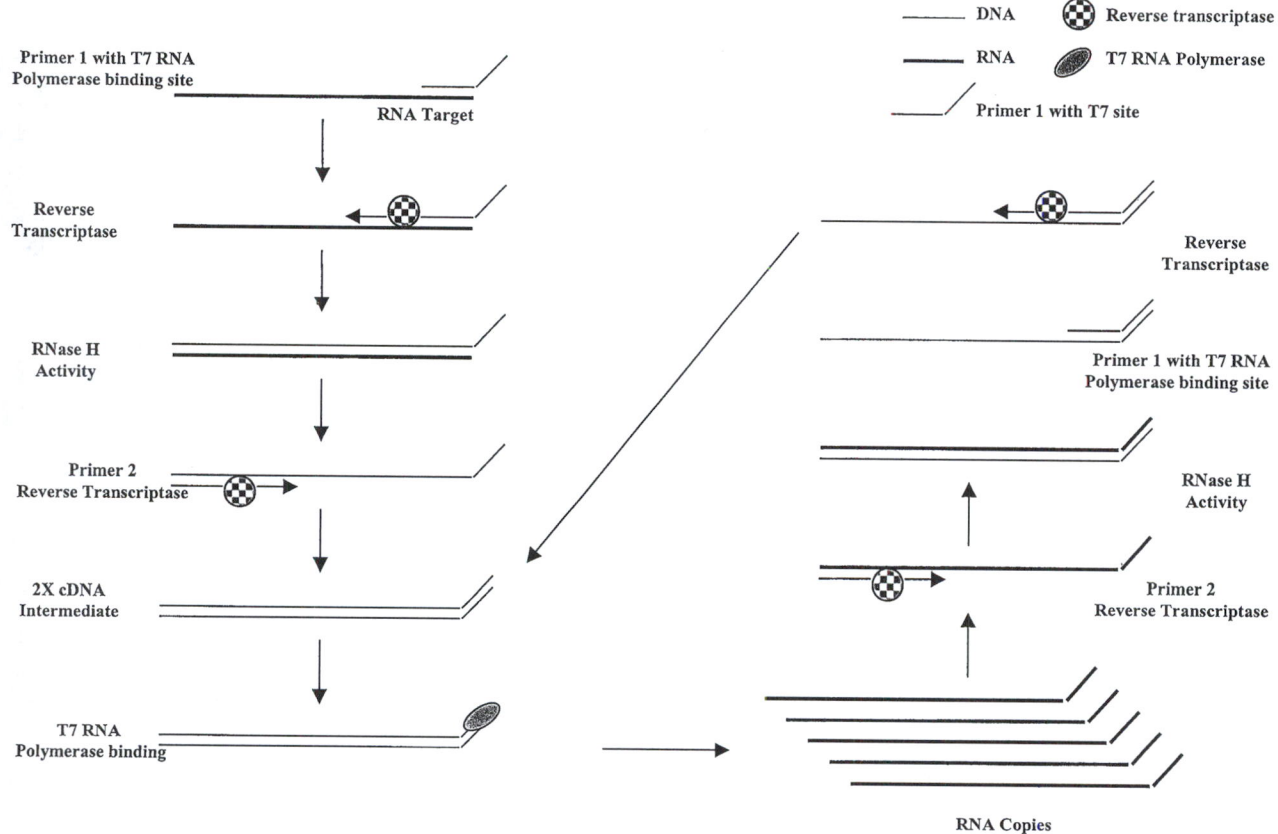

FIGURE 5 TAS. The initial steps in the reaction involve formation of cDNAs from the target RNA by using oligonucleotide primers, one of which contains a T7 binding site. RNase H activity (a separate enzyme in NASBA, associated with the reverse transcriptase in TMA) degrades the initial strands of target RNA in the RNA-DNA hybrids after they have served as templates for the initial primer. The second primer then primes the initial single-stranded cDNAs, resulting in the formation of double-stranded cDNAs with one strand capable of serving as the transcription template for T7 RNA polymerase. This results in the synthesis of numerous copies of RNA. These RNAs serve as templates for synthesis of more cDNA intermediates. These cDNAs lead to the synthesis of more copies of RNA which then reenter the cycle.

Although NASBA involves several enzymes and a complex series of reactions, individual steps in the reaction are invisible to the user. Advantages of NASBA include very rapid kinetics and an isothermal environment of 41°C. NASBA is especially useful for the amplification of single-stranded RNA targets. PCR amplification of mRNA requires isolation of RNA and/or pretreatment of the samples with DNase prior to the reverse transcription and amplification. With NASBA, because reaction conditions are maintained at temperatures that do not extensively denature DNA, the DNA is largely inaccessible to the NASBA machinery, and no pretreatment steps are necessary. While NASBA is well suited for amplification of single-stranded RNA, it is a more complicated procedure when it comes to the amplification of double-stranded DNA. For DNA amplification, heat denaturation steps are required in the initial stages of the reaction in order to generate the necessary amplification intermediates. Despite this potential shortcoming, NASBA has been used successfully to amplify DNA targets (32).

TMA

TMA is an RNA amplification system developed and patented by Gen-Probe (48). The procedure is very similar to NASBA, with the exception that only two enzymes are involved. The procedure is an isothermal reaction that uses one oligonucleotide primer, with an RNA polymerase binding site, to a specific target sequence of rRNA. This primer and a reverse transcriptase together generate cDNA molecules (Fig. 5). RNase H activity inherent in the reverse transcriptase degrades the RNA template from the cDNA, leaving a single-stranded cDNA. A second oligonucleotide primer initiates copying of the cDNA strand by the reverse transcriptase to made a double-stranded DNA template. The double-stranded DNA molecules produced act as intermediates in the TMA process. RNA polymerase binds to the polymerase binding site at one end of the cDNA intermediate and transcribes one strand of the molecule into thousands of RNA copies. These RNA copies feed back into the reaction, leading to more cDNA intermediates which in turn lead to thousands more RNA copies (Fig. 5). Detection of the amplified rRNA is done in solution using a labeled DNA probe via Gen-Probe's chemiluminescence-based HPA. The level of RNA-DNA hybrids formed is determined using a instrument to detect the light emitted during the chemiluminescence reaction. TMA is widely used for the direct detection of *Mycobacterium tuberculosis* in respiratory specimens (25, 39).

In this assay, sonication is used to lyse the mycobacteria and 12- by 75-mm tubes are used for amplification and detection. Because of all the handling involved, the *M. tuberculosis* TMA kit does not work as easily with large numbers of specimens as some other nucleic acid amplification assays, and it may be prone to cross contamination between specimens. Great care in the performance of the assay must be exercised in order to prevent cross contamination and possible false-positive results. TMA is a procedure that can potentially be applied to many molecular diagnostic assays, not just for *M. tuberculosis* and *Chlamydia trachomatis*, in the clinical laboratory (41).

SDA

SDA was developed and patented by Becton Dickinson, Inc., in 1991 (54, 111, 112). SDA is an isothermal DNA amplification procedure that uses specific primers, a DNA polymerase, and a restriction endonuclease to achieve exponential amplification of the target. Published reports claim ≈10^7-fold amplification of the target following a 2-h reaction (111). The key technology behind SDA is the generation of site-specific nicks by the restriction endonuclease *Bso*BI. The site-specific nicks are utilized by an exonuclease-deficient DNA polymerase (*Bst* DNA polymerase) to displace the nicked strand of DNA, generating a single-stranded DNA target for synthesis primers. At the same time, *Bst* DNA polymerase utilizes the remaining template strand to generate a new strand of DNA. Normally, restriction enzyme cleavage produces double-stranded DNA products, which would not be the proper template for SDA. However, if α-thio-substituted nucleotides (dCTPαS; one of the oxygen molecules in the triphosphate moiety has been replaced with sulfur) are used to synthesize a double-stranded, hemiphosphorothioated DNA recognition site for restriction enzyme cleavage, the restriction enzyme is capable of cleaving only the unmodified strand, while the hemiphosphorothioated strand remains unbroken. dCTPαS is the key base in SDA because it is responsible for transforming the original target sequence into the hemiphosphorothioate form, which is resistant to restriction endonuclease cleavage. This results in a nick being formed in the unmodified primers used to initiate SDA, with the hemiphosphorothioated strand serving as a template for DNA synthesis by *Bst* DNA polymerase at the site of the nick (Fig. 6). SDA can be thought of as a two-part reaction (111). The initial rounds of the reaction transform the original target sequence into the hemiphosphorothioate form with nickable *Bso*BI sites at each end. The second part of the reaction involves the exponential amplification of the transformed target sequence.

Although the SDA reaction is a complex one, individual reaction steps occur simultaneously and do not require attention once the reaction has been initiated. With the exception of the initial 95°C denaturation step, SDA is isothermal and requires no specialized laboratory equipment other than a controlled environment of 37°C. In addition, SDA can be applied to either single- or double-stranded DNA. With SDA, a limit to the size of the target DNA that can be efficiently amplified has been observed. For Becton Dickinson's FDA-approved *C. trachomatis* and *N. gonorrhoeae* SDA assay, the DNA targets are both around 100 bp in length (54). While this may not result in a serious functional limitation of SDA, it may complicate postamplification decontamination procedures if these are utilized (75).

POSTAMPLIFICATION DETECTION

One of the reasons nucleic acid-based amplification assays are becoming more commonplace in the clinical laboratory is that more convenient methods for detecting the reaction products are being developed. Although several different procedures are available for the detection of the products from these assays, the choice of a postamplification detection procedure depends upon several factors, including (i) the type of amplification system used, i.e., target, probe, or signal amplification; (ii) the extent of heterogeneity in the sample being detected; (iii) the need for detection of rare sequence variants in the amplified product; (iv) the requirement for sequence confirmation of the amplification product; and (v) the equipment required (72, 116). Target amplification procedures probably provide the simplest products for postamplification detection. Not only are there frequently large amounts of product, but also the sequence of product is homogeneous, reducing the complexity of detection and allowing the use of less stringent hybridization conditions than would be required if there were other sequences at similar concentrations in the mixture. Less stringent hybridization conditions may be critical to the detection of targets that contain multiple sequence variants.

In this edition of the manual there is no discussion of agarose gel and blotting-based amplification product detection procedures. These procedures are obsolete for most clinical laboratory assays and have been replaced by more rapid and less labor-intensive product detection methods that are discussed below. Those who are interested in these procedures can review earlier editions of the manual and other references (77). In addition, dedicated procedures for the detection of amplified products following nucleic acid amplification, such as reverse dot blots, are discussed only briefly because these methods are being replaced with real-time nucleic acid amplification assays where the product is detected concurrently with the ongoing amplification. Real-time nucleic acid detection systems are discussed below.

Amplification Product Capture—Reverse Dot Blot

The amplification product capture procedure is based on a modified solution-phase hybridization technique that incorporates the use of amplification primers biotinylated on their 5′ ends (116). This type of amplification product detection procedure is frequently called a reverse dot blot because, unlike a dot blot where the nucleic acid to be probed is immobilized to a solid support and the probe is free in solution, the probe itself is actually attached to a solid support and the nucleic acid to be probed is free in solution (94). In systems commonly used in the clinical laboratory, capture probes specific for a certain amplified target nucleic acid are attached to the wells of a 96-well microtiter plate or to magnetic beads (14, 56). However, unlike in typical solid-phase hybridization, the capture probes are only tethered at one end and have considerable freedom to twist and turn in the hybridization buffer. Because of the freedom of movement available to the capture probes, hybridization reactions can occur at rates that rival those of true solution-phase hybridizations. Amplified DNA with its biotinylated 5′ end is allowed to hybridize to the capture probes. After the unbound DNA is washed away, avidin-horseradish peroxidase is added, and it binds to the biotin incorporated into amplified DNA. A chromogenic substrate is then added to detect the amplified DNA colorimetrically.

DNA detection systems of this type are attractive for use in the clinical laboratory because no radioactive isotopes are involved and often microtiter plates or magnetic bead-based systems are used that depend on familiar laboratory instrumentation. In addition, capture systems of this type can be developed to allow simultaneous assaying with multiple

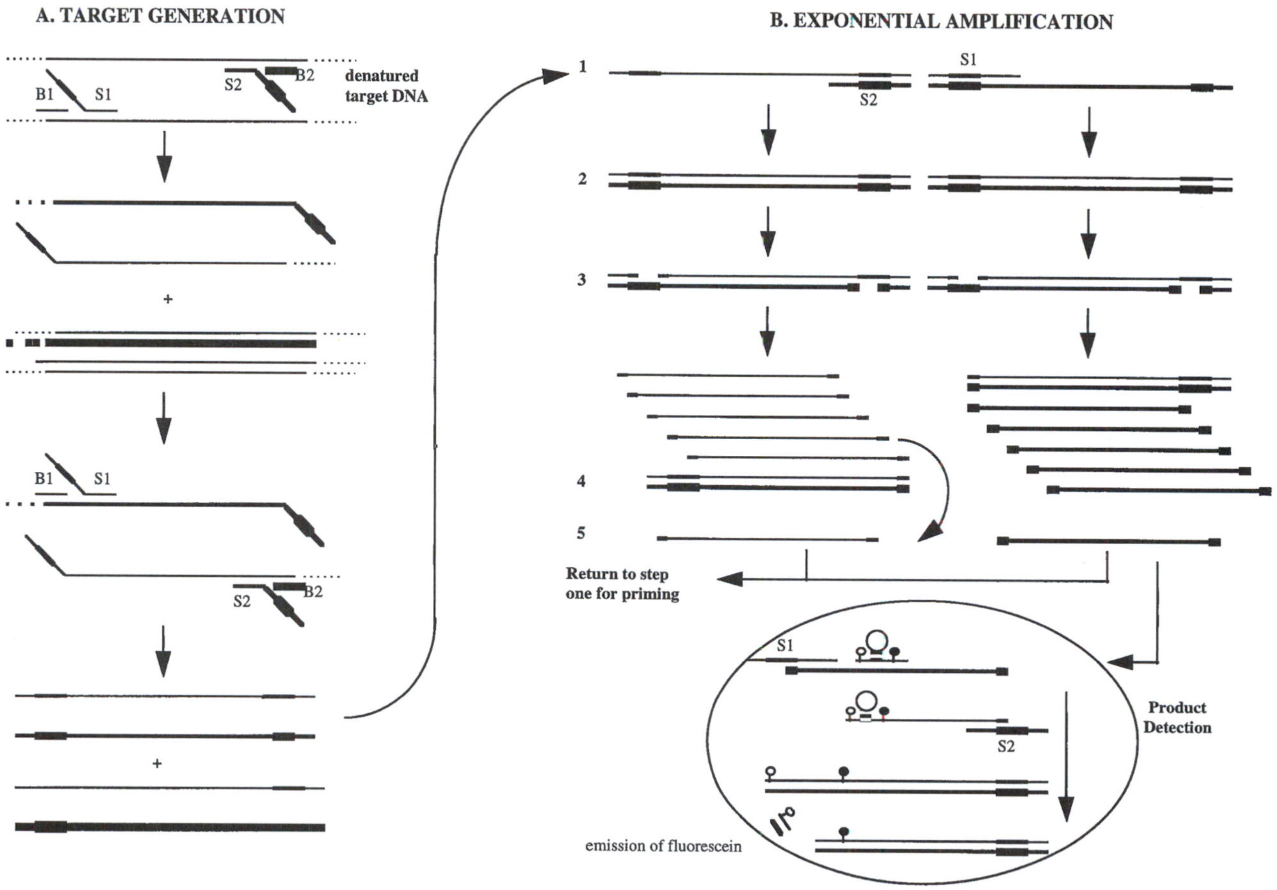

A. TARGET GENERATION

B. EXPONENTIAL AMPLIFICATION

FIGURE 6   SDA. The initial rounds of the reaction (A) transform the original target sequence into the hemiphosphorothioate form with nickable *Bso*BI sites at each end that enter into the second part of the reaction (B), which involves exponential amplification of the transformed target sequence. In reaction part A, sample DNA is denatured at 95°C in the presence of an excess of four specific primers that define the target sequence. Two primers, S1 and S2, contain unmodified *Bso*BI recognition sites at their 5′ ends and specific target-binding sequences at their 3′ ends. S1 and S2 bind opposite strands of DNA flanking the target region. The other two primers, B1 and B2, are target-binding primers only, without a restriction endonuclease recognition sequence, and bind opposite strands of DNA immediately upstream of primers S1 and S2. The incorporation of primers B1 and B2 concomitantly generates a product with defined ends during the reaction and eliminates the need for restriction enzyme cleavage of the sample DNA prior to SDA. Following the addition of the primers, the reaction mixture is allowed to cool to 37°C, and *Bst* DNA polymerase and *Bso*BI are added in excess together with dATP, dGTP, dTTP, and dCTPαS. The *Bst* DNA polymerase activity now extends all four primers simultaneously (A). Primers S1 and S2 form complementary strands of modified DNA that contain unmodified *Bso*BI sites at their 5′ ends. B1 and B2 prime the same strands and displace the newly synthesized strands primed with S1 and S2, producing new strands of DNA with defined ends that start immediately upstream of the S1 and S2 binding sites. Now S1 and B1 bind to the displaced strand initially primed with S2, while S2 and B2 bind to the displaced strand initially primed with S1 (A). Extension and displacement reactions on these templates produce two defined fragments with a hemiphosphorothioate *Bso*BI site at each end. Copies of the original target DNA containing hemiphosphorothioate *Bso*BI ends have now been generated (A, bottom). These copies now enter the second, and prominent, part of the SDA reaction (B). Following priming and extension from S1 and S2, a double-stranded fragment of a specific size that contains a *Bso*BI site on each end that is susceptible to nicking (remember that S1 and S2 primers contain unmodified *Bso*BI recognition sites at their 5′ ends) is generated. Repeated cycles of nicking, *Bst* DNA polymerization and strand displacement, and priming of the displaced strands with S1 and S2 result in exponential amplification of target DNA. For product detection, the fluorogenic probe (large circle) binds to one strand of amplified DNA and its 3′ end is extended simultaneously with the amplification (S1) probe for that strand. The extended fluorogenic probe is displaced by the product from the amplification (S1) probe. The extended fluorogenic probe is now bound by the opposite-strand primer (S2) and is copied. The copying of the fluorogenic probe forces the stem-loop structure apart and creates a double-stranded *Bso*BI site, which is flanked by both FAM (small open circle) and ROX (small solid circle). The *Bso*BI site in the fluorogenic probe lacks the dCTPαS at the nucleotide position of *Bso*BI cleavage. As a result, *Bso*BI cuts clean through the two strands of DNA and liberates FAM from the quencher. Now fluorescent emission from FAM can be detected.

probes, which avoids the need to use separate amplification reactions for multiple probings.

HPA

HPA detection systems are based on the use of a chemiluminescent DNA probe and hold considerable promise (67, 81). HPA is a proprietary procedure from Gen-Probe which is used to detect the amplified product from their TMA assay. In HPA, an acridinium ester-labeled DNA probe that is hybridized to amplified target RNA is protected from alkaline hydrolysis and upon addition of peroxides will emit detectable light. However, in its unhybridized form, the attached acridinium ester is not protected and is hydrolyzed to a form that does not emit light. HPA does not require the binding of amplified RNA to a solid support by RNA capture or other means, it can be performed in about an hour, the excess unbound DNA probe does not need to be removed, and it has a sensitivity of 10^{-16} to 10^{-18} mol (10^4 to 10^7 copies) of target RNA. However, because HPA is proprietary technology, it is not widely available.

Real-Time Product Detection

While the detection systems described below could be read following PCR (or some other nucleic acid amplification technique) by using a fluorescent plate reader, the true power of the technology is realized when it is done using an instrument that is capable of real-time detection of the PCR product (27, 33, 92). Real-time detection is when the fluorescence emission of the reporter probe (driven by the PCR product accumulation, for example) is monitored cycle by cycle. Real-time PCR utilizes one instrument (thermal cycler/signal detector) for both amplification and product detection. There is no transferring of the PCR products into a plate to be read in a fluorescence reader, and there is no agarose gel or other postamplification product detection system to run. A very important advantage of real-time detection is that once the amplification reactions have been prepared, each tube remains closed throughout the PCR amplification and detection process. The closed system associated with real-time detection greatly reduces the risk of laboratory contamination with PCR products. Additional advantages of real-time detection over older methods include the ability to quantitate a wider concentration of target, increased precision, increased accuracy, reduced hands-on time, fewer reagents and instruments required, and shorter turnaround times. The advantages real-time detection offers compared to other postamplification product detection systems in use today are so overwhelming that they cannot be ignored.

Fluorescent resonance energy transfer (FRET), or some close facsimile of this, is the principle behind the real-time detection technology in use today (19, 55, 103). FRET is an energy transfer between two dye molecules in close proximity, one acting as a donor and the other acting as an acceptor. The acceptor molecule can be either another fluorescent dye molecule or a nonfluorescent dark quencher molecule. These molecules used in real-time amplification assays are attached to short DNA probes specific for the target sequence of interest. The efficiency of energy transfer between the dyes depends upon the physical distance between them and the degree of overlap between the emission spectrum of the donor dye and the absorption spectrum of the acceptor dye/quencher. When the molecules are close, following excitation with the appropriate wavelength of light, energy is transferred from the donor dye to an acceptor dye/quencher without the emission of fluorescence. As a result, the donor dye fluorescence is quenched, and the acceptor dye/quencher

is excited, resulting in either fluorescent light of a different emission wavelength than the donor dye or heat. When the dyes are distant, following excitation with the appropriate wavelength of light, energy transfer is sharply reduced or eliminated and the donor dye emits the energy via a specific wavelength of fluorescent light that differs from that of the acceptor dye/quencher. Real-time DNA probes incorporating dark quenchers have become very popular because they have a broad absorption spectrum with lower background fluorescence. These characteristics lead to assays with increased sensitivity and allow the use of multiple reporter dyes with the same dark quencher. There are numerous fluorescence-based real-time detection systems available today. Only a few of the more popular ones are discussed below.

TaqMan

The $5' \rightarrow 3'$ exonuclease-based detection assay developed by Holland et al., now called TaqMan, allows real-time PCR detection of the target sequence (34). This method employs the $5' \rightarrow 3'$ exonuclease activity of *Taq* to generate a specific detectable product concomitantly with amplification (69) (Fig. 7). Fluorescent energy transfer is the principle behind TaqMan detection technology (19, 55, 103). A special reporter probe designed to hybridize within the target sequence is added to the PCR amplification mixture. The reporter probe contains 6-carboxyfluorescein (FAM) as a reporter dye covalently linked to the 5' end. A quencher dye, such as 6-carboxytetramethylrhodamine (TAMRA) or a nonfluorescent dark quencher, is covalently linked close to the 3' end of the probe. This probe is not involved in the amplification reaction and is phosphorylated on its 3' end to prevent extension by *Taq*. Because of the close proximity of the quencher dye to the reporter dye, the reporter dye fluorescence is suppressed. Annealing of this reporter probe to one of the PCR product strands during the course of amplification generates a target-specific substrate suitable for exonuclease cleavage. During DNA extension from a PCR primer, the $5' \rightarrow 3'$ exonuclease activity of *Taq* cleaves 5'-terminal nucleotides off the bound reporter probe in essentially a nick translation reaction and frees the FAM reporter from the quencher (50). The free FAM reporter now emits fluorescence. The cleavage of the reporter probe does not affect the emission of the quencher (if it has any). Even in a high background of genomic DNA, labeled-probe degradation occurs only in a target-specific fashion. Since the exonuclease activity of *Taq* acts only if the fluorogenic probe is annealed to the target, the increase in fluorescence is proportional to the amount of PCR product produced and because of this proportionality, this system is readily capable of performing quantitative determinations of the amount of target nucleic acid in the amplification reaction.

This detection system differs from a traditional PCR procedure only by the addition to the amplification reaction of a fluorogenic reporter probe. One requirement for this detection method is that the reporter probe must bind to target before extension from a PCR primer blocks the binding site. If the annealing temperature of the reporter probe is close to or below the annealing temperature of the upstream amplification primer, there is a greater chance that the amplification primer will be extended before the reporter probe has bound to the target. This would result in inefficient label release and could lead to a false-negative result. This problem may be overcome by varying the relative concentrations of amplification primers and reporter probe, by manipulating the sequence and length of the reporter probe, or by using more stable base analogs.

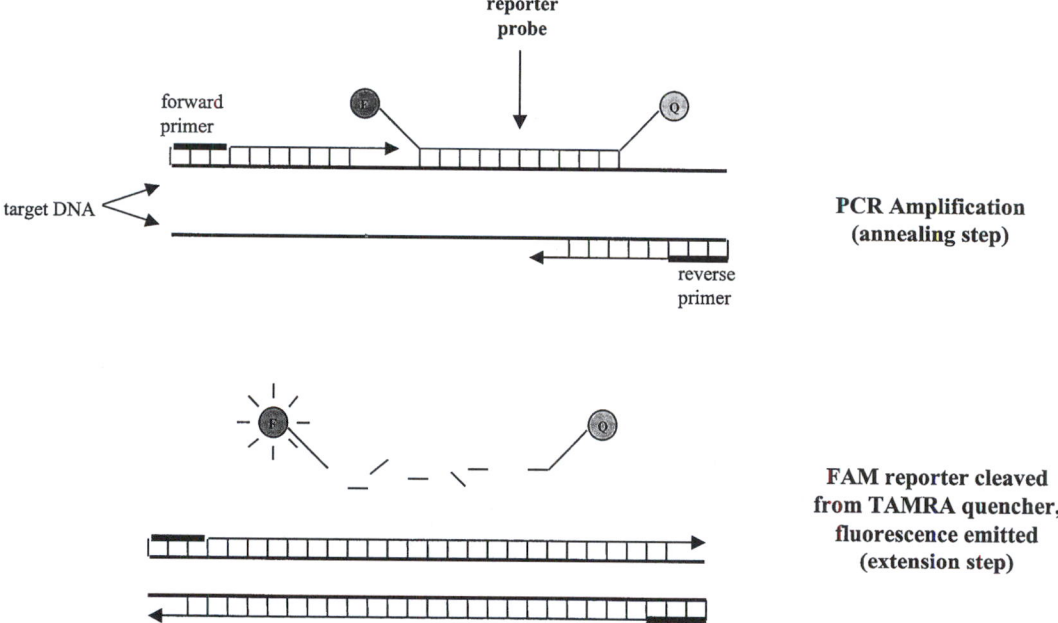

FIGURE 7   TaqMan. Annealing of the reporter probe to one specific strand of the PCR product during the course of amplification generates a target-specific substrate suitable for exonuclease cleavage. During DNA extension from a PCR primer, the 5′ → 3′ exonuclease activity of *Taq* cleaves 5′-terminal nucleotides off the bound reporter probe and frees the FAM reporter (F) from the TAMRA quencher (Q). The free FAM reporter now emits fluorescence.

Molecular Beacons

Another popular way to realize real-time PCR detection in a nucleic acid amplification assay is through the use of molecular beacons (107, 108). Like in TaqMan, a "FRET-like" transfer is the key to molecular beacons. Molecular beacons are single-stranded DNA hairpin-shaped reporter probes with an internally quenched reporter dye whose fluorescence is restored when the probe binds to a target nucleic acid (Fig. 8). Molecular beacons are designed so the loop portion of the molecule is the probe sequence complementary to PCR product. The stem is formed by the annealing of the complementary sequences on the ends of the probe

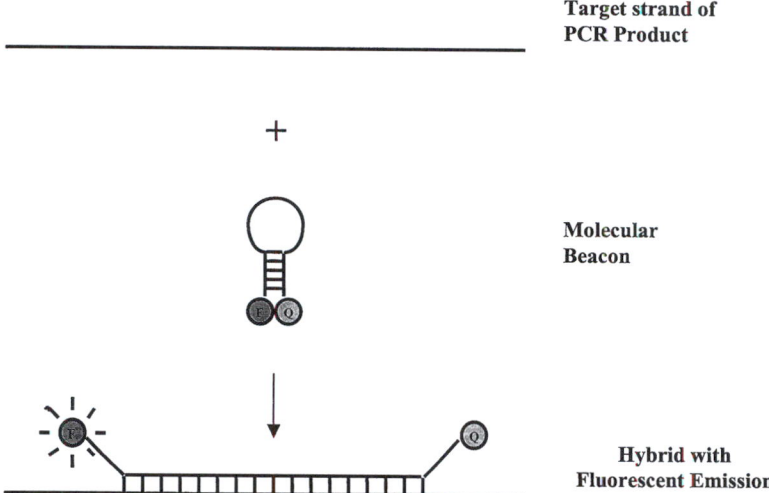

FIGURE 8   Molecular beacons. During the denaturation step of PCR, the target DNA and the stem-loop of the molecular beacon denature. As the temperature is lowered to allow annealing of PCR primers, the molecular beacon hybridizes to one specific strand of the PCR product. This conformational change that occurs during hybridization forces the stem apart and causes the fluorescent dye (F) to move away from the quencher (Q), leading to fluorescence. When the temperature is raised for primer extension, the molecular beacons dissociate from their targets and do not interfere with PCR.

sequence. The fluorescent dye is attached to the end of one arm and a quencher is attached to the end of the other arm. The stem keeps these two moieties in close proximity to each other, causing the fluorescence to be quenched by energy transfer. In molecular beacons the quencher is typically a nonfluorescent molecule, such as 4-([4′-dimethylamino-phenyl]azo)-benzoic acid, that serves as a universal quencher for many fluorescent dyes used in molecular beacons. The quencher emits the energy that it receives from the fluorescent dye as heat so the probe is unable to fluoresce. During the denaturation step of PCR, the molecular beacons assume a random coil configuration and fluoresce. As the temperature is lowered to allow annealing of PCR primers, stem-loop structures form rapidly, preventing fluorescence. However, when the molecular beacon hybridizes to a target molecule, it forms a structure that is longer and more stable than the stem-loop structure of the unhybridized probe. This conformational change forces the stem apart and causes the fluorescent dye to move away from the quencher, leading to fluorescence. When the temperature is raised for primer extension, the molecular beacons dissociate from their targets and do not interfere with PCR. A new hybridization takes place in the annealing step of every PCR cycle, and the intensity of the resulting fluorescence indicates the amount of accumulated PCR product. Like TaqMan, molecular beacons can detect multiple targets in the same solution when different-colored fluorescent dyes are used on the probes (107). Unlike a TaqMan probe, molecular beacons fluoresce specifically only when the probe is hybridized (annealing step of a PCR cycle) to its target molecule.

The selection of a DNA sequence to be used in a molecular beacon depends upon several parameters. For best results, molecular beacons should be targeted to the middle of the PCR product of interest. The length of the stem sequences should be chosen so that a stem is formed at the annealing temperature of the specific PCR in which the molecular beacon is to be used. The stem sequences should hybridize only to each other and not to the probe portion of the molecular beacon. The length of the loop sequence should be chosen so that the probe-PCR product hybrid is stable at the annealing temperature of the specific assay. Owing to their stem-loop structure, the recognition of targets by molecular beacons is more specific than traditional DNA probes, so single-nucleotide differences between probe targets can be readily detected using melting-curve analysis (6). Since molecular beacons remain intact throughout the amplification process, unlike TaqMan probes, they can be utilized in melting-curve analysis. Following completion of target amplification, melting-curve analysis is done by slowly raising the temperature to 95°C and measuring the decrease in fluorescence as the molecular beacon is "melted off" the target. Melting-curve analysis is a very simple way to detect mutations in the target DNA. Molecular beacons melt away at higher temperatures when they match the target DNA perfectly and at a lower temperature when there is even just a single-base mismatch between the probe and target DNA.

Hybridization Probes

The probe system used in many molecular assays built for the Roche LightCycler real-time PCR instrument is called hybridization probes. This system involves two separate individually labeled DNA probes that both target a region of one strand of the amplified product. Specific binding of these two probes places them next to one another in a tail-to-head arrangement (Fig. 9). The 5′ probe is the donor probe and has a fluorescein reporter dye at its 3′ end. The 3′ probe is the acceptor probe and has a LightCycler Red reporter dye at its 5′ end and is phosphorylated at its 3′ end to prevent elongation during PCR. During the denaturing step of a PCR cycle, the hybridization probes (just like the PCR primers) are free in solution. During the annealing step, the probes will hybridize to an internal sequence of one specific stand of the amplified product and be positioned next to one another. This results in the reporter dyes being brought into very close proximity with each other. The fluorescein reporter dye is specifically excited and the excitation is transferred (FRET) to the acceptor LightCycler Red reporter. The fluorescein emission is quenched by the close LightCycler Red dye. The LightCycler Red reporter dye becomes excited and emits a red fluorescence that is measured by the instrument at the end of each annealing step. When the temperature is raised for the extension step of the assay, an exonuclease-deficient thermostable DNA polymerase starts elongation from the PCR primer on the strand that the hybridization probes are bound to and the hybridization probes are displaced. At the end of the elongation phase, the PCR product is double stranded again and the hybridization probes are back in solution. A new hybridization by the hybridization probes takes place in the annealing step of every PCR cycle, and the intensity of the resulting fluorescence indicates the amount of accumulated PCR product. Like TaqMan and molecular beacons, hybridization probes can detect multiple targets in the same solution when different-colored fluorescent dyes are used on the probes (107). Since hybridization probes remain intact throughout the amplification process, they can be utilized in melting-curve analysis to detect mutations in the target DNA.

Because each probe has only a single label, hybridization probes are frequently touted as being easier to synthesize, purify, and characterize than dually labeled probes. However, there are several factors that must be considered when contemplating the use of these probes. Cost is something to keep in mind. You are paying for synthesis, labeling, and purification of two probes that are typically 20 to 30 bases each. Also, instead of working out the sequence requirements and annealing conditions for one reporter probe, you have to work it out for two. The melting temperature (T_m) of the hybridization probes should be 5 to 10°C higher than the T_m of the PCR primers. The optimum T_m between the two hybridization probes depends upon how they are used. For basic detection of an amplified product, the T_ms of the probes should be within 2°C of each other. For detection of mutations in the amplified product, the best results are obtained when the difference between the T_ms of the hybridizations probes is 5 to 10°C. The probe with the lowest T_m (called the sensor probe when detecting a mutation) should be the donor probe and should be positioned directly over the mutation of interest. In addition to calculating the T_ms for the probes, you have to determine how far apart from one another the hybridization probes should bind. The distance required between donor reporter dye and acceptor reporter dye for efficient FRET depends upon the fluorophores that are used to make the hybridization probes. Typically the hybridization probes are designed so that they hybridize from 1 to 5 nucleotides apart. However, some studies suggest that the probes should be a minimum of 5 nucleotides apart to prevent close contact quenching and to maximize emission from the acceptor probe (57).

Real-Time Detection Used in SDA

The real-time detection system utilized in Becton Dickinson's *C. trachomatis*/*N. gonorrhoeae* SDA kit is a hybrid with some

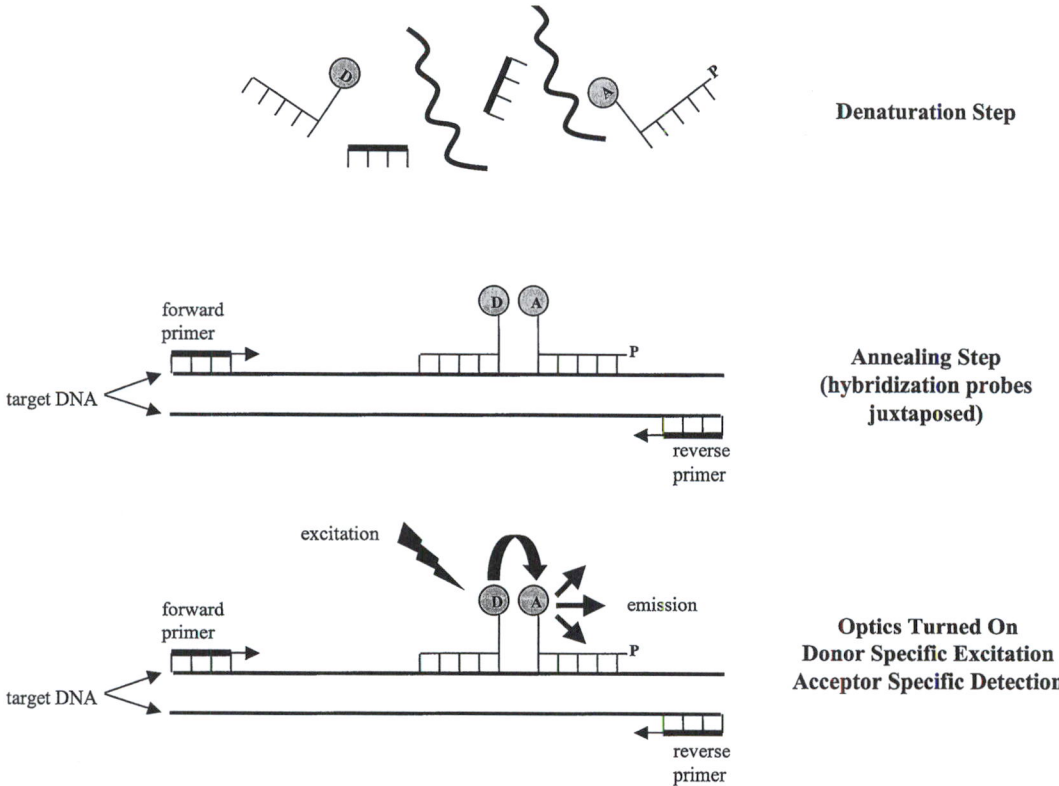

FIGURE 9 Hybridization probes. Two separate fluorescently labeled probes (the donor probe is labeled at the 3′ end with fluorescein [probe D] and the acceptor probe is labeled at the 5′ end with LightCycler Red 640 [probe A]) are juxtaposed tail to head upon specifically binding to one strand of the PCR product during the annealing phase of PCR. An excitation wavelength of light specific for the donor probe only is produced during annealing. The acceptor probe absorbs resonance energy from the donor probe and emits fluorescence, with emission collection only being done in the acceptor range.

features of molecular beacons, some features of TaqMan, and some features found in both (54). Like for TaqMan and molecular beacons, fluorescent energy transfer is the principle behind SDA real-time detection (55). The SDA reaction contains a single-stranded DNA fluorogenic probe with FAM as a reporter dye covalently linked to the 5′ end. A quencher dye, rhodamine (ROX), is covalently linked close to the middle of the fluorogenic probe. The area between the two dyes includes a stem-loop structure, making the fluorogenic probe similar in conformation to a molecular beacon (Fig. 6). The loop contains the recognition sequence for the BsoBI restriction endonuclease used in SDA. However, the BsoBI recognition sequence in the fluorogenic probe contains dCTP, not dCTPαS. The fluorogenic probe also contains a target-specific sequence 3′ to the ROX. In its native form, the FAM and ROX dyes are proximal to each other such that excitation of FAM leads to transfer of the emitted energy to ROX. The result is that very little emission from excited fluorescein is detected. As SDA product accumulates, the fluorogenic probe binds to one strand of amplified DNA and its 3′ end is extended simultaneously with the amplification (S1) probe for that strand. The extended fluorogenic probe is displaced by the product from the amplification (S1) probe. The extended fluorogenic probe is now capable of being bound by the opposite-strand primer (S2) and is copied. The copying of the fluorogenic probe forces the stem-loop structure apart and creates a double-stranded BsoBI site, which is flanked by both FAM and ROX. The BsoBI site in the fluorogenic probe

lacks the dCTPαS at the nucleotide position of BsoBI cleavage. As a result, BsoBI cuts clean through the two strands of DNA and liberates FAM from the quencher (mechanism similar to TaqMan). Now fluorescence emission from FAM can be detected. The detection steps occur simultaneously with SDA, making a real-time detection process similar to TaqMan and molecular beacons. Real-time detection in the C. trachomatis/N. gonorrhoeae kit is very important because no SDA product inactivation system is included. Real-time detection allows the amplification reactions to remain closed throughout the SDA procedure. The closed amplification reactions significantly reduce (but do not totally eliminate) the risk of contamination of the laboratory with amplified product. This detection system will undoubtedly be utilized in other SDA assays developed by Becton Dickinson.

Real-Time PCR Instruments

To realize the full potential of real-time PCR, an instrument is required that can do the thermal cycling as well as the concurrent amplification product detection. As described above, fluorescence-based product detection is typically how real-time PCR is done. Currently, there are numerous instruments on the market that are capable of doing real-time PCR. They differ markedly in terms of cost, complexity, capability, cycling speed, utility in the clinical laboratory, and space requirements. It is beyond the scope of this chapter to provide a detailed comparison of the many real-time PCR instruments available today. However, Table 1 lists some of the more popular real-time PCR instruments that are available in the United States today and compares some of their basic features. All of these instruments are capable of doing basic real-time PCR, using some or all of the real-time detection systems listed above, and graphically displaying the results. The fluorescent dyes supported by the real-time PCR instruments vary depending upon the manufacturer. In addition, features such as the ability to custom select excitation and emission filters depend upon the manufacturer. All of the instruments in Table 1 are capable of doing conventional PCR; however, the ease of recovery of the amplified product varies depending upon the amplification tube used by the manufacturer. Some of the instruments listed in Table 1 may be better suited than others for use in the clinical laboratory. Roche and Cepheid both produce real-time PCR instruments that are being extensively marketed for use in the clinical laboratory. In addition, both of these companies have some FDA-approved diagnostic kits available for use in the clinical laboratory as well as an ever-expanding number of ASRs. The reader should check with representatives of these companies for the latest information on the availability of kits and reagents.

The basic design is similar among real-time PCR instruments (Fig. 10). They consist of a computer and software to run the instrument and analyze the data, a thermal cycler for nucleic acid amplification, and an optical system to excite the fluorescent reporter molecules together with an emission detector. The optical systems used by the various manufacturers of real-time PCR instruments do vary. It is important for potential buyers to determine which instrument best fits their needs. One nice thing about these machines is that the space requirements for real-time PCR instruments have decreased significantly as new instruments have been introduced. They now should be able to be accommodated by all but the most crowded of clinical laboratories. However, when considering space requirements for the instrument, remember that a computer is required to run the instrument and a printer may be needed to generate hard copies of the results.

DNA SEQUENCE ANALYSIS IN THE CLINICAL LABORATORY

The application of nucleic acid sequencing technology to problems in medicine is starting to come of age (40). The utilization of sequencing to aid in the diagnosis and management of disease will be a major growth area in the clinical laboratory in the coming years. As the utility of sequencing information becomes more appreciated, and the sequencing hardware and software become more readily available and easier to use, more and more laboratories will incorporate this technology into their routine testing.

Sanger's dideoxy chain termination procedure has become the most popular sequencing method in use today (96). This procedure takes advantage of two properties of DNA polymerases: (i) their ability to synthesize faithfully a complementary copy of a single-stranded DNA template and (ii) their ability to use $2',3'$-dideoxynucleoside triphosphates as bases. $2',3'$-Dideoxynucleoside triphosphates resemble

TABLE 1 Comparison of basic features of five real-time PCR instruments

Feature	Roche LightCycler 2.0	Cepheid SmartCycler II	Stratagene Mx3000P	Applied Biosystems 7500	Bio-Rad iCycler iQ
Tube	Glass capillary tube	Proprietary reaction tube	Conventional 0.2-ml PCR tube	Conventional 0.2-ml PCR tube	Conventional 0.2-ml tube
Optics	Blue LED excitation, photohybrid detection, detects six different spectral bands	High-intensity LED excitation, silicon photodetectors, filters to excite/detect four different spectral bands	Tungsten halogen lamp excitation, scanning photo-multiplier tube detector, user-selected filters to excite/detect four different spectral bands	Tungsten halogen lamp excitation, charge-coupled device camera detector, filters to excite/detect five different spectral bands	Tungsten halogen lamp excitation, filters to excite/detect five different spectral bands
Probe capability	SYBR Green I, TaqMan, Molecular beacons, Hybridization probes	SYBR Green I, TaqMan, Molecular beacons	SYBR Green I, TaqMan, Molecular beacons	SYBR Green I, TaqMan, Molecular beacons	SYBR Green I, TaqMan, Molecular beacons
Thermal cycling system/capacity	Ambient temp based, forced air, 32 reactions	Ambient temp based, I-CORE modules, 16 reactions	Ambient temp based, 96-well block	Peltier based, 96-well block	Peltier based, 96-well block
Cycling speed capability	Very fast	Fast	Similar to conventional PCR	Similar to conventional PCR	Similar to conventional PCR
Relative price	***	**	**	***	***
Ease of conventional PCR	Not particularly easy	Somewhat easy	Very easy	Very easy	Very easy
Availability of FDA-approved kits and ASRs	Yes	Yes	No	No	No

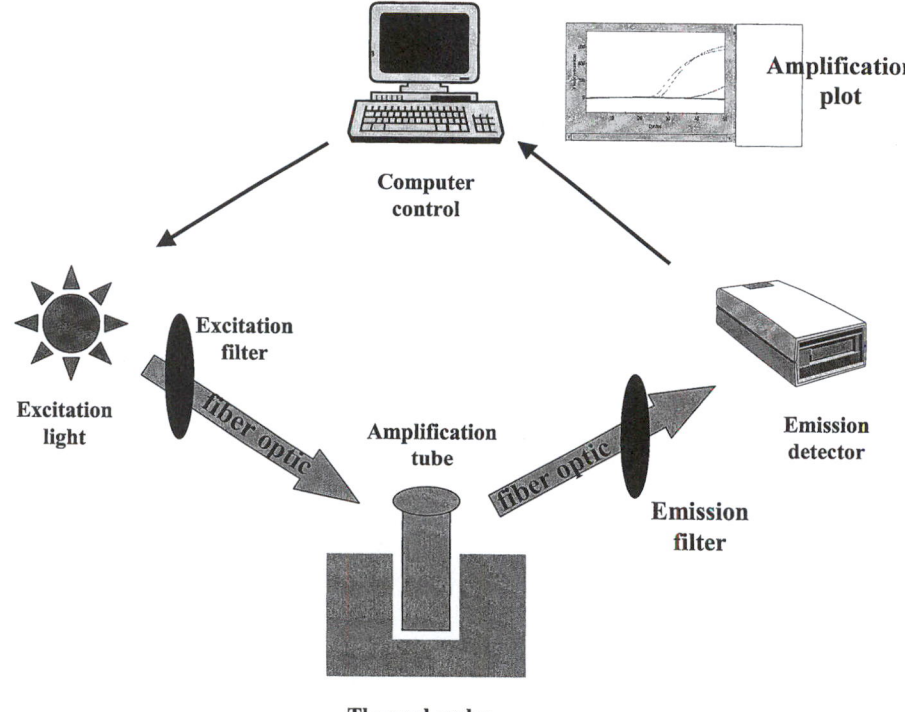

FIGURE 10 Basic components of a real-time nucleic acid amplification instrument. A computer and associated software run the instrument and analyze the amplification data. A thermal cycler provides the cycling temperature conditions for nucleic acid amplification. The optical system includes components to excite the fluorescent reporter molecules, together with an emission detector.

2′-deoxynucleoside triphosphates except that they lack a 3′-OH group (Fig. 11). They can be added to an extending strand of DNA, but they cannot be added onto and therefore serve as chain terminators. Initiation of DNA synthesis requires a primer (short single-stranded piece of DNA) that binds to the strand of DNA to be copied, resulting in the copy strand of DNA being synthesized downstream from the primer. One commonly used version of the Sanger DNA sequencing protocol is carried out in a single tube in the presence of four 2′-deoxynucleoside triphosphates (dA, dC, dG, and dT), specific primer, single-stranded template DNA, and DNA polymerase. Also included in the mixture is a limiting amount of four 2′,3′-dideoxynucleoside triphosphates (ddA, ddC, ddG, and ddT), each coupled to a different-colored fluorescent dye (28). The concentration of the 2′,3′-dideoxynucleoside triphosphates is much lower than the concentration of 2′-deoxynucleoside triphosphates. The 2′,3′-dideoxynucleoside triphosphates randomly terminate the extending DNA fragments at one of the four nucleotides. When the sequencing reaction is finished, the reaction tube contains a population of partially synthesized DNA molecules, each having a common 5′ end (designated by the DNA primer used) but each varying in length to a base-specific 3′ end. The sequencing mixture is then cleaned up to remove any unincorporated dye terminators, and the DNA fragments are denatured and then separated by electrophoresis in a sequencing gel or by capillary gel electrophoresis. The labeled DNA bands are revealed by laser light. Each dye attached to a terminator 2′,3′-dideoxynucleoside triphosphate emits light at a different wavelength when excited by the laser; thus, all four colors (and therefore all four bases) can be distinguished in a single gel lane or capillary tube. The sequence is read directly from the gel in the sequencing instrument, starting with the fastest-moving (smallest) fragment at the bottom and moving up the gel. As you move up the gel each fragment is one base longer than the preceding fragment, thus revealing the DNA sequence. In capillary gel electrophoresis the sequence is read as the fragments reach the end of the capillary, starting with the fastest-moving (smallest) fragment. The sequencing information is then loaded directly into a computer. Direct electronic entry of sequence data eliminates the tedious and error-prone entry of the DNA sequence by manual methods. Review and editing of the DNA sequence generated by the computer can be easily done by evaluating the electropherograms generated by the sequencing analysis software.

Sanger's dideoxy sequencing protocol requires a single-stranded DNA template (96). In traditional DNA sequencing the fragment of DNA to be sequenced is inserted into the polycloning region of the M13mp series of vectors (62). M13mp is a genetically engineered *E. coli* bacteriophage that contains a single-stranded circular molecule of DNA. Growing up M13mp with the inserted DNA to be sequenced generates large quantities of single-stranded DNA template. While M13mp has been used for many years, and is still used today for the generation of single-stranded template DNA for sequencing, it is much too cumbersome for routine use in the clinical laboratory. A much simpler procedure for DNA sequencing combines features of PCR with the Sanger dideoxy sequencing procedure. This procedure has been termed "cycle sequencing" and allows ready sequencing of double-stranded PCR products (76, 86, 87). Today, when sequencing is done in the clinical laboratory, cycle sequencing is most often the procedure used. Cycle sequencing involves linear amplification of DNA using one specific

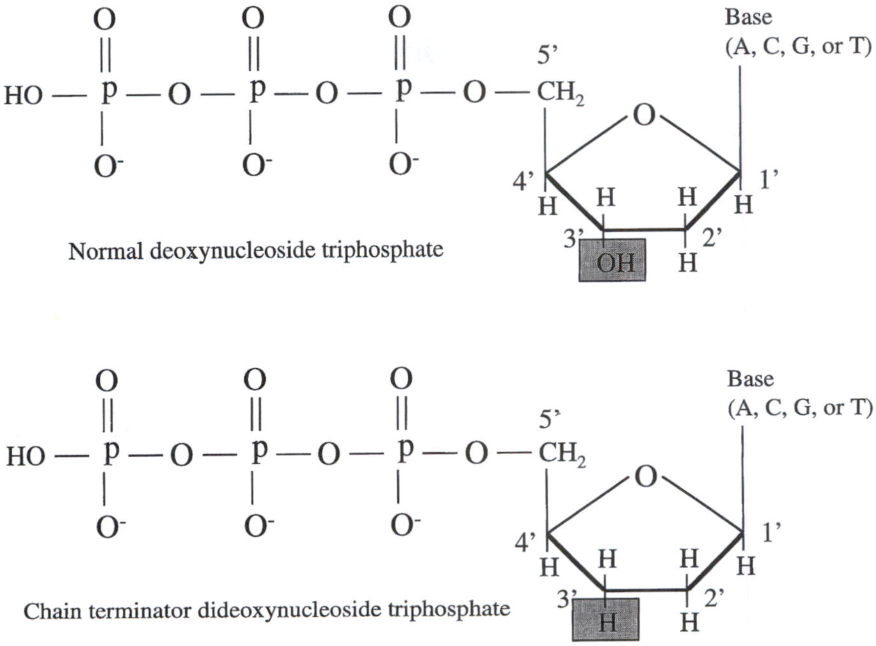

Normal deoxynucleoside triphosphate

Chain terminator dideoxynucleoside triphosphate

FIGURE 11 Bases used in Sanger's dideoxy chain termination procedure.

primer targeted to a region of the PCR product to be sequenced. Cycle sequencing is typically carried out as described above, with the exceptions that a double-stranded PCR product serves as template DNA and a thermostable DNA polymerase is used for DNA synthesis (76, 86, 87). The reaction mixture is subjected to 20 to 40 cycles of denaturation, annealing, and extension, resulting in the synthesis of new DNA from the sequencing primer. During the denaturation phase of the cycle the double-stranded DNA template is denatured to single-stranded fragments. Cooling the reaction to the primer annealing temperature allows the

sequencing primer to bind to one of the strands of target DNA. Raising the temperature to the extension temperature allows the thermostable DNA polymerase to extend the copy strand of DNA. During extension, the 2′,3′-dideoxynucleoside triphosphates randomly terminate the extending DNA fragments at one of the four nucleotides. Following the sequencing reaction, the sequencing mixture is cleaned up to remove any unincorporated dye terminators, and the DNA fragments are denatured and then separated by electrophoresis in a sequencing gel or by capillary gel electrophoresis (Fig. 12). The labeled DNA bands are identified

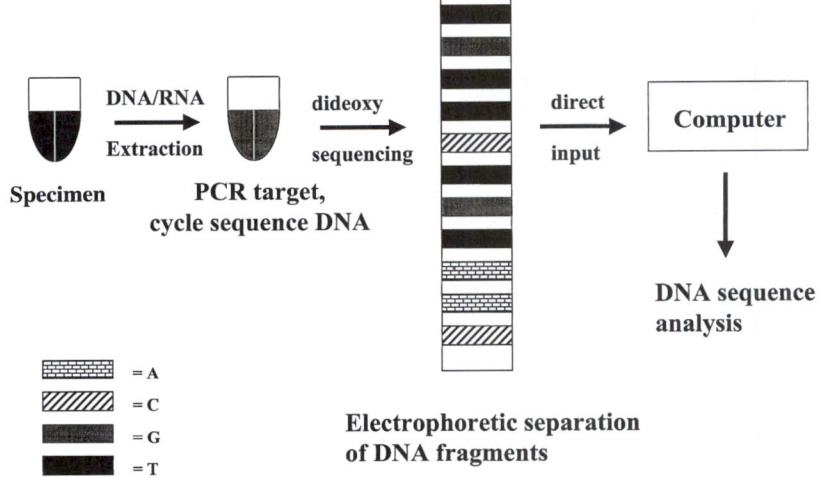

FIGURE 12 Cycle sequencing-based procedure. DNA or RNA to be sequenced is extracted from the sample of interest, and PCR is used to amplify the target to be sequenced. Once the target has been cleaned up it is used as template in a dideoxy-based cycle sequencing reaction. An automated sequencer determines the composition of the sequence template based upon different-colored fluorescent chain terminators and directly enters the sequence data into a computerized workstation, where data analysis is completed.

using a laser light source and detector system as described above. Depending upon the template DNA, cycle sequencing reactions routinely extend 200 to 600 bases from the primer. The major advantage of cycle sequencing is that it permits direct sequencing of double-stranded DNA without many of the inconveniences associated with conventional DNA sequencing (cloning DNA to be sequenced and isolating single-stranded M13 DNA). Several additional advantages are also associated with cycle sequencing. The elevated reaction temperature used in cycle sequencing reduces false stops induced by template secondary structure and decreases background caused by nonspecific primer binding because of the higher-stringency conditions. In addition, high-G+C-content DNA is sequenced with greater accuracy because of the higher temperatures associated with cycle sequencing. The denaturation step also frees template DNA from newly synthesized cDNA strands, making them available as templates for subsequent rounds of priming and extension; thus, less DNA is required in cycle sequencing than in a standard dideoxy sequencing reaction.

Very thin polyacrylamide gels formerly were used to separate DNA fragments and determine the sequence of template DNA. However, their use is very time-consuming and labor-intensive. Although 36 to 96 sequencing reactions can be run on a single gel, a new gel is required for each run of sequencing reactions. Capillary gel electrophoresis systems eliminate the need for repeated pouring of gels and many other sequencing gel-associated preparation steps (20, 43, 83). Capillary systems are replacing many polyacrylamide gel-based systems in use today. Because of the inherent difficulty in loading specimens into small capillaries, these instruments come with autoloaders. The capillary systems used in these sequencing instruments differ among manufacturers. Some capillary systems automatically inject fresh separation material into the capillary before each run, while other systems reuse the capillaries after a regeneration cycle has been completed. For ease of setup and operation, capillary electrophoresis instruments have become standard platforms in most laboratories. Until relatively recently, the cost of the capillary sequencing instruments was quite high, and some had only had one capillary. However, there are several models of capillary instruments available today, covering a wide range of prices. Depending upon your needs, you can purchase capillary instruments with from 8 to 96 working capillaries. The system that can run 96 sequencing reactions at once utilizes a 96-well thermal cycler microplate format. The 96-well format provides an easy interface between the thermal cycler, where cycle sequencing is done, and the capillary sequencing instrument. Another concern voiced about some capillary electrophoresis systems is that the length of DNA that can be analyzed is shorter than that obtained from the same type of reactions sequenced using polyacrylamide gels (63). However, with improvements that have been made to the capillary systems and the gel matrix used for DNA fragment separation there is now little, if any, difference in the read length between polyacrylamide gels and the capillary electrophoresis systems.

MOLECULAR ARRAYS

Molecular arrays are ordered sets of unique DNA probe molecules attached to a solid support (99). Arrays consist of a few different probes to hundreds of thousands of different DNA probes. Each individual probe goes on the array at a precisely defined location on the substrate. The identity of the DNA molecule fixed to each substrate never changes.

Molecular arrays evolved from Southern's work in the 1970s that demonstrated that labeled DNA molecules (called probes today) could be used to interrogate DNA molecules attached to a solid support (100). The Southern blot was a very simple molecular array utilizing one DNA probe. The strategy of the molecular arrays today parallels that of a reverse dot blot, because the probe is immobilized, not the target as in a Southern blot. In general, molecular arrays are described as macroarrays or microarrays, the difference being the size of the DNA probe spots. Macroarrays contain probe spot sizes of about 300 μm or larger and can be easily imaged by existing gel and blot scanners. Microarrays have probe spot sizes typically less than 200 μm in diameter, and these arrays usually contain thousands to hundreds of thousands of probes. Two commonly used methods to produce microarrays are "printing" (spotting) and in situ synthesis procedures such as photolithography, ink-jet, or maskless array synthesis (1, 12, 13, 21, 30, 36, 52, 53, 68). With printed microarrays, about 10,000 DNA probes (PCR products from cDNAs) can be printed onto a microscope slide using high-speed robotics (Fig. 13) (13, 21). Microarrays synthesized by in situ procedures can contain up to 400,000 distinct DNA probes, each in its own 20-μm^2 region, depending upon the technology used. Unlike printed microarrays, in situ microarrays utilize short DNA probes (oligonucleotides typically 8 to up to 90 bases in length) and not PCR products from cDNAs (12, 30, 36, 52, 53, 68).

Two key innovations have led to the practical use of microarrays. First, the use of nonporous substrates, such as glass or silica, has facilitated miniaturization and fluorescence-based detection (99). The second innovation was the development of methods for high-density spatial synthesis of short DNA probes, such as photolithography, ink-jet technology, and maskless array synthesizers (36, 53, 68). Glass or silica has a number of practical advantages over porous membranes such as nylon or nitrocellulose for use in microarrays. Because liquid cannot penetrate the surface of glass or silica, target nucleic acids can find immediate access to the probes without diffusing into pores, thus speeding the rate of hybridization. The washing step which follows hybridization is also unimpeded by diffusion, speeding up the procedure and improving reproducibility. The flatness, rigidity, and transparency of glass or silica improve image analysis, as the locations of the probes can be much better defined than they are on a nylon membrane. High image definition is critical because of the very small scale associated with microarrays. The physical rigidity associated with glass or silica allows their incorporation into cartridges or flow cells for automated processing, which is essential for development of high-throughput assays. Microarrays, with their thousands of probes that determine cDNA binding, allow enormous amounts of data to be collected in a single experiment.

Microarrays are used for two major applications: (i) determination of DNA sequences and mutation detection and (ii) genome-scale determination of gene expression. For DNA sequence analysis it is important that the hybridization between target and probe is able to discriminate a single mismatched base pair; this high degree of discrimination is possible only with short probes (12, 30, 53, 71). Precise sequence discrimination is less important for gene expression microarrays, but in this case, quantitative measurement of gene expression over a wide dynamic range is important. Printed microarrays and high-density spatial microarrays are both commonly used for gene expression assays, while sequencing assays have largely been the province of high-density spatial

MAKING THE ARRAY

PREPARING THE TARGET

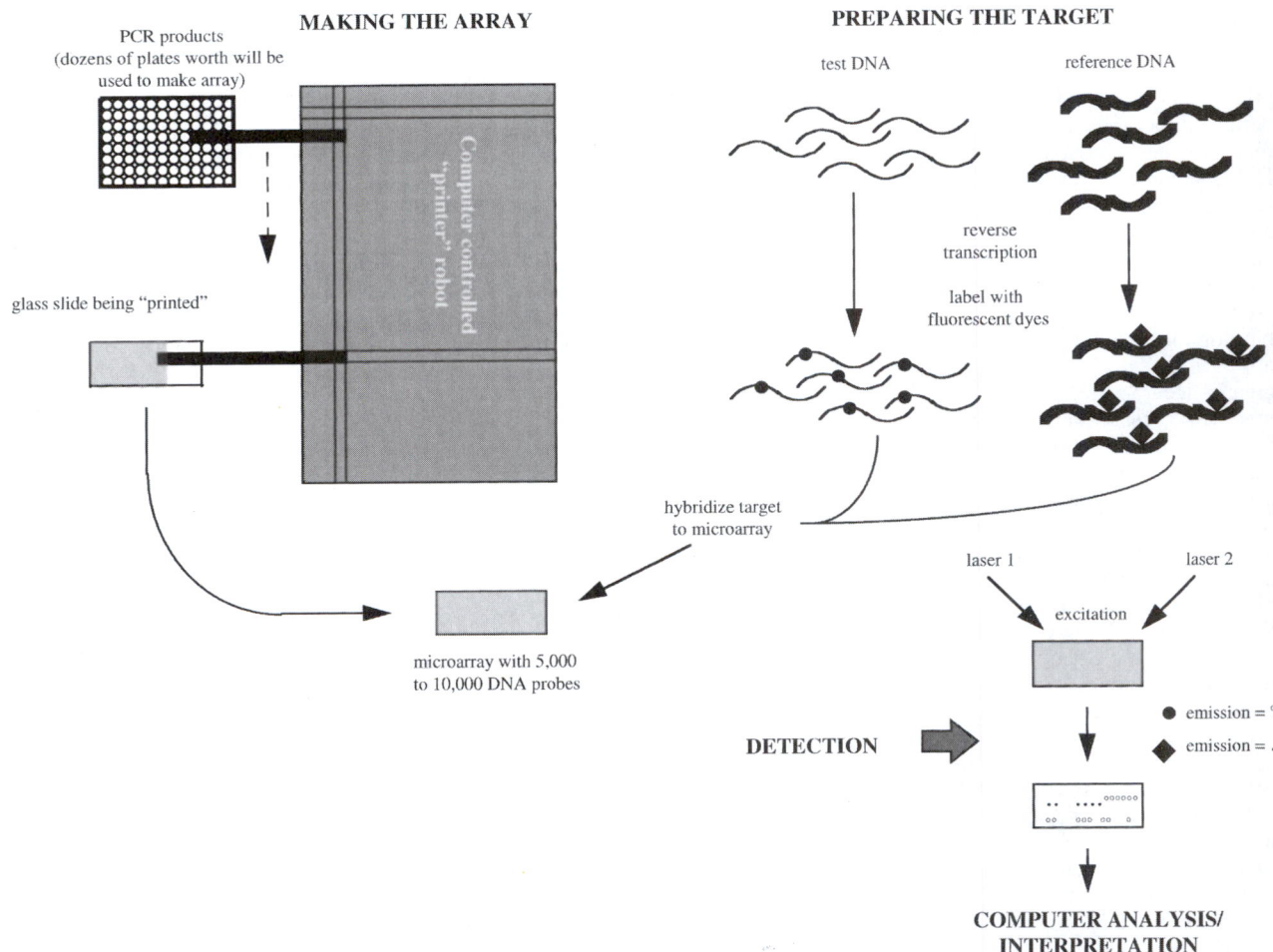

FIGURE 13 Expression array schema. Templates for genes of interest are obtained from DNA clones and amplified by PCR. Following purification, the aliquots (≈5 nl) are "printed" on glass microscope slides using a high-speed computer-controlled robot that draws the capture probes from a microtiter plate (left side of figure). Total RNA synthesized from test cDNA (stimulated T cells, for example) and control cDNA (unstimulated T cells) is labeled with different-colored fluorescent dyes during a single round of reverse transcription (right side of figure). The labeled test RNAs are pooled and allowed to hybridize under stringent conditions to the capture probes on the microarray. Laser excitation of the fluorescent dyes yields an emission of known spectra, which is measured using a scanning confocal laser microscope. Data from a single hybridization experiment are viewed as a normalized ratio comparing the intensity of the signal between the two dyes. Significant deviations from background are indicative of increased or decreased levels of gene expression relative to the control sample.

oligonucleotide microarrays. Genome-scale gene expression microarrays are the most commonly used today. An experiment with a single microarray can provide researchers information on thousands of genes simultaneously or thousands of bases of DNA sequence—a dramatic increase in throughput from methods previously available. Today, researchers are able to purchase arrays with probes to thousands of human or mouse genes as well as expression arrays covering the complete genomes of hundreds of different bacteria. The challenge is no longer in the development of microarrays, but in developing experimental designs to exploit the full power of microarrays. Microarray technology has the potential to be as revolutionary to biological research as PCR technology. The potential for microarrays seems virtually limitless (42, 113).

An ingenious microarray that is finding utility in the clinical laboratory today is manufactured by Affymetrix, Inc.,

using their proprietary, light-directed chemical synthesis process called photolithography (Fig. 14) (12, 30, 52, 53, 58, 106). This process combines solid-phase chemical synthesis with photolithographic synthesis techniques employed in the semiconductor industry. Short DNA probes are generated in situ on a glass substrate by combining standard DNA synthesis protocols with phosphoramidite reagents modified with photolabile 5′-protecting groups. Spatially addressable synthesis is accomplished through selective photodeprotection of substrate areas, utilizing a photolithographic mask set in a process similar in principle to that utilized in computer chip manufacturing. These deprotected areas are then activated for chemical coupling. Selective deprotection of multiple areas containing a distinct DNA sequence allows for the simultaneous stepwise synthesis of numerous different short probes. Any probe can be synthesized at any discrete, specified

A.

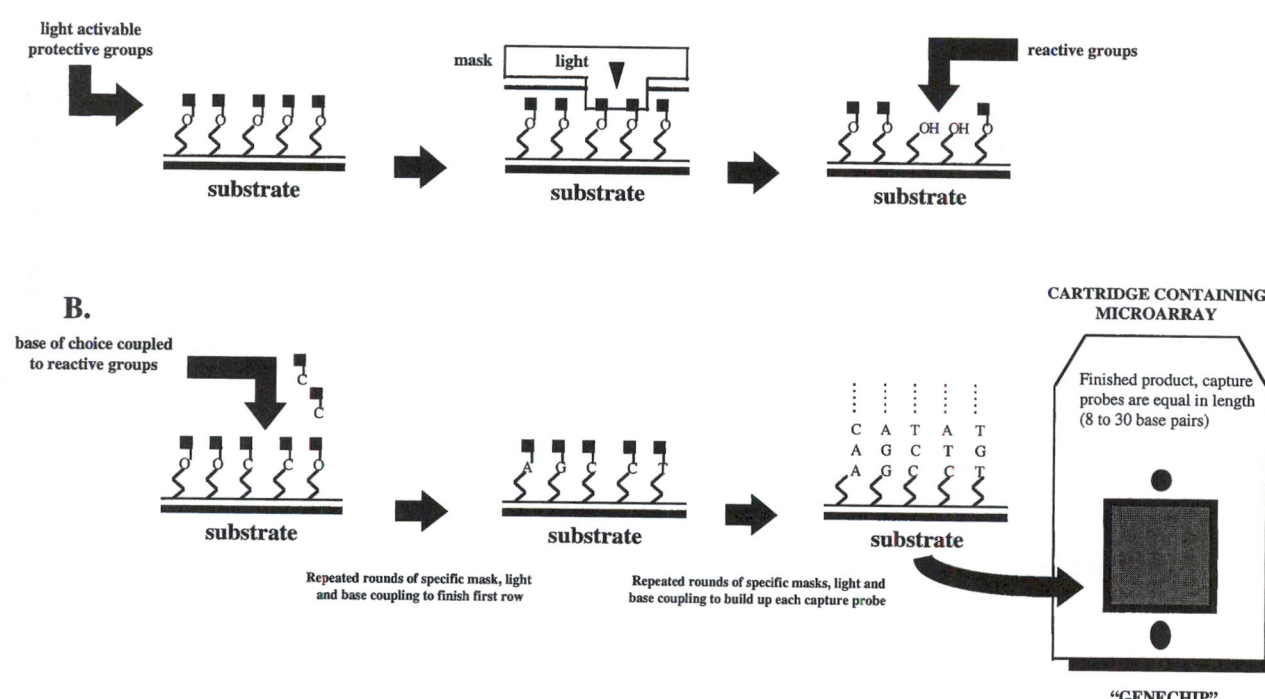

B.

FIGURE 14 Photolithography. (A) A 1.2- by 1.2-cm glass substrate with photoprotected linker groups. Areas of the glass substrate are selectively illuminated by light passing through a photolitho-graphic mask. Deprotected areas are activated. (B) With nucleoside incubation, chemical coupling occurs at activated positions. This process is repeated until the desired set of probes is obtained. This type of microarray is called a GeneChip. The microarray is placed into a cartridge to facilitate its use in a hybridization assay.

location in the array, and any set of probes composed of the four nucleotides can be synthesized in a maximum of $4N$ cycles where N is the length of the longest probe in the array. For example, the entire set of 10^5 20-nucleotide probes, or any desired subset, can be synthesized in only 80 coupling cycles. Multiple high-density microarrays are synthesized simultaneously on a large glass wafer. The wafers are then punched out into individual microarrays that are packaged in plastic cartridges. The cartridges protect the array from the environment and serve as flow cells for automated hybridization and laser scanning. Affymetrix has termed their high-density microarrays GeneChips. Each GeneChip contains from 10,000 to 400,000 different short DNA probes on a 1.2- by 1.2-cm glass wafer. The number of probes that can be put on a chip is limited only by the physical size of the array and the achievable photolithographic resolution (12). The number of probes needed on a chip depends upon the function of the chip. It is staggering to comprehend that the precise sequence and location of each probe on a GeneChip microarray are known. Following hybridization the chip is scanned using a laser scanner (Fig. 15). The fluorescent reporter groups emit light that is proportional to the stringency of hybridization at each probe. Probes with nothing bound emit no light, while probes bound with a perfectly matching target nucleic acid emit 5 to 35 times more light than probes bound with a target nucleic acid that is mismatched by only one base (53). Currently, an Affymetrix GeneChip (Roche AmpliChip CYP450) is FDA approved and available for human cytochrome P450 gene mutation analysis (15). The

Affymetrix instrument on which the cytochrome P450 GeneChip is run has also been FDA approved. Other GeneChips for clinical use are in development.

UTILIZATION OF MOLECULAR TESTS IN THE CLINICAL LABORATORY

Just a few years ago, DNA probes and nucleic acid amplification techniques were used only in a relatively few high-volume microbiology, histocompatibility, and human genetics laboratories. In these early years molecular tests typically occupied their own niche in the laboratory and did not replace any conventional procedures. Because of their cost and complexity they were only used where they could produce results that could not be duplicated by any other method. However, the application of molecular procedures has become far more common in recent years and will continue to expand rapidly in the coming years. This virtual explosion of molecular utilization is fueled by many factors. These include more readily available reagents, both FDA-approved reagents and ASRs, the shift to real-time amplification technologies, more choices of automated specimen processing instrumentation, competition leading to decreases in the costs of reagents, the advent of more choices of amplification technology, the virtual elimination of the need for radioactive nucleotides for reporter probes, the scaling up of molecular procedures allowing high-volume analysis, and the volumes of scientific literature demonstrating that these procedures are the "gold standard" for diagnosing many types of

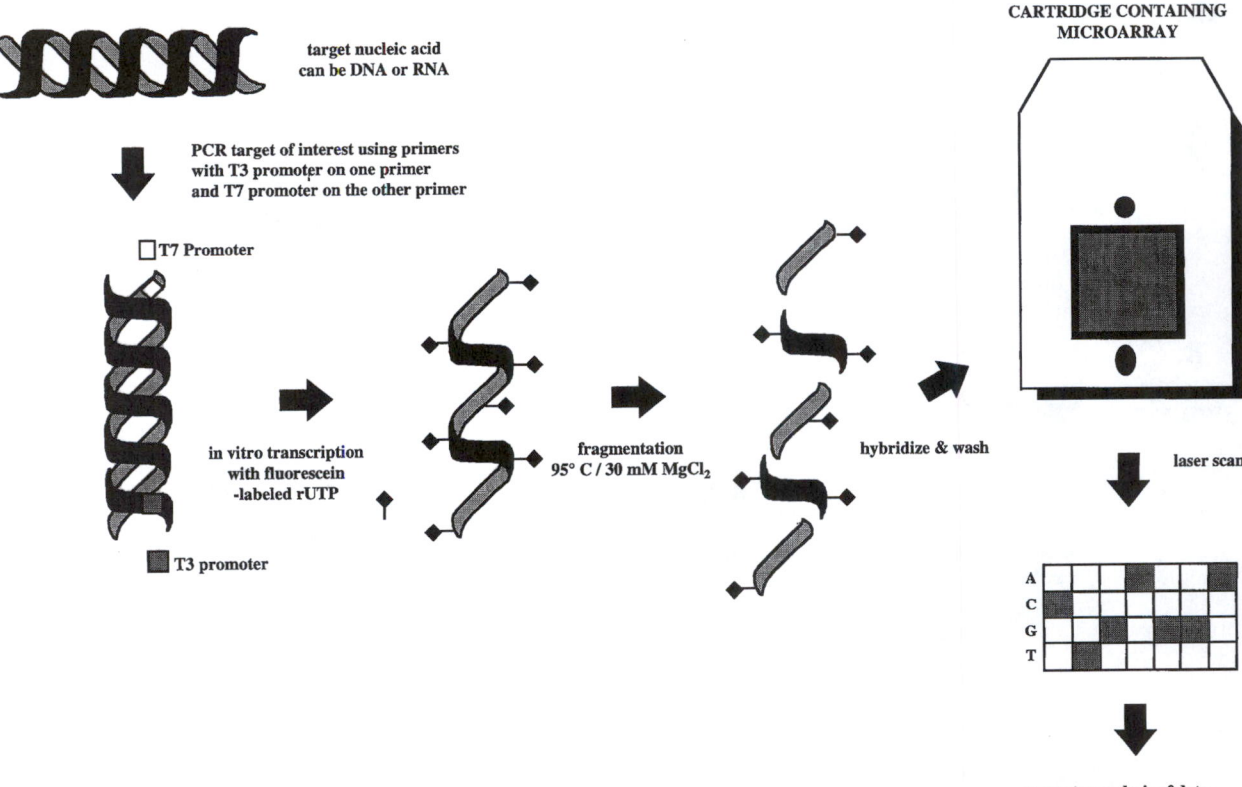

target nucleic acid
can be DNA or RNA

PCR target of interest using primers
with T3 promoter on one primer
and T7 promoter on the other primer

☐ T7 Promoter

in vitro transcription
with fluorescein
-labeled rUTP

☐ T3 promoter

fragmentation
95° C / 30 mM MgCl₂

hybridize & wash

CARTRIDGE CONTAINING
MICROARRAY

laser scan

A						
C						
G						
T						

computer analysis of data

FIGURE 15 Protocol for using the GeneChip. Target DNA or RNA is amplified by PCR using primers with a T3 RNA polymerase promoter sequence in one and a T7 RNA polymerase promoter sequence in the other. The PCR product is transcribed (DNA → RNA) using T7 or T3 RNA polymerase in the presence of fluorescein-labeled rUTP. The fluorescein-labeled RNA is fragmented by heating (95°C for 30 min) in the presence of 30 mM MgCl₂. The labeled and fragmented RNA is hybridized to the GeneChip and then analyzed by laser scanning and computer analysis of the resulting fluorescence.

infections and diseases. Today we see molecular tests replacing more conventional technology in the clinical laboratory, and this trend will only continue. *C. trachomatis* and *N. gonorrhoeae* testing is an excellent example of nucleic acid amplification-based testing replacing more conventional technology in the clinical laboratory. The competitive price, superior sensitivity, and relatively easy procedures have led to widespread use of amplification-based testing for *C. trachomatis* and *N. gonorrhoeae* (18, 97, 105).

At this writing, the number of nucleic acid amplification-based procedures that have been approved for use by the FDA exceeds 40 and continues to grow. The number of available ASRs is also growing very fast. A new landmark in molecular diagnostics was reached in early 2005 with FDA approval of the first microarray-based diagnostic test (Roche AmpliChip CYP450). Because of the widespread applicability of molecular technology to many areas of laboratory testing, it is certain that many more commercial molecular kits and reagents of all types will continue to be developed at a rapid pace. It is difficult to compare molecular technology with conventional immunology procedures such as enzyme immunoassay, immunoprecipitation, immunohistology, and flow cytometry with regard to such parameters as ease of use, cost, and appropriateness. This is because one rarely is faced with choosing a method for a particular test where all the available procedures produce the same result with equivalent sensitivity, specificity, accuracy, and precision. Certainly,

more costly molecular diagnostic procedures should not be used to replace procedures currently in place that have been proven to be cost-effective, rapid, sensitive, and reliable. It is important to remember that despite all their sensitivity and speed, nucleic acid amplification procedures will not replace conventional immunological procedures in all situations. This is because the results from nucleic acid amplification procedures mean different things than those from many immunology-based tests. For example, nucleic acid amplification procedures determine if DNA or RNA from a particular organism is present in the specimen. They reveal nothing about the viability of the organism (nucleic acid amplification techniques are capable of detecting DNA from dead organisms) or whether the organism is involved in an infectious process. Serology that clearly demonstrates a rise in titer of antibody to a specific organism strongly suggests involvement in infection.

When making the decision to utilize molecular diagnostic procedures, the institution must take into consideration all the benefits that the new technology may offer (90). The decision should not be based solely on a laboratory price comparison between the conventional assay and a molecular assay. Instead, the decision should take into account the impact new diagnostic technology will have on clinical practice and patient management and the cost savings associated with it. For example, the direct detection of *C. trachomatis* in poor-quality specimens using amplification technology would lead to more positive results than conventional procedures and better patient management (18). The costs saved by selecting the appropriate antibiotic therapy and preventing infectious complications associated with untreated *C. trachomatis* infections are part of the cost-benefit equation that must be considered when evaluating the use of molecular diagnostic assays. In some cases, in order for the benefits of molecular testing to outweigh their inherent costs, the procedures must be integrated into the assessment of the total patient management picture to realize the impact they have on clinical and financial outcomes. Major financial and patient outcome benefits are achievable because of the ability of molecular tests to replace or reduce the use of less sensitive and less specific tests and cause a decrease in the use of unnecessary diagnostic procedures and ineffective therapies.

FUTURE OF MOLECULAR TECHNOLOGY IN CLINICAL IMMUNOLOGY

Nucleic acid probes, amplification technology, sequencing technology, and microarrays represent some of the greatest advances in the clinical immunology laboratory since the introduction of the flow cytometer. As molecular diagnostics become more widely available, their use in the immunology laboratory will only increase. In the near term, the major application of molecular techniques will be for diagnosis and monitoring the progression of hematological diseases and in histocompatibility testing. In addition, clinical studies have demonstrated that molecular techniques provide prognostic information that directly influences treatment choices in acute leukemia cases. Looking further out into the future, the use of molecular tests will probably lead to further subdivision of the neoplasms that are presently being diagnosed and generate more clinically useful information. The advent of gene therapy will make the identification of specific molecular targets (e.g., the type of junctional species in the *bcr/abl* gene translocation) particularly important so the appropriate therapy can be selected. These applications of molecular technology will only proceed at greater speed in the coming years due to advanced automated analysis using microarrays.

For nucleic acid amplification technology, the most significant challenge that must be addressed with these techniques is false positivity due to contaminating nucleic acids (61, 72, 73, 74, 75, 78). It is absolutely essential that the issue of contamination control be addressed and the integrity of the amplification assay results be ensured. "An ounce of prevention is worth a pound of cure" is especially applicable here; once clinicians have lost faith in a laboratory procedure it can be very difficult to regain. The availability of well-established amplification product inactivation procedures and, especially, the use of closed real-time product detection systems have smoothed the way for more widespread use of this technology in the clinical laboratory (47, 75).

The ability to partially or fully automate molecular diagnostic procedures is another key factor in determining how large a role these procedures will play in the near future (72). Because of their complexity, the high cost of reagents, and the amount of labor involved, many molecular-biology-based tests were very expensive to perform. However, these limitations are rapidly declining because of the production of more automated instrumentation at lower costs by more manufacturers, the availability of more FDA-approved kits, and greatly simplified procedures through the use of real-time target amplification instrumentation. The use of target amplification technology coupled with microarrays will lead to entire assays being done on a small chip. The aim of these miniaturized systems is to create devices that will perform the same assays as are currently carried out in large molecular laboratories much more simply, faster, and at lower cost. Early versions of this all-in-one system can be found in the Gen-Probe Tigris DTS, the Cepheid GeneXpert, and the IQuum Liat System. For a limited number of assays these instruments do the specimen processing, nucleic acid amplification, and product detection (84). Instruments such as these greatly simplify molecular analysis, leaving the operator to just make sure that the appropriate specimen and reagents are being used for the test. In many ways the early years of molecular assays in the clinical laboratory are very similar to early years of immunoassays in the clinical laboratory. The first immunoassays were laborious, expensive, and used exclusively in the research laboratory. But as advances were made in the technology that simplified and automated the procedures, immunoassays became a commonplace in the clinical laboratory.

An especially important challenge that lies ahead for molecular technology in the clinical laboratory is in the area of education (73). Clinical laboratory science training programs at all levels will need to provide more in-depth instruction in molecular diagnostic procedures. Clinical immunologists must be willing to acquire new skills or they may relinquish control of diagnostic molecular biology to laboratory sections that are perceived by some to be more technology oriented, but with little vested interest in immunology. For example, some DNA probe-based tests for infectious diseases are currently being performed in chemistry laboratories. This is due in part to the perception by the manufacturers and laboratory administrators that microbiologists and immunologists are unfamiliar with performing tests based upon nucleic acid chemistry and so they believe that this testing should fall within the realm of the clinical chemist. Undoubtedly, the clinical chemists will be glad to fill this role. The American Association for Clinical Chemistry, through its American Board of Clinical Chemistry, is now offering board certification in molecular diagnostics. Only through education and the ability to meet new challenges will clinical immunologists be able to control the use of molecular techniques and practice of molecular diagnostics in the clinical immunology laboratory.

REFERENCES

1. **Albert, T. J., J. Norton, M. Ott, T. Richmond, K. Nuwaysir, E. F. Nuwaysir, K.-P. Stengele, and R. D. Green.** 2003. Light-directed $5' \rightarrow 3'$ synthesis of complex oligonucleotide microarrays. *Nucleic Acids Res.* **31:**e35.
2. **Arnheim, N., T. White, and W. E. Rainey.** 1990. Application of PCR: organismal and population biology. *BioScience* **40:**174–182.
3. **Arnold, L. J., Jr., P. W. Hammond, W. A. Wiese, and N. C. Nelson.** 1989. Assay formats involving acridinium-ester-labeled DNA probes. *Clin. Chem.* **35:**1588–1594.
4. **Aspinall, S., A. D. Steele, I. Peenze, and M. J. Mphahlele.** 1995. Detection and quantitation of hepatitis B virus DNA: comparison of two commercial hybridization assays with polymerase chain reaction. *J. Viral Hepat.* **2:**107–111.
5. **Bieche, I., P. Onody, I. Laurendeau, M. Olivi, D. Vidaud, R. Lidereau, and M. Vidaud.** 1999. Real-time reverse transcription-PCR assay for future management of ERBB2-based clinical applications. *Clin. Chem.* **45:**1148–1156.
6. **Bonnet, G., S. Tyagi, A. Libchaber, and F. R. Kramer.** 1999. Thermodynamic basis of the enhanced specificity of structured DNA probes. *Proc. Natl. Acad. Sci. USA* **96:**6171–6176.

7. **Britten, R. J., and E. H. Davidson.** 1985. Hybridization strategy, p. 3–14. *In* B. D. Hames and S. J. Higgins (ed.), *Nucleic Acid Hybridization: a Practical Approach.* IRL Press, Oxford, United Kingdom.

8. **Brown, T.** 1993. Southern blotting, p. 2.9.1–2.9.15. *In* F. M. Ausubel, R. Brent, R. E. Kingston, D. D. Moore, J. G. Seidman, and K. Struhl (ed.), *Current Protocols in Molecular Biology,* vol. 1. John Wiley & Sons, New York, N.Y.

9. **Brown, T.** 1993. Dot and slot blotting of DNA, p. 2.9.15–2.9.20. *In* F. M. Ausubel, R. Brent, R. E. Kingston, D. D. Moore, J. G. Seidman, and K. Struhl (ed.), *Current Protocols in Molecular Biology,* vol. 1. John Wiley & Sons, New York, N. Y.

10. **Brown, T.** 1993. Analysis of RNA by Northern and slot blot hybridization, p. 4.9.1–4.9.14. *In* F. M. Ausubel, R. Brent, R. E. Kingston, D. D. Moore, J. G. Seidman, and K. Struhl (ed.), *Current Protocols in Molecular Biology,* vol. 1. John Wiley & Sons, New York, N.Y.

11. **Castle, P. E., A. T. Lorincz, D. R. Scott, M. E. Sherman, A. G. Glass, B. B. Rush, S. Wacholder, R. D. Burk, M. M. Manos, J. E. Schussler, P. Macomber, and M. Schiffman.** 2003. Comparison between prototype hybrid capture 3 and hybrid capture 2 human papillomavirus DNA assays for detection of high-grade cervical intraepithelial neoplasia and cancer. *J. Clin. Microbiol.* **41:**4022–4030.

12. **Chee, M., R. Yang, E. Hubbell, A. Berno, X. C. Huang, D. Stern, J. Winkler, D. J. Lockhart, M. S. Morris, and S. P. Fodor.** 1996. Assessing genetic information with high-density DNA arrays. *Science* **274:**610–614.

13. **Cheung, V. G., M. Morley, F. Aguilar, A. Massimi, R. Kucherlapati, and G. Childs.** 1999. Making and reading microarrays. *Nat. Genet.* **21**(1 Suppl.)**:**15–19.

14. **Chevrier, D., S. R. Rasmussen, and J.-L. Guesdon.** 1993. PCR product by quantification by non-radioactive hybridization procedures using an oligonucleotide covalently bound to microwells. *Mol. Cell. Probes* **7:**187–197.

15. **Chou, W.-H., F.-X. Yan, D. K. Robbins-Weilert, T. B. Ryder, W. W. Liu, C. Perbost, M. Fairchild, J. De Leon, W. H. Koch, and P. J. Wedlund.** 2003. Comparison of two CYP2D6 genotyping methods and assessment of genotype-phenotype relationships. *Clin. Chem.* **49:**542–551.

16. **Collins, M. L., B. Irvine, D. Tyner, E. Fine, C. Zayati, C. Chang, T. Horn, D. Anle, J. Detmer, L. Shen, J. Kolberg, S. Bushnell, M. S. Urdea, and D. D Ho.** 1997. A branched DNA signal amplification assay for quantitation of nucleic acid targets below 100 molecules/ml. *Nucleic Acids Res.* **25:**2979–2984.

17. **Compton, J.** 1990. Nucleic acid sequence-based amplification. *Nature* (London) **350:**91–92.

18. **Dicker, L. W., D. J. Mosure, W. C. Levine, C. M. Black, and S. M. Berman.** 2000. Impact of switching laboratory tests on reported trends in Chlamydia trachomatis infections. *Am. J. Epidemiol.* **151:**430–435.

19. **Didenki, V. V.** 2001. DNA probes using fluorescence resonance energy transfer (FRET): designs and applications. *BioTechniques* **31:**1106–1121.

20. **Dovichi, N. J.** 1997. DNA sequencing by capillary electrophoresis. *Electrophoresis* **18:**2393–2399.

21. **Duggan, D. J., M. Bittner, Y. Chen, P. Meltzer, and J. M. Trent.** 1999. Expression profiling using cDNA microarrays. *Nat. Genet.* **21**(1 Suppl.)**:**10–14.

22. **Dyson, N. J.** 1991. Immobilization of nucleic acids and hybridization analysis, p. 111–156. *In* T. A. Brown (ed.), *Essential Molecular Biology: a Practical Approach,* vol. 2. IRL Press, Oxford, United Kingdom.

23. **Eisenstein, B. I.** 1990. The polymerase chain reaction: a new method of using molecular genetics for medical diagnosis. *N. Engl. J. Med.* **322:**178–183.

24. **Fahrlander, P. D., and A. Klausner.** 1988. Amplifying DNA probe signals: a "Christmas Tree" approach. *Bio/Technology* **6:**1165–1168.

25. **Fairfax, M. R.** 1996. Evaluation of the Gen-Probe amplified *Mycobacterium tuberculosis* direct test. *Am. J. Clin. Pathol.* **106:**594–599.

26. **Farthing, A., P. Masterson, W. P. Mason, and K. H. Vousden.** 1994. Human papillomavirus detection by hybrid capture and its possible clinical use. *J. Clin. Pathol.* **47:**649–652.

27. **Gelmini, S., C. Orlando, R. Sestini, G. Vona, P. Pinzani, L. Ruocco, and M. Pazzagli.** 1997. Quantitative polymerase chain reaction homogenous assay based on the use of fluorogenic probes for the measurement of c-erbB-2 oncogene amplification. *Clin. Chem.* **43:**752–758.

28. **Griffin, H. G., and A. M. Griffin.** 1993. DNA sequencing. Recent innovations and future trends. *Appl. Biochem. Biotechnol.* **38:**147–159.

29. **Guatelli, J. C., K. M. Whitfield, D. Y. Kwoh, K. J. Barringer, D. D. Richman, and T. R. Gingeras.** 1990. Isothermal, in vitro amplification of nucleic acids by multienzyme reaction modeled after retroviral replication. *Proc. Natl. Acad. Sci. USA* **87:**1874–1878.

30. **Hacia, J. G., L. C. Brody, M. S. Chee, S. P. Fodor, and F. S. Collins.** 1996. Detection of heterozygous mutations in BRCA1 using high density oligonucleotide arrays and two-colour fluorescence analysis. *Nat. Genet.* **14:**441–447.

31. **Hankin, R. C.** 1992. In situ hybridization: principles and applications. *Lab. Med.* **23:**764–770.

32. **Haydock, P. V., and S. A. Kochik.** 1993. 3SR detection of *Chlamydia trachomatis,* p. 242–246. *In* D. H. Persing, T. F. Smith, F. C. Tenover, and T. J. White (ed.), *Diagnostic Molecular Microbiology: Principles and Applications.* American Society for Microbiology, Washington, D.C.

33. **Heid, C. A., J. Stevens, K. J. Livak, and P. M. Williams.** 1996. Real time quantitative PCR. *Genome Res.* **6:**986–994.

34. **Holland, P. M., R. D. Abramson, R. Watson, and D. H. Gelfand.** 1991. Detection of specific polymerase chain reaction product by utilizing the 5′ to 3′ exonuclease activity of *Thermus aquaticus* DNA polymerase. *Proc. Natl. Acad. Sci. USA* **88:**7276–7280.

35. **Hubbard, R. A.** 2003. Human papillomavirus testing methods. *Arch. Pathol. Lab. Med.* **127:**940–945.

36. **Hughes, T. R., M. Mao, A. R. Jones, J. Burchard, M. J. Marton, K. W. Shannon, S. M. Lefkowitz, M. Ziman, J. M. Schelter, M. R. Meyer, S. Kobayashi, C. Davis, H. Dai, Y. D. He, S. B. Stephaniants, G. Cavet, W. L. Walker, A. West, E. Coffey, D. D. Shoemaker, R. Stoughton, A. P. Blanchard, S. H. Friend, and P. S. Linsley.** 2001. Expression profiling using microarrays fabricated by an ink-jet oligonucleotide synthesizer. *Nat. Biotechnol.* **19:**342–347.

37. **Hunsaker, W. R., H. Badri, M. Lombardo, and M. L. Collins.** 1989. Nucleic acid hybridization assays employing dA-tailed capture probes. II. Advanced multiple capture methods. *Anal. Biochem.* **181:**360–370.

38. **Iftner, R., and L. L. Villa.** 2003. Human papillomavirus technologies. *J. Natl. Cancer Inst. Monogr.* **31:**80–88.

39. **Jonas, V., M. J. Alden, J. I. Curry, K. Kamisango, C. A. Knott, R. Lankford, J. M. Wolfe, and D. F. Moore.** 1993. Detection and identification of *Mycobacterium tuberculosis* directly from sputum sediments by amplification of rRNA. *J. Clin. Microbiol.* **31:**2410–2416.

40. **Kant, J. A.** 1995. Direct DNA sequencing in the clinical laboratory. *Clin. Chem.* **41:**1407–1409.

41. **Keiichi, K., C. Kamogawa, M. Sumi, S. Goto, A. Hirao, F. Gonzales, K. Yasuda, and S. Iino.** 1999. Quantitative detection of hepatitis B virus by transcription-mediated amplification and hybridization protection assay. *J. Clin. Microbiol.* **37:**310–314.

42. **Khan, J., M. L. Bittner, Y. Chen, P. S. Meltzer, and J. M. Trent.** 1999. DNA microarray technology: the anticipated impact on the study of human disease. *Biochim. Biophys. Acta* **1423:**M17–M28.

43. **Kheterpal, I., and R. A. Mathies.** 1999. Capillary array electrophoresis DNA sequencing. *Anal. Chem.* **71:**31A–37A.

44. **Konnick, E. Q., M. Erali, E. R. Ashwood, and D. R. Hillyard.** 2005. Evaluation of the COBAS Amplicor HBV Monitor assay and comparison with the Ultrasensitive HBV Hybrid Capture 2 assay for quantitation of hepatitis B virus DNA. *J. Clin. Microbiol.* **43:**596–603.

45. **Kwiatkowski, R. W., V. Lyamichev, M. de Arruda, and B. Neri.** 1999. Clinical, genetic, and pharmacogenetic applications of the Invader assay. *Mol. Diagn.* **4:**353–364.

46. **Kwoh, D. Y., G. R. Davis, K. M. Whitfield, H. L. Chappelle, L. J. DiMichele, and T. R. Gingeras.** 1989. Transcription-based amplification system and detection of amplified human immunodeficiency virus type 1 with a bead-based sandwich hybridization format. *Proc. Natl. Acad. Sci. USA* **86:**1173–1177.

47. **Kwok, S.** 1990. Procedures to minimize PCR-product carryover, p. 142–145. *In* M. A. Innis, D. H. Gelfand, J. J. Sninsky, and T. J. White (ed.), *PCR Protocols: a Guide to Methods and Applications.* Academic Press, Inc., San Diego, Calif.

48. **La Rocco, M. T., A. Wanger, H. Ocera, and E. Macias.** 1994. Evaluation of a commercial rRNA amplification assay for direct detection of Mycobacterium tuberculosis in processed sputum. *Eur. J. Clin. Microbiol. Dis.* **13:**726–731.

49. **Ledford, M., K. D. Friedman, M. J. Hessner, C. Moehlenkamp, T. M. Williams, and R. S. Larson.** 2000. A multi-site study for detection of the factor V (Leiden) mutation from genomic DNA using a homogeneous invader microplate fluorescence resonance energy transfer (FRET) assay. *J. Mol. Diagn.* **2:**97–104.

50. **Lee, L. G., C. R. Connel, and W. Bloch.** 1993. Allelic discrimination by nick translation PCR with fluorogenic probes. *Nucleic Acids Res.* **21:**3761–3766.

51. **Levi, K., and K. J. Towner.** 2003. Detection of methicillin-resistant *Staphylococcus aureus* (MRSA) in blood with the EVIGENE MRSA detection kit. *J. Clin. Microbiol.* **41:**3890–3892.

52. **Lipshutz, R. J., S. P. Fodor, T. R. Gingeras, and D. J. Lockhart.** 1999. High density synthetic oligonucleotide arrays. *Nat. Genet.* **21**(1 Suppl.)**:**20–24.

53. **Lipshutz, R. J., D. Morris, M. Chee, E. Hubbel, M. J. Kozal, N. Shah, N. Shen, R. Yang, and S. P. Fodor.** 1995. Using oligonucleotide probe arrays to access genetic diversity. *BioTechniques* **19:**442–447.

54. **Little, M. C., J. Andrews, R. Moore, S. Bustos, L. Jones, C. Embres, G. Durmowicz, J. Harris, D. Berger, K. Yanson, C. Rostkowski, D. Yursis, J. Price, T. Fort, A. Walters, M. Collis, O. Llorin, J. Wood, F. Failing, C. O'Keefe, B. Scrivens, B. Pope, T. Hansen, K. Marino, K. Williams, and M. Boenisch.** 1999. Strand displacement amplification and homogenous real-time detection incorporated in a second-generation DNA probe system, BDProbe TecET. *Clin. Chem.* **45:**777–784.

55. **Livak, K., S. J. A. Flood, J. Marmaro, W. Giusti, and K. Deetz.** 1995. Oligonucleotides with fluorescent dyes at opposite ends provide a quencher probe system useful for detecting PCR product and nucleic acid hybridization. *PCR Methods Applic.* **4:**357–362.

56. **Loeffelholz, M. J., C. A. Lewinski, S. R. Silver, A. P. Purohit, S. A. Herman, D. A. Buonagurio, and E. A. Dragon.** 1992. Detection of *Chlamydia trachomatis* in endocervical specimens by polymerase chain reaction. *J. Clin. Microbiol.* **30:**2847–2851.

57. **Marras, S. A. E., F. R. Kramer, and S. Tyagi.** 2002. Efficiencies of fluorescence resonance energy transfer and

contact-mediated quenching in oligonucleotide probes. *Nucleic Acids Res.* **30:**e122.

58. **Matsuzaki, H., S. Dong, H. Loi, X. Di, G. Liu, E. Hubbell, J. Law, T. Berntsen, M. Chadha, H. Hui, G. Yang, G. C. Kennedy, T. A. Webster, S. Cawley, P. S. Walsh, K. W. Jones, S. P. Fodor, and R. Mei.** 2004. Genotyping over 100,000 SNPs on a pair of oligonucleotide arrays. *Nat. Methods* **1:**109–111.

59. **Matthews, J. A., and J. Kricka.** 1988. Analytical strategies for the use of DNA probes. *Anal. Biochem.* **169:**1–25.

60. **Mayer, S. P., J. Giamelli, C. Sandoval, A. S. Roach, M. Fevzi Ozkaynak, O. Tugal, G. Rovera, and S. Jayabose.** 1999. Quantitation of leukemia clone-specific antigen gene rearrangements by a single-step PCR and fluorescence-based detection method. *Leukemia* **13:**1843–1852.

61. **McCreedy, B. J., and T. H. Callaway.** 1993. Laboratory design and work flow, p. 149–159. *In* D. H. Persing, T. F. Smith, F. C. Tenover, and T. J. White (ed.), *Diagnostic Molecular Microbiology: Principles and Applications.* American Society for Microbiology, Washington, D.C.

62. **Messing, J.** 1993. M13 cloning vehicles: their contribution to DNA sequencing, p. 9–22. *In* H. G. Griffin and A. M. Griffin (ed.), *DNA Sequencing Protocols.* Humana, Totowa, N.J.

63. **Mullikin, J. C., and A. A. McMurray.** 1999. Sequencing the genome, fast. *Science* **283:**1867–1868.

64. **Mullis, K., F. Faloona, S. Scharf, R. Saiki, G. Horn, and H. Erlich.** 1986. Specific enzymatic amplification of DNA in vitro: the polymerase chain reaction. *Cold Spring Harbor Symp. Quant. Biol.* **51:**263–273.

65. **Mullis, K. B.** 1990. The unusual origin of the polymerase chain reaction. *Sci. Am.* **262:**56–65.

66. **Mullis, K. B., and F. A. Faloona.** 1987. Specific synthesis of DNA *in vitro* via a polymerase-catalyzed reaction. *Methods Enzymol.* **155:**335–350.

67. **Nelson, N. C., and D. L. Kacian.** 1990. Chemiluminescent DNA probes: a comparison of the acridinium ester and dioxetane detection systems and their use in clinical diagnostic assays. *Clin. Chim. Acta* **194:**73–90.

68. **Nuwaysir, E. F., W. Huang, T. J. Albert, J. Singh, K. Nuwaysir, A. Pitas, R. Richmond, T. Gorski, J. P. Berg, J. Ballin, M. McCormick, J. Norton, T. Pollock, T. Sumwalt, L. Butcher, D. Porter, M. Molla, C. Hall, F. Blattner, M. R. Sussman, R. L. Wallace, F. Cerrina, and R. D. Green.** 2002. Gene expression analysis using oligonucleotide arrays produced by maskless photolithography. *Genome Res.* **12:**1749–1755.

69. **Orlando, C., P. Pinzani, and M. Pazzagli.** 1998. Developments in quantitative PCR. *Clin. Chem. Lab. Med.* **36:**255–269.

70. **Palva, A., and M. Ranki.** 1985. Microbial diagnosis by nucleic acid sandwich hybridization. *Clin. Lab. Med.* **5:**475–490.

71. **Pease, A. C., D. Solas, E. J. Sullivan, M. T. Cronin, C. P. Holmes, and S. P. Fodor.** 1994. Light-generated oligonucleotide arrays for rapid DNA sequence analysis. *Proc. Natl. Acad. Sci. USA* **91:**5022–5026.

72. **Persing, D. H.** 1991. Polymerase chain reaction: trenches to benches. *J. Clin. Microbiol.* **29:**1281–1285.

73. **Persing, D. H.** 1993. Diagnostic molecular microbiology: current challenges and future direction. *Diagn. Microbiol. Infect. Dis.* **16:**159–163.

74. **Persing, D. H.** 1993. In vitro nucleic acid amplification techniques, p. 51–87. *In* D. H. Persing, T. F. Smith, F. C. Tenover, and T. J. White (ed.), *Diagnostic Molecular Microbiology: Principles and Applications.* American Society for Microbiology, Washington, D.C.

75. **Persing, D. H., and G. D. Cimino.** 1993. Amplification product inactivation methods, p. 105–121. *In* D. H. Persing, T. F. Smith, F. C. Tenover, and T. J. White (ed.), *Diagnostic*

Molecular Microbiology: Principles and Applications. American Society for Microbiology, Washington, D.C.

76. **Phear, G., and J. Harwood.** 1994. Direct sequencing of PCR products. *Methods Mol. Biol.* **31:**247–256.

77. **Podzorski, R. P.** 2004. Gel electrophoresis, Southern hybridization, and restriction fragment length polymorphism analysis, p. 273–280. *In* D. H. Persing, F. C. Tenover, J. Versalovic, Y.-W. Tang, E. R. Unger, D. A. Relman, and T. J. White (ed.), *Molecular Microbiology: Diagnostic Principles and Practice.* American Society for Microbiology, Washington, D.C.

78. **Podzorski, R. P., and D. H. Persing.** 1993. PCR: the next decade. *Clin. Microbiol. Newsl.* **15:**137–143.

79. **Podzorski, R. P., and D. H. Persing.** 1995. Molecular detection and identification of microorganisms, p. 130–157. *In* P. R. Murray, E. J. Baron, M. A. Pfaller, F. C. Tenover, and R. H. Yolken (ed.), *Manual of Clinical Microbiology,* 6th ed. American Society for Microbiology, Washington, D.C.

80. **Podzorski, R. P., and D. H. Persing.** 1995. Molecular methods for the detection and identification of viral pathogens. *J. Histotechnol.* **18:**225–232.

81. **Pollard-Knight, D., C. A. Read, M. J. Downes, L. A. Howard, M. R. Leadbetter, S. A. Pheby, E. McNaughton, A. Syms, and M. A. W. Brady.** 1990. Nonradioactive nucleic acid detection by enhanced chemiluminescence using probes directly labeled with horseradish peroxidase. *Anal. Biochem.* **185:**84–89.

82. **Poulsen, A. B., R. Skov, and L. V. Pallesen.** 2003. Detection of methicillin resistance in coagulase-negative staphylococci and in staphylococci directly from simulated blood cultures using the EVIGENE MRSA detection kit. *J. Antimicrob. Chemother.* **51:**419–421.

83. **Quesda, M. A.** 1997. Replacement polymers in DNA sequencing by capillary electrophoresis. *Curr. Opin. Biotechnol.* **8:**82–93.

84. **Raja, S., J. Ching, L. Xi, S. J. Hughes, R. Chang, W. Wong, W. McMillian, W. E. Gooding, K. S. McCarty, Jr., M. Chestney, J. D. Luketich, and T. E. Godfrey.** 2005. Technology for automated, rapid, and quantitative PCR or reverse transcription-PCR clinical testing. *Clin. Chem.* **51:**882–890.

85. **Ranki, M., A. Palva, M. Virtanen, M. Laaksonen, and H. Soderlund.** 1983. Sandwich hybridization as a convenient method for detection of nucleic acids in crude samples. *Gene* **21:**77–85.

86. **Rao, V. B.** 1994. Direct sequencing of polymerase chain reaction-amplified DNA. *Anal. Biochem.* **216:**1–14.

87. **Rapley, R. (ed.).** 1996. *PCR Sequencing Protocols.* Humana, Totowa, N.J.

88. **Reddy, K. J., and M. Gilman.** 1993. Preparation of bacterial RNA, p. 4.4.1–4.4.7. *In* F. M. Ausubel, R. Brent, R. E. Kingston, D. D. Moore, J. G. Seidman, and K. Struhl (ed.), *Current Protocols in Molecular Biology,* vol. 1. John Wiley & Sons, New York, N.Y.

89. **Romano, J. W., B. van Gemen, and T. Kievits.** 1996. A novel, isothermal detection technology for qualitative and quantitative HIV-1 measurements. *Clin. Lab. Med.* **16:**89–103.

90. **Ross, J. S.** 1999. The impact of molecular diagnostic tests on patient outcomes. *Clin. Lab. Med.* **19:**815–831.

91. **Ryan, D., B. Nuccie, and D. Arvan.** 1999. Non-PCR-dependent detection of the factor V Leiden mutation from genomic DNA using a homogenous invader microtiter plate assay. *Mol. Diagn.* **4:**135–144.

92. **Ryncarz, A. J., J. Goddard, A. Wald, M. L. Huang, B. Roizman, and L. Corey.** 1999. Development of a high-throughput quantitative assay for detecting herpes simplex virus DNA in clinical samples. *J. Clin. Microbiol.* **37:**1941–1947.

93. **Saiki, R. K.** 1989. The design and optimization of the PCR, p. 7–22. *In* H. A. Erlich (ed.), *PCR Technology: Principles and Applications for DNA Amplification.* Stockton Press, New York, N.Y.

94. **Saiki, R. K., P. S. Walsh, C. H. Levenson, and H. A. Erlich.** 1989. Genetic analysis of amplified DNA with immobilized sequence-specific oligonucleotide probes. *Proc. Natl. Acad. Sci. USA* **86:**6230–6234.

95. **Sanchez-Pescador, R., M. S. Stempien, and M. S. Urdea.** 1988. Rapid chemiluminescent nucleic acid assays for detection of TEM-1 β-lactamase-mediated penicillin resistance in *Neisseria gonorrhoeae* and other bacteria. *J. Clin. Microbiol.* **26:**1934–1938.

96. **Sanger, F., S. Nicklen, and A. R. Coulson.** 1977. DNA sequencing with chain-terminating inhibitors. *Proc. Natl. Acad. Sci. USA* **74:**5463–5467.

97. **Schachter, J.** 1997. DFA, EIA, PCR, LCR, and other technologies: what tests should be used for diagnosis of chlamydia infections. *Immunol. Investig.* **26:**157–161.

98. **Sia, I. G., J. A. Wilson, M. J. Espy, C. V. Paya, and T. F. Smith.** 2000. Evaluation of the COBAS AMPLICOR CMV MONITOR test for detection of viral DNA in specimens taken from patients after liver transplantation. *J. Clin. Microbiol.* **38:**600–606.

99. **Southern, E., K. Mir, and M. Shchepinov.** 1999. Molecular interactions on microarrays. *Nat. Genet.* **21**(1 Suppl.):5–9.

100. **Southern, E. M.** 1975. Detection of specific sequences among DNA fragments separated by gel electrophoresis. *J. Mol. Biol.* **98:**503–517.

101. **Strickler, J. D., and C. D. Copenhaver.** 1990. In situ hybridization in hematology. *Am. J. Clin. Pathol.* **93**(suppl.):544–548.

102. **Sun, X. W., A. Ferenczy, D. Johnson, J. P. Koulos, O. Lungu, R. M. Richart, and T. C. Wright, Jr.** 1995. Evaluation of the hybrid capture human papillomavirus deoxyribonucleic acid detection test. *Am. J. Obstet. Gynecol.* **173:**1432–1437.

103. **Szollosi, J., S. Damjanovich, and L. Matyus.** 1998. Application of fluorescence resonance energy transfer in the clinical laboratory: routine and research. *Cytometry* **15:**159–179.

104. **Tenover, F. C., and E. R. Unger.** 1993. Nucleic acid probes for detection and identification of infectious agents, p. 3–25. *In* D. H. Persing, T. F. Smith, F. C. Tenover, and T. J. White (ed.), *Diagnostic Molecular Microbiology: Principles and Applications.* American Society for Microbiology, Washington, D.C.

105. **Thejls, H., J. Gnarpe, H. Gnarpe, P. G. Larsson, J. J. Platz-Christensen, L. Ostergaard, and A. Victor.** 1994. Expanded gold standard in the diagnosis of *Chlamydia trachomatis* in a low prevalence population: diagnostic efficacy of tissue culture, direct immunofluorescence, enzyme immunoassay, PCR and serology. *Genitourin. Med.* **70:**300–303.

106. **Trojan, L., A. Schaff, A. Steidler, M. Haak, G. Thalmann, T. Knoll, N. Gretz, P. Alken, and M. S. Michel.** 2005. Identification of metastasis-associated genes in prostate cancer by genetic profiling of human prostate cancer cell lines. *Anticancer Res.* **25:**183–191.

107. **Tyagi, S., D. P. Bratu, and F. R. Kramer.** 1998. Multicolor molecular beacons for allele discrimination. *Nat. Biotechnol.* **16:**49–53.

108. **Tyagi, S., and F. R. Kramer.** 1996. Molecular beacons: probes that fluoresce upon hybridization. *Nat. Biotechnol.* **14:**303–308.

109. **Urdea, M. S., T. Fultz, T. J. Anderson, M. Running, J. A. Hamren, S. Ahle, and C. A. Chang.** 1991. Branched amplification multimers for the sensitive, direct detection of human hepatitis viruses. *Nucleic Acids Symp. Ser.* **24:**197–200.

110. **Vogelstein, B., and K. W. Kinzler.** 1999. Digital PCR. *Proc. Natl. Acad. Sci. USA* **96:**9236–9241.

111. **Walker, G. T., M. L. Fraiser, J. L. Schram, M. C. Little, J. G. Nadeau, and D. P. Malinowski.** 1992. Strand displacement amplification—an isothermal, *in vitro* DNA amplification technique. *Nucleic Acids Res.* **20:**1691–1696.

112. **Walker, G. T., M. C. Little, J. G. Nadeau, and D. D. Shank.** 1992. Isothermal *in vitro* amplification of DNA by a restriction enzyme/DNA polymerase system. *Proc. Natl. Acad. Sci. USA* **89:**392–396.

113. **Watson, A., A. Mazumder, M. Stewart, and S. Balasubramanian.** 1998. Technology for microarray analysis of gene expression. *Curr. Opin. Biotechnol.* **9:**609–614.

114. **Wetmur, J. G.** 1991. DNA probes: applications of the principles of nucleic acid hybridization. *Crit. Rev. Biochem. Mol. Biol.* **26:**227–259.

115. **White, T. J.** 1993. Amplification product detection methods, p. 138–148. *In* D. H. Persing, T. F. Smith, F. C. Tenover, and T. J. White (ed.), *Diagnostic Molecular Microbiology: Principles and Applications.* American Society for Microbiology, Washington, D.C.

116. **White, T. J., R. Madej, and D. H. Persing.** 1992. The polymerase chain reaction for the diagnosis of infectious diseases. *Adv. Clin. Chem.* **29:**161–196.

117. **Wiedbrauk, D. L.** 1992. Molecular methods for virus detection. *Lab. Med.* **23:**737–742.

118. **Wolcott, M. J.** 1992. Advances in nucleic acid-based detection methods. *Clin. Microbiol. Rev.* **5:**370–386.

IMMUNOGLOBULIN METHODS

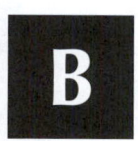

VOLUME EDITOR
ROBERT G. HAMILTON
SECTION EDITOR
DAVID F. KEREN

Introduction

DAVID F. KEREN

6

Section B examines the topics of immunoglobulin production by gene rearrangements, the measurement of immunoglobulins, identification of monoclonal protein products by serum protein electrophoresis and immunofixation, detection of oligoclonal bands in cerebrospinal fluid, and characterization of cryoglobulin, cryofibrinogen, and pyroglobulins.

The chapter by Kipps (chapter 7) examines the genes that code for immunoglobulins. Immunoglobulin heavy-chain constant-region exons, heavy-chain variable-region genes, and light-chain gene complexes are each described. Immunoglobulin gene rearrangements are then discussed in detail, with a focus on their expression in ontogeny and the mechanisms of heavy-chain class switching that generate antibody diversity. Detection methods for immunoglobulin gene rearrangements involving PCR methods and an anchored-reverse transcriptase PCR–enzyme-linked immunosorbent assay are overviewed in the final section of this chapter.

Warren (chapter 8) overviews how the immunoglobulin structure is related to its function and the utility of serum viscosity evaluations. Practical methods for the measurement of immunoglobulins in the clinical laboratory are then described, with a focus on nephelometry, immunoturbidimetry, and the more classic radial immunodiffusion and Laurell rocket techniques. A new method is presented that uses affinity-purified antibodies in a nephelometric format to measure serum free light chains. This method has been useful in detecting light-chain myeloma, AL (light-chain-associated) amyloidosis, and nonsecretory myeloma. The clinical uses of these techniques to identify patients with congenital or acquired humoral immunodeficiency and polyclonal and monoclonal increases in gamma globulin are reviewed. Finally, the ability of high-molecular-weight immunoglobulins to increase viscosity is discussed, along with currently available viscometers.

In chapter 9, Keren and Humphrey review the technical details and clinical applications of serum and urine protein electrophoresis. First, the relevance of protein structure to migration of immunoglobulins and other proteins in an electrophoretic field is discussed. This is followed by an overview of techniques used for gel electrophoresis and capillary zone electrophoresis on serum and urine, complete with details for specimen processing, quality control, and quality assurance. Descriptions of the major proteins identified are presented along with several case examples—including possible causes for false-positive and false-negative results. Finally, detection and measurement of monoclonal proteins in the serum and urine are reviewed in detail.

Katzmann and Kyle (chapter 10) present a thorough review of characterization of monoclonal gammopathies in serum and urine by immunofixation and immunosubtraction. They describe the use of isoelectric focusing with immunoblotting as a useful technique to evaluate cerebrospinal fluid for the presence of oligoclonal bands. They provide details of the methodological background of these techniques and a practical approach to interpret monoclonal gammopathies that takes into account the type and amount of the monoclonal protein present as well as the background of nonmonoclonal immunoglobulins. Artifacts that can cause false-positive results are described. Newer methods such as immunosubtraction and Penta gel (Sebia, Norcross, Ga.) immunofixation are presented as possible alternatives to standard immunofixation. The Mayo Clinic database is used to provide definitive information on the occurrence of the monoclonal gammopathies.

Gorevic and Galanakis (chapter 11) present the state of the art for detecting and measuring cryoglobulins, cryofibrinogenemia, and pyroglobulins. This timely chapter includes details on the importance of hepatitis C virus in both type II and III cryoglobulins. Many practical suggestions are made about the importance of proper handling in the identification and characterization of these temperature-critical samples. The discussion of cryofibrinogens emphasizes their heterogeneity and reviews the clinical indications for their detection. Lastly, pyroglobulins that lack the clinical manifestations of cryoglobulins but can confound laboratory findings in heat-based assays such as those used to inactivate complement are overviewed.

Immunoglobulin Genes

THOMAS J. KIPPS

7

IMMUNOGLOBULIN MOLECULES

Introduction

Immunoglobulins are a heterogeneous group of glycoproteins produced by B lymphocytes and plasma cells. A single person can synthesize 10 million to 100 million different immunoglobulin molecules, each having distinct antigen-binding specificities. This great diversity in the so-called humoral immune system allows us to generate antibodies specific for a variety of substances, including synthetic molecules not naturally present in our environment. Despite the diversity in the specificities of antibody molecules, the binding of an antibody to an antigen initiates a limited series of biologically important effector functions, such as complement activation and/or adherence of the immune complex to receptors on leukocytes (32). Resolution of immunoglobulin structure has revealed how these molecules can have such great diversity in antigen-binding activities while maintaining conserved effector functions, such as complement activation.

Basic Immunoglobulin Structure

The basic unit of the immunoglobulin molecule is composed of two identical heavy chains and two identical light chains. These four polypeptides are held together by disulfide bonds and noncovalent interactions (15, 89). The amino-terminal domains (110 to 120 amino acids) of the heavy and light chains are designated the variable regions, because their primary structures vary markedly among different immunoglobulin molecules (33). The carboxy-terminal domains, however, are referred to as constant regions, because their primary structures are the same among immunoglobulins of the same class or subclass. The amino acids in the light- and heavy-chain variable regions interact to form an antigen-binding site (15, 25). Each four-chain immunoglobulin basic unit has two identical binding sites. The constant-region domains of the heavy and light chains provide stability for the immunoglobulin molecule. The heavy-chain constant regions also mediate the specific effector functions of the different immunoglobulin classes (Table 1) (31).

There are two classes of immunoglobulin light chains, the κ and λ light chains, that differ in the amino acid sequences of the constant-region domains. The ratio of κ to λ chains in adult plasma is 2:1. The main purpose of the light-chain constant region may be to allow for proper assembly and release of an intact immunoglobulin molecule. Soon after synthesis, the antibody light-chain constant region associates with the nascent immunoglobulin heavy chain, releasing the latter from the immunoglobulin-binding protein, or BiP. BiP is a heat shock protein that, in the absence of antibody light chain, binds the first constant-region domain of the newly synthesized heavy chain, thereby retaining the heavy-chain polypeptide in the cell's endoplasmic reticulum (45).

Heavy-Chain Isotypes

Five major classes of immunoglobulin molecules—immunoglobulin G (IgG), IgA, IgM, IgD, and IgE—correspond to the five classes of heavy-chain isotypes (γ, α, μ, δ, and ε). The immunoglobulin molecule of each isotype can contain either a κ or a λ light chain but not both. The physical properties of each of these classes of immunoglobulin molecules are summarized in Table 1.

IgG

IgG is the most abundant of immunoglobulins found in adult plasma, accounting for approximately 80% of the total immunoglobulin. IgG is the predominant antibody produced during a secondary immune response. IgG molecules can penetrate extravascular spaces and cross the placental barrier to provide immunity to the fetus. These molecules have a four-chain 150-kDa immunoglobulin structure with a hinge region that can be attacked by proteolytic enzymes such as papain and pepsin, allowing for separation of the antigen-binding fragment(s), Fab or F(ab)$_2$, from the crystalizable or constant fragment (Fc) of the antibody molecule. Receptors for the Fc (FcR) allow effector cells to recognize target cells coated with a specific antibody (68).

There are four subclasses of IgG: IgG1, IgG2, IgG3, and IgG4. Each subclass has a particular heavy-chain constant region and has different effector functions (31). The most abundant class is IgG1, which accounts for approximately 65% of the total IgG in the plasma. Of the IgG subclasses, IgG1 binds best to FcRI (CD64) and FcRII (CD32), with affinities (K_d) of 10^{-8} M and 5×10^{-7} M, respectively. IgG1 and IgG3 bind equally well to FcRIII (CD16), with a K_d of 2×10^{-6} M. FcRIII is the FcR expressed by natural killer cells (NK cells, or K cells) that mediate antibody-dependent cell-mediated cytotoxicity. Proteins of the IgG4 or IgG2 subclass bind poorly to FcRI (CD64) or FcRII (CD32) and do not bind to FcRIII (CD16) at all. The average half-life of circulating IgG molecules is about 21 days.

TABLE 1 Physical properties of human immunoglobulins

Heavy-chain class (isotype)	Heavy-chain subclasses	No. of heavy-chain domains	Secretory form(s)	Molecular mass (Da)	Antigen-binding valency	Concn (mg/ml) in serum	% of total immunoglobulins
IgG (γ)	γ1, γ2, γ3, γ4	4	Monomer	150,000	2	8–16	80
IgA (α)	α1, α2	4	Monomer, dimer	160,000 (monomer)	2 (monomer)	1.4–4.0	13
				400,000 (secretory protein)	4 (secretory protein)		
IgM (μ)		5	Pentamer	900,000	10	0.5–2.0	6
IgD (δ)		4	Monomer	180,000	2	0–0.4	1
IgE (ε)		5	Monomer	190,000	2	17–450	0.002

IgA

The IgA molecules constitute 13% of the total plasma immunoglobulins. There are two major classes of IgA molecules, designated IgA1 and IgA2, with IgA1 being the more abundant (85% of total IgA in plasma). The half-life of IgA molecules is about 6 days.

IgA antibodies are synthesized during a secondary immune response and contribute to mucosal immunity (9, 43, 54). IgA antibodies are the primary antibodies in saliva, tears, and colostrum and in the fluids of the gastrointestinal, respiratory, and urinary tracts. These secreted immunoglobulins consist of an IgA dimer bound to the joining (J)-chain polypeptide and a secretory protein with a molecular mass of 70 to 80 kDa. The J chain is required for proper hepatic transport of IgA (59). The secretory component is actually part of an FcR for dimeric IgA that is synthesized not by B cells but rather by epithelial cells of organs such as the intestine. This protein facilitates the transport of the IgA protein across the epithelial cell and may protect the secreted IgA molecule from proteolytic digestion by enzymes in the intestinal lumen. Since these molecules do not cross the placenta barrier and do not easily bind to cell surfaces, their main role may be to prevent foreign substances from binding to mucosal surfaces and entering the blood.

IgM

The IgM immunoglobulins comprise about 6% of the immunoglobulins in adult plasma. These molecules have very high molecular weights (thus, they are called macroglobulins), and they are formed by the linking of five identical immunoglobulin units by disulfide bonds and a J chain. IgM is the predominant class found during a primary immune response. The IgM molecules do not cross the placenta and do not enter into extravascular spaces; however, they fix complement more efficiently than the monomeric IgG molecules. The half-life of IgM molecules in plasma is approximately 6 days. In addition, monomeric IgM is the main immunoglobulin expressed on B cells.

IgD

The IgD molecules constitute only 1% of the plasma immunoglobulins and they are expressed on B cells with IgM. These immunoglobulins do not cross the placenta and do not easily penetrate extravascular spaces. However, IgD molecules are found in relatively high concentrations in umbilical cord blood. IgD molecules are thought to function as B-cell membrane receptors for antigens and may help in the recruitment of B cells for specific antigen-driven responses (70).

IgE

IgE has been called a reaginic antibody to denote its association with immediate hypersensitivity. IgE antibodies constitute a very small percentage of the total plasma immunoglobulins (0.002%). Although four human IgE isoforms can be produced by alternative splicing of the epsilon primary transcript (47), the isoforms appear to have similar functions. Plasma IgE levels may increase (5 to 20 times the baseline) in parasitic infections and children with atopic diseases. The Fc portion of the IgE molecule can bind to high-affinity receptors on the surfaces of basophils and mast cells. The cross-linking of IgE antibody by an allergen can induce the release of vasoactive amines; proteases; lipid-derived inflammatory mediators; and cytokines such as tumor necrosis factor alpha, gamma interferon, and interleukins 1, 3, 4, 5, and 6 (see section M, this volume). Studies indicate that the microenvironment of mucosal tissues in allergic disease favors class switching to IgE (21).

IMMUNOGLOBULIN GENE COMPLEXES

Immunoglobulin Heavy-Chain Gene Complex

Immunoglobulin Heavy-Chain Constant-Region Exons
The heavy-chain gene complex is located at band q32 on the long arm of chromosome 14 (39). This complex is composed of approximately 50 functional heavy-chain variable-region genes (V_H genes), more than 120 nonfunctional V_H pseudogenes, 25 functional diversity (D) segments, 6 functional heavy-chain J-region (J_H) minigenes, and exons encoding the constant regions (C genes) for each of the immunoglobulin heavy-chain isotypes (37, 51, 72). The order (5′→3′) of the genes encoding each of the immunoglobulin heavy-chain isotypes is C_μ, C_δ, $C_\gamma 3$, $C_\gamma 1$, $C_\epsilon 2$ (a nonfunctional pseudogene), $C_\alpha 1$, C_γ (a nonfunctional pseudogene), $C_\gamma 2$, $C_\gamma 4$, $C_\epsilon 1$, and $C_\alpha 2$ (Fig. 1). The exons encoding the heavy-chain constant regions and each associated intronic switch region are as depicted in Fig. 1. These exons are labeled and pseudogenes are also indicated in the figure.

Immunoglobulin V_H Genes
The V_H gene segments map within a region of approximately 1,100 kb in size that is telomeric to the J_H and constant-region exons (Fig. 1). Each V_H gene can be assigned to one of seven V_H gene subgroups. Each subgroup comprises V_H genes with more than 80% nucleic acid sequence homology. Genes of the $V_H 1$, $V_H 5$, and $V_H 7$ subgroups have similarities

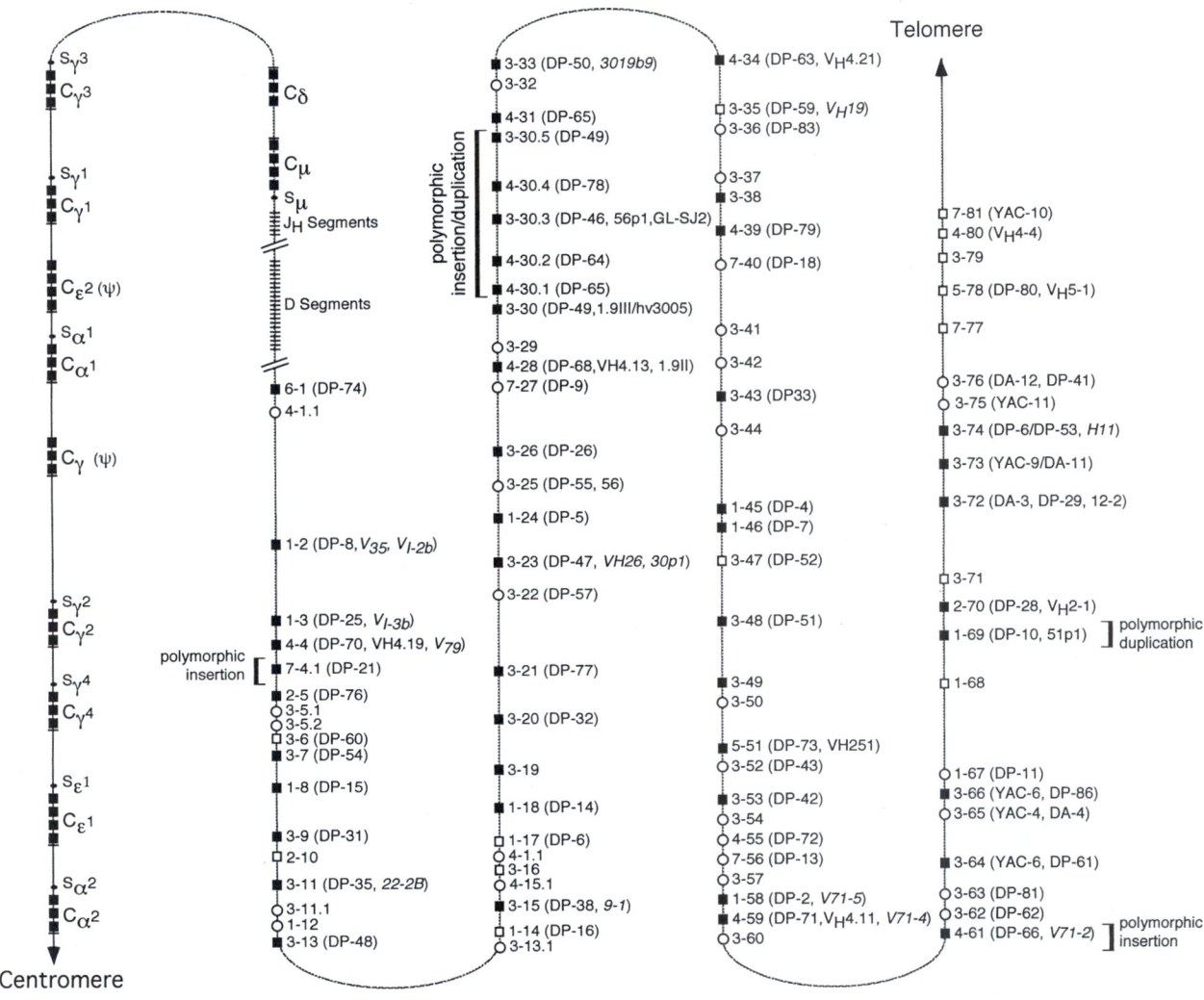

FIGURE 1 Immunoglobulin heavy-chain gene complex. The heavy-chain exons encoding the constant regions are represented by black boxes, and the associated intronic switch (S) regions are indicated by lines. A ψ next to the heavy-chain isotype designation indicates that the gene is a pseudogene. J_H segments and D segments are indicated by lines. Each V_H gene locus is labeled on the right of each symbol. Identified polymorphic insertions and/or duplications are indicated with brackets. Black squares represent V_H gene loci that are known to be functional. White circles represent V_H pseudogenes. At the ends of the line connecting the symbols are arrows that indicate the direction to the centromere or the telomere. The white boxes denote loci that apparently are functional V_H genes but that rarely, if at all, are expressed into protein. The arrows indicate the direction of transcription of the gene segments.

in primary structure, suggesting a common ancestral origin in evolution, whereas the V_H2, V_H4, and V_H6 families share similarities that allow them to be classified into a different clan (7, 38). The V_H3 genes constitute their own discrete clan.

The immunoglobulin V_H genes of each subgroup, except the immunoglobulin V_H6 gene, are interspersed throughout the immunoglobulin heavy-chain locus. By convention, the loci of each of the various V_H genes are assigned a number corresponding to the V_H gene subgroup followed by a hyphen and then the rank order distance from the heavy-chain D segments on chromosome 14 (Fig. 1). The immunoglobulin V_H6 subgroup has only one functional V_H

gene. Since this is the first V_H gene telomeric to the D segments, this gene is called V_H6-1 (Fig. 1). There are an additional 50 loci that have been identified as functional V_H genes (83) (Fig. 1). The largest subgroup is V_H3, with 22 to 24 functional genes. The next largest are the V_H1 and V_H4 subgroups, each with 8 to 11 functional genes. The V_H2, V_H5, and V_H7 subgroups each have one to three functional genes. Of the 51 functional V_H genes, there are four V_H loci that may have noncoding-region defects that preclude their translation into protein and/or have V_H genes that are expressed at very low frequency relative to other V_H genes (Fig. 1). Also, interspersed among the functional V_H genes are several nonfunctional pseudogenes (Fig. 1).

The extent of identified genetic polymorphism varies among the different immunoglobulin V_H gene loci. Some immunoglobulin V_H gene loci, e.g., V_H6-1, V_H5-51, and V_H4-34, are highly conserved (65, 73). Indeed, the single-copy immunoglobulin V_H6 gene, V_H6-1, is conserved even among higher primates (52). Other loci have been used to identify genetic polymorphic variations. These allelic variations are of two different types. The first type of genetic polymorphism is the classic form in which there are two or more alleles at a single locus, each differing from one another in one or more nucleotide bases. For example, 1.9III and hv3005 differ from each other at several nucleotide bases and have only 98.8% overall homology (98.3% coding-sequence homology), but are alleles of locus V_H3-30. The second type of allelic variation results from duplications, insertions, and/or deletions of whole segments of immunoglobulin V_H genes within the immunoglobulin heavy-chain gene complex. Duplication of an immunoglobulin V_H gene(s) results in some haplotypes' having identical immunoglobulin V_H genes belonging to distinct loci, each possibly differing from their respective alleles by one or more nucleotide base substitutions. For example, there may be an insertion in and about locus V_H3-30, in part consisting of another copy of this gene. As a result, alleles of V_H3-30, e.g., 1.9III and hv3005, also may be alleles of locus V_H3-30.5 in haplotypes containing this insertion. On the other hand, some haplotypes are missing gene loci altogether. For example, allele frequencies for hv3005 (V_H3-30b) and 1.9III (V_H3-30) in the Caucasian population are 0.19 and 0.72, respectively (56). An additional haplotype(s) with an allele frequency of 0.08 lacks either 1.9III or hv3005 and thus apparently is a blank haplotype for this locus. Genetic disequilibrium also is noted for certain groups of V_H genes in a given haplotype. For example, 56p1 (V_H3-30.3) is an insertion or deletion element that has been observed only with haplotypes carrying one or two copies of 1.9III. The V Base website (http://vbase.mrc-cpe.cam.ac.uk/), the international ImMunoGeneTics information system (http://imgt.cines.fr:8104/), and the international ImMunoGeneTics project of the European Bioinformatics Institute (http://www.ebi.ac.uk/imgt/) provide Internet databases and listings of V_H gene maps and alleles.

The relative expression level of each functional V_H gene is not uniform. Certain V_H genes, e.g., V_H3-23, V_H4-34, and V_H1-69, are overexpressed relative to other V_H genes (56, 74). Each of seven V_H3 genes (V_H3-23, V_H3-30, V_H3-30b, V_H3-30.3, V_H3-33, V_H3-15, and V_H3-11) accounts for 8 to 20% of the V_H3 gene rearrangements, whereas the remaining functional V_H3 genes contribute to less than 3% of the rearrangements. Some of the V_H genes that encode a disproportionate share of the immunoglobulin expressed by normal adults also are polymorphic. For example, the V_H genes V_H4-31 and, to a lesser extent, V_H30.4 are deleted in some persons but, when present, encode a significant proportion of the heavy-chain repertoire (56).

Immunoglobulin Light-Chain Gene Complexes

κ Light-Chain Complex

The κ light-chain gene complex is contained within band p12 on the short arm of chromosome 2 (Fig. 2). This gene complex consists of approximately 40 functional κ light-chain variable-region genes ($V_κ$ genes), more than 30 nonfunctional $V_κ$ pseudogenes, 5 $J_κ$ segments, 1 constant-region exon, and 1 κ-deleting element (Kde) (Fig. 2) (34, 82).

The $V_κ$ genes in the κ light-chain gene complex are found in two regions centromeric to the $J_κ$ and $C_κ$ exons,

each region spanning approximately 500 kb. Approximately 800 kb separates the two regions (Fig. 2). The region proximal to $J_κ$ and $C_κ$, designated the p region, contains 40 $V_κ$ gene segments (B3 → B1, L13 → L1, A30 → A15, and O18 → O11), and the distal region, designated the d region, contains 36 gene segments (O1 → O10, A1 → A14, and L14 → L25). Thirty-two of the 76 $V_κ$ genes are pseudogenes (Fig. 2). The d region apparently arose through duplication of a large portion of the p region (47). Consequently, there are 33 pairs of $V_κ$ genes that have 95 to 100% nucleic acid sequence homology, accounting for 66 of the 76 $V_κ$ genes in the κ light-chain complex (92). The $V_κ$ genes can be grouped further into four clusters, A, B, L, and O, three of which (A, L, and O) are duplicated and found in both the $J_κ$-proximal p region and the $J_κ$-distal d region. The B cluster, containing $V_κ$ genes B1, B2 (EV15), and B3 (DPK26), is found only in the $J_κ$-proximal p region.

The $V_κ$ genes in the κ light-chain gene complex can be categorized into three main subgroups (1 to 3) and several smaller subgroups (4, 5, 6, and 7) based on nucleotide sequence homology (28, 44). The largest subgroup is $V_κ$1, with 21 functional genes (Fig. 2). The next largest subgroups are $V_κ$2, with 11 functional genes, and $V_κ$3, with 7. There are three functional genes in the $V_κ$6 subgroup, and one each in the $V_κ$4 and $V_κ$5 subgroups. The $V_κ$7 subgroup has only one nonfunctional pseudogene.

As in the V_H locus, there are several prominent alleles identified in the $V_κ$ gene locus. The $V_κ$ genes coding for segments O12, L4, and L16 (humkv328/humkv328h2) each have several alleles, some with open reading frames and others with stop codons (10, 41). Moreover, the $V_κ$A2 gene also is polymorphic, with some alleles having defective promoters that preclude their translation into protein. Inheritance of such defective $V_κ$A2 alleles has been associated with an increased risk for serious infection with type b *Haemophilus influenzae*, suggesting that the polymorphic variations in the germ line repertoire can influence the susceptibility to infectious disease (16).

As with the immunoglobulin V_H genes, the expression of $V_κ$ genes is not uniform. Eleven of the nearly 30 known functional $V_κ$ genes encode most of the κ light-chain variable regions expressed in the normal adult repertoire (10). Moreover, of the 44 genes that are potentially functional, only 28 have been found commonly to encode κ light-chain variable regions (Fig. 2) (10, 41). This raises the possibility that some of the potentially functional $V_κ$ genes have defects that preclude their ability to undergo light-chain gene rearrangement or to be translated into protein. Alternatively, these genes may have an extremely low expression frequency.

λ Light-Chain Gene Complex

The λ light-chain gene complex is located at band q11.12 on the long arm of chromosome 22. These λ constant-region genes are telomeric to the λ variable-region genes. Originally, the isotypes they encoded were designated Mcg$^+$, Ke$^-$ Oz$^-$, Ke$^-$ Oz$^+$, and Ke$^+$ Oz$^-$, depending on their reactivity with Mcg, Kern, and Oz antisera that were raised against λ Bence Jones proteins of patients with multiple myeloma (26). These isotypes are now designated $C_λ$1, $C_λ$2, $C_λ$3, and $C_λ$7, respectively. In total, there are 7 to 10 $C_λ$ genes telomeric to the $V_λ$ genes, depending on the haplotype (20, 87). Each $C_λ$ gene is associated with its own $J_λ$ segment. The most prevalent haplotype contains four functional $C_λ$ genes ($C_λ$1, $C_λ$2, $C_λ$3, and $C_λ$7, encoding the Mcg, Ke$^-$ Oz$^-$, Ke$^-$ Oz$^+$, and Ke$^+$ Oz$^-$ isotypes, respectively) and three pseudogenes ($C_λ$4, $C_λ$5, and $C_λ$6) (Fig. 2) (11, 87).

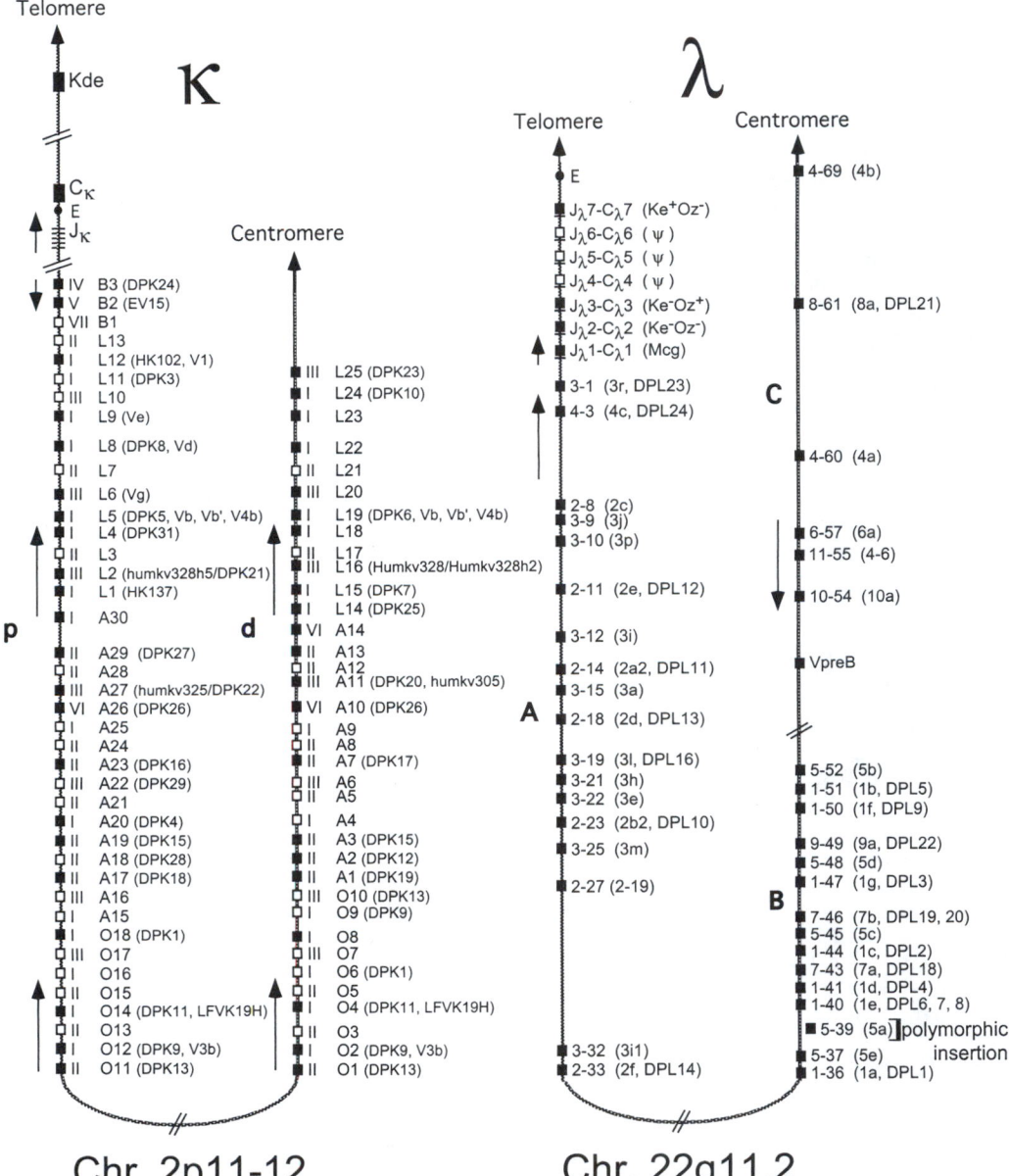

FIGURE 2 Immunoglobulin light-chain gene complexes. The left panel depicts the κ light-chain gene complex on chromosome (Chr) 2p11-12. The black rectangles in this figure represent the Kde or the C_κ constant-region exon as indicated to the right of each rectangle. The J_κ segments are indicated by lines labeled "J_κ." The κ light-chain enhancer (labeled E) is located between the J_κ segments and the C_κ exon. The V_κ genes that can encode functional κ light-chain variable regions are represented by black boxes, and the V_κ pseudogenes are indicated by white boxes. Immediately adjacent to and to the right of each box is a Roman numeral that denotes the subgroup to which the respective V_κ gene belongs, followed by its designated name. The arrows indicate the direction of transcription of the gene segments. A *p* is used to label the proximal arm of the V_κ gene complex, and *d* is used to label the distal arm. The right panel depicts the λ light-chain gene complex on chromosome 22q11.2. The black boxes represent functional J_λ-C_λ exons, whereas white boxes represent J_λ-C_λ pseudogenes. Each of the J_λ-C_λ exon pairs is indicated to the right of each symbol. Each V_λ gene is represented by a black box. To the right of each box is a tentative designation indicating the subgroup (first number) followed by a number indicating the rank order of the particular V_λ in the λ light-chain gene complex. The V_λ genes are organized into three clusters, designated A, B, and C, that are indicated to the left of each cluster. The gene encoding VpreB is located near the C cluster. The direction to the telomere or the centromere is as indicated at the top. The arrows indicate the direction of transcription of the gene segments.

There are about 41 functional V_λ genes and more than 30 nonfunctional V_λ pseudogenes that are arranged into 10 subgroups (35, 64, 91). Each subgroup comprises V_λ genes with more than 75% nucleotide sequence homology (6, 64) (Fig. 2). Like that of the κ light-chain locus, the sequence organization suggests that large DNA duplications contributed to the generation of the germ line repertoire of V_λ gene segments (35). The V_λ genes are clustered into three large DNA segments located within 860 kb of the J_λ and C_λ genes (18, 35, 91). The cluster most proximal to the J_λ-C_λ exons, designated cluster A, comprises 18 functional V_λ genes, belonging mostly to the $V_\lambda 2$ and $V_\lambda 3$ gene subgroups, designated 3-1 (3r, DPL23) through 2-33 (2f, DPL14) in Fig. 2. The next cluster, cluster B, contains 15 functional V_λ genes of the $V_\lambda 1$, $V_\lambda 5$, $V_\lambda 7$, and $V_\lambda 9$ gene subgroups, designated 1-36 (1a, DPL1) through 5-52 (5b). The third cluster, cluster C, contains six functional V_λ genes of the $V_\lambda 4$, $V_\lambda 6$, $V_\lambda 8$, $V_\lambda 10$, and $V_\lambda 11$ gene subgroups, designated 10-54 (10a) through 4-69 (4b) (Fig. 2). As in the other immunoglobulin gene complexes, there are multiple nonfunctional pseudogenes interspersed between these functional V_λ genes in all three clusters. Also, located on the telomeric end of these clusters is the exon encoding VpreB.

As noted for the relative expression of individual V_H and V_κ genes, the expression of individual V_λ genes appears to be nonrandom. V_λ genes of the $V_\lambda 1$ and $V_\lambda 3$ subgroups are used most frequently. These subgroups encode approximately 44 and 40%, respectively, of the λ light-chain immunoglobulins in normal adult sera (1). This proportionate representation apparently is not observed in B-cell plasmacytic disorders. Although the $V_\lambda 2$ subgroup was identified for 3% of the λ light-chain immunoglobulins in normal adult sera, it accounted for 40% of the λ Bence Jones proteins and 60% of the λ macroglobulins from patients with Waldenström macroglobulinemia in one survey (1).

IMMUNOGLOBULIN GENE REARRANGEMENT

Immunoglobulin Gene Rearrangement and Expression in Ontogeny

As B cells develop, they generally first rearrange their immunoglobulin heavy-chain genes (84). One or more D segments rearranges to become juxtaposed with a single J_H element. This generates a D-J_H complex that then may rearrange with any one of some 50 functional V_H genes.

Subsequently, gene rearrangements occur within the light-chain gene complexes. One of the 40 functional V_κ genes rearranges with any one of five J_κ segments. Should these gene rearrangements fail to generate a functional V_κ-J_κ exon, the Kde generally rearranges to a site in or immediately downstream of the V_κ-J_κ exon, thus deleting the κ light-chain constant-region exon (22). Many of the V_κ genes in the p region are in the orientation opposite that of the J_κ segments, thus requiring that the V_κ exons in this region undergo inversion during immunoglobulin gene rearrangement (Fig. 2). Subsequent to κ light-chain gene rearrangement, one of the functional V_λ exons can rearrange with any one of the four functional J_κ-C_λ exons to generate a gene that can encode a λ light chain (Fig. 3) (87).

Precursor B cells that have only D and J_H elements rearranged are referred to as progenitor B cells, or pro-B cells. The term pre-B cells is reserved for precursor B cells that have completed immunoglobulin heavy-chain gene rearrangement and have a functional V_H-D-J_H complex.

Both pro-B cells and pre-B cells generally have immunoglobulin light-chain loci in the germ line configuration.

Nevertheless, pre-B cells express small amounts of immunoglobulin μ chains in association with "surrogate" λ light chains. One of these surrogate λ light chains is called λ_5. λ_5 has similarity with known C_λ light-chain domains (53). Another surrogate λ light chain is called VpreB, because it resembles a variable-region domain but bears an extra N-terminal protein sequence. Both proteins are encoded by genes located on chromosome 22. The λ_5 gene is situated within a λ-like locus that is telomeric to the true λ light-chain locus. The VpreB gene is located within the cluster of immunoglobulin V_λ genes defined by breakpoints of chromosomal translocations found in a few leukemias and lymphomas (53). VpreB and λ_5 pair with the μ heavy chains to form a primitive immunoglobulin receptor that may be expressed on the surface membrane of the developing pre-B cell together with CD79a and CD79b (80). Monoclonal antibodies that recognize λ_5 or VpreB specifically bind to pre-B cells and can react with B-lineage acute lymphocytic leukemias (86).

Expression of the surrogate light chains plays a critical role in normal B-cell development. This is underscored by studies on transgenic mice that lack functional λ_5 genes (40). In these mice, B-cell development in the marrow is blocked at the pre-B-cell stage, thereby markedly reducing the numbers of functional mature B lymphocytes in the blood and lymphoid tissues (8). Similarly, humans that have inactivating mutations in the λ_5 genes on both alleles of chromosome 22 have agammaglobulinemia and markedly reduced numbers of B cells (57).

Under normal conditions, a B lymphocyte or plasma cell synthesizes only one species of light chain and heavy chain, even though the cell has two different sets of each of the immunoglobulin gene complexes that initially undergo seemingly independent immunoglobulin gene rearrangements. This is achieved by limiting each B-cell clone to the expression of only one immunoglobulin heavy-chain allele and one light-chain allele. This phenomenon is called allelic exclusion. Although some B-cell leukemias may lack allelic exclusion and express both immunoglobulin alleles (66), allelic exclusion generally is observed with most B-cell tumors.

Genetic Basis for Immunoglobulin Gene Rearrangement

Each germ line V gene, D element, and J segment is flanked by recognition sequences that are required for site-specific recombination. These sequences typically consist of a conserved palindromic heptamer (e.g., 5' CACAGTG 3'), a nonconserved spacer of 12 or 23 bp, and an A/T-rich nonamer (5' ACAAAAACC 3') (46). Joining occurs between segments flanked by recognition sequences with unequal spacers (19, 77, 84). This is referred to as the 12/23 joining rule. Because all segments of a particular type (e.g., V gene segments) are flanked by one type of signal sequence and all the segments to which they should be joined (e.g., J segments) are flanked by the opposite type of signal sequence, the 12/23 rule ensures that the joining will be restricted to events that could be biologically productive. Although each spacer varies in sequence, the length of each spacer is conserved and corresponds to one or two turns of the DNA double helix. Each spacer serves to bring the heptamer and nonamer sequences to the same side of the DNA helix, where they both can be bound by a protein complex that catalyzes recombination. These heptamer-spacer-nonamer sequences are often called recombination signal sequences, or RSS (19, 77).

HEAVY CHAIN

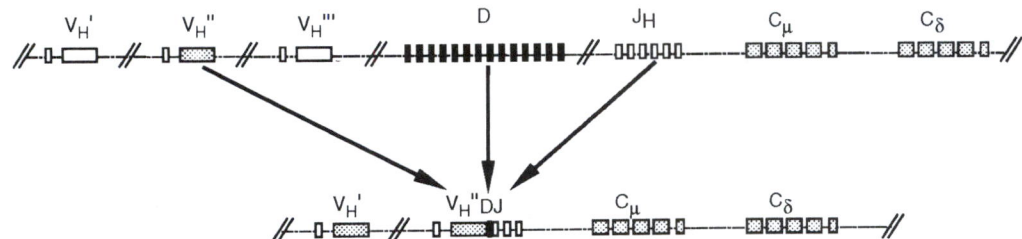

KAPPA CHAIN

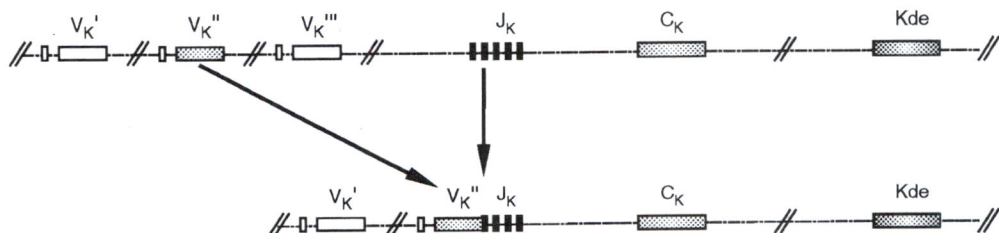

LAMBDA CHAIN

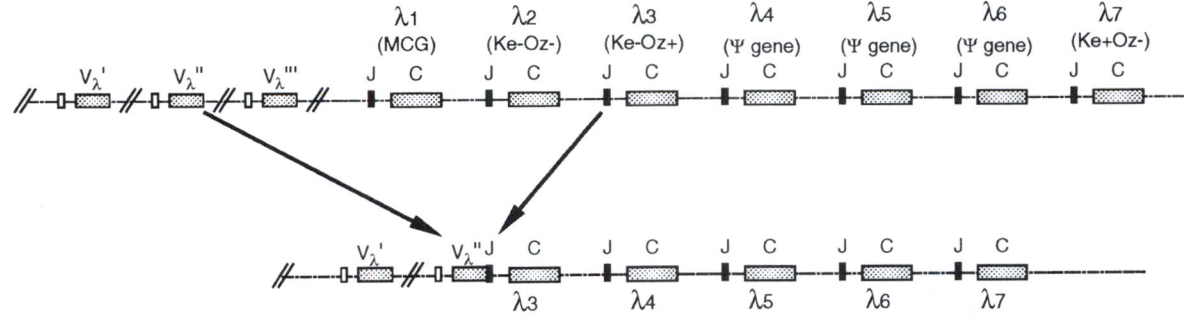

FIGURE 3 Immunoglobulin gene rearrangement. Diagonal double lines indicate that there is a large distance between flanking genes depicted as rectangular boxes (not drawn to scale). Depicted on the left side of each immunoglobulin gene complex are exemplary immunoglobulin V_H genes (V_H', V_H'', and V_H'''), immunoglobulin κ light-chain genes ($V_κ'$, $V_κ''$, and $V_κ'''$), or immunoglobulin λ light-chain genes ($V_λ'$, $V_λ''$, and $V_λ'''$). D designates the diversity gene segments of the antibody heavy-chain locus. J_H, $J_κ$, and $J_λ$ indicate the joining gene segments of the antibody heavy chain, κ light chain, and λ light chain, respectively. $C_μ$ and $C_δ$ are the constant-region exons of the μ and δ heavy chains, respectively. Below each is a possible immunoglobulin gene rearrangement comprising a V_H-D-J_H segment for the antibody heavy-chain gene or a $V_κ$-$J_κ$ or a $V_λ$-$J_λ$ segment for the κ or λ light-chain gene, respectively. Below the representative λ constant-region loci in row C are listed the names of the lambda nonallelic genetic markers, Mcg, Ke⁻ Oz⁻, Ke⁻ Oz⁺, and Ke⁺ Oz⁻, on $C_λ1$, $C_λ2$, $C_λ3$, and $C_λ7$, respectively. As indicated, $C_λ4$, $C_λ5$, and $C_λ6$ are pseudogenes (ψ gene) that do not encode protein.

Somatic V-region gene recombination involves introduction of double-stranded DNA breaks at RSS, juxtaposition of the broken ends, and then religation through a process called nonhomologous DNA end joining (NHEJ). The commonest mode of recombination involves the looping out and deletion of the DNA between two gene segments on the same chromosome. The 12- and 23-mer-spaced RSS are brought together by interactions between proteins that specifically recognize the length of the spacer between the heptamer and nonamer signals, thus accounting for the 12/23 joining rule (19, 77). The two DNA molecules then are broken and religated (23). The ends of the heptamer sequences are joined precisely in a head-to-head configuration to form a signal joint in a circular piece of DNA that then is lost from the genome when the cell divides. However, when the RSS are oriented in the same direction along the chromosome, the segments undergo recombination via inversion, in which case the intervening DNA is retained.

The first cleavage step requires a specialized heterodimeric endonuclease encoded by *RAG-1* and *RAG-2* (60, 61). The RAG-1 endonuclease has sequence similarities to bacterial topoisomerases that catalyze the breakage and rejoining of DNA. *RAG-1* and *RAG-2* are coexpressed normally only in developing lymphocytes that are undergoing receptor gene rearrangement. Mice with either of these genes knocked out cannot undergo immunoglobulin or T-cell receptor gene rearrangements and consequently fail to produce mature B or T lymphocytes (75). Mutations that impair but do not completely abolish the function of *RAG-1* or *RAG-2* in humans result in a form of combined immune deficiency called Omenn syndrome (88).

The RAG-1/RAG-2 endonuclease recognizes either the 12-mer-spaced or the 23-mer-spaced RSS and then introduces double-stranded DNA breaks. After introducing these breaks, the RAG-1/RAG-2 complex remains bound to the DNA. Mutations that affect the ability of the RAG proteins to bind and to maintain the broken ends in a stable postcleavage complex can lead to misrepair of the double-stranded breaks, thereby enhancing the risk for oncogenic chromosomal aberrations (29, 85). Involved in the processing and juxtaposition of these double-stranded breaks are several proteins, including the high-mobility-group proteins 1 and 2 (HMG1 and HMG2). HMG1 and HMG2 are widely expressed, abundant nuclear proteins that bind and bend DNA without sequence specificity, thereby playing an important role in the assembly of nucleoprotein complexes involved in DNA repair and transcription (81). HMG1 may facilitate the bending of the DNA to allow for the components of one double-stranded break-RAG complex to bind and to cleave the DNA at a different RSS, thus bringing together two disparate RSS in accordance with the 12/23 joining rule (19, 77).

The double-stranded break-RAG complex also binds at least six other proteins, including Ku70, Ku80, DNA-dependent protein kinase (DNA-PK), XRCC4, DNA ligase IV (Lig4), and Artemis (48). DNA-PK is a serine-threonine protein kinase that is activated by DNA double-stranded breaks and is essential for the normal repair of DNA breaks induced by ionizing radiation, chemical agents, or VDJ recombination (49, 79). Mice that are deficient in DNA-PK can make only trivial amounts of immunoglobulin or T-cell receptors and are called severe combined immunodeficiency mice, or SCID mice (36). Mice deficient in Artemis have a "leaky" SCID phenotype and develop some T and B cells in later life (79). Ku-deficient mice also are deficient in T and B cells but have small stature and other nonimmunologic defects, suggesting that the Ku proteins also play important roles in normal development (24, 63). Defects in mice resulting from mutations in either Ku, XRCC4, Lig4, Artemis, or DNA-PK genes predispose to lymphoma (2, 4).

The process of recombination allows for the generation of junctional diversity in the sequences of the rearranged gene segments. DNA ends generated by the RAG-1/RAG-2 endonuclease cleavage reaction are each fused by the NHEJ pathway involving the proteins listed in the preceding paragraphs. The hairpinned termini of gene segments that give rise to the coding joint are each subsequently cleaved at random sites by an endonuclease. Cleavage of a hairpin away from its apex generates an overhanging flap, which, if incorporated into the joint, results in the addition of palindromic nucleotides that contribute to junctional diversity. The opened hairpin ends can be modified further by nucleases that can remove a self-complementary overhang or cut further

into the original coding sequence. In addition, a lymphocyte-specific enzyme, terminal deoxynucleotidyl transferase, can add non-template-encoded nucleotides (42). Finally, additional junctional diversity comes from the nucleolytic activities that remove potential coding-end nucleotides prior to the final ligation of the DNA breaks into one intact recombination joint (23).

Heavy-Chain Class Switching

During differentiation, a single B lymphocyte can synthesize heavy chains with different constant regions coupled to the same variable region (76). As pre-B cells develop into mature B cells, intact IgM monomers are inserted into the plasma membrane, followed by IgD molecules with the same antigen-binding specificity. The IgM and IgD constant-region genes are closely linked in embryonic DNA and may be transcribed together. The differential splicing of the transcript allows the simultaneous synthesis of the two immunoglobulin heavy chains from a single species of RNA.

The switch from IgM to IgG, IgA, or IgE requires active transcription of the downstream constant-region exons encoding the switched immunoglobulin isotype. This requires prior interaction of B lymphocytes with an antigen or mitogen and ligation of CD40 via the ligand for CD40 (CD154) expressed by activated T cells. Patients with inherited defects in CD40 or CD154 have an immune deficiency syndrome (hyper-IgM syndrome type I) characterized by normal to high serum levels of IgM and extremely low serum levels of other immunoglobulin isotypes (14, 17). Interleukins provided by antigen-reactive T lymphocytes strongly influence (i) which B cells differentiate into IgM-secreting plasma cells and (ii) which B cells switch their immunoglobulin heavy-chain isotype, e.g., to IgG or IgA (3, 76).

Immunoglobulin class-switching recombination (CSR) occurs in or near the α switch region upstream of the μ gene and any one of the switch regions of the other heavy-chain isotype genes (Fig. 1). The μ switch region, designated S_μ, consists of approximately 150 repeats of the sequence $(GAGCT)_n(GGGGGT)$, where n is generally three but can be as many as seven. The sequences of the other switch regions (S_γ, S_α, and S_ε) are similar in that they also contain repeats of the GAGCT and GGGGGT sequences. The switch in heavy-chain classes results from DNA recombination between S_μ and S_γ, S_α, or S_ε accompanied by the deletion of intervening DNA segments and the apposition of the previously rearranged variable-region gene next to the new constant-region gene.

In contrast to VDJ recombination, which occurs mostly in the G_0 and/or G_1 stage of the cell cycle, CSR seems to require DNA replication. Also, unlike VDJ recombination, CSR also requires expression of activation-induced deaminase (AID), an enzyme expressed in activated B cells that also is required for somatic hypermutation (see "Generation of Antibody Diversity," below) (27, 58). Patients with inherited defects in AID have an immune deficiency syndrome (hyper-IgM syndrome type II) characterized by relatively high serum levels of IgM, and negligible serum levels of other immunoglobulin isotypes (69). AID is expressed in germinal centers of the lymph nodes and spleen, the sites where CSR takes place in B cells activated in response to an antigen (50). AID most likely deaminates the closely positioned cytosines (dC) in the S-region DNA, converting the dC into uracils (dU), which in turn are removed by uracil-DNA glycosylase (UNG). The importance of UNG is underscored by patients who have inherited defects in this enzyme, resulting in an autosomal recessive form of the hyper-IgM immune deficiency syndrome similar to that of patients with inherited defects in AID (30, 33). The abasic sites generated by UNG are cleaved by apurinic/apyrimidinic endonuclease, resulting in closely positioned staggered nicks in the DNA that may result in double-stranded DNA breaks (5). The end-processing, repair, and joining mechanisms for these DNA breaks apparently involve mechanisms and proteins similar to those involved in NHEJ used for VDJ recombination. Because the CSR occurs in the intron between the variable-region exon and the exon encoding the first constant-region domain, this process does not generate mutations in the regions encoding the variable or constant regions of the newly generated immunoglobulin heavy chain (90).

GENERATION OF ANTIBODY DIVERSITY

Several mechanisms contribute to the generation of diversity among immunoglobulin polypeptide variable regions (84). These are (i) the presence in the germ line of multiple V, J, and D gene segments; (ii) the random joining of these DNA segments to produce a complete variable-region exon; (iii) uncorrected errors made during the recombination process; (iv) the coming together of the heavy- and light-chain polypeptides to produce a complete immunoglobulin monomer capable of binding an antigen; and (v) somatic mutations within the rearranged DNA segments themselves. The last of these occurs through a process called somatic hypermutation.

Somatic hypermutation is not active in all B cells and cannot be triggered merely by mitogen-induced B-cell activation. However, during discrete stages of B-cell differentiation, expressed immunoglobulin V genes can incur new mutations at rates as high as 10^{-3} base changes per base pair per generation over several cell divisions, particularly during the secondary immune response to an antigen. Hypermutations begin on the 5′ ends of rearranged V genes downstream of the transcription initiation site and continue through the V gene and into the 3′-flanking region before tapering off. As such, the mutations are clustered in the region spanning from 300 bp 5′ of the rearranged variable-region exon to approximately 1 kb 3′ of the rearranged minigene J segment. Mutations frequently are clustered around hot spots defined by the primary DNA sequence. The sequence RGYW (R, purine [A or G]; Y, pyrimidine [C or T]; W, A or T) and its complement, for example, are hot spots for mutation that are conserved among species (55, 71).

Somatic hypermutation requires the activity of AID through a process that has some similarity to CSR (13). In addition to having the hyper-IgM immune deficiency syndrome type II, patients that have inherited defects in AID have B cells that lack the capacity to undergo somatic hypermutation (58). As with CSR, somatic hypermutation requires active transcription of the genes undergoing mutation. AID most likely deaminates the dC in the region encompassing the rearranged variable-region gene, converting the dC into dU, which are converted into T after DNA replication, giving rise to CG-to-T or -A transitions. Alternatively, the dU are removed by UNG, resulting in abasic sites that subsequently may be cleaved by apurinic/apyrimidinic endonuclease. The removal of uracil generates staggered nick cleavage of the DNA. Repair of these staggered nicks may involve low-fidelity DNA synthesis, giving rise to frequent mutations. DNA-cleaving enzymes and DNA repair enzymes (e.g., mismatch repair enzymes, base excision repair enzymes, proteins involved in NHEJ, etc.) form a complex called the mutasome that also apparently binds the target DNA to reduce

its tendency to incur complete double-stranded DNA breaks. As a consequence of this process, mostly transitional mutations are introduced at high frequencies into the expressed immunoglobulin V genes, as well as into other transcriptionally active genes with hot spots that can serve as a substrate for AID, UNG, and the mutasome (55, 78). Subsequent selection of the B cell and its daughter cells that express mutated V genes encoding an immunoglobulin variable region with improved fitness for binding antigen allows for "affinity maturation" of the antibodies expressed during the immune response to antigen (62). Such selection enhances the frequency of nonconservative base substitutions in the DNA sequences encoding the complementarity-determining regions that serve as the contact sites for antigen binding (12).

DETECTION OF IMMUNOGLOBULIN GENE REARRANGEMENTS

Analysis for immunoglobulin gene rearrangements can detect clonal immunoglobulin gene rearrangements. Immunoglobulin gene rearrangement irreversibly alters the genomic DNA of the developing B cell and its descendant daughter cells. Because of the many different immunoglobulin gene rearrangements possible, a B cell's particular type of immunoglobulin gene rearrangement can serve as a clonal marker.

Southern Blot Hybridization

The Southern blot hybridization technique frequently is used to examine for clonal immunoglobulin gene rearrangement secondary to an abnormal expansion of cells from a single B-cell clone. In this technique, genomic DNA is cleaved at specific sites with a restriction enzyme(s) to generate restriction fragments of various sizes that can be resolved with respect to length via agarose gel electrophoresis. After electrophoresis, the DNA fragments inside the gel are denatured and then blotted onto a nitrocellulose or nylon membrane. The membrane then is hybridized to a ^{32}P-radiolabeled probe specific for a region of the immunoglobulin gene of interest. Polyclonal B-cell populations reveal nonrearranged germ line bands in Southern blot analysis, as each B-cell clone contributes to only a small fraction of the total genomic DNA isolated from normal lymphoid tissue. However, if the population is monoclonal, non-germ line bands will be observed using probes specific for sites contiguous to the site of recombination (i.e., the J_H region). Such non-germ line bands indicate that the lymphoid tissue contains an expansion of one B-cell clone.

PCR

More-sensitive methods for detecting immunoglobulin gene rearrangements, such as PCR, can be used to examine for residual cells of a malignant B-cell clone following antitumor therapy. PCR using sense-strand oligonucleotide primers corresponding to an immunoglobulin V gene subgroup (Table 2) together with antisense-strand oligonucleotide primers corresponding to the relevant J-region or constant-region exon can amplify the rearranged V gene in genomic DNA or cDNA, respectively.

Because these gene segments are separated by large stretches of intervening DNA in germ line DNA, PCR with genomic DNA and primers specific for a V gene subgroup and the J gene segment(s) will fail to amplify any immunoglobulin genes unless the genes have first undergone rearrangement. However, after immunoglobulin gene rearrangement, the variable-region gene leader sequence

TABLE 2 Oligonucleotide primers corresponding to the sense strand of the leader sequences of each of the major V gene subgroups

Gene	Primer sequence[a]
V_H genes	
V_H1a	CAGGT(G/T)CAGCTGGTGCAG
V_H1b	CAGGTCCAGCTTGTGCAG
V_H1c	(G/C)AGGTCCAGCTGGTACAG
V_H1d	CA(A/G)ATGCAGCTGGTGCAG
V_H2a	CAGATCACCTTGAAGGAG
V_H2b	CAGGTCACCTTGA(A/G)GGAG
V_H3a	GA(A/G)GTGCAGCTGGTGGAG
V_H3b	CAGGTGCAGCTGGTGGAG
V_H3c	GAGGTGCAGCTGTTGGAG
V_H4a	CAG(C/G)TGCAGCTGCAGGAG
V_H4b	CAGGTGCAGCTACAGCAG
V_H5	GA(A/G)GTGCAGCTGGTGCAG
V_H6	CAGGTACAGCTGCAGCAG
V_H7	CAGGT(C/G)CAGCTGGTGCAA
V_κ genes	
$V_\kappa1a$	(A/G)ACATCCAGATGACCCAG
$V_\kappa1b$	G(A/C)CATCCAGTTGACCCAG
$V_\kappa1c$	GCCATCC(A/G)GATGACCCAG
$V_\kappa2a$	GATATTGTGATGACCCAG
$V_\kappa2b$	GAT(A/G)TTGTGATGACTCAG
$V_\kappa3a$	GAAATTGTGTTGAC(A/G)CAG
$V_\kappa3b$	GAAATAGTGATGACGCAG
$V_\kappa3c$	GAAATTGTAATGACACAG
$V_\kappa4a$	GACATCGTGATGACCCAG
$V_\kappa5a$	GACATCGTGATGACCCAG
$V_\kappa6a$	GAAATTGTGCTGACTCAG
$V_\kappa6b$	GATGTTGTGATGACACAG
V_λ genes	
$V_\lambda1a$	
$V_\lambda1b$	CAGTCTGTGCTGACTCAG
$V_\lambda1c$	CAGTCTGTG(C/T)TGACGCAG
$V_\lambda2$	CAGTCTGTCGTGACGCAG
$V_\lambda3a$	CAGTCTGCCCTGACTCAG
$V_\lambda3b$	TCCTATG(A/T)GCTGACTCAG
$V_\lambda3c$	TCCTATGAGCTGACACAG
$V_\lambda3d$	TCCTATGAGCTGATGCAG
$V_\lambda4$	CAGC(C/T)TGTGCTGACTCAA
$V_\lambda5$	CAG(C/G)CTGTGCTGACTCAG
$V_\lambda6$	AATTTTATGCTGACTCAG
$V_\lambda7$	CAG(A/G)CTGTGGTGACTCAG
$V_\lambda8$	CAGACTGTGGTGACCCAG
$V_\lambda4/9$	C(A/T)GCCTGTGCTGACTCAG
$V_\lambda10$	CAGGCAGGGCTGACTCAG

[a] Positions at which either of two nucleotides is used to represent most, if not all, of the V genes in a given subgroup are indicated in parentheses.

primers and J primers anneal to sites that are separated by fewer than 400 bp, making PCR straightforward. It should be noted that PCR on genomic DNA with primers specific for a V gene subgroup and a constant-region exon will not amplify rearranged immunoglobulin genes because the distance between the J segment and the immunoglobulin constant-region exon is too large. Such primer pairs are better suited for amplifying cDNA derived from the immunoglobulin transcripts from which the intron separating the J region and the constant-region exon are deleted through RNA processing and splicing.

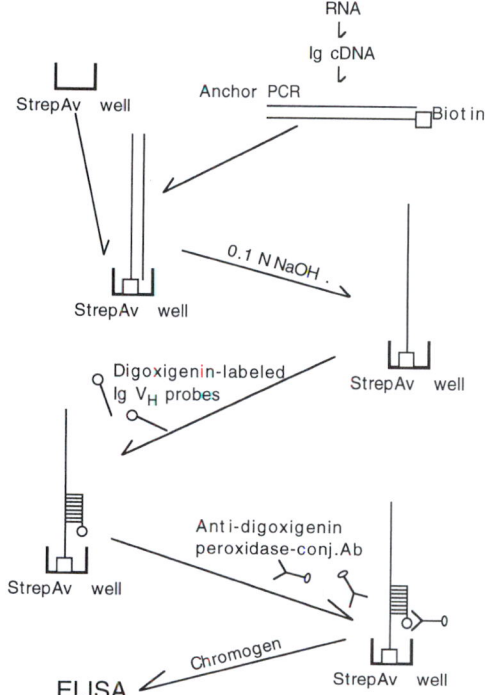

FIGURE 4 Schematic representation of the PCR-ELISA technique. Following anchored PCR, a nested PCR attaches a biotin molecule (white box) to the antisense strand of the PCR product. This allows the strand to bind to streptavidin (StrepAv)-coated wells of an ELISA plate. The sense strand is removed by alkaline wash, allowing for hybridization of the tethered antisense strand with digoxigenin-labeled immunoglobulin V_H oligonucleotide probes (represented by the ball and stick figures). Hybridized and bound oligonucleotides then are detected using peroxidase-conjugated antidigoxigenin antibodies (anti-digoxigenin peroxidase-conj. Ab). The peroxidase-conjugated antibodies are developed with chromogen, and the plates are read using an ELISA plate reader.

Resolution of the junctional sequences in the rearranged immunoglobulin genes expressed by a tumor can provide a specific tumor marker. This marker can be used to examine for any tumor-derived immunoglobulin gene fragments amplified by PCR performed on genomic DNA of lymphoid tissue. Such methods are highly sensitive, allowing for detection of minimal residual disease in lymphoid tissue that otherwise harbors no detectable pathologic or immunophenotypic trace of a residual tumor.

Anchored Reverse Transcriptase PCR-ELISA

Another method for assessing immunoglobulin V gene expression is the anchored reverse transcriptase PCR–enzyme-linked immunosorbent assay (ELISA). This method can be used to assess the expressed immunoglobulin repertoire of monoclonal or polyclonal B-cell populations (67). With this technique, the expressed genes are amplified uniformly regardless of polymorphism and/or somatic mutations, since the cDNA is G tailed and used in a primary PCR with a poly(C) anchor sense primer and an immunoglobulin constant-region antisense primer. The amplified cDNA then is used as the template for a secondary nested PCR that increases the specificity of the overall PCR and that generates a final PCR product having a biotin molecule attached to the 5' end of the antisense strand. This allows the antisense strand to become tethered to avidin-coated polystyrene ELISA plates. Digoxigenin-labeled oligonucleotides specific for subgroup or V gene consensus sequences of the sense strand of the PCR product are used to probe the tethered and alkali-denatured antisense strand. Because of the digoxigenin label, the probe that hybridizes with the tethered antisense strand can be detected using alkaline phosphatase-conjugated antidigoxigenin antibodies. The latter can be detected by adding a chromogen and then by reading the change in optical density of the reaction mixture with an ELISA plate reader (Fig. 4). The frequency of each gene or gene subgroup then can be calculated by dividing the concentration of each immunoglobulin gene product by the total concentration of immunoglobulin V genes.

REFERENCES

1. Abe, M., S. Ozaki, D. Wolfenbarger, M. deBram-Hart, D. T. Weiss, and A. Solomon. 1994. Variable-region subgroup distribution among lambda-type immunoglobulins in normal human serum. *J. Clin. Lab. Anal.* **8:**4–9.
2. Bassing, C. H., H. Suh, D. O. Ferguson, K. F. Chua, J. Manis, M. Eckersdorff, M. Gleason, R. Bronson, C. Lee, and F. W. Alt. 2003. Histone H2AX: a dosage-dependent suppressor of oncogenic translocations and tumors. *Cell* **114:**359–370.
3. Calame, K. L., K. I. Lin, and C. Tunyaplin. 2003. Regulatory mechanisms that determine the development and function of plasma cells. *Annu. Rev. Immunol.* **21:**205–230.
4. Celeste, A., S. Difilippantonio, M. J. Difilippantonio, O. Fernandez-Capetillo, D. R. Pilch, O. A. Sedelnikova, M. Eckhaus, T. Ried, W. M. Bonner, and A. Nussenzweig. 2003. H2AX haploinsufficiency modifies genomic stability and tumor susceptibility. *Cell* **114:**371–383.
5. Chen, X., K. Kinoshita, and T. Honjo. 2001. Variable deletion and duplication at recombination junction ends: implication for staggered double-strand cleavage in class-switch recombination. *Proc. Natl. Acad. Sci. USA* **98:** 13860–13865.
6. Chuchana, P., A. Blancher, F. Brockly, D. Alexandre, G. Lefranc, and M. P. Lefranc. 1990. Definition of the human immunoglobulin variable lambda (IGLV) gene subgroups. *Eur. J. Immunol.* **20:**1317–1325.
7. Cook, G. P., and I. M. Tomlinson. 1995. The human immunoglobulin VH repertoire. *Immunol. Today* **16:**237–242.
8. Corcos, D., O. Dunda, C. Butor, J. Y. Cesbron, P. Lorès, D. Bucchini, and J. Jami. 1995. Pre-B-cell development in the absence of lambda 5 in transgenic mice expressing a heavy-chain disease protein. *Curr. Biol.* **5:**1140–1148.
9. Corthesy, B., and J. P. Kraehenbuhl. 1999. Antibody-mediated protection of mucosal surfaces. *Curr. Top. Microbiol. Immunol.* **236:**93–111.
10. Cox, J. P., I. M. Tomlinson, and G. Winter. 1994. A directory of human germ-line V kappa segments reveals a strong bias in their usage. *Eur. J. Immunol.* **24:**827–836.
11. Dariavach, P., G. Lefranc, and M. P. Lefranc. 1987. Human immunoglobulin C lambda 6 gene encodes the Kern+Oz-lambda chain and C lambda 4 and C lambda 5 are pseudogenes. *Proc. Natl. Acad. Sci. USA* **84:**9074–9078.
12. Dorner, T., S. J. Foster, H. P. Brezinschek, and P. E. Lipsky. 1998. Analysis of the targeting of the hypermutational machinery and the impact of subsequent selection on the distribution of nucleotide changes in human VHDJH rearrangements. *Immunol. Rev.* **162:**161–171.
13. Dudley, D. D., J. Chaudhuri, C. H. Bassing, and F. W. Alt. 2005. Mechanism and control of V(D)J recombination versus class switch recombination: similarities and differences. *Adv. Immunol.* **86:**43–112.
14. Durandy, A., P. Revy, and A. Fischer. 2004. Human models of inherited immunoglobulin class switch recombination and somatic hypermutation defects (hyper-IgM syndromes). *Adv. Immunol.* **82:**295–330.
15. Edelman, G. M. 1991. Antibody structure and molecular immunology. *Scand. J. Immunol.* **34:**1–22.
16. Feeney, A. J., M. J. Atkinson, M. J. Cowan, G. Escuro, and G. Lugo. 1996. A defective Vκ A2 allele in Navajos which may play a role in increased susceptibility to Haemophilus influenzae type b disease. *J. Clin. Investig.* **97:** 2277–2282.
17. Ferrari, S., and A. Plebani. 2002. Cross-talk between CD40 and CD40L: lessons from primary immune deficiencies. *Curr. Opin. Allergy Clin. Immunol.* **2:**489–494.
18. Frippiat, J. P., S. C. Williams, I. M. Tomlinson, G. P. Cook, D. Cherif, D. Le Paslier, J. E. Collins, I. Dunham, G. Winter, and M. P. Lefranc. 1995. Organization of the human immunoglobulin lambda light-chain locus on chromosome 22q11.2. *Hum. Mol. Genet.* **4:**983–991.
19. Gellert, M. 1997. Recent advances in understanding V(D)J recombination. *Adv. Immunol.* **64:**39–64.
20. Ghanem, N., P. Dariavach, M. Bensmana, J. Chibani, G. Lefranc, and M. P. Lefranc. 1988. Polymorphism of immunoglobulin lambda constant region genes in populations from France, Lebanon and Tunisia. *Exp. Clin. Immunogenet.* **5:**186–195.
21. Gould, H. J., B. J. Sutton, A. J. Beavil, R. L. Beavil, N. McCloskey, H. A. Coker, D. Fear, and L. Smurthwaite. 2003. The biology of IGE and the basis of allergic disease. *Annu. Rev. Immunol.* **21:**579–628.
22. Graninger, W. B., P. L. Goldman, C. C. Morton, S. J. O'Brien, and S. J. Korsmeyer. 1988. The kappa-deleting element. Germline and rearranged, duplicated and dispersed forms. *J. Exp. Med.* **167:**488–501.
23. Grawunder, U., R. B. West, and M. R. Lieber. 1998. Antigen receptor gene rearrangement. *Curr. Opin. Immunol.* **10:**172–180.
24. Gu, Y., J. Sekiguchi, Y. Gao, P. Dikkes, K. Frank, D. Ferguson, P. Hasty, J. Chun, and F. W. Alt. 2000. Defective embryonic neurogenesis in Ku-deficient but not DNA-dependent protein kinase catalytic subunit-deficient mice. *Proc. Natl. Acad. Sci. USA* **97:**2668–2673.
25. Harris, L. J., S. B. Larson, K. W. Hasel, J. Day, A. Greenwood, and A. McPherson. 1992. The three-dimensional structure of an intact monoclonal antibody for canine lymphoma. *Nature* **360:**369–372.
26. Hilschmann, N. 1987. The immunoglobulin receptor. *Behring Inst. Mitt.* **1987:**98–99.
27. Honjo, T., K. Kinoshita, and M. Muramatsu. 2002. Molecular mechanism of class switch recombination: linkage with somatic hypermutation. *Annu. Rev. Immunol.* **20:**165–196.
28. Huber, C., E. Huber, A. Lautner-Rieske, K. F. Schable, and H. G. Zachau. 1993. The human immunoglobulin kappa locus. Characterization of the partially duplicated L regions. *Eur. J. Immunol.* **23:**2860–2867.
29. Huye, L. E., M. M. Purugganan, M. M. Jiang, and D. B. Roth. 2002. Mutational analysis of all conserved basic amino acids in RAG-1 reveals catalytic, step arrest, and joining-deficient mutants in the V(D)J recombinase. *Mol. Cell. Biol.* **22:**3460–3473.
30. Imai, K., G. Slupphaug, W. I. Lee, P. Revy, S. Nonoyama, N. Catalan, L. Yel, M. Forveille, B. Kavli, H. E. Krokan, H. D. Ochs, A. Fischer, and A. Durandy. 2003. Human uracil-DNA glycosylase deficiency associated with profoundly impaired immunoglobulin class-switch recombination. *Nat. Immunol.* **4:**1023–1028.
31. Jefferis, R., J. Lund, and M. Goodall. 1995. Recognition sites on human IgG for Fc gamma receptors: the role of glycosylation. *Immunol. Lett.* **44:**111–117.

32. **Joiner, K. A., L. F. Fries, and M. M. Frank.** 1987. Studies of antibody and complement function in host defense against bacterial infection. *Immunol. Lett.* **14**:197–202.

33. **Kavli, B., S. Andersen, M. Otterlei, N. B. Liabakk, K. Imai, A. Fischer, A. Durandy, H. E. Krokan, and G. Slupphaug.** 2005. B cells from hyper-IgM patients carrying UNG mutations lack ability to remove uracil from ssDNA and have elevated genomic uracil. *J. Exp. Med.* **201**:2011–2021.

34. **Kawasaki, K., S. Minoshima, E. Nakato, K. Shibuya, A. Shintani, S. Asakawa, T. Sasaki, H. G. Klobeck, G. Combriato, H. G. Zachau, and N. Shimizu.** 2001. Evolutionary dynamics of the human immunoglobulin kappa locus and the germline repertoire of the Vkappa genes. *Eur. J. Immunol.* **31**:1017–1028.

35. **Kawasaki, K., S. Minoshima, E. Nakato, K. Shibuya, A. Shintani, J. L. Schmeits, J. Wang, and N. Shimizu.** 1997. One-megabase sequence analysis of the human immunoglobulin lambda gene locus. *Genome Res.* **7**:250–261.

36. **Khanna, K. K., and S. P. Jackson.** 2001. DNA double-strand breaks: signaling, repair and the cancer connection. *Nat. Genet.* **27**:247–254.

37. **Kipps, T. J.** 1997. Human B cell biology. *Int. Rev. Immunol.* **15**:243–264.

38. **Kirkham, P. M., F. Mortari, J. A. Newton, and H. W. Schroeder, Jr.** 1992. Immunoglobulin VH clan and family identity predicts variable domain structure and may influence antigen binding. *EMBO J.* **11**:603–609.

39. **Kirsch, I. R., C. C. Morton, K. Nakahara, and P. Leder.** 1982. Human immunoglobulin heavy chain genes map to a region of translocations in malignant B lymphocytes. *Science* **216**:301–303.

40. **Kitamura, D., A. Kudo, S. Schaal, W. Muller, F. Melchers, and K. Rajewsky.** 1992. A critical role of lambda 5 protein in B cell development. *Cell* **69**:823–831.

41. **Klein, R., and H. G. Zachau.** 1995. Expression and hypermutation of human immunoglobulin kappa genes. *Ann. N. Y. Acad. Sci.* **764**:74–83.

42. **Komori, T., A. Okada, V. Stewart, and F. W. Alt.** 1993. Lack of N regions in antigen receptor variable region genes of TdT-deficient lymphocytes. *Science* **261**:1171–1175.

43. **Lamm, M. E., J. G. Nedrud, C. S. Kaetzel, and M. B. Mazanec.** 1995. IgA and mucosal defense. *APMIS* **103**:241–246.

44. **Lautner-Rieske, A., C. Huber, A. Meindl, W. Pargent, K. F. Schable, R. Thiebe, I. Zocher, and H. G. Zachau.** 1992. The human immunoglobulin kappa locus. Characterization of the duplicated A regions. *Eur. J. Immunol.* **22**:1023–1029.

45. **Lee, Y. K., J. W. Brewer, R. Hellman, and L. M. Hendershot.** 1999. BiP and immunoglobulin light chain cooperate to control the folding of heavy chain and ensure the fidelity of immunoglobulin assembly. *Mol. Biol. Cell* **10**:2209–2219.

46. **Lewis, S. M.** 1994. The mechanism of V(D)J joining: lessons from molecular, immunological, and comparative analyses. *Adv. Immunol.* **56**:27–150.

47. **Lyczak, J. B., K. Zhang, A. Saxon, and S. L. Morrison.** 1996. Expression of novel secreted isoforms of human immunoglobulin E proteins. *J. Biol. Chem.* **271**:3428–3436.

48. **Ma, Y., U. Pannicke, K. Schwarz, and M. R. Lieber.** 2002. Hairpin opening and overhang processing by an Artemis/DNA-dependent protein kinase complex in nonhomologous end joining and V(D)J recombination. *Cell* **108**:781–794.

49. **Ma, Y., K. Schwarz, and M. R. Lieber.** 2005. The Artemis:DNA-PKcs endonuclease cleaves DNA loops, flaps, and gaps. *DNA Repair* (Amsterdam) **4**:845–851.

50. **Maclennan, I. C.** 2005. Germinal centers still hold secrets. *Immunity* **22**:656–657.

51. **Matsuda, F., K. Ishii, P. Bourvagnet, K. Kuma, H. Hayashida, T. Miyata, and T. Honjo.** 1998. The complete nucleotide sequence of the human immunoglobulin heavy chain variable region locus. *J. Exp. Med.* **188**:2151–2162.

52. **Meek, K., T. Eversole, and J. D. Capra.** 1991. Conservation of the most JH proximal Ig VH gene segment (VHVI) throughout primate evolution. *J. Immunol.* **146**:2434–2438.

53. **Melchers, F., H. Karasuyama, D. Haasner, S. Bauer, A. Kudo, N. Sakaguchi, B. Jameson, and A. Rolink.** 1993. The surrogate light chain in B-cell development. *Immunol. Today* **14**:60–68.

54. **Mestecky, J., C. Lue, and M. W. Russell.** 1991. Selective transport of IgA. Cellular and molecular aspects. *Gastroenterol. Clin. North Am.* **20**:441–471.

55. **Michael, N., T. E. Martin, D. Nicolae, N. Kim, K. Padjen, P. Zhan, H. Nguyen, C. Pinkert, and U. Storb.** 2002. Effects of sequence and structure on the hypermutability of immunoglobulin genes. *Immunity* **16**:123–134.

56. **Milner, E. C., W. O. Hufnagle, A. M. Glas, I. Suzuki, and C. Alexander.** 1995. Polymorphism and utilization of human VH genes. *Ann. N. Y. Acad. Sci.* **764**:50–61.

57. **Minegishi, Y., E. Coustan-Smith, Y. H. Wang, M. D. Cooper, D. Campana, and M. E. Conley.** 1998. Mutations in the human lambda5/14.1 gene result in B cell deficiency and agammaglobulinemia. *J. Exp. Med.* **187**:71–77.

58. **Muramatsu, M., K. Kinoshita, S. Fagarasan, S. Yamada, Y. Shinkai, and T. Honjo.** 2000. Class switch recombination and hypermutation require activation-induced cytidine deaminase (AID), a potential RNA editing enzyme. *Cell* **102**:553–563.

59. **Niles, M. J., L. Matsuuchi, and M. E. Koshland.** 1995. Polymer IgM assembly and secretion in lymphoid and non-lymphoid cell lines: evidence that J chain is required for pentamer IgM synthesis. *Proc. Natl. Acad. Sci. USA* **92**:2884–2888.

60. **Oettinger, M. A., D. G. Schatz, C. Gorka, and D. Baltimore.** 1990. RAG-1 and RAG-2, adjacent genes that synergistically activate V(D)J recombination. *Science* **248**:1517–1523.

61. **Oettinger, M. A., B. Stanger, D. G. Schatz, T. Glaser, K. Call, D. Housman, and D. Baltimore.** 1992. The recombination activating genes, RAG 1 and RAG 2, are on chromosome 11p in humans and chromosome 2p in mice. *Immunogenetics* **35**:97–101.

62. **Ollila, J., and M. Vihinen.** 2005. B cells. *Int. J. Biochem. Cell. Biol.* **37**:518–523.

63. **Ouyang, H., A. Nussenzweig, A. Kurimasa, V. C. Soares, X. Li, C. Cordon-Cardo, W. Li, N. Cheong, M. Nussenzweig, G. Iliakis, D. J. Chen, and G. C. Li.** 1997. Ku70 is required for DNA repair but not for T cell antigen receptor gene recombination in vivo. *J. Exp. Med.* **186**:921–929.

64. **Pallarès, N., J. P. Frippiat, V. Giudicelli, and M. P. Lefranc.** 1998. The human immunoglobulin lambda variable (IGLV) genes and joining (IGLJ) segments. *Exp. Clin. Immunogenet.* **15**:8–18.

65. **Pascual, V., and J. D. Capra.** 1991. Human immunoglobulin heavy-chain variable region genes: organization, polymorphism, and expression. *Adv. Immunol.* **49**:1–74.

66. **Rassenti, L. Z., and T. J. Kipps.** 1997. Lack of allelic exclusion in B cell chronic lymphocytic leukemia. *J. Exp. Med.* **185**:1435–1445.

67. **Rassenti, L. Z., H. Kohsaka, and T. J. Kipps.** 1995. Analysis of immunoglobulin V_H gene repertoire by an anchored PCR-ELISA. *Ann. N. Y. Acad. Sci.* **764**:463–473.

68. **Ravetch, J. V., and S. Bolland.** 2001. IgG Fc receptors. *Annu. Rev. Immunol.* **19**:275–290.

69. **Revy, P., T. Muto, Y. Levy, F. Geissmann, A. Plebani, O. Sanal, N. Catalan, M. Forveille, R. Dufourcq-Labelouse,**

A. Gennery, I. Tezcan, F. Ersoy, H. Kayserili, A. G. Ugazio, N. Brousse, M. Muramatsu, L. D. Notarangelo, K. Kinoshita, T. Honjo, A. Fischer, and A. Durandy. 2000. Activation-induced cytidine deaminase (AID) deficiency causes the autosomal recessive form of the hyper-IgM syndrome (HIGM2). *Cell* **102:**565–575.

70. **Roes, J., and K. Rajewsky.** 1993. Immunoglobulin D (IgD)-deficient mice reveal an auxiliary receptor function for IgD in antigen-mediated recruitment of B cells. *J. Exp. Med.* **177:**45–55.

71. **Rogozin, I. B., N. E. Sredneva, and N. A. Kolchanov.** 1996. Somatic hypermutagenesis in immunoglobulin genes. III. Somatic mutations in the chicken light chain locus. *Biochim. Biophys. Acta* **1306:**171–178.

72. **Ruiz, M., N. Pallarès, V. Contet, V. Barbi, and M. Lefranc.** 1999. The human immunoglobulin heavy diversity (IGHD) and joining (IGHJ) segments. *Exp. Clin. Immunogenet.* **16:**173–184.

73. **Sanz, I., P. Kelly, C. Williams, S. Scholl, P. Tucker, and J. D. Capra.** 1989. The smaller human VH gene families display remarkably little polymorphism. *EMBO J.* **8:**3741–3748.

74. **Sasso, E. H., T. Johnson, and T. J. Kipps.** 1996. Expression of the Ig VH gene 51p1 is proportional to its germline gene copy number. *J. Clin. Investig.* **97:**2074–2080.

75. **Shinkai, Y., G. Rathbun, K. P. Lam, E. M. Oltz, V. Stewart, M. Mendelsohn, J. Charron, M. Datta, F. Young, and A. M. Stall.** 1992. RAG-2-deficient mice lack mature lymphocytes owing to inability to initiate V(D)J rearrangement. *Cell* **68:**855–867.

76. **Stavnezer, J., and C. T. Amemiya.** 2004. Evolution of isotype switching. *Semin. Immunol.* **16:**257–275.

77. **Steen, S. B., L. Gomelsky, S. L. Speidel, and D. B. Roth.** 1997. Initiation of V(D)J recombination in vivo: role of recombination signal sequences in formation of single and paired double-strand breaks. *EMBO J.* **16:**2656–2664.

78. **Storb, U., H. M. Shen, N. Michael, and N. Kim.** 2001. Somatic hypermutation of immunoglobulin and non-immunoglobulin genes. *Philos. Trans. R. Soc. Lond. B* **356:**13–19.

79. **Taccioli, G. E., A. G. Amatucci, H. J. Beamish, D. Gell, X. H. Xiang, M. I. Torres Arzayus, A. Priestley, S. P. Jackson, A. Marshak Rothstein, P. A. Jeggo, and V. L. Herrera.** 1998. Targeted disruption of the catalytic subunit of the DNA-PK gene in mice confers severe combined immunodeficiency and radiosensitivity. *Immunity* **9:**355–366.

80. **ten Boekel, E., T. Yamagami, J. Andersson, A. G. Rolink, and F. Melchers.** 1999. The formation and selection of cells expressing preB cell receptors and B cell receptors. *Curr. Top. Microbiol. Immunol.* **246:**3–10.

81. **Thomas, J. O., and A. A. Travers.** 2001. HMG1 and 2, and related "architectural" DNA-binding proteins. *Trends Biochem. Sci.* **26:**167–174.

82. **Tomlinson, I. M., J. P. Cox, E. Gherardi, A. M. Lesk, and C. Chothia.** 1995. The structural repertoire of the human V kappa domain. *EMBO J.* **14:**4628–4638.

83. **Tomlinson, I. M., G. Walter, J. D. Marks, M. B. Llewelyn, and G. Winter.** 1992. The repertoire of human germline VH sequences reveals about fifty groups of VH segments with different hypervariable loops. *J. Mol. Biol.* **227:**776–798.

84. **Tonegawa, S.** 1993. The Nobel Lectures in Immunology. The Nobel Prize for Physiology or Medicine, 1987. Somatic generation of immune diversity. *Scand. J. Immunol.* **38:**303–319.

85. **Tsai, C. L., A. H. Drejer, and D. G. Schatz.** 2002. Evidence of a critical architectural function for the RAG proteins in end processing, protection, and joining in V(D)J recombination. *Genes Dev.* **16:**1934–1949.

86. **Tsuganezawa, K., N. Kiyokawa, Y. Matsuo, F. Kitamura, N. Toyama-Sorimachi, K. Kuida, J. Fujimoto, and H. Karasuyama.** 1998. Flow cytometric diagnosis of the cell lineage and developmental stage of acute lymphoblastic leukemia by novel monoclonal antibodies specific to human pre-B-cell receptor. *Blood* **92:**4317–4324.

87. **Vasicek, T. J., and P. Leder.** 1990. Structure and expression of the human immunoglobulin lambda genes. *J. Exp. Med.* **172:**609–620.

88. **Villa, A., S. Santagata, F. Bozzi, L. Imberti, and L. D. Notarangelo.** 1999. Omenn syndrome: a disorder of Rag1 and Rag2 genes. *J. Clin. Immunol.* **19:**87–97.

89. **Virella, G., and A. C. Wang.** 1993. Immunoglobulin structure. *Immunol. Ser.* **58:**75–90.

90. **Wang, C. L., and M. Wabl.** 2004. DNA acrobats of the Ig class switch. *J. Immunol.* **172:**5815–5821.

91. **Williams, S. C., J. P. Frippiat, I. M. Tomlinson, O. Ignatovich, M. P. Lefranc, and G. Winter.** 1996. Sequence and evolution of the human germline V lambda repertoire. *J. Mol. Biol.* **264:**220–232.

92. **Zachau, H. G.** 1993. The immunoglobulin kappa locus-or-what has been learned from looking closely at one-tenth of a percent of the human genome. *Gene* **135:**167–173.

Immunoglobulin Quantification and Viscosity Measurement

JEFFREY S. WARREN

8

Quantification of intact immunoglobulins has proven useful in the evaluation of patients with suspected immunodeficiency syndromes, B-cell and plasma cell neoplastic diseases, allergic conditions, and chronic inflammatory and autoimmune disorders. The armamentarium of quantitative immunoglobulin assays was initially extended by the development of immunoglobulin light-chain assays and more recently by the development of free (unbound) immunoglobulin light-chain assays. Despite important advances in immunoglobulin and light-chain quantification methods, there remain technical complexities that can influence proper clinical usage. Equally important, even when measurements are straightforward, is the need for a thorough understanding of the clinical indications for, and limitations to, immunoglobulin measurement.

Viscosity is the resistance of a fluid to flow. A wide variety of clinical conditions can affect the viscosity of blood (25). While abnormalities of the formed elements of blood (e.g., polycythemia and extreme leukocytosis) can result in clinically significant hyperviscosity, the overwhelmingly most common explanation for hyperviscosity is an abnormality in structure and/or concentration of immunoglobulin. There are several methods available for the measurement of whole-blood, plasma, and serum viscosity. It is important to understand the uses and limitations of whole-blood, plasma, and serum viscosity measurements and how each is reported.

This chapter is divided into three sections. The first section provides a brief review of immunoglobulin structure, important because of its direct relevance to quantitative immunoglobulin measurement. The second section provides a review of assay methods, issues related to quality control and assurance, and test validation, as well as a brief discussion of the clinical application of immunoglobulin measurements. A new development since the 6th edition of this manual has been the advent of free-light-chain assays. Finally, the third section addresses both technical and clinical aspects of viscosity measurement.

IMMUNOGLOBULIN STRUCTURE

Knowledge of immunoglobulin structure is important to understanding measurements of intact immunoglobulins and free light chains as well as in clinical viscometry. Basic antibody function (i.e., antigen binding) was recognized for years before the elucidation of immunoglobulin structure (1).

Early studies of antibody binding to highly purified carbohydrate antigens led to the deduction that antibody was composed of protein. The development of clinical electrophoresis led to the further recognition that antibody migrated largely within the gamma region of serum proteins, hence the names "gamma globulin" and "immunoglobulin" (34). In 1952, Colonel Ogden Bruton, a pediatrician, used serum protein electrophoresis to evaluate a boy suffering from recurrent bacterial infections (6). Recognition that the gamma fraction of protein was absent, coupled with the boy's favorable response to injections of gamma globulin from healthy humans, supported the conclusion that this serum fraction was important in host defense and led to the definition of a specific immunodeficiency syndrome (Bruton's agammaglobulinemia). Recognition of monoclonal immunoglobulins as the uniform product of clonal proliferations of neoplastic B lymphocytes and plasma cells was important in the understanding of such diseases as multiple myeloma and Waldenström's macroglobulinemia.

In contrast to serum alpha and beta globulins, which are composites of structurally homogeneous proteins (e.g., alpha-1 antiproteinase, transferrin, and complement protein 3), immunoglobulins are structurally heterogeneous (11, 17). This structural heterogeneity is accounted for at several levels. There are five major immunoglobulin classes, each different in both structure and function (Table 1). Subclasses within immunoglobulin G (IgG) (Table 2), IgA, and IgM also contribute to immunoglobulin heterogeneity, as do allotypic variations in both heavy- and light-chain structure. Overwhelmingly, however, the great heterogeneity of structure reflects the vast array of different amino acid sequences within the variable and hypervariable regions of immunoglobulin molecules. One of the pivotal scientific advances in the history of immunology was the elucidation of the molecular mechanisms responsible for the generation of antibody and immunoglobulin diversity (35) (see chapter 7). It is important to remember these different levels as contributors to the structural heterogeneity of immunoglobulins because they warrant consideration both in the quantitation of polyclonal immunoglobulins by class (e.g., total IgG or IgM) and in the quantitation of monoclonal immunoglobulins (e.g., in patients with multiple myeloma). The general structure of an intact immunoglobulin molecule includes two heavy chains (gamma, alpha, mu, delta, or epsilon), two light chains (kappa or lambda) (Table 1),

TABLE 1 Characteristics of immunoglobulins

Nomenclature	IgG	IgA	IgM	IgD	IgE
Heavy-chain class	Gamma	Alpha	Mu	Delta	Epsilon
Heavy-chain subclasses	1, 2, 3, 4	1, 2	1, 2		
Light-chain types	Kappa and lambda	Kappa and lambda	Kappa and lambda	Kappa and lambda	Kappa and lambda
Physical characteristics					
Molecular mass (Da)	143,000–160,000	159,000–447,000	900,000	177,000–185,000	187,000–200,000
Sedimentation coefficient					
(Svedberg units)	6.7–7.0	7.5–9.0	18–19	6.9–7.0	7.9–8.0
Functional characteristics					
Serum half-life (days)	7–23	5–6	5	2–8	1–5
Complement fixation[a]	+	−	+ +	−	−
Placental transfer[a]	+	−	−	−	−
Reaginic activity[a]	±	−	−	−	+ +

[a] ±, borderline; +, present; + +, strong activity; −, no activity.

and bridging disulfide bonds (chapter 7). Within each heavy and light chain are N-terminal variable and hypervariable (antigen-binding) domains and C-terminal constant domains. Antibody structure is best understood in the context of the genetic and molecular bases for structural and functional diversity (chapter 7).

Pioneering studies of antibody structure, carried out in the 1950s and 1960s (11, 28, 30), provided important insight into antibody function and resulted in immunoglobulin subunit nomenclature that is still in use. In 1958, Porter (30) digested rabbit gamma globulin with the enzyme papain. Separation of the digestion products on the basis of charge density revealed two identical antigen-binding fragments (Fab) and one fragment that could be crystallized (Fc). The Fab fragments had sedimentation coefficients of 3.5S. The fact that the Fc fragment could be crystallized provided evidence that it was biochemically homogeneous. Digestion of purified antibody with pepsin yielded a different set of fragments. The largest, which has a sedimentation coefficient of 5S, had an antigen-binding valence of 2, hence its designation, F(ab')$_2$. Reduction of the disulfide bonds that held F(ab')$_2$ fragments intact led to the formation of two fragments that resembled Fab. In 1961, Edelman and Poulik reported that reduction of intact immunoglobulin molecules led to the formation of two so-called "heavy" chains and two so-called "light" chains (11).

As noted above, the Fab domains of immunoglobulin molecules are structurally variable and responsible for antigen binding. In contrast, the Fc domain determines the biological function of a given immunoglobulin molecule. As summarized in Table 1, the biological functions of immunoglobulins are diverse, including such characteristics as complement fixation (e.g., IgG and IgM), placental transfer (IgG), high-affinity

cytophilic binding to mast cells (IgG4 and IgE), etc. (28). IgM generally circulates as a pentamer that consists of five covalently linked IgM monomers with an antigen-binding valence of 10. IgA occurs as a monomer in serm weighing 160,000 Da with a valence of 2. In secretions, IgA can occur as a multimer, usually a dimer.

Light chains (kappa and lambda) each possess an N-terminal 110-amino-acid variable region and a C-terminal 107-amino-acid constant domain. By analogy, heavy chains (gamma, alpha, mu, epsilon, and delta) each possess a 110-amino-acid N-terminal variable region and, depending on the particular class, >330-amino-acid constant regions. Structurally apposed light- and heavy-chain variable regions form an antigen-binding site. It is useful to think of the antigen-binding (Fab) region of an immunoglobulin molecule as a hand that grasps a uniquely shaped doorknob (antigen). Finally, as alluded to above, the genetic and molecular bases for immunoglobulin structure and antibody diversity have been studied intensively (chapter 7) (15, 35). Kappa light chains are encoded on chromosomal band 2p11, lambda light chains are encoded on 22q11, and the heavy-chain loci are encoded on chromosome 14. A highly regulated series of DNA recombination and splicing steps are required to generate intact immunoglobulin molecules (15, 35). Immunoglobulins are produced only by B lymphocytes and plasma cells.

IMMUNOGLOBULIN CLASSES

IgG is the predominant class of serum immunoglobulins. More than 60% of circulating IgG is IgG1, with IgG2, IgG3, and IgG4, in that order, present in decreasing concentrations (Table 2) (31). Except for IgG3, which has a serum half-life of 1 week, the IgG subclasses have half-lives of 2 to 3 weeks. IgG antibodies comprise the most important effector class of molecules in a secondary or anamnestic humoral immune response. Among large populations of B lymphocytes that express different cell surface IgG molecules, high-avidity antigen binding provides a selective advantage for clonal proliferation (14). As a result, as a humoral immune response "matures," higher proportions of IgG antibodies exhibit a high degree of antigenic specificity.

IgA is the most important immunoglobulin in the mucosal host defense system. Mucosal IgA exists chiefly as dimers covalently linked by J chains (14). A 60-kDa peptide called the secretory piece is necessary for IgA to be secreted by the various types of epithelial cells that line the mucosa.

TABLE 2 Characteristics of IgG subclasses

Property	IgG1	IgG2	IgG3	IgG4
Concn in serum (g/liter)	1.8–7.8	1.0–4.6	0.3–1.4	0.08–1.8
Half-life (days)	14–23	14–23	7–8	14–23
Complement fixation	Strong	Weak	Strong	None
Phagocyte binding (via Fc receptors)	Yes	No	Yes	No
Associated with allergies	No	No	No	Yes

IgA, like all immunoglobulins, is produced by B lymphocytes and plasma cells but is transported across mucosal epithelial layers (from the abluminal to the luminal side). As noted in Table 1, IgA exists as IgA1 and IgA2, the former being present in a higher concentration in serum and each having a half-life of 4 to 5 days.

Serum IgM circulates chiefly in the form of pentamers. Each monomeric subunit includes two mu heavy chains, which in turn each possess an extra constant-region domain. As a result, pentameric IgM has a molecular mass of approximately 900 kDa. IgM is the first immunoglobulin class to be expressed on B cells during lymphocyte development, and it is the predominant immunoglobulin class in a primary humoral response (14).

IgD circulates in very low concentrations. Like IgM, B-cell surface IgD is expressed early in lymphocyte development (14). Monomeric IgD consists of two heavy chains (each 62 kDa) and two identical kappa or lambda light chains. The biological role of serum IgD is unknown, and clinical measurement of IgD has no value except for the rare patient with either an IgD-secreting neoplasm (e.g., multiple myeloma) or the equally rare patient with a familial hyper-IgD fever syndrome.

The clinical use of IgE measurements is discussed in greater detail in section M, which describes allergic diseases. Serum IgE molecules circulate as monomers that consist of two epsilon chains that each weigh 70 kDa and two identical kappa or lambda light chains. Like IgM, IgE contains an extra constant-region domain. While IgE is normally present in low concentrations, elevated IgE concentrations are seen in a wide variety of allergic and autoimmune diseases. In contrast to total IgE measurements, antigen-specific IgE measurements are widely used in the evaluation and management of patients with specific atopic disorders. Cytophilic IgE binds to mast cells and basophils via very high affinity Fcε receptors. Activation of such cells via IgE-specific antigen binding results in the rapid release of vasoactive mediators that can cause localized swelling and/or a generalized, sometimes life-threatening reaction (anaphylaxis) (14, 16).

MEASUREMENT OF IMMUNOGLOBULINS

Quantification of IgG, IgA, and IgM in clinical laboratories is currently almost exclusively performed by automated nephelometric or immunoturbidimetric assay systems (8). Application of nephelometry and immunoturbidimetry to immunoglobulin measurement represents a trend away from more labor-intensive manual methods such as radial immunodiffusion (RID) and the Laurell rocket technique (18). Likewise, most serum kappa and lambda light-chain measurements and total IgE measurements are also carried out using automated nephelometric or dedicated immunoturbidimetric assay systems (9). In contrast, more than 20% of clinical laboratories that participated in the 2004 College of American Pathologists proficiency testing survey program used a RID method for IgG subclass measurements, and nearly all laboratories that measured total IgD employed a RID assay (8).

Nephelometric assays are based on rate reactions in which antigen, in this case an immunoglobulin such as IgG, is injected into a reaction chamber with an antigen-specific antibody (13). As antigen-antibody complexes form in suspension, they are interrogated with an intense light source. Photons are reflected (30° to 90°) from the immune complexes, where they are quantified with a photomultiplier tube. The rise in light signal intensity as a function of time

(in milliseconds) is determined by the concentrations of antigen and antibody. Rate nephelometers are sophisticated instruments that perform duplicate assays, can exhibit high throughput, and are programmed to employ multiple dilutions of antigen or antibody, thus allowing for a near-optimal precipitin-forming rate reaction. While rate nephelometers are quite accurate, abberant results can occur as the result of antigen excess effects. This may be particularly pronounced when measuring an analyte that has a relatively low normal concentration (e.g., IgG4 subclass). Such antigen excess effects can fail the instrument-derived antigen excess check. When measuring IgG subclasses it is a useful check to add up the concentrations of all four subclasses to see if their total approximates the total IgG concentration. Immunoturbidimetric assays are formatted similarly, but rather than relying upon the quantitation of reflected light, they rely on the blockade light transmission (180°) through the suspension of immune complexes being formed by antigen and reagent antibody (29, 33).

Nephelometric and immunoturbidimetric assay systems have had a large economic impact on clinical laboratories because they are automated, can be used to assay many different analytes with a single platform, and allow higher throughput. As a result, employment of these methods yields a lower cost per test in laboratories that process significant volumes.

RID assays entail addition of reagent antibody to warm (50°C) agarose while it is in the liquid state (12, 27). Liquefied antibody-containing agarose is poured into a flat plastic container and allowed to cool to room temperature. Wells are then cut into the solidified agarose. Standard dilutions of known concentrations of antigen, in this case, immunoglobulin such as IgG, are placed into multiple wells. Serum samples that contain patient IgG to be measured are placed in other wells. As the antigen (IgG) diffuses in all directions from the wells, a visible antigen-antibody precipitin reaction forms where antigen and antibody reach equivalence. The concentration of the unknown analyte, in this case serum IgG, can be calculated by comparing the diameter of the precipitin ring to those of the standard curve generated by the serially diluted known concentrations of antigen added to different wells. Typically, a 5-$\log_{10}$ dilution standard curve is employed (12, 29). The diameters measured from precipitin rings formed by patient samples can be interpolated from the standard curve. RID offers the advantages that it is simple and requires very little equipment. The major disadvantages are that RID assays are manual, take 16 to 48 h to run, and are often very expensive. Technical artifacts attributable to lipids or monomeric IgM or IgA can lead to inaccurate results. When reagent antibody is monoclonal, as in the many IgG subclass assays, the per-test cost can be extraordinarily high. Inherent in RID immunoglobulin assays are higher coefficients of variation than those observed for nephelometric and immunoturbidimetric methods (greater than 10% versus less than or equal to 7.9%).

The Laurell rocket technique is very similar to RID except that the diffusion phase of the assay is accelerated from hours (typically 16 to 48) to minutes by the application of an electrophoretic field (26). While the end point is still the formation of a precipitin line (antigen-antibody complexes in agarose), the geometry is changed from a circle to that of a rocket-shaped arc, hence the designation "rocket." With the Laurell technique, the height of the precipitin rocket is proportional to the antigen concentration. As in the RID technique, a standard curve is constructed by running multiple known dilutions of a standard antigen preparation. Again, immunoglobulin concentrations in patient samples are calculated based on interpolation from the standard curve. While Laurell rocket electrophoresis is faster than RID, the remaining shortcomings still apply.

FREE-LIGHT-CHAIN MEASUREMENT

The detection of free monoclonal immunoglobulin light chains in serum and/or urine is fraught with technical and practical challenges. Identification of free monoclonal light chains in the serum of patients with multiple myeloma or light-chain (AL)-type amyloidosis is limited, especially early in the course of the disease, because these proteins, by virtue of their low molecular mass (less than 25,000 Da), are filtered by the glomerulus and subsequently reabsorbed by the proximal tubular epithelial cells. Accordingly, serum protein electrophoresis may reveal no apparent abnormality. The diagnostic yield is increased substantially by also screening urine for such Bence Jones proteins (monoclonal free light chains). Again, low concentrations of Bence Jones proteins may be missed early in disease because proximal tubular reabsorption of such clonal proteins is relatively efficient either until the quantities of protein increase and exceed the reabsorptive capacity of the tubular epithelium or until tubular damage (acquired Fanconi syndrome) occurs and there is increased excretion of Bence Jones proteins.

Bradwell et al. (4) developed a highly sensitive immunoassay for the quantification of free immunoglobulin light chains in both urine and serum. Affinity-purified antibodies that react specifically with free light chains, but not bound light chains, are linked to the surface of latex particles which in turn form aggregates when incubated with free light chains. Employment of such particles in automated immunoturbidimetric analyzers has led to the development of a robust assay system that can be used in clinical practice. Because free kappa and lambda (polyclonal) light chains are normally present in serum and urine, it is necessary to report results of the free-light-chain assay in terms of a ratio of free kappa to free lambda. The existence of a significant clonal increase in either free kappa or free lambda light chains will distort this ratio.

The serum and urine free-light-chain assays have been proposed to be useful as a screening test, as a means to monitor response to therapy, and as a means to assess disease progression and/or relapse (3). In addition, a recent study suggests that this assay yields an abnormal free kappa/lambda ratio for most patients with nonsecretory myelomas (10). Finally, the presence of Bence Jones proteins (clonal free light chains in urine) in patients with monoclonal gammopathy of undetermined significance has been reported to predict a greater risk of progression to myeloma (2).

The addition of sensitive and specific free-light-chain assays to the armamentarium of laboratory tests available for the diagnosis and management of patients suspected to have myeloma, Waldenström's macroglobulinemia, monoclonal gammopathy of undetermined significance, B-cell leukemias and lymphomas, and AL-type amyloidosis is an exciting prospect. It will be critical for clinical studies to address specific potential applications of these assays. Particular attention will need to be paid to comparisons between free-light-chain assays and optimally used "traditional" assays. For example, it will be appropriate to compare sensitivities and specificities of free-light-chain assays to those of serum *and* urine immunofixation assays, not serum *or* urine immunofixation assays. Likewise, it will be important to assess the impact of sensitive free-light-chain assays on outcomes for patients. Serum and urine free-light-chain assays are Food and Drug Administration cleared for use in the diagnosis and monitoring of patients with B-cell and plasma cell neoplasms and collagen vascular diseases such as systemic lupus erythematosus (3). However, important utilization questions remain to be answered.

CLINICAL ASPECTS OF IMMUNOGLOBULIN MEASUREMENT

Serum immunoglobulin concentrations vary widely in children and adults (19). Very low concentrations of IgG, IgA, and IgM are observed in the sera of healthy infants approximately 6 months after birth. Immunoglobulin concentrations in a newborn are nearly equal to those observed in adults as a result of transplacental passage from the mother. These immunoglobulin concentrations then decline to a nadir at approximately 6 months of age. Normal ranges of immunoglobulins rise progressively until adult concentrations are reached during adolescence. It is important to apply age-specific reference ranges when one interprets quantitative immunoglobulin measurements in prepubertal children.

There are a variety of congenital and acquired immunodeficiency disorders that are characterized by hypogammaglobulinemia (14). Depending upon the underlying etiology and accompanying abnormalities, humoral immunodeficiency syndromes are often accompanied by specific clinical findings and/or manifestations. In general, patients with humoral immunoglobulin deficiencies are at risk for bacterial infections caused by high-grade encapsulated bacteria such as *Streptococcus pneumoniae* and *Haemophilus influenzae* (23). Detailed discussion of humoral immunodeficiency syndromes is beyond the scope of this chapter. Children suspected of suffering from Bruton's (X-linked) agammaglobulinemia and adults suspected of suffering from common variable immunodeficiency will typically exhibit markedly subnormal concentrations of IgG, IgA, and IgM in serum. The most common congenital humoral immunodeficiency disorder is selective IgA deficiency, which affects approximately 1 in 700 adults (14). Many of these patients are asymptomatic, but some suffer from recurrent mucosal infections and/or autoimmune phenomena. A subset of selective IgA deficiency patients exhibit concomitant IgG subclass deficiency. Aggressive treatment of patients with various neoplastic and autoimmune diseases has resulted in many individuals with acquired humoral immunodeficiencies. Like patients with congenital humoral immunodeficiency disorders, these individuals are at risk of high-grade bacterial infections. Likewise, multiple myeloma is frequently accompanied by both the presence of a monoclonal immunoglobulin spike (M protein) and suppression of polyclonal gamma globulin (see below).

A vast array of chronic inflammatory and infectious diseases is accompanied by polyclonal increases in immunoglobulin concentration. In these settings there is usually value in specific quantitative measurements of IgG, IgA, or IgM. Serum protein electrophoresis, accompanied by a densitometric measurement of the total gamma globulin concentration, will usually suffice as a means to assess the humoral immune system and to rule out the possibility of an underlying monoclonal gammopathy.

The great majority of patients with multiple myeloma and Waldenström's macroglobulinemia have monoclonal increases in immunoglobulins in serum, urine, or both (21). Serum and urine protein electrophoresis and immunofixation are important in the establishment of the presence of such an M protein (19–22, 24). Typically, smaller paraprotein immunoglobulin spikes are frequently seen in patients with B-cell lymphoproliferative conditions (e.g., chronic lymphocytic leukemia), monoclonal gammopathy of undetermined significance, AL-type amyloidosis, M-protein-associated peripheral neuropathy, and posttransplantation lymphoproliferative disorder. In many cases, the presence of a monoclonal protein will be obvious when serum or urine protein electrophoresis is performed. Performance of serum and/or urine immunofixation allows maximal sensitivity and will allow identification of the M protein. It is important to remember that many patients with light-chain-type myeloma will not exhibit a serum M-protein spike but will possess urine Bence Jones proteins (18, 21, 24). Once an M protein is identified and characterized, densitometric quantification of the spike remains the best available means by which to monitor the monoclonal protein (7, 22). As discussed above, the precise clinical roles for free monoclonal light-chain assays remain to be clearly defined.

VISCOSITY MEASUREMENT

Viscosity is the resistance of a fluid to flow. Abnormalities of the formed elements of blood (e.g., increased red blood cell mass, decreased red blood cell deformability, and changes in properties and/or numbers of white blood cells) or abnormalities in plasma proteins (e.g., increased immunoglobulin concentration) can cause hyperviscosity. While emerging technologies such as laser Doppler velocimetry and mass-detecting sensors (32) promise to change clinical viscometry, most laboratories continue to employ either Ostwald, Wells-Brookfield, or falling-drop viscometers.

Ostwald viscometers are based on the relationship between fluid viscosity and the rate of flow through a fixed wall narrow-bore tube. The greater the viscosity of either anticoagulated whole blood, plasma, or serum, the lower the rate of flow. Typically, the flow rate of the sample of interest is compared to a standard (e.g., that of water). The Wells-Brookfield viscometer employs a stationary plate (sample cup) and a cone (needle) that is rotated within the cup by an electric meter at a constant speed and temperature (5). The fluid sample is placed in the cup in which the cone rotates. The greater the viscosity of the fluid, the greater the torque generated. In turn, the torque is measured with a torque meter and translated into "viscosity." Falling-drop viscometry is based on the fact that particulates fall more slowly through a viscous fluid than through a less viscous fluid. Viscosity of biological samples is typically reported in centipoise; normal plasma viscosity is approximately 1.35 to 1.85 cP. Water exhibits a viscosity of 1.0 cP at 37°C. Whole-blood viscosity can also be expressed as "equivalent hematocrit of whole blood viscosity," which is the viscosity equivalent to that exhibited by anticoagulated whole blood at the given hematocrit. Clinical interpretation of "equivalent hematocrit" requires an actual hematocrit measurement for comparison. For example, a patient with hyperviscosity due to a high concentration of a monoclonal paraprotein might exhibit a hematocrit equivalent of 55% and an actual hematocrit of 40%. In this case the "excess" viscosity would be attributable to the paraprotein. Conversely, a patient with polycythemia and hyperviscosity might exhibit a hematocrit equivalent of whole-blood viscosity of 55% and an actual hematocrit of 55%. In this case, the "excess" viscosity would be attributable to the increase in red blood cell mass. Charts are available that display the mathematical relationship between hematocrit and viscosity of whole blood (5).

CLINICAL ASPECTS OF VISCOSITY MEASUREMENT

The most common cause of hyperviscosity is the presence of a paraprotein. More than 80% of cases of hyperviscosity are associated with Waldenström's macroglobulinemia and an IgM paraprotein. IgM molecules have a high molecular weight as well as a shape that increases their intrinsic viscosity. IgA paraproteins, less commonly, IgG paraproteins, and, rarely, monoclonal light chains can also result in hyperviscosity (25). Increases in red blood cell mass (e.g., polycythemia), abnormal deformability of red blood cells (e.g., hemoglobinopathies), and very high white blood cell counts (e.g., chronic lymphocytic leukemia) can result in increases in whole-blood viscosity. As alluded to above, hyperviscosity attributable to a paraprotein would increase both whole-blood and plasma or serum viscosity, while abnormalities of formed elements affect whole-blood viscosity but not plasma or serum viscosity.

Symptoms and signs of hyperviscosity include fatigue, blurred vision, headache, tinnitus, decreased hearing, vertigo, paresthesias, segmental dilation of retinal veins, retinal hemorrhage, mucosal bleeding, nystagmus, ataxia, somnolence, stupor, and coma (25). Individual patients exhibit different thresholds, but symptoms and signs of hyperviscosity typically occur when whole-blood viscosity exceeds 4 cP. Serum protein electrophoresis, immunofixation, a complete blood count with differential, and review of a peripheral blood smear will nearly always elucidate the underlying cause of hyperviscosity. In the great majority of cases of clinically significant hyperviscosity, the underlying etiology has previously been established (e.g., Waldenström's macroglobulinemia and multiple myeloma).

REFERENCES

1. **Abbas, A. K., and C. A. Janeway, Jr.** 2000. Immunology: improving on nature in the twenty-first century. *Cell* **100:** 129–138.
2. **Baldini, L., A. Guffanti, B. M. Cesana, M. Colombi, O. Chiorboli, I. Damilano, and A. T. Maiolo.** 1996. Role of different haematological variables in defining the risk of malignant transformation in monoclonal gammopathy. *Blood* **87:**912–918.
3. **The Binding Site, Ltd.** 2003. *Serum Free Light Chain Analysis*, p. 1–6. The Binding Site Ltd., Birmingham, United Kingdom.
4. **Bradwell, R. M., H. D. Carr-Smith, G. P. Mead, L. X. Tang, P. J. Showell, M. T. Drayson, and R. Drew.** 2001. Highly sensitive automated immunoassay for immunoglobulin free light chains in serum and urine. *Clin. Chem.* **47:**673–680.
5. **Brookfield Engineering Laboratories, Inc.** 2003. More solutions to sticky problems, p. 1–17. Brookfield Engineering Laboratories, Inc., Middleboro, Mass.
6. **Bruton, O. C.** 1952. Agammaglobulinemia. *Pediatrics* **9:**722–727.
7. **Bush, D., and D. F. Keren.** 1992. Over- and underestimation of monoclonal gammopathies by quantification of kappa- and lambda-containing immunoglobulins in serum. *Clin. Chem.* **38:**315–316.
8. **College of American Pathologists.** 2004. *CAP Survey S2-B, 2004.* College of American Pathologists, Chicago, Ill.
9. **College of American Pathologists.** 2004. *CAP Survey SE-B, 2004.* College of American Pathologists, Chicago, Ill.
10. **Drayson, M., L. X. Tang, R. Drew, G. P. Mead, H. Carr-Smith, and A. R. Bradwell.** 2001. Serum free light chain measurements for identifying and monitoring patients with non-secretory multiple myeloma. *Blood* **97:**2900–2902.
11. **Edelman, G. M., and M. D. Poulik.** 1961. Studies on structural units of the gamma globulins. *J. Exp. Med.* **113:**867–884.

12. **Fahey, J., and E. M. McKelvey.** 1965. Quantitative determination of serum immunoglobulins in antibody-agar plates. *J. Immunol.* **94:**84–91.

13. **Finely, P. R.** 1982. Nephelometry: principles and clinical laboratory applications. *Lab. Management* **20**(9):34.

14. **Goronzy, J. J., and C. M. Weyand.** 2004. The innate and adaptive immune systems, p. 208–217. *In* L. Goldman and D. Ausiello (ed.), *Cecil Textbook of Medicine,* 22nd ed. The W. B. Saunders Co., Philadelphia, Pa.

15. **Honjo, T.** 1982. Immunoglobulin genes. *Annu. Rev. Immunol.* **1:**489–512.

16. **Ishizaka, K.** 1989. Regulation of IgE biosynthesis. *Hospital Pract.* **9:**51–60.

17. **Kabat, E. A.** 1976. *Structural Concepts in Immunology and Immunochemistry,* 2nd ed. Holt, Rinehart, and Winston, New York, N.Y.

18. **Keren, D. F.** 1999. Procedures for the evaluation of monoclonal immunoglobulins. *Arch. Pathol. Lab. Med.* **123:**126–132.

19. **Keren, D. F.** 1998. Quantitative, electrophoretic, and immunochemical characterization of immunoglobulins and serum proteins, p. 57–65. *In* R. M. Nakamura, C. L. Burek, L. Cook, J. D. Folds, and J. L. Sever (ed.), *Clinical Diagnostic Immunology: Protocols in Quality Assurance and Standardization.* Blackwell Science, Victoria, Australia.

20. **Keren, D. F.** 1994. *High-Resolution Electrophoresis and Immunofixation,* 2nd ed. Butterworth-Heineman, Boston, Mass.

21. **Keren, D. F., R. Alexanian, J. A. Goeken, P. D. Gorevic, R. A. Kyle, and R. H. Tomar.** 1999. Guidelines for clinical and laboratory evaluation of patients with monoclonal gammopathies. *Arch. Pathol. Lab. Med.* **123:**106–107.

22. **Keren, D. F., A. C. DiSante, and S. L. Bordine.** 1986. Densitometric scanning of high-resolution electrophoresis of serum: methodology and clinical application. *Am. J. Clin. Pathol.* **85:**348–352.

23. **Kornfeld, S. J., R. N. Haire, and S. J. Strong.** 1997. Extreme variation in X-linked agammaglobulinemia phenotype in a three-generation family. *J. Allergy Clin. Immunol.* **100:**702–706.

24. **Kyle, R. A.** 1999. Sequence of testing for monoclonal gammopathies. Serum and urine assays. *Arch. Pathol. Lab. Med.* **123:**114–118.

25. **Kyle, R. A., and S. V. Rajkumar.** 2004. Plasma cell disorders, p. 1184–1195. *In* L. Goldman and D. Ausiello (ed.), *Cecil Textbook of Medicine,* 22nd ed. The W. B. Saunders Co., Philadelphia, Pa.

26. **Laurell, C.** 1975. The use of electroimmunoassay for determining specific proteins as a supplement to agarose gel electrophoresis. *J. Clin. Pathol. Suppl.* **6:**22–26.

27. **Mancini, G., A. O. Carbonara, and J. F. Heremans.** 1965. Immunochemical quantitation of antigens by single radial immunodiffusion. *Immunochemistry* **2:**235–254.

28. **McPherson, R. A.** 2001. Laboratory evaluation of immunoglobulin function and humoral immunity, p. 878–891. *In* J. B. Henry (ed.), *Clinical Diagnosis and Management by Laboratory Methods,* 20th ed. The W. B. Saunders Co., Philadelphia, Pa.

29. **Nakamura, R. M., E. S. Tucker, and J. H. Carlson.** 1991. Immunoassays in the clinical laboratory, p. 848–884. *In* J. B. Henry (ed.), *Clinical Diagnosis and Management by Laboratory Methods,* 17th ed. The W. B. Saunders Co., Philadelphia, Pa.

30. **Porter, R. R.** 1959. The hydrolysis of rabbit gamma globulin and antibodies with crystalline papain. *Biochem. J.* **73:**119–126.

31. **Shearer, M. H., R. D. Dark, J. Chodosh, and R. C. Kennedy.** 1999. Comparison and characterization of immunoglobulin G subclasses among primate species. *Clin. Diagn. Lab. Immunol.* **6:**953–958.

32. **Shin, S., and D.-Y. Keum.** 2002. Measurement of blood viscosity using mass-sensing sensor. *Biosensors Bioelectronics* **17:**383–388.

33. **Tiffany, T. O.** 1999. Fluorometry, nephelometry, and turbidimetry, p. 94–112. *In* C. A. Burtis and E. R. Ashwood (ed.), *Teitz Textbook of Clinical Chemistry.* The W. B. Saunders Co., Philadelphia, Pa.

34. **Tiselius, A.** 1932. A new apparatus for electrophoretic analysis of colloidal mixtures. *Trans. Faraday Soc.* **33:**524–531.

35. **Tonegawa, S.** 1983. Somatic generation of antibody diversity. *Nature* **302:**575.

Clinical Indications and Applications of Serum and Urine Protein Electrophoresis

DAVID F. KEREN AND RICHARD L. HUMPHREY

9

Serum and urine protein electrophoreses are performed to detect and measure monoclonal gammopathies (M proteins). In effect, serum and urine protein electrophoreses provide an immunochemical "biopsy" of the humoral immune system. However, a wide variety of other clinically relevant information is also available from examination of the proteins demonstrated from these studies. This chapter reviews basic principles of electrophoresis, the types of apparatus that are available, quality control and quality assurance procedures, and costs involved with the procedure and provides a wide variety of patterns with recommended interpretations.

BACKGROUND ON PROTEIN STRUCTURE

Electrophoresis of serum and urine in the clinical laboratory takes advantage of the fact that each protein has its own unique structure. Proteins are composed of amino acids, each of which contain a basic amino group ($-NH_2$), an acidic group ($-COOH$), and a sequence that is specific to each amino acid, referred to as an R group (Fig. 1). The R groups may be acidic or basic and vary in size from a single hydrogen atom, to linear or branched hydrocarbon chains, to a complex double-ring structure. The complex structural and charge characteristics of these amino acids and the unique amino acid sequence of each protein determine the position that the protein migrates to upon electrophoresis (15).

The primary structure of a protein results when amino acids connect to one another by linking the amino group of one amino acid to the carboxyl group of the next. While this covalent peptide bond is formed, a water molecule is released (Fig. 2). The resulting linear chain of amino acids is a polypeptide containing a free amino group at one end (N terminus) and a free carboxyl group at the other end (C terminus). The amino acid composition of each protein is determined by the information encoded in the individual's DNA.

As the polypeptide chains of amino acids form, a simple secondary structure is created by folding along one dimension and is held together primarily by hydrogen bonds. These may take the form of random coils, an alpha-helix, or a beta sheet. A three-dimensional tertiary structure forms as a result of several types of attachment: hydrogen bonds, disulfide bonds, van der Waals forces, and hydrophobic bonds. In more complex molecules, such as immunoglobulins, a quaternary structure forms when several polypeptide chains link together. For instance, consider the immunoglobulin M (IgM) molecule. Though classified as a single protein, it consists of 10 identical heavy chains, 10 identical light chains, and 1 joining chain, combining for a molecular mass of about 900 kDa. Finally, many proteins have carbohydrate groups attached (glycosylated) covalently. These carbohydrate groups stabilize the protein's conformation and in some circumstances help to protect it from digestion (13, 15).

Following synthesis of the protein, posttranslational modifications which convey heterogeneity to the protein may occur. These include phosphorylation, N-terminal acylation, side-chain acylation, sulfation of tyrosine, C-terminal α-amidation of glycine, and γ-carboxylation of glutamic acid (15). The ability of electrophoretic techniques to detect subtle changes in charge is illustrated by the second band that is seen in heterozygotes for $α_1$ antitrypsin variants due to substitution of a single amino acid of a different charge (Fig. 3).

The charge on the protein molecule and, consequently, its migration on serum and urine protein electrophoresis are determined both by its constituent amino acids and by the pH of the buffer used for the electrophoresis. Each protein may be defined by its isoelectric point (pI), the pH at which its positive and negative charges are equal and hence migration does not occur. At the pH of agarose gel electrophoresis, the algebraic sum of the protein's positive and negative charges determines the protein's migration. This allows the laboratory to separate the major proteins into unique bands and fractions that can be used to identify a wide variety of clinical conditions.

PRINCIPLES OF PROTEIN ELECTROPHORESIS

The first studies of serum protein electrophoresis were performed entirely in a fluid-based system devised by Arne Tiselius, winner of the 1948 Nobel Prize in Chemistry, called moving boundary electrophoresis (25). In that regard, it is similar to the most recently available technique of capillary zone electrophoresis (CZE). In his system, Tiselius layered a mixture of proteins on a buffer in a U-shaped tube with electrodes at each end of the U. The migration of the proteins through the electrical field was detected by a sensitive Schlieren band optical system. With this technique, the major protein fractions of albumin, alpha, beta, and gamma globulins were defined.

$$H_2N - \underset{\underset{R}{|}}{\overset{\overset{H}{|}}{C}} - COOH$$

FIGURE 1 General structure of an amino acid.

Zone Electrophoresis

In the late 1930s, to improve separation and allow direct visualization of the major protein fractions, filter paper was deployed as the first support medium. The filter paper was placed between two reservoirs of buffer with electrodes at each end. The protein solution was carefully applied to the filter paper, and after electrophoresis the major bands were visualized by use of a protein dye. However, the addition of this support medium introduced new variables, such as the texture of the medium, which provided resistance (that would vary according to the brand and lot) to protein migration, as well as charge effects due to endosmotic flow (19). The latter reflected the fact that the support medium itself contained a net negative charge that could not migrate, and as a consequence, the positive buffer ions would flow toward the cathode. The result was that weakly anionic proteins were pulled cathodally from the application point.

The use of cellulose acetate and agarose, which started in the 1950s and was vastly improved in the 1970s with the development of techniques with higher resolution, began techniques that are used today. These clear support media allow rapid electrophoresis, crisp separation of major protein fractions, and densitometric scanning to measure the protein fractions (18).

The simplicity of separation in a fluid-based system has been revisited in the past decade with the development of CZE. In this procedure, instead of a large, glass U-shaped tube, thin fused silica capillaries, about 25 μm in diameter, are the vessels through which the proteins pass. The narrow

$$H_2N - \underset{\underset{R1}{|}}{\overset{\overset{H}{|}}{C}} - COOH \ + \ H_2N - \underset{\underset{R2}{|}}{\overset{\overset{H}{|}}{C}} - COOH$$

$$\downarrow$$

$$H_2N - \underset{\underset{R1}{|}}{\overset{\overset{H}{|}}{C}} - \overset{\overset{O}{\|}}{C} - \underset{\underset{H}{|}}{\overset{\overset{H}{|}}{N}} - \underset{\underset{H}{|}}{\overset{\overset{R2}{|}}{C}} - COOH \ + \ H_2O$$

FIGURE 2 Peptide bond formation between two amino acids.

capillaries create a huge negatively charged surface area that results in a strong endosmotic flow toward the cathode. At a strong alkaline pH, the proteins are pulled by the endosmotic flow past a UV detector (using a 200- or 215-nm wavelength) that records the amount of each protein fraction on an electropherogram (resembling a densitometric scan) and is able to convert the values to a virtual gel image (6, 14, 20, 21).

Unfortunately, while this mode of detection is efficient, it also detects other substances that absorb at those UV wavelengths. So far, the most frequent causes of false-positive deflections in the electropherogram have been radiocontrast dyes and occasionally antibiotics (3, 7, 8, 10). Radiocontrast dyes and some antibiotics can produce suspicious bands anywhere from the transthyretin (prealbumin) area through the γ region (Table 1).

One key feature of the evolution in electrophoresis systems has been the improvement in resolution. With the development of clear cellulose acetate gels in the 1950s, densitometric scans could distinguish five major protein fractions, with the bands in each fraction being relatively

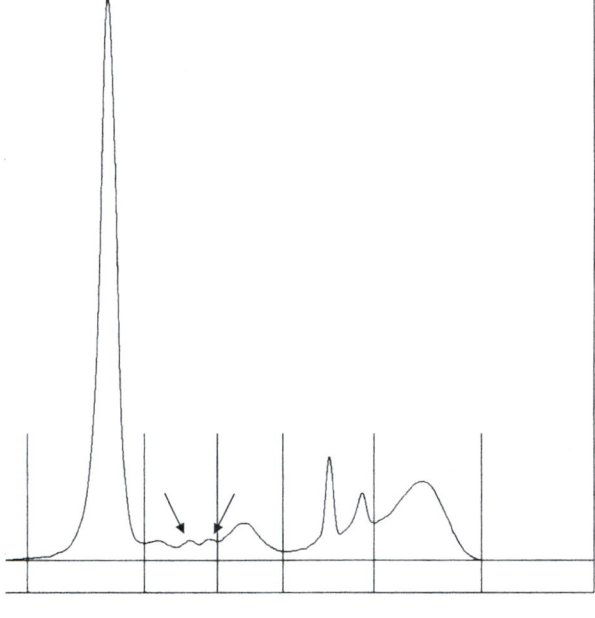

ALBUMIN	53.8		4.57	
ALPHA 1	5.4		0.46	
ALPHA 2	6.7		0.57	
BETA	13.2		1.12	+
GAMMA	21.0	++	1.79	+++

Reference Ranges

	Rel %		g/dL	
ALBUMIN	52.6	- 68.9	3.80 -	5.20
ALPHA 1	3.6	- 8.1	0.30 -	0.60
ALPHA 2	5.3	- 12.2	0.40 -	0.90
BETA	8.3	- 14.3	0.60 -	1.10
GAMMA	8.2	- 18.6	0.60 -	1.40

TP: 6.40 - 8.20   A/G: 1.20 - 2.20

FIGURE 3 Serum electropherogram for a patient who is heterozygous for α_1 antitrypsin (PIMS). Rel, relative; TP, total protein; A/G, albumin-to-globulin ratio.

TABLE 1 Locations of radiocontrast spikes in CZE[a]

Location	Name	Substance
Prealbumin	Bilisegrol	Meglumine iotroxate
α_2 globulin		
Anodal	Gastrografin	Sodium-meglumine
	Urangiografin	Meglumine amidotrizoate
Mid-region	Telebrix	Ioxitaalamic acid
	Xenetix	Iobitridol
Cathodal	Iopamiro	Ioamidol
	Omnitrast and Omnipaque	Iohexol
	Ultravist	Iopromide
β_2 globulin		
Anodal	Hexabrix	Sodium-meglumine ioxaglate
Mid-region	Optiray	Ioversol
	Iomeron	Iomeprol

[a] Data are from the work of Arranz-Peña et al. (3).

diffuse. Further improvements enhanced the ability to distinguish small M proteins or genetic variants (such as α_1 antitrypsin) that were difficult or impossible to see by previous techniques (Fig. 4). Improvements have included enclosed systems that prevent evaporation of buffer, helping to keep the ionic concentration of the buffer constant; the addition of calcium lactate to buffer; the use of thin gels; and the use of cooling devices to control heat production.

Guidelines for the diagnosis of monoclonal gammopathies recommend use of electrophoretic systems that provide crisp separation of the β_1 from the β_2 region and which are able to recognize M proteins at concentrations as low as 0.05 gm/dl in the γ region (2, 16).

With currently available manual agarose systems, excess moisture needs to be removed from the surface of the gel prior to application of the sample. After blotting, in most manual systems, 3 to 5 µl of sample is applied to uniform narrow slits in a plastic template. However, with semiautomated systems, the samples may be placed in a well connected to special paper that wicks the sample to its sharp edge, which is applied directly to the surface of the gel. With some urine samples with particulate matter and serum with IgM monoclonal gammopathies, there have been reports of poor application (7, 17). The manufacturer recommends centrifuging the urine in such cases and observing that the paper moistens all the way to the sharp edge. In addition, we recommend always comparing the total protein value with the observed migration to help in preventing false negatives.

Laboratories should establish their own reference ranges when adopting these techniques. While the different methods provide similar numbers, significant differences have been reported (Table 2) (9). The largest differences between the agarose gel technique and CZE occur in the α_1 region for both men and women. These differences in part reflect the considerable improvement in detection of α lipoprotein and α_1 acid glycoprotein (orosomucoid) by CZE. Nonetheless, as long as the appropriate ranges are established for each technique, there should be good agreement in the interpretation of the results obtained (22).

QUALITY CONTROL AND QUALITY ASSURANCE

Specimen Requirements for Serum

For serum testing, the blood sample should be drawn into a Vacutainer tube without anticoagulant. After clotting, the serum is separated and stored at 4°C for up to 72 h. Although serum can be used after 72 h, C3 will deteriorate, changing the quantity of protein in the β_2 region of the electrophoresis. If the sample is to be held longer than 72 h before electrophoresis, freezing the sample at −20°C preserves the C3 for future study.

Proper samples are important because interferences can provide special problems for interpretation. Hemolysis will provide a broadly migrating band in the α_2-β region reflecting the presence of hemoglobin-haptoglobin complexes. This may obscure or even mimic an M protein in this region. Lipemic samples may not absorb effectively into a gel and may not be taken up by the thin capillaries used in CZE. Centrifuge and insert the pipette below the floating lipid

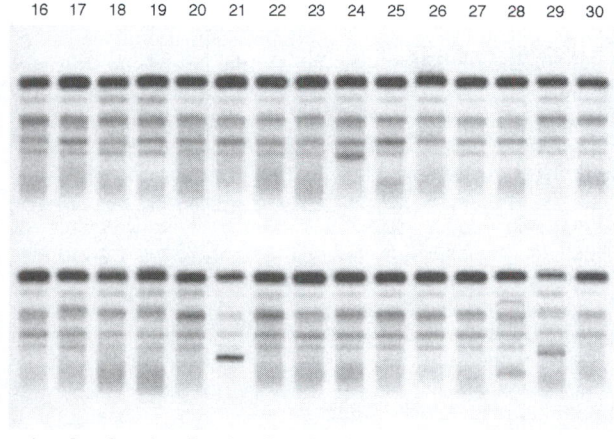

FIGURE 4 Serum protein electrophoresis on the semiautomated Sebia Hydragel 30 β_1-β_2 gel demonstrating sharp bands and a crisp separation of the β_1 (transferrin) band from the β_2 (C3) band. Samples 6, 13, 14, 24, and 25 have suspicious bands that all proved to be M proteins by immunofixation. In sample 24, the M protein (an IgA κ) migrated in the same location as the C3 (β_2) band. By comparing this band to the other C3 bands on this gel, the increase becomes more obvious.

TABLE 2 Comparison of serum protein intervals by agarose gel electrophoresis and CZE[a]

Group and fraction	Protein concn range (g/dl)	
	Agarose gel electrophoresis	CZE
Men		
Albumin	4.19–5.36	4.17–5.23
α_1	0.13–0.27	0.26–0.45
α_2	0.38–0.70	0.34–0.64
β	0.65–1.14	0.58–0.95
γ	0.49–1.21	0.53–1.32
Women		
Albumin	4.0–5.11	3.74–4.98
α_1	0.14–0.28	0.26–0.51
α_2	0.41–0.69	0.39–0.64
β	0.65–1.00	0.55–0.87
γ	0.49–1.21	0.53–1.32

[a] Data modified from those of Bossuyt et al. (9).

layer to procure the sample. To prevent interference from lipemic samples, the patient should be fasting.

Specimen Requirements for Urine

An early-morning void collected into a container without preservative is adequate for screening for the presence of monoclonal free light chains (MFLC, or Bence Jones protein) (11). The urine should be stored at 4°C until electrophoresis. Prior to electrophoresis, the sample should be concentrated to optimize the detection of MFLC. The amount of concentration necessary depends on the protein concentration of the urine. Usually, a 50- to 100-times concentration is sufficient for urine samples with relatively small amounts of protein. One approach is to place the urine sample into a commercial ultrafiltration concentrating device and allow it to be concentrated for a set period of time (one of our laboratories uses 4 h). Samples with small amounts of protein will be concentrated more rapidly, up to 100 times, whereas samples with high protein concentration will be concentrated much less. If the patient is known to have an M protein in the serum and/or an MFLC in the urine, a carefully timed 24-h urine sample should be collected in a container without preservative. Collection of the sample is key to obtaining accurate and reproducible information about the M protein. Patients should be instructed to note the time when they are ready to start their collection, to empty their bladder, and to discard this first voiding. All subsequent voidings are then saved and added to the collection. The next day, at the same time, finish the collection by including the final bit of urine in the 24-h sample. While this seems excessively compulsive, if the first sample is included, it may be including urine that has been in the bladder for as long as 8 h (effectively making this a 32-h collection). The container should be refrigerated at 4°C during the collections and until the collection is delivered to the laboratory to minimize deterioration of proteins and growth of microorganisms. The 24-h collection is needed in order to quantify the amount of MFLC, which is used in the estimation of tumor burden and the response to therapy.

Internal Controls

Each protein electrophoresis gel should have an internal control sample run on it. The percentage of protein in each fraction should be recorded and compared day to day. Even with urine protein electrophoresis, serum controls are recommended because normal urine contains only trivial amounts of protein and would not serve as an adequate estimation of the migration of proteins on the gel. The controls should be evaluated for migration positions of the major bands and for the amount of protein in each region. One convenient way to do this is by using a Levey Jennings chart (Fig. 5). For CZE systems, each channel should have such samples performed, because the separation characteristics will differ slightly from one capillary to the next.

Avoiding False-Positive Results

Unexplained bands from the α through the γ region may represent an M protein. However, before they are interpreted as being M proteins, this diagnosis should be secured by immunofixation (see chapter 10). As mentioned above, in CZE, interference from radiocontrast dyes and some antibiotics gives deflections that may be misinterpreted as M proteins (Fig. 6). Some of these, such as sulfamide sulfamethoxazole, produce a small deflection at the anodal end of albumin which would not be confused with an M protein (8, 10). Others, such as piperacillin-tazobactam (Tazocin; Wyeth), can produce a peak in the γ region. These interfering substances may be removed by desalting or use of activated charcoal (3, 5). In both CZE and gel-based electrophoresis, other proteins can produce bands that are not immunoglobulins but which do mimic an M protein. Fibrinogen, C-reactive protein, C3 variants, transferrin variants, hemoglobin-haptoglobin complexes, and markedly elevated levels of β lipoprotein can all be confused with an M protein. We recommend that all bands suspected of being M proteins be confirmed by immunofixation or immunosubtraction (see chapter 10) before being reported. One inexpensive way of ensuring that the suspected M protein is an immunoglobulin and not another interfering protein or radiocontrast dye is to use a single-lane pentavalent (anti-IgG, -IgA, -IgM, -κ, -λ) in the same serum (15). If the suspected band does not precipitate (forming an immunofixed band) with that reagent, it is not consistent with an immunoglobulin or M protein (Fig. 7).

When performing immunofixation, the specificity of the reagent antisera needs to be confirmed with each new lot. The study of the antisera should include both serum and plasma. Even though plasma is not the specimen that is

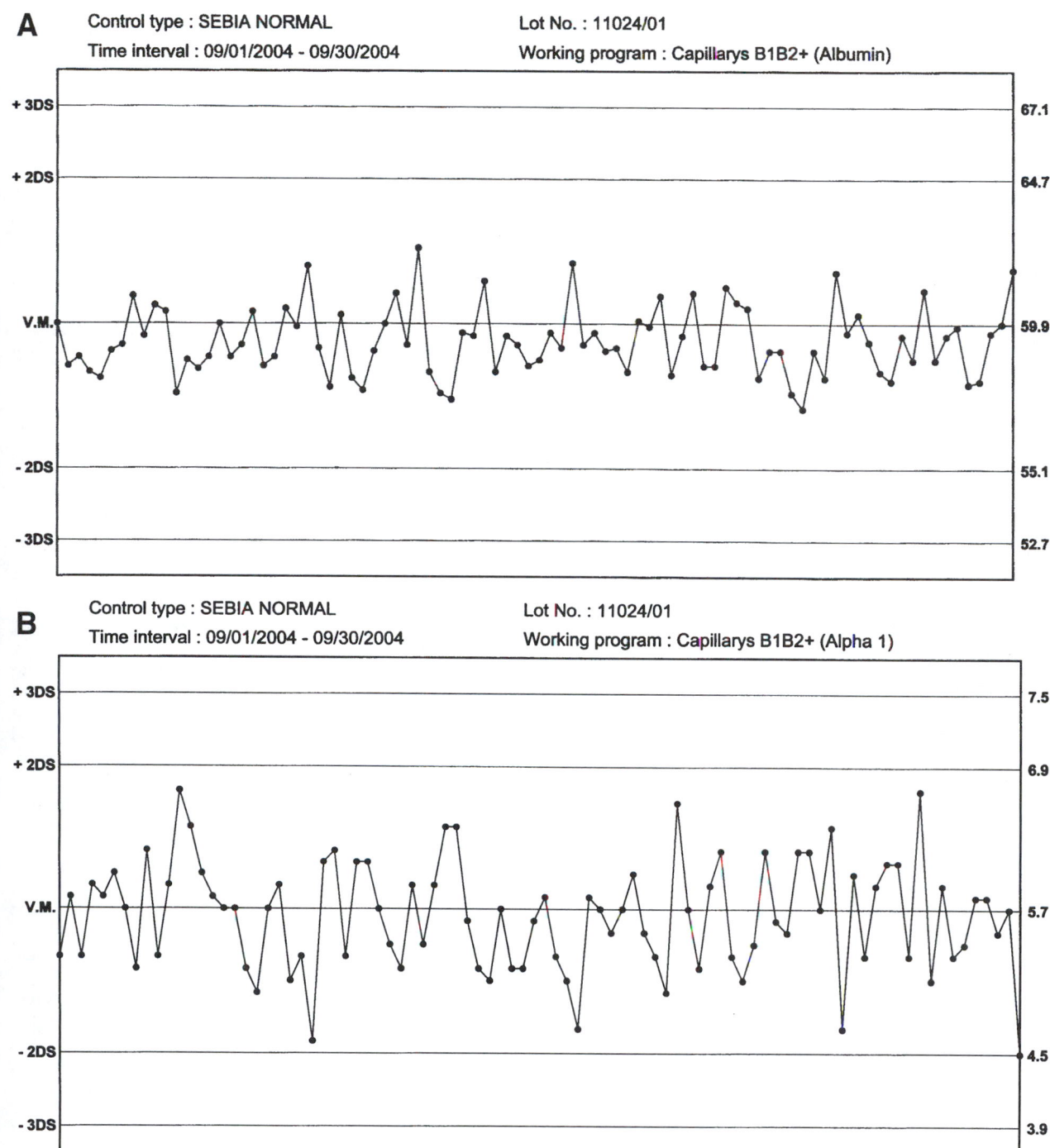

FIGURE 5 Levey Jennings charts for albumin for the month of September 2004 (top) and the α_1 fraction for the same run (bottom). More variation is seen in the α_1 fraction because of the smaller percentage of proteins present in this fraction. Nonetheless, no sample is beyond 2DS (2 standard deviations) and no trend of high or low values is evident. V.M., median value.

recommended for use, occasionally fibrinogen will be present due to the presence of anticoagulation therapy, inadequate time for the specimen to clot before the serum was removed from the clot, or drawing of the sample into a tube containing an anticoagulant. If the reagent antiserum against immunoglobulin contains reactivity for fibrinogen, a false-positive result may be recorded (23).

Good quality assurance requires coordination of all available laboratory information for the patient. A file is set up for the patient the first time that an M protein is detected in the serum or in the urine. The patient's current sample should be correlated with previous studies by using this file, for several reasons. First, the migrations of the M protein should be compared. If there is any change in migration, identification of

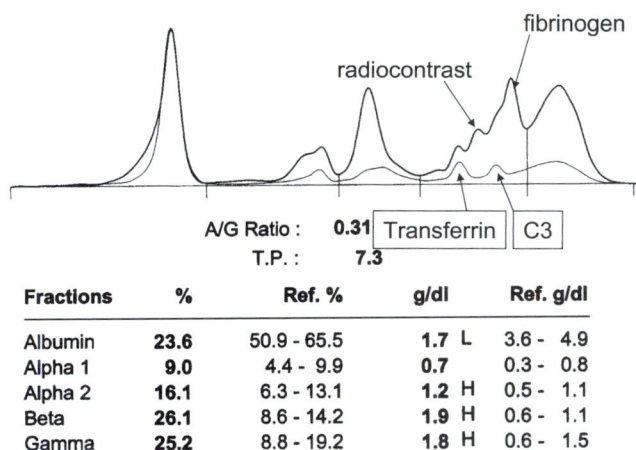

Fractions	%	Ref. %	g/dl		Ref. g/dl
Albumin	23.6	50.9 - 65.5	1.7	L	3.6 - 4.9
Alpha 1	9.0	4.4 - 9.9	0.7		0.3 - 0.8
Alpha 2	16.1	6.3 - 13.1	1.2	H	0.5 - 1.1
Beta	26.1	8.6 - 14.2	1.9	H	0.6 - 1.1
Gamma	25.2	8.8 - 19.2	1.8	H	0.6 - 1.5

A/G Ratio: **0.31** T.P.: **7.3**

FIGURE 6 A complex electropherogram pattern with a normal pattern underlaid to show the normal positions of the β-region bands. The abnormal serum shows hypoalbuminemia and anodal slurring of albumin, and the four peaks in the β region are labeled. The fibrinogen was identified by immunofixation, and the radiocontrast dye was indicated by both the lack of a band in that region by immunofixation for IgG, IgA, IgM, κ, and λ and a telephone call indicating that the patient had been given a radiocontrast dye (Table 1). Ref., reference; T.P., total protein; A/G, albumin/globulin.

the patient sample should be confirmed. If this matches, the identification of the M protein should be confirmed immunologically (by immunofixation or immunosubtraction). When a new and different M protein from that seen in the original study is identified, the clinician should be contacted to determine if the patient has had extensive chemotherapy and/or stem cell transplantation. Occasionally, new M proteins can appear in the context of these events. Otherwise, the appearance of a new M protein is distinctly unusual, so we recommend another sample to confirm that a mislabeling at the time of the sample draw has not occurred.

If the migration of the M protein matches that of the previous serum or urine sample, the amount of the M protein should be measured. The amount of the M protein is recorded on the report along with a statement as to whether it has increased, decreased, or remained unchanged since the previous sample.

Comment is also made about the remaining normal gamma globulins (Fig. 8). Suppression of the gamma globulins can be a negative prognostic indicator and, if severe enough, may predispose the patient to infections, possibly requiring gamma globulin replacement therapy (26). If the

M protein is in the gamma globulin region, our laboratory subtracts the M-protein value from the total gamma region. If the remaining gamma globulin is 0.25 g/dl or less, we comment that the normal gamma globulins are suppressed. This number derives from earlier data noting that patients with common variable immunodeficiency disease have clinical problems when the gamma globulin region is below this level. If the M-protein is in another region (α or β), the total gamma globulin is looked at to see if it is below 0.25 g/dl.

The patient's file is reviewed to see if the patient has had a recent urine sample. If the patient has a known MFLC, a follow-up urine sample is indicated periodically (depending on the aggressiveness of the process and/or therapy) to monitor the tumor burden and to help estimate the degree of damage to the nephron. Patients with monoclonal gammopathy of undetermined significance should have periodic urine and serum electrophoresis, depending on clinical judgment.

Recently, the availability of free light-chain (FLC) testing in serum and urine has been shown to be useful both in the initial detection of MFLC and in monitoring of patients with light-chain disease. The measurement of the FLC may be able to replace the 24-h urine collection to follow tumor burden in such cases after demonstration of the clonality of the process by immunofixation.

The use of external quality assurance proficiency testing is essential to compare the results from one laboratory with those of others who are using the same system in the detection of M proteins, and also to allow gauging of the effectiveness of one manufacturer's electrophoretic system to correctly identify an abnormality versus the systems provided by other manufacturers.

Cost-Effectiveness of Testing

Cost is related mainly to the number of samples assayed per day and selection of the most appropriate type of equipment used for the number of tests performed. For laboratories with relatively small volumes (two to four serum samples per day), it may be worthwhile to consider sending the test to a reference laboratory and using the resources of the laboratory for higher-volume testing or required stat testing. Laboratories

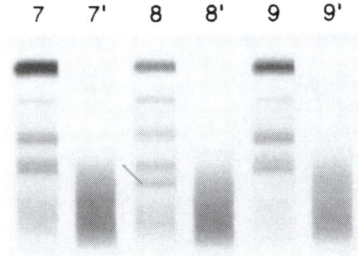

7   7'   8   8'   9   9'

FIGURE 7 Results for three serum samples. For each sample, there are two lanes; the lane on the left is a serum protein electrophoresis fixed with acid, and the lane on the right is an immunofixation with antipentavalent antisera (anti-IgG, IgA, IgM, κ, and λ). The sample in lane 8 shows a band (arrow) that does not react with antipentavalent antisera; it is fibrinogen.

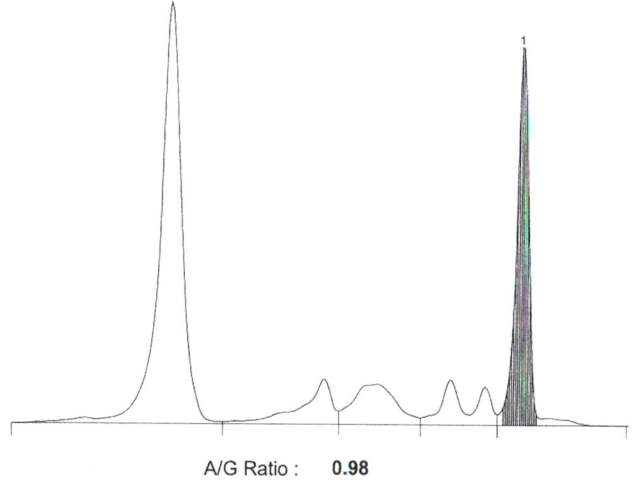

| | A/G Ratio : | 0.98 | | |
| | T.P. : | 7.8 | | |

Fractions	%	Ref. %	g/dl	Ref. g/dl
Albumin	49.6	50.9 - 65.5	3.9	3.6 - 4.9
Alpha 1	7.4	4.4 - 9.9	0.6	0.3 - 0.8
Alpha 2	9.4	6.3 - 13.1	0.7	0.5 - 1.1
Beta	7.4	8.6 - 14.2	0.6	0.6 - 1.1
Gamma	26.2	8.8 - 19.2	2.0 H	0.6 - 1.5
1	24.7		1.9	

FIGURE 8 An electropherogram with a prominent M-protein spike and suppression of the normal gamma globulin. The spike measures 1.9 g/dl, and the total gamma globulin is 2.0 g/dl. Only 0.1 g/dl is accounted for by the gamma globulin not measured in the M-protein spike. T.P., total protein; A/G, albumin/globulin; Ref., reference.

with larger volumes (5 to 10 per day) may wish to use a manual assay. Although this testing is relatively inefficient, it would allow for a more rapid turnaround time. With a volume of about 20 samples per day, a semiautomated method would decrease technologist time. At volumes of 40 or more samples per day, the bar-coded, automated CZE systems are highly efficient, with excellent resolution.

PROTEINS IDENTIFIED IN SERUM PROTEIN ELECTROPHORESIS

By use of agarose or acetate electrophoresis, serum proteins were classified as the five major regions identified by electrophoresis: albumin, α_1, α_2, β, and γ. However, we now can recognize several specific major proteins by electrophoresis (Fig. 9).

A tiny transthyretin (formerly named prealbumin) band may be seen in systems with superior resolution (Fig. 9). It is a 55-kDa protein that is used mainly to assess the nutritional status of patients with protein calorie malnutrition. The normal concentration in serum (20 to 40 mg/dl) is too low to be reliably evaluated by serum protein electrophoresis; therefore, measurements are usually performed by nephelometry.

Albumin is the main serum protein. It is a 69-kDa protein that is responsible for the osmotic effect of serum proteins and serves as a transport protein for a wide variety of molecules. An innocuous variant, bisalbuminemia, is occasionally seen. Analbuminemia is a rare condition in which patients do surprisingly well. Occasionally, the latter patients require diuretics to control mild edema, and some have had elevated cholesterol levels.

α_1 lipoprotein (high-density lipoprotein) is better evaluated by specific biochemical methods, but it may be seen on serum protein electrophoresis. In gel-based techniques, it usually accounts for the faint, diffusely staining broad band between the α_1-antitrypsin band and albumin. By CZE, it migrates in the α_1 region.

α_1 acid glycoprotein is a heavily glycosylated acute-phase reactant protein that migrates just anodal to α_1 antitrypsin. With its usual concentration of 50 to 150 mg/dl and heavy glycosylation, it is either barely visible or not seen on normal samples. However, with acute-phase reactions, it is seen on the anodal side of α_1 antitrypsin. Because the glycosylation

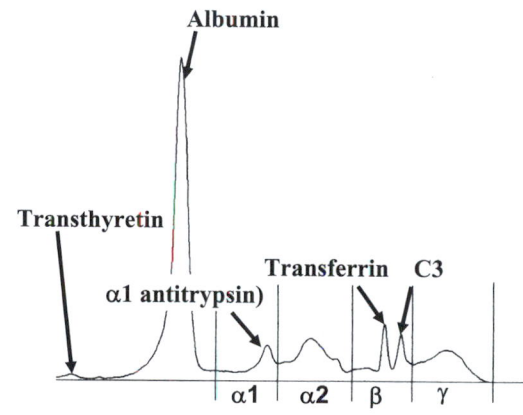

FIGURE 9 Serum electropherogram with major protein bands noted, as well as globulin regions.

interferes with protein staining, it is not seen well by gel-based methods; however, CZE methods show it to advantage as an anodal shoulder to the α_1 antitrypsin band in patients with an acute-phase reaction.

α_1 antitrypsin is a 52-kDa protein that is a member of the serine protease inhibitors (serpins) that function to inhibit a wide variety of proteases, including trypsin. This important protease inhibitor (PI) is usually present as PIMM (the normal homozygous type). However, there are several genetic variants. The Z variant and S variant are secreted in decreased amounts and are ineffective in inhibiting proteases. These variants in their homozygous form predispose the patient to emphysema and cirrhosis. The α_1 region must be carefully inspected to be certain that the α_1 antitrypsin band is present with appropriate migration (Fig. 10).

α_2 macroglobulin is a huge, 720-kDa molecule that is a member of the thiol ester plasma proteins and functions as a protease inhibitor. Despite this, it is not an acute-phase protein. Its level is elevated in patients with nephrotic syndrome due to its large size and increased synthesis in those patients.

Haptoglobin is the other major α_2-region protein. It binds free hemoglobin and exists in various forms that have a mass of between 86 and 900 kDa. The 1-1 genotype protein migrates slightly anodal to α_2 macroglobulin, the 2-1 genotype protein completely overlaps α_2 macroglobulin, and the 2-2 protein is slightly cathodal to α_2 macroglobulin. It is decreased in hemolysis and increased as an acute-phase reactant.

Transferrin, the major β_1-region molecule, is a 76.5-kDa protein that transports nonheme ferric iron. During acute-phase reactions, this protein decreases in concentration. In serum it contains two complex carbohydrate chains, each of which has a sialic acid residue. Cerebrospinal fluid contains both this form of transferrin and one that lacks the sialic acid residues. The latter fraction of transferrin migrates in the β_2 region and has been used to distinguish leakage of cerebrospinal fluid from nasal or aural secretions.

β_1 lipoprotein (low-density lipoprotein) is better evaluated by specific biochemical methods, but it may be seen in the β region (with gel-based systems) or α region (by capillary zone methods). It is an enormous molecule, with a mass of 2,750 kDa.

C3, the third component of complement and the only one readily visualized by serum protein electrophoresis, is the major β_2-region molecule. It consists of a 110-kDa α-chain and a 75-kDa β-chain. The level of C3 becomes elevated late in an acute-phase reaction. As mentioned above, if the sample is not stored properly, it is the first serum protein to break down.

Fibrinogen is the 340-kDa protein present in plasma but not in normal serum (Fig. 6 and 7). However, if the patient is anticoagulated, the sample is drawn into a tube containing an anticoagulant, or the serum is separated before clotting is completed, the sample may have enough residual fibrinogen to give a band in the β-γ region that can be confused with an M protein.

C-reactive protein is a 135-kDa protein that migrates in the γ region. Its name derives from its ability to react with the capsular polysaccharide of *Streptococcus pneumoniae*. It is an early indicator of an acute-phase reaction, best measured by nephelometric techniques.

Immunoglobulins migrate mainly in the β and γ regions. IgG is the main serum immunoglobulin (700 to 1,600 mg/dl). It is a 160-kDa protein, typically with a γ migration. It consists of four subclasses: IgG1, IgG2, IgG3, and IgG4. A polyclonal increase in the IgG4 subclass on occasion may mimic an M protein (Fig. 11). Such polyclonal increases can be

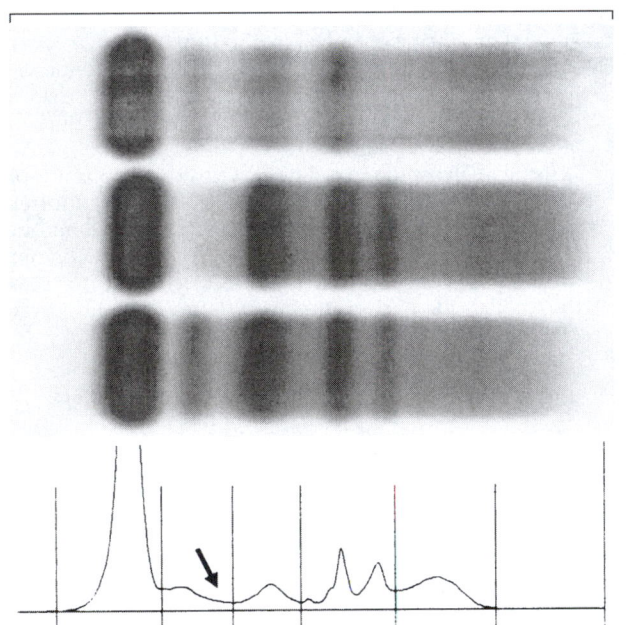

Fraction	Rel %	g/dL
ALBUMIN	63.8	4.47
ALPHA 1	6.7	0.47
ALPHA 2	5.8	0.41
BETA	12.8	0.89
GAMMA	11.0	0.77

Reference Ranges

	Rel %	g/dL
ALBUMIN	52.6 - 68.9	3.80 - 5.20
ALPHA 1	3.6 - 8.1	0.30 - 0.60
ALPHA 2	5.3 - 12.2	0.40 - 0.90
BETA	8.3 - 14.3	0.60 - 1.10
GAMMA	8.2 - 18.6	0.60 - 1.40

TP: 6.40 - 8.20   A/G: 1.20 - 2.20

FIGURE 10 Serum protein electrophoresis gel with three samples. The middle sample is deficient in α_1 antitrypsin (a ZZ variant). This can be seen by the lack of the α_1 antitrypsin band compared to the samples above and below it. The electropherogram is the CZE pattern from the same case. Note that while the α_1 antitrypsin band is absent, the measurement of the α_1 region shows a normal amount of α_1 globulin. This reflects the measurement of proteins involved with α_1 lipoprotein and orosomucoid. Rel, relative; TP, total protein; A/G, albumin/globulin.

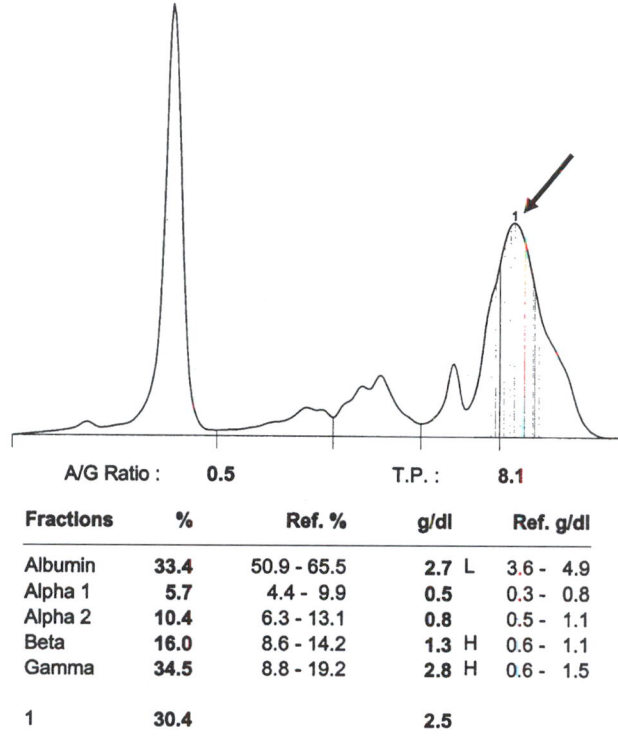

A/G Ratio :	0.5		T.P. :	8.1	
Fractions	**%**	**Ref. %**	**g/dl**	**Ref. g/dl**	
Albumin	33.4	50.9 - 65.5	2.7 L	3.6 - 4.9	
Alpha 1	5.7	4.4 - 9.9	0.5	0.3 - 0.8	
Alpha 2	10.4	6.3 - 13.1	0.8	0.5 - 1.1	
Beta	16.0	8.6 - 14.2	1.3 H	0.6 - 1.1	
Gamma	34.5	8.8 - 19.2	2.8 H	0.6 - 1.5	
1	30.4		2.5		

FIGURE 11 Electropherogram demonstrating a massive polyclonal increase in IgG4 subclass (arrow) (proven by immunofixation). Ref., reference; T.P., total protein; A/G, albumin/globulin.

distinguished from M proteins by performing an immunofixation. IgM migrates in the β-γ region (40 to 230 mg/dl). It is a 900-kDa molecule that exists as a pentamer. It is the earliest immunoglobulin to respond to antigenic stimulation but does not appear to have a memory response. IgA in the serum exists mainly as a 160-kDa monomer (70 to 400 mg/dl), but in mucosal secretions it exists mainly as a dimer attached to a secretory component (380 kDa). IgD is present mainly on the surface of lymphocytes and is present only in small quantities in the serum (0 to 8 mg/dl). IgE is present mainly on the surface of mast cells and basophils. Serum concentrations are measured only for patients with allergies and in the extremely rare cases of IgE myeloma (see chapter 107).

PATTERN INTERPRETATION FOR SERUM

Although the main purpose of serum protein electrophoresis is the detection of M proteins, several other protein patterns that can be detected may be of clinical use. Some of these findings were mentioned above with regard to each major protein; however, others that depend upon a pattern of reactivity are reviewed here.

Liver Disease Pattern

In patients with cirrhosis, synthesis of hepatocyte-derived proteins such as albumin and transferrin is decreased. As shown in the capillary zone electropherogram in Fig. 12, this usually forms a stepwise increase from the α_2 region through the γ region. However, due to inflammation and rerouting of blood around the liver, the levels of other proteins may be increased. Typically, the serum demonstrates hypoalbuminemia (there may be anodal slurring of the albumin band if the bilirubin level is increased). There is β-γ bridging due to a polyclonal

increase in IgA, and a broad increase in the γ region reflecting the polyclonal increase in IgG.

Protein Loss Patterns

With nephrotic syndrome, loss of protein occurs through damaged glomeruli. The serum shows hypoalbuminemia, low or low-normal levels of α_1 globulin, and elevated levels of α_2 globulin due to retention of its large molecules (α_2 macroglobuin and haptoglobin) in the serum; the β region may be increased due to elevated levels of β_1 lipoprotein, and there may be low-normal gamma globulin levels or hypogammaglobulinemia due to loss of IgG into the urine (Fig. 13).

In protein-losing enteropathy, damage to the gastrointestinal tract such as occurs in gluten-losing enteropathy (celiac disease), the serum demonstrates findings similar to those of the nephritic syndrome with hypoalbuminemia, hypogammaglobulinemia, and occasionally elevated levels of α_2 macroglobulin.

Milder patterns of protein loss may result in only decreased albumin and gamma globulin. Because most serum protein electrophoresis is performed for patients for whom an M protein is in the differential diagnosis, when we see these findings, we recommend performing a urine immunofixation to rule out MFLC.

Acute-Phase Pattern

Acute-phase reaction is the result of recent damage that may occur due to disease such as infection and inflammation, or it may result from therapeutic measures such as surgery. In the serum, largely due to the effect of interleukin-6, there is a decrease in albumin and transferrin (β_1 globulin) with an increase in α_1 acid glycoprotein (orosomucoid), α_1 antitrypsin, and haptoglobin. In the mid- to fast-γ region, depending on the electrophoresis system being used, the C-reactive protein band may be seen. Later in the course of the inflammation, C3

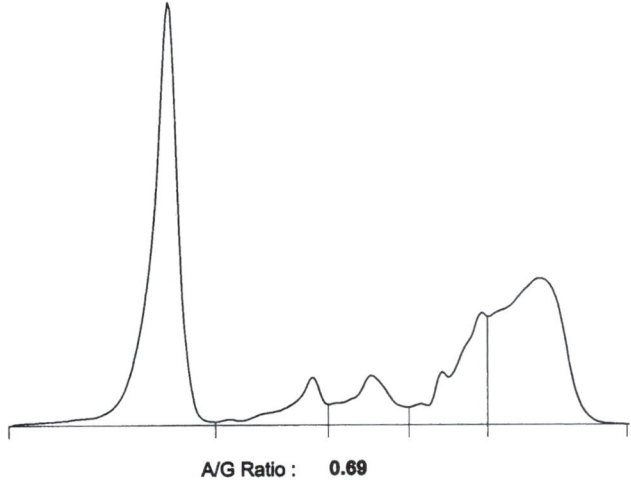

Fractions	%	Ref. %	g/dl	Ref. g/dl
Albumin	40.9	50.9 - 65.5	2.2 L	3.6 - 4.9
Alpha 1	5.8	4.4 - 9.9	0.3	0.3 - 0.8
Alpha 2	7.3	6.3 - 13.1	0.4 L	0.5 - 1.1
Beta	13.7	8.6 - 14.2	0.7	0.6 - 1.1
Gamma	32.3	8.8 - 19.2	1.7 H	0.6 - 1.5

A/G Ratio: 0.69
T.P.: 5.4

FIGURE 12 Electropherogram demonstrating a cirrhosis pattern. Ref., reference; L, low value; H, high value; T.P., total protein.

increases. A somewhat similar pattern is seen in pregnancy and in patients receiving estrogen therapy, except that in the estrogen effect pattern a normal albumin level and an elevated transferrin level accompany the increase in α_1 antitrypsin and haptoglobin.

Hypogammaglobulinemia is never normal in an adult. When the total γ-region value falls below the normal range of 2 standard deviations set in our laboratories, we note that hypogammaglobulinemia is present. This may be seen in a variety of conditions, such as common variable immunodeficiency

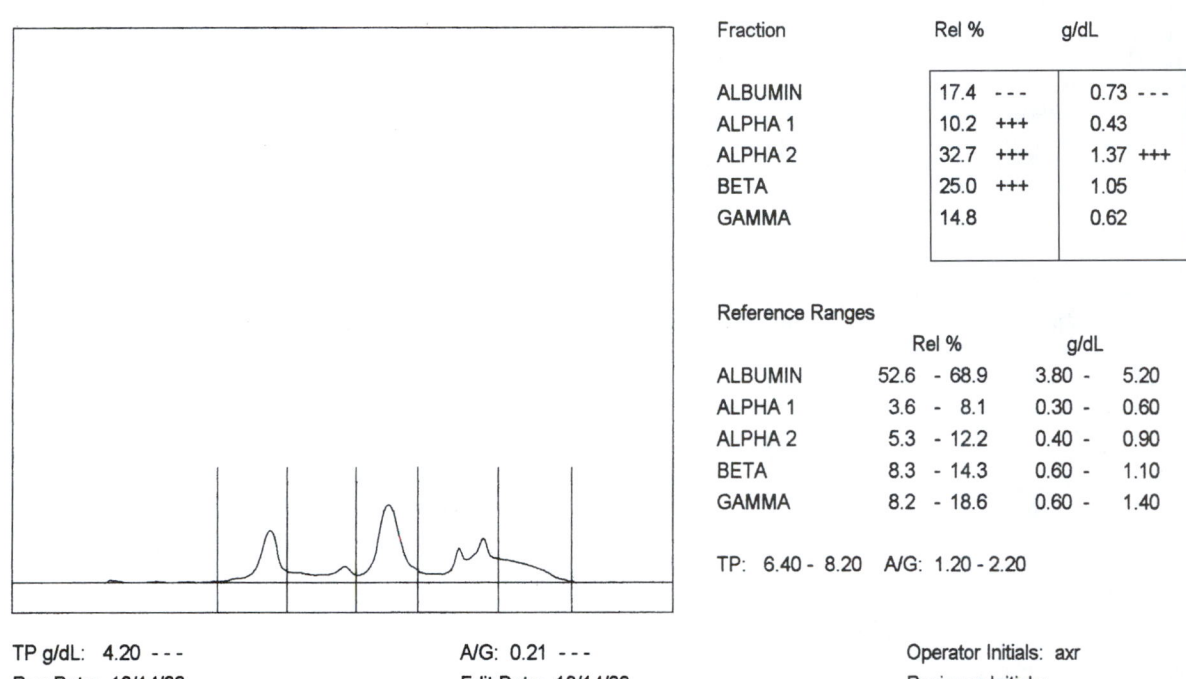

Fraction	Rel %		g/dL	
ALBUMIN	17.4	---	0.73	---
ALPHA 1	10.2	+++	0.43	
ALPHA 2	32.7	+++	1.37	+++
BETA	25.0	+++	1.05	
GAMMA	14.8		0.62	

Reference Ranges

	Rel %		g/dL	
ALBUMIN	52.6	- 68.9	3.80 -	5.20
ALPHA 1	3.6	- 8.1	0.30 -	0.60
ALPHA 2	5.3	- 12.2	0.40 -	0.90
BETA	8.3	- 14.3	0.60 -	1.10
GAMMA	8.2	- 18.6	0.60 -	1.40

TP: 6.40 - 8.20   A/G: 1.20 - 2.20

TP g/dL: 4.20 - - -   A/G: 0.21 - - -   Operator Initials: axr
Run Date: 10/14/99   Edit Date: 10/14/99   Reviewer Initials:

FIGURE 13 Electropherogram demonstrating a protein loss pattern. TP, total protein; A/G, albumin/globulin; Rel, relative.

disease, chronic lymphocytic leukemia, well-differentiated lymphocytic lymphoma, light-chain disease, and nonsecretory myeloma, and in patients who are receiving chemotherapy. The patient should have a urine protein electrophoresis and immunofixation performed to rule out the presence of MFLC. Amyloid AL (light-chain-associated amyloid) can sometimes be seen in cases of hypogammaglobulinemia. Measurement of the serum FLC has been shown to help in detecting both cases of AL and cases of nonsecretory myeloma (1, 12). Hypogammaglobulinemia is not a normal finding in the elderly.

Detection of M Proteins in Serum

Most M proteins belong to the IgG subclass and migrate in the γ region (Fig. 4, samples 13 and 25). Since the normal IgG migrates broadly throughout the slow β and γ region, even small M proteins at as low as 0.05 to 0.1 g/liter (especially in the presence of hypogammaglobulinemia) can be detected in systems with high-quality resolution (Fig. 14). Identification of the M protein requires immunologic demonstration that the M-protein band is made up of only one heavy-chain type and one light-chain type. Immunofixation and immunosubtraction are the two methods we recommend for this (see chapter 10).

M proteins, especially those of the IgA (Fig. 4, sample 24) and IgM (Fig. 4, sample 6) classes, are commonly detected in the β region. These can be more challenging to detect because of the presence of the three major proteins in that region: β_1 lipoprotein (in gel-based methods), transferrin, and C3. This is when electrophoresis systems of high-quality resolution can be especially helpful. When we see protein level elevations in the β region on densitometry (or electropherogram, in the case of CZE) that are unexplained by β-γ bridging (such as in the cirrhosis pattern), immunofixation or immunosubtraction is indicated to rule out an M protein. Occasionally, M proteins will appear as a shoulder to one of the other bands, or even migrate directly on top of the band, producing an aberrantly large C3 or transferrin band.

Rarely, M proteins may migrate in the α_2 region. These are very difficult to detect because of the higher concentration of the proteins that normally migrate there. This is one reason why a negative serum protein electrophoresis does not rule out the presence of a detectable serum M protein. When serum protein electrophoresis is negative for a patient for whom having an M protein is strongly suspected, an immunofixation of the serum and urine should be performed.

Measurement of Serum M Proteins

With the better-resolution systems, the lower limit of detection of M proteins has been estimated at about 50 mg/dl (4, 24). Detection of small M proteins can be clinically significant. These proteins may indicate early detection of what will prove over time to be a typical myeloma. Differentiation between myeloma and monoclonal gammopathy of unknown significance requires careful follow-up of the patient by the clinician and period laboratory studies. Small M proteins may be seen in patients with light-chain myeloma, IgD myeloma, IgE myeloma, amyloid AL, and other B-cell lymphoproliferative processes such as chronic lymphocytic lymphoma or well-differentiated lymphocytic lymphoma. Once an M protein has been detected and characterized immunologically, it should be measured to allow follow-up. For M proteins that are clearly distinguishable from other proteins, we recommend measuring the M-protein band itself by densitometry (for gel-based systems) or by use of the electropherogram (for CZE). We place the demarcation for the M protein at the notch it forms with the normal immunoglobulins (Fig. 14). For M proteins that migrate in the β or α_2 regions, where other proteins are present, it is a judgment call as to whether the M protein is distinguishable from the other proteins in the region. If one can make this distinction, this measurement will usually be better for monitoring of patients with M proteins than a measurement by nephelometry of the total immunoglobulin of that class. The M-protein measurement excludes most of the polyclonal immunoglobulins, whereas the nephelometric measurement will include them, obscuring to some degree changes in the M protein on subsequent measurements.

PATTERN INTERPRETATION FOR URINE

In 50- to 100-fold-concentrated urine samples, albumin in small amounts may be seen in a variety of conditions. Normally, up to 150 mg of total protein (mostly albumin) may be detected during 24 h. The amount may be increased following strenuous exercise and in patients with diabetes.

Mild glomerular damage will demonstrate the moderate-size major serum proteins that normally do not pass effectively through the glomerular barrier (Fig. 15). As long as the tubular reabsorptive function is intact, no, or little, faintly staining protein will be seen in the α_2 and β regions. When the capacity for the tubules to reabsorb 1 g of protein in 24 h is exceeded, small bands will be seen in these regions, along with faintly staining γ region. With severe nonselective renal disease, a pattern that resembles that of serum

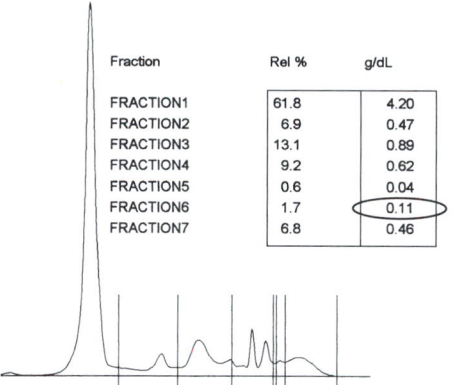

Fraction	Rel %	g/dL
FRACTION1	61.8	4.20
FRACTION2	6.9	0.47
FRACTION3	13.1	0.89
FRACTION4	9.2	0.62
FRACTION5	0.6	0.04
FRACTION6	1.7	0.11
FRACTION7	6.8	0.46

FIGURE 14 Electropherogram demonstrating a tiny M protein (0.11 g/dl). This tiny M protein turned out to indicate λ light-chain disease with a massive monoclonal FLC in the urine. Rel, relative.

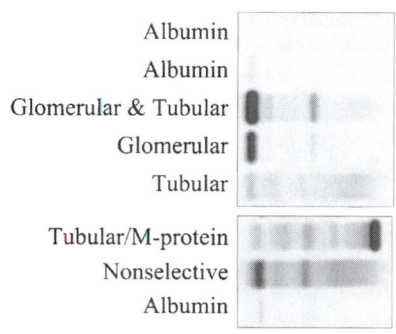

FIGURE 15 Several urine protein electrophoretic patterns for concentrated urine samples.

protein electrophoresis excluding, to a lesser extent, the large molecules in the α_2 region is found.

If only the tubules are damaged, the large amounts of small serum proteins that pass through the glomerulus will not be reabsorbed and will appear in the urine. Typically, one will find a small amount of albumin and numerous bands of various sizes in the α_1, α_2, and β and γ regions (Fig. 15). After the interpreter gets used to the usual bands of tubular proteinuria, if a band is found in a different location an immunofixation should be performed to rule out the presence of MFLC.

When a large excess of a relatively small molecule is present, such as in a patient with myoglobinuria, if the amount excreted is greater than the tubular reabsorptive capacity, an overflow proteinuria pattern is seen. This situation must be studied by immunofixation to rule out the possibility that the band represents an M protein.

Detection of M Proteins in the Urine

MFLC (Bence Jones proteins) typically occur as monomers (22 kDa) and dimers (44 kDa), both of which pass into the urine. Uncommonly, they exist as tetramers that are too large to pass through the normal glomerular capillaries and into the glomerular filtrate.

An early-morning void or a 24-h urine sample is the best specimen in which to look for MFLC. Alternatively, or in addition, measurement of FLC in serum via new nephelometric techniques may also be able to detect MFLC (see chapter 8). Once MFLC have been demonstrated by electrophoresis and documented by immunofixation or FLC measurements, they should be monitored by measuring the MFLC peak on the densitometric scan of a 24-h urine collection. Because urine immunofixation electrophoresis can be informative even when the spike cannot be seen by urine protein electrophoresis, some laboratories use a semiquantitative method of comparing very small quantities of MFLC by grading the density of the band on a scale of 1 to 4. Alternatively, FLC measurements have been suggested as a possible technique. These have the advantage that serum measurements can be made, avoiding the necessity to collect a 24-h urine sample. However, FLC measurements are a relatively new technique and need to be related to the immunofixation results for each case.

Although CZE techniques to detect MFLC have been described, they are not yet commonly used in clinical laboratories. Therefore, this discussion will focus on gel-based results.

MFLC and M proteins may migrate anywhere from the α through the γ region on urine protein electrophoresis (Fig. 15). Once one becomes familiar with the common patterns of glomerular and tubular proteinuria discussed above, unusual bands will become apparent. This is more difficult with tubular proteinuria and its many bands from small proteins which are not reabsorbed than with glomerular proteinuria.

For optimal detection of MFLC, we recommend performing immunofixation and urine protein electrophoresis on all samples. For the initial detection of MFLC, we review our files on the patient to see if there is a known M protein in the serum. If so, that information is used to determine the antisera we use to evaluate the urine. We always use anti-κ and anti-λ but would in addition use antisera of the heavy-chain isotype demonstrated in the serum (γ, α, μ, δ, or ϵ).

Commonly, both the intact M protein and the MFLC can be found in the urine of a patient with multiple myeloma. The urine immunofixation is compared to the urine protein electrophoresis to determine which band is the MFLC. This band is measured by densitometry of the urine protein

electrophoresis. The concentration of the total protein in the urine is used with this measurement and the volume of 24-h urine to determine the amount of the MFLC per 24 h as follows: MFLC/24 h = (total protein concentration [mg/ml]) × (ml/24 h) × % MFLC by densitometry.

The record of the urine protein electrophoresis and immunofixation is stored in a file with the serum protein and immunofixation results. This allows correlation of the current results with previous results and on occasion can catch a mislabeled sample.

CLINICAL APPLICATIONS

Serum and urine protein electrophoreses are not general screening techniques. They are employed to detect M proteins in patients suspected of harboring plasma cell and B-lymphocyte proliferative disorders. We recommend that both urine and serum be studied for patients suspected of having an M protein.

In addition to M proteins, however, performance of serum and urine protein electrophoresis often detects a wide variety of other abnormalities that can provide useful clinical information, as described above. Therefore, attention to all regions of the electrophoretic pattern is needed, and such abnormalities are included in the final report.

The presence of a band suspected of being an M protein requires immunological characterization (see chapter 10). Also, measurement of the immunoglobulin isotype, and in some cases the FLC, may be useful for monitoring of the patient (see chapter 8).

REFERENCES

1. Abraham, R. S., J. A. Katzmann, R. J. Clark, A. R. Bradwell, R. A. Kyle, and M. A. Gertz. 2003. Quantitative analysis of serum free light chains. A new marker for the diagnostic evaluation of primary systemic amyloidosis. *Am. J. Clin. Pathol.* **119:**274–278.
2. Aguzzi, F., J. Kohn, C. Petrini, and J. T. Whicher. 1986. Densitometry of serum protein electrophoretograms. *Clin. Chem.* **32:**2004–2005.
3. Arranz-Peña, M. L., M. Gonzalez-Sagrado, A. M. Olmos-Linares, N. Fernandez-Garcia, and F. J. Martin-Gil. 2000. Interference of iodinated contrast media in serum capillary zone electrophoresis. *Clin. Chem.* **46:**736–737.
4. Bienvenu, J., M. S. Graziani, F. Arpin, H. Bernon, C. Blessum, C. Marchetti, G. Righetti, M. Somenzini, G. Verga, and F. Aguzzi. 1998. Multicenter evaluation of the Paragon CZE 2000 capillary zone electrophoresis system for serum protein electrophoresis and monoclonal component typing. *Clin. Chem.* **44:**599–605.
5. Blessum, C. R., N. Khatter, and S. C. Alter. 1999. Technique to remove interference caused by radio-opaque agents in clinical capillary zone electrophoresis. *Clin. Chem.* **45:**1313.
6. Bossuyt, X. 2003. Separation of serum proteins by automated capillary zone electrophoresis. *Clin. Chem. Lab. Med.* **41:**762–772.
7. Bossuyt, X. 2004. Interferences in clinical capillary zone electrophoresis of serum proteins. *Electrophoresis* **25:**1485–1487.
8. Bossuyt, X., and W. E. Peetermans. 2002. Effect of piperacillin-tazobactam on clinical capillary zone electrophoresis of serum proteins. *Clin. Chem.* **48:**204–205.
9. Bossuyt, X., G. Schiettekatte, A. Bogaerts, and N. Blanckaert. 1998. Serum protein electrophoresis by CZE 2000 clinical capillary electrophoresis system. *Clin. Chem.* **44:**749–759.

10. **Bossuyt, X., J. Verhaegen, G. Marien, and N. Blanckaert.** 2003. Effect of sulfamethoxazole on clinical capillary zone electrophoresis of serum proteins. *Clin. Chem.* **49:**340–341.

11. **Brigden, M. L., E. D. Neal, M. D. McNeely, and G. N. Hoag.** 1990. The optimum urine collections for the detection and monitoring of Bence Jones proteinuria. *Am. J. Clin. Pathol.* **93:**689–693.

12. **Drayson, M., L. X. Tang, R. Drew, G. P. Mead, H. Carr-Smith, and A. R. Bradwell.** 2001. Serum free light-chain measurements for identifying and monitoring patients with nonsecretory multiple myeloma. *Blood* **97:**2900–2902.

13. **Johnson, A. M., E. M. Rohlts, and L. M. Silverman.** 1999. Proteins, p. 477–540. *In* C. Burtis and E. R. Ashwood (ed.), *Tietiz Textbook of Clinical Chemistry.* W.B. Saunders, Philadelphia, Pa.

14. **Katzmann, J. A., R. Clark, E. Sanders, J. P. Landers, and R. A. Kyle.** 1998. Prospective study of serum protein capillary zone electrophoresis and immunotyping of monoclonal proteins by immunosubtraction. *Am. J. Clin. Pathol.* **110:**503–509.

15. **Keren, D. F.** 2003. *Protein Electrophoresis in Clinical Diagnosis.* Arnold, London, United Kingdom.

16. **Keren, D. F., R. Alexanian, J. A. Goeken, P. D. Gorevic, R. A. Kyle, and R. H. Tomar.** 1999. Guidelines for clinical and laboratory evaluation of patients with monoclonal gammopathies. *Arch. Pathol. Lab. Med.* **123:**106–107.

17. **Keren, D. F., R. Gulbranson, and S. J. Ebrom.** 2004. False-negative urine protein electrophoresis by semiautomated gel electrophoresis. *Clin. Chem.* **50:**933–934.

18. **Kohn, J.** 1957. A cellulose acetate supporting medium for zone electrophoresis. *Clin. Chim. Acta* **2:**297–304.

19. **Kunkel, H. G., and A. Tiselius.** 1951. Electrophoresis of proteins on filter paper. *J. Gen. Physiol.* **35:**39–118.

20. **Le Bricon, T., E. Launay, P. Houze, D. Bengoufa, B. Bousquet, and B. Gourmel.** 2002. Determination of poorly separated monoclonal serum proteins by capillary zone electrophoresis. *J. Chromatogr. B Analyt. Technol. Biomed. Life Sci.* **775:**63–70.

21. **Luraschi, P., E. D. Dea, and C. Franzini.** 2003. Capillary zone electrophoresis of serum proteins: effects of changed analytical conditions. *Clin. Chem. Lab. Med.* **41:**782–786.

22. **Petrini, C., M. G. Alessio, L. Scapellato, S. Brambilla, and C. Franzini.** 1999. Serum proteins by capillary zone electrophoresis: approaches to the definition of reference values. *Clin. Chem. Lab. Med.* **37:**975–980.

23. **Register, L. J., and D. F. Keren.** 1989. Hazard of commercial antiserum cross-reactivity in monoclonal gammopathy evaluation. *Clin. Chem.* **35:**2016–2017.

24. **Smalley, D. L., R. P. Mayer, and M. F. Bugg.** 2000. Capillary zone electrophoresis compared with agarose gel and immunofixation electrophoresis. *Am. J. Clin. Pathol.* **114:**487–488.

25. **Tiselius, A.** 1959. Introduction, p. xv–xx. *In* M. Bier (ed.), *Electrophoresis: Theory, Methods and Applications.* Academic Press, New York, N.Y.

26. **Walchner, M., and M. Wick.** 1997. Elevation of CD8$^+$ CD11b$^+$ Leu-8$^-$ T cells is associated with the humoral immunodeficiency in myeloma patients. *Clin. Exp. Immunol.* **109:**310–316.

Immunochemical Characterization of Immunoglobulins in Serum, Urine, and Cerebrospinal Fluid

JERRY A. KATZMANN AND ROBERT A. KYLE

10

The characterization of immunoglobulins spans a spectrum of methods, including molecular analysis of gene usage and rearrangement; quantitation of immunoglobulin heavy chains as well as intact and free light chains; qualitative assessment and characterization of clonality; and identification of abnormalities that may be clinically significant, such as hyperviscosity syndrome, cryoglobulinemia, and amyloidosis (AL). This chapter focuses on qualitative methods for the assessment and characterization of clonality. The methods include nondenaturing agarose gel electrophoresis (AGE) with immunofixation, capillary zone electrophoresis (CZE) with immunosubtraction, and isoelectric focusing with immunoblotting. All three methods can be used to identify monoclonal, oligoclonal, and polyclonal immunoglobulin populations and to identify the heavy and/or light chains contained in the population. Immunofixation electrophoresis (IFE) and immunosubtraction electrophoresis (ISE) are diagnostic tools used for the identification of monoclonal gammopathies and, conversely, for the confirmation of polyclonal hypergammaglobulinemia. Isoelectric focusing with immunoblotting is a cerebrospinal fluid (CSF) diagnostic test for the identification of oligoclonal bands (OCB) in multiple sclerosis (MS).

MONOCLONAL GAMMOPATHIES

The monoclonal gammopathies (dysproteinemias or paraproteinemias) are characterized by the proliferation of a single clone of plasma cells that produces an immunologically homogeneous protein commonly referred to as a monoclonal protein or a paraprotein. It is important to identify monoclonal proteins and to be able to distinguish between increases in monoclonal and polyclonal immunoglobulins (19–21). Monoclonal immunoglobulins are associated with a clonal process that is malignant or potentially malignant, whereas an increase in polyclonal immunoglobulins is due to an inflammatory or reactive process (22).

All immunoglobulins are products of clonal plasma cells. In a normal immune response, each of the thousands of immunoglobulin clonotypes produced by the plasma cell clones is present in relatively small proportion. The normal immune response is therefore described as polyclonal. Monoclonal gammopathies are a group of disorders that include plasma cell and B-lymphoid proliferative disorders and are defined by the expansion of a plasma cell clone. The secreted immunoglobulin from the expanded plasma cell clone results in a detectable monoclonal immunoglobulin (12). The monoclonal gammopathies include a spectrum of diseases, from ones that may have little clinical significance to ones that may be rapidly fatal. These include multiple myeloma (MM), Waldenström's macroglobulinemia, smoldering MM, monoclonal gammopathy of undetermined significance (MGUS), primary systemic AL, lymphoproliferative diseases, and plasmacytomas. The distribution of these diseases in the Mayo Clinic practice from 1960 through 2003 is listed in Table 1. During this interval, our dysproteinemia practice identified 31,479 monoclonal gammopathies. The most common of the monoclonal gammopathies is MGUS, but the hallmark monoclonal gammopathy is MM. MM is a malignant plasma cell disorder that resides in the bone marrow and causes multiple osteolytic lesions. Patients often present with bone pain or fractures due to these bone lesions. The monoclonal immunoglobulin produced by the malignant plasma cell clone was one of the first serological tumor markers. The identification of a monoclonal immunoglobulin in serum (or urine) is an indicator of the expansion of the clone of plasma cells and, depending on the clinical presentation, triggers a series of additional laboratory tests to confirm the diagnosis of a monoclonal gammopathy. In addition to monoclonal immunoglobulin being a diagnostic tool for the identification of monoclonal gammopathies such as MM, the amount of monoclonal immunoglobulin can be quantitated and used as a surrogate marker to monitor the plasma cell population.

METHOD BACKGROUND

Analysis of serum or urine for monoclonal proteins requires a sensitive, rapid, and simple screening method that detects the presence of a monoclonal protein and also requires a specific assay to confirm the clonality and identify the heavy-chain class and light-chain type. High-resolution agarose gel protein electrophoresis (PEL) and CZE fulfill the requirements for a screening procedure for detection of monoclonal proteins (17, 18, 20). IFE in agarose or ISE with CZE is needed to confirm the presence of the monoclonal protein and determine its type.

Nondenaturing PEL systems such as cellulose acetate, agarose gel, and CZE separate proteins on the basis of charge and size. Five serum fractions have traditionally been identified

TABLE 1 Distribution of plasma cell proliferative disorders at Mayo Clinic, 1960 to 2003[a]

Type of monoclonal gammopathy	% of cases
MGUS	61
MM	17
Primary systemic AL	9
Lymphoproliferative disease	3
Smoldering myeloma	4
Solitary or extramedullary plasmacytoma	2
Macroglobulinemia	2
Other	2

[a] From the Mayo Clinic Dysproteinemia Data Base. $n = 31,479$.

by PEL: albumin, α_1, α_2, β, and γ. In a normal serum separated by agarose gel PEL, the γ fraction will have a broad, Gaussian distribution (Fig. 1). The distribution of immunoglobulins through the γ fraction is predominantly due to charge differences on the different immunoglobulin clono-

types. In the IFE results illustrated in Fig. 1, it can be seen that the immunoglobulin G (IgG) migration pattern corresponds to the PEL γ fraction. In the serum of a patient with a monoclonal gammopathy, the increased monoclonal immunoglobulin migrates in a restricted area of migration in the electrophoresis pattern (Fig. 2). All patients with a localized band on PEL require IFE or ISE to confirm the monoclonal protein and to determine its heavy-chain class and/or light-chain type. The IFE reactivity in Fig. 2 indicates that the restricted electrophoretic migration is due to an IgG (γ) heavy chain and an associated λ light chain. It is this restricted heavy-chain migration on the gel and the associated migration of only one light-chain type that identify and characterize the monoclonal immunoglobulin heavy- and light-chain types. The monoclonal fraction (M-spike) from the serum PEL quantitates the amount of the monoclonal protein.

Plasma cells produce immunoglobulin heavy and light chains which are assembled into the intact immunoglobulin molecules. In order to ensure proper assembly, there is an approximately 40% excess of light chain produced. Unlike

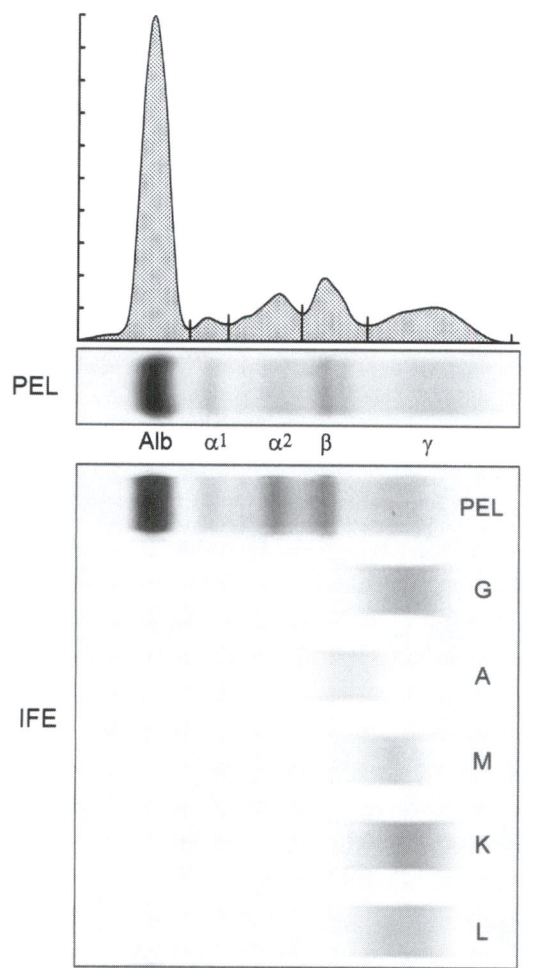

FIGURE 1 PEL and IFE of normal serum. (Top) PEL gel scan and electrophoretogram with the albumin (Alb), α_1, α_2, β, and γ fractions. (Bottom) IFE gel scan. Lanes were immunofixed with antisera to γ (G), α (A), μ (M), κ (K), and λ (L). The distribution of normal serum immunoglobulins is illustrated.

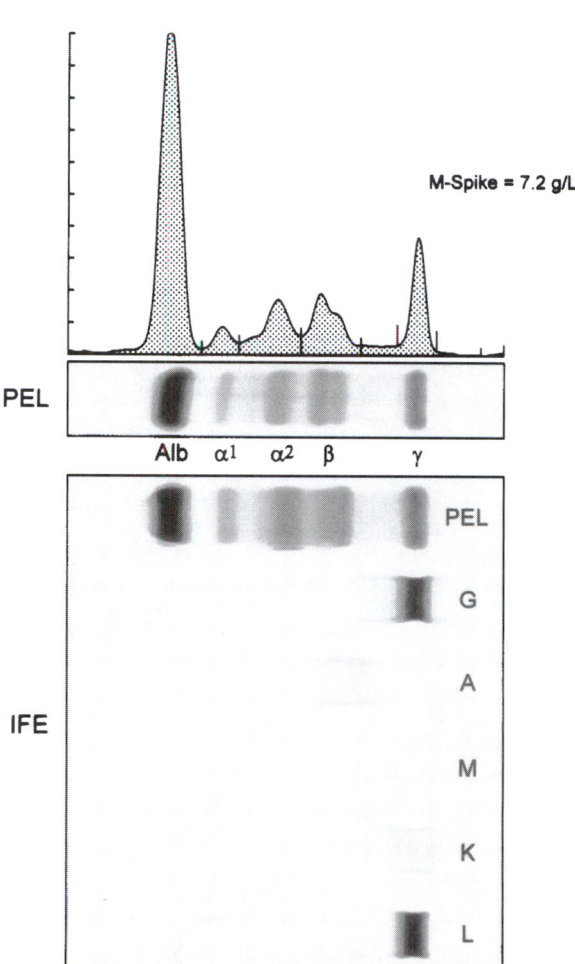

FIGURE 2 PEL and IFE of a serum containing a monoclonal protein. The PEL indicates that the M-spike equals 7.2 g/liter, and the IFE indicates that it is a monoclonal IgG λ protein. The γ and λ bands are sharp and comigrate. There is very little polyclonal immunoglobulin in this serum sample. Alb, albumin; lanes G to L, as defined in the legend to Fig. 1.

the secreted intact immunoglobulins, the free light chains are rapidly cleared from serum (32, 33). The light chains are cleared and metabolized by the kidneys within hours of secretion. In healthy individuals, the light chains are catabolized and are not readily apparent by urine PEL. As patients become proteinuric, however, both heavy and light chains can be detected by PEL and IFE. In patients with monoclonal gammopathies, the excess monoclonal free light-chain production may often be detected in urine. In IgG myeloma, for example, approximately three-fourths of patients have an excess of light chains that are excreted and detected in the urine as Bence Jones proteinuria (24). The immunofixation assay for urine studies is identical to the serum assay except that urine samples with low protein content need to be concentrated to increase the detection sensitivity.

IFE and ISE are required for confirmation and characterization of monoclonal proteins identified by PEL. In addition, it should be emphasized that even when PEL is negative, IFE may detect small monoclonal proteins. In the absence of a localized band on serum and/or urine PEL, IFE should still be performed if MM, macroglobulinemia, AL, solitary or extramedullary plasmacytomas, or a related disorder is suspected.

MONOCLONAL PROTEINS

Most patients with monoclonal gammopathies have a detectable monoclonal heavy and light chain in the serum, and some have a detectable monoclonal urinary protein as well. In some patients, however, heavy chains are not produced by the plasma cells. Table 2 lists the distribution of monoclonal serum proteins detected in the Mayo Clinic practice from 1960 through 2003. During this time, 28,249 monoclonal proteins were detected. Most of the monoclonal proteins were IgG, IgM, and IgA molecules, and there were a small number of monoclonal IgD and IgE immunoglobulins. There were, however, significant numbers (5%) of serum monoclonal proteins in which monoclonal light chains were detected but which had no associated heavy chain. Because the free light chains are so readily cleared from the serum, patients with these disorders often show small or undetectable M-spikes on serum PEL. The monoclonal free light-chain diseases, however, represent very significant disorders. Although monoclonal free light chains represented 5% of all the monoclonal gammopathies, light-chain MM (LCMM) accounted for 20% of the MM cases (Table 3). This overrepresentation of free light chains in MM (20%) versus all monoclonal gammopathies (5%) emphasizes the importance of confirming small serum PEL abnormalities by IFE. It can also be seen in Table 3 that

TABLE 2 Monoclonal serum proteins detected at Mayo Clinic, 1960 to 2003[a]

Type of protein	%
IgG	60.5
IgM	17
IgA	13
IgD	0.5
IgE	0.0001
Biclonal	4
Light chain only	5

[a] From the Mayo Clinic Dysproteinemia Data Base. $n = 28,249$.

TABLE 3 Monoclonal serum proteins: newly diagnosed MM[a]

Type of protein	%
IgG	52
IgA	21
IgM	0.5
IgD	2
Biclonal	2
Free light chain only	20
Nonsecretory myeloma	2.8

[a] From Kyle et al. (24). $n = 1,027$.

nearly 3% of MM patients have no detectable monoclonal heavy chain or light chain (6, 30, 35). These nonsecretory-MM patients have large numbers of plasma cells in the bone marrow, and most of these patients have clonal plasma cells with cytoplasmic κ or λ light chain, indicating a secretory defect. A small number of these nonsecretory-myeloma patients, however, have no detectable cytoplasmic immunoglobulin in their plasma cells and are nonproducers. Although not listed in Table 3, there are also rare monoclonal gammopathy patients who produce a portion of the heavy chain but no light chain. These disorders include γ, α, and μ heavy-chain disease.

One final point should be taken from Table 2. Four percent of the detected monoclonal gammopathies are biclonal gammopathies. In these patients, there are two separate expanded clones of plasma cells. The PEL may show two M-spikes, and the immunofixation will show two different heavy and light chains with different mobilities (Fig. 3). The presence of two monoclonal proteins is clinically no different

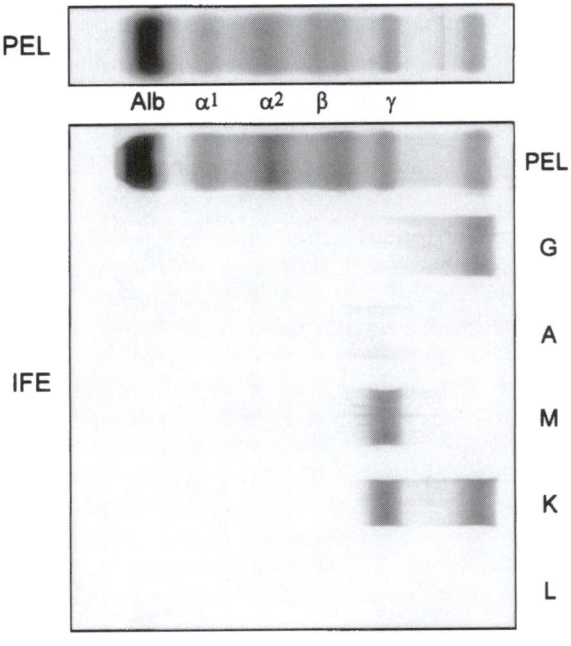

FIGURE 3 PEL gel scan and IFE of a serum containing a biclonal gammopathy. The PEL gel contains two discrete bands in the γ fraction. The IFE indicates that there is a γ band with a corresponding κ band plus a μ band with a corresponding κ band. The biclonal gammopathy contains a monoclonal IgG κ and a monoclonal IgM κ protein. Lanes G to L, as defined for Fig. 1.

from a monoclonal gammopathy (25). Above 50 years of age, monoclonal gammopathies are detected in the general population at a rate of 3% (26). If a monoclonal protein occurs in 3% of the population over age 50, we can expect that 3% of these individuals will have a second "monoclonal" protein. In addition, we can predict that 0.09% of monoclonal gammopathies will actually be triclonal gammopathies.

IFE

IFE is the composite of the two separate procedures of PEL and immunofixation. Proteins are first separated by electrophoresis in a nondenaturing agarose gel, and then an antiserum is applied to precipitate the proteins of interest. Soluble proteins are washed away, and the immunoprecipitate is visualized with a protein stain. There are a number of reagent sets that are available from commercial vendors. These assay kits provide agarose gels, diluent, electrophoresis buffer, antisera, wash buffer, stain, and destaining solution as well as the application system for applying sample and antisera to the gel. In a single assay, the patient serum or urine is usually applied to six lanes of the gel and electrophoresed so that all six lanes have the proteins separated in an identical manner. Fixative solution is added to a single lane to precipitate all the proteins. This is the PEL lane and serves as the reference lane for all the proteins. The remaining five lanes are overlaid with antiserum to γ, α, μ, κ, or λ chains in order to precipitate the specific immunoglobulins. The soluble proteins are washed out of the gel, and the immunoprecipitated proteins are visualized with acid violet stain and compared to the reference lane. In the IFE shown in Fig. 1, it can be seen that the IgG migration pattern corresponds almost exactly to the shape of the γ fraction, whereas the IgA and IgM immunoglobulins migrate predominantly in the fast-γ region and the interface of the β and γ fractions. Because IgG is normally present in serum in much higher concentrations than IgA or IgM, the distribution of the κ and λ light-chain reactivity corresponds to the distribution of the IgG population. In addition, the κ lane appears denser than the λ lane as a reflection of the increased concentration of κ immunoglobulins compared to λ. The commercial reagent sets are available in gel configurations that allow the analysis of samples from one, two, four, or nine patients on a single gel. The entire process from sample application to stained IFE gel takes approximately 1.5 h.

Serum IFE

Serum samples should be collected and stored refrigerated until analyzed. Refrigerated samples are stable for at least 2 weeks and can be stored frozen indefinitely. Serum samples are often diluted for application to the IgG lane, and a lesser dilution is used for the other gel lanes. In the Sebia Hydragel system, the serum for the IgG lane is diluted 1:6 and the sera for the other five lanes (PEL, α, μ, κ, and λ) are diluted 1:3. If the serum is hypogammaglobulinemic (γ fraction or total immunoglobulins, <0.5 g/dl), the IFE may need to be performed with undiluted serum applied to the gel in order to sufficiently visualize the immunoglobulins. Conversely, if the serum has marked polyclonal hypergammaglobulinemia (γ fraction or total immunoglobulins, >4 g/dl), the serum may need to be diluted further in order to see through the dense protein stain.

The evaluation of PEL and IFE gels is a qualitative skill that takes experience for correct interpretation. The agarose gels should always be examined directly by the interpreter. As illustrated in Fig. 1, normal serum samples show broad, homogeneous staining in all the lanes. Perhaps most importantly, the κ and λ lanes show identical staining distributions. Some monoclonal proteins have a broad distribution on PEL and can be confused with a polyclonal immunoglobulin pattern, but the light-chain distribution shows only κ or λ associated with the increased heavy-chain staining pattern. Conversely, large increases in polyclonal immunoglobulin concentrations may appear to have restricted migration on PEL and may be confused with a monoclonal gammopathy. Large polyclonal increases in immunoglobulins may occur in patients with chronic active hepatitis, connective tissue disorders, or chronic lymphoproliferative disease. The distribution of κ and λ migration on IFE should always be examined carefully.

Patients with hypogammaglobulinemia will have faintly staining γ fractions, and those with polyclonal hypergammaglobulinemia will have darkly staining γ fractions. Because undiluted hypogammaglobulinemic sera may be applied to the gels, the gels may have an artifact at the point of application that represents material that does not enter the agarose. This type of artifact is recognized by noting that all lanes contain stained material at the point of application. Because of the high protein content of polyclonal hypergammaglobulinemic sera as well as the potential for rheumatoid factors in these sera, they may also exhibit a point-of-application artifact. In addition, these polyclonal hypergammaglobulinemic samples often contain multiple faint, fuzzy areas of nonhomogeneous distribution in many of the lanes. These most likely represent the "tips" of the polyclonal responses. The presence of these multiple bands in polyclonal hypergammaglobulinemic sera should be interpreted as artifact and not reported as small monoclonal proteins.

Most monoclonal protein bands are straightforward to identify and interpret (Fig. 2). The bands are dark and narrow, and there is a heavy-chain band and either a κ or λ light-chain band but not both. The IFE bands have the same migration as the band in the PEL lane. The most difficult samples to interpret are sera that contain very small, fuzzy heavy- and light-chain bands within a polyclonal background (Fig. 4). Because all immunoglobulins are clonal products and because our analytic procedures have become very sensitive, we can identify small clones that may have no clinical significance. If a serum free light-chain assay and/or urine IFE has ruled out a monoclonal free light chain, it is better to report these diffuse bands as unable to rule out a small monoclonal protein. If the small monoclonal protein is clearly present (as in Fig. 4) but is too small to fractionate as an M-spike on PEL, our laboratory reports the result as a small monoclonal protein within a polyclonal background. This makes it clear to the clinician that the monoclonal protein is too small to be quantitated and is not equal to the quantitation of the γ fraction.

In our practice, approximately 90% of the monoclonal proteins identified by IFE contain a single monoclonal heavy chain and corresponding light chain (Table 2). In 4% of the identified monoclonal gammopathies, there is a second monoclonal protein identified (biclonal gammopathy). In the biclonal gammopathy illustrated in Fig. 3, the IFE contains a γ heavy-chain band and a μ heavy-chain band, and each has a corresponding κ light-chain band. If, however, the two heavy-chain and the two light-chain bands are identical, they should not be reported as a biclonal gammopathy unless migration of one is cathodal and that of the second is anodal. If the bands are identical IgM molecules, they are most likely monomeric and pentameric IgM (7S and 19S), and if they are identical IgA or IgG molecules, they are most likely

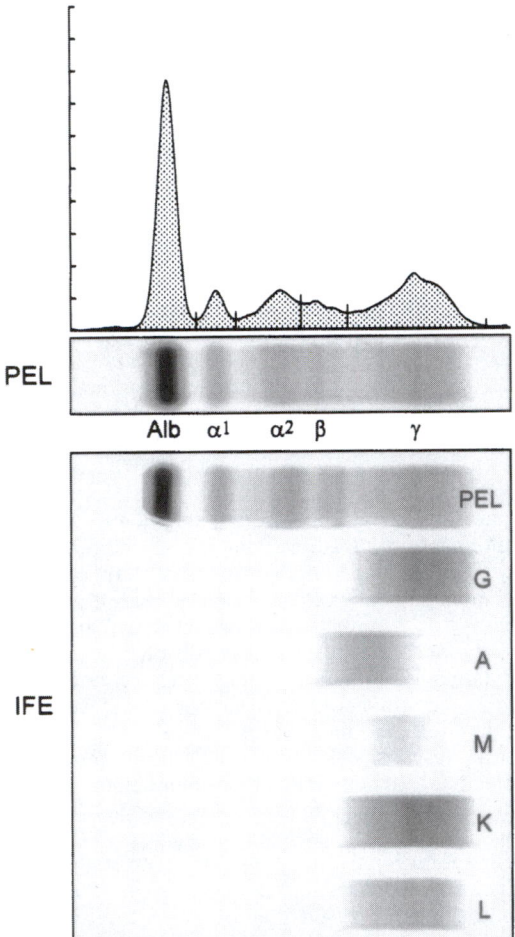

FIGURE 4 PEL and IFE of a serum containing a small monoclonal IgG κ protein. The protein is too small to be fractionated and quantitated as an M-spike. The γ fraction contains mostly polyclonal immunoglobulin, and the PEL electrophoretogram shows a small bump on top of the γ fraction. The PEL gel scan contains a small, fuzzy band corresponding to the asymmetry in the electrophoretogram, and the IFE shows some corresponding increased, restricted reactivity in the γ and κ lanes. Lanes G to L, as defined for Fig. 1.

monomers and dimers. The biclonal gammopathies are clinically identical to the monoclonal gammopathies, and most of these patients will be diagnosed with biclonal gammopathy of undetermined significance. The size of each individual M-spike should be separately monitored for disease activity. In the case of a monoclonal protein that circulates as a monomer and polymer, the sum of the peaks should be used to monitor disease activity.

Monoclonal free light chains represent the other 5% of the monoclonal gammopathies. Sera with monoclonal light chains will show a discrete κ or λ band on IFE, and there will be no corresponding γ, α, or μ heavy chain (Fig. 5). Although IgD monoclonal proteins are uncommon and IgE monoclonal proteins are very rare, any monoclonal free light-chain result should be confirmed by retesting the sample by IFE using antisera to δ and ε in the lanes usually reserved for γ, α, and μ (Fig. 6). Monoclonal free light chains usually do not accumulate in the serum and may

have a small M-spike or no M-spike (Fig. 5). In spite of this small serum abnormality, monoclonal free light chains are often associated with serious disease. The light-chain diseases include LCMM, AL, and light-chain deposition disease. Although monoclonal free light chains represent 5% of all monoclonal proteins identified in our practice, they account for 20% of the monoclonal proteins found in MM patients. Monoclonal free light chains are uncommon in MGUS and are associated predominantly with MM or AL. The recognition and reporting of a monoclonal free light chain should therefore be done cautiously. If the light-chain band on IFE is very faint and fuzzy or if the light-chain band is distinct but has a corresponding faint, fuzzy heavy-chain band, the report should suggest that a small monoclonal protein or a monoclonal free light chain cannot be excluded. Follow-up tests of urine IFE and serum free light chains should be recommended.

Serum IFE Clinical Significance

The identification of a serum monoclonal protein suggests the possibility of a diagnosis of a number of monoclonal gammopathies. Most of these are clinical diagnoses, but the

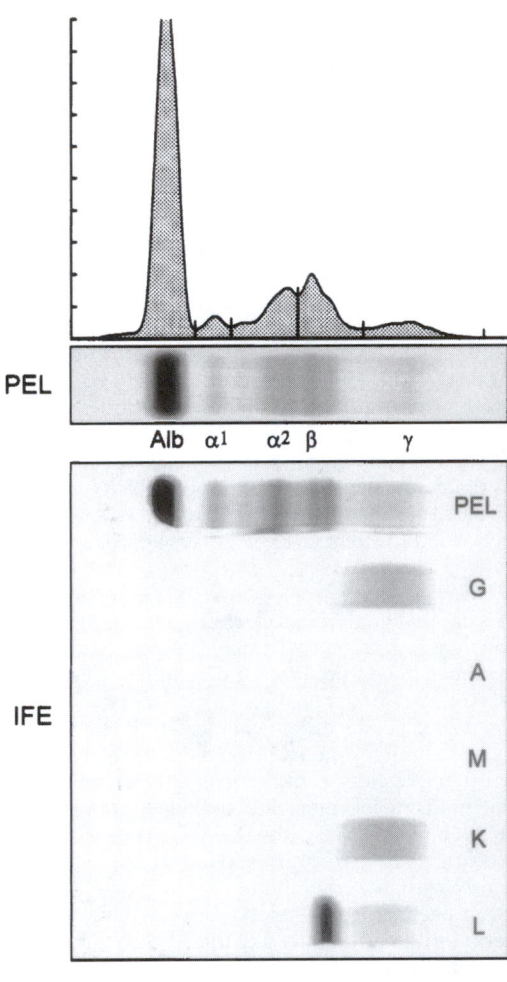

FIGURE 5 PEL and IFE of a serum specimen from a patient with LCMM. Although this patient has myeloma, there is no obvious PEL abnormality. The IFE, however, clearly shows a discrete λ band with no corresponding γ, α, or μ reactivity. Lanes G to L, as defined for Fig. 1.

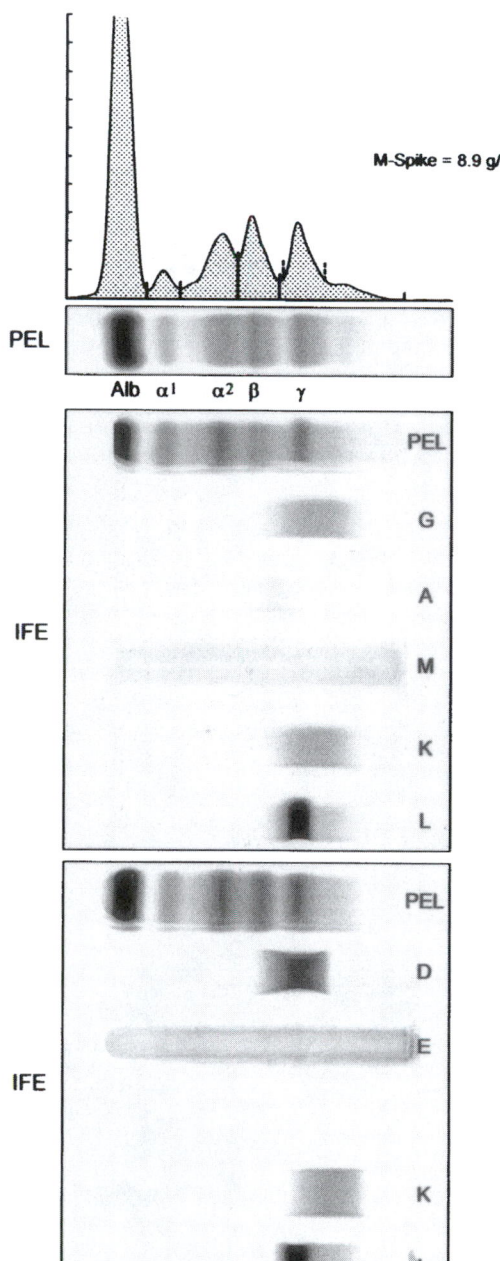

FIGURE 6 PEL and IFE of a serum from a patient with an IgD myeloma. The PEL contains a small M-spike that has a corresponding λ band as determined by IFE. The IFE was repeated with antisera to κ, λ, δ (D), and ε (E) and indicated that the monoclonal protein is an IgD λ immunoglobulin. Lanes G to L, as defined for Fig. 1.

background. In addition, we suggest that the studies be repeated in 6 to 12 months. Repeat testing allows the identification of those cases in which a very early monoclonal process was present during the initial PEL and IFE, and a significant increase in the M-spike will be detected in the second sample.

If the monoclonal protein is an IgG or IgA and is a quantifiable M-spike that is <3 g/dl, our laboratory reports that the result is consistent with MGUS, early myeloma, or AL. The order of the report indicates the relative frequency of each group of diseases, and the three diseases represent three categories of monoclonal gammopathies that the clinician needs to consider: (i) diseases such as MGUS or smoldering myeloma that should be observed but not treated; (ii) malignant diseases such as MM, lymphoma, plasma cell leukemia, or plasmacytomas; and (iii) diseases of protein structure such as AL, light-chain deposition disease, or cryoglobulinemia. If the IgG or IgA M-spike is >3 g/dl, the result is consistent with MM.

If the monoclonal protein is an IgM that is <3 g/dl, our laboratory reports that the result is consistent with MGUS, early macroglobulinemia, or lymphoproliferative disease. If the IgM M-spike is >3 g/dl, the IFE result is consistent with Waldenström's macroglobulinemia.

If the monoclonal protein is an IgD or free κ or λ light chain, our laboratory reports that the result is consistent with MM or AL. A 24-h urine monoclonal protein study should be suggested for any patient who has a serum monoclonal free light chain or monoclonal IgD, as well as for IgG, IgA, or IgM M-spikes >1.5 g/dl (21). Some laboratories suggest urine monoclonal protein studies for all patients with a monoclonal serum protein.

Serum Artifacts

As described above, sera with very low or very high immunoglobulin concentrations or γ fractions may need to be retested at different dilutions in order to evaluate the IFE.

The presence of fibrinogen or hemoglobin may cause the artifactual identification of an M-spike on PEL. Fibrinogen migrates in the fast-γ region and has the appearance of an M-spike on PEL. Analysis by IFE, however, shows no monoclonal immunoglobulin corresponding to the PEL band (Fig. 7). If a fast-γ band is identified in a patient with no previous history of a fast-γ monoclonal protein, the PEL report should be delayed until the sample is tested for fibrinogen and/or the IFE results are known. Samples can be checked for fibrinogen by the addition of 10 μl of thrombin (topical USP, 1,000 U/ml) to 200 μl of serum and incubation of the sample for 15 min at 37°C. If a fibrin clot forms, the supernatant should be retested by PEL. Some samples have sufficient anticoagulant that addition of thrombin will not remove the entire fibrinogen peak. In addition to reporting no monoclonal protein detected by IFE, the report should indicate that the γ fraction may be increased due to the presence of fibrinogen. Depending on the particular AGE system, hemoglobin-haptoglobin complexes migrate in the β or α fractions. If a fuzzy extra β/α band is identified on PEL, the sample should be examined for hemolysis (Fig. 8).

The presence of a very sharp band in each lane at the point of application indicates nonspecific staining that is due to protein not entering the agarose gel. This point of application may represent immunoglobulin aggregates or cryoglobulins, and the sample should be retested after treatment of the sample with a reducing agent such as dithiothreitol (DTT) and warming. A 0.5 M solution of DL-DTT in water

laboratory may want to suggest the possible clinical significance of the PEL and IFE results. If the monoclonal protein is an intact immunoglobulin (IgG, IgA, or IgM) but is too small to be fractionated as an M-spike on PEL, our laboratory does not associate a potential diagnosis with the report. These small abnormalities are reported as small monoclonal proteins within a normal (or polyclonal hypergammaglobulinemic, hypogammaglobulinemic, or β-fraction)

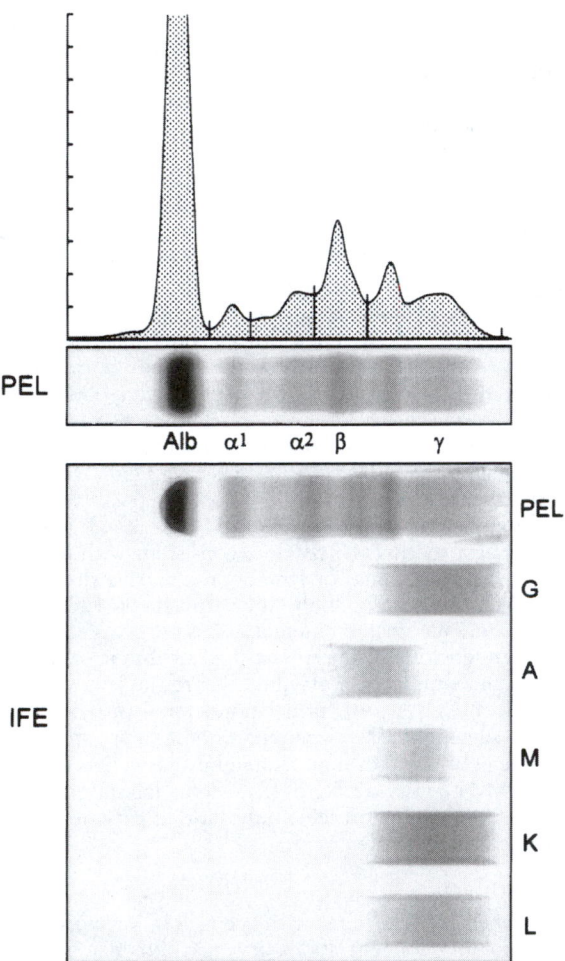

FIGURE 7 PEL and IFE of a sample containing fibrinogen. The PEL contains a fast-γ peak that is indistinguishable from a small monoclonal protein. The IFE shows no corresponding heavy- or light-chain bands. Lanes G to L, as defined for Fig. 1.

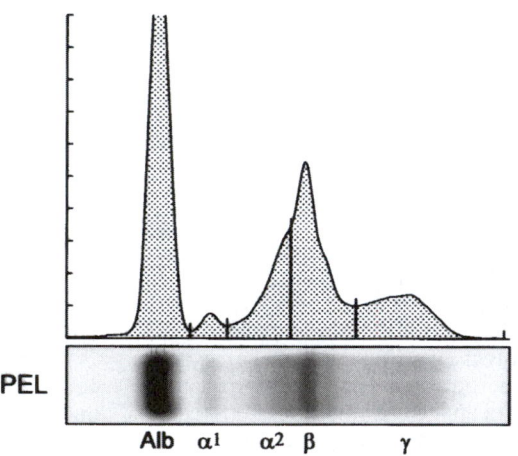

FIGURE 8 PEL of a hemolyzed serum sample. The gel scan appears to contain a small monoclonal protein in the α_2-β region. Alb, albumin.

can be stored up to 1 year at −20°C. Twenty microliters of the DTT solution is added to 80 μl of serum, and the mixture is vortexed and incubated at 37°C for 15 min. The reduced serum sample should be retested.

Very large M-spikes are sometimes difficult to completely wash out of the gel. A large IgG κ monoclonal protein, for example, may have dark, sharp bands in the γ and κ lanes but may also cause fuzzy, faint reactivity in the α, μ, and λ lanes due to the inability to remove the large amount of soluble protein in the narrow region of the M-spike. In addition to causing this "shadow" artifact, large IgG peaks (>3 g/dl) may migrate so sharply on PEL that the binding of stain in the center of the peak is saturated. The quantitation of the M-spike by PEL will be lower than the quantitative immunoglobulin measurement and thus may not reflect changes in concentration due to therapy or progression. Nephelometry should be suggested to assist in patient monitoring (Fig. 9).

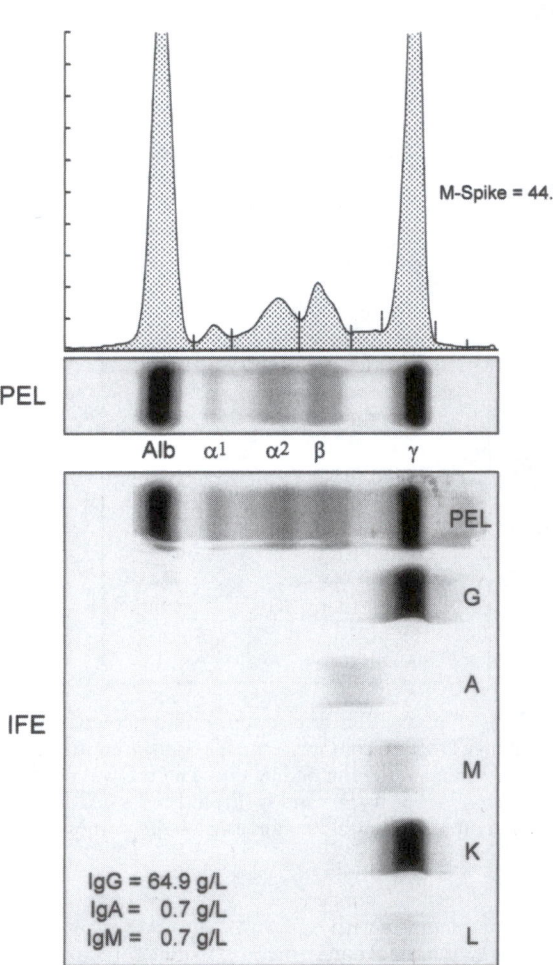

FIGURE 9 PEL, IFE, and quantitative immunoglobulins of a serum sample that contains a large IgG κ M-spike. The large, narrow IgG band has saturated the amount of stain in the PEL agarose gel. The M-spike is 44.9 g/liter, whereas the IgG nephelometric quantitation is 50% higher at 64.9 g/liter. Alb, albumin; lanes G to L, as defined for Fig. 1.

Quality Control

New reagent lots should be tested against sera with known monoclonal proteins before being used for routine testing. In addition, antisera should be tested with a plasma sample to ensure no cross-reactivity with fibrinogen. A sample containing a monoclonal protein of known immunotype should be tested each day. If a patient sample that has been previously immunotyped is part of the workload, that sample may serve as a daily control. The gels should be reviewed with respect to the sharpness of the AGE bands and the correlation of the IFE bands with the AGE M-spike. IFE gels that are too faint or too dense should be repeated with the appropriate dilution. The IFE gels are reviewed in our laboratory by two independent observers.

In addition to the internal laboratory controls, external proficiency challenges are available for identification and characterization of monoclonal proteins. The College of American Pathologists proficiency program supplies challenges on a quarterly basis, and its summary reports allow laboratories to compare their performance with that of other laboratories as well as with those of other methods and reagents from different manufacturers.

Urine IFE

Because light chains may accumulate in the urine, the presence of a monoclonal immunoglobulin light chain in the urine may be seen in almost any of the monoclonal gammopathies. For patients with LCMM, urine PEL and IFE are the major diagnostic and monitoring assays. Patients for whom a monoclonal light chain in the serum, a monoclonal IgD, or any intact monoclonal immunoglobulin M-spike that is >1.5 g/dl is detected should have 24-h urine monoclonal protein studies ordered. Although urine IFE is recommended for patients with a serum M-spike of >1.5 g/dl (21), patients with smaller serum M-spikes may have a large amount of light-chain immunoglobulin in the urine. Many laboratories perform urine monoclonal protein studies for all patients with a serum monoclonal protein. In addition, urine IFE should be performed for patients in whom MM, Waldenström's macroglobulinemia, AL, or light-chain deposition disease is suspected, even if the routine urinalysis is negative for protein. It is not uncommon for the urine to have a normal total protein result and no abnormality on urine PEL but still have a monoclonal light chain detected by IFE. Conversely, patients for whom a monoclonal protein is identified in the urine should have serum studies ordered.

The assessment of urine samples by IFE is similar to serum IFE. The major difference is the need to concentrate urine samples to achieve an appropriate protein concentration. Because of the very large range of urine protein concentrations, the urine IFE test has more stringent sample preparation requirements than serum IFE. Final concentrations of urine protein should ideally be between 2,000 and 8,000 mg/dl. This means that samples with protein concentrations of <16 mg/dl should be maximally concentrated (200×). Centrifugal concentrators allow rapid concentration of urine samples with minimal loss of protein. Our laboratory uses Vivaspin concentrators which are centrifuged at 5,000 rpm until the urine specimens reach final concentration. The polyethersulfone membrane has a 10,000-molecular-weight cutoff and retains most urinary proteins. Urine samples collected with acetic acid, hydrochloric acid, or sodium carbonate should not be accepted for analysis, and samples collected in toluene should have the toluene aspirated before concentration.

Urine samples should be collected and stored refrigerated until analyzed. Urine specimens that are collected with no preservatives are stable for 3 days at room temperature and for 14 days refrigerated or frozen. Urine samples collected with toluene or thymol as a preservative are stable at room temperature for 7 days. Most of the observed instabilities relate to urine samples with low protein content and monoclonal proteins that are at the detection limit of the assay. Large monoclonal protein peaks will be detectable beyond these limits. The limit of detection for urinary monoclonal proteins is 0.5 to 2.6 mg/dl. These limits are 10- to 20-fold lower than the detection limit for serum, and the difference is a reflection of the lack of polyclonal background in many urine samples and of the urine concentration step.

The evaluation of urine IFE gels is similar to that of serum gels. In urine specimens with low protein concentration and with no monoclonal proteins, we may see sufficient staining to identify broad κ and λ reactivity with identical staining distribution. If the gels are too light to visualize any κ and λ reactivity and the urine is already concentrated 100 to 200 times, the assay result should be reported as no monoclonal protein detected. If the gel is too densely stained to evaluate whether there is restricted migration, the assay should be repeated with a lower concentration of the urine sample. As for serum, small abnormalities within a polyclonal background are the most difficult to interpret. Small bands may be less distinct in urine than in serum, and it is important to compare the κ and λ reactivities for differences in distribution. As in serum, however, identification and characterization of most monoclonal proteins in urine is usually straightforward on IFE (Fig. 10). Many samples with monoclonal proteins in the urine have a single monoclonal light-chain band with no corresponding heavy-chain band. Two discrete light-chain bands of either the κ or the λ type may be present, and these are due to the presence of monomers and dimers of the monoclonal light chain. Often, however, there is a second, small monoclonal light-chain band with a corresponding heavy-chain band. Our laboratory reports these results as a monoclonal light chain plus an immunoglobulin fragment. The paired heavy and light chains usually have the same migration as the serum monoclonal protein and are most likely intact immunoglobulin.

Urine IFE Clinical Significance

A urinary monoclonal light chain in an M-peak of >1 g/24 h is consistent with a diagnosis of MM or macroglobulinemia (Fig. 10). In patients with MM, there are a large number of monoclonal plasma cells in the bone marrow and a large amount of monoclonal protein is usually produced. Any excess free light chain that is produced has a short half-life in serum and accumulates in the urine. The amount of excess free light chain is, of course, most dramatic in LCMM. In patients with LCMM, the serum may have a small M-spike, whereas the urine will contain a large M-spike and very little other protein.

A small amount of monoclonal light chain in the presence of proteinuria (>3 g/24 h) which is predominantly albumin is consistent with AL or light-chain deposition disease (Fig. 11) (23). In these diseases, there are usually small numbers of monoclonal plasma cells in the bone marrow and a small amount of monoclonal light chain is produced. The monoclonal free light chains, however, may be deposited as amyloid fibrils or may deposit in the glomerulus, causing light-chain deposition disease. The resultant organ damage results in proteinuria that is predominantly albumin and contains only a small amount of monoclonal light chain.

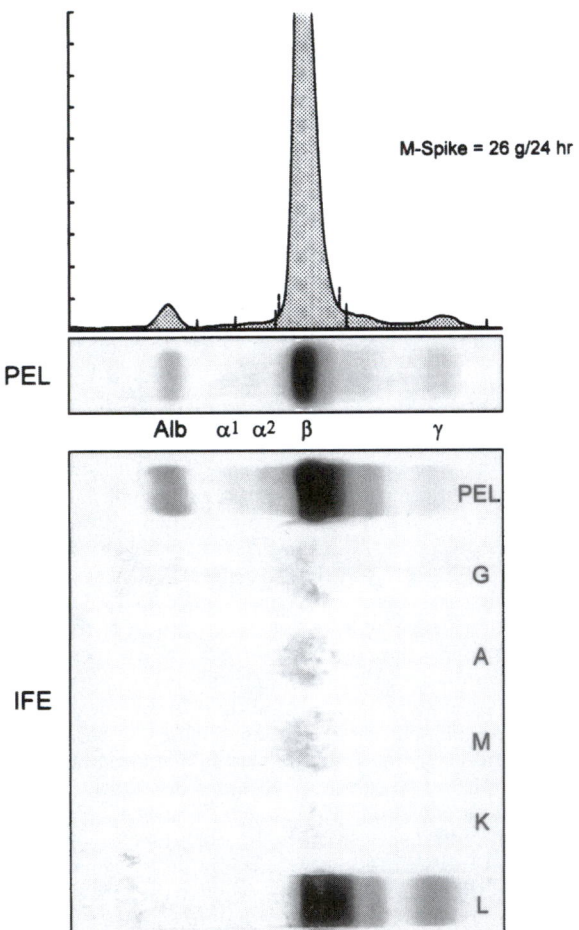

FIGURE 10 PEL and IFE of urine from a patient with LCMM. The PEL shows a large M-spike in the β fraction. The IFE shows a dense λ band corresponding to the M-spike. In addition, there are small amounts of additional λ reactivity in the γ fraction that most likely represent multimers of the monoclonal λ protein. Alb, albumin; lanes G to L, as defined for Fig. 1.

Urine Artifacts

As described above, inadequate concentration of urine specimens may result in false negatives, and overly concentrated urine samples will give high background staining if large amounts of polyclonal immunoglobulins are present. This makes interpretation impossible.

Interfering substances are more commonly identified in urine than in serum by PEL. As in serum, the presence of hemoglobin will result in a band in the α region on PEL, and as with sera, these samples should be examined for their red color. If hemoglobin is present, the report should indicate hemolysis. Other reported interfering substances have included radiographic dyes, antibiotics, and proteins such as myoglobin, lysozyme, and β2 microglobulin. Reports of newly identified monoclonal protein bands on PEL should be delayed until confirmed by IFE.

Artifacts at the point of application are more common in urine than in serum. These are usually caused by insoluble material other than immunoglobulin aggregates. The shadow artifacts caused by large M-spikes are also more common in urine than in serum and need to be recognized as such (Fig. 10).

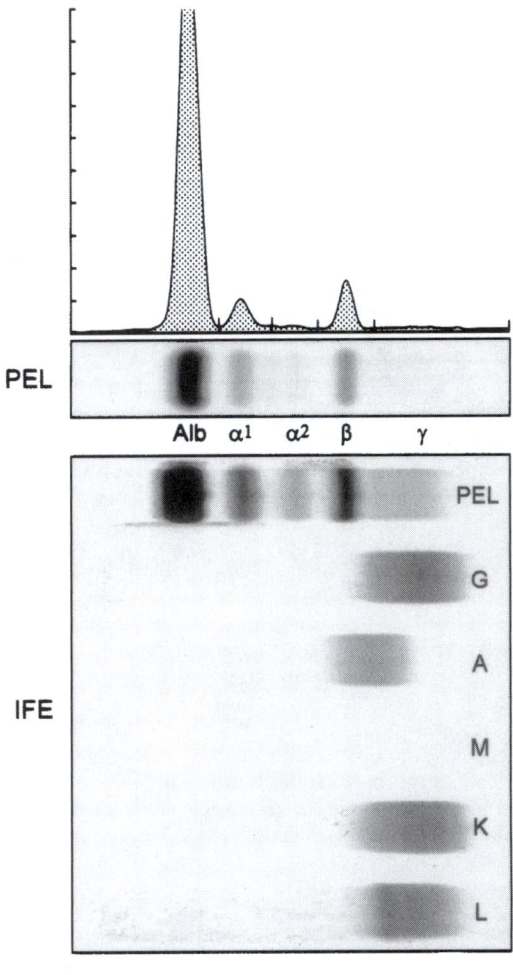

FIGURE 11 PEL and IFE of urine from a patient with primary systemic AL. The urine contains 5 g of protein per 24-h collection. The PEL shows mostly albumin and no apparent monoclonal protein. The IFE shows a faint λ band in the fast-γ region. Alb, albumin; lanes G to L, as defined for Fig. 1.

Because monoclonal gammopathies are uncommon in people under the age of 40, IFE of urine is rarely indicated for patients <30 years of age. In addition, IFE of urine specimens is not useful for general screening without a clinical suspicion of plasma cell dyscrasia.

SERUM ISE

Because of increased sensitivity and shorter turnaround time, IFE has replaced immunoelectrophoresis as the preferred method for characterization of monoclonal proteins. CZE been shown to be a rapid procedure that can be automated for the clinical laboratory, and because of its high resolution, it is slightly more sensitive than AGE (2, 3, 13, 16, 18). CZE may therefore eventually replace AGE as a method of screening for serum M-spikes. The ISE procedure is an addition to the basic CZE method.

The small sample volume required for CZE makes ISE possible for routine characterization of M-spikes. Like CZE, ISE is rapid and automated, but it is not as sensitive as IFE. ISE detects only abnormalities that are apparent on PEL. In the ISE procedure, an M-spike is identified by CZE, the serum is then incubated with various antisera, and the sample is reanalyzed by CZE to determine which specific antiserum removed the electrophoretic abnormality. In addition to ISE being automated and rapid, it may show which light chains are associated with which heavy chains in sera in which two monoclonal proteins comigrate. The disadvantage of ISE is that in order to "immunosubtract" an abnormality, there must first be an abnormality detected by CZE. Small monoclonal proteins that are not detected by electrophoresis but which would be detected by IFE are therefore not able to be identified by ISE. Because some small serum abnormalities may represent very serious clinical disease, ISE cannot be the only method used by a laboratory for detection and characterization of monoclonal proteins.

Almost a decade ago, Beckman introduced a clinical laboratory CZE instrument that was dedicated to PEL and ISE. The Paragon CZE 2000 has seven capillaries and an automated loader for patient serum samples and has been evaluated for its use in the detection of monoclonal proteins. In a comparison study of 1,518 serum samples, we found that agarose gel PEL had a sensitivity and specificity for monoclonal protein detection of 91 and 99%, respectively, whereas CZE had a sensitivity and specificity of 95 and 99%, respectively (16). The increased sensitivity was due to increased resolution in the β region as well as increased resolution of small monoclonal proteins within a polyclonal background. The increased resolution included sera from a small number of patients with monoclonal free light chains that were positive by IFE but negative by agarose PEL. In spite of the increased resolution and sensitivity, the specificity appears to be the same for the two procedures. Recently, Sebia has also introduced a CZE system for PEL in the clinical laboratory.

Because of the automation and the small volumes passing through the capillary tubes, it is feasible to use this method for ISE. The Beckman system uses solid-phase reagents that are packaged for use on the Paragon instrument. The process uses solid-phase beads that are either bare or coupled with antisera that are specific for either γ, α, μ, κ, or λ chains. The beads are contained in a reaction chamber that has six wells (one for each bead type). The loader aliquots patient serum into each well, incubates the reaction chamber, aspirates the supernatants, and then performs CZE on each supernatant. The electrophoretograms from the original serum sample and from the absorbed samples are compared to determine which antiserum removed the abnormality. The Sebia instrument and reagent set employs a similar approach except that the antisera are modified to migrate on CZE in an area that is outside the standard serum fractions. Any patient immunoglobulin that combines with the antisera will therefore be removed from the electrophoresis pattern. These ISE reagent sets are not configured to identify IgD or IgE monoclonal proteins, nor are they configured for analysis of urine samples.

The ISE patterns for a normal serum sample are illustrated in Fig. 12. The PEL pattern shows the resolution of the β fraction into two distinct peaks. This increased resolution allows the identification of some abnormalities that are hidden in the AGE β fraction. The "subtraction" of IgG results in almost total removal of the γ fraction except for the fast-γ region where IgA and IgM migrate. The anti-κ and anti-λ reagents decrease the γ fraction by approximately two-thirds and one-third, respectively. The use of anti-IgA and anti-IgM decreases the background under the β fraction and the β/γ region, respectively. Results for an abnormal serum sample are shown in Fig. 13. The anti-IgG reagent

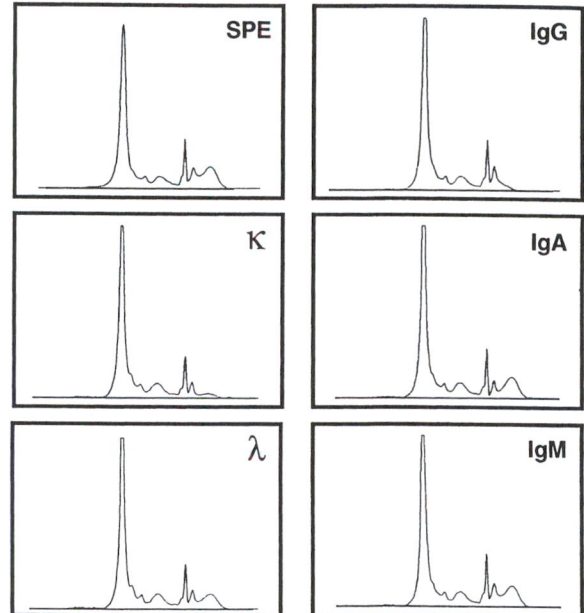

FIGURE 12 ISE of a normal serum sample. The CZE pattern is shown in the upper left panel (SPE, serum protein electrophoresis). The upper right panel shows the CZE pattern after subtraction of IgG from the sample. Except for the remaining IgM and IgA near the β fraction, almost the entire γ fraction is removed. The IgA panel shows the CZE after subtraction of IgA, and the troughs surrounding the β fraction now appear closer to the baseline. The κ and λ panels show the reduction in the γ fraction after removal of the immunoglobulins that contain κ or λ light chains.

removes the M-spike as well as the polyclonal portion of the γ fraction. The anti-κ reagent removes the M-spike as well as a portion of the polyclonal γ fraction. The ISE procedure works well when an abnormality is detected by capillary electrophoresis. In addition to being rapid and automated, the method is not subject to point-of-application artifacts and can detect biclonal gammopathies that comigrate on IFE. γ, κ, and λ bands that comigrate on IFE, for example, may represent IgG κ and IgG λ proteins or may represent an intact IgG monoclonal protein plus a monoclonal free light chain. The ISE procedure or a free light-chain assay will clarify this type of IFE result.

The most important limitation of ISE is that small monoclonal proteins that are not identified by electrophoresis are not able to be characterized. If ISE is used to immunotype monoclonal proteins identified by PEL, an IFE procedure must also be used to screen sera that have normal electrophoretic patterns but for which IFE has been ordered. In addition, IFE for δ and ε heavy chains needs to be performed on samples with a newly identified monoclonal free light chain.

The use of the Sebia Hydragel IF Penta for normal PEL patterns is one approach to complementing the use of CZE with ISE. Although serum samples with normal electrophoretic patterns require IFE for monoclonal gammopathy screening, there will be a low incidence of monoclonal proteins in these samples. The Penta-gel system uses antisera that are a blend of the five specificities used in IFE (anti-γ, -α, -μ, -κ, and -λ). If the single-lane Penta IFE shows a restricted band, then the IFE must be repeated for the sample with all five antisera in separate gel lanes. Depending on

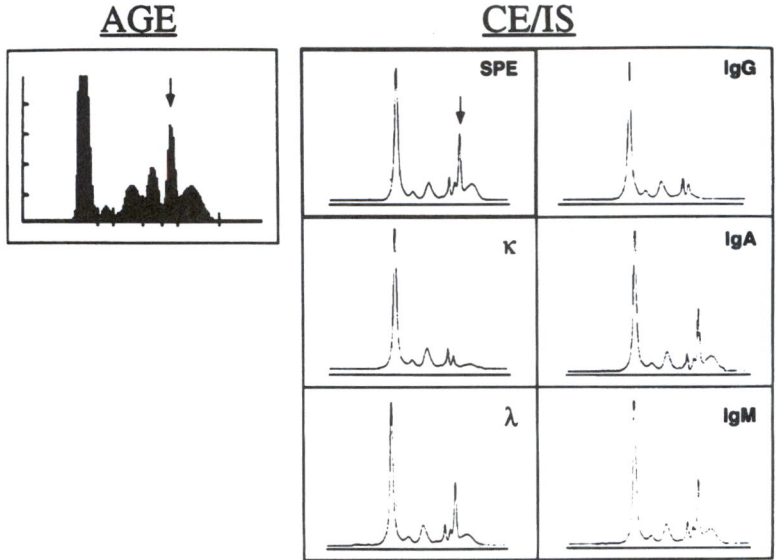

FIGURE 13 Immunosubtraction of a serum sample from a patient with an IgG κ monoclonal protein. The M-spike is apparent by AGE and CZE. After subtraction, the M-spike is removed with antiserum to IgG and κ. Note that the polyclonal portion of the γ fraction is also removed by the IgG reagent and is reduced by the κ and λ reagents. CE/IS, capillary electrophoresis/immunosubtraction; SPE, serum protein electrophoresis.

the volume and mix of cases, this approach may be an efficient approach for identifying and characterizing monoclonal proteins by ISE and IFE.

Quality Control

New reagent lots should be tested against sera with known monoclonal proteins before being used for routine testing. A commercial triclonal control is supplied by Beckman. A sample containing a monoclonal protein of known isotype should be tested each day. If a patient sample that has been previously isotyped is part of the workload, that sample may serve as a daily control. The electrophoretograms for each patient should be reviewed to ensure that all the capillaries gave consistent patterns.

HEAVY-CHAIN DISEASE

Although rare, there are monoclonal immunoglobulins that are composed of truncated heavy chains and contain no immunoglobulin light chain (9, 31, 35). These are often Fc regions with molecular masses that range between 27 and 49 kDa. The serum IFE will show a heavy-chain band, but there is no corresponding light-chain abnormality. Because the heavy-chain peptide is truncated, the heavy chain is also detected in the urine. When immunoelectrophoresis was the common method for characterization of monoclonal proteins, the lack of sensitivity made it necessary to use other methods to confirm the absence of the light chain. As a group, these methods were termed immunoselection (10, 34). In these procedures, antisera to κ and λ are incorporated into an AGE gel prior to sample application. When the serum sample is applied, any molecules containing light chains will be precipitated near the application point and only free heavy chains will electrophorese away from the origin. In normal serum, IFE with anti-heavy-chain specificity will then result in reactivity near the origin, but for heavy-chain disease patients there will be an additional band that has migrated away from the origin. As IFE procedures have replaced

immunoelectrophoresis, the increased sensitivity has made immunoselection unnecessary. Although a monoclonal protein in heavy-chain disease is not always apparent on PEL, ISE is an immunoselection method that can be used for heavy-chain disease samples that contain a visible electrophoretic abnormality. The monoclonal band in γ heavy-chain disease is often broad and not clearly localized on PEL. Localized PEL bands have never been seen in α heavy-chain disease, and hypogammaglobulinemia is often the only prominent feature on PEL of μ heavy-chain disease.

CSF OLIGOCLONAL BANDING

The diagnosis of MS is based predominantly on clinical and radiological findings, but CSF laboratory tests are used to support the diagnosis and are especially useful for patients with unusual presentations (11, 28). The concentration of immunoglobulins is increased in the CSF of patients with inflammatory diseases of the central nervous system, such as MS, neurosyphilis, and acute inflammatory polyradiculoneuropathy (15, 29). This increase in gamma globulins in the CSF of MS patients is due to increased intrathecal synthesis of immunoglobulins (5). Because serum proteins cross the blood-brain barrier, it is important to ascertain whether the gamma globulins are synthesized in the CSF or are derived from the serum. The two most commonly used laboratory tests for CSF-specific immunoglobulin synthesis in MS are oligoclonal banding and the CSF IgG index. OCB have been reported to be positive for 75 to 90% of patients with MS, and the CSF IgG index is positive for 70 to 80% (4, 7, 14, 27). The use of both tests increases the sensitivity to 90 to 95% (27). Although these tests are not specific for MS, they provide useful supportive data when MS is part of the differential diagnosis and when the presentation is unusual.

As described above, the normal polyclonal migration pattern of serum gamma globulins on AGE results in a homogeneous, Gaussian distribution, and monoclonal proteins migrate as a distinct, discrete band. The repertoire of

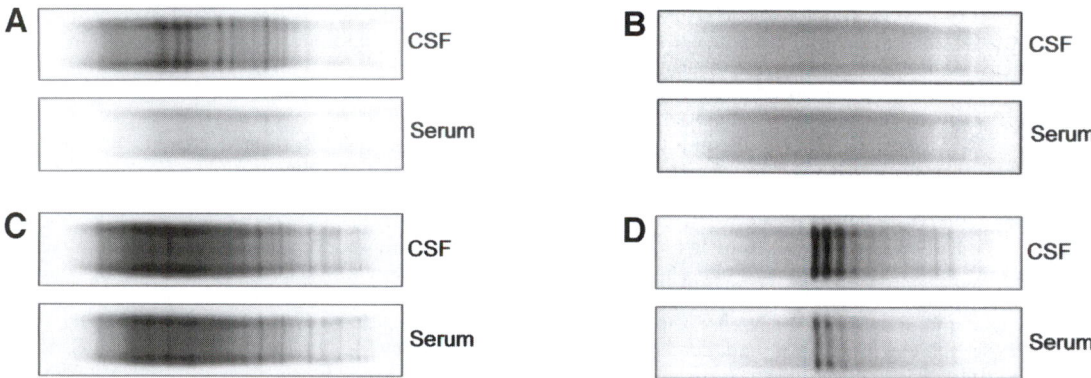

FIGURE 14 IEF with IgG immunoblotting of paired CSF-serum samples. (A) Positive oligoclonal banding result for an MS patient. The CSF contains more than four IgG OCB that are not seen in the serum. (B) Negative result with no IgG bands detected in the CSF or serum. (C) Negative result with no IgG bands that are CSF specific. (D) Banding pattern obtained with a sample that contains a monoclonal protein.

immunoglobulins within the CSF of patients with MS, however, is of such restricted heterogeneity that the electrophoretic pattern does not show a normal continuous distribution. The γ region contains multiple faint bands reflecting the limited number of plasma cell clones. The detection of these OCB within the CSF (but not in a paired serum sample) is interpreted as representing increased CSF-specific immunoglobulin synthesis and is supportive of the diagnosis of MS.

Isoelectric focusing with immunoblotting has been reported to be more sensitive than high-resolution AGE for OCB detection in MS patients (1, 28). In our own studies comparing isoelectric focusing with IgG immunoblotting to high-resolution AGE, the isoelectric focusing had a sensitivity and specificity of 90 and 94%, respectively, compared to a sensitivity and specificity of 60 and 96%, respectively, for AGE (8). It is this increased diagnostic sensitivity that has led to the switch from AGE to isoelectric focusing.

Our laboratory uses gels and reagents from Helena Laboratories for isoelectric focusing and IgG immunoblotting detection of OCB. The isoelectric focusing agarose gel has a pH gradient from 3 to 10. Five microliters of serum diluted 60-fold and 5 μl of unconcentrated CSF are each applied to the gel. After electrophoresis, the separated proteins are transferred to a nitrocellulose membrane and blotted with an anti-IgG peroxidase conjugate. The OCB that are visualized in this assay are much fainter and less distinct than monoclonal bands detected in serum or urine by IFE. A band is considered positive if it is detected in the CSF but not in the serum. Many laboratories interpret two or more CSF-specific bands as consistent with MS. Our validation studies have indicated that most patients with MS have eight or more CSF-specific bands in this reagent system, whereas most non-MS patients have three or fewer CSF-specific bands. We therefore interpret four or more bands as consistent with MS. Results for a paired CSF and serum sample from an MS patient are shown in Fig. 14A. The CSF has more than 10 IgG bands, and the serum contains no discrete IgG bands. Two negative results are shown in Fig. 14B and C. The first CSF-serum pair has no IgG bands. The second CSF-serum pair has no CSF-specific IgG bands, since the banding pattern for the CSF is exactly mirrored by the serum banding pattern. Results for a CSF-serum paired sample from a patient with a monoclonal gammopathy are

shown in Fig. 14D. The monoclonal protein is detected in the serum and CSF, and the laddered pattern is typical for the distribution of a monoclonal protein on isoelectric focusing.

Although OCB are difficult to interpret and count, the isoelectric focusing procedure results in sharper bands that are easier to identify than OCB on AGE. In addition, positive CSF samples usually have only two CSF bands as determined by AGE but more than eight CSF bands as determined by isoelectric focusing. The higher number of CSF bands in positive samples makes the interpretation of the gels easier.

Quality Control

Every gel should contain a positive CSF sample with a known number of bands. The gel is acceptable if band resolution, separation, and staining allow identification of the appropriate number of bands. The number of bands detected in the control should be within one band of the target. All gels should be read independently by two readers. If the two readers do not agree on the test interpretation (e.g., positive versus negative), then a third reader should be consulted. Because of the difficulty in interpreting these gels, all members of the laboratory should participate in periodic blind challenges to standardize gel interpretation.

REFERENCES

1. **Andersson, M., J. Alvarez-Cermeno, G. Bernardi, I. Cogato, P. Fredman, P. Frederiksen, S. Fredrikson, P. Gallo, L. M. Grimaldi, M. Gronning, et al.** 1994. Cerebrospinal fluid in the diagnosis of multiple sclerosis: a consensus report. *J. Neurol. Neurosurg. Psychiatry* **57:**897–902.
2. **Bienvenu, J., M. S. Graziani, F. Arpin, H. Bernon, C. Blessum, C. Marchetti, G. Righetti, M. Somenzini, G. Verga, and F. Aguzzi.** 1998. Multicenter evaluation of the Paragon CZE 2000 capillary zone electrophoresis system for serum protein electrophoresis and monoclonal protein typing. *Clin. Chem.* **44:**599–605.
3. **Bossuyt, X., A. Bogaerts, G. Schiettekatta, and N. Blanckaert.** 1998. Detection and classification of paraproteins by capillary immunofixation/subtraction. *Clin. Chem.* **44:**760–764.
4. **Cavuoti, D., L. Baskin, and I. Jialal.** 1998. Detection of oligoclonal bands in cerebrospinal fluid by immunofixation electrophoresis. *Am. J. Clin. Pathol.* **109:**585–588.

5. Cowdrey, G. N., P. G. Tasker, B. J. Gould, M. Rice-Oxley, and G. B. Firth. 1993. Isoelectric focusing in an immobilized pH gradient for the detection of intrathecal IgG in cerebrospinal fluid: sensitivity and specificity for the diagnosis of multiple sclerosis. *Ann. Clin. Biochem.* **30:**463–468.

6. Dreicer, R., and R. Alexanian. 1982. Nonsecretory multiple myeloma. *Am. J. Hematol.* **13:**313–318.

7. Ebers, G. C., and D. W. Paty. 1980. CSF electrophoresis in one thousand patients. *Can. J. Neurol. Sci.* **7:**275–280.

8. Fortini, A. S., E. L. Sanders, B. G. Weinshenker, and J. A. Katzmann. 2003. Cerebrospinal fluid oligoclonal bands in the diagnosis of multiple sclerosis. Isoelectric focusing with IgG immunoblotting compared with high-resolution agarose gel electrophoresis and cerebrospinal fluid IgG index. *Am. J. Clin. Pathol.* **120:**672–675.

9. Franklin, E. C. 1975. γ- and μ-heavy chain diseases and related disorders. *J. Clin. Pathol.* **28**(Suppl. 6 [*Assoc. Clin. Pathol.*]):65–71.

10. Geraci, L., G. Merlini, A. Spadano, S. Di Matteo, G. Torlontano, and E. Ascari. 1985. Alpha heavy chain disease: report of two cases. *Haematologica* **70:**431–436.

11. Gerson, B., S. R. Cohen, I. M. Gerson, and G. H. Guest. 1981. Myelin basic protein, oligoclonal bands, and IgG in cerebrospinal fluid as indicators of multiple sclerosis. *Clin. Chem.* **27:**1974–1977.

12. Gutman, A. B. 1948. The plasma proteins in disease. *Adv. Protein Chem.* **4:**155–250.

13. Henskens, Y., J. de Winter, M. Pekelharing, and G. Ponjee. 1998. Detection and identification of monoclonal gammopathies by capillary electrophoresis. *Clin. Chem.* **44:**1184–1190.

14. Hershey, L. A., and J. L. Trotter. 1980. The use and abuse of the cerebrospinal fluid IgG profile in the adult: a practical evaluation. *Ann. Neurol.* **8:**426–434.

15. Kabat, E. A., H. Landow, and D. H. Moore. 1942. Electrophoretic patterns of concentrated cerebrospinal fluid. *Proc. Soc. Exp. Biol. Med.* **49:**260–263.

16. Katzmann, J. A., R. Clark, E. Sanders, J. P. Landers, and R. A. Kyle. 1998. Prospective study of serum protein capillary zone electrophoresis and immunotyping of monoclonal proteins by immunosubtraction. *Am. J. Clin. Pathol.* **110:**503–509.

17. Keren, D. F. 2003. *Protein Electrophoresis in Clinical Diagnosis.* Arnold Publishing, London, United Kingdom.

18. Keren, D. F. 1998. Capillary zone electrophoresis in the evaluation of serum protein abnormalities. *Am. J. Clin. Pathol.* **110:**248–252.

19. Keren, D. F., R. Alexanian, J. A. Goeken, P. D. Gorevic, R. A. Kyle, and R. H. Tomar. 1999. Guidelines for clinical and laboratory evaluation of patients with monoclonal gammopathies. *Arch. Pathol. Lab. Med.* **123:**106–107.

20. Keren, D. F., J. S. Warren, and J. B. Lowe. 1998. Strategy to diagnose monoclonal gammopathies in serum: high-resolution electrophoresis, immunofixation, and kappa/lambda quantification. *Clin. Chem.* **34:**2196–2201.

21. Kyle, R. A. 1999. Sequence of testing for monoclonal gammopathies. *Arch. Pathol. Lab. Med.* **123:**114–118.

22. Kyle, R. A., R. C. Bieger, and G. J. Gleich. 1970. Diagnosis of syndromes associated with hyperglobulinemia. *Med. Clin. N. Am.* **54:**917–938.

23. Kyle, R. A., and M. A. Gertz. 1995. Primary systemic amyloidosis: clinical and laboratory features in 474 cases. *Semin. Haematol.* **32:**45–59.

24. Kyle, R. A., M. A. Gertz, T. E. Witzig, J. A. Lust, M. Q. Lacy, A. Dispenzieri, R. Fonseca, S. V. Rajkumar, J. R. Offord, D. R. Larson, M. E. Plevak, T. M. Therneau, and P. R. Greipp. 2003. Review of 1027 patients with newly diagnosed multiple myeloma. *Mayo Clin. Proc.* **78:**21–33.

25. Kyle, R. A., R. A. Robinson, and J. A. Katzmann. 1981. The clinical aspects of biclonal gammopathies. Review of 57 cases. *Am. J. Med.* **71:**999–1008.

26. Kyle, R. A., T. M. Therneau, S. V. Rajkumar, J. R. Offord, D. R. Larson, M. F. Plevak, and L. J. Melton III. 2003. Prevalence of monoclonal gammopathy of undetermined significance (MGUS) among Olmsted County, MN residents 50 years of age. *Blood* **102:**934a (A3476).

27. Lunding, J., R. Midgard, and C. A. Vedeler. 2000. Oligoclonal bands in cerebrospinal fluid: a comparative study of isoelectric focusing, agarose gel electrophoresis, and IgG index. *Acta Neurol. Scand.* **102:**322–325.

28. Petereit, H. F., and W. D. Heiss. 2002. New diagnostic criteria for multiple sclerosis. *Ann. Neurol.* **51:**533–534.

29. Poser, C. M. 1985. Multiple sclerosis and other diseases of the white matter, p. 996–1006. *In* R. B. Conn (ed.), *Current Diagnosis*, 7th ed. W. B. Saunders Company, Philadelphia, Pa.

30. Rubio-Felix, D., M. Giralt, M. P. Giraldo, J. M. Martinez-Penuela, F. Oyarzabal, F. Sala, and A. Raichs. 1987. Nonsecretory multiple myeloma. *Cancer* **59:**1847–1852.

31. Seligmann, M. 1975. Alpha-chain disease. *J. Clin. Pathol.* **28**(Suppl. 6 [*Assoc. Clin. Pathol.*]):72–76.

32. Solomon, A. 1976. Bence Jones proteins and light chains of immunoglobulins. *N. Engl. J. Med.* **294:**17–23.

33. Solomon, A. 1985. Light chains of human immunoglobulins. *Methods Enzymol.* **116:**101–121.

34. Sun, T., S. Peng, and L. Narurkar. 1994. Modified immunoselection technique for definitive diagnosis of heavy-chain disease. *Clin. Chem.* **40:**664.

35. Wahner-Roedler, D. L., T. E. Witzig, L. L. Loehrer, and R. A. Kyle. 2003. γ-Heavy chain disease. Review of 23 cases. *Medicine* **82:**236–250.

Cryoglobulins, Cryofibrinogenemia, and Pyroglobulins

PETER D. GOREVIC AND DENNIS GALANAKIS

11

CRYOGLOBULINS

Background

Cryoglobulinemia is one of a group of syndromes which are characterized by the induction of clinical and/or laboratory abnormalities by cold. Cryoglobulins are immunoglobulins (Igs) that precipitate out of solution below core body temperatures, either as a single isotype (simple cryoglobulins) or as immune complexes in which both antibody and antigen are Igs (mixed cryoglobulins). In some instances, cryoglobulinemia may coexist with other related but usually distinct forms of cold hypersensitivity, such as Raynaud's phenomenon, cold agglutinin activity, or cold-dependent activation of complement (14).

Simple cryoglobulins may be either an intact Ig or a cryoprecipitable Ig light chain (type I cryoglobulins) and are always clonal in terms of electrophoretic mobility or variable-region amino acid sequence. In mixed cryoglobulins, the antibody is almost always IgM (occasionally IgA), which may be monoclonal (type II) or polyclonal (type III) (5). The antigen in mixed cryoglobulins is usually polyclonal IgG, though in some instances the IgG may be oligoclonal when analyzed as to subclass or as revealed by immunoblotting, immunofixation, or two-dimensional gel electrophoresis (24). Mixed cryoglobulins are therefore cold-precipitable rheumatoid factors (RFs), with the serum often being positive when standard assays for IgM antiglobulin activity are used. Many type II RFs have a predilection for the $C\gamma2$-$C\gamma3$ interface of the Fc portion of IgG and react with the binding site for staphylococcal protein A. The complexing of the two isotypes of Ig in mixed cryoglobulins is prerequisite for in vitro cryoprecipitation; the binding affinity of the IgM RF and stoichiometry of complexes formed by mixed cryoglobulins are significantly influenced by temperature (4, 23). The relative frequencies of the different types of cryoglobulins seen in a clinical immunology laboratory will vary significantly with the type of diseases sampled or referred for analysis, and depending on how carefully sera are processed prior to study; the latter is particularly of concern in screening for type III cryoglobulins, which are generally present only at low levels and may require larger volumes of serum for analysis (Table 1).

Concept

The decision to test a serum sample for cryoglobulins may be based on the knowledge that the patient has a specific known or suspected disease, be dictated by the evaluation of a particular clinical manifestation, or be carried out to clarify other abnormalities that have been uncovered in the course of a laboratory evaluation for another purpose. Type I cryoglobulinemia may be suspected in the presence of a known plasma cell dyscrasia (e.g., multiple myeloma or Waldenström's macroglobulinemia), immunochemical evidence of a monoclonal Ig (M-spike) or Ig light chain (Bence Jones protein) in serum and/or urine (see chapters 9 and 10), or clinical evidence of hyperviscosity or ischemic vasculopathy. Type II cryoglobulinemia should be considered in B-cell neoplastic states that may be associated with RF and other autoimmune phenomena, in Sjögren's syndrome, and in chronic inflammatory liver diseases, particularly due to infection by hepatitis C virus (HCV) (7). Type III cryoglobulins have been associated with a wide variety of chronic infectious and autoimmune diseases, many of which are characterized by hyperimmunization and/or hyperglobulinemia. The presence of mixed cryoglobulins may be suggested by purpura or documented cutaneous vasculitis, clinical findings of or biopsy-proven glomerulonephritis, unexplained neuropathy or hepatitis, a positive RF in serum, or markedly depressed C4 levels (14) (Table 2).

Other laboratory abnormalities may be consequences of the physicochemical properties of the cryoglobulins or reflect polyclonal B-cell activation or clonal B-cell proliferation often associated with these disorders. Since cryoprecipitation does not occur at core body temperatures and may begin within minutes of the cooling of serum, it is especially important to consider ex vivo artifacts in the interpretation of laboratory data for patients affected by these syndromes. Most important of these is the handling of the serum before separation, which can significantly affect quantitation, especially when the endpoint is to assess the effect of therapy by comparison of serial specimens. Others may be introduced in the handling of biopsy specimens, during measurements of serum viscosity (9), or by cooling of anticoagulated blood in processing for the Coulter Counter (Table 3). The first

TABLE 1 Classification of cryoglobulins

Type	Frequency (%)	% at concn of:		
		<1 mg/ml	1–5 mg/ml	>5 mg/ml
Simple (type I)	5–38	10	30	60
IgG, IgM, or IgA				
Ig light chain				
Mixed				
Monoclonal (type II)	14–72	20	40	40
Polyclonal (type III)	23–54	80	20	0

clinical description of cryoglobulinemia in a patient with multiple myeloma in 1933 by Wintrobe was based on the recognition of an apparently copious buffy coat fraction in an individual known to be cytopenic due to bone marrow replacement. In more recent experience, failure to recognize pseudoleukocytosis or pseudothrombocytosis due to a high-thermal-amplitude cryoglobulin during treatment with cytotoxic agents can significantly compromise care (11) (Fig. 1).

Procedures

Proper handling of blood samples is the single most important variable determining the success rate for identifying cryoglobulinemia and the most difficult to achieve. In our experience, the best results have been obtained when the screen for cryoprecipitation is carried out by the individual in direct contact with the patient (i.e., physician, house staff, or technician) and proper attention is given to the importance of separating serum from whole blood at 37°C. Although less sensitive and specific than other tests for gammopathy or immune-complex disease, analysis of serum for cryoprecipitation has the advantage of simplicity, requires minimal equipment, and is therefore very cost efficient. It is also an excellent teaching instrument for students and other trainees, as all that is required is a "warm heart" (to keep the sample close to core body temperature and minimize ex vivo cryoprecipitation before separation), a refrigerator (in which to observe the sample overnight), and a source of warm running water (to prove that any precipitate that forms can be redissolved on warming). Since cryoglobulins often come out of solution within 24 to 48 h, many sera can be efficiently screened within 1 or 2 days of collection, allowing the clinician to rapidly make further decisions regarding additional workup.

Isolation, Quantitation, and Characterization of Cryoglobulins

1. Collect 10 to 20 ml of blood (2 red-top tubes) and keep at 37°C for 30 to 60 min prior to separation. To ensure that cryoprecipitation does not occur ex vivo, the blood may be placed in a thermos kept at this temperature or put into a 37°C water bath prior to centrifugation. Patients previously found to have high levels of cryoglobulin may require smaller volumes for serial studies, and those suspected of having type III cryoglobulins may require larger volumes for analysis. Occasionally, gel formation in the syringe or Vacutainer tube may occur as the initial manifestation of cryoprecipitation (see also below). Serum is separated from the clot by centrifuging the clot warm for 10 min at 2,500 rpm (1,500 × g). Following separation, it should be carefully inspected for lipemia, which may complicate the visual inspection of the sample for cryoprecipitation over the several hours following collection. Serum thus collected antiseptically, or to which a drop of sodium azide (0.1 g/liter) is added to prevent bacterial overgrowth, may be safely sent by overnight mail (even at room temperature) to a reference laboratory for detailed characterization.

2. Cryoglobulins are grossly apparent on visual inspection down to the range of 50 to 100 µg/ml, depending on the volume of the serum sample submitted for analysis. Type I cryoglobulins are often apparent as flocculent, occasionally crystalline precipitates that are usually observed within 24 h of separation. Cryocrystalglobulins can be characterized by light microscopy, using Giemsa or hematoxylin and eosin stains, as dense-structured inclusions or extracellular material on staining with osmium and uranyl acetate for electron microscopy, or as non-Congo red-binding birefringence visualized by polarizing microscopy. Type III cryoglobulins are

TABLE 2 Disease, clinical,[a] and laboratory associations

Type of cryoglobulin	Associations		
	Disease(s)[b]	Clinical	Laboratory
I	Macroglobulinemia, myeloma, idiopathic	Necrosis, Raynaud's phenomenon, acrocyanosis	M-spike, increase in viscosity, cryocrystals
II	HCV infection, Sjögren's syndrome, CLL, lymphoma, macroglobulinemia	Purpura, neuropathy, keratoconjunctivitis	RF, nephritis, hepatitis, decrease in C4
III	Chronic infections, autoimmune disease	Vasculitis	RF, nephritis

[a] Reversible cyanosis of the helices of the ears and livedoid vasculitis are characteristic of IgG type I cryoglobulinemia, whereas purpura due to leukocytoclastic angiitis is characteristic of type II IgMκ-IgG cryoglobulins.
[b] Idiopathic, no apparent underlying disease; CLL, chronic lymphocytic leukemia.

TABLE 3 Laboratory abnormalities in cryoglobulinemia

Abnormality

Direct effects
  Cryoprecipitation
    Cryogel formation
    Cryocrystalglobulins
  Hyperviscosity
    Present only with cooling
    Accentuated by cooling

Immunochemical findings
  Normal (frequent with type III)
  Hyperglobulinemia
    Diffuse elevation or M-spike on serum protein electrophoresis
    Elevation of a specific isotype (IgG, IgA, or IgM) or subclass (type I)
    Increased high (19S)- and low (7S)-molecular-weight IgM (type II)
    Skewing of the normal (2/1) κ:λ ratio of Ig light chains (types I and II)
  Hypoglobulinemia
    Diffuse (occasionally with type II)
    Noncryoglobulin isotypes (type I)

Clonal markers of B cells
  Monoclonal gammopathy
  Clonal populations of B cells revealed by surface Ig
    Peripheral blood (heavy- and light-chain determinants)
    Lymphoid aggregates in bone marrow (type II)
  Evidence of Ig gene rearrangement

Antibody activity and immune complex formation
  19S IgM antiglobulins (RFs) (types II and III)
    IgA (type II) or IgG (type I) RF
  Elevated levels of circulating immune complexes, especially assays based on C1q binding activity
  Antinuclear antibodies (see chapters 112–115)
  Antiviral antibodies (Epstein-Barr virus, HBV, HCV)

Hypocomplementemia
  Classical or alternative pathway activation as a manifestation of specific diseases (e.g., lupus)
  In vivo/ex vivo activation by cryoprecipitates
  Selective depression of C4
  Cold-dependent activation independent of cryoprecipitation

Ex vivo artifacts (avoid by testing at 37°C)
  Increased erythrocyte sedimentation rate
  Pseudoleukocytosis
  Pseudothrombocytosis
  Cryoprecipitation in biopsy material

Associated abnormalities
  Proteinuria, hematuria, pyuria, casts
  Abnormal liver function tests

usually gelatinous and may take up to a week to be fully apparent. Consequently, serum samples are observed at 4°C for 7 days after collection. This analysis may be facilitated by measurement of turbimetry (e.g., using a jacketed spectrophotometer cuvette at 630 nm) at 15-min intervals or by cryoprecipitation from hypotonic media. The kinetics of cryoprecipitation are quite variable, depending on the individual sample and the concentration of cryoglobulin present (10). This may reflect in part different mechanisms for cryoprecipitation, including lag periods overcome by nucleation events (14, 15). We have observed little variability when the kinetics of cryoprecipitation of serum, plasma, or isolated cryoglobulins have been compared by turbimetric analysis (Fig. 2).

3. Positive sera are spun down in a refrigerated (4°C) centrifuge (Sorvall) at 3,000 rpm for 15 min, and the supernatant is removed for further analysis. The pellet is vortexed six times with 5 to 10 ml of ice-cold 0.15 M saline, each time spinning out the precipitate for 15 min at 3,000 rpm; contaminating red blood cells may be lysed hypotonically. Finally, the sample is suspended in warm saline (1/10 to 1 volume of the initial serum) and incubated at 37°C for 1 h. Ideally, there should be complete dissolution of the precipitate with shaking. If this does not occur, the presence of fibrin or bacterial contamination should be considered; warm-insoluble precipitate should be spun out at 37°C (3,000 rpm for 10 minutes) and the supernatant should again be cooled to 4°C and observed for cryoprecipitation.

4. The concentration of cryoglobulin can be determined as a cryocrit or as an absolute concentration of protein back-calculated for the initial volume of serum. Cryocrits are appropriate for serial measurements in individual patients (provided that the method is carefully reproduced between samples) and for the purposes of general comparison. Exact protein

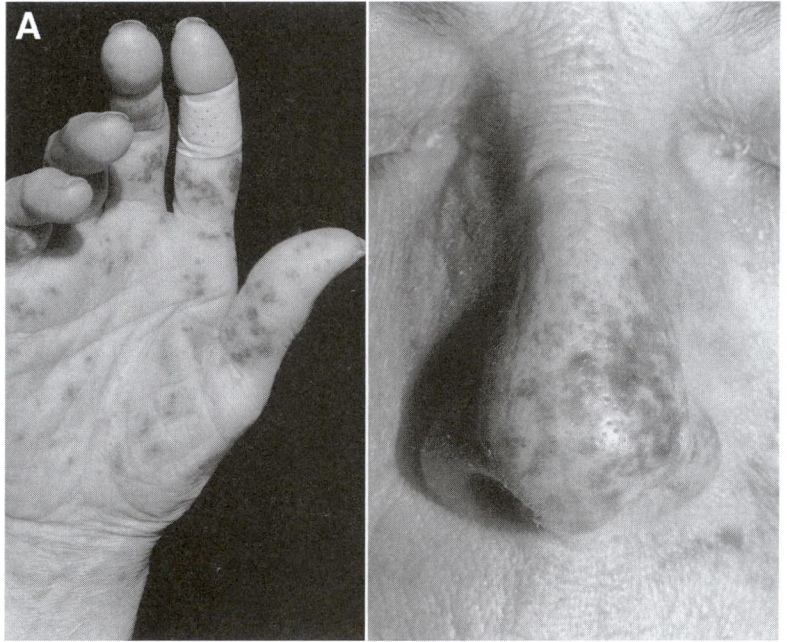

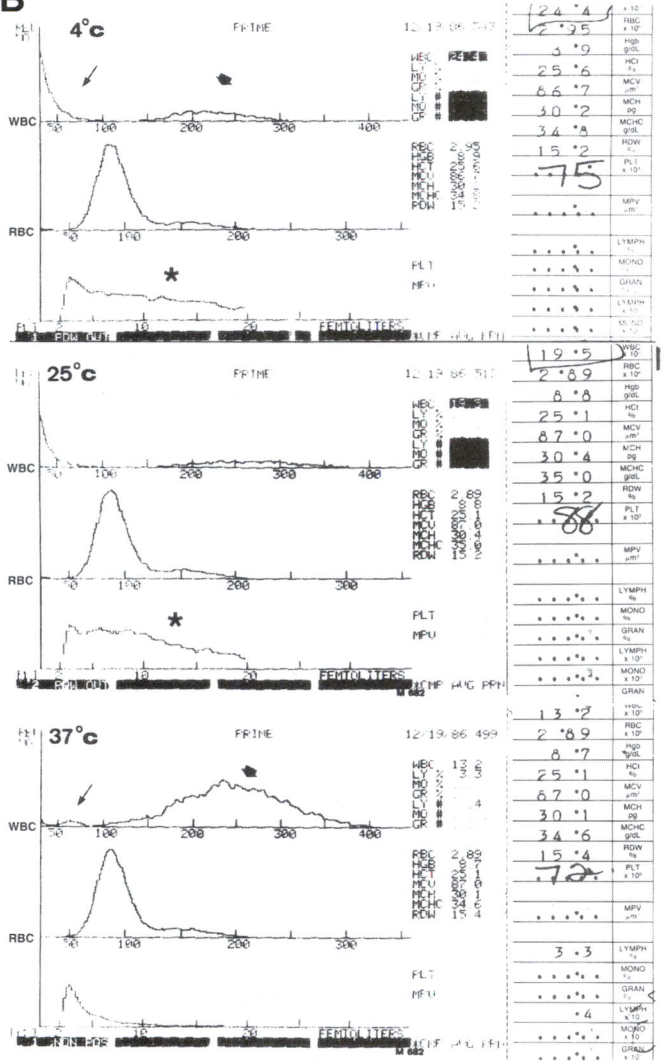

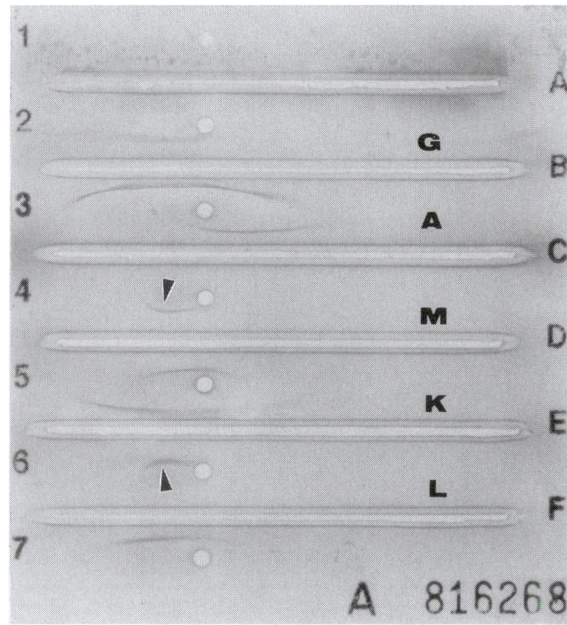

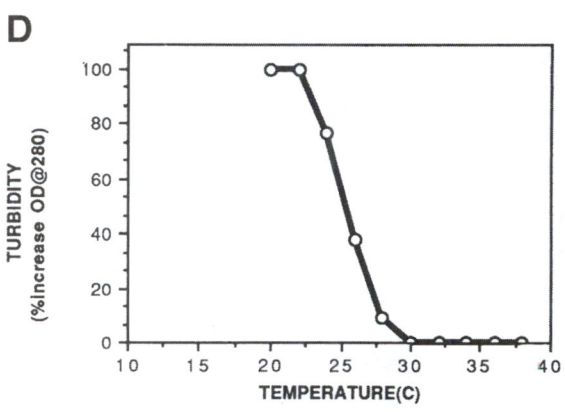

measurements are more accurate and can be compared to quantitation of specific Ig isotypes in serum, isolated cryoglobulins, and serum supernatant obtained following cryoprecipitation. To obtain a cryocrit, an aliquot of the initial warm serum is used to fill a disposable Wintrobe tube to the 10-mm mark. The tube is kept vertical at 4°C for the time determined above for cryoprecipitation and then centrifuged cold at 2,000 rpm (2,000 × g) for 30 min; the percent total volume occupied by the pellet is then obtained by visual inspection. The total protein content of isolated cryoglobulin (rigorously washed as described above) is determined in our laboratory by the Bradford method, using the Coomassie protein assay (Pierce bicinchoninic acid protein assay). In some instances, repeated warming and cryoprecipitation lead to significant loss of material, and therefore quantitation is defined in terms of the initial isolation protocol for consistency.

5. Warmed dissolved cryoprecipitate is characterized by immunochemical analysis, in our laboratory first by double diffusion in agar (Ouchterlony plates) and then by agarose gel immunofixation electrophoresis (IFE) (see chapter 9). In addition to defining type I cryoglobulins, immunofixation may reveal the clonality of the IgM component, or the oligoclonality of the IgG components, of mixed cryoglobulins. Since the monoclonal components of type II cryoglobulins are almost invariably IgM(κ), the percent contribution of clonal IgM to total IgM present in a mixed cryoglobulin can either be estimated by correlating the contribution of a clonal band to total immunoreactive IgM on a strip developed with anti-μ antiserum with one developed with anti-κ antiserum by visual inspection or be more formally quantitated by densitometry.

6. Other modalities which have been utilized include the following. (i) Immunoblot analysis with anti-heavy-chain or anti-light-chain antisera of cryoglobulins separated under nondenaturing conditions on 4% polyacrylamide gels (which can also be used to demonstrate 7S IgM in serum) or on composite agarose polyacrylamide gels. Immunoblotting combined with IFE can be performed on as little as 10 μg of material, can distinguish type II from type III mixed cryoglobulins, and may be particularly effective for the demonstration of the oligoclonality of each component of the complex. (ii) Two-dimensional gel electrophoresis, run under denaturing and reducing conditions in order to dissociate mixed cryoglobulins and separate Ig heavy and light chains by molecular weight and isoelectric focusing point. Two-dimensional polyacrylamide gel electrophoresis (PAGE) may be more sensitive than IFE for the demonstration of B-cell clonality in patients with cryoglobulinemia and has been combined with Fourier transform-ion cyclotron resonance mass spectrometry for the high-resolution analysis of cryoglobulin constituents (8, 24). (iii) Capillary zone electrophoresis,

which has been adapted in some laboratories for the rapid characterization of cryoprecipitates, may be particularly useful for type III cryoglobulins because of the sensitivity of the technique. Subtraction analysis of the gamma globulin curve before and after cryoprecipitation can be used as an alternative to protein and Ig determinations for quantitation (16).

7. The relative contributions of the different components of mixed cryoglobulins may be determined immunochemically by standard techniques (i.e., radial immunodiffusion or, more commonly, nephelometry) if sufficient material is available (see chapter 8). This may be used to confirm the nature of mixed cryoglobulins and to show selective enhancement of specific antibody activity in cryoprecipitates compared to that in serum but is rarely of clinical significance. The power of this type of analysis has been significantly expanded in research studies through the use of capture enzyme-linked immunosorbent assays (ELISAs) that employ both isotype- and idiotype-specific antibodies (21). Since most mixed cryoglobulins remain cryoprecipitable in the pH range of 5.0 to 8.5, they can be dissociated under, e.g., acid conditions, and IgM can be separated from IgG and quantitated after ion-exchange chromatography or passage through specific immunoabsorbents (e.g., protein G columns) or size fractionated by high-pressure liquid chromatography or fast protein liquid chromatography.

Assays for Specific Antibody Activities, Antigens, or Detection of Nucleic Acid

1. Mixed cryoglobulins contain IgM RF activity when tested by either standard assays or more sensitive techniques (e.g., binding of radiolabeled aggregated IgG). Unlike rheumatoid arthritis, cryoglobulin RF activity, particularly in HCV-associated disease, is not associated with antibodies to cyclic citrullinated peptide. Although both cryoprecipitable and noncryoprecipitable RF activity can be detected, occasional testing of RF activity in serum may be invalid because it has been lost due to cryoprecipitation of a high-thermal-amplitude (i.e., one that rapidly cryoprecipitates above room temperature) mixed cryoglobulin (Fig. 1).

2. Individual case reports and small series have shown enrichment of a number of specific antibody activities, including binding to antigens such as IgG or HCV recombinant proteins, in cryoglobulins associated with specific disease states (14). Most of these antibodies (e.g., HCV antibodies [HCVAbs]) are associated with the IgG fraction of mixed cryoglobulins and can be quantitated by ELISA, which should be normalized for total IgG quantitated in cryoglobulin relative to serum (21, 23). In some instances, we have found that a specific antibody activity was in fact not concentrated in the isolated cryoglobulin, as was the case for a patient with a type 1 IgG(κ) cryoglobulin without

FIGURE 1 Cryoglobulinemia was initially missed in a patient with cutaneous vasculitis documented by biopsy of a purpuric lesion on the right second digit (A, left panel). Because of deteriorating status, including renal failure, she was treated with high doses of steroids and then cytotoxic agents, with apparently poor response in terms of an expected drop in leukocyte count. One weekend, while still in the intensive care unit, the patient was noted to have developed nasal purpura in the distribution of a cold-air oxygen mask (A, right panel). The Coulter histograms obtained at 4, 25, and 37°C (B) display the leukocyte (top), erythrocyte (middle), and platelet (bottom) panels. The leukocyte panel shows small lymphocytes to the left (thin arrow) and larger polymorphonuclear leukocytes and monocytes to the right (thick arrow), with the ordinate displaying percent total cells; the platelet panels at 4 and 25°C are unusual in having a long tail (*) after the expected narrow peak. Pseudoleukocytosis and pseudothrombocytosis are revealed at 37°C, which shows (i) all the leukocytes to be polymorphonuclear, with few lymphocytes, as expected for a patient on high-dose corticosteroids; and (ii) a narrow platelet peak. Both findings are reflected in the manual counts (B, right). Recognition of this artifact led to identification of a type II cryoglobulin with RF activity, with restricted IgM and κ arcs by immunoelectrophoresis (C, arrowheads) and a high thermal amplitude of cryoprecipitation (D). OD, optical density.

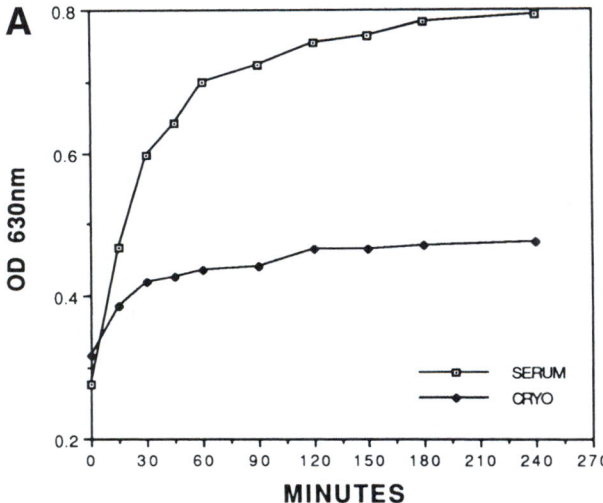

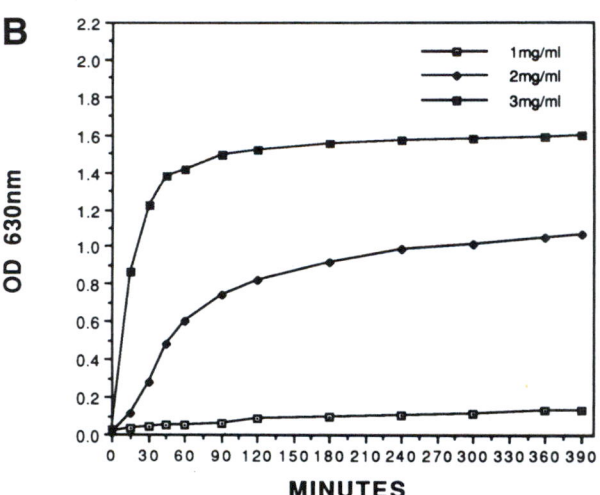

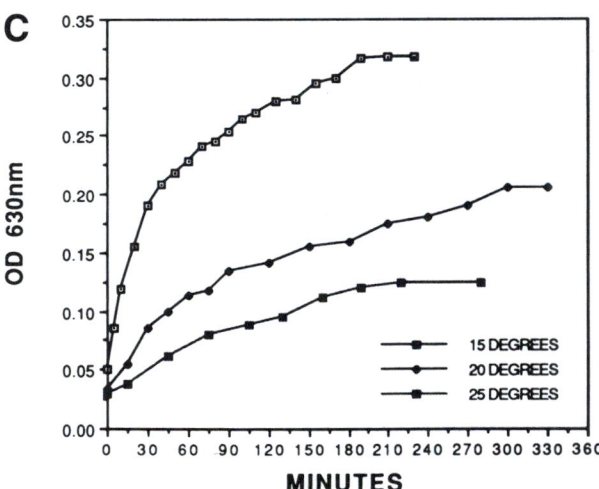

FIGURE 2 Kinetics of cryoprecipitation, assessed by turbimetric analysis, for a type II cryoglobulin, comparing serum and isolated cryoglobulin (A), different concentrations of isolated cryoglobulin (B), and different temperatures of cryoprecipitation (C). OD, optical density.

instrinsic HCVAb activity who developed HCV infection during the course of his illness.

3. The nature of mixed cryoglobulins as immune complexes in chronic infection by HBV and HCV is indicated by reports of selective enrichment of both antigens (e.g., HBV surface and HCV core antigens) and specific antibody activity in some isolated cryoprecipitates (14). Current experience is that 60 to 80% of type II cryoglobulins in patients with the syndrome of mixed cryoglobulinemia (purpura, arthralgias, and renal disease) are associated with evidence of HCV infection, assessed by anti-HCV antibody activity and/or amplification of specific nucleic acid by PCR following reverse transcription (RT) (1). In our laboratory, HCVAb activity is assessed by recombinant immunoblot assay and the presence of HCV RNA is determined initially by RT-PCR using nested primers framing conserved sequences in the 5′ untranslated region of the viral genome. The recombinant immunoblot assay for HCVAb measures primarily IgG antibody to HCV antigens. Controls include known positive and RF-positive, HCVAb-negative sera; RT-PCR is also carried out with positive and negative samples, with care taken to control for carryover contamination (see chapter 83). HCV copy number can be more accurately determined by commercially available quantitative assays, including those using competitive PCR (e.g., the Roche Amplicor system) or direct capture of viral RNA by complementary branched DNA (Chiron). The lower limits of detection for these assays are 600 and 615 IU of HCV RNA per ml, respectively. Quantitative assays may be used to demonstrate selective enrichment of HCV RNA in cryoprecipitates (reported as being more frequent than enrichment of HCVAb), in some instances when the serum supernatant is negative or below the level of detection of the particular assay, and to follow the clinical course and the effect of therapy with alpha interferon (IFN-α) (20). HCV genotype analysis is commercially available and may be used as one variable to anticipate the efficacy of therapy with IFN-α; however, its value for the evaluation of mixed cryoglobulinemia and other autoimmune manifestations of chronic infection is uncertain (12).

New HCV assays are likely to enhance the sensitivity and specificity of measurements of cryoglobulins associated with extrahepatic diseases associated with chronic infection. These include the quantitation of hepatitis core antigen (18) and real-time PCR assays for HCV RNA and replicative intermediate (negative strand) (17). The former may be assayed by ELISA (Chiron-Ortho Clinical Diagnostics) and has been found to be concentrated in isolated cryoprecipitates (22); the latter may prove to be a more sensitive marker for occult HCV infection in cryoglobulinemia (6) and as a criterion for productive infection by virus in extrahepatic sites.

Complement Measurements in Cryoglobulinemia

Sera from type II mixed cryoglobulinemia patients typically have low antigenic levels of the early components of complement (see chapter 12), with relatively normal levels of C3 and factor B. Measurements are best made at 37°C in order to minimize artifacts introduced by ex vivo cryoprecipitation or activation by other complexes that may occur over time at 4°C. Serial studies have shown that hypocomplementemia correlates only poorly with symptomatology or cryoglobulin levels. Most patients with type I cryoglobulinemia have normal complement levels, though occasional instances in which complement activation occurs and has been shown to be directly due to cryoprecipitate formation have been well described. In type III cryoglobulinemia, complement measurements may reflect abnormalities prevalent in the underlying disease (e.g., lupus erythematosus) or among the subset of patients predisposed to develop cryoglobulinemia (e.g., rheumatoid vasculitis or primary Sjögren's syndrome).

In sera manifesting cold-dependent activation of complement (CDAC), a similar profile of low 50% hemolytic complement value and poorly hemolytic C4 with normal hemolytic C5 to C9 is seen at 4°C, with normal values being obtained for EDTA-treated plasma and for serum kept at 37°C. In contradistinction to cryoglobulinemia, C1q and C4 antigenic levels are normal. CDAC may be consequent to HCVAb-monoclonal RF complexes with differing stoichiometry, may be present in sera that do not contain detectable cryoprecipitates, and appears to correlate somewhat with liver damage and response to treatment with IFN-α (25). CDAC, RF, cryoglobulinemia, and elevated levels of IgM-containing immune complexes are all prevalent in HCV infection.

Conclusions

Although many clinical laboratories offer cryoglobulin determinations, rarely is testing rigorously carried out, and there is considerable interlaboratory variability. The most common sources of error are (i) false-negative results due to loss of cryoprecipitate during storage and (ii) false-positive results, usually due to residual fibrin in the sample and failure to demonstrate redissolution of material with warming. In most instances, cryoglobulins are readily apparent by visual inspection of the specimen at 1 to 3 days. Many have thermal amplitudes characterized by 10^3- to 10^4-fold decreases in solubility occurring over a relatively restricted (<10°C) temperature range, which may be significantly influenced by the level of cryoprotein in the sample. Detailed characterization can be achieved by using standard immunochemical techniques modified to be carried out above the temperature of cryoprecipitation.

Intralaboratory Quality Control and Interlaboratory Proficiency Testing

1. Serum must be obtained from blood that is clotted at body temperature; whole blood that is allowed to cool or placed at 4°C before separation should not be accepted.

2. A sample size of 1 to 3 ml of serum may be adequate to screen for type I or II cryoglobulins but is inadequate for type III cryoglobulins; for type III, 5 to 10 ml of serum should be required. Smaller sample volumes should be rejected, especially if a protocol that requires aliquoting of the specimen is followed.

3. Serum samples obtained from patients who are receiving heparin or other anticoagulants are not acceptable for cryoglobulin determinations (see below).

4. Complement and HCV RNA measurements should not be performed on serum that has been allowed to cryoprecipitate; they should be carried out on parallel samples of blood appropriately processed for these determinations.

5. A positive cryoprecipitate formed at 4°C may be defined by complete solubilization when warmed to body temperature or by comparison to a sterile aliquot of the same specimen kept at this temperature.

6. Whereas a cryocrit determination may be made for a centrifuged aliquot of serum cooled in a calibrated hematocrit tube, reflex cryoglobulin characterization requires rigorous washing of the cryoprecipitate.

7. Reflex testing may include immunofixation, Ig quantitation, and nephelometric evaluation for RF activity.

CRYOFIBRINOGENS

Background

In the older literature, the term "cryofibrinogenemia" was used to describe a related phenomenon of cryoprecipitation in plasma that is distinct from cryoglobulinemia but which may be associated with thromboembolic disease, vasculopathy, and occasionally connective tissue diseases. Whereas cryoglobulins precipitate in both cooled plasma and serum, cryofibrinogens are seen only in plasma. A more accurate description of this phenomenon might be abnormal or pathologic fibrinemia, which is observed as a precipitate when citrated plasma is left at 4°C for several or more hours or overnight and reflects the presence of abnormal levels of soluble fibrinogen-fibrin complexes; such cryoprecipitates often redissolve at higher temperatures (e.g., 37°C) and contain, in addition, major amounts of fibronectin, in and of itself a cryoprecipitable protein (Fig. 3). Thus, cryofibrinogenemia is a misnomer and actually describes cold-precipitable complexes of fibrin and fibrinogen which also contain fibronectin. These may occur (i) when blood drawing is slow, allowing thrombin generation ex vivo; (ii) in any condition in which increased levels of fibrin occur (e.g., chronic intravascular coagulation); or (iii) in certain dysfibrinogenemias, because the fibrin generated in these conditions is poorly or not at all coagulable at ambient or physiologic temperatures but may polymerize in the cold. This last occurrence is rare and can be ruled out by the presence of a normal plasma thrombin time.

Concept

The decision to test a plasma sample for cryofibrinogenemia may be suggested by clinical features of severe cold intolerance (e.g., Raynaud's phenomena or cold urticaria) or evidence of thrombotic vasculopathy that cannot be explained by antiphospholipid autoantibodies, clotting factor deficiencies, or relevant mutations (see chapter 118). It may be part of a more general evaluation for causes of purpura, disseminated thrombohemorrhagic coagulopathy, or other thromboembolic disorders; in major surgery or trauma during the intraoperative or immediate postoperative period; or evaluation of skin necrosis, chronic leg ulcers, or gangrene. Cryofibrinogenemia may be associated with neoplastic states (notably, multiple myeloma, various solid malignancies, and leukemia) and IgA nephropathy and is rarely familial; it has also been described in the absence of clearcut underlying disease and in about 3% of random blood samples from hospitalized patients or asymptomatic healthy blood donors (2).

Two examples of pathologic fibrinemia follow.

Case 1

A 14-year-old girl was evaluated for cold-sensitive vasculitic purpura, mainly of the extremities. The condition had become so severe that she required home tutoring throughout the year to avoid cold exposure. Her condition was monitored by measuring her plasma cryocrit, the column of insoluble material formed when citrated plasma was incubated at 4°C and centrifuged. This value rose markedly during exacerbations of her disease and decreased following each plasmapheresis treatment. Cryoprecipitate that formed when plasma was frozen and thawed at 4°C was also measured as another indicator of cryoprecipitable plasma protein. Relative to those of healthy donors, and to other patient plasmas with similarly elevated fibrinogen levels, her level of cryoprecipitable protein was at least threefold higher during a quiescent period. Her isolated fibrinogen was functionally normal, as was that obtained from her parents. Her protease-free serum, alone or with added

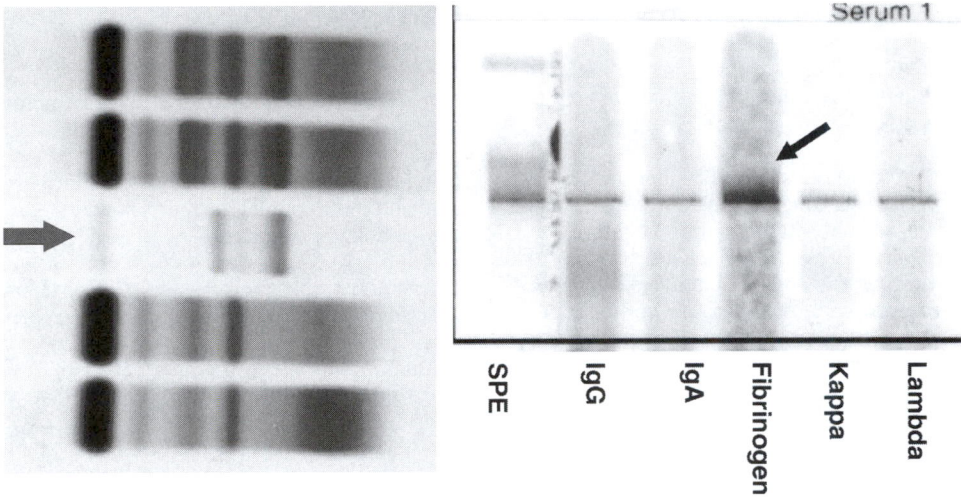

FIGURE 3 Isolated washed cryofibrinogen (arrows) visualized by agarose gel electrophoresis (left) and immunofixation (right). Gel electrophoresis reveals some residual albumin toward the anode, fibronectin in the β region, an origin artifact, and fibrinogen, compared to serum samples in the upper and lower lanes. In the immunofixation on the right, an origin artifact is seen in all lanes due to precipitation on the cold gel. However, the antifibrinogen lane shows increased precipitate, thereby characterizing this as fibrinogen. (Figure generously provided by D. Keren.)

fibrin-depleted fibrinogen isolated from her plasma or from that of a normal donor, did not form a cryoprecipitate.

Case 2

A 42-year-old man was referred for cryogel formation, occurring each time blood was drawn by venipuncture (Fig. 4). He was known to have chronic hepatitis due to HCV and had achieved only limited response to various regimens of IFN-α and ribavirin. Other significant clinical features were visual changes; purplish blotching, notably involving the forehead; and erectile dysfunction. The initial coagulation profile disclosed a prolonged thrombin time and only partial correction when equal volumes of his plasma and normal donor plasma were mixed. Serial plasma dilutions yielded

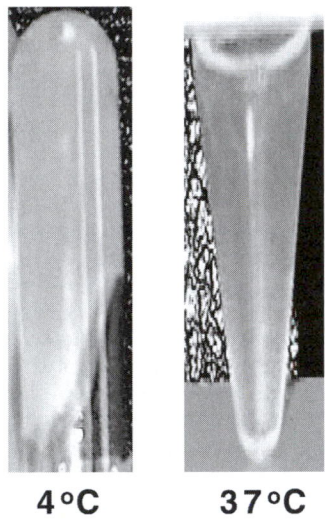

4°C   **37°C**

FIGURE 4 Reversible cryogel formation at 4°C (tube inverted) and 37°C (liquid).

abnormally increasing thrombin times, consistent with the acquired dysfibrinogenemia of hepatic disorders. There was no family history of dysfibrinogenemia.

Repeated evaluations showed that drawn blood rapidly formed a gel-like material at 4°C that did not fully dissolve when rewarmed to 37°C; this gel did not contain significant Ig as determined by either Ouchterlony analysis or sodium dodecyl sulfate-PAGE. After removal of this gel, no further cryoprecipitation was observed; similarly, when plasma was clotted by addition of thrombin at 37°C and the clot was synerized and removed after several hours, his serum formed no additional cryoprecipitate when left at 4°C. By contrast, the level of citrated plasma cryoprecipitate obtained by conventional freeze-thawing was approximately threefold higher than that of normal controls.

All of the patient's symptoms improved following plasmapheresis but recurred progressively within 2 weeks or so, requiring repeat treatments. During the first few plasmaphereses, the intravenous line to the cell separator, as well as the plasma line to the disposal container, began to occlude with visible strands of clot; frequent flushing of the lines with normal saline was only partially successful in overcoming this obstacle. The problem was solved by incorporating 6 to 10 U of heparin/ml in the citrate anticoagulant solution used during the procedure. The patient's plasma formed abnormally increased amounts of precipitate when left at 4°C overnight, whether obtained before plasmapheresis or after the procedure from the removed plasma. For testing, his serum was rendered protease-free by addition of hirudin (20 U/ml), aprotinin (50 U/ml), and phenylmethylsulfonyl fluoride (100 μM); soluble fibrin was depleted by incubation of fibrinogen solutions at 4°C, pH 6.4, and an ionic strength of 0.1 overnight followed by removal of formed precipitates by centrifugation at 4°C. Such protease-free serum formed no cryoprecipitate with or without added fibrinogen that had been depleted of its soluble fibrin.

In subsequent weeks, the patient was placed on coumadin, and heparin was stopped; plasmapheresis was continued uneventfully over several months and eventually stopped without recurrence of symptoms.

Interpretation

In the first patient, pathologic fibrinemia was clearly related to the inflammatory vascular lesions and could be used as an index to follow the activity of the disease and response to treatment. In the second patient, fibrinemia may have resulted from the delayed clearance of activated coagulant factors that is prevalent among patients with chronic liver disease. Paradoxically, dysfibrinogenemia may have contributed to the abnormal levels of circulating fibrin by allowing higher levels of soluble fibrinogen-fibrin complexes to accumulate, as fibrin monomers are normally soluble in high fibrinogen excess under physiologic conditions. Whether dysfibrinogenemia is congenital or acquired, such plasma often has a greater maximal capacity for soluble fibrin owing to defective coagulability or incoagulability of abnormal fibrinogen molecules.

Procedures

1. To screen for cryofibrinogenemia, simultaneous normal and patient plasma samples are collected in citrate, ideally containing an added inhibitor of thrombin generation ex vivo (see below), at 37°C and allowed to stand overnight at 4°C. It is important *not* to collect plasma in EDTA, because this agent will inhibit cryoprecipitation of fibrin-fibrinogen complexes. Also important, blood should *not* be collected in heparin unless its concentration is ≤2 U/ml of collected plasma, since much higher concentrations can induce cryoprecipitation. This is related to heparin-fibronectin interactions with some fibrinogen and fibrin in the cryoprecipitate (see step 6 below). Blood should be collected rapidly, and sufficient anticoagulant (e.g., 3.8% sodium citrate) should be added to avoid in vitro induction of fibrin formation. For best results, low concentrations of heparin (see below) or hirudin (1 to 5 U/ml) should be added to the citrate before blood collection in order to inactivate any thrombin following collection. Since cryoglobulins will also precipitate out of plasma, the presence of a cryofibrinogen will be suggested by the absence of a comparable precipitate in a paired sample of serum (13).

2. To evaluate fibrinemia (cryofibrinogenemia), procedures involving EDTA-collected blood should not be used (see specific recommendations below). The essential reason is that EDTA prevents fibrinogen-fibrin cryoprecipitation. Soluble fibrin in plasma can be measured by using commercially available kits; those using either tissue plasminogen activator-based or monoclonal antibody-based assays are increasingly used, the latter being technically more convenient. A double-antibody assay (Organon Teknika) which uses a fibrin-specific antibody directed to γ-chain residues 312 to 324 and another antibody specific for the carboxy-terminal end of the α chain or another similar test is preferred. Since the latter epitope is lost when fibrin is degraded, this assay also distinguishes between intact and degraded forms. Care must be taken to draw blood so as to avoid ex vivo fibrin formation (see above), as specified in the manufacturer's instructions. In one report, levels of 13 to 105 ng/ml were found in healthy individuals of widely differing ages.

3. Two alternative methods may be used to measure cryoprecipitable protein. One is to allow citrated plasma to remain undisturbed overnight (or at least 6 h and preferably >24 h) on ice or at 4°C, centrifuge the plasma cold, and measure the insoluble column as a percentage of the total volume (cryocrit). This method, though imprecise, is useful when fibrinemia is pronounced. The second option is to freeze the platelet-poor plasma shortly after harvesting in a self-defrosting freezer (−8 to 20°C) overnight (or at least 6 h) and then thaw it at 4°C overnight. Centrifugation at cold temperatures yields insoluble material, which can then be suspended in ice-cold buffered saline and washed several times to remove noncryoprecipitable proteins. More exhaustive washing may progressively remove fibronectin as well. The final pellet is solubilized at 37°C or in 6 M urea; protein content is determined by diluting an aliquot in 6 M urea and measuring the absorbance at 280 nm, which is compared to a control. For conversion to milligrams of protein, an extinction coefficient (1%, 1 cm, 280 nm) of 14 or 15 can be used, since the two major proteins (i.e., 80 to 90% of the total content), fibrinogen-fibrin and fibronectin, have coefficients of 15.5 and 14, respectively (5).

4. Fibrin-fibrinogen complexes in most, if not all, dysfibrinogenemic individuals can be quantified by harvesting the cryoprecipitate obtained from frozen and thawed plasma. The exception may be the very rare homozygous individuals with dysfibrinogenemia whose fibrinogen is incoagulable. In such an instance, plasma may not form cryoprecipitate, and measurement of fibrinogen antigen or activity is useful. This is best done by using a clotting and/or an antigen-based assay, as high Ig levels may significantly affect heat precipitation, clot mass, or turbidity-based assays for fibrinogen. Though little information other than case reports is available, it seems likely that paraproteinemias can significantly affect heat-based fibrinogen assays and that fibrinemia may complicate the interpretation of heat-based assays for Ig (see below).

5. Commonly not appreciated is the ex vivo fibrinemia resulting from the use of blood cell separators in which the standard anticoagulant is citrate. By measuring cryoprecipitate content, which is fibrin concentration dependent, we observed up to five times more fibrin in plasmapheresis plasma than in plasma from a blood donation which was harvested and frozen within 2 h. Similarly, a very slow withdrawal of blood dramatically increases cryoprecipitable protein relative to that in rapidly drawn blood. If serum is harvested from such samples prematurely, it will subsequently form cryoprecipitates (i.e., at 4°C) which may be erroneously interpreted as cryoglobulins. Its failure to redissolve at 37°C is a strong clue that this is cross-linked fibrin gel rather than cryoglobulin. A reasonable precaution is to allow whole blood to clot for at least 6 h at 37°C, remove the clot, and observe for another hour or so to ascertain that no further clot forms before serum is harvested to be tested for cryoglobulins. To confirm that no fibrinogen remains, one can perform a commercially available fibrinogen assay with the patient serum and a normal control serum, preferably a pool from several or more donors.

6. If cryoglobulin analysis is carried out for patients who are receiving heparin anticoagulation, or on samples collected during plasmapheresis in which heparin has been administered, it is also important to be aware of the possibility of cryoprecipitation due to complexes between heparin and fibronectin, if heparin is present in sufficient concentration; in addition, fibronectin itself is cold insoluble. Thus, heparin induces or enhances cryoprecipitate formation. Here, the presence of fibrinogen in the complexes is a secondary and variable event; the relative content of fibrinogen and fibronectin in isolated cryoprecipitates can be assessed by immunoblot analysis using monospecific antisera to these proteins (3). Although at in vivo therapeutic concentrations (i.e., <1 U of heparin/ml) this effect may be negligible, the heparin content of blood samples may range up to 5 or more U/ml, at which level it can significantly induce cryoprecipitation.

Conclusions

Cryofibrinogenemia may result from elevated levels of fibrin-fibrinogen complexes in plasma, be a manifestation of dys-fibrinogenemia, be secondary to cold insolubility of fibronectin, or, rarely, result from complexing with mono-clonal antifibrinogen antibodies; in addition, fibronectin can form cold-insoluble complexes with Ig in various disease states (e.g., fibrillary glomerulonephritis). A search for cry-ofibrinogenemia may be dictated by unexplained thrombo-hemorrhagic coagulopathy or cold-dependent purpura; it may also be dictated by the finding of characteristic pathol-ogy, occurring in various affected organs, as for example an occlusive thrombotic diathesis due to eosinophilic deposits within vessel lumina, extending into the intima, which may be associated with a granulomatous vasculitic component. Cryofibrinogenemia can be screened by cryoprecipitating or freeze-thawing plasma collected in citrate that contains an inhibitor of thrombin generation and is most convincing in the absence of coexisting cryoglobulinemia. It is important not to collect blood in EDTA or in high concentrations of heparin (see below), since the former interferes with cryo-precipitate formation and the latter (depending on the heparin concentration in plasma) may enhance cryoprecipi-tate formation; this needs to be carefully considered in the performance of serial studies to assess the effect of treatment in individual patients.

Anticoagulant-Related Recommendations

An optimal tube for collecting plasma for cryofibrinogen determination is not commercially available. Conse-quently, the clinical utility of this test is limited because of lack of sensitivity. In the practice setting, it could be argued, for example, that a cryofibrinogen determination might potentially be useful in detecting only markedly positive patients (e.g., cold-sensitive vasculitis) and for monitoring such a patient's clinical course or a therapeutic response.

1. A thrombin or thrombin generation inhibitor should inhibit ex vivo thrombin activity but not enhance cryopre-cipitation. To achieve this, the usual citrate tube can contain the added inhibitor (e.g., low concentrations of heparin). It is important that blood be collected and mixed rapidly with this citrate-inhibitor solution. If such a heparin-citrate mix is used, the heparin concentration in harvested plasma should be ~0.5 to 2 U/ml. For this calculation, it can be assumed that most, if not all, blood heparin will remain in the plasma.

2. Always collect a control serum sample from the same draw.

3. Commercially available tubes: citrate tubes can be used with the knowledge that they have the disadvantage of unpredictable ex vivo thrombin generation and therefore falsely enhanced or positive cryoprecipitate formation. This is particularly so in a prolonged blood draw. EDTA tubes should not be used. Heparin tubes: a currently popular 7-ml-capacity tube has 90 U of heparin (Vacutainer; Becton Dickinson). The resulting concentration in collected plasma is approxi-mately 20 U/ml, far too high, and should not be used. It may cause heparin-induced cryoprecipitate formation that is not fibrin or fibrinogen related.

4. Validation: to institute and validate such a test, an analytical second step is needed. Among the choices (vide supra), immunofixation is a reasonable analytical procedure.

5. Volumes of plasma to be observed at 4°C for 3 days must be at least 3 ml.

PYROGLOBULINEMIA

Background

Pyroglobulins are Igs that precipitate irreversibly as a gel when serum is heated to 56 to 60°C for 30 min; by contrast, heat precipitation of Bence Jones proteins under similar conditions is reversible. Pyroglobulins are invariably single-component proteins and constitute <1% of monoclonal gammopathies overall and ~6% of Waldenström's macroglobulins.

Concept

Pyroglobulins of every Ig isotype (including IgD and IgE) have been reported in association with multiple myeloma, lymphoproliferative diseases, and plasma cell leukemia. Unlike the case for cryoglobulins, their occurrence has not been associated with specific clinical manifestations, although high levels of these proteins may also cause hyper-viscosity or coagulopathies.

Procedure

1. Pyroglobulins precipitate when warmed to 56°C and do not redissolve on heating to 100°C. They are usually apparent as an M-spike on serum protein electrophoresis which significantly decreases, or completely disappears, after pyroprecipitation. Serum immunofixation will thus define the specific monoclonal component forming the pyroglobu-lin, and this can be confirmed by sodium dodecyl sulfate-PAGE of the isolated material.

2. As noted above, fibrinogen and fibrin and their core proteins are also heat precipitable at these temperatures. Any remaining fibrinogen and/or fibrin due to dysfibrinogenemia or an incompletely clotted blood sample and their split prod-ucts (typically containing the thermally sensitive D domain) will also form irreversible precipitates at 56°C. To control for this, serum can be treated with 2 or more μU of thrombin per ml and allowed to stand for 1 to 2 h at 37°C; any clots formed can be removed by syneresis before heating to 56°C.

3. Unlike cryoglobulins, pyroglobulin formation is usu-ally not significantly inhibited by the pH range 3 to 9 or by changes in the ionic strength of the solution. Similarly, the effects of reducing (e.g., 2-mercaptoethanol) or dissociating (e.g., Triton X-100) agents on this phenomenon are variable. Occasionally, single patients have been described to have both cryoglobulins and pyroglobulins.

Conclusion

Recognition of the laboratory phenomenon of pyroglobu-linemia has importance as a potentially confounding factor for heat-based assays used to inactivate complement or to measure fibrinogen levels. Proper identification of a pyroglobulin as being a monoclonal component may in turn lead to the diagnosis of macroglobulinemia or plasma cell dyscrasia.

REFERENCES

1. **Agnello, V., and F. G. De Rosa.** 2004. Extrahepatic disease manifestations of HCV infection: some current issues. *J. Hepatol.* **40:**341–352.
2. **Amdo, T. D., and J. A. Welker.** 2004. An approach to the diagnosis and treatment of cryofibrinogenemia. *Am. J. Med.* **116:**332–337.
3. **Blain, H., P. Cacoub, L. Musset, N. Costedoat-Chalumeau, C. Silberstein, O. Chosidow, P. Godeau, C. Frances, and J. C. Piette.** 2000. Cryofibrinogenemia: a study of 49 patients. *Clin. Exp. Immunol.* **120:**253–260.

4. Brandau, D. T., P. A. Trautman, B. L. Steadman, E. Q. Lawson, and C. R. Middaugh. 1986. The temperature-dependent stoichiometry of mixed cryoimmunoglobulins. *J. Biol. Chem.* **16:**16385–16391.

5. Brouet, J. C., J. P. Clauvel, F. Danon, M. Klein, and M. Seligmann. 1974. Biologic and clinical significance of cryoglobulins. *Am. J. Med.* **57:**775–788.

6. Casato, M., D. Lilli, G. Donato, M. Granata, V. Conti, G. Del Giudice, D. Rivanera, C. Scagnolari, G. Antonelli, and M. Fiorilli. 2003. Occult hepatitis C virus infection in type II mixed cryoglobulinaemia. *J. Viral Hepat.* **10:**455–459.

7. Dammacco, F., D. Sansonno, C. Piccoli, F. A. Tucci, and V. Racanelli. 2001. The cryoglobulins: an overview. *Eur. J. Clin. Invest.* **31:**628–638.

8. Damoc, E., N. Youhnovski, D. Crettaz, J. D. Tissot, and M. Przybylski. 2003. High resolution proteome analysis of cryoglobulins using Fourier transform-ion cyclotron resonance mass spectrometry. *Proteomics* **3:**1425–1433.

9. Della Rossa, A., A. Tavoni, and S. Bombardieri. 2003. Hyperviscosity syndrome in cryoglobulinemia: clinical aspects and therapeutic considerations. *Semin. Thromb. Hemost.* **29:**473–477.

10. Di Stasio, E., P. Bizzarri, M. Bove, M. Casato, B. Giardina, M. Fiorilli, A. Galtieri, and L. P. Pucillo. 2003. Analysis of the dynamics of cryoaggregation by light-scattering spectrometry. *Clin. Chem. Lab. Med.* **41:**152–158.

11. Fohlen-Walter, A., C. Jacob, T. Lecompte, and F.-J. Lesesve. 2002. Laboratory identification of cryoglobulinemia from automated blood cell counts, fresh blood samples, and blood films. *Am. J. Clin. Pathol.* **117:**606–614.

12. Gad, A., E. Tanaka, A. Matsumoto, A. el-Hamid Serwah, K. Ali, F. Makledy, A. el-Gohary, K. Orii, A. Ijima, A. Rokuhara, K. Yoshizawa, Z. Nooman, and K. Kiyosawa. 2003. Factors predisposing to the occurrence of cryoglobulinemia in two cohorts of Egyptian and Japanese patients with chronic hepatitis C infection: ethnic and genotypic influence. *J. Med. Virol.* **70:**594–599.

13. Galanakis, D. K. 1995. Plasma cryoprecipitation studies: major increase in fibrinogen yield by albumin enrichment of plasma. *Thrombosis Res.* **78:**303–313.

14. Gorevic, P. D. 2001. Cryopathies: cryoglobulins and cryofibrinogenemia, p. 1002–1022. *In* K. F. Austen, M. M. Frank, J. P. Atkinson, and H. Cantor (ed.), *Samter's Immunologic Diseases*, 6th ed., vol. 2. Lippincott Williams & Wilkins, Baltimore, Md.

15. Grey, H. M., and P. F. Kohler. 1973. Cryoimmunoglobulins. *Semin. Hematol.* **10:**87–112.

16. Jonsson, M., J. Carlson, J. O. Jeppsson, and P. Simonsson. 2001. Computer-supported detection of M-components and evaluation of immunoglobulins after capillary electrophoresis. *Clin. Chem.* **47:**110–111.

17. Komurian-Pradel, F., M. Perret, B. Deiman, M. Sodoyer, V. Lotteau, G. Paranhos-Baccala, and P. Andre. 2004. Strand specific quantitative real-time PCR to study replication of hepatitis C virus genome. *J. Virol. Methods* **116:**103–106.

18. Krajden, M., R. Shivji, K. Gunadasa, A. Mak, G. McNabb, M. Friesenhahn, D. Hendricks, and L. Comanor. 2004. Evaluation of the core antigen assay as a second-line supplemental test for diagnosis of active hepatitis C virus infection. *J. Clin. Microbiol.* **42:**4054–4059.

19. Lawson, E. Q., D. T. Brandau, P. A. Trautman, S. E. Aziz, and C. R. Middaugh. 1987. Kinetics of the precipitation of cryoimmunoglobulins. *Mol. Immunol.* **24:**897–905.

20. Naarendorp, M., U. Kallemuchikkal, G. J. Nuovo, and P. D. Gorevic. 2001. Longterm efficacy of interferon-alpha for extrahepatic disease associated with hepatitis C virus infection. *J. Rheumatol.* **28:**2466–2473.

21. Sansonno, D., A. R. Iacobelli, V. Cornacchiulo, G. Lauletta, M. A. Distasi, P. Gatti, and F. Dammacco. 1996. Immunochemical and biomolecular studies of circulating immune complexes isolated from patients with acute and chronic hepatitis C virus infection. *Eur. J. Clin. Invest.* **26:**465–475.

22. Sansonno, D., G. Lauletta, L. Nisi, P. Gatti, F. Pesola, N. Pansini, and F. Dammacco. 2003. Non-enveloped HCV core protein as constitutive antigen of cold-precipitable immune complexes in type II mixed cryoglobulinaemia. *Clin. Exp. Immunol.* **133:**275–282.

23. Schott, P., F. Polzien, A. Muller-Issberner, G. Ramadori, and H. Hartmann. 1998. In vitro reactivity of cryoglobulin IgM and IgG in hepatitis C virus-associated mixed cryoglobulinemia. *J. Hepatol.* **28:**17–26.

24. Tissot, J.-D., F. Invernizzi, J. A. Schifferli, F. Spertini, and P. Schneider. 1999. Two-dimensional electrophoretic analysis of cryoproteins: a report of 335 samples. *Electrophoresis* **20:**606–613.

25. Wei, G., S. Yano, T. Kuroiwa, K. Hiromura, and A. Maezawa. 1997. Hepatitis C virus (HCV)-induced IgG-IgM rheumatoid factor (RF) complex may be the main causal factor for cold-dependent activation of complement in patients with rheumatic disease. *Clin. Exp. Immunol.* **107:**83–88.

COMPLEMENT

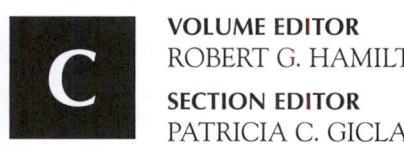

VOLUME EDITOR
ROBERT G. HAMILTON
SECTION EDITOR
PATRICIA C. GICLAS

Analysis of Complement in the Clinical Laboratory

PATRICIA C. GICLAS

12

The serum complement system represents an important effector arm of the innate, or "nonspecific," immune response in vertebrates. Complement provides a fast-acting mechanism for the identification and removal of foreign substances before the more specific arms of the adaptive immune system can come into play. Among other important roles of complement is the clearance of immune complexes, effete cells, and the cellular debris that results from damaged tissues. Complement activation contributes to many of the symptoms associated with inflammation, including local changes in blood flow and the influx of inflammatory cells into the affected area. If uncontrolled, complement activation presents a danger that can result in tissue damage and loss of function or death. Learning the reason for a patient's low complement is becoming easier with the advent of more specific methods of evaluation, including the ability to differentiate between acquired and inherited deficiency.

Many clinical laboratories have shied away from the analysis of complement, due in large part to the lability of the system and the special handling that samples require if the results are to be reliable. Although with overnight shipping of frozen specimens and more commonly available ultracold freezer storage ($-60°C$ and below) mishandling of specimens is not a major problem in today's laboratory, care should still be taken to ensure that the referring laboratory has the appropriate information for sample collection and preservation. The previous editions of this manual included methods for analysis of complement that remain valid and are a source of methods not described in this volume. The chapters to follow provide information about some methods of analysis to be used for screening tests that are necessary to perform before deciding which specific tests are required for diagnosis of a complement deficiency.

ACTIVATION PATHWAYS

The classical pathway (CP) was the first to be discovered and the first for which the action of its components was described. The alternative pathway (AP) is more primitive in the evolutionary sense and includes a unique "amplification loop" that enables far more C3 cleavage than is possible with the other pathways. The lectin pathway (LP) bypasses C1 of the CP but makes use of C4 and C2 to form a C3-cleaving enzyme. As can be seen from comparing these pathways in Fig. 1, they share the same terminal, or late,

components (C3 and C5 to C9) as well as many similar proteins in the activation mechanisms. After an initial pathway-specific "recognition" event, activation occurs in an enzyme cascade that results in production of physiological effects. The key event in complement activation is deposition of C3b on the activator's surface, the central event in all of the activation pathways.

Activation seldom involves only one pathway. If enough C3b is deposited on the activator or other surfaces in the area by the CP or LP, the AP will also become involved. Small immune complexes that bind C1q are the usual activators of the CP, but large, insoluble ones activate the AP. There are other substances that also bind and activate C1q, such as lipid A of bacterial lipopolysaccharide, monosodium urate crystals, subcellular membranes, and some enveloped viruses. CP activation can also occur through interaction of C1q and C-reactive protein that is complexed with pneumococcal C polysaccharide. The binding of the pattern recognition lectins, mannose-binding lectin, or ficolin to the appropriate sugar residues on bacterial surfaces leads to activation of the LP. Complex polysaccharides such as yeast cell walls (zymosan), high-molecular-weight inulin, Sephadex, cellulose acetate, and bacterial cell walls provide appropriate surfaces for AP activation. Even without the involvement of the complement pathways, cleavage of C3 or C5 by enzymes of the contact coagulation system (e.g., XIIa and Kallikrein), from inflammatory cells (e.g., elastase and cathepsin G) or from bacteria, can produce active C3a and C5a, and presumably deposit C3b that could initiate the amplification loop of the AP.

MEASUREMENT OF COMPLEMENT

In the previous edition of this manual, I discussed the value of performing the CH50 and AH50 assays as the first step in complement analysis when a deficiency is suspected. Chapter 14, by Seelen et al., describes functional assays for CP, AP, and LP activity that can be done at the same time, thus adding an additional dimension to the screen. Once it has been determined that a defect in one pathway is present, the appropriate tests can be done to determine whether a single component is missing (e.g., genetic deficiency) or several components are affected (e.g., depletion by activation). The function of mannose-binding lectin can be evaluated more extensively by the

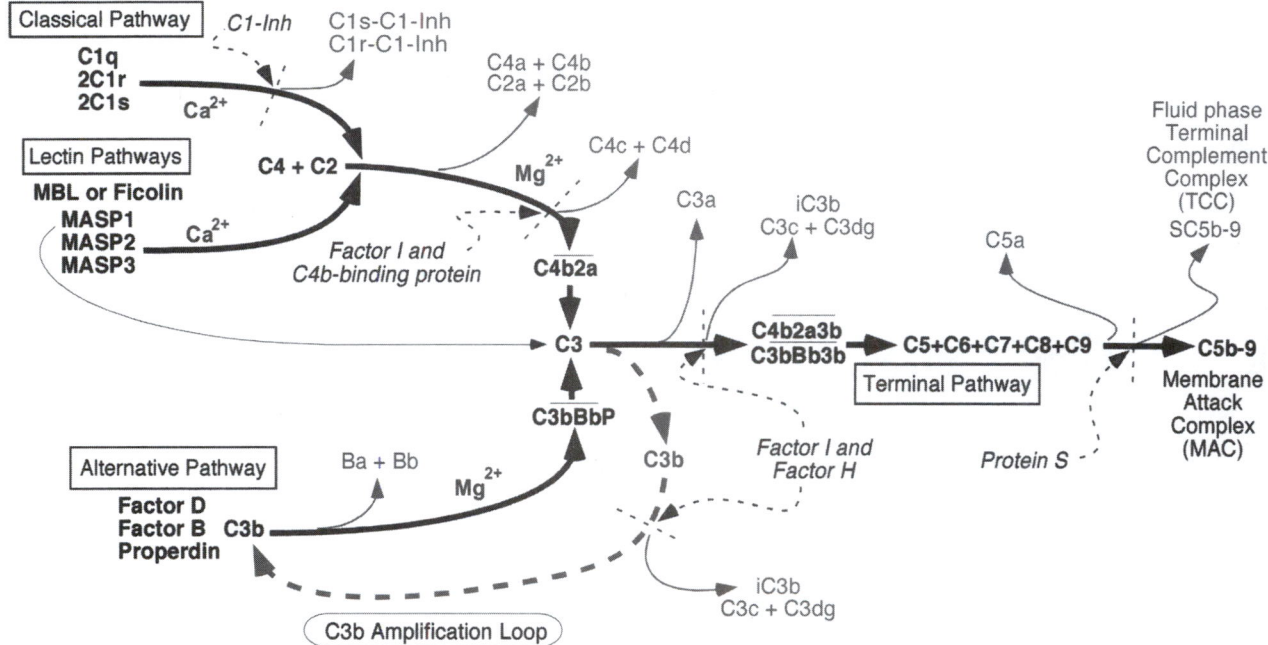

FIGURE 1 CP, LP, and AP of the human complement system, showing the control steps and where some of the biologically active split products are produced.

method described in chapter 15, by Gadjeva and Thiel. For other tests to quantitate individual components of any of the pathways, the reader should consult the previous editions of this manual.

BIOLOGICAL ACTIVITIES OF COMPLEMENT FRAGMENTS

The symptoms of inflammation associated with complement activation are due to a limited number of biologically active complement split products that are produced by the enzymatic cascade. The anaphylatoxins C3a and C5a can interact with their specific receptors on many cell types. Some of their effects include alterations in local blood flow through increased dilation and permeability of small vessels and smooth muscle contraction (e.g., guinea pig ileum and tracheal rings and estrous rat uterus) as well as upregulation of adhesion molecules on endothelial and white blood cell surfaces. Systemic effects on blood pressure, heart rate, and oxygen perfusion have been noted in animal models of complement activation. Neutrophils, monocytes, macrophages, eosinophils, and mast cells can be enticed to perform many of their tricks (e.g., chemotaxis and mediator and enzyme release) by these complement fragments. An inactivator of the anaphylatoxins, serum carboxypeptidase N, rapidly cleaves the C-terminal arginase from C3a and C5a, rendering them unable to interact appropriately with their receptors. $C5a_{desArg}$ retains some chemotactic activity, but neither $C3a_{desArg}$ nor $C5a_{desArg}$ has the ability to induce enzyme release or the other functions associated with anaphylatoxin activity. The assays available for measurement of these peptides are directed against the desArg forms since these are the ones that are found in the circulation. It should be noted that C4a, once grouped with the anaphylatoxins, has not been found to interact with either the C3a or C5a receptor, and a specific C4a receptor has not been found to date.

Complement split products (C4a, C3a, C5a, iC3b, C4d, SC5b-9, and Bb, as well as others) can be measured by enzyme immunoassay or radioimmunoassay methods or by changes in electrophoretic mobility or size. These tests are very sensitive and can pick up activation of less than 1% of the parent component. Analysis of complement split products, including $C3a_{desArg}$ and $C5a_{desArg}$, can give valuable insight into pathological processes taking place during a disease state. These assays are extremely useful in determining whether complement activation is occurring and by which pathway(s), thus providing information about the underlying pathological mechanism. Chapter 16, by Baldwin, describes the application of complement analysis in diagnosing acute and chronic transplant rejection.

In addition to the enzymes and other components of the activation pathways, there are a number of important proteins that control the cascade. Among these, C1-esterase inhibitor is responsible for stopping the uncontrolled activation of the CP and also acts as a control for certain enzymes of the coagulation system. Deficiencies of this protein result in the condition of hereditary or acquired angioedema, and a number of new therapies are being developed to specifically treat the acute symptoms of hereditary and acquired angioedema. The major control of the AP occurs through the action of two proteins that stop the cleavage of C3. Another important control protein is factor H, which binds to C3b in either the classical or alternative C3 convertase enzyme and is required before factor I can cleave and inactivate the C3b. While the gross absence of either of these proteins has long been associated with severe depletion of C3 and subsequent pyogenic infections in the affected individual, more recently, subtle changes in the protein structure of factor H and its cell-associated counterpart, membrane cofactor protein (CD46), have been associated with atypical hemolytic-uremic syndrome. The analysis of these proteins and their genes in this devastating disease is discussed in chapter 13 by Strain et al.

It should be noted that complement is appearing daily in the literature of immunology in many contexts that were once considered the domain of the cellular immunologist, e.g., interactions with B-cell and T-cell functions as basic as the induction of antibody responses and memory cell retention. Its involvement in such diverse processes as asthma, early pregnancy loss or low birth weight, and age-related macular degeneration makes us realize how little we know about this ancient and intriguing system. No doubt additional interactions will be discovered in the coming years and give even more importance to the laboratory evaluation of the complement system.

Molecular and Clinical Evaluation of Atypical Hemolytic Uremic Syndrome

LISA STRAIN, JUDITH A. GOODSHIP, AND TIMOTHY H. J. GOODSHIP*

13

ATYPICAL HUS

The hemolytic uremic syndrome (HUS) consists of the triad of a microangiopathic hemolytic anemia, thrombocytopenia, and acute renal failure (43). Most commonly, this is associated with a preceding diarrheal illness, often due to infection with *Escherichia coli* O157 (19). Less frequently, there is no preceding diarrheal illness, and hence this form of the disease is known as atypical HUS. This can be either sporadic or, when more than one member of a family is affected, familial. In both sporadic and familial HUS, the disease can be recurrent. The clinical features of the syndrome are due to the development of platelet-rich microthrombi in small vessels. This particularly affects the glomeruli of the kidney, causing acute renal failure. Recovery of renal function is uncommon in atypical HUS, and many patients require long-term renal replacement therapy. While dialysis is often successful, recurrence of the disease in renal allografts is seen in approximately 50% of patients (21).

ATYPICAL HUS AND COMPLEMENT FACTOR H

Recent findings for both the familial and the sporadic forms of the disease suggest that atypical HUS is a disease of complement dysregulation. Familial HUS was first described in 1956; both autosomal dominant and recessive forms of inheritance have been reported (2, 12, 13). In 1998, linkage to a cluster of genes on chromosome 1 (the so-called regulators of complement activation [RCA] cluster) that encode proteins important in the control of complement activity was established. Warwicker et al. studied three families with HUS and established linkage in the affected individuals to the RCA cluster (44). The first RCA gene examined in these families was the gene for factor H. This is because there had been previous reports of an association between familial HUS and factor H deficiency (24, 28, 33, 39). Factor H shares a basic structure with other proteins encoded by the genes of the RCA cluster. Such proteins consist largely of multiple contiguous homologous modules called complement control protein modules (CCPs), also known as short consensus repeats or sushi domains (reviewed in reference 14). Each factor H CCP is approximately 60 amino acids in length and possesses 10 to 18 highly conserved residues. Four cysteines form two disulfide bridges to give the CCP a loop-within-a-loop characteristic structure. The CCPs house the sites for interaction with C3b and C4b and thus complement regulation.

Warwicker et al. found a mutation in the exon encoding CCP 20 in one of the families but not in the other two (44). Since then, there have been a series of reports documenting the association between atypical HUS and factor H mutations (3, 4, 7, 21, 26, 31, 45). These studies show that between 15 and 30% of patients with atypical HUS (both familial and sporadic) have a factor H mutation. The majority of the mutations, especially in adults, are missense, with a normal factor H level. These mutations tend to cluster in the C-terminal region of the molecule, an area known to be important for binding to C3b and anionic surfaces (27) (Fig. 1A). Such mutations result in impaired protection of host surfaces against complement activation (17, 25, 35). Other mutations in factor H predisposing to HUS are associated with either complete or partial factor H deficiency, and they are distributed throughout the gene (Fig. 1B).

Three pieces of evidence suggested that other complement genes apart from the gene for factor H were involved in the pathogenesis of atypical HUS.

1. Only 15 to 30% of patients have a factor H mutation.
2. Two of the original three families whose defect mapped to the RCA cluster (44) did not have a factor H mutation.
3. In our HUS panel, several patients who exhibited evidence of overactivity of the alternative complement pathway, such as a low C3 level, did not have a factor H mutation (31).

To take this further, other candidate genes involved in the regulation of complement activation have been examined, including those for membrane cofactor protein (MCP) (CD46) and factor I.

MCP

MCP is widely expressed on the surface of almost every human cell except erythrocytes (8, 10, 11, 18, 20). Together with serine protease factor I, it degrades C3b and C4b bound to the cell surface (1, 6, 15, 23, 37, 38). This proteolytic event is known as cofactor activity.

Structurally, MCP consists of four alternatively spliced isoforms that coexist on most cells (5, 16, 30, 34). The extracellular domain is composed of four CCPs. Following this is an

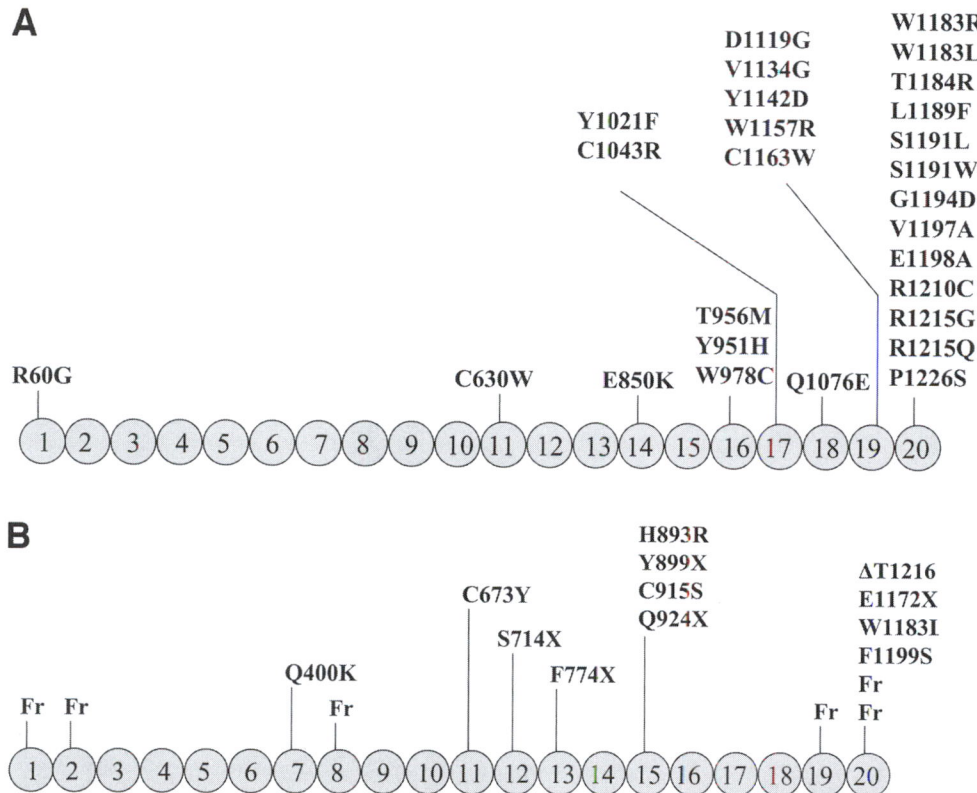

FIGURE 1 Factor H mutations associated with HUS are identified above the corresponding CCP. (A) Missense mutations with normal factor H levels. (B) Mutations associated with factor H deficiency (Fr, frameshift; X, premature stop codon; Δ, deletion). The amino acid numbering includes the 18-amino-acid signal peptide.

O-glycosylated region rich in serines, threonines, and prolines, the STP region, which is alternatively spliced. There are either 14 or 29 amino acids in the STP region, depending on the splicing in or out of STP exon B. The STP region is followed by a juxtamembranous region of 12 amino acids of unknown function, which is followed by a hydrophobic transmembrane domain and cytoplasmic anchor. The cytoplasmic tail of MCP is also alternatively spliced (the 16-amino-acid CYT-1 and the 23-amino-acid CYT-2) and mediates signaling events (16). The MCP gene is located within the RCA cluster on chromosome 1 with 14 exons spanning ~43 kb.

Because MCP lies within the RCA cluster on chromosome 1, it was considered as a candidate gene in the two families from Warwicker's original linkage study in which a factor H mutation had not been found (44). In one family, mutation screening showed no abnormality. In the other, a heterozygous 6-bp deletion (GACAGT) in the exon encoding CCP4, resulting in the loss of two amino acids (ΔD237/S238), was detected in affected individuals (32). In this family, three male siblings were affected at the ages of 27, 31, and 35 years (29). C3 levels at presentation were normal, and there was no recovery of renal function. Subsequently, all three received a cadaver renal transplant, with no recurrence of HUS in the allograft. Fluorescence-activated cell sorter (FACS) analysis of peripheral blood mononuclear cells (PBMCs) from an affected individual demonstrated reduced expression of MCP, and C3b binding studies of PBMC lysates revealed ~50% reduction in C3b binding. Mutant MCP constructs were evaluated after

transfection into Chinese hamster ovary (CHO) cells. Western blot, flow cytometry, cell surface labeling (biotinylation), and pulse-chase analysis all showed that the mutant protein was retained intracellularly. Noris et al. have also described a family in which two siblings were affected by HUS (22). The female patient was first affected at the age of 16 months and had recurrent episodes of HUS, eventually resulting in end-stage renal failure requiring dialysis. Her brother had two episodes of HUS at the age of 9, from which he made a complete recovery. Mutation screening in both revealed a heterozygous 2-bp deletion in MCP exon 7, which encodes CCP4. This results in a premature stop codon and was associated with reduced expression of MCP on PBMCs (22). The functional effect of this mutation is therefore similar to the deletion mutation and results in half of the normal level of cell surface expression of MCP.

Following the finding of the MCP deletion mutation (ΔD237/S238), a panel of other HUS families in whom a factor H mutation had not been found (31) were examined. In two families, a transition (T822C) resulting in a serine-to-proline change, S206P, in the exon encoding CCP4 was found. In one family, two brothers were affected at the ages of 8 and 15. In both, renal function recovered. The two affected individuals in this family were heterozygous for the S206P substitution. In the other family, one male and one female sibling were affected. Again, both made a complete recovery. The affected individuals in this family were homozygous for the substitution, their parents being first-degree relatives. For the affected individuals from both families, FACS analysis revealed that the levels of MCP expression in PBMCs were normal. C3b binding was ~50% reduced in affected heterozygotes and undetectable in affected homozygotes. The functional consequences of the S206P substitution were studied in CHO cells expressing this mutant. All the studies undertaken showed that the mutant protein's ability to interact with C3b was severely impaired (32). Cells bearing the mutation demonstrated less inhibition of C3b deposition. The mutant protein exhibited almost total loss of reactivity to the MCP monoclonal antibody GB24 that blocks C3b binding. C3b binding was diminished, and C3b cofactor activity was abolished. However, C4b binding and cofactor activity were unaffected. This mutation, therefore, had a very specific effect on alternative pathway regulation.

FACTOR I

Besides abnormalities of soluble and membrane-bound RCA, mutations in factor I in atypical HUS have recently been described. Factor I is a soluble regulatory serine protease of the complement system which cleaves three peptide bonds in the alpha-chain of C3b and two bonds in the alpha-chain of C4b, thereby inactivating these proteins. The protein is a heterodimer with a molecular weight (MW) of about 88,000 which consists of a noncatalytic heavy chain (MW, 50,000) which is linked to a catalytic light chain (MW, 38,000) by a disulfide bond. The protein is synthesized as a single-chain precursor of 565 amino acids, predominantly in the liver. Four basic amino acids are then excised from the precursor prior to secretion of the heterodimer. Like many of the complement proteins, factor I has a modular structure. The heavy chain contains two low-density lipoprotein receptor domains, a CD5 domain, and a module found only in factor I and complement proteins C6 and C7. The factor I gene is located on chromosome 4q25 and spans 63 kb (40). It comprises 13 exons, and there is a strong correlation between the exonic organization of the gene and the modular structure of the protein. The light chain of factor I, which is the serine proteinase region of the molecule, is encoded in five exons. The genomic organization of the enzymatic part of factor I is similar to that of trypsin. The gene structure is unusual in that the first exon is small, 86 bp, and it is separated from the rest of the gene by a large first intron of 36 kb. Factor I deficiency has been described previously in approximately 30 kindreds and is usually associated with a predisposition to pyogenic infection (41, 42). Fremeaux-Bacchi et al. have recently described three mutations in factor I in atypical HUS (9). They screened the coding sequence of factor I in 6 familial and 19 sporadic cases of HUS. In two cases, heterozygous nonsense mutations led to a premature stop codon (G456X and W528X). Both of these had approximately half-normal antigenic factor I levels, and in the third, which had normal factor I levels, there was a heterozygous missense mutation in exon 13 (A1600T) which leads to the substitution of an aspartic acid residue by valine (D506V). Factor I levels were normal. D506 is a highly conserved residue in the catalytic site of factor I, and its substitution is likely to be functionally significant.

CLINICAL EVALUATION OF THE PATIENT WITH ATYPICAL HUS

The diagnosis of HUS should be suspected for any patient presenting with the aforementioned triad of a microangiopathic hemolytic anemia, thrombocytopenia, and acute renal failure. The same triad is also a feature of thrombotic thrombocytopenic purpura (TTP), a syndrome in which neurological and systemic manifestations such as fever are also seen at presentation. Distinction of the two is based on the predominant presenting feature, renal involvement in HUS versus neurological involvement in TTP. The triad of presenting features can also be seen as a secondary manifestation of systemic lupus erythematosis, systemic sclerosis, antiphospholipid antibody syndrome, malignant hypertension, cobalamin C disease, and human immunodeficiency virus infection. Appropriate investigations should be undertaken to exclude these. An evaluation of complement activation should be undertaken as outlined above. However, it has been shown that factor H and MCP mutations can be present without evidence of complement activation. Consideration should therefore be given to undertaking mutation screening of the genes for factor H, MCP, and factor I.

MOLECULAR EVALUATION OF FACTOR H, MCP, AND FACTOR I

Table 1 summarizes the methods that can be used to detect mutations within or near the genes for factor H, MCP, and factor I. The two techniques most frequently used for mutation scanning are denaturing high-performance liquid chromatography (DHPLC) and single-strand conformation polymorphism (SSCP). DHPLC is based on heteroduplex analysis in which mutant and wild-type sequences present in a PCR product are heated and allowed to reanneal slowly. This results in the formation of four species of DNA: two heteroduplexes and two homoduplexes. These DNAs have altered mobility compared to the wild-type sequence, and this is seen as a time shift or variant pattern on DHPLC. In SSCP, the PCR amplicon is denatured, snap-cooled, and electrophoresed in a nondenaturing polyacrylamide gel. The single-stranded DNA assumes a three-dimensional conformation which is dependent on the primary sequence and secondary structure, and this results in altered migration patterns compared to the wild-type pattern. The disadvantages of these scanning methods are that neither can detect homozygous changes and the sensitivity is not greater than 95%. In addition, all variant patterns have to be sequenced to fully characterize the nature of the change. Sequencing PCR amplicons directly without prior mutation scanning can be costly, but the sensitivity of detection approaches 100%. With the wide availability of automated fluorescent sequencers and robotic liquid handling, direct sequencing is increasingly becoming the method of choice for mutation detection. If the exon-specific primers have a 5' N13* (N13 forward GTAGCGCGACGGCCAGT, N13 reverse CAGGGCGCAGCGATGAC) (modified M13) tag, then all sequencing reactions can be carried out with a common forward primer and a common reverse primer. Genomic DNA is sequenced, with each exon being amplified with approximately 20 bp of flanking intron. Care has to be taken in designing primers to amplify the exons coding for the C-terminal exons of factor H because of the close homology with the factor H-related proteins (46). Genomic DNA is extracted from peripheral blood by standard methods and then amplified by PCR with exon-specific primers and annealing temperatures as reported previously (9, 31, 32). PCR products are purified by use of magnetic microparticles (AMPure; Agencourt Biosciences) to remove unincorporated deoxynucleoside triphosphates, primers, and salts. Sequencing reactions are carried out by dye terminator cycle sequencing using either exon-specific primers or N13 primers, purification with magnetic microparticles

TABLE 1 Methods for mutation detection[a]

Method	Advantage(s)	Disadvantage(s)
Southern blot, hybridize to cDNA probe	Only way to determine major deletions and rearrangements	Laborious, expensive Needs several μg of DNA
Sequencing	Detects all changes Mutations fully characterized	Expensive
Heteroduplex gel mobility	Very simple Cheap	Sequences of <200 bp only Limited sensitivity Does not reveal position of change
DHPLC	Quick, high throughput Quantitative	Expensive equipment Does not reveal position of change
SSCP	Simple, cheap	Sequences of <200 bp only Does not reveal position of change
DGGE	High sensitivity	Choice of primers is critical Expensive primers Does not reveal position of change
Chemical mismatch cleavage	High sensitivity Shows position of change	Toxic chemicals Experimentally difficult
PTT	High sensitivity for chain-terminating mutations Shows position of change	Chain-terminating mutations only Expensive, difficult technique Usually needs RNA
Quantitative PCR	Detects heterozygous deletions	Expensive
Microarrays	Quick High throughput Might detect and define all changes	Expensive Limited range of genes

[a]DGGE, denaturing gradient gel electrophoresis; PTT, protein truncation test. Reproduced with permission from *Human Molecular Genetics* (38a).

(CleanSeq; Agencourt Biosciences), and then electrophoresis on a fluorescent 16-capillary sequencer (Beckman CEQ 8000). The resulting electropherograms are checked for homozygous and heterozygous base changes by use of an automated sequence analysis package (Mutation Surveyor [50]; SoftGenetics LLC). This program has a trace difference component in which the test electropherogram is subtracted from the normal electropherogram and base changes are seen as peaks rising above the background. One disadvantage of both sequencing and mutation scanning, however, is that large deletions and duplications or other large-scale rearrangements will not be detected, so some method of dosage analysis is required. MLPA (multiplex ligation-dependent probe amplification) is a relatively new method for detecting deletions and duplications in a simple two-stage procedure and gives dosage information for up to 45 exons in one test (36). Conventional dosage analysis can also be carried out with a fluorescent multiplex PCR, but a limited number of exons can be tested in this way.

REFERENCES

1. **Barilla-LaBarca, M. L., M. K. Liszewski, J. D. Lambris, D. Hourcade, and J. P. Atkinson.** 2002. Role of membrane cofactor protein (CD46) in regulation of C4b and C3b deposited on cells. *J. Immunol.* **168:**6298–6304.
2. **Berns, J. S., B. S. Kaplan, R. C. Mackow, and L. G. Hefter.** 1992. Inherited hemolytic uremic syndrome in adults. *Am. J. Kidney Dis.* **19:**331–334.
3. **Buddles, M. R., R. L. Donne, A. Richards, J. Goodship, and T. H. Goodship.** 2000. Complement factor H gene mutation associated with autosomal recessive atypical hemolytic uremic syndrome. *Am. J. Hum. Genet.* **66:**1721–1722.
4. **Caprioli, J., P. Bettinaglio, P. F. Zipfel, B. Amadei, E. Daina, S. Gamba, C. Skerka, N. Marziliano, G. Remuzzi, and M. Noris.** 2001. The molecular basis of familial hemolytic uremic syndrome: mutation analysis of factor H gene reveals a hot spot in short consensus repeat 20. *J. Am. Soc. Nephrol.* **12:**297–307.
5. **Cole, J. L., G. A. Housley, Jr., T. R. Dykman, R. P. MacDermott, and J. P. Atkinson.** 1985. Identification of an additional class of C3-binding membrane proteins of human peripheral blood leukocytes and cell lines. *Proc. Natl. Acad. Sci. USA* **82:**859–863.
6. **Devaux, P., D. Christiansen, M. Fontaine, and D. Gerlier.** 1999. Control of C3b and C5b deposition by CD46 (membrane cofactor protein) after alternative but not classical complement activation. *Eur. J. Immunol.* **29:**815–822.
7. **Dragon-Durey, M. A., V. Fremeaux-Bacchi, C. Loirat, J. Blouin, P. Niaudet, G. Deschenes, P. Coppo, F. W. Herman, and L. Weiss.** 2004. Heterozygous and homozygous factor H deficiencies associated with hemolytic uremic syndrome or membranoproliferative glomerulonephritis: report and genetic analysis of 16 cases. *J. Am. Soc. Nephrol.* **15:**787–795.
8. **Endoh, M., M. Yamashina, H. Ohi, K. Funahashi, T. Ikuno, T. Yasugi, J. P. Atkinson, and H. Okada.** 1993. Immunohistochemical demonstration of membrane cofactor protein (MCP) of complement in normal and diseased kidney tissues. *Clin. Exp. Immunol.* **94:**182–188.
9. **Fremeaux-Bacchi, V., M. Dragon-Durey, J. Blouin, C. Vigneau, D. Kuypers, B. Boudailliez, C. Loirat, E. Rondeau, and W. Fridman.** 2004. Complement Factor I: a susceptibility gene for atypical hemolytic-uremic syndrome. *J. Med. Genet.* **41:**e84.

10. Ichida, S., Y. Yuzawa, H. Okada, K. Yoshioka, and S. Matsuo. 1994. Localization of the complement regulatory proteins in the normal human kidney. *Kidney Int.* **46:**89–96.

11. Johnstone, R. W., B. E. Loveland, and I. F. McKenzie. 1993. Identification and quantification of complement regulator CD46 on normal human tissues. *Immunology* **79:**341–347.

12. Kaplan, B. S., R. W. Chesney, and K. N. Drummond. 1975. Hemolytic uremic syndrome in families. *N. Engl. J. Med.* **292:**1090–1093.

13. Kaplan, B. S., and P. Kaplan. 1992. Hemolytic uremic syndrome in families, p. 213–225. *In* B. S. Kaplan, R. S. Trompeter, and J. L. Moake (ed.), *Hemolytic Uremic Syndrome and Thrombotic Thrombocytopenic Purpura.* Marcel Dekker, New York, N.Y.

14. Kirkitadze, M. D., and P. N. Barlow. 2001. Structure and flexibility of the multiple domain proteins that regulate complement activation. *Immunol. Rev.* **180:**146–161.

15. Kojima, A., K. Iwata, T. Seya, M. Matsumoto, H. Ariga, J. P. Atkinson, and S. Nagasawa. 1993. Membrane cofactor protein (CD46) protects cells predominantly from alternative complement pathway-mediated C3-fragment deposition and cytolysis. *J. Immunol.* **151:**1519–1527.

16. Liszewski, M. K., T. C. Farries, D. M. Lublin, I. A. Rooney, and J. P. Atkinson. 1996. Control of the complement system. *Adv. Immunol.* **61:**201–283.

17. Manuelian, T., J. Hellwage, S. Meri, J. Caprioli, M. Noris, S. Heinen, M. Jozsi, H. P. Neumann, G. Remuzzi, and P. F. Zipfel. 2003. Mutations in factor H reduce binding affinity to C3b and heparin and surface attachment to endothelial cells in hemolytic uremic syndrome. *J. Clin. Invest.* **111:**1181–1190.

18. McNearney, T., L. Ballard, T. Seya, and J. P. Atkinson. 1989. Membrane cofactor protein of complement is present on human fibroblast, epithelial, and endothelial cells. *J. Clin. Invest.* **84:**538–545.

19. Moake, J. L. 2002. Thrombotic microangiopathies. *N. Engl. J. Med.* **347:**589–600.

20. Nakanishi, I., A. Moutabarrik, T. Hara, M. Hatanaka, T. Hayashi, T. Syouji, N. Okada, E. Kitamura, Y. Tsubakihara, M. Matsumoto, et al. 1994. Identification and characterization of membrane cofactor protein (CD46) in the human kidneys. *Eur. J. Immunol.* **24:**1529–1535.

21. Neumann, H. P., M. Salzmann, B. Bohnert-Iwan, T. Mannuelian, C. Skerka, D. Lenk, B. U. Bender, M. Cybulla, P. Riegler, A. Konigsrainer, U. Neyer, A. Bock, U. Widmer, D. A. Male, G. Franke, and P. F. Zipfel. 2003. Haemolytic uraemic syndrome and mutations of the factor H gene: a registry-based study of German speaking countries. *J. Med. Genet.* **40:**676–681.

22. Noris, M., S. Brioschi, J. Caprioli, M. Todeschini, E. Bresin, F. Porrati, S. Gamba, and G. Remuzzi. 2003. Familial haemolytic uraemic syndrome and an MCP mutation. *Lancet* **362:**1542–1547.

23. Oglesby, T. J., C. J. Allen, M. K. Liszewski, D. J. White, and J. P. Atkinson. 1992. Membrane cofactor protein (CD46) protects cells from complement-mediated attack by an intrinsic mechanism. *J. Exp. Med.* **175:**1547–1551.

24. Ohali, M., H. Shalev, M. Schlesinger, Y. Katz, L. Kachko, R. Carmi, S. Sofer, and D. Landau. 1998. Hypocomplementemic autosomal recessive hemolytic uremic syndrome with decreased factor H. *Pediatr. Nephrol.* **12:**619–624.

25. Pangburn, M. K. 2002. Cutting edge: localization of the host recognition functions of complement factor H at the carboxyl-terminal: implications for hemolytic uremic syndrome. *J. Immunol.* **169:**4702–4706.

26. Pérez-Caballero, D., C. González-Rubio, M. E. Gallardo, M. Vera, M. López Trascasa, S. Rodríguez de Córdoba, and P. Sánchez-Corral. 2001. Clustering of missense mutations in the C-terminal region of factor H in atypical hemolytic uremic syndrome. *Am. J. Hum. Genet.* **68:**478–484.

27. Perkins, S. J., and T. H. J. Goodship. 2002. Molecular modelling of the C-terminal domains of factor H of human complement. A correlation between haemolytic uraemic syndrome and a predicted heparin binding site. *J. Mol. Biol.* **316:**217–224.

28. Pichette, V., S. Querin, W. Schurch, G. Brun, G. Lehnernetsch, and J. M. Delage. 1994. Familial hemolytic-uremic syndrome and homozygous factor-H deficiency. *Am. J. Kidney Dis.* **24:**936–941.

29. Pirson, Y., C. Lefebvre, C. Arnout, and C. Van Ypersele de Strihou. 1987. Hemolytic uremic syndrome in three adult siblings: a family study and evolution. *Clin. Nephrol.* **28:**250–255.

30. Post, T. W., M. K. Liszewski, E. M. Adams, I. Tedja, E. A. Miller, and J. P. Atkinson. 1991. Membrane cofactor protein of the complement system: alternative splicing of serine/threonine/proline-rich exons and cytoplasmic tails produces multiple isoforms that correlate with protein phenotype. *J. Exp. Med.* **174:**93–102.

31. Richards, A., M. R. Buddles, R. L. Donne, B. S. Kaplan, E. Kirk, M. C. Venning, C. L. Tielemans, J. A. Goodship, and T. H. J. Goodship. 2001. Factor H mutations in hemolytic uremic syndrome cluster in exons 18–20, a domain important for host cell recognition. *Am. J. Hum. Genet.* **68:**485–490.

32. Richards, A., E. J. Kemp, M. K. Liszewski, J. A. Goodship, A. K. Lampe, R. Decorte, M. H. Muslumanoglu, S. Kavukcu, G. Filler, Y. Pirson, L. S. Wen, J. P. Atkinson, and T. H. J. Goodship. 2003. Mutations in human complement regulator, membrane cofactor protein (CD46), predispose to development of familial hemolytic uremic syndrome. *Proc. Natl. Acad. Sci. USA* **100:**12966–12971.

33. Roodhooft, A. M., R. H. McLean, E. Elst, and K. J. Van Acker. 1990. Recurrent hemolytic uremic syndrome and acquired hypomorphic variant of the third component of complement. *Pediatr. Nephrol.* **4:**597–599.

34. Russell, S. M., R. L. Sparrow, I. F. McKenzie, and D. F. Purcell. 1992. Tissue-specific and allelic expression of the complement regulator CD46 is controlled by alternative splicing. *Eur. J. Immunol.* **22:**1513–1518.

35. Sanchez-Corral, P., D. Perez-Caballero, O. Huarte, A. M. Simckes, E. Goicoechea, M. Lopez-Trascasa, and S. Rodriguez De Cordoba. 2002. Structural and functional characterization of factor H mutations associated with atypical hemolytic uremic syndrome. *Am. J. Hum. Genet.* **71:**1285–1295.

36. Schouten, J. P., C. J. McElgunn, R. Waaijer, D. Zwijnenburg, F. Diepvens, and G. Pals. 2002. Relative quantification of 40 nucleic acid sequences by multiplex ligation-dependent probe amplification. *Nucleic Acids Res.* **30:**e57.

37. Seya, T., and J. P. Atkinson. 1989. Functional properties of membrane cofactor protein of complement. *Biochem. J.* **264:**581–588.

38. Seya, T., J. R. Turner, and J. P. Atkinson. 1986. Purification and characterization of a membrane protein (gp45-70) that is a cofactor for cleavage of C3b and C4b. *J. Exp. Med.* **163:**837–855.

38a. Strachan, T., and A. P. Read (ed.). 2003. *Human Molecular Genetics*, 3rd ed. Garland Science, London, United Kingdom.

39. Thompson, R. A., and M. H. Winterborn. 1981. Hypocomplementaemia due to a genetic deficiency of beta-1H globulin. *Clin. Exp. Immunol.* **46:**110–119.

40. Vyse, T. J., G. P. Bates, M. J. Walport, and B. J. Morley. 1994. The organization of the human complement factor I gene (IF): a member of the serine protease gene family. *Genomics* **24:**90–98.

41. Vyse, T. J., B. J. Morley, I. Bartok, E. L. Theodoridis, K. A. Davies, A. D. Webster, and M. J. Walport. 1996. The molecular basis of hereditary complement factor I deficiency. *J. Clin. Invest.* **97:**925–933.

42. Vyse, T. J., P. J. Spath, K. A. Davies, B. J. Morley, P. Philippe, P. Athanassiou, C. M. Giles, and M. J. Walport. 1994. Hereditary complement factor I deficiency. *Q. J. Med.* **87:**385–401.

43. Warwicker, P., and T. H. J. Goodship. 2003. Haemolytic uraemic syndrome, p. 407–410. *In* D. A. Warrell, T. M. Cox, J. D. Firth, and E. J. Benz, Jr. (ed.), *Oxford Textbook of Medicine.* Oxford University Press, Oxford, United Kingdom.

44. Warwicker, P., T. H. J. Goodship, R. L. Donne, Y. Pirson, A. Nicholls, R. M. Ward, and J. A. Goodship. 1998. Genetic studies into inherited and sporadic haemolytic uraemic syndrome. *Kidney Int.* **53:**836–844.

45. Ying, L., Y. Katz, M. Schlesinger, R. Carmi, H. Shalev, N. Haider, G. Beck, V. C. Sheffield, and D. Landau. 1999. Complement factor H gene mutation associated with autosomal recessive atypical hemolytic uremic syndrome. *Am. J. Hum. Genet.* **65:**1538–1546.

46. Zipfel, P. F., T. S. Jokiranta, J. Hellwage, V. Koistinen, and S. Meri. 1999. The factor H protein family. *Immunopharmacology* **42:**53–60.

An Enzyme-Linked Immunosorbent Assay-Based Method for Functional Analysis of the Three Pathways of the Complement System

M. A. SEELEN, A. ROOS, J. WIESLANDER, AND M. R. DAHA

14

BACKGROUND

The complement system has a crucial role in innate immune defense against invading microorganisms and can be activated by the classical pathway (CP), the alternative pathway (AP), and the mannose-binding lectin (MBL) pathway (MP) (8). Initiation of the complement system generates a cascade of enzymatically activated proteins and is associated with the initiation of the terminal complement pathway and formation and deposition of the terminal C5b-9 complement complex, also termed the membrane attack complex. Furthermore, activation of the complement system generates opsonic components of complement, facilitating the phagocytosis of microorganisms by phagocytes (1).

The CP is activated by binding of C1q to, e.g., immunoglobulins present on microorganisms or by direct binding to apoptotic cells. The AP can be directly activated by invading microorganisms. The MP is also directly activated, via carbohydrate moieties present on the surface of invading microbes.

For assessment of the functional activity of the classical and alternative pathways, hemolysis of erythrocytes by complement activation via either the CP (CH50) or the AP (AP50) is used in most laboratories. Functional enzyme-linked immunosorbent assay (ELISA)-based procedures for the classical and alternative pathways have been developed on the basis of previously reported methods (2, 7). Also, for assessment of the functional activity of the MP, hemolytic assays have been developed.

Direct hemolysis of erythrocytes coated with mannan and indirect hemolysis of chicken erythrocytes, as innocent bystander cells, have been used (3, 4). In both assays, exogenous mannan-binding-lectin-associated serine proteases (MASP) and/or additional complement factors have to be added to the assay system to permit erythrocyte lysis. Furthermore, both types of assays are difficult to perform on a routine basis for clinical use and do not exclude participation of the CP in the assay. Petersen et al. (6) introduced an ELISA-based assay with mannan-coated plates to evaluate the activity of the MBL-MASP complex. In this assay, sera are incubated in high-ionic-strength buffer to prevent interference from CP activation by antimannan antibodies. The activity of the MBL-MASP complex is assessed in a second step with exogenously added purified C4. In clinical practice, it would be helpful to assess the functional activity of the whole MP, from MBL through to C9, without the use of

additional complement sources. Such ELISA-based procedures using mannan-coated plates have been developed (5, 7), and it has been recently demonstrated that the contribution of the CP in such an assay can be prevented by addition of an inhibitory antibody directed against C1q (7).

A combination ELISA has been developed at Wieslab (Lund, Sweden), in collaboration with European academic partners, to assess the functional activity of the CP, AP, and MP.

ASSAY

The methods to assess pathway activity of the CP, AP, and MP are ELISA based. All three assays are delivered as one ELISA system. Strips of wells for CP evaluation are precoated with immunoglobulin M, strips for AP determination are coated with lipopolysaccharide, and strips for the MP are coated with mannan. Sera should be diluted 1/101 for the CP and MP assays and 1/18 for the AP assay. Specific buffers containing Mg^{2+} and Ca^{2+} for the CP and MP and a buffer containing Mg-EGTA for the AP are used to ensure that activation of only one of the pathways can occur. Activation of the CP in the MP assay, by naturally occurring antibodies directed against mannan, is inhibited by specific anti-C1q antibodies.

SAMPLES

Samples: Blood samples are to be collected under sterile conditions in red-top tubes, without serum separator. A minimum of 5 ml of whole blood is recommended. Allow blood to clot for 60 to 65 min at room temperature (20 to 25°C). Centrifuge clotted blood samples in a refrigerated centrifuge, and transfer cell-free serum to a clean tube. Sera should be handled in such a way that in vitro complement activation is prevented. Sera should be frozen at $-70°C$ in tightly sealed sterile tubes for extended storage and should be frozen and thawed preferably only once but at most three times and should not be older than 1 year. Plasma samples cannot be used. A 30-μl serum sample is required for the assay of all three pathways.

MATERIALS AND REAGENTS

Kit components and storage of reagents:

A foil pack with a desiccation sachet including four blue-colored ELISA well strips for the CP, coated with

124

human immunoglobulin M; four green-colored strips for the MP, coated with mannan; and four red-colored strips for the AP, coated with lipopolysaccharide

10 ml of diluent CP, labeled blue

10 ml of diluent MP, labeled green

10 ml of diluent AP, labeled red

13 ml of conjugate alkaline phosphatase-labeled antibodies to C5b-9 (blue)

13 ml of substrate solution, ready to use

30 ml of wash solution, 30× concentrated

0.2-ml negative control, containing human serum

0.2-ml positive control, containing freeze-dried human serum

The reagents should be stored at 2 to 8°C. The positive control should be stored at −20°C.

Washing solution: A 30× concentrated washing solution is provided. A 30-ml volume of solution should be diluted in 870 ml of distilled water. When stored at 2 to 8°C, the diluted wash solution is stable until the date of expiry of the kit. Before use, the solution should be at room temperature.

EQUIPMENT AND INSTRUMENTS

Precision pipettes with disposable tips

Water bath at 37°C

Ice bath

Washer for strips, absorbent tissue, tubes, and timer

Microplate spectrophotometer with 405-nm filter

PREPARATION OF SAMPLES

Positive control: A positive control is provided in the kit. Gently tap down all lyophilized material to the bottom of the vial and remove the cap. Immediately add 200 μl of distilled water and replace the cap. Allow the vial to stand on ice for 5 min and gently shake or vortex occasionally until completely dissolved. The reconstituted positive control can be stored for 4 h prior to use if kept at 2 to 8°C or on ice. It can be frozen at −70°C and thawed once.

Serum samples: Partially thaw frozen sera by briefly placing them in a 37°C water bath with gentle mixing. After partially thawing, immediately place the tubes in an ice bath and leave them on ice until the dilution step.

Procedure 1: Dilution of Samples

CP

Dilute the serum samples, positive control, and negative control 1/101 with diluent for CP, provided in the kit in a vial with a blue label (500 μl + 5 μl of serum). The diluted serum can be left at room temperature for 60 min before analysis.

MP

Dilute the serum samples, positive control, and negative control 1/101 with diluent for MP, provided in the kit in a vial with a green label (500 μl + 5 μl of serum). The diluted serum *must* be left at room temperature for >15 min before analysis but not longer than 60 min.

AP

Dilute the serum samples, positive control, and negative control 1/18 with diluent for AP, provided in the kit in a vial with a red label (340 μl + 20 μl of serum). The diluted serum can be left at room temperature for 60 min before analysis.

Procedure 2: Incubation of Samples

In duplicate, pipette 100 μl of the following per well:

Diluent alone, as a blank

Positive control

Negative control

Patient serum

The best order of sample addition to the plate is shown in Table 1. Incubate the plate for 60 to 70 min at 37°C with a lid.

Procedure 3: Washing

Empty all wells and wash the plate three times with 300 μl of washing solution, filling and emptying the wells each time. After the last wash, empty the wells by tapping the strip on an absorbent tissue.

Procedure 4: Adding Conjugate

Add 100 μl of conjugate to each well, and incubate the plate for 30 min at room temperature. The conjugate, containing alkaline phosphatase-labeled antibodies to C5b-9, is used for all three pathways.

Procedure 5: Washing

See procedure 3.

TABLE 1 Diagram for placement of the diluted sera from patients and controls in the assay plate

Row	Contents of indicated column[a]											
	CP				MP				AP			
	1	2	3	4	5	6	7	8	9	10	11	12
A	BL	PS2	PS6	PS10	BL	PS2	PS6	PS10	BL	PS2	PS6	PS10
B	BL	PS2	PS6	PS10	BL	PS2	PS6	PS10	BL	PS2	PS6	PS10
C	PC	PS3	PS7	PS11	PC	PS3	PS7	PS11	PC	PS3	PS7	PS11
D	PC	PS3	PS7	PS11	PC	PS3	PS7	PS11	PC	PS3	PS7	PS11
E	NC	PS4	PS8	PS12	NC	PS4	PS8	PS12	NC	PS4	PS8	PS12
F	NC	PS4	PS8	PS12	NC	PS4	PS8	PS12	NC	PS4	PS8	PS12
G	PS1	PS5	PS9	PS13	PS1	PS5	PS9	PS13	PS1	PS5	PS9	PS13
H	PS1	PS5	PS9	PS13	PS1	PS5	PS9	PS13	PS1	PS5	PS9	PS13

[a] BL, blank; PC, positive control; NC, negative control; PS, patient serum.

Procedure 6: Addition of Substrate

Add 100 μl of substrate solution to each well, and incubate the plate for 30 min at room temperature. Read the absorbance at 405 nm on a microplate reader. (A 100-μl volume of 5 mM EDTA per well can be used as stop solution. Read the absorbance of the wells within 60 min.)

Procedure 7: Calculation of Result

Subtract the absorbance of the blank from all other samples. The absorbance of the positive control should be >1, and that of the negative control should be <0.2.

The negative and positive controls can be used in a semiquantitative way. Pathway activity can be calculated as follows: activity = 100% × (mean A_{405} of sample − mean A_{405} of negative control)/(mean A_{405} of standard serum − mean A_{405} of negative control).

It is recommended that each laboratory establish its own reference level and cutoff value for deficiencies.

PREANALYTICAL CONCERNS

Collection and Storage of Samples

With the combined assay, the functional activity of the three pathways of complement activation can be assessed. Because the functional activity is being assessed, it is important that no in vitro complement consumption occurs when the samples are collected. Serum should be stored at −70°C in tightly sealed tubes and not be frozen and thawed more than once. Storage at −70°C for more than one year can influence functional activity.

Storage of Assay

The complement kit should be stored at 2 to 8°C and not be used after the expiry date. The positive control, provided as lyophilized material, should be stored at −20°C.

All solutions should be equilibrated to room temperature (20 to 25°C) before analysis.

ANALYTICAL CONCERNS

The positive control serum should be stored at −20°C. After thawing, serum samples should be kept on ice during performance of the assay. Serum samples from patients should be stored at −70°C and thawed only just before the test is performed and should not be frozen and thawed more than once. Sera diluted for one test should not be used again. Let all solutions equilibrate to room temperature (20 to 25°C).

The diluted serum sample for the MP must be left at room temperature for >15 min and no longer than 60 min prior to analysis. The time periods for the different incubations should be kept accurately.

POSTANALYTICAL CONCERNS

The controls are intended to monitor for substantial reagent failure. It is recommended that each laboratory establish its own reference level and cutoff value for deficiencies. The individual patient complement pathway activity cannot be used as a measure of disease severity, as it may vary from patient to patient. The test results are dependent on the quality of the serum samples.

TEST VALIDATION

Sera from healthy blood donors were tested in the three assays (n = 120). The intra-assay variation for the three pathways was below 7%, whereas the interassay variation was below or equal to 20%. The normal reference range in the sera was calculated for the CP, AP, and MP. Because of the limited variation of complement activity between different sera, particularly in the CP but also in the AP, a cutoff value for normal pathway activity could be defined as the mean value of activity minus two times the standard deviation. This approach resulted in 2.5% of the healthy population falling below the cutoff value for normal complement activity. The cutoff value for the CP was calculated to be 74%, and that for the AP was calculated to be 39%. Because of the variation in MBL concentration in the normal healthy population, which is mainly genetically determined, there is a large variation in MP activity. Therefore, an arbitrary minimum level for normal MP activity was set at 10% of the standard, which corresponded to MBL concentrations below 300 ng/ml.

PITFALLS AND TROUBLESHOOTING

Because collection and storage of samples are of crucial importance in functional complement assays and the handling is not always correct, the in-house accuracy results should always be used in combination with clinical symptoms. When inappropriate handling of serum samples is suspected, the test should be repeated. Tests with results just above or below the cutoff value are best repeated.

INTERPRETATION OF RESULTS

The level of complement activity evaluated by functional assays takes into account the rate of synthesis, degradation, and consumption of complement components. Decreased functional activity can be the result of a complement deficiency or an ongoing process leading to complement consumption. With the use of this combined ELISA system, the three pathways for complement activation can be assessed at the same time. The possible deficiencies of components leading to reduced functional activity can be detected by using the combined test results of the three pathways (Table 2). For further evaluation of deficiency of a single complement component, other assays are available.

CONCLUSION

For clinicians suspecting a deficiency in innate immunity in patients with, for example, recurrent severe infections or systemic autoimmune diseases, analysis of the complement system is important. The ELISA-based kit presented in this chapter provides the tools to screen the three pathways of

TABLE 2 Determination of possible complement deficiency by combination of the test results from the three assays

Complement deficiency	ELISA result[a]		
	CP	AP	MP
C1q, C1r, C1s,	↓	=	=
C4, C2	↓	=	↓
C3	↓	↓	↓
Factor B, D, properdin	=	↓	=
MBL, MASP-2	=	=	↓
C5, C6, C7, C8, C9	↓	↓	↓
C1 inhibitor	↓	↓	↓
Factor H and I	↓	↓	↓

[a] Decreased (↓) or normal (=) functional pathway activity.

complement activation for possible deficiencies. By using the results from the three assays, it is possible to detect the possible complement components responsible for reduced functional activity. The levels of these individual components can subsequently be evaluated.

REFERENCES

1. **Aderem, A., and D. M. Underhill.** 1999. Mechanisms of phagocytosis in macrophages. *Annu. Rev. Immunol.* **17:**593–623.
2. **Fredrikson, G. N., L. Truedsson, and A. G. Sjoholm.** 1993. New procedure for the detection of complement deficiency by ELISA. Analysis of activation pathways and circumvention of rheumatoid factor influence. *J. Immunol. Methods* **166:**263–270.
3. **Ikeda, K., T. Sannoh, N. Kawasaki, T. Kawasaki, and I. Yamashina.** 1987. Serum lectin with known structure activates complement through the classical pathway. *J. Biol. Chem.* **262:**7451–7454.
4. **Kuipers, S., P. C. Aerts, A. G. Sjoholm, T. Harmsen, and H. van Dijk.** 2002. A hemolytic assay for the estimation of functional mannose-binding lectin levels in human serum. *J. Immunol. Methods* **268:**149–157.
5. **Minchinton, R. M., M. M. Dean, T. R. Clark, S. Heatley, and C. G. Mullighan.** 2002. Analysis of the relationship between mannose-binding lectin (MBL) genotype, MBL levels and function in an Australian blood donor population. *Scand. J. Immunol.* **56:**630–641.
6. **Petersen, S. V., S. Thiel, L. Jensen, R. Steffensen, and J. C. Jensenius.** 2001. An assay for the mannan-binding lectin pathway of complement activation. *J. Immunol. Methods* **257:**107–116.
7. **Roos, A., L. H. Bouwman, J. Munoz, T. Zuiverloon, M. C. Faber-Krol, F. C. Fallaux-van den Houten, N. Klar-Mohamad, C. E. Hack, M. G. Tilanus, and M. R. Daha.** 2003. Functional characterization of the lectin pathway of complement in human serum. *Mol. Immunol.* **39:**655–668.
8. **Walport, M. J.** 2001. Complement. First of two parts. *N. Engl. J. Med.* **344:**1058–1066.

Evaluation of the Mannan-Binding Lectin Pathway of Complement Activation

MIHAELA GADJEVA AND STEFFEN THIEL

15

Mannan-binding lectin (MBL) activates the complement system and therefore triggers an innate antimicrobial defense mechanism. Events in the MBL pathway of complement activation involve the binding of MBL to patterns of carbohydrate structures presented on the surface of microorganisms and the following activation of the proenzymes of the complement system. MBL selectively binds to sugars, e.g., mannose, glucose, L-fucose, and N-acetylglucosamine, with low affinity. To obtain physiologically relevant high-avidity interaction with MBL they must be clustered, e.g., as binding occurs on the surface of the microorganisms. In circulation, MBL is found in complex with serine protease zymogens: MASP-1 (MBL-associated serine protease-1), MASP-2, and MASP-3. The MBL-MASP complex also contains a nonenzymatic protein, MAp19. The functions of the different MASPs remain to be determined, but there is some knowledge as to the function of MASP-2. Upon binding of the MBL complex to its ligands, MASP-2 autoactivates and then proteolytically cleaves complement components C4 and C2 to generate the C3 convertase C4bC2b.

TECHNOLOGY

The protocols described here are useful for routine quantification of MBL and evaluation of the MBL pathway activity in clinical samples. The assays are based on the robust, highly sensitive and reproducible time-resolved immunofluorometric assay (TRIFMA). TRIFMAs are similar to enzyme-linked immunosorbent assays (ELISAs), with the only difference being the type of labeling of detecting molecules. Instead of enzyme-linked antibodies or streptavidin, Eu^{3+} is used to label antibodies or streptavidin. In the ELISA, a colorimetric reaction is monitored, while in the TRIFMAs, fluorescence is detected. The assay can easily be changed to an ELISA format by changing the label of the developing reagent to the relevant enzyme; e.g., if an ELISA setup is preferred, enzyme-linked streptavidin can be used instead of Eu^{3+}-labeled streptavidin. This step is followed by use of the relevant substrate solution.

QUANTIFICATION OF MBL

Different approaches have been used to measure the MBL concentration in plasma or serum (11, 12, 26). The recommended assays in this chapter focus on two approaches. The first is based on a modification of the conventional sandwich ELISA, in which microtiter wells are coated with anti-MBL antibody and then incubated with dilutions of plasma or serum and the amount of bound MBL is measured by using europium-labeled anti-MBL antibody (MBL antigen assay) (Fig. 1A). The second assay quantifies MBL on the basis of its lectin-binding activity (lectin assay), in which microtiter wells are coated with mannan instead of anti-MBL antibody (Fig. 1B) (27). The two assays produce comparable results ($r = 0.97$); however, the sensitivities of the assays differ. The MBL antigen assay is more sensitive (down to 2 ng of MBL/ml of plasma) than the lectin assay (10 ng/ml). Both assays demonstrate a high degree of reproducibility.

MBL ANTIGEN ASSAY

Sample Requirement

Both serum and plasma (EDTA, citrate, or heparin) samples may be used because the high NaCl concentration in the sample buffer inhibits coagulation. If serum is used, the blood is allowed to coagulate at room temperature (RT) for 2 h before centrifugation and removal of the serum. Serum aliquots are stored at $-80°C$ until use. The assay is not influenced by possible variations of other serum factors, e.g., complement factor C4, C1q, or C1 inhibitor. The assay can be performed with commercially available reagents.

Materials and Reagents

- 96-well microtiter plates (437958; FluoroNunc, Kamstrup, Denmark)
- Coating anti-MBL antibody of choice (e.g., monoclonal antibody [MAb] 131-1; Immunolex, Copenhagen, Denmark)
- Detection antibody: biotinylated anti-MBL antibody of choice (e.g., MAb 131-1 [Immunolex], biotinylated by using reagents from, e.g., Pierce [Lausanne, Switzerland])
- Streptavidin-Eu^{3+} (Wallac Oy/Perkin Elmer, Turku, Finland)
- Time-resolved fluorometer, e.g., 1232 DELFIA fluorometer (Wallac Oy)
- Phosphate-buffered saline (PBS): 0.23 g of NaH_2PO_4 (anhydrous; 1.9 mM), 1.15 g of Na_2HPO_4, 9 g of NaCl. Adjust the pH to 7.4 and the volume to 1 liter.

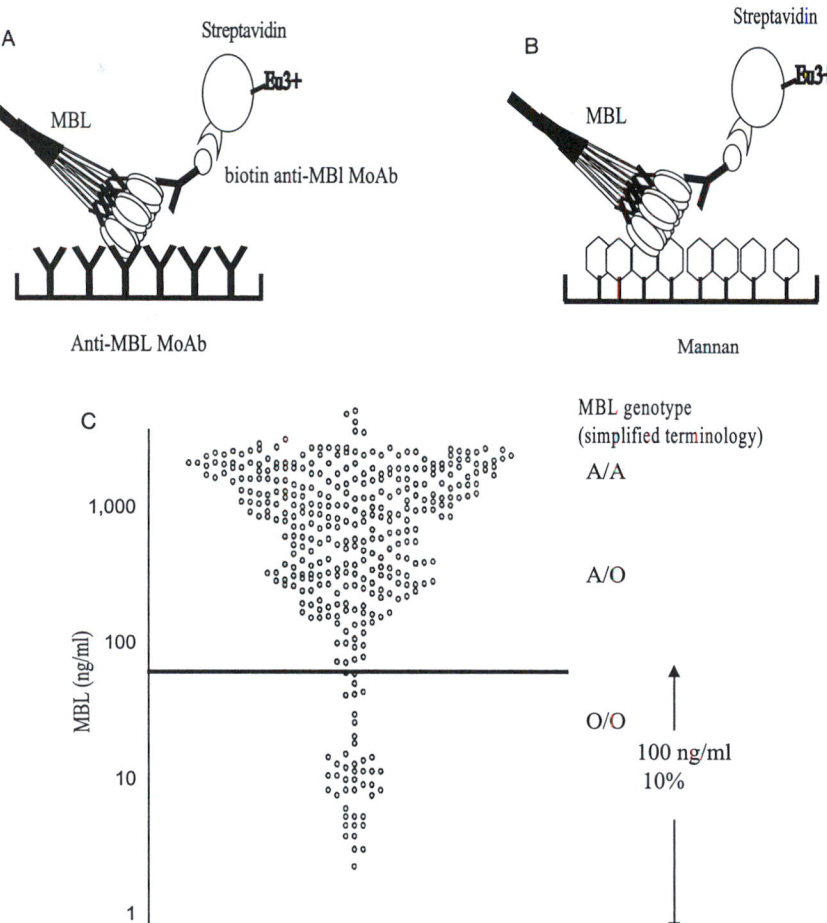

FIGURE 1 Quantification of MBL. (A) Quantification by the antigen assay. MBL is captured in the microtiter well by anti-MBL MAb and then detected by a biotinylated anti-MBL MAb. (B) Quantification by the lectin assay. MBL is captured in the microtiter well by mannan (high-affinity ligand for MBL) and is detected by biotinylated anti-MBL MAb. In both the antigen and the lectin assays, the biotinylated anti-MBL MAb step is followed by incubation with Eu^{3+}-labeled streptavidin. (C) Histogram showing levels of MBL in plasma. MBL levels correlate with MBL polymorphisms. For illustrative purposes, the genotypes are given in a simplified form, as follows: A/A, wild-type gene, excluding XA/XA; A/O, heterozygotes for the mutations in exon 1 and in the promoter region, including also XA/XA; and O/O, homozygote mutants and compound heterozygote mutants. Individual MBL levels are represented as circles. Approximately 10% of the population appears to have MBL levels below 100 ng/ml, which can be recognized as deficiency.

MBL binding buffer: 20 mM Tris, 1 M NaCl, 0.05% Triton X-100, 10 mM $CaCl_2$, 15 mM NaN_3, 1-mg/ml human serum albumin (HSA) or bovine serum albumin, 100 μg of heat-aggregated human immunoglobulin G (IgG)/ml. Adjust pH to 7.4. Store at RT. The heat-aggregated human IgG is made by heating a solution of human IgG (at 10 μg/ml) at 63°C for 30 min and then subjecting it to centrifugation at 1,000 × g; the supernatant is used as heat-aggregated IgG.

Blocking buffer: dissolve 1 mg of HSA per ml in 10 mM Tris–145 mM NaCl–15 mM NaN_3 (pH 7.4). Store at 4°C.

Washing buffer: 10 mM Tris, 145 mM NaCl, 0.05% Tween 20, 5 mM $CaCl_2$. Adjust pH to 7.4. Store at RT.

Enhancement solution: mix 5.7 ml of CH_3COOH with potassium hydrogen phthalate to reach a pH of 3.2. Add 1 ml of Triton X-100, and adjust the volume

to 1 liter with distilled H_2O. Store at 4°C. Before use, add 2 μl of 15 μM 2-naphthoyltrifluoracetate (2-NTA)–50 μM tri-o-octylphosphine oxide (TOPO) per ml of CH_3COOH–potassium hydrogen phthalate (pH 3.2). Store at 4°C.

Protocol

1. Coat the wells of the microtiter plate with 0.5 μg of anti-MBL MAb 131-1 per ml in 100 μl of PBS and incubate at 20°C overnight in a moist chamber.

2. Empty the wells and block the wells with 200 μl of *blocking buffer* per well. Incubate the plate for 1 h at 20°C. After incubation, wash the plates three times with Tris-buffered saline (TBS) (100 mM Tris-Cl [pH 7.5], 0.9% NaCl)–0.05% Tween 20.

If the plates are to be stored for later use, add 200 μl of TBS per well and store them at 4°C in a moist chamber.

3. Dilute samples in *MBL binding buffer* and incubate in a moist chamber overnight at 4°C. Wash three times with *washing buffer*.

Usually 100-fold sample dilution is sufficient.

4. Detect with biotinylated anti-MBL antibody 131-1. Dilute the biotinylated antibodies in *washing buffer* (use 100 μl/well) and incubate for 1 to 2 h at 20°C in a moist chamber. Wash the wells three times with *washing buffer*.

5. Develop with streptavidin-Eu³⁺ by diluting streptavidin-Eu³⁺ appropriately in TBS–0.05% Tween 20–25 μM EDTA and incubate the plates for 1 to 2 h at 20°C in a moist chamber. After incubation, wash the plates three times in *washing buffer*.

6. Read the plate on a DELFIA fluorometer after you have added 200 μl of enhancement solution per well and shaken the plate for 5 min before reading.

LECTIN ASSAY

The lectin assay protocol describes the quantification of MBL as a lectin. It involves a modification of the previous protocol, in which the coating of the plate with anti-MBL MAb is substituted by coating with mannan.

Additional Materials and Reagents

Mannan (M7504; Sigma, St. Louis, Mo.)

Coating buffer: 15 mM Na_2CO_3, 35 mM $NaHCO_3$, 15 mM NaN_3. Adjust the pH to 9.6. Store at RT.

1. Coat a FluoroNunc 96-well plate with 100 μl of mannan per well at 10 μg/ml diluted in *coating buffer* and incubate at 20°C overnight in a moist chamber.

2. Follow steps 2 to 6 from the main protocol.

Note that MBL is a calcium-dependent lectin; thus, all buffers for dilution or washing contain 5 mM $CaCl_2$. The only solution that does not contain calcium is the buffer for the dilution of the Eu^{3+}-labeled reagent (step 5, main protocol), which contains 25 μM EDTA to lower the background in the assays due to traces of free europium in the Eu^{3+}-labeled reagents.

MBL-MASP COMPLEX ACTIVITY ASSAY

The MBL-MASP complex activity assay permits determination of the MBL complex activity in serum or plasma samples and may therefore be used to evaluate the clinical implications of MBL pathway-mediated complement activation (Fig. 2) (21). The assay determines the ability of the serum to lead to deposition of C4b onto a mannan-coated surface.

Additional Materials and Reagents

Human complement C4 (A402; Quidel, San Diego, Calif.). Note that complement C4 can be easily purified from human plasma by conventional laboratory techniques as described elsewhere (3).

Biotinylated anti-human C4 antibodies, e.g., rabbit anti-human C4 (DAKO, Glostrup, Denmark). The biotinylation is carried out by using reagents from, e.g., Pierce.

The contents of the *coating buffer, blocking buffer, washing buffer*, and *MBL binding buffer* are similar to the ones described for the two assays above.

TBS

1. Coat the wells with 10-μg/ml mannan (100 μl/well diluted in *coating buffer*) and incubate the plate at 20°C overnight in a moist chamber.

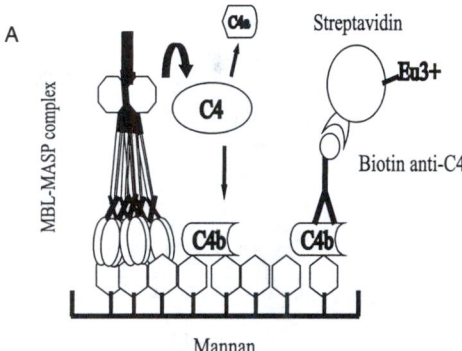

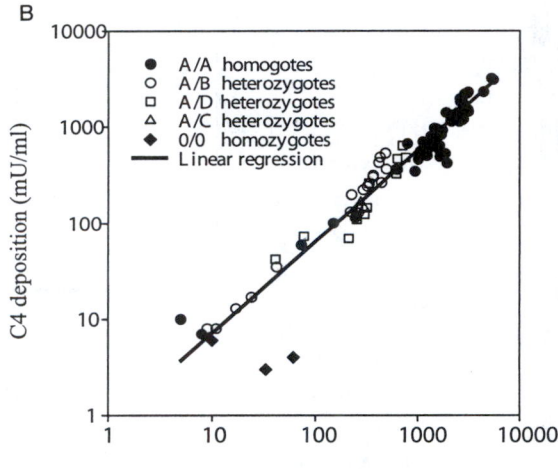

FIGURE 2 MBL pathway activity assay. (A) Schematic representation of the MBL-MASP pathway activity assay. MBL-MASP complexes bind to the mannan-coated microtiter wells. MASP-2 cleaves C4, splitting it into C4a and C4b. The C4b covalently deposits on mannan, and the bound C4b can be detected by use of biotinylated anti-C4 antibodies followed by streptavidin-Eu³⁺. (B) Relationship between C4 deposition activity and the MBL concentration in 100 normal plasma specimens. The genotypes of each individual are indicated. Linear regression, $r = 0.96$.

2. Block the plate with 200 μl of *blocking buffer* per well. Incubate for 1 h at 20°C. After incubation, wash the plates three times with *washing buffer*.

If the plates are to be stored for later use, add 200 μl of TBS per well and store them at 4°C in a moist chamber.

3. Dilute samples in *MBL binding buffer* and incubate in a moist chamber overnight at 4°C. Wash three times with washing buffer.

Usually 200-fold sample dilution is adequate.

4. Add 0.5 μg of human C4 per ml diluted in *washing buffer*, incubate the plates for 1.5 h at 37°C, and then wash the plates three times with washing buffer.

5. Detect with 0.2-μg/ml biotinylated anti-human C4 diluted in washing buffer by incubating the plate for 1 h at RT.

6. Follow steps 5 and 6 from the main protocol.

QUANTIFICATION OF MASP-2

Activation of the complement system through the MBL pathway relies on the activity of MASP-2. MASP-2 is capable of activation of C4 and is found in circulation in complex with MBL or ficolins (L-ficolin and H-ficolin). Here, we describe an assay for quantification of plasma or serum MASP-2 (Fig. 3A) (16).

Sample Requirements

EDTA-plasma, heparin-plasma, or serum samples can be used in the assay.

Materials and Reagents

96-well microtiter plates (437958; FluoroNunc)

Coating anti-MASP-2 antibody (e.g., MAb 85B, from the Department of Medical Microbiology and Immunology, University of Aarhus [16])

Detection antibody: biotinylated anti-MASP-2 antibody (e.g., MAb 6G12, from the Department of Medical Microbiology and Immunology, University of Aarhus [16], biotinylated with reagents from, e.g., Pierce)

Streptavidin-Eu^{3+} (Wallac Oy)

Time-resolved fluorometer, e.g., 1232 DELFIA fluorometer

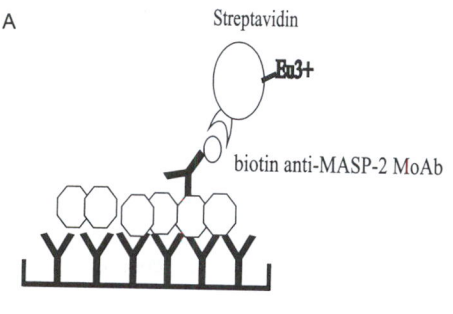

A

Streptavidin

Eu3+

biotin anti-MASP-2 MoAb

Anti-MASP-2 MoAb

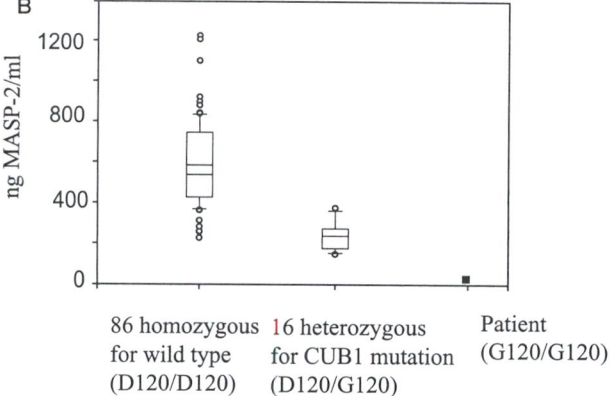

B

FIGURE 3 Quantification of MASP-2. (A) Schematic representation of MASP-2 assay. MASP-2 is captured on the anti-MASP-2 MAb-coated microtiter wells and detected by biotinylated anti-MASP-2 MAb. (B) Concentrations of MASP-2 in 100 healthy individuals. The individuals were genotyped for the presence of the MASP-2 D120G mutation and grouped according to the allele. A total of 86 individuals carried the wild-type allele, and the concentration of MASP-2 varied between 200 and 1,200 ng/ml. The 16 heterozygous individuals had less MASP-2 (between 50 and 400 ng/ml). While both the wild-type and the heterozygous groups consisted of healthy blood donors, the single individual homozygous for the G120 polymorphism was a patient (24) who had no detectable levels of MASP-2.

MASP-2 binding buffer: 10 mM Tris, 1 M NaCl, 0.05% Tween 20, 10 mM EDTA, 15 mM NaN$_3$, 0.01% heat-aggregated human IgG. Adjust pH to 7.4. Store at RT.

TBS

1. Coat the wells of the microtiter plate with 0.5-μg/ml anti-MASP-2 MAb (8B5) in 100 μl of PBS and incubate the plate at 20°C overnight in a moist chamber.

2. Empty the wells and block the wells with 200 μl of *blocking buffer* per well. Incubate the plates for 1 h at 20°C. After incubation, wash the plates three times with TBS–0.05% Tween 20.

If the plates are to be stored for later use, add 200 μl of TBS per well and store them at 4°C in a moist chamber.

3. Dilute plasma or serum samples in *MASP-2 binding buffer* and incubate in a moist chamber overnight at 4°C. Wash the plates three times with *washing buffer*.

The MASP-2 binding buffer contains a high salt concentration (1 M NaCl) and EDTA to ensure the dissociation of MBL-MASP and MBL-ficolin complexes.

4. Detect with 1 μg of biotinylated anti-MASP-2/MAp19 antibody (6G12) per ml. Dilute the biotinylated antibody in TBS–0.05% Tween 20–5 mM CaCl$_2$–0.01% heat-aggregated human IgG–0.01% (vol/vol) bovine serum. Use 100 μl/well, and incubate the plates for 1 to 2 h at 20°C in a moist chamber. Wash the wells three times with *washing buffer*.

5. Develop with streptavidin-Eu^{3+} by diluting streptavidin-Eu^{3+} appropriately in TBS–0.05% Tween 20–25 μM EDTA, and incubate the plates for 1 to 2 h at 20°C in a moist chamber. After incubation, wash the plates three times in TBS–0.05% Tween 20–5 mM CaCl$_2$.

6. Read the plate on a DELFIA fluorometer after you have added 200 μl of enhancement solution per well and shaken the plate for 5 min before reading.

COMMENTARY

Quantification of MBL

The quantification of MBL based on the described antigen assay and lectin assay is highly reproducible. It is advisable to include internal standards as controls in each assay. We usually use samples of plasma with known high (e.g., 1,586 ng of MBL/ml), medium (e.g., 224 ng of MBL/ml) and low (e.g., 17 ng of MBL/ml) MBL concentrations. We also include fivefold dilutions of standard plasma for the calibration curve. We have calculated the interassay coefficients of variation for the lectin assay to be 15, 9, and 12%, respectively, for high-, medium-, and low-MBL concentration internal standards, whereas for the antigen assay the the interassay coefficients of variation are 8, 8, and 11%, respectively.

The possible influence of rheumatoid factor, which may bind to IgG-coated wells and increase the background of the assay by cross-linking the capture and development antibodies, is eliminated by the inclusion of heat-aggregated IgG in the relevant buffer.

Note that at least three commercially available MBL antigen quantification assays exist, e.g., from HyCult Biotechnology, Uden, The Netherlands; Immunolex; and Dobeel Corp., Seoul, Korea.

MBL levels in plasma vary between 0 and 5 μg/ml (Fig. 1A). The MBL deficiency, often defined as circulating MBL levels below 100 ng/ml, is a common complement deficiency (Fig. 1C). In Caucasians, the frequency of MBL deficiency is between 5 and 10%. The level of MBL in the blood is influenced by single-nucleotide polymorphisms (SNPs) in the

MBL gene (*mbl2*) (28), e.g., in the promoter region (X or Y) and in exon 1 (B, C, and D; A is the wild type). The mutations in exon 1 lead to disruption of the Gly-Xaa-Yaa pattern of the collagen region. Such a disordered collagen helix appears to act like a dominant feature and results in decreased circulating levels of MBL. Due to linkage disequilibrium between the SNPs, seven distinct haplotypes exist in humans, four of which (YB, YC, YD, and XA) dictate low serum MBL levels (Fig. 1C) (13). Individuals with structural gene mutations have profoundly low levels of MBL, individuals heterozygous for the mutations have normal to low levels, and wild-type individuals have normal levels. The TRIFMAs, described here, yield data that correlate well with the MBL genotyping. Similar results may be obtained by ELISA (15).

MBL is a pattern recognition molecule which binds numerous bacteria, viruses, and fungi and activates the complement cascade. The MBL deficiency can be an important modulator in a disease setting or may by itself cause disease. A few examples of low MBL levels modulating disease progression are presented below. For a more extensive review, please see, e.g., reference 4. Pediatric patients with infections and with suspected immunodeficiencies have increased frequencies of MBL variant alleles (8, 25). Since patients with a suppressed cellular immune system, e.g., due to chemotherapy treatment, have higher numbers of infections and since some of those patients tend to suffer from uncommon bacterial infections, such patient groups have been studied for associations between infections and MBL levels. Bacteremia and pneumonia were associated with decreased MBL levels in chemotherapy-treated hematology patients (22), and a correlation between longer periods of fever and lower levels of MBL were noted among children with hematologic malignancies (18). Similarly, the presence of alleles giving rise to low MBL levels was found to be associated with bacterial, viral, and fungal infections in patients after treatment with myoablative bone marrow transplantation conditioning regimens (17).

Another group of patients whose immune system may be suppressed is critically ill patients admitted to the intensive care unit (ICU). Systemic inflammatory response syndrome (SIRS) may render the patients partly immunocompromised and may in some cases progress to sepsis and septic shock. When the frequencies of variant alleles in such patients were compared, it was concluded that higher levels of MBL may be important for avoiding sepsis and septic shock (6). Lower MBL levels were observed in the group of nonsurvivors than in those who survived admission to ICUs (9). Among the patients of the pediatric ICU, the MBL gene polymorphisms with low levels in serum were associated with a greatly increased risk of developing SIRS and of progression from infection to sepsis and septic shock (5).

Regarding MBL levels and viral infections, conflicting data on the associations with human immunodeficiency virus (HIV) infections have been published, showing either significantly more cases of MBL deficiency among HIV-infected patients (7, 19, 23) or a lack of correlation between MBL levels and susceptibility to HIV infection (10, 14). Regarding fungal infections, reduced levels of MBL were correlated with recurrent vaginal candidiases (1). MBL avidly binds *Aspergillus fumigatus*, and chronic necrotizing aspergillosis has been shown to be associated with polymorphisms of the MBL gene, as there was a significant increase in MBL-D allele carriers among the patient group (2).

Among systemic lupus erythematosus (SLE) patients, the presence of variant alleles is associated with increased disease activity and increased risk of infection, and homozygosity for

variant alleles increases the risk for arterial thrombosis in SLE patients (20).

MBL Pathway Activity Assay

The activity of the MBL pathway is measured by C4 deposition on mannan-coated wells (Fig. 2). The C4 deposition is triggered by the formation of active MBL-MASP complexes, which cleave C4 and lead to exposure of the internal thioester bond in the C4 molecule, followed by covalent deposition of C4 on the mannan. The classical pathway activity, which can also result in C4 activation, is inhibited by the high-ionic-strength buffer used in the assay, as the binding of C1q to immune complexes is inhibited and proteases C1r and C1s are eluted from C1 complex. The activation of C4 by MASP-2 is inhibited by the high ionic strength, and therefore the assay requires subsequent incubation with purified C4 in an isotonic buffer. Published evidence indicates that the MBL pathway activity determined with this assay reflects the activity of MASP-2 in the MBL-MASP complexes. The specific activity of the lectin pathway may be determined as the ratio of milliunits of MBL per milliliter, with a standard serum set to 1,000 mU/ml. If both the MBL levels and the MBL pathway activity are measured, the specific activity can be determined as a ratio of milliunits of MBL per microgram. The deposition of C4 correlates with the deposition of MBL (Fig. 2B). This is observed when plasma from individuals who are homozygous for the wild-type MBL allele A or plasma from individuals heterozygous for the MBL polymorphisms is tested for C4b deposition and MBL concentration (Fig. 2B). The only obvious deviation from the regression line appears when plasma from individual homozygotes for the structural mutations is tested.

Quantification of MASP-2 Assay

On the basis of the MASP-2 assay described above, the MASP-2 levels in 97 healthy Danish blood donors were determined (16). The MASP-2 levels ranged from 170 to 11,196 ng/ml, with a mean of 530 ng/ml. Unlike MBL deficiency, which is fairly common, the MASP-2 deficiency appears less frequent. A polymorphic structural variant of the MASP-2 gene was described for a patient with recurrent bacterial infections and SLE manifestation (24). The mutation led to diminished MASP-2 levels in circulation (Fig. 3B). Since MASP-2 forms complexes with ficolins, it is possible that the consequences of the MASP-2 deficiency will be more severe than those of the MBL deficiency. We recommend testing for MASP-2 deficiency in patients with recurrent bacterial infections, for whom the contribution of the MASP-2 deficiency to the susceptibility to infection may be crucial.

REFERENCES

1. Babula, O., G. Lazdane, J. Kroica, W. J. Ledger, and S. S. Witkin. 2003. Relation between recurrent vulvovaginal candidiasis, vaginal concentrations of mannose-binding lectin, and a mannose-binding lectin gene polymorphism in Latvian women. *Clin. Infect. Dis.* **37:**733–737.
2. Crosdale, D. J., K. V. Poulton, W. E. Ollier, W. Thomson, and D. W. Denning. 2001. Mannose-binding lectin gene polymorphisms as a susceptibility factor for chronic necrotizing pulmonary aspergillosis. *J. Infect. Dis.* **184:**653–656.
3. Dodds, A. W. 1993. Small-scale preparation of complement components C3 and C4. *Methods Enzymol.* **223:**46–61.

4. Eisen, D. P., and R. M. Minchinton. 2003. Impact of mannose-binding lectin on susceptibility to infectious diseases. *Clin. Infect. Dis.* **37:**1496–1505.

5. Fidler, K. J., P. Wilson, J. C. Davies, M. W. Turner, M. J. Peters, and N. J. Klein. 2004. Increased incidence and severity of the systemic inflammatory response syndrome in patients deficient in mannose-binding lectin. *Intensive Care Med.* **30:**1438–1445.

6. Garred, P., J. Strom, L. Quist, E. Taaning, and H. O. Madsen. 2003. Association of mannose-binding lectin polymorphisms with sepsis and fatal outcome, in patients with systemic inflammatory response syndrome. *J. Infect. Dis.* **188:**1394–1403.

7. Garred, P., H. O. Madsen, U. Balslev, B. Hofmann, C. Pedersen, J. Gerstoft, and A. Svejgaard. 1997. Susceptibility to HIV infection and progression of AIDS in relation to variant alleles of mannose-binding lectin. *Lancet* **349:**236–240.

8. Garred, P., H. O. Madsen, B. Hofmann, and A. Svejgaard. 1995. Increased frequency of homozygosity of abnormal mannan-binding-protein alleles in patients with suspected immunodeficiency. *Lancet* **346:**941–943.

9. Hansen, T. K., S. Thiel, P. J. Wouters, J. S. Christiansen, and G. Van den Berghe. 2003. Intensive insulin therapy exerts antiinflammatory effects in critically ill patients and counteracts the adverse effect of low mannose-binding lectin levels. *J. Clin. Endocrinol. Metab.* **88:**1082–1088.

10. Heggelund, L., T. E. Mollnes, T. Ueland, B. Christophersen, P. Aukrust, and S. S. Froland. 2003. Mannose-binding lectin in HIV infection: relation to disease progression and highly active antiretroviral therapy. *J. Acquir. Immune Defic. Syndr.* **32:**354–361.

11. Ikeda, K., T. Sannoh, N. Kawasaki, T. Kawasaki, and I. Yamashina. 1987. Serum lectin with known structure activates complement through the classical pathway. *J. Biol. Chem.* **262:**7451–7454.

12. Kuipers, S., P. C. Aerts, A. G. Sjoholm, T. Harmsen, and H. van Dijk. 2002. A hemolytic assay for the estimation of functional mannose-binding lectin levels in human serum. *J. Immunol. Methods* **268:**149–157.

13. Lipscombe, R. J., M. Sumiya, J. A. Summerfield, and M. W. Turner. 1995. Distinct physicochemical characteristics of human mannose binding protein expressed by individuals of differing genotype. *Immunology* **85:**660–667.

14. Malik, S., M. Arias, C. Di Flumeri, L. F. Garcia, and E. Schurr. 2003. Absence of association between mannose-binding lectin gene polymorphisms and HIV-1 infection in a Colombian population. *Immunogenetics* **55:**49–52.

15. Minchinton, R. M., M. M. Dean, T. R. Clark, S. Heatley, and C. G. Mullighan. 2002. Analysis of the relationship between mannose-binding lectin (MBL) genotype, MBL levels and function in an Australian blood donor population. *Scand. J. Immunol.* **56:**630–641.

16. Moller-Kristensen, M., J. C. Jensenius, L. Jensen, N. Thielens, V. Rossi, G. Arlaud, and S. Thiel. 2003. Levels of mannan-binding lectin-associated serine protease-2 in healthy individuals. *J. Immunol. Methods* **282:**159–167.

17. Mullighan, C. G., S. Heatley, K. Doherty, F. Szabo, A. Grigg, T. P. Hughes, A. P. Schwarer, J. Szer, B. D. Tait, L. B. To, and P. G. Bardy. 2002. Mannose-binding lectin gene polymorphisms are associated with major infection following allogeneic hemopoietic stem cell transplantation. *Blood* **99:**3524–3529.

18. Neth, O., I. Hann, M. W. Turner, and N. J. Klein. 2001. Deficiency of mannose-binding lectin and burden of infection in children with malignancy: a prospective study. *Lancet* **358:**614–618.

19. Nielsen, S. L., P. L. Andersen, C. Koch, J. C. Jensenius, and S. Thiel. 1995. The level of the serum opsonin, mannan-binding protein in HIV-1 antibody-positive patients. *Clin. Exp. Immunol.* **100:**219–222.

20. Ohlenschlaeger, T., P. Garred, H. O. Madsen, and S. Jacobsen. 2004. Mannose-binding lectin variant alleles and the risk of arterial thrombosis in systemic lupus erythematosus. *N. Engl. J. Med.* **351:**260–267.

21. Petersen, S. V., S. Thiel, L. Jensen, R. Steffensen, and J. C. Jensenius. 2001. An assay for the mannan-binding lectin pathway of complement activation. *J. Immunol. Methods* **257:**107–116.

22. Peterslund, N. A., C. Koch, J. C. Jensenius, and S. Thiel. 2001. Association between deficiency of mannose-binding lectin and severe infections after chemotherapy. *Lancet* **358:**637–638.

23. Senaldi, G., E. T. Davies, M. Mahalingam, J. Lu, A. Pozniak, M. Peakman, K. B. Reid, and D. Vergani. 1995. Circulating levels of mannose binding protein in human immunodeficiency virus infection. *J. Infect.* **31:**145–148.

24. Stengaard-Pedersen, K., S. Thiel, M. Gadjeva, M. Moller-Kristensen, R. Sorensen, L. T. Jensen, A. G. Sjoholm, L. Fugger, and J. C. Jensenius. 2003. Inherited deficiency of mannan-binding lectin-associated serine protease 2. *N. Engl. J. Med.* **349:**554–560.

25. Summerfield, J. A., S. Ryder, M. Sumiya, M. Thursz, A. Gorchein, M. A. Monteil, and M. W. Turner. 1995. Mannose binding protein gene mutations associated with unusual and severe infections in adults. *Lancet* **345:**886–889.

26. Super, M., R. J. Levinsky, and M. W. Turner. 1990. The level of mannan-binding protein regulates the binding of complement-derived opsonins to mannan and zymosan at low serum concentrations. *Clin. Exp. Immunol.* **79:**144–150.

27. Thiel, S., M. Moller-Kristensen, L. Jensen, and J. C. Jensenius. 2002. Assays for the functional activity of the mannan-binding lectin pathway of complement activation. *Immunobiology* **205:**446–454.

28. Turner, M. W. 2003. The role of mannose-binding lectin in health and disease. *Mol. Immunol.* **40:**423–429.

Complement in Transplant Rejection

WILLIAM M. BALDWIN III

16

Better reagents have led to an increased appreciation of the association between complement activation in transplants and poor outcome (7, 19). As diagnostic markers, products of complement activation have two attractive attributes related to the fact that activation of complement proceeds through a series of enzymatic steps resulting in multiple cleavage products. First, each enzymatic step is capable of amplifying the number of molecules that are cleaved. Second, the cleavage process reveals cryptic epitopes that allow the activated products to be distinguished from the unactivated precursors. In addition, activation products from two complement components, namely, C4 and C3, have the unusual property of covalently binding to protein and carbohydrate substrates. All of these properties distinguish complement activation products from some of the molecules that activate complement, such as antibodies. Antibodies themselves are not readily detected in tissue sections because only transient binding of a small number of antibodies to tissue is required to activate exponentially larger amounts of complement.

This chapter will examine the advantages and disadvantages of various reagents to complement as applied to the diagnosis of different types of rejection in transplants.

SELECTION AND INTERPRETATION OF DIAGNOSTIC REAGENTS TO COMPLEMENT IN ALLOTRANSPLANTS

Deposits of Complement in Tissue Biopsies

Examination of biopsies from organ transplants provides the most direct assessment of pathological processes jeopardizing the transplant. Stains for complement components in the organ transplant offer direct evidence of the location, distribution, and extent of complement activation at the site of injury. The different components of complement that have been used as markers of antibody-mediated rejection in transplants will be discussed in their order of activation by antibodies as shown in Fig. 1.

Polyclonal and Monoclonal Antibodies to C1q

The activation of complement by antibodies occurs primarily through the classical pathway. Because C1 is the first component of the classical pathway of complement activation, it has long been used as a marker of antibody activation of complement. Polyclonal and monoclonal antibodies to detect

C1q, the subcomponent of C1 that actually binds to antibodies, are available (Fig. 1). These are frequently applied in renal pathology and dermatopathology to detect immune complexes. There are several drawbacks to C1q as a marker of rejection, however. The most serious drawback relates to sensitivity. In order to bind, one C1q molecule requires at least a pair of immunoglobulin G (IgG) antibodies (Fig. 1A). This means that there are actually fewer C1q molecules than IgG molecules to detect. Moreover, the C1q molecules that are bound to antibodies depart when antibodies release from antigen or are shed from a cell surface (Fig. 1C).

In addition to sensitivity, there are theoretical problems of specificity. It is now clear that antibody is not the only ligand that is bound by C1q. C1q can also bind to phosphatidylcholine and sphingomyelin, which are exposed on plasma membranes of apoptotic or ischemic cells, or to the surface of virally infected cells. The presence of receptors for C1q on endothelial cells raises the possibility that immune complexes containing C1q could result in antigen-independent deposition of C1q on endothelium. However, these reactions are usually less diffuse, and in the case of immune complexes, the pattern is usually granular rather than linear.

As predicted by these theoretical considerations, C1q has not proved to be a sensitive marker of antibody-mediated rejection in practice.

Polyclonal and Monoclonal Antibodies to C4d

The tissue-bound split products of C4 are significantly more sensitive than C1q as a marker of antibody-mediated inflammation. Because each activated C1 molecule can enzymatically cleave many C4 molecules, more C4 split products are available to be detected. One study found that for each C1 molecule there were about 28 C4b fragments deposited on the cell membrane (16). The covalent binding of C4b and its further-split products to tissues results in extended half-lives (Fig. 1C). The result of greater quantities and longer half-lives is that C4b and its further-split product C4d are detected more easily than C1q or antibodies in biopsies. Another advantage that results from the enzymatic cleavage of C4 is that neo-epitopes are exposed on the split products. Monoclonal antibodies produced to these neoantigens are specific for the activated split product and not the intact precursor.

C4d, the final split product of C4, has been the most widely reported marker for humoral immune responses to

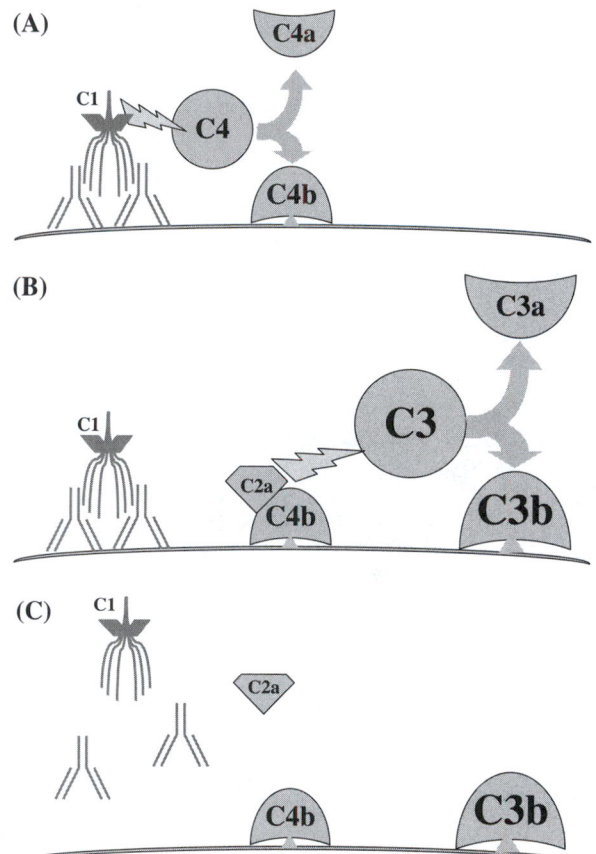

FIGURE 1 Activation of the early complement components by antibodies. (A) A pair of IgG antibodies is bound by C1 through the C1q subcomponent, and the enzymatic C1r and C1s subcomponents are activated to cleave C4 into C4a and C4b. C4b can bind covalently to a membrane protein and provide an anchor for C2, which is then cleaved. (B) The complex of C4bC2a enzymatically cleaves C3 into C3a and C3b. C3b is structurally homologous to C4b and can bind covalently to a membrane protein. (C) The covalently bound split products of C4 and C3 remain attached to the cell membrane after the antibody, C1, and C2a have dissociated from the membrane. (The sizes of the symbols for C4b and C3b are intended to reflect the potential for larger quantities of C3 than C4 activation products.)

transplants (7, 19). Therefore, the mechanism that produces C4d is worth reviewing. C4d represents the end product of a regulatory mechanism that evolved to prevent damage to autologous tissues during complement activation. The small C4d fragment results when factor I cleaves C4b twice, once on either side of the covalent bond. Factor I requires a cofactor, such as membrane cofactor protein (MCP) (CD46) or complement receptor 1 (CR1), to cleave C4b (Fig. 2). MCP is widely distributed on cells, including leukocytes and vascular endothelial cells. In contrast, CR1 is expressed on erythrocytes and leukocytes, including neutrophils and macrophages. The fluid-phase complement regulatory protein, C4-binding protein (C4bp), can also interact with cell-associated C4b and may also be found in regions of coagulation through its ability to bind to protein S. The rapid enzymatic cleavage of C4b by factor I makes C4d a more stable marker of complement activation than C4b. In fact, the monoclonal antibody used to detect C4d (Quidel, San Diego, Calif.)

actually detects an epitope expressed on C4b as well as C4d. As a result, both C4d and any remaining C4b are detected by this reagent.

The use of the monoclonal antibody to C4d has been limited to frozen tissue sections. This limitation has been circumvented by the development of a polyclonal antibody that can be used in formalin-fixed and paraffin-embedded tissues (available from Biomedica Gruppe, Vienna, Austria). The polyclonal antibody was produced by immunizing a rabbit with a synthetic 15-amino-acid peptide that coincides with a loop segment of C4d that is not shared by C3d (20). This reagent has proved to be very useful in biopsies for which no frozen tissue is available. However, detection of C4d in fixed tissues is less sensitive than in frozen sections. In addition, there are difficulties with high background and nonspecific staining of the edges of the biopsies ("edge effects").

The pattern and strength of staining are important for the interpretation of the results (Fig. 3). In biopsies from renal transplants, antibodies to major histocompatibility antigens (HLA in humans) or major blood group antigens are associated with diffuse, linear staining of the peritubular capillaries (7, 8, 13, 15, 19, 23). Arterial endothelial cells are variably involved. This pattern may reflect in part the distribution of both the target antigens and complement regulatory proteins. For example, class II major histocompatibility antigens, such as HLA-DR, are expressed constitutively on capillary and venous endothelium, but not arterial endothelium. However, HLA-DR

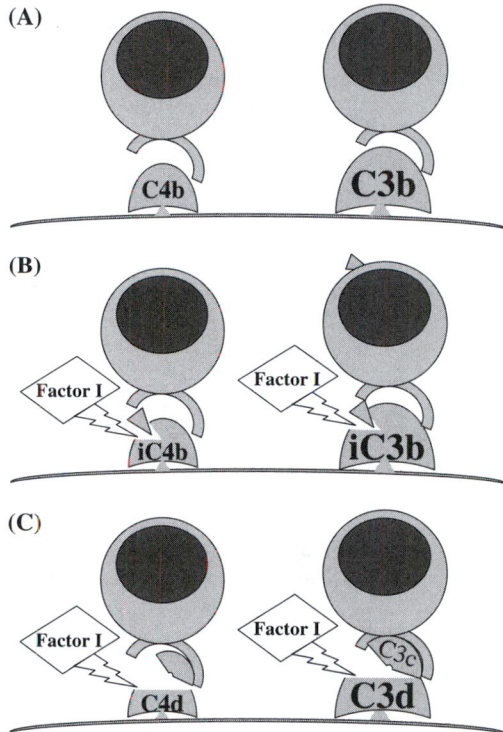

FIGURE 2 Regulation of C4b and C3b by circulating factor I and leukocytes expressing CR1. (A) CR1, which is expressed by leukocytes, associates with C4b or C3b, allowing factor I to cleave C4b and C3b. (B) The first enzymatic cleavage leaves iC4b or iC3b attached to the cell membrane. (C) Factor I then enzymatically cleaves iC4b or iC3b, and C4d and C3d remain covalently bound to the cell membrane. (As in Fig. 1, the sizes of the symbols for C4b and C3b are intended to reflect the potential for larger quantities of C3 than C4 activation products.)

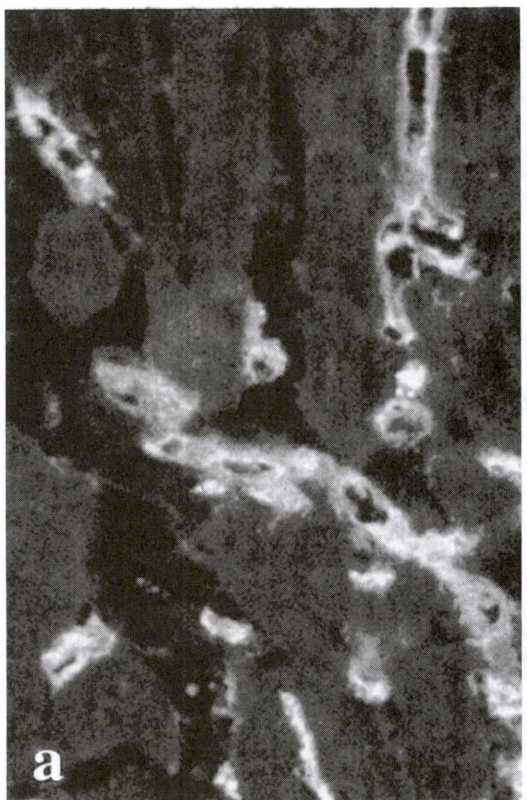

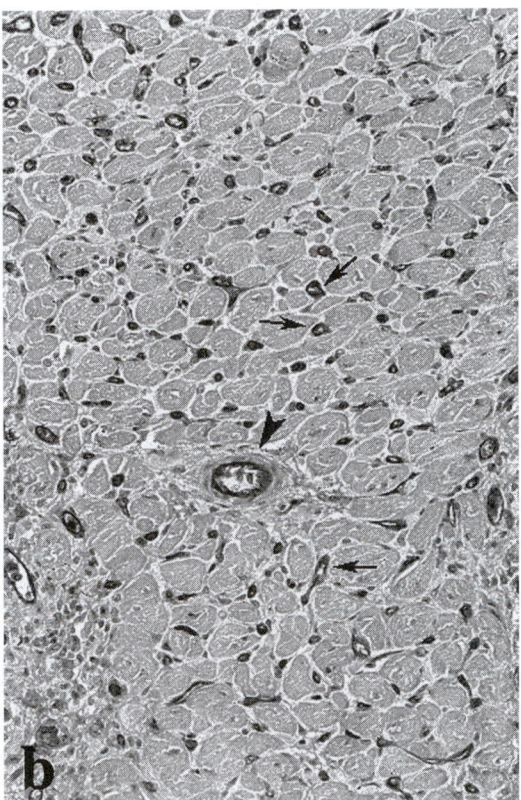

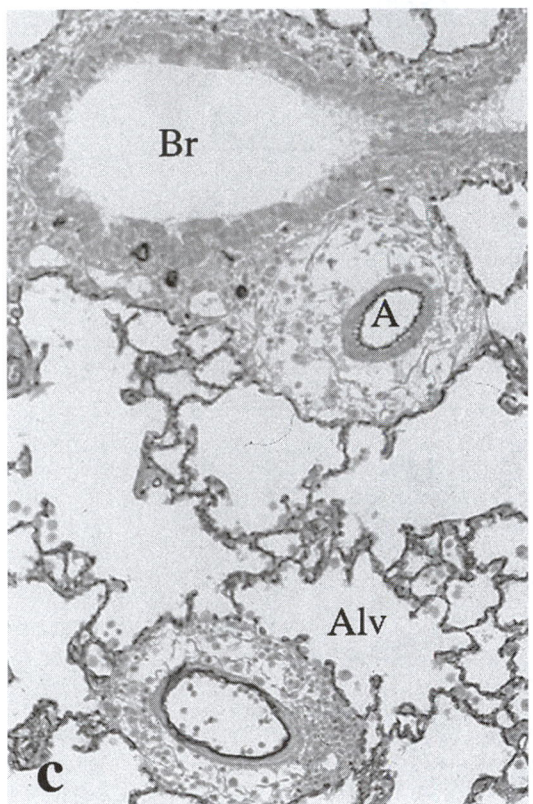

FIGURE 3 Examples of C4d and C3d deposition in organ transplants. (a) Immunofluorescent stain for C3d in an endomyocardial biopsy from a human heart transplant (magnification, ×64). The capillaries have diffuse linear staining. (b) Immunoperoxidase stain for C4d in an experimental cardiac allograft in a rat (magnification, ×16). C4d is deposited in an artery (arrowhead) as well as all of the capillaries (small arrows point to examples). (c) Immunoperoxidase stain for C4d in an experimental lung allograft in a rat (magnification, ×16). The alveolar (Alv) capillaries are stained, as are the endothelial cells of arteries (A), capillaries, and veins adjacent to the bronchiole (Br). (Fluorescein isothiocyanate signal appears white and immunoperoxidase signal appears black in these black-and-white photographs.)

antigens are upregulated by arterial endothelial cells as well as by tubular epithelial cells in sites of inflammation (15).

Fewer studies of C4d have been reported for other organ transplants. In cardiac transplants, antibody-mediated rejection is associated with strong linear staining of capillaries for C4d, but this staining pattern has also been found in patients without detectable antibodies to HLA or clinical evidence of cardiac dysfunction (1).

Although C4d is frequently proposed to be a specific marker for antibody-mediated activation of complement, C4 is also activated by mannose-binding lectin (MBL). MBL activates complement in the innate immune system by recognizing carbohydrate structures on pathogens, but it can also bind to plasma membranes of apoptotic or ischemic cells (9).

The most rigorous criteria for diagnosing antibody-mediated rejection do not rely exclusively on C4d as a marker. Rather, these criteria include three additional parameters: (i) detection of circulating antibodies to donor antigens, (ii) demonstration of marginated neutrophils or macrophages in the capillaries of the transplant, and (iii) correlation with clinical evidence of graft dysfunction (19).

Polyclonal and Monoclonal Antibodies to C3 Split Products

Because C3 and C4 are both members of the alpha 2-macroglobulin family (5), the activation and regulation of C3 produce split products that are homologous to C4 split products (Fig. 2). C3d is the final membrane-bound split product of the regulation of C3b by factor I and a cofactor such as factor H, CR1, or MCP. C3d has been compared to C4d as a marker of complement activation (1). Like C4d, C3d is covalently bound to tissues. Monoclonal antibodies to C3d are also specific for activated C3 because the epitope recognized is cryptic in uncleaved C3.

There are two major theoretical advantages of C3d as a marker for complement activation. The first is that quantitatively more C3 than C4 can be activated because there is more substrate available and there is an amplification loop that sustains C3 activation. About twice as much C3 as C4 is present normally in the circulation (1.3 and 0.6 mg/ml, respectively), and these levels can be doubled by increased hepatic production in response to acute-phase reactions. In inflammatory sites, macrophages can produce additional C4 and C3. Once C3 is activated by any mechanism, a large supply of C3 is available as a substrate for an amplification loop, in which C3b activates more C3 through factor B (see Fig. 1 in chapter 12).

The second advantage of C3d as a marker is that the split products of C3 have more biological activities than their C4 counterparts. C3b, iC3b, and C3d are the primary ligands for CR1, CR3, and CR2, respectively. Like CR1, CR3 is expressed on neutrophils, macrophages, and subsets of T lymphocytes. CR2 is part of a major second signaling pathway for antibody production by B lymphocytes. Although C4b is also a ligand for CR1, C4d does not bind CR2 (22). Therefore, the regulation steps for C4b that result in C4d deposition could terminate the complement cascade without activation of C3 or proinflammatory consequences. As a result, cases in which C4d is deposited in the absence of significant activation of C3 would be predicted to be associated with little or no complement-mediated injury (1, 18). In fact, this situation may account for the striking amounts of C4d found in well-functioning major-blood-group-incompatible renal transplants (8, 23). The capacity of renal transplants to function well in the presence of circulating antibodies has been termed "accommodation" (10). The demonstration that C4 is activated indicates that the circulating antibodies do bind to the transplant and initiate activation of complement. Therefore, C3d might be a particularly valuable marker in evaluating the progress of complement activation in blood group-incompatible renal transplants.

There are practical and theoretical reasons that C4d has been advocated as a better marker for antibody-mediated rejection than C3d. The practical advantage of C4d is that normal renal tissue contains less C4d than C3d. In healthy kidneys, C3d is found in the tubular basement membrane and mesangium, particularly in biopsies from older animals or humans. In spite of this extraneous staining, C3d has been found to be a useful marker in some studies of renal transplant biopsies (12). Although prominent staining of the media of arterioles for C3d occurs frequently in endomyocardial biopsies (1), this does not present a diagnostic problem.

The theoretical assertion that has been advanced for C4d as a marker for antibody-mediated responses is that it decreases false-positive reactions due to complement activation by the alternative pathway. However, in antibody-mediated immunity, the alternative pathway serves fundamentally as an amplification loop for the classical pathway, and this is one of the reasons that C3 split products can be deposited in larger amounts than C4 split products.

Polyclonal and monoclonal antibodies to other split products of C3 have also been applied in the diagnostic evaluation of tissue biopsies, but these reagents have disadvantages. The intermediate split product iC3b has the disadvantage of being short-lived. Moreover, iC3b may be more involved with down regulation of immune responses through its function as the primary ligand for CR3 on T lymphocytes as well as macrophages (reviewed in reference 10).

The use of antibodies to C3c offers even fewer advantages because C3c is the portion of iC3b that is cleaved away to produce C3d (Fig. 2C). As such, C3c does not remain bound to the membrane after being cleaved.

Polyclonal and Monoclonal Antibodies to C5b-9

The terminal five components of complement attach to each other in succession to form the membrane attack complex (MAC), which increases cell permeability. Polyclonal and monoclonal antibodies to neoantigens that are created as the complex is formed have been produced. MAC should be the best indicator that enough complement has been activated to exceed the multiple regulatory proteins capable of truncating the complement cascade after C4 or C3 activation. With currently available reagents, however, MAC has proven to be an insensitive indicator (2). This lack of sensitivity is probably related to the fact that MAC is deposited in limited quantities and sublytic amounts of MAC can be cleared rapidly from cell membranes. Regulatory proteins, such as CD59, limit the assembly of MAC on the surface of endothelial cells. Clearance of sublytic amounts of MAC occurs through an endocytic and exocytic response that removes the segments of membrane containing MAC.

Quality Control of Complement Assays Related to Tissue Biopsies

Quality controls have to be performed on the tissue substrate as well as on the reagents and methods used for the detection of complement. The extremely small tissue samples that are obtained from transplants by percutaneous needle biopsy procedures or biotomes on catheters can be inadequate, quantitatively or qualitatively. The biopsies may provide inadequate amounts of parenchyma or may contain tissue damaged during procurement. Hematoxylin and eosin stains of adjacent tissue sections are useful to control for the quality of the tissue. The use of isotype-matched control antibodies is helpful to determine artifactual staining due to crushed tissue or edge effect. The small size of the transplant biopsies precludes their use as routine controls for the quality or dilution profiles of reagents. Larger specimens from kidneys with deposits of immune complexes can be used to establish optimal dilutions for the primary and secondary antibodies. For this purpose, renal specimens from patients with systemic lupus erythematosis can be useful as positive controls.

Soluble Products of Complement Activation in Serum, Urine, or Bronchoalveolar Lavage Specimens

Activation of the complement cascade produces many split products that do not bind to tissues or that are released from tissues. These fluid-phase products can be detected in plasma, serum, urine, and bronchoalveolar lavage samples. Enzyme-linked immunosorbent assay kits are available to quantitate soluble split products in fluids (Quidel, San Diego, Calif.). C3a, C3c, soluble C4d (sC4d), sC3d, and soluble C5b-8 or -9 (sC5b-8 or -9) are among the most frequently measured soluble complement products. C4a, C3a, and C5a are fluid-phase reactants that are produced by the enzymatic activation of C4, C3, and C5, respectively (Fig. 1B). Regulation of C3b by factor I produces the soluble split product C3c (Fig. 2C). Excess C4b and C3b that fail to bind to protein are hydrolyzed and can be the source of soluble split products, such as sC4d and sC3d. Activation through the amplification loop of the alternative pathway results in the presence of Bb in the plasma. Finally, various forms of MAC that fail to insert into plasma membranes can be detected as sC5b-8 or -9.

Plasma

Diagnostic tests that require only blood samples are appealing because they are much less invasive than biopsies from organ transplants. Theoretically, this approach might also circumvent the sampling error inherent in taking minute pieces of tissue from organs, in which the rejection process may not be diffuse. Finally, avoiding repeated trauma to the transplant could reduce nonspecific inflammation in the organ.

The major disadvantage of testing plasma is the lack of specificity. Many confounding variables can alter the levels of markers in the circulation. In the first decades after transplantation became a successful therapeutic modality, elevated levels of complement split products were detected in the serum as the result of infection as well as rejection (6). More recent studies have confirmed this finding. One study of patients with renal transplants identified C4b, C4d, C3b, and C3d bound to C-reactive protein in the first days after transplantation (26).

Testing of serum can lead to even more sources of artifact. Coagulation enzymes can cleave C3, C4, and C5 and generate excess fragments in a relatively unpredictable fashion (24). Moreover, ex vivo activation of complement occurs frequently in samples containing immune complexes, certain drugs, or other contaminants. This is especially true of cryoglobulins that are barely detectable by other methods. Therefore, it is recommended that samples be collected as EDTA-plasma and frozen as soon after centrifugation as possible.

Urine

Urine provides a sample that reflects the inflammatory events in renal transplants more directly. Several reports have indicated that elevated levels of soluble complement split products can be detected in the urine during rejection episodes (2). Obviously, these assays cannot be applied during periods of anuria or oligurea, such as when there is delayed graft function after transplantation. Nonetheless, this is an approach that deserves further investigation.

Bronchoalveolar Lavage

Currently, most lung transplants are evaluated by periodic bronchoscopic exams that include an infusion and retrieval of saline referred to as bronchoalveolar lavage. This procedure is invasive, but the sample is focused on the most susceptible tissue in the transplanted lung. Elevated levels of split products of complement are found during rejection (14). However, the appropriate method of accounting for effects of dilution has not been established (4).

TYPES OF COMPLEMENT-MEDIATED INJURY IN ALLOTRANSPLANTS

Hyperacute Rejection

Hyperacute rejection is the most unambiguous example of complement-mediated injury to transplants. This type of rejection was first recognized in renal transplants by three groups of investigators between 1966 and 1969 (11, 17, 25). This devastatingly rapid type of rejection occurs within minutes to hours after blood flow is restored to the grafted kidney. Immunohistological studies demonstrated that antibodies and complement components were deposited in the transplant. Consequently, hyperacute rejection was quickly attributed to the action of antibodies and complement.

After early reports established a link between antibodies and hyperacute rejection, a "crossmatch test" was devised by Patel and Terasaki to test for the offending antibodies (17). The screening method consisted of mixing leukocytes from the prospective donor with serum from the prospective recipient and then adding a source of complement to demonstrate lysis. After the institution of this test, hyperacute rejection of allografts was almost eliminated.

In hyperacute rejection, complement activation is initiated by large amounts of antibody binding to antigens on the endothelial cells of the transplanted organ. The most characteristic features of hyperacute rejection can be predicted from our knowledge of complement. Prominent inflammatory manifestations of complement activation in hyperacute rejection include (i) recruitment and activation of numerous neutrophils, (ii) disruption of vascular integrity resulting in edema and hemorrhage, and (iii) activation of coagulation leading to fibrin deposition and thrombosis. The relative intensities of these features depend upon the quantities and qualities of the antibodies and their target antigens. Both antibodies to major histocompatibility complex antigens (HLA in humans) and antibodies to the major blood group antigens (A and B) can cause hyperacute rejection because these antigens are expressed in high concentrations on vascular endothelial cells.

Acute Rejection

Until recently, acute rejection was often cited as an example of pure cell-mediated immunity. This classification was based largely on experimental animal studies, but the vast majority of experimental transplants are performed with young, healthy (even pathogen-free) donor and recipient animals. Unless specifically under study, previous surgical interventions, blood transfusions, trauma, and prolonged ischemia are all avoided or introduced under highly controlled and isolated circumstances. Unfortunately, in clinical transplantation, the recipient by definition is suffering from the final stages of organ failure, and the organ most often comes from a donor who has died from a traumatic injury. Therefore, the recipient has frequently undergone previous surgical interventions or blood transfusions, the donor has experienced major trauma, and the organ has been subjected to ischemia. All of these variables can affect the function and survival of transplants adversely by increasing the initial recognition of the transplanted organ through complement-mediated processes. More recent animal experiments have provided evidence to support the clinical observations that complement contributes to the rejection process (1, 21).

Antibodies to major histocompatibility complex antigens can be elicited by previous blood transfusions, pregnancies, or transplants. If this sensitization is below the threshold of the crossmatch test used, then hyperacute rejection may be avoided, but the risk of antibody-mediated rejection is increased. Sensitization from previous pregnancies is especially pertinent when a kidney is transplanted to a wife from her husband or to a mother from her child. In these cases, complement deposition can be a prominent feature of the rejection process (3). Obviously, the incidence of antibody-mediated immunity will be related to the composition of the population of patients selected for transplantation. In some studies, a majority of the "steroid-resistant" acute rejections may have an antibody-mediated component (13). These acute rejection episodes often occur within the first weeks or months after transplantation in presensitized patients. In unsensitized patients, acute rejection episodes can occur years after transplantation (1, 15).

Chronic Rejection

Chronic loss of graft function is not due solely to immune causes. Instead, the chronic lesions in organ allografts represent repair and remodeling processes that are the final common response to many types of tissue injury. For example, the proliferative vascular lesions that characterize chronic dysfunction of renal and cardiac allografts have some similarities to ordinary arteriosclerosis. The vascular lesions in transplants are generally more extensive and uniform in distribution than in ordinary arteriosclerosis, but this may just represent the more widespread injury of the immunologically incompatible tissue. Both types of vascular lesions are currently thought to involve inflammatory processes.

The use of C4d and C3d as markers for diagnosis or prognosis of chronic graft dysfunction is under investigation. It is evident already that these markers are not as closely associated with chronic pathology in transplants. This is not unexpected, because the events that initiate chronic repair and remodeling may be resolved and even the covalently bound complement split products can be cleared from the membrane of endothelial cells before the repair processes impair organ function.

SUMMARY

Complement can be a useful adjunct in diagnosing and directing treatment of transplant rejection. Currently, the tissue-associated final split products of C4b and C3b, namely, C4d and C3d, are the most useful markers of antibody-mediated rejection. Both C4d and C3d offer the advantages of being produced in large amounts and binding covalently to tissues. Monoclonal antibodies to neoantigens on C4d and C3d that are not accessible in the unactivated precursors are available. Although these markers have provided significant diagnostic advances for organ transplantation, appropriate interpretation

requires additional information, including testing for circulating antibodies to donor antigens and correlation with clinical evidence of graft dysfunction.

I am supported by National Institutes of Health grants R01-AI42387 and P01-HL56091.

REFERENCES

1. **Baldwin, W. M., III, E. K. Kasper, A. A. Zachary, B. A. Wasowska, and E. R. Rodriguez.** 2004. Beyond C4d: other complement related diagnostic approaches to antibody-mediated rejection. *Am. J. Transplant.* **4:**311–318.
2. **Bechtel, U., R. Scheuer, R. Landgraf, A. Konig, and H. E. Feucht.** 1994. Assessment of soluble adhesion molecules (sICAM-1, sVCAM-1, sELAM-1) and complement cleavage products (sC4d, sC5b-9) in urine. *Transplantation* **58:**905–911.
3. **Bohmig, G. A., H. Regele, M. D. Saemann, M. Exner, W. Druml, J. Kovarik, W. H. Horl, G. J. Zlabinger, and B. Watschinger.** 2000. Role of humoral immune reactions as target for antirejection therapy in recipients of a spousal-donor kidney graft. *Am. J. Kidney Dis.* **35:**667–673.
4. **Dargaville, P. A., M. South, P. Vervaart, and P. N. McDougall.** 1999. Validity of markers of dilution in small volume lung lavage. *Am. J. Respir. Crit. Care Med.* **160:**778–784.
5. **Dodds, A. W., and S. K. Law.** 1998. The phylogeny and evolution of the thioester bond-containing proteins C3, C4 and alpha 2-macroglobulin. *Immunol. Rev.* **166:**15–26.
6. **Fearon, D. T., M. R. Daha, T. B. Strom, J. M. Weiler, C. B. Carpenter, and K. F. Austen.** 1977. Pathways of complement activation in membranoproliferative glomerulonephritis and allograft rejection. *Transplant. Proc.* **9:**729–739.
7. **Feucht, H. E.** 2003. Complement C4d in graft capillaries—the missing link in the recognition of humoral alloreactivity. *Am. J. Transplant.* **3:**646–652.
8. **Fidler, M. E., J. M. Gloor, D. J. Lager, T. S. Larson, M. D. Griffin, S. C. Textor, T. R. Schwab, M. Prieto, S. L. Nyberg, M. B. Ishitani, J. P. Grande, P. A. Kay, and M. D. Stegall.** 2004. Histologic findings of antibody-mediated rejection in ABO blood-group-incompatible living-donor kidney transplantation. *Am. J. Transplant.* **4:**101–107.
9. **Jordan, J. E., M. C. Montalto, and G. L. Stahl.** 2001. Inhibition of mannose-binding lectin reduces postischemic myocardial reperfusion injury. *Circulation* **104:**1413–1418.
10. **King, K. E., D. S. Warren, M. Samaniego-Picota, S. Campbell-Lee, R. A. Montgomery, and W. M. Baldwin III.** 2004. Antibody, complement and accommodation in ABO-incompatible transplants. *Curr. Opin. Immunol.* **16:**545–549.
11. **Kissmeyer-Nielsen, F., S. Olsen, V. P. Petersen, and O. Fjeldborg.** 1966. Hyperacute rejection of kidney allografts associated with pre-existing humoral antibodies against donor cells. *Lancet* **ii:**662–665.
12. **Kuypers, D. R., E. Lerut, P. Evenepoel, B. Maes, Y. Vanrenterghem, and B. Van Damme.** 2003. C3D deposition in peritubular capillaries indicates a variant of acute renal allograft rejection characterized by a worse clinical outcome. *Transplantation* **76:**102–108.
13. **Mauiyyedi, S., and R. B. Colvin.** 2002. Humoral rejection in kidney transplantation: new concepts in diagnosis and treatment. *Curr. Opin. Nephrol. Hypertens.* **11:**609–618.
14. **Miller, G. G., L. Destarac, A. Zeevi, A. Girnita, K. McCurry, A. Iacono, J. J. Murray, D. Crowe, J. E. Johnson, M. Ninan, and A. P. Milstone.** 2004. Acute humoral rejection of human lung allografts and elevation of C4d in bronchoalveolar lavage fluid. *Am. J. Transplant.* **4:**1323–1330.

15. Nickeleit, V., and M. J. Mihatsch. 2003. Kidney transplants, antibodies and rejection: is C4d a magic marker? *Nephrol. Dial. Transplant.* **18:**2232–2239.

16. Ollert, M. W., J. V. Kadlec, K. David, E. C. Petrella, R. Bredehorst, and C. W. Vogel. 1994. Antibody-mediated complement activation on nucleated cells. A quantitative analysis of the individual reaction steps. *J. Immunol.* **153:**2213–2221.

17. Patel, R., and P. I. Terasaki. 1969. Significance of the positive crossmatch test in kidney transplantation. *N. Engl. J. Med.* **280:**735–739.

18. Platt, J. L. 2002. C4d and the fate of organ allografts. *J. Am. Soc. Nephrol.* **13:**2417–2419.

19. Racusen, L. C., R. B. Colvin, K. Solez, M. J. Mihatsch, P. F. Halloran, P. M. Campbell, M. J. Cecka, J. P. Cosyns, A. J. Demetris, M. C. Fishbein, A. Fogo, P. Furness, I. W. Gibson, D. Glotz, P. Hayry, L. Hunsickern, M. Kashgarian, R. Kerman, A. J. Magil, R. Montgomery, K. Morozumi, V. Nickeleit, P. Randhawa, H. Regele, D. Seron, S. Seshan, S. Sund, and K. Trpkov. 2003. Antibody-mediated rejection criteria—an addition to the banff 97 classification of renal allograft rejection. *Am. J. Transplant.* **3:**708–714.

20. Regele, H., M. Exner, B. Watschinger, C. Wenter, M. Wahrmann, C. Osterreicher, M. D. Saemann, N. Mersich, W. H. Horl, G. J. Zlabinger, and G. A. Bohmig. 2001. Endothelial C4d deposition is associated with inferior kidney allograft outcome independently of cellular rejection. *Nephrol. Dial. Transplant.* **16:**2058–2066.

21. Sacks, S. H., P. Chowdhury, and W. Zhou. 2003. Role of the complement system in rejection. *Curr. Opin. Immunol.* **15:**487–492.

22. van den Elsen, J. M., A. Martin, V. Wong, L. Clemenza, D. R. Rose, and D. E. Isenman. 2002. X-ray crystal structure of the C4d fragment of human complement component C4. *J. Mol. Biol.* **322:**1103–1115.

23. Warren, D. S., A. A. Zachary, C. J. Sonnenday, K. E. King, M. Cooper, L. E. Ratner, R. S. Shirey, M. Haas, M. S. Leffell, and R. A. Montgomery. 2004. Successful renal transplantation across simultaneous ABO incompatible and positive crossmatch barriers. *Am. J. Transplant.* **4:**561–568.

24. Wiggins, R. C., P. C. Giclas, and P. M. Henson. 1981. Chemotactic activity generated from the fifth component of complement by plasma kallikrein of the rabbit. *J. Exp. Med.* **153:**1391–1404.

25. Williams, G. M., D. M. Hume, R. P. Hudson, Jr., P. Morris, K. Kano, and F. Milgrom. 1968. "Hyperacute" renal-homograft rejection in man. *N. Engl. J. Med.* **279:**611–618.

26. Wolbink, G. J., M. C. Brouwer, S. Buysmann, I. J. ten Berge, and C. E. Hack. 1996. CRP-mediated activation of complement in vivo: assessment by measuring circulating complement–C-reactive protein complexes. *J. Immunol.* **157:**473–479.

FLOW CYTOMETRY

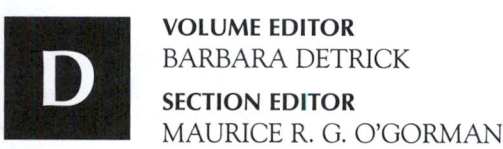

VOLUME EDITOR
BARBARA DETRICK
SECTION EDITOR
MAURICE R. G. O'GORMAN

Introduction

MAURICE R. G. O'GORMAN

Since the last edition of the *Manual of Clinical Laboratory Immunology* (6th edition, 2002), clinical flow cytometry has grown and evolved significantly in three general areas: (i) established flow cytometry applications have improved in their efficiency and proficiency; (ii) new applications have been developed and adopted; and (iii) a whole new field of molecular-based flow cytometry applications has emerged and several applications are rapidly evolving towards use in the clinical and diagnostic laboratories. In an effort to capture the burgeoning field of clinical flow cytometry, the chapters presented here are divided into two sections. The first is current application, which encompasses updates in established procedures as well as new procedures that have been recently adopted. The second section is more innovative, with applications combining molecular methodologies and flow cytometry. Below is a brief summary of the chapters in this section as well as a quick review of clinical flow cytometry applications that were not addressed in this edition of the *Manual*.

FLOW CYTOMETRY

The opening chapter in this section, compiled by Lance and Patricia Hultin, provides a general introduction to clinical flow cytometry as well as up-to-date information on reagents, instrumentation, safety, quality control, and the procedures utilized for measurement of absolute T-lymphocyte subsets in human immunodeficiency virus (HIV)-infected patients. Instrument and reagent quality control, single-platform absolute counting, and novel markers in HIV infection are a few of the areas addressed. The next chapter, by Jiachun Kung and Eric Hsi, describes new "nontraditional" clinical flow procedures that have been developed for the diagnosis of paroxysmal nocturnal hemoglobinuria and the assessment of circulating fetal red cells, T-cell receptor Vβ repertoire, and various platelet markers. The chapter on immunophenotyping of leukemia and lymphoma, written by Brent Wood, provides detailed information required to perform multicolor immunophenotyping, descriptions of normal and abnormal expression of surface markers, lists of antibodies used in the diagnosis of leukemia and lymphoma, and histograms exemplifying the specific principles and practices reviewed in the chapter.

Stem cell transplant is no longer a rare procedure performed only at highly specialized institutions. With the advent of cord blood banking, new safer stem cell transplant protocols, and numerous new clinical trials, accurate enumeration of stem cells in a variety of products has become an essential procedure for an increasing number of institutions. Robert Sutherland and coauthors complete the current clinical applications with an up-to-date review of the standards for the enumeration of hematopoietic stem cells.

The second part of this section presents new and emerging techniques in flow cytometry. The chapter by Elisabeth Paietta reviews the status of currently recognized phenotypic correlates of genetic abnormalities in leukemia and lymphoma. The recognition of specific phenotypic patterns that correlate with genetic abnormalities ultimately improves both the accuracy and speed of diagnosis. The development of reagents containing specific peptide antigen in the context of the antigen-presenting molecules has led to an entirely new tool for the measurement of antigen-specific lymphocytes. John Altman describes many of the practical details with respect to flow cytometric applications of tetramers for the detection of antigen-specific T cells. In addition to a general staining protocol, sample and instrument requirements, reagent availability, reagent providers, etc., this chapter presents the reader with a comprehensive introduction to this rapidly emerging application. In the last chapter, Bruce Patterson provides the background, technology, and clinical applications of several promising new procedures that combine molecular biology technologies (for the detection of specific targets) and flow cytometry (for the specific detection of the cell population harboring the target). This area is currently practiced by only a few highly specialized laboratories but has significant potential as the individual applications are validated and the process becomes more standardized.

OTHER APPLICATIONS

As part of this introduction, I would like to review briefly two applications that are currently being performed in clinical flow cytometry laboratories but, due to space limitations, were not covered in specific chapters in this volume.

Flow Cytometry for the Diagnosis of X-Linked Hyper IgM Syndrome

The X-linked hyper immunoglobulin M (IgM) syndrome is a combined immune deficiency resulting from mutations in the genes encoding the CD40 ligand (CD154). Clinically, the disease presents with infections usually associated with humoral immune deficiency, although there is some evidence of cellular immune deficiency, as most patients suffer from pneumonia caused by *Pneumocystis carinii*. The CD40 ligand is expressed primarily on activated CD4-positive T cells and is responsible for inducing immunoglobulin class switching in B lymphocytes from IgM to IgG, IgA, and IgE. Patients' immunoglobulin levels often reveal elevated IgM with very low to absent detection of all other immunoglobulin classes.

A diagnostic flow cytometry screening test has been developed for the rapid detection of CD40 ligand expression abnormalities (9). Briefly, whole blood is stimulated with a phorbol ester and a calcium ionophore (the up-regulation of CD40 ligand is strongly dependent on calcium) for 4 h, after which the sample is labeled with a cocktail of monoclonal

antibodies to detect T-helper cells (CD3 and CD8) using a negative gating strategy. (Since the CD4 molecule is modulated off of the cell surface with this stimulation protocol, the CD4$^+$ T cells are analyzed by setting the gate around the CD3$^+$CD8$^-$ population.) The level of expression of CD40 ligand on the activated T cells is then assessed. This assay has been used routinely in our laboratory for the diagnosis of hyper IgM patients (see Fig. 1), to investigate CD40 ligand expression in HIV-infected children (8), and to assess functional immune reconstitution following bone marrow transplant (7) of hyper IgM patients (Fig. 2).

Flow Cytometry Applications in Allergy

Currently, the most commonly utilized laboratory methods for laboratory diagnosis of allergy involve the detection of allergen-specific IgE. Although the latter test methods have become very popular (and many have been cleared by the

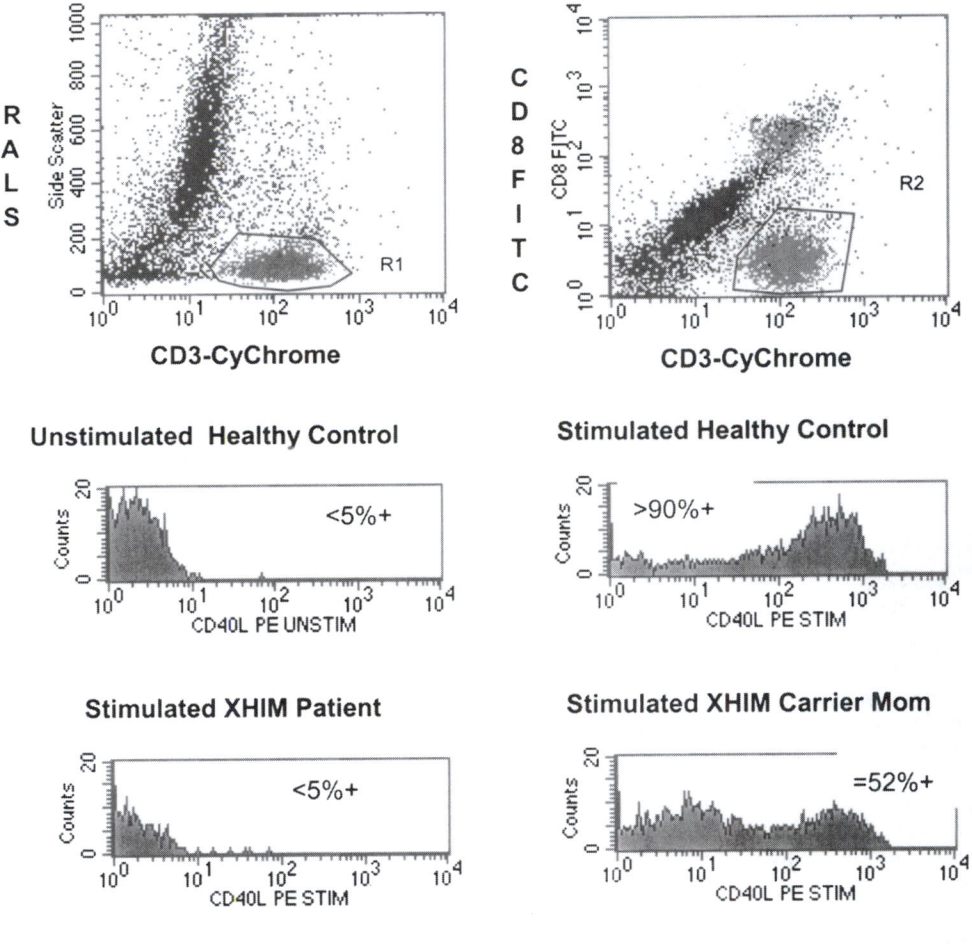

FIGURE 1 Measurement of CD40 expression on CD4$^+$ T cells. CD4$^+$ T cells are gated indirectly by first gating (R1) on CD3$^+$ T cells (in the histogram of right-angle light scatter [RALS] versus CD3 and then gating (R2) on CD3$^+$CD8$^-$ T cells. The level of expression of CD40 ligand is then measured on the events that satisfy both of these gates (R1 and R2) as percent positive (number of events expressing fluorescence above an isotype control antibody). Shown below are the results on CD40 ligand expression levels of resting CD4$^+$ T cells in whole blood from a healthy control and on vitro-activated CD4$^+$ T cells in whole blood obtained from a healthy control, a patient diagnosed with the hyper IgM (XHIM) syndrome, and an XHIM carrier mother as labeled above.

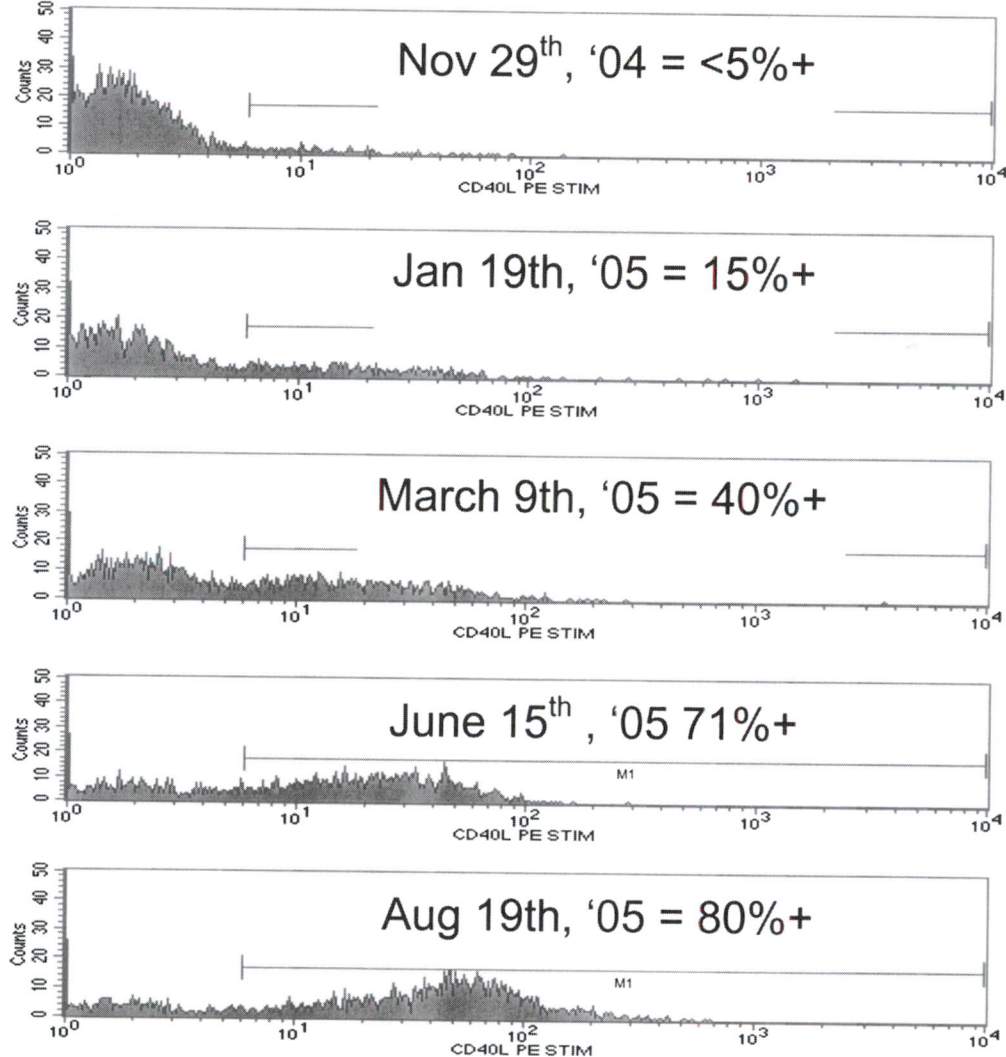

FIGURE 2 CD40 ligand expression on CD4+ T cells, illustrating functional immune reconstitution in an XHIM patient transplanted with peripheral blood stem cells from an HLA identical donor sibling. Transplant date was 14 October 2004. Gating was performed as illustrated in Fig. 1.

U.S. Food and Drug Administration for in vitro diagnostic use), they do not indicate a functional relationship between allergen and disease. The skin test remains the "gold standard" for the detection of a functional allergic response; however, flow cytometry, specifically the assessment of basophil activation markers, is rapidly emerging as a viable alternative. The basis of the procedure is very simple. If basophils are sensitized in vivo with allergen-specific IgE, exposure to the allergen in vitro will initiate basophil degranulation (activation) which can be assessed by the increased expression of either CD63 or CD203c on the cell surface. Numerous publications have documented the validity of these methods (1) as well as their utility in the detection of latex allergy, insect venoms, local foods, and pollens (2–6, 10). The availability of a kit (Orpegen, Heidelberg, Germany) that includes buffers, the appropriate antibodies, and a mixture of grass pollens and food allergens has provided a platform for several laboratories to develop additional allergen-specific tests. The method is relatively simple. Briefly: whole blood is incubated for a specified amount of time with the allergen(s) of interest

as well as a negative control (buffer only). The activation process is stopped by completing the remainder of the procedure on ice. Whole blood is labeled with CD63 (activation marker) and anti-IgE (used to detect basophils). Another marker that has been utilized by several investigators due to its more restricted circulating leukocyte expression (on basophils only) is CD203c. This marker is constitutively expressed, and its level is increased upon activation of the basophils. Ronald Harbeck of the National Jewish Center in Denver, Colo. (personal communication), has recently exploited this phenomenon to detect functional antibody in patients with idiopathic chronic urticaria. Some (approximately 40%) patients with a diagnosis of chronic urticaria have a circulating antibody (IgG) which reacts with the high-affinity IgE receptor (or the IgE molecule) expressed on mast cells and basophils. Detection of this antibody has traditionally been via the autologous serum skin test (injection of the patient's serum causes a characteristic wheal and flare response) or the histamine release assay. In Harbeck's laboratory, patient serum is incubated with appropriate donor basophils, and the change in cell surface CD203c expression is assessed relative to negative (buffer only), strong positive (anti-Fc$_\varepsilon$ receptor), and moderate positive (f-Met-Leu-Phe) controls. In chronic urticaria patients, up-regulation of basophil cell surface CD203c expression in this flow cytometry assay indicates a significant correlation with both the histamine release assay and the autologous serum skin test (presented in part at the 16th annual meeting of the Association of Medical Laboratory Immunology, Denver, Colo., 2005). Improved standardization of the allergens used for in vitro testing combined with improvements in the procedures will lead to an increased adoption of this testing modality in the near future.

Two other broad areas involving flow cytometry were not specifically addressed in this section. The use of flow cytometry in "array" testing, or so-called "multiplex" testing, is addressed in the chapter by Daniel Remick, "Multiplex Cytokine Assays" (chapter 39), where the advantages and technical aspects of multiplex testing by flow cytometry are elegantly covered. The other area not included in this section is DNA ploidy and cell cycle analyses. The excellent coverage of DNA content flow cytometry in the previous edition of the *Manual* and the lack of significant new developments in this field justified the omission of this subject from the present edition.

It was not long ago that the clinical flow cytometry community was worried that the emergence of quantitative viral loads in HIV would replace CD4 T-cell enumeration and lead to a decrease in clinical applications involving flow cytometry. This section should convince you that a decrease in clinical flow cytometry application was never realized. In fact, quite the opposite has developed, as several novel applications are being developed and are poised for adoption in clinical diagnostic laboratories.

REFERENCES

1. Boumiza, R., A. L. Debard, and G. Monneret. 2005. The basophil activation test by flow cytometry: recent developments in clinical studies, standardization and emerging perspectives. *Clin. Mol. Allergy* 3:9.

2. Eberlein-Konig, B., J. Rakoski, H. Behrendt, and J. Ring. 2004. Use of CD63 expression as marker of in vitro basophil activation in identifying the culprit in insect venom allergy. *J. Investig. Allergol. Clin. Immunol.* 14:10–16.

3. Erdmann, S. M., B. Sachs, A. Schmidt, H. F. Merk, O. Scheiner, S. Moll-Slodowy, I. Sauer, R. Kwiecien, B. Maderegger, and K. Hoffmann-Sommergruber. 2005. In vitro analysis of birch-pollen-associated food allergy by use of recombinant allergens in the basophil activation test. *Int. Arch. Allergy Immunol.* 136:230–238.

4. Erdmann, S. M., B. Sachs, R. Kwiecien, S. Moll-Slodowy, I. Sauer, and H. F. Merk. 2004. The basophil activation test in wasp venom allergy: sensitivity, specificity and monitoring specific immunotherapy. *Allergy* 59:1102–1109.

5. Gyimesi, E., S. Sipka, K. Danko, E. Kiss, B. Hidvegi, M. Gal, J. Hunyadi, B. Irinyi, and A. Szegedi. 2004. Basophil CD63 expression assay on highly sensitized atopic donor leucocytes—a useful method in chronic autoimmune urticaria. *Br. J. Dermatol.* 151:388–396.

6. Hemery, M. L., B. Arnoux, H. Dhivert-Donnadieu, M. Rongier, E. Barbotte, R. Verdier, and P. Demoly. 2005. Confirmation of the diagnosis of natural rubber latex allergy by the Basotest method. *Int. Arch. Allergy Immunol.* 136:53–57.

7. Jacobsohn, D. A., K. M. Emerick, P. Scholl, H. Melin-Aldana, M. O'Gorman, R. Duerst, and M. Kletzel. 2004. Non-myeloablative hematopoietic stem cell transplant for X-linked hyper-immunoglobulin M syndrome with cholangiopathy. *J. Pediatr.* 113:e122–127.

8. O'Gorman, M. R., B. DuChateau, M. Paniagua, J. Hunt, N. Bensen, and R. Yogev. 2001. Abnormal CD40 ligand (CD154) expression in human immunodeficiency virus-infected children. *Clin. Diagn. Lab. Immunol.* 8:1104–1109.

9. O'Gorman, M. R., D. Zaas, M. Paniagua, V. Corrochano, P. R. Scholl, and L. M. Pachman. 1997. Development of a rapid whole blood flow cytometry procedure for the diagnosis of X-linked hyper-IgM syndrome patients and carriers. *Clin. Immunol. Immunopathol.* 85:172–181.

10. Paris-Kohler, A., P. Demoly, L. Persi, B. Lebel, J. Bousquet, and B. Arnoux. 2000. In vitro diagnosis of cypress pollen allergy using cytofluorometric analysis of basophils (Basotest). *J. Allergy Clin. Immunol.* 105:339–345.

Flow Cytometry-Based Immunophenotyping Method and Applications

LANCE HULTIN AND PATRICIA HULTIN

18

The immunophenotype of a cell describes the collection of antigens expressed on or inside the cell. Flow cytometry is a very efficient immunophenotyping tool because it can measure multiple antigens simultaneously, rapidly providing accurate measures of the percentage of cells with a particular phenotype and the absolute number of these cells per volume of blood, and can be used to quantify the number of antigens on a per-cell basis. The reactivity of specific monoclonal antibodies (MAbs) to cell surface antigens is used to subtype leukocytes into distinct lineages and differentiation and activation states. There are numerous applications, including leukemia and lymphoma typing, enumerating CD34-positive stem cells, evaluating immune reconstitution, and monitoring cancer therapies and immunodeficiency diseases. These applications are discussed throughout this manual.

The field of human immunodeficiency virus (HIV) disease in particular has broadened our understanding of the immune system and has driven many of the improvements in immunophenotyping methods. HIV type 1 (HIV-1) infection causes a rapid, profound decrease in CD4 T-cell numbers and an expansion of CD8 T-cell levels during the first 12 to 18 months of HIV-1 disease (9, 27). Some donors continue to lose CD4 T cells rapidly and progress to AIDS, while others maintain relatively stable CD4 T-cell numbers and remain AIDS free for years. During this chronic phase of HIV-1 disease the decline in CD4 T-cell numbers can be slow: it can last more than 10 to 15 years. Homeostatic mechanisms maintain relatively stable T-cell numbers during this time. Prior to the development of AIDS, homeostatic mechanisms fail and there is further decline in CD4 T cells accompanied by a decline in CD8 T-cell numbers on average 2 years prior to the onset of AIDS (18). CD4 T-cell levels are used to stage HIV disease progression, are prognostic for the development of AIDS, and are used to monitor responses to antiretroviral therapy. Centers for Disease Control and Prevention (CDC) guidelines stage HIV-1 disease by CD4 T-cell level into three groups: >500 CD4 cells/mm^3, or >28% CD4 cells within lymphocytes; 200 to 500 CD4 cells/mm^3, or 14 to 28% CD4 cells; and <200 CD4 cells/mm^3, or <14% CD4 cells (3).

The goal of this chapter is to provide a broad description of the principles of flow cytometric immunophenotyping; to provide specific methods for lymphocyte enumeration, with particular emphasis on CD4 T-cell counting; and to review quality assurance issues that improve the accuracy and reproducibility of overall immunophenotyping results.

PRINCIPLES OF FLOW CYTOMETRY

A flow cytometer is an instrument that measures the scattered and fluorescent light derived from cells as they pass via a fluid stream through the intersection of a light source. The light source is typically a laser beam operating at one specific wavelength (e.g., 488 nm), suitable for exciting dye molecules. Scattered laser light characterizes the size and granularity of the cell, enabling the operator to distinguish the smaller, less granular lymphocytes from the other leukocytes found in whole blood. This process is called scatter gating. The fluorescent light is derived from dye molecules (fluorochromes) conjugated to MAbs that bind very specifically to cell surface antigens.

Samples for immunophenotyping are prepared by incubation with fluorochrome-labeled MAbs, and red blood cells are removed by lysis to prepare the sample for analysis on the flow cytometer. The cytometer draws up the cell suspension and injects the sample inside a carrier stream of isotonic saline solution to form a laminar flow. The sample stream is constrained by the carrier stream and thus hydrodynamically focused so that the cells pass single file through the intersection of the laser light source. For clinical flow cytometers, this process happens inside a flow cell or cuvette. At this time detectors collect the scattered and fluorescent light. The forward scatter (FSC) detector is placed in the direct path of the light source. Larger cells scatter more light than smaller cells. The remaining light is usually collected orthogonally (90°) from the light source (25). This side scatter (SSC) and fluorescent light is collected through a microscope objective (fluorescence collection lens) that focuses the light to the fluorescent detectors. Some newer systems use fiber optic cables to direct the light to these detectors. The collected light is passed through optical filters to direct specific wavelengths of light to the appropriate detectors. The filters are designed to maximize collection of light derived from a specific fluorochrome while minimizing collection of light from the other fluorochromes used to stain the cells. For example, a 530- ± 30-nm band-pass filter is used to collect the fluorescence emission of fluorescein isothiocyanate (FITC) and minimize contaminating light from phycoerythrin (PE), which has a maximum emission at 575 nm.

The detectors are photomultiplier tubes (PMT). When the fluorescence light reaches the PMT, it creates an electrical current that is converted to a voltage pulse. How the voltage pulse is processed from this point on varies depending on the manufacturer and the age of the instrument. Subsequently, the magnitude of the voltage output from the PMT is quantified and digitized for collection and storage by the computer system. It is important to note that the magnitude of voltage pulse is related not only to the amount of light reaching the PMT but also to the voltage setting of the PMT. The voltage setting of the PMT is a critical step of instrument setup, as discussed below. Clearly, if the sample stream is too wide, the flow cell is dirty, or the laser light source or collection lenses are not focused properly, the light measurements derived from the cells may be reduced and more variable. This is why proper daily instrument setup and daily quality control are important aspects of flow cytometry.

MAbs

MAbs are created by the fusion of B-cell tumors and primary B cells previously selected to make antibodies to only one epitope of a specific antigen. These hybridomas, as they are called, then produce large quantities of epitope-specific antibody. The specificity of MAbs greatly improved the accuracy and reproducibility of immunophenotyping compared to those obtained with polyclonal antisera and thus facilitated the rapid expansion of flow cytometry studies to elucidate the association of cellular phenotype and immune diseases. The nomenclature used to define the reactivity of MAbs is the cluster of differentiation (CD) nomenclature (7). Different MAb clones that bind to the same antigen are designated with the same CD name (e.g., all CD3 MAbs bind to the T-cell receptor).

Many cell surface molecules are responsible for specific functional activities, explaining the association of cellular phenotype with the lineage or differentiation state of the cell. There is an ever-increasing availability of MAbs directly conjugated to a variety of fluorochromes that will provide more in-depth analysis of leukocyte subsets. Useful fluorochromes are constrained by the availability of a reliable excitation source. The 488-nm laser line is most commonly used for excitation of FITC, PE, PerCP, and the tandem fluorochromes PE-Cy5, PE-Texas red, and PE-CY7. A second laser, operating at ~635 nm, is available on some clinical flow cytometers and is used to excite allophycocyanin and allophycocyanin-CY7.

With this vast array of MAb and fluorochrome choices, it is important to recognize potential sources of variation.

Different clones may differ in staining or variably affect cellular function because they may bind to different epitopes on the antigen. The same MAb clone conjugated with two different fluorochromes may yield disparate results. This is especially true for weakly staining markers. In multicolor experiments, some MAb fluorochrome combinations can interfere with the fluorescence emission of another dye molecule and can even turn a positive reactivity into a negative one. Tandem conjugates are especially prone to show interaction with other fluorochromes. T-cell subsetting panels provided by manufacturers for in vitro diagnostic work are designed to avoid these issues. However, when developing a specific research panel in the laboratory, a thorough review of the published literature is perhaps the most important first step prior to undertaking new studies.

Precise identification of most lymphocyte subsets requires the combination of at least two different MAbs, each conjugated with a different dye molecule. Table 1 lists the accepted antibody combinations used to define the main lymphocyte subsets assessed in HIV-infected patients. The table is arranged into categories of two-, three-, and four-color MAb combinations. The number of colors simply means the number of different fluorochromes that the cytometer is capable of measuring simultaneously.

INSTRUMENTATION

Current clinical flow cytometry equipment includes less expensive two-color instruments dedicated to absolute counting, three- and four-color cytometers capable of utilizing bead-based, single-platform (SPT) absolute-counting methodology, and, finally, five- and six-color instrumentation which permits more in-depth immunophenotyping and the ability to perform multiple assays in one tube, saving time and reagents while using less cellular material. Cytometer selection therefore depends on which types of clinical assays will be performed and on whether the cytometer will be used for more complex research studies. A cytometer with at least three-color capability is recommended because it allows addition of the pan-leukocyte antibody CD45 to the original two-color basic immunophenotyping panel. Four-color cytometers permit simultaneous enumeration of CD4 and CD8 T-cell subsets or simultaneous measurement of T-, B-, and NK-cell subsets. Advanced five- and six-color cytometers permit in-depth measurement of naïve, memory, and activated lymphocyte subsets and improve studies of rare cell types, such as enumeration of antigen-specific T cells in HIV-1 vaccine studies, NK T-cell studies, and dendritic-cell studies. At this point, it is not yet clear whether such detailed immunophenotyping

TABLE 1 MAb panels for HIV immunophenotyping

Recommended MAb(s) for panel type[a]			Result
Two color[b]	Three color[c]	Four color[c]	
Isotype control			Background staining
CD45 and CD14			Lymphocyte purity and recovery
CD3 and CD4	CD3, CD4, and CD45	CD3, CD4, CD8, and CD45	CD4 T cells
CD3 and CD8	CD3, CD8, and CD45		CD8 T cells
CD3 and CD19[d]	CD3, CD19, and CD45[d]	CD3, CD19, CD16/CD56, and CD45[d]	B cells
CD3 and CD16/CD56	CD3, CD16/CD56, and CD45		NK cells

[a]Recommended panels of MAbs to derive CD4 and CD8 T-cell results. Each tube contains two, three, or four antibodies as indicated (3).
[b]Light scatter gating.
[c]CD45/SSC gating.
[d]For pediatric specimens, as recommended by the AIDS Clinical Trials Group (3).

will lead to improved clinical care. The most recent advance in modern five- and six-color cytometers is digital signal processing. With replacement of logarithmic amplifier signal processing with more linear digital signal processing, the within-laboratory fluorescence should more accurately reflect changes in antigen density that may accompany disease or treatment and fluorescence standardization between laboratories should also improve. This is especially true for studies that utilize markers that stain dimly or markers that are not clearly bimodal, like the activation markers CD38, HLA-DR, CD95, and CD45RA, a marker used for enumerating naïve T cells. However, proper utilization of modern five- and six-color digital cytometers is not a trivial endeavor and requires an increased diligence in antibody fluorochrome selection and instrument quality control procedures.

IMMUNOPHENOTYPING PROCEDURES

The goal of a flow cytometry laboratory is to develop methods that generate accurate, reproducible immunophenotyping results that are comparable across laboratories. The sections below describe the general sample preparation, instrument setup, sample acquisition, analysis, and quality control procedures used to achieve this goal. Stepwise protocols are provided for running the preferred three- and four-color basic immunophenotyping panel using lyse/no-wash (LNW) sample preparation. The LNW method also permits SPT absolute counting. A second protocol is provided for laboratories that perform more advanced immunophenotyping (Table 2), using MAbs that must be used in lyse/wash (LW) sample procedures prior to running on the cytometer.

Specimen Collection and Storage

Whole blood is collected into tubes containing EDTA, the anticoagulant of choice for samples processed within 30 h of collection. Heparin and acid-citrate-dextrose can also used for immunophenotyping but have not been validated for all methods. Heparin is preferred when the sample age exceeds 30 h. Blood should be stored at room temperature (20 to 25°C) prior to specimen staining. The blood specimen must be well mixed (5 min on a rocker) before being pipetted into the staining tubes. Hemolyzed or clotted specimens are rejected (4, 20).

Biosafety

Universal precautions outlining safe practices for the handling of blood are widely available and should be consulted (2). Practices relating to the biosafety of processing samples for flow cytometry have been published and are recommended (23). Briefly, laboratory personnel should wear lab coats and gloves. The use of sharps and glass should be avoided to the extent that is possible. Specific to processing samples for flow cytometry, the following hazards should be guarded against. Aerosols are created during the numerous vortexing and centrifugation steps throughout specimen processing. Working within a biosafety cabinet and attaching the safety lids to centrifugation buckets will protect against these hazards. Be sure to uncap centrifuge buckets in the safety cabinet! The use of a sample handling device which can be loaded with sample tubes inside the biosafety cabinet and attached to the flow cytometer for automated processing reduces sample handling and samples can be safely vortexed throughout sample acquisition. All of the lysing procedures outlined below include fixation, shown to inactivate HIV, but other hazards, such as hepatitis virus, may still exist. It is generally recommended that flow cytometer waste tanks be treated with bleach so that when full, the bleach will comprise 10% of the final volume. When disposing of waste, be aware that sodium azide is contained in most commercially available antibodies and staining buffer preparations

TABLE 2 Expanded T-cell panels for HIV immunophenotyping

Cell type	Phenotype(s)	MAb combination	Comments
Naïve CD4 T cells	CD45RA+ CD27+	CD45RA/CD27/CD3/CD4	CD3+ excludes CD4dim monocytes.
	CD45RA+ CD28+	CD45RA/CD28/CD3/CD4	CD27+ or CD28+ improves naïve purity by excluding CD45RA+ CD27− CD28− cells.
RTE[b] enriched naïve CD4 T cells	CD45RA+ CD31+	CD45RA/CD31/CD3/CD4	CD31 subset naïve CD4 T cells.
Peripheral expanded CD4 T cells	CD45RA+ CD31−	CD45RA/CD31/CD4/CD27	CD27+ improves naïve purity.
Naïve CD8 cells T cells	CD45RA+ CD27+	CD45RA/CD27/CD3/CD8	CD3+ excludes CD8dim NK cells.
	CD45RA+ CD28+	CD45RA/CD28/CD3/CD8	Naïve cells are bright for CD45RA; CD45RA+ CD27+ CD28+ can improve purity.
CTL[c] enriched CD8 T cells	CD28−, CD57+	CD28/CD3/CD8 CD57/CD3/CD8	Perforin+ cells are primarily CD28−.
Senescent CD4 and CD8 T cells	CD28−, CD57+	CD57/CD3/CD4/CD8 CD3/CD28/CD4/CD8	Cultured CD57+ cells fail to replicate. Shorter telomeres in CD28− and CD57+ cells.
Activated CD4 T cells	HLA-DR+ CD38+ HLA-DR+ CD38−	HLA-DR/CD38/CD3/CD4	Elevated mostly in late HIV-1 disease; prognostic in late HIV-1.
Activated CD8 T cells	HLA-DR+ CD38bright	HLA-DR/CD38/CD3/CD8	Elevated throughout HIV-1 disease.
Activated memory CD8 T cells	CD38bright CD45RO+	CD3/CD38/CD8/CD45RO	Prognostic in early and late HIV-1; quantifying CD38 improves power.

[a]Recommended panels of MAbs to subset differentiation/activation state of CD4 and CD8 T cells.
[b]RTE, recent thymic emigrant.
[c]CTL, cytotoxic T lymphocyte.

and can become explosive if left to accumulate in drainage pipes, so it is necessary to flush well with water after disposal. A notebook of material safety data sheets that is easily available for reference should be maintained. Most importantly, laboratories must have clear protocols outlined for personnel to follow in the event of exposure to potentially hazardous material.

Basic Immunophenotyping Panel with Three- and Four-Color LNW Sample Preparation and Bead-Based SPT Absolute Counting

CD4 T-cell levels are important measures for staging HIV-1 disease and predicting disease progression. In HIV-1-infected adults the CD4 T-cell absolute count is the most useful measure of disease progression, while in children CD4 T-cell percentage is preferred because of high variability in lymphocyte counts (6). The conventional method for determining the absolute CD4 T-cell count (CD4 T cells per cubic millimeter of blood) is referred to as a dual-platform method because it is obtained by multiplying the absolute lymphocyte count (lymphocytes per cubic millimeter), derived from a hematology analyzer, by the CD4 T-cell percentage, derived from the flow cytometer. The variation in hematology-derived absolute lymphocyte counts across different analyzers and the inability to produce reliable counts for aged samples (>24 h old) have led to development of SPT absolute-count methods. SPT refers to flow cytometry methods that do not require a hematology analyzer. The Centers for Disease Control and Prevention guidelines for performing CD4 T-cell determinations using the dual-platform (1997) and SPT (2003) methodologies are published (4, 5).

The CD45 gating method is used for the basic three- and four-color immunophenotyping panels. The addition of the pan-leukocyte marker, CD45, to the original two-color immunophenotyping panel has greatly improved the precision of the lymphocyte gate for the clinical laboratory (24). Refer to Table 1 for approved staining panels. The CD45 lymphocyte gating method permits the use of LNW sample preparation methods. CD45 gating combined with the LNW method improves lymphocyte recovery compared to that of the older light scatter gating methods. The LNW sample preparation method does not utilize a centrifugation step and therefore avoids two main pitfalls of older methods: cell loss and formation of cellular aggregates. LNW methods also allow for SPT absolute counting. Pipetting precision is critical when absolute counts are to be determined. Variability can be greatly reduced by use of reverse pipetting. Reverse pipetting is a technique in which more sample is drawn up into the pipette tip than the measured amount to be dispelled. Pipettes must be maintained and calibrated to ensure accurate results (5). Below are two commercially available SPT protocols.

Method 1: FACS Lysing Solution Used With or Without TruCOUNT Tubes Containing Lyophilized Bead Pellet

1. Add 20 μl of premixed Becton Dickinson (San Jose, Calif.), Tritest (three color) or Multitest (four color) reagent cocktail to a standard 12- by 75-mm tube or, when absolute counts are desired, to a TruCOUNT tube.

2. Add 50 μl of well-mixed whole blood, vortex gently, and incubate for 15 min at room temperature (RT) in the dark.

3. Add 450 μl of 1× FACS lysing solution, gently vortex, and incubate for 15 min at RT in the dark. Keep samples at RT in the dark prior to running the test. Vortex well just prior to acquisition on the cytometer.

Method 2: Coulter IMMUNOPREP Lysing System With or Without FlowCount Beads

1. Add 100 μl of well-mixed whole blood to the bottom of a 12- by 75-mm tube.

2. Add 10 μl of CYTO-STAT MAb reagent to the blood and vortex.

3. Incubate for approximately 10 min at RT in the dark.

4. Prepare stained specimens with the IMMUNOPREP reagent system utilizing Q-Prep, TQ Prep, Multi Q-Prep, or FP 1000 processing according to the manufacturer's directions for the removal of red blood cells and fixation.

5. When performing SPT absolute counting, pipette 100 μl of FlowCount fluorospheres to each tube just prior to acquisition on the flow cytometer.

Establishing LNW Instrument Settings

Cytometer manufacturers provide easy, software-driven procedures for determining initial instrument settings and daily quality control and compensation settings for performing basic whole-blood immunophenotyping specific for either LNW or LW sample preparation procedures. Briefly, dye-labeled and unlabeled beads are run on the cytometer. PMT voltages are automatically adjusted to place the fluorescence of the unlabeled bead into the manufacturer-established target channel, and then the fluorescence intensity of the dye-labeled beads is determined to validate that a minimum separation of the positive and negative beads exists. The software also measures the noise level of scatter signals to verify that the number of nonbead debris events is low and will not interfere with leukocyte scatter resolution. The software program adjusts compensation and flags results that are below manufacturer specifications. What is compensation? Each fluorescence detector is assigned to measure light from a particular fluorochrome that is defined by the optical filters; however, light emitted by other fluorochromes may also be detected. This spillover of fluorescence is often referred to as spectral overlap, and the removal of the nondesired fluorescence is referred to as compensation. For example, fluorescent light from fluorochrome one (FITC) can reach the detector designed to measure fluorochrome two (PE). This is because the fluorescence emission spectrum of FITC extends out beyond a wavelength of 600 nm and thus overlaps into the detection range assigned to PE, ~562 to 588 nm. Compensation subtracts the percentage of fluorescence derived from spectral overlap from the total amount of fluorescence that reaches the detector. The percentage of FITC fluorescence that reaches the PE detector, for instance, is usually around 20%. It is recommended that scatter settings and compensation be fine-tuned with a stained whole-blood sample. For use of manufacturer-derived instrument settings with LNW samples, visual confirmation that the relevant stained lymphocyte populations are retained within the appropriate analysis region is usually all that is necessary. For example, confirm that the CD3$^+$ CD4$^-$ population is retained within the lower right analysis region and that the CD3$^+$CD4$^+$ population is retained within the upper right region as shown in Fig. 1B. Perform similar examinations of the lymphocyte clusters for each MAb combination and refer to Fig. 1. Notice how the CD3$^+$CD8$^-$ population (lower right region) in Fig. 1C has an amount of PE fluorescence similar to that of the CD3$^-$ CD8$^-$ population (lower left region). Accurate, reproducible basic immunophenotyping

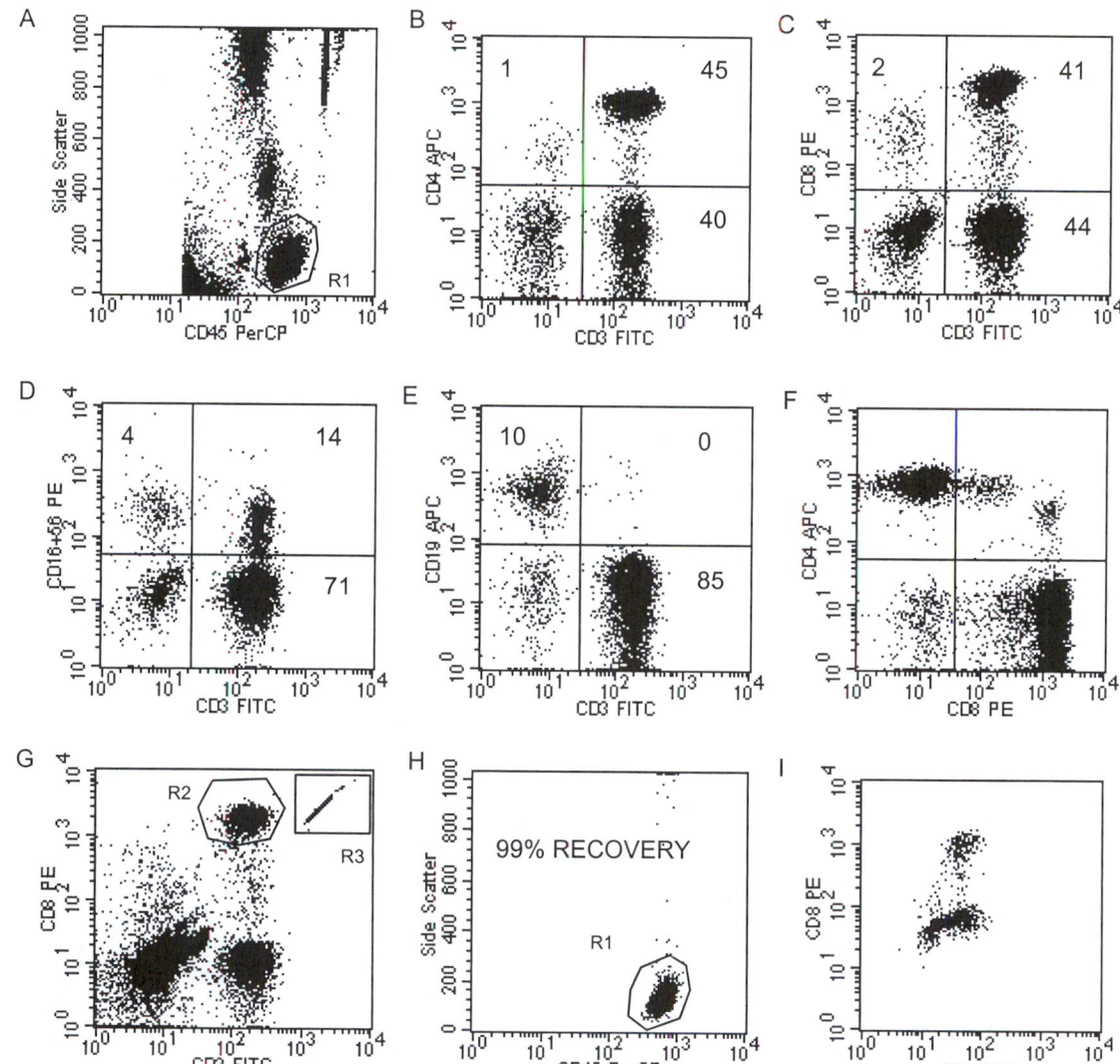

FIGURE 1 LNW sample preparation. Plot A demonstrates optimal CD45 lymphocyte gating with SSC adjusted to reveal distinct leukocyte populations. Plots B, C, D, and E show lymphocyte subsets with the R1 gate applied and cursor settings guided by the negatively stained populations. Results would be reported as follows: CD4 = 45%, CD8 = 41%, NK cells = 4%, and B cells = 10%. The total T-cell percentage (CD3) is 85% in both tubes sampled, providing confidence in the overall result. Plot F is gated on CD45+ CD3+ lymphocytes, illustrating the additional information available when the four-color immunophenotyping panel is used. Plot G is an ungated display of FL1 versus FL2 used for two different applications. The R3 gating region enumerates counting beads for SPT absolute-count determinations. The R2 gating region includes all CD8+ stained events, which are then backgated through the original lymphocyte gate (R1) in plot H to determine recovery for quality assurance. Finally, plot I shows a sample that bound antibody nonspecifically. This staining artifact was successfully corrected for reporting subset percentages by restaining an aliquot of washed blood.

results are produced when manufacturer-defined instrument setup is combined with the manufacturer-supplied MAb and the LNW sample preparation procedure. These methods are highly recommended, as they have been extensively validated. It is important to record the instrument's PMT voltages each day to spot changes in instrument performance. These data are graphed in a Levey-Jennings plot. Time is plotted on the x axis and PMT voltages are plotted on the y axis for each detector. Upper and lower boundaries are usually set 5% above and below the mean PMT voltage for each

detector. When PMT voltages drift beyond the established boundaries, the cytometer should be serviced to correct the problem and preclude absolute instrument failure or compromised immunophentyping results. Some laboratories also monitor the coefficients of variation (CVs) using highly uniform particles with known low CVs. Elevated CVs may indicate more subtle performance issues, such as fluidic problems in the absence of large PMT changes. For a more detailed description of instrument setup consult the individual manufacturer's procedures.

Data Acquisition

The data acquisition screen for LNW, CD45 gated sample preparations should display the leukocyte populations using a CD45-versus-SSC plot. Optimal leukocyte resolution is verified and an analysis region is set on the CD45-positive, low-SSC lymphocyte population. A stop counter is set to collect a minimum of 2,500 lymphocytes. An ungated plot of FL1 versus FL2 is created to monitor absolute-counting beads, if applicable. If TruCOUNT beads are used, the instrument threshold must be set on the FL3 detector since the beads are smaller than lymphocytes and risk being excluded when an FSC threshold is applied. Additional plots of the relevant stained lymphocyte populations, e.g., CD3 versus CD4 or CD3 versus CD8, are gated on the lymphocytes and displayed to review the staining quality. An example of identifying poor staining is shown in Fig. 1I. The sample had to be restained using a prewash in phosphate-buffered saline to remove a serum component that interferes with staining.

Data Analysis

The basis of accurate lymphocyte analysis is the establishment of a valid lymphocyte gate. Two important criteria for determining the quality of a lymphocyte gate are purity and recovery. Purity is the percentage of cells in the gate that are lymphocytes. Contamination of the lymphocyte gate is most often caused by monocytes and basophils. Recovery describes the proportion of all lymphocytes that have been included in the lymphocyte gate. Poor recovery is often caused by formation of cellular aggregates or by creating a lymphocyte gate that is too small. Small or "tight" lymphocyte gates frequently exclude dim CD45-staining B cells. A small lymphocyte gate may achieve high purity at the cost of low recovery.

Step-by-Step Three-Color Analysis

1. To simplify the description of analysis steps, the MAb combination of CD3-FITC, CD4-PE, and CD45-PerCP is used as an example. Display an ungated plot of CD45 versus SSC and set an analysis region around the CD45-positive, low-SSC cluster (Fig. 1A). The gate should be set to capture all lymphocytes, including any dim CD45 B cells and more granular NK lymphocytes. Non-CD45-staining debris should easily be excluded from the lymphocyte gate, and effective purities should approach 100%.

2. Display a plot of CD3 versus CD4 that includes only those cells within the CD45 lymphocyte gate (Fig. 1B). Set quadrant cursors (analysis regions) to separate the lymphocyte populations into distinct positive and negative clusters to derive the percentage of CD3$^+$ CD4$^+$ T cells. Record cell counts when performing SPT counting.

3. The CD3-versus-CD4 tube is used to assess the CD3$^-$ CD4^{dim} monocyte contamination. Monocyte contamination should be adjusted to ≤3%.

4. Display the relevant plots for the remaining tubes in the panel gated on lymphocytes (CD3 versus CD8, CD3 versus CD16$^+$ CD56, and CD3 versus CD19). Quadrant markers may need to be adjusted slightly between tubes to effectively separate the populations, since the positions of stained clusters may vary slightly. Example plots of the complete basic immunophenotyping panel are shown in Fig. 1A to E.

Backgating and Other Quality Assurance Procedures

Purity for the CD45 gating method is estimated as 100% minus the monocyte contamination. An estimate of lymphocyte recovery is a little trickier for CD45 lymphocyte gating. Some investigators suggest that recovery can be estimated by adding the percentages obtained for the major lymphocyte markers, T cells plus B cells plus NK cells; however, this method does not prove that all lymphocytes were included in the gate. If a restrictive gate is drawn that excludes dim CD45 B cells, for example, the B-cell percentage will obviously be lower and the T-cell and NK-cell percentages will be correspondingly higher, with the sum of T cells plus B cells plus NK cells still approaching 100%. An effective method to confirm recovery of T-cell and B-cell populations is called "backgating." Backgating is the practice of projecting a lineage-gated population back through the original lymphocyte gate. An example of backgating CD3$^+$ CD8$^+$ T cells is shown in Fig. 1. Figure 1G shows an ungated display of CD3 versus CD8. A lineage gate is set on the CD8 T-cell cluster and is projected back through the CD45 lymphocyte gate (Fig. 1H). This method should be used to confirm the recovery of CD4 and CD8 T cells and CD19$^+$ B cells. The method is not effective for NK cells because the NK cell marker CD16 is also expressed by monocytes and granulocytes. Backgating methods can reveal other problems, such as cellular aggregates, dying cells, and blast cells.

Four-Color Analysis

The four-color T-cell panel uses the MAb combination CD3, CD4, CD8, and CD45. The staining and analysis are performed the same as for the three-color method described above. In addition to reducing the panel from two tubes to one, saving sample processing time, reagents, and expense, the T-cell subsets, if desired, are resolved with additional information. By displaying a CD8-versus-CD4 plot that is gated on CD3$^+$ T cells, three novel T-cell types and one staining artifact might be resolved (Fig. 1F). The additional T-cell subsets are the CD4$^-$ CD8$^-$ CD3$^+$, CD4^{bright} CD8^{dim} CD3$^+$, and CD4^{dim} CD8^{bright} CD3$^+$. Cell sorting experiments can demonstrate that the CD8^{bright} CD4^{bright} CD3$^+$ cells are mostly cellular aggregates of CD4 and CD8 T cells. Four-color analysis can therefore be used to validate quality control checks that flag samples where the CD4 and CD8 T cells do not add up to the total frequency of CD3-positive lymphocytes (22).

Despite the improved clarity achieved with four-color immunophenotyping, T-cell subset percentages are reported the same way as in two- and three-color analysis, namely, CD3$^+$ CD4$^+$ lymphocytes are graded as CD4 T cells and CD3$^+$ CD8$^+$ lymphocytes are graded as CD8 T cells.

Absolute-Count Determinations

Follow the above steps for three- and four-color analysis. Create an ungated plot of either CD3 versus CD4 or CD3 versus CD8, and draw a gate around the bead population (Fig. 1G). Display statistics to determine the number of beads counted.

The absolute count is calculated as the ratio of analyzed cellular events to bead events multiplied by the ratio of total bead count to blood sample volume. For example, (8,400 CD4 T cells/10,000 beads) × (51,225 beads/50 μl) = 860 CD4 cells/mm^3.

SPT versus Dual-Platform Absolute Counting

The interlaboratory CD4 T-cell count CV for the TruCOUNT bead method (Becton Dickinson) was reported as 9%, compared to 16% for the dual-platform method, and the interlaboratory CV for CD4 T-cell counts was 10% for the TetraOne method (Beckman Coulter, Miami, Fla.), compared to 18% for the dual-platform method. These reports also indicated that the intralaboratory variation was slightly lower (CV, 1 to 3% lower) for SPT (1, 21, 24). Absolute counts for overnight samples appear to be more stable, and fewer samples fail to meet quality control criteria using the SPT. Therefore, SPTs are more suitable for quality assurance testing that relies on samples shipped overnight. There can also be bias in absolute counts between the SPT and dual-platform methods depending on which hematology analyzer is used, so comparative studies should be performed. The SPT bead methodology is less variable and is preferred, especially for interlaboratory studies. Many of the published reports demonstrating higher variation for dual platform versus SPT used older sample preparation and lymphocyte gating methodologies for generating the T-cell percentage portion of the dual-platform absolute count. These older methods, discussed below, include the LW staining method and scatter gating, which clearly contribute to the overall variability of the dual-platform method. Generating the CD4 T-cell percentage portion of the dual-platform method using newer LNW and CD45 lymphocyte gating should reduce the overall variability in absolute counting using the dual-platform method; however, this approach clearly does not control for variation across hematology analyzers. The dual-platform method is still very valuable, especially for laboratories that process samples in less than 24 h, because the intralaboratory variation is relatively low and the counting beads add a significant cost to the assay. *The bead-based methods have been independently validated in multicenter studies and are Food and Drug Administration cleared for in vitro diagnostic use.*

Alternate LW Staining Methods

The LW procedure is used primarily for research studies that use novel panels of MAbs that are not specifically titrated for the LNW procedure. An example is the enumeration of naïve or memory T cells and activation marker expression on various lymphocyte subpopulations. The panel should include appropriate isotype-matched controls and a tube (CD45 and CD14) to assess the quality of the FSC-versus-SSC lymphocyte gate. The LW method uses excess MAb to ensure saturation of antigen and then removes the excess unbound dye-labeled MAb by washing to reduce background fluorescence, thereby optimizing the resolution of stained cells from unstained cells. The LW method can also be used for dual-platform absolute counts when appropriate reagents are not available.

LW Staining Procedures

A. Part one: antibody incubation
1. Add appropriate amounts of MAb to 12- by 75-mm round-bottom tubes (typically 5 to 20 μl depending on fluorochrome conjugate and manufacturer).
2. Add 100 μl of whole blood and vortex tubes, watching for proper mixing and blood droplets that may remain unmixed on the sides of the tubes.
3. Incubate for 30 min in the dark at RT.
4. Next, the stained samples are lysed, washed, and fixed. The procedures for lysing and fixing vary depending on the erythrocyte lysing method; two methods are provided.

B. Part two: erythrocyte lysing and fixation procedures
1. For FACSlyse erythrocyte lysing/fixing reagent
   a. Add 2 ml of 1× FACSlyse, vortex immediately (~5 s), and incubate for 10 min in the dark (do not exceed 12 min).

b. Centrifuge cells at $300 \times g$ for 5 min (Becton Dickinson recommends RT) and aspirate the supernatant, taking care not to aspirate cells.
   c. Vortex pellet gently, add 2 ml of wash buffer, and spin at $300 \times g$ for 5 min.
   d. Aspirate supernatant, vortex gently, and add 0.5 ml of 1% formaldehyde solution. Vortex cells again.

2. For alternate ammonium chloride erythrocyte lysing reagent
   a. Add 2 ml of 1× ammonium chloride lysing solution, vortex immediately (~5 s), and incubate for 5 min in the dark.
   b. Centrifuge cells at $300 \times g$ for 5 min (use centrifuge temperature of 4°C to inhibit lysing) and aspirate supernatant, taking care not to aspirate cells.
   c. Repeat steps a and b, except reduce second lysing to 3 min.
   d. Aspirate supernatant, vortex gently, and add 0.5 ml of protein-free phosphate-buffered saline with 1% formaldehyde (pH 7.2). Vortex cells again; allow fixation to stabilize for 10 min. Store samples in the dark at 4°C, if not processing samples immediately.

The LW protocols are suitable for the majority of research antigens routinely assayed in the clinical laboratory; however, some antigens may require specific modifications of the basic methods. Variations in staining of problem antigens (chemokine receptors and adhesion molecules) may include choice of blood anticoagulant, blood storage time, prewashing of the blood prior to staining to remove serum factors, MAb concentration, time and temperature of MAb incubation, and selection of fluorochrome (10).

Establishment of Initial LW Instrument Settings and Daily Quality Control

Initial instrument detector settings can be established with stained whole-blood samples. FSC and SSC detector settings are adjusted to optimize leukocyte resolution. A lymphocyte gate is set and the fluorescent plots are displayed for each fluorescence detector. Cells stained with fluorochrome-labeled CD4 MAb can be used to optimize PMT voltages for each detector. Voltages are set to place the unstained cells on scale and in the first decade of the scale. Voltages are adjusted to maximize the separation of the negative and positive median fluorescence intensities (signal-to-noise ratio). PMT voltages must not be too low or the PMT will not function linearly. PMT voltages that are too high can increase the CVs of the fluorescence distribution and effectively reduce the cytometer's ability to resolve dimly staining populations. Once optimal PMT voltages are established using CD4 T-cell staining, it is recommended to validate sensitivity using a dimly staining marker like CD56. The next step is to run a stable fluorescent particle such as chicken red blood cells (BioSure, Grass Valley, Calif.) at the same PMT voltages to establish target channels for daily instrument setup. On subsequent days the particles are run and PMTs are adjusted to place the median fluorescence into the established target channel. The CV and PMT voltages are recorded for each detector on a log sheet and plotted as a Levey-Jennings plot to monitor instrument stability. Finally, compensation is set using stained biological controls at these exact fluorescence PMT settings. More extensive descriptions of instrument performance and quality control issues are available in *Current Protocols in Cytometry* (12).

Setting Compensation

Compensation is dependent on a number of factors, particularly PMT voltage settings, fluorescence emission spectra, and optical-filter combinations, and therefore must be performed after setting PMT voltages. Compensation for LW samples is typically set using a series of single-stained samples stained with one of each fluorochrome being used for the research panel. The brightest-staining MAb (such as CD8) is typically used to avoid the possibility of under compensation.

The stepwise procedure is as follows.

1. A sample stained with CD8-FITC is gated on lymphocytes and displayed on a plot of FITC versus PE.
2. Analysis regions are set (quadrants) to separate the positive and negative populations. The median PE fluorescence is measured for the negative and positive populations.
3. Compensation is adjusted so that the amount of PE fluorescence in the FITC-positively stained cells is equal to PE fluorescence in the negatively stained cells.
4. This process is repeated for each fluorochrome.

Sample Acquisition

Samples are typically acquired with the threshold set on FSC to exclude residual red cells and debris. An FCS-versus-SSC plot is displayed to assess sample condition by observing the three distinct white blood cell populations of lymphocytes, monocytes, and granulocytes, as seen in Fig. 2A. The FSC and SSC instrument settings should be adjusted to maximize this distinction. A stop counter should be set to collect sufficient numbers of the population of interest, e.g., CD4 or CD8 T cells (typically 2,500). Additional plots with the lymphocyte gate applied should be displayed to validate the quality of staining for all MAbs being measured.

Data Analysis

Analysis begins with evaluating the quality of the lymphocyte gate and setting the positive and negative analysis regions with an isotype control. An example of enumerating naïve CD4 T cells is provided.

A. Step 1: measuring the purity and recovery of the lymphocyte gate
   1. To measure purity, set an FSC-versus-SSC lymphocyte gate as displayed in Fig. 2A, R1. Lymphocytes have low FSC and low SSC.
   2. Display a plot of CD45 versus CD14; set analysis regions (quadrants) to enumerate the CD45^{bright} CD14^{negative} lymphocyte population to determine the lymphocyte purity (Fig. 2B). Maintain monocyte contamination at $\leq$3%. Optimize purity at $\geq$95%.
   3. To measure recovery, display a second plot of CD45 versus CD14 that is ungated, creating an analysis region around the CD45^{bright} CD14^{negative} lymphocyte population (Fig. 2C, R2).
   4. Display a second plot of FSC versus SSC that displays the original lymphocyte region, R1, but that is gated on cells in analysis region 2 (Fig. 2D). To determine lymphocyte recovery, create a statistical view to enumerate the percentage of bright CD45$^+$ CD14$^-$ cells contained within the R1 scatter gate.
   5. The scatter gate is then adjusted to optimize recovery to $\geq$95%.
   6. The lymphocyte gate is optimized for recovery and purity with the CD45 CD14 tube. This gate is used for analysis of the remaining tubes in the panel.

B. Step 2: setting cursors with isotype controls to establish negative staining region
   1. Display plots for each of the relevant markers to be measured with the region 1 lymphocyte gate applied.
   2. Set analysis regions to measure $\geq$99% in the negative quadrant (quadrant 3). Occasionally, binding will occur nonspecifically in the isotype control tube, indicating that it may also occur with the corresponding MAbs in the panel. In this event the nonspecific staining observed in the isotype control tube can then be subtracted from that in the corresponding tubes.

C. Step 3: sample analysis using the example of CD45RA/ CD27/CD4/CD3 four-color-stained sample
   1. Create an FSC-versus-SSC plot and apply the lymphocyte gate optimized in step 1 above.
   2. Create a plot to display CD3 versus CD4 gated on lymphocytes.
   3. Create an analysis region to select the CD3$^+$ CD4$^+$ T cells. This region must be combined with the lymphocyte gate to establish a gate that includes only CD3$^+$ CD4$^+$ lymphocytes (G2).
   4. Create a second plot of CD45RA versus CD27 gated on CD3$^+$ CD4$^+$ lymphocytes.
   5. Set quadrant markers as established in step 2 above and as shown in Fig. 2H. The naïve CD4 T cells are in the upper right region (CD45RA$^+$ CD27$^+$).

Backgating and Other Quality Assurance Issues

Scatter gating and LW sample preparation are much more likely to produce suboptimal lymphocyte purities and recoveries than are CD45 gating and the LNW sample preparation. Minimum purity standards for LW methods are recommended at 90%; however, in practice 95% purities are achievable with good sample preparation (4). Samples that do not meet these standards should be retested. Monocytes (CD45^{dim} CD14$^+$), basophils (CD45^{dim} CD14$^-$) and red cell debris (CD45$^-$) are the usual contaminants of the lymphocyte gate. Samples with elevated numbers of lysing resistant or nucleated red blood cells can result in substandard purities that cannot be improved by repeated staining. In this event, it may be necessary to correct all lymphocyte subset percentages from this specimen based on the purity of the lymphocyte gate. For example, if the original CD4 T-cell percentage is 20% and the lymphocyte purity is 86%, the corrected CD4 T-cell percentage would equal 20% divided by 0.86, or 23%. Correcting data by lymphocyte purity is problematic because it assumes that the lymphocyte gate is not biased toward exclusion of a particular lymphocyte subset and that the purity and recovery are the same for all tubes in the panel. This is often NOT the case. For example, in a sample where the correlated light scatter profiles do not reveal a distinct lymphocyte population, the tendency is to set a restrictive lymphocyte gate in the area of the debris, which tends to bias recovery toward T cells and away from smaller B cells. Backgating CD19$^+$ B cells can confirm this bias. In other samples the backgating technique identifies a cell preparation artifact called "escapees" (10). Escapees are aptly named because they are made up of cell aggregates, often CD8 cells that due to their high SSC signal escape from the original lymphocyte gate (Fig. 2E and F). For these reasons it is recommended that only samples with purities below 92% be corrected. Backgating the relevant lineage markers in the research panel will ensure their inclusion in the lymphocyte gate and is a preferred practice. Elevated

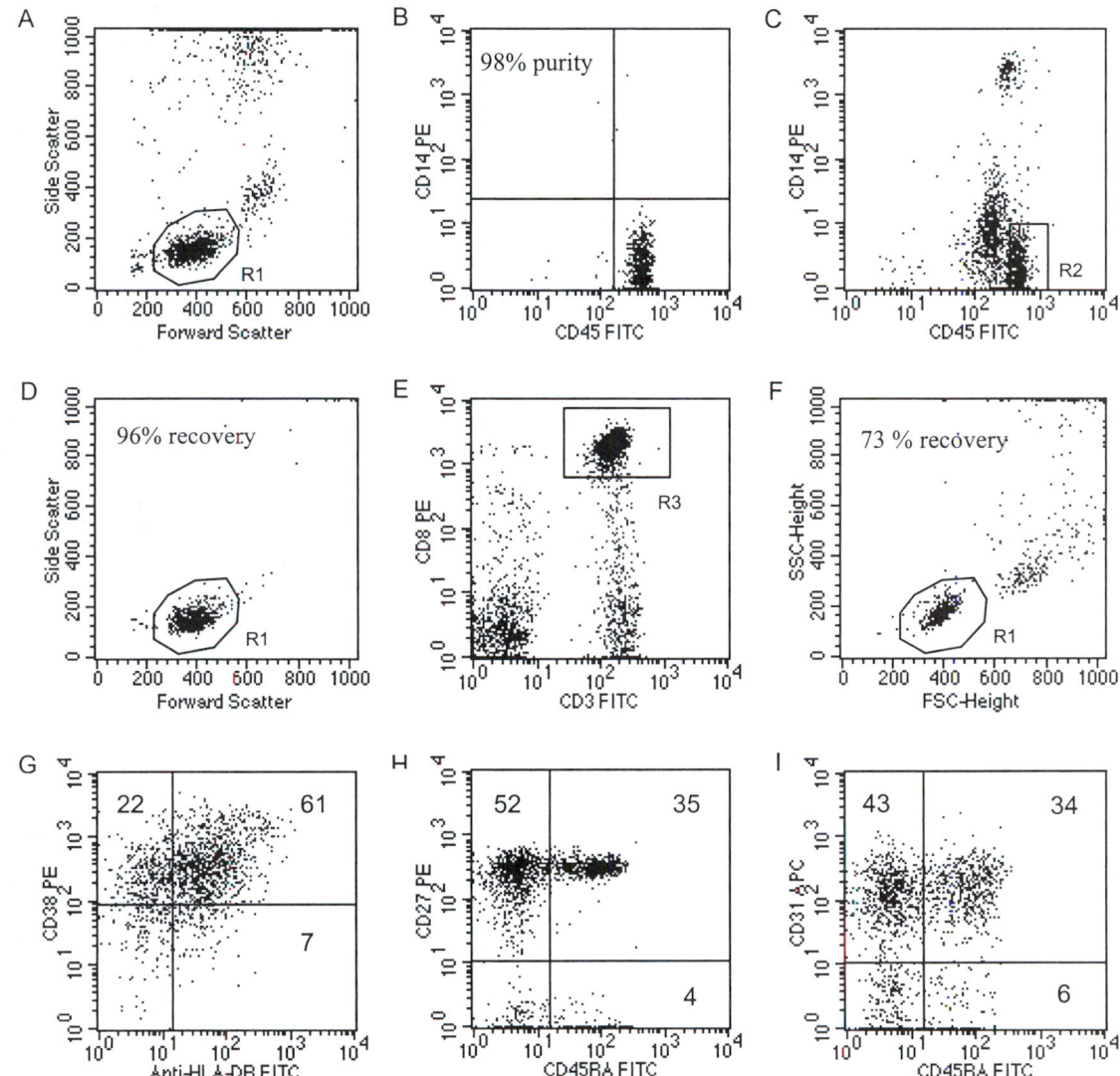

FIGURE 2 LW sample preparation. Plots A, B, C, and D are analyzed together to establish an FSC-versus-SSC lymphocyte gate with the highest purity and recovery of lymphocytes. Plots E and F show poor backgating of CD8+ stained events due to cell clumping (escapees). Plot G measures elevated coexpression of HLA-DR versus CD38 gated on CD3+ CD8+ lymphocytes from an HIV-1-infected donor. Plots H and I use CD45RA in combination with either CD27 (H) or CD31 (I) to define CD4+ naïve cells.

numbers of dead cells that have higher SSC can also be identified with this method.

Alternate SPT Absolute-Count Methods

The FACSCount system (Becton Dickinson) is a unique bead-based method that uses a no-lyse procedure. The inter-laboratory CV in CD4 T-cell counts is reported to be less than 10% (17). The FACSCount is ideal for some laboratories because it does not require flow cytometry experience and is less expensive. It is a dedicated absolute counter that does not provide the versatility of MAb panels and cannot determine percentages within the lymphocyte population required for pediatric samples. The volumetric methodology was previously validated against dual-platform methods using the OrthoCytoron flow cytometer, which is no longer commercially available. At least two new volumetric systems have recently been developed, the Guava PCA system,

primarily for use in resource-poor countries, and the Partec CyFlow. These systems have not yet been approved in the United States for in vitro diagnostic use, and publications from independent multicenter studies are not currently available. Data for the Guava system have been submitted to the Food and Drug Administration for approval. Absolute counting is facilitated by use of a precision syringe-driven pump to accurately determine the volume of prepared sample that is measured. The blood sample is stained with a cocktail of CD4-PE and the tandem conjugate CD3-PE-CY5, and erythrocytes are removed using an LNW method. Precise measurement of all reagents is critical because the dilution of blood to lysing reagent (1:20) is used for calculation of the absolute count. The instrument uses a green diode laser to excite the dyes PE and PE-CY5 and to generate FSC measurement. The system does not currently derive the percentage of CD4 or CD8 T cells within the lymphocyte population; however, this capability is under development using the MAb combination of CD45 and CD4.

The CyFlow system by Partec can generate absolute counts by a novel electrode method. When the sample volume in a tube containing the stained cells drops below the upper electrode in the tube the counting begins, and when the sample dips below the lower electrode the counting stops. The precise volume of sample between electrodes is 200 μl, so the absolute count can be generated based on a dilution factor.

T-CELL ALTERATIONS IN HIV-1 DISEASE

There are phenotypic changes in CD4 cells through the chronic phase of HIV-1 disease that may include a slight decrease in expression of CD45RO, CD28, and CD27, with slight increases in the expression of CD45RA, CD57, and HLA-DR; however, these phenotypic changes do not appear to contribute prognostic power beyond the enumeration of CD4 T-cell numbers alone and do not reflect the profound decrease that is observed in assays of CD4 T-cell function. More pronounced phenotypic alterations are seen in late HIV-1 disease. A study involving participants with advanced HIV-1 disease (<50 CD4 cells/mm³) demonstrated a significant increase in expression of the activation markers CD95, HLA-DR, and CD38 on CD4 T cells compared to uninfected controls and that elevated CD38 but not HLA-DR or CD95 expression was strongly associated with a shorter (<6 month) versus longer (>18 month) survival time ($P = 0.002$). Although the level of naïve cells as measured by dual expression of CD45RA and CD62L was greatly diminished in advanced HIV-1 disease, this was not associated with shorter versus longer survival ($P = 0.338$) (8). Subtyping of CD4 T cells following highly active antiretroviral therapy treatment is relevant for assessing immune reconstitution. The proportion of naïve CD4 T cells is usually determined by dual expression of CD45RA and either CD62L, CD27, or CD28. Although most CD45RA⁺ CD4 T cells are considered naïve, a small percentage (1 to 5%) of CD45RA⁺ cells do not express CD62L, CD27, or CD28 and are not considered naïve (Fig. 2H) (11). Early studies used CD45RA in combination with CD62L to measure naïve T cells; however, due to variable loss of the CD62L antigen on cryopreserved lymphocytes, CD27 and CD28 are now more commonly used. Another marker, CD31, provides additional information about the replicative history of naïve CD4 T cells that may be useful for studies designed to assay the contribution of the thymus to CD4 T-cell reconstitution (14). CD45RA⁺ CD31⁻ naïve cells contain about one-eighth the level of T-cell receptor excision circles (TREC) that CD45RA⁺ CD31⁺ naïve cells contain, suggesting that they are a consequence of homeostasis-driven peripheral expansion. TREC are a molecular measurement of the replicative history of T cells such that populations of cells with high levels of TREC are considered more enriched in recent thymic emigrants than are populations of cells with low TREC levels, which are enriched in peripherally expanded naïve cells.

The phenotypic alterations of CD8 T cells are more profound in early and late HIV-1 disease than observed for CD4 T cells. Alterations include a decrease in naïve CD8 T cells as measured by the dual expression of CD45RA and CD62L and elevations in the memory cell marker CD45RO. The cells expressing markers associated with cytotoxic function (CD57⁺ and CD28⁻) and cell activation (HLA-DR, CD38, and CD95) are also increased. Elevated levels of CD38 expression have been shown to be prognostic for time to AIDS and death in several studies (15, 16). In early HIV-1

disease (median length of infection = 2.8 years) the prognostic significance of CD38 expression was similar to that of HIV-1 plasma viral load, and as the duration of infection increased (median length of infection = 8.7 years), CD38 antigen density was more predictive of AIDS development than CD4 T-cell count or viral load. These prognostic studies on CD38 expression demonstrate that measurement of antigen density can be more relevant than grading cells as positive or negative. In the study of advanced disease described above, elevated expression of CD38 on CD8 T cells was strongly associated ($P = 0.002$) and CD95 was marginally associated ($P = 0.006$) with shorter versus longer survival (8). The study group used for the prognostic studies described above consisted primarily of male Caucasians. Testing these observations on different populations based on age, race, and gender is an area of importance. Other studies have demonstrated that CD38 expression on CD8 cells is predictive of CD4 T-cell loss in a mostly minority, female adolescent population and that CD38 expression predicts virologic failure in HIV-1-infected children receiving antiretroviral therapy (26). The Adult AIDS Clinical Trial Group reported that high pretreatment CD8 T-cell activation levels predicted virologic failure ($P = 0.046$) (19). The methods used to determine CD38 expression on CD8 cells, however, vary across studies. Standardized and more simplified methods of antigen quantitation may help improve and extend this important work so that measurement of CD38 on CD8 cells becomes broadly available to clinical laboratories (13).

REFERENCES

1. **Brando, B., D. Barnett, G. Janossy, F. Mandy, B. Autran, G. Rothe, B. Scarpati, G. D'Avanzo, J. L. D'Hautcourt, R. Lenkei, G. Schmitz, A. Kunkl, R. Chianese, S. Papa, and J. W. Gratama for the European Working Group on Clinical Cell Analysis.** 2000. Cytofluorometric methods for assessing absolute numbers of cell subsets in blood. *Cytometry* 42:327–346.
2. **Centers for Disease Control.** 1988. Perspectives in disease prevention and health promotion update: universal precautions for prevention of transmission of human immunodeficiency virus, hepatitis B virus and other bloodborne pathogens in health-care settings. *Morb. Mortal. Wkly. Rep.* 37:377–388.
3. **Centers for Disease Control.** 1992. 1993 revised classification system for HIV infection and expanded case definition for AIDS among adolescents and adults. *Morb. Mortal. Wkly. Rep.* 41:1–19.
4. **Centers for Disease Control and Prevention.** 1997. 1997 revised guidelines for performing CD4⁺ T cell determinations in persons infected with human immunodeficiency virus (HIV). *Morb. Mortal. Wkly. Rep.* 46:1–29.
5. **Centers for Disease Control and Prevention.** 2003. Guidelines for performing single-platform absolute CD4⁺ determinations with CD45 gating in persons infected with human immunodeficiency virus. *Morb. Mortal. Wkly. Rep.* 52:1–13.
6. **Giorgi, J. V.** 1996. Phenotype and function of T-cells in HIV disease, p. 181–199. *In* S. Gupta (ed.), *Immunology of HIV Infection.* Plenum Press, New York, N.Y.
7. **Giorgi, J. V., L. Boumsell, and B. Autran.** 1995. Reactivity of T-cell section monoclonal antibodies with circulating CD4⁺ and CD8⁺ T cells in HIV disease and following in vitro activation, p. 446–461. *In* S. Schlossman, L. Boumsell, W. Gilks, J. Harlan, T. Kishimoto, C. Morimoto, J. Ritz, S. Shaw, R. Silverstein, T. Springer, T. Tedder, and R. Todd (ed.), *Leukocyte Typing V: White Cell Differentiation Antigens.* Oxford University Press, Oxford, United Kingdom.

8. Giorgi, J. V., L. E. Hultin, J. A. McKeating, T. D. Johnson, B. Owens, L. P. Jacobson, R. Shih, J. Lewis, D. J. Wiley, J. P. Phair, S. M. Wolinsky, and R. Detels. 1999. Shorter survival in advanced human immunodeficiency virus type 1 infection is more closely associated with T lymphocyte activation than with plasma virus burden or virus chemokine coreceptor usage. *J. Infect. Dis.* **179:**859–870.

9. Giorgi, J. V., A. M. Kesson, and C. C. Chou. 1992. Immunodeficiency and infectious diseases, p. 174–181. *In* N. R. Rose, E. C. deMacario, J. L. Fahey, H. Friedman, and G. M. Penn (ed.), *Manual of Clinical Laboratory Immunology*, 4th ed. American Society for Microbiology, Washington, D.C.

10. Giorgi, J. V., and A. Landay. 1994. HIV infection: diagnosis and disease progression evaluation, p. 437–455. *In* Z. Darzynkiewicz, J. P. Robinson, and H. A. Crissman (ed.), *Methods in Cell Biology.* Academic Press, Orlando, Fla.

11. Hamann, D., P. A. Baars, M. H. G. Rep, B. Hooibrink, S. R. Kerkhof-Garde, M. R. Klein, and R. A. W. van Lier. 1997. Phenotypic and functional separation of memory and effector human CD8+ T cells. *J. Exp. Med.* **186:**1407–1418.

12. Hoffman, A. 1997. Standardization, calibration, and control in flow cytometry, p. 31–319. *In* J. P. Robinson, Z. Darzynkiewicz, P. N. Dean, L. G. Dressler, P. S. Rabinovitch, C. C. Stewart, H. J. Tanke, and L. L. Wheeless (ed.), *Current Protocols in Cytometry.* John Wiley & Sons, Inc., New York, N.Y.

13. Iyer, S., L. E. Hultin, J. A. Zawadzki, K. A. Davis, and J. V. Giorgi. 1998. Quantitation of CD38 expression using Quantibrite beads. *Cytometry* **33:**206–212.

14. Kimmig, S., G. K. Przybylsky, C. A. Schmidt, K. Laurisch, B. Mowes, A. Radbruch, and A. Thiel. 2002. Two subsets of naïve T helper cells with distinct T cell receptor excision circle content in human adult peripheral blood. *J. Exp. Med.* **195:**789–794.

15. Liu, Z., W. G. Cumberland, L. E. Hultin, A. H. Kaplan, R. Detels, and J. Giorgi. 1998. CD8+ T-lymphocyte activation in HIV-1 disease reflects an aspect of pathogenesis distinct from viral burden and immunodeficiency. *J. Acquir. Immune Defic. Syndr. Hum. Retrovirol.* **18:**332–340.

16. Liu, Z., W. G. Cumberland, L. E. Hultin, H. E. Prince, R. Detels, and J. V. Giorgi. 1997. Elevated CD38 antigen expression on CD8+ T-cells is a stronger marker for the risk of chronic HIV disease progression to AIDS and death in the multicenter AIDS cohort study than CD4+ cell count, soluble immune activation markers, or combinations of HLA-DR and CD38 expression. *J. Acquir. Immune Defic. Syndr. Hum. Retrovirol.* **16:**83–92.

17. Lopez, A., I. Carogol, J. Candeias, N. Villamor, P. Echaniz, F. Ortuno, A. Sempere, K. Strauss, and A. Orfao. 1999. Enumeration of CD4+ T-cells in the peripheral blood of HIV-infected patients: an interlaboratory study of the FACSCount system. *Cytometry* **38:**231–237.

18. Margolick, J. B., A. Munoz, A. Donnenberg, L. P. Park, N. Galai, J. V. Giorgi, M. R. G. O'Gorman, and J. Ferbas. 1995. Failure of T-cell homeostasis preceding AIDS in HIV infection. *Nat. Med.* **1:**674–680.

19. Mildvan, D., R. J. Bosch, R. S. Kim, J. Spritzler, D. W. Haas, D. Kuritzkes, J. Kagan, M. Notka, V. DeGruttola, M. Moreno, and A. Landay. 2004. Immunophenotypic markers and antiretroviral therapy (IMART) cell activation and maturation help predict treatment response. *J. Infect. Dis.* **189:**1811–1820.

20. National Committee for Clinical Laboratory Standards. 1998. *Clinical Applications of Flow Cytometry. Quality Assurance and Immunophenotyping of Peripheral Blood Lymphocytes.* H42-A. National Committee for Clinical Laboratory Standards, Wayne, Pa.

21. Reimann, K. A., M. R. G. O'Gorman, J. Spritzler, C. L. Wilkening, D. E. Sabath, K. Helm, D. E. Campbell, and the NIAID DAIDS New Technologies Evaluation Group. 2000. Multisite comparison of CD4 and CD8 T-lymphocyte counting by single- versus multiple-platform methodologies:evaluation of Beckman Coulter Flow-Count fluorospheres and the tetraONE system. *Clin. Diagn. Lab. Immunol.* **7:**344–351.

22. Schenker, E. L., L. E. Hultin, K. D. Bauer, J. Ferbas, J. B. Margolick, and J. V. Giorgi. 1993. Evaluation of a dual-color flow cytometry immunophenotyping panel in a multicenter quality assurance program. *Cytometry.* **14:**307–317.

23. Schmid, I., A. Kunkl, and J. K. A. Nicholson. 1999. Biosafety considerations for flow cytometric analysis of human immunodeficiency virus-infected samples. *Cytometry.* **38:**195–200.

24. Schnizlein-Bick, C. T., J. Spritzler, C. L. Wilkening, J. K. A. Nicholson, M. R. G. O'Gorman, Site Investigators, and the NIAID DAIDS New Technologies Evaluation Group. 2000. Evaluation of TruCount absolute-count tubes for determining CD4 and CD8 cell numbers in human immunodeficiency virus-positive adults. *Clin. Diagn. Lab. Immunol.* **7:**336–343.

25. Shapiro, H. M. 2003. *Practical Flow Cytometry*, 4th ed. John Wiley & Sons, Hoboken, N.J.

26. Wilson, C. M., J. H. Ellenberg, S. D. Douglas, A. B. Moscicki, and C. A. Holland. 2004. CD8+ CD38+ T-cells but not HIV type 1 RNA viral load predict CD4+ T-cell loss in a predominantly minority female HIV+ adolescent population. *AIDS Res. Hum. Retrovir.* **20:**263–269.

27. Zaunders, J., A. Carr, L. McNally, R. Penny, and D. A. Cooper. 1995. Effects of primary HIV-1 infection on subsets of CD4+ and CD8+ T lymphocytes. *AIDS* **9:**561–566.

Nontraditional Clinical Applications: Paroxysmal Nocturnal Hemoglobinuria Testing, Fetal Red Cell Testing, T-Cell Receptor Vβ Analysis, and Platelet Analysis by Flow Cytometry

JIACHUN X. KUNG AND ERIC D. HSI

19

Flow cytometric immunophenotyping has several well-accepted applications. Determination of lymphocyte subsets in the diagnosis and monitoring of human immunodeficiency virus infection became the first major application that made flow cytometry an economically viable and medically necessary component of most large clinical laboratories. With dependence of modern classification schemes on immunophenotype, it has also become an indispensable part of the routine evaluation of leukemias and lymphomas. Immunophenotyping panels are generally focused upon lineage assignment and documentation of B-cell clonality. Specific phenotypic patterns are also assessed since they can be useful in classification of these disorders.

Flow cytometry is also beginning to be more widely used in other areas of hematologic malignancies, such as a diagnostic adjunct for myelodysplastic syndromes. Multiparameter flow cytometry is also making inroads into the detection of minimal residual disease. These applications can still be considered investigational. In this chapter we focus on four less common clinical applications of flow cytometry: paroxysmal nocturnal hemoglobinuria (PNH), T-cell receptor Vβ (TCR Vβ) analysis, fetal hemoglobin (Hgb F)detection, and platelet surface marker and functional testing.

PNH

PNH is an acquired hemolytic anemia due to a clonal hematopoietic stem cell mutation in the phosphatidylinositol glycan class A gene located on chromosome X. This leads to the inability to synthesize the glycosylphosphatidylinositol (GPI) anchor that binds numerous proteins to the cell membranes (3–5). The critical missing membrane proteins are complement-regulating surface proteins, which include decay-accelerating factor (CD55), homologous restriction factor or C8 binding protein, and the membrane inhibitor of reactive lysis (CD59). These proteins normally interact with complement proteins, particularly C3b and C4b, and dissociate the convertase complexes of the classic and alternative pathways. This interrupts complete activation of complement and thus protects cells from inappropriate complement-mediated lysis. Other cell surface molecules are absent in PNH, and many are listed in Tables 1 and 2 (29).

Three PNH red blood cell (RBC) phenotypes are recognized due to variations in genetic defects that can result in PNH. These are types I, II, and III, which exhibit normal, moderate, and severe complement sensitivities, respectively.

Clinical manifestations of intravascular hemolysis include the breakdown of RBCs with the release of hemoglobin into the urine, which is indicated by distinct dark-colored urine. Classically this occurs in the first morning urine due to concentration of hemoglobin in the urine overnight, which produces the dark color. This feature is a major symptom in PNH patients, with 84% of patients having hemoglobinuria as a chief symptom (28). Lack of GPI-linked proteins on other cell types leads to other manifestations. For example, complement activation plays a role in excessive platelet activation, microparticle formation, and elevated levels in plasma of leukocyte-derived tissue factor, which results in increased risk of thrombosis (23, 33, 42, 76). This is, in fact, a major source of morbidity and mortality in PNH patients (28, 51).

Classical clinical tests for PNH are aimed at demonstrating the presence of RBCs that are exceptionally sensitive to the hemolytic action of complement compared to normal RBCs (25, 26). These are the sucrose hemolysis test, which serves as a screening test, followed by the more specific acidified serum (Ham's) test. With Ham's test, a false-positive test result can be seen in congenital dyserythropoietic anemia, type II (hereditary erythroblastic multinuclearity with positive acidified serum tests). These patients have a negative sucrose hemolysis (sugar water) test. In addition, a false-negative Ham's test can also occur, and the sucrose water test is more sensitive but less specific for PNH. Neither of these assays is sensitive for small PNH populations (as may occur after an active phase of the disease and transfusion in which few PNH RBCs remain) and cannot be used to assess the size of the PNH clone.

Flow cytometry is becoming the preferred method for assessing blood samples for the presence of PNH clones (24). This method offers greater sensitivity and specificity than classical tests in identifying patients with PNH. Furthermore, flow cytometry tests are capable of easily detecting low levels of PNH cells (on the order of 1 to 2% in our experience) in a sample. Analysis of nonerythrocyte populations also allows one to detect PNH cells more easily in patients undergoing hemolysis or in the setting of recent transfusion. PNH granulocytes, in contrast to PNH RBCs, have a normal life span and so the percentage of abnormal granulocytes more accurately reflects the size of the PNH clone (10).

TABLE 1 CD markers for GPI-anchored proteins

Protein[a]	CD marker	Lineage
Endotoxin-binding protein receptor	CD14	Monocytes
Low-affinity IgG Fc receptor	CD16	Neutrophils, T cells
GPI-sialoglycoprotein	CD24	Neutrophils, B cells
GPI-anchored glycoprotein	CD48	Lymphocytes, monocytes
Campath-1 antigen	CD52	Lymphocytes
DAF	CD55	All
LFA-3	CD58	Lymphocytes, erythrocytes
MIRL	CD59	All
Selectin ligand	CD66b	Granulocytes
Ecto-5'-nucleotidase	CD73	Lymphocytes
uPAR	CD87	Monocytes, granulocytes, T cells, NK cells
Thy-1	CD90	Lymphocytes
JMH blood group antigen	CD108	Lymphocytes, erythrocytes
gp 170 kDa	CD109	T cells, platelets
Pre-B, thymocyte growth signal	CD157	Pre-B, pre-T, monocyte, granulocyte

[a]IgG, immunoglobulin G; DAF, decay-accelerating factor; LFA-3, lymphocyte function-associated antigen 3; MIRL, membrane inhibitor of reactive lysis; uPAR, urokinase plasminogen activator receptor; gp, glycoprotein.

Flow cytometry tests are capable of distinguishing types of PNH cells. Type I cells express normal amounts of GPI-linked antigens, type II cells display intermediate expression levels, and type III cells completely lack these antigens. The amounts of these types of cells vary from patient to patient. In a recent analysis, approximately 60% of patients displayed all three types of erythrocytes and 34% of patients showed types I and III, with less than 5% type II (61). Finally, flow cytometry allows quantitation of the PNH clone as a percentage of the total cells in the specimen. Some authors have correlated the amount of the clone with clinical parameters (1, 57). For example, Nishimura and colleagues suggest that decreasing populations of PNH cells are correlated with bone marrow failure (57). Moyo et al. have correlated increasing PNH clone size with risk of thrombosis (51).

There is a lack of consensus on specific methods for analyzing specimens for PNH clones. In general, most authors would state that at least two GPI-linked proteins should be absent on a cell type for one to conclude that a PNH clone is present (29, 61). Ideally, this should be done in a multicolor format to simultaneously assess the same cell (Fig. 1 and 2). One reason for this requirement is to exclude congenital deficiencies of some of these markers, such as CD55 or CD59 (60, 77). The Inab phenotype (congenital lack of the Cromer blood group, located on CD55) has been reported, and these patients lack other evidence of PNH (60). CD59 deficiency has also been reported, although patients appear symptomatic (77).

The PNH assay is unusual since a positive result is *decreased or absence of* reactivity to directly labeled monoclonal antibodies. This can cause some difficulties in cases in which clear separation from type I, II, or III cells is not apparent, making definitive threshold setting difficult. CD59 is preferable for distinguishing between these cell types since it is expressed at a density 10-fold greater than that of CD55 (30).

A kit is commercially available with control beads that assist operators in setting a threshold for lack of expression of CD55 and CD59 (32). These two antigens are analyzed on erythrocytes and neutrophils. A disadvantage of this kit is its reliance on single-color (fluorescein isothiocyanate [FITC]) analysis of the key antigens. Because clinical experience with PNH samples will be limited in most individual laboratories due to the rarity of the disorder, such a "standardized" kit may be useful, although individual laboratories must still validate the assay (32). Using definitions supplied by the manufacturer, the minimum sensitivity for this assay is 3% PNH cells. However, we have found that in

TABLE 2 Parameters used for gating specific cell types and GPI-linked proteins for PNH screening

Lineage	Cell markers useful for gating	CDs for GPI protein
RBCs		
Reticulocytes	Thiazole orange, LS[a]	CD59, CD58, CD55
Erythrocytes	Glycophorin A, LS	CD59, CD58, CD55
Leukocytes		
Neutrophils	CD33, LS	CD66b, CD24, CD16
Monocytes	CD33, LS	CD14, CD48
Granulocytes	CD11b, LS	CD16, CD55, CD59
Lymphocytes		
T	CD3, LS	CD48, CD52
B	CD19	CD24
Progenitor cells	CD34, CD45	CD59
Platelets	CD41, CD42, CD61, LS	CD55

[a]LS, light scatter.

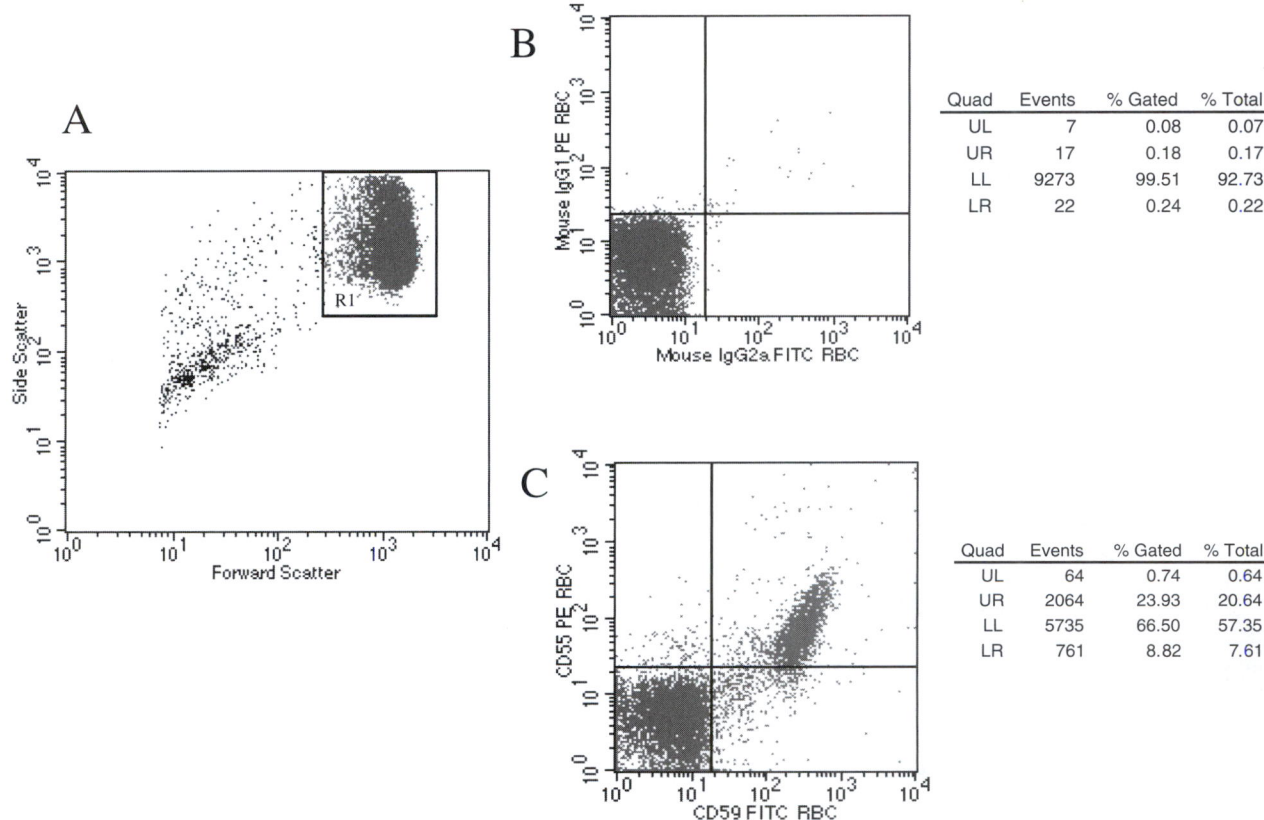

FIGURE 1 PNH analysis of RBCs. (A) Light scatter gating of RBCs; (B) isotype control; (C) dual-color CD55 and CD59 staining identifies CD55⁻ CD59⁻ RBCs in a PNH patient.

our specimens, the 3% threshold was a bit low, particularly for CD59 on granulocytes when clinical diagnosis of PNH was used as the standard. Dual reagents are available that allow simultaneous assessment of CD55 and CD59 expression on erythrocytes and granulocytes. Analysis for dually negative cells increases sensitivity and specificity in our experience.

In addition to CD55 and CD59, other antigens recommended by many authors include CD66b and CD16 on neutrophils and CD14 on monocytes (1, 24, 1, 27, 32, 61, 62). The latter can be problematic in our experience due to the wide distribution of expression intensity and the difficulty in collecting enough events in specimens with a relatively low monocyte count. These white cell antigens can be paired with CD45 and CD13; this allows for specific gating using CD45, side scatter, and CD13 expression characteristics. CD66b is highly expressed on granulocytes and is suitable for diagnostic purposes.

Detection of a large population of PNH-type cells with these assays in the appropriate clinical setting, such as significant intravascular hemolysis, is diagnostic of PNH. However, interpretation of low levels of these cells in subclinical patients (no evidence of PNH) can be problematic since GPI-deficient clones can be detected in patients with marrow failure syndromes such as aplastic anemia, myelodysplasia, or other clonal bone marrow disorders (34, 45). The significance of such a finding is uncertain; however, it has been reported that patients with bone marrow failure syndrome and minor PNH clones respond to immunotherapy (74). Consequently, it is best to merely report the presence or absence of a PNH clone and its relative abundance. Correlation by the ordering

physician with the clinical findings may help stratify patients into one of three categories: classical PNH, PNH with bone marrow failure syndrome, or subclinical (laboratory PNH) (The International PNH Interest Group, unpublished data). Because of variation in the size of the clone, multiple analyses for a single patient may be needed to confirm the presence of a PNH clone. Due to possible time-dependent loss of antigen expression, a freshly (<24 h) drawn EDTA-anticoagulated specimen is required for appropriate analysis. An example protocol follows.

PNH Staining Protocol (55)

1. Patient sample: EDTA-anticoagulated blood (<24 h old, preferably <12 h).
2. For erythrocytes:
   a. Use 10 μl of 1:10-diluted whole blood in phosphate-buttered saline (PBS).
   b. Incubate for 15 min at room temperature with anti-CD59-FITC and anti-CD59-phycoerythrin (anti-CD59-PE) antibodies (clones MEM54 and MEM140-30; Research Diagnostics, Flanders, N.J.).
   c. Wash once with PBS.
   d. Pellet cells and resuspend with 0.5 ml of PBS for erythrocytes (instead of PBS, incubate for 15 min with 0.5 ml of thiazol orange or Recticount for reticulocytes).
   e. Analyze within 2 h (or place at 4 to 10°C for overnight storage). Dually negative cells should be enumerated.

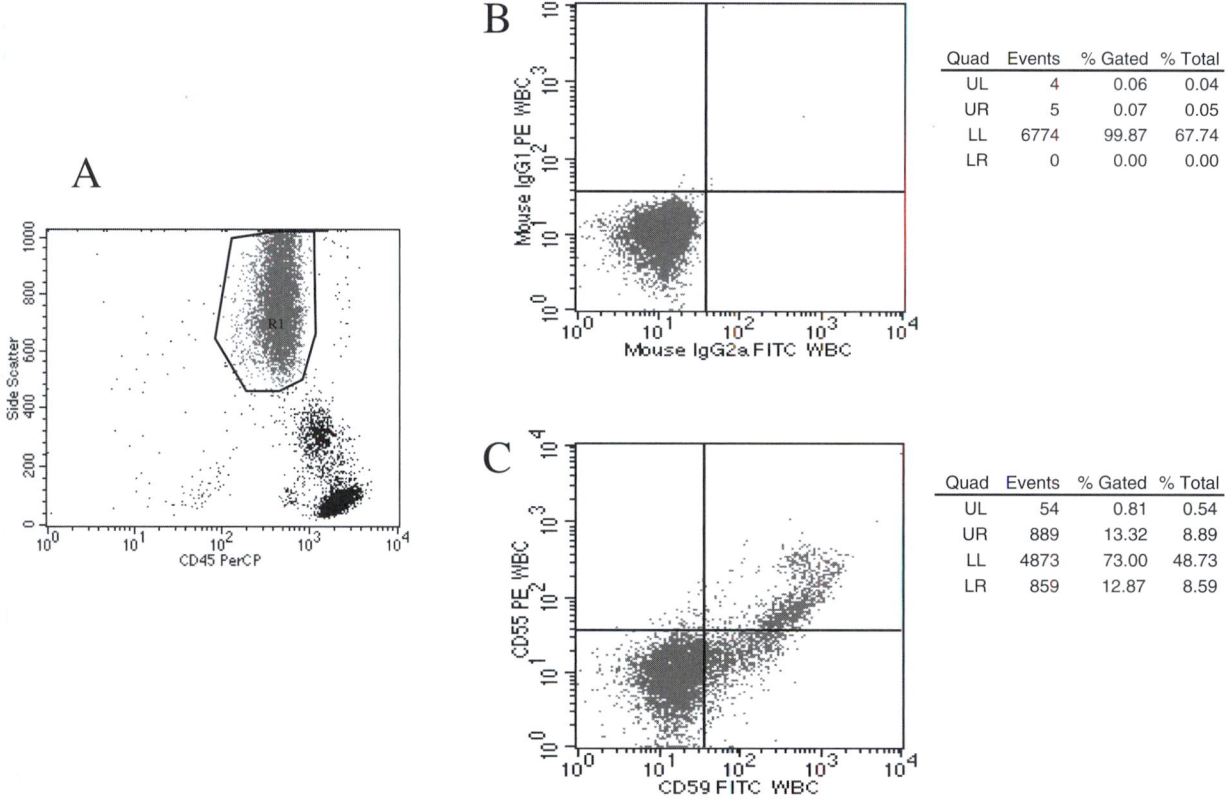

Quad	Events	% Gated	% Total
UL	4	0.06	0.04
UR	5	0.07	0.05
LL	6774	99.87	67.74
LR	0	0.00	0.00

Quad	Events	% Gated	% Total
UL	54	0.81	0.54
UR	889	13.32	8.89
LL	4873	73.00	48.73
LR	859	12.87	8.59

FIGURE 2 PNH analysis of neutrophils. (A) CD45 and light scatter gating of neutrophils; (B) isotype control; (C) two-color CD55 and CD59 staining identifies CD55$^-$ CD59$^-$ neutrophils in PNH patient.

Notes

1. Avoid heparinized plasma since it causes platelet aggregation.

2. Use isotype controls.

3. Perform the test within 24 h after sample collection.

4. Lyse RBCs for leukocyte analysis (otherwise use whole blood for RBCs and platelets).

5. For leukocytes, incubate 50 μl of whole blood with 20 μl of antibodies to CD66b-FITC, CD13-PE, CD45-PerCP, and CD14-allophycocyanin for 15 min (CD66b clone 80H3 from Beckman-Coulter [Hialeah, Fla.] and remaining antibodies from BD Biosciences[San Jose, Calif.]). Lyse erythrocytes and wash with PBS as described above. Analyze granulocyte gate (CD45$^+$ CD13$^+$ CD14$^-$ high side scatter) looking for CD66b-negative cells. CD14 can be used to enumerate monocytes using CD45 side scatter gating but is more difficult in our experience.

6. The lower limit of detection of PNH cells should be determined in each laboratory using normal volunteer samples.

Interferences to stained cells can occur from other cells:

- Erythrocytes: white blood cells and macrothrombocytes
- Neutrophils: eosinophils and immature myeloid progenitors (CD16$^+$ or CD24$^+$)
- Lymphocytes: RBCs, normoblasts, macrothrombocytes, and basophils
- Monocytes: difficult to define by light scattering
- Platelets: require particle-free solutions

Most recently, a fluorescently labeled inactive variant of aerolysin (FLAER) has been shown to be sensitive and specific for assessment of GPI-linked protein deficiency in PNH patients (9). Aerolysin is a toxin produced by *Aeromonas hydrophila* and has the property of binding to GPI anchors; thus, it is useful in identifying PNH cells by lack of binding. Type III PNH cells are completely resistant to lysis by the active toxin (32). It more effectively identifies GPI-deficient nucleated cells than RBCs because of a higher fluorescent signal intensity in the former than in the latter. Flow cytometric assays using FLAER may prove to be a widely used method for identifying PNH cells in the near future. The United Kingdom National Quality Assessment Service has preliminarily tested stabilized PNH samples that may be helpful in assessing performance and developing standardized procedures.

TCR Vβ ANALYSIS BY FLOW CYTOMETRY

T cells recognize antigens via clonally distributed TCR heterodimers, of which the vast majority are composed of α and β chains and a small subset (1 to 5%) carry the alternative γ and δ chains. Demonstration of monoclonal rearrangement of these TCR genes plays a central role in the diagnosis of T-cell malignancy. Classical techniques such as Southern blot hybridization and PCR have enabled monoclonal T-cell proliferations to be detected reliably in clinical samples. (68, 70).

Southern blot analysis is the "gold standard" method for investigation of T-cell clonality, with a sensitivity level in the range of 1 to 5% of clonal cells in the total infiltrate.

Southern blotting using TCR Jβ probes is a reliable and sensitive (fewer false negatives) method but requires a long preparation time and large amounts of high-quality DNA in order to obtain results. PCR-based methods for assessing TCR Vβ or Vγ rearrangement have become popular, and VJγ PCR has become widely used in clinical laboratories. These PCR assays are relatively quick (on the order of days), and assays for TCR-γ rearrangement can be adapted for use in paraffin-embedded tissues. However, the limited repertoire of the Vγ locus, which is attractive from the perspective of consensus primer design, makes false positives possible. The diversity and complexity of the Vβ gene locus require the use of numerous primers in multiplex formats, and false negatives due to lack of consensus primer binding remain a possibility (68, 70). Optimal analysis of PCR products requires capillary gel electrophoresis or heteroduplex analysis (68). Extensive development and validation testing of agreed-upon consensus PCR primers and methods are ongoing for these molecular methods (68).

In recent years, monoclonal antibody reagents specific to various TCR-β family V regions have become available. Since the TCRβ V genes can be divided into functional families, one can use these reagents to assess the TCR repertoire in peripheral blood T cells. Just as immunoglobulin light-chain restriction (kappa and lambda) can be used as a surrogate for B-cell clonality, so too can skewing or restriction of TCR Vβ family expression patterns. In order to facilitate this, commercially available antibodies to 24 specificities covering 19 TCR Vβ families have been combined in a multicolor flow cytometry format to allow assessment of TCR Vβ usage. This format accounts for approximately 70% of T cells in peripheral blood, and normal ranges for each family in healthy volunteers have been determined (67).

The use of Vβ flow cytometry in diagnosing T-cell chronic lymphoproliferative disorders in blood has been assessed (2, 37, 38). Clear overrepresentation of a particular Vβ family can be used as a surrogate for molecular studies for TCR gene rearrangements when one suspects a T-cell lymphoproliferative disorder on clinical and morphological grounds (Fig. 3). Likewise, accounting for only a fraction of T cells using this kit (less than 50%) can also be taken as evidence for a clonal T-cell proliferation. Beck et al. found a 100% sensitivity and 88% specificity for T-cell lymphoproliferative disorders in blood in their study (2). No clear association with a particular disease entity and Vβ family usage has been found. As with all ancillary testing for clonality in lymphoid malignancies, these results should be considered in clinical context. For example, restricted Vβ expression was seen in 2 of 16 control samples (patients presenting with a concern of a lymphoproliferative disorder who ultimately were not found to have a lymphoproliferative disorder) that were also confirmed to be monoclonal by TCR-γ PCR analysis (2). Examples of monoclonal T-cell populations in the elderly or in certain clinical situations such as autoimmune disorders have been documented (20, 59). In addition to assisting in primary diagnosis, TCR Vβ flow cytometry has also been used to monitor therapy in patients with cutaneous T-cell lymphoma. Given its limited sensitivity, it is unlikely that TCR Vβ flow cytometry will have a large role in residual disease detection. The following details a sample protocol.

TCR Vβ Staining Protocol (IOTest Beta Mark Manufacturer's Protocol)

1. Prepare peripheral blood with anticoagulant (EDTA preferred).

2. Incubate blood sample with appropriate antibody for 20 min at room temperature (in the dark, IOTest Beta Mark TCR Vβ Repertoire kit [Beckman-Coulter] and anti-CD3).

3. Lyse erythrocytes.

4. Fix cells and then wash and resuspend them for analysis.

Notes

1. Stain cells with appropriate isotypic conjugated antibodies to serve as controls (for fluorescence limits of background).

2. Lymphocyte gate set with forward scatter (size parameter):

   a. For TCR Vβ usage, one can select for total CD3+ T cells or dual CD3+ CD4+ and CD3+ CD8+ T cells using appropriate gating antibodies.

   b. The manufacturer supplies normal ranges for peripheral blood. A good control is a summation of total T-cell percentage accounted for in the Vβ analysis. A very small number suggests an aberrant population using a Vβ family not detected by the kit reagents. A number greater than 100% suggests a problem with background or analysis thresholds.

Hgb F MEASUREMENT BY FLOW CYTOMETRY

Detection of Hgb F in RBCs has several clinical applications. The most common method is the Kleihauer-Betke test (KBT), which enumerates Hgb F-containing cells based on their relative resistance to acid elution (39). In this test, RBCs are fixed on a slide and exposed to a citric acid sodium phosphate buffer solution that elutes Hgb A but leaves Hgb F in fetal RBCs. Slides are stained with hematoxylin and eosin and a manual count of fetal cells is performed as percentage of RBCs (39). This test has many disadvantages, including its manual nature, subjectivity, limited sensitivity, and high coefficient of variation.

Flow cytometric analysis of Hgb F is superior to the KBT. In this assay, RBCs are permeabilized, stained with fluorescent antibodies to Hgb F, and analyzed by flow cytometry. Determination of Hgb F by flow cytometry has several clinical applications, including the diagnosis and quantitation of fetomaternal hemorrhage (FMH) (11, 14, 44, 56), determining the cellular distribution of Hgb F in adult RBCs (so-called F cells) in various hemoglobinopathies (31), and monitoring therapies aimed at increasing Hgb F, such as in hydroxyurea therapy for sickle cell disease (17, 46, 52, 54).

Much of the effort in developing flow cytometry assays has focused on detecting and quantitating fetal RBCs in maternal blood for the detection and quantitation of FMH (11, 14, 36, 53, 56). Detection of fetal cells can confirm the diagnosis of FMH, and quantitation can guide therapy to prevent maternal alloimmunization to RhD antigen in RhD-negative mothers. These assays show improved sensitivity (as low as 0.02%), precision, and linearity over manual methods (14, 44, 56). Chen and colleagues summarized College of American Pathology survey data showing markedly superior performance of laboratories performing FMH determinations by flow cytometry compared to traditional methods. In a sample made to simulate values close to the 0.6% level, which triggers an additional therapy with Rh immune globulin, approximately 50% of laboratories failed to correctly identify the specimens by traditional methods, while most laboratories correctly identified them by flow cytometry (11). A U.S. Food and Drug

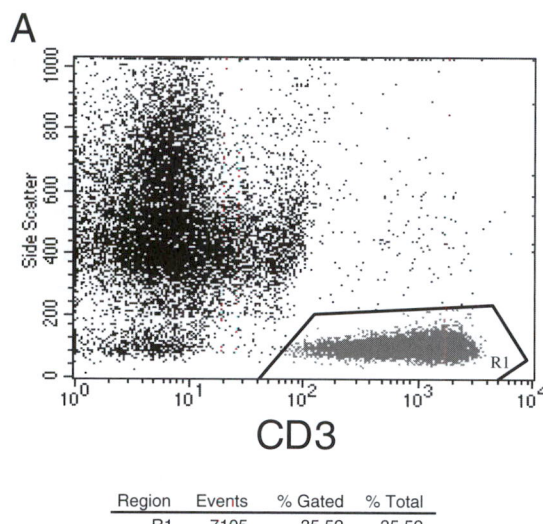

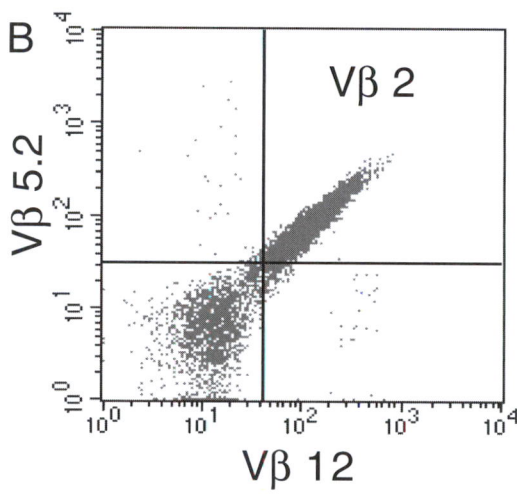

Region	Events	% Gated	% Total
R1	7105	35.52	35.52

Quad	Events	% Gated	% Total
UL	102	1.54	0.51
UR	4312	64.97	21.56
LL	2036	30.68	10.18
LR	187	2.82	0.94

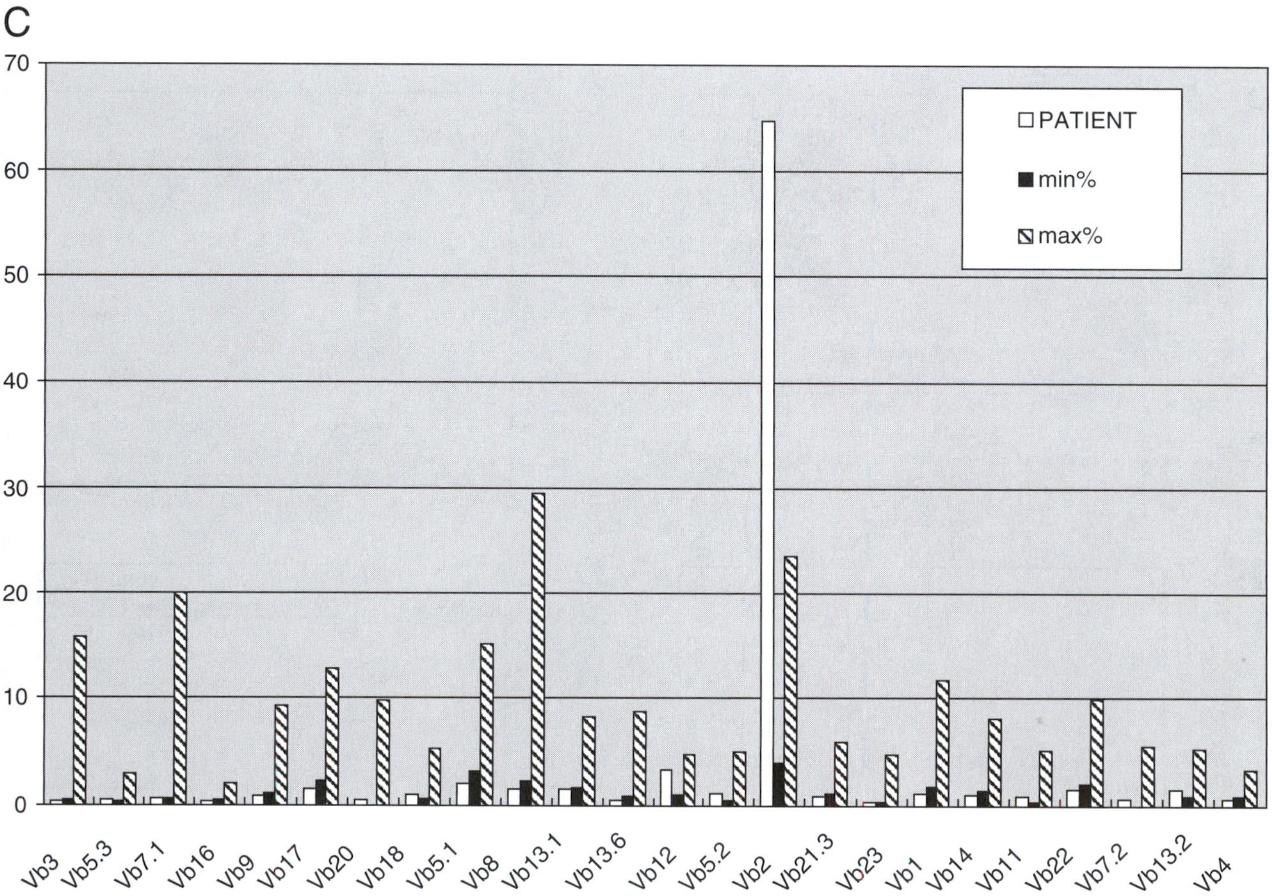

C

FIGURE 3 Vβ analysis, T large granular lymphocyte leukemia. (A) CD3 gating for analysis. More specific CD4 or CD8 gating may also be done. (B) Dot plot analysis of T-cell gate with Vβ 12 FITC, Vβ 5.2 PE, and Vβ 2 PE/FITC. (C) Bar graph of Vβ expression showing marked overexpression of Vβ 2.

Administration-approved test is now available for this assay. High and low controls are also available for this assay but can also be made using cord blood to spike adult blood samples. This assay specifies procedures for specimen preparation, fixation, staining, data acquisition, and analysis (Fig. 4) (http://www.caltag.com/pdf/L13011.pdf).

Of note, gating strategies have been devised to assist with finding small numbers of fetal RBCs by gating out autofluorescent leukocytes that might contaminate a light scatter RBC gate and are currently recommended by the manufacturer (36, 53, 75). This method suggests that the operator first draw a light scatter gate around erythrocytes and then visualize the gated cells on an FL2-versus-FL1 plot (FITC-conjugated anti-Hgb F). This allows one to exclude autofluorescent cells in FL2 that also show FL1 signal. This procedure results in increased sensitivity. Wide use of flow cytometry for this application may change the opinion of clinicians regarding the use (or lack thereof) of the KBT in managing FMH (15, 16, 66). Familiarity with the variability of F cells, which can at times be strongly positive in some settings, such as thalassemia or other hemoglobinopathy, is needed so that one does not mistake such cells for FMH (36, 35). The following is an example protocol.

Fetal Cell Staining Protocol (65) (Manufacturer Protocol)

1. Prepare EDTA whole blood, less than 30 h old.
2. Use 10 μl of whole blood fixed with 0.5% glutaraldehyde for 10 min; wash 3× in PBS–0.1% bovine serum albumin (BSA).
3. Permeabilize cells with 0.1% Triton X-100 in PBS for 3 to 5 min at room temperature, and wash once in PBS–0.1% BSA.
4. Resuspend in 0.5 ml of PBS–0.1% BSA. Add together 10 μl of cell suspension, 5 μl of anti-Hgb F, and 70 μl of PBS–0.1% BSA. Incubate for 15 min in the dark.
5. Wash with PBS–0.1% BSA, and resuspend in 0.5 ml of PBS–0.1% BSA with 1% formaldehyde.

Notes

1. Patient sample is to be assayed within 20 h.
2. For control cells, a commercially available reagent may be used (Fetatrol) or a control can be made using umbilical cord and adult blood dilutions.
3. The gating strategy to remove autofluorescent cells is important for optimal assay sensitivity.

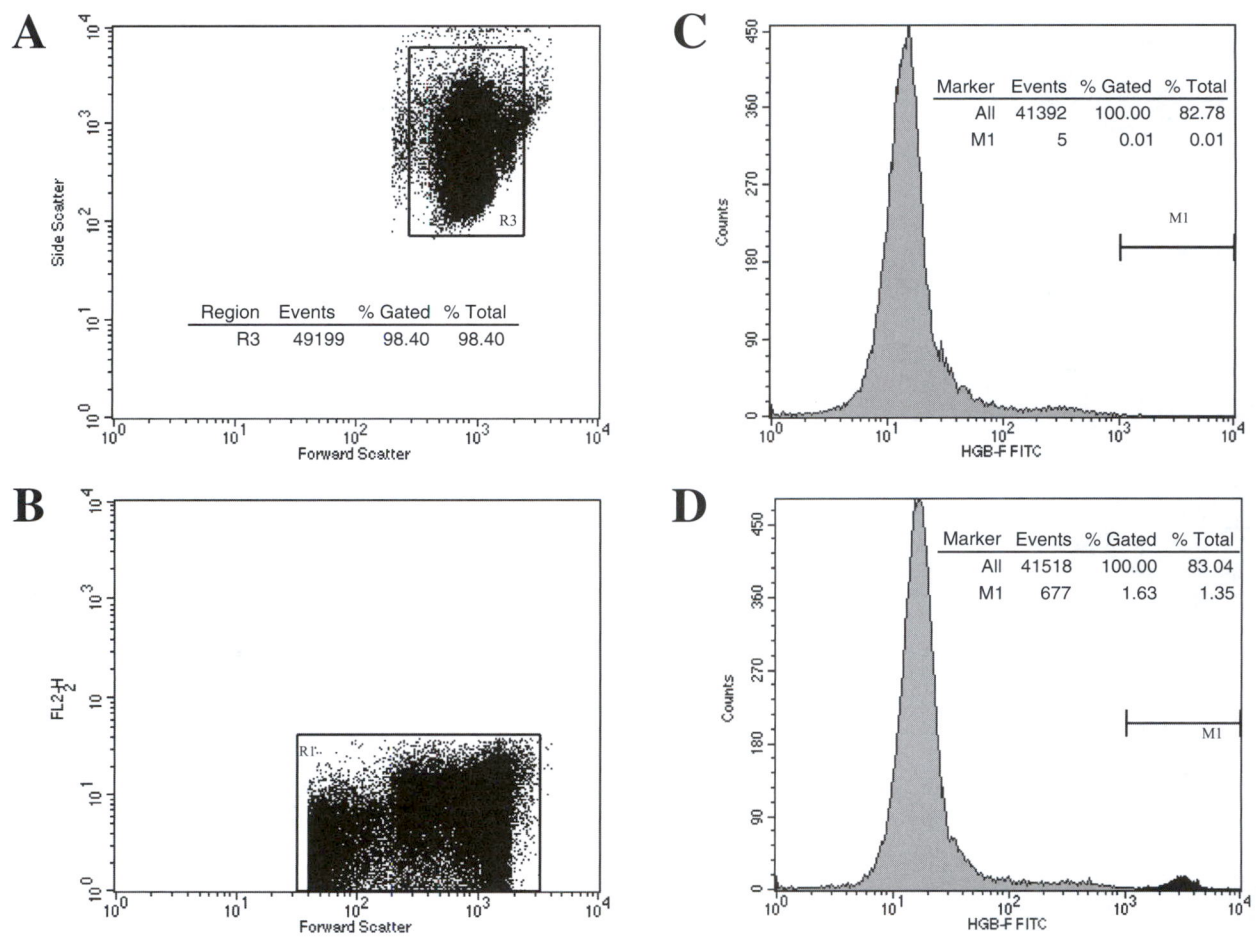

FIGURE 4 Hgb F testing. (A) Forward and side scatter gating of RBCs. (B) Cells with high FL2 are excluded from acquisition to avoid problems with autofluorescence. (C) Case with no detectable fetal RBCs. (D) Case with 1.6% fetal RBCs.

Practical issues regarding availability (or lack thereof) of this test during off-hours of the laboratory need to be addressed with clinical services, and a KBT may need to be retained in the laboratory as a backup method.

PLATELET ANALYSIS

Structural and functional defects in platelets can lead to a variety of bleeding disorders. Standard clinical tests have been developed to assess platelet function, including bleeding time and platelet aggregometry (41). The traditional bleeding time test is fraught with variability and poor reproducibility, since it is dependent on platelet number and function, fibrinogen concentration, operator technique, patient cooperation, skin temperature, skin quality, incision size, and the site of incision. Platelet aggregometry, performed either by impedance using whole blood or by turbidimetry using platelet-rich plasma, evaluates platelet-platelet binding and agonist-induced platelet activation. Results of these tests are affected by medication, age of sample, processing temperature, stirring rate, and platelet count. Aggregometry may show whether platelet reactivity is affected by a particular clinical condition but is unable to determine the activation status of platelets, or to detect distinct subpopulations of platelets, or to measure the extent of activation of individual platelets.

Development of commercially available antibodies to relevant platelet antigens permits the discrimination between activated and resting platelets and permits platelet receptor quantitation (40, 44, 49). A small amount of whole blood (about 10 μl per tube) is needed, and there is minimal sample manipulation prior to analysis. The following paragraphs describe current usage of flow cytometry in diagnosing and monitoring platelet disorders.

Patients with diseases involving genetic abnormalities in platelet surface receptors exhibit aggregation anomalies (44, 58, 64). Glanzmann's thrombasthenia results from mutations in the genes for GPIIb and GPIIIa, thereby preventing the aggregation of platelets in response to fibronectin, fibrinogen, von Willebrand factor (vWF), and vitronectin. The absence of GPIIb and GPIIIa is traditionally confirmed via sodium dodecyl sulfate-polyacrylamide gel electrophoresis of radiolabeled platelet proteins. However, with the availability of antibodies to GPIIb and GPIIIa, flow cytometry offers a more efficient and non-radioactive method for detecting the deficiency concurrently on all desired cellular populations (Fig. 5). With Bernard-Soulier disease, there is defective expression of the GPIb-GPIX-GPV complex (the platelet receptor for vWF) and a lack of response to ristocetin (41). Flow cytometry can be performed to scan for deficiencies in GPIbα, GPIX, and GPV, using the appropriate platelet identifiers (GPIIb and GPIIIa) (see Table 3) (13, 63). Other disorders in this category are the Gray platelet syndrome and May-Hegglin anomaly (MYH9-related disease) (48). Flow cytometry studies have shown that the platelets in gray platelet syndrome have abnormal expression of CD62 (P-selectin) on the surface and in the alpha granule (41).

Platelet dense granule storage pool disease results from a deficiency of dense granules or a defect in granule release via

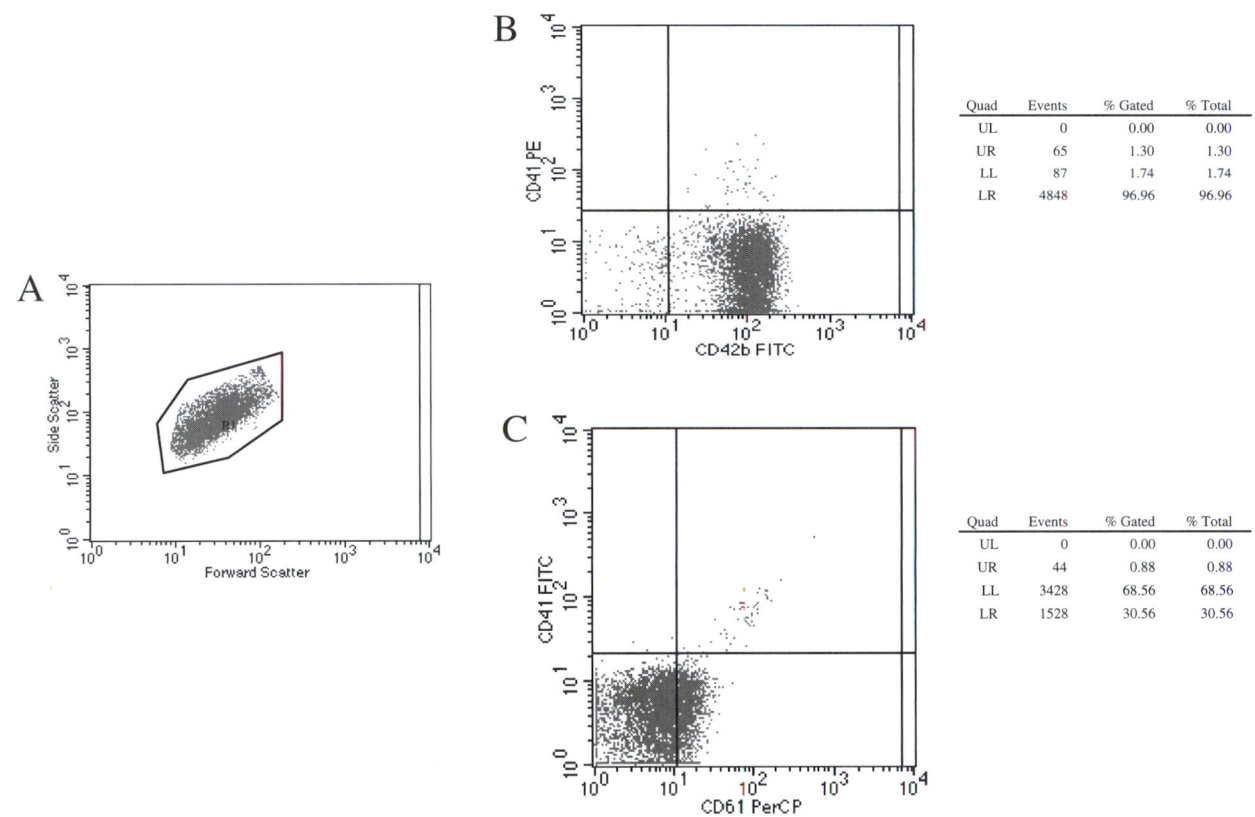

Quad	Events	% Gated	% Total
UL	0	0.00	0.00
UR	65	1.30	1.30
LL	87	1.74	1.74
LR	4848	96.96	96.96

Quad	Events	% Gated	% Total
UL	0	0.00	0.00
UR	44	0.88	0.88
LL	3428	68.56	68.56
LR	1528	30.56	30.56

FIGURE 5 Platelet flow cytometry surface analysis. (A) Light scatter gating of platelets; (B) loss of expression of CD41; and (C) marked decrease in CD61 expression. These features are consistent with Glanzmann's thrombasthenia.

TABLE 3 Platelet markers

Platelet protein[a]	Marker
Tetraspan-associated molecule	CD9
LFA-1, integrin alpha	CD11a
Lactocylceramide	CDw17
Integrin beta chain	CD29
PECAM-1	CD31
IgG Fc receptor (FcγRII)	CD32
GPIIIb	CD36
GPIIb	CD41
vWF receptor	CD42
Leukosialin	CD43
gp, 85–200 kDa	CD44
VLA-1 alpha chain	CD49
ICAM-3	CD50
Integrin alpha	CD51
Tetraspan family	CD53
DAF	CD55
LFA-3	CD58
MACIF	CD59
9-O-acetyl GD3	CDw60
GPIIIa	CD61
Selectins (E, L, P)	CD62
Activated platelet gp	CD63
Sialomucin	CD68
AIM	CD69
gp, 72–86 kDa	CD84
gp, 100–120 kDa	CD107
PDGF receptor	CD140
Thrombomodulin	CD141
gp, 32 kDa	CD151

[a]LFA-1, lymphocyte function-associated antigen 1; IgG, immunoglobulin G; gp, glycoprotein; DAF, decay-accelerating factors; PDGF, platelet-derived growth factor.

platelet activation (41). Hereditary and congenital forms such as Hermansky-Pudlak syndrome and δ-storage pool disease and acquired forms such as in myeloproliferative or rheumatologic disorders exist. Clinical diagnosis is supported by monitoring uptake of mepacrine (a fluorescent molecule that is rapidly taken up and localized to dense granules) into dense granules of platelets and its loss with dense granules release upon stimulation (Fig. 6) (22,72). This is more reproducible with flow cytometry than with fluorescent microscopy (6, 49). If the granule release deficiency is a function of a defect in epinephrine or collagen receptor, then confirmation via flow cytometry can be obtained by scanning for either receptor. The following is an example protocol for surface marker expression and analysis of granule release.

Platelet Staining Protocol (from Reference 49; Cleveland Clinic Protocol)

1. Use citrated whole blood or citrated platelet-rich plasma. A simultaneous sample from normal donor should be run with the patient sample as a control.
2. Set up tubes as in Table 4.
   Reagents
   CD41a, CD42b, CD49b, CD36, CD29 (Beckman-Coulter)
   CD61, CD62P, CD42a (BD Biosciences)
   Mepacrine (Q3251; Sigma Chemical, St. Louis, Mo.): 0.1 M solution (10× working stock) in Dulbecco PBS without Ca^{2+} or Mg^{2+}

Staining medium (9.9 ml of Dulbecco PBS + 100 μl of newborn calf serum [Sigma])
ADP stock (A2754; Sigma): working solution of 45 mg of ADP in 0.5 ml of distilled H_2O (dH_2O); store at 2 to 8°C
Thrombin (T9135; Sigma): one vial diluted with 0.5 ml of dH_2O; store at 2 to 8°C
RGDS (A9041; Sigma): 10 mg diluted with 1 ml of Dulbecco PBS; store at 2 to 8°C
3. Surface staining
   a. Add 100 μl of staining medium to tubes 1 through 7.
   b. Add 5 μl of each appropriate antibody to each tube (Table 4).
   c. Prepare a separate tube containing 50 μl of ADP and 20 μl of RGDS. Label this tube "Platelet activation."
   d. Add 10 μl of whole blood to tubes 1–6 and 450 μl of whole blood to the tube labeled "Platelet activation." Incubate for 15 min at room temperature in the dark.
   e. After 15 min, add 500 μl of cold 1% paraformaldehyde to tubes 1 to 6.
   f. Add 10 μl of "Platelet activation" tube to tube 7 and incubate for 15 min at room temperature in the dark. Add 500 μl of cold 1% paraformaldehyde to tube 7. This serves to determine whether platelets are capable of being activated.
4. Store refrigerated until ready for data acquisition (up to 48 h).

Mepacrine Staining Protocol (from Reference 49; Cleveland Clinic Protocol)

Mepacrine testing should be done with a normal control sample to confirm thrombin activation and mepacrine uptake.

1. In a separate tube, dilute 50 μl of sample blood with 1.95 ml of staining medium.
2. Add 10 μl of mepacrine and 5 μl of appropriate antibody to tubes 8 and 9.
3. Add 250 μl of diluted blood from step 1 to tubes 8 and 9 and incubate for 30 min at 37°C (water bath).
4. Label two blank tubes "8 post incubation" and "9 post incubation." Add 950 μl of Dulbecco PBS to each tube.
5. Remove 50-μl aliquots of incubated blood from tubes 8 and 9 and add to tubes "8 post incubation" and "9 post incubation," respectively. Immediate acquire data. The "8 post incubation" tube will serve as the control for inadvertent activation of platelets and "9 post incubation" will serve as a baseline for mepacrine uptake.
6. Take 500 μl of sample from tube 9 and place in tube 10. Add 20 μl of thrombin to tube 10 and incubate for 15 min at room temperature. Acquire data immediately. This serves to determine mepacrine release.

Interpretive guidelines

Surface Staining

Antibody	Reference range
CD41a (GPIIb/GPIIIa) fibrinogen receptor	95 to 100%
CD61 (GPIIIa) fibrinogen receptor	95 to 100%
CD42b (GPIb) vWF receptor	95 to 100%
CD42a (GPIX)	92 to 100%
CD36 collagen receptor	95 to 100%
CD49b (GPIa) collagen receptor	69 to 100%
CD29 (GPIIa) collagen receptor	95 to 100%

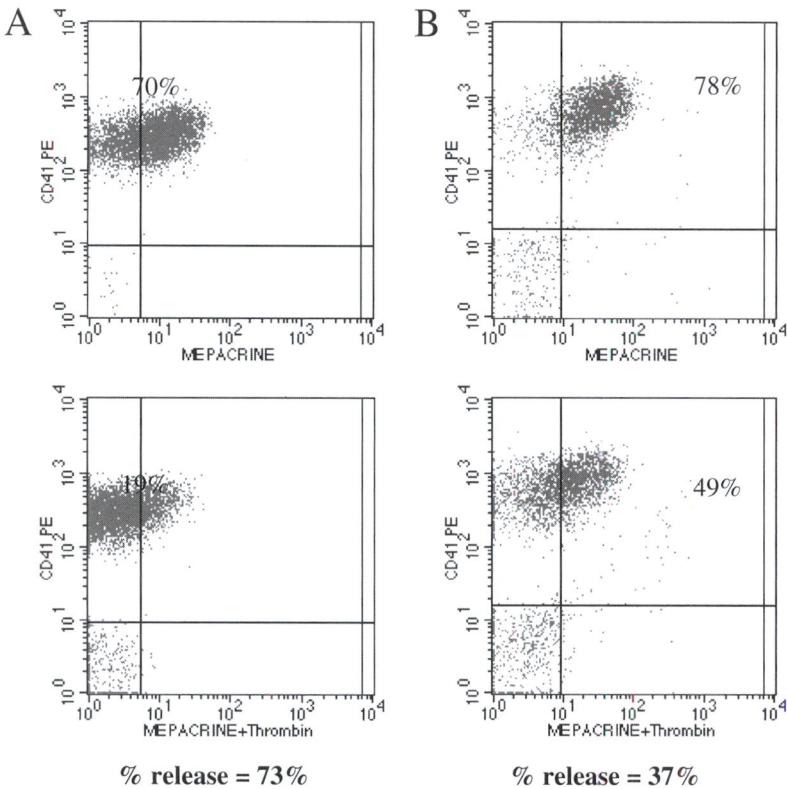

$$\% \text{ release} = 73\% \qquad \% \text{ release} = 37\%$$

FIGURE 6 Mepacrine release as a measure of granule function. (A) Platelets loaded with mepacrine show normal fluorescence uptake (upper panel) which decreases upon thrombin activation and granule release (lower panel). (B) Abnormal (decreased) mepacrine release compared to normal.

Mepacrine Uptake and Release

Percent release = [(percent M_u − percent $M_{thrombin}$)/ percent M_u] × 100, where M_u is mepacrine uptake and $M_{thrombin}$ is percent of mepacrine left in tube 10.

Parameter	Reference range
Mepacrine uptake	54 to 84%
Mepacrine release	58 to 93%
CD62P (P-selectin)	0 to 12%
CD62P + ADP	33 to 86%

Notes (mepacrine portion of panel)

1. No fixing is required, since fixing prevents mepacrine uptake.
2. Mepacrine fluorescence decreases with time. Immediate analysis is required.
3. Dilution of sample blood minimizes platelet aggregation.
4. Platelet-specific antibodies can be used as a gating tool (such as CD61).
5. Carefully monitor the light scattering aspects of the platelets since they can be large or small. Large platelets from

TABLE 4 Tube setup for platelet staining protocol

Tube	FITC	PE	PerCP	Comment
1[a]	Auto	Auto	Auto	
2	CD42b	CD41a	CD42a	
3	CD49b		CD61	
4	CD29		CD61	
5	CD36		CD61	
6	CD41a	CD62P	CD61	Platelet (Plt) activation negative control
7	CD41a	CD62P	CD61	Platelet activation positive control, ADP/RGDS added
8	CD41a	CD62P		
9	Mepacrine	CD41a		
10				Thrombin added for platelet activation and mepacrine increase

[a]A negative control tube is unstained (autofluorescence).

giant platelet syndrome can be mistaken for RBCs or lymphocytes, and thus a platelet identifier is requisite.

6. Specimens should be scheduled with the laboratory so that patient and normal patient control specimens can be drawn immediately prior to processing.

7. Overall interpretation requires knowledge of the clinical setting and recent history of medications that might interfere with platelet function, such as nonsteroidal anti-inflammatory drugs.

Idiopathic thrombocytopenic purpura is primarily a disease of increased peripheral platelet destruction, with most patients carrying antibodies to specific platelet membrane glycoproteins, resulting in splenic sequestration and phagocytosis by mononuclear macrophages (12, 41). Destruction of the circulating platelets, combined with inadequate platelet production by bone marrow megakaryocytes, results in the decreased platelet count. The presence of platelet-associated antibodies (PAIgs) can be ascertained by flow cytometry (18). However, because of issues of sensitivity and specificity of PAIgs, clinical guidelines do not require demonstration of such antibodies (21). Thus, flow cytometry-based assays for PAIg have not become part of routine clinical assays in most laboratories.

Circulating activated platelets have been reported for several diseases, including myeloproliferative disorders, thrombocythemia, hypertension, cardiovascular diseases, diabetes, and polycythemia (38, 40). Flow cytometry using annexin V binding to the exposed aminophospholipids can be employed to monitor the activation process of the platelets during disease progression and treatment, such as for patients undergoing coronary angioplasty and stent implantation (71). Similarly, platelet activation studies have shown that patients with ischemic cerebrovascular disease display excessive platelet and/or endothelial cell activation (47). Furthermore, reticulated platelets (youngest circulating platelets) can be selectively assayed by staining the platelets with thiazole orange (an RNA dye) and gating against platelet-specific markers (e.g., CD42 or CD41) (49). The measurement of reticulated platelets can be used in the assessment of patients with idiopathic thrombocytopenic purpura and assessing bone marrow recovery after chemotherapy or transplantation (7, 19, 74). The latter studies are not routinely performed in our clinical laboratory.

REFERENCES

1. **Alfinito, F., L. Del Vecchio, S. Rocco, P. Boccuni, P. Musto, and B. Rotoli.** 1996. Blood cell flow cytometry in paroxysmal nocturnal hemoglobinuria: a tool for measuring the extent of the PNH clone. *Leukemia* **10:**1326–1330.

2. **Beck, R. C., S. Stahl, C. L. O'Keefe, J. P. Maciejewski, K. S. Theil, and E. D. Hsi.** 2003. Detection of mature T-cell leukemias by flow cytometry using anti-T-cell receptor V beta antibodies. *Am. J. Clin. Pathol.* **120:**785–794.

3. **Bessler, M., P. Hillmen, L. Longo, L. Luzzatto, and P. J. Mason.** 1994. Genomic organization of the X-linked gene (PIG-A) that is mutated in paroxysmal nocturnal haemoglobinuria and of a related autosomal pseudogene mapped to 12q21. *Hum. Mol. Genet.* **3:**751–757.

4. **Bessler, M., P. J. Mason, P. Hillmen, and L. Luzzatto.** 1994. Mutations in the PIG-A gene causing partial deficiency of GPI-linked surface proteins (PNH II) in patients with paroxysmal nocturnal haemoglobinuria. *Br. J. Haematol.* **87:**863–866.

5. **Bessler, M., P. J. Mason, P. Hillmen, T. Miyata, N. Yamada, J. Takeda, L. Luzzatto, and T. Kinoshita.** 1994. Paroxysmal nocturnal haemoglobinuria (PNH) is caused by somatic mutations in the PIG-A gene. *EMBO J.* **13:**110–117.

6. **Billio, A., C. Moeseneder, G. Donazzan, A. Triani, N. Pescosta, and P. Coser.** 2001. Hermansky-Pudlak syndrome: clinical presentation and confirmation of the value of the mepacrine-based cytofluorimetry test in the diagnosis of delta granule deficiency. *Haematologica* **86:**220.

7. **Briggs, C., S. Kunka, D. Hart, S. Oguni, and S. J. Machin.** 2004. Assessment of an immature platelet fraction (IPF) in peripheral thrombocytopenia. *Br. J. Haematol.* **126:**93–99.

8. **Brodsky, R. A., G. L. Mukhina, S. Li, K. L. Nelson, P. L. Chiurazzi, J. T. Buckley, and M. J. Borowitz.** 2000. Improved detection and characterization of paroxysmal nocturnal hemoglobinuria using fluorescent aerolysin. *Am. J. Clin. Pathol.* **114:**459–466.

9. **Brodsky, R. A., G. L. Mukhina, K. L. Nelson, T. S. Lawrence, R. J. Jones, and J. T. Buckley.** 1999. Resistance of paroxysmal nocturnal hemoglobinuria cells to the glycosylphosphatidylinositol-binding toxin aerolysin. *Blood* **93:**1749–1756.

10. **Brubaker, L. H., L. J. Essig, and C. E. Mengel.** 1977. Neutrophil life span in paroxysmal nocturnal hemoglobinuria. *Blood* **50:**657–662.

11. **Chen, J. C., B. H. Davis, B. Wood, and M. J. Warzynski.** 2002. Multicenter clinical experience with flow cytometric method for fetomaternal hemorrhage detection. *Cytometry* **50:**285–290.

12. **Cines, D. B., and V. S. Blanchette.** 2002. Immune thrombocytopenic purpura. *N. Engl. J. Med.* **346:**995–1008.

13. **Cohn, R. J., G. G. Sherman, and D. K. Glencross.** 1997. Flow cytometric analysis of platelet surface glycoproteins in the diagnosis of Bernard-Soulier syndrome. *Pediatr. Hematol. Oncol.* **14:**43–50.

14. **Davis, B. H., S. Olsen, N. C. Bigelow, and J. C. Chen.** 1998. Detection of fetal red cells in fetomaternal hemorrhage using a fetal hemoglobin monoclonal antibody by flow cytometry. *Transfusion* **38:**749–756.

15. **Dhanraj, D., and D. Lambers.** 2004. The incidences of positive Kleihauer-Betke test in low-risk pregnancies and maternal trauma patients. *Am. J. Obstet. Gynecol.* **190:**1461–1463.

16. **Dupre, A. R., J. C. Morrison, J. N. Martin, Jr., R. C. Floyd, and P. G. Blake.** 1993. Clinical application of the Kleihauer-Betke test. *J. Reprod. Med.* **38:**621–624.

17. **Epstein, N., M. Epstein, A. Boulet, E. Fibach, and G. P. Rodgers.** 1996. Monoclonal antibody-based methods for quantitation of hemoglobins: application to evaluating patients with sickle cell anemia treated with hydroxyurea. *Eur. J. Haematol.* **57:**17–24.

18. **Fabris, F., R. Scandellari, M. L. Randi, G. Carraro, G. Luzzatto, and A. Girolami.** 2002. Attempt to improve the diagnosis of immune thrombocytopenia by combined use of two different platelet autoantibodies assays [sic] (PAIgG and MACE). *Haematologica* **87:**1046–1052.

19. **Figuerres, E., M. Olszewski, and M. Kletzel.** 2001. A flow cytometric technique using thiazole orange to detect platelet engraftment following pediatric stem-cell transplants. *Cytotherapy* **3:**277–283.

20. **Fitzgerald, J. E., N. S. Ricalton, A. C. Meyer, S. G. West, H. Kaplan, C. Behrendt, and B. L. Kotzin.** 1995. Analysis of clonal CD8+ T cell expansions in normal individuals and patients with rheumatoid arthritis. *J. Immunol.* **154:**3538–3547.

21. **George, J. N., S. H. Woolf, G. E. Raskob, J. S. Wasser, L. M. Aledort, P. J. Ballem, V. S. Blanchette, J. B. Bussel, D. B. Cines, J. G. Kelton, A. E. Lichtin, R. McMillan, J. A. Okerbloom, D. H. Regan, and I. Warrier.** 1996. Idiopathic thrombocytopenic purpura: a practice guideline developed by explicit methods for the American Society of Hematology. *Blood* **88:**3–40.

22. **Gordon, N., J. Thom, C. Cole, and R. Baker.** 1995. Rapid detection of hereditary and acquired platelet storage pool deficiency by flow cytometry. *Br. J. Haematol.* **89:**117–123.

23. **Gralnick, H. R., M. Vail, L. P. McKeown, P. Merryman, O. Wilson, I. Chu, and J. Kimball.** 1995. Activated platelets in paroxysmal nocturnal haemoglobinuria. *Br. J. Haematol.* **91:**697–702.

24. **Hall, S. E., and W. F. Rosse.** 1996. The use of monoclonal antibodies and flow cytometry in the diagnosis of paroxysmal nocturnal hemoglobinuria. *Blood* **87:**5332–5340.

25. **Hartmann, R. C., and D. E. Jenkins.** 1966. The "sugar-water" test for paroxysmal nocturnal hemoglobinuria. *N. Engl. J. Med.* **275:**155–157.

26. **Hartmann, R. C., D. E. Jenkins, Jr., and A. B. Arnold.** 1970. Diagnostic specificity of sucrose hemolysis test for paroxysmal nocturnal hemoglobinuria. *Blood* **35:**462–475.

27. **Hernandez-Campo, P. M., M. Martin-Ayuso, J. Almeida, A. Lopez, and A. Orfao.** 2002. Comparative analysis of different flow cytometry-based immunophenotypic methods for the analysis of CD59 and CD55 expression on major peripheral blood cell subsets. *Cytometry* **50:**191–201.

28. **Hillmen, P., S. M. Lewis, M. Bessler, L. Luzzatto, and J. V. Dacie.** 1995. Natural history of paroxysmal nocturnal hemoglobinuria. *N. Engl. J. Med.* **333:**1253–1258.

29. **Hillmen, P., and S. J. Richards.** 2000. Implications of recent insights into the pathophysiology of paroxysmal nocturnal haemoglobinuria. *Br. J. Haematol.* **108:**470–479.

30. **Holguin, M. H., L. A. Wilcox, N. J. Bernshaw, W. F. Rosse, and C. J. Parker.** 1989. Relationship between the membrane inhibitor of reactive lysis and the erythrocyte phenotypes of paroxysmal nocturnal hemoglobinuria. *J. Clin. Investig.* **84:**1387–1394.

31. **Hoyer, J. D., C. S. Penz, V. F. Fairbanks, C. A. Hanson, and J. A. Katzmann.** 2002. Flow cytometric measurement of hemoglobin F in RBCs: diagnostic usefulness in the distinction of hereditary persistence of fetal hemoglobin (HPFH) and hemoglobin S-hPFH from other conditions with elevated levels of hemoglobin F. *Am. J. Clin. Pathol.* **117:**857–863.

32. **Hsi, E. D.** 2000. Paroxysmal nocturnal hemoglobinuria testing by flow cytometry. Evaluation of the REDQUANT and CELLQUANT kits. *Am. J. Clin. Pathol.* **114:**798–806.

33. **Hugel, B., G. Socie, T. Vu, F. Toti, E. Gluckman, J. M. Freyssinet, and M. L. Scrobohaci.** 1999. Elevated levels of circulating procoagulant microparticles in patients with paroxysmal nocturnal hemoglobinuria and aplastic anemia. *Blood* **93:**3451–3456.

34. **Iwanaga, M., K. Furukawa, T. Amenomori, H. Mori, H. Nakamura, K. Fuchigami, S. Kamihira, H. Nakakuma, and M. Tomonaga.** 1998. Paroxysmal nocturnal haemoglobinuria clones in patients with myelodysplastic syndromes. *Br. J. Haematol.* **102:**465–474.

35. **Iyer, R., B. McElhinney, N. Heasley, M. Williams, and K. Morris.** 2003. False positive Kleihauer tests and unnecessary administration of anti-D immunoglobulin. *Clin. Lab. Haematol.* **25:**405–408.

36. **Janssen, W. C., and J. J. Hoffmann.** 2002. Evaluation of flow cytometric enumeration of foetal erythrocytes in maternal blood. *Clin. Lab. Haematol.* **24:**89–92.

37. **Johnson, P. R., R. C. Tait, E. B. Austin, K. H. Shwe, and D. Lee.** 1995. Flow cytometry in diagnosis and management of large fetomaternal haemorrhage. *J. Clin. Pathol.* **48:**1005–1008.

38. **Kappelmayer, J., B. Nagy, Jr., K. Miszti-Blasius, Z. Hevessy, and H. Setiadi.** 2004. The emerging value of P-selectin as a disease marker. *Clin. Chem. Lab. Med.* **42:**475–486.

39. **Kleihauer, E., and H. B. K. Braun.** 1957. Demonstration of fetal hemoglobin in erythrocytes of a blood smear. *Klin. Wochenschr.* **35:**637–638.

40. **Knight, C. J., M. Panesar, C. Wright, D. Clarke, P. S. Butowski, D. Patel, A. Patrineli, K. Fox, and A. H. Goodall.** 1997. Altered platelet function detected by flow cytometry. Effects of coronary artery disease and age. *Arterioscler. Thromb. Vasc. Biol.* **17:**2044–2053.

41. **Kottke-Marchant, K., and G. Corcoran.** 2002. The laboratory diagnosis of platelet disorders. *Arch. Pathol. Lab. Med.* **126:**133–146.

42. **Liebman, H. A., and D. I. Feinstein.** 2003. Thrombosis in patients with paroxysmal nocturnal hemoglobinuria is associated with markedly elevated plasma levels of leukocyte-derived tissue factor. *Thromb. Res.* **111:**235–238.

43. **Lima, M., J. Almeida, A. H. Santos, T. M. dos Anjos, M. C. Alguero, M. L. Queiros, A. Balanzategui, B. Justica, M. Gonzalez, J. F. San Miguel, and A. Orfao.** 2001. Immunophenotypic analysis of the TCR-Vbeta repertoire in 98 persistent expansions of CD3(+)/TCR-alphabeta(+) large granular lymphocytes: utility in assessing clonality and insights into the pathogenesis of the disease. *Am. J. Pathol.* **159:**1861–1868.

44. **Linden, M. D., A. L. Frelinger III, M. R. Barnard, K. Przyklenk, M. I. Furman, and A. D. Michelson.** 2004. Application of flow cytometry to platelet disorders. *Semin. Thromb. Hemost.* **30:**501–511.

45. **Maciejewski, J. P., C. Rivera, H. Kook, D. Dunn, and N. S. Young.** 2001. Relationship between bone marrow failure syndromes and the presence of glycophosphatidyl inositol-anchored protein-deficient clones. *Br. J. Haematol.* **115:**1015–1022.

46. **Marcus, S. J., T. R. Kinney, W. H. Schultz, E. E. O'Branski, and R. E. Ware.** 1997. Quantitative analysis of erythrocytes containing fetal hemoglobin (F cells) in children with sickle cell disease. *Am. J. Hematol.* **54:**40–46.

47. **McCabe, D. J., P. Harrison, I. J. Mackie, P. S. Sidhu, G. Purdy, A. S. Lawrie, H. Watt, M. M. Brown, and S. J. Machin.** 2004. Platelet degranulation and monocyte-platelet complex formation are increased in the acute and convalescent phases after ischaemic stroke or transient ischaemic attack. *Br. J. Haematol.* **125:**777–787.

48. **Mhawech, P., and A. Saleem.** 2000. Inherited giant platelet disorders. Classification and literature review. *Am. J. Clin. Pathol.* **113:**176-190.

49. **Michelson, A. D.** 1996. Flow cytometry: a clinical test of platelet function. *Blood* **87:**4925–4936.

50. **Morice, W. G., T. Kimlinger, J. A. Katzmann, J. A. Lust, P. J. Heimgartner, K. C. Halling, and C. A. Hanson.** 2004. Flow cytometric assessment of TCR-Vbeta expression in the evaluation of peripheral blood involvement by T-cell lymphoproliferative disorders: a comparison with conventional T-cell immunophenotyping and molecular genetic techniques. *Am. J. Clin. Pathol.* **121:**373–383.

51. **Moyo, V. M., G. L. Mukhina, E. S. Garrett, and R. A. Brodsky.** 2004. Natural history of paroxysmal nocturnal haemoglobinuria using modern diagnostic assays. *Br. J. Haematol.* **126:**133–138.

52. **Mundee, Y., N. C. Bigelow, B. H. Davis, and J. B. Porter.** 2001. Flow cytometric method for simultaneous assay of foetal haemoglobin containing red cells, reticulocytes and foetal haemoglobin containing reticulocytes. *Clin. Lab. Haematol.* **23:**149–154.

53. **Nance, S. J., J. M. Nelson, P. A. Arndt, H. C. Lam, and G. Garratty.** 1989. Quantitation of fetal-maternal hemorrhage by flow cytometry. A simple and accurate method. *Am. J. Clin. Pathol.* **91:**288–292.

54. **Navenot, J. M., T. Merghoub, R. Ducrocq, J. Y. Muller, R. Krishnamoorthy, and D. Blanchard.** 1998. New method for quantitative determination of fetal hemoglobin-containing red blood cells by flow cytometry: application to sickle-cell disease. *Cytometry* **32:**186–190.

55. **Nebe, T., J. Schubert, K. Gutensohn, and H. Schrezenmeier.** 2003. Flow cytometric analysis of GPI-deficient cells for the diagnosis of paroxysmal nocturnal hemoglobinuria (PNH). *Lab. Medizin* **27**(7–8):257–265.

56. **Nelson, M., K. Zarkos, H. Popp, and J. Gibson.** 1998. A flow-cytometric equivalent of the Kleihauer test. *Vox Sang.* **75**:234–241.

57. **Nishimura, J., Y. Kanakura, R. E. Ware, T. Shichishima, H. Nakakuma, H. Ninomiya, C. M. DeCastro, S. Hall, A. Kanamaru, K. M. Sullivan, H. Mizoguchi, M. Omine, T. Kinoshita, and W. F. Rosse.** 2004. Clinical course and flow cytometric analysis of paroxysmal nocturnal hemoglobinuria in the United States and Japan. *Medicine* (Baltimore) **83**:193–207.

58. **Noris, P., A. Pecci, F. Di Bari, M. T. Di Stazio, M. Di Pumpo, I. F. Ceresa, N. Arezzi, C. Ambaglio, A. Savoia, and C. L. Balduini.** 2004. Application of a diagnostic algorithm for inherited thrombocytopenias to 46 consecutive patients. *Haematologica* **89**:1219–1225.

59. **Posnett, D. N., R. Sinha, S. Kabak, and C. Russo.** 1994. Clonal populations of T cells in normal elderly humans: the T cell equivalent to "benign monoclonal gammapathy." *J. Exp. Med.* **179**:609–618.

60. **Reid, M. E., G. Mallinson, R. B. Sim, J. Poole, V. Pausch, A. H. Merry, Y. W. Liew, and M. J. Tanner.** 1991. Biochemical studies on red blood cells from a patient with the Inab phenotype (decay-accelerating factor deficiency). *Blood* **78**:3291–3297.

61. **Richards, S. J., A. C. Rawstron, and P. Hillmen.** 2000. Application of flow cytometry to the diagnosis of paroxysmal nocturnal hemoglobinuria. *Cytometry* **42**:223–233.

62. **Rotoli, B., M. Bessler, F. Alfinito, and L. Del Vecchio.** 1993. Membrane proteins in paroxysmal nocturnal haemoglobinuria. *Blood Rev.* **7**:75–86.

63. **Sachs, U. J., H. Kroll, A. C. Matzdorff, H. Berghofer, J. A. Lopez, and S. Santoso.** 2003. Bernard-Soulier syndrome due to the homozygous Asn-45Ser mutation in GPIX: an unexpected, frequent finding in Germany. *Br. J. Haematol.* **123**:127–131.

64. **Seri, M., A. Pecci, F. Di Bari, R. Cusano, M. Savino, E. Panza, A. Nigro, P. Noris, S. Gangarossa, B. Rocca, P. Gresele, N. Bizzaro, P. Malatesta, P. A. Koivisto, I. Longo, R. Musso, C. Pecoraro, A. Iolascon, U. Magrini, S. J. Rodriguez, A. Renieri, G. M. Ghiggeri, R. Ravazzolo, C. L. Balduini, and A. Savoia.** 2003. MYH9-related disease: May-Hegglin anomaly, Sebastian syndrome, Fechtner syndrome, and Epstein syndrome are not distinct entities but represent a variable expression of a single illness. *Medicine* (Baltimore) **82**:203–215.

65. **Setty, B. N., S. Kulkarni, C. D. Dampier, and M. J. Stuart.** 2001. Fetal hemoglobin in sickle cell anemia: relationship to erythrocyte adhesion markers and adhesion. *Blood* **97**:2568–2573.

66. **Towery, R., T. P. English, and D. Wisner.** 1993. Evaluation of pregnant women after blunt injury. *J. Trauma* **35**:731–735.

67. **van Den, B. R., P. P. Boor, E. G. van Lochem, W. C. Hop, A. W. Langerak, I. L. Wolvers-Tettero, H. Hooijkaas, and J. J. van Dongen.** 2000. Flow cytometric analysis of the Vbeta repertoire in healthy controls. *Cytometry* **40**:336–345.

68. **van Dongen, J. J., A. W. Langerak, M. Bruggemann, P. A. Evans, M. Hummel, F. L. Lavender, E. Delabesse, F. Davi, E. Schuuring, R. Garcia-Sanz, J. H. van Krieken, J. Droese, D. Gonzalez, C. Bastard, H. E. White, M. Spaargaren, M. Gonzalez, A. Parreira, J. L. Smith, G. J. Morgan, M. Kneba, and E. A. Macintyre.** 2003. Design and standardization of PCR primers and protocols for detection of clonal immunoglobulin and T-cell receptor gene recombinations in suspect lymphoproliferations: report of the BIOMED-2 Concerted Action BMH4-CT98-3936. *Leukemia* **17**:2257–2317.

69. **van Dongen, J. J., and I. L. Wolvers-Tettero.** 1991. Analysis of immunoglobulin and T cell receptor genes. Part I. Basic and technical aspects. *Clin. Chim. Acta* **198**:1–91.

70. **van Dongen, J. J., and I. L. Wolvers-Tettero.** 1991. Analysis of immunoglobulin and T cell receptor genes. Part II. Possibilities and limitations in the diagnosis and management of lymphoproliferative diseases and related disorders. *Clin. Chim. Acta* **198**:93–174.

71. **Vidal, C., C. Spaulding, F. Picard, F. Schaison, J. Melle, S. Weber, and M. Fontenay-Roupie.** 2001. Flow cytometry detection of platelet procoagulation activity and microparticles in patients with unstable angina treated by percutaneous coronary angioplasty and stent implantation. *Thromb. Haemost.* **86**:784–790.

72. **Wall, J. E., M. Buijs-Wilts, J. T. Arnold, W. Wang, M. M. White, L. K. Jennings, and C. W. Jackson.** 1995. A flow cytometric assay using mepacrine for study of uptake and release of platelet dense granule contents. *Br. J. Haematol.* **89**:380–385.

73. **Wang, C., B. R. Smith, K. A. Ault, and H. M. Rinder.** 2002. Reticulated platelets predict platelet count recovery following chemotherapy. *Transfusion* **42**:368–374.

74. **Wang, H., T. Chuhjo, S. Yasue, M. Omine, and S. Nakao.** 2002. Clinical significance of a minor population of paroxysmal nocturnal hemoglobinuria-type cells in bone marrow failure syndrome. *Blood* **100**:3897–3902.

75. **Warzynski, M. J., and J. L. Roys.** 2004. Improving laboratory practice: looking at fetal hemoglobin histograms. *Cytometry* **58B**:61–64.

76. **Wiedmer, T., S. E. Hall, T. L. Ortel, W. H. Kane, W. F. Rosse, and P. J. Sims.** 1993. Complement-induced vesiculation and exposure of membrane prothrombinase sites in platelets of paroxysmal nocturnal hemoglobinuria. *Blood* **82**:1192–1196.

77. **Yamashina, M., E. Ueda, T. Kinoshita, T. Takami, A. Ojima, H. Ono, H. Tanaka, N. Kondo, T. Orii, and N. Okada.** 1990. Inherited complete deficiency of 20-kilodalton homologous restriction factor (CD59) as a cause of paroxysmal nocturnal hemoglobinuria. *N. Engl. J. Med.* **323**:1184–1189.

Immunophenotyping of Leukemia and Lymphoma by Flow Cytometry

BRENT LEE WOOD

20

The diagnosis and classification of lymphoma and leukemia have improved greatly over the past two decades, in part due to the widespread application of immunophenotypic studies to hematopoietic neoplasms. As a result, flow cytometric and immunocytochemical studies have become increasingly important in the initial evaluation and subsequent posttherapeutic monitoring of leukemia and lymphoma. The impact of immunophenotypic studies is reflected by their incorporation into current leukemia and lymphoma classifications, beginning with the Revised European-American Lymphoma classification in 1994 (33) and, more recently, in the proposed World Health Organization (WHO) classification (32) (see Tables 1 to 3). An important component of both of these classifications is the stratification of hematopoietic neoplasms by their lineage, i.e., B cell, T cell, or myeloid, and degree of differentiation, features which are in part immunophenotypically defined. Additionally, a number of specific entities are in large part defined by their immunophenotypic profile, e.g., chronic lymphocytic leukemia. Reflecting this importance, guidelines for the use of flow cytometry in the clinical laboratory for the immunophenotyping of leukemic cells have been published (65), and a National Institutes of Health-sponsored conference on the flow cytometric analysis of leukemia and lymphoma was convened in 1995 to attempt standardization of clinical practice (15). Despite these efforts, flow cytometric immunophenotyping of leukemia and lymphoma remains poorly standardized, and significant variation exists between laboratories in terms of methods of specimen preparation, panels of reagents used, methods of data analysis, and reporting of results.

The medical indications for the use of flow cytometric leukemia and lymphoma immunophenotyping in a clinical setting continue to be defined, but three general areas have been identified (21). (i) At a minimum, flow cytometry allows improved reproducibility in the diagnosis and classification of hematopoietic neoplasms, particularly for chronic lymphoproliferative disorders and acute leukemias, and is widely used for this purpose. (ii) Additionally, flow cytometry can evaluate for the presence of biological parameters associated with therapeutic response or outcome, for example, an increased proliferative rate in neoplastic plasma cells (70) or increased CD38 or Zap-70 expression by the neoplastic cells in chronic lymphocytic leukemia (19, 20), immunophenotypic features both associated with a poorer clinical outcome. (iii) Finally, the presence of residual neoplastic cells following therapy can be detected by flow cytometry with a sensitivity down to 0.01% of cells analyzed. Increasing evidence suggests that the persistence of small residual neoplastic populations after therapy is of clinical significance, and the topic continues to be an active area of investigation (17).

INSTRUMENT SETUP AND SPECIMEN PREPARATION

The general principles and procedures for instrument setup and specimen handling are similar to those used for lymphocyte immunophenotyping (64), as discussed in the previous chapter, and are only summarized here, with an emphasis on areas of particular importance to leukemia and lymphoma immunophenotyping.

Biohazard Precautions

Universal biohazard precautions should be used with all specimens, as is standard clinical laboratory practice. This should include the use of laboratory coats and gloves by all laboratory personnel, biological safety cabinets or similar containment devices for specimen manipulation, and avoidance of sharp or potentially sharp materials. Following specimen preparation and prior to analysis, a fixative such as 0.5 to 2% (vol/vol) paraformaldehyde or formaldehyde is commonly added both to stabilize the specimen if analysis is delayed and to inactivate potentially infectious agents. Most current benchtop flow cytometers used in the clinical laboratory are closed systems, unlike cell sorters or older flow cytometers, so aerosolization during analysis is not an important issue. Additional protection during disposal of instrument waste may be provided by the routine addition of bleach at a final concentration of 10% to the instrument's waste receptacle.

Instrument Setup

Optimization and standardization of instrument performance on a daily basis are very important in the immunophenotypic analysis of leukemia and lymphoma (84). Unlike lymphocyte immunophenotyping, where the antigens detected generally result in relatively bright and consistent fluorescence intensities between samples, the intensity of antigen expression on neoplastic cells is highly variable. Consequently, it is critical that the instrumentation be capable of reliably resolving a wide range of fluorescence intensities in a reproducible manner. On a daily basis, stable optical alignment should be verified using brightly fluorescent microbeads with low and well-defined coefficients of variation (CV), and optimization should be performed if the CV exceed expected values. Fluorescence intensity must also be standardized by adjusting photomultiplier tube (PMT) voltages to provide a consistent level of fluorescence using a stable fluorescence standard, typically a single brightly fluorescent microbead. The PMT voltage should have been initially set so that the autofluorescence of the least autofluorescent population of interest fills the first decade of the logarithmic scale. In actual practice, no significant changes in PMT voltages should be required on a day-to-day basis, and if significant variation is seen, instrument maintenance is required. It is also important to verify the instrument's ability to resolve low-level fluorescence from background noise, a process accomplished by comparing the autofluorescence of unstained lymphocytes to a nonfluorescent bead. On a periodic basis, either weekly or monthly, the linearity of the system should also be verified by using a series of microbeads having defined fluorescence intensities that range from zero to very bright. Linear regression analysis of measured versus actual fluorescence not only confirms the linearity of the system but also provides additional information on the level of instrument noise, the minimum level of fluorescence the instrument is capable of resolving, and the number of decades of fluorescence detected. Such evaluation should be a scheduled part of the routine instrument quality control program.

Multiple fluorochromes, generally three to five, are commonly used simultaneously in the analysis of leukemia and lymphoma. Since most fluorochromes used in flow cytometry have overlapping emission spectra, determination of the fluorescence due to a single fluorochrome requires subtraction of a portion of the signals produced by each of the other fluorochromes from the measured signal, a process performed on the linearized data and termed compensation. The appropriate amount of each signal to subtract, i.e., compensation coefficients, may be represented by an $n \times n$-dimensional matrix where n is the number of fluorochromes. Consequently, as the number of fluorochromes used increases, the number of compensation coefficients that must be determined increases geometrically.

The correct determination of the compensation coefficients is critical for the resolution of weakly fluorescent signals, i.e., low-level antigen expression, and for consistent fluorescence intensities when antibodies are used in multiple combinations (78). To determine the compensation coefficients, a sample is individually labeled with a series of fluorescent molecules or antibodies, one for each fluorochrome to be used, having spectral characteristics identical to those that are to be assayed. The intensity of the fluorescent signal used must be at least as bright as the brightest signal to be measured for each fluorochrome. Antibody capture beads may be used for this purpose but are not entirely equivalent to fresh cells, and settings generated by their use should be confirmed using cells. As each labeled sample is run through the instrument, the compensation coefficients are adjusted to give identical medians between the positive and negative populations for each combination of fluorochromes. The use of mean values, either arithmetic or geometric, while common, is not appropriate since the populations are not normally distributed and often contain outliers that unduly influence the mean. This form of "hardware" compensation can be quite laborious when more than three fluorochromes are used simultaneously, as the number of parameters to evaluate increases dramatically and interactions between the parameters can be surprisingly nonintuitive. In addition, when tandem conjugate dyes, e.g., phycoerythrin (PE)-Texas red, PE-Cy5, etc., are used, the spectral characteristics of the dyes can vary significantly between lots, requiring separate compensation coefficients for each lot of these reagents. For these reasons, "software" compensation methods have been developed which are rapid, offer the ability to save and conveniently apply tube-specific compensation settings, and give superior quality compensation (2). The newer generation of flow cytometers has software compensation incorporated into their systems, although third-party software is also available for offline compensation and analysis. Regardless of the compensation method used, the appropriateness of the compensation settings should be validated daily by the visual inspection of data.

Specimen Handling

Immunophenotyping of leukemia and lymphoma may be performed on any specimen from which a single cell suspension can be generated, including peripheral blood, bone marrow, lymph node, body fluids, tissue, etc. Peripheral blood and bone marrow specimens must be anticoagulated; EDTA, heparin, and acid-citrate-dextrose (ACD) are the anticoagulants most frequently used. Heparin and ACD offer improved stability when the specimen is greater than 12 to 24 h old, as specimens in EDTA will show a progressive loss of myeloid cells. However, ACD should not be used for bone marrow specimens, as it may cause viability problems related to change in pH (86). Specimens should generally be stored at room temperature (16 to 28°C) prior to analysis, although refrigeration will retard degradation when analysis must be delayed.

Specimens containing large numbers of erythrocytes, particularly peripheral blood and bone marrow, require erythrocyte removal to allow efficient analysis of white blood cells. Historically, density gradient centrifugation with Ficoll-Hypaque was used to generate a cell suspension enriched for lymphocytes and/or blasts. While still sometimes used in a research setting, this method results in the selective loss of some cell populations (76) and has largely been replaced by erythrocyte lysis techniques using a variety of commercial and noncommercial preparations (18), of which ammonium chloride is the most common. Current recommended methods involve the addition of antibodies to an aliquot of blood or marrow, followed by erythrocyte lysis, and washing with a buffered salt solution such as phosphate-buffered saline to remove cell debris, the lysing reagent, and unbound antibody. This method allows for rapid specimen preparation and is convenient to use in the clinical laboratory. However, the binding of certain antibodies may be differentially affected by lysing reagents, resulting in either increased or, more commonly, decreased binding depending on the antibodies and lysing reagents involved (57). Addition of a small amount of fixative, i.e., 0.25 to 0.5% formaldehyde, during lysis can minimize these changes and stabilize the specimen. In addition, the degree of erythrocyte lysis may vary between tubes, sometimes dramatically, and serum must be washed away prior to antibody addition for samples in which immunoglobulin light-chain antibodies are to be used. Consequently, a common variation of this method involves performing bulk erythrocyte lysis on a large volume of the specimen followed by washing, aliquoting, addition of antibodies, and washing. This method eliminates the effect of the lysing reagent on antibody binding, allowing more reproducible binding, and allows consistent specimen processing for all antibodies used, including immunoglobulin light-chain antibodies. This is provided that the lysing reagent does not result in the destruction of antigenic sites, an infrequent problem. However, erythrocyte lysis does result in some destruction of white blood cells, particularly neutrophils, and the activation of some cell populations, such as monocytes, which then may nonspecifically bind antibodies and result in increased background, as well as altering the native expression patterns of some antigens. Additionally, certain tandem fluorochromes, in particular Cy7-containing tandems, may show degradation with this method of sample preparation. All erythrocyte lysis methods also result in some loss of nucleated red cell precursors, distorting the composition of the sample evaluated, particularly for bone marrow. Consequently, an ideal system for erythrocyte removal has not yet been developed.

Tissue specimens are best collected and transported in tissue culture medium (RPMI 1640) at either room temperature or 4°C, if analysis will be delayed. The sample is then disaggregated to form a single cell suspension, either by mechanical dissociation or by enzymatic digestion. Mechanical dissociation is preferred and is accomplished by the use of either a scalpel and forceps, needle and syringe, or wire mesh screen (13) followed by filtration through a fine-gauge wire mesh screen. Antibodies can then be added to the resulting suspension and processed as usual.

Data Acquisition

It is important during acquisition of the sample to collect enough events to allow detection of populations of the desired frequency. For populations that represent a large percentage of the total, relatively few total events need to be acquired, while the converse is true for infrequent populations. Consequently, unless the operator monitors the data in real time and terminates acquisition when a population of interest is well defined, one must decide before acquisition how many events will be collected. One strategy is to collect a specified number of events of some subpopulation of interest, e.g., 10,000 lymphocyte events. This guarantees that a sufficient number of events will be acquired for that subpopulation, but since the frequency of that subpopulation can vary significantly between samples, the total number of events collected and acquisition time can vary tremendously. Also, if an unexpected abnormal population is detected, the number of events may be insufficient for analysis. An alternative method is to acquire a consistent total number of events to achieve a desired degree of sensitivity; e.g., if the ability to detect a population having a frequency of 0.1% is desired and 100 events is determined to be adequate for confident identification, then 100,000 total ungated events would need to be collected. The precision of such a measurement can be estimated from Poisson statistics, given that the $CV = \sqrt{N}/N$ where N is the number of events in the population. This approach allows for consistency in both the number of events collected and acquisition time with little interaction from the operator, but it will collect an unnecessarily large number of events when the population of interest has a high frequency and will result in generally longer acquisition times. A third alternative is to screen the sample with a limited panel of reagents and perform gated acquisition on a subpopulation of interest as a second step, generally on a second separately prepared aliquot. In gated acquisition, only events within the gate of interest are collected and all others are excluded from the listmode file, a strategy primarily used to reduce the size of the resulting listmode file when examining populations of low frequency. However, as a consequence, any events outside of the acquisition gate are not present at analysis and the determination of population frequencies is not possible without reference to the initial screening aliquot. In addition, the expenditure of reagents and preparation time may be significantly increased and the overall work flow becomes recursive, making laboratory operation less efficient.

Instrument carryover of material between samples can become an important consideration when populations of low frequency are evaluated. Many instruments have a manufacturer's specification for carryover of roughly 1%, although most instruments will perform better than this if properly maintained. However, the accumulation of material in instrument tubing does occur to some degree and can manifest as sporadically increased carryover or ultimately as a "plug." This sporadic carryover can result in the appearance of unusual subpopulations of low frequency, depending on the combination of reagents in the preceding sample, and lead to erroneous analysis. To minimize this, a small amount of water may be run through the instrument between each aliquot of sample until the count rate returns to a normal background level.

A final consideration is the rate of sample aspiration. While it is desirable to acquire samples as quickly as is reasonably possible to minimize the use of instrument time, certain instruments are not capable of accurately evaluating specimens at rates over roughly 1,000 events/sec. In addition, at increased sample event rates, the phenomenon of coincidence, i.e., the occurrence of two particles simultaneously in the laser path, becomes increasingly frequent and the use of coincidence correction techniques becomes mandatory.

PATTERNS OF ANTIGEN EXPRESSION

The detection of hematopoietic malignancies by flow cytometry relies on the principle that neoplastic cells express antigens in patterns recognizably different from those of normal hematopoietic cells. Antigen expression in normal cells is tightly regulated, with each antigen following a predictable pattern of expression during cell maturation and activation. In neoplastic cells, this pattern of expression is altered in nonrandom ways that differ from normal, allowing the identification, quantitation, and immunophenotypic characterization of the abnormal population. Patterns of abnormal antigen expression that commonly occur include the following: (i) a gain of antigens not normally expressed by the cell type or lineage (if the abnormally expressed antigen is characteristically expressed by another lineage, this is termed lineage infidelity); (ii) asynchronous antigen expression where antigens normally present on a given cell lineage are expressed at inappropriate times during maturation or activation; (iii) abnormally increased or decreased levels of normal antigens, which in some cases may be entirely absent; and (iv) abnormally homogeneous expression of one or more antigens by a population that normally exhibits more heterogeneous expression. Together, these abnormalities give rise to abnormal maturational patterns or populations that are commonly visualized using two-parameter dot plots. Consequently, the flow cytometric analysis of hematopoietic neoplasms involves a thorough knowledge of the normal patterns of antigen expression on hematopoietic subpopulations, as well as a knowledge of the patterns of expression commonly seen on the ever-expanding variety of hematopoietic neoplasms.

Patterns of Normal Antigen Expression

B-cell maturation occurs largely in the bone marrow through a series of discrete stages characterized by increasing intensity of CD45 expression, gradual acquisition of the mature B-cell antigens CD20, CD21, and CD22 and immunoglobulin light chains, and loss of immature antigens such as CD34, terminal deoxynucleotidyl transferase (TdT), and CD10 (51, 52, 54). Expression of bright HLA-DR and moderate CD19 are present throughout maturation, with some variability in intensity. The least mature stage shows the lowest level of CD45 and expresses both CD34 and nuclear TdT with bright CD10, slightly decreased HLA-DR and CD19, low CD22, and no expression of CD20 or surface or cytoplasmic immunoglobulins. The second stage shows a loss of CD34 and nuclear TdT with a mild reduction in CD10, acquisition of variable CD20 and brighter CD22, an increase in CD45, and slightly increased CD19. Immunoglobulins are acquired at this stage as cytoplasmic immunoglobulin M and are subsequently expressed in combination with kappa or lambda light chains on the surface with maturation. The final stage shows a loss of CD10; further increases in CD20, CD22, and surface immunoglobulins; and the brightest expression of CD45, with a slight decrease in CD19. At all stages, the degree of right-angle light scatter is quite low, although larger forms with a variable degree of increased forward and side scatter are present. Myeloid-associated antigens such as CD13 and CD33 are not usually expressed at any stage of B-cell maturation but may be seen at a very low level in immature stages in some cases.

Mature B cells are present largely in lymph nodes but may be seen in lower numbers in peripheral blood and bone marrow. They are characterized by the expression of bright CD45, the B-cell antigens CD19, CD20, CD21, and CD22, and surface light chains (35). Mature B-cell populations normally consist of a mixture of subsets expressing either surface kappa or lambda light chains with a relatively constant kappa/lambda ratio of 1.4. Within lymph nodes, there is often a discrete subset exhibiting expression of low-level CD10 and brighter CD20 and CD45 corresponding to a subset of germinal center B cells. Populations with this immunophenotype are not normally found in marrow or peripheral blood. Plasma cells represent the terminal stage of B-cell maturation and have a unique immunophenotype characterized by decreased expression of many mature B-cell antigens, including CD45, CD19, and surface light chains, with a complete loss of CD20, and very bright expression of the activation antigen CD38 (31, 92).

T-cell maturation occurs predominantly in the thymus through a series of discrete stages (28). The least mature T cells are characterized by the expression of the pan-T-cell antigens CD2, CD5, and CD7 in combination with expression of CD34 and nuclear TdT. In the subsequent common thymocyte stage of maturation, the cells acquire the coexpression of CD4 and CD8 in conjunction with cytoplasmic CD3 and the common thymocyte antigen CD1a, and they lose expression of CD34 and TdT. Subsequently, the T cells begin to express either CD4 or CD8 in combination with surface CD3 and lose expression of CD1a, the immunophenotype seen in mature T cells. A population of mature T cells normally consists of a mixture of cells expressing either CD4 or CD8 in a relatively constant ratio of between 1:1 and 3:1. The CD4- and CD8-positive subsets also exhibit slight differences in their expression of some pan-T-cell antigens, including generally decreased expression of CD3 and CD5 on the CD8 T cells and more variable expression of CD7 on the CD4 T cells (91). Upon activation, shifts in the intensity of a variety of these antigens may be seen, in addition to the acquisition of additional antigens, such as HLA-DR, CD25, and CD69. These findings apply largely to T cells expressing the αβ form of the T-cell receptor, which represent the majority of mature lymphocytes. However, a small subset of T cells expressing the γδ T-cell receptor is also often present in increased numbers in reactive states and is characterized by a mature T-cell immunophenotype with expression of brighter CD3, variably decreased CD5, variable low-level CD56, and either no CD4 or CD8 or variable low-level CD8 (36, 62).

NK cells represent a lymphocyte population closely related to T cells, but with a distinct immunophenotype which includes the expression of bright CD7, intermediate CD2, low variable CD8 αα-homodimer, and coexpression of CD56, CD11b, and CD16, without the expression of other mature T-cell antigens, including CD3, CD5, or CD4 (28). NK cells also typically exhibit slightly decreased CD45 and slightly increased right-angle light scatter relative to other lymphocytes.

In contrast to lymphocytes, myeloid cells exhibit a more continuous pattern of antigen expression during maturation (90, 93). Myeloid blasts are readily identifiable by their decreased expression of CD45, mildly increased right-angle side scatter, and expression of intermediate CD34, variable CD13, variable CD33, variable HLA-DR, variable CD38 and CD133, and low CD117. These blasts do not express more mature myeloid antigens such as CD11b, CD14, CD15, or CD16. As the blasts mature to promyelocytes, they exhibit markedly increased right-angle light scatter, gain increased autofluorescent background, begin to express the more mature myeloid antigens CD64 and CD15, and lose expression of HLA-DR, CD34, and CD117. Further maturation toward mature neutrophils results in the increased expression of CD45, CD11b, and CD15, slightly decreased right-angle light scatter and expression of CD64 and CD33, and abrupt acquisition of increasingly bright CD16 at roughly the metamyelocyte stage. CD13 exhibits a variable pattern of expression, with expression at an intermediate level on blasts, increased expression on promyelocytes, and decreased expression through the myelocyte stage, followed by a marked increase with maturation to mature neutrophils. Mature neutrophils are characterized by the expression of bright CD11b, CD13, CD15, and CD16 and low CD33, CD14, and CD10.

Monocytes also mature from the myeloid blasts but retain a lower degree of right-angle light scatter than the neutrophilic lineage (90, 93). Mature monocytes are characterized by the expression of bright CD45, HLA-DR, CD11b, CD14, CD33, CD36, and CD64, with variable CD13 and low-level expression of CD15 and CD16. Immature monocytic forms exhibit patterns of antigen expression intermediate between blasts and mature monocytes, particularly with decreased expression of CD14, CD36, and CD45. CD56 is typically not expressed on immature or mature monocytes but may be seen in some reactive conditions.

Eosinophils have increased right-angle light scatter, with expression of bright CD11b and CD45, low CD33, and low CD15 and no expression of CD16 (90). Basophils are easy to identify by their relatively low right-angle light scatter, slightly decreased level of CD45 relative to lymphocytes, and expression of intermediate CD13 and CD33 without significant HLA-DR, CD15, CD16, or CD117 (95, 99). Most cells have an immunophenotype similar to that of basophils but are characterized by bright CD117 expression and increased right-angle light scatter (23, 24).

Patterns of Abnormal Antigen Expression

Most hematopoietic neoplasms have characteristic immunophenotypic profiles that allow for their detection. In some cases, the immunophenotypic profiles are specific enough to allow definitive classification using flow cytometric data alone (37). However, significant variability in antigen expression exists within each category, and proper diagnosis depends on the recognition of overall immunophenotypic patterns and not on the rigid application of these profiles. As a corollary, caution should be used in making a diagnosis or classification based on the abnormal expression of a single antigen.

Acute Leukemia

Acute leukemia is diagnosed when more than 20% (WHO criteria) (33) or 30% (French-American-British cooperative group [FAB] criteria) (4) of all nucleated cells in either bone marrow or peripheral blood are abnormal blasts. These leukemias are further subdivided based on their lineage of differentiation into acute myeloid leukemia (AML) or acute lymphoblastic leukemia (ALL), and ALL is further subdivided by lineage, with approximately 75 to 80% of ALLs being of B-cell origin and 20 to 25% being of T-cell origin. These subclassifications have therapeutic implications, and flow cytometry plays an important role in their diagnosis and classification.

AML is a clonal proliferation of abnormal myeloid blasts that in many cases retain a limited ability to differentiate along a neutrophilic, monocytic, erythroid, and/or megakaryocytic lineage. AML is more common in adults than children and in many cases is thought to arise from an underlying myelodysplastic syndrome (MDS) (34). The subclassification of AML historically has used primarily morphological criteria in combination with limited cytochemical staining to assign a predominant lineage of differentiation, the FAB classification (4). However, this method has limited clinical significance and influence on therapeutic decision making. More recently, cytogenetic findings have come to play an increasingly important role in AML subclassification and prognostication, and characteristic chromosomal translocations have been associated with differences in prognosis and response to therapeutic regimens (53) (see Table 1). Flow cytometric immunophenotyping is not formally included in current classification systems, but it does show characteristic findings in certain subsets of AML and is commonly used to confirm lineage.

Most AMLs have an immunophenotype similar to that of normal myeloid blasts, with the expression of the early myeloid antigens CD13 and CD33 in combination with HLA-DR, CD34, CD117, and low to intermediate CD45 (11, 55, 56, 75, 83, 94). However, the pattern of antigen expression on abnormal myeloid blasts may be more homogeneous than the usual variable expression of these antigens on normal maturing myeloid blast populations, consistent with their clonal nature. In addition, the intensity of these antigens is often abnormally increased or decreased to absent. The abnormal expression by myeloid blasts of more mature myeloid antigens such as CD11b or CD15 is seen in some cases, and expression of one or more antigens normally expressed on B or T lymphocytes, i.e., CD7, CD2, CD4, CD19, or CD56, occurs relatively frequently.

Certain subtypes of AML have been associated with characteristic immunophenotypic findings. Acute promyelocytic leukemia [AML-M3; t(15;17) AML] characteristically shows an absence of HLA-DR expression, as is seen in normal promyelocytes, with variably increased right-angle light scatter, frequent expression of CD2, and variable to absent

TABLE 1 WHO classification of AML

Classification
AML with cytogenetic abnormalities
t(8;21)(q22;q22) AML1(CBFa)/ETO
t(15;17)(q22;q11-12) PML/RAR-a
inv(16)(p13q22) or t(16;16)(p13;q11) CBFb/MYH11X
11q23 (MLL) abnormalities
AML with multilineage dysplasia (two or more lines)
Prior MDS
No prior MDS
AML and MDS therapy related
Alkylating agent related
Epipodophyllotoxin related
Other
AML, not otherwise categorized
AML with minimal differentiation
AML without maturation
AML with maturation
Acute myelomonocytic leukemia
Acute monocytic leukemia
Acute erythroid leukemia
Acute basophilic leukemia
Acute panmyelosis with myelofibrosis

expression of CD15 and CD34 (40, 67). AML containing t(8;21) is associated with the expression of bright CD34, and low nuclear TdT is associated with coexpression of CD19 and/or CD56 (71). AMLs having monocytic differentiation (AML-M4 and -M5) are often associated with a spectrum of differentiated forms between the low-CD45-positive myeloid blasts and more brightly CD45-positive mature monocytes, with the mature forms often increased in number. Monocytic blasts may also show bright CD33 and expression of one or more monocyte-associated antigens such as CD64, CD36, CD14 (highly specific but not sensitive), and CD4 (highly sensitive but not specific) (42). Acute megakaryocytic leukemia (AML-M7) generally shows the expression of the platelet antigens CD61 and/or CD41, although care must be taken to exclude the possibility of activated platelets adherent to the blasts as a cause for false positivity (5).

Precursor B-cell lymphoblastic leukemia/lymphoma (ALL of B-cell lineage) is composed of a clonal proliferation of immature B cells having an immunophenotype similar to that of its normal counterpart, i.e., expression of CD19, CD22, CD10, HLA-DR, CD34, and nuclear TdT and decreased CD45 and variable CD20 without surface light chains (10, 25, 97) (see Fig. 1). However, the neoplasm is generally relatively homogeneous in composition and often lacks the presence of discrete maturational stages characteristic of normal B-cell maturation. In addition, the intensity of one or more normal antigens is typically altered, with a common finding being increased CD10 or abnormally decreased or absent CD45, particularly in pediatric patients, for whom the latter abnormality may be correlated with prognosis (10). Often, antigenic combinations not seen during normal B-cell development are present (asynchronous expression). The low or absent expression of both CD9 and CD20 in ALL of B-cell lineage has been associated with the presence of t(12;21), a good prognostic feature (9). The myeloid antigens CD13 and CD33 may be abnormally coexpressed in a significant subset of pediatric (72) and adult (73) cases of ALL, without apparent clinical significance.

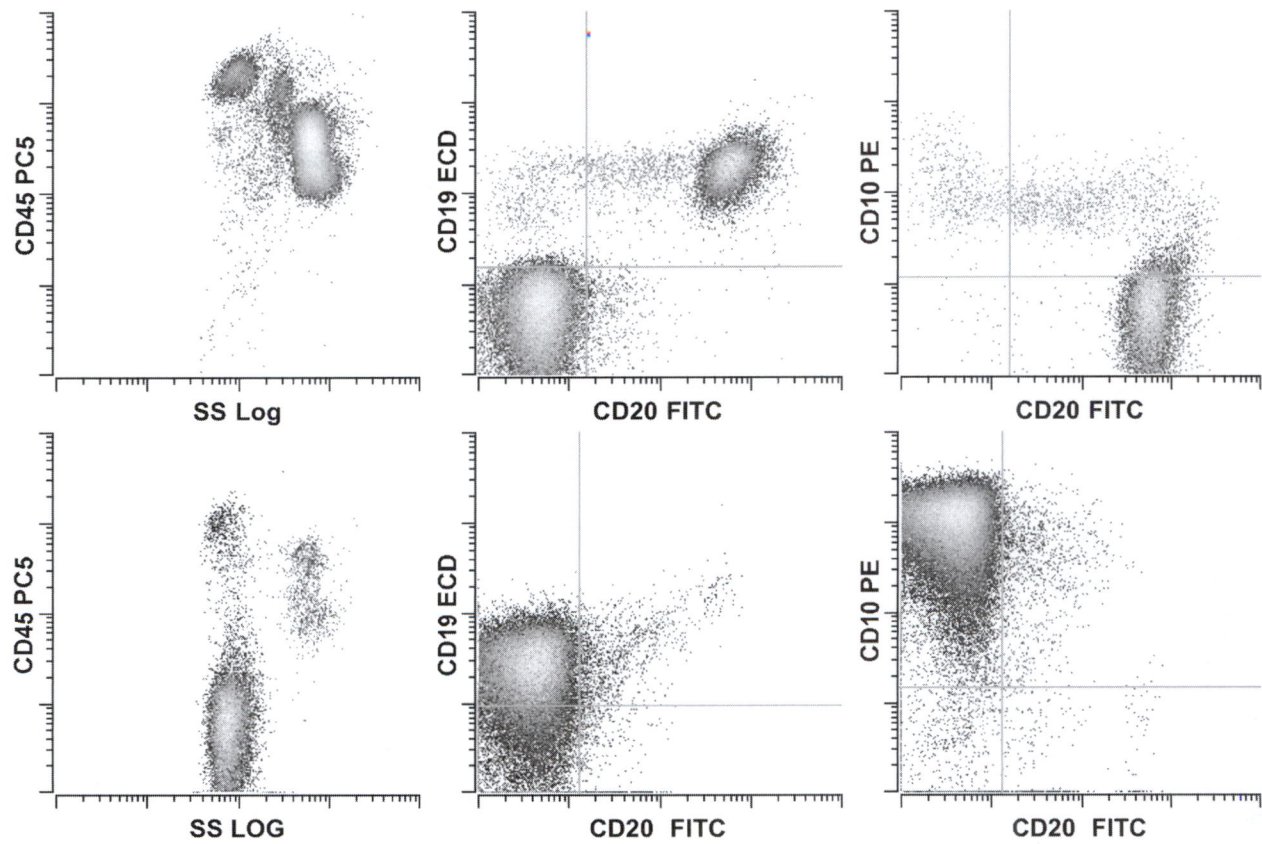

FIGURE 1 Normal B-cell maturation (upper row) versus precursor B-cell lymphoblastic leukemia/lymphoma (lower row). The dot plots display white blood cells (left), lymphocytes (center), or B cells (right). Note the small number of B-cell precursors in normal bone marrow relative to the large abnormal B-cell population lacking CD45 expression (bottom left) in the patient with leukemia. The abnormal B cells also show decreased expression of CD19 (bottom center) and increased CD10 without normal maturational acquisition of CD20 (bottom right). FITC, fluorescein isothiocyanate.

Precursor T-cell lymphoblastic leukemia/lymphoma (ALL of T-cell lineage) is composed of a clonal proliferation of immature T cells having an immunophenotype similar to that of a normal thymic counterpart (39). In contrast to that in normal thymus, the neoplastic population appears to be relatively homogeneous, often with an immunophenotype that does not correspond completely to any normal stage of maturation. Most cases express the early T-cell antigens CD2, CD5, and CD7 at some, often abnormal, level. CD4 and CD8 are usually both absent or coexpressed, in the latter case often in combination with CD1a, and surface CD3 is absent or weak, with invariable positivity for cytoplasmic CD3. CD45 is often expressed at a level higher than seen in immature B cells but slightly lower than seen in mature lymphocytes. Nuclear TdT and CD34 may also be present and can help confirm the immature nature of the process, if present. Given that the immunophenotype may be similar to that of normal thymocytes, one must be cautious about making this diagnosis in material from an anterior mediastinal mass, as the lymphocytic component of a thymoma may appear to be somewhat similar.

Mixed-lineage leukemia is an ill-defined concept, but it is minimally characterized by some authors as the expression of at least two myeloid and at least two lymphoid antigens on leukemic blasts. In most cases, examination of the overall surface immunophenotype and/or evaluation for lineage-associated cytoplasmic antigen expression, i.e., myeloperoxidase for myeloid, CD22 or CD79a for B cell, or CD3 for T cell, is able to assign a predominant lineage (16, 30, 59). Consequently, this designation should be used only for cases where the lineage remains uncertain after complete immunophenotyping including cytoplasmic antigen detection. A rare form of acute leukemia containing separate discrete subsets of abnormal myeloid and lymphoid blasts can occur and is better termed acute bilineage leukemia.

The analysis of MDSs by flow cytometry has recently been evaluated, and a number of abnormalities of surface antigen expression on blasts and maturing myeloid cells have been described (22, 46, 98) (see Fig. 2). High-grade myelodysplasia (refractory anemia with excess blasts in the WHO classification) is a precursor to AML and is characterized by the presence of between 5 and 20% blasts with at least two of three marrow cell lineages exhibiting abnormal morphological findings. Consequently, high-grade MDS is usually readily identifiable by the presence of an increased myeloid blast population having an abnormal immunophenotype similar to those seen in AML, but which represents less than 20% of the nucleated cells. Consequently, the overall flow cytometric approach to MDS mirrors that used for AML. In addition, the maturing myeloid forms may show

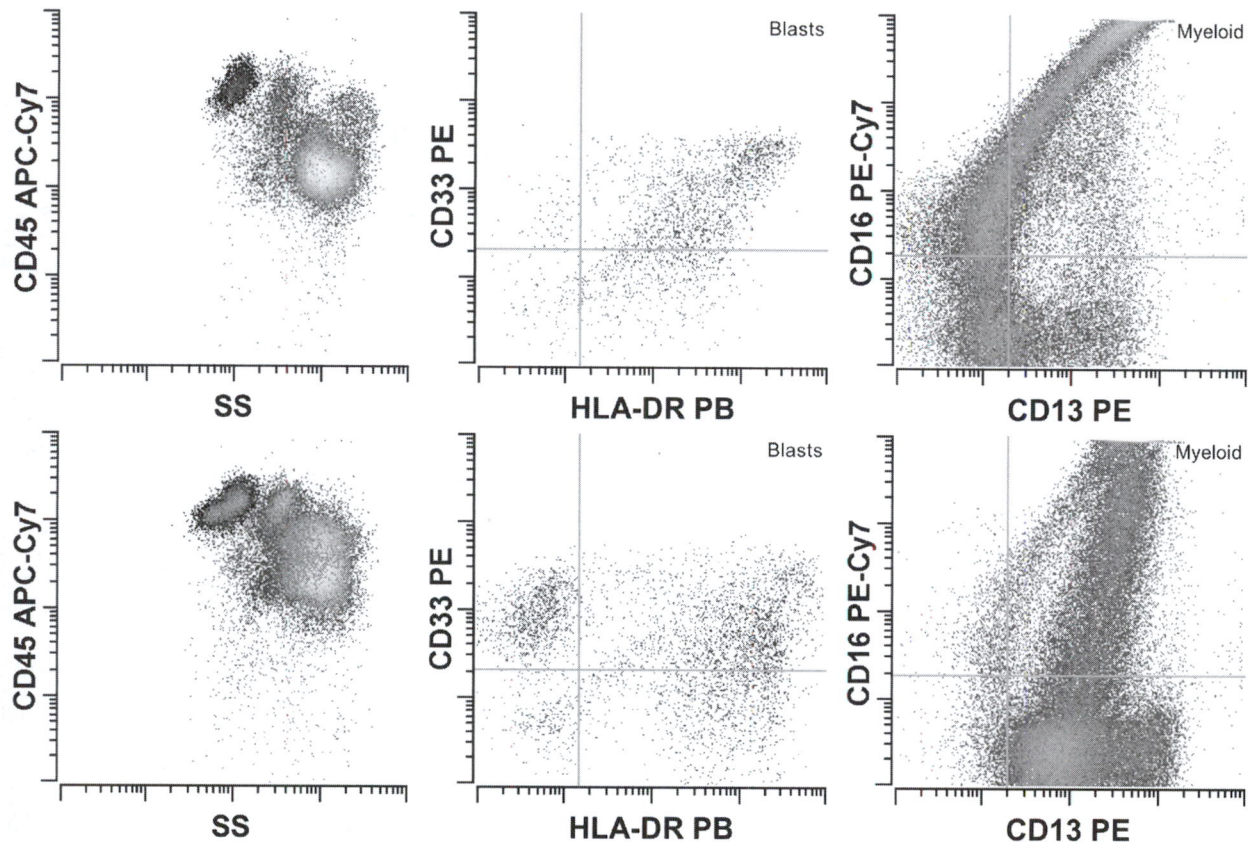

FIGURE 2 Normal myeloid maturation (upper row) versus MDS (lower row). The dot plots display white blood cells (left), blasts (center), or maturing myeloid cells (right). Note the decrease in side scatter on the maturing myeloid population in myelodysplasia, as indicated by the shift of the maturing myeloid cells to the left so that they overlap the monocytes. The blasts (center) show an increase in HLA-DR expression, and the maturing myeloid cells (right) show an aberrant expression pattern of CD13 and CD16 in myelodysplasia. Note the small number of myeloid cells having normal maturation in the background. SS, side scatter; PB, Pacific Blue.

decreased right-angle light scatter corresponding to morphological hypogranularity, increased numbers of immature forms with increased CD45, asynchronous expression of maturational myeloid antigens CD11b, CD13, CD15, CD33, and CD16, and/or abnormal expression of nonmyeloid antigens such as CD56. The monocytic population may exhibit similar abnormalities, with expression of CD56 being relatively common but not specific. Low-grade myelodysplasia (refractory anemia with or without ringed sideroblasts in the FAB classification) is a more heterogeneous category predominantly characterized by unexplained anemia with minimal morphological abnormalities. While abnormalities similar to those seen in high-grade MDS may be present, blasts are not significantly increased in number and the erythroid lineage is predominantly affected so the myeloid cells may not show demonstrable abnormalities, including myeloid blasts. Rates of proliferation and apoptosis are quite high in low-grade myelodysplasia and decline with progression to higher-grade myelodysplasia (68).

Myeloproliferative disorders have not been well studied by flow cytometry, but abnormalities similar to those seen in MDS can be identified in some cases (45). Myeloid blasts are not generally increased in number but may show immunophenotypic abnormalities, and abnormal CD56 expression on maturing myeloid and monocytic forms is relatively common, particularly in chronic myeloid leukemia (CML) (48). The findings are often subtle, and few data exist to support flow cytometry as a primary method for the diagnosis of these disorders. However, acute leukemia may arise from myeloproliferative disorders as a result of transformation over time, an inevitable occurrence with CML but relatively infrequent otherwise. Blast crisis of CML may be of either lymphoid or myeloid lineage, an important therapeutic distinction, with a higher incidence of cases showing mixed myeloid and lymphoid surface antigen expression (38).

Non-Hodgkin's Lymphoma

Non-Hodgkin's lymphomas are neoplasms composed of clonal proliferations of mature B cells, T cells, or NK cells. Current classification systems stratify lymphomas in part on their morphological and/or immunophenotypic similarities to normal components of the immune system (32, 33) (see Tables 2 and 3). Given the complexity of the immune system, the variety of immunophenotypic alterations that may be seen with activation, and the similarity of neoplastic lymphoid immunophenotypes to normal counterparts, the demonstration of clonality is an important part of the diagnosis of these disorders. However, it is critical to recognize

TABLE 2 WHO classification of B-cell neoplasms

Classification
Precursor B-cell neoplasms
Precursor B-lymphoblastic leukemia/lymphoma (ALL)
Mature B-cell neoplasms
B-cell CLL/SLL
B-cell prolymphocytic leukemia
Lymphoplasmacytic lymphoma
Splenic marginal-zone lymphoma
Hairy cell leukemia
Plasma cell myeloma/plasmacytoma
Extranodal marginal-zone B-cell lymphoma of MALT type
Nodal marginal-zone B-cell lymphoma
Follicular lymphoma
Mantle cell lymphoma
Diffuse large B-cell lymphoma
Mediastinal large B-cell lymphoma
Primary-effusion lymphoma
Burkitt's lymphoma/leukemia

that the members of the immune system normally undergo clonal expansion as part of the immune response, and consequently, clonality does not necessarily equate with malignancy for lymphocytic proliferations (44).

The flow cytometric demonstration of clonality can be achieved most easily for B-cell neoplasms (14, 26). A normal mature B-cell population consists of a mixture of cells expressing immunoglobulins with either surface kappa or lambda light chains in a ratio of roughly 1.4:1. Consequently, the identification of a discrete B-cell population showing expression of either only kappa or lambda light chains is evidence for clonality. A common technique is to calculate the kappa-to-lambda ratio for the total B cells and compare this with numerical cutoffs determined from the examination of a series of normal or reactive lymphoid tissues (27). More sophisticated mathematical procedures have also been used with minimal improvement on this basic idea (3, 74). While these methods successfully identify the presence of B-cell

TABLE 3 WHO classification of T-cell and NK-cell neoplasms

Classification
Precursor T-cell neoplasms
Precursor T-lymphoblastic lymphoma/leukemia (ALL)
Mature T-cell neoplasms
T-cell prolymphocytic leukemia
T-cell granular lymphocytic leukemia
Aggressive NK-cell leukemia
Adult T-cell lymphoma/leukemia
Extranodal NK/T-cell lymphoma, nasal type
Enteropathy-type T-cell lymphoma
Hepatosplenic γδ T-cell lymphoma
Subcutaneous panniculitis-like T-cell lymphoma
Mycosis fungoides/Sézary syndrome
Anaplastic large-cell lymphoma, cutaneous type
Peripheral T-cell lymphoma, not otherwise characterized
Angioimmunoblastic T-cell lymphoma
Anaplastic large-cell lymphoma, systemic type

lymphoma when the clonal population represents the majority of the B cells in the specimen, it has poor sensitivity when the clonal population represents a smaller subset of the B cells, a relatively common occurrence (82). Another method is to overlay single-parameter histograms for kappa and lambda light-chain expression and look for differences in the distribution of intensity that can herald the presence of a clonal subpopulation. While this method is more sensitive, it requires that kappa and lambda be evaluated using the same fluorochrome and hence must be set up in separate tubes, making it difficult to account for nonspecific and/or Fc receptor-mediated immunoglobulin binding. Such undesirable light-chain binding can readily be accounted for by the inclusion of both kappa and lambda in the same tube of reagents. All methods are significantly improved by the incorporation of additional light scatter and immunophenotypic information obtained from multiparametric flow cytometry. At a minimum, this should include the presence of a B-cell-lineage antigen, i.e., CD19 or CD20, in every tube containing light-chain antibodies (49). The analysis of such data is best performed by the visual examination of two-parameter histograms to attempt the detection of discrete abnormal subpopulations rather than relying on numerical cutoffs.

In addition to the determination of clonality, a variety of characteristic abnormal immunophenotypes have been described for B-cell lymphoproliferative disorders that aid in their classification. In B-cell chronic lymphocytic leukemia/small lymphocytic lymphoma (CLL/SLL), the abnormal B cells express the T-cell-lineage-associated antigen CD5 in combination with dim CD20, dim CD22, dim surface light chain, and moderate to bright CD23, with little to no expression of FMC7 (41, 61, 96). The expression of CD38 and/or Zap-70 on the neoplastic B cells has been associated with a poorer prognosis in recent studies (13, 54). Mantle cell lymphoma has a similar immunophenotype but is characterized by coexpression of CD5 with brighter CD20, CD22, and surface light chains than seen in CLL/SLL, with bright expression of FMC7 and a lack of CD23 (96). Hairy cell leukemia has a diagnostic immunophenotype which includes increased forward- and right-angle light scatter and bright expression of CD19, CD20, CD22, and surface light chains, with coexpression of CD103, CD25, and bright CD11c (60, 77). Follicle center cell lymphoma has a somewhat variable immunophenotype but often exhibits mildly decreased expression of CD19, bright CD20, CD38, and variable light chains, with coexpression of the follicle center-associated antigen CD10 detectable in 60% of the cases (1). Marginal-zone and lymphoplasmacytoid lymphomas lack characteristic immunophenotypes at present. Large B-cell lymphomas are a heterogeneous category but generally show increased forward- and right-angle light scatter with light-chain expression of variable intensity, including occasionally a complete loss of surface light chains. Burkitt's lymphoma/leukemia has an immunophenotype similar to that seen in follicle center lymphoma, including the frequent expression of CD10.

The determination of clonality by flow cytometry has recently been described for T-cell or NK-cell neoplasms, utilizing T-cell receptor Vβ subset or killer inhibition receptor subset antibodies, respectively (50, 63). However, their diagnosis most frequently depends on the demonstration of abnormal immunophenotypes, usually the gain or loss in intensity of an antigen normally expressed by that cell type (29, 69). Most peripheral T-cell lymphomas arise from the CD4-positive mature T-cell subset, although CD8-positive forms are occasionally seen (58). In mycosis fungoides/Sézary syndrome, the abnormal mature T cells characteristically express CD4 with a loss of CD7, a memory T-cell immunophenotype (6, 43). However, considerable variability in the expression of all mature T-cell antigens may be seen, and this disorder cannot be distinguished from other peripheral T-cell lymphomas by immunophenotype alone. Hepatosplenic γδ T-cell lymphoma can be readily identified by an immunophenotype similar to that of its normal counterpart and its expression of the γδ T-cell receptor, in contrast to the expression of the αβ form seen in most other peripheral T-cell lymphomas (81). Large granular lymphocytic leukemia is typically composed of a proliferation of CD8-positive mature T cells (CD3 positive) having variably decreased expression of CD5 with variable expression of cytotoxic antigens, including CD57 and, less consistently, CD16 and/or CD56 (47). The less common NK-cell form of large granular lymphocytic leukemia, now termed aggressive NK-cell leukemia, has a typical NK-cell immunophenotype, commonly with the abnormal expression of CD2, CD7, CD11b, or CD16 and/or CD56, without expression of the T-cell antigens CD3 and CD5. Considerable care must be taken when using immunophenotypic findings to diagnose T- and NK-cell neoplasms, as both populations may possess a variety of small reactive clonal subpopulations with unusual immunophenotypes and a variety of activation states having immunophenotypic alterations which can be mistaken for neoplasia.

Plasma cell neoplasms characteristically express moderate to bright CD38 with decreased to absent CD45, absent CD19, surface or, more commonly, cytoplasmic light-chain restriction, and coexpression of CD56 in 60% of the cases (66, 80). Similar to normal plasma cells, they lack expression of CD20. Abnormalities of DNA ploidy are also common in plasma cell myeloma and may be detected by flow cytometry in combination with immunophenotypic studies to enhance the identification of abnormal plasma cell populations.

REAGENT SELECTION

The construction of panels of reagents for the diagnosis of hematopoietic neoplasms requires the balancing of multiple, sometimes conflicting, objectives (88). Antibodies commonly used for the diagnosis of acute leukemia and non-Hodgkin's lymphoma are listed in Tables 4 and 5. The selection of reagents is largely determined by three basic considerations: the number of simultaneous fluorophores used, the availability of reagents, and the strategy used for population identification. In general, weakly expressed antigens should be coupled with bright fluorophores to maximize their detection, and conversely, brightly expressed antigens should be coupled with weaker fluorophores to maintain the expected range of fluorescence within the dynamic range of the instrument.

The number of simultaneous fluorochromes used is in part determined by the instrument which will be used, with most current instruments allowing up to four simultaneous fluorochromes and more advanced instruments allowing six or more. In general, the greater the number of fluorochromes used, the more specifically one can identify normal and abnormal populations of cells, particularly when they represent small percentages of the total. However, this comes at the cost of increasing technical complexity for both instrument setup and data analysis. The advent of simplified single-laser and multilaser benchtop instruments, the availability of both hardware and software methods to deal with

TABLE 4 Antibodies commonly used in the diagnosis of acute leukemia

Designation	Specificity
CD1	Common thymocyte, early T cells, Langerhans cells
CD2	Pan T cell, NK cells
CD3	Mature pan T cell
CD4	Helper/inducer T cells
CD5	Pan T cell, subset of B cells
CD7	Pan T cell, 25% of AML
CD8	Cytotoxic/suppressor T cell
CD10	Immature B cells, mature granulocytes
CD11b	Maturing myeloid cells
CD13	Myeloid cells
CD14	Maturing monocytes
CD15	Maturing myeloid cells
CD16	Granulocytes, NK cells
CD19	Pan B cell
CD20	Maturing B cells
CD22	Maturing B cells
CD33	Myeloid cells
CD34	Immature hematopoietic cells, stem cell
CD41	Glycoprotein IIb/IIIa, platelets, and megakaryocytes
CD45	Leukocyte common antigen
CD56	NK cells, some stem cell disorders
CD61	Glycoprotein IIb/IIIa, platelets, and megakaryocytes
CD64	Monocytes, activated granulocytes
CD117	Myeloid and erythroid blasts
CD133	Immature hematopoietic cells, stem cell
HLA-DR	Myeloid blasts, B cells, activated T cells

TABLE 5 Antibodies commonly used in the diagnosis of non-Hodgkin's lymphoma

Designation	Specificity
CD1	Common thymocyte, early T cells, Langerhans cells
CD2	Pan T cell, NK cells
CD3	Mature pan T cell
CD4	Helper/inducer T cells
CD5	Pan T cell, subset of B cells
CD7	Pan T cell
CD8	Cytotoxic/suppressor T cell
CD10	Immature and germinal center B cells
CD11c	Hairy cell leukemia, some marginal-zone lymphoma
CD19	Pan B cell
CD20	Maturing B cells
CD22	Maturing B cells
CD23	Activated B cells
CD38	Plasma cells
CD45	Leukocyte common antigen
CD56	NK cells
CD79b	B cells
CD103	Hairy cell leukemia
FMC7	B-cell lymphoma other than CLL/SLL
Kappa light chain	Mature B cells
Lambda light chain	Mature B cells

compensation, and a proliferation of software for off-line data analysis have greatly simplified these tasks. Consequently, it has been recommended that a minimum of three simultaneous fluorochromes, in addition to two light scatter parameters, be used for the diagnosis of hematopoietic neoplasms, with four fluorochromes preferred.

In a three-color analysis, the commonly used fluorochromes are fluorescein isothiocyanate, PE, and either PE-Cy5 or PerCP-Cy5.5. PE-Cy5 produces a brighter signal than PerCP-Cy5.5 but is a tandem conjugate dye and requires more compensation due to variable PE emission/leakage. A large number of antibodies are now available in these fluorochromes from a variety of manufacturers, with the exception of PerCP-Cy5.5, allowing a wide variety of useful antibody combinations. The additional fluorochrome used in a four-color combination depends largely on instrumentation, with PE-Texas red used on single-laser instruments and allophycocyanin (APC) used on dual-laser instruments. PE-Texas red is a tandem dye that is difficult to manufacture reproducibly with low PE leakage and requires significant compensation due to a high degree of spectral overlap with both PE and PE-Cy5 or PerCP-Cy5.5. However, an increasing number of useful antibodies are available in PE-Texas red. The use of APC avoids the compensation and manufacturing difficulties of PE-Texas red, as it is not a tandem conjugate dye but requires a different excitation wavelength, provided by a second laser (633 nm), minimizing spectral overlap with dyes excited by the primary laser (488 nm). However, the secondary laser will partially excite the Cy5 component of PE-Cy5, requiring interlaser compensation, a problem avoided by the use of PerCP-Cy5.5. A variety of antibodies are now available in APC. Current strategies for >4-color analysis include additional dyes such as Pacific blue, Alexa 594, Alexa 700, APC-Cy7, PE-Cy7, and/or PE-Cy5.5 with those already discussed, but these are restricted by limited reagent availability. Few laboratories currently utilize >4-color techniques for routine analysis of hematopoietic neoplasms, but this will change as new multilaser benchtop analyzers are developed and reagents become more available (79).

Three general approaches for the use of antibody panels have been described (88). In the first, a comprehensive panel of antibodies is run, which will answer most relevant questions. This provides extensive information and saves some time, as additional reagents are rarely required, but it may use unnecessary reagents and cannot be used on samples having limited numbers of cells. Another approach is to use a minimal screening panel containing a limited number of reagents, followed by a secondary panel to address specific issues raised in the initial screen. The recursive nature of this approach may be more economical for reagents, but it is lengthier and may be relatively insensitive for the detection of small abnormal populations. A more directed approach may be used where reagents are selected to address specific questions based on clinical and/or morphological information. However, this assumes that the information provided is correct, and unsuspected abnormalities may not be identified. This approach may be the only possible option for a sample with a limited number of cells.

Finally, the strategy used for normal and abnormal population identification is critical for panel construction, and a number are in common use. These strategies are not necessarily mutually exclusive, and often more than one must be used. However, no consensus exists as to optimal combinations of reagents for this purpose. Commonly, one or more fluorescent reagents are included in each tube of a panel to specifically facilitate the identification of a subpopulation of cells that are further characterized by the remaining reagents in that tube. These reagents may identify general subpopulations of cells, e.g., blasts using CD45 in combination with side scatter, or specifically identify a cell lineage, e.g., CD19 for B cells or CD3 for T cells. To allow tracking of the subpopulation between multiple tubes, the reagent(s) used for population identification must be included in every tube used for characterization of that population. This results in some unavoidable redundancy in panel construction. For the further characterization of the identified population, it is important to create combinations of reagents that emphasize normal patterns of maturation for the population, providing internal controls against which an abnormal population can be assessed. The inclusion of combinations of reagents to detect both aberrant maturational antigen expression, either of degree or of maturational stage, and the expression of non-lineage-associated antigens is desirable. However, it may be difficult to design an optimal panel that will address all these concerns in all situations. It is most important that the operator be familiar with the properties of each antibody combination used, on both normal and abnormal populations.

DATA ANALYSIS

The analysis of flow cytometric data for diagnosis of hematopoietic neoplasms involves identification of normal and abnormal populations within a multiparametric data space typically involving at least six dimensions (7). As multidimensional spaces are difficult to visualize for more than three dimensions, analysis commonly relies largely on the visual inspection of multiple one- and two-dimensional scatterplots or histograms. For a given tube assayed, the number of two-dimensional histograms that should be examined to completely evaluate the data space represents all possible two-parameter combinations, i.e., $\Sigma(n - 1)$, where n is the number of parameters evaluated. This results in a rather large number of histograms to evaluate when higher-order multiparametric data are collected. In practice, this process is often simplified by examining only histograms containing combinations of parameters that are felt to be informative, with the associated risk of occasionally overlooking populations that were not anticipated.

Analysis may be restricted to subpopulations of interest by a process termed "gating," whereby the operator encircles a population of interest on a histogram with an electronic line or "gate" and restricts further analysis to that subpopulation of events. Combinations of gates may be created using Boolean logic as a powerful way to more specifically identify subsets of events. Despite the power of these methods, it is advisable to initially examine data ungated before proceeding to more restrictive gating strategies, as populations of interest could be entirely excluded by the premature application of gating. This is particularly important when evaluating for the presence of hematopoietic neoplasms, as the immunophenotype and light scatter properties of the population of potential interest are often unknown. Once a population of interest has been identified, more sophisticated gating is useful to improve the purity of the population being evaluated.

One of the gating strategies inherited from lymphocyte subset analysis is the use of light scatter properties alone to identify populations of interest, i.e., forward- versus right-angle side scatter. While for simple specimens such as lymph node or peripheral blood this might be adequate in some situations, the method is clearly inadequate for more complex specimens such as bone marrow, as significant overlap exists for light scatter properties of normal and abnormal populations (89) (see Fig. 3). Consequently, fluorescent reagents are often included in reagent panels to improve population identification, often creating redundancy between tubes within a panel.

One common method is the use of antibodies to CD45 in combination with right-angle light scatter (see Fig. 4). This method allows the separation of nucleated cell populations into six basic groups: mature lymphocyte, maturing monocyte, maturing myeloid, myeloblast, immature lymphocyte (lymphoblast), and red blood cell (Fig. 4) (8, 87). While this method is very useful for a preliminary identification of populations in complex specimens, particularly for the identification of blasts, often populations identified by this method are not entirely pure and other reagents must be used to confirm their identity. This is particularly true for lymphocyte subpopulations where CD45 versus side scatter does not discriminate between B cells, T cells, or NK cells and often adds little useful information. Consequently, CD45 versus side-scatter population identification is of the greatest utility in the diagnosis of acute leukemia and myelodysplasia and is less useful in the diagnosis of lymphoma. This approach also relies on the assumption that neoplastic populations retain a pattern of light scatter and CD45 expression similar to that of their normal counterparts, an assumption that is not valid in some cases.

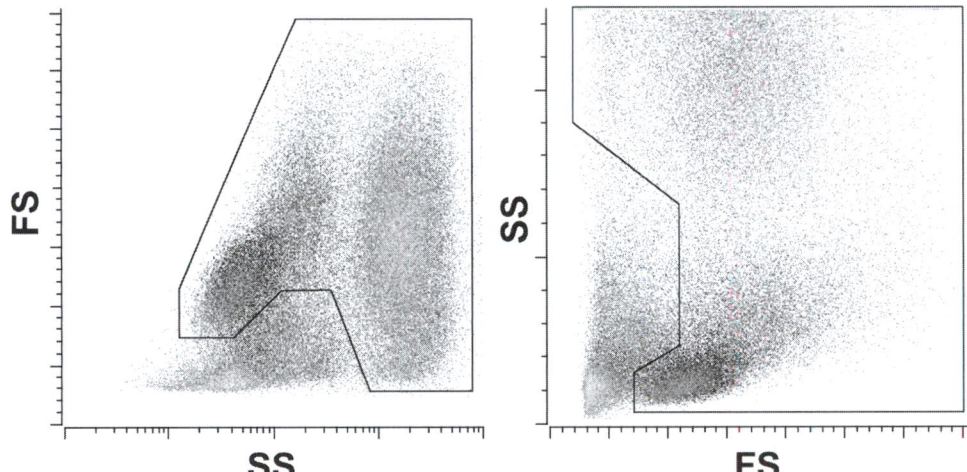

FIGURE 3 Forward-scatter (FS) versus side-scatter (SS) display of normal bone marrow using either logarithmic (left) or linear (right) SS as commonly displayed. The axes may be reversed depending upon the operator's preference. The dark line encloses the viable white blood cells. Note the difficulty in resolving the low FS and SS populations, i.e., lymphocytes, lymphoblasts, and myeloblasts, relative to CD45 versus SS gating of the same sample in Fig. 2. The very low scatter events lying outside the dark lines represent unlysed erythrocytes and degenerating cells.

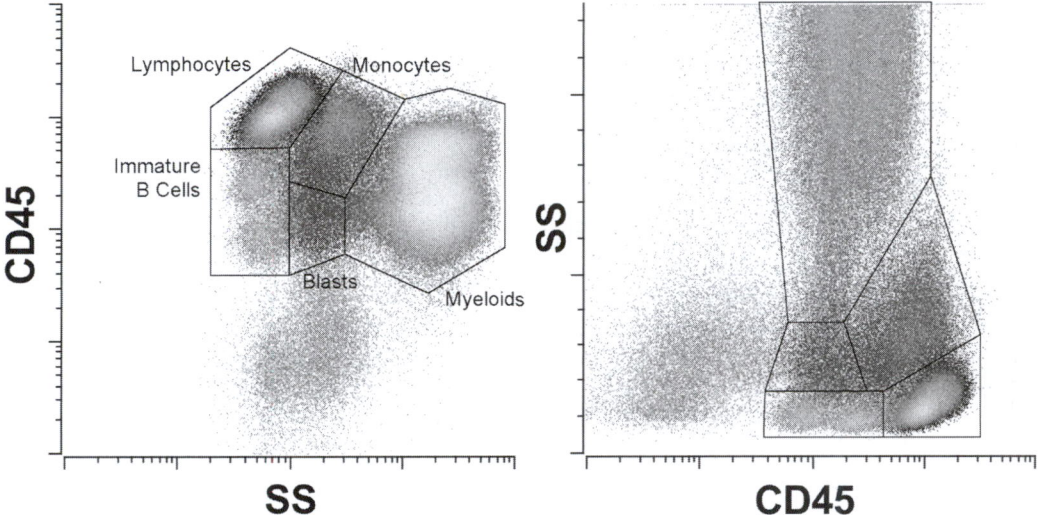

FIGURE 4 CD45 versus side-scatter (SS) gating of normal bone marrow using either logarithmic (left) or linear (right) SS as commonly displayed. Note that the use of logarithmic SS results in tighter clustering of the populations having higher SS, in particular the myeloid cells. The ungated cells with low to negative CD45 represent unlysed erythrocytes.

However, such deviation from these expected patterns may itself be useful to detect the presence of abnormal populations. Particular care must be taken to not overlook the presence of CD45-negative hematopoietic neoplasms such as myeloma, pediatric ALL, or, occasionally, anaplastic large-cell lymphoma using this approach.

Another common method of population identification is the use of lineage-associated antigens to more specifically isolate subpopulations such as B cells with CD19, T cells with CD3, blasts with CD34, etc. (85). In this approach, the three parameters available to uniquely identify populations of interest are the lineage-associated antigen used, forward scatter, and right-angle light scatter. This approach is particularly well suited for the analysis of lymphoma, as it allows more specific dissection of lymphocyte subpopulations (see Fig. 5). However, caution should be used when one relies on the expression of any single antigen for the detection of abnormal populations. In a given case, the neoplastic population may exhibit a complete loss of the antigen used for lineage detection, even for relatively consistently expressed antigens such as CD19 on B cells. This can result in a failure to detect the presence of an abnormal population if care is not taken. Consequently, it is

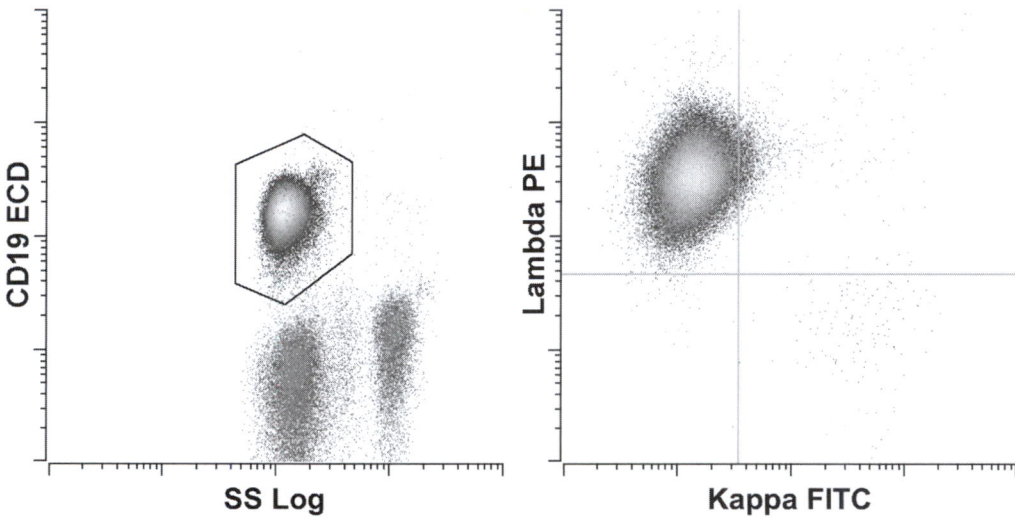

FIGURE 5 Lineage-specific gating of peripheral blood using CD19 to identify the B-cell population (left). The additional presence of both kappa and lambda light chains in the tube allows the ability to specifically analyze the B-cell population and demonstrate a sizeable clonal B-cell population having lambda light-chain restriction (right). Note the presence of a very small subset of polyclonal B cells having brighter light-chain expression. SS, side scatter; FITC, fluorescein isothiocyanate.

advisable to use at least two lineage-associated antigens within a panel when this approach is used.

Given that neoplastic populations may have an unpredictably wide variety of abnormal immunophenotypes that in some cases deviate markedly from normal, it is prudent to use more than one of the above approaches in some combination when one analyzes multiparametric flow cytometry data. The validity of assumptions inherent in any single method of analysis may be cross-checked using one or more other methods.

DATA REPORTING

The reporting of data resulting from flow cytometric analysis should focus on providing information relevant to those submitting the sample for analysis, generally clinicians or pathologists. Flow cytometric analysis is not a well-standardized procedure, and this is reflected in a variety of reporting methods. Components which should be present in every report include patient demographic information, including relevant clinical information and reason for flow cytometric analysis, sample source, specimen number, dates collected and received, antibodies used, description of data resulting from analysis, and an interpretation of the findings (12). The viability of the specimen should be included in the report if low enough to potentially compromise the analysis. The manner in which analysis results have been historically reported includes a list of antibodies used with the corresponding percentage positive for some population of interest. This format does not generally provide meaningful data for those reading the report, as it is often difficult to determine which distinct populations were identified, whether their immunophenotypes were normal or abnormal, and what the intensity of antigen expression was, and it obscures possible relationships between the parameters. A population-based method of reporting using simple text descriptions is capable of presenting all of the above findings in a manner that is more understandable to those reading the report and is strongly preferred. The inclusion of representative histograms in the report may provide useful information in some cases, but it must be weighed against the labor required. An interpretation of the significance of the findings should be present in all reports and may include a differential diagnosis. It is critical that flow cytometric results be interpreted in light of the patient's clinical setting and in conjunction with other laboratory findings to determine their true clinical significance. It is important to recognize that flow cytometric analysis of hematopoietic neoplasms is not a simple or standardized procedure and requires the involvement and critical judgment of professional laboratory personnel, a fact that should be recognized by appropriate signatures on the final report.

REFERENCES

1. **Almasri, N. M., J. A. Iturraspe, and R. C. Braylan.** 1998. CD10 expression in follicular lymphoma and large cell lymphoma is different from that of reactive lymph node follicles. *Arch. Pathol. Lab. Med.* **122:**539–544.

2. **Bagwell, C. B., and E. G. Adams.** 1993. Fluorescence spectral overlap compensation for any number of flow cytometry parameters. *Ann. N. Y. Acad. Sci.* **677:**167–184.

3. **Bagwell, C. B., E. J. Lovett, and K. A. Ault.** 1988. Localization of monoclonal B-cell populations through the use of Komogorov-Smirnov D-value and reduced chi-square contours. *Cytometry* **9:**469–476.

4. **Bennett, J. M., D. Catovsky, M. T. Daniel, G. Flandrin, D. A. Galton, H. R. Gralnick, and C. Sultan.** 1976. Proposals for the classification of the acute leukaemias. French-American-British (FAB) co-operative group. *Br. J. Haematol.* **33:**451–458.

5. **Betz, S. A., K. Foucar, D. R. Head, I. M. Chen, and C. L. Willman.** 1992. False-positive flow cytometric platelet glycoprotein IIb/IIIa expression in myeloid leukemias secondary to platelet adherence to blasts. *Blood* **79:**2399–2403.

6. **Bogen, S. A., D. Pelley, M. Charif, M. McCusker, H. Koh, F. Foss, M. Garifallou, C. Arkin, and D. Zucker-Franklin.** 1996. Immunophenotypic identification of Sezary cells in peripheral blood. *Am. J. Clin. Pathol.* **106:**739–748.

7. **Borowitz, M. J., R. Bray, R. Gascoyne, S. Melnick, J. W. Parker, L. Picker, and M. Stetler-Stevenson.** 1997. U.S.-Canadian Consensus recommendations on the immunophenotypic analysis of hematologic neoplasia by flow cytometry: data analysis and interpretation. *Cytometry* **30:**236–244.

8. **Borowitz, M. J., K. L. Guenther, K. E. Shults, and G. T. Stelzer.** 1993. Immunophenotyping of acute leukemia by flow cytometric analysis. Use of CD45 and right-angle light scatter to gate on leukemic blasts in three-color analysis. *Am. J. Clin. Pathol.* **100:**534–540.

9. **Borowitz, M. J., J. Rubnitz, M. Nash, D. J. Pullen, and B. Camitta.** 1998. Surface antigen phenotype can predict TEL-AML1 rearrangement in childhood B-precursor ALL: a Pediatric Oncology Group study. *Leukemia* **12:**1764–1770.

10. **Borowitz, M. J., J. Shuster, A. J. Carroll, M. Nash, A. T. Look, B. Camitta, D. Mahoney, S. J. Lauer, and D. J. Pullen.** 1997. Prognostic significance of fluorescence intensity of surface marker expression in childhood B-precursor acute lymphoblastic leukemia. A Pediatric Oncology Group study. *Blood* **89:**3960–3966.

11. **Bradstock, K., J. Matthews, E. Benson, F. Page, and J. Bishop.** 1994. Prognostic value of immunophenotyping in acute myeloid leukemia. Australian Leukaemia Study Group. *Blood* **84:**1220–1225.

12. **Braylan, R. C., S. K. Atwater, L. Diamond, J. M. Hassett, M. Johnson, P. G. Kidd, C. Leith, and D. Nguyen.** 1997. U.S.-Canadian Consensus recommendations on the immunophenotypic analysis of hematologic neoplasia by flow cytometry: data reporting. *Cytometry* **30:**245–248.

13. **Braylan, R. C., and N. A. Benson.** 1989. Flow cytometric analysis of lymphomas. *Arch. Pathol. Lab. Med.* **113:**627–633.

14. **Braylan, R. C., N. A. Benson, and J. Iturraspe.** 1993. Analysis of lymphomas by flow cytometry. Current and emerging strategies. *Ann. N. Y. Acad. Sci.* **677:**364–378.

15. **Braylan, R. C., M. J. Borowitz, B. H. Davis, G. T. Stelzer, and C. C. Stewarte.** 1997. U.S.-Canadian Consensus recommendations on the immunophenotypic analysis of hematologic neoplasia by flow cytometry. *Cytometry* **30:**213–274.

16. **Buccheri, V., E. Matutes, M. J. Dyer, and D. Catovsky.** 1993. Lineage commitment in biphenotypic acute leukemia. *Leukemia* **7:**919–927.

17. **Campana, D.** 2003. Determination of minimal residual disease in leukemia patients. *Br. J. Haematol.* **121:**823–838.

18. **Carter, P. H., S. Resto-Ruiz, G. C. Washington, S. Ethridge, A. Palini, R. Vogt, M. Waxdal, T. Fleisher, P. D. Noguchi, and G. E. Marti.** 1992. Flow cytometric analysis of whole blood lysis, three anticoagulants, and five cell preparations. *Cytometry* **13:**68–74.

19. **Crespo, M., F. Bosch, N. Villamor, B. Bellosillo, D. Colomer, M. Rozman, S. Marcé, A. López-Guillermo, E. Campo, and E. Montserrat.** 2003. ZAP-70 expression as a surrogate for immunoglobulin-variable-region mutations in chronic lymphocytic leukemia. *N. Engl. J. Med.* **348:**1764–1775.

20. **Damle, R. N., T. Wasil, F. Fais, F. Ghiotto, A. Valetto, S. L. Allen, A. Buchbinder, D. Budman, K. Dittmar,**

J. Kolitz, S. M. Lichtman, P. Schulman, V. P. Vinciguerra, K. R. Rai, M. Ferrarini, and N. Chiorazzi. 1999. Ig V gene mutation status and CD38 expression as novel prognostic indicators in chronic lymphocytic leukemia. *Blood* **94**:1840–1847.

21. Davis, B. H., K. Foucar, W. Szczarkowski, E. Ball, T. Witzig, K. A. Foon, D. Wells, P. Kotylo, R. Johnson, C. Hanson, and D. Bessman. 1997. U.S.-Canadian Consensus recommendations on the immunophenotypic analysis of hematologic neoplasia by flow cytometry: medical indications. *Cytometry* **30**:249–263.

22. Elghetany, M. T. 1998. Surface marker abnormalities in myelodysplastic syndromes. *Haematologica* **83**:1104–1115.

23. Escribano, L., B. Diaz-Agustin, P. Bravo, R. Navalon, J. Almeida, and A. Orfao. 1999. Immunophenotype of bone marrow mast cells in indolent systemic mast cell disease in adults. *Leuk. Lymphoma* **35**:227–235.

24. Escribano, L., A. Orfao, J. Villarrubia, B. Diaz-Agustin, C. Cervero, A. Rios, J. L. Velasco, J. Ciudad, J. L. Navarro, and J. F. San Miguel. 1998. Immunophenotypic characterization of human bone marrow mast cells. A flow cytometric study of normal and pathological bone marrow samples. *Anal. Cell. Pathol.* **16**:151–159.

25. Farahat, N., D. Lens, A. Zomas, R. Morilla, E. Matutes, and D. Catovsky. 1995. Quantitative flow cytometry can distinguish between normal and leukaemic B-cell precursors. *Br. J. Haematol.* **91**:640–646.

26. Fukushima, P. I., P. K. Nguyen, P. O'Grady, and M. Stetler-Stevenson. 1996. Flow cytometric analysis of kappa and lambda light chain expression in evaluation of specimens for B-cell neoplasia. *Cytometry* **26**:243–252.

27. Geary, W. A., H. F. Frierson, D. J. Innes, and D. E. Normansell. 1993. Quantitative criteria for clonality in the diagnosis of B-cell non-Hodgkin's lymphoma by flow cytometry. *Mod. Pathol.* **6**:155–161.

28. Ginaldi, L., N. Farahat, E. Matutes, M. De Martinis, R. Morilla, and D. Catovsky. 1996. Differential expression of T cell antigens in normal peripheral blood lymphocytes: a quantitative analysis by flow cytometry. *J. Clin. Pathol.* **49**:539–544.

29. Ginaldi, L., E. Matutes, N. Farahat, M. De Martinis, R. Morilla, and D. Catovsky. 1996. Differential expression of CD3 and CD7 in T-cell malignancies: a quantitative study by flow cytometry. *Br. J. Haematol.* **93**:921–927.

30. Hanson, C. A., M. Abaza, S. Sheldon, C. W. Ross, B. Schnitzer, and L. M. Stoolman. 1993. Biphenotypic leukaemia: immunophenotypic and cytogenetic analysis. *Br. J. Haematol.* **84**:49–60.

31. Harada, H., M. M. Kawano, N. Huang, Y. Harada, K. Iwato, O. Tanabe, H. Tanaka, A. Sakai, H. Asaoku, and A. Kuramoto. 1993. Phenotypic difference of normal plasma cells from mature myeloma cells. *Blood* **81**:2658–2663.

32. Harris, N. L., E. S. Jaffe, J. Diebold, G. Flandrin, H. K. Muller-Hermelink, J. Vardiman, T. A. Lister, and C. D. Bloomfield. 1999. The World Health Organization classification of neoplastic diseases of the hematopoietic and lymphoid tissues. Report of the Clinical Advisory Committee meeting, Airlie House, Virginia, November, 1997. *Ann. Oncol.* **10**:1419–1432.

33. Harris, N. L., E. S. Jaffe, H. Stein, P. M. Banks, J. K. C. Chan, M. L. Cleary, G. Delsol, C. De Wolf-Peeters, B. Falini, K. C. Gatter, T. M. Grogan, P. G. Isaacson, D. M. Knowles, D. Y. Mason, H.-K. Muller-Hermelink, S. A. Pileri, M. A. Piris, E. Ralfkiaer, and R. A. Warnke. 1994. A revised European-American classification of lymphoid neoplasms: a proposal from the International Lymphoma Study Group. *Blood* **84**:1361–1392.

34. Head, D. R. 1996. Revised classification of acute myeloid leukemia. *Leukemia* **10**:1826–1831.

35. Hoffkes, H. G., G. Schmidtke, M. Uppenkamp, and U. Schmucker. 1996. Multiparametric immunophenotyping of B cells in peripheral blood of healthy adults by flow cytometry. *Clin. Diagn. Lab. Immunol.* **3**:30–36.

36. Inghirami, G., B. Y. Zhu, L. Chess, and D. M. Knowles. 1990. Flow cytometric and immunohistochemical characterization of the gamma/delta T-lymphocyte population in normal human lymphoid tissue and peripheral blood. *Am. J. Pathol.* **136**:357–367.

37. Jennings, C. D., and K. A. Foon. 1997. Recent advances in flow cytometry: applications to the diagnosis of hematologic malignancy. *Blood* **90**:2863–2892.

38. Khalidi, H. S., R. K. Brynes, L. J. Medeiros, K. L. Chang, M. L. Slovak, D. S. Snyder, and D. A. Arber. 1998. The immunophenotype of blast transformation of chronic myelogenous leukemia: a high frequency of mixed lineage phenotype in "lymphoid" blasts and a comparison of morphologic, immunophenotypic, and molecular findings. *Mod. Pathol.* **11**:1211–1221.

39. Khalidi, H. S., K. L. Chang, L. J. Medeiros, R. K. Brynes, M. L. Slovak, J. L. Murata-Collins, and D. A. Arber. 1999. Acute lymphoblastic leukemia. Survey of immunophenotype, French-American-British classification, frequency of myeloid antigen expression, and karyotypic abnormalities in 210 pediatric and adult cases. *Am. J. Clin. Pathol.* **111**:467–476.

40. Khalidi, H. S., L. J. Medeiros, K. L. Chang, R. K. Brynes, M. L. Slovak, and D. A. Arber. 1998. The immunophenotype of adult acute myeloid leukemia: high frequency of lymphoid antigen expression and comparison of immunophenotype, French-American-British classification, and karyotypic abnormalities. *Am. J. Clin. Pathol.* **109**:211–220.

41. Kilo, M. N., and D. M. Dorfman. 1996. The utility of flow cytometric immunophenotypic analysis in the distinction of small lymphocytic lymphoma/chronic lymphocytic leukemia from mantle cell lymphoma. *Am. J. Clin. Pathol.* **105**:451–457.

42. Krasinskas, A. M., M. A. Wasik, M. Kamoun, R. Schretzenmair, J. Moore, and K. E. Salhany. 1998. The usefulness of CD64, other monocyte-associated antigens, and CD45 gating in the subclassification of acute myeloid leukemias with monocytic differentiation. *Am. J. Clin. Pathol.* **110**:797–805.

43. Kuchnio, M., E. A. Sausville, E. S. Jaffe, T. Greiner, F. M. Foss, J. McClanahan, P. Fukushima, and M. A. Stetler-Stevenson. 1994. Flow cytometric detection of neoplastic T cells in patients with mycosis fungoides based on levels of T-cell receptor expression. *Am. J. Clin. Pathol.* **102**:856–860.

44. Kussick, S. J., M. Kalnoski, R. M. Braziel, and B. L. Wood. 2004. Prominent clonal B-cell populations identified by flow cytometry in histologically reactive lymphoid proliferations. *Am. J. Clin. Pathol.* **121**:464–472.

45. Kussick, S. J., and B. L. Wood. 2003. Four-color flow cytometry identifies virtually all cytogenetically abnormal bone marrow samples in the workup of non-CML myeloproliferative disorders. *Am. J. Clin. Pathol.* **120**:854–865.

46. Kussick, S. J., and B. L. Wood. 2003. Using 4-color flow cytometry to identify abnormal myeloid populations. *Arch. Pathol. Lab. Med.* **127**:1140–1147.

47. Lamy, T., and T. P. Loughran, Jr. 1999. Current concepts: large granular lymphocyte leukemia. *Blood Rev.* **13**:230–240.

48. Lanza, F., S. Bi, G. Castoldi, and J. M. Goldman. 1993. Abnormal expression of N-CAM (CD56) adhesion molecule on myeloid and progenitor cells from chronic myeloid leukemia. *Leukemia* **7**:1570–1575.

49. Letwin, B. W., P. K. Wallace, K. A. Muirhead, G. L. Hensler, W. H. Kashatus, and P. K. Horan. 1990. An improved clonal excess assay using flow cytometry and B-cell gating. *Blood* **75**:1178–1185.

50. Lima, M., J. Almeida, A. H. Santos, M. dos Anjos Teixeira, M. C. Alguero, M. L. Queiros, A. Balanzategui, B. Justica, M. Gonzalez, J. F. San Miguel, and A. Orfao. 2001. Immunophenotypic analysis of the TCR-Vbeta repertoire in 98 persistent expansions of CD3(+)/TCR-alphabeta (+) large granular lymphocytes: utility in assessing clonality and insights into the pathogenesis of the disease. *Am. J. Pathol.* **159:**1861–1868.

51. Loken, M. R., V. O. Shah, K. L. Dattilio, and C. I. Civin. 1987. Flow cytometric analysis of human bone marrow. II. Normal B lymphocyte development. *Blood* **70:**1316–1324.

52. Loken, M. R., V. O. Shah, Z. Hollander, and C. I. Civin. 1988. Flow cytometric analysis of normal B lymphoid development. *Pathol. Immunopathol. Res.* **7:**357–370.

53. Lowenberg, B., J. R. Downing, and A. Burnett. 1999. Acute myeloid leukemia. *N. Engl. J. Med.* **341:**1051–1062.

54. Lucio, P., A. Parreira, M. W. van den Beemd, E. G. van Lochem, E. R. van Wering, E. Baars, A. Porwit-MacDonald, E. Bjorklund, G. Gaipa, A. Biondi, A. Orfao, G. Janossy, J. J. van Dongen, and J. F. San Miguel. 1999. Flow cytometric analysis of normal B cell differentiation: a frame of reference for the detection of minimal residual disease in precursor-B-ALL. *Leukemia* **13:**419–427.

55. Macedo, A., A. Orfao, M. Gonzalez, M. B. Vidriales, M. C. Lopez-Berges, A. Martinez, and J. F. San Miguel. 1995. Immunological detection of blast cell subpopulations in acute myeloblastic leukemia at diagnosis: implications for minimal residual disease studies. *Leukemia* **9:**993–998.

56. Macedo, A., A. Orfao, M. B. Vidriales, M. C. Lopez-Berges, B. Valverde, M. Gonzalez, M. D. Caballero, F. Ramos, M. Martinez, J. Fernandez-Calvo, et al. 1995. Characterization of aberrant phenotypes in acute myeloblastic leukemia. *Ann. Hematol.* **70:**189–194.

57. Macey, M. G., D. A. McCarthy, T. Milne, J. D. Cavenagh, and A. C. Newland. 1999. Comparative study of five commercial reagents for preparing normal and leukaemic lymphocytes for immunophenotypic analysis by flow cytometry. *Cytometry* **38:**153–160.

58. Macon, W. R., and K. E. Salhany. 1998. T-cell subset analysis of peripheral T-cell lymphomas by paraffin section immunohistology and correlation of CD4/CD8 results with flow cytometry. *Am. J. Clin. Pathol.* **109:**610–617.

59. Matutes, E., R. Morilla, N. Farahat, F. Carbonell, J. Swansbury, M. Dyer, and D. Catovsky. 1997. Definition of acute biphenotypic leukemia. *Haematologica* **82:**64–66.

60. Matutes, E., R. Morilla, K. Owusu-Ankomah, A. Houliham, P. Meeus, and D. Catovsky. 1994. The immunophenotype of hairy cell leukemia (HCL). Proposal for a scoring system to distinguish HCL from B-cell disorders with hairy or villous lymphocytes. *Leuk. Lymphoma* **14** (Suppl. 1):57–61.

61. Matutes, E., K. Owusu-Ankomah, R. Morilla, J. Garcia Marco, A. Houlihan, T. H. Que, and D. Catovsky. 1994. Immunological profile of B-cell disorders and proposal of a scoring system for the diagnosis of CLL. *Leukemia* **8:**1640–1645.

62. McClanahan, J., P. I. Fukushima, and M. Stetler-Stevenson. 1999. Increased peripheral blood gamma delta T-cells in patients with lymphoid neoplasia: a diagnostic dilemma in flow cytometry. *Cytometry* **38:**280–285.

63. Morice, W. G., P. J. Kurtin, P. J. Leibson, A. Tefferi, and C. A. Hanson. 2003. Demonstration of aberrant T-cell and natural killer-cell antigen expression in all cases of granular lymphocytic leukaemia. *Br. J. Haematol.* **120:**1026–1036.

64. National Committee for Clinical Laboratory Standards. 1992. *Clinical Applications of Flow Cytometry: Quality Assurance and Immunophenotyping of Peripheral Blood Lymphocytes.* NCCLS document H42-T, vol. 9, no. 13.

National Committee for Clinical Laboratory Standards, Villanova, Pa.

65. National Committee for Clinical Laboratory Standards. 1998. *Clinical Applications of Flow Cytometry: Immunophenotyping of Leukemic Cells.* Approved guideline. NCCLS document H43-A, vol. 18, no. 8. National Committee for Clinical Laboratory Standards, Wayne, Pa.

66. Ocqueteau, M., A. Orfao, J. Almeida, J. Blade, M. Gonzalez, R. Garcia-Sanz, C. Lopez-Berges, M. J. Moro, J. Hernandez, L. Escribano, D. Caballero, M. Rozman, and J. F. San Miguel. 1998. Immunophenotypic characterization of plasma cells from monoclonal gammopathy of undetermined significance patients. Implications for the differential diagnosis between MGUS and multiple myeloma. *Am. J. Pathol.* **152:**1655–1665.

67. Orfao, A., M. C. Chillon, A. M. Bortoluci, M. C. Lopez-Berges, R. Garcia-Sanz, M. Gonzalez, M. D. Tabernero, M. A. Garcia-Marcos, A. I. Rasillo, J. Hernandez-Rivas, and J. F. San Miguel. 1999. The flow cytometric pattern of CD34, CD15 and CD13 expression in acute myeloblastic leukemia is highly characteristic of the presence of PML-RAR alpha gene rearrangements. *Haematologica* **84:**405–412.

68. Parker, J. E., K. L. Fishlock, A. Mijovic, B. Czepulkowski, A. Pagliuca, and G. J. Mufti. 1998. 'Low-risk' myelodysplastic syndrome is associated with excessive apoptosis and an increased ratio of pro- versus anti-apoptotic bcl-2-related proteins. *Br. J. Haematol.* **103:**1075–1082.

69. Picker, L. J., L. M. Weiss, L. J. Medeiros, G. S. Wood, and R. A. Warnke. 1987. Immunophenotypic criteria for the diagnosis of non-Hodgkin's lymphoma. *Am. J. Pathol.* **128:**181–201.

70. Pope, B., R. Brown, J. Gibson, and D. Joshua. 1999. The bone marrow plasma cell labeling index by flow cytometry. *Cytometry* **38:**286–292.

71. Porwit-MacDonald, A., G. Janossy, K. Ivory, D. Swirsky, R. Peters, K. Wheatley, H. Walker, A. Turker, A. H. Goldstone, and A. Burnett. 1996. Leukemia-associated changes identified by quantitative flow cytometry. IV. CD34 overexpression in acute myelogenous leukemia M2 with t(8;21). *Blood* **87:**1162–1169.

72. Preti, H. A., Y. O. Huh, S. M. O'Brien, M. Andreeff, S. T. Pierce, M. Keating, and H. M. Kantarjian. 1995. Myeloid markers in adult acute lymphocytic leukemia. Correlations with patient and disease characteristics and with prognosis. *Cancer* **76:**1564–1570.

73. Pui, C. H., J. E. Rubnitz, M. L. Hancock, J. R. Downing, S. C. Raimondi, G. K. Rivera, J. T. Sandlund, R. C. Ribeiro, D. R. Head, M. V. Relling, W. E. Evans, and F. G. Behm. 1998. Reappraisal of the clinical and biologic significance of myeloid-associated antigen expression in childhood acute lymphoblastic leukemia. *Clin. Oncol.* **16:**3768–3773.

74. Ratech, H., and S. Litwin. 1989. Surface immunoglobulin light chain restriction in B-cell non-Hodgkin's malignant lymphomas. *Am. J. Clin. Pathol.* **91:**583–586.

75. Reading, C. L., E. H. Estey, Y. O. Huh, D. F. Claxton, G. Sanchez, L.W. Terstappen, M. C. O'Brien, S. Baron, and A. B. Deisseroth. 1993. Expression of unusual immunophenotype combinations in acute myelogenous leukemia. *Blood* **81:**3083–3090.

76. Renzi, P., and L. C. Ginns. 1987. Analysis of T cell subsets in normal adults. Comparison of whole blood lysis technique to Ficoll-Hypaque separation by flow cytometry. *Immunol. Methods* **98:**53–56.

77. Robbins, B. A., D. J. Ellison, J. C. Spinosa, C. A. Carey, R. J. Lukes, S. Poppema, A. Saven, and L. D. Piro. 1993. Diagnostic application of two-color flow cytometry in 161 cases of hairy cell leukemia. *Blood* **82:**1277–1287.

78. **Roederer, M.** 2001. Spectral compensation for flow cytometry: visualization artifacts, limitations, and caveats. *Cytometry* **45:**194–205.

79. **Roederer, M., S. De Rosa, R. Gerstein, M. Anderson, M. Bigos, R. Stovel, T. Nozaki, D. Parks, L. Herzenberg, and L. Herzenberg.** 1997. 8 color, 10-parameter flow cytometry to elucidate complex leukocyte heterogeneity. *Cytometry* **29:**328–339.

80. **Ruiz-Arguelles, G. J., and J. F. San Miguel.** 1994. Cell surface markers in multiple myeloma. *Mayo Clin. Proc.* **69:**684–690.

81. **Sallah, S., S. V. Smith, L. C. Lony, P. Woodard, J. L. Schmitz, and J. D. Folds.** 1997. Gamma/delta T-cell hepatosplenic lymphoma: review of the literature, diagnosis by flow cytometry and concomitant autoimmune hemolytic anemia. *Ann. Hematol.* **74:**139–142.

82. **Samoszuk, M. K., M. Krailo, Q. H. Yan, R. J. Lukes, and J. W. Parker.** 1985. Limitations of numerical ratios for defining monoclonality of immunoglobulin light chains in B-cell lymphomas. *Diagn. Immunol.* **3:**133–138.

83. **San Miguel, J. F., A. Martinez, A. Macedo, M. B. Vidriales, C. Lopez-Berges, M. Gonzalez, D. Caballero, M. A. Garcia-Marcos, F. Ramos, J. Fernandez-Calvo, M. J. Calmuntia, J. Diaz-Mediavilla, and A. Orfao.** 1997. Immunophenotyping investigation of minimal residual disease is a useful approach for predicting relapse in acute myeloid leukemia patients. *Blood* **90:**2465–2470.

84. **Schwartz, A., G. E. Marti, R. Poon, J. W. Gratama, and E. Fernandez-Repollet.** 1998. Standardizing flow cytometry: a classification system of fluorescence standards used for flow cytometry. *Cytometry* **33:**106–114.

85. **Segal, G. H., M. G. Edinger, M. Owen, M. McNealis, P. Lopez, A. Perkins, M. D. Linden, A. J. Fishleder, M. H. Stoler, and R. R. Tubbs.** 1991. Concomitant delineation of surface Ig, B-cell differentiation antigens, and HLADR on lymphoid proliferations using three-color immunocytometry. *Cytometry* **12:**350–359.

86. **Stelzer, G. T., G. Marti, A. Hurley, P. McCoy, Jr., E. J. Lovett, and A. Schwartz.** 1997. U.S.-Canadian Consensus recommendations on the immunophenotypic analysis of hematologic neoplasia by flow cytometry: standardization and validation of laboratory procedures. *Cytometry* **30:**214–230.

87. **Stelzer, G. T., K. E. Shults, and M. R. Loken.** 1993. CD45 gating for routine flow cytometric analysis of human bone marrow specimens. *Ann. N. Y. Acad. Sci.* **677:**265–280.

88. **Stewart, C. C., F. G. Behm, J. L. Carey, J. Cornbleet, R. E. Duque, S. D. Hudnall, P. E. Hurtubise, M. Loken, R. R. Tubbs, and S. Wormsley.** 1997. U.S.-Canadian Consensus recommendations on the immunophenotypic analysis of hematologic neoplasia by flow cytometry: selection of antibody combinations. *Cytometry* **30:**231–235.

89. **Sun, T., R. Sangaline, J. Ryder, K. Gibbens, C. Rollo, S. Stewart, and C. Rajagopalan.** 1997. Gating strategy for immunophenotyping of leukemia and lymphoma. *Am. J. Clin. Pathol.* **108:**152–157.

90. **Terstappen, L. W., Z. Hollander, H. Meiners, and M. R. Loken.** 1990. Quantitative comparison of myeloid antigens on five lineages of mature peripheral blood cells. *J. Leukoc. Biol.* **48:**138–148.

91. **Terstappen, L.W., S. Huang, and L. J. Picker.** 1992. Flow cytometric assessment of human T-cell differentiation in thymus and bone marrow. *Blood* **79:**666–677.

92. **Terstappen, L.W., S. Johnsen, I. M. Segers-Nolten, and M. R. Loken.** 1990. Identification and characterization of plasma cells in normal human bone marrow by high-resolution flow cytometry. *Blood* **76:**1739–1747.

93. **Terstappen, L. W., and M. R. Loken.** 1990. Myeloid cell differentiation in normal bone marrow and acute myeloid leukemia assessed by multi-dimensional flow cytometry. *Anal. Cell. Pathol.* **2:**229–240.

94. **Terstappen, L. W., M. Safford, S. Konemann, M. R. Loken, K. Zurlutter, T. Buchner, W. Hiddemann, and B. Wormann.** 1992. Flow cytometric characterization of acute myeloid leukemia. Part II. Phenotypic heterogeneity at diagnosis. *Leukemia* **6:**70–80.

95. **Toba, K., T. Koike, A. Shibata, S. Hashimoto, M. Takahashi, M. Masuko, T. Azegami, H. Takahashi, and Y. Aizawa.** 1999. Novel technique for the direct flow cytofluorometric analysis of human basophils in unseparated blood and bone marrow, and the characterization of phenotype and peroxidase of human basophils. *Cytometry* **35:**249–259.

96. **Tworek, J. A., T. P. Singleton, B. Schnitzer, E. D. Hsi, and C. W. Ross.** 1998. Flow cytometric and immunohistochemical analysis of small lymphocytic lymphoma, mantle cell lymphoma, and plasmacytoid small lymphocytic lymphoma. *Am. J. Clin. Pathol.* **110:**582–589.

97. **Weir, E. G., K. Cowan, P. LeBeau, and M. J. Borowitz.** 1999. A limited antibody panel can distinguish B-precursor acute lymphoblastic leukemia from normal B precursors with four color flow cytometry: implications for residual disease detection. *Leukemia* **13:**558–567.

98. **Wells, D. A., M. Benesch, M. R. Loken, C. Vallejo, D. Myerson, W. M. Leisenring, and H. J. Deeg.** 2003. Myeloid and monocytic dyspoeisis as determined by flow cytometric scoring in myelodysplastic syndrome correlates with the IPSS and with outcome after hematopoietic stem cell transplantation. *Blood* **102:**394–403.

99. **Willheim, M., H. Agis, W. R. Sperr, M. Koller, H. C. Bankl, H. Kiener, G. Fritsch, W. Fureder, A. Spittler, W. Graninger, O. Scheiner, H. Gadner, K. Lechner, G. Boltz-Nitulescu, and P. Valent.** 1995. Purification of human basophils and mast cells by multistep separation technique and mAb to CDw17 and CD117/c-kit. *J. Immunol. Methods* **182:**115–129.

Standardized Flow Cytometry Assays for Enumerating Hematopoietic Stem Cells

D. ROBERT SUTHERLAND, IAN CHIN-YEE,
MICHAEL KEENEY, AND JAN GRATAMA

21

HEMATOPOIETIC STEM/PROGENITOR CELLS EXPRESS THE CD34 ANTIGEN

An important phenotypic characteristic of the stem/progenitor cells in marrow and peripheral blood responsible for multilineage engraftment in the transplant setting was initially established in the late 1980s, when it was demonstrated that the 1 to 3% of marrow leukocytes that expressed the cell surface antigen CD34 (11) contained the majority of CFU activity for myeloid and erythroid lineages and also contained cells exhibiting the phenotypic properties of primitive lymphoid cells. Berenson et al., using a novel CD34 antibody called 12.8 (4) that uniquely cross-reacted with a similar subset of baboon marrow cells, conclusively demonstrated that the CD34 antigen not only was expressed on a variety of lineage-committed progenitors but also was expressed on true hematopoietic stem cells that could reconstitute long-term multilineage hematopoiesis in lethally irradiated animals. Subsequent studies on human subjects have firmly established that CD34+-cell transplants are safe, durable, and generally therapeutically effective.

Confirming earlier data obtained using colony-forming cell assays, CD34+ cells can be found in the peripheral blood of healthy individuals but are extremely rare (range, 0.01 to 0.1%). However, the use of chemotherapy and/or cytokines to "mobilize" CD34+ cells (28) has greatly facilitated the use of peripheral blood stem cells (PBSC) versus marrow for both autotransplantation and, more recently, allotransplantation (reviewed in reference 33). This increased use of PBSC evolved in the absence of any consensus means to monitor the engraftment potential of the stem cell product. Recent studies have indicated that umbilical cord blood (CB) also represents a rich source of CD34+ hematopoietic stem/progenitor cells, and consequently, there has been a proliferation of CB banks worldwide (8). Methods of collection, processing (with or without T-cell depletion), and cryopreservation have similarly proliferated without a rapid, reliable, and standardized method to measure the effects of such manipulations on the engraftment potential of the postthawed CB product.

CLINICAL ISSUES IN ENUMERATING STEM CELLS BY FLOW CYTOMETRY

Currently, the enumeration of CD34+ stem/progenitor cells by flow cytometry represents the most clinically useful surrogate marker of graft adequacy and provides crucial information to the transplant physician. Most transplant centers determine graft adequacy based on the number of CD34+ cells per kilogram of patient body weight. Over the last few years, the "recommended" minimum number of CD34+ cells has fallen from about 10^7/kg to around 2×10^6 to 2.5×10^6/kg, although a full consensus on the latter figure has not yet been reached (35). In addition to determining yield, the number of CD34+ cells mobilized to the peripheral blood is also a predictor of the success of apheresis, and thus an increasing number of centers use peripheral blood CD34+-cell counts to monitor online the yield of CD34+ cells (22). Accurately timing the harvesting of CD34+ cells may be particularly important for patients who have poor bone marrow function or who have received extensive prior therapy. For such poor mobilizers, daily measurements of the CD34+-cell concentration in the circulation to optimize timing of stem cell collections may have merit (29). Early collection of stem cells may be especially useful, for example in heavily pretreated myeloma patients, given the reported increase in malignant-cell contamination of apheresis products noted on later collection days (12).

More recently, there has been a shift in interest from the minimum number of stem cells required to attempts to maximize the CD34+-cell dose, a factor which has been shown by several investigators to correlate inversely with time to engraftment of neutrophils and platelets (37). Furthermore, rapid reengraftment may correlate with not only total CD34+-cell dose but also the presence or absence of certain specific subsets of CD34+ cells (25). The clinical interest in subset analysis of rare populations of CD34+ cells adds to the complexity of this assay and adds demands on the clinical flow cytometry laboratory. Ultimately, the number of viable CD34+ cells (or subsets thereof) actually reinfused to patients is the most clinically important variable determining graft success or failure. A systematic evaluation of viable stem cells from the time of collection to actual reinfusion would be ideal to quality assure these products. We envision this process to involve measurements of peripheral blood CD34+ cells in patients to "time" apheresis, to evaluate the yield of viable cells postcollection, and to evaluate the number of viable CD34+ cells postcryopreservation actually infused.

To be clinically relevant, any flow cytometric assay must meet the following criteria. (i) It must correlate with a clinically meaningful outcome, such as time to multilineage

187

engraftment. (ii) It must be applicable for the different stem cell products, i.e., peripheral blood, CB, and bone marrow. (iii) It must provide timely results (less than 2 h) and must be reproducible between institutions. (iv) It should be sufficiently flexible to permit more sophisticated qualitative analysis of CD34$^+$ subsets using a multiparametric approach. (v) It should be able to determine the viability of the target (i.e., CD34$^+$) population. (vi) It should be a single-platform assay (see below).

TECHNICAL ISSUES IN THE ENUMERATION OF CD34$^+$ CELLS BY MULTIPARAMETER FLOW CYTOMETRY

CD34 Antigen: Structural Considerations and Choice of Fluorochromes

The CD34 antigen is a heavily glycosylated mucin-like molecule, the structural characteristics of which have important implications for the choice of an appropriate CD34 antibody clone for flow-based enumeration techniques (21, 30). Due to their dependence on terminal sialic acids, which are only found on the most fully glycosylated/processed forms of CD34, class I antibodies generate the most aberrant data in clinical samples, whereas class II and class III reagents detect similar, if not identical, numbers of CD34$^+$ cells in a wide variety of normal and abnormal samples (31). Thus, for accurate enumeration of rare CD34$^+$ cells in hematopoietic samples, it is important to use a CD34 antibody that detects all glycosylation variants of the molecule, i.e., class II or class III antibodies (14, 31, 33).

It is generally advantageous to utilize an antibody conjugated to the brightest fluorochrome excitable, i.e., phycoerythrin (PE), by an argon laser-based flow cytometer. After parallel analysis of a large number of normal blood, cytokine-mobilized peripheral blood, CB, and normal marrow samples, as well as of CD34$^+$ cell lines that fail to express some class I CD34 epitopes, it is our experience that commercially made PE conjugates of the clones QBEnd10, 8G12, Birma K3, and 581 can be utilized with confidence (31). As detailed elsewhere, if fluorescein isothiocyanate (FITC) conjugates of CD34 antibodies have to be used, only class III reagents such as HPCA2 and 581 can be recommended since these reagents detect numbers of CD34$^+$ cells in parallel analyses of clinical samples using the ISHAGE protocol (see below) that are similar, if not identical, to those detected by their PE-conjugated versions (31). Although we have tested a variety of other CD34 antibody conjugates in two-, three-, and four-color combinations, some of these conjugates are not suitable for all applications or instrument platforms (10, 14, 21, 31, 33) and should be rigorously evaluated alongside currently validated reagents before introduction into the clinical laboratory. Overall, it is critical to select an appropriate CD34 antibody clone that retains high specificity and avidity of binding after conjugation to the designated fluorochrome.

CD45 Antigen: Structural Considerations and Choice of Fluorochromes

Several protocols have been developed that use CD45 antibodies to gate total nucleated white blood cells, this number serving as the denominator in the calculation of percent CD34$^+$ cells. For such protocols, it is important that pan-CD45 antibodies that detect not just all isoforms, but all glycoforms, of this mucin-like molecule are used. In this respect, the clones J33, T29/33, and HLE-1 can be used with confidence (14, 31, 33). Note, however, that the PerCP

conjugate of HLE-1, while usable on benchtop cytometers equipped with low-powered lasers, can be problematic if used on cell sorters equipped with higher-powered lasers. Of note, a very small fraction of CD34$^+$ cells that do not express CD45 comprises endothelial cells, which have been reported in increased numbers in the blood of patients with solid tumors (23). Although other pan-CD45 antibodies can be used for CD34$^+$ stem cell enumeration, the selected reagent should be carefully evaluated prior to routine use in clinical protocols.

MEASURING CD34$^+$ CELLS BY FLOW CYTOMETRY: TWO-PLATFORM METHODS

While flow cytometric enumeration of CD34$^+$ cells represents the most clinically useful assay of graft assessment, the assays that were initially developed were insufficiently robust, and interinstitutional variability in particular was problematic (6, 18). One source of variability was the method used by many transplant centers to determine the absolute number of CD34$^+$ cells per kilogram of patient body weight. Traditionally, this number was obtained by determining the percent CD34$^+$ cells by flow cytometry and multiplying it by the absolute leukocyte count (LKC) as determined by an automated hematology analyzer (hence the name "two-platform" methodology).

Siena et al. (28) were the first to describe a flow cytometric method to measure percent CD34$^+$ cells in mobilized peripheral blood. This method was initially based on mononuclear cell enrichment by density gradient centrifugation, followed by staining with the class I CD34 antibody MY10 using indirect immunofluorescence. The subsequent development of what was called the Milan protocol (27) was due to the availability around 1990 of class III CD34 antibodies, such as 8G12, that could be conjugated with FITC and, later, with PE without loss of reactivity. The protocol utilized whole-blood staining and lyse-and-wash sample processing, while the gating strategy utilized simple forward-angle (FSC) versus side-angle (SSC) light scatter above an FSC threshold or discriminator to set a denominator. An isotype-matched control was used to set the positive analysis region for CD34$^+$ cells. In the CD34 antibody-stained sample, the number of events that stained brighter than the control and exhibited low to intermediate SSC were counted and used as the numerator in the calculation of percent CD34$^+$ cells. A minimum of 50 CD34$^+$ events were counted in a list mode file of 50,000 events.

Although a number of minor developments were subsequently incorporated to improve the Milan method (18), the inherent difficulties in enumerating bona fide CD34$^+$ cells in increasingly diverse sources of hematopoietic stem cells led to the development of more sophisticated methods utilizing multiparameter gating strategies. The first two-color strategy was developed by Bender et al. (3); in this method, CD45-FITC is used in addition to CD34-PE. CD45 staining was used to establish a more stable denominator by enumerating only nucleated white blood cells in the denominator. CD45$^+$ events were then analyzed in a manner similar to the Milan protocol using an isotype and analysis of CD34 staining versus SSC to enumerate CD34$^+$ cells.

While the above protocols were generally capable of analyzing fresh peripheral blood and apheresis samples, they were inadequate for the accurate enumeration of CD34$^+$ cells in other sources of hematopoietic stem cells, or shipped or otherwise-manipulated samples of less than pristine quality. The approach proposed by Owens and Loken (26) incorporated the nuclear dye 7-amino-actinomycin D (7-AAD) to exclude dead cells, a CD14 antibody to exclude monocytes, and a CD34 antibody to identify CD34$^+$ cells. A plot of CD14-FITC versus SSC was generated from the live cell gate (7-AAD-negative events) to exclude monocytes. From this histogram, a third plot of CD34-PE versus SSC was generated and compared to an immunoglobulin G (IgG)-PE control versus SSC as in the Milan protocol. Both dim and bright CD34$^+$ events were included in the calculation. CD34$^+$ events were expressed as a percentage of total nucleated cells (live plus dead) based on an FSC-versus-SSC plot.

The Dutch Cooperative Study Group on Immunophenotyping of Haematological Malignancies (16) developed a three-color protocol based on LDS-751 and CD14, CD66e, and CD34 antibodies. LDS-751 stains DNA and RNA, and gating on FSC versus LDS-751 allows discrimination between nucleated cells and debris, unlysed erythrocytes, and platelets. Monocytes (CD14$^+$) and granulocytes (CD66e$^+$) were then excluded from further analysis, after which the stem cells were identified as dim or bright CD34$^+$ cells in a CD34-versus-SSC dot plot. Nonspecific staining was analyzed using identical gate settings on a control staining in which the CD34 monoclonal antibody (MAb) was replaced by an isotype control MAb, and any nonspecifically stained events were subtracted from the CD34 result.

CD34$^+$-CELL ENUMERATION USING SEQUENTIAL BOOLEAN GATING

As already indicated, accurate enumeration of rare events such as CD34$^+$ cells in heterogeneous clinical samples by flow cytometry represents a serious challenge for both clinical and research laboratories. Cytometers measure events, whether they are white cells, red cells, platelets, dead cells, or debris. Therefore, to eliminate nonleukocytes and debris from the analysis and generate a much more stable denominator against which to measure CD34$^+$ cells, we used CD45 as a counterstain as described previously (3). However, we also took advantage of the prior observations of Borowitz et al. (5) indicating that leukemic blast cells, which exhibit light scatter properties generally similar to those of lymphocytes, express lower levels of CD45 on their surfaces, thus providing a means of delineating lymphocytes from normal blast cells using this surface marker. Just as lymphocytes, monocytes, and granulocytes form discrete clusters on analysis of CD45 staining versus SSC (5), so do CD34$^+$ cells. Thus, a sensitive and accurate multiparameter flow methodology was devised that utilizes the maximum information available of four parameters: FSC and SSC and CD34 and CD45 staining. These four parameters were combined in a sequential or Boolean gating strategy that was usable on a variety of sources of hematopoietic stem cells (32). Thereafter, this basic protocol was incorporated into a set of clinical guidelines constructed for the International Society of Hematotherapy and Graft Engineering (ISHAGE), nowadays called the International Society for Cellular Therapy, to enumerate CD34$^+$ cells in peripheral blood and apheresis products (31).

The original methodology (32) at the heart of the ISHAGE protocol (31) is very sensitive, being capable of detecting 10 to 20 CD34$^+$ cells per 100,000 CD45$^+$ nucleated white blood cells. The method is highly specific when appropriate pan-CD45 antibodies (that detect all isoforms and glycoforms) and CD34 conjugates (that detect all CD34 glycoforms) are used (see below). It is quick and can be performed on a variety of single- and dual-laser flow cytometers, with only basic software being required for data analysis. The basic ISHAGE protocol can be used to enumerate CD34$^+$ cells in a variety of normal hematopoietic tissues, including marrow and CB as well as abnormal clinical samples from a variety of disease states. CD34$^+$ cells selected from both normal and abnormal marrow, CB, and peripheral blood samples can also be assessed for purity using this flexible method (34).

BASIC ISHAGE PROTOCOL AND GATING STRATEGY

The ISHAGE protocol and critical issues relating to the enumeration of CD34$^+$ cells have been published in detail elsewhere (14, 31, 33). Briefly, as shown in Fig. 1 with a CB sample, the first gate (region 1 [R1]) is established from a plot of CD45 staining versus SSC. As indicated above, this approach allows, during analysis of the list mode data file, the exclusion of red cells, platelets, and other debris commonly found in hematopoietic samples, especially those prepared by lysis–no-wash methods. Sufficient events are acquired in R1 (histogram A) that at least 100 CD34$^+$ cells are displayed in the lymph-blast region, R4 (histogram D). The acquired cells are then sequentially displayed on a plot of CD34 staining versus SSC (histogram B) and R2 is adjusted to include dim and bright CD34$^+$ events with low to intermediate SSC. The events gated by both R1 and R2 are then displayed in turn on a plot of CD45 fluorescence versus SSC (histogram C), and true CD34$^+$ cells form a cluster characterized by low CD45 staining (relative to lymphocytes) and low to intermediate SSC. It is this cluster that determines the size and location of gating R3. Excluded from this gated cluster (R3) are platelet aggregates, nonspecifically stained lymphocytes, monomyeloid cells, and debris. The cells gated within R1, R2, and R3 are then displayed on a light scatter plot to confirm that the selected events fall into a generic lymph-blast region (R4) that is precisely set to include events no smaller than small lymphocytes.

One controversial issue that arose in the early development of the ISHAGE protocols was whether all specifically stained, nonmalignant CD34$^+$ cells express low levels (at least) of CD45 molecules. To address this and other technical issues related to instrument setup and to optimize the gating regions, two additional "housekeeping" plots have been added to the original four-plot strategy. As shown in Fig. 1, R5 on plot A is set precisely to include only lymphocytes (bright CD45, low SS) and these lymphocytes are displayed on plot F (FSC versus SSC). This helps to establish the minimum size range for the lymph-blast region (R4 on histogram F and its duplicate on histogram D), and when appropriately set, nonspecifically stained debris, platelets, and some dead cells, if present and not fully excluded by the previous gates, can generally be excluded. This region also helps to confirm that the forward-angle light scatter (FALS) discriminator and FALS detector volts/gain are adequately set. The discriminator (or FSC threshold) is set to ensure that even the smallest CD45$^+$ lymphocytes scatter above it. FALS volts/gain is adjusted so that the smallest lymphocytes scatter around channel 200 of a 1,024-by-1,024 linear dot plot. After determining the appropriate discriminator setting, R1 is positioned on plot A to include all CD45$^+$ events. The lower extremity of R1 is set low enough to include all dim CD45-positive events (histogram E is used as a guide). Histogram E (CD34-PE versus CD45-FITC staining) helps to establish the lower limit of CD45 expression such that

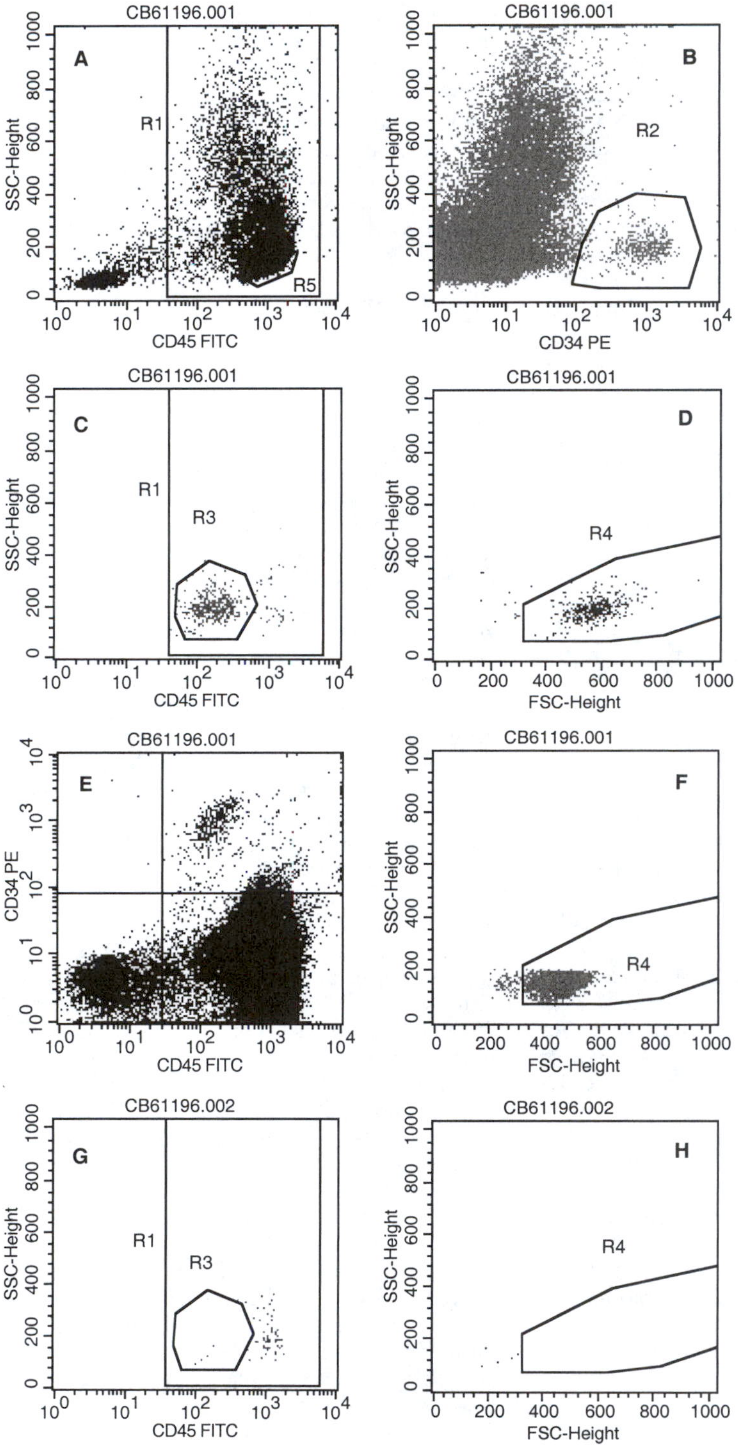

Basic ISHAGE Protocol

CD34PE/CD45FITC (A-F)

File: CB61196.001
Gate: G1
Gated Events: 60378
Total Events: 65000

Gate	Events	% Gated
G1	60378	100.00
G2	451	0.75
G3	406	0.67
G4	393	0.65

IgG1PE/CD45FITC (G-H)

File: CB61196.001
Gate: G1
Gated Events: 60378
Total Events: 65000

Gate	Events	% Gated
G1	60378	100.00
G2	451	0.75
G3	406	0.67
G4	393	0.65

FIGURE 1 Enumeration of CD34$^+$ cells in a CB sample stained with CD34-PE and CD45-FITC (clones 581 and J33, respectively; Immunotech-Coulter) using the basic ISHAGE protocol (31). Plot A is gated on all events, plot B is gated on R1 events, plot C is gated on R1 and R2 events, and plot D is gated on R1, R2, and R3 events. Plot E is gated on all events, and plot F is gated lymphocytes back-scattered from R5 (plot A) to ensure optimal placement of lymph-blast region R4 as described previously (31). Plots G and H show the same sample stained with isotype control IgG1-PE and CD45-FITC. Only two plots (equivalent to plots C and D) are shown for the control sample. No events satisfying the gating criteria of plots A to D are found in R4 of plot H. Gate statistics are obtained from plot B (CD45$^+$ events).

potential CD34$^+$ cells (that express low levels of CD45) are not excluded. The absolute CD34$^+$-cell count is obtained by multiplying this value by the absolute LKC, obtained from an automated hematology analyzer.

Basic ISHAGE Protocol Calculation

$$\frac{\text{no. of CD34}^+ \text{ events (R4)}}{\text{no. of CD45}^+ \text{ events (R1)}} \times \text{LKC } (\times 10^9/\text{liter}) \times 1,000$$

$$= \text{no. of CD34}^+ \text{ cells} \times 10^6/\text{liter}$$

ISOTYPE CONTROLS

Given the sequential gating strategy at the heart of the ISHAGE method, we reasoned that the use of isotype control antibodies to set the positive analysis region for CD34$^+$ cells would be inappropriate. Thus, the same gating regions that were established for the CD34/CD45-stained sample (Fig. 1, plots A to D) are used to analyze the IgG1/CD45 control sample. In virtually all situations, including samples containing significant numbers of dead cells, few, if any, events are detected. An example of this analysis is shown in Fig. 1. Although only the last two plots (G and H) are shown, the gate statistics indicate that while 66 events were stained by the isotype control in R2 of plot F (not shown), none appear in R4 of plot H. We have, however, seen some isotype controls that stain more events in R2 than the CD34 antibody in specific samples. Even then, due to the sequential gating strategy used in this protocol, it is unusual for any of these events to find their way into R4. Indeed, studies of a large number of normal hematopoietic samples have shown that the sequential gating approach best delineates specific from nonspecific staining and that traditional isotype controls provide no useful information regarding the levels of nonspecific staining in the flow cytometric analysis of rare events, such as CD34$^+$ cells (reviewed in reference 19). Thus, a distinguishing characteristic of the ISHAGE protocol is that the sequential gating strategy used eliminates the need to use an isotype-matched control antibody to set the positive cell analysis region for CD34$^+$ cells (14, 33). In support of this strategy, the European Working Group on Clinical Cell Analysis (EWGCCA) concluded (13) that control staining for nonspecific antibody binding for cell surface marker analysis is redundant because of the Boolean gating strategies used in modern protocols such as ISHAGE, its single-platform variant.

SINGLE-PLATFORM ABSOLUTE CD34$^+$-CELL COUNTING

The use of two-platform methods to obtain the absolute CD34$^+$-cell count is prone to error, particularly if the sample is not in fresh condition, since platelet aggregates, dead cells, and other debris can compromise the accuracy of the absolute LKC and the accuracy of the flow analysis. Furthermore, the variable presence of nucleated red blood cells in CB and other samples leads to an overestimate of the absolute CD34$^+$-cell count. By incorporating a known number of fluorescent counting beads in the flow cytometric analysis, an absolute CD34$^+$-cell count can be generated directly on a flow cytometer, thus eliminating the need for a nucleated-cell count as performed by a hematology analyzer. Assessment of the ratio between the number of beads and CD34$^+$ cells counted allows the direct calculation of the absolute CD34$^+$-cell count. This approach is used by BD

Biosystems (BDB) (San Jose, Calif.) in their TruCOUNT tubes, in the single-platform variant of the ISHAGE protocol (20), and by Beckman-Coulter (Miami, Fla.) in their Stem-Kit assay. Regardless of which of these single-platform assays is used, accurate pipetting of samples (for sample dilution or aliquoting purposes) is required. For the single-platform ISHAGE protocol and Stem-Kit assays, accurate pipetting of the beads is also critical.

ISHAGE Single Platform Including Viability Assessment

The basic ISHAGE method was modified to include a known number of Flow-Count fluorospheres (Beckman-Coulter), and ammonium chloride lysis–no-wash sample processing was adopted. These modifications combine the accuracy and sensitivity provided by the sequential gating strategy of the original ISHAGE protocol with the capability to generate an absolute CD34$^+$-cell count directly from a flow cytometer (20) and form the basis of the Stem-Kit from Beckman-Coulter (see below). As shown in Fig. 2, from list mode data acquired on a BDB FACScan cytometer, from a diluted sample of a 24-h-old apheresis pack, the number of CD34$^+$ cells is determined as described above using gating R1 to R4 (gate 4 in gate statistics) and compared with the total number of singlet beads counted (concentration supplied by manufacturer) in the same list mode file. In the example shown, total beads are gated in R6 of plot E and displayed on plot G (time versus FSC). Using Boolean gating logic, singlet beads are then gated in R7 (G7 in gate statistics). The calculation involved in generating an absolute CD34$^+$-cell count per microliter is as follows: (no. of CD34$^+$ cells $\times$ bead concentration $\times$ DF)/no. of singlet beads, where the number of CD34$^+$ cells is determined from gate 4 (R1 through R4), the bead concentration is specified per lot, DF is the sample dilution factor, and the singlet bead count is determined from gate 7 (R6 and R7). This value is multiplied by the apheresis pack volume (in liters) to convert this value to an absolute CD34$^+$-cell number $\times 10^6$ per apheresis pack.

As detailed above and elsewhere, for absolute counting of CD34$^+$ cells using bead-based methods, accurate pipetting of sample and beads is critical to the reliability of the assay (14, 20, 33). In our standardized assay, 100 μl of sample and 100 μl of counting beads are used (33).

The addition of the viability dye 7-AAD to the single-platform ISHAGE method permits the determination of the absolute numbers of viable and nonviable CD34$^+$ cells from a sample (20). The ability to perform such sophisticated analysis has clinical utility in the accurate measurement of viable CD34$^+$ cells in packs that may have been manipulated (e.g., purged), potentially damaged by shipping to another site for analysis, or otherwise inappropriately handled prior to analysis. An example of how the 7-AAD is incorporated into the ISHAGE single-platform method is shown in Fig. 2, plot H. In the example shown, dead cells (7-AAD$^+$) are gated in R8 and subtracted, using logical gating, from the other analysis gates. An absolute viable CD34$^+$ cell count of 117/μl is obtained. When the 7-AAD$^+$ cells (dead cells) are not excluded (by removing gate R8) as shown in Fig. 3, and the gating R4 is adjusted on plot F to include all lymphocytes (live plus dead) from R5, a total absolute CD34$^+$-cell count of 162/μl is obtained.

The essential components and fine technical details of the "single-platform ISHAGE with viability protocol" (20) are embodied in the basic protocol constructed for *Current Protocols in Cytometry* (CPC) (14; updated in reference 33).

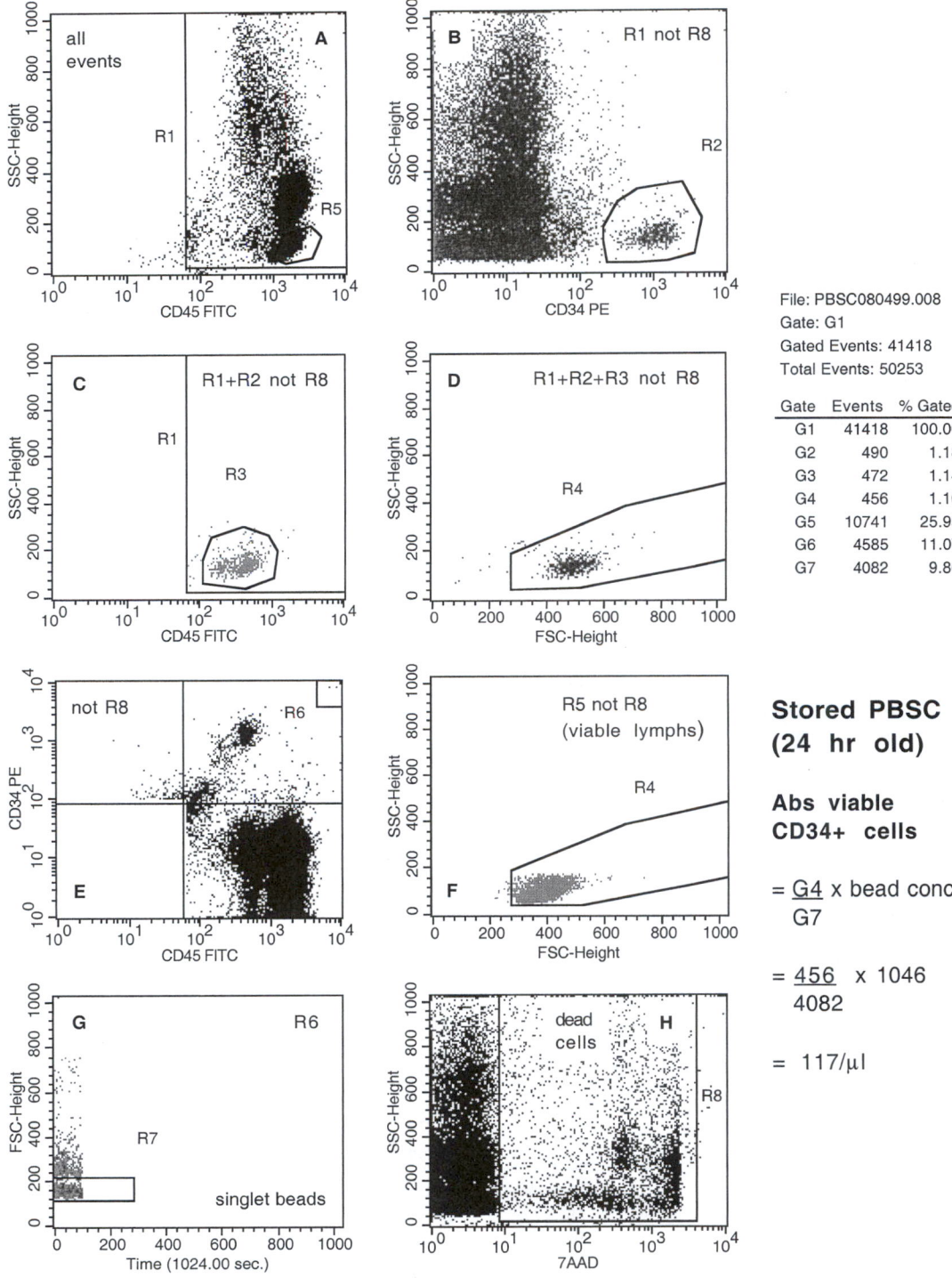

File: PBSC080499.008
Gate: G1
Gated Events: 41418
Total Events: 50253

Gate	Events	% Gated
G1	41418	100.00
G2	490	1.18
G3	472	1.14
G4	456	1.10
G5	10741	25.93
G6	4585	11.07
G7	4082	9.86

Stored PBSC (24 hr old)

Abs viable CD34+ cells

$$= \frac{\underline{G4}}{G7} \times \text{bead conc}$$

$$= \frac{456}{4082} \times 1046$$

$$= 117/\mu l$$

FIGURE 2 Absolute viable CD34+-cell counting using the single-platform ISHAGE protocol (14, 20, 33) performed on 100 μl of a 24-h-old PBSC sample stained with CD34-FITC and CD45-PE. After 25 min, the sample was lysed with 2 ml of NH₄Cl containing 1 μg of 7-AAD. After 10 min at room temperature, 100 μl of Flow-Count beads was added and the sample was analyzed immediately as described previously (14, 20). Dead cells (7-AAD⁺) gated in R8 and were removed from analysis by logical gating as depicted in plots B, C, D, and F. A total of 456 viable CD34⁺ cells were counted in gate 4 (not R8 and R1 through R4), 4,082 beads were counted in gate 7 (R6 and R7), and the assayed bead concentration was 1,046/μl. The sample contains 117 viable CD34⁺ cells/μl.

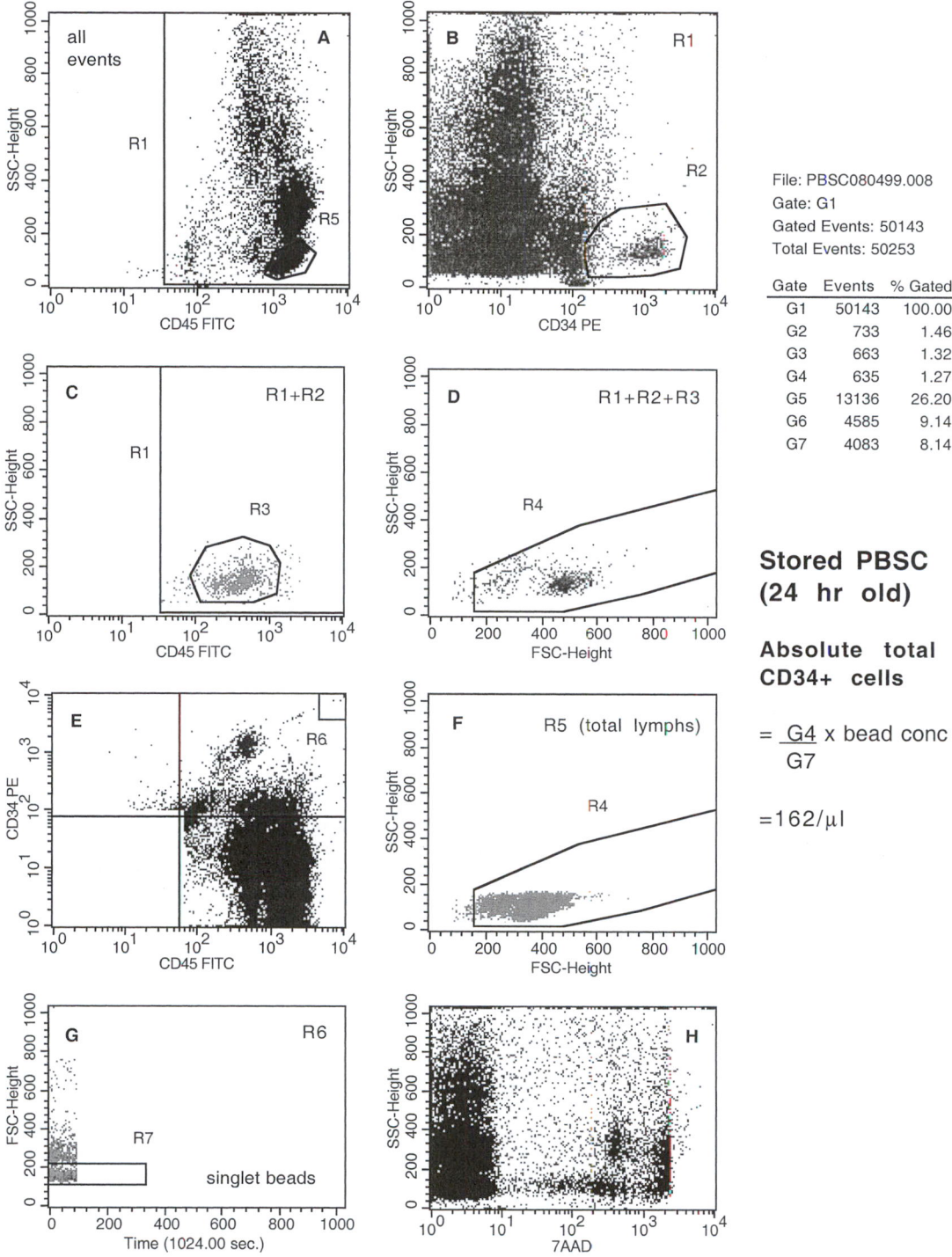

File: PBSC080499.008
Gate: G1
Gated Events: 50143
Total Events: 50253

Gate	Events	% Gated
G1	50143	100.00
G2	733	1.46
G3	663	1.32
G4	635	1.27
G5	13136	26.20
G6	4585	9.14
G7	4083	8.14

Stored PBSC (24 hr old)

Absolute total CD34+ cells

$$= \frac{G4}{G7} \times \text{bead conc}$$

$$= 162/\mu l$$

FIGURE 3 Importance of removing dead cells in accurate enumeration of CD34$^+$ cells by the single-platform ISHAGE protocol. The list mode file from the same 24-h-old sample as shown in Fig. 2 was analyzed without prior removal of nonviable (7-AAD$^+$) cells. Note that most nonviable CD34$^+$ cells and nonviable lymphocytes (plots D and F, respectively) form a second cluster characterized by lower FSC compared to their viable equivalents shown on the corresponding plots of Fig. 2. The sample contains 162 total CD34$^+$ cells/μl.

They are also embodied in the recommendations from the EWGCCA (13), the British Protocol for CD34+-cell enumeration (2), and the German reference protocol (17), among others.

Like earlier versions of the ISHAGE protocols, the single-platform derivatives have been developed to work on both Beckman-Coulter and BDB flow cytometers. However, there are minor technical differences in the way the assay is set up on the different instruments (detailed in references 14 and 33). Briefly, there are two main differences. On single-laser instruments with only three photomultiplier tubes such as the BDB FACScan, the counting beads are visualized using FSC versus time. Since the beads are detected as smaller events than lymphocytes on BDB instruments, the FSC threshold has to be lowered so as not to exclude the beads. As shown in Fig. 2, plot G, the singlet beads appear around channel 160, whereas the viable lymphocytes shown in plot F are found above channel 280. On the Coulter Epics XL and FC500 instruments, the beads appear above channel 800, so there is no need to adjust the FALS discriminator from its normal setting, just below the smallest lymphocytes (14, 20). However, it is our recent experience that certain stabilized samples that are routinely distributed for quality assurance or proficiency testing purposes exhibit reduced FSC properties. For the analysis of such samples, it is advisable to increase the FSC gain of the Coulter instruments to ensure that all CD45+ leukocytes are included in the list mode file. Although the counting beads can be detected on the Coulter Epics XL and FC500 using the same parameters of FSC versus time, the presence of a fourth photomultiplier tube on this single-laser instrument allows the counting beads to be detected in the FL3 channel of the instrument (on an FL3-versus-time plot) while the 7-AAD is detected in the FL4 channel (equivalent to the FL3 channel of the FACScan) (14, 20).

The Stem-Kit Assay

The Stem-Kit from Beckman-Coulter utilizes ISHAGE gating criteria to identify CD34+ cells. The kit also contains a CD45-FITC/CD34 (isoclonic) control to enumerate nonspecifically stained events. In this control, unconjugated CD34 antibody is present in large excess to block specific staining of PE-labeled CD34 present at the same concentration as the test. However, given the selectivity of the sequential gating strategy utilized in this protocol, we have not found that the isoclonic control makes a significant contribution to the accuracy and reliability of the assay (20) and, therefore, consider it to be redundant (reviewed in reference 19).

Beckman-Coulter has also developed Stem-Trol control cells, stabilized KG1a cells that have been modified to present the CD34 and CD45 epitopes at densities similar to those found on normal CD34+ hematopoietic cells. The inclusion of Stem-Trol cells is useful in determining and monitoring the accuracy of the pipetting steps of the single-platform method. As this material can be diluted in peripheral blood, it can also be used as a process control, undergoing staining and lysis exactly as performed on the test samples (20). Their staining pattern with respect to CD34 and CD45 reagents can be used as an extra internal control to ensure that the FL1, FL2, and light scatter parameters of the cytometer are adequately set (20).

Beckman-Coulter has developed a software package that automates instrument setup and compensation as well as automated data acquisition and analysis of samples prepared with the Stem-Kit. This software has been developed specifically for use on the Coulter Epics XL and, more recently, FC500 instruments.

ISHAGE Single Platform Using TruCOUNT Tubes

As described by Brocklebank and Sparrow (7), it is also possible to perform the ISHAGE protocol using TruCOUNT absolute counting tubes (BD Biosciences), instead of Flow-Count microspheres. In this setting, due to the small size of the beads, a threshold cannot be set on FSC, necessitating its setting on a fluorescence parameter. An advantage of this approach is that it eliminates the requirement to carefully suspend and pipette the counting beads. However, accurate pipetting is still required if any predilution of the sample is required, as well as for the delivery of the sample into the TruCOUNT tube. An example of the single-platform ISHAGE protocol performed on TruCOUNT tubes is shown in Fig. 4. A threshold was set on FL1 (CD45-FITC). Note that for TruCOUNT tubes, all beads (singlets and doublets, etc.) have to be counted (Fig. 4, plot G, R7), in contrast to the singlet bead count that is collected for Flow-Count beads.

Benefits of Single-Platform CD34+-Cell Enumeration

By including an internal reference bead in the analysis, CD45 positivity is no longer used as a denominator in the calculation of absolute CD34+ cells. Thus, controversial issues such as whether the true denominator is nucleated white blood cells (CD45+ events) or total nucleated cells can be avoided. Instead, the characteristic CD45 expression of CD34+ cells is used solely as part of the sequential gating strategy to accurately identify bona fide CD34+ cells. It must be stressed that focused training is highly recommended for laboratory staff adopting single-platform flow methodologies. As shown in an EWGCCA multicenter trial (1), consistently reproducible results were obtained between multiple centers only after adequate training and monitoring of performance. Notwithstanding the critical requirement for accurate pipetting in single-platform assays, addition of counting beads has the advantage of eliminating the potential introduction of errors in calculating the absolute CD34+-cell count inherent in two-platform methodologies (10, 14, 20). The cytometrist need not be concerned about the presence of nucleated red blood cells, platelet aggregates, and dead cells, which can be counted as leukocytes by some automated hematology analyzers. While the presence of significant numbers of nucleated red cells (that play no role in engraftment) in apheresis samples is quite rare, they are often abundant in CB collections, and single-platform analysis can significantly increase the accuracy of the absolute CD34+-cell number in the latter.

QUALITY ASSURANCE OF CD34+-CELL ENUMERATION

Flow cytometric analysis of CD34+ cells offers a potential means to quality assure all aspects of stem cell processing from mobilization to reinfusion. By analyzing list mode data by a variety of different gating strategies, Chang and Ma demonstrated that gating strategies were a major contributing factor to result variability (9). For an individual sample, the use of different gating strategies could produce as much as a twofold variation in results. In their study, only one gating strategy, the ISHAGE protocol, gave reproducible results from all centers of within ±10% of the median CD34+-cell value on both peripheral blood and PBSC collections.

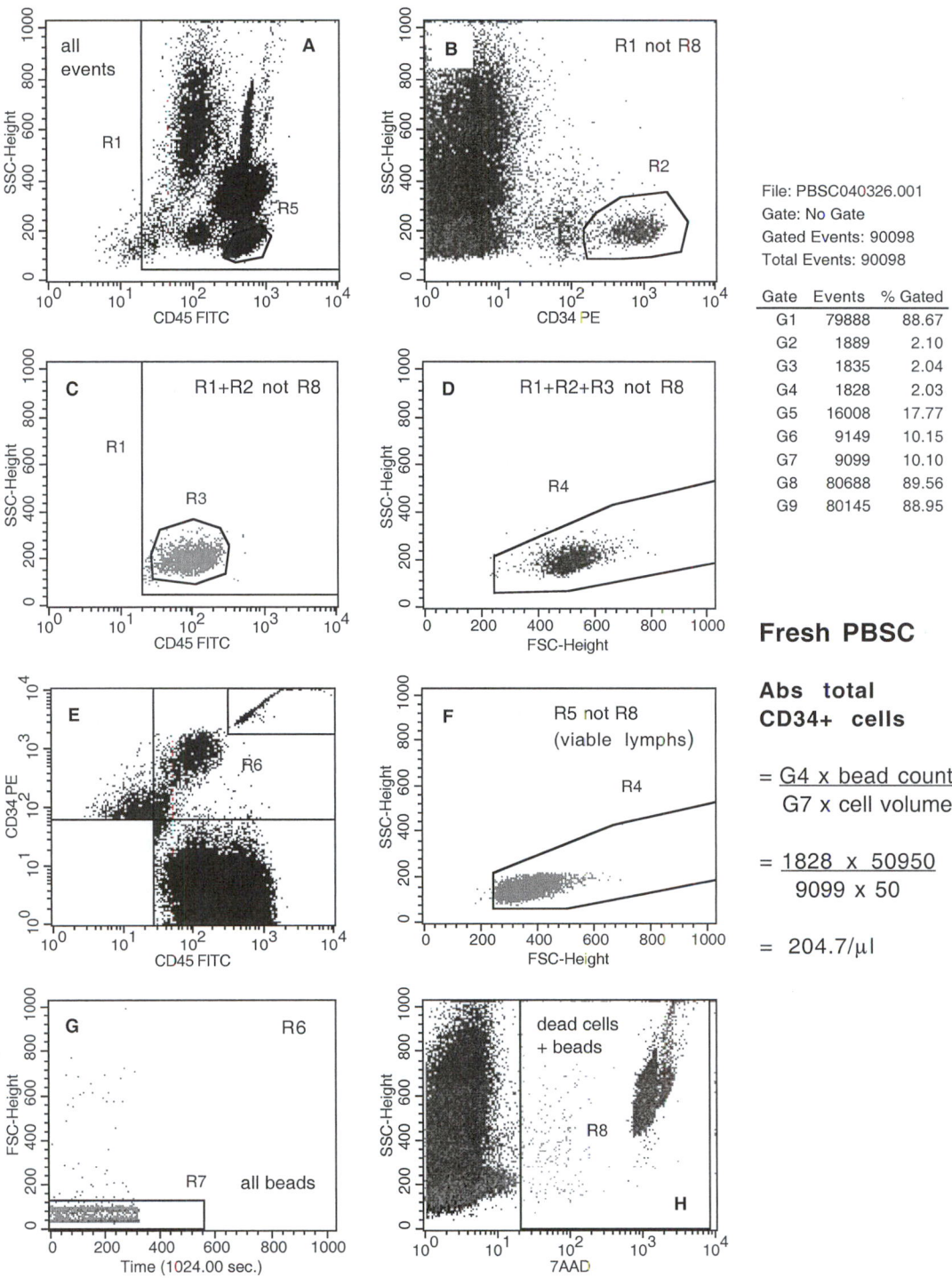

File: PBSC040326.001
Gate: No Gate
Gated Events: 90098
Total Events: 90098

Gate	Events	% Gated
G1	79888	88.67
G2	1889	2.10
G3	1835	2.04
G4	1828	2.03
G5	16008	17.77
G6	9149	10.15
G7	9099	10.10
G8	80688	89.56
G9	80145	88.95

Fresh PBSC

Abs total CD34+ cells

$$= \frac{\text{G4} \times \text{bead count}}{\text{G7} \times \text{cell volume}}$$

$$= \frac{1828 \times 50950}{9099 \times 50}$$

$$= 204.7/\mu l$$

FIGURE 4 Absolute viable CD34⁺-cell counting with the ISHAGE single-platform protocol using TruCOUNT tubes. Fifty microliters of a fresh peripheral blood sample was stained with CD45-FITC and CD34-PE in a TruCOUNT tube. A threshold was established on FL1 (CD45-FITC) because the size of the TruCOUNT beads precludes the use of an FSC threshold. The total number of beads in the list mode file is obtained from gate 7 (R6 and R7). Gate statistics are obtained from plot A (all events). The sample contains 205 viable CD34⁺ cells/μl.

Initial experience, however, with interlaboratory studies using various methodologies on shared samples reveals poor reproducibility, with coefficients of variation (CVs) ranging from 3 to 235% (13). As reported by Johnsen et al. (18), the CVs of list mode data on stained and fixed samples sent to 28 laboratories ranged from 10 to 18%. For two fresh samples shipped overnight the CVs were 38 and 34. However, for the 10 most active transplant labs the CVs for the fresh samples were 29 and 16%. A North American multicenter study report (6) showed unacceptable variability among 10 participating laboratories, with improved but still unacceptable variation between 3 Cytometry Associates laboratories using a common protocol. In the first Canadian Laboratory Provincial Testing Program quality assurance send-out for CD34+ stem/progenitor cell enumeration by flow cytometry, 9 of 11 labs had CVs of 14 and 18% for preserved whole-blood samples with CD34+-cell counts of 20 and 40/μl, respectively. All labs used either ISHAGE or ISHAGE-based Stem-Kit methodology (unpublished data). In a study undertaken by the EWGCCA using the single-platform ISHAGE protocol (14, 20), CVs of <10% were obtained by the majority of participating labs on a long-term stabilized blood sample with a target CD34+-cell value of 170/μl (1). In a more recent study involving 36 participants from the Benelux countries, similar CVs were obtained. In contrast, the lowest between-laboratory CVs using dual-platform techniques were 16% (Benelux) and 21% (United Kingdom National Quality Assessment Service) (15). Thus, the experience with CD34+-cell counting confirms that the use of a common standardized protocol and targeted training, where needed, is able to significantly increase reproducibility and reduce variation between laboratories.

IMMUNOPHENOTYPIC CHARACTERIZATION OF CD34+ SUBSETS

While the total number of viable CD34+ cells is the most clinically relevant parameter in determining reengraftment, the ability to reconstitute the human hematopoietic system probably lies within a very primitive subset of this population that does not express lineage-associated antigens (Lin− phenotype) but expresses the CD90/Thy-1 antigen (24, 34). Rapid multilineage engraftment was observed in the human transplant setting with as few as 8×10^5 highly purified Lin− CD34+ Thy-1+ PBSC-derived cells (25). Other studies that employed sophisticated animal models of human hematopoiesis have indicated that the AC133/CD133+ subset of CD34+ cells is also enriched in candidate hematopoietic stem cells (38).

Further standardizing an assay to perform subset analysis is even more problematic since most antigens used to identify subsets of CD34+ cells are not expressed on discrete, nonoverlapping populations, but instead are expressed on populations that display a continuum of antigen density from negative to weakly positive. The approach we have developed in concert with the EWGCCA (detailed in references 14 and 33) makes use of the autofluorescence of the gated CD34+ cells to define the lower FL intensity limit of the positive analysis region, following which the experimentally stained sample is to be analyzed (Fig. 5). Though this will not completely account for low-level nonspecific binding of the PE-conjugated antibody to CD34+ cells, it still greatly improves the ability to standardize the analysis of weakly stained subsets of CD34+ cells (14, 33). In the example shown in Fig. 5, a fresh PBSC sample was stained with a combination of CD34-FITC and CD45–PE-Cy5. Bona fide CD34+ cells were

identified and gated per the ISHAGE protocol in R4 of plot D and displayed on a bivariate plot of CD34-FITC versus FL2 (plot E). Since no antibody-PE conjugate is present in this sample, the natural fluorescence, or autofluorescence, in the PE (FL2) channel of the gated CD34+ cells is used to establish the subset positive gating region for the CD90/Thy-1–PE-stained sample shown in plot G. All gating regions remain identical between the two (and any subsequent) tubes. On a technical note, it is crucial to the intra- and interinstitutional reliability of the data generated that the flow cytometer be properly set up and compensated. As shown in plots F and H, respectively, the fluorescence of lymphocytes (gated from the CD45-versus-SSC plot A [not shown]) from the unstained control (plot F) and the CD90/Thy-1–PE-stained sample (plot H) are essentially identical in the FL2 channel (apart from a small number of lymphocytes that have stained specifically with CD90, in keeping with known characteristics of a small subset of T cells). These plots not only demonstrate proper instrument setup and fluorescence compensation but also show that the CD90 antibody used is optimally titrated. Also shown in Fig. 5 are the CD133+ (plot J) and CD33+ (plot K) subsets of CD34+ cells.

DOES ENUMERATING CD34+ SUBSETS HAVE CLINICAL UTILITY?

Whether enumerating specific CD34+ subsets has utility as a predictor of rapid reengraftment remains somewhat controversial. Since several studies have shown that the rate of platelet engraftment is generally rapid in patients given at least 5×10^6 CD34+ cells per kg (37), it is unlikely that monitoring subsets in patients receiving this target dose (or greater) will provide any additional clinical information. At the Toronto Hospital, we monitored CD34+ subsets on those patients in whom the target value of 5×10^6 CD34 cells per kg was unlikely to be met. In this way, we hoped to enumerate specific subsets that correlated best with speed of engraftment. Subsets enumerated included CD90/Thy-1, AC133, CD38lo, CD33lo, and, on selected samples, CD109+ and CD117+. Analysis to date shows, however, that all patients transplanted with CD34+ cells in the range of 2×10^6 to 5×10^6/kg engrafted platelets and neutrophils by days 12 to 14 (unpublished observations). Therefore, it would appear that performing accurate enumeration of CD34+ cells is perhaps more relevant to predicting platelet engraftment than is the qualitative composition of the CD34+ cells, at least for patients receiving at least 2×10^6 to 2.5×10^6 CD34 cells/kg. In light of this analysis, it may be informative to analyze subsets only in patients whose collections are in the range of 1×10^6 to 3×10^6/kg. Thus, potential clinical applications for CD34+-subset analysis might include evaluating poor mobilizers with inadequate or marginal CD34 collections in addition to measuring qualitative differences in response to different cytokine regimens and quality assuring selected stem cell products during cell processing.

CD34+-CELL SUBSETS IN BACKUP MARROW OF POOR MOBILIZERS

A number of studies have indicated that the use of backup bone marrow cells does not improve engraftment in patients who failed to mobilize sufficient CD34+ PBSC, perhaps suggesting that poor PBSC mobilization is indicative of poor marrow function (36). We analyzed backup marrow from a number of patients who had failed to mobilize an adequate number of CD34+ PBSC. As shown in Fig. 6, using a sample

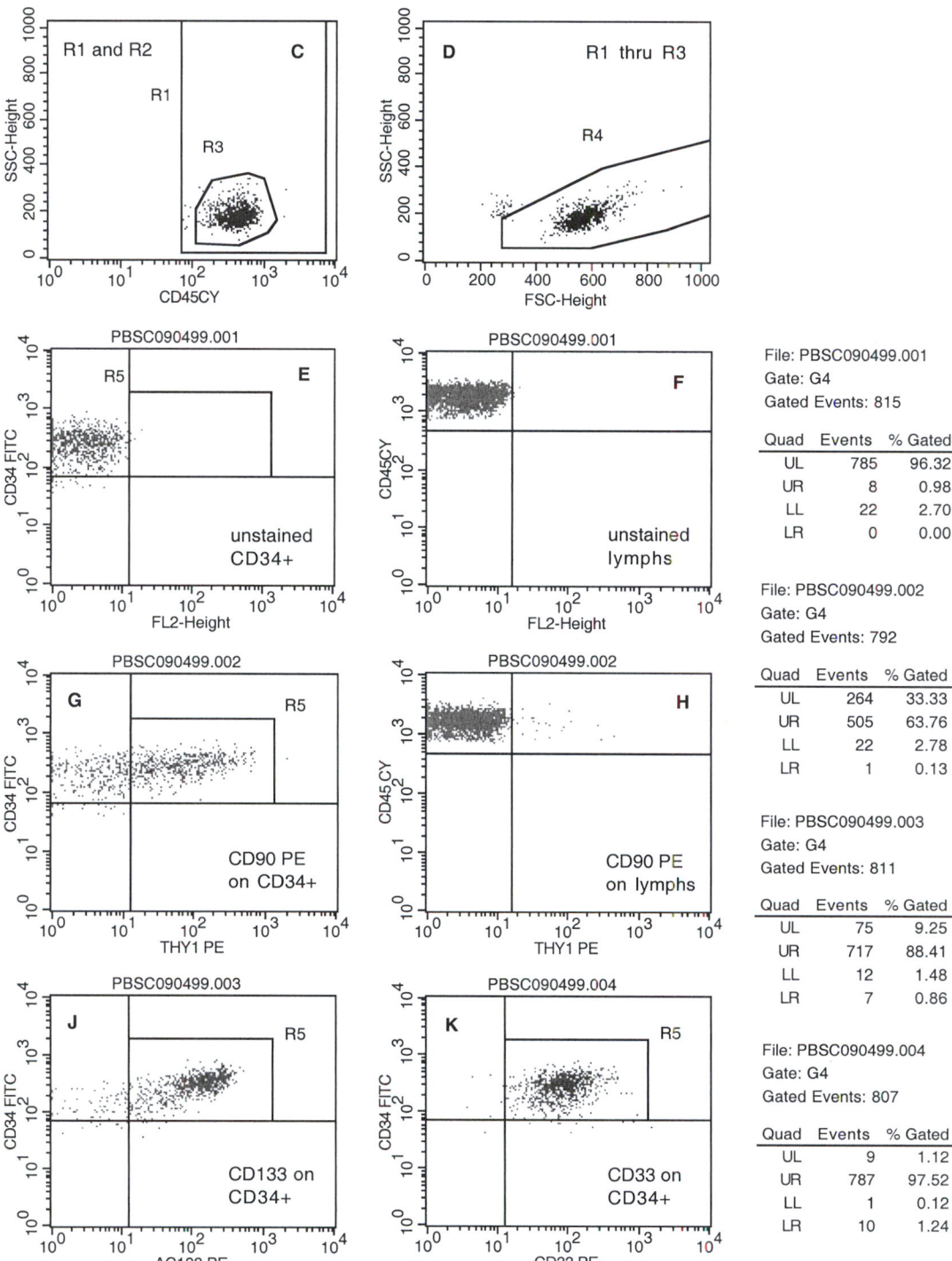

FIGURE 5 Identifying CD34+-cell subsets using the CPC support protocol (33) and PBSC sample stained with CD34-FITC and CD45–PE-Cy5. CD34+ cells (1.01% of the gated CD45+ events) were identified as described for Fig. 1, plots A to D (plots A and B not shown), and displayed on CD34 versus FL2 to establish positive cell analysis R5 (plot E). Plot F displays gated lymphocytes (from plot B) on a CD45-versus-FL2 plot. Note that the back-scattered lymphocytes have autofluorescence similar to that of gated CD34+ cells (plot E) and cluster parallel with the horizontal axis, indicating optimized FL2/FL3 fluorescence compensation. Plots G and H show the staining of CD34+ cells and lymphocytes, respectively, with CD90/Thy-1–PE. Plots J and K show the staining of the CD34+ cells with CD133-PE and CD33-PE, respectively.

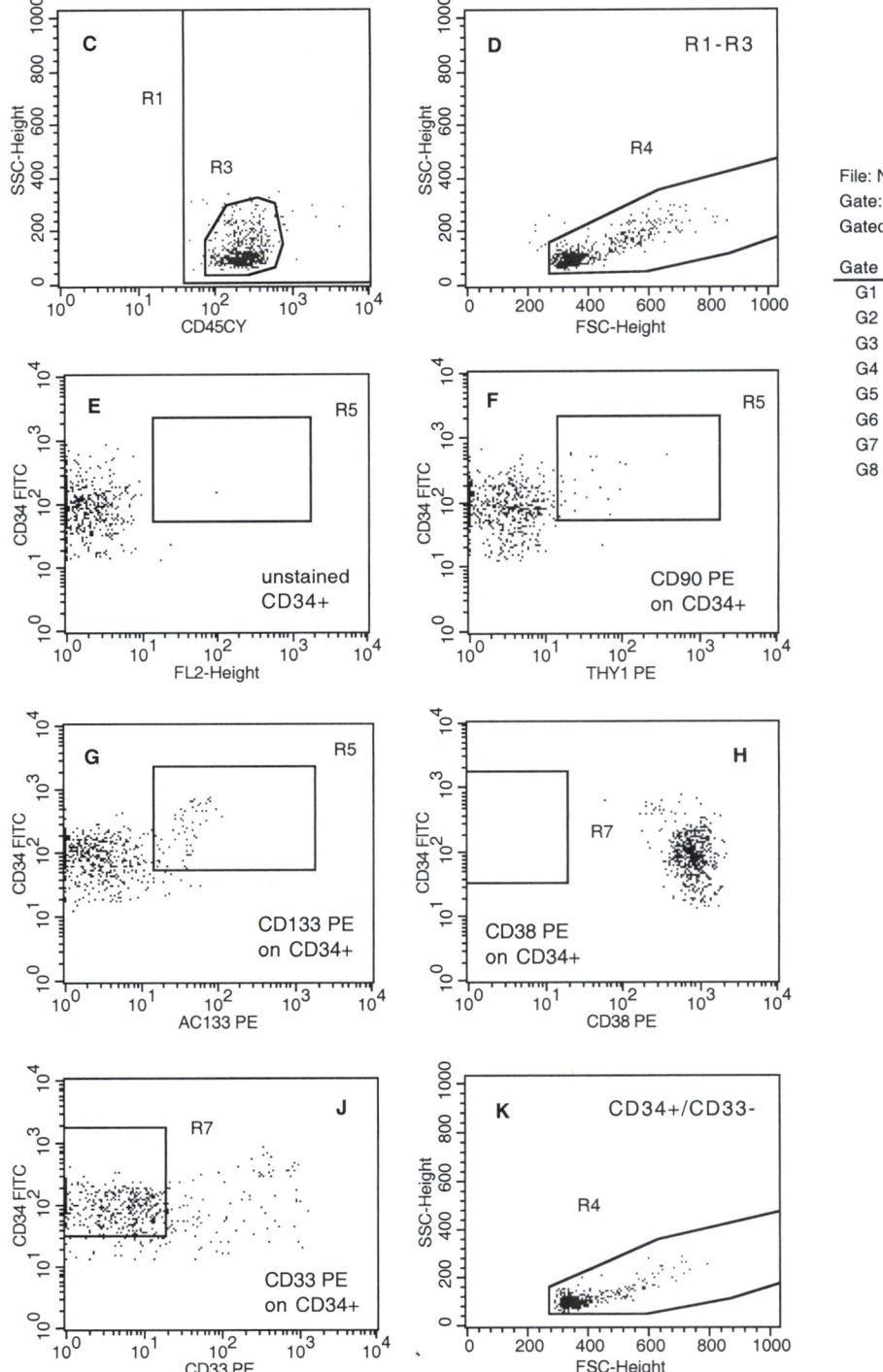

File: NGBM220499.003
Gate: G1
Gated Events: 27776

Gate	Events	% Gated
G1	27776	100.00
G2	595	2.14
G3	568	2.04
G4	559	2.01
G5	0	0.00
G6	3122	11.24
G7	504	1.81
G8	0	0.00

FIGURE 6   Identifying CD34$^+$-cell subsets in the marrow of a poor mobilizer. CD34$^+$ cells (2.00% of the total CD45$^+$ events in G4) are identified in plots A to D (A and B not shown). The majority of CD34$^+$ cells exhibit light scatter characteristics of prelymphoid cells. An unstained control (no PE conjugate) of the gated CD34$^+$ cells from R4 was used to establish gating R5 (plot E). Plots F, G, H, and J show the staining of gated CD34$^+$ cells with CD90/Thy-1, AC133, CD38, and CD33, respectively. The lower right plot shows the light scatter of the CD34$^+$ CD33$^-$ cells.

from a patient with acute myelogenous leukemia, CD34$^+$ cells were gated as described above (plots A to D), and strikingly, as shown in plot D, a majority of the CD34$^+$ cells identified exhibited the characteristics of pre-B cells (i.e., low FSC and SSC signals). When subset analysis was performed using Thy-1, AC133, CD38, and CD33 (plots G, H, J, and K, respectively), there was a demonstrable lack of CD34$^+$ cells exhibiting the composite phenotype of primitive candidate stem cells, with very few CD34$^+$ cells expressing the CD34^{bright} Thy-1$^+$ AC133$^+$ CD38^{dull} phenotype. Additionally, virtually all CD34$^+$ CD33$^{dull/negative}$ cells exhibited the light scatter of lymphoid progenitors. It will be interesting to monitor the engraftment kinetics of such patients should they indeed undergo transplantation with these marrow samples.

SUMMARY

Over the last few years, the number of clinical applications for stem cell transplantation has expanded considerably. At the same time, stem cell collections have been obtained from increasingly diverse sources, including marrow, peripheral blood, and CB, for use in both autologous and allogeneic transplantation. In addition, an increasing array of ex vivo manipulations has been developed to engineer the graft to suit specific clinical requirements. Included in the latter are positive selection techniques to purify CD34$^+$ cells and negative purging techniques to remove residual tumor cells in the autologous setting, or T lymphocytes in the allogeneic setting. Finally, there is widespread interest in the development of clinically useful ex vivo expansion methodologies and gene therapy protocols. As the clinical utility of both unmanipulated and manipulated stem cell products expands, it is critical that robust technologies are developed to accurately monitor the consequences of such procedures on the engraftment potential of the stem cell products. Thus, the graft assessment protocol (i.e., CD34$^+$-cell enumeration by flow cytometry) must be capable of measuring CD34$^+$ cells accurately in a variety of sources of stem cell products without the added expense of redundant isotype controls. It must also be able to distinguish viable CD34$^+$ cells from nonviable CD34$^+$ cells, from nonviable non-CD34$^+$ cells, and from other nonspecifically stained debris. The single-platform variant should be robust enough that viable CD34$^+$ cells can be accurately measured in postcryopreserved samples. Furthermore, the chosen protocol must be flexible enough that, for example, in the allotransplant setting, residual T lymphocytes can be enumerated (33), or in the autologous setting, specific subsets of CD34$^+$ cells can be enumerated (33). In the autologous setting, it may be possible to detect the differential mobilization of specific subsets of CD34$^+$ cells by different growth factor cocktails, or measure the cell cycling status of CD34$^+$ cells and their subsets after mobilization. At present, it is our view that the methodologies based on the original ISHAGE protocol (31) and updated in CPC (14, 33) represent the most accurate and flexible protocols currently available to both clinical and research laboratories for the analysis of the increasingly wide variety of normal and abnormal hematopoietic samples.

REFERENCES

1. **Barnett, D., V. Granger, J. Kraan, L. Whitby, J. T. Reilly, S. Papa, and J. W. Gratama.** 2000. Reduction of intra- and interlaboratory variation in CD34+ stem cell enumeration using stable test material, standard protocols and targeted training. CD34 Task Force of the European Working Group of Clinical Cell Analysis (EWGCCA). *Br. J. Haematol.* **108:**784–792.

2. **Barnett, D., G. Janossy, A. Lubenko, E. Matutes, A. Newland, and J. T. Reilly.** 1999. Guideline for the flow cytometric enumeration of CD34+ haematopoietic stem cells. Prepared by the CD34+ haematopoietic stem cell working party. General Haematology Task Force of the British Committee for Standards in Haematology. *Clin. Lab. Haematol.* **21:**301–308.

3. **Bender, J. G., K. Unverzagt, and D. Walker.** 1994. Guidelines for determination of CD34+ cells by flow cytometry: application to the harvesting and transplantation of peripheral blood stem cells, p. 31–43. *In* E. Wunder, H. Sovalat, P. R. Henon, and S. Serke (ed.), *Hematopoietic Stem Cells: the Mulhouse Manual.* AlphaMed Press, Dayton, Ohio.

4. **Berenson, R. J., R. G. Andrews, W. I. Bensinger, D. Kalamasz, G. Knitter, C. D. Buckner, and I. D. Bernstein.** 1988. Antigen CD34-positive marrow cells engraft lethally irradiated baboons. *J. Clin. Investig.* **81:**951–955.

5. **Borowitz, M. J., K. L. Guenther, K. E. Schultz, and G. T. Stelzer.** 1993. Immuno-phenotyping of acute leukemia by flow cytometry: use of CD45 and right angle light scatter to gate on leukemic blasts in three color analysis. *Am. J. Clin. Pathol.* **100:**534–540.

6. **Brecher, M. E., L. Sims, J. Schmitz, T. Shea, and S. A. Bentley.** 1996. North American multicenter study on flow cytometric enumeration of CD34+ hematopoietic stem cells. *J. Hematother.* **5:**227–236.

7. **Brocklebank, A. M., and R. L. Sparrow.** 2001. Enumeration of CD34+ cells in cord blood: a variation on a single-platform flow cytometric method based on the ISHAGE gating strategy. *Cytometry* **46:**254–261.

8. **Cairo, M. S., and J. E. Wagner.** 1997. Placental and/or umbilical cord blood: an alternative source of hematopoietic stem cells for transplantation. *Blood* **90:**4665–4678.

9. **Chang, A., and D. D. F. Ma.** 1996. The influence of flow cytometric gating strategy on the standardization of CD34+ cell quantitation: an Australian multicenter study. *J. Hematother.* **5:**605–616.

10. **Chin-Yee, I., M. Keeney, L. Anderson, R. Nayar, and D. R. Sutherland.** 1997. Current status of CD34+ cell analysis by flow cytometry: the ISHAGE Guidelines. *Clin. Immunol. Newsl.* **17:**21–29.

11. **Civin, C., T. Trischman, M. J. Fackler, I. Bernstein, H. Buhring, L. Campos, M. F. Greaves, M. Kamoun, D. Katz, P. Lansdorp, T. Look, B. Seed, D. R. Sutherland, R. Tindle, and B. Uchanska-Zeigler.** 1989. Summary of CD34 cluster workshop section, p. 818–825. *In* W. Knapp, B. Dorken, W. R. Gilks, E. P. Rieber, R. E. Schmidt, H. Stein, and A. E. G. K. von dem Borne (ed.), *Leucocyte Typing IV.* Oxford University Press, Oxford, United Kingdom.

12. **Gazitt, Y., E. Tian, B. Barlogie, C. L. Reading, D. H. Vesole, S. Jagannath, J. Schnell, R. Hoffman, and G. Tricot.** 1996. Differential mobilization of myeloma cells and normal hematopoietic stem cells in multiple myeloma following treatment with cyclophosphamide and GM-CSF. *Blood* **87:**805–811.

13. **Gratama, J., A. Orfao, D. Barnett, B. Brando, A. Huber, G. Janossy, H. E. Johnsen, M. Keeney, G. E. Marti, F. Preijers, G. Rothe, S. Serke, D. R. Sutherland, C. E. Van Der Schoot, G. Schmitz, and S. Papa for the European Working Group on Clinical Cell Analysis.** 1998. Flow cytometric enumeration of CD34+ hematopoietic progenitor cells. *Cytometry* **34:**128–142.

14. **Gratama, J. W., M. Keeney, and D. R. Sutherland.** 1999. Enumeration of CD34+ hematopoietic stem and progenitor cells, p 6.4.1–6.4.22. *In* J. P. Robinson, Z. Darzynkiewicz,

P. N. Dean, A. R. Hibbs, A. Orfao, P. S. Rabinovitch, and L. L. Wheeless (ed.), *Current Protocols in Cytometry*. John Wiley and Sons Inc., New York, N.Y.

15. **Gratama, J. W., J. Kraan, M. Keeney, D. R. Sutherland, V. Granger, and D. Barnett.** 2003. Validation of the single-platform ISHAGE method for CD34+ hematopoietic stem and progenitor cell enumeration in an international multicenter study. *Cytotherapy* **5:**55–65.

16. **Gratama, J. W., J. Kraan, W. Levering, D. R. Van Bockstaele, G. T. Rijkers, and C. E. Van der Schoot.** 1997. Analysis of variation in results of CD34+ hematopoietic progenitor cell enumeration in a multicenter study. *Cytometry* **30:**109–117.

17. **Gutensohn, K., I. Carrero, W. Krueger, N. Kroeger, P. Schafer, K. Luedemann, and P. Kuehnl.** 1999. Semi-automated flow cytometric analysis of CD34-expressing hematopoietic cells in peripheral blood progenitor cell apheresis products. *Transfusion* **39:**1220–1226.

18. **Johnsen, H. E., J. Baech, and K. Nicolajsen.** 1999. Validation of the Nordic flow cytometry standard for CD34+ cell enumeration in blood and autografts: report from the third workshop. *J. Hematother.* **8:**15–28.

19. **Keeney, M., I. Chin-Yee, J. W. Gratama, and D. R. Sutherland.** 1998. Perspectives: isotype controls in the analysis of lymphocytes and CD34+ stem/progenitor cells by flow cytometry—time to let go! *Cytometry* **34:**280–283.

20. **Keeney, M., I. Chin-Yee, K. Weir, J. Popma, R. Nayar, and D. R. Sutherland.** 1998. Single platform flow cytometric absolute CD34+ cell counts based on the ISHAGE Guidelines. *Cytometry* **34:**61–67.

21. **Lanza, R., L. Healy, and D. R. Sutherland.** 2001. Structural and functional features of the CD34 antigen: an update. *J. Biol. Regulators Homeostatic Agents* **15:**1–13.

22. **Luider, J., C. Brown, S. Selinger, D. Quinlan, L. Karlsson, D. Ruether, D. Stewart, J. Klassen, and J. A. Russell.** 1997. Factors influencing yields of progenitor cells for allogeneic transplantation: optimization of G-CSF dose, day of collection, and duration of leukapheresis. *J. Hematother.* **6:**575–580.

23. **Mancuso, P., A. Burlini, G. Pruneri, A. Goldhirsch, G. Martinelli, and F. Bertolini.** 2001. Resting and activated endothelial cells are increased in the peripheral blood of cancer patients. *Blood* **97:**3658–3661.

24. **Murray, L., B. Chen, A. Galy, S. Chen, R. Tushinski, N. Uchida, R. Negrin, G. Tricot, S. Jagannath, D. Vesole, B. Barlogi, R. Hoffman, and A. Tsukamoto.** 1985. Enrichment of human hematopoietic stem cell activity in the CD34+Thy1+Lin− subpopulation from mobilized peripheral blood. *Blood* **85:**368–378.

25. **Negrin, R. S., K. Atkinson, T. Leemhuis, E. Hanania, C. Juttner, D. Tierney, W. W. Hu, L. J. Johnston, J. A. Shizuru, K. E. Stockerl-Goldstein, K. G. Blume, I. L. Weissman, S. Bower, R. Baynes, R. Dansey, C. Karanes, W. Peters, and J. Klein.** 2000. Transplantation of highly purified CD34+Thy-1+ hematopoietic stem cells in patients with metastatic breast cancer. *Biol. Blood Marrow Transplant.* **6:**262–271.

26. **Owens, M. A., and M. R. Loken.** 1995. Peripheral blood stem cell quantitation, p. 111–127. *In* M. A. Owens and M. R. Loken (ed.), *Flow Cytometric Principles for Clinical Laboratory Practice*. Wiley-Liss, New York, N.Y.

27. **Siena, S., M. Bregni, B. Brando, N. Belli, F. Ravagnani, L. Gandola, A. C. Stern, P. M. Lansdorp, G. Bonadonna, and A. M. Gianni.** 1991. Flow cytometry for clinical estimation of circulating hematopoietic progenitors for autologous transplantation in cancer patients. *Blood* **77:**400–409.

28. **Siena, S., M. Bregni, B. Brando, F. Ravagnani, G. Bonadonna, and A. M. Gianni.** 1989. Circulation of CD34+ hematopoietic stem cells in the peripheral blood of high-dose cyclophosphamide-treated patients: enhancement by intravenous recombinant human granulocyte-macrophage colony-stimulating factor. *Blood* **74:**1905–1914.

29. **Stewart, A. K., K. Imrie, A. Keating, S. Anania, R. Nayar, and D. R. Sutherland.** 1995. Optimizing the CD34+ Thy-1+ stem cell content of peripheral blood collections. *Exp. Hematol.* **23:**1619–1627.

30. **Sutherland, D. R., and A. Keating.** 1992. The CD34 antigen: structure, biology and potential clinical applications. *J. Hematother.* **1:**115–129.

31. **Sutherland, D. R., L. Anderson, M. Keeney, R. Nayar, and I. Chin-Yee.** 1996. The ISHAGE guidelines for CD34+ cell determination by flow cytometry. *J. Hematother.* **5:**213–226.

32. **Sutherland, D. R., A. Keating, R. Nayar, S. Anania, and A. K. Stewart.** 1994. Sensitive detection and enumeration of CD34+ cells in peripheral blood and cord blood by flow cytometry. *Exp. Hematol.* **22:**1003–1010.

33. **Sutherland, D. R., M. Keeney, and J. W. Gratama.** 2003. Enumeration of CD34+ hematopoietic stem and progenitor cells, p. 6.4.1–6.4.23. *In* J. P. Robinson, Z. Darzynkiewicz, P. H. Dean, L. G. Dressler, P. S. Rabinovitch, C. S. Stewart, H. J. Tanke, and L. L. Wheeless (ed.), *Current Protocols in Cytometry*. John Wiley and Sons Inc., New York, N.Y.

34. **Sutherland, D. R., E. L. Yeo, A. K. Stewart, R. Nayar, R. DiGiusto, R. Hoffman, E. D. Zanjani, and L. J. Murray.** 1996. Identification of CD34+ subsets following glycoprotease selection: engraftment of CD34+/Thy-1+/Lin− stem cells in fetal sheep. *Exp. Hematol.* **24:**795–806.

35. **To, L. B., D. N. Haylock, P. J. Simmons, and C. A. Juttner.** 1997. The biology and clinical uses of blood stem cells. *Blood* **89:**2233–2258.

36. **Watts, M. J., A. M. Sullivan, D. Leverett, A. J. Peniket, A. R. Perry, C. D. Williams, S. Devereux, A. H. Goldstone, and D. C. Linch.** 1995. Back-up bone marrow is frequently ineffective in patients with poor peripheral-blood stem-cell mobilization. *J. Clin. Oncol.* **16:**1554–1560.

37. **Weaver, C. H., B. Hazelton, R. Birch, P. Palmer, C. Allen, L. Schwartzberg, and W. West.** 1995. An analysis of engraftment kinetics as a function of CD34 cell content of peripheral blood progenitor collections in 692 patients after the administration of myeloablative chemotherapy. *Blood* **86:**3961–3969.

38. **Yin, A. H., S. Miraglia, E. D. Zanjani, G. Almeida-Porada, M. Ogawa, A. G. Leary, J. Olweus, J. Kearney, and D. W. Buck.** 1997. AC133, a novel marker for human hematopoietic stem and progenitor cells. *Blood* **90:**5002–5012.

Phenotypic Correlates of Genetic Abnormalities in Acute and Chronic Leukemias

ELISABETH PAIETTA

22

The first classification of the acute leukemias in 1976 relied exclusively on the evaluation of cell size, granularity, nuclear shape, cytoplasmic appearance, cytochemical reactions, and dysplastic features of cells surrounding the "leukemic blast." Leukemia diagnostics have come a long way since then. Today, the lineage affiliation of a leukemic cell is accurately defined by multiparameter flow cytometry and prognostically relevant chromosome aberrations are revealed by standard and molecular cytogenetic analyses. In selected cases, researchers have even succeeded in not only elucidating but also reversing the oncogenic mechanism, such as in acute promyelocytic leukemia (APL). APL has become the paradigm for the ultimate goal of leukemia diagnosis: to be able to tell an oncologist what targeted therapy a patient is a candidate for, based on the detection of a specific genotype. APL, furthermore, reflects the major change in criteria that nowadays are or should be used to subclassify leukemias in general. Diagnosis based on similarities in cellular structures has been replaced by outcome-based classifications.

The history of APL (12) goes back to the 1970s, when leukemias with hypergranular morphologies were unified under the French-American-British classification of morphology and cytochemistry (FAB) (69) as FAB M3. In a variant form, M3v, hypergranulated cells were found in bone marrow and circulating leukemic cells had monocytoid features. The description of a balanced translocation between chromosomes 15 and 17 as the hallmark of APL subsequently confirmed the accuracy of the morphologic diagnosis. Only 1 to 2% of non-M3 acute myeloid leukemia (AML) patients express the promyelocytic leukemia protein (PML) retinoic acid receptor α (RARα) gene, the gene fusion product that results at the molecular level from the t(15;17)(q22;q21) translocation. Yet there is a subset of patients in whom, despite the presence of M3 morphology, the t(15;17) translocation cannot be demonstrated (60). While all variant APL translocations involve the RARα gene on chromosome 17, its partner gene in the translocation varies.

Previously, the morphologic diagnosis of APL sufficed and could be, but did not have to be, confirmed by karyotyping. With the introduction of effective, APL-specific therapy with all-*trans* retinoic acid (ATRA), however, it became unacceptable to misdiagnose a patient with APL. When it was realized that the differentiation block in APL resulted from transcriptional repression of the retinoic acid signaling pathway due to histone deacetylase activities, it was postulated that histone deacetylase-mediated gene silencing might be a general mechanism of leukemogenesis, at least in AML associated with chromosomal translocations that affect genes encoding transcription factors (57, 61). At the same time, it became clear that in some of the variant APL translocations, ATRA failed to alleviate the transcriptional repression. Thus, it was important to diagnose not just APL but ATRA-responsive APL and this had to happen as quickly as possible after a patient's presentation since ATRA was found to reverse the life-threatening disseminated intravascular coagulation typical of APL (17). Although ideally positioned to confirm the diagnosis of APL, cytogenetic analysis can take 3 to 4 days and may occasionally fail; on the other hand, amplification of aberrant gene sequences by PCR is a method not available to everybody and beset by its own problems.

Because of the unique morphologic appearance of hypergranular leukemic promyelocytes, the heterogeneity invariably introduced in all other FAB classes due to subjective interpretation of cellular features by morphologists largely does not exist in M3 disease. To be able to compare antigen expression patterns in a group of homogenous patients, at least by morphology analysis, was a huge advantage when flow cytometrists started to look for an APL-specific immunophenotype. Indeed, the typical negativity of APL cells for HLA-DR and CD34 was recognized ~20 years ago. Still, it was not until 2004 that an antigen profile was established that reliably served as a surrogate for the t(15;17) or the PML/RARα gene and which held up for most of the cytogenetic (molecular) variants (54). Deviations from this profile, such as expression of the neural cell adhesion molecule CD56, proved to offer prognostic information that was not provided by any other diagnostic parameter. If results of flow cytometric tests, which take about 2 h, "are consistent with the diagnosis of APL," subsequent confirmation of this diagnosis by molecular studies is highly recommended; at the very least, flow cytometry results can exclude APL.

But challenges do remain; a priori resistance to ATRA and variable response durations in responsive patients suggest that an even more refined subclassification of APL is needed. Internal tandem duplications (ITD) of the *FLT3* gene that constitutively activate the FLT3 receptor tyrosine kinase (TK) are found in almost 40% of APL cases; they are associated with hyperleukocytosis and possibly with inferior outcome, although definitive studies are pending.

Recently, *FLT3* ITD have been shown to cooperate with the *PML/RARα* gene in the development of APL in a murine model, suggesting that mutant *FLT3* represents the necessary second pathogenetic "hit" in this disease (34). In non-APL AML, *FLT3* gene mutations are the most common genetic aberration. Given their potential prognostic implications, it would be advantageous to be able to predict *FLT3* ITD through other cellular features. Kussick et al. (37) described a small subpopulation of non-APL AMLs (<5% of cases) in which the lack of HLA-DR, CD34, and CD133 (antigenic properties also seen in APL) in association with a normal karyotype predicted *FLT3* ITD. In acute lymphoid leukemia (ALL), activating *FLT3* gene mutations identify a rare patient subset with a unique immunophenotype of immature T lymphoblasts that express the CD117/KIT TK (55). These data suggest that genotypic alterations leading to constitutively activated FLT3 TK may indeed affect the overall phenotype of the leukemic cells.

The basic hypothesis of surrogate marker profiles is that individual genetic lesions result in characteristic distortions of the cellular phenotype with some predictable consistency that can be exploited by sophisticated immunophenotyping.

METHODOLOGIC PREREQUISITES AND KNOWLEDGE

Morphologic Evaluation of Peripheral Blood and Bone Marrow Smears

Access to a microscope and to a hematology laboratory that routinely prepares bone marrow or peripheral blood smears and Wright-Giemsa staining is required. Bone marrow smears must be prepared before the aspirate is mixed with anticoagulant.

Traditionally, morphologic and cytochemical analyses (in particular, those using peroxidase and esterase stains) were the predominant processes utilized in diagnosis. Major drawbacks were the subjectivity and inaccuracy associated with microscopic examination of specimens, a lack of prognostic power of morphology-based classification of leukemia subgroups, and a low level of sensitivity for the detection of blast cells during clinical remission. Today, analysis of antigen expression profiles, cytogenetics, and genetic information has, for the most part, supplanted morphology analysis. Still, examination of both peripheral blood and bone marrow smears is an important first step in the workup for any leukemia patient. Furthermore, the main criterion for the generally accepted definition of remission continues to be the percentage of blast cells present as recognized by morphology. The original FAB classification criteria (5, 69) were recently supplemented with pertinent data on chromosomal and molecular associations in the 2001 World Health Organization (WHO) classification system for hematopoietic tumors (31).

Multiparameter Flow Cytometry and Interpretation of Results

Access to a flow cytometer or to a clinical laboratory or core facility with staff that performs multiparameter flow cytometry with three- or four-fluorochrome combinations is required for the application of flow cytometry to leukemia diagnosis. In addition, a pathologist or cell biologist trained in the interpretation of normal and leukemic hematopoietic antigen expression profiles should be available for the interpretation of flow cytometry data. The choice of anticoagulant in the collection of peripheral blood or bone marrow for flow

cytometry is insignificant. As a side note, controversy exists as to whether the choice of anticoagulants does matter when cells are isolated for the purpose of nucleic acid preparation. (For instance, heparin, the anticoagulant most widely used in clinics, has been condemned by many molecular biologists, although others have found no effect on nucleic acid quality or specific transcript levels.) If samples from one patient are to be used for both flow cytometry and nucleic acid isolation, one should perform appropriate control testing with the anticoagulants used to ensure that they do not impair the aspect of the project that deals with DNA or RNA.

All samples are to be kept sterile. If specimens are to be stored or shipped, they can be kept at 10 to 15°C, without freezing, for 48 to 96 h. Leukemic blasts are considerably hardier than normal cells, and antigen expression does not change during prolonged time periods under appropriate storage conditions. Whole specimens can be stained for flow cytometry; mononuclear cells must be isolated (by density gradient centrifugation) before cells are frozen in a viable state in the presence of dimethyl sulfoxide (10%) and 50 to 90% fetal bovine serum; the serum concentration increases with the granularity of blast cells. Should viability be low after thawing, one must consider the selective retrieval of leukemia subpopulations (47).

Antibodies are grouped in clusters of designation (CD); if at least two antibodies show identical reactivity patterns and are proven to recognize the same antigen, a new cluster is designated. Clusters may be split based on selective reactivities of certain antibodies with a modified version of the antigen. For instance, the CD15 cluster is subdivided since some antibodies recognize the sialylated CD15 antigen (CD15s) while others recognize only the asialo form (CD15). Since the early 1980s, CDs have been established through international meetings, with the last two such meetings held in Harrogate, United Kingdom, in June 2000 (43) and in Adelaide, Australia, in December 2004.

Attention needs to be paid to quality control of flow cytometer performance, the choice of antibodies and of fluorochromes, the design of most informative antibody panels, and the mode of analysis, particularly the fact that data should be reported exclusively for the abnormal cell population (47).

In terms of data reporting, there are two philosophies of flow cytometry that in the minds of many are mutually exclusive. One concept teaches the use of a quantitative approach that reports the percentage of blast cells binding a given antibody; the other relies on quantitative fluorescence and reports fluorescence intensities as a reflection of antigen density on the cell surface. It is imperative that every laboratory establish its own optimal conditions of antibody performance. Despite its importance, quality control of flow cytometer and antibody performance, unfortunately, is not well standardized (47). Choice of antibodies and fluorochromes, staining, and erythrocyte lysing and fixation conditions, as well as flow cytometer settings, will largely affect flow cytometry data. For intracellular antigens, permeabilization and fixation conditions will determine whether an antigen is detected or not. The best example is the failure to detect nuclear expression of terminal transferase (TdT) in leukemic myeloblasts when suboptimal conditions and antibodies are used (50). Experience should guide the decision of when to report the percentage of staining blast cells or the fluorescence intensity. Some antibodies invariably stain all cells from a given lineage but vary markedly in their intensity of staining between normal and malignant cells, suggesting variable antigen densities (e.g., those of CD20 and CD22 on normal versus chronic lymphocytic leukemia [CLL]

B lymphocytes); for other antigens, the fraction of cells binding the antibody will contain the diagnostic information (e.g., the percentage of CD34$^+$ or CD117$^+$ cells in any acute leukemia).

Standard Cytogenetic Analysis and FISH

Access to a cytogenetics laboratory with well-trained cytogeneticists is required for standard cytogenetic analysis and fluorescence in-situ hybridization (FISH). Specimens for cytogenetic analysis are prepared in the same manner as those for flow cytometry, and bone marrow is preferred over peripheral blood. Most cytogenetic laboratories have optimized their processing techniques on specimens drawn in sodium heparin; one truly contraindicated anticoagulant is EDTA (purple-top tubes). At the same time, EDTA should be avoided for the collection of leukemic blasts (especially lymphoblasts), as it can introduce vacuoles into the cytoplasm and confuse the morphology analyses. Samples should be set up within 24 h of collection; if stored, they should be stored at room temperature. AML, ALL, or chronic myelogenous leukemia (CML) tissues should be cultured for 24 h without mitogens before processing. Samples from CLL require stimulation by B-cell mitogens (B-cell CLL) or T-cell mitogens (T-cell CLL) for cell division to occur (22).

To see distinct chromosomes under the microscope, cells must be dividing. This prerequisite is a limiting factor when the abnormal cells have low mitotic indices or very few blast cells are present (in remission) so that normal dividing cells outnumber cells with an abnormal karyotype. FISH is one way to overcome this obstacle. FISH uses fluorochrome-labeled nucleic acid probes and detects abnormalities both in interphase (nondividing) and in metaphase (dividing) cells (25). CLL, multiple myeloma, and plasma cell leukemia are paradigms for diseases in which low mitotic activity prompts the use of interphase FISH. The specific probes used determine which aberrations are detected. In CLL, a series of recurrent genomic aberrations correlates with survival (16); because interphase FISH analysis has a greater chance of detecting these aberrations than standard cytogenetics (given the low mitotic rate of CLL cells), it is the method of choice for determining chromosomal abnormalities in CLL.

FISH has increased sensitivity compared to standard cytogenetic analysis. With optimal strategies, e.g., the use of dual color/dual fusion (D)-FISH, one abnormal cell can be detected in 6,000 normal cells (15). Although such high sensitivity is not important at the time of diagnosis, when the proportion of leukemic cells, by definition, must exceed 20% in the diagnostic tissue, it is essential when FISH is used for the detection of minimal residual disease (MRD); at least three abnormal cells should be seen among a total of 6,000 normal cells prior to concluding the presence of MRD (14). Aside from its higher sensitivity, FISH can detect deletions in chromosomes involved in reciprocal chromosomal translocations (see below).

The consensus is that if cytogenetic abnormalities are absent, at least 20 metaphases must be viewed before the patient is considered to have normal cytogenetics. Given that leukemias with apparently normal karyotypes represent a biologically very heterogenous group, there is major emphasis on categorizing them into subsets with prognostic implications, e.g., based on mutations of the FLT3 gene, which in non-APL AML occur preferentially in cases with normal cytogenetics (35).

A clone is defined by the presence of two metaphases that share the same chromosome abnormality, unless the change involves loss of a chromosome, in which case three such cells are required (22). In a follow-up specimen, however, one metaphase may be considered a remnant of the original clone. Otherwise, single abnormal metaphases do not count as clonal cytogenetic abnormalities; if they present a specific aberration known to be associated with leukemia, e.g., t(9;22) or t(8;21), FISH or PCR analysis targeted at that aberration is recommended. In most cases, the leukemic cells contain one primary clone with or without additional (secondary) aberrations that result from clonal evolution. Patients with two distinct cytogenetic clones are rare. The International System for Human Cytogenetic Nomenclature in 1995 established a uniform code for designating both constitutional and acquired chromosome abnormalities and for reporting results obtained by FISH. For details on the preparation of metaphase spreads, banding techniques, and quality assurance, etc., the reader is referred to a few excellent publications (15, 22).

At the time of leukemia diagnosis, conventional cytogenetic analysis should be performed, as this method reveals all chromosomal abnormalities that are present. In a large portion of patients, karyotypic aberrations do not lend themselves to either FISH or PCR analysis, because specific probes are not (yet) available. However, if a patient is found to have a genetic lesion that can be monitored by these techniques, they can be very helpful for detecting MRD during clinical remission (71). It is important to remember that if one monitors patients during their clinical course by FISH or PCR targeted at their initial genetic lesions only, clonal evolution or the occurrence of new cytogenetic abnormalities will be missed. An example are CML patients treated with imatinib in whom the development of clonal cytogenetic abnormalities in BCR/ABL-negative cells would have been missed had conventional cytogenetic analysis not been performed in some of these cases (9).

Molecular Consequences of Chromosome Translocations and the Creation of Novel Fusion Genes

Chromosome translocations can have two distinct effects at the molecular level: either the inopportune activation of an unaltered gene or the creation and transcription of a novel gene. The first process occurs predominantly in lymphoid malignancies. The translocation places a transcriptionally silent gene under the control of the promoter of a transcriptionally very active gene, e.g., immunoglobulin or T-cell-receptor genes in B or T lymphocytes, respectively. This leads to the inappropriate transcription of a normal gene. Since those deregulated genes encode proteins involved in normal cellular growth and/or differentiation, particularly transcription factors (proteins that bind to specific DNA sequences, thereby stimulating or suppressing the expression of other genes), inappropriate expression results in uncontrolled cellular proliferation.

Alternatively, balanced translocations, interstitial chromosome deletions, or inversions can lead to the creation of novel, leukemogenic fusion genes. At each of the chromosomal breakpoints, a critical gene is disrupted [e.g., the ABL gene on chromosome 9 and the BCR gene on chromosome 22 in the t(9;22)(q34;q11.2)]; fragments of the two genes are brought together as a result of the translocation. Two hybrid fusion genes are created, one on each of the two chromosomes partnering in the translocation [e.g., BCR/ABL on the derivative chromosome 22 and ABL/BCR on the derivative chromosome 9, resulting from the (9;22) translocation]. Even if both chimeric genes are transcribed, only one is usually suspected as the transforming gene, based on gene sequences preserved in the fusion product and its in vitro activities. The altered properties of the chimeric proteins may predict their leukemogenic effects, e.g., the constitutive TK activity of BCR/ABL proteins that are localized exclusively in the cytoplasm, which contrasts with the tightly regulated activity of the normal ABL TK that shuttles between the nucleus and the cytoplasm (36).

Examples for this type of translocation are numerous among the leukemias. The novel fusion proteins are the only true leukemia-specific antigens. Antibodies to a few of these unique proteins exist but have not found widespread use as diagnostic tools; rather, they may be attractive targets for novel therapies. The deregulated BCR/ABL TK, the product of the t(9;22), is the best example for effective therapy through inhibition of the aberrant gene product, for instance, with imatinib (13). Targets for imatinib other than BCR/ABL are therapeutically relevant molecules in myeloid disorders (56).

Since several balanced translocations and the corresponding chimeric gene products have been associated with clinical response in leukemia, modern classification systems have incorporated them as hallmarks of distinct leukemia subtypes (31).

FISH analysis has found large deletions at breakpoints of reciprocal chromosomal translocations. Best characterized, to date, are deletions on either chromosome 9 or 22 of the t(9;22), which, at least in CML, are independent indicators of rapid progression to blast crisis and shorter survival. It is possible that loss of a critical region, involving loss of a tumor suppressor gene, confers a growth or survival advantage or results in an increase in genomic instability. There is strong evidence that similar deletions may exist in other leukemia translocations [e.g., inv(16) and t(8;21)] (30).

PCR Amplification

Balanced translocations, which appear identical by standard cytogenetic analysis, can be genetically very complex. This may be due to chromosome deletions that require FISH for detection (see above) or to differences in the genomic breakpoints that produce structurally and biologically distinct fusion products. Genetic variability may also derive from alternative splicing of fusion transcripts. Specific primer pairs, or combinations thereof, allow for the identification of such genetic variants. For instance, several BCR/ABL oncogenes exist that vary in the amount of BCR gene included; the encoded proteins are associated with distinct clinical and biologic features and may confer distinct prognoses (39, 72). Another example are the more than a dozen different CBFβ/MYH11 fusion messages that are generated by the inversion of chromosome 16 [inv(16)(p13q22)]; in these isoforms, the portion of the MYH11 gene that participates in the creation of the fusion product can vary (11). When combined with the existence of large deletions in the CBFβ gene (30), the complexity of this allegedly simple inversion becomes apparent.

Chromosomal aberrations can be monitored by PCR if the gene sequences affected by the aberrations have been identified, as the sequences are required to serve as templates for primer construction. The PCR technique is an essential tool for (i) subgrouping of patients with apparently identical chromosome abnormalities according to genetic variants and (ii) monitoring of the actual state of remission. In the near future, the definition of "remission" will have to be revisited, particularly for diseases in which the presence of MRD, in the absence of clinical and hematologic symptoms, is confirmed to have treatment implications (45). One caveat to the use of PCR for MRD monitoring relates to the finding of several of these presumably leukemogenic fusion genes in healthy individuals (6).

Cryptic Chromosome Translocations

Rare cryptic translocations derive from submicroscopic insertions of genes, yielding a molecular result identical to that of the common translocations; FISH or PCR can detect them. Whether cryptic translocations, in general, confer the same prognostic significance as visible ones has not yet been established.

The (12;21)(p13;q22) translocation that results in the TEL/AML1, also called ETV6/RUNX1, gene fusion is an exceptional chromosomal aberration in that it is always cryptic. It is the most common genetic rearrangement found in children with precursor B-lineage ALL and associated with excellent prognosis; on the other hand, this fusion transcript is rarely found in adult disease (52).

PRESENTLY ACCEPTED DIAGNOSTIC CLASSIFICATION OF HEMATOLOGIC MALIGNANCIES

The WHO Classification of Hematopoietic Tumors published in 2001 (31) represents the first worldwide comprehensive classification of the hematologic malignancies. The WHO system took the stand of compiling established classification approaches into one; at the same time, new information (e.g., cytogenetics) was incorporated and some subcategories that appeared to be outdated were selectively deleted (e.g., L1 and L2 morphological subgroups in ALL were combined). The committee members decided that sorting neoplasms according to associated prognoses was neither practical nor necessary and could be misleading.

The WHO proposal created novel diagnostic subclasses based on clinically relevant cytogenetic abnormalities and their molecular equivalents, such as t(9;22)(q34;q11.2) (BCR/ABL); t(v;11q23) (rearranged mixed-lineage leukemia [MLL] gene), with "v" standing for one of approximately 50 different translocation partners (genes); t(1;19) (q23;p13.3) (PBX1/E2A); t(12;21)(p13;q22) (TEL/AML1); hyperdiploid, and hypodiploid karyotypes in ALL. AML was subgrouped into (i) AML with recurrent cytogenetic abnormalities, t(8;21)(q22;q22) (AML1/ETO), inv(16) (p13q22) or t(16;16)(p13;q22) (CBFβ/MYH11), t(15;17) (q22;q12) (PML/RARα), and AML with 11q23 abnormalities (rearranged MLL gene); (ii) AML with multilineage dysplasia; (iii) therapy-related AML/myelodysplastic syndrome; and (iv) the largest group of all, AML not otherwise categorized but subdivided into the old FAB morphology categories.

The fifth WHO category for AML comprises "acute leukemia of ambiguous lineage"; to recognize such leukemias, the WHO system advocated the use of scoring systems in the interpretation of immunophenotypic data (31). More than 20 years ago, Bettelheim and Paietta (7, 49) introduced the terms "biphenotypic" and "mixed leukemias" to describe ambiguous cases in which TdT-positive lymphoblasts expressed the myeloid surface antigen CD15 and in which leukemia populations appeared to consist of cells with distinct lineage affiliations, respectively. Even though these terms were understandable back then, in the earliest days of monoclonal antibodies to hematopoietic antigens and in the pre-flow (cytometry) era, their creation was unfortunate. Despite new knowledge and much better technology, these diagnostic terms have persisted as viable parts even of the new WHO classification and are widely abused based primarily on flawed data interpretation. It is now known that in up to 60% of ALL cases, the lymphoblasts express one to two myeloid antigens. The pattern of distribution of myeloid antigens in ALL varies with the stage of maturation of the lymphoblasts [myeloid antigens CD33 and CD13 in CD10$^+$ early pre-B-ALL and myeloid antigens CD65(s) and CD15(s) in CD10$^-$ undifferentiated pro-B-ALL] (48). Alternatively, TdT and other lymphoid-associated antigens can be expressed by leukemic myeloblasts. The B-lymphoid antigen CD19, for instance, is part of the surrogate marker profile for t(8;21) AML (see below).

Neither the finding of myeloid antigens in ALL nor that of lymphoid antigens in AML per se signifies lineage ambiguity; most notably, it does not affect clinical outcome, unless these antigens form part of a marker profile typical of a prognostic genetic lesion. For instance, expression of CD33 and CD13 in early pre-B-ALL is frequently associated with the presence of *BCR/ABL* transcripts (see below); the *BCR/ABL* transcript, reflecting t(9;22)(q34;q11.2), the Philadelphia chromosome, is found in ~30% of adult ALL cases and is the strongest negative prognostic indicator in this disease (27).

In at least 95% of acute leukemias, a single dominant lineage affiliation can be established through the detection of one of three lineage-*specific* antigens, myeloperoxidase, intracytoplasmic CD22 (cCD22), or intracytoplasmic CD3 (cCD3), for the myeloid, B, or T lineage, respectively. It is essential that myeloperoxidase be tested simultaneously with cCD3 or cCD22 in leukemic blasts that are gated flow cytometrically either through side scatter versus CD45 or through the use of a gating antibody, such as CD34 or CD117. Leukemia populations with truly biphenotypic features are rare and manifest themselves through dual expression of two lineage-*specific* antigens in the same cell, e.g., myeloperoxidase and cCD3, as seen in some cases of CD117$^+$ ALL (55). Unfortunately, these essential antigens are intracellular and thus still present a technical challenge to many flow cytometrists. It is important to remember that CD22 and CD3 can be found on the surfaces of mature B and T lymphocytes, respectively; control staining of the cell surface and gating exclusively on abnormal cells are absolute prerequisites for meaningful results.

To rely solely on standard cytogenetics is problematic when one considers that in national cooperative group adult leukemia trials up to 40% of patients have either normal, invalid, or no cytogenetic results. The WHO proposal failed to appreciate the potential of immune profiles to serve as surrogates for clinically relevant genetic defects in the absence of cytogenetic and/or molecular information.

INTERRELATIONSHIPS OF THE VARIOUS DIAGNOSTIC LABORATORY DISCIPLINES

While the various diagnostic disciplines should work together, compensate for one another's weaknesses, and eventually provide an overall diagnosis, individual diagnostic parameters are often not predictive of one another or even directly comparable. An example is the assumption that a patient who, according to blast immunophenotyping, has differentiated AML must have blasts with FAB M2 morphology. Similarly, blasts appearing to have monocytoid features under the microscope may not necessarily express CD11b and/or CD14, two prototype monocytic antigens. Both immunophenotyping and morphologic evaluation yield significant, but independent, pieces of information. Only in rare circumstances, e.g., in hypergranular APL, will a unique immunophenotype be consistently associated with a particular morphologic appearance.

There are some who believe that gene expression profiling, with its potential to measure the relative abundances of thousands of transcripts and provide information on the transcriptional activity of leukemic cells on a genomic scale (29), may soon replace other diagnostic disciplines, particularly if combined with protein analyses. Although gene expression arrays benefit from established basic leukemia biology, they can focus on areas in which conventional methods have failed, such as diseases devoid of standard prognostic indicators (e.g., leukemias with normal cytogenetics); the first promising results along these lines have been reported (e.g., references 8 and 70). As part of their prospective ability to elucidate molecular pathways that sustain the growth and survival of the various leukemic cells, gene expression analyses have great potential for discovering novel therapeutic targets; such discoveries may eventually lead to a leukemia classification system based on response to target-specific therapy.

Morphology Versus Immunophenotype

The best example of cooperation between morphologic evaluation and immunophenotyping was the creation of FAB class M0, the subtype with the least morphologic differentiation (69). That M0 leukemias belong to the myeloid lineage is based primarily on the detection of the myeloperoxidase protein through antibody binding; cytochemical staining fails to yield a positive reaction because the myeloperoxidase precursor that is present in these undifferentiated cells lacks enzymatic activity. If myeloperoxidase cannot be detected, affiliation with the myeloid lineage depends on the detection of CD33 and CD13 in the absence of lymphoid-specific antigens (53).

In APL, despite the presence of the same cytogenetic aberration, t(15;17), the hypogranular variant (M3v) demonstrates some immunophenotypic features distinct from those of M3: the stem cell antigen CD34, HLA-DR, and the T-cell antigen CD2 are commonly expressed by M3v leukemic promyelocytes, and antibody to the common leukocyte antigen CD45 binds with fluorescence intensity higher than that seen in M3 cells (54). Grimwade et al. (26) speculated that APL cells that expressed the CD2 antigen were derived from progenitors with T-lineage potential and thus earlier in differentiation than CD2$^-$ APL cells. This suggestion is based on their finding that in CD2$^+$ APL cells the *CD2* locus demonstrates chromatin features identical to those of T cells. The expression of CD2 is the strongest indicator for M3v APL (or APL with the S-transcript isoform of *PML/RARα*; see next section). It is important to remember that CD2 is rarely found in AML. The only other AML subtype famous for occasional CD2 expression is inv(16) AML (1). The distinction between CD2$^+$ APL and inv(16) AML is based on the lack of CD11a, CD18, and CD133 in the former (54).

CD2 expression can override all other immunophenotypic "rules" in the characterization of APL. If CD2 expression on leukemic myeloblasts is unequivocally demonstrated, it is recommended that these blast cells be subjected to molecular analysis for *PML/RARα*, irrespective of the cells' morphology or other immunophenotypic features.

Immunophenotyping Versus Cytogenetic and Molecular Analysis

In APL, differential breakpoints in the *PML* gene lead to either the L (long; bcr1)-, S (short; bcr3)-, or V (variable; bcr2)-transcript isoform of *PML/RARα*. The recently described surrogate marker profile for *PML/RARα* APL, HLA-DR^{Low} CD11a^{Low} CD18^{Low} (54), is applicable to all three molecular isoforms (Fig. 1). In terms of specific

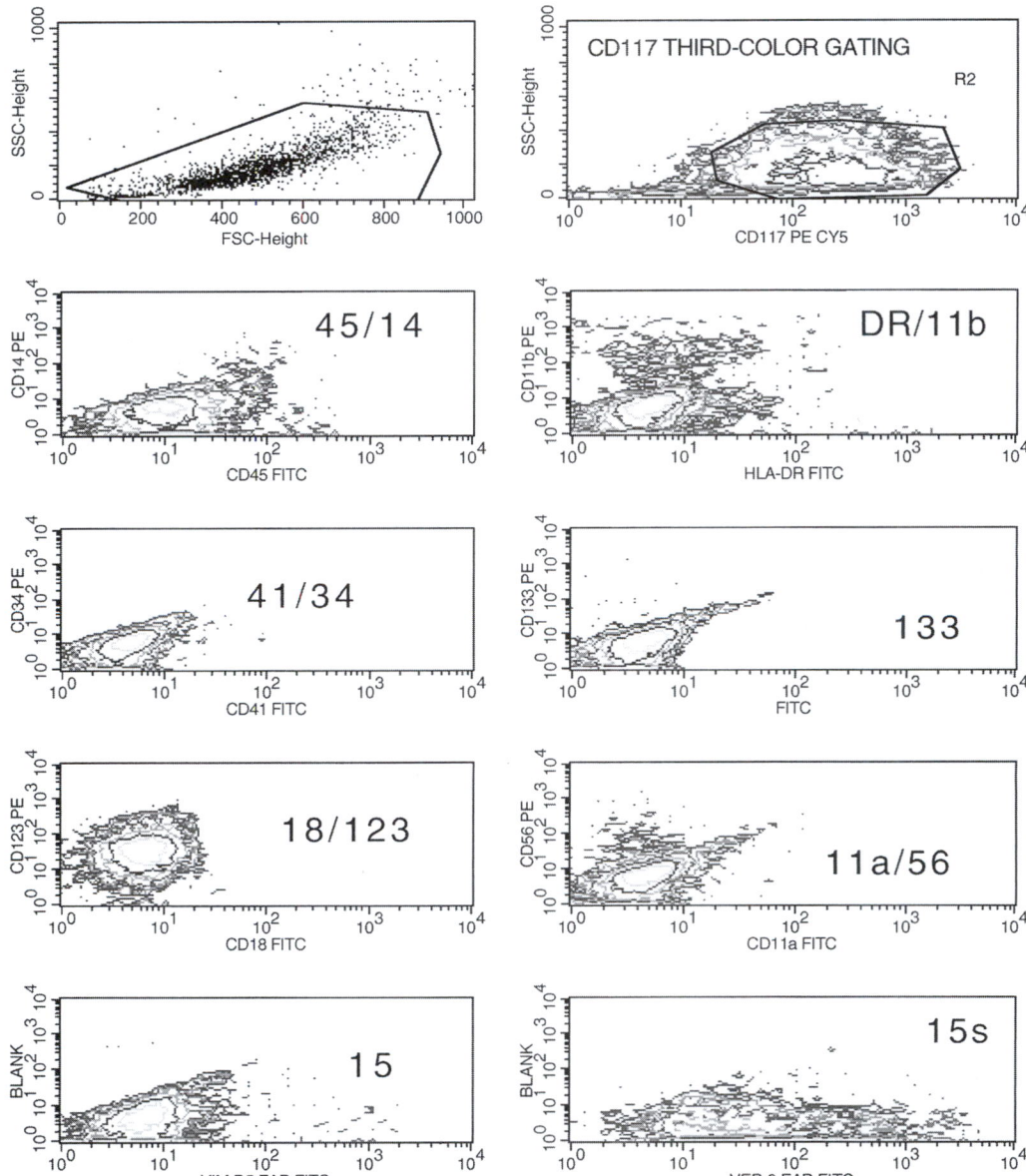

FIGURE 1 Typical antigen profile of *PML/RARα*-positive APL (for all L- and V-form and many S-form cases and for all M3 and some M3v morphologies). The scattergram in the left upper corner characterizes all cells present by size (forward scatter [FSC]) and granularity (side scatter [SSC]). A gate is set around all cells of interest. In the contour plot to the right, the leukemic promyelocytes are gated on the basis of CD117 expression (R2), whereby cells are stained with CD117 conjugated to phycoerythrin-cyanin 5 (PE CY5); this CD117-PE CY5 antibody is added to every antibody combination so that gating can be limited to leukemic cells. All subsequent contour plots show antigen expression only on gated leukemic promyelocytes. Such or similar gating strategy should always be applied in order to eliminate the inclusion of normal cells in the evaluation of antigen expression patterns. In all contour plots, data along the *x* axes reflect cells stained with antibodies conjugated to fluorescein isothiocyanate (FITC). Along the *y* axes are data for cells stained with antibodies conjugated to phycoerythrin (PE). Any blasts, which bind both FITC- and PE-antibodies in a given combination, appear in the right upper quadrant of the contour plot. For each contour plot, single or double antibodies tested (in addition to CD117) are indicated; CD clusters for all antibodies tested are written into the contour plots. Fluorescence intensity, a measure of antigen density, is usually expressed by the mean fluorescence channel of the cell population stained with the specific antibody of interest (along the *x* or *y* axis) divided by the mean fluorescence channel of the negative isotype control (mean fluorescence intensity or mean fluorescence intensity ratio).

antigenic features, the L- and V-form diseases are indistinguishable but clearly separable from S-isoform APL. Only in S-form disease do leukemic promyelocytes express CD34, CD2, and CD56. CD56, the neural cell adhesion molecule, has been associated with poor clinical outcome in APL (48). Note that, although the presence of CD2 and/or CD56 on a patient's leukemic promyelocytes is highly suggestive of the S isoform because these antigens are never seen in L- or V-isoform disease, there are a large number of S-isoform patients who lack these antigens. CD34 expression may be associated with the molecular isoform or the microgranular morphologic variant (see above). The density of the CD34 antigen is significantly lower on the surfaces of leukemic promyelocytes than on non-APL myeloblasts (46).

While CD56 expression in AML is not uncommon, the expression of the T-cell-affiliated antigen CD2 by leukemic myeloblasts is rarely observed, provided that antigen expression is viewed on gated leukemic cells exclusively. CD2 expression by myeloid leukemic cells, therefore, should raise the immediate suspicion of APL. The only other AML subtype that frequently demonstrates CD2 expression is AML associated with $CBF\beta/MYH11$ [inv(16)(p13q22)] (1). This is an important though not well-appreciated association, given that inv(16) is a subtle cytogenetic abnormality that is easily missed.

The t(9;22)(q34;q11) encodes various isoforms of the BCR/ABL fusion gene that resides in the Philadelphia chromosome, the derivative chromosome 22. All BCR/ABL proteins share similar carboxy-terminal ABL TK domains but differ in the portions of the BCR protein included in the fusion product. In the majority of CML cases and in one-third of BCR/ABL-positive ALL cases, the break within the BCR gene occurs in the major breakpoint cluster region (M-bcr), resulting, when joined with a portion of c-ABL from chromosome 9, in a b2a2 or b3a2 fusion transcript encoding a protein of 210,000 daltons (p210$^{BCR-ABL}$). A break in the minor breakpoint cluster region (m-bcr) forms the e1a2 transcript encoding a 190,000-dalton protein (p190$^{BCR-ABL}$) found mostly in BCR/ABL-positive ALL (39, 72). Lymphoblasts express specific antigenic features dependent upon which BCR/ABL isoform they contain (e.g., the myeloid antigen combination CD33+CD13 and CD25 expression are much more frequent in p210$^{BCR-ABL}$ lymphoblasts) (E. Paietta et al., Blood 100[11]:755a, abstr. no. 2990, 2002). This finding suggests that the two major isoforms affect distinct target cells of transformation.

Cytogenetic Versus Molecular Analysis

Whether or not patients with molecular but not chromosomal evidence of certain genetic lesions are to be considered identical in terms of outcome is still in question. In pediatric and adult T-lineage ALL, overexpression of the transcription factor HOX11 can occur in the absence of the cytogenetic aberration that is linked to the activation of the HOX11 gene, namely, translocations involving 10q24; despite the lack of visible chromosomal rearrangements, the favorable outcome associated with HOX11 overexpression is preserved (18, 19).

The situation is different with t(8;21)(q22;q22), a translocation associated with favorable prognosis in AML; patients who lacked this translocation as determined by standard cytogenetic analysis or FISH but who were found to express its molecular product, the AML1/ETO fusion gene, did substantially more poorly than cytogenetically t(8;21)-positive patients (63).

Gene Profiling Versus All Other Diagnostic Disciplines

Recent results from gene expression profiling suggest that the two morphologic subtypes of APL, M3 and M3v, are clearly separable. Schoch et al. proposed that the difference might lie in the higher frequency of FLT3 gene mutations in M3v (64).

In pediatric B-lineage ALL, conventional differentiation stages, such as early pre-B-ALL (CD10$^+$; negative for intracytoplasmic μ chains) versus pre-B-ALL (positive for intracytoplasmic μ chains), do not elicit strong enough gene signatures to stand out in comparison with those of chromosomal translocations (21, 62). Of particular interest are specific gene profiles that correlate with response to therapy and survival outside of standard diagnostic criteria (e.g., references 10, 21, and 68), as they highlight the limitations of present classification systems, particularly in terms of clinical relevance.

SURROGATE MARKER PROFILES FOR GENETIC LESIONS

PML/RARα-Positive APL and Its Variants

APL with M3 (or M3v) morphology is the only AML subtype to date for which morphology and immunophenotype agree. Early definitions were limited in their ability to distinguish APL from other AML subtypes, such as natural killer (NK) cell AML, an important distinction considering that NK AML is unresponsive to ATRA (reviewed in reference 46). The newest definition (54) reliably identifies t(15;17)(q22;q21) APL based predominantly on the following: (i) lack of HLA-DR and CD133, two antigens expressed at differentiation levels more immature than that of promyelocytes during normal myelopoiesis; (ii) absence of several adhesive molecules, such as the leukocyte integrins CD11a (α$_L$ subunit of the leukocyte function-associated antigen 1 [LFA-1]), CD18 (β$_2$ subunit of LFA-1), and CD11b (α$_M$ subunit of Mac-1 integrin); (iii) low expression of carbohydrate structures which serve as ligands for other adhesion molecules (CD65s and CD15); and (iv) faint expression of CD45, the common leukocyte antigen, and of CD38, a bifunctional ectoenzyme catalyzing both the synthesis and the hydrolysis of cyclic ADP-ribose and involved in cell adhesion to the endothelium. With respect to CD15, it is important to realize that leukemic promyelocytes express CD15 in its sialylated form. Therefore, although CD15s antibodies, such as VEP-9 in Fig. 1, will readily stain APL cells, CD15 antibodies that lack reactivity with the sialylated antigen, such as VIM-D5, will not (46, 54).

In addition to the PML/RARα fusion gene, which accounts for >98% of APL cases, a common segment of the 5'-truncated RARα gene has been found to fuse with alternative genes (60). Because such variant translocations are rare, clinical information regarding the responsiveness of associated diseases to ATRA is scarce; recurrent cases of promyelocyte leukemia zinc finger (PLZF)/RARα leukemia, derived from t(11;17)(q23;q21), appear to lack ATRA responsiveness, and nucleophosmin (NPM)/RARα APL, derived from t(5;17)(q35;q21), is ATRA responsive. Despite their low frequency, the limited immunophenotypic observations available suggest that the main characteristic features of PML/RARα APL cells hold up for all presently known variant APL translocations that involve rearrangement of the RARα gene (E. Paietta, unpublished results), i.e., HLA-DR$^{-/Low}$ CD34$^{-/Low}$ CD11a$^-$ CD18$^-$ CD15s$^+$/CD15$^-$. Novel variant RARα fusion genes keep appearing in the literature, for which ATRA sensitivity in individual cases appears to vary.

Two pieces of evidence should prompt the search for the presence of an alternative *RARα* fusion gene in a patient, (i) the finding of APL-specific immunophenotypic features in a patient negative for *PML/RARα* and (ii) cytogenetic evidence of chromosome 17 abnormalities in such a patient. Occasionally, slight variations from the typical APL profile may be found. Gallagher et al., for instance, found weak expression of CD133 in only the second case of signal transducer and activator of transcription b (*STATb*)/*RARα*-positive leukemia (R. E. Gallagher et al., *Blood* **104**[11]:821a, abstr. no. 3005, 2004). If confirmed in further cases, this antigenic peculiarity may serve as a diagnostic tool for this particular APL variant.

The controversy regarding the expression of CD117 by APL cells deserves mentioning. CD117, the stem cell factor receptor KIT, is expressed by normal hematopoietic precursor cells and appears to be lost prior to maturation of normal myeloblasts into promyelocytes (48). The erroneous view that leukemic promyelocytes are equally negative for CD117 could only recently be rectified. The intensity of CD117 staining of leukemic promyelocytes is sometimes very low and can be recognized only by comparison with negative staining of normal cells contaminating the leukemic sample (54). Due to its constant expression by APL cells, CD117 is an excellent tool for the monitoring of residual APL cells posttreatment.

One more word of caution: some flow cytometry books promise a characteristic scattergram for APL, reflecting cells of large size (high forward-angle light scatter [FSC]) with a high degree of granularity (high 90°-angle scatter or side scatter [SSC]). While it is correct that scatter patterns of hypergranular APL cells are different from those of M3v cells, the scatter signal can be quite variable and misleading (54).

AML1/ETO-Positive AML

Translocation (8;21)(q22;q22) is one of the most common recurring cytogenetic abnormalities in AML and is thus considered to represent its own subtype in the WHO classification (31). The two genes involved in this translocation are *AML1* (now called *RUNX1*), a gene encoding a transcription factor on chromosome 21q22.3, and the *Eight-Twenty-One* gene (*ETO*, also called *MTG8*) on chromosome 8q22 (40). This AML subtype is an example of core binding factor (CBF) leukemias; inv(16)(p13q22) AML is another example of a CBF AML.

The immunophenotype of t(8;21) AML allows for a correct prediction of this genetic aberration (20). The distinctive features are expression of CD19, a B-lineage-associated antigen, and of CD56, the neural cell adhesion molecule, by CD34+ myeloblasts. The presence of CD56 may explain the increased incidence of granulocytic sarcomas observed in this disease. While the CD19/CD56 marker profile is invariably associated with t(8;21) AML, a substantial portion of t(8;21) patients lack either one or both of these discriminating antigens. In such cases, low expression of the integrin CD11a is a very helpful diagnostic tool. With the exception of t(8;21) AML or t(15;17) APL (and its variants), >90% of AMLs demonstrate strong expression of CD11a. The low expression of CD11a in t(8;21) AML is explained by the inhibition of CD11a promoter activity through the AML1/ETO fusion product (58). Figure 2 compares two cases of differentiated AML (FAB M2), one being *AML1/ETO* negative (Fig. 2A) and the other *AML1/ETO* positive (Fig. 2B). Note that CD7, a T-lineage-affiliated antigen frequently expressed by leukemic myeloblasts, is never expressed in AML1/ETO AML.

In CD13- and/or CD33-negative t(8;21) cases (2, 48), CD19 expression can lead to misdiagnosis as ALL; simultaneous detection of cCD22 and myeloperoxidase in the same cell is an essential tool in the differential diagnosis. Remember that dual absence of myeloperoxidase and cCD22 in such a case is consistent with AML. This marker combination is particularly relevant since CD19+ t(8;21) AMLs frequently coexpress PAX5, a B-lineage-associated transcription factor (67). The markers CD34 and CD133 discriminate between CD11a^Low^ t(8;21) AML and APL.

BCR/ABL-Positive ALL

In 1997, expression of CD25, the α-chain of the interleukin-2 receptor (IL-2R), was reported to predict the presence of *BCR/ABL* fusion transcripts, representative of the (9;22) translocation, in ALL (51). This initial observation, based on data from 144 patients, was subsequently confirmed with 485 adult ALL cases in the Eastern Cooperative Oncology Group Phase III trial, E2993, with a 29% incidence of *BCR/ABL* positivity (Paietta et al., ASH abstract, 2002). Although the final analysis of these data must await closure of the E2993 study, CD25 remained the most predictive marker in the interim analysis, with other antigenic features only aiding in the surrogate marker profile for *BCR/ABL*-positive lymphoblasts: CD25^High^ CD34^High^ CD33+CD13+. This profile is significantly different from that of *BCR/ABL*-negative disease ($P < 0.0001$) and is considerably more specific than those previously suggested for *BCR/ABL*-positive ALL, which relied on antigens shared by *BCR/ABL*-positive and *BCR/ABL*-negative lymphoblasts (28). Most strikingly, the higher the fraction of CD25-expressing lymphoblasts, the lower the likelihood of complete remission and the shorter the disease-free survival in *BCR/ABL*-positive ALL.

BCR/ABL-positive lymphoblasts express not only CD25, the α-chain, but also CD132, the γ-chain of the IL-2R, while lacking CD122, the β-chain. Since the presence of all three components of the high-affinity IL-2R is a prerequisite for IL-2-mediated transduction of growth signals, the physiologic role of this partial IL-2R in *BCR/ABL*-positive ALL and reasons for its prognostic implications remain unclear.

CD117/KIT-Positive ALL

CD117 in leukemia immunophenotyping is considered more specific for the myeloid lineage than CD33 or CD13 (48). Early hematopoietic progenitor cells express CD117, the stem cell factor receptor KIT (41). During normal lymphopoiesis, CD117/KIT is expressed by a fraction of CD34+ CD3- CD4- CD8- (triple-negative) thymocytes. In normal T-cell progenitors, expression of CD117/KIT coincides with that of CD135, the FLT3 receptor TK that is activated by the FLT3 ligand; FLT3 and CD117/KIT share extensive structural homology (39).

CD117/KIT expression by leukemic lymphoblasts is rare and mostly (albeit not exclusively) associated with the T-cell phenotype. Recently, CD117/KIT-positive T-lineage ALL was characterized as an immunophenotypically distinct subtype, frequently associated with myeloid morphologic features, including the presence of Auer rods (55). CD117+ lymphoblasts are surface CD3-, CD34+, CD62L+, CD56-, CD2+, CD7+, CD1a-, CD5-, CD4/CD8-, and TdT positive, expressing one myeloid antigen, CD13. This profile fits the most immature category of T-lineage ALL (4, 18), resembling multipotent thymic precursors. The lack of CD5 expression must be particularly emphasized since it is unique to this subtype of T-lineage ALL.

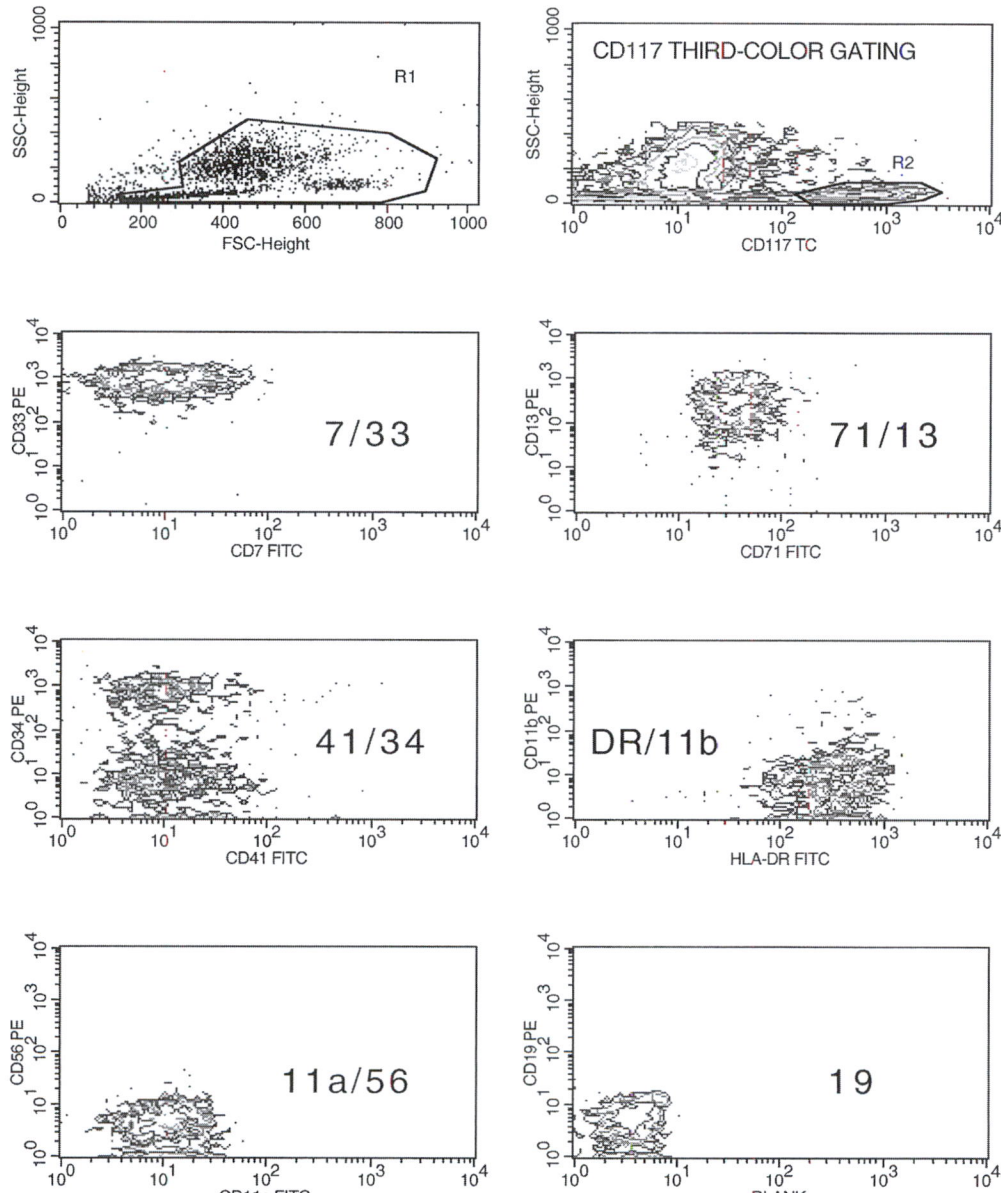

FIGURE 2 Differential antigen expression profiles of differentiated AMLs dependent upon the presence of the *AML1/ETO* fusion gene. The first panel demonstrates antigen expression in a case of differentiated AML with a normal karyotype (AML-M2), negative for *AML1/ETO*. A small percentage of blast cells was gated by CD117 staining (R2) and analyzed. In comparison, the second panel demonstrates a typical surrogate marker profile for *AML1/ETO*-positive AML. While this case represents a differentiated AML with FAB M2 morphology, many cases with *AML1/ETO* present with a rather undifferentiated phenotype, occasionally CD33 negative. Note the high expression of CD34, which is typical for this AML subtype, the absence of CD11a, the partial expression of CD56, and the weak albeit definite presence of CD19. One more observation of importance is that *AML1/ETO*-positive AML does not involve expression of CD7 on the leukemic myeloblasts. SSC, side scatter; FSC, forward scatter; R1, gating of all white cells excluding debris; R2, gating on CD117+ leukemic myeloblasts within R1. TC, third color; PE, phycoerythrin; FITC, fluorescein isothiocyanate; PerCP, peridinin chlorophyll protein. Antibody combinations are written as CDs into the contour plots.

CD117/KIT-positive ALL cases show a high frequency of *FLT3* gene mutations, either ITD or point mutations. *FLT3* is otherwise rarely mutated in leukemic lymphoblasts; only B-lineage ALLs containing *MLL* gene rearrangements have previously been found to demonstrate *FLT3* mutations (3). Thus, CD117/KIT expression in T-lineage ALL might be considered a surrogate marker for *FLT3* gene mutations.

Table 1 gives an overview of currently known surrogate marker profiles for genetic lesions in the acute leukemias.

Antigen-Specific and Gene-Specific Therapy

"Treatment by design" is what Larson et al. (38) called the novel approaches to leukemia and lymphoma therapy that take advantage of phenotypic (due to antigens) or genotypic

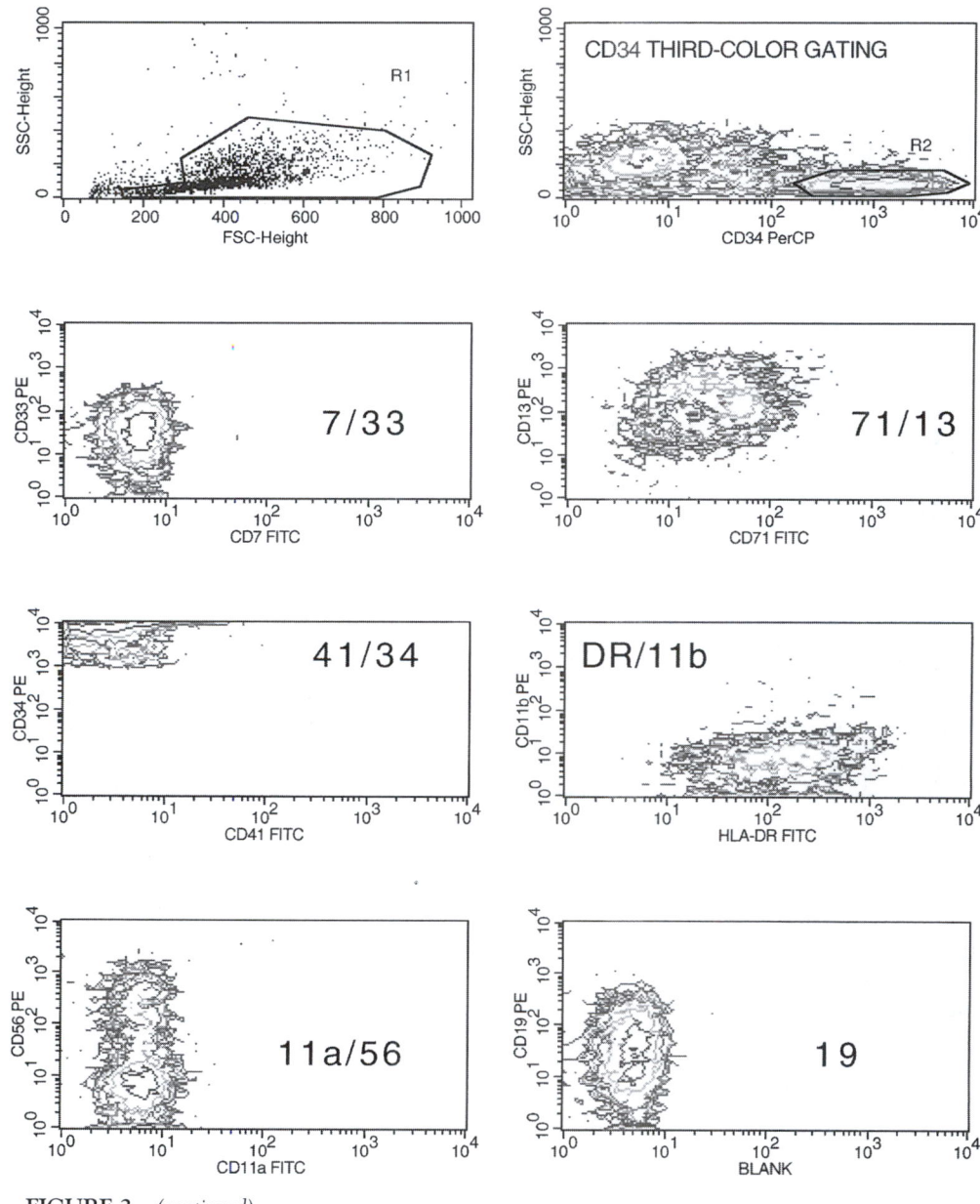

FIGURE 2 (continued)

(due to perturbed signal transduction pathways) features of malignant cells.

Monoclonal antibodies depend on the presence of the specific antigens that they recognize for their activity. In addition, at least for gemtuzumab ozogamicin, the CD33 antibody linked to the cytotoxic drug calicheamicin, antigen-independent endocytosis has been found to provide a nonspecific uptake mechanism, presenting a rationale for the treatment of both CD33⁺ and CD33⁻ malignancies (32). Once bound to the cell surface, antibodies per se can induce direct signaling in the malignant cells, which may result, for instance, in apoptosis (programmed cell death) or mediate antibody-directed cellular cytotoxicity (e.g., antibodies to the B-lineage antigen CD20 or to CD52, an antigen expressed by most B and T lymphocytes), or the antibody may be conjugated and function as a vehicle delivering immunotoxins or chemotherapeutic agents (e.g., antibodies to the myeloid

antigen CD33) or radiation (e.g., antibodies to CD20, CD22, or CD33 conjugated with various radioemitters, such as ¹³¹I or ⁹⁰Y) to the target cells. Bispecific antibodies target leukemia-associated antigens and activating antigens simultaneously on cytotoxic effector cells or may otherwise potentiate the signaling events that will eventually lead to inhibition of leukemia cell growth (24, 33, 44, 66). One disadvantage is that antibodies also attach to the corresponding antigen when it is expressed by nonleukemic cells; furthermore, high levels of circulating soluble antigens reduce the bioavailability and thus the efficacy of the administered antibody.

Multidrug resistance (MDR) is the ability of tumor cells to survive exposure to various chemotherapeutic drugs due to the presence of membrane transporter molecules, such as P-glycoprotein (Pgp) or the multidrug-resistance-related proteins (MRPs). Strategies to disable Pgp, at least to date, have yielded conflicting and less than convincing clinical

TABLE 1 Established surrogate marker profiles for genetic lesions in acute leukemia[a]

Phenotype	Diagnosis	Antigenic characteristics
PML/RARα	APL (M3; all L and V form, some S form)	HLA-DR$^-$ CD11a$^-$ CD18$^-$ CD133$^-$ CD45^{Low} CD38^{Low} CD34^{Low} CD15s^{High} CD15^{Low}
	APL (M3v; S form)	As above, except HLA-DR$^{Low-High}$ CD34$^{Low-High}$ CD2^{High} CD56$^{Low-High}$
X/RARα	Variant APLs	As above, with occasional slight variations, such as CD133^{Low} in STATb/RARα-positive APLs
AML1/ETO	AML	Myeloid phenotype (often undifferentiated; CD33$^-$); CD34^{High} CD19$^{Low-High}$ CD56$^{Low-High}$
CBFβ/MYH11	AML	Myeloid phenotype; CD2^{High}
BCR/ABL	Adult ALL (p190/p210)	CD25^{High} CD34^{High} CD33+CD13^{High} (usually CD10^{High} cytoplasmic mu$^-$)
Mutant FLT3	Adult T-cell ALL	CD117^{High} CD34^{High} CD5$^-$ CD7^{High} CD2^{High} cCD3^{High} CD4/CD8$^-$ CD13^{High}

[a] The description of antigen expression as negative ($-$), low, or high refers both to intensity of fluorescence and percentage of blast cells expressing the antigen. Negative indicates the virtual absence of antibody binding by the leukemic cells beyond the level in the negative isotype control; low can refer either to subset of leukemic cells binding the antibody or to the entire blast cell population binding the antibody with low fluorescence; high indicates expression of the antigen by the majority of blast cells at high density. X/RARα, fusion proteins in which X represents variable partner genes.

results (42); yet, these membrane transporter molecules deserve mentioning in the context of antigen-targeted therapy. Aside from demonstrating the presence of Pgp and other MDR proteins, flow cytometry can confirm the functional integrity of these proteins as drug efflux pumps and thus establish the MDR status of leukemia populations. Furthermore, at least in AML, expression of CD34 correlates positively with Pgp function.

Gene mutations that are associated with cellular transformation present other attractive targets for therapy. I have already mentioned the efficacy of therapeutic doses of ATRA in reversing the perturbed histone acetylation and chromatin remodeling induced by the RARα-fusion proteins expressed uniquely in APL (57, 61). An analogous pathogenetic mechanism has been elucidated for CBF leukemias, such as those associated with AML1/ETO, CBFβ/MYH11, and TEL/AML1 fusions. Like RARα, CBF, the heterodimeric transcription factor with components AML1 and CBFβ, is essential for normal hematopoietic development; unlike RARα, CBF does not bind any ligand. But analogous to the action of PML/RARα, the loss of CBF function from the leukemic fusion products leads to active suppression of transcription by maintaining the histones in a deacetylated conformation and making DNA inaccessible to transcription induction. Using histone deacetylase inhibitors may, therefore, be a rather general strategy to overcome leukemic transformation due to disruption of chromatin-remodeling mechanisms (23, 61).

Whether or not FLT3 gene mutations represent the primary genetic event in cellular transformation is irrelevant for therapy. What is important is that FLT3 mutations result in the constitutive activation of the FLT3 TK and that inhibitors of this activity have shown clinical efficacy (23, 59). The best evidence that targeted inhibition of aberrant TK signaling can be an effective therapeutic intervention has been obtained in CML and other diseases that respond to treatment with imatinib mesylate, the BCR/ABL TK inhibitor (13, 56). The downstream targets of constitutively activated TK molecules, such as STAT proteins that become activated through constitutive phosphorylation, may also provide rational targets for therapeutic interventions (59, 65).

The principle of targeted therapy, as attractive and promising as it is, requires much more understanding of transforming molecular events and perturbed signaling pathways than the simple administration of indiscriminately cytotoxic chemotherapy. Developing phenotypic profiles as surrogates for underlying genetic aberrations is clinically useful only if

antileukemic therapy is available that targets any component of the disturbed molecular pathways associated with these genetic lesions. PML/RARα-positive APL is the paradigm for a leukemia subtype for which a surrogate marker profile is clinically valid given the availability of genotype-specific therapy (ATRA). As the list of known therapeutic targets grows, undoubtedly as the result of gene expression profiling and similar techniques, the role of surrogate antigen profiles will grow, as they can predict the efficacy of targeted approaches in lieu of expensive, time-consuming, and not always accessible gene expression analyses.

REFERENCES

1. Adriaansen, H. J., P. A. W. te Boekhorst, A. M. Hagemeijer, C. E. van der Schoot, H. R. Delwel, and J. J. M. van Dongen. 1993. Acute myeloid leukemia M4 with bone marrow eosinophilia (M4Eo) and inv(16)(p13q22) exhibits a specific immunophenotype with CD2 expression. *Blood* 81:3043–3051.
2. Arber, D. A., C. Glackin, G. Lowe, L. J. Medeiros, and M. L. Slovak. 1997. Presence of t(8;21)(q22;q22) in myeloperoxidase-positive, myeloid surface antigen-negative acute myeloid leukemia. *Am. J. Clin. Pathol.* 107:68–73.
3. Armstrong, S. A., A. L. Kung, M. E. Mabon, L. B. Silverman, R. W. Stam, M. L. Den Boer, R. Pieters, J. H. Kersey, S. E. Sallan, J. A. Fletcher, T. R. Golub, J. D. Griffin, and S. J. Korsmeyer. 2003. Inhibition of FLT3 in MLL: validation of a therapeutic target identified by gene expression based classification. *Cancer Cell* 3:173–183.
4. Asnafi, V., K. Beldjord, E. Boulanger, B. Comba, P. Le Tutour, M.-H. Estienne, F. Davi, J. Landman-Parker, P. Quartier, A. Buzyn, E. Delabesse, F. Valensi, and E. Macintyre. 2003. Analysis of TCR, pTα, and RAG-1 in T-acute lymphoblastic leukemias improves understanding of early human T-lymphoid lineage commitment. *Blood* 101:2693–2703.
5. Bain, B. J. 2003. *Leukaemia Diagnosis: a Guide to the FAB Classification.* Blackwell Scientific Publications Ltd., Oxford, United Kingdom.
6. Bäsecke, J., F. Griesinger, L. Trümper, and G. Brittinger. 2002. Leukemia- and lymphoma-associated genetic aberrations in healthy individuals. *Ann. Hematol.* 81:64–75.
7. Bettelheim, P., E. Paietta, O. Majdic, H. Gadner, J. D. Schwarzmeier, and W. Knapp. 1982. Expression of a myeloid marker on TdT-positive acute lymphocytic leukemic cells: evidence by double-fluorescence staining. *Blood* 60:1392–1396.

8. Bullinger, L., K. Döhner, E. Bair, S. Fröhling, R. F. Schlenk, R. Tibshirani, H. Döhner, and J. R. Pollack. 2004. Use of gene-expression profiling to identify prognostic subclasses in adult acute myeloid leukemia. *N. Engl. J. Med.* **350:**1605–1616.

9. Bumm, T., C. Müller, H.-K. Al-Ali, K. Krohn, P. Shepherd, E. Schmidt, S. Leiblein, C. Franke, E. Hennig, T. Friedrich, R. Krahl, D. Niederwieser, and M. W. N. Deininger. 2003. Emergence of clonal cytogenetic abnormalities in Ph⁻ cells in some CML patients in cytogenetic remission to imatinib but restoration of polyclonal hematopoiesis in the majority. *Blood* **101:**1941–1949.

10. Chiaretti, S., X. Li, R. Gentleman, A. Vitale, M. Vignetti, F. Mandelli, J. Ritz, and R. Foa. 2004. Gene expression profile of adult T-cell acute lymphocytic leukemia identifies distinct subsets of patients with different response to therapy and survival. *Blood* **103:**2771–2778.

11. Costello, R., D. Sainty, P. Lecine, A. Cusenier, M.-J. Mozziconacci, C. Arnoulet, D. Maraninchi, J.-A. Gastaut, J. Imbert, M. Lafage-Pochitaloff, and J. Gabert. 1997. Detection of CBFβ/MYH11 fusion transcripts in acute myeloid leukemia: heterogeneity of cytological and molecular characteristics. *Leukemia* **11:**644–650.

12. Degos, L. 2003. The history of acute promyelocytic leukemia. *Br. J. Haematol.* **122:**539–553.

13. Deininger, M., E. Buchdunger, and B. J. Druker. 2005. The development of imatinib as a therapeutic agent for chronic myeloid leukemia. *Blood* **105:**2640–2653.

14. Dewald, G. W. 2002. Interphase FISH studies for chronic myeloid leukemia, p. 311–342. *In* Y. S. Fan (ed.), *Methods in Molecular Biology*, vol. 204. *Molecular Cytogenetics: Protocols and Applications*. Humana Press, Totowa, N.J.

15. Dewald, G. W., S. R. Brockman, and S. F. Paternoster. 2004. Molecular cytogenetic studies for hematological malignancies, p. 69–112. *In* W. G. Finn and L. C. Peterson (ed.), *Hematopathology in Oncology*. Kluwer Academic Publications, Dordrecht, The Netherlands.

16. Döhner, H., S. Stilgenbauer, A. Benner, E. Leupolt, A. Kröber, L. Bullinger, K. Döhner, M. Bentz, and P. Lichter. 2000. Genomic aberrations and survival in chronic lymphocytic leukemia. *N. Engl. J. Med.* **343:**1910–1916.

17. Dombret, H., M. L. Scrobohaci, M. T. Daniel, J. M. Miclea, S. Castaigne, C. Chomienne, P. Fenaux, and L. Degos. 1995. In vivo thrombin and plasmin activities in patients with acute promyelocytic leukemia (APL): effect of all-trans retinoic acid (ATRA) therapy. *Leukemia* **9:**19–24.

18. Ferrando, A. A., D. S. Neuberg, J. Staunton, M. L. Loh, C. Huard, S. C. Raimondi, F. G. Behm, C. H. Pui, R. Downing, D. G. Gilliland, E. S. Lander, T. R. Golub, and A. T. Look. 2002. Gene expression signatures define novel oncogenic pathways in T cell acute lymphoblastic leukemia. *Cancer Cell* **1:**75–87.

19. Ferrando, A. A., D. S. Neuberg, R. K. Dodge, E. Paietta, R. A. Larson, P. H. Wiernik, J. M. Rowe, M. A. Caligiuri, C. D. Bloomfield, and A. T. Look. 2004. Prognostic importance of HOX11 oncogene expression in adults with T-cell acute lymphoblastic leukemia. *Lancet* **363:**535–536.

20. Ferrara, F., and L. Del Vecchio. 2002. Acute myeloid leukemia with t(8;21)/AML1/ETO: a distinct biological and clinical entity. *Haematologica* **87:**306–319.

21. Fine, B. M., M. Stanulla, M. Schrappe, M. Ho, S. Viehmann, J. Harbott, and L. M. Boxer. 2004. Gene expression patterns associated with recurrent chromosomal translocations in acute lymphoblastic leukemia. *Blood* **103:**1043–1049.

22. Gersen, S. L., and M. B. Keagle. 2005. *The Principles of Clinical Cytogenetics*. Humana Press, Totowa, N.J.

23. Gilliland, D. G., and M. S. Tallman. 2002. Focus on acute leukemias. *Cancer Cell* **1:**417–420.

24. Gökbuget, N., and D. Hoelzer. 2004. Treatment with monoclonal antibodies in acute lymphoblastic leukemia: current knowledge and future prospects. *Ann. Hematol.* **83:**201–205.

25. Gozzetti, A., and M. M. Le Beau. 2000. Fluorescence in situ hybridization: uses and limitations. *Semin. Hematol.* **37:**320–333.

26. Grimwade, D., S. V. Outram, R. Flora, S. J. Ings, A. R. Pizzey, R. Morilla, C. F. Craddock, D. C. Linch, and E. Solomon. 2002. The T-lineage-affiliated CD2 gene lies within an open chromatin environment in acute promyelocytic leukemia cells. *Cancer Res.* **62:**4730–4735.

27. Hölzer, D., and N. Gökbuget. 2003. Diagnosis and treatment of adult acute lymphoblastic leukemia, p. 273–305. *In* P. Wiernik, J. Dutcher, J. Goldman, and R. Kyle (ed.), *Neoplastic Diseases of the Blood*, 4th ed. Cambridge University Press, Cambridge, United Kingdom.

28. Hrušak, O., and A. Porwit-MacDonald. 2002. Antigen expression patterns reflecting genotypes of acute leukemias. *Leukemia* **16:**1233–1258.

29. Hubank, M. 2004. Gene expression profiling and its application in studies of hematological malignancy. *Br. J. Haematol.* **124:**577–594.

30. Huntly, B. J. P., A. Bench, and A. R. Green. 2003. Double jeopardy from a single translocation: deletions of the derivative chromosome 9 in chronic myeloid leukemia. *Blood* **102:**1160–1168.

31. Jaffe, E. S., N. L. Harris, H. Stein, and J. W. Vardiman. 2001. *Pathology and Genetics of Tumours of Haematopoietic and Lymphoid Tissues*. IARC Press, Lyon, France.

32. Jedema, I., R. M. Y. Barge, V. H. J. van der Velden, B. A. Nijmeijer, J. J. M. van Dongen, R. Willemze, and J. H. F. Falkenburg. 2004. Internalization and cell cycle-dependent killing of leukemic cells by Gemtuzumab Ozogamicin: rationale for efficacy in CD33-negative malignancies and endocytic capacity. *Leukemia* **18:**316–325.

33. Johnson, P. W. M., and M. J. Glennie. 2001. Rituximab: mechanisms and applications. *Br. J. Cancer* **85:**1619–1623.

34. Kelly, L. M., J. L. Kutok, I. R. Williams, C. L. Boulton, S. M. Amaral, D. P. Curley, T. J. Ley, and D. G. Gilliland. 2002. PML/RARα and FLT3-ITD induce an APL-like disease in a mouse model. *Proc. Natl. Acad. Sci. USA* **99:**8283–8288.

35. Kottaridis, P. D., R. E. Gale, and D. C. Linch. 2003. FLT3 mutations and leukemia. *Br. J. Haematol.* **122:**523–538.

36. Kurzrock, R., H. M. Kantarjian, B. J. Druker, and M. Talpaz. 2003. Philadelphia chromosome-positive leukemias: from basic mechanisms to molecular therapeutics. *Ann. Intern. Med.* **138:**819–830.

37. Kussick, S., D. L. Stirewalt, H. S. Yi, K. M. Sheets, E. Pogosova-Agadjanyan, S. Braswell, T. H. Norwood, J. P. Radich, and B. L. Wood. 2004. A distinctive nuclear morphology in acute myeloid leukemia is strongly associated with loss of HLA-DR expression and FLT3 internal tandem duplication. *Leukemia* **18:**1591–1598.

38. Larson, R. A., G. Q. Daley, C. A. Schiffer, P. Porcu, C.-H. Pui, J.-P. Marie, L. S. Steelman, F. E. Bertrand, and J. A. McCubrey. 2003. Treatment by design in leukemia, a meeting report, Philadelphia, Pennsylvania, December 2002. *Leukemia* **17:**2358–2382.

39. Laurent, E., M. Talpaz, H. Kantarjian, and R. Kurzrock. 2001. The BCR gene and Philadelphia chromosome-positive leukemogenesis. *Cancer Res.* **61:**2343–2355.

40. Licht, J. D. 2001. AML1 and the AML1-ETO fusion protein in the pathogenesis of t(8;21) AML. *Oncogene* **20:**5660–5679.

41. Lyman, S. D., and S. E. W. Jacobsen. 1988. C-kit ligand and Flt3 ligand: stem/progenitor cell factors with overlapping yet distinct activities. *Blood* **91:**1101–1134.

42. Mahadevan, D., and A. F. List. 2004. Targeting the multidrug resistance-1 transporter in AML: molecular regulation and therapeutic strategies. *Blood* **104:**1940–1951.

43. Mason, D., P. André, A. Bensussan, C. Buckley, C. Civin, E. Clark, M. de Haas, S. Goyert, M. Hadam, D. Hart, V. Hořejší, Y. Jones, S. Meuer, J. Morrissey, R. Schwartz-Albiez, S. Shaw, D. Simmons, L. Turni, M. Uguccioni, E. van der Schoot, E. Vivier, and H. Zola. 2001. *Leucocyte Typing VIII.* Oxford University Press, New York, N.Y.

44. Mavromatis, B., and B. D. Cheson. 2003. Monoclonal antibody therapy in chronic lymphocytic leukemia. *J. Clin. Oncol.* **21:**1874–1881.

45. Paietta, E. 2002. Assessing minimal residual disease (MRD) in leukemia: a changing definition and concept? *Bone Marrow Transplant.* **29:**459–465.

46. Paietta, E. 2003. Expression of cell surface antigens in APL, p. 369–385. *In* M. S. Tallman (ed.), *Bailliere's Best Practice and Research: Clinical Haematology,* vol. 16, no. 3. *Acute Promyelocytic Leukemia.* Harcourt Publishers Ltd., London, United Kingdom.

47. Paietta, E. 2003. How to optimize multiparameter flow cytometry for leukemia/lymphoma diagnosis, p. 671–683. *In* E. Paietta (ed.), *Bailliere's Best Practice and Research: Clinical Haematology,* vol. 16, no. 4. *Immunophenotyping in Leukemia and Lymphoma.* Harcourt Publishers Ltd., London, United Kingdom.

48. Paietta, E. 2003. Immunobiology of acute leukemia, p. 194–231. *In* P. Wiernik, J. Dutcher, J. Goldman, and R. Kyle (ed.), *Neoplastic Diseases of the Blood,* 4th ed. Cambridge University Press, Cambridge, United Kingdom.

49. Paietta, E., P. Bettelheim, J. D. Schwarzmeier, D. Lutz, O. Majdic, and W. Knapp. 1983. Distinct lymphoblastic and myeloblastic populations in TdT positive acute myeloblastic leukemia: evidence by double-fluorescence staining. *Leukemia Res.* **7:**301–307.

50. Paietta, E., J. Racevskis, J. M. Bennett, and P. H. Wiernik. 1993. Differential expression of terminal transferase (TdT) in acute lymphocytic leukemia expressing myeloid antigens and TdT positive acute myeloid leukemia as compared to myeloid antigen negative acute lymphocytic leukemia. *Br. J. Haematol.* **84:**416–422.

51. Paietta, E., J. Racevskis, D. Neuberg, J. M. Rowe, A. H. Goldstone, and P. H. Wiernik. 1997. Expression of CD25 (interleukin-2 receptor α chain) in adult acute lymphoblastic leukemia predicts for the presence of BCR/ABL fusion transcripts: results of a preliminary laboratory analysis of ECOG/MRC intergroup study E2993. *Leukemia* **11:**1887–1890.

52. Paietta, E., and P. Papenhausen. 2001. Cytogenetic alterations and related molecular consequences in adult leukemia, p. 161–190. *In* P. H. Wiernik (ed.), *American Cancer Society Atlas of Clinical Oncology: Adult Leukemias.* B. C. Decker Inc., Hamilton, Canada.

53. Paietta, E., D. Neuberg, J. M. Bennett, G. Dewald, J. M. Rowe, P. A. Cassileth, L. Cripe, M. S. Tallman, and P. H. Wiernik. 2003. Low expression of the myeloid differentiation antigen CD65s, a feature of poorly differentiated AML in older adults: study of 711 patients enrolled in ECOG trials. *Leukemia* **17:**1544–1550.

54. Paietta, E., O. Goloubeva, D. Neuberg, J. M. Bennett, R. Gallagher, J. Racevskis, G. Dewald, P. H. Wiernik, and M. S. Tallman. 2004. A surrogate marker profile for PML/RARα expressing acute promyelocytic leukemia and the association of immunophenotypic markers with morphologic and molecular subtypes. *Clin. Cytometry* **59B:**1–9.

55. Paietta, E., A. A. Ferrando, D. Neuberg, J. M. Bennett, J. Racevskis, H. Lazarus, G. Dewald, J. M. Rowe, P. H. Wiernik, M. S. Tallman, and A. T. Look. 2004. Activating *FLT3* mutations in CD117/KIT positive T-cell acute lymphoblastic leukemia. *Blood* **104:**558–560.

56. Pardanani, A., and A. Tefferi. 2004. Imatinib targets other than bcr/abl and their clinical relevance in myeloid disorders. *Blood* **104:**1931–1939.

57. Pitha-Rowe, I., W. J. Petty, S. Kitareewan, and E. Dmitrovsky. 2003. Retinoid target genes in acute promyelocytic leukemia. *Leukemia* **17:**1723–1730.

58. Puig-Kröger, A., T. Sánchez-Elsner, N. Ruiz, E. J. Andreu, F. Prosper, U. B. Jensen, J. Gil, P. Erickson, H. Drabkin, Y. Groner, and A. L. Corbi. 2003. RUNX/AML and C/EBP factors regulate CD11a integrin expression in myeloid cells through overlapping regulatory elements. *Blood* **102:**3252–3261.

59. Ravandi, F., M. Talpaz, and Z. Estrov. 2003. Modulation of cellular signaling pathways: prospects for targeted therapy in hematological malignancies. *Clin. Cancer Res.* **9:**535–550.

60. Redner, R. L. 2002. Variations on the theme: the alternate translocations in APL. *Leukemia* **16:**1927–1932.

61. Redner, R. L., and J. M. Liu. 2005. Leukemia fusion proteins and co-repressor complexes: changing paradigms. *J. Cell. Biochem.* **94:**864–869.

62. Ross, M. E., X. Zhou, G. Song, S. A. Shurtleff, K. Girtman, W. K. Williams, H.-C. Liu, R. Mahfouz, S. C. Raimondi, N. Lenny, A. Patel, and J. R. Downing. 2003. Classification of pediatric acute lymphoblastic leukemia by gene expression profiling. *Blood* **102:**2951–2959.

63. Sarriera, J. E., M. Albitar, Z. Estrov, C. Gidel, R. Aboul-Nasr, T. Manshouri, S. Kornblau, K.-S. Chang, H. Kantarjian, and E. Estey. 2001. Comparison of outcome in acute myelogenous leukemia patients with translocation (8;21) found by standard cytogenetic analysis and patients with AML1/ETO fusion transcript found only by PCR testing. *Leukemia* **15:**57–61.

64. Schoch, C., A. Kohlmann, S. Schnittger, B. Brors, M. Dugas, S. Mergenthaler, W. Kern, W. Hiddemann, R. Eils, and T. Haferlach. 2002. Acute myeloid leukemias with reciprocal rearrangements can be distinguished by specific gene expression profiles. *Proc. Natl. Acad. Sci. USA* **99:**10008–10013.

65. Sternberg, D. W., and D. G. Gilliland. 2004. The role of signal transducer and activator of transcription factors in leukemogenesis. *J. Clin. Oncol.* **22:**361–371.

66. Tallman, M. S. 2002. Monoclonal antibody therapies in leukemias. *Semin. Hematol.* **39:**12–19.

67. Tiacci, E., S. Pileri, A. Orleth, R. Pacini, A. Tabarrini, F. Frenguelli, A. Liso, D. Diverio, F. Lo Coco, and B. Falini. 2004. PAX5 expression in acute leukemias: higher B-lineage specificity than CD79a and selective association with t(8;21)-acute myelogenous leukemia. *Cancer Res.* **64:**7399–7404.

68. Tsutsumi, S., T. Taketani, K. Nishimura, X. Ge, T. Taki, K. Sugita, E. Ishii, R. Hanada, M. Ohki, H. Aburatani, and Y. Hayashi. 2003. Two distinct gene expression signatures in pediatric acute lymphoblastic leukemia with MLL rearrangements. *Cancer Res.* **63:**4882–4887.

69. Tuzuner, N. N., and J. M. Bennett. 2003. Classification of the acute leukemias: cytochemical and morphological considerations, p. 176–193. *In* P. Wiernik, J. Dutcher, J. Goldman, and R. Kyle (ed.), *Neoplastic Diseases of the Blood,* 4th ed. Cambridge University Press, Cambridge, United Kingdom.

70. Valk, P. J. M., R. G. W. Verhaak, M. A. Beijen, C. A. J. Erpelinck, S. Barjesteh van Waalwijk van Doorn-Khosrovani, J. M. Boer, H. B. Beverloo, M. M. Moorhouse, P. J. van der Spek, B. Löwenberg, and R. Delwel. 2004. Prognostically useful gene-expression profiles in acute myeloid leukemia. *N. Engl. J. Med.* **350:**1617–1628.

71. van der Velden, V. H. J., A. Hochhaus, G. Cazzaniga, T. Szczepanski, J. Gabert, and J. J. M. van Dongen. 2003. Detection of minimal residual disease in hematologic malignancies by real-time quantitative PCR: principles, approaches, and laboratory aspects. *Leukemia* **17:** 1013–1034.

72. Wilson, G. A., E. A. Vandenberghe, R. C. Pollitt, D. C. Rees, A. C. Goodeve, I. R. Peake, and J. T. Reilly. 2000. Are aberrant BCR-ABL transcripts more common than previously thought? *Br. J. Haematol.* **111:**1109–1111.

Multimeric Major Histocompatibility Complex Reagents for the Detection and Quantitation of Specific T-Cell Populations

JOHN D. ALTMAN

23

T cells play essential effector and regulatory roles in adaptive immune responses. Helper T cells expressing the CD4 coreceptor are required to support effective humoral immune memory—including generation of memory B cells and long-lived, antibody-secreting plasma cells, as well as antibody affinity maturation—and activation of pathways that allow macrophages to kill intracellular bacteria and parasites. Cytotoxic T cells expressing the CD8 coreceptor kill virus-infected cells as well as many tumors. In addition to their roles in pathogen clearance and tumor surveillance, both helper and cytotoxic T cells play roles in immunopathologies such as systemic and organ-specific autoimmunity, contact dermatitis, asthma, and atopy. All T cells express immunoglobulin-like antigen receptors that are the product of somatic gene rearrangements and that recognize peptides bound to major histocompatibility complex (MHC) molecules expressed on the antigen-presenting cell surface. The peptide ligands of MHC molecules are generated by proteolytic processing of proteins that are synthesized endogenously—such as tumor-associated or viral proteins—or outside the presenting cell and brought in through endocytic pathways. The endogenous pathway is largely associated with presentation on class I MHC molecules, which are recognized by CD8$^+$ T cells, while the exogenous pathway is associated with presentation on class II MHC molecules, which are recognized by CD4$^+$ T cells. In humans, the MHC molecules are also commonly referred to as HLA molecules, or human leukocyte antigens.

Efforts to manipulate T-cell responses for a preventative or therapeutic end—such as by inducing new antigen-specific T-cell populations through vaccination, or induction of tolerance in an existing autoreactive population of T cells—are predicated upon the ability to accurately measure quantitative and qualitative aspects of antigen-specific T-cell responses by using in vitro assays. For example, there are now several examples where clinical responses to tumor vaccines are significantly correlated with the magnitude of the induced T-cell response (14, 37), and recent efforts to develop preventative vaccines for human immunodeficiency virus (HIV) (23, 29), malaria (6), and tuberculosis (23, 35) have focused upon the induction of strong, pre-existing T-cell responses.

Through the mid-1990s, nearly all in vitro assays of antigen-specific T cells required moderate to extensive in vitro expansion of low-frequency populations of precursors in order to provide a population of cells large enough to measure in bulk assays such as the chromium release assay for cytotoxic T cells or the tritiated thymidine incorporation assay for T-cell proliferation (once the most common assay for helper T-cell function). For accurate measurements of T-cell immunity as it exists in vivo, the act of in vitro expansion creates at least two significant problems. First, the efficiency of the expansion is highly variable and therefore the results are semiquantitative at best. Second, the stimuli required for in vitro expansion of specific T cells unavoidably alter their phenotype, inducing changes in the patterns of cell surface molecules involved in crucial functions such as cell adhesion and trafficking, as well as potentially altering effector functions such as cytokine secretion profiles.

Starting in the mid-1990s, sensitive new assays have been developed that permit detection of antigen-specific T cells at the single-cell level, largely eliminating the requirement for in vitro expansion (34). These assays fall into two broad classes: functional and antigen binding. Functional assays at the single-cell level require short-term stimulation with antigen, generally for time periods between 4 and 24 h, during which proliferation is minimal, followed by detection of effector molecules—for example, cytokines (50), CD40L (10), or granule-associated transmembrane proteins such as CD107 (7)—using either flow cytometry (31, 54) or ELISpot assays (11, 28). In contrast, antigen-binding methods employ engineered multimers of soluble MHC/peptide complexes labeled with appropriate fluorophores that are used as if they were antibodies in flow cytometry or in situ staining of tissue sections (25). The engineered multimers come in at least three distinct flavors: (i) enzymatically biotinylated MHC/peptide complexes can be mixed with fluorescently labeled streptavidin to create MHC tetramers (3); (ii) the cDNA for an MHC protein can be genetically fused to an immunoglobulin G heavy chain of Fc domain to create MHC dimers (16); and (iii) MHC molecules can be fused to a self-assembling coiled-coil domain to create MHC pentamers.

The MHC tetramer version was the first to be described and has the largest publication record behind it. Identification of antigen-specific T cells by antigen-binding methods requires no assumptions with respect to the potential functions of the target cells. While this is sometimes a drawback, since T-cell effector functions are often the most relevant correlate to a particular disease state or to disease prevention, the antigen-binding methods can be combined with functional assays and often serve as the best measure of the total T-cell population specific for a defined MHC/peptide epitope. Antigen-binding methods provide two additional unique advantages: (i) they are the most direct method for assessing complex, multiparameter cell phenotypes by flow cytometry and (ii) they are the only practical method for detection of so-called dysfunctional cells, which often arise during chronic exposure to antigens such as tumors or persisting viruses such as HIV and hepatitis C virus. Although tetramers are the focus of this chapter, the other MHC multimers are apparently functionally equivalent. In addition, this chapter will focus on flow cytometry applications of tetramers, their most common use. Tissue staining with MHC tetramers has been demonstrated and promises to be very powerful as more examples appear (14, 17, 24, 33, 38, 39, 49), but it is beyond the scope of this chapter.

TECHNOLOGY AND INSTRUMENTATION FOR HLA TETRAMER ANALYSIS OF ANTIGEN-SPECIFIC T-CELL RESPONSES

Tetramer Reagents—Suppliers

The major commercial supplier of MHC tetramer reagents is the Immunomics division of Beckman Coulter, Inc. (http://www.immunomics.com), which sells them under the iTag trade name. The list of available reagents includes a number of HLA-A and -B class I alleles, several HLA-DR and -DP class II alleles, and a small selection of MHC alleles in other species such as the mouse and the rhesus macaque.

The National Institutes of Health (NIH) has also established a Tetramer Core Facility (http://www.niaid.nih.gov/reposit/tetramer/index.html) that prepares and distributes custom reagents to researchers throughout the world, focusing on reagents not available from Beckman Coulter. (The author of this chapter is the director of the NIH facility, which is located at Emory University in Atlanta, Ga.) The NIH facility currently offers a larger selection of alleles, especially for studies in nonhuman species, including a number of nonclassical MHC proteins such as HLA-E and CD1d. In addition, the NIH facility will prepare custom expression vectors for alleles that are not already available.

Tetramer Reagents—Expression

An extended discussion of the production of tetramer reagents is beyond the scope of this chapter. This section presents some key highlights and points to key references.

Classical class I MHC/peptide complexes are nearly always produced by in vitro folding of antigenic peptides together with denaturant-solubilized subunits expressed in *Escherichia coli* as inclusion bodies (2). In contrast, while *E. coli*-based in vitro folding methods work for some class II alleles, most alleles apparently cannot be produced this way. The reason for the strikingly different success rate for in vitro folding of class I and class II proteins is not well understood, but it may be related to the difference in quaternary structure of the peptide-binding groove, which in class I proteins is formed from a single chain but in class II proteins requires coming together of two separate protein chains. As a consequence, a variety of alternative eukaryotic expression systems for class II proteins have been developed, all providing correctly folded proteins secreted into culture supernatants. Many of these systems fuse complementary leucine

zipper motifs to the carboxy termini of the MHC protein chains in order to promote heterodimerization (22), and some employ covalent attachment of antigenic peptide ligands to the amino terminus of the class II β chain (27). Insect cell systems seem to be the most popular (40) and have been increasingly refined (15), but mammalian-based cell culture systems have also been described (13).

The nonclassical class I proteins are a heterogeneous group, and the expression systems used to produce them defy generalization. In vitro folding methods work well for proteins such as HLA-E, -F, and -G, some of which have known peptide ligands (1), but insect cell systems seem to be more efficient for molecules such as CD1d (32), which binds to glycolipids.

Variant Tetramer Reagents

The CD8 coreceptor is known to bind to a site in the α3 domain of class I MHC molecules, and therefore it is not surprising that the CD8 molecule itself contributes to class I tetramer binding to specific cells (21a). A number of investigators have taken advantage of this observation and have shown that mutant tetramers will bind to "high"- but not "low"-avidity populations of T cells (8, 9, 57); this approach may be particularly valuable for characterization of tumor-specific responses, where high-avidity T cells specific for the relevant tumor antigens may have been deleted during thymic development.

Fluorophores Used for Tetramers

By far the most popular fluorophore labels for MHC tetramers are the algae-derived phycobiliproteins R-phycoerythrin and allophycocyanin. Conjugates of these fluorescent proteins with streptavidin are widely available, and these fluorophores provide some of the best signal-to-noise ratios on most flow cytometers. The R-phycoerythrin label is excited by common argon lasers operating at 488 nm, while the allophycocyanin label requires a red laser operating between 633 and 647 nm. Tetramers labeled with other fluorophores have been described and are in fact required when tetramers are combined with some experimental protocols, such as flow–fluorescent in situ hybridization (Flow-FISH) methods for telomere-length determination (44).

Supporting Antibody Reagents

MHC tetramer stains are nearly always combined with an anti-CD3 antibody as well as either a CD8 antibody (for class I tetramers) or a CD4 antibody (for class II tetramers). These antibodies are widely available from multiple suppliers. There have been reports that some antibody clones specific for these molecules can inhibit tetramer binding (12, 21), probably through steric interference. It is worthwhile to examine several different antibody clones if interference is suspected.

MHC tetramer stains are also combined with a nearly infinite array of antibodies to obtain additional phenotypic information about the target population, such as the expression levels of a diverse array of cell surface markers such as CD62L (the lymph node homing receptor), CD28, CD45RA, CD27, or CCR7, or intracellular markers such as perforin, granzyme B, or Ki67. Tetramers can also be combined with reagents that assess T-cell function, such as cytokines produced after T-cell stimulation (5), though these protocols are often finicky due to down-regulation of surface T-cell receptors induced by stimulation.

Sample Requirements

HLA tetramer staining for flow cytometry can be performed using relevant single-cell suspensions from any source.

Whole blood and Ficoll gradient-purified peripheral blood mononuclear cells (PBMC) are the most common sample types from human subjects, but it is possible to perform tetramer staining on samples from tissue biopsies, including lymph nodes (47), tumors (52), liver (18), lung (51), and even lesions from delayed-type hypersensitivity reactions (14). HLA tetramer staining of in vitro expanded cultures, cell lines, and T-cell clones is also commonly used (40) and can be used to back-calculate precursor frequencies (40) when combined with the CFSE method for tracking cell division (30). (CFSE stands for carboxyfluorescein succinimidyl ester; though this is the common name, it is more appropriately called CFDA-SE, for carboxyfluorescein diacetate, succinimidyl ester.) This chapter focuses on methods employing whole blood and freshly isolated PBMC.

Any assay requiring a blood sample immediately raises questions of which of the three common anticoagulants—heparin, EDTA, or acid citrate dextrose—should be used for blood collection. In general, high-quality tetramer stains may be obtained when any of these anticoagulants are used, especially when the samples are stained less than 24 h after collection. When given a choice, my laboratory has a slight preference for EDTA.

The volume of blood or the number of cells required for the assay is dependent upon the frequency of the target cell population. When the target cell population exceeds 0.1% of the relevant T-cell subset (CD4$^+$ cells when using class II tetramers; CD8$^+$ cells when using class I tetramers), the assay can be performed on as little as 100 μl of whole blood or 10^6 PBMC; for detection of target cell populations in the range of 0.01 to 0.1%, up to 1 ml of blood or 5×10^6 PBMC can be used. In general, background noise limits reliable detection of cell populations below 0.01% of T cells, though extraordinarily skilled investigators working with especially clean samples and reagents can achieve reliable detection down to frequencies of 0.001%.

Additional sample aliquots are often used for negative controls and for setting instrument compensations. Negative control samples—for example, samples stained with an irrelevant control tetramer—should be the same size as the test samples. Sample aliquots for fluorescent compensation settings should be at least 100 μl of blood or 10^6 cells for each antibody used in the experiment. Note that the samples used for compensation settings need not be from the same individual as the test sample, and when sample sizes from an individual are limiting (such as in clinical trial samples), compensation samples should be set up with more easily obtained cells. Very recently, antibody capture beads have been introduced as an alternative for preparation of compensation samples (e.g., BD CompBeads; BD Biosciences, San Jose, Calif.), and cells are no longer required at all.

INSTRUMENT REQUIREMENTS

A flow cytometer with a minimum of three fluorescent channels is required for collection of data from HLA tetramer-stained cells. One channel is required for the tetramer, a second is required for an anti-CD3 antibody, and a third is required for an antibody specific for the coreceptor on the relevant target population—e.g., anti-CD4 when using class II tetramers and anti-CD8 when using class I tetramers. Most three-color instruments, such as the no-longer-available FACScan from BectonDickinson, use a single argon laser with a wavelength of 488 nm.

For the past 8 years, my lab has acquired most of its tetramer data on a four-color FACSCalibur instrument

from BDBiosciences. Most often, we use the additional channel to obtain additional phenotypic information about the target population, as noted above. Of course, on a four-color instrument, all of these phenotypic parameters must be analyzed one at a time in separately stained samples. Alternatively, the fourth channel could be used as an exclusion channel, where one or more reagents are used that are known to bind to cells other than the lineage of interest. For example, the iMASC Antibody Gating Kit for class I tetramers, from the Immunomics division of Beckman Coulter, contains antibodies specific for B cells (anti-CD19), granulocytes and monocytes (anti-CD13), and anti-CD4, all labeled with the same fluorophore (PC5). Exclusion gating can often reduce background noise and may permit more reliable analyses of low-frequency populations. Four-color instruments are available with a single argon laser such as the EPICS XL from Coulter, or with two lasers (an argon and a red diode laser) such as the FACSCalibur from BDBiosciences. When using tetramers labeled with the allophycocyanin dye, an instrument equipped with a red laser, operating near 635 nm, is required.

In the past several years, new so-called multicolor flow cytometers such as the LSR-II (BDBiosciences) and the Cyan from DakoCytomation (Fort Collins, Colo.) have been introduced that are capable of measuring up to 17 colors, depending upon the instrument configuration (42). The additional colors can be used for at least two distinct purposes: (i) they enable studies in which multiple cell phenotypes can be measured in the same sample, and (ii) they make it possible to include several distinct tetramers with distinct peptide epitopes (and maybe HLA alleles), each labeled with a separate fluorophore.

In addition to the flow cytometer, a variety of standard laboratory equipment—tabletop centrifuges, pipettes, vortex mixers, microscopes and hemacytometers, etc.—is required.

PROTOCOLS

Background on the General Protocol

The protocols used for standard MHC tetramer staining are identical in all essential details to those used for common antibody staining. As noted in "Sample Requirements," above, whole blood, PBMC, or other single-cell suspensions may be used. The notes in this chapter will focus on whole-blood stains; only simple and standard adaptations are required for other sample types.

Three of the most important parameters in MHC tetramer staining protocols are temperature, staining time, and reagent titer. Whole-blood stains are nearly always performed at room temperature. When PBMC are used, some groups have reported better results when staining at 37°C (55)—especially for class II tetramers (8a)—though excellent results may still be obtained at temperatures down to 4°C. Staining times should be optimized in each system, and they are in the range of 10 to 60 min; this parameter should certainly be standardized.

The optimal titer of a tetramer reagent should be determined in preliminary experiments, starting at a final tetramer concentration of about 25 μg/ml, and performing a two- or threefold dilution series. The optimal titer is often a compromise between the concentration required to achieve saturation and optimal separation from the "bulk" background population, and that required to minimize the frequency of "outlier" populations, which may be characterized as "noise," rather than background. In practice, the optimal titer often provides "baseline" but less than maximum separation between the positive and negative staining populations. Commercial reagents usually come with suggested titers, but these should be tested in each laboratory.

Appropriate controls for tetramer staining remain a surprisingly vexing issue, especially for work with human samples. T-cell lines or clones of an appropriate specificity often constitute a suitable positive control, but they are not always available, certainly not commercially. Cryopreserved PBMC from an individual previously shown to have cells that stain with a specific tetramer can be used; of course, these are not a renewable resource, though large numbers can be obtained by leukapheresis, though this is also not always convenient or possible. Barring either of these possibilities, the only practical approach requires omission of desired positive controls.

Negative controls are a more simple matter. It is possible to perform the equivalent of an isotype control by staining with an irrelevant tetramer composed of the same MHC allele, loaded with a peptide that the subject does not respond to. This is often less valuable than seems logical, as the control reagent could fail for a variety of reasons. Alternatively, it is possible to stain samples from an individual not previously exposed to the antigen of interest, either matched or mismatched at the HLA allele corresponding to the tetramer. In practice, when performing stains with whole blood samples that contain low to moderate frequencies of relevant antigen-specific cells, the sample itself contains abundant internal negative controls, and it is not necessary to perform additional negative control stains. This approach works quite well when the tetramer stain is very bright (as is often the case), but less well when the intensity of the tetramer-positive population is only moderately greater than the background on genuine nonspecific cells in the same sample. Finally, in some cases the most valuable control for tetramer staining is a sample stained with all of the reagents used in the test sample except for the tetramer itself. This sample, known as a "fluorescence-minus-one" or FMO control, allows for the most precise definition of cells that have fluorescence above background levels (45).

A General Tetramer Staining Protocol

The following steps constitute a general tetramer staining protocol. Individual details, such as the staining volumes, can be varied by knowledgeable investigators.

1. Prepare a 20× stock of a relevant tetramer in ice-cold fluorescence-activated cell sorter (FACS) buffer (2% fetal bovine serum plus 0.1% sodium azide in phosphate-buffered saline). See the notes above on determination of optimal titers.

2. Add 10 μl of the 20× tetramer stock to the bottom of a 12- by -75-mm FACS tube. Add additional antibody reagents as required or desired.

3. Add 200 μl of whole blood and vortex for 5 s.

4. Incubate at room temperature in the dark for 20 to 30 min.

5. Add 2 ml of 1× FACS Lyse solution (Becton Dickinson) and vortex thoroughly. Red blood cell lysis products from other suppliers may be used, but they should be carefully tested.

6. Incubate at room temperature for 10 min in the dark.

7. Pellet the cells by centrifugation for 5 min at $300 \times g$.

8. Carefully decant or aspirate the supernatant.

9. Disrupt the cell pellet by vortexing for 5 min.

10. Wash the cells.

a. Add 2 ml of ice-cold FACS buffer to the disrupted pellet.

b. Vortex for 5 s.

c. Pellet the cells by centrifugation for 5 min at $300 \times g$.

d. Carefully aspirate or decant the supernatant.

e. Disrupt the pellet by vortexing for 5 s.

11. Repeat step 10 to further reduce the number of outlier events.

12. Add 300 μl of Ultrapure 2% formaldehyde (diluted from a 10% stock obtained from PolySciences) in phosphate-buffered saline and vortex for 5 s.

13. Acquire the data on a flow cytometer within 24 h. Keep the samples protected from light as much as is practical before and during acquisition.

Compensation Controls

Basic protocols for fluorescence compensation controls have been described (46), and except for a few brief notes, the topic is beyond the scope of this chapter. Briefly, the same antibodies that are used in combination with the tetramers can be used as single stains for compensation controls, especially for lineage-specific markers such as CD3, CD4, or CD8. Usually, the low frequency of antigen-specific populations precludes practical use of the tetramer stain itself as a compensation control. Instead, as a compensation control for the tetramer stain, an antibody specific for a lineage-specific marker such as CD8 should be substituted. As noted in "Sample Requirements," above, the cells used for compensation controls need not come from the same individual as the test samples, and antibody capture beads can be substituted for cells. Capture beads for tetramers are not available, though in some cases the beads could be stained with an unlabeled anti-HLA antibody such as W6/32, followed by secondary staining with a tetramer.

Data Acquisition

The flow cytometer should be set up according to the manufacturer's recommendations and standard protocols, with particular attention paid to the setting of appropriate voltages on the photomultiplier tubes for each fluorescence channel. The appropriate protocol for setting up instrument compensation depends upon the available instrument and software. On analog instruments such as the FACSCalibur, the compensation setting must be adjusted manually before acquisition of data from test samples. In contrast, on new digital instruments such as the LSR-II or the FACSCanto, a data file (containing at least 20,000 relevant events) should be acquired for each of the compensation control samples, and the compensation matrix is then calculated by appropriate instrument software; in this case, uncompensated data are stored, and the compensation matrix can be applied either during or after acquisition.

Following instrument setup, data from the test samples are finally acquired. Since tetramers are usually used to detect low-frequency populations, it is often necessary to acquire a large number of events. For a typical sample, we attempt to acquire 100,000 to 200,000 lymphocyte-gated events, or more if the population frequency is below 0.05% of CD3$^+$ cells. Data are stored in industry-standard flow cytometry standard (FCS) format.

DATA ANALYSIS

The FCS-formatted data files from tetramer staining experiments can be analyzed by any of the common software packages, including those provided by the instrument manufacturers, or by third parties. We favor the FlowJo software package from TreeStar, Inc., but any package will do.

Standard approaches to gating are used when analyzing tetramer staining data. The steps for one very common approach—illustrated in Color Plate 1—are:

1. Plot FSC (forward scatter) versus SSC (side scatter) and set a gate around the lymphocyte-sized cell population.
2. For lymphocyte-gated cells, plot CD3 versus CD8 and set a gate on the CD3$^+$CD8$^+$ population.
3. For cells that are both lymphocyte sized and CD3$^+$CD8$^+$, plot the phenotypic parameter (CD11a in Color Plate 1) versus the tetramer stain (HLA-B7/EBV.RPP in Color Plate 1), and set a gate on the tetramer$^+$ population.

Color Plate 1 illustrates two different displays for the data; in panel A, the "pseudo-color dot plot" format is used, while in panel B, black and white contour plots are used, with the "show-outlier" option turned on for the final plot of CD11a versus tetramer. It is almost always necessary to use a data display that shows tetramer-stained cells as dots, since the frequency of the tetramer-positive population is usually below the 5% level required for the most common settings for contours in most flow cytometry data analysis software packages.

The final gate on the tetramer-positive cells in Color Plate 1 illustrates decisions that are typically made in the analysis of tetramer staining data. The gate is set on a tight cluster of cells that are all CD11a^{hi} and have nearly the same tetramer staining intensity. There are additional outlier events that appear to have tetramer staining intensity slightly above the main clusters of clearly tetramer-negative cells, but since these cells are not tightly clustered and are of lower intensity than the clearly tetramer-positive population, they have been omitted from the analysis.

The frequency of tetramer-positive cells should be reported as a fraction of the major lineage subset used to define them. In the example in Color Plate 1, this would be CD3$^+$CD8$^+$ lymphocytes. If it is necessary to omit either the CD3 or CD8 stain—for example, to accommodate an additional phenotypic marker—then the frequency should be reported as a fraction of either CD3$^+$ or CD8$^+$ cells.

When tetramer-positive data are phenotyped with two or more markers, the use of overlay plots can be very helpful in displaying the data. An example is shown in Color Plate 2, where the phenotype of the bulk CD8^{hi} population is shown in the orange "zebra-plot" format, while the tetramer-positive population is presented as an overlay of blue dots. The overlay plots allow the simultaneous display of two phenotypic parameters for tetramer-positive cells, but at the cost of losing the display of the intensity of the tetramer stain.

In all of the examples above, the relative frequency of tetramer-positive cells is reported with either CD3$^+$CD8$^+$ (Color Plate 1) or CD8^{hi} (Color Plate 2) cells in the denominator. In some cases, it may be more desirable to report absolute numbers of tetramer-positive cells per volume of blood, and single-platform methods for doing so have recently been introduced (19).

INTERPRETATION

The interpretation of tetramer staining data is as diverse as the different types of immune responses to which the technique is applied. When tetramers are used to analyze prophylactic vaccine experiments (48) or vaccine clinical trials, the interpretation of both the numbers and phenotypes of the detected antigen-specific cells is relatively straightforward: at some time between 1 and 2 weeks after vaccination, the frequency of tetramer-positive cells rises from an undetectable level to a peak, at which point the tetramer-positive cells often have a highly activated phenotype that is typical of effector T cells (e.g., CD38$^+$, HLA-DR$^+$, perforin$^+$, granzyme B$^+$, etc.). Over the next several weeks, the frequency of the tetramer-positive cells decreases and they lose their activated phenotype, especially if the antigen in the vaccine is completely cleared. Analysis of prophylactic vaccine responses is by far the simplest scenario.

When MHC tetramers are used to analyze T-cell responses to natural viral infections, at least five complications arise: (i) it is often impossible to establish the time of infection, so the kinetics of the response cannot be determined; (ii) many viruses chronically persist, either at a high level, such as HIV or hepatitis C virus, or in a latent form with periodic (and undetected) reactivation, such as with the herpesviruses cytomegalovirus and Epstein-Barr virus (EBV); (iii) chronic exposure to antigen can lead to deletion of specific T cells, functional inactivation, or T-cell-receptor down-regulation (58); (iv) for all viruses, especially those that do not persist, there is a significant likelihood of repeated exposure; and (v) in all cases, viral variants may arise that have epitopes that are closely related, but not identical, to those used in the tetramer (or those that were in the pathogen present during the primary immune response). These factors are also present for other infectious pathogens, such as *Mycobacterium tuberculosis*. As a consequence of all of these complications, early attempts to correlate disease states with some tetramer measurement—such as an inverse correlation of the frequency of HIV-specific CD8$^+$ T cells with HIV viral load (41) or an association of the failure of HIV-specific cells to clear HIV with a dysfunctional phenotype of tetramer-positive cells (4)—are now regarded with caution (53). Extended discussions of many of these complications are available in several excellent and recent reviews (26, 56).

Interpretation of data using tetramers to analyze tumor- and auto-antigen-specific cells is as complex as for persistent viruses, for many of the same reasons. The most serious complications are the difficulty in accounting for the effects of chronic antigen exposure, which may lead to functional inactivation or purging of the repertoire of high-affinity T cells specific for tumor antigens by induction of peripheral tolerance (36); in addition, the repertoire of tumor-specific cells is in many cases strongly influenced by a process of negative selection during thymic development (20). Only in the most favorable cases has it been possible to correlate data from tetramer staining experiments with clinical responses (14, 37).

Despite the difficulties noted above, antigen-binding methods for the identification of antigen-specific T cells promise to play an ever-expanding role in clinical immunology. Every year, more T-cell epitopes are mapped (43), which increases the range of responses to which the technique might be applied. In addition, immunotherapies that attempt to reactivate or alter the functional activities of antigen-specific cells will continue to rely upon tetramer staining methods to provide the crucial identification of the specific targets of potential therapies.

I thank Lily Wang and Adam Toenes for preparation of the HLA-B7/EBV.RPP tetramer, and Suzanne Mertens for the FACS data.

REFERENCES

1. **Allan, D. S., E. J. Lepin, V. M. Braud, C. A. O'Callaghan, and A. J. McMichael.** 2002. Tetrameric

complexes of HLA-E, HLA-F, and HLA-G. *J. Immunol. Methods* **268**:43–50.

2. **Altman, D., and M. Davis.** 2003. MHC-peptide tetramers to visualize antigen-specific T cells, p. 17.3.1–17.3.33. *In* E. Bierer et al. (ed.), *Current Protocols in Immunology*. John Wiley & Sons, Inc., New York, N.Y.

3. **Altman, J. D., P. A. Moss, P. J. Goulder, D. H. Barouch, M. G. McHeyzer-Williams, J. I. Bell, A. J. McMichael, and M. M. Davis.** 1996. Phenotypic analysis of antigen-specific T lymphocytes. *Science* **274**:94–96.

4. **Appay, V., D. F. Nixon, S. M. Donahoe, G. M. Gillespie, T. Dong, A. King, G. S. Ogg, H. M. Spiegel, C. Conlon, C. A. Spina, D. V. Havlir, D. D. Richman, A. Waters, P. Easterbrook, A. J. McMichael, and S. L. Rowland-Jones.** 2000. HIV-specific CD8(+) T cells produce antiviral cytokines but are impaired in cytolytic function. *J. Exp. Med.* **192**:63–75.

5. **Appay, V., and S. L. Rowland-Jones.** 2002. The assessment of antigen-specific CD8+ T cells through the combination of MHC class I tetramer and intracellular staining. *J. Immunol. Methods* **268**:9–19.

6. **Ballou, W. R., M. Arevalo-Herrera, D. Carucci, T. L. Richie, G. Corradin, C. Diggs, P. Druilhe, B. K. Giersing, A. Saul, D. G. Heppner, K. E. Kester, D. E. Lanar, J. Lyon, A. V. Hill, W. Pan, and J. D. Cohen.** 2004. Update on the clinical development of candidate malaria vaccines. *Am. J. Trop. Med. Hyg.* **71**:239–247.

7. **Betts, M. R., J. M. Brenchley, D. A. Price, S. C. De Rosa, D. C. Douek, M. Roederer, and R. A. Koup.** 2003. Sensitive and viable identification of antigen-specific CD8+ T cells by a flow cytometric assay for degranulation. *J. Immunol. Methods* **281**:65–78.

8. **Bodinier, M., M. A. Peyrat, C. Tournay, F. Davodeau, F. Romagne, M. Bonneville, and F. Lang.** 2000. Efficient detection and immunomagnetic sorting of specific T cells using multimers of MHC class I and peptide with reduced CD8 binding. *Nat. Med.* **6**:707–710.

8a. **Cameron, T. O., P. J. Norris, A. Patel, C. Moulon, E. S. Rosenberg, E. D. Mellins, L. R. Wedderburn, and L. J. Stern.** 2002. Labeling antigen-specific CD4(+) T cells with class II MHC oligomers. *J. Immunol. Methods* **268**:51–69.

9. **Choi, E. M.-L., J.-L. Chen, L. Wooldridge, M. Salio, A. Lissina, N. Lissin, I. F. Hermans, J. D. Silk, F. Mirza, M. J. Palmowski, P. R. Dunbar, B. K. Jakobsen, A. K. Sewell, and V. Cerundolo.** 2003. High avidity antigen-specific CTL identified by CD8-independent tetramer staining. *J. Immunol.* **171**:5116–5123.

10. **Cohen, G. B., A. Kaur, and R. P. Johnson.** 2005. Isolation of viable antigen-specific CD4 T cells by CD40L surface trapping. *J. Immunol. Methods* **302**:103–115.

11. **Czerkinsky, C., G. Andersson, H. P. Ekre, L. A. Nilsson, L. Klareskog, and O. Ouchterlony.** 1988. Reverse ELISPOT assay for clonal analysis of cytokine production. I. Enumeration of gamma-interferon-secreting cells. *J. Immunol. Methods* **110**:29–36.

12. **Daniels, M. A., and S. C. Jameson.** 2000. Critical role for CD8 in T cell receptor binding and activation by peptide/major histocompatibility complex multimers. *J. Exp. Med.* **191**:335–346.

13. **Day, C. L., N. P. Seth, M. Lucas, H. Appel, L. Gauthier, G. M. Lauer, G. K. Robbins, Z. M. Szczepiorkowski, D. R. Casson, R. T. Chung, S. Bell, G. Harcourt, B. D. Walker, P. Klenerman, and K. W. Wucherpfennig.** 2003. Ex vivo analysis of human memory CD4 T cells specific for hepatitis C virus using MHC class II tetramers. *J. Clin. Investig.* **112**:831–842.

14. **de Vries, I. J., M. R. Bernsen, W. J. Lesterhuis, N. M. Scharenborg, S. P. Strijk, M.-J. Gerritsen, D. J. Ruiter, C. G. Figdor, C. J. Punt, and G. J. Adema.** 2005. Immunomonitoring tumor-specific T cells in delayed-type hypersensitivity skin biopsies after dendritic cell vaccination correlates with clinical outcome. *J. Clin. Oncol.* **23**:5779–5787.

15. **Fourneau, J. M., H. Cohen, and P. M. van Endert.** 2004. A chaperone-assisted high yield system for the production of HLA-DR4 tetramers in insect cells. *J. Immunol. Methods* **285**:253–264.

16. **Greten, T. F., J. E. Slansky, R. Kubota, S. S. Soldan, E. M. Jaffee, T. P. Leist, D. M. Pardoll, S. Jacobson, and J. P. Schneck.** 1998. Direct visualization of antigen-specific T cells: HTLV-1 Tax11-19-specific CD8(+) T cells are activated in peripheral blood and accumulate in cerebrospinal fluid from HAM/TSP patients. *Proc. Natl. Acad. Sci. USA* **95**:7568–7573.

17. **Haanen, J. B., M. G. van Oijen, F. Tirion, L. C. Oomen, A. M. Kruisbeek, F. A. Vyth-Dreese, and T. N. Schumacher.** 2000. In situ detection of virus- and tumor-specific T-cell immunity. *Nat. Med.* **6**:1056–1060.

18. **He, X. S., B. Rehermann, F. X. López-Labrador, J. Boisvert, R. Cheung, J. Mumm, H. Wedemeyer, M. Berenguer, T. L. Wright, M. M. Davis, and H. B. Greenberg.** 1999. Quantitative analysis of hepatitis C virus-specific CD8(+) T cells in peripheral blood and liver using peptide-MHC tetramers. *Proc. Natl. Acad. Sci. USA* **96**:5692–5697.

19. **Heijnen, I. A., D. Barnett, M. J. Arroz, S. M. Barry, M. Bonneville, B. Brando, J. L. D'hautcourt, F. Kern, T. H. Tötterman, E. W. Marijt, D. Bossy, F. W. Preijers, G. Rothe, J. W. Gratama, and the European Working Group on Clinical Cell Analysis.** 2004. Enumeration of antigen-specific CD8+ T lymphocytes by single-platform, HLA tetramer-based flow cytometry: a European multicenter evaluation. *Cytometry B Clin. Cytom.* **62**:1–13.

20. **Hernández, J., P. P. Lee, M. M. Davis, and L. A. Sherman.** 2000. The use of HLA A2.1/p53 peptide tetramers to visualize the impact of self tolerance on the TCR repertoire. *J. Immunol.* **164**:596–602.

21. **Hoffmann, T. K., V. S. Donnenberg, U. Friebe-Hoffmann, E. M. Meyer, C. R. Rinaldo, A. B. DeLeo, T. L. Whiteside, and A. D. Donnenberg.** 2000. Competition of peptide-MHC class I tetrameric complexes with anti-CD3 provides evidence for specificity of peptide binding to the TCR complex. *Cytometry* **41**:321–328.

21a. **Holman, P. O., E. R. Walsh, and S. C. Jameson.** 2005. Characterizing the impact of CD8 antibodies on class I MHC multimer binding. *J. Immunol.* **174**:3986–3991.

22. **Kalandadze, A., M. Galleno, L. Foncerrada, J. L. Strominger, and K. W. Wucherpfennig.** 1996. Expression of recombinant HLA-DR2 molecules. Replacement of the hydrophobic transmembrane region by a leucine zipper dimerization motif allows the assembly and secretion of soluble DR alpha beta heterodimers. *J. Biol. Chem.* **271**: 20156–20162.

23. **Kaufmann, S. H., and A. J. McMichael.** 2005. Annulling a dangerous liaison: vaccination strategies against AIDS and tuberculosis. *Nat. Med.* **11**:S33–44.

24. **Kita, H., X. S. He, and M. E. Gershwin.** 2003. Application of tetramer technology in studies on autoimmune diseases. *Autoimmun. Rev.* **2**:43–49.

25. **Klenerman, P., V. Cerundolo, and P. R. Dunbar.** 2002. Tracking T cells with tetramers: new tales from new tools. *Nat. Rev. Immunol.* **2**:263–272.

26. **Klenerman, P., and A. Hill.** 2005. T cells and viral persistence: lessons from diverse infections. *Nat. Immunol.* **6**:873–879.

27. **Kozono, H., J. White, J. Clements, P. Marrack, and J. Kappler.** 1994. Production of soluble MHC class II proteins with covalently bound single peptides. *Nature* **369**:151–154.

28. Lalvani, A., R. Brookes, S. Hambleton, W. J. Britton, A. V. Hill, and A. J. McMichael. 1997. Rapid effector function in CD8+ memory T cells. *J. Exp. Med.* **186:**859–865.

29. Letvin, N. L. 2005. Progress toward an HIV vaccine. *Annu. Rev. Med.* **56:**213–223.

30. Lyons, A. B., J. Hasbold, and P. D. Hodgkin. 2001. Flow cytometric analysis of cell division history using dilution of carboxyfluorescein diacetate succinimidyl ester, a stably integrated fluorescent probe. *Methods Cell. Biol.* **63:** 375–398.

31. Maino, V. C., and H. T. Maecker. 2004. Cytokine flow cytometry: a multiparametric approach for assessing cellular immune responses to viral antigens. *Clin. Immunol.* **110:**222–231.

32. Matsuda, J. L., O. V. Naidenko, L. Gapin, T. Nakayama, M. Taniguchi, C.-R. Wang, Y. Koezuka, and M. Kronenberg. 2000. Tracking the response of natural killer T cells to a glycolipid antigen using CD1d tetramers. *J. Exp. Med.* **192:**741–754.

33. McGavern, D. B., U. Christen, and M. B. Oldstone. 2002. Molecular anatomy of antigen-specific CD8(+) T cell engagement and synapse formation in vivo. *Nat. Immunol.* **3:**918–925.

34. McMichael, A. J., and C. A. O'Callaghan. 1998. A new look at T cells. *J. Exp. Med.* **187:**1367–1371.

35. McShane, H., A. A. Pathan, C. R. Sander, S. M. Keating, S. C. Gilbert, K. Huygen, H. A. Fletcher, and A. V. Hill. 2004. Recombinant modified vaccinia virus Ankara expressing antigen 85A boosts BCG-primed and naturally acquired antimycobacterial immunity in humans. *Nat. Med.* **10:**1240–1244.

36. Molldrem, J. J., P. P. Lee, S. Kant, E. Wieder, W. Jiang, S. Lu, C. Wang, and M. M. Davis. 2003. Chronic myelogenous leukemia shapes host immunity by selective deletion of high-avidity leukemia-specific T cells. *J. Clin. Invest.* **111:**639–647.

37. Molldrem, J. J., P. P. Lee, C. Wang, K. Felio, H. M. Kantarjian, R. E. Champlin, and M. M. Davis. 2000. Evidence that specific T lymphocytes may participate in the elimination of chronic myelogenous leukemia. *Nat. Med.* **6:**1018–1023.

38. Moore, A., J. Grimm, B. Han, and P. Santamaria. 2004. Tracking the recruitment of diabetogenic CD8+ T-cells to the pancreas in real time. *Diabetes* **53:**1459–1466.

39. Muraro, P. A., K.-P. Wandinger, B. Bielekova, B. Gran, A. Marques, U. Utz, H. F. McFarland, S. Jacobson, and R. Martin. 2002. Molecular tracking of antigen-specific T cell clones in neurological immune-mediated disorders. *Brain* **126:**20–31.

40. Novak, E. J., A. W. Liu, G. T. Nepom, and W. W. Kwok. 1999. MHC class II tetramers identify peptide-specific human CD4(+) T cells proliferating in response to influenza A antigen. *J. Clin. Investig.* **104:**R63–R67.

41. Ogg, G. S., X. Jin, S. Bonhoeffer, P. R. Dunbar, M. A. Nowak, S. Monard, J. P. Segal, Y. Cao, S. L. Rowland-Jones, V. Cerundolo, A. Hurley, M. Markowitz, D. D. Ho, D. F. Nixon, and A. J. McMichael. 1998. Quantitation of HIV-1-specific cytotoxic T lymphocytes and plasma load of viral RNA. *Science* **279:**2103–2106.

42. Perfetto, S. P., P. K. Chattopadhyay, and M. Roederer. 2004. Seventeen-colour flow cytometry: unravelling the immune system. *Nat. Rev. Immunol.* **4:**648–655.

43. Peters, B., J. Sidney, P. Bourne, H. H. Bui, S. Buus, G. Doh, W. Fleri, M. Kronenberg, R. Kubo, O. Lund, D. Nemazee, J. V. Ponomarenko, M. Sathiamurthy, S. P. Schoenberger, S. Stewart, P. Surko, S. Way, S. Wilson, and A. Sette. 2005. The design and implementation of the immune epitope database and analysis resource. *Immunogenetics* **57:**326–336.

44. Plunkett, F. J., M. V. D. Soares, N. Annels, A. Hislop, K. Ivory, M. Lowdell, M. Salmon, A. Rickinson, and A. N. Akbar. 2001. The flow cytometric analysis of telomere length in antigen-specific CD8+ T cells during acute Epstein-Barr virus infection. *Blood* **97:**700–707.

45. Roederer, M. 2001. Spectral compensation for flow cytometry: visualization artifacts, limitations, and caveats. *Cytometry* **45:**194–205.

46. Roederer, M. 2002. Compensation in flow cytometry, p. 1.14.1–1.14.20. *In* J. P. Robinson et al. (ed.), *Current Protocols in Cytometry.* John Wiley & Sons, New York, N.Y.

47. Romero, P., P. R. Dunbar, D. Valmori, M. Pittet, G. S. Ogg, D. Rimoldi, J.-L. Chen, D. Lienard, J.-C. Cerottini, and V. Cerundolo. 1998. Ex vivo staining of metastatic lymph nodes by class I major histocompatibility complex tetramers reveals high numbers of antigen-experienced tumor-specific cytolytic T lymphocytes. *J. Exp. Med.* **188:**1641–1650.

48. Seth, A., I. Ourmanov, M. J. Kuroda, J. E. Schmitz, M. W. Carroll, L. S. Wyatt, B. Moss, M. A. Forman, V. M. Hirsch, and N. L. Letvin. 1998. Recombinant modified vaccinia virus Ankara-simian immunodeficiency virus gag pol elicits cytotoxic T lymphocytes in rhesus monkeys detected by a major histocompatibility complex class I/peptide tetramer. *Proc. Natl. Acad. Sci. USA* **95:**10112–10116.

49. Skinner, P. J., M. A. Daniels, C. S. Schmidt, S. C. Jameson, and A. T. Haase. 2000. Cutting edge: in situ tetramer staining of antigen-specific T cells in tissues. *J. Immunol.* **165:**613–617.

50. Suni, M. A., V. C. Maino, and H. T. Maecker. 2005. Ex vivo analysis of T-cell function. *Curr. Opin. Immunol.* **17:**434–440.

51. Tully, G., C. Kortsik, H. Höhn, I. Zehbe, W. E. Hitzler, C. Neukirch, K. Freitag, K. Kayser, and M. J. Maeurer. 2005. Highly focused T cell responses in latent human pulmonary *Mycobacterium tuberculosis* infection. *J. Immunol.* **174:**2174–2184.

52. Valmori, D., V. Dutoit, D. Liénard, D. Rimoldi, M. J. Pittet, P. Champagne, K. Ellefsen, U. Sahin, D. Speiser, F. Lejeune, J. C. Cerottini, and P. Romero. 2000. Naturally occurring human lymphocyte antigen-A2 restricted CD8+ T-cell response to the cancer testis antigen NY-ESO-1 in melanoma patients. *Cancer Res.* **60:**4499–4506.

53. van Lier, R. A., I. J. ten Berge, and L. E. Gamadia. 2003. Human CD8(+) T-cell differentiation in response to viruses. *Nat. Rev. Immunol.* **3:**931–939.

54. Waldrop, S. L., C. J. Pitcher, D. M. Peterson, V. C. Maino, and L. J. Picker. 1997. Determination of antigen-specific memory/effector CD4+ T cell frequencies by flow cytometry: evidence for a novel, antigen-specific homeostatic mechanism in HIV-associated immunodeficiency. *J. Clin. Investig.* **99:**1739–1750.

55. Whelan, J. A., P. R. Dunbar, D. A. Price, M. A. Purbhoo, F. Lechner, G. S. Ogg, G. Griffiths, R. E. Phillips, V. Cerundolo, and A. K. Sewell. 1999. Specificity of CTL interactions with peptide-MHC class I tetrameric complexes is temperature dependent. *J. Immunol.* **163:**4342–4348.

56. Wherry, E. J., and R. Ahmed. 2004. Memory CD8 T-cell differentiation during viral infection. *J. Virol.* **78:**5535–5545.

57. Wooldridge, L., H. A. van den Berg, M. Glick, E. Gostick, B. Laugel, S. L. Hutchinson, A. Milicic, J. M. Brenchley, D. C. Douek, D. A. Price, and A. K. Sewell. 2005. Interaction between the CD8 coreceptor and major histocompatibility complex class I stabilizes T cell receptor-antigen complexes at the cell surface. *J. Biol. Chem.* **280:**27491–27501.

58. Zajac, A. J., J. N. Blattman, K. Murali-Krishna, D. J. D. Sourdive, M. Suresh, J. D. Altman, and R. Ahmed. 1998. Viral immune evasion due to persistence of activated T cells without effector function. *J. Exp. Med.* **188:**2205–2213.

In Situ Gene Amplification and Hybridization Assays: Disease Monitoring Applications Using Flow Cytometry

BRUCE K. PATTERSON

24

Since the discovery of PCR, the diagnostic field has followed the pathway of taking tissues (plasma, blood, and tissue biopsy samples), preparing nucleic acids (DNA, RNA, or total), and amplifying genes of interest. Lost in the process are the characteristics of the cells from which these genes originated. The loss of this important information has profound implications in the areas of infectious diseases and oncology. The ideal situation in diagnostics would be if one could in a sensitive and specific manner detect certain disease-causing genes, including infectious agents, without destroying the cells. Maintaining the integrity of the cells not only allows one to assess the characteristics of a cell expressing a particular disease-causing gene (e.g., human papillomavirus [HPV] E6 or E7 mRNA expression in a dysplastic or cancerous squamous epithelial cell) but also allows one to enrich for rare cells of interest using antibodies in a multiparameter approach, for example. From a diagnostic perspective, the detection of genes and proteins within a cell would need to be high throughput on a user-friendly platform capable of an expanded menu. All of the aforementioned attributes of an extremely powerful molecular diagnostics platform reside in flow cytometry. In the following sections, I describe multiple approaches of performing molecular biology in a cell. Most importantly, I also describe how to use these assays to gain a better understanding of disease processes and ultimately how these assays can be adopted in clinical laboratories to provide the most comprehensive information on response to a variety of therapies.

MOLECULAR BIOLOGY IN THE CELL: ACCESSING THE TARGET WITHIN

Intracellular detection of nucleic acids, proteins, and phosphoepitopes is performed in research laboratories using a variety of different agents to gain access into the cell while preserving the integrity of the cell. Ideally, these agents should preserve the target of choice, such as DNA, RNA, or proteins, including those subject to phosphorylation. Many of the current fixation and permeabilization reagents fail to preserve all of these macromolecules though they perform well for a particular application. Though consideration of all the best attributes of cell fixation extends beyond the scope of this chapter and they are covered more completely in other reviews (27), a fixative called

PermiFlow approaches the ideal fixative described above. This reagent preserves cell surface and intracellular antigenicity, while maintaining the integrity of DNA and RNA and the phosphorylation state of phosphoepitopes. This fixative is used in many of the applications described herein. In summary, maintenance of the target of interest and protocol simplicity is critical in the clinical application of in situ methodology.

Procedure

Collect a 10-ml venous blood sample aseptically by venipuncture using standard procedures. One hundred microliters of sample per test is required when performing analysis using whole blood. Blood samples should not be refrigerated. For testing using a peripheral blood mononuclear cell (PBMC) preparation derived by differential density centrifugation, 10 ml of whole blood is sufficient for approximately 20 analyses. Centrifuge the 10-ml blood sample at $300 \times g$ for 10 min at room temperature ($25 \pm 5°C$). Discard the plasma layer, which will appear cloudy due to the presence of platelets. Transfer the buffy coat layer (1 to 1.5 ml per 10 ml of whole blood) with a Pasteur pipette to a disposable test tube (10-ml volume). Bring to a volume of 7 ml with room temperature $1\times$ phosphate-buffered saline (PBS). Mix well and transfer to a 15-ml conical centrifuge tube. Underlay 3 to 5 ml of Ficoll-Paque to the cell suspension in the conical centrifuge tube. Do not disturb the interface between the sample and the Ficoll-Paque. Centrifuge at $400 \times g$ for 30 min at room temperature. Mononuclear cells should form a visible, clean interface between the plasma and the Ficoll-Paque. Within 5 min of centrifugation, collect the mononuclear cells from the PBS–Ficoll-Paque interface with a Pasteur pipette and transfer to a 15-ml conical centrifuge tube. Resuspend the mononuclear cells in a 10-ml conical centrifuge at $400 \times g$ for 5 min at room temperature. Aspirate carefully and remove the supernatant. Repeat once. Resuspend the mononuclear cells in 2 ml of $1\times$ PBS and determine the cell number with a hemocytometer or an automated cell counter. Adjust the mononuclear cell density to 5×10^6 cells/ml in $1\times$ PBS. Deliver 10 µl (or typical volume for the reagent in use) of antibody specific for markers expressed on the cell surface to the bottom of each appropriately labeled test tube, except the control tube. Add the appropriate volume of isotype-matched control antibody to the control tube.

Note: Most cell surface-expressed antigens remain immunoreactive after treatment with PermiFlow (Invirion, Inc., Frankfort, Mich.). Therefore, in some instances it may be appropriate to first treat the cells with PermiFlow, wash with wash buffer (1× PBS, pH 7.4), and then incubate simultaneously with antibodies to cell surface and intracellular antigens. Add 100 µl of a single-cell suspension (5 × 10⁶ cells/ml in 1× PBS, pH 7.4) to each tube and vortex gently. Incubate for 20 min at room temperature. Collect the cells by centrifugation at 400 × g for 5 min at room temperature and aspirate the supernatant. Add 0.5 ml of 1× PermiFlow directly to each tube, vortex, and incubate for 40 min at room temperature. Note: For in situ hybridization or in situ PCR, incubate for 1 to 18 h (see procedures below). Collect the cells by centrifugation at 400 × g for 5 min at room temperature and aspirate the supernatant. Resuspend the cell pellet in 1.0 ml of 1× PBS, pH 7.4. Centrifuge at 400 × g for 5 min at room temperature and discard the supernatant. Deliver 10 µl (or typical volume for the reagent in use) of antibody specific for intracellular antigens to the bottom of each appropriately labeled test tube, except the control tube. Add the appropriate volume of isotype-matched control antibody to the control tube. Vortex gently and incubate for 40 min at room temperature. Wash the cells with wash buffer and centrifuge. Resuspend the cells in 1.0 ml of 1× PBS, pH 7.4, and analyze by flow cytometry according to the manufacturer's instructions.

Clinical Considerations

Clinical Utility of In Situ Gene Detection: The Virology Model

Viruses can be categorized as RNA or DNA, and since they infect cells, the viral diagnostics area is a true test of molecular diagnostics. To date, the majority of diagnostic tests consist of detection of virus in plasma or lysed cells by solution-based amplification assays such as PCR, transcription-mediated amplification, strand displacement amplification, branched DNA (bDNA), or nucleic acid-based sequence amplification. The power of being able to detect DNA or RNA in cells is illustrated in Fig. 1 using human immunodeficiency virus type 1 (HIV-1) as a diagnostic model system. In HIV-1-infected individuals, T lymphocytes can be free of virus (Fig. 1, far left), be defectively infected (DNA⁺, RNA⁻) and incapable of producing virus (Fig. 1, second from left), be latently infected (DNA⁺, RNA⁻), and replication competent (Fig. 1, second from right), or be productively infected (DNA⁺, RNA⁺), producing viral particles (Fig. 1, far right). Eradication of HIV-1, which was thought to be possible early in the epidemic, would involve clearing the virus and virally infected cells from individuals, thus producing an overall loss of DNA-containing cells (long arrow). Eradication of DNA-containing cells could be monitored using an in situ amplification assay such as real-time PCR in situ, as is discussed below. Presently, however, antiretroviral therapy actually produces a latent-like phenotype in cells;

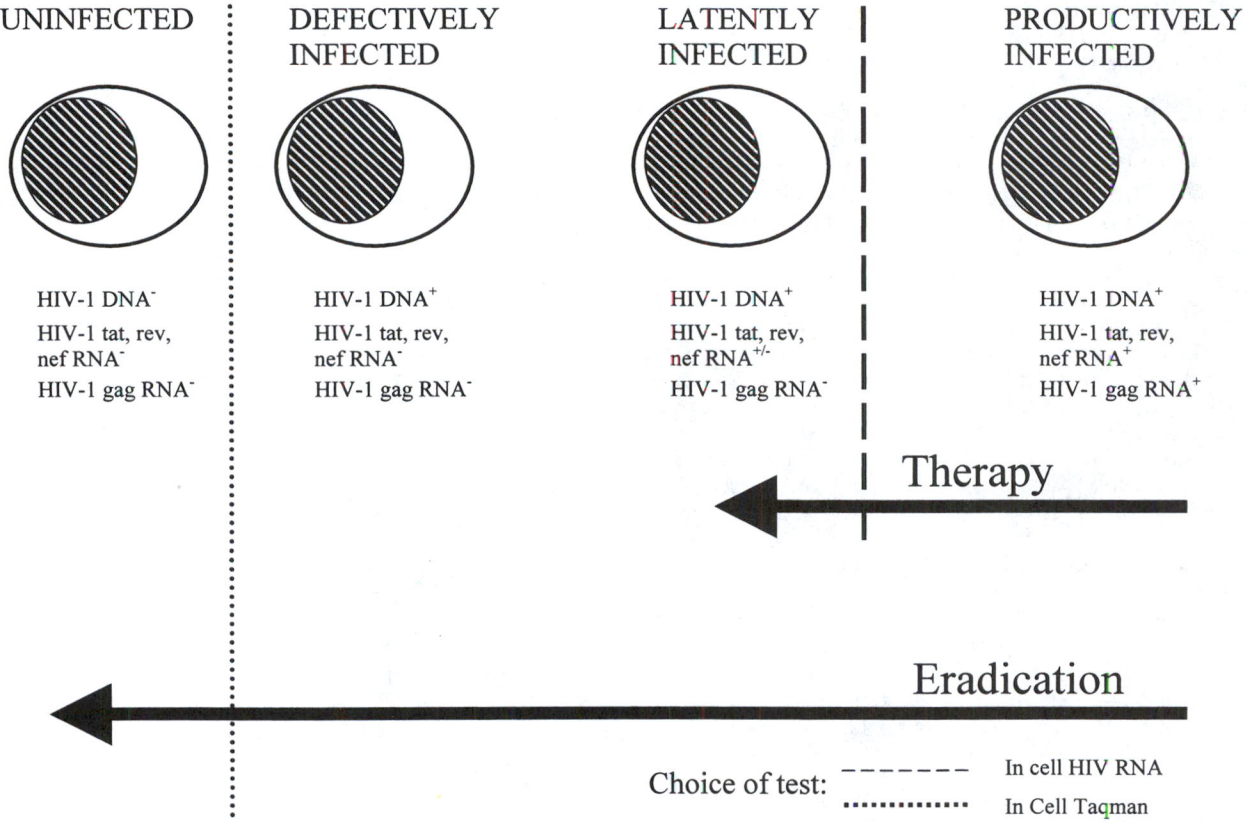

FIGURE 1 Schematic of the HIV-1 life cycle in T lymphocytes and the ideal tests to determine the response to therapy.

that is, cells contain HIV-1 DNA but do not express HIV-1 RNA. The preferred assay in this instance would be one that can monitor production of HIV-1 RNA in cells, given that cells containing HIV-1 DNA will remain relatively stable throughout the course of disease.

AMPLIFICATION TECHNIQUES PRIOR TO IN SITU HYBRIDIZATION

Detection of single-copy DNA and low-abundance mRNA was greatly facilitated in the cell with the advent of in situ PCR soon after the discovery of PCR and the thermal stable polymerase from *Thermus aquaticus* (*Taq* polymerase) (4, 10, 16, 17, 19, 25, 34, 37, 41). The powerful combination of single-copy detection in cells combined with the high-throughput cellular analysis platform of flow cytometry led to the elucidation that HIV-1 infected enough cells to account for the severe immune destruction leading to AIDS (10, 34). This assay was used clinically in several studies monitoring changes in HIV-1 DNA-containing cells during therapy (12, 28, 30, 37). Subsequent work described the combination of cell surface immunophenotyping and in situ PCR by flow cytometry and ultimately real-time PCR (TaqMan) in situ and flow cytometry (30, 31). As opposed to the simpler and quantitative fluorescence in situ hybridization, in situ PCR using flow cytometry still awaits a compelling diagnostic application. Further, HIV/AIDS treatment strategies have yet to reduce the HIV-1 DNA burden in patients, though reducing replication and viral load is now a routine goal of antiretroviral therapy.

Other in situ amplification strategies exist and fall into three categories: target amplification, signal amplification, and signal generation (27, 36). Although these technologies have been generally used for slide-based analyses, adaptation to flow cytometry could also be performed.

3SR In Situ

Self-sustained sequence replication (3SR) is an isothermal amplification strategy that exploits the activities of three enzymes in the reaction mixture. In situ 3SR (IS-3SR) is based on the use of primers with attached RNA polymerase initiation sites and the combination of three different enzymes in the same reaction mixture (DNA polymerase, RNase H, and RNA polymerase), resulting in accumulation of target mRNA through the combination of reverse transcription, DNA synthesis, and in vitro transcription (18). IS-3SR assay shows significantly less amplification efficiency than in situ PCR. So far, IS-3SR has only successfully been applied to cells in suspension and not to tissue sections.

In situ transcription and oligonucleotide-primed in situ labeling (PRINS) are methods used for the detection of mRNA involving the use of an mRNA-complementary primer, reverse transcription, and labeled nucleotides to produce labeled cDNA within a cell (43). However, similarly to the 3SR reaction, potential mispriming or nonspecific incorporation of labeled nucleotides may yield nonspecific results or increased background staining, although probably at a significantly lower level than in techniques applying DNA polymerase enzymes. In situ transcription has so far not found broad acceptance in the field of in situ detection of mRNA.

bDNA In Situ

bDNA technology has been used extensively to measure nucleic acids in serum, plasma, or digested cells and has recently been adapted for the in situ detection of DNA or RNA. The bDNA in situ hybridization method to detect nucleic acids is a signal amplification technology, as mentioned previously, rather than a target amplification like in situ PCR or IS-3SR (35). mRNA and DNA can be detected with similar sets of probes, with the only difference being the requirement for denaturation if the target of interest is double-stranded DNA. Similar to the bDNA assay in nucleic acids extracted from plasma or serum, cells are incubated with a prehybridization solution, hybridized with target probes, and then detected with a series of oligonucleotide probes for signal amplification. In most iterations of this technology, the reagents include a preamplifier, amplifier, and alkaline phosphatase-conjugated probe or probes. This in situ bDNA method is very specific and quantitative at the cellular level, which is an attribute lacking for other target amplification procedures. In situ bDNA, however, is not very sensitive compared with target and probe amplification methods. This lack of sensitivity may be related to the ability of the branched molecule to diffuse in and out of a permeabilized cell.

TaqMan In Situ Assay or FISNA

Unlike some of the target amplification approaches that require too many steps to be clinically useful, TaqMan in situ assay or fluorescence 5′ nuclease assay (or FISNA) requires only a few steps and little "hands-on" time. Because this is by definition a fluorescence-based assay, FISNA has already been adapted for use on a flow cytometer (Fig. 2) (31). One application in particular deserves mention as a potential clinical tool. Like PCR in situ hybridization, FISNA can be used to detect cells containing HIV-1 DNA (2, 23, 26, 40). Though therapies that actually reduce the HIV-1 DNA burden have yet to be developed, this assay is still useful for identifying cellular reservoirs capable of producing viral particles. Further, this technology has been used on tissue sections to identify HIV-1 reservoirs that remain following highly active antiretroviral therapy (Fig. 3) (26).

Procedure

Adherent cells or PBMCs (1×10^6 to 2×10^6 cells/reaction) are washed in PBS twice before fixation in PermiFlow

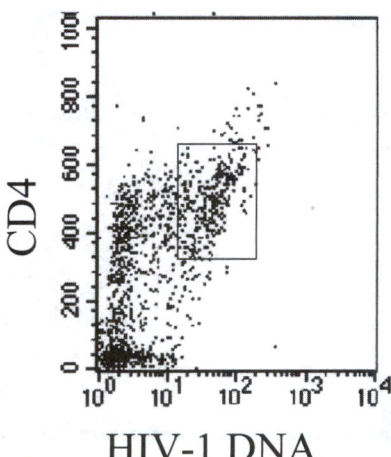

FIGURE 2 Representative dot plot of simultaneous immunophenotyping for CD4 and real-time PCR in situ (FISNA) detecting cells containing HIV-1 DNA. Biotinylated or 2,4-dinitrophenol (DNP)-conjugated antibodies survive the thermocycling process (30).

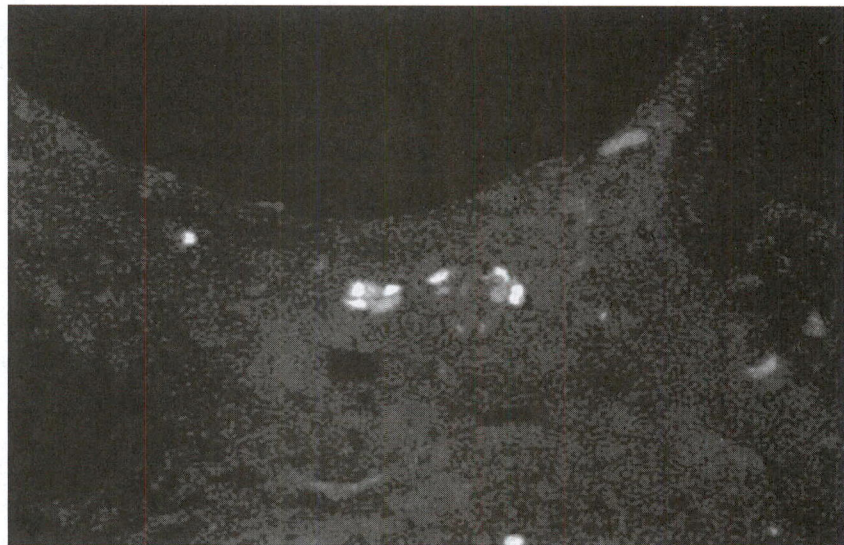

FIGURE 3 Representative laser confocal image analysis of real-time PCR in situ (FISNA) detecting cells in the prostate containing HIV-1 DNA following long-term therapy with antiretroviral drugs. These data suggest that reservoirs of HIV-1 DNA-containing cells are not necessarily cleared by long-term therapy (26).

(Invirion, Inc.). Cells are fixed for 1 to 18 h, and HIV-1 *gag* DNA is detected by TaqMan (real-time PCR) in situ or by FISNA. The cells are washed once in 1× PCR buffer without cations (Mg or Mn) and pelleted by centrifugation (600 × g). The PCR is performed in cell suspension (1× PCR buffer II; 0.35 mM $MgCl_2$; 200 μM each of dATP, dCTP, dGTP, and dTTP; 200 μM each of *gag* primers SK38/SK39 [sequences 5'-ATAATCCACCTATCCCAGTAGGAGAAAT-3' {SK38} and 5'-TTTGGTCCTTGTCTTATGTCCAGAATGC-3' {SK39}]; 100 nM *gag* probe FTSK19 [sequence 5'-ATCCTGGATTAAATAAAATAGTAAGAATGTATAGC CCTAC-3'-TAMRA]; and 10 U of AmpliTaq DNA polymerase Gold. Using the GeneAmp PCR System 2400 (PE Applied Biosystems, Foster City, Calif.), reaction tubes are heated to 95°C for 5 min followed by 30 cycles consisting of 94°C for 45 s and 56°C for 2 min, followed by a 15°C soak. The cells are thereafter washed in PBS and analyzed by flow cytometry or laser confocal microscopy. Autofluorescence can be quenched by incubation with trypan blue. The cutoff values are determined based on fluorescence emitted from noninfected cells.

CLINICAL APPLICATION OF ULTRASENSITIVE FLUORESCENCE IN SITU HYBRDIZATION

One of the most important applications of in situ hybridization clinically is for the detection of infectious diseases, in particular those caused by viruses (1, 7, 8, 15, 20–22, 24, 28, 29, 33, 38, 42). Viruses replicate in cells, not in plasma, which the majority of diagnostic tests use as sample. This raises the question of why one of the most powerful cell analysis tools, flow cytometry, is not being used to determine the response of virus replication to antiviral therapy. Unlike PCR in situ hybridization or some of the other in situ amplification techniques previously discussed, fluorescence in situ hybridization offers quantitative information at both the cellular level and the cell population level, making these assays useful for monitoring viral replication clinically (3, 5, 13, 21, 28, 29). For example, one can use fluorescence equivalent bead standards

and the number of fluorochromes per viral copy to calculate the number of copies of HIV-1 expressed in a particular cell (3). Further, the cytometer will determine the number of cells expressing a detectable amount of virus in a heterogeneous cell population such as blood or a liquid-based cervical cytology specimen as described below. As is the case with HIV-1, in situ hybridization combined with immunophenotyping yields additional information on the inhibition of viral replication by drugs or other therapeutics within certain cellular reservoirs (Fig. 4) (1, 13, 21, 28, 29, 33).

HIV

Detection of HIV replication in cells has immediate and important clinical significance. It has been proposed that the diagnostic goal of HIV therapy should be the minimization of viral replication with the hope that HIV evolution is minimized and the prospect of developing drug resistance or immune escape mutations ultimately is minimized (44). Several studies determined that HIV-1 replication can persist in cells in the presence of an undetectable plasma viral load (11, 29, 44). These studies suggested that the diagnostic goal just described can be achieved by combining plasma viral load determinations with a cytometry-based assessment of HIV-1 replication in both T lymphocytes and monocytes/macrophages (29). In fact, Patterson et al. previously showed that HIV-1 replicates in distinct subpopulations of T cells and monocytes/macrophages (Fig. 4) (29). In the T-cell compartment, HIV-1 predominantly replicated in activated, memory T cells with the CD4+ CD45RO+ HLA-DR+ phenotype. Similarly, HIV-1 predominantly replicates in the CD14$_{lo}$ CD16$_{hi}$ subpopulation of monocytes (Fig. 5). Monitoring these two cellular compartments as well as the plasma provides additional, clinically useful information when the results are reported together (Fig. 5). When persistent viral replication exists in cells despite undetectable plasma viral load, additional agents such as hydroxyurea and the drug Abacavir have been shown to provide additional suppression of HIV-1 replication (14, 32).

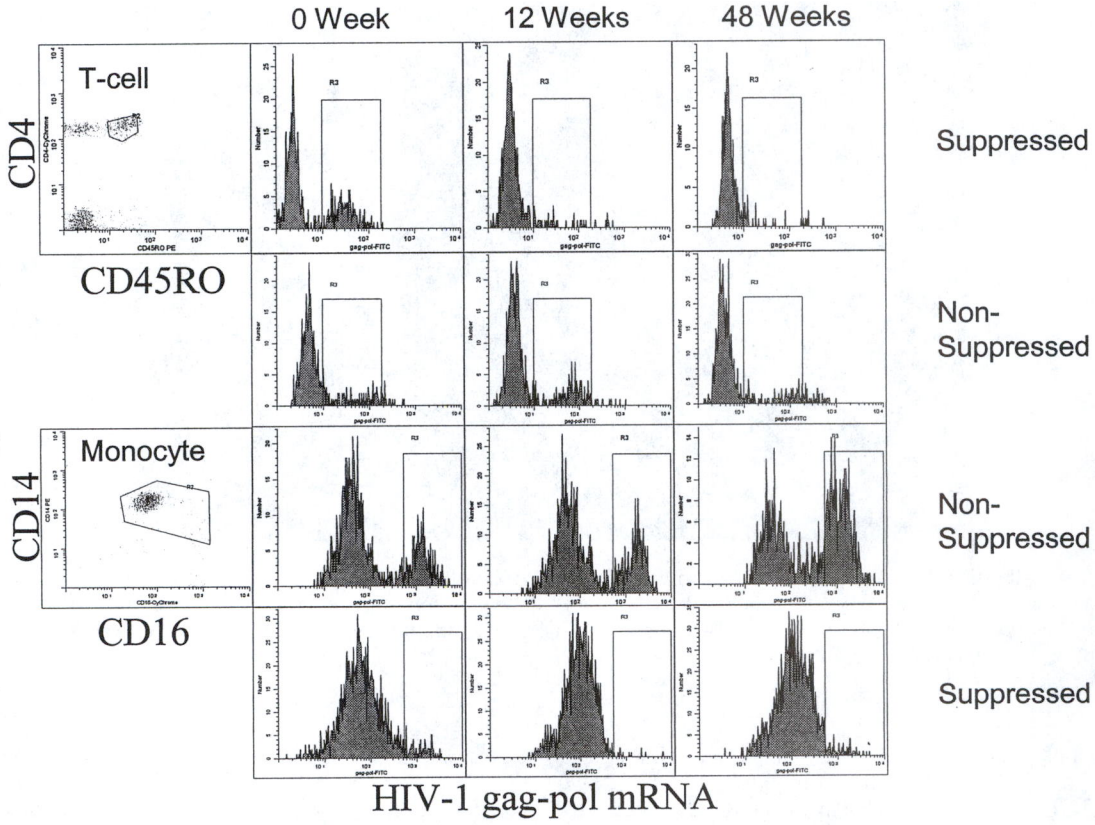

FIGURE 4 Monitoring HIV-1 replication in patients on highly active antiretroviral therapy by simultaneous immunophenotyping and ultrasensitive fluorescence in situ hybridization in T lymphocytes (CD4+ CD45RO+) and in monocytes/macrophages (CD14/CD16).

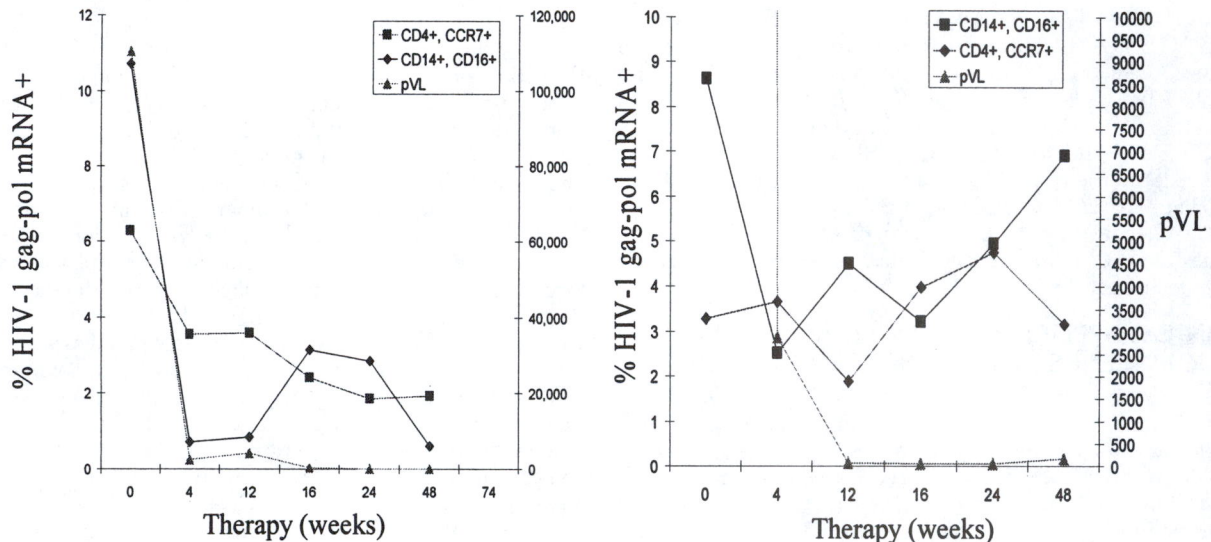

FIGURE 5 Combining plasma viral load (pVL) and simultaneous immunophenotyping and ultrasensitive fluorescence in situ hybridization in T lymphocytes (CD4+ CD45RO+) and in monocytes/macrophages (CD14/CD16) to determine response of multiple tissue compartments to highly active antiretroviral therapy. This extremely powerful test bundle identifies individuals with a maximal response to therapy in all compartments (left) and those individuals with persistent viral replication (in cells) despite undetectable plasma viral load (right). As one might predict for an individual with persistent viral replication, plasma viral load increased during the course of therapy.

The development of HIV-1 entry inhibitors, most notably the CCR5 inhibitors, will present an exciting opportunity for cell-based diagnostics. These compounds target one of the major coreceptors (in addition to CD4) used by HIV-1 to gain entry into susceptible target cells. In preclinical and early clinical studies, these compounds were shown to have little effect on plasma viral load as they prevent entry of HIV-1 into uninfected cells. These compounds will be used as frontline therapy against HIV-1 and as such will need to be assessed for their efficacy. Additional concern exists in the field due to the possibility that using CCR5 inhibitors will select for viral isolates that can use the other major HIV-1 coreceptor, CXCR4, a phenomenon termed "tropism shift" (6). Isolates that use CXCR4 have been shown to be more virulent than isolates that use CCR5 alone (6). Detection of this tropism shift is another application best suited for cell-based diagnostics as demonstrated in Fig. 6.

Procedure

Simultaneous flow cytometric analysis of intracellular HIV-1 RNA and cellular immunophenotyping of PBMCs were done as previously described (1, 13, 21, 28, 29, 33). Duplicate samples containing 5×10^4 to 1×10^6 cells were labeled with optimal concentrations of a T-cell (CD4, CD45RO) cocktail (Invirion, Inc.) or a monocyte/macrophage (CD14/CD16) cocktail (Invirion, Inc.) and incubated for 20 min at room temperature. The cells were washed with PBS, fixed, and permeabilized by the addition of 300 μl of PermiFlow (Invirion, Inc.). The cells were permeabilized for at least 60 min and up to 18 h. The cells were then washed twice in PBS, pH 7.4, and once in 2× SSC (1× SSC is 0.15 m NaCl plus 0.015 m sodium citrate). The cells were then resuspended in 100 μl of hybridization buffer containing a cocktail of 5-carboxyfluorescein-labeled oligonucleotide probes specific for HIV gag-pol mRNA (ViroTect In Cell HIV Detection System; Invirion, Inc.) at 43°C for 30 min. The cells were washed for 5 min at low stringency and then at high stringency for 30 min at 43°C. Multiparameter

three-color analysis was then performed on labeled cells in a Coulter XL or BD FACSCalibur flow cytometer.

HPV and Cervical Cancer Screening

Cervical cancer affects approximately 15,000 women per year in the United States and more than 450,000 women worldwide, though the exact number may be greater because of the lack of screening in developing nations. The Papanicolaou (Pap) smear has been the standard of care in the United States for more than 50 years, resulting in a significant decline in deaths due to cervical cancer during this time. More than 99% of cervical squamous cell carcinomas are due to infection by oncogenic genotypes of HPV such as HPV types 16, 18, 31, and 33, among others. HPV detection has been performed by a broad menu of molecular techniques, including hybrid capture (liquid hybridization), genotype-specific PCR, in situ hybridization, and in situ PCR. Most HPV assays, such as type-specific PCR and Hybrid Capture II, detect the presence of HPV L1 DNA from oncogenic types despite the fact that only a minority of women infected with oncogenic types of HPV will progress to cancer. The holy grail of HPV diagnostics is to find the "molecular switch" that defines when transformation of the cell has occurred. Most of the literature suggests that this molecular switch involves the overexpression of the E6 and E7 oncogenes, usually as a result of HPV integration into the chromosomal DNA (39). PCR for E6 and E7 mRNA has been used with some success; however, PCR for E6 and E7 mRNA is difficult to interpret, as some E6 and E7 mRNA is expressed in normal cells. For example, if mRNA from 1 million cells from a liquid-based cervical cytology (Pap) specimen were placed in a PCR for E6 or E7 quantification and the assay determined that 1 million copies of E6 or E7 mRNA were present, the clinician would not know if 1 million cells were making 1 copy per cell or 1,000 cells were producing 1,000 copies per cell. Simultaneous immunophenotyping and ultrasensitive fluorescence in situ hybridization can be used to detect cells in liquid-based cervical cytology specimens to detect the upregulation of E6 and E7 mRNA in cells undergoing transformation (9, 24). Use of this assay on a flow cytometer (Fig. 7) or a capillary-based cytometer (Fig. 8) is a powerful tool to detect cells in which HPV has "switched on" the viral oncogenes E6 and E7.

Procedure

A 1-ml aliquot was removed from a liquid-based cervical cytology specimen (PreservCyt [Cytyc, Boxborough, Mass.] or SurePath [Tripath Imaging, Durham, N.C.]). The cells were pelleted by centrifugation at 400 × g and washed once in PBS, pH 7.4. Cells were resuspended in 100 μl of PBS, pH 7.4, and stained with a 1:10 dilution of phycoerythrin (PE)-conjugated anti-CAM 5.2 and PE-Cy5-conjugated anti-CD16 (BD Pharmingen, San Diego, Calif.). The cells were then incubated at 4°C for 20 min in the dark. Following incubation, the cells were fixed and permeabilized in PermiFlow (Invirion, Inc.) for 1 h at ambient temperature. Following fixation and permeabilization, the cells were washed once in PBS, pH 7.4, pelleted by centrifugation at 400 × g, washed again in 2× SSC, and pelleted by centrifugation. HPV fluorescence in situ hybridization for E6 and E7 mRNA was performed by resuspending the cells in a hybridization mixture consisting of 5× SSC, 30% formamide, and 100 μg of sheared salmon sperm DNA per ml and a cocktail of 5'- and 3'-labeled oligonucleotide probes (HPV OncoTect; Invirion, Inc.). Hybridization was performed at 37°C for 30 min and

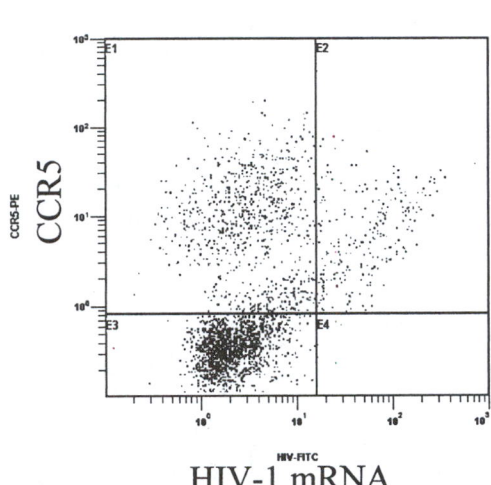

HIV-1 mRNA

FIGURE 6 Simultaneous detection of the HIV-1 coreceptor CCR5 and HIV-1 replication. This combination can be used to monitor response to HIV-1 entry and CCR5 inhibitors. Combining this with CXCR4 in a third color will allow the monitoring of potential tropism shifts.

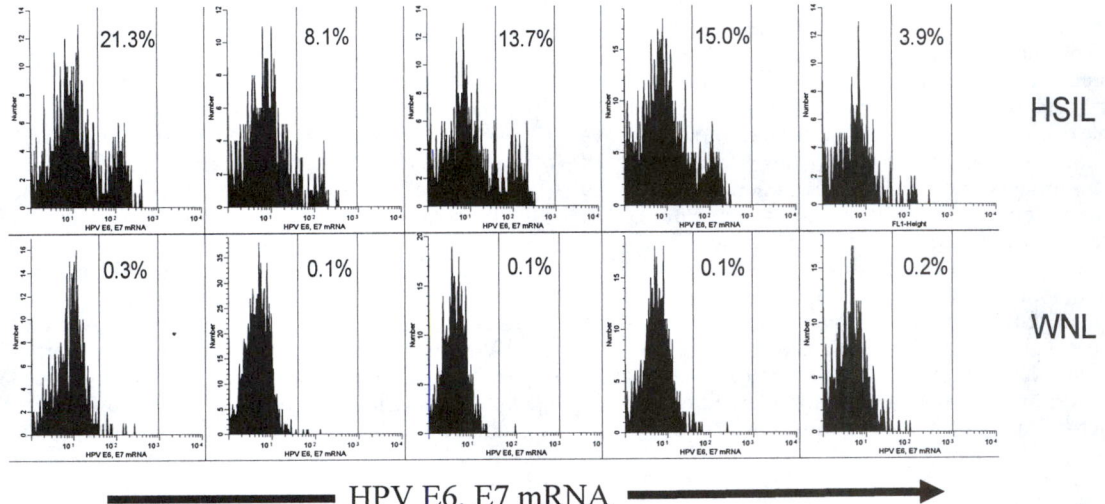

FIGURE 7 In situ detection of HPV E6 and E7 mRNA in cervical cytology samples from women with high-grade squamous intraepithelial lesions (HSIL) and women without cytologic abnormalities (WNL). The difference in the percentage of E6 and E7 mRNA-expressing cells is highly statistically significant (24).

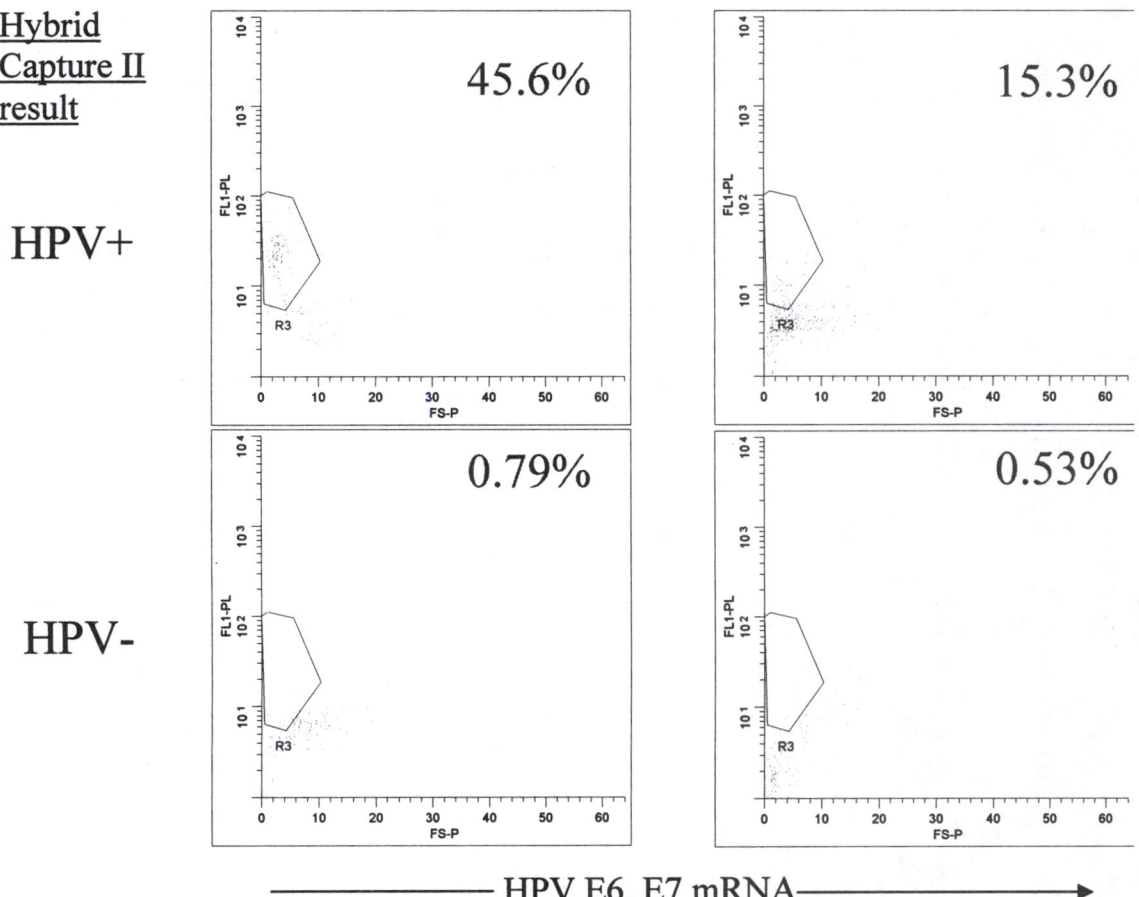

FIGURE 8 Ultrasensitive fluorescence in situ hybridization detection of HPV E6 and E7 mRNA expression in liquid-based cervical cytology samples. Hybrid Capture II high-risk HPV-positive samples (top row) and Hybrid Capture II high-risk HPV-negative samples were hybridized and run on a Guava Technologies PCA-96 capillary cytometer.

was followed by a 5-min wash in 2× SSC–0.1% Triton X-100 and a 15-min wash in 0.1% SSC–0.1% Triton X-100. The cells were resuspended in PBS, pH 7.4, with 2% fetal calf serum for flow cytometric analysis.

SUMMARY

Currently, cell-based diagnostics make up a small fraction of the diagnostics market. Cell-based diagnostics that guide therapy to viral infections and cancer much like the her-2/Herceptin model for breast cancer will continue to grow in popularity. The ability to perform molecular biological and immunological analyses in situ will greatly accelerate this growth. Hybrid instruments that incorporate the attributes of a flow cytometer with the imaging of a confocal microscope are currently available and will begin to find a place in clinical laboratories. At the very least, however, clinical applications of cytometry are beginning to extend beyond leukemia/lymphoma immunophenotyping to other fields, such as virology, where high-throughput analysis of intracellular events is critical for the diagnosis and management of infected individuals.

REFERENCES

1. **Al-Harthi, L., J. Voris, B. K. Patterson, S. Becker, J. Eron, K. Y. Smith, R. D'Amico, D. Mildvan, J. Snidow, B. Pobiner, L. Yau, and A. Landay.** 2004. Evaluation of the impact of highly active antiretroviral therapy on immune recovery in antiretroviral naive patients. *HIV Med.* **5:**55–65.

2. **Behbahani, H., A. Landay, B. K. Patterson, P. Jones, J. Pottage, M. Agnoli, J. Andersson, and A. L. Spetz.** 2000. Normalization of immune activation in lymphoid tissue following highly active antiretroviral therapy. *J. Acquir. Immune. Defic. Syndr.* **25:**150–156.

3. **Behbahani, H., E. Popek, P. Garcia, J. Andersson, A. L. Spetz, A. Landay, Z. Flener, and B. K. Patterson.** 2000. Up-regulation of CCR5 expression in the placenta is associated with human immunodeficiency virus-1 vertical transmission. *Am. J. Pathol.* **157:**1811–1818.

4. **Brodie, S. J., D. A. Lewinsohn, B. K. Patterson, D. Jiyamapa, J. Krieger, L. Corey, P. D. Greenberg, and S. R. Riddell.** 1999. In vivo migration and function of transferred HIV-1-specific cytotoxic T cells. *Nat. Med.* **5:**34–41.

5. **Collins, K. B., B. K. Patterson, G. J. Naus, D. V. Landers, and P. Gupta.** 2000. Development of an in vitro organ culture model to study transmission of HIV-1 in the female genital tract. *Nat. Med.* **6:**475–479.

6. **Connor, R. I., K. E. Sheridan, D. Ceradini, S. Choe, and N. R. Landau.** 1997. Change in coreceptor use correlates with disease progression in HIV-1-infected individuals. *J. Exp. Med.* **185:**621–628.

7. **Crouch, J., D. Leitenberg, B. R. Smith, and J. G. Howe.** 1997. Epstein-Barr virus suspension cell assay using in situ hybridization and flow cytometry. *Cytometry* **29:**50–57.

8. **Doherty, T. M., C. Chougnet, M. Schito, B. K. Patterson, C. Fox, G. M. Shearer, G. Englund, and A. Sher.** 1999. Infection of HIV-1 transgenic mice with Mycobacterium avium induces the expression of infectious virus selectively from a Mac-1-positive host cell population. *J. Immunol.* **163:**1506–1515.

9. **Dyson, N., P. M. Howley, K. Munger, and E. Harlow.** 1989. The human papilloma virus-16 E7 oncoprotein is able to bind to the retinoblastoma gene product. *Science* **243:**934–937.

10. **Embretson, J., M. Zupancic, J. Beneke, M. Till, S. Wolinsky, J. L. Ribas, A. Burke, and A. T. Haase.** 1993. Analysis of human immunodeficiency virus-infected tissues by amplification and in situ hybridization reveals latent and permissive infections at single-cell resolution. *Proc. Natl. Acad. Sci. USA* **90:**357–361.

11. **Furtado, M. R., D. S. Callaway, J. P. Phair, K. J. Kunstman, J. L. Stanton, C. A. Macken, A. S. Perelson, and S. M. Wolinsky.** 1999. Persistence of HIV-1 transcription in peripheral-blood mononuclear cells in patients receiving potent antiretroviral therapy. *N. Engl. J. Med.* **340:**1614–1622.

12. **Gibellini, D. E., M. C. Re, G. Furlini, and P. M. LaPlaca.** 1997. Flow cytometry analysis of an in situ PCR for the detection of human immunodeficiency virus type-1 (HIV-1) proviral DNA. *Methods Mol. Biol.* **71:**113–122.

13. **Gupta, P., K. B. Collins, D. Ratner, S. Watkins, G. J. Naus, D. V. Landers, and B. K. Patterson.** 2002. Memory CD4⁺ T cells are the earliest detectable human immunodeficiency virus type 1 (HIV-1)-infected cells in the female genital mucosal tissue during HIV-1 transmission in an organ culture system. *J. Virol.* **76:**9868–9876.

14. **Havlir, D. V., M. C. Strain, M. Clerici, C. Ignacio, D. Trabattoni, P. Ferrante, and J. K. Wong.** 2003. Productive infection maintains a dynamic steady state of residual viremia in human immunodeficiency virus type 1-infected persons treated with suppressive antiretroviral therapy for five years. *J. Virol.* **77:**11212–11219.

15. **Janes, M. S., B. J. Hanson, D. M. Hill, G. M. Buller, J. Y. Agnew, S. W. Sherwood, W. G. Cox, K. Yamagata, and R. A. Capaldi.** 2004. Rapid analysis of mitochondrial DNA depletion by fluorescence in situ hybridization and immunocytochemistry: potential strategies for HIV therapeutic monitoring. *J. Histochem. Cytochem.* **52:**1011–1018.

16. **Koffron, A. J., M. Hummel, B. K. Patterson, S. Yan, D. B. Kaufman, J. P. Fryer, F. P. Stuart, and M. I. Abecassis.** 1998. Cellular localization of latent murine cytomegalovirus. *J. Virol.* **72:**95–103.

17. **Komminoth, P., A. A. Long, R. Ray, and H. J. Wolfe.** 1992. In situ polymerase chain reaction detection of viral DNA, single-copy genes, and gene rearrangements in cell suspensions and cytospins. *Diagn. Mol. Pathol.* **1:**85–97.

18. **Komminoth, P., and M. Werner.** 1997. Target and signal amplification: approaches to increase the sensitivity of in situ hybridization. *Histochem. Cell Biol.* **108:**325–333.

19. **Korber, B. T., K. J. Kunstman, B. K. Patterson, M. Furtado, M. M. McEvilly, R. Levy, and S. M. Wolinsky.** 1994. Genetic differences between blood- and brain-derived viral sequences from human immunodeficiency virus type 1-infected patients: evidence of conserved elements in the V3 region of the envelope protein of brain-derived sequences. *J. Virol.* **68:**7467–7481.

20. **Lalli, E., D. Gibellini, S. Santi, and A. Facchini.** 1992. In situ hybridization in suspension and flow cytometry as a tool for the study of gene expression. *Anal. Biochem.* **207:**298–303.

21. **Lange, C. G., Z. Xu, B. K. Patterson, K. Medvik, B. Harnisch, R. Asaad, H. Valdez, S. J. Lee, A. Landay, J. Lieberman, and M. M. Lederman.** 2004. Proliferation responses to HIVp24 during antiretroviral therapy do not reflect improved immune phenotype or function. *AIDS* **18:**605–613.

22. **Lizard, G., M. C. Chignol, Y. Chardonnet, C. Souchier, M. Bordes, D. Schmitt, and J. P. Revillard.** 1993. Detection of human papillomavirus DNA in CaSki and HeLa cells by fluorescent in situ hybridization. Analysis by flow cytometry and confocal laser scanning microscopy. *J. Immunol. Methods* **157:**31–38.

23. **Lore, K., A. Sonnerborg, J. Olsson, B. K. Patterson, T. E. Fehniger, L. Perbeck, and J. Andersson.** 1999. HIV-1 exposed dendritic cells show increased pro-inflammatory

cytokine production but reduced IL-1ra following lipopolysaccharide stimulation. *AIDS* **13**:2013–2021.

24. **Narimatsu, R., and B. K. Patterson.** 2005. High-throughput cervical cancer screening using intracellular human papillomavirus E6 and E7 mRNA quantification by flow cytometry. *Am J. Clin. Pathol.* **123**:716–723.

25. **Nuovo, G. J., G. A. Gorgone, P. MacConnell, M. Margiotta, and P. D. Gorevic.** 1992. In situ localization of PCR-amplified human and viral cDNAs. *PCR Methods Applic.* **2**:117–123.

26. **Paranjpe, S., J. Craigo, B. Patterson, M. Ding, P. Barroso, L. Harrison, R. Montelaro, and P. Gupta.** 2002. Subcompartmentalization of HIV-1 quasispecies between seminal cells and seminal plasma indicates their origin in distinct genital tissues. *AIDS Res. Hum. Retrovir.* **18**:1271–1280.

27. **Patterson, B. K. (ed.).** 2000. *Techniques in the Quantitative Localization of Gene Expression.* Springer-Verlag, New York, N.Y.

28. **Patterson, B. K., D. J. Carlo, M. H. Kaplan, M. Marecki, S. Pawha, and R. B. Moss.** 1999. Cell-associated HIV-1 messenger RNA and DNA in T-helper cell and monocytes in asymptomatic HIV-1-infected subjects on HAART plus an inactivated HIV-1 immunogen. *AIDS* **13**:1607–1611.

29. **Patterson, B. K., M. A. Czerniewski, J. Pottage, M. Agnoli, H. Kessler, and A. Landay.** 1999. Monitoring HIV-1 treatment in immune-cell subsets with ultrasensitive fluorescence-in-situ hybridisation. *Lancet* **353**:211–212.

30. **Patterson, B. K., C. Goolsby, V. Hodara, K. L. Lohman, and S. M. Wolinsky.** 1995. Detection of CD4+ T cells harboring human immunodeficiency virus type 1 DNA by flow cytometry using simultaneous immunophenotyping and PCR-driven in situ hybridization: evidence of epitope masking of the CD4 cell surface molecule in vivo. *J. Virol.* **69**:4316–4322.

31. **Patterson, B. K., D. Jiyamapa, E. Mayrand, B. Hoff, R. Abramson, and P. M. Garcia.** 1996. Detection of HIV-1 DNA in cells and tissue by fluorescent in situ 5′-nuclease assay (FISNA). *Nucleic Acids Res.* **24**:3656–3658.

32. **Patterson, B. K., S. McCallister, M. Schutz, J. N. Siegel, K. Shults, Z. Flener, and A. Landay.** 2001. Persistence of intracellular HIV-1 mRNA correlates with HIV-1-specific immune responses in infected subjects on stable HAART. *AIDS* **15**:1635–1641.

33. **Patterson, B. K., V. L. Mosiman, L. Cantarero, M. Furtado, M. Bhattacharya, and C. Goolsby.** 1998. Detection of HIV-RNA-positive monocytes in peripheral blood of HIV-positive patients by simultaneous flow cytometric analysis of intracellular HIV RNA and cellular immunophenotype. *Cytometry* **31**:265–274.

34. **Patterson, B. K., M. Till, P. Otto, C. Goolsby, M. R. Furtado, L. J. McBride, and S. M. Wolinsky.** 1993.

Detection of HIV-1 DNA and messenger RNA in individual cells by PCR-driven in situ hybridization and flow cytometry. *Science* **260**:976–979.

35. **Player, A. N., L. P. Shen, D. Kenny, V. P. Antao, and J. A. Kolberg.** 2001. Single-copy gene detection using branched DNA (bDNA) in situ hybridization. *J. Histochem. Cytochem.* **49**:603–612.

36. **Qian, X., and R. V. Lloyd.** 2003. Recent developments in signal amplification methods for in situ hybridization. *Diagn. Mol. Pathol.* **12**:1–13.

37. **Re, M. C., G. Furlini, D. Gibellini, M. Vignoli, E. Ramazzotti, E. Lolli, S. Ranieri, and P. M. La.** 1994. Quantification of human immunodeficiency virus type 1-infected mononuclear cells in peripheral blood of seropositive subjects by newly developed flow cytometry analysis of the product of an in situ PCR assay. *J. Clin. Microbiol.* **32**:2152–2157.

38. **Rochet, V., L. Rigottier-Gois, S. Rabot, and J. Dore.** 2004. Validation of fluorescent in situ hybridization combined with flow cytometry for assessing interindividual variation in the composition of human fecal microflora during long-term storage of samples. *J. Microbiol. Methods* **59**:263–270.

39. **Scheffner, M., B. A. Werness, J. M. Huibregtse, A. J. Levine, and P. M. Howley.** 1990. The E6 oncoprotein encoded by human papillomavirus types 16 and 18 promotes the degradation of p53. *Cell* **63**:1129–1136.

40. **Spetz, A. L., B. K. Patterson, K. Lore, J. Andersson, and L. Holmgren.** 1999. Functional gene transfer of HIV DNA by an HIV receptor-independent mechanism. *J. Immunol.* **163**:736–742.

41. **Spira, A. I., P. A. Marx, B. K. Patterson, J. Mahoney, R. A. Koup, S. M. Wolinsky, and D. D. Ho.** 1996. Cellular targets of infection and route of viral dissemination after an intravaginal inoculation of simian immunodeficiency virus into rhesus macaques. *J. Exp. Med.* **183**:215–225.

42. **Stowe, R. P., M. L. Cubbage, C. F. Sams, D. L. Pierson, and A. D. Barrett.** 1998. Detection and quantification of Epstein-Barr virus EBER1 in EBV-infected cells by fluorescent in situ hybridization and flow cytometry. *J. Virol. Methods* **75**:83–91.

43. **Wilkens, L., J. Tchinda, P. Komminoth, and M. Werner.** 1997. Single- and double-color oligonucleotide primed in situ labeling (PRINS): applications in pathology. *Histochem. Cell Biol.* **108**:439–446.

44. **Zhang, L., B. Ramratnam, K. Tenner-Racz, Y. He, M. Vesanen, S. Lewin, A. Talal, P. Racz, A. S. Perelson, B. T. Korber, M. Markowitz, and D. D. Ho.** 1999. Quantifying residual HIV-1 replication in patients receiving combination antiretroviral therapy. *N. Engl. J. Med.* **340**:1605–1613.

FUNCTIONAL CELLULAR ASSAYS

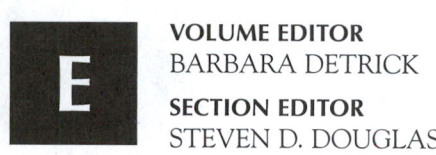

VOLUME EDITOR
BARBARA DETRICK

SECTION EDITOR
STEVEN D. DOUGLAS

Introduction

STEVEN D. DOUGLAS

25

A number of advances in basic immunology, molecular biology, and cellular physiology have resulted in major developments in cellular immunologic assays relevant to clinical and diagnostic immunology. The application of these techniques in research and clinical laboratories has led to their high sensitivity and specificity. These techniques afford the clinical immunology laboratorians, the clinical allergists and immunologists, and physicians in allied specialties with assays and techniques which make possible the precise diagnoses of primary and secondary disorders of the immune system. The chapters presented in this section incorporate newer diagnostic assays that have come into use since the previous edition of this manual. Furthermore, new chapters have been added for detection and measurement of T-cell responses to antigens and mitogens and assays for B-cell function and humoral immune responses. Shacklett and Nixon describe methodology for enzyme-linked immunospot assays (ELISPOT) for the detection of antigen-specific CD8 T cells. Several methods for enhancing ELISPOT sensitivity, assay validation, and interpretation are listed in tabular form. The potential clinical utility of this assay in infectious disease, autoimmunity, and cancer immunotherapy is extensive. International efforts are under way to standardize ELISPOT methodology for large-scale human immunodeficiency virus vaccine trials. Other examples include screening for tuberculosis and monitoring of clinical trials for melanoma therapeutics. McCloskey et al. describe four assays for apoptosis. These include the subdiploid method, DNA strand breaks (terminal deoxynucleotidyltransferase-mediated duTP-biotin nick end labeling method), detection with translocated phosphatidylserine (annexin V method), and a more recently developed method involving detection of cells using active caspases. Krogstad has added new details on real-time PCR assays for T-cell receptor excision circles and quantitation of recent thymic migrants. The chapter by Whiteside provides methodology for the assessment of natural killer cell activity in humans, and a figure delineates the conceptual interactions between "activation" and "inhibitory" natural killer cell markers. There is an expanded need for cellular immunologic assays for vaccine assessment in international clinical trials. Standardization of these techniques is essential. Cox et al. provide considerable detail for assay validation, and technical issues related to cell storage and viability, which are relevant and crucial for international vaccine studies. This important chapter provides details for specimen collection, lymphocyte function, CD4 and CD8 T-cell responses, and assays in developing countries. Cryopreservation is also dealt with in detail in the chapter by Weinberg. A new chapter by Currier examines T-cell activation and cell signaling, focusing on early events associated with T-cell activation and clinical application, namely, the identification of genetic signaling defects and signaling defects associated with immunosuppression or malignancy. Procedures are presented for measuring CD69, early cell activation; receptor expression after T-cell activation; and intracellular calcium cell signaling. Nahm and Lorenz provide assays for B cells and antibodies; in particular, these include bactericidal opsonophagocytosis and whole-blood lymphocyte proliferation. The chapter further provides background for the diagnosis of primary and secondary defects in B cells. O'Gorman's chapter provides methodology for the assessment of myeloid and monocytic cell function for the clinical immunology laboratory. Heyworth and Curnutte present approaches for molecular diagnosis of chronic granulomatous disease. There is direct application of these assays in clinical medicine related to primary and secondary immune deficiency, autoimmunity, hematology, rheumatology, transplantation, and a wide array of clinical disorders. These chapters afford a segue toward precise cellular immunologic diagnoses of these important clinical conditions.

Delayed-Type Hypersensitivity Skin Testing

THERON McCORMICK AND WILLIAM T. SHEARER

26

Cell-mediated immunity (CMI) provides the principal immunologic mechanism against a host of intracellular microbiologic agents, including many viruses, fungi, protozoa, and parasites. Screening of this arm of the immune system often begins with delayed-type hypersensitivity (DTH) skin testing. This test is a widely available, cost-effective, and relatively simple tool for assessing the integrity of CMI. Once properly placed, a positive response to DTH skin testing indicates intact CMI, while a negative response may represent either a possible defect in CMI, a lack of previous exposure or an inability to respond. In this chapter, a brief discussion of the molecular mechanism of action and a survey of the different implementation tools, as well as test interpretation, is provided. In addition, the clinical implications of DTH skin testing in disease diagnosis and screening (i.e., tuberculosis) and the monitoring of specific disease progression (i.e., human immunodeficiency virus [HIV]) will be reviewed.

BIOLOGY

The DTH reaction occurs in several steps after the antigen has been introduced intracutaneously. The ensuing inflammatory response is an intact recall response initiated by memory T cells that involves a coordinated process of cytokine and chemokine secretion and cellular infiltration (15). The reaction begins with the uptake and initial processing of the antigen by antigen-presenting cells, such as dendritic cells and/or monocytes (31). During the tuberculin reaction, the antigen is processed in the context of major histocompatibility complex (MHC) class II molecules and presented to naïve CD4$^+$ T cells. In particular, skin-derived dendritic cells are among the first cells to display peptides in the antigen-MHC class II complex (25). Generally, soluble antigens do not enter the MHC class I pathway; therefore, CD8$^+$ T cells have minimal or no contribution to this reaction (27).

Cytokines are derived from this interaction, particularly interleukin-12 (IL-12), IL-18, and gamma interferon (IFN-γ), serving to drive the T helper cells to a Th1 CD4$^+$ profile (47). By 4 to 6 h a lymphocytic and basophilic infiltrate is present in the perivascular area. When the tuberculin reaction is used as a model, 75 to 90% of the mononuclear cells in the perivascular aggregates are CD4$^+$ T lymphocytes and monocytes, with subsequent dermal interstitial infiltration by 12 to 24 h (40). The swelling at the skin testing site can be seen within 24 to 48 h after challenge but becomes most intense between 48 and 72 h (28). IFN-γ, tumor necrosis factor alpha, IL-1, and IL-6 are detected in the dermis within 48 h and are sustained for 7 days after testing (7, 39). Of note, in mice, the cellular response to DTH tends to be predominantly neutrophilic, with reaction elucidation requiring much higher concentrations of antigen than in humans (10). Also, IFN-γ is required for the development of stress-induced DTH in mice (11).

METHODS AND IMPLEMENTATION: MANTOUX METHOD OF SKIN TESTING

DTH skin testing is routinely performed by the Mantoux method. In the Mantoux method, an individual antigen is selected and administered intradermally. Appropriate antigen(s) should be selected on the basis of the likelihood of the individual's exposure. Concentrations and availability of commonly used antigens are shown in Table 1. In general, the lower concentration is preferred for the initial testing in order to avoid a possible severe DTH reaction. Subsequently, the more concentrated form of antigen can be administered if the initial testing is negative.

The ventral surface of the forearm is the preferred site for testing. A 27-gauge needle containing 0.1 ml of antigen should be used for injection into the superficial layers of the dermis (approximately 1 to 2 mm under the epidermis), resulting in a small bleb on the skin 7 to 10 mm in diameter. A distance of at least 3 cm (1.2 in.) between antigens should prevent an incorrect reading in case of large DTH reactions. Syringes without excess airspace at the tip are preferred for accurate delivery of antigens. Two methods of needle insertion can be employed: a bevel-up or a bevel-down method, with the former being more widely used. It is unclear whether DTH testing by these two methods differs in outcome. A study comparing the bevel-up and the bevel-down methods using 0.03 ml of sterile saline per injection showed that the bevel-down method caused less bleeding and discomfort at the site and was more time-efficient in the delivery of multiple injections (24). Trained health professionals should read DTH reactions within 48 to 72 h of testing. The largest diameter of the induration should be recorded. An induration of 5 mm or more in response to a single antigen is considered sufficient evidence for intact CMI. Individuals who do not respond are considered anergic. In our institution, DTH is

TABLE 1 Common antigens for DTH skin testing by the Mantoux method

Antigen	Concn. used for DTH skin testing[a]	Pharmaceutical supplier(s) (examples)
PPD	5 TB/0.1 ml	Aventis-Pasteur, Swiftwater, Pa.
C. albicans	1:10 or 1:100 dil (wt/vol)	Allermed, San Diego, Calif.; Hollister-Stier, Spokane, Wash.
Trichophyton	1:30 or 1:100 dil (wt/vol)	Hollister-Stier, Spokane, Wash.
Tetanus	1:10 dil (wt/vol)	Aventis-Pasteur, Swiftwater, Pa.
Mumps	40 CFU/ml	Aventis-Pasteur, Swiftwater, Pa.

[a]TB, tuberculin units; dil, dilution.

performed with a panel of tetanus (1:10), purified protein derivative (PPD) of *Mycobacterium tuberculosis*, and *Candida albicans* (1:20 and 1:200) antigen as shown in Fig. 1. The rates of positive response with this panel for HIV-positive and HIV-negative individuals are approximately 70 and 80%, respectively. Sensitivity does not increase with the addition of another recall antigen (22). Anergic individuals with strong clinical suspicion of a CMI defect should have peripheral blood obtained for the in vitro lymphoproliferative assay (LPA) to mitogens and antigens. Otherwise, DTH skin testing using tetanus (1:10) and *Candida* (1:20) antigen should be repeated in 3 to 6 months. In cases where antigen avoidance is crucial, such as in immunosuppressed patients in the transplantation setting, trans vivo DTH testing has been proposed for CMI screening (4). This described method involves the injection of human peripheral blood mononuclear cells combined with a set amount of antigen into murine pinnae, with induration measurement within 48 h.

FACTORS THAT MAY AFFECT DTH RESULT

Correct handling and storage of antigens are important in maintaining the efficacy of the reagents and, thus, accurate results. Similar antigens from different sources may produce variable results; therefore, they may not be comparable, especially when serial testing is performed (30). DTH skin testing with two antigens (yeast cell suspension and polysaccharide antigens) from the same strains of *Candida* can produce discordant results in up to 20% of individuals (14). Placement of DTH skin tests and reading of results require trained personnel. Loss of antigens during needle insertion and injection into the deep dermal layers can result in false-negative results. Interpretation of a large wheal reaction as a positive DTH response is not uncommon. Care should be taken in ensuring that only the widest part of the induration is recorded. Positive DTH responses can also develop as a result of repeat testing. This phenomenon is known as the booster effect (32). It should not occur if at least 3 months

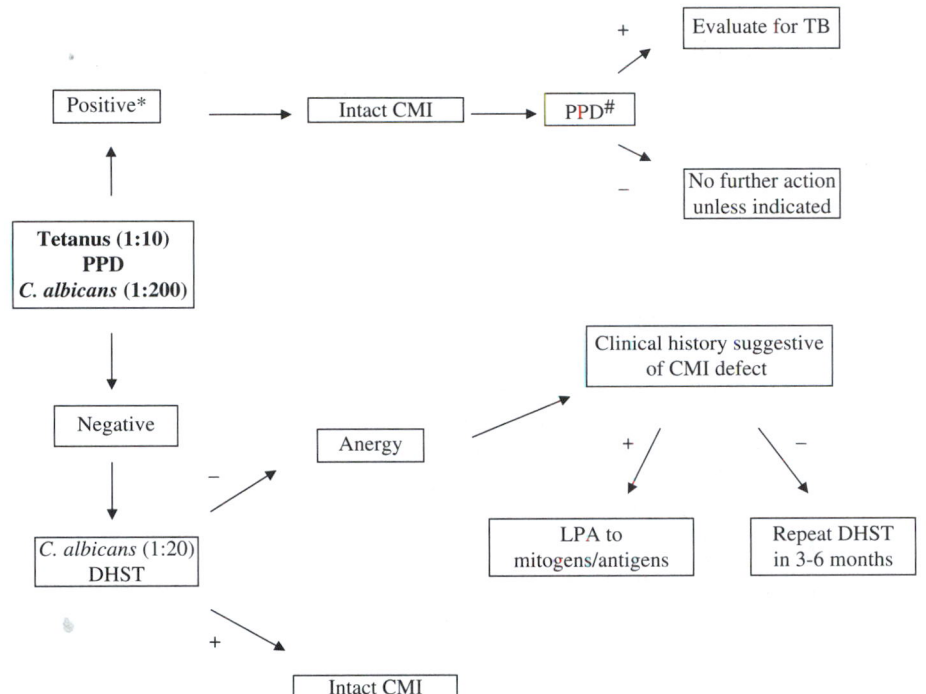

FIGURE 1 Suggested procedure for DTH skin testing by the Mantoux method. A positive reaction (*) is signaled by an induration of ≥5 mm in response to a single antigen or an induration of ≥2 mm in response to at least two antigens; a PPD-positive reaction (#) is signaled by an induration of ≥10 mm except in HIV-infected individuals and children at high risk for tuberculosis (induration, ≥5 mm). DHST, DTH skin testing; TB, tuberculosis.

is allowed between tests. The type and dose of antigens may influence such occurrences as well. For instance, DTH testing with *Candida* antigens resulted in a positive response in only 9% of HIV-infected individuals within 1 week of antiretroviral therapy, whereas no response was seen with mumps antigen, *Trichophyton*, or PPD (9).

Awareness of conditions that may affect the DTH response is critical for accurate assessment (Table 2). As an example, acute influenza infection can cause transient impairment of CMI. Reversion of a negative *Candida* DTH skin test was documented for such subjects after 17 days of infection (45). Also, significant alcohol consumption, such as is seen in people with alcoholism, decreases the sensitivity of detection of a DTH response (46). Patients with primary immunodeficiency disorders involving CMI typically show no DTH responses. Some hereditary and metabolic disorders can cause secondary CMI defects and thus are associated with failure to respond to DTH testing (2). Decreased DTH responses are seen in chronic obstructive pulmonary disease patients with poor lung function (12). Prolonged use of systemic corticosteroids has been known to depress CMI and, thus, DTH in patients. However, when one of the more potent inhaled corticosteroids, fluticasone, was used in a double-blind, placebo-controlled study, after 28 days of inhaled therapy, DTH skin responses were not affected (13). There are no current studies reporting a depression of DTH response after a period exceeding 2 months on high-dose inhaled corticosteroids. With regard to childhood immunizations, the measles vaccine can temporarily suppress tuberculin reactivity; thus, a tuberculin skin test should either be placed at the same time as the measles, mumps, and rubella vaccine or postponed for 4 to 6 weeks (1). Also, in the elderly, DTH cutaneous responses to recall bacterial and fungal antigens are reduced in frequency and size (6).

CORRELATION OF DTH SKIN TESTING AND LPA

Another assessment of CMI is performed by using the in vitro LPA. This test entails the proliferation of lymphocytes in response to antigens to which the individual has previously been sensitized. In general, LPA results correspond to those obtained with in vivo DTH skin testing. More specifically, correlation between responses produced by DTH skin testing and LPA depends on the type of antigen, the level of CMI impairment of the subject, and the criteria used in defining a positive response. In HIV-negative individuals, correlation between DTH and LPA responses to frequently exposed recall antigens is excellent (48, 49). However, in a study of an HIV-infected population, the baseline DTH skin testing response to *Candida* antigen was found to be absent while the LPA response to *Candida* antigen was relatively intact (9). After 12 weeks of highly active antiretroviral therapy (HAART), LPA responses to *Candida* normalized to those of control subjects, while only 30% of patients showed a response by DTH skin testing (9). Figure 2 shows the results of a different study revealing concordance between improved DTH (68%) and LPA (57%) responses to tetanus after 48 weeks or more of HAART (48). The differences between the results of these two studies may be due partly to the higher cutpoint (≥10 mm) for defining positive DTH reactions in the former study compared to the latter (≥5 mm). Earlier reports have suggested better correlation between LPA and DTH results when a cutpoint of <5 mm is used (35). Concordance of improvement in DTH and LPA

TABLE 2 Conditions associated with decreased response to DTH skin testing

Condition
Physiologic
Young age
Pregnancy
Primary immunodeficiencies
T-cell defects: DiGeorge syndrome
Combined T- and B-cell defects
Common variable immunodeficiencies
Hereditary diseases
Down syndrome
Thalassemia
Metabolic diseases
Uremia and dialysis
Liver disease
Protein-calorie malnutrition, nutrient deficiencies, and eating disorders
Diabetes mellitus
Infectious diseases
Acute viral infection, especially measles, varicella, and influenza
Bacterial pneumonia
HIV
Medications
Corticosteroids
Chemotherapeutic agents
Anticoagulants
Others
Chronic obstructive pulmonary disease

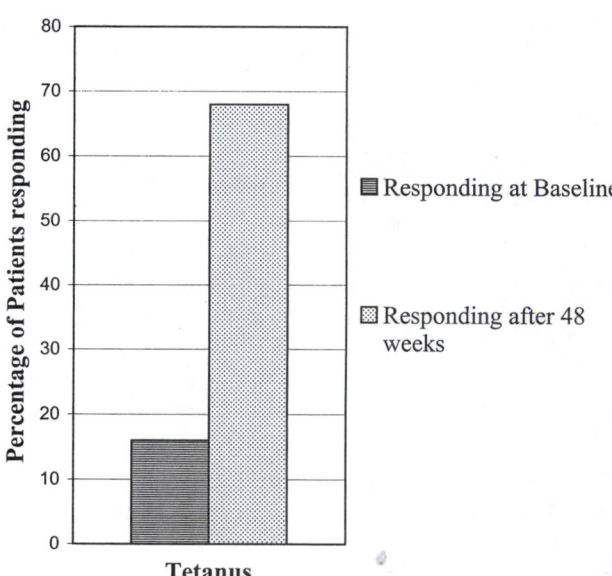

FIGURE 2 Percentage of patients having a baseline DTH response (induration, >5 mm) and developing an increase in DTH response (at least a 5-mm increase from baseline) to a given antigen after 48 weeks or more of HAART. The total numbers of patients evaluated for tetanus at baseline, week 6, week 18, and any time after baseline were 31, 23, 23, and 31, respectively. Adapted from reference 48.

responses to a specific antigen following treatment was superior for HIV-infected individuals who had CD4$^+$ T-cell counts of 250/μl or more (49). Immune recovery following HAART can be observed better with the LPA response in patients with relatively lower CD4$^+$ T-cell counts than with the DTH response. In the assessment of the CMI response to recombinant gp160 immunization in asymptomatic HIV-infected patients, the sensitivity of DTH skin testing compared to LPA was 75% (26). Recovery of DTH to a battery of recall antigens correlated well with improved LPA responses to anti-CD2, anti-CD28, and anti-CD3 (33).

CLINICAL IMPLICATIONS OF DTH

DTH skin testing is a practical screening measure for assessing the integrity of CMI. Abnormal DTH responses can signify an associated CMI defect in conditions such as frequent infections, autoimmunity, and malignancy. DTH skin testing is also useful for patients with known immune deficiency. Primary immunodeficient patients who fail to respond to DTH with ubiquitous antigens can experience a predisposition to infections from intracellular pathogens. DTH skin testing is especially helpful in the assessment and management of HIV-infected patients (16). Development of anergy in these individuals predicts disease progression, whereas loss of anergy indicates disease improvement and response to treatment. In addition, DTH skin testing can also aid in the diagnosis of many bacterial and fungal infections such as tuberculosis, leishmaniasis, histoplasmosis, blastomycosis, and aspergillosis. Of these, clinical utility in the diagnosis of tuberculosis is perhaps the most well known. Furthermore, DTH can aid in the assessment of CMI responses to vaccines. For instance, it was used to assess cellular response to HIV type 1 Tat protein immunization in HIV-positive individuals (20).

ASSESSMENT OF CMI

In the healthy HIV-negative population, anergy is typically seen in <5% of individuals; however, prevalence of anergy as high as 15% in such study subjects has been reported (8, 22, 43). In HIV-infected individuals, prevalence of anergy typically ranges between 20 and 50% (8, 29, 34, 36, 41, 42). A noted example of the use of DTH in determining anergy is shown in a large study of 358 HIV-negative and 721 HIV-positive women (29). In Table 3, a comparison of percentages of nonreactivity to Candida, tetanus, or mumps antigens using cutpoints of 1 to 5 mm is shown. The percent nonreactivity was the highest with mumps antigen and the lowest with

tetanus antigen, irrespective of HIV status or cutpoints. The difference between nonreactivity in HIV-negative and HIV-positive women was best distinguished by use of the tetanus antigen. Across the board, cutpoints of 1 and 2 mm did not differ in their ability to define anergy. However, raising the cutpoint from 2 to 5 mm did increase the percentage of nonreactivity, regardless of antigens or HIV status. In Table 4, percentages of nonreactivity to different combinations of two antigens and to all three antigens with cutpoints of 1 to 5 mm are shown. Tetanus and mumps antigen testing had the highest reactivity of all the combinations in HIV-negative women. The best identification of anergy in both the HIV-negative and the HIV-positive populations was achieved by using all three antigens and cutpoints of either 1 or 2 mm (Table 4). With this guideline, 90 and 60% of HIV-negative and HIV-positive women, respectively, responded to one or more antigens. Due to the difficulty in measuring the small induration size of 1 mm, 2 mm was recommended as the best cutpoint for establishing anergy.

In HIV-infected individuals, response to DTH skin testing, including the number of positive antigens and the summed response, correlates directly with CD4$^+$ T-cell numbers and clinical stages of HIV disease (3, 17, 35). Klein et al. demonstrated the correlation between DTH responses and numbers of CD4$^-$ T cells in HIV-infected women (29). The inability to respond to a single antigen differed significantly among the subjects in each CD4$^+$ T-cell group, with response seen in patients with CD4 counts higher than 200/μl. In general, women with higher CD4$^+$ T-cell counts were more likely to have a DTH response. Similarly, women in the lower CD4$^+$ T-cell count group (≤200/μl) had significantly lower percentages of DTH reactivity.

DIAGNOSIS OF M. TUBERCULOSIS DISEASE

Prevalence of positive PPD reactions varies among different population groups. The highest prevalence is seen in intravenous drug users, homeless persons, HIV-infected persons, and immigrants from Asia, Africa, and South America (1). In a mixed population of HIV-positive and HIV-negative individuals, a history of a positive PPD reaction predicted subsequent positive testing for 70% of subjects (42).

In general, development of an induration of 10 mm or more in response to PPD is considered a positive reaction, except in HIV-infected individuals and children at high risk for tuberculosis, for whom an induration of 5 mm or more is considered significant. Children with histories of close contact with patients with tuberculosis or immunosuppressive

TABLE 3 Effect of varying induration cutpoint on DTH testing among 721 HIV-seropositive and 358 HIV-seronegative at-risk women[a]

Induration, cutpoint (mm)[b]	Candida			Tetanus			Mumps		
	HIV$^-$	HIV$^+$	OR (95% CI)[c]	HIV$^-$	HIV$^+$	OR (95% CI)	HIV$^-$	HIV$^+$	OR (95% CI)
<1	181 (50.6)	497 (68.9)	2.2 (1.7–2.8)	78 (21.8)	444 (61.6)	5.8 (4.3–7.7)	101 (28.2)	483 (67.0)	5.2 (3.9–6.8)
<2	182 (50.8)	498 (69.1)	2.2 (1.7–2.8)	78 (21.8)	447 (62.0)	5.9 (4.4–7.8)	102 (28.5)	484 (67.1)	5.1 (3.9–6.8)
<3	190 (53.1)	522 (72.4)	2.3 (1.8–3.0)	81 (22.6)	466 (64.6)	6.2 (4.7–8.4)	112 (31.3)	498 (69.1)	4.7 (3.7–6.4)
<4	209 (58.4)	539 (74.8)	2.1 (1.6–2.8)	85 (23.7)	482 (66.9)	6.7 (5.0–8.9)	155 (43.3)	564 (78.2)	4.7 (3.6–6.2)
<5	223 (62.3)	575 (79.8)	2.4 (1.8–3.2)	91 (25.4)	501 (69.5)	6.7 (5.0–8.9)	155 (43.3)	564 (78.2)	4.7 (3.6–6.2)

[a]Reprinted from reference 29, with permission of the publisher.
[b]Reaction size defining lack of DTH response.
[c]OR, odds ratio; CI, confidence interval.

TABLE 4 Rates of cutaneous anergy by HIV status: effect of varying number of antigens and induration cutpoint[a]

Anergy cutpoint (mm)[b] and antigens tested	No. (%) of nonreactive women		
	HIV− (n = 358)	HIV+ (n = 721)	OR (95% CI)[c]
<1			
Candida and tetanus	50 (14.0)	335 (46.5)	5.4 (3.8–7.6)
Candida and mumps	70 (19.6)	372 (51.6)	4.4 (3.2–6.0)
Tetanus and mumps	46 (12.8)	355 (49.2)	6.6 (4.6–9.4)
Candida, tetanus, and mumps	34 (9.5)	293 (40.6)	6.5 (4.4–9.8)
<2			
Candida and tetanus	50 (14.0)	339 (47.0)	5.5 (3.9–7.8)
Candida and mumps	70 (19.6)	374 (51.9)	4.4 (3.2–6.1)
Tetanus and mumps	46 (12.8)	358 (49.7)	6.7 (4.7–9.6)
Candida, tetanus, and mumps	34 (9.5)	297 (41.2)	6.7 (4.5–10.0)
<3			
Candida and tetanus	52 (14.5)	359 (49.8)	5.8 (4.1–8.3)
Candida and mumps	77 (21.5)	393 (54.5)	4.4 (3.2–5.9)
Tetanus and mumps	49 (13.7)	384 (53.3)	7.2 (5.1–10.2)
Candida, tetanus, and mumps	36 (10.1)	317 (44.0)	7.0 (4.7–10.4)
<4			
Candida and tetanus	60 (16.8)	381 (52.8)	5.6 (4.0–7.7)
Candida and mumps	96 (26.8)	422 (58.5)	3.9 (2.9–5.2)
Tetanus and mumps	55 (15.4)	413 (57.3)	7.4 (5.3–10.4)
Candida, tetanus, and mumps	42 (11.7)	343 (47.6)	6.8 (4.7–9.9)
<5			
Candida and tetanus	65 (18.2)	417 (57.8)	6.2 (4.5–8.5)
Candida and mumps	116 (32.4)	471 (65.2)	3.9 (3.0–5.2)
Tetanus and mumps	60 (16.8)	443 (61.4)	7.9 (5.7–11.0)
Candida, tetanus, and mumps	47 (13.1)	380 (52.7)	7.4 (5.2–10.6)

[a]Reprinted from reference 29 with prior permission from the publisher.
[b]Reaction size defining lack of DTH response.
[c]OR, odds ratio; CI, confidence interval.

conditions are considered at high risk for tuberculosis infection (1). Of note, individuals with disseminated tuberculosis may not react to PPD placement. In the United States, where native-born individuals are not routinely immunized with *Mycobacterium bovis* (i.e., Bacille Calmette-Guerin [BCG]), prior immunization with BCG does not alter the criteria for PPD interpretation, since most adult immigrants were immunized as children and are likely no longer sensitized. Nevertheless, persistent positive responses to PPD at 1 to 3 years after BCG immunization have been seen. This may pertain to immigrants from countries where repeated BCG immunization is employed (23).

The revised recommendation by the Centers for Disease Control and Prevention no longer requires DTH for recall antigens (anergy testing) with PPD testing in HIV-infected individuals (5). This recommendation is based partly on the lack of statistical significance in the reduction of tuberculosis in PPD-negative, anergic individuals who were on isoniazid prophylaxis (18). In addition, HIV-positive patients generally have a brisk response to PPD when infected with tuberculosis and may selectively react to PPD without any reaction to recall antigens (19, 34). The lack of antigen standardization and the multiple factors resulting in variations in DTH results have led to difficulties in interpreting anergy testing results (5). However, determination of anergy has important clinical implications in the detection of tuberculosis in the HIV-infected population. Anergic HIV-infected

individuals are at higher risk for active tuberculosis than nonanergic individuals (42). In the large cohort of HIV-infected women discussed above, individuals who reacted to one or more control antigens (*Candida*, tetanus, and mumps) were four to six times more likely to react to PPD (29). When all three antigens and a 2-mm cutpoint were used, anergy was seen in only 9.5% of HIV-negative women but in 40% of HIV-positive women (29). With the same criteria, the rates of positive PPD reaction were 1.4 and 5.8% in anergic and nonanergic HIV-positive women, respectively. However, among HIV-negative women, the rates of positive PPD reaction did not differ according to whether or not the women were anergic. The benefits of anergy testing in this study have been supported by others (21, 33, 37, 44). Therefore, careful consideration of performing anergy testing in conjunction with tuberculin testing in a population at high risk for tuberculosis (HIV-positive patients) should be made. In the HIV-negative population, there is no clear recommendation regarding placement of control antigens with PPD testing. Nevertheless, PPD testing alone appears to be an accurate screening test for tuberculosis (38).

CONCLUSIONS

DTH skin testing provides a practical tool in the assessment of CMI. It can be used to establish defects in CMI, predict progression of and monitor HIV disease, test responses to vaccines, and diagnose bacterial and fungal infections. For valid interpretation of DTH testing, the skin test placement and accuracy of the skin test reading as well as various health factors need to be taken into consideration. Lastly, DTH correlates well with the more specific in vitro LPA, and it remains the recommended initial screening tool for CMI on the basis of its ease of use and inexpensiveness.

Special thanks are due to Terri L. Raburn for providing information regarding antigens and DTH skin test placement. This work was supported in part by National Institutes of Health General Clinical Research Center grant RR-00188, Pediatric AIDS Clinic Trial Group grant AI 27551, Women and Infants Transmission Study grant HD 41983, Training Program for Clinical Research on AIDS grant T32-AI 07456, Cardiac Status of HAART Exposed Infants of HIV-Infected Mothers grant HL 72705, Sleep Studies in HIV+ Older Children and Adolescents grant HL 79533, Center for AIDS Research grant P30 AI 36211, and the David Fund and the Immunology Research Fund of Texas Children's Hospital.

REFERENCES

1. **American Academy of Pediatrics.** 2003. Tuberculosis, p. 541–562. *In* G. Peter (ed.), *Red Book: Report of the Committee on Infectious Diseases,* 24th ed. American Academy of Pediatrics, Elk Grove Village, Ill.
2. **Ananworanich, J., and W. T. Shearer.** 2001. Immune deficiencies in congenital and metabolic diseases, p. 42.1–42.10. *In* R. R. Rich, T. A. Fleisher, W. T. Shearer, B. Kotzin, and H. Schroeder (ed.), *Clinical Immunology: Principles and Practice,* 2nd ed. Harcourt Publishing Ltd., London, United Kingdom.
3. **Blatt, S. P., C. W. Hendrix, C. A. Butzin, T. M. Freeman, W. W. Ward, R. E. Hensley, G. P. Melcher, D. J. Donovan, and R. N. Boswell.** 1993. Delayed-type hypersensitivity skin testing predicts progression to AIDS in HIV-infected patients. *Ann. Intern. Med.* **119:**177–184.
4. **Carrodeguas, L., C. G. Orosz, W. J. Waldman, D. D. Sedmak, P. W. Adams, and A. M. Vanbuskirk.** 1999. Trans vivo analysis of human delayed-type hypersensitivity reactivity. *Hum. Immunol.* **60:**640–651.
5. **Centers for Disease Control and Prevention.** 1997. Anergy skin testing and preventive therapy for HIV-infected persons: revised recommendation. *Morb. Mortal. Wkly. Rep.* **46:**1–10.
6. **Chandra, R. K.** 2002. Nutrition and the immune system from birth to old age. *Eur. J. Clin. Nutr.* **56** (Suppl. 3)**:**s73–s76.
7. **Chu, C. Q., M. Field, F. Andrew, D. Haskard, M. Feldmann, and R. N. Maini.** 1992. Detection of cytokines at the site of tuberculin-induced delayed-type hypersensitivity in man. *Clin. Exp. Immunol.* **90:**522–529.
8. **Colebunders, R. L., I. Lebughe, N. Nzila, D. Kalunga, H. Francis, R. Ryder, and P. Piot.** 1989. Cutaneous delayed-type hypersensitivity in patients with human immunodeficiency virus infection in Zaire. *J. Acquir. Immune Defic. Syndr.* **2:**576–578.
9. **Connick, E., M. M. Lederman, B. L. Kotzin, J. Spritzler, D. R. Kuritzkes, M. St. Clair, A. D. Sevin, L. Fox, M. Heath-Chiozzi, J. M. Leonard, F. Rousseau, J. D'Arc Roe, A. Martinez, H. Kessler, and A. Landay.** 2000. Immune reconstitution in the first year of potent antiretroviral therapy and its relationship to virologic response. *J. Infect. Dis.* **181:**358–363.
10. **Crowe, A. J.** 1975. Delayed hypersensitivity in the mouse. *Adv. Immunol.* **20:**97.
11. **Dhabbar, F. S., A. R. Satoskar, H. Bluethmann, J. R. David, and B. S. McEwen.** 2000. Stress-induced enhancement of skin immune function: a role for γ-interferon. *Proc. Natl. Acad. Sci. USA* **97:**2846–2851.
12. **Dhalen, I., E. Lindberg, C. Janson, and G. Stalenheim.** 1999. Delayed type of hypersensitivity and late allergic reactions in patients with stable COPD. *Chest* **116:**1625–1631.
13. **England, R. W., J. S. Nugent, K. W. Grathwohl, L. Hagan, and J. M. Quinn.** 2003. High dose inhaled Fluticasone and delayed hypersensitivity skin testing. *Chest* **1234:**1014–1017.
14. **Fava-Netto, C., W. Gambale, J. Croce, C. R. Paula, and S. de C. Fava.** 1996. Candidin: comparison of two antigens for cutaneous delayed hypersensitivity testing. *Rev. Inst. Med. Trop. Sao Paulo* **38:**397–399.
15. **Fleisher, T. A., and J. B. Oliveira.** 2004. Functional and molecular evaluation of lymphocytes. *J. Allergy Clin. Immunol.* **114:**227–234.
16. **French, M. A. H., P. U. Cameron, G. Grimsley, L. A. Smyth, and R. L. Dawkins.** 1990. Correction of human immunodeficiency virus-associated depression of delayed-type hypersensitivity (DTH) after zidovudine therapy: DTH, CD4+ T-cell numbers, and epidermal langerhans cell density are independent variables. *Clin. Immunol. Immunopathol.* **55:**86–96.
17. **Gordin, F. M., P. M. Hartigan, N. G. Klimas, S. B. Zolla-Pazner, M. S. Simberkoff, and J. D. Hamilton.** 1994. Delayed-type hypersensitivity skin tests are an independent predictor of human immunodeficiency virus disease progression. *J. Infect. Dis.* **169:**893–897.
18. **Gordin, F. M., J. P. Matts, C. Miller, L. S. Brown, R. Hafner, S. L. John, M. Klein, A. Vaughn, C. L. Besch, G. Perez, S. Szabo, and W. El-Sadr.** 1997. A controlled trial of isoniazid in persons with anergy and human immunodeficiency virus infection who are at high risk for tuberculosis. Terry Beirn community programs for clinical research on AIDS. *N. Engl. J. Med.* **337:**315–320.
19. **Gourevitch, M. N., D. Hartel, E. E. Schoenbaum, and R. S. Klein.** 1996. Lack of association of induration size with HIV infection among drug users reacting to tuberculin. *Am. J. Respir. Crit. Care Med.* **154:**1029–1033.
20. **Gringeri, A., E. Santagostino, M. Muca-Perja, P. M. Mannucci, J. F. Zagury, B. Bizzini, A. Lachgar, M. Carcagno, J. Rappaport, M. Criscuolo, W. Blattner, A. Burney, R. C. Gallo, and D. Zagury.** 1998. Safety and immunogenicity of HIV-1 Tat toxoid in immunocompromised HIV-1 infected patients. *J. Hum. Virol.* **1:**293–298.
21. **Heubner, R. E., M. F. Schein, C. A. Hall, and S. A. Barnes.** 1994. Delayed-type hypersensitivity anergy in human immunodeficiency virus-infected persons screened for infection with *Mycobacterium tuberculosis. Clin. Infect. Dis.* **19:**26–32.
22. **Hickie, C., I. Hickie, D. Silove, D. Wakefield, and A. Lloyd.** 1995. Delayed-type hypersensitivity skin testing: normal values in the Australian population. *Int. J. Immunopharmacol.* **17:**629–634.
23. **Hoft, D. F., and J. M. Tennant.** 1999. Persistence and boosting of Bacille Calmette-Guerin-induced delayed-type hypersensitivity. *Ann. Intern. Med.* **131:**32–36.
24. **Howard, A., P. Mercer, H. C. Nataraj, and B. C. Kang.** 1997. Bevel-down superior to bevel-up in intradermal skin testing. *Ann. Allergy Asthma Immunol.* **78:**594–596.
25. **Itano, A. A., S. J. McSorley, R. L. Reinhardt, B. D. Ehst, E. Ingulli, A. Rudensky, and M. K. Jenkins.** 2003. Distinct dendritic cell populations sequentially present antigen to CD4 T cells and stimulate different aspects of cell-mediated immunity. *Immunity* **19:**47–57.
26. **Katzenstein, D. A., S. Kundu, J. Spritzler, B. R. Smoller, P. Haszlett, F. Valentine, and T. C. Merigan.** 1999. Delayed-type hypersensitivity to recombinant HIV envelope glycoprotein (rgpl60) after immunization with homologous antigen. *J. Acquir. Immune Defic. Syndr.* **22:**341–347.
27. **Kaufmann, S. H. E.** 2003. Immunity to intracellular bacteria, p. 1229–1261. *In* W. E. Paul (ed.), *Fundamental*

Immunology, 5th ed. Lippincott Williams & Wilkins, Philadelphia, Pa.

28. **Kay, A. B., J. Ravetch, J. G. J. van de Winkel, and S. J. Galli.** 1999. Allergy and hypersensitivity, p. 461–488. *In* C. A. Janeway, P. Travers, and M. Walport (ed.), *Immunobiology: the Immune System in Health and Disease*, 4th ed. Elsevier Science Ltd./Garland Publishing, London, United Kingdom.

29. **Klein, R. S., T. Flanigan, P. Schuman, D. Smith, and D. Vlahov.** 1999. Criteria for assessing cutaneous anergy in women with or at risk for HIV infection. *J. Allergy Clin. Immunol.* **103:**93–98.

30. **Klein, R. S., J. Sobel, T. Flanigan, D. Smith, and J. B. Margolick.** 1999. Stability of cutaneous anergy in women with or at high risk for HIV infection. *J. Acquir. Immune Defic. Syndr. Hum. Retrovirol.* **20:**238–244.

31. **Kobayashi, K., K. Kaneda, and T. Kasama.** 2001. Immunopathogenesis of delayed-type hypersensitivity. *Microsc. Res. Tech.* **15:**241–245.

32. **Lesourd, B. M., A. Wang, and R. Moulias.** 1985. Serial delayed cutaneous hypersensitivity skin testing with multiple recall antigens in healthy volunteers: booster effect study. *Ann. Allergy* **55:**729–735.

33. **Maas, J. J., M. T. L. Roos, I. P. M. Keet, E. A. M. Mensen, A. Krol, J. Veenstra, P. T. A. Schellekens, S. Jurriaans, R. A. Coutinho, and F. Miedema.** 1998. In vivo delayed-type hypersensitivity skin test anergy in human immunodeficiency virus type I infection is associated with T cell nonresponsiveness in vitro. *J. Infect. Dis.* **178:**1024–1029.

34. **Markowitz, N., N. I. Hansen, T. C. Wilcosky, P. C. Hopewell, J. Glassroth, P. A. Kvale, B. T. Mangura, D. Osmond, J. M. Wallace, M. J. Rosen, and L. B. Reichman.** 1993. Tuberculin and anergy testing in HIV-seropositive and HIV-seronegative persons. *Ann. Intern. Med.* **119:**185–193.

35. **Miller, S. D., and H. E. Jones.** 1974. Correlation of lymphocyte transformation with tuberculin skin-test reactivity. *Am. Rev. Respir. Dis.* **107:**530–538.

36. **Miller, W. C., N. M. Thielman, N. Swai, J. P. Cegielski, J. Shao, D. Ting, J. Mlalasi, D. Manyenga, and G. J. Lallinger.** 1996. Delayed-type hypersensitivity testing in Tanzania adults with HIV infection. *J. Acquir. Immune Defic. Syndr.* **12:**303–308.

37. **Mofenson, L. M., E. M. Rodriguez, R. Hershow, H. E. Fox, S. Landesman, R. Tuomala, C. Diaz, E. Daniels, and D. Brambilla.** 1995. *Mycobacterium tuberculosis* infection in pregnant and nonpregnant women infected with HIV in the women and infants transmission study. *Arch. Intern. Med.* **155:**1066–1072.

38. **Morrow, R., J. Fanta, and S. Kerlin.** 1997. Tuberculosis screening and anergy in a homeless population. *J. Am. Board Fam. Pract.* **10:**1–5.

39. **Pais, T. F., R. A. Silva, B. Smedegaard, R. Appelberg, and P. Anderson.** 1998. Analysis of T cells recruited during delayed-type hypersensitivity to purified protein derivative (PPD) versus challenge with tuberculosis infection. *Immunology* **95:**69–75.

40. **Platt, J. L., B. W. Grant, A. A. Eddy, et al.** 1983. Immune cell populations in cutaneous delayed-type hypersensitivity. *J. Exp. Med.* **58:**1227.

41. **Sears, S. D., R. Fox, R. Brookmeyer, R. Leavitt, and B. F. Polk.** 1987. Delayed hypersensitivity skin testing and anergy in a population of gay men. *Clin. Immunol. Immunopathol.* **45:**177–183.

42. **Selwyn, P. A., B. M. Sckell, P. Alcabes, G. H. Friedland, R. S. Klein, and E. E. Schoenbaum.** 1992. High risk of active tuberculosis in HIV-infected drug users with cutaneous anergy. *JAMA* **268:**504–509.

43. **Shearer, W. T., R. H. Buckley, R. J. M. Engler, A. F. Finn, T. A. Fleisher, T. M. Freeman, H. G. Herrod, A. I. Levinson, M. Lopez, R. R. Rich, S. I. Rosenfeld, and L. J. Rosenwasser.** 1996. Practice parameters for the diagnosis and management of immunodeficiency. *Ann. Allergy Asthma Immunol.* **76:**282–294.

44. **Shearer, W. T.** 1999. Monitoring cellular immune function in HIV infection by the delayed hypersensitivity skin test: alternative to the CD4+ T-cell count? *J. Allergy Clin. Immunol.* **103:**26–28.

45. **Skoner, D. P., B. L. Angelini, A. Jones, J. Seroky, W. J. Doyle, and P. Fireman.** 1996. Suppression of in vivo cell-mediated immunity during experimental influenza A virus infection of adults. *Int. J. Pediatr. Otorhinolaryngol.* **20:** 143–153.

46. **Smith, A. J., U. Vollmer-Conna, B. Bennett, I. B. Hickie, and A. R. Lloyd.** 2004. Influences of distress and alcohol consumption on the development of a delayed-type hypersensitivity skin test response. *Psychosom. Med.* **664:** 614–619.

47. **Trinchieri, G.** 1995. Interleukin 12: a proinflammatory cytokine with immunoregulatory functions that bridge innate resistance and antigen-specific adaptive immunity. *Annu. Rev. Immunol.* **13:**251–276.

48. **Valdez, H., K. Y. Smith, A. Landay, E. Connick, D. R. Kuritzkes, H. Kessler, L. Fox, J. Spritzer, J. Roe, M. B. Lederman, H. M. Lederman, T. G. Evans, M. Heath-Chiozzi, M. M. Lederman, and the ACTG 375 Team.** 2000. Response to immunization with recall and neoantigens after prolonged administration of an HIV-1 protease inhibitor-containing regimen. *AIDS* **14:**11–21.

49. **Wendland, T., H. Furrer, P. L. Vernazza, K. Frutig, A. Christen, L. Matter, R. Malinverni, and W. J. Pichler.** 1999. HAART in HIV-infected patients: restoration of antigen-specific CD T-cell responses in vitro is correlated with CD4 memory T-cell reconstitution, whereas improvement in delayed type hypersensitivity is related to a decrease in viraemia. *AIDS* **13:**1857–1862.

Cryopreservation of Peripheral Blood Mononuclear Cells

ADRIANA WEINBERG

27

The utility of cryopreserved peripheral blood mononuclear cells (PBMC) in clinical and diagnostic immunology is widely recognized. The use of cryopreserved PBMC offers multiple advantages for in vitro studies. The ability to batch specimens permits significant cost reductions through efficient utilization of labor and reagents and permits testing of multiple samples in a single run, thus avoiding interassay variability and providing more meaningful comparisons in longitudinal studies (3, 4).

Immunologic assays on cryopreserved PBMC provide important end points for large clinical trials of highly active antiretroviral therapy (HAART). The incidence of end-organ disease in human immunodeficiency virus (HIV)-infected patients has dramatically fallen since the introduction of HAART. The use of cryopreserved PBMC for the studies of immune reconstitution in these patients permits the selection of samples from well-characterized study subjects (1).

Transportation of frozen PBMC to laboratories for highly specialized tests has certain advantages over shipping of fresh blood (8). Certain populations of blood cells have a limited life span outside the human body, whereas cryopreserved PBMC are stable for prolonged periods when adequately stored or shipped in liquid nitrogen tanks.

Tests developed after the collection of clinical samples can be applied to cryopreserved PBMC. This allows for utilization of archived samples obtained from well-characterized study subjects to answer new scientific questions and avoids costly and unnecessary repetition of clinical studies (2).

Finally, cryopreserved PBMC are used to treat congenital or iatrogenic immune defects. For example, ex vivo generation of anti-cytomegalovirus (anti-CMV) and anti-Epstein-Barr virus cytotoxic T lymphocytes (CTL) can be used to protect stem cell transplant recipients.

The utility of cryopreserved cells depends on the viability and function retention of PBMC after freezing and thawing (7). To achieve optimal results in this respect, technical aspects are critical, but the intrinsic fragility of PBMC subpopulations can also play a role.

TECHNICAL ASPECTS OF PBMC CRYOPRESERVATION

The goal of the cryopreservation is to freeze and thaw the PBMC without compromising cell viability. Cryoprotective agents are essential in order to avoid water crystals and cell burst with freezing. Both glycerol and dimethyl sulfoxide (DMSO) can provide this function, but only DMSO has been extensively studied for cryopreservation of PBMC. Other critical steps of the cryopreservation procedure include inhibition of cell metabolism while in the presence of DMSO, rate-controlled freezing to avoid cell dehydration, rapid thawing, and resuspension in serum-containing medium, which protects the cells against osmotic trauma.

Ficoll-Hypaque-separated PBMC are washed at 4°C, counted, and resuspended at 10^7 PBMC/ml in cold fetal calf serum containing 10% DMSO. The cell suspension is aliquoted into cryovials kept on ice, which are then inserted into a Nalgene Mr. Frosty freezing apparatus or a Cryomed freezing chamber (2). The cells are gradually cooled at a rate of -1°C/min during the first 24 h and are then transferred into liquid nitrogen tanks for prolonged storage. For thawing, the cryovials are incubated with agitation in a 37°C water bath until almost all the cryovial content has become fluid. The cell suspension is then transferred to a 15-ml polypropylene conical tube, and warm RPMI containing 10% fetal calf or human AB serum is slowly added, at a rate of approximately 1 ml/min for the first 5 min, and then another 5 to 10 ml of medium is rapidly added. Benzonase (Novagen) or other DNases can be added to the thawing medium to avoid excessive clumping. While the use of these products may improve PBMC recovery, it does not affect viability or function. Thawed cells are washed two or three times by centrifugation, counted, and assessed for viability before being used in immunologic assays.

FUNCTIONAL ASSAYS USING CRYOPRESERVED PBMC

Lymphoproliferative Assays

Lymphoproliferative responses measure mainly CD4-dependent immune responses. Severely impaired CD4 responses confer broad immunodeficiency. More subtle CD4 deficits impair defenses against certain pathogens, such as viruses, mycobacteria, yeasts, and certain protozoa, that are highly dependent on cell-mediated immunity.

Several studies compared responder cell frequency and lymphocyte proliferation assays (LPAs), traditionally used to assess CD4 responses, with cryopreserved versus fresh PBMC collected from immunocompromised patients or healthy

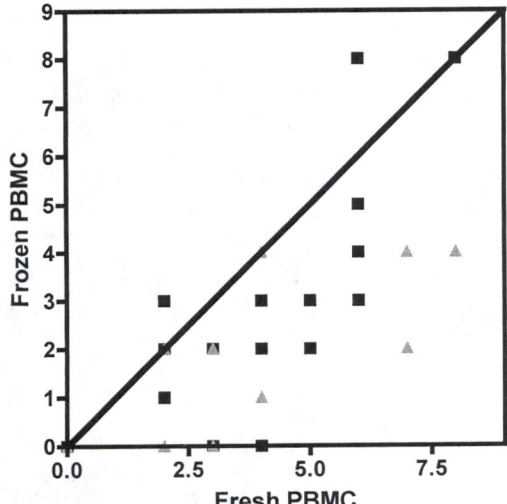

FIGURE 1 CMV-specific responder cell frequency (RCF) in cryopreserved versus fresh PBMC from HIV-infected patients (gray triangles) and uninfected controls (solid squares). The diagonal represents the slope of equivalence between fresh- and frozen-cell assays.

hosts. These investigations showed that antigen- and mitogen-induced proliferation of fresh and frozen cells was highly correlated, despite the loss of responders or decrease in stimulation indices in cryopreserved cells compared with fresh cells (Fig. 1). In Fig. 1, which shows a plot correlating CMV-specific responders in fresh and frozen PBMC, the majority of the data points fall below the line of equivalency, illustrating the loss of responders in cryopreserved preparations.

The viability of cryopreserved PBMC significantly affects the results of proliferative assays. The studies of normal hosts and HIV-infected patients illustrated in Fig. 2 show that a viability of ≥70% of cryopreserved PBMC is necessary to reproduce the LPA results obtained with fresh cells. In contrast, LPA responses of PBMC with a viability of <70% increase or decrease with the viability of the cell preparation, introducing a variable that is extraneous to the status of the cell donor. In addition, cell recovery of cryopreserved PBMC and CD4 cell numbers of the donor do not affect the result of lymphoproliferative responses in cryopreserved PBMC in comparison with fresh cells.

Cytotoxic Assays

Defenses against viral infections and malignancies rely predominantly on cyotoxic immune responses. Several studies of bone marrow transplant patients have shown that protective

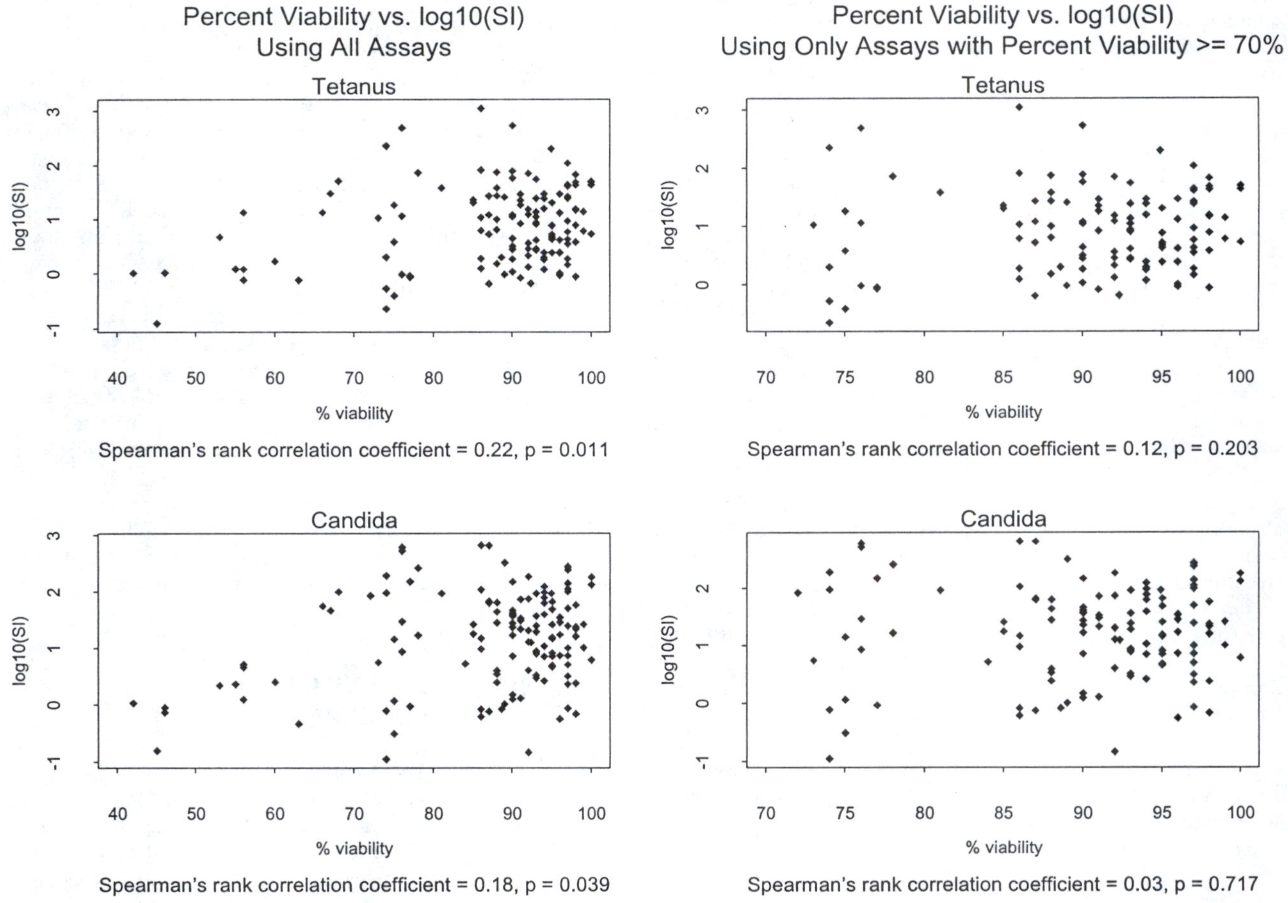

Percent Viability vs. log10(SI) Using All Assays

Tetanus

Spearman's rank correlation coefficient = 0.22, p = 0.011

Candida

Spearman's rank correlation coefficient = 0.18, p = 0.039

Percent Viability vs. log10(SI) Using Only Assays with Percent Viability >= 70%

Tetanus

Spearman's rank correlation coefficient = 0.12, p = 0.203

Candida

Spearman's rank correlation coefficient = 0.03, p = 0.717

FIGURE 2 Effect of viability on cryopreserved PBMC LPA results. Data were derived from samples from HIV-infected patients. The column on the left shows that when all samples were analyzed, the LPA results significantly increased with greater viability. A breakpoint in the distribution pattern can be observed at a viability of 70%. The column on the right shows that when only samples with a viability of ≥70% were analyzed, the LPA results were independent of the PBMC viability. SI, stimulation index.

immunity against CMV coincides with the return of specific CTL. Exogenous generation and transfusion of specific CTL can protect immunocompromised hosts against several viral infections and malignancies.

CTL activity of cryopreserved PBMC is comparable to that in fresh-cell assays. The use of cryopreserved PBMC allows for better scheduling of these complex assays which involve effector and target preparation.

Natural killer (NK) cell activity, in contrast to CTL, is more labile to freezing and thawing. Several investigators, but not all, have found significant losses of NK cell-mediated lysis following cryopreservation. Because of these conflicting data, the use of cryopreserved PBMC for NK cell assays is not recommended, unless carefully controlled experiments validate this procedure in the individual laboratory.

Cytokine-Based Assays

Cell-mediated responses are modulated by cytokines released by mononuclear phagocytes, NK cells, and T lymphocytes. These cytokines, which regulate many cell surface recognition molecules and affect the recruitment of inflammatory cells into an area of infection, are likely to play a pivotal role in the expression of cell-mediated immunity. PBMC produce a range of cytokines in tissue culture following mitogen and antigen stimulation, which have been used to characterize their functional status.

Inducible-cytokine assays measure the amount of cytokine released by stimulated PBMC in the culture supernatant. Studies of HIV-infected patients and uninfected controls show that gamma interferon (IFN-γ) production is essentially the same in fresh and cryopreserved PBMC (Fig. 3). There are conflicting data on interleukin 2 (IL-2) levels in frozen versus fresh cell cultures, and more studies are necessary to clarify this subject (6). However, the rank order correlation between either IFN-γ or IL-2 released by cryopreserved cells compared with fresh cells is highly significant, indicating that inducible-cytokine assays of cryopreserved cells are suitable for comparative analyses of the immune response, such as longitudinal observations.

Single-cell intracellular cytokine assays use flow cytometry to enumerate antigen- or mitogen-stimulated PBMC that synthesize cytokines. The single-cell intracellular cytokine assays provide a sensitive and specific indication of the cell mediated response. Furthermore, the single-cell assay can analyze the phenotype of the cytokine-producing cells, thus further characterizing the immune response. To date, the findings with frozen PBMC in these assays are similar to those for the inducible-cytokine assays; i.e., there is a strong correlation between the results with fresh and cryopreserved PBMC. However, additional studies are needed in order to fully evaluate the utility of frozen cells for these assays.

The enzyme-linked immunospot assay (ELISPOT) is yet another format for measuring cytokine-producing cells. This assay detects captured cytokines diffusing from single antigen- or mitogen-stimulated cells. The assay is extremely sensitive and versatile. It can be performed with fractionated PBMC, such as purified CD8 or CD4 cells. ELISPOT has traditionally measured IFN-γ-producing responder cells but can be adapted to detect other cytokines. The IFN-γ ELISPOT is commonly performed on cryopreserved PBMC because the results are comparable to those obtained with fresh cells and there are considerable cost savings when assays are done in batches.

SURFACE MARKERS ON CRYOPRESERVED PBMC

Immune Phenotyping by Flow Cytometry

Enumeration of PBMC subsets by flow cytometry provides important information on the immune capacity of the host. As such, flow cytometry-based immune phenotyping is a standard procedure in the evaluation of immunodeficiency disorders. The distribution of major surface markers, such as CD3, CD4, CD8, CD19, and CD14, is essentially unchanged by cryopreservation (4, 5). The percentages of T-cell subsets in fresh and cryopreserved PBMC typically show statistically significant correlations, despite the fact that fresh-cell assays are typically performed with whole blood, whereas frozen-cell assays use PBMC separated by Ficoll-Hypaque. The percentage of cells bearing certain immune phenotypic markers (CD4, CD8, etc.) was stable over many decades of frozen PBMC storage in the multicenter AIDS cohort study (MACS) cohort (3). As with the LPA, cell recovery does not influence the distribution of T-cell phenotypes in cryopreserved PBMC. Furthermore, results of phenotyping of cryopreserved PBMC are stable across a wide range of baseline CD4 cell numbers, demonstrating the robustness of this complex procedure.

Cell membrane markers used for advanced immunophenotyping, such as CD21, CD22, CD28, CD38, HLA DR, CD95 (Fig. 4A), and CD45RA and RO, are well preserved during the freezing and thawing processes. In contrast, CD62L, which is commonly used for the identification of naïve T-cell populations, is present in significantly smaller amounts on the surface of cryopreserved PBMC than on fresh PBMC (Fig. 4B). Hence, it is desirable to avoid the use of anti-CD62L monoclonal antibodies for advanced immunophenotyping of cryopreserved PBMC.

T-Cell Receptor Vβ Repertoire

Definition of the T-cell receptor repertoire has become increasingly prevalent in studies of the maturation and senescence of the immune system. These assays can provide valuable information about immune deficiency stages and immune restoration. Flow cytometry- and PCR-based methods are

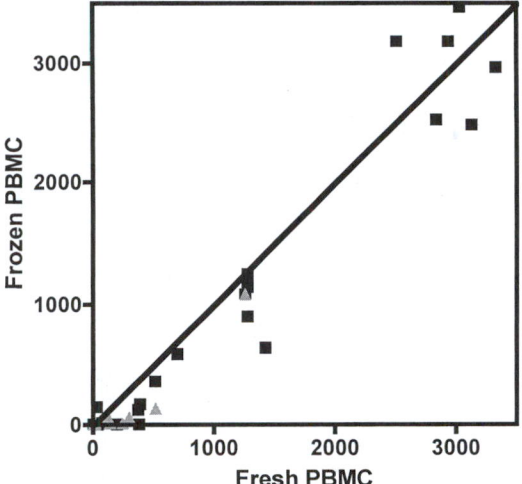

FIGURE 3 CMV-specific IFN-γ in cryopreserved versus fresh PBMC from HIV-infected patients (gray triangles) and uninfected controls (solid squares). The diagonal represents the slope of equivalence between the fresh- and frozen-cell assays.

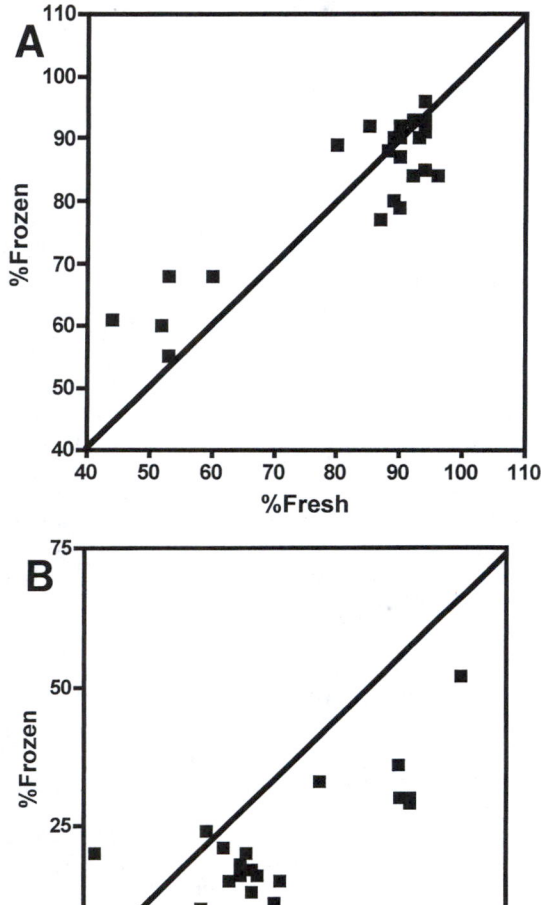

used for T-cell receptor characterization. The two techniques seem to yield similar results when performed with fresh and cryopreserved PBMC.

Anne Sevin (deceased) performed the statistical analysis of the data presented in Fig. 2 and prepared the illustration.

REFERENCES

1. **Autran, B., G. Carcelain, T. S. Li, C. Blanc, D. Mathez, R. Tubiana, C. Katlama, P. Debre, and J. Leibowitch.** 1997. Positive effects of combined antiretroviral therapy on CD4+ T cell homeostasis and function in advanced HIV disease. *Science* **277**:112–116.

2. **Hviid, L., G. Albeck, B. Hansen, T. G. Theander, and A. Talbot.** 1993. A new portable device for automatic controlled-gradient cryopreservation of blood mononuclear cells. *J. Immunol. Methods* **157**:135–142.

3. **Kleeberger, C. A., R. H. Lyles, J. B. Margolick, C. R. Rinaldo, J. P. Phair, and J. V. Giorgi.** 1999. Viability and recovery of peripheral blood mononuclear cells cryopreserved for up to 12 years in multicenter study. *Clin. Diagn. Lab. Immunol.* **6**:14–19.

4. **Reimann, K. A., M. Chernoff, C. Wilkening, C. Nickerson, A. Landay, and the ACTG Immunology Advanced Technology Laboratories.** 2000. Preservation of lymphocyte immunophenotype and proliferative responses in cryopreserved peripheral blood mononuclear cells from HIV-1-infected donors: implications for multicenter clinical trials. *Clin. Diagn. Lab. Immunol.* **7**:352–359.

5. **Sleasman, J. W., B. H. Leon, L. F. Aleixo, M. Rojas, and M. M. Goodenow.** 1997. Immunomagnetic selection of purified monocyte and lymphocyte populations from peripheral blood mononuclear cells following cryopreservation. *Clin. Diagn. Lab. Immunol.* **4**:653–658.

6. **Ventakaraman, M.** 1992. Cryopreservation-induced enhancement of interleukin-2 production in human peripheral blood mononuclear cells. *Cryobiology* **29**:165–174.

7. **Weinberg, A., L. Zhang, D. Brown, A. Erice, B. Polsky, M. S. Hirsch, S. Owens, and K. Lamb for ACTG Team 360.** 2000. Viability and functional activity of cryopreserved mononuclear cells. *Clin. Diagn. Lab. Immunol.* **7**:714–716.

8. **Weinberg, A., R. Betensky, L. Zhang, and G. Ray.** 1998. Effect of shipment, storage, anticoagulant and cell separation on lymphoproliferative responses in HIV-infected patients. *Clin. Diagn. Lab. Immunol.* **5**:804–807.

FIGURE 4 Effect of cryopreservation on flow cytometric immune phenotyping. Data were derived from HIV-infected subjects. Cell membrane markers CD95 (A) and CD62L (B) were used. The diagonal represents the slope of equivalence between the fresh- and frozen-cell assays, which give identical results.

Methods for Detection of Antigen-Specific T Cells by Enzyme-Linked Immunospot Assay (ELISPOT)

BARBARA L. SHACKLETT AND DOUGLAS F. NIXON

28

CD3[+] CD8[+] T-cell receptor (TCR) αβ thymus-derived T cells form the major effector cell component of the immune response against a viral infection. Naïve CD8[+] T cells encounter antigen, expand, and divide, and effector cells mediate a range of antiviral functions. After the acute viral infection is contained, the number of active effector cells declines but antigen-specific memory CD8[+] T cells persist, ready to expand rapidly upon reexposure to antigen. Most CD8[+] antigen-specific T cells recognize viral antigen as a peptide presented by a major histocompatibility complex (MHC) class I molecule. The TCR of the antigen-specific CD8[+] cell interacts with the MHC class I viral peptide complex on the surface of the antigen-presenting cell.

Antigen-specific CD8[+] T cells can be detected by identification of a specific TCR which will interact with a unique MHC class I peptide complex or functionally through effector activities after stimulation with specific antigen. The traditional method for the detection of antigen-specific CD8[+] T cells has been the ^{51}Cr release assay. This assay detects the ability of an effector cell population to lyse a target cell population labeled with the gamma emitter [51]Cr. Over the past few years, other assays have been developed to study the antigen-specific CD8[+] T-cell response. These are generally easier to use and have become standard in the field. The assay most widely utilized is the enzyme-linked immunospot assay (ELISPOT). This assay detects the secretion of cytokine after specific stimulation, usually with a specific peptide or recombinant vaccinia virus with a foreign gene insert. The sensitivity of the assay has been estimated as 50 or fewer antigen-specific T cells per 10^6 lymphocytes, at least 1 log_{10} more sensitive than traditional limiting dilution analysis or bulk ^{51}Cr release assay (20).

The ELISPOT was first described in 1983 as an alternative to plaque-forming assays for the detection of antibody-secreting cells (9). In the initial report, spleen cells from immunized mice were incubated in antigen-coated, 96-well polystyrene plates. After removal of the cells, bound antibodies were detected by an immunoenzyme procedure. In areas of the plate where antibody production had occurred, the substrate was deposited in circular zones (spots), which could then be enumerated with the naked eye (9). It was not long before the ELISPOT was modified for the detection of cytokine-secreting T cells, by use of nitrocellulose membranes and cytokine-specific monoclonal antibodies (MAbs) (8). A survey of the recent literature reveals that ELISPOT is now widely used to detect T-cell responses to autoantigens, tumor antigens, and antigens from a variety of infectious agents. ELISPOT has also become the method of choice for rapid mapping of T-cell epitopes (1, 3).

ELISPOT PROTOCOL

The protocol given below is for the detection and enumeration of gamma interferon (IFN-γ)-secreting T cells from human immunodeficiency virus type 1 (HIV-1)-infected subjects after specific stimulation of peripheral blood mononuclear cells (PBMC) with recombinant vaccinia viruses (rVVs) expressing HIV-1 gene products (16). This assay may be adapted for use with synthetic peptides, including overlapping peptide pools, as described elsewhere (1, 3).

Day 1: Coating of ELISPOT Plates

1. Mix 25 μl of anti-IFN-γ MAb clone 1-DIK (1 mg/ml; Mabtech no. 3420-3) with 5 ml of sodium bicarbonate buffer (pH 9.6) (2.93 g of $NaHCO_3$, 1.59 g of Na_2CO_3, and 0.2% NaN_3 in a volume of 1 liter of H_2O, sterile filtered). (Note that some laboratories use standard phosphate-buffered saline [PBS] as a coating buffer.)

2. Add 50 μl of the above primary antibody solution to each well of a sterile MultiScreen 96-well filtration plate (Millipore no. MAHA S4510), ensuring that the bottom of each well is entirely covered; refrigerate at 4°C overnight. ELISPOT plates with hydrophobic polyvinylidene fluoride membranes may also be used; consult manufacturers' recommendations for use of these plates.

Note: coated plates must be left in the refrigerator for a minimum of 5 h or can remain at 4°C for up to 5 days before proceeding to the next step.

Day 2: Addition of Cells and Stimulating Antigen

3. Invert the plate to discard unbound primary antibody and pat down firmly onto paper towels to remove excess liquid from wells. Using a multichannel pipettor, add 200 μl of PBS (Cellgro) to each well. Avoid touching the bottom of wells with pipette tips. Invert the plate to discard liquid, and again pat down firmly onto paper towels. Repeat the above washing step with PBS three more times. (Note: plates may also be washed with a hand-held squirt bottle.)

4. Mix 5 ml of heat-inactivated pooled human serum (Biowhittaker) with 45 ml of RPMI 1640 (Cellgro), and subject to sterile filtration. Add 50 μl of the above blocking

solution to each well and incubate the plate at 37°C under 5% CO_2 for 1 h.

5. While the plate is incubating in blocking solution, prepare cells for addition to the plate. Either fresh or frozen PBMC can be used. Usually 1×10^5 to 2×10^5 cells are required per well, and each condition is assayed in triplicate (for example, an assay in which responses to the HIV antigens Env, Gag, Pol, and Nef are being measured will require 4×3 wells in addition to triplicate background and one positive control well [4 additional wells]; if the optimal 2×10^5 cells are added per well, 3.2×10^6 cells are required). Frozen cells can be thawed, or fresh PBMC can be isolated from whole blood; the cells are washed three times in RPMI 1640 supplemented with 15% fetal calf serum and resuspended in 5% pooled human serum solution (same as blocking solution in step 4) at a concentration of 1×10^5 to 2×10^5 cells per 100 μl.

6. After the 1-h incubation in step 4, add 100 μl of cell suspension to each well. It is not necessary to remove the blocking solution.

7. If using rVV to stimulate cells, add to appropriate wells at a multiplicity of infection of 2. Note: for consistency it is recommended that all rVVs be diluted to the same concentration; a versatile concentration is 2×10^8 rVVs/ml. If using peptide to stimulate cells, add peptide so that the final concentration of the peptide in each well (150 μl total volume) is 10 μg/ml. For a positive control, add phytohemagglutinin (PHA) to the well so that the final concentration of PHA is 10 μg/ml. Incubate the plate at 37°C under 5% CO_2 for 1 h. (If not using vaccinia viruses, incubate overnight at 37°C under 5% CO_2 and then proceed to step 9.)

8. If using vaccinia viruses, add 30 μl of filtered fetal calf serum (Gemini Bioproducts) to each well. Return the plate to the incubator at 37°C under 5% CO_2 and incubate overnight (14 to 20 h).

Day 3: Assay Development

9. Aspirate the contents of each well, being careful not to touch the membrane at the bottom of the well. Add 200 μl of 0.05% Tween solution to each well (250 μl of Tween 20, 500 ml of PBS). Invert the plate to discard washing solution and pat firmly on paper towels to remove excess liquid from wells. Repeat the washing step three more times.

10. Mix 5 μl of biotin-conjugated anti-IFN-γ MAb clone 7-B6-1 (1 mg/ml; Mabtech no. 3420-6) with 5 ml of PBS (Cellgro). Add 50 μl of the above secondary antibody solution to each well and incubate the plate at 37°C under 5% CO_2 for 2 h.

11. Twenty minutes before the end of the 2-h incubation, prepare the avidin-peroxidase complex solution (Vectastain ABC kit, Vector Laboratories Elite PK-6100 Standard). Add 1 drop each of solutions A and B to 5 ml of 0.1% Tween solution (the washing solution used in step 12). This complex must be prepared at least 20 min prior to use.

12. Invert the plate to discard unbound secondary antibody and pat firmly on paper towels to remove excess

liquid from wells. Add 200 μl of 0.1% Tween solution to each well (500 μl of Tween 20, 500 ml of PBS). Discard the wash solution as described above and repeat the washing step three more times.

13. Add 50 μl of this ABC solution (prepared in step 11) to each well and incubate the plate at room temperature on a flat surface for 1 h.

14. Wash the wells four times as in step 12.

15. Add 50 μl of stable diaminobenzidine (DAB) (ResGen/Invitrogen no. 750118) to each well. Incubate at room temperature for 5 min on a flat surface.

16. Invert the plate to discard DAB into sink. Rinse the wells thoroughly with tap water three times. Remove the plastic underdrain, wipe the back of the plate gently with absorbent paper towels, and allow the plate to air dry. Count spots under an inverted microscope or with the aid of an automated reader (AID, Autoimmun Diagnostika, distributed by Cell Technology, Inc., Columbia, Md.).

17. Analyze ELISPOT data by subtracting the average number of spot-forming cells (SFC) in triplicate background wells (stimulated by media alone) from the average number of SFC in test wells. Convert the result to SFC per 10^6 cells by multiplying by 5 (in the case of 2×10^5 cells/well) or 10 (in the case of 1×10^5 cells/well).

METHODS OF ENHANCING ELISPOT SENSITIVITY

In an effort to increase the sensitivity of ELISPOT, several groups have developed modifications of the standard protocol involving the addition of exogenous cytokines, costimulatory antibodies, or antigen-presenting cells. A partial listing of these methods is given in Table 1; for additional details, the references should be consulted.

QUALITY CONTROL AND ASSAY VALIDATION

The ELISPOT is relatively new, and considerable methodological variation exists among laboratories. However, in recent years, there has been an effort to standardize procedures in view of initiating large-scale clinical trials (4, 12, 13, 18, 20).

As a positive control for cytokine release, many laboratories rely on polyclonal stimuli (PHA or staphylococcal enterotoxin B). However, these reagents may give rise to a nearly confluent lawn of spots. Recently, Currier et al. introduced a control peptide pool consisting of 23 peptides derived from influenza virus, cytomegalovirus, and Epstein-Barr virus, corresponding to known CD8 epitopes restricted by a variety of MHC class I alleles (7). This pool, known as CEF (cytomegalovirus–Epstein-Barr virus–flu), is recognized by approximately 85% of the general population and is available through the National Institutes of Health AIDS Research and Reference Reagent Program (http://www.aidsreagent.org).

The quality of ELISPOT results may be affected by cell viability, cell concentration, addition of antigen-presenting cells,

TABLE 1 Methods of enhancing ELISPOT sensitivity

Method	Comments	Reference(s)
Costimulatory antibodies	May increase background	Ott et al. (19)
Monocyte-derived dendritic cells	Mature dendritic cells are more efficient than immature dendritic cells	Larsson et al. (17)
B cells	May increase background	Altfeld et al. (2)
IL-7, IL-15	May increase background	Calarota et al. (5), Chitnis et al. (6), Jennes et al. (14)

TABLE 2 Parameters influencing ELISPOT variability

Parameter	Comments	Reference(s)
Background	Assays with background of >120 SFC/10⁶ cells considered invalid	Mwau et al. (18)
Cell no. (PBMC)	Optimal no. is 2×10^5/well	Russell et al. (20)
Cryopreservation	Average recovery, 60%; viability, 90%. Positive responses remain detectable. Magnitude of responses is diminished. Controlled stepwise freezing is optimal.	Russell et al. (20) Russell et al. (20) Mwau et al. (18) Mwau et al. (18)
Detection threshold	50 SFC/10⁶ PBMC (0.005%)	Russell et al. (20)
ELISPOT reader	Automated readers superior to manual counting	Herr et al. (11), Janetzki et al. (13)
Incubation time	16–20 h	Russell et al. (20)
Peptide preparations	Dimethyl sulfoxide, <1%. Optimal length: 15-mers. Effect of concn: 2 μg/ml adequate; 5–10 μg/ml maximal; 20 μg/ml inhibitory. Peptides should be filtered.	Mwau et al. (18), Russell et al. (20) Russell et al. (20) Russell et al. (20) Karlsson et al. (15)
Vaccinia viruses	Titer on susceptible cell line. Routinely verify expression of foreign protein by Western blotting.	Larsson et al. (16)

source of stimulating antigen, length of stimulating peptides, dimethyl sulfoxide content of peptide preparations, infectivity of vaccinia virus stocks, operator variability, reader variability, and numerous other factors. These issues are addressed in detail by several recent reports, as shown in Table 2.

INTERPRETING ELISPOT DATA: ESTABLISHING BACKGROUND LEVELS AND IDENTIFYING POSITIVE RESPONSES

Statistical methods for evaluating ELISPOT results and determining the appropriate positive cutoff have varied considerably between laboratories. Although many research laboratories continue to rely on empirical approaches, several recent reviews have addressed the need to standardize ELISPOT data analysis for phase I and II clinical trials. A summary of statistical methods reported in the recent literature is given in Table 3.

RESEARCH AND CLINICAL APPLICATIONS OF THE ELISPOT

Since the first reports describing the T-cell ELISPOT nearly 20 years ago, ELISPOT has been used to detect T-cell responses to autoantigens, tumor antigens, and antigens from a variety of infectious agents including bacteria, viruses, and protozoa. An expanding variety of individual antibodies, matched reagent sets, detection reagents, and complete kits are now manufactured commercially, and new ELISPOT products are continuing to be introduced at a rapid rate. As of this writing, reagent sets and/or kits are commercially available to assess the following molecules: interleukin 1β (IL-1β), IL-2, IL-4, IL-5, IL-8, IL-10, IL-12, IL-13, IL-16, IFN-γ, granulocyte-macrophage colony-stimulating factor, tumor necrosis factor alpha, transforming growth factor β, RANTES/CCL5, MIG/CXCL9, granzyme B, perforin, and sFAS ligand. However, the majority of these assays are currently limited to research settings.

Nevertheless, as ELISPOT technology becomes more accessible, sponsors of phase I and II clinical trials are expected to become increasingly reliant on this sensitive, rapid method to assess T-cell responses. ELISPOT is now widely utilized in research on infectious diseases, autoimmunity, and cancer immunotherapy. As novel vaccines and immunotherapies move into the development pipeline, ELISPOTs will require standardization and validation appropriate to large-scale clinical trials. International efforts

TABLE 3 Methods of analyzing ELISPOT data

Data analysis method	Reference
Empirical approaches	
Positive response: >3× mean of negative control wells and >50 SFC/10⁶ PBMC	Addo et al. (1)
Positive response: >2× mean of background wells and >20 SFC/10⁶ PBMC	Currier et al. (7)
Positive response: >5 more SFC/well than in negative controls and >2× mean of negative control wells	Ewer et al. (10)
Positive response: >2× average of background wells and >50 SFC/10⁶ PBMC	Mwau et al. (18)
Statistical approaches	
Unpaired *t* test to determine whether SFC are significantly greater in test wells than controls	Herr et al. (11)
Exact binomial test to determine whether SFC are significantly greater in test wells than controls	Russell et al. (20)
Comparison of several statistical methods; a permutation-based criterion using a resampling adjustment for multiple comparisons is recommended	Hudgens et al. (12)

are already under way to standardize ELISPOT methodology for large-scale HIV vaccine trials (12, 18, 20). Other areas currently under development include an ELISPOT-based screen for tuberculosis (10) and ELISPOTs to monitor clinical trials for melanoma therapeutics (4). Standardization and validation of any bioassay is a lengthy process and will require many multicenter studies. As ELISPOT readers continue to improve and statistical methods achieve broader acceptance, the trend towards increasing standardization is likely to accelerate rapidly within the next few years.

REFERENCES

1. Addo, M. M., X. G. Yu, A. Rathod, D. Cohen, R. L. Eldridge, D. Strick, M. N. Johnston, C. Corcoran, A. G. Wurcel, C. A. Fitzpatrick, M. E. Feeney, W. R. Rodriguez, N. Basgoz, R. Draenert, D. R. Stone, C. Brander, P. J. Goulder, E. S. Rosenberg, M. Altfeld, and B. D. Walker. 2003. Comprehensive epitope analysis of human immunodeficiency virus type 1 (HIV-1)-specific T-cell responses directed against the entire expressed HIV-1 genome demonstrates broadly directed responses, but no correlation to viral load. *J. Virol.* **77:**2081–2092.

2. Altfeld, M. A., A. Trocha, R. L. Eldridge, E. S. Rosenberg, M. N. Phillips, M. M. Addo, R. P. Sekaly, S. A. Kalams, S. A. Burchett, K. McIntosh, B. D. Walker, and P. J. Goulder. 2000. Identification of dominant optimal HLA-B60- and HLA-B61-restricted cytotoxic T-lymphocyte (CTL) epitopes: rapid characterization of CTL responses by enzyme-linked immunospot assay. *J. Virol.* **74:**8541–8549.

3. Anthony, D. D., and P. V. Lehmann. 2003. T-cell epitope mapping using the ELISPOT approach. *Methods* **29:**260–269.

4. Asai, T., W. J. Storkus, and T. L. Whiteside. 2000. Evaluation of the modified ELISPOT assay for gamma interferon production in cancer patients receiving antitumor vaccines. *Clin. Diagn. Lab. Immunol.* **7:**145–154.

5. Calarota, S. A., M. Otero, K. Hermanstayne, M. Lewis, M. Rosati, B. K. Felber, G. N. Pavlakis, J. D. Boyer, and D. B. Weiner. 2003. Use of interleukin 15 to enhance interferon-gamma production by antigen-specific stimulated lymphocytes from rhesus macaques. *J. Immunol. Methods* **279:**55–67.

6. Chitnis, V., R. Pahwa, and S. Pahwa. 2003. Determinants of HIV-specific CD8 T-cell responses in HIV-infected pediatric patients and enhancement of HIV-gag-specific responses with exogenous IL-15. *Clin. Immunol.* **107:**36–45.

7. Currier, J. R., E. G. Kuta, E. Turk, L. B. Earhart, L. Loomis-Price, S. Janetzki, G. Ferrari, D. L. Birx, and J. H. Cox. 2002. A panel of MHC class I restricted viral peptides for use as a quality control for vaccine trial ELISPOT assays. *J. Immunol. Methods* **260:**157–172.

8. Czerkinsky, C., G. Andersson, H. P. Ekre, L. A. Nilsson, L. Klareskog, and O. Ouchterlony. 1988. Reverse ELISPOT assay for clonal analysis of cytokine production. I. Enumeration of gamma-interferon-secreting cells. *J. Immunol. Methods* **110:**29–36.

9. Czerkinsky, C. C., L. A. Nilsson, H. Nygren, O. Ouchterlony, and A. Tarkowski. 1983. A solid-phase enzyme-linked immunospot (ELISPOT) assay for enumeration of specific antibody-secreting cells. *J. Immunol. Methods* **65:**109–121.

10. Ewer, K., J. Deeks, L. Alvarez, G. Bryant, S. Waller, P. Andersen, P. Monk, and A. Lalvani. 2003. Comparison of T-cell-based assay with tuberculin skin test for diagnosis of Mycobacterium tuberculosis infection in a school tuberculosis outbreak. *Lancet* **361:**1168–1173.

11. Herr, W., B. Linn, N. Leister, E. Wandel, K. H. Meyer zum Buschenfelde, and T. Wolfel. 1997. The use of computer-assisted video image analysis for the quantification of CD8^{+} T lymphocytes producing tumor necrosis factor alpha spots in response to peptide antigens. *J. Immunol. Methods* **203:**141–152.

12. Hudgens, M. G., S. G. Self, Y. L. Chiu, N. D. Russell, H. Horton, and M. J. McElrath. 2004. Statistical considerations for the design and analysis of the ELISpot assay in HIV-1 vaccine trials. *J. Immunol. Methods* **288:**19–34.

13. Janetzki, S., S. Schaed, N. E. Blachere, L. Ben-Porat, A. N. Houghton, and K. S. Panageas. 2004. Evaluation of Elispot assays: influence of method and operator on variability of results. *J. Immunol. Methods* **291:**175–183.

14. Jennes, W., L. Kestens, D. F. Nixon, and B. L. Shacklett. 2002. Enhanced ELISPOT detection of antigen-specific T cell responses from cryopreserved specimens with addition of both IL-7 and IL-15—the Amplispot assay. *J. Immunol. Methods* **270:**99–108.

15. Karlsson, R. K., W. Jennes, K. Page-Shafer, D. F. Nixon, and B. L. Shacklett. 2004. Poorly soluble peptides can mimic authentic ELISPOT responses. *J. Immunol. Methods* **285:**89–92.

16. Larsson, M., X. Jin, B. Ramratnam, G. S. Ogg, J. Engelmayer, M. A. Demoitie, A. J. McMichael, W. I. Cox, R. M. Steinman, D. Nixon, and N. Bhardwaj. 1999. A recombinant vaccinia virus based ELISPOT assay detects high frequencies of Pol-specific CD8 T cells in HIV-1-positive individuals. *AIDS* **13:**767–777.

17. Larsson, M., D. T. Wilkens, J. F. Fonteneau, T. J. Beadle, M. J. Merritt, R. G. Kost, P. A. Haslett, S. Cu-Uvin, N. Bhardwaj, D. F. Nixon, and B. L. Shacklett. 2002. Amplification of low-frequency antiviral CD8 T cell responses using autologous dendritic cells. *AIDS* **16:**171–180.

18. Mwau, M., A. J. McMichael, and T. Hanke. 2002. Design and validation of an enzyme-linked immunospot assay for use in clinical trials of candidate HIV vaccines. *AIDS Res. Hum. Retroviruses* **18:**611–618.

19. Ott, P. A., B. R. Berner, B. A. Herzog, R. Guerkov, N. L. Yonkers, I. Durinovic-Bello, M. Tary-Lehmann, P. V. Lehmann, and D. D. Anthony. 2004. CD28 costimulation enhances the sensitivity of the ELISPOT assay for detection of antigen-specific memory effector CD4 and CD8 cell populations in human diseases. *J. Immunol. Methods* **285:**223–235.

20. Russell, N. D., M. G. Hudgens, R. Ha, C. Havenar-Daughton, and M. J. McElrath. 2003. Moving to human immunodeficiency virus type 1 vaccine efficacy trials: defining T cell responses as potential correlates of immunity. *J. Infect. Dis.* **187:**226–242.

Evaluation of the T-Cell Receptor Repertoire

SAVITA PAHWA

29

During the process of differentiation in the thymus, T cells undergo rearrangement of their T-cell receptor (TCR) genes and mature into single positive cells of either the CD4+ or the CD8+ phenotype. Approximately 95% of the peripheral blood T cells bear the αβ TCR, while the remaining bear the γδ TCR. The TCR structure, repertoire generation, and interaction with antigen have been extensively studied (2, 9–11, 16, 41). The αβ TCR is a heterodimer composed of two polypeptide chains, α and β (Fig. 1). In humans, the genes of the α chain are located on chromosome 14 and those of the β chain are on chromosome 7. The function of the TCR is to confer antigen recognition capacity to T cells; CD4 and CD8 T cells recognize antigens that are presented as processed peptides in association with major histocompatibility complex class II and class I molecules, respectively (11). The entire 685-kb β-chain gene locus has been sequenced (42). Twenty-six TCR Vβ families have been described on the basis of sequence homology (2), and some Vβ families are further divided into subfamilies, e.g., Vβ 5, which is divided into 5.1 and 5.2 (also referred to as 5S1 or 5S2, respectively, where "S" stands for "segment"). The simplified structure of the β chain consists of V-D-J-C segments that correspond to variable, diversity, joining, and constant regions, respectively. In the α chain, the D segment is absent. For the β chain, 47 Vβ, 2 Dβ, and 13 Jβ segments have been identified, and for the α chain, 42 Vα and 61 Jα segments are known. The V-D-J recombination events in the β chain and the V-J recombination events of the α chain together form the basis of genetic diversity of the TCR, generating a repertoire size of 10^{15} different TCR αβ dimers (24).

For study of the TCR repertoire, analysis of the Vβ chain affords the most practical approach. The variable regions of α and β chains contain relatively stable and hypervariable regions. The hypervariable regions of α and β chains together form three complimentarity-determining regions, referred to as CDR1, CDR2, and CDR3, of which CDR3 is the most hypervariable. The fine antigen specificity of the TCR is dependent primarily on the CDR3 region of the β chain, which lies close to the antigenic peptide (8). The CDR3 region of the β chain is formed by the D segment and parts of the V and J segments (see Fig. 2). It is sandwiched between the conserved amino acid motifs -Y-(L/F)-C-A-S- of the V segment at the 5' end and -F-G-X-G- of the J segment at the 3' end (37). The V-D and D-J junctions, designated N, contain one to six nucleotides (9), resulting in CDR3 segments of various lengths ranging between 5 and 15 amino acid residues.

TCR Vβ REPERTOIRE IN HEALTH AND DISEASE

A complete TCR repertoire is developed by 24 weeks of gestation, and the CDR3 segments in both CD4 and CD8 T-cell subsets are fully mature at the time of birth (37, 43). Perturbations in the TCR repertoire may occur due to the loss, underexpression, or expansion of one or more T-cell clones, in particular Vβ families. Alterations in the peripheral T-cell repertoire have been previously reported for healthy individuals (21, 35, 40, 47) and individuals in diseased states (6, 12, 27, 39, 48, 49, 52). The perturbations seen in healthy subjects are few and relatively stable and may arise due to chronic stimulation with antigens of known or unknown origin (47), following vaccination (23) and with aging (44). Tumor-infiltrating lymphocytes have been shown to have a distinctive TCR Vβ repertoire profile (45). In pathologic conditions, the perturbations may be extensive, e.g., in human immunodeficiency virus (HIV) infection (7, 17), involving both CD4 and CD8 T cells. Clonal expansions, particularly involving CD8 T cells, have been described for the acute and chronic phases of HIV infection in adults and children (17, 27, 49). Clones responsive to antigens of interest (25) can be tracked, and somatic mutations have been observed in sequenced PCR products of appropriate Vβ families (3). Following therapy, a perturbed Vβ profile can normalize, as in hairy cell leukemia (28).

METHODS FOR ANALYZING THE TCR Vβ REPERTOIRE

General Considerations

The TCR Vβ repertoire can be analyzed by different methods, including PCR (18, 30), heteroduplex PCR analysis (50, 51, 53), and flow cytometry (26). Anchor PCR analysis (30) amplifies the entire gene segment of the known and unknown families of the TCR repertoire but fails to resolve fine specificity of the CDR3 segment or the Vβ gene usage. In the heteroduplex assay, the amplified cDNA forms a duplex, and the output may compromise the fine specificity of each Vβ family in comparison to that determined by the CDR3 length analysis. TCR repertoire analysis by flow cytometry utilizes monoclonal antibodies (MAbs) against the TCR β chains and has the advantage of coupling the identification of TCR Vβ families with phenotypic characterization of T cells. However, the

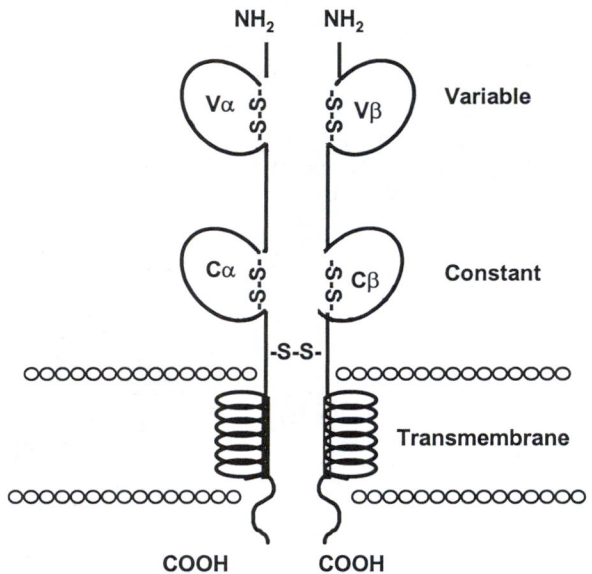

FIGURE 1 Organization of the αβ TCR showing the constant, transmembrane, and variable regions of the α and β chains.

method is limited by the availability of MAbs and its inability to determine diversity and restrictions in TCR gene usage, as is feasible by PCR analysis.

For analysis of TCR CDR3 lengths by PCR, the number of PCRs or probes needed to detect all Vβ genes can be cumbersome, especially when multiple samples need to be analyzed. Several groups have applied the multiplex PCR method for the analysis of TCR genes (1, 15, 18, 33, 39). In this chapter, we will update methods (4) for assessment of the TCR Vβ repertoire in peripheral blood by CDR3 length spectratyping by multiplex PCR and with MAbs by flow cytometry. Other methods, viz., Southern blotting, semiquantitative PCR, anchor PCR, and heteroduplex analysis, are briefly discussed below (for a summary, see Table 4).

TCR Vβ CDR3 Length Analysis by PCR

Principle
The CDR3 segments within each Vβ family vary from 5 to 15 amino acids in length, and this variation can be examined by resolving the PCR products on the basis of their size. Of the

26 Vβ families, Vβ 10 and Vβ 19 are pseudogenes (42, 54) and are excluded from analysis. The PCR is performed with Vβ-specific forward primers and a ^{32}P-labeled or fluorescently labeled Cβ-R reverse primer. In the multiplex PCR, for each reaction, two or more Vβ primers are used in combination on the basis of their product sizes. Figure 2 shows examples of the β-chain regions selected for use in the design of primers for the CDR3 length analysis. CDR3 length analysis of the TCR Vβ repertoire can be performed with peripheral blood T cells as well as T cells isolated from other sites. It is advisable to examine purified populations of CD4 and CD8 T-cell subsets because the perturbations can be strikingly different in the two subsets. Analyses can also be performed with purified T-cell subpopulations within the CD4 and CD8 T-cell subsets, e.g., naive and memory T-cell subsets.

Steps for Performing TCR Vβ CDR3 Length Analysis
The major steps in the CDR3 length analysis for the TCR Vβ repertoire include isolation of T-cell populations of interest, RNA extraction, cDNA synthesis, and the multiplex PCR.

Sample Collection, Storage, and Processing to Isolate T-Cell Subsets from Peripheral Venous Blood
Whole blood is collected by venipuncture into a tube containing an anticoagulant such as heparin, acid-citrate-dextrose, or EDTA. A blood volume of 5 to 8 ml is required, based upon the age of the subject and CD4 and CD8 T-cell counts; usually less blood is required from younger children and infants because of higher lymphocyte counts. The blood can be processed up to 24 h after the draw if left at room temperature. Anticoagulated blood samples can be shipped at room temperature for overnight delivery to the laboratory performing this assay. Peripheral blood mononuclear cells (PBMCs) are isolated from the blood by standard methods. T-cell subsets of interest are purified either by fluorescence activated cell sorting or by immunomagnetic separation. T-cell subsets may be immunomagnetically separated from PBMCs by using commercially available magnetizable polystyrene bead reagents (e.g., from Miltenyi Biotec, Dynal Corp. or StemCell Technologies) coated with specific MAbs as described elsewhere (31). The aim should be to obtain highly purified subpopulations (>98% purity); purity of the isolated cells should be checked by flow cytometry. We have used 40 μl of Dynal beads for positive selection of an estimated 10⁶ CD4 or CD8 T cells in PBMC samples. For the PCR assay, a concentration of 10⁶ cells of each T-cell subset is optimal. Cryopreserved PBMCs may be used if cells are recovered with ≥95% viability.

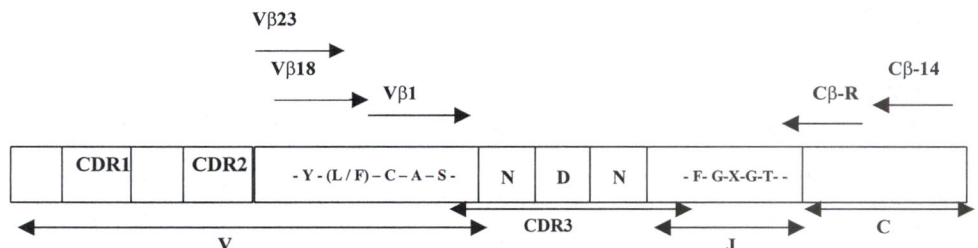

FIGURE 2 Schematic representation of the β-chain transcript of the TCR. For CDR3 length analysis PCR, a nested reverse Cβ-R primer is used in combination with multiplexed forward Vβ primers. The locations of one set of Vβ primers (set A), primer Cβ-R for PCR and reverse primer Cβ-14 for reverse transcription, are indicated (single-headed arrows). -Y-(L/F)-C-A-S- and -F-G-X-G-T-, the amino acid residues that flank the CDR3 region of the β chain of the TCR. The V, CDR3, J, and C regions are also indicated (double-headed arrows).

RNA Extraction

Equipment and reagents.

Microcentrifuge with a capacity of ≥12,000 × g (14,000 rpm) (Eppendorf)

Vortex mixer

UV range spectrophotometer

2-ml screw-cap microtubes with conical bottom (Sarstedt, Newton, N.C.)

TRI reagent (Sigma, St. Louis, Mo.)

Chloroform, molecular biology grade (Sigma)

Isopropanol, molecular biology grade (Sigma)

Glycogen (Glycoblue; Ambion, Austin, Tex.)

Ethanol, molecular biology grade (Sigma)

Molecular-biology-grade water (Ambion)

75% ethanol (75 ml of ethanol plus 25 ml of molecular-biology-grade water)

Procedure. Lyse the cells by addition of TRI reagent (200 μl for ≤10⁶ cells) while the cells are attached to beads and vortex at full speed for 20 s. The lysate can be stored at −80°C or processed immediately for RNA extraction. Thaw the cell lysate if frozen previously, and bring it to room temperature and vortex. To the cell lysate in TRI reagent, add chloroform (0.2 ml of chloroform/ml of TRI reagent). After the cell lysate is mixed vigorously with chloroform for 20 s, allow the mixture to stand for 10 min at room temperature and centrifuge at high speed (12,000 × g) for 15 min. The mixture separates into three phases. Transfer the top aqueous phase into a separate Eppendorf tube without disturbing the interphase. The interphase can be discarded or used to isolate DNA and protein for other use. Add glycogen at a concentration of 75 μg/ml of the aqueous phase and mix by gentle vortexing to enhance the precipitation of RNA. Glycogen is particularly useful when dealing with low (<10⁶) cell numbers. Add an equal volume of chilled isopropanol to the aqueous phase, and leave the tube at −20°C overnight for precipitating RNA. On the next day, centrifuge at high speed (12,000 × g or 14,000 rpm) for 15 min to pellet the RNA precipitate, and discard the supernatant. In the same manner, wash the RNA twice with 500 μl of 75% ethanol. Dissolve the RNA pellet in molecular-biology-grade water (Ambion), using ~10 μl/≤4 × 10⁶ starting cells. Determine the optical density of the RNA solution in a spectrophotometer at wavelengths of 260 and 280 nm (at 260 nm, 1 optical density unit = 37 μg of RNA per ml). The ratio A_{260}/A_{280} should be ≥1.7. The dissolved RNA can be stored at −80°C until used. Repeated freezing and thawing of RNA should not be done.

Newer commercial kits (e.g., RNeasy, Qiagen) have greatly simplified the process for RNA extraction and do not require phenol-chloroform extraction.

Reverse Transcription for cDNA Synthesis

The reverse transcriptase (RT) enzyme uses RNA-dependent DNA polymerase activity to synthesize cDNA from an RNA template. The cDNA may be synthesized with oligo(dT) or TCR-specific C-region (Cβ-14) primers. The following protocol uses a constant-region primer (Cβ-14) that specifically reverse transcribes the TCR transcripts from total cellular RNA. Typically, murine leukemia virus (MuLV) RT is used in a 60-μl cDNA synthesis reaction volume for 0.5 μg of RNA. For smaller amounts of RNA (<0.5 μg), the MuLV RT reaction volume is scaled down to 30 μl or the Omniscript RT kit (Quiagen, Valencia, Calif.) may be used

instead, as described below. Up to 100 RNA samples can be processed at a time by one individual.

Reagents for MuLV RT.

Test RNA

MuLV RT enzyme (Gibco BRL, Rockville, Md.)

5× buffer (supplied with the enzyme)

0.1 M dithiothreitol (DTT) solution, supplied with the enzyme

DEPC (diethyl pyrocarbonate)-treated molecular-biology-grade water (Ambion)

Cβ-14 primer for reverse transcription

RNasin (PE Biosystems, Foster City, Calif.)

Deoxynucleoside triphosphates (dNTPs) (Gene Amp dNTP set containing dATP, dCTP, dGTP, and dTTP [PE Biosystems])

Reagents for Omniscript RT.

Omniscript RT kit (Quiagen), which contains the reagents 10× buffer, dNTP mix, water, and Omniscript RT

Additional reagents needed: RNasin and primer Cβ-14, as desribed above

Procedure for reverse transcription using MuLV RT.

1. Prepare a 10 mM dNTP mix with equal volumes (10 mM each) of dATP, dGTP, dCTP, and dTTP (Gene Amp dNTPs). The dNTP mix is prepared in bulk and stored at −20°C in aliquots.

2. In a 200-μl PCR amplification tube, add test RNA in a 10-μl volume.

3. Heat the RNA to 65°C for 10 min and then place it immediately on ice to avoid secondary structure formation.

4. During these 10 min, prepare the following 50-μl mix for each RNA sample in an Eppendorf tube and place on ice:

5× first-strand buffer	12.0 μl
10 mM dNTP mixture	6.0 μl
0.1 M DTT	12.0 μl
Primer Cβ-14 (5 pmol/μl)	2.0 μl
RNasin (20 U/μl)	3.0 μl
MuLV RT (200 U/μl)	1.0 μl
DEPC-treated water	14.0 μl

5. Add the mixture described above to the tube containing RNA on ice to give a total volume of 60 μl.

6. Place the tube in a thermocycler; reverse transcription for cDNA synthesis is performed at 42°C for 1 h followed by 95°C for 5 min followed by 4°C for 5 min.

7. The synthesized cDNA can be stored at −20°C for several months before PCR amplification. Do not repeatedly freeze and thaw the cDNA.

Procedure for reverse transcription using the Omniscript RT kit. This method is useful for RNA quantities of <0.5 μg. Follow the steps described above as for the MuLV RT procedure but use 4 μl of Cβ-14 and mix the other reagents in the volumes specified by the manufacturer to give a final reaction volume of 40 μl instead of 60 μl. The temperature conditions for cDNA synthesis are the same as those for MuLV RT.

Multiplex PCR for CDR3 Length Analysis

The multiplex PCR may be performed with fluorescently or radioactively labeled primers. In the radioactive method, the PCR products are resolved on a sequencing polyacrylamide gel and the spectratype is analyzed with a phosphorimager. In the PCR with fluorescent primers, the products are resolved on an automated DNA sequencer that directly computes the size and area of the peaks representing the CDR3 segments. The two labeling methods give comparable results (33), but the fluorescent approach is preferred because it is less labor-intensive. Variations in the fluorescent PCR have been developed to further reduce the complexity. Both approaches are described here. The basic steps are the same for the two methods and include labeling of the Cβ primer (with P32 or fluorescent dyes), preparation of the multiplex Vβ primer sets, preparation of the master mix, and PCR of the cDNA. A simplified flow sheet for these protocols is shown in Fig. 3.

Radioactive Multiplex PCR Steps

Steps in the radioactive PCR consist of labeling of the Cβ-R primer, performing of the PCR, and resolution of the PCR products on a sequencing gel.

Equipment and reagents.

Aluminum-backed sequencing gel equipment with each well having at least a 10-μl loading capacity and wedged by spacers (0.2 to 0.4 mm)

Push-column beta-shield device (Stratagene, La Jolla, Calif.) with push columns (Stratagene), for purification of labeled probe

Thermocycler

Gel dryer

0.2-ml PCR tubes

Water baths (37 and 65°C)

T4 polynucleotide kinase (T4PNK) (Gibco)

5× kinase forward reaction buffer (supplied with the enzyme)

Molecular-biology-grade water (Ambion)

[γ-^{32}P]ATP (10 mCi/ml; NEN, Boston, Mass.)

1× STE buffer (100 mM NaCl, 20 mM Tris [pH 7.5], 10 mM EDTA)

AmpliTaq Gold polymerase enzyme, stored at −20°C (PE Biosystems)

AmpliTaq Gold buffer (supplied with the enzyme)

25 mM MgCl$_2$ (supplied with the enzyme)

TCR Vβ primers and unlabeled Cβ-R primers (Table 1) obtained in lyophilized form from either a commercial source or a core facility

^{32}P-labeled Cβ-R primer (described below)

4× gel loading dye (0.05 g of NaOH, 9.5 ml of formamide, 5 mg of bromophenol blue, and 5 mg of xylene cyanol, 10-ml final volume with molecular-biology-grade water and stored at 4°C)

Hyperfilm-MP (Amersham, Piscataway, N.J.)

Labeling of primer Cβ-R. Primer Cβ-R is labeled in a forward reaction using [γ-^{32}P]ATP and T4PNK. The steps are outlined below.

1. Prepare stock solutions of the unlabeled Cβ primer by reconstitution in molecular-biology-grade water to a concentration of 100 pmol/μl and store at −20°C until use.

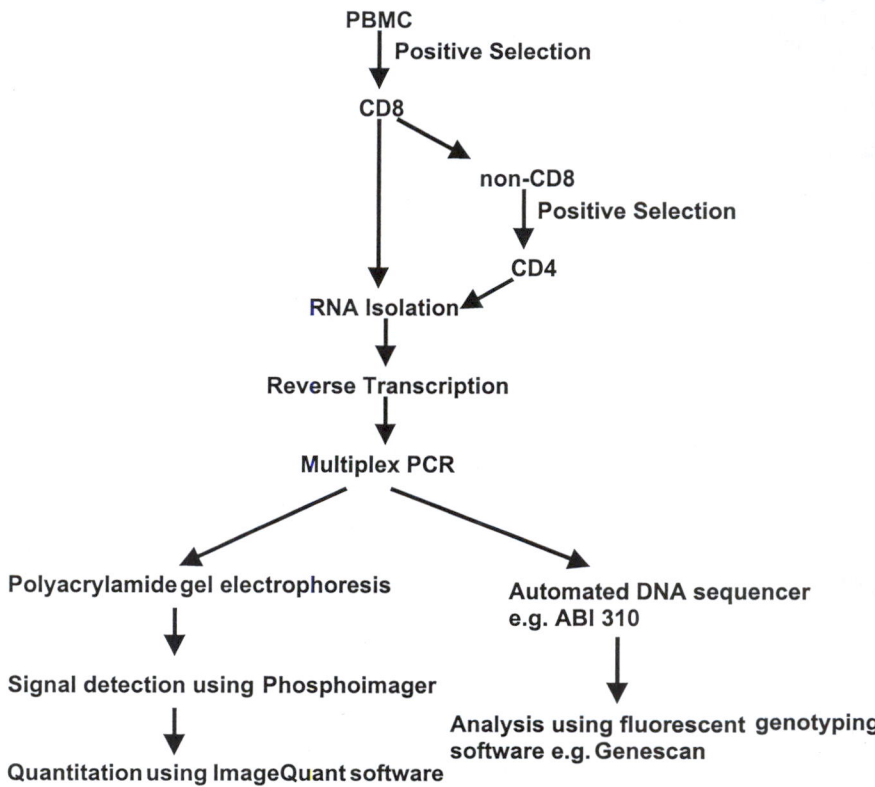

FIGURE 3 Flow chart indicating various steps for the CDR3 length analysis of CD4 and CD8 T cells by the radioactive and fluorescent multiplex PCR methods.

2. Mix the following reagents in an Eppendorf tube and spin for a few seconds:

Cβ-R (100 pmol /μl)	1.0 μl
5× T4 kinase buffer	4.0 μl
[γ-^{32}P]ATP (10 mCi/ml)	4.0 μl
Water	10.0 μl
T4PNK	1.0 μl
Total volume	20.0 μl

3. Incubate the above mixture at 37°C (in a water bath) for 10 min and then incubate for another 10 min at 65°C (in a water bath). Stop the reaction with 50 μl of 1× STE buffer, and purify the labeled primer by passing it through a push column according to the manufacturer's instructions. This step yields ~0.7 pmol of labeled Cβ-R per μl.

Preparation of Vβ primer and Cβ-R primer working sets. A list of the primers used for the PCR is given in Table 1. In the multiplex PCR, one to three primers are mixed in sets A to L, as follows: A (Vβ 1, Vβ 18, Vβ 23), B (Vβ 2, Vβ 4, Vβ 8), C (Vβ 3c, Vβ 13.1), D (Vβ 5.2, Vβ 5.1), E (Vβ 6, Vβ 20), F (Vβ 7, Vβ 22), G (Vβ 9, Vβ 16), H (Vβ 11, Vβ 12), I (Vβ 15, Vβ 13.2), J (Vβ 14, Vβ 17), K (Vβ 24), and L (Vβ 21). The final concentration of each primer is 2.5 pmol/μl. Stock solutions of the lyophilized primers (Vβ and Cβ-R) are prepared by reconstituting each primer in water to a concentration of 100 pmol/μl and are stored as 100-μl aliquots at −20°C until use. To prepare working solutions for the three-primer mixes (sets A and B), prepare 7.5 pmol of each primer per μl by adding 46.25 μl of molecular-biology-grade water to 3.75 μl of the stock solution. For the remaining Vβ primers

and Cβ primer, prepare 5 pmol of each primer per μl by adding 47.5 μl of molecular-biology-grade water to 2.5 μl of the stock solution of the Vβ primer. For multiplexing primer sets (A to J), the working solutions of relevant primers are mixed in equal volumes. For K (Vβ 24) and L (Vβ 21), the 5-pmol/μl solution is used. The prepared multiplex sets may be stored at −20°C in 100-μl aliquots. Prepare the Cβ-R working set from 100-pmol/μl stock solution at 5 pmol/μl by adding 47.5 μl of molecular-biology-grade water to 2.5 μl of the stock solution of the Cβ primer, and store it at −20°C in 100-μl aliquots.

Preparation of the master mixture. To avoid handling of small volumes, prepare sufficient master mixture for 14 tubes before use. The master mixture is prepared for a 12.5-μl PCR mixture. In a 2-ml Eppendorf tube, mix the following reagents:

AmpliTaq Gold buffer	17.5 μl
MgCl$_2$ (25 mM)	14.0 μl
dNTPs (10 mM mixture)	14.0 μl
Cβ-R (0.7 pmol/μl, labeled)	8.4 μl
Cβ-R (5 pmol/μl, unlabeled)	5.6 μl
Water	93.63 μl
cDNA	14.0 μl
AmpliTaq Gold polymerase	1.0 μl
Total volume	168.13 μl

Mix well by gentle vortexing, and place the mixture on ice.

Add 11.5 μl of the master mixture to each of the tubes A through L containing 1 μl of Vβ mix. This gives a final PCR volume of 12.5 μl.

TABLE 1 Primers used for reverse transcription-PCR

Vβ family	Primer sequence	Location[a]
Vβ 1	5'-CAA CAG TTC CCT GAC TTG CAC-3'	84
Vβ 2	5'-TCA ACC ATG CAA GCC TGA CCT-3'	86
Vβ 3	5'-TCT AGA GAG AAG AAG GAG CGC-3'	86
Vβ 4	5'-CAT ATG AGA GTG GAT TTG TCA TT-3'	122
Vβ 5S1	5'-TTC AGT GAG ACA CAG AGA AAC-3'	135
Vβ 5S2	5'-CCT AAC TAT AGC TCT GAG CTG-3'	75
Vβ 6	5'-AGG CCT GAG GGA TCC GTC TC-3'	81
Vβ 7	5'-CTG AAT GCC CCA ACA GCT CTC-3'	86
Vβ 8	5'-TAC TTT AAC AAC AAC GTT CCG-3'	144
Vβ 9	5'-AAA TCT CCA GAC AAA GCT CAC-3'	84
Vβ 11	5'-ACA GTC TCC AGA ATA AGG ACG-3'	90
Vβ 12	5'-GAC AAA GGA GAA GTC TCA GAT-3'	117
Vβ 13S1	5'-GAC CAA GGA GAA GTC CCC AAT-3'	117
Vβ 13S2	5'-GTT GGT GAG GGT ACA ACT GCC-3'	135
Vβ 14	5'-TCT CGA AAA GAG AAG AGG AAT-3'	84
Vβ 15	5'-GTC TCT CGA CAG GCA CAG GCT-3'	87
Vβ 16	5'-GAG TCT AAA CAG GAT GAG TCC-3'	132
Vβ 17	5'-CAC AGA TAG TAA ATG ACT TTC AG-3'	137
Vβ 18	5'-GAG TCA GGA ATG CCA AAG GAA-3'	117
Vβ 20	5'-TCT GAG GTG CCC CAG AAT CTC-3'	111
Vβ 21	5'-GAT ATG AGA ATG AGG AAG CAG-3'	143
Vβ 22	5'-CAG AGA AGT CTG AAA TAT TCG A-3'	122
Vβ 23	5'-TCA TTT CGT TTT ATG AAA AGA TGC-3'	146
Vβ 24	5'-AAA GAT TTT AAC AAT GAA GCA GAC-3'	129
Cβ-14	5'-CTC AGC TCC ACG TG-3'	
Cβ-R	5'-CTT CTG ATG GCT CAA ACA C-3'	

[a] The CDR3 region encompasses residues 95 to 106. Location indicates the nucleotide distance of the 5' end of the primer from codon 95.

PCR amplification.

1. Place the tubes containing the Vβ primer sets and the master mixture in the thermocycler.

2. Heat at 95°C for 12 min for activation of AmpliTaq Gold.

3. Set for 35 cycles for the PCR as specified: 94°C for 30 s for denaturation, 55°C for 30 s for annealing, and 72°C for 1 min for extension.

4. Follow by heating at 72°C for 10 min for final extension.

5. Maintain at 4°C until the next step.

Polyacrylamide gel electrophoresis: running the gel.

1. Mix 6 μl of the PCR product from each tube with 2 μl of gel loading dye and run the mixture in 12 separate lanes corresponding to sets A to L on a 6% acrylamide gel using 1× TBE (Tris-borate-EDTA) buffer. The procedure for running gels described in *Current Protocols in Immunology* (36) can be followed. Continue the run until the second dye (xylene cyanol) front reaches approximately 1 in. from the end.

2. Dry the gel in the gel dryer at 80°C for 45 min to 1 h. Check with a Geiger counter to ensure the presence of signals. Place the gel and film in a cassette at −70°C overnight. Develop the film the next day or after a longer time if the signal intensity is weak. Carefully mark and cut the area of interest and reexpose the gel to the phosphorimager for quantitation.

3. In the phosphorimager, using ImageQuant software or software with similar capabilities, analyze the intensity of signals generated by bands in each Vβ family by marking them with a rectangle that includes all the bands in that family (Fig. 4). If the PCR products lie close to each other, e.g., Vβ 11 and Vβ 12, be careful not to include bands from the adjacent family. The readout is a spectratype showing the CDR3 bands as peaks in each Vβ family.

Fluorescent Multiplex PCR Steps

Equipment and reagents.

Automated DNA sequencer such as the ABI 310 genetic analyzer or other equipment with similar capabilities

AmpliTaq Gold polymerase

AmpliTaq Gold buffer (10×)

10 mM dNTP mixture (see above)

25 mM MgCl₂

cDNA

DEPC-treated or molecular-biology-grade water

Vβ upstream primer sets (prepared as explained for radioactive PCR)

Fluorescently tagged Cβ-R primer (5.0 pmol/μl) (PE Biosystems), tagged to 6-carboxyfluorescein (6-FAM) (blue), tetrachloro 6-carboxyfluorescein (TET) (green), and hexachloro 6-carboxyfluorescein (HEX) (yellow) dyes and stored in dark tubes to protect the contents from light

POP4 polymer (performance-optimized polymer 4) and 10× buffer (PE Biosystems)

Deionized molecular-biology-grade formamide (Sigma)

Make 1-ml aliquots and store at −20°C. Standard molecular size markers (35 to 350 bp) coupled to a red fluorescent dye (6-carboxytetramethyl-rhodamine [TAMRA]; Genescan 350 Tamra; PE Biosystems) are also used. It is important to avoid working in excessive light and to not expose any of the fluorescent products to bright light for long periods.

Preparation of master mixture. Prepare sufficient quantity for 14 tubes. In a 2-ml Eppendorf tube, mix the following reagents:

AmpliTaq Gold buffer	17.5 μl
2.5 mM dNTP mix	14.0 μl
25 mM MgCl₂	14.0 μl
cDNA	14.0 μl
AmpliTaq Gold polymerase	1.0 μl
DEPC-treated water	93.7 μl
Total volume	154.2 μl

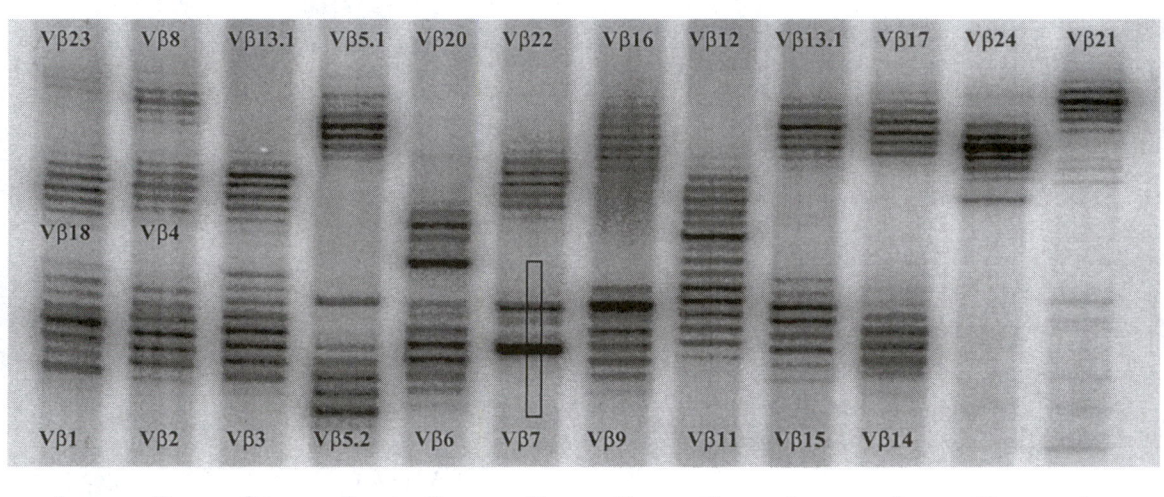

FIGURE 4 CDR3 length analysis of the Vβ chain of TCR showing radiolabeled PCR products resolved by polyacrylamide gel electrophoresis. The figure shows an example of dominance of Vβ 7 from CD8 T cells of a healthy subject. The Vβ7 family (rectangle) is shown as an example of the step for further analysis with ImageQuant software.

Preparation of Vβ primer and Cβ-R primer working sets.

1. Label a set of 12 PCR tubes A through L. Add 1 μl of each Vβ primer mix to the tubes.

2. Vortex the master mixture gently, and aliquot 51.4 μl of the master mixture into each of three Eppendorf tubes labeled "blue," "green," and "yellow" and kept on ice.

3. Add 7 μl each of primer Cβ-R (5.0 pmol/μl) labeled with the blue, green, or yellow dye to the three tubes above corresponding to each dye color. Gently vortex the mixture after adding the fluorescent primers.

4. Add 11.5 μl of the master mixture plus fluorescently labeled Cβ-R from the blue, green, and yellow tubes to tubes A to L containing Vβ primers as follows: blue to tubes A, D, G, and J; green to tubes B, E, H, and K; and yellow to tubes C, F, I, and L. Spin the tubes briefly, or flick firmly if strips are used.

PCR amplification.

1. Perform the PCR under the conditions described above for the radioactive method. Maintain the tubes at 4°C and keep them protected from light until the next step.

2. Prepare a set of four sterile Eppendorf tubes labeled 1 to 4 and add 7 μl of water to each tube. Mix 1 μl of PCR product from the 12 tubes labeled A to L with the tubes labeled 1 to 4 as follows: tube A, B, and C products, tube 1; tube D, E, and F products, tube 2; tube G, H, and I products, tube 3; and tube J, K, and L products, tube 4. This step achieves 1:10 dilution of each PCR product.

3. Prepare another set of four tubes labeled 1 to 4, each containing 0.5 μl of Genescan 350 Tamra standard and 12 μl of deionized formamide. Add 1 μl of the diluted PCR product from tubes 1 to 4 to the corresponding tubes 1 to 4. Denature the contents of the tubes at 95°C for 5 min, and immediately place the tubes on an ice-water bath for at least 5 min.

Running the sample on a genetic analyzer. Training (provided by the manufacturer) is required to operate the ABI 310 genetic analyzer equipment. Prepare the instrument by using a capillary (47 cm by 50 μm; marked green). Filter "c" is used for the 6-FAM, TET, HEX, and TAMRA combination. Launch the ABI 310 collection software, and prepare the sample sheet by entering the appropriate information. In the injection list, set the instrument for a 24-min run and a 5-s injection time for each sample. Load and run the samples. The raw data are collected by the ABI Prism 310 collection software and simultaneously analyzed by the Genescan software. After the run is complete, open the run folder through the Genescan software, define new standards, and analyze the data in the "analysis control" window. Raw data are then visualized in the "results control" window.

Variation of the Fluorescent Multiplex PCR Using Labeled Vβ Primers

Recently, a variation of the fluorescent multiplex method for TCR Vβ CDR3 length spectratyping has been described (14, 39), in which the Vβ primers instead of Cβ-R are labeled with fluorescent probes. This method simplifies the earlier method by reducing the number of PCR tubes from 12 to 7, reduces assay time, and improves the resolution. The Vβ primers are divided into three groups and labeled with the fluorescent dyes 6-FAM, TET, and HEX, as shown in Table 2. The fluorescently tagged Vβ primers are then mixed in seven sets, in tubes A to G as follows: A (Vβ 1, 2, 5.1, 5.2), B (Vβ 6, 7, 8, 9, 16), C (Vβ 12, 13.1, 13.2), D (Vβ 11, 20, 15), E (Vβ 3, 21, 17, 24), F (Vβ 14, 18, 23), and G (Vβ 4, 22). Each multiplex PCR mixture contains 1 μl of cDNA, 1 μl of each TCR Vβ primer, 2 μM Cβ-R, 1 mM (each) dNTPs, 2 mM MgCl$_2$, and 1 U of AmpliTaq Gold DNA polymerase in a final reaction volume of 12.5 μl. For the Vβ 2, 7,

TABLE 2 Primers used for TCR Vβ analysis with fluorescently labeled Vβ primers[a]

Dye	TCR Vβ family	Sequence	Amplicon size (bp)	Tube
6-FAM	Vβ 1	5'-CAA CAG TTC CCT GAC TTG CAC-3'	185–214	A
	Vβ 4	5'-CAT ATG AGA GTG GAT TTG TCA TT-3'	222–251	G
	Vβ 8	5'-TAC TTT AAC AAC AAC GTT CCG-3'	248–277	B
	Vβ 14	5'-TCT CGA AAA GAG AAG AGG AAT-3'	185–211	F
	Vβ 18	5'-GAG TCA GGA ATG CCA AAG GAA-3'	220–246	F
	Vβ 6	5'-AGG CCT GAG GGA TCC GTC TC-3'	182–211	B
	Vβ 12	5'-GAC AAA GGA GAA GTC TCA GAT-3'	219–248	C
	Vβ 11	5'-ACA GTC TCC AGA ATA AGG ACG-3'	186–218	D
	Vβ 3	5'-TCT AGA GAG AAG AAG GAG CGC -3'	185–214	E
	Vβ 21	5'-GAT ATG AGA ATG AGG AAG CAG-3'	242–280	E
TET	Vβ 2	5'-TCA ACC ATG CAA GCC TGA CCT-3'	182–220	A
	Vβ 5S1	5'-TTC AGT GAG ACA CAG AGA AAC-3'	238–267	A
	Vβ 7	5'-CTG AAT GCC CCA ACA GCT CTC-3'	188–220	B
	Vβ 13S1	5'-GAC CAA GGA GAA GTC CCC AAT-3'	218–247	C
	Vβ 20	5'-TCT GAG GTG CCC CAG AAT CTC-3'	212–244	D
	Vβ 17	5'-CAC AGA TAG TAA ATG ACT TTC AG-3'	235–270	E
	Vβ 16	5'-GAG TCT AAA CAG GAT GAG TCC-3'	229–261	B
HEX	Vβ 23	5'-TCA TTT CGT TTT ATG AAA AGA TGC-3'	248–277	F
	Vβ 24	5' -AAA GAT TTT AAC AAT GAA GCA GAC-3'	232–261	E
	Vβ 15	5'-GTC TCT CGA CAG GCA CAG GCT-3'	188–214	D
	Vβ 22	5'-CAG AGA AGT CTG AAA TAT TCG A-3'	221–250	G
	Vβ 5S2	5'-CCT AAC TAT AGC TCT GAG CTG-3'	176–214	A
	Vβ 9	5'-AAA TCT CCA GAC AAA GCT CAC-3'	185–217	B
	Vβ 13S2	5'-GTT GGT GAG GGT ACA ACT GCC-3'	236–271	C
None	Cβ-R	5'-CTT CTG ATG GCT CAA ACA C-3'		

[a]In this method, the Vβ primers were labeled with appropriate fluorescent tags as described in the text. For multiplexing primers, see materials and methods.

13.1, and 17 primers, it was determined that the labeled primers had to be mixed with unlabeled primers at a ratio of 3:1 in order to prevent disproportionately high signal intensity. The PCR conditions are 94°C for 12 min for enzyme activation followed by 35 cycles of 94°C for 20 s, 58°C for 20 s, and 72°C for 30 s and finally 1 cycle of 72°C for 10 min. The PCRs can be carried out on a PTC-225 Peltier thermal cycler (M J Research, San Franciso, Calif.).

Quality Control

Controls for radioactive as well as fluorescent PCRs can be established by storing adequate amounts of cDNA that can be repeatedly used. For quality assurance purposes, sufficient master mixture should be made for a given batch of samples and should be tested with the control cDNA.

Cautionary Notes

- RNA needs to be handled with care to prevent degradation. RT is sensitive to mechanical damage; therefore, vortexing should be avoided. The enzyme is temperature sensitive, so it should not be taken from the freezer until it is ready to use and should be kept on ice when not at −20°C. Do not leave on ice for >5 min.

- For longer storage of RNA, Superasin (Ambion) at 1 U/μl may be used to dissolve the RNA. If the cells for RNA extraction need to be stored for more than a year, then the use of "RNA later" from Ambion may be considered. The reagent is reported to be capable of extracting intact RNA even if the cells are left at 25°C for a week or −80°C for archival storage.

- The dNTPs should not be exposed to bright light or room temperature, as these result in hydrolysis of the dNTPs. Avoid repeated freezing and thawing of dNTPs, since it has been shown that after three to five freeze-thaw cycles the PCR can fail (22).

- The fluorescent Cβ primers or PCR products should not be exposed to bright light for longer periods, as that leads to quenching.

- Inadequate cell numbers may result in erroneous data (38). In our hands, the lowest cell number (purified CD4 or CD8 T cells) which can give reliable results is 0.5×10^6.

- If a large number of assays need to be performed, it is advisable to make the master mixture (containing PCR buffer, MgCl$_2$, dNTP mix, water, and Vβ primer) in bulk and freeze it at −20°C until it is used. It is convenient to use 50% of the recommended water in this mixture and use the remaining 50% for making the cDNA mixture to prevent handling of small volumes while preparing the cDNA mixture. For fluorescent PCRs, the fluorescent Cβ primers may also be added to the mixture as appropriate. The cDNA, the remaining 50% of the water, the Cβ primer (for radioactive assay), and the *Taq* polymerase must be mixed fresh on the day the PCR is performed. The PCR products should not be discarded until the data have been examined. In the fluorescent PCR, if the signal intensities are below detection limits, then the same PCR products can be rediluted to achieve a 1:4 dilution instead of a 1:10 dilution. The diluted sample should then be mixed with the deionized formamide and size standards as described above and the sample should be run with an injection time of 10 s instead of 5 s.

- In circumstances in which high background levels are encountered, use of a runoff PCR can be considered (7).

Data Interpretation and Analysis

Examples of the TCR repertoire spectratype obtained on a sequencing gel or the fluorescent equipment are shown in Fig. 4 and 5, respectively. Bands in the sequencing gel are converted into peaks by the ImageQuant software and give information similar to that of the fluorescent PCR but without the CDR3 sizes that are computed by the automated DNA sequencer. Each band or peak represents one or a set of T-cell clones bearing the same CDR3 length. In most instances, each peak represents a mixture of clones with different amino acid compositions. Within a TCR Vβ family, the difference between each successive band or peak is three nucleotides, i.e., one amino acid (40). Analysis of the TCR Vβ repertoire has not been standardized for the clinical laboratory. An unperturbed polyclonal repertoire for any Vβ family is represented by a set of peaks or bands distributed in a Gaussian pattern, with the highest-intensity CDR3 segment lying in the center. A "normal" profile of an unperturbed repertoire for CD4 and CD8 T cells can be generated with umbilical cord blood T cells (Fig. 5A) (17) and can be used as the standard against which the test sample is evaluated. Deviation from this Gaussian pattern is termed perturbation, skewing, or restrictions and results from either overrepresentation, underrepresentation, or absence of one or more CDR3 segments (38).

Counting the number of "peaks" that represent CDR3 lengths in each family is a simple approach for examination of each Vβ family. The peaks are distinct and are easy to identify (Fig. 5). Each CDR3 segment is represented by a particular size, which varies only slightly between individuals. Thus, all the "peaks" in the Vβ 1 family lie in the 186- to 210-bp range. In order to count the peaks in the fluorescent PCR readout, it is important to adjust the signal intensity (y-axis scale) to that of the highest peak in that Vβ family. For example, in Fig. 5A, the families Vβ 1, 2, 3, 5.2, 5.1, 6, 7, 9, 12, 13.2, 17, 24, and 21 are appropriately scaled, while for the remaining, i.e., Vβ 18, 23, 4, 8, 13.1, 20, 22, 16, 11, 15, and 14, the intensity needs to be adjusted to 1,000 or less. In a normal representation, each Vβ family exhibits a Gaussian pattern with ~6 to 12 peaks, with the exception of Vβ 23, which shows ~4 to 6 peaks.

A normal control range may be established by studying a group of cord blood samples or samples from age-matched healthy controls. A reduction in the number of peaks compared to that of the control range thus represents restrictions in the repertoire. One cannot rely solely on counting peaks, as peak numbers may remain in the normal range despite loss of the Gaussian pattern (e.g., Vβ 9 in Fig. 5B) or may remain in the normal range in the presence of dominance of particular segments (e.g., Vβ 2 in Fig. 5B). A more objective approach is to estimate the degree of perturbation in relation to a standard control by statistical methods (7, 17, 38). A control profile can be obtained by calculating the average distribution of samples obtained from normal cord blood. Areas occupied by each set of CDR3 segments within each TCR Vβ family are used for computing the distribution. For example, each Vβ profile may be measured as a frequency histogram (17), which is then translated into a relative frequency probability distribution, where the total area is 1. Differences in the distribution profiles between the test and control samples are used to estimate the degree of perturbation. Thus, for the test sample, perturbation in each TCR Vβ family and an estimate of average perturbation in the total repertoire can be determined.

All Vβ families in a T-cell population are not equally expressed. The usage of Vβ families also varies between individuals and with the state of T-cell activation (32). In the

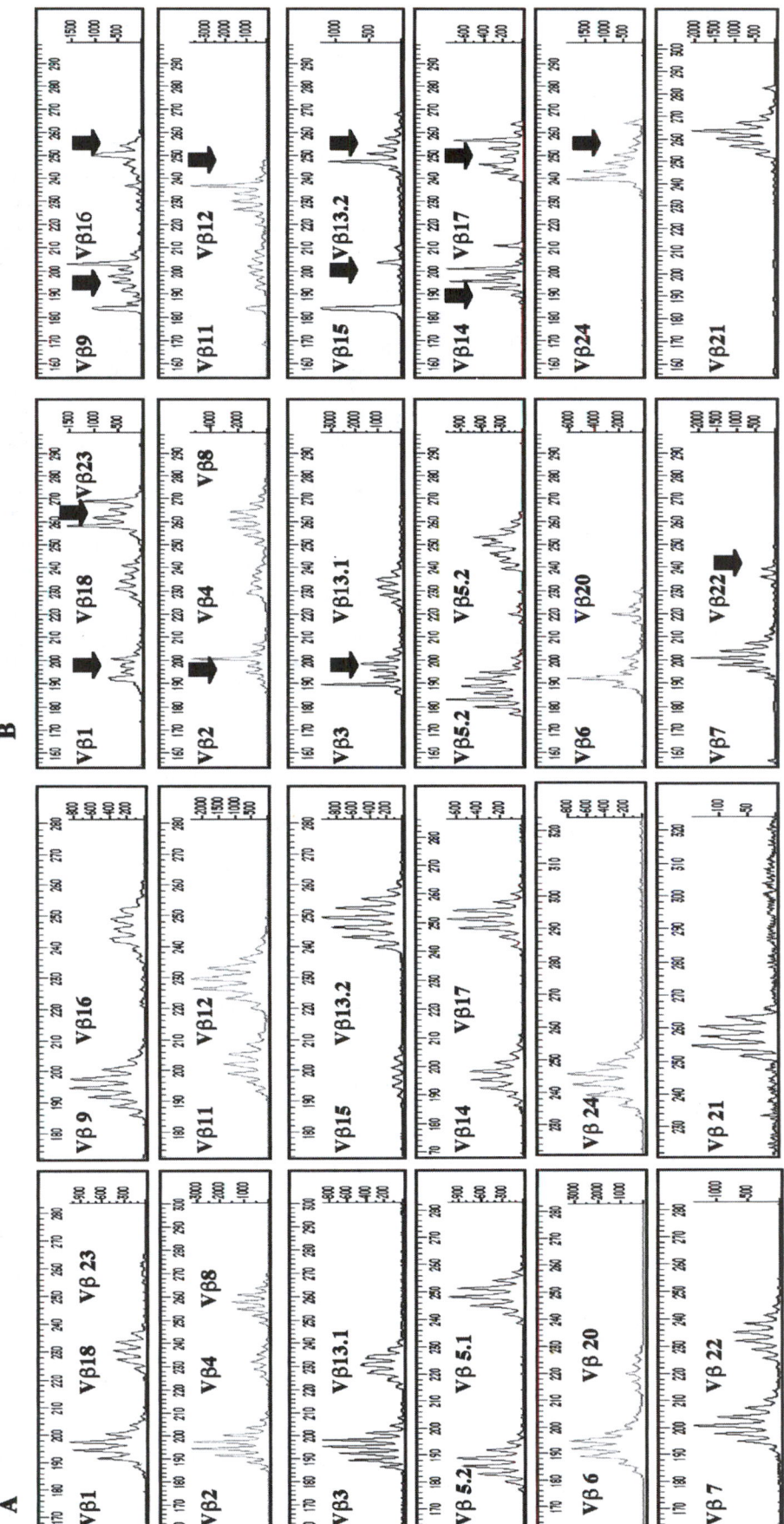

FIGURE 5 CDR3 spectratype generated after the fluorescent PCR products were resolved on an automated DNA sequencer (ABI 310). The x axis for each set represents the size of the PCR product, and the y axis represents the signal intensity. (A) TCR repertoire of cord blood CD4 T cells showing normal Gaussian patterns for all Vβ families. (B) TCR repertoire of peripheral blood CD8 T cells from an HIV-infected child, showing perturbation (arrows).

peripheral blood, Vβ 15, 16, and 23 are used less frequently, while Vβ 1, 2, 3, 4, 5, 7, and 8 are reported to be present at a higher frequency. Precaution should be taken while interpreting the data under specific experimental settings, as the Vβ primers differ in their ability to proportionally amplify their targets (19). If one band or peak is strongly expressed (Vβ 9 in Fig. 4 and Vβ 2 in Fig. 5B), the likelihood of clonal expansions or dominance should be considered. Arbitrary criteria have been established (18) for suspected clonal dominance on the basis of the expression of a single dominant peak with a signal intensity of ≥50% of the total intensity of the other CDR3 segments in that particular Vβ family. Determination of clonality requires further testing to identify the sequence of the dominant clones.

Note that some perturbations may be present in healthy subjects. Large restrictions in the repertoire, the absence of one or more Vβ families, or frequent changes with the appearance and disappearance of perturbations in one or more Vβ families are indicative of ongoing immune responses or changes in the peripheral T-cell compartments.

Assessment of Clonality

A PCR product of a Vβ family that exhibits dominance, as discussed above, may be directly sequenced by using the Vβ-specific primer and the Cβ primer. The presence of a single sequence is suggestive of clonal expansion (18, 40). This sequence helps identify the preferred usage of the Jβ segment and the sequence of the CDR3 regions. However, more than one expanding clone may utilize the same CDR3 segments, or, alternatively, more than one CDR3 segment in one Vβ family may exhibit dominance (Vβ 7 in Fig. 4 and Vβ 14 in Fig. 5B) within that Vβ family. In such cases, the direct sequencing approach is not useful, and to confirm clonality the frequency with which a particular clone is present must be determined. For this task, the PCR product should be cloned in an appropriate vector and sequenced to determine the frequency with which different clones are expressed (17). The sequencing is performed by standard protocols (20). Once the clonotype is defined by sequencing, clonotypic primers can be designed to monitor the persistence or loss of a particular clone over time.

Analysis of the TCR Vβ Repertoire by Flow Cytometry

Flow cytometry allows a quantitative estimate of the expression of the TCR Vβ families at the protein level with MAbs. Fluorescently tagged MAbs that specifically recognize the idiotypic determinants on the variable regions of each Vβ family are used for the analysis (13). As it is a flow cytometry-based assay, it is amenable to multiparameter analyses (34, 46) using other reagents in combination, as needed. Thus, Vβ family usage in CD4 or CD8 T-cell subsets can be studied without sample manipulation. This assay is less labor-intensive and can be performed by a trained flow cytometry operator without special training. The drawbacks of the flow cytometric approach are that it does not provide information about the TCR Vβ repertoire diversity and perturbations that are more precisely defined by CDR3 length analysis.

Equipment and Reagents

Flow cytometer with the ability to analyze four colors

Sterile polystyrene round tubes (12 by 75 mm) (Falcon, BD BioSciences, San Diego, Calif.)

Hanks balanced salt solution (HBSS) without Ca or Mg and phenol red (Biowhitaker, Walkersviller, Md.)

Fluorescent conjugated MAbs for TCR Vβ families, T-cell subsets, and isotype controls (stored at 4°C protected from light)

Coulter lysing buffer (Coulter Corp., Miami, Fla.)

Coulter fixative (Coulter)

CD4-phycoerythrin-cytochrome 5 (CD4-PC5) and CD8-allophycocyanin (CD8-APC) (Immunotech) MAbs

Isotype controls for these reagents include immunoglobulin G2a (IgG2a)-fluorescein isothiocyanate (FITC) and IgG1-phycoerythrin (PE) (BD Biosciences).

Staining Protocol

Each laboratory needs to standardize its staining combination and choice of MAbs. Depending on the number of parameters being studied and the capacity of the cytometer, it is advisable to include anti-CD3 MAb in the panel. A possible format is to perform four-color analysis with two TCR Vβ antibodies as well as antibodies for CD4 and CD8 in each tube. The fluorochrome label could be FITC and PE for TCR Vβ antibodies, PC5 for CD4, and APC for CD8. The panel of TCR Vβ antibodies from Immunotech is shown in Table 3.

1. For each sample, label twelve polystyrene tubes (12 by 75 mm) A to K for the panel of antibodies shown in Table 3 and one isotype control.
2. To each tube, add 100 μl of heparinized whole blood.
3. Add 10 μl of IgG2a-FITC and IgG1-PE isotype MAbs to the isotype tube and 10 μl of each TCR-specific reagent (A to K, Table 3) to the appropriate labeled tube.
4. Add 5 μl each of CD4 and CD8 MAbs to all the tubes.
5. Vortex the tubes gently, and incubate them for 10 min in the dark at room temperature.
6. Add 3 ml of HBSS, vortex the tubes gently, and centrifuge the tubes at 300 × g for 5 min.
7. Aspirate the supernatant and add 1 ml of Coulter lysing buffer (for experimentation, dilute 1:25 with HBSS freshly before use) to each tube.

TABLE 3 Panel of Vβ-specific MAbs

Reagent	Specificity	Fluorochrome	Clone
A	Vβ 3	FITC	CH92
	Vβ 7	PE	ZOE
B	Vβ 9	PE	FIN9
	Vβ 16	FITC	TAMAYA1.2
C	Vβ 20	FITC	ELL1.4
	Vβ 5.1	PE	IMMU157
D	Vβ 13.1	PE	IMMU222
	Vβ 13.6	FITC	JU74.3
E	Vβ 5.2	PE	36213
	Vβ 2	FITC	MPB2D5
F	Vβ 23	PE	AF23
	Vβ 21.3	FITC	IG125
G	Vβ 11	PE	C21
	Vβ 14	FITC	CAS1.1.3
H	Vβ 22	PE	IMMU546
	Vβ17	FITC	E17.5F3
I	Vβ 8.1 and 8.2	PE	56C5
	Vβ 18	FITC	BA62
J	Vβ 1	PE	BLB37.2
	Vβ 21.3	FITC	1G125
K	Vβ 12	FITC	VER2.32.1
	Vβ 5.3	PE	3D11

TABLE 4 Methods for assessing the TCR repertoire

Method	Purpose	Reference(s)
Southern blotting	TCR gene rearrangement at different stages of T-cell development	19
Semiquantitative PCR	Quantitative estimation of TCR Vβ usage	3
Anchor PCR	Amplification of known as well as unknown TCR transcripts	19
Heteroduplex analysis	Assessment of clonality	31, 35
CDR3 length analysis	Global assessment (qualitative) of TCR Vβ gene usage and diversity at CDR3 length level	
Flow cytometry	Quantitative estimation of TCR Vβ usage; allows simultaneous phenotypic and functional characterization	9

8. Vortex the tubes gently, and incubate them for 2 min at room temperature.

9. Add 250 μl of Coulter fixative and vortex the tubes again.

10. Add 2 ml of HBSS, gently vortex the tubes, and centrifuge the tubes at $300 \times g$ for 5 min at room temperature.

11. Aspirate the supernatant and resuspend it in 3 ml of HBSS wash buffer.

12. Centrifuge the tubes again at $300 \times g$ for 5 min at room temperature.

13. Aspirate the supernatant, gently tap out the pellet, and resuspend the pellet in 250 μl of 1% paraformaldehyde.

14. Store the mixture at 4°C and protect it from light until it is analyzed.

15. Analysis should be performed after 2 h or anytime thereafter within 7 days of sample processing.

Sample Analysis

The instrument should be set up for compensation. The percentages of each Vβ family can be calculated by gating on lymphocyte subsets. The accuracy of the cell count depends on the number of events counted and the frequency of the subset analyzed. Since the Vβ families may constitute as little as 0.5% of the T cells, counting of at least 10^4 events is recommended (13). A standard range for the expression of the TCR repertoire can be established by using cord blood or age-matched controls, depending on the experimental settings. The 5th and 95th percentiles can be used to calculate the normal range. Increased Vβ expression suggests that a particular Vβ family is expanded but does not necessarily imply clonal expansion. Clonality can be confirmed only by CDR3 length analysis, followed by sequencing of the PCR products.

Other Methods for Evaluation of TCR Vβ Repertoire

Southern blotting can be used for assessment of TCR Vβ and Jβ segments (Table 4). The extracted DNA is treated with a set of restriction enzymes. The products of digestion are separated by agarose gel electrophoresis, blotted onto a nylon membrane, and probed with a set of labeled Jβ probes (29). The method yields information about TCR gene rearrangement at various stages of T-cell development. This method is particularly useful in examining maturation arrest and lineage commitment in lymphoid malignancies.

Vβ gene usage can also be determined by using the semiquantitative PCR technique (5). In this method, the RNA is reverse transcribed with random hexanucleotides. The cDNA is coamplified with 5'-labeled Vβ and 3'-labeled Cβ specific primers and primers for TCR Cα as an internal control. The ratio of Vβ to Cα is used to normalize the data and estimate the Vβ usage. This method gives a quantitative estimate of the Vβ usage.

Anchor PCR (29, 30) generates information about all the known and unknown Vβ families since it does not use the specific Vβ primers. In this method, cDNA is synthesized from total RNA and its 5' end is tagged with a poly(G) tail. A PCR is then performed using an upstream poly(C) primer and a downstream TCR C-region-specific primer. The products are then cloned in appropriate vectors and sequenced to characterize the CDR3 region.

Heteroduplex analysis is a sensitive and useful way to assess clonality (5, 16, 47). Here, the amplified PCR products are denatured and randomly reannealed in the presence of carrier DNA of the specific Vβ family. The reannealed products are electrophoresed on a polyacrylamide gel and stained with ethidium bromide. Smearing of the products on the gel suggests a polyclonal repertoire, while single and distinct bands reflect oligoclonality. Sequencing of the PCR product is required for confirmation of clonal expansions.

This work was supported by grant HD37345 from the National Institutes of Health. I acknowledge Thomas McClosky, Surendra Charan, Monica Kharbanda, and Vivek Chitris for helpful information and comments.

REFERENCES

1. **Akatsuka, Y., E. Martin, A. Madonik, A. Barsoukov, and J. Hansen.** 1999. Rapid screening of T-cell receptor (TCR) variable gene usage by multiplex PCR: application for assessment of clonal composition. *Tissue Antigens* **53:**122–134.

2. **Arden, B., S. P. Clark, D. Kabelitz, and T. W. Mak.** 1995. Human T-cell receptor variable gene segment families. *Immunogenetics* **42:**455–500.

3. **Cheynier, R., S. Henrichwark, and S. Wain-Hobson.** 1998. Somatic hypermutation of the T cell receptor V beta gene in microdissected splenic white pulps from HIV-1-positive patients. *Eur. J. Immunol.* **28:**1604–1610.

4. **Chitnis, V., and S. Pahwa.** 2002. Evaluation of the T-cell receptor repertoire, p. 244–255. *In* N. R. Rose, R. G. Hamilton, and B. Detrick (ed.), *Manual of Clinical Laboratory Immunology*, 6th ed. ASM Press, Washington, D.C.

5. **Choi, Y. W., B. Kotzin, L. Herron, J. Callahan, P. Marrack, and J. Kappler.** 1989. Interaction of Staphylococcus aureus toxin "superantigens" with human T cells. *Proc. Natl. Acad. Sci. USA* **86:**8941–8945.

6. **Choi, I. H., Y. J. Chwae, W. S. Shim, D. S. Kim, D. H. Kwon, J. D. Kim, and S. J. Kim.** 1997. Clonal expansion of CD8+ T cells in Kawasaki disease. *J. Immunol.* **159:**481–486.

7. **Connors, M., J. A. Kovacs, S. Krevat, J. C. Gea-Banacloche, M. C. Sneller, M. Flanigan, J. A. Metcalf,**

R. E. Walker, J. Falloon, M. Baseler, I. Feuerstein, H. Masur, and H. C. Lane. 1997. HIV infection induces changes in CD4+ T-cell phenotype and depletions within the CD4+ T-cell repertoire that are not immediately restored by antiviral or immune-based therapies. *Nat. Med.* **3:**533–540.

8. Davis, M. M., J. J. Boniface, Z. Reich, D. Lyons, J. Hamp, B. Arden, and Y. Chin. 1998. Ligand recognition by alpha beta T cell receptors. *Annu. Rev. Immunol.* **16:**523–544.

9. Davis, M., and Y. Chien. 1999. T-cell antigen receptor, p. 341–366. *In* W. Paul (ed.), *Fundamental Immunology.* Lippincott-Raven Publishers, New York, N.Y.

10. Davis, M. M., D. Lyons, J. D. Altman, M. McHeyzer-Williams, J. Hampl, J. Boniface, and Y. Chien. 1997. T cell receptor biochemistry, repertoire selection and general features of TCR and Ig structure. *Ciba Found. Symp.* **204:**94–100.

11. Ehrich, E. W., B. Devaux, E. Rock, J. Jorgensen, M. Davis, and Y. Chien. 1993. T cell receptor interaction with peptide/major histocompatibility complex (MHC) and superantigen/MHC ligands is dominated by antigen. *J. Exp. Med.* **178:**713–722.

12. Eiraku, N., R. Hingorani, S. Ijichi, K. Machigashira, P. K. Gregersen, J. Monteiro, K. Usuku, S. Yashiki, S. Sonoda, M. Osame, and W. W. Hall. 1998. Clonal expansion within CD4+ and CD8+ T cell subsets in human T lymphotropic virus type I-infected individuals. *J. Immunol.* **161:**6674–6680.

13. Faint, J. M., D. Pilling, A. N. Akbar, G. D. Kitas, P. A. Bacon, and M. Salmon. 1999. Quantitative flow cytometry for the analysis of T cell receptor Vbeta chain expression. *J. Immunol. Methods* **225:**53–60.

14. Fernandes, S., S. Chavan, V. Chitnis, N. Kohn, and S. Pahwa. 2005. Simplified fluorescent multiplex PCR method for evaluation of the T cell receptor (TCR) Vβ chain repertoire. *Clin. Diagn. Lab. Immunol.* **12:**477–483.

15. Fodinger, M., H. Buchmayer, I. Schwarzinger, I. Simonitsch, K. Winkler, U. Jager, R. Knobler, and C. Mannhalter. 1996. Multiplex PCR for rapid detection of T-cell receptor-gamma chain gene rearrangements in patients with lymphoproliferative diseases. *Br. J. Haematol.* **94:**136–139.

16. Frank, S. J., I. Engel, T. Rutledge, and F. Letourneur. 1991. Structure/function analysis of the invariant subunits of the T cell antigen receptor. *Semin. Immunol.* **3:**299–311.

17. Gorochov, G., A. U. Neumann, A. Kereveur, C. Parizot, T. Li, C. Katlama, M. Karmochkine, G. Raguin, B. Autran, and P. Debre. 1998. Perturbation of CD4+ and CD8+ T-cell repertoires during progression to AIDS and regulation of the CD4+ repertoire during antiviral therapy. *Nat. Med.* **4:**215–221.

18. Gregersen, P. K., R. Hingorani, and J. Monteiro. 1995. Oligoclonality in the CD8+ T cell population: analysis using a multiplex PCR assay for CDR3 length. *Ann. N. Y. Acad. Sci.* **756:**19–27.

19. Grunewald, J., and H. Wigzell. 1996. T-cell expansions in healthy individuals. *Immunologist* **4:**97–102.

20. Gussoni, E., M. A. Panzara, and L. Steinman. 2000. Evaluating T cell receptor gene expression by PCR, p. 10.26. *In* J. E. Coligan, A. M. Kruisbeek, D. H. Margulies, E. M. Shevach, and W. Strober (ed.), *Current Protocols in Immunology.* John Wiley & Sons, New York, N.Y.

21. Halapi, E., M. Jeddi-Tehrani, A. Blucher, R. Andersson, P. Rossi, H. Wigzell, and J. Grunewald. 1990. Diverse T-cell receptor CDR3 length patterns in human CD4+ and CD8+ T lymphocytes from newborns and adults. *Scand. J. Immunol.* **49:**149–154.

22. Henegariu, O., N. A. Heerema, S. R. Dlouhy, G. H. Vance, and P. H. Vogt. 1997. Multiplex PCR: critical parameters and step-by-step protocol. *BioTechniques* **23:**504–511.

23. Hingorani, R., I. H. Choi, P. Akolkar, B. Gulwani-Akolkar, R. Pergolizzi, J. Silver, and P. K. Gregersen. 1993. Clonal predominance of T cell receptors within the CD8+ CD45RO+ subset in normal human subjects. *J. Immunol.* **151:**5762–5769.

24. Jores, R., and T. Meo. 1993. Few gene segments dominate the T cell receptor beta-chain repertoire of the human thymus. *J. Immunol.* **151:**6110–6122.

25. Kalams, S. A., R. P. Johnson, A. K. Trocha, M. J. Dynan, H. S. Ngo, R. T. D'Aquila, J. T. Kurnick, and B. D. Walker. 1994. Longitudinal analysis of T cell receptor (TCR) gene usage by human immunodeficiency virus 1 envelope-specific cytotoxic T lymphocyte clones reveals a limited TCR repertoire. *J. Exp. Med.* **179:**1261–1271.

26. Kharbanda, M., T. W. McCloskey, R. Pahwa, and S. Pahwa. 2003. Alterations in T cell receptor Vβ repertoire of CD8 T lymphocytes in HIV infected children. *Clin. Diagn. Lab. Immunol.* **10:**53–58.

27. Kharbanda, M., S. Than, V. Chitnis, M., Sun, S. Chavan, S. Bakshi, and S. Pahwa. 2000. Patterns of CD8 T cell clonal dominance and response to antiretroviral therapy in HIV infected children. *AIDS* **14:**2229–2238.

28. Kluin-Nelemans, H. C., M. G. Kester, L. van de Corput, P. P. Boor, J. E. Landegent, J. J. van Dongen, R. Williams, and J. H. Frederik Falkberg. 1998. Correction of abnormal T-cell receptor repertoire during interferon-α therapy in patients with hairy cell leukemia. *Blood* **91:**4224–4231.

29. Litwin, V., and S. Plaeger. 1997. Methods for the identification of the T cell antigen receptor, p. 304–312. *In* N. R. Rose, E. Conway de Macario, J. D. Folds, H. C. Lane, and R. M. Nakamura (ed.), *Manual of Clinical Laboratory Immunology,* 5th ed. ASM Press, Washington, D.C.

30. Loh, E. Y., J. Elliott, S. Cwirla, L. Lanier, and M. Davis. 1989. Polymerase chain reaction with single-sided specificity: analysis of T cell receptor delta chain. *Science* **243:**217–220.

31. Lou, C. C., K. J. Cunniffe, and M. R. Garovoy. 1997. Histocompatibility testing by immunological methods: humoral assays, p. 1093. *In* N. R. Rose, E. Conway de Macario, J. D. Folds, H. C. Lane, and R. M. Nakamura (ed.), *Manual of Clinical Laboratory Immunology,* 5th ed. ASM Press, Washington, D.C.

32. Maguire, J. E., S. A. McCarthy, A. Singer, and D. S. Singer. 1990. Inverse correlation between steady-state RNA and cell surface T cell receptor levels. *FASEB J.* **4:**3131–3134.

33. Maslanka, K., T. Piatek, J. Gorski, M. Yassai, and J. Gorski. 1995. Molecular analysis of T cell repertoires. Spectratypes generated by multiplex polymerase chain reaction and evaluated by radioactivity or fluorescence. *Hum. Immunol.* **44:**28–34.

34. McMichael, A. J., and C. A. O'Callaghan. 1998. A new look at T cells. *J. Exp. Med.* **187:**1367–1371.

35. Monteiro, J., R. Hingorani, I. Choi, J. Silver, R. Pergolizzi, and P. Gregersen. 1995. Oligoclonality in the human CD8+ T cell repertoire in normal subjects and monozygotic twins: implications for studies of infectious and autoimmune diseases. *Mol. Med.* **1:**614–624.

36. Morrison, S. L. 2000. Double stranded DNA sequence analysis, p. 10.25. *In* J. E. Coligan, A. M. Kruisbeek, D. H. Margulies, E. M. Shevach, and W. Strober (ed.), *Current Protocols in Immunology.* John Wiley & Sons, New York, N.Y.

37. Moss, P. A., and J. I. Bell. 1995. Sequence analysis of the human αβ T-cell receptor CDR3 region. *Immunogenetics* **42:**10–18.

38. Mugnaini, E. N., T. Egeland, A. M. Syversen, A. Spurkland, and J. E. Brinchmann. 1999. Molecular analysis of the complementarity determining region 3 of the human T cell receptor beta chain. Establishment of a

reference panel of CDR3 lengths from phytohaemagglutinin activated lymphocytes. *J. Immunol. Methods* **223:**207–216.

39. **Pahwa, S., V. Chitnis, R. Mitchell, S. Fernandez, A. Chandrasekharan, C. Wilson, and S. Douglas.** 2003. CD4+ and CD8+ T cell receptor repertoire perturbations with normal levels of T cell receptor excision circles in HIV infected therapy naive individuals. *AIDS Res. Hum. Retroviruses* **19:**487–495.

40. **Pannetier, C., J. Even, and P. Kourilsky.** 1995. T-cell repertoire diversity and clonal expansions in normal and clinical samples. *Immunol. Today* **16:**176–181.

41. **Rosenberg, W. M., P. A. Moss, and J. I. Bell.** 1992. Variation in human T cell receptor V beta and J beta repertoire: analysis using anchor polymerase chain reaction. *Eur. J. Immunol.* **22:**541–549.

42. **Rowen, L., B. F. Koop, and L. Hood.** 1996. The complete 685-kilobase DNA sequence of the human β T cell receptor locus. *Science* **272:**1755–1762.

43. **Schelonka, R. L., F. M. Raaphorst, D. Infante, E. Kraig, J. M. Teale, and A. J. Infante.** 1998. T cell receptor repertoire diversity and clonal expansion in human neonates. *Pediatr. Res.* **43:**396–402.

44. **Schwab, R., P. Szabo, J. S. Manavalan, M. E. Weksler, D. N. Posnett, C. Pannetier, P. Kourilsky, and J. Even.** 1997. Expanded CD4+ and CD8+ T cell clones in elderly humans. *J. Immunol.* **158:**4493–4499.

45. **Sensi, M., and G. Parmiani.** 1995. Analysis of TCR usage in human tumors: a new tool for assessing tumor-specific immune responses. *Immunol. Today* **16:**588–595.

46. **Sewell, W. A., M. E. North, A. D. Webster, and J. Farrant.** 1997. Determination of intracellular cytokines by flowcytometry following whole-blood culture. *J. Immunol. Methods* **209:**67–74.

47. **Shen, D., L. Doukhan, S. Kalams, and E. Delwart.** 1998. High-resolution analysis of T-cell receptor beta-chain repertoires using DNA heteroduplex tracking: generally stable, clonal CD8+ expansions in all healthy young adults. *J. Immunol. Methods* **215:**113–121.

48. **Soudeyns, H., P. Champagne, C. L. Holloway, G. U. Silvestri, N. Ringuette, J. Samson, N. Lapointe, and R. P. Sekaly.** 2000. Transient T cell receptor beta-chain variable region-specific expansions of CD4+ and CD8+ T cells during the early phase of pediatric human immunodeficiency virus infection: characterization of expanded cell populations by T cell receptor phenotyping. *J. Infect. Dis.* **181:**107–120.

49. **Than, S., M. Kharbanda, V. Chitnis, S. Bakshi, P. K. Gregersen, and S. Pahwa.** 1999. Clonal dominance patterns of CD8 T cells in relation to disease progression in HIV-infected children. *J. Immunol.* **162:**3680–3686.

50. **Uematsu, Y.** 1991. A novel and rapid cloning method for the T-cell receptor variable region sequences. *Immunogenetics* **34:**174–178.

51. **Wack, A., D. Montagna, P. Dellabona, and G. Casorati.** 1996. An improved PCR-heteroduplex method permits high sensitivity detection of clonal expansions in complex T cell populations. *J. Immunol. Methods* **196:**181–192.

52. **Wagner, U. G., K. Koetz, C. M. Weyand, and J. J. Goronzy.** 1998. Perturbation of the T cell repertoire in rheumatoid arthritis. *Proc. Natl. Acad. Sci. USA* **95:**14447–14452.

53. **Yoshioka, T., T. Matsutan, S. Iwagami, Y. Tsuruta, T. Kaneshige, T. Toyosaki, and R. Suzuki.** 1997. Quantitative analysis of the usage of human T cell receptor alpha and beta chain variable regions by reverse dot blot hybridization. *J. Immunol. Methods* **201(2):**145–155.

54. **Zeng, W., S. Nakao, H. Takamatsu, A. Yachie, A. Takami, Y. Kondo, N. Sugimori, H. Yamazaki, Y. Miura, S. Shiobara, and T. Matsuda.** 1999. Characterization of T-cell repertoire of the bone marrow in immune-mediated aplastic anemia: evidence for the involvement of antigen-driven T-cell response in cyclosporine-dependent aplastic anemia. *Blood* **93:**3008–3016.

Molecular Diagnosis of Chronic Granulomatous Disease

PAUL G. HEYWORTH AND JOHN T. CURNUTTE

30

BACKGROUND

Chronic granulomatous disease (CGD) is an uncommon primary immunodeficiency caused by defects in the genes encoding any one of four protein components of the phagocyte NADPH oxidase. This complex enzyme system, also known as the respiratory burst oxidase, is composed of gp91-*phox* and p22-*phox*, which are integral membrane proteins and together form flavocytochrome b_{558}, the redox center of the enzyme; the soluble proteins, p40-*phox*, p47-*phox*, and p67-*phox*; and the small GTP-binding protein, Rac. In normal activated phagocytes, the enzyme assembles at the plasma and phagosomal membranes and catalyzes the one-electron reduction of oxygen to form superoxide. Although superoxide itself has little microbicidal activity, its toxic derivatives (e.g., hydrogen peroxide, hypohalous acids, and hydroxyl radical) are potent microbicides and are important for killing many invading microorganisms. CGD is characterized by an absence or severely diminished levels of superoxide generation, and affected individuals suffer from severe, recurrent, sometimes fatal bacterial and fungal infections.

The minimum incidence of CGD in the United States was estimated at between 1 per 200,000 and 1 per 250,000 live births (based on a national registry of patients [21]), and most patients (~75%) are diagnosed before the age of 5 years. Mutations in *CYBB* (chromosome Xp21.1), the gene encoding gp91-*phox*, account for approximately 70% of all cases of CGD. This form of the disease is inherited in an X-linked recessive manner, and, as predicted by the genetics, the vast majority of patients are male. The three other CGD subtypes have an autosomal recessive mode of inheritance, with cases equally distributed between males and females. The most common of these is caused by defects in the p47-*phox* gene, *NCF-1* (on chromosome 7q11.23), which accounts for about 20% of cases. Defects in the p67-*phox* gene, *NCF-2* (on chromosome 1q25), and in the p22-*phox* gene, *CYBA* (on chromosome 16q24), each account for approximately 5% of cases. These subtypes of CGD are referred to as X91, A47, A67, and A22 CGD, with addition of the superscripts $^+$, $^-$, or ^{0} to indicate a normal level, a reduced level, or an absence of the affected oxidase component, respectively.

This chapter focuses on defining the CGD subtype and identifying the specific genetic defect. (The initial diagnosis of CGD is discussed in another chapter.) Before genetic analysis of CGD patients is performed, it is advisable to identify the affected protein component to pinpoint the defective gene. In most cases of CGD (~90%), the affected protein component is undetectable. Consequently, immunoblot analysis of neutrophil extracts with antibodies specific for each of the components provides a relatively straightforward way of narrowing down the identity of the defective gene. Spectroscopic analysis of neutrophil extracts for flavocytochrome b_{558} can also be used to distinguish between defects arising in membrane-bound and cytosolic proteins. An absence of p47-*phox* or of p67-*phox* determined by immunoblotting can confidently be interpreted as identifying the defective gene as *NCF-1* or *NCF-2*, respectively. However, for diagnostic purposes, note that the subunits of flavocytochrome b_{558} are interdependent for full maturation and expression, with the result that the absence of one subunit (gp91-*phox* or p22-*phox*) leads to the secondary absence or greatly diminished levels of the other.

It is also important to note that approximately 5% of X-linked CGD cases (and one case each of A22 and A67 CGD) evaluated to date are caused by missense mutations (or short in-frame deletions) that lead to the expression of normal amounts of apparently inactive protein. An additional 10% of X91 CGD patients have low but detectable levels of flavocytochrome b_{558} (as determined by either immunoblotting or spectroscopy [see below]), which can be either nonfunctional or, in a few cases, very weakly active. Therefore, immunoblotting by itself does not always provide a definitive answer. In the absence of both flavocytochrome subunits, a distinction between different CGD subtypes usually can be made by looking for a mosaic pattern of NADPH oxidase activity (e.g., by the nitroblue tetrazolium slide test or flow cytometry using dihydrorhodamine or dichlorofluorescein) in female relatives of the patient. Such a pattern of mosaicism is indicative of a carrier of X-linked disease. However, failure to identify the mother as an X-linked carrier does not rule out an X-linked origin, since more than 10% of defects in *CYBB* appear to arise from new mutations in germ line cells. Carriers of autosomal recessive CGD are more difficult to detect since their phagocytes stain normally in the nitroblue tetrazolium slide test and usually show rates of superoxide generation which are within the normal range. Carriers of A22 and A67 CGD are most easily identified unambiguously once the mutation has been identified in the proband. Detection of carriers of A47 CGD with a high degree of confidence is problematic because genomes of all normal individuals include at least one, and in most cases two, highly homologous p47-*phox* pseudogenes that bear the ΔGT mutation prevalent in this form of the disease.

For recent, comprehensive reviews of CGD and NADPH oxidase, see references 6, 9, 14, 17, 19, 20, and 21.

IDENTIFICATION OF THE AFFECTED NADPH OXIDASE SUBUNIT

Concept

Since the affected oxidase subunit is absent in most cases of CGD (exceptions are noted above), the subtype often can be identified by using two complementary approaches: reduced-minus-oxidized difference spectroscopy and immunoblot analysis of neutrophil extracts. The use of spectroscopy relies on the fact that gp91-*phox* and p22-*phox* together form flavocytochrome b_{558}, a heme-containing protein that has a characteristic absorbance spectrum. In most (but not all) cases of CGD in which either the gp91-*phox* or the p22-*phox* gene is affected, flavocytochrome b_{558} is absent. Immunoblot analysis can also be used to determine (or confirm) an absence of these two components and to establish the presence or absence of p47-*phox* and p67-*phox*. Antibodies to one or more of the four *phox* proteins, p47-*phox*, p67-*phox*, p22-*phox*, and gp91-*phox*, are commercially available from BD Biosciences, Santa Cruz Biotechnology, and Upstate Biotechnology. Antibodies to all the *phox* proteins may also be available from individual investigators. As with all antibodies used for diagnostic purposes, each should be validated with samples from unaffected individuals and patients of known CGD subtype, under the specific set of conditions to be used.

Sample Requirements

Spectroscopic and immunoblot analyses require neutrophils purified from a minimum of 30 and 10 ml of blood, respectively. Blood should be collected into and immediately mixed with sodium heparin or specially formulated acid-citrate-dextrose (0.14 M citric acid, 0.20 M sodium citrate, 0.22 M glucose; mix 1 part acid-citrate-dextrose with 5 parts blood) as an anticoagulant and stored at 4°C. A sample from a normal control individual (not a family member) should be collected at the same time. Neutrophils should be purified within 24 h of drawing blood.

Flavocytochrome b_{558} Detection

Reduced-Minus-Oxidized Difference Spectroscopy (2, 5)

Sample
The sample consists of a pellet(s) of 10^7 neutrophils.

Reagents

100 mM KH_2PO_4 (pH 7.25) (phosphate buffer)
2% (vol/vol) Triton X-100 in phosphate buffer
Sodium dithionite crystals (store desiccated)

Equipment
Sensitive UV-visible recording spectrophotometer and semimicro (1-ml) cuvettes are needed.

Method

1. Resuspend the neutrophil pellet in 400 μl of Triton X-100 in phosphate buffer, and thoroughly disperse by repeated aspiration using a 200-μl micropipettor tip.

2. Incubate on ice for 5 min.
3. Centrifuge at 27,000 × *g* for 20 min at 4°C.
4. Carefully transfer 350 μl of the supernatant to a semi-micro cuvette, add 400 μl of phosphate buffer, and mix by inversion.
5. Record the oxidized (untreated) spectrum of the sample between 600 and 400 nm, using phosphate buffer as a reference.
6. Reduce the sample with a few crystals (~200 μg) of sodium dithionite, and mix by inversion.
7. Record the reduced spectrum as described above.
8. Subtract the oxidized spectrum from the reduced spectrum, and plot the result.
9. Calculate the flavocytochrome b_{558} content from the height of the peak at 427 nm according to the formula (A_{427} − A_{413})/106,000 = molar concentration of flavocytochrome b_{558} heme. To convert this concentration to picomoles of heme per milliliter, multiply by 10^9; multiply by 0.75 to account for the actual volume in the cuvette; and finally multiply by 400/350, since only 350 μl of the original 400-μl extract was used. This calculation gives the amount of flavocytochrome b_{558} heme (in picomoles) in the original pellet of 10^7 neutrophils.

Controls
Compare the patient spectrum with that of a normal control sample collected at the same time.

Pitfalls
Contamination of the sample with traces of hemoglobin will cause the appearance of absorption bands that closely resemble flavocytochrome b_{558}, even if no flavocytochrome b_{558} is present. Therefore, great care should be taken during the hemolysis steps of neutrophil purification to ensure that all erythrocytes are removed.

As discussed at the beginning of this chapter, some missense mutations in *CYBB* (and one known mutation in *CYBA*) can lead to the expression of normal levels of nonfunctional protein. In these rare cases, the presence of flavocytochrome b_{558} is not informative in deciding which gene is affected.

Interpretation
Normal values for flavocytochrome b_{558} are 74 ± 13 pmol of heme/10^7 cells. Female carriers of X-linked CGD generally have approximately half of this value (Fig. 1), but there is some variability, depending on the degree of skewing of X-chromosome inactivation. In most cases, patients deficient in either gp91-*phox* or p22-*phox* have undetectable levels of flavocytochrome b_{558} and the absence of the absorbance bands at 558, 530 and 427 nm is clear (Fig. 1).

Immunoblotting of Neutrophil Extracts

Sodium Dodecyl Sulfate-Polyacrylamide Gel Electrophoresis (SDS-PAGE) and Immunoblotting (1, 3, 12)

Sample
The sample consists of purified neutrophils from the patient and a normal control, suspended in cold phosphate-buffered saline (PBS) at 10^7 cells/ml.

Reagents

PBS (pH 7.4)

Stock solution of the protease inhibitor diisopropylfluorophosphate (DFP)

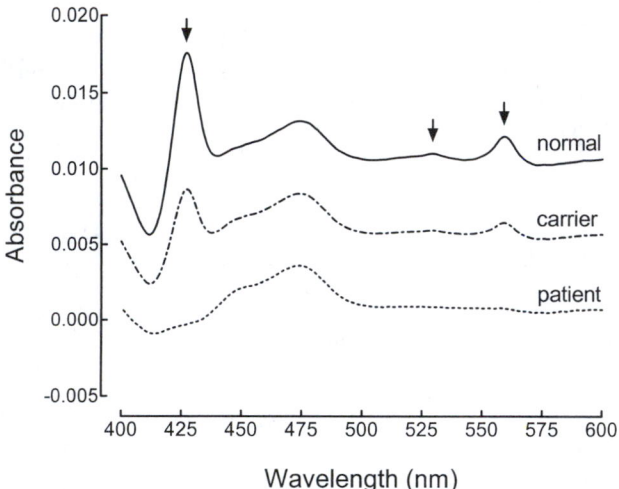

FIGURE 1 Reduced-minus-oxidized difference spectra of Triton X-100 extracts of neutrophils from a patient with X-linked CGD, his mother (carrier), and a normal control. The absorbance bands at 427, 530 and 559 nm, characteristic of flavocytochrome b_{558}, are indicated (arrows). The broad absorbance band around 470 nm is due to myeloperoxidase. The spectra have been manually offset for clarity.

SDS-PAGE sample buffer

10% polyacrylamide gels and electrophoresis buffer

Polyvinylidene difluoride or nitrocellulose membrane

Primary antibodies against gp91-*phox*, p22-*phox*, p47-*phox*, and p67-*phox*; secondary antibodies conjugated to an appropriate detection agent

Equipment

An electrophoresis unit, blotting apparatus, and power supply are required.

Method

1. Treat purified neutrophils with DFP at a final concentration of 5 mM for 10 min at 4°C, wash once in PBS, and resuspend in PBS in a screw-cap tube at 10^7 cells/ml. Prepare patient and normal control samples at the same time.

2. Pellet cells in 1-ml aliquots by centrifugation for either a single ~8-s pulse in a microcentrifuge set at full speed, or 6 min at $250 \times g$ and 4°C.

3. Remove as much of the PBS as possible without disturbing the cell pellet, and immediately add 1 ml of SDS-PAGE sample buffer to the pellet. Mix rapidly by repeated aspiration with a 1-ml micropipette tip. (The sample will be slightly stringy.)

4. Place the tube in a boiling-water bath for 5 min.

5. If samples are not to be immediately subjected to SDS-PAGE, store them at −80°C until use.

6. Run 40 to 60 μl of each sample on a 10% acrylamide gel, and transfer to a polyvinylidene difluoride or nitrocellulose membrane, using standard electrophoresis and transfer protocols.

7. Detect proteins by using primary antibodies to each oxidase component and appropriate secondary antibodies. Dilutions will have to be determined empirically, depending on the antibody titer and the detection method used.

Controls

Prepare and process a neutrophil extract from a normal individual, preferably from blood shipped with the test sample.

Pitfalls

p67-*phox* is particularly susceptible to proteolysis; therefore, neutrophils should be prepared from freshly drawn blood samples and DFP or a commercially available protease inhibitor cocktail should be used.

Although the protein core of gp91-*phox* has a predicted molecular mass of 65 kDa, it is heavily glycosylated and migrates on SDS-PAGE as a very broad and rather diffuse band (or series of bands) between ~70 and 120 kDa.

Interpretation

As discussed above, the absence of either flavocytochrome b_{558} subunit, gp91-*phox* or p22-*phox*, leads to the secondary absence of the other subunit. An absence of these subunits therefore implies X91⁰ or A22⁰ CGD. Consideration of the sex of the patient, family history, and/or carrier status of the mother may provide further information about the mode of inheritance and therefore the CGD subtype. An absence of p47-*phox* or p67-*phox* identifies the subtype as A47⁰ or A67⁰ CGD, respectively.

IDENTIFICATION OF SPECIFIC GENE DEFECTS

Concept

The molecular defects that cause the X91, A22, and A67 forms of CGD are highly heterogeneous in nature, with many of them being family specific. In contrast, in A47⁰ CGD, a single defect has been found on ~94% of alleles examined. In addition to confirming the CGD subtype, the identification of specific mutations can provide important information for detecting or confirming carriers among patients' family members and for prenatal diagnosis in affected families.

Detection of Mutations in the gp91-*phox* Gene (*CYBB*)

Once genomic DNA has been isolated, single-strand conformational polymorphism (SSCP) analysis can be used initially to examine the 13 exons of the gene, in order to identify the region likely to contain a mutation. Once identified, the exon can be analyzed by direct sequencing. About 160 bp of the 5' regulatory region of the gene is amplified together with exon 1. Exon 9 is amplified and analyzed in two fragments.

Preparation of DNA

Isolate genomic DNA from 3 to 5 ml of whole blood anticoagulated with EDTA, using any one of several commercially available kits. The Puregene DNA isolation kit (Gentra Systems, Inc., Minneapolis, Minn.) gives good results. Alternatively, an automated DNA extractor can be used.

SSCP Analysis

Sample

The sample consists of genomic DNA isolated from whole blood (see "Preparation of DNA" above).

Reagents

SSCP dye: 2 ml of 0.5 M EDTA (pH 8.0), 250 μl of 20% SDS, 10 mg of xylene cyanol, 10 mg of bromophenol blue. Add formamide to give a final volume of 50 ml. Store at −20°C.

Master mix (volumes given are for each reaction tube; multiply by the number of reactions to be run): 5 μl of 10× Perkin-Elmer PCR buffer II (Perkin-Elmer Applied Biosystems, Foster City, Calif.), 5 μl of 25 mM MgCl₂, 2.5 μl of a mix of four deoxynucleoside triphosphates (dNTPs) each at 2.5 mM, 0.5 μl of AmpliTaq, 11 μl of sterile ultrapure H₂O.

Oligonucleotide primers at 180 ng/ml (sequences are given in the SSCP column in Table 1)

Tris-borate-EDTA (TBE) buffer

20% TBE gels, 15-well (no. EC-63155; Novex, San Diego, Calif.) or similar

SYBR Green II gel stain (Molecular Probes, Eugene, Oreg.); for each gel, dilute 5 μl of SYBR Green II in 50 ml of 1× TBE.

Equipment
A Novex ThermoFlow or similar unit is required.

Method

1. Dilute patient and control DNA samples to a concentration of 500 ng/25 μl; 8 μg (in 400 μl) will be enough for 14 PCRs.

2. Place 14 PCR tubes on ice for each DNA sample to be analyzed (one tube per exon except for exon 9, which is amplified in two reactions).

3. Aliquot 0.5 μl of each primer into the bottom of the appropriate PCR tube (two primers per tube).

4. Aliquot 2.5 μl of 1 M KCl into the exon 6 and exon 13 PCR tubes.

5. Pipette 24 μl of master mix into each PCR tube.

6. Pipette 500 ng (in 25 μl) of each DNA sample into the bottom of each PCR tube, pipetting up and down gently three times.

7. Amplify by PCR under these conditions: an initial denaturation for 5 min at 94°C, followed by 30 cycles of 30 s at 94°C, 30 s at 58°C, and 30 s at 72°C, followed by a 7-min extension at 72°C; hold at 4°C.

8. For SSCP analysis with the ThermoFlow unit, set the refrigerated circulator to 12°C; this will yield a buffer temperature of 14 to 15°C. Fill the core of the ThermoFlow with 1× TBE buffer. Set the power supply to 2 h 20 min, 300 V, 30 mA, and 10 W. Circulate until the buffer is at the desired temperature.

9. Aliquot 10 μl of SSCP dye into each one of 14 fresh PCR tubes, and add 2 μl from the completed amplification reactions. Heat the tubes to 94°C for 4 min in a thermocycler, and rapidly cool them in a bath of ice slush for at least 3 min.

10. Remove any bubbles from the wells, and load the samples.

11. When the run is complete, stain the gel with SYBR Green II.

Pitfalls
Not all mutations lead to observable shifts on the gel. SSCP analysis identified the affected exon in about 90% of gp91-*phox*-deficient CGD patients evaluated by us and others (7, 14). If mutations are undetectable by SSCP analysis, a complete set of PCR-amplified fragments can be sequenced (see the following procedure).

Interpretation
Figure 2 shows a stained gel from SSCP analysis of exons 1 through 7 of CYBB and shows a shift in exon 1. For ease of comparison, patient and control samples for each exon were run side by side. Exon 1 of the patient's *CYBB* gene was subsequently found to contain an insertion of four nucleotides (see the following procedure). An absence of PCR product for one or more exons may indicate a large deletion in the patient's gene.

Amplification and Sequencing of Specific CYBB Exons from Genomic DNA (14, 18)

Sample
The sample consists of genomic DNA isolated from whole blood (see "Preparation of DNA" above). PCR amplicons from SSCP analysis (see the previous procedure) can be sequenced directly, but they do not always provide sufficient unambiguous sequence for the detection of a mutation localized to the 5' or 3' end of the fragment.

Reagents
The procedure requires amplification buffer (e.g., 10× Perkin-Elmer PCR buffer) containing 0.125 mM each dNTP, 90 ng of each specific primer, 2.5 U of AmpliTaq polymerase, and 500 ng of genomic DNA, in a total volume of 50 μl. The primers used are indicated in Table 1 (Amplification).

Equipment
A thermocycler and automatic sequencer are required (alternatively, manual sequencing can be used).

Method

1. Amplify the exons under these conditions: initial denaturation for 3 min at 94°C, followed by 30 cycles of 30 s at 94°C, 30 s at 58°C, and 30 s at 72°C, followed by a 7-min extension at 72°C.

2. Purify the amplified fragments by using a QIAquick PCR purification kit (Qiagen, Valencia, Calif.) or the equivalent, as specified by the manufacturer.

3. Sequence the fragments in both directions with the ABI Prism BigDye Terminator cycle-sequencing ready reaction kit (Perkin-Elmer). Set up sequencing reaction mixtures as follows: 2 μl of ready reaction premix, 3 μl of 5× sequencing buffer, 10 ng of sequencing primer (Table 1), and 2 μl of PCR product in a 20-μl total reaction volume. Purify the sequencing reaction products in 96-well MicroAmp trays by precipitation with 80 μl of 75% isopropanol before analysis.

Controls
Samples of DNA from unaffected individuals should always be run in parallel.

Pitfalls
As with other genes, not all mutations are exonic or at intron-exon borders; some may be found in regulatory regions of the gene or within introns. Analysis of mRNA may be informative when intronic mutations cause splicing errors.

CYBB contains a number of polymorphisms that should not be confused with disease-causing mutations. Some known polymorphisms in CYBB are tabulated in reference 7, but others may exist.

Sequencing of exon 6 can be problematic. If a clean sequence is not obtained, use a nested PCR protocol and primers 6LA2 and 6RA3 for the second reaction.

Detection of large deletions in female carriers can be problematic due to the presence of the normal allele.

TABLE 1 Oligonucleotide primers for PCR amplification of *CYBB*

Name[a]	Nucleotide sequence[b]	SSCP	Amplification	Sequencing
−425LA	gcaaggctatgaatgctgttc		*	
1RA2	gctttggtctattttagttcc		*	
−181LB2	tgtagttgttgaggtttaaag	*		*
1RB2	caagataaccccagaagtcagag	*		*
2LA	gacttgggaagtcctgaccc		*	
2RA	ccagccaatattgcatggga	*	*	
2LB	tgactccagtcttgtgtggaatc	*		*
2RB	atattgcatgggatgg			*
3LA	tggtgtgtggcctcatgctaag	*	*	
3RA	gatggcctttgaaaattagagg	*		
3RA2	ctagataatggcttggctca		*	
3LB	gaagtggggacagggcatattc			*
3RB2	agctggaatcctcccaaatca			*
4LA6	actgcatctctctgaacctcag		*	
4RA4	catatccaaccaccacttaatc		*	
4LA5	gatacagtttgcagggtggtc	*		*
4RA3	ggtatctatgaatagagggaac	*		*
5LA2	tgtcccagaaacccagcttac		*	
5RA2	gagaggtcttcactcactgaaatc		*	
5LB	gttcatacccttcattctctttg	*		*
5RB2	gtcctcaattgtaatggcctagag	*		*
6LA2	gcgacatgtgtgtgtgtg		*	
6RA4	gcatcctgcctagaaattgag		*	
6LB2	gtgtgtgtgtgtgtgtttat	*		*
6RA3	ggacatgaaatccttcacttcag	*		*
7LA2	aatttaatttcctattactaaatgatctggac	*	*	*
7RA	agacacaggttaaagattgt		*	
7RB2	gtcagtaatgaaactgtaataacaac	*		*
8LA	ctccctctgaatattttgttatc	*	*	
8RA2	gttagacactgaccactagtaatta	*	*	
8LB	taccacttaatgtatctc			*
8RB2	ccactagtaattactaaacc			*
9LA	ccatatgacactaaaaaggc	*	*	
9.5RA	CGATGCGGATATGGATACT	*	*	
9LB	ggaaaaatgtcatttccagac			*
9.5RB	ACTAAAGAAGTCTTCCTCA			*
9.5LA	TGGAAGTGGGACAATACA	*	*	
9RA	agctatttagtgccattttcctga	*	*	
9.5LB2	CTGGAGTGGCACCCTTTTAC			*
9RB2	ctcatatacgttggtaatatg			*
10LA2	ggaagcacccaatagataca		*	
10RA	tcttcacttcccatggtctct		*	
10LA	actctgaagagcaagacatctc			*
10RA2	tgctctaaggccctccga			*
10LB	acatctctgtaactatctcctc	*		
10RB2	ggccctccgataaatgaaag	*		
11LA2	gaattccacatggtaatgctgatag	*	*	
11RA2	agccctgtcactatggaaggac	*	*	
11LB2	gatagggcctgccaaatataatc			*
11RB5	actatggaaggacctgagcc			*
12LA	tgtatgtgcttttacagaatgtctc		*	
12LB3	acagaatgtctctttttttttctgaatt	*		*
12RA2	tgccgctttggcagatgcaagc	*	*	*
13LA	cgggaaattcacctacctgc		*	
13RA2	agcattatttgagcatttggc		*	
13LB	tgtagacatctcatcccaaag	*		*
13RB	agcatttggcagcacaacccac	*		*

[a] The initial number indicates the exon for which the primer is used; negative numbers represent primers in the 5′ untranslated region used for amplification and sequencing of this region together with exon 1.
[b] Lowercase letters are used for intronic primers, and uppercase letters are used for primers within exon 9.

exon: 1 2 3 4 5 6 7

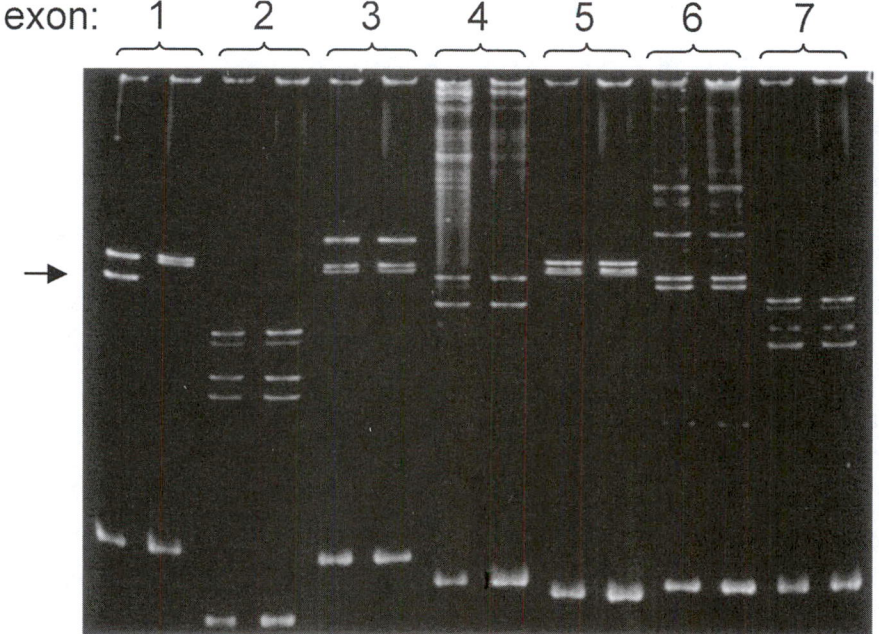

FIGURE 2 SSCP analysis of exons 1 through 7 of the *CYBB* gene. After electrophoresis of amplified and denatured DNA, the gel was stained with SYBR Green II. In each bracketed pair of lanes, the patient sample is on the left and the normal control is on the right. In the analysis shown, exon 1 of the patient contained an aberrant band (arrow); for all the other exons, the control and patient single-strand bands were the same. A four-nucleotide insertion was subsequently identified in exon 1 of this patient's *CYBB* gene. Nondenatured, double-stranded DNA appears at the bottom of the gel.

Interpretation

The *CYBB* sequence from the patient should be compared with the *CYBB* sequence from an unaffected individual and with the published sequence (GenBank accession no. NM-000397).

Detection of Mutations in the p22-*phox* Gene (CYBA)

For identifying mutations in CYBA, the gene can be amplified by PCR using paired synthetic oligonucleotide primers specific for each of the six exons of the gene (Table 2).

TABLE 2 Oligonucleotide primers for PCR amplification and sequencing of CYBA

Name[a]	Nucleotide sequence	Primer used for:	
		Amplification	Sequencing
1LA	ccagccgggttcgtgtc	*	*
1RA2	tggcgccccacttccccaccctgt	*	*
2LA8	ggtggcccacagtaggtagagaa	*	*
2RA8	gctcactgtgaagtggctcccca	*	
2RA6	cgcccaccccagcctcag		*
3LA	ctgagctgggctgttcctt	*	*
3RA	ccacccaaccctgtgagc	*	*
4LA2	cagcaaaggagtcccgagt	*	
4RA2	ggaaaaacactgaggtaagt	*	
4LA	caaaggagtcccgagtgg		*
4RB	gtggctcctgtccaggca		*
5LA	ccctgggtctgcagtctgcct	*	
5RA	cccaggctcacacttgctccca	*	
5LB	cctgagactttgttggcct		*
5RB	ggcttcaagggccatgcgtgt		*
6LA5	cctctctgagtggcagtcaca	*	
6RA3	cggccttcgctgcgttta	*	
6LB	cctgtcccagggcccta		*
6RB	atgcaggtgggtgcacct		*

[a] The initial number indicates the exon for which the primer is used.

Amplification and Sequencing of *CYBA* from Genomic DNA (4, 15)

Sample

The sample consists of genomic DNA isolated from whole blood (as described above in "Preparation of DNA" in the *CYBB* section).

Reagents

The procedure requires amplification buffer [33.5 mM Tris-HCl (pH 8.8), 8.3 mM $(NH_4)_2SO_4$, 3.35 mM $MgCl_2$, 85 μg of bovine serum albumin per ml, 5% dimethyl sulfoxide], containing 0.125 mM each dNTP, 90 ng of each specific primer, 2.5 U of AmpliTaq polymerase, and 500 ng of genomic DNA, in a total volume of 50 μl. The primers used are indicated in Table 2 (Amplification).

Equipment

A thermocycler and automatic sequencer are required (alternatively, manual sequencing can be used).

Method

1. Amplify the exons under these conditions: for exons 1, 2, 3, and 5, do an initial denaturation for 3 min at 94°C, followed by 30 cycles of 5 s at 94°C and 1 min at 70°C, followed by a 7-min extension at 72°C. For exons 4 and 6, do an initial denaturation for 3 min at 94°C, followed by 30 cycles of 30 s at 94°C, 15 s at 63°C, and 30 s at 72°C, followed by a 7-min extension at 72°C.

2. Purify and sequence amplified DNA fragments as described above for *CYBB*, using the primers indicated in Table 2 (Sequencing).

Controls

Samples of DNA from unaffected individuals should always be run in parallel.

Pitfalls

CYBA contains a number of polymorphisms that should not be confused with disease-causing mutations. Known polymorphisms are documented in reference 4.

As with other genes, not all mutations are exonic or at intron-exon borders; some may be found in regulatory regions of the gene or within introns. Analysis of mRNA may be informative when intronic mutations cause splicing errors.

Detection of large deletions can be problematic in heterozygotes.

Interpretation

The *CYBA* sequence from the patient should be compared with the *CYBA* sequence from an unaffected individual and with the published sequence (GenBank accession no. M21186 and J03774).

Detection of Mutations in the p47-*phox* Gene (NCF-1)

More than 90% of all A47 CGD patients analyzed to date are homozygous for the deletion of GT from the normal GTGT at the beginning of exon 2 (ΔGT/ΔGT genotype). Therefore, once an absence of p47-*phox* protein has been established for a patient, the initial molecular analysis can focus on the amplification and sequencing of exon 2, using primers 2LB2 and 2RB2 (Table 3), to determine if the patient has this prevalent genotype.

Amplification and Sequencing of *NCF-1* Exon 2 for the Common GT Deletion (8, 11, 16)

Sample

The sample consists of genomic DNA isolated from whole blood (as described above in "Preparation of DNA" in the *CYBB* section).

Reagents

The reagents are the same as for the amplification and sequencing of *CYBB* (see above).

Equipment

A thermocycler and automated sequencer are required (alternatively, manual sequencing can be used).

Method

1. For amplification of the exon, perform an initial denaturation for 3 min at 94°C, followed by 30 cycles of 30 s at 94°C, 30 s at 62°C, and 30 s at 72°C, followed by a 7-min extension at 72°C.

2. Purify and sequence amplified DNA fragments as described above for *CYBB*, using the primers in Table 3.

Controls

A sample of DNA from an unaffected individual should always be amplified and sequenced in parallel. A negative control sample (containing no DNA or DNA from a patient known to be homozygous for ΔGT) can be useful, in the event that the normal (GTGT) sequence is seen in a p47-*phox*-deficient patient (see "Pitfalls"). This control will exclude the possibility of normal-DNA contamination of buffers, primers, etc.

Pitfalls

The appearance of ΔGT- and GTGT-containing sequence (see "Interpretation") in a patient who is known to be deficient in p47-*phox* (<10% of A47 CGD patients) indicates the presence of a mutation other than ΔGT on one allele or both alleles of *NCF-1*. Allele-specific PCR strategies that amplify only GTGT-containing sequence have been developed. These prevent coamplification of pseudogene DNA and facilitate identification of the rare, non-ΔGT mutations.

TABLE 3 Oligonucleotide primers for PCR amplification and sequencing of exon 2 of *NCF-1*

Name	Sequence	Primer used for:	
		Amplification	Sequencing
2LB2	gtgcacacagcaaagcctct	*	*
2RB2	ctaaggtccttcccaaagggt	*	*

TABLE 4 Oligonucleotide primers for PCR amplification and sequencing of *NCF-2*

Name[a]	Nucleotide sequence	Primer used for:	
		Amplification	Sequencing
5'LA1	catcactttgtaagccaggaacc	*	
1RA2	ccacccctgttctgtggca	*	
5'LB3	gttcccctacccaaaggc		*
1RB	cctccctggtgataatgaca		*
2LA	ggcccagaaagtgaacac	*	
2RA	ctccccagaggttaggttt	*	
2LB	ctgctaggggagacgctc		*
2RB	attggggttgagaatcataat		*
3LA2	ctgggcaccacagggagcta	*	
3RA2	caccaagcccgcaacactga	*	
3LB2	tggctcatctcacacctcct		*
3RB2	tgggtttctctctgaaatc		*
4LA2	gctgcatttatttctccatc	*	*
4RA2	atccagccatgatcccctcct	*	*
5LA2	ggcaccttgatttggagtag	*	
5RA	atggcatgtcctctgaga	*	
5LB	ttttatgtttgcggtctgt		*
5RB	tccagtgacatcctctcaac		*
6LA3	gggcttctatgtggttatctcaa	*	
6RA3	ccacaaggaggctaccctcttct	*	
6LA	cgtcaccccattttcac		*
6RA	tcccaccttgctccacat		*
7LA2	ctagggcatgagcaaagag	*	
7RA	aggagcccttacaatcag	*	
7LB	agaagaatggaaacagtgc		*
7RB	tctctcgaattgaatgctt		*
8LA	ttctggaagaatgctcaaat	*	
8RA	ccccaccttcatcttctt	*	
8LB2	tagccgtttgttgtctct		*
8RB	cctttcttgccatcagc		*
9-10L[b]	ccaggcaggctcagtgtcat	*	
9-10R[b]	catctcaaggcgggctcaag	*	
9LA	ctggctccaagttcagtg		*
9RA	caaagaaggcagcagatact		*
10LA	tgtgggtactgatgagca		*
10RA	tcctgacaacacctctttt		*
11LA	gtgtttccccacatccac	*	
11RA2	aaggcagggagaggaact	*	
11LB2	gcctgggaactttgaatg		*
11RB	cagggagagaactcagga		*
12LA	ccctatttgaagaggttt	*	
12RA	atgtctgtggttgatagcc	*	
12LB	attcaccatcttcttttg		*
12RB	ccatcttctaccacttga		*
13-14L[b]	caagggttgggctaaaggac	*	
13-14R[b]	caggtaaaagggaggcagag	*	
13LA	tgatccaggatgttgagagaa		*
13RA2	gcacaaggttcccactgta		*
14LA	atggttttgtgatgatgtt		*
14RA	acagaaggtgcttgataaat		*
15LA	atttcgctgtttcctta	*	*
15RA	ttgaccttgtttctgcta	*	*
16LA	aagggtgaccgataacaaat	*	
16RA	ctcagagcaagaaacaggat	*	
16LB	agccagacagggtaatct		*
16RB	gcagaagggtgctaaatc		*

[a] The initial number indicates the exon for which the primer is used; primers designated 5' are in the 5' untranslated region and used for amplification and sequencing of this region together with exon 1.

[b] Exons 9 and 10 and exons 13 and 14 are amplified in single reactions and then sequenced separately (introns 9 and 13 are very short).

A detailed description of these protocols is beyond the scope of this chapter, but they are fully documented in references 8 and 11.

The identification of carriers (GTGT/ΔGT) among family members of ΔGT/ΔGT A47 CGD patients remains highly problematic, since the genomes of all normal individuals include at least one, and in most cases two, highly homologous p47-*phox* pseudogenes that bear the common ΔGT mutation.

Interpretation

In normal controls, a double sequence is seen after the initial GT at the start of exon 2, due to coamplification of the normal functional gene and p47-*phox* pseudogenes. A47 CGD patients who are homozygous for the common mutation (ΔGT/ΔGT) will show only ΔGT sequence at this position. The GenBank Accession numbers for p47-*phox* cDNA are M25665 and M26193.

Detection of Mutations in the p67-*phox* Gene (NCF-2)

For identifying mutations in *NCF-2*, the gene can be amplified by PCR using paired synthetic oligonucleotide primers specific for each of the 16 exons of the gene (Table 4).

Amplification and Sequencing of *NCF-2* from Genomic DNA (10, 13)

Sample

The sample consists of genomic DNA isolated from whole blood (as described above in "Preparation of DNA" in the *CYBB* section).

Reagents

The reagents are the same as for the amplification and sequencing of *CYBB* (see above). The primers used are indicated in Table 4 (Amplification).

Equipment

A thermocycler and automated sequencer are required (alternatively, manual sequencing can be used).

Method

1. Amplify the exons under these conditions: initial denaturation for 3 min at 94°C, followed by 30 cycles of 30 s at 94°C, 30 s at 58°C, and 30 s at 72°C, followed by a 7-min extension at 72°C.
2. Purify and sequence amplified DNA fragments as described above for *CYBB*, using the sequencing primers in Table 4.

Controls

Samples of DNA from unaffected individuals should always be run in parallel.

Pitfalls

NCF-2 contains a number of polymorphisms that should not be confused with disease-causing mutations. Known polymorphisms are tabulated in reference 4, but others may exist.

As with other genes, not all mutations are exonic or at intron-exon borders; some may be found in regulatory regions of the gene or within introns. Analysis of mRNA may be informative when intronic mutations cause splicing errors.

Interpretation

The *NCF-2* sequence from the patient should be compared with the *NCF-2* sequence from an unaffected individual and with the published sequence (GenBank accession no. M32011).

REFERENCES

1. **Clark, R. A., H. L. Malech, J. I. Gallin, H. Nunoi, B. D. Volpp, D. W. Pearson, W. M. Nauseef, and J. T. Curnutte.** 1989. Genetic variants of chronic granulomatous disease: prevalence of deficiencies of two discrete cytosolic components of the NADPH oxidase system. *N. Engl. J. Med.* **321:**647–652.
2. **Cross, A. R., F. K. Higson, O. T. G. Jones, A. M. Harper, and A. W. Segal.** 1982. The enzymic reduction and kinetics of oxidation of the cytochrome b_{-245} of neutrophils. *Biochem. J.* **204:**479–485.
3. **Cross, A. R., P. G. Heyworth, J. Rae, and J. T. Curnutte.** 1995. A variant X-linked chronic granulomatous disease patient (X91+) with partially functional cytochrome b. *J. Biol. Chem.* **270:**8194–8200.
4. **Cross, A. R., D. Noack, J. Rae, J. T. Curnutte, and P. G. Heyworth.** 2000. Hematologically important mutations: the autosomal recessive forms of chronic granulomatous disease (first update). *Blood Cells Mol. Dis.* **26:**561–565.
5. **Curnutte, J. T., R. Kuver, and P. J. Scott.** 1987. Activation of neutrophil NADPH oxidase in a cell-free system: partial purification of components and characterization of the activation process. *J. Biol. Chem.* **262:**5563–5569.
6. **Heyworth, P. G., J. T. Curnutte, and J. A. Badwey.** 1999. Structure and regulation of the NADPH oxidase of phagocytic leukocytes: insights from chronic granulomatous disease, p. 165–191. *In* C. N. Serhan and P. A. Ward (ed.), *Molecular and Cellular Basis of Inflammation.* Humana Press Inc., Totowa, N.J.
7. **Heyworth, P. G., J. T. Curnutte, J. Rae, D. Noack, D. Roos, E. van Koppen, and A. R. Cross.** 2001. Hematologically important mutations: X-linked chronic granulomatous disease—second update. *Blood Cells Mol. Dis.* **27:**16–26.
8. **Heyworth, P. G., D. Noack, and A. R. Cross.** 2002. Identification of a novel *NCF-1* (p47-*phox*) pseudogene not containing the signature GT deletion: significance for detection of A47⁰ chronic granulomatous disease carrier detection. *Blood* **100:**1845–1851.
9. **Heyworth, P. G., A. R. Cross, and J. T. Curnutte.** 2003. Chronic granulomatous disease. *Curr. Opin. Immunol.* **15:**578–584.
10. **Noack, D., J. Rae, A. R. Cross, J. Munoz, S. Salmen, J. A. Mendoza, N. Rossi, J. T. Curnutte, and P. G. Heyworth.** 1999. Autosomal recessive chronic granulomatous disease caused by novel mutations in *NCF-2*, the gene encoding the p67-*phox* component of phagocyte oxidase. *Hum. Genet.* **105:**460–467.
11. **Noack, D., J. Rae, A. R. Cross, B. A. Ellis, P. E. Newburger, J. T. Curnutte, and P. G. Heyworth.** 2001. Autosomal recessive chronic granulomatous disease caused by defects in *NCF-1*, the gene encoding the phagocyte p47-*phox*: mutations not arising in the *NCF-1* pseudogenes. *Blood* **97:**305–311.
12. **Parkos, C. A., M. C. Dinauer, A. J. Jesaitis, S. H. Orkin, and J. T. Curnutte.** 1989. Absence of both the 91 kD and 22 kD subunits of human neutrophil cytochrome b in two genetic forms of chronic granulomatous disease. *Blood* **73:**1416–1420.
13. **Patiño, P. J., J. Rae, D. Noack, R. W. Erickson, J. Ding, D. Garcia de Olarte, and J. T. Curnutte.** 1999. Molecular characterization of autosomal recessive chronic granulomatous disease caused by a defect of the NADPH oxidase component p67-*phox*. *Blood* **94:**2505–2514.
14. **Rae, J., P. E. Newburger, M. C. Dinauer, D. Noack, P. J. Hopkins, R. Kuruto, and J. T. Curnutte.** 1998. X-linked

chronic granulomatous disease: mutations in the *CYBB* gene encoding the gp91-*phox* component of respiratory-burst oxidase. *Am. J. Hum. Genet.* **62:**1320–1331.

15. **Rae, J., D. Noack, P. G. Heyworth, B. A. Ellis, J. T. Curnutte, and A. R. Cross.** 2000. Molecular analysis of nine new families with chronic granulomatous disease caused by mutations in *CYBA*, the gene encoding p22-*phox*. *Blood* **96:**1106–1112.

16. **Roesler, J., J. T. Curnutte, J. Rae, D. Barrett, P. Patiño, S. J. Chanock, and A. Görlach.** 2000. Recombination events between the p47-*phox* gene and its highly homologous pseudogenes are the main cause of autosomal recessive chronic granulomatous disease. *Blood* **95:**2150–2156.

17. **Roos, D., and J. T. Curnutte.** 1999. Chronic granulomatous disease, p. 353–374. *In* H. D. Ochs, C. I. E. Smith, and J. M. Puck (ed.), *Primary Immunodeficiency Diseases: a Molecular and Genetic Approach.* Oxford University Press, New York, N.Y.

18. **Roos, D., M. De Boer, F. Kuribayashi, C. Meischl, R. S. Weening, A. W. Segal, A. Åhlin, K. Nemet, J. P. Hossle, E. Bernatowska-Matuszkiewicz, and H. Middleton-Price.** 1996. Mutations in the X-linked and autosomal recessive forms of chronic granulomatous disease. *Blood* **87:**1663–1681.

19. **Segal, B. H., T. L. Leto, J. I. Gallin, H. L. Malech, and S. M. Holland.** 2000. Genetic, biochemical, and clinical features of chronic granulomatous disease. *Medicine* (Baltimore) **79:**170–200.

20. **Vignais, P. V.** 2002. The superoxide-generating NADPH oxidase: structural aspects and activation mechanism. *Cell. Mol. Life Sci.* **59:**1428–1459.

21. **Winkelstein, J. A., M. C. Marino, R. B. Johnston, Jr., J. Boyle, J. Curnutte, J. I. Gallin, H. L. Malech, S. M. Holland, H. Ochs, P. Quie, R. H. Buckley, C. B. Foster, S. J. Chanock, and H. Dickler.** 2000. Chronic granulomatous disease—report on a national registry of 368 patients. *Medicine* (Baltimore) **79:**155–169.

Clinical Evaluation of Myeloid and Monocytic Cell Functions

MAURICE R. G. O'GORMAN

31

Granulocytes (predominantly polymorphonuclear leukocytes) and monocytes collectively form the major components of the innate or nonadaptive immune system and are the main cells involved in inflammatory processes. Monocytes are also intimately involved in the adaptive immune response, but these functions will not be discussed in detail in this chapter. Their functions are both diverse and complex, and although they share many functions, these subsets represent very distinct cell lineages. Granulocytes (of which neutrophils or polymorphonuclear leukocytes represent >90%) are far more abundant than monocytes (approximately 60 to 70% of circulating leukocytes, compared with 1 to 6% for monocytes), and they have a much shorter half-life (approximately 1 to 3 days) than monocytes (weeks to months). Both cell types are derived from precursors in the bone marrow. In a 24-h period, the bone marrow of an average individual produces over 100 billion granulocytes. Most common clinical problems are manifested when the circulating granulocytes fall below critical levels (neutropenia). There are, however, specific clinical manifestations in which granulocytes or monocytes are present in normal numbers but are deficient in one or more of their functions.

With the implicit understanding that monocytes and granulocytes represent distinct cell lineages, this chapter will review laboratory procedures which can be utilized to assess their functions and phenotypes. Clinical assays used for the assessment of cell surface marker expression (defining specific cell lineages and functions), cellular activation, binding, directed migration (chemotaxis), endocytosis and/or phagocytosis, and finally killing (collectively referred to as phagocytic cell function) will be reviewed. Although there is a complete armamentarium of laboratory procedures which have been utilized to investigate phagocytic cell functions, few are practical enough to be implemented in a routine clinical use laboratory setting. In this chapter, assays which have proven to be adaptable for routine clinical use or have potential for increased utility in a clinical context will be reviewed. It is no coincidence that the majority of the procedures described are performed on a flow cytometer. The multiparametric nature of this technology for assessing single cells, the availability of flow cytometers in most clinical laboratories, and the increased commercial availability of probes, dyes, monoclonal antibody reagents, and kits developed to assess specific physiologic processes make flow cytometry the ideal clinical tool for the assessment of phagocytic cell functions.

Eosinophils and basophils complete the peripheral myeloid cell subsets. Eosinophil function will not be addressed here, and basophil function will be briefly described in the context of allergy in the last section of this chapter.

CLINICAL INDICATIONS FOR THE ASSESSMENT OF PHAGOCYTIC CELL FUNCTIONS

The principal clinical manifestation of neutropenia or abnormal phagocyte function is repeated bacterial infections. If a patient has a history of repeated bacterial infections, is not neutropenic, and has no abnormalities in either immunoglobulin (antibody) or complement, then abnormalities in phagocytic cell function should be assessed. Disorders involving abnormalities in phagocytic cell function, although rare, lead to profound morbidity. The laboratory can provide specific information leading to a diagnosis and, in most cases, effective therapeutic options. For young infants, the development of whole-blood assays which require very small blood samples has simplified the assessment of phagocytic cell functions. The clinical entities necessitating an evaluation of granulocyte and monocyte function are quite varied. For example, pediatric patients with repeat infections, slow wound healing, and delayed umbilical cord separation may be evaluated in the laboratory for abnormalities in microbial killing (for a diagnosis of chronic granulomatous disease [CGD]) or abnormalities in adhesion molecule expression (for a diagnosis of leukocyte adhesion deficiency type 1 [LAD-1]). With the current options of bone marrow transplantation, gene therapy, and immunotherapy protocols, laboratories are playing increasingly important roles in monitoring and assessing patients' responses to therapy. The laboratory can provide information on engraftment of functional cells following bone marrow transplantations, the frequency of circulating transfected cells in the peripheral blood of patients enrolled in gene therapy protocols, and the efficacy of immune modulatory therapy.

Monocytes play a key role in the innate immune response but are also centrally involved in the initiation and regulation of adaptive humoral and cell-mediated immune responses. Monocytes process and present antigens during the initiation of specific immune responses and are intimately involved in the induction, activation, and differentiation of B cells to immunoglobulin-secreting cells and of T cells to cytotoxic T cells. They act both directly via cell-cell contact and indirectly via the secretion of cytokines and chemokines. Although these functions are clearly central for the elaboration of a normal immune response, the assessment of the latter is currently relegated to specialized research laboratories and will not be discussed further in this chapter.

MONOCYTE AND GRANULOCYTE ISOLATION

Monocytes

It is well recognized that any physical manipulation of the monocyte subset alters its normal resting state. Physical isolation procedures may also lead to the selective loss of specific monocyte subsets. As they circulate in the peripheral blood, monocytes can be induced by a variety of stimuli to adhere to the vascular endothelium and migrate into various tissues, where they differentiate into specialized cells, collectively referred to as macrophages, for example, Kupfer cells in the liver, microglial cells in the central nervous system, and synovial cells in the joint capsule. With the appropriate stimuli, monocytes can also be induced to differentiate into dendritic cells. Although many studies have utilized isolated and purified monocytes and granulocytes in order to investigate their functions (for procedures on the isolation of monocytes and macrophages, refer to the appropriate chapters in previous volumes of this text [4, 7]), it is more desirable to assess their functions directly in whole blood if and when possible. Nonphysical or so-called analytical isolation

of monocytes can be performed based on the innate physical properties of these cells, as detected in a flow cytometer (Fig. 1). It is more effective, however, to identify monocytes by a combination of cell surface markers and light scatter properties, for example, CD14 and right-angle light scatter (Fig. 1). Defining lineage-specific surface markers for monocytes remains an area of significant debate, as evidenced by a conference convened in the fall of 1999 entitled "Definition of Human Blood Monocytes" (21). Although there was no clear consensus regarding the best marker to encompass all monocyte subpopulations, the summary was stated as "...the enumeration of the total monocytes with CD14 and CD16 antibodies is state of the art at this point in time." With the combination of CD14 and CD16 antibodies, specific monocyte subsets have been identified. For example, CD14$^+$ CD16$^-$ cells have been reported to function as dendritic cell precursors (19), and CD14$^+$ CD16$^+$ cells are elevated in patients with sepsis, psoriasis, or atopic dermatitis; in neonates; and in human immunodeficiency virus-infected patients with neurological involvement (18). The major population of blood monocytes is strongly positive for CD14 (CD14^{++}) and negative for CD16$^-$. More recently, a combination of monoclonal antibodies which included CD163 with either CD14 or CD64 conjugated to the same fluorochrome was reported to increase the detection of all monocytes by flow cytometry (20). This combination has not been widely adopted, and the increased cost of adding an additional marker must be considered in the context of the gains in clinical significance achieved.

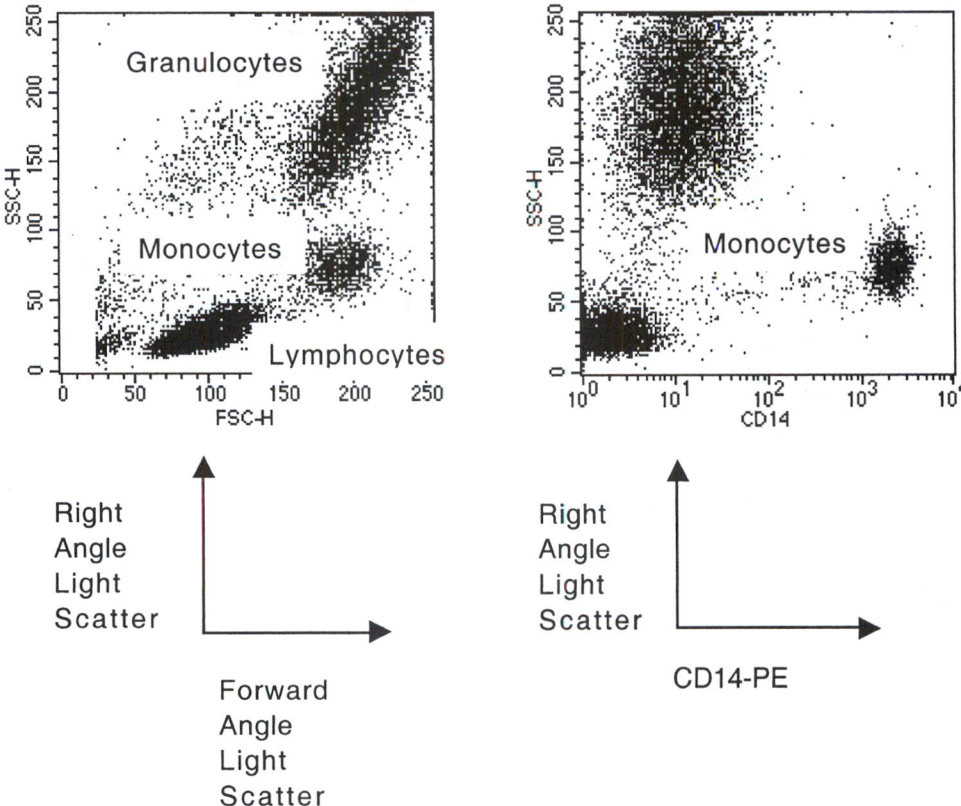

FIGURE 1 Two-dimensional dot plots illustrating the separation of monocytes and granulocytes (and lymphocytes) by their inherent light-scattering properties (forward-angle light scatter versus right-angle light scatter) (left) or the combination of a light-scattering property (right-angle light scatter) and a specific lineage-defining surface antigen (CD14-PE) (right).

PMN (Neutrophils)

Polymorphonuclear leukocytes (PMN) generate very distinct light scatter properties and can easily be identified on a correlated histogram of right-angle light scatter versus forward- or near-forward-angle light scatter (Fig. 2). Like monocytes, PMN express specific patterns of surface markers; for example, CD33 is useful for differentiating PMN from monocytes because each cell type expresses characteristic levels of expression (Fig. 2). HLA-DR is also helpful for differentiating granulocytes from monocytes, since PMN are HLA-DR negative while monocytes are positive for this marker. Other markers which are useful for assessing lineage restriction as well as the activation status of these phagocytic cells are the immunoglobulin G (IgG) Fc receptor molecules, CD16, CD32, and CD64 (for more information on Fc receptors, see references 5 and 13). Resting PMN express CD16 and CD32. PMN express CD64 during development and after specific stimulation, but CD64 is absent from the cell surface by the time mature PMN are released into the circulation. Circulating monocytes express CD32 and CD64, but upon differentiation into macrophages, monocytes express CD16. In summary, monocytes can be most accurately and completely assessed by surface labeling with a combination of CD14 and CD163, while PMN are easily identified on the basis of characteristic light scatter properties and also by their characteristic cell surface levels of CD33.

ASSESSMENT OF PHAGOCYTIC CELL FUNCTION

Once monocytes or PMN have been "analytically isolated" or "gated" on the flow cytometer, various functional parameters can be assessed. In vivo, in response to appropriate stimuli, phagocytes quickly adhere to and migrate out of the vasculature. Early changes following cellular activation include an increase in the expression of adhesion markers and immunoglobulin Fc receptors. Surface marker upregulation is quickly followed by the rolling, adhesion, and directed migration of cells out of the vasculature, through the endothelium, and towards the inflammatory focus (chemotaxis). Once the cells arrive at their target foci, they adhere to (via adhesion molecules and Fc receptors), engulf (via phagocytosis), and through various oxidative and nonoxidative mechanisms, kill and degrade invading microorganisms. The next sections will review clinical assays for the assessment of each of these functions.

Upregulation of Adhesion Molecules

In vivo, inflammatory mediators at or near the site of inflammation, such as complement fragments, endogenous lipid mediators, and chemokines such as interleukin-8 (IL-8) and monocyte chemoattractant protein 1, cause granulocytes and monocytes to leave the circulation. Before they extravasate from the blood vessels, however, they undergo a series of well-regulated adhesion steps. First, the cells slow down and roll

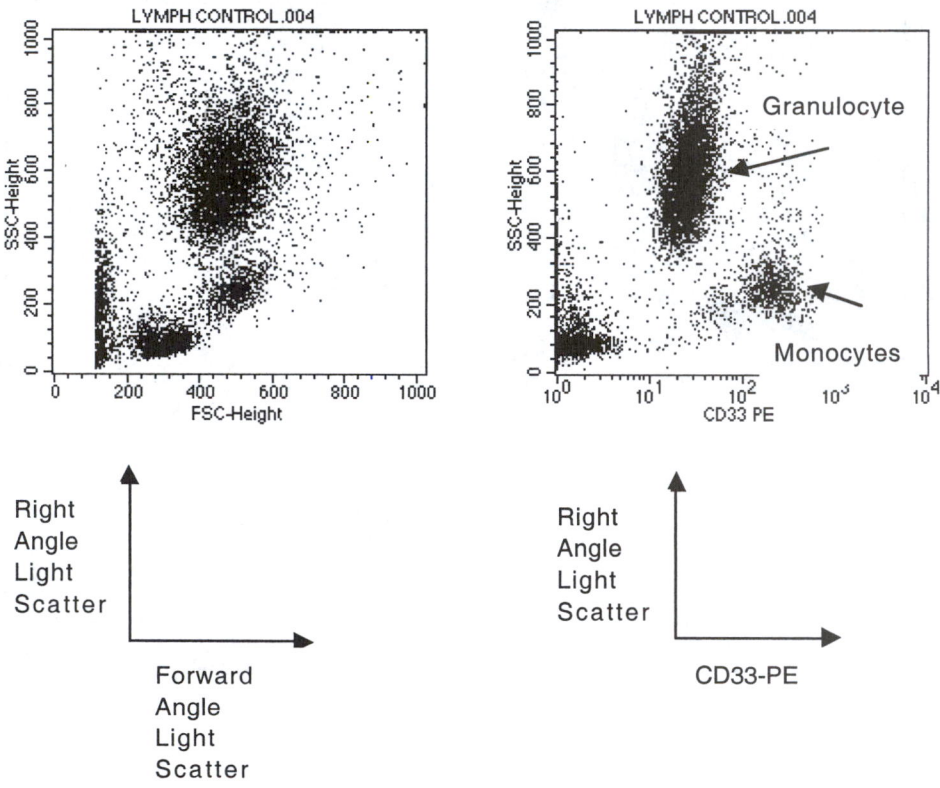

FIGURE 2 Two-dimensional dot plots illustrating the inherent light-scattering properties of monocytes and granulocytes (left) as in Fig. 1. (Right) For the same tube, the same populations were visualized on the basis of right-angle light scatter (*y* axis) versus the level of cell surface CD33-PE expression (*x* axis). Note the high level of expression of CD33 on monocytes, the less densely expressed levels of CD33 on granulocytes, and the negative expression on lymphocytes.

along the endothelium, primarily via low-avidity interactions between the sialylated Lewis X antigen (CD15s) on the phagocytes and the CD62 selectin family molecules on the endothelium, before they eventually stop if activated appropriately. Stopping and extravasation involve high-avidity interactions between the β1 and β2 integrin families of adhesion molecules on the phagocytic cell surface and the appropriate counterreceptors (e.g., ICAM-1 and CD54) on the endothelium. In vitro, the β2 leukocyte integrins CD11a, CD11b, and CD11c (α chains) and CD18 (the common β chain) can be induced to increase on the cell surface within minutes after stimulation with phorbol esters. Patients with abnormalities in the expression of the β2 leukocyte integrins (resulting from mutations within the gene coding for CD18) suffer from a disease referred to as LAD-1. Clinically, these patients are characterized as having delayed umbilical cord separation, nonpurulent bacterial and fungal infections (despite persistent leukocytosis), and periodontitis or gingivitis. Patients with abnormalities in the expression of sialyl-Lewis X (CD15s) have a similar clinical presentation, and this disorder is referred to as LAD-2 (9). In the next section, a clinical laboratory procedure for the measurement of the β2 leukocyte integrins on resting and in vitro-activated PMN developed as a clinical laboratory screening test for the diagnosis of LAD-1 is described.

Measurement of β2 Leukocyte Adhesion Molecule Upregulation in Whole Blood as a Screening Test for the Diagnosis of LAD-1

CD11a (LFA-1) is expressed on all leukocytes, and CD11b and CD11c are expressed on monocytes, granulocytes, and NK cells. There are commercially available monoclonal antibodies to each of these cell surface markers which represent the α-chain components of the β2 leukocyte integrin subfamily. In addition, there are monoclonal antibodies available to the common β chain, CD18. None of the α chains are expressed on the cell surface without CD18. Our laboratory has developed an abbreviated and simplified procedure to measure the expression of the β2 leukocyte integrins on granulocytes (or other cell subsets) in whole blood (17) as a screening test for the diagnosis of LAD-1.

It is important that the expression of β2 leukocyte integrins on the PMN of LAD-1 patients is significantly reduced on both resting and in vitro-activated cells. Of the β2 leukocyte integrins, CD11b is the most densely expressed and also displays the largest increase upon stimulation, which makes this marker the most sensitive marker for the assessment of LAD-1 (Fig. 3). The other β2 leukocyte integrins, i.e., CD11a, CD11c, and CD18, have characteristic patterns of expression on lymphocytes, granulocytes, and monocytes and can also be assessed by utilizing the same protocol (17). These procedures can be performed on very young infants and require a minimal amount of blood, which may also be advantageous for monitoring gene therapy and bone marrow transplant patients.

Briefly, 900 μl of phosphate-buffered saline (PBS) and 100 μl of EDTA-anticoagulated whole blood are added to each of three tubes, labeled "1," "2," and "3," and mixed well. Next, 15 μl of phorbol myristate acetate (PMA) (final concentration, 100 μg/ml) is added to tube 3. All tubes are incubated at 37°C in a shaking water bath for 15 min. After this time, the tubes are centrifuged at 300 × g for 5 min, the supernatants are removed, the cells are resuspended, and 20 μl of an IgG2a-phycoerythrin (PE) (Becton Dickinson) isotype control is added to tube 1, while 20 μl of the monoclonal antibody CD11b-PE (Leu-15; Becton Dickinson) is added to tubes 2 and 3. The tubes are allowed to incubate at room

temperature for an additional 15 min and then 2 ml of lysing solution is added to each tube (FACSlyse; Becton Dickinson), vortexed, and allowed to stand for 10 min. After this time period, samples are centrifuged at 300 × g for 5 min and washed two times with PBS containing 1% fetal bovine serum and 0.25% sodium azide. After the last wash, cells are resuspended in 1% paraformaldehyde. Alignment and other quality control parameters for setting up the flow cytometer are performed per daily routine (see chapter 18). On a dot plot displaying forward-angle light scatter versus right-angle light scatter, an electronic gate is drawn around the granulocyte subpopulation, and PE fluorescence (CD11b-PE) is evaluated. On a FACScan or FACScalibur instrument (Becton Dickinson), this is the FL2 parameter. Tube 1 (isotype control) serves as the control for background fluorescence (i.e., nonspecific as well as Fc receptor binding) and is used to optimize the FL2 parameter by setting the voltages on the photomultiplier tube (FL2) such that the entire peak of FL2 fluorescence is contained within the first decade (Fig. 3, top histogram at right). Note that the level of fluorescence emitted by the granulocyte population labeled with the isotype control is significantly higher than the level of fluorescence emitted by the lymphocyte population incubated with the same isotype control reagents. Once the flow cytometer is optimized, 10,000 events are collected as list mode data. The second tube (i.e., unstimulated cells labeled with CD11b) is then analyzed. This represents the baseline level of CD11b expressed on granulocytes. Note that normal resting granulocytes express significant levels of CD11b (Fig. 3, middle histogram at right). Tube 3 (i.e., PMA-stimulated CD11b-PE-stained cells) is run last, and for healthy persons, the level of CD11b should be significantly higher than that observed on resting PMN (Fig. 3, bottom histogram at right). The level of expression of CD11b is recorded as the mean fluorescent channel (MFC), which is proportional to the actual number of CD11b molecules expressed on the cell surface. Cell surface molecule upregulation can then be assessed either relative to the isotype control (MFC of CD11b on monocytes in tube 2 [baseline] or tube 3 [activated]/MFC of tube 1 [isotype control]) or relative to the level of CD11b expressed on resting (unstimulated) cells (MFC of CD11b on monocytes in tube 3 [activated]/MFC of CD11b on monocytes in tube 2 [baseline]).

This procedure can be used to measure the baseline and activation levels of other inducible adhesion markers expressed on granulocytes or monocytes (e.g., CD18, CD11a, and CD11c). In addition to PMA, other stimuli can be used, for example, opsonized zymosan (0.4 mg/ml) as well as f-Met-Leu-Phe (10^{-5} M) for particulate- versus receptor-mediated activation, respectively. In our laboratory, by using a 4-decade log scale from channel 1 to channel 10,000, we have observed the following ranges (MFCs for the 10th and 90th percentiles) of CD11b expression for a population of healthy adults. For the IgG2a isotype control, the range is 2 to 10; for resting CD11b-PE, the range is 28 to 153; and for in vitro PMA-activated PMN, the range is 263 to 1,135. Note that cells can express CD11b at levels higher than these ranges and that this is normal and not consistent with a diagnosis of LAD-1, but rather is indicative of normal in vivo activation. Only a profound decrease in the expression of CD11b (and all other β2 integrins) on both resting and in vitro activated PMN is consistent with a diagnosis of LAD-1. Laboratories should establish their own normal ranges.

Immunoglobulin Fc Receptor Upregulation

Of the three Fcγ receptors, CD16, CD32, and CD64, CD64 has the most potential for routine clinical use. Resting

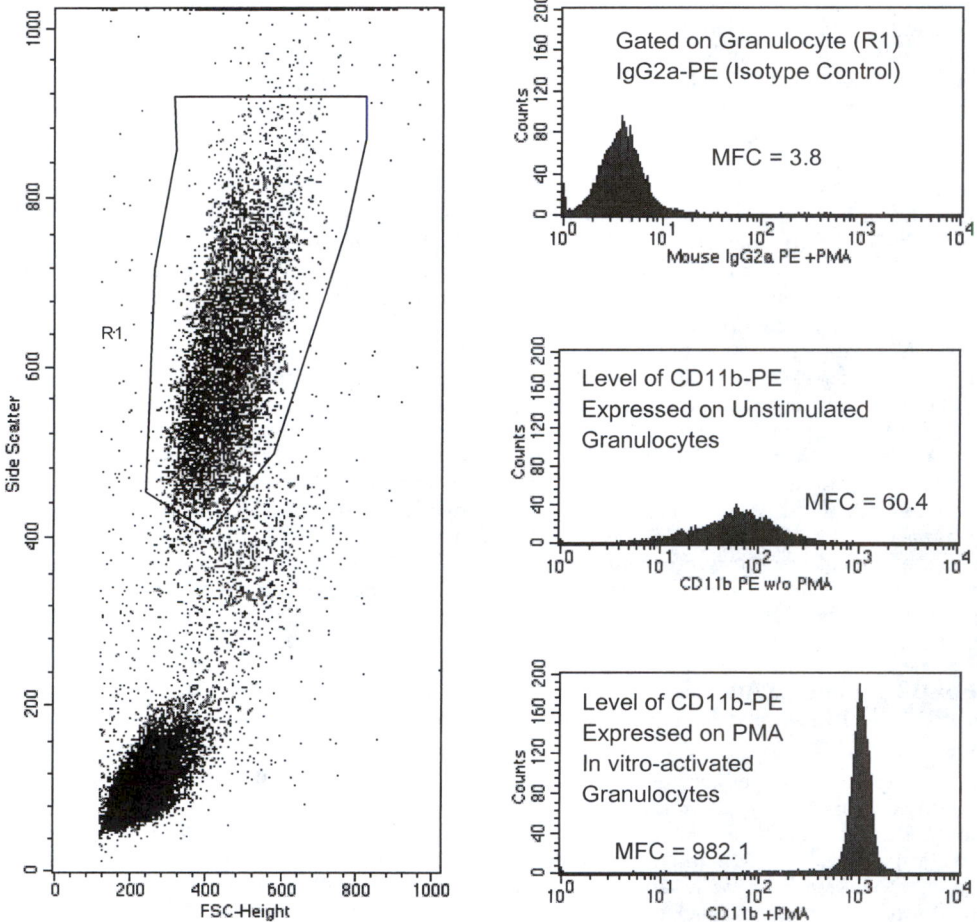

FIGURE 3 Summary of the results of a flow cytometric screening assay for the dignosis of LAD-1. The large dot plot represents the light-scattering characteristics of lysed whole blood and is used to electronically gate the granulocyte population (R1). The events in this gate are then evaluated for the surface expression of CD11b. The top histogram on the right shows the expression level of the isotype control antibody (negative control), which is used as a positive versus negative discriminatory set (so that the granulocyte population is contained within the first decade on a 4-decade log scale). The middle histogram on the right illustrates the level of expression of CD11b-PE on resting unstimulated granulocytes. The bottom histogram on the right indicates the level of expression of CD11b-PE on granulocytes which have been stimulated in vitro with a phorbol ester (PMA; for details, see the text). Results are expressed in MFC. Note the level of expression of CD11b on resting PMN (MFC = 60.4) relative to that of the isotype control (MFC = 3.8) and to the level achieved after in vitro stimulation (MFC = 982.1). These results would be consistent with normal expression and not with a diagnosis of LAD-1 (15).

granulocytes and monocytes obtained from healthy individuals express very low levels of CD64 on the cell surface, but the number of CD64 molecules is rapidly upregulated during infections and in patients with active systemic vasculitis. In vitro, CD64 is rapidly upregulated on granulocytes and monocytes in response to gamma interferon, granulocyte colony-stimulating factor (but not granulocyte-macrophage colony-stimulating factor), and IL-12. Cross-linking of CD64 triggers an oxidative burst as well as antibody-dependent cytotoxicity, so it is assumed that upregulation in vivo is physiologically significant (5). The assay for upregulation of CD64 originally reported and developed by Bruce Davis and colleagues (1, 4, 5) is slowly gaining attention in the clinical community, as evidenced by an increase in the number of reports of its applications in the literature. It has been reported that 95% of granulocytes obtained from individuals with a bacterial

infection (with a documented positive culture) expressed cell surface CD64 above the normal range (6). The measurement of CD64 upregulation on monocytes or granulocytes provides a unique laboratory measurement in circumstances where confirmation of an acute inflammatory process may influence patient management. Additionally, monitoring of monocyte and/or granulocyte CD64 levels in patients receiving gamma interferon has been used to ascertain compliance and to modify the dose scheduling (11, 12). CD64 expression is elevated in rheumatoid arthritis patients, and changes in the level of expression have been used to assess responses to therapy in this patient population (3). The level of CD64 expressed on granulocytes in vivo has also been reported to be useful for distinguishing between acute inflammatory autoimmune disease and systemic infections (2). A kit-based assay for the assessment of CD64 expression on granulocytes has been codeveloped by Trillium Diagnostics and Verity Software House, is manufactured by R&D Systems (Minneapolis, Minn.), and is currently being reviewed by the Food and Drug Administration for clearance as an in vitro diagnostic test (B. Davis, personal communication).

Chemotaxis

Chemotaxis assays are complex, time-consuming, and very rarely performed in clinical laboratories. The assays that are performed have not changed in several years, and the reader is referred to another reference (4) for a review of these procedures. A kit-based assay for the assessment of chemotaxis activity by flow cytometry is available from Orpegen Inc. (Heidelberg, Germany).

PHAGOCYTOSIS

Phagocytosis is a complex physiological process involving the engulfment and internalization of material bearing appropriate surface molecules. The measurement of phagocytosis is confounded by the difficulty of differentiating bound from internalized material, regardless of whether this process is evaluated by microscopy or flow cytometry (10). The procedure below assesses phagocytosis by flow cytometry and differentiates between surface-bound and internalized particles.

Whole-Blood Flow Cytometric Assessment of Phagocytosis

The method described below is commercially available as a kit (Orpegen) and includes an optional procedure to exclude from analysis cells with bound bacteria that have not been internalized (i.e., phagocytosed) (14). Fresh heparinized whole blood is recommended, as citrate and EDTA reduce phagocytosis. Briefly, whole blood is cooled in an ice water bath for 15 min and 100 μl is added to the bottom of each of two 5-ml polystyrene tubes. A cooled (15 min in an ice bath) Escherichia coli preparation (fluorescein isothiocyanate [FITC]-labeled E. coli preopsonized with immunoglobulin and complement from pooled sera) is mixed well, 20 μl is added to the whole blood and vortexed, and one tube is incubated at 37°C in a shaking (2 Hz) water bath for 10 min while the other tube remains on ice as the negative control (no phagocytosis occurs at 0°C). At the end of the incubation period, the samples are removed and immediately placed in ice in order to stop phagocytosis. Ice-cold quenching solution (100 μl) is added to each sample and vortexed. This step significantly reduces the fluorescence emitted by any bacteria adhering to the cell surface but not yet internalized. Samples are then washed two times with 3 ml of cold (4°C) wash solution, and after the last wash, the supernatants are discarded, the pellet is resuspended, and 2 ml of prewarmed (room temperature) 1× lysing solution is added. Samples are then incubated at room temperature for 20 min. This step lyses the red blood cells and fixes the remaining leukocytes. After the lysis step, samples are washed once more, and 100 μl of DNA staining solution is added. The samples are vortexed, incubated for 10 min at 0°C, and then analyzed on a flow cytometer (or under a fluorescence microscope) within 30 min. (In the instructions in the package insert, a FacScan [Becton Dickinson] flow cytometer is referred to.) During acquisition, red fluorescence (FL2) in a histogram of FL2 versus cell count is displayed, and a "live" acquisition gate is set on the events which display a level of fluorescence equivalent to the DNA content of human DNA diploid cells. This procedure excludes from analysis

debris, bacterial aggregates, and unlysed red blood cells which may have the same scatter parameters as leukocytes. At least 15,000 leukocytes (events) are acquired. Forward-angle light scatter versus right-angle light scatter is displayed for analysis, and a gate is drawn around the monocyte or granulocyte population (this can be facilitated by a three-color staining procedure with a PE-labeled CD14 or CD33 monoclonal antibody for monocytes and granulocytes, respectively) (Fig. 1 and 2). An evaluation of the percentage of cells having phagocytosed the E. coli is performed with the FL1 parameter (FITC). The percentage of FITC-positive cells is then determined, as well as the mean fluorescence intensity (a correlate of the number of bacteria per cell). Each laboratory should determine its own normal ranges. It must be noted that the bacteria provided are already opsonized; however, an additional effect is achieved by the plasma products present in whole blood. This should be acknowledged when working with cells which are not present in whole blood (i.e., purified granulocyte and purified monocyte populations will not show the same level of phagocytic activity). Additionally, the assay was established to provide a ratio of bacteria to cells of 25:1, with a white blood cell count of 8,000/μl, or 40:1, with a white blood cell count of 5,000/μl. Counts above or below these values, e.g., in pediatric samples, require a correction for the amount of bacteria being added. Color compensation for spectral overlap may be adjusted by using the following two controls: one tube contains FITC-labeled phagocytosed bacteria only, i.e., no DNA stain, and one tube contains the DNA stain only, i.e., no FITC-labeled bacteria (an optional third tube would contain the PE-labeled antibody only). The flow cytometer must be calibrated and checked each time the assay is performed by placing a stably fluorescent bead into the same channel before each run and checking that position after each run.

KILLING

Following adherence and phagocytosis, digested microorganisms are killed by a variety of oxidative and nonoxidative mechanisms. Microbicidal killing assays represent the "gold standard" for the assessment of phagocytic killing function, but these assays are very complex and time-consuming (take days) and are performed only in very specialized laboratories (4). The generation of reactive oxygen intermediates (ROI) which occurs in response to a variety of stimuli, including phagocytosis, represents one of the most significant mechanisms of intracellular killing. The NADPH oxidase system is responsible for the generation of ROI, and patients with mutations in the genes coding for this enzyme suffer from very severe and potentially fatal infections as well as other complications as a result of the formation of large granulomas. This disorder, CGD, can be screened for in vitro. The procedure described below is a whole-blood flow cytometry assay which detects the elaboration of ROI following in vitro activation of the NADPH oxidase system. In the presence of peroxidases and hydrogen peroxide, appropriately stimulated PMN (or monocytes/macrophages) oxidize the preloaded nonfluorescent dye dihydrorhodamine-123 (DHR-123) to rhodamine-123, which makes it brightly fluorescent and amenable to measurement on a flow cytometer. The granulocytes of patients with either the autosomal or the X-linked form of CGD as well as granulocytes (expressing the mutated X chromosome) obtained from females who carry the X-linked form of CGD fail to generate hydrogen peroxide when stimulated and can be easily and reliably identified in this assay by their inability to generate a positive fluorescent signal.

Whole-Blood Flow Cytometry for the Measurement of ROI

The whole-blood flow cytometry procedure for the measurement of ROI was developed for use as a clinical whole-blood assay, requires minimal blood, is relatively easy to perform, and has been widely adopted as a diagnostic screening test for CGD (16). Briefly, 100 μl of whole blood is added to each of three 5-ml polystyrene tubes and diluted with 900 ml of Ca^{2+}- and Mg^{2+}-free PBS. Optimally titrated DHR-123 is added (25 μl) to two of the tubes, one tube is stimulated, and one tube is left unstimulated (negative background control). All of the tubes are then incubated at 37°C in a shaking water bath for 15 min. Note that the DHR-123 is diluted from a stock in dimethylformamide to 5 mg/ml and stored frozen at −70°C (stable for up to 1 year), and all subsequent dilutions are done in PBS (working concentration, 45 μg/ml; final concentration, 1.125 μg/ml). Next, 10 μl of PMA (final concentration, 100 μg/ml; Sigma, St. Louis, Mo.) is added to one of the tubes containing DHR-123, and again all tubes are incubated for 15 min in a 37°C water bath. Note that PMA is initially diluted in dimethyl sulfoxide for a stock concentration of 1 mg/ml and then diluted in PBS to a working concentration of 10 μg/ml. After the last incubation, the samples are centrifuged at 400 × g for 5 min, the supernatants are discarded, the cells are resuspended, and an ammonium chloride-based lysing solution is added in order to lyse the red blood cells. Samples are mixed vigorously and left for 10 min at room temperature in the dark. After this incubation, the samples are washed two times with PBS and resuspended in 1 ml of 1% paraformaldehyde. Samples are run on a flow cytometer, and 10 to 15,000 events are acquired. For analysis, a histogram of forward-angle light scatter versus right-angle light scatter is displayed, and a gate is drawn around the monocytes or granulocytes (Fig. 4). On most analytical flow cytometers, the fluorescence can be measured in either the FL1 or FL2 photomultiplier tube. Analysis is expressed as the MFC, which is a correlate of the amount of DHR-123 that is oxidized and therefore an indirect measure of the level of ROI generated. The amount of fluorescence emitted by granulocytes is expressed as the normal oxidative index (NOI), which is calculated by dividing the MFC of the stimulated cells (plus DHR-123 and PMA) by that of the unstimulated cells (DHR-123 only). In our laboratory, the level of response obtained in whole blood from healthy individuals (NOI) is always >30. Conversely, patients with a diagnosis of CGD have an NOI which is <10. X-linked carriers of CGD will have two populations of granulocytes, one normal, i.e., with an NOI of >30, and one abnormal, with an NOI similar to that observed for a patient with CGD. Whole blood anticoagulated with either heparin or EDTA can be used, but note that if samples are to be kept for longer periods (up to 48 h), heparin is recommended.

Intracellular Staining

There have been significant improvements recently in the ability to detect intracellular antigens by flow cytometry. Although the current clinical applications for detecting intracellular antigens are limited, it is conceivable that in the future there will be an increased demand for this type of analysis. For example, it may be desirable to measure the ability of phagocytes to elaborate specific cytokines or cytokine inhibitors in response to provocative stimuli.

Currently, it is possible to identify rare patients with myeloperoxidase deficiency by measuring the intracellular levels of myeloperoxidase. It is important that patients with a complete myeloperoxidase deficiency can have a false-positive test for the diagnosis of CGD (15). It is recommended that patients with a positive screening test for CGD by either the DHR-123 assay or the dichlorodihydrofluorescein diacetate (DCFH-DR) assay who clinically do not appear to have a diagnosis of CGD be screened for the presence of myeloperoxidase by the use of intracellular staining protocols. For details of intracellular staining protocols, see the chapter on immunophenotyping.

Basophil Activation as a Measure of IgE-Dependent Allergen-Specific Responses in Allergic Patients

Flow cytometry allows for a relatively simple alternative to the time-consuming two-step process of measuring basophil degranulation in vitro (incubation and then measurement of specific mediators). The ability to measure basophil activation in response to an in vitro challenge with allergens has the potential to become a routine assay in the clinical laboratory. We have utilized a Basotest kit manufactured and distributed by Orpegen. (As a known positive control for tree pollen allergy myself, I can attest to the fact that the assay did in fact correctly identify sensitization to a seven-tree pollen combination and not to a mite preparation.) A recent review covers this area relatively comprehensively, discussing technical issues (CD63 versus CD203c, allergen concentrations, native versus recombinant allergens, etc.) as well as various laboratories' experiences with this relatively new flow cytometry procedure (8). A summary of the applications and test sensitivities and specificities of flow cytometric methods for detecting basophils is presented in Table 1 (8). Although this methodology is early in its development and will require more validation through clinical trials, it is an exciting avenue with potential applications not only in diagnosis but also in the monitoring of immunotherapy. Briefly, the principle of the assay is as follows. The assay is performed with sodium heparin-anticoagulated whole blood. If the patient is known to have high IgE levels, the blood should be washed once prior to the initiation of the assay. The whole blood is usually incubated at 37°C for 20 min with an appropriate stimulation buffer (IL-3) that increases the sensitization of the basophils without inducing degranulation. An appropriate concentration of the potential allergen(s) and positive (e.g., f-MetLeuPhe) and negative (pyrogen-free dilution buffer) controls are then incubated with the whole blood at 37°C for approximately 20 min. After this incubation, the samples are put on ice and labeled with a combination of antibodies against IgE (to allow for gating on basophils) and the appropriate activation marker (CD63 or CD203c) on ice and in the dark. After the labeling procedure, the red cells are lysed, the sample is washed at least one time, and the cells are fixed. Whole blood can be held for up to 24 h, and prepared samples should be analyzed within 2 h of red cell lysis. Analysis is accomplished by setting a gate around the low-right-angle light scatter, high anti-IgE-positive cells and measuring the expression of the basophil activation marker. The background or negative control sample is used to set the discrimination marker. The normal range for the positive controls should be established in each laboratory and then used to validate whether the test is performing properly or not prior to the analysis of patient samples. This test has the potential to become a valuable addition to allergy and/or immunology laboratories, but more clinical trial experience and better allergen preparations must be available before this assay becomes widely applicable.

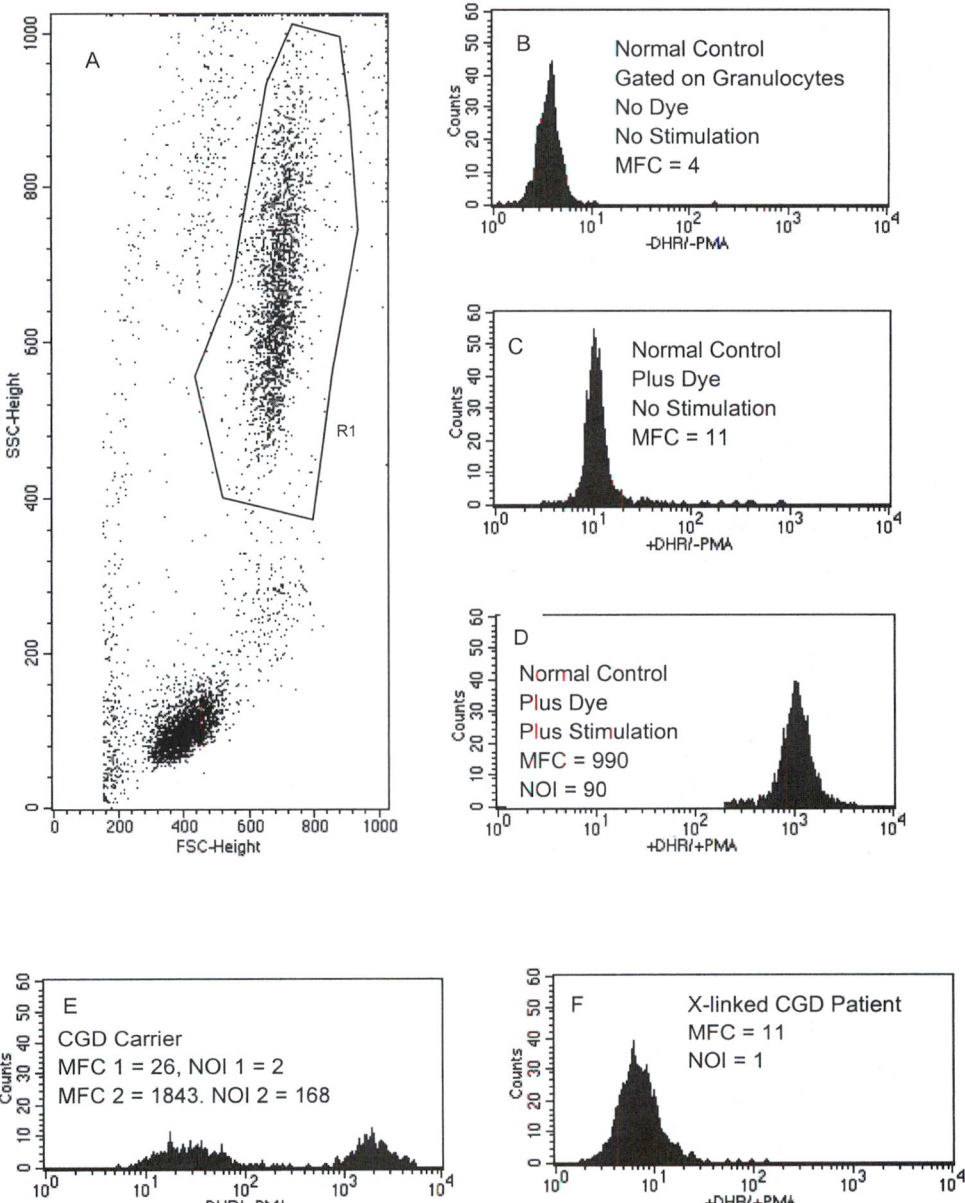

FIGURE 4 Summary of the flow cytometry procedure used to screen patients suspected of having CGD. The results illustrated are for a healthy control (D), an X-linked CGD carrier (E), and a CGD patient (F). The large two-dimensional dot plot on the left (A) illustrates the innate light scatter properties of lysed whole blood, with an electronic gate (R1) drawn around the granulocyte cluster. The histogram on the top right (B) represents the innate fluorescence emitted by granulocytes which have not been incubated with the oxidation-sensitive dye DHR-123; this tube is used to establish the baseline fluorescence settings for the flow cytometer. Histogram C represents gated granulocytes which have been incubated with the dye (DHR-123) but which have not been stimulated (baseline oxidative state). Histogram D represents granulocytes which have been incubated with the dye and which have been stimulated in vitro with PMA (see the text for details). Note that the NOI, which is the geometric MFC of the granulocyte population in histogram D (MFC = 990) divided by the MFC of the granulocytes in histogram C (MFC = 11), is 90, which is consistent with normal expression (i.e., an NOI of >30). Note that in histogram E, there are two populations of cells expressing different levels of fluorescence, one with an NOI of 2 (abnormal) and the other with an NOI of 168. This result is consistent with an X-linked CGD carrier status. The last histogram (F) illustrates an example of the results obtained for a patient with a diagnosis of CGD (note that the NOI [2] is significantly less than 30).

TABLE 1 Sensitivity and specificity of flow cytometric analysis of in vitro allergen-activated basophils[a]

Allergen	Gold standard or reference test[b]	n	Sensitivity (%)	Specificity (%)	Reference value
Cypress pollen	Hx + SPT + NC	34	91	100	71
Lolium perenne	Hx + SPT+IgE	51	93.3	98.4	86
House dust mite	Hx + SPT+IgE	53	93.3	98.4	86
Apple-mediated oral allergy syndrome	Hx	26	100[c]	100[c]	73
Pollen-associated food	Hx	29	≥85	≥80	72
Hevea latex	Hx + SPT+IgE	29	93.1	91.7	49
	Hx + SPT	43	93.0	100	70
Muscle relaxants	Hx	21	64	100	74
β-Lactam antibiotics	Hx + SPT	58	50	93.3	50
Metamizol	Hx ± SPT	26	42.3	100	89
Serum of patients with chronic urticaria[d]	Hx + ASST	20	70	65	53

[a] Reprinted from reference 8 with permission of the publisher.

[b] Hx, history; SPT, skin-prick test; NC, nasal challenge; ASST, autologous serum skin test (i.e., intradermal injection of autologous serum).

[c] According to data for control individuals without birch pollinosis. The basophil activation test was also positive for 7 of 20 patients with birch pollinosis but without a history of apple allergy.

[d] With the use of atopic donor basophils.

REFERENCES

1. Akerley, W. L., P. M. Guyre, and B. H. Davis. 1991. Neutrophil activation through high-affinity Fc-gamma receptors using monomeric antibody with unique properties. Blood 77:607–615.

2. Allen, E., A. C. Bakke, M. Z. Purtzer, and A. Deodhar. 2002. Neutrophil CD64 expression: distinguishing acute inflammatory autoimmune disease from systemic infections. Ann. Rheum. Dis. 61:522–525.

3. Bunescu, A., P. Seideman, R. Lenkei, K. Levin, and N. Egberg. 2004. Enhanced Fc gamma receptor I, alphaMbeta2 integrin receptor expression by monocytes and neutrophils in rheumatoid arthritis: interaction with platelets. J. Rheumatol. 31:2347–2355.

4. Campbell, D. E., and S. D. Douglas. 1997. Phagocytic cell functions. Oxidation and chemotaxis, p. 320–328. In R. E. Rose, E. C. Conway de Macario, J. D. Folds, H. C. Lane, and R. M. Nakamura (ed.), Manual of Clinical Laboratory Immunology, 5th ed. ASM Press, Washington, D.C.

5. Davis, B. H. 1996. Quantitative neutrophil CD64 expression: promising diagnostic indicator of infection or systemic acute inflammatory response. Clin. Immunol. Newsl. 16:121–130.

6. Davis, B. H., N. C. Bigelow, J. T. Churnutte, and K. Ornvold. 1995. Neutrophil CD64 expression: potential diagnostic indicator of acute inflammation and therapeutic monitor of interferon-gamma therapy. Lab. Hematol. 1:3–12.

7. Djeu, J. Y. 1992. Monocyte/macrophage functions, p. 231–239. In N. R. Rose, E. Conway De Macario, J. L. Fahey, H. Friedman, and G. M. Penn (ed.), Manual of Clinical Laboratory Immunology, 4th ed. American Society for Microbiology, Washington, D.C.

8. Ebo, D. G., M. M. Hagendorens, C. H. Bridts, A. J. Schuerwegh, L. S. De Clerck, and W. J. Stevens. 2004. In vitro allergy diagnosis: should we follow the flow? Clin. Exp. Allergy 34:332–339.

9. Etzioni, A., M. Frydman, S. Pollack, I. Avidur, M. L. Phillips, J. C. Paulson, and R. Gershoni-Baruch. 1992. Recurrent severe infections caused by a novel leukocyte adhesion deficiency. N. Engl. J. Med. 327:1789–1792.

10. Giaimis, J., Y. Lombard, P. Poindron, and C. D. Muller. 1994. Flow cytometry distinction between adherent and phagocytized yeast particles. Cytometry 17:173–178.

11. Goulding, N. J., S. M. Knight, J. L. Godolphin, and P. M. Guyre. 1992. Increase in neutrophil Fc gamma receptor I expression following interferon gamma treatment in rheumatoid arthritis. Ann. Rheum. Dis. 51:465–468.

12. Huizinga, T. W., C. E. Van Der Schoot, D. Roos, and R. S. Weening. 1991. Induction of neutrophil Fc-gamma receptor I expression can be used as a marker for biologic activity of recombinant interferon-gamma in vivo. Blood 77:2088–2089. (Letter.)

13. McKenzie, S. E., and A. D. Schrieber. 1988. Fc-gamma receptors in phagocytes. Curr. Opin. Hematol. 5:16–21.

14. Nebe, C. T. 1993. Phagocytic activity of monocytes and granulocytes, p. 181–182. In J. P. Robinson (ed.), Handbook of Flow Cytometry Methods. Liss Inc., New York, N.Y.

15. O'Gorman, M. R. G., A. R. Cross, T. Lowe, D. Osborn, S. Kasuga, and J. D. Harris. 1998. "Pseudo CGD" incorrect flow cytometry based diagnosis of CGD due to myeloperoxidase (MPO) deficiency: a case report. Cytometry 34:301.

16. O'Gorman, M. R. G., and V. Corrochano. 1995. Rapid whole-blood flow cytometry assay for diagnosis of chronic granulomatous disease. Clin. Diagn. Lab. Immunol. 2:227–232.

17. O'Gorman, M. R. G., A. C. McNally, D. C. Anderson, and B. L. Myones. 1993. A rapid whole blood lysis technique for the diagnosis of moderate or severe leukocyte adhesion deficiency (LAD). Ann. N. Y. Acad. Sci. 67:427–430.

18. Pulliam, L., R. Gascon, M. Subblebine, D. McGuire, and M.S. McGrath. 1997. Unique monocyte subset in patients with AIDS dementia. Lancet 349:692–695.

19. Thomas, R., and P. E. Lipsky. 1994. Human peripheral blood dendritic cell subsets. Isolation and characterization of precursor and mature antigen-presenting cells. J. Immunol. 153:4016–4028.

20. Zarev, P. V., and B. H. Davis. Comparative study of monocyte enumeration by flow cytometry: improved detection by combining monocyte-related antibodies with anti-CD163. Lab. Hematol. 10:24–31.

21. Ziegler-Heitbrock, H. W. 2000. Definition of human blood monocytes. J. Leukoc. Biol. 67:603–606.

Flow Cytometric Detection and Quantification of Apoptotic Cells

THOMAS W. McCLOSKEY, BARBARA N. PHENIX, AND SAVITA PAHWA

32

Interest in apoptosis has increased dramatically during the past 10 years, despite the fact that it was first observed over a century ago (31) and was conceptualized during ancient Greek times (13). Once the widespread biological significance of this process became apparent, investigators began to study cell death as it related to both hyperplastic and hypoplastic disease. Dysregulation of the apoptotic pathway can result in diseases of aberrant cell numbers, including cancer and AIDS. As pathways which regulate apoptosis continue to be discovered, the ability to modulate it becomes very real; such an achievement could have tremendous medical implications.

In 1971, Kerr (26) described a process of cell death called shrinkage necrosis, the initial events of which were cytoplasmic condensation and compaction of nuclear chromatin followed by nuclear fragmentation. The next year, a landmark paper by Kerr et al. (27) named this cell death cascade apoptosis. These investigators noted that apoptotic bodies and mitotic figures coexisted in tumors, and they had the foresight to speculate that hyperplasia might result from decreased cell death rather than increased cell division. Programmed cell death is a normal, physiological event which occurs without inflammation, so nontargeted bystander cells are not harmed. It is the body's mechanism for eliminating cells which are no longer needed or potentially injurious. Often referred to as cell suicide, an initiating trigger is required, after which the entire series of events leading to its own demise are carried out by the cell itself. Apoptosis is a critical component of normal embryonic development (5) which plays a prominent role in the formation of the nervous (52) and immune (61) systems. After maturation, it also plays a role in maintaining homeostasis, as it occurs naturally at the end of the life span of differentiated cells. Recent evidence has brought to light the function of death inducers, such as Fas ligand (which binds to the receptor Fas [CD95]), in protecting immune privileged sites (4).

However, alterations in cell survival contribute to several human diseases (57), including those of either cell accumulation or cell depletion. As a result of the intensive investigation in this field in recent years, numerous mammalian and viral regulatory proteins which interact with apoptotic pathways have been identified (15, 29, 35, 38), leading to potential therapeutic implications for cancer (40). Since the deletion of self-reactive leukocytes is beneficial for the host, dysregulated cell death is reported to be involved in autoimmune disease (49). Increased peripheral lymphocyte apoptosis has emerged as an important pathogenic factor during human immunodeficiency virus (HIV) infection (19, 46); in fact, our understanding of the immune system's interaction with both viral (51) and bacterial (60) pathogens may unveil cell death as a critical variable determining an effective host response.

The intensive research conducted thus far has led to an enhanced understanding of the cellular processes involved in apoptosis (Fig. 1) and the diseases in which dysregulated cell death plays a role (reviewed in reference 14). The interaction of death receptors with their respective ligands is an important area of investigation which has discovered multiple death-inducing molecules. Much progress has been made in clarifying intracellular signal transduction pathways following triggering at the cell surface (reviewed in reference 2). Physiological cell death is a highly regulated process which may be determined by the balance of pro- and antiapoptotic molecules within the cell (reviewed in reference 23), leading to cells that are either prone to die or protected from death. In addition, chemical or radiation exposure which disrupts the DNA may initiate deletion of a particular cell or, alternatively, may activate DNA repair mechanisms. Recently, the important role of mitochondria (reviewed in reference 22) as central players in several major pathways of apoptosis has been elucidated.

The characteristic series of events typical of apoptosis are generally cell membrane blebbing, chromatin condensation, and fragmentation of DNA. Such distinguishing features are visible microscopically, particularly in DNA-stained samples observed under a fluorescence microscope. Thus, visual determination and quantification of apoptosis in a sample should accompany flow cytometric measurement. Many of these features can be utilized to resolve apoptotic cells cytometrically. After the diffusion of fragmented chromatin, DNA content measurements can distinguish apoptotic from live cells by detection of a subdiploid population. Strand breaks within the DNA molecule can be fluorescently tagged via an enzymatic reaction by the terminal deoxynucleotidyl transferase-mediated dUTP nick end labeling (TUNEL) method. The exposure of phosphatidylserine is an apoptotic event which can be revealed by the specific binding of annexin. Activation of the caspase cascade can be detected by using fluorescence-based techniques. Each of these features of apoptotic cells has been taken advantage of to allow the resolution of dying cells within a heterogeneous sample.

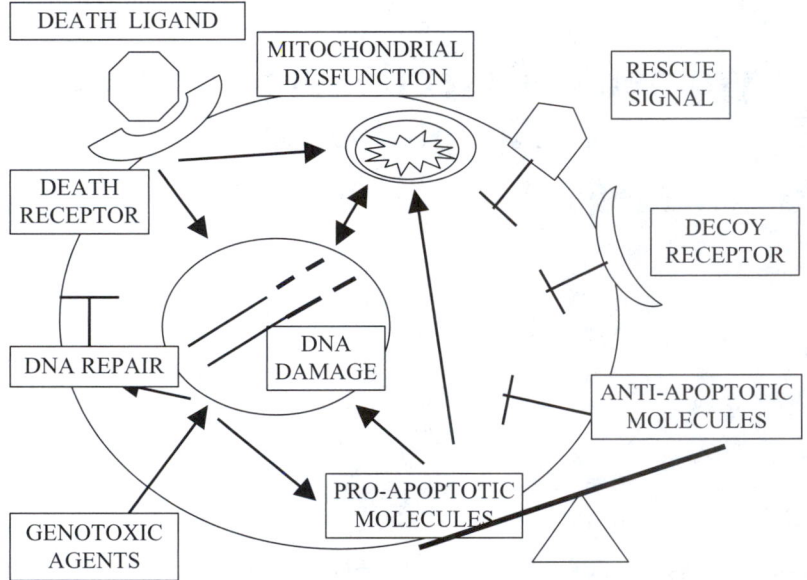

FIGURE 1 Major mechanisms for regulation of cell death. Cell death pathways may involve (i) the interaction between a cell surface receptor capable of signaling for apoptosis and its ligand; (ii) DNA damage, after which chromosome repair or cell deletion mechanisms may commence; (iii) alterations in the mitochondria, which are major cellular organelles involved in the decision for replication or elimination; and (iv) an imbalance in apoptotic regulatory molecules, such as those in the Bcl-2 family.

METHODS FOR DETECTION OF APOPTOSIS

As interest in apoptosis has increased due to its pivotal role in many fields of cell biology, the requirement for clinical assessment has also risen. For example, it may be important to know the percentage of cells which are dying for a disease characterized by increased lymphocyte apoptosis, such as HIV infection (8, 36). In addition, confirmation of the primary immunodeficiency Canale-Smith syndrome (autoimmune lymphoproliferative syndrome) (12, 16, 50) requires a demonstration of reduced apoptosis in response to Fas stimulation. A determination of the in vitro sensitivity of cancer cells to apoptosis may be helpful for selection of the most appropriate chemotherapeutic regimen for treatment (6).

The study of apoptosis is being increasingly applied to many different cell types (e.g., hepatocytes, neurons, cardiac myocytes, etc.). The methods described here are approaches to investigate apoptosis in lymphocytes. For investigations of lymphocyte apoptosis in the peripheral circulation, blood should be collected by venipuncture into sterile Vacutainer tubes containing anticoagulant. Blood samples should be processed as soon as possible and no later than 6 h after blood draw and should be maintained at room temperature until the time of processing. Peripheral blood mononuclear cells are isolated by standard techniques (as discussed elsewhere in this manual) and then processed for the evaluation of lymphocyte apoptosis per the objectives of the study (see "Important Considerations" in this chapter). The methods discussed here refer to the analysis of apoptotic cells in the sample of interest by utilizing flow cytometry, which has emerged as a technology well suited to quantifying dying cells (11, 43). Many of the events of cell death can be detected by using fluorescent dyes or fluorochrome-conjugated reagents and can be measured by flow cytometry.

Detection of Cells with Reduced DNA Content (Subdiploid Method)

One of the hallmarks of the process of apoptosis is the activation of endonucleases. Fragmented chromatin results in cells with a diminished total DNA content, a characteristic which can be utilized to tag these cells within a mixed population (Fig. 2). By utilizing nucleic acid-specific dyes such as propidium iodide, apoptotic cells can be distinguished from live cells within the same sample (42). This assay is applicable to both human cell lines (24) and primary isolates (36).

Reagents

Ethanol (100%; Pharmco Products, Brookfield, Conn. [www.pharmco-prod.com/products.html])

Propidium iodide (50-μg/ml stock; Molecular Probes, Eugene, Oreg. [www.probes.com])

RNase (1-mg/ml stock; Sigma, St. Louis, Mo. [www.sigma.com])

Procedure

1. Centrifuge samples and aspirate supernatant.

2. Resuspend pellet in 0.5 ml of Hanks balanced salt solution (HBSS), vortex, add 1.5 ml of ethanol, and vortex.

3. Incubate for 1 h at 4°C.

4. Centrifuge samples and aspirate supernatant. (Note that higher centrifuge speeds may be required after ethanol fixation.)

5. Add the following to the pellet: 250 μl of Hanks balanced salt solution, 250 μl of RNase, and 500 μl of propidium iodide.

6. Incubate the mixture for 15 min at room temperature and then maintain the mixture at 4°C in the dark until flow cytometric analysis (Fig. 3). The time after fixation for optimal analysis should be determined for each system, as

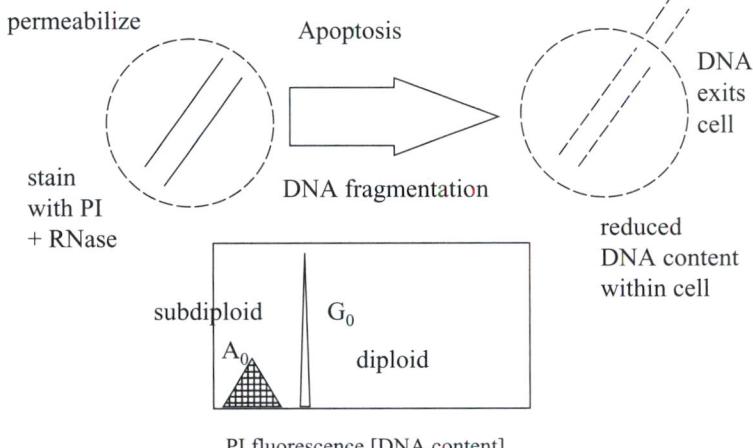

FIGURE 2 Rationale for subdiploid apoptosis assay. A hallmark of apoptosis is the activation of endonuclease, resulting in the fragmentation of cellular DNA. Samples are fixed and permeabilized with ethanol, which allows DNA fragments to escape past the plasma membrane. Staining with propidium iodide (PI) and measuring the DNA content flow cytometrically reveal a population with reduced DNA content representing apoptotic cells. (Inset) Apoptotic cells are a distinct population with reduced fluorescence (shaded population).

additional fragmented DNA will continue to diffuse out of cells (for approximately 24 to 48 h).

Assay Interpretation and Pitfalls

Apoptotic cells are visible as a distinct peak with a reduced fluorescence intensity compared to that of the live cells located in the G_0 peak. The conventional flow cytometric thought process of locating the diploid peak and then measuring those cells with greater fluorescence (cycling cells) must be dismissed. Instead, the goal here is to locate those cells with reduced fluorescence and to distinguish them from

other "events" which may also have reduced fluorescence. Tight coefficients of variation for the G_0 peak are essential for this assay. The machine alignment should be checked and set carefully. Samples should be run at low differential pressures to maximize the resolution of apoptotic and intact cells. Nucleic acid dyes with differing binding properties work equally well in this assay (39, 56).

Careful gating and analysis are essential in order to achieve accurate measurements when using the subdiploid assay. Samples are initially gated on light scatter and then on a doublet discrimination histogram of peak versus integral (height versus area on some instruments) fluorescence to exclude clumps. The discriminator (threshold) setting on the machine should be adjusted for propidium iodide fluorescence equal to 25% of the G_0 peak (e.g., if the G_0 peak is set at channel 400, the cytometer should be triggered on red fluorescence corresponding to channel 100). The rationale governing this setting is that apoptotic cells (A_0) will possess slightly less DNA than intact cells. Although this conservative analysis scheme may miss some late-stage apoptotic cells, it will exclude from the measurement many potentially confounding events, such as apoptotic bodies, mitochondria, and nuclear and cellular fragments, all of which would erroneously elevate the observed percentage of apoptosis. Thus, incorrect levels of apoptosis may be enumerated by the inclusion of noncellular events in the apoptotic region of the histogram and their counting as apoptotic cells. These data are always collected on a linear fluorescence scale.

The subdiploid assay is highly recommended as an initial assay for a simple evaluation of apoptosis. The major advantages of this method include its ease, similarity to familiar assays of the cell cycle, and low cost, and in addition, following flow cytometric analysis, samples can be spun down onto slides and examined by fluorescence microscopy (note that improved cellular morphology for microscopic examination may be obtained by splitting samples and making slides prior to fixation and staining). Apoptotic cells are readily detectable due to membrane blebbing or condensed and fragmented chromatin. These visual results can be compared

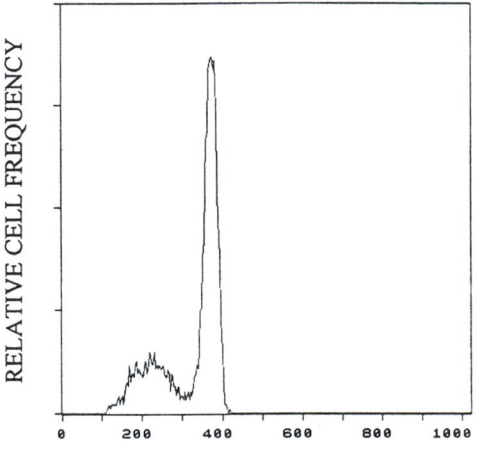

FIGURE 3 Representative histogram of subdiploid method for assay of apoptosis. Peripheral blood mononuclear cells (PBMC) from an HIV-infected child were cultured for 3 days and then processed by the subdiploid assay. Cells with reduced DNA content compared to G_0 cells are clearly visible.

to those obtained with the cytometer for accuracy of gating and analysis regions. The drawbacks of this method are its incompatibility with monoclonal antibody labeling, as those subsets undergoing apoptosis in a mixed population cannot be determined, and that caution must be exercised to exclude noncellular events which have subdiploid levels of fluorescence from the final analysis.

Assay Variations

Instead of allowing fragmented chromatin to diffuse from permeabilized cells, a citrate-based buffer can be utilized to extract it (as described in reference 20). Another variation on this assay utilizes hypotonic lysis to isolate free nuclei (42), after which a similar analysis is performed. This procedure may be useful in circumstances where cell adherence is a problem, as free nuclei can be released. However, the ability to differentiate apoptotic nuclei from debris by measuring light scatter is compromised compared to that of the whole-cell assay.

Detection of Cells with DNA Strand Breaks (TUNEL Method)

The TUNEL method (Fig. 4) is based on the enzyme-mediated insertion of nucleotides into DNA strand breaks which are present in apoptotic cells (21). The use of fluorochrome-conjugated nucleotides offers a single-step procedure (30). The TUNEL method is recommended for its outstanding sensitivity and specificity, as it has demonstrated excellent agreement with fluorescence microscopy for both cell lines ($r = 0.98$; $P = 0.0001$) and isolated lymphocytes ($r = 0.75$; $P = 0.0001$) (34). TUNEL assays have been facilitated by the introduction of kits by various manufacturers.

Reagents

Apo-Direct TUNEL kit (Phoenix Flow Systems, San Diego, Calif. [www.phnxflow.com])

Permeafix fixation and permeabilization reagent (Ortho Diagnostic Systems, Raritan, N.J. [www.ortho.com])

Procedure

1. Cells are incubated for 40 min at room temperature with Permeafix.
2. Samples are centrifuged, the supernatant is removed, and cells are resuspended in 1 ml of wash buffer.
3. Samples are centrifuged, the supernatant is removed, and cells are resuspended in 50 µl of TUNEL labeling solution containing the following (in each tube): 10 µl of TdT reaction buffer, 0.75 µl of TdT enzyme, 8 µl of fluorescein-dUTP, and 32 µl of distilled H_2O (note that a useful negative control is obtained following incubation in labeling solution in which the enzyme has been omitted).
4. Incubate samples with TUNEL labeling solution for 60 min at 37°C.
5. Add 1 ml of rinse buffer to each tube.
6. Centrifuge, aspirate the supernatant, and resuspend the cells in rinse buffer.
7. Analyze by flow cytometry (Fig. 5).

Assay Interpretation and Pitfalls

Apoptotic cells labeled by TUNEL are visible as a distinct population with increased fluorescence intensity compared to the live cells present in the tube. This assay depends on an enzyme-mediated insertion of labeled nucleotides; appropriate enzyme function should be verified. This may be accomplished by the use of negative and positive control cells (prefixed cells, either nonapoptotic or partially apoptotic), which are provided with the kit and should be prepared for each experiment. These cells demonstrate both the absence of nonspecific labeling in live cells and the presence of specific labeling in known apoptotic cells. Quantification of the percentage of TUNEL-positive cells among the positive control cells can be useful for daily quality control of the assay. This method is also reliant on adequate permeabilization of the sample. Thus, when problems are encountered during use of the TUNEL procedure, the permeabilization step should be checked. An appropriate and useful control sample is prepared by omitting the enzyme but subjecting

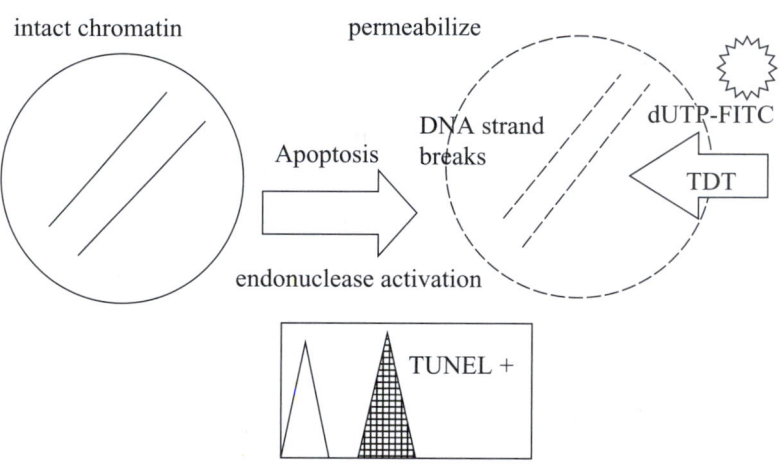

FIGURE 4 Rationale for TUNEL apoptosis assay. Endonuclease activation during apoptosis results in DNA strand breaks. Samples are fixed and permeabilized. The enzyme terminal deoxynucleotidyl transferase inserts fluorescently labeled nucleotides, allowing the resolution of apoptotic from live cells. (Inset) Apoptotic cells exhibit an increased fluorescence intensity compared to live cells (shaded population). FITC, fluorescein isothiocyanate.

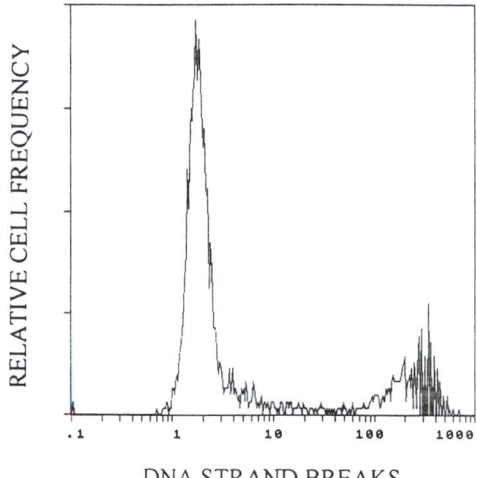

DNA STRAND BREAKS

FIGURE 5 Representative histogram of TUNEL assay. PBMC from an HIV-infected child were cultured for 3 days, prepared by the TUNEL method, and analyzed flow cytometrically. Apoptotic cells exhibit a bright fluorescence intensity.

the sample to all other steps of the procedure. A biological variable affecting this assay is the number of DNA strand breaks that the apoptotic cells possess, which will determine the ability to resolve them from live cells. It is possible, therefore, that early apoptotic cells with minimal chromatin damage will not incorporate enough fluorescence to allow detection.

Assay Variations

Alternative reagents available for the fixation and permeabilization step include (i) paraformaldehyde-FACS Perm (Becton Dickinson, San Jose, Calif. [www.bdfacs.com]), (ii) Cytofix/Cytoperm (Pharmingen, San Diego, Calif. [www.pharmingen.com]), (iii) Fix and Perm (Caltag, Burlingame, Calif. [www.caltag.com]), (iv) Intraprep (Coulter, Miami, Fla. [www.coulter.com]), (v) paraformaldehyde-ethanol, and (vi) paraformaldehyde-saponin. (Note that single-step fixation and permeabilization reagents may enhance cell recovery.) This assay is compatible with monoclonal antibody labeling of surface antigens (Fig. 6). Cells are labeled prior to fixation and then processed as described above.

Detection of Cells with Translocated Phosphatidylserine (Annexin V Method)

The annexin V assay (Fig. 7) for the detection of apoptosis is based on the exposure of phosphatidylserine on the outer plasma membrane (33, 59). This phospholipid is normally sequestered in the inner cell membrane exclusively, and its translocation acts as an important signal for the clearance of deceased cells (32). Fluorochrome-conjugated annexin is capable of binding phosphatidylserine, thus allowing the detection of apoptotic cells.

Reagents

Annexin binding buffer (Pharmingen [www.pharmingen.com])

Fluorescein-conjugated annexin V (Pharmingen [www.pharmingen.com])

Paraformaldehyde (Electron Microscopy Sciences, Fort Washington, Pa. [www.emsdiasum.com/ems])

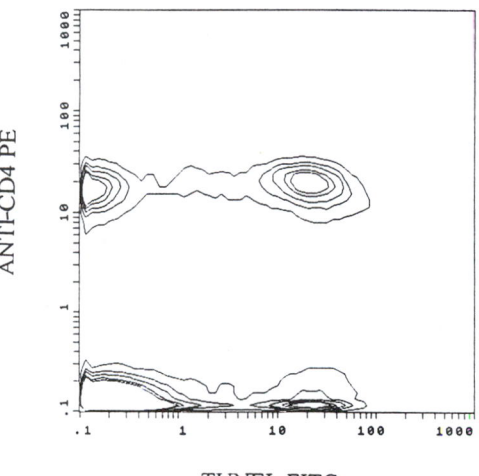

TUNEL FITC

FIGURE 6 Determination of DNA strand breaks within a specific subpopulation. PBMC from an HIV-infected child were cultured for 3 days. The sample was then labeled with an anti-CD4–phycoerythrin (PE) monoclonal antibody, fixed and permeabilized in Ortho Permeafix, and then subjected to the TUNEL procedure. This experimental design allows the quantification of apoptotic CD4 cells.

Procedure

1. Suspend cells in 1 ml of binding buffer.
2. Centrifuge the sample, aspirate the supernatant, and resuspend the cells in 100 μl of binding buffer.
3. Add 5 μl of annexin, vortex, and incubate for 10 min at room temperature.
4. Add 1 ml of binding buffer, centrifuge, remove the supernatant, and resuspend the cells in binding buffer.
5. The sample may be analyzed on a flow cytometer immediately or fixed in 1% paraformaldehyde (Fig. 8).

Assay Interpretation and Pitfalls

Apoptotic cells revealed by the annexin assay will exhibit an increased fluorescence intensity compared to that of the live cells in the same sample. This assay depends on the presence of two distinct populations in the test sample, since otherwise it is difficult to determine the background fluorescence. A drawback of this method is the lack of a control molecule to determine nonspecific binding of annexin, and thus a continuous distribution of annexin fluorescence is problematic.

Any sample manipulation which results in damage to the cell membrane may allow annexin binding to live cells. The inclusion of propidium iodide in this assay is often used to detect such cells, but cells in the late stages of apoptosis will also admit propidium iodide through their membranes and should rightfully be included in a count of total apoptosis. Thus, careful sample preparation is a prerequisite for accurate quantification of apoptosis by the annexin method. Simultaneous assessments of annexin binding and propidium iodide exclusion may be used to determine early from late apoptosis, if that is the intent of the investigator.

The binding of annexin to phosphatidylserine is a calcium-dependent process, thus requiring calcium-enriched buffers. This assay has the unique attribute of detecting apoptotic cells without the requirement of fixation. The potential exists for phosphatidylserine-expressing cells to be sorted, placed back in culture, and subsequently reassayed.

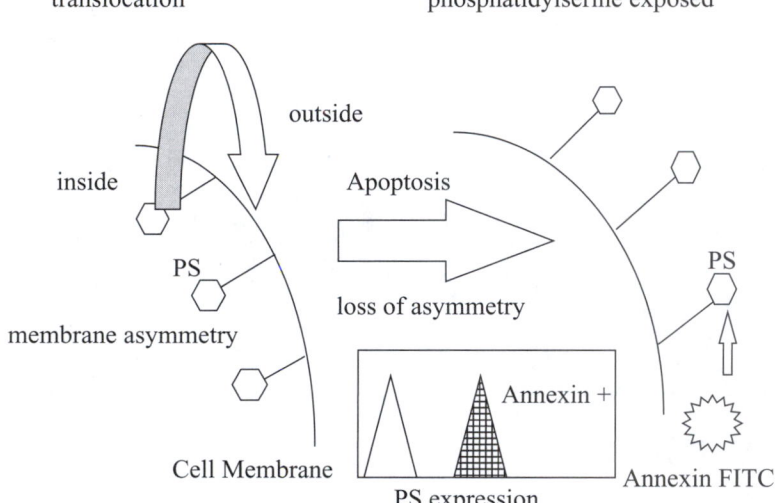

FIGURE 7 Rationale for annexin V apoptosis assay. In live cells, a state of membrane asymmetry exists in which phosphatidylserine (PS) is sequestered in the inner portion of the plasma membrane. During apoptosis, phosphatidylserine translocates to the outer cell membrane. Fluorochrome-conjugated annexin V binds specifically, thus tagging apoptotic cells. (Inset) Annexin-positive cells exhibit enhanced fluorescence compared to live cells (shaded population).

Assay Variations

This procedure is compatible with monoclonal antibody labeling (Fig. 9). Fluorochrome-conjugated antibodies can be added simultaneously at the annexin binding step. For samples in which contaminating erythrocytes may present a problem, the lysis of red cells with commercial reagents and/or the use of a fixative which eliminates red cells may be incorporated (as described in reference 34).

Detection of Cells Containing Active Caspases

The execution of apoptosis consistently involves the activation of a family of cysteine aspartyl proteases, termed caspases.

Caspases cleave their target proteins at specific aspartate residues and are important mediators of the apoptosis cascade (1, 41). Caspases exist as inactive zymogens and are processed in cells undergoing apoptosis by self-proteolysis and/or cleavage by other proteases (9, 58). Several methods currently exist for the detection of active caspases. Antibodies to active caspases (anti-active caspase-3; Beckman Coulter) bind to a conformational epitope that is exposed by activation-induced cleavage of procaspase 3 (7). Cell-permeative fluorogenic caspase substrates (28, 47) such as those from Phiphilux, Oncoimmunin, College Park, Md.,

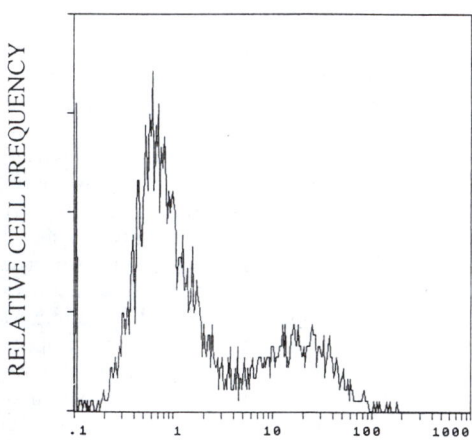

PHOSPHATIDYLSERINE EXTERNALIZATION

FIGURE 8 Representative histogram for detection of apoptosis by annexin method. PBMC from an HIV-infected child were cultured for 3 days, prepared by the annexin method, and analyzed by flow cytometry. Phosphatidylserine-expressing cells are distinguishable from live cells as a separate peak.

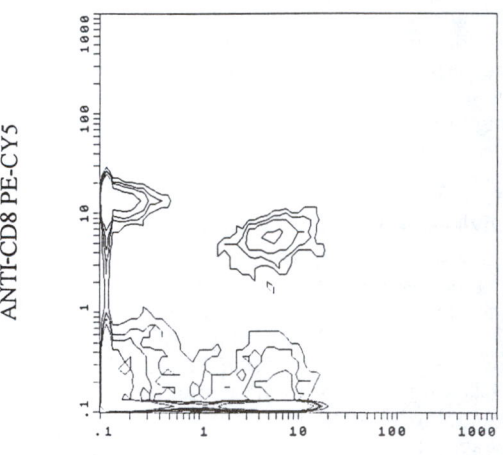

ANNEXIN FITC

FIGURE 9 Determination of phosphatidylserine exposure within a specific subpopulation. PBMC from a healthy adult were cultured for 3 days. The sample was labeled with anti-CD8–phycoerythrin-cyanine 5 (PE-CY5) and annexin fluorescein, washed, and fixed. Subsequent analysis allows the quantification of apoptosis within the CD8 subset.

and fluorescent inhibitors of caspases (10, 54) such as those from Molecular Probes both allow for the identification of intracellular caspase activity (Fig. 10).

Reagents

Vybrant FAM caspase-3 and -7 assay kit (Molecular Probes [www.probes.com])

Procedure

1. Resuspend 10^6 cells in 1 ml of culture medium.
2. Add 10 μl of 30× fluorescent inhibitor of caspases (FLICA) working solution directly to 300 μl of cell suspension. Mix.
3. Incubate for 60 min at 37°C and 5% CO_2, with protection from light. Mix during incubation to prevent settling.
4. Add 2 ml of 1× wash buffer.
5. Pellet cells by centrifugation. Discard the supernatant and resuspend cells in 1 ml of wash buffer.
6. Pellet cells by centrifugation. Discard the supernatant and resuspend cells in 400 μl of wash buffer.
7. Analyze on a flow cytometer with a 488-nm excitation wavelength and green emission immediately or fix in 1% paraformaldehyde for later analysis.

Assay Interpretation and Pitfalls

Apoptotic cells containing active caspase-3 or -7 will exhibit an increased fluorescence intensity compared to that of the live cells in the same sample. This assay depends on the presence of two distinct populations in the test sample; otherwise; it is difficult to determine the background fluorescence. A potential drawback of this method is that interactions with other cellular sites may contribute to the signal intensity of nonapoptotic cells (48).

Hoechst 33342 and propidium iodide are also included in the Vybrant FAM caspase-3 and -7 assay kit, allowing for additional evaluations of membrane permeability and the cell cycle. However, samples may not be fixed if these additional reagents are to be used. The potential exists for active caspase-expressing cells to be sorted, placed back in culture, and subsequently reassayed.

Assay Variations

The Vybrant FAM caspase-3 and -7 assay procedure is compatible with monoclonal antibody labeling. Fluorochrome-conjugated antibodies may be added after the washing step (step 6). Resuspend the cell pellet in an appropriate volume of phosphate-buffered saline and follow regular surface labeling protocols. This kit may also be used in conjunction with other apoptosis detection reagents, such as red-excited annexin V-allophycocyanin.

USE OF JURKAT CELLS AS CONTROLS FOR APOPTOSIS ASSAYS

Negative and positive controls are necessary to characterize the assay system as well as to verify its consistency. Negative controls may consist of primary isolates (e.g., peripheral blood lymphocytes) from healthy individuals or cell lines in growth phase. These should be cells that exhibit no signs of deterioration, which additionally should be checked for viability by a trypan blue assay. Positive control cells may be produced within the laboratory. The acute T-cell leukemia cell line Jurkat is readily induced to undergo apoptotic cell death. Jurkat T lymphocytes (clone E6-1; ATCC TIB-152) may be obtained from the American Type Culture Collection (Manassas, Va. [www.atcc.org]).

Reagents

RPMI 1640 culture medium (Whittaker Bioproducts, Walkersville, Md. [www.biowhittaker.com])

Fetal calf serum (Hyclone Laboratories, Logan, Utah [www.hyclone.com])

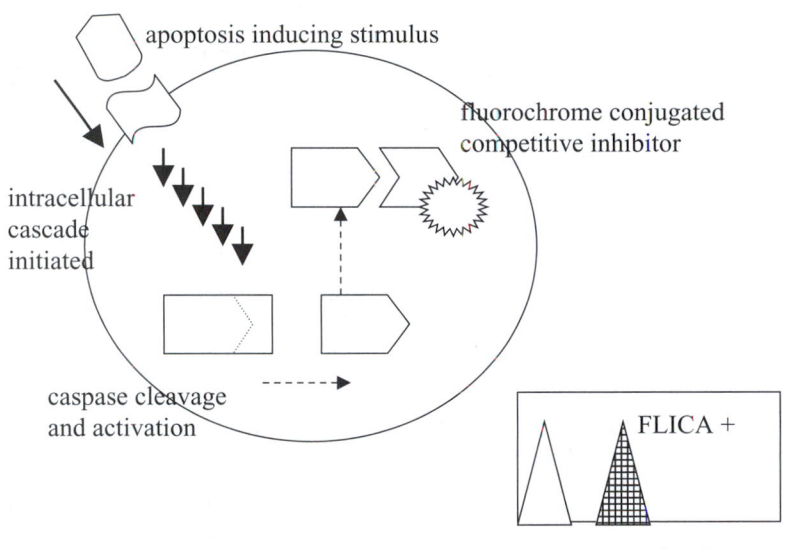

FIGURE 10 Rationale for caspase apoptosis assay. A cell encounters an apoptosis-inducing stimulus, which initiates a cascade of intracellular events. Among these events in caspase-dependent apoptosis are the cleavage and activation of caspase enzymes. The fluorescent inhibitor of caspases (FLICA) is able to compete with the natural ligand and bind to activated caspase. (Inset) Cells can be analyzed by flow cytometry, and apoptotic cells will be detectable via their increased fluorescence.

L-Glutamine (Whittaker Bioproducts [www.biowhit-taker.com])

Penicillin-streptomycin (Whittaker Bioproducts [www.biowhittaker.com])

CD95 antibody (clone CH-11 [immunoglobulin M]; Upstate Biotechnology, Lake Placid, N.Y. [www.upstatebiotech.com])

Procedure

1. Maintain Jurkat cells in RPMI 1640 medium with 10% fetal calf serum, 2 mM L-glutamine, 100 U of penicillin G/ml, and 100 μg of streptomycin/ml. Set up 12- by 75-mm tubes with 10^6 cells/ml.

2. Add anti-CD95 (100 ng/ml) antibody to tubes and incubate for 2 to 4 h at 37°C. (Time course data are available in reference 34.)

3. Harvest cells and apply apoptosis assay for quantification of cell death.

IMPORTANT CONSIDERATIONS

Initial ventures for the detection, quantification, and characterization of apoptotic cells should address the following issues. In what cell type is apoptosis occurring? Which method is most applicable? What are the kinetics of the death process, i.e., is a period of cell culture required before apoptosis can be detected? What are appropriate negative and positive controls? How can the presence of apoptosis be verified in the test sample?

Regarding cell type, there is a major difference between performing apoptosis assays with cell lines and performing them with primary isolates. Cell lines consist of one cell type and are homogeneous in nature. In contrast, a sample isolated from a subject may have contaminating cell types along with the cells of interest. This issue ties in with method selection. For a mixed sample, a method must be chosen which has the potential to simultaneously utilize another parameter to mark the cells of interest. For example, for the measurement of T-lymphocyte apoptosis in a human peripheral blood sample, the TUNEL method combined with labeling for anti-CD3 would be an appropriate choice. It is also critical to ensure that the cell isolation method does not differentially select for live or apoptotic cells. For example, adherent cells undergoing apoptosis may disengage themselves and could be lost during a wash procedure, or a centrifugation step may fragment dying cells without affecting healthy cells. These events would result in erroneous measurement of the percentage of apoptotic cells.

Careful consideration should be given to the kinetics of cell death. Each flow cytometric assay takes a snapshot in time, i.e., it measures the percentage of apoptotic cells (by the characteristic being used to detect them) in the total number of cells that the instrument senses. Thus, the assay does not provide information on the cumulative amount of cell death which has occurred, but rather that in process at the time of assay. For an in vitro model system, such as a cell line induced to undergo apoptosis, a time course study can be performed over several hours to determine the peak response. For primary cells, the detection of maximal levels of cell death may require ex vivo culturing for one to several days (36, 45). Cell counts provide useful information during culture periods because they yield an estimate of the total number of cells lost. Furthermore, the question of timing becomes even more important if the experimental design is attempting to estimate in vivo levels of deceased cells. Can apoptosis be detected immediately in freshly isolated cells? The assay chosen for this application is critical, as in vivo clearance of apoptotic cells is very efficient, making their detection difficult. Can samples be obtained in one laboratory and then shipped to another for apoptosis assessment? Results obtained through testing by the AIDS Clinical Trials Group suggest that shipping influences apoptosis.

The choice of controls is critical, both for assurance that the assay is performing as expected and for the detection of biological variability. As outlined earlier, Jurkat cells serve as a readily prepared positive control for apoptosis. However, depending on the experimental design, an investigator may wish to include both negative and positive control samples for the cell type of interest. Therefore, one requires a known live sample of the cell type under study as well as an induced apoptotic sample. Any discussion of controls naturally leads to the important issue of verification of results. Since cellular, and especially nuclear, morphology is the defining characteristic of apoptotic cell death, microscopy remains the method of choice for verifying apoptosis results. Fluorescence microscopy following staining of the sample with a DNA dye such as propidium iodide will allow the direct quantification of apoptotic cells within the sample. In addition, it may reveal artifacts which might account for unexpected flow cytometric results. It is important to bear in mind that flow cytometers do not quantify apoptosis; they measure fluorescence, and it is left to the operator to interpret the data.

ALTERNATIVE METHODOLOGY

Four flow cytometric assays for apoptosis have been presented. These methods performed well in a multiassay comparison study (34). In contrast, since apoptotic cells are generally able to maintain membrane integrity, trypan blue dye exclusion is not recommended as a means of apoptosis quantification. Many other methods have been reported, including the detection of changes in the mitochondrial membrane potential (62), the use of Hoechst in combination with propidium iodide or 7-amino actinomycin D (53, 55), the use of flow cytometric light-scatter parameters (44), and the use of the Apo 2.7 monoclonal antibody (63). Depending on the experimental design, these alternative methods may prove useful. For example, changes in the mitochondrial membrane potential are thought to be among the earliest events in apoptosis. However, time-dependent assays using live cells are inherently more difficult to perform.

Besides allowing for the detection of apoptosis itself, many reagents are available for the flow cytometric investigation of the molecules involved in cell death, including both cell membrane-associated and cytoplasmic molecules. For example, monoclonal antibodies against members of the Fas and Bcl-2 families of proteins are readily attainable. Cytokines, which are often important accessories in apoptosis initiation, are evaluable by the use of fluorochrome-conjugated immunoglobulins. The increasing availability of these reagents continues to open new avenues for apoptosis research by flow cytometry. In addition to advances in reagent technology, the laser scanning cytometer (3) represents novel instrumentation suitable for the quantification and investigation of apoptosis. The expression of genes involved in apoptosis may be evaluated at the DNA and mRNA levels by using appropriate assays described elsewhere in this book.

PRECAUTIONS IN DATA INTERPRETATION

Systems have been reported in which apoptosis occurs in an atypical fashion. For example, model systems of cell death have been described in which cells do not exhibit decreased DNA content (17), do not label with the TUNEL reaction (37), and do not express phosphatidylserine (18). These reports emphasize the importance of verifying data obtained with any single method. Microscopic evaluation, a positive control of death induction in the test system, and the use of more than one method may be required to validate apoptosis data.

CONCLUSIONS

The appreciation of the fact that a complete understanding of the cell cycle includes knowledge of physiological cell death has generated tremendous research interest in the process of apoptosis and has led to the development of many assays for examining apoptosis. The consideration of potential variables and artifacts, microscopic examinations of samples, and the choice of method stand as critical components in the successful investigation of apoptosis.

Our increased understanding of the role of apoptosis in cell biology has elevated it to a place of important stature in both science and medicine. Its significance is underscored by its tremendous evolutionary conservation, as baculoviral inhibitors of apoptosis are capable of interaction with mammalian caspases (25). Furthermore, as evidenced by the deletion of autoreactive clones in the human thymus, apoptosis is essential for life. Dysregulated cell death, however, such as the rising apoptosis associated with AIDS progression, is clearly associated with pathogenesis. The potential to treat human disease via manipulation of apoptotic pathways holds great promise, and as the elucidation of both protective and inductive cell death signaling mechanisms continues, such possibilities approach realization.

This work was supported by grants AI28281 and DA05161 from the National Institutes of Health.

REFERENCES

1. **Alnemri, E. S., D. J. Livingston, D. W. Nicholson, G. Salvesen, N. A. Thornberry, W. W. Wong, and J. Yuan.** 1996. Human ICE/CED-3 protease nomenclature. *Cell* **87:**171.
2. **Ashkenazi, A., and V. M. Dixit.** 1998. Death receptors: signaling and modulation. *Science* **281:**1305–1308.
3. **Bedner, E., X. Li, W. Gorczyca, M. R. Melamed, and Z. Darzynkiewicz.** 1999. Analysis of apoptosis by laser scanning cytometry. *Cytometry* **35:**181–195.
4. **Bellgrau, D., and R. C. Duke.** 1999. Apoptosis and CD95 ligand in immune privileged sites. *Int. Rev. Immunol.* **18:**547–562.
5. **Brill, A., A. Torchinsky, H. Carp, and V. Toder.** 1999. The role of apoptosis in normal and abnormal embryonic development. *J. Assist. Reprod. Genet.* **16:**512–519.
6. **Campana, D.** 1994. Applications of cytometry to study acute leukemia: in vitro determination of drug sensitivity and detection of minimal residual disease. *Cytometry* **18:**68–74.
7. **Campos, L., O. Sabido, A. Viallet, C. Vasselon, and D. Guyotat.** 1999. Expression of apoptosis controlling proteins in acute leukemia cells. *Leuk. Lymphoma* **33:**499–509.
8. **Chavan, S. J., S. L. Tamma, M. Kaplan, M. Gersten, and S. G. Pahwa.** 1999. Reduction in T cell apoptosis in patients with HIV disease following antiretroviral therapy. *Clin. Immunol.* **93:**24–33.
9. **Cryns, V., and J. Yuan.** 1998. Proteases to die for. *Genes Dev.* **12:**1551–1570.
10. **Darzynkiewicz, Z., E. Bedner, P. Smolewski, B. W. Lee, and G. L. Johnson.** 2002. Detection of caspase activation in situ by fluorochrome labeled inhibitors of caspases (FLICA). *Methods Mol. Biol.* **203:**289–299.
11. **Darzynkiewicz, Z., G. Juan, X. Li, W. Gorczyca, T. Murakami, and F. Traganos.** 1997. Cytometry in cell necrobiology: analysis of apoptosis and accidental cell death (necrosis). *Cytometry* **27:**1–20.
12. **Drappa, J., A. K. Vaishnaw, K. E. Sullivan, J. L. Chu, and K. B. Elkon.** 1996. Fas gene mutations in the Canale-Smith Syndrome, an inherited lymphoproliferative disorder associated with autoimmunity. *N. Engl. J. Med.* **335:**1643–1649.
13. **Esposti, M. D.** 1998. Apoptosis: who was first. *Cell Death Differ.* **5:**719.
14. **Fadeel, B., S. Orrenius, and B. Zhivotovsky.** 1999. Apoptosis in human disease: a new skin for the old ceremony? *Biochem. Biophys. Res. Commun.* **266:**699–717.
15. **Fadeel, B., B. Zhivotovsky, and S. Orrenius.** 1999. All along the watchtower: on the regulation of apoptosis regulators. *FASEB J.* **13:**1647–1657.
16. **Fisher, G. H., F. J. Rosenberg, S. E. Strauss, J. K. Dale, L. A. Middleton, A. Y. Lin, W. Strober, M. J. Lenardo, and J. M. Puck.** 1995. Dominant interfering Fas gene mutations impair apoptosis in a human autoimmune lymphoproliferative syndrome. *Cell* **81:**935–946.
17. **Fournel, S., L. Genestier, J. P. Rouault, G. Lizard, M. Flacher, O. Assossou, and J. P. Revillard.** 1995. Apoptosis without decrease of cell DNA content. *FEBS Lett.* **367:**188–192.
18. **Frey, T.** 1997. Correlated flow cytometric analysis of terminal events in apoptosis reveals the absence of some changes in some model systems. *Cytometry* **28:**253–263.
19. **Goldberg, B., and R. B. Stricker.** 1999. Apoptosis and HIV infection: T cells fiddle while the immune system burns. *Immunol. Lett.* **70:**5–8.
20. **Gong, J., F. Traganos, and Z. Darzynkiewicz.** 1994. A selective procedure for DNA extraction from apoptotic cells applicable for gel electrophoresis and flow cytometry. *Anal. Biochem.* **218:**314–319.
21. **Gorczyca, W., J. Gong, and Z. Darzynkiewicz.** 1993. Detection of DNA strand breaks in individual apoptotic cells by the in situ terminal deoxynucleotidyl transferase and nick translation assays. *Cancer Res.* **53:**1945–1951.
22. **Green, D. R., and J. C. Reed.** 1998. Mitochondria and apoptosis. *Science* **281:**1309–1312.
23. **Gross, A., J. M. McDonnell, and S. J. Korsmeyer.** 1999. Bcl-2 family members and the mitochondria in apoptosis. *Genes Dev.* **13:**1899–1911.
24. **Hotz, M. A., F. Traganos, and Z. Darzynkiewicz.** 1992. Changes in nuclear chromatin related to apoptosis or necrosis induced by the DNA topoisomerase II inhibitor fostriecin in MOLT-4 and HL-60 cells are revealed by altered DNA sensitivity to denaturation. *Exp. Cell Res.* **201:**184–191.
25. **Huang, Q., Q. L. Deveraux, S. Maeda, G. S. Salvesan, H. R. Stennicke, B. D. Hammock, and J. C. Reed.** 2000. Evolutionary conservation of apoptosis mechanisms: lepidopteran and baculoviral inhibitors of apoptosis proteins are inhibitors of mammalian caspase 9. *Proc. Natl. Acad. Sci. USA* **97:**1427–1432.
26. **Kerr, J. F. R.** 1971. Shrinkage necrosis: a distinct mode of cellular death. *J. Pathol.* **105:**13–20.
27. **Kerr, J. F. R., A. H. Wyllie, and A. R. Currie.** 1972. Apoptosis: a basic biological phenomenon with wide ranging implications in tissue kinetics. *Br. J. Cancer* **26:**239–257.
28. **Komoriya, A., B. Z. Packard, M. J. Brown, M. L. Wu, and P. A. Henkart.** 2000. Assessment of caspase activities

in intact apoptotic thymocytes using cell permeable fluorogenic caspase substrates. *J. Exp. Med.* **191**:1819–1828.

29. **Krilov, L. R., T. W. McCloskey, S. H. Harkness, L. Pontrelli, and S. Pahwa.** 2000. Alterations in apoptosis of cord and adult peripheral blood mononuclear cells induced by in vitro infection with RSV. *J. Infect. Dis.* **181**:349–353.

30. **Li, X., F. Traganos, M. R. Melamed, and Z. Darzynkiewicz.** 1995. Single step procedure for labeling DNA strand breaks with fluorescein- or bodipy-conjugated deoxynucleotides: detection of apoptosis and bromodeoxyuridine incorporation. *Cytometry* **20**:172–180.

31. **Majno, G., and I. Joris.** 1995. Apoptosis, oncosis, and necrosis: an overview of cell death. *Am. J. Pathol.* **146**:3–15.

32. **Marguet, D., M. F. Luciani, A. Moynault, P. Williamson, and G. Chimini.** 1999. Engulfment of apoptotic cells involves the redistribution of membrane phosphatidylserine on phagocyte and prey. *Nat. Cell Biol.* **1**:454–456.

33. **Martin, S. J., C. P .M. Reutelingsperger, A. J. McGahon, J. A. Rader, R. C. A. A. van Schie, D. M. LaFace, and D. R. Green.** 1995. Early redistribution of plasma membrane phosphatidylserine is a general feature of apoptosis regardless of the initiating stimulus: inhibition by overexpression of Bcl-2 and Abl. *J. Exp. Med.* **182**:1545–1556.

34. **McCloskey, T. W., S. Chavan, S. M. L. Tamma, and S. Pahwa.** 1998. Comparison of seven quantitative assays to assess lymphocyte cell death during HIV infection: measurement of induced apoptosis in anti-Fas treated Jurkat cells and spontaneous apoptosis in PBMC from children infected with HIV. *AIDS Res. Hum. Retrovir.* **14**:1413–1422.

35. **McCloskey, T. W., M. Ott, E. Tribble, S. A. Khan, S. Teichberg, M. O. Paul, S. Pahwa, E. Verdin, and N. Chirmule.** 1997. Dual role of HIV Tat in regulation of apoptosis in T cells. *J. Immunol.* **158**:1014–1019.

36. **McCloskey, T. W., N. Oyaizu, M. Coronesi, and S. Pahwa.** 1994. Use of a flow cytometric assay to quantitate apoptosis in human lymphocytes. *Clin. Immunol. Immunopathol.* **71**:14–18.

37. **McKenna, S. L., T. Hoy, J. A. Holmes, J. A. Whittaker, H. Jackson, and R. A. Padua.** 1998. Flow cytometric apoptosis assays indicate different types of endonuclease activity in hematopoietic cells and suggest a cautionary approach to their quantitative use. *Cytometry* **31**:130–136.

38. **Miller, D. K.** 1999. Activation of apoptosis and its inhibition. *Ann. N. Y. Acad. Sci.* **886**:132–157.

39. **Myc, A., F. Traganos, J. Lara, M. R. Melamed, and Z. Darzynkiewicz.** 1992. DNA stainability in aneuploid breast tumors: comparison of four DNA fluorochromes differing in binding properties. *Cytometry* **13**:389–394.

40. **Negoescu, A.** 2000. Apoptosis in cancer: therapeutic implications. *Histol. Histopathol.* **15**:281–297.

41. **Nicholson, D. W., and N. A. Thornberry.** 1997. Caspases: killer proteases. *Trends Biochem. Sci.* **22**:299–306.

42. **Nicoletti, I., G. Migliorati, M. C. Pagliacci, F. Grignani, and C. Riccardi.** 1991. A rapid and simple method for measuring thymocyte apoptosis by propidium iodide staining and flow cytometry. *J. Immunol. Methods* **139**:271–279.

43. **Ormerod, M. G.** 1998. The study of apoptotic cells by flow cytometry. *Leukemia* **12**:1013–1025.

44. **Ormerod, M. G., F. Paul, M. Cheetham, and X. M. Sun.** 1995. Discrimination of apoptotic thymocytes by forward light scatter. *Cytometry* **21**:300–304.

45. **Oyaizu, N., T. W. McCloskey, M. Coronesi, N. Chirmule, V. S. Kalyanaraman, and S. Pahwa.** 1993. Accelerated apoptosis in PBMC from HIV infected patients and in CD4 crosslinked PBMC from normal individuals. *Blood* **82**:3392–3400.

46. **Oyaizu, N., and S. Pahwa.** 1996. Lymphocyte apoptosis in HIV infection, p. 133–151. *In* S. Gupta (ed.), *Immunology of HIV Infection.* Plenum Medical Book Company, New York, N.Y.

47. **Packard, B. Z., D. D. Toptygin, A. Komoriya, and L. Brand.** 1997. Design of profluorescent protease substrates guided by exciton theory. *Methods Enzymol.* **278**:15–23.

48. **Pozarowski, P., X. Huang, D. H. Halicka, B. Lee, G. Johnson, and Z. Darzynkiewicz.** 2003. Interactions of fluorochrome labeled caspase inhibitors with apoptotic cells: a caution in data interpretation. *Cytometry* **55A**:50–60.

49. **Ravirajan, C. T., V. Pittoni, and D. A. Isenberg.** 1999. Apoptosis in autoimmune diseases. *Int. Rev. Immunol.* **18**:563–589.

50. **Rieux-Laucat, F., F. LeDeist, C. Hivroz, I. A. G. Roberts, K. M. Debatin, A. Fischer, and J. P. deVillartay.** 1995. Mutations in Fas associated with human lymphoproliferative syndrome and autoimmunity. *Science* **268**:1347–1349.

51. **Roulston, A., R. C. Marcellus, and P. E. Branton.** 1999. Viruses and apoptosis. *Annu. Rev. Microbiol.* **53**:577–628.

52. **Sastry, P. S., and K. S. Rao.** 2000. Apoptosis and the nervous system, *J. Neurochem.* **74**:1–20.

53. **Schmid, I., C. H. Uittenbogaart, and J. V. Giorgi.** 1994. Sensitive method for measuring apoptosis and cell surface phenotype in human thymocytes by flow cytometry. *Cytometry* **15**:12–20.

54. **Smolewski, P., J. Grabarek, J. B. W. Lee, G. L. Johnson, and Z. Darzynkiewicz.** 2002. Kinetics of HL-60 cell entry to apoptosis during treatment with TNF-alpha or camptothecin assayed by the stathmo apoptosis method. *Cytometry* **47**:143–149.

55. **Sun, X. M., R. T. Snowden, D. N. Skilleter, D. Dinsdale, M. G. Ormerod, and G. M. Cohen.** 1992. A flow cytometric method for the separation and quantitation of normal and apoptotic thymocytes. *Anal. Biochem.* **204**:351–356.

56. **Telford, W. G., L. E. King, and P. J. Fraker.** 1992. Comparative evaluation of several DNA binding dyes in the detection of apoptosis associated chromatin degradation by flow cytometry. *Cytometry* **13**:137–143.

57. **Thompson, C. B.** 1995. Apoptosis in the pathogenesis and treatment of disease. *Science* **267**:1456–1462.

58. **Thornberry, N. A., and Y. Lazebnik.** 1998. Caspases: enemies within. *Science* **281**:1312–1316.

59. **Vermes, I., C. Haanen, H. Steffens-Nakken, and C. Reutelingsperger.** 1995. A novel assay for apoptosis: flow cytometric detection of phosphatidylserine expression on early apoptotic cells using fluorescein labeled annexin V. *J. Immunol. Methods* **184**:39–51.

60. **Weinrauch, Y., and A. Zychlinsky.** 1999. The induction of apoptosis by bacterial pathogens. *Annu. Rev. Microbiol.* **53**:155–187.

61. **Yang, Y., and J. D. Ashwell.** 1999. Thymocyte apoptosis. *J. Clin. Immunol.* **19**:337–349.

62. **Zamzami, N., P. Marchetti, M. Castedo, C. Zanin, J. L. Vayssiere, P. X. Petit, and G. Kroemer.** 1995. Reduction in mitochondrial potential constitutes an early irreversible step of programmed lymphocyte death in vivo. *J. Exp. Med.* **181**:1661–1672.

63. **Zhang, C., Z. Ao, A. Seth, and S. F. Schlossman.** 1996. A mitochondrial membrane protein defined by a novel monoclonal antibody preferentially detected in apoptotic cells. *J. Immunol.* **157**:3980–3987.

Quantification of Recent Thymic Emigrants: T-Cell-Receptor Excision Circles

PAUL KROGSTAD

33

The thymus is the site of differentiation of bone marrow-derived precursors into mature CD4[+] and CD8[+] T cells. In the absence of thymic development, as in complete DiGeorge syndrome, there is an absence of mature blood T cells, resulting in profound immunodeficiency. The peripheral T-cell populations are established by birth, and postnatal thymectomy does not cause overt immunodeficiency. Since thymic weight begins to decrease after puberty, it was long assumed that the thymus is active early in life, declining substantially in early adulthood. However, recent anatomic and functional studies have demonstrated that the differentiation of new T cells within the thymus (thymopoiesis) continues well into adulthood (6, 10, 13), exhibiting a gradual age-related decline. Moreover, postnatal thymectomy has been associated with lower levels of T cells (7).

Several clinical developments have come together to heighten interest in identifying parameters of thymopoiesis. Among these are the elucidation of the nature of several primary immunodeficiencies, the use of more potent chemotherapeutic regimens for the treatment of cancer, and the demonstration that multidrug regimens for human immunodeficiency virus (HIV) infection produce improvement of immune function in many individuals (10, 16, 17). The changes in T-cell populations seen during highly active antiretroviral therapy (HAART) for HIV infection are particularly provocative. Significant increases in the number of circulating CD4[+] T cells are seen in 50% or more of children and adults treated with HAART (10, 15). However, a significant number of patients with an excellent virological response to HAART (that is, complete suppression of detectable viremia) show no discernible increase in CD4[+] T-cell numbers, while others demonstrate immunologic improvements (an increase in CD4[+] T-cell populations) that are discordant with the virological response (the presence of ongoing viremia) (3, 15).

METHODS FOR QUANTIFICATION OF THYMOPOIESIS

In chickens, blood lymphocytes may be identified as recent thymic emigrants (RTEs) by the use of antibodies that react with the cell surface marker chT1 (14). No similar phenotypic marker of mammalian RTEs has been identified, but the differential and mutually exclusive expression of two isoforms of CD45 (CD45RO and CD45RA) has been used to distinguish naïve T cells from those which have undergone proliferation in response to antigenic stimulation. In particular, naïve CD4 and CD8 T cells exhibit cell surface expression of CD45RA, CD27, CD62L, and other markers, while CD45RO expression is seen on memory T cells (4). This simple model has been complicated by the observation that CD45RO cells can revert to the expression of CD45RA (1, 8, 10). As an additional confounding factor, CD45RA T cells are long-lived (21). Consequently, the simple enumeration of CD45RA[+] T cells does not provide a clear measure of thymopoiesis.

Methods have recently been developed to quantify RTEs based on the use of quantitative PCR detection of DNA molecules generated during rearrangement of the gene loci encoding the α and β chains of the T-cell receptor (TCR) during T cell differentiation. This process involves the excision of DNA fragments that persist in cells as circular extrachromosomal molecules, termed TCR rearrangement excision circles (TRECs) or TCR deletion circles (5, 24). The initial step in productive recombination at the TCR α chain locus (TCRA) involves deletion of the TCR δ gene locus (TCRD) embedded within it. End-to-end ligation of recombination signal sequences produces a TREC with a unique nucleotide sequence termed the signal joint (Fig. 1). Subsequently, an additional recombination event brings the variable (V) and joining (J) segments of the TCRA into contiguity, producing a coding-joint TREC. Although stable, these TRECs are not replicated (and therefore are not truly episomes) and are diluted by cellular division (5).

The observation that the excision events involved in the production of functional α chains are identical in 70% of αβ T cells (22) led to the development of straightforward PCR-based strategies to quantify these αTRECs. Douek et al. (5) initially described a quantitative-competitive PCR assay employing internal standards bearing an internal deletion in the signal joint and coding joint sequences. This method was successfully used to characterize the age-dependent decrease in thymopoiesis, to investigate the role of the thymus in the expansion of the peripheral blood T-lymphocyte pool in HIV infection during HAART (5), and to evaluate the success of transplantation of thymus tissue in complete DiGeorge syndrome (17). Since then, a similar approach with real-time PCR methods has been used to quantify TRECs, and they have been shown to serve as an independent predictor of the progression of disease following transfusion-related HIV infection (2, 9, 18, 24). Moreover, TRECs have been shown to be

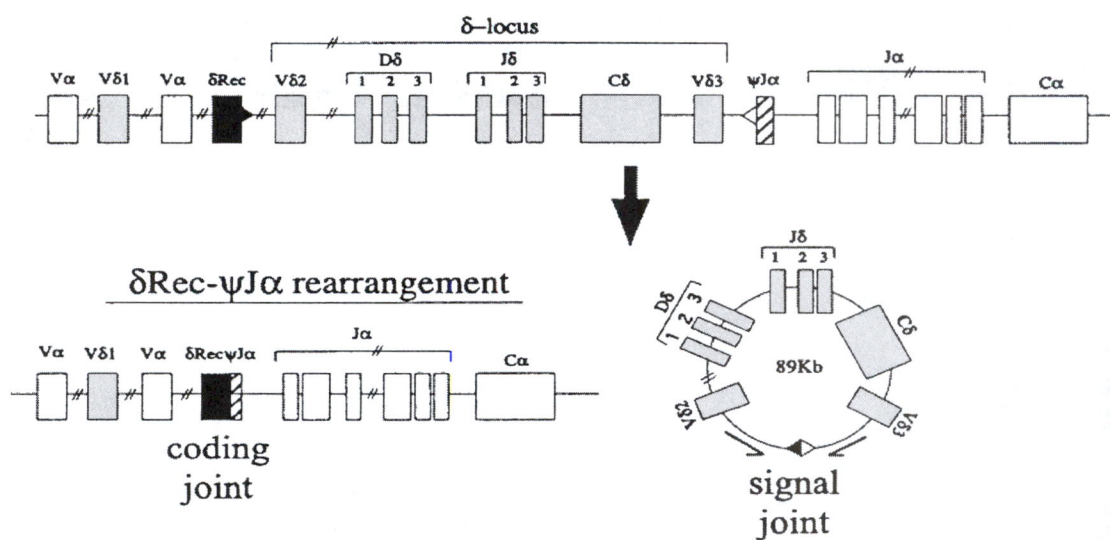

FIGURE 1 Production of αTREC. The TCRD locus is shown embedded within TCRA. Recombination releases an 89-kbp signal-joint TREC containing a distinctive sequence that may be detected by oligonucleotide primers spaced approximately 180 bp from either side of the joint. A second recombination event brings the Vα and Jα sequences into contiguity, releasing a second TREC containing the coding joint (not shown). (Modified from reference 24 with permission of the publishers.)

diminished or absent following thymectomy performed during pediatric cardiothoracic surgery or during adulthood to ameliorate the manifestations of myasthenia gravis (7, 20).

PCR quantification of TRECs derived from TCR β chain locus rearrangement has also been described and has been used to provide additional evidence that the differentiation of T cells with a diverse TCR repertoire continues until late adulthood (19). Moreover, rearrangement of the TCRB locus occurs during the early, double-positive phase of T-cell maturation, in which thymocytes express both CD4 and CD8. Proliferation occurs during subsequent steps of maturation, leading to intrathymic dilution of TCRB-derived TRECs. In addition, the methods employed to detect these βTRECs are more complex. For these and other reasons, αTRECs are seen as the optimal target for quantitation (11).

METHODS FOR QUANTITATION OF αTRECs

Separation of CD4+ and CD8+ T Cells (Optional)
The quantitation of TRECs may be performed with unsorted cells or with subpopulations of cells purified by fluorescent cell sorting, magnetic bead separation (5), panning, or other techniques. In view of its high yield and relative simplicity, magnetic cell sorting with CD4 and CD8 microbeads and positive selection columns is often used.

Magnetic Cell Sorting Method

1. Rapidly thaw cryopreserved peripheral blood mononuclear cells in a 37°C water bath and immediately dilute the cells in 8 to 10 ml of complete medium (RPMI medium with 20% fetal bovine serum).
2. Pellet the cells by low-speed centrifugation, resuspend them in 100 μl of ice-cold medium, and transfer the suspension to a 1.5-ml microcentrifuge tube.

3. Label the cells by the addition of 2 μl of CD4 MultiSort microbeads (Miltenyi Biotec) and incubate the mixture at 4°C for 12 min. Stop the labeling reaction after 12 min by the addition of 500 μl of complete medium.
4. Pass labeled cells through a MACS MS+ separation column (Miltenyi Biotec). Rinse the column twice with 500 μl of complete medium. After collecting the eluate, remove the column from the magnet and place it in a 1.5-ml conical tube. Flushing the column with 1 ml of complete medium yields the CD4+ cells.
5. To obtain CD8+ cells, collect the eluate while the column is on the magnet by incubating the column with 20 μl of MACS MultiSort release reagent for 10 min at 4°C. To stop the action of the release reagent, add approximately 5 ml of complete medium. Centrifuge the solution at 300 × g for 10 min, resuspend the cell pellet in 68 μl of medium, and add 30 μl of MultiSort Stop reagent. Then, add 2 μl of CD8+ microbeads and incubate the mixture for 12 min. CD8+ cells are obtained by passing the mixture through the MACS MS+ separation column as described above.
6. The purity of the cells obtained in this fashion is examined by flow cytometry using conventional methods. We routinely obtain a purity of >80% CD4+ or CD8+ T cells from aliquots of cryopreserved peripheral blood mononuclear cells.

Preparation of Cell Lysate for PCR
Suitable approaches to the preparation of cellular lysates include the disruption of cells with a lysis buffer containing 7 M urea followed by phenol and ethanol extraction (23), the use of commercial nucleic acid preparation reagents such as Trizol (Gibco BRL) or TriReagent (Molecular Research Center, Cincinnati, Ohio) (5), and the preparation of a crude DNA lysate as described below.

1. Purified CD4+ or CD8+ cells are washed with phosphate-buffered saline and pelleted by low-speed centrifugation,

and the cells are resuspended in PCR-grade proteinase K (100 μg/ml; 100 μl per 100,000 cells) (Boehringer Mannheim) in 0.5 mM EDTA.

2. Incubate the cells at 56°C for a minimum of 1 h, and then inactivate the protease by incubating the cells at 95°C in a dry bath incubator for 15 min.

3. Centrifuge the cells briefly at full speed (10,000 to 16,000 × g for 3 to 5 min) in a microcentrifuge to pellet cell debris and transfer the supernatant to a new tube.

PCR Quantitation by Radioisotope Method

A. PCR setup. Assemble reaction mixtures containing the following reagents:
   1. 5 μl of DNA lysate
   2. 4 pmol each of the SJ1 and SJ2 primers (Table 1)
   3. 0.5 U of Platinum *Taq* polymerase (Gibco)
   4. 2 to 5 μCi of [α-^{32}P]dCTP (3,000 Ci/mmol)
   5. 2.5 μl of 10× PCR buffer (200 mM Tris-HCl [pH 8.4], 500 mM KCl)
   6. 1.8 mM MgCl$_2$
   7. 200 μM dideoxynucleotide triphosphates (including dCTP)
   8. Deionized water to bring the final volume to 25 μl
B. In a DNA thermal cycler, denature the samples at 95°C for 5 min and perform 24 to 35 cycles of amplification as follows:
   1. Denaturation at 94°C for 30 s
   2. Annealing at 60°C for 30 s
   3. Extension at 72°C for 35 s
C. The total cellular DNA from the lysate must be quantitated by a second method. If nucleic acids have been purified by using agents that remove cellular proteins, a spectrophotometric estimation of the amount of chromosomal DNA may be satisfactory. Alternatively, PCR detection of a cellular gene such as β-globin may be employed, as previously described (23).
D. Electrophoresis. PCR products are prepared for electrophoresis by the addition of 5 μl of 6× loading buffer (0.2% xylene cyanol, 0.2% bromophenol blue, 50% sucrose [wt/vol], 100 mM EDTA [pH 7.4]). Equal amounts of each reaction mixture (5 to 15 μl) are separated through a nondenaturing 6% polyacrylamide gel. The radiolabeled PCR products are detected and quantified by use of a phosphorimager with appropriate imaging software (e.g., ImageQuant [Amersham Pharmacia Biotechnology]).
E. Calculation of TRECs. For quantification of the number of TRECs in test samples, a standard curve is constructed by amplifying in parallel a set of reaction mixtures containing 0, 10^1, 10^2, 10^3, and 10^4 copies of a cloned signal joint sequence (see below). A linear relationship generally

may be found between the $\log_{10}$-transformed signal intensity and 10^1 to 10^4 TRECs with 22 to 25 cycles of amplification. Interpolation along this standard curve is used to determine the number of TRECs in test samples. Prior to beginning the analysis of samples, the number of cycles of amplification needed to produce a linear standard curve must be determined for a given thermocycler.

Real-Time PCR Quantitation

As noted above, Douek et al. initially described a quantitative-competitive PCR approach to quantify αTRECs. Subsequently, Sempowski et al. (20) and others (24) described real-time molecular beacon-based PCR methods to quantify signal joint and cellular DNA sequences. The molecular beacon approach obviates the gel electrophoresis and phosphorimager detection steps described above. We present below a slight modification of the protocol presented by Sempowski et al. that we have used to quantify αTRECs (7) by using a spectrofluorometric thermocycler (ABI PRISM 7700; Applied Biosystems, Foster City, Calif.) (18).

A. PCR setup. Assemble reaction mixtures containing the following reagents:
   1. 5 μl of DNA lysate
   2. Platinum *Taq* buffer (200 mM Tris-HCl [pH 8.4], 500 mM KCl) (2.5 μl)
   3. 50 mM MgCl$_2$ (1.75 μl)
   4. 10 mM dioxynucleoside triphosphates (0.5 μl)
   5. 12.5 μM 5′ forward primer (1 μl) (Table 1)
   6. 12.5 μM 3′ reverse primer (1 μl) (Table 1)
   7. 5 μM TREC probe (1 μl) (Table 1)
   8. 25 μM Rox internal reporter dye (5-carboxy-x-rhodamine, succinimidyl ester) (0.5 μl)
   9. Platinum *Taq* (Gibco Life Sciences) (5 U/μl; 0.125 μl)
   10. Deionized water to bring the final volume to 25 μl
B. In an ABI PRISM 7700 thermal cycler, denature samples at 95°C for 5 min and perform 40 cycles of amplification as follows:
   1. Denaturation at 95°C for 30 s
   2. Annealing at 60°C for 60 s
   3. The instrument should be set to record the fluorescence emission during the annealing phase of each cycle. The cycle threshold is set to the level at which all positive control reactions demonstrate exponential DNA amplification.
C. The total cellular DNA from the lysate must be quantitated by a second method. If nucleic acids have been purified by using agents that remove cellular proteins, a spectrophotometric estimation of the amount of chromosomal DNA is satisfactory. Alternatively, PCR detection of a cellular gene may be employed. Following the protocol for TREC amplification, we

TABLE 1 PCR primer and probe sequences

Primer or probe	Sequence (5′ → 3′)
Radiolabeled PCR	
SJ1	AAA GAG GGC AGC CCT CTC CAA GGC AAA
SJ2	AGG CTG ATC TTG TCT GAC ATT TGC TCC G
Real-time PCR	
Forward primer	CACATCCCTTTCAACCATGCT
Reverse primer	GCCAGCTGCAGGGTTTAGG
Probe	FAM-ACACCTCTGGTTTTTGTAAAGGTGCCCACT-TAMRA[a]

[a]FAM, 6-carboxyfluorescein; TAMRA, 6-carboxytetramethylrhodamine.

amplify sequences found in the CCR5 chemokine receptor gene by using the following primer-probe combination supplied by D. Douek (18): forward primer, 5′-TACCTGCTCAACCTGGCCAT-3′; reverse primer, 5′-TTCCAAAGTCCCACTGGGC-3′; 5 μM probe (1 μl), 5′-FAM-TTTCCTTCTTACTGTCCCCTTCT GGGCTC-TAMRA-3′. A standard curve is established by using fivefold dilutions of human peripheral blood lymphocyte DNA to generate samples containing 750 ng to 1.2 μg/5 μl. These standards and test samples are analyzed in duplicate, and the mean DNA quantity is used for data analysis.

D. Calculation of TRECs. All samples are analyzed in triplicate. TREC values for the unknown samples are determined by interpolation along a standard curve produced by linear regression to correlate the cycle threshold values and TREC copy numbers (see below). The mean of the triplicate TREC values is used for data analysis; the coefficient of variation is generally <20%. TREC data are reported as number of TREC per million cells, using an estimate of 8 μg of DNA per 1 million peripheral blood mononuclear cells.

Negative and Positive Controls

αTRECs are not present in CEM, HUT78, MT2, and other T-cell lines (reference 24 and our unpublished data). DNAs prepared from these cell lines in parallel with test samples are used as a negative control for TREC PCR. Buffer blanks are used as additional negative controls.

For the production of a cloned standard for TREC quantitation, the primers SJ1 and SJ2 are used to amplify TREC sequences from 0.1 to 0.5 μg of peripheral blood mononuclear cell DNA (40 cycles of amplification under the conditions described above). The 395-bp product of this amplification is extracted from an ethidium bromide-stained 1.2% agarose gel and ligated into a TA cloning vector (Invitrogen Corp., Carlsbad, Calif.) according to the manufacturer's specifications. The product should be sequenced to determine that it contains the features of a signal joint and a sequence matching the primers SJ1 and SJ2 (5, 22, 24). Once the sequence has been confirmed, the plasmid is digested with EcoRI to release the fragment, which is purified by gel electrophoresis and diluted in tRNA (prepared at 10 μg/ml in TE buffer [10 mM Tris-HCl, pH 8.0, 1 mM EDTA]) or salmon sperm DNA (20 μg/ml) to produce a set of standards at known concentrations. For the radioisotope-labeled PCR approach, we use standards for the range of 10^1 to 10^4 TREC copies/5 μl. For the real-time PCR method, we use 10-fold dilutions covering the range of 10^1 to 10^6 TREC copies/5 μl.

Technical Pitfalls

As with any PCR-based assay, extreme caution must be applied to minimize the possibility of contamination of reagents, micropipettes, and other equipment with DNA carried over from a prior amplification or DNA from the standards. The accurate quantitation of TREC molecules necessitates that the cloned standard be prepared by using plasmid DNA that has been fastidiously prepared and carefully quantified by spectrophotometry. In particular, the optical density at 260 nm of the plasmid standard stock should be measured at several dilutions prior to the preparation of standards. The input DNA in cell lysates should be quantified, especially if cells cannot accurately be counted prior to preparation of the lysate. The concentration of cellular DNA

can be determined by PCR quantitation of β-globin or CCR5 gene sequences, as described above.

Interpretation

The methods described above yield reproducible data over a broad dynamic range. High TREC concentrations have been associated with changes in T-cell populations after the transplantation of thymic tissue in patients with DiGeorge syndrome and, in some cases, after HAART for HIV infection (5, 17, 24). Moreover, recent data suggest that TREC values may prove to be a useful predictor of disease progression for HIV infection (9). Nonetheless, TREC data must be interpreted with caution. Physiological changes and pathophysiological processes that alter T-cell proliferation and survival are likely to affect this parameter of thymic output (11, 12).

REFERENCES

1. Bell, E. B., and S. M. Sparshott. 1990. Interconversion of CD45R subsets of CD4 T cells in vivo. *Nature* **348**:163–166.
2. Chavan, S., B. Bennuri, M. Kharbanda, A. Chandrasekaran, S. Bakshi, and S. Pahwa. 2001. Evaluation of T cell receptor gene rearrangement excision circles after antiretroviral therapy in children infected with human immunodeficiency virus. *J. Infect. Dis.* **183**:1445–1454.
3. Deeks, S. G. 2003. Treatment of antiretroviral-drug-resistant HIV-1 infection. *Lancet* **362**:2002–2011.
4. De Rosa, S. C., L. A. Herzenberg, and M. Roederer. 2001. 11-color, 13-parameter flow cytometry: identification of human naive T cells by phenotype, function, and T-cell receptor diversity. *Nat. Med.* **7**:245–248.
5. Douek, D. C., R. D. McFarland, P. H. Keiser, E. A. Gage, J. M. Massey, B. F. Haynes, M. A. Polis, A. T. Haase, M. B. Feinberg, J. L. Sullivan, B. D. Jamieson, J. A. Zack, L. J. Picker, and R. A. Koup. 1998. Changes in thymic function with age and during the treatment of HIV infection. *Nature* **396**:690–695.
6. Flores, K. G., J. Li, G. D. Sempowski, B. F. Haynes, and L. P. Hale. 1999. Analysis of the human thymic perivascular space during aging. *J. Clin. Invest.* **104**:1031–1039.
7. Halnon, N., B. Jamieson, M. Plunkett, C. Kitchen, T. Pham, and P. Krogstad. 2004. Thymic function and impaired maintenance of peripheral T cell populations in children with congenital heart disease and surgical thymectomy. *Pediatr. Res.* **57**:42–48.
8. Hargreaves, M., and E. B. Bell. 1997. Identical expression of CD45R isoforms by CD45RC⁺ "revertant" memory and CD45RC⁺ naive CD4 T cells. *Immunology* **91**:323–330.
9. Hatzakis, A., G. Touloumi, R. Karanicolas, A. Karafoulidou, T. Mandalaki, C. Anastassopoulou, L. Zhang, J. J. Goedert, D. D. Ho, and L. G. Kostrikis. 2000. Effect of recent thymic emigrants on progression of HIV-1 disease. *Lancet* **355**:599–604.
10. Haynes, B. F., M. L. Markert, G. D. Sempowski, D. D. Patel, and L. P. Hale. 2000. The role of the thymus in immune reconstitution in aging, bone marrow transplantation, and HIV-1 infection. *Annu. Rev. Immunol.* **18**:529–560.
11. Hazenberg, M. D., M. C. Verschuren, D. Hamann, F. Miedema, and J. J. van Dongen. 2001. T cell receptor excision circles as markers for recent thymic emigrants: basic aspects, technical approach, and guidelines for interpretation. *J. Mol. Med.* **79**:631–640.
12. Hellerstein, M. K. 1999. Measurement of T-cell kinetics: recent methodologic advances. *Immunol. Today* **20**:438–441.
13. Jamieson, B. D., D. C. Douek, S. Killian, L. E. Hultin, D. D. Scripture-Adams, J. V. Giorgi, D. Marelli, R. A. Koup, and J. A. Zack. 1999. Generation of functional thymocytes in the human adult. *Immunity* **10**:569–575.

14. **Kong, F., C. H. Chen, and M. D. Cooper.** 1998. Thymic function can be accurately monitored by the level of recent T cell emigrants in the circulation. *Immunity* **8:**97–104.
15. **Ledergerber, B., M. Egger, M. Opravil, A. Telenti, B. Hirschel, M. Battegay, P. Vernazza, P. Sudre, M. Flepp, H. Furrer, P. Francioli, and R. Weber.** 1999. Clinical progression and virological failure on highly active antiretroviral therapy in HIV-1 patients: a prospective cohort study. Swiss HIV Cohort Study. *Lancet* **353:**863–868.
16. **Mackall, C. L., T. A. Fleisher, M. R. Brown, M. P. Andrich, C. C. Chen, I. M. Feuerstein, M. E. Horowitz, I. T. Magrath, A. T. Shad, S. M. Steinberg, et al.** 1995. Age, thymopoiesis, and CD4+ T-lymphocyte regeneration after intensive chemotherapy. *New Engl. J. Med.* **332**(3):143–149.
17. **Markert, M. L., A. Boeck, L. P. Hale, A. L. Kloster, T. M. McLaughlin, M. N. Batchvarova, D. C. Douek, R. A. Koup, D. D. Kostyu, F. E. Ward, H. E. Rice, S. M. Mahaffey, S. E. Schiff, R. H. Buckley, and B. F. Haynes.** 1999. Transplantation of thymus tissue in complete DiGeorge syndrome. *New Engl. J. Med.* **341**(16):1180–1189.
18. **Pham, T., M. Belzer, J. A. Church, C. Kitchen, C. M. Wilson, S. D. Douglas, Y. Geng, M. Silva, R. M. Mitchell, and P. Krogstad.** 2003. Assessment of thymic activity in human immunodeficiency virus-negative and -positive adolescents by real-time PCR quantitation of T-cell receptor rearrangement excision circles. *Clin. Diagn. Lab. Immunol.* **10:**323–328.
19. **Poulin, J. F., M. N. Viswanathan, J. M. Harris, K. V. Komanduri, E. Wieder, N. Ringuette, M. Jenkins, J. M. McCune, and R. P. Sekaly.** 1999. Direct evidence for thymic function in adult humans. *J. Exp. Med.* **190:**479–486.
20. **Sempowski, G., J. Thomasch, M. Gooding, L. Hale, L. Edwards, E. Ciafaloni, D. Sanders, J. Massey, D. Douek, R. Koup, and B. Haynes.** 2001. Effect of thymectomy on human peripheral blood T cell pools in myasthenia gravis. *J. Immunol.* **166:**2808–2817.
21. **Tough, D. F., and J. Sprent.** 1995. Life span of naive and memory T cells. *Stem Cells* **13**(3):242–249.
22. **Verschuren, M. C., I. L. Wolvers-Tettero, T. M. Breit, J. Noordzij, E. R. van Wering, and J. J. van Dongen.** 1997. Preferential rearrangements of the T cell receptor-delta-deleting elements in human T cells. *J. Immunol.* **158:**1208–1216.
23. **Zack, J. A., S. J. Arrigo, S. R. Weitsman, A. S. Go, A. Haislip, and I. S. Chen.** 1990. HIV-1 entry into quiescent primary lymphocytes: molecular analysis reveals a labile, latent viral structure. *Cell* **61:**213–222.
24. **Zhang, L., S. R. Lewin, M. Markowitz, H. H. Lin, E. Skulsky, R. Karanicolas, Y. He, X. Jin, S. Tuttleton, M. Vesanen, H. Spiegel, R. Kost, J. van Lunzen, H. J. Stellbrink, S. Wolinsky, W. Borkowsky, P. Palumbo, L. G. Kostrikis, and D. D. Ho.** 1999. Measuring recent thymic emigrants in blood of normal and HIV-1-infected individuals before and after effective therapy. *J. Exp. Med.* **190**(5):725–732.

Measurement of NK-Cell Activity in Humans

THERESA L. WHITESIDE

34

Natural killer (NK) cells comprise a morphologically distinct subset of lymphocytes which have the capability to spontaneously kill virally infected or transformed targets but spare most normal cells (7). Recent studies have indicated that NK cells are capable of mediating the killing of susceptible targets by several distinct mechanisms, of secreting a broad spectrum of cytokines, and of extravasating as well as entering tissue sites, including premalignant and malignant tissues (8). In contrast to other immune effector cells, e.g., T lymphocytes, NK cells mediate cytotoxicity under conditions that do not require prior immunization or antigen sensitization (7). The process of target recognition by NK cells seems to involve unique sets of receptors present on the NK-cell surface, including "killing inhibitory receptors" (KIRs), which interact with major histocompatibility complex (MHC) ligands, and NK-cell-activating receptors (NKARs) interacting with non-MHC ligands on target cells (Fig. 1).

The NK cell recognizes a "self" peptide complexed with MHC class I molecules on the surface of a target cell and turns off its lytic machinery. In other words, the NK cell is poised not to kill "self"; the NK cell is only able to kill its target when an inhibitory signal is absent, especially when its activating receptors are signaling (Fig. 1). Ligands for activating C-type lectin-like receptors (e.g., NKG2D and CD94/NKG2) or natural cytotoxicity receptors (e.g., NK p30, NK p44, and NK p46) are expressed by target cells that are susceptible to NK cell lysis (2, 6). For example, many tumor cell targets susceptible to NK-cell-mediated cytotoxicity express NK-cell-activating ligands such as the MHC class I chain-related molecules MICA and MICB or UL-16 binding proteins, which bind to NKG2D receptors on NK cells (6). Tumors that down-regulate MICA and MICB expression tend to be resistant to NK-cell-mediated lysis. This highly sophisticated receptor-driven recognition system ensures that normal cells are spared and only targets that are altered are eliminated. The alterations that may be recognized by NK cells and result in lysis typically involve a down-regulation or loss of MHC class I molecules, which often occurs in tumor cells or virally infected targets. Also, genetic changes that are likely to lead to the expression of new antigens on the cell surface or to a reduction or absence of self epitopes on target cells are recognized by NK cells. Therefore, the killing of susceptible targets by NK cells is a highly regulated process involving negative signaling by KIRs, which recognize specific self peptides in the context of MHC class I molecules, as well as positive signaling by NKARs upon interaction with their ligands (Fig. 1). In short, NK cells discriminate between normal and abnormal targets by balancing positive and negative signals through their activating and inhibitory receptors. It is important, however, that cytokine-activated NK cells (e.g., lymphokine-activated killer [LAK] cells) lose this selectivity in killing, and by bypassing negative signals, proceed to kill a broad array of target cells. Also, NK cells express a variety of the tumor necrosis factor family ligands and up-regulate these molecules upon activation, so in addition to perforin- and granzyme-mediated lysis, they are capable of inducing apoptosis in targets endowed with corresponding death receptors, such as FasR, TRAILR, and TNFR1 (5).

The role of NK cells in innate immunity has been well recognized. Recent data suggest that in addition to their lytic functions, NK cells are involved in a variety of biologically important pathways, which include facilitating hematopoiesis, modulating neuroimmunologic processes, mediating immunoregulation, influencing fetal development, and engaging in interactions with a variety of tissue cells at the site of tumor growth or tissue injury (7, 8). The biologic importance of NK cells provides a strong rationale for measuring their numbers and function during health and disease. In most cases, NK activity is determined in the peripheral blood and only rarely in the target tissue, largely because it is difficult to isolate NK cells from diseased tissues in humans. In rare instances when this was done, information about tissue-infiltrating NK cells indicated that substantial phenotypic and functional differences may exist between circulating and tissue-infiltrating human NK cells (8). For example, NK cells residing in the liver are activated and have the phenotype of LAK cells, while NK cells isolated from tumors are functionally impaired (8). NK cells present in the peripheral circulation of healthy donors are in the resting stage, although during disease NK activity is frequently altered, and the extent of this alteration may be of clinical and scientific importance.

CONCEPT

Although many modifications of assays measuring NK activity have been developed recently, the 4-h ^{51}Cr-release assay using K562 leukemia cells as targets still remains a prototype NK-cell assay. Many of the newer cytotoxicity assays are

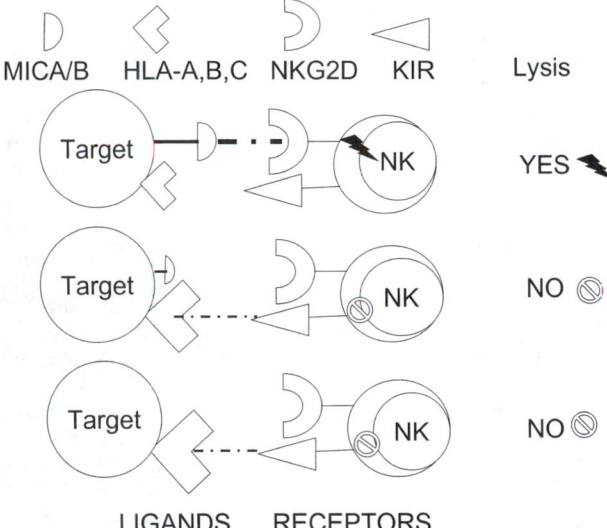

MICA/B	HLA-A,B,C	NKG2D	KIR	Lysis

LIGANDS   RECEPTORS

FIGURE 1 Interactions between NK cells and targets that are NK-cell sensitive or resistant. Targets expressing NK-cell-activating ligands, such as MICA and MICB, in conjunction with a down-regulated expression of HLA-A, -B, and -C molecules are sensitive to killing by NK cells expressing inhibitory receptors (KIRs) and activating receptors (NKARs), such as NKG2D. However, targets that have lost the expression of MICA and MICB and express normal levels of HLA-A, -B, and -C are resistant to lysis by NK cells. Positive and negative signals resulting in target cell lysis and the absence of lysis, respectively, are indicated.

based on flow cytometry and are nonradioactive. Therefore, they may be preferable to ^{51}Cr-release assays. However, these newer procedures have not been validated by comparisons with the ^{51}Cr-release assay and are not uniformly accepted. For these reasons, the ^{51}Cr-release assay is described here in detail, with a focus on its reliability, reproducibility, and result interpretation. The assay involves the coincubation of effector cells with ^{51}Cr-labeled target cells in triplicate wells of a 96-well microtiter plate at various effector-to-target (E:T) ratios, followed by the determination of levels of radioactivity released from lysed target cells into the supernatants. It is essential to emphasize that this assay measures just one of many NK-cell functions and that it may not be the best or even the most biologically relevant assay available today. Nevertheless, until the flow-based multiparameter assays are validated, the ^{51}Cr-release procedure remains the "gold standard." It has been the most widely used assay, and much experience has accumulated to define its attributes and limitations. In combination with flow cytometry for the enumeration of cells expressing the NK-cell phenotype, the assay can provide a quantitative estimate of NK-cell function during human health and disease.

PROCEDURES

Sample Requirements
About 10 ml of heparinized venous blood (one full green-top Vacutainer tube) or suspensions of NK cells isolated from body fluids or tissues are needed for NK-cell enumeration and assay. This translates into 10×10^6 peripheral blood mononuclear cells (PBMC), which are recovered by Ficoll-Hypaque centrifugation performed under standard conditions. More

venous blood should be obtained from individuals who are leukopenic. Blood should be drawn in the morning to avoid diurnal variation and should be processed as soon after phlebotomy as possible. Blood samples that are shipped to a reference laboratory require special handling: an overnight carrier must be used and specimens traveling in ambient (25°C) temperature must reach their destinations within 24 h of collection.

The NK-cell assay must be performed with fresh, not cryopreserved, cells. The cryopreservation of effector cells, even when performed under optimized conditions and using a rate-control freezing device, significantly and unpredictably decreases NK activity. We have compared the NK activities of fresh and cryopreserved PBMC from the same individuals and have encountered differences as large as 100%, although PBMC from certain individuals can be cryopreserved without such losses in cytolytic function. Since one cannot a priori decide or predict the degree of such loss, either freshly separated PBMC or NK cells freshly separated from body fluids or tissues are used as effector cells in this assay.

Materials and Reagents

Effector cells: PBMC or NK cells separated from heparinized body fluids

RPMI medium supplemented with 5% (vol/vol) fetal bovine serum, referred to as RPMI-5

Trypan blue solution for viable cell counts

5 mCi of Na^{51}CrO$_4$/ml (specific activity, 250 to 900 mCi/ml)

Suspension of ^{51}Cr-labeled K562 cells in RPMI-5 medium containing 5×10^4 cells/ml

5% (vol/vol) solution of Triton X-100 in phosphate-buffered saline

10-ml round-bottomed polypropylene snap-cap tubes

96-well round-bottomed sterile microtiter plates (e.g., Costar)

15-ml conical polypropylene tube

1-ml tuberculin syringe with 25-gauge needle

Equipment and Instrumentation

Eight-channel micropipettor capable of delivering 100-μl aliquots

Disposable micropipette tips

Sorvall RT-6000 centrifuge with H-1000B rotor (or equivalent) and microplate carriers

Gamma scintillation counter and counting tubes

An area designated for radioisotope use and disposal of ^{51}Cr

Procedure

1. For each effector cell suspension to be tested, determine the number of viable cells by trypan blue exclusion. Transfer each cell suspension to a separate 10-ml round-bottomed polypropylene snap-cap tube, and by using RPMI-5 medium warmed to room temperature, adjust the suspension to have a cell concentration appropriate for achieving the desired starting E:T ratio. The E:T ratio will vary depending on the potency of the effector cells. If resting NK cells (e.g., in PBMC) are tested, then a starting E:T ratio of 50:1 is recommended. In this case, the suspension of PBMC should be adjusted to 2.5×10^6 cells/ml. For LAK cells, the starting E:T ratio may be 6:1, and the starting cell suspension should be adjusted to 3.125×10^5 cells/ml.

2. Gently vortex the first starting suspension of effector cells. Deliver 200 μl of the suspension into each of triplicate wells in row B (B1, B2, and B3) of a microtiter plate. Follow the same procedure with all other starting suspensions, placing cells in triplicate wells in rows C to H. Up to seven different effector cell suspensions can be tested in one microtiter plate. Be careful to label each row carefully to identify the starting cell suspension. Row A is used for preparing control wells.

3. To each of the wells in columns 4 to 12 of rows B to H, add 100 μl of RPMI-10 medium, using an eight-channel micropipettor with seven tips attached.

4. Using the eight-channel micropipettor with seven tips attached, remove 100-μl aliquots from well 1 in rows B to H and transfer them to well 4 in rows B to H. Mix thoroughly by pipetting up and down with the micropipettor, remove 100-μl aliquots, and transfer them to well 7 in rows B to H. Mix thoroughly, remove 100-μl aliquots, and transfer them to well 10 in rows B to H. Mix thoroughly, remove 100-μl aliquots from well 10, and discard. Repeat this serial twofold dilution process for well 5 in rows B to H, with transfers of 100-μl aliquots to wells 8 and 11. Then, starting with well 6 in rows B to H, transfer 100-μl aliquots to wells 9 and 12. Note that it is not necessary to change pipette tips while performing these twofold dilutions of effector cells. This format allows for the testing of four different E:T ratios, with each tested in triplicate, as follows: 50:1 in wells 1 to 3, 25:1 in wells 4 to 6, 12.5:1 in wells 7 to 9, and 6.25:1 in wells 10 to 12.

5. Using the micropipettor with eight fresh tips attached, add 100 μl of target cell suspension to each well in rows A to H. Target cells are labeled with ^{51}Cr prior to the NK-cell assay (see below).

6. Add 100 μl of RPMI-5 medium to wells 1 to 6 in row A (spontaneous release controls) and then add 100 μl of Triton X solution to wells 7 through 12 in row A (maximal release controls).

7. Cover the microplate with a lid and centrifuge it for 3 min at $200 \times g$ (1,000 rpm in an H-1000B rotor with a microplate carrier) at room temperature without using a brake. Transfer the microplate to a humidified 37°C CO_2 incubator (5% CO_2 in air) and incubate it for 4 h.

8. After the incubation, remove 50 or 100 μl of the supernatant (without disturbing the cell pellet!) from each well by using the eight-channel micropipettor. Transfer the supernatants to prelabeled counting tubes. A cell harvesting system (e.g., Skatron) can be used and is recommended.

9. Measure the radioactivity in each harvested supernatant (from all control and experimental wells) by using a gamma counter.

10. Calculate the percent specific lysis (activity of NK or LAK cells) according to the following formula:

$$\% \text{ specific lysis} = 100 \times \frac{(\text{mean experimental cpm} - \text{mean spontaneous-release cpm})}{(\text{mean maximal-release cpm} - \text{mean spontaneous-release cpm})}$$

Labeling of Target Cells with ^{51}Cr

Cultured tumor cells such as K562 cells or a leukemia cell line should be in the logarithmic phase of growth. The cell viability is always checked by trypan blue exclusion prior to labeling and should be ≥75%.

1. On the day of the assay, determine the number of viable tumor cells and transfer 2×10^6 to 10×10^6 viable cells to a 15-ml conical polypropylene tube. Centrifuge the cells for 5 min at $200 \times g$ (1,000 rpm in a Sorvall RT 6000 centrifuge with an H-1000B rotor) at room temperature. Decant the supernatant.

2. By using a 1-ml tuberculin syringe with a 25-gauge needle, transfer an aliquot of 5-mCi/ml $Na^{51}CrO_4$ containing 100 μCi of ^{51}Cr to the cell pellet. For best results, a ^{51}Cr solution that is no more than 1 to 2 weeks past its maximum activity date should be used.

3. Mix the cells gently and incubate them for 1 h at 37°C in a 5% CO_2 incubator. Rotate the tube gently every 15 min to mix the cells.

4. Wash the cells at least twice, each time adding 10 ml of RPMI-5 medium, centrifuging the mixture for 5 min at $200 \times g$, and then decanting the supernatant into a radioactive liquid waste container. Finally, suspend the cells in 10 ml of RPMI-5 medium.

5. Determine the number of viable cells by using trypan blue exclusion, adjust the concentration of cells to 5×10^4/ml, and then check the radioactivity of the labeled cells by placing 0.1 ml of the final cell suspension into a vial or tube and counting for 1 min with a gamma scintillation counter. Labeling is satisfactory when the cell suspension incorporates 0.2 to 1.5 cpm per cell.

Controls

The NK-cell assay includes several different types of controls, as follows:

Assay controls: maximal-^{51}Cr-release controls and spontaneous-^{51}Cr-release controls (see above).

Intra-assay controls: fresh PBMC from a healthy donor are tested in row B as well as row H.

Interassay controls: cryopreserved, thawed, and pretested PBMC from three different selected healthy donors, who are known to have low, medium, and high levels of NK activity and whose PBMC cryopreserve well, are tested every time the assay is performed. These three cell samples are monitored for NK activity over weeks or months, providing a measure of the assay's reproducibility.

Biologic variability controls: fresh PBMC from the same healthy donors are obtained repeatedly at various time intervals and used to chart the biologic variability in NK-cell activity over time.

Quality Control and Quality Assurance

Criteria for an acceptable NK-cell assay are defined on the basis of intra-assay and interassay variability, which must be established for every laboratory. For an NK-cell assay to be accepted or rejected, a quality control program has to be in effect. This program should involve the following components:

The definition of intra-assay as well as interassay variability, based on the continually monitored performance of fresh as well as cryopreserved control cells, as described above.

Continued maintenance and frequent (every 6 months) analysis of the control cell performance to confirm that the assay is in control.

Strict adherence to the standard operating procedure (SOP) and written documentation of changes that may be introduced.

The formulation and availability of written criteria for assay acceptance or rejection.

The establishment of a proficiency program, with an exchange of samples between several laboratories.

Quality assurance for the NK-cell assay is particularly important. Handling of samples and the quality of effector cells are likely to have a major impact on the results. Therefore, it is essential to document in writing any departure from the SOP for sample collection or delivery to the testing laboratory as well as from the SOP for assay performance. Quality assurance is also concerned with the quality of target cells and their ability to spontaneously release the radioactive label. Cultured K562 cells must be in the logarithmic phase of growth to perform optimally as target cells. Radioactivity counts depend on the gamma counter's performance, and thus routine maintenance checks and control radioactive counts need to be regularly performed and documented in writing.

Pitfalls and Troubleshooting

NK-cell assays are not easy to perform reliably, and they require considerable effort to implement and interpret. The most difficult single problem with cytotoxicity assays employing tumor cell targets is the unacceptably high level of spontaneous release of ^{51}Cr (i.e., >5%). While careful culturing and frequent splitting of nonadherent K562 target cells to maintain them in the logarithmic phase of growth tend to control the problem, it is likely that it will appear periodically. We tend to resort to a newly thawed batch of cryopreserved target cells to correct this problem. A new batch of target cells is put in culture at about 2- to 3-month intervals. It is also important to perform mycoplasma assays on K562 target cells with regularity to avoid artifacts due to mycoplasma infections. The second perennial problem is a lack of assay reliability from day to day, which originates from unpredictable losses in NK activity. Such losses may be due to specimen handling, including the time elapsed between the cell harvest and testing, or to biologic variability, which cannot be controlled. For a number of healthy donors tested for NK activity repeatedly over a period of several months in our laboratory, significant biologic variability was observed. For this reason, designations of low, normal, or high NK activity for an individual should be based on three, not one, assays performed over time. In clinical trials, patients generally serve as their own baseline controls, and drug-related changes from the baseline are computed. Samples for NK activity assays are drawn in the morning to avoid diurnal variations. Samples arriving at the laboratory after an overnight shipment need to be processed and tested immediately. Shipments should be carried out in ambient temperatures, and green-top tubes, not separated mononuclear cells in medium, should be shipped. There is generally a loss of NK activity in specimens shipped or stored overnight, which varies from 10 to 25%. It is best to avoid shipping and to perform NK-cell assays on freshly harvested morning specimens, adhering as strictly as possible to the SOP. The third common problem concerns the interpretation of results. NK-cell assays performed at a single E:T ratio are not meaningful. At least four E:T ratios should be included in the assay to allow for the construction of a lytic curve defining a relationship between the percent specific lysis and the E:T ratio. For acceptable NK-cell assays, this curve is linear.

Interpretation

While the results of NK-cell assays are expressed as percentages of specific lysis at various E:T ratios, it is more convenient to present these results in lytic units (LU). This type of data transformation is especially useful when comparisons between the levels of lysis mediated by different effector cells tested at multiple E:T ratios are performed. Instead of comparing lytic curves, which is inconvenient, it is possible to transform the specific lysis data into a single number which accurately reflects the ability of a batch of effector cells to kill 20% of a predetermined number of target cells (4). A computer program for the calculation of LU is available from the reference laboratories engaged in NK-cell measurements, or LU can be calculated manually as described by Bryant et al. (1). Briefly, an LU is defined as the number of effector cells required to lyse a specific percentage, usually 20%, of a predetermined standard number (T_{STD}) of target cells (e.g., the T_{STD} could be 5×10^3). Assume that 20% lysis of 5×10^3 target cells occurs at the 12:1 E:T ratio. Multiplying this E:T ratio by the number of targets in the assay (5,000) shows that 6.0×10^4 effectors are required to lyse 20% of the targets. Thus, one LU consists of 6.0×10^4 effector cells. However, to allow a measure of lytic activity that increases with the level of cytotoxicity, the results are generally reported as the number of LU contained in a specified number of effector cells (E_{STD}); commonly, E_{STD} is chosen to equal 10^7 effector cells. These calculations can be expressed by the following formula:

$$\text{number of LU}/10^7 \text{ effector cells} = \frac{E_{STD}}{(E:T_{20})(T_{STD})}$$

$$= \frac{10^7}{(E:T_{20})(5 \times 10^3)}$$

where $E:T_{20}$ is the E:T ratio at which 20% of the target cells are killed.

The results of NK-cell assays performed with PBMC cannot be adequately interpreted unless a simultaneous estimation of the absolute number of NK cells present in the peripheral circulation is made and the results are expressed on a per-NK-cell basis. This is because the NK-cell assay does not discriminate between a high level of lytic activity mediated by a few NK cells and one mediated by many NK cells that are present in a particular batch of PBMC tested for NK activity. By the same token, the enumeration of NK cells in the circulation is not indicative of NK activity. Few NK cells can be highly effective at mediating lysis, and many NK cells may have only weak activity. Thus, assays of NK activity should be accompanied by NK-cell enumeration. A simultaneous measure by flow cytometry of the percentage of CD56$^+$ CD16$^+$ NK cells in the PBMC followed by a calculation of their absolute number (for which the white blood cell and differential lymphocyte counts must be available) is necessary to be able to express the units of NK activity per NK cell. Alternatively, fluorospheres (Flow-count fluorospheres; Beckman Coulter, Miami, Fla.) can be used to determine by flow cytometry the absolute number of CD56$^+$ CD16$^+$ NK cells among the PBMC present in the assay. Results presented in LU per NK cell are more meaningful than those expressed either as the percent specific lysis or LU alone, because they account for the actual number of NK cells responsible for the measured activity. In my laboratory, NK activity and NK-cell enumeration are offered as a panel, and both are routinely performed on all specimens. Of course, when the assay is performed with purified NK cells, this calculation is unnecessary.

NK cells can be subdivided into two functionally distinct populations on the basis of CD56 and CD16 expression on the cell surface (3). Approximately 90% of NK cells are CD56^{dim} CD16^{bright}, express abundant KIRs, and are highly cytotoxic. The remaining 10% are CD56^{bright} CD16$^{dim/neg}$. These NK cells have the ability to produce high levels of immunoregulatory cytokines, such as tumor necrosis factor alpha, but express few KIRs and are poorly cytotoxic. This phenotypic and functional heterogeneity of NK cells probably reflects their various maturation stages, and it considerably complicates the analysis of the NK-cell repertoire during disease, where one or another NK-cell subset may be preferentially expanded. The clinical significance of the two NK-cell subsets may be that CD56^{dim} cells represent cytotoxic effector cells, while CD56^{bright} NK cells play an immunoregulatory role due to their ability to produce cytokines (3).

NK activity may vary substantially among healthy individuals, and therefore it is necessary to establish a normal range of NK activity by testing PBMC from many different donors who are presumably representatives of the general population in a particular geographic area. For example, in my laboratory, a mid-80% range for normal NK activity is 53 to 301 LU$_{20}$/10^7 cells based on 140 individual determinations. While establishing a normal range for NK activity, it is important to consider both the age and sex of the blood donors. Generally, NK activity in males is significantly higher than that in females (i.e., males [n = 49] have a median activity of 201 LU$_{20}$/10^7 cells, while females [n = 103] have a median activity of 115 LU$_{20}$/10^7 cells), as determined in my laboratory. There is some statistical evidence that NK activity increases with age, but in my laboratory, this trend is not significant. In an individual, the level of NK activity tends to be stable over time, provided that this individual remains healthy and is not experiencing severe or prolonged stress or taking medications known to alter NK activity.

CONCLUSIONS

Measurements of NK activity are difficult to perform in a clinical laboratory setting. They require considerable expertise, constant vigilance, and extensive quality control and quality assurance. Consequently, the assay is relatively costly. While the use of transformed data simplifies interpretation, it also creates concerns about data manipulation. The format of data presentation may vary from one institution to another, and minor variations in the SOP might account for the lack of interlaboratory agreement. There is no NK-cell proficiency program in effect, and each laboratory is responsible for defining its own criteria for assay acceptance or rejection.

A variety of nonradioactive assays have been developed to measure NK activity, as alluded to earlier. These assays measure either secretory-type killing, and thus may be equivalent to the ^{51}Cr-release assay, or nonsecretory killing (apoptosis), which can also be mediated by NK cells (9). The results of the latter tend not to correlate with those of ^{51}Cr-release assays. On the other hand, when ^{51}Cr-release assays have been used for serial monitoring, relatively poor correlations between NK activity and clinical responses have been observed in many cases. This is not surprising in view of the current knowledge about NK cells. These effector cells can perform multiple functions, utilize more than one mechanism of killing to eliminate susceptible targets, and secrete multiple cytokines upon activation. Therefore, the biologic relevance of any one in vitro assay for NK activity is not clear at present, and future measurements of NK activity are likely to include assays for measuring a broader range of NK-cell functions.

REFERENCES

1. **Bryant, J., R. Day, T. L. Whiteside, and R. B. Herberman.** 1992. Calculation of lytic units for the expression of cell-mediated cytotoxicity. *J. Immunol. Methods* **146:**91–103.
2. **Burshtyn, D. N., and E. O. Long.** 1997. Regulation through inhibitory receptors: lessons for natural killer cells. *Trends Cell Biol.* **7:**473–479.
3. **Cooper, M. A., T. A. Fehniger, and M. A. Caligiuri.** 2001. The biology of human natural killer-cell subsets. *Trends Immunol.* **22:**633–640.
4. **Friberg, D., J. L. Bryant, and T. L. Whiteside.** 1996. Measurements of natural killer (NK) activity and NK cell quantification. *Methods* **9:**316–326.
5. **Kashii, Y., R. Giorda, R. B. Herberman, T. L. Whiteside, and N. L. Vujanovic.** 1999. Constitutive expression and role of the TNF family ligands in apoptotic killing of tumor cells by human NK cells. *J. Immunol.* **163:**5358–5366.
6. **Lanier, L. L.** 2003. Natural killer cell receptor signaling. *Curr. Opin. Immunol.* **15:**308–314.
7. **Trinchieri, G.** 1989. Biology of natural killer cells. *Adv. Immunol.* **47:**187–376.
8. **Vujanovic, N. L., P. Basse, R. B. Herberman, and T. L. Whiteside.** 1996. Antitumor function of natural killer cells and control of metastases. *Methods* **9:**394–408.
9. **Vujanovic, N. L., S. Nagashima, R. B. Herberman, and T. L. Whiteside.** 1996. Nonsecretory apoptotic killing by human NK cells. *J. Immunol.* **157:**1117–1126.

Cellular Immune Assays for Evaluation of Vaccine Efficacy

JOSEPHINE H. COX, MARK deSOUZA, SILVIA RATTO-KIM, GUIDO FERRARI, KENT J. WEINHOLD, AND DEBORAH L. BIRX

35

It is estimated that routine immunization with currently licensed vaccines against polio, diphtheria, whooping cough, tetanus, and measles could prevent 3 million annual deaths worldwide. Tuberculosis (TB), malaria, and human immunodeficiency virus (HIV), for which no effective vaccines are available, are responsible for 7 million deaths per year worldwide. Most of these deaths occur in developing countries, where the economic impact of endemic diseases is immense and the need for vaccines is most pressing. Vaccines for approximately 100 different bacterial and viral organisms are currently under development, with current progress ranging from basic research and development through phase I to III clinical trials (23, 49).

Vaccine development now increasingly draws on the expanded understanding of the immune mechanisms involved in preventing or controlling viral, bacterial, and parasitic infections (13). In the 20th century, successful vaccines were produced against many acute viral and bacterial infections. The challenge facing current vaccinologists is how to develop vaccines to control chronic persisting or recurrent diseases like TB and HIV, hepatitis C virus, and human papillomavirus infections (3). A greater understanding of the immune response, particularly of cell-mediated immune responses in malaria, TB, HIV, and cancer patients, will lead to improved vaccine design (2, 5, 26, 36, 37, 52). Currently, in vitro analyses of cellular immune responses are being used for assessments of the efficacy of therapeutic and prophylactic vaccines, for clinical diagnosis, and for studies of immune regulation (21, 34, 41, 53, 56, 57).

Concurrent with progress in vaccine design, there is a need for sophisticated cellular immunologic testing at specialized centralized laboratories, at clinical sites involved in vaccine trials, or on-site in developing countries. There has been a dramatic increase in the number of countries and institutions involved in vaccine trials in the past 5 years (34, 37, 54). Both privately and publicly funded organizations have focused some of their primary efforts toward a worldwide approach for testing vaccines.

With the increase in institutions involved in vaccine testing, there is a need for collaborative efforts that focus on the reproducibility of measuring immune responses across organizations. Previously, cellular assessments of immunity were performed with nonstandardized reagents and with protocols that were different from laboratory to laboratory. As a consequence, performance characteristics differed from laboratory to laboratory, making it almost impossible to compare the immunogenicity of one vaccine to that of another. In a study of 11 laboratories that used standard operating procedures and common reagents, there was a larger-than-expected discordance in the outcome of an enzyme-linked immunospot (ELISPOT) assay (11). The publicly funded Partnership for AIDS Vaccine Evaluation (PAVE [www.hiv-pave.org]) and the privately funded Enterprise organization (www.glf.org) are organizations leading the effort toward the standardization of cell processing, sample storage, and immunogenicity assessments at the preclinical and clinical stages of vaccine development (27). The requirements for standardizing cellular immunology assays, cell processing, and cell freezing are seen as necessities by various regulatory agencies because they will allow quicker interagency and interlaboratory comparisons for making the best informed decisions on which candidate vaccines will be worth sponsoring for advanced development. Table 1 lists organizations involved in validating immunogenicity assays for human vaccine trials. The transfer of technically demanding assays to developing countries is necessary, or alternatively, samples need to be processed, stored, and then shipped to central laboratories for testing. This chapter was compiled by authors who have been involved in HIV vaccine testing for 15 years and have been collaborating with or have worked in laboratories in both developed and developing countries.

PROCESSING AND COLLECTION OF PBMC FROM WHOLE BLOOD

The assessment of T-cell function may be affected by procedures, beginning with the blood draw and through cell separation, cryopreservation, storage, and thawing prior to the assays. Additionally, the time from blood collection to actual processing for lymphocyte separation is critical. Different procedures for collection and separation of peripheral blood mononuclear cells (PBMC) are shown in Table 2, along with their potential advantages and disadvantages.

When conducting cellular immunology assays, the integrity of the PBMC, especially the cellular membranes, is critical for success. A correct cellular separation process yields a pure, highly viable population of mononuclear cells consisting of lymphocytes and monocytes, with minimal red blood cell and platelet contamination, that retains optimum functional capacity. The standard method for the separation

TABLE 1 Organizations involved in validating immunogenicity assays for human vaccine trials

Organization	Website	Role
British Association of Research Quality Assurance	www.barqa.com	Assists in the understanding, interpretation, and implementation of national and international regulations covering good laboratory practice (GLP), good clinical practice (GCP) and good manufacturing practice (GMP).
U.S. Food and Drug Administration	www.FDA.org	U.S. body regulating safety of all vaccine products as well as GLP, GCP, and GMP compliance.
Clinical and Laboratory Standards Institute (formerly NCCLS)	www.clsi.org	Nonpartisan body that facilitates the development and availability of useful, accurate medical services, including criteria for validating immunogenicity assays.
National Association of Testing Authorities, Australia	www.nata.asn.au	Australia's GLP compliance monitoring authority; a private, nonprofit company owned and governed by its members and by representatives from industry, government, and professional bodies.

of PBMC is the use of Ficoll-Hypaque gradients, as originally described by Boyum (6). A high degree of technical expertise is required to execute the procedure. Two new types of collection vessels that are available commercially have greatly simplified PBMC separation and are applicable for vaccine studies because of their ease of use and potential for automation (10).

Protocol 1. Separation of PBMC by Using CPTs

Vacutainer cell preparation tubes (CPTs; Becton Dickinson [http://www.bd.com/vacutainer/products/molecular/citrate/procedures.asp]) provide a convenient, single-tube system for the collection and separation of mononuclear cells from whole blood. Blood is drawn into the CPT and can be immediately centrifuged, allowing the gel to form a stable barrier between the anticoagulated blood and Ficoll. The

separated blood can then be transported at ambient temperature to the processing and/or storage laboratory. This step reduces the risk of sample contamination and eliminates the need for additional tubes and processing reagents. In many instances, in particular when biosafety level 2 safety cabinets are not available on-site, the CPT method is useful because the centrifugation step can be done on-site and the remaining processing steps can be performed after shipment to a central laboratory within the shortest time possible, optimally within 8 h. The central laboratory can complete cell processing in a biosafety level 2 cabinet and set up functional assays or cryopreserve the samples as needed. The simplicity of the CPT separation method gives it superior technical reliability in our hands over the Ficoll-Hypaque method and is the method of choice for our phase III vaccine trial in Thailand, despite the increased cost associated with the

TABLE 2 Stages and variables in the separation and cryopreservation of PBMC from whole blood

Procedure or technology	Equipment or reagent	Advantage(s)	Disadvantage(s)
PBMC collection	Heparin	Greater cellular stability than EDTA	Impacts DNA isolation; plasma from whole blood cannot be used for PCR-based assays
	EDTA		Time-dependent negative impact on T-cell responses
	Sodium citrate	Greater cellular stability than EDTA	
PBMC separation	Standard Ficoll		Technically challenging, time-consuming
	CPTs	Rapid, technically easy, with less interperson variability; blood is drawn into the same tube that is used for separation	Subject to temperature fluctuations manifested by gel deterioration and contamination in PBMC fraction
	Accuspin or Leucosep tubes	Rapid, technically easy, with less interperson variability	
PBMC cryopreservation	Nalgene "Mr. Frosty" freezer	Cheap, technically easy	Lack of ability to monitor temperature
	Controlled-rate freezer	Accurate temperature control; the temperature is monitored and recorded	Expensive, requires a supply of LN
Counting	Hemacytometer	Cheap	Subjective counting procedure
	Automated counter	Accurate	Some automated counters do not have the capacity to count viable cells; expensive

method. The CPT method reduces interperson variability related to removing the PBMC layer from Ficoll and thus allows for uniformly higher cell yields.

Note that CPTs are sensitive to excessive temperature fluctuations, resulting in deterioration of the gel, which impacts successful cellular separation. This is a particularly serious problem in tropical countries, where ambient storage temperatures may be >25°C. Following PBMC separation, one may macroscopically observe the presence of gel spheres in the cellular layer which are very difficult to distinguish from the actual PBMC. This has been observed after storage at temperatures of >25°C. Where possible, the tubes should be stored at temperatures no higher than 25°C. Once the tubes are filled with blood, the temperatures should be kept between 18 and 25°C. Blood-filled CPTs should under no circumstances be stored on ice or next to an ice pack. It is recommended that they be separated from any ice packs by bubble wrap or another type of insulation within a cooler so that temperature fluctuations are kept to a minimum.

Materials and Reagents

Vacutainer CPTs (Becton Dickinson)

Sterile phosphate-buffered saline (PBS) without Ca^{2+} and Mg^{2+}, supplemented with antibiotics (penicillin and streptomycin)

Sterile RPMI medium containing 2% fetal bovine serum (FBS) and supplemented with antibiotics

Method

Specimens should be centrifuged as soon as possible after collection. The manufacturer recommends that the initial centrifugation step (see below) to separate the lymphocytes should occur within 2 h. The plasma and leukocytes, which are then separated from the red blood cells by the gel barrier, can be mixed by inversion, and processing should be completed within 8 h of the first centrifugation. The specimens should be put into a cooler box and transported at room temperature (18 to 25°C) to the processing laboratory.

1. Spin tubes at room temperature (18 to 25°C) in a horizontal rotor (with a swinging-bucket head) for a minimum of 20 min and a maximum of 30 min at a relative centrifugal force (RCF or g) of 1,500 with the brake off. To calculate the revolutions per minute (rpm), use the following calculation, where r is the radial distance from the centrifuge's center post to the tube bottom (in centimeters):

$$\text{rpm speed setting} = \sqrt{\frac{\text{RCF} \times 100,000}{1.12 \times r}}$$

2. Remove the tubes from the centrifuge and pipette the entire contents of each tube above the gel into a 50-ml tube. This tube will now contain both PBMC and undiluted plasma. An additional centrifugation step will allow the removal of undiluted plasma, if desired. Wash each CPT with 5 ml of PBS–1% penicillin–streptomycin (Pen/Strep). This wash step will remove cells from the top of the gel plug. Combine these cells with the cells removed from the tube. This wash increases the yield of cells as much as 30 to 40%.

3. Spin down this tube at 1,600 rpm for 15 to 20 min at room temperature with the brake on.

4. Resuspend the PBMC pellet in RPMI with 2% FBS, and wash it one more time to remove contaminating platelets. PBMC are counted and cryopreserved or used, as required.

Protocol 2. Separation of PBMC by Using Accuspin or Leucosep Tubes

More recently, Leucosep and Accuspin tubes have become available. Further information on Leucosep tubes is available at www.gbo.com, and information on Accuspin tubes is available at www.sigmaaldrich.com; the working principles of these tubes are the same. The tubes are separated into two chambers by a porous barrier made of highly transparent polypropylene. This biologically inert barrier allows the elimination of the laborious overlaying of the sample material over Ficoll. The barrier allows the separation of the sample material added to the top from the separation medium (Ficoll added to the bottom). The tubes are available in two sizes (15 and 50 ml) and may be purchased with or without Ficoll. There is an advantage of buying the tubes without Ficoll in that they can be stored at room temperature rather than refrigerated. This may be an important problem if cold space is limiting or the cold chain is difficult; also, the expiration date of the Ficoll will not affect the tube expiration. The following procedure describes the separation method for Leucosep tubes that are not prefilled with Ficoll-Hypaque. The Accuspin procedure is virtually identical.

Note that whole blood can be diluted 1:2 with a balanced salt solution. While this dilution step is not necessary, it can improve the separation of PBMC and enhance the PBMC yield. The procedure is performed by using aseptic technique.

Materials and Reagents

Accuspin or Leucosep tubes

Ficoll-Hypaque

Sterile PBS without Ca^{2+} and Mg^{2+}, supplemented with antibiotics (Pen/Strep)

Sterile RPMI medium containing 2% FBS and supplemented with antibiotics

Method

1. Warm the separation medium (Ficoll-Hypaque) to room temperature and keep it protected from light.

2. Fill the Leucosep tubes with separation medium, using 3 ml for 14-ml tubes and 15 ml for 40-ml tubes.

3. Close the tubes and centrifuge them at 1,000 × g (see protocol 1 for g-to-rpm conversion) for 30 s at room temperature.

4. Pour whole blood or diluted blood into the tubes, using 3 to 6 ml for 14-ml tubes and 15 to 30 ml for 50-ml tubes.

5. Centrifuge the tubes for 10 min at 1,000 × g or for 15 min at 800 × g in a swinging-bucket rotor with the centrifuge brake off.

6. After centrifugation, the sequence of layers from top to bottom should be as follows:
   1. Plasma and platelets
   2. Enriched PBMC fraction
   3. Separation medium
   4. Porous barrier
   5. Separation medium
   6. Pellet (erythrocytes and granulocytes)

7. Plasma can be collected to within 5 to 10 mm of the enriched PBMC fraction and further processed or stored for additional assays.

8. Harvest the enriched PBMC, wash them with 10 ml of PBS containing 1% Pen/Strep, and centrifuge them at 250 × g for 10 min.

9. Resuspend the PBMC pellet in RPMI with 2% FBS and wash it one more time to remove contaminating platelets. PBMC are counted and cryopreserved or used, as required.

EFFECT OF CELL SEPARATION AND ANTICOAGULANT ON LYMPHOCYTE SUBTYPES

We conducted experiments to determine the effect of the time from blood draw to processing on cell subsets within the white blood cell component and on PBMC purity (defined as lymphocytes plus monocytes/lymphocytes plus monocytes plus neutrophils plus eosinophils plus basophils). Whole blood was collected into two sodium citrate-containing CPTs from each of 20 subjects who gave informed consent (9 females and 11 males) and was processed within 2 and 30 h of collection according to the standard operating procedure described above (protocol 1). Following processing, a complete blood differential was obtained by using automated technology. As shown in Fig. 1, the lymphocyte population was diminished, while the neutrophil and monocyte populations were increased, as the time to processing of whole blood increased. The PBMC purity decreased, from 92% within 2 h of collection to 80% 30 h after collection. Cell viability measurements by trypan blue exclusion were identical for the two time points.

In a separate experiment, we assessed the effect of the time from collection to processing on the proportions of lymphocyte subsets (total T cells, CD4 and CD8 T cells, B cells, and NK cells). Subsets were assessed by two-color flow cytometry. Whole blood was collected into sodium citrate-containing CPTs from 19 HIV-seronegative Thai subjects who gave informed consent (10 females and 9 males). Two tubes were collected per subject. The first tube was processed as described previously within 2 h of collection, and the second tube was processed 24 to 26 h after collection. Flow cytometry was conducted on the enriched PBMC fraction. Delayed processing had little impact on the percentages of the various lymphocyte subsets, although with the exception of B and NK cells, there was a general decrease with the longer time from collection to processing (Fig. 2).

We compared the viability and percentages of lymphocytes and neutrophils after processing of paired samples (from 20 subjects) of whole blood collected into citrate-containing CPTs and acid citrate dextrose tubes and transferred to Leucosep tubes. PBMC separation with both tube types was conducted by using the manufacturers' protocols. Figure 3 shows that the data were comparable for the three parameters measured, although the overall percentage of lymphocytes was marginally higher with Leucosep tubes than with CPT separation for 19 of 20 subjects tested.

LYMPHOCYTE FUNCTION ASSAYS FOR VACCINE TRIALS

Flow cytometric analyses of lymphocyte subpopulations, as well as cell viability tests, are not necessarily indicative of cell function. Therefore, in addition to monitoring PBMC viability and recovery, it is also important to examine T-cell function. The last 10 years have seen a change in how lymphocyte function can be measured. Sophisticated assays are now available to dissect the fine specificities and functions of lymphocytes. Such assays include lymphocyte proliferation assays (LPAs), cytotoxic T-cell (CTL) assays, ELISPOT assays, tetramer assays, intracellular cytokine secretion (ICS) assays, and polychromatic flow cytometry assays (19, 22, 30, 32, 48).

CTL assays and LPAs do not directly measure the frequency of precursor cells in the peripheral circulation. Cells in culture may expand at different rates, some may undergo antigen-induced apoptosis, and others may not expand under these conditions. The classic CTL assays and LPAs allowed the measurement of two important functions, namely, the ability to lyse relevant target cells and the ability to proliferate in response to antigen, respectively. With a limiting dilution format, they also allowed an estimate of the precursor-T-cell frequency. The advantages of the ELISPOT, ICS, and tetramer assays are that they are quantitative and directly measure the frequency of T cells circulating in the

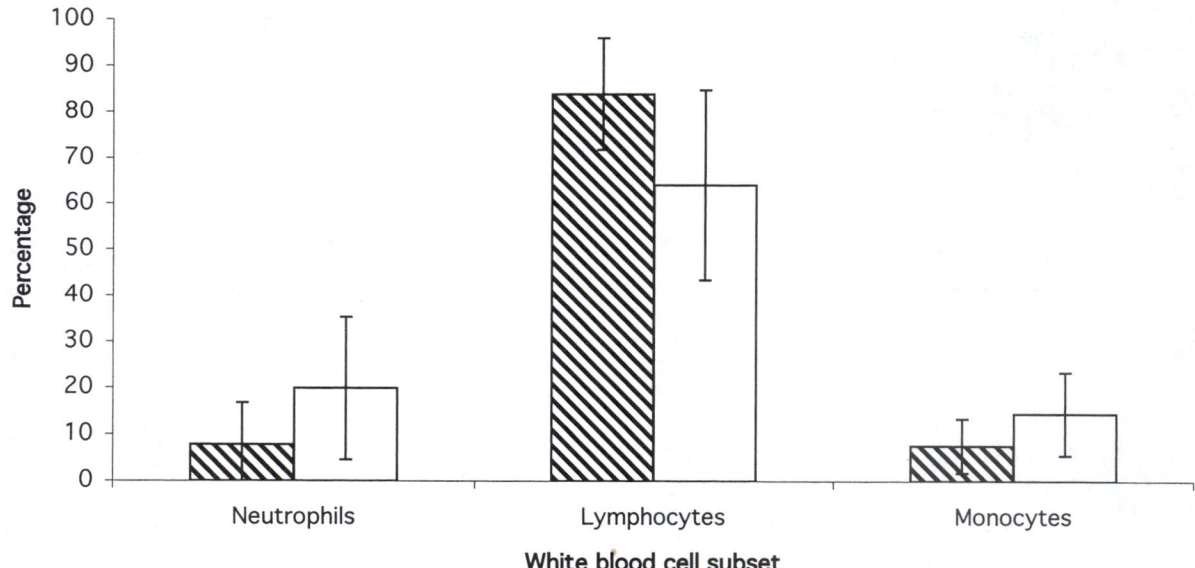

FIGURE 1 Effect of time to processing of whole blood on white blood cell subsets. Whole blood was collected from 20 subjects into CPTs (two per subject) and stored at 22 to 25°C for 2 and 30 h prior to processing. Hatched bars, 2 h; white bars, 30 h.

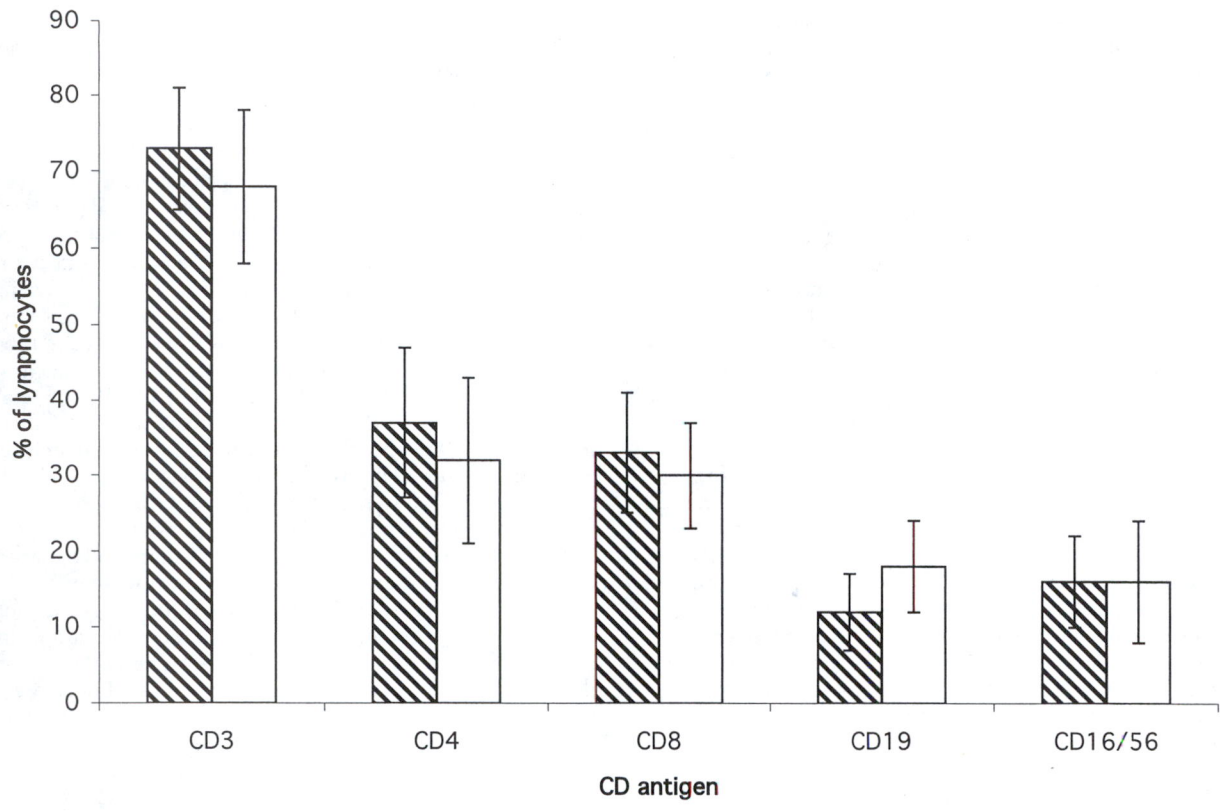

FIGURE 2 Effect of time to processing of whole blood on lymphocyte subsets. Whole blood was collected from 19 subjects into CPTs (two per subject) and stored at 22 to 25°C prior to PBMC separation and measurements of lymphocyte subsets by flow cytometry. Hatched bars, 2 h; white bars, 30 h.

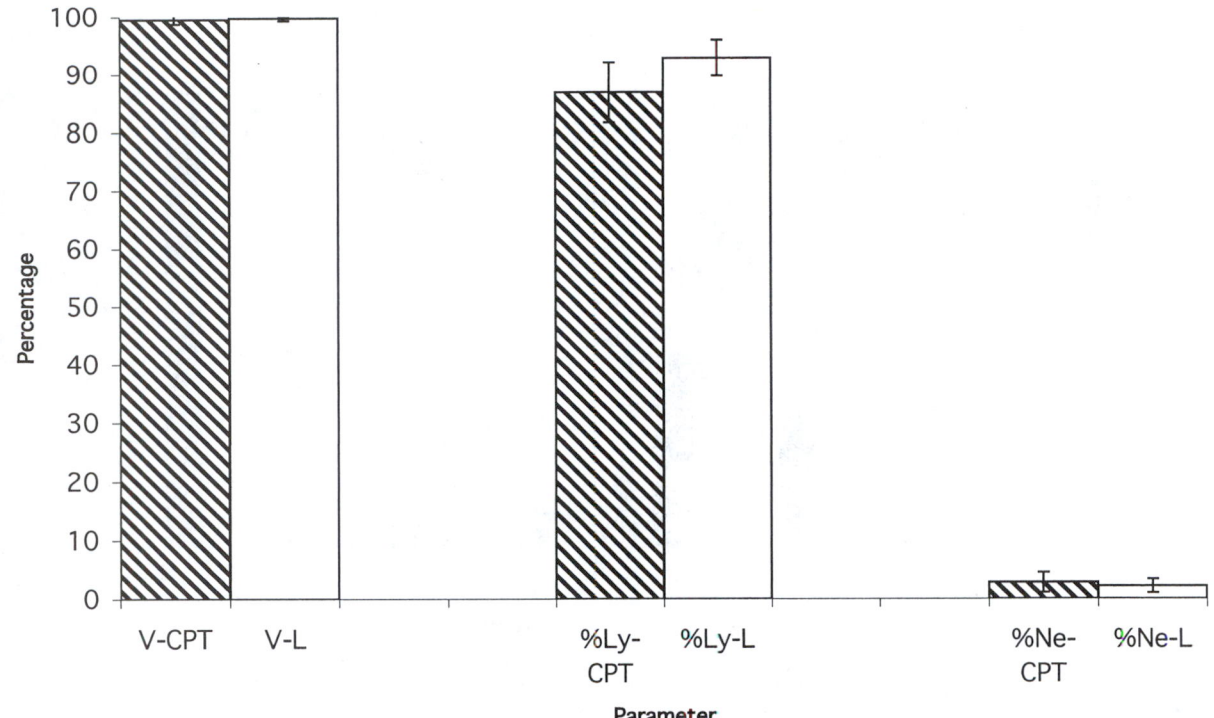

FIGURE 3 Comparison of viability (V), percent lymphocytes (%Ly), and percent neutrophils (%Ne) of PBMC following separation of paired samples from 20 subjects by using CPTs and Leucosep (L) tubes. Hatched bars, CPTs; white bars, Leucosep tubes.

blood without any further in vitro manipulation. It should be pointed out that none of these assays are able in their present forms to measure simultaneously all possible effector mechanisms of CD8+ or CD4+ T-cell populations. Each assay has its limitations, but it is not really known for any given disease which is likely to be the main effector mechanism that correlates with protection or vaccine efficacy (30, 45). Hence, it is important to evaluate as many cell functions as possible and to stay up-to-date with the rapidly expanding field of cellular immunology assays.

There is no doubt that ELISPOT and, most recently, ICS assays are becoming the cellular assessment tools of choice. This is because cryopreserved PBMC can be used, allowing batch testing of samples and thereby decreasing interassay variation and increasing the possibility of automation of the procedures (10). A description of each of these assays is outside the scope of this chapter, but these methods are presented elsewhere in this manual (chapters 27 and 28).

Because HIV vaccine candidates entering human phase I trials are increasingly being conducted multinationally, there is a need for the standardization of these assays. ELISPOT and ICS assays will aid in the determination of the best candidate vaccine to move forward into phase II or III testing. This selection should be based on comparative immunogenicity analyses of the potential vaccines tested. The wide use of standardized reagents, assay kits, and protocols for ELISPOT and ICS assays will allow intergroup assay comparisons among laboratories and among the different vaccines tested.

Effect of Time to Cell Separation and Anticoagulant on Lymphocyte Function

CD8+ T-Cell Functions

Whole-blood samples left too long in the presence of anticoagulants or at nonphysiologic temperatures adversely affect the PBMC separation process and may also cause changes which can subsequently affect PBMC function (4, 11, 60). Several laboratories within the PAVE network have now described that there is a dramatic effect on the number of gamma interferon (IFN-γ)-secreting cells if PBMC are not processed in a timely fashion (within 8 h). A peptide pool consisting of 23 cytomegalovirus, Epstein-Barr virus, and influenza virus (CEF) epitopes was used to directly quantify the integrity of PBMC and the number of IFN-γ-secreting cells when PBMC were separated from whole blood at different times after collection (12). For an evaluation of the effect of the time to cell separation on cell functions, whole blood from 12 individuals was collected in tubes containing sodium heparin anticoagulant, and processing of the blood was either performed immediately or after overnight storage of the blood at approximately 25°C. The ELISPOT assay was then performed immediately after PBMC separation. Eight of the freshly isolated PBMC samples secreted IFN-γ in response to the CEF epitope pool. When whole blood was stored overnight prior to the separation of PBMC, six of the eight PBMC samples had a marked reduction in the number of IFN-γ-secreting spot-forming cells (SFC). Three samples exhibited a more than fivefold reduction, and three had a one- to twofold reduction in the number of IFN-γ-secreting SFC (Fig. 4). One of the responders changed to a nonresponder, with a 25-fold decrease in response, from 123 to 5 CEF epitope-specific SFC/10⁶ cells. The responder with the highest CEF epitope response was the least susceptible to the effects of a delay in processing. For this patient, there were 2,789 and 3,056 CEF epitope-specific SFC per 10⁶ PBMC for blood processed immediately and overnight after cryopreservation, respectively (data not shown). The data suggest that low to moderate responders are the most susceptible to delays in processing and that delays may substantially affect the interpretation of vaccine

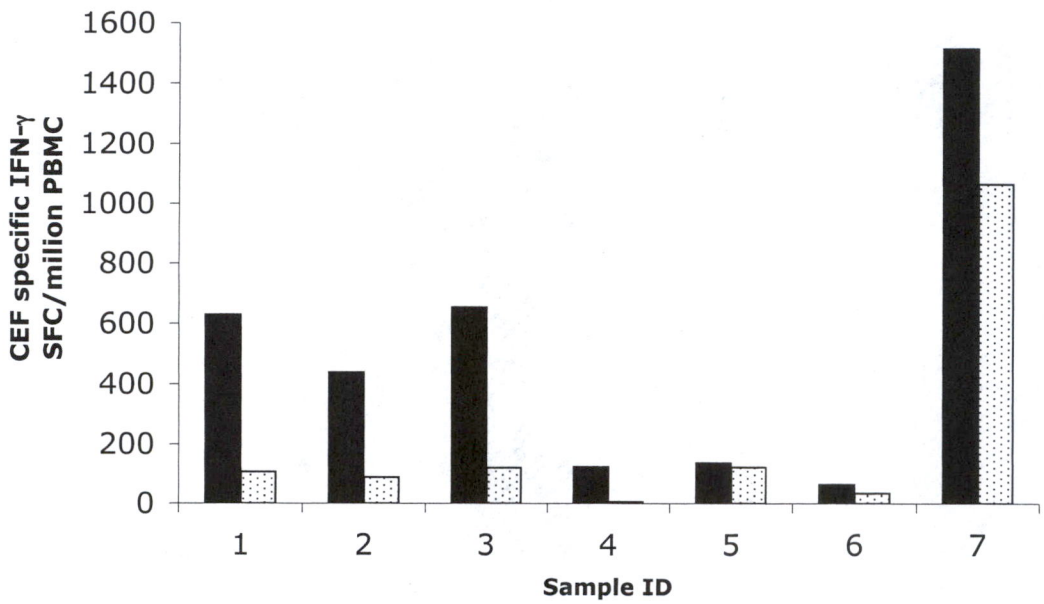

FIGURE 4 Time to processing affects production of IFN-γ. The processing of seven blood samples and ELISPOT assay setup were either performed immediately (solid bars) or after overnight storage of blood at room temperature in a safety cabinet (stippled bars). PBMC were stimulated with a pool of CEF peptides. The average number of background SFC attributable to PBMC only was subtracted.

immunogenicity. The optimal time frame for the collection of blood samples and the processing, separation, and cryopreservation of PBMC is <8 h or the same day as blood collection.

The effect of three different anticoagulants on T-cell function was measured by an ELISPOT assay. All 10 samples were processed within 6 h of collection, and the secretion of IFN-γ in response to the CEF epitope pool was examined. Figure 5 shows that equivalent CEF responses were obtained regardless of the anticoagulant used. A Kruskall-Wallis test revealed that there were no significant differences among the CEF-induced responses ($P = 0.58$).

CD4+ T-Cell Functions

The standard LPA measures antigen-induced cell division. Cells (usually PBMC) are incubated in the presence of various concentrations of an antigen (specific) or mitogen (nonspecific) stimulus of interest. After a period of 2 to 7 days, tritiated thymidine is added to the cultures for 6 to 24 h. The amount of tritiated thymidine incorporated into the cells is measured by liquid scintillation counting and reflects the proliferation of cells in response to the mitogen or antigen. LPAs are straightforward and robust. Lymphoproliferative responses of different samples can be compared by using a stimulation index (SI). The SI is the ratio of the scintillation counts obtained in the presence of antigen to the counts obtained in the presence of culture medium alone. Comparable lymphoproliferative responses of fresh PBMC separated with CPTs or Ficoll-Hypaque have been documented (61). In our own studies in Thailand, six HIV-1-seronegative subjects had comparable lymphoproliferative responses to a mitogen and an antigen. The median SIs of PBMC separated with Ficoll and CPTs in response to phytohemagglutinin were 34 (4 to 65) and 52 (8 to 211), respectively (ranges are given in parentheses). The median SIs in response to tetanus toxin were identical (4), with ranges of 1 to 55 and 2 to 89 for Ficoll and CPTs, respectively. Heparin

and citrate anticoagulants do not appear to adversely affect lymphoproliferative responses (61).

Summary of Critical Issues for Processing and Collection of PBMC

To optimize and standardize blood collection and processing procedures that will yield functionally intact T cells, follow these guidelines:

- Limit the time between blood draw and processing to <8 h.
- Avoid extremes of temperature during cell shipment and processing.
- Minimize red blood cell and platelet contamination by the use of good technique and multiple washing steps.
- Use the correct centrifugation speed for PBMC separation.
- Heparin and sodium citrate anticoagulants appear to be interchangeable for use in immunology assays. However, for some molecular assays (e.g., assays of HIV viral load), a sodium citrate anticoagulant is recommended.
- Batch test and perform quality assurance and quality control for all antigens and mitogens in each assay prior to use on precious samples.
- All batches of media, ELISPOT plates, serum, and wash buffers as well as antibodies and detection reagents should be tested prior to conducting assays.

EFFECT OF CRYOPRESERVATION ON IMMUNE FUNCTION ASSAYS

For successful cellular immunology studies, the viability, recovery, and function of PBMC need to be optimal. There are clear advantages to being able to batch assays from multiple time points from a clinical trial, but this requires the cryopreservation of PBMC in a manner that maintains their functional capabilities. One study analyzed the integrity of ~600 cryopreserved samples collected and processed within 5 to 24 h of collection from four different sites in the Multicenter AIDS Cohort Study (28). Approximately one-third of the samples were from HIV-1-seronegative individuals, and two-thirds were from HIV-1-seropositive individuals. The median number of viable cells recovered was about 50% of the total number stored, and the median viability was at least 90%. Cells were stored for up to 12 years, and during this time period the percent cell viability stayed remarkably stable, with few differences between the sites (Fig. 6). The viability of the cells was >85% in 519 of 596 specimens tested. Other studies have documented similar findings (42, 59). On the other hand, the viable-cell recovery rate over time has been shown to be quite variable. In a study by Kleeberger et al. (28), the median number of total cells recovered per vial was 7.75×10^6 (range, 1×10^6 to 25×10^6) for an input cell number of 10×10^6 cells (Fig. 7). For one of our Thai studies, PBMC from HIV-1-seronegative patients enrolled in a vaccine trial were processed and cryopreserved at two geographically separate sites (Bangkok and Chiang Mai). The samples from Chiang Mai were shipped to a central immunology laboratory in Bangkok in aliquots of 5 million cells/vial. PBMC from both sites were thawed and tested in an LPA at the AFRIMS Department of Retrovirology cellular immunology laboratory. The mean cell recovery of PBMC per vial for samples from Bangkok was 5.08 million cells (range, 1.33 to 8.67 million) and that for samples from Chiang Mai was 3.25 million cells (range, 1.67 to 6.33 million). Seventy-eight samples from each site were tested.

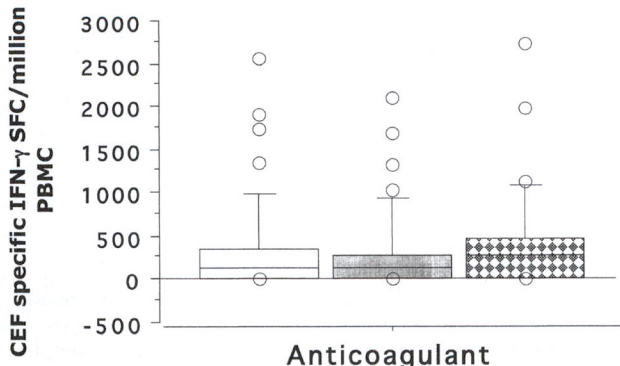

FIGURE 5 The effect of three different anticoagulants on T-cell function was measured by an ELISPOT assay. White box, heparin; shaded box, EDTA; stippled box, acid citrate dextrose. Ten samples were processed within 6 h of collection, and the secretion of IFN-γ in response to the CEF epitope pool was examined. The data are shown with a box plot of IFN-γ-secreting SFC/million PBMC. The box plot shows the distribution of values; from the top to bottom, lines are drawn parallel to the x axis, indicating the 95th, 75th, 50th (median), 25th, and 5th percentiles. A Kruskall-Wallis test revealed that there were no significant differences between the CEF-induced responses in PBMC collected in heparin, EDTA, and acid citrate dextrose.

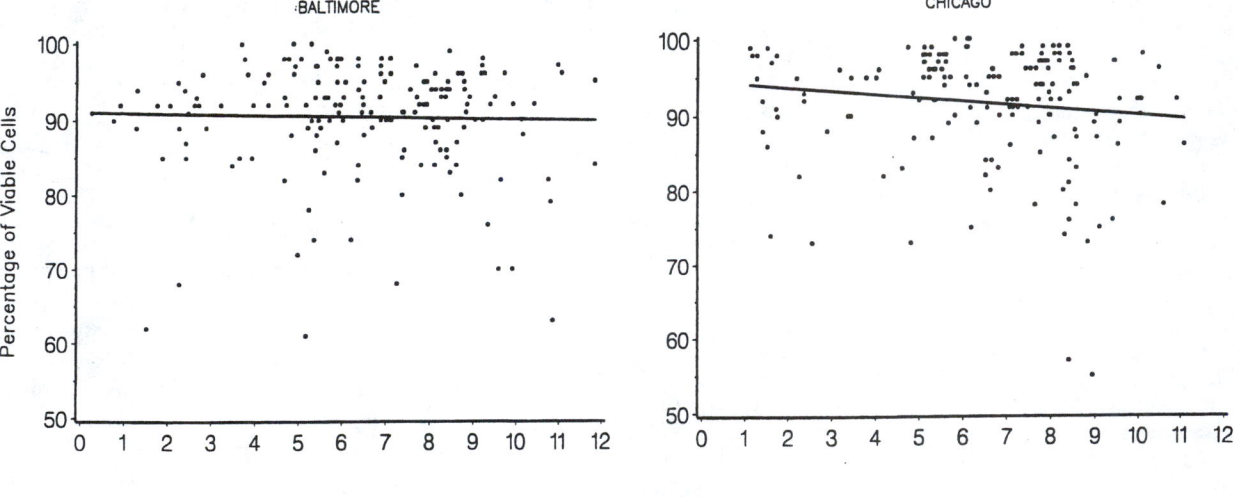

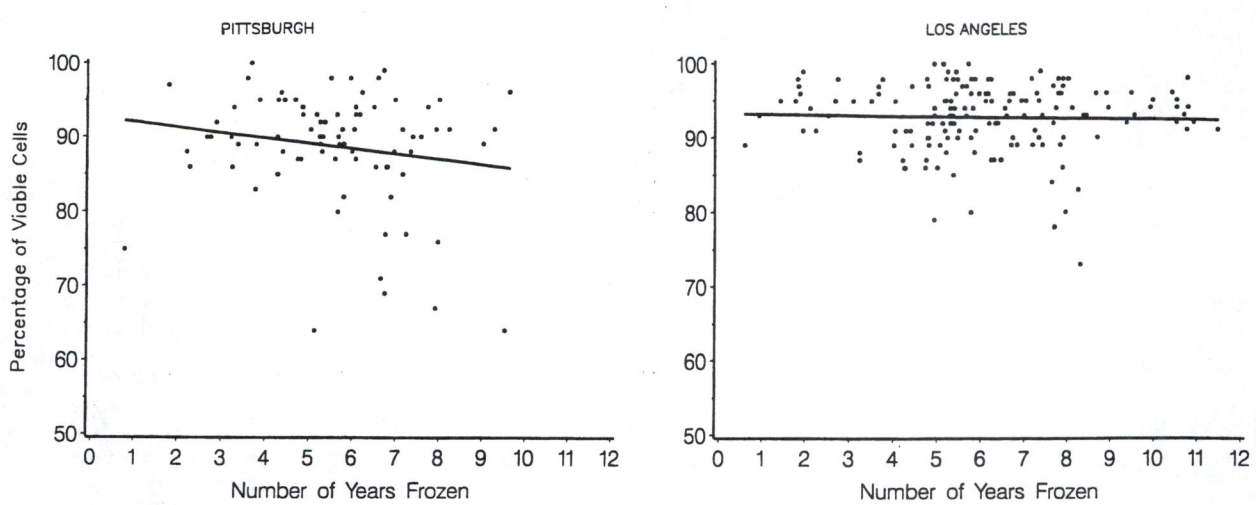

FIGURE 6 Percent viability of stored PBMC over time, indicated by center. PBMC were thawed, and their viability was assessed by a trypan blue exclusion technique. (Reproduced with permission from reference 28.)

The reasons for the variability in cell recovery rates can come from several sources, including (i) errors in counting, (ii) different methods of freezing, (iii) different methods of thawing cells, (iv) the number of centrifugation and washing steps between thawing counting, (v) the length and type of storage conditions, (vi) the origin of the PBMC, and (vii) storage and shipping conditions. Since the goal of cryopreservation is to allow batch testing of samples to be performed, it is critical to limit the variability in the above parameters and thus to optimize cell function, viability, and recovery.

Effect of Different Shipping Methods on Immune Function Assays

After optimizing the cell processing, separation, and cryopreservation techniques, it is essential that cells are shipped correctly so that a deterioration of function does not occur during shipment. In some instances, it is necessary to ship specimens to a central laboratory, mainly if the equipment and reagents for processing are not readily available on-site. Currently, two methods of shipment are widely used: samples are placed on dry ice or in specially constructed liquid nitrogen (LN) cryoshippers such as MVE vapor shippers (www.chartbiomed.com). The LN in the MVE shipper is absorbed into a specially designed foam liner. LN is released slowly to ensure that vapor-phase LN is present inside the shipping container. Samples can be kept at a consistent temperature of ≤−140°C for periods of 10 to 18 days, depending on the size of the shipper. Ongoing work is being done to evaluate the function of PBMC that are cryopreserved and shipped on dry ice (−70°C) and stored for long periods in LN, thus avoiding too many shifts in temperature. Moving PBMC up and down a temperature gradient may be detrimental to cell viability, recovery, and function. Relocating PBMC from LN (–180°C) to dry ice (−70°C) and back to LN may impair

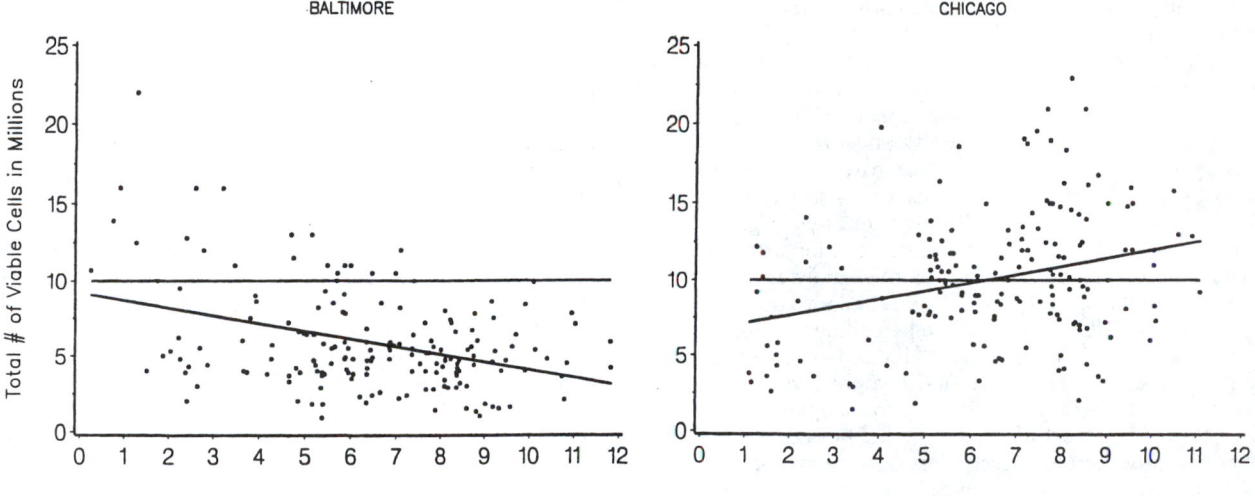

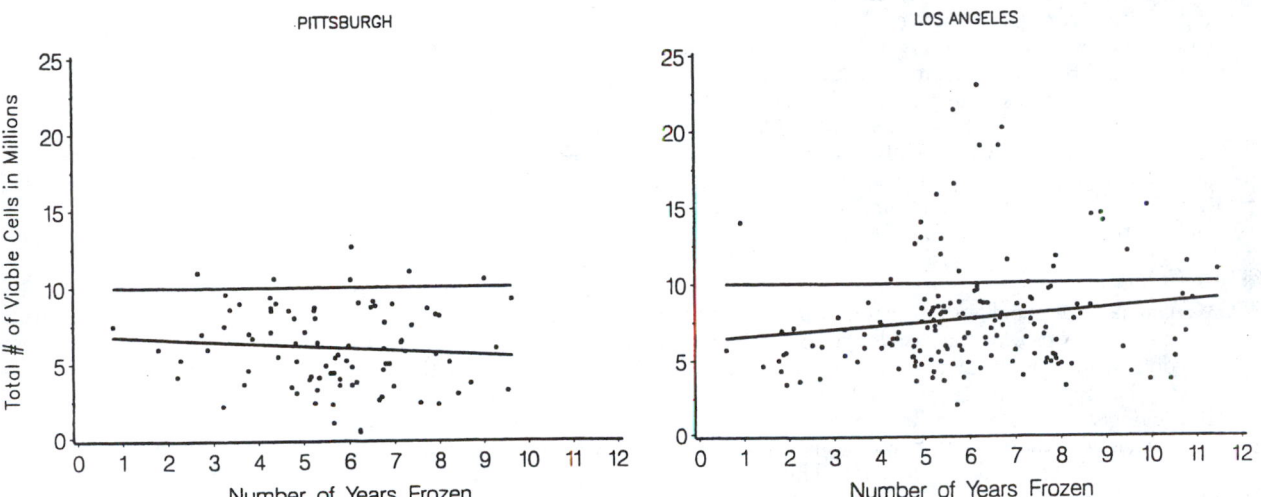

FIGURE 7 Viable cell recovery over time, indicated by center. Reference lines at 10^7 cells mark the original numbers of PBMC stored per vial. (Reproduced with permission from reference 28.)

PBMC function (J. H. Cox, L. Galley, et al., unpublished data). For the long-term storage of cells, the use of vapor-phase LN is the optimal method.

Summary of Critical Issues for Cryopreservation and Shipping of PBMC

To optimize and standardize cryopreservation and shipping that will yield functionally intact T cells, follow these guidelines:

- Use a slow freezing procedure to bring the temperature of the cells down to $\sim -140°C$.
- Nalgene "Mr. Frosty" or controlled-rate freezers provide optimal and comparable results.
- Store and ship cells in vapor-phase LN at $-140°C$ or lower.
- Avoid fluctuations in the temperature.
- Long-term storage should be done in vapor-phase LN or at temperatures below $-140°C$.

USE OF CRYOPRESERVED PBMC FOR CELLULAR IMMUNE ASSAYS

Provided that the viability, recovery, and functional integrity of PBMC are optimal, a comprehensive series of cellular immunoassays can be performed. The sections below describe our experience with individual assays and provide information regarding which assays can be performed with fresh and frozen PBMC. The results are collated from data collected over a 10-year period in our laboratories in both the United States and Thailand.

CD4 T-Cell Assay by LPA

For LPAs, well-cryopreserved PBMC can be used (43, 50, 55). In one of our studies, 141 HIV-1-infected individuals 18 to 60 years of age with CD4 counts of >400 cells/mm³ were enrolled in a double-blind placebo-controlled safety and efficacy therapeutic vaccine trial for HIV infection. Heparinized whole blood was collected prior to vaccination, and after Ficoll separation, PBMC were used for LPAs.

Proliferation assays were performed with fresh PBMC from patients whose clinical visits were at local cell-processing sites. PBMC collected at remote sites were cryopreserved and shipped to our laboratory, where they were assayed at a later date. The proliferative responses of PBMC from HIV-infected individuals to a range of concentrations of HIV-1 Env gp160, HIV-1 Gag p24, tetanus toxoid, diphtheria toxoid, *Candida albicans,* and mitogens were assessed. A positive response was defined as an SI of ≥5 for any antigen at any concentration. Although there were occasional statistically significant differences in comparative analyses (data not shown), results for fresh PBMC were similar to those for cryopreserved PBMC (Table 3). The percentages of responders to mitogens, recall antigens, and HIV antigens were consistent for comparisons of fresh and cryopreserved PBMC. In general, values obtained with frozen samples were lower than those obtained with fresh samples, but the percentages of antigen and mitogen responders were comparable.

In a very careful study by Schiller et al., the extent of T-cell proliferation in response to HIV-1 Gag antigen in fresh and cryopreserved PBMC from HIV-1-seropositive and -seronegative patients was examined (55). The inter-assay variation was very low, and regression analyses showed a strong positive correlation between the SIs obtained in assays in which two aliquots of cryopreserved PBMC each from six different HIV-1-infected subjects were tested. Generally, the SIs for fresh samples were higher than those for cryopreserved samples, and when a cutoff of 5 was used, 11 of 24 assays performed with fresh PBMC had an SI above the cutoff and 13 of 24 assays performed with cryopreserved PBMC had an SI above the cutoff. Similar results have been obtained in other laboratories (51, 61).

CD8 T-Cell Assays

CD8[+] T lymphocytes are able to mediate a variety of effector mechanisms and may provide the basis for protective immunity against a diverse array of infectious pathogens and tumors. For this reason, current vaccine strategies have been directed towards eliciting strong CD8[+] T-cell responses. The chromium release assay has been the assay of choice for many years for the evaluation of CD8[+] T-cell cytotoxicity. This technically demanding assay needs to be performed on fresh cells if the samples are from individuals receiving an HIV vaccine. It has been demonstrated by many laboratories, including ours, that the sensitivity and reproducibility of the assay are lost once the PBMC are frozen (9). Because of the complexity and difficulties associated with performing CTL assays, most institutions involved in vaccine trials no longer perform this assay, although the Walter Reed group and the U.S. HIV Vaccine Trials Network have deployed this assay at international sites with

optimal results (7, 24, 44, 58). In our experiences, the most difficult component of the chromium release assay is the importation and disposal of radioactive chromium. For a discussion of the use of CTL assays in vaccine trial settings, the previous edition of this manual and additional references should be consulted (8, 9, 35).

The ELISPOT assay can be used with fresh and cryopreserved specimens, and under ideal conditions, fresh and cryopreserved PBMC have been shown to have similar functional activities (12, 29, 39, 53, 57). ELISPOT and ICS assays are being standardized and compared across laboratories, and their performance characteristics are being established. As these assays become available and standardized, their usefulness for the detection of human immune responses in the field will become clearer (11). Since these assays all measure different aspects of the CD8[+] T-cell response, the correlations between vaccine efficacy, cytolytic effector function, the release of IFN-γ, and tetramer binding will need to be defined (15, 30, 33, 40, 45, 53, 62). A thorough review of methods for detecting CD8 T-lymphocyte function by ELISPOT, tetramer, and ICS assays is provided elsewhere in this volume (chapter 28). It should also be noted that major histocompatibility class II tetramers have now been developed and that they, along with intracellular cytokine assays, allow the ability to more directly measure CD4[+] T-cell responses in vitro.

EVALUATION OF CELLULAR IMMUNE RESPONSES IN DEVELOPING COUNTRIES

The advantages of conducting vaccine studies in the country of interest are numerous, with the most important being that the relevant population for vaccine or therapeutic intervention is being evaluated on-site. The influences of host genes, health and nutrition status, and disease burden of patients are taken into consideration by conducting studies in-country. The additional advantages of performing testing on-site are: (i) it avoids the problem of having to use cryopreserved samples if fresh samples provide better reproducibility and sensitivity, (ii) it avoids problems associated with shipping valuable samples, (iii) it facilitates the transfer of technologies and a build-up of human capacity and the physical infrastructure, (iv) it allows investigators from developing countries to test samples from their own country, (v) laboratories involved in such studies can train and employ staff from within their country, providing economic benefits and other incentives, and (vi) national health authorities can gain valuable experience by testing investigative phase I vaccine trials prior to commitments to larger intervention studies. Sophisticated cellular immunology studies can be done in developing countries, as exemplified

TABLE 3 Lymphoproliferative responses in fresh and cryopreserved PBMC from HIV-1-infected individuals

Antigen or mitogen	Concn range (μg/ml)	% responders (SI of >5)	
		Fresh PBMC (*n* = 76)	Cryopreserved PBMC (*n* = 65)
gp160 Env	0.4–6.2	34	32
p24 Gag	12.5–25	52	32
Phytohemagglutinin	0.5–2	100	100
Pokeweed mitogen	0.6–2.5	97	100
Concanavalin A	5–20	100	100
Tetanus toxoid	1.6–6.5[a]	75	73
Diphtheria toxoid	5.8–23[a]	70	56

[a] Concentration is given in limits of flocculation (L.f.).

by several recent vaccine trials conducted by us and other groups (16, 34, 44, 54).

T-cell responses elicited by vaccines may differ in geographically and genetically diverse populations as a result of variations in the distribution of T-cell subtypes and phenotypes, HLA types, disease burdens, antivaccine vector responses, and other iatrogenic factors. Listed below are some of the issues that may influence the elicitation of T-cell responses in diverse populations.

- Viral or parasite variation: vaccines may need to be tailored to circulating strains or variants present in the population (17, 47). Reagents for testing the immunogenicity of vaccines need to match the vaccine strains.
- Regional and tribal HLA types may influence responses to vaccines (25, 46).
- Vaccine-induced T-cell responses may be influenced by other host factors, such as the microbe burden, nutritional status, and host immunogenetic influences (1, 18, 38).

Other Considerations for Conducting Vaccine Trials in Developing Countries

Field studies and vaccine efficacy trials present a huge undertaking, both for sponsoring international agencies and for the developing countries involved. A thorough review of these issues is beyond the scope of this article, but the reader can refer to some excellent review articles (2, 14, 20, 31). In addition, it cannot be emphasized enough that consideration and respect are of paramount importance between the sponsoring country and the country in which the studies are being conducted. Possible issues to take into consideration may include the following:

- Confidentiality and ethical issues may arise.
- The blood volume that participants are willing to provide is often less than that expected for U.S. trials.
- Compliance issues are likely to be a problem when people have poor transportation options or come from remote areas.
- The ability to accurately convey the study rationale in a different language.
- Difficulties may exist in transporting samples from field sites to the central laboratory.
- Seasonal droughts and monsoons may significantly affect compliance.
- The use of isotopes for immunology assays poses problems for availability and disposal.

Obtaining Equipment and Supplies

The enormous cost of purchasing and shipping equipment to developing countries necessitates that careful consideration is given to setting up a new laboratory to ensure that compatible and reliable equipment is purchased. One of the greatest problems with conducting immunologic assays in developing countries is that the special equipment and reagents required for these tests are not routinely carried by the manufacturer's local agent. Local agents tend to carry supplies that are necessary for clinical assays, such as routine hematology. Hence, there is a need for careful planning for the acquisition of equipment and reagents. Since the first edition of this chapter was written, this issue has dramatically improved as more and more vaccine trials are being conducted overseas. Many biotechnology companies have deployed not only sales representatives but also technical representatives at overseas sites.

With respect to equipment, one must first consider the voltage employed by the country in which the equipment is to be used. Our experience in Thailand underscores the need to stress the voltage requirement (often more than once!) with equipment companies when ordering from the United States. While transformers may be an alternative for many pieces of small laboratory equipment such as microscopes, they generally lead to a poor performance of larger equipment such as centrifuges. The second major consideration is the continuity of the power supply, and a backup fuel generator is often essential for critical equipment. Protection against electrical power surges with uninterrupted power source regulators is a critical component for all pieces of equipment used in the field. The number of overseas representatives of laboratory equipment companies has increased over the last few years, but the cost of purchasing the equipment in-country is often higher due to customs duties. Many international groups have opted to purchase equipment at their headquarters and then ship it to the overseas laboratories. Although this is cheaper in the short term, it often voids the warranty for service in-country. Receiving equipment internationally can take up to 1 year from the date of purchasing. One should estimate at least a 1-year lag time before functional capabilities are in place. The ease of maintaining equipment is also an important consideration. While many scintillation counters are becoming more automated, this feature is useless in the field if there is no one in the country to service the equipment. Service engineers from Europe or the United States are likely to be required, with increased cost and time considerations. This is particularly pertinent to large equipment such as scintillation counters, where shipment of the equipment to the manufacturer for repair is not an option because it is too costly. In the event of scintillation counter failure, one has the advantage with the LPA of being able to freeze the plate due to the long half-life of tritiated thymidine. However, for CTL assays using ^{51}Cr, the short half-life of the isotope (<1 month) may preclude this step.

Equipment such as refrigerators with glass doors is particularly convenient for laboratory personnel, but in tropical countries, where the laboratory temperature tends to be marginally higher than those in the United States and Europe, this type of door puts extra work on the compressor, leading to a more rapid deterioration of the equipment. Similarly, if there is an electricity failure, which may result in laboratory temperatures of up to 35°C, the rate of heat loss from a glass-door-refrigerator is more rapid than that from a refrigerator with an insulated metal door, often reaching room temperature within 30 min. Low-temperature freezers (−70°C or less) generate a great deal of heat, thereby putting extra work on the compressors, and hence it is a good idea to consider a designated air-conditioned room for freezers. Provided that LN is readily available within the country, LN freezers are often a better means for storing PBMC than electric freezers, as maintenance is minimal. Given the high cost and unreliability of the supply of LN from commercial vendors in many developing countries, laboratories may wish to invest in their own LN plant. The storage capacity can be in excess of 100 liters, with the start-up time to full LN production being only 10 min. There are several commercial options for this process, including Stirling Cryogenics (www.stirling.nl). The plant requires a separate housing structure of approximately 3 by 3 m and can be installed with on-site operator training in 7 days.

In many developing countries, particularly those that rely heavily on imported materials, one must consider the time that equipment and reagents may be held in customs and excise prior to their release, as it may exceed 1 month.

Many of the problems with ordering equipment also pertain to the ordering of reagents. The ordering of reagents also has the additional constraint of expiration dates. Many reagents may have a long expiration date, but others, such as CD-Chex, a CD4$^+$ T-cell flow cytometry control reagent, do not. Hence, one may have to establish a link with a laboratory in the United States or Europe for shipments of these reagents. Additionally, the required storage temperature of the reagents must be considered. Appropriate shipping documents must be sent at the time of shipment to the laboratory to ensure that the customs department is notified about proper storage of the supplies in the event of a delay in processing.

The quality of water in the country in which the assays are to be conducted must be taken into consideration as well. While one may have the necessary filtration system, quality assurance of the water may be problematic if there is not a laboratory capable of conducting coliform counts and silicon testing of the water supply. Filters used in deionizing systems in developing countries typically need to be replaced sooner than those in the United States. Another point of concern is the adequate drainage of buildings in developing countries, so that high-volume sink drainage goes to a septic tank or sewer and not directly into the water table. While it is more costly to order premade media because of the requirement of greater refrigeration capabilities, this is the best choice for quality control and quality assurance issues.

Many cellular immunology assays require the use of radioactive materials. One must be cognizant of the procedures for handling radioactive materials in each developing country because the regulations concerning shipping, use, and disposal of these reagents may differ from those in developed countries.

In our experience, the best way to establish cellular immunology assay capability in the field is to have laboratory personnel from the sponsoring country conduct site visits to the country where laboratory infrastructures are being built. Visits need to be made to clinical and university laboratories to ascertain what equipment and reagents are in use, are serviceable, and are readily available on-site (with particular attention to the time intervals between ordering and receipt). The need to learn about rules and regulations concerning the use of radioactive isotopes is critical. In addition, sponsoring countries should allow personnel from the developing countries to train in their laboratory facilities, especially if they will be involved in the execution of cellular immunology assays. A period of no less than 3 months is recommended. A major dilemma faced by investigators from one country operating in another is at what point national laboratory guidelines from the vaccine trial support country should be implemented. These questions can only be answered by dialogues with those who will conduct the assays and representatives from the necessary local regulatory agencies.

Summary of Equipment and Supply Requirement Issues

- Customs duty and tax fees in addition to shipping fees for equipment and supplies are likely to be imposed.
- Permits are required for shipping infectious materials internationally (International Air Transportation Association [www.IATA.org]).
- Refrigerators, freezers, and incubators may have problems with maintaining temperatures where the ambient temperature often exceeds 25°C.
- Problems are likely to be encountered with equipment service contracts and general equipment maintenance.
- For local purchases, a petty cash account in-country should be established.
- Special requirements for the power and voltage supply to laboratory equipment must be considered.
- Backup power and voltage regulators are usually necessary.
- Water quality and water sanitation and drainage issues are important.
- Laboratory safety (chemical, biological, and radiological) standards need to be set to the same level as those in developed countries.

This chapter is dedicated to all the laboratory research assistants and their supervisors who have labored over thousands of CTL, ELISPOT, LPA, and ICS assays in support of HIV vaccine development and to the volunteers who have donated time and specimens to the cause of HIV vaccine development.

The opinions or assertions contained herein are the private views of the author and are not to be construed as official or as reflecting true views of the Department of the Army or the Department of Defense.

REFERENCES

1. **Ahmed, R. K., G. Biberfeld, and R. Thorstensson.** 2005. Innate immunity in experimental SIV infection and vaccination. *Mol. Immunol.* **42:**251–258.
2. **Aidoo, I., and I. Udhayakumar.** 2000. Field studies of cytotoxic T lymphocytes in malaria infections: implications for malaria vaccine development. *Parasitol. Today* **16:**50–56.
3. **Berzofsky, J. A., J. D. Ahlers, J. Janik, J. Morris, S. Oh, M. Terabe, and I. M. Belyakov.** 2004. Progress on new vaccine strategies against chronic viral infections. *J. Clin. Investig.* **114:**450–462.
4. **Betensky, R. A., E. Connick, J. Devers, A. Landav, M. Nokta, S. Plaeger, H. Rosenblatt, J. L. Schmitz, F. Valentine, D. Wara, A. Weinberg, and H. M. Lederman.** 2000. Shipment impairs lymphocyte proliferative responses to microbial antigens. *Clin. Diagn. Lab. Immunol.* **7:**759–763.
5. **Blattman, J. N., and P. D. Greenberg.** 2004. Cancer immunotherapy: a treatment for the masses. *Science* **305:**200–205.
6. **Boyum, A.** 1968. Isolation of mononuclear cells and granulocytes from human blood. *Scand. J. Clin. Lab. Investig.* **21:**77–89.
7. **Cao, H., P. Kaleebu, D. Hom, J. Flores, D. Agrawal, et al.** 2003. Immunogenicity of a recombinant human immunodeficiency virus (HIV)-canarypox vaccine in HIV-seronegative Ugandan volunteers: results of the HIV Network for Prevention Trials 007 Vaccine Study. *J. Infect. Dis.* **187:** 887–895.
8. **Carruth, L., T. Greten, C. Murray, M. Castro, S. Crone, W. Pavlat, J. Schneck, and R. Siliciano.** 1999. An algorithm for evaluating human cytotoxic T lymphocyte responses to candidate AIDS vaccines. *AIDS Res. Hum. Retrovir.* **15:**1021–1034.
9. **Cox, J., M. deSouza, S. Ratto-Kim, G. Ferrari, K. Weinhold, and D. Birx.** 2002. Accomplishing cellular immune assays for evaluation of vaccine efficacy in developing countries; p. 301–315. *In* N. R. Rose, R. G. Hamilton, and B. Detrick, (ed.), *Manual of Clinical Laboratory Immunology,* 6th ed. ASM Press, Washington, D.C.
10. **Cox, J. H., G. Ferrari, R. T. Bailer, and R. A. Koup.** 2004. Automating procedures for processing, cryopreservation, storage and manipulation of human peripheral blood mononuclear cells. *J. Assoc. Lab. Automat.* **9:**16–23.
11. **Cox, J. H., G. Ferrari, S. Kalams, W. Lopaczynski, N. Oden, M. P. D'Souza, and ECS Group.** 2005. Results

of an ELISPOT proficiency panel conducted in 11 laboratories participating in international human immunodeficiency virus type 1 vaccine trials. *AIDS Res. Hum. Retrovir.* **21**:68–81.

12. **Currier, J., E. Kuta, E. Turk, L. Earhart, L. Loomis-Price, S. Janetzki, G. Ferrari, D. Birx, and J. Cox.** 2002. A panel of MHC class I restricted viral peptides for use as a quality control for vaccine trial ELISPOT assays. *J. Immunol. Methods* **260**:157–172.

13. **Esser, M. T., R. D. Marchese, L. S. Kierstead, L. G. Tussey, F. Wang, N. Chirmule, and M. W. Washabaugh.** 2003. Memory T cells and vaccines. *Vaccine* **21**:419–430.

14. **Excler, J. L., and C. Beyrer.** 2000. HIV vaccine development in developing countries. Are efficacy trials feasible? *J. Hum. Virol.* **3**:193–214.

15. **Flanagan, K., E. Lee, M. Gravenor, W. Reece, B. Urban, T. Doherty, K. Bojang, M. Pinder, A. Hill, and M. Plebanski.** 2001. Unique T cell effector functions elicited by Plasmodium falciparum epitopes in malaria-exposed Africans tested by three T cell assays. *J. Immunol.* **167**:4729–4737.

16. **Garber, D. A., G. Silvestri, and M. B. Feinberg.** 2004. Prospects for an AIDS vaccine: three big questions, no easy answers. *Lancet Infect. Dis.* **4**:397–412.

17. **Gaschen, B., J. Taylor, K. Yusim, B. Foley, F. Gao, D. Lang, V. Noritsky, B. Haynes, B. H. Hahn, T. Bhattacharya, and B. Korber.** 2002. Diversity considerations in HIV-1 vaccine selection. *Science* **296**:2354–2360.

18. **Gonzalez, E., H. Kulkarni, H. Bolivar, A. Mangano, R. Sanchez, G. Catano, R. J. Nibbs, B. I. Freeman, M. P. Quinones, M. J. Bamshad, K. K. Murthy, B. H. Rovin, W. Bradley, R. A. Clark, S. A. Anderson, R. J. O'Connell, B. K. Agon, S. S. Ahuja, R. Bologna, L. Sen, M. J. Dolan, and S. K. Ahuja.** 2005. The influence of CCL3L1 gene-containing segmental duplications on HIV-1/AIDS susceptibility. *Science* **307**:1434–1440.

19. **Gratama, J. W., and F. Kern.** 2004. Flow cytometric enumeration of antigen-specific T lymphocytes. *Cytometry* **58A**:79–86.

20. **Halloran, M., R. Anderson, R. Azevedo-Neto, W. Bellini, O. Branch, M. Burke, M. Compans, K. Day, L. Gooding, S. Gupta, J. Katz, O. Kew, H. Keyserling, R. Krause, A. Lal, E. Massad, A. McLean, P. Rosa, P. Rota, P. Wiener, S. Wynn, and D. Zanetla.** 1998. Population biology, evolution, and immunology of vaccination and vaccination programs. *Am. J. Med. Sci.* **315**:76–86.

21. **Hamilton, R.** 1994. The clinical immunology laboratory of the future. *Clin. Chem.* **40**:2186–2192.

22. **Hickling, J.** 1998. Measuring human T-lymphocyte function. *Exp. Rev. Mol. Med.* [Online.] www.ermm.cbcu.cam.ac.uk/.

23. **Jordan, W.** 2002. The Jordan Report 20th Anniversary. Accelerated development of vaccines. National Institute of Allergy and Infectious Diseases, Bethesda, Md. [Online.] http://www.niaid.nih.gov/dmid/vaccines/jordan20/.

24. **Kantakamalakul, W., J. Cox, U. Kositanont, S. Siritantikorn, K. Limbach, D. L. Birx, P. Thongcharoen, and P. Puthavathana.** 2001. CTL responses to vaccinia virus antigens but not HIV-1 subtype E envelope protein seen in HIV-1 seronegative Thais. *Asian Pac. J. Allergy Immunol.* **19**:17–22.

25. **Kaslow, R. A., C. Rivers, J. Tang, T. J. Bender, P. A. Goepfert, R. El Habib, K. Weinhold, and M. J. Mulligan.** 2001. Polymorphisms in HLA class I genes associated with both favorable prognosis of human immunodeficiency virus (HIV) type 1 infection and positive cytotoxic T-lymphocyte responses to ALVAC-HIV recombinant canarypox vaccines. *J. Virol.* **75**:8681–8689.

26. **Kaufmann, S. H.** 2002. Protection against tuberculosis: cytokines, T cells, and macrophages. *Ann. Rheum. Dis.* **61** (Suppl. 2):54–58.

27. **Klausner, R. D., A. S. Fauci, L. Corey, G. J. Nabel, H. Gayle.** 2003. The need for a global HIV vaccine enterprise. *Science* **300**:2036–2039.

28. **Kleeberger, C., R. Lyles, J. Margolick, C. Rinaldo, J. Phair, and J. Giorgi.** 1999. Viability and recovery of peripheral blood mononuclear cells cryopreserved for up to 12 years in a multicenter study. *Clin. Diagn. Lab. Immunol.* **6**:14–19.

29. **Kreher, C. R., M. T. Dittrich, R. Guerkov, B. O. Boehm, and M. Tary-Lehmann.** 2003. CD4+ and CD8+ cells in cryopreserved human PBMC maintain full functionality in cytokine ELISPOT assays. *J. Immunol. Methods* **278**:79–93.

30. **Lieberman, J.** 2004. Tracking the killers: how should we measure CD8 T cells in HIV infection? *AIDS* **18**:1489–1493.

31. **Mahoney, R., and J. Maynard.** 1999. The introduction of new vaccines into developing countries. *Vaccine* **17**:646–652.

32. **Maino, V. C., and H. T. Maecker.** 2004. Cytokine flow cytometry: a multiparametric approach for assessing cellular immune responses to viral antigens. *Clin. Immunol.* **110**:222–231.

33. **Mashishi, T., and C. M. Gray.** 2002. The ELISPOT assay: an easily transferable method for measuring cellular responses and identifying T cell epitopes. *Clin. Chem. Lab. Med.* **40**:1–7.

34. **McConkey, S., W. Reece, V. Moorthy, D. Webster, S. Dunachie, et al.** 2003. Enhanced T-cell immunogenicity of plasmid DNA vaccines boosted by recombinant modified vaccinia virus Ankara in humans. *Nat. Med.* **9**:729–735.

35. **McElrath, M., R. Siliciano, and K. Weinhold.** 1997. HIV type 1 vaccine-induced cytotoxic T cell responses in phase I clinical trials: detection, characterization, and quantitation. *AIDS Res. Hum. Retrovir.* **13**:211–216.

36. **McMichael, A., and T. Hanke.** 2002. The quest for an AIDS vaccine; is the CD8+ T-cell approach feasible? *Nat. Immunol.* **2**:283–291.

37. **McMichael, A., and T. Hanke.** 2003. HIV vaccines 1983–2003. *Nat. Med.* **9**:874–880.

38. **McNicholl, J. M., M. V. Downer, V. Udhayakumar, C. A. Alper, and D. L. Swerdlow.** 2000. Host-pathogen interactions in emerging and re-emerging infectious diseases: a genomic perspective of tuberculosis, malaria, human immunodeficiency virus infection, hepatitis B, and cholera. *Annu. Rev. Public Health* **21**:15–46.

39. **Mwau, M., I. Cebere, J. Sutton, P. Chikoti, N. Winstone, et al.** 2004. A human immunodeficiency virus 1 (HIV-1) clade A vaccine in clinical trials: stimulation of HIV-specific T-cell responses by DNA and recombinant modified vaccinia virus Ankara (MVA) vaccines in humans. *J. Gen. Virol.* **85**:911–919.

40. **Mwau, M., A. McMichael, and T. Hanke.** 2002. Design and validation of an enzyme-linked immunospot assay for use in clinical trials of candidate HIV vaccines. *AIDS Res. Hum. Retrovir.* **18**:611–618.

41. **Nakamura, R., and D. Bylund.** 1994. Factors influencing changes in the clinical immunology laboratory. *Clin. Chem.* **40**:2193–2204.

42. **Nicholson, J., B. M. Jones, G. Cross, and J. McDougal.** 1984. Comparison of T and B cell analyses on fresh and aged blood. *J. Immunol.* **73**:29–40.

43. **Nitayaphan, S., C. Khamboonruang, N. Sirisophana, P. Morgan, J. Chiu, A. Duliege, C. Chuenchitra, T. Supapongse, K. Rungruengthanakit, M. deSouza, J. Mascola, K. Boggio, S. Ratto-Kim, L. Markowitz, D. Birx, V. Suriyanon, J. McNeil, A. Brown, and R. Michael.** 2000. A phase I/II trial of HIV SF2 gp120/MF59 vaccine in seronegative Thais. *Vaccine* **18**:1448–1455.

44. **Nitayaphan, S., P. Pitisuttithum, C. Karnasuta, C. Eamsila, M. de Souza, et al.** 2004. Safety and immunogenicity of an

HIV subtype B and E prime-boost vaccine combination in HIV-negative Thai adults. *J. Infect. Dis.* **190:**702–706.

45. **Pantaleo, G., and R. A. Koup.** 2004. Correlates of immune protection in HIV-1 infection: what we know, what don't know and what we should know. *Nat. Med.* **10:**806–810.

46. **Paris, R., S. Bejrachandra, C. Karnasuta, D. Chandanayingyong, W. Kunachiwa, et al.** 2004. HLA class I serotypes and cytotoxic T-lymphocyte responses among human immunodeficiency virus-1-uninfected Thai volunteers immunized with ALVAC-HIV in combination with monomeric gp120 or oligomeric gp160 protein boosting. *Tissue Antigens* **64:**251–256.

47. **Peeters, M., C. Toure-Kane, and J. N. Nkengasong.** 2003. Genetic diversity of HIV in Africa: impact on diagnosis, treatment, vaccine development and trials. *AIDS* **17:**2547–2560.

48. **Perfetto, S. P., P. K. Chattopadhyay, and M. Roederer.** 2004. Seventeen-colour flow cytometry: unravelling the immune system. *Nat. Rev. Immunol.* **4:**648–655.

49. **Plotkin, S.** 2003. Vaccines, vaccination, and vaccinology. *J. Infect. Dis.* **187:**1349–1359.

50. **Ratto-Kim, S., K. Sitz, R. Garner, J. Kim, C. Davis, N. Aronson, N. Ruiz, K. Tencer, R. Rodfield, and D. Birx.** 1999. Repeated immunization with recombinant gp160 human immunodeficiency virus (HIV) envelope protein in early HIV-1 infection: evaluation of the T cell proliferative response. *J. Infect. Dis.* **179:**337–344.

51. **Reimann, K., M. Chernoff, C. Wilkening, C. Nickerson, and A. Landay.** 2000. Preservation of lymphocyte immunophenotype and proliferative responses in cryopreserved peripheral blood mononuclear cells from human immunodeficiency virus type 1-infected donors: implications for multicenter clinical trials. The ACTG Immunology Advanced Technology Laboratories. *Clin. Diagn. Lab. Immunol.* **7:**352–359.

52. **Robinson, H.** 2002. New hope for an AIDS vaccine. *Nat. Rev. Immunol.* **2:**239–250.

53. **Russell, N. D., M. G. Hudgens, R. Ha, C. Havenar-Daughton, and M. J. McElrath.** 2003. Moving to HIV-1 vaccine efficacy trials: defining T cell responses as potential correlates of immunity. *J. Infect. Dis.* **187:**226–242.

54. **Sandstrom, E., and D. Birx.** 2002. HIV vaccine trials in Africa. *AIDS* **16:**S89–S95.

55. **Schiller, D., J. Binley, K. Roux, C. Adamson, I. Jones, H. Krausslich, A. Hurley, M. Markowitz, and J. Moore.** 2000. Parameters influencing measurement of the Gag antigen-specific T-proliferative response to HIV type 1 infection. *AIDS Res. Hum. Retrovir.* **16:**259–271.

56. **Shearer, G., and M. Clerici.** 1994. In vitro analysis of cell-mediated immunity: clinical relevance. *Clin. Chem.* **40:**2162–2165.

57. **Smith, J. G., X. Liu, R. M. Kaufhold, J. Clair, and M. J. Caulfield.** 2001. Development and validation of a gamma interferon ELISPOT assay for quantitation of cellular immune responses to varicella zoster virus. *Clin. Diagn. Lab. Immunol.* **8:**871–879.

58. **Spearman, P.** 2003. HIV vaccine development: lessons from the past and promise for the future. *Curr. HIV Res.* **1:**101–120.

59. **Venkataraman, M., and M. Westerman.** 1986. Susceptibility of human T cells, T-cell subsets, and B cells to cryopreservation. *Cryobiology* **23:**199–208.

60. **Weinberg, A.** 2005. Cryopreservation of peripheral blood mononuclear cells, p. 220–223. *In* N. R. Rose, R. G. Hamilton, and B. Detrich (ed.), *Manual of Clinical Laboratory Immunology*, 6th ed. ASM Press, Washington, D.C.

61. **Weinberg, A., R. Betensky, L. Zhang, and G. Ray.** 1998. Effect of shipment, storage, anticoagulant, and cell separation on lymphocyte proliferation assays for human immunodeficiency virus-infected patients. *Clin. Diagn. Lab. Immunol.* **5:**804–807.

62. **Whiteside, T. L., Y. Zhao, T. Tsukishiro, E. M. Elder, W. Gooding, and J. Baar.** 2003. Enzyme-linked immunospot, cytokine flow cytometry, and tetramers in the detection of T-cell responses to a dendritic cell-based multipeptide vaccine in patients with melanoma. *Clin. Cancer Res.* **9:**641–649.

T-Lymphocyte Activation and Cell Signaling

JEFFREY R. CURRIER

36

The early consequences of T-cell activation are a succession of intracellular biochemical events resulting in a tyrosine kinase cascade, phosphorylation of linker proteins, assembly of the signalosome, cytoskeletal reorganization, formation of the immunological synapse, activation of transcription factors, and rapid expression of new cell surface molecules. Measurement of these events can be used to assess a number of clinically relevant parameters, such as the current state of immune competence, the presence and number of activated T cells, and the capacity for antigen-specific and antigen-nonspecific responsiveness. T-cell activation is a prerequisite for all subsequent functional activities of T cells (e.g., cytokine production and proliferation and target cell cytolysis) and hence can be indirectly assessed by many methods covered elsewhere in this manual (see other chapters in section E). This chapter focuses upon methods that measure early events associated directly with T-cell activation. Historically, the presence in tissue or body fluids of T cells with various activated phenotypes has been used as a clinical correlate of progression of many autoimmune and infectious diseases. Activation of T cells directly ex vivo in an antigen-independent or antigen-dependent manner also has important clinical applications. Typically, antigen-independent activation of T cells ex vivo is performed to assess the current state of immunocompetence as a result of either immunosuppressive therapy, possession of a genetically linked immunodeficiency, or the presence of an infectious agent. Antigen-dependent (or antigen-specific) activation of T cells can be used to demonstrate either that a patient's T cells and antigen-presenting cells (APCs) are capable of acting in concert to initiate an immune response or that prior sensitization to a specific antigen has occurred. The initiation of T-cell activation is brought about by a remarkably complex cell-cell interaction between a T cell and an APC. Central to this interaction is the T-cell receptor (TCR), which binds to major histocompatibility complex (MHC) molecules and short peptide antigens on the surface of the APC. The interaction of a large number of accessory, adhesion, and costimulatory molecules contributes to T-cell activation by formation of the "immunological synapse" which increases the avidity of the TCR-MHC interaction and initiates independent signal transduction events (15, 20, 27). A review of the signaling events associated with T-cell activation is presented here. To present a sufficiently broad overview, the details of each aspect of T-cell signaling are necessarily limited; however, for

greater detail the reader is referred to comprehensive reviews cited throughout the text.

TCR STRUCTURE AND RECOGNITION

The TCR is a multisubunit complex composed of six different polypeptide chains: α, β, γ, δ, ε, and ζ. The TCR α and β chains form a disulfide-linked heterodimer and confer the specificity of ligand binding. By virtue of genetic rearrangement, germ line-encoded Vα, Jα, and Cα and Vβ, Dβ, Jβ, and Cβ segments recombine to form millions of TCR αβ variants, each with different molecular specificities (16). Crystal structure analysis has confirmed that the molecular specificity of the TCR is conferred by the solvent-exposed membrane-distal variable regions of the α and β chains (19). The ligand for this receptor is a complex of short peptide antigens (generated by intracellular processing of self-proteins or foreign pathogens), bound noncovalently to class I or class II MHC molecules on the surface of an APC (43). The noncovalently associated subunits of the TCR complex are the monomorphic γ, δ, ε, and ζ chains (formally designated CD3). The TCR ζ chain exists predominantly as a ζζ homodimer, but in some cases ζ and its splice variant η exist in the TCR complex as a ζη heterodimer. An important characteristic of the TCR complex is that it links the exquisite specificity of the polymorphic TCR αβ heterodimer with transmembrane signal transduction mediated by the cytoplasmic domains of the invariant CD3 subunits and the TCR γ, δ, ε, and ζ chains (2, 5, 31).

TYROSINE KINASE CASCADE AND PHOSPHORYLATION OF LINKER PROTEINS

Ligation of the TCR complex to its cognate peptide-MHC counterpart or with particular anti-CD3 monoclonal antibodies (MAbs) initiates the process of T-cell activation and delivers the primary signal for the activation of resting T cells. The earliest biochemical events elicited by T-cell activation are the phosphorylation of proteins in the TCR-CD3 complex and the activation and interaction of Syk and Src family protein tyrosine kinases (PTKs) (8, 44). Within seconds of TCR stimulation the cytoplasmic tails of the TCR and CD3 γ, δ, ε, and ζ chains are phosphorylated on specific immunoreceptor tyrosine-based activation motifs (ITAMs) by the CD4 or CD8 coreceptor-associated Src family kinase

Lck. A highly ordered sequential phosphorylation of six tyrosines of the TCR ζ ITAMs is dependent upon the strength of TCR occupancy. Recruitment of a Syk family kinase (most notably ZAP-70 and Syk itself) to this complex by the interaction of its Src homology 2 domain with the phosphorylated TCR ζ and CD3 chains results in its transphosphorylation by Lck (24). The multiple-tyrosine-phosphorylated ZAP-70/Syk family has a crucial role in TCR activation. Self-phosphorylated ZAP-70 serves as a scaffold for recruiting positive and negative regulators of TCR signaling such as α-tubulin, Sam-68, Vav-1, VHR, Shc, Grb-2, LAT, and SLP-76 (23, 24). The last two adapter proteins play a pivotal role in TCR signaling, as they serve as nucleation points for higher-order macromolecular structures referred to as the signalosome (9, 28). Once phosphorylated by Syk kinases, LAT and SLP-76 participate in coupling the TCR to Ca^{2+} mobilization, Ras-signaling pathways, and NFAT-dependent interleukin-2 (IL-2) production. Importantly, LAT is palmitoylated, which targets it (and the molecules it recruits) to glycolipid-enriched microdomains known as lipid rafts. Recruitment of the tyrosine-phosphorylated TCR to lipid rafts is a critical step in T-cell activation and presumably concentrates the downstream signaling machinery in close proximity, facilitating enzymatic activity and molecular scaffold formation (18, 28). Redistribution of the TCR to lipid rafts also sequesters negative regulatory phosphatases away from the TCR (22). The selective disruption of lipid rafts results in attenuation of activation and signal transduction in T cells, further underscoring their importance.

SECONDARY MESSENGER MOBILIZATION

The net result of this tyrosine phosphorylation cascade is the activation of the key enzyme phospholipase C-γ1 (PLC-γ1) and the formation of complexes containing the Src homology 3-binding adapter proteins LAT, Grb2, Sos, SLP-76, and Vav complex (24). Once recruited to the lipid rafts of the plasma membrane, PLC-γ1 cleaves membrane phospholipids and releases the intracellular second messengers inositol 1,4,5-triphosphate (IP$_3$) and diacylglycerol (DAG) (4, 26). IP$_3$ has the critical role of regulating the transient mobilization of intracellular calcium ([Ca^{2+}]$_i$) stores from the endoplasmic reticulum. This early [Ca^{2+}]$_i$ flux is short-lived (on the order of several minutes only) and requires an additional trans-membrane Ca^{2+} flux from outside the cell to inside to maintain the persistence required for IL-2 gene transcription (37). This effect can be directly mimicked in vitro by the calcium ionophore ionomycin. DAG activates the proto-oncogene Ras via its direct interaction with one of the protein kinase C (PKC) family kinases. In concert with several adapter proteins (such as Shc, Grb-2, Sos, SLP-76, and Vav) which are activated or recruited by the Syk kinases and LAT, the activation of Ras by PKC then results in downstream activation of the serine-threonine kinase pathway (39). This key enzyme cascade in turn directly regulates key nuclear events involved in gene transcription and T-cell growth. The stimulation of T cells in vitro with phorbol esters (e.g., phorbol myristate acetate [PMA]) induces the rapid activation of both PKC and Ras. The transmission of signals from Ras and PKC to the nucleus involves the regulation of the ubiquitous mitogen-activated protein (MAP) kinase pathway (9, 24, 39). The concerted activity of both PMA and ionomycin can therefore imitate many of the early molecular consequences of TCR-dependent T-cell activation.

A second important pathway involving inositol lipid metabolism occurs immediately after TCR engagement. The enzyme phosphatidylinositol-3-hydroxyl kinase (PI3K) is weakly activated when the TCR alone is stimulated, but optimal activation occurs only when TCR and the costimulatory molecule CD28 are both triggered. CD28 regulation of PI3K depends upon its recruitment to the plasma membrane via interaction with the tyrosine-phosphorylated cytoplasmic domain of CD28. All of the downstream targets of phospho-inositides generated by PI3K are not yet well defined; however, they include members of the Tec/Itk PTK family (29). The pleckstrin homology domains of the Tec/Itk family and several important serine-threonine kinases can bind the products of PI3K. The binding of the products of PI3K to pleckstrin homology domains couples cell surface receptors to a diverse array of signal transduction pathways (41).

As a consequence of the early signal transduction events discussed above, many biochemical and physiological changes occur in activated T cells. Most of the biochemical events that occur in T cells immediately following activation are shared with many other cell types in response to external stimuli. These events include the activation of kinases and initiation of signaling cascades (as discussed above), changes in cytoplasmic pH, ion flux, and changes in cyclic nucleotide levels. An increase in cellular pH has been observed in T-cell lines following mitogenic activation and is presumably mediated by the plasma membrane Na$^+$/H$^+$ antiporter in response to inositol phosphate hydrolysis. Transient fluxes in cyclic nucleotides (cyclic AMP and cyclic GMP) have also been observed in mitogen-activated T cells. The specific role, if any, of cyclic nucleotides in T-cell activation is not yet defined; however, their role in regulating a variety of cellular functions in many cell types is well documented.

T cells, like many cell types, have an electrochemical gradient across their plasma membrane. The transient hyperpolarization and depolarization of this gradient have been observed immediately following T-cell activation and include the transport of Na$^+$, K$^+$, Cl$^-$, and Ca^{2+} ions. The measurement of [Ca^{2+}]$_i$ flux is significant for assessing T-cell activation because of its central role in the initiation of IL-2 gene transcription, an event specific to activated T cells. As discussed earlier, the intracellular second messenger IP$_3$ accounts for the transient increase in [Ca^{2+}]$_i$ (first minutes of T-cell activation), but sustained increases in [Ca^{2+}]$_i$ (typically several hours after initial T-cell activation) require a transmembrane flux from outside the cell. This is provided by a non-voltage-gated Ca^{2+} transmembrane channel that opens when intracellular stores are depleted and closes when they are replenished. The functional consequences of increased [Ca^{2+}]$_i$ flux include polarization of the cytoskeleton and cooperation with Ras and MAP kinase pathways for the activation of IL-2 gene transcription. The calcium phosphatase calcineurin is an essential link in the synergized activities of [Ca^{2+}]$_i$ flux and the MAP kinase pathways. Critically, calcineurin is the target of the immunosuppressive drugs cyclosporine and FK506. These drugs form a complex with cytosolic calcineurin and inhibit calcium-mediated signal pathways in T cells.

The ability to conveniently measure [Ca^{2+}]$_i$ flux in ex vivo mitogen-activated T cells allows for rapid assessment of the overall state of a patient's T-cell competence. For the activation of naive T cells to occur there is a formal requirement for a second, or costimulatory, signal in addition to the TCR-derived signal. In most instances this signal is delivered via the CD28 molecule on the surface of the T cell upon interaction with either of its ligands, the B7-1 and B7-2 molecules, on the surface of professional APCs (1). The biochemical mechanism by which CD28 transduces its signal remains ill defined, but its cytoplasmic tail alone is sufficient to mediate the signals required for costimulating IL-2 gene transcription. Memory T cells, or T cells that have been previously activated in vivo, have a less stringent requirement for functional activation but in general still require a second signal. This signal may be delivered either via a soluble factor such as a cytokine or by a cell surface molecule on the APC. The absence of a costimulatory signal in conjunction with a TCR-derived signal leads to a nonfunctional, or anergic, state in the target T cell. The function of costimulation in the priming phase of an immune response is presumably to ensure that antigenic peptides that are recognized are nonself peptides presented only by professional APCs (3).

Activation of T cells may also be accomplished independently of the TCR and CD28. Cross-linking the CD2 surface molecules of T cells with specific antibody pairs can initiate a signaling cascade and induce cytokine production, cytolytic activity, and proliferation. CD2 is a cell surface glycoprotein expressed on all mature peripheral T cells in humans (46). The natural ligand for CD2 is CD58 (LFA-3), which is expressed on many cell types, including APCs. The interaction of CD2 and CD58 regulates the response of T cells to antigen and augments cytokine production and proliferation. In common with the TCR activation pathway, CD2 cross-linking activation requires the presence of a functional CD3ζ chain. CD2 has a unique mechanism of engagement of intracellular machinery based on proline-rich motifs which bypasses members of the ZAP-70/Syk family, which are not phosphorylated by this mode of activation (40). CD2 can substitute for CD28 as a costimulatory molecule for inducing many functions of T cells, including cytokine synthesis, cell proliferation, and target cell recognition.

CYTOSKELETAL REORGANIZATION AND CONSEQUENCES OF EARLY SIGNAL TRANSDUCTION EVENTS

Subsequent to and in some cases concomitant with the immediate biochemical consequences of T-cell activation, many specialized cellular responses occur. The reorientation and redistribution of the cytoskeleton constitute an important consequence of T-cell activation, since they are closely linked to functional outcome. As discussed earlier, the phosphorylation of TCR ITAMs following TCR engagement serves as a focal point for cytoskeletal reorientation and formation of the microtubule-organizing center (13, 17, 33). This new layer of complexity in TCR signaling has been termed the immunological synapse or supramolecular activation complex (14, 25, 33, 42). During an antigen-dependent response a rapid accumulation of actin cytoskeletal proteins occurs at the interface of the APC–T-cell interaction. The potential functional consequence of microtubule-organizing center reorientation is to properly orient and localize T-cell responses. In the case of helper T cells, newly synthesized cytokines would be delivered toward the relevant APC, and in the case of cytotoxic T cells this would result in the focused secretion of prepackaged cytolytic granule constituents towards the target cell. Activation of the cytolytic mechanism is also dependent upon $[Ca^{2+}]_i$ flux, and as with cytokine gene transcription it can be mimicked by the synergized activity of PMA and ionomycin.

Gene activation and transcription are a common response to receptor-mediated signal transduction in many cell types. Following T-cell activation a specific set of responsive genes becomes transcriptionally active. This subset includes both newly synthesized genes and genes that are already expressed but are now up-regulated and expressed at higher concentrations. The immediate-early response genes represent the first wave of T-cell activation-induced genes, and their activation may be detected within minutes of receiving an appropriate stimulus. The immediate-early response genes do not rely upon protein synthesis for expression; however, many later response genes do rely upon protein synthesis for their activation. In fact, many of the early response genes are transcription factors for late response genes which mediate complex cellular functions such as the progression to the cell cycle (e.g., T-cell proliferation) and acquisition of differentiated functions (e.g., memory cells with polarized cytokine production profiles). As far as the practical measurement of early T-cell activation is concerned, the most important response genes are cell surface receptors. Receptors of various functions appear on the surface of activated T cells at different times and in different concentrations. The kinetics of expression may vary from within minutes to hours and even days after activation, indicating that different mechanisms of transcriptional regulation are operative. The kinds of T-cell surface receptors up-regulated upon activation include adhesion molecules, accessory molecules for modifying immune responses, cytokine receptors, nutrient receptors, and many molecules with still-undefined functions. In addition, new antigenic epitopes may be revealed on existing cell surface molecules, indicating that translational and posttranslational regulation of protein expression is also modified upon T-cell activation.

MEASUREMENT OF T-CELL ACTIVATION IN CLINICAL APPLICATIONS

The development, activation, and normal function of T cells are all dependent on the ability to signal properly through TCR, to transmit such signals, and to respond appropriately to these signals. The importance of each of these outcomes, particularly with respect to its clinical relevance and practicality of measurement, will now be discussed. Genetic defects affecting expression of important surface receptors or any of the signaling pathways may be manifested as one of the many different forms of inherited immunodeficiency (11, 38). Signaling defects in T cells may also be associated with malignancy; however, these are often manifestations of the negative effects of tumors on the host immune system (45). Immunodeficiency may also be acquired transiently as the result of an immunosuppressive therapy (e.g., cyclosporine) or as the long-term consequence of infectious disease (e.g., AIDS resulting from human immunodeficiency virus type 1 [HIV-1] infection). Assessment of inherited immunodeficiency can be performed by in vitro antigen-independent T-cell activation using surface receptor-specific MAbs or pharmacological agents which mimic T-cell activation (e.g., PMA and ionomycin) and by measuring calcium flux and/or surface receptor up-regulation. A lack of calcium flux would indicate a defect in early signal transduction, while normal calcium flux and decreased up-regulation of surface receptor expression would indicate a downstream defect in receptor signaling.

Defects affecting the termination of T-cell activation and growth may result in systemic autoimmune disease. Measurement of the activation status of T cells isolated directly from peripheral blood can give an indication of the presence of systemic autoimmune disease. The chronic expression of early or late activation markers can be conveniently measured with minimal handling required. Localized autoimmune diseases may be assessed with either peripheral T cells or cells biopsied from the site of inflammation.

The subsequent antigen-dependent activation of these cells in vitro and measurement of functional outcomes such as intracellular calcium flux and surface receptor up-regulation can then be used to monitor sensitization to a specific antigen.

PROCEDURES

Method 1. Measurement of Receptor Function in Early Cell Activation: CD69 Activation Assay

The CD2 receptor plays an important role in TCR activation by binding to the ligand CD58 (LFA-3) and optimizing the complex interaction between the TCR complex and the MHC-peptide complex on the APC (12, 46). In addition, cross-linking this receptor independent of the TCR complex interaction can induce intracellular calcium release and up-regulate the early activation marker molecule, CD69. The CD69 molecule is a 34-kDa dimeric glycoprotein expressed early after activation and is present on B and T cells as well as a variety of hematopoietic cells (48). For this reason genetic defects or infectious diseases that may affect early cell signaling events can be measured. For example, early-stage HIV-1-positive individuals showed impaired CD69 induction after stimulation with anti-CD2/2R (35). Anti-CD2/2R is a mixture of two MAbs that recognize different epitopes on the CD2 molecule and therefore produces cross-linking of the receptor (30, 32). Figure 1 shows a three-color staining analysis of CD69 expression in CD3+ CD4+ lymphocytes in unlysed whole-blood preparations from an HIV-1-seronegative individual, an HIV-infected individual with a CD69 response in the normal range, and an HIV-infected individual with a low CD69 response to stimulation with anti-CD2/2R MAbs. This figure demonstrates the use of

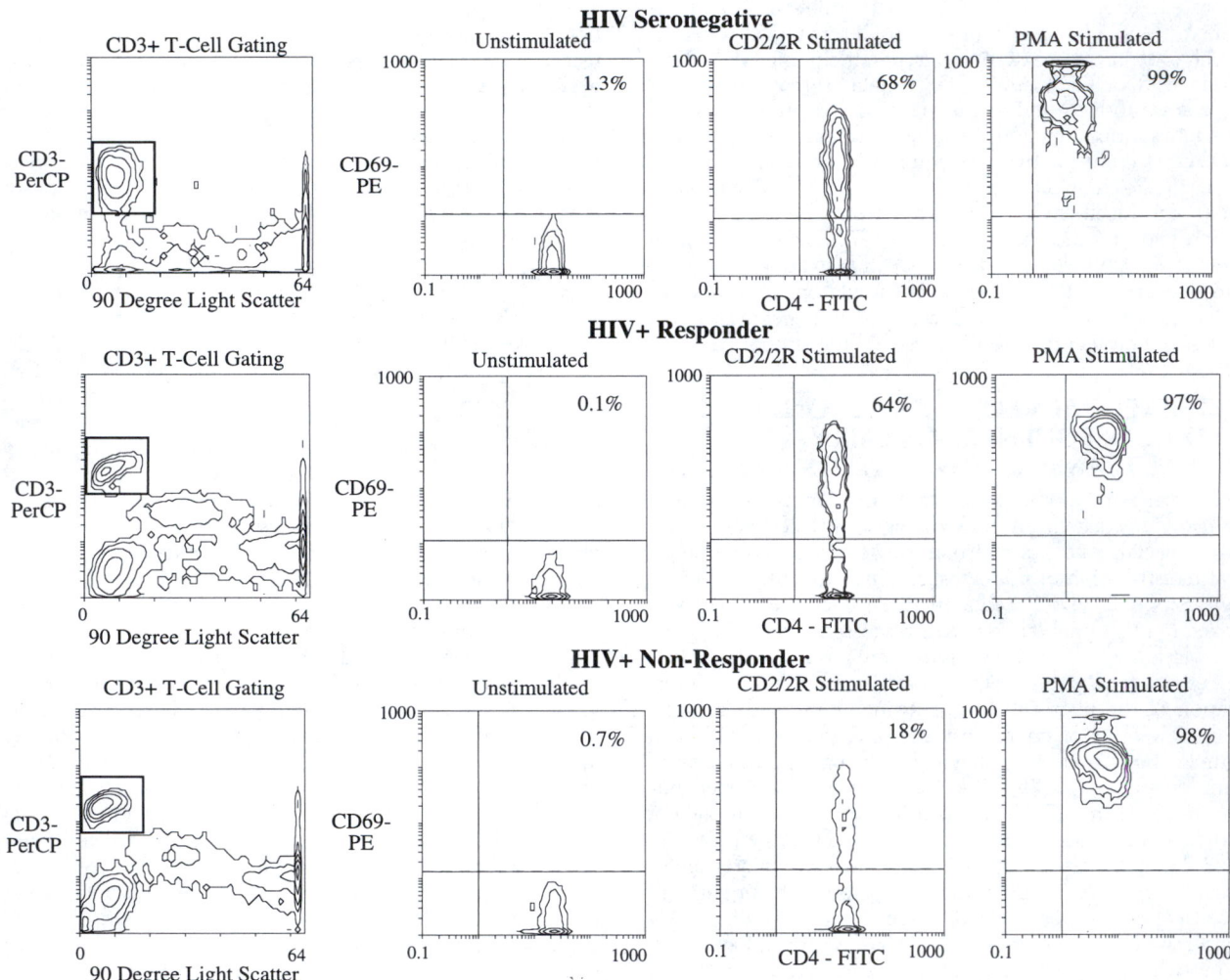

FIGURE 1 Three-color analysis of CD69 expression in CD3+ CD4+ lymphocytes in unlysed whole-blood preparations from an HIV-1-seronegative individual (top panels), an HIV-infected individual with a CD69 response in the normal range (middle panels), and an HIV-infected individual with a low CD69 response to stimulation with anti-CD2/2R MAbs (bottom panels). T cells were gated as 90° light scatter, and CD3 staining was carried out (left panels). CD69 expression was measured in CD3+ CD4+ lymphocytes cultured for 4 h in medium alone, with a stimulatory anti-CD2/2R MAb combination, or with PMA (right panels). PMA will spontaneously activate all cells within this time period and is considered the positive control.

CD69 percentage to measure the reduced signaling that occurs through the CD2 receptor in some patients with early-stage HIV-1 infection.

Sample Requirements

Ten milliliters of whole blood was collected from patients in heparin-treated Vacutainer tubes and processed within 2 to 4 h. Cell viability must be greater than 95% or additional reagents are required to identify the nonapoptotic or membrane-damaged cells.

Materials and Reagents

CD2/2R MAb mixture (Becton Dickinson Corp.): Dilute to a final concentration of 5 µg/ml per 10^6 cells.

Isotype controls, CD4-fluorescein isothiocyanate (CD4-FITC), CD8-FITC, CD69-phycoerythrin (CD69-PE), and CD3-PerCP (Becton Dickinson Corp.): Dilute to a final concentration of 5 µg/ml per 10^6 cells.

PMA (Sigma Chemical Co.): Dilute stock with dimethyl sulfoxide (DMSO) and use at a final concentration of 100 ng/ml.

Wash buffer: Dilute 0.1% bovine serum albumin and 0.1% sodium azide in phosphate-buffered saline (PBS) (without Ca^{2+} or Mg^{2+} ions).

Coulter-Immunolyse (Beckman-Coulter Corp.): Make a 1:20 dilution of Coulter-Immunolyse with cold PBS (without Ca^{2+} or Mg^{2+} ions).

1% Formaldehyde: Add 2.5 ml of 20% buffered formaldehyde (Tousimis Research Corporation) to 47.5 ml of PBS.

Vacutainer tubes (Becton Dickinson Corp.) or equivalent blood collection system

Equipment and Instrumentation

Flow cytometer: Elite-ESP (Beckman-Coulter) equipped with a 488-nm argon laser and five photomultiplier tubes (PMT2, PMT3, PMT4, and PMT5) in addition to a solid-state light scatter detector (FALS). The 488-nm monochromatic light excites all conjugates in the assay: FITC, PE, and PerCP. All data are stored in list-mode file format (FCS), and complete analysis is performed using Flow-JO software (Tree Star, Inc.).

Standard water bath capable of reaching and maintaining 37°C

Procedure

1. Collect 10 ml of whole blood in heparin-treated Vacutainer tubes and process within 2 to 3 h.
2. Mix 100 µl of whole blood with anti-CD2/2R MAb (5 µg/ml) in a 12- by 75-mm test tube.
3. Cap all tubes and incubate for 4 h in a 37°C water bath.
4. Add 2 ml of cold wash buffer and centrifuge at $400 \times g$ for 5 min.
5. Resuspend cell pellet in 240 µl of wash buffer and 20 µl of each clone tested to a total volume of 300 µl per tube. Stain cells with the following combinations: immunoglobulin G (IgG)-FITC, IgG-PE, and IgG-PerCP; CD4-FITC, CD69-PE, and CD3-PerCP; and CD8-FITC, CD69-PE, and CD3-PerCP.
6. Incubate at 4°C for 30 min.
7. Add 2 ml of cold wash buffer and centrifuge at $400 \times g$ for 5 min.

8. Remove all supernatant from cell pellet and vortex in remaining buffer. Add 1 ml of cold Coulter-Immunolyse to each tube for 2 min and vortex. Red blood cells (RBCs) should be completely lysed if a clear solution is observed.
9. Add 250 µl of Coulter-Immunolyse fixative and vortex.
10. Add 2 ml of wash buffer and centrifuge for 5 min at $400 \times g$. Repeat wash twice using 2 ml of wash buffer.
11. Remove supernatant and resuspend cell pellet in 200 µl of PBS and 200 µl of 1% formaldehyde. Incubate at 4°C for at least 2 h.
12. Place each sample on a flow cytometer and collect 5,000 gated events within the CD3+ gate and store as a list-mode file (FCS).
13. Using Flow-JO analysis software, gate on the CD3+ T cells and measure the percentage of cells which are CD4+ (or CD8+) and CD69+.

Controls and Calculations
Positive control: PMA-activated cells

1. Mix 100 µl of whole blood with 100 µl of PMA to a final concentration of 100 ng/ml in a 12- by 75-mm test tube.
2. Cap all tubes and incubate for 4 h in a 37°C water bath.
3. Add 2 ml of cold wash buffer and centrifuge at $400 \times g$ for 5 min.
4. Resuspend cell pellet in 240 µl of wash buffer and 20 µl of each clone tested to a total volume of 300 µl per tube. Stain cells with the following combinations: IgG-FITC, IgG-PE, and IgG-PerCP; CD4-FITC, CD69-PE, and CD3-PerCP; and CD8-FITC, CD69-PE, and CD3-PerCP.

Isotype control: These clones (IgG1-FITC, IgG1-PE, and IgG1-PerCP) provide the general location of cursors to define the negative and positive regions of test clones.

Standardization, Quality Control, and Quality Assurance
Determining a kinetic curve will require an evaluation of time with the various stimulants used. In general, a 4- to 6-h analysis is needed to determine the linearity of the surface expression of CD69 (Fig. 2). In this example the kinetics of CD69 expression on CD4+ T cells are illustrated. Whole blood from an HIV-1-seronegative subject (Fig. 2A) and an HIV-1-infected patient (Fig. 2B) was cultured without further stimulus or stimulated with soluble anti-CD2 MAb, bead-bound anti-CD3 MAb, or PMA. Flow cytometric measurements were performed on cells stained with anti-CD3, anti-CD4, and anti-CD69 MAbs. The percentage of cells positive for CD69 was calculated for cells in the CD3+ CD4+ gate. Results are shown from a representative HIV-1-seronegative individual and an HIV-infected patient with a depressed CD69 response.

Interpretation
Individuals whose percentages of T cells (CD4 or CD8) are below 2 standard deviations of those of healthy uninfected individuals are considered nonresponders. Each stimulant used to activate lymphocytes and measure the level of CD69 expression should be evaluated by a kinetic curve over 4 to 6 h as described in the standardization section.

Method 2. Measurement of Receptor Expression after T-Cell Activation: Quantitative Fluorescent Receptor Expression Assay

In addition to the percentages of cells which can change in response to infectious diseases or vaccine stimuli, the expression

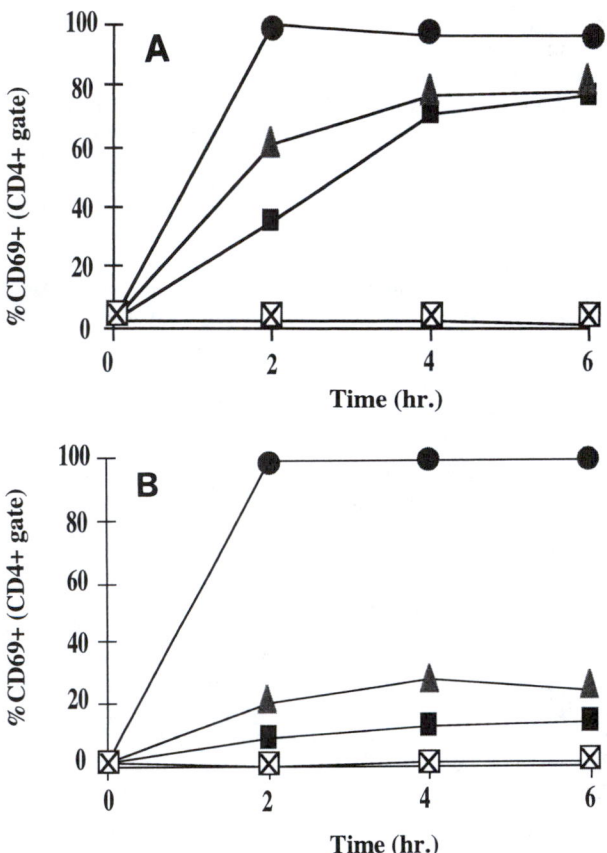

FIGURE 2 Kinetics of CD69 expression on CD4⁺ T cells. Whole blood from an HIV-1-seronegative individual (A) and an HIV-infected patient (B) was cultured without further stimulus (⊠) or stimulated with soluble anti-CD2 MAb (■), bead-bound anti-CD3 MAb (▲), or PMA (●). At the indicated times, flow cytometric measurements were performed on cells stained with anti-CD3, anti-CD4, and anti-CD69 MAbs. The percentage of cells positive for CD69 was calculated for cells in the CD3⁺ CD4⁺ gate. Five uninfected controls and five HIV-infected patients were studied. Results shown are from a representative HIV-1-seronegative individual and an HIV-infected patient with a depressed CD69 response.

of receptors, which are generally tightly controlled by the release of cytokines and other proteins, can be up-regulated or down-regulated in response to these protein signals. Viruses have evolved mechanisms to evade the immune response by interfering with intracellular trafficking and cell surface expression of important immune receptors such as MHC class I or II molecules, cytokines, and chemokines. For example, the Nef protein produced by HIV can down-regulate the expression of HLA class I and CD4 molecules on the cell surface (7, 10). During an ongoing immune response, lymphocytes can express many activation markers at various expression levels. In general, this group includes CD95 (FAS), CD38, CD26, CD25, and many of the chemokine receptors (CXCR4, CCR3, and CCR5). In this example, the up-regulation of the activation receptor CD38 on the surface of the CD8⁺ T cells is correlated with a poor prognosis and a more rapid progression in HIV disease (21, 36). The measurement of this expression can be performed by comparing

changes (median intensity) of the CD8⁺ CD38⁺ T cells of infected individuals (Fig. 3A and B) to a standard curve (Fig. 3C) as described below. Additionally, highly active antiretroviral therapy down-regulates the level of CD38 expression (47). Thus, a change in receptor expression might indicate changes in disease progression or an effective method to monitor the treatment course.

Sample Requirements

Collect 10 ml of whole blood in heparin-treated Vacutainer tubes and process within 6 to 8 h. Cell viability must be greater than 95% or additional reagents are required to identify the nonapoptotic or membrane-damaged cells.

Materials and Reagents

Wash buffer: Dilute 0.1% bovine serum albumin and 0.1% sodium azide in PBS.

Coulter-Immunolyse (Beckman-Coulter Corp.): Make a 1:20 dilution of Coulter-Immunolyse with cold PBS (without Ca²⁺ or Mg²⁺ ions).

Isotype controls, CD4-FITC, CD8-FITC, and CD3-PerCP (Becton Dickinson Corp.): Dilute to a final concentration of 5 μg/ml per 10⁶ cells.

CD38-PE (1:1; Becton Dickinson Corp.): Dilute to a final concentration of 5 μg/ml per 10⁶ cells. This reagent is designed to produce a protein/fluorescence ratio of 1.0. This means that one antibody molecule is conjugated with only one fluorochrome, making this reagent ideal for quantitative fluorescence analysis.

Equipment and Instrumentation

Flow cytometer: Elite-ESP (Beckman-Coulter) equipped with a 488-nm argon laser and five photomultiplier tubes (PMT1, PMT2, PMT3, PMT4, and PMT5) in addition to a solid-state light scatter detector (FALS). The 488-nm monochromatic light excites all conjugates in the assay: FITC, PE, and PerCP. All data are stored in list-mode file format (FCS), and complete analysis is performed using Flow-JO software (Tree Star, Inc.).

Procedure

1. Collect 10 ml of whole blood in heparin-treated Vacutainer tubes.

2. Mix 100 μl of whole blood with the indicated clone combinations (5 μg/ml) in a 12- by 75-mm test tube to a total volume of 300 μl with PBS as follows: tube 1, IgG1-FITC, IgG1-PE, and IgG1-PerCP (isotype control); tube 2, CD8-FITC, CD38-PE, and CD3-PerCP.

3. Incubate tubes at 4°C for 30 min.

4. Add 2 ml of cold wash buffer and centrifuge at 400 × g for 5 min. Repeat wash one additional time.

5. Remove all supernatant from cell pellet and vortex in remaining buffer. Add 1 ml of cold Coulter-Immunolyse to each tube for 2 min and vortex. RBCs should be completely lysed as determined by observing a clear solution.

6. Add 250 μl of Coulter-Immunolyse fixative and vortex.

7. Add 2 ml of wash buffer and centrifuge for 5 min at 400 × g. Repeat wash twice using 2 ml of wash buffer.

8. Remove supernatant and resuspend cell pellet in 200 μl of PBS and 200 μl of 1% formaldehyde. Incubate at 4°C overnight.

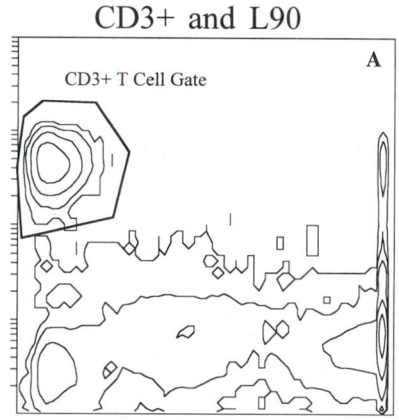

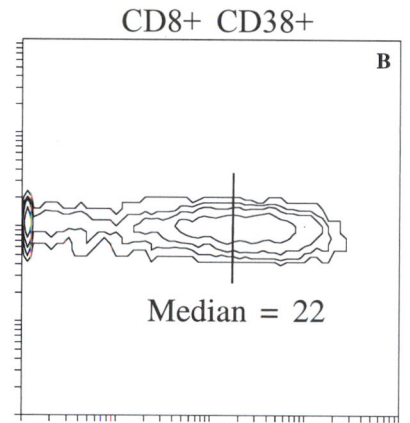

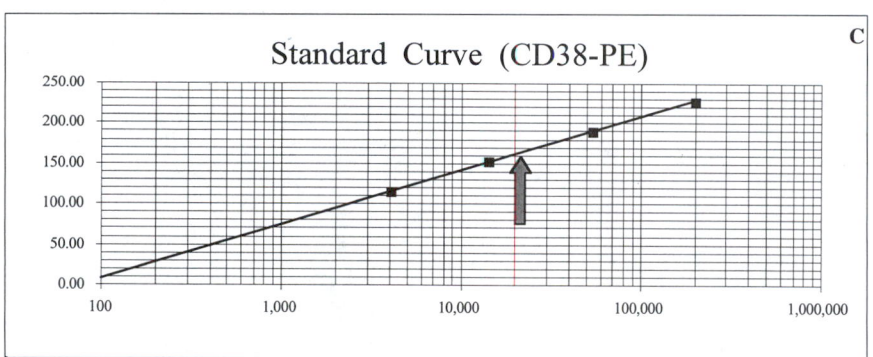

FIGURE 3 Representative histograms show the measurement of the CD38 intensity from CD3$^+$ CD8$^+$ T cells. (A) T-cell gate population (CD3$^+$ cells) on a side scatter-versus-CD3 histogram; (B) CD38 median measured on a CD38-versus-CD8 histogram; (C) calibration curve of antibody binding capacity values versus histogram channel number (scale, 0 to 255). Median channel number (relative linear channel) is converted to a 256-standard channel number and then read from the calibration curve (C) to determine the antibody binding capacity. In this example, a median channel measurement of 22 was determined to represent an antibody binding capacity of 21,272.

9. Using Flow-JO analysis software, gate on the CD3$^+$ T cells and measure the median value of cells which are CD8$^+$ and CD38$^+$. Each median value is compared to the standard curve (as described below) to calculate the receptor expression.

Controls and Calculations

Isotype control: These clones (IgG1-FITC, IgG1-PE, and IgG1-PerCP) provide the general location of cursors to define the negative and positive regions of test clones.

Positive control: The Daudi cell culture lines are cancer cells expressing high levels of CD38. These cells are available commercially (PanBIO INDX, Inc.) as a fixed stable product, which when stained with anti-CD38 provides a reproducible positive control.

Standardization, Quality Control, and Quality Assurance

QSC standard curve: Quantum Simply Cellular (QSC) beads have a standardized amount of goat anti-mouse clone on the surface to capture reacting mouse clone added to these beads. Figure 3C shows the typical standard curve produced by the procedure listed below.

Shown is a plot of the median values versus each bead intensity as assigned by the product insert.

1. Mix 280 μl of QSC beads with 20 μl of anti-CD38 MAb (final concentration, 5 μg/ml) in a 12- by 75-mm test tube.
2. Incubate for 30 min at 4°C.
3. Add 2 ml of PBS and centrifuge at 400 × *g* for 5 min.
4. Resuspend in 150 μl of PBS and 150 μl of 1% formaldehyde.
5. Acquire at least 2,000 total counts of data on the flow cytometer and run the analysis in the Flow-JO software. Plot the median values versus each bead intensity as assigned by the product insert.

Interpretation

The sensitivity of the quantitative fluorescence is based on the use of the standard curve as described in the standardization section. Tolerance ranges for each receptor can be defined by the measurements based on healthy, uninfected individuals. Median channel values obtained from the flow cytometer can be translated into receptor expression using the standard curve and compared to the normal range. Values outside of 2 standard deviations from the median (median values obtained, usually ca. 10 to 20 measurements) are considered significant.

Method 3. Measurement of T-Cell Activation Function: Intracellular Calcium Cell Signaling Assay

As discussed in detail in the introduction, the measurement of ligand binding to specific cell surface receptors is a complex but highly organized event. One of the best-studied examples is TCR complex binding to a specific peptide-MHC complex on the APCs. After these cell surface events occur, PTKs sequentially activate PLC-γ1. This active enzyme forces the hydrolysis of phosphotidylinositol 4,5-bisphosphate, causing an increase in IP₃. Within seconds following stimulation of the TCR or other surface receptors a substantial increase in IP₃ is observed. This molecule acts as a secondary messenger to increase the intracellular calcium levels as well as PKC from the stores associated with the endoplasmic reticulum. Increases in calcium cause activation of genes whose products are involved in the transcription of DNA sequences such as the IL-2 gene. In this method the calcium measured results from the increase that occurs after cell surface events have occurred and in general

indicates a cell committed to the lymphocyte activation process. The outcome of the committed cell process may be the secretion of cytokines such as IL-2, chemokines, or hormones involved in cell growth.

In this example (Fig. 4), the binding of chemokines to specific cell surface receptors, such as the interaction of SDF-1 with CXCR4, increases intracellular calcium levels. The consequence of this increase can influence the release of soluble cytokines, which can increase the surface expression of chemokine receptors. Increases in chemokine synthesis and secretion can have dramatic effects on lymphocyte trafficking and the immune response (6, 34). The well-known fluorescent dye INDO-1 can be transported through the cell membrane and once in the cytoplasm is converted by cell esterases into the active form, INDO-1-a. This active form interacts with free calcium, causing a change in the fluorescent properties of this dye. In resting cells, where very little free calcium is measurable (<200 nM), the dye exhibits high blue light emission and low UV light emission, making the violet/blue

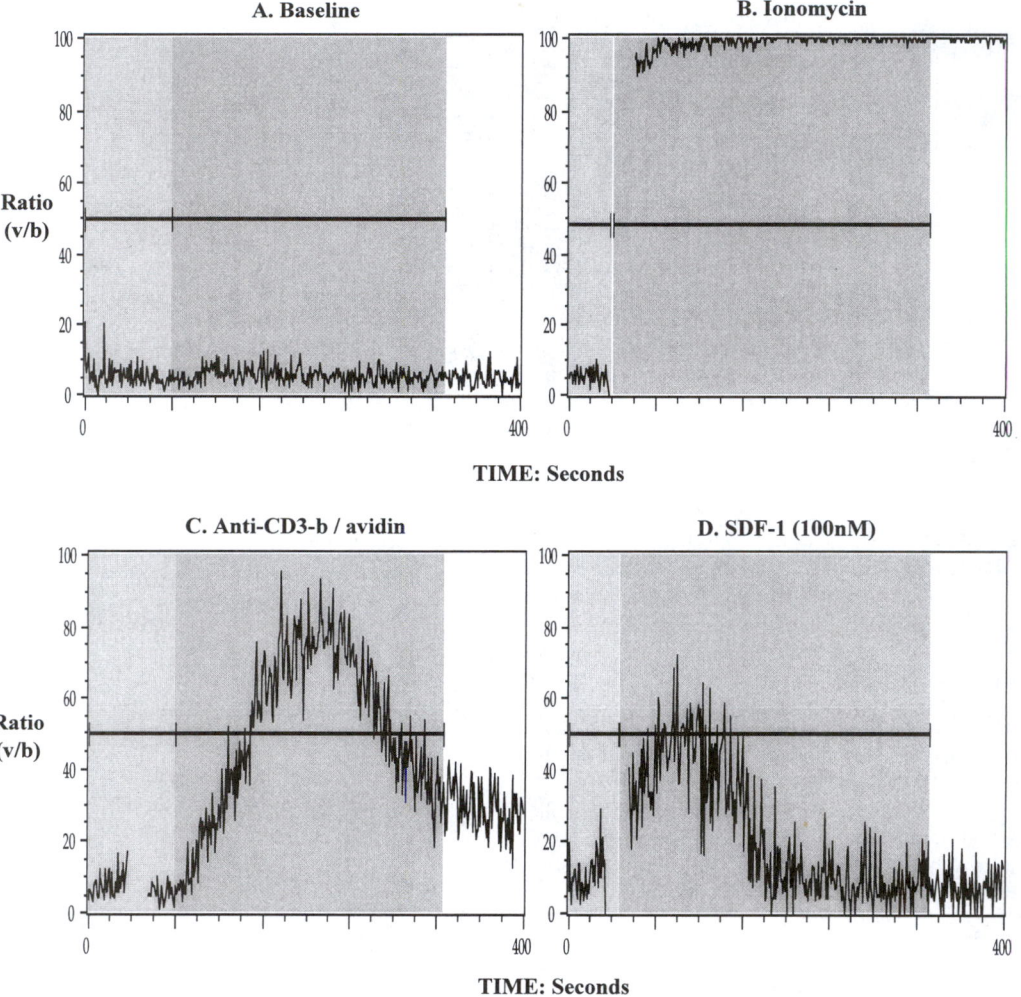

FIGURE 4 Representative calcium assay graphics showing the measurement of the v/b ratio versus time. The first cursor indicates the resting phase, and the second cursor represents the responding phase. (A) Baseline curve with no stimulation added; (B) INDO-1-labeled cells stimulated with ionomycin (2 μg); (C) INDO-1-labeled cells stimulated with avidin after pretreatment of cells with anti-CD3 (see control section for details); (D) INDO-1-labeled cells stimulated with SDF-1 (100 nM) after 7 days of cell activation.

(v/b) ratio low. However, upon cell activation and release of free calcium (<200 nM) the v/b ratio is increased, indicating calcium binding to INDO-1 dye and changing the spectral characteristics (e.g., low blue light emission and high UV light emission).

Sample Requirements

Collect whole blood (40 ml) in heparin-treated Vacutainer tubes and process within 2 to 4 h. Cell viability must be greater than 95% or additional reagents are required to identify the nonapoptotic or membrane-damaged cells.

Materials and Reagents

Prepare Pluronic/INDO working solution.

1. Reconstitute a 50-μg ampoule of INDO-1 AM (Molecular Probes) with 50 μl of DMSO. Mix well by pipetting and incubate for 2 min at room temperature (RT). INDO-1 is both hygroscopic and light sensitive, so this reagent must be made fresh for each use.

2. Add 25 μl of the 20% Pluronic F-127 stock. Mix well by pipetting and incubate for 2 min at RT. (Note: Heat under hot tap water to resolve into a clear liquid before use.)

3. Add 62.5 μl of the fetal calf serum stock. Mix well by pipetting and incubate for 2 min at RT.

4. Keep at RT and protect from light; reagent will remain stable for 24 h.

INDO medium (Hanks balanced salt solution [HBSS] with Ca^{2+} and Mg^{2+} ions and 1% fetal calf serum): add 0.5 ml of fetal calf serum into a final volume of 50 ml of HBSS (with Ca^{2+} and Mg^{2+} ions). If HBSS does not contain Ca^{2+} and Mg^{2+} ions, add 0.07 g of CaCl$_2$ and 0.07 g of MgSO$_4 \cdot$ 8H$_2$O in 500 ml of HBSS. Stored at 4°C, the reagent is stable for 1 month.

Pluronic F-127 solution: Prepare a 20% (wt/vol) stock solution in DMSO (Sigma Chemical Co.). Store at 4°C and protect from light. Dissolve reagent gels at RT by placing under hot tap water until all dissolved. Reagent will remain stable for 6 months at 4°C.

Stocks of MIP-1β, eotaxin, and SDF-1β (R&D Systems Inc.) are frozen at concentrations of 50 μg/ml (2,700 nM) in 50-μl volumes in 0.1% fetal calf serum (heat inactivated) in sterile PBS. Dilute stocks with INDO medium to make a working concentration of 22.2 μg/ml (1,200 nM) by adding 62.5 μl of INDO medium into 50 μl of stock ligand (R&D Systems Inc.).

Streptavidin (Southern Biotechnology Corp.): Add 20 μl of a stock concentration of 1,000 μg/ml or 40 μg per

cell activation. Note: This control may not work in some cell lines.

Ionomycin (working concentration = 1 mg/ml [molecular weight, 747.1]; Sigma Chemical Co.): Use 2 μl (3 μM) per cell activation.

CD3-biotin (Becton Dickinson Corp.): Dilute to a final concentration of 5 μg/ml per 10^6 cells.

Phytohemagglutinin: Dilute to a final concentration of 100 μg/ml in sterile culture medium (Gibco BRL).

Ficoll-Hypaque (Sigma Chemical Co.): Sterile lymphocyte density medium; use undiluted.

IL-2 (R&D Systems Inc.): Dilute to 20 U/ml in sterile culture medium.

Culture medium: Mix the reagents shown in Table 1 in a sterile container. Store at 4°C for 1 month.

Equipment and Instrumentation

Flow cytometer: Elite-ESP (Beckman-Coulter Corp.) equipped with a 488-nm argon laser, a 325-nm HeCad laser, gated AMP, and five photomultiplier tubes (PMT1, PMT2, PMT3, PMT4, and PMT5) in addition to a solid-state light scatter detector (FALS). The 488-nm monochromatic argon laser excites all conjugated MAbs in the assay: FITC, PE, and PerCP. The 325-nm HeCad laser excites the active form of the INDO-1 dye. All data are stored in listmode file format (FCS), and complete analysis is performed using Flow-JO software (Tree Star, Inc.).

Procedure

1. Collect 40 ml of whole blood in heparin-treated Vacutainer tubes and process within 4 to 6 h.

2. Centrifuge Vacutainers at 600 × g for 20 min and remove leukocytes located on top of the RBC fraction (i.e., the buffy coat layer). Dilute this fraction 1:2 with sterile PBS and overlay onto 5 ml of Ficoll-Hypaque. Centrifuge at 600 × g for 30 min at RT. Remove lymphocyte layer (middle layer), dilute 1:2 with sterile PBS, and centrifuge at 400 × g for 5 min.

3. Resuspend cells in culture medium containing phytohemagglutinin (50 μg/ml) and IL-2 (20 U/ml); culture cells for 3 days at 37°C in 5% CO$_2$. After 3 days in culture, replace medium with culture medium containing IL-2 (20 U/ml) and culture for an additional 4 days.

4. Add 10 × 10^6 cells to a 15-ml conical tube, wash twice in INDO medium, and resuspend cells in 1 ml of INDO medium. Note: Use at least 0.25 × 10^6 to 1.0 × 10^6 cells per reaction; ideally 500,000 cells should be used.

TABLE 1 Culture medium reagents (Gibco BRL) required for the protocol

Reagent (concn)	Vol (ml)	Concn (%)	Final concn
Fetal calf serum (sterile filtered)	100	10	10% (vol/vol)
Penicillin (10,000 U/ml) +	10	1	100 U/ml
streptomycin (10,000 μg/ml)			100 μg/ml
Gentamicin (40 mg/ml)	2.5	1	100 μg/ml
Glutamine (200 mM)	10	1	2 mM
RPMI 1640	877.5	NA^a	NA
Total	1,000		

^{a}NA, not applicable.

5. Add 7 μl of Pluronic/INDO working solution to 1 ml of cells. Note: Since time to activation is critical (complete activation within 2 h from the addition of the dye), samples should be staggered by 40 min. Keep samples on ice until the INDO dye is added.

6. Incubate at 31°C for 40 min. Note: Time and incubation periods are important in that the cell esterases must convert the entire enzyme into the active form. For this reason, time studies are necessary to determine this critical step. Generally, for most cells 40 min will be long enough; however, cells like monocytes will process the stain faster because of the increase in active esterases with these cells.

7. Wash twice (400 × g for 5 min) in INDO medium.

8. Add enough medium to adjust the cell concentration to 10^6/ml (example: if cells are at a concentration of 10 × 10^6/ml, add 9 ml of INDO medium). Remove 500 μl per reaction (500,000 cells). Cells are now ready for analysis. Hold on ice no longer than 2 h before activation.

9. Incubate 500 μl of INDO-loaded cells (0.5 × 10^6) at 37°C for 5 min.

10. Run on flow cytometer for at least 30 s for background analysis (unstimulated fraction) before pausing to add stimulant.

11. After 30 s add stimulant to achieve the final concentrations shown in Tables 2 and 3 for each activation.

12. From saved listmode files, complete analysis using the Flow-JO software program. Report percentage of cells responding over baseline of the unstimulated cell fraction.

Controls and Calculations

CD3 staining for biological positive control: This control determines the intact nature of the cell signaling proteins and thus after cross-linking with avidin acts as a positive control.

1. Resuspend 0.5 × 10^6 cells in 500 μl of INDO medium and label this tube as the CD3 control.

2. Add 40 μl of anti-CD3-biotin clone (final concentration, 5 μg/ml).

3. Place on ice in the dark for 20 min.

4. Add 2 ml of INDO medium and centrifuge at 400 × g for 5 min.

5. Wash once with 2 ml of INDO medium and centrifuge at 400 × g for 5 min.

6. Resuspend in 500 μl of INDO medium before analysis.

Alignment of the HeCad Laser

Using the standard blue beads (324/421; Molecular Probes), dilute 1/1,000 with PBS (or until the rate of 300/s can be established), and run using the calcium protocol and filters as described by the protocol, except the 325LP should be substituted for the 381BP filter. With this filter in place light should be collected in both the violet and blue photomultiplier tube

parameters (simulating positive signal detection). When the 381BP filter is in place only blue light will be observed (simulating baseline signal detection). Hence, this controls for both alignment and the ability of the instrument to measure UV light (Color Plate 3).

Unstimulated or baseline negative control: INDO-loaded cells run for the first 30 s before any stimulant is added provide a negative control as well as an internal control.

Calculations

INDO-1 AM: Molecular mass is 1,009.9 g/mol. One vial contains 0.05 mg. The total diluent volume in Pluronic/INDO working solution is 0.1375 ml; use 7.0 μl of working solution in 1 ml of cell suspension.

The molarity (in millimoles per liter) of INDO-1 AM in the Pluronic/INDO working solution is calculated as follows: 0.05 mg/(1,009.9 g/mol × 0.1375 ml × 10^{-3} liter/ml) = 0.05/0.13886 = 0.36.

The final concentration (molarity) (in millimoles per liter) of INDO-1 AM in the cell loading mixture is calculated as follows: (0.007 ml × 0.36 mM)/1 ml = 0.00255, or 2.55 μM. Thus, the final concentration of INDO-1 AM in the cell loading mixture is 2.55 μM.

The concentration of Pluronic F-127 in stock solution is 20% (0.025 ml of Pluronic F-127 stock solution in Pluronic/INDO working solution). The total diluent volume in Pluronic/INDO working solution is 0.1375 ml. Use 7.0 μl of working solution in 1 ml of cell suspension. The concentration (Z) of Pluronic F-127 in the Pluronic/INDO working solution is calculated as follows: (0.025 ml × 20%)/0.1375 ml = 3.636%.

The final concentration (Z) of Pluronic F-127 in the cell loading mixture is calculated as follows: (0.007 ml × 3.636%)/1 ml = 0.025%.

The final concentration of MIP-1β = 128 nM.

The final concentration of SDF-1β = 125 nM.

Standardization, Quality Control, and Quality Assurance

To standardize the mean calcium peak response, by using the formula below, the mean peak response can be translated into calcium concentration (nanomolar). It is important to note that the dissociation constant (K_d) varies dramatically as a function of temperature, pH, and ionic strength. Hence, it is critical to keep these parameters consistent from test to

TABLE 2 Experimental nanomolar equivalents for final concentrations of stimulants

Final concn (μg/ml)	Equivalent concn (nM)	
	SDF-1	MIP-1β
1	125	128
0.5	62.5	64
0.1	12.5	12.8

TABLE 3 Chemokine test layout

Stimulant	Vol required (μl)	Final concn	Expected result
INDO medium	NA[a]	NA	Negative control
Streptavidin	20	40 μg/ml	Positive control
SDF-1	100	100 nM	Test
MIP-1β	100	100 nM	Test
Eotaxin	100	100 nM	Test
Ionomycin	2	2 μg/ml	Positive control

[a] NA, not applicable.

test and experiment to experiment to use this calculation. In this equation the K_d is the effective dissociation constant (250 nM at 37°C, pH 7.05), and R, R_{min}, and R_{max} are the fluorescence intensity ratio (v/b) values at test, zero, and saturating levels of calcium, respectively. S_{f2}/S_{b2} is the ratio of blue or green fluorescence intensity of the calcium-free and bound dyes. Since this term is a constant that depends primarily on the filters used for the INDO-1 analysis, it can be considered equivalent to 1 when using the same instrument for the calcium determination. The R_{min} can be determined by using certified blank beads (Flow Cytometry Standards Corp.) and calculating the intensity ratio (v/b). Finally, the R_{max} can be determined by the addition of the calcium ionosphere ionomycin to INDO-1-loaded cells as follows: $[Ca^{2+}] = K_d \times (R - R_{min})/(R_{max} - R) \times S_{f2}/S_{b2}$.

Interpretation

The resting cell concentration of free calcium is approximately 200 nM, with less than 5% of total cells above baseline. Percentages greater than 5% or calcium concentrations two times more than the baseline are considered to indicate responding cells. These values can be compared to those from a normal group to determine significance ($n = 20$) with each stimulant used.

Quality Control and Quality Assurance

Tube-to-tube reproducibility: With addition of anti-CD3 to each test sample the total number of CD3$^+$ T cells can be determined. The acceptable tolerance is 5% between tubes within the same run. In the calcium assay, reproducibility can be determined by using the baseline fluorescence intensity ratio (v/b). The tolerance on these values should be within 5% of each run.

Lot-to-lot reproducibility of MAb: MAbs can be tested against a normal cell line, which is fixed to maintain stability (CD Chex cell control; Streck Laboratories). In general, the percentage or the intensity of fluorescence can be monitored from lot to lot with a tolerance ±10% from defined ranges provided in the product insert.

Microscopic examination: After staining samples or loading cells with INDO-1 dye, a sample can be observed under a fluorescence microscope for correct fluorescence. As an example, cells stained with CD38-PE should appear yellow, while cells stained with CD4-FITC should appear green. In the calcium assay, cells stained with INDO-1 in the active form should appear blue under a mercury arc lamp with a UV filter setup.

College of American Pathologists surveys: Cell proficiency surveys can test both accuracy and reproducibility of immunophenotyping. However, there is currently no proficiency program available for the calcium assay.

Pitfalls and Troubleshooting

The more common problems found in the above-mentioned assays and the corrective actions are listed in Table 4.

TABLE 4   Problems and corrective actions

Problem	Corrective action
High angle interference in the forward scatter vs. L90 light scatter pattern	Suspect RBC contamination from unlysed cells. Check expiration date on lysis reagent and correct dilution. Run autofluorescent control to check lysis reagent before adding to test samples.
Limited cell recovery after separation on Ficoll-Hypaque	Suspect failure to use this density medium at RT. Warm Ficoll-Hypaque to RT before adding cells and centrifuge at RT.
Loss of CD4 on the surface of T cells after exposure to PMA	Suspect kinetic issue or concentration of PMA. A loss of CD4 will occur after PMA treatment due to the activation of PKC. This is generally observed with longer incubation times and higher concentrations of phytohemagglutinin. If longer time is needed, adding monensin (2 μM) to the culture will inhibit this process.
Loss of cells or inconsistent CD3$^+$ T cells from tube to tube	Suspect cells may be lost due to low centrifuge speed. Increase speed for all cell washes to 400 × g and centrifuge for at least 5 min at 4°C.
Decreased number or loss of INDO-1-positive cells	Suspect incubation time or temperature. Most cells will be completely loaded with the active form of INDO-1 at 40 min. Check using a fluorescence microscope equipped with UV filters. Active dye will fluoresce blue after exposure to UV irradiation.
No violet or blue light emission but cells are INDO-1 positive	Suspect UV laser alignment. Repeat HeCad laser alignment procedure as outlined in the control section.
High INDO-1 background fluorescence	Suspect tubing is contaminated with previously run stimulant. Replace tubing and wash between runs with DMSO-distilled H$_2$O and INDO medium. Additionally, run all ionomycin controls at the end of all test samples.
Ionomycin control is negative	Suspect cells are not loaded correctly or INDO-1 dye reagent has expired. Load cells with INDO-1 within a 2-h window of analysis and prepare INDO-1 dye from frozen stock on the day of analysis.

REMARKS AND CONCLUSIONS

The combined use of flow cytometry and evolving technologies, such as gene microarray systems and proteomics, will tremendously increase our understanding in the field of T-lymphocyte activation and signaling.

REFERENCES

1. Acuto, O., S. Mise-Omata, G. Mangino, and F. Michel. 2003. Molecular modifiers of T cell antigen receptor triggering threshold: the mechanism of CD28 costimulatory receptor. *Immunol. Rev.* **192**:21–31.
2. Alarcon, B., D. Gil, P. Delgado, and W. W. Schamel. 2003. Initiation of TCR signaling: regulation within CD3 dimers. *Immunol. Rev.* **191**:38–46.
3. Appleman, L. J., and V. A. Boussiotis. 2003. T cell anergy and costimulation. *Immunol. Rev.* **192**:161–180.
4. Bonvini, E., K. E. DeBell, M. C. Veri, L. Graham, B. Stoica, J. Laborda, M. J. Aman, A. DiBaldassarre, S. Miscia, and B. L. Rellahan. 2003. On the mechanism coupling phospholipase Cgamma1 to the B- and T-cell antigen receptors. *Adv. Enzyme Regul.* **43**:245–269.
5. Call, M. E., J. Pyrdol, M. Wiedmann, and K. W. Wucherpfennig. 2002. The organizing principle in the formation of the T cell receptor-CD3 complex. *Cell* **111**:967–979.
6. Campbell, D. J., G. F. Debes, B. Johnston, E. Wilson, and E. C. Butcher. 2003. Targeting T cell responses by selective chemokine receptor expression. *Semin. Immunol.* **15**:277–286.
7. Chen, B. K., R. T. Gandhi, and D. Baltimore. 1996. CD4 down-modulation during infection of human T cells with human immunodeficiency virus type 1 involves independent activities of *vpu*, *env*, and *nef*. *J. Virol.* **70**:6044–6053.
8. Chu, D. H., C. T. Morita, and A. Weiss. 1998. The Syk family of protein tyrosine kinases in T-cell activation and development. *Immunol. Rev.* **165**:167–180.
9. Clements, J. L. 2003. Known and potential functions for the SLP-76 adapter protein in regulating T-cell activation and development. *Immunol. Rev.* **191**:211–229.
10. Collins, K. L., B. K. Chen, S. A. Kalams, B. D. Walker, and D. Baltimore. 1998. HIV-1 Nef protein protects infected primary cells against killing by cytotoxic T lymphocytes. *Nature* **391**:397–401.
11. Cooper, M. D., L. L. Lanier, M. E. Conley, and J. M. Puck. 2003. Immunodeficiency disorders. *Hematology (Am. Soc. Hematol. Educ. Progr.)* **2003**:314–330.
12. Damle, N. K., K. Klussman, G. Leytze, A. Aruffo, P. S. Linsley, and J. A. Ledbetter. 1993. Costimulation with integrin ligands intercellular adhesion molecule-1 or vascular cell adhesion molecule-1 augments activation-induced death of antigen-specific CD4+ T lymphocytes. *J. Immunol.* **151**:2368–2379.
13. Das, V., B. Nal, A. Roumier, V. Meas-Yedid, C. Zimmer, J. C. Olivo-Marin, P. Roux, P. Ferrier, A. Dautry-Varsat, and A. Alcover. 2002. Membrane-cytoskeleton interactions during the formation of the immunological synapse and subsequent T-cell activation. *Immunol. Rev.* **189**:123–135.
14. Davis, D. M., and M. L. Dustin. 2004. What is the importance of the immunological synapse? *Trends Immunol.* **25**:323–327.
15. Davis, D. M., T. Igakura, F. E. McCann, L. M. Carlin, K. Andersson, B. Vanherberghen, A. Sjostrom, C. R. Bangham, and P. Hoglund. 2003. The protean immune cell synapse: a supramolecular structure with many functions. *Semin. Immunol.* **15**:317–324.
16. Davis, M. M., and P. J. Bjorkman. 1988. T-cell antigen receptor genes and T-cell recognition. *Nature* **334**:395–402. (*Erratum*, **335**:744.)
17. Finkelstein, L. D., and P. L. Schwartzberg. 2004. Tec kinases: shaping T-cell activation through actin. *Trends Cell Biol.* **14**:443–451.
18. Fuller, C. L., V. L. Braciale, and L. E. Samelson. 2003. All roads lead to actin: the intimate relationship between TCR signaling and the cytoskeleton. *Immunol. Rev.* **191**:220–236.
19. Garcia, K. C., L. Teyton, and I. A. Wilson. 1999. Structural basis of T cell recognition. *Annu. Rev. Immunol.* **17**:369–397.
20. Gascoigne, N. R., and T. Zal. 2004. Molecular interactions at the T cell-antigen-presenting cell interface. *Curr. Opin. Immunol.* **16**:114–119.
21. Giorgi, J. V., Z. Liu, L. E. Hultin, W. G. Cumberland, K. Hennessey, and R. Detels. 1993. Elevated levels of CD38+ CD8+ T cells in HIV infection add to the prognostic value of low CD4+ T cell levels: results of 6 years of follow-up. The Los Angeles Center, Multicenter AIDS Cohort Study. *J. Acquir. Immune Defic. Syndr.* **6**:904–912.
22. Horejsi, V. 2003. The roles of membrane microdomains (rafts) in T cell activation. *Immunol. Rev.* **191**:148–164.
23. Hornstein, I., A. Alcover, and S. Katzav. 2004. Vav proteins, masters of the world of cytoskeleton organization. *Cell Signal* **16**:1–11.
24. Huang, Y., and R. L. Wange. 2004. T cell receptor signaling: beyond complex complexes. *J. Biol. Chem.* **279**:28827–28830.
25. Jacobelli, J., P. G. Andres, J. Boisvert, and M. F. Krummel. 2004. New views of the immunological synapse: variations in assembly and function. *Curr. Opin. Immunol.* **16**:345–352.
26. Katan, M., R. Rodriguez, M. Matsuda, Y. M. Newbatt, and G. W. Aherne. 2003. Structural and mechanistic aspects of phospholipase Cgamma regulation. *Adv. Enzyme Regul.* **43**:77–85.
27. Krogsgaard, M., J. B. Huppa, M. A. Purbhoo, and M. M. Davis. 2003. Linking molecular and cellular events in T-cell activation and synapse formation. *Semin. Immunol.* **15**:307–315.
28. Lindquist, J. A., L. Simeoni, and B. Schraven. 2003. Transmembrane adapters: attractants for cytoplasmic effectors. *Immunol. Rev.* **191**:165–182.
29. Lucas, J. A., A. T. Miller, L. O. Atherly, and L. J. Berg. 2003. The role of Tec family kinases in T cell development and function. *Immunol. Rev.* **191**:119–138.
30. Maino, V. C., M. A. Suni, and J. J. Ruitenberg. 1995. Rapid flow cytometric method for measuring lymphocyte subset activation. *Cytometry* **20**:127–133.
31. Malissen, B. 2003. An evolutionary and structural perspective on T cell antigen receptor function. *Immunol. Rev.* **191**:7–27.
32. Mardiney, M., III, M. R. Brown, and T. A. Fleisher. 1996. Measurement of T-cell CD69 expression: a rapid and efficient means to assess mitogen- or antigen-induced proliferative capacity in normals. *Cytometry* **26**:305–310.
33. Miletic, A. V., M. Swat, K. Fujikawa, and W. Swat. 2003. Cytoskeletal remodeling in lymphocyte activation. *Curr. Opin. Immunol.* **15**:261–268.
34. Moser, B., M. Wolf, A. Walz, and P. Loetscher. 2004. Chemokines: multiple levels of leukocyte migration control. *Trends Immunol.* **25**:75–84.
35. Perfetto, S. P., T. E. Hickey, P. J. Blair, V. C. Maino, K. F. Wagner, S. Zhou, D. L. Mayers, D. St. Louis, C. H. June, and J. N. Siegel. 1997. Measurement of CD69 induction in

the assessment of immune function in asymptomatic HIV-infected individuals. *Cytometry* **30:**1–9.

36. **Perfetto, S. P., J. D. Malone, C. Hawkes, G. McCrary, B. August, S. Zhou, R. Garner, M. J. Dolan, and A. E. Brown.** 1998. CD38 expression on cryopreserved CD8+ T cells predicts HIV disease progression. *Cytometry* **33:**133–137.

37. **Randriamampita, C., and A. Trautmann.** 2004. Ca2+ signals and T lymphocytes: new mechanisms and functions in Ca2+ signalling. *Biol. Cell* **96:**69–78.

38. **Simonte, S. J., and C. Cunningham-Rundles.** 2003. Update on primary immunodeficiency: defects of lymphocytes. *Clin. Immunol.* **109:**109–118.

39. **Sommers, C. L., L. E. Samelson, and P. E. Love.** 2004. LAT: a T lymphocyte adapter protein that couples the antigen receptor to downstream signaling pathways. *Bioessays* **26:**61–67.

40. **Sunder-Plassmann, R., and E. L. Reinherz.** 1998. A p56lck-independent pathway of CD2 signaling involves Jun kinase. *J. Biol. Chem.* **273:**24249–24257.

41. **Takesono, A., R. Horai, M. Mandai, D. Dombroski, and P. L. Schwartzberg.** 2004. Requirement for Tec kinases in chemokine-induced migration and activation of Cdc42 and Rac. *Curr. Biol.* **14:**917–922.

42. **Taner, S. B., B. Onfelt, N. J. Pirinen, F. E. McCann, A. I. Magee, and D. M. Davis.** 2004. Control of immune responses by trafficking cell surface proteins, vesicles and lipid rafts to and from the immunological synapse. *Traffic* **5:**651–661.

43. **Unanue, E. R.** 2002. Perspective on antigen processing and presentation. *Immunol. Rev.* **185:**86–102.

44. **van Leeuwen, J. E., and L. E. Samelson.** 1999. T cell antigen-receptor signal transduction. *Curr. Opin. Immunol.* **11:**242–248.

45. **Whiteside, T. L.** 1999. Signaling defects in T lymphocytes of patients with malignancy. *Cancer Immunol. Immunother.* **48:**346–352.

46. **Wilkins, A. L., W. Yang, and J. J. Yang.** 2003. Structural biology of the cell adhesion protein CD2: from molecular recognition to protein folding and design. *Curr. Protein Pept. Sci.* **4:**367–373.

47. **Wilkinson, J., J. J. Zaunders, A. Carr, and D. A. Cooper.** 1999. CD8+ anti-human immunodeficiency virus suppressor activity (CASA) in response to antiretroviral therapy: loss of CASA is associated with loss of viremia. *J. Infect. Dis.* **180:**68–75.

48. **Ziegler, S. F., F. Ramsdell, and M. R. Alderson.** 1994. The activation antigen CD69. *Stem Cells* **12:**456–465.

Functional Assays for B Cells and Antibodies

MOON H. NAHM AND ROBIN G. LORENZ

37

The primary cells of the adaptive immune system are T cells, B cells, and natural killer cells. These lymphocytes assist the host in eliminating both intracellular pathogens (T cells) and extracellular pathogens (B cells and antibodies) through B-cell–T-cell interactions, as well as interactions with cells and molecules of the innate immune system. B cells recognize foreign antigen by the B-cell receptor (BCR), a membrane-bound immunoglobulin generated through a complex genetic recombination process (3). The BCR recognizes conformational protein antigens, as well as nonprotein antigens. Two types of B cells have been described based on expression of cell surface molecules and function. B1 (CD5[+]) B cells are thought to be a more "natural" type of B cell which responds to T-cell-independent forms of antigen (i.e., bacterial polysaccharides) (22, 25). B2 B cells respond to T-cell-dependent antigens, such as the more classical protein antigens tetanus and diphtheria toxoids. Both classes of B cells respond to BCR binding of foreign antigen by proliferation, differentiation into antibody-secreting plasma cells, and formation of memory B cells.

The function of the humoral immune response differs depending on the class of antibody produced and the differentiation state of the B cell. Naive B cells express CD19, CD20, and surface immunoglobulin M (IgM) and IgD (Table 1). After BCR stimulation, B cells become memory cells or plasma cells. These cells express unique antigens. In addition, immunoglobulin class switching occurs and IgG, IgA, or IgE is produced. Each of these immunoglobulin classes has distinct functions. IgM can bind pathogens and activate complement. IgG can directly neutralize bacterial toxins, block adhesion of pathogens, and also activate complement. IgA can also neutralize toxins and block adhesion of pathogens, but it functions primarily at mucosal sites, while IgE plays a role in the immune response to parasites. After BCR stimulation, the immunoglobulin produced by B cells also increases its affinity for antigen, therefore improving the functionality of the humoral response.

Primary defects in the humoral components of the immune response are usually recognized by such clues as frequent development of infections early in life and difficulty in clearance of infections. The type of infection will often clue the clinician in to a possible B-cell or antibody defect (Table 2). In addition, frequent or incompletely cleared infections are also often a clue (Table 2). Primary immunodeficiencies are covered in greater detail in chapter 101.

A more immediate concern to most physicians is the increasing incidence of secondary immune deficiencies due to infections such as human immunodeficiency virus (covered in chapter 95), cancer (multiple myeloma), chronic renal failure, autoimmune processes, or posttransplantation immunosuppression.

In some patients, the absence of B-cell function is clear because B cells are undetectable. In many cases, patients may have B cells but their function is abnormal because the B cells are either tolerized or anergic. There is also a need to measure functionality of antibodies since not all antibodies are protective. A very young child may produce ineffective antibodies. Elderly persons may produce ineffective pneumococcal antibodies, and human immunodeficiency virus patients may make ineffective antibodies. The ineffective antibodies may express inappropriate isotypes or V regions, resulting in low-avidity antibodies or the inability to activate complement.

APPROACHES FOR ASSESSING B-CELL FUNCTION

A complete blood count (CBC) is often the first test performed in the evaluation of the humoral immune response. However, the CBC is clearly not a good screening test, as often the total lymphocyte count in humoral immunodeficiencies is normal or only slightly decreased. Therefore, the next step in the evaluation of a possible humoral immunodeficiency is the measurement of serum antibody concentrations.

In Vivo B-Cell Function

Immunoglobulins

The most direct measure of in vivo B-cell function is immunoglobulin secretion by plasma cells. Serum immunoglobulins are most commonly measured by automated nephelometry (described in detail in chapter 8). The immunoglobulins routinely measured in serum are IgG, IgA, and IgM. The normal ranges for serum immunoglobulins vary depending on both the age and gender of the individual (8). A significant seasonal variation in serum IgA levels has also been described (40). In addition to the measurement of total serum immunoglobulin concentrations, levels of subclasses of IgG and IgA can also be determined by automated nephelometry. Patients have been reported to have deficiencies of one or

TABLE 1 B-cell markers used in flow cytometry

Marker	B-cell population
CD19	Early B cells to B-cell blasts
CD20	Pre-B cells to B-cell blasts
CD23	Activated B cells
CD27	Memory B cells
CD5	B1 B cells
Surface IgM	Immature, mature, and memory B cells
Surface IgD.	Mature and memory B cells
Surface IgG, IgA, and IgE	Isotype-switched memory B cells
CD138 (syndecan 1)	Plasma cells

more subclasses of IgG even when they have normal levels of total serum IgG. However, the true biological significance of IgG subclass deficiencies remains controversial (7, 21). The rate of bacterial infections is increased in some individuals with low serum IgG2 concentrations but not in others, e.g., Wiskott-Aldrich syndrome patients (27). Therefore, it is more clinically significant to measure functional levels of serum antibody to typical vaccine components, such as tetanus, diphtheria, pneumococcus or *Haemophilus influenzae* type b (for protein antigens refer to chapter 52, and for polysaccharides refer to chapter 51).

The presence of antibodies against vaccine components, detected by random sampling, is indicative of an intact humoral immune system in children who have received their vaccines. If titers of immunoglobulins against common vaccine antigens are low, then specific antigen challenge should be performed. Serum samples are obtained before and 2 to 3 weeks after vaccination. The paired sera are then tested simultaneously, and a patient is considered to have mounted an adequate response if a fourfold or greater rise in specific titer is seen. This type of challenge can be performed either with polysaccharide vaccines (pneumococcal or meningococcal vaccines) or with neo-protein antigens such as bacteriophage ϕX174 or keyhole limpet hemocyanin (4, 13, 29).

In addition to the measurement of serum immunoglobulins against vaccine antigens, the levels of B1 B-cell production of anti-A or anti-B isohemagglutinin IgM antibodies can also be investigated. The presence of these T-cell-independent antibodies against blood group antigens depends on both the age of the patient and the patient's blood group (i.e., no

TABLE 2 Associations with humoral or B-lymphocyte deficiencies

Infectious agents
   Streptococcus pneumoniae
   Streptococcus pyogenes
   Haemophilus influenzae
   Ureaplasma urealyticum
   Giardia lambia

Clinical conditions
   Recurrent otitis
   Recurrent pharyngitis
   Recurrent sinusitis
   Recurrent bronchitis
   Recurrent conjunctivitis

antibodies are seen in the serum of blood type AB individuals). As IgM is produced by the newborn, this type of testing can be performed earlier than testing for vaccine-induced immunoglobulins. A normal titer is at least 1:8 (11).

Peripheral Blood B Cells

The actual number of B cells in the peripheral blood cannot be determined by the CBC. B cells can, however, be identified through the use of flow cytometry (see chapter 18, this volume). In this technique, cells are characterized by their expression of cell surface markers and the percentage and absolute number of B cells expressing certain immunophenotypes are compared to age-matched reference values (36). The most classic B-cell surface markers are CD19 and CD20 (Table 1). CD19 is a critical signal transduction molecule that regulates B-lymphocyte development, differentiation, and activation. Its expression is seen on B cells from the earliest recognizable B-lineage (early immunoglobulin gene rearrangements) to B-cell blasts. However, the expression is lost upon plasma cell maturation. CD20 is expressed on B cells from the pre-B stage to the B-cell lymphoblast stage but is not found on early B-cell progenitors or plasma cells. In general, CD19$^+$ CD20$^+$ cells constitute between 5 and 10% of the total peripheral blood lymphocyte pool. Upon antigen activation, a number of cell surface markers are detected on B cells (Table 1). The presence or absence of these markers can be useful in the evaluation of B-cell deficiencies in patients. One recent example is the absence of CD27$^+$ IgD$^-$ IgM$^-$ mature class-switched memory B cells in X-linked hyper-IgM syndrome and a subpopulation of patients with common variable immunodeficiency (1, 30, 39). It has also recently been reported that flow cytometry can be used to identify antigen-specific B cells, using the fact that the BCR can be "stained" by its specific antigen (37).

In Vitro B-Cell Function

Flow cytometric analysis of B-cell populations is only useful to identify defects in the actual numbers of B cells. In order to identify functional abnormalities, additional studies must be undertaken. The classic evaluation of B-cell function is through isolating peripheral blood lymphocytes from the patient and culturing them with agents known to activate normal B cells. This assay is known as the lymphocyte proliferation assay (LPA) (14, 35). In the LPA, either whole blood or purified peripheral blood mononuclear cells (PBMC) are cultured with a variety of stimulants to determine the B-cell response. The cells are cultured with the stimulants for 3 to 7 days, and the effects of this activation can be measured by cellular proliferation and antibody secretion. The agents that specifically activate B cells are listed in Table 3. B cells can also be exposed to protein antigens such as tetanus toxoid, and then specific antibody (and isotype) secretion into the media can be characterized. As the amount of antibody secreted is small, these levels cannot be detected by nephelometry, and enzyme-linked immunosorbent assay (ELISA) or ELISPOT must be used instead (see chapter 28, this volume). As LPAs are not available in most clinical immunology laboratories, this testing must often be performed on patient samples that are shipped to a specialized testing facility. This sample transport introduces a significant concern regarding sample integrity, as the testing requires live, functional B cells for accuracy. Many laboratories performing LPAs consequently require a normal sample to be shipped with the patient sample, to control for transport issues.

TABLE 3 In vitro activators for B-cell proliferation and immunoglobulin production

Activator[a]	Target	Dose range	Source[c]	Reference
SAC	BCR	0.004%	Calbiochem	9
Anti-IgM	BCR	10 μg/ml	BioRad	10
PWM	—[b]	1–10 μg/ml	Sigma	16
Tetanus toxoid	BCR	1–20 μg/ml	Wyeth	16

[a] SAC, *Staphylococcus aureus* Cowan I; PWM, pokeweed mitogen.
[b] PWM requires T cells to be present for its mitogenic effect on B cells; therefore, it is not a specific assay of B-cell function.
[c] Multiple sources exist for some products.

Cellular Proliferation

The ability of B cells to proliferate in response to stimulation in the LPA is usually presented as the stimulation index (SI). Currently the proliferative response is measured by the incorporation of tritiated thymidine ([³H]thymidine) into DNA of replicating cells. Therefore, the SI is expressed as the counts per minute of the stimulated wells divided by the counts per minute of the control wells (wells with patient B cells but no stimulus). A second method of reporting is the net counts per minute, which are the counts per minute of the stimulated wells minus the counts per minute of the control wells. An alternative method for the measurement of proliferation in the LPA is the analysis of the cell cycle by flow cytometry (2). In this readout of proliferation, stimulated and control cells are permeabilized and stained with propidium iodide, and the cells in the S phase of the cell cycle are counted. Normal ranges for proliferation in the LPA have been difficult to establish due to a high degree of variability in this assay secondary to different culture conditions in each laboratory. Therefore, the LPA is best utilized as a qualitative indicator of lymphocyte function, rather than a quantitative assay.

Secretion of Soluble Mediators

In addition to proliferation, stimulation of B cells in the LPA induces B cells to produce and secrete immunoglobulins. Measurement of mitogen- or antigen-induced immunoglobulin secretion will assess whether the immunoglobulin class or isotype of interest is produced in the amounts expected by age or disease state. The total culture levels of immunoglobulins are assayed by ELISA (see chapter 28, this volume). The amount of immunoglobulins produced can also be assayed at the single-cell level by ELISPOT. This assay is most useful to determine antigen-specific B-cell frequency, which is not determined by proliferation or total immunoglobulin assays.

APPROACHES FOR ASSESSING ANTIBODY FUNCTION

Antibodies provide protection to the host in various ways. Antibodies can neutralize toxins (e.g., tetanus toxin), neutralize viruses, prevent the adhesion of bacteria to the host cells, kill bacteria in the presence of complement, and opsonize bacteria for phagocytes (19). Consequently, a variety of assays can be used to measure antibody function. While antibody function assays can be performed with experimental animals, in vivo assays are impractical and thus in vitro assays are widely used. As examples of in vitro antibody function assays, we describe in vitro bactericidal assays and in vitro opsonization assays in detail below.

Bactericidal Assays

In bactericidal assays, antiserum is mixed with bacteria and complement. The antibodies bind to the bacteria and activate complement. The activation of the complement damages the bacterial surface and results in their death. The number of surviving bacteria can be determined by plating a sample of reaction mixture on an agar plate. Then, by testing the bactericidal properties of the serum samples at multiple dilutions, one can determine the dilution that kills half of the bacteria.

Generally, the complement-mediated bactericidal mechanism does not kill gram-positive bacteria, although there are exceptional cases (15). This mechanism is primarily relevant in the study of antibodies to gram-negative bacteria, which have thin walls. This assay method has been extensively used in developing meningococcal vaccines (38). Studies with meningococcal antibodies have shown that the animal source of the complement can influence the results. For example, generally rabbit serum produces higher bactericidal titers than human serum. In case of antibodies to group B meningococcus, human complement may detect antibodies to subcapsular antigens, but rabbit complement may detect antibodies to the capsule itself (38).

A major technical problem associated with the use of the bactericidal assay is determining the number of surviving bacteria. The classical approach is to plate the sample on an agar plate and count the bacterial colonies. This method is too tedious to use with a large number of samples. Although an effort has been made to automate the counting of bacterial colonies, other investigators have explored the use of dyes that either develop a color or become fluorescent in proportion to the number of live bacteria (20, 26, 31).

Opsonophagocytosis Assays

Opsonophagocytosis is the primary protective mechanism of antibodies against gram-positive bacteria. Various methods have been developed to measure the opsonizing capacity of antibodies in vitro. The classical approach is to perform an opsonophagocytic killing assay (18). In this assay, the bacteria are opsonized (coated) with antibodies and complement. Then the bacteria are exposed to phagocytes for phagocytosis and killing. The number of surviving bacteria is then determined. To rapidly determine the phagocytosis of bacteria, a new approach has recently been developed. In this approach, target bacteria are made fluorescent and the uptake of bacteria by phagocytes is measured with a flow cytometer (17, 24). Fluorescent bacteria can be prepared by chemically tagging a fluorochrome or by inserting a gene for a fluorescent protein.

Opsonophagocytosis assays have been extensively studied for use during the development of pneumococcal vaccines. Since pneumococcal vaccines induce antibodies against 7 to 23 different serotypes, there is a need to develop functional assays that can simultaneously study antibodies to multiple serotypes. The multiplex assays would reduce not only the amount of work but also the need for expensive reagents and precious serum samples. One approach is to use target bacteria labeled with different fluorochromes that flow cytometers can differentiate (23). A flow cytometer-based assay can then be used to identify the uptake of different target bacteria.

Another approach, the antibiotic resistance strategy, uses target bacterial species with different antibiotic resistances (6, 18, 28). For instance, one bacterial species can be susceptible to penicillin but resistant to streptomycin. The other can be susceptible to streptomycin but resistant to penicillin. If these two bacterial species are mixed and tested together, the number of surviving bacteria of each species can be determined by using agar plates containing different antibiotics. This strategy is simpler to use and has been used successfully for up to seven different target bacteria (6). With automation of colony counting, the antibiotic sensitivity strategy may be simpler to adopt.

The increased use of functional assays has shown the importance of standardization. In the past, the Centers for Disease Control and Prevention has coordinated a collaborative study to demonstrate that functional assays can be standardized if various aspects of the assays (e.g., protocol and reagents) can be carefully controlled (33). For opsonization assays, phagocytes can vary. For instance, peripheral blood granulocytes can differ depending on the donor's genetic traits (e.g., Fc receptor allele) or health status. Thus, the use of a cell line such as HL-60 has been promoted. A recent study showed that even the source of the cell line must be standardized because samples of a cell line from different sources appear to have different biological properties (12).

METHODOLOGIES

In Vitro Whole-Blood LPA

Materials and Reagents

RPMI 1640 (1×) liquid with L-glutamine, containing 10% human AB serum (heat inactivated for 1 h at 56°C)

Penicillin and streptomycin (P/S) (100×; 5,000 U of penicillin per ml and 5,000 μg of streptomycin per ml) liquid

Pokeweed mitogen (Sigma Chemical Co., St. Louis, Mo.) dissolved in phosphate-buffered saline (PBS) and kept frozen at −20°C at a concentration of 1 mg/ml. Keep frozen in small aliquots and use a fresh aliquot for each assay.

Tritiated thymidine ([³H]thymidine) sterile, aqueous solution

96-well round-bottomed tissue culture plates with lids (sterile)

Scintillation fluid

Pipette tips (sterile)

Ficoll-Hypaque (density, 1.077 g/liter)

PBS

15-ml conical centrifuge tubes

Serological pipettes (sterile)

Class II laminar-flow biosafety hood

CO_2 incubator with >95% humidity

Cell harvester

Pipetters and pipette aid

Procedure

1. Obtain a fresh heparinized venous blood sample. The sample should be held at room temperature (RT) prior to analysis and should be analyzed within 24 h of draw. A normal healthy control should be drawn at the same time as the patient sample and treated in a similar manner.

2. Dilute fresh heparinized blood 1:2 with sterile PBS and place in a 15-ml sterile conical centrifuge tube.

3. Underlay the Ficoll-Hypaque solution, using 3 ml of Ficoll-Hypaque per 10 ml of blood-PBS mixture.

4. Centrifuge for 20 min at 400 × g in a refrigerated centrifuge at 18 to 20°C, with no brake.

5. Harvest the PBMC from the interface using a sterile pipette and wash three times in PBS (200 × g, 10 min, 18 to 20°C).

6. Resuspend PBMC in RPMI 1640–10% AB serum, with P/S and glutamine at 10^6 live cells/ml. Use PBMC within 1 h. Viability can be ascertained by trypan blue exclusion.

7. In a sterile hood, add 100 μl of each antigen/mitogen concentration being tested to each well. This needs to be done in triplicate.

8. Add 100 μl of the diluted PBMC to each well.

9. Put on the sterile lid and place the plate in a CO_2 incubator at 37°C with 5% CO_2. To measure cell proliferation, incubate for 3 days for mitogens and 6 to 7 days for recall antigens.

10. To determine cell proliferation by [³H]thymidine incorporation, on the morning of day 3, each well is pulsed with 0.5 μCi of [³H]thymidine in 20 μl of RPMI 1640 (no serum). After 6 h the cells are harvested on fiberglass filters using a cell harvester. The filters are placed into scintillation fluid and counted on a beta scintillation counter. Triplicates are averaged and the SI is reported.

11. To assay for total antibody production, the assays are incubated for 7 days at 37°C with 5% CO_2. Remove the culture supernatant and use for ELISA determination (see chapter 28, this volume).

H. influenzae Type b

This procedure was adapted from the protocol of S. Romero-Steiner et al. used by the Centers for Disease Control and Prevention (32, 34).

Materials and Reagents

Microtiter plate (round bottom)

Cryovial

Chocolate II agar plates (catalog no. 21169-21267; Becton Dickinson)

Fildes enrichment (catalog no. 220810; BBL, Sparks, Md.) (see note 1 of assay notes at end of the procedure)

Brain heart infusion (BHI) broth

BHI broth with 2% Fildes enrichment (5)

Hanks' buffer with Ca^{2+} and Mg^{2+} (Life Technologies)

Dilution buffer: Hanks' buffer with Ca and Mg and 2% Fildes enrichment

Bacteria: *H. influenzae* type b strain Eagan or GB3292

Newborn rabbit serum for complement (Pel-Freez, Brown Deer, Wis.)

CBER standard serum (lot 1983). A serum standard from the Food and Drug Administration with 70 μg of antibody per ml is available.

Gamma globulin (Bayer, Elkhart, Ind.) for quality control purposes

Procedure for Preparing Bacteria

1. Inoculate *Haemophilus* bacteria onto a chocolate II agar plate and incubate the plate overnight (16 h) at 37°C in a 5% CO_2 atmosphere.

2. Transfer about 10 isolated bacterial colonies to 20 ml of BHI broth with 2% Fildes enrichment in a 50-ml glass vial and incubate at 37°C and 5% CO_2 until the optical density at 600 nm becomes 0.4 to 0.5 (note 2).

3. Add 3 ml of sterile glycerol to the bacterial culture (20 ml). Mix well. Dispense 0.5 ml into each cryovial.

4. Quickly freeze all cryovials (except one) at −70°C. Once frozen, store the vials at −70°C until use. The non-frozen vial will be used in step 5.

5. Determine the bacterial recovery from frozen vials. (It should be greater than 80%.)

    a. Thaw a vial of frozen bacteria (step 4).

    b. Dilute both the unfrozen and thawed bacteria (step 4) 10^{-6}-, 10^{-7}-, and 10^{-8}-fold in dilution buffer.

    c. Plate 100 μl from each dilution onto a chocolate II agar plate.

    d. Incubate the plates overnight at 37°C in a candle jar.

    e. Count the colonies.

    f. Determine the ratio of the number of thawed bacteria to the number of unfrozen bacteria. The ratio should be >0.8.

6. Determine the dilution necessary to get about 1,000 CFU per 20 μl.

    a. Prepare six tubes with 0.9 ml of dilution buffer.

    b. Rapidly thaw an aliquot of bacteria.

    c. Add 100 μl of thawed bacteria to 1 ml of dilution buffer. Perform 10-fold serial dilutions by transferring 100 μl.

    d. Plate 10 μl in triplicate onto a chocolate II agar plate.

    e. Incubate the plates overnight at 37°C in a candle jar.

    f. Count the colonies and determine the average.

    g. Determine the dilution factor required to yield 1,000 CFU/20 μl.

Assay Procedure (note 4)

1. Perform twofold serial dilutions (8 or 10 dilutions) of antisera with dilution buffer.

2. Add 10 μl of diluted antiserum to duplicate wells of a microtiter plate.

3. Thaw an aliquot of bacteria.

4. Dilute the thawed bacteria in dilution buffer to prepare 1,000 CFU/20 μl.

5. Add 20 μl of the diluted bacterial suspension.

6. Incubate at 37°C for 15 min in a 5% CO_2 incubator.

7. Add 25 μl of baby rabbit complement (note 3).

8. Add 25 μl of dilution buffer.

9. Incubate the plates at 37°C for 60 min in a 5% CO_2 incubator.

10. Plate 5 μl of the reaction mixture onto a chocolate II agar plate.

11. Incubate the plates at 37°C in 5% CO_2 for 16 h.

12. Count the surviving bacteria.

13. Determine the serum dilution that kills ≥50% of the bacteria.

Assay Notes

Note 1: Fildes enrichment is a peptic digest of sheep blood. It is rich in hemin and NAD. Although 5% supplement is usually used (5), we found that 2% supplement is sufficient for bactericidal assays.

Note 2: Bacteria will be in the exponential phase of growth. It takes about 2 to 3 h. The broth acquires an amber color.

Note 3: Complement lots should be qualified prior to use in the assay. Both active and heat-inactivated baby rabbit complement is used to show that no bacterial killing is found during a 1-h incubation period.

Note 4: Serum growth controls (all reagents except complement source) should be included when the serum source is unknown or it is suspected to contain antibiotics or any other inhibitory substances.

Double Serotype Opsonophagocytic Killing Assay

The procedure for the double serotype opsonophagocytic killing assay was adapted from that described by Kim et al. (18).

Materials and Reagents

Tissue culture flask, vent cap (T-75 cm²) (no. 430641; Corning)

Tissue culture flask, vent cap (T-150 cm²) (no. 430825; Corning)

Microtiter plate (round bottom) (no. 3799; Costar)

Square petri dish (100 by 15 cm) (no. 08-757-10K; Fisher)

N,N-Dimethylformamide (DMF) (no. D131-1; Fisher)

2,3,5,-Triphenyltetrazolium chloride (TTC) (no. T-8877; Sigma)

Streptomycin sulfate (no. S-6501; Sigma)

Optochin (ethylhydrocupreine hydrochloride) (no. E-9876; Sigma)

Todd-Hewitt broth (no. 249240; Difco)

Yeast extract (no. 212750; Difco)

Bacto Agar (no. 214010; Difco)

10× Hanks' balanced salt solution (HBSS) (without Ca, Mg, or phenol red) (no. 14185-052; Gibco BRL)

10× HBSS (with Ca and Mg, without phenol red) (no. 14065-056; Gibco BRL)

RPMI 1640 (no. MT 10-040-CMRF; CellGro)

P/S (100×) (no. 15140-148; Gibco [Invitrogen])

GlutaMax-1 (100×) (no. 35050-061; Gibco [Invitrogen])

Fetal bovine serum (FBS; Fetalclone 1) (no. SH30080.03; HyClone)

Baby rabbit complement (no. 31038-100; Pel-Freez)

HL-60 cell line (CCL-240; American Type Culture Collection)

Target bacteria: These are shown in Table 4 (*target pneumococci are available from the NIH Respiratory Pathogen Reference Laboratory at* the University of Alabama at Birmingham, Birmingham, Ala.).

World Health Organization pneumococcal assay validation sera: These are available from D. Goldblatt in London, England.

−70°C ethanol: Keep a beaker with 400 ml of ethanol at −70°C for freezing bacteria.

Streptomycin stock solution: Prepare a 100-mg/ml stock solution in water. Make 1-ml aliquots and store at −20°C.

Optochin stock solution: Prepare a 5-mg/ml stock solution in water. Make 1-ml aliquots and store at −20°C.

Glycerol stock: Mix 20 ml of water and 100 g of glycerol. Autoclave and store at RT.

1% Sterile gelatin stock solution: Add 1 g of gelatin to 100 ml of water. Autoclave and store at RT.

Overlay agar: Add 15 g of Todd-Hewitt broth, 2.5 g of yeast extract, and 3.75 g of Bacto Agar to 500 ml of water. Autoclave and store at RT.

Todd-Hewitt–yeast broth (THY broth): Add 30 g of Todd-Hewitt broth and 5 g of yeast extract to 1 liter of water. Autoclave and store at 4°C.

Todd-Hewitt–yeast extract agar plate (THYA plate): Add 15 g of Todd-Hewitt broth, 2.5 g of yeast extract, and 7.5 g of Bacto Agar to 500 ml of water. Autoclave and let it cool down (to about 56°C). Pour 12 ml into a square petri dish and allow the plates to cool to RT. Store at 4°C in a humidified chamber for up to 1 month.

TTC stock solution for overlay agar: Dissolve 1 g of TTC in 100 ml of water, filter sterilize (0.22 μm pore size), and store at 4°C protected from light (up to 2 months). Warm the TTC stock solution to RT to dissolve any precipitate before use.

Procedures

Procedure for Routine HL-60 Cell Propagation

1. Add 100 ml of the tissue culture medium (RPMI 1640 with 1% L-glutamine plus 10% FBS + 1× P/S) with HL-60 cells (~10^5 cells/ml) to a T-75 cm^2 flask.

TABLE 4 Pneumococcal strains used as targets for the opsonization assay

Serotype	Name
4	OREP4
6A	OREP6A
6B	STREP6B
9V	STREP9V
14	OREP14
18C	OREP18C
19A	STREP19A
19F	OREP19F
23F	STREP23F

2. Place the flasks in an incubator (37°C, 5% CO_2, see note 6); they can lie flat or upright.

3. When the cells become confluent, split the culture 10× (e.g., 10 ml of cells/90 ml of fresh medium).

4. The feeding cycle is ~2 to 3 days.

Procedure for HL-60 Cell Differentiation

1. Centrifuge the HL-60 cells at 1,200 rpm (Sorvall, RT-7 with RTH-250 rotor) for 5 to 10 min at RT. Remove **ALL** of the supernatant (to completely remove any antibiotics).

2. Gently resuspend the cell pellet in the differentiating medium (RPMI 1640 with 1% L-glutamine + 10% FBS + DMF [0.8%, vol/vol]) and adjust the concentration to ~4 × 10^5 cells/ml.

3. Add 100 ml of the cell suspension to a T-150 cm^2 flask.

4. Incubate the flask in an incubator (37°C, 5% CO_2; see note 6) for 5 to 6 days; it can lie flat or upright. Do not feed the culture during this period.

5. Two flasks will usually yield enough differentiated cells to prepare four to six microtiter assay plates at ~150:1 (HL-60 cells to bacteria).

Procedure for Preparing Target Bacteria

1. Inoculate bacteria onto a blood agar plate and incubate overnight at 37°C in a candle jar (note 1). Pneumococci yield alpha-hemolytic colonies that can be identified by a green halo surrounding the colony.

2. Transfer ~10 isolated colonies to each of 10 tubes containing 10 ml of THY broth. Incubate for 3 to 6 h in a 37°C water bath until the top 150 μl of the culture broth has an optical density at 600 nm of 0.2 to 0.4.

3. Harvest the top 2 ml of the broth from each of the 10 tubes and pool (the pool will be 20 ml).

4. Add 7.6 ml of the 80% sterile glycerol and 20 ml of THY broth to the 20-ml bacterial pool. Dispense 0.5-ml aliquots into cryovials.

5. Do **NOT** freeze one vial, which will be used in step 6. Quickly freeze all the remaining cryovials in 95% ethanol kept at −70°C, and store the vials frozen at −70°C until used. The frozen vials can be stored up to ~18 months.

6. Determine whether the viability of frozen bacteria is greater than 80% using the unfrozen aliquot from step 5.

7. Determine the dilution necessary to get about 100 CFU/5 μl on THYA plates (note 2).

Procedure for the Double Serotype Opsonization Assay

1. Incubate the serum samples to be tested at 56°C for 30 min to inactivate the endogenous complement.

2. Dry the THYA plates by removing the lids and placing the plates in a laminar-flow hood for 30 to 60 min (see note 4). After plates are dry, replace lid to prevent overdrying, and keep at RT until needed.

3. Prepare opsonization buffer B by mixing 35 ml of sterile water, 5 ml of 10× Hanks' buffer (with Ca^{2+} and Mg^{2+}), 5 ml of 1% gelatin, and 5 ml of FBS. Prepare 1× HBSS (without Ca^{2+}, Mg^{2+}, or phenol red) and 1× HBSS (with Ca^{2+} and Mg^{2+}, without phenol red).

4. Locate (but do not remove) the frozen bacteria and complement in the −70°C freezer.

5. Prepare the microtiter assay plates (see note 7 for an example of assay setup).

    a. Add 20 μl of opsonization buffer B to rows A through G, columns 1 through 12. Also, add 20 μl of opsonization buffer B to row H, columns 1 and 2, but **NOT** to row H, columns 3 through 12.

    b. Add 30 μl of heat-inactivated serum samples (in duplicate) to row H, columns 3 through 12, according to the template. Perform threefold serial dilutions by transferring 10 μl from row H to G, mixing, and transferring 10 μl from row G to F, etc. Serum samples added to row H are undiluted. Serum samples yielding a high titer may have to be retested at a higher starting dilution.

6. Rapidly thaw an aliquot of each of the two frozen bacterial strains and dilute them according to the dilution factors calculated earlier in opsonization buffer B. Add 10 μl of the bacterial mixture to each well, including all control wells.

7. Incubate the microtiter plates at RT for 30 min without shaking.

8. During this time, take the complement out of the freezer to thaw. Also, melt the overlay agar in a microwave and place in 56°C water bath until needed (note 5).

9. Also, during this incubation, prepare the differentiated HL-60 cells.

    a. Transfer the DMF-differentiated HL-60 cells from the culture flasks to 50-ml centrifuge tubes.

    b. Centrifuge the HL-60 cells at 1,200 rpm (e.g., Sorvall, RT-7 with RTH-250 rotor) for 5 min at RT.

    c. Remove the supernatant and wash the cells with 1× HBSS (without Ca^{2+} or Mg^{2+}) by centrifugation as described above.

    d. Remove the supernatant and wash the cells with 1× HBSS (with Ca^{2+} and Mg^{2+}) by centrifugation as described above.

    e. Remove the supernatant, and suspend the cells at 10^7 cells/ml in opsonization buffer B. Keep the cells at RT until needed.

10. Following the 30-min incubation (step 7 above), add 10 μl of complement to the appropriate wells (add 10 μl of opsonization buffer B to the appropriate control wells).

11. Add 40 μl of HL-60 cells to the appropriate wells (add 40 μl of opsonization buffer B to the appropriate control wells).

12. Incubate the microtiter plates on a shaker (400 rpm) for 60 min at 37°C.

13. After the incubation period, place the microtiter plates on ice (to stop the phagocytic process).

14. Plate 5 μl of reaction mixture from each well onto two THYA plates (one plate will receive overlay containing optochin and the second plate will receive overlay containing streptomycin). Using a multichannel pipette, remove 5 μl from each well in an eight-well column, and apply as eight 5-μl spots to THYA plates on the left side, center, and right side of the plate (for a total of three microtiter plate columns, or 24 individual wells). Tilt the plates to the right to shape the spot into a small strip of fluid (~1.5 to 2 cm long).

15. Leave the plates at RT for 10 to 20 min to let the excess fluid seep into the agar.

A

	Row Letter	Column Number							Sample Dilution
		1	2	3 & 4	5 & 6	7 & 8	9 & 10	11 & 12	
	A	Bac. Only	Bac.+HL60	1/2187	1/2187	1/2187	1/2187	1/2187	
	B	Bac. Only	Bac.+HL60	1/729	1/729	1/729	1/729	1/729	
	C	Bac. Only	Bac.+HL60	1/243	1/243	1/243	1/243	1/243	
	D	Bac. Only	Bac.+HL60	1/81	1/81	1/81	1/81	1/81	
	E	Bac.+Comp.	Bac.+Comp.+HL60	1/27	1/27	1/27	1/27	1/27	
	F	Bac.+Comp.	Bac.+Comp.+HL60	1/9	1/9	1/9	1/9	1/9	
	G	Bac.+Comp.	Bac.+Comp.+HL60	1/3	1/3	1/3	1/3	1/3	
	H	Bac.+Comp.	Bac.+Comp.+HL60	Neat	Neat	Neat	Neat	Neat	
		Controls		Sample 1	Sample 2	Sample 3	Sample 4	Sample 5	

B

	Row Letter	Column Number						Sample Dilution
		1 & 2	3 & 4	5 & 6	7 & 8	9 & 10	11 & 12	
	A	1/2187	1/2187	1/2187	1/2187	1/2187	1/2187	
	B	1/729	1/729	1/729	1/729	1/729	1/729	
	C	1/243	1/243	1/243	1/243	1/243	1/243	
	D	1/81	1/81	1/81	1/81	1/81	1/81	
	E	1/27	1/27	1/27	1/27	1/27	1/27	
	F	1/9	1/9	1/9	1/9	1/9	1/9	
	G	1/3	1/3	1/3	1/3	1/3	1/3	
	H	Neat	Neat	Neat	Neat	Neat	Neat	
		Sample 6	Sample 7	Sample 8	Sample 9	Sample 10	Sample 11	

FIGURE 1 Setup template for assay with multiple plates. (A) First plate arrangement. (B) Additional plate arrangement.

16. Divide equally the overlay agar (56°C) into two containers. Add TTC to a final concentration of 25 μg/ml to each container of overlay agar (note 3).

17. To one container of overlay agar, add optochin to a final concentration of 1.5 μg/ml. Add 12 ml of this overlay per plate to one replicate of the THYA plates spotted in step 14 above.

18. To the other container of overlay agar, add streptomycin to a final concentration of 150 μg/ml. Add 12 ml of this overlay per plate to the second replicate of the THYA plates spotted in step 14 above.

19. After the overlay has solidified (~30 min), place the plates, right side up, in a candle jar and incubate them for 16 to 18 h at 37°C. Colonies that grow on the THYA plates with the optochin overlay are bacteria of the optochin-resistant serotype, and those that grow on the THYA plates containing streptomycin are bacteria of the streptomycin-resistant serotype.

20. Count colonies and calculate the opsonization titer. The opsonization titer is the final dilution of serum that gives half the number of colonies as the complement/HL-60 control wells. If an undiluted serum sample killed 50% of the available bacteria but the next dilution (1/3) killed 0% of the available bacteria, then the opsonization titer is 4 [e.g., $1/(20/80) = 4$, where 20 is the volume of serum in microliters and 80 is the total volume of the reaction in microliters].

Assay Notes

Note 1: To maintain the integrity of the pneumococcal bacterial stock cultures, remove the stock vial(s) containing bacteria from the freezer, quickly remove a fleck of ice from the stock vial, and immediately streak onto a blood agar plate. Replace the stock vial into the freezer promptly.

Note 2: Baby rabbit complement and/or HL-60 cells can influence the number of viable bacterial cells. Their effect must be determined ahead of time and should be considered in calculating the final dilution of bacteria used in the opsonophagocytic killing assay.

Note 3: TTC turns red upon heating and should **NOT** be added before autoclaving or before reheating in a microwave oven. Add TTC to the agar after it cools to ~56°C.

Note 4: Drying the THYA plates for the correct amount of time is very important. Usually 30 to 60 min is sufficient, although drying times vary depending on the humidity in the air. Underdrying the plates results in an excess number of colonies around the perimeter of the spot. This can affect the counting of the colonies. Overdrying the plates can cause the spots to run together when the plates are tilted.

Note 5: Use a microwave oven to reheat the agar slowly to avoid boiling and accidental burns.

Note 6: It is important to maintain the CO_2 concentration at ~5%, as HL-60 cells are sensitive to subtle pH changes that can occur when the percent CO_2 changes. It is recommended that the percent CO_2 be checked regularly with an outside reference (such as a FYRITE gas analyzer produced by Bacharach, Pittsburgh, Pa.).

Note 7: A setup template for a typical assay involving multiple plates is shown in Fig. 1. Note that control wells are found only on the first plate.

REFERENCES

1. **Agematsu, K., T. Futatani, S. Hokibara, N. Kobayashi, M. Takamoto, S. Tsukada, H. Suzuki, S. Koyasu, T. Miyawaki, K. Sugane, A. Komiyama, and H. D. Ochs.** 2002. Absence of memory B cells in patients with common variable immunodeficiency. *Clin. Immunol.* **103:**34–42.

2. **Aguilar, P., E. Renoult, L. Jarrosson, M. N. Kolopp-Sarda, C. P. Mathieu, G. C. Faure, M. Kessler, M. C. Bene, C. Kohler, and A. Kennel De March.** 2003. Anti-HBs cellular immune response in kidney recipients before and 4 months after transplantation. *Clin. Diagn. Lab. Immunol.* **10:**1117–1122.

3. **Alam, R., and M. Gorska.** 2003. 3. Lymphocytes. *J. Allergy Clin. Immunol.* **111:**S476–S485.

4. **Balmer, P., J. North, D. Baxter, E. Stanford, A. Melegaro, E. B. Kaczmarski, E. Miller, and R. Borrow.** 2003. Measurement and interpretation of pneumococcal IgG levels for clinical management. *Clin. Exp. Immunol.* **133:**364–369.

5. **Bergeron, M. G., P. Simard, and P. J. Provencher.** 1987. Influence of growth medium and supplement on growth of *Haemophilus influenzae* and on antibacterial activity of several antibiotics. *J. Clin. Microbiol.* **25:**650–655.

6. **Bogaert, D., M. Sluijter, R. De Groot, and P. W. Hermans.** 2004. Multiplex opsonophagocytosis assay (MOPA): a useful tool for the monitoring of the 7-valent pneumococcal conjugate vaccine. *Vaccine* **22:**4014–4020.

7. **Buckley, R. H.** 2002. Immunoglobulin G subclass deficiency: fact or fancy? *Curr. Allergy Asthma Rep.* **2:**356–360.

8. **Buckley, R. H., S. C. Dees, and W. M. O'Fallon.** 1968. Serum immunoglobulins. I. Levels in normal children and in uncomplicated childhood allergy. *Pediatrics* **41:**600–611.

9. **Butch, A. W., K. A. Macke, M. G. Scott, M. Inkster, and M. H. Nahm.** 1989. Mitogen-induced human IgG subclass expression. II. IgG1 and IgG3 subclasses are preferentially stimulated by a combination of *Staphylococcus aureus* Cowan I and pokeweed mitogen. *Hum. Immunol.* **24:**207–218.

10. **Butch, A. W., and M. H. Nahm.** 1992. Functional properties of human germinal center B cells. *Cell. Immunol.* **140:**331–344.

11. **Carneiro-Sampaio, M. M., A. S. Grumach, and A. Manissadjian.** 1991. Laboratory screening for the diagnosis of children with primary immunodeficiencies. *J. Investig. Allergol. Clin. Immunol.* **1:**195–200.

12. **Fleck, R. A., S. Romero-Steiner, and M. H. Nahm.** 2005. Use of HL-60 cell line to measure opsonic capacity of pneumococcal antibodies. *Clin. Diagn. Lab. Immunol.* **12:**19–27.

13. **Fleisher, T. A., and J. B. Oliveira.** 2004. Functional and molecular evaluation of lymphocytes. *J. Allergy Clin. Immunol.* **114:**227–234; quiz 235.

14. **Folds, J. D., and J. L. Schmitz.** 2003. 24. Clinical and laboratory assessment of immunity. *J. Allergy Clin. Immunol.* **111:**S702–S711.

15. **Fusco, P. C., J. W. Perry, S. M. Liang, M. S. Blake, F. Michon, and J. Y. Tai.** 1997. Bactericidal activity elicited by the beta C protein of group B streptococci contrasted with capsular polysaccharides. *Adv. Exp. Med. Biol.* **418:**841–845.

16. **James, S. P.** 2004. Measurement of basic immunologic characteristics of human mononuclear cells, p. 7.10.1–7.10.6. *In* J. E. Coligan, A. M. Kruisgeek, D. H. Margulies, E. M. Shevach, and W. Strober (ed.), *Current Protocols in Immunology.* John Wiley & Sons, New York, N.Y.

17. **Jansen, W. T., M. Vakevainen-Anttila, H. Kayhty, M. Nahm, N. Bakker, J. Verhoef, H. Snippe, and A. F. Verheul.** 2001. Comparison of a classical phagocytosis assay and a flow cytometry assay for assessment of the phagocytic capacity of sera from adults vaccinated with a pneumococcal conjugate vaccine. *Clin. Diagn. Lab. Immunol.* **8:**245–250.

18. **Kim, K. H., J. Yu, and M. H. Nahm.** 2003. Efficiency of a pneumococcal opsonophagocytic killing assay improved by multiplexing and by coloring colonies. *Clin. Diagn. Lab. Immunol.* **10:**616–621.

19. **Langermann, S., S. Palaszynski, M. Barnhart, G. Auguste, J. S. Pinkner, J. Burlein, P. Barren, S. Koenig, S. Leath, C. H. Jones, and S. J. Hultgren.** 1997. Prevention of mucosal *Escherichia coli* infection by FimH-adhesin-based systemic vaccination. *Science* **276:**607–611.

20. **Lin, J. S., M. K. Park, and M. H. Nahm.** 2001. Chromogenic assay measuring opsonophagocytic killing capacities of antipneumococcal antisera. *Clin. Diagn. Lab. Immunol.* **8:**528–533.

21. **Maguire, G. A., D. S. Kumararatne, and H. J. Joyce.** 2002. Are there any clinical indications for measuring IgG subclasses? *Ann. Clin. Biochem.* **39:**374–377.

22. **Martin, F., and J. F. Kearney.** 2001. B1 cells: similarities and differences with other B cell subsets. *Curr. Opin. Immunol.* **13:**195–201.

23. **Martinez, J., T. Pilishvili, S. Barnard, J. Caba, W. Spear, S. Romero-Steiner, and G. M. Carlone.** 2002. Opsonophagocytosis of fluorescent polystyrene beads coupled to *Neisseria meningitidis* serogroup A, C, Y, or W135 polysaccharide correlates with serum bactericidal activity. *Clin. Diagn. Lab. Immunol.* **9:**485–488.

24. **Martinez, J. E., S. Romero-Steiner, T. Pilishvili, S. Barnard, J. Schinsky, D. Goldblatt, and G. M. Carlone.** 1999. A flow cytometric opsonophagocytic assay for measurement of functional antibodies elicited after vaccination with the 23-valent pneumococcal polysaccharide vaccine. *Clin. Diagn. Lab. Immunol.* **6:**581–586.

25. **McHeyzer-Williams, M. G.** 2003. B cells as effectors. *Curr. Opin. Immunol.* **15:**354–361.

26. **Mountzouros, K. T., and A. P. Howell.** 2000. Detection of complement-mediated antibody-dependent bactericidal activity in a fluorescence-based serum bactericidal assay for group B *Neisseria meningitidis. J. Clin. Microbiol.* **38:**2878–2884.

27. **Nahm, M. H., R. M. Blaese, M. J. Crain, and D. E. Briles.** 1986. Patients with Wiskott-Aldrich syndrome have normal IgG2 levels. *J. Immunol.* **137:**3484–3487.

28. **Nahm, M. H., D. E. Briles, and X. Yu.** 2000. Development of a multi-specificity opsonophagocytic killing assay. *Vaccine* **18:**2768–2771.

29. **Noroski, L. M., and W. T. Shearer.** 1998. Screening for primary immunodeficiencies in the clinical immunology laboratory. *Clin. Immunol. Immunopathol.* **86:**237–245.

30. **Piqueras, B., C. Lavenu-Bombled, L. Galicier, F. Bergeron-van der Cruyssen, L. Mouthon, S. Chevret, P. Debre, C. Schmitt, and E. Oksenhendler.** 2003. Common variable immunodeficiency patient classification based on impaired B cell memory differentiation correlates with clinical aspects. *J. Clin. Immunol.* **23:**385–400.

31. **Rodriguez, T., M. Lastre, B. Cedre, J. del Campo, G. Bracho, C. Zayas, C. Taboada, M. Diaz, G. Sierra, and O. Perez.** 2002. Standardization of *Neisseria meningitidis* serogroup B colorimetric serum bactericidal assay. *Clin. Diagn. Lab. Immunol.* **9:**109–114.

32. **Romero-Steiner, S., J. Fernandez, C. Biltoft, M. E. Wohl, J. Sanchez, J. Feris, S. Balter, O. S. Levine, and G. M. Carlone.** 2001. Functional antibody activity elicited by fractional doses of *Haemophilus influenzae* type b conjugate vaccine (polyribosylribitol phosphate-tetanus toxoid conjugate). *Clin. Diagn. Lab. Immunol.* **8:**1115–1119.

33. **Romero-Steiner, S., C. Frasch, N. Concepcion, D. Goldblatt, H. Kayhty, M. Vakevainen, C. Laferriere, D. Wauters, M. H. Nahm, M. F. Schinsky, B. D. Plikaytis, and G. M. Carlone.** 2003. Multilaboratory evaluation of a viability assay for measurement of opsonophagocytic antibodies specific to the capsular polysaccharides of *Streptococcus pneumoniae. Clin. Diagn. Lab. Immunol.* **10:**1019–1024.

34. **Romero-Steiner, S., W. Spear, N. Brown, P. Holder, T. Hennessy, P. Gomez De Leon, and G. M. Carlone.** 2004. Measurement of serum bactericidal activity specific for *Haemophilus influenzae* type b by using a chromogenic and fluorescent metabolic indicator. *Clin. Diagn. Lab. Immunol.* **11:**89–93.

35. **Scott, M. G., and M. H. Nahm.** 1984. Mitogen-induced human IgG subclass expression. *J. Immunol.* **133:**2454–2460.

36. **Shearer, W. T., H. M. Rosenblatt, R. S. Gelman, R. Oyomopito, S. Plaeger, E. R. Stiehm, D. W. Wara, S. D. Douglas, K. Luzuriaga, E. J. McFarland, R. Yogev, M. H. Rathore, W. Levy, B. L. Graham, and S. A. Spector.** 2003. Lymphocyte subsets in healthy children from birth through 18 years of age: the Pediatric AIDS Clinical Trials Group P1009 study. *J. Allergy Clin. Immunol.* **112:**973–980.

37. **Thiel, A., A. Scheffold, and A. Radbruch.** 2004. Antigen-specific cytometry—new tools arrived! *Clin. Immunol.* **111:**155–161.

38. **Vermont, C., and G. van den Dobbelsteen.** 2002. *Neisseria meningitidis* serogroup B: laboratory correlates of protection. *FEMS Immunol. Med. Microbiol.* **34:**89–96.

39. **Warnatz, K., A. Denz, R. Drager, M. Braun, C. Groth, G. Wolff-Vorbeck, H. Eibel, M. Schlesier, and H. H. Peter.** 2002. Severe deficiency of switched memory B cells (CD27(+)IgM(−)IgD(−)) in subgroups of patients with common variable immunodeficiency: a new approach to classify a heterogeneous disease. *Blood* **99:**1544–1551.

40. **Weber-Mzell, D., P. Kotanko, A. C. Hauer, U. Goriup, J. Haas, N. Lanner, W. Erwa, I. A. Ahmaida, S. Haitchi-Petnehazy, M. Stenzel, G. Lanzer, and J. Deutsch.** 2004. Gender, age and seasonal effects on IgA deficiency: a study of 7293 Caucasians. *Eur. J. Clin. Investig.* **34:**224–228.

CYTOKINES AND CHEMOKINES

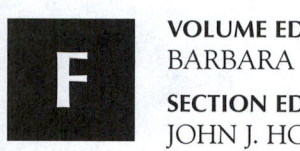

VOLUME EDITOR
BARBARA DETRICK
SECTION EDITOR
JOHN J. HOOKS

Introduction

JOHN J. HOOKS

38

Fifty years ago, Issacs and Lindenman first described the interferons as soluble molecules secreted by cells. When cells or a whole organism, such as an embryonating hen egg, were treated with interferon, virus replication was depressed. The field of cytokine biology and the related molecules, including chemokines and adhesion molecules, has come a long way from these early beginnings.

Today it is almost impossible to discuss normal homeostasis, development, or pathologic processes without including a description of cytokines, chemokines, and adhesion molecules. These multifunctional proteins exert biological properties which suggest a key role in hematopoiesis, immunity, infectious disease, tumorigenesis, homeostasis, tissue repair, and cellular development and growth. Because of their major participatory role in nearly all pathophysiologic processes and their therapeutic potential, there is a need to identify and measure cytokines, chemokines, and adhesion molecules. In the clinical laboratory, cytokine assessment has been used to monitor disease progression and activity. In addition, the increasing use of cytokines and cytokine antagonists as therapeutic modalities requires the measurement of cytokine levels to determine the pharmacokinetics of the administered molecule. In the research laboratory, the measurement of cytokine gene expression is currently being explored with the hope that this approach will offer clues to better define the mechanisms of cytokine action in disease processes.

This section encompasses reviews on cytokines and chemokines. The intent of this section is to provide the reader with an up-to-date description of appropriate ways to detect gene and/or protein expression of these molecules. We begin with an introductory chapter by Daniel Remick. In the 6th edition of this Manual, Remick provided a detailed overview of the varied forms of analysis of cytokines, focusing on protein analysis and bioassays of cytokines and cytokine receptors. In this 7th edition, Remick has focused on the newer multiplex technologies that are rapidly becoming available for laboratory analysis. Two of the newer technologies, flow cytometry and molecular analysis, have been assigned separate chapters. Ghanekar, Maecker, and Maino identify the utility of flow cytometric analysis of cytokines and cytokine receptors in chapter 40. They identify some of the recent advances with multiwell plate loaders for flow

cytometers. Chapter 41, by Kruse and Rieckmann, provides insight into approaches to monitor molecular analysis of cytokines and cytokine receptors. They focus on improvements of the recently developed real-time quantitative PCR. These methods provide high sensitivity and allow quantification of minute amounts of mRNA in small samples due to the exponential amplification of the target sequence and the generation of fluorescent molecules that are detected during the amplification reaction. Chapter 42, by Medoff and Luster, is devoted to an in-depth analysis of chemokines and chemokine receptors. This is clearly a rapidly developing area of study: analysis of chemokines continues to provide insight into the pathophysiology of several inflammatory diseases. The final chapter, by Andrew Pachner, contains new material not covered in previous editions and reflects the growing importance of cytokine therapy. Pachner identifies the various ways to monitor the development of antibody to cytokine therapy, with an emphasis on IFN-β therapy for multiple sclerosis.

In addition to the chapters included in this section, chapters incorporating discussions on cytokines, chemokines, or adhesion molecules can be found throughout this Manual. For example, section E incorporates several chapters that review various aspects of interactions among these molecules and selected cells of the immune system. O'Gorman addresses phagocytic cell function (chapter 31), McCloskey et al. focus on apoptosis (chapter 32), and Whiteside talks about NK cell assays (chapter 34). Likewise, in section Q, Reinsmoen and Zeevi (chapter 138) identify cytokines in their evaluation of cellular immune responses in transplantation. Also within that section, novel molecular approaches to detect cytokine and chemokine gene expression are extensively reviewed by Hartono et al. (chapter 139). They demonstrate a correlation of molecular detection of cytokines with rejection in solid organ transplantation.

This wide distribution and interest in cytokines, chemokines, and adhesion molecules reinforces the concept that these molecules are an integral part of a variety of immune cell functions. The immunology laboratory, with effective quality control and quality assurance programs, is in a unique position to provide the medical community with accurate identification and quantitation of these important bioregulatory molecules.

Multiplex Cytokine Assays

DANIEL G. REMICK

39

Cytokines are low-molecular-weight proteins representing important components of the inflammatory and immune responses (36). In response to external stimuli, they are rapidly induced and secreted into the extracellular milieu. In some situations, cytokines are constitutively present. Cytokines exert numerous biological activities which are critical for host defense, physiologic responses to stress, and immune surveillance. The world of cytokine biology has exploded in the past decades. It can be said without hyperbole that cytokines are critical from birth (gestation) (4) to death (apoptosis) (20).

Given the wide range of activities induced by cytokines, there is great interest in accurate measurement of these critical mediators. It is important to know if the cytokines are present during a particular disease process since they may potentially serve as a target for therapy (35). Conversely, there may be value in documenting that cytokines are depressed during a disease state such that the appropriate therapy is administration of exogenous cytokines such as granulocyte colony-stimulating factor. Clear evidence of the interest in measuring cytokines is demonstrated by the numerous companies which prepare and market kits for quantifying levels of cytokines.

Since there are numerous cytokines, a final biological outcome may not be dependent upon a single cytokine. Indeed, it has been reported that the ratio of cytokines to cytokine inhibitors provides the best documentation for progression of disease (1, 2). The best insights into the disease state will probably be achieved when multiple parameters are analyzed and assessed. As in making a clinical diagnosis, as much information as possible is needed in order to arrive at the correct determination for the precise disease process.

As a result of these issues, multiplex cytokine assays are beginning to be developed which will allow measurement of several cytokines simultaneously. While some of these assays were described over 5 years ago, they are beginning to mushroom into the commercial sector. As will be discussed further below, flow cytometric array assays are now marketed by more than 10 separate vendors. The technology has developed to the point that papers are now being written which directly compare the different kits from different vendors (17).

While this book chapter will examine measurement of cytokines, it should be borne in mind that this technology is not limited to measuring only these inflammatory mediators. Indeed, virtually any molecule that exhibits a specific interaction with another molecule may be measured by either a traditional enzyme-linked immunosorbent assay (ELISA) or a multiplex assay. Whether the interaction is a ligand-receptor interaction, a nucleic acid-protein interaction (3), or the traditional antibody-antigen interaction, the multiplex technology may be adapted to allow measurement (50). The principal consideration is the specificity of the interaction, such that the results are specific for measuring the analyte in question.

This chapter will explore both traditional ELISAs and the newer multiplexed assays. For each of the methods, I will examine the technology, instrumentation, and data analysis. Pitfalls that may arise with the assay will be explored to provide a better understanding of the limitations of the technique in question.

TRADITIONAL ELISA

I will begin with an explanation of the traditional ELISA. This is done because most of the newer assays are still based on the same antibody-antigen interaction that is most easily understood through examination of a single ELISA for a single cytokine. Virtually all ELISAs are based on the concept that a specific antibody will recognize a specific antigen. This concept dates back to the pioneering work of Yalow and Berson, who discovered that an antibody could recognize insulin (49). This single finding revolutionized the process for the detection and quantification of specific analytes.

Most commercially available ELISAs are based on a sandwich, or two-antibody, technique. A simpler method is the direct ELISA. For this assay, the antigen is bound directly to the surface of the microtiter well in the plate (Fig. 1). An antibody which specifically detects the cytokine in question is applied to the plate. For purposes of illustration, I use the cytokine interleukin 6 (IL-6) in the schematic figures. There are multiple methods for detecting the antibody bound to the antigen. The antibody may be directly conjugated to an enzyme such as horseradish peroxidase. An enzymatic reaction will occur within the well of the microtiter plate. Alternatively, the antibody may be detected by a second antibody. For example, the first antibody may be a mouse monoclonal antibody which recognizes human IL-6. The second antibody may then be a goat anti-mouse antibody which has been labeled with horseradish peroxidase. An alternative method for detecting the primary antibody is

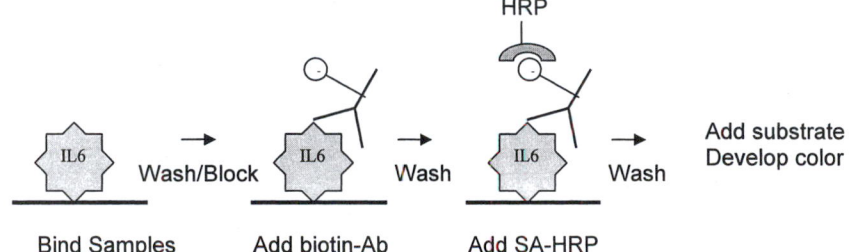

FIGURE 1 Direct ELISA. In the direct ELISA, the analyte is first bound to the bottom of the microtiter well. In this example, the analyte is IL-6. Unbound IL-6 is washed away, and excess protein binding sites are blocked in order to reduce background. In the next step, biotin-labeled antibody (biotin-Ab) directed against IL-6 is added; the small circle represents the biotin moiety directly attached to the antibody. After washing, streptavidin (SA) conjugated to horseradish peroxidase (HRP) is added and a final wash is performed. Following addition of a colorimetric substrate, the color develops. The intensity of the color development is directly proportional to the amount of IL-6 in the first step.

to attach a biotin moiety to the antibody. Streptavidin conjugated to horseradish peroxidase is applied next. For all of these assays, the enzyme conjugated to the detection moiety develops color. The process follows a fairly simple equation in which more antigen present results in more antibody binding which results in greater concentrations of the enzyme which results in stronger color development.

For the sandwich ELISA, there is a slight modification. First, an antibody is bound to the surface of the microtiter well (Fig. 2). This antibody has specificity for the cytokine which will be detected, in this case IL-6. The sample is then applied to the well, and the IL-6 binds to the antibody. During washing, all the proteins which are not IL-6 should be washed away. The only entity remaining in the well should be the IL-6 bound to the antibody. Subsequent development steps are similar to those for the direct ELISA described above.

There are several critical elements in developing a sensitive and specific ELISA. The same critical elements apply to multiplexing assays, but again these elements are more easily understood when a single cytokine is considered. First and foremost, the primary factor driving the sensitivity and specificity is the quality of the antibodies (26, 47). There is simply no substitute for having high-quality antibodies for the assay. As a specific example, antibodies are available which detect the precursor form of IL-1β but not the mature, processed form (7, 8). This may result in gross underestimation of the total amount of IL-1β present in cell lysates, because the antibodies selected for detection may not be optimal. In many situations, the antibodies have already been matched for the development of a sandwich ELISA. With a few simple techniques, it is possible to buy these antibodies and establish ELISAs for the detection of cytokines in one's own laboratory (25). In this regard, the commercial vendors are excellent sources of good-quality reagents.

Another important aspect is the selection of the proper blocking reagent. After the antigen or the antibody has been applied to the plate, it is important that nonspecific binding sites on the plate are blocked. In my experience, it is not possible to predict the optimal blocking reagent and testing needs to be done in order to determine which reagent will work the best. The "matrix" of the sample may also affect the best blocking reagent. For example, in tissue culture supernatants, the protein content is extremely low compared to that in organ homogenates or plasma. A blocking reagent such as bovine serum albumin which works quite

well for tissue culture supernatants may be suboptimal for measuring cytokines in human plasma. Testing different blocking reagents, which are available from the commercial vendors, will generally produce a low background.

Different enzymes may be conjugated to the detection moiety, whether it is an antibody or streptavidin. Horseradish peroxidase is the most commonly used enzyme, but alkaline phosphatase may also be used.

A number of substrates may be used in the assay; the substrate will depend upon the enzyme used for detection. The color development reagents are available from a number of commercial vendors, and they may be purchased already prepared. It is also possible to buy the individual reagents necessary for the substrate preparation and assemble one's own color detection components. This results in significant cost savings compared to purchasing already prepared material and in my hands results in similar sensitivity and specificity (25). Several authors have reported that the use of chemiluminescent reagents results in greater sensitivity (18, 27, 31, 39). I have found that careful attention to the details of the assay will allow the development of an ELISA using the colorimetric reagents that has better sensitivity than the chemiluminescent assays and also results in significant cost savings (41).

Once the assay has been completed, it is necessary to calculate the results. Typically, the readout from an ELISA reader is the absorbance measured at a specific wavelength. If a fluorescent or chemiluminescent detection reagent has been used, then relative light units are the output. Regardless of the output, the actual concentrations of the cytokine in the sample are determined by comparison to a standard curve. There are several commercial software programs available which will perform these calculations. These programs may come bundled with the plate reader, or one may purchase separate, stand-alone software. Examples of data analysis are presented later in this chapter.

This has been a brief overview of the traditional ELISA, an assay run literally in hundreds of labs thousands of times every week. This assay is robust and relatively straightforward and has exquisite sensitivity and specificity. Given the tremendous utility of measuring a single cytokine, a natural extension is to measure multiple cytokines.

SEQUENTIAL ELISA

One easy method for measuring multiple cytokines in a single sample is to perform a sequential ELISA. In most biological

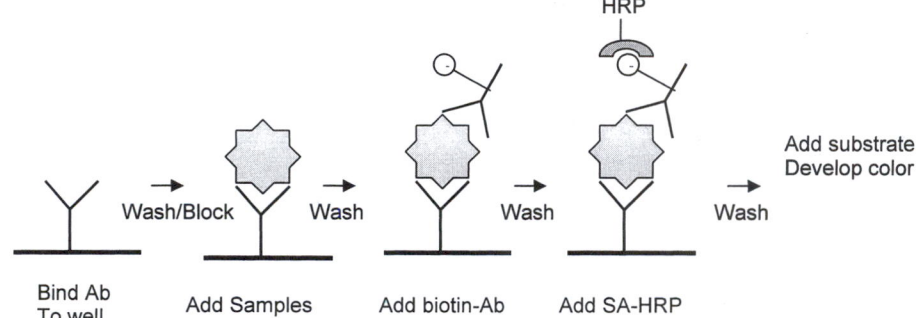

FIGURE 2 Indirect or sandwich ELISA. This ELISA shares many features with the assay described in the legend to Fig. 1. The major difference is in the first step, in which an antibody (Ab) directed against the analyte is bound to the bottom of the microtiter well. This antibody is termed the capture or coating antibody. Following addition of the analyte, the biotin-labeled detection antibody (biotin-Ab) is applied, followed by horseradish peroxidase (HRP)-conjugated streptavidin (SA-HRP). Color development proceeds, and the intensity of the color is directly related to the amount of the analyte. This is termed a sandwich ELISA because the analyte is sandwiched between two antibodies.

samples, multiple cytokines are present simultaneously. The antibody directed against the cytokine which is present on the plate should react only with its specific cytokine. When the sample containing multiple cytokines is added to the microtiter well, only the cytokine recognized by the antibody will remain bound on the plate (Fig. 3). Therefore, when the sample is removed, all of the other cytokines will be taken away and will be available for detection by another ELISA. Thus, it is possible to measure the cytokines in sequence by stretching the sample to detect multiple cytokines. In fact, a basic description of this technique has been published previously (28). I also found in my laboratory that it is possible to do sequential ELISAs and detect several cytokines simultaneously (my unpublished data).

The sequential ELISA still has several pitfalls. First, the sample volume necessary is still greater than that used in most multiplex assays. Second, the amount of time required to measure each one of the cytokines is not reduced in the sequential ELISA, so there is no cost savings with regards to time. Third, if there is potential cross-reactivity of the antibodies, then measurement of the first cytokine will result in an overestimate of the amount of that cytokine present and measurement of the next cytokine in the sequence will result in an underestimate of the amount of that cytokine present. Despite these caveats, the sequential ELISA is a method that is available to anyone who is presently running ELISAs.

PLATE-BASED MICRO-ELISAS

None of the previously described techniques using traditional ELISA plates measure multiple cytokines at once. The breakthrough in technology comes about when several cytokines may be detected simultaneously from a small sample volume. The first report demonstrating the feasibility of this approach was published in 1999 (22). This publication documented the ability to detect up to eight different analytes simultaneously in a single well. The analytes that the researchers detected were immunoglobulins derived from different species, such as rabbit, guinea pig, and human. The detection was achieved by placing very small amounts of these immunoglobulins in the bottom of a 96-well glass-bottom plate. The amount of immunoglobulin that was placed on the bottom of a well was approximately 200 pl.

This is in contrast to a typical ELISA, in which the bottom of the entire well is coated with a single antibody directed against a single cytokine, with a volume of approximately 100 µl. Therefore, the amount of antibody used for detection is 500,000 times smaller in the microarray assay than in the traditional ELISA. I will discuss in greater detail below how the use of a smaller volume of antibody does not result in lower signal intensity.

An individual spot of the immunoglobulin was designated as an element, and six-by-six arrays of these elements were printed onto the bottom of each well. Four identical arrays could be printed, resulting in the deposition of up to 144 elements. Precise control of the locations of the individual elements is necessary so that the locations can be appropriately mapped to the later images.

Each one of the immunoglobulins affixed to the glass bottoms of the wells was then detected with the appropriate biotinylated secondary antibody. For this assay, alkaline phosphatase was used as the detection enzyme. This enzyme results in color development in the region of the spot. A charge-coupled device (CCD) camera was used to record the image. Typically, special modifications to the CCD camera are made, including the addition of specialized hardware and cooling to improve the optical image. Additionally, a black Teflon mask is usually applied around the individual wells to prevent scatter of the light from one well to the next.

Once the image has been captured, the intensity of the individual spot is mapped back to its precise location. Since each element detects a single cytokine, the intensity of an element is directly proportional to the concentration of the cytokine. Similar to the method in traditional ELISA, a standard curve is prepared with a separate set of wells. The intensity of the color, or the number of relative light units if fluorescence or chemiluminescence has been utilized, is compared back to the standard curve to determine the concentration of the analyte in question.

Although the technique described in this initial publication was used only to measure immunoglobulins, which are present in high concentrations and relatively easy to detect, the innovation was the simultaneous measurement of multiple discrete molecules within the same well (22). This served as a launching point for the development of other assays.

Shortly after this report was published, another study used a 96-well plate to detect three separate molecules

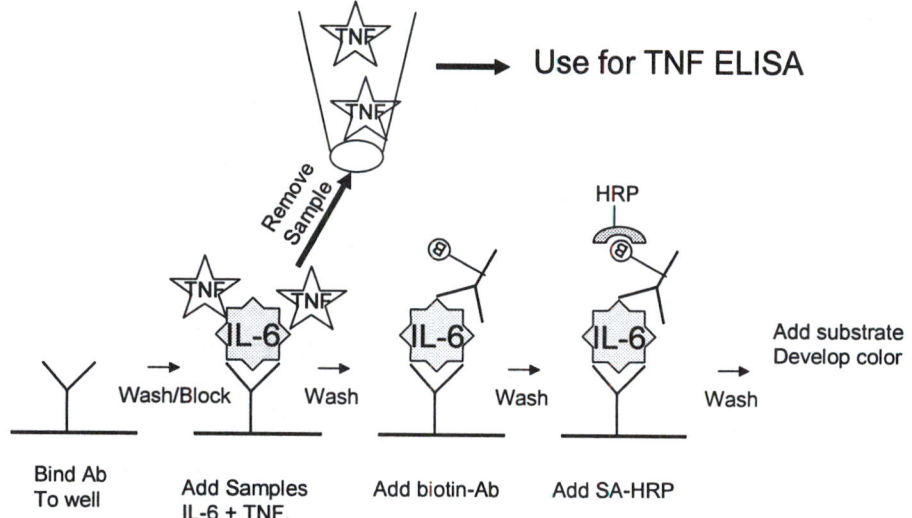

FIGURE 3 Sequential ELISA. A sample containing a mixture of cytokines is applied to an IL-6 ELISA. IL-6 binds to the anti-IL-6 antibody attached to the bottom of the well. When the sample is removed, cytokines which are not IL-6, such as tumor necrosis factor (TNF), may be used in a subsequent ELISA. Ab, antibody; B, biotin moiety; biotin-Ab, biotin-labeled antibody; HRP, horseradish peroxidase; SA-HRP, horseradish peroxidase-conjugated streptavidin.

simultaneously (48). In this study, prostate-specific antigen, prostate-specific antigen bound to α_1-antitrypsin, and IL-6 were measured at the same time. The report carefully compared the results of the protein microarray with the results obtained from a traditional ELISA. The results were surprisingly consistent, especially when one considers that the researchers included serum samples from patients. However, the sensitivity of the individual determinations was not exceptional.

Another report published in the same year from a commercial vendor showed that this technology could be used to detect multiple human cytokines (23). In this study, the sensitivity was very close to that observed in a traditional ELISA. This initial study had three-by-three arrays of the monoclonal antibodies detecting seven different cytokines. More recent iterations of this technology have detected far more cytokines.

As one can imagine, when one is working with extremely small sample volumes the printing of the arrays is a critical issue. The deposition of the small sample volumes must be uniform, and the alignment must be extremely precise (10). There are several manufacturers of spotters. In many situations, spotters that have been used for the preparation of DNA microarrays may be successfully used for protein applications. These are typically contact type printers, where a quill tip is dipped into the protein solution and the solution is dotted onto the substrate. While these work quite well for nucleic acid microarrays, better results are typically obtained with noncontact printers. In one extremely novel and low-cost approach, a standard ink jet printer was used for depositing the antibodies (38).

The substrate onto which the antibodies are spotted is also important. Nucleic acids spot quite well onto glass slides, but antibodies are not optimally placed onto glass. The surface of the glass slide may be derivatized in order to improve binding of the antibodies (10). Alternatively, the antibodies may be spotted onto other substrates such as nitrocellulose which have a high protein binding capacity. Other membranes

are also suitable. For 96-well plates, traditional ELISA plates may be used since these have already been developed and tested for binding of antibodies. A potential disadvantage is that it may be difficult to spot onto the bottom of the 96-well plate.

Since only a small amount of antibody is spotted and the spot is extremely small, the immediate concern is that the signal intensity would be extremely small. In fact, the signal intensity may be greater with the smaller amounts of antibody. In a traditional ELISA, the antibodies spread across the bottom of the entire plate. Once the analyte binds to the antibody, the signals also spread across the entire plate. In contrast, with the microarrays, the antibodies are usually at higher concentrations. This is shown schematically in Fig. 4. In this figure, each of the black dots represents an antibody to IL-6 which has been coupled with IL-6 and subsequently detected. If the same amount of one analyte (IL-6) is bound to the same number of antibodies but the antibodies are now more closely spaced, the resulting signal intensity will be higher.

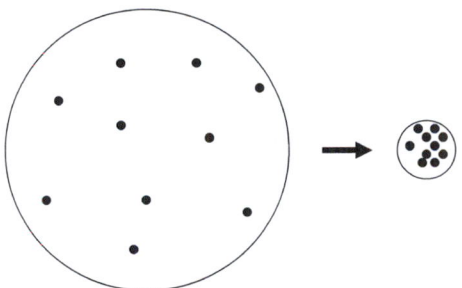

FIGURE 4 Increase in signal intensity with smaller spot size. On the left, each black dot represents the analyte bound to an antibody, which spreads across the entire well. On the right, the same number of antibodies are bound to the analyte, but they now occupy a smaller space, with a resulting increase in signal intensity.

Special Equipment Required

Spotting device. Accurately placing each of the individual spots into the well of the microtiter plate requires a high-quality spotting device. This device must be one capable of accurately and reproducibly placing the capture antibody in a precise location. Additionally, because of the depth of the microtiter plate, the robotic arm doing the plating must have pipette tips able to clear the tops of the wells. This problem does not occur with the glass slide-based arrays, as will be discussed below. As previously described, noncontact printers provide the most uniform arrays when working with proteins. This is a rapidly changing market, and the investigator should carefully research the spotters available on the market before purchase. Alternatively, plates may be purchased from a commercial vendor with the antibodies to the individual cytokines already placed in the bottoms of the wells. Presently there is only one commercial vendor selling the arrays in a microtiter plate format (Pierce; http://www.piercenet.com). The plates may be purchased off the shelf, or custom arrays may be ordered. The product is sold under the name Searchlight. Another vendor for plate-based microarrays is Meso Scale Discovery (42).

Detection equipment. Microarray assays are run using a colorimetric reagent, and a CCD camera is used to record the image. This is a high-quality camera which is specially modified in order to reduce background and provide a greater range of sensitivity and specificity.

MEMBRANE-BOUND-ANTIBODY ARRAYS

A series of recent papers have been published which describe technology capable of detecting multiple cytokines in a relatively simple format (9, 11, 12, 19). The authors have manually arrayed antibodies to several cytokines on a membrane. Simplicity of design represents an attractive feature of this methodology. In the initial study, several important steps were evaluated to arrive at the optimal conditions for the assay. Some of the parameters that were studied include the concentrations of antibodies and the best membranes for use.

For this type of assay, there are multiple antibodies directed against specific cytokines bound to a membrane. Each antibody is spotted onto the membrane in a different location, and the location is determined by the map. Diluted samples are placed onto the membrane, which is then incubated for 1 h. Following washing, a cocktail of detection antibodies is placed onto the membrane. After washing again, the detection reagent is added and the spots representing the individual cytokines are detected by chemiluminescence. X-ray film, or a phosphorimager, may be used to determine the intensity of the individual spots.

Advantages to this technology are that it is easily performed in virtually any laboratory. The incubation may be done in a simple six-well tissue culture dish, and the cytokines are arrayed on a membrane about the size of a postage stamp.

A significant disadvantage to this technology is a lack of quantification. In most other multiplexed assays, standard curves are generated and the concentration of an individual cytokine is determined from the standard curve. Without a standard curve, it is difficult to perform the precise quantification necessary for many scientific investigations of cytokine biology. Additionally, published results from our laboratory have shown that the sensitivity of the membranes is at least 2 logs lower than that of the traditional ELISA for several cytokines (5).

Special Equipment Required

X-ray film processor or phosphorimager. X-ray film may be used to capture the relative intensities of the individual spots, or this step may be done more quantitatively using the phosphorimager. Most institutions have an X-ray film processor available from molecular biology experiments in which Northern blots were developed, so it may not be accurate to consider this as special equipment.

GLASS SLIDES WITH MICROARRAYS

Glass slides have been extensively used for gene chip analysis. For traditional gene chips, portions of nucleic acid are spotted onto the slide. Each bit of nucleic acid coats a specific gene, as reviewed in reference 29. A similar format is used for the protein microarrays; however, instead of placing nucleic acid sequences onto slides and performing DNA hybridization, a compound is placed onto the slide which will interact with a specific protein. Typically, this means that an antibody directed against cytokines is placed on the individual slide, and that is the method that I will describe here.

The antibodies used for the protein microarrays are usually those which have already been demonstrated to be effectively employed in an ELISA format. These antibodies typically have been screened to determine that they have appropriate sensitivity. Additionally, when the antibodies are purchased from commercial vendors, they have frequently been tested against multiple different cytokines to ensure appropriate specificity. A careful examination of the antibody description supplied by the company will allow one to determine if cross-reactivity may represent a potential problem.

For protein microarrays, the capture antibody is placed onto the slide. The surface of the glass slide may be altered to enhance the binding of the antibody. Alternatively, a matrix may be applied to the surface of the cell to enhance the antibody binding. A number of different coatings are available for this purpose, although one of the simpler solutions is to affix nitrocellulose membranes to the surface of the slide. Nitrocellulose has a high protein binding affinity and will avidly capture the antibody (45). However, appropriate blocking reagents must be used in order to prevent a high background resulting from nonspecific binding of other proteins. Several different blocking reagents are available, but there is frequently a trade-off with these reagents. The trade-off arises because though one blocking reagent may be optimal for one antibody pair, a different blocking reagent is optimal for another antibody pair. In other words, the best blocking reagent for detecting tumor necrosis factor may be bovine serum albumin and the best blocking reagent for the antibodies detecting IL-6 may be casein. As in the traditional ELISA, a significant amount of trial and error is necessary in order to arrive at the appropriate combination of reagents.

Once the slide has been blocked, the detection antibodies are added. Because the assay is in a multiplex format, all of the detecting antibodies are added all at once in a cytokine antibody detection cocktail. Usually these antibodies have a biotin moiety attached to them in order to improve the sensitivity of the signal. Each of the individual antibodies needs to be appropriately titered in order to achieve a strong signal with low background. It is also important to keep the antibodies at the correct concentrations in order to prevent cross-reactivity. If an antibody is present in too high a concentration, it is possible that there will be a loss of specificity.

Virtually all of the slide microarray formats detect the antibodies through the use of fluorescent tags. These fluorescent reagents are directly attached to steptavidin, which binds to the biotin attached to the detection antibody. The slide is then read in a glass slide reader by using the same equipment used for the gene chip array work. Similar software is also employed in order to properly align the individual spots and quantitate the intensity of the signal. An example of a spotted microarray is shown in Fig. 5, which was directly obtained from the image obtained from the glass slide reader.

The fluorescent tags most commonly used to determine the intensity of the spots are the cyanine (Cy) dyes. These dyes are extremely stable and emit with a bright intensity. Two principal dyes are used, Cy3, which has an emission maximum at 563 nm, and Cy5, which has an emission maximum at 662 nm. These dyes may be used together since the spectra essentially do not overlap.

When the cytokines are detected in the multiplex format, antibody specificity becomes an even more critical issue. Even slight cross-reactivity between individual antibodies may result in false-positive signals. Rigorous testing must be performed in order to document that the antibodies detect only that against which they are directed. This testing may be

accomplished in the multiplex format by running the entire assay and detecting the presence of a cocktail of cytokines. In this cocktail of cytokines, one of the cytokines will be left out. In the multiplex assay which detects 18 different cytokines, 19 different cocktails will need to be prepared. One of these will have all of the cytokines present, and the fluorescence intensity for each individual cytokine will be determined. The remaining 18 cocktails will each have one of the cytokines intentionally left out. When these cocktails are run on the microarray, the intensity should be virtually nonexistent for the cytokines which are missing. Fig. 6 represents an example of this type of study for examining cross-reactivity. In this example, the cocktail was prepared with 17 different cytokines, although the microarray was designed to detect 18 cytokines. The missing cytokine for this assay was IL-12. As can be observed, no signal was detected from any of the spots that were arrayed with the antibodies detecting IL-12. This demonstrates that this assay has the appropriate level of specificity. Similar results were obtained in the other studies in which the individual cytokines were deleted.

After the intensity of the individual spots has been quantified, data analysis becomes the next important critical issue. In order to efficiently manage the information, the

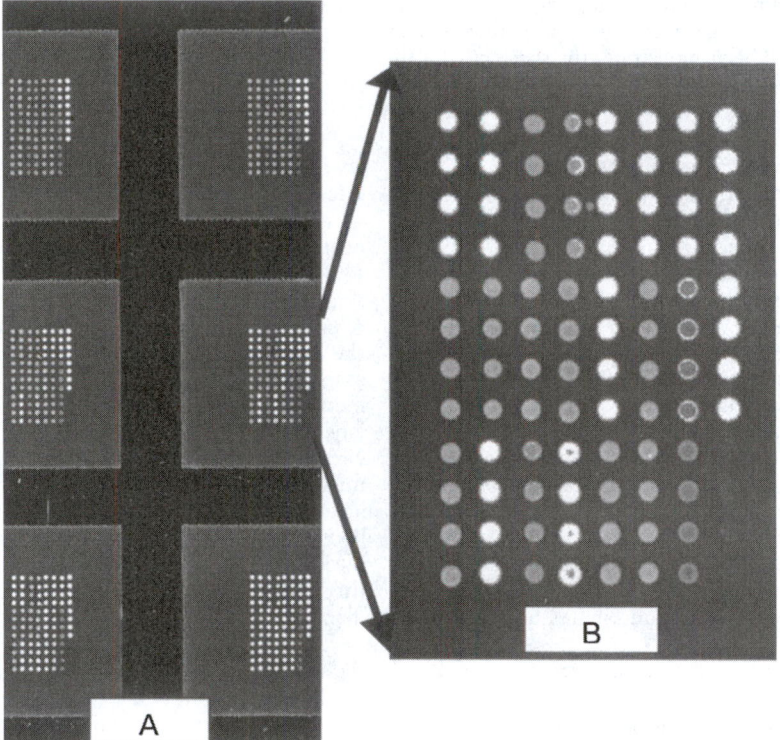

FIGURE 5 Example of a microarray. Panel A shows six individual nitrocellulose pads arranged on a glass slide. Each pad has been spotted in an 8-by-12 format. The black area between the pads is the place where a silicon gasket was adhered to the surface to allow each of the wells to function individually, similar to the way in which an individual well in a 96-well plate is independent from its neighbors. The antibodies have been spotted in an identical manner onto each of the nitrocellulose pads. Panel B is an enlarged picture of one of the individual pads and highlights the detail of the spots. The antibodies have been spotted in quadruplicate on the pad in a vertical fashion. Each individual spot has a diameter of 150 μl, and the distance between the spot is 300 μm. The total volume delivered to each spot was 350 to 367 pl. In the far-right column of spots, those in the top eight positions are extremely bright and the lower four have virtually no signal. This line of eight plus four spots may be used for alignment of the protein chip. The intensity of the individual spots may be quantified and used to determine the cytokine concentration in the sample. This image shows excellent reproducibility of the quadruple spots.

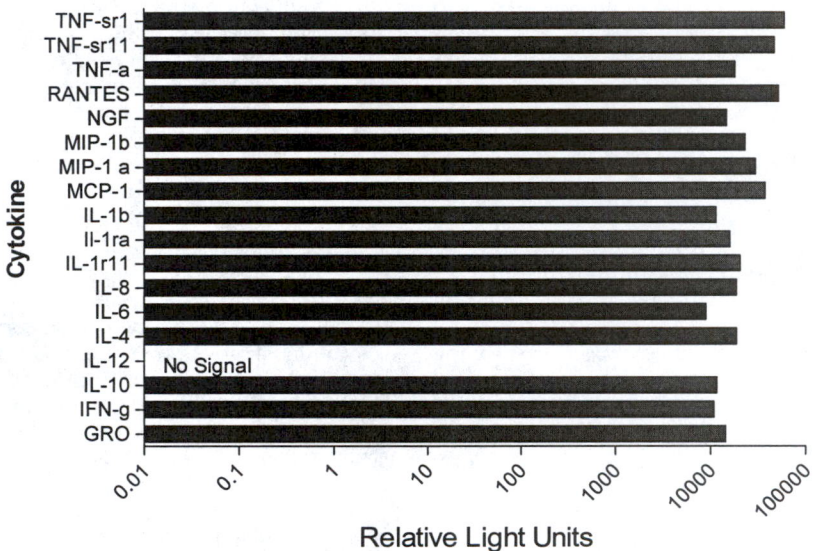

FIGURE 6 Specificity of the microarray. For this microarray, 18 different cytokines were tested. A cocktail containing recombinant cytokines was prepared, but IL-12 was not added to the cocktail. There is a strong signal from all the other cytokines, but no fluorescence was observed on the array for IL-12. This demonstrates the specificity for the array.

software needs to generate a mathematical model of the standard curve. The concentrations of the cytokines in the unknown samples are then calculated by referring back to the model of the standard curve.

There are multiple mathematical models that may be used to generate the appropriate fit for the standard curve. The same set of data may be analyzed by different iterations of the standard curve. For example, the data may be analyzed by plotting the number of relative light units (i.e., fluorescence intensity) versus the concentration of the cytokine. A simple linear expression may then be used to draw a straight line through the points. Alternatively, the data may be graphed on a log-log scale, and again, a straight line may be fitted to the points. I have had the most success using the concentration of the cytokine on a log scale and the fluorescence intensity on a linear scale. Examination of the graph usually shows an S-shaped or sigmoidal-type curve. Software is available which automates and reduces the time necessary for data analysis.

Examples of a standard curve prepared from the multiplex assay for the cytokine IL-8 are shown in Fig. 7. The exact same standard curve was subjected to different mathematical models to determine the one which would yield the optimum performance. As can be observed, plotting the information on a log-linear scale and using polynomial regression result in the highest correlation between the standard curve and the actual data.

Another level of data analysis is needed when substantial amounts of information are collected: analysis of the biological significance of the findings. In contrast to gene chip data, where only the relative abundances of different genes are determined, the actual levels of the cytokines have been measured. The levels may be important because previous publications have indicated that elevated levels of some cytokines are associated with worse prognosis. For example,

levels of IL-6 in plasma predict outcome in mouse models of infection (37, 46).

A modification of the slide-based microarray method has been developed which allows amplification of the signal (40). The same sandwich type ELISA is used, but the detection antibody contains a small fragment of a DNA primer. A circular piece of DNA hybridizes to the primer conjugated to the antibody, and the circular piece of DNA is used for the amplification step. Amplification occurs when DNA polymerase is incubated with the sample in the presence of labeled nucleotides. As the DNA polymerase works on the circular piece of nucleic acid, an elongated string of labeled nucleic acid is generated. With this method, researchers were able to measure up to 75 cytokines. However, because of antibody cross-reactivity, it was necessary to separate the samples into two separate reaction mixtures. This helps to illustrate the point, raised previously, that the major limitation for many of these methods is specificity of the antibodies.

There is another variation that is used with the glass slides, a method that compares normal to abnormal samples but does not quantify the amount of protein present. For this type of assay, samples are obtained from healthy sources and also from those in altered states. Altered-state sources may be patients who have disease or may be tissue or stimulated cells. All of the proteins from one sample are labeled with one color; for example, the normal samples may be labeled in green. All of the diseased or altered-state samples are labeled with a second color, such as red. The proteins from the normal and the diseased or altered-state samples are then mixed together. In this situation, there is a mixture of red and green molecules in the same tube.

As a specific example, one could take tissue culture supernatants from endotoxin-stimulated macrophages to represent the altered state and label these in red. Among these proteins would be IL-6. Tissue culture supernatant from unstimulated

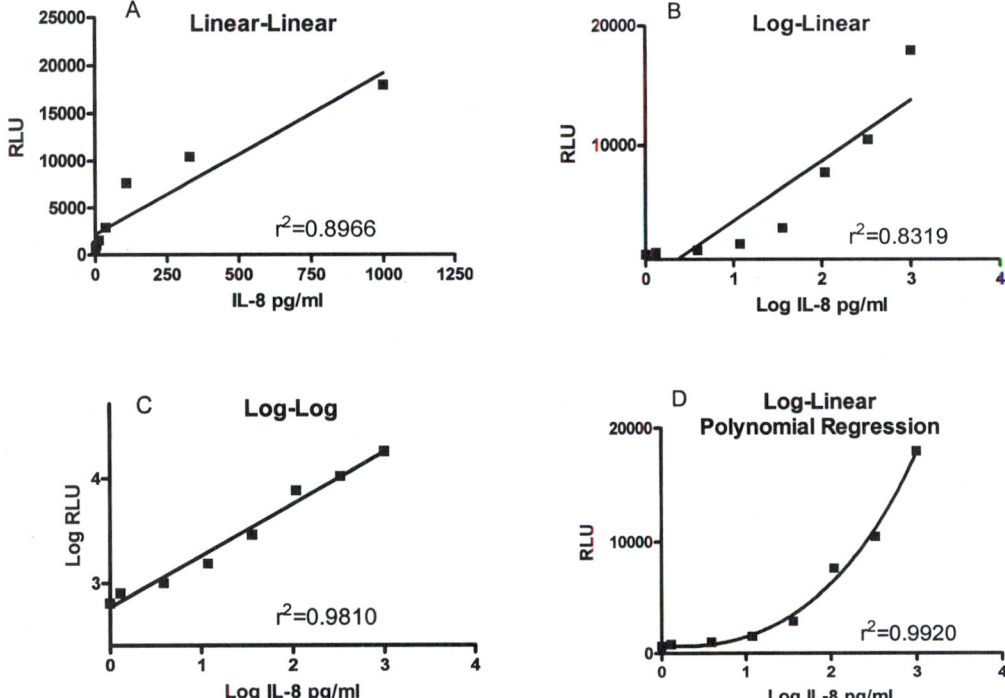

FIGURE 7 Mathematical modeling of the standard curve. Data from a microarray standard curve were used to generate a mathematical model for calculations for unknown samples. In panel A, the number of relative light units (RLU) and the concentration of the cytokine (IL-8) were plotted on a linear-linear scale. The correlation coefficient (r^2) was not very precise. In panel B, the concentration of the IL-8 was plotted on a log scale and the number of RLU was plotted on a linear scale. This resulted in even worse correlation. In panel C, both the number of RLU and the IL-8 concentration were plotted on a log scale and a very good linear regression could be fitted. However, the optimal modeling of the curve was obtained when the number of RLU was plotted on a linear scale, the IL-8 concentration was plotted on a log scale, and a fourth-order polynomial regression line was used. The results for all four panels were obtained using the same data from the IL-8 standard curve, but similar results are observed with most other cytokines.

cells would represent the control state and in this situation would be labeled in green. Both of these protein samples would compete for binding to the antibodies which had been placed on the slide. In this specific example, there would be a large amount of IL-6 labeled in red because the stimulated cells would secrete a large amount of IL-6. Normal, unstimulated cells would have very low concentrations of IL-6, and there would be virtually no IL-6 labeled in green. When the samples were placed on the slide, the IL-6-specific antibodies would be occupied mostly by red IL-6. Looking at the ratio between the red and green proteins would reveal the relative up or down regulation in the disease or altered state. For this example, the results would predict that lipopolysaccharide up regulates IL-6. This approach has been used successfully in several experiments and has been used specifically to demonstrate that certain proteins become up regulated following radiation treatment (43).

Special Equipment Required

Spotter. A high-quality spotter is required in order to prepare the microarrays. It is possible to obtain acceptable results using the same type of equipment used to prepare slides for gene chip studies. However, for spotting of proteins, noncontact printing generally results in better-quality arrays. Commercial companies presently produce prespotted slides with the capture antibodies already spotted onto the slides. Two such companies are Proteoplex (http://www.proteoplex.com) and Schleicher and Scheull (Fast slides). Custom arrays may also be prepared by commercial vendors.

Detection equipment. The glass slide may be read in a glass slide reader, or there are commercial services that will read the slides.

CAPILLARY ELECTROPHORESIS

A recent paper has described a novel method for rapidly detecting cytokines. In a special apparatus, antibodies directed to specific analytes were placed in the injection ports, where they were permanently bound (32). The samples containing the cytokines were then added, and all the bound proteins were labeled with Alexa Fluor 633. Electrophoresis was performed by lowering the pH, which dissociated the labeled cytokine from the antibody. The retention time determined the cytokine, and the intensity of the label correlated with the concentration. The entire process was very rapid and could be completed in just a few minutes. Additionally, the sample volume required for the assay was only a few microliters. By using this technology, six cytokines could be quantitated in less than 2 min. However, the chemistry of coupling the antibodies and performing the electrophoresis and detection presently is beyond the capabilities of most laboratories.

BEAD ARRAY ASSAYS

Bead array assays are rapidly becoming the rage in cytokine measurement. The first papers hinting at the capabilities of using a flow cytometer to measure cytokines were published more than 10 years ago (6, 21). There are several commercial vendors marketing the bead array assays. The assays may generally be divided into two groups, those that utilize the Luminex platform and the assays designed by BD Biosciences. The differences between these two types of assays will be described in greater detail below. The bead array assays may be used to measure proteins such as cytokines and immunoglobulins. Additionally, they have been used extensively for the development of assays for examining polymorphisms in genetic material (13, 14). HLA typing has been revolutionized by the adaptation of this technology (30).

Bead array assays for the measurement of cytokines are all based on the standard antibody cytokine interactions already described. They are represented schematically in Fig. 8. The first and most important step in the bead array assay is finding a specific antibody that may be conjugated to the bead. The quality of the antibody drives the sensitivity and specificity of the assay, as with virtually all immunoassays. The steps are similar to the basic steps shown in Fig. 2 for a sandwich ELISA. As the first step, the capture antibody is conjugated to the bead. This bead mixture is then incubated with the samples containing the cytokines. After the cytokines are bound to the capture antibody, a biotinylated detection antibody is added, followed by streptavidin which is coupled to a fluorescent probe. The entire mixture is then run on a flow cytometer. Although this is a simple description of the overall assay, several features allow the assay to be performed rapidly and in a multiplexed manner.

The beads are an important part of the overall assay since they are the component that allows the samples to be run in a multiplexed manner (15). There are two variations on the way the individual beads are detected. In the first version, which is used by BD Biosciences, a single fluorescent molecule is incorporated into the beads (24). The beads are distinguished by the various amounts of the fluorescent probe inside the beads. Careful manufacturing allows the individual groups of beads to be distinguished from one another. For this example, the antibodies to IL-6 would be conjugated to

bead set 1 and the antibodies to tumor necrosis factor would be conjugated to bead set 2. When these beads are mixed together, the fluorescence intensity of the fluorochrome inside each bead indicates whether one is analyzing tumor necrosis factor or IL-6. Up to six different sets of beads may be distinguished with this method.

The other method for discriminating among the individual bead sets involves mixing two different fluorescent dyes in various mixtures. The individual groups of beads are then differentiated based on two-color analysis. The groups of beads may be clumped according to the relative intensities of the two separate fluorochromes. Similar to the method for the assay previously described, one group of beads is conjugated to antibodies to tumor necrosis factor and a separate group of beads is conjugated to antibodies to IL-6. Up to 100 different discrete sets of beads may be differentiated on the basis of the various concentrations of the two fluorescent dyes. This is the technology used with the Luminex platform. There are several commercial vendors who manufacture the beads conjugated to the antibodies, but all of them use the Luminex equipment. An example of an assay run using the Luminex platform is shown in Fig. 9.

We have described how the individual beads are grouped, but how does the quantification of the cytokines occur? Quantification takes place through the measurement of the intensity of the fluorescent tag attached to streptavidin. As in the traditional ELISA, the intensity of the signal is directly related to how much detection antibody has attached to the cytokine. A standard curve with several concentrations of cytokines is prepared and run in the assay. Fig. 10 shows an example of the standard curve with mouse IL-1β. The steps that are involved with the precise measurement of the cytokine include, first, the detection of the groups of the beads. The intensity of the streptavidin fluorescent tag for each group of beads is then assayed and compared to the standard curve in order to determine the concentrations of the cytokines within the sample. In Fig. 9, there are 22 individual groups of beads which may be assayed, which indicates that there are 22 individual groups or individual cytokines that may be measured in this multiplexed assay.

There are several advantages to the bead array assays. First, it is possible to perform the assays without washing the beads, limiting many of the time-consuming and tedious steps in a traditional ELISA (15, 44). It is possible to do these assays without washing because the fluorescence intensity of only the molecules bound to the beads is measured, not the intensity of everything in the solution. In

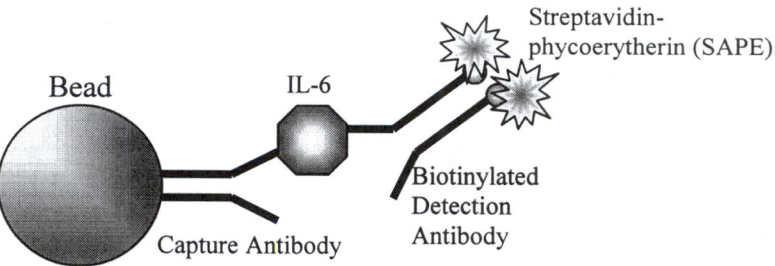

FIGURE 8 Schematic representation of the principle of a flow cytometric bead-based assay. The capture antibody specific for the analyte, in this example IL-6, is attached to a bead. The IL-6 binds to this antibody, which is then followed by a detection antibody which is biotinylated. Streptavidin conjugated to phycoerythrin is then added, and the entire complex is analyzed with the flow cytometer.

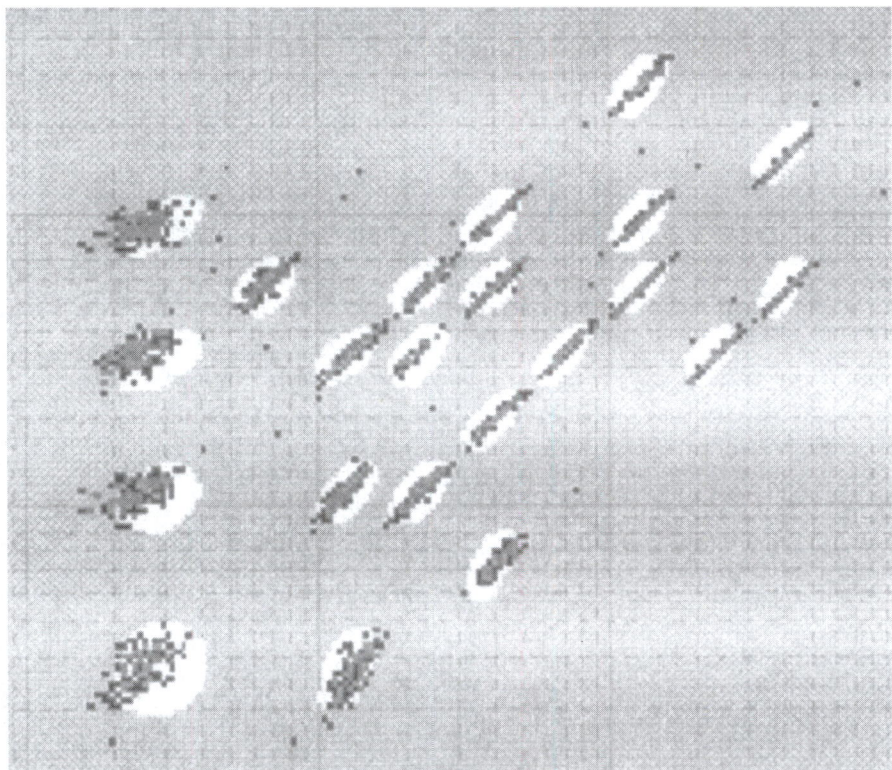

FIGURE 9 Example of the readout from a bead-based flow cytometry assay. In this example, the individual beads have different concentrations of two fluorescent dyes. The groups of beads are detected on the basis of the fluorescence intensities. The individual dots represent individual beads, and the darker-colored dots are doublets. The clear areas around collections of beads indicate those areas used for analysis. In this example, 22 individual cytokines have been detected. The intensity of the fluorescence of each individual bead is captured in a third fluorescent channel and compared to the standard curve in order to determine the concentration of the cytokine.

a traditional ELISA, the fluorescence intensity or color is measured in the well. Unless unbound antibodies are washed away, the background will be extremely high. In the bead array assay, the flow cytometer will analyze the group of beads to determine the specific fluorescence intensity and not the overall fluorescence intensity.

A second significant advantage is that up to 100 discrete groups of beads may be analyzed; thus, up to 100 different cytokines may be measured in a multiplexed assay. The major limitation is obtaining antibody with sufficient specificity in order to prevent cross-reactivity.

Many of the steps for the bead array assays may be automated, which is a third distinct advantage of this methodology. Automated sampling of each of the discrete wells used for an individual sample may be done, allowing walk-away ease of use.

Finally, the volume of sample required to measure multiple cytokines is extremely small. This is an advantage of any of the multiplexed assays, which generally require smaller sample volumes than the traditional ELISA. Even use of the sequential ELISA requires a larger sample volume than that typically used in a bead array assay.

At the present time, the range of bead array assays available for the Luminex platform is much greater than that of any other presently available array assay. In fact, there are at least 75 different identified cytokines that may be measured by using this platform. The cytokines include those of

human, rat, and mouse. Additionally, this technology may be used for allergy testing, tissue typing, detection of cardiac markers and cancer markers, and diagnosis of infectious diseases. The bead array assays have been successfully used to measure cytokines in human plasma (33), though

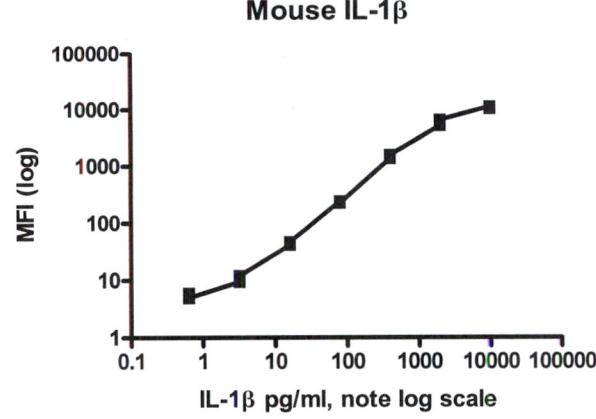

FIGURE 10 Example of a standard curve generated from the bead-based flow cytometry assay. In this example, a standard curve using recombinant mouse IL-1β is displayed. MFI, mean fluorescence intensity.

appropriate caution must be observed with plasma or serum samples (34).

Special Equipment Required

Preparation of Beads

While it is possible to conjugate the antibodies to the purchased beads, in reality this is technically difficult to do. Presently, most investigators will find it necessary to rely upon commercial sources for the conjugated beads. Fortunately, there are several vendors in the marketplace at the present time. This is encouraging news for investigators, since it is not likely that all of the vendors would terminate manufacturing of beads at the same time. Inevitably as the market matures, there will be fewer vendors, but the strong will survive such that those companies with excellent technical assistance, range of reagents, and ease of use will continue to sell products. The fact that several companies are marketing their products for the bead array assays also indicates that business analysts have determined that there is a robust market available for their wares. Again, this increases enthusiasm among investigators since the technology is more likely to persist. Additionally, the technology has been used to detect more than just cytokines. As a result, the flow cytometry apparatus is more widely available since it can be used for multiple applications.

By working with the vendors, it is possible to have custom-prepared sets of beads. The companies are pleased to conjugate specific antibodies to the beads and then multiplex the reagents into kits for the customer. Provided that there is an appropriate antibody available, there is really no limitation on what is available.

Flow Cytometry

For some of the commercial kits, it is not necessary to have a special, dedicated instrument. Any standard flow cytometer may be used for measuring cytokines provided that the appropriate software has been employed. Since many institutions already have flow cytometers which have been used for routine cell work, there is no real additional expense for running the assays. If the investigator desires to purchase a Luminex instrument, this will be a substantial additional cost.

COST COMPARISON

A true comparison of different multiplexed formats requires a delineation of the costs involved. I performed such analysis using a bead array assay based on the Luminex platform in contrast with a conventional ELISA which would be performed in the sequential format. For the ELISA, the cost remains essentially the same for each cytokine that is measured. However, in the bead array the cost decreases with the number of cytokines that are measured. This savings comes about as the cost of the kits decreases as the number of cytokines multiplexed increases. The cost analysis is carefully delineated in Table 1. The analysis was carefully constructed to include the time of a skilled technician as well as the cost of reagents. When the ELISA is performed, the major component of the cost is the salary of the person who actually performs the assay. The cost analysis was based on a single technician being able to process five plates of samples per day. Five plates of samples would amount to measuring approximately 200 samples for a single cytokine per day. When calculating the cost for the beads, I based the cost on the use of only a single well of the 96-well plate for each sample. Many investigators would use two individual wells to

TABLE 1 Cost analysis for cytokine measurements[a]

Parameter	Assay	
	ELISA	Beads array
No. of cytokines	1	17
Vol (μl)	50	50
Cost per sample (dollars)	1.95	59
Cost per cytokine (dollars)	1.95	1.87–3.31
Lower limit of detection	1–10	1–10
Range (logs)	3	3
Expandability	Not expandable	Expandable

[a] The cost of measuring cytokines by traditional ELISA, used in the sequential format, is directly compared to the cost of doing a bead array assay. Included in these costs are the necessary reagents, including buffers, antibodies, and kits purchased from the manufacturer. Also included is the time of a technician, assuming that the technician could test up to five full plates (about 200 samples) per day. The cost of this time is also included in cost analysis for the bead assays.

measure a sample, and the cost would proportionally increase. As can be observed in Table 1, the total cost for measuring a single cytokine by ELISA is about $2, whereas the same sample run in a multiplexed assay would cost about $59.

However, the cost decreases as the number of cytokines which are measured increases. This is delineated in Table 2, demonstrating that there is a sliding scale for the cost of measuring cytokines in a single sample. When approximately 17 cytokines are measured, it is less expensive to use the bead array assay than to perform multiple ELISAs. Again, it must be borne in mind that the cost of doing the ELISA principally involves the time of a technician and that has been included in the cost calculation.

There is one significant cost which has not been included in these analyses, that of the capital equipment necessary to perform some of these assays. Specifically, I did not include the cost of a plate reader, a flow cytometer, or a Luminex platform. Typically, these large pieces of equipment are purchased through capital funds and may be considered a fixed cost for the assays. In other words, if one cytokine is measured there is still the cost of buying a flow cytometer and this cost is the same if one runs 100,000 cytokines.

Issues concerning the sample volumes necessary to run the individual assays also become important. These are especially critical when dealing with rodents such as mice from which only a small volume of plasma may be obtained. Since only a single sample is required to run the multiplexed assay, the bead array assays or the spotted arrays consume significantly less sample volume than even a sequential ELISA. The amounts of sample necessary to run several different cytokines are listed in Table 3.

TABLE 2 Sliding-scale cost of measuring cytokines[a]

No. of cytokines	Cost (dollars) for:	
	ELISA	Bead array assay
4	7.80	13.25
6	11.70	19.28
14	27.30	27.95
17	33.15	31.79

[a] As the number of cytokines measured in a multiplexed assay increases, the cost decreases. The cost per cytokine per assay remains relatively fixed in the ELISA format, but as more antibodies are multiplexed to different sets of beads, the bead array assay decreases in cost. At about 17 cytokines, the bead array assay becomes more cost-effective than the ELISA.

TABLE 3 Sample volumes required for performing assays[a]

No. of cytokines	Vol (μl) needed for:	
	ELISA	Bead array
1	50	25
6	75	25
20	145	25

[a] As the number of cytokines measured increases, the sample volume necessary for the ELISA increases while that for the bead array assays remains static. The calculation of the sample volumes for the ELISA assumes that the assay is being performed in sequential manner.

While this cost analysis was performed for measuring cytokines in a bead array assay, similar comments may be made regarding an alternative multiplexed format such as the spotted arrays on glass slides or spotted arrays in a 96-well plate. Additionally, analysis of issues such as the purchase of capital equipment and the amount of a technician's time necessary to perform the assays would probably give similar results. Specifically, as more cytokines are measured, the cost per cytokine would go down for the multiplexed assay and would remain the same, of course, for the sequential ELISA. Additionally, the sample volume would remain static for a spotted microarray.

CONCLUSIONS

Multiplex assays for measuring cytokines are rapidly becoming standard across the world. A clear indicator of the enthusiasm for these assays may be found in the large number of companies which are presently producing and manufacturing multiplex cytokine kits. There are several platforms that are available for measuring the cytokines, and the market is not yet sufficiently mature to conclusively address which of these offers the best speed, sensitivity, and specificity and the lowest cost. At the risk of attempting to predict the future, it is probably safe to say only that multiplex assays are here to stay.

This work has been supported in part by NIH grants GM44918, GM50401, and GM62119.

Assistance with preparation of the graphs and manuscript was kindly provided by Shannon Copeland and Javed Siddiqui.

REFERENCES

1. **Akalin, H., A. C. Akdis, R. Mistik, S. Helvaci, and K. Kilicturgay.** 1994. Cerebrospinal fluid interleukin-1 beta/interleukin-1 receptor antagonist balance and tumor necrosis factor-alpha concentrations in tuberculous, viral and acute bacterial meningitis. *Scand. J. Infect. Dis.* **26:**667–674.
2. **Atwell, D. M., K. P. Grichnik, M. F. Newman, J. G. Reves, and W. T. McBride.** 1998. Balance of proinflammatory and antiinflammatory cytokines at thoracic cancer operation. *Ann. Thorac. Surg.* **66:**1145–1150.
3. **Brody, E. N., M. C. Willis, J. D. Smith, S. Jayasena, D. Zichi, and L. Gold.** 1999. The use of aptamers in large arrays for molecular diagnostics. *Mol. Diagn.* **4:**381–388.
4. **Chaouat, G., N. Ledee-Bataille, S. Dubanchet, S. Zourbas, O. Sandra, and J. Martal.** 2004. TH1/TH2 paradigm in pregnancy: paradigm lost? Cytokines in pregnancy/early abortion: reexamining the TH1/TH2 paradigm. *Int. Arch. Allergy Immunol.* **134:**93–119. (First published 17 May 2004; doi:10.1159/000.74300.)
5. **Copeland, S., J. Siddiqui, and D. Remick.** 2004. Direct comparison of traditional ELISAs and membrane protein arrays for detection and quantification of human cytokines. *J. Immunol. Methods* **284:**99–106.
6. **Frengen, J., R. Schmid, B. Kierulf, K. Nustad, E. Paus, A. Berge, and T. Lindmo.** 1993. Homogeneous immunofluorometric assays of alpha-fetoprotein with macroporous, monosized particles and flow cytometry. *Clin. Chem.* **39:**2174–2181.
7. **Herzyk, D. J., A. E. Berger, J. N. Allen, and M. D. Wewers.** 1992. Sandwich ELISA formats designed to detect 17 kDa IL-1 beta significantly underestimate 35 kDa IL-1 beta. *J. Immunol. Methods* **148:**243–254.
8. **Herzyk, D. J., and M. D. Wewers.** 1993. ELISA detection of IL-1 beta in human sera needs independent confirmation. False positives in hospitalized patients. *Am. Rev. Respir. Dis.* **147:**139–142.
9. **Huang, R. P.** 2001. Detection of multiple proteins in an antibody-based protein microarray system. *J. Immunol. Methods* **255:**1–13.
10. **Huang, R. P.** 2003. Protein arrays, an excellent tool in biomedical research. *Front. Biosci.* **8:**d559–d576.
11. **Huang, R. P.** 2001. Simultaneous detection of multiple proteins with an array-based enzyme-linked immunosorbent assay (ELISA) and enhanced chemiluminescence (ECL). *Clin. Chem. Lab. Med.* **39:**209–214.
12. **Huang, R. P., R. Huang, Y. Fan, and Y. Lin.** 2001. Simultaneous detection of multiple cytokines from conditioned media and patients' sera by an antibody-based protein array system. *Anal. Biochem.* **294:**55–62.
13. **Iannone, M. A., J. D. Taylor, J. Chen, M. S. Li, P. Rivers, K. A. Slentz-Kesler, and M. P. Weiner.** 2000. Multiplexed single nucleotide polymorphism genotyping by oligonucleotide ligation and flow cytometry. *Cytometry* **39:**131–140.
14. **Iannone, M. A., J. D. Taylor, J. Chen, M. S. Li, F. Ye, and M. P. Weiner.** 2003. Microsphere-based single nucleotide polymorphism genotyping. *Methods Mol. Biol.* **226:**123–134.
15. **Kellar, K. L., and J. P. Douglass.** 2003. Multiplexed microsphere-based flow cytometric immunoassays for human cytokines. *J. Immunol. Methods* **279:**277–285.
16. [Reference deleted.]
17. **Khan, S. S., M. S. Smith, D. Reda, A. F. Suffredini, and J. P. McCoy, Jr.** 2004. Multiplex bead array assays for detection of soluble cytokines: comparisons of sensitivity and quantitative values among kits from multiple manufacturers. *Cytometry* **61B:**35–39.
18. **Lewkowich, I. P., J. D. Campbell, and K. T. HayGlass.** 2001. Comparison of chemiluminescent assays and colorimetric ELISAs for quantification of murine IL-12, human IL-4 and murine IL-4: chemiluminescent substrates provide markedly enhanced sensitivity. *J. Immunol. Methods* **247:**111–118.
19. **Lin, Y., R. Huang, N. Santanam, Y. G. Liu, S. Parthasarathy, and R. P. Huang.** 2002. Profiling of human cytokines in healthy individuals with vitamin E supplementation by antibody array. *Cancer Lett.* **187:**17–24.
20. **Martinon, F., and J. Tschopp.** 2004. Inflammatory caspases: linking an intracellular innate immune system to autoinflammatory diseases. *Cell* **117:**561–574.
21. **McHugh, T. M.** 1994. Flow microsphere immunoassay for the quantitative and simultaneous detection of multiple soluble analytes. *Methods Cell Biol.* **42:**575–595.
22. **Mendoza, L. G., P. McQuary, A. Mongan, R. Gangadharan, S. Brignac, and M. Eggers.** 1999. High-throughput microarray-based enzyme-linked immunosorbent assay (ELISA). *BioTechniques* **27:**778–780, 782–786, 788.
23. **Moody, M. D., S. W. Van Arsdell, K. P. Murphy, S. F. Orencole, and C. Burns.** 2001. Array-based ELISAs for high-throughput analysis of human cytokines. *BioTechniques* **31:**186–190, 192–194.
24. **Morgan, E., R. Varro, H. Sepulveda, J. A. Ember, J. Apgar, J. Wilson, L. Lowe, R. Chen, L. Shivraj, A. Agadir,**

R. Campos, D. Ernst, and A. Gaur. 2004. Cytometric bead array: a multiplexed assay platform with applications in various areas of biology. *Clin. Immunol.* **110:**252–266.

25. **Nemzek, J. A., J. Siddiqui, and D. G. Remick.** 2001. Development and optimization of cytokine ELISAs using commercial antibody pairs. *J. Immunol. Methods* **255:**149–157.

26. **Nielsen, U. B., and B. H. Geierstanger.** 2004. Multiplexed sandwich assays in microarray format. *J. Immunol. Methods* **290:**107–120.

27. **Obenauer-Kutner, L. J., S. J. Jacobs, K. Kolz, L. M. Tobias, and R. W. Bordens.** 1997. A highly sensitive electro-chemiluminescence immunoassay for interferon alfa-2b in human serum. *J. Immunol. Methods* **206:**25–33.

28. **O'Connor, K. A., A. Holguin, M. K. Hansen, S. F. Maier, and L. R. Watkins.** 2004. A method for measuring multiple cytokines from small samples. *Brain Behav. Immun.* **18:**274–280.

29. **Olson, J. A., Jr.** 2004. Application of microarray profiling to clinical trials in cancer. *Surgery* **136:**519–523.

30. **Pei, R., J. Lee, T. Chen, S. Rojo, and P. I. Terasaki.** 1999. Flow cytometric detection of HLA antibodies using a spectrum of microbeads. *Hum. Immunol.* **60:**1293–1302.

31. **Petrovas, C., S. M. Daskas, and E. S. Lianidou.** 1999. Determination of tumor necrosis factor-alpha (TNF-alpha) in serum by a highly sensitive enzyme amplified lanthanide luminescence immunoassay. *Clin. Biochem.* **32:**241–247.

32. **Phillips, T. M.** 2004. Rapid analysis of inflammatory cytokines in cerebrospinal fluid using chip-based immunoaffinity electrophoresis. *Electrophoresis* **25:**1652–1659.

33. **Prabhakar, U., E. Eirikis, and H. M. Davis.** 2002. Simultaneous quantification of proinflammatory cytokines in human plasma using the LabMAP assay. *J. Immunol. Methods* **260:**207–218.

34. **Prabhakar, U., E. Eirikis, M. Reddy, E. Silvestro, S. Spitz, C. Pendley II, H. M. Davis, and B. E. Miller.** 2004. Validation and comparative analysis of a multiplexed assay for the simultaneous quantitative measurement of Th1/Th2 cytokines in human serum and human peripheral blood mononuclear cell culture supernatants. *J. Immunol. Methods* **291:**27–38.

35. **Remick, D. G.** 2003. Cytokine therapeutics for the treatment of sepsis: why has nothing worked? *Curr. Pharm. Des.* **9:**75–82.

36. **Remick, D. G., and J. S. Friedland (ed.).** 1997. *Cytokines in Health and Disease*, 2nd ed., revised and expanded. Marcel Dekker, Inc., New York, N.Y.

37. **Remick, D. G., G. R. Bolgos, J. Siddiqui, J. Shin, and J. A. Nemzek.** 2002. Six at six: interleukin-6 measured 6 h after the initiation of sepsis predicts mortality over 3 days. *Shock* **17:**463–467.

38. **Roda, A., M. Guardigli, C. Russo, P. Pasini, and M. Baraldini.** 2000. Protein microdeposition using a conventional ink-jet printer. *BioTechniques* **28:**492–496.

39. **Rongen, H. A., H. M. van der Horst, A. J. van Oosterhout, A. Bult, and W. P. van Bennekom.** 1996. Application of xanthine oxidase-catalyzed luminol chemiluminescence in a mouse interleukin-5 immunoassay. *J. Immunol. Methods* **197:**161–169.

40. **Schweitzer, B., S. Roberts, B. Grimwade, W. Shao, M. Wang, Q. Fu, Q. Shu, I. Laroche, Z. Zhou, V. T. Tchernev, J. Christiansen, M. Velleca, and S. F. Kingsmore.** 2002. Multiplexed protein profiling on microarrays by rolling-circle amplification. *Nat. Biotechnol.* **20:**359–365.

41. **Siddiqui, J., and D. G. Remick.** 2003. Improved sensitivity of colorimetric compared to chemiluminescence ELISAs for cytokine assays. *J. Immunoassay Immunochem.* **24:**273–283.

42. **Spieles, G., E. Grossi, A. Kishbaugh, K. Johnson, R. Calamunci, G. Sigal, S. Leytner, and J. N. Wohlstadter.** 2004, posting date. *Multiplex Measurements of Cytokines in High Density Formats Using Multi-Array Technology.* [Online.] http://www.meso-scale.com/CatalogSystemWeb/WebRoot/literature/applications/pdf/MultiplexCyt_2003.pdf.

43. **Sreekumar, A., M. K. Nyati, S. Varambally, T. R. Barrette, D. Ghosh, T. S. Lawrence, and A. M. Chinnaiyan.** 2001. Profiling of cancer cells using protein microarrays: discovery of novel radiation-regulated proteins. *Cancer Res.* **61:**7585–7593.

44. **Swartzman, E. E., S. J. Miraglia, J. Mellentin-Michelotti, L. Evangelista, and P. M. Yuan.** 1999. A homogeneous and multiplexed immunoassay for high-throughput screening using fluorometric microvolume assay technology. *Anal. Biochem.* **271:**143–151.

45. **Tonkinson, J. L., and B. A. Stillman.** 2002. Nitrocellulose: a tried and true polymer finds utility as a post-genomic substrate. *Front. Biosci.* **7:**c1–c12.

46. **Turnbull, I. R., P. Javadi, T. G. Buchman, R. S. Hotchkiss, I. E. Karl, and C. M. Coopersmith.** 2004. Antibiotics improve survival in sepsis independent of injury severity but do not change mortality in mice with markedly elevated interleukin 6 levels. *Shock* **21:**121–125.

47. **Vignali, D. A.** 2000. Multiplexed particle-based flow cytometric assays. *J. Immunol. Methods* **243:**243–255.

48. **Wiese, R., Y. Belosludtsev, T. Powdrill, P. Thompson, and M. Hogan.** 2001. Simultaneous multianalyte ELISA performed on a microarray platform. *Clin. Chem.* **47:**1451–1457.

49. **Yalow, R. S., and S. A. Berson.** 1959. Assay of plasma insulin in human subjects by immunological methods. *Nature* **184:**1648–1649.

50. **Zhu, H., and M. Snyder.** 2003. Protein chip technology. *Curr. Opin. Chem. Biol.* **7:**55–63.

Monitoring of Immune Response Using Cytokine Flow Cytometry

SMITA A. GHANEKAR, HOLDEN T. MAECKER, AND VERNON C. MAINO

40

The emergence of highly sensitive quantitative antigen-specific-T-cell assays during the last 10 years has dramatically enhanced our understanding of the immune response at the single-cell level. The most widely used of these assays include the enzyme-linked immunospot (ELISPOT) assay, assays using major histocompatibility complex (MHC) oligomers, and cytokine flow cytometry (CFC) or intracellular cytokine staining (ICS) assays. Each of these methods has distinct advantages and limitations. MHC oligomers (e.g., tetramers) can be used to rapidly assess frequencies of T cells specific for defined peptide antigens by using flow cytometry (1, 4). However, this method is limited to analysis of single-peptide specificities and is restricted to single MHC alleles, making this approach impractical to evaluate responses to multiple antigenic peptides or proteins in heterogeneous populations. An alternative assay for detecting antigen-specific T cells based on cytokine expression is the ELISPOT assay (2). ELISPOT is a useful non-flow cytometric method for rapidly screening large numbers of samples for the presence of antigen-specific-cytokine-producing cells. However, because the ELISPOT assay cannot simultaneously determine the phenotype of the antigen-reactive populations, this approach has limited value in defining the heterogeneity of the immune response.

Because flow cytometry assays offer multiparametric assessments of minimally manipulated cells without a need for presorting or preenrichment, CFC has become an integral tool for assessment of immune function. CFC assays can be used to evaluate responses to complex antigens as well as peptides or peptide mixes (6, 9). Low levels of background staining achieved by use of an optimized procedure and high-quality reagents for fixation, permeabilization, and intracellular staining facilitate confident quantitation of low-frequency events in response to any protein (for CD4+ T cells) or peptides (CD4+ and CD8+ T cells). The CFC assay can also be applied to a variety of other cell types, including NK cells, monocytes, and dendritic cells, to unfold functional events associated with innate immunity. Because of its more quantitative and informative output, increasing numbers of researchers involved in vaccine clinical trials for diseases such as cancer and AIDS in addition to bacterial and parasitic infections are using CFC for detection of antigen-specific T cells in peripheral blood mononuclear cells (PBMC) as well as whole blood (3, 4, 10, 12, 15, 17, 18). In this chapter, we describe the optimized methods for CFC that offer increased throughput and robustness compared to the method described previously (8).

CONCEPT

The basic principle of the CFC assay is that whole blood or PBMC are activated with a specific antigen in the presence of a secretion inhibitor such as brefeldin A (BFA) or monensin for a short duration (6 h). The activated cells are then fixed and permeabilized to enable fluorophore-conjugated anti-cytokine antibodies to enter the cell and bind to the intracellular cytokines. Staining with a subset-specific cellular marker(s) can be performed at the same time as intracellular staining for markers such as CD3, CD4, and CD8 or before fixation of the cells when antibodies directed against fixation-sensitive epitopes are used. After acquisition of cells with the use of a flow cytometer, the cells of interest are gated and cytokine-positive cells are reported as a percent positive response after subtraction of the background value (percent positive in the absence of a stimulus or the presence of an irrelevant stimulus).

In order to bring together the high-content benefit of flow cytometry and the high-throughput aspect of ELISPOT, the CFC assay has recently been optimized for a multiwell format (19) from an originally devised tube format (8, 20, 21). The samples in the plates can then be acquired using a multiwell-plate loader connected to the flow cytometer. Dynamic gating strategies that account for sample-to-sample staining variability can simplify data analysis and improve the reproducibility of the results. In addition, use of lyophilized reagents (both activation agents and staining antibody cocktails) in the multiwell plates can simplify the assay further by preventing errors in assay setup and lot-to-lot variations in reagents, which are a concern for large trials. The procedural details to be discussed in this chapter include recommendations for sample type and handling, choice of antigen(s) and plates, and the gating strategy for this improved CFC format using cytomegalovirus (CMV) pp65 peptide mix as a model antigen.

PROCEDURE

Instructions for Processing Reagents

SEB

Add 2 ml of sterile phosphate-buffered saline (PBS) directly to a 1-mg vial of staphylococcal enterotoxin B (SEB; positive activation control; Sigma). Cap the vial and shake to dissolve all the powder. Store this stock solution at 4°C. On the day of use, prepare working stock by diluting 1:10 in sterile PBS.

Peptides

Dissolve single peptides in dimethyl sulfoxide at a concentration of 2 mg/ml. Freeze aliquots of 5 μl each at −80°C. On the day of use, prepare working stock by diluting 1:10 in sterile PBS to achieve a final concentration of 2 μg/ml.

Peptide Mixes

CMV pp65 and human immunodeficiency virus (HIV) Gag-p55 peptide mixes (15 amino acid residues in length, overlapping by 11 amino acid residues each) have been described previously (9). These peptide mixes are also available commercially (BD Biosciences, San Jose, Calif.). Store small aliquots of these peptide mixes at −80°C and dilute in sterile PBS on the day of use to achieve a final concentration of approximately 2 μg/ml/peptide.

BFA

Dissolve BFA (Sigma) powder at 5 mg/ml in dimethyl sulfoxide and store frozen as 20-μl aliquots. Just before use, dilute 1:10 in PBS and use at a 10-μg/ml final concentration.
BD FACS Lysing Solution and BD FACS Permeabilizing Solution 2
Dilute BD FACS lysing solution and BD FACS permeabilizing solution 2 (each 10×) in deionized water to make a 1× working solution. Store at room temperature.

Paraformaldehyde

Dilute a 10% solution of paraformaldehyde 1:10 in 1 × PBS. Store at 4°C.

Wash Buffer

The wash buffer consists of 0.5% bovine serum albumin and 0.1% NaN₃ in PBS. Store at 4°C.

Complete RPMI 1640 Medium

Supplement sterile RPMI 1640 medium with 10% sterile heat-inactivated fetal bovine serum and 1% sterile antibiotic-antimycotic (cRPMI). Store at 4°C.

CFC PROTOCOL FOR DETECTION OF ANTIGEN-SPECIFIC T CELLS BY USING PBMC IN A 96-WELL-PLATE FORMAT

The 96-well-plate format protocol is recommended for antigenic stimulation of freshly isolated as well as cryopreserved PBMC. The flow chart for plate-based CFC is depicted in Fig. 1, and a representative analysis of one of the PBMC samples (from a CMV-seropositive donor) stimulated with the pp65 peptide mix is shown in Fig. 2A.

PBMC Preparation

Fresh PBMC

1. Blood should be collected in tubes with sodium heparin and used within 8 h after being drawn for better quality of cells. PBMC can be harvested from blood by using Ficoll-Hypaque solution according to the manufacturer's instructions. Alternatively, PBMC can be harvested by centrifugation of blood that is collected in cell preparation tubes (Vacutainer CPT, BD Vacutainer).

2. Prepare a working concentration of 5 × 10⁶ PBMC/ml in room-temperature cRPMI. Check for clumps and remove

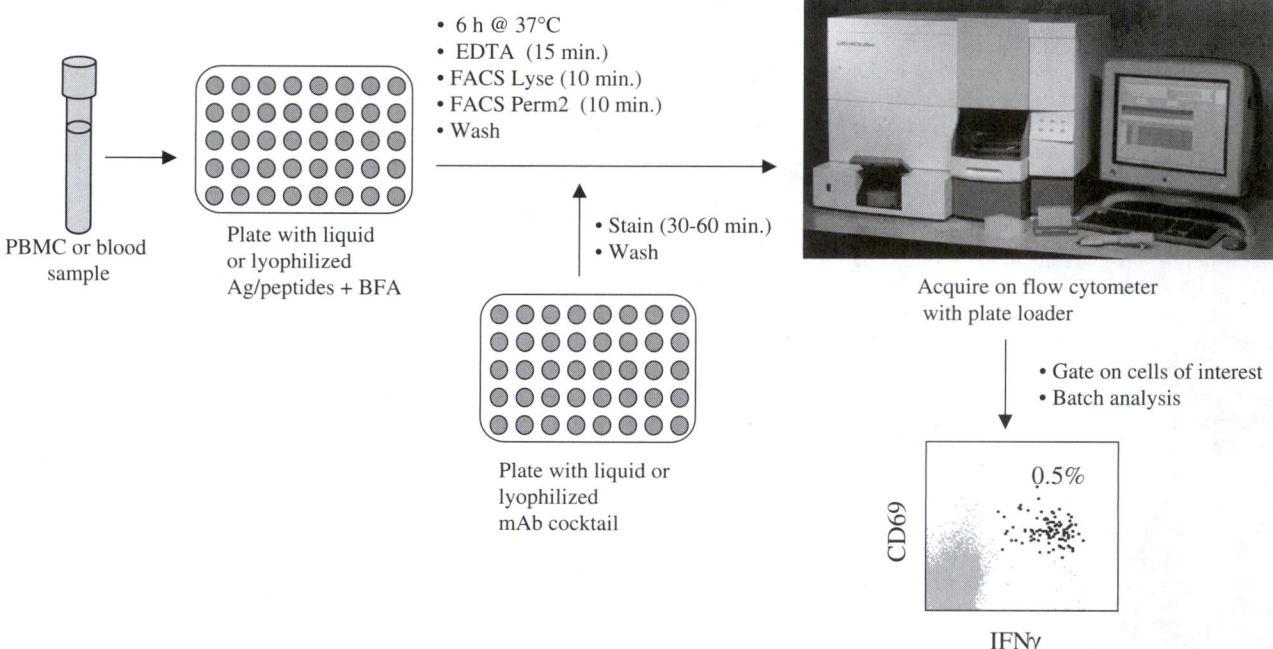

FIGURE 1 Flow chart of plate-based CFC assay. PBMC or whole blood is added to appropriate plate(s) as described in the text. After 6 h of incubation at 37°C, the cells are processed as described in the protocol. After staining with mAb cocktails for CFC, the cells are acquired on a flow cytometer using a plate loader and the data are batch analyzed. Ag, antigen; FACS Lyse, BD FACS, lysing solution; FACS Perm 2, BD FACS permeabilizing solution 2.

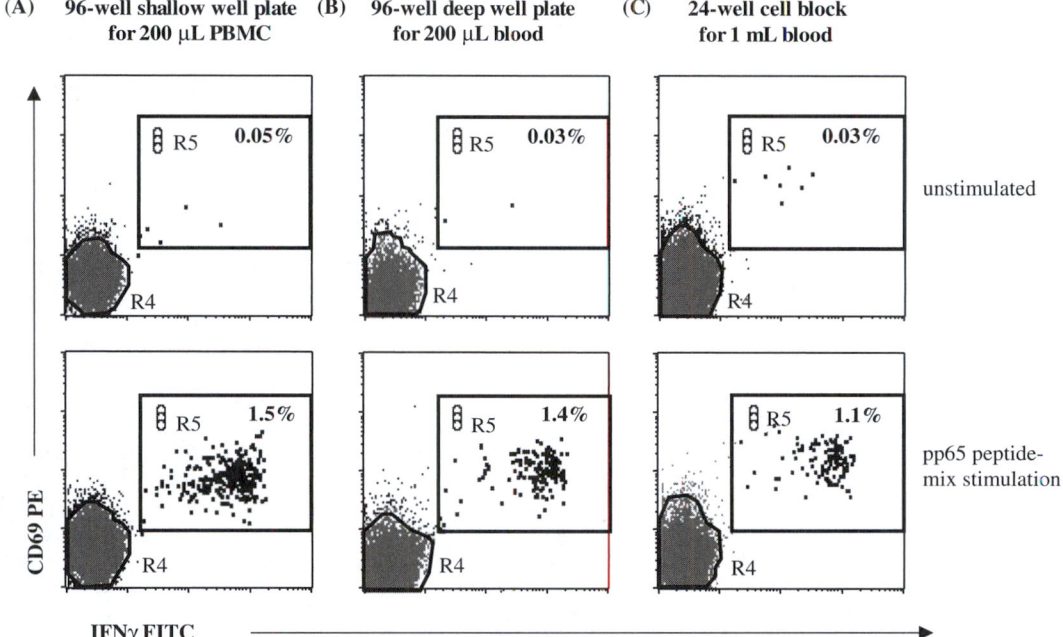

(A) 96-well shallow well plate for 200 μL PBMC **(B)** 96-well deep well plate for 200 μL blood **(C)** 24-well cell block for 1 mL blood

unstimulated

pp65 peptide-mix stimulation

CD69 PE

IFNγ FITC

FIGURE 2 Representative four-color flow cytometric analysis of plate-based CFC. PBMC 10^6 (A), 200 μl of whole blood (B), or 1 ml of whole blood (C) from a CMV-seropositive donor was stimulated (or not) with the pp65 peptide mix in a 96-well shallow-well plate, a 96-well deep-well plate, or a 24-well deep-well block, respectively. Samples were processed as described in the "Procedure." The plots were gated on CD3$^+$ CD8$^+$ lymphocytes. Responses and staining intensities of IFNγ$^+$ CD69$^+$ cells were comparable in all three assays. R4, snap-to region to identify double-negative population; R5, manually drawn region around cytokine$^+$ CD69$^+$ cells.

them with a pipette tip or a cell strainer. Proceed with PBMC activation (see below).

Cryopreserved PBMC

1. Cryopreserved PBMC should be thawed at 37°C and diluted and washed using warm medium (22 to 37°C cRPMI).

2. Resuspend cells at a final working concentration of 5×10^6 PBMC/ml in cRPMI. Make sure to remove any clumps if present.

3. Plate 200 μl/well in a polypropylene V-bottom or polystyrene U-bottom 96-well plate (Falcon; BD Discovery Labware). This will result in a concentration of 10^6 cells per well (we have tested 5×10^5 to 2×10^6 cells per well with equivalent results). Prepare additional wells for manual compensation, if desired.

4. Incubate the covered plate at 37°C for 12 to 18 h.

PBMC Activation

1. Prepare working stock solutions of activating reagents.

2. Label three tubes "NS" (for nonstimulated control), "SEB," and "Peptide." Prepare stimulation reagents in bulk by combining costimulatory monoclonal antibodies (mAbs) CD28 and CD49d (recommended when a whole antigen instead of peptides is used), a stimulus (add nothing to the nonstimulated control), BFA, and PBS in the appropriately labeled tubes. Add appropriate amounts of PBS to bring the volume to 20 μl per well for each condition on the plate; use at least one extra well to account for fluid loss. An example is given in the matrix shown in Table 1.

3. Add 200 μl of fresh PBMC to the wells containing appropriate stimuli, or add appropriate stimuli to PBMC that have rested overnight. Mix well by pipetting.

4. Incubate the covered plate for 6 h at 37°C. Following incubation, cells may be held in the sealed plate at 4 or 18°C for up to 18 h.

5. Add 20 μl of 20mM EDTA to each well and incubate for 15 min at room temperature. Mix the cell suspension well with a pipette.

6. Centrifuge the plate at $250 \times g$ for 5 min; aspirate the supernatant with a manifold (7-mm-diameter multiwell-plate aspirator manifold; V&P Scientific Inc., San Diego, Calif.). Keep the plate flat while aspirating to avoid loosening the pellet. Insert the manifold fully into the plate and hold until no more liquid is aspirated; approximately 30 μl will remain in the wells. Resuspend cells in 100 μl of 1× BD FACS lysing solution. Incubate at room temperature for 10 min. For batch processing of longitudinal study samples, cells may be frozen at this point. Place the sealed plate, containing cells in FACS lysing solution, in a −80°C freezer. When ready to stain, thaw the plate at 37°C and continue as described below.

TABLE 1 Example of stimulus preparation per well

Condition	Amt (μl) of:			Total volume (μl)
	Stimulus	BFA	PBS	
No stimulus	0	4	16	20
SEB stimulation	4	4	12	20
Peptide stimulation	5	4	11	20

Permeabilization and Staining of Activated Cells

1. Add 100 µl of wash buffer to each well and centrifuge at 500 × g for 5 min. The cell density decreases after treatment with BD FACS lysing solution, requiring a higher centrifugation speed to pellet the cells.

2. Aspirate the supernatant and resuspend cells in 200 µl of 1 × BD FACS permeabilizing solution 2. Incubate at room temperature for 10 min.

3. Centrifuge at 500 × g for 5 min. Aspirate the supernatant.

4. Resuspend the cell pellet in 200 µl of wash buffer and centrifuge at 500 × g for 5 min. Aspirate the supernatant and repeat this wash step one additional time to ensure complete removal of the permeabilizing solution. This helps to avoid background staining of the negative population.

5. Add staining mAbs to each well (e.g., BD FastImmune gamma interferon [IFN-γ]–CD69–CD4–CD3 cocktail or FastImmune IFN-γ–CD69–CD8–CD3 cocktail; BD Biosciences) and mix by pipetting. Add single-color mAbs to compensation control wells, if used.

6. Incubate the plate at room temperature for 30 to 60 min in the dark.

7. Add 175 µl of cold wash buffer and centrifuge at 500 × g for 5 min, aspirate the supernatant, and use a pipette to resuspend the cells.

8. Repeat step 7 two times with 200 µl of wash buffer. Because of the small well volume, these extra washes are recommended to reduce the background staining.

9. Resuspend the pellet with 200 µl of cold 1% paraformaldehyde.

10. Keep the plate at 4°C in the dark until acquisition using a plate loader on a flow cytometer, which should be performed within 24 h.

CFC PROTOCOL FOR DETECTION OF ANTIGEN-SPECIFIC T CELLS USING HEPARINIZED BLOOD IN A DEEP-WELL-PLATE FORMAT

The deep-well-plate format protocol is recommended for antigenic stimulation of whole blood. Deep-well plates are used because processing of whole blood after activation requires a higher volume of lysis reagent than that of PBMC for complete lysis of red blood cells. For blood volumes of up to 200 µl, use a 96-well deep-well plate (BD Discovery Labware), and for activation of up to 1 ml of blood, use 24-well deep-well blocks (Qiagen, Hilden, Germany). Blood should be drawn into tubes containing heparin as an anticoagulant and used within 8 h after being drawn. Representative analysis of a blood sample (from a CMV-seropositive donor) stimulated with the CMV pp65 peptide mix is shown in Fig. 2B.

Whole-Blood Activation

Preparation of stimuli and activation of blood are the same as described above for the PBMC assay (PBMC activation steps 1 through 5) except that heparinized whole blood is added to the wells of a deep-well plate containing appropriate stimuli. After treatment of samples with 200 µl of EDTA per well, resuspend cells in 1.5 ml of 1× BD FACS lysing solution. Incubate at room temperature for 10 min. For batch processing of longitudinal study samples at a later time, pellet the cells by centrifugation, remove the supernatant, resuspend cells in the remaining volume of the liquid, and place the

sealed plate in a −80°C freezer. When ready to stain, thaw the plate at 37°C and continue as described below.

Permeabilization and Staining of Activated Blood

1. Add 1.5 ml of wash buffer to each well and centrifuge at 500 × g for 5 min. The cell density decreases after treatment with BD FACS lysing solution, requiring a higher centrifugation speed to pellet the cells.

2. Aspirate the supernatant using a 35-mm-diameter multiwell-plate aspirator manifold (V&P Scientific Inc.) and resuspend the cells in 1 ml of 1 × BD FACS permeabilizing solution 2. Incubate at room temperature for 10 min.

3. Centrifuge at 500 × g for 5 min. Aspirate the supernatant.

4. Resuspend the cell pellet in 1.5 ml of wash buffer and centrifuge at 500 × g for 5 min. Aspirate the supernatant using a manifold and repeat this wash step one additional time to ensure complete removal of permeabilizing solution, thus avoiding background staining of the negative population.

5. Add staining mAbs to each well (e.g., BD FastImmune IFN-γ–CD69–CD4–CD3 cocktail or BD FastImmune IFN-γ–CD69–CD8–CD3 cocktail; BD Biosciences) and mix by pipetting. Add single-color mAbs to compensation control wells, if used.

6. Incubate the plate at room temperature for 30 to 60 min in the dark.

7. Add 1.5 ml of wash buffer and centrifuge at 500 × g for 5 min; aspirate the supernatant and pipette the pellet to resuspend cells.

8. Repeat step 7 one time with 1.5 ml of wash buffer.

9. Resuspend the pellet with 200 µl of cold 1% paraformaldehyde. Keep the plate at 4°C in the dark until acquisition using a plate loader on a flow cytometer, which should be performed within 24 h. The cells can be transferred from a deep-well plate into a shallow-well plate before acquisition if the plate loader does not accept deep-well plates.

Acquisition and Gating

1. Set up the flow cytometer photomultiplier tube and compensation values either automatically by using calibration beads and appropriate calibration software or manually by using cells treated the same way as the samples and either unstained or stained individually with each of the fluorochromes (e.g., CD8-fluorescein isothiocyanate [FITC], CD8-phycoerythrin [PE], CD8-peridinin chlorophyll protein-Cy 5.5 [PerCP-Cy5.5], and CD8-allophycocyanin [CD8-APC]). Unstained cells can be used to adjust the photomultiplier tube settings of the flow cytometer, followed by compensation using single-stained controls.

2. Acquire at least 20,000 relevant (CD4+ or CD8+) events, preferably 40,000 in order to obtain high power and confidence levels for comparisons of small antigen-specific responses to unstimulated controls.

3. Display of the data, gating strategy for reporting the percent response, and data interpretation have been described in detail earlier (8). The cells are first gated by drawing a region around lymphocytes, followed by another region around CD3+ CD4+ or CD3+ CD8+ cells. Then a logical gate containing lymphocytes and CD4 or CD8 cells is applied to cytokine-versus-CD69 plots (e.g., IFN-γ–FITC versus CD69-PE). Even though this is a short-term assay, expression levels of CD3, CD4, and CD8 are down-regulated on activated cells. Thus, it is important to include those down-regulated cells when drawing a region around these populations.

4. A response region is then drawn around the IFN-γ⁺ CD69⁺ population (Fig. 3, R5) from a positive control sample, and this region is copied to the plots for other samples. The percentage of gated cells within this region is obtained from region statistics for each of the plots and reported after subtracting the response of an unstimulated control.

Dynamic Gating and Analysis of CFC Data

Gating of flow cytometry data for analysis is a frequent source of assay variation, especially in rare-event assays such as CFC where antigen-specific responses may be as low as 0.1%. Relatively minor differences resulting from subjective gating can quantitatively affect CFC results, since cytokine-positive cells are not distributed symmetrically within the CD3⁺, CD4⁺, or CD8⁺ cell populations. By using a software package that contains a cluster-finding algorithm (e.g., Snap-To gating), much of the subjectivity in gating can be avoided. Such an algorithm allows gating to be both dynamic and unbiased in that it can automatically track populations that might be displaced from one sample to another without requiring user input. It can also provide consistency in results, as size and movement of the gated regions can be set and tethered regions can be created to identify rare populations by their relative positions with respect to more dense populations. We have designed templates for CFC analysis that utilize Snap-To and tethered regions to identify the required cell populations and report a percentage of cytokine⁺ CD69⁺ cells (Fig. 3).

Batch processing of the data using such an analysis template and automatic export of statistical results to a spreadsheet can both save time and prevent errors. In our laboratory, results obtained with expert manual gating were highly correlated with those obtained using a dynamic gating template for analysis of samples stimulated with the CMV pp65 peptide mix, the HIV p55 peptide mix, or SEB (19).

Performance of Lyophilized Antigens and Lyophilized Antibodies in CFC Assays

In situations where large numbers of samples need to be evaluated, e.g., in vaccine immune response-monitoring studies, it is desirable to minimize time and errors that may occur in assay setup and processing. One way to achieve this is to use preconfigured plates with lyophilized reagents (antigens as well as antibody cocktails). This method will also avoid lot-to-lot variations in the reagents in addition to issues with cold storage, as lyophilized reagents provide prolonged stability at room temperature.

We have optimized the process of using lyophilized antigens and lyophilized antibody cocktails for CFC assays of both PBMC and whole blood. The comparison of lyophilized reagents to liquid reagents in a CFC assay using pp65 peptide mix-activated blood resulted in highly significant correlation in the frequency of the response and staining intensity (Fig. 4). Using lyophilized reagents for activation as well as for staining, researchers in our laboratory have obtained

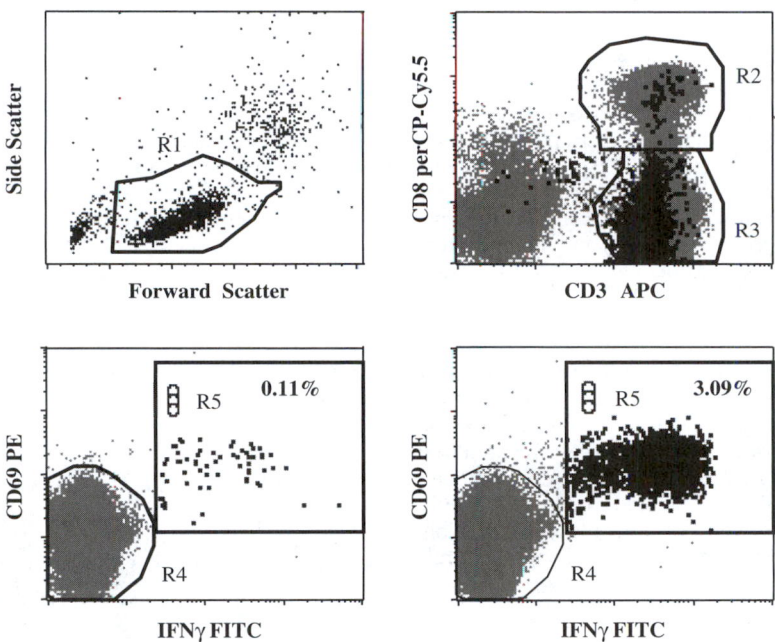

FIGURE 3 Example of CFC data analysis using dynamic gating. Analysis templates are typically defined using a positive control sample (e.g., SEB-activated PBMC or blood). R1 (lymphocytes based on forward- and right-angle light scatter), R2 (CD3⁺ CD8⁺ cells), and R3 (CD3⁺ CD8⁻, i.e., CD3⁺ CD4⁺ cells) are all Snap-To regions. The sizes and the movement of R2 and R3 are maximized to automatically include activated cells that have down-regulated CD3 and CD8 (bold dots) and to track the "roaming" populations that may be a result of variations in reagents, donors, and instrument settings. In the lower left plot that is gated on CD3⁺ CD8⁺ cells (R1 and R2), R4 is another Snap-To region (double-negative population) that is tethered to manually drawn region R5 that identifies cytokine-positive events (rare-event response region). The plot on the lower right is gated on CD3⁺ CD8⁻ cells (R1 and R3), and regions R4 and R5 are selected, copied, and pasted onto this plot. The percentage of gated events in R5 is reported.

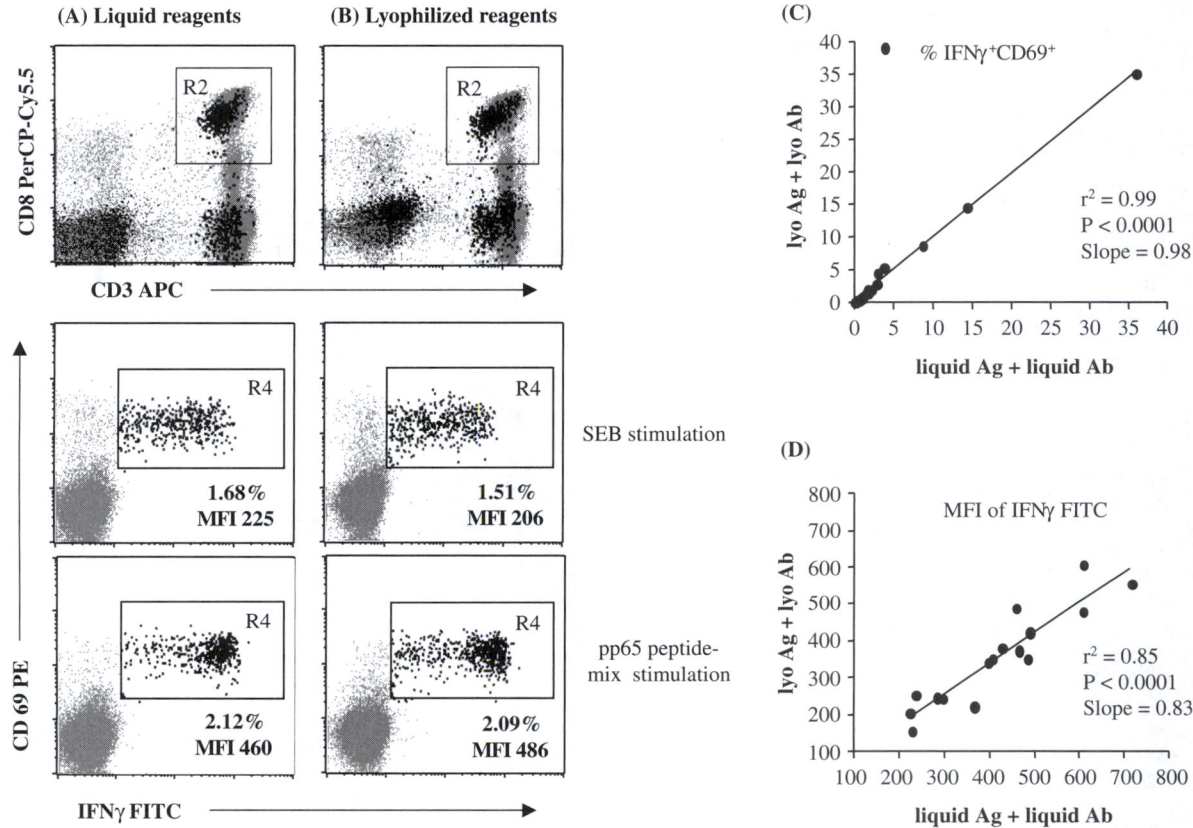

FIGURE 4 Performance of lyophilized reagents in CFC. Whole blood from a CMV-seropositive donor was activated with either liquid (column A) or lyophilized (column B) SEB or the pp65 peptide mix. The cells were processed as per the procedure described in the text. Cells were stained with either liquid (column A) or lyophilized (column B) cocktail containing IFN-γ–FITC, CD69–PE, CD8–PerCP-Cy5.5, and CD3–APC. Comparable frequencies (percent positive) and staining intensities (mean fluorescence intensity [MFI]) of CD3, CD8, IFN-γ, and CD69 were observed with both sets of reagents. Significant correlation between liquid and lyophilized reagents was observed in terms of percent positive (C) and staining intensities (D) of responding cells (CD4+ and CD8+ gated; $n = 8$). R2, region to identify CD8+ T cells; R4, region to identify cytokine+ CD69+ cells; lyo, lyophilized; Ag, antigen; Ab, antibody.

CD4 and CD8 T-cell response ranges of normal healthy donors to antigens such as SEB, CMV lysate, the CMV pp65 peptide mix, and a variety of cancer antigens (M. Inokuma and H. T. Maeker, unpublished results). Use of (i) lyophilized reagents for the CFC assay, (ii) a dynamic gating template for automated data analysis, and (iii) batch export of statistics saved a considerable amount of time, making it possible to acquire CFC data from a large number of donors in a relatively short time.

CONTROLS

Detailed description of the appropriate positive and negative controls for CFC assays has been published previously (8). In this chapter, we describe the use of two additional controls that utilize lyophilized cells to ensure the quality of the assay. One type of control is cells lyophilized after activation, lysis, and permeabilization that may be reconstituted, washed, and stained (Fig. 5B). Another type is cells lyophilized after going through the entire process, including staining, that may be reconstituted, washed, and analyzed on the cytometer by the user (Fig. 5C). The former serves as a staining control and the latter can be used as a positive

control to check the instrument setup. These lyophilized cell controls perform as well as nonlyophilized cells in the CFC assay (Fig. 5).

STANDARDIZATION OF CFC ASSAY

Complexity of the assay, in addition to biological variation of activated samples, tends to increase the variability in functional assays. We have observed intra-assay variability within 10% and interassay variability within 25% when the assays were performed as described previously, using tubes and liquid reagents for activation and staining and manual gating of the flow data (14). In order to be able to compare data from multisite clinical trials, it is important that the assay design is well controlled with regard to reagents, gating, and use of proper controls to reduce inadvertent errors. When 11 different laboratories used the procedures described here with lyophilized antigen and antibody reagents in plates, the interassay variation in antigen-specific responses of CD4 and CD8 T cells averaged 14% (11). This variation was significantly lower than that in another study performed by six different laboratories using liquid reagents and manual gating; the coefficient of variation was

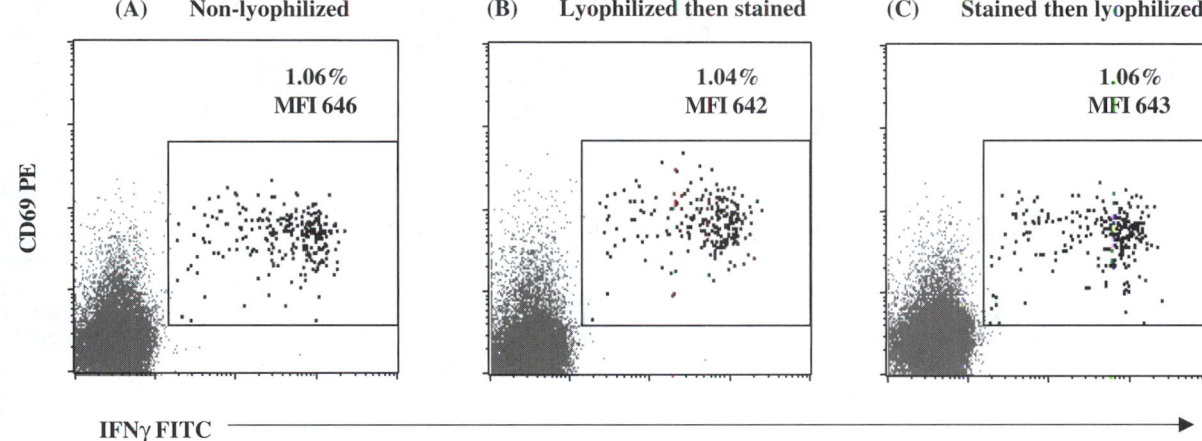

FIGURE 5 Use of lyophilized cells as process controls. CMV pp65 peptide mix-activated whole blood was lysed or fixed and permeabilized according to the protocol, and three aliquots were processed as described below. (A) Nonlyophilized. The first aliquot was stained with IFN-γ–FITC–CD69–PE–CD8–peridinin chlorophyll protein–Cy5.5–CD3–allophycocyanin, washed twice, and analyzed immediately. (B) Lyophilized then stained. The second aliquot was lyophilized, reconstituted in wash buffer, washed once, and then stained as described above. (C) Stained then lyophilized. The third aliquot was stained as described for panel, A, lyophilized, reconstituted in wash buffer, washed once, and then analyzed. Equivalent frequencies and staining intensities of responding cells were obtained for all three sets of cells.

40% but was reduced to 33% when data were analyzed using a template designed with dynamic gates (M. Suni and H. T. Maecker, unpublished data).

TROUBLESHOOTING TIPS AND NOTES

A guide to troubleshooting for CFC assays has been published (8) that addresses problems such as poor cell recovery, low or no levels of cytokine-positive cells, poor staining intensity, and high background levels, etc. When the assay is performed in plates, some additional measures need to be taken.

1. Use of appropriate-length multiwell aspirators is required for consistent assay performance in terms of cell yields and quality of staining.

2. Because the plates cannot be vortexed, it is important to mix the cell suspension several times with a multichannel pipette while avoiding cross-contamination of wells.

3. In order to avoid sample-to-sample carryover that may occur during acquisition using a plate loader, it is recommended that strong positive control stimuli (e.g., SEB or phorbel myristate acetate plus ionomycin) be placed in the wells towards the end of the plate.

4. For CFC assays using whole blood from HIV-positive donors, there may be a need to use more than 200 μl of blood per well because of lower CD4+-T-cell counts. In such a situation, 24-well deep-well plates should be used for activation of up to 1 ml of whole blood per well. The size of wells in these plates allows for use of 8 ml of FACS lysing solution and higher wash volumes than the 96-well plate formats for subsequent washes.

REMARKS AND CONCLUSION

We have described how plate-based CFC assays for both whole blood and PBMC can increase the throughput that is a necessity for immune-response monitoring in clinical trials. As shown in Fig. 2, CFC assays performed using (i) PBMC in shallow-well plates (ii) whole blood in 96-well deep-well plates, or (iii) whole blood in 24-well deep-well blocks in parallel resulted in comparable frequencies of IFNγ⁺ CD69⁺ cells and IFN-γ staining intensities. Plate-based CFC allows for activation, processing, and staining in a single plate, reducing the labor required and the cell loss that results from sample transfers (19). In addition, batch analysis using dynamic gating improves reproducibility of the results and lowers subjectivity in gating, facilitating standardization and robust assay performance. CFC assays can be used efficiently to detect more than one cytokine (e.g., IFN-γ, interleukin-2, and tumor necrosis factor alpha) per stimulus by using six-color or eight-color analysis (16). All these characteristics of plate-based CFC provide the benefits of high-content information and higher efficiency of detection than that of ELISPOT assays, with comparable throughput (5, 7, 13). In fact, current National Institutes of Health clinical trials for HIV vaccines will be using this CFC assay format as part of their routine immune-response monitoring. Increasing usage of plate-based CFC in multisite clinical trials will undoubtedly accelerate the search for a surrogate biomarker(s) of vaccine efficacy.

We thank Maria Suni for optimizing procedures and providing data and Laurel Nomura for editing the manuscript.

REFERENCES

1. **Altman, J. D., P. A. Moss, P. J. Goulder, D. H. Barouch, M. G. McHeyzer-Williams, J. I. Bell, A. J. McMichael, and M. M. Davis.** 1996. Phenotypic analysis of antigen-specific T lymphocytes. *Science* **274:**94–96.

2. **Czerkinsky, C. C., L. A. Nilsson, H. Nygren, O. Ouchterlony, and A. Tarkowski.** 1983. A solid-phase enzyme-linked immunospot (ELISPOT) assay for enumeration of specific antibody-secreting cells. *J. Immunol. Methods* **65:**109–121.

3. **Ghanekar, S. A., and H. T. Maecker.** 2003. Cytokine flow cytometry: multiparametric approach to immune function analysis. *Cytotherapy* **5:**1–6.

4. **Gratama, J. W., and F. Kern.** 2004. Flow cytometric enumeration of antigen-specific T lymphocytes. *Cytometry* **58A:**79–86.

5. **Karlsson, A. C., J. N. Martin, S. R. Younger, B. M. Bredt, L. Epling, R. Ronquillo, A. Varma, S. G. Deeks, J. M. McCune, D. F. Nixon, and E. Sinclair.** 2003. Comparison of the ELISPOT and cytokine flow cytometry assays for the enumeration of antigen-specific T cells. *J. Immunol. Methods* **283:**141–153.

6. **Kern, F., N. Faulhaber, C. Frommel, E. Khatamzas, S. Prosch, C. Schonemann, I. Kretzschmar, R. Volkmer-Engert, H. D. Volk, and P. Reinke.** 2000. Analysis of CD8 T cell reactivity to cytomegalovirus using protein-spanning pools of overlapping pentadecapeptides. *Eur. J. Immunol.* **30:**1676–1682.

7. **Kuzushima, K., Y. Hoshino, K. Fujii, N. Yokoyama, M. Fujita, T. Kiyono, H. Kimura, T. Morishima, Y. Morishima, and T. Tsurumi.** 1999. Rapid determination of Epstein-Barr virus-specific CD8(+) T-cell frequencies by flow cytometry. *Blood* **94:**3094–3100.

8. **Maecker, H. T., L. J. Picker, and V. C. Maino.** 2002. Flow cyotmetric analysis of cytokines, p. 338–346. *In* N. R. Rose, R. G. Hamilton, and B. Detrick (ed.), *Manual of Clinical Laboratory Immunology,* 6th ed. ASM Press, Washington, D.C.

9. **Maecker, H. T., H. S. Dunn, M. A. Suni, E. Khatamzas, C. J. Pitcher, T. Bunde, N. Persaud, W. Trigona, T. M. Fu, E. Sinclair, B. M. Bredt, J. M. McCune, V. C. Maino, F. Kern, and L. J. Picker.** 2001. Use of overlapping peptide mixtures as antigens for cytokine flow cytometry. *J. Immunol. Methods* **255:**27–40.

10. **Maecker, H. T., and V. C. Maino.** 2003. T cell immunity to HIV: defining parameters of protection. *Curr. HIV Res.* **1:**249–259.

11. **Maecker, H. T., A. Rinfret, P. D'Souza, J. Darden, E. Roig, C. Landry, P. Hayes, J. Birungi, O. Anzala, M. Garcia, A. Harari, I. Frank, R. Baydo, M. Baker, J. Holbrook, J. Ottinger, L. Lamoreaux, C. L. Epling, E. Sinclair, M. A. Suni, K. Punt, S. Calarota, S. El-Bahi, G. Alter, H. Maila, E. Kuta, J. Cox, C. Gray, M. Altfeld, N. Nougarede, J. Boyer, L. Tussey, T. Tobery, B. Bredt, M. Roederer, R. Koup, V. C. Maino, K. Weinhold, G. Pantaleo, J. Gilmour, H. Horton, and R. P. Sekaly.** 24 June 2005, posting date. Standardization of cytokine flow cytometry assays. *BMC Immunol.* **6:**13. [Online.] doi: 10.1186/1471-2172-6-13.

12. **Maino, V. C., and H. T. Maecker.** 2004. Cytokine flow cytometry: a multiparametric approach for assessing cellular immune responses to viral antigens. *Clin. Immunol.* **110:**222–231.

13. **Moretto, W. J., L. A. Drohan, and D. F. Nixon.** 2000. Rapid quantification of SIV-specific CD8 T cell responses with recombinant vaccinia virus ELISPOT or cytokine flow cytometry. *AIDS* **14:**2625–2627.

14. **Nomura, L. E., J. M. Walker, and H. T. Maecker.** 2000. Optimization of whole blood antigen-specific cytokine assays for CD4(+) T cells. *Cytometry* **40:**60–68.

15. **Reece, W. H., M. Pinder, P. K. Gothard, P. Milligan, K. Bojang, T. Doherty, M. Plebanski, P. Akinwunmi, S. Everaere, K. R. Watkins, G. Voss, N. Tornieporth, A. Alloueche, B. M. Greenwood, K. E. Kester, K. P. McAdam, J. Cohen, and A. V. Hill.** 2004. A CD4(+) T-cell immune response to a conserved epitope in the circumsporozoite protein correlates with protection from natural Plasmodium falciparum infection and disease. *Nat. Med.* **10:**406–410.

16. **Roederer, M., J. M. Brenchley, M. R. Betts, and S. C. De Rosa.** 2004. Flow cytometric analysis of vaccine responses: how many colors are enough? *Clin. Immunol.* **110:**199–205.

17. **Shinn, A. H., N. C. Bravo, H. T. Maecker, and J. W. Smith.** 2003. TNF-alpha detection using a flow cytometric assay to determine cellular responses to anthrax vaccine. *J. Immunol. Methods* **282:**169–174.

18. **Sun, P., R. Schwenk, K. White, J. A. Stoute, J. Cohen, W. R. Ballou, G. Voss, K. E. Kester, D. G. Heppner, and U. Krzych.** 2003. Protective immunity induced with malaria vaccine, RTS,S, is linked to Plasmodium falciparum circumsporozoite protein-specific CD4+ and CD8+ T cells producing IFN-gamma. *J. Immunol.* **171:**6961–6967.

19. **Suni, M. A., H. S. Dunn, P. L. Orr, R. de Laat, E. Sinclair, S. A. Ghanekar, B. M. Bredt, J. F. Dunne, V. C. Maino, and H. T. Maecker.** 2 Sept. 2003, posting date. Performance of plate-based cytokine flow cytometry with automated data analysis. *BMC Immunol.* **4:**9. [Online.] doi: 10.1186/1471-2172-4-9.

20. **Suni, M. A., L. J. Picker, and V. C. Maino.** 1998. Detection of antigen-specific T cell cytokine expression in whole blood by flow cytometry. *J. Immunol. Methods* **212:**89–98.

21. **Waldrop, S. L., C. J. Pitcher, D. M. Peterson, V. C. Maino, and L. J. Picker.** 1997. Determination of antigen-specific memory/effector CD4+ T cell frequencies by flow cytometry: evidence for a novel, antigen-specific homeostatic mechanism in HIV-associated immunodeficiency. *J. Clin. Investig.* **99:**1739–1750.

Molecular Analysis of Cytokines and Cytokine Receptors

NIELS KRUSE AND PETER RIECKMANN

41

REAL-TIME QUANTITATIVE PCR

Background

During the last decades, analysis of cytokines and cytokine receptor research have gathered much interest. Numerous methods have been developed for the detection and quantification of cytokines and cytokine receptors, which may be detected at either the protein or the mRNA level (see Table 1). For quantification at the protein level, enzyme-linked immunosorbent assays, biological assays, and extracellular as well as intracellular cytokine staining (31) have been widely used. Problems with protein quantification derive from the low concentrations of cytokines and cytokine receptors present in the blood or other body fluids and the minor amounts secreted into cell culture supernatants, especially if cells are not stimulated. Furthermore, detectability of cytokine proteins in plasma may be hampered by specific and nonspecific cytokine inhibitors (5). Higher sensitivity is obtained when the expression of mRNAs coding for cytokines and cytokine receptors is utilized. Quantification of cytokine mRNA expression is possible by using Northern blotting (4), RNase protection assays (24), in situ hybridization (30), and quantitative PCR. Although Northern blotting and RNase protection assays have been shown to give excellent quantitative results, these techniques are very labor-intensive and require large amounts of starting material (1). Furthermore, the sensitivity of these assays is rather low as indicated by a detection limit of 10^5 mRNA copies (12). In situ hybridization allows not only for more-sensitive quantification of mRNA (12) but also, in combination with immunocytochemistry, for identification of the expressing cell type (13). The most sensitive assay for quantification of mRNA molecules available today is reverse transcription of mRNA into cDNA in combination with PCR (RT-PCR) (8). With this technique, even single molecules of specific mRNAs were reported to be detectable due to the exponential amplification of target molecules (23), and reproducible quantitative results can be obtained with copy numbers as low as 50 molecules (14, 15, 29).

In this chapter, we will focus on improvements of the recently developed real-time quantitative PCR (7, 9) that has been used in our laboratory for a couple of years in comparison to other available techniques (14, 15). The methods described allow quantification of minute amounts of mRNA in small samples due to the exponential amplification of the target sequence and the generation of fluorescent molecules that are detected during the amplification reaction.

Analysis of Cytokine and Cytokine Receptor Expression in Cell Culture and Tissue

Gene expression can be analyzed in tissues or cell culture systems. The real-time RT-PCR has been evaluated for the quantification of mRNA expression in cell culture systems (e.g., peripheral blood mononuclear cells, dendritic cells, and cerebral endothelial cell cultures of different species), tissues (those of the central and peripheral nervous systems), and whole blood (fresh and stored frozen). Depending on the starting material, the procedure of RNA purification has to be optimized and may vary considerably. As RNA molecules are subject to degradation by ubiquitous RNases, special emphasis has to be placed on preserving the integrity of the molecules during isolation and storage. We recommend immediately dissolving the tissue and cell culture material in a buffer containing guanidine thiocyanate and β-mercaptoethanol to denature proteins and inactivate RNases. If possible, samples should be snap-frozen in liquid nitrogen and stored at −80°C until use. For quantification of RNA or DNA in blood samples, devices for transportation to specialized laboratories have been developed that preserve the integrity of the nucleic acids (e.g., PAXgene blood RNA or DNA system from QIAGEN) even if stored at room temperature.

Concept

Principle of PCR

PCR is suitable to specifically amplify target sequences by a millionfold. A typical amplification reaction mixture includes a sample of RNA, cDNA, or DNA (the template), two sequence-specific oligonucleotide primers, deoxynucleoside triphosphates, reaction buffer, magnesium, and a thermostable DNA polymerase. PCRs are performed in thermal cyclers, which take the reaction mixture through a series of different temperatures. Incubation of the reaction mixture at 95°C leads to denaturation and unfolding of the target sequence. Lowering the temperature to 40 to 60°C allows the oligonucleotide primers to specifically anneal to the template and prime the amplification reaction. At temperatures between 60 and 72°C, thermostable DNA polymerases elongate the primers and amplify the target sequence. Under

TABLE 1 Comparison of methods for quantification of cytokine and cytokine receptor mRNA expression[a]

Method	Amt of RNA required	Sensitivity	Labor intensity	Post-PCR steps required	Dynamic range	Kinetic control required	High-throughput application	Coamplification with internal standards
Northern blotting	Large	Low	High	NA		No	No	
RNase protection assay	Large	Low	High	NA		No	No	
In situ hybridization RT-PCR	Small	High	High	NA		No	No	
Semiquantitative PCR	Small	High	High	Yes	Narrow	No	No	No
Quantitative PCR								
Competitive	Small	High	High	Yes	Narrow	No	No	Yes
Real-time	Small	High	Low	No	Wide	Yes	Yes	No
cDNA arrays	Small	High	Low	NA	Narrow	No	Yes	NA

[a] NA, not applicable.

optimal conditions, each cycle theoretically doubles the number of template molecules. A recent development in PCR technology was the invention of real-time PCR based on the 5′ nuclease assay (10). PCR are performed in real-time thermocyclers from various companies (e.g., Applied Biosystems, Stratagene, Roche, BioRad, MJ Research, Incyte, Smartcycler, and Corbett). These machines can be classified into flexible and high-throughput systems. The flexible systems allow the user to run up to 96 temperature profiles per run, and most high-throughput thermocyclers allow only one temperature profile per run. Furthermore, the instruments differ considerably in ramping and therefore in the time required for analysis.

The compositions of the real-time PCR assay mixtures differ from the mixture described above in that a third oligonucleotide (an internal probe) is added to the reaction mixture and anneals to the template between the oligonucleotide primers. The probe is labeled with a reporter dye at the 5′ end and a quencher dye at the 3′ end. Furthermore, the 3′ end is phosphorylated to prevent elongation by the DNA polymerase. When the probe is intact, the proximity of the reporter dye to the quencher dye results in suppression of the reporter dye fluorescence, primarily by Föster-type fluorescent resonance energy transfer (FRET) (6, 18). During PCR amplification, the DNA polymerase displaces the probe from the template and cleaves it by its 5′→3′ nuclease activity. Both dyes now become separated, FRET does not work anymore, and the reporter dye fluorescence can now be detected. A schematic representation of the reaction is shown in Fig. 1. The amount of reporter fluorescence generated is directly proportional to the number of template molecules as one probe molecule is cleaved for each double strand synthesized. Fig. 2 illustrates the increase in reporter fluorescence during the amplification reaction.

During PCR with the ABI PRISM 7700 sequence detection system, all PCR assay mixtures are sequentially excited every 7 s by an argon laser. The light is directed through fiber-optic cables to the tubes. The fluorescence emission is collected from each well and transferred through a system of lenses, filters, and a dichroic mirror to a spectrograph. Here the light is separated across a charge-coupled device camera. A computer collects the fluorescent signals from the camera and applies analysis algorithms. In addition to the described double-dye oligonucleotide probes for sequence-specific detection, several other formats have been developed. These include molecular beacons, scorpions, hybridization, and

Elipse probes. (An overview is given at http://www.eurogentec.com/code/en/page_07.asp?Page = 409.)

Sequence-unspecific detection is obtained by using SYBR Green I. This initially nonfluorescent dye intercalates into DNA double strands and fluoresces upon light activation. A potential drawback of this detection method is that

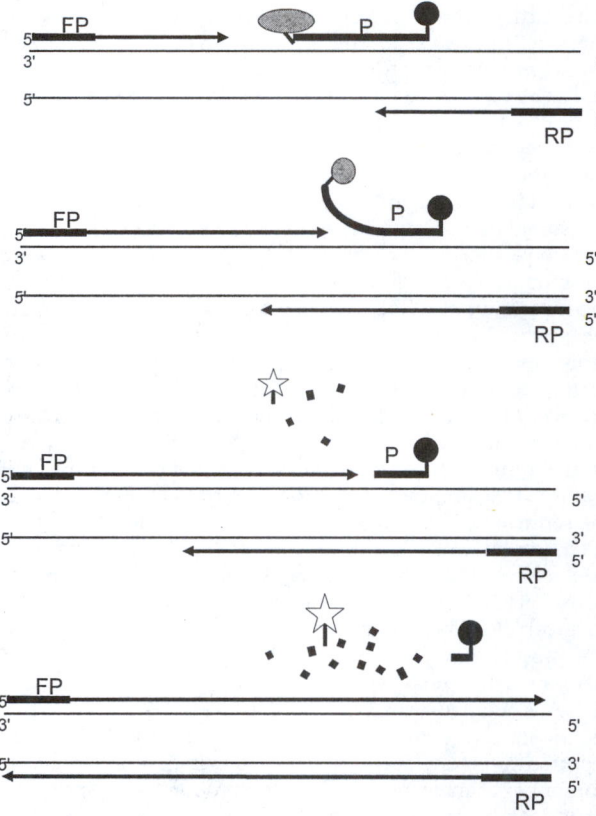

FIGURE 1 Schematic representation of the quantification reaction. Fluorescence signals are generated during the PCR as, upon elongation of one primer, the internal probe is first displaced from the template strand and then cleaved by the *Taq* DNA polymerase. Separation of reporter and quencher dye leads to detectable amounts of reporter fluorescence. F, sense primer; R, antisense primer; P, probe.

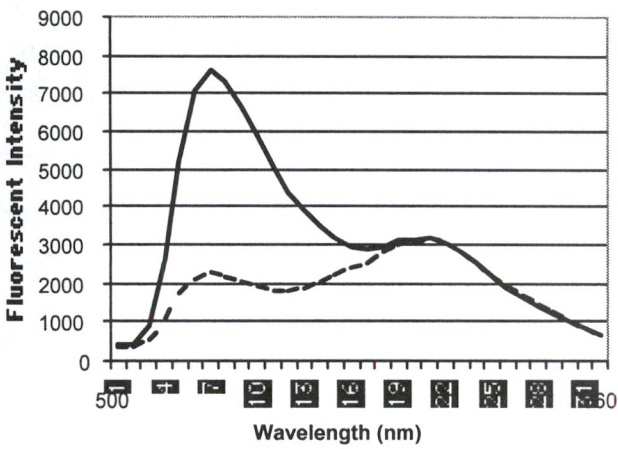

FIGURE 2 Increase in reporter dye fluorescence during amplification reactions. Fluorescence intensities are measured in cycles 5 (dashed line) and 40 (solid line) in the range of 500 to 660 nm. While the TAMRA signal at 580 nm is hardly changed, the FAM signal at 535 nm strongly increases due to separation of reporter and quencher dyes by probe cleavage.

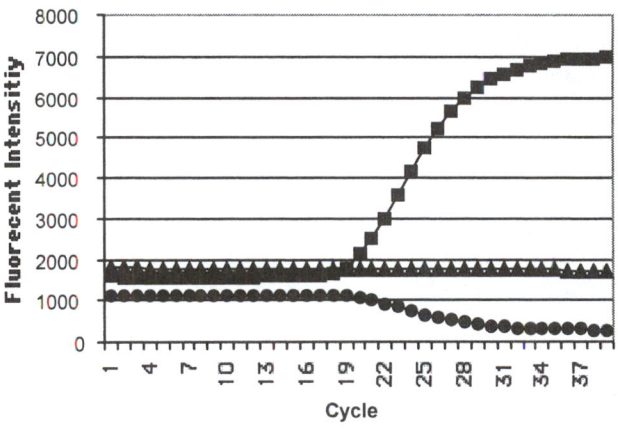

FIGURE 3 Multicomponent view. The changes in FAM, (squares), ROX (triangles), and TAMRA (circles) fluorescence intensities during PCR are shown. ROX serves as a passive reference dye and remains unchanged during PCR. The fluorescence of FAM, as the reporter dye, increases during PCR due to separation from the quencher upon probe cleavage. The TAMRA fluorescence decreases during PCR due to reduced energy transfer from the reporter dye after probe cleavage.

unspecifically amplified sequences as well as primer dimers contribute to the signal. For this reason, a melting curve analysis has to be performed after the PCR is run in order to quantify the amount of specific product.

Predeveloped Assays

Predeveloped assays are available from several vendors. With these assays, the labor-intensive establishment and optimization of quantitative real-time PCR assays is no longer neccessary. The assays are developed in such a way that the sequence of interest and a housekeeping gene from the sample are amplified in separate wells. The results are then subjected to a mathematical calculation in order to determine the concentration difference in a pathological or stimulated sample in relation to a standard sample (see below). Most of the assays developed thus far show comparable amplification efficiencies. Therefore, many targets can be amplified and quantified from a single sample in parallel.

Kinetic Control of Amplification Reaction

Real-time PCR enables control of reaction kinetics. An example is given in Fig. 3. The multicomponent view illustrates the change in fluorescence energies of the different dyes contained in the reaction mix. 6-Carboxy-X-rhodamine (ROX) serves as a passive reference dye to control for pipetting errors. It should give a straight line at the same level for all assays within one experiment. 6-Carboxyfluorescein (FAM) and 6-carboxytetramethylrhodamine (TAMRA) are the reporter and quencher dyes, respectively, covalently attached to the probe molecules. During the first cycles, only a few probe molecules are cleaved and the ratio of the dye intensities does not change significantly. During cycles 3 to 15, the sequence detection system software calculates the mean and standard deviation of the FAM fluorescence. Addition of 10 standard deviations to the mean is defined as the threshold level. Fluorescence intensity has to exceed this threshold value to be regarded as significant. As during the exponential phase of the amplification reaction, as the cleaved probe molecules accumulate, FAM fluorescence increases and

TAMRA fluorescence decreases due to reduced FRET. Increase in FAM fluorescence should be as high as possible to allow sensitive detection of template molecules.

Procedure

Preparation of RNA (Total RNA or mRNA)

RNA can be used either as total RNA or as mRNA. Preparation of total RNA has the advantage that, in case of RNase contamination of mRNA, due to the high concentration of rRNA and tRNA the target RNA sequence is relatively protected against degradation. During preparation, it is essential to immediately inactivate RNases contained in the tissue or cells. RNases are usually inactivated by guanidine thiocyanate in combination with β-mercaptoethanol. Guanidine thiocyanate is a strong denaturing agent. It efficiently lyses cells or tissues and denatures proteins. β-Mercaptoethanol acts by reducing disulfide bridges. For purification of RNA, several methods have been developed. Most of them are based on separation of RNA from contaminating DNA and proteins by phenol-chloroform extraction. After mixing and centrifugation, DNA is concentrated in the phenol phase, proteins are concentrated in the interphase, and RNAs are concentrated in the upper aqueous phase. RNAs are further purified from the aqueous phase by alcohol precipitation and several washing steps. Besides the procedure described, numerous kits are commercially available for RNA preparation from different tissues and cell populations. These kits often contain resin-based separation materials and are nontoxic, and the procedures are fast and less laborious. Up to 96 samples can be processed in parallel.

Preparation of Standards

Decisions should be made about what kind of standard should be used for quantification of cytokine mRNAs. Standards may be either cRNA reverse transcribed in vitro (25) or cDNAs cloned into a plasmid vector (cDNA standards) (14, 15). Using cRNA as a standard allows absolute quantification of mRNA expression if known amounts of cRNA are prepared and reverse transcribed in parallel with sample mRNAs and used to generate standard curves. This procedure controls for RNA recovery and efficiency of reverse transcription in different samples. However, one has to keep in mind that if multiple mRNAs are to be quantified, cRNAs for each target sequence have to be processed, which may impact the comparability between individual cytokine quantifications. With the use of cDNA standards, one does not control for RNA recovery and efficiency of reverse transcription. Therefore, only relative quantification is possible. We routinely use cDNA standards as we usually quantify multiple mRNAs in our samples. If the standards are handled appropriately and reverse transcription has initially been optimized, the results from different experiments are comparable and highly reproducible.

For preparation of standards, cDNAs encompassing the entire coding sequence should be cloned into a plasmid vector. This method has the advantage that, during establishment of new quantitative assays, one often has to try several oligonucleotide combinations in order to find a combination sensitive and specific for target cDNA and not prone to interfere with genomic DNA. Sequence identity has to be confirmed by sequencing because even single base pair exchanges may critically impact the optimal hybridization conditions for the internal probe that determines quantification efficacy. Furthermore, in several instances nucleotide sequences derived from databases may harbor single nucleotide exchanges due to naturally occurring polymorphisms within the population. An alternative method for relative quantification is used in predeveloped assays from several companies. These rely on the comparative cycle threshold (C_T) or $\Delta\Delta C_T$ method (22). One or multiple genes of interest (target) and an appropriate endogenous control from a sample are amplified in two separate assays. For both sequences, the C_T is determined. ΔC_T is calculated as follows: $C_{Tendogenous\ control}$ − $C_{Tgene\ of\ interest}$. A calibrator sample is treated similarly. The expression of the gene of interest in a sample is then normalized to its expression in the calibrator sample by calculating $\Delta\Delta C_T$ as follows: $\Delta\Delta C_T = \Delta C_{Tsample} - \Delta C_{Tcalibrator}$. The amount of target normalized to the endogenous control and relative to the calibrator sample is $2^{\Delta\Delta CT}$.

Synthesis of cDNA [Oligo(dT), Random Hexanucleotide, and Sequence-Specific Oligonucleotide Priming]

Different methods have been applied for the synthesis of cDNAs from purified total RNA or mRNA. Reverse transcription may be primed by oligo(dT) oligonucleotides (14, 15), random hexanucleotides (20), or sequence-specific oligonucleotides (32). While reverse transcription with sequence-specific oligonucleotides should lead to reverse transcription of only the respective mRNA, both oligo(dT) and random hexanucleotides prime reverse transcription of a mixture of mRNAs. Oligo(dT) restricts reverse transcription to poly(A)$^+$ mRNAs, whereas random hexanucleotides prime reverse transcription of all RNAs, including rRNA and tRNA, both of which allow cDNA preparation for multiple-target amplification.

Choice of Oligonucleotides for Amplification and Quantification

To prevent amplification of genomic DNA, oligonucleotide primers should anneal to different exons separated by long introns. Higher specificity may be obtained if at least one oligonucleotide anneals to the mRNA template at an exon-exon boundary (Fig. 4). Several software packages are

available to analyze physicochemical characteristics of oligonucleotide sequences such as melting temperature (T_m), G+C content, secondary structure, and primer dimer formation, etc. We routinely use PrimerExpress software (PerkinElmer). This software automatically chooses combinations of oligonucleotide primers and a corresponding internal probe according to predefined parameters. The T_m of the oligonucleotide primers should be 58 to 60°C. The G+C content should be 30 to 80%. The higher the G+C content, the shorter the oligonucleotide will be for a given T_m. For quantitative assays, the T_m of the probe sequence should be approximately 10°C above the primer T_m. Extensive secondary-structure formation and primer dimer formation should be avoided. The probe sequence must not start with a G since guanidine serves as a quencher for reporter dyes. Runs of five or more identical nucleotides are to be avoided. If possible, the probe sequence with a low G/C ratio should be used. The last five nucleotides at the 3′end of the oligonucleotide primer should not include more than two G's plus C's to improve priming specificity. Alternatively, Web-based programs are available from several companies. During recent years, several databases of validated oligonucleotides for quantitative PCR have appeared on the Web (http://appliedbiosystems.com/catalog/myab/StoreCatalog/products/CategoryDetails.jsp?hierarchyID=101&category3rd=111951&trail=0; https://www1.qiagen.com/Products/PCR/QuantiTect/Search/Default.aspx; https://catalog.invitrogen.com/index.cfm?fuseaction=viewCatalog.viewProductDetails&sku=108M01&productDescription=953; http://medgen.ugent.be/rtprimerdb).

Specificity for mRNA templates may be validated by using genomic DNA as a template. No fluorescence signal should be generated in this amplification reaction. To exclude significant depletion of oligonucleotides by contaminating genomic DNA, defined amounts of cDNA and cDNA with a contaminating amount of genomic DNA (e.g., 50 ng, corresponding to roughly 8,500 copies of genomic DNA) should be amplified in separate reactions. C_Ts for both reactions should be the same. This guarantees that contaminating genomic DNA has no influence on the results of mRNA quantification. An example is shown in Fig. 5.

Amplicons should be as short as possible. Real-time PCR works best with amplicon sizes of 50 to 150 bp. Figure 6 illustrates the effect of amplicon size on amplification efficiency. Figure 6A shows the amplification plots of interleukin-2 (IL-2) cDNA standards amplified with oligonucleotide primers IL2S and IL2AS (Fig. 4), and Fig. 6B shows the amplification plots of the same template with primers IL2S2 and IL2AS2 (Fig. 4). Both quantifications were performed with the same internal IL-2 probe (Fig. 4). The amplification plots differ in that amplification with primers IL2S2 and IL2AS2 gives a much steeper amplification plot than that with primers IL2S and IL2AS. This demonstrates that during PCR with primers IL2S2 and IL2AS2 the number of cleaved probe molecules per cycle is much larger than it is during PCR with primers IL2S and IL2AS, and therefore the efficiency of amplification is higher. Amplification efficiency can be calculated from the slope of the standard curve according to the following equation:

$$\%\ \text{Efficiency} = [10^{(-1/\text{slope})} - 1] \times 100$$

In Fig. 7, the standard curves for the experiment from Fig. 6 are shown. As easily seen for defined amounts of target molecules, the threshold for detection of fluorescence is reached much earlier with primers IL2S2 and IL2AS2 than with the original primers. The slopes of the curves were −3,622

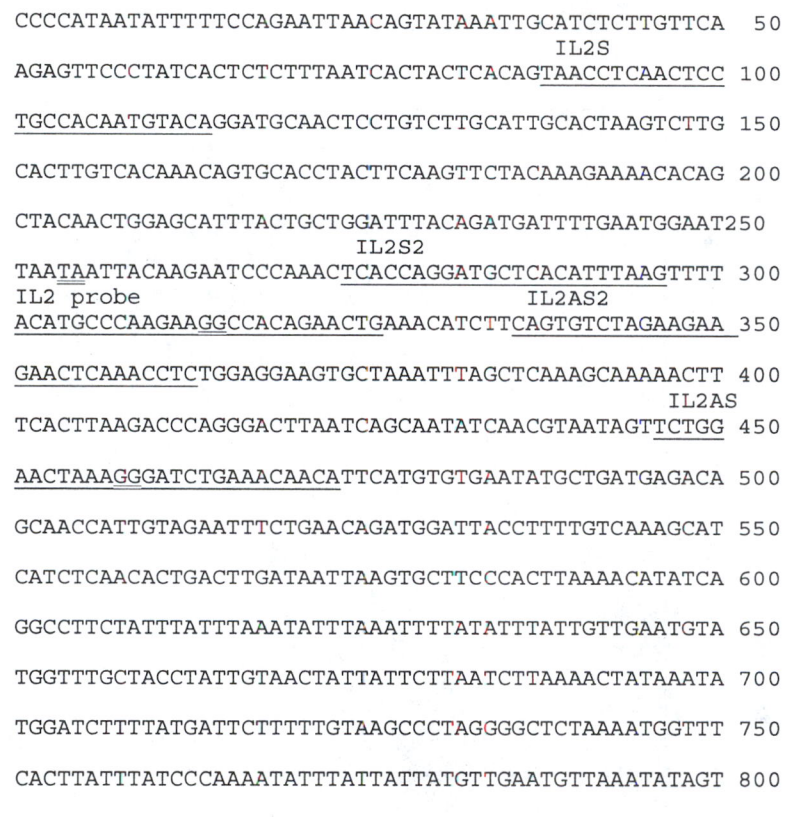

```
CCCCATAATATTTTTCCAGAATTAACAGTATAAATTGCATCTCTTGTTCA 50
                                        IL2S
AGAGTTCCCTATCACTCTCTTTAATCACTACTCACAGTAACCTCAACTCC 100

TGCCACAATGTACAGGATGCAACTCCTGTCTTGCATTGCACTAAGTCTTG 150

CACTTGTCACAAACAGTGCACCTACTTCAAGTTCTACAAAGAAAACACAG 200

CTACAACTGGAGCATTTACTGCTGGATTTACAGATGATTTTGAATGGAAT 250
                                        IL2S2
TAATAATTACAAGAATCCCAAACTCACCAGGATGCTCACATTTAAGTTTT 300
IL2 probe                               IL2AS2
ACATGCCCAAGAAGGCCACAGAACTGAAACATCTTCAGTGTCTAGAAGAA 350

GAACTCAAACCTCTGGAGGAAGTGCTAAATTTAGCTCAAAGCAAAACTT 400
                                        IL2AS
TCACTTAAGACCCAGGGACTTAATCAGCAATATCAACGTAATAGTTCTGG 450

AACTAAAGGGATCTGAAACAACATTCATGTGTGAATATGCTGATGAGACA 500

GCAACCATTGTAGAATTTCTGAACAGATGGATTACCTTTTGTCAAAGCAT 550

CATCTCAACACTGACTTGATAATTAAGTGCTTCCCACTTAAAACATATCA 600

GGCCTTCTATTTATTTAAATATTTAAATTTTATATTTATTGTTGAATGTA 650

TGGTTTGCTACCTATTGTAACTATTATTCTTAATCTTAAAACTATAAATA 700

TGGATCTTTTATGATTCTTTTTGTAAGCCCTAGGGGCTCTAAAATGGTTT 750

CACTTATTTATCCCAAAATATTTATTATTATGTTGAATGTTAAATATAGT 800

ATCTATGTAGATTGGTTAGTAAAACTATTTAATAAATTTGATAA
```

FIGURE 4 Nucleotide sequence of human IL-2 cDNA (HSIL2R). Sequence characteristics must be taken into account when oligonucleotide probes are chosen for quantification. Here, the cDNA sequence for human IL-2 is shown with exon boundaries double underlined and oligonucleotide binding sites underlined. The names of the oligonucleotides are indicated at the starting nucleotides. Note that the IL-2 probe spans an exon boundary.

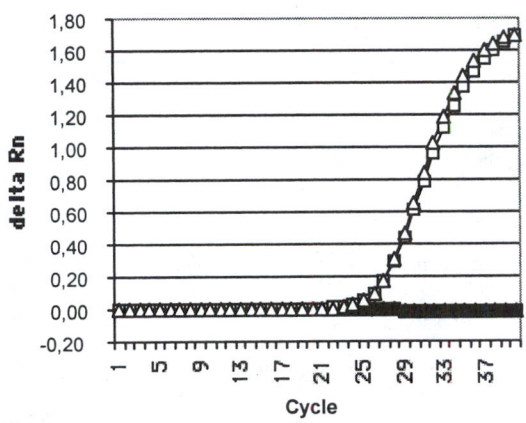

FIGURE 5 Specificity of oligonucleotide primers for cDNA. Means of results in three amplification plots for no-template controls (solid squares), cDNA (open squares), genomic DNA (solid triangles), and coamplified cDNA and genomic DNA (open triangles) are shown. The amplification of NTC and genomic DNA does not generate a fluorescence signal. The amplification of cDNA and cDNA plus genomic DNA results in identical amplification plots. Delta Rn, normalized reporter fluorescence (see text).

(Fig. 7A) and −3,559 (Fig. 7B), which indicates 89 and 91% amplification efficiency, respectively. Short amplicons have the advantage that the rate of incorporation of wrong nucleotides is reduced. Furthermore, with a short distance between primer and probe, one ensures that the first polymerase molecule attached to the primer cleaves the probe, as roughly 60 nucleotides are incorporated into the growing strand before the polymerase molecule detaches from the template.

Optimization of Reaction Conditions (MgCl₂ and Oligonucleotide Concentration)

The performance of amplification reactions is affected to a large extent by the concentrations of magnesium ions and oligonucleotide primers. Usually, specificity of primer annealing increases with decreasing magnesium ion concentration. With real-time PCR, specificity in terms of amplification of only the correct sequence is not the major goal, since hybridization and cleavage of the internal probe guarantee specificity of target quantification. In contrast, one should try to make the reaction as sensitive as possible, i.e., to get the lowest C_T for a given template concentration. To achieve this, the first step in optimization of the reaction conditions is to test several magnesium ion concentrations in increments of 0.5 or 1.0 mM in the range of 2 to 9 mM. The concentration giving the lowest C_T is used for the next step, optimization of oligonucleotide primer concentration.

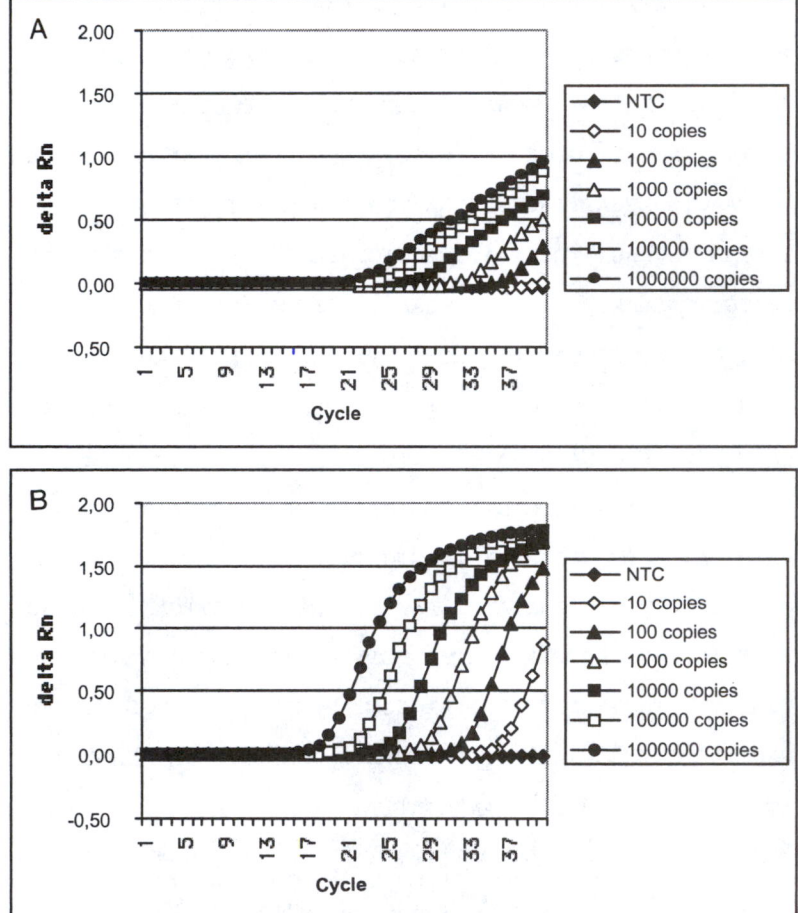

FIGURE 6 Amplification of IL-2 plasmid standards with two different oligonucleotide combinations. IL-2 plasmid standard molecules (10 to 10⁶) were amplified with oligonucleotides IL2S and IL2AS (A) or IL2S2 and IL2AS2 (B) within one experiment. The oligonucleotide binding sites are shown in Fig. 4. With both primer combinations, the same probe (IL-2 probe) was used. Note that usage of oligonucleotides IL2S2 and IL2AS2 results in steeper amplification plots and higher fluorescence intensities. NTC, no-template controls; delta Rn, normalized reporter fluorescence.

Forward and reverse primers are titrated in a checkerboard dilution in the range of 100 to 300 (or 900) nM final concentrations. Again, one is interested in the concentration giving the lowest C_T for a given template concentration. For these experiments, the probe concentration can be kept at 100 nM. A further point of interest is the slope of the amplification plots. This should be as steep as possible because the more labeled probes that are cleaved within one cycle, the higher the efficiency of the amplification reaction (Fig. 6).

Evaluation of Experimental Results

After data analysis is performed, plotting the input number of standard molecules against the C_T determined to detect the respective fluorescence signal generates a plot. This provides the standard curve for the experiment. For unknown samples, the C_T for each sample is detected and transmitted to the computer. The sequence detection software now takes each C_T from the unknown samples to calculate the amount of starting copy number in the assay by comparing individual C_T to those of the standard curve (Fig. 7).

Controls

As data from the real-time PCR are continuously recorded, a retrospective quantitative analysis of the amplification process may be performed. Data analysis starts with a view at the amplification plots of the PCR. The increase in fluorescence intensity for all reactions is displayed on the monitor. This enables the researcher to judge if all reactions were performed with equal efficiencies. Variations in efficiency can easily be detected by changes in amplification profiles. Comparison of C_Ts for defined standard concentrations allows for comparison of different experiments. If quantitative experiments are properly standardized, C_Ts for the standard concentrations yield comparable results within a range of ≤8%. All quantitative determinations should be performed at least in triplicate. The sequence detection software allows assignment of replicates within the experiments. After data analysis, the experimental report constitutes a table with the number of molecules determined in each assay as well as the mean and standard deviations of results for the triplicates.

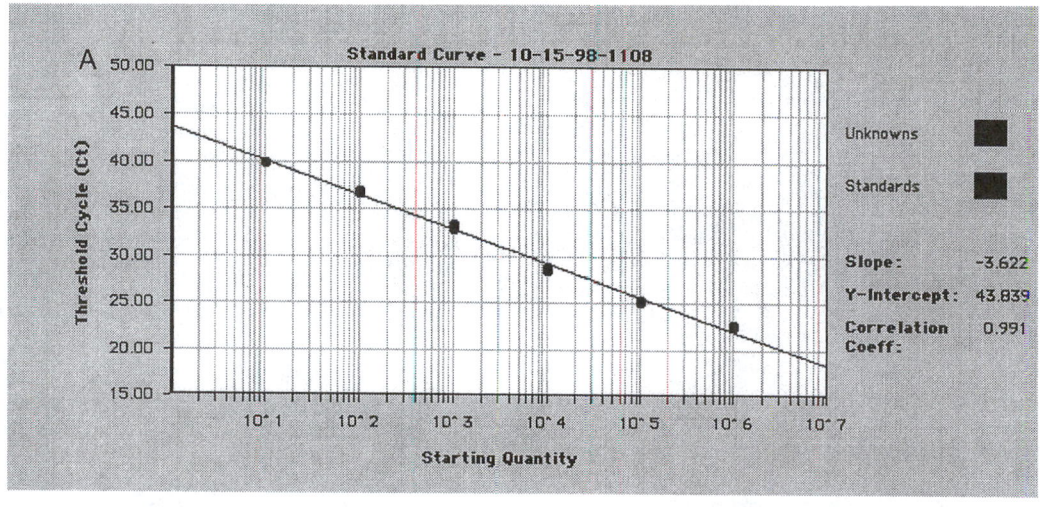

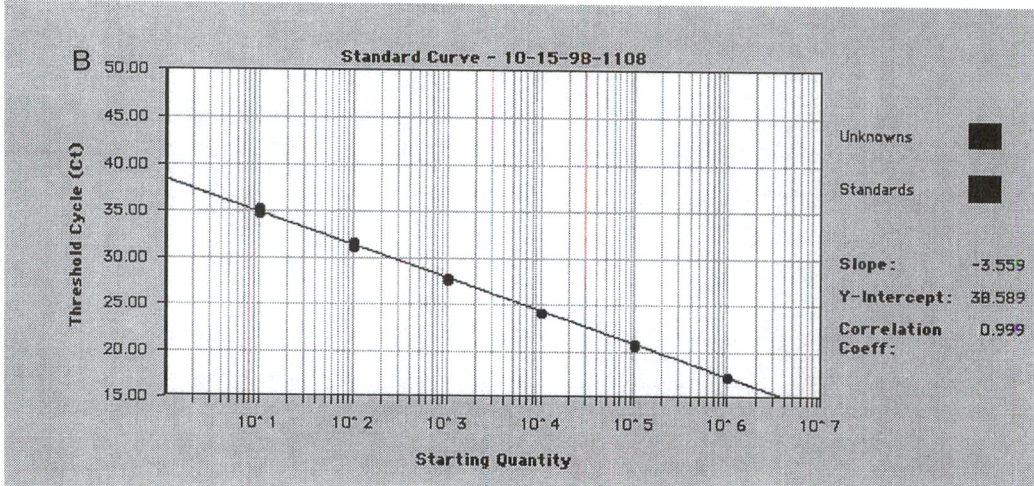

FIGURE 7 IL-2 standard curves generated with two different oligonucleotide combinations. IL-2 plasmid standard molecules (10 to 10^6) were amplified with oligonucleotides IL2S and IL2AS (A) or IL2S2 and IL2AS2 (B) within one experiment. The oligonucleotide binding sites are shown in Fig. 4. With both primer combinations, the same probe (IL-2 probe) was used. Note that usage of oligonucleotides IL2S2 and IL2AS2 results in earlier detection of significant fluorescence, i.e., higher sensitivity. Coeff., coefficient.

Standardization, Pitfalls, and Troubleshooting

In order to achieve a high reproducibility of quantitative analysis, all experimental procedures should be highly standardized as much as possible. Within one study, all reagents required should be purchased from the same vendor, if possible from the same lot. If different lots have to be used, the comparability of results should be verified. In the case of quantitative PCR assays, we sometimes found significantly variable amplification efficiencies with different oligonucleotide batches. The plasmid standards should be stored as aliquots of defined concentrations. Dilution series of standards should be prepared freshly. Freezing of plasmid standard dilution series is not recommended since repetitive freezing and thawing may lead to degradation of DNA molecules.

Application

Real-time PCR is a valuable tool for research and clinical applications. Minor variations in cytokine expression under physiological conditions are often not detectable with enzyme-linked immunosorbent assay techniques. The high sensitivity of the exponential amplification of target molecules (mRNA or DNA) and the high reproducibility of the real-time PCR makes this technique an ideal tool to analyze even minor changes in mRNA concentrations in clinical samples. Serial analysis of cytokine mRNA expression in whole-blood samples has been performed with excellent reproducibility (15).

Differential quantitative expression of cytokine mRNAs in cultures of human purified peripheral blood mononuclear cells and endothelial cells stimulated with various agents has been analyzed in our laboratory. These studies demonstrated that significant changes in mRNA expression can be detected as early as 4 h after initiation of the cultures. The amount of mRNA correlates with the secretion of protein into the culture supernatant (16). Therefore, physiological changes in cytokine mRNA expression can be detected much earlier than changes in protein expression.

ALLELIC DISCRIMINATION PCR

Background

Genetic disorders and drug responses may be critically determined by small variations within functional relevant parts of the genome (11, 19). About 0.1% of the nucleotides are changed between the two chromosomes of a diploid cell (3, 17). These changes are known as single nucleotide polymorphisms (SNPs). Methods used for the analysis of SNPs include, among others, restriction fragment length polymorphism (28), single-strand confirmation polymorphism (31), and sequencing (2). All these techniques are time-consuming and require multiple post-PCR steps that limit the number of samples that can be analyzed per day. For large-scale SNP analysis, routine applications, and pharmacological research, methods are warranted that are reliable, easy to perform, and suitable for automation. The 5′ nuclease assay offers the possibility of analyzing hundreds of samples per day without the need for any post-PCR processing. A major advantage of allelic discrimination PCR is that the amplification of the target sequences may be performed in any thermocycler. The ABI PRISM 7700 sequence detection system is required only for establishing the optimal reaction conditions and measuring the amount of fluorescence generated during amplification in a plate read mode.

Concept

Principle of Allelic Discrimination Using Oligonucleotides Labeled with Fluorescent Dyes

Real-time PCR also allows for allelic discrimination of SNPs in genomic DNA samples (21, 26, 27). Internal probes labeled with different reporter dyes for each allele are used within one reaction (e.g., probe 1 labeled with FAM for the wild-type allele and probe 2 labeled with TET (6-carboxy-2′,4,7,7′-tetrachlorofluuprecein) for the mutant allele). Depending on the haplotype, either probe 1 or probe 2 is cleaved if homozygous DNA is present. If heterozygous DNA is present, both probes are cleaved. If the wrong probe is hybridized to the template, the mismatch within the probe sequence introduces so much instability that upon initial strand displacement by the DNA polymerase the incorrect probe floats away before cleavage while the correct probe sticks to the template and gets cleaved. The sequence detection system software automatically makes allele calls by calculating the ratio of fluorescence intensities for probe 1 and probe 2 for each DNA sample. DNA homozygous for allele 1 should give a high FAM/TET ratio, and DNA homozygous for allele 2 should give a low FAM/TET ratio. Heterozygous DNA should give a FAM/TET ratio of approximately 1.

Procedure

Preparation of DNA

Numerous kits are commercially available for preparation of genomic DNA from different sources. Most easily, DNA can be prepared from blood cells. One milliliter of whole blood is sufficient to yield good-quality genomic DNA for several hundred allelic discrimination reactions.

Preparation of Standards

DNA fragments comprising the polymorphic position of interest and the primer binding sites should be cloned into a plasmid vector. The sequence identity should be confirmed by sequence analysis.

Choice of Oligonucleotides for Amplification and Detection

The physicochemical characteristics of the oligonucleotides should be as described above for quantitative assays with the only exception that the T_m of the internal probes should be approximately 7°C above the primer T_m. For successful allelic discrimination, it is extremely important that T_ms for both probes be as similar as possible to achieve comparable annealing efficiencies and differentiate as little as one base pair exchange.

Optimization of Reaction Conditions (MgCl$_2^-$ and Oligonucleotide Concentrations and Annealing Temperature)

The aim of optimizing the reaction conditions for allelic discrimination PCR is to increase cleavage of the correct internal probe and concurrently decrease cleavage of the false internal probe. Allelic discrimination PCR usually works with 5 mM Mg^{2+}. Oligonucleotide primer concentrations are titrated in a checkerboard test at concentrations of 50, 300, and 900 nM with 100 nM final concentrations of both internal probes. The concentrations giving the lowest C_T and the highest delta Rn values should be used for further experiments. (Delta Rn is the ratio of the fluorescence emission intensity of the reporter dye to the fluorescence emission intensity of the passive reference dye minus baseline.) Next, the internal probe concentration is titrated at concentrations of 50, 100, and 200 nM with the fixed primer concentration determined before. This test serves to find the conditions for best discrimination between the two alleles, i.e., the highest ratios between the fluorescence signals generated by cleavage of the matching and the mismatching probes. Improvement of discrimination can be obtained by changing the annealing temperature in 1°C increments. An example of increase in fluorescence intensities obtained in an allelic discrimination experiment is given in Fig. 8.

Evaluation of Experimental Results

Figure 9 presents the results from an allelic discrimination experiment. In this experiment, the internal probe specific for the wild-type allele at position −308 of the human tumor necrosis factor alpha (TNF-α) promoter (TNFα−308G) was labeled with TET as the reporter dye. The internal probe for the mutant allele (TNFα−308A) was labeled with FAM as the reporter dye. It is expected that in the presence of homozygous wild-type DNA the TET-labeled probe is preferentially cleaved, giving rise to significant TET fluorescence and, if any, very little FAM fluorescence. In the presence of homozygous mutant DNA, significant FAM fluorescence with little TET fluorescence should be generated. Heterozygous DNA, due to cleavage of both probes, should give increases in both fluorescence signals. Based on the data from the standards run within the experiment, the sequence detection software generates a plot of FAM versus TET fluorescence for the standards and the unknown DNA samples. As clearly visible from Fig. 9, three populations are distinguished according to the amount of FAM and TET fluorescence generated during amplification. Samples giving a high TET/FAM ratio are identified as homozygous GG, and those giving a high FAM/TET ratio are identified as homozygous AA. Heterozygous DNAs give intermediate ratios.

Remarks and Conclusions

Real-time PCR can be regarded as a state-of-the-art technique to investigate the expression of cytokine and cytokine receptor mRNA in different tissues or experimental or clinical settings. Several advantages of the system described in

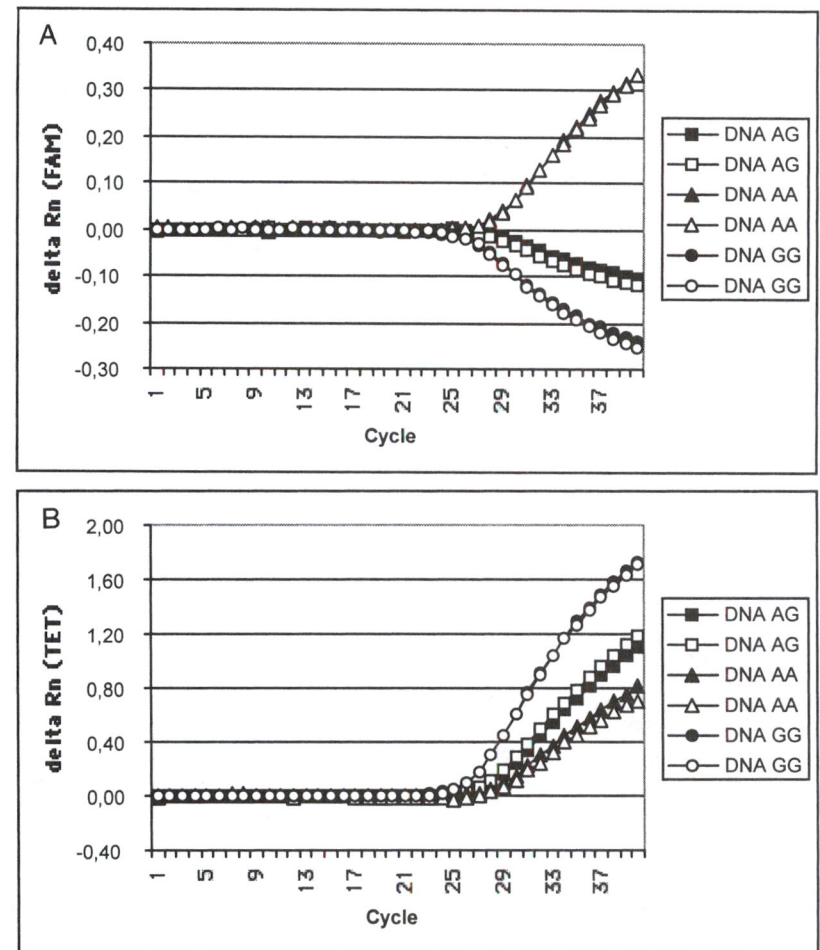

FIGURE 8 Increase in FAM (A) and TET (B) fluorescence during PCR amplification of different TNF-α haplotypes. Three different haplotypes of the human TNF-α promotor (DNA AG, DNA AA, and DNA GG) were amplified in the presence of two different internal probes. One is labeled with TET and specific for the wild type (TNFα-308G), the other is labeled with FAM and specific for the mutant promotor (TNFα-308A). If homozygous DNA TNFα-308A is present, the FAM fluorescence gives the higher intensity. If homozygous DNA TNFα-308G is present, the FAM fluorescence gives the lower intensity. The opposite holds true for the TET fluorescence. Heterozygous DNA in both cases gives intermediate intensities. Delta Rn, normalized reporter fluorescence (see text).

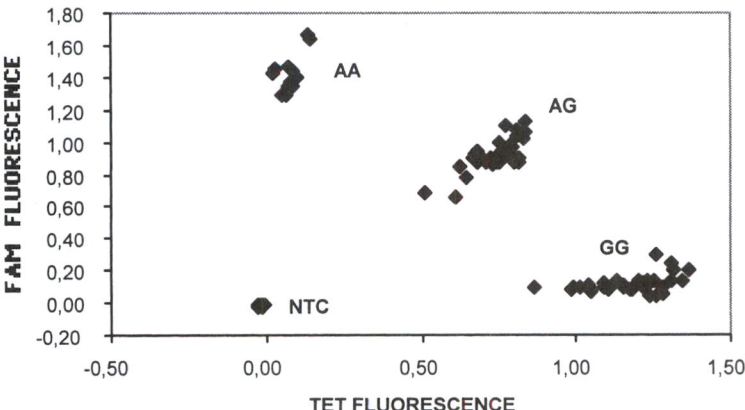

FIGURE 9 Identification of TNF-α haplotypes by allelic discrimination PCR. After PCR, the FAM and TET fluorescence intensities were determined for each sample. Plotting FAM fluorescence against TET fluorescence revealed different populations representing three haplotypes. High TET and low FAM intensities identify wild-type alleles; high FAM and low TET intensities identify mutant alleles. Heterozygous DNA gives intermediate results. NTC, no-template controls.

this chapter include its broad applicability, high sensitivity, wide dynamic range, and ease of adaptation to almost every field of interest (e.g., analysis of mRNA expression in research and clinical settings, detection of bacterial or viral infection, detection of contamination in dairy products, and determination of point mutations in genomewide screenings, etc.), as well as the potential for online control of reaction kinetics to verify the likelihood of results. A major advantage of the real-time PCR is its application as a high-throughput analytical system in routine diagnostics and research, as, in contrast to other conventional PCR-based techniques, no post-PCR processing of the reaction products is required.

REFERENCES

1. **Benveniste, O., M. Martin, F. Villinger, and D. Dormont.** 1998. Techniques for quantification of cytokine mRNAs. *Cytokines Cell. Mol. Ther.* **4:**207–214.
2. **Braun, N., U. Michel, B. P. Ernst, R. Metzner, A. Bitsch, F. Weber, and P. Rieckmann.** 1996. Gene polymorphism at position −308 of the tumor-necrosis-factor-alpha (TNF-alpha) in multiple sclerosis and its influence on the regulation of TNF-alpha production. *Neurosci. Lett.* **215:**75–78.
3. **Cooper, D. N., B. A. Smith, H. J. Cooke, S. Niemann, and L. Schmidtke.** 1985. An estimate of unique DNA sequence heterozygosity in the human genome. *Hum. Genet.* **69:**201–205.
4. **Dallman, M. J., R. A. Montgomery, C. P. Larson, A. Wanders, and A. F. Wells.** 1991. Cytokine gene expression: analysis using Northern blotting, polymerase chain reaction and in situ hybridization. *Immunol. Rev.* **119:**163–179.
5. **Delarche, C., and S. Chollet-Martin.** 1999. Plasma cytokines: what we are measuring. *Curr. Opin. Clin. Nutr. Metab. Care* **2:**475–479.
6. **Föster, V. T.** 1948. Zwischenmolekulare energiewanderung und fluoreszenz. *Ann. Phy. (Leipzig)* **2:**55–75.
7. **Gibson, U. E. M., C. A. Heid, and P. M. Williams.** 1996. A novel method for real time quantitative RT-PCR. *Genome Res.* **6:**995–1001.
8. **Gilliland, G., S. Perrin, K. Blanchard, and F. Bunn.** 1990. Analysis of cytokine mRNA and DNA: detection and quantitation by competitive polymerase chain reaction. *Proc. Natl. Acad. Sci. USA* **87:**2725–2729.
9. **Heid, C. A., J. Stevens, K. J. Livak, and P. M. Williams.** 1996. Real time quantitative PCR. *Genome Res.* **6:**986–994.
10. **Holland, P. M., R. D. Abramson, R. Watson, and D. H. Gelfand.** 1991. Detection of specific polymerase chain reaction product by utilizing the 5→3 endonuclease activity of *Thermus aquaticus* DNA polymerase. *Proc. Natl. Acad. Sci. USA* **88:**7276–7280.
11. **Housman, D., and F. D. Ledley.** 1998. Why pharmacogenomics? Why now? *Nat. Biotechnol.* **16:**492–493.
12. **Innis, M. A., D. H. Gelfand, J. J. Sninsky, and T. J. White (ed.).** 1990. *PCR Protocols: a Guide to Methods and Applications.* Academic Press, New York, N.Y.
13. **König, A., V. Krenn, R. Gillitzer, J. Glockner, E. Janssen, F. Gohlke, J. Eulert, and H. K. Muller-Hermelink.** 1997. Inflammatory infiltrate and interleukin-8 expression in the synovium of psoriatic arthritis—an immunohistochemical and mRNA analysis. *Rheumatol. Int.* **17:**159–168.
14. **Kruse, N., M. Pette, K. Toyka, and P. Rieckmann.** 1997. Quantification of cytokine mRNA expression by RT PCR in samples of previously frozen blood. *J. Immunol. Methods* **210:**195–203.
15. **Kruse, N., M. Greiff, N. F. Moriabadi, L. Marx, K. V. Toyka, and P. Rieckmann.** 2000. Variations in cytokine

mRNA expression during normal human pregnancy. *Clin. Exp. Immunol.* **119:**317–322.
16. **Kruse, N., N. F. Moriabadi, K. V. Toyka, and P. Rieckmann.** 2001. Characterization of early immunological responses in primary responses of differentially activated human peripheral mononuclear cells. *J. Immunol. Methods* **247:**131–139.
17. **Kwok, P. Y., Q. Deng, H. Zakeri, S. L. Taylor, and D. A. Nickerson.** 1996. Increasing the information content of STS-based genome maps: identifying polymorphisms in mapped STSs. *Genomics* **31:**123–126.
18. **Lakowicz, J. R.** 1993. *Principles of Fluorescence and Spectroscopy,* p. 303–339. Plenum Press, New York, N.Y.
19. **Lander, E., and L. Kruglyak.** 1995. Genetic dissection of complex traits: guidelines for interpreting and reporting linkage results. *Nat. Genet.* **11:**241–247.
20. **Lindsey, J. W., and L. Steinman.** 1993. Competitive PCR quantification of CD4, CD8, ICAM-1, VCAM-1, and MHC class II mRNA in the central nervous system during development and resolution of experimental allergic encephalomyelitis. *J. Neuroimmunol.* **48:**227–234.
21. **Livak, K. J., J. Marmaro, and J. A. Todd.** 1995. Towards fully automated genome-wide polymorphism screening. *Nat. Genet.* **9:**341–342. (Letter.)
22. **Livak, K. J., and T. D. Schmittgen.** 2001. Analysis of relative gene expression data using real-time quantitative PCR and the $2^{-\Delta\Delta CT}$ method. *Methods* **25:**402–408.
23. **Lockey, C., E. Otte, and Z. Long.** 1998. Real-time fluorescence detection of a single DNA molecule. *BioTechniques* **24:**744–746.
24. **Lowry, R. P., K. Wang, B. Venooij, and D. Harcus.** 1989. Lymphokine transcription in vascularised mouse heart grafts: effects of "tolerance" induction. *Transplant. Proc.* **21:**72–73.
25. **Martell, M., J. Gomez, J. I. Esteban, S. Sauleda, J. Quer, B. Cabot, R. Esteban, and J. Guardia.** 1999. High-throughput real-time reverse transcription-PCR quantitation of hepatitis C virus RNA. *J. Clin. Microbiol.* **37:**327–332.
26. **Mäurer, M., N. Kruse, R. Giess, K. Kyriallis, K. V. Toyka, and P. Rieckmann.** 1999. Gene polymorphism at position −308 of the human tumor necrosis factor α promotor is not associated with disease progression in multiple sclerosis patients. *J. Neurol.* **246:**949–954.
27. **Mäurer, M., N. Kruse, R. Giess, K. V. Toyka, and P. Rieckmann.** 2000. Genetic variation at position −1082 of the human interleukin 10 (IL10) promotor and the outcome of multiple sclerosis. *J. Neuroimmunol.* **104:**98–100.
28. **Messer, G., U. Spengler, M. C. Jung, G. Honold, K. Blomer, G. R. Pape, G. Riethmuller, and E. H. Weiss.** 1991. Polymorphic structure of the tumor necrosis factor (TNF) locus: an NcoI polymorphism in the first intron of the human TNF-beta gene correlates with a variant amino acid in position 26 and a reduced level of TNF-beta production. *J. Exp. Med.* **173:**209–219.
29. **Morrison, T. B., J. J. Weis, and C. T. Wittwer.** 1998. Quantification of low-copy transcripts by continous SYBR Green I monitoring during amplification. *BioTechniques* **24:**954–959.
30. **Navikas, V., B. He, J. Link, M. Haglund, M. Söderström, S. Fredrikson, A. Ljungdahl, B. Höjeberg, B. Qiao, T. Olsson, and H. Link.** 1996. Augmented expression of tumour necrosis factor-α and lymphotoxin in mononuclear cells in multiple sclerosis and optic neuritis. *Brain* **119:**213–223.
31. **Selvakumar, N., B. C. Ding, and S. M. Wilson.** 1997. Separation of DNA strands facilitates detection of point mutations by PCR-SSCP. *BioTechniques* **22:**604–606.
32. **Souazé, F., A. Ntodou-Thomé, C. Y. Tran, W. Rostène, and P. Forgez.** 1996. Quantitative RT-PCR: limits and accuracy. *BioTechniques* **21:**280–285.

Chemokine and Chemokine Receptor Analysis

BENJAMIN D. MEDOFF AND ANDREW D. LUSTER

42

BACKGROUND

Overview

The active movement of leukocytes towards a site of antigen challenge, infection, or tissue damage represents a central aspect of the establishment of both the inflammatory and the immune responses (78, 106). The movement of cells towards a chemical gradient of a particular stimulus or chemotactic factor is called chemotaxis. Chemotactic factors which induce the directional movement of leukocytes include the chemokines, a superfamily of proteins 8 to 10 kDa in size, which signal chemotaxis through seven-transmembrane G protein-coupled cell surface receptors (GPCRs) (6, 40, 66, 78, 106, 108). In this chapter, the methodological approaches to studying the role of chemokines and chemokine receptors in the physiology of immune and inflammatory responses will be described. Although assays of chemokines or chemokine receptors have yet to be used for widespread clinical applications, this chapter will discuss the role of these proteins in the pathophysiology of several inflammatory diseases and suggest potential clinical uses for these proteins.

Chemokines and Chemokine Receptors: Basic Principles

Chemokines

Approximately 50 chemokines which share 20 to 70% homology in amino acid sequence have now been identified (6, 40, 66, 78, 106, 108) (Table 1). Chemokines share the common function of attracting leukocytes to sites of an inflammatory or immune response. Chemokine families are defined on the basis of the spacing of the first two cysteine amino acids in the mature protein. Based on this criteria, four families of chemokines exist. In α, or CXC, chemokines, the cysteine residues are separated by a single amino acid. A further subdivision of CXC chemokines relates to the presence or absence of the sequence glutamic acid-lysine-arginine (ELR) near the N terminus of the protein. In general, ELR CXC chemokines chemoattract neutrophils whereas non-ELR CXC chemokines attract lymphocytes. In β, or CC, chemokines, the cysteine residues are adjacent to each other. There are two chemokines that do not fit into these two categories: the so-called C chemokine, lymphotactin, which has only one proximal cysteine residue, and the

CXXXC chemokine, fractalkine, which has three intervening amino acids between the two proximal cysteine residues. Fractalkine is also unique in that it is expressed as a cell surface glycoprotein with the chemokine domain sitting on top of a mucin-like stalk and has both transmembrane and cytoplasmic domains.

It has recently been proposed that the chemokines be given numerical names, like the interleukins and the chemokine receptors (144). In the proposed nomenclature, CC chemokines are named CCLn, for CC chemokine ligand, where n is the number that corresponds to the gene symbol number given to each chemokine as it was mapped and designated SCYn for small secreted cytokine. Likewise, the CXC chemokines are named CXCLn, for CXC chemokine ligands.

Chemokine Receptors

All chemokines signal via seven transmembrane-spanning GPCRs (114, 137), which are named by a numbering system based on the type of chemokines to which they bind (Table 1). GPCRs are a highly versatile group of proteins which have evolved to sense subtle changes in concentration gradients and are involved in signal transduction for vision, olfaction, hormone reception, and neurotransmission in addition to directional cell movement (33, 87, 134). The GPCRs as signal transducers of chemotaxis appear to be highly conserved in evolution, being present on amoebae and slime molds, and are involved in the signaling of chemotaxis in these simple eukaryotes.

GPCRs consist of an extracellular N terminus, an intracellular C terminus, and seven transmembrane-spanning regions (114, 137). Chemokine binding to the extracellular portion of the receptor results in intracytoplasmic signaling, which is mediated in part through heterotrimeric G proteins of the $G\alpha i$ subclass. Chemokines may present to chemokine receptors in both the liquid and solid phases (109). Chemokine receptor binding occurs with both the chemokine in solution and the chemokine bound to the matrix and cell surface glycosaminoglycans (5, 124, 125). The binding of chemokine to receptor results in a complex signaling cascade, which may result in directed cell movement, cell activation, differentiation, and/or cell proliferation (6, 78, 106). Activation of chemokine receptors is usually accompanied by a transient rise in the level of intracellular calcium. The G protein is itself coupled to a number

TABLE 1 Chemokines and receptors

Designation	Chemokine	Receptor
CXC		
CXCL1	GRO-α (MGSA)	CXCR2
CXCL2	GRO-β (MIP-2α)	CXCR2
CXCL3	GRO-γ (MIP-2β)	CXCR2
CXCL4	PF4	Unknown
CXCL5	ENA-78 (LIX)	CXCR2
CXCL6	GCP-2	CXCR1, CXCR2
CXCL7	NAP-2	CXCR2
CXCL8	IL-8	CXCR1, CXCR2
CXCL9	MIG	CXCR3
CXCL10	IP-10 (crg-2, mob-1)	CXCR3
CXCL11	I-TAC	CXCR3
CXCL12	SDF-1	CXCR4
CXCL13	BLC (BCA-1)	CXCR5
CXCL14	BRAK	Unknown
CXCL15	Lungkine (mouse only)	Unknown
CXCL16		CXCR6
CC		
CCL1	I-309 (TCA3)	CCR8
CCL2	MCP-1	CCR2
CCL3	MIP-1α	CCR1, CCR5
CCL4	MIP-1β	CCR5
CCL5	RANTES	CCR1, CCR3, CCR5
CCL6	C-10 (MRP-1) (mouse only)	Unknown
CCL7	MCP-3 (Fic, MARC)	CCR2, CCR3
CCL8	MCP-2	CCR1, CCR2, CCR3, CCR5
CCL9/10	MIP-1γ (MRP-2, CCF18, mouse only)	CCR1
CCL11	Eotaxin	CCR3
CCL12	MCP-5	CCR2
CCL13	MCP-4	CCR2, CCR3, CR5
CCL14	HCC-1	CCR1
CCL15	Leukotactin-1 (HCC-2, MIP-5)	CCR1, CCR3
CCL16	HCC-4 (NCC-4, LEC)	CCR1
CCL17	TARC	CCR4
CCL18	DC-CK1 (PARC, AMAC-1, MIP-4)	Unknown
CCL19	ELC (MIP-3β, Exodus-3)	CCR7
CCL20	MIP-3α (LARC, Exodus-1)	CCR6
CCL21	SLC (Exodus-2, 6CKine, TCA4)	CCR7
CCL22	MDC (STCP-1, ABCD-1)	CCR4
CCL23	MPIF1 (MIP-3)	Unknown
CCL24	Eotaxin-2 (MPIF-2)	CCR3
CCL25	TECK	CCR9
CCL26	Eotaxin-3 (MPIF-2)	CCR3
CCL27	CTAK	CCR10
C		
XCL1	Lymphotactin, SCM-1α	XCR1
XCL2	SCM-1β	XCR1
CX3C		
CX3CL1	Fractalkine (neurotactin)	CX3CR1

of downstream intracytoplasmic signal transduction pathways, including those involving protein kinase C (PKC), tyrosine kinases, and phosphatidylinositol 3-kinase (PI 3-kinase) (34, 125) (Fig. 1). The direct link between these signal transduction pathways and the activation of the cytoskeletal machinery involved in cell motility is not known. However, Rho proteins, which are known to be involved in actin-dependent processes, are thought to be involved in linking chemokine receptor activation to activation of the cytoskeletal machinery (27, 70, 115).

Role of Chemokines and Chemokine Receptors in Disease

Overview

The attraction of leukocytes to sites of inflammation and infection is an essential component of the host response to disease. Chemokines and chemokine receptors have been shown to be an integral part of this process and have been implicated in the pathophysiology of many infectious diseases and inflammatory disorders (78). Although chemokines are

Chemokines

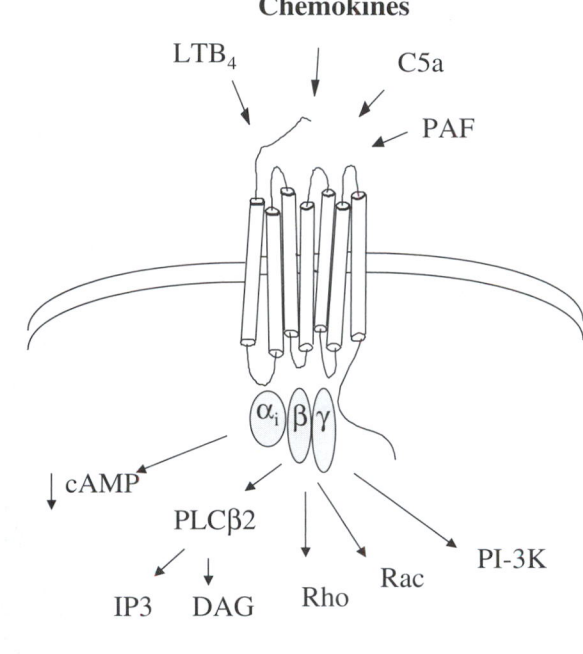

FIGURE 1 Chemokine receptor signal transduction. Chemokine receptors are a subfamily of seven-transmembrane-spanning GPCRs. They are coupled to heterotrimeric G proteins of the Gi subclass, which are distinguished by their pertussis toxin sensitivity. Chemokine receptor activation leads to the stimulation of multiple signal transduction pathways, including the activation of PI 3-kinase (PI-3K) and phospholipase C, leading to the generation of inositol triphosphates, intracellular calcium release, and PKC activation. Chemokine signaling also induces the upregulation of integrin affinity and the activation of Rho, leading to cytoskeletal reorganization. Agonist-stimulated receptors also activate G protein receptor kinases, which leads to receptor phosphorylation, arrestin binding, G protein uncoupling (desensitization), and clathrin-mediated receptor endocytosis (internalization). LTB$_4$, leukotriene B4; C5a, complement fragment 5a; PAF, platelet activating factor; cAMP, cyclic AMP; PLC β2, phospholipase C β2; DAG, diacylglycerol.

clearly important for the ability of the host to control infections, they can also be detrimental in certain inflammatory conditions, such as asthma and atherosclerosis, in which inflammatory cells are recruited into sites in the body and cause the development of an inflammatory infiltrate and damage to the site (32). The chemokine-chemokine receptor axis likely participates in the pathophysiology of these diseases by leading to the pathologic accumulation and activation of leukocytes in affected tissues. In such disorders, it has been suggested that the chemokine-chemokine receptor axis could be used both as a diagnostic tool and as a therapeutic target for controlling the inflammation. The following section will highlight the role of chemokines and their receptors in four different inflammatory conditions, namely, atherosclerosis, arthritis, asthma, and transplantation. The potential clinical applications of assays for chemokine and chemokine receptor expression will be discussed.

Atherosclerosis

Atherosclerosis is the underlying process in coronary artery disease and peripheral vascular disease, two of the most common causes of morbidity and mortality in the United States. It is believed that atherosclerotic lesions develop in response to repeated insults to the arterial wall. Inflammation is a critical component in this process (72), and prominent leukocyte recruitment occurs in almost every stage of lesion development from the appearance of the fatty streak lesion to the formation of complex plaques (118). Immunohistochemical analysis of atherosclerotic lesions reveals that approximately 80% of leukocytes in the atheroma are monocytes/macrophages while T lymphocytes (predominantly memory cells) make up 5 to 20% of the inflammatory infiltrate (40). The recruited monocytes and T lymphocytes are thought to play a key role in the pathogenesis of atherosclerotic plaque, and thus the molecular signals that attract these cells into the lesions are likely important for lesion formation (40, 82). The expression of multiple chemokines has been shown to be upregulated in human atherosclerotic lesions (Table 2).

In addition, studies with mouse models of atherosclerosis have shown that deletion of the chemokine CCL2/monocyte chemoattractant protein 1 (MCP-1) or the chemokine receptors CCR2 and CXCR2 leads to significant reductions in macrophage recruitment into vessel walls and decreased formation of atherosclerotic lesions. These data strongly support a role for chemokines in the development of atherosclerosis.

Based on these data, one could potentially utilize the expression levels of these chemokines as a noninvasive marker of atherosclerosis or as a tool to assess disease through molecular imaging techniques (55, 140). Several studies now exist demonstrating a correlation between atherosclerosis and levels of MCP-1 in serum (26, 38, 94); however, the use of this information for testing in humans has not been widely adopted.

RA

Rheumatoid arthritis (RA) is a chronic inflammatory disease of the joints that can lead to long-term joint destruction with severe disability in affected patients. The underlying pathology is notable for prominent leukocyte infiltration of the synovial tissue of the joints. The majority of cells recruited into the synovium are neutrophils and mononuclear leukocytes that presumably help propagate the inflammation and joint destruction. Chemokine expression studies

TABLE 2 Chemokines identified in human atherosclerotic lesions

Chemokine	Cellular source(s)^a	Reference
CCL2/MCP-1	Macrophage, SMC, EC	91
CCL13/MCP-4	Macrophage, EC	12
CCL5/RANTES	T cells, EC	139
CCL18/pulmonary and activation-regulated chemokine	Macrophage	99
CCL19/MIP-3β	Macrophage, SMC	99
CXCL8/IL-8	Macrophage	133
CXCL12/SDF-1	Macrophage, SMC, EC	3
CXCL10/IP-10	Macrophage, SMC, EC	82
CXCL9/MIG	Macrophage, EC	82
CXCL11/I-TAC	Macrophage, EC	82

^{a}SMC, smooth muscle cell; EC, endothelial cell.

have shown markedly increased levels of certain chemokines in synovial tissue from patients with RA compared to those in tissue from normal joints. Both CC (i.e., CCL3/macrophage inflammatory protein 1α[MIP-1α], CCL5/RANTES, and CCL2/MCP-1) and CXC (i.e., CXCL10/gamma interferon-inducible protein 10 [IP-10], CXCL8/interleukin-8 [IL-8], and CXCL5/epithelial neutrophil-activating peptide 78 [ENA-78]) chemokines are expressed in fibroblasts and macrophages in the synovia of RA patients (54, 60-62, 104). Consistent with this chemokine expression, synovial fluid T cells recovered from patients with active RA express high levels of the chemokine receptors CCR5 and CXCR3 (73). In addition, patients who are homozygous for a null mutation in the CCR5 gene have fewer swollen joints and less morning stiffness than RA patients with the normal alleles (39). Finally, studies with animal models of arthritis have demonstrated that inhibition of CCR2, CCR1, CCR5, CXCR2, CXCL8, and CXCL5 attenuates joint swelling and leukocyte infiltration (4). These data clearly show that chemokines are important mediators of the joint inflammation seen in this disease (Table 3) (122).

Measurement of chemokine expression in serum could be used as a surrogate to quantify the degree of inflammation in the joints. In one study, higher levels of CCL3/MIP-1α, CXCL8/IL-8, and CXCL5/ENA-78 in sera were found in patients with active RA than in those with inactive disease (61, 62, 65). Presently, there are only limited studies looking at the role of measurements of chemokine and chemokine receptor function or levels in RA. However, the therapeutic role of chemokine inhibition is being explored with at least one chemokine antagonist in clinical trials for RA.

Asthma

Asthma is one of the most common chronic diseases in the world, with an incidence in excess of 5% of the population. It is characterized by chronic inflammation of the airways that in most cases is allergic in nature. Experimental studies with animal models and humans suggest that inhalation of an allergen initiates a cascade of events that lead to the recruitment of eosinophils, neutrophils, lymphocytes, and mast cells into the airways (21). Chemokines have been implicated as important mediators of this cellular recruitment (Table 4) and are likely crucial for the development of

allergic inflammation in the airways (77, 79). Data from bronchoalveolar lavage and lung biopsy studies have demonstrated the upregulation of the chemokines CCL11/eotaxin-1, CCL24/eotaxin-2, CCL7/MCP-3, CCL13/MCP-4, CCL5/RANTES, CCL17/thymus and activation-regulated chemokine (TARC), CCL22/macrophage-derived chemokine (MDC), and CXCL10/IP-10 in patients, during asthma attacks or after allergen challenge (78). Some of these chemokines recruit eosinophils and others affect T-cell trafficking. Animal models of asthma suggest that no single chemokine controls all aspects of cell trafficking into the airway; rather, multiple chemokines likely work in a sequential and redundant manner to orchestrate the inflammation (80).

As in the other diseases profiled in this chapter, measurements of chemokine and chemokine receptor levels are not widely used in asthma; however, there are several scenarios in which such measurements may be useful. For instance, currently clinicians monitor the effectiveness of therapy in people with asthma based on symptom reporting and crude measures of lung function. Acute exacerbations of asthma are life-threatening complications of this disorder that can often occur rapidly. In addition, it is hypothesized that long-term low-grade inflammation that can be missed with routine monitoring may lead to scarring of the airways and permanent changes in lung function. Unfortunately, the available technology does not allow us to easily measure the degree of airway inflammation and thus predict a patient's risk of exacerbation or airway scarring or remodeling. Chemokine expression in the lung or blood could be used as a reliable noninvasive marker of inflammation in the airways and thus would be of great value in the management of asthma. The technology to measure chemokine levels in exhaled breath condensates is available and has been used in limited studies for measurements in children with asthma (71). In addition, expectorated sputum or serum has been used in assays to measure chemokine levels and predict exacerbation in patients (67, 123). Finally, allergic asthma can often be confused with related disorders such as emphysema, bronchiolitis, and eosinophilic bronchitis. These disorders have different forms of airway inflammation and thus may have different profiles of expressed chemokines. Therefore, it may be possible to use the chemokine or chemokine receptor profiles of samples from the lung or serum to accurately diagnose a

TABLE 3 Chemokines and chemokine receptors with importance in RA based on human and animal studies (122)

Chemokine receptor	Ligand(s)	Reference(s)
CXC chemokine receptors		
CXCR1	CXCL8/IL-8	63
CXCR2	CXCL8/IL-8, CXCL5/ENA-78, CXCL1/GRO-α	46, 61–63
CXCR3	CXCL10/IP-10, CXCL9/MIG	93
CXCR4	CXCL12/SDF-1	90
CC chemokine receptors		
CCR1	CCL3/MIP-1α, CCL5/RANTES	60, 120
CCR2	CCL2/MCP-1	42, 45, 50
CCR3	CCL5/RANTES	120
CCR5	CCL5/RANTES, CCL3/MIP-1α	39, 93, 98, 120
CCR6	CCL20/MIP-3α	83
CCR10	CCL2/MCP-1	42, 45, 50
CX$_3$C chemokine receptors		
CX$_3$CR1	CX$_3$CL1/fractalkine	112

TABLE 4 Chemokines and chemokine receptors with importance in asthma based on human and animal studies (142)

Chemokine receptor	Ligand(s)	Reference(s)
CXC chemokine receptors		
CXCR1	CXCL8/IL-8	30
CXCR2	CXCL8/IL-8	30
CXCR3	CXCL10/IP-10	85, 86
CXCR4	CXCL12/SDF-1	75
CC chemokine receptors		
CCR1	CCL3/MIP-1α, CCL5/RANTES	86, 142
CCR2	CCL2/MCP-1, CCL8/MCP-2, CCL7/MCP-3, CCL13/MCP-4	69, 86, 142
CCR3	CCL5/RANTES, CCL7/MCP-3, CCL13/MCP-4, CCL11/eotaxin-1, CCL24/eotaxin-2, CCL26/eotaxin-3	86, 142
CCR4	CCL17/TARC, CCL22/MDC	142
CCR5	CCL5/RANTES	142
CCR6	CCL20/MIP-3α	76
CX$_3$C chemokine receptors		
CX$_3$CR1	CX$_3$CL1/fractalkine	102

patient with airway inflammation. The use of measurements of markers of inflammation such as chemokines may have a large impact on the diagnosis and management of asthmatics.

Organ Transplantation

Organ transplantation is often the only effective treatment for the large number of patients with end-stage kidney, liver, heart, or lung disease. Although a transplant is often life-saving therapy, it ushers in a new set of problems and diseases for the organ recipient. These include increased risk of infection (including opportunistic infections), organ ischemia-reperfusion injury, acute rejection, and chronic organ dysfunction from chronic rejection. These processes involve recruitment of leukocytes into the transplanted organs, with neutrophil recruitment dominating in infections and ischemia-reperfusion injury and lymphocyte and monocyte recruitment involved in rejection. Chemokine expression has been clearly shown to be important in all of these processes (Table 5) and represents a potential therapeutic target to prevent these complications of transplantation (31).

Chemokine expression in infections of organs has been well documented and depends on the nature of the microbe infecting the host (78, 128). Organ ischemia-reperfusion injury, acute rejection, and chronic rejection lead to increased expression of multiple chemokines that are surprisingly similar in all organs after transplantation (31). However, organ-specific differences do exist, so one cannot fully generalize the response to all transplanted organs (1). In the limited studies looking at chemokine expression following human organ transplantation, the expression of CXCL8/IL-8 has been associated with ischemia-reperfusion injury (28) and CCL5/RANTES, CCL2/MCP-1, CCL3/MIP-1α, CCL4/MIP-1β, CXCL9/monokine induced by gamma interferon (MIG), CXCL10/IP-10, and CXCL11/interferon-inducible T-cell alpha chemoattractant (I-TAC) have been associated with acute rejection (8-11, 28, 29, 143). In chronic rejection of lungs, CXCL8/IL-8, CCL5/RANTES, CXCL9/MIG, CXCL10/IP-10, CXCL11/I-TAC, and CCL2/MCP-1 are upregulated and may be predictive of the development of this complication (10, 100).

TABLE 5 Chemokines and chemokine receptors with importance in transplantation based on human and animal studies (31)

Chemokine receptor	Ligand(s)	Reference(s)
CXC chemokine receptors		
CXCR1	CXCL8/IL-8	28, 100
CXCR2	CXCL8/IL-8	28, 100
CXCR3	CXCL9/MIG, CXCL10/IP-10, CXCL11/I-TAC	10, 11, 57
CXCR4	CXCL12/SDF-1	35, 41
CC chemokine receptors		
CCR1	CCL3/MIP-1α, CCL5/RANTES	37
CCR2	CCL2/MCP-1	1, 9
CCR5	CCL5/RANTES	2, 8
CCR6	CCL20/MIP-3α	64, 107
CX$_3$C chemokine receptors		
CX$_3$CR1	CX$_3$CL1/fractalkine	51, 105

Frequent episodes of acute rejection and untreated low-grade rejection are thought to lead to chronic organ dysfunction, which is the major limiting factor in long-term graft survival. Thus, the ability to better detect these processes could have a major impact on the management of posttransplant patients. The expression of specific chemokines during episodes of acute rejection or low-grade chronic rejection may be a biomarker of inflammation and may allow better detection of these processes. Monitoring for occult infections with chemokine expression would also be of use for the transplant population. Although no large studies have utilized measurements of chemokines for monitoring of transplant patients, the ability to measure chemokine levels in serum, urine, or sputum makes this a potential future indication for the technology.

Methodological Approaches

Overview

Since inflammatory and immune cell localization appears to be central to the pathogenesis of a wide variety of diseases, numerous avenues for studying the role of chemokines and chemokine receptors have emerged. These techniques follow a logical progression from the characterization of the inflammatory or immune cell infiltrate through the measurement of chemokine and chemokine receptor distribution in diseased tissues, the establishment of in vitro models of chemotaxis, and in vivo dissection of the role of chemokines in animal models of the disease process. This series of approaches has enabled the definition of the role of chemokine-chemokine receptor-driven immune and inflammatory cell localization in a variety of diseases.

Analysis of the Cellular Infiltrate and Chemokine-Chemokine Receptor Milieu

The first step towards understanding whether localization of immune or inflammatory cells influences a disease process is to define the cellular composition of the infiltrate seen in sites in the body which are affected by the disease. This may be best done by one of two methods, immunohistochemistry of tissue sections or staining of cellular preparations obtained from disaggregated pathological specimens. There are a large number of monoclonal antibodies which enable the definition of subpopulations of immune and inflammatory cells and the characterization and quantitation of chemokine and chemokine receptor expression (95, 132).

Monoclonal antibodies that are reactive to specific antigens expressed on T cells, B cells, monocytes/macrophages, dendritic cells, neutrophils, eosinophils, and basophils-mast cells can be utilized to detect these cells or specific subsets of these cells in frozen sections by using immunohistochemical techniques. The immunoperoxidase technique, utilizing the avidin-biotin complex, has excellent sensitivity, and stained slides can be mounted and stored permanently. In addition, sections can be counterstained with hematoxylin and eosin, for example, to provide additional morphologic information. Serial sectioning allows the assessment of three-dimensional relationships between subsets of immune and inflammatory cells within tissue specimens. Appropriate isotype controls should be run with experimental immunostaining to establish levels of background nonspecific staining.

Fluorescent conjugated monoclonal antibodies targeting specific cell surface molecules can be similarly used to establish the cellular makeup of a tissue infiltrate (95). Tissue samples can be physically disaggregated and then passed through a sterile sieve. Mononuclear cell preparations can

then be stained with monoclonal antibodies, and the immunophenotypes of cell populations can be determined by fluorescence-activated cell sorter-based flow cytometry. Up to 12 different fluorochromes can be used, depending on the number of available lasers, to define cell subpopulations. Again, appropriate isotype antibody controls should be used to establish background and nonspecific staining.

A third aspect of analysis of a cellular infiltrate is the determination of levels of chemokine or chemokine receptor expression. A combination of methods can be used, including RNA in situ hybridization, immunohistochemistry, quantitative reverse transcriptase PCR, enzyme-linked immunosorbent assay (ELISA) or protein multiplexing technology, and flow cytometry (16, 121). Monoclonal antibodies directed against a number of chemokines suitable for use in staining of tissue sections, ELISA, or protein multiplexing have been defined. These antibodies can be used as a basis for measuring chemokine protein concentrations from tissue lysates and fluid collections. A number of different chemokines can now be detected by sandwich ELISAs. Some of these ELISAs are now commercially available as kits. Initially, microtiter plates are coated with the capture antibody and nonspecific protein binding is adsorbed with goat serum or bovine serum albumin. Chemokine-containing samples are then added to the wells of the plate, and this step is followed by exposure to a second enzyme-conjugated antibody. Similarly, these chemokine-specific monoclonal antibodies are also available conjugated to a fluorochrome or to fluorescent bead arrays, which allows them to be used to assess intracellular chemokine levels in permeablized cells or to assess the levels of multiple chemokines simultaneously in various biologic samples, both by utilizing flow cytometry technology. Monoclonal antibodies specific for individual chemokine receptors are also commercially available and are used to determine the expression of chemokine receptors on individual cells in situ or those isolated from inflammatory tissue or fluid via immunohistochemistry or flow cytometry.

Analysis of Chemotactic Responses: In Vitro Assays

Having defined the chemokine and chemokine receptor expression in the diseased tissue, one can examine the chemotactic responses of the specific leukocyte subpopulations to chemokines. A variety of transmigration assays exist which exploit the ability of migratory cells to polarize and migrate in response to a chemotactic gradient. The in vivo correlate of in vitro transmigration is thought to be the migration of cells towards sites of tissue injury, pathogen invasion, and/or immune challenge. Cells to be used in the transmigration assays can be derived from a number of sources, including the diseased tissue itself or purified subpopulations of inflammatory and immune cells isolated from the peripheral blood.

Boyden Chamber

The Boyden chamber designed in 1962 represents the original system by which the chemotactic responses of cells can be quantitated (19). The assembly consists of two chambers, an upper and a lower one, separated by a polycarbonate filter of standard pore size. The chemokine, dissolved in medium containing a low percentage of serum or 0.5% bovine serum albumin, is loaded into the lower chamber. A fixed number of indicator cells in suspension in an identical medium are loaded into the upper chamber. The unit is then sealed and incubated at 37°C for 2 to 3 h. Transmigration is then assessed in two ways. The polycarbonate membrane is carefully removed from the assembly, and the cells which are adhered to the underside of the filter are quantitated following staining with Giemsa. Alternatively, the cells which have transmigrated into the lower chamber are counted using a hemocytometer and the proportion of migrating cells is determined. Ultimately, a so-called checkerboard analysis of chemotaxis can be performed in which every chemokine concentration in the lower chamber is considered in relation to every tested concentration of the chemokine in the upper chamber. Chemotaxis is defined as cell movement towards increasing chemokine concentration. Chemokinesis refers to random or nondirectional cell movement in response to a stimulus. In the checkerboard analysis, chemotaxis is measured when there is a greater concentration of chemokine in the lower chamber than in the upper one and chemokinesis is measured when the concentrations of chemokines are equivalent on both sides of the membrane (Fig. 2). Modifications of the standard Boyden chamber have been made, including one using an image analyzer to quantitate the number of cells which migrate in response to a chemokinetic agent (36, 101).

Transwell Assays

More recently, transmigration assays have been performed in a transwell system (15). In this assembly, each lower

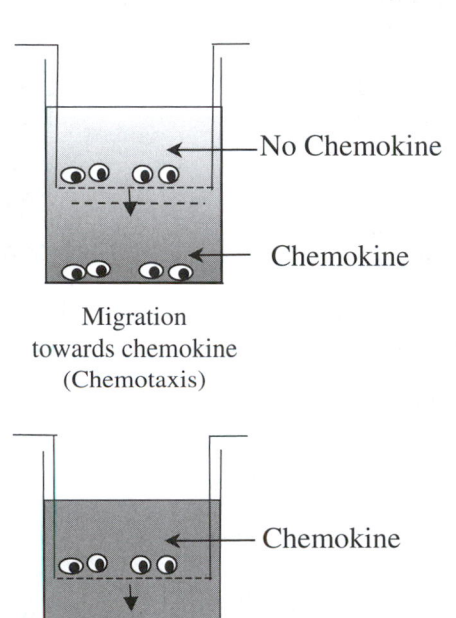

Migration
towards chemokine
(Chemotaxis)

Random movement in response to the
chemokine in the absence of a gradient
(Chemokinesis)

FIGURE 2 Transmigration assay system. Positive, negative, and absent gradients of a chemokine are established in order to assess chemotaxis (movement towards a chemokine) and chemokinesis (random movement of cells in response to a chemokine in the absence of a gradient). Cells are plated into the upper chamber of the transwell system or Boyden chamber, and the proportion of migrating cells is determined by accurate counting of cells which migrate to the lower chamber. The upper and lower chambers are separated by a polycarbonate membrane of standard pore size (between 3 and 8 μm), dependent on the migrating cell type.

chamber is associated with an independently removable upper chamber containing the polycarbonate membrane of fixed pore size. A checkerboard analysis of chemotaxis can be similarly performed with the transwell system. The Boyden chamber appears to be markedly better for analyzing granulocyte movement with a polycarbonate membrane of 3-μm pore size, whereas transwells containing membranes with a 5- or 8-μm pore size have proven to be useful for quantitating mononuclear cell migration. Several modifications of transmigration assays have been designed. These include the assessment of transmigration through a layer of cells grown on the transwell membrane. Transmigration of lymphocytes, eosinophils, or monocytes through an endothelial cell layer has been assessed by this means (14). Transmigration systems allow the further phenotypic characterization of responding cell subpopulations from a complex mixture of input cells. By using flow cytometry, cells which transmigrate can be phenotypically compared with those that do not (56, 119). Automated quantitation of transmigration has been achieved by loading cells to be tested with a vital fluorescent dye, such as CMFDA (5-chloromethylfluorescein diacetate) or acridine orange, and then using a fluorescent plate reader to quantitate the number of cells in the lower chamber (25, 88). A further modification of the fluorescent plate reader technique includes the ability to read the kinetic changes associated with transmigration into the lower chamber over time.

Direct Visualization

Measurement of transmigration with a Boyden chamber or transwell assay can be confirmed using time lapse video microscopy (Fig. 3) (97). The active movement of cells is viewed with a video camera as the cells respond to gradients of a chemokinetic agent. A continuous gradient of chemokine or a point source of chemokine can be used to manipulate the directional movement of cells. Cell movement can also be tracked using digital video, and images can be analyzed for cell polarization and speed of movement towards a chemokine source by using leukocytes or organisms such as *Dictyostelium* spp. (59, 92, 116, 131).

Adhesion Assays

The migratory response of immune cells in vivo involves a rapid adhesive event in which the circulating cell is stimulated to firmly adhere to the endothelial surface over which it flows and rolls and is necessary for a cell to undergo diapedesis into an immune organ or an inflammatory site (66, 78, 106). This event is triggered by chemokines and involves the upregulation of integrin affinity on leukocytes. This aspect of cell migration can be studied in vitro using a static adhesion assay or dynamically using a flow chamber to visualize the adhesion of leukocytes to endothelial cell monolayers. In the latter systems, endothelial cell layers are established on coverslips, fluorescently labeled leukocytes are passed over these monolayers at controlled flow rates, and the number of cells rolling or sticking to the endothelial layer is determined using image analysis and digitized time lapse video microscopy. In vivo flow systems have been designed which use intravital microscopy to visualize and quantitate the adhesion and transmigration of fluorescently labeled leukocytes in the vasculature of living animals (14).

Analysis of Chemotactic Responses: In Vivo Assays and Imaging

Several systems have been developed to assess leukocyte infiltration into specific anatomical sites in vivo. Chemokines can be injected intradermally, subcutaneously,

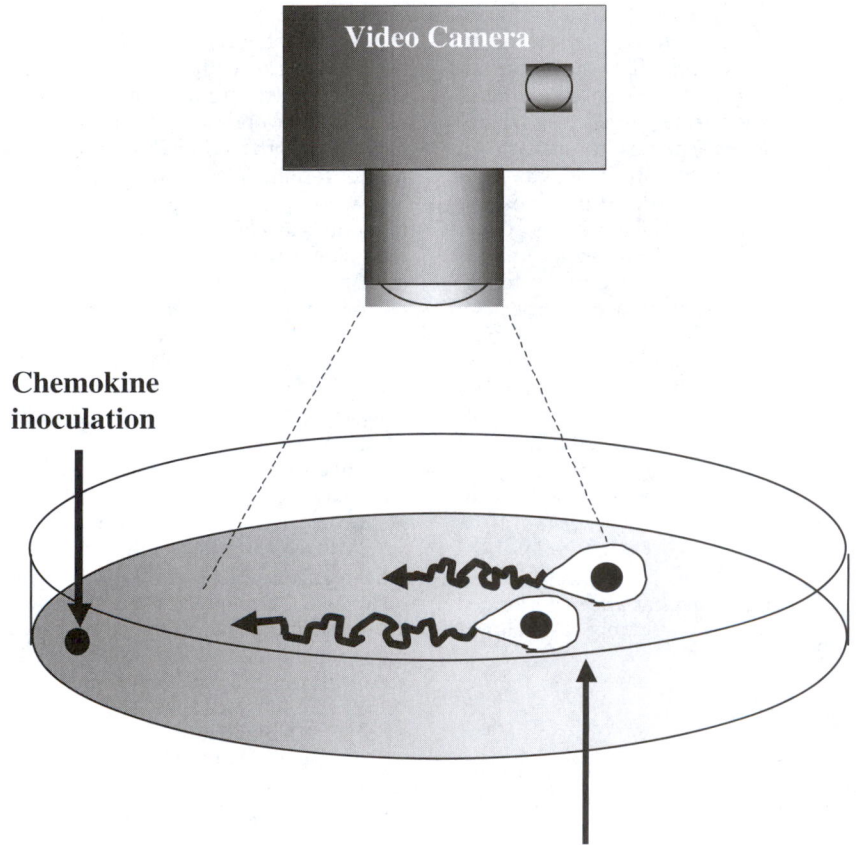

FIGURE 3 Digitized time lapse photography of cells moving in the presence of a gradient of a chemokine. Positive and negative gradients of a chemokine can be established in methylcellulose as previously described (52). Cells are plated into methylcellulose, and a gradient is established by inoculating the methylcellulose at a fixed point with the chemokine. Cells are then visualized migrating in response to the gradient by using time lapse video microscopy.

or intraperitoneally, and the leukocyte infiltration thus caused can be quantified. Recruitment of endogenous leukocytes or adoptively transferred leukocytes can be assessed in this manner. Leukocytes can be labeled ex vivo with radiolabels, such as indium-111 (48, 49), or with fluorescent dyes such as green fluorescent protein (GFP) or CMFDA (141). In addition, monoclonal antibodies exist that can recognize adoptively transferred antigen-specific T cells or allelic markers. A transgenic mouse has been engineered in which the vast majority of T cells express a T-cell receptor (TCR) which binds ovalbumin (OVA). This specific TCR chain can itself be detected using a monoclonal antibody (23, 117). T cells reactive to a specific antigen can be quantitated and the localization of adoptively transferred OVA-specific T cells in specific anatomic sites can be detected by immunostaining for OVA-specific TCRs.

New technology known as molecular imaging allows scientists to assay several different aspects of chemokine biology in intact organisms. It is now possible to evaluate, with imaging, the distribution of injected chemokines as well as track the movement of cells in response to chemokines or inflammation (136). This is a rapidly developing field that utilizes techniques of molecular and cell biology, advanced

imaging technology, and highly specific probes that serve as sources for the imaging signal. Specifically, whole-body imaging of animals or humans after injection of radiolabeled chemokines or bioluminescent cells allows localization of the labeled material to specific organs and areas of the body. Whole-body imaging of radioactive material or light generated deep within the body is now feasible in laboratory animals and potentially in humans, representing an exciting new tool for studying chemokine biology.

Analysis of Signal Transduction Associated with Active Cell Movement

The signal transduction events activated by ligand binding controlling leukocyte migration are not entirely defined and involve many different signaling pathways. A dramatic polarization of the cell occurs in response to a chemotactic gradient, which is the result of asymmetric signal transduction and the establishment of intracellular molecular gradients. While all of the molecular details remain to be elucidated, certain signaling molecules appear to play important roles in chemokine-induced cell movement. Chemokine receptors are coupled to the Gi subfamily of G proteins and pertussis toxin, which ADP-ribosylates and irreversibly inactivates the Gα subunits of the αi class, inhibiting the majority of chemokine-induced effects on leukocytes, including chemotaxis, calcium flux, and integrin activation (7). Other signaling events activated by the majority of chemokine receptors include the activation of phospholipase C, leading to generation of inositol triphosphates, intracellular calcium release, and PKC activation. Inhibition of chemokine-induced chemotaxis by wortmannin implicates PI 3-kinase in chemokine receptor signal transduction. Mouse strains engineered with a null mutation in the p110 subunit of PI 3-kinase γ have defects in chemokine-induced neutrophil and macrophage migration, confirming the importance of this enzyme in directed leukocyte movement (52). Phorbol myristate acetate activation of integrins implicates PKC as a potential mediator by which chemokines activate integrins. Chemokine signaling also leads to guanine nucleotide exchange on Rho, indicating the activation of Rho (70). Rac and Rho are small GTP binding proteins that are involved in controlling cell locomotion through regulation of actin cytoskeletal rearrangement leading to membrane ruffling and pseudopod formation.

The first and most immediate indication of a signal being transduced in relation to chemokine-induced signaling is a measurable rise in intracellular calcium concentration. The calcium flux is transient and may be detected using several methods (20, 24, 43, 129, 130). Cells are examined by using cuvette-based techniques, which assess calcium flux in populations of cells, and flow cytometry-based systems, which assess individual cell calcium flux responses to chemokines. The emission ratio dyes such as indo-1 and fura-2 are commonly used for flow cytometry-based and cuvette-based methods, respectively. Cells to be tested, including monocytes and lymphocytes, are loaded with ionic calcium binding dyes. Cells are then exposed to sequential pulses of a chemokine, and the change in intracytoplasmic fluorescence is monitored. Control substances include ionomycin, which selectively causes a large calcium flux since it serves as a calcium ion channel in the membrane. EDTA can be used to deplete all calcium from the medium and hence eradicate any cell-related calcium flux. Modifications have been made in order to determine the calcium flux in single cells. Adherent cells on a single slide can be visualized and loading of calcium dyes and intracytoplasmic changes in calcium concentrations can be monitored directly under a fluorescent microscope with an associated image analyzer.

Activation of additional signal transduction pathways can be meaured in cells in response to activation by chemokines (53). Adenylate cyclase assays, phosphoinositide turnover, protein kinase activation, and assays of protein tyrosine kinase activity have all been utilized to measure chemokine receptor activation.

Although the precise mechanistic link between chemokine receptor activation and the activation of the cytoskeletal machinery which induces cellular migration remains unknown, the polymerization of filamentous F-actin has been used as a measure of chemokine-induced functional signaling (126, 138). Intracellular F-actin polymerization can be quantitated using fluorescein isothiocyanate-labeled phalloidin and flow cytometry (103). This technique has been especially useful for assaying small numbers of responding cells. Polymerized F-actin can also be visualized in cells by using confocal microscopy in conjunction with a fluorescently labelled monoclonal antibody directed against F-actin. Studies have revealed that signal transduction occurring after exposure to a chemokinetic gradient results in the polarization of the cell's cytoskeletal elements and the polymerization of activated actin at the leading edge of a cell's newly formed pseudopodia. The Arp2/3 complex has recently been shown to colocalize with and nucleate sites of actin polymerization. A recently engineered GFP-Arp2/3 fusion protein has been used to visualize sites of actin polymerization in the advancing pseudopods of migrating cells by using phase-contrast fluorescent time lapse photography (135). A time lapse fluorescent microscope with a digital spot camera can be used to visualize the polarization of actin polymerization and pseudopod formation in cells transduced with the GFP-Arp2/3 construct and exposed to gradients of chemokines.

Animal Models To Assess the Role of Chemokines and Chemokine Receptors in Development and Disease

The above-mentioned techniques provide data which suggest how chemokines and their receptors may play a role in immune and inflammatory cell function in health and disease. Genetically modified mice in which the gene for a specific chemokine or chemokine receptor has been deleted or is overexpressed in a tissue-specific manner have been used to study both physiological and pathological processes. The effect of neutralization of a specific chemokine or chemokine receptor by specific antibodies on disease processes has also been utilized. These animal models currently provide the cornerstone for determining functional roles of chemokines and chemokine receptors in vivo (17, 74, 81, 89, 110, 111).

The role of chemokines and their receptors in vivo is complex. In an attempt to correlate in vitro determinations of chemokine activities and chemokine receptor expression with in vivo physiology and pathology, gene-targeted mice which fail to express a chemokine or chemokine receptor have been created by selective homologous recombination (110, 111). The phenotype of the so-called knockout is then compared to that of wild-type mice under physiological and pathological conditions. The generation of knockout mice involves the introduction of a mutant gene into embryonic stem cells in vitro and the selection for homologous recombination at the desired locus, which results in the deletion of a specific gene. Animals are then produced which are homozygous for the deleted gene. Embryonic, fetal, and neonatal development is then examined in these mice with a targeted disruption of both wild-type alleles in order to determine whether the gene deletion has effects on embryogenesis, hematopoiesis, or immunologic abnormalities, such as thymic development. In the adult mouse inflammatory and immune responses can be examined. Knockout mice corresponding to more than 10 of the chemokines and all of the chemokine receptors have been developed (96). So far, only the deletion of the stromal cell-derived factor 1 (SDF-1) and CXCR4 genes has been shown to be embryonically lethal and is associated with severe neurological, cardiological, and hematological abnormalities (81, 89). In contrast, fetal development is not affected in other chemokine-chemokine receptor knockouts, such as those not expressing eotaxin, MCP-1, and CCR2 (17, 74, 111). However, resting levels of eosinophils in the murine jejunum are reduced in the eotaxin knockout mouse, which indicates a physiological role for this chemokine in the homeostatic trafficking of eosinophils (84, 111).

Many important roles for chemokines and their receptors have been elucidated in experiments using knockouts and inhibitory antibodies. Different aspects of the host response to infectious pathogens have been shown to be dependent on neutrophil-active chemokines and their receptors, such as MIP-2 and CXCR2 (22), monocyte-active chemokines and their receptors, such as MCP-1 and CCR2 (68, 128), T-cell-active chemokines and their receptors, such as IP-10 (58), and NK cell-active chemokines, such as MIP-1α (113). Likewise, individual chemokine receptor knockouts have revealed an important role for this family of molecules in inflammatory and autoimmune diseases and allograft transplantation. For example, attenuated immunopathology has been noted in MCP-1 knockout and CCR2 knockout mice in models of atherosclerosis (18, 44) and glomerulonephritis (13, 127). Decreased inflammatory responses and increased allograft survival have been noted in CCR1 (17) and CXCR3 (47) knockouts. These in vivo experiments have revealed the significant role of individual chemokines and chemokine receptors in the immune and inflammatory responses that could not be appreciated by in vitro assays that implicated apparent functional redundancy.

CONCLUSIONS

The Boyden chamber stood as the singular system for quantitating leukocyte migration in response to chemokinetic agents for more than 20 years. However, in the past 5 years, and since the discovery of the chemokine-chemokine receptor superfamilies, there has been a considerable expansion in the number of methodological approaches available to scientists for quantitation of cell migration. These techniques vary widely, from phase-contrast fluorescent digital video microscopy to examine individual cell movement in response to chemokines to the use of knockout mice to delineate the effects of specific chemokines and chemokine receptors in vivo. These diverse methodological approaches have revealed an intricate world of immune and inflammatory cell localization, which appears to be critical to the pathophysiology of a wide variety of disease processes ranging from allergic lung inflammation to atherosclerosis to the way in which the immune system handles infectious agents such as *Toxoplasma gondii*.

During the next 10 years, we should expect to see a further expansion in the methodological approaches to studying the roles of chemokines and chemokine receptors, and this expansion should itself lead to a greater understanding of human diseases and the development of novel therapeutic approaches in order to combat them.

REFERENCES

1. **Abdi, R., T. K. Means, T. Ito, R. N. Smith, N. Najafian, M. Jurewicz, V. Tchipachvili, I. Charo, H. Auchincloss, Jr., M. H. Sayegh, and A. D. Luster.** 2004. Differential role of CCR2 in islet and heart allograft rejection: tissue specificity of chemokine/chemokine receptor function in vivo. *J. Immunol.* **172:**767–775.
2. **Abdi, R., R. N. Smith, L. Makhlouf, N. Najafian, A. D. Luster, H. Auchincloss, Jr., and M. H. Sayegh.** 2002. The role of CC chemokine receptor 5 (CCR5) in islet allograft rejection. *Diabetes* **51:**2489–2495.
3. **Abi-Younes, S., A. Sauty, F. Mach, G. K. Sukhova, P. Libby, and A. D. Luster.** 2000. The stromal cell-derived factor-1 chemokine is a potent platelet agonist highly expressed in atherosclerotic plaques. *Circ. Res.* **86:**131–138.
4. **Ajuebor, M. N., M. G. Swain, and M. Perretti.** 2002. Chemokines as novel therapeutic targets in inflammatory diseases. *Biochem. Pharmacol.* **63:**1191–1196.
5. **Ali, S., A. C. Palmer, B. Banerjee, S. J. Fritchley, and J. A. Kirby.** 2000. Examination of the function of RANTES, MIP-1alpha, and MIP-1beta following interaction with heparin-like glycosaminoglycans. *J. Biol. Chem.* **275:**11721–11727.
6. **Baggiolini, M.** 1998. Chemokines and leukocyte traffic. *Nature* **392:**565–568.
7. **Becknew, S.** 1997. G-protein activation by chemokines. *Methods Enzymol.* **298:**309–326.
8. **Belperio, J. A., M. D. Burdick, M. P. Keane, Y. Y. Xue, J. P. Lynch III, B. L. Daugherty, S. L. Kunkel, and R. M. Strieter.** 2000. The role of the CC chemokine, RANTES, in acute lung allograft rejection. *J. Immunol.* **165:**461–472.
9. **Belperio, J. A., M. P. Keane, M. D. Burdick, J. P. Lynch III, Y. Y. Xue, A. Berlin, D. J. Ross, S. L. Kunkel, I. F. Charo, and R. M. Strieter.** 2001. Critical role for the chemokine MCP-1/CCR2 in the pathogenesis of bronchiolitis obliterans syndrome. *J. Clin. Investig.* **108:**547–556.
10. **Belperio, J. A., M. P. Keane, M. D. Burdick, J. P. Lynch III, Y. Y. Xue, K. Li, D. J. Ross, and R. M. Strieter.** 2002. Critical role for CXCR3 chemokine biology in the pathogenesis of bronchiolitis obliterans syndrome. *J. Immunol.* **169:**1037–1049.
11. **Belperio, J. A., M. P. Keane, M. D. Burdick, J. P. Lynch III, D. A. Zisman, Y. Y. Xue, K. Li, A. Ardehali, D. J. Ross, and R. M. Strieter.** 2003. Role of CXCL9/CXCR3 chemokine biology during pathogenesis of acute lung allograft rejection. *J. Immunol.* **171:**4844–4852.
12. **Berkhout, T. A., H. M. Sarau, K. Moores, J. R. White, N. Elshourbagy, E. Appelbaum, R. J. Reape, M. Brawner, J. Makwana, J. J. Foley, D. B. Schmidt, C. Imburgia, D. McNulty, J. Matthews, K. O'Donnell, D. O'Shannessy, M. Scott, P. H. Groot, and C. Macphee.** 1997. Cloning, in vitro expression, and functional characterization of a novel human CC chemokine of the monocyte chemotactic protein (MCP) family (MCP-4) that binds and signals through the CC chemokine receptor 2B. *J. Biol. Chem.* **272:**16404–16413.
13. **Bird, J. E., M. R. Giancarli, T. Kurihara, M. C. Kowala, M. T. Valentine, P. H. Gitlitz, D. G. Pandya, M. H. French, and S. K. Durham.** 2000. Increased severity of glomerulonephritis in C-C chemokine receptor 2 knockout mice. *Kidney Int.* **57:**129–136.
14. **Black, D.** 2000. Endothelial cell chemotaxis assays. *Methods Mol. Biol.* **138:**121–127.
15. **Bleul, C. C., R. C. Fuhlbrigge, J. M. Casasnovas, A. Aiuti, and T. A. Springer.** 1996. A highly efficacious lymphocyte chemoattractant, stromal cell-derived factor 1 (SDF-1). *J. Exp. Med.* **184:**1101–1119.
16. **Bonecchi, R., G. Bianchi, P. P. Bordignon, D. D'Ambrosio, R. Lang, A. Borsatti, S. Sozzani, P. Allavena, P. A. Gray, A. Mantovani, and F. Sinigaglia.** 1998. Differential expression of chemokine receptors and chemotactic responsiveness of type 1 T helper cells (Th1s) and Th2s. *J. Exp. Med.* **187:**129–134.
17. **Boring, L., J. Gosling, S. W. Chensue, S. L. Kunkel, R. V. Farese, Jr., H. E. Broxmeyer, and I. F. Charo.** 1997. Impaired monocyte migration and reduced type 1 (Th1) cytokine responses in C-C chemokine receptor 2 knockout mice. *J. Clin. Investig.* **100:**2552–2561.
18. **Boring, L., J. Gosling, M. Cleary, and I. F. Charo.** 1998. Decreased lesion formation in CCR2−/− mice reveals a role for chemokines in the initiation of atherosclerosis. *Nature* **394:**894–897.
19. **Boyden, S.** 1962. The chemotactic effect of mixtures of antibody and antigen on polymorphonuclear leucocytes. *J. Exp. Med.* **115:**453–466.
20. **Buser, R., and A. E. Proudfoot.** 2000. Calcium mobilization. *Methods Mol. Biol.* **138:**143–148.
21. **Busse, W. W., and R. F. Lemanske, Jr.** 2001. Asthma. *N. Engl. J. Med.* **344:**350–362.
22. **Cacalano, G., J. Lee, K. Kikly, A. M. Ryan, S. Pitts-Meek, B. Hultgren, W. I. Wood, and M. W. Moore.** 1994. Neutrophil and B cell expansion in mice that lack the murine IL-8 receptor homolog. *Science* **265:**682–684.

23. **Carbone, F. R., S. J. Sterry, J. Butler, S. Rodda, and M. W. Moore.** 1992. T cell receptor alpha-chain pairing determines the specificity of residue 262 within the Kb-restricted, ovalbumin257-264 determinant. *Int. Immunol.* **4:**861–867.

24. **Cobbold, P. H., and T. J. Rink.** 1987. Fluorescence and bioluminescence measurement of cytoplasmic free calcium. *Biochem. J.* **248:**313–328.

25. **Das, A. M., M. N. Ajuebor, R. J. Flower, M. Perretti, and S. R. McColl.** 1999. Contrasting roles for RANTES and macrophage inflammatory protein-1 alpha (MIP-1 alpha) in a murine model of allergic peritonitis. *Clin. Exp. Immunol.* **117:**223–229.

26. **de Lemos, J. A., D. A. Morrow, M. S. Sabatine, S. A. Murphy, C. M. Gibson, E. M. Antman, C. H. McCabe, C. P. Cannon, and E. Braunwald.** 2003. Association between plasma levels of monocyte chemoattractant protein-1 and long-term clinical outcomes in patients with acute coronary syndromes. *Circulation* **107:**690–695.

27. **del Pozo, M. A., M. Vicente-Manzanares, R. Tejedor, J. M. Serrador, and F. Sanchez-Madrid.** 1999. Rho GTPases control migration and polarization of adhesion molecules and cytoskeletal ERM components in T lymphocytes. *Eur. J. Immunol.* **29:**3609–3620.

28. **De Perrot, M., Y. Sekine, S. Fischer, T. K. Waddell, K. McRae, M. Liu, D. A. Wigle, and S. Keshavjee.** 2002. Interleukin-8 release during early reperfusion predicts graft function in human lung transplantation. *Am. J. Respir. Crit. Care Med.* **165:**211–215.

29. **De Perrot, M., K. Young, Y. Imai, M. Liu, T. K. Waddell, S. Fischer, L. Zhang, and S. Keshavjee.** 2003. Recipient T cells mediate reperfusion injury after lung transplantation in the rat. *J. Immunol.* **171:**4995–5002.

30. **De Sanctis, G. T., J. A. MacLean, S. Qin, W. W. Wolyniec, H. Grasemann, C. N. Yandava, A. Jiao, T. Noonan, J. Stein-Streilein, F. H. Green, and J. M. Drazen.** 1999. Interleukin-8 receptor modulates IgE production and B-cell expansion and trafficking in allergen-induced pulmonary inflammation. *J. Clin. Investig.* **103:**507–515.

31. **DeVries, M. E., K. A. Hosiawa, C. M. Cameron, S. E. Bosinger, D. Persad, A. A. Kelvin, J. C. Coombs, H. Wang, R. Zhong, M. J. Cameron, and D. J. Kelvin.** 2003. The role of chemokines and chemokine receptors in alloantigen-independent and alloantigen-dependent transplantation injury. *Semin. Immunol.* **15:**33–48.

32. **DeVries, M. E., L. Ran, and D. J. Kelvin.** 1999. On the edge: the physiological and pathophysiological role of chemokines during inflammatory and immunological responses. *Semin. Immunol.* **11:**95–104.

33. **Dryer, L.** 2000. Evolution of odorant receptors. *Bioessays* **22:**803–810.

34. **Dustin, M. L., and A. C. Chan.** 2000. Signaling takes shape in the immune system. *Cell* **103:**283–294.

35. **Eitner, F., Y. Cui, K. L. Hudkins, and C. E. Alpers.** 1998. Chemokine receptor (CXCR4) mRNA-expressing leukocytes are increased in human renal allograft rejection. *Transplantation* **66:**1551–1557.

36. **Falk, W., R. H. Goodwin, Jr., and E. J. Leonard.** 1980. A 48-well micro chemotaxis assembly for rapid and accurate measurement of leukocyte migration. *J. Immunol. Methods* **33:**239–247.

37. **Gao, W., P. S. Topham, J. A. King, S. T. Smiley, V. Csizmadia, B. Lu, C. J. Gerard, and W. W. Hancock.** 2000. Targeting of the chemokine receptor CCR1 suppresses development of acute and chronic cardiac allograft rejection. *J. Clin. Investig.* **105:**35–44.

38. **Garlichs, C. D., S. John, A. Schmeisser, S. Eskafi, C. Stumpf, M. Karl, M. Goppelt-Struebe, R. Schmieder, and W. G. Daniel.** 2001. Upregulation of CD40 and CD40 ligand (CD154) in patients with moderate hypercholesterolemia. *Circulation* **104:**2395–2400.

39. **Garred, P., H. O. Madsen, J. Petersen, H. Marquart, T. M. Hansen, S. Freiesleben Sorensen, B. Volck, A. Svejgaard, and V. Andersen.** 1998. CC chemokine receptor 5 polymorphism in rheumatoid arthritis. *J. Rheumatol.* **25:**1462–1465.

40. **Gersxten, R. E., F. Mach, A. Sauty, A. Rosenzweig, and A. D. Luster.** 2000. Chemokines, leukocytes, and atherosclerosis. *J. Lab. Clin. Med.* **136:**87–92.

41. **Goddard, S., A. Williams, C. Morland, S. Qin, R. Gladue, S. G. Hubscher, and D. H. Adams.** 2001. Differential expression of chemokines and chemokine receptors shapes the inflammatory response in rejecting human liver transplants. *Transplantation* **72:**1957–1967.

42. **Gong, J. H., L. G. Ratkay, J. D. Waterfield, and I. Clark-Lewis.** 1997. An antagonist of monocyte chemoattractant protein 1 (MCP-1) inhibits arthritis in the MRL-lpr mouse model. *J. Exp. Med.* **186:**131–137.

43. **Grynkiewicz, G., M. Poenie, and R. Y. Tsien.** 1985. A new generation of Ca^{2+} indicators with greatly improved fluorescence properties. *J. Biol. Chem.* **260:**3440–3450.

44. **Gu, L., Y. Okada, S. K. Clinton, C. Gerard, G. K. Sukhova, P. Libby, and B. J. Rollins.** 1998. Absence of monocyte chemoattractant protein-1 reduces atherosclerosis in low density lipoprotein receptor-deficient mice. *Mol. Cell* **2:**275–281.

45. **Hachicha, M., P. Rathanaswami, T. J. Schall, and S. R. McColl.** 1993. Production of monocyte chemotactic protein-1 in human type B synoviocytes. Synergistic effect of tumor necrosis factor alpha and interferon-gamma. *Arthritis Rheum.* **36:**26–34.

46. **Halloran, M. M., J. M. Woods, R. M. Strieter, Z. Szekanecz, M. V. Volin, S. Hosaka, G. K. Haines III, S. L. Kunkel, M. D. Burdick, A. Walz, and A. E. Koch.** 1999. The role of an epithelial neutrophil-activating peptide-78-like protein in rat adjuvant-induced arthritis. *J. Immunol.* **162:**7492–7500.

47. **Hancock, W. W., B. Lu, W. Gao, V. Csizmadia, K. Faia, J. A. King, S. T. Smiley, M. Ling, N. P. Gerard, and C. Gerard.** 2000. Requirement of the chemokine receptor CXCR3 for acute allograft rejection. *J. Exp. Med.* **192:**1515–1520.

48. **Hanto, D. W., U. T. Hopt, R. Hoffman, and R. L. Simmons.** 1982. Lymphocyte recruitment, regional blood flow, and vascular permeability at sites of allogeneic cellular interactions. *J. Immunol.* **129:**2437–2443.

49. **Hanto, D. W., U. T. Hopt, R. Hoffman, and R. L. Simmons.** 1982. Recruitment of unsensitized circulating lymphocytes to sites of allogeneic cellular interactions. *Transplantation* **33:**541–546.

50. **Harigai, M., M. Hara, T. Yoshimura, E. J. Leonard, K. Inoue, and S. Kashiwazaki.** 1993. Monocyte chemoattractant protein-1 (MCP-1) in inflammatory joint diseases and its involvement in the cytokine network of rheumatoid synovium. *Clin. Immunol. Immunopathol.* **69:**83–91.

51. **Haskell, C. A., W. W. Hancock, D. J. Salant, W. Gao, V. Csizmadia, W. Peters, K. Faia, O. Fituri, J. B. Rottman, and I. F. Charo.** 2001. Targeted deletion of CX(3)CR1 reveals a role for fractalkine in cardiac allograft rejection. *J. Clin. Investig.* **108:**679–688.

52. **Hirsch, E., V. L. Katanaev, C. Garlanda, O. Azzolino, L. Pirola, L. Silengo, S. Sozzani, A. Mantovani, F. Altruda, and M. P. Wymann.** 2000. Central role for G protein-coupled phosphoinositide 3-kinase gamma in inflammation. *Science* **287:**1049–1053.

53. **Horuk, R. (ed.).** 1997. *Methods in Enzymology,* vol. 288. *Chemokine Receptors.* Academic Press, San Diego, Calif.

54. Hosaka, S., T. Akahoshi, C. Wada, and H. Kondo. 1994. Expression of the chemokine superfamily in rheumatoid arthritis. *Clin. Exp. Immunol.* **97**:451–457.

55. Jaffer, F. A., and R. Weissleder. 2004. Seeing within: molecular imaging of the cardiovascular system. *Circ. Res.* **94**:433–445.

56. Jourdan, P., J. P. Vendrell, M. F. Huguet, M. Segondy, J. Bousquet, J. Pene, and H. Yssel. 2000. Cytokines and cell surface molecules independently induce CXCR4 expression on CD4+ CCR7+ human memory T cells. *J. Immunol.* **165**:716–724.

57. Kao, J., J. Kobashigawa, M. C. Fishbein, W. R. MacLellan, M. D. Burdick, J. A. Belperio, and R. M. Strieter. 2003. Elevated serum levels of the CXCR3 chemokine ITAC are associated with the development of transplant coronary artery disease. *Circulation* **107**:1958–1961.

58. Khan, I. A., J. A. MacLean, F. S. Lee, L. Casciotti, E. DeHaan, J. D. Schwartzman, and A. D. Luster. 2000. IP-10 is critical for effector T cell trafficking and host survival in Toxoplasma gondii infection. *Immunity* **12**:483–494.

59. Kim, J. Y., J. A. Borleis, and P. N. Devreotes. 1998. Switching of chemoattractant receptors programs development and morphogenesis in Dictyostelium: receptor subtypes activate common responses at different agonist concentrations. *Dev. Biol.* **197**:117–128.

60. Koch, A. E., S. L. Kunkel, L. A. Harlow, D. D. Mazarakis, G. K. Haines, M. D. Burdick, R. M. Pope, and R. M. Strieter. 1994. Macrophage inflammatory protein-1 alpha: a novel chemotactic cytokine for macrophages in rheumatoid arthritis. *J. Clin. Investig.* **93**:921–928.

61. Koch, A. E., S. L. Kunkel, L. A. Harlow, D. D. Mazarakis, G. K. Haines, M. D. Burdick, R. M. Pope, A. Walz, and R. M. Strieter. 1994. Epithelial neutrophil activating peptide-78: a novel chemotactic cytokine for neutrophils in arthritis. *J. Clin. Investig.* **94**:1012–1018.

62. Koch, A. E., S. L. Kunkel, M. R. Shah, S. Hosaka, M. M. Halloran, G. K. Haines, M. D. Burdick, R. M. Pope, and R. M. Strieter. 1995. Growth-related gene product alpha: a chemotactic cytokine for neutrophils in rheumatoid arthritis. *J. Immunol.* **155**:3660–3666.

63. Koch, A. E., M. V. Volin, J. M. Woods, S. L. Kunkel, M. A. Connors, L. A. Harlow, D. C. Woodruff, M. D. Burdick, and R. M. Strieter. 2001. Regulation of angiogenesis by the C-X-C chemokines interleukin-8 and epithelial neutrophil activating peptide 78 in the rheumatoid joint. *Arthritis Rheum.* **44**:31–40.

64. Krukemeyer, M. G., J. Moeller, L. Morawietz, B. Rudolph, U. Neumann, T. Theruvath, P. Neuhaus, and V. Krenn. 2004. Description of B lymphocytes and plasma cells, complement, and chemokines/receptors in acute liver allograft rejection. *Transplantation* **78**:65–70.

65. Kullich, W. C., and G. Klein. 1998. High levels of macrophage inflammatory protein-1alpha correlate with prolactin in female patients with active rheumatoid arthritis. *Clin. Rheumatol.* **17**:263–264.

66. Kunkel, S. L. 1999. Through the looking glass: the diverse in vivo activities of chemokines. *J. Clin. Investig.* **104**:1333–1334.

67. Kurashima, K., N. Mukaida, M. Fujimura, J. M. Schroder, T. Matsuda, and K. Matsushima. 1996. Increase of chemokine levels in sputum precedes exacerbation of acute asthma attacks. *J. Leukoc. Biol.* **59**:313–316.

68. Kuziel, W. A., S. J. Morgan, T. C. Dawson, S. Griffin, O. Smithies, K. Ley, and N. Maeda. 1997. Severe reduction in leukocyte adhesion and monocyte extravasation in mice deficient in CC chemokine receptor 2. *Proc. Natl. Acad. Sci. USA* **94**:12053–12058.

69. Lamkhioued, B., E. A. Garcia-Zepeda, S. Abi-Younes, H. Nakamura, S. Jedrzkiewicz, L. Wagner, P. M. Renzi, Z. Allakhverdi, C. Lilly, Q. Hamid, and A. D. Luster. 2000. Monocyte chemoattractant protein (MCP)-4 expression in the airways of patients with asthma. Induction in epithelial cells and mononuclear cells by proinflammatory cytokines. *Am. J. Respir. Crit. Care Med.* **162**:723–732.

70. Laudanna, C., J. J. Campbell, and E. C. Butcher. 1996. Role of Rho in chemoattractant-activated leukocyte adhesion through integrins. *Science* **271**:981–983.

71. Leung, T. F., G. W. Wong, F. W. Ko, C. W. Lam, and T. F. Fok. 2004. Increased macrophage-derived chemokine in exhaled breath condensate and plasma from children with asthma. *Clin. Exp. Allergy* **34**:786–791.

72. Libby, P., and P. M. Ridker. 2004. Inflammation and atherosclerosis: role of C-reactive protein in risk assessment. *Am. J. Med.* **116** (Suppl. 6A):9S–16S.

73. Loetscher, M., P. Loetscher, N. Brass, E. Meese, and B. Moser. 1998. Lymphocyte-specific chemokine receptor CXCR3: regulation, chemokine binding and gene localization. *Eur. J. Immunol.* **28**:3696–3705.

74. Lu, B., B. J. Rutledge, L. Gu, J. Fiorillo, N. W. Lukacs, S. L. Kunkel, R. North, C. Gerard, and B. J. Rollins. 1998. Abnormalities in monocyte recruitment and cytokine expression in monocyte chemoattractant protein 1-deficient mice. *J. Exp. Med.* **187**:601–608.

75. Lukacs, N. W., A. Berlin, D. Schols, R. T. Skerlj, and G. J. Bridger. 2002. AMD3100, a CxCR4 antagonist, attenuates allergic lung inflammation and airway hyperreactivity. *Am. J. Pathol.* **160**:1353–1360.

76. Lukacs, N. W., D. M. Prosser, M. Wiekowski, S. A. Lira, and D. N. Cook. 2001. Requirement for the chemokine receptor CCR6 in allergic pulmonary inflammation. *J. Exp. Med.* **194**:551–555.

77. Lukacs, N. W., R. M. Strieter, S. W. Chensue, and S. L. Kunkel. 1996. Activation and regulation of chemokines in allergic airway inflammation. *J. Leukoc. Biol.* **59**:13–17.

78. Luster, A. D., S. Abi-Younes, and A. Tager. 2000. Chemokines and disease, p. 339–382. *In* M. E. Rothenberg (ed.), *Chemokines in Allergic Disease*. Marcel Dekker AG, New York, N.Y.

79. Luster, A. D., R. D. Cardiff, J. A. MacLean, K. Crowe, and R. D. Granstein. 1998. Delayed wound healing and disorganized neovascularization in transgenic mice expressing the IP-10 chemokine. *Proc. Assoc. Am. Physicians* **110**:183–196.

80. Luster, A. D., and A. M. Tager. 2004. T-cell trafficking in asthma: lipid mediators grease the way. *Nat. Rev. Immunol.* **4**:711–724.

81. Ma, Q., D. Jones, P. R. Borghesani, R. A. Segal, T. Nagasawa, T. Kishimoto, R. T. Bronson, and T. A. Springer. 1998. Impaired B-lymphopoiesis, myelopoiesis, and derailed cerebellar neuron migration in CXCR4- and SDF-1-deficient mice. *Proc. Natl. Acad. Sci. USA* **95**:9448–9453.

82. Mach, F., A. Sauty, A. S. Iarossi, G. K. Sukhova, K. Neote, P. Libby, and A. D. Luster. 1999. Differential expression of three T lymphocyte-activating CXC chemokines by human atheroma-associated cells. *J. Clin. Investig.* **104**:1041–1050.

83. Matsui, T., T. Akahoshi, R. Namai, A. Hashimoto, Y. Kurihara, M. Rana, A. Nishimura, H. Endo, H. Kitasato, S. Kawai, K. Takagishi, and H. Kondo. 2001. Selective recruitment of CCR6-expressing cells by increased production of MIP-3 alpha in rheumatoid arthritis. *Clin. Exp. Immunol.* **125**:155–161.

84. Matthews, A. N., D. S. Friend, N. Zimmermann, M. N. Sarafi, A. D. Luster, E. Pearlman, S. E. Wert, and M. E. Rothenberg. 1998. Eotaxin is required for the baseline level of tissue eosinophils. *Proc. Natl. Acad. Sci. USA* **95**:6273–6278.

85. Medoff, B. D., A. Sauty, A. M. Tager, J. A. Maclean, R. N. Smith, A. Mathew, J. H. Dufour, and A. D. Luster. 2002. IFN-gamma-inducible protein 10 (CXCL10)

contributes to airway hyperreactivity and airway inflammation in a mouse model of asthma. *J. Immunol.* **168**:5278–5286.

86. Miotto, D., P. Christodoulopoulos, R. Olivenstein, R. Taha, L. Cameron, A. Tsicopoulos, A. B. Tonnel, O. Fahy, J. J. Lafitte, A. D. Luster, B. Wallaert, C. E. Mapp, and Q. Hamid. 2001. Expression of IFN-gamma-inducible protein; monocyte chemotactic proteins 1, 3, and 4; and eotaxin in TH1- and TH2-mediated lung diseases. *J. Allergy. Clin. Immunol.* **107**:664–670.

87. Mombaerts, P., F. Wang, C. Dulac, R. Vassar, S. K. Chao, A. Nemes, M. Mendelsohn, J. Edmondson, and R. Axel. 1996. The molecular biology of olfactory perception. *Cold Spring Harbor Symp. Quant. Biol.* **61**:135–145.

88. Moshfegh, A., G. Hallden, and J. Lundahl. 1999. Methods for simultaneous quantitative analysis of eosinophil and neutrophil adhesion and transmigration. *Scand. J. Immunol.* **50**:262–269.

89. Nagasawa, T., S. Hirota, K. Tachibana, N. Takakura, S. Nishikawa, Y. Kitamura, N. Yoshida, H. Kikutani, and T. Kishimoto. 1996. Defects of B-cell lymphopoiesis and bone-marrow myelopoiesis in mice lacking the CXC chemokine PBSF/SDF-1. *Nature* **382**:635–658.

90. Nanki, T., K. Hayashida, H. S. El-Gabalawy, S. Suson, K. Shi, H. J. Girschick, S. Yavuz, and P. E. Lipsky. 2000. Stromal cell-derived factor-1-CXC chemokine receptor 4 interactions play a central role in CD4+ T cell accumulation in rheumatoid arthritis synovium. *J. Immunol.* **165**:6590–6598.

91. Nelken, N. A., S. R. Coughlin, D. Gordon, and J. N. Wilcox. 1991. Monocyte chemoattractant protein-1 in human atheromatous plaques. *J. Clin. Investig.* **88**:1121–1127.

92. Parent, C. A., B. J. Blacklock, W. M. Froehlich, D. B. Murphy, and P. N. Devreotes. 1998. G protein signaling events are activated at the leading edge of chemotactic cells. *Cell* **95**:81–91.

93. Patel, D. D., J. P. Zachariah, and L. P. Whichard. 2001. CXCR3 and CCR5 ligands in rheumatoid arthritis synovium. *Clin. Immunol.* **98**:39–45.

94. Piemonti, L., G. Calori, A. Mercalli, G. Lattuada, P. Monti, M. P. Garancini, F. Costantino, G. Ruotolo, L. Luzi, and G. Perseghin. 2003. Fasting plasma leptin, tumor necrosis factor-α receptor 2, and monocyte chemoattracting protein 1 concentration in a population of glucose-tolerant and glucose-intolerant women: impact on cardiovascular mortality. *Diabetes Care* **26**:2883–2889.

95. Ponath, P., N. Kassam, and S. Qin. 2000. Monoclonal antibodies to chemokine receptors. *Methods Mol. Biol:* **138**:231–242.

96. Power, C. A. 2003. Knock out models to dissect chemokine receptor function in vivo. *J. Immunol. Methods* **273**:73–82.

97. Poznansky, M. C., I. T. Olszak, R. Foxall, R. H. Evans, A. D. Luster, and D. T. Scadden. 2000. Active movement of T cells away from a chemokine. *Nat. Med.* **6**:543–548.

98. Rathanaswami, P., M. Hachicha, M. Sadick, T. J. Schall, and S. R. McColl. 1993. Expression of the cytokine RANTES in human rheumatoid synovial fibroblasts. Differential regulation of RANTES and interleukin-8 genes by inflammatory cytokines. *J. Biol. Chem.* **268**:5834–5839.

99. Reape, T. J., K. Rayner, C. D. Manning, A. N. Gee, M. S. Barnette, K. G. Burnand, and P. H. Groot. 1999. Expression and cellular localization of the CC chemokines PARC and ELC in human atherosclerotic plaques. *Am. J. Pathol.* **154**:365–374.

100. Reynaud-Gaubert, M., V. Marin, X. Thirion, C. Farnarier, P. Thomas, M. Badier, P. Bongrand, R. Giudicelli, and P. Fuentes. 2002. Upregulation of chemokines in bronchoalveolar lavage fluid as a predictive marker of post-transplant airway obliteration. *J. Heart Lung Transplant.* **21**:721–730.

101. Richards, K. L., and J. McCullough. 1984. A modified microchamber method for chemotaxis and chemokinesis. *Immunol. Commun.* **13**:49–62.

102. Rimaniol, A. C., S. J. Till, G. Garcia, F. Capel, V. Godot, K. Balabanian, I. Durand-Gasselin, E. M. Varga, G. Simonneau, D. Emilie, S. R. Durham, and M. Humbert. 2003. The CX3C chemokine fractalkine in allergic asthma and rhinitis. *J. Allergy Clin. Immunol.* **112**:1139–1146.

103. Riviere, C., F. Subra, K. Cohen-Solal, V. Cordette-Lagarde, R. Letestu, C. Auclair, W. Vainchenker, and F. Louache. 1999. Phenotypic and functional evidence for the expression of CXCR4 receptor during megakaryocytopoiesis. *Blood* **93**:1511–1523.

104. Robinson, E., E. C. Keystone, T. J. Schall, N. Gillett, and E. N. Fish. 1995. Chemokine expression in rheumatoid arthritis (RA): evidence of RANTES and macrophage inflammatory protein (MIP)-1 beta production by synovial T cells. *Clin. Exp. Immunol.* **101**:398–407.

105. Robinson, L. A., C. Nataraj, D. W. Thomas, D. N. Howell, R. Griffiths, V. Bautch, D. D. Patel, L. Feng, and T. M. Coffman. 2000. A role for fractalkine and its receptor (CX3CR1) in cardiac allograft rejection. *J. Immunol.* **165**:6067–6072.

106. Rollins, B. J. 1997. Chemokines. *Blood* **90**:909–928.

107. Ross, D. J., A. M. Cole, D. Yoshioka, A. K. Park, J. A. Belperio, H. Laks, R. M. Strieter, J. P. Lynch III, B. Kubak, A. Ardehali, and T. Ganz. 2004. Increased bronchoalveolar lavage human beta-defensin type 2 in bronchiolitis obliterans syndrome after lung transplantation. *Transplantation* **78**:1222–1224.

108. Rossi, D., and A. Zlotnik. 2000. The biology of chemokines and their receptors. *Annu. Rev. Immunol.* **18**:217–242.

109. Rot, A. 1993. Neutrophil attractant/activation protein-1 (interleukin-8) induces in vitro neutrophil migration by haptotactic mechanism. *Eur. J. Immunol.* **23**:303–306.

110. Rothenberg, M. E. 2000. Chemokine knockout mice. *Methods. Mol. Biol.* **138**:253–257.

111. Rothenberg, M. E., J. A. MacLean, E. Pearlman, A. D. Luster, and P. Leder. 1997. Targeted disruption of the chemokine eotaxin partially reduces antigen-induced tissue eosinophilia. *J. Exp. Med.* **185**:785–790.

112. Ruth, J. H., M. V. Volin, G. K. Haines III, D. C. Woodruff, K. J. Katschke, Jr., J. M. Woods, C. C. Park, J. C. Morel, and A. E. Koch. 2001. Fractalkine, a novel chemokine in rheumatoid arthritis and in rat adjuvant-induced arthritis. *Arthritis Rheum.* **44**:1568–1581.

113. Salazar-Mather, T. P., J. S. Orange, and C. A. Biron. 1998. Early murine cytomegalovirus (MCMV) infection induces liver natural killer (NK) cell inflammation and protection through macrophage inflammatory protein 1alpha (MIP-1alpha)-dependent pathways. *J. Exp. Med.* **187**:1–14.

114. Sallusto, F., C. R. Mackay, and A. Lanzavecchia. 2000. The role of chemokine receptors in primary, effector, and memory immune responses. *Annu. Rev. Immunol.* **18**:593–620.

115. Sanchez-Madrid, F., and M. A. del Pozo. 1999. Leukocyte polarization in cell migration and immune interactions. *EMBO J.* **18**:501–511.

116. Servant, G., O. D. Weiner, P. Herzmark, T. Balla, J. W. Sedat, and H. R. Bourne. 2000. Polarization of chemoattractant receptor signaling during neutrophil chemotaxis. *Science* **287**:1037–1040.

117. Shepherd, D. M., E. A. Dearstyne, and N. I. Kerkvliet. 2000. The effects of TCDD on the activation of ovalbumin (OVA)-specific DO11.10 transgenic CD4(+) T cells in adoptively transferred mice. *Toxicol. Sci.* **56:**340–350.

118. Shin, W. S., A. Szuba, and S. G. Rockson. 2002. The role of chemokines in human cardiovascular pathology: enhanced biological insights. *Atherosclerosis* **160:**91–102.

119. Simson, L., and P. S. Foster. 2000. Chemokine and cytokine cooperativity: eosinophil migration in the asthmatic response. *Immunol. Cell Biol.* **78:**415–422.

120. Snowden, N., A. Hajeer, W. Thomson, and B. Ollier. 1994. RANTES role in rheumatoid arthritis. *Lancet* **343:**547–548.

121. Sozzani, S., P. Allavena, G. D'Amico, W. Luini, G. Bianchi, M. Kataura, T. Imai, O. Yoshie, R. Bonecchi, and A. Mantovani. 1998. Differential regulation of chemokine receptors during dendritic cell maturation: a model for their trafficking properties. *J. Immunol.* **161:**1083–1086.

122. Szekanecz, Z., J. Kim, and A. E. Koch. 2003. Chemokines and chemokine receptors in rheumatoid arthritis. *Semin. Immunol.* **15:**15–21.

123. Taha, R. A., S. Laberge, Q. Hamid, and R. Olivenstein. 2001. Increased expression of the chemoattractant cytokines eotaxin, monocyte chemotactic protein-4, and interleukin-16 in induced sputum in asthmatic patients. *Chest* **120:**595–601.

124. Tanaka, Y., D. H. Adams, S. Hubscher, H. Hirano, U. Siebenlist, and S. Shaw. 1993. T-cell adhesion induced by proteoglycan-immobilized cytokine MIP-1 beta. *Nature* **361:**79–82.

125. Tanaka, Y., D. H. Adams, and S. Shaw. 1993. Proteoglycans on endothelial cells present adhesion-inducing cytokines to leukocytes. *Immunol. Today* **14:**111–115.

126. Tenscher, K., B. Metzner, E. Schopf, J. Norgauer, and W. Czech. 1996. Recombinant human eotaxin induces oxygen radical production, Ca(2+)-mobilization, actin reorganization, and CD11b upregulation in human eosinophils via a pertussis toxin-sensitive heterotrimeric guanine nucleotide-binding protein. *Blood* **88:**3195–3199.

127. Tesch, G. H., A. Schwarting, K. Kinoshita, H. Y. Lan, B. J. Rollins, and V. R. Kelley. 1999. Monocyte chemoattractant protein-1 promotes macrophage-mediated tubular injury, but not glomerular injury, in nephrotoxic serum nephritis. *J. Clin. Investig.* **103:**73–80.

128. Traynor, T. R., W. A. Kuziel, G. B. Toews, and G. B. Huffnagle. 2000. CCR2 expression determines T1 versus T2 polarization during pulmonary Cryptococcus neoformans infection. *J. Immunol.* **164:**2021–2027.

129. Tsien, R. Y. 1980. New calcium indicators and buffers with high selectivity against magnesium and protons: design, synthesis, and properties of prototype structures. *Biochemistry* **19:**2396–2404.

130. Tsien, R. Y., T. J. Rink, and M. Poenie. 1985. Measurement of cytosolic free Ca^{2+} in individual small cells using fluorescence microscopy with dual excitation wavelengths. *Cell Calcium* **6:**145–157.

131. van Es, S., D. Wessels, D. R. Soll, J. Borleis, and P. N. Devreotes. 2001. Tortoise, a novel mitochondrial protein, is required for directional responses of Dictyostelium in chemotactic gradients. *J. Cell Biol.* **152:**621–632.

132. Waldmann, T. A. 1991. Monoclonal antibodies in diagnosis and therapy. *Science* **252:**1657–1662.

133. Wang, N., I. Tabas, R. Winchester, L. E. Ravalli, L. E. Rabbani, and A. Tall. 1996. Interleukin 8 is induced by cholesterol loading of macrophages and expressed by macrophage foam cells in human atheroma. *J. Biol. Chem.* **271:**8837–8842.

134. Wank, S. A. 1998. G protein-coupled receptors in gastrointestinal physiology. I. CCK receptors: an exemplary family. *Am. J. Physiol.* **274:**G607–G613.

135. Weiner, O. D., G. Servant, M. D. Welch, T. J. Mitchison, J. W. Sedat, and H. R. Bourne. 1999. Spatial control of actin polymerization during neutrophil chemotaxis. *Nat. Cell. Biol.* **1:**75–81.

136. Weissleder, R., and U. Mahmood. 2001. Molecular imaging. *Radiology* **219:**316–333.

137. Wells, T. N., C. A. Power, and A. E. Proudfoot. 1998. Definition, function and pathophysiological significance of chemokine receptors. *Trends Pharmacol. Sci.* **19:**376–380.

138. Westlin, W. F., J. M. Kiely, and M. A. Gimbrone, Jr. 1992. Interleukin-8 induces changes in human neutrophil actin conformation and distribution: relationship to inhibition of adhesion to cytokine-activated endothelium. *J. Leukoc. Biol.* **52:**43–51.

139. Wilcox, J. N., N. A. Nelken, S. R. Coughlin, D. Gordon, and T. J. Schall. 1994. Local expression of inflammatory cytokines in human atherosclerotic plaques. *J. Atheroscler. Thromb.* **1** (Suppl. 1):S10–S13.

140. Winter, P. M., A. M. Morawski, S. D. Caruthers, R. W. Fuhrhop, H. Zhang, T. A. Williams, J. S. Allen, E. K. Lacy, J. D. Robertson, G. M. Lanza, and S. A. Wickline. 2003. Molecular imaging of angiogenesis in early-stage atherosclerosis with alpha(v)beta3-integrin-targeted nanoparticles. *Circulation* **108:**2270–2274.

141. Xie, H., Y. C. Lim, F. W. Luscinskas, and A. H. Lichtman. 1999. Acquisition of selectin binding and peripheral homing properties by CD4(+) and CD8(+) T cells. *J. Exp. Med.* **189:**1765–1776.

142. Ying, S., and A. B. Kay. 2000. Chemokines in allergic asthma, p. 383–401. *In* M. E. Rothenberg (ed.), *Chemokines in Allergic Disease.* Marcel Dekker AG, New York, N.Y.

143. Zhao, D. X., Y. Hu, G. G. Miller, A. D. Luster, R. N. Mitchell, and P. Libby. 2002. Differential expression of the IFN-gamma-inducible CXCR3-binding chemokines, IFN-inducible protein 10, monokine induced by IFN, and IFN-inducible T cell alpha chemoattractant in human cardiac allografts: association with cardiac allograft vasculopathy and acute rejection. *J. Immunol.* **169:**1556–1560.

144. Zlotnik, A., and O. Yoshie. 2000. Chemokines: a new classification system and their role in immunity. *Immunity* **12:**121–127.

Laboratory Monitoring of Cytokine Therapy

ANDREW R. PACHNER

43

Cytokines, anticytokine antibodies, and cytokine receptors, available as recombinant proteins, are becoming increasingly utilized by physicians to treat a variety of diseases, particularly autoimmune diseases. These medications, cytokine-based therapies (CBTs), a subclass of a group of therapeutic agents called "biologics," have a significant role in therapy. However, there are also major problems with their use, including high cost, immunogenicity, adverse effects, and unknown mechanisms of action. Because of this, laboratory monitoring for drug efficacy as well as for antidrug antibodies and side effects has increasingly become a focus of investigation. Laboratory monitoring for all of the cytokine therapies currently available (see Table 1) is beyond the scope of this chapter. Also not covered in this review is pretherapy genetic testing, which has been studied as a means of increasing the likelihood of positive therapeutic response or decreasing the likelihood of adverse events (18). I instead focus on general strategies, as well as on monitoring for two cytokine therapies, beta interferon (IFN-β) and infliximab.

The goal of laboratory monitoring for cytokine therapies is to maximize the efficacy and minimize adverse effects of these agents. The optimal monitoring strategy will depend on the characteristics of the specifics of the therapy, but general strategies can be identified. In IFN-β therapy for multiple sclerosis (MS), many of these general strategies have been utilized with significant benefit to MS patients. In other CBTs, monitoring has not been as extensively utilized.

GENERAL STRATEGIES OF LABORATORY MONITORING OF CBTs

Mechanisms of Action of CBTs

Cytokines bind to specific receptors on the surface of their target cells, triggering signal transduction with subsequent upregulation of specific genes (Fig. 1). These agents tend to have a relatively narrow spectrum of action and are thus considered "smart bombs," able to effectively suppress the "bad guys" and not affect the "good guys." Because efficacy is dependent upon activation of specific receptors, an understanding of the receptors is essential, i.e., their patterns of expression, ligand binding characteristics, signal transduction molecules, pattern of induced gene activation, etc. These details are imperfectly understood for most CBTs.

Because of the lack of knowledge about it, the mechanism of action in human disease is speculative. A good example is IFN-β therapy of MS. Interferons are a heterogeneous class of molecules which share the ability to protect cells from viral lysis. IFN-α and -β are classed as type 1 interferons, while IFN-γ is considered a type 2 interferon. The type 1 interferons bind to the IFN-α/β receptor, also called IFNAR, while IFN-γ binds to its own receptor. Binding of IFN-β to the IFNAR results in signal transduction, activation of kinases, and activation of transcription factors, with subsequent increases in the levels of the mRNAs and proteins. The MxA gene is an example of such a gene (see below). IFN-β was initially tested in MS in pursuit of the hypothesis that the disease was virally linked and that an antiviral therapy such as IFN-β would ameliorate the natural history of the disease (21). The viral hypothesis has not been completely invalidated, but most researchers now believe that IFN-β induces a change in the immune/inflammatory system in such a way that "harmful" inflammation is decreased. A large body of literature exists on possible mechanisms of IFN-β in MS (6, 11, 12, 45), but speculation is rampant and hard data are sparse. Whatever proves to be the operative mechanism of action, at this point, IFN-β is used as a therapy in MS without a firm understanding of how it works.

Similar considerations apply to tumor necrosis factor (TNF) blockers, used extensively in rheumatoid arthritis (RA) and inflammatory bowel disease. A variety of cell types secrete TNF-α as a 17-kDa soluble protein which then aggregates, forming trimers. The trimers bind to two receptors: p55 TNF receptor 1 and the p75 TNF receptor. TNF-α also induces other cytokines, such as interleukin 1 (IL-1) and IL-6. Another action of TNF-α is to increase leukocyte migration by inducing expression of adhesion molecules by both leukocytes and endothelial cells. Infliximab (Remicade; Centocor) is an intravenously administered chimeric monoclonal immunoglobulin G1 (IgG1) specific to TNF. It is composed of human constant and murine variable regions.

The multitude of TNF blockers currently available have as their putative mechanism of action blockade of TNF binding to the TNF receptor. Infliximab binds specifically and with high affinity to human TNF-α, but its precise mechanism of action in RA or Crohn's disease is not known. Mere neutralization of TNF is not the main therapeutic effect, at least in Crohn's disease, since other TNF-α blockers

TABLE 1 Partial list of cytokines available for therapy in the autumn of 2004

Cytokine or cytokine receptor	Disease(s)	Company(ies)	Year of launch (United States)
IFN-α (Infergen, Intron, PegIntron, Alferon, Pegasys, Roferon)	Hepatitis C, melanoma, leukemia, lymphoma, condyloma acuminatum, Kaposi's sarcoma	Numerous	
IFN-β (Betaseron, Avonex, Rebif)	MS	Berlex, Biogen, Serono	1993
IL-2 (aldesleukin [Proleukin])	Melanoma, renal cell cancer	Chiron	1998
IFN-γ-1b (Actimmune)	Chronic granulomatous disease/osteopetrosis	InterMune	2000
GM-CSF[a] (sargramostim [Leukine])	Reconstitution after chemotherapy	Immunex	1995
TNFR[b] IgG1 (etanercept [Enbrel])	RA, JRA[c], psoriatic arthritis, ankylosing spondylitis	Immunex-Wyeth	1998
Anti-TNF antibody (adalimumab [Humira], infliximab [Remicade])	RA, Crohn's disease	Abbott, Centocor	2002
CD-11a (efalizumab [Raptiva])	Psoriasis	Genentech	2003
LFA-3–IgG (alefacept [Amevive])	Psoriasis	Biogen	2003
IL-1 (anakinra [Kineret])	RA	Amgen	2001
G-CSF (pegfilgrastim [Neulasta], filgrastim [Neupogen])	Reconstitution after chemotherapy	Amgen	1991

[a]GM-CSF, granulocyte-macrophage colony-stimulating factor.
[b]TNFR, TNF receptor.
[c]JRA, juvenile RA.
[d]G-CSF, granulocyte colony-stimulating factor.

are equally able to neutralize yet have little or no effect. Although there are a number of hypotheses (e.g., decreased expression of adhesion molecules or acceleration of apoptosis of TNF-α-bearing cells), none have been widely accepted, and the explanation for differences in efficacy of the various TNF-α-lowering agents is not known.

Monitoring of CBT Effect: General Principles

There are two major types of laboratory measures used to monitor CBTs: biomarkers of disease and cytokine-induced molecules. Biomarkers of disease are assays used to monitor disease activity, are not specific for the CBT, and can be used to monitor any therapy for the disease. Examples include

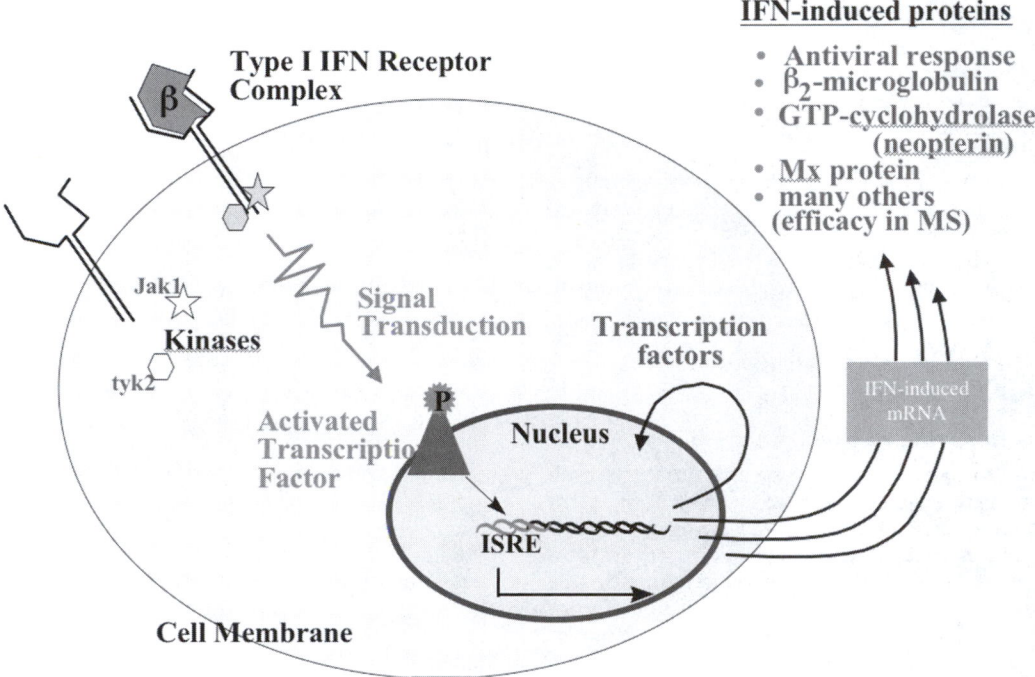

FIGURE 1 Diagram of cellular effects of IFN-β as a prototype of a CBT. The cellular response to IFN-β is a prototype system in which receptor binding by the cytokine results in upregulation of a host of early, intermediate, and late genes, with complex downstream effects.

sedimentation rate and rheumatoid factor measurement in RA or C-reactive protein in inflammatory bowel disease (23). Biomarkers of disease are extensively dealt with in other chapters of this manual and are not discussed here. Cytokine-induced molecules are relatively specific markers of cytokine induction and represent expected responses ideally linked to the therapy's mode of action. MxA is such a marker in IFN-β therapy for MS.

Most cytokines during their natural function have their effect over a short distance. In other words, they are released by one cell and act upon a nearby cell so that their concentrations in serum are low or not measurable. Thus, when CBTs are injected it is assumed that they will achieve effective concentrations at the appropriate location of optimal action, and that these concentrations will be uniform from individual to individual. Unfortunately, with many CBTs, the subject of therapy is a black box in which a drug is injected and a clinical effect is assessed; this "black box" nature of therapy presents serious problems in identifying biomarkers. An example is IFN-β therapy for MS. Within an hour after injection the drug is not detectable in blood. The target cell mediating the drug effect is unknown; many different cell types have IFNARs and can respond to IFN-β. These facts, combined with the fact that MS is a highly variable disease requiring hundreds of trial subjects to show a therapeutic effect for a given treatment, make it very difficult to assess the drug's effect in any one patient, and they underline the need for biomarkers of drug efficacy.

Because of this lack of a firm understanding of the mechanism of action of CBTs, efficacy monitoring is not highly developed for most biologicals. Ideally, we would be able to measure multiple products of genes which (i) are sensitive and specific for the CBT, (ii) are highly correlated with the expected molecular effect of the cytokine on gene products critical for the disease, and (iii) represent bioactivity of the CBT at various levels of its mechanism, from interaction with cell surface receptors to activation of necessary downstream gene products. This ideal has not been reached for any CBTs, but the currently available monitoring assays closest to the ideal involve monitoring of genes upregulated after injection of IFN-β, described at length below.

Monitoring of Immunogenicity: General Principles

During development of biologicals by pharmaceutical companies, efforts are made to minimize immunogenicity. However, as summarized recently by Schellekens (41), the immunogenicity of a product in humans is not predictable from structural analyses and animal studies. Even during clinical trials, immunogenicity may be underestimated if the antibody assays are not reliable. Such a situation occurred for anti-IFN-β therapy in the treatment of MS. In the pivotal study of IFN-β therapy for MS (19), anti-IFN-β antibodies were measured but the assays used were unreliable, and there was considerable variability in readings. This resulted in a highly confusing picture, and the problems with immunogenicity of the product were thus overlooked.

The need for high quality in assays for antibiological antibodies induced during therapy cannot be overstated, since both underdiagnosis and overdiagnosis create problems for clinicians. Antibodies to recombinant proteins used in therapy can cause serious side effects by inactivating both the injected and the native protein. This was demonstrated to be potentially fatal in pure red cell aplasia

in patients treated with recombinant erythropoietin who developed antierythropoietin antibodies (5, 46). At a minimum, antibodies can lead to loss of bioactivity of the injected CBT, a state known as antibody-mediated decreased bioactivity (ADB) (25). Assays for antibodies to CBTs are generally developed to address two different aspects of antibody function: binding and neutralization.

Binding-antibody (BAb) assays are generally faster, more sensitive, and more inexpensive than other assays. Enzyme-linked immunosorbent assay (ELISA) technology can be used, which allows for the screening of hundreds of samples in a few hours in an automated fashion. Other methodologies to detect BAbs include immunoprecipitation assays and blotting methods. Careful attention must be paid in the development of these assays to a number of factors which contribute to imprecision in BAb assays, especially in ELISAs. These have been well summarized recently by Bendtzen (1). For instance, some cytokines which are adhered to solid phase become partially denatured, creating neoepitopes not found in the recombinant molecule. These neoepitopes will then serve as antigens in ELISAs, creating false positivity. Conversely, partial denaturation of the antigen will also result in destruction of some epitopes for true BAbs, leading to potential false negativity. For instance, in ELISAs measuring anti-IFN-β BAbs, adhering IFN-β directly to plastic plates by using highly alkaline coating buffers results in both false positivity and false negativity (31), making this method of coating plates for anti-IFN-β ELISAs highly unreliable. However, the many advantages of ELISA technology make this technique highly desirable if methodologically feasible. Thus, a modified ELISA has proven to be highly useful in the monitoring of MS patients treated with IFN-β (27); in this assay, IFN-β is captured in liquid phase by a monoclonal anti-IFN-β antibody adhered to the plate (4) and then reacted with the patient's serum and developing reagents. BAb assays are ideal for screening for biologically relevant antibodies, but they tend to detect low-affinity antibodies. Thus, BAb assays can be positive for patients in whom there is no interference with CBT therapeutic effect, i.e., false positive.

For an antibody assay that more closely correlates with ADB, neutralizing-antibody (NAb) assays are used. NAbs are unlikely to be false positive; i.e., patients in whom NAbs are positive are likely to be receiving incomplete benefit from the medication. They measure the ability of the patient's serum to neutralize a biological effect of the CBT. For IFN-β, the standard NAb assay is performed by adding serum to IFN-β and then to a layer of IFN-β-responsive cells, with subsequent exposure to a virus which kills unprotected cells, described at more length below. For the TNF blocker infliximab, no NAb assay is available. NAb assays are advantageous in being more highly correlated with clinical measures, but they tend to be difficult and much more expensive than BAb assays.

MONITORING OF IFN-β THERAPY

Monitoring of Efficacy

Activation of the IFNAR as a Measure of Effect of Anti-IFN-β Antibodies

Neurologists prescribe IFN-β for their MS patients with the assumption that bioactivity of the drug will be maintained with repeated injection. However, many patients injecting the drug develop anti-IFN-β antibodies, and these anti-IFN-β antibodies can interfere with bioactivity, inducing a state known as ADB. In this situation, antibodies developed against the drug prevent the binding of the drug to its specific receptor, leading to lack of activation of the IFNAR after the patient injects the drug. Because of this, in those patients in whom ADB is suspected, bioactivity measurements, measuring activation of IFN-β-inducible genes, are increasingly being used as a direct measure of whether IFN-β is stimulating the IFNAR, the receptor critical for IFN-β function. IFNAR binding with subsequent signal transduction is a necessary first step for IFN-β action in MS. If bioactivity is maintained, each injection of IFN-β results in the strong upregulation of the MxA gene, which is IFN-β inducible, in the blood. MxA is a cytoplasmic protein (47) with a molecular mass of about 75 kDa which has intrinsic GTPase activity blocking viral replication, and it is encoded by the Mx1 gene, located on chromosome 21q22.3. Other genes, such as those for 2′,5′-oligoadenylate synthetase (28), neopterin (8), and viperin (7), are also upregulated after IFN-β injection, but MxA has proven to be the most robust and widely used marker.

Bioactivity measurements using IFN-β-induced MxA mRNA or MxA protein have been performed in both cross-sectional and longitudinal studies of MS patients (2, 3, 9, 10, 27, 28, 32, 43). Blood is obtained 12 h after IFN-β injection, at which time a strong MxA mRNA signal is detectable in patients without high levels of anti-IFN-β antibodies. The three commercially IFN-β preparations have similar doses of IFN-β with each injection, approximately 6 to 9 mIU of IFN-β, so the MxA mRNA levels induced are similar. RNA is obtained as whole RNA, and the reliability of the assay is dependent on the quality of the RNA, since RNA is an unstable molecular species. Thus, the methodology of RNA purification for these assays is critical. In order to ensure optimal RNA quality, we have utilized the PAXgene purification system, developed by Becton Dickinson, for our version of the MxA mRNA measurement, which we call the gene expression of MxA.

Once RNA is purified, reverse transcription is performed using the SuperScript First-Strand Synthesis System for reverse transcription-PCR (Life Technologies, Grand Island, N.Y.). cDNA is then subjected to real-time PCR analysis using the PE Applied Biosystems Taqman system; a 6-carboxyfluorescein- or 6-carboxytetramethylrhodamine-labeled probe is used for either MxA or glyceraldehyde-3-phosphate dehydrogenase (GAPDH) in separate tubes. We have utilized plasmids containing the sequence of MxA and GAPDH in order to standardize our assay. We then express the values obtained for any particular patient as a normalization ratio, a ratio of expression of MxA of the patient relative to that of a healthy control, with each measurement indexed to the GAPDH RNA level.

When this method is used for a large group of healthy controls, a normal distribution of values is obtained with the mean at 1 (Fig. 2A). When this method is used for a large group of MS patients with low or absent anti-IFN-β antibody levels in blood samples obtained 12 h after injection, a normal distribution of values is obtained with the mean at 17 (27) (Fig. 2B). GEM values expressed as the normalization ratios obtained for the same patient over time are very stable as long as anti-IFN-β antibody levels are absent or low.

The results of the GEM assay are highly dependent on the level of anti-IFN-β antibodies. Four stages of the relationship between antibody assays and bioactivity measured by GEM can be identified (Fig. 3) in those patients who develop significant levels of antibodies. In the first stage, which occurs in the first few months after initiation of therapy, NAbs are absent, and bioactivity is normal. In the second stage, as NAbs rise, bioactivity decreases. In the third stage, which can last for years if the patient continues IFN-β injections, NAbs remain positive and bioactivity is decreased or absent. In the fourth stage, which occurs in an unknown but significant percentage of patients with ADB, usually those taking IFN-β-1b rather than IFN-β-1a, NAb levels spontaneously decrease and bioactivity increases despite continued injection.

Prolonged periods of ADB result in a loss of clinical efficacy of IFN-β, particularly in those measures of MS activity responsive to IFN-β therapy, such as gadolinium-enhancing lesions on magnetic resonance imaging or relapse rates (20, 34, 39). The clinical effects of the loss of efficacy are much more difficult to identify in MS relative to other diseases in which CBTs have been used, because of the incomplete response of patients to IFN-β and the highly variable progression and relapse rate in MS. This has prompted some clinicians to claim that "the effects of IFNβ NAb on clinical efficacy are incompletely understood" (50). However, most investigators in the field believe that adequate evidence exists to conclude that levels of NAbs high enough to substantially lower bioactivity as measured by MxA assays will lead to significant diminution or loss of therapeutic efficacy (13, 25).

Monitoring of IFN-β-Induced Genes Important in MS Pathogenesis

Although the MxA gene is an IFN-β-induced gene in MS patients, there is no evidence that MxA is important in MS pathogenesis. Thus, the MxA gene is an excellent gene for measuring IFNAR activation and monitoring the effect of anti-IFN-β antibodies, and its induction is a necessary condition for effect of IFN-β in MS, but it may not be a sufficient condition for treatment effect. Other molecules, like IL-10 (37, 38, 49), may be directly linked to the therapeutic effect. Efforts are underway to identify IFN-β-inducible genes important for the therapeutic effect (22, 48).

Immunogenicity

Assays for antibodies which neutralize the ability of IFN-β to protect susceptible cell lines from viral lysis were the first antibody assays to be used for MS patients treated with IFN-β. Such assays, called cytopathic-effect assays (14, 15), are currently the standard in the field. In the most popular version of this assay, the A549 cell line, a human lung carcinoma line, is the target, and encephalomyocarditis virus is used to lyse the cells. Cell death is measured using a vital dye, and the assay is considered positive when addition of a 1:20 dilution of patient serum is able to result in cell death by interfering with the protective effect of IFN-β. An alternative assay which is increasingly being used is the NAb-MxA test (36). In this more recently developed assay, the readout is measurement of production of an IFN-β-inducible protein, MxA, by a cell line; A549 cells can also be used as the cell line for this assay. Cells exposed to IFN-β preincubated with serum devoid of NAbs will make high levels of MxA, while cells exposed to IFN-β preincubated with serum with NAbs present will not produce MxA. In both assays, the NAbs exert their effect by binding to IFN-β in such a way as to prevent its ability to bind to the IFNAR; IFNAR-activated signal transduction leads to both protection from viral lysis and production of MxA. NAb assays, like all antibody assays, have both strengths and weaknesses. Positives are that these

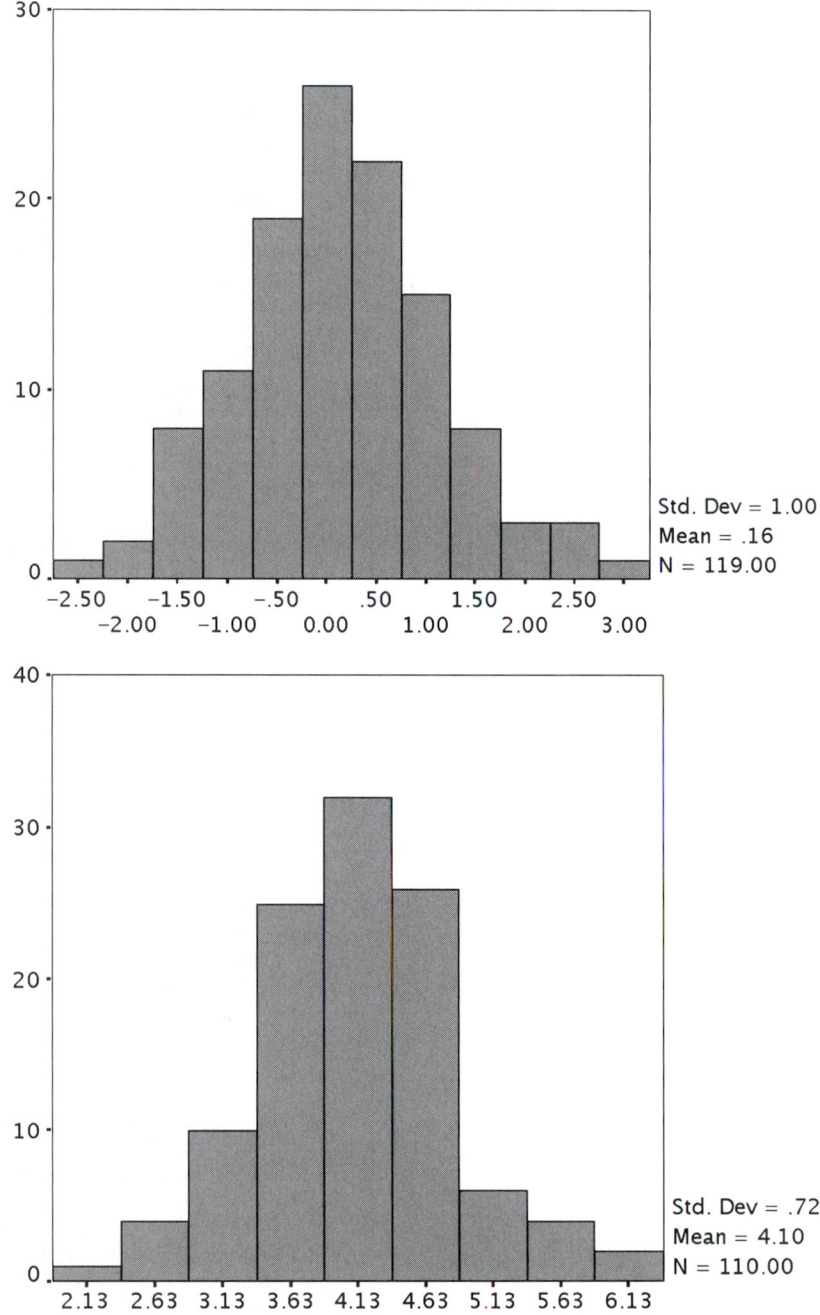

FIGURE 2 Histograms of gene expression of MxA (GEM) in controls without IFN-β injection (top) and MS patients 12 h after IFN-β injection (bottom). The x axis represents log$_2$ of normalization ratios, i.e., 2 to the power ($\Delta\Delta Ct$) where $\Delta\Delta Ct$ is (Ct of MxA – Ct of GAPDH) for sample minus (Ct of MxA – Ct of GAPDH) for normal control. The y axis represents number of patients. The expected response after injection is a strong increase in level of MxA mRNA as detected by real-time reverse transcription-PCR. In this group of patients the MS patients had a mean of over 16-fold increase in MxA mRNA after injection.

assays are now relatively well standardized and correlate quite well with loss of clinical efficacy. However, disadvantages are that they are difficult technically, cumbersome, and quite expensive. Also, because they are based on responses of cell lines, any serum constituents that affect the cells will lead to problems in the assay.

Increasingly, BAb assays for anti-IFN-β antibodies are being used as screening assays. BAb assays test for all antibodies that bind at a range of affinities to IFN-β; serum samples that have low or absent binding levels are negative for NAbs and do not require further analysis (31, 33). In the capture ELISA technique initially developed by Brickelmaier

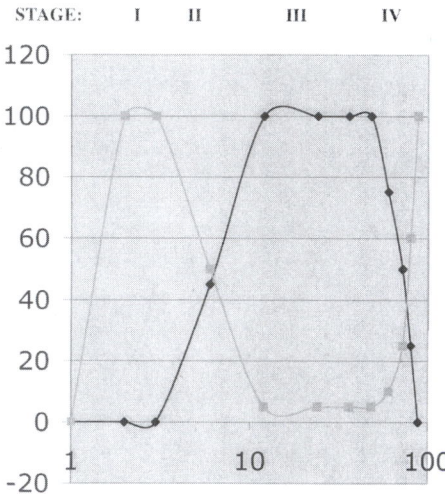

FIGURE 3 Stages of ADB in IFN-β-treated MS patients. Four stages can be identified in the interplay between antibody and bioactivity of IFN-β as measured by the GEM assay. ◆, Nab level (%); ■, bioactivity (%). The y axis represents percent maximal response, and the x axis represents months post initiation of therapy.

et al. (4), a monoclonal anti-IFN-β antibody, adhered to the plate, is used to capture the antigen, IFN-β, and then the solid phase is incubated sequentially with serum, conjugated antibody, and the developing reagent. The test was initially shown to be reliable for a small number of samples from patients treated with Avonex, an IFN-β-1a preparation. Our laboratory subsequently demonstrated that the assay could accurately assess antibody response in a large number of patients treated with all three IFN-β preparations (31). BAb assays have also been used successfully in screening for NAbs in clinical trial specimens (35, 39).

MONITORING OF INFLIXIMAB THERAPY

Infliximab-Sensitive Genes

Unlike IFN-β, infliximab, as a monoclonal antibody to TNF-α, does not have a receptor for its action and thus does not directly upregulate gene expression. Because it is designed to block TNF-α, one might assume that its effect can be measured by documenting decreased expression of TNF-α in the peripheral blood, but this assumption would not be correct. TNF-α, IL-6, and IL-1β were not significantly decreased by infliximab therapy, but acute-phase proteins such as cyclic AMP receptor protein and haptoglobin were decreased (24). At this point, there are no well-accepted biomarkers for infliximab direct action, either for assessment of the effect of anti-infliximab antibodies or for therapeutic effect.

Recent reports on infliximab in Crohn's disease provided an interesting potential biomarker. Ten Hove et al. (42) found that infliximab induced apoptosis of lamina propria T lymphocytes in patients with Crohn's disease but did not influence expression of activation markers, homing receptors, memory cells, Fas expression, or Bax/Bcl-2 expression on peripheral blood T lymphocytes from these patients. In an extension study from this group, Van den Brande et al. (44) investigated why infliximab is clinically effective in

Crohn's disease, while a related TNF blocker, etanercept (Enbrel), is not; etanercept is a dimeric fusion protein consisting of the extracellular portion of the p75 TNF receptor linked to the Fc domains of human IgG1. They found the two drugs to be equally effective in in vitro bioassays of TNF neutralization; however, infliximab was able to induce apoptosis of lamina propria T lymphocytes, while etanercept was not. These data indicate that biomarkers of drug efficacy may need to utilize biopsies of inflamed tissue rather than peripheral blood lymphocytes, a not-surprising situation when one considers the compartmentalization of the immune response and the normally short range of action of cytokines.

Infliximab Immunogenicity

The immunogenicity problems with infliximab (17, 40) are not as well studied as with IFN-β, possibly because of the very different ways in which these CBTs are used. Antibodies to infliximab are measured using a double-antigen ELISA in which infliximab serves as the detection and capture reagent. All immunoglobulin isotypes and subclasses can be detected. Anti-infliximab antibodies can occur in as many as 30% of patients, despite the concurrent use of immunosuppressives such as methotrexate in these patients. Antibodies to infliximab are associated with a more rapid reduction in serum infliximab concentrations from postinfusion peak levels and an impaired clinical response. Also, delayed infusion reactions, characterized by myalgias, arthralgias, fever, rash, pruritus, dysphagia, urticaria, sore throat, headache, and facial, hand, or lip edema, may occur 3 to 12 days after infusion; these reactions are felt to be likely due to anti-infliximab antibodies (16).

SUMMARY

CBTs are a subclass of biologicals that have profound biological effects, many of which are poorly understood. These drugs are recent additions to therapy, and consequently, we are still relatively early in a growth curve about their optimal use. Monitoring of their effects is going to be important for many reasons. One of the major reasons is that these therapies tend to be highly immunogenic and the optimal approach for identification of antidrug antibodies and their potential to neutralize drug effects needs to be identified. Another reason is the high cost of these biologicals, which makes optimal use critical. Unfortunately, pharmaceutical companies which invest a great deal in the development of these drugs are reluctant to invest even more in working on optimal techniques for monitoring immunogenicity and drug effect. This situation leaves a vacuum after these drugs become available, which is filled only very slowly as problems with the therapies surface and the medical community attempts to solve them. For example, in 2005, 12 years after IFN-β came to the market in the United States for therapy of MS, there is still no standardized assay for anti-IFN-β antibodies and no clearly effective treatment options for the many patients who have high titers of NAbs with no therapeutic effect (26, 29, 30). It is hoped that robust assays for therapeutic efficacy and for immunogenicity will be developed more effectively in the future after the launch of other CBTs.

REFERENCES

1. **Bendtzen, K.** 2003. Anti-IFN BAb and NAb antibodies; a minireview. *Neurology* **61:**S6–S10.
2. **Bertolotto, A., F. Gilli, A. Sala, L. Audano, A. Castello, U. Magliola, F. Melis,** and **M. T. Giordana.** 2001.

Evaluation of bioavailability of three types of IFNb in multiple sclerosis patients by a new quantitative-competitive-PCR method for MxA quantification. *J. Immunol. Methods* **256**:141–152.

3. Bertolotto, A., F. Gilli, A. Sala, M. Capobianco, S. Malucchi, E. Milano, F. Melis, F. Marnetto, R. L. Lindberg, R. Bottero, A. Di Sapio, and M. T. Giordana. 2003. Persistent neutralizing antibodies abolish the interferon beta bioavailability in MS patients. *Neurology* **60**:634–639.

4. Brickelmaier, M., P. S. Hochman, R. Baciu, B. Chao, J. H. Cuervo, and A. Whitty. 1999. ELISA methods for the analysis of antibody responses induced in multiple sclerosis patients treated with recombinant interferon-β. *J. Immunol. Methods* **227**:121–135.

5. Casadevall, N., J. Nataf, B. Viron, A. Kolta, J. J. Kiladjian, P. Martin-Dupont, P. Michaud, T. Papo, V. Ugo, I. Teyssandier, B. Varet, and P. Mayeux. 2002. Pure red-cell aplasia and antierythropoietin antibodies in patients treated with recombinant erythropoietin. *N. Engl. J. Med.* **346**:469–475.

6. Chan, A., R. Seguin, T. Magnus, C. Papadimitriou, K. V. Toyka, J. P. Antel, and R. Gold. 2003. Phagocytosis of apoptotic inflammatory cells by microglia and its therapeutic implications: termination of CNS autoimmune inflammation and modulation by interferon-beta. *Glia* **43**(3):231–242.

7. Chin, K.-C., and P. Cresswell. 2001. Viperin (cig5), an IFN-inducible antiviral protein directly induced by human cytomegalovirus. *J. Immunol.* **98**:15125–15130.

8. Cook, S. D., J. R. Quinless, A. Jotkowitz, P. Beaton, and The Neutralizing Antibody Study Group. 2001. Serum IFN neutralizing antibodies and neopterin levels in a cross-section of MS patients. *Neurology* **57**:1080–1084.

9. Deisenhammer, F., I. Mayringer, J. Harvey, E. Dilitz, T. Gasse, D. Stadlbauer, M. Reindl, and T. Berger. 2000. A comparative study of the relative bioavailability of different interferon beta preparations. *Neurology* **54**:2055–2060.

10. Deisenhammer, F., M. Reindl, J. Harvey, T. Gasse, E. Dilitz, and T. Berger. 1999. Bioavailability of interferon beta 1b in MS patients with and without neutralizing antibodies. *Neurology* **52**:1239–1243.

11. Feng, X., D. Yau, C. Holbrook, and A. T. Reder. 2002. Type I interferons inhibit interleukin-10 production in activated human monocytes and stimulate IL-10 in T cells: implications for Th1-mediated diseases. *J. Interferon Cytokine Res.* **22**:311–319.

12. Floris, S., S. R. Ruuls, A. Wierinckx, S. M. van der Pol, E. Dopp, P. H. van der Meide, C. D. Dijkstra, and H. E. De Vries. 2002. Interferon-beta directly influences monocyte infiltration into the central nervous system. *J. Neuroimmunol.* **127**:69–79.

13. Giovannoni, G., F. E. Munschauer III, and F. Deisenhammer. 2002. Neutralising antibodies to interferon beta during the treatment of multiple sclerosis. *J. Neurol. Neurosurg. Psychiatry* **73**:465–469.

14. Grossberg, S. E., Y. Kawade, M. Kohase, and J. P. Klein. 2001. The neutralization of interferons by antibody. II. Neutralizing antibody unitage and its relationship to bioassay sensitivity: the tenfold reduction unit. *J. Interferon Cytokine Res.* **21**:743–755.

15. Grossberg, S. E., Y. Kawade, M. Kohase, H. Yokoyama, and N. Finter. 2001. The neutralization of interferons by antibody. I. Quantitative and theoretical analyses of the neutralization reaction in different bioassay systems. *J. Interferon Cytokine Res.* **21**:729–742.

16. Han, P. D., and R. D. Cohen. 2004. Managing immunogenic responses to infliximab: treatment implications for patients with Crohn's disease. *Drugs* **64**:1767–1777.

17. Hanauer, S. B., C. L. Wagner, M. Bala, L. Mayer, S. Travers, R. H. Diamond, A. Olson, W. Bao, and P. Rutgeerts. 2004. Incidence and importance of antibody responses to infliximab after maintenance or episodic treatment in Crohn's disease. *Clin. Gastroenterol. Hepatol.* **2**: 542–553.

18. Hosford, D. A., E. H. Lai, J. H. Riley, C. F. Xu, T. M. Danoff, and A. D. Roses. 2004. Pharmacogenetics to predict drug-related adverse events. *Toxicol. Pathol.* **32**(Suppl. 1):9–12.

19. IFNB Multiple Sclerosis Study Group. 1993. Interferon beta-1b is effective in relapsing-remitting multiple sclerosis. *Neurology* **43**:655–661.

20. IFNB Multiple Sclerosis Study Group and the University of British Columbia MS/MRI Analysis Group. 1996. Neutralizing antibodies during treatment of multiple sclerosis with interferon beta-1b: experience during the first three years. *Neurology* **47**:889–894.

21. Jacobs, L., J. O'Malley, A. Freeman, and R. Ekes. 1981. Intrathecal interferon reduces exacerbations of multiple sclerosis. *Science* **214**:1026–1028.

22. Koike, F., J. Satoh, S. Miyake, T. Yamamoto, M. Kawai, S. Kikuchi, K. Nomura, K. Yokoyama, K. Ota, T. Kanda, T. Fukazawa, and T. Yamamura. 2003. Microarray analysis identifies interferon beta-regulated genes in multiple sclerosis. *J. Neuroimmunol.* **139**:109–118.

23. Louis, E., S. Vermeire, P. Rutgeerts, M. De Vos, A. Van Gossum, P. Pescatore, R. Fiasse, P. Pelckmans, H. Reynaert, G. D'Haens, M. Malaise, and J. Belaiche. 2002. A positive response to infliximab in Crohn disease: association with a higher systemic inflammation before treatment but not with −308 TNF gene polymorphism. *Scand. J. Gastroenterol.* **37**:818–824.

24. Martinez-Borra, J., C. Lopez-Larrea, S. Gonzalez, D. Fuentes, A. Dieguez, E. M. Deschamps, J. M. Perez-Pariente, A. Lopez-Vazquez, R. de Francisco, and L. Rodrigo. 2002. High serum tumor necrosis factor-alpha levels are associated with lack of response to infliximab in fistulizing Crohn's disease. *Am. J. Gastroenterol.* **97**: 2350–2356.

25. Pachner, A. 2003. Anti-IFNβ antibodies in IFNβ-treated MS patients: summary. *Neurology* **61**(Suppl. 5):1–5.

26. Pachner, A. 2004. Anti-interferon antibodies: surprises and lessons. *Lancet Neurol.* **3**:515.

27. Pachner, A., D. Dail, E. Pak, and K. Narayan. 2005. The importance of measuring IFNβ bioactivity: monitoring in MS patients and the effect of anti-IFNβ antibodies. *J. Neuroimmunol.* **166**:180–188.

28. Pachner, A., K. Narayan, N. Price, M. Hurd, and D. Dail. 2003. MxA gene expression analysis as an interferon-beta bioactivity measurement in patients with multiple sclerosis and the identification of antibody-mediated decreased bioactivity. *Mol. Diagn.* **7**:17–25.

29. Pachner, A. R. 1997. Anticytokine antibodies in beta interferon-treated MS patients and the need for testing: plight of the practicing neurologist. *Neurology* **49**:647–650.

30. Pachner, A. R. 2001. Measurement of antibodies to interferon beta in patients with multiple sclerosis. *Arch. Neurol.* **58**:1299–1300.

31. Pachner, A. R. 2003. An improved ELISA for screening for neutralizing anti-IFN-beta antibodies in MS patients. *Neurology* **61**:1444–1446.

32. Pachner, A. R., A. Bertolotto, and F. Deisenhammer. 2003. Measurement of MxA mRNA or protein as a

biomarker of IFNbeta bioactivity: detection of antibody-mediated decreased bioactivity (ADB). *Neurology* **61**(Suppl. 5):S24–S26.

33. Pachner, A. R., J. Oger, and J. Palace. 2003. The measurement of antibodies binding to IFNbeta in MS patients treated with IFNbeta. *Neurology* **61**(Suppl. 5):S18–S20.

34. PRISMS-4. 2001. Long-term efficacy of interferon-beta-1a in relapsing MS. *Neurology* **56**:1628–1636.

35. PRISMS Study Group. 1998. Randomised double-blind placebo-controlled study of interferon beta-1a in relapsing remitting multiple sclerosis. *Lancet* **352**:1498–1504.

36. Pungor, E., Jr., J. G. Files, J. D. Gabe, L. T. Do, W. P. Foley, J. L. Gray, J. W. Nelson, E. Nestaas, J. L. Taylor, and S. E. Grossberg. 1998. A novel bioassay for the determination of neutralizing antibodies to IFN-beta1b. *J. Interferon Cytokine Res.* **18**:1025–1030.

37. Rudick, R. A., R. M. Ransohoff, J. C. Lee, R. Peppler, M. Yu, P. M. Mathisen, and V. K. Tuohy. 1998. In vivo effects of interferon beta-1a on immunosuppressive cytokines in multiple sclerosis. *Neurology* **50**:1294–1300.

38. Rudick, R. A., R. M. Ransohoff, R. Peppler, S. VanderBrug Medendorp, P. Lehmann, and J. Alam. 1996. Interferon beta induces interleukin-10 expression: relevance to multiple sclerosis. *Ann. Neurol.* **40**:618–627.

39. Rudick, R. A., N. A. Simonian, J. A. Alam, M. Campion, J. O. Scaramucci, W. Jones, M. E. Coats, D. E. Goodkin, B. Weinstock-Guttman, R. M. Herndon, M. K. Mass, J. R. Richert, A. M. Salazar, F. E. Munschauer III, D. L. Cookfair, J. H. Simon, and L. D. Jacobs for the Multiple Sclerosis Collaborative Research Group (MSCRG). 1998. Incidence and significance of neutralizing antibodies to interferon beta-1a in multiple sclerosis. *Neurology* **50**:1206–1208.

40. Rutgeerts, P., G. Van Assche, and S. Vermeire. 2004. Optimizing anti-TNF treatment in inflammatory bowel disease. *Gastroenterology* **126**:1593–1610.

41. Schellekens, H. 2002. Bioequivalence and the immunogenicity of biopharmaceuticals. *Nat. Rev.* **1**:457–462.

42. ten Hove, T., C. van Montfrans, M. P. Peppelenbosch, and S. J. van Deventer. 2002. Infliximab treatment induces apoptosis of lamina propria T lymphocytes in Crohn's disease. *Gut* **50**:206–211.

43. Vallittu, A. M., M. Halminen, J. Peltoniemi, J. Ilonen, I. Julkunen, A. Salmi, J. P. Eralinna, and the Finnish Beta-Interferon Study Group. 2002. Neutralizing antibodies reduce MxA protein induction in interferon-beta-1a-treated MS patients. *Neurology* **58**:1786–1790.

44. Van den Brande, J. M., H. Braat, G. R. van den Brink, H. H. Versteeg, C. A. Bauer, I. Hoedemaeker, C. van Montfrans, D. W. Hommes, M. P. Peppelenbosch, and S. J. van Deventer. 2003. Infliximab but not etanercept induces apoptosis in lamina propria T-lymphocytes from patients with Crohn's disease. *Gastroenterology* **124**:1774–1785.

45. Van Weyenbergh, J., J. Wietzerbin, D. Rouillard, M. Barral-Netto, and R. Liblau. 2001. Treatment of multiple sclerosis patients with interferon-beta primes monocyte-derived macrophages for apoptotic cell death. *J. Leukoc. Biol.* **70**:745–748.

46. Verhelst, D., J. Rossert, N. Casadevall, A. Kruger, K. U. Eckardt, and I. C. Macdougall. 2004. Treatment of erythropoietin-induced pure red cell aplasia: a retrospective study. *Lancet* **363**:1768–1771.

47. von Wussow, P., D. Jakschies, H. K. Hochkeppel, C. Fibich, L. Penner, and H. Deicher. 1990. The human intracellular Mx-homologous protein is specifically induced by type I interferons. *Eur. J. Immunol.* **20**:2015–2019.

48. Wandinger, K. P., C. S. Sturzebecher, B. Bielekova, G. Detore, A. Rosenwald, L. M. Staudt, H. F. McFarland, and R. Martin. 2001. Complex immunomodulatory effects of interferon-beta in multiple sclerosis include the upregulation of T helper 1-associated marker genes. *Ann. Neurol.* **50**:349–357.

49. Williams, G. J., and P. L. Witt. 1998. Comparative study of the pharmacodynamic and pharmacologic effects of Betaseron and Avonex. *J. Interferon Cytokine Res.* **18**:967–975.

50. Wolinsky, J. S., K. V. Toyka, L. Kappos, and S. E. Grossberg. 2003. Interferon-beta antibodies: implications for the treatment of MS. *Lancet Neurol.* **2**:528.

IMMUNOHISTOLOGY AND IMMUNOPATHOLOGY

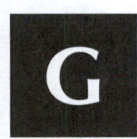

VOLUME EDITOR
ROBERT G. HAMILTON

SECTION EDITOR
RUSSELL H. TOMAR

Introduction

RUSSELL H. TOMAR

44

The contemporary practice of anatomic pathology is intertwined with and unthinkable without the contributions of immunohistochemistry. Since our last edition, more antigens have been shown to add value to the diagnosis, prognosis, and treatment processes associated with more tissues and more diseases. The techniques have been refined and increasingly standardized; the instrument continues to improve; the interpretations are more precise and sophisticated.

Major enhancements are on the immediate horizon. The instrumentation not only to perform immunohistochemical assays but also to evaluate histopathological slides in general is becoming more automated, which has shortened turnaround times. Enhancements in the technology will increase the utilization and value of the assays discussed in this section. The increased understanding and application of molecular methods will undoubtedly alter the practice not only of pathology but also of many other subspecialty areas, including surgery, gynecology, oncology, hematology, and gastroenterology.

Section G provides an overview of present practice and insights into the future of immunohistology and immunopathology measurements. The chapter by Roche et al. reviews general immunohistochemistry principles. Setty et al. then discuss the use of molecular biology methods on tissues. The chapter by Shidham and Kajdacsy-Balla covers the diagnostic and prognostic applications of immunohistochemistry. Finally, Collins et al. discuss immunofluorescence methods for the diagnosis of renal and skin diseases.

Immunohistochemistry: Principles and Advances

PATRICK C. ROCHE, ERIC D. HSI, AND BOURKE L. FIRFER

45

Immunohistochemistry (IHC) has become indispensable for detection, classification, and management of neoplasms in the daily practice of surgical pathology and increasingly so in cytopathology. Automation and the increasing availability of primary and secondary antibodies have augmented this revolution. In addition, tissue may now be examined for nucleic acid components, thereby enhancing diagnostic sensitivity and specificity.

The implementation of the Food and Drug Administration (FDA) ruling on the classification of immunohistochemical reagents and kits (1) is a significant occurrence that is familiar to many who deal with IHC and other areas such as flow cytometry. This ruling has led to the classification of the majority of immunohistochemical reagents as "analyte-specific reagents" (32, 33) and as class I medical devices, exempting them from premarket notification. This is permitted because IHC staining results are incorporated into the surgical pathology report as one part of the entire diagnostic evaluation. The IHC results are not stand-alone results. A few immunostains such as estrogen receptor (ER) and progesterone receptor are considered class II devices. These immunostains have no routine morphologic correlates but do have substantial and accepted scientific validation. Class III devices include immunostains that are not considered part of the surgical pathology diagnostic process and may result in a stand-alone report to a physician. Such tests require premarket notification and specific FDA approval. An example is the FDA-approved HercepTest for determination of Her2 protein overexpression as an indication for trastuzumab (Herceptin) therapy.

The FDA ruling essentially permits IHC laboratories to continue operating as they have been. Manufacturers must now label the antibody reagents they sell for diagnostic use (but for which they have not sought FDA clearance) as analyte-specific reagents. The manufacturers have the responsibility of following "good manufacturing practices" to ensure that antibodies are of consistent high quality and have the specificity that is claimed. However, all surgical pathology reports that incorporate IHC results are required to contain a statement indicating that the individual laboratory (not the manufacturer of the reagent) has the ultimate responsibility for ensuring the quality of the immunostaining (31). Thus, the laboratory director has the responsibility to utilize high-quality immunostains and to document their performance.

The intention of this chapter is to present current, practical methods that are applicable for performance of quality immunostains in the modern automated IHC laboratory. A review of the many different staining systems available today is beyond the scope of this chapter, although some are specifically mentioned by way of example.

SPECIMEN PROCESSING FOR PARAFFIN SECTION IHC

The importance of tissue fixation for the outcome of immunohistochemical staining is commonly recognized but cannot be overemphasized. In most pathology laboratories, neutrally buffered formalin is the routine fixative of choice. It is relatively inexpensive, easy to prepare, and produces excellent morphological preservation without shrinkage artifacts. The exact mechanism by which formaldehyde fixes tissues is not fully known but does involve cross-linking of reactive sites within and between protein molecules via hydroxymethylene bridges (41). Calcium ions have also been implicated in cross-link formation (20). The cross-links are believed to be responsible for masking antibody-binding epitopes and to be a major cause of lack of sensitivity in paraffin section IHC. Other fixatives (such as alcohol) that are considered less damaging to tissue antigenicity have been promoted as substitutes for formalin (4), but there has been little movement away from neutrally buffered formalin as the routine fixative in the daily practice of pathology. Instead, there have been increasing research and development focused on antigen recovery in formalin-fixed tissues in order to improve immunohistochemical staining.

In spite of its inherent detrimental effects on antigenicity and IHC, a proper and consistent protocol for fixation with neutrally buffered formalin is imperative for high-quality IHC. Formaldehyde is commercially available as a concentrated (37 to 40%) solution, and 10% neutrally buffered formalin is made by 1:10 dilution of the concentrate with phosphate-buffered saline (PBS; 50 mM phosphate, 0.9% NaCl [pH 7.2 to 7.4]), resulting in a final formaldehyde concentration of 3.7 to 4.0%. Ideally, tissue samples that are approximately 1.0 by 1.0 by 0.3 cm are placed in a cassette and immersed in 20 times the volume of freshly prepared formalin buffer for a minimum of 12 h and a maximum of 24 h. In practice, larger pieces are usually processed, but the tissue should not be forced into the cassette, and the smaller the size, the better and more thorough the fixation. If the specimens cannot be processed into paraffin blocks after 24 h of fixation in formalin, they should be transferred into 70% ethanol for holding until the tissue can be put on the processor. Prolonged exposure to formalin results in excessive cross-link formation and increasing loss of antigenicity (2, 3, 10). After they are properly fixed and embedded in a paraffin block, tissue specimens appear to retain antigenicity for decades (25).

Paraffin tissue sections for IHC are usually cut at a thickness of 4 to 6 μm. In order to retain sections on the glass microscope slide throughout the staining process, it is necessary to use slides that have been specially treated to increase their adhesive properties. Erie Scientific Company (Portsmouth, N.H.) produces slides that are treated with aminoalkyl silane and known as SuperFrost Plus. These slides are also generically referred to as charged or silanized slides and adhere to tissue sections through a combination of electrostatic and hydrophobic interactions. Although not used as commonly, glass slides treated with poly-L-lysine to increase their adhesive properties are another option. Storage of cut sections on microscope slides for use in IHC is still a subject of debate. At issue is the reported loss of reactivity of certain antigens, including p53 and Her2, when cut sections have been stored at room temperature. This phenomenon may be more pronounced when tissue is fixed in alcohol-supplemented formalin (14). For some laboratories, positive control sections or sections for research studies must be cut in advance and stored for subsequent use. If for practical reasons this is the case, sections should not be heated or melted down but just allowed to air dry on the slides. They should be stored in a closed slide box in a cool location or at 4°C if possible. Immediately prior to staining, slides can be placed in a 60°C oven for 60 min to melt excess paraffin and promote stronger adherence to the slides. Sections are then deparaffinized, hydrated through graded ethanols, and blocked for endogenous peroxidase.

SPECIMEN PROCESSING FOR FROZEN-SECTION IHC

Optimal preservation of cellular antigens and tissue morphology occurs if tissue is frozen rapidly, in a relatively cryoprotected fashion, and ice crystal formation is prevented. Properly snap-frozen tissue can also be used for molecular genetic studies and for mRNA extraction and analysis. Since all fresh tissue should be considered infectious, it should be handled with gloves in a biological hood with universal precautions. Specimens for freezing should first be trimmed of excess adipose and connective tissue and then divided with a scalpel or scissors into pieces that are no larger than 1.5 cm^2 in surface area and 0.5 cm in thickness. Prior to freezing, tissue specimens can be collected and transported in 4°C balanced salt solution or tissue culture medium such as minimal essential medium or RPMI 1640. Specimens in such liquid media must be handled and transported at 4°C to slow autolysis of the tissue and should be delivered to the laboratory for freezing within 1 h of surgical excision.

In preparation for freezing and storage, prepare all containers and slides (i.e., imprints) as needed with patient name, identification number, date, and tissue source. A 24-by-24-mm disposable base mold (Allegiance Healthcare Corporation, McGaw Park, Ill.) can be used for actual tissue freezing, and PolyCons (4-cm diameter by 1.5-cm height; Madan Plastics, Inc., Cranford, N.J.) can be used for storage of frozen specimens. Rapid freezing is accomplished by immersion of the specimen in an isopentane (2-methylbutane) bath that has

been precooled with either liquid nitrogen (−135 to −140°C) or dry ice (−30°C). Alternatively (and more conveniently), a refrigerated (lowest temperature, −52°C) quick-freezing tissue bath (Histobath; Shandon, Inc., Pittsburgh, Pa.) containing isopentane can be used and is designed for constant operation.

Prior to freezing, blot the tissue on a fresh absorbent towel (do not use gauze) to remove excessive liquid medium. Dispense a small amount of Tissue-Tek optimal cutting temperature (OCT) compound (Sakura Finetek U.S.A., Inc., Torrance, Calif.) into the bottom of a disposable base mold, place the tissue in the OCT layer, and then cover the entire specimen with OCT compound until the base mold's lower chamber has been completely filled. Grasp the edge of the base mold with a surgical clamp or forceps, and slowly submerge the base mold into precooled isopentane until it is completely immersed. Allow to freeze for 20 to 30 s and remove from the isopentane bath, then pop the frozen OCT compound-tissue block out of the base mold by using a twisting action at the ends of the base mold. Excess freezing compound can be trimmed away with a scalpel or single-edged razor blade. The frozen OCT compound-tissue block can then be placed into a labeled PolyCon for storage in a −70 to −80°C ultracold freezer until sectioned.

Cut frozen sections on a cryostat at a thickness of 4 to 5 μm and place on appropriately labeled charged (silanized) slides. Dry the sections in a 37°C oven for 15 min and then place in 4°C high-performance liquid chromatography-grade acetone (in a refrigerator or cooler) for 10 min. Remove slides from the acetone and fan dry for 10 min. If immunostaining is not to be performed immediately, the dried sections can be placed in a storage box and kept at room temperature in an electronic desiccator for up to 7 days. If longer storage of sections is required, the slides should be tightly wrapped in aluminum foil and stored at −70 to −80°C. When ready for staining, slides that have been stored in the freezer must be allowed to come to room temperature BEFORE they are unwrapped. Equilibration to room temperature prior to unwrapping prevents condensation from accumulating or freezing on the section, either of which can compromise morphology and immunoreactivity.

Immediately before immunostaining, sections are fixed in a freshly prepared 1% paraformaldehyde–PBS solution for 10 min. This fixative solution is prepared from a stock 10% solution of paraformaldehyde. Proper preparation of the 10% paraformaldehyde solution is critical and should be performed as detailed in Table 1.

A 1% paraformaldehyde solution is made by dilution of the 10% stock with PBS. All sections for immunostaining, EXCEPT those that are to be stained for κ and λ light chains, are fixed for 10 min at room temperature in the 1% paraformaldehyde solution. Slides are then rinsed in several changes of tap water and placed in a Tris-buffered saline solution for 5 min. Sections that are to be immunostained for κ and λ light chains are fixed a second time in 4°C acetone for 5 min, air dried with a fan for 10 min, and hydrated for 1.5 min in PBS. Sections are then fixed in 1% paraformaldehyde for **1 min**, rinsed in tap water, and placed in Tris-buffered saline for 5 min. The shorter fixation time for slides destined to be immunostained for κ and λ light chains is necessary for optimal detection of cell surface-associated immunoglobin. Both manual and automated IHC can be performed with frozen sections, but the buffers that are used must contain only a minimal amount (0.025%) of nonionic detergent (e.g., Tween 20) in order to maintain nuclear and cellular detail.

TABLE 1 Protocol for preparation of 10% paraformaldehyde stock solution[a]

1. Weigh out 100 g of paraformaldehyde powder into a 2-liter beaker.
2. Add 800 ml of distilled water to the beaker.
3. Place the beaker on a hot plate or stirrer. Slowly heat to 58°C (about 30 min), stirring constantly. Heat for 15 min at 58°C. DO NOT OVERHEAT.
4. Add **2 to 5 drops of 5N NaOH.** The solution will clear. Let cool for 30 min.
5. Pour the solution into a graduated cylinder. Add distilled water to 1 liter. Mix by inversion three times.
6. Filter the solution into a dark reagent bottle. This solution is good for 1 month at room temperature.

[a] This entire procedure should be done in a fume hood.

HEAT-INDUCED EPITOPE AND ANTIGEN RETRIEVAL TECHNIQUES

The most significant advance in the field of IHC in the past decade is perhaps the development and refinement of heat-induced epitope retrieval, also referred to as antigen retrieval. In the first application of antigen retrieval to tissue sections in 1991, Shi et al. (30) showed that the sensitivity of immunohistochemical staining could be increased by high-temperature heating of sections in a heavy-metal solution by using a microwave. Since that initial report, a variety of different retrieval solutions and sources have been used to enhance the immunoreactivity of formalin-fixed paraffin sections. Excellent reviews and reports have been published on this subject in the past 5 years (7, 11, 18, 27, 28, 35), and readers are referred to these for comprehensive discussions regarding the different permutations of this important technique.

Analogous to formaldehyde fixation, the mechanism for heat-induced antigen retrieval is also not completely established. A high temperature (100°C) is necessary for epitope unmasking and reportedly may work by disrupting of protein-protein cross-links (30, 34, 42) and/or cross-links involving calcium ions (20), increasing tissue permeability, and unfolding or refolding protein antigens (6, 19). The source of heating does not appear to be critical as successful results have been obtained with microwave ovens, water baths, autoclaves, pressure cookers, and vegetable steamers (35). What does appear to be important is the maximum temperature achieved and the length of time sections are exposed to that temperature. In general, exposure of sections to 100°C for a minimum of 20 min is recommended and will produce adequate immunohistochemical staining for most antibodies. Surprisingly, this treatment does not significantly change tissue morphology but can cause a decrease in the intensity of hematoxylin staining of nuclei (18). A protocol for heat-induced antigen retrieval using a vegetable steamer is presented in Table 2.

A variety of antigen retrieval solutions have been used successfully, and include citrate buffer at pH 3 to 6, Tris-HCl at pH 8 to 10 (with or without urea), and EDTA solutions at pH 8 to 9 (21, 27-29). For most antibodies, the staining intensity changes little over a pH range of 2 to 10, and therefore, 10 mM citrate buffer, pH 6.0, or 100 mM Tris-HCl, pH 8, is commonly used. In our experience, antigen retrieval in 1 mM EDTA, pH 8.0, produces superior staining of most nuclear antigens, including ER, progesterone receptor, p53, MIB-1, TdT, MLH-1, MSH-2, and MSH-6. Others have reported similar findings for a variety of cytoplasmic antigens (23). However, EDTA solutions also tend to cause increased cytoplasmic background staining in some tissues, especially liver, kidney, and adrenal cortex, presumably due to retrieved endogenous biotin (5). This increased staining can be eliminated by a biotin blocking step.

EVALUATION OF PRIMARY ANTIBODIES

Frequently, different antibodies from several different sources are available for use against a particular antigen, and selection of a particular antibody clone should be an informed choice. Often there are assessments in the literature that can provide guidance in this decision. As an example, comparison of different antibodies against p53 in fixed tissues has demonstrated differences in reactivities that impact the prognostic significance of p53 expression in breast cancer (12), with the pAb1801 and DO7 antibodies reported to be more effective than others tested. A comprehensive review of differences in reactivities of antibody clones with particular antigens is beyond the scope of this chapter. However, it is critical that the user be familiar with the recent literature regarding specific antibodies in order to avoid, or at least be informed of, potential problems specific to an individual clone.

Most antibodies used in a clinical IHC laboratory are commercially available and have well-characterized specificities. For analyte-specific reagents, it is assumed that good manufacturing practices have been followed and that the antibody will likely perform as advertised. Usually, prior peer-reviewed literature also exists and can be used to acquire a realistic review of the performance of the antibody in a particular diagnostic setting. This information will provide the user with a good foundation from which to start antibody dilutions and antigen retrieval methods. The manufacturer's technical service representatives can also be contacted for this information, but details on diagnostic utility will not be available. Many vendors now offer their analyte-specific reagent antibodies as prediluted reagents optimized for immunohistochemical staining. The use of prediluted reagents is becoming a common practice and can limit the flexibility when the stain is being established in a particular laboratory. One concern related to the antibody is that it may be diluted so that it works on optimally fixed tissues in the manufacturer's own immunostaining system but it may be too diluted for cases in which suboptimally processed tissue is evaluated or a less-sensitive detection system is used. Whenever possible, undiluted primary antibody is preferable.

The immunohistochemist should also note whether the antibody is polyclonal versus monoclonal and pay attention to the species and isotype of the primary antibody. Polyclonal antibodies have high-affinity clones within them, allowing for substantial dilution (often greater than 1:1,000), but also can have problems with increased background, requiring extra blocking steps. Knowing the species and isotype will prevent problems in which an inappropriate suboptimal secondary antibody is used. An example in which the isotype makes a difference is the LeuM1 clone (anti-CD15), an immunoglobulin M mouse monoclonal antibody that has been shown to have superior performance when anti-immunoglobulin M is used as the secondary antibody.

TABLE 2 Protocol for steam heat-induced antigen retrieval

1. Sections are mounted on charged slides, deparaffinized, hydrated through graded alcohols, and blocked for endogenous peroxidase activity.
2. Ten to fifteen minutes prior to the completion of step 1, the lower chamber of a Black & Decker Handy Steamer Plus is filled with 1,000 ml of distilled water. A reagent reservoir containing 200 ml of 10 mM sodium citrate, pH 6.0, or 1 mM EDTA, pH 8.0, is placed in the upper chamber of the steamer, and the timer is turned to the maximum time setting.
3. After the distilled water in the lower chamber has reached a full boil (usually 10 to 15 min), carefully open the steamer cover by holding it with both hands, rotating it clockwise one-quarter turn and draining, and then pulling back slowly away from the steamer.
4. Place the slides into the hot antigen retrieval solution and cover the steam chamber.
5. Steam slides for 30 min without opening the steamer cover. Time the steaming period with an independent lab timer (the timer on the steamer is inaccurate).
6. Open the steamer cover by holding it with both hands, rotating it clockwise one-quarter turn and draining, and then pulling back slowly away from the steamer.
7. Remove the reagent reservoir containing slides and place the reservoir with slides on the counter. Allow to stand for 5 min.
8. Rinse slides in cool running tap water for 1 min or long enough to thoroughly rinse slides free of retrieval solution.
9. Begin the immunohistochemical staining protocol.

CONTROL TISSUES

Selection of appropriate positive and negative control tissues is critical for evaluation and validation of immunohistochemical stains. The lack of standardized tissue makes it important for the immunohistochemist to select specimens that reflect the intended diagnostic use of the antibody and also the different fixation and processing conditions that are used in the laboratory. This point is made abundantly clear to us on a daily basis. The Cleveland Clinic, Cleveland, Ohio, uses Hollande's fixative and Mayo Clinic, Rochester, Minn., uses B-5 fixative for lymphoid tissues and bone marrow core biopsy specimens due to the excellent detailing of nuclear morphology that these fixatives produce. However, problems can arise when IHC is attempted with these tissues and the staining protocols have been optimized for formalin-fixed tissues. Therefore, we must also procure positive and negative control tissues fixed in Hollande's or B-5, as well as tissue fixed in neutrally buffered formalin. Positive control tissue is easy to obtain if the target antigen is present in normal tissues but can be difficult to find when the antigen is expressed only in certain tumors. An example of the latter case is the anaplastic lymphoma kinase protein recognized by anaplastic lymphoma kinase 1. This antigen is present in only a percentage of anaplastic large-cell lymphomas (9), and therefore a laboratory may be obligated to obtain control material from other accredited laboratories or to use cell lines known to overexpress the protein in order to establish conditions for diagnostic use (detection of anaplastic large-cell lymphoma).

OPTIMIZING CONDITIONS FOR IMMUNOREACTIVITY

Numerous factors can be manipulated and adjusted in order to optimize immunohistochemical staining. Some of the most commonly altered variables are antibody dilution, duration of primary antibody incubation, choice and concentration of secondary reagent, antigen retrieval buffer, incubation temperature, choice of detection system, and addition of amplification steps. Checkerboard approaches to optimizing staining have been advocated in which each variable is systematically altered while all other variables remain constant (28). However, the large number of variables just listed would require an unrealistic number of slides to be stained and evaluated. Since most automated stainers have limited temperature control and have optimized secondary reagents and detection chemistries, the immunohistochemist is left

primarily with adjustments of antibody dilution, primary incubation time, and antigen retrieval method. These limitations dramatically decrease the number of test slides required to evaluate a particular antibody.

In general, the lower the dilution, the more intense the staining for a given incubation time. However, use of highly concentrated antibodies may result in a prozone effect, causing a decreased intensity of staining. Nonspecific staining can also become a problem at higher concentrations of primary antibody. Longer incubation times (1 h to overnight) may permit greater dilutions of primary antibodies. However, since some automated stainers operate in a batch mode, the adjustments that can be made to incubation times may be limited (<30 min). If prolonged incubations are required, they are best performed "off-line."

As discussed previously, the most significant advance in IHC in the last 10 years is the development of heat-induced antigen retrieval (27, 30). Antigen retrieval enables antibodies that might previously have performed only in frozen tissues to be reactive in fixed tissues and has greatly expanded the number of antibodies that can now be applied to paraffin-embedded tissue (8). The increase in sensitivity afforded by antigen retrieval also can result in cost savings for the laboratory since higher dilutions of primary antibody may be used and more tests per vial can be performed with this technique than with previous methods. Most antibodies demonstrate an increase in staining intensity when antigen retrieval is used. However, some antibodies may perform better in acidic citrate-based buffers and many perform better in alkaline EDTA-based buffers (21). Further, some antibodies such as Epstein-Barr Virus latent membrane protein 1 and CD21 perform best with the use of enzyme digestion as the method of antigen retrieval. There appears to be no way to predict the behavior of a particular antibody, and conditions must be determined empirically. Several studies have looked at a fairly broad range of antibodies and can serve as a guide to the immunohistochemist (6, 8, 21, 40).

Increased sensitivity for detecting antigens can also be associated with increased detection of false-positive signals due to nonspecific staining. In particular, endogenous biotin or biotin-binding activity can be retrieved, causing false-positive granular cytoplasmic reactions (5). An example was the erroneous report of inhibin staining in hepatocellular carcinomas that was subsequently demonstrated to be due to endogenous biotin (13, 17). Biotin or biotin-binding activity can be eliminated by a blocking step consisting of the application of free avidin after that of primary antibody followed by the application of free biotin (5, 42). Blocking kits are available from several commercial vendors, including Dako Corporation (Carpenteria, Calif.) and Vector Laboratories (Burlingame, Calif.). Other potential causes of false-positive staining include endogenous peroxidase activity in horseradish peroxidase-based systems and endogenous phosphatase in alkaline phosphatase-based systems. Both activities can be minimized by blocking steps with hydrogen peroxide and levamisole, respectively (16, 22).

DETECTION SYSTEMS

Numerous methods are presently available for detecting bound primary antibodies. Most are enzyme-based techniques using either horseradish peroxidase or alkaline phosphatase, but peroxidase methods appear to be favored for most automated immunostainers in clinical laboratories. Examples include the peroxidase-antiperoxidase (PAP) method, the enzyme-labeled streptavidin-biotin (LSAB) technique, and the avidin-biotin complex (ABC) method. These are three-layer techniques involving a primary antibody, an appropriately specific secondary antibody, and the enzyme-containing tertiary reagent. In the case of the PAP method, the secondary antibody is unlabeled and added in excess so that it binds both the primary antibody and the soluble enzyme-antibody (PAP) complex that comprises the third layer. The antibody species in the PAP complex must therefore be the same as the primary antibody. For the LSAB and ABC techniques, the secondary antibody is covalently conjugated with biotin (biotinylated) and must recognize and bind only the primary antibody. The third layer of LSAB or ABC then binds tightly to the biotin.

The long-established indirect method uses secondary antibodies directly conjugated with peroxidase or alkaline phosphatase to bind primary antibody. This two-step method is simple and quick but also considerably less sensitive than the three-step detection systems described above. More recently, secondary antibodies conjugated to a dextran polymer backbone containing a large number of enzyme molecules (~100) have become commercially available (EnVision Systems; Dako Corporation). This new generation of secondary antibody conjugates permit two-step techniques that have sensitivities approaching those of the three-layer methods (26). The system is biotin free and therefore does not display nonspecific staining associated with biotin-binding proteins or endogenous biotin.

Newer catalyzed signal amplification or catalyzed reporter deposition techniques generate extreme sensitivity to which most users are not accustomed (15). Typically, these are five-step, peroxidase-based procedures that involve (i) application of primary antibody, (ii) application of a biotinylated secondary antibody, (iii) application of ABC-peroxidase, (iv) application of biotinyl tyramide and hydrogen peroxide (H_2O_2), and (v) application of peroxidase-labeled streptavidin. In the presence of the free radicals generated by ABC-peroxidase and H_2O_2, the biotinyl tyramide is activated and covalently attaches to locally available free amino groups. The reaction essentially results in a biotin "lawn" in the vicinity of the antigen and primary antibody. Peroxidase-labeled streptavidin binds to the numerous attached biotin molecules, and the slide is then routinely developed with chromogen and H_2O_2. A drawback to this methodology relative to other techniques is the additional time required for multiple incubation steps and the higher level of nonspecific staining that may accompany the dramatic increase in sensitivity.

Chromogen selection is also important. Peroxidase systems generally use 3,3'-diaminobenzidine (DAB; brown) or 3-amino-9-ethylcarbazole (AEC; red) chromogens. For alkaline phosphatase systems, BCIP (5-bromo-4-chloro-3-indolylphosphate)-nitroblue tetrazolium may be used to yield a blue-purple product or fast red–naphthol AS-TR phosphate may be used to produce a red-pink product. Choice may be influenced by personal preference (red versus blue versus brown), contrast with the counterstain (hematoxylin versus methyl green), incubation time (peroxidase-DAB reacts faster, allowing for a shorter incubation time, than phosphatase-fast red), sensitivity, safety issues (DAB is a carcinogen), and technical issues (AEC is soluble in organic solvents and cannot be used with xylene-based permanent mounting medium). DAB is a reliable chromogen that produces crisp, well-localized reactions that are permanent. At Mayo Clinic, DAB is used for nuclear antigens in paraffin sections and for all antigens in frozen-section immunostains related to lymphoma phenotyping. AEC (red) has traditionally been the chromogen of choice at Mayo Clinic for membrane and cytoplasmic antigens in paraffin sections because of the excellent color contrast with a light hematoxylin counterstain. A drawback to the use of AEC, however, is the solubility of AEC in organic solvents and the requirement for aqueous mounting media.

Techniques for performing double and triple immunoenzyme staining on tissue specimens can also be useful for the simultaneous visualization of two or more different antigens in paraffin-embedded or frozen tissue. Two or more different chromogen substrates are used to detect multiple cellular epitopes present in a tissue specimen. This technique can be particularly useful in applications involving quantitative analysis, for example, comparing the ratio of two cell populations in tissues (39), determining the spatial or morphometric relationships of disparate cell lines in tissue, and confirming the presence of coexpression of certain antigens within a single cell population. The details of the procedures and protocols for multiple immunoenzyme staining techniques are available from other sources (36–38).

SUMMARY

In this chapter, we have focused on present methods of IHC that are essential to the generation of quality stains. We have also discussed recent advances that have improved the sensitivity and versatility for paraffin section immunostains. Chief among these is the incorporation of antigen retrieval techniques into the daily practice of the IHC laboratory. With the increasing utilization of automated immunostainers, a moderate amount of standardization is now possible, both within an individual laboratory and among laboratories using similar reagents and equipment. Encouraging data are emerging from the United Kingdom's national external quality assessment scheme for immunocytochemistry (23). Using fixed breast tumors from multiple different laboratories, we found that in a central laboratory, routine procedures could be 90 to 100% efficient at demonstrating ER expression. The assay made use of the anti-ER 1D5 clone with pressure cooker antigen retrieval. Thus, variations in tissue processing at different laboratories did not seem to be a limiting factor in accurately determining ER statuses of breast cancers. In a companion study (24), there was good concordance among different laboratories when tumors expressed high or moderate levels of ER. Most participating laboratories used either the 1D5 or 6F11 clones with heat-induced antigen retrieval. However, there was still considerable interlaboratory variation for tumors that expressed low levels of ER, with significant false-negative rates (30 to 60%). Ultimately, the performance of a particular immunostain is the responsibility of the medical director of the laboratory. National proficiency testing programs such as those conducted by the CAP can be helpful with issues related to standardization of staining procedures (including specimen processing, antigen retrieval, detection systems, and antibody selection) and interpretation.

REFERENCES

1. **Anonymous.** 1998. Medical devices: classification/reclassification of immunohistochemistry reagents and kits—FDA. Final rule. *Fed. Regist.* **63:**30132–30142.
2. **Battifora, H.** 1991. Assessment of antigen damage in immunohistochemistry. The vimentin internal control. *Am. J. Clin. Pathol.* **96:**669–671.
3. **Battifora, H., and M. Kopinski.** 1986. The influence of protease digestion and duration of fixation on the immunostaining of keratins. A comparison of formalin and ethanol fixation. *J. Histochem. Cytochem.* **34:**1095–1100.
4. **Bostwick, D. G., N. al Annouf, and C. Choi.** 1994. Establishment of the formalin-free surgical pathology laboratory. Utility of an alcohol-based fixative. *Arch. Pathol. Lab. Med.* **118:**298–302.
5. **Bussolati, G., P. Gugliotta, M. Volante, M. Pace, and M. Papotti.** 1997. Retrieved endogenous biotin: a novel marker and a potential pitfall in diagnostic immunohistochemistry. *Histopathology* **31:**400–407.
6. **Cattoretti, G., S. Pileri, C. Parravicini, M. H. Becker, S. Poggi, C. Bifulco, G. Key, L. D'Amato, E. Sabattini, E. Feudale, et al.** 1993. Antigen unmasking on formalin-fixed, paraffin-embedded tissue sections. *J. Pathol.* **171:**83–98.
7. **Chan, J. K.** 2000. Advances in immunohistochemistry: impact on surgical pathology practice. *Semin. Diagn. Pathol.* **17:**170–177.
8. **Cuevas, E. C., A. C. Bateman, B. S. Wilkins, P. A. Johnson, J. H. Williams, A. H. Lee, D. B. Jones, and D. H. Wright.** 1994. Microwave antigen retrieval in immunocytochemistry: a study of 80 antibodies. *J. Clin. Pathol.* **47:**448–452.
9. **Falini, B., S. Pileri, P. L. Zinzani, A. Carbone, V. Zagonel, C. Wolf-Peeters, G. Verhoef, F. Menestrina, G. Todeschini, M. Paulli, M. Lazzarino, R. Giardini, A. Aiello, H. D. Foss, I. Araujo, M. Fizzotti, P. G. Pelicci, L. Flenghi, M. F. Martelli, and A. Santucci.** 1999. ALK+ lymphoma: clinico-pathological findings and outcome. *Blood* **93:**2697–2706.
10. **Fox, C. H., F. B. Johnson, J. Whiting, and P. P. Roller.** 1985. Formaldehyde fixation. *J. Histochem. Cytochem.* **33:**845–853.
11. **Gown, A. M.** 2004. Unmasking the mysteries of antigen or epitope retrieval and formalin fixation. *Am. J. Clin. Pathol.* **121:**172–174.
12. **Horne, G. M., J. J. Anderson, D. G. Tiniakos, G. G. McIntosh, M. D. Thomas, B. Angus, J. A. Henry, T. W. Lennard, and C. H. Horne.** 1996. p53 protein as a prognostic indicator in breast carcinoma: a comparison of four antibodies for immunohistochemistry *Br. J. Cancer* **73:**29–35.
13. **Iezzoni, J. C., S. E. Mills, T. J. Pelkey, and M. H. Stoler.** 1999. Inhibin is not an immunohistochemical marker for hepatocellular carcinoma. An example of the potential pitfall in diagnostic immunohistochemistry caused by endogenous biotin. *Am. J. Clin. Pathol.* **111:**229–234.
14. **Jacobs, T. W., J. E. Prioleau, I. E. Stillman, and S. J. Schnitt.** 1996. Loss of tumor marker-immunostaining intensity on stored paraffin slides of breast cancer. *J. Natl. Cancer Inst.* **88:**1054–1059.
15. **King, G., S. Payne, F. Walker, and G. I. Murray.** 1997. A highly sensitive detection method for immunohistochemistry using biotinylated tyramine. *J. Pathol.* **183:**237–241.
16. **Li, C. Y., S. C. Ziesmer, and O. Lazcano-Villareal.** 1987. Use of azide and hydrogen peroxide as an inhibitor for endogenous peroxidase in the immunoperoxidase method. *J. Histochem. Cytochem.* **35:**1457–1460.
17. **McCluggage, W. G., P. Maxwell, A. Patterson, and J. M. Sloan.** 1997. Immunohistochemical staining of hepatocellular carcinoma with monoclonal antibody against inhibin. *Histopathology* **30:**518–522.
18. **McNicol, A. M., and J. A. Richmond.** 1997. Optimizing immunohistochemistry: antigen retrieval and signal amplification. *J. Histochem. Cytochem.* **45:**327–343.
19. **Montero, C., E. Chi-Ahumada, S. Chavez-Porras, and M. Gutierrez.** 2000. Application of the critical molar concentration concept to heat-mediated antigen retrieval in immunohistochemistry. *Histochem. J.* **32:**111–114.
20. **Morgan, J. M., H. Navabi, K. W. Schmid, and B. Jasani.** 1994. Possible role of tissue-bound calcium ions in citrate-mediated high-temperature antigen retrieval. *J. Pathol.* **174:**301–307.
21. **Pileri, S. A., G. Roncador, C. Ceccarelli, M. Piccioli, A. Briskomatis, E. Sabattini, S. Ascani, D. Santini, P. P. Piccaluga, O. Leone, S. Damiani, C. Ercolessi, F. Sandri, F. Pieri, L. Leoncini, and B. Falini.** 1997. Antigen retrieval techniques in immunohistochemistry: comparison of different methods. *J. Pathol.* **183:**116–123.
22. **Ponder, B. A., and M. M. Wilkinson.** 1981. Inhibition of endogenous tissue alkaline phosphatase with the use of alkaline phosphatase conjugates in immunohistochemistry. *J. Histochem. Cytochem.* **29:**981–984.
23. **Rhodes, A., B. Jasani, A. J. Balaton, and K. D. Miller.** 2000. Immunohistochemical demonstration of oestrogen and progesterone receptors: correlation of standards achieved on in house tumours with that achieved on external quality assessment material in over 150 laboratories from 26 countries. *J. Clin. Pathol.* **53:**292–301.
24. **Rhodes, A., B. Jasani, D. M. Barnes, L. G. Bobrow, and K. D. Miller.** 2000. Reliability of immunohistochemical demonstration of oestrogen receptors in routine practice: interlaboratory variance in the sensitivity of detection and evaluation of scoring systems. *J. Clin. Pathol.* **53:**125–130.
25. **Roche, P. C.** 1998. Antigen stability in stored paraffin sections. *CAP Today* **12:**59–61.
26. **Sabattini, E., K. Bisgaard, S. Ascani, S. Poggi, M. Piccioli, C. Ceccarelli, F. Pieri, G. Fraternali-Orcioni, and S. A. Pileri.** 1998. The EnVision++ system: a new immunohistochemical method for diagnostics and research. Critical comparison with the APAAP, ChemMate, CSA, LABC, and SABC techniques. *J. Clin. Pathol.* **51:**506–511.
27. **Shi, S. R., R. J. Cote, and C. R. Taylor.** 1996. Antigen retrieval immunohistochemistry: past, present, and future. *Biotech. Histochem.* **71:**190–196.
28. **Shi, S. R., R. J. Cote, C. Yang, C. Chen, H. J. Xu, W. F. Benedict, and C. R. Taylor.** 1997. Development of an optimal protocol for antigen retrieval: a "test battery" approach exemplified with reference to the staining of retinoblastoma protein (pRB) in formalin-fixed paraffin sections. *Histopathology* **31:**400–407.
29. **Shi, S. R., R. J. Cote, L. Young, S. A. Imam, and C. R. Taylor.** 1999. Use of pH 9.5 Tris-HCl buffer containing 5% urea for antigen retrieval immunohistochemistry. *Am. J. Clin. Pathol.* **111:**445–448.
30. **Shi, S. R., M. E. Key, and K. L. Kalra.** 1991. Antigen retrieval in formalin-fixed, paraffin-embedded tissues: an enhancement method for immunohistochemical staining based on microwave oven heating of tissue sections. *J. Histochem. Cytochem.* **39:**741–748.

31. **Swanson, P. E.** 1999. Labels, disclaimers, and rules (oh, my!). Analyte-specific reagents and practice of immunohistochemistry. *Am. J. Clin. Pathol.* **111:**445–448.

32. **Taylor, C. R.** 1999. FDA issues final rule for classification and reclassification of immunochemistry reagents and kits. *Am. J. Clin. Pathol.* **111:**443–444.

33. **Taylor, C. R.** 1998. Report from the Biological Stain Commission: FDA issues final rule for classification/reclassification of immunochemistry (IHC) reagents and kits. *Biotech. Histochem.* **73:**175–177.

34. **Taylor, C. R., and S. R. Shi.** 1997. Immunohistochemistry: principles and practice, p. 369–379. *In* N. R. Rose, E. Conway de Macario, J. D. Folds, H. C. Lane, and R. M. Nakamura (ed.), *Manual of Clinical Laboratory Immunology*, 5th ed. ASM Press, Washington, D.C.

35. **Taylor, C. R., S. R. Shi, C. Chen, L. Young, C. Yang, and R. J. Cote.** 1996. Comparative study of antigen retrieval heating methods: microwave, microwave and pressure cooker, autoclave, and steamer. *Histochem. Cell Biol.* **105:**253–260.

36. **Van der Loos, C. M.** 1999. *Immunoenzyme Multiple Staining Methods*. Bios Scientific Publishers Limited, Oxford, United Kingdom.

37. **Van der Loos, C. M., J. van den Oord, P. K. Das, and H. J. Houthoff.** 1988. Use of commercially available monoclonal antibodies for immunoenzyme double staining. *Histochem. J.* **20:**409–413.

38. **Van der Loos, C. M., A. E. Becker, and J. J. van den Oord.** 1993. Practical suggestions for successful immunoenzyme double staining experiments. *Histochem. J.* **25:**1–13.

39. **Van der Loos, C. M., M. M. Marijianowski, and A. E. Becker.** 1994. Quantification in immunohistochemistry: the measurement of the ratios of collagen types I and II. *Histochem. J.* **26:**347–354.

40. **von Wasielewski, R., M. Werner, M. Nolte, L. Wilkens, and A. Georgii.** 1994. Effects of antigen retrieval by microwave heating in formalin-fixed tissue sections on a broad panel of antibodies. *Histochemistry* **102:**165–172.

41. **Werner, M., R. Von Wasielewski, and P. Komminoth.** 1996. Antigen retrieval, signal amplification and intensification in immunohistochemistry. *Histochem. Cell Biol.* **105:**253–260.

42. **Wood, G. S., and R. Warnke.** 1981. Suppression of endogenous avidin-binding activity in tissues and its relevance to biotin-avidin detection systems. *J. Histochem. Cytochem.* **29:**1196–1204.

Use of Molecular Biology Methods on Tissues

SUMAN SETTY, CHUNG-CHE (JEFF) CHANG,
AND ANDRÉ A. KAJDACSY-BALLA

46

Molecular diagnostic techniques have become important tools in pathology over the last decade, and giant strides are expected to continue to occur during the next few years as well. Tumors that appear to be very similar by light microscopy and immunohistochemistry analyses can still have very divergent outcomes and responses to therapy. The burgeoning field of molecular biomarkers has helped differentiate malignancies that need more aggressive or more specific therapy. Pathology has finally arrived at a point where the first tumor-specific molecular therapeutic targets have been identified. This chapter does not cover the details of most of these methods, but it will provide an overview of several examples of molecular biology applications in this rapidly advancing field.

Not all present biomarkers can be detected in tissues that are routinely available in pathology laboratories. There is an ongoing effort to adapt techniques that work well with fresh, unfixed tissues to specimens such as formalin-fixed paraffin-embedded needle biopsy material and cytology smear material. Fluorescent in situ hybridization (FISH) is an example of a test that has been successfully used in the clinical laboratory.

Today, most leukemias and lymphomas are characterized by specific chromosomal translocations or chromosomal lesions (Table 1). Molecular methodologies such as Southern blotting, PCR, FISH, reverse transcription PCR (RT-PCR) including real-time PCR, and molecular arrays have been applied to detect genetic lesions and to aid in the detection, determination of prognoses, and classification of malignancies. FISH and RT-PCR are particularly good for the detection of chromosomal lesions with widely dispersed breakpoints within large introns (3). For example, t(2;5) and t(9;22) translocations of chromosomes are found in anaplastic large-cell lymphoma and chronic myelogenous leukemia, respectively.

Additionally, molecular diagnostic techniques facilitate the detection and determination of prognoses of solid tumors. For example, detection of the t(X;18) translocation facilitates the diagnosis of synovial sarcoma. FISH for *HER-2/neu* gene amplification in breast carcinoma facilitates therapeutic decision making. In recent times, the thrust has been towards detecting markers of genetic susceptibility function by detecting polymorphisms associated with disease predisposition. For example, genetic polymorphism in the cytochrome P-450 gene CYP1A can explain higher-than-average individual ability to metabolize procarcinogens in cigarette smoke, leading to a greater risk of carcinoma.

About a quarter of patients with mammary carcinoma have up-regulated expression of the HER-2/neu gene and protein (20). Semiquantitation by immunohistochemistry detects a large percentage of these cases. However, a small fraction of the results of protein studies fall into the equivocal category and require in situ hybridization (ISH) studies to detect amplification when present. ISH assays can be performed on archival paraffin-embedded tissues (17, 23). ISH is a morphologic approach to genetic testing in which a fluorochrome (FISH)- or chromogen (chromogenic ISH [CISH])-tagged DNA probe is hybridized either to a metaphase or interphase preparation of chromosomes released from cells or to a tissue section. A fluorescent microscopic signal is obtained when the probe selectively attaches to the gene-specific complementary DNA. A second probe labeled with a different color attaches to the chromosome 17 centromere. The presence of only two signals for *HER-2/neu* per cell is indicative of an unamplified state. The presence of more than two signals argues for amplification. A control probe for chromosome 17 is used to rule out aneuploidy in the tumor by determining the ratio of the *HER-2/neu* to the chromosome 17 signals. The use of various fluorophores or chromogens on the same section facilitates the reading of the slides. For example, in breast cancer, two signals for chromosome 17 and five signals for *HER-2/neu* in the same cell are interpreted to indicate *HER-2/neu* amplification.

Additionally, ISH assays can detect deletions, amplifications, or duplications of chromosomal loci. ISH studies can also detect disease recurrence in cytological material and body fluids. For example, the Vysis Urovision test detects aneuploidy for chromosomes 3, 7, and 17 in urine specimens as an adjunct to detection of cytologic atypia that occurs in bladder cancer.

The CISH method using type-specific primers or pools of high-risk-associated and low-risk-associated primers for human papillomavirus (HPV) detects intracellular virus. CISH is commonly performed on residual material from liquid-based cervical Papanicolaou test material.

HPV-associated carcinomas of the head and neck, lung, and cervix have different mechanisms associated with carcinogenesis, but they may have a common feature, the presence of HPV DNA integrated into the host cell genome. The resulting up-regulation of viral E6 and E7 proteins leads to immortalization of the cells and resulting HPV-associated dysplasia or cancer (14). Detection of HPV in precursor

TABLE 1 Correlation of genetic lesions and immunohistochemical (IHC) markers

Type of lymphoma	Genetic lesion(s)	IHC marker(s)[a]	Reliability of IHC marker(s)
Mucous-associated lymphoid tissue lymphoma	t(1;14) (BCL10/IGH), t(11;18) (API2/MALT1)	BCL-10	Variable
Mantle cell lymphoma	t(11;14) (BCL1/IGH)	Cyclin D1 (Bcl-1)	Variable
Follicular lymphoma	t(14;18) (BCL2/IGH)	Bcl-2	Excellent
Burkitt's lymphoma	t(8;14) (c-MYC/IGH), variants	CD10$^+$ phenotype, MIB1 100%, Bcl-2$^-$ phenotype	Excellent
Anaplastic large-cell lymphoma	t(2;5) (ALK/NPM), variants	ALK (cytoplasmic and nuclear), ALK (only cytoplasmic)	Excellent

[a]ALK, anaplastic lymphoma kinase; MIB1, approaching 100% of neoplastic cells with nuclear graining of MIB1 (a polycation marker).

lesions is a screening tool for bringing women with a predisposition for cervical carcinoma to attention. The screening of cervical cytology (Papanicolaou smear) has led to early detection and treatment of squamous lesions (21). One of the clinical algorithms calls for DNA testing for the high-risk HPV types that are associated with a higher-than-average likelihood of development of carcinoma. The "gold standard" is the PCR-based assay using consensus-degenerate MY09-MY11 or GP5+-GP6+ primers followed by restriction digestion for typing of the HPV (19). The ISH method provides the pathologist with a visual tool to complete a cytological interpretation. A nonvisual method which uses RNA-DNA hybridization is commercially available (Digene Corp., Gaithersburg, Md.).

Molecular techniques are used for detecting the presence of and quantitating the sequences found in organisms responsible for predisposition to disease. They may also be used for predicting drug responses (pharmacogenomics), detecting carrier states and the presence of genetic conditions, tumor typing, determining prognoses, detecting tumors, and assessing tumor responses to drugs. PCR may be used for detection of *Mycobacterium tuberculosis* in tissues and quantitation of target molecules such as human immunodeficiency virus and hepatitis C virus DNA.

Ligase chain reaction and similar techniques are presently used for the detection of microorganisms in tissues by labeling the oligonucleotides with organism-specific sequences. This process can also be used for detection and quantitation of the expression of specific genes in tissues.

OTHER EXAMPLES OF MOLECULAR TESTING FOR HISTOLOGIC DIAGNOSIS

Detection of polymorphic genomic DNA with differences in restriction fragment lengths is the basis of the tests used by forensic laboratories and those used for the study of disease-causing mutations. This method may also be used for the identification of the tissue of origin of "floaters" in surgical pathology blocks. Floaters are small fragments of tissue that accidentally float from one specimen to another during gross tissue sectioning, processing, and slide preparation. Sometimes it becomes impossible to distinguish a floater from tissue that really belongs to the patient in question. Comparison of the patterns of DNA digestion with a panel of restriction enzymes reveals a distinctive pattern for the tissue in question. It is possible to determine whether the tissue in question belongs to the patient or to a different patient being studied in the same histology batch.

Mutation Analysis

Genetic mutations may be clinically silent or result in disease. Germ line mutations may be transmitted to offspring. Mutations in tumor suppressor genes have been likened to a car running on one flat tire. A second mutation results in the loss of function of both alleles, possibly resulting in unregulated growth.

Somatic mutations are of significance in the development of neoplasms via their impact on cell cycle, growth, and differentiation. Certain diseases are associated with a single known mutation, but others, such as cystic fibrosis, are associated with more than 100 mutations and therefore require comprehensive testing. The "gold standard" test would be DNA sequencing in such situations to detect all possible known mutations or new mutations. Cystic fibrosis transmembrane conductance regulator mutation analysis for carrier screening of a panel of 25 mutations is presently recommended by the American College of Medical Genetics (8). Recent studies have attempted the use of oral mucosa cytologic material for screening.

Hereditary and Familial Cancer Syndromes

Hereditary and familial cancer syndromes usually occur in a dominant manner but may also occur through multifactorial inheritance due to the inheritance of multiple low-frequency alleles. Mutations of breast cancer susceptibility genes *BRCA1* and *BRCA2* are identified in about 3% of breast cancer cases (16). Individuals with Li-Fraumeni syndrome (12) inherit one mutant *p53* allele and are therefore predisposed to malignancy, especially when a subsequent hit leads to inactivation of the other allele. They develop tumors at an earlier age than their counterparts without the mutant allele and may have multiple malignancies of the breast and brain, as well as sarcoma and leukemia.

Colorectal cancers can be characterized as those with or without underlying polyposis syndromes. The study of familial adenomatous polyposis has demonstrated the presence of adenomatous polyposis coli gene mutations in 5q21.

Therapeutic Target Detection

The study of molecular pathways of carcinogenesis has highlighted various molecules that are now therapeutic targets. A part of this approach is individualized study of tumor specimens. Clinical trial data on patient outcomes are often put together with protein expression data to determine the thresholds for labeling protein expression as positive or negative. An example of a therapeutic target is HER-2/neu, a member of the tyrosine kinase receptor family. Another example is epidermal growth factor receptor, also a member of the tyrosine kinase receptor family, which is expressed in colon carcinoma. Recent regimens of treatment of late-stage colon carcinoma with antibodies to epidermal growth factor receptor require immunohistochemical studies of tissue to detect the presence of tumor expression.

Gene Expression Profiling

The ability to test the expression of 1,000 to 40,000 genes simultaneously with microarray technology has significantly changed our approach to the analysis of tumors. Instead of comparing different tumors one gene at a time, advances in bioinformatics have made it possible to find out combinations of genes that characterize a specific tumor. This approach of gene profiling has been successfully used to reclassify tumors according to clusters of gene expression. For example, van de Vijver et al. (24) have found a gene expression "signature" that can serve as a predictor of survival of breast cancer patients much more reliably than histological morphology and individual immunohistochemistry staining. Recently, high-throughput genomic approaches such as gene expression profiling by cDNA microarray have shown promising results in detecting different prognostic groups of soft-tissue tumors. In a pilot study using cDNA microarray and cluster analysis, the gene expression profiles of different types of soft-tissue tumors correctly discriminated patients who survived from those who did not, with P values of less than 0.0001 (10). Notably, none of the existing prognostic factors, including histologic type and response to therapy, were as reliable for predicting the survival of these patients (10). Once gene expression signatures are discovered, there is always a need for subsequent validation. After this is accomplished, commercial companies prepare smaller gene arrays that have only the genes of interest (usually fewer than 100). These specific arrays can be used clinically to predict response to therapy and outcome. The main advantage of this approach is the ability to sort out which patients need additional therapy immediately after surgery and which ones do not. Avoiding excessive therapy for patients who are unlikely to have tumor recurrence would decrease the inconvenience and the side effects of unnecessary treatment.

Microdissection as a Preparative Method for Molecular Testing

It is easy to perform molecular testing with tissues that contain a very large percentage of the cell type of interest. For example, if one is interested in comparing heart muscle with skeletal muscle, there is only a small percentage of contaminating cells such as those of vessels and nerves and therefore there is no need to tease out muscle cells for study. On the other hand, if one is interested in comparing expression patterns of genes in type I and type II skeletal muscles, then a method to separate these cells before analysis becomes necessary. This is also true when one wants to separate stromal cells from epithelial cancer cells in preparation for comparison among different types of cancers. Methods used for obtaining relatively pure cell populations include flow cytometry, density gradient-based cell separation, and for tissues in histological sections, either blunt manual microdissection with an inverted microscope and a lancet or laser microdissection. Several commercial instruments for microdissection are available, and these are capable of isolating even one individual cell from a tissue section. These instruments usually have an inverted microscope, an infrared laser, a control unit for the laser, a controlled mechanical stage for the glass

slide, and a digital camera. The cells of interest are cut out of the tissue with the laser and collected in a flask for subsequent RNA, DNA, or protein extraction. One may need to apply nucleic acid amplification to these cells, depending on the number of cells collected and also on the final application. For more-detailed descriptions of methods of and caveats on microdissection, one may refer to several publications and comprehensive monographs on this subject (e.g., reference 15), as well as commercial instrument manuals.

TMAs

A relatively simple method of examining hundreds of tissue sections in one experiment is the use of tissue microarrays (TMAs) (9). TMA has brought histotechnology into the "omics," high-throughput style. Tens to hundreds of minute tissue cores from different patient samples (0.6 to 2.0 mm in diameter) are neatly arranged on each glass slide. For example, slides can be used for immunohistochemical studies and ISH. The advantages of this method are many. Reagents are less expensive, all experiments can be performed in one run, interassay variation is avoided, there is less depletion of paraffin-embedded tissues, tissues can be obtained from departments of pathology from multiple institutions, and the tissue blocks can be returned to the original hospital archives. Studies have shown that adequate sampling is not an issue, and TMAs may even improve sampling by avoiding interpretation bias. A whole section of a tumor may have a small focus of positivity for a marker while the random areas selected for TMA may all be negative. This result correlates better with overall tumor prognosis. However, there are also clear disadvantages of this method over conventional slide methods. These include the initial cost of a tissue microarrayer, the need for a solution to formidable bioinformatics issues that result from increasing the number of samples, and greater difficulty in correlating staining results with the original histological findings. Methods for constructing TMAs from needle biopsy material, cell cultures, and frozen samples have expanded the applications of this technology. These "tissue chips" have helped researchers to keep up with the volume of research data on possible markers generated by genomics and proteomics laboratories. Fulfilling of the promise of TMA is still in its first steps, as methods of high-speed automated quantitative analysis are slowly developed. Important issues to remember when starting to build TMAs are the learning curve associated with using the instrument, the rapid oxidation of antigenic sites when unstained slides are exposed to ambient air, and bioinformatics management of the annotated common data elements for each tissue core, etc. TMA technology is of limited utility in the diagnostic histology laboratory, and TMAs have been mostly used for immunohistochemical slide control samples and for preparation of multi-institutional quality assurance slides.

Detection of Lymphomas and Leukemias

The detection of acute lymphoid leukemias and lymphomas is done in part by determining the clonalities of neoplastic lymphocytes, i.e., rearrangement of immunoglobulin (Ig) heavy-chain and light-chain genes (B-cell clonality) and T-cell receptor (TCR) genes (T-cell clonality) (13). Southern blotting remains the "gold standard" for this type of determination. However, this method requires fresh or frozen tissues or cells, large amounts of DNA, and a long period of hands-on time and has become a second-line test. This method has 1 to 5% sensitivity (i.e., 1 to 5 neoplastic cells/100 nucleated cells can be detected). The most common target genes are those of the Ig heavy chain, the Ig κ light chain, and TCRβ. PCR-based methodologies with the advantage of using fresh, frozen, or formalin-fixed tissues or cells are faster and less labor-intensive and have become the first-line methods in clinical laboratories for clonality testing. PCR methods use consensus primers targeting highly conserved sequences of different J or V segments of Ig heavy-chain or TCR genes to amplify clonally rearranged Ig heavy-chain or TCR genes. The sensitivity is at 1 clonal B or T cell detected/100 B or T cells with the routine method and can be significantly increased by using clone-specific probes to the range of 1 clonal cell in 10,000 to 1 million normal cells. The major weakness of the PCR method is the tendency for false-negative results due to imperfect consensus primers. Therefore, negative results should be confirmed by Southern blotting whenever possible. The majority of lymphomas and leukemias can be further classified by their characteristic chromosomal lesions (2, 13). Some of these lesions can be detected by immunohistochemical markers as shown in Table 1.

The major limitation of clonality testing using the chromosomal lesions or Ig-TCR gene rearrangement is the false-positive rate. Pseudoclonality associated with Ig gene rearrangement has been seen in cases of small biopsy specimens with a paucity of lymphocytes, helicobacter pylori-induced gastritis, hepatitis C, human immunodeficiency virus infection and other viral infections, Sjögren's syndrome, and rheumatoid arthritis. Pseudoclonality associated with TCR gene rearrangement has been seen in cases of immune system reconstitution post-hematopoietic stem cell transplantation, immune response to tumors, and clonal dermatitis. Furthermore, most of the characteristic chromosomal translocations occurring in hematopoietic malignancies are also observed in healthy individuals when highly sensitive PCR-based assays are applied. Other important limitations include false-negative results due to sampling or technical issues and lineage infidelity (i.e., Ig heavy-chain rearrangement may occur in T-cell malignancies). Therefore, it is necessary to correlate molecular testing results with immunophenotyping results for accurate lineage determination.

Presently molecular diagnostic techniques are considered as second-line tools for clinical detection of hematopoietic malignancies due to the above-mentioned limitations. Morphology analysis and immunophenotyping remain the "gold standards" for diagnosis and classification. However, in difficult cases with inconclusive morphology and immunophenotyping results, molecular diagnostic techniques can be important for reaching an accurate diagnosis. Examples of ambiguous results include atypical reactive interfollicular infiltrate versus T-cell lymphoma (clonal TCR gene rearrangement analysis favoring the latter), follicular lymphoma with marginal zone (monocytoid) differentiation versus marginal zone lymphoma with follicular colonization (IgH-BCL2 translocation favoring the former), and atypical lymphoid infiltrate of gastric mucosa versus extranodal marginal zone B-cell lymphoma [t(11;18) translocation favoring the latter].

Besides being used for diagnostic applications, molecular diagnostic techniques can provide important prognostic information in cases of lymphomas and leukemias. For example, t(8;21), t(15;17), and inv(16) are associated with good prognosis, and t(9;22) is associated with poor prognosis in acute myeloid leukemia (2). The *FLT3* mutation has become the most common identifiable genetic abnormality in acute myeloid leukemia and an important poor-prognosis indicator (7). In acute lymphoid leukemia, t(12;21) is not detected by conventional cytogenetics, but with the use of FISH, RT-PCR, or Southern blotting, it is an important good-prognosis indicator while t(9;22) and mixed-lineage leukemia gene

rearrangement [t(4;11)] serve as poor-prognosis indicators (2). In B-cell chronic lymphocytic leukemia, patients with mutated IgH genes (correlating with a CD38⁻, Zap70⁻ phenotype) have better prognoses than those with IgH genes without mutations, correlating with CD38⁺ (>30% of neoplastic cells expressing CD38) and Zap70⁺ (>20% of neoplastic cells expressing Zap70) phenotypes, which have poor prognoses (18).

Detection of Soft Tissue Tumors

Similar to those associated with hematopoietic malignancies, most genetic abnormalities associated with soft-tissue tumors are chromosomal translocations resulting in novel fusion proteins (5). These fusion proteins often affect transcription factors, resulting in a disruption of transcription regulation. This disruption may lead to activation of inappropriate genes or inappropriate repression of some genes. The fusion genes can also serve as targets for the molecular detection of respective tumors and the development of targeted therapy.

Molecular diagnostic techniques, particularly RT-PCR and FISH, have become important tools to detect the characteristic fusion genes associated with soft-tissue tumors. These molecular techniques require only a minimal amount of tissue. This is particularly important when managing needle core biopsy specimens, which are becoming the most common type of specimens in the pathology laboratory. In the majority of cases, the evaluation of morphology and immunohistochemical studies may be sufficient for diagnosis. However, in difficult cases such as that of monophasic synovial sarcoma with a spindle-cell pattern, molecular genetics can be employed.

The specificity of fusion genes, although reasonably high, is not absolute. Thus, most authorities concur that conventional morphological assessment, supplemented by ancillary techniques including molecular studies, remains the standard diagnostic approach. A good example is that of *TPM3-ALK* and *CLTC-ALK* gene fusions, which have been recently identified in both inflammatory myofibroblastic tumors and anaplastic large-cell lymphomas.

In addition to their diagnostic applications, molecular studies may further provide important prognostic information for each specific soft-tissue tumor. Anderson et al. reported the translocation t(2;13)/*PAX3-FKHR* to be an adverse prognostic factor in alveolar rhabdomyosarcoma (1). In contrast, t(1;13)/*PAX7-FKHR* was associated with a favorable prognosis and was more frequently observed in younger patients with relatively localized disease (1). Sorensen et al. (22) reported that, among the patients with metastatic alveolar rhabdomyosarcoma, bone marrow involvement was significantly higher in *PAX3-FKHR*-positive patients (22).

PROGNOSTIC SIGNIFICANCE OF DETECTION AND QUANTITATION OF MINIMAL RESIDUAL DISEASE IN LEUKEMIAS, LYMPHOMAS, AND SOFT-TISSUE TUMORS

The sensitivity and specificity of the PCR and RT-PCR protocols have provided evidence for the existence of minimal disease which cannot be detected by physical, morphologic, or radiographic examination. Cumulative data have demonstrated that most patients still harbor a significant tumor burden after resection of tumors or establishment of complete clinical remission of leukemias (4). When patients with Ewing's sarcoma or primitive neuroectodermal tumors were studied using RT-PCR, about 50% of patients with metastatic or relapsed disease had blood or marrow samples positive for the *EWS–FLI-1* transcripts and approximately 25% of patients without clinically metastatic disease did so as well. Other RT-PCR methods to detect minimal alveolar rhabdomyosarcoma and synovial sarcoma disease and desmoplastic small round cell tumors have also been described (5). In patients with chronic myeloid leukemia, rising or persistently high levels of *BCR-ABL* (*BCR-ABL:ABL* ratio of >0.02% or >100 *BCR-ABL* transcripts/μg of RNA), determined by quantitative RT-PCR, in two sequential specimens obtained more than 4 months following stem cell transplantation are predictive of overt clinical relapse (11). Similarly, by using real-time quantitative PCR to quantify the amount of t(14;18)(q32;q21) cells, it was recently observed that a measurable tumor load of ≥0.01% after stem cell transplantation may predict subsequent relapse of follicular lymphoma (4). Furthermore, studies have shown that treating chronic myeloid leukemia patients before overt clinical relapse of disease can improve survival of such patients after stem cell transplantation (6). Quantification of minimal residual disease may lead to new therapeutic avenues to improve patient outcome. However, the clinical and therapeutic significance of minimal disease remains to be evaluated for most cancers.

REFERENCES

1. **Anderson, J., T. Gordon, A. McManus, T. Mapp, S. Gould, A. Kelsey, H. McDowell, R. Pinkerton, J. Shipley, K. Pritchard-Jones, U.K. Children's Cancer Study Group, and the U. K. Cancer Cytogenetics Group.** 2001. Detection of the PAX3-FKHR fusion gene in paediatric rhabdomyosarcoma: a reproducible predictor of outcome? *Br. J. Cancer* **85**:831–835.

2. **Bagg, A.** 2003. Clinical applications of molecular genetic testing in hematologic malignancies: advantages and limitations. *Hum. Pathol.* **34**:352–358.

3. **Bridge, J. A., J. Liu, V. Weibolt, K. S. Baker, D. Perry, R. Kruger, S. Qualman, F. Barr, P. Sorensen, T. Triche, and R. Suijkerbuijk.** 2000. Novel genomic imbalances in embryonal rhabdomyosarcoma revealed by comparative genomic hybridization and fluorescence in situ hybridization: an intergroup rhabdomyosarcoma study. *Genes Chromosomes Cancer* **27**:337–344.

4. **Chang, C. C., C. Bredeson, M. Juckett, B. Logan, and C. A. Keever-Taylor.** 2003. Tumor load in patients with follicular lymphoma post stem cell transplantation may correlate with clinical course. *Bone Marrow Transplant.* **32**:287–291.

5. **Chang, C. C., and V. B. Shidham.** 2003. Molecular genetics of pediatric soft tissue tumors: clinical application. *J. Mol. Diagn.* **5**:143–154.

6. **Dazzi, F., R. M. Szydlo, and J. M. Goldman.** 1999. Donor lymphocyte infusions for relapse of chronic myeloid leukemia after allogeneic stem cell transplant: where we now stand. *Exp. Hematol.* **27**:1477–1486.

7. **Gilliland, D. G., and J. D. Griffin.** 2002. The roles of FLT3 in hematopoiesis and leukemia. *Blood* **100**:1532–1542.

8. **Grody, W. W., G. R. Cutting, K. W. Klinger, C. S. Richards, M. S. Watson, and R. J. Desnick.** 2001. Laboratory standards and guidelines for population-based cystic fibrosis carrier screening. *Genet. Med.* **3**:149–154.

9. **Kononen, J., L. Bubendorf, A. Kallioniemi, M. Barlund, P. Schraml, S. Leighton, J. Torhorst, M. J. Mihatsch, G. Sauter, and O. P. Kallioniemi.** 1998. Tissue microarrays for high-throughput molecular profiling of tumor specimens. *Nat. Med.* **4**:844–847.

10. **Ladanyi, M., W. C. Chan, T. J. Triche, and W. L. Gerald.** 2001. Expression profiling of human tumors: the end of surgical pathology? *J. Mol. Diagn.* **3**:92–97.

11. **Lin, F., F. van Rhee, J. M. Goldman, and N. C. Cross.** 1996. Kinetics of increasing BCR-ABL transcript numbers in chronic myeloid leukemia patients who relapse after bone marrow transplantation. *Blood* **87**:4473–4478.

12. **Malkin, D., F. P. Li, L. C. Strong, J. F. Fraumeni, Jr., C. E. Nelson, D. H. Kim, J. Kassel, M. A. Gryka, F. Z. Bischoff, and M. A. Tainsky.** 1990. Germ line p53 mutations in a familial syndrome of breast cancer, sarcomas, and other neoplasms. *Science* **250**:1233–1238.

13. **Medeiros, L. J., and J. Carr.** 1999. Overview of the role of molecular methods in the diagnosis of malignant lymphomas. *Arch. Pathol. Lab. Med.* **123**:1189–1207.

14. **Munoz, N., F. X. Bosch, S. de Sanjose, R. Herrero, X. Castellsague, K. V. Shah, P. J. Snijders, C. J. Meijer, and the International Agency for Research on Cancer Multicenter Cervical Cancer Study Group.** 2003. Epidemiologic classification of human papillomavirus types associated with cervical cancer. *N. Engl. J. Med.* **348**:518–527.

15. **Murray, G., and S. Curran (ed.).** 2005. *Laser Capture Microdissection Methods and Protocols.* Humana Press, Towata, N.J.

16. **Nathanson, K. N., R. Wooster, and B. L. Weber.** 2001. Breast cancer genetics: what we know and what we need. *Nat. Med.* **7**:552–556.

17. **Park, K., J. Kim, S. Lim, S. Han, and J. Y. Lee.** 2003. Comparing fluorescence in situ hybridization methods to determine the HER-2/neu status in primary breast carcinoma using tissue microarray. *Mod. Pathol.* **16**:937–943.

18. **Rassenti, L. Z., L. Huynh, T. L. Toy, L. Chen, M. J. Keating, J. G. Gribben, D. S. Neuberg, I. W. Flinn, K. R. Rai, J. C. Byrd, N. E. Kay, A. Greaves, A. Weiss, and T. J. Kipps.** 2004. ZAP-70 compared with immunoglobulin heavy-chain gene mutation status as a predictor of disease progression in chronic lymphocytic leukemia. *N. Engl. J. Med.* **351**:893–901.

19. **Resnick, R. M., M. T. Cornelissen, D. K. Wright, G. H. Eichinger, H. S. Fox, J. ter Schegget, and M. M. Manos.** 1990. Detection and typing of human papillomavirus in archival cervical specimens by DNA amplification with consensus primers. *J. Natl. Cancer Inst.* **82**:1477–1484.

20. **Slamon, D. J., W. Godolphin, L. A. Jones, J. A. Holt, S. G. Wong, D. E. Keith, W. J. Levin, S. G. Stuart, J. Udove, and A. Ullrich.** 1989. Studies of the HER-2/neu proto-oncogene in human breast and ovarian cancer. *Science* **244**:707–712.

21. **Solomon, D., and M. Schiffman.** 2004. Have we resolved how to triage equivocal cervical cytology? *J. Nat. Cancer Inst.* **96**:250–251.

22. **Sorensen, P. H., J. C. Lynch, S. J. Qualman, R. Tirabosco, J. F. Lim, H. M. Maurer, J. A. Bridge, W. M. Crist, T. J. Triche, and F. G. Barr.** 2002. PAX3-FKHR and PAX7-FKHR gene fusions are prognostic indicators in alveolar rhabdomyosarcoma: a report from the children's oncology group. *J. Clin. Oncol.* **20**:2672–2679.

23. **Tanner, M., D. Gancberg, A. Di Leo, D. Larsimont, G. Rouas, M. J. Piccart, and J. Isola.** 2000. Chromogenic in situ hybridization: a practical alternative for fluorescence in situ hybridization to detect HER-2/neu oncogene amplification in archival breast cancer samples. *Am. J. Pathol.* **157**:1467–1472.

24. **van de Vijver, M. J., Y. D. He, L. J. van't Veer, H. Dai, A. A. Hart, D. W. Voskuil, G. J. Schreiber, J. L. Peterse, C. Roberts, M. J. Marton, M. Parrish, D. Atsma, A. Witteveen, A. Glas, L. Delahaye, T. van der Velde, H. Bartelink, S. Rodenhuis, E. T. Rutgers, S. H. Friend, and R. Bernards.** 2002. A gene-expression signature as a predictor of survival in breast cancer. *N. Engl. J. Med.* **347**:1999–2009.

Immunohistochemistry: Diagnostic and Prognostic Applications

VINOD B. SHIDHAM AND ANDRÉ A. KAJDACSY-BALLA

47

By revolutionizing the cytomorphological and histomorphological evaluation of human tissue, immunostaining is altering the diagnosis and treatment of an increasing number of diseases. Although initially investigators had only polyclonal antibodies and immunofluorescence as tools, progressive technological advances such as the use of hybridomas, flow cytometry, cytogenetics, and solid-tissue immunostaining have led to reclassification of certain tumors based on the expression patterns of specific cellular antigens. Immunostaining is being applied to aid in the classification and differentiation of neoplasms by using antibodies to lineage-specific proteins such as vimentin, cytokeratin, and S-100 protein.

Advances in production of monoclonal antibodies and techniques for immunostaining sections of formalin-fixed, paraffin-embedded tissue for light microscopy have greatly accelerated these developments (6). Various antigen retrieval methods such as heat-induced epitope retrieval (13) and molecular biology approaches which predict peptide sequences based on the DNA sequences in newly identified target genes have advanced the field further. This chapter highlights the basic principles of immunostaining for light microscopy in brief and discusses the diagnostic and prognostic applications of immunostaining.

ANTIGENS

Computerized programs can predict immunogenic sequences of target molecules to allow for the genetic engineering of peptides for the production of polyclonal antibodies. Semipurified proteins or recombinant proteins are commonly used for producing monoclonal antibodies, which are most commonly reactive with nonlinear conformational epitopes. The epitopes may be destroyed if proteins are digested, denatured, or modified by a cross-linking fixative such as formalin which causes alterations in protein folding patterns.

Formalin fixation is a major barrier for immunohistochemistry. With formalin treatment, methyl group cross-linking frequently destroys the epitope by unfolding the protein. It can also mask the desired epitope by cross-linking it with adjacent proteins. Therefore, many monoclonal antibodies that work well for fresh tissues are frequently rendered useless for paraffin-embedded fixed tissues. Another problem with aqueous formalin solutions is the formation of methoxy alcohol derivative with little aldehyde in the solution, leading to a slowdown of the fixation process (only 1 mm of tissue/h). This slowdown results in the fixation of tissue predominantly along the surface, with autolysis in the central portion, which is eventually fixed by alcohol during the dehydration steps.

Pretreatment of sections (prior to treatment with a primary antibody) with various proteolytic enzymes (papain, trypsin, and pepsin, etc.) may unmask epitopes and facilitate detection. Cross-linking may also be reversed by heating tissue sections in aqueous citrate buffer, resulting in the recovery of epitope reactivity (2, 13). These technical advances have increased the possibility of many monoclonal antibodies to be used with archived tissue sections (23).

The need for immunohistochemical evaluation, including analysis and quantification, is increasing. A quantitative approach to immunostaining is significantly limited because of variations in the types of fixatives, pHs of the fixatives, durations of fixation, temperatures of fixation, and storage conditions. Improved standardization of fixation methods, automated immunostaining, and image analysis are likely to improve the global interpretation of tissue subjected to immunohistochemistry.

ANTIBODIES

Polyclonal rather than monoclonal antibodies are more likely to detect antigens in which some but not all of the epitopes have been masked or denatured. Although wider in their spectrum of reactivity than monoclonal antibodies, polyclonal antibodies usually have less selectivity, resulting in frequent nonspecific staining. The usual practice is to raise polyclonal antibodies against synthetic peptides and increase specificity by peptide absorption. The amount of polyclonal antibodies that can be recovered from any one immunized animal is limited. In addition, there is considerable lot to lot variation in polyclonal antibody reagents.

Murine monoclonal antibodies are uniquely specific in their reactivity with a particular epitope. The recent availability of hybridoma technology for the production of rabbit monoclonal antibodies may further enhance the quality and sensitivity of immunostaining, because rabbit antibodies have stronger affinities than murine antibodies (20). By using a cocktail of several unique monoclonal antibodies, one may enhance the spectrum of reactivity without compromising specificity (18).

DETECTION SYSTEMS

Immunostaining may be performed on tissue sections (immunohistochemistry) or cytology smear specimens (immunocytochemistry). It may be performed as one step, with a primary antibody conjugated directly with an indicator system, or two steps, with a primary antibody followed by a secondary antibody conjugated with an indicator system.

There are a number of methods for the detection of antibodies bound to their specific target antigens. Commonly, heavy-chain-specific, anti-Fc secondary antibodies are conjugated directly with reactive substances, such as biotin. This allows for the detection of numerous specific primary antibodies by using the same secondary antibody system. Biotin is detected by streptavidin, linked to one of several indicator enzymes such as horseradish peroxidase, alkaline phosphatase, or glucose oxidase, which then reacts with a substrate, producing an insoluble colored product visible by light microscopy. It is possible to investigate multiple antigens simultaneously by using primary antibodies of different heavy-chain classes, immunoglobulin A (IgA), IgG, and IgM, with different epitope specificities to first attach to the antigens of interest. Each secondary anti-heavy-chain antibody will have its own detection substances with different visual color development patterns (3, 16).

A polymer backbone labeled with an indicator enzyme such as horseradish peroxidase or alkaline phosphatase may be conjugated to either primary antibodies (Zymed cytokeratin rapid immunohistochemistry kit; Zymed Laboratories, Inc., South San Francisco, Calif.) or secondary antibodies (PowerVision+ [ImmunoVision Technologies Co., Brisbane, Calif.] and EnVision and EnVision+ systems [DakoCytomation, Carpinteria, Calif.]). This provides an amplified biotin-free detection system with high sensitivity and fewer steps than conventional methods.

CONTROLS

As the reagents used and the targets evaluated are mostly proteins, they are subject to nonspecific binding, degradation, and cross-reactivity. It is important to monitor the process with negative and positive controls. There are two methods for negative controls. The antibody to be used may be reacted with the target antigen prior to immunostaining. More commonly, the primary antibody may be replaced by another antibody of the same idiotype but different specificity.

The positive controls may be tissue sections or cytology smear specimens with proven immunoreactivity with the test antigen. The positive controls should ideally be treated in a fashion identical to that of the test material with reference to steps such as fixation, tissue smear specimen processing, and antigen retrieval. Generally, one positive control is sufficient for a particular immunostaining run utilizing automated procedures. In order to avoid errors introduced by failures of mechanical delivery, these positive controls should preferably be placed on the same slide as the test specimen. This is relatively easy for tissue sections but may not be feasible for cytology smear specimens, depending on the method of smear preparation. Tissue "sausages" or tissue microarrays with several control tissues, including ones fixed at different times, are used as positive controls by some laboratories. Positive controls for cytology may be the smear specimens prepared from lesions with known immunoreactivity for a particular antigen or from smear specimens from cell lines with known immunoreactivity patterns. Positive control smear specimens should be processed and fixed using methods identical to those used for test smear specimens. The fixed smears may

then be dehydrated without staining, cleared, and covered with glass coverslips using mounting medium similar to that used for permanent sections (15, 17, 19). Such coverslipped unstained smears are stable at room temperatures of 70 to 80°F as positive controls for commonly used immunomarkers (19).

Ubiquitous antigens may serve as internal controls to establish the stability of antigens after fixation and tissue processing. Vimentin is a stable antigen in formalin-fixed tissue sections and thus may be used to evaluate unevenly fixed tissue blocks by evaluating only those areas with vimentin reactivity for other specific antigens. The lack of reactivity for such an internal control indicates a need to modify the immunostaining protocol by, for example, incorporating pretreatment of the sections by enzyme digestion or heat-induced epitope retrieval. Although vimentin is considered to be a reliable internal control for formalin-fixed, paraffin-embedded tissue sections, it may not be applicable to all methods of fixation and processing. As reported previously (17), vimentin immunoreactivity deteriorates in air-dried smear specimens after rehydration in saline and postfixation in alcoholic formalin but other markers are stable (17).

Nonspecific binding may be reduced by preincubating the sections with milk or with Igs of the same species and type as the secondary antibody used. Preincubation with streptavidin may be necessary for biotin-rich tissues, especially when one is using heat-induced epitope retrieval, which may greatly enhance the intrinsic biotin reactivity (2).

INTERPRETATION

The chromogen's color indicates the presence of the antigen in question. In general, the intensity of immunoreactivity should be comparable to that seen with the positive control. This is important for certain immunomarkers such as CD117 (c-kit), which may be interpreted spuriously as positive when only faint immunostaining is seen.

The location of the marker within the cell helps in interpretation. Some examples of immunomarkers with diagnostic nuclear reactivity are estrogen receptor (ER), progesterone receptor (PR), androgen receptor, S-100 protein, microphthalmia transcription factor, thyroid transcription factor 1 (TTF-1), MyoD1, β catenin (for desmoid), and calretinin (for mesothelial cells). The appearance of these markers in the cytoplasm alone may be confusing, but suggests nonspecific or nondiagnostic staining.

Some immunostaining patterns are typical for a particular lesion (see Table 1). Examples include the canalicular immunostaining pattern associated with polyclonal carcinoembryonic antigen (pCEA) in hepatocellular carcinoma, the concentric fibrillar immunostaining pattern associated with cytokeratins in mesothelial cells, the peripheral microvillous immunostaining pattern associated with HBME-1 and epithelial membrane antigen (EMA) in mesothelial cells, the membranous immunostaining pattern associated with Her2/neu in mammary carcinoma, the membranous pattern associated with E-cadherin in mammary ductal carcinoma, and the dot-like paranuclear globular immunoreactivity pattern associated with cytokeratin in desmoplastic small round cell and Merkel cell tumors.

APPLICATIONS

Textbooks (1), journals (e.g., *Applied Immunohistochemistry* and *Molecular Morphology*), and websites (Immunoquery; http://www.ipox.org) are invaluable tools for keeping up with

TABLE 1 Typical immunoreactivity (antigen expression) patterns of a few types of tumors[a]

Tumor type(s)	Immunoreactivity (antigen expression) pattern(s)
Biliary tract, mucinous ovarian, and transitional cell ca	CyK 20+, CyK 7+
Gastric tumor	CyK 20−, CyK 7+, MUC5AC+
Breast, lung, endometrial, and nonmucinous ovarian ca	CyK 20−, CyK 7+
Colon ca	CyK 20+, CyK 7−, diffuse pCEA+, MUC5AC−
Hepatocellular ca	pCEA+ (canalicular-pattern), AFP+, MUC5AC−
Cholangiocarcinoma	pCEA− (or diffusely+), AFP−, CyK7+, MUC5AC+
Thyroid, endometrial, mesothelioma, and renal ca	Coexpression of Vim and CyK
Breast and nonmucinous ovarian ca	ER/PR/AR+
Small cell ca	+ For neuroendocrine markers (synaptophysin, chromogranin, CD56)
Merkel cell ca	Globular CyK20+, + for neuroendocrine markers
Thyroid ca	Vim+, CyK+, thyroglobulin+
Prostate ca	PSAP+, PSA+, CEA−
Choriocarcinoma	HCG+
Seminoma	PLAP+
Mesothelioma	Vim+, CyK 5+, nuclear calretinin+, CEA− (or focal)
GIST	CD117+, CD34+
Desmoplastic small round cell tumor	CyK+ (globular), desmin+ (globular), Vim+/−
Prostatic adenocarcinoma versus transitional cell ca	PSA/PSA/Leu7+ versus CyK 903 (34βE12)+
Small cell lung ca versus Merkle cell ca	TTF-1+ versus CyK 20+
Thyroid ca versus medulary ca of thyroid	Thyroglobulin+ versus calcitonin+
Stromal tumors versus leiomyosarcoma	CD10+ versus SMA+
Breast ca versus colon ca	ER/PR/AR/CyK 7+ versus CyK 20+
Ovarian mucinous ca versus appendiceal mucinous ca	CyK 7+ versus CyK 20+ and Cdx2+
Hepatocellular ca versus cholangiocarcinoma	pCEA+ (canalicular), hepar+, albumin+ versus pCEA− (canalicular), hepar−, albumin−
Mesothelioma versus lung ca	Calretinin+ (nuclear) versus TTF-1+ (nuclear)

[a] Ca, carcinoma; CyK, cytokeratin; MUC5AC, mucin 5 subtypes A and C; AR, androgen receptor; PSAP, prostate-specific acid phosphatase; PSA, prostate-specific antigen; Vim, vimentin; HCG, human chorionic gonadotropin; PLAP, placental alkaline phosphatase; SMA, smooth muscle actin; AFP, alpha-1 fetoprotein; +, positive; −, negative.

the rapidly changing field of immunohistochemistry diagnostic and prognostic applications. The areas in which immunostaining might be used for such applications may be categorized as follows: differential diagnosis, evaluation using therapeutic predictive markers, evaluation using prognostic markers, evaluation for dysplasia and malignancy, and intraoperative evaluation.

Differential Diagnosis

Immunohistochemistry is commonly used to aid in the differential diagnosis of neoplasms, particularly those classified as poorly differentiated. The undifferentiated neoplasms may be grouped morphologically into four categories: small blue cell tumors, large cell tumors, pleomorphic tumors, and spindle cell tumors. Figure 1 shows a simplified algorithm to be applied with reference to morphological features and clinical details (7, 10, 14, 23). This algorithm may be modified and updated further depending on future additions to and improvements in the ever expanding list of immunomarkers.

Up to 20% of neoplasms present as metastases with an unknown primary. The search for the primary site is a time-consuming, expensive, and often fruitless process. In rare cases, it may not be found even after a complete autopsy. Immunomarkers have contributed greatly to the resolution of this challenge. For example, coordinate expression of

cytokeratins 7 and 20 may help in determining the primary sites of metastatic lesions (23). In addition, all epithelial neoplasms express cytokeratins; however, expression of the nontrichogenic cytokeratins follows a site-specific pattern. Similarly, different types of mucins, along with cytokeratins, facilitate the diagnostic algorithm for interpretation of gastrointestinal tract cancers (7).

Immunostaining has also been effectively used for the detection of small metastatic lesions in sentinel lymph nodes (SLNs) for identification of melanoma (16), mammary carcinoma (22), Merkel cell tumor (21), and other tumors. It may also be helpful for identification of surgical margins such as in cases of carcinoma of the stomach and for detection and confirmation of various microorganisms such as cytomegalovirus and polyoma virus and of other substances such as amyloid.

Evaluation Using Therapeutic Predictive Markers

A therapeutic predictive marker is used to help guide therapy. The best known therapeutic predictive makers are ER and PR in breast carcinoma (11), the growth factor receptor Her-2/neu in breast carcinoma (12), CD117 in gastrointestinal stromal tumors (GIST) (8), and epidermal growth factor receptor in several different tumors (9).

The presence of nuclear ER and PR favors a positive response to estradiol antagonist treatment (12). These markers

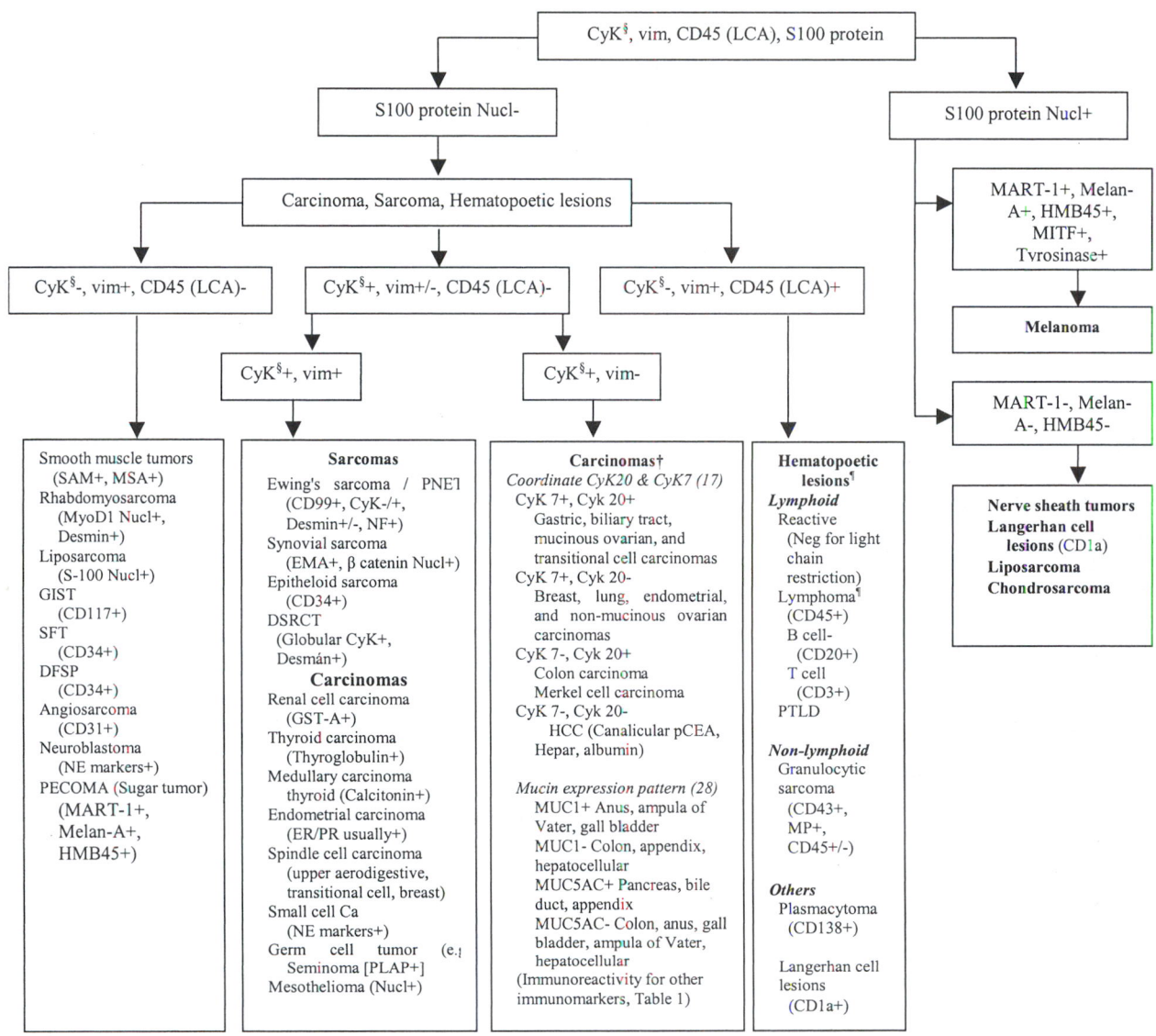

FIGURE 1 Algorithm for immuohistochemical evalution of tumors—to be interpreted with reference to morphology and clinical details (7, 14, 23). §, For covering a wider spectrum of cytokeratins (CyK), cytokeratin–Lu-5 or a cocktail of cytokeratin AE1/AE3 and CAM5.2 is preferred. ¶, The list of hematopoietic lesions is partial and abbreviated (for details, see reference 14 and other specific literature). †, For details, see specific references including reference 7 and 23.

are assayed routinely in breast cancers. Patients with tumors with 10% or more nuclei positive for ER or PR are more likely to respond to hormonal therapy. A variety of methods have been used to quantify results by image analysis with evolving automation.

Due to the amplification of the Her-2/neu gene, ErbB-2 (HER-2) tyrosine kinase receptor, a member of the epidermal growth factor family of receptors, is overexpressed in approximately 30% of breast carcinomas. Humanized antibody Herceptin (Genentech, Inc., South San Francisco, Calif.) has demonstrated benefits in women with advanced breast cancer who did not respond to conventional chemotherapy. Although the impact of ErbB-2 has been studied for 20 years, its importance was accelerated when the humanized antibody (Herceptin) was developed. Her-2/neu protein is expressed in

the cell membrane and can be demonstrated by immunohistochemistry as a marker with a membranous immunostaining pattern. In cases with equivocal immunohistochemistry results, gene amplification can be demonstrated by the use of labeled nuclear probes with in situ hybridization, either fluorescent in situ hybridization or chromogenic in situ hybridization.

Virtually all GIST are associated with mutations of the c-kit oncogene with expression of CD117 (c-kit). This association is extremely helpful for the detection of GIST (8). Imatinib mesylate (STI571; Gleevec) is a potent, specific inhibitor of c-kit (CD117) used in chronic myeloid leukemia. It has demonstrated significant therapeutic effects in cases with unresectable and metastatic malignant GIST. The relationship of CD117 to imatinib mesylate in other tumors is being evaluated.

Other agents such as gefitinib (Iressa; ZD1839) and lapatinib (GlaxoSmithKline, Research Triangle Park, N.C.) are inhibitors of epidermal growth factor receptor (ErbB-1 tyrosine kinase receptor) expressed in the cytoplasm and membranes of cells from several different tumors.

Evaluation Using Prognostic Markers

Examples of prognostic markers include proliferation and cell cycle proteins (such as Ki-67, p53, and retinoblastoma protein), various growth factors and their receptors, molecules involved in apoptosis (Bcl-2), proteases and their inhibitors (including tissue metalloproteinase inhibitor), and adhesion molecules (such as cadherins and integrins).

Knowledge about the prognostic significance of each marker will continue to be updated as the follow-up data from an increasing number of studies become available (4). Association such as that of poor prognosis with the immunoexpression of vimentin in breast and renal cell carcinomas is expected to emerge.

Evaluation for Dysplasia and Malignancy

Although rare, in some situations immunostaining may facilitate interpretation of dysplasia (through detection of p16 in cervical dysplasia [5]) and malignancy (through detection of monoclonal antibody for CEA in minimal deviation endocervical adenocarcinoma versus normal endocervical mucosa and S-100A6 immunoreactivity in normal nevi versus rare or weak immunoreactivity in melanoma). Other approaches such as the use of p53 immunoreactivity in serous cavity fluids and in urine have been studied for detecting neoplastic cells.

Intraoperative Evaluation

Rapid intraoperative immunocytochemical evaluation facilitates improved management in a variety of clinical situations. The most practical application is the rapid intraoperative immunocytochemical evaluation of SLNs for detection of cutaneous melanoma (19). The imprint smear specimens can be immunostained by using a standardized protocol in 17 min (19). If the SLNs are positive for melanoma micrometastases, the surgeon can proceed with completion of regional lymphadenectomy during the same anaesthetic session, thus eliminating the need for additional surgery at a later date. This has obvious financial and social benefits with improved quality of patient care. If indicated, the same principle may be applied for the evaluation of SLNs for breast carcinoma, Merkel cell tumor, and many other malignancies in the future.

Rapid intraoperative immunocytochemical evaluation can also be applied for the evaluation of the imprint smears of surgical margins of carcinomas, especially in fatty tissues such as breast. Frozen sections of such tissues are technically difficult to assess for micrometastases due to significant artifacts and blank holes in the sections.

We thank Carl Becker, Richard Komorowski, Petio Kotov, Lakshmy Parameswaran, and Vladimir Osipov for reviewing the manuscript. We also thank Glen Dawson (American Society for Clinical Pathology) and Jeanette Bjerke for checking the manuscript. We appreciate their input and criticisms.

REFERENCES

1. **Dabbs, D. J. (ed.).** 2002. *Diagnostic Immunohistochemistry.* Churchill Livingstone, Philadelphia, Pa.
2. **Fan, Z., V. Clark, and R. B. Nagle.** 1997. An evaluation of enzymatic and heat epitope retrieval methods for the immunohistochemical staining of intermediate filaments. *Appl. Immunol.* **5:**49–58.
3. **Grogan, T. M., C. Rangel, L. Rimza, J. Rybski, and R. Zehab.** 1995. Clinical and research applications of rapid kinetic-mode automated double labeled immunohistochemistry and in situ hybridization. *Adv. Pathol.* **8:**79–100.
4. **Henson, D. E., L. P. Fielding, D. L. Grignon, D. L. Page, M. E. Hammond, G. Nash, N. M. Pettigrew, F. Gorstein, R. V. Hutter, et al.** 1995. College of American Pathologists Conference XXVI on clinical relevance of prognostic markers in solid tumor. Summary. *Arch. Pathol. Lab. Med.* **119:**1109–1112.
5. **Klaes, R., T. Friedrich, D. Spitkovsky, R. Ridder, W. Rudy, U. Petry, G. Dallenbach-Hellweg, D. Schmidt, and M. von Knebel Doeberitz.** 2001. Overexpression of p16(INK4A) as a specific marker for dysplastic and neoplastic epithelial cells of the cervix uteri. *Int. J. Cancer* **92:**276–284.
6. **Koehler, G., and C. Milstein.** 1975. Continuous cultures of fused cells secreting antibody of predefined specificity. *Nature* **256:**495–497.
7. **Lee, M. J., H. S. Lee, W. H. Kim, Y. Choi, and M. Yang.** 2003. Expression of mucins and cytokeratins in primary carcinomas of the digestive system. *Mod. Pathol.* **16:**403–410.
8. **Logrono, R., D. V. Jones, S. Faruqi, and M. S. Bhutani.** 2004. Recent advances in cell biology, diagnosis, and therapy of gastrointestinal stromal tumor (GIST). *Cancer Biol. Ther.* **3:**251–258.
9. **Marquez, A., R. Wu, J. Zhao, J. Tao, and Z. Shi.** 2004. Evaluation of epidermal growth factor receptor (EGFR) by chromogenic in situ hybridization (CISH) and immunohistochemistry (IHC) in archival gliomas using bright-field microscopy. *Diagn. Mol. Pathol.* **13:**1–8.
10. **Nielsen, T. O., R. B. West, S. C. Linn, O. Alter, M. A. Knowling, J. X. O'Connell, S. Zhu, M. Fero, G. Sherlock, J. R. Pollack, P. O. Brown, D. Botstein, and M. van de Rijn.** 2002. Molecular characterisation of soft tissue tumours: a gene expression study. *Lancet* **359:**1301–1307.
11. **Pertschuk, L. P., D. S. Kim, K. Nayer, J. G. Feldman, K. B. Eisenberg, A. C. Carter, Z. T. Rong, W. L. Thelmo, J. Fleisher, and G. L. Greene.** 1990. Immunocytochemical estrogen and progestin receptor assays in breast cancer with monoclonal antibodies. Histopathologic, demographic, and biochemical correlations and relationship to endocrine response and survival. *Cancer* **66:**1663–1670.
12. **Ross, J. S., and J. A. Fletcher.** 1998. The her-2/neu oncogene in breast cancer: prognostic factor, predictive factor, and target for therapy. *Oncologist* **3:**237–252.
13. **Shi, S. R., R. J. Cote, and C. R. Taylor.** 1997. Antigen retrieval immunohistochemistry: past, present, and future. *J. Histochem. Cytochem.* **39:**741–748.
14. **Shidham, V. B.** 2004. Respiratory cytology, p. 273–356. *In* B. F. Atkinson (ed.), *Atkinson Atlas of Diagnostic Cytopathology,* 2nd ed. W. B. Saunders Company, Philadelphia, Pa.
15. **Shidham, V. B., P. F. Lindholm, A. Kajdacsy-Balla, C. Chang, and R. Komorowski.** 2000. Methods of cytology smear preparation and fixation: effect on the immunoreactivity of commonly used anti-cytokeratin antibody AE1/AE3. *Acta Cytologica* **44:**1015–1022.
16. **Shidham, V. B., D. Qi, S. Acker, B. Kampalath, C. Chang, V. George, and R. Komorowski.** 2001. Evaluation of micrometastases in sentinel lymph nodes of cutaneous melanoma: higher diagnostic accuracy with Melan-A and MART-1 compared to S-100 protein and HMB-45. *Am. J. Surg. Pathol.* **25:**1039–1046.
17. **Shidham, V. B., C. C. Chang, R. N. Rao, R. Komorowski, and M. Chivukula.** 2003. Immunostaining of cytology smears: a comparative study to identify the most suitable method of smear preparation and fixation with reference to commonly used immunomarkers. *Diagn. Cytopathol.* **29:**217–221.
18. **Shidham, V. B., D. Qi, R. Rao, S. Acker, C. Chang, B. Kampalath, G. Dawson, J. Macchi, and R. Komorowski.** 7 May 2003, posting date. Improved immunohistochemical evaluation of micrometastases in sentinel lymph nodes of cutaneous melanoma with MCW melanoma cocktail—a

mixture of monoclonal antibodies to MART-1, Melan-A, and tyrosinase. *BMC Cancer* **3:**15. [Online.] doi: 10. 1186/1471-2407-3-15.

19. **Shidham, V. B., R. Komorowski, G. Dawson, S. Kaul, C. C. Chang, and V. Macias.** 6 Aug. 2004, posting date. Optimization of immunostaining protocol for rapid intraoperative evaluation of imprint smears of melanoma sentinel lymph nodes with "MCW melanoma cocktail." *CytoJournal* **1:**2. [Online.] doi: 10. 1186/1742-6413-1-2.

20. **Spieker-Polet, H., P. Sethupathi, P. C. Yam, and K. L. Knight.** 1995. Rabbit monoclonal antibodies: generating a fusion partner to produce rabbit-rabbit hybridomas. *Proc. Natl. Acad. Sci. USA* **92:**9348–9352.

21. **Su, L. D., L. Lowe, C. R. Bradford, A. I. Yahanda, T. M. Johnson, and V. K. Sondak.** 2002. Immunostaining for cytokeratin 20 improves detection of micrometastatic Merkel cell carcinoma in sentinel lymph nodes. *J. Am. Acad. Dermatol.* **46:**661–666.

22. **Viale, G., A. Sonzogni, G. Pruneri, F. Maffini, M. Masullo, P. Dell'Orto, and G. Mazzarol.** 2004. Histopathologic examination of axillary sentinel lymph nodes in breast carcinoma patients. *J. Surg. Oncol.* **85:**123–128.

23. **Wang, N. P, S. Zee, R. Zarbo, C. Bacchi, and A. Gown.** 1995. Coordinate expression of cytokeratins 7 and 20 defines unique subsets of carcinomas. *Appl. Immunohistochem.* **3:**99–107.

Immunofluorescence Methods in the Diagnosis of Renal and Skin Diseases

A. BERNARD COLLINS, ROBERT B. COLVIN, CARLOS H. NOUSARI,
AND GRANT J. ANHALT

48

Immunofluorescence is a well-established technique for the detection of antigens in tissue sections or cell suspensions (6, 7, 11, 29, 40). Since its development in 1941 by Albert Coons at Harvard Medical School to demonstrate the presence of pneumococcal antigens in tissue (15), immunofluorescence has become a crucial tool in the diagnosis and determination of prognoses of immunologically mediated kidney (12, 28, 38–40) and skin (1, 5, 6, 8, 16) diseases. Direct immunofluorescence (defined as the application of specific antibodies to detect specific antigens in tissue) is a sensitive and simple technique for the detection of tissue-bound immunoglobulins (Igs), complement components, and fibrin-fibrinogen in cases of glomerulonephritis and autoimmune or immunologically mediated mucocutaneous disorders. In the kidney, many forms of primary glomerulonephritis are characterized by deposition of immunoreactants in distinctive diagnostic patterns. The primary renal targets are the glomerulus, the proximal tubules, and the interstitium. In many skin diseases, demonstration of Ig or complement deposition in specific structures in the dermis and epidermis is an essential criterion for accurate diagnosis. For the skin, we will focus primarily on the immunofluorescence findings in bullous and connective tissue disorders, vasculitides, and other mucocutaneous conditions, for which this immunohistochemistry technique can provide useful diagnostic information. This chapter will also emphasize the common immunofluorescence techniques used for diagnosis and interpretation with kidney and skin biopsy specimens.

TISSUE FOR IMMUNOFLUORESCENCE

Kidney

Renal tissue submitted for immunofluorescence studies is usually obtained from percutaneous needle biopsies, surgical wedge biopsies, or nephrectomies. A hand lens (magnification, × 7) or dissecting microscope is useful to determine if the tissue specimen contains glomeruli. The complete diagnostic work-up for renal tissue includes electron microscopy (33), direct immunofluorescence (11), and light microscopy studies (40). Percutaneous needle biopsy specimens, which usually range in length from 0.5 to 2.0 cm, can be divided in such a manner as to ensure that adequate tissue is available for the three-part study. The division of a closed and surgical (wedge) renal biopsy specimen is illustrated in Collins (11). Briefly, a 1-mm portion is cut from each end of the core and placed immediately in Karnovsky's fixative (33) for electron microscopy studies. The remainder of the core is divided longitudinally. One half is frozen for direct immunofluorescence studies, and the other half is placed into 10% buffered formalin for light microscopic studies.

Skin

For skin specimens used for immunofluorescence studies, the proper choice of a biopsy site is critical to maximize the probability of obtaining diagnostic information. In most if not all cases of bullous skin diseases, namely, those autoimmune in nature, biopsy specimens should be obtained from perilesional tissue (Fig. 1). A 3- to 4-mm punch biopsy specimen from inflamed but unblistered skin adjacent to a blister is most useful. Blistered lesional skin is the most common cause of negative results. Skin biopsy specimens from sites too distant from the blistering can also cause negative results. However, there are exceptions when examination of lesional tissue is required (Fig. 2). For the diagnosis of pemphigoid, pemphigus, linear IgA bullous disease, epidermolysis bullosa acquisita (EBA), and dermatitis herpetiformis, the tissue sample should be taken from inflamed but unblistered skin. For the diagnosis of connective tissue diseases, vasculitis, lichen planus, erythema multiforme, and porphyria (55), the biopsy specimen should come from the lesional skin.

While renal tissue obtained at autopsy may be suitable for direct immunofluorescence, skin undergoes postmortem autolysis and nonspecifically traps serum proteins. This leads to difficulty in interpretation due to high background staining.

TISSUE-HANDLING AND -FREEZING PROCEDURE: RENAL AND SKIN BIOPSY SPECIMENS

Tissue for immunofluorescence studies should be obtained fresh and kept moist until rapidly frozen or snap-frozen. If freezing can be performed within 20 to 30 min for renal biopsy specimens and within 24 h for skin biopsy specimens, the tissue can be kept on a saline-moistened piece of gauze or filter paper in a closed vial or small petri dish. For longer delay times (due to transport) or as an alternative to freezing, the specimen can be put into Michel's immunofluorescence transport medium. Increasingly, it is standard practice

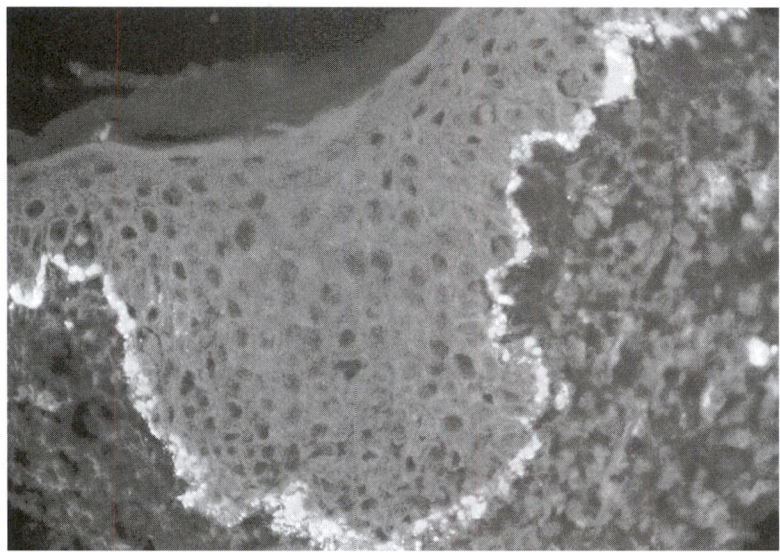

FIGURE 1 Direct immunofluorescence of a skin biopsy specimen. There is granular IgG deposition along the basement membrane zone. This pattern is characteristic of that seen in connective tissue disease-associated interface dermatitis, including lupus erythematosus.

to use Michel's medium (41, 45) for all skin biopsy specimens. The medium is composed of an 85% saturated solution of ammonium sulfate, the protease inhibitor N-ethylmaleimide, and magnesium sulfate, in citrate buffer, pH 7.25 (available commercially from Zeus Scientific Inc., Raritan, N.J.). The solution is stable at room temperature but must be kept in a tightly capped container to prevent absorption of CO_2 and acidification. The ammonium sulfate reversibly denatures all proteins in the biopsy specimen. Specimens stored in the transport medium are stable for at least 2 to 4 weeks at room temperature. Immunofluorescence results for the skin are usually identical to those obtained for snap-frozen tissue (41), but kidney specimens frequently have increased background. When the specimen is received in the laboratory, the ammonium sulfate is removed by placing the tissue into the wash solution (three 10-min washes; Zeus Scientific Inc.). Although it is standard procedure to use repeated, brief washings for other tissues, often in the case of skin specimens, high levels of background fluorescence can be reduced by more-prolonged washes, such as three times for 1 h or overnight at 4°C.

The renatured skin biopsy specimen is then oriented and embedded in optimal cutting temperature (OCT) compound (Tissue-Tek; Miles Laboratories, Inc., Elkhart, Ind.)

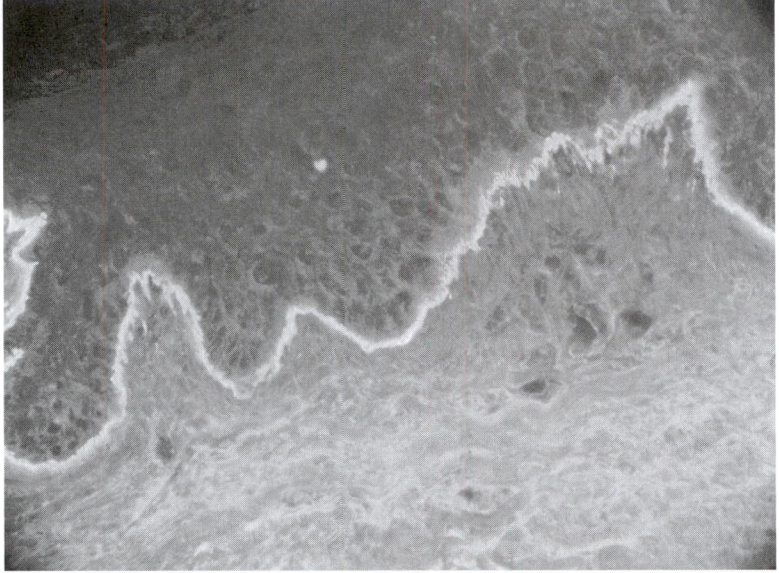

FIGURE 2 Direct immunofluorescence of a skin biopsy specimen. There is fine linear wavy IgG deposition along the basement membrane zone. This pattern is characteristic of that seen in bullous pemphigoid.

contained in a small aluminum foil "bullet" formed by wrapping a layer of foil around the bottom of a serum Vacutainer tube. The bullet is frozen by dipping it into liquid nitrogen, the foil is peeled off, and the OCT compound block is mounted on the cryostat chuck.

Renal tissue is frozen by immersing properly oriented tissue into a small amount of OCT compound, a water-soluble resin (Miles Laboratories, Inc., Naperville, Ill.), on a precooled metal chuck in a cryostat and spraying gently with MCB Tissue Freeze (Matheson, Coleman and Bell Manufacturing Chemists, Norwood, Ohio). Tissue is ready for sectioning in less than 3 min.

Many of the difficulties in immunofluorescence studies are related to tissue-handling techniques, suboptimal freezing procedures, or inappropriate frozen storage conditions. If tissue is allowed to freeze too slowly, ice crystal formation can occur, causing structural disruption.

STORAGE CONDITIONS FOR FROZEN SPECIMENS

Frozen specimens should be stored frozen at $-70°C$ in a small plastic bag with as little air as possible. At $-70°C$, it is possible to store blocks for long periods, often for years, and still obtain adequate results. Tissue can be stored at $-20°C$, but at this temperature the duration of satisfactory preservation usually does not exceed several months. Frozen tissue deteriorates during storage, usually from ice crystal formation or desiccation.

FIXATION

Most diagnostic studies using direct immunofluorescence techniques are performed with unfixed frozen tissue sections, since many antigens can be altered or destroyed by fixation. However, the demonstration of the presence of some cytoplasmic antigens, such as viral antigens, for diagnostic purposes may require fixation. The optimal fixation conditions must be empirically determined for each antigen of interest. Fixation may also cause the physical redistribution of some antigens. For example, in anti-neutrophil cytoplasmic antibody (ANCA) assays, alcohol fixation of the neutrophil slide preparation causes the myeloperoxidase contained in the primary azurophilic granules of neutrophils to redistribute to a perinuclear or nuclear location (19).

FROZEN-TISSUE SECTIONING

Frozen kidney tissue sections for direct immunofluorescence should be cut in a cryostat at a thickness of 2 to 4 mm. The frozen blocks of tissue should be equilibrated in the cryostat at -25 to $-20°C$ before frozen sectioning. The tissue sections are picked up on single-end SuperFrost/Plus glass slides (Fisher Scientific, Pittsburgh, Pa.) to facilitate labeling and decrease the chance that tissue will be lost by wiping off of the wrong side. The tissue attaches because the slides are at a higher temperature than the tissue and are positively charged, reducing the likelihood of washing off the tissue. Furthermore, the Plus slide pretreatment eliminates the time-consuming need for coating slides with albumin, glue, poly-L-lysine, or 3-aminopropyltriethoxysilane (27, 30). An initial frozen tissue section is stained using a 1% toluidine blue solution in order to determine whether glomeruli are contained in the tissue section. If so, sections are cut for the routine direct immunofluorescence panel. If the specimen is small, a circle is cut around the tissue with a diamond or aqueous insoluble pencil,

since it can be difficult to find the tissue on the slide after coverslips are placed on the tissue sections.

Three sections are placed on each slide and either air dried and stained immediately or stored frozen at $-20°C$ in a slide box covered with aluminum foil or plastic wrap. Storing slides overnight allows more effective organization of technical time. Frozen skin biopsy specimens are sectioned at a thickness of 5 μm in a cryostat at $-20°C$, stained with a rapid tissue stain (such as Multiple Stain; Polysciences, Warrington, Pa.) to ensure proper orientation, and mounted on albumin-coated slides. For skin biopsy specimens, five slides are prepared with three tissue sections on each slide.

DIRECT IMMUNOFLUORESCENCE

Principle

In the direct immunofluorescence technique, frozen tissue sections are incubated at room temperature in a moist chamber using well-characterized fluorochrome-conjugated antibodies. After incubation, the unbound labeled antibody is washed from the tissue sections, the slides are placed on coverslips, and the bound labeled antibody is detected by examination and interpretation using a fluorescence microscope.

Evaluation of skin and renal tissues by direct immunofluorescence usually entails examination of the frozen sections of specimens for deposition of Igs, complement components, and fibrin detected by using fluorescein-labeled monospecific antibodies directed against these immunoreactants. However, in 1989 Fogazzi et al. (20) reported a method for performing direct immunofluorescence with formalin-fixed, paraffin-embedded renal tissue after treatment of the sections with the proteolytic enzyme pronase. They found comparable results when the intensities, distribution patterns, and locations of immunoreactants were compared to those obtained with direct immunofluorescence performed with frozen tissue sections from patients with the same disorders, namely, IgA nephropathy and membranous and proliferative lupus nephritis. Subsequently, they studied more than 500 renal cases with this technique and found good correlation between the direct immunofluorescence results obtained with the two methods. In our laboratory, we have confirmed the results obtained with the technique in cases of IgA nephropathy, membranous postinfectious glomerulonephritis, and lupus nephritis. The technique is more time-consuming, expensive, and complex than using frozen tissue but provides a sensitive alternative when only paraffin-embedded material is available for diagnostic studies.

Immunoperoxidase techniques have been explored as an alternative methodology, but in almost all bullous diseases and cases of glomerulonephritis, immunofluorescence techniques are more sensitive and accurate (6, 40).

Staining Procedure

Renal and skin biopsy specimens are routinely stained with a panel of IgG fractions of fluorescein-labeled monospecific antisera to IgG, IgA, IgM, C3, C1q, fibrin-fibrinogen, κ and λ light chains, and, in the case of renal biopsy specimens, albumin as a negative control.

1. Prior to staining, cryostat sections (2 to 5 μm) are air dried for 30 min at room temperature to maximize adherence. Afterward, slides are washed for 5 min in 0.01 M sodium-phosphate buffered saline (PBS)–0.15 M NaCl (pH 7.3) to remove unbound serum proteins which contribute to background staining. The slides are loaded into a staining rack of a Tissue-Tek II (Miles Laboratories) slide-staining

unit, which is placed on a clinical rotator adjusted to give gentle stirring.

2. After washing, one slide at a time is removed, the excess PBS is blotted from around the tissue section, and 50 to 100 µl of appropriately diluted fluorescein conjugate is applied to the tissue section while it is still moist. A drop of conjugate should be added just above the tissue section, and to ensure that the conjugate covers the entire specimen, the slide should be gently tipped to one side and then the other. The slides are then incubated for 30 min at room temperature in a moist, level chamber or in petri dishes containing a moistened piece of filter paper. It is essential that tissue remain moistened after being hydrated to avoid problems with background staining.

3. After incubation, the slides are tipped to one side to allow the excess conjugate to run off and the slides are washed as in step 1 in PBS four times for 5 to 10 min each time to remove unbound fluorochrome-labeled conjugate from the section.

4. The excess PBS is blotted from around the specimen, and the moistened tissue is placed on a coverslip with mounting medium. For skin tissue sections, it is necessary to mount the sections with a medium containing compounds to reduce fluorescence burnout, such as Permafluor (Shandon Lipshaw, Pittsburgh, Pa.), mixed with 0.3 M diazabicycloctane and triethylenediamine (Sigma Chemical Co., St. Louis, Mo.) and buffered to pH 10.00 with 2 M glycine (31). For kidney tissue sections, Aqua-Mount (Lerner Labs, Pittsburgh, Pa.) is used as a mounting medium.

5. The slides are examined using a fluorescence microscope with epi-illumination equipment, which consists of barrier and excitation filters contained in a dichroic mirror package, to allow the visualization of fluorescein.

C4d Staining of Renal Allografts

In addition to being stained with the routine direct immunofluorescence panel, allograft kidney biopsy specimens are stained for C4d as a marker of antibody-mediated rejection by using a three-step immunofluorescence technique (14). Diffuse staining of C4d in peritubular capillaries (Fig. 3) has been shown to be associated with circulating antibodies to donor HLA class I and class II antigens in acute and chronic rejection (14, 36, 37).

Use of NaCl-Induced Split-Skin Biopsy Specimens

In subepidermal blistering diseases, it is often possible to infer precise diagnoses from localization of the in vivo bound Igs. Most commonly, this involves differentiating bullous pemphigoid and its variants (in which IgG is bound to epidermal hemidesmosomal proteins) from EBA (in which IgG is bound to dermal type VII collagen) or antiepiligrin mucous membrane pemphigoid (in which IgG is bound to laminin type V and epiligrin and also localized to the dermal surface) (22).

This procedure may be useful when IgG is detected along the epidermal basement membrane zone after standard preparation of a punch biopsy specimen. The biopsy specimen is thawed at room temperature from the OCT compound block, and the dermis is trimmed to a thickness of <1 mm. (It is important to have as thin a dermal remnant as possible to aid in the salt splitting step.) The punch biopsy specimen is then placed in 20 to 30 ml of 1M NaCl dissolved in water for 48 to 72 h at 4°C. At the end of this time, the biopsy specimen is washed briefly in tissue wash solution to remove excess salt and separation through the lamina lucida may be induced by manually peeling the epidermis from the dermis. The epidermis is then placed back on top of the dermis, reembedded in OCT compound, and stained using the routine immunofluorescence technique. Occasionally, even after adequate incubation in 1 M NaCl, the epidermis will not easily separate from the dermis. In such cases, the biopsy specimen should be immersed in PBS at 56°C for 30 to 45 s and cooled and afterward the epidermis should be easily separated. Care must be taken to keep the temperature at 56°C, since at 60°C Igs will be irreversibly denatured.

In bullous pemphigoid, the IgG will localize to the basilar surfaces of the epidermal cells, on the roof of the induced

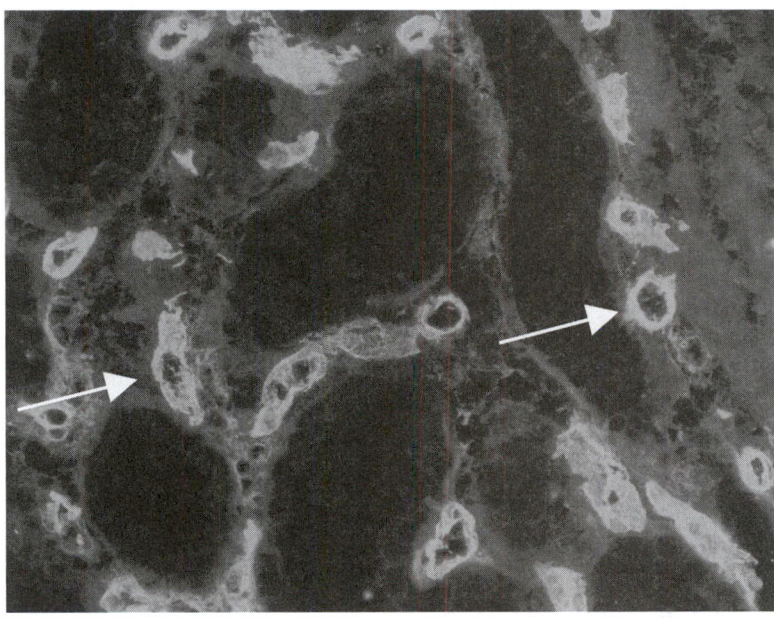

FIGURE 3 Acute humoral rejection of a renal allograft. A three-step immunofluorescence technique shows diffuse C4d deposition (arrow) in peritubular capillaries.

blister; in EBA and antiepiligrin cicatricial pemphigoid, IgG will be found solely on the dermal side after the induced separation (22, 34, 61). This split-skin technique cannot distinguish between EBA and antiepiligrin cicatricial pemphigoid, because dermal staining is observed in both disorders (18). However, because bullous pemphigoid is far more common than these other two diseases, this technique often helps determine if the deposits are epidermal or dermal, thus eliminating the need for less readily available immunochemical techniques (such as immunoblotting, antigen-specific enzyme-linked immunosorbent assay [ELISA], and immunoprecipitation of epidermal extracts, which employ serum autoantibodies). Additionally, in pemphigoid and EBA, circulating serum autoantibodies are not detectable in as many as 50% of cases and immunochemical techniques cannot be performed (34, 42, 61). In cases without circulating autoantibodies, the only way of differentiating these disorders would be the far more difficult and expensive technique of direct immunoelectron microscopy. In some cases, when autoantibodies are not detectable by routine techniques, they can be detected by antigen-specific ELISAs. ELISAs for the detection of circulating antibodies to desmogleins 3 and 1 in pemphigus vulgaris and foliaceus patients (2, 10, 26) as well as those for the detection of antibodies to the NCA16 epitope of the BP180 antigen in bullous pemphigoid patients (35, 51) have been recently and rapidly used as an important complementary tool for management of these diseases. However, a critical correlation of ELISA results with the clinical findings and results of routine histology and immunofluorescence testing, direct and indirect, is essential to rendering an accurate diagnosis and prognosis (4, 9, 23, 62).

INDIRECT IMMUNOFLUORESCENCE

Indirect immunofluorescence is used to detect circulating autoantibodies with tissue specificity. These include antiglomerular basement (anti-GBM) and anti-tubular basement antibodies in renal disease (13, 40, 59) and bullous pemphigoid and pemphigus antibodies in skin disease (5, 7). Anti-GBM antibodies are now detected in our laboratory using Western blot analysis (see chapter 125, this volume) and/or ELISA. Patterns of reactivity of ANCA, both cytoplasmic ANCA and perinuclear ANCA, can be detected by indirect immunofluorescence, but confirmation using antigen-specific immunoassays for proteinase 3 and myeloperoxidase is required (44).

MOUNTING MEDIUM

The simplest mounting medium for immunofluorescence preparations is the one described by Coons et al. (15), which contains 9 parts glycerol and 1 part PBS. One disadvantage is that it requires that the perimeter of the coverslip be sealed using nail polish or permount, which can be troublesome to contain.

Another mounting medium, preferred by many laboratories, is polyvinyl alcohol-glycerol-PBS (50). It immobilizes the coverslip by forming a semisolid gel when it sets and allows storage for several weeks at 4°C without significant loss of fluorochrome intensity. Polyvinyl alcohol (Monsanto, St. Louis, Mo.) is a water-soluble resin. Available as Gelvatol, grade 20 to 30, it was previously referred to as Elvanol (E. I. Du Pont de Nemours and Company, Wilmington, Del.) by Goldman (24). This preparation is available commercially under the name of Aqua-Mount (Lerner Laboratories).

For most purposes, the pH of mounting medium should be neutral. However, the pH of mounting medium can be adjusted to achieve more intense fluorescence or to emphasize one color over another, which is particularly helpful in performing double staining. The green fluorescence of fluorescein is quenched at lower pHs, which accents the visualization of the red fluorescence of rhodamine; at high alkaline pHs, both fluorochromes fluoresce yellow. If slides are mounted in Gelvatol or Aqua-Mount and stored without light exposure at 4°C or frozen, the fluorescence can be preserved for at least 4 to 8 weeks and longer if the staining is intense.

Rapid fading of fluorescence after excitation is a serious limitation of immunofluorescence preparations, since it restricts reexamination of slides for further evaluation. To ensure that sufficient sections are available for interpretation and reevaluation, several can be placed on the same slide or staining can be done in duplicate. Photography can also be used to document results.

The fading of immunofluorescence slides is related to a combination of factors, including photochemical reactions, fluorochrome oxidation, and the physical and chemical properties of the fluorescein isothiocyanate (FITC) conjugate. As mentioned previously, it may be necessary to mount the specimens with a medium containing compounds to reduce fluorescence burnout, such as Permafluor (Shandon Lipshaw). The addition of reducing agents such as p-phenylenediamine and n-propylgallate to the mounting medium also retards fading (48, 56). These reducing agents are thought to suppress photodecomposition in the excited state of the fluorochrome. They have little quenching effect on rhodamine emission, which is an important consideration in double-labeling studies.

QUALITY CONTROL

Fluorescein-conjugated antibodies are available from commercial sources. The conjugate should be diluted according to the manufacturer's recommendations. Optimal dilutions of the fluorochrome conjugates are determined empirically using known positive and negative controls. The range of working dilutions for direct immunofluorescence studies using fluorochrome-labeled conjugates is usually 1:5 to 1:40 (or about 50 to 150 mg of protein/ml). The range of working dilutions for direct immunofluorescence is usually lower than that for indirect immunofluorescence because of the amplification effect. The appropriate dilution should be determined by checkerboard titrations as described by Beutner et al. (6). The correct dilution of individual lots of antibody conjugates can be estimated by determining the end-point precipitation against normal serum in Ouchterlony double immunodiffusion. The working dilution should be two to four times that of the greatest dilution that produces a precipitin line in the Ouchterlony plate after 24 h. If the dilution estimated by this method varies greatly from the manufacturer's recommendations, dilutions of the conjugate can be tested with a known positive biopsy specimen and visually inspected for optimal signal-to-background fluorescence. In any case, the laboratory should run known positive and negative tissue controls to validate the working dilutions.

The negative tissue controls for skin biopsy specimens should be sections from normal skin and should be incubated with each of the fluorescein conjugates. An additional single control specimen of normal skin, washed only with PBS and viewed without exposure to any fluorescein conjugate, should be prepared. This helps in evaluation of nonspecific fluorescence and autofluorescence from the tissue, usually not necessary in direct immunofluorescence with kidney specimens.

ANTIBODY SPECIFICITY

Specificity is an important prerequisite for the FITC-labeled antisera or antibodies used in immunofluorescence studies. Many commercial suppliers sell monospecific fluorochrome-labeled reagents that produce satisfactory results. However, confirmation of specificity and sensitivity is the responsibility of the user. Commercial suppliers of antibodies usually provide information about the specificity and sensitivity of the fluorochrome-labeled antisera, including the results of Ouchterlony immunodiffusion studies or immunoelectrophoresis analysis (46, 54). It should be noted that these techniques are not sufficiently sensitive to detect minor contaminating antibodies.

The best method for determining the specificities of FITC-labeled antisera used in diagnostic immunofluorescence kidney studies is to assess their reactivities with known positive and negative tissue controls. For example, a renal biopsy specimen from a patient with membranous glomerulonephritis that has previously been shown to contain only IgG but not IgA is very helpful in defining the specificity of a new lot of FITC-labeled anti-human IgA. Specificity can sometimes be established by blocking or absorption studies (46, 54). To block staining, the tissue is incubated with unlabeled specific antibody prior to being incubated with the specific fluorochrome-labeled antibody. Although this sometimes results in diminished fluorescence, complete prevention of staining is rarely seen. In the second approach, the tissue is incubated with specific conjugated antibody after it has been absorbed with antigen coupled to an insoluble matrix such as cyanogen-bromide-activated Sepharose-CL4B particles (21). Positive controls for Igs can include touch preparations and frozen tissue sections of tonsil or small intestine. Another useful approach is to compare old lots of antisera to new ones with respect to their abilities to detect a known antigen in archival positive cases. Rigorous proof of antibody specificity, although often required in research applications, is usually not necessary in diagnostic studies, particularly if one has evidence of specificity of a particular reagent by either immunodiffusion or electrophoresis and the reactivity and the lack of reactivity with positive and negative tissue controls, respectively.

Polyclonal antibody preparations may contain extraneous antibodies, such as anti-nuclear antibodies, because the antigenic preparation used for immunization can be contaminated with nuclear fragments. Unwanted antibodies can be removed by incubation of the antiserum with appropriate insoluble preparations, such as tissue homogenates or washed red blood cells (43). It is necessary to use insoluble antigens, since soluble complexes cannot be removed effectively by centrifugation and may bind to the tissue. One method of insolubilizing proteins is to conjugate them to cyanogen-bromide-activated Sepharose particles (Pharmacia, Uppsala, Sweden) (21).

Even antibodies directed against a purified macromolecular protein may have undesirable reactivities. For example, if intact human IgG is used to immunize an animal, the resultant antiserum will usually detect all classes of Igs because they share light chains. Such reactivity can be removed by absorbing the antibody with a preparation of light chains, as is done in the preparation of commercially available heavy-chain-specific antisera (21, 43). Cross-species antigenic similarity of Igs can result in problems in indirect immunofluorescence studies: for instance, goat anti-rabbit IgG may cross-react with human IgG. If, for example, one is attempting to detect human IgG in immune deposits by using antibodies of rabbit and goat origin as the primary and secondary antibodies, respectively, it is essential that the goat anti-rabbit IgG be absorbed with human IgG until no cross-reactivity remains. It is wise to include a control slide with deposits of human IgG, which is incubated with normal rabbit serum (diluted to the same extent as the antiserum) followed by FITC-labeled goat anti-rabbit IgG. Positive staining indicates that the goat antibodies have not been properly absorbed.

FLUORESCENCE MICROSCOPES

Fluorescence microscopy depends on the principle that certain molecules, such as fluorescein, have electrons that are readily excited to unstable higher energy states by absorbing photons of light of certain energies (32, 43). When these electrons return to a more stable energy state, they release the stored energy as light, but at a lower energy level and a longer wavelength.

This loss of energy is emitted as fluorescent light. An excitation filter is chosen to provide incident photons of optical energy at the correct wavelength, and a barrier filter is chosen to block most of the photons of excitation energy and allow only those with lower energies (the fluorescent or emitted photons) to pass through. Fluorescein is maximally excited at around 490 nm and has a peak emission at around 510 to 517 nm. FITC interference and excitation filters take advantage of the strong absorption of fluorescein at 490 nm, and when combined with a barrier filter, they block energy with a wavelength of less than 500 nm. This combination of filters results in an apple green color with fluorescein-labeled antibodies. Rhodamine is maximally excited at 500 nm, with peak emission at 580 nm, and appears cherry red with the appropriate corresponding excitation and barrier filters (24, 43).

Tissues or cells stained with fluorescein conjugates can be examined with fluorescence microscopes equipped with appropriate excitation and barrier filters. The optics is fully described by Nairn (43). The most commonly used system is that of epi-illumination, composed of a vertical illuminator and dichroic mirrors, developed by Ploem (49). The dichroic mirrors serve as both excitation and barrier filters, since they allow the passage of excitation energy in one direction and emission energy in the other. One limitation of epi-illumination is that the intensity of light at lower magnifications is considerably less than with a dark-field condenser. Another problem is that fluorescence signals of structures above or below the plane of focus result in a background glow or halo effect. This can interfere with interpretation and is frequently more of a concern with cell suspension preparations than with tissue sections. Reduction of these out-of-focus signals can be accomplished by using laser confocal microscopy (57, 58, 60) and digital deconvolution immunofluorescence studies (3, 17, 52, 53), usually not necessary for diagnostic applications but more useful for research purposes. Despite these disadvantages, there are several advantages of epi-illumination over transmitted illumination using a dark-field condenser: (i) no oil is needed; (ii) the intensity of illumination is constant, once the objective is focused so that the brightnesses of staining of different specimens can be more reliably compared; and (iii) viewing can be combined with standard-phase microscopy, which is important for cell suspension studies and for definition of morphological detail in tissue sections, and examination in double-staining studies is easier because of interchangeable FITC and rhodamine dichroic filter systems.

The light source for most fluorescence microscopes is a high-pressure mercury lamp. Illumination is very important, since the brightness of fluorescence depends on the light source, the efficiency of the fluorochrome in converting incident light into fluorescent light, and the concentration of the fluorochrome in the specimen.

EXAMINATION OF SLIDES AND EVALUATION AND RECORDING OF STAINING RESULTS

Preferably, slides should be examined on the day of staining, and a detailed record of the results should be kept on worksheets. Positive and negative controls should be run with each biopsy specimen until one gains confidence in the specificity of staining with a given fluorochrome-labeled reagent. Unexpected findings should always be confirmed before results are reported.

The fluorescence staining should be described according to location, extent, pattern, and intensity. For the glomerulus, examples of location are the mesangium (Color Plate 4) and the capillary wall, and for the skin, examples are the basement membrane zone and the intraepidermal layer. The extent of the staining should be described, usually by the terms focal or diffuse in immunofluorescence studies of the kidney. Sometimes it may be necessary to counterstain the section with 0.01% Evans blue or to stain adjacent sections with toluidine blue in order to determine the exact location of immunofluorescence staining, since morphology can sometimes be difficult to visualize. In addition to location and extent of staining, the pattern must be described. A granular pattern (Color Plate 5) is suggestive of immune complex deposition, whereas a linear pattern (Color Plate 6) is characteristic of autoantibodies bound to basement membranes, as in anti-GBM disease or bullous pemphigoid. Intensity is assessed in a subjective manner, usually on a graded scale of 0 to 4+. There is often a need to compare relative intensities of positive and background staining in control slides, particularly in screening for autoantibodies. Many factors affect intensity, principally the antiserum characteristics (dilution, avidity, and fluorescein/protein [F/P] ratio), the thickness of the section, and the light path and filter system of the fluorescence microscope.

PHOTOGRAPHY

Photography is the only permanent record one has of the immunofluorescence findings. Many immunopathology laboratories are now using a digital camera interfaced with a computer to capture fluorescence images for documentation of results. One of the most significant advantages digital imaging offers over 35-mm photography is permanent electronic storage of the image. Fewer images are required for documentation, and the costs of photographic and darkroom supplies are eliminated. Alternatively, a 35-mm camera interfaced with the fluorescence microscope can be used for documentation. Black-and-white Tri-X film (American Standards Association [ASA] 400) and high-speed Ektachrome film (ASA 400, 800, or 1,000) for color slides are recommended. Rapid processing and pushing to a higher ASA rating is possible for Ektachrome film. Exposure time is determined empirically. Cameras with automatic exposure

meters should have spot metering. Average exposure times vary from 5 to 10 s for fast (ASA 400) black-and-white film and from 30 to 60 s for ASA 400 color film. A log book in which exposure times are recorded may be useful in determining subsequent correct exposure times.

PROBLEMS AND PITFALLS

Fluorescent Reagents

High background staining often results from antibodies that are too heavily conjugated with fluorescein (F/P molar ratio, >4); these molecules adhere nonspecifically to tissue because of their net negative charge. High background staining may also be the result of partial drying of tissue sections after the staining procedure has begun. The best reagents for tissue staining are IgG fractions of FITC- or tetramethyl rhodamine isocyanate-labeled antisera recovered by DEAE-cellulose chromatography from the sera of animals that have been immunized with highly purified immunogens (25). They should contain two to four molecules of FITC per molecule of IgG. More highly labeled antisera, with F/P ratios greater than 2, are usually more suitable for detecting cell surface antigens in cell suspension studies using flow cytometry analysis.

Polyclonal monospecific fluorescein-labeled IgG antisera are available from a number of commercial companies and are generally satisfactory for diagnostic purposes. If conjugation is necessary, the dialysis method of Goldman (24) is recommended. This method of conjugation results in conjugates with low F/P ratios. Commercial conjugates are sometimes supplied in a lyophilized form and require reconstitution with distilled water or in a diluent supplied by the manufacturer, or they may come already reconstituted. Data from the supplier should include documentation of specificity, total protein concentration, antibody concentration, and the F/P ratio.

The undiluted stock antisera or antibodies can be stored at 4°C or aliquoted into volumes of 0.1 to 0.5 ml and stored frozen at −20°C until ready to be diluted. Storage should be according to the conditions specified by the manufacturer. Monoclonal antibodies are particularly sensitive to denaturation due to freeze-thawing and should be stored at 4°C or aliquoted and stored at −70°C. It is necessary to centrifuge conjugates just before using (10,000 × g for 15 min) to remove the aggregates that form as a result of storage.

Interpretation, Nonspecific Fluorescence, Autofluorescence, and Specific Fluorescence

Many proteins and structures in skin autofluoresce, and recognizing this background fluorescence is an important acquired interpretive skill. For example, elastin, elastin microfibrils, and collagen autofluoresce rather strongly. In skin, actinic damage causes a progressive increase in background fluorescence, especially along the basement membrane and around dermal blood vessels, that can obscure or even mimic specific Ig deposition. Lipofuscin granules in the sweat gland epithelium also autofluoresce orange, and the quantity of lipofuscin increases with age. In inflammatory skin lesions, vascular leakage can cause granular deposition of Igs and complement components that can mimic the findings in vasculitis cases. These changes are especially frequent in biopsy specimens from the lower extremities, presumably due to increased venous hydrostatic pressure.

Autofluorescence, caused by fluorescence found intrinsically in the tissue, is usually recognized by its color, which is generally yellow or orange with the usual FITC filter system and is easily distinguishable from the apple green of fluorescein. Examination of an unstained section can be helpful in judging autofluorescence.

As already noted, nonspecific fluorescence from a non-immunologic reaction of fluorescein-conjugated antibody with the tissue most often results from the use of FITC-labeled antibodies that are too heavily conjugated with fluorescein. Several methods can be used to remove highly charged negative molecules. The simplest involves absorption of the conjugate with tissue powder, prepared by acetone treatment and drying at 37°C (43). Alternatively, highly conjugated molecules can be removed by anion exchange (DEAE) chromatography (24, 43). Further fractionation is usually not necessary, since commercial conjugates that have already been chromatographed to obtain fractions with F/P ratios of 2 to 4 are available from a number of sources. Highly charged molecules usually precipitate in conjugates during storage at 4°C, and background or nonspecific staining may disappear in time. Other methods that can be used to prevent nonspecific fluorescence include the addition of a negatively charged molecule, such as bovine serum albumin, which competes with the conjugate for binding sites in the tissue, and prestaining of the tissue with a negative dye, such as Evans blue. Usually these procedures are not necessary for diagnostic studies. Nonspecific fluorescence can also be due to the presence of free fluorochrome in the conjugate, which can be removed by dialysis against PBS or by gel filtration using a Sephadex G-25 column (24). Another mechanism by which antibodies can bind nonspecifically to tissues or to cells in suspensions is by reaction of the Fc receptor on the surfaces of cells or of anti-IgG antibodies with aggregated IgG. Aggregated protein can be removed by ultracentrifugation (100,000 × g for 45 min). Binding by Fc receptor activity can be excluded by the use of F(ab')$_2$ or Fab fragments, both of which are available commercially for a variety of antisera. Alternatively, these fragments can be prepared by either pepsin or papain digestion, respectively, according to the method of Parham (47). F(ab')$_2$ or Fab fragments are only occasionally required for tissue immunofluorescence studies.

Specific fluorescence observed in tissue is reported with consideration of the following features: (i) the morphology and distribution of the deposits (most important is distinguishing true linear deposition from granular or globular deposits, and less important is the focal or continuous distribution of the deposition); (ii) the nature of the immunoreactant(s) detected, for example IgG versus IgA; and (iii) the localization of the deposition (for example, it is critical to distinguish between deposition of IgG on the epidermal cell surface as seen in pemphigus and deposition along the basement membrane as seen in bullous pemphigoid). As described previously, for basement membrane zone deposition, the ultrastructural localization of the immunoreactant can be inferred by salt splitting the biopsy specimen and observing the localization after epidermal separation. For a more complete description of specific fluorescence findings in skin diseases, see chapter 123, this volume.

REFERENCES

1. **Ahmed, A. R., and T. T. Provost.** 1979. Incidence of a positive lupus band test using sun-exposed and unexposed skin. *Arch. Dermatol.* **115:**228–229.
2. **Amagai, M., A. Komai, T. Hashimoto, Y. Shirakata, K. Hashimoto, T. Yamada, Y. Kitajima, K. Ohya, H. Iwanami, and T. Nishikawa.** 1999. Usefulness of enzyme-linked immunosorbent assay using recombinant desmogleins 1 and 3 for serodiagnosis of pemphigus. *Br. J. Dermatol.* **140:**351–357.
3. **Arndt-Jovin, D. J., M. Robert-Nicoud, S. J. Kaufman, and T. M. Jovin.** 1985. Fluorescence digital imaging microscopy in cell biology. *Science* **230:**247–256.
4. **Arteaga, L. A., P. S. Prisayanh, S. J. Warren, Z. Liu, L. A. Diaz, M. S. Lin, and Cooperative Group on Fogo Selvagem Research.** 2002. A subset of pemphigus foliaceus patients exhibits pathogenic autoantibodies against both desmoglein-1 and desmoglein-3. *J. Investig. Dermatol.* **118:**806–811.
5. **Beutner, E., and R. Jordan.** 1964. Demonstration of skin antibodies in sera of pemphigus vulgaris patients by indirect immunofluorescent staining. *Proc. Soc. Exp. Biol. Med.* **117:**505–510.
6. **Beutner, E., V. Kumar, S. Krajny, and T. Chorzelski.** 1987. Defined immunofluorescence in immunodermatology, p. 3–40. *In* E. Beutner, T. Chorzelski, and V. Kumar (ed.), *Immunopathology of the Skin*, 3rd ed. John Wiley & Sons, New York, N.Y.
7. **Beutner, E., R. Nisengar, and B. Albini.** 1983. Defined immunofluorescence and related cytochemical methods. *Ann. N. Y. Acad. Sci.* **420:**28–54.
8. **Burnham, T., T. Neblett, and G. Fine.** 1963. The application of fluorescent antibody technique to the investigation of lupus erythematosus and various dermatoses. *J. Investig. Dermatol.* **41:**541–556.
9. **Bystryn, J. C., A. Akman, and D. Jiao.** 1252. Limitations in enzyme-linked immunosorbent assays for antibodies against desmogleins 1 and 3 in patients with pemphigus. *Arch. Dermatol.* **138:**1252–1253.
10. **Cheng, S. W., M. Kobayashi, K. Kinoshita-Kuroda, A. Tanikawa, M. Amagai, and T. Nishikawa.** 2002. Monitoring disease activity in pemphigus with enzyme-linked immunosorbent assay using recombinant desmogleins 1 and 3. *Br. J. Dermatol.* **147:**261–265.
11. **Collins, A.** 1995. Immunofluorescence, p. 699–709. *In* R. Colvin, A. Bhan, and R. McCluskey (ed.), *Diagnostic Immunopathology*, 2nd ed. Raven Press, New York, N.Y.
12. **Collins, A., A. Bhan, J. L. Dienstag, R. Colvin, G. J. Haupert, I. Mushahwar, and R. T. McCluskey.** 1983. Hepatitis B immune complex glomerulonephritis: simultaneous glomerular deposition of hepatitis B surface and e antigens. *Clin. Immunol. Immunopathol.* **26:**137–153.
13. **Collins, A., and R. Colvin.** 2002. Kidney and lung disease mediated by anti-glomerular basement membrane antibodies: detection by western blot analysis, p. 1049–1053. *In* N. Rose, R. Hamilton, and B. Detrick (ed.), *Manual of Clinical Laboratory Immunology*, 6th ed. ASM Press, Washington, D.C.
14. **Collins, A. B., E. E. Schneeberger, M. A. Pascual, S. L. Saidman, W. W. Williams, N. Tolkoff-Rubin, A. B. Cosimi, and R. B. Colvin.** 1999. Complement activation in acute humoral renal allograft rejection: diagnostic significance of C4d deposits in peritubular capillaries. *J. Am. Soc. Nephrol.* **10:**2208–2214.
15. **Coons, A., H. Creech, R. Jones, and E. Berliner.** 1942. The demonstration of pneumococcal antigen in tissues by the use of fluorescent antibody. *J. Immunol.* **45:**159–170.
16. **Dahl, M.** 1983. Usefulness of direct immunofluorescence in patients with lupus erythematosus. *Arch. Dermatol.* **119:**1010–1017.
17. **DiGiuseppi, J., R. Inman, A. Ishihara, K. Jacoben, and B. Herman.** 1985. Applications of digitized fluorescence microscopy to problems in cell biology. *BioTechniques* **3:**394–403.
18. **Domloge-Hultsch, N., G. J. Anhalt, W. R. Gammon, Z. Lazarova, R. Briggaman, M. Welch, D. A. Jabs, C. Huff, and K. B. Yancey.** 1994. Antiepiligrin cicatricial

pemphigoid: a subepithelial bullous disorder. *Arch. Dermatol.* **130**:1521–1529.

19. **Falk, R., and J. Jennette.** 1988. Anti-neutrophil cytoplasmic autoantibodies with specificity for myeloperoxidase in patients with systemic vasculitis and idiopathic necrotizing and crescentic glomerulonephritis. *N. Engl. J. Med.* **318**:1651–1657.

20. **Fogazzi, G. B., M. Bajetta, G. Banfi, and M. Mihatsch.** 1989. Comparison of immunofluorescent findings in kidney after snap-freezing and formalin fixation. *Pathol. Res. Pract.* **158**:225–230.

21. **Fuchs, S., and M. Sela.** 1986. Immunoadsorbents, p. 16.1–16.5. *In* D. Weir (ed.), *Handbook of Experimental Immunology*, vol. 1. Blackwell Scientific Publications, Oxford, United Kingdom.

22. **Gammon, W., C. Kowaleski, and T. Chorzelski.** 1990. Direct immunofluorescence studies of sodium chloride-separated skin in the differential diagnosis of bullous pemphigoid and epidermolysis bullosa acquisita. *J. Am. Acad. Dermatol.* **22**:664–670.

23. **Giudice, G. J., K. C. Wilske, G. J. Anhalt, J. A. Fairley, A. F. Taylor, D. J. Emery, R. G. Hoffman, and L. A. Diaz.** 1994. Development of an ELISA to detect anti-BP180 autoantibodies in bullous pemphigoid and herpes gestationis. *J. Investig. Dermatol.* **102**:878–881.

24. **Goldman, M.** 1968. *Fluorescent Antibody Methods.* Academic Press, Inc., New York, N.Y.

25. **Harlow, E., and D. Lane.** 1988. *Antibodies: a Laboratory Manual*, p. 53–138. Cold Spring Harbor Laboratory, Cold Spring Harbor, N.Y.

26. **Harman, K. E., P. T. Seed, M. J. Gratian, B. S. Bhogal, S. J. Challacombe, and M. M. Black.** 2001. The severity of cutaneous and oral pemphigus is related to desmoglein 1 and 3 antibody levels. *Br. J. Dermatol.* **144**:775–780.

27. **Henderson, C.** 1989. Aminoalkylsilane: an inexpensive simple preparation for slide adhesion. *J. Histotechnol.* **12**:123–124.

28. **Hepinstall, R.** 1992. *Pathology of the Kidney.* Little, Brown & Co., Boston, Mass.

29. **Hijmans, W., and M. Schaeffer (ed.).** 1975. *Annals of the New York Academy of Sciences*, vol. 254. *Fifth International Conference on Immunofluorescence and Related Staining Techniques.* New York Academy of Sciences, New York, N.Y.

30. **Huang, W., S. Gibson, P. Facer, J. Gu, and J. Polak.** 1983. Improved section adhesion for immunochemistry using high molecular weight polymers of L-lysine as a slide coating. *Histochemistry* **77**:275–279.

31. **Johnson, G., R. Davidson, and G. McNammeeke.** 1982. Fading of immunofluorescence during microscopy. A study of the phenomenon and its remedy. *J. Immunol. Methods* **55**:231–242.

32. **Johnson, G., and E. Holborrow.** 1986. Preparation and use of fluorochrome conjugates, p. 28.1–28.15. *In* D. Weir (ed.), *Handbook of Experimental Immunology*, vol. 1. Blackwell Scientific Publications, Oxford, United Kingdom.

33. **Karnovsky, M.** 1965. A formaldehyde-glutaraldehyde fixation of high osmolality for use in electron microscopy. *J. Cell Biol.* **27**:137–138.

34. **Kelly, S., and F. Wojnarowska.** 1988. The use of chemically split tissue in the detection of circulating anti-basement membrane zone antibodies in bullous pemphigoid and cicatricial pemphigoid. *Br. J. Dermatol.* **118**:31–40.

35. **Kobayashi, M., M. Amagai, K. Kuroda-Kinoshita, T. Hashimoto, Y. Shirakata, K. Hashimoto, and T. Nishikawa.** 2002. BP180 ELISA using bacterial recombinant NC16a protein as a diagnostic and monitoring tool for bullous pemphigoid. *J. Dermatol. Sci.* **30**:224–232.

36. **Mauiyyedi, S., M. Crespo, A. B. Collins, E. E. Schneeberger, M. A. Pascual, S. L. Saidman, N. E. Tolkoff-Rubin, W. W. Williams, F. L. Delmonico, A. B.** Cosimi, and R. B. Colvin. 2002. Acute humoral rejection in kidney transplantation. II. Morphology, immunopathology, and pathologic classification. *J. Am. Soc. Nephrol.* **13**:779–787.

37. **Mauiyyedi, S., P. D. Pelle, S. Saidman, A. B. Collins, M. Pascual, N. E. Tolkoff-Rubin, W. W. Williams, A. A. Cosimi, E. E. Schneeberger, and R. B. Colvin.** 2001. Chronic humoral rejection: identification of antibody-mediated chronic renal allograft rejection by C4d deposits in peritubular capillaries. *J. Am. Soc. Nephrol.* **12**:574–582.

38. **McCluskey, R., and A. Bhan.** 1981. Immune complexes and renal diseases, p. 302–308. *In* A. Fauci (ed.), *Clinics in Immunology and Allergy.* W. B. Saunders Co., London, United Kingdom.

39. **McCluskey, R., and A. Collins.** 1983. The value of immunofluorescence in the study of renal disease, p. 302–308. *In* E. Beutner, R. Nisengard, and B. Albini (ed.), *Defined Immunofluorescence and Related Cytochemical Methods.* New York Academy of Sciences, New York, N.Y.

40. **McCluskey, R., A. Collins, and J. Niles.** 1995. Kidney, p. 109. *In* R. Colvin, A. Bhan, and R. McCluskey (ed.), *Diagnostic Immunopathology*, 2nd ed. Raven Press, New York, N.Y.

41. **Michel, B., Y. Milner, and K. David.** 1973. Preservation of tissue-fixed immunoglobulins in skin biopsies of patients with lupus erythematosus and bullous diseases—preliminary report. *J. Investig. Dermatol.* **59**:449–452.

42. **Mutasim, D., G. Anhalt, and L. Diaz.** 1987. Linear immunofluorescence staining of the cutaneous basement membrane zone produced by pemphigoid antibodies: the result of hemidesmosomes staining. *J. Am. Acad. Dermatol.* **16**:75–82.

43. **Nairn, R.** 1976. *Fluorescent Protein Tracing.* Churchill Livingstone, Edinburgh, United Kingdom.

44. **Niles, J., G. Pan, A. Collins, T. Shannon, S. Skates, R. Fienberg, M. Arnaout, and R. McCluskey.** 1991. Antigen-specific radioimmunoassays for antineutrophil cytoplasmic antibodies in the diagnosis of rapidly progressive glomerulonephritis. *J. Am. Soc. Nephrol.* **1**:27–36.

45. **Nisengar, R., M. Blaszczyk, T. Chorzelski, and E. Beutner.** 1978. Immunofluorescence of biopsy specimens: comparison of methods of transportation. *Arch. Dermatol.* **114**:1329–1332.

46. **Ouchterlony, O., and L. Nilsson.** 1986. Immunodiffusion and immunelectrophoresis, p. 32.1–32.15. *In* D. Weir (ed.), *Handbook of Experimental Immunology*, vol. 1. Blackwell Scientific Publications, Oxford, United Kingdom.

47. **Parham, P.** 1986. Preparation purification of active fragments from mouse monoclonal antibodies, p. 14.1–14.23. *In* D. Weir (ed.), *Handbook of Experimental Immunology*, vol. 1. Blackwell Scientific Publications, Oxford, United Kingdom.

48. **Platt, J., and A. Michael.** 1983. Retardation of facing and enhancement of intensity of immunofluorescence by p-phenylenediamine. *J. Histochem. Cytochem.* **31**:840–842.

49. **Ploem, J.** 1967. The use of a vertical illuminator with interchangeable dichroic mirrors for fluorescence microscopy with incidental light. *Z. Wiss. Mikrosk.* **68**:129–142.

50. **Rodriquez, J., and F. Deinhardt.** 1960. Preparation of a semi-permanent mounting medium for fluorescent antibody studies. *Virology* **12**:316–371.

51. **Sakuma-Oyama, Y., A. M. Powell, N. Oyama, S. Albert, B. S. Bhogal, and M. M. Black.** 2004. Evaluation of a BP180-NC16a enzyme-linked immunosorbent assay in the initial diagnosis of bullous pemphigoid. *Br. J. Dermatol.* **151**:126–131.

52. **Savolainen, S., K. Liewendahl, M. T. Syrjala, and J. Gripenberg.** 1992. Platelet splenic transit times in idiopathic thrombocytopenic purpura. Compartmental vs. noncompartmental model. *Int. J. Hematol.* **55**:81–87.

53. **Shakur, Y., M. Wilson, L. Pooley, M. Lobban, S. L. Griffiths, A. M. Campbell, J. Beattie, C. Daly, and M. D. Houslay.** 1995. Identification and characterization of the type-IVA cyclic AMP-specific phosphodiesterase RD1 as a membrane-bound protein expressed in cerebellum. *Biochem. J.* **306:**801–809.

54. **Stites, D.** 1982. Clinical laboratory methods for detection of antigens and antibodies, p. 325–365. *In* D. Stites, J. Stobo, H. Fudenberg, and J. Wells (ed.), *Basic and Clinical Immunology.* Lange, Los Altos, Calif.

55. **Study, C.** 1975. Uses for immunofluorescence tests of skin and sera. *Arch. Dermatol.* **11:**371–381.

56. **Valnes, K., and P. Brandtzaeg.** 1985. Retardation of immunofluorescence during microscopy. *J. Histochem. Cytochem.* **33:**755–761.

57. **White, J., W. Amos, and M. Fordham.** 1987. An evaluation of confocal versus conventional imaging of biological structures by fluorescence light microscopy. *J. Cell Biol.* **105:**41–48.

58. **Wijnaendts van Resandt, R., H. Marsman, R. Kaplan, J. Davoust, E. Stelzer, and R. Striker.** 1985. Optical fluorescence microscopy in three dimensions: microtomoscopy. *J. Microsc.* **138:**29–34.

59. **Wilson, C. B.** 1980. Radioimmunoassay for anti-glomerular basement membrane antibodies, p. 376–379. *In* N. Rose and H. Friedman (ed.), *Manual of Clinical Immunology,* 2nd ed. American Society for Microbiology, Washington, D.C.

60. **Wilson, T.** 1990. *Confocal Microscopy.* Academic Press, London, United Kingdom.

61. **Woodley, D.** 1990. Immunofluorescence on salt-split skin for the diagnosis of epidermolysis bullous acquisita. *Arch. Dermatol.* **126:**229–231.

62. **Zillikens, D., J. M. Mascaro, P. A. Rose, Z. Liu, S. M. Ewing, F. Caux, R. G. Hoffmann, L. A. Diaz, and G. J. Giudice.** 1997. A highly sensitive enzyme-linked immunosorbent assay for the detection of circulating anti-BP180 autoantibodies in patients with bullous pemphigoid. *J. Investig. Dermatol.* **109:**679–683.

INFECTIOUS DISEASES CAUSED BY BACTERIA, MYCOPLASMAS, CHLAMYDIAE, AND RICKETTSIAE

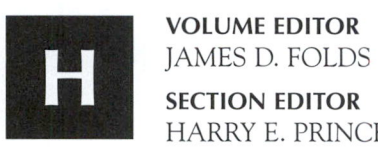

VOLUME EDITOR
JAMES D. FOLDS
SECTION EDITOR
HARRY E. PRINCE

Introduction

HARRY E. PRINCE

49

The chapters in this section describe a variety of methods and their applications for detecting infections caused by bacteria, mycoplasmas, chlamydiae, rickettsiae, and bartonellae. Most of these methods are designed to measure organism-specific antibodies; in many situations, antibody detection is still one of the most effective tools available for identifying the infecting pathogen (e.g., *Borrelia burgdorferi*, *Bartonella henselae*, and *Legionella pneumophila*). Similarly, assessment of vaccine efficacy still relies heavily on demonstrating the postvaccination presence of antibodies recognizing intrinsic components (e.g., polysaccharides of *Streptococcus pneumoniae* and *Neisseria meningitidis*) or secreted products (e.g., tetanus and diphtheria toxins) of the relevant organisms. The methods cover the entire historical range of antibody assays, ranging from gel diffusion and agglutination to complement fixation and indirect immunofluorescence to enzyme-linked immunosorbent assays and Western blotting (2).

In addition to antibody detection methods, procedures for assessing cellular immune responses to selected pathogens (e.g., *Mycobacterium tuberculosis*) are discussed. Both in vivo assays (e.g., skin testing) and in vitro assays (e.g., gamma interferon secretion) for detecting cell-mediated immune reactivity are presented.

Also described in this section are antigen detection assays, which utilize organism-specific polyclonal or monoclonal antibodies as capture and/or indicator reagents. Such assays range from direct fluorescent assays for visualization of whole organisms (e.g., *Treponema pallidum*) to enzyme immunoassays for detecting specific antigens (e.g., *Helicobacter pylori* and *Vibrio cholerae* antigens in stool).

Molecular methods for pathogen detection are increasingly performed under the auspices of the clinical immunology laboratory. Thus, relevant descriptions of such procedures are presented in this section where appropriate. Of particular note are the clinically relevant assays for detecting mycoplasmas and ureaplasmas, toxin-producing strains of *Escherichia coli*, and rickettsial infections.

A notable addition to section H in this edition is the inclusion of a chapter discussing laboratory tools useful for diagnosing *Bordetella pertussis* infections. Over the last several years, we have witnessed a profound increase in the number of recognized pertussis cases, particularly in adults (3). As increased awareness of the prevalence of pertussis reaches the general physician community, it is important to provide information on the serologic tests useful in diagnosing the illness and how these tests are interpreted.

Section H also contains a new chapter reflecting changes in our world since the last edition was published, namely, the use of anthrax as an agent of bioterrorism in the autumn of 2001 (1). This new chapter discusses assays performed at facilities that are part of the Laboratory Response Network and provides valuable practical information on specimen collection and transport.

REFERENCES

1. **Centers for Disease Control and Prevention.** 2001. Update: investigation of bioterrorism-related anthrax and interim guidelines for clinical evaluation of persons with possible anthrax. *Morb. Mortal. Wkly. Rep.* **50:** 941–948.
2. **Sever, J. L.** 1997. Major technological advances affecting clinical and diagnostic immunology. *Clin. Diagn. Lab. Immunol.* **4:**1–3.
3. **von Konig, C. H., S. Halperin, M. Riffelmann, and N. Guiso.** 2002. Pertussis in adults and infants. *Lancet Infect. Dis.* **2:**744–750.

Diagnostic Methods for Group A Streptococcal Infections

ANITA SHET AND EDWARD KAPLAN

50

Group A streptococcus, previously known as *Streptococcus pyogenes*, is a major human pathogen orchestrating a litany of infections, including common illnesses such as pharyngitis, impetigo, and scarlet fever, as well as life-threatening conditions like rheumatic fever, necrotizing fasciitis, and streptococcal toxic shock syndrome. Unique to group A streptococci is the predilection of the organisms to promote autoimmunity that results in serious nonsuppurative sequelae such as rheumatic fever/rheumatic heart disease and acute glomerulonephritis. An unexplained resurgence of severe group A streptococcal infections has been observed in the United States and Europe since the mid-1980s (1, 3) and has heightened public concern, largely because no vaccine is available, and resistance to certain antibiotics, such as macrolides, has recently emerged. Thus, there is great emphasis on the importance of accurate diagnosis of group A streptococcal infections.

Group A streptococci belong to the genus *Streptococcus*, which consists of gram-positive aerobic bacteria that microscopically appear as pairs or chains. Common to these organisms is a peptidoglycan cell wall. Based on carbohydrate antigens associated with this cell wall, Rebecca Lancefield classified beta-hemolytic streptococci into 20 serogroups, A to H and K to V (25). Furthermore, in 1928, Lancefield devised an elegant serotyping system for classifying group A streptococci based on a heat-stable surface protein called M protein (22). The ability to differentiate serotypes (and later *emm* types) of M protein allowed epidemiological association with specific infections. For example, the concept of distinct throat and skin strains arose from epidemiological studies during which it became evident that there are certain M types with a tendency to cause throat infection and rheumatic fever (M1, M3, M5, M6, M18, and M19 are termed "rheumatogenic") (14, 33), others with the propensity to cause impetigo/pyoderma and glomerulonephritis (M2, M12, M49, M57, M59, and M60 are termed "nephritogenic"), and many that are associated with invasive streptococcal infections.

Following careful clinical observation, the laboratory confirmation of acute group A streptococcal infections may be accomplished by the following:

- Microbiological culture and identification
- Rapid streptococcal antigen detection tests
- Group A streptococcal antibody tests

MICROBIOLOGICAL CULTURE AND IDENTIFICATION

A properly obtained and adequately processed culture (e.g., throat or wound swab) remains the "gold standard" for confirming the presence of group A streptococci. Typical group A streptococcal colonies grown in standard 5% sheep blood agar plates are surrounded by a clear hemolytic (beta-hemolytic) zone. Presumptive identification of group A streptococci is made by demonstrating a clear zone of inhibition around special bacitracin disks containing 0.04 IU of bacitracin. Definitive identification is done by cell wall carbohydrate grouping, which involves group A carbohydrate extraction using formamide or hydrochloric acid, followed by an antigen-antibody reaction. This precipitation reaction is done in capillary tubes using streptococcal antigen extract and group-specific antisera (commercially available or obtained from reference laboratories) (15). Rapid grouping methods involving the principle of latex agglutination (Streptex; Wellcome Diagnostics) have now largely replaced traditional grouping techniques.

M-Protein Serotyping

The M protein is a major virulence factor of group A streptococci. Antigenic differences within the hypervariable region at the N terminus constitute the basis for the Lancefield serological classification for group A streptococci. Identification of M types is accomplished using a precipitation reaction between M-protein antigen and type-specific antiserum. The antisera against the M-protein antigens are produced with whole-cell streptococcal (killed) vaccines used to immunize rabbits. M-protein antigen is extracted from streptococci using Lancefield's hot hydrochloric acid method (15). More than 80 different M types were identified by this method (23). Many group A streptococcal isolates were deemed nontypeable because of lack of expression of M protein, because of lack of reactivity of the M protein with available antisera, or, importantly, due to previously unidentified M proteins. Alternate methods for group A streptococcal characterization include the use of T-antigen agglutination and opacity factor type determination (13, 35).

Molecular Approaches to Characterization of Group A Streptococci

emm Typing

The labor-intensive nature of traditional M serotyping and the presence of nontypeable strains have led to widespread utilization of *emm* sequence typing as a method of identification of M-protein types. *emm* typing consists of sequencing the 5′ end of the group A streptococcal *emm* gene (which encodes M protein) by rapid PCR analyses using nucleotide primer pairs. The standard detailed procedure may be obtained at the Centers for Disease Control and Prevention website, http://www.cdc.gov/ncidod/biotech/strep/protocols.htm. Studies have shown excellent correlation between known M serotypes and *emm* types identified by this approach (9). There are currently 124 recognized M genotypes (9).

PFGE

Pulsed-field gel electrophoresis (PFGE) is a useful method of molecular analysis that has been used for epidemiological studies (16). Group A streptococcal DNA is treated with a restriction enzyme (*Sma*I is typically used) to generate DNA fragments, which may be separated by alternating electric fields to obtain unique patterns. These patterns may be compared during an epidemiological outbreak to study clonality or relatedness. However, there is no universally accepted PFGE typing nomenclature.

RAPID STREPTOCOCCAL ANTIGEN DETECTION TESTS FOR GROUP A STREPTOCOCCI

Rapid streptococcal antigen tests have overcome the inherent overnight delay associated with the culture method for identification of group A streptococci and have allowed clinicians to make management decisions based on laboratory data shortly after examining the patient (12). The principle of rapid antigen tests involves an acid extraction step to solubilize streptococcal group-specific cell wall carbohydrate, followed by an antigen-antibody reaction step to identify its presence. Early rapid tests used the principle of latex agglutination; in these cases group-specific rabbit immunoglobulin G (IgG) was bound to latex particles. When extracted streptococcal group antigen is mixed with these IgG-coated latex particles, visible agglutination is detected and recorded as a positive test for the presence of group A streptococcus. Further development led to more sensitive tests using the enzyme immunoassay method. Another technique for rapid antigen tests uses optical immunoassay technology and has been reported by some to offer increased sensitivity (12).

Molecular Approach to Rapid Streptococcal Antigen Detection Tests

The two latest commercially available rapid antigen detection tests employ molecular biology methods. The first is a chemiluminescent single-stranded DNA probe that detects specific rRNA sequences unique to group A streptococci and is a nucleic acid hybridization test (Group A Streptococcus Direct Test; Gen-Probe, Inc., San Diego, Calif.) (11). The second molecular rapid test combines the features of rapid PCR and real-time detection of amplified target streptococcal DNA (LightCycler Strep-A assay; Roche Applied Science, Indianapolis, Ind.) (32).

SEROLOGICAL TESTS: THE HUMAN IMMUNE RESPONSE TO GROUP A STREPTOCOCCAL ANTIGENS

The human host infected with group A streptococci produces a plethora of specific antibodies directed against both somatic and extracellular streptococcal antigens. These immune responses are summarized in Table 1. The extracellular antigens are products released by group A streptococci, whereas the cellular (or somatic) antigens form an integral part of the organism and are usually exposed on its surface (Fig. 1). Most authorities believe that compared to only a single titer of a particular streptococcal antibody, a rising titer from an acute-phase to a convalescent-phase serum sample is a more accurate reflection of a previous streptococcal infection (8). Ideally, the paired sera, obtained approximately 4 weeks apart, should be assayed simultaneously in order to demonstrate a significant rise in titer. As paired sera may be more difficult to obtain in practice, a single serum sample obtained during the illness that exceeds the upper limit of normal (ULN) is considered strongly supporting evidence of a preceding group A streptococcal infection. The ULN is defined as that titer exceeded by 20% of a normal population (34). The immune response is also influenced by myriad factors, and these are reviewed in Table 2 (17, 29).

ASO

Of the two hemolysins produced by group A streptococci, streptolysin S and streptolysin O, only the latter is antigenic. Streptolysin O acts on red blood cell membranes, inducing lysis of cells, but it also can bind to cholesterol in membranes of all eukaryotic cells. Antibody to this enzyme neutralizes its hemolytic activity. Although the anti-streptolysin O (ASO) antibody is thought to be composed of IgG, IgA (5), and IgM during the initial streptococcal infection stage (31), this has not been carefully examined in recent years. This antibody has not been shown to have a protective role against future group A streptococcal infections in the host.

Clinical Indications

The ASO test measures the host immune response to streptolysin O produced by group A streptococci and provides

---

TABLE 1 Host immune response to group A streptococcal infection

Streptococcal serological test	Antigen
Extracellular streptococcal antigen response	
ASO	Streptolysin O
Anti-DNase B	DNase B
Anti-streptococcal hyaluronidase[a]	Hyaluronidase
Antistreptokinase[a]	Streptokinase
Anti-NADase[a]	NADase
Cellular (somatic) antigen response	
M-protein antibody[a]	Type-specific M protein
Anti-A-carbohydrate[a]	Group A carbohydrate
Anti-streptococcal C5a peptidase[a]	Streptococcal C5a peptidase (group A)

[a] Not commercially available but currently used in research and reference laboratories.

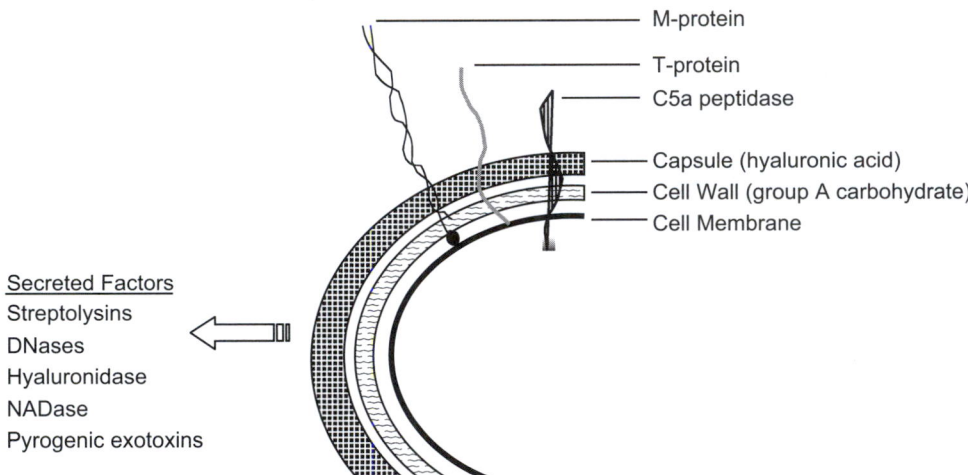

FIGURE 1 Schematic diagram of cellular and extracellular antigens of group A streptococci.

serological evidence for preceding group A streptococcal infection. The ASO test is primarily used to provide evidence of preceding streptococcal infection in patients suspected of having acute rheumatic fever or acute glomerulonephritis following throat infections. However, in acute glomerulonephritis following skin infections, it is uncommon to see an immune response to streptolysin O. The use of the ASO titer for diagnosis of an acute uncomplicated group A streptococcal infection is rarely, if ever, indicated.

ASO: Classic Hemolytic Method

The classic ASO test is based on neutralization of the hemolytic activity of the streptolysin O toxin in the presence of erythrocytes by specific ASO antibodies in the serum. The absence of specific serum antibodies or a negative ASO test would result in persistence of residual unneutralized streptolysin O and is demonstrated by hemolysis of added erythrocytes.

Specimens

Peripheral blood collected in a plain glass tube is allowed to clot. Serum is separated from clotted blood and further clarified by centrifugation of erythrocytes at $500 \times g$ for 5 min. Clear serum is transferred to a sterile storage vial and may be stored at 4°C for up to a week. For longer storage, a temperature of −70°C should be used. For shipping purposes, it is preferable to separate the serum prior to shipping.

Equipment

Equipment includes 96-well microtiter plates, micropipette and tips, multichannel pipette, test tubes, conical centrifuge tubes, and microtiter plate reading platform with mirror.

Reagents

ASO buffer: phosphate-buffered saline (commercially available, or prepare by dissolving 7.4 g of NaCl, 3.17 g of KH_2PO_4, and 1.8 g of Na_2HPO_4 in 1,000 ml of distilled water). Add 1 g of gelatin and heat to dissolve. When cooled, adjust pH to 6.5 to 6.7. Autoclave and store at 4°C.

Streptolysin O reagent (commercially available): Rehydrate using manufacturer's instructions, and use within 15 min.

ASO standards: three internal control human sera of known antibody titer (high, medium, and low titers). These can be obtained from reference laboratories.

Defibrinated erythrocytes: rabbit erythrocytes or human type O/Rh-negative fresh erythrocytes. Wash cells twice with normal saline and then with ASO buffer. Centrifuge after each wash for 10 min at $400 \times g$. Draw off supernatant and continue washing until supernatant is clear. After the final wash, resuspend erythrocytes in ASO buffer to make a 5% suspension (0.75 ml of erythrocytes and 14.25 ml of ASO buffer).

Serum dilutions: Stock dilution of 1:25 may be made by adding 0.1 ml of test or control sera and 2.4 ml of ASO buffer. This stock is inactivated at 56°C for 30 min. Further dilutions of 1:30 and 1:40 may be made as follows: 1:30 dilution, add 0.2 ml of ASO buffer and 1 ml of 1:25 stock serum dilution, and 1:40 dilution, add 0.3 ml of ASO buffer and 0.5 ml of 1:25 stock serum dilution.

TABLE 2 Factors that can influence serological response to group A streptococcal infection

Specific influence	Comment
Age of patient	Highest titers seen in children between ages 6 and 12 yr
Geography	Populations living in areas with a high incidence of streptococcal infections have higher titers (20, 21)
Site of infection (ASO only)	Higher ASO response seen in poststreptococcal upper respiratory infections than in poststreptococcal skin infections (17)
Season of the year	Titers are higher during winter and early spring months
Prompt antibiotic treatment	Reduces the streptococcal antibody response (29)

Procedure

The microtiter plate may be divided into eight sections of three by four wells, which would enable seven different serum samples to be assayed. Add 25 μl of ASO buffer to each well, except the erythrocyte control well, which should receive 50 μl. Now add 25 μl of patient's serum dilutions (1:25, 1:30, and 1:40) to the first three wells of the first row. Complete loading of all seven serum samples and control sera in the corresponding first row may be done at this point. Then make twofold serial dilutions with a multichannel pipette by transferring 25 μl row by row down the plate, discarding the 25 μl that is removed from the last row of wells. After the twofold dilutions have been completed, add 25 μl of ASO buffer to every well. Then add 25 μl of the freshly reconstituted streptolysin O reagent to all wells except the erythrocyte control well. Incubate the plate for 30 min at 37°C. Then add 25 μl of the erythrocyte suspension to every well, and reincubate for 45 min at 37°C. Centrifuge the plate at $400 \times g$ for 5 min. Place the plate on the plate reader, using a fluorescent lamp as a source of light, and examine wells for hemolysis. The last well (highest dilution) without hemolysis is noted. The ASO titer of a serum sample is equal to the reciprocal of this dilution and is expressed as Todd units or international units (depending on whether the streptolysin reagent used is the Todd standard or the World Health Organization international standard, respectively).

Interpretation

The ASO test result is considered interpretable only if the streptolysin O control well shows total hemolysis or if the erythrocyte control well shows no hemolysis, and if the reference serum standards yield titers that differ by no more than 1 dilution from the designated titer for that serum. The assay endpoint is the last well with the highest dilution showing no hemolysis. For paired acute- and convalescent-phase sera assayed simultaneously, a difference of 0.2 log or a difference of two wells between the titers of the two sera is accepted as a minimum for a significant difference. If one serum sample is assayed, the elevated titer should exceed the ULN, as described above. Table 3 shows the age-stratified ULNs of ASO and anti-DNase B in children and adults residing in the United States (20, 21). Ideally, these values must be established separately within each population and geographic area. In patients with group A streptococcal infections, the ASO response can usually be demonstrated after 1 week, with the maximal response being reached 3 to 6 weeks after the infection (19). The ASO titer may begin to decline 6 to 8 weeks after infection, although in some patients the titer may remain elevated for indefinite periods (19). About 20% of infected individuals do not respond with elevated ASO titers (34). Thus, a negative ASO test alone cannot be used to rule

out rheumatic fever or other streptococcal sequelae, and additional antibody tests (e.g., anti-DNase B test) may be used. False elevation of ASO titer may occur due to the presence of lipids in serum, which can act as nonspecific inhibitors of streptolysin O. Freezing and thawing of sera may destabilize lipoproteins, which may alter the titer. Group C and G streptococcal infections can also result in elevated titers, as these groups produce streptolysin O.

More recently, alternative methods for ASO determination have become commercially available. Latex agglutination is one such method, in which latex particles coated with streptolysin O can react with ASO antibodies in the serum. Agglutination occurs when the level of antibody in serum is greater than 200 IU/ml. The advantages of this method include quick testing time and decreased complexity in its execution. However, documentation on the accuracy and precision of the assay is incomplete.

ASO Determinations Using Nephelometry

Nephelometry has been introduced as a simple, rapid procedure for quantitative measurement of ASO titers. The principle of nephelometry is based on the ability to measure the rate of increase in light intensity scattered from particles suspended in solution as a result of complexes formed during an antigen-antibody reaction (6, 7, 28). In the performance of the ASO test, purified recombinant streptolysin O is added to the patient's serum. ASO in the serum sample binds with recombinant streptolysin O, forming complexes resulting in an increase in light scatter that is converted into a peak rate signal. This signal is a function of the serum ASO concentration. Following calibration, the signal is converted to concentration units by the analyzer. All reagents and instrumentation are supplied by the manufacturer (Beckman Coulter IMMAGE Immunochemistry System) (6, 7). Results are reported in ASO international units (per milliliter) and are extrapolated from values measured by the classic hemolytic method previously described.

Comment: Nephelometry has replaced the classic hemolytic method for streptococcal antibody determination in many clinical laboratories. This is an automated method, and less technical expertise is required in its performance. It is also less expensive when performed in large numbers. At present, data regarding correlation between the nephelometric and hemolytic methods are incomplete (17, 27). Furthermore, comprehensive definition of a significant rise in ASO titer and data regarding the ULNs for different populations have yet to be determined independently using nephelometry.

Anti-DNase B Test

Of the four DNases (DNases A, B, C, and D) produced by group A streptococci, DNase B is the most immunogenic following infection (34). Clinical indications for the performance of the anti-DNase B test are essentially those cited for the ASO test. However, unlike ASO, infection of the skin produces a brisk anti-DNase B response. Thus, the anti-DNase B test is more reliable than the ASO test in providing evidence for a preceding streptococcal infection in patients with sequelae following pyoderma (17). The anti-DNase B test is also used as an additional streptococcal antibody test for patients with suspected rheumatic fever who may show no ASO response after upper respiratory tract infection.

Classic Methyl Green Dye anti-DNase B Test

The classic anti-DNase B assay is based on the fact that antibodies to DNase B neutralize the enzymatic activity of DNase B, preventing it from depolymerizing DNA that has

TABLE 3 Examples of age-stratified ULNs of ASO and anti-DNase B in children and adults residing in United States: a guideline

Age (yr)	ULN	
	ASO	Anti-DNase B
2–5	120–160[a]	240–320[a]
6–9	240[a]	480–640[a]
10–12	320[a]	480–640[a]
13–15	170[b]	170[b]
Adult	85[b]	85[b]

[a] From reference 20.
[b] From reference 21.

been coupled to an indicator dye. DNase activity can be detected by incubating the enzyme with calf thymus DNA, which is conjugated to methyl green dye. The DNA-dye complex remains greenish unless the enzyme degrades the DNA, in which case the substrate then turns colorless. The reciprocal of the highest dilution of serum that shows definite inhibition of enzyme activity represents the antibody titer for that serum.

Reagents

Tris dilution buffer: Dissolve 1,021 g of Tris, 362 mg of $MgSO_4$, 333 mg of $CaCl_2$, and 1 g of gelatin in 1,000 ml of distilled water. Heat to dissolve gelatin, cool, and adjust pH to 7.6.

Tris inactivation buffer: Add 0.6 g of NaCl to 100 ml of Tris buffer, mix, and filter with a Millipore membrane. Store at 4°C.

Anti-DNase B standards, DNase B, calf thymus DNA, methyl green dye, and imidazole: commercially available.

Serum dilutions: as described for the ASO method using Tris buffer. Stock dilution may be inactivated at 63°C for 30 min.

Procedure

The microtiter plate may be divided into eight sections of three by four wells, which would enable six test sera and two control sera to be assayed. Add 25 μl of Tris buffer to each well, except the DNA substrate control well, which should receive 50 μl. Now add 25 μl of patient's serum dilutions (1:25, 1:30, and 1:40) to the first three wells of the first row. Complete loading of all six test sera and control sera in the corresponding first row may be done at this point. Then make twofold serial dilution with a multichannel pipette by transferring 25 μl row by row down the plate, discarding the 25 μl that is removed from the last row of wells. After the twofold dilutions have been completed, add 25 μl of DNase B to all wells except the DNA-methyl green substrate well. Incubate the plate for 15 min at 37°C. Then add 50 μl of DNA-methyl green substrate to every well, and reincubate for 20 h at 37°C. Read and record the results.

Interpretation

DNase activity on the DNA-methyl green conjugate is reflected by digestion of DNA and depolymerization of the colored complex, resulting in loss of blue-green color in the substrate. This represents the end point of antibody neutralization (27). The color gradation is assigned a range from 0 (no color) to 4+ (strongest color). The enzyme control should be 0 and the substrate control should be 4+. The last well (highest dilution) with a reading of 4+ or 3+ is the end point, and the reciprocal of its titer represents the anti-DNase B value in units per milliliter.

Anti-DNase B: Nephelometry

Anti-DNase B can also be quantitated by nephelometry. The principles are the same as described above; purified DNase B is added to serum to form immune complexes that result in change in light scatter, which is subsequently measured (6, 7). As before, the results are reported in units per milliliter, which are extrapolated from values obtained by the classic method. As with ASO measurements, further studies to correlate the two methods for anti-DNase B measurement need to be performed, especially in defining a ULN and a significant rise in anti-DNase B titer.

Anti-A-Carbohydrate Test

Studies have suggested a specific correlation between persistence of serum antibody against group A carbohydrate and the presence of rheumatic carditis and rheumatic mitral valve disease, with elevated levels of anti-A-carbohydrate being reported for individuals with rheumatic heart disease (2). At present only a very few laboratories are performing this test, and these determinations are for research purposes. Information about required reagents and the procedure for performing the anti-A-carbohydrate test may be obtained from the literature (4).

Group A Streptococcal Antihyaluronidase Test

The streptococcal antihyaluronidase determination is an enzyme neutralization test in which the antigen used is streptococcal hyaluronidase elaborated by the bacteria (26). However, this test is no longer commercially available and is now usually performed only in reference or research laboratories.

Anti-M-Protein Antibodies

Following group A streptococcal infection, the host produces antibodies against type-specific streptococcal M protein. These antibodies have opsonic properties and have been shown to correlate with protection against group A streptococcal infection (24). M-protein antibodies appear slowly, over a period of several months. These antibodies have been shown to consist of both IgA and IgG subclasses that play a role in inhibiting streptococcal adherence to pharyngeal cells and in preventing internalization of the organism into pharyngeal epithelial cells, respectively (10). The indirect bactericidal test is used for detecting the antibodies and is based on the antiphagocytic effect of streptococcal M protein and its neutralization by type-specific antibody (15). This test is used only in research laboratories, especially in studies of M-protein vaccines, and has limited clinical use.

Other streptococcal antibody tests are streptokinase and NADase, but the availability of these is limited to research laboratories. The recently reported antibody to group A streptococcal C5a peptidase (30) has been shown to parallel the rise of ASO during acute streptococcal pharyngitis, but at the present time this is a research test with limited clinical applicability.

CONCLUSION

Several microbiological tests are available for accurate diagnosis of group A streptococcal infection. While classic culture methods remain the "gold standard" for determining the presence of group A streptococci, rapid antigen detection methods have gained popularity in many clinical settings due to their efficiency and ease of performance. However, a confirmatory group A streptococcal culture is still recommended as a backup for a negative rapid antigen test result. It should be emphasized that the most common clinically used streptococcal antibody tests (ASO and anti-DNase B) provide evidence only for a preceding group A streptococcal infection. Together with clinical findings the tests may support the diagnosis of sequelae to group A streptococcal infection, but they are not by themselves diagnostic of these clinical conditions.

REFERENCES

1. **Active Bacterial Core Surveillance.** Active Bacterial Core Surveillance (ABCs) Report, group A streptococcus, 2003—preliminary. Emerging Infections Program Network, http://www.cdc.gov/ncidod/dbmd/abcs/survreports.htm (Accessed 2 October 2004.)

2. **Appleton, R. S., B. E. Victorica, D. Tamer, and E. M. Ayoub.** 1985. Specificity of persistence of antibody to the streptococcal group A carbohydrate in rheumatic valvular heart disease. *J. Lab. Clin. Med.* **105:**114–119.

3. **Ayoub, E. M.** 1992. Resurgence of rheumatic fever in the United States. The changing picture of a preventable illness. *Postgrad. Med.* **92:**133–136, 139–142.

4. **Ayoub, E. M., and E. Harden.** 1997. Immune response to streptococcal antigens: diagnostic methods, p. 409–417. *In* P. R. Murray, E. J. Baron, M. A. Pfaller, F. C. Tenover, and R. H. Yolken (ed.), *Manual of Clinical Microbiology*, 7th ed. American Society for Microbiology, Washington, D. C.

5. **Barbosa, S. F., P. M. Nakamura, and S. Hoshino-Shimizu.** 1996. Detection of antibody isotypes to streptolysin O by dot ELISA. *Braz. J. Med. Biol. Res.* **29:**763–767.

6. **Beckman Coulter IMMAGE Immunohistochemistry Systems.** Antideoxyribonuclease O: chemistry information sheet. April 2004. http://www.beckman.com/customersupport/IFU/cis/988630/AB/EN_ASO.pdf. (Accessed 15 September 2004.)

7. **Beckman Coulter IMMAGE Immunohistochemistry Systems.** Antideoxyribonuclease B: chemistry information sheet. http://www.beckman.com/customersupport/IFU/cis/988630/AB/EN_DNB.pdf. (Accessed 15 September 2004.)

8. **Dajani, A., K. Taubert, P. Ferrieri, and S. Shulman for the Committee on Rheumatic Fever, Endocarditis, and Kawasaki Disease of the Council on Cardiovascular Disease in the Young, The American Heart Association.** 1995. Treatment of acute streptococcal pharyngitis and prevention of rheumatic fever: a statement for health professionals. *Pediatrics* **96:**758–764.

9. **Facklam, R. F., D. R. Martin, M. Lovgren, D. R. Johnson, A. Efstratiou, T. A. Thompson, S. Gowan, P. Kriz, G. J. Tyrrell, E. Kaplan, and B. Beall.** 2002. Extension of the Lancefield classification for group A streptococci by addition of 22 new M protein gene sequence types from clinical isolates: emm103 to emm124. *Clin. Infect. Dis.* **34:**28–38.

10. **Fluckiger, U., K. F. Jones, and V. A. Fischetti.** 1998. Immunoglobulins to group A streptococcal surface molecules decrease adherence to and invasion of human pharyngeal cells. *Infect. Immun.* **66:**974–979.

11. **GenProbe.** Group A Streptococcus Direct Test. Product information sheet, 2001. Gen-Probe Inc., San Diego, Calif. http://www.gen-probe.com/pdfs/pi/103887.pdf. (Accessed 15 September 2004.)

12. **Gerber, M. A., and S. T. Shulman.** 2004. Rapid diagnosis of pharyngitis caused by group A streptococci. *Clin. Microbiol. Rev.* **17:**571–580, table of contents.

13. **Johnson, D., and E. Kaplan.** 1993. A review of the correlation of T-agglutination patterns and M-protein typing and opacity factor production in the identification of group A streptococci. *J. Med. Microbiol.* **38:**311–315.

14. **Johnson, D., D. Stevens, and E. Kaplan.** 1992. Epidemiologic analysis of group A streptococcal serotypes associated with severe systemic infections, rheumatic fever, or uncomplicated pharyngitis. *J. Infect. Dis.* **166:**374–382.

15. **Johnson, D. R., E. L. Kaplan, J. Sramek, R. Bicova, J. Havlicek, H. Havlickova, J. Motlova, and P. Kriz.** 1996. Laboratory diagnosis of group A streptococcal infections. World Health Organization, Geneva, Switzerland.

16. **Johnson, D. R., J. T. Wotton, A. Shet, and E. L. Kaplan.** 2002. A comparison of group A streptococci from invasive and uncomplicated infections: are virulent clones responsible for serious streptococcal infections? *J. Infect. Dis.* **185:**1586–1595.

17. **Kaplan, E., B. Anthony, S. Chapman, E. Ayoub, and L. Wannamaker.** 1970. The influence of the site of infection on the immune response to group A streptococci. *J. Clini. Investig.* **49:**1405–1414.

18. **Kaplan, E., S. Chan, P. Ness, and R. Creager.** 1992. Quantitation of ASO titers using rate nephelometry in comparison to the classical hemolytic inhibition assay. *Proc. 32nd Intersci. Conf. Antimicrob. Agents Chemother.*, abstr. 1128.

19. **Kaplan, E., P. Ferrieri, and L. Wannamaker.** 1974. Comparison of the antibody response to streptococcal cellular and extracellular antigens in acute pharyngitis. *J. Pediatr.* **84:**21–28.

20. **Kaplan, E. L., C. D. Rothermel, and D. R. Johnson.** 1998. Antistreptolysin O and anti-deoxyribonuclease B titers: normal values for children ages 2 to 12 in the United States. *Pediatrics* **101:**86–88.

21. **Klein, G. C., C. N. Baker, and W. L. Jones.** 1971. "Upper limits of normal" antistreptolysin O and antideoxyribonuclease B titers. *Appl. Microbiol.* **21:**999–1001.

22. **Lancefield, R.** 1928. The antigenic complex of streptococcus haemolyticus. I. Demonstration of a type-specific substance in extracts of streptococcus haemolyticus. *J. Exp. Med.* **47:**91–103.

23. **Lancefield, R. C.** 1962. Current knowledge of type-specific M antigens of group A streptococci. *J. Immunol.* **89:**307–313.

24. **Lancefield, R. C.** 1959. Persistence of type specific antibodies in man following infection with group A streptococci. *J. Exp. Med.* **110:**271–292.

25. **Lancefield, R. C.** 1933. A serological differentiation of human and other groups of hemolytic streptococci. *J. Exp. Med.* **57:**571–595.

26. **Murphy, R. A.** 1972. Improved antihyaluronidase test applicable to the microtitration technique. *Appl. Microbiol.* **23:**1170–1171.

27. **Nelson, J., E. Ayoub, and L. Wannamaker.** 1968. Streptococcal anti-deoxyribonuclease B: micro-technique determination. *J. Lab. Clin. Med.* **71:**867–873.

28. **Pacifico, L., G. Mancuso, E. Properzi, G. Ravagnan, A. M. Pasquino, and C. Chiesa.** 1995. Comparison of nephelometric and hemolytic techniques for determination of antistreptolysin O antibodies. *Am. J. Clin. Pathol.* **103:**396–399.

29. **Rantz, L. A., P. J. Boisvert, and W. W. Spink.** 1946. Hemolytic streptococcal sore throat: antibody response following treatment with penicillin, sulphadiazine, and salicylates. *Science* **103:**352–353.

30. **Shet, A., E. L. Kaplan, D. R. Johnson, and P. P. Cleary.** 2003. Immune response to group A streptococcal C5a peptidase in children: implications for vaccine development. *J. Infect. Dis.* **188:**809–817.

31. **Sonozaki, H., S. Takizawa, and M. Torisu.** 1970. Immunoglobulin analysis of anti-streptolysin-O antibody. *Clin. Exp. Immunol.* **7:**519–531.

32. **Uhl, J. R., S. C. Adamson, E. A. Vetter, C. D. Schleck, W. S. Harmsen, L. K. Iverson, P. J. Santrach, N. K. Henry, and F. R. Cockerill.** 2003. Comparison of LightCycler PCR, rapid antigen immunoassay, and culture for detection of group A streptococci from throat swabs. *J. Clin. Microbiol.* **41:**242–249.

33. **Wannamaker, L.** 1970. Differences between streptococcal infections of the throat and of the skin. *N. Engl. J. Med.* **282:**23–31, 78–85.

34. **Wannamaker, L., and E. Ayoub.** 1960. Antibody titers in acute rheumatic fever. *Circulation* **21:**598–614.

35. **Widdowson, J., W. Maxted, and D. Grant.** 1970. The production of opacity in serum by group A streptococci and its relationship with the presence of M antigen. *J. Gen. Microbiol.* **61:**343–353.

Immune Responses to Polysaccharide and Conjugate Vaccines

CARL E. FRASCH

51

Most invasive bacterial disease in humans results from encounters with encapsulated bacterial pathogens. For this reason polysaccharide (PS) vaccines have been licensed for protection against several serious bacterial infections, including those caused by *Neisseria meningitidis, Streptococcus pneumoniae, Haemophilus influenzae* type b (Hib), and *Salmonella enterica* serovar Typhi. A problem with most native PSs is that they induce a poor immune response in children under 2 years of age, making young children particularly susceptible to invasive disease caused by these organisms. For this reason, conjugate vaccines were developed. The first conjugate against Hib was licensed in 1987. While Hib, meningococcal, and pneumococcal conjugate vaccines are now in general use in young children, PS vaccines are still widely used in older children and adults. The antibody responses to the Hib, meningococcal, pneumococcal, and typhoid Vi PSs are discussed below, whether induced by immunization with PS or conjugate vaccines.

The presently U.S.-licensed bacterial PS and conjugate vaccines are listed in Tables 1 and 2 and are the focus of this chapter. Estimation of antibody concentrations and measurements of functional antibody are critical to our understanding of PS-induced immunity. Information on quantitative immunoassays for anti-PS antibodies is presented. Discussions of methods for functional assays are presented in another chapter of this book.

IMMUNOLOGY OF THE ANTIBODY RESPONSE TO BACTERIAL PSs

Serum antibody in concert with the complement system plays a central role in protection against invasive diseases caused by encapsulated bacterial pathogens, whether primarily by direct killing (bactericidal antibody) or by opsonophagocytosis (opsonic antibody).

The humoral immune response to bacterial PSs is clonally restricted compared to the response to protein antigens. Within individual adults the serum antibody response to pneumococcal and other PSs derives from a small number of dominant B-cell clones. The reason is likely that PSs express relatively few epitopes that would not be recognized as self. A clonally restricted immune response means that any one individual will likely have an antibody response restricted to a very small number of epitopes on any given PS.

A widely held premise is that PSs are T-cell-independent immunogens and thus do not induce immunologic memory.

This is based largely upon studies with short-lived animal species (mostly mice) and young children. While a single exposure to a PS vaccine may not induce immunologic memory, there is evidence for immunologic memory responses to bacterial PSs in adults (5). Epitopes present on a bacterial PS can be widely shared among different cross-reactive PS structures, and repeated exposure to epitopes on these PS structures can induce immunologic memory. Unlike children, adults have had repeated exposure to meningococcal and pneumococcal PSs complexed with other bacterial components, and this repeated exposure appears to induce B-cell memory. In children, immunization with a PS-protein conjugate vaccine primes for a booster response upon reexposure to the bacterium-associated PS (43, 70). By comparison, adults generally respond to a similar magnitude to PS presented as either the native PS or a conjugate, though conjugates generally stimulate somewhat higher antibody concentrations (68).

QUANTITATION OF ANTI-PS ANTIBODIES BY ELISA

In an assessment of naturally occurring levels of antibody to encapsulated bacteria and evaluation of the immune response to PS or conjugate vaccines, one should consider both antibody quantitation and measures of biological (functional) activity. Quantitation of anti-PS antibody is important, because as the type-specific antibody concentration increases, the risk of invasive disease on a population basis due to that bacterial strain decreases. The functional activity measured should correlate with a known mechanism of protection.

Antibody concentrations should be determined using conditions such that immunoglobulin G (IgG) specific for a serogroup or serotype is measured. This requires careful control of assay conditions, use of purified PSs, and application of cross-absorptions to verify antibody specificity. The enzyme-linked immunosorbent assay (ELISA) is now the most commonly used method for quantitation of antibody concentration. Where possible these concentrations should be measured as micrograms of specific antibody per milliliter. To facilitate accurate and comparable quantitative anti-Hib, antimeningococcal, and antipneumococcal antibody measurements in different laboratories, reference sera have been produced and characterized (21, 46, 54), and they are now in international use. Antibody concentrations in these reference sera are shown in Table 3.

TABLE 1 Bacterial PS vaccines licensed in the United States

Vaccine type	Manufacturer	PS(s) included	Dose
Meningococcal	Aventis Pasteur	A, C, Y, W135	50 μg/PS
Pneumococcal	Merck & Co.[a]	1, 2, 3, 4, 5, 6B, 7F, 8, 9N, 9V, 10A, 11A, 12F, 14, 15B, 17A, 18C, 19F, 19A, 20, 22F, 23F, 33F	25 μg/PS
Typhoid	Aventis Pasteur	Vi	25 μg

[a] In December 2002, Wyeth Vaccines discontinued production of their pneumococcal 23-valent PS vaccine.

TABLE 2 Bacterial PS-protein conjugate vaccines licensed in the United States

Vaccine type	Manufacturer	PS(s) included	Dose
Hib	Aventis Pasteur Wyeth Merck & Co.	b	7.5–10 μg/PS
Pneumococcal	Wyeth	4, 6B, 9V, 14, 18C, 19F, 23F	2 μg/PS (4 μg for 6B)
Meningococcal[a]	Baxter Chiron Wyeth	C	10 μg
	Aventis Pasteur	A, C, Y, w13S	4 μg/PS

[a] The meningococcal conjugate was first licensed in the United Kingdom, and only the 4-valent conjugate is licensed in the United States.

TABLE 3 Human reference sera for ELISA[a]

Bacterial species	Serum designation	PS type/group	Antibody concn (μg/ml)			Reference
			IgG	IgM	IgA	
H. influenzae	1983	b	60.9	3.5	5.6	46
N. meningitidis	CDC1992	A	91.8	23.9	20.1	21
		C	24.1	2.0	5.9	21
		Y	31.8	2.9	3.7	21
		W135	16.2	1.4	2.5	21
S. pneumoniae	89SF	1	6.3	1.7	1.4	54
		2	12.2	5.1	3.9	52
		3	2.4	0.6	4.3	54
		4	4.1	1.4	1.2	54
		5	5.8	4.2	1.2	54
		6B	16.9	3.0	1.5	54
		7F	5.2	1.9	1.1	54
		8	5.1	2.0	2.0	52
		9N	7.8	2.4	2.1	52
		9V	6.9	1.6	1.7	54
		10A	6.8	3.9	1.2	52
		11A	6.4	1.0	0.9	52
		12F	1.7	1.4	0.4	52
		14	27.8	1.2	1.9	54
		15B	16.6	1.6	3.2	52
		17F	10.1	1.7	0.8	52
		18C	4.5	1.3	0.8	54
		19A	18.6	2.3	3.3	52
		19F	13.0	3.2	2.0	54
		20	8.7	1.7	0.6	52
		22F	10.1	3.1	3.6	52
		23F	8.1	0.7	1.3	54
		33F	11.9	2.6	2.5	52

[a] Internationally recognized sera used for quantitation of anti-PS antibodies in human sera.

The human Hib reference serum, lot 1983, is a serum pool from 15 adult plasma donors who were immunized with the purified Hib PS (61). These adults received the Hib PS vaccine as part of a three-vaccine immunization series for preparation of bacterial PS immune globulin, also called BPIG. Plasma recovered from these individuals was converted to serum and then pooled. The resulting pool contained 70.0 μg of total anti-Hib PS antibody per ml, determined by comparison with an earlier Hib reference serum, Stan Klein, using a radioimmunoassay method.

The meningococcal PS reference serum pool, CDC1992, was prepared from plasma obtained from 18 adults that received the ACYW135 PS vaccine (21). A total of 24 adults at the Centers for Disease Control and Prevention were immunized with the Aventis Pasteur PS vaccine Menomune. Test sera were obtained after vaccination and assayed for anti-meningococcal PS antibody by ELISA. Eighteen of the individuals were then subjected to plasmapheresis. The pooled plasma was converted to serum. Antibody assignments were made using the cross-standardization method described by Concepcion and Frasch (15).

The pneumococcal PS reference serum pool, 89SF (also called 89S), was prepared from plasma obtained from 17 adults immunized with the 23-valent pneumococcal PS vaccine produced by Lederle Laboratories. These plasma units were selected from among units from 68 immunized plasma donors as being high in anti-pneumococcal PS antibody. The donors were originally immunized to produce BPIG (61), but their plasma units were used instead to produce the reference serum 89S described by Quataert et al. (54). The plasma units were pooled and then converted to serum. Antibody assignments were made by using a reference antigen capture ELISA, the reference antigen being immunoglobulin molecules from the U.S. National Reference Preparation of serum proteins, batch IS 1644, which were captured by light chain-specific antibody previously attached to the ELISA plates. Isotype-specific second-antibody–enzyme conjugates were used. Some antibody concentrations for selected pneumococcal types were confirmed by quantitative precipitation (54). Concepcion and Frasch later confirmed most of the results of Quataert et al. using a cross-standardization ELISA method (15).

General ELISA Method for Bacterial PS

It is important to absorb the PS to the plastic surface of the microtitration plate such that the PS retains its native conformation. Pyrogen-free water should be used for preparation of the antigen coating solution to avoid nonspecific antibody binding to lipopolysaccharides. The most straightforward approach would be to use the native PS as the coating antigen, but PSs do not absorb to plastic surfaces as efficiently as proteins. Since PSs are essentially never 100% pure, one should use the minimum amount necessary for antigen coating to obtain sufficient signal and sensitivity. To be able to use low concentrations of the native PS and yet have uniform attachment, Arakere and Frasch utilized methylated human serum albumin (mHSA) to facilitate attachment of negatively charged PSs and those having hydrophobic groups. The chemical treatment used to prepare the mHSA converts nearly all free carboxyl groups to methyl groups, leaving the protein positively charged and hydrophobic due to the methyl groups (3). One to 5 μg of PS per ml can be used when a negatively charged PS is admixed with mHSA for plate coating, whereas direct absorption of the PS may require 10 to 20 μg of PS per ml and uniform well-to-well attachment may not be achieved.

Another approach to attaching bacterial PSs to ELISA plates with high binding efficiency is to use chemically modified PSs (conjugates), as has been done for Hib (52). However, a potential problem with this approach is possible generation of new antibody-reactive epitopes. This has been shown to be the case with some pneumococcal PSs and the group B streptococcal type III PS (7). In general it is best to avoid activation methods that have the potential to break carbon-carbon bonds, as occurs when sodium periodate is used to create the reactive aldehyde groups needed for attachment of the PS to the amino groups of a protein or peptide.

Historically, Hib PS antibodies have been measured by radioimmunoassay, but the recommended assay method is now an ELISA based upon the method described by Phipps et al. (52). This ELISA utilizes Hib oligosaccharides conjugated by reductive amination to human serum albumin (also called HbO-HA) and has been standardized (45). The reference serum is lot 1983 with 70 μg of total anti-Hib PS antibody per ml. The isotype breakdown within the total antibody is as follows: IgG, 60.9 μg/ml; IgA, 5.6 μg/ml; and IgM, 3.5 μg/ml.

The limit of antibody detection using the HbO-HA ELISA is approximately 0.05 μg/ml. An alternative approach for coating the 96-well ELISA plate is to use a mixture of 5 μg of native Hib PS per ml and 2.5 μg of mHSA per ml in phosphate-buffered saline, pH 7.4. The mechanism of PS attachment using mHSA is a combination of hydrophobic and charge interactions between the PS and mHSA (3). Using the mHSA method with the native PS, the limit of anti-PS antibody quantitation is approximately 0.15 μg/ml.

PS antigens used in ELISA are often taken from bulk PS stocks used in production of licensed PS vaccines and are thus purified to the purity requirements for the vaccine. In general, the requirements are <1 to 2% contamination for both protein and nucleic acids. The Hib, meningococcal, and serovar Typhi PSs will also contain small amounts of lipopolysaccharide, while the pneumococcal PSs will contain about 5% of a common PS, the C PS, relative to the type PS content. For this reason it is critical that an anti-PS ELISA be carefully evaluated for specificity. This should be done by absorption with a heterologous type PS from the same bacterial species. For example, one can use meningococcal group Y PS to determine the specificity of meningococcal group C PS antibodies. The heterologous PS should remove less than 20% of the antibody reactivity. To achieve the required specificity it may be necessary to preabsorb the sera with the heterologous PS. It is likely that the specificity of measurements of antibody to the meningococcal and Vi PSs could be improved by preabsorption with meningococcal and serovar Typhi lipopolysaccharides, respectively.

To achieve the needed specificity in the pneumococcal ELISA it is necessary to absorb test sera with purified C PS and with a heterologous pneumococcal PS (16). The heterologous PS that has generally been used is the type 22F PS. C PS absorption removes most of the non-type-specific cross-reacting antibody, but the 22F PS removes antibodies to another common antigen, possibly the site of covalent attachment of the C PS to the type PS. In my laboratory, I am able to avoid the preadsorption steps by the addition of about 1 to 2 μg of the absorbent(s) per ml to the buffer used to dilute the serum samples, with subsequent overnight incubation of the test sera on antigen-coated plates. A detailed ELISA protocol for the pneumococcal ELISA can be downloaded from the website http://www.vaccine.uab.edu.

FUNCTIONAL ASSAYS FOR ANTI-PS ANTIBODY

Use of functional assays is important, and the functional assay used should be a surrogate for the known protective function of anti-PS antibodies, either naturally induced or stimulated by vaccination. The methodology for the bactericidal and opsonophagocytic assays is described by Nahm and Lorenz in chapter 37 of this volume.

Although the words *correlate* and *surrogate* are at times used interchangeably, this is not correct. A correlate is when two variables are related where variation in one is accompanied by a linear variation in the other. A surrogate takes the place of something else. In the case of meningococcal disease it is clear that protection is mediated by the presence of bactericidal antibody, but not necessarily only by such antibodies, and that anti-PS antibodies are sufficient to protect against disease. Thus, in vitro measurements of bactericidal antibody can be considered a surrogate for in vivo protection. Furthermore, we know that anti-PS antibody is bactericidal in vitro and that these antibodies are largely IgG. From this, measuring the amount of anti-PS IgG antibody by ELISA is a correlate of protection and will correlate with bactericidal antibody titers.

The presence or induction of bactericidal antibody is predictive of protection against meningococcal disease. The studies by Goldschneider et al. showed that the presence of detectable bactericidal antibodies using human serum as the complement source was sufficient to protect against invasive serogroup-specific meningococcal disease (26). A group C meningococcal conjugate vaccine is licensed in a number of countries (not the United States) for use in infants and children. The approval was based upon the ability of the group C conjugate vaccine to induce bactericidal antibodies (10). During the United Kingdom clinical evaluation of the vaccine, the investigators utilized a bactericidal assay using baby rabbit serum as the complement source and were able to define bactericidal titers that predicted protection against group C meningococcal disease. Bactericidal titers of <1:8 reliably predicted susceptibility, and titers of 1:128 or greater were highly predictive of protection. Prevalence studies of meningococcal serogroup C bactericidal antibody in the United Kingdom showed an inverse relationship between disease incidence and prevalence of bactericidal antibody akin to the classic studies by Goldschneider et al. (26, 66). Thus, using rabbit complement, antibody titers of 1:8 or greater correlated best on a population basis with low disease incidence.

Serotype-specific opsonic antibodies protect against invasive pneumococcal disease, but little information is available regarding the amount of opsonic antibody needed for protection. Similarly, it is likely that serum bactericidal antibody against the Vi PS protects against typhoid fever, but the relevant titer has not been established (56).

INTERPRETATION OF ANTIBODY RESPONSE DATA FOR SPECIFIC BACTERIAL PSs

Hib PS

Hib was the leading cause of invasive bacterial disease in children under the age of 5 years in most industrialized countries prior to the introduction of conjugate vaccines in 1987 (9, 60). Then approximately 1 in 200 children by the age of 5 years had developed Hib meningitis, septicemia, or epiglottitis and 5 to 8% died, despite effective antimicrobial therapy. Of the survivors, 20 to 30% had some form of lasting sequelae. More than half of all children who develop invasive Hib disease in industrialized countries have meningitis. Hib disease is now rare in the United States and other countries.

A number of investigators have shown the Hib capsule to be a major virulence factor. Antibodies to the capsular PS are bactericidal and opsonize the bacteria for phagocytic killing (17). In a field trial performed in Finland in 1974, the presence of antibodies induced by a Hib PS vaccine correlated with protection (51). The Finnish trial helped show that the minimum protective level of anti-Hib PS antibodies at the time of exposure was about 0.15 µg/ml. This estimate was originally based on calculations of the amount of anti-Hib antibody in agammaglobulinemic children just prior to receipt of an immune globulin injection (55). In the Finnish trial an anti-Hib PS antibody titer of ≥1.0 µg/ml following vaccination with unconjugated Hib PS vaccine was associated with long-term protection against invasive Hib disease (9, 51). Although the relevance of this antibody threshold to clinical protection after immunization with a conjugate vaccine is not known, this level continues to be considered indicative of long-term protection. Although both the geometric mean titer using a standardized ELISA and the rate of seroconversion to 1 µg/ml are used to compare different Hib conjugate vaccines, the seroconversion rate is more important since it is an indication of the percentage of vaccinees expected to have long-term protection.

The nonconjugated Hib PS, like most PSs, is capable of stimulating B lymphocytes to produce antibody without help of T lymphocytes (T-cell-independent response) (64). Responses to protein antigens are augmented by helper T lymphocytes (T cell dependent). Covalent attachment of the Hib PS to a protein carrier converted the T-cell-independent PS into a T-cell-dependent antigen. The ability of a conjugate to recruit helper T lymphocytes into the immune response helps explain why an infant responds to the Hib conjugate vaccine but not to the PS on primary immunization (18). The T-cell-dependent nature of the immune response also results in induction of immunologic memory, leading to an anamnestic or booster response on reexposure to the native PS (28). Other features of a T-cell-dependent response, such as predominance of IgG1 in young children and affinity maturation, are also seen with conjugate vaccines (64).

Bactericidal titers in postvaccination sera against Hib are strongly correlated with the affinity or functional avidity of the sera (59). Those children with low-affinity antibody after immunization showed little increase in bactericidal activity. Although there was a direct and significant correlation between bactericidal activity and functional avidity, a wide range of anti-Hib PS antibody concentrations were found to have equivalent bactericidal titers, indicating that multiple factors contribute to the observed bactericidal titer (59). However, the in vivo biological importance of antibody avidity is not clear.

Meningococcal PS

N. meningitidis is a leading cause of bacterial meningitis in the United States, with an incidence of about 1/100,000 population, and is the leading cause of meningitis in Europe and Africa. The endemic rates in Europe are about 4 or 5/100,000 and about 20/100,000 in sub-Saharan Africa. The rates are highest in young children. In the United Kingdom the rate in 1999, prior to introduction of the group C conjugate vaccine, was 50/100,000 in children 1 to 4 years of age (47). Meningococcal meningitis and meningococcemia have a case fatality rate of about 10%. Serogroups A, B, C, and Y account for more than 90% of meningococcal disease worldwide, and nonencapsulated strains are essentially avirulent. The major problem that *N. meningitides* presents is its ability to cause outbreaks and epidemics. This is particularly a problem in sub-Saharan Africa, where in 1996 an epidemic in the West African countries of Burkina Faso, Mali, Niger, and Nigeria resulted in over 200,000 cases, with 20,000 deaths (14). In addition, about 20% of survivors have permanent sequelae such as deafness or loss of extremities.

Meningococcal PS vaccines were developed in the 1960s and licensed in the United States and France in 1975. These vaccines were the first purified component bacterial vaccines. The two formulations generally available are the AC vaccine, produced in Europe, and the ACYW135 vaccine, produced mostly in the United States by Aventis Pasteur. These vaccines are recommended for use in individuals 2 years of age and older who may be at increased risk of meningococcal disease.

A problem with the group C PS vaccine component, not evident with the group A PS, is that reimmunization induces lower antibody concentrations than does primary immunization. This hyporesponsiveness was evident in toddlers and adults when age-matched groups received a second compared to a primary group C PS immunization (27, 42).

Each of the four meningococcal PSs included in the vaccine contains O-acetyl groups. The critical role of the O-acetyl groups in the group A PS for induction of bactericidal antibodies has now been shown (6). De-O-acetylated group A PS no longer reacted with antibodies in postvaccination sera, and a de-O-acetylated group A PS-tetanus toxoid vaccine induced only low levels of bactericidal antibody.

The presence of O-acetyl groups is not important for induction of bactericidal antibodies to group C (24), and unpublished studies from the 1970s by investigators at the National Institute of Public Health in The Netherlands indicated the same for the Y and W135 PSs. About 10% of clinical isolates of group C meningococci are O-acetyl negative (3). Studies comparing O-acetyl-positive and -negative group C conjugate vaccines showed the O-acetyl-negative vaccine to be more immunogenic (11).

Protection against meningococcal disease is mediated largely by serum bactericidal antibodies. Prior to development of antibiotics and effective vaccines, the mortality rate of untreated meningococcal disease was between 60 and 80% (23). Introduction of serum therapy shortly after 1900 using hyperimmune horse sera reduced the mortality to between 13 and 30% in treated patients, depending upon how promptly serum therapy was initiated. The success of this therapy demonstrated very early the central role of humoral antibody in protection against meningococcal bacteremia and meningitis.

The critical role of bactericidal antibodies has been further demonstrated in a number of ways. (i) The highest incidence of meningococcal disease occurs in individuals between 6 and 12 months of age. This age has the lowest bactericidal antibody levels. (ii) Studies with U.S. Army recruits in the mid-1960s showed a direct correlation between susceptibility to meningitis and absence of serum bactericidal antibodies (26). In prospective studies, Goldschneider et al. (26) showed that disease occurred only among individuals lacking measurable bactericidal antibodies. (iii) Individuals deficient in complement component C5, C6, C7, or C8 have a significantly increased susceptibility to invasive meningococcal infection, even though they may have high levels of antimeningococcal antibodies. (iv) A correlation has been shown between the efficacy of meningococcal PS vaccines and induction and persistence of bactericidal antibodies.

Meningococcal PSs induce opsonic antibodies. In fact, the earliest name for the organism was *Diplococcus intracellularis meningitidis*, based upon the frequent observation of meningococci within polymorphonuclear leukocytes in Gram-strained cerebrospinal fluid samples. Roberts showed that immunization of adults with the group AC PS vaccine induced opsonic antibodies and that these antibodies were mostly IgG (57).

The antibody response to the meningococcal PSs is age dependent. Like other PSs, they are T-cell-independent immunogens, and the ability to respond to such immunogens shows age maturation. The natural development of antibodies to the group A and C meningococcal PSs showed a progressive increase with age, antibodies to group A developing more rapidly, due in large part to more prevalent cross-reacting PSs (25). Adult levels of naturally acquired antibodies to group A are achieved by 12 to 14 years of age. Naturally occurring peak levels of antibody to the group C PS occur at an older age. With administration of AC PS vaccines to children, mature adult-type responses were seen by 10 to 12 years of age (25, 36).

A single dose of either the meningococcal group A or group C PS does not induce protective antibody responses in the majority of infants until about 2 years of age. The group A PS does, however, prime for a booster-type response when given to infants, and a two-dose immunization schedule induced complete protection in children under 1 year of age in New Zealand (38).

The minimum protective concentration of anti-meningococcal PS antibodies has not been determined, but Gold estimates the level to be about 2 μg/ml (25). He based this estimation on a number of observations: (i) most adults have >2 μg/ml and have bactericidal activity, (ii) patients at the time of hospital admission with meningococcal disease have <2 μg of anti-PS antibody per ml, and finally (iii) protection against group A meningococcal disease was observed in infants in whom vaccination induced a geometric mean anti-A PS concentration of 2 μg/ml or more. Burian et al. have estimated the protective level of naturally acquired group A meningococcal PS antibody to be 1 μg/ml or greater, by comparing antibody levels by age with age-specific incidence of disease and with antibody levels in acute-phase sera from patients with meningococcal group A (12). The antibody assays for the studies of both Gold and Burian et al. were done by radioimmunoassay in the laboratory of Emil Gotschlich.

Relatively little has been done to ascertain the relative importance of IgG versus IgM antibodies in protection against meningococcal disease, but most of the bactericidal antibody resides in the IgG fraction (62).

Pneumococcal PS

S. pneumoniae (pneumococcus) is a pathogen that affects both children and adults worldwide, but it is particularly a problem at the extremes of life. The pneumococcus colonizes the upper respiratory tract and can cause disseminated disease (bacteremia and meningitis), pneumonia, upper respiratory infections (including sinusitis), and otitis media. In children, the peak incidence of invasive disease occurs by 12 to 15 months of age. It is the most common cause of bacterial pneumonia and otitis media. Annually, an estimated 1.2 million deaths due to pneumococcal pneumonia occur worldwide in children less than 5 years of age (49). Prior to introduction of the pneumococcal conjugate vaccine in the United States, there were an estimated 3,000 cases of meningitis, 50,000 cases of bacteremia, 500,000 cases of pneumonia, and 7 million cases of otitis media each year (13).

Pneumococci are subdivided into more than 90 different serotypes based upon antigenic and structural differences among the surface capsular PSs. According to the Danish identification system, these types are included within 47 groups, members of each group being antigenically related. Some groups, such as 1, 3, 5, and 14, contain a single serotype, while other groups, such as 19, contain multiple serotypes, for example, 19F, 19A, 19B, and 19C. While there are many different serotypes, about 30 types account for most pneumococcal disease. Among young children in the United States, 7 types account for over 80% of invasive pneumococcal disease, while 11 types account for most invasive disease in children worldwide.

Protection against pneumococcal disease is antibody mediated. The critical role of antibody and opsonophagocytosis in protection against pneumococcal disease can be deduced from those defects in host immunity that predispose individuals to invasive pneumococcal infection (31). Defects in antibody production (hypogammaglobulinemia), complement activity (C2 or C3 deficiency), or phagocytic function (anatomic or functional asplenia, as in sickle cell disease) all result in increased susceptibility to pneumococcal disease.

Antibody to the capsular PS is protective, and antibody to one serotype PS does not provide protection against another, except among some serotypes within a group. Zysk et al. found that anti-C PS antibodies were significantly lower among patients (median age, 54 years) with invasive pneumonia and meningitis than in healthy adults (71). However, the predisposition to develop invasive pneumococcal disease in those lacking an immune response to C PS is not clear, because others have shown that anti-C PS antibody is not opsonic (69).

The first well-controlled pneumococcal vaccine efficacy trial was conducted by MacLeod et al. and published in 1945 (44). Their vaccine contained 50 to 70 μg of each of four pneumococcal types, and 8,500 military recruits received the vaccine while 8,500 received saline. Within 2 weeks there were no more cases of pneumonia due to the four types in the immunized group. The two vaccine groups had the same number of cases of pneumonia due to types not immunized against, showing that protection was type specific.

The currently licensed 23-valent pneumococcal PS vaccine was approved in 1983 for use in individuals 2 years of age and older. The primary recommendation was for use in adults aged 65 years and older and in high-risk children, especially those with sickle cell disease. The vaccine contains 25 μg of each serotype PS per dose (575 μg of total PS). See Table 1 for pneumococcal type PSs included in the vaccine.

As seen with other PS vaccines, there is a clear age-related maturation apparent in the ability to respond to the pneumococcal 23-valent PS vaccine. The pneumococcal PSs are poorly immunogenic and fail to induce protective antibody levels in children <2 years of age. Those serotypes most associated with disease in young children, types 6A/6B, 14, 19F, and 23F, are the least immunogenic in this age group (37). For this reason conjugate vaccines were developed against the 7 to 11 most common pediatric pneumococcal types. The first pneumococcal conjugate vaccine was the 7-valent (4, 6B, 9V, 14, 18C, 19F, and 23F) product Prevnar, produced by Wyeth Vaccines, and was licensed in the United States in 2000.

The ability to respond to the different native pneumococcal PS types increases with age. Studies on age-related development of pneumococcal PS antibodies show that there is a marked increase in antibody synthesis between 12 and 18 months of age (63). For most pneumococcal types, adult level responses are generally observed by 15 years of age (Fig. 1). However, for some types, adult level responses to pneumococcal PSs occur by 8 to 10 years of age (19, 50). The antibody responses to types 14 and 23F reach adult levels by 13 to 15 years of age.

The pneumococcus is associated with high morbidity and mortality among the elderly. The ability of the pneumococcal PS vaccine to elicit a functional antibody response was found to be markedly reduced in the elderly compared to young adults (58). In the study by Romero-Steiner et al., a group of

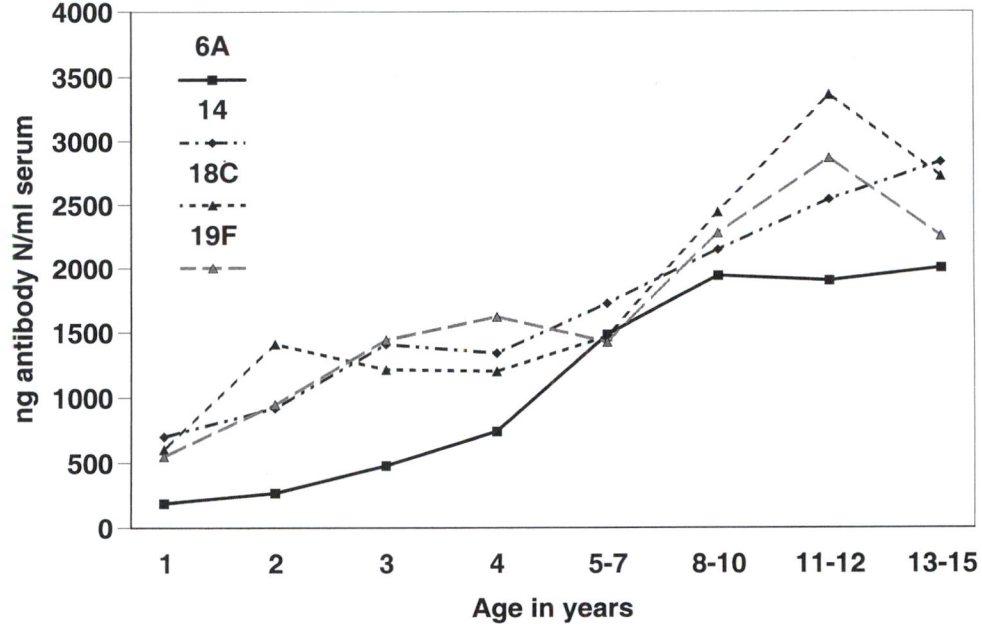

FIGURE 1 Age-related maturation in antibody response to PSs. Antibody response to four serotypes upon immunization with the pneumococcal PS vaccine in children from 1 to 15 years of age was measured.

mostly female elderly subjects (mean age, 85 years) was immunized with the 23-valent PS vaccine. Their immune responses were measured by ELISA and opsonophagocytic assays and compared to those of a control group of younger adults (mean age, 37 years). As observed in other studies, the ability to respond decreased with age, but those 63 to 79 years of age had an IgG antibody response to vaccination very similar to that of younger adults. However, a striking difference was seen in that the elderly had much lower opsonophagocytic titers following immunization than did younger adults. The IgG antibodies from elderly individuals were found to have a much lower avidity than those from young adults. Thus, the critical measure is not total antibody but functional antibody titers.

Antibody avidity affects the antibody concentration needed to induce opsonophagocytic killing of pneumococci (67). High-avidity IgG antibodies against pneumococcal types 6B and 23F were significantly more effective in mediating opsonophagocytosis on a weight basis than lower-avidity antibodies.

An efficacy trial was conducted in northern California for the 7-valent pneumococcal conjugate vaccine Prevnar (8). The vaccine contains 2 μg/dose for types 4, 9V, 14, 18C, 19F, and 23F and 4 μg/dose for type 6B. The trial involved about 37,000 infants, approximately half of whom received Prevnar. The efficacy against serotypes included in the vaccine was 97.4% (95% confidence interval, 83 to 100%) compared to the control group that received a meningococcal group C conjugate vaccine. To obtain an estimate of protective IgG antibody levels the 97% efficacy was compared to antibody concentrations achieved by approximately 97% of the infants after dose 3 at 7 months of age (30). Most vaccinated infants had >0.18 μg of IgG antibody per ml.

For most of the serotypes in Prevnar there is a good correlation between IgG antibody concentrations determined by ELISA and opsonic titers when the sera were preadsorbed with both C PS and 22F PS (16, 30). The proportion of vaccinated individuals achieving a threshold IgG antibody concentration can be used as a correlate of protection. However, serological criteria that may predict efficacy against invasive pneumococcal disease are not precise concentrations, but rather estimates or threshold levels that predict protection on a population basis. It is likely that higher antibody concentrations are needed to protect against pneumonia or otitis media (22).

In the absence of serotype-specific efficacy estimates for invasive pneumococcal disease, it is not possible to define specific serological criteria for each serotype. For this reason we must rely upon one antibody threshold applicable to all serotypes. Since there were vaccine failures for serotype 19F, an antibody threshold of 0.4 μg/ml has been derived for this serotype (30). Thus, a conservative threshold estimate applicable to most pneumococcal serotypes causing invasive disease in young children can be 0.5 μg of IgG per ml as predictive of protection at the time of exposure.

Comparing the immunoglobulin isotypes, IgG is clearly the predominant protective antibody against invasive pneumococcal infections. The major anti-pneumococcal PS IgG isotype in adults is IgG2, while the response in young children is IgG1 (2, 41). The switch from a predominantly IgG1 to a IgG2 response begins after 2 years of age, and older adults have a negligible IgG1 response to the pneumococcal PS vaccine (41). Adults possessing the G2m(n) immunoglobulin allotype have significantly higher postimmunization levels of antibody to various pneumococcal serotypes than do individuals lacking this allotype (41). G2m(n) is an allotype antigen of IgG2 subclass heavy chains. Interestingly, IgG2 makes up only about 20 to 30% of total serum IgG but accounts for the majority of pneumococcal PS-specific antibody.

Substantial IgM antibody is induced by vaccination with the pneumococcal PS vaccine, even in the face of a strong IgG response (29). Anti-pneumococcal IgM antibodies are opsonic.

A recent report documents that the pneumococcal PS vaccine induced capsular serotype-specific mucosal secretory IgA (sIgA) in breast milk is opsonic (22a). The sIgA induced complement-dependent killing of pneumococci by phagocytosis, but it is not clear how the sIgA activates complement. Janoff et al. showed that the majority of pneumococcal PS-specific serum IgA was polymeric and this polymeric IgA induced type-specific complement-dependent killing of pneumococci (4, 29).

Typhoid Vi PS

S. enterica serovar Typhi is the etiologic agent of typhoid fever and is the only *Salmonella* serovar that has a capsular PS. Further, only Vi-positive strains of serovar Typhi invade the blood and cause typhoid fever. Approximately 33 million cases of typhoid fever, with 500,000 deaths, are estimated to occur each year worldwide, mostly in developing countries (20).

The Vi PS typhoid vaccine is produced as a liquid vaccine by Aventis Pasteur. The recommended dose is 25 μg. It is recommended for individuals as a traveler's vaccine beginning at 2 years of age. Studies showed that either 25 or 50 μg of Vi PS elicited fourfold or greater rises in serum antibody concentrations in 95% of adults from either the United States or France (1, 33), where preimmunization levels were low, whereas in South Africa the seroconversion rate was 75% (33). A booster immunization basically restored post-first-dose antibody levels. These Vi PS antibody levels were all measured by radioimmunoassay.

In Nepal, where the attack rate in individuals 5 to 44 years of age was 16.2/1,000, the Vi PS vaccine given as a single 25-μg dose had an efficacy of 75% measured 17 months after vaccination (1). This study clearly showed that serum antibodies to the Vi PS were sufficient to protect against typhoid fever. In South Africa the protective efficacy was measured out to 3 years postvaccination (34).

The Vi PS vaccine is clearly superior to the old inactivated whole-cell vaccines, based upon both safety and effectiveness against typhoid fever. The efficacy of the whole-cell vaccine was 50 to 60% and of relatively short duration (53). The other currently available typhoid vaccine is the attenuated live oral Ty21a strain of serovar Typhi, formulated as enteric coated capsules. This vaccine requires three doses to achieve 60 to 70% protection in children and adults (39).

Keitel and colleagues have estimated that the protective level of Vi PS serum antibodies is 1.5 μg/ml (32). A single dose induced about 80% seroconversion to this level in healthy American adults. About 3 years after immunization the percentage of vaccinees with 1.5 μg or more of antibody per ml declined to 38%, compared to 1% of individuals having 1.5 μg/ml or more before immunization. Reimmunization restored the initial postvaccination antibody levels (32).

Concerning the age-related immune response to the Vi PS, immunogenicity studies in areas of endemicity, including Nepal and Indonesia, show little evidence of an age-related antibody response down to 2 years of age (1, 53). Interestingly, adults in the United States developed increases (fourfold) in antibody similar to those in adults in areas of endemicity, suggesting that previous exposure to the Vi PS does not seem to be necessary for a good immune response.

The mechanism by which the anti-capsular PS antibodies protect against typhoid fever is not entirely clear (56). Typhoid fever is not a diarrheal disease, but a blood infection. The bacteria must invade the blood and to do so must be encapsulated (54). Antibodies to the Vi PS likely protect by complement-mediated lysis, as is found with other blood-invasive gram-negative bacteria (39). The most important antibody isotype is IgG. It is known that the presence of O-acetyl groups on the Vi PS is essential for induction of protective antibody (65).

Subsequent to licensure of the typhoid Vi Ps vaccine, a Vi PS-protein conjugate vaccine was developed (35). This vaccine was shown to be more immunogenic in young children than the Vi PS vaccine. The conjugate was evaluated for efficacy in Vietnamese children 2 to 5 years of age (40). The efficacy was 91.5% (95% confidence interval, 77.1 to 96.6%) in these children.

REFERENCES

1. **Acharya, I. L., C. U. Lowe, R. Thapa, V. L. Gurubacharya, M. B. Shrestha, M. Cadoz, D. Schulz, J. Armand, D. A. Bryla, B. Trollfors, et al.** 1987. Prevention of typhoid fever in Nepal with the Vi capsular polysaccharide of *Salmonella typhi*. A preliminary report. *N. Engl. J. Med.* **317:**1101–1104.
2. **Ambrosino, D. M., G. Schiffman, E. C. Gotschlich, P. H. Schur, G. A. Rosenberg, G. G. DeLange, E. van Loghem, and G. R. Siber.** 1985. Correlation between G2m(n) immunoglobulin allotype and human antibody response and susceptibility to polysaccharide encapsulated bacteria. *J. Clin. Investig.* **75:**1935–1942.
3. **Arakere, G., and C. E. Frasch.** 1991. Specificity of antibodies to O-acetyl-positive and O-acetyl-negative group C meningococcal polysaccharides in sera from vaccinees and carriers. *Infect. Immun.* **59:**4349–4356.
4. **Barrett, D. J., A. J. Ammann, S. Stenmark, and D. W. Wara.** 1980. Immunoglobulin G and M antibodies to pneumococcal polysaccharides detected by enzyme-linked immunosorbent assay. *Infect. Immun.* **27:**411–417.
5. **Baxendale, H. E., Z. Davis, H. N. White, M. B. Spellerberg, F. K. Stevenson, and D. Goldblatt.** 2000. Immunogenetic analysis of the immune response to pneumococcal polysaccharide. *Eur. J. Immunol.* **30:**1214–1223.
6. **Berry, D. S., F. Lynn, C. H. Lee, C. E. Frasch, and M. C. Bash.** 2002. Effect of O acetylation of *Neisseria meningitidis* serogroup A capsular polysaccharide on development of functional immune responses. *Infect. Immun.* **70:**3707–3713.
7. **Bhushan, R., B. F. Anthony, and C. E. Frasch.** 1998. Estimation of group B streptococcus type III polysaccharide-specific antibody concentrations in human sera is antigen dependent. *Infect. Immun.* **66:**5848–5853.
8. **Black, S., H. Shinefield, B. Fireman, E. Lewis, P. Ray, J. R. Hansen, L. Elvin, K. M. Ensor, J. Hackell, G. Siber, F. Malinoski, D. Madore, I. Chang, R. Kohberger, W. Watson, R. Austrian, K. Edwards, and Northern California Kaiser Permanente Vaccine Study Center Group.** 2000. Efficacy, safety and immunogenicity of heptavalent pneumococcal conjugate vaccine in children. *Pediatr. Infect. Dis. J.* **19:**187–195.
9. **Booy, R., and E. R., Moxon.** 1993. *Haemophilus influenzae* type b. *Arch. Dis. Child.* **68:**440–441.
10. **Borrow, R., N. Andrews, D. Goldblatt, and E. Miller.** 2001. Serological basis for use of meningococcal serogroup C conjugate vaccines in the United Kingdom: reevaluation of correlates of protection. *Infect. Immun.* **69:**1568–1573.
11. **Bramley, J. C., T. Hall, A. Finn, R. B. Buttery, D. Elliman, S. Lockhart, R. Borrow, and I. G. Jones.** 2001. Safety and immunogenicity of three lots of meningococcal

12. **Burian, V., E. Gotschlich, P. Kuzemenska, and E. Svandova.** 1977. Naturally occurring antibodies to *Neisseria meningitidis*. *Bull. W.H.O.* **55:**653–657.
13. **Centers for Disease Control and Prevention.** 1997. Prevention of pneumococcal disease: recommendations of the Advisory Committee on Immunization Practices (ACIP). *Morb. Mortal. Wkly. Rep.* **46:**1–24.
14. **Chippaux, J. R., H. Debois, and R. Saliou.** 2002. A critical review of control strategies against meningococcal meningitis epidemics in sub-Saharan African countries. *Infection* **30:**216–224.
15. **Concepcion, N., and C. E. Frasch.** 1998. Evaluation of previously assigned antibody concentrations in pneumococcal polysaccharide reference serum 89SF by the method of cross-standardization. *Clin. Diagn. Lab. Immunol.* **5:**199–204.
16. **Concepcion, N. F., and C. E. Frasch.** 2001. Pneumococcal type 22F polysaccharide absorption improves the specificity of a pneumococcal-polysaccharide enzyme-linked immunosorbent assay. *Clin. Diagn. Lab. Immunol.* **8:**266–272.
17. **Deveikis, A., J. Ward, and K. S. Kim.** 1988. Functional activities of human antibody induced by the capsular polysaccharide or polysaccharide-protein conjugate vaccines against *Haemophilus influenzae* type b. *Vaccine* **6:**14–18.
18. **Dintzis, R. Z.** 1994. Structure/function relationships in vaccines, p. 111–127. *In* R. W. Ellis and D. M. Granoff (ed.), *Development and Clinical Uses of Haemophilus b Conjugate Vaccines*. Marcel Dekker, New York, N.Y.
19. **Douglas, R. M., J. C. Paton, S. J. Duncan, and D. J. Hansman.** 1983. Antibody response to pneumococcal vaccination in children younger than five years of age. *J. Infect. Dis.* **148:**131–137.
20. **Edelman, R., and M. M. Levine.** 1986. Summary of an international workshop on typhoid fever. *Rev. Infect. Dis.* **8:**329–349.
21. **Elie, C. M., P. K. Holder, S. Romero-Steiner, and G. M. Carlone.** 2002. Assignment of additional anticapsular antibody concentrations to the Neisseria meningitidis group A, C, Y, and W-135 meningococcal standard reference serum CDC1992. *Clin. Diagn. Lab. Immunol.* **9:**725–726.
22. **Esposito, S., and N. Principi.** 2003. Effect of conjugate pneumococcal vaccine on recurrent acute otitis media. *Lancet* **362:**1080–1081.
22a. **Finn, A., Q. B. Zhang, L. Seymour, C. Fasching, E. Pettitt, and E. N. Janoff.** 2002. Induction of functional secretory IgA responses in breast milk by pneumococcal capsular polysaccharides. *J. Infect. Dis.* **186:**1422–1429.
23. **Frasch, C. E.** 1995. Meningococcal vaccines: past, present and future, p. 245–283. *In* K. Cartwright (ed.), *Meningococcal Disease*. Wiley, New York, N.Y.
24. **Glode, M. P., E. B. Lewin, A. Sutton, C. T. Le, E. C. Gotschlich, and J. B. Robbins.** 1979. Comparative immunogenicity of vaccines prepared from capsular polysaccharides of group C *Neisseria meningitidis* O-acetyl-positive and O-acetyl-negative variants and *Escherichia coli* K92 in adult volunteers. *J. Infect. Dis.* **139:**52–59.
25. **Gold, R.** 1979. Immunogenicity of meningococcal polysaccharides in man, p. 121–150. *In* J. A. Rudbach and P. J. Baker (ed.), *Immunology of Bacterial Polysaccharides*. Elsevier, Amsterdam, The Netherlands.
26. **Goldschneider, I., E. C. Gotschlich, and M. S. Artenstein.** 1969. Human immunity to the meningococcus. II. Development of natural immunity. *J. Exp. Med.* **129:**1327–1348.
27. **Granoff, D. M., R. K. Gupta, R. B. Belshe, and E. L. Anderson.** 1998. Induction of immunologic refractoriness in adults by meningococcal C polysaccharide vaccination. *J. Infect. Dis.* **178:**870–874.

28. Granoff, D. M., S. J. Holmes, M. T. Osterholm, J. E. McHugh, A. H. Lucas, E. L. Anderson, R. B. Belshe, J. L. Jacobs, F. Medley, and T. V. Murphy. 1993. Induction of immunologic memory in infants primed with *Haemophilus influenzae* type b conjugate vaccines. *J. Infect. Dis.* 168:663–671.

29. Janoff, E. N., C. Fasching, J. M. Orenstein, J. B. Rubins, N. L. Opstad, and A. P. Dalmasso. 1999. Killing of *Streptococcus pneumoniae* by capsular polysaccharide-specific polymeric IgA, complement, and phagocytes. *J. Clin. Investig.* 104:1139–1147.

30. Jodar, L., J. Butler, G. Carlone, R. Dagan, D. Goldblatt, H. Kaeyhty, K. Klugman, B. Plikaytis, G. Siber, R. Kohberger, I. Chang, and T. Cherian. 2003. Serological criteria for evaluation and licensure of new pneumococcal conjugate vaccine formulations for use in infants. *Vaccine* 21:3265–3272.

31. Johnson R. B., Jr. 1981. The host response to invasion by *Streptococcus pneumoniae*: protection and the pathogenesis of tissue damage. *Rev. Infect. Dis.* 3:282–288.

32. Keitel, W. A., N. L. Bond, J. M. Zahradnik, T. A. Cramton, and J. B. Robbins. 1994. Clinical and serological responses following primary and booster immunization with *Salmonella typhi* Vi capsular polysaccharide vaccines. *Vaccine* 12:195–199.

33. Klugman, K. P., I. T. Gilbertson, H. J. Koornhof, J. B. Robbins, R. Schneerson, D. Schulz, M. Cadoz, and J. Armand. 1987. Protective activity of Vi capsular polysaccharide vaccine against typhoid fever. *Lancet* ii:1165–1169.

34. Klugman, K. P., H. J. Koornhof, J. B. Robbins, and N. N. Le Cam. 1996. Immunogenicity, efficacy and serological correlate of protection of *Salmonella typhi* Vi capsular polysaccharide vaccine three years after immunization. *Vaccine* 14:435–438.

35. Kossaczka, Z., F. Y. Lin, V. A. Ho, N. T. Thuy, P. Van Bay, T. C. Thanh, H. B. Khiem, D. D. Trach, A. Karpas, S. Hunt, D. A. Bryla, R. Schneerson, J. B. Robbins, and S. C. Szu. 1999. Safety and immunogenicity of Vi conjugate vaccines for typhoid fever in adults, teenagers, and 2- to 4-year-old children in Vietnam. *Infect. Immun.* 67:5806–5810.

36. Law, B. J., T. Rosenberg, N. E. MacDonald, F. E. Ashton, J. C. Huang, W. J. King, W. J. Ferris, and G. J. Gray. 1998. Age-related immunogenicity of meningococcal polysaccharide vaccine in Aboriginal children and adolescents living in a Northern Manitoba reserve community. *Pediatr. Infect. Dis. J.* 17:860–864.

37. Leinonen, M., A. Sakkinen, R. Kalliokoski, J. Luotonen, M. Timonen, and P. H. Makela. 1986. Antibody response to 14-valent pneumococcal capsular polysaccharide vaccine in pre-school age children. *Pediatr. Infect. Dis.* 5:39–44.

38. Lennon, D., B. Gellin, D. Hood, L. Voss, H. Heffernan, and S. Thakur. 1992. Successful intervention in a group A meningococcal outbreak in Auckland, New Zealand. *Pediatr. Infect. Dis. J.* 11:617–623.

39. Levine, M. M., C. Ferreccio, R. E. Black, and R. Germanier. 1987. Large-scale field trial of Ty21a live oral typhoid vaccine in enteric-coated capsule formulation. *Lancet* i:1049–1052.

40. Lin, F. Y., V. A. Ho, H. B. Khiem, D. D. Trach, P. V. Bay, T. C. Thanh, Z. Kossaczka, D. A. Bryla, J. Shiloach, J. B. Robbins, R. Schneerson, and S. C. Szu. 2001. The efficacy of a *Salmonella typhi* Vi conjugate vaccine in two- to five-year-old children. *N. Engl. J. Med.* 344:1263–1269.

41. Lottenbach, K. R., C. M. Mink, S. J. Barenkamp, E. L. Anderson, S. M. Homan, and D. C. Powers. 1999. Age-associated differences in immunoglobulin G1 (IgG1) and IgG2 subclass antibodies to pneumococcal polysaccharides following vaccination. *Infect. Immun.* 67:4935–4938.

42. MacDonald, N. E., S. A. Halperin, B. J. Law, L. E. Danzig, and D. M. Granoff. 2000. Can meningococcal C conjugate vaccine overcome immune hyporesponsiveness induced by previous administration of plain polysaccharide vaccine? *JAMA* 283:1826–1827.

43. MacDonald, N. E., S. A. Halperin, B. J. Law, B. Forrest, L. E. Danzig, and D. M. Granoff. 1998. Induction of immunologic memory by conjugated vs. plain meningococcal C polysaccharide vaccine in toddlers—a randomized controlled trial. *JAMA* 280:1685–1689.

44. MacLeod, C. M., R. G. Hodges, M. Heidelberger, and W. G. Bernhard. 1945. Prevention of pneumococcal pneumonia by immunization with specific capsular polysaccharides. *J. Exp. Med.* 82:445–465.

45. Madore, D. V., P. Anderson, B. D. Baxter, G. M. Carlone, K. M. Edwards, R. G. Hamilton, P. Holder, H. Kayhty, D. C. Phipps, C. C. Peeters, R. Schneerson, G. R. Siber, J. I. Ward, and C. E. Frasch. 1996. Interlaboratory study evaluating quantitation of antibodies to *Haemophilus influenzae* type b polysaccharide by enzyme-linked immunosorbent assay. *Clin. Diagn. Lab. Immunol.* 3:84–88.

46. Madore, D. V., C. L. Johnson, D. C. Phipps, Pennridge Pediatric Associates, M. G. Myers, R. Eby, and D. H. Smith. 1990. Safety and immunogenicity of *Haemophilus influenzae* type b oligosaccharide-CRM$_{197}$ conjugate vaccine in infants aged 15 to 23 months. *Pediatrics* 86:527–534.

47. Miller, E., D. Salisbury, and M. Ramsay. 2001. Planning, registration, and implementation of an immunisation campaign against meningococcal serogroup C disease in the UK: a success story. *Vaccine* 20(Suppl.1):S58–S67.

48. Reference deleted.

49. Ostroff, S. M. 1999. Continuing challenge of pneumococcal disease. *Lancet* 353:1201–1202.

50. Paton, J. C., I. R. Toogood, R. A. Cockington, and D. Hansman. 1986. Antibody response to pneumococcal vaccine in children aged 5 to 15 years. *Am. J. Dis. Child.* 140:135–138.

51. Peltola, H., H. Kayhty, M. Virtanen, and P. H. Makela. 1984. Prevention of Haemophilus influenzae type b bacteremic infections with the capsular polysaccharide vaccine. *N. Engl. J. Med.* 310:1561–1566.

52. Phipps, D. C., J. West, R. Eby, M. Koster, D. V. Madore, and S. A. Quataert. 1990. An ELISA employing a *Haemophilus influenzae* type b oligosaccharide-human serum albumin conjugate correlates with the radioantigen binding assay. *J. Immunol. Methods* 135:121–128.

53. Plotkin, S. A., and N. Bouveret-Le Cam. 1995. A new typhoid vaccine composed of the Vi capsular polysaccharide. *Arch. Intern. Med.* 155:2293–2299.

54. Quataert, S. A., C. S. Kirch, L. J. Wiedl, D. C. Phipps, S. Strohmeyer, C. O. Cimino, J. Skuse, and D. V. Madore. 1995. Assignment of weight-based antibody units to a human antipneumococcal standard reference serum, lot 89-S. *Clin. Diagn. Lab. Immunol.* 2:590–597.

55. Robbins, J. B., J. C. Parke, R. Schneerson, and J. K. Whisnant. 1973. Quantitative measurement of "natural" and immunization-induced *Haemophilus influenzae* type b capsular polysaccharide antibodies. *Pediatr. Res.* 7:103–110.

56. Robbins, J. D., and J. B. Robbins. 1984. Reexamination of the protective role of the capsular polysaccharide (Vi antigen) of *Salmonella typhi*. *J. Infect. Dis.* 150:436–449.

57. Roberts, R. B. 1970. The relationship between group A and group C meningococcal polysaccharides and serum opsonins in man. *J. Exp. Med.* 131:499–513.

58. Romero-Steiner, S., D. M. Musher, M. S. Cetron, L. B. Pais, J. E. Groover, A. E. Fiore, B. D. Plikaytis, and

G. M. Carlone. 1999. Reduction in functional antibody activity against *Streptococcus pneumoniae* in vaccinated elderly individuals highly correlates with decreased IgG antibody avidity. *Clin. Infect. Dis.* **29:**281–288.

59. Schlesinger, Y., D. M. Granoff, and The Vaccine Study Group. 1992. Avidity and bactericidal activity of antibody elicited by different *Haemophilus influenzae* type b conjugate vaccines. *JAMA* **267:**1489–1494.

60. Shapiro, E. D., and J. I. Ward. 1991. The epidemiology and prevention of disease caused by *Haemophilus influenzae* type b. *Epidemiol. Rev.* **13:**113–142.

61. Siber, G. R., D. M. Ambrosino, J. McIver, T. J. Ervin, G. Schiffman, S. Sallan, and G. F. Grady. 1984. Preparation of human hyperimmune globulin to *Haemophilus influenzae* b, *Streptococcus pneumoniae*, and *Neisseria meningitidis. Infect. Immun.* **45:**248–254.

62. Skevakis, L., C. E. Frasch, J. M. Zahradnik, and R. Dolin. 1984. Class-specific human bactericidal antibodies to capsular and noncapsular surface antigens of *Neisseria meningitidis. J. Infect. Dis.* **149:**387–396.

63. Soininen, A., H. Pursiainen, T. Kilpi, and H. Kaeyhty. 2001. Natural development of antibodies to pneumococcal capsular polysaccharides depends on the serotype: association with pneumococcal carriage and acute otitis media in young children. *J. Infect. Dis.* **184:**569–576.

64. Stein, K. E. 1992. Thymus-independent and thymus-dependent responses to polysaccharide antigens. *J. Infect. Dis.* **165:**S49–S52.

65. Szu, S. C., X. R. Li, A. L. Stone, and J. B. Robbins. 1991. Relation between structure and immunologic properties of the Vi capsular polysaccharide. *Infect. Immun.* **59:**4555–4561.

66. Trotter, C., R. Borrow, N. Andrews, and E. Miller. 2003. Seroprevalence of meningococcal serogroup C bactericidal antibody in England and Wales in the pre-vaccination era. *Vaccine* **21:**1094–1098.

67. Usinger, W. R., and A. H. Lucas. 1999. Avidity as a determinant of the protective efficacy of human antibodies to pneumococcal capsular polysaccharides. *Infect. Immun.* **67:**2366–2370.

68. Van Parijs, B. A. 2004. Review of pneumococcal conjugate vaccine in adults: implications on clinical development. *Vaccine* **22:**1362–1371.

69. Vitharsson, G., I. Jonsdottir, S. Jonsson, and H. Valdimarsson. 1994. Opsonization and antibodies to capsular and cell wall polysaccharides of *Streptococcus pneumoniae. J. Infect. Dis.* **170:**592–599.

70. Zepp, F., H. J. Schmitt, A. Kaufhold, A. Schuind, M. Knuf, P. Habermehl, C. Meyer, H. Bogaerts, M. Slaoui, and R. Clemens. 1997. Evidence for induction of polysaccharide specific B-cell memory in the 1st year of life: plain *Haemophilus influenzae* type b-PRP (Hib) boosters children primed with a tetanus-conjugate Hib-DTPa-HBV combined vaccine. *Eur. J. Pediatr.* **156:**18–24.

71. Zysk, G., G. Bethe, R. Nau, D. Koch, V. C. D. H. Von Bassewitz, H. P. Heinz, and R. R. Reinert. 2003. Immune response to capsular polysaccharide and surface proteins of *Streptococcus pneumoniae* in patients with invasive pneumococcal disease. *J. Infect. Dis.* **187:**330–333.

Corynebacterium diphtheriae and Clostridium tetani: Immune Response and Diagnostic Methods

MARTHA L. LEPOW AND PATRICIA A. HUGHES

52

Corynebacterium diphtheriae and *Clostridium tetani* are responsible for important diseases. Tetanus is caused by introduction of *C. tetani* from soil through contaminated wounds, while diphtheria results from airborne infection from infected cases. In both instances it is a potent exotoxin that is responsible for clinical disease. The toxin of *C. tetani* is so potent that the lethal dose may not be of sufficient strength to stimulate antibody production. In both instances formalin-inactivated toxins have been used for universal immunization. For children they are combined with pertussis vaccine, and adults are given both together at a reduced dose of diphtheria toxoid. In September 2005, two new vaccines containing combined acellular pertussis, diphtheria, and tetanus vaccines were licensed.

DIPHTHERIA

Diphtheria is an acute communicable disease of the nasopharynx, larynx, and trachea with complications involving the heart and peripheral nerves and kidney; it has been known since antiquity. Although largely controlled through immunization in the United States, cases do occur sporadically in the United States and elsewhere in the Western world. Recent epidemics have occurred in some countries of the former Soviet Union (9, 12).

The Organism and Pathogenesis

C. diphtheriae is a gram-positive rod with one end being wider, giving it a club-shaped appearance. On culture, characteristic bands or granules appear. On smears the organisms assume a parallel appearance. There are four different biotypes, but no difference in disease is noted among them.

The exotoxin produced by *C. diphtheriae* is the most important pathogenic factor. Toxin production which results from a nonlytic infection by one of a series of related bacteriophages containing a genetic sequence encoding toxin transmission may be facilitated by local tissue damage resulting from the toxin. The *tox* gene is part of a multiple bacterial gene operon, and the entire operon is under the control of a repressor gene, *dtx*, which in the presence of iron binds to and inhibits the *tox* gene. Toxin is produced only under low-iron conditions.

Diphtheria toxin is a polypeptide with a molecular weight of approximately 58,000. It is secreted as a proenzyme requiring enzymatic cleavage into fragments A and B to become active. Fragment B is responsible for attachment to and presentation of the host cell, and although it is not toxic by itself, it is the antigen responsible for clinical immunity. After penetration of the cell, fragments A and B are detached and fragment A, the toxin, inhibits protein synthesis and results in cell death.

On mucous membranes, the toxin causes local cell death with membrane formulation and remote manifestations in the myocardium, central nervous system, and kidney. Clinical immunity is dependent upon antibodies to the toxin, and formalinized toxin (toxoid) is the active immunizing agent.

Assays for Antitoxin Levels

Several laboratory assays are available. In vitro neutralization assays are based on capabilities of serum containing diphtheria toxin antibodies to neutralize the cytopathogenic effect of diphtheria toxin on the tissue culture system of Vero cells derived from African green monkey kidney cells (7). Neutralization assays are very accurate in this system but are available only in research laboratories. Levels of 1.0 IU and above are associated with long-term protection.

Several enzyme-linked immunosorbent assays (ELISAs) capable of detecting specific immunoglobulin G (IgG) have been developed; however, false-positive results may occur due to recognition of nonneutralizing antibodies. Results of ELISAs may not correlate well with toxin-neutralizing assays.

Recently a delayed-fluorescence immunoassay has been used to determine diphtheria antitoxin levels in human serum. This has been evaluated in vivo in neutralization tests performed with rabbits and has been shown to be superior to Vero cells on sera with titers below 0.02 μg/ml (3).

In the first international meeting of the WHO European Laboratory Working Group on Diphtheria in 1994, it was agreed that the in vitro toxin neutralization assay on Vero cells is the most appropriate method for measurement of diphtheria antitoxin antibodies. In vitro assays such as ELISA and passive hemagglutination (PHA) assays are required to provide comparison with toxin neutralization assays.

Clinical Manifestations

The disease most commonly presents with gradual onset over 1 to 2 days as a membranous pharyngitis with confluent exudate over the tonsils and soft palate, with a moderate fever. Laryngeal diphtheria occurs concomitantly with inspiratory stridor and hoarseness. Transmission is through the respiratory route. Nasal and cutaneous diphtheria are rare manifestations. Cases of diphtheria are reportable to local health departments.

Complications associated with the toxin occur within a few days, and it is important to establish a diagnosis quickly with culture so that treatment can be instituted. Effective treatment includes early administration of an equine diphtheria antitoxin (DAT), although toxin which has already entered the host cell cannot be affected by antitoxin. The Centers for Disease Control and Prevention has recently procured an equine DAT product from Instituto Butantan in Brazil. It can be provided to physicians caring for patients with respiratory diphtheria under a Food and Drug Administration investigational new drug protocol. Skin testing is mandatory, and treatment for acute reactions must be available. Serum sickness can occur with large doses of antitoxin. A novel approach to passive immunity may be the development of a modified diphtheria toxin receptor molecule to bind diphtheria toxin (4).

Penicillin or erythromycin can be given to clear the organisms from cases or for eradication of the carrier state. There is little evidence for use of antitoxin in carriers.

Active Immunization

In the early 20th century, it was discovered that a balanced mixture of toxin and antitoxin could be used to successfully immunize susceptible persons. Diphtheria toxoid was subsequently developed, and by the mid-1940s diphtheria toxoid was combined with tetanus toxoid and whole-cell pertussis vaccines (DPT). Adsorption of all three onto an aluminum salt for intramuscular use came soon after, which enhanced immunogenicity. Universal immunization with the combined vaccine was well under way in the 1950s. Recently, acellular pertussis vaccine has replaced whole-cell pertussis vaccine, and a schedule of five doses, with administration at 2, 4, 6, and 15 to 18 months and 4 to 6 years constitutes the childhood schedule (1). Older children and adults receive DT with a lower concentration of diphtheria toxoid in order to prevent more severe local reactions.

After three doses of diphtheria toxoid almost all infants will have developed anti-diphtheria toxoid titers at 0.01 IU/ml, which is the minimal protective level. During the past few years immunization programs in the former Soviet Union have resulted in 90% efficacy (7).

A combined vaccine consisting of DT acellular pertussis (DTACP) together with inactive poliovirus vaccine and hepatitis B virus vaccine has become available for immunization of infants up to 6 months of age, and others may be in the pipeline to decrease the number of injections required for young infants. In the future efforts will be made to reduce reactogenicity of components of DTACP (8).

A diphtheria toxoid from CR 197, a mutant nontoxogenic strain of *C. diptheriae*, has been conjugated to capsular polysaccharides of *Haemophilus influenzae* type b, seven types of pneumococcus, and four types of meningococcus, resulting in enhanced immunity to the antigens and longer persistence of antibody. A booster effect has been observed for diphtheria antibody following administration of the polyvalent pneumococcal conjugate vaccines.

TETANUS

Introduction

The Organism and Its Exotoxins

C. tetani is a gram-positive, spore-forming motile anaerobic bacillus. Although considered a strict anaerobe, it can be cultured in a range of temperatures and in a variety of media used in growing anaerobes. Spores may persist in soil for months or years. Animals can carry *C. tetani* in their feces.

Exotoxins of *C. tetani*

C. tetani produces two exotoxins, tetanolysin and the neurotoxin tetanospasmin, which is responsible for the manifestations of the disease. It is one of the most potent known toxins, and the minimal lethal dose in humans is estimated to be <2.5 μg/kg of body weight. Formalinization detoxifies the toxin while retaining its immunogenicity.

Pathogenesis

Infection usually begins with the inoculation of spores through the epithelium. Wounds accompanied by tissue injury and necrosis (with or without aerobic organisms) leading to low oxygen concentration allow spores to germinate and bacilli to replicate. Toxin produced locally reaches the central nervous system via lymphatics and along neurons.

Diagnosis

The diagnosis is clinical, supported by an appropriate epidemiological setting. The illness presents as trismus, nuchal rigidity, and dysphagia accompanied by spasms of major muscle groups. Today with universal effective immunization, clinical tetanus rarely occurs and is seen in the elderly and in neonates in parts of the world where the umbilical stump is treated with soil which then constitutes a portal of entry for spores. Antitoxic antibodies are protective in prevention of infection, and treatment is mainly supportive.

Methods for Measuring Antitoxin

Although reliable methods of measuring antitoxic neutralizing antibodies have existed for many years for tetanus antitoxin, regular clinical laboratories rarely maintain the capability of determining tetanus antitoxin levels because they are of no use in diagnosis or treatment of the acute disease. They are also time-consuming and are mainly used as research tools.

The most reliable method for determining tetanus antitoxin levels is in vivo neutralization of toxin which depends upon antibodies of the IgG class. The mouse neutralization assay is the most widely used (2), and this method is described below.

PHA has good correlation with neutralization tests. This detects IgM and IgG antibodies, and since only IgG is active in neutralization tests, low levels of early antibody (IgM) may not be active (8).

An ELISA can be used for the determination of serum tetanus antitoxin levels (10). It is a simple test, is relatively inexpensive, and can detect antitoxin of specific immunoglobulin types. The titer may be higher with ELISA than with neutralization assays, especially for recently immunized people, suggesting the presence of low-avidity antibodies.

ELISA has in some hands proven to be as sensitive as the neutralization test for the detection of antitoxin, but there are problems in reproducibility. Despite the ability of the ELISA to detect IgG antitoxin, which presumably contains all of the toxin-neutralizing activity, differences in binding activity and neutralization have occurred. At this time, ELISAs should be employed for screening but not for determining the specific titer of antibody.

Counterimmunoelectrophoresis can be used for the detection of tetanus antitoxin (13), but because of its relative insensitivity, this method is useful only in screening sera containing relatively high levels (>7.0 IU/ml) of antitoxin. A solid-phase radioimmunoassay has also been described for the detection of tetanus antitoxin (5), but no comparisons with in vivo neutralization tests have been reported.

It is recommended that in a clinical laboratory, where values for individual patients are important, the more reliable mouse neutralization test should be used. There is no tissue culture method available for the titration of tetanus toxin or antitoxin.

Natural Immunity and Response to Disease

It is unclear whether humans can develop circulating antibody to tetanus in the absence of vaccination or disease. Intestinal colonization could result in such protection. The exotoxin of *C. tetani* is so potent and the lethal dose so small that survivors of the disease will rarely develop significant antibody titers.

Immune Response to Tetanus Toxoids

Injection of tetanus toxoid, which is one of the most effective immunizing agents in use today, regularly evokes antitoxic antibodies. A circulating neutralizing antibody titer of 0.01 IU/ml is protective against disease.

In 1944, following success of tetanus toxoid immunization during World War II, routine inoculation in childhood was recommended by the American Academy of Pediatrics. Shortly thereafter, tetanus toxoid was combined with diphtheria toxoid and whole-cell inactivated pertussis organisms (DTP), and this combination became the standard immunization protocol for infants and children up to 7 years of age. As of January 2000 acellular pertussis vaccines have replaced whole-cell vaccine in formulations with diphtheria and tetanus (6). For older children and adults, only diphtheria and tetanus toxoid are recommended, and the quantity of diphtheria toxoid is lower (Td) in order to avoid serious reactions. In the United States aluminum hydroxide, aluminum phosphate, or alum is used as an adjuvant. These allow an adequate immune response with fewer doses than with fluid preparations.

Infant Immunization Schedule

Three doses of vaccine at 2, 4, and 6 months are recommended, with a booster at age 12 to 18 months and again at 5 years. This regimen will ensure nearly 100% durable protection. A minimum of two doses is necessary for stimulation of measurable protective levels of tetanus antibody.

For unimmunized older children and adults, two doses four or more weeks apart will produce tetanus antitoxin levels of >0.01 IU/ml, but a booster dose should be given 6 to 12 months later. Td vaccination is recommended every 10 years to maintain immunity to both tetanus and diphtheria. With these regimens, tetanus has largely been eliminated. Persons who have recovered from tetanus should be immunized because the natural disease may not be protective. The World Health Organization recommendation for tetanus immunization of women of childbearing age is two doses 2 months apart in parts of the world where neonatal tetanus still occurs.

Care of Tetanus-Prone Wounds

For wounds contaminated with soil or feces or where there is devitalized tissue (e.g., burns or puncture wounds), a booster dose of vaccine is usually given if the immunization status is unknown or more than 5 years has elapsed since the last dose.

Passive antibody is also recommended as a single dose of human tetanus immune globulin (TIG) (250 U) in a separate site if the immunization status of the patient is not known. If TIG is unavailable, equine antitoxin (3,000 to 5,000 U) can be used after skin testing. Epinephrine must be available in case of anaphylaxis, and if the skin test is positive, desensitization may be required. This product is not available in the United States. Because of a variable immune response, individuals with symptomatic human immunodeficiency virus infection should receive passive antibody (TIG) for all tetanus-prone wounds regardless of immunization status (11).

Treatment of Disease

Currently a single dose of human TIG is given at diagnosis to bind circulating toxin. Wound debridement and antibiotics as well as supportive care are needed.

Standardization of Commercially Produced Tetanus Toxoid

In North America the available preparations are given as 0.5-ml doses intramuscularly. The toxoid content of commercial products is assessed by flocculation with standard antitoxin and is measured in units termed the limits of flocculation. Potency is determined by animal bioassays: for the fluid preparation, immunized guinea pigs are tested for survival after a toxin challenge; for precipitated toxoid, a serum pool from immunized guinea pigs must exceed 2 IU/ml (8).

CLINICAL USE OF ANTITOXIN LEVELS

There are few indications for the determination of tetanus antitoxin levels. Diagnosis and therapy are determined on the basis of clinical symptoms and exposure history. A possible clinical use could be to determine the antitoxin level before using tetanus antitoxin for therapy. If 0.01 IU of antitoxin is present prior to treatment, the diagnosis of tetanus would surely be in doubt. On the other hand, the absence of antitoxin in serum after a clinical illness compatible with tetanus does not rule out the diagnosis because the quantity of toxin producing disease may not be sufficient to stimulate antibody formation.

For population surveys of immune status to tetanus, one of the more rapid but less quantitative tests commercially available such as PHA or ELISA can be used (8). Probably the most frequent need for these assays today is in connection with studies of immunocompetence in infants and young children. The response to tetanus toxoid after three or four doses is of practical use where B-cell activity is being measured.

METHOD FOR ANTIBODY DETERMINATION

Titration of Tetanus Antitoxin by the Mouse Toxin Neutralization Test

The procedure for titration of tetanus antitoxin is based on the capacity of tetanus antitoxin to protect mice from death after subcutaneous injection of tetanus toxin. The following procedure is based on the method of Barile et al. (2).

The sample of tetanus toxin to be used must first be titrated against a standard tetanus antitoxin to determine the L+/1,000 toxin dose. The L+/1,000 dose is the least amount of tetanus toxin which when mixed with 0.001 U of antitoxin and injected subcutaneously into mice in a volume of 0.5 ml causes the death of all mice by 96 h.

Female mice, 15 to 18 g, are used since males tend to fight. Any strain may be used, but strain and source should not be changed once the titration procedure has been established. Preliminary estimation of the L+/1,000 dose of toxin can be made in groups of four to six mice. In all mouse tests, pool all mice needed for the test, including the controls, and distribute them randomly into the groups required.

Phosphate-buffered saline (0.067 M, pH 7.4) containing 0.2% gelatin is used as the diluent for all reagents.

For the initial screening test to estimate the L+/1,000 dose of toxin, add constant volumes of standard antitoxin containing 0.004 antitoxin units (AU)/ml to a series of 8 to 10 tubes. Prepare a series of three- to fivefold dilutions of tetanus toxin, and add an equal volume to each tube of antitoxin. Shake the mixtures gently, incubate them for 1 h at room temperature, and then keep the mixtures at 4 to 8°C until the time of injection.

Inject 0.5 ml of each toxin-antitoxin mixture subcutaneously in the right inguinal fold of 4 to 10 mice per dose, using 26-gauge, 3/8-in. needles. Each injection contains 0.001 AU. Observe for 96 h and record the number of deaths. The smallest dose of toxin which kills all mice is the approximate L+/1,000 dose. (The corresponding toxin dilution contained 4 L+/1,000 doses per ml.)

To ascertain a more precise L+/1,000 dose, repeat the test using narrower increments of toxin and 4 to 10 mice per toxin dose. Since tetanus toxin produces very precise and reproducible results in mice, good results may be obtained by using a very narrow range of doses. Increments of 5% over a twofold range can be used successfully.

For serum titrations, test sera should be inactivated at 56°C for 30 min. Constant volumes of 2- to 10-fold dilutions of serum are dispensed into test tubes (13 by 100 mm). To each tube add an equal volume of toxin containing 1 L+/1,000 dose per ml. Each mouse thus receives 1 L+/4,000 dose of toxin per injection volume of 0.5 ml (one-fourth of an L+/1,000 dose). Run a concurrent L+/1,000 titration of the toxin against standard antitoxin as described above, using the same pool of mice. One group of mice should also receive the toxin test dose (1 L+/1,000 dose per ml) mixed with an equal volume of diluent. For serum titrations, groups of two to four mice per serum dilution give satisfactory results. The test is considered satisfactory if the concurrent L+/1,000 dose of toxin is within 25% of the test dose.

The results are interpreted as follows: if all mice are protected by undiluted serum but all die at the 1:10 dilution, then 0.25 ml of the undiluted serum contained >0.00025 AU and 0.25 ml of the 1:10 dilution contained <0.00025 AU. Thus, the serum contained >0.001 but <0.01 AU/ml. For purposes of calculation, such a serum can be assigned a value equal to the logarithmic mean of the values, or 0.003 AU/ml. For more precise titration, narrower increments of test sera can be used or the level of testing can be shifted by using multiples or fractions of the L+/1000 dose of toxin.

REAGENTS

U.S. standard samples of equine tetanus antitoxin are supplied to qualified laboratories by the Center for Biologics Evaluation and Research, Rockville, Md. The quantity of antitoxin is indicated in the label on the vial.

These samples are to be used by the receiving laboratory in preparing and standardizing its own reference stock.

Antitoxin may be purchased from pharmaceutical houses or state laboratories, which prepare tetanus antitoxins for prophylactic or therapeutic use. Such antitoxins must be precisely standardized against the official U.S. standard preparation before they can be used as reference reagents for the mouse neutralization tests. Tetanus immune globulin of human origin can be purchased from several pharmaceutical companies and then standardized against the standard reagent for use in ELISAs.

REFERENCES

1. **American Academy of Pediatrics.** 2003. *Report of the Committee on Infectious Diseases*, p. 614–616. American Academy of Pediatrics, Elk Grove, Ill.
2. **Barile, M. F., M. C. Hardegree, and M. Pittman.** 1970. Immunization against neonatal tetanus in New Guinea. 3. The toxin neutralization test as used in the immunization schedules in New Guinea. *Bull. W. H. O.* **43:**453–459.
3. **Bonin, E., M. Tiru, H. Hallander, and U. Bredberg-Raden.** 1999. Evaluation of single and dual antigen delayed fluorescence immunoassay in comparison to an ELISA and the in vivo toxin neutralization test for detection of diphtheria toxin antibodies. *J. Immunol. Methods* **230:**131–140.
4. **Cha, J., J. S. Brooke, M. Y. Chang, and L. Eidels.** 2002. Receptor based antidote for diphtheria. *Infect. Immun.* **70:**2344–2350.
5. **Dow, B. C., A. Barr, R. J. Crawford, and R. Mitchell.** 1983. A solid-phase radioimmunoassay for detection of tetanus antibody. *Med. Lab. Sci.* **40:**73–74.
6. **Edwards, K. M., and M. D. Decker.** 1997. Combination vaccines consisting of acellular pertussis vaccines. *Pediatr. Infect. Dis. J.* **16**(Suppl.):S97–S102.
7. **Efstratiou, A., and P. A. Maple.** 1994. *WHO Manual for the Laboratory Diagnosis of Diphtheria*. Publication ICP-EPI 038. World Health Organization, Geneva, Switzerland.
8. **Gupta, R. A., S. C. Maheshwari, and H. Sing.** 1984. The titration of tetanus antitoxin. III. A comparative evaluation of indirect hemagglutination and toxin neutralization titers of human sera. *J. Biol. Stand.* **12:**145–149.
9. **Hardy, I. R. B., S. Dittman, and R. W. Sutter.** 1996. Current situation and control strategies for resurgence of diphtheria in newly independent states of the former Soviet Union. *Lancet* **347:**1739–1744.
10. **Melville-Smith, M. E., V. A. Seagroatt, and J. T. Watkins.** 1983. A comparison of enzyme-linked immunosorbent assay (ELISA) with the toxin neutralization test in mice as a method for the estimation of tetanus antitoxin in human sera. *J. Biol. Stand.* **11:**137–144.
11. **Wassilak, G. F., W. A. Orenstein, and R. W. Sutter.** 1999. Tetanus toxoid, p. 441–473. *In* S. A. Plotkin and E. A. Mortimer, Jr. (ed.), *Vaccines*, 3rd ed. The W. B. Saunders Co., Philadelphia, Pa.
12. **Wharton, M., and C. Vitek.** 2004. Diphtheria toxoid, p. 211–228. *In* S. A. Plotkin and W. A. Orenstein (ed.), *Vaccines*, 4th ed. W. B. Saunders Co., Philadelphia, Pa.
13. **Winsnes, R., and G. Christiansen.** 1979. Quantification of tetanus antitoxin in human sera. II. Comparison of counterimmunoelectrophoresis and passive hemagglutination with toxin neutralization in mice. *Acta Pathol. Microbiol. Scand. Sect. B* **87:**197–200.

Immunologic Methods for Diagnosis of Infections Caused by Diarrheagenic *Enterobacteriaceae* and *Vibrionaceae*

MARCELA F. PASETTI, JAMES P. NATARO, AND MYRON M. LEVINE

53

The families *Enterobacteriaceae* and *Vibrionaceae* encompass a heterogeneous group of gram-negative organisms. Many members of these families are normal colonizers of the human intestinal tract (e.g., *Escherichia coli* strains) or may cause transient asymptomatic infections. Alterations of the immune system or breakdown in normal epithelial or mucosal barriers to infection may render these organisms virulent. Under such circumstances, they may cause bacteremia, meningitis, or infections of the urinary tract, skin, and soft tissues. However, certain members of these two families possess virulence factors that render them primary pathogens for the human intestinal tract. The consequences of infection with these agents are predominantly, but not necessarily, limited to diarrhea.

Members of the *Enterobacteriaceae* family associated with acute diarrheal disease include diarrheagenic *E. coli* and *Salmonella* and *Shigella* spp. There are six distinct categories of *E. coli* generally recognized as causative agents of diarrheal disease: enterotoxigenic *E. coli* (ETEC), enteroinvasive *E. coli* (EIEC), enteropathogenic *E. coli* (EPEC), enterohemorrhagic *E. coli* (EHEC), enteroaggregative *E. coli* (EAEC), and diffusely adherent *E. coli* (23, 40). Pathogenic isolates from each category tend to be clonal groups that fall within distinct somatic O (lipopolysaccharide [LPS]) and H (flagellar) serotypes (23). Within the *Vibrionaceae* family, *Vibrio cholerae* strains of serogroups O1 and O139 are the major agents of watery diarrhea.

The organisms chosen for discussion in this chapter are recognized as major public health concerns because of their significant contribution to morbidity and mortality in both children and adults in less developed and industrialized countries. In developing countries, diarrheagenic *E. coli*, particularly ETEC, isolates are the second most common cause of dehydrating diarrhea (after rotavirus) in infants and toddlers (40), while *V. cholerae* remains a major cause of epidemic diarrhea in South Asia and sub-Saharan Africa (28). In industrialized countries, these organisms are responsible for infections primarily in travelers, although some of them cause disease in institutional settings and among day care attendees (28).

Although acute diagnosis of infections with some of these agents has traditionally been made by microbiological isolation and serotyping of strains, this conventional approach may not be practical or even reliable for the following reasons: (i) the virulent *E. coli* strains are indistinguishable from normal flora by conventional bacteriology; (ii) some pathogens, such as EHEC, may no longer be retrievable at the time of disease presentation; (iii) optimal bacteriological specimens may be technically difficult to obtain (acute or chronic infection with *Salmonella enterica* serovar Typhi, for example); (iv) a bacteriology laboratory may not be available (or may not be well prepared) during acute outbreak situations, particularly in developing countries; and (v) bacteriological isolation may be too slow to allow timely clinical or public health intervention. Although O-antigen serogrouping may help to presume the category of diarrheagenic *E. coli*, this is not a reliable method of definitive diagnosis. Strains of *E. coli*, for example, that have the same O antigen may have virulence markers that put them into distinct categories. Thus, diarrheagenic O111 isolates may be either EPEC or EHEC. In addition, organisms that do not fall into the traditional EPEC O:H serotypes may possess some virulence characteristics of EPEC strains. For this reason, it is important to characterize and identify organisms based on their genetic virulence determinants and/or phenotypic expression of these virulence determinants. Improved, rapid immunologic and molecular methods for diagnosis of enteric infections can be important tools for clinical care and for public health action.

ENTEROBACTERIACEAE

EHEC

EHEC strains cause diarrhea that may progress to bloody diarrhea (hemorrhagic colitis); 5 to 10% of these cases may progress to hemolytic-uremic syndrome (HUS), a severe complication characterized by the triad of hemolytic anemia, thrombocytopenia, and acute renal failure (40). Up to 40% of patients with HUS develop long-term renal dysfunction, and 3 to 5% die during the acute phase of the disease. It has been suggested that the use of antibiotics for treatment of EHEC diarrheal illness may actually increase the risk for developing HUS (40). Consequently, it is critical to have adequate rapid diagnostic methods to identify disease caused by EHEC strains.

The principal EHEC serotype that causes disease in the United States and much of the industrialized world is O157:H7. Other EHEC serotypes implicated as causes of HUS include O26:H11, O4:NM (nonmotile), O111:H8, O111:NM, and O145:NM. These EHEC strains possess one or more phage-encoded Shiga toxins (Stx1 and Stx2) (also known as verocytotoxins), an ~ 60-MDa virulence plasmid, and a chromosomal pathogenicity island (the locus of enterocyte effacement [LEE]), all of which contribute to virulence (23, 40).

Detection of Stx by Cytotoxicity

Demonstration of cytotoxicity for Vero cells remains the "gold standard" method to detect Stx-producing strains in fecal samples (4, 24). HeLa cells can also be used, although they lack the preferred Stx2 cell surface receptor and therefore may be less sensitive than Vero cells (44). In these assays, serial dilutions of filtered stool supernatants are incubated in cell monolayers (in 96-well plates) and examined for cytopathic effect 48 to 72 h later. Cytotoxicity is usually examined under the microscope or can be quantified by colorimetric methods. Positive samples should be retested in the presence of Stx-specific antibodies to confirm the specificity of the cytotoxic effect. The success of the assay is limited by the number of bacteria in the fecal samples (44, 45); it is known that 1 week after the onset of diarrhea, two-thirds of HUS patients no longer excrete *E. coli* O157 or other causative EHEC organisms in their stools (40). Results may also be influenced by the amount and potency of the Stx secreted and the degree to which it is released from the bacterial cells (44). Nonetheless, cytotoxicity tests are extremely sensitive and free fecal toxin can be detected even though stool cultures are negative. This assay, however, is labor-intensive and time-consuming. Although more than 200 serotypes of *E. coli* produce Stx, most of these do not contain the LEE pathogenicity island and are not associated with human disease (23). Thus, for proper diagnosis of EHEC, detection of Stx should be accompanied by the demonstration of EHEC virulence factors.

Detection of Stx Antigen

A number of immunoassays that detect Stx1 and Stx2 in fecal samples have been described (4, 24, 44). Most of them consist of a sandwich enzyme-linked immunosorbent assay (ELISA) that uses monoclonal antibody (MAb) or affinity-purified polyclonal antibodies immobilized to the microplate to capture Stx in the specimens, which is revealed with Stx-specific antibodies labeled with an enzyme or using an appropriate secondary antiserum. There are commercially available ELISA kits (4) to detect Stx (e.g., Premier EHEC from Meridian Biosciences, Inc., Cincinnati, Ohio, and ProSpect Stx *E. coli* microplate assay from Alexon-Trend, Ramsey, Minn.). Results from these tests are influenced by the amount of bacteria in fecal samples and their capacity to produce toxin; for this reason, specimens should be obtained as early as possible in the course of infection. The Premier EHEC test has a sensitivity of 100% and a specificity of 99.7%, in comparison with fecal EHEC isolation using sorbitol-MacConkey (SMAC) agar, the culture method routinely used in clinical laboratories (4). The ProSpecT assay was also found to be highly sensitive and specific (100%) compared to SMAC agar, and the values are similar to those reported for the Premier EHEC technique (16). A reverse passive latex agglutination test to detect Stx1 and Stx2 (VTEC-RPLA "Seiken" from Denka Seiken, Tokyo, Japan) is commercially available. According to the manufacturer, the VTEC-RPLA has a limit of detection of 1 ng of toxin per ml and is 100% sensitive and 100% specific for Stx detection compared with the Vero cell assay. To reiterate, detection of both Stx and virulence factors is needed to confirm EHEC infection.

Detection of O157 LPS Antigen

Expression of O157 antigen can be assessed by agglutination of sorbitol-negative *E. coli* colonies from SMAC agar cultures (24). However, some O157 strains which ferment sorbitol have emerged as causes of human disease, and these strains are missed by this diagnostic procedure (4). Sandwich ELISAs have been described that detect O157 antigen in fecal samples. These assays have similar or higher sensitivity compared with the culture of organisms on SMAC agar and can detect sorbitol-fermenting strains (24). There are several *E. coli* O157 immunoassay detection kits commercially available (*E. coli* O157 latex test from Denka Seiken; ImmunoCard *E. coli* O157 from Meridian Biosciences, Inc.; *E. coli* O157 antigen detection microwell ELISA from Biotech Trading Partners, Encinitas, Calif.; and *E. coli* antigen detection by Diagnostic Automation, Calabasas, Calif.). The usefulness of these methods is limited by the fact that most patients are no longer excreting O157 EHEC in stools at the time of clinical presentation of HUS. There may also be cross-reactivity between O157 LPS and LPSs of other bacteria. Because nontoxigenic isolates of *E. coli* O157 have been reported (40), these assays must be considered primary screening methods that require confirmation by culture and/or demonstration of Stx production. It must also be emphasized that EHEC of serotypes other than O157:H7 are emerging as agents responsible for HUS, outbreaks and sporadic causes of HUS, and the clinical features of these cases are identical to those caused by Stx+ O157:H7 strains (44).

Molecular Methods To Detect EHEC Strains

In the late 1980s and early 1990s, hybridization using DNA probes to detect virulence determinants, such as the 60-MDa EHEC virulence plasmid and genes encoding Stx1 and Stx2, was a sensitive and specific technique to diagnose EHEC infections. These probes were used to test large numbers of stool *E. coli* isolates by hybridization (4, 24, 40). The sequencing of EHEC virulence genes now permits the design of primers for amplification using PCR (23, 40, 43). For example, Stx+ O157 strains have been distinguished from non-EHEC strains by amplifying a variable sequence on the 3′ portion of the *eae* gene (a component of the LEE pathogenicity island that encodes the bacterial adhesin intimin) either alone or combined with Stx genes (40, 43). PCR kits for detection of Stx+ *E. coli* are commercially available (e.g., ZipLys Bacto from ZipGen Inc., Solon, Ohio). PCR can also differentiate serogroups O157, O111, and O113 by using primers directed to the genetic loci (*rfb* regions) involved in O-antigen biosynthesis (43). Two other genetic markers associated with O157:H7 Stx+ *E. coli* strains, *fliCh7*, which encodes the H7 antigen, and *uidA*, responsible for the β-glucoronidase-negative phenotype of O157:H7 strains, have been used for PCR assays (40, 43). A system that allows identification of *Salmonella*, *Shigella*, and *E. coli* O157:H7 with sensitivity to detect as few as 3 to 50 CFU was recently developed (32). This system combines common PCR, seminested PCR, and random amplification polymorphic DNA (RAPD) analysis, using universal primers of enteric pathogens located in the *uidA* gene, primers for *ipaH* from *Shigella*, *eae* from *E. coli*, and the most conserved fragment, 16S rRNA, for *Salmonella* (32). PCR techniques are rapid and can be applied to crude lysates or DNA extracts from single colonies, broth cultures, feces, or food. They are extremely sensitive and specific, as the identity of the amplified product can be confirmed by ethidium bromide staining after separation in agarose gel electrophoresis, by restriction analysis, and by DNA probe. PCR analysis has an advantage over the serological methods to detect EHEC Stx, other virulence factors, or LPS, since it can be combined to identify the toxin type, other specific virulence genes, or genes associated with serogroups. A multiplex PCR assay combining specific primers for the *eae*, *bfp*, *stII*, and *lt* virulence genes that allows detection of EHEC, EPEC, and ETEC in a single reaction was used in an epidemiological study to evaluate the incidence of *E. coli* diarrheal infections in pediatric patients in Chile (56). This multiplex PCR can differentiate *E. coli* strains in cases of HUS, food-borne diarrheal disease outbreaks, and cases of sporadic enterocolitis or diarrhea (56). Despite its high sensitivity, however, even PCR may be unable to detect bacteria in the late course of the disease due to the low number of organisms present. In addition, stools may contain substances that interfere with PCR, thereby decreasing its sensitivity. Sometimes the results may be difficult to interpret, as the genotype profile observed may correspond to more than one organism (43). Whereas molecular techniques were once regarded as sophisticated, labor-intensive, and reserved for research laboratories, they are being increasingly adopted by large clinical laboratories.

Detection of Serum Antibodies to *E. coli* O157 LPS

Detection of immunoglobulin M (IgM), IgG, and IgA antibodies specific for O157 LPS has emerged as a useful, popular, and reliable tool for clinical diagnosis of O157 infection associated with HUS, especially when stool cultures are negative (9, 44). Children with HUS caused by O157 EHEC mount a rapid IgM response to O157 LPS that can be readily measured by ELISA (9). IgG antibodies, which may be detected early in the course of HUS caused by O157, persist for several months after disease onset. LPS antibodies measured by ELISA in serum samples or saliva (described below) may also serve to determine exposure to *E. coli* O157 in epidemiological surveys and to evaluate the extent of outbreaks. Several other techniques have been described to measure serum LPS antibodies, including immunoblotting, agglutination, and indirect hemagglutination, and the results obtained appear to be in close agreement (9, 24, 44). We describe the O157 ELISA, since we consider it one of the most practical and useful techniques.

Reagents

O157 LPS antigen can be extracted from a clinical isolate using the hot water-phenol method (9). Antigen preparations need to be free from protein and nucleic acid contamination. The optimal concentration of antigen should be determined by standard ELISA checkerboard titration, coating plates with different amounts of antigen and testing them with known positive and negative control sera during the standardization of the assay (13). The usual range of LPS coating concentrations is 1 to 10 μg/ml. Coating buffer is sodium bicarbonate, pH 9.6. Washing buffer is phosphate-buffered saline (PBS), pH 7.4, with 0.05% Tween 20 (PBST). Blocking solution is 10% nonfat dry milk in PBS, pH 7.4 (PBSM). Horseradish peroxidase (HRP)-labeled goat anti-human IgG (MP [formerly ICN Biomedicals], Aurora, Ohio) is used as secondary antibody; the appropriate dilution needs to be established in checkerboard titrations (13) (usually around 1:5,000). The diluent for serum and secondary antibody is 10% nonfat dry milk in PBS, pH 7.4, with 0.05% Tween 20 (PBSTM). The substrate solution is (3,5,3′,5′)-tetramethylenebenzidine (TMB) microwell peroxidase (Kirkegaard and Perry Laboratories [KPL], Gaithersburg, Md.).

Procedure

This technique follows a standard indirect ELISA procedure for detection of serum antibodies (13). ELISA plates (Immulon II; ThermoLabsystems) are incubated with 100 μl of antigen solution for 3 h at 37°C, washed, and blocked overnight at 4°C with 250 μl (full wells) of blocking solution (PBSM). Note that milk should be properly dissolved. After each incubation, plates are washed six times with washing buffer (PBST), soaking plates for 2 min between washes; the residual wash fluid is removed from the wells by tapping the inverted plate on absorbent paper. Proper washing is critical to minimize background signals. After plates are washed, serum samples are added at the appropriate dilution and incubated for 1 h at 37°C. When the antibody titer of the sample is unknown, starting dilutions of 1:100 or 1:1,000 are recommended for screening. Further twofold dilutions are made in the plate until row G; the last row (H) is usually reserved for blanks. Additional runs using different dilutions may be needed in order to obtain a linear dose-response curve of absorbance versus serum dilutions. Conjugate is added in a 100-μl volume, and plates are incubated for 1 h at 37°C. Substrate solution is prepared by following instructions from the manufacturer, added to the washed plates in a 100-μl volume, and incubated in an ELISA rotator for 15 min at room temperature in darkness. Color development is stopped by adding 100 μl of 1 M phosphoric acid. Absorbance is read immediately at 405 nm. The following controls should be included in each assay. (i) Blanks consisting of coated wells in which serum samples are replaced by the diluent should be used; the rest of the reagents, such as conjugate, substrate, and stop solution, as well as procedures are maintained. (ii) A calibrated positive control, which can be prepared from a pool of serum samples with a high LPS antibody titer, should be used. The titer of this calibrated control is established during the calibration of the assay; it must be run in each assay to confirm reproducibility. (iii) A calibrated negative control, usually prepared from a pool of negative samples, should be used; this control allows assessment of reproducibility in each assay and confirmation of the cutoff value for positive samples.

Endpoint antibody titers can be calculated as follows. Mean absorbance values for blank wells are subtracted from all individual absorbance values. Mean absorbance values (from duplicate wells) for the different serum dilutions are analyzed by linear regression. An endpoint titer is calculated through regression parameters as the inverse of the serum dilution that produces an absorbance value of 0.2 above the blank.

Results and Interpretation

Each laboratory must determine an appropriate cutoff value for positive samples as the mean absorbance produced by control (e.g., negative) samples + 3 standard deviations. A high proportion of patients infected with O157 strains have elevated acute-phase levels of serum antibody to O157 LPS; healthy controls have a low seropositivity rate.

Remarks

High titers even in a single sample at the time of acute disease is considered a reliable indicator of current or very recent infection (9, 24). O157 LPS serology was shown to be consistently more sensitive than bacterial isolation or Stx serology (24). Serodiagnosis is less valuable when serum is obtained several months after clinical disease, due to the rapid decrease of antibody titers. Another limitation of this method is that healthy people living in areas where EHEC strains are prevalent may have increased baseline O157 LPS titers. Indirect hemagglutination assays detecting O157 LPS antibodies have also been used for serological diagnosis of

E. coli O157 infections (6). Early studies showed that using a cutoff of $\geq$1:4,096, the indirect hemagglutination assay has a sensitivity of 81 to 91% and a specificity of 94 to 100% (6, 44). These studies examined samples from children with HUS during the acute and postacute phases; samples from children with diarrhea but who did not develop HUS were used as controls (6).

EHEC organisms belonging to serogroups other than O157 may also cause HUS and bloody diarrhea (40). Thus, if possible, clinical samples that are seronegative for O157 LPS should be tested against common non-O157 serogroups (e.g., O26, O55, O111, and O128, available from Sigma Chemical Co., St. Louis, Mo.). It should be noted that *E. coli* O157 shares epitopes with other gram-negative organisms, such as *Yersinia enterocolitica* O9, *V. cholerae* non-O1, *Citrobacter freundii*, *Brucella abortus*, and *Salmonella* spp. This fact limits the specificity of serodiagnosis based on antibodies that bind O157 antigens (9); thus, highly purified LPS antigens must be used to minimize cross-reactions.

Detection of Salivary Antibodies to *E. coli* O157 LPS

A few studies have demonstrated that saliva-based immunoassays offer a reliable, noninvasive method for the diagnosis of *E. coli* O157 infection in patients (including children) with enteropathic HUS (9, 36), particularly small and severely anemic children. In one study, paired serum and saliva samples from 22 children with HUS collected during acute disease and the convalescent phase and 44 age-matched controls were tested for O157 LPS IgM and IgA antibodies by ELISA (36). Increased O157 LPS IgM and IgA titers were found in saliva of all HUS patients with stool cultures positive for Stx$^+$ *E. coli* O157 and from four of five HUS patients for whom stool cultures were negative. The saliva antibody titers showed a strong correlation with titers in serum. In Stx$^+$ *E. coli* O157 culture-confirmed cases, the sensitivity of the ELISA was 92% for saliva IgM and IgA, based on the first available sample, and 100 and 92%, respectively, when subsequent samples were included. The specificities were 98% for IgM and 100% for IgA. Saliva- and oral fluid-based assays are increasingly being used for diagnosis and prediction of disease progression (10). Since oral fluid collection is a simple, noninvasive procedure and oral fluid antibodies accurately reflect serum antibody levels, one may expect the use of such assays to become increasingly popular for diagnosis in children.

Detection of Antibodies to Stx and EHEC Virulence Factors

The presence of serum neutralizing antibodies to the Stxs has been reported for patients with HUS (9, 44). But the specificity of these responses has been questioned, since Stx-neutralizing antibodies (mostly to Stx2) have also been found in sera from healthy individuals (9). Another limitation of this method is that only a minority of patients with proven Stx-producing *E. coli* infection exhibit detectable serum antibodies to the respective toxin type (9). Paton and Paton showed by Western blot analysis that convalescent-phase sera from patients with HUS caused by LEE-positive strains reacted with an important EHEC virulence determinant, Tir, the translocated intimin receptor that is inserted by the bacterium into host cells (45). Another study confirmed the presence of strong antibody responses to Tir in all patients with diarrhea or HUS caused by EHEC as early as 8 days after onset of illness and for at least 2 months following acute disease (33). Brazilian mothers and children had antibodies to Tir in colostrum and serum (50). The clinical specificity of this assay, however, is

not known since Tir is also an important virulence factor of EPEC. Immune responses to other products of the LEE locus, such as intimin and the secreted protein EspB, have also been demonstrated in patients infected with O157 EHEC (33, 40). Although titers of antibodies against these virulence factors may be lower than those against LPS, evidence indicates that they are expressed during acute disease and the host can still recognize them.

ETEC

ETEC strains producing heat-labile toxin (LT) and/or heat-stable toxin (STa and STb) are common agents of dehydrating diarrhea among young children in developing countries and are a major cause of traveler's diarrhea (40). Approximately 50% of clinical ETEC strains produce LT with or without ST. ST, of which STa is most commonly seen in human infections, is not immunogenic. LT is antigenically and functionally similar to cholera toxin (CT) of *V. cholerae* O1 and O139 and is highly immunogenic (40). The expression of these toxins is plasmid mediated, as is the expression of the fimbrial colonization factors (CFAs) that mediate attachment to intestinal mucosa. CFA/I represents a single antigenic type of fimbrial antigen, while CFA/I and CFA/IV constitute families of fimbrial antigens. All CFA/II strains contain the common coli surface antigen 3 (CS3), alone or with CS1 or CS2. CFA/IV-producing ETEC strains express CS6 either alone or in conjunction with CS4 or CS5. These virulence factors are usually associated with a limited number of serotypes of *E. coli*; however, due to the multiple serotypes involved, serotyping of isolates is of only limited value in the diagnosis of ETEC infections and should be limited to epidemiological studies.

Diagnosis of acute ETEC infections requires the detection of LT, ST, or toxin genes in isolated strains. Since ETEC strains may produce either or both toxins, immunologic identification of ETEC strains must detect them both. Simple immunologic assays, such as agglutination and ELISAs, to detect LT and ST have been described.

The STa detection assay described below utilizes STa-specific MAbs (54). STa produced by *E. coli* isolates competes with adsorbed STa for binding to the antibody. A similar ST competitive ELISA using synthetic peptide toxin bound to microtiter plates and toxin-specific MAb is commercially available from Denka Seiken.

The LT detection assay uses GM1 ganglioside, a receptor for LT, adsorbed to microtiter plates that captures free LT in the specimens (49). A latex test to detect LT is available from Denka Seiken; the manufacturer reports a limit of detection of approximately 1 to 2 ng/ml and 100% correlation to the classical Y1 bioassay.

Retrospective analysis can be made for some ETEC infections by measuring antibodies to LT and CFAs. However, the LT antibody assay is limited since about one-third of diarrhea-causing ETEC strains express only ST. In addition, there exists significant antigenic cross-reactivity between LT and CT that needs to be considered. ELISAs to measure antibodies to ETEC CFAs in serum and intestinal fluids have been developed and used to assess the immunogenicity of vaccine candidates (1). However, the many fimbrial antigens prevalent on ETEC strains that cause disease in humans and the lack of availability of reagents limit their usefulness in seroepidemiological studies.

Detection of ETEC LT by GM1 ELISA

The GM1 assay enables the detection of LT produced by *E. coli* clinical isolates. It is useful for diagnosis of clinical cases.

Reagents

E. coli is grown in Casamino Acid-yeast extract medium containing, per liter, 20 g of Casamino Acids (Difco Laboratories, Detroit, Mich.), 6 g of yeast extract (Difco), 2.5 g of NaCl, 8.71 g of K_2HPO_4, 2.5 g of glucose, and 1 ml of trace salts (containing 5% $MgSO_4 \cdot 7H_2O$, 0.5% $MnCl_2 \cdot 4H_2O$, and 0.5% $FeCl_2$), pH adjusted to 8.5. The essential requirements for optimal LT production are glucose and trace salts, which increase LT production by 40 to 90%. In addition, lincomycin (4.5% final concentration) is added to the culture to release LT from the periplasmic space, significantly increasing the amount of LT that can be detected in culture. The coating antigen is GM1 ganglioside (Sigma). Coating buffer is 0.1 M PBS, pH 7.2. Washing buffer is PBS–0.05% Tween 20. Blocking buffer is PBS–5% fetal calf serum (FCS). Hyperimmune rabbit anti-LT (or anti-CT) antibody produced against purified enterotoxin is used as detector antibody, along with alkaline phosphatase or HRP-labeled anti-rabbit IgG (KPL). Substrate is TMB (KPL).

Procedure

Microtiter plates are coated overnight at room temperature with 100 µl of GM1 solution (1 µg/ml) or PBS (control) in different rows and blocked for 1 h at 37°C. Culture medium is added to all wells (200 µl) and test strains are inoculated in duplicate into the GM1-coated and control wells. Plates are incubated for 24 h on a rotary shaking platform at 37°C. *E. coli* LT is used as a positive control in a range of concentrations, and PBS is used as a negative control. After incubation, plates are washed six times with PBST and incubated with anti-LT (or anti-CT) antiserum diluted in PBST containing 1% FCS (100 µl/well). Plates are then washed, incubated with a conjugate secondary antibody (100 µl/well) for 1 h at 37°C, washed again, and incubated with substrate. The reaction is stopped and absorbance values are measured.

Results and Interpretation

The mean absorbance value of the control wells is subtracted from absorbance values of test wells. Each laboratory should establish a cutoff value based on absorbance values from non-LT-producing strains. This assay has been shown to be 97% sensitive and 100% specific compared to the Y1 adrenal cell assay (49). The limit of detection is approximately 1 to 7 ng of purified LT per ml (49).

Remarks

This assay can be read visually, maintaining high levels of accuracy. LT can also be detected using sandwich ELISAs, with LT-specific antibodies attached to microtiter plates.

Detection of STa by Competitive Binding ELISA

Detection of STa from culture supernatants of *E. coli* isolates is valuable for clinical diagnosis, epidemiological studies, and assessing ETEC vaccine candidates.

Reagents

Purified STa is conjugated to bovine serum albumin (BSA) (Sigma) using 1-ethyl-3-(3 dimethylaminopropyl)-carbodiimide (Bio-Rad Laboratories, Richmond, Calif.) at a coupling ratio of 5:1, STa to BSA. The STa to specific MAb (no. 20C1B8; Genetic Diagnostics, Great Neck, N.Y.) is diluted in 0.1% BSA–PBS. HRP-labeled goat anti-mouse IgG (Roche, Indianapolis, Ind.) is used as a secondary antibody at optimal dilution (around 1:1,000). Coating buffer is sodium bicarbonate buffer, pH 9.6. Washing buffer is PBST. Blocking buffer is PBS with 1% BSA. Substrate is TMB (KPL).

Procedure

The optimal coating concentration for STa-BSA antigen and the optimal dilution for MAb and anti-mouse conjugate must be determined using standard checkerboard titrations (13). The recommended STa-BSA coating concentration is 1 µg/ml; MAb concentrations range from 5 to 100 ng/ml. Plates are coated with STa-BSA for 18 h at 4°C, washed, and blocked for 2 h at 37°C. Strains are grown in a Casamino Acid-yeast extract medium as described above. MAb (100 µl) mixed with STa alone (0.5 to 10 ng/ml) or with different dilutions of unknown samples (100 µl) are allowed to equilibrate at room temperature for 5 to 10 min before being added to the plate. Plates are incubated for 1 h at 37°C, washed, and incubated again with 100 µl of secondary antibody at the appropriate dilution. Plates are washed again and substrate is added. Specific absorbance values are determined by subtracting from the absorbance values of the test wells the mean absorbance of control wells. Controls must include (i) coated wells that will have added diluent in lieu of samples (and all other reagents), (ii) samples and only secondary detector antibody (no STa-MAb), and (iii) uncoated wells with all the rest of the reagents.

Results and Interpretation

Absorbance values measured for different concentrations of STa are analyzed by linear regression. Strains are considered positive when a culture supernatant tested yields a ≥65% reduction in absorbance (from that measured in the absence of competing toxin). A quantitative measurement of STa present in a sample is obtained by interpolation of its absorbance value in the standard curve.

Remarks

Changes in temperature and incubation time may affect the kinetics of the reaction, influencing the sensitivity of the assay. The sensitivity of this assay is 3 to 10 pg of toxin (54). There is no cross-reactivity with LT, CT, or staphylococcal enterotoxin B. Similar competitive inhibition ELISAs that use STa chemically linked to other protein carriers, such as the B subunit of LT or CT, have been described to enhance ST binding to the solid phase via GM1.

Molecular Methods To Detect ETEC Strains

Molecular diagnostic techniques became available early on to detect ETEC strains (40). Comparison of LT detection immunoassays with early membrane-based DNA hybridization assays with LT probes has shown more than 95% concordance of results. In these studies, however, as many as 10% of isolates that were positive by hybridization techniques did not produce phenotypically detectable LT. Similar to the DNA probes for LT, oligonucleotide hybridization assays to detect STa plasmid genes show a high rate of concordance with ELISA techniques. In studies comparing competitive ELISA with hybridization for the STa gene, the ELISA detected STa production in 94% of probe-positive strains (54). Hybridization assays to identify ETEC strains with probes that detect ST, LT, and CFA/I, CS1 to CS8, CS12 to CS15, CS17 to CS19, and CS22 have been described (52). Further refinement in molecular methods for the detection of ETEC gave rise to PCR and multiplex PCR that can detect ETEC in stool specimens with enhanced sensitivity over bacteriological culture (40). A real-time PCR assay using primers and hybridization probes for simultaneous detection of LT and ST (STa and STb) genes has been described; this technique is 10^2 to 10^3 times more sensitive than block-cycle PCR assays, allowing the detection of 10^5 to 10^6 CFU of ETEC per g without enrichment (48).

Measurement of IgG Anti-LT by ELISA

Because of the antigenic cross-reactivity between LT of ETEC and CT of *V. cholerae*, simple measurement of antibody responses against LT alone is not sufficient for the accurate diagnosis of ETEC infection in the absence of bacterial isolation from stool. However, differences in the magnitude of the antibody responses against CT and LT antigens can be used to differentiate between infections caused by CT$^+$ *V. cholerae* strains and LT$^+$ ETEC strains (31). This approach can also be used for seroepidemiological studies or to assess immune responses to new vaccine candidates.

Reagents

Purified *E. coli* LT is used as a coating antigen. Detector antibody is HRP-labeled goat anti-human IgG (ICN Biomedicals) diluted in PBSTM. The working dilution is selected during calibration of the assay. Coating buffer is PBS, pH 7.4. The rest of the reagents are the same as described for O157 LPS ELISA.

Procedure

The optimal antigen coating concentration is determined by checkerboard titration using different amounts of LT in the presence of positive and negative calibrated control sera (13). A number of assays report that the optimal LT coating concentration was 1 μg/ml (from a 0.1- to 10-μg/ml range tested) (31). The recommended starting dilution for samples of unknown titer is 1:25. The ELISA procedure is similar to that described above.

Results and Interpretation

For the diagnosis of ETEC infections caused by LT$^+$ strains, the most reliable way to prove causality is to test both pre- and postinfection serum samples. A fourfold rise in titer of paired sera is considered a positive response. If only a single serum sample is available, high levels of LT IgG antibody can only give evidence of recent exposure to LT. Even though there are antigenic similarities between CT and LT, one can discriminate between infections caused by LT$^+$ ETEC and CT$^+$ *V. cholerae* by the magnitude of antibody response between LT and CT. While LT antitoxin levels fall after 3 months of infection, high CT titers persist during the convalescent period (31). Nevertheless, it is possible to establish a cutoff level of LT for diagnosis of recent (within the previous 3 months) ETEC infection (31). Data derived from wild-type challenge studies with nonimmune North American subjects have shown the presence of a significant level of antitoxin as early as day 10 postchallenge, peaking at day 21 postchallenge (31). Using appropriately timed paired specimens, this assay can detect approximately 80% of both clinical and subclinical LT$^+$ ETEC infections. When only single specimens are available, this assay can accurately detect a recent LT$^+$ ETEC infection (within the last 6 months) with a sensitivity above 80% and a specificity of 100%, using the CT/LT ratio described above.

Remarks

The need to discriminate between CT- and LT-specific antibody responses makes the immunologic detection of LT$^+$ ETEC infections difficult for a nonresearch laboratory. These assays are most reliable for diagnosis of an individual case when paired sera are available. Consequently, this assay is mainly used for seroepidemiological studies or to assess immunogenicity of vaccine candidates.

EPEC

EPEC strains are clonal pathogens that harbor both chromosomal and plasmid-mediated virulence determinants (23, 40). Typical EPEC strains carry both a chromosomally encoded LEE, which mediates a complex signal transduction phenotype on the target epithelial cell, and the EPEC adherence factor plasmid (EAF), which encodes the principal EPEC adhesin. The attaching and effacing histopathology (visualized by electron microscopy) that is conferred by the LEE is accompanied by cytoskeletal rearrangement, perturbation of signal transduction cascades, activation of inflammatory and secretory responses, and opening of the epithelial tight junction fence. The essential components of the LEE include a type III secretion apparatus and a series of protein effectors that are thereby injected into the target cell. Among these are Tir, which activates target cell signal transduction and serves as the epithelial receptor for intimin, a ca. 94-kDa bacterial outer membrane protein. Interaction of intimin with Tir mediates adherence and colonization as well as the attaching and effacing phenotype.

Identification of several LEE genes or their products has been used in EPEC diagnosis, particularly the gene encoding intimin (*eae*) (40). It should be recognized, however, that an *eae* homologue is also present in EHEC. Several diarrheal outbreaks have been linked to atypical EPEC carrying the LEE but no other recognizable virulence genes. Thus, the presence of *eae* or other LEE-borne genes or products cannot be considered definite evidence of an organism being an enteric pathogen. Identification of a typical EPEC strain requires identification of both the LEE and the EAF plasmid.

Two diagnostic genetic targets for the EAF have been well substantiated: the original EPEC probe, derived empirically from the plasmid of strain E2348/69, and the gene corresponding to the major pilin subunit of the bundle-forming pilus (*bfpA*). They yield similar sensitivity and specificity in the detection of EPEC strains (40). Both gene probes and PCR have been described for *eae* and EAF plasmid-borne genes, and the performance of these assays is essentially equivalent. Multiplex PCR assays have been described recently which permit simultaneous detection of *eae* and EAF genes, often in combination with other gene targets, such as *bfpA*; this method offers great potential for detection of EPEC in conjunction with other diarrheagenic *E. coli* strains (41).

The HEp-2 adherence assay can be used to identify EPEC, recognized by their specific localized, microcolony adherence pattern (40). However, the test must be performed using rigorous standards and is best interpreted by a trained observer. In addition, cultivation of cells for use in diagnosis is cumbersome and likely to delay timely diagnosis.

EAEC and EIEC

EAEC is an emerging diarrheal pathogen that is important in three epidemiological scenarios: infant diarrhea in both developing and industrialized countries, diarrhea of travelers from industrialized to developing countries, and persistent diarrhea in human immunodeficiency virus-infected patients (23, 40). Though EAEC strains are classically defined by the presence of a characteristic stacked-brick pattern of adherence to HEp-2 cells, this phenotype is nonspecific and can be considered only suggestive of the presence of a true enteric pathogen. Recently, the designation "typical EAEC" has been offered to describe organisms harboring a series of virulence-related genes under the control of the gene activator AggR. Thus, identification of one or more AggR-controlled loci is highly suggestive of pathogenic EAEC strains. Diagnostic tests for the AggR regulon include detection of the *aggR* plasmid-borne gene itself; both genetic probes and PCR have been shown to offer excellent sensitivity and specificity for *aggR* detection (40). Results generated by *aggR* detection are similar to those produced by the first EAEC probe (variously called the AA or CVD 432 probe), now shown to detect the *aatA* gene under the control of AggR. Several multiplex PCR assays have been described to detect typical EAEC along with other diarrheagenic pathotypes (41). EIEC strains are similar to *Shigella* spp. at the genetic and pathogenetic level. EIEC strains are best detected using DNA probes or PCR for the target genes of *Shigella*, including the *ipaH* locus and the *ial* locus (14).

Shigella

Shigella flexneri and *Shigella dysenteriae* are responsible for about 15% of all deaths attributable to diarrhea in children younger than 5 years of age in developing countries; *Shigella sonnei* is also encountered in industrialized nations, particularly in specialized settings such as day care centers (28). *Shigella* infections occur primarily in children 6 months to approximately 5 years of age; illness peaks in toddlers and preschool children 12 to 47 months of age. However, adults from industrialized countries who travel to areas of high endemicity are also susceptible to diarrheal infection with these agents. Thus, *Shigella* is often the second most important cause of traveler's diarrhea in surveys. Since *Shigella* invades the mucosa of the distal small intestine and colon, the full-blown clinical disease can progress to overt bacillary dysentery, marked by gross blood and mucus in diarrheal stools, systemic toxicity, high fever, abdominal pain, and tenesmus. The diarrhea is watery for about 24 h but then decreases in volume. Acute diagnosis of shigellosis is primarily made by bacteriological isolation. However, because *Shigella* may be difficult to isolate or facilities for culturing may not be available, serological assays may be helpful in retrospective diagnosis. Serum antibody responses are primarily directed against two surface antigens: LPS and invasion plasmid antigens (IpaB, IpaC, and IpaD). Cohen et al. reported a significant correlation between levels of *Shigella* LPS IgG and resistance to shigellosis (11). This group also proposed the use of a single high serum *Shigella* LPS IgA determination as a potentially reliable indicator of recent symptomatic and asymptomatic *Shigella* infection. IgM shows a pattern similar to that of IgA, except that it has a much lower convalescence increase. Following exposure to these strains, serum antibody responses directed against Ipas are not as frequently detected as LPS responses. IpaB and IpaC are the most immunogenic antigens (25), and Ipa-specific secretory IgA antibodies can be detected following dysentery. In cases of *S. dysenteriae* type 1 infection, measurement of antibodies to Stx by ELISA has been found to be unhelpful diagnostically because few infected individuals generate responses (29).

Herein we describe a general format for an indirect ELISA which can be used to measure both LPS IgG and IgA for all *Shigella* groups. Antibody responses can be helpful in diagnosing *Shigella* infection retrospectively, although IgA antibodies are more transient, peaking at 2 weeks after infection and declining to baseline by approximately 2 months.

Molecular Methods To Detect *Shigella* Strains

DNA probes detecting portions of the three *ipa* genes (*ipaB*, *ipaC*, and *ipaD*) were described early as indicators of invasive dysentery bacilli. However, the spontaneous loss of invasion plasmids seen in *Shigella* may produce false-negative results. The same group later developed a probe for the *ipaH* gene, a multiple-copy element found in the large invasion plasmid and the chromosome (55).

PCR techniques have been used to detect *Shigella* in stool samples amplifying target sequences of *ial*, *ipaH* (14), and *rfc* (20). In a study carried out in India, the *ipaH* PCR assay was approximately 100-fold more sensitive than the colony hybridization assay and the conventional culture and could identify a number of nontypeable *Shigella* strains (Sh OUT), which otherwise would have remained undiagnosed (14). Although highly sensitive to detect organisms directly from stool samples, PCR amplifying *ial* and *ipaH* sequences cannot distinguish EIEC from *Shigella* or one *Shigella* species from another. Serotype-specific primers derived from the *rfc* genes allowed for the first time differentiation among *Shigella* serotypes (e.g., *S. sonnei*, *S. flexneri*, and *S. dysenteriae* type 1) (20). Furthermore, a multiplex PCR containing the same *rfc*-specific primers can efficiently identify the most prominent *Shigella* serotypes in raw stool samples from acute diarrheal patients (20).

Measurement of *Shigella* LPS IgG by ELISA

ELISA to measure *Shigella* LPS IgG is most useful for retrospective diagnosis of infection in immunologically naive individuals, especially for *S. sonnei* and *S. dysenteriae*. However, because multiple serotypes exist for *S. flexneri* and *Shigella boydii*, serological diagnosis is useful only if a particular serotype is suspected. The assay is also useful to assess *Shigella* vaccines in clinical trials, since LPS IgG antibodies correlate with protection from homologous wild-type challenge.

Sample Requirements

Although optimum collection times are preinfection (as in the case of serum samples obtained prior to travel) and 21 to 28 days postinfection, access to preinfection serum is unusual in clinical practice. Sera from the acute phase (i.e., at the time of presentation) and convalescent phase (4 weeks after) are more likely to be available but may be less useful to detect a seroconversion, especially for people living in areas where *Shigella* is endemic. For example, approximately 65% of culture-confirmed *S. dysenteriae* type 1 infections could be detected in Thai individuals by evaluating acute- and convalescent-phase serum samples; however, 25% of the subjects had such high titers in their acute-phase sera (obtained 7 to 14 days after disease onset) that seroconversion could not be demonstrated from comparison of the acute- and convalescent-phase sera (29). A single serum sample can be useful for previously nonexposed subjects such as travelers, if that sample is obtained within 3 weeks to 3 months of the onset of diarrhea.

Reagents and Procedure

Shigella LPS is purified using hot water-phenol extraction. The appropriate coating concentration should be determined by checkerboard titration (13). Coating concentrations range between 2 and 10 μg/ml. Reagents and procedures are the same as described for O157 LPS ELISA.

Results and Interpretation

A cutoff for positive response can be established by testing a large number of known negative serum samples. To maximize the specificity of the assay, accounting for cross-reactive antibodies, convalescent-phase sera from individuals with known culture-proven *Shigella* infections should be tested using LPS preparations from heterologous *Shigella* serotypes (*S. sonnei* and *S. flexneri* 2a in the case of *S. dysenteriae* infection, for example) and cutoff values should be adjusted accordingly.

Measurement of anti-LPS antibodies by ELISA using paired acute- and convalescent-phase sera has a sensitivity of 60 to 85% and a specificity between 85 and 100% based on culture-proven cases (29). When a single specimen is available (obtained within 3 weeks to 3 months of onset of diarrhea), the sensitivity and specificity of this assay to determine infection are slightly lower, 60 to 70% and 80 to 90%, respectively. Measurement of serum antibodies to LPS and Ipa antigens is useful to assess immune responses to vaccine candidates (25).

S. enterica Serovar Typhi

Typhoid fever is a systemic infection that results from the ingestion of *S. enterica* serovar Typhi and uptake into the gut-associated lymphoid tissues. In successive steps, the bacilli reach draining lymph nodes, enter the lymph and then the blood circulation, and ultimately attain their intracellular niche in fixed macrophages of the reticuloendothelial system. After an incubation period of 8 to 14 days a secondary bacteremia occurs, accompanied by a stepwise increase in fever, headache, and abdominal pain. The case fatality rate in untreated typhoid fever is 10 to 20%. From 1 to 6% of acutely infected individuals, depending on age and sex, can develop chronic infections of the gallbladder that may persist throughout life. These chronic biliary carriers intermittently excrete organisms in their stool and serve as an epidemiological reservoir of infection. Typhoid fever is endemic in many developing areas of the world and is a risk for travelers to such areas.

Isolating the organism from blood, bone marrow, or duodenal aspirate in cases of acute infection or from bile or stool from chronic carriers provides a definitive diagnosis. However, bacteriological culture has limitations. The yield from blood cultures is 70 to 80% during the first week of fever and steadily decreases thereafter. Bacteriological isolation of *Salmonella* can take several days (it is much more rapid if automated blood culture systems are used), and the sensitivity of cultures can be influenced by previous antibiotic treatment, inadequate sampling, and the low level of bacteremia (1 to 10 organisms per ml of blood). Sensitivity can be increased by culturing bone marrow samples; however, bone marrow collection is an invasive procedure that is not suitable for routine use. Culturing of stools is not practical for large-scale screening to identify chronic carriers.

There is a long history of serodiagnosis of acute typhoid fever, going back to the agglutination tests of the late 19th century. Modern serodiagnosis is based on measurement of specific anti-serovar Typhi LPS and flagellar H antibodies. Commercial kits for the diagnosis of typhoid fever include the Multi-Test Dip-S-Tick (PANBIO INDX, Inc., Baltimore, Md.), TyphiDot (Malaysian Biodiagnostic Research SDN BHD, Singapore, Malaysia), and TUBEX (IDL Biotech, Sollentuna, Sweden). The Multi-Test Dip-S-Tick tests for five pathogens, including serovar Typhi. It consists of a dipstick that detects IgM or IgG against serovar Typhi LPS, H, and capsular polysaccharide Vi antigens. The TyphiDot is a dot enzyme immunoassay that qualitatively detects either IgM or IgG antibodies against a serovar Typhi outer membrane protein. TUBEX is a semiquantitative inhibition latex agglutination test to detect IgM antibodies to the O9 antigen. Olsen et al. evaluated the performance of these three commercial kits in comparison with the Widal test for Vietnamese patients, considering blood culture as the gold standard. They found that overall, TUBEX and TyphiDot exhibited the most promising results, with ~79% sensitivity and 89% specificity (42). ELISAs that measure H and LPS antibodies are commonly used (39, 47) and are described below. Detection of antibodies to the Vi capsular polysaccharide is helpful as a screening test for identification of chronic carriers, since only about 20% of subjects with acute typhoid fever exhibit increased levels of IgG anti-Vi antibodies, whereas over 90% of chronic carriers exhibit high titers of Vi antibodies (34).

Detection of H and O Antibodies by Agglutination (Widal Tests)

The Widal tests, which measure agglutinating antibodies to serovar Typhi H and LPS antigens, are the classic assays for serodiagnosis of acute typhoid fever (27, 47). Although the validity of these tests for the serological diagnosis of typhoid fever in areas where typhoid is endemic has been questioned, they are widely used throughout the world; therefore, it is important to discuss their usefulness and limitations. Only the tube dilution method for H antigen agglutination is described here, since the assay using LPS antigen is very similar (27).

Reagents

For the LPS agglutination assay, a suspension of serovar Typhi adjusted to a standardized concentration is used. The infecting strain is used during outbreaks; otherwise, clinical laboratories use a nonflagellated serovar Typhi O-901 strain containing LPS W (Difco). For the H-agglutination assay, exposed H antigen from formalinized whole-cell *Salmonella enterica* serovar Virginia (10^{10}/ml) is used (27). Serovar Virginia has the identical flagellar antigen as serovar Typhi but has distinct O antigens and does not express Vi. Serum samples and H antigen are diluted in 0.85% NaCl.

Procedure

Serum samples in serial twofold dilutions (starting at 1:20) are incubated with an equal volume of H (diluted 1:10) overnight in a 45°C water bath. Each tube is examined for agglutination against a black background in a well-lighted area. A positive test will exhibit flocculent agglutination, similar in appearance to cotton balls. The amount of agglutination is graded according to clarity of the supernatant and amount and size of flocculence: 4+ agglutination has a clear supernatant and large flocculent clumps, 3+ agglutination is similar to 4+ except that clumps are smaller, 2+ agglutination has a cloudy supernatant with small clumps of cells, 1+ agglutination has a cloudy supernatant with very fine clumps of agglutinated cells, and 0 grading reveals a cloudy supernatant with cells appearing as a smooth button in the bottom of the test tube. The O antigen, being somatic, produces a coarse, compact, and granular agglutination, whereas H antigen, being flagellar, brings about a larger, loose agglutination. Turbid or contaminated sera should not be used for testing. The endpoint titer is the last serum dilution that exhibits a 3+ or 4+ agglutination of cells. Positive and negative calibrated control sera are included in each run. The sera for positive controls used in the assays were obtained from patients with bacteriologically confirmed acute typhoid fever obtained at the time of hospital presentation (27). Negative controls were obtained from age-matched healthy patients from an area of nonendemicity.

Results and Interpretation

The reading of agglutination can be difficult, and the reliability of the results is correlated with the experience of the reader. When acute- and convalescent-phase serum samples are available, a fourfold rise in titer is considered a positive response and believed to be a reliable indicator of infection when the clinical picture is compatible with typhoid fever. This is true for both travelers and people living in areas where infection is endemic. However, the development of agglutination antibodies in people with bacteriologically proven infection is variable, ranging from 25 to 100%, depending on the degree of illness and the time the second serum sample was collected. As expected, those patients with more severe illness and from whom serum samples were taken within 2 months of onset are more likely to have a serological response (75 to 100%). Since peak titers occur approximately 2 to 3 weeks after onset of illness, samples obtained much earlier may yield negative results. Agglutination results are more variable for LPS than for H antibodies since other *Salmonella* organisms (such as *Salmonella enterica* serovar Enteriditis) that cause disease in humans share antigenic LPS determinants with serovar Typhi. Titers considered positive vary depending on geographic area and the laboratory performing the assay but usually are in the range of ≥1:40 to ≥1:400 (27). Using a cutoff of 1:160 as indicative of infection, for example, yields a sensitivity of 46%, with a specificity of 98%; 1:80 gives a sensitivity of 66% but a specificity of 94%; and 1:40 gives a sensitivity of 90% and a specificity of 85% (27).

Although the Widal test requires acute- and convalescent-phase serum samples, usually only one serum sample taken at the time of clinical presentation is available for evaluation. In such cases, however, a single Widal test has no diagnostic value, since even high titers may be due to other *Salmonella* species, rather than serovar Typhi; a high prevalence of antibodies has also been found among healthy individuals in areas of endemicity (27). Results may also be difficult to interpret for people receiving antibiotic treatment.

Remarks

Standardization of this assay is extremely important. It can be performed in large laboratories with experienced personnel used to run samples from areas of endemicity, but it is not recommended to diagnose the infrequent case of acute typhoid fever. Recipients of both oral and parenteral typhoid vaccines can also have a positive Widal result.

Measurement of LPS and H Antibodies by ELISA

Measurement of LPS antibody and H antibody levels by ELISA may have diagnostic potential for acute typhoid fever for patients from areas where the disease is endemic (21, 39, 47).

Reagents

Serovar Typhi LPS is commercially available (Sigma). Flagellar H antigen can be purified by a bulk shearing method from the rough serovar Typhi strain Ty2R or from serovar Virginia. The appropriate coating concentration should be determined by checkerboard titration (13). Usually, coating concentrations range between 2 and 10 μg/ml (39, 53). The rest of the reagents are the same as for above-described ELISAs to measure LPS antibodies.

Procedure

Tacket et al. describe a standard indirect ELISA procedure to measure serum antibodies to serovar Typhi LPS (53); a number of similar techniques have been reported elsewhere (21). The procedure is identical to that used for detection of antibodies to O157 LPS, except that plates are coated with serovar Typhi LPS or H. Serum samples of unknown titer may be added at a 1:25 starting dilution, and further serial twofold dilutions are made in the plate. A higher starting dilution (e.g., 1:1,000 to 1:10,000) is recommended for screening of samples collected in areas of endemicity or from potentially infected individuals.

Results and Interpretation

Nardiello et al. showed that the IgM ELISA test is as specific as the Widal test (using a cutoff of 1:160) in identifying acutely infected individuals; a strong correlation was demonstrated between LPS titers obtained by both methods, yet the ELISA was significantly more sensitive (39). Others have confirmed the higher sensitivity of the LPS IgM ELISA than the Widal test when used with a single acute-phase serum sample and have proposed its use for diagnosis of typhoid fever in patients with suspected infection but whose blood cultures are negative (21). As with the Widal method, this assay is helpful only within the first month of clinical presentation.

Remarks

Detection of LPS IgM (21) or combined LPS IgM and IgG antibodies (47) has been proposed as one of the most sensitive methods to diagnose acute typhoid fever. In areas where typhoid is endemic, however, preexisting high levels of IgG against LPS and H antigens, particularly in adults, preclude an accurate interpretation of the results (27). In such cases, detection of IgM antibodies may be more suitable because they not only arise early in the course of infection but also fall off rapidly, whereas IgG antibodies can persist in the absence of ongoing infection. Measurement of LPS-specific IgG and IgA antibody levels has been helpful to assess immune responses following vaccination (53).

As a noninvasive diagnostic alternative, an ELISA was developed to measure serovar Typhi-specific IgA antibodies in a single salivary sample. This test had a sensitivity of 83% and a specificity of 97% compared with culture-confirmed cases, with maximum efficiency during the first 2 to 3 weeks of fever, enabling detection of acute infection (18).

In Chilean field trials with Ty21a vaccine, vaccine formulations and immunization schedules that produced the highest levels of protection also elicited the strongest rises in LPS antibody (26). Thus, LPS seroconversion was an immunologic correlate of protection. Nevertheless, there is no evidence that LPS antibodies actually mediate protection; they may merely serve as a proxy for other immune responses that do mediate protection.

Measurement of Vi Antibodies by ELISA in Chronic Carriers

Since humans are the only reservoir of serovar Typhi, identification of chronic carriers may be useful to control typhoid fever outbreaks. Most individuals with chronic infection develop high levels of antibodies to the Vi capsule. Chronic carriers of serovar Typhi can be identified by measuring the levels of IgG antibodies against Vi by ELISA (34).

Reagents and Procedure

Purified Vi is used as a coating antigen. The optimal antigen concentration is determined by checkerboard titration (13). The usual range of coating concentrations is 1 to 2 μg/ml (34, 53). The rest of the reagents and procedure are the same as described for ELISAs above.

Results and Interpretation

A similar ELISA that detects Vi antibodies was 86% sensitive and 95% specific in identifying carriers using serum samples from known chronic carriers, noninfected individuals, and people with acute typhoid fever (34).

Remarks

The licensed live attenuated typhoid vaccine Ty21a neither expresses Vi antigen nor elicits Vi antibodies; therefore, it does not produce false-positive results for vaccinated individuals. The parenteral Vi vaccine, however, has over a 90% rate of Vi seroconversion in vaccinated individuals, and therefore assessment of the chronic state by means of Vi antibody testing in such individuals would not be reliable.

Molecular Methods To Detect Serovar Typhi

Early molecular methods included Vi-specific DNA probe to detect serovar Typhi among freshly isolated bacteria and in clinical specimens followed by enrichment. Highly specific and sensitive PCR and nested techniques have been successfully used to detect serovar Typhi by amplification of the dH flagellin gene in blood samples from patients with acute typhoid fever (38) or by amplification of Vi antigen gene fragments (17). A PCR was developed for diagnosis of typhoid fever by amplification of *hilA*, a regulatory gene found in pathogenicity island 1 of *Salmonella* spp. (51), which is important for the regulation of the type III secretion apparatus, involved in the invasion of enterocytes. The sensitivity, specificity, positive predictive value, and negative predictive value of the *hilA* PCR with blood samples were all 100%, and these values were 97 to 100% for PCR with fecal samples. Hirose and colleagues developed a multiplex PCR with primers for O, H, Vi antigen genes, *tyv* (*rfbE*), *prt* (*rfbS*), *fliC-d*, *fliC-a*, and *viaB* for rapid identification of *S. enterica* serovars Typhi and Paratyphi A; all clinical isolates examined were accurately identified by this assay (19).

VIBRIONACEAE

V. cholerae O1

V. cholerae O1 strains producing CT cause cholera gravis, a disease clinically characterized by voluminous watery diarrhea leading to severe dehydration and death if left untreated. Clinical O1 isolates from cholera patients express CT, the principal virulence factor responsible for intestinal water and electrolyte loss due to the enzymatic activity of the toxin A subunit. The seventh pandemic of cholera, caused by the El Tor biotype, has been spreading across the world since the 1960s; it started in Asia, spread throughout that continent and then Africa, and finally moved to South and Central America in the 1990s. Among individuals infected with *V. cholerae* O1 El Tor, only a small number proceed to develop cholera gravis. Thus, El Tor strains often cause milder diarrhea and asymptomatic infection. Milder illness caused by these strains cannot easily be differentiated from other causes of gastroenteritis in areas where cholera is endemic.

In persons with a clinical presentation suggestive of cholera, rehydration treatment should never be withheld in order to make a diagnosis. Laboratory diagnosis is important primarily for epidemiological and public health control purposes. A definitive clinical diagnosis has traditionally relied on the bacteriological isolation of *V. cholerae* from stool, with isolates screened for agglutination with O1 antiserum.

The O1 serogroup is divided into three serotypes, Inaba, Ogawa, and Hikojima (rare), which are differentiated from each other based on the presence of three antigenic factors, so-called A, B, and C. All three serotypes contain the A factor, Inaba strains contain the A and C antigens, and Ogawa strains contain A, B, and a small amount of C. Poly- and monovalent O1 (Inaba and Ogawa) antisera for serotyping of bacteriological isolates are readily available for clinical laboratories (Oxoid/Denka Seiken Co. Japan). Antibody-based detection systems for O1 antigen offer a rapid diagnostic approach using whole-stool samples without the need for culture. Assays to detect CT from whole-stool and culture isolates have clinical applicability and are also discussed.

Natural cholera infection gives rise to a high level of enduring antibacterial and antitoxin immune responses that protect against illness (30). Antibody detection assays have been very useful in retrospective diagnosis of cholera infections, epidemiological studies, and assessment of vaccine-induced immunity (30). Popular current assays include serum vibriocidal antibody testing and ELISA to measure anti-CT IgG.

Rapid Immunologic Assays for Direct Detection of V. cholerae O1

Different rapid agglutination tests were developed to detect *V. cholerae* O1 antigens, including agglutination of latex beads (7) and coagglutination using heat-killed *Staphylococcus aureus* (e.g., Cholera-Screen) (12). In these assays the agglutinating support (latex beads or heat-killed *S. aureus*) is coated with specific antibodies against *V. cholerae* O1 antigen; agglutination occurs when capture antibodies bind cholera antigens. These tests are simple and inexpensive and provide results faster than conventional methods. They have higher sensitivity (100%) than bacterial culture and specificity (100%) with regard to asymptomatic controls (7). A *V. cholerae* O1 latex test is available from Denka Seiken. The latex particles are coated with a MAb to cell wall antigen of O1 serogroups. Additional reagents are included in this kit for subtyping. The manufacturer indicates that this test has a sensitivity of 100% for culture confirmation and 65% for point-of-care screening of stool samples. A commercial colloidal gold-based sandwich immunoassay is commercially available to identify O1 strains (Cholera-SMART Cholera O1 from New Horizons Diagnostics Corp., Columbia, Md.). This assay uses a colloidal gold-labeled MAb specific for the A antigen of O1 LPS; after binding the antigen, the complex diffuses and is captured and concentrated by a detector polyclonal antibody that concentrates the gold, forming a pink to red spot. The level of detection of the Cholera-Screen and Cholera-SMART assays using pure cultures of *V. cholerae* O1 is approximately 10^5 to 10^6 CFU/ml (12). These assays have been found to be highly sensitive (>90%) and 100% specific to detect O1 strains in stool samples from infected individuals. In areas where cholera is endemic, stool specimens have yielded positive O1 results for 20 to 25% of *V. cholerae* O1 culture-negative specimens. This finding suggests that O1 antigen is present in stools of infected individuals either as nonviable organisms or as free antigen. In many instances, positive antigen results in the absence of cultured microorganisms were confirmed by serological evidence of infection (vibriocidal antibodies) (7, 12).

CT Antigen Detection Systems

Since CT and LT are antigenically similar, antigen detection systems for CT using whole stools without culture isolation of the organism, such as the ELISA, also detect some LT-producing ETEC strains and thus are less useful clinically. In addition, in the absence of isolated organisms, CT detection will not differentiate between cholera caused by O1 or O139 strains. However, if *V. cholerae* O1 strains are isolated from the stool, CT production can be confirmed using a latex agglutination assay, a GM1-based antigen capture immunoassay similar to the one described for LT detection, or specific gene probes for the *ctx* genes encoding CT. A latex agglutination kit is commercially available (VET-RPLA; Denka Seiken); this test has a sensitivity of 97% and a specificity of 100% compared with a sandwich ELISA. CT agglutination kit results with clinical *V. cholerae* isolates from areas where cholera is not endemic should be confirmed by a reference laboratory due to the possibility of false negatives. Immuno-assays with increased sensitivity for CT detection using GM1 or antibody capture systems coupled with novel detection systems such as to biosensors have been described.

Serum Vibriocidal Antibodies

The functional capacity of serum antibodies to kill bacteria in the presence of complement can be measured by assay. The assay is most useful for diagnosis of recent cholera infections in outbreak situations in areas where cholera is not endemic or in previously unexposed individuals living in areas where cholera is endemic. It is useful for the diagnosis of cases of symptomatic cholera caused by V. cholerae O1, regardless of age, in areas of endemicity. However, it is less useful for assessing recent V. cholerae O1 exposures and asymptomatic infections in adults from areas where cholera is endemic because continued exposure results in the acquisition of antibodies with age, and secondary vibriocidal responses upon reinfection may not be elicited.

Procedure

Two days before the test, V. cholerae Inaba strain 89 and Ogawa strain 79 are plated on blood agar and incubated overnight at 37°C. Their identities should be confirmed by agglutination with specific antiserum, using PBS as a negative control. Organisms are then transferred onto a brain heart infusion (BHI) agar plate and incubated overnight at 37°C. On the day of assay, a BHI agar plate should be inoculated for confluent growth and incubated for 4 h at 37°C. Organisms should be harvested with 1.5 ml of PBS and the bacterial suspension adjusted to a concentration of 1.5×10^9 CFU/ml using a calibrated curve of absorbance versus CFU. The antigen preparation is diluted 1:20 in cold PBS containing 1:10 guinea pig complement (Sigma) and kept at 4°C to preserve complement activity. The 96-well plate should be turned so that rows A to H are on the top and columns 1 to 12 are on the side. Serum samples diluted 1:10 in sterile PBS are added in 50-μl volumes to the first row and in 25-μl volumes to the last row. PBS is then added to the remaining wells from rows 2 to 11. Note that sera should not be heat inactivated since doing so could alter the functional capacity of antibodies. Twofold dilutions are made from rows 1 to 11. Antigen is added to wells except to row 12, which is used as a serum control. Plates are shaken for 1 to 2 min and incubated for 1 h at 37°C. BHI broth (150 μl) is then added to the entire plate and incubated for 3 to 4 h at 37°C. The final readings are made after overnight refrigeration. There should be a clear distinction between the turbid fluid in the wells in which the vibrios had grown out and the crystal-clear yellowish fluid in those wells in which the organisms had been killed and lysed. Calibrated positive and negative controls are included in each assay.

Results and Interpretation

An endpoint titer of vibriocidal activity is determined as the highest dilution of serum that inhibits bacterial growth. The reproducibility of this assay depends on the activity of the complement and the bacterial suspension used. A decrease of 1 log in bacterial concentration can result in a two- to four-fold titer increase. The use of paired sera is most helpful, with a fourfold rise in titer of acute- to convalescent-phase samples indicative of exposure. However, since the peak response occurs 10 days after infection, reflecting the presence of IgM as the primary isotype responsible for vibriocidal activity in naive individuals, acute-phase serum samples need to be obtained at the time of clinical presentation to be most useful. For those living in areas where cholera is endemic and for cholera-naive individuals, a single serum sample obtained within 2 weeks of clinical presentation is most reliable. In these situations, a titer of $\geq 1,280$ is indicative of recent O1 infection. For people with a single V. cholerae O1 exposure in areas where cholera is not endemic, vibriocidal titers return to baseline in approximately 6 months (30).

Remarks

The majority of the vibriocidal response is directed against the V. cholerae LPS, although it may also include activity against protein antigens of the bacterial surface (30). This causes cross-reactive responses seen as an increase of vibriocidal activity against both Ogawa and Inaba serotypes after exposure to a single serotype. The magnitude of the antibody response, typically higher for the infecting serotype, can be used to differentiate them. Secondary vibriocidal responses are more difficult to elicit on subsequent O1 exposures, especially if no overt clinical disease occurs and active mucosal immunity is present. Seroepidemiological studies in Bangladesh and Pakistan in the early 1960s showed that the best correlation of protective immunity against clinical cholera is the serum vibriocidal antibodies (30). These studies reported a rise in vibriocidal antibody with age, with an impressive inverse relationship between the geometric mean vibriocidal titer and the incidence of disease. It is believed that serum vibriocidal antibodies, rather than being the actual mediator of protection, are surrogate markers for mucosal immunity, such as intestinal secretory IgA, which might protect the gastrointestinal mucosa by preventing colonization by cholera organisms after ingestion (30). Measurement of vibriocidal responses following vaccination has been used to assess vaccine immunogenicity. Unfortunately, individuals from areas where cholera is endemic who already have serum vibriocidal activity may not mount a secondary vibriocidal response after immunization.

Measurement of Anti-CT IgG by ELISA

Measurement of anti-CT IgG by ELISA is most useful for seroepidemiological studies of cholera or to measure CT responses in individuals from areas where cholera is not endemic who are exposed to wild-type cholera (outbreaks) or vaccine strains.

Procedure

The procedure is the same as that described above for the detection of LT antibodies by ELISA, except that purified CT (List Biological Laboratories, Campbell, Calif.) is used as a coating antigen. Another method to measure CT antibodies is GM1 ganglioside ELISA (31). However, when purified reagents are used, results are the same whether the antigens are used to coat the plate directly or used to coat the GM1 receptor attached to the plate (31).

Results and Interpretation

Because individuals with cholera infection may have cross-reactive antibodies to LT, serodiagnosis of recent cholera infection requires the detection of both LT and CT antibodies. Higher CT titers are seen in the majority of individuals with recent cholera infection in areas where cholera is endemic (31).

Remarks

In contrast to LT antibody responses, which are transient, antibodies to CT remain elevated for several years after infection, precluding the use of this assay as a marker for recent infection in areas of endemicity. However, it is very useful for seroepidemiological purposes. Infection with *V. cholerae* O139 strains in nonimmune individuals elicits antitoxin antibody; therefore, assays to detect anti-CT IgG antibody will not discriminate between infections caused by O1 or O139 strains.

V. cholerae O139 Bengal

In 1993, a new variant of *V. cholerae* that was clinically indistinguishable from toxigenic *V. cholerae* O1 yet had new surface antigens appeared in the Indian subcontinent; this strain has reemerged recently (15). This epidemic pathogen belongs to a new serogroup, O139, and is called O139 Bengal to identify its place of origin. From this initial site, the organism has spread to cause sporadic outbreaks in Pakistan, Nepal, China, Thailand, and other neighboring countries. It contains the principal virulence factors, CT and Tcp, which make it similar to the O1 strains. However, it does not produce the O1 LPS; rather, it produces a single unique O antigen attached to the LPS core surrounded by polymerized O-antigen repeat units forming a capsule. The majority of cases in these areas where *V. cholerae* O1 is endemic are in adults, suggesting that preexisting O1 immunity does not protect against O139 infection.

Detection of *V. cholerae* O139 Antigens

A number of rapid immunoassays that could be useful in remote settings have been proposed as reliable alternatives to bacterial culture to diagnose *V. cholerae* O139 infection. Coagglutination assays have been developed to detect *V. cholerae* O139 in a 4-h enrichment culture and in stool samples (46). In enrichment culture, this test had 100% sensitivity and specificity, with no cross-reaction with *V. cholerae* O1 antigen or coliform enterobacteria. With watery diarrhea samples the coagglutination test had 92% sensitivity (with a limit of detection of 10^7 CFU/ml), 100% specificity, and 100% positive and 95% negative predictive values (46). A dot blot ELISA using O139 LPS MAbs was developed to detect *V. cholerae* O139 in watery stools. This assay showed high sensitivity and specificity (100 and 96.3%, respectively) compared with the conventional bacterial isolation method using a large number of stool samples (8). A one-step immunochromatographic dipstick test for rapid detection of *V. cholerae* O1 and O139 from stool samples was developed. In areas where cholera is endemic the specificity of the O1 and O139 dipsticks ranged between 84 and 100% and the sensitivity ranged from 94.2 to 100%. A subsequent study with hospitalized patients with diarrhea showed that the dipsticks had enhanced sensitivity and specificity (>92 and 91%, respectively) when used with enriched rectal swabs rather than stool samples (5). An assay to detect *V. cholerae* O1 and O139 strains using purified outer membrane proteins and polyclonal antibodies was described (37). This assay can be used with whole stools and is capable of detecting 10^6 and 10^8 CFU/ml in a dot as well as regular ELISA format. A Cholera- and Bengal-SMART direct fluorescence kit to detect *V. cholerae* O1 and O139 strains in stool specimens is available from New Horizons Diagnostics.

Measurement of O139 Vibriocidal Antibodies

Vibriocidal assays developed for *V. cholerae* O1 strains need to be modified for non-O1 strains because the capsule reduces the effectiveness of complement-mediated antibody attachment and bacterial lysis. To solve this problem, Losonsky et al. adapted the vibriocidal assay using capsule-deficient mutants such as Tn*phoA* insertion mutant 2L of fully encapsulated strain AI-1837, which retains the LPS but not the capsule (35). This assay was used to measure bactericidal antibodies after administration of wild-type or attenuated *V. cholerae* O139. The responses observed, however, were very low and did not correlate with immune status upon rechallenge. Moreover, low-level vibriocidal activity was detected in sera obtained 7 days after experimental wild-type challenges with *V. cholerae* O1, *S. flexneri* 2a, EPEC, and EAEC (35), probably due to cross-reactive antibody. Others have used a spontaneous O139 colony variant of a disease-causing strain with low levels of capsule production in a microplate assay. These assays require a smaller inoculum (1 to 2 $\log_{10}$/ml lower), use of Mg^{2+} in the sample diluent, and an amount of complement carefully determined to avoid antibody-independent bacterial lysis. To more accurately determine endpoints, plates can be read spectrophotometrically, calculating, for example, 70% inhibition growth (2). Preexposure bactericidal titers measured with a recently described microplate assay showed a significant inverse correlation with bactericidal response subsequent to vaccination with an oral, inactivated, bivalent O1/O139 vaccine, or after O139 disease (2). A quantitative bactericidal assay in tubes that uses fully encapsulated clinical strains at a small bacterial inoculum (2×10^3 cells/ml) and increased complement activity (10%) has been described; this test allowed detection of bactericidal responses in 9 of 11 cases of O139 disease (3).

Molecular Methods To Detect *V. cholerae* O1 and O139

In order to cause diarrhea, *V. cholerae* strains belonging to serogroups O1 and O139 require genes for CT (*ctx*), TcpA, and central regulatory protein ToxR. A number of DNA probes are available to detect the *ctx* genes (22). DNA fragment probes have levels of sensitivity of approximately 10^3 CFU/g of stool. PCR techniques, however, by amplifying the genetic signal, can increase the sensitivity at least 100-fold. PCR and multiplex PCR targeting a number of different genes have been used for epidemiological studies (15). These techniques detect the presence of genes specific for *V. cholerae* biotypes, including *tcpA*, *ctx*, and *rstR*. A multiplex PCR (ezAmp Octaplex Cholera; Centre for Medical Innovations & Technology Development, Kelatan, Malaysia) is commercially available; this assay is designed to amplify genes for all serogroups (O1, O139, non-O1 and non-O139, El Tor, and classical biotype), toxin genes, and O139-specific *rfb*. These genetic techniques are limited to research laboratories but have great potential applicability, particularly in screening environmental sources such as water and food as vectors for transmission of toxigenic *V. cholerae*.

REFERENCES

1. **Ahren, C., C. Wenneras, J. Holmgren, and A. M. Svennerholm.** 1993. Intestinal antibody response after oral immunization with a prototype cholera B subunit-colonization factor antigen enterotoxigenic *Escherichia coli* vaccine. *Vaccine* **11:**929–934.
2. **Attridge, S. R., C. Johansson, D. D. Trach, F. Qadri, and A. M. Svennerholm.** 2002. Sensitive microplate assay for detection of bactericidal antibodies to *Vibrio cholerae* O139. *Clin. Diagn. Lab. Immunol.* **9:**383–387.
3. **Attridge, S. R., F. Qadri, M. J. Albert, and P. A. Manning.** 2000. Susceptibility of *Vibrio cholerae* O139 to antibody-dependent, complement-mediated bacteriolysis. *Clin. Diagn. Lab. Immunol.* **7:**444–450.
4. **Bettelheim, K. A., and L. Beutin.** 2003. Rapid laboratory identification and characterization of verocytotoxigenic

(Shiga toxin producing) *Escherichia coli* (VTEC/STEC). *J. Appl. Microbiol.* **95**:205–217.

5. **Bhuiyan, N. A., F. Qadri, A. S. Faruque, M. A. Malek, M. A. Salam, F. Nato, J. M. Fournier, S. Chanteau, D. A. Sack, and N. G. Balakrish.** 2003. Use of dipsticks for rapid diagnosis of cholera caused by *Vibrio cholerae* O1 and O139 from rectal swabs. *J. Clin. Microbiol.* **41**:3939–3941.

6. **Bitzan, M., and H. Karch.** 1992. Indirect hemagglutination assay for diagnosis of *Escherichia coli* O157 infection in patients with hemolytic-uremic syndrome. *J. Clin. Microbiol.* **30**:1174–1178.

7. **Carillo, L., R. H. Gilman, R. E. Mantle, N. Nunez, J. Watanabe, J. Moron, V. Quispe, and A. Ramirez-Ramos and the Loyaza Cholera Working Group in Peru.** 1994. Rapid detection of *Vibrio cholerae* O1 in stools of Peruvian cholera patients by using monoclonal immunodiagnostic kits. *J. Clin. Microbiol.* **32**:856–857.

8. **Chaicumpa, W., P. Srimanote, Y. Sakolvaree, T. Kalampaheti, M. Chongsa-Nguan, P. Tapchaisri, B. Eampokalap, P. Moolasart, G. B. Nair, and P. Echeverria.** 1998. Rapid diagnosis of cholera caused by *Vibrio cholerae* O139. *J. Clin. Microbiol.* **36**:3595–3600.

9. **Chart, H., and C. Jenkins.** 1999. The serodiagnosis of infections caused by Verocytotoxin-producing *Escherichia coli*. *J. Appl. Microbiol.* **86**:731–740.

10. **Choo, R. E., and M. A. Huestis.** 2004. Oral fluid as a diagnostic tool. *Clin. Chem. Lab. Med.* **42**:1273–1287.

11. **Cohen, D., M. S. Green, C. Block, R. Slepon, and I. Ofek.** 1991. Prospective study of the association between serum antibodies to lipopolysaccharide O antigen and the attack rate of shigellosis. *J. Clin. Microbiol.* **29**:386–389.

12. **Colwell, R. R., J. A. Hasan, A. Huq, L. Loomis, R. J. Siebeling, M. Torres, S. Galvez, S. Islam, M. T. Tamplin, and D. Bernstein.** 1992. Development and evaluation of a rapid, simple, sensitive, monoclonal antibody-based coagglutination test for direct detection of *Vibrio cholerae* O1. *FEMS Microbiol. Lett.* **76**:215–219.

13. **Crowther, J. R.** 2001. *The Elisa Guidebook.* Humana Press Inc., Totowa, N.J.

14. **Dutta, S., A. Chatterjee, P. Dutta, K. Rajendran, S. Roy, K. C. Pramanik, and S. K. Bhattacharya.** 2001. Sensitivity and performance characteristics of a direct PCR with stool samples in comparison to conventional techniques for diagnosis of *Shigella* and enteroinvasive *Escherichia coli* infection in children with acute diarrhoea in Calcutta, India. *J. Med. Microbiol.* **50**:667–674.

15. **Faruque, S. M., N. Chowdhury, M. Kamruzzaman, Q. S. Ahmad, A. S. Faruque, M. A. Salam, T. Ramamurthy, G. B. Nair, A. Weintraub, and D. A. Sack.** 2003. Reemergence of epidemic *Vibrio cholerae* O139, Bangladesh. *Emerg. Infect. Dis.* **9**:1116–1122.

16. **Gavin, P. J., L. R. Peterson, A. C. Pasquariello, J. Blackburn, M. G. Hamming, K. J. Kuo, and R. B. Thomson, Jr.** 2004. Evaluation of performance and potential clinical impact of ProSpecT Shiga toxin *Escherichia coli* microplate assay for detection of Shiga toxin-producing *E. coli* in stool samples. *J. Clin. Microbiol.* **42**:1652–1656.

17. **Hashimoto, Y., Y. Itho, Y. Fujinaga, A. Q. Khan, F. Sultana, M. Miyake, K. Hirose, H. Yamamoto, and T. Ezaki.** 1995. Development of nested PCR based on the *viaB* sequence to detect *Salmonella typhi*. *J. Clin. Microbiol.* **33**:775–777.

18. **Herath, H. M.** 2003. Early diagnosis of typhoid fever by the detection of salivary IgA. *J. Clin. Pathol.* **56**:694–698.

19. **Hirose, K., K. Itoh, H. Nakajima, T. Kurazono, M. Yamaguchi, K. Moriya, T. Ezaki, Y. Kawamura, K. Tamura, and H. Watanabe.** 2002. Selective amplification of *tyv* (*rfbE*), *prt* (*rfbS*), *viaB*, and *fliC* genes by multiplex

20. **Houng, H. S., O. Sethabutr, and P. Echeverria.** 1997. A simple polymerase chain reaction technique to detect and differentiate *Shigella* and enteroinvasive *Escherichia coli* in human feces. *Diagn. Microbiol. Infect. Dis.* **28**:19–25.

21. **House, D., J. Wain, V. A. Ho, T. S. Diep, N. T. Chinh, P. V. Bay, H. Vinh, M. Duc, C. M. Parry, G. Dougan, N. J. White, T. T. Hien, and J. J. Farrar.** 2001. Serology of typhoid fever in an area of endemicity and its relevance to diagnosis. *J. Clin. Microbiol.* **39**:1002–1007.

22. **Iyer, L., J. Vadivelu, and S. D. Puthucheary.** 2000. Detection of virulence associated genes, haemolysin and protease amongst *Vibrio cholerae* isolated in Malaysia. *Epidemiol. Infect.* **125**:27–34.

23. **Kaper, J. B., J. P. Nataro, and H. L. Mobley.** 2004. Pathogenic *Escherichia coli*. *Nat. Rev. Microbiol.* **2**:123–140.

24. **Karch, H., M. Bielaszewska, M. Bitzan, and H. Schmidt.** 1999. Epidemiology and diagnosis of Shiga toxin-producing *Escherichia coli* infections. *Diagn. Microbiol. Infect. Dis.* **34**:229–243.

25. **Kotloff, K. L., M. F. Pasetti, E. M. Barry, J. P. Nataro, S. S. Wasserman, M. B. Sztein, W. D. Picking, and M. M. Levine.** 2004. Deletion in the *Shigella* enterotoxin genes further attenuates *Shigella flexneri* 2a bearing guanine auxotrophy in a phase 1 trial of CVD 1204 and CVD 1208. *J. Infect. Dis.* **190**:1745–1754.

26. **Levine, M. M., J. Galen, C. O. Tacket, E. M. Barry, M. F. Pasetti, and M. B. Sztein.** 2004. Attenuated strains of *Salmonella enterica* serovar Typhi as live oral vaccines against typhoid fever, p. 479–486. *In* M. M. Levine, J. B. Kaper, R. Rappuoli, M. A. Liu, and M. F. Good (ed.), *New Generation Vaccines*. Marcel Dekker, Inc., New York, N.Y.

27. **Levine, M. M., O. Grados, R. H. Gilman, W. E. Woodward, R. Solis-Plaza, and W. Waldman.** 1978. Diagnostic value of the Widal test in areas endemic for typhoid fever. *Am. J. Trop. Med. Hyg.* **27**:795–800.

28. **Levine, M. M., and O. S. Levine.** 1994. Changes in human ecology and behavior in relation to the emergence of diarrheal diseases, including cholera. *Proc. Natl. Acad. Sci. USA* **91**:2390–2394.

29. **Levine, M. M., J. McEwen, G. Losonsky, M. Reymann, I. Harari, J. E. Brown, D. N. Taylor, A. Donohue-Rolfe, D. Cohen, and M. Bennish.** 1992. Antibodies to shiga holotoxin and to two synthetic peptides of the B subunit in sera of patients with *Shigella dysenteriae* 1 dysentery. *J. Clin. Microbiol.* **30**:1636–1641.

30. **Levine, M. M., and N. F. Pierce.** 1992. Immunity and vaccine development, p. 285–327. *In* D. Barua and W. B. Greenough III (ed.), *Cholera*. Plenum Medical Book Company, New York, N.Y.

31. **Levine, M. M., C. R. Young, R. E. Black, Y. Takeda, and R. A. Finkelstein.** 1985. Enzyme-linked immunosorbent assay to measure antibodies to purified heat-labile enterotoxins from human and porcine strains of *Escherichia coli* and to cholera toxin: application in serodiagnosis and seroepidemiology. *J. Clin. Microbiol.* **21**:174–179.

32. **Li, J. W., X. Q. Shi, F. H. Chao, X. W. Wang, J. L. Zheng, and N. Song.** 2004. A study on detecting and identifying enteric pathogens with PCR. *Biomed. Environ. Sci.* **17**:109–120.

33. **Li, Y., E. Frey, A. M. Mackenzie, and B. B. Finlay.** 2000. Human response to *Escherichia coli* O157:H7 infection: antibodies to secreted virulence factors. *Infect. Immun.* **68**:5090–5095.

34. **Losonsky, G. A., C. Ferreccio, K. L. Kotloff, S. Kaintuck, J. B. Robbins, and M. M. Levine.** 1987. Development and evaluation of an enzyme-linked immunosorbent assay for serum Vi antibodies for detection

of chronic *Salmonella typhi* carriers. *J. Clin. Microbiol.* **25**:2266–2269.

35. **Losonsky, G. A., Y. Lim, P. Motamedi, L. E. Comstock, J. A. Johnson, J. G. Morris, Jr., C. O. Tacket, J. B. Kaper, and M. M. Levine.** 1997. Vibriocidal antibody responses in North American volunteers exposed to wild-type or vaccine *Vibrio cholerae* O139: specificity and relevance to immunity. *Clin. Diagn. Lab. Immunol.* **4**:264–269.

36. **Ludwig, K., E. Grabhorn, M. Bitzan, C. Bobrowski, M. J. Kemper, I. Sobottka, R. Laufs, H. Karch, and D. E. Muller-Wiefel.** 2002. Saliva IgM and IgA are a sensitive indicator of the humoral immune response to *Escherichia coli* O157 lipopolysaccharide in children with enteropathic hemolytic uremic syndrome. *Pediatr. Res.* **52**:307–313.

37. **Martinez-Govea, A., J. Ambrosio, L. Gutierrez-Cogco, and A. Flisser.** 2001. Identification and strain differentiation of *Vibrio cholerae* by using polyclonal antibodies against outer membrane proteins. *Clin. Diagn. Lab. Immunol.* **8**:768–771.

38. **Massi, M. N., T. Shirakawa, A. Gotoh, A. Bishnu, M. Hatta, and M. Kawabata.** 2003. Rapid diagnosis of typhoid fever by PCR assay using one pair of primers from flagellin gene of *Salmonella typhi. J. Infect. Chemother.* **9**:233–237.

39. **Nardiello, S., T. Pizzella, M. Russo, and B. Galanti.** 1984. Serodiagnosis of typhoid fever by enzyme-linked immunosorbent assay determination of anti-*Salmonella typhi* lipopolysaccharide antibodies. *J. Clin. Microbiol.* **20**:718–721.

40. **Nataro, J. P., and J. B. Kaper.** 1998. Diarrheagenic *Escherichia coli. Clin. Microbiol. Rev.* **11**:142–201.

41. **Nguyen, T. V., P. Le Van, C. Le Huy, K. N. Gia, and A. Weintraub.** 2005. Detection and characterization of diarrheagenic *Escherichia coli* from young children in Hanoi, Vietnam. *J. Clin. Microbiol.* **43**:755–760.

42. **Olsen, S. J., J. Pruckler, W. Bibb, T. M. Nguyen, M. T. Tran, T. M. Nguyen, S. Sivapalasingam, A. Gupta, T. P. Phan, T. C. Nguyen, V. C. Nguyen, D. C. Phung, and E. D. Mintz.** 2004. Evaluation of rapid diagnostic tests for typhoid fever. *J. Clin. Microbiol.* **42**:1885–1889.

43. **Paton, A. W., and J. C. Paton.** 2003. Detection and characterization of STEC in stool samples using PCR, p. 45–54. *In* D. Philpott and F. Ebel (ed.), *E. coli Shiga Toxin Methods and Protocols.* Humana Press Inc., Totowa, N.J.

44. **Paton, J. C., and A. W. Paton.** 1998. Pathogenesis and diagnosis of Shiga toxin-producing *Escherichia coli* infections. *Clin. Microbiol. Rev.* **11**:450–479.

45. **Paton, J. C., and A. W. Paton.** 2003. Methods for detection of STEC in humans, p. 9–26. *In* D. Philpott and F. Ebel (eds.), *E. coli Shiga Toxin Methods and Protocols.* Humana Press Inc., Totowa, N.J.

46. **Qadri, F., A. Chowdhury, J. Hossain, K. Chowdhury, T. Azim, T. Shimada, K. M. Islam, R. B. Sack, and M. J. Albert.** 1994. Development and evaluation of rapid monoclonal antibody-based coagglutination test for direct detection of *Vibrio cholerae* O139 synonym Bengal in stool samples. *J. Clin. Microbiol.* **32**:1589–1590.

47. **Quiroga, T., M. Goycoolea, R. Tagle, F. Gonzalez, L. Rodriguez, and L. Villarroel.** 1992. Diagnosis of typhoid fever by two serologic methods. Enzyme-linked immunosorbent assay of antilipopolysaccharide of *Salmonella typhi* antibodies and Widal test. *Diagn. Microbiol. Infect. Dis.* **15**:651–656.

48. **Reischl, U., M. T. Youssef, H. Wolf, E. Hyytia-Trees, and N. A. Strockbine.** 2004. Real-time fluorescence PCR assays for detection and characterization of heat-labile I and heat-stable I enterotoxin genes from enterotoxigenic *Escherichia coli. J. Clin. Microbiol.* **42**:4092–4100.

49. **Ristaino, P. A., M. M. Levine, and C. R. Young.** 1983. Improved GM1-enzyme-linked immunosorbent assay for detection of *Escherichia coli* heat-labile enterotoxin. *J. Clin. Microbiol.* **18**:808–815.

50. **Sanches, M. I., R. Keller, E. L. Hartland, D. M. Figueired, M. Batchelor, M. B. Martinez, G. Dougan, M. M. Careiro-Sampaio, G. Frankel, and L. R. Trabulsi.** 2000. Human colostrum and serum contain antibodies reactive to the intimin-binding region of the enteropathogenic *Escherichia coli* translocated intimin receptor. *J. Pediatr. Gastroenterol. Nutr.* **30**:73–77.

51. **Sanchez-Jimenez, M. M., and N. Cardona-Castro.** 2004. Validation of a PCR for diagnosis of typhoid fever and salmonellosis by amplification of the *hilA* gene in clinical samples from Colombian patients. *J. Med. Microbiol.* **53**:875–878.

52. **Steinsland, H., P. Valentiner-Branth, H. M. Grewal, W. Gaastra, K. K. Molbak, and H. Sommerfelt.** 2003. Development and evaluation of genotypic assays for the detection and characterization of enterotoxigenic *Escherichia coli. Diagn. Microbiol. Infect. Dis.* **45**:97–105.

53. **Tacket, C. O., M. F. Pasetti, M. B. Sztein, S. Livio, and M. M. Levine.** 2004. Immune responses to an oral typhoid vaccine strain that is modified to constitutively express Vi capsular polysaccharide. *J. Infect. Dis.* **190**:565–570.

54. **Thompson, M. R., R. L. Jordan, M. A. Luttrell, H. Brandwein, J. B. Kaper, M. M. Levine, and R. A. Giannella.** 1986. Blinded, two-laboratory comparative analysis of *Escherichia coli* heat-stable enterotoxin production by using monoclonal antibody enzyme-linked immunosorbent assay, radioimmunoassay, suckling mouse assay, and gene probes. *J. Clin. Microbiol.* **24**:753–758.

55. **Venkatesan, M. M., J. M. Buysse, and D. J. Kopecko.** 1989. Use of *Shigella flexneri ipaC* and *ipaH* gene sequences for the general identification of *Shigella* spp. and enteroinvasive *Escherichia coli. J. Clin. Microbiol.* **27**:2687–2691.

56. **Vidal, R., M. Vidal, R. Lagos, M. Levine, and V. Prado.** 2004. Multiplex PCR for diagnosis of enteric infections associated with diarrheagenic *Escherichia coli. J. Clin. Microbiol.* **42**:1787–1789.

Serologic and Molecular Diagnosis of *Helicobacter pylori* Infection and Eradication

BRUCE E. DUNN AND SUHAS H. PHADNIS

54

CLINICAL PRESENTATION AND OUTCOMES OF INFECTION WITH *HELICOBACTER PYLORI*

Helicobacter pylori is a gram-negative, microaerophilic spiral bacterium which is recognized as the primary cause of chronic gastritis in humans. *H. pylori* infection is an essential contributing factor in the development of duodenal and gastric ulcers except in cases of nonsteroidal anti-inflammatory drug use and Zollinger-Ellison syndrome. The most convincing evidence supporting the role of *H. pylori* as an essential factor in the development of gastric and duodenal ulcers comes from clinical studies which have demonstrated that eradication of *H. pylori* infection eliminates ulcer recurrence (19).

H. pylori is distributed worldwide; the prevalence of infection in adults ranges from 30% in developed countries to more than 90% in developing countries. In developing countries, the infection is acquired primarily in childhood and, unless treated, persists for life (15, 19). In developed countries, the prevalence of infection increases with age. Improvements in hygiene in developed countries have probably resulted in reduction of *H. pylori* infection rates within the younger population. Persistent infection with *H. pylori* is a significant risk factor for the development of gastric carcinoma and gastric mucosa-associated lymphoid tissue lymphoma. The prevalence of *H. pylori* infection, gastritis, and gastric carcinoma increases with age, is inversely related to socioeconomic status, and declines in successive generations in developed countries. In contrast, a definite association between *H. pylori* infection and nonulcer dyspepsia has not been established, although a subset of individuals with dyspepsia may have symptoms related to *H. pylori* infection (15, 19).

A consensus panel convened by the National Institutes of Health in 1994 recommended that all individuals with gastric or duodenal ulcers who are infected with *H. pylori* receive antimicrobial therapy in addition to traditional antiulcer medications as primary therapy for ulcer disease, whether at initial presentation or at the time of recurrence (15, 19). Empiric anti-*H. pylori* therapy is generally considered inappropriate and should not be substituted for diagnostic evaluation and diagnosis-guided therapy. Success or failure of treatment cannot be determined reliably until 4 weeks or more after cessation of antimicrobial therapy (15).

GENETIC HETEROGENEITY OF *H. PYLORI*

Rapid advances in molecular genetic methods have allowed the elucidation of the complete genome sequences of two different *H. pylori* strains. In addition, DNA sequencing of a number of defined regions, along with other genetic techniques, has shown a high degree of heterogeneity among *H. pylori* strains, perhaps due to frequent genetic exchange between strains. With the notable exception of the CagA status of the infecting strain, little is known about the impact of strain heterogeneity on serologic detection methods.

The CagA protein, which is highly immunogenic, is one of the most widely studied virulence factors of *H. pylori*. The *cagA* gene is one of the genes in the *cag* pathogenicity island (26). The severity of *H. pylori*-related disease is correlated with the presence of the *cag* pathogenicity island. The CagA protein is injected into gastric epithelial cells by a type IV secretion mechanism; once in these cells, it becomes tyrosine phosphorylated and mediates changes in the host cell signal transduction pathways and actin skeleton reorganization (26). Another important virulence factor, vacuolating cytotoxin (VacA), is so named because it causes vacuolization of cultured eukaryotic cells (17). The *vacA* gene encodes a 140-kDa toxin precursor and is present in all strains. However, its expression is transcriptionally regulated; therefore, only about 50% of all strains express the toxin. Epidemiological studies have shown an increased risk of developing gastric or peptic ulcers and/or gastric carcinoma in patients infected with *cagA*- and *vacA*-positive strains (28, 29).

METHODS FOR DETECTION OF *H. PYLORI*

A variety of techniques are available for the diagnosis of *H. pylori* infection. In large part, due to the significant potential and actual clinical impact of *H. pylori* infection, the number of commercial tests available to diagnose infection has proliferated significantly over the past several years. In this chapter the tests are discussed generically rather than listed specifically. These methods can be categorized into two broad categories. The first involves invasive assays, which require the availability of gastric tissue obtained by endoscopic biopsy for histological examination, culture, molecular assays such as PCR, and biopsy urease tests. The second involves noninvasive assays, which detect either an

TABLE 1   Diagnostic tests for detection of *H. pylori*

Test	Requirement for endoscopy	Advantages	Disadvantages	Approximate sensitivity and specificity (%)
Histology	Yes	Allows evaluation of the type and degree of inflammation and direct observation of bacteria	Results may be variable, depending on pathologist experience; multiple biopsies recommended	>90, >90
Culture	Yes	Allows identification of antibiotic-resistant isolates	Variable results, depending on laboratory experience; considerable risk of false-negative results	>75, 100
Biopsy urease test (e.g., CLO test)	Yes	Rapid, inexpensive; endoscopic method of choice	May be falsely negative immediately after antibiotic treatment or during treatment with omeprazole	>90, >95
Urea breath tests (^{14}C and ^{13}C UBT[a])	No	Responds rapidly to eradication of *H. pylori*, noninvasive; breath samples can be sent to reference laboratories	^{14}C UBT involves radiation exposure; ^{13}C UBT requires specialized equipment (mass spectrometer) but is preferred when multiple tests are required.	>95, >95
Stool antigen	No	Noninvasive, available commercially; potentially responds rapidly to bacterial eradication	Guidelines required for follow-up after antimicrobial therapy	>90, >95
Serology	No	Noninvasive, inexpensive, available commercially	Prolonged delays before antibody levels decrease	>95, >90
Urine antibody	No	Noninvasive, potentially inexpensive	Methods require further standardization	>80, >80
Molecular tests	Depends on specimen	Allow sensitive detection of *H. pylori* and specific virulence markers	Not well standardized or available in clinical laboratories	Variable

[a] UBT, urea breath test.

immunologic response (e.g., specific antibodies directed against *H. pylori*), metabolic products of *H. pylori* urease activity (urea breath test), bacterial antigens, or nucleic acid present in stool or urine. The most common diagnostic tests for detection of *H. pylori* infection are summarized in Table 1. Molecular methods not only permit highly sensitive detection of *H. pylori* but also allow detailed characterization of the infecting strain by detection and analysis of virulence-associated genes. Local validation of diagnostic tests is important since, in addition to characteristics of the tests themselves, other factors such as local prevalence of *H. pylori* infection influence the predictive value of the tests.

Invasive Tests

Histologic examination allows evaluation of the type and degree of inflammation and direct observation of bacteria, if present. *H. pylori* can be difficult to detect on hematoxylin-and-eosin-stained slides. Thus, special stains such as the Warthin-Starry stain, in which darkly stained spiral bacteria appear prominent on a lightly colored background, are frequently employed, despite the technical demands and higher cost involved.

Microbiological culture of *H. pylori* is the most specific diagnostic method, but the sensitivity of culture is usually significantly lower than that of other methods. There are several reasons for this low sensitivity. The patchy distribution of *H. pylori* in gastric mucosa can lead to endoscopic sampling error, resulting in false-negative cultures. In addition, isolation of *H. pylori* is technically demanding and

requires proper specimen transport, specific medium, and microaerophilic growth conditions. Isolation of the organism is highly recommended, however, when antimicrobial susceptibility testing of *H. pylori* is desired.

An important characteristic of *H. pylori* that forms the basis of several diagnostic tests is the ability of the bacterium to produce large amounts of the enzyme urease. Urease catalyzes the hydrolysis of urea to ammonia and bicarbonate. This reaction causes an increase in the pH of the surrounding medium, which can be detected by a pH indicator dye. Thus, the presence of urease activity, and hence of *H. pylori*, is heralded by a color change in the indicator. Commercial biopsy urease tests are available which provide a medium in which to incubate gastric biopsy specimens to detect the presence of preformed urease and hence of *H. pylori*. Results are available within 2 to 24 h, depending on the test and conditions used. Compared with histologic and culture methods, biopsy urease tests are the endoscopic method of choice for rapid diagnosis of *H. pylori* infection on the basis of low cost and excellent sensitivity and specificity (14).

Once the biopsy specimen is obtained, the bacteria present within the specimen can be used for molecular assays without the need for bacterial culture. PCR-based molecular assays have been developed to detect *H. pylori*-specific DNA from gastric biopsies and from paraffin-embedded tissues. Additionally, *cagA* and *vacA* genotyping of *H. pylori* strains is possible using such specimens. However, DNA-based assays remain relatively time-consuming and expensive for routine clinical laboratory application.

Noninvasive Tests

Urea breath testing involves oral administration of urea which has been labeled with a carbon isotope. In infected individuals, urea is metabolized to ammonia and bicarbonate; the latter is excreted in the breath as labeled carbon dioxide. The amount of labeled carbon dioxide which is excreted can then be quantified. The [^{14}C]urea breath test involves radiation exposure but has the advantage that it can be performed in a relatively large number of laboratories equipped to detect such radioactivity. In contrast, the [^{13}C]urea breath test uses a nonradioactive isotope of urea, which requires a specialized mass spectrometer to detect $^{13}CO_2$ in the breath sample (5). The [^{13}C]urea breath test is preferred when repeated testing is required on an individual. Urea breath testing is an excellent noninvasive method by which to evaluate successful eradication of H. pylori, since it reflects active bacterial metabolism and responds rapidly to changes in H. pylori infection status. Many referral centers now accept urea breath samples for analysis of $^{13}CO_2$ at moderate expense. In selected circumstances, urea breath testing is well suited as the method of choice for follow-up of antimicrobial therapy (5).

Enzyme immunoassays for detection of H. pylori antigens in feces (H. pylori stool antigen test) have been developed commercially. As the next-most-common test after urea breath testing, stool antigen tests have been recommended for noninvasive diagnosis of H. pylori before and after eradication therapy (10, 15). In general, the sensitivity of the polyclonal antibody-based stool antigen tests varies from 57 to 96% in different studies. Recent improvements appear to have increased the sensitivity (73 to 95%) of a modified stool antigen test by replacing polyclonal antibodies with a specific monoclonal antibody. In a pretreatment setting, a commercial polyclonal antibody-based stool antigen test showed a sensitivity of 84 to 94% and a specificity of 90 to 100% compared to urea breath testing. In a posttreatment setting comparing the results of the polyclonal stool antigen test to those obtained using urea breath testing, nearly 8% of the patients gave discordant or indeterminate results with the two tests. Thus, the polyclonal stool antigen test appears to be less accurate than the urea breath test (23). However, compared with urea breath testing 4 to 6 weeks posttherapy, the monoclonal stool antigen test was more specific (88.6%) than was the polyclonal test (77.1%) but the specificities were similar (95 to 97%) (12). Continued progress in increasing the sensitivity of the stool antigen testing may lead to a robust noninvasive test to monitor eradication of H. pylori after antimicrobial therapy. However, the unpleasantness of the stool collection procedure may limit acceptance of this assay by patients.

Enzyme-Linked Immunosorbent Assays

Infection with H. pylori results in a systemic immune response characterized by circulating specific immunoglobulins (immunoglobulin G [IgG], IgA, and, acutely, IgM) (2). Spontaneous eradication of H. pylori infection rarely occurs. Thus, the presence of H. pylori-specific antibodies is indirect evidence of active infection (15).

Enzyme-linked immunosorbent assay (ELISA) methodology is considered the optimal approach to test for H. pylori antibodies because such tests are noninvasive, simple to perform, rapid, and cost-effective compared to endoscopic biopsy. Further, serologic testing allows "global" sampling of gastric mucosal infection whereas biopsy-based assays allow only localized sampling of the gastric mucosa. The choice of antigen is critical for the success of ELISA. In general, four types of antigen have been used for detection of H. pylori-specific anti-

bodies (23, 24). These preparations include crude antigens such as whole cells and whole-cell sonicates, cell fractions such as glycine extracts and heat-stable antigens, component-enriched antigenic fractions such as urease and the 120-kDa protein associated with vacuolating cytotoxic activity, and specific recombinant antigens such as CagA. The sensitivities and specificities of several of the enriched antigen preparations typically exceed 95%. While analysis of whole-cell preparations of H. pylori by sodium dodecyl sulfate-polyacrylamide gel electrophoresis reveals a large number of polypeptides, generally no more than about 25 protein antigens are recognized by immunoblotting using sera from infected individuals. There is significant heterogeneity in the specificity of these antibodies. As shown by a variety of techniques, very few, if any, antigens are recognized by all positive sera. Among the most commonly recognized antigens are the 62- and 30-kDa subunits of urease and the 58-kDa homolog of the Cpn60 family of heat shock proteins (HspB). Considering the genetic heterogeneity of H. pylori strains, it is generally thought that use of pooled extracts from multiple and genetically diverse strains as antigen preparations for detection of antibody will improve diagnostic performance. A significant fraction of individuals infected with H. pylori also produce serum and local antibodies directed against the 120-kDa CagA protein and the 89-kDa VacA protein. Antibodies directed against CagA and/or VacA protein antigen have a strong association with the severity of gastritis and with gastric cancer (9, 14).

The possibility of false-negative serologic test results for H. pylori has to be considered for any individual with an impaired immune response, e.g., the elderly, dialysis patients, immunosuppressed individuals, and organ recipients. In addition, chronic nonsteroidal anti-inflammatory drug treatment may suppress infection and decrease the sensitivity of serologic tests. False-negative results may also occur during the first few weeks of infection if methods are used which detect only IgG or IgA.

Value of Analysis of Specific Immunoglobulin Classes

In general, measurement of H. pylori-specific IgM levels has not proven useful in the clinical laboratory. A number of studies have evaluated the relative value of detecting H. pylori-specific IgG and IgA. Detection of H. pylori-specific IgA alone is generally less sensitive than detection of specific IgG antibodies alone (14). Testing for the presence of H. pylori-specific IgA in addition to IgG may increase test sensitivity slightly. However, the specificity of H. pylori-specific IgA appears to be at least equal to that of H. pylori-specific IgG (24). Individuals who have IgA but not IgG antibodies against H. pylori are uncommon.

Stability of H. pylori-Specific Antibody Levels in Untreated Individuals

Infection with H. pylori is chronic, and the host retains the capacity to respond to infection. As a result, circulating levels of specific IgG and IgA in H. pylori-infected individuals typically remain elevated for years, if not an entire lifetime, in the absence of bacterial eradication.

H. pylori-Specific Antibodies in Body Fluids Other than Serum

In an attempt to eliminate the need for venipuncture, diagnostic tests have been developed for the detection of IgG and IgA antibodies in saliva and urine (21,27). Studies using urine-based ELISA for detection of IgG antibodies against H. pylori have been conducted (13, 27). Such studies have shown sensitivity between 82 and 90% and specificity between 68 and 82%. The ease of obtaining specimens is an obvious advantage of using urine as a source of IgG antibodies against *H. pylori* infection, especially in children.

Effect of Eradication of *H. pylori* on Antibody Levels

In untreated individuals with *H. pylori* infection, specific IgG and IgA antibody levels generally remain elevated. After successful bacterial eradication, specific antibody levels may decrease to as little as 50% of the pretreatment value within 6 months (14). However, specific antibodies may persist for years even after eradication of *H. pylori*. Some antigens, in particular the 120-kDa CagA protein, induce very persistent antibodies. Serology is, therefore, a potentially problematic method for the follow-up of treatment response. If *H. pylori* is suppressed but not eradicated, antibody levels may transiently decrease as antigen load falls but eventually rise to pretreatment levels.

Immunoblot Analysis

Immunoblot analysis of whole-cell lysates of *H. pylori* permits a detailed analysis of antibody profiles and is useful for identifying immunologic responses to specific antigens. However, beyond research studies, immunoblot technology is of limited utility for several reasons. First, antibodies in some patients infected by specific strains of *H. pylori* may not recognize antigens if a single strain of *H. pylori* is used in the immunoblot assay. Second, the resolution of the immunoblot is limited, permitting only about 25 distinctive bands to be detected. It may be difficult to distinguish between antigens with similar molecular sizes. Finally, since immunoblot assays are labor-intensive and semiquantitative, this type of assay is not suitable for automation or for screening large collections of sera. One new commercial immunoblot method showed high sensitivity (99%) and specificity (98%) compared with three other methods (18). However, when CagA antibodies were determined by this assay, false-positive reactions were detected in patients infected with CagA-negative strains and in individuals not infected with *H. pylori* (18, 21).

Rapid Serologic Tests

Over the past several years, a number of rapid near-patient tests have been marketed to detect antibodies to *H. pylori* in untreated individuals. These rapid tests are generally based on latex agglutination or flowthrough membrane-based enzyme immunoassays. Serum, plasma, or whole blood can be tested. Most of these tests detect IgG antibodies. While some studies have shown acceptable sensitivity and specificity, many qualitative rapid antibody tests have been clearly inferior to quantitative ELISAs. The use of rapid tests has not been recommended in Europe (15). The present authors recommend that if near-patient testing for *H. pylori* is to be instituted, the results of such tests must be correlated with results of serologic tests from the local reference laboratory, on a select group of well-characterized patients, before the test is accepted for widespread clinical use.

Serologic Tests for Children

Pediatric iron deficiency may be due to otherwise asymptomatic *H. pylori* gastritis (4). While the stool antigen test and [^{13}C]urea breath testing were the methods of choice for diagnosis and "test for cure" of *H. pylori* in Europe in 2003, these tests have not become accepted standards of care in the United States (4). Upper endoscopy and biopsy remain the gold standard for diagnosis of pediatric infection in the United States. Variable results have been reported for ELISAs used to detect *H. pylori* infection in children.

Molecular Methods

Over the past several years, a variety of molecular techniques have been developed to detect *H. pylori*, determine susceptibility to clarithromycin, and serve as tools for strain typing. A major limitation of PCR-based detection methods for *H. pylori* is the inability to distinguish between living and dead organisms. Thus, residual DNA may potentially be detected by PCR even after successful eradication of *H. pylori*. While molecular methods have been applied to the detection of *H. pylori*, such methods have not yet been applied systematically to testing the eradication of *H. pylori* after antimicrobial therapy.

PCR is as sensitive as culture in detecting *H. pylori* in gastric biopsy specimens (11). PCR has the advantage of allowing the detection of virulence factors such as *cagA*, *vacA* alleles, and other factors such as *iceA*. Real-time PCR has been used to estimate the gastric mucosal density of *H. pylori* (8). Chisholm et al. developed a multiplex PCR technique to detect *vacA* alleles in a single step (3). The latter authors reported perfect correlation with the genotypes determined directly in gastric biopsy specimens and in the *H. pylori* isolates cultured from the specimens. "Fingerprinting" of *H. pylori* strains can be performed on gastric biopsy specimens directly using PCR-restriction fragment length polymorphism without having to culture bacteria. Real-time PCR using TaqMan technology has been applied to determine the bacterial load of *H. pylori* in the gastric mucosa. A good correlation was obtained with results obtained using the urea breath test (8). PCR has been used to detect the presence of *H. pylori* in tissues other than gastric biopsy specimens as well.

Molecular methods have been developed to detect resistance of *H. pylori* to clarithromycin by using cultured isolates or gastric biopsy specimens directly. Clarithromycin resistance is due to single point mutations in the peptidyltransferase region of the 23S rRNA gene (1, 6, 16, 25); hence, detection of such mutations is well suited to PCR analysis. More recently, real-time PCR protocols have been developed which allow the detection of clarithromycin resistance-associated point mutations on the 23S rRNA (20).

PCR tests have been developed to detect *H. pylori* in human feces (7, 10). There are a number of potential limitations to the PCR method for detection of *H. pylori* in stool specimens. (i) False-negative results may occur due to the presence of PCR inhibitors or to genetic variability. (ii) False-positive results may occur by contamination or nonspecific amplification of human genomic DNA. (iii) PCR detection of *H. pylori* has not yet been standardized and is not generally available. However, when appropriate steps are taken to purify DNA in fecal specimens by using various biochemical, immunological, and physical steps prior to PCR amplification, the sensitivity and specificity of stool-based PCR for detection of *H. pylori* can approach 100% in the appropriate research setting (7). One-step PCR protocols have been developed using radiolabeled primers, an efficient extraction protocol, and 80 cycles of amplification to genotype *vacA* and detect *cagA* in stool specimens of *H. pylori*-infected children (28).

USE OF SEROLOGIC TESTING

Clinical Indications

As noted above, an accurate diagnosis of the presence of *H. pylori* infection should precede antimicrobial therapy. Routine serologic follow-up of patients after treatment for *H. pylori* infection is not recommended, since no clear guidelines have been established to quantify the reduction of antibody level which is correlated with bacterial eradication, outside of the research setting.

Specimens

Generally, serum can be collected using standard phlebotomy techniques. There are no dietary restrictions prior to collection of the serum sample. Typically, no more than 10 μl of serum is needed to perform a single test.

Procedure

A variety of ELISA kits are available from manufacturers in North America and Europe. A general outline of methods involved in detection of *H. pylori*-specific IgG antibodies by ELISA testing is provided below. All procedures described in the package insert must be followed exactly as described for the particular test kit being used. In typical commercial ELISA kits, antigen is attached to the surface of microtiter plate wells, diluted serum is added to individual wells, and the *H. pylori*-specific IgG antibody, if present, binds to the antigen. All unbound antibody is washed away, and enzyme-conjugated anti-human IgG is added. The enzyme conjugate binds to the antibody complex. Excess enzyme conjugate is then washed away, and substrate is added. Bound enzyme conjugate begins a hydrolytic reaction. After a specified period, the enzyme reaction is stopped. The results are read by a spectrophotometer, which gives an indirect measurement of the amount of *H. pylori*-specific IgG antibody present in the serum.

Results and Interpretation

Typically, ELISA kits have a predetermined cutoff for absorbance values considered to be positive or negative. There is usually a range of absorbance values between which the reading is considered equivocal. It is recommended by many manufacturers that specimens giving equivocal results be retested. If the retest result is also equivocal, the report should be reported as "equivocal" and the sample should be retested by an alternate method or with a new serum specimen drawn after an interval of at least 4 weeks.

Commercial ELISAs are designed for use in the qualitative detection of *H. pylori*-specific IgG antibodies in human serum. Such tests typically assess the serologic status by using a single serum specimen per individual and are intended to be used as an aid in the diagnosis of *H. pylori* infection in individuals with gastrointestinal symptoms. Virtually all individuals infected with *H. pylori* possess IgG antibodies. Because infection with *H. pylori* is so prevalent and because it may be asymptomatic, many individuals apparently free of gastrointestinal symptoms exhibit *H. pylori*-specific antibodies. The prevalence of *H. pylori* antibodies increases with age. *H. pylori* antibodies are found in men and women at approximately equal rates. Blacks, Hispanics, and persons born outside of the United States tend to show higher rates of infection with *H. pylori*.

Technical Limitations

Typically, icteric, lipemic, hemolyzed, or heat-inactivated serum may cause erroneous results; such samples should be avoided if possible.

A positive test result indicates that the individual has antibodies to *H. pylori*.

Such a result does not indicate that any existing symptoms are necessarily due to *H. pylori* infection. In the absence of prior therapy to eradicate *H. pylori* infection, the positive test result very probably indicates active infection with *H. pylori*. However, in the absence of an adequate

patient history, a single positive test result does not differentiate between active and past infection.

A negative serologic test result indicates that the individual does not have detectable levels of antibody to *H. pylori*. If a sample is drawn too early during *H. pylori* infection, IgG antibodies may not be present.

Use of Specific Antigens in ELISA

The most important factor in using immunological methods for identifying VacA-specific antibodies by ELISA is the antigen preparation used to detect circulating antibodies. VacA protein is quite diverse among *H. pylori* strains and is broadly classified as *s1/m1* or *s2/m2* type. While commercial kits are available for detection of VacA antibodies by using immunoblot assays, most ELISA studies have been developed with purified or enriched VacA protein fractions; this is a time-consuming and expensive approach (22). The availability of recombinant VacA protein will help to make the VacA ELISA more widely available.

At least one commercial assay is available which uses recombinant CagA protein to detect CagA-specific IgG. This assay also uses anti-human IgG monoclonal antibody enzyme conjugate to detect the presence of specific IgG. The assay has been automated to operate in a high-speed walkaway analyzer for 96-well ELISAs.

Limitations of Serologic Assays in Monitoring Eradication

There are two basic limitations to the clinical utility of serology in monitoring the eradication of *H. pylori* infection. First, baseline and follow-up sera must be analyzed at the same time to minimize assay variability. Significant variability may result from assaying sera at different times or using different lots of reagent. Therefore, pretreatment sera must be saved to be analyzed along with posttherapy samples. This limitation requires that pretreatment specimens be saved for up to 12 months. The second limitation is that serology must be monitored for at least 3 months (and for 6 to 9 months in many cases) before a significant decrease in antibody concentration is observed. Depending on the clinical circumstances, this may represent an unacceptable delay. The percent decrease in the concentration of *H. pylori*-specific IgG which indicates eradication of infection in an individual patient has not been clearly established.

When using serologic analysis in the evaluation of treatment success under controlled conditions, the absolute concentrations of *H. pylori*-specific IgG antibodies in the serum are less important than are the changes in concentrations from the pretreatment level. For example, over 60% of individuals from whom *H. pylori* was eradicated continued to have seropositive IgG levels (index value, >1.0) at 6, 9, and 12 months despite demonstrating a 20% reduction in antibody concentration. Thus, a single serum specimen from such an individual would appear to reflect active infection with *H. pylori* in the absence of an adequate clinical history.

In summary, ELISAs for detection of *H. pylori*-specific antibodies are sensitive, specific, and cost-effective in untreated individuals. The major limitation of such tests is the lack of a rapid, clear serologic response to eradication of bacterial infection. Molecular tests have been developed which preclude culture and allow direct, sensitive detection of *H. pylori* and specific virulence factors thereof in a variety of biological specimens. Much work remains to be done to standardize molecular assays so that they can be applied generally to the diagnosis of *H. pylori* infection and eradication.

REFERENCES

1. **Alarcon, T., A. E. Vega, D. Domingo, M. J. Martinez, and M. Lopez-Brea.** 2003. Clarithromycin resistance among *Helicobacter pylori* strains isolated from children: prevalence and study of mechanism of resistance by PCR-restriction fragment length polymorphism analysis. *J. Clin. Microbiol.* **41:**486–499.

2. **Bergy, B., P. Marchildon, J. Peacock, and F. Megraud.** 2003. What is the role of serology in assessing *Helicobacter pylori* eradication? *Aliment. Pharmacol. Ther.* **18:**635–639.

3. **Chisholm, S. A., E. L. Teare, B. Patel, and R. J. Owen.** 2002. Determination of *Helicobacter pylori* VacA allelic types by single-step multiplex PCR. *Lett. Appl. Microbiol.* **35:**42–46.

4. **Crone, J., and B. D. Gold.** 2004. *Helicobacter pylori* infection in pediatrics. *Helicobacter* **9**(Suppl. 1)**:**49–56.

5. **Graham, D. Y., A. R. Opekun, F. Hammoud, Y. Yamaoka, R. Reddy, M. S. Osato, and H. M. El-Zimaity.** 2003. Studies regarding the mechanism of false negative urea breath tests with proton pump inhibitors. *Am. J. Gastroenterol.* **98:**1005–1009.

6. **Hao, Q., Y. Li, Z. J. Zhang, Y. Liu, and H. Gao.** 2004. New mutation points in 23S rRNA gene associated with *Helicobacter pylori* resistance to clarithromycin in northeast China. *World J. Gastroenterol.* **10:**1075–1077.

7. **Kabir, S.** 2004. Detection of *Helicobacter pylori* DNA in feces and saliva by polymerase chain reaction: a review. *Helicobacter* **9:**115–123.

8. **Kobayashi, D., Y. Eishi, T. Ohkusa, T. Ishige, T. Suzuki, J. Minami, T. Yamada, T. Takizawa, and M. Koike.** 2002. Gastric mucosal density of *Helicobacter pylori* estimated by real-time PCR compared with results of urea breath test and histological grading. *J. Med. Microbiol.* **51:**305–311.

9. **Krah, A., S. Miehlke, K. P. Pleissner, U. Zimny-Arndt, C. Kirsch, N. Lehn, T. F. Meyer, P. R. Jungblut, and T. Aebischer.** 2004. Identification of candidate antigens for serologic detection of *Helicobacter pylori*-infected patients with gastric carcinoma. *Int. J. Cancer* **108:**456–463.

10. **Lehmann, F. S., and C. Beglinger.** 2003. Current role of *Helicobacter pylori* stool tests. *Digestion* **68:**119–123.

11. **Lehours, P., A. Ruskone-Fourmestraux, A. Lavergne, A. Cantet, and F. Megraud.** 2003. Which test to use to detect *Helicobacter pylori* infection in patients with low grade gastric mucosa-associated lymphoid tissue lymphoma? *Am. J. Gastroenterol.* **98:**291–295.

12. **Leodolter, A., U. Peitz, M. P. Ebert, K. Agha-Amiri, and P. Malfertheiner.** 2002. Comparison of two enzyme immunoassays for the assessment of *Helicobacter pylori* status in stool specimens after eradication therapy. *Am. J. Gastroenterol.* **97:**1682–1686.

13. **Leodolter, A., D. Vaira, F. Bazzoli, K. Schutze, A. Hirschl, F. Megraud, and P. Malfertheiner.** 2003. European multicentre validation trial of two new non-invasive tests for the detection of *Helicobacter pylori* antibodies: urine-based ELISA and rapid urine test. *Aliment. Pharmacol. Ther.* **18:**927–931.

14. **Makristathis, A., A. M. Hirschl, P. Lehours, and F. Megraud.** 2004. Diagnosis of *Helicobacter pylori* infection. *Helicobacter* **9**(Suppl. 1)**:**7–14.

15. **Malfertheiner, P., F. Megraud, C. O'Morain, and the European *Helicobacter pylori* Study Group (EHPSG).** 2002. Current concepts in the management of *Helicobacter pylori* infection—the Maastricht 2-2000 Consensus Report. *Aliment. Pharmacol. Ther.* **16:**167–180.

16. **Matsumura, M., Y. Hikiba, K. Ogura, G. Togo, I. Tsukuda, K. Ushikawa, Y. Shiratori, and M. Omata.** 2001. Rapid detection of mutations in the 23S rRNA gene of *Helicobacter pylori* that confers resistance to clarithromycin treatment to the bacterium. *J. Clin. Microbiol.* **39:**691–695.

17. **Megraud, F.** 2001. Impact of *Helicobacter pylori* virulence in the outcome of gastroduodenal diseases: lessons from the microbiologist. *Dig. Dis.* **19:**99–103.

18. **Monteiro, L., B. Bergey, N. Gras, and F. Megraud.** 2002. Evaluation of the performance of the Helico Blot 2.1 as a tool to investigate the virulence properties of *Helicobacter pylori*. *Clin. Microbiol. Infect.* **8:**676–679.

19. **National Institutes of Health Consensus Conference.** 1994. *Helicobacter pylori* in peptic ulcer disease. *JAMA* **272:**65–69.

20. **Oleastro, M., A. Menard, A. Santos, H. Lamouliatte, L. Monteiro, P. Barthelemy, and F. Megraud.** 2003. Real-time PCR assay for rapid and accurate detection of point mutations conferring resistance to clarithromycin in *Helicobacter pylori*. *J. Clin. Microbiol.* **41:**397–402.

21. **Park, C. Y., Y. K. Cho, T. Kodama, H. M. El-Zimaity, M. S. Osato, D. Y. Graham, and Y. Yamaoka.** 2002. New serological assay for detection of putative *Helicobacter pylori* virulence factors. *J. Clin. Microbiol.* **40:**4753–4756.

22. **Perez-Perez, G. I., R. M. Peek, J. C. Atherton, M. J. Blaser, and T. L. Cover.** 1999. Detection of anti-VacA antibody response in serum and gastric juice samples using types 1/ma and s2/m2 *Helicobacter pylori* VacA antigens. *Clin. Diagn. Lab. Immunol.* **6:**489–493.

23. **Perri, F., G. Manes, M. Neri, D. Vaira, and G. Nardone.** 2002. *Helicobacter pylori* antigen stool test and ^{13}C-urea breath test in patients after eradication treatments. *Am. J. Gastroenterol.* **97:**2756–2762.

24. **Rautelin, H., P. Lehours, and F. Megraud.** 2003. Diagnosis of *Helicobacter pylori* infection. *Helicobacter* **8**(Suppl. 1)**:**13–20.

25. **Ribeiro, M. L., M. M. Gerrits, Y. H. Benvengo, M. Berning, A. P. Godoy, E. J. Kuipers, S. Mendonca, A. H. van Vliet, J. Pedrazzoli, Jr., and J. G. Kusters.** 2004. Detection of high-level tetracycline resistance in clinical isolates of *Helicobacter pylori* using PCR-RFLP. *FEMS Immunol. Med. Microbiol.* **40:**57–61.

26. **Segal, E. D., J. Cha, J. Lo, S. Falkow, and L. S. Tompkins.** 1999. Altered states: involvement of phosphorylated CagA in the induction of host cellular growth changes by *Helicobacter pylori*. *Proc. Natl. Acad. Sci. USA* **96:**14559–14564.

27. **Shimizu, T., Y. Yarita, H. Haruna, K. Kaneko, Y. Yamashiro, R. Gupta, A. Anazawa, and K. Suzuki.** 2003. Urine-based enzyme-linked immunosorbent assay for the detection of *Helicobacter pylori* antibodies in children. *J. Paediatr. Child Health* **39:**606–610.

28. **Sicinschi, L. A., P. Correa, L. E. Bravo, and B. G. Schneider.** 2003. A positive assay for identification of cagA negative strains of *Helicobacter pylori*. *J. Microbiol. Methods* **55:**625–633.

29. **Sokic-Milutinovic, T., T. Wex, V. Todorovic, T. Milosavljevic, and P. Malfertheiner.** 2004. Anti-CagA and Anti-VacA antibodies in *Helicobacter pylori*-infected patients with and without peptic ulcer disease in Serbia and Montenegro. *Scand. J. Gastroenterol.* **3:**222–226.

Detection of Antibodies to *Legionella*

PAUL H. EDELSTEIN

55

Legionnaires' disease is a type of bacterial pneumonia caused by the legionellae (15). *Legionella pneumophila* causes more than 90% of cases of Legionnaires' disease, with *L. pneumophila* serogroup 1 (SG1) being responsible for about 85 to 95% of the cases of community-acquired Legionnaires' disease (4, 31). Determination of the levels of antibody to *L. pneumophila* was one of the first methods used to diagnose Legionnaires' disease and was especially valuable when culture diagnosis was at a primitive stage. Serologic testing is now a second-line test because of the length of time required for seroconversion, its relatively low sensitivity, and the low specificity of seroconversion for antigens other than *L. pneumophila* SG1. The major use of this test is for epidemiologic purposes, such as outbreak investigations, research purposes, and to complement other diagnostic tests. Other immunologic tests used to diagnose Legionnaires' disease include detection of bacteria in respiratory tract samples using immunofluorescent microscopy and detection of *L. pneumophila* SG1 antigenuria by enzyme-linked immunosorbent assay (ELISA) or immunochromatographic assay (13–15). Culture of respiratory tract specimens is an excellent but insensitive method to diagnose Legionnaires' disease, while urinary antigen detection is the most useful test for diagnosing *L. pneumophila* SG1 infection. Molecular methods for diagnosis, such as PCR, have been successfully used on a research basis, and a newly introduced commercial DNA amplification and detection test for *L. pneumophila* (BD ProbeTek ET *Legionella pneumophila*) has great promise. This chapter describes antibody testing because it is still very widely used and is of major importance for epidemiologic and research studies.

HISTORY OF AND CONTROVERSIES SURROUNDING ANTIGEN PREPARATION

McDade and Shepard, the test originators, used live yolk sac-grown bacteria; this method was subsequently adopted and modified by Harrison and Taylor, who used Formalin-killed yolk sac-grown bacteria (20, 27). Centers for Disease Control (CDC) workers then switched to heat-killed plate-grown bacteria, which had equivalent sensitivity to that of the original McDade and Shepard antigen (27). Heating is the antigen inactivation method used in the United States, whereas Formalin-inactivated yolk sac-grown bacteria was preferentially used in the European Community. Use of the

Harrison-Taylor preparation gave an exceptionally low background frequency of elevated titers (1 to 3% at a titer of 16), as opposed to the 1 to 20% frequency (titer of 128) with use of the CDC antigen (20, 27). The relative performance of the two antigen preparations was not studied for large numbers of specimens, but if seroconversion was used as a diagnostic criterion, there was probably little difference. Some commercial North American laboratories provide Formalin-fixed plate-grown antigen, which is not equivalent to the yolk sac-grown one. There is currently no public or private supplier of the yolk sac-grown Formalin-fixed antigen.

The CDC method uses antigen suspended in yolk sac, whereas none of the North American commercial laboratories producing Food and Drug Administration (FDA)-cleared kits for antibody detection use yolk sac, nor is yolk sac itself commercially available. The non-FDA-cleared Focus Technologies antigen is Formalin fixed and suspended in yolk sac (Focus Technologies, personal communication, July 2004). Yolk sac helps the antigen to adhere to the slide and prevents bacterial aggregation, and its use may affect antibody titers. Yolk sac is also used in the CDC method for making the first serum dilution, to decrease autofluorescence. Yolk sac omission in commercial kits may therefore affect the interpretive criteria.

A very important point is that validation studies of the CDC and Harrison-Taylor methods utilized only *L. pneumophila* SG1 antigen (20, 27). This antigen is very specific, much more so than that of other serogroups and other *Legionella* spp. The interpretive criteria developed for these antigens cannot be applied to other antigen preparations, regardless of serogroup and species. Elevated titers of antibody to other *L. pneumophila* serogroups and *Legionella* species are more common among healthy blood donors than are those of antibody to *L. pneumophila* SG1 (5, 29). Because of this, neither CDC nor British Public Health Laboratories routinely perform testing for other serogroups and species. Laboratories are strongly advised against routine testing for antibody to other serogroups and species unless an adequate local control population is available to determine the specificity of testing and unless appropriate interpretive criteria are used. An adequate control population should encompass not only healthy blood donors but also patients with bacteriologically confirmed pneumonia not caused by *Legionella*. Unfortunately, many commercially available indirect immunofluorescent-antibody (IFA) kits sold in the

United States contain polyvalent antigen, so the results of positive screening tests must be confirmed by using a mono-specific assay kit or home-made reagents.

TEST SENSITIVITY AND SPECIFICITY

When seroconversion to heat-killed *L. pneumophila* SG1 is defined as a fourfold increase in titer from ≤32 to ≥128, the sensitivity is in the range of 70 to 80%, provided that up to 9 weeks is allowed for antibody levels to rise (27). Using different criteria, the Formalin-fixed antigen had similar sensitivity (20). Of note, the test sensitivity is lower for epidemic disease, about 50%, presumably because convalescent-phase sera are not collected at later time points (11, 12). The sensitivity of seroconversion to other antigens in the case of infections caused by other serogroups and species is unknown. Because of cross-reactive antibody formation, a significant but not precisely known proportion (possibly around 50%) of patients with non-*L. pneumophila* SG1 infection will demonstrate seroconversion to *L. pneumophila* SG1 (29). The specificity of seroconversion to *L. pneumophila* SG1 ranges from 99 to 99.9%; for other serogroups and species, it ranges from 90 to 95% (29). This makes seroconversion to *L. pneumophila* SG1 highly predictive of disease even in low-prevalence populations, but it makes seroconversion to other serogroups and species nonspecific when pretest probabilities are below 20%. Once positive due to Legionnaires' disease, antibody levels fall to a background level in 3 to 10 years (10).

RATE OF SEROCONVERSION AND USE OF SINGLE RATHER THAN PAIRED SAMPLES

Up to 9 weeks may be required to develop a significant rise in titer in those who seroconvert (27). About 25% of patients seroconvert in week 1 of illness, 50% seroconvert in week 2, 75% seroconvert in week 3, 90% seroconvert in week 4, and the remaining 10% of patients seroconvert during weeks 6 to 9. Thus, testing of paired sera drawn during the first 2 weeks of illness has only about a 40% (50% of 80%) chance of yielding a positive result in patients with Legionnaires' disease. The Harrison-Taylor antigen apparently has a higher early yield, with 30 to 40% of patients developing elevated titers, but not necessarily seroconversion, after the first week of illness (20). Because of high background antibody levels (1 to 20%) in North America, unpaired serum testing is often of low specificity and should not be done. The low specificity of single antibody titers as high as 1:256 (*L. pneumophila* SG1 heated antigen) has been documented by Plouffe et al. (25). It is exceptionally important that serum specimens be tested in parallel when testing for seroconversion. Otherwise, in the process of testing specimens on different days, the normal 1 two-fold dilution variability of testing that occurs from day to day could either mask a fourfold rise or produce apparent titer changes that are not real.

High single titers are often used in the investigation of known outbreaks of Legionnaires' disease. In this case, the very high pretest probability of disease makes single-serum testing useful. Serum antibody to *L. pneumophila* SG1 heat-killed antigen at a titer of ≥1,024 is often used as "presumptive" evidence of Legionnaires' disease in outbreak settings. Recently, detection of single elevated levels of immunoglobulin M (IgM) to *L. pneumophila* SG1 heat-killed antigen has been used to detect epidemic-disease patients with otherwise negative antibody tests (12, 18). The specificity of elevated IgM levels in this setting is not known with certainty but may be around 93 to 99%, with a sensitivity of around 70% (12). In an epidemic setting, where pretest probability may be as high as 50%, the positive predictive value of a single elevated IgM or IgGAM test is about 89 to 98%, an epidemiologically helpful level of certainty. However, in the setting of sporadic disease, the positive predictive value of such a positive test is only about 18 to 60%, a dubious level of certainty for clinical purposes.

USE OF POLYVALENT ANTIGENS

More than 60 different *Legionella* serogroups have been described to date. Patients infected with some *Legionella* serogroups may not demonstrate antibody to other serogroups. In one study, about 60% of seroconversions were missed by workers screening sera by using only *L. pneumophila* SG1 antigen; it is unknown how many patients with missed seroconversions actually had Legionnaires' disease and how many had cross-reactive antibody to other bacteria (29).

The failure to detect seroconversions with non-*L. pneumophila* antigens led to the use of polyvalent pools of antigens for screening purposes (16, 27). Very good correlation between monovalent and polyvalent antigen results were observed for *L. pneumophila* SG1 disease, but no negative control sera were tested. A subsequent study examined the specificity of multiple polyvalent pools; overall, the specificity of seroconversion was estimated to be 96% (29). Unfortunately, the control groups did not contain sera from patients with infections caused by organisms known to be cross-reactive. These studies led to the use of multiple polyvalent pools, for which proper studies of correlation of results with monovalent antigens have not been performed and for which specificity is not well established but probably is low. Fallon and Abraham found that the specificity of an *L. pneumophila* SG1 to SG4 polyvalent antigen was quite good when judged against reactivity with monovalent antigens but that it was not perfect, and they recommended that the polyvalent pool be used only for screening purposes and that all high antibody titers be checked with the monovalent components (16). I have found that at least 25% of seroconversions to four different polyvalent antigen pools did not prove to be genuine when the sera were retested with the monovalent components (P. Edelstein, unpublished observations). In most of these cases, patients had nosocomial pneumonia caused by *Pseudomonas* and other gram-negative bacteria, a group of patients not tested by the CDC workers. Because of this, it is mandatory to confirm polyvalent seroconversions by using the monovalent components. A better policy is to avoid the use of such pools completely and to use only *L. pneumophila* SG1 antigen as discussed above. Use of this antigen alone should enable a serologic diagnosis of the majority (65 to 70%) of cases of Legionnaires' disease (26). A case can be made for the use of such pools for screening purposes in epidemiologic investigations, providing that adequate control populations are studied and that monovalent antigen preparations are used once the epidemic strain becomes known.

DETERMINATION OF INFECTING SEROGROUP

It is often not possible to determine the serogroup or species causing infection by using antibody responses (27). For example, in one outbreak caused by *L. pneumophila* SG1, some patients had marked antibody responses to other *Legionella* species and serogroups (17). Thus, the use of relative antibody titers to determine the infecting type of bacterium can be misleading.

ANTIBODY IMMUNOGLOBULIN TYPE

Antibody to *L. pneumophila* during and after infection may be composed of either IgA, IgG, IgM, or various combinations of the three immunoglobulin classes (1, 3, 20, 28). It has been demonstrated that tests for *L. pneumophila* antibody must examine for all three of the immunoglobulin classes for optimal sensitivity. IgM antibody can persist for considerable lengths of time, making impossible the distinction of new from old disease by determining IgM antibody levels. Unfortunately, some commercial kits for IFA testing do not use a secondary antibody proven to react with IgM or IgA antibodies to *L. pneumophila*.

AGGLUTINATION ASSAYS

A rapid microagglutination assay is used in the European Community to detect early rises in levels of antibody to *L. pneumophila* SG1 (20). The advantage of this over immunofluorescence microscopy is the slightly more rapid appearance of agglutinating antibodies and the ability to test a large number of specimens more easily. The specificity of such testing is estimated to be 97 to 99%, with a sensitivity of about 80% (20). About 40% of people who eventually seroconvert have agglutinating antibodies detected during the first week of infection (20). The Michigan State Department of Community Health Laboratory uses a multivalent hemagglutination assay which has been well validated only for the detection of antibodies to *L. pneumophila* SG1 (21, 30).

ELISAS

Extensive studies of the performance of ELISAs for the measurement of *L. pneumophila* antibody have not been performed. Sonicated whole bacterium and purified lipopolysaccharide appear to be the best antigens for use in this assay (1, 3). Detection of specific IgA antibodies may also increase the sensitivity and specificity of the ELISA (3).

Several enzyme immunoassay (EIA) kits that measure *L. pneumophila* antibodies are commercially available and are manufactured or sold by Wampole Laboratories and Zeus Diagnostics. These kits screen for IgM and IgG antibodies to *L. pneumophila* SG1 to SG6. The sensitivity of the kits for measurement of antibody to *L. pneumophila* SG2 to SG6 is unknown, but they do appear to be reasonably sensitive in comparison to the IFA method (70 to 90%) for the estimation of SG1 antibodies (19). Test specificities are about 98%. These tests are designed to detect relatively high IFA titers, in the range of 1:128 to 1:256. Of note, the IFA technique detects IgA antibody, which is apparently not detected by ELISA; this has the potential to decrease ELISA sensitivity (28). The Serion Classic EIA test A kit is used in Europe but has not been FDA cleared, in contrast to the Zeus and Wampole EIA kits. Detailed published studies of the performance of the Serion EIA test A kit are unavailable, but use of the kit in a large outbreak of Legionnaires' disease caused by *L. pneumophila* SG1 showed the sensitivity to be 62%, about the same as that observed historically for IFA testing in the same setting (11). The specificity of the Serion EIA in patients with pneumonia not caused by *Legionella*

spp. is unknown, but its age-related normative values have been determined (6). Since all the EIA kits use a pool of serogroups, a positive EIA result can be the result of cumulative low-level antibodies to different serogroups, as has been observed for the IFA method using multiple antigens (16). Because of this, the positive predictive accuracy of a positive EIA result may be low. The predictive value of a positive Wampole assay is about 90%; in other words, about 90% of EIA-positive or indeterminate sera will have IFA titers (heat-killed antigen) of ≥64, with most being >64 (Edelstein, unpublished). All positive EIA results should be confirmed by use of the IFA test with an *L. pneumophila* SG1 antigen (19). The best use of the EIA test is as a screening assay of convalescent-phase sera (19). Any such sera yielding positive or indeterminate results can then be tested in parallel with the acute-phase serum by the IFA method. Using this scheme, about 10% of serum pairs so selected are positive for a significant change in IFA titer (Edelstein, unpublished). A recent comparison of the sensitivity of the Wampole and Zeus EIA kits versus a home-made polyvalent IFA test showed the EIAs to be about 24% sensitive, in striking contrast to prior studies and FDA submission data; this may be because of nonspecificity of the IFA results or, less likely, because of poor detection of IgA antibodies by the ELISA kits (22).

CROSS-REACTIVE ANTIBODY

Cross-reactive antibody is occasionally found in patients with non-*Legionella* infections. These infections have included pneumonia and bacteremias caused by *Pseudomonas*, *Haemophilus*, *Mycobacterium*, gram-negative enteric rods, *Bordetella*, *Chlamydia*, *Rickettsia*, and *Bacteroides* (reviewed in references 2 and 9). Most problematic are pseudomonas infections, especially when antibody to *Legionella* antigens other than *L. pneumophila* SG1 is measured (9, 20). Up to 25% of people with *Campylobacter jejuni* enteritis have cross-reactive antibodies to *L. pneumophila* (7, 8, 23). Bornstein et al. found that cross-reactive antibodies to yolk sac-grown Formalin-fixed *L. pneumophila* SG1 were very rare (ca. 0.4%) in sera collected from patients with tuberculosis or non-*Legionella* pneumonia. However, as many as 10% of patients with tuberculosis had cross-reactive antibodies to other *Legionella* serogroups and species (5). Using similar antigen preparations, McIntyre et al. found that 193 patients with other causes of pneumonia had no appreciable titer (<16) of antibody to *L. pneumophila* SG1 antigen, whereas 21 (11%) had elevated convalescent-phase titers (>16) of antibodies to a number of other *Legionella* antigens (24). Taylor and Harrison found the specificity of their *L. pneumophila* SG1 antigen to be near 100% when testing presumably late-phase sera collected from 317 patients with a variety of bacterial infections not caused by *Legionella*. The only exception involved sera collected from 2 of 26 patients with *Pseudomonas* infections, both of whom had positive but low (titer of 16) antibody titers (20).

BLOCKING ANTIGEN

Because of the cross-reactivity noted above, Wilkinson and colleagues absorbed serum with an *Escherichia coli* "blocking antigen" to remove cross-reactive antibody, somewhat analogous to the absorption step used in syphilis serologic testing (28). It is unclear whether this absorption removes only nonspecific antibodies and what criteria should be used to evaluate the serologic results of testing before and after the use of this blocking antigen (2). Boswell and colleagues have also proposed using a *C. jejuni* blocking antigen (23). Because of its uncertain utility, the blocking antigen has been little used by most laboratories and probably adds little to this test.

CLINICAL INDICATIONS

Detection of *L. pneumophila* SG1 serum antibody is indicated in suspected cases of Legionnaires' disease or Pontiac fever. Pontiac fever is an acute, nonfatal febrile illness associated with *Legionella* but not proven to be caused by it. In the majority of cases, it is most appropriate to freeze acute-phase serum and to test it in parallel with a convalescent-phase serum sample only if a clinical or laboratory diagnosis has not been made by other means. Antibody testing used to diagnose Pontiac fever often requires testing of sera from matched controls. Investigations of outbreaks of pneumonia or research studies may be indications for testing single serum specimens.

SUMMARY

1. Only paired sera which have been collected at least 2 weeks, and preferably 6 to 9 weeks, apart should be accepted for serologic testing.

2. All specimens from the same patient must be tested together for optimal results.

3. Except for epidemiologic surveys, with well-matched negative control populations, testing should be done with *L. pneumophila* SG1 antigen only.

4. To obtain results that can be related to CDC results, heat-fixed Philadelphia 1 strain antigen should be used and suspended in yolk sac and the first serum dilution should be made in yolk sac diluent.

METHODS

Principles of the IFA Procedure

The IFA test measures the level of antibody to bacteria fixed to multiple wells of a microscope slide. Serially diluted serum ("primary antibody") is added to the slide wells containing the fixed bacteria and incubated to allow adherence of serum to the bacteria. The slide is then washed to remove any unbound serum. Antibody to human globulins that is conjugated with fluorescein isothiocyanate ("secondary antibody") is added to the slide and allowed to react with the bound primary antibody. Excess secondary antibody is then washed off. The presence of secondary antibody is detected by observation of the slide using a microscope equipped with a UV light source and the proper filters. Wells with sufficient bound secondary antibody contain fluorescent bacteria, whereas wells containing little secondary antibody (because of poor binding of primary antibody to the bacteria) contain very few or no fluorescent bacteria. The actual concentration of antibody is determined by ascertaining the serum dilutions at which there is bright staining of the bacterial cells.

Specimen Requirements, Collection, Transport, and Storage

A 4-ml volume of blood collected in a tube without anticoagulants is required for testing. The blood specimen can be transported to the laboratory at ambient temperatures but protected from freezing. On arrival at the laboratory, blood should be allowed to clot at room temperature. The serum is separated by centrifugation at 500 to 1,000 × *g* and removed from the clot promptly. Serum separation should be done within a day of specimen collection; this period can be prolonged by storage of the clotted specimen at 5°C. Once the serum has been separated, it should be stored at 5°C until aliquoted for low-temperature storage. *Legionella* antibodies are relatively stable, such that serum can be transported at temperatures above freezing without significant antibody loss. Freeze-thawing may reduce antibody titers, necessitating aliquoting of samples before testing so that more than one comparative test can be performed on the same specimen without loss of antibody.

The serum specimen is aliquoted into at least three glass or plastic freezer vials that will withstand storage at −70°C. The filled vials are stored at −70°C. If low-temperature freezing is not possible, the vials should be stored at the lowest possible temperature and freeze-thaw cycles should be avoided.

Serum samples should be collected at the onset of illness and every 2 to 4 weeks afterward for a total of 8 to 9 weeks. Testing of single specimens should not be performed routinely, regardless of the stage of illness. In epidemic situations, testing of acute-phase specimens may be helpful, but this practice should be confined to such instances. The minimum number of specimens required is two, drawn at least 2 weeks apart. Exceptions to the requirement for two specimens include patients with pneumonia of more than 2 months' duration and spot prevalence epidemiologic surveys when a control population is used.

The most cost-efficient method of testing is to test only the convalescent-phase sera at a dilution of 1:64. If this is positive, then both acute- and convalescent-phase sera can be further tested at the same time. If it is negative, there is no need to test the acute-phase serum. Although unpaired serum specimens should not ordinarily be tested, screening should be done at a dilution of 1:512 if they are tested. An alternative screening approach is to first screen the convalescent-phase sera by using one of the commercial ELISA kits; all specimens giving positive or equivocal results in the assay are then tested in parallel with the acute-phase serum in the IFA test. This second strategy can be cost- and time-effective if a large number of samples must be tested. About 1 to 2 h of hands-on time and about 3 to 4 h of total time is required to screen 90 samples using the ELISA kits, whereas two to four times the amount of time is required to screen the same number of specimens using the IFA method. In addition, usually only about 1 to 10% of convalescent-phase sera from patients suspected of having Legionnaires' disease are positive in the ELISA screening, greatly reducing the number of IFA assays that have to be set up.

Materials

Serum

Serum to be tested (minimum volume, 20 μl)

Positive control serum for antigen to be tested (minimum volume, 20 μl)

Anti-human globulin (IgG, IgA, and IgM) conjugated with fluorescein isothiocyanate, at its working dilution (this is available from a number of commercial sources; the working dilution for each lot has to be determined; for example, the working dilution of Kirkegaard and Perry goat anti-human globulin, catalog no. 02-1-07, lot no. UH065, is 1:25 in my assay; minimum volume is 0.3 to 0.4 ml total for two samples and the controls)

Supplies and Equipment

Multiwell Teflon-coated glass slides, 6 or 12 wells per slide, staggered, 5-mm-diameter wells

Glass coverslips, no. 1 thickness (40 by 60 mm)

Disposable, nonsterile glass tubes (12 by 75 mm), seven per specimen, or nonsterile 96-well microtiter plates

Pasteur pipettes, 5 in. (13 cm) long, disposable and nonsterile

Micropipette tips, nonsterile

Calibrated micropipettes, capable of dispensing 50, 100, and 750 µl

Glass staining dish with stainless steel rack or Coplin jar

Covered plastic or metal box with an interior slide rack, large enough to hold at least three slides (a 150-mm-diameter petri dish with wooden sticks on the bottom can be used) (this is referred to as a moisture chamber in the instructions; during all incubations the chamber should be kept humid inside by covering its bottom with wet paper towels)

Air incubator, preferably humidified, set at 35 to 37°C

Microscope equipped with an epi-illumination UV source (HBO 50 to HBO 200) and proper filters for fluorescein isothiocyanate (oculars should be in the range of 10× to 12.5×, and the objective should be 20× to 40× [oil, water, or dry], with a total magnification of about ×250 to ×500)

Reagents

Bacterial antigen suspension (minimum volume, 0.2 ml for one specimen and two controls)

3% yolk sac suspension in phosphate-buffered saline (PBS) (minimum volume, 1.5 ml for one specimen and two controls)

PBS, 0.01 M (pH 7.6), 0.5 liter

PBS, 0.01 M (pH 7.6), filter sterilized, 2 ml (for reconstituting lyophilized conjugate, if required)

Wash bottle containing PBS

Distilled or deionized water

Bicarbonate-buffered glycerol mounting fluid (pH 9). Use of antifade mounting media is not required and may decrease intensity and titer.

Controls

A negative and a positive control are used for each run. The positive control uses a serum specimen of known high titer, usually 512. Positive and negative control sera for *L. pneumophila* SG1 are commercially available, although they are of variable quality. It is sometimes better to use aliquoted human serum of known titer than to use commercially available antisera. It is difficult to obtain good control sera for other serogroups and species. Two approaches are possible for a negative control. The best one is to use serum of a known low titer, such as 32. A negative monkey control serum is available for *L. pneumophila* serogroups 1 to 6 but has not been extensively tested for any other antigens. Normal blood donors can often be used as the source of a negative control serum. A non-serum-containing negative control, such as PBS, can be used to help troubleshoot assay problems but is not routinely needed. This nonserum control is used to detect nonspecific binding of the secondary antibody to the antigen (antigen, PBS instead of serum, and conjugate) and autofluorescence of the antigen (antigen, PBS instead of serum, but no conjugate).

Procedure

Preparation of Slides

1. Store the microscope slides at −20°C to prevent the masking from coming loose. Thaw them at room temperature, and then dust them lightly with lint free tissues. **If commercially prepared antigen coated slides are being used, skip this step and the next step.**

2. Make sure that the antigen is evenly suspended by mixing with a vortex mixer. Apply 1 drop of the antigen to each well of the slides with a Pasteur pipette, and then immediately suck back as much solution as possible, leaving only a fine film on the slide. Air dry for 30 minutes. **Do not heat fix, as this will agglutinate the antigen and invalidate the assay.**

Dilution of Sera

1. Label seven test tubes with the specimen identification number and with the final serum dilution (16 to 1,024). Also, label tubes for the positive and negative control sera. Put the tubes in order in a rack, with the lowest dilution on the far left. Add 100 µl of PBS to all of the tubes except for the ones marked 16. These dilutions can also be carried out in a 96-well microtiter tray, using half the volumes specified for the tube method and mixing with a multichannel pipette or plate shaker.

2. Make an initial 1:16 dilution of serum in 3% yolk sac-PBS solution. You can do this by adding 50 µl of serum and 750 µl of the yolk sac diluent to the tube marked 16; for smaller volumes of serum, use 20 µl of serum and 300 µl of diluent. Vortex mix this tube.

3. Add 100 µl of the 1:16 dilution of serum to the test tube marked 32, and vortex mix briefly. Using a new pipette tip, add 100 µl of the 1:32 dilution to the tube marked 64, and vortex mix briefly. Continue this until you have made the 1:1,024 dilution of serum, changing the pipette tip each time.

Addition of Sera and Conjugate to Slides

1. Using a Pasteur pipette, add 1 drop of the 1:32 to 1:1,024 dilutions of the patient sera and the control sera to the wells of their respective slides. The drops should be added to the slides in decreasing order starting with the 1:1,024 dilution. In this way, one pipette can be used per specimen. The entire dilution should be expelled before pipetting the next lower dilution. The drop should cover the entire well of the antigen slide. It is most useful to place both acute- and convalescent-phase sera on the same slide, since this will allow ready comparison.

2. Place the slides flat on racks in the moisture chamber, cover the chamber, and incubate at 35 to 37°C for 30 min.

3. Remove the slides one at a time from the moisture chamber, and rinse each one with a stream of PBS from a squeeze bottle. The slide should be held horizontally and the stream of PBS should be directed gently downward to avoid rinsing different dilutions of the specimen together. Place the slides in the racks in glass rinsing dishes (Coplin jars); avoid touching the slides together. Fill the dishes with PBS, and incubate them for 10 min at room temperature.

4. Empty the PBS out of the dishes, and replace it with distilled water twice for 15 to 30 s each time.

5. Remove the slides from the rinsing dishes, and blot each slide dry with bibulous paper; alternatively, the slides can be left to air dry.

6. If required, reconstitute the anti-human conjugate with the filter-sterilized PBS (pH 7.6), and vortex mix until the solution is clear.

7. Add a drop of conjugated secondary antibody (ca. 8 to 20 μl) to each well of the dry slides, which have been placed on racks in the wet chamber. Since secondary antibody may be expensive, as little as 7 to 8 μl can be used; the pipette tip is then used to break the surface tension and allow the small drop to distribute evenly over the well. Using smaller conjugate volumes is more labor-intensive than use of a larger volume, which can be added as a free-flowing drop. The conjugate should fill the wells completely.

8. Cover the chamber, and incubate at 35 to 37°C for 30 min.

9. Repeat steps 3 to 5 above.

10. Mount coverslips with glycerol mounting medium. Care should be taken to use a minimum amount of glycerol for confluency to avoid leakage around the edges of the slides.

Reading the Slides

The prepared slides should be examined using a fluorescence microscope equipped as stated above. The 10× objective should be used initially to locate the antigen circle in the well. When this is achieved, the circle should be examined using the 20× to 40× objective. A 20× objective can be just as accurate as a 40× objective, especially if a 12.5× or 15× ocular is used; practice is required for correct reading with the smaller objective, but the end result is a shorter reading time, less affected by photobleaching. It is important that the UV light source be changed on a regular schedule (e.g., every 150 h for an HBO 100 bulb) to maintain relatively constant light intensity. Different results will be obtained for each type of light source, magnification, kinds of objective (immersion type, numerical aperture, flatness of field, and color correction), and filters. Also, there is often observer-to-observer variability of ±1 dilution. Reading of the end points with each microscope should be done with reference to the positive control serum used with the antigens and conjugate. The only commercially available positive control serum is of monkey origin and has been highly diluted. The end point of this control serum is not clear-cut, and the fluorescence tends to be very weak at the stated titer. Record the brightness of the staining at each dilution. The degree of staining intensity is based on the overall appearance of the smear. Specifically, a single bright area in an otherwise dimly fluorescent well should be ignored, as should fluorescent bits of yolk sac and filamentous bacterial cells that have a fluorescence intensity different from the majority of other bacteria in the well. Novices to this procedure should pay special attention to the appearance and fluorescence intensity of negative controls, especially wells containing bacteria, PBS, and secondary antibody. Otherwise, wells containing nonfluorescing but visible bacteria may be mistakenly thought to contain dimly fluorescent bacteria.

Scoring Fluorescence Intensity

4+ = maximal fluorescence; brilliant yellow-green staining of bacterial cells

3+ = bright yellow-green staining

2+ = definite but dim yellow-green staining

1+ = barely visible yellow-green staining

Negative = absence of yellow-green specific fluorescence

Serum titration end point (titer): the reciprocal of the highest dilution of serum giving 1+ fluorescence of at least half the number of *Legionella* bacteria in the field

Quality Control Testing

Each day the test is performed, tests of positive and negative controls must be carried out. The control sera should give the expected titers within one twofold dilution. If a negative control serum is not used, the negative control wells of conjugate plus antigen and of antigen alone must have been read as negative. If the control results are not within acceptable limits, the run must be repeated.

Test Interpretation

Providing that the results of quality control tests are acceptable and that sera were tested in parallel, a fourfold rise in titer to ≥128 from the acute to the convalescent phase provides evidence of a recent infection for *L. pneumophila* SG1. A single high titer of ≥256 is compatible with no disease, past disease, or current disease; however, an *L. pneumophila* SG1 antibody titer of ≥1,024 is very unlikely to be found in the normal population and could reasonably be interpreted to be compatible with past or, more likely, current disease. A single negative serum specimen is compatible with current or past disease and failure to produce antibody or with nondisease. The interpretation, or definition, of elevated high titers or seroconversion for antigens other than *L. pneumophila* SG1 is uncertain.

Antigen Preparation for Indirect Fluorescent-Antibody Test

Materials and Equipment

Bent glass rod or Pasteur pipette, sterile
Pasteur pipettes, sterile
16- by 120-mm glass screw-cap test tubes, sterile
10-ml volumetric pipettes, sterile
1-ml volumetric pipettes, sterile
Micropipette tips, sterile
Hot plate
Beaker for boiling-water bath
Bacteriological loop
Microcentrifuge
Micropipettor
Microcentrifuge tubes, sterile
Spectrophotometer cuvettes, 1-cm cell width
Spectrophotometer set at 660-nm wavelength

Reagents

Sterile distilled water
Buffered charcoal yeast extract α (BCYEα) and blood agar plates
Filter-sterilized PBS (pH 7.6), 0.01 M
0.5% yolk sac in PBS containing 0.05% sodium azide
Legionella strain to be used as antigen (Table 1)

Procedure

Monovalent-Antigen Preparation

1. Maintain sterility throughout the procedure to avoid bacterial contamination of the antigen suspension.

TABLE 1 *Legionella* strains used for IFA antigens

Species and serogroup	Strain
L. pneumophila serogroup 1	Philadelphia 1
L. pneumophila serogroup 2	Togus 1
L. pneumophila serogroup 3	Bloomington 2
L. pneumophila serogroup 4	Los Angeles 1
L. pneumophila serogroup 5	Dallas 1E
L. pneumophila serogroup 6	Chicago 2
L. pneumophila serogroup 7	Chicago 8
L. pneumophila serogroup 8	Concord 3
L. pneumophila serogroup 9	IN 23
L. dumoffii	TEX-KL
L. longbeachae serogroup 1	WADS 80-537B
L. longbeachae serogroup 2	Tucker 1
L. micdadei	TATLOCK

Appropriate biosafety precautions must be used, including using a class II biosafety cabinet for preparing the antigen. Once the antigen has been boiled, it may be safely handled outside the safety cabinet. Streak *Legionella* for confluent growth on a single BCYEα plate. Incubate for 48 to 72 h at 35°C in a humidified air incubator. Harvest the growth when it is confluent but not heavy; some strains may require longer periods of incubation than others. Examine a wet mount of the harvested antigen to determine the fraction of filamentous cells present; if these constitute more than 5% of the cells present, the preparation will not be optimal. To reduce the frequency of cellular filaments, harvest younger growth and make certain that the incubator is well humidified (>85% relative humidity) and that the BCYEα medium is fresh. Some strains of non-*L. pneumophila* species (e.g., *L. gormanii* and *L. sainthelensi*) may require a 3 to 5% CO$_2$ atmosphere for optimal growth without excessive filament formation. It is extremely important to use the specified strains, since aberrant results may occur when other strains are used.

2. Add 1 to 2 ml of sterile distilled water to the culture plate, and gently rub the growth off the plate with a bent Pasteur pipette. Transfer the suspension to a screw-cap sterile test tube. Subculture a loopful of the suspension to a blood agar plate to check for contamination by other bacteria; incubate for 3 days at 35°C in 5% CO$_2$ before reading. Discard the suspension if contamination is detected.

3. Place the tube containing the bacterial suspension in a boiling-water bath (not a dry heating block) for 15 min.

4. Centrifuge the tube contents for 1 minute in a microcentrifuge tube at ca. 14,000 × g.

5. Discard the supernatant fluid, and resuspend the bacterial cell sediment in 2 ml of sterile distilled water.

6. Prepare 1:100, 1:200, 1:400, and 1:800 dilutions of the resuspended organism in filter-sterilized PBS.

7. Check the optical densities (OD) of the antigen dilutions, using a spectrophotometer set at 660 nm, using PBS or distilled water as a blank. The desired OD for the working antigen suspension is 0.09 ± 0.01. Determine approximately which dilution of antigen will give this OD, by graphical means; make this dilution, and recheck the OD. You may have to make several other dilutions near this approximate value to get the OD right.

8. Make a working dilution of antigen in 0.5% yolk sac, from the original washed boiled suspension, that corresponds to the dilution determined in the step above. A 5- to 10-ml volume of suspension is adequate for several hundred assays. Save the undiluted suspension for future use.

9. Check for contamination of the working antigen suspension by streaking a loopful of the suspension on a blood agar plate. Examine the plate after 2 days of incubation at 35°C in 5% CO$_2$. Discard the suspension if contamination is detected.

Polyvalent-Antigen Preparation

1. Choose the four strains of *Legionella* which are to be used together as polyvalent antigen. Prepare each strain separately as for monovalent antigen. Use the procedure described above, through step 7 (determination of the dilution required to give an optical density of 0.09 ± 0.01).

2. For each strain, using the 0.5% yolk sac as diluent, make a dilution twice as concentrated as that determined to be needed for monovalent antigen.

3. Pool equal-volume aliquots of the double-strength dilutions of the four strains into one test tube. This is the polyvalent antigen. Each of the four strains is now represented by organisms at one-half the concentration that would be provided in a monovalent antigen.

4. Follow step 9 above.

Quality Control

1. Determine that the bacterium from which the prepared antigen is made is of the correct serogroup by staining it with monovalent antibody specific to that serogroup. This need be done only once, providing that the stock bacterial strain is handled correctly.

2. Determine that the new antigen preparation gives results with positive and negative control antisera that agree within one twofold dilution of their stated titer. There should be about 300 to 500 organisms per ×350 magnification field.

Storage and Shelf Life

Store the working dilution and undiluted antigen suspensions at 5°C. The shelf life of the diluted suspension is about 2 to 3 months, while that of the undiluted suspension is highly variable but as long as 6 months to 1 year. New lots of working dilutions can be made from the undiluted suspension until quality control testing with positive and negative control sera gives results that are out of range.

Preparation of 3% Yolk Sac Diluent

Materials and Equipment

Embryonated hen eggs, 12 to 14 days old, three

10% povidone iodine

70% isopropyl alcohol

Forceps, two pairs, sterile

Petri dish, 150-mm diameter, sterile

Egg candling light

Food blender with sterile glass jar, or sterile tissue grinder

PBS (pH 7.6), 0.01 M, filter sterilized, containing 0.05% sodium azide, 300 ml

Cotton gauze, sterile

Flask, 500 ml, sterile

Procedure

1. Candle the eggs to be certain that the embryos are alive (indicated by movement, with extensive blood vessel formation).

2. Paint the top of the egg with the povidone iodine, and allow it to dry completely. Remove the iodine by

painting the egg with the isopropyl alcohol, and allow it to dry completely.

3. With the closed pointed ends of the forceps, make a small hole in the egg tops. Enlarge the holes with the forceps so that the top 25% of the egg shell has been removed. Invert the eggs over a petri dish bottom so that the egg contents fall into the dish; you may need to use your forceps to effect complete removal.

4. Using blunt dissection, separate the yolk sacs from the rest of the egg contents, and transfer them to the inverted petri dish lid. Make a small tear in the yolk sacs, and allow their contents to drain freely.

5. Transfer the yolk sacs to the tissue grinder or homogenizer, and add an equal volume of PBS. Blend or grind until homogeneous.

6. Filter the yolk sac homogenate through two layers of the sterile gauze into the sterile flask. Add 300 ml of PBS. This will make a roughly 3% solution.

7. Culture a small portion of the 3% suspension on a blood agar plate to check for sterility. Discard the lot if not sterile.

8. To make a 0.5% solution, dilute the 3% solution in PBS containing 0.05% sodium azide.

Quality Control

It is best to perform quality control tests in parallel with an old lot of yolk sac. The titers of negative and positive control sera should be within their specified range. The bacterial antigen suspended in the new lot of yolk sac should be uniformly adherent to slides without large clumps of yolk sac.

Shelf Life and Storage Conditions

Store at 5°C and handle aseptically. The yolk sac suspension is of highly variable stability, from 3 months to over 20 years.

Glycerol Mounting Fluid

A high-pH mounting fluid must be used for fluorescein isothiocyanate, since the fluorescence intensity is pH dependent; the optimal pH for maximal brightness is 9, and the pH used should not be below 8. Mounting medium is commercially available from a number of vendors.

Reagents

Glycerol (glycerin), reagent grade
Sodium bicarbonate (NaHCO$_3$), reagent grade
Sodium carbonate (Na$_2$CO$_3$), reagent grade
Deionized or distilled water, 100 ml

Procedure

1. Make stock 0.5 M buffer by adding 0.22 g of Na$_2$CO$_3$ and 4.00 g of NaHCO$_3$ to a beaker. Add 100 ml of water, and mix until completely dissolved. Check the pH, which should be 9.0 ± 0.1. If the pH is below 8.9, add a small amount of Na$_2$CO$_3$, while stirring, until the pH is correct.

2. Add 5 ml of buffer to 45 ml of glycerol, and stir to dissolve.

Quality Control

Check the pH of the buffered glycerol monthly. Discard if the pH is less than 8. Check clarity daily, and discard if the solution is cloudy.

Storage and Shelf Life

Store the buffered glycerol at room temperature. The shelf life is 2 to 4 months. The stock buffer solution should be stored in a closed high-quality glass (Pyrex type) or plastic container at 5°C for up to 6 months, as long as it remains clear and the pH is acceptable.

APPENDIX

Reagent Suppliers

IFA and ELISA kits

Focus Technologies (not FDA cleared)
Cypress, CA 90630
Phone: (800) 445-0185
http://www.focustechnologies.com

Serion Immunodiagnostica (not FDA cleared)
Würzburg, Germany
http://virion-serion.de

Trinity Biotech
Wicklow, Ireland
(multiple distributors)
http://www.trinitybiotech.com

Wampole Laboratories
Cranbury, NJ 08512
Phone: (800) 257-9525 or (609) 655-6000
http://www.wampolelabs.com

Zeus Scientific
P.O. Box 38
Raritan, NJ 08869
Phone: (800) 286-2111 or (908) 526-3744
http://www.zeusscientific.com

Multiwell microscope slides (12-well staggered, Teflon coated, catalog no. 10-188)

Cel-Line Associates, Inc.
Portsmouth, NH 03801
Phone: (800) 258-0834 or (603) 431-8410
http://www.cel-line.com

Secondary antibody

Sold by a large number of suppliers, including Kirkegaard & Perry, Cappel, and Sigma

REFERENCES

1. **Bangsborg, J. M.** 1997. Antigenic and genetic characterization of *Legionella* proteins: contributions to taxonomy, diagnosis and pathogenesis. *APMIS* (Suppl.) **70:**1–53.
2. **Bangsborg, J. M., A. Friss-Møller, C. Rechnitzer, N. Høiby, and K. Lind.** 1988. The *E. coli* immunosorbent as used in serodiagnosis of *Legionella* infections studied by crossed immunoelectrophoresis. *APMIS* **96:**177–184.
3. **Bangsborg, J. M., G. H. Shand, K. Hansen, and J. B. Wright.** 1994. Performance of four different indirect enzyme-linked immunosorbent assays (ELISAs) to detect specific IgG, IgA, and IgM in Legionnaires' disease. *APMIS* **102:**501–508.
4. **Benin, A. L., R. F. Benson, and R. E. Besser.** 2002. Trends in Legionnaires disease, 1980-1998: declining mortality and new patterns of diagnosis. *Clin. Infect. Dis.* **35:**1039–1046.
5. **Bornstein, N., N. Janin, G. Bourguignon, M. Surgot, and J. Fleurette.** 1987. Prevalence of anti-*Legionella* antibodies in a healthy population and in patients with tuberculosis or pneumonia. *Pathol. Biol.* (Paris) **35:**353–356.
6. **Boshuizen, H. C., J. W. den Boer, H. de Melker, J. F. Schellekens, M. F. Peeters, J. A. van Vliet, and M. A. Conyn-van Spaendonck.** 2003. Reference values for the

SERION classic ELISA for detecting *Legionella pneumophila* antibodies. *Eur. J. Clin. Microbiol. Infect. Dis.* **22:**706–708.

7. **Boswell, T. C.** 1996. Serological cross reaction between legionella and campylobacter in the rapid microagglutination test. *J. Clin. Pathol.* **49:**584–586.

8. **Boswell, T. C., and G. Kudesia.** 1992. Serological cross-reaction between *Legionella pneumophila* and campylobacter in the indirect fluorescent antibody test. *Epidemiol. Infect.* **109:**291–295.

9. **Collins, M. T., F. Espersen, N. Høiby, S. N. Cho, A. Friss-Møller, and J. S. Reif.** 1983. Cross-reactions between *Legionella pneumophilla* (serogroup 1) and twenty-eight other bacterial species, including other members of the family *Legionellaceae. Infect. Immun.* **39:**1441–1456.

10. **Darelid, J., S. Lofgren, B. E. Malmvall, M. A. Olinder-Nielsen, G. Briheim, and H. Hallander.** 2003. *Legionella pneumophila* serogroup 1 antibody kinetics in patients with Legionnaires' disease: implications for serological diagnosis. *Scand. J. Infect. Dis.* **35:**15–20.

11. **den Boer, J. W., E. P. Yzerman, J. Schellekens, K. D. Lettinga, H. C. Boshuizen, J. E. Van Steenbergen, A. Bosman, S. Van den Hof, H. A. Van Vliet, M. F. Peeters, R. J. van Ketel, P. Speelman, J. L. Kool, and M. A. Conyn-van Spaendonck.** 2002. A large outbreak of Legionnaires' disease at a flower show, the Netherlands, 1999. *Emerg. Infect. Dis.* **8:**37–43.

12. **De Ory, F., J. M. Echevarria, C. Pelaz, A. Tellez, M. A. Mateo, and J. Lopez.** 2000. Detection of specific IgM antibody in the investigation of an outbreak of pneumonia due to *Legionella pneumophila* serogroup 1. *Clin. Microbiol. Infect.* **6:**64–69.

13. **Domínguez, J. A., N. Galí, L. Matas, P. Pedroso, A. Hernandez, E. Padilla, and V. Ausina.** 1999. Evaluation of a rapid immunochromatographic assay for the detection of *Legionella* antigen in urine samples. *Eur. J. Clin. Microbiol. Infect. Dis.* **18:**896–898.

14. **Domínguez, J. A., N. Galí, P. Pedroso, A. Fargas, E. Padilla, J. M. Manterola, and L. Matas.** 1998. Comparison of the Binax *Legionella* urinary antigen enzyme immunoassay (EIA) with the Biotest *Legionella* urine antigen EIA for detection of *Legionella* antigen in both concentrated and nonconcentrated urine samples. *J. Clin. Microbiol.* **36:**2718–2722.

15. **Edelstein, P. H.** 1993. Legionnaires' disease. *Clin. Infect. Dis.* **16:**741–749.

16. **Fallon, R. J., and W. H. Abraham.** 1982. Polyvalent heat-killed antigen for the diagnosis of infection with *Legionella pneumophila. J. Clin. Pathol.* **35:**434–438.

17. **Fallon, R. J., and R. E. Johnston.** 1987. Heterogeneity of antibody response in infection with *Legionella pneumophila* serogroup 1. *J. Clin. Pathol.* **40:**569–572.

18. **Fry, A. M., M. Rutman, T. Allan, H. Scaife, E. Salehi, R. Benson, B. Fields, S. Nowicki, M. K. Parrish, J. Carpenter, E. Brown, C. Lucas, T. Horgan, E. Koch, and R. E. Besser.** 2003. Legionnaires' disease outbreak in an automobile engine manufacturing plant. *J. Infect. Dis.* **187:**1015–1018.

19. **Harrison, T. G., N. Doshi, G. Hallas, and R. C. George.** 1999. *Legionella pneumophila* antibody assays. An evaluation of commercial kits and reagents for the estimation of *Legionella pneumophila* antibody levels, p. 1–40. Respiratory and Systemic Infection Laboratory, Central Public Health Laboratory, Colindale, England.

20. **Harrison, T. G., and A. G. Taylor.** 1988. The diagnosis of Legionnaires' disease by estimation of antibody levels, p. 113–135. *In* T. G. Harrison and A. G. Taylor (ed.), *A Laboratory Manual for Legionella.* John Wiley & Sons, Ltd., Chichester, England.

21. **Lennette, D. A., E. T. Lennette, B. B. Wentworth, M. L. French, and G. L. Lattimer.** 1979. Serology of Legionnaires' disease: comparison of indirect fluorescent antibody, immune adherence hemagglutination, and indirect hemagglutination tests. *J. Clin. Microbiol.* **10:**876–879.

22. **Malan, A. K., T. B. Martins, T. D. Jaskowski, H. R. Hill, and C. M. Litwin.** 2003. Comparison of two commercial enzyme-linked immunosorbent assays with an immunofluorescence assay for detection of *Legionella pneumophila* types one to 6. *J. Clin. Microbiol.* **41:**3060–3063.

23. **Marshall, L. E., T. C. Boswell, and G. Kudesia.** 1994. False positive legionella serology in campylobacter infection: campylobacter serotypes, duration of antibody response and elimination of cross-reactions in the indirect fluorescent antibody test. *Epidemiol. Infect.* **112:**347–357.

24. **McIntyre, M., J. B. Kurtz, and J. B. Selkon.** 1990. Prevalence of antibodies to 15 antigens of *Legionellaceae* in patients with community-acquired pneumonia. *Epidemiol. Infect.* **104:**39–45.

25. **Plouffe, J. F., T. M. File, Jr., R. F. Breiman, B. A. Hackman, S. J. Salstrom, B. J. Marston, B. S. Fields, and the Community Based Pneumonia Incidence Study Group.** 1995. Reevaluation of the definition of Legionnaires' disease: use of the urinary antigen assay. *Clin. Infect. Dis.* **20:**1286–1291.

26. **Reingold, A. L., B. M. Thomason, B. J. Brake, L. Thacker, H. W. Wilkinson, and J. N. Kuritsky.** 1984. *Legionella* pneumonia in the United States: the distribution of serogroups and species causing human illness. *J. Infect. Dis.* **149:**819.

27. **Wilkinson, H. W.** 1983. Status of serologic tests for *Legionella* antigen and antibody at the Centers for Disease Control. *Zentbl. Bakteriol. Mikrobiol. Hyg. A* **255:**3–7.

28. **Wilkinson, H. W., C. E. Farshy, B. J. Fikes, D. D. Cruce, and L. P. Yealy.** 1979. Measure of immunoglobulin G-, M-, and A-specific titers against *Legionella pneumophila* and inhibition of titers against nonspecific, gram-negative bacterial antigens in the indirect immunofluorescence test for legionellosis. *J. Clin. Microbiol.* **10:**685–689.

29. **Wilkinson, H. W., A. L. Reingold, B. J. Brake, D. L. McGiboney, G. W. Gorman, and C. V. Broome.** 1983. Reactivity of serum from patients with suspected legionellosis against 29 antigens of *Legionellaceae* and *Legionella*-like organisms by indirect immunofluorescence assay. *J. Infect. Dis.* **147:**23–31.

30. **Yonke, C. A., H. E. Stiefel, D. L. Wilson, and B. B. Wentworth.** 1981. Evaluation of an indirect hemagglutination test for *Legionella pneumophila* serogroups 1 to 4. *J. Clin. Microbiol.* **13:**1040–1045.

31. **Yu, V. L., J. F. Plouffe, M. C. Pastoris, J. E. Stout, M. Schousboe, A. Widmer, J. Summersgill, T. File, C. M. Heath, D. L. Paterson, and A. Chereshsky.** 2002. Distribution of *Legionella* species and serogroups isolated by culture in patients with sporadic community-acquired legionellosis: an international collaborative survey. *J. Infect. Dis.* **186:**127–128.

Immunologic Methods for Diagnosis of Spirochetal Diseases

VICTORIA POPE, MARY D. ARI, MARTIN E. SCHRIEFER, AND PAUL N. LEVETT

56

BIOLOGIC CHARACTERISTICS OF THE ORDER *SPIROCHAETALES*

The bacteria that comprise the order *Spirochaetales* (Table 1) have in common a helical shape and two or more axial filaments (periplasmic flagella) permanently wound around a cytoplasmic cylinder and enclosed by an outer sheath (3). Although enclosed and not in contact with the environment, as are the flagella of other bacteria, the flagella of the spirochetes still rotate to produce the characteristic corkscrew movement of the organisms, enabling them to move through environments of relatively high viscosity, such as intracellular space, that block the flagellar motion of other bacteria. Nine genera are found within the order (3, 16), but only three contain human pathogens. They differ morphologically in thickness, length, number of spirals, and spiral depth. All seven genera within the family *Spirochaetaceae* lack the hooked end of the family *Leptospiraceae*. The spirochetes differ in their nutritional requirements as well (Table 1). Some species, such as *Borrelia hermsii*, grow in vitro on artificial media with little difficulty (16), whereas others, such as the subspecies of *Treponema pallidum*, are extremely difficult or impossible to culture in vitro. Even though growth requirements vary greatly within the same genera, species differentiation is not usually based on growth characteristics but rather on disease manifestation (treponemes), animal or vector tropism (borreliae), or antigenic and serologic relationships or DNA relatedness (3, 4) (leptospires).

Clinical Characteristics

Three genera, *Treponema*, *Borrelia*, and *Leptospira*, contain pathogenic spirochetes (Table 2) (3, 16). Only named species clearly shown to cause disease in humans are included in Table 2. All spirochetal diseases share remarkable similarities in clinical manifestations, including spirochetemia early in the course of the disease, dissemination of spirochetes to body organs, skin lesions, one or more stages of disease frequently interrupted by periods of latency, and neurologic and cardiac involvement (34). Syphilis is the most common spirochetal disease in the United States, with the most recent estimate being 32,871 newly reported cases in 2002. About 100 cases of leptospirosis and 20 cases of tick-borne relapsing fever are reported in the United States each year.

Etiologic Diagnosis

For the spirochetal diseases, direct dark-field microscopic examination often provides an immediate means of presumptive diagnosis. If a specific fluorescein-, alkaline phosphatase-, or peroxidase-labeled conjugate is used, the identification is definitive. *Borrelia burgdorferi*, the subspecies of *T. pallidum*, and *Treponema carateum* may be detected in skin lesions. *T. pallidum* subspecies *pallidum*, *B. burgdorferi*, and *Leptospira* spp. may be detected in biopsied material from organs or tissues and in some body fluids. The *Borrelia* species causing relapsing fever may be detected by dark-field examination of blood or Giemsa staining of a blood smear. With the exception of the pathogenic *Treponema* spp. and some noncultivable species of *Borrelia*, culture may also provide a preliminary diagnosis.

Serologic tests (Table 3) play a primary role in the diagnosis of syphilis and provide a presumptive diagnosis for leptospirosis but are only emerging as aids in the diagnosis of relapsing fever. Syphilis, borreliosis, and leptospirosis have many serodiagnostic assay methods in common. However, each of these test procedures has been modified for a specific etiologic agent and may play a different role in the diagnosis of that particular disease. Therefore, the test procedures are described for a specific disease rather than in general terms.

Collection of Specimens for Serologic Tests

In general, serum is the specimen of choice. Plasma or cerebrospinal fluid (CSF) may be an appropriate sample for some of the serologic tests. If serum samples are to be stored, use a mechanical pipetting device to carefully transfer serum to a labeled storage tube. Samples should be stored at 4 to 8°C if they are to be tested within a few days; otherwise, storage at -20°C is preferred. Freeze-thawing should be avoided. Single serum samples are appropriate for syphilis testing, but both acute- and convalescent-phase serum samples should be collected for leptospirosis. Tubes containing specimens should always be stored upright. When shipping a sample to a reference laboratory, secure the top and seal it with tape or Parafilm. Place the tube containing the sample in a container, with absorbent tissue impregnated with germicide. Place specimen documentation around the outside of this sealed container, and place both in a container that cannot be crushed during shipment.

TABLE 1 Characteristics of the order *Spirochaetales*

Organism	Habitat	Distinguishing features
Spirochaetaceae	Worldwide	Utilize carbohydrates or amino acids as carbon and energy sources; do not utilize long-chain fatty acids or alcohols
Spirochaeta	Free-living in aquatic environments	Utilize carbohydrates as carbon and energy sources
Cristispira	Digestive tract of mollusks	Crest or ridge (crista) on protoplasmic cylinder
Treponema	Mouth, intestinal tract, and genital area of humans and animals	Utilize carbohydrates and amino acids as carbon and energy sources
Borrelia	Rodents, reptiles, bats, birds, armadillos, monkeys, humans, horses, and ruminants	Stain with aniline dyes; arthropod vector borne; microaerophilic
Serpulina	Intestinal tract of pigs	Growth on tryptose blood agar
Brachyspira	Intestinal tract of humans	Growth on tryptose blood agar
Anguilina	Intestinal tract of humans, and pigs	
Leptospiraceae	Worldwide	Utilize long-chain fatty acids or long-chain fatty alcohols as carbon and energy sources
Leptospira	Free-living in surface water and moist soil, or animal and human host associated	One or both ends hooked
Leptonema	Worldwide	Intracytoplasmic tubules; growth in Trypticase soy broth without blood

TABLE 2 Spirochetal diseases of humans

Etiologic agent	Disease	Mode of transmission	Geographical distribution
Treponema species			
T. pallidum subsp.			
pallidum	Syphilis	Sexual	Worldwide
pertenue	Yaws	Contact with lesion	Tropical climates
endemicum	Nonvenereal endemic syphilis (bejel)	Contact with lesion or lesion material	Middle East, Africa, Southeast Asia, and former Yugoslavia
T. carateum	Pinta	Contact with lesion	Tropical climates of South America
Borrelia species			
recurrentis	Relapsing fever	Louse	Europe, Asia, Africa, possibly South America
caucasica	Relapsing fever	Tick	Caucasus to Iraq
crocidurae	Relapsing fever	Tick	Africa, Near East, Central Asia
duttoni	Relapsing fever	Tick	Africa
hermsii	Relapsing fever	Tick	Western United States, Canada
hispanica	Relapsing fever	Tick	Spain, Portugal, Morocco, Algeria, Tunisia
latyschewii	Relapsing fever	Tick	Iran, Central Asia
mazzotti	Relapsing fever	Tick	Mexico, Guatemala
parkeri	Relapsing fever	Tick	Western United States
persica	Relapsing fever	Tick	Middle East, Central Asia
turicatae	Relapsing fever	Tick	United States, Mexico
venezuelensis	Relapsing fever	Tick	Central and South American
burgdorferi	Lyme disease	Tick	Northern hemisphere
afzelii	Lyme disease	Tick	Eurasia
garinii	Lyme disease	Tick	Eurasia
Leptospira species			
interrogans	Leptospirosis	Zoonoses	Worldwide
borgpetersenii	Leptospirosis	Zoonoses	Worldwide
santarosai	Leptospirosis	Zoonoses	Worldwide
inadai	Leptospirosis	Zoonoses	Worldwide
noguchi	Leptospirosis	Zoonoses	Worldwide
weilii	Leptospirosis	Zoonoses	Worldwide
kirschneri	Leptospirosis	Zoonoses	Worldwide
meyeri	Leptospirosis	Zoonoses	Worldwide
alexanderi	Leptospirosis	Zoonoses	China

TABLE 3 Tests for diagnosis of spirochetal diseases

Disease	Assay method	Test	Use
Syphilis	Flocculation (cardiolipin, lecithin, cholesterol antigen)	Venereal Disease Research Laboratory (VDRL) slide; unheated serum reagin (USR); RPR 18-mm-circle card test; toluidine red unheated serum test (TRUST)	Serologic screening; treatment monitoring; presumptive diagnosis
	Hemagglutination	*T. pallidum* hemagglutination assay	Confirmation of screening test results
	Agglutination	TP-PA	Confirmation of reactive screening test results
	Direct microscopic examination	Dark-field microscopy	Visualization of treponemes in lesion exudates
	DFA (monoclonal or absorbed polyclonal antibody-*T. pallidum* conjugate)	DFA-TP	Definitive diagnosis of *T. pallidum* in lesion material or tissue sample
	IFA (polyclonal antibody-human conjugate, human gamma chain-specific conjugate, *T. pallidum* antigen)	FTA-ABS FTA-ABS DS	Confirmation of reactive screening test results
	Immunoassays	ELISA, Western blot	Confirmation of reactive screening test results
	Molecular antigen detection methods	PCR	Detection of *T. pallidum* in ulcers, CSF, blood
Leptospirosis	Indirect hemagglutination	IHA	Serologic screening in early stages of disease
	Agglutination	Macroscopic slide agglutination test	Serologic screening
	Agglutination lysis	MAT	Serologic screening and confirmation of other screening assays
	Immunohistochemistry (anti-*Leptospira* conjugate)	Immunochemistry for *Leptospira*	Detection of leptospires in formalin-fixed tissues
	Immunoassays	ELISA, Dip-S-Ticks, LEPTO dipstick	Serologic screening
Borreliosis	Direct microscopic examination	Dark-field microscopy; Wright- or Giemsa-stained blood smears	Screening blood to visualize borrelia
	Immunoassays	IFA; ELISA; Western blotting	Serologic screening

METHODS

Syphilis

For the laboratory-assisted diagnosis of syphilis, each test method (antigen detection, screening tests, and confirmatory tests) has a role in the diagnosis of syphilis and may be used singly or in combination with other tests, depending on the stage of syphilis or the patient population studied.

DFA-TP Test

Clinical indications

The direct fluorescent-antibody test for *T. pallidum* (DFA-TP) (19) is a practical alternative to dark-field microscopy and is the most specific means of diagnosing syphilis in most clinical laboratories. The demonstration of *T. pallidum* in lesion material or tissue in primary, secondary, early congenital, or infectious early latent stages constitutes a positive diagnosis for syphilis. All genital lesions should be examined for *T. pallidum*, even if the lesion is atypical and the individual does not belong to a population considered at high risk. In persons who are members of a high-risk group, all lesions, including oral, anal, and skin lesions, should be examined, because the lesions of syphilis can resemble lesions related to various conditions from psoriasis to Lyme disease to human

immunodeficiency virus (HIV) infection. The DFA-TP examination of tissue and body fluids is particularly valuable in the diagnosis of congenital syphilis. Specimen sources include (but are not limited to) amniotic fluid, placenta, umbilical cord, mucous patches, nasal discharge, and skin lesions. In the diagnosis of tertiary or late-stage syphilis, DFA-TP plays a lesser role; however, the CSF, brain biopsy tissue, aqueous humor, synovial fluid, and tissue from gummas may serve as specimen sources.

Equipment

Fluorescence microscope assembly

Slide board or holder

Moist chamber

35 to 37°C incubator

Bibulous paper

Adjustable micropipettors able to deliver 30 μl

Rubber bulbs, approximately 2-ml capacity

Disposable capillary pipettes, 5.75 in. (ca. 14.6 cm) long

Microscope slides, 1 by 3 in. (ca. 2.5 by 7.6 cm), frosted end, approximately 1 mm thick

Coverslips, no. 1, 22 by 22 mm

Reagents

Sterile distilled water

Phosphate-buffered saline (PBS), pH 7.2

PBS, pH 7.2, with 2% Tween 80

Methanol, reagent grade

Mounting medium (one part buffered saline [pH 7.2] plus nine parts reagent grade glycerol)

Fluorescein isothiocyanate (FITC)-labeled anti-*T. pallidum* globulin that has been absorbed with the non-pathogenic *Treponema phagendenis* biotype Reiter treponeme and demonstrated to stain only *T. pallidum* after absorption, or FITC-labeled monoclonal antibody to *T. pallidum*

Sample Preparation

Body fluids, exudates, or macerated tissue.

1. Body fluids, lesion exudates, suspensions of macerated tissue, or other materials should be well mixed with a disposable pipette and rubber bulb to ensure even distribution of material.

2. If quantity allows, organisms in spinal fluids and aqueous humor fluids should be concentrated by centrifugation ($17,300 \times g$ for 30 min). Supernatant fluid is carefully removed, and slides are made from the sediment.

3. Smears prepared in the clinic should be air dried. If they are being shipped to a reference laboratory, they should be mailed without fixation.

Tissue sections.

1. Cut sections from paraffin-embedded tissues at 2 μm, attach to slides with gelatin in a 44°C flotation water bath, and dry in an oven at 60°C for 20 min.

2. Deparaffinize tissue sections in two 3-min changes of xylene.

3. Rehydrate tissue by passage through two changes of absolute alcohol, 95% ethyl alcohol, and 80% ethyl alcohol, respectively, and place in PBS (pH 7.2).

4. Treat deparaffinized slides in one of the following ways.
(a) NH₄OH treatment
  (i) Flood deparaffinized tissue sections on microscope slides for 3 min with PBS (pH 7.2) containing 1% NH₄OH.
  (ii) Wash the slides for 10 min in 3% Tween 80 in PBS, and rinse in two 5-min changes of PBS.
  (iii) Rinse briefly in distilled water. Blot dry around tissue borders.
(b) Trypsin treatment
  (i) Flood deparaffinized tissue sections on microscope slides with PBS (pH 7.2) containing 0.25% trypsin (1:250 trypsin; ICN Biochemicals).
  (ii) Place slides in a moist chamber, and incubate at 37°C for 30 min.
  (iii) Rinse slides in three 5-min changes of PBS.
(c) Microwave treatment
  (i) Place slides in glass slide holder. Place holder in microwavable container that will hold 500 ml. Add 500 ml of PBS (pH 7.2).
  (ii) Place in microwave set on high. Boil for 5 min.
  (iii) Remove from microwave, and allow to cool for 5 min. Remove slides, and briefly rinse them in PBS.

Controls

Positive control. Smears made from FTA-ABS antigen or testicular impression smears made from *T. pallidum*-infected rabbits must be included. If tissue sections are the samples being stained, a section from an infected tissue should be used.

Negative control. Smears made from washed nonpathogenic Reiter treponeme cultures, freshly obtained human mouth treponemes, or washed *T. denticola* biotype microdentium cultures may be included.

Procedure for Staining

Exudates.

1. Spread approximately 10 μl of test material within each circle or 1-cm area of clean, grease-free slide, and allow to air dry. If possible, four smears should be prepared for each specimen.

2. Fix the slides in 100% methanol for 10 s. All slides from an individual patient must be handled separately throughout the staining process.

3. Cover each circle with approximately 30 μl of diluted conjugate or with a sufficient amount to cover the smear, and place the slides in a moist chamber at 35 to 37°C for 30 min.

4. Rinse the slides individually with PBS, and cover the slides, placed on a staining rack, with PBS for a total of 10 min. Follow with a brief final rinse in distilled water. Reactive controls and nonreactive controls may be rinsed in the same staining dish.

5. Drain the slides to remove excess water. Blot areas outside of the smears with bibulous paper if necessary. Place a very small drop of mounting medium on each circle, and apply a coverslip. (The mounting medium should be dropped from a disposable capillary pipette. Discard any medium left in the pipette.)

Tissues.

1. Dilute the FITC-labeled anti-treponemal monoclonal conjugate in 2% Tween 80 in PBS containing a 1:20,000 concentration of Evans blue dye.

2. Cover tissue sections with 30 μl of the diluted conjugate.

3. Place slides in a moist chamber for 30 min at 35 to 37°C.

4. Rinse slides in two 5-min changes of PBS, briefly rinse in distilled water, allow to drain, and blot along the edge to remove any residual water.

5. Place a very small drop of mounting medium on each circle, and cover with a no. 1 coverslip. (The mounting medium should be dropped from a disposable capillary pipette. Discard any medium left in the pipette.)

Reading Test Results

1. Use a microscope equipped with UV and tungsten light sources for observations. When an HBO-200 mercury bulb is used, a BG-12 exciter filter or a KP490 filter may be used in combination with an OG-1 barrier filter (K510 or K530).

2. A 45× high-dry objective is used for scanning the area, and a 100×/1.25 oil immersion objective is used for verification. (For fluorescent-antibody [FA] testing with transmitted illumination, the oil immersion objective must be fitted with a funnel stop or equipped with a built-in iris diaphragm.)

3. Scan the complete smear or tissue section. If definite evidence of typical fluorescing treponemes is observed, verify morphology using a 100× oil immersion objective.

Reporting Results

1. If FITC-stained treponemes are observed, report: "Treponemes, immunologically specific for *T. pallidum*, were observed by direct immunofluorescence."

2. If no treponemes were observed, report: "No treponemes were observed by direct immunofluorescence."

Precautions and Potential Problems

During the fixation and rinsing of smears, treponemes may be washed off the slides, particularly the control slides, and can adhere to other smears. Therefore, smears from patients must be handled individually to prevent *T. pallidum* organisms from adhering to nonreactive smears, resulting in a false-positive report. If staining dishes are used for controls, they must be cleaned after each use.

Failure to demonstrate *T. pallidum* from a syphilitic lesion may be caused by the age or condition of the lesion, treatment of the patient before the specimen was taken, or, most commonly, poor technique in collecting the specimen.

If a precipitate occurs in the labeled globulin, the precipitate should be removed, because artifacts about the same size as *T. pallidum* may interfere with the correct reading of the slide. This can occur with staining of both lesion and biopsy material. Poor technique in processing tissues and prior treatment of the patient adversely affect DFA-TP staining in tissues.

Rapid Plasma Reagin (RPR) 18-mm-Circle Card Test

Clinical Indications

Humoral antibodies, both immunoglobulin M (IgM) and IgG, as detected by the nontreponemal test for syphilis, usually do not appear until 1 to 4 weeks after the primary chancre has formed. Thus, the sensitivities of the tests may vary in primary syphilis according to time the blood is drawn after lesion formation. However, within 2 months, as the lesion begins to resolve spontaneously, all nontreponemal tests are 100% reactive. Because the disseminated lesions of the secondary stage take many forms, the nontreponemal tests are used to distinguish the lesions of syphilis from those of other infections or conditions. In addition, serologic tests for syphilis may be the only means of identifying individuals with untreated syphilis during the latent periods of infection.

Reactive nontreponemal test results should be quantitated. The titer of the nontreponemal tests will decrease with adequate treatment. When an individual is treated during the primary or secondary stage of a first infection with *T. pallidum*, the titer should show a 2-dilution decline after treatment, usually within 6 months. Patients who are treated in the latent or late stages of syphilis, have had more than one infection with syphilis, or are infected with HIV frequently show a more gradual decline in titer. Persistent seroreactivity does not necessarily signify treatment failure. However, a 2-dilution or fourfold increase in titer usually indicates a treatment failure or a reinfection.

Kit

Kits for the RPR 18-mm-circle card test (19), the most commonly used nontreponemal test, contain test antigen,

disposable 20-gauge needle, antigen-dispensing bottle, plastic-coated test cards, and disposable sampling straws-spreaders or stirrers. Some kits also contain control serum samples with specified reactivities of reactive, minimally reactive, and nonreactive.

Control Serum Samples

The reactive, minimally reactive, and nonreactive control sera are used to test the antigen suspension each day of use to confirm optimal reactivity before routine testing is performed and are not intended to be used as reading standards. Only RPR card antigen suspensions that produce the established reactivity pattern of the control serum samples should be used. The minimal reactive control is the most critical and is the first indicator of problems with the antigen, such as deterioration, which reduces reactivity.

Equipment

Mechanical rotator with fixed speed or adjustable to 100 ± 2 rpm circumscribing a circle 2 cm (3/4 in.) in diameter on a horizontal plane.

Humidity cover. Any convenient cover containing a moistened blotter or sponge can be used to cover cards during rotation.

Safety pipetting device. Must deliver 0.05 ml (50 μl) of reagent for use in the quantitative test and may also be used for the qualitative test.

Light source for reading test results. A high-intensity lamp can be used.

Reagents

0.9% saline. A 900-mg portion of dry sodium chloride (ACS) is used for each 100 ml of distilled water.

Diluent. A 1:50 dilution of serum nonreactive for syphilis prepared in 0.9% saline should be used in the quantitative procedure for making 1:32 and higher dilutions of serum specimens.

Antigen. Antigen suspension is stored in ampules or in the antigen-dispensing bottle at 2 to 8°C. An unopened ampule of antigen is stable until the expiration date. Antigen suspension in the plastic dispensing bottle (stored at 2 to 8°C) is stable for 3 months or until the expiration date, whichever is earlier. The suspension must not be used beyond the expiration date. A new lot of antigen suspension should be tested in parallel with a reference reagent to verify that it is of standard reactivity before it is placed in routine use.

Qualitative Test

Note: All flocculation tests for syphilis are affected by room temperature. For reliable and reproducible results, control serum samples, RPR card test antigen suspension, and test specimens must be at room temperature, 23 to 29°C (73 to 85°F), when tests are performed.

1. With a dispensing or an automatic pipetting device that delivers 0.05 ml (50 μl), place 50 μl of serum onto an 18-mm circle of the RPR test card.

2. With the reverse end of the dispensing device or with a toothpick, spread the specimen to fill the entire circle. Take care not to allow the serum to spread beyond the confines of the circle. Use a clean spreader for each sample.

3. Gently resuspend the RPR antigen suspension. Hold the dispensing bottle in a vertical position, and add exactly 1 free-falling drop (1/60 ml) of suspension to each test area containing serum.

4. Place the card on a mechanical rotator under a humidity cover.

5. Rotate for 8 min at 100 rpm.

6. Read the test reactions in the wet state under a high-intensity light source immediately after removing the card from the rotator. Read the test without magnification. To better differentiate minimally reactive from nonreactive serum, immediately after rotation tilt the card to about 30° from horizontal and briefly rotate the card manually.

7. Report the results as follows.

Reactive: Characteristic clumping of the RPR card antigen from slight but definite (minimally reactive) to marked and intense (reactive).

Nonreactive: No clumping of RPR card antigen or only slight "roughness."

Note: Results are reported as reactive or nonreactive regardless of the degree of reactivity. Slight but definite flocculation should always be reported as reactive.

Specimens giving any degree of reactivity should be quantitated. Rough nonreactive results should also be quantitated to identify possible prozone reactions.

8. On completion of the daily tests, remove the needle, rinse it with distilled or deionized water, and air dry. (Avoid wiping the needle because this removes the silicone coating.) Recap the dispensing bottle, and store it in the refrigerator.

Quantitative Test

1. For each specimen to be tested, place 50 μl of 0.5% saline onto circles 2 through 5. Do not spread the saline.

2. Using a safety pipetting device, place 50 μl of serum specimen onto circles 1 and 2.

3. Mix the saline and the specimen in circle 2 by drawing the mixture up and down in the safety pipettor eight times. Avoid the formation of bubbles. Continue making serial dilutions through circle 5. Discard 50 μl from circle 5.

4. Using a clean stirrer for each specimen, start at the highest dilution (1:16, circle 5), and with the broad end of the stirrer, spread the serum dilution within the confines of the circle. Repeat this action using the same sampling stirrer in circles 4, 3, 2, and 1.

5. Gently resuspend the RPR card antigen suspension in the dispensing bottle. Hold the antigen suspension bottle in a vertical position, dispense 1 or 2 drops to clear the needle of air, and then place exactly 1 free-falling drop (1/60 ml) of antigen suspension onto each test area.

6. Place the card on the rotator under a humidity cover. Rotate for 8 min at 100 rpm.

7. Read the test reactions as described in step 6 of the qualitative test (above).

8. Report results in terms of the highest dilution giving any reactivity, in accordance with the examples in Table 4.

9. If the highest dilution tested (1:16) is reactive, proceed as follows:

(a) Prepare a 1:50 dilution (2.0%) of nonreactive serum in 0.9% saline (this is to be used for making 1:32 and higher dilutions of specimens to be quantitated).

(b) Prepare a 1:16 dilution of the test specimen by adding 100 μl of the specimen to 1.5 ml of 0.9% saline. Mix thoroughly.

(c) Place 50 μl of the 1:50 nonreactive serum in circles 2, 3, 4, and 5 of an RPR card.

TABLE 4 Reporting results of the RPR card test on serum (quantitative test)[a]

Reaction with undiluted serum (1:1)	Reaction at serum dilution of:				Report
	1:2	1:4	1:8	1:16	
Rm	N	N	N	N	Reactive, 1:1 dilution or undiluted only
R	R	N	N	N	Reactive, 1:2 dilution
R	R	Rm	N	N	Reactive, 1:4 dilution
R	R	R	R	N	Reactive, 1:8 dilution

[a]Abbreviations: N, nonreactive; R, reactive; Rm, minimally reactive.

(d) Place 50 μl of the 1:16 dilution of the test specimen onto circles 1 and 2.

(e) Using the same pipettor, make serial twofold dilutions, and complete the test as described under steps 2 through 8 (RPR card quantitative test). Higher dilutions may be prepared, if necessary, in a similar manner.

Note: All dilutions may be made on the card if the 1:50 nonreactive serum is used as the diluent from circle 6 (1:32) on.

Interpretation of Results

Interpretation of the results must be based on the population being tested and the stage of syphilis suspected. When the nontreponemal tests are used as a screening test in a low-risk population, all reactive results should be confirmed with a treponemal test.

In pregnancy, irrespective of reports in the literature of false-positive results in the nontreponemal test in expectant mothers, reactive results should be confirmed with a treponemal test, and if it is reactive, the patient should be treated unless she has documented adequate treatment and declining antibody titers. In congenital syphilis, at birth the nontreponemal tests for syphilis measure passively transferred maternal IgG as well as infant IgM. If the nontreponemal test titer for the infant is higher than that of the mother, some clinicians interpret these results as indicative of congenital syphilis, but infants with congenital syphilis frequently have a titer lower than the mother's titer.

Precautions and Potential Problems

Most of the problems in nontreponemal test performance can be avoided if instructions for test performance, reagent control, and general quality control are carefully followed. Test results with plasma specimens improperly collected, e.g., collection tube only partially filled, or with specimens tested more than 24 h after collection can appear as minimally reactive. Cord blood samples may also react in this manner. Because of these problems, the use of plasma and/or cord serum should be restricted to special testing situations.

Problems which cannot always be avoided result in test misinterpretation by the physician as well as the laboratory. Prozone reactions occur in 1 to 2% of patients with secondary syphilis. These specimens may exhibit a nonreactive pattern which is slightly granular or "rough" or show an atypical appearance. On dilution, the reactivity increases and then decreases as the end-point titer is approached. All tests with a rough appearance should be quantitated to render a dilution that will surpass the prozone.

Another problem is that of false-positive results, which occur in the general population at a rate of between 1 and

2% regardless of the nontreponemal test used. In populations of intravenous drug users, more than 10% of the sera may give false-positive test results. Acute false-positive reactions lasting less than 6 months usually occur after various febrile diseases, shortly after vaccinations, and during pregnancy. Chronic false-positive reactions are more often associated with autoimmune diseases such as arthritis and lupus, the aging process, or chronic infections such as leprosy. False-positive titers are usually less than 1:8, but low titers are also seen in latent and late syphilis and high-titer false-positive results are associated with intravenous drug use and lymphomas. False-positive test results may be excluded through repetition of the test, confirmation with a treponemal test, and subsequent testing of a second specimen.

Test misinterpretation most often results from (i) failure to recognize that a variation of ±1 dilution is inherent in most serologic tests, (ii) failure to establish the true positivity of test results, and (iii) failure to obtain adequate patient history. A particular error which leads to misinterpretation involves using more than one nontreponemal test to monitor treatment. Initially, all serum samples should be tested in a qualitative nontreponemal test. The same nontreponemal test should be used for subsequent quantitative testing, since up to a fourfold difference in end-point titer may result with certain serum samples when they are tested by different nontreponemal tests.

TP-PA Test

Clinical Indications

The need to perform a treponemal test is related to the results of the nontreponemal test. Treponemal tests should be performed when clinical signs or patient history disagree with the nontreponemal test result. In general, only when late syphilis is suspected should the treponemal test be performed when the nontreponemal test is nonreactive. The *T. pallidum* particle agglutination (TP-PA) test (19) is more widely used than the fluorescent treponemal antibody-absorption test for confirmatory testing of nontreponemal test results or clinical impression.

Equipment

Safety pipetting devices capable of delivering 100 and 25 µl
Pipettes, 1.0 ml serologic, for reconstituting reagents
Vibratory shaker
Polystyrene microplates with U-shaped wells
Tray viewer (optional)

Reagents

All reagents are supplied in the kits (Fujirebio America, Inc., Wilmington, Del.).

Controls

A positive control, which is serially diluted, and a negative control are included in each test run. The sensitized and unsensitized particles are monitored for nonspecific agglutination, and each sample is tested with sensitized and unsensitized particles to check for anti-*T. pallidum* antibodies and nonspecific antibodies that may cause false positive reactions.

Procedure

Four wells are required for each patient sample and negative control run in the test (eight wells for reactive control). Wells 1 and 2 are for dilution of the sample, well 3 is for the unsensitized particles, and well 4 (wells 4 to 8 for the reactive control) is for the sensitized particles.

1. Add 100 µl of the sample diluent to well 1 and 25 µl to wells 2 to 4 (2 to 8 for the reactive control).
2. Using a micropipettor, add 25 µl of patient sample or control to well 1.
3. Mix the contents of well 1 by filling and discharging the micropipette five or six times. Using the micropipette, transfer 25 µl of the diluted serum sample from well 1 to well 2. Mix the contents of well 2, and transfer 25 µl to well 3. Mix the contents of well 3, and transfer 25 µl to well 4. Mix the contents of well 4, and discard 25 µl. (For the reactive control, continue the procedure through well 8 and discard 25 µl from well 8.)
4. Add 1 drop (25 µl) of unsensitized particles to well 3 and 1 drop (25 µl) of sensitized particles to well 4 (wells 4 to 8 for the reactive control) using the droppers supplied in the kit.
5. Repeat the process for each patient sample.
6. Mix the contents of the wells thoroughly by placing on a vibratory mixer for 30 s or tap the plate sharply several times with a finger. Cover the plate with a microplate cover or empty microplate. Allow the plate to sit undisturbed at room temperature for 2 h before reading. Alternatively, the plate can incubate overnight and be read the next morning.
7. Place the plate on a flat surface against a white background to observe the agglutination pattern for each well. A plate viewer may be used to aid visualization of the reaction. Observe the agglutination pattern for each patient and control well. Ensure that the well containing the unsensitized particles is nonreactive. Record the agglutination according to the criteria in Table 5.

Interpretation of Results

Treponemal tests vary in their reactivity in early primary syphilis. Reactivity in these tests appears at approximately the same time as reactivity in nontreponemal tests. In secondary and latent stages of syphilis, the treponemal tests are usually 100% reactive. The sensitivity declines somewhat in the late stage of syphilis to about 95%. In approximately 84% of cases of syphilis, once the treponemal tests are reactive they remain reactive for life. Treponemal tests are qualitative and are not recommended for monitoring of reinfection or the efficacy of treatment. In babies with possible congenital syphilis, all treponemal tests that detect IgG antibodies may be reactive. Passively transferred maternal IgG treponemal antibodies should be catabolized and undetectable in uninfected infants by the age of 12 to 18 months.

TABLE 5 Reporting system for TP-PA test

Initial test reading	Repeat test reading	Report
2 to 4 +		Reactive
1+	>1+	Reactive
	1+	Minimally reactive[a]
	<1+	Nonreactive
<1+		Nonreactive
N[b]		Nonreactive

[a] In the absence of historical or clinical evidence of treponemal infection, this test result should be considered equivocal. A second specimen should be obtained 1 to 2 weeks after the initial specimen and submitted to the laboratory for serologic testing.
[b] N, nonreactive.

Precautions and Potential Problems

Inadequate mixing of the microplate after all the regents are added, disturbance of the plate during the incubation step, the presence of dirt or dust in any of the wells of the microplate, or use of V-shaped or flat-bottom wells instead of U-shaped wells may affect the results of the test.

The TP-PA test is not intended for routine use as a screening procedure. The greatest value is to distinguish true-positive nontreponemal results from false-positive results and to establish the diagnosis of late latent or late syphilis. Problems arise when these tests are used as screening procedures, especially in low-prevalence populations, because about 1% of the general population will have false-positive results. False-positive results in the treponemal tests are often transient, and their cause is unknown.

When the treponemal test results and clinical opinion disagree, the treponemal test should be repeated and additional clinical history information should be obtained. If the disagreement persists, the specimen should be sent to a reference laboratory for additional confirmatory tests. The final diagnosis depends on clinical judgment.

EIA

There are at least two types of enzyme immunoassay (EIA) on the market. One uses sonicated treponemes, and the other uses cloned antigens. The procedures for the two tests differ slightly, but in general the antigen is coated on the wells of a microtiter plate. A dilution of serum is added, and the plates are incubated at 37°C for a specific period (usually about 30 min). The plates are washed, and conjugate is added. After a 30-min incubation, the plates are again washed and an enzyme substrate is added. If the serum sample contains antibodies to *T. pallidum*, a color reaction takes place. The reaction is halted by the addition of a stop reagent, and the plates are then read at 450 nm on a microplate reader. The tests offer the advantages of being able to be automated, having an objective interpretation of results, and having a hard copy of the results automatically printed.

The EIAs were originally cleared by the Food and Drug Administration for confirmatory testing, but one test has received clearance as a screening test. A disadvantage of using the EIA as a screening test is that because it is a treponemal test, it will remain reactive for life in approximately 84% of all persons who have ever had syphilis. As with all serologic tests, there is also some nonspecificity, although for treponemal tests it is generally only around 1%. When it is used as a screening test, all reactive results must be followed up with a nontreponemal test. This will help determine whether an active case of syphilis is present and will give a baseline titer for determining treatment efficacy if a new case of syphilis has been detected. Because the test can be automated, large numbers of samples can be tested by fewer technicians than when manual procedures are used. In some populations, such as intravenous drug users or people with autoimmune diseases, there will also be fewer false-positive results when the EIA is used for screening, because antitreponemal antibodies rather than anti-cardiolipin antibodies are being detected. In addition, prozone reactions are eliminated because the detection method is dependent on attachment of antibodies rather than on flocculation.

Molecular Biology-Based Techniques

Molecular biology-based techniques, using unique sequences of *T. pallidum* DNA, are being used to detect the spirochete for definitive diagnosis and for typing of subspecies and strains of *T. pallidum*. None of the procedures being used are currently available commercially, nor is there any universal technique for either detection or subtyping.

PCR

PCR can be used on CSF or blood, lesion exudates, or tissues to detect the presence of *T. pallidum* (25, 29). There is no standardized method or target. The target used at the Centers for Disease Control and Prevention is the polymerase A (*polA*) (25) gene. PCR has advantages over some of the other antigen detection methods such as DFA-TP. PCR does not depend on the organisms being alive or intact, and fewer organisms can be detected than when using DFA-TP or dark-field microscopy (25). Because the methods are not commercially available, PCR is generally restricted to the larger laboratories. The procedure is not cleared by the Food and Drug Administration; therefore, it must be considered an experimental procedure.

Subtyping

Subtyping for *T. pallidum* done at the Centers for Disease Control and Prevention is based on two genes that exhibit intrastrain variability, the genes encoding the acidic repeat protein (*arp*) and the *T. pallidum* repeat (*tpr*) protein (31). The method appears to be useful for epidemiologic purposes. The number of repeats of *arp* varies from 4 to 25 in different strains of *T. pallidum*. The *trp* gene has several unique MseI restriction fragment length polymorphism patterns labeled a to g. Using a combination of the number of *arp* repeats (4 to 25) and *tprJ* restriction fragment length polymorphism patterns (a to g), a workable, discriminating typing scheme has been developed (31). Using this system, the Nichols strain is determined to be subtype 14a. In addition to differentiating among strains of *T. pallidum*, the typing scheme distinguishes the various pathogenic treponemes from each other. This could potentially be useful in areas of the world where the endemic treponematoses exist.

The *tpr* family of genes is composed of three subfamilies of genes: subfamily I (*tprC*, *tprD*, *tprF*, and *tprI*), subfamily II (*tprE*, *tprG*, and *tprJ*), and subfamily III (*tprA*, *tprB*, *tprH*, *tprK*, and *tprL*). *tprK* has also been used to differentiate different strains of *T. pallidum* as well as the various subspecies based on size heterogeneity in the central portions of the hydrophilic domain (6).

Leptospirosis

Most leptospiral infections are subclinical or of mild severity and may go unrecognized. The clinical presentation is difficult to distinguish from dengue, malaria, influenza, and many other diseases characterized by fever, headache, and myalgia. Icteric leptospirosis is a more severe disease characterized by rapid progression and may include liver, pulmonary, cardiac, and ocular involvement. A diagnosis of leptospirosis should also be considered in cases of unexplained jaundice, aseptic meningitis, and fever of unknown origin. Diagnosis is usually made based on the patient's clinical history, exposure history, and laboratory results. Members of some occupations are at a higher risk than the rest of the population, but recreational and hurricane or extensive flooding-related water exposures have recently become significant (18, 28, 35). The disease is fatal in 5 to 30% of all cases.

Leptospirosis can be diagnosed by detection of the organism by microscopy; culture of blood, CSF, or urine; or DNA amplification (from serum, urine, or tissues) (21). Definitive diagnosis of leptospirosis is made by isolation of leptospires from tissue or body fluids, but leptospires grow slowly on initial isolation and culture is therefore often not useful in patient management. Most cases are therefore diagnosed by serology. However, serology cannot be used to determine the infecting serovar. This can be done only by isolation and serotyping of the organism.

Antibodies are detectable in blood about 5 to 7 days after onset of symptoms. The microscopic agglutination test (MAT) is the reference method for serologic diagnosis (11). However, the MAT is relatively insensitive when acute-phase samples are tested (7). Because of the complexity of the MAT, rapid screening tests for detection of antileptospiral IgM antibodies in acute infection have been developed, and some of these are commercially available. The diagnostic tests discussed in this chapter are the MAT, which is the standard against which all other serologic tests for leptospirosis are evaluated, and two screening tests, the IgM dot enzyme-linked immunosorbent assay (ELISA) (1, 23) and the IgM ELISA (1, 40). These assays have been extensively evaluated for use in the diagnosis of leptospirosis (21).

MAT

Clinical Indications

The MAT detects agglutinating antibodies and is considered the standard reference test for the diagnosis of leptospirosis. Agglutinating antibodies are directed against surface antigens of leptospires and are of both IgM and IgG classes. Antibodies can be detected approximately 1 week after onset of symptoms and reach maximum titers usually within 4 weeks. The use of paired sera, drawn at least 1 week apart, is required to confirm a diagnosis of leptospirosis. A fourfold increase in titer between paired sera indicates recent exposure. Low titers may persist for years after exposure, so a low titer in a single serum sample is insufficient evidence from which to make a diagnosis of leptospirosis, but a single titer of 1:800 is generally considered diagnostic in areas of endemic infection. In regions where leptospirosis is not endemic, the threshold titer for a presumptive diagnosis may be correspondingly lower.

Antibodies in serum may cross-react with several different serovars in the MAT (paradoxical reaction), particularly in acute-phase specimens (20). As the immune response matures, the cross-reactivity lessens and the test becomes relatively serogroup specific; for this reason, a battery of antigens, composed of serovars that each represent a different serogroup, is used. The serovars generally included are listed in the MAT methods section (see below). If the patient has been outside the United States recently, serovars endemic to the places visited should be included since antibodies to these may not be detected by the standard battery of antigens. The test is generally done using live spirochetes, but formalin-killed leptospires may also be used. If the latter are used, titers are lower and the reactivity is somewhat less specific (20). Regardless of which antigens are used, the MAT cannot be used to determine the infecting serovar because the test uses only 12 to 19 of the more than 200 known serovars. The antigens listed below detect antibodies to most serovars.

The MAT may be run with either human or animal sera. It is used in epidemiologic studies or outbreaks to determine the potential source of infection.

Equipment

Multichannel pipettors, 50 and 100 μl, and tips
96-well flat-bottom microtiter plates
Dark-field microscope with 10× long-working-distance objective and standard-working-distance objective
Glass microscope slides (for checking antigens)

Pipettes and pipetting devices (pipettor, rubber bulb)
Test tubes: 16- by 125-mm screw cap and 12- by 100-mm cork stoppered
Monitek model 21 nephelometer or 0.5 McFarland turbidity standard (a spectrophotometer is used in some laboratories to measure transmittance)

Reagents

Antisera. Antiserum is needed for each corresponding serovar (antigen) used in the assay. These antisera are used as homologous controls for each antigen and should have titers of ≥1:3,200 to the corresponding antigen. Antisera are available commercially from Difco Laboratories or the National Veterinary Services Laboratories, Ames, Iowa.

Antigens. A panel of serovars relevant to the testing area should be used. Commonly the panel consists of the following serovars: Alexi, Australis, Autumnalis, Ballum, Bataviae, Borincana, Bratislava, Canicola, Celledoni, Copenhageni or Icterohaemorrhagiae, Cynopteri, Djasiman, Georgia, Grippotyphosa, Javanica, Mankarso, Pomona, Pyrogenes, Tarassovi, and Wolffi.

Maintenance of culture

1. Serovars previously mentioned are grown in PLM-5 broth (Intergen Co., Purchase, N.Y.). Cultures can be grown in milk bottles (250 ml bottles).
2. Maintain cultures by transferring them weekly, using a 10% inoculum, and incubating at 30°C. The frequent transfer helps prevent excessive clumping.

Antigen preparation. Antigens for the MAT are live cell suspensions prepared from 4- to 7-day-old PLM-5 broth cultures.

1. Check cultures for use in the test by dark-field microscopy for clumping and contamination. Do not use contaminated cultures. Clumps can sometimes be dispersed by shaking.
2. With a sterile 10-ml pipette, transfer 10 ml of 4- to 7-day-old culture to a 16- by 125-mm screw-cap tube.
3. Measure the turbidity with a turbidity meter/nephelometer calibrated for the 0.5 McFarland standard. Alternatively, turbidity can be estimated visually against the 0.5 McFarland standard.
4. If necessary, dilute with sterile PBS to adjust the turbidity of each cell suspension to match the turbidity of the 0.5 McFarland standard or to measure in the range of 45 to 79 on the nephelometer.
5. After the cell suspensions have been adjusted to the appropriate turbidity, shake them vigorously to disperse any aggregates. Centrifuge cultures at 1,500 to 2,000 × g for 15 min to sediment any large clumps, and set them aside until ready to use.

Homologous Titer Determination

Test all antigens against their homologous antisera weekly. The titer obtained should be within a twofold dilution of the known titer of the homologous antiserum. If the titer is not within the acceptable range, the antigen should not be used. Three 96-well plates are required for the homologous titer determination.

1. Make an initial 1:50 dilution of antisera. Dispense 100 μl into the first wells (column 1) of each row of a microtiter plate.
2. Using 50-μl volume transfers, make a serial twofold dilution of antisera in PBS starting with a 1:50 dilution. Use

one row for each homologous serum. The last wells (column 12) should contain only PBS.

3. Add 50 μl of homologous antigen to all wells for each corresponding antiserum.

4. Tap plates gently to mix, and incubate at ambient temperature for 1.5 to 2 h. Read reactions by dark-field microscopy at a magnification of ×100, and grade on a scale of 0 to 4+. The end point is the dilution that gives 50% agglutination.

Screening Procedure

Each unknown specimen is screened against all the serovars on the antigen panel. Map out a block of wells to accommodate all specimens to be tested, including controls for each antigen, on 96-well microtiter plates. For example, a 96-well plate can be used to screen 45 specimens plus 3 controls (48 wells) against 2 antigens.

1. Make a 1:50 dilution of the patient's serum by adding 60 μl of serum to 3.0 ml of PBS (pH 7.2). Heat inactivate the diluted serum at 56°C for 30 min. Positive (homologous) and negative control sera are also diluted 1:50 (5 μl of control serum to 250 μl of PBS).

2. Screen serum samples by placing 50 μl of diluted serum into wells of 96-well flat-bottom microtiter plates. To screen eight serum samples (five unknowns and three controls) against 20 antigens, two microtiter plates (eight wells, or a column per antigen) are required.

3. For each antigen, allow wells for the positive control, a negative control, and antigen control. The antigen control well contains PBS instead of serum to check for nonspecific agglutination of the antigen.

Note: A set of controls (negative, positive, and antigen) is required per antigen for every test run.

4. After all the serum samples have been added to the plate, add 50 μl of antigen, one per column, to all the serum samples and the controls. This is now a 1:100 dilution of serum.

5. Gently mix the contents of the plates, cover, and allow the plates to sit at room temperature for 90 min to 2 h.

6. Read the plates under a dark-field microscope, using a l0× long-working-distance objective and a 10× eyepiece.

7. Any well with at least 50% agglutination (2+), provided that the antigen control has no agglutination or only a roughness, is considered reactive.

Confirmatory Procedure

For confirmation, each serum sample with a positive agglutination reaction in the screening test should be subjected to determination of its titer against the antigens for which it is positive. Careful planning is required to map out test plates. Group all serum samples positive by each antigen to the same block of wells, using a row (12 wells) for each serum sample tested. *Note:* Titer determinations can also be done per column (eight wells) if generally specimens do not have very high titers.

1. Place 50 μl of PBS in wells of columns 2 to 12 on a microtiter plate, and place 100 μl of the serum dilution in the first well.

2. Using 50-μl volume transfers, make twofold dilutions through column 11. Discard the last 50 μl. Wells of column 12 serve as the antigen control.

3. After the serum is diluted, add 50 μl of antigen to each well.

4. Repeat steps 1 to 3 for each antigen with which the patient's serum reacted in the screen.

5. The titer is the last dilution that shows a 2+ (50%) or greater agglutination.

Note: The agglutination pattern differs from one serovar to the next. Sera that were reactive in the screening test may be nonreactive when subjected to titer determination.

Quality Control

Positive controls (homologous antisera) are included to ensure that the right antigens are used. Homologous serum titers should be within a twofold dilution of their established titer. Antigen controls are included in the assay to check for autoagglutination. The antigen control should not have more than a 1+ reaction. The negative control should not have more than a 1+ reaction.

Interpretation of Results

1. Results are reported as the reciprocal of the titer for each antigen that was reactive with that serum.

2. Titers of ≥1:100 are considered positive.

3. Nonspecific reactions may occur due to unknown factors in the patient's serum. If all or most of the sera tested are reactive with a particular antigen at the 1:100 (or screening) dilution, the antigen is too sensitive and should not be included in the run.

Precautions and Potential Problems

As mentioned above, an excessively sensitive antigen can give false-positive results. Nonspecific agglutination in the antigen control may also occur. If agglutination of ≤1+ occurs, then the end-point titer is the highest serum dilution with 3+ agglutination. Prozone reactions occasionally occur with high-titer sera. All serum samples should be treated as potentially infectious and handled using universal precautions.

A serum sample may test falsely nonreactive if the patient has been exposed to a serovar not commonly found in the home geographic area. Therefore, it is important to know the patient's travel history so that serovars representative of those geographic areas may be included in the screening test. Each laboratory must establish its own baseline antibody levels, especially in areas of endemic infection.

Cross-reactions (sometimes with significant seroconversion) have been observed with serum from patients with syphilis, relapsing fever, Lyme disease, legionellosis, viral hepatitis, and Epstein-Barr virus infection (1). Therefore, results should be interpreted with caution.

Dot ELISA Dipstick

Clinical Indications

The IgM dot ELISA is a qualitative screening test; therefore, confirmation of results is recommended. The assay detects antibodies earlier than do the agglutination assays (indirect hemagglutination assay and MAT) (1, 23) and is ideal for use when only a few specimens are tested at a time. The dot ELISA dipstick (INDX Dip-S-Ticks; PANBIO Inc., Columbia, Md.) uses a genus-specific antigen (*Leptospira biflexa* serovar Patoc) dispensed as discrete dots on a solid membrane. The patient sample is added to diluent containing Prosorb-G, which adsorbs the IgG in the test serum. Diluted serum reacts with the antigens on the assay strip, and alkaline phosphatase-conjugated anti-human immunoglobulin reacts with the bound antibodies from the patient's serum, eliminating competitive inhibition of IgM binding by IgG. The test is intended as a screening test for the diagnosis of acute infection. The presence of antibody is considered suggestive of active *Leptospira* infection.

Equipment

Dry-heat bath or water bath with racks, adjustable to 50°C. *Note*: If a water bath is used, caution is required to prevent water from getting into the reaction cuvettes.

Accurate micropipette (10 µl) and serologic pipettes

Cup or beaker to serve as the clarifier vessel

Distilled or deionized water to be used as the clarifier

Timer

Absorbent toweling to blot dry the assay strips

Materials

INDX Dip-S-Ticks kit. The kit contains assay strips, sample diluent, enhancer, anti-human immunoglobulin conjugate, enzyme substrate (5-bromo-4-chloro-3-indolyl phosphate and *p*-nitro blue tetrazolium), reaction cuvettes, positive control serum, and negative control serum.

Test Procedure

1. Bring all reagents and serum samples to room temperature.
2. Label assay strips with corresponding patient identifier.
3. Remove and label (1 to 4) four reaction cuvettes (RC-1 to RC-4) per sample. Place in rack in a 50°C water bath.
4. Place 2 ml of appropriate reagent in the corresponding reaction cuvette:
   (a) To RC-1, add 2 ml of diluent.
   (b) To RC-2, add 2 ml of enhancer.
   (c) To RC-3, add 2 ml of conjugate.
   (d) To RC-4, add 2 ml of developer.
5. Add sufficient distilled or deionized water to the clarifier vessel to adequately cover the window of the assay strip when it is immersed.
6. Allow the reaction cuvettes to sit for 10 min to equilibrate all reagents to 50°C. During this step, specimens may be added (step 7).
7. Add 10 µl of patient serum or heparinized plasma specimen to the corresponding cuvette labeled RC-1.
8. Prewet the assay strip by immersing it in clarifier vessel for 2 to 4 min.
9. Using 10 to 15 quick up-and-down motions with the assay strip, mix the diluent and patient sample thoroughly in RC-1. Let stand for 5 min.
10. Remove assay strip from RC-1, and swish in the clarifier vessel. Use a swift back-and-forth motion for 6 to 10 s, allowing for optimal washing of the assay strip membrane window.
11. Dispose of used distilled water in the clarifier vessel, and replace with fresh distilled water.
12. Place assay strip in RC-2. Mix thoroughly by using 6 to 10 quick up-and-down motions. Let strip stand in RC-2 for 5 min.
13. Remove strip from RC-2 and rinse in clarifier vessel as described in steps 10 and 11.
14. Place strip in RC-3. Mix thoroughly by using 6 to 10 up-and-down motions. Let strip stand in RC-3 for the length of time indicated on the kit master label.
15. Remove assay strip and rinse as in step 10. Allow assay strip to remain in the clarifier vessel for 5 min. Dispose of used distilled water, and replace with fresh distilled water.
16. Place assay strip in RC-4. Mix thoroughly using 6 to 10 quick up-and-down motions. Let strip stand in RC-4 for 5 min.
17. Remove assay strip from RC-4 and swish in clarifier vessel as described in step 10.
18. Blot assay strip, and allow to air dry. Do not use artificial methods, other than a fan, to dry the strips. Borderline specimens cannot be interpreted until the assay strip has been allowed to dry completely.

Quality Control

The top two membrane windows on the assay strip contain reagent controls. The top dot is a positive reagent control and must be positive for the assay to be valid. The second dot is a reagent negative control and must be negative for the assay to be valid. Positive and negative control sera included should also yield the desired results for the assay to be valid.

Interpretation of Results

Reactions are graded from 1 to 4 according to the number of reactive dots that appear. The dots should be easily seen; they have a distinct border, and the outer perimeter of the window must be white to pale gray. Results are interpreted as the number of reactive dots: 0 to 1 for negative, 2 to 2.5 for borderline positive, and 3 to 4 for strongly positive. Specimens showing a borderline positive reaction should be further tested with an additional specimen collected later or confirmed by MAT. A negative reaction does not eliminate the diagnosis of leptospirosis in a symptomatic patient. A convalescent-phase specimen, collected at least 7 days later, should be tested for patients whose acute-phase specimens are negative. A positive result for the second sample implies seroconversion but should be confirmed by MAT.

Precautions and Potential Problems

The dot ELISA dipstick assay is designed as a screening test. Results must be considered in conjunction with epidemiologic factors, clinical findings, exposure in regions of endemic infection, and other laboratory results. Lipemic, hemolyzed, or contaminated sera may interfere with the assay; these specimens should not be used. All sera demonstrating a weakly positive result should be referred to a reference laboratory for confirmation using the MAT. Although this is an IgM assay, positive results do not necessarily reflect recent or acute infection since IgM is known to persist for months or years following recovery (7). Cross-reactions have been observed with sera positive for Epstein-Barr Virus and HIV (1).

IgM ELISA

The IgM ELISA exhibits high sensitivity while maintaining a high specificity (1, 22). The assay is useful as a screening tool for testing few specimens or large numbers of specimens and has been especially valuable in the investigation of outbreaks. This is a solid-phase assay in which IgM present in serum binds to leptospiral antigen attached to the polystyrene surface of the microwell. Peroxidase-conjugated anti-human IgM reacts with the antigen-bound antibody. The detection system is a colorless substrate, tetramethyl benzidine plus hydrogen peroxide, which is hydrolyzed by the enzyme, and the chromogen changes to a blue color. The color intensity is directly related to the concentration of anti-*Leptospira* IgM antibodies in the test sample.

Materials

The Leptospira IgM ELISA kit (PANBIO Inc., Columbia, Md.) contains antigen-coated plates (12 8-well strips), wash buffer concentrate, serum diluent, horseradish peroxidase-conjugated anti-human IgM, tetramethyl benzidine substrate (TMB), stop solution, positive control serum, cutoff calibrator serum, and negative control serum.

Equipment

Micropipettes (10-μl single, 100-μl multichannel) and serologic pipettes

Deionized water

Microplate washing system

Microplate reader with 450-nm filter

Test tubes or dilution block for serum dilution

Solution basin

Timer

Graduated cylinder

Test Procedure

All reagents must be equilibrated to ambient temperature before the assay is begun. Microwells should not be removed from their bag until after they have reached ambient temperature.

1. Remove the required number of microwell strips, and insert into the holder. Five microwells are required for controls (one positive, one negative, and calibrator in triplicate).

2. Using appropriate tubes, make a 1:100 dilution of patient and control sera.

3. Mix and pipette 100 μl of diluted test, calibrator, and control sera into their respective wells.

4. Cover and incubate plates for 30 min at 37°C.

5. Wash six times with diluted wash buffer by repeatedly aspirating well contents and filling each well with 350 μl of wash fluid. After the final wash, discard contents of well and tap plate on blotting paper to get rid of any moisture left.

Note: Automated plate washers can be programmed to perform this wash cycle. Ensure all channels on the washer are open for efficient washing.

6. Pipette 100 μl of horseradish peroxidase-conjugated anti-human IgM into each well, cover the plate, and incubate for 30 min at 37°C.

7. Wash six times as described in step 5.

8. Pipette 100 μl of TMB to each well, cover, and incubate for 10 min at ambient temperature, timing from the first addition. A blue color will develop.

9. Pipette 100 μl of stop solution to each well and mix well. The color changes to yellow.

10. Within 30 min of completion of the assay, read the absorbance of each well at a wavelength of 450 nm, using automatic ELISA reader.

Note: If a dual-wavelength spectrometer is being used, set the reference filter between 600 and 650 nm.

Quality Control

Each kit contains a cutoff calibrator, positive control, and negative control sera. Acceptable values for the sera are found on the specification sheet packaged with each kit. The test is invalid if the absorbance readings of the controls and/ or the calibrator do not meet the specifications.

Interpretation of Results

PANBIO units are calculated by dividing the unknown specimen absorbance by the mean absorbance of the cutoff calibrator and multiplying by 10. Results are reported as negative, equivocal, or positive.

Negative: <9 PANBIO units indicates no evidence of IgM antibodies.

Equivocal: 9 to 11 PANBIO units is suggestive of possible infection, and retesting of the specimen and a second specimen taken at a later date is recommended.

Positive: >11 PANBIO units indicates presence of IgM antibodies and is suggestive of recent or past exposure to leptospires.

Note: If a negative or equivocal result is obtained and there is a strong suspicion of leptospirosis clinically, a second specimen taken 7 to 14 days later should be tested.

Potential Problems and Precautions

Results should be interpreted in conjunction with other laboratory and clinical findings. This assay is designed as a screening test; therefore, confirmation of positive and equivocal specimens by the MAT is recommended.

The design of this assay potentially allows competitive inhibition of IgM binding in the presence of high levels of IgG; therefore, false-negative results are possible. Although this is an IgM assay, positive results do not necessarily reflect recent or acute infection since IgM is known to persist for months or years following recovery (7). Cross-reactions in this assay have been observed with sera positive for autoimmune disease, cytomegalovirus, HIV, group C *Neisseria meningitidis*, and viral hepatitis (1).

Molecular Biology-Based Techniques

Diagnosis

Several PCR assays have been described for amplification of leptospiral DNA (20). However, few of these assays have been evaluated in experiments with human (5, 27) or veterinary (14, 39) populations. Real-time assays, which offer greater analytical sensitivity and more rapid diagnosis, have recently been described (24, 36). Primers, probes, and targets for some PCR assays used for human diagnosis are shown in Table 6.

Identification and Subtyping

Because of the difficulty in serologic identification of leptospires (20) many molecular subtyping techniques have been applied to the identification and subtyping of the genus *Leptospira* (37). Pathogenic leptospires are now classified into several species determined by DNA reassociation (4), and strains of some serovars are found in multiple species (21), so it is no longer adequate to know the identity of a serovar in order to understand its pathogenic potential and likely epidemiology. Both species and serovar identity must be determined.

The most widely applicable approach for species determination is 16S rRNA sequencing (17). Of the numerous molecular methods evaluated for subtyping, only pulsed-field gel electrophoresis has sufficient potential for standardization (15).

Borreliosis

Borreliae pathogenic to humans are the agents of louse-borne (epidemic) relapsing fever (LBRF), tick-borne (endemic) relapsing fever (TBRF) and Lyme disease. Human relapsing-fever infections occur throughout tropical and temperate regions with the possible exception of Australia, New Zealand, and the southwestern Pacific. Lyme disease, which has recently emerged as a leading vector-borne disease in the northern hemisphere, is discussed separately in the chapter on *Borrelia burgdorferi*.

Humans are the only known reservoir of the LBRF spirochete, *Borrelia recurrentis*, and outbreaks involving many thousands of people were common in the first half of the 20th century in parts of Europe, Africa, South America, and Asia. The disease is still prevalent in Africa, most notably in Sudan and Ethiopia. Because of the close association of the louse

TABLE 6 PCR assays for diagnosis of leptospirosis in humans

Target	Specificity	Primers	Probe	Format	Sensitivity	Reference(s)
secY	*L. interrogans* *L. meyeri* *L. borgpetersenii* *L. weilii* *L. noguchii* *L. santarosai*	G1 (5′-TGAATC GCTGTATAAAAGT-3′) and G2 (5′-GG AAAACAAATGGTC GGAAG-3′)	G195-28 [5′-A (G/A)ATGATCG GCAT(T/C) ACGTT(T/C) GC(A/G)CCGTT-3′]	Conventional PCR + hybridization	~10 cells/ml	2, 13
flaB	*L. kirschneri*	B64-I (5′-ACTAACTG AGAAACTTCTAC-3′) and B64-II (5′-TCCTTAA GTCAACCTATGA-3′)	B88-29 (5′-CTCTG AACGATCT CAT GAGTTTCCTGGAG-3′)	Conventional PCR + hybridization	~10 cells/ml	2, 13
rrs	Genus *Leptospira*	A (5′-GGCGGCGCGTC TTAAACATG-3′) and B (5′-TTCCCCCCA TTGAGCAAGATT-3′)	289-bp probe, internal to target sequence	Conventional PCR + dot blot hybridization	~10 cells/ml	26

vector, *Pediculus humanus humanus*, and the human reservoir, epidemic outbreaks are associated with conditions of overcrowding, malnutrition, and poor hygiene. Case fatality rates range from greater than 40% in untreated epidemic outbreaks to less than 5% in treated cases. It is unclear if virulence factors play a role in the higher mortality rates commonly associated with large epidemic outbreaks or whether this outcome is reflective of generally poorer patient management under these circumstances.

TBRF is caused by infection with any one of 11 *Borrelia* species (Table 2). These spirochetes are transmitted by soft ticks of the genus *Ornithodoros*. Species designations of the relapsing-fever spirochetes are often based on their vector tick species (e.g., *Borrelia hermsii* is transmitted by *Ornithodoros hermsi*). In contrast to LBRF, TBRF is usually a zoonotic disease cycling between ticks and their rodent hosts. Because of the extreme dependence of these ticks on their animal hosts, humans are only rarely exposed to the vector ticks. The distribution of endemic foci includes the western United States, British Columbia, Mexico, Central and South America, much of Africa, Europe, and Asia. Cases in the United States are typically sporadic, although common-source clusters of 6 to 62 cases have been reported in Washington, Arizona, California, and Colorado (10). These clusters typically involve rodent-infested cabins left vacant for periods just prior to human occupation and exposure. Vector ticks are also found in caves and burrows of owls and snakes associated with rodent and other animal inhabitants or their nesting materials. The nocturnal, brief (5 to 30 min), and usually painless feeding habits of the vector ticks are responsible for low recall of tick exposure. Thus, unless a history of lodging in rodent-infested dwellings or of wilderness or cave exposure is noted, the disease is rarely suspected during the initial febrile episode. The disease is reportable in 12 western states: Arizona, California, Colorado, Idaho, Montana, Nevada, New Mexico, Oregon, Texas, Utah, Washington, and Wyoming. In addition to these states, cases have been reported from Ohio and Oklahoma. Between 1990 and 2000, 247 cases were reported in the United States. However, due to its frequent misdiagnosis and the lack of systematic reporting, the incidence of TBRF is unknown. Case fatality rates range from 2 to 8%.

The clinical presentations of LBRF and TBRF are similar, although LBRF tends to be more severe (9, 10). The incubation periods range from 4 to 18 days (average of 8 days) and are followed by the sudden onset of fever, headache, shaking chills, and myalgia and arthralgia. Other symptoms include nausea, vomiting, anorexia, dry cough, photophobia, neck pain, eye pain, and confusion. Thrombocytopenia is common to both diseases, although bleeding complications (epistaxis, subconjunctival hemorrhage, and petechial hemorrhage) are much more frequently associated with LBRF. The febrile period lasts for 3 to 7 days. A skin rash with variable appearance, rarely resembling erythema migrans associated with Lyme disease, has been detected in 28% of relapsing-fever patients. After an afebrile period of several days to weeks, a relapse occurs. The number of relapses is variable and is affected by antibiotic therapy. Most untreated LBRF patients suffer one relapse, but the occurrence of three or more relapses is rare. In untreated TBRF, 3 to 5 relapses (range, 0 to 13) are common. The severity and duration of the relapse generally decrease with each subsequent episode, while the afebrile interval is extended. Numbers of circulating spirochetes also diminish with each relapse, and spirochetes are rarely observed or recovered during afebrile periods.

Diagnosis of relapsing fever is largely dependent on obtaining a detailed travel history for the several weeks prior to onset of illness. If a history of risk exposure in an area of endemic infection is given, a blood smear should be examined. Blood samples must be collected during a febrile period, and the presence of spirochetes is considered diagnostic. Spirochetes are observed in approximately 70% of cases. Failure to demonstrate spirochetes does not rule out relapsing fever, and alternative culture or serologic approaches may confirm or support the diagnosis. Both LBRF and TBRF spirochetes are capable of crossing the placenta in pregnant women. Fetal infection, even in the absence of apparent maternal disease or in the face of maternal disease resolution, may result in an overwhelming spirochetemia and abortion.

The sporadic nature of relapsing fever and the spontaneous antigenic variation of the spirochetes have minimized and complicated efforts to develop serodiagnostic assays (33). Nonetheless, substantial progress has been made toward the understanding of regulation of antigen expression, and several specific markers, both genetic and antigenic, have been identified. In experimentally infected mice, each relapse is associated with the expression of a novel surface antigen designated variable major protein (VMP). Twenty-six VMPs and associated serotypes originating from a mouse infection with a single relapsing-fever spirochete have been described.

Direct Detection and Isolation of Borreliae

Detection in Blood

The most direct and simple approach to laboratory confirmation of relapsing-fever infection is by microscopy. Spirochetemias of greater than 10^8 organisms/ml of blood are common during early febrile periods of TBRF and LBRF and enable microscopic detection. The large size (5 to 25 μm in length and 0.2 to 0.5 μm in width) of spirochetes and their coiling (3 to 10 spirals; average, 5 to 7) facilitate identification with magnifications of ×400 to ×1,000. Additionally, spirochetes may be concentrated up to 100-fold by buffy coat preparations (38).

Spirochetes may be visualized in peripheral blood wet mounts by dark-field microscopy or in fixed and stained preparations by bright-field microscopy. In live wet mounts (anticoagulated blood diluted 1:1 with saline), the corkscrew motility of spirochetes is readily detected under dark-field microscopy. Alternatively, Wright- or Giemsa-stained thick or thin blood smears (Fig. 1) also afford visualization of spirochetes. Thick blood smears should be dehemoglobinized for 10 to 20 s with 6% acetic acid in ethanol before being stained.

For all microscopic detection of spirochetemia, it is crucial that blood be collected during a febrile episode. Analysis of multiple blood smears collected during the febrile period significantly increases the likelihood of spirochete observation. However, as the level of spirochetemia diminishes with each subsequent relapse, attempts to visually confirm spirochete presence become less fruitful. Examination of stained thick smears is recommended during later relapses or whenever thin smears are negative. Phenotypic variations in borreliae (number and size of coils as well as overall spirochete length) are affected by environmental and culture conditions, and species are not readily discriminated on the basis of morphology.

Molecular Biology-Based Detection

Molecular biology-based techniques analyzing amplified signature gene sequences from borreliae have been developed and widely utilized to establish taxonomic relationships, further our understanding of the life cycles of spirochetes, and identify vaccine candidates. Diagnostic application of these analytic approaches has focused largely on the confirmation of Lyme disease infection. Due to the comparatively small numbers of Lyme borreliae in any infected tissue source compared to TBRF and LBRF spirochetes in blood, the molecular biology-based diagnosis of relapsing fever has not received much attention. Nonetheless, there are clinical situations, such as afebrile periods and later relapses, in which circulating spirochete numbers are diminished, where highly sensitive molecular biology-based detection tests may find application and utility. A number of specific gene targets have been identified (30, 32). Standardization of protocols and multicenter evaluation of test performance will greatly facilitate a broader application of molecular biology-based diagnostic approaches to relapsing fever.

Animal Inoculation

Although most laboratories are not equipped to perform animal inoculation for the propagation of relapsing-fever spirochetes, this approach is sensitive and relatively simple. Weanling mice or rats are inoculated intraperitoneally with 0.1 to 0.2 ml of anticoagulated patient blood or a blood clot triturated in an equal volume of saline. Spirochetes may be observed in smears of peripheral blood from test animals as soon as 3 days postinoculation. Since infected animals experience phasic spirochetemias, smears should be examined daily for up to 15 days. Animal inoculation and subsequent analysis of blood smears are often more sensitive for detecting relapsing-fever spirochetes than is direct examination or culturing of patient blood. It is highly recommended during later relapses, when spirochetemias may be very low.

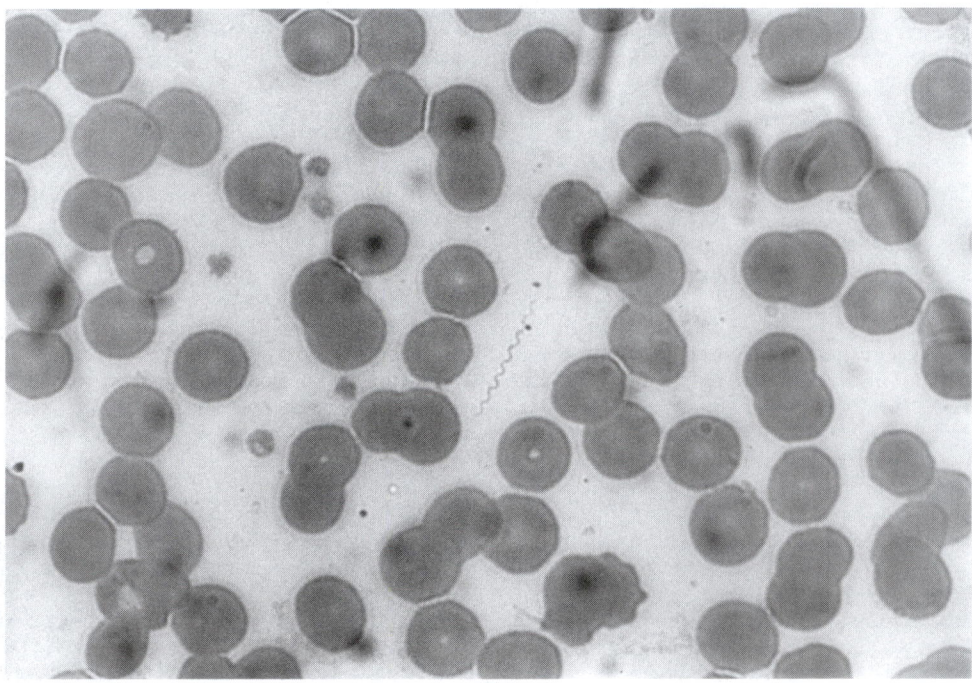

FIGURE 1 *B. hermsii* in a Giemsa-stained human peripheral blood smear. Magnification, ×1,000.

Detection by Culture

In addition to demonstration of spirochetes by animal inoculation, direct culture of relapsing-fever spirochetes is possible. Barbour-Stoenner-Kelly II (BSK-II) medium is most commonly used, and a commercial formulation is available (BSK-H; Sigma Chemical Co., St. Louis, Mo.). Optimal growth is obtained under microaerophilic conditions at temperatures between 30 and 37°C. Generation times of approximately 12 h are common at 35°C. Cultures should be seeded with 0.1 to 0.2 ml of patient blood or a suspension of a triturated blood clot. If culture medium is not on hand, weanling mice may be inoculated with the blood sample or blood may be stored or transported at 4°C for several days until medium is obtained. Borreliae are resistant to rifampin (50 μg/ml), phosphomycin (100 μg/ml), and amphotericin B (10 μg/ml), and these antibiotics may be added to the culture medium to minimize contamination by other bacteria and fungi. Dark-field microscopy of culture wet mounts is utilized to confirm the presence of spirochetes.

Indirect Detection of Borreliae

Although serologic assays detecting antibody responses to spirochetal infection have not been fully standardized or widely practiced, several approaches may be used to support the initial diagnosis. Serologic tests include indirect fluorescent-antibody assay (IFA), ELISA, and Western immunoblotting. It must be noted that seroconversion is rarely demonstrated during the first febrile episode and that prompt antibiotic therapy may abrogate the antibody response. Thus, while positive results in any of these assays may strongly support the clinical diagnosis of relapsing fever, negative results are inconclusive.

Detailed protocols for cell growth, harvest, and antigen preparation have been reported, and stock cultures of *B. hermsii* (serotype C) are available from the American Tissue Type Collection. Additional relapsing-fever spirochete isolates are available from the reference collection of the Centers for Disease Control and Prevention, Division of Vector-Borne Infectious Diseases, in Fort Collins, Colo. For ELISA, whole-cell lysates of *B. hermsii* are used as antigen sources and assay cutoffs are based on patient serum reactivity in relation to a set of negative and positive control samples. Western immunoblot analysis of sera from relapsing-fever patients has also been reported, and patients typically demonstrate increasing IgM and IgG reactivity to an expanding number of antigens during the first few weeks postinfection (12).

In Western blots, IFA, and ELISA, which utilize whole-cell spirochete lysates as antigen sources, antibody cross-reactivity is observed among patients with Lyme disease, syphilis and other treponemal diseases, and leptospiral infections. Absorption of relapsing-fever serum with heterologous antigens indicates that relapsing-fever-specific seroconversion does occur. Antibody responses to one antigen, glycerophosphodiester phosphodiesterase, have been reported to enable the sensitive detection of both TBRF and LBRF infections and are not observed in infections with the closely related Lyme disease spirochete (32). Further evaluation and standardization of assays utilizing this antigen may justify its greater use. Despite the utility of laboratory diagnostic tests, the importance of a detailed case history and clinical presentation in the diagnosis of relapsing-fever borreliosis cannot be overemphasized.

REFERENCES

1. Bajani, M. D., D. A. Ashford, S. L. Bragg, C. W. Woods, T. Aye, R. A. Spiegel, B. D. Plikaytis, B. A. Perkins, M. Phelan, P. N. Levett, and R. S. Weyant. 2003. Evaluation of four commercially available rapid serologic tests for diagnosis of leptospirosis. *J. Clin. Microbiol.* **41:**803–809.
2. Bal, A. E., C. Gravekamp, R. A. Hartskeerl, J. De Meza-Brewster, H. Korver, and W. J. Terpstra. 1994. Detection of leptospires in urine by PCR for early diagnosis of leptospirosis. *J. Clin. Microbiol.* **32:**1894–1898.
3. Baranton, G., and I. G. Old. 1995. The spirochaetes: a different way of life. *Bull. Inst. Pasteur* **93:**63–95.
4. Brenner, D. J., A. F. Kaufmann, K. R. Sulzer, A. G. Steigerwalt, F. C. Rogers, and R. S. Weyant. 1999. Further determination of DNA relatedness between serogroups and serovars in the family *Leptospiraceae* with a proposal for *Leptospira alexanderi* sp. nov. and four new *Leptospira* genomospecies. *Int. J. Syst. Bacteriol.* **49:**839–858.
5. Brown, P. D., C. Gravekamp, D. G. Carrington, H. Van de Kemp, R. A. Hartskeerl, C. N. Edwards, C. O. R. Everard, W. J. Terpstra, and P. N. Levett. 1995. Evaluation of the polymerase chain reaction for early diagnosis of leptospirosis. *J. Med. Microbiol.* **43:**110–114.
6. Centurion-Lara, A., C. Godornes, C. Castro, W. C. van Voorhis, and S. A. Lukehart. 2000. The *tprK* gene is heterogeneous among *Treponema pallidum* strains and has multiple alleles. *Infect. Immun.* **68:**824–831.
7. Cumberland, P. C., C. O. R. Everard, and P. N. Levett. 1999. Assessment of the efficacy of the IgM enzyme-linked immunosorbent assay (ELISA) and microscopic agglutination test (MAT) in the diagnosis of acute leptospirosis. *Am. J. Trop. Med. Hyg.* **61:**731–734.
8. Cumberland, P. C., C. O. R. Everard, J. G. Wheeler, and P. N. Levett. 2001. Persistence of anti-leptospiral IgM, IgG and agglutinating antibodies in patients presenting with acute febrile illness in Barbados 1979–1989. *Eur. J. Epidemiol.* **17:**601–608.
9. Dennis, D. T., and N. B. Hayes. 2004. Relapsing fever, p. 991–995. *In* D. L. Kasper, E. Braunwald, A. S. Fauci, S. L. Hauser, D. L. Longo, and J. L. Jameson (ed.), *Harrison's Principles of Internal Medicine,* 16th ed. McGraw Hill, New York, N.Y.
10. Dworkin, M. S., P. C. Shoemaker, C. L. Fritz, M. E. Dowell, and D. E. Anderson, Jr. 2002. The epidemiology of tick-borne relapsing-fever in the United States. *Am. J. Trop. Med. Hyg.* **66:**753–758.
11. Faine, S., B. Adler, C. Bolin, and P. Perolat. 1999. *Leptospira and Leptospirosis,* 2nd ed. MedSci, Melbourne, Australia.
12. Fritz, C. L., L. R. Bronson, C. R. Smith, M. E. Schriefer, J. R. Tucker, and T. G. Schwan. 2004. Isolation and characterization of *Borrelia hermsii* associated with two foci of tick-borne relapsing-fever in California. *J. Clin. Microbiol.* **42:**1123–1128.
13. Gravekamp, C., H. Van de Kemp, M. Franzen, D. Carrington, G. J. Schoone, G. J. Van Eys, C. O. Everard, R. A. Hartskeerl, and W. J. Terpstra. 1993. Detection of seven species of pathogenic leptospires by PCR using two sets of primers. *J. Gen. Microbiol.* **139:**1691–1700.
14. Harkin, K. R., Y. M. Roshto, J. T. Sullivan, T. J. Purvis, and M. M. Chengappa. 2003. Comparison of polymerase chain reaction assay, bacteriologic culture, and serologic testing in assessment of prevalence or urinary shedding of leptospires in dogs. *J. Am. Vet. Med. Assoc.* **222:**1230–1233.
15. Herrmann, J. L. 1993. Genomic techniques for identification of *Leptospira* strains. *Pathol. Biol.* **41:**943–950.
16. Holt, J. G., N. R. Krieg, P. H. A. Sneath, J. T. Staley, and S. T. Williams (ed.). 1994. The spirochetes, p. 27–37. *In* W. R. Hensyl (ed.), *Bergey's Manual of Systemic Bacteriology,* 9th ed. The Williams & Wilkins Co., Baltimore, Md.
17. Hookey, J. V. 1993. Characterization of *Leptospiraceae* by 16S DNA restriction length polymorphisms. *J. Gen. Microbiol.* **139:**1681–1689.

18. **Ko, A. I., M. Galvao Reis, C. M. Ribeiro Dourado, W. D. Johnson, L. W. Riley, and the Salvador Leptospirosis Study Group.** 1999. Urban epidemic of severe leptospirosis in Brazil. *Lancet* **354:**820–825.

19. **Larsen, S. A., V. Pope, R. E. Johnson, and E. J. Kennedy, Jr. (ed.).** 1998. *A Manual of Tests for Syphilis*, 9th ed. American Public Health Association, Washington, D.C.

20. **Levett, P. N.** 2003. *Leptospira* and *Leptonema*, p. 929–936. *In* P. R. Murray, E. J. Baron, J. H. Jorgensen, M. A. Pfaller, and R. H. Yolken (ed.), *Manual of Clinical Microbiology*, 8th ed. ASM Press, Washington, D.C.

21. **Levett, P. N.** 2001. Leptospirosis. *Clin. Microbiol. Rev.* **14:**296–326.

22. **Levett, P. N., and S. L. Branch.** 2002. Evaluation of two enzyme-linked immunosorbent assay methods for detection of immunoglobulin M antibodies in acute leptospirosis. *Am. J. Trop. Med. Hyg.* **66:**745–748.

23. **Levett, P. N., S. L. Branch, C. U. Whittington, C. N. Edwards, and H. Paxton.** 2001. Two methods for rapid serological diagnosis of acute leptospirosis. *Clin. Diagn. Lab. Immunol.* **8:**349–351.

24. **Levett, P. N., R. E. Morey, R. L. Galloway, D. E. Turner, A. G. Steigerwalt, and L. W. Mayer.** 2005. Detection of pathogenic leptospires by real-time quantitative PCR *J. Med. Microbiol.* **54:**45–49.

25. **Liu, H., B. Rodes, C.-Y. Chen, and B. Steiner.** 2001. New tests for syphilis: rational design of a PCR method for detection of *Treponema pallidum* in clinical specimens using unique regions of the DNA polymerase I gene. *J. Clin. Microbiol.* **39:**1941–1946.

26. **Merien, F., P. Amouriaux, P. Perolat, G. Baranton, and I. Saint Girons.** 1992. Polymerase chain reaction for detection of *Leptospira* spp. in clinical samples. *J. Clin. Microbiol.* **30:**2219–2224.

27. **Merien, F., G. Baranton, and P. Pérolat.** 1995. Comparison of polymerase chain reaction with microagglutination test and culture for diagnosis of leptospirosis. *J. Infect. Dis.* **172:**281–285.

28. **Morgan, J., S. L. Bornstein, A. M. Karpati, M. Bruce, C. A. Bolin, C. C. Austin, C. W. Woods, J. Lingappa, C. Langkop, B. Davis, D. R. Graham, M. Proctor, D. A. Ashford, M. Bajani, S. L. Bragg, K. Shutt, B. A. Perkins, and J. W. Tappero.** 2002. Outbreak of leptospirosis among triathlon participants and community residents in Springfield, Illinois, 1998. *Clin. Infect. Dis.* **34:**1593–1599.

29. **Orle, K. A., C. A. Gates, D. H. Martin, B. A. Body, and J. B. Weiss.** 1996. Simultaneous PCR detection of *Haemophilus ducreyi*, *Treponema pallidum*, and herpes simplex virus types 1 and 2 from genital ulcers. *J. Clin. Microbiol.* **34:**49–54.

30. **Picken, R.N.** 1992. Polymerase chain reaction primers and probes derived from flagellin gene sequences for specific detection of the agents of Lyme disease and North American relapsing-fever. *J. Clin. Microbiol.* **30:**99–114.

31. **Pillay, A., H. Liu, C. Y. Chen, B. Holloway, A. W. Sturm, B. Steiner, and S. A. Morse.** 1998. Molecular subtyping of *Treponema pallidum* subspecies *pallidum*. *Sex. Transm. Dis.* **25:**408–414.

32. **Porcella, S. F., S. J. Raffel, M. E. Schrumph, M. E. Schriefer, D. T. Dennis, and T.G. Schwan.** 2000. Glycerophosphodiester phosphodiesterase (GlpQ) of *Borrelia recurrentis* and its use for serodiagnosis of louse-borne relapsing-fever. *J. Clin. Microbiol.* **38:**3561–3571.

33. **Rich, S. M., S. A. Sawyer, and A. G. Barbour.** 2000. Antigen polymorphism in *Borrelia hermsii*, a clonal pathogenic bacterium. *Proc. Natl. Acad. Sci. USA* **98:** 15038–15043.

34. **Schmid, G. P.** 1989. Epidemiology and clinical similarities of human spirochetal diseases. *Rev. Infect. Dis.* **2:** 51460–51469.

35. **Sejvar, J., E. Bancroft, K. Winthrop, M. J. Bettinger, M. Bajani, S. Bragg, K. Shutt, R. Kaiser, N. Marano, T. Popovic, J. Tappero, D. Ashford, L. Mascola, D. Vugia, B. Perkins, and N. Rosenstein.** 2003. Leptospirosis in "Eco-challenge" athletes, Malaysian Borneo, 2000. *Emerg. Infect. Dis.* **9:**702–707.

36. **Smythe, L. D., I. L. Smith, G. A. Smith, M. F. Dohnt, M. L. Symonds, L. J. Barnett, and D. B. McKay.** 2002. A quantitative PCR (TaqMan) assay for pathogenic *Leptospira* spp. *BMC Infect. Dis.* **2:**13.

37. **Terpstra, W. J.** 1992. Typing *Leptospira* from the perspective of a reference laboratory. *Acta Leiden.* **60:**79–87.

38. **Van Dam, A. P., T. Van Gool, J. C. F. M. Wetsteyn, and J. Dankert.** 1999. Tick-borne relapsing-fever imported from West Africa: diagnosis by quantitative buffy coat analysis and in vitro culture of *Borrelia corcidurae*. *J. Clin. Microbiol.* **37:**2027–2030.

39. **Wagenaar, J., R. L. Zuerner, D. Alt, and C. A. Bolin.** 2000. Comparison of polymerase chain reaction assays with bacteriologic culture, immunofluorescence, and nucleic acid hybridization for detection of *Leptospira borgpetersenii* serovar *hardjo* in urine of cattle. *Am. J. Vet. Res.* **61:**316–320.

40. **Winslow, W. E., D. J. Merry, M. L. Pirc, and P. L. Devine.** 1997. Evaluation of a commercial enzyme-linked immunosorbent assay for detection of immunoglobulin M antibody in diagnosis of human leptospiral infection. *J. Clin. Microbiol.* **35:**1938–1942.

Lyme Disease: Serologic Assays for Antibodies to *Borrelia burgdorferi*

BARBARA J. B. JOHNSON

57

Lyme disease is the most common tick-borne bacterial disease in the northern hemisphere (5, 23). The disease is caused by three genomic groups or genospecies of *Borrelia burgdorferi* sensu lato: *B. burgdorferi* sensu stricto, *Borrelia garinii*, and *Borrelia afzelii*. Only *B. burgdorferi* sensu stricto is known to cause Lyme disease in North America, whereas all three genospecies are responsible for the disease in Europe. *B. garinii* and *B. afzelii* but not *B. burgdorferi* sensu stricto have been isolated from patients in Japan, China, and eastern Russia. Eight other genospecies within the sensu lato complex have been identified. Of these eight, there is some anecdotal evidence that *Borrelia valaisiana*, *Borrelia lusitaniae*, and spirochetes related to *Borrelia bissettii* also are pathogenic to humans (reviewed in reference 20).

In 2003, more than 21,200 new cases of Lyme disease were reported to the Centers for Disease Control and Prevention (CDC) in the United States (5). The risk of exposure to *B. burgdorferi*-infected ticks in the United States depends on geographic area and is highly focal. Most cases of Lyme disease are reported in northeastern, mid-Atlantic, and north central states. Twelve states—Connecticut, Delaware, Maine, Maryland, Massachusetts, Minnesota, New Hampshire, New Jersey, New York, Pennsylvania, Rhode Island, and Wisconsin—account for 95% of cases reported nationally. Although few European countries have official surveillance systems for Lyme disease, the World Health Organization reports that Lyme disease increases in incidence from west to east, with the highest estimated incidences in central eastern Europe, especially Austria and Slovenia. There also is a gradient of increasing incidence from south to north, with higher rates in Scandinavia. Lyme disease is widespread in the forested areas of the Russian Federation, ranging from the Baltic region to the Far East (20). Since the probability of Lyme disease in a patient depends on the risk of having received a bite from a *B. burgdorferi*-infected tick, knowledge of the geographic distribution of documented human cases and of the circumstances of a patient's tick exposure is diagnostically useful.

Lyme disease spirochetes are transmitted by ticks of the genus *Ixodes* (18, 20). The tick vectors in North America are *Ixodes scapularis* (deer tick) in the northeastern and north central regions and *Ixodes pacificus* (western black-legged tick) in the Pacific northwest. *Ixodes ricinus* and *Ixodes persulcatus* are responsible for the transmission of *Borrelia* in Europe and Asia. The major incidence of early Lyme disease coincides with the seasonal feeding activity of nymphal vector ticks, usually from April to September. Late manifestations of the disease may occur throughout the year. *I. scapularis* ticks are slow feeders, requiring several days for engorgement and more than 24 h of attachment before the spirochetes are effectively transmitted. *Ixodes ricinus* ticks may transmit *B. afzelii* earlier in the course of feeding than *I. scapularis* transmits *B. burgdorferi* sensu stricto. An expanding erythematous skin lesion, erythema migrans, develops at the site of the tick bite 7 to 9 days following tick engorgement in about 80% of patients. Weeks to months later, some untreated individuals develop abnormalities of the nervous system, heart, and joints. Since the hallmark of the disease, erythema migrans, may be absent or atypical in appearance and signs and symptoms of the disease may be nonspecific, laboratory tests play an important role in the diagnosis of Lyme disease.

Serology is the most useful type of laboratory test that is widely available to support a clinical diagnosis of Lyme disease. Positive serologic test results, however, should not be used by themselves to establish this diagnosis. A patient's clinical history, physical signs and symptoms, and risk of exposure to infected ticks are essential components of a clinical diagnosis (3, 18, 19). An American College of Physicians expert panel has defined the conditions of appropriate use of laboratory testing as when the pretest probability of Lyme disease in a patient is estimated to be between 0.20 and 0.80 (19). A patient with erythema migrans exposed to tick bite in an area where Lyme disease is endemic is considered to have a pretest probability of greater than 0.80. Laboratory testing is not recommended, and the patient should be treated with antibiotics. A patient with nonspecific findings such as headache, fatigue, and malaise is considered to have a pretest probability for Lyme disease of less than 0.20. Laboratory testing of samples from such patients also is not recommended, since testing will result in more false-positive results than true positives.

When serologic testing is appropriate, the Association of Public Health Laboratories (APHL, formerly ASTPHLD) and CDC recommend a two-test protocol (1, 4). Serum specimens first should be evaluated by a sensitive enzyme immunoassay (EIA) or immunofluorescent assay (IFA). Specimens found to be positive or indeterminate (also called borderline or equivocal) by this first test should be evaluated further by a standardized Western blot procedure.

Specimens found to be negative by a sensitive EIA or IFA need not be tested further. During the first month of infection, both immunoglobulin M (IgM) and IgG antibody responses should be determined. After 1 month of infection, the antibody responses of most untreated patients with Lyme disease will have switched class from IgM to IgG. Since most patients have an IgG response after 1 month, the finding of only IgM antibodies in a patient with prolonged illness should not be used by itself to establish a diagnosis of Lyme disease. It may be a false-positive result, especially since the specificity of IgM assays is not as high as that of IgG tests (7, 15, 19).

The usefulness of serology depends on the stage of Lyme disease (Table 1). During the first few weeks of infection by *B. burgdorferi*, serum antibody responses are often undetectable, even by the most sensitive tests (2). This is the period when most patients develop erythema migrans, so the false-negative serologic results occur mainly in patients who should be treated but not tested. If early Lyme disease is suspected when erythema migrans is atypical or absent, testing of both acute- and convalescent-phase serum samples may be of value, although negative results will not rule out the diagnosis. After patients with early Lyme disease are treated with antibiotics for 8 to 12 days, the sensitivity of serology with convalescent-phase serum reaches 70 to 80% (2, 7–10). About 20 to 30% of patients treated for early Lyme disease do not develop an antibody response, suggesting that early initiation of antibiotic therapy may abort the immune response (2, 8).

If the signs and symptoms of Lyme disease are not recognized early and appropriately treated, *Borrelia* may disseminate to the major organ systems. Later-stage Lyme disease may develop weeks to months after tick bite and affect the nervous system, the joints and, uncommonly, the heart. Patients with later-stage disease, particularly those with arthritis, have a strong humoral response with a predominance of IgG antibodies. Most patients with neuroborreliosis also have serum antibodies, and some also have intrathecally produced antibodies in the cerebrospinal fluid (CSF) (17).

After successful antibiotic therapy, most patients have a slowly declining antibody titer. However, antibody titer to whole-cell antigens cannot be used to monitor a patient's response to therapy. Some patients, especially those with a strong IgG response, may remain seropositive for years following successful antibiotic therapy. The IgM response may persist as well; therefore, the presence of IgM antibodies is not definitive proof of recent infection (3, 15, 18).

The false-positive rate for the first test of two-tiered testing of samples from healthy blood donors is about 2 to 5% (4% for the data set in Table 1). Other spirochetes—such as the agents of syphilis, leptospirosis, and tick-borne relapsing fever—elicit antibodies that cross-react with *B. burgdorferi* antigens. Patients infected (or previously infected) with these spirochetes have high rates of false-positive test results. About 6 to 7% of patients with inflammatory disorders within the differential diagnosis of Lyme disease (for example, rheumatoid arthritis) also have false-positive reactions (Table 1). Immunoblotting significantly improves the specificity of serologic testing (Table 1) (1, 3, 6–9, 15, 18, 19).

A strain used as an antigen in a serologic test should express appropriate amounts of the immunoreactive proteins of diagnostic interest. Since *B. burgdorferi* sensu lato is genetically diverse, strain choice may affect test performance (11). Ideally, serum samples from patients should be tested for reactivity with antigens appropriate for the geographic area where patients were exposed to infected ticks, since there are antigenic differences between genospecies of borreliae.

TABLE 1 Performance of serologic tests for detecting antibodies to *B. burgdorferi* sensu stricto in serum[a]

Serum sample classification	No. of samples	ELISA results[b]				Two-tiered results for ELISA plus Western blot[b]			
		No. with results		Se (%)	Sp (%)	No. with results		Se (%)	Sp (%)
		+ or ±	−			+	−		
Lyme disease	280	236	44	84		189	91	68	
Acute (erythema migrans)	80	47	33	60		30	50	38	
Early convalescent	106	96	10	91		71	35	67	
Early neurologic	15	15	0	100		13	2	87	
Early neurologic convalescent	11	11	0	100		9	2	82	
Arthritis	33	32	1	97		32	1	97	
Arthritis convalescent	24	24	0	100		23	1	96	
Late neurologic	11	11	0	100		11	0	100	
Diseases other than Lyme disease	559	52	507		91	5	554		99
Anti-nuclear antibody positive	116	7	109		93	2	114		98
Healthy blood donors	257	11	246		96	0	257		100
Leptospirosis	10	3	7		70	0	10		100
Multiple sclerosis	10	0	10		100	0	10		100
Rheumatoid arthritis and/or rheumatoid factor positive	109	6	103		94	1	108		99
Syphilis[c]	43	17	26		60	0	43		100
Tick-borne relapsing fever	14	8	6		43	2	12		86

[a]Patients in the United States. Adapted from data in references 2 and 10.

[b]Automated VIDAS immunoassay for IgM and IgG antibody to *B. burgdorferi* whole-cell antigens (BioMérieux Vitek); Se, sensitivity; Sp, specificity; +, positive; −, negative; ±, equivocal.

[c]Includes samples that were positive for anticardiolipin antibodies and/or rapid plasma reagin reaction.

Large differences in the accuracy of EIAs in detecting serum antibodies have not been observed, however, when antigens from various sensu stricto strains have been compared (1, 14). Apparently, immunodominant epitopes are sufficiently widely shared that antigens from numerous strains are appropriate for use in EIAs. With some individual specimens, however, antigen choice may affect the determination of diagnostically significant levels of antibody.

Serologic testing in Europe is complicated by the fact that three genospecies of *B. burgdorferi* may be sympatric. Differences among these three groups of strains may result in diverse immune responses in patients infected in Europe. At present, various testing approaches, including EIAs and immunoblots using whole-cell antigens, indirect and antibody-capture EIAs using morphologically intact flagella, and assays based on purified recombinant proteins, are employed. A framework for immunoblot interpretation has been developed, but there is no single set of criteria that performs equally well in laboratories across Europe (16, 22).

Efforts by APHL and the CDC to standardize immunoblot interpretation in the United States have resulted in the recognition of 10 proteins as particularly useful in the serodiagnosis of *B. burgdorferi* sensu stricto infection (1, 4, 7, 8). Of these 10 proteins, 3 currently are scored in the interpretation of IgM immunoblots: OspC (apparent molecular mass, 21 to 25 kDa, depending on the *B. burgdorferi* strain and gel system used for separation of proteins), BmpA (39 kDa), and FlaB (41 kDa). If bands corresponding to two of the preceding three proteins are present, an IgM blot is considered to be positive (8). Seven additional proteins are scored in IgG immunoblots, which are usually named by their apparent molecular masses: 18, 28, 30, 45, 58, 66, and 93 kDa (the last one is also referred to as 83 kDa or 100 kDa in some laboratories). The 18-kDa antigen is DbpA; the 45-kDa antigen comigrates with Bbk32 and may be identical to it. An IgG immunoblot is considered to be positive if antibody reactivity with 5 of the 10 scored proteins is present (7).

The level of expression of the 10 proteins currently recommended to be scored in immunoblots will affect test sensitivity. Three strains have been demonstrated to be particularly well suited for use as *B. burgdorferi* sensu stricto antigens: 2591, low-passage 297, and low-passage B31. Some strains are deficient in OspC or the 39-kDa protein, for example, particularly after many passages in in vitro culture (1, 7). Adequate production of all 10 diagnostic antigens should be verified by immunoblotting with calibrating monoclonal antibodies and serum samples.

Newer, simpler technologies have been developed and are undergoing evaluation as potential alternatives to two-tiered serologic testing. The most promising tests are based on VlsE antigen or a synthetic peptide that reproduces a 26-amino-acid portion of VlsE (2, 12, 13). At this writing, the U.S. Food and Drug Administration has cleared a test based on the peptide antigen for use as the first test in a two-tiered protocol.

METHODS

EIA

Specimens and Controls

Specimens for serologic tests must be taken aseptically and preferably refrigerated until assayed. When necessary, samples may be frozen, but freeze-thaw stress of serum should be avoided. IgM antibodies are particularly vulnerable to freeze-thaw damage. Gloves should always be worn, and specimens should be handled with the precautions extended to any human body fluid (universal precautions).

An essential part of test development is establishing positive and negative cutoff values. Patient samples are compared with reference ranges established by using panels of controls. To identify negative controls, a large number of serum samples (preferably more than 100) from healthy donors not known to have a history of exposure to *B. burgdorferi* should be tested individually. Once a large number of samples have been evaluated, a small subset of them can be randomly selected for use on a given EIA plate. Statistical methods should be applied first to exclude samples with atypically high or low optical densities (ODs) from the large set of samples from which negative controls are randomly selected (9). In the protocol below, healthy blood donors ($n = 116$) were screened to determine the range of reactivity in the control population. Specimens with ODs that were >1.5 times the interquartile range over the third quartile or ODs that were <1.5 times this range below the first quartile ("outliers") were eliminated from the group of negative controls ($\sim$10% of the specimens). Six serum samples were selected randomly from the remaining 90% of healthy donor specimens for use on each EIA plate. A sufficient volume of these controls should be available for long-term use and to determine test reproducibility over time. Negative control samples should not be pooled (physically mixed). The OD of the pool will probably be lower than the ODs of the individual samples.

Positive-control serum samples from patients with well-characterized Lyme disease are required, preferably four samples that possess a range of anti-*B. burgdorferi* antibody levels from low to high. Investigators may obtain reference quantities of positive-control serum samples suitable for assessing antibodies to *B. burgdorferi* sensu stricto from the Diagnostic and Reference Laboratory, CDC, Fort Collins, Colo. (phone 970-221-6400).

Instruments, Equipment, and Labware

Incubator (35°C)

High-speed centrifuge, rotors, centrifuge bottles and tubes

Filter apparatus with filters (pore size, 0.22 μm, and "prefilter")

Sonicator

Spectrophotometer

Polystyrene microtiter plates, 96 wells, flat-bottom (Immulon II [Dynex Technologies] or equivalent)

Micropipettors, single and multichannel, plus appropriate tips

Refrigerator (4°C)

Microtiter plate washer

Microtiter plate reader capable of reading at 405 nm

Reagents

Culture medium for *B. burgdorferi* (BSK supplemented with 6% [vol/vol] trace hemolyzed rabbit serum)

Cell wash solution (10 mM Tris HCl [pH 8.2], 150 mM NaCl, 5 mM CaCl$_2$ or phosphate-buffered saline [PBS] plus 5 mM MgCl$_2$), chilled on ice

Protein assay kit (bicinchoninic acid assay, Pierce; Bio-Rad [Richmond, Calif.] assay, or equivalent)

Tris-buffered saline (TBS = 13 mM Tris HCl, 3 mM Tris base [pH 7.4], 140 mM NaCl, 2.7 mM KCl)

Tween 20

Distilled water

Carbonate plate-coating buffer (90 mM NaHCO$_3$, 60 mM Na$_2$CO$_3$ [pH 9.6])

Carbonate substrate buffer (23 mM NaHCO$_3$, 25 mM Na$_2$CO$_3$, 0.1 M MgCl$_2$ [pH 9.8])

Plate-washing solution (TBS-T = TBS plus 0.05% Tween 20)

Blocking buffer (15 mM NaCl, 10 mM Tris HCl [pH 7.5], 0.05% Tween 20, 3% fetal bovine serum)

Goat anti-human IgM alkaline phosphatase-conjugated antibody (Kirkegaard & Perry Laboratories, Gaithersburg, Md.) or equivalent

Goat anti-human IgG alkaline phosphatase-conjugated antibody (Kirkegaard & Perry) or equivalent

Goat anti-human IgG-IgM alkaline phosphatase-conjugated antibody (Jackson ImmunoResearch Laboratories, West Grove, Pa.) or equivalent

Substrate for alkaline phosphatase (2 mg of *p*-nitrophenyl phosphate per ml)

Cell Growth and Antigen Preparation

1. Grow *B. burgdorferi* cells in BSK culture medium (21) at 35°C under microaerophilic conditions to late log phase (approximately 10^8 cells per ml). To do this, start a 1-liter culture in a sterile glass bottle by inoculation with 1 to 5 ml of a highly motile miniculture started from a frozen, low-passage stock. With serial passage, borreliae lose plasmids encoding proteins of diagnostic importance. It is critical to make and maintain primary frozen stocks for production of antigens. Incubate cells in tightly capped vessels that have minimal air space. Document that *B. burgdorferi* was free of contaminating microorganisms by culture of samples of the seed stock and of the bacterial suspension collected immediately before harvest. Four bacteriologic media should be inoculated to detect possible contamination: brain heart infusion broth, Trypticase soy agar slants, thioglycolate medium, and Sabouraud dextrose agar slants. Hold one of each test specimen at room temperature and another at 37°C, with the exception of the Sabouraud dextrose agar, which can be incubated at room temperature only. Hold quality control test specimens for 2 weeks, then examine them by microscopy to verify the absence of contaminating cell growth.

2. Harvest borreliae while they are in late log phase of growth (after about 7 days; growth rate is strain and passage dependent). To do this, decant cultures into centrifuge bottles, and pellet the cells at 10,000 × *g* for 20 min at 20°C. Discard supernatants as biohazard waste. Immediately place cell pellets on ice to reduce protease activity.

3. Wash cells to remove residual culture medium, particularly bovine serum albumin. To do this, suspend cells in cell wash solution, a cold isotonic buffer supplemented with divalent cations to reduce loss of borrelial lipoproteins from the cell surface. For each wash, disperse the pellet gently. If necessary, allow the pellet to soak in wash buffer on ice (up to ca. 15 min) to facilitate dispersion of the pellet without lysis of the cells. Centrifuge the cells again at 10,000 × *g* for 20 min at 4°C. Wash and collect the cells a second time. Suspend the cells in cold TBS at a concentration of 1 × 10^9 to 2 × 10^9 cells per ml.

4. Sonicate the cell suspension on ice until the cells are completely lysed (typically requires three 20-s intervals at intermediate power). Verify cell lysis by microscopy.

5. Filter sonicate through 0.22-μm-pore-size filter. Aliquots can be frozen and stored at −70°C for at least 1 year.

6. Determine protein concentration of the sonicate by using a protein assay kit.

Procedure

1. Dilute antigen in carbonate coating buffer to a concentration of 1 μg of protein per 100 μl.

2. Add 100 μl of antigen to each well of microtiter plate. Investigators developing an assay with a strain of *Borrelia* other than the B31 described here should perform titrations to determine the concentration of whole-cell proteins that produces the highest ratio of ODs between positive and negative control samples.

3. Incubate covered plates overnight (16 to 18 h) at 4°C.

4. Wash wells five times with about 400 μl of TBS-T each, add 300 μl of blocking buffer, and hold plates for 1 h at room temperature. Wash the wells five times again.

5. Add 100 μl of each serum sample diluted 1:500 in blocking buffer to duplicate wells and blocking buffer alone to background control wells. The appropriate dilution factor for serum is determined by twofold serial dilution of positive and negative control samples. The dilution giving the highest ratio between the ODs of the positive and negative controls is selected. The optimum dilution depends on the class(es) of antibodies to be detected. This protocol is for detecting IgG and IgM together.

6. Incubate plates, covered, for 1 h at room temperature.

7. Wash wells five times with TBS-T.

8. Add 100 μl of anti-human IgG plus IgM conjugated to alkaline phosphatase, appropriately diluted in TBS-T. Optimal working dilutions must be determined previously. *Examples:* IgG-IgM conjugate is diluted 1:10,000, IgG conjugate is diluted 1:20,000, and IgM conjugate is diluted 1:7000.

9. Incubate plates, covered, for 1 h.

10. Wash wells five times with TBS-T.

11. Add 100 μl of substrate solution in carbonate buffer, and develop for 0.5 h. Development time is determined by how long it takes for positive controls to reach expected OD readings (20 to 60 min).

12. Stop color development with 5 N NaOH (100 μl/well).

13. Read OD at 405 nm (minus the OD at 630 nm) with a microplate reader.

Results and Interpretation

The mean of the OD for each patient sample is calculated and compared with reference ranges previously established for healthy blood donors. A serum specimen is considered positive if the OD is 3 standard deviations (SD) above the mean absorbance of the control samples from the six healthy donors. The mean + 1 SD of the six negative controls is the negative cutoff value. Indeterminate values are between 1 and and 3 SD of the mean. All positive and indeterminate samples should be further tested by Western blotting.

IFA

An IFA can be used for testing serum, CSF, and other body fluids for the presence of antibodies to *B. burgdorferi*. IFA was the first test to be used to detect antibodies to *B. burgdorferi*, but it is less commonly used than EIA because it requires a skilled and experienced microscopist and cannot be automated for testing large numbers of samples. Reading and interpretation of IFA results are subjective, so interlaboratory standardization of results is difficult.

Specimens and Controls

The specimens are the same as for the EIA (see above). Positive controls yielding strong and weak fluorescence, as well as a negative control, should be run on each slide.

Instruments, Equipment, and Labware

Fluorescence microscope: microscope, ARC lamp with UV light source (xenon or mercury bulb), filter appropriate for fluorescein, 40× high dry objective for scanning, 63×/1.40 oil immersion objective for titer determinations

Dark-field microscope for determining viability of culture (preferred) or phase-contrast microscope

Microscope slides (fluorescent antibody slides, 25 by 75 mm, with 12 5-mm wells)

Moist slide chamber for incubations

Slide-rinsing jar

Coverslips, 24 by 50 mm

Micropipettor capable of 2-μl delivery and tips

Micropipettor capable of 100-μl delivery and tips

Microtiter plates, polystyrene U-bottomed

Incubator, 37°C

Reagents

Acetone, for antigen fixation

PBS (pH 7.2), sterile, to wash cells and dilute them

Positive control serum sample

Negative control serum sample

Antibody conjugate labeled with fluorescein (goat anti-human IgM, IgG, or IgM-IgG fluorescein isothiocyanate conjugate). Prepare and store master stock as specified by the manufacturer. Prepare working dilution, generally 1:200, in PBS–1% bovine serum albumin before use.

Mounting medium (preferably glycerol-based medium formulated to retard photobleaching of fluorochromes or 9 ml of glycerol plus 1 ml of PBS)

Distilled water

Clear fingernail polish with applicator brush

Cells

Select a genospecies of *B. burgdorferi* known to circulate in the geographic area where patients were potentially exposed to infected ticks. In North America, the type strain of *B. burgdorferi* sensu stricto, B31, is an appropriate choice. To detect antibodies to European *Borrelia* species, strains such as *B. garinii* PBi or 20047, *B. afzelii* strains PKo or PGau, or local isolates are suitable.

Grow cells at 35°C until log phase (approximately 10^8 cells per ml). Harvest cells by centrifugation at 10,000 × *g*, and thoroughly wash them three times with PBS–5 mM $MgCl_2$. Resuspend washed cells in PBS so that a small drop of cell suspension fixed on a slide yields approximately 100 cells per field when viewed under oil immersion. The number of cells per field of view under the microscope should be as consistent as possible from slide to slide. These concerns also apply to antigen slides obtained from commercial suppliers.

Procedure for Analysis of Serum

1. Apply antigen preparation to slides (approximately 10 μl per well), and allow them to air dry at room temperature.

Fix cells on slides in acetone for 15 min, and then air dry again. Slides may be wrapped in aluminum foil and frozen at −20°C for storage of up to 6 months.

2. Make serial twofold dilutions of negative and positive control serum samples and patient serum in PBS in a microtiter plate. Dilute patient serum to 1:512.

3. Place 10 μl of undiluted and diluted patient sera into 9 wells. Place 10 μl of the 1:4 dilution of the negative and positive controls into three other wells.

4. Incubate slides in a moist chamber at 37°C for 60 min.

5. Rinse slides in PBS, and dry them in air.

6. Apply 10 μl of the appropriately diluted goat anti-human immunoglobulin-fluorescein isothiocyanate conjugate to each well.

7. Incubate slides in a moist chamber at 37°C for 60 min.

8. Rinse slides in PBS.

9. Rinse slides in distilled water and air dry them.

10. Place a small drop of mounting fluid on each slide, and apply a coverslip.

11. Seal all edges with nail polish and air dry (optional if slide will be read immediately).

12. Scan slide using high dry objective. Read results using oil immersion objective.

Results and Interpretation

Titer is defined as the reciprocal of the highest dilution of sample at which the fluorescence has decreased by 50%. Negative and weak and strong positive controls should be run on each slide and should always yield their expected results. Established values for positive samples may vary from laboratory to laboratory but are generally 256 or higher.

Since the interpretation of IFA results is subjective, rigorous proficiency and quality control procedures are critical to ensure test reliability. An experienced microscopist can often distinguish false-positive reactions by the beaded fluorescent staining pattern of the cells. Positive results should be confirmed by Western immunoblotting

Western Immunoblotting

The Western blot is used to supplement positive and indeterminate EIA or IFA results. It should not be used for initial testing because it is not quantitative.

Specimens and Controls

The specimens are the same as for the EIA. Three human serum controls should be run with each set of samples: a strongly positive control, a weakly positive control to standardize blot development time, and a negative control. Calibration controls (mouse monoclonal antibodies recognizing diagnostically important antigens) should be run individually when the procedure is first set up. Pooled monoclonal antibodies may be run subsequently to establish a calibration "ladder." Monoclonal antibodies suitable for calibration of diagnostic immunoblots are available from the Diagnostic and Reference Laboratory, Division of Vector-Borne Infectious Diseases, CDC. These reagents include antibodies that recognize the following *B. burgdorferi* sensu stricto antigens: Decorin-binding protein A (P18), OspC (P21-P24, depending on strain), OspA (P31), OspB (P34), P35, FlaA (P37), BmpA (P39), FlaB (P41), VlsE1 (P43), GroEL (P62), P66, and P93.

Instruments, Equipment, and Supplies

Dounce homogenizer

Power supply for electrophoresis, capable of delivering 40 mA at constant current

Power supply for electroblotting capable of delivering 1 A at constant current

Polyacrylamide gel slab electrophoresis apparatus, with wide sample slot and lanes for molecular weight standards

Micropipettor or Hamilton syringe, 50 μl, for loading antigen

Electroblotting apparatus to transfer proteins from gel to membrane

Nitrocellulose sheets, 0.2-μm pore size (Schleicher & Schuell [Keene, N.H.], BA 83)

Membrane cutter (Matrix 1201, Kinematic Automation, Twain Harte, Calif., or equivalent) or scalpel and shallow cutting tray

Immunoblot incubation tray, 40 channel (MarDx Diagnostics, Carlsbad, Calif.), or disposable incubation trays, 8 channel (Schleicher & Schuell)

Glass pans (Pyrex)

Lab markers, permanent alcohol or waterproof

Reagents

TE buffer (10 mM Tris HCl [pH 8], 1 mM EDTA), sterile

Protein assay kit (bicinchoninic acid assay, Pierce; Bio-Rad assay or equivalent)

Sample buffer, 2× concentration (125 mM Tris-HCl [pH 6.8], 4.0% sodium dodecyl sulfate, 20% glycerol, 200 mM dithiothreitol, 0.01% bromophenol blue)

30% acrylamide–0.8% bisacrylamide solution

Sodium dodecyl sulfate, electrophoresis grade

Ammonium persulfate

N,N,N′,N′-Tetramethylenediamine (TEMED)

Trizma base

Glycine

Sodium chloride

Glycerol

Dithiothreitol

Bromophenol blue

Molecular weight standards, unstained

Molecular weight standards, prestained (Bio-Rad or equivalent)

Methanol, acetone-free

Gel transfer buffer (3.03 g of Trizma base, 14.4 g of glycine [pH 8.3], 400 ml of methanol, distilled water to 2 liters [final volume])

Amido black ink stain solution (0.1 g of amido black, 45 ml of methanol, 45 ml of distilled H₂O, 10 ml of glacial acetic acid)

Goat anti-human IgG conjugated to alkaline phosphatase (Kirkegaard & Perry or equivalent)

Goat anti-human IgM conjugated to alkaline phosphatase (Kirkegaard & Perry or equivalent)

Goat anti-mouse IgG conjugated to alkaline phosphatase (Kirkegaard & Perry or equivalent)

Instant dry milk (Carnation or equivalent)

TBS as in EIA protocol above

BLOTTO (0.5% instant dry milk in TBS)

Tween 20

TBS-T solution

Nitroblue tetrazolium (NBT)

5-Bromo-4-chloro-3-indolylphosphate (BCIP)

N,N-Dimethylformamide (DMF)

NBT solution (1.13 g of NBT in 10.5 ml of DMF and 4.5 ml of distilled water; freeze in 0.8-ml aliquots at −20°C)

BCIP solution (0.75 g of BCIP in 15 ml of DMF; freeze in 0.6-ml aliquots at −20°C)

Magnesium chloride (MgCl₂·6H₂O)

Developing buffer (12.11 g of Trizma base, 5.84 g of NaCl, 10.17 g of MgCl₂·6H₂O, 1 liter of distilled water; adjust pH to 9.5 with concentrated HCl).

Developing solution (200 ml of developing buffer, 1 aliquot of BCIP [0.6 ml], plus 1 aliquot of NBT [0.8 ml]; add BCIP and NBT to developing buffer 5 min prior to use.

Cells and Antigen Preparation

1. Grow cells, harvest, and wash as described above for the EIA.

2. Resuspend pellet in TE buffer with a sterile Dounce homogenizer (approximately 3.0 ml of TE buffer/0.1 g [wet weight] of cells).

3. Determine protein concentration, adjust to 2 mg/ml with TE buffer, and add an equal volume of sample buffer. Mix thoroughly, and boil for 2 min in closed tubes. Divide sample stock (1 mg/ml) into convenient portions, and store at −70°C.

Procedure

The procedure for preparing and running polyacrylamide gels and formulas of the solutions used for this are described elsewhere in this volume. Electroblotting of gels and immunoprobing of Western blots are also described. A detailed guideline for Western blot assay for antibodies to *B. burgdorferi* has been developed by the Clinical and Laboratory Standards Institute (formerly NCCLS) through its formal consensus process. A copy of Approved Guideline M34-A may be purchased (www.nccls.org). A brief outline of immunoblotting procedures is given here.

1. Prepare a 12% polyacrylamide resolving gel or a linear gradient gel from 7.5 to 15%. Top the resolving gel with a 4% polyacrylamide stacking gel. A larger size range of antigens is resolved in 7.5 to 15% gradient gels, but the antigens of greatest diagnostic interest can be well separated in a 12% gel. Either a large-gel (16-cm format) or mini-gel apparatus may be used, provided that adequate physical separation of the antigens to be scored is obtained. The conditions below are for a large-format gel, 1.5 mm thick. Antigen loads should be adjusted proportionately for smaller gels.

2. For each gel, use a comb that produces a large trough (111 mm) for the antigen and two small lanes (6 mm) for the molecular weight standards (one unstained, one prestained). With a micropipettor, load 4 μg of the molecular weight standard into the small lane. Load antigen (150 μg of protein per gel) into the large lane, using a 50-μl Hamilton syringe.

3. To each gel, apply 40 mA of current for about 3 h until dye front reaches the bottom of the gel. (This current is appropriate for the large-format gel under discussion; use conditions specified by the manufacturer for the gel rig selected.)

4. Remove the gel(s), and equilibrate it in 300 ml of transfer buffer for 15 min by gentle agitation on a shaker.

5. Transfer the antigens in the gel to nitrocellulose paper by electrotransfer at 100 mA for 1 h for the system described

(use conditions specified by the manufacturer of the electroblotter selected).

6. With a scalpel, cut off sections containing the molecular weight standards and small strips containing antigen from each side of the blot. The remaining center piece may be dried and stored for up to 1 month.

7. Stain the sections described in step 6 (except the prestained markers) with amido black stain for 3 min, rinse with water, destain with methanol-acetic acid solution, and rinse again with water. These stained sections will be used to identify specific protein bands in the immunoblots. The prestained strip is used to monitor protein separation during electrophoresis.

8. To rewet a dried blot (the center piece), incubate it in 200 ml of 0.5% Tween 20–PBS for 30 min.

9. Block the blot by incubation in BLOTTO for 1 h.

10. Incubate the blot in TBS-T solution for 45 min.

11. Draw a line at the top of the blot before cutting it, to assist in alignment of strips later. Cut the blot into strips (3 mm wide) with a membrane cutter or by hand with a scalpel, and number them sequentially.

12. Incubate strips in a multichannel tray with serum samples or calibrating monoclonal antibodies for 1 h in 2 ml of BLOTTO with 20 μl of serum per channel (1:100) or in an incubation tray (allow serum and BLOTTO to mix before adding the strips).

13. Wash each strip twice in 2 ml of TBS-T solution for 5 min each time.

14. Incubate each strip for 1 h in 2 ml of BLOTTO containing the appropriate diluted goat anti-human IgG and/or IgM conjugate. Strips used for calibration by reaction with mouse monoclonal antibodies should be incubated with goat anti-mouse IgG conjugate.

15. Wash each strip twice in 2 ml of TBS-T solution for 5 min each time.

16. Wash each strip twice in 2 ml of TBS for 5 min each time.

17. Wash each strip once in developing buffer for 5 min.

18. Develop each strip in 2 ml of developing solution for 10 to 15 min until the weakly reactive positive control band becomes visible.

19. Rinse each strip twice in distilled water for 10 min. Dry between sheets of filter paper.

20. Align the probed strips with the amido black-stained sections containing antigen and standards, and tape together.

Results and Interpretation

The specificity of Lyme disease serodiagnosis is greatly improved through the use of the Western blot to supplement positive or indeterminate results of a sensitive EIA or IFA. An IgM blot is considered positive if two or more of three bands (OspC, ca. 21 to 24 kDa, depending on strain; BmpA, 39 kDa; FlaB, 41 kDa) are present. An IgG immunoblot is considered positive if 5 of 10 bands (18, 21 to 24 [OspC], 28, 30, 39, 41, 45, 58, 66, and 93 kDa) are present. Monoclonal antibodies should be used to calibrate blots to aid in the correct scoring of blot bands. It is unusual that a patient with active Lyme disease will have only a positive IgM immunoblot after 4 to 6 weeks of infection; the likelihood of a false-positive test result should be considered.

Caution

Western immunoblotting is a labor-intensive, time-consuming, and technically demanding procedure. Care should be exercised in establishing the appropriate dilution of the serum samples and conjugate and in determining the developing

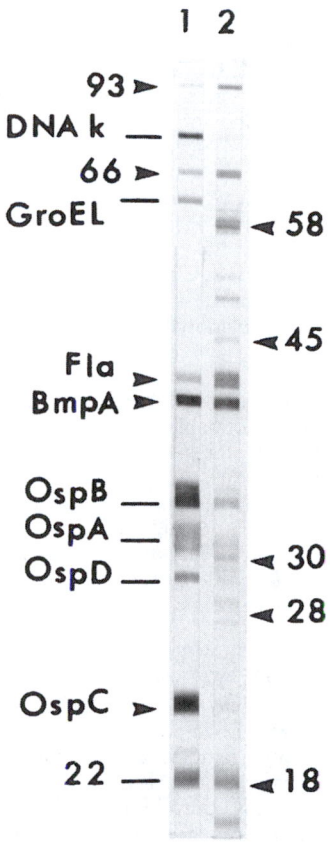

FIGURE 1 Example of immunoblot calibration. Lanes: 1, monoclonal antibodies defining selected antigens of *B. burgdorferi* B31 separated in a linear sodium dodecyl sulfate-polyacrylamide gel (Marblot; MarDx Diagnostics, Carlsbad, Calif.); 2, human serum (IgG) reactive with the 10 antigens scored in the currently recommended criteria for blot interpretation. Arrowheads mark the bands recommended for scoring; lines indicate other calibrating antibodies. Molecular masses are in kilodaltons.

times. Failure to carefully determine these conditions may lead to either false-positive or false-negative results. Immunoblots must be calibrated with monoclonal or polyclonal antibodies reactive with antigens of diagnostic importance, as well as with molecular weight standards (Fig. 1). Calibration is important, since the apparent molecular mass of some proteins of *B. burgdorferi*, such as OspC, vary depending on the *B. burgdorferi* strain and the gel electrophoresis system used. Reading of blots involves judgment that develops with experience. A common source of false-positive blots is scoring of very faint bands. In the United States, the Food and Drug Administration has cleared several commercial immunoblot kits. Monoclonal antibody calibration controls also should be used with commercial immunoblots.

REFERENCES

1. **Association of State and Territorial Public Health Laboratory Directors and the Centers for Disease Control and Prevention.** 1995. Recommendations, p. 1–5. *In Proceedings of the Second National Conference on the Serologic Diagnosis of Lyme Disease.* Association of State and Territorial Public Health Laboratory Directors, Washington, D.C.

2. **Bacon, R., B. J. Biggerstaff, M. E. Schriefer, R. D. Gilmore, Jr., M. T. Philipp, A. C. Steere, G. P. Wormser, A. R. Marques, and B. J. B. Johnson.** 2003. Serodiagnosis of Lyme disease by kinetic enzyme-linked immunosorbent assay using recombinant VlsE1 or peptide antigens of *Borrelia burgdorferi* compared with 2-tiered testing using whole-cell lysates. *J. Infect. Dis.* **187:**1187–1199.

3. **Bunikis, J., and A. G. Barbour.** 2002. Laboratory testing for suspected Lyme disease. *Med. Clin. North Am.* **86:**311–340.

4. **Centers for Disease Control and Prevention.** 1995. Recommendations for test performance and interpretation from the Second National Conference on the Serologic Diagnosis of Lyme Disease. *Morb. Mortal. Wkly. Rep.* **44:**590–591.

5. **Centers for Disease Control and Prevention.** 2004. Reported cases of notifiable diseases, by geographic division and area—United States, 2003. *Morb. Mortal. Wkly. Rep.* **53:**688–696.

6. **Craven R. B., T. J. Quan, R. E. Bailey, R. Dattwyler, R. W. Ryan, L. H. Sigal, A. C. Steere, B. Sullivan, B. J. Johnson, D. T. Dennis, and D. J. Gubler.** 1996. Improved serodiagnostic testing for Lyme disease: results of a multicenter serologic evaluation. *Emerg. Infect. Dis.* **2:**136–140.

7. **Dressler, F., J. A. Whalen, B. N. Reinhardt, and A. C. Steere.** 1993. Western blotting in the serodiagnosis of Lyme disease. *J. Infect. Dis.* **167:**392–400.

8. **Engstrom, S. M., E. Shoop, and R. C. Johnson.** 1995. Immunoblot interpretation criteria for serodiagnosis of early Lyme disease. *J. Clin. Microbiol.* **33:**419–427.

9. **Johnson, B. J. B., K. E. Robbins, R. E. Bailey, B-L. Cao, S. L. Sviat, R. B. Craven, L. W. Mayer, and D. T. Dennis.** 1996. Serodioagnosis of Lyme disease: accuracy of a two-step approach using a flagellin-based ELISA and immunoblotting. *J. Infect. Dis.* **174:**346–353.

10. **Johnson, B. J. B., B. J. Biggerstaff, R. M. Bacon, and M. E. Schriefer.** 2004. Cost-effectiveness of peptide-antigen immunoassays for Lyme disease. *J. Infect. Dis.* **189:**1962–1964.

11. **Kaiser, R.** 2000. False-negative serology in patients with neuroborreliosis and the value of employing different borrelial strains in serological assays. *J. Med. Microbiol.* **49:**911–915.

12. **Lawrenz, M. B., J. M. Hardham, R. T. Owens, J. Nowakowski, A. C. Steere, G. P. Wormser, and S. J. Norris.** 1999. Human antibody responses to VlsE antigenic variation protein of *Borrelia burgdorferi*. *J. Clin. Microbiol.* **37:**3997–4004.

13. **Liang, F. T., A. C. Steere, A. R. Marques, B. J. B. Johnson, J. N. Miller, and F. T. Philipp.** 1999. Sensitive and specific serodiagnosis of Lyme disease by enzyme-linked immunosorbent assay with a peptide based on an immunodominant conserved region of *Borrelia burgdorferi* VlsE. *J. Clin. Microbiol.* **37:**3990–3996.

14. **Magnarelli, L. A., J. F. Anderson, R. C. Johnson, R. B. Nadelman, and G. P. Wormser.** 1994. Comparison of different strains of *Borrelia burgdorferi* sensu lato used as antigens in enzyme-linked immunosorbent assays. *J. Clin. Microbiol.* **32:**1154–1158.

15. **Reed, K.** 2002. Minireview. Laboratory testing for Lyme disease: possibilities and practicalities. *J. Clin. Microbiol.* **40:**319–324.

16. **Robertson, J., E. Guy, N. Andrews, B. Wilske, P. Anda, M. Granstrom, U. Hauser, Y. Moosmann, V. Sambri, J. Schellekens, G. Stanek, and J Gray.** 2000. A European multicenter study of immunoblotting in serodiagnosis of Lyme borreliosis. *J. Clin. Microbiol.* **38:**2097–2102.

17. **Steere, A. C., V. P. Berardi, K. E. Weeks, E. L. Logigian, and R. Ackerman.** 1990. Evaluation of the intrathecal antibody response to *Borrelia burgdorferi* as a diagnostic test for Lyme neuroborreliosis. *J. Infect. Dis.* **161:**1203–1209.

18. **Steere, A. C., J. Coburn, and L. Glickstein.** 2004. The emergence of Lyme disease. *J. Clin. Investig.* **113:**1093–1101.

19. **Tugwell, P., D. T. Dennis, A. Weinstein, G. Wells, B. Shea, G. Nichol, R. Haywood, R. Lightfoot, P. Baker, and A. C. Steere.** 1997. Laboratory evaluation in the diagnosis of Lyme disease. *Ann. Intern. Med.* **127:**1109–1123.

20. **Wang, G., A. P. van Dam, I. Schwartz, and J. Dankert.** 1999. Molecular typing of *Borrelia burgdorferi* sensu lato: taxonomic, epidemiological, and clinical implications. *Clin. Microbiol. Rev.* **12:**633–653.

21. **Wang, G., R. Iyer, S. Bittker, D. Cooper, J. Small, G. P. Wormser, and I. Schwartz.** 2004. Variations in Barbour-Stoenner-Kelly culture medium modulate infectivity and pathogenicity of *Borrelia burgdorferi* clinical isolates. *Infect. Immun.* **72:**6702–6706.

22. **Wilske, B., L. Zoller, V. Brade, H. Eiffert, U. B. Göbel, G. Stanek, and H.-W. Pfister.** 2000. MIQ 12 Lyme-Borreliose, p. 1–59. *In* H. Mauch, R. Lütticken and S. Gatermann (ed.), *Qualitätsstandards in der mikrobiologisch-infektiologischen Diagnostik*. Urban & Fischer Verlag, Munich, Germany. (Translated into English at http://NRZ-Borrelien.lmu.de/miq-lyme/index.html.)

23. **World Health Organization.** 2004. Tick-borne bacterial infections, p. 54–66. *In The Vector-Borne Human Infections of Europe: Their Distribution and Burden on Public Health.* WHO Regional Office for Europe, Copenhagen, Denmark.

Immunological Tests in Tuberculosis and Leprosy

GRAHAM H. BOTHAMLEY

58

Tuberculosis is one of the most common of the serious bacterial infections. Approximately one-third of the human population has been infected with *Mycobacterium tuberculosis*, and there are 8 million notified cases with about 2.6 million deaths each year. Culture of the tubercle bacillus remains an absolute requirement for the diagnosis of tuberculosis. The identification of mycobacterial genes using PCR has achieved the sensitivity of culture techniques, and the problems of reliability have been largely overcome (20). However, at least one-third of patients with tuberculosis do not have a positive culture. In these patients, the diagnosis rests on an immunologic response, most notably the delayed hypersensitivity reaction to tuberculin, with histological evidence and/or a response to antituberculosis drug treatment. Blood tests based on gamma interferon production are now used routinely in some parts of the world. Serology, also described here, may become complementary to T-cell-based assays.

The association between infection with human immunodeficiency viruses (HIV) and tuberculosis has become increasingly important. Unfortunately, the very nature of this combination implies that immunological tests will be of limited value in the diagnosis of coexistent tuberculosis. The value of tuberculin testing in HIV-positive individuals is discussed.

The diagnosis of leprosy is clinical. The cardinal criteria are anesthetic skin patches and thickened nerves; acid-fast bacilli are found in skin smears in patients with multibacillary (lepromatous) leprosy. Despite a substantial fall in the point prevalence of leprosy from 5.4 million in 1985 to below 1 million in 1998, due to the almost universal implementation of multidrug therapy with rifampin, clofazimine, and dapsone, the annual incidence of leprosy remains unchanged (5). The lepromin test is rarely of diagnostic help but can confirm the polarity of leprosy, whether lepromatous or tuberculoid, and thereby can be of prognostic value. Indeterminate leprosy, perhaps the earliest clinically apparent form of the disease, lacks the distinctive immunological features which indicate polarity. Serological tests have also found no role in the clinical management of leprosy. Preventive treatment for close contacts with subclinical infection, a diagnosis made immunologically on the basis of reaction to antigens of *Mycobacterium leprae*, is not widely used.

The clinical spectrum in tuberculosis and leprosy is broad. Tuberculosis can be divided into primary and postprimary disease depending on the absence or presence, respectively, of preexisting immunity. Primary tuberculosis occurs most frequently in children, affecting mediastinal lymph nodes with or without a primary focus visible on the chest radiograph and occasionally progressing to more significant, disseminated disease such as tuberculous meningitis, renal involvement, and osteomyelitis. Postprimary tuberculosis is characterized in young adults by pulmonary cavitation that leads to infectious tuberculosis and a sputum smear displaying large numbers of tubercle bacilli. Less severe forms of postprimary tuberculosis, such as pleural effusions and smear-negative pulmonary disease, may also occur. The presentation of tuberculosis in elderly patients is frequently atypical. An inverse relationship between cell-mediated and humoral immunity has been described for different forms of tuberculosis and is the essential discriminator between lepromatous and tuberculoid leprosy. This relationship reflects a dichotomy in T-helper-cell function that is characterized by the secretion of different cytokines. This broad spectrum of disease and immunological reactivity in mycobacterial disease is responsible for both the value of immunological tests and the difficulties in their interpretation.

TUBERCULOSIS

Tuberculin Skin Testing

Tuberculin

Measurement of the delayed hypersensitivity reaction to extracts from *M. tuberculosis* has been performed for more than a century. Old tuberculin, the first reagent used in skin testing, was prepared by autoclaving and filtering autolyzed 8-week-old liquid cultures of *M. tuberculosis*. The protein content of this preparation, purified first with trichloroacetic acid and later with ammonium sulfate, was termed purified protein derivative (PPD). A large batch of PPD produced by Florence Seibert in 1939 (PPD-S) has become the international standard. Subsequent preparations have equivalent biological reactivity and contain a detergent (0.05% Tween 80) to prevent adsorption. The concentration of these tuberculin preparations is determined such that 0.1 ml will be biologically equivalent to 0.1 μg of PPD-S (5 tuberculin units). This amount of tuberculin gives maximal sensitivity with minimal adverse reactions.

Clinical Indications and Methods

Tuberculin testing can be used to increase the suspicion of tuberculosis (e.g., in patients with symptoms consistent with tuberculosis or in those with abnormal chest radiographs) or as a screening test (e.g., for contacts of tuberculosis patients or for those with a high risk of tuberculosis through concurrent disease, social circumstances, or country of birth). For each tuberculin test, it is necessary to clearly record the technique, dose and nature of tuberculin, and size of the reaction in millimeters.

Mantoux Test

The Mantoux test is used for diagnostic purposes and in documenting skin test conversion in individuals regularly exposed to tuberculosis. PPD (0.1 ml) is injected just beneath the surface of the skin of the forearm with a 1-ml syringe and a 26- or 27-gauge needle. The skin becomes pale and elevated, with a characteristic "peau d'orange" appearance, if the solution has been injected intradermally (Color Plate 7); a subcutaneous injection will not produce these characteristic features. The test result should be read at 48 to 72 h. The extent of erythema gives greater sensitivity and specificity and was measured in the past, but observer error was significant in reading the results for patients with dark skin. Induration is now the measure of choice. The edge of induration can be determined by using a ballpoint pen, and the diameter should be measured across the long axis of the forearm.

Multiple-Puncture Tests

Multiple-puncture tests are less widely used but are valuable in screening because of their ease of administration. The Heaf test is performed by using a six-prong head through a film of tuberculin solution (20 mg/ml), using a spring release action to penetrate the skin surface with a disposable head. The reaction is read at 48 to 72 h as millimeters of induration, or a grading system is used. The absence of any reaction or minute puncture scars with slight erythema but no induration is termed grade 0, and individual papules indicate grade 1 (Color Plate 8); both of these are considered negative. Positive reactions include grade 2, when the six papules coalesce to form a ring of induration; grade 3, a combined weal 5 to 10 mm in diameter; and grade 4, in which the induration is >10 mm or there is vesiculation of the response. Multiple-puncture test results are frequently read after 7 days. Because the quantity of tuberculin introduced by multiple-puncture methods is variable, a confirmatory Mantoux test is recommended unless vesiculation is present.

The tine test is similar but uses a disposable plastic holder with a stainless steel disk with four prongs dipped in old tuberculin. The disk is applied to the volar aspect of the forearm for 1 s with sufficient pressure to produce four visible puncture sites and a circular depression of the skin from the plastic base. The reaction is read at 48 to 72 h, and ≥2 mm of palpable induration is considered comparable to a 5-mm induration in the Mantoux technique. A positive reaction of ≥5 mm is thought to be equivalent to a Mantoux reaction of 10 mm, but Mantoux testing is recommended for indurations between 2 and 4 mm.

Interpretation of the Tuberculin Test

Interpretation of the tuberculin response requires the clear separation of reactions due to tuberculosis from those arising for other reasons. Epidemiological evidence from populations with no history of household contact with tuberculosis has established the distribution of tuberculin reactivity in infected and uninfected individuals (9). In the United States, data from naval recruits suggested that no person with tuberculosis would have a Mantoux reaction of <5 mm but that the number of incorrectly classified subjects would be smallest if an induration of ≥10 mm was used in diagnosis. Therefore, a positive Mantoux test was defined as an area of induration of >10 mm 48 to 72 h after the administration of 5 tuberculin units (0.1 μg in 0.1 ml of PPD-S or biological equivalent). The sensitivity of a test is the percentage of people with the condition who have a positive test; the specificity of a test is the percentage of people without the condition who have a negative test. The sensitivity of the tuberculin test is ~89% and the specificity is 85% when these criteria are used in a population which has not received *Mycobacterium bovis* BCG vaccination (9). In areas where tuberculosis is endemic, the sensitivity and specificity of tuberculin testing both fall (e.g., 61 and 64% in Indonesia when a cutoff of 15 mm is used [2]), with a corresponding fall in the positive predictive value. In general, the larger the reaction, the more likely it is that tuberculosis is present. However, clinical considerations determine the importance of failing to make a diagnosis of tuberculosis. As a result, a positive test is defined by both diameter of induration and context of the test (Table 1). There is about 15% variability

TABLE 1 Definition of a positive tuberculin test[a]

Diam of induration (mm)	Clinical situation
>5	Patients in contact with tuberculosis
	Patients with concurrent HIV infection
	Patients with clinical or radiographic evidence of tuberculosis
	Patients with organ transplants or otherwise immunosuppressed
>10	Individuals suspected of having tuberculosis
	Persons from areas where tuberculosis is common
	Intravenous-drug users
	Persons with social reasons for exposure to tuberculosis
	Residents of long-term-care facilities (including prisons)
	Persons with medical conditions which increase the risk of tuberculosis
	Children younger than 4 years exposed to a smear-positive index case
>15	Patients with no known risk factor for tuberculosis
	Patients from areas where false-positive tuberculin reactions are common, e.g., southern United States

[a] Data from reference 1.

with the Mantoux test; that is, a concurrent test would place the subject in a different diagnostic category (7). Readers show an unconscious bias toward 10- and 15-mm measurements (18).

A recent skin test conversion is defined in a person 35 years of age or younger as a ≥10-mm increase in induration and in a person older than 35 years as a ≥15-mm increase over a 2-year period.

Not all individuals who react to tuberculin are infected with tubercle bacilli. Cross-reactivity with environmental mycobacteria causes a significant number of positive reactions and explains the geographical variability of tuberculin testing. Tuberculin reactivity develops after BCG vaccination, but the diameter of induration is usually smaller than in patients with tuberculosis. In BCG-vaccinated subjects, a positive skin test (>10 mm) can be attributed to tuberculosis if there is contact with a patient who has tuberculosis, if there is a family history of tuberculosis or a high incidence of tuberculosis in the person's country of origin, or if the subject was vaccinated a long time before the tuberculin test (6). In BCG-vaccinated patients with tuberculosis, an accelerated reaction to tuberculin can be observed at 6 h (2).

Concurrent infections, immunosuppression due to drugs, nutrition, age, stress, and disease are the most common causes of a false-negative response to tuberculin (1). More importantly, the tuberculin skin test can be negative in patients with active tuberculosis, although tuberculin positivity returns with treatment. Interestingly, erythema and induration can be suppressed in responsive subjects by hypnotic suggestion (2). Histological examination shows substantial numbers of inflammatory cells at the site of the tuberculin test even when there is no visible induration in patients with leprosy or sarcoidosis and in those treated with steroids (2). Tuberculin reactivity declines with age. Repeated testing after a week can be helpful both in patients with suspected tuberculosis and in older persons. This "booster" or "recall" phenomenon occurs most commonly in those older than 55 years but is unusual in individuals older than 75 years. Technical failures due to subcutaneous rather than intradermal injection or to administration of <0.1 ml are common problems. Tuberculin testing itself does not induce delayed hypersensitivity.

Allergic reactions to the diluent (phosphate-buffered saline), preservative (phenol), and detergent (Tween 80) are unknown. Some reactions may ulcerate, and topical hydrocortisone cream or intradermal triamcinolone can reduce these symptoms. Lymphangitis, regional lymphadenitis, and fever are recorded and most often respond to aspirin.

Conclusions

Most individuals infected with the tubercle bacillus will contain the infection and do not develop overt disease. Tuberculin testing reveals existing cellular immunity but can only suggest a probability of active disease. Culture of M. tuberculosis remains essential in the diagnosis of tuberculosis. Tuberculin tests can be interpreted only in the context of the patient and the prevailing epidemiology of mycobacterial exposure. Attempts have been made to improve the specificity of the delayed hypersensitivity reaction by using selected antigens, but none are as yet commercially available.

Cytokines

Cell-mediated immunity acts directly by cytoxicity toward infected cells and indirectly by secretion of cytokines that permit the proliferation of cells engaged in the immune response (e.g., interleukin-2 [IL-2]) or activation of other effector cells (e.g., gamma interferon and IL-12 toward macrophages). Diagnostic tests for tuberculosis have therefore been designed with specific antigens to stimulate cytokine production by cells from peripheral blood (Table 2).

Gamma Interferon Secretion in Response to Antigenic Stimulation

The QuantiFERON-TB test (Cellestis Inc., Valencia, Calif.) was based on earlier findings in cattle, which showed that M. bovis infection could be detected by measuring gamma interferon in whole blood stimulated with tuberculin (24). Aliquots of blood (1 ml) are stimulated with tuberculin or an equivalent product made from M. avium, with saline as a negative control and phytohemagglutinin (PHA) as a positive control. Samples are incubated for 16 to 24 h at 37°C, and then 200 to 300 μl of plasma is removed without disturbing settled red blood cells. Plate wells are coated with 50 μl of a conjugate (which binds gamma interferon), and then 50 μl of plasma is incubated in each well for 60 min at room temperature. After the plates are washed, a second antibody to gamma interferon with a color detection system (100 μl of substrate) is incubated for 30 min at room temperature, after which the reaction is stopped and absorbance is measured. The kit comes with analytical software, which will determine whether the test is positive by using the criteria

- absorbance from wells stimulated by tuberculin (T) minus absorbance from wells with normal saline control (C), divided by absorbance from wells stimulated by M. avium extract (A) minus C [(T − C) divided by (A − C)] ≥ 0.15 and
- (T − C) − (A − C) divided by (T − C) ≥ 0.10, using the same notation.

  Reactivity to M. avium was defined as
- (A − C) divided by (PHA response − C) ≥ 0.20 and
- (T − C) − (A − C) divided by (T − C) < −0.1.

The assay was considered void if there was no response to PHA (i.e., PHA − C < 0.5). Comparison with tuberculin testing showed discordance related to prior BCG vaccination and reactivity toward M. avium (18). The test is currently recommended for patients with an increased risk of latent tuberculosis infection and has received Food and Drug Administration approval (19). Patients with active tuberculosis are more likely and those with treated tuberculosis are less likely to have a positive QuantiFERON-TB test than a positive tuberculin reaction (11).

Understanding the molecular biology of M. tuberculosis has advanced the quest for a more specific test for tuberculosis. The genomes of pathogenic strains of M. tuberculosis and M. bovis BCG differ by a deletion of eight open reading frames known as RD1. This region includes the early secreted antigen of tuberculosis of 6 kDa (ESAT-6) and the culture filtrate protein of 10 kDa (CFP-10). There is a member of each of the PE and PPE families (characterized by recurring motifs of proline [P] and glutamine [E] in the N terminus of these proteins) and four other proteins. These proteins have therefore been proposed as specific antigens for distinguishing between infection with M. tuberculosis and BCG vaccination. A new test, based on measuring the gamma interferon response to overlapping peptides derived from the sequences of ESAT-6 and CFP-10 and using colloidal gold to increase the sensitivity of detection of gamma interferon (QuantiFERON-GOLD), has been developed and is currently available for research purposes from the manufacturer of QuantiFERON-TB.

TABLE 2 Summary of diagnostic value of cytokine-based and serological tests

Antigen or assay	Sensitivity and 95% confidence intervals (%) for[a]:			
	Smear-positive pulmonary tuberculosis	Smear-negative pulmonary tuberculosis	Extrapulmonary tuberculosis	Child tuberculosis
Gamma interferon				
ESAT-6 5-day cell culture supernatant	33.3 (17.9–48.7)	47.8 (41.6–54.0)		ND[c]
ESAT-6 ELISPOT	ND	88.7 (83.1–93.2)[b]		0.7 (58.4–79.5)[b]
CFP-10 5-day cell culture supernatant	72.9 (64.2–80.1)[b]	63.0 (55.6–70.4)		ND
CFP-10 ELISPOT	ND	80.0 (69.9–91.1)[b]		ND
T SPOT-TB	96.5 (88.3–98.9)[b,f]		ND	80.7 (68.6–88.8)[b]
QuantiFERON-GOLD	85.4 (77.3–91.0)[g]	76 (56.4–88.4)[g]	92.3 (66.1–98.2)[g]	ND
Antibody to				
38 kDa	62.2 (59.2–65.2)	50.0 (46.7–53.3)	ND	85.7 (70.0–100)
TB72 monoclonal antibody competition	76.7 (72.1–81.3)	59.9 (52.6–67.2)	76.7 (66.0–86.4)	16.7 (0–33.9)[d]
81 kDa	63.5 (53.3–73.7)[b]	51.3 (40.2–62.4)[b]	ND	ND
30 kDa/antigen 6	57.1 (50.5–63.7)	27.0 (18.7–35.3)	ND	ND
16 kDa	51.7 (60.7–42.7)	49.4 (57.0–41.8)	25.6 (16.1–35.1)[e]	33.3 (11.5–55.1)
19 kDa	40.4 (32.9–47.9)	33.6 (25.3–41.9)	32.5 (24.0–41.0)	ND
CFP-10	27.6 (22.0–33.2)	ND	ND	ND
ESAT-6	22.7 (5.2–40.2)	17.3 (7.0–27.6)	ND	ND

[a] The cutoff titer was calculated as the mean +2 standard deviations of control values, i.e., a defined specificity of 95%. Confidence intervals have been calculated from the sensitivity and the number of patients tested, combining studies.

[b] Only a single group has been responsible for the data, but this may include multiple publications.

[c] ND, no data.

[d] Sensitivity using cutoff titers derived from adult control values.

[e] Tuberculous meningitis only.

[f] Sensitivity, 91.7% (64.0 to 98.1%).

[g] Specificity, 88.2% (64.6 to 94.4%) in one study.

Enumeration of Gamma Interferon-Secreting Cells

The ELISPOT (enzyme-linked immunosorbent spot-forming cell) technique was first used in 1983 to identify antibody-secreting cells by using anti-immunoglobulin antibodies linked to peroxidase, and the assay was adapted 5 years later to the enumeration of gamma interferon-secreting cells (10). This technique has been applied to overlapping peptides from ESAT-6 and CFP-10 as a diagnostic test (15). Polyvinylidene difluoride-backed 96-well plates (MAIP S 45; Millipore, Bedford, Mass.) are coated with 15 μg of anti-gamma-interferon monoclonal antibody (1-DIK; Mabtech, Stockholm, Sweden) per ml overnight at 4°C. The plates are washed with RPMI 1640 and blocked for 1 h with RPMI 1640 supplemented with L-glutamine, ampicillin and gentamicin, and 10% heat-inactivated pooled human AB serum. Peripheral blood mononuclear cells are separated from whole blood on a Ficoll-Hypaque gradient and washed three times in supplemented medium, and then 5×10^5 cells are added to each well in 100 μl of supplemented medium containing peptides at 2 μmol/liter in duplicate or triplicate wells. A positive control with PHA and a negative control without peptide are used as standards. Assay mixtures are incubated overnight in 5% CO_2, the contents are shaken off, and the wells are washed six times with phosphate-buffered saline (PBS)–0.05% Tween 20 (PBST). A 100-μl volume of a different monoclonal antibody to gamma interferon (7-B6-1; Mabtech) labeled with biotin at 1 μg/ml is then added to each well, the plates are incubated for 3 h at room temperature, and the wells are washed six times with PBST. Spots are developed using streptavidin-alkaline phosphatase conjugate for 2 h followed, after washing, with 100 μl of chromogenic substrate for 30 min and further washing to halt the reaction. Spots are counted under ×20 magnification, and only large spots with fuzzy borders are scored. A positive score requires at least five more spots than the negative control and a number at least twice that of the negative control. This assay has been developed into a commercial test (SPOT-TB; Immunotec, Oxford, United Kingdom) and is available currently for clinical use in the United Kingdom.

The HIV pandemic has clearly shown the importance of CD4$^+$ T cells in containing tuberculous infection. Studies of mice in which the genes for gamma interferon or IL-12 and their receptors have been deleted have confirmed the importance of these cytokines in resisting the development of tuberculosis after aerosol challenge. Genetic analysis of human families with an increased susceptibility for mycobacterial infections has shown similar defects within the pathways initiated by these cytokines. These data suggest that tests based on gamma interferon might better detect individuals with a protective response to tuberculosis rather than those who will develop or have developed disease, unless exposure to the tubercle bacilli leads inevitably to disease in the setting of propitious circumstances within the human host. The immunological spectrum of tuberculosis suggests that complementary tests based on Th2 responses (i.e., measurement of IL-4 to RD1 antigens or antibody responses) may be important to obtain a high diagnostic sensitivity.

Serology

Clinical Indications

Patients with infectious tuberculosis may have symptoms for 2 or 3 months before diagnosis and may frequently present to hospital services with nonspecific complaints. A serological test, which could make an early diagnosis, perhaps even before a chest radiograph is obtained, would be valuable in restricting the transmission of tuberculosis. Patients who have smear-negative pulmonary tuberculosis, reactivation, or extrapulmonary disease (particularly tuberculous meningitis) and children with tuberculosis would also benefit from a serodiagnostic test which could increase the suspicion of tuberculosis.

From these clinical indications, it is apparent that few serological studies have been performed in a manner relevant to clinical practice. Common errors include the use of healthy subjects rather than patients with suspected tuberculosis in whom an alternative diagnosis is reached as controls, biased selection and enrollment of patients, and failure to analyze test performance by sputum smear status and site of disease. Other problems include the small numbers studied, leading to wide confidence intervals for sensitivity and specificity. Many of the near-patient tests require interpretation by the reader, and repeatability has not been demonstrated.

Purified Antigens

The selection of antigens for serological tests is defined by the need for specificity. Many mycobacterial antigens are cross-reactive. The specificity of the RD1 antigens ESAT-6 and CFP-10 has been noted. Historically, antigens specific for M. tuberculosis have been identified by using preabsorbed hyperimmune serum or monoclonal antibodies. Four independent groups identified the same antigen with a relative molecular mass of 38 kDa by these methods. The recombinant antigen is available through the World Health Organization (WHO) and forms the basis of commercial kits (Omega Diagnostics and ICT Diagnostics). The sensitivity of antibody to this antigen in smear-positive pulmonary tuberculosis has been explored by several groups and remains the greatest of the sensitivities of the 25 antigens tested to date (Table 2).

Most researchers agree that a serological test for tuberculosis will require several antigens. Starting with the 38-kDa antigen, patients who are seronegative for this antigen are positive to antigens such as the 16-kDa, CFP-10, Mtb8.4, Mtb48, Mtb81, and MPT32 antigens. These antigens have been combined as a multiepitope polyprotein, which is being currently investigated as a serological agent (14). Antibody to the 14-kDa (16-kDa) and ESAT-6 antigens has been associated with latent tuberculous infection (3, 22).

Monoclonal Antibodies

Monoclonal antibodies are used widely in all aspects of clinical immunology and microbiology. An animal is immunized with an antigen or mixture of antigens, and plasma cells are harvested from the spleen and fused to a malignant cell to produce a potentially immortal hybrid, which secretes antibody of a single specificity. Monoclonal antibodies to M. tuberculosis (and M. leprae) have been defined in WHO-sponsored workshops by their ability to bind to extracts from other mycobacterial species and/or their specificity for these pathogenic mycobacteria. Several monoclonal antibodies with defined specificity for M. tuberculosis are available through WHO. These reagents have been used to prepare purified antigens by affinity chromatography or to select clones expressing the recombinant protein (3). Even highly cross-reactive proteins may have species-restricted epitopes, and a competition assay can measure antibody levels which overlap with the binding site of the monoclonal antibody.

Methods

ELISA with Purified Antigens

The enzyme-linked immunoassay (ELISA) has become an integral part of the methodology of the immunology laboratory (17). Microtiter wells are coated with an antigen at a concentration at which maximal binding occurs (usually within the range of 1 to 10 μg/ml). Nonspecific binding is blocked by incubating the wells with bovine serum albumin or milk, often containing 0.05% Tween 20. A fixed dilution (e.g., 1:100) or a series of dilutions of sera are incubated in duplicate or triplicate microtiter wells, and after being washed, the wells are incubated with anti-human immunoglobulin G (IgG)-peroxidase or IgG-alkaline phosphatase conjugate. After another washing of the wells, antibody titers are determined by color development with chromogens such as tetramethylbenzidine or o-phenylenediamine. Antibody titers are recorded as the absorbance (optical density) after the reaction has been halted by a change in pH. Wells not coated with the purified antigen act as a negative control, and wells containing hyperimmune serum which displays maximal binding to the purified antigen act as a positive control. Some serum samples show excessive nonspecific binding despite the blocking step, and for serum dilutions of <1:100, the absorbance of a negative control for each serum dilution must be subtracted from the absorbance of the complete assay. Antibody titers should also be compared to the maximal absorbance of a standard hyperimmune serum in order to correct for any variability in the procedure or reagents.

Competition Assays

The preparation of large quantities of a purified antigen requires an enormous investment. Monoclonal antibodies are more readily obtained and can measure antibody titers by competing with human sera for binding to antigens. There is no need to purify individual mycobacterial antigens. Wells are coated with a soluble extract of M. tuberculosis. After nonspecific binding is blocked with bovine serum albumin or milk containing 0.05% Tween 20, human serum is incubated in duplicate or triplicate wells in serial dilutions. A dilution of the monoclonal antibody which will give 90% of the maximal binding in the absence of competing human serum is then added to the wells (the human serum is not removed by washing prior to this step). The monoclonal antibody either can be conjugated directly to peroxidase or can be detected using an antiserum to the class of antibody specific for the animal from which the monoclonal antibody was prepared, e.g., mouse anti-IgG (γ-chain specific)-peroxidase conjugate for a mouse IgG monoclonal antibody (23). The presence of the monoclonal antibody is then detected with a chromogen and hydrogen peroxide as with the ELISA technique. The nature of the competition assay gives a high sensitivity because low dilutions of sera can be employed without raising the problems of background interference.

Immunochromatographic assays. Near-patient tests are based on lateral-flow techniques where the antigen is immobilized on a nitrocellulose membrane. As the serum passes the antigen and forms an immune complex, anti-human IgG labeled with colloidal gold reacts with the antibody from the serum and creates a visible line. The main problem with these assays is the variable density of the observed reaction and hence the potential for observer error. These assays are available as preformed kits.

Reliability

Serological tests have improved greatly in terms of specificity and reproducibility and compare well with those for other infectious diseases, especially in patients with smear-positive pulmonary tuberculosis (Table 2). False-negative results have been attributed to HLA restriction, when antigens of such restricted specificity are used, and to the presence of circulating immune complexes, which are rapidly removed from the bloodstream. The use of a collection of antigens or epitopes defined by monoclonal antibodies improves the sensitivity of serological tests. Although tuberculosis is characterized by cell-mediated immunity, the development of significant disease is associated with a change in T-helper-cell phenotype to one which encourages antibody production. Different antigens evoke more of an antibody response in patients with early or primary tuberculosis than in those with more extensive disease (3). False-positive serological results occur in patients with lepromatous leprosy and have been attributed to T-cell priming by prior exposure to tuberculosis. False-positive results have not been demonstrated in patients with nontuberculous mycobacterial disease for antigens currently under investigation. The clinical circumstances of false-positive results would probably not cause any difficulty in the interpretation of these tests.

LEPROSY

Delayed Hypersensitivity

Lepromin and Leprosin

M. leprae cannot be cultured in vitro, and therefore there is no material equivalent to tuberculin, which is derived from the culture filtrate of M. tuberculosis. In the 1920s, Mitsuda prepared lepromin from heat-sterilized bacilliferous tissue from lepromatous leprosy patients. Attempts to purify this material involved differential centrifugation (National Institute of Medical Research, Mill Hill, London; lepromin-H) and, later, extraction of bacilli with chloroform (Dharmendra lepromin). M. leprae can multiply within the nine-banded armadillo, and this material forms the basis of the WHO preparation lepromin-A. Standardization was achieved by bacterial count such that preparations contain 4×10^6 to 16×10^6 bacilli per 0.1 ml of inoculum. Leprosin is a soluble filtered sonicate of leprosy bacilli derived from armadillos which has been sterilized by exposure to 2.5 megarads from a cobalt-60 source; this material is standardized by using a protein concentration of 10 µg/ml.

Clinical Indications and Methods

Lepromin testing is not of value in the diagnosis of leprosy. However, in borderline leprosy and as indeterminate leprosy progresses, the presence of a positive delayed hypersensitivity reaction indicates progression toward the tuberculoid form of the disease. A large response also occurs in the majority of individuals living in areas where leprosy is endemic. Lepromatous leprosy usually occurs in the lepromin-negative population. The test is performed by injecting 0.1 ml of lepromin intradermally into the upper arm over the deltoid muscle.

Interpretation of the Lepromin Test

Two types of delayed hypersensitivity reaction can be elicited by lepromin: the Fernandez reaction and the classical Mitsuda reactions.

Fernandez Reaction

The Fernandez reaction occurs after 48 to 96 h, is essentially similar to the tuberculin reaction, and is thought to be a response to soluble extrabacillary antigens. There is marked variability in the amount of this soluble material in different preparations and a corresponding variability in positive reactions. In general, very few healthy persons, even those who give a positive Mitsuda reaction, will develop an early reaction. The frequency of positive responses is related to the degree of contact with leprosy patients, so that many household contacts of a lepromatous leprosy patient will give an early reaction to lepromin. Only patients with tuberculoid leprosy have a Fernandez reaction. Measurement of the diameter of the reaction has no clinical significance.

Mitsuda Reaction

The Mitsuda reaction is the more classical measurement of delayed hypersensitivity to lepromin. It appears as an indurated nodule 7 to 10 days after intradermal injection and can persist for more than a month. The delay has been attributed to the release of antigens from within the leprosy bacillus; leprosin coupled to liposomes produces a similarly delayed reaction. As many as 70% of healthy individuals living in countries where leprosy is rare will give a small positive reaction, and this figure rises to 90% in areas where leprosy is endemic. Again, in leprosy patients, a positive reaction occurs only in those with tuberculoid rather than lepromatous features. An area of induration with a diameter of ≥5 mm is widely accepted as a positive reaction; the lesion can progress through superficial necrosis, ulceration, and scarring.

Leprosin

Leprosin is a soluble extract of leprosy bacilli and gives the equivalent of a Fernandez reaction, i.e., almost no reaction in healthy individuals and patients with lepromatous leprosy. However, leprosin also fails to evoke a response in at least half of those with tuberculoid leprosy.

Thus, delayed hypersensitivity can indicate the prognosis of patients with leprosy by confirming their polarity, whether lepromatous or tuberculoid. If household contacts of leprosy patients have no reaction to lepromin, they could be considered for preventive therapy.

Serology

Clinical Indications

The ease of clinical diagnosis of leprosy makes a serological test for leprosy superfluous. As with the lepromin test, antibody levels can be used to distinguish between lepromatous and tuberculoid leprosy. Antibody levels correlate well with the bacterial index and might be helpful in judging the duration of chemotherapy (21). Some studies have suggested that seropositivity in contacts of leprosy patients indicates an increased likelihood of developing leprosy at a later stage, but these studies lack confirmation.

Phenolic Glycolipid

Phenolic glycolipid was identified from M. leprae sonicates and proved to have a unique trisaccharide component not found in other mycobacterial species. The crude extract is hydrophobic, and so conventional ELISA techniques are difficult to use. Synthesis of the trisaccharide and conjugation of its inherent terminal disaccharide to bovine serum albumin provided reagents that were more readily incorporated into the standard ELISA. If wells are coated with the phenolic glycolipid and nonspecific binding is blocked with an irrelevant protein plus 0.05% Tween 20, then sera can be added at serial dilutions or at a fixed 1:300 dilution. After the wells are washed, IgM binding is measured using anti-human anti-IgM (μ-chain specific)-peroxidase conjugate and developed with chromogens. Absorbance (optical density) is related to the amount of IgM antibody, and positive titers have an absorbance of >0.2. As before, subtraction of absorbances measured with the same dilutions of serum on uncoated plates improves accuracy, and a standard high control is especially valuable for correcting any plate-to-plate variation.

Monoclonal Antibody-Based Tests

A competition assay using the ML04 monoclonal antibody which binds to an M. leprae-specific epitope on a 35-kDa antigen gives a sensitivity similar to, if not greater than, that of phenolic glycolipid in leprosy patients. The method is the same as with serodiagnostic competition assays for tuberculosis, except that the wells are coated with a soluble extract of M. leprae. Levels of anti-35-kDa antibody show a strong correlation with bacterial load and can be used to monitor effective chemotherapy (18).

BCG VACCINATION

Bacillus Calmette-Guérin (BCG)

BCG was first derived from M. bovis attenuated by serial culture at the Pasteur Institute in Lille, France. The original BCG strain was not derived from a single colony but from a whole culture and was therefore, strictly speaking, not a strain at all. The continuous subculturing of BCG has subsequently given rise to a number of different strains that can be identified by variations in their virulence toward guinea pigs and their ability to induce tuberculin sensitivity. However, widely disparate vaccines have given similar efficacies in the prevention of tuberculosis (e.g., Danish BCG and a vaccine derived from M. microti). Two BCG vaccines are licensed for use in the United States, namely, the Glaxo strain (Quad Pharmaceuticals, Inc., Indianapolis, Ind.) and the Tice strain (Bionetics Research, Inc., Chicago, Ill., or Antigen Supply House, Northridge, Calif.) (6). BCG vaccines have been given to more than 3 billion individuals and are the world's most widely used vaccines. The adjuvant properties of BCG vaccines may be exploited by the incorporation of recombinant genes into BCG to provide immunity to a number of different infectious diseases.

Efficacy of Vaccination

BCG vaccines were first used against human tuberculosis in France in 1921. A number of controlled trials of BCG were conducted in the 1930s but gave inconsistent results. Examination of randomized controlled trials and case-control or household contact studies has shown a beneficial effect, albeit with a wide variation in efficacy (12). A meta-analysis of studies, which included random allocation of subjects for BCG vaccination and measured the number of cases and/or deaths due to tuberculosis, also demonstrated significant benefit from BCG vaccination in preventing active tuberculosis (8). The overall relative risks for tuberculosis and for death due to tuberculosis were 0.49 (95% confidence interval, 0.34 to 0.70) and 0.29 (95% confidence interval, 0.16 to

0.53), respectively, in those who received BCG vaccination compared to nonvaccinated subjects. The protective effects were 64% against tuberculous meningitis (i.e., relative risk of 0.36 for BCG-vaccinated individuals) and 78% against disseminated tuberculosis. Much of the variation among the different trials was associated with geographic latitude and study validity score.

Four controlled trials have shown that BCG vaccination is effective against the development of leprosy, and in one trial in which both tuberculosis and leprosy were studied (Chingleput, India), benefit was confined to the prevention of leprosy (12).

Clinical Indications

Most nations (except the United States and The Netherlands) recommend routine BCG vaccination for the prevention of tuberculosis. The WHO recommends a single dose at birth as part of the Extended Program on Immunization. In the United Kingdom, neonatal vaccination is recommended in areas where the incidence of tuberculosis is >40/100,000 (i.e., London) and vaccination at 13 years is recommended elsewhere, whereas in Eastern Europe, multiple doses of BCG vaccine are given throughout childhood. In the United States, BCG vaccination is recommended for groups in which the incidence of tuberculosis is >1% per year, for tuberculin-negative infants and children who are exposed to infectious tuberculosis and cannot take isoniazid, and for tuberculin-negative children exposed to multiple-drug-resistant tuberculosis. BCG vaccination is also given to household contacts of leprosy patients in Cuba and Venezuela, and recent studies recommend a wider use in the prevention of leprosy. BCG should not be given to individuals with immunodeficiency from whatever cause, whether familial, due to concurrent disease (e.g., HIV infection or malignancy), or drug induced.

Procedure

BCG vaccines should be reserved for persons whose tuberculin skin test reaction to 5 TU is negative. Data from countries where tuberculosis is endemic suggest that a tuberculin skin test is not necessary in children younger than 10 years before vaccination. Intradermal injection of BCG is superior to other methods such as multiple puncture, scarification, jet injection, and the use of a bifurcated needle and is recommended for the Glaxo strain. Percutaneous injection (Tice strain) gives adequate results in terms of induced tuberculin sensitivity but may produce an abscess or unsightly scar. A dose-dependent relationship between the amount of BCG and the protective effect can be demonstrated in animals. The human immune response is also dose dependent in terms of induced tuberculin sensitivity, size of local reaction, and incidence of regional lymphadenitis. The dose recommended by WHO is 0.1 ml containing 0.75 mg of BCG per ml (100,000 to 300,000 CFU) or half this dose for children younger than 1 year. BCG is a live vaccine and consequently requires greater care than tuberculin in storage and administration. A 5-min exposure to tropical sunlight reduces the number of culturable particles by 99%. Freeze-dried vaccine has a lower viability than liquid preparations but can be prepared in bulk in a standard form, keeps better after distribution, and is therefore specified as the required form of BCG vaccine. The vaccine should be refrigerated when not in use and then reconstituted, protected from exposure to light, and used within 8 h. The vaccine is drawn up in a 1-ml syringe and injected with a short-bevel 25-gauge needle just beneath the surface of the skin at the level of the insertion of the deltoid muscle. A weal of about 7 mm should be produced. Normally, a local reaction appears after 2 to 6 weeks. It begins with a small papule that slowly increases in size and may discharge purulent material to leave a shallow ulcer. This lesion heals after 1 to 3 months, with the formation of a small scar. Dry permeable dressings may be used to cover the ulcer, but impermeable dressings delay healing and can be recommended only for short periods. An early reaction to the vaccine suggests the possibility of tuberculosis (see below). Inspection of the vaccination site after 6 weeks is suggested to ensure that the vaccination has been successful and that no severe reactions have occurred.

Complications from BCG vaccination are variously estimated at 1 to 10% (4) and 15 per million vaccinations (16). Lymphadenitis accounts for approximately two-thirds of the reported complications, followed by local ulceration and keloid scarring. Keloid scarring can be minimized by not using the upper deltoid region of the arm and, in susceptible persons, using an alternative site which is more readily concealed. Disseminated BCG may occur with otitis media, osteomyelitis, and cutaneous "tuberculosis." Dissemination is particularly common in persons with a defect in cell-mediated immunity and is responsible for the small number of deaths (3 per billion vaccinations [16]) attributed to BCG vaccination worldwide.

HIV Infection and BCG

Disseminated BCG disease may occur after vaccination in patients with AIDS. The WHO recommends BCG vaccination for children in areas where HIV infection and tuberculosis are common unless the children have symptoms of AIDS (6). HIV infection is difficult to assess in the infant who may be seropositive because of maternal antibodies. If it occurs, BCG dissemination can be effectively treated with antituberculous chemotherapy, but, clearly, the prognosis is poor. In populations in which tuberculosis is rare, BCG vaccination should not be given to persons suspected of being infected with HIV.

Use as a Diagnostic Test

In persons with tuberculosis, the response to BCG vaccine is accelerated (13). Malnutrition and disseminated tuberculosis (as with tuberculous meningitis and miliary disease) reduce the sensitivity of the tuberculin skin test and are common features of child tuberculosis. Following a report by WHO in 1964, BCG as a diagnostic test for childhood tuberculosis was evaluated in India. In children with tuberculosis but without a visible BCG scar, a papule of >5 mm in diameter appeared within 24 to 48 h (compared to the normal 2 to 3 weeks) and a pustule appeared in the next 3 to 5 days. Reactions may begin as early as 6 h. A delayed reaction occurs in malnourished children but is still earlier than expected. BCG vaccination is especially effective in preventing primary tuberculosis (see above), and the use of BCG as a diagnostic test in areas where tuberculosis is endemic has the advantage of vaccinating the unprotected population as well as confirming the clinical suspicion of active disease.

CLINICAL VALUE OF TESTS OTHER THAN IN DIAGNOSIS

Chemoprophylaxis

The tuberculin response remains a key test in deciding who should receive preventive treatment with isoniazid. Despite the potentially toxic effects of this drug, epidemiological evidence promotes the use of preventive therapy in those with recent contact with tuberculosis and in persons with abnormal chest radiographs consistent with previous tuberculosis. The definition of tuberculin positivity in the light of the clinical situation restricts the need for isoniazid treatment in subjects with no known exposure to tuberculosis (Table 1). The incidence of isoniazid-induced hepatitis has been estimated to be 10.3 in 1,000, with a mortality of 0.06%. Immunological markers which could predict the persons who are most likely to develop tuberculosis, perhaps by HLA phenotype (DR15) or the human equivalent of the Bcg^s phenotype, could further restrict the use of isoniazid to those who would gain the greatest benefit from this treatment. Enumerating cells from peripheral blood which secrete gamma interferon in response to peptide epitopes of ESAT-6 may be helpful in indicating the patients infected with M. tuberculosis (15), but its value in comparison with tuberculin skin testing remains uncertain.

Compliance with Treatment

A large number of serological studies have shown that there is an early increase in antibody levels immediately following the start of treatment for tuberculosis (3). Levels of antibody to the 16-kDa antigen rise when the lack of effective treatment has been sufficient to allow tubercle bacilli to multiply again in numbers that can be detected by sputum culture (4). Antibody levels are slow to rise in patients infected with isoniazid-resistant strains of tubercle bacilli (4). Immunological markers might be valuable in assessing significant problems in the treatment of tuberculosis, whether adherence or drug resistance.

Reactivation

In patients with radiographic evidence of self-healed tuberculosis, reactivation may occur. Estimates suggest a breakdown rate of 1 to 5% per year. One study suggested that the development of detectable antimycobacterial antibody coincides with reactivation and that serological assessment of patients with radiographic evidence of healed tuberculosis might define a population which requires treatment for tuberculosis (3).

Nontuberculous Mycobacteria

The epidemiology of infection with nontuberculous mycobacteria has changed radically as infection with HIV progresses. Infection with the M. avium-M. intracellulare complex (MAC) is particularly common, and empirical therapy for both tuberculosis and MAC is often given to immunosuppressed patients while the results of culture are awaited. Detection of species-specific mycobacterial DNA following amplification by PCR will become the preferred means of early distinction between the two species. Tests involving species-restricted monoclonal antibodies were used briefly, but the requirement for culture to obtain material for testing means that the new test has insufficient advantage over the detection of mycobacterial DNA directly in clinical specimens.

Epidemiological studies have shown a high frequency of MAC in the southern United States and have been cited to explain the variation in tuberculin sensitivity. Skin testing with soluble antigens from different mycobacterial species has enjoyed some favor but has no certain clinical application. One group suggested that the observed reduction in responses to other mycobacterial sensitins in patients with tuberculosis compared to healthy controls indicates a lack of immune responsiveness to "common antigens" or perhaps a focusing of the immune response on the invading pathogen.

CONCLUSION

Tuberculin testing remains the most widely employed immunological test for the diagnosis of tuberculous infection. Tests based on cellular immunity and the secretion of gamma interferon have shown significant progress and are used routinely in some parts of the world. Serological tests may have a complementary role and remain the basis for near-patient tests.

APPENDIX

Sources of Materials

Tuberculin PPD solution for the Mantoux test

Parke-Davis, Morris Plains, N.J.

Tuberculin PPD multiple-puncture devices

Lederle Laboratories, Division of American Cyanamid Co., Wayne, N.J.
Parke-Davis (see above)
Sclavo Inc., Wayne, N.J.

Tuberculin OT multiple-puncture devices

Lederle Laboratories (see above)
Mérieux Institute Inc., P.O. Box 523980, Miami, Fla.

BCG vaccines

Strain Glaxo (Quad Pharmaceuticals Inc., Indianapolis, Ind.)
Strain Tice (Bionetics Research Inc., Chicago, Ill., and Antigen Supply House, Northridge, Calif.)

Cytokine assays

QuantiFERON-TB and QuantiFERON-GOLD (Cellestis Inc., Valencia, Calif.)

ELISPOT assays

T SPOT-TB (Oxford Immunotec Ltd., Abingdon, United Kingdom)

Serological tests

Pathozyme TB Complex Plus, recombinant 38- and 16-kDa antigens (Omega Diagnostics Ltd., Alva, United Kingdom)

REFERENCES

1. **American Thoracic Society and Centers for Disease Control and Prevention.** 2000. Targeted tuberculin testing. *Am. J. Respir. Crit. Care Med.* **161:**S221–S247.
2. **Beck, J. S.** 1991. Skin changes in the tuberculin test. *Tubercle* **72:**81–87.
3. **Bothamley, G. H.** 1995. Serological diagnosis of tuberculosis. *Eur. Respir. J.* **8**(Suppl. 20):676s–688s.
4. **Bothamley, G. H.** 2004. Epitope-specific antibody levels demonstrate recognition of new epitopes and changes in titer but not affinity during treatment of tuberculosis. *Clin. Diagn. Lab. Immunol.* **11:**942–951.
5. **Britton, W. J., and D. N. Lockwood.** 2004. Leprosy. *Lancet* **363:**1209–1219.
6. **Centers for Disease Control.** 1988. Use of BCG vaccines in the control of tuberculosis: a joint statement by the ACIP and the Advisory Committee for the Elimination of Tuberculosis. *JAMA* **260:**2983–2991.
7. **Chaparas, S. D., H. M. Vandiviere, I. Melvin, G. Koch, and C. Becker.** 1985. Tuberculin test: variability with the Mantoux procedure. *Am. Rev. Respir. Dis.* **132:**175–177.
8. **Colditz, G. A., T. F. Brewer, C. S. Berkey, M. E. Wilson, E. Burdick, H. V. Fineberg, and F. Mosteller.** 1994. Efficacy of BCG vaccine in the prevention of tuberculosis. Meta-analysis of the published literature. *JAMA* **271:**698–702.
9. **Comstock, G. W., T. M. Daniel, D. E. Snider, P. Q. Edwards, P. C. Hopewell, and H. M. Vandiviere.** 1981. The tuberculin skin test. *Am. Rev. Respir. Dis.* **124:**356–363.
10. **Czerkinsky, C., G. Andersson, H. P. Ekre, L. A. Nilsson, L. Klareskog, and O. Ouchterlony.** 1988. Reverse ELISPOT assay for clonal analysis of cytokine production. I. Enumeration of gamma-interferon-secreting cells. *J. Immunol. Methods* **110:**29–36.
11. **Fietta, A., F. Meloni, A. Cascina, M. Morosini, M. Marena, P. Troupioti, P. Mangiarotti, and L. Casali.** 2003. Comparison of a whole-blood interferon-γ assay and tuberculin skin testing in patients with active tuberculosis and individuals at high or low risk of *Mycobacterium tuberculosis* infection. *Am. J. Infect. Control* **31:**347–353.
12. **Fine, P. E. M., and L. C. Rodrigues.** 1990. Modern vaccines. Mycobacterial diseases. *Lancet* **335:**1014–1020.
13. **Göçmen, A., N. Kiper, Ü. Ertan, Ö. Kalayci, and U. Özçlik.** 1994. Is the BCG test of diagnostic value in tuberculosis? *Tubercle Lung Dis.* **75:**54–57.
14. **Houghton, R. L., M. J. Lodes, D. C. Dillon, L. D. Reynolds, C. H. Day, P. D. McNeill, R. C. Hendrickson, Y. A. W. Skeiky, D. P. Sampaio, R. Badaro, K. P. Lyashchenko, and S. G. Reed.** 2002. Use of multiepitope polyproteins in serodiagnosis of active tuberculosis. *Clin. Diagn. Lab. Immunol.* **9:**883–891.
15. **Lalvani, A., A. A. Pathan, H. McShane, R. J. Wilkinson, M. Latif, C. P. Conlon, G. Pasvol, and A. V. S. Hill.** 2001. Rapid detection of *Mycobacterium tuberculosis* infection by enumeration of antigen specific T cells. *Am. J. Respir. Crit. Care Med.* **163:**824–828.
16. **Lotte, A., O. Wasz-Höckert, N. Poisson, N. Dumitrescu, M. Verron, and E. Couvet.** 1984. BCG complications. Estimates of the risks among vaccinated subjects and statistical analysis of their main characteristics. *Adv. Tuberc. Res.* **21:**107–193.
17. **Mahon, J. B., and M. A. Chernesky.** 1999. Immunoassays for the diagnosis of infectious diseases, p. 202–210. *In* P. R. Murray, E. J. Baron, M. A. Pfaller, F. C. Tenover, and R. H. Yolken (ed.), *Manual of Clinical Microbiology*, 7th ed. ASM Press, Washington, D.C.
18. **Mazurek, G. H., P. A. LoBue, C. L. Daley, J. Bernardo, A. A. Lardizabel, W. R. Bishai, M. F. Iademarco, and J. S. Rothel.** 2001. Comparison of a whole-blood interferon-g assay with tuberculin skin testing for detecting latent *Mycobacterium tuberculosis* infection. *JAMA* **286:**1740–1747.
19. **Mazurek, G. H., and M. E. Villarino.** 2002. Guidelines for using the QuantiFERON®-TB test for diagnosing latent *Mycobacterium tuberculosis* infection. *Morb. Mortal. Wkly. Rep.* **51:**1–5.
20. **Podzorski, R. P., and D. H. Persing.** 1995. Molecular detection and identification of microorganisms, p. 130–157. *In* P. R. Murray, E. J. Baron, M. A. Pfaller, F. C. Tenover, and R. H. Yolken (ed.), *Manual of Clinical Microbiology*, 6th ed. ASM Press, Washington, D.C.
21. **Roche, P. W., W. J. Britton, S. S. Faibus, K. D. Naupane, and W. J. Theuvenet.** 1993. Serological monitoring of the response to chemotherapy in leprosy patients. *Int. J. Lepr.* **61:**35–43.
22. **Silva, V. M., G. Kanaujia, M. L. Gennaro, and D. Menzies.** 2003. Factors associated with a humoral response to ESAT-6, 38 kDa and 14 kDa in patients with a spectrum of tuberculosis. *Int. J. Tuberc. Lung Dis.* **7:**478–484.
23. **Wilkins, E., G. Bothamley, and P. Jackett.** 1991. A rapid, simple enzyme immunoassay for detection of antibody to individual epitopes in the serodiagnosis of tuberculosis. *Eur. J. Clin. Microbiol. Infect. Dis.* **10:**559–563.
24. **Woods, P. R., L. A. Corner, and P. Plackett.** 1990. Development of a simple rapid in vitro cellular assay for bovine tuberculosis based on the production of gamma interferon. *Res. Vet. Sci.* **49:**46–49.

Mycoplasma: Immunologic and Molecular Diagnostic Methods

KEN B. WAITES, MARY B. BROWN, AND JERRY W. SIMECKA

59

Mycoplasmas and ureaplasmas are members of a unique group of organisms (class *Mollicutes*) that are characterized by their small genomes, lack of cell walls, sterols in cell membranes, and complex nutritional requirements. The role of *Mycoplasma* and *Ureaplasma* species in human diseases was largely underappreciated until recent years, and as a result, most diagnostic laboratories ignored them. Because of their complex nutritional requirements as well as their adaptation to the host during infection, these fastidious organisms can be difficult and time-consuming to culture from patient samples. However, there are improved methods for detection, including PCR detection assays, serologic assays, and commercially available growth media, but these are still limited compared to the products for other organisms.

Several organisms in the class *Mollicutes* are associated with human disease. The best-known mycoplasma disease in humans is *Mycoplasma pneumoniae* respiratory disease, and it remains a leading cause of respiratory illness worldwide. Some members of the *Mollicutes* are also significant causes of urogenital tract disease; these include *Mycoplasma genitalium*, *Ureaplasma* species, and *Mycoplasma hominis*. A number of other mycoplasma infections occur in humans, which in some instances may also contribute to disease. Thus, mycoplasmas are emerging as primary etiologic agents in a number of human diseases. Additional evidence supports their role in exacerbation of other diseases. As diagnostic approaches become better established and more frequently used by clinical laboratories, the impact of this unique group of infectious agents in humans is likely to become better appreciated.

The purpose of this chapter is to discuss the advantages and disadvantages of current molecular and serologic diagnostic techniques for mycoplasmal and ureaplasmal infections. Established approaches to the detection of *M. pneumoniae*, *Ureaplasma*, *M. genitalium*, and *M. hominis* infections are discussed. A majority of the discussion focuses on *M. pneumoniae*, but many of the same principles and limitations of detection also apply to the other members of the *Mollicutes*.

MYCOPLASMA PNEUMONIAE

M. pneumoniae occurs endemically and epidemically in persons of all age groups. The most frequent clinical syndrome is tracheobronchitis, often accompanied by upper respiratory tract symptoms. Typical symptoms can persist for weeks to months and include hoarseness, fever, cough, sore throat, headache, chills, coryza, and general malaise (10). *M. pneumoniae* may occur in up to 20% of adults requiring hospitalization for community-acquired pneumonias in the United States (26) and probably an even greater proportion of those not requiring hospitalization. The incubation period is 1 to 3 weeks, and spread throughout households often occurs. *M. pneumoniae* can persist in the respiratory tract for several months after initial infection and sometimes for years in hypogammaglobulinemic persons (10, 36). Some people may experience extrapulmonary complications including skin rashes, pericarditis, hemolytic anemia, arthritis, meningoencephalitis, and peripheral neuropathy.

Serology

Historically, serology was the most common laboratory means of diagnosis of *M. pneumoniae* respiratory tract infections. It has the advantages of not requiring viable microorganisms, of allowing easy acquisition of small amounts of serum for storage and testing, and of having the availability of many different commercially available assays. *M. pneumoniae* has both lipid and protein antigens which elicit antibody responses in clinical infections that can be detected after about 1 week of illness, peaking at 3 to 6 weeks, followed by a gradual decline, allowing the use of several different serologic assays based on different antigens and technologies. Although serology is a historically common and useful approach to the diagnosis of mycoplasma infection, its use alone has several potential disadvantages.

One disadvantage of serology is that ideally both acute- and convalescent-phase sera need to be tested in order to confirm seroconversion. Measurement of immunoglobulin M (IgM) and IgG levels in paired specimens collected 2 to 3 weeks apart is optimal for the most accurate diagnosis of recent or current *M. pneumoniae* infection, especially in adults older than 40 years, in whom an IgM response may be minimal or absent, presumably because of reinfection (37). A fourfold or greater rise in antibody titer indicates a current or recent infection. The duration of the IgM response can be variable; it usually peaks after about 3 weeks and then gradually declines. However, IgM antibodies can last for several weeks in some cases, further complicating the interpretation of serologic data in diagnosis of acute *M. pneumoniae* infection and making it risky to base a diagnosis on the analysis of a single serum specimen for IgM. Detection of IgA responses may be a better approach to diagnosis. M. *pneumoniae* is primarily a pathogen of mucosal surfaces, and therefore IgA antibodies are produced early in infection. Serum IgA levels also decrease sooner, since the half-life of IgA in serum is short. Thus, IgA may perhaps be more reliable and useful for diagnosis of acute infection than IgM; however, few commercial tests include reagents for the detection of *Mycoplasma*-specific IgA.

One of the first serologic indicators used in diagnosis of M. *pneumoniae* infection is the presence of cold agglutinins, which does not rely on *Mycoplasma*-specific antibody responses. Cold agglutinins are IgM antibodies that agglutinate human erythrocytes at 4°C. They occur in association with M. *pneumoniae* infection in about 50% of cases within a few days, and their levels remain elevated for about 6 weeks. One hypothesis is that cold agglutinins result from cross-reactive autoantibodies against the I antigen of human erythrocytes. Another is that they develop directly as a result of antigenic alteration of erythrocytes caused by M. *pneumoniae* infection.

Performance of a qualitative "bedside cold-agglutinin test" involves placing 1 ml of anticoagulated blood in a cup of crushed ice for several minutes and then visually examining it for agglutination. On warming, the agglutination will resolve, but repeating the cooling procedure can reproduce it. A positive test for a patient in whom mycoplasmal infection is strongly suspected may have some clinical value. A more precise test is to determine the cold-agglutinin titer by reacting 0.1 ml of doubling dilutions of patient sera with 0.1 ml of a 1% suspension of washed human type O erythrocytes in a microtiter plate and determining the highest dilution at which agglutination occurs after 30 min of incubation at 4°C. Titers of 64 to 128 or a fourfold or greater rise in titer suggest a recent M. *pneumoniae* infection, and the magnitude of the cold-agglutinin response may correlate directly with the severity of pulmonary disease. Detection of cold agglutinins is generally not recommended for the diagnosis of M. *pneumoniae* infection since cold agglutinins are associated with a wide variety of conditions, such as viral infections and collagen vascular diseases, and, more importantly, specific serologic assays are now widely available.

Complement fixation (CF) was the major diagnostic technique used to measure M. *pneumoniae*-specific serum antibodies for many years. Seroconversion, defined as a four-fold change in titer, measured in paired sera collected 2 to 4 weeks apart and assayed simultaneously, provides the greatest diagnostic accuracy. However, CF measures mainly the early IgM response and is unable to differentiate the other antibody classes. In addition, CF has limited sensitivity and specificity because the glycolipid antigen mixture used is not specific for M. *pneumoniae* and may be found in other microorganisms, as well as human tissues and even plants. Cross-reactions with other organisms, most notably M. *genitalium* (21), are well recognized, and false-positive results due to cross-reactive autoantibodies induced by acute inflammation from other unrelated causes may occur. To help overcome the problem with cross-reactivity, confirmation of positive CF results using Western blotting can be done, but this adds to the time and cost. Commercial assays for detection of M. *pneumoniae* antibodies by Western immunoblotting are available in Europe (Virotech, Rüsselheim, Germany) but not yet in the United States.

Most clinical laboratories have replaced CF with techniques of greater sensitivity and specificity. Numerous assay formats have been developed over the past several years and

sold as commercial kits. Commercial kits are often evaluated using CF as the reference method. However, considering its lack of antibody class distinction and its cross-reactivity with other microorganisms, CF is not really suitable as a reference standard. Many of these tests, however, have not been fully evaluated and compared. In addition, the extent to which newer commercial serologic assays for M. *pneumoniae* will cross-react with M. *genitalium* or other mycoplasma was not established with certainty, but this seems less likely to be a problem than with CF.

An in-depth discussion of various types of commercial M. *pneumoniae* antibody assays and a comparative analysis of them based on published studies is available in a recent review (41). Table 1 summarizes the three most popular types of serologic assays used to detect M. *pneumoniae* infection that have been developed commercially. These are indirect immunofluorescence, particle agglutination, and enzyme immunoassays (EIAs).

Experience with EIAs dates back to the 1970s, and these assays are now the most widely used techniques for measuring antibodies against M. *pneumoniae*. A review of Food and Drug Administration-approved diagnostic tests reveals at least a dozen different M. *pneumoniae* EIAs marketed in the United States over the past several years, all of which are described as having either moderate or high complexity according to CLIA (Clinical Laboratory Improvement Act) classification. EIAs are more sensitive for detecting acute infection than is culture and can be comparable in sensitivity to PCR, provided that sufficient time has elapsed since infection for antibody to develop and that the patient has a functional immune system. Although most EIAs are sold as 96-well microtiter plate formats, some can be obtained as breakaway microwell strips, which allow smaller numbers of sera to be tested economically.

There are two EIAs packaged as qualitative membrane-based procedures for the detection of single test specimens. These are truly rapid EIAs (taking 10 min or less) and are simple to perform. The Meridian ImmunoCard (Meridian Diagnostics, Cincinnati, Ohio) is an IgM-only assay that is simple to read and is especially useful for testing pediatric samples. However, as discussed above, there are limitations in interpreting the results of IgM-only assays. The Remel EIA (Remel Laboratories, Lenexa, Kans.) is a membrane-based assay that detects IgM and IgG simultaneously. Although acute- and convalescent-phase sera should be tested quantitatively for both IgG and IgM for greatest diagnostic accuracy, the practical value of the qualitative single point-of-care tests offered by both kits is lost if paired specimens are required. Thus, these single point-of-care tests can be useful if the potential limitations are considered in the diagnosis.

Molecular Biology-Based Techniques

The attention focused on nucleic acid amplification techniques, such as PCR, has largely eclipsed earlier interest in nonamplified antigen detection or DNA hybridization systems. Numerous studies since the late 1980s using simulated clinical specimens, animal models, and clinical trials have validated the ability of the PCR assay to detect M. *pneumoniae*, often in conjunction with serology and/or culture (for example, see reference 8). The same types of clinical specimens that can undergo culture, such as throat swabs, nasopharyngeal swabs, sputum, and other sterile tissues or body fluids, can also be tested by the PCR assay. Additional advantages of PCR assays are that they can be used to detect mycoplasmas in tissue that has already been processed for

TABLE 1 Major commercial serologic test kits for M. *pneumoniae* in United States

Assay format	Antibodies measured	Equipment required	Comments and limitations
EIA	IgM, IgG, or IgA separately	Spectrophotometer/ EIA reader	EIAs are typically performed using a microtiter plate format in which antigens are adsorbed onto the polystyrene surface. Dilutions of test serum are added to the wells and incubated. Antibodies bound to the solid-phase antigen are visualized by using enzyme-labeled conjugates directed against the primary antibody and substrate read in a spectrophotometer. The amount of conjugate reacting is proportional to the levels of antibody present. EIAs have the advantages of requiring very small serum volumes (<100 μl), are adaptable to testing larger or small numbers of specimens, and can be made isotype specific.
Membrane EIA	IgM or IgG separately	None	Membrane EIAs are rapid, qualitative, point-of-care procedures designed for testing single serum specimens. A permeable membrane or filter paper is impregnated with antigen to which serum is added. This step is followed by addition of anti-human IgG or IgM enzyme conjugate. Development of color after enzyme substrate is added constitutes a positive test. Lipemic or hemolyzed serum samples will interfere with results.
Particle agglutination (PA)	IgG or IgM separately or simultaneously	None	PA tests utilize latex or gelatin as carrier particles coated with antigen that are incubated with test serum. If specific antibodies are present, the particles agglutinate, resulting in a visible reaction. PA products may provide qualitative results that can be visualized on a card or quantitative data read in a microtiter plate format. PA assays do not offer any advantages over other techniques such as EIAs or IFAs, except possibly their ease and simplicity of performance.
Indirect immunofluorescence (IFA)	IgG or IgM separately	Fluorescence microscope	Antigen is fixed to glass slides. Specific antibody is detected in dilutions of test serum after staining with anti-human IgM or IgG fluorochrome conjugate. Results can be affected by the presence of rheumatoid factor and high M. *pneumoniae*-specific IgG antibody levels. Additional procedures to validate IgM results are needed in these settings. IFA provides quantitative data but interpretation is very subjective.

histologic examination or in cultures that are contaminated so that culture is impossible (35, 40). Furthermore, PCR assays generally require only one specimen, can be completed in 1 day, may give positive results earlier in infection than serology does, and do not require viable organisms.

Most PCR-based techniques are somewhat similar and do not differ in principle from PCR assays used for detection of other microorganisms. Although most approaches focus on amplifying sequences of *Mycoplasma* genomic DNA, RNA-based amplification has also been used. Specific advantages of RNA-based amplification techniques are the high sensitivity that can be achieved due to the large number of rRNA copies per mycoplasmal cell and the fact that its detection is more indicative of viable mycoplasmas in a clinical sample (6). Table 2 lists selected original references of M. *pneumoniae* nucleic acid amplification assays that describe different target regions of the genome. However, it is difficult to compare the results of one study utilizing PCR directly with another because of the different specimen types, DNA extraction and amplification techniques, primer selection, and reference

standards used for comparison. Additional technical information, primer sequences, and tabulations of various nucleic acid amplification assays according to respiratory specimen tested or to publication with or without validation data are available in recent publications on this topic (6, 23, 27).

Comparison of the PCR technique with culture has yielded varied results, and large-scale experience with M. *pneumoniae* is still limited. In view of the enhanced analytical sensitivity of the PCR assay over culture, a positive PCR result together with negative culture can be easily

TABLE 2 Gene target used in M. *pneumoniae* nucleic acid amplification assays

Gene target	PCR product size (bp)	Reference(s)
ATPase operon gene	144	3
P1 adhesin gene	153–466	7, 15, 31
16S RNA	277	38
tuf gene	950	24

explained. However, in a situation of a negative PCR assay with a positive culture, the presence of inhibitors or some other technical problem with the PCR assay must be considered. Interestingly, PCR inhibition is much more likely to occur with nasopharyngeal aspirates than with throat swabs, according to one study (32). In support, another study (8) found that sputum was more likely to be PCR positive than were nasopharyngeal specimens, throat swabs, or throat washes. Sometimes dilution of samples overcomes inhibition of PCR due to a reduction in inhibitors during the reaction, but this is at the cost of diminished sensitivity because the nucleic acid is diluted along with any inhibitors. To overcome this problem, there are commercial reagents for nucleic acid purification that are effective in removing most inhibitors of amplification in PCR assays. Thus, the type of sample and its preparation influence the ability to detect mycoplasma infection using the PCR assay.

PCR results may not always correspond with serologic test results. For example, elderly adults with pneumonia might have age-related impairment in immunity, resulting in low serologic responses after M. *pneumoniae* infection (8). A positive PCR test together with a negative serologic test could also mean that the specimen was collected too soon in the course of the illness to allow sufficient time for antibody to develop. PCR results may also be negative as soon as 24 h following antibiotic treatment, whereas serologic results remain positive. Based on the discussion above, there are further reasons for positive serologic data when concomitant PCR testing is negative.

Despite the issues in comparing PCR with serology and culture, there is justifiable concern when PCR is used as the sole means of detection for surveillance purposes without being accompanied by culture, serology, or clinical data. It is not known with certainty whether there is a specific threshold quantity of M. *pneumoniae* in respiratory tract tissues that can differentiate colonization versus infection. Therefore, relying solely on a positive result by PCR may overestimate the clinical importance of M. *pneumoniae* as a pathogen if the population sampled has a high carriage rate and because of the propensity of this organism to cocirculate with other bacterial and viral pathogens.

Further refinements to traditional PCR assays are needed. These improvements could include the development of multiplex PCR tests to detect other atypical pathogens such as *Chlamydophila pneumoniae* simultaneously with M. *pneumoniae*, which may make PCR assays more attractive and practical for routine use in diagnostic laboratories. A number of products are currently in clinical trials, but no diagnostic products are being sold commercially in the United States thus far. Ideally, the development of multiplex assays that also provide quantitative information would be useful. In support, Hardegger et al. (12) found that a real-time PCR assay was equal to a conventional nested PCR in its sensitivity of detection of M. *pneumoniae* in clinical samples, allowing for quantitation of the amplified product during PCR and reduction in hands-on time. Tests of this nature may eventually turn out to be the most valuable for M. *pneumoniae* diagnosis since they might be able to take into account the potential confounding effect of a prolonged low-level carrier state in healthy persons. Thus, until PCR assays can be standardized, made available at a reasonable cost, and sold commercially as complete diagnostic kits suitable for use in hospital-based or other reference laboratories, this method of diagnosis is unlikely to achieve widespread use in the detection of M. *pneumoniae* infection for clinical as opposed to epidemiological purposes in the United States.

Recommended Diagnostic Approach to *M. pneumoniae* Disease

Clinical manifestations, radiographic presentation, and general laboratory tests are not sufficiently specific to allow the differentiation of M. *pneumoniae* infection from infections caused by other common microorganisms, and more specific laboratory methods are needed to confirm the diagnosis. This situation is complicated further by the fact that mycoplasmal respiratory infections often coexist with infections caused by several other respiratory pathogens (39). Mild respiratory infection suspected to be due to M. *pneumoniae* may not require a microbiological diagnosis to guide patient management. Furthermore, most of the diagnostic methods currently available for the detection of M. *pneumoniae* infections are somewhat better suited for use in epidemiological studies, as opposed to direct management of individual patients, due to their prolonged turnaround time, limited availability, and high cost. However, attempts to detect M. *pneumoniae* infection are justified in the event of an outbreak of illness in which M. *pneumoniae* is suspected or any infection that is of sufficient severity as to require hospitalization, especially in patients with an immune deficiency or underlying condition that may contribute to an unfavorable outcome.

The ideal diagnostic strategy will take advantage of both serology and PCR, since culture is laborious, time-consuming, insensitive, and expensive. There are several factors imposing limitations on the use of serology as a sole means of diagnosing M. *pneumoniae* infections. However, the single point-of-care tests, such as those marketed by Remel and Meridian, can be useful, particularly for use with pediatric patients, after considering the potential problems of serology alone. PCR assays are promising due to their analytical sensitivity and specificity, but the results can be confounded by the presence of a carrier state. Therefore, the use of serology combined with PCR can overcome many of the limitations of each approach alone in diagnosis, but the expense has to be considered along with the lack of standardized commercially available PCR assays.

UREAPLASMA UREALYTICUM AND *UREAPLASMA PARVUM*

Ureaplasma spp. are implicated in a number of human urogenital infections. *Ureaplasma* was proven to cause nongonococcal urethritis in experimental infection studies of humans. Demonstrating their role in disease is complicated by the high carriage rate of the microbe in the lower genital tract of asymptomatic, healthy women. Most recently, colonization of the placenta and/or amniotic fluid with *Ureaplasma* spp. has been associated with histologic chorioamnionitis and premature birth (42). Importantly, colonization of the neonate was linked to the development of chronic lung disease (20).

Originally thought to have two biovars composed of 14 serotypes, *Ureaplasma* is now recognized as two species: U. *parvum* (formerly biovar 1; serovars 1, 3, 6, and 14) and U. *urealyticum* (formerly biovar 2; serovars 2, 4, 5, and 7 to 13). Although some serovars are more fastidious than others, most *Ureaplasma* species are relatively easy to culture and develop classic colonies on A7 or A8 agar (commercially available from Remel Laboratories) within 2 to 3 days.

Serology

Although several EIA protocols have been published, no commercial product is available in the United States. The EIA does not differentiate between U. *parvum* and

U. urealyticum, and other approaches, such as monoclonal antibody capture assays, microimmunofluorescence, growth inhibition, and metabolic inhibition, were used to detect serovar differences. As with *M. pneumoniae,* seroconversion, a fourfold rise in titer, or change in subclass-specific response may be useful. However, serology has never been used to any significant degree for the diagnosis of ureaplasmal infections in a clinical setting.

Molecular Biology-Based Techniques

The same principles, limitations, and considerations that were discussed for *M. pneumoniae* also apply to the detection of *Ureaplasma* species. Furthermore, not all PCR assays differentiate between the two newly recognized species of *Ureaplasma.* The newest molecular biology-based tools permit the identification of species as well as limited determination of serovars (17, 18, 29). However, it is presently unclear if there are differences in the pathogenic potential of the two *Ureaplasma* species or between the different serovars, and therefore, species- and serovar-specific assays are limited to epidemiologic studies and are currently not necessary in clinical diagnosis.

The most commonly tested samples from adults include urine, urethral swabs, vaginal swabs, endocervical swabs, placental or endometrial tissues, amniotic fluid, and, more rarely, synovial fluid. Synovial fluid has a particular problem in that some samples appear to be inhibitory for PCR assays and therefore false-negative results can occur. Due to high carriage rates, vaginal swabs are of limited clinical significance for *Ureaplasma.* Urethral swabs from males are more informative than are those from females. In addition, first-void urine is a frequent sample used for PCR, but again there is the inherent caveat that first-void urine may reflect transient contamination rather than a clinically significant finding. For neonates, both transtracheal aspirates and nasopharyngeal lavages can be informative, but the results from nasopharyngeal lavages can be confounded by transient colonization due to passage through the birth canal.

Ureaplasma-specific primers were developed to target several different genes; the most commonly used are the urease, multiple-band antigen, and 16S rRNA genes (Table 3).

At least one commercial PCR test is based on the urease gene (Maxim Biotech, Inc., San Francisco, Calif.). However, extensive field-testing data and comparisons with other test systems have not been done, and this assay does not appear to differentiate between species or among serovars. Multiplex PCR assays have also been developed for the genital mycoplasmas, including *U. urealyticum* and *U. parvum.* A recent approach incorporated hybridization with specific labeled probes to standard PCR reactants in a microtiter plate format (25, 30, 43). This system has the advantage of using a single primer pair to amplify the 16S rRNA target from the major genital mycoplasmal species as well as the two ureaplasmal species, followed by a probe specific to each of the species. In addition, detailed protocols were developed by using real-time PCR. The advantages to real-time PCR are that the reactions can be completed rapidly and are quantitative, allowing an estimation of microbial load. Thus, PCR tests to detect ureaplasmas need further field evaluation, but ongoing efforts to improve and standardize PCR approaches are likely to lead to more specific and cost-effective diagnostic methods.

Recommended Diagnostic Approach

Since none of the serologic assays are available commercially, most clinical laboratories depend on the use of culture. The recommended 10B broth and A8 agar are available commercially. Although PCR assays need to be fully validated, they may be of great value when combined with culture, particularly in high-risk situations such as cultures of amniotic fluid or neonatal specimens. Research laboratories are strongly encouraged to use PCR assays that permit the differentiation of the two species of *Ureaplasma.*

MYCOPLASMA GENITALIUM

M. genitalium is a very fastidious, slow-growing mycoplasma first identified in 1981 from the urethras of men with urethritis. Its role in human disease is just now becoming apparent, mainly as a result of epidemiological studies that have used PCR to detect infections. Despite the increased awareness of the pathogenic potential of *M. genitalium,* there are

TABLE 3 Examples of PCR-based assays and gene targets for detection of urogenital mycoplasmas

Genital *Mycoplasma* species detected	Assay (references)	Target gene (references)	Clinical samples tested
Ureaplasma species	PCR	Urease (42), 16S rRNA (28)	Amniotic fluid, synovial fluid, endocervical swab, urine, urethral swab, placenta and membranes, endometrium
U. parvum and *U. urealyticum*	PCR (17, 19); PCR and microtiter plate hybridization (25, 30, 43); PCR-single strand conformation polymorphism analysis (29)	16S rRNA (25), urease (30), MBA (17, 29), 16S rRNA-23S rRNA intergenic spacers (19)	Urethral swab, urine, endocervical swab, endotracheal aspirate, nasopharyngeal aspirate, amniotic fluid, synovial fluid
M. genitalium	Real-time PCR (4, 14, 16); PCR (2, 16); PCR + liquid hybridization (9, 43)	16S rRNA (16, 43), *MgPa*/P140, Adhesin (2, 9), GyrA (4)	Urine, urethral swab, vaginal swab, endocervical swabs, synovial fluid
M. hominis	RT-PCR (1); PCR (33); PCR microtiter plate hybridization (43)	*gap* (1), 16S rRNA (33, 43)	Urine, blood, wound abscess, vaginal swab, endocervical swab, placenta and membranes, endometrium, amniotic fluid, synovial fluid

very few clinical isolates of the microbe because of the extremely fastidious nature of the microbe. This mycoplasma is believed to play a role in some cases of cervicitis and pelvic inflammatory disease in women and in urinary tract infections in both men and women.

Serology

A microimmunofluorescence assay for M. *genitalium* was developed as a research tool and shown to detect antibody responses in men with nongonococcal urethritis and women with salpingitis (11). This method is rapid, reproducible, and quite sensitive and specific, with less cross-reactivity with M. *pneumoniae* than is seen with other methods. EIA protocols using LAMP antigens were applied to population studies, and the results were confirmed by Western blotting (2). LAMP antigens have limited cross-reactivity with M. *pneumoniae*, and the EIA platform is more amenable to large-scale testing than is Western blot analysis. However, these assays are not available outside of specialized research laboratories and therefore cannot be recommended at this time for diagnostic purposes.

Molecular Biology-Based Techniques

Perhaps more than for any other mycoplasma, molecular biology-based techniques have played the critical and indeed defining role in diagnosis of M. *genitalium* infections. M. *genitalium* is notoriously difficult to culture, perhaps in part because of its ability to persist in the intracellular environment but also because of its fastidious growth requirements. The sites that are sampled, preparation of DNA template material, and conventional PCR approaches are basically identical to those used for M. *pneumoniae*, U. *urealyticum*, and U. *parvum*. The 16S rRNA (13, 16, 43) gene is a common target, as is the M. *pneumoniae* P1 adhesin homolog, *MgPa* (9, 14). Both multiplex PCR and real-time PCR assays were developed for the genital mycoplasmas (14, 16, 25, 43). Although presently unavailable, several commercial kits are currently in the development stage. Because of the extraordinary difficulty in obtaining culture-based confirmation of the presence of M. *genitalium* in clinical samples, it is especially critical that PCR assays be stringently controlled and monitored. Ideally, a positive PCR result should be confirmed by a second PCR assay using an unrelated target gene.

Recommended Diagnostic Approach

The recommended approaches to and considerations for diagnosis of M. *genitalium* infections have been recently reviewed (2). The major consideration is that one single test or combination of tests is not adequate. The difficulty in cultivation, coupled with the recent findings that suggest more variability in both PCR and EIA than was originally believed to occur, strongly suggests that the true incidence of M. *genitalium* infection may be underestimated.

MYCOPLASMA HOMINIS

Like *Ureaplasma* species and M. *genitalium*, M. *hominis* is associated with urogenital infections. However, unlike *Ureaplasma* species, detection of M. *hominis* in the vagina is of clinical significance since this microbe is a component of the suite of bacteria associated with bacterial vaginosis. M. *hominis* is also more closely linked to systemic diseases, including pyelonephritis, postpartum fever and endometritis, meningitis, bacteremia, and wound infections. Like *Ureaplasma* species, M. *hominis*, although slow growing, is relatively easy to cultivate and can be isolated using commercial

SP4 agar and broth or 10B broth and A8 agar (Remel Laboratories). Classic "fried-egg" colonies can be observed within 3 to 7 days.

SEROLOGY

As with the other urogenital mycoplasmas, no commercial serological assays are available in the United States. The most recent EIA is based on LAMP antigens (22) and is more broadly cross-reactive among different M. *hominis* strains than are assays using cell lysates as antigens (5). Confirmation by immunoblot analysis is also appropriate. Seroepidemiology to determine exposure to M. *hominis* within a population can be done with a single serum sample; however, for diagnostic purposes, paired acute- and convalescent-phase sera are likely to be more informative. As is the case for ureaplasmas, clinical experience using serology for diagnosis of M. *hominis* infections is scant.

Molecular Biology-Based Techniques

The molecular biology-based techniques and considerations are essentially the same as for the other mycoplasmal species. The most common target gene is 16S rRNA, and both multiplex PCR and real-time PCR assays have been developed (1, 25, 34, 43). Because of the relative ease of cultivation, standardization and validation of the PCR assays can be more easily achieved. Commercial PCR assays are under development and may be available in the future.

Recommended Diagnostic Approach

Since none of the serologic or molecular assays are available commercially, most clinical laboratories will have to depend on culture using specific procedures designed to recover these organisms. Use of Columbia blood agar or blood culture systems such as BacT/Alert is strongly discouraged because the number of false-negative results would be significant and culture results would therefore be unreliable.

REFERENCES

1. **Baczynska, A., H. F. Svenstrup, J. Fedder, S. Birkelund, and G. Christiansen.** 2004. Development of real-time PCR for detection of *Mycoplasma hominis*. *BMC Microbiol.* **4:**35.
2. **Baseman, J. B., M. Cagle, J. E. Korte, C. Herrera, W. G. Rasmussen, J. G. Baseman, R. Shain, and J. M. Piper.** 2004. Diagnostic assessment of *Mycoplasma genitalium* in culture-positive women. *J. Clin. Microbiol.* **42:**203–211.
3. **Bernet, C., M. Garret, B. de Barbeyrac, C. Bebear, and J. Bonnet.** 1989. Detection of *Mycoplasma pneumoniae* by using the polymerase chain reaction. *J. Clin. Microbiol.* **27:**2492–2496.
4. **Blaylock, M. W., O. Musatovova, J. G. Baseman, and J. B. Baseman.** 2004. Determination of infectious load of *Mycoplasma genitalium* in clinical samples of human vaginal cells. *J. Clin. Microbiol.* **42:**746–752.
5. **Brown, M. B., G. H. Cassell, W. M. McCormack, and J. K. Davis.** 1987. Measurement of antibody to *Mycoplasma hominis* by an enzyme-linked immunoassay and detection of class-specific antibody responses in women with postpartum fever. *Am. J. Obstet. Gynecol.* **156:**701–708.
6. **Daxboeck, F., R. Krause, and C. Wenisch.** 2003. Laboratory diagnosis of *Mycoplasma pneumoniae* infection. *Clin. Microbiol. Infect.* **9:**263–273.
7. **de Barbeyrac, B., C. Bernet-Poggi, F. Febrer, H. Renaudin, M. Dupon, and C. Bebear.** 1993. Detection of *Mycoplasma pneumoniae* and *Mycoplasma genitalium* in clinical samples by polymerase chain reaction. *Clin. Infect. Dis.* **17**(Suppl. 1):S83–S89.

8. Dorigo-Zetsma, J. W., R. P. Verkooyen, H. P. van Helden, H. van der Nat, and J. M. van den Bosch. 2001. Molecular detection of *Mycoplasma pneumoniae* in adults with community-acquired pneumonia requiring hospitalization. *J. Clin. Microbiol.* **39:**1184–1186.

9. Dutro, S. M., J. K. Hebb, C. A. Garin, J. P. Hughes, G. E. Kenny, and P. A. Totten. 2003. Development and performance of a microwell-plate-based polymerase chain reaction assay for *Mycoplasma genitalium*. *Sex. Transm. Dis.* **30:**756–763.

10. Foy, H. M. 1993. Infections caused by *Mycoplasma pneumoniae* and possible carrier state in different populations of patients. *Clin. Infect. Dis.* **17**(Suppl. 1):S37–S46.

11. Furr, P. M., and D. Taylor-Robinson. 1984. Microimmunofluorescence technique for detection of antibody to *Mycoplasma genitalium*. *J. Clin. Pathol.* **37:**1072–1074.

12. Hardegger, D., D. Nadal, W. Bossart, M. Altwegg, and F. Dutly. 2000. Rapid detection of *Mycoplasma pneumoniae* in clinical samples by real-time PCR. *J. Microbiol. Methods* **41:**45–51.

13. Jensen, J. S., E. Bjornelius, B. Dohn, and P. Lidbrink. 2004. Comparison of first void urine and urogenital swab specimens for detection of *Mycoplasma genitalium* and *Chlamydia trachomatis* by polymerase chain reaction in patients attending a sexually transmitted disease clinic. *Sex. Transm. Dis.* **31:**499–507.

14. Jensen, J. S., E. Bjornelius, B. Dohn, and P. Lidbrink. 2004. Use of TaqMan 5' nuclease real-time PCR for quantitative detection of *Mycoplasma genitalium* DNA in males with and without urethritis who were attendees at a sexually transmitted disease clinic. *J. Clin. Microbiol.* **42:**683–692.

15. Jensen, J. S., J. Sondergard-Andersen, S. A. Uldum, and K. Lind. 1989. Detection of *Mycoplasma pneumoniae* in simulated clinical samples by polymerase chain reaction. Brief report. *APMIS* **97:**1046–1048.

16. Jurstrand, M., J. S. Jensen, H. Fredlund, L. Falk, and P. Molling. 2005. Detection of *Mycoplasma genitalium* in urogenital specimens by real-time PCR and by conventional PCR assay. *J. Med. Microbiol.* **54:**23–29.

17. Knox, C. L., and P. Timms. 1998. Comparison of PCR, nested PCR, and random amplified polymorphic DNA PCR for detection and typing of *Ureaplasma urealyticum* in specimens from pregnant women. *J. Clin. Microbiol.* **36:**3032–3039.

18. Kong, F., Z. Ma, G. James, S. Gordon, and G. L. Gilbert. 2000. Molecular genotyping of human *Ureaplasma* species based on multiple-banded antigen (MBA) gene sequences. *Int. J. Syst. Evol. Microbiol.* **50:**1921–1929.

19. Kong, F., X. Zhu, W. Wang, X. Zhou, S. Gordon, and G. L. Gilbert. 1999. Comparative analysis and serovar-specific identification of multiple-banded antigen genes of *Ureaplasma urealyticum* biovar 1. *J. Clin. Microbiol.* **37:**538–543.

20. Kotecha, S., R. Hodge, J. A. Schaber, R. Miralles, M. Silverman, and W. D. Grant. 2004. Pulmonary *Ureaplasma urealyticum* is associated with the development of acute lung inflammation and chronic lung disease in preterm infants. *Pediatr. Res.* **55:**61–68.

21. Lind, K. 1982. Serological cross-reactions between "*Mycoplasma genitalium*" and *M. pneumoniae*. *Lancet* **ii:**1158–1159.

22. Lo, S. C., R. Y. Wang, T. Grandinetti, N. Zou, C. L. Haley, M. M. Hayes, D. J. Wear, and J. W. Shih. 2003. *Mycoplasma hominis* lipid-associated membrane protein antigens for effective detection of *M. hominis*-specific antibodies in humans. *Clin. Infect. Dis.* **36:**1246–1253.

23. Loens, K., D. Ursi, H. Goossens, and M. Ieven. 2003. Molecular diagnosis of *Mycoplasma pneumoniae* respiratory tract infections. *J. Clin. Microbiol.* **41:**4915–4923.

24. Luneberg, E., J. S. Jensen, and M. Frosch. 1993. Detection of *Mycoplasma pneumoniae* by polymerase chain reaction and nonradioactive hybridization in microtiter plates. *J. Clin. Microbiol.* **31:**1088–1094.

25. Maeda, S., T. Deguchi, H. Ishiko, T. Matsumoto, S. Naito, H. Kumon, T. Tsukamoto, S. Onodera, and S. Kamidono. 2004. Detection of *Mycoplasma genitalium*, *Mycoplasma hominis*, *Ureaplasma parvum* (biovar 1) and *Ureaplasma urealyticum* (biovar 2) in patients with non-gonococcal urethritis using polymerase chain reaction-microtiter plate hybridization. *Int. J. Urol.* **11:**750–754.

26. Marston, B. J., J. F. Plouffe, T. M. File, Jr., B. A. Hackman, S. J. Salstrom, H. B. Lipman, M. S. Kolczak, R. F. Breiman and The Community-Based Pneumonia Incidence Study Group. 1997. Incidence of community-acquired pneumonia requiring hospitalization. Results of a population-based active surveillance Study in Ohio. *Arch. Intern. Med.* **157:**1709–1718.

27. Murdoch, D. R. 2003. Nucleic acid amplification tests for the diagnosis of pneumonia. *Clin. Infect. Dis.* **36:**1162–1170.

28. Perni, S. C., S. Vardhana, I. Korneeva, S. L. Tuttle, L. R. Paraskevas, S. T. Chasen, R. B. Kalish, and S. S. Witkin. 2004. *Mycoplasma hominis* and *Ureaplasma urealyticum* in midtrimester amniotic fluid: association with amniotic fluid cytokine levels and pregnancy outcome. *Am. J. Obstet. Gynecol.* **191:**1382–1386.

29. Pitcher, D., M. Sillis, and J. A. Robertson. 2001. Simple method for determining biovar and serovar types of *Ureaplasma urealyticum* clinical isolates using PCR-single-strand conformation polymorphism analysis. *J. Clin. Microbiol.* **39:**1840–1844.

30. Povlsen, K., J. S. Jensen, and I. Lind. 1998. Detection of *Ureaplasma urealyticum* by PCR and biovar determination by liquid hybridization. *J. Clin. Microbiol.* **36:**3211–3216.

31. Ramirez, J. A., S. Ahkee, A. Tolentino, R. D. Miller, and J. T. Summersgill. 1996. Diagnosis of *Legionella pneumophila*, *Mycoplasma pneumoniae*, or *Chlamydia pneumoniae* lower respiratory infection using the polymerase chain reaction on a single throat swab specimen. *Diagn. Microbiol. Infect. Dis.* **24:**7–14.

32. Reznikov, M., T. K. Blackmore, J. J. Finlay-Jones, and D. L. Gordon. 1995. Comparison of nasopharyngeal aspirates and throat swab specimens in a polymerase chain reaction-based test for *Mycoplasma pneumoniae*. *Eur. J. Clin. Microbiol. Infect. Dis.* **14:**58–61.

33. Schaeverbeke, T., H. Renaudin, M. Clerc, L. Lequen, J. P. Vernhes, B. De Barbeyrac, B. Bannwarth, C. Bebear, and J. Dehais. 1997. Systematic detection of mycoplasmas by culture and polymerase chain reaction (PCR) procedures in 209 synovial fluid samples. *Br. J. Rheumatol.* **36:**310–314.

34. Stellrecht, K. A., A. M. Woron, N. G. Mishrik, and R. A. Venezia. 2004. Comparison of multiplex PCR assay with culture for detection of genital mycoplasmas. *J. Clin. Microbiol.* **42:**1528–1533.

35. Talkington, D. F., W. L. Thacker, D. W. Keller, and J. S. Jensen. 1998. Diagnosis of *Mycoplasma pneumoniae* infection in autopsy and open-lung biopsy tissues by nested PCR. *J. Clin. Microbiol.* **36:**1151–1153.

36. Taylor-Robinson, D., A. D. Webster, P. M. Furr, and G. L. Asherson. 1980. Prolonged persistence of *Mycoplasma pneumoniae* in a patient with hypogammaglobulinaemia. *J. Infect.* **2:**171–175.

37. Thacker, W. L., and D. F. Talkington. 2000. Analysis of complement fixation and commercial enzyme immunoassays for detection of antibodies to *Mycoplasma pneumoniae* in human serum. *Clin. Diagn. Lab. Immunol.* **7:**778–780.

38. van Kuppeveld, F. J., K. E. Johansson, J. M. Galama, J. Kissing, G. Bolske, E. Hjelm, J. T. van der Logt, and W. J. Melchers. 1994. 16S rRNA based polymerase chain

reaction compared with culture and serological methods for diagnosis of *Mycoplasma pneumoniae* infection. *Eur. J. Clin. Microbiol. Infect. Dis.* **13:**401–405.

39. **Waites, K. B.** 2003. New concepts of *Mycoplasma pneumoniae* infections in children. *Pediatr. Pulmonol.* **36:**267–278.

40. **Waites, K. B., C. M. Bebear, J. A. Robertson, D. F. Talkington, and G. E. Kenny.** 2001. *Cumitech 34, Laboratory Diagnosis of Mycoplasmal Infections.* Coordinating ed., F. Nolte. American Society for Microbiology, Washington, D.C.

41. **Waites, K. B., and D. F. Talkington.** 2004. *Mycoplasma pneumoniae* and its role as a human pathogen. *Clin. Microbiol. Rev.* **17:**697–728.

42. **Yoon, B. H., R. Romero, J. H. Lim, S. S. Shim, J. S. Hong, J. Y. Shim, and J. K. Jun.** 2003. The clinical significance of detecting *Ureaplasma urealyticum* by the polymerase chain reaction in the amniotic fluid of patients with preterm labor. *Am. J. Obstet. Gynecol.* **189:**919–924.

43. **Yoshida, T., S. Maeda, T. Deguchi, T. Miyazawa, and H. Ishiko.** 2003. Rapid detection of *Mycoplasma genitalium*, *Mycoplasma hominis*, *Ureaplasma parvum*, and *Ureaplasma urealyticum* organisms in genitourinary samples by PCR-microtiter plate hybridization assay. *J. Clin. Microbiol.* **41:**1850–1855.

Chlamydial Infections

LEE ANN CAMPBELL, CHO-CHOU KUO, AND CHARLOTTE A. GAYDOS

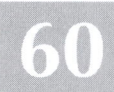

Chlamydiae are obligate intracellular bacteria, which cause many diseases in animals and humans. This chapter will focus on the diagnosis of human infections.

CHLAMYDIA TRACHOMATIS

C. trachomatis is divided into two biovars, namely, biovars trachoma and lymphogranuloma venereum (LGV) (22). The trachoma biovar causes ocular and urogenital infections. Trachoma is the leading cause of preventable blindness (22). Urogenital infections are sexually transmitted and may be transmitted to infants during birth by infected mothers, causing acute neonatal conjunctivitis and infantile pneumonia. *C. trachomatis* infections are among the most common sexually transmitted diseases among young adults and adolescents (7). The LGV biovar causes LGV.

Introduction and Epidemiology

C. trachomatis genital infections are associated with many syndromes, including cervicitis, urethritis, pelvic inflammatory disease, infertility, and ectopic pregnancy in females, and urethritis, proctitis, and epididymitis in males (7). The population prevalence in young adults is 5 to 20% (6). Up to 80 to 90% of infected women and >50% of infected men are asymptomatic (1), which creates a public health problem in disease control. Widespread screening of high-risk individuals has been recommended (7). More than 50 million cases occur worldwide, and 3 to 4 million cases occur in the United States annually (7).

Serovars of *C. trachomatis*

Eighteen serovars are recognized. The trachoma serovars are A, B, Ba, and C, the genital serovars are D to K, and the LGV serovars are L_1 to L_3. Serovars can be distinguished by serology or by genetic typing of the major outer membrane protein (MOMP) gene. Serotyping differentiation is not usually important for treatment, since the antibiotic susceptibility patterns are the same. If LGV is suspected, serovar determination should be done to guide treatment, which needs to be performed for a longer period for cases of LGV.

Diagnosis of *C. trachomatis*

Culture

The cell line most commonly used for the culture of *C. trachomatis* is McCoy cells, but others have also been used (HeLa, HEp-2, and monkey kidney cells). Since cell culture is difficult and not often available in clinical labs, it is rarely used except for sexual abuse cases and medical legal matters. Culture sensitivity compared to molecular techniques can range from 50 to 100% (an average of 85%), while culture specificity is 100% (29, 30). Culture procedures are as described below for *Chlamydia pneumoniae*, except that the preferred cell line for *C. trachomatis* is McCoy cells and the incubation time is 2 days for biovar LGV and 3 days for biovar trachoma. After incubation, the cells are fixed, stained with a fluorescein-conjugated monoclonal antibody, and read for the presence of inclusions using an epifluorescence microscope. Commercial monoclonal antibodies for either the genus-specific lipopolysaccharide or the species-specific epitope on the *C. trachomatis* MOMP are available.

Nonculture Tests

A direct cytological examination of clinical specimens for the detection of elementary bodies (EBs) can be done by direct fluorescent antibody (DFA) staining (1). The specimen swab is rolled onto a glass slide, air dried, and fixed with methanol. A fluorescein-conjugated monoclonal antibody is applied to the slide. After incubation, a coverslip is mounted with mounting medium and the slide is read for the presence of EBs with an epifluorescence microscope at a magnification of ×1,000. This test requires a trained microscopist and has a sensitivity of 80 to 85% with a specificity of 98 to 99% compared to culture (22).

Antigen detection using an enzyme immunoassay (EIA) was used before the advent of molecular tests and is still the most common nonculture detection test for *C. trachomatis* (1). Table 1 shows a comparison of the sensitivities and specificities of diagnostic tests. Methods for improving EIA sensitivity include retesting samples which give values close to the cutoff value (negative gray-zone value) by EIA and confirming the results with DFA staining or amplified testing (http://www.aphl.org/docs/NCCNGZTesting).

Serology

The microimmunofluorescence (micro-IF) test has been the "gold standard" for the detection of antibodies against chlamydiae (5). The assay is useful for population studies but not for the diagnosis of *C. trachomatis* disease in adults. It has been widely used for the diagnosis of *C. pneumoniae* (see below).

TABLE 1 Sensitivity and specificity of diagnostic tests for the detection of *C. trachomatis*

Diagnostic method or sample type	Sensitivity (%)	Specificity (%)
Tissue culture	70–85	100
DFA staining	80–85	>99
EIA	53–76	95
Hybridization (Pace2)	65–83	99
LCR		
Cervical	94.4–96.4	99.5–100
Female urine	93–98	99–100
Male urine	96.4	94–100
PCR (COBAS)		
Cervical	89.7	99.4
Female urine	89.2	99.0
Male urine	90.3	98.4
SDA		
Cervical	92.8	98.1
Female urine	80.5	98.4
Male urine	93.1	93.8
TMA		
Cervical	94.2	97.6
Female urine	94.7	98.9
Male urine	97.0	99.1
Male urethral	95.2	98.2

New Molecular Diagnostic Tests for Detection of *C. trachomatis*

Nonamplification Tests

The first molecular test, the nucleic acid probe hybridization test, which uses DNA-RNA hybridization to detect chlamydial RNA, is commercially available (GenProbe, San Diego, Calif.) and widely used (2). Recently, the Digene hybrid capture II CT-ID test (Digene, Silver Spring, Md.) was introduced. This test amplifies the detection signal, not nucleic acids. It has had limited evaluation, but in one study with cervical specimens, the sensitivity and specificity were 95.4 and 99.0%, respectively (15). It has not yet been evaluated with urine specimens.

NAATs

Nucleic acid amplification tests (NAATs) comprise the standard testing modality with the highest sensitivities. These tests include PCR (Roche Molecular Diagnostics, Indianapolis, Ind.), ligase chain reaction (LCR; Abbott Laboratories, Abbott Park, Ill.), transcription-mediated amplification (TMA; APTIMA; GenProbe), and strand displacement amplification (SDA; ProbeTec; Becton Dickinson, Sparks, Md.). All have >90% sensitivity and high specificities (Table 1) (11, 29, 30) and are approved by the Food and Drug Administration (FDA) for the detection of *C. trachomatis*. All except the LCR test, which has been taken off the market, are commercially available for use with cervical and urethral swabs or urine specimens. The TMA test is no longer produced and has been replaced by the APTIMA Combo2 assay (14). The lower specificities (Table 1) of this assay may be artificial, as this assay may be more sensitive than other NAATs, and the confirmation of uniquely positive samples by another NAAT can be problematic.

Unique positive results can be confirmed by using another primer set with the same assay (11, 14).

Comparisons and Validation of New Tests

Calculations of the sensitivity and specificity of new tests can be problematic when a new test is more sensitive than the older test to which it is being compared. "Discrepant analysis" of samples by performing a third, "tiebreaker," test has been used to confirm unique positive results but has been criticized as slightly biasing upward the sensitivity and specificity of the new test (16). In evaluating a new NAAT, there is probably an inherent underestimate of specificity since the new test may identify more true-positive results (11).

NAATs can be used to define the infected patient gold standard to evaluate chlamydia diagnostic tests. Using data from a large clinical trial comparing results from three different assays, Martin et al. determined that the use of any "two-tests-positive-out-of-three" definition resulted in estimates that were as good as or better than those based on the use of any other definition of the infected patient gold standard and provided the best combinations of sensitivity and specificity estimates (23).

Inhibitors

Specimens may contain inhibitors to amplification. Some inhibitors are labile and disappear upon retesting, diluting, or heating. The prevalence of inhibitors ranges from 1.8 to 2.6% for female and male urine samples to 19% for cervical samples. A failure to amplify the nonspecific amplification control in commercial NAATs indicates the presence of inhibitors in the specimen (http://www.aphl.org/docs/NCCInhibitorsofAmplification).

Contamination Issues

The contamination of laboratories with amplification products (amplicons) from previous PCRs can cause false-positive results. Besides recommendations of using barrier-filter pipette tips and dedicated rooms and equipment for preamplification and postamplification procedures, monitoring on a monthly basis of environmental amplicon contamination in each area where procedures are performed is recommended. The "swipe test" is performed by using a sterile NAAT sampling swab. Twenty to 30 laboratory and equipment surfaces should be sampled. The swab should be moistened with sterile molecular-grade water, used to wipe the desired area, placed into the test's transport buffer or tube, and processed as a NAAT. If an amplicon is found, the area should be cleaned with a 5 to 10% bleach solution, wiped with 70% ethanol, and retested. This should be repeated until the test is negative.

Point-of-Care Tests and Leukocyte Esterase (LE) Test

Several rapid point-of-care tests, which are performed while the patient waits for results, have been introduced. These include an individual, single-use device (optical immunoassay; Biostar Inc., Boulder, Colo.). These tests have low sensitivities (50 to 70% or less) and cannot be recommended for general use. If their sensitivities can be improved, they will be useful in settings, such as homeless shelters and detention centers, where the patient may not return for test results.

The LE test is a rapid dipstick test for use with urine specimens to determine the presence of polymorphonuclear leukocyte esterase. This nonspecific test diagnoses urethritis but cannot determine the specific cause because it only detects polymorphonuclear leukocytes. The sensitivity of the LE test for *C. trachomatis* varies from 31 to 100%, and its specificity ranges from 83 to 100% (1). This test is used to screen adolescent males and should not be used for testing specimens from women or older men (1). The LE test may be useful for screening asymptomatic men to determine who should be screened with more sensitive and specific tests (1).

New Types of Specimens for Detection of *C. trachomatis*

Because of the improved sensitivities of new NAATs, other specimens, including first-void urines from both men and women and vaginal or vulvar swabs, are useful for diagnosis (20, 26). Because urines are easily obtainable, noninvasive specimens, they offer a great advantage for large public health screening programs, for which cervical or urethral specimens cannot be obtained (13). Additionally, urine specimens are acceptable to asymptomatic individuals and those who are unwilling to have a medical examination. Because a clinician is not required for urine collection, cost savings are also generated (19). Studies have reported the successful use of self-administered vaginal swabs, but this specimen type is not yet FDA approved, except for use in the APTIMA Combo2 assay (25, 31). The usefulness of noninvasive specimens has made nontraditional sites (e.g., schools, prisons, and shopping malls) attractive for screening programs.

Choice of Diagnostic Test, Specimen, and Venue for Testing

Often, only symptomatic persons or contacts of infected patients will seek care. Symptomatic patients should receive a pelvic examination, with a sample taken for a NAAT, as recommended by the Centers for Disease Control and Prevention (CDC) as the test of choice (6). For asymptomatic infections, traditional approaches leave a large population that would not ordinarily get tested. Because physical examinations are not required for urine or vaginal swabs, the use of self-obtained specimens for testing with NAATs has enhanced the use of nontraditional sites for screening programs. For the screening of asymptomatic persons, only a NAAT can be used because none of the older tests have the necessary sensitivity.

Need for Confirmation of Positive Tests

Because of potential lower positive predictive values (i.e., <90%) of NAAT results for low-prevalence populations, where the test specificity is <100%, the CDC has recommended the use of an additional test for persons with positive screening test results (6). Approaches for the additional test include testing a second specimen with a different test that uses a different target, testing the original specimen with a different test that uses a different target or format, repeating the original test on the original specimen with a blocking antibody or competitive probe, or repeating the original test on the original specimen (6). The need for confirmatory testing is controversial and requires more definitive studies.

Tests of Cure versus Rescreening

The CDC does not routinely recommend doing a test of cure (25). Because DNA may persist for about 2 weeks after treatment, retesting by a NAAT should be done after 21 days (12).

Cost Considerations

Even though NAATs are more expensive than older nonculture tests, they are more cost-effective for use with women for preventing sequelae associated with chlamydia infections (19). If a woman does not have a pelvic exam because it is not indicated, the clinician should obtain a urine specimen or self-administered vaginal swab for amplification testing.

Recommendations for Screening and Rescreening

In the United States, the CDC recommends that all sexually active adolescent women be screened for *C. trachomatis* infection at least annually (7). Annual screening of sexually active women 20 to 25 years of age and of older women with new or multiple sex partners is recommended (5). Previously infected women are at a high risk and should be rescreened 3 to 4 months after treatment (7).

Influences of New Diagnostic Tests on Prevalence and Epidemiology

The introduction of the NAATs has resulted in a dramatic increase in estimates of the population prevalence of *C. trachomatis* infection (7). In 2000, 702,093 *C. trachomatis* infections were reported to the CDC, which was an increase from 78.5 cases per 100,000 persons in 1987 to 404.0 per 100,000 (7). Caution must be exercised in interpreting prevalence trends since the use of a more sensitive test can result in an increase in the number of positive tests with no real increase in the true infection prevalence.

Topics on laboratory diagnosis, including specimen rejection criteria, negative-gray-zone supplemental testing, and guidelines for test verification, can be found on the Association of Public Health Laboratories website (http://www.aphl.org/chlamydia_lab.cfm).

C. PNEUMONIAE

Introduction and Epidemiology of *C. pneumoniae*

C. pneumoniae is a human respiratory pathogen. The first isolate, TW183, was obtained from the conjunctiva of a Taiwanese child in 1965 (21). The association of TW183 with respiratory tract infections was discovered by serology during an outbreak of pneumonia in military conscripts in Finland, and the first respiratory isolate was obtained in Seattle from a university student with pharyngitis (21). The species *C. pneumoniae* was established in 1989 based on antibody reactivity, EB ultrastructure, and DNA homology (21). Recently, *C. pneumoniae* and *Chlamydia psittaci* were designated as a separate genus, *Chlamydophila*; however, this designation remains controversial (10, 27).

Approximately 50% of adults have antibodies against *C. pneumoniae* (21). Antibodies against *C. pneumoniae* are rare in children under the age of 5 in the United States, increase sharply from ages 5 through 14, at an increment of 6 to 8%, and continue to increase in adulthood to a prevalence of approximately 75% in the elderly. Most people are infected and reinfected throughout their life.

Transmission occurs via respiratory secretions, and secondary transmission is rare (21). The incubation period is about 3 weeks, which is longer than that for other respiratory pathogens.

Diseases Caused by *C. pneumoniae*

C. pneumoniae causes 10% of pneumonia and 5% of bronchitis and sinusitis cases in adults (21). Asymptomatic infections and mildly symptomatic illnesses are the most common outcomes. *C. pneumoniae* is associated with other diseases, such as asthmatic bronchitis, asthma exacerbation, and chronic obstructive pulmonary disease (21).

The most widely studied association of *C. pneumoniae* with a chronic disease has been that with coronary artery disease and other atherosclerotic syndromes (4). Evidence of an association includes an increased risk of cardiovascular disease (CVD) for individuals with antibodies against *C. pneumoniae*, detection of the organism in approximately 50% of atherosclerotic lesions, but not in healthy tissue, by immunocytochemistry (ICC) and PCR, and isolation of the organism from atheromatous tissue. Both in vitro and in vivo studies with animal models support a role for *C. pneumoniae* in CVD, although this has not been definitively determined (4).

Classical Methods for Diagnosis of *C. pneumoniae* Infection

Culture

The identification of cell lines that are more susceptible to *C. pneumoniae* infection than those classically used for *C. trachomatis* culture was critical to the successful culturing of *C. pneumoniae*. These include HL (human line) and Hep-2 cells (5).

Handling and Storage of Specimens

C. pneumoniae is sensitive to temperature and to freezing and thawing. Adding sucrose and glutamic acid to potassium phosphate buffer best preserves the organism's viability. Two useful storage media are SPG and 2SP (Table 2). Slow freezing preserves viability better than quick freezing. Infectivity is reduced by 23% when specimens are kept in a refrigerator (4°C) for 0.5 to 4 h and frozen at −75°C (5) but by 61% if specimens are frozen immediately. It is not necessary to freeze the samples if isolation can be done within 24 h. For thawing, organisms should be quickly thawed in lukewarm water (no higher than 37°C).

Specimen Collection

Samples for the diagnosis of a respiratory infection are usually collected from the nasopharynx (infants) or throat (older children and adults) by use of a standard swab. Sputum is difficult to process for cell culture isolation and is not a specimen of choice. Bronchoalveolar lavage fluid can be used.

Rarely, tissue samples from surgery or autopsy may be tested. Tissues should be homogenized by use of a tissue homogenizer or a mortar and pestle in SPG or 2SP medium, coarse tissue debris removed by low-speed centrifugation, and the supernatants used for culture.

Early reports demonstrating *C. pneumoniae* in peripheral blood mononuclear cells (PBMC) at a high frequency for patients undergoing coronary angiography (59%) and for blood donors (46%) by PCR raised the possibility that *C. pneumoniae* DNA in PBMC might serve as a surrogate

marker for *C. pneumoniae* in CVD (3). However, in a review of 18 studies, the overall prevalence of *C. pneumoniae* DNA in patients with CVD was 14.3%, compared to 8.5% for controls (28). Most PBMC preparation methods use 8-ml CPT tubes (BD Vacutainer Systems, Franklin Lakes, N.J.), which are centrifuged to separate the white cell layer out at $3,000 \times g$ for 10 min at room temperature. The cell layer should be removed and frozen at −70°C or placed on dry ice within 10 min. The use of a QIAamp DNA extraction kit (Qiagen, Valencia, Calif.) is common.

Culture Medium

Eagle's minimal essential medium supplemented with 10% fetal calf serum, antibiotics (gentamicin or streptomycin and vancomycin), and a fungicide (amphotericin B or mycostatin) is commonly used. Cycloheximide (0.6 to 1.0 µg/ml) is added to enhance chlamydial growth. Fast-growing cells require more cycloheximide (1.0 µg/ml for HeLa cells) than slow-growing cells (0.6 to 0.8 µg/ml for HL cells).

Isolation Procedure

Cell monolayers are prepared in 24- or 96-well culture plates or 1-dram shell vials. For the identification of inclusions, a round coverslip (12-mm diameter) is placed in the well or vial. Freshly prepared (24-h) monolayers are more susceptible than older ones. Plating 1×10^5 to 2×10^5 cells per well (24-well plate) or vial produces a confluent monolayer overnight.

Inoculation

The culture medium is removed before inoculation, and the cell monolayers are washed once with Hanks balanced salt solution. One- to two-tenths of a milliliter of inoculum is inoculated into each well or vial. A small inoculum volume gives a higher infection efficiency than a large volume. For an enhancement of infectivity, cultures are centrifuged at $900 \times g$ for 60 min at room temperature. The inoculum is removed, and culture medium is added (1 ml per well [24-well plates] or vial or 0.2 ml per well [96-well plates]). At least three wells or vials are inoculated. One is used for the detection of inclusions, and the remaining two are harvested for passage. Cultures are incubated at 35°C in a CO_2 incubator (open vessel culture) or a dry incubator (sealed culture) for 3 days.

Passages

After incubation, one coverslip is stained for the detection of inclusions, and the remaining two wells or vials are harvested for passage. The harvested material is used to inoculate three fresh monolayers. Two passages are recommended to determine whether a sample is positive or negative (9). The keys to successful passaging are "slow expansion" and the use of the minimum inoculum volume. For harvest, minimal essential medium is removed, and the cell monolayer is scraped off the vial with a plastic Pasteur pipette in a small volume (0.5 ml per two vials) of SPG or 2SP medium. Vial cultures can also be harvested by vortexing with glass beads. Although harvested cells can be used for passaging without further processing, sonication (20 s) increases the release of intracellular organisms.

Inclusion Detection

Inclusions are detected by fluorescent-antibody (FA) staining using a genus- or *C. pneumoniae*-specific monoclonal antibody conjugated with fluorescein isothiocyanate. If a genus-specific antibody is first used to detect all chlamydiae, each positive culture is then stained with a *C. pneumoniae*-specific antibody.

TABLE 2 Storage media for *C. pneumoniae*

Medium or component	Formula (component, amt or concn)
SPG	Sucrose, 75 g; KH$_2$PO$_4$, 0.52 g; Na$_2$HPO$_4$, 1.22 g; glutamic acid, 0.72 g; H$_2$O to 1 liter; pH, 7.4–7.6
2SP	Sucrose, 68.47 g; KH$_2$PO$_4$, 0.6 g; K$_2$HPO$_4$, 2.83 g; H$_2$O to 1 liter; pH, 7.4–7.6
Antibiotics	Gentamicin (10 µg/ml), or vancomycin + streptomycin (100 µg/ml each), for antibacterial activity; add amphotericin (25 µg/ml) or mycostatin (25 U/ml) for antifungal activity

Nonculture Methods

Swab Samples

Two direct detection methods, FA staining and EIA using C. pneumoniae-specific monoclonal antibodies, have been evaluated. FA staining is not sufficiently sensitive and specific for C. pneumoniae, and EIA has not been sufficiently evaluated with clinical specimens to make any recommendation.

Tissue Samples

C. pneumoniae has been detected in formalin-fixed tissues by the standard ICC avidin-biotinylated immune complex method (4). By counterstaining with hematoxylin, histology can be examined. A positive tissue control and a tissue control stained with an irrelevant antibody should be included. To avoid false-positive results from nonspecific background staining or artifacts, the staining pattern should be noted. An intracytoplasmic granular staining pattern of macrophages, endothelial cells, or smooth muscle cells is considered positive, while a homogenous staining pattern is suspect (9).

PCR (see relevant section below) is useful for the diagnosis of chronic C. pneumoniae infection because isolation is rare at this stage.

Sensitivity of Detection Methods

The sensitivity of cell culture for the diagnosis of serologically confirmed acute C. pneumoniae respiratory infection is about 60% (5). In one study, the sensitivity of PCR for diagnosis from throat swabs taken during acute respiratory infections was 95% for isolation- and serology-positive patients and 46% during the chronic stage for seropositive, isolation-negative patients (5). All isolation-negative and seronegative patients were negative by PCR.

Serology

The serological diagnosis of chlamydial infection was originally done by the complement fixation (CF) test, which uses boiled whole EBs as the antigen and is genus specific. The micro-IF test for serology and typing of C. trachomatis isolates was developed by S.-P. Wang in 1970 and subsequently modified for the serodiagnosis of C. pneumoniae (5, 21). Although micro-IF has revealed only one C. pneumoniae serotype, a peptide-based C. pneumoniae enzyme-linked immunosorbent assay (ELISA) specific for serology is difficult because the epitope is conformational.

Antigen Preparation

Cell culture-grown organisms are purified by Hypaque-76 (Nycomed, Inc., Princeton, N.J.) density gradient purification, resuspended in 0.02% formalin, and stored at 4°C ($\sim 10^9$ EB particles in stock solution). Formalin-fixed EBs are stable for many years at 4°C. An ~100% infected T155 culture flask yields 1×10^8 to 2×10^8 EBs after purification.

Formalin-Fixed Yolk Sac Membrane Homogenate

A homogenate of yolk sac membranes is used as an adhesin to bind EBs to the microscope slide. Yolk sac membranes are harvested from 13-day-old chick embryos. The yolk is drained, and the membranes are kept in a petri dish in a refrigerator overnight to drain off more yolk. Membranes are homogenized in phosphate-buffered saline (PBS) by use of a blender or mortar and pestle and washed a few times with PBS. Egg yolk adhered to the centrifuge tube is wiped off with cotton swabs after each centrifugation.

Stock suspensions of yolk sac homogenates (40% [wt/vol]) are stored at −20°C. Equal volumes (0.1 ml) of EBs and 2 to 3% yolk sac membrane homogenate in 0.02% formalin are mixed, sonicated, kept at 4°C, and used within a week to avoid aggregation. The optimal EB concentration is determined by micro-IF using a positive serum.

Test Procedure

Dip pen points (e.g., Hunter Fine Pens #104; Hunt Manufacturing, Statesville, N.C.) are used to dot the antigen onto a microscope slide. A template with four by four equidistant dots spaced 5 mm apart is placed under the slide to guide antigen application. To assist in reading, the microscope stage is marked with fluorescent paint to locate the antigen positions when the slide is centered. More than one antigen can be placed over each of 16 spots, e.g., if duplicate readings are desired or if different serovars or species are included. If more than one antigen is placed in the area of the spot, care should be taken that the antigens do not fuse with each other. Slides are air dried and fixed with acetone for 15 min at room temperature.

Twofold serum dilutions starting at 1:8 are prepared in a 96-well microtiter plate. Each dilution is applied to the antigen dot by use of a bacteriology loop and incubated in a moist chamber at 37°C for 30 min. Antibody dilutions are applied from the highest to lowest dilutions. Slides are rinsed by dipping and draining slides in a series of four beakers of 0.01 M PBS followed by three beakers of distilled water and then air dried at room temperature. Fluorescein isothiocyanate-conjugated anti-human immunoglobulin (Ig) and the counterstain rhodamine-conjugated bovine albumin or Evans blue (0.05%) are applied to each dot. Slides are incubated in a moist chamber for 30 min at 37°C, washed with PBS and distilled water, and air dried. A coverslip is mounted with FA mounting fluid.

Reading Slides

Only crisp, bright, apple-green fluorescence associated with distinctive EB particles is considered positive. Dull fluorescence associated with unevenly distributed particles without clear EB morphology is considered negative. The end point or titer is defined as the highest serum dilution with an unequivocal positive reaction. The simultaneous testing of paired sera is recommended. When a large number of sera are tested, it is more practical to screen sera first at a single dilution of 1:8. Positive sera are then titrated to determine the end points.

Interference of Rheumatoid Factor

Sera from patients with IgG autoantibodies against IgM may cross-react with the anti-C. pneumoniae IgM antibody. Thus, a positive result for IgM antibodies against C. pneumoniae should be retested after rheumatoid factor is removed by use of a commercial kit, such as Gullsorb (Meridian Diagnostic Corp., Cincinnati, Ohio).

Criteria of Serological Diagnosis

The serodiagnosis of acute C. pneumoniae respiratory infection has been based on the antibody kinetics of paired sera. Because the appearance of antibody during primary infection is often delayed, the paired sera should be collected 3 weeks instead of 2 weeks apart as with other infectious agents. For the micro-IF test, current or acute infection has been defined as follows: (i) seroconversion, (ii) fourfold titer rise, or (iii) IgM titer of ≥16 or IgG titer of ≥512. The presence of chronic antibodies has been defined as an IgG titer of 8 to 256. For the genus-reactive CF test, the presence of acute antibodies has been defined as a fourfold titer rise or a titer of ≥64.

ELISA Serology

ELISA serology using C. pneumoniae EBs as the antigen has been applied for the measurement of serum antibodies but lacks sensitivity and specificity. Variability among different commercial kits has been reported (18). Other disadvantages are that ELISA results are often based on a single dilution, reported as positive or negative based on an arbitrarily determined optical density cutoff point, and not standardized among different kits.

Development of Molecular Diagnostic Techniques

Although culture remains the gold standard for the diagnosis of acute infection, alternative methods are needed for detecting the organism during chronic disease. Although many in-house PCR methods have been developed, the literature is confounded by reports of methods that have not been standardized or validated by comparison to established methods. Of the few multicenter studies analyzing different PCR tests on the same specimens, all have found interlaboratory variations in diagnosis (e.g., see reference 8). Additional factors contributing to discrepant results are different sample collection, preparation, processing, and DNA extraction methods, a lack of appropriate controls, and no confirmation of results (9). In 2001, the CDC and the Laboratory Centre for Disease Control in Canada convened a workshop to address the standardization of methods. The recommendations are summarized as follows. Only four PCR assays, targeting a PstI fragment, rRNA, and MOMP genes, met the following criteria for a validated assay: (i) validation by more than two outside laboratories for sensitivity and specificity, using "spiked" specimens and clinical specimens; (ii) a sensitivity of <1 inclusion-forming unit (IFU); and (iii) documentation of specificity. Swab specimens should be placed in transport medium and stored as described previously. The aliquot should be centrifuged at ~18,000 × g for 15 min and processed for DNA extraction. Positive controls (DNA dilutions to <10 ng of DNA or <10 IFU) should be used. Negative controls consisting of water in place of the clinical specimen should be run on at least every fifth extraction.

A positive step toward PCR standardization has been the development and testing of a commercial kit, the LCx research-use-only PCR developed by Abbot Laboratories. In a multicenter study comparing LCx to validated assays, the results of the LCx test were promising, as (i) a 100% sensitivity was reported for positive samples with more than one copy of DNA per microliter of specimen, in contrast to those of in-house PCRs, which ranged from 54 to 94%; (ii) no false-positive results were observed with negative specimens; and (iii) LCx results were reproducible (8).

Real-time PCR assays have been developed in research laboratories but are not yet standardized for use in the clinical laboratory. The advantages of these assays are their sensitivity, decreased possibility of contamination, and ability to quantify DNA. A recent study tested 355 samples by real-time PCR, nested PCR, and touchdown enzyme time-released PCR and found real-time PCR to be sensitive and specific (17).

Impact of Nonculture Methods

The recurrent theme for C. pneumoniae diagnosis is the dire need for commercially available, user-friendly, standardized tests. The multilaboratory studies that have been done have shown variations in both micro-IF serology and PCR results (8, 24). The key impact of these methods has been the association of the organism with clinical syndromes. It is imperative that personnel performing micro-IF, ICC, or culture are trained in correct interpretation by individuals skilled in the art. Investigators should not use in-house tests that have not been compared to validated methods when investigating the disease spectrum of C. pneumoniae, as there are examples in the literature where controversial and unsubstantiated associations have been noted.

OTHER CHLAMYDIA SPECIES

Introduction and Epidemiology

Originally, C. psittaci was a heterogenous group comprised of pathogens of primarily birds and nonhuman mammals. It has now been separated into five species, C. psittaci, C. pecorum, C. feli, C. abortus, and C. caviae (10). Transmission to humans of species infecting nonhuman mammals is rare, with only a few cases of abortion reported for women who worked with C. abortus-infected sheep. Avian strains (C. psittaci) are virulent to humans and cause severe pneumonia accompanied by systemic symptoms known as psittacosis (5). Transmission occurs by the airborne route, either by direct contact with birds or by the inhalation of dust contaminated with excreta of infected birds. Cases of psittacosis are still reported from households owning birds. The largest reservoirs of infection in North America and Europe have been turkeys, ducks, and pigeons, which puts poultry breeders and processing workers at risk. Transmission from person to person has been suggested but not proven. The incubation time is usually 7 to 14 days but can range from 4 to 28 days (5).

C. psittaci is resistant to desiccation and remains viable for a month at room temperature but is destroyed within 3.5 to 5 min at 56°C. Proper cooking of poultry eliminates any risk. There have not been any reports of food-borne transmission.

Diagnosis

Culture

The diagnosis of C. psittaci infection is commonly done by cell culture isolation and serology, as described for other Chlamydia spp. Various cell lines have been used for the isolation of C. psittaci because C. psittaci grows much better than C. trachomatis and C. pneumoniae. Specimens for isolation can be throat swabs, bronchoalveolar lavage fluid, or PBMC.

Nonculture Tests

The rapid diagnosis of C. psittaci pneumonia has been reported for the use of direct immunofluorescent antibody staining of respiratory secretions. In-house PCR tests have also been developed.

Serology

The group-reactive CF test is often used for the detection of serum antibodies in patients suspected of C. psittaci infection because the infecting C. psittaci strain is unknown and strain-specific antigens are not available. The micro-IF test has been shown to detect type-specific antibodies to C. psittaci in human sera and can be used for typing isolates (5). For micro-IF testing of C. psittaci, paired sera should be taken at the onset of symptoms and 2 weeks after the first specimen.

REFERENCES

1. **Black, C. M.** 1997. Current methods of laboratory diagnosis of *Chlamydia trachomatis* infections. *Clin. Microbiol. Rev.* **10:**160–184.

2. **Black, C. M., J. M. Marrazzo, R. E. Johnson, E. W. I. Hook, R. B. Jones, T. A. Green, J. Schachter, W. E. Stamm, G. Bolin, M. E. St. Louis, and D. H. Martin.** 2002. Head-to-head multicenter comparison of DNA probe and nucleic acid amplification tests for *Chlamydia trachomatis* in women performed with an improved reference standard. *J. Clin. Microbiol.* **40:**3757–3763.

3. **Boman, J., S. Soderberg, J. Forsberg, L. S. Birgander, A. Allard, K. Persson, E. Jidell, U. Kumlin, P. Juto, A. Waldenstrom, and G. Wadell.** 1998. High prevalence of *Chlamydia pneumoniae* DNA in peripheral blood mononuclear cells in patients with cardiovascular disease and in middle-aged blood donors. *J. Infect. Dis.* **178:**274–277.

4. **Campbell, L. A., and C.-C. Kuo.** 2004. *Chlamydia pneumoniae*, an infectious risk factor for atherosclerosis? *Nat. Med. Rev. Microbiol.* **2:**23–32.

5. **Campbell, L. A., J. Marazzo, W. E. Stamm, and C.-C. Kuo.** 2001. Chlamydiae, p. 795–821. *In* N. Cimolai (ed.), *Laboratory Diagnosis of Bacterial Infections.* Marcel Dekker, Inc., New York, N.Y.

6. **Centers for Disease Control and Prevention.** 2002. Screening tests to detect *Chlamydia trachomatis* and *Neisseria gonorrhoeae* infections—2002. *Morb. Mortal. Wkly. Rep.* **51** (RR-15):1–38.

7. **Centers for Disease Control and Prevention.** 2003. Sexually transmitted disease surveillance, 2002. Centers for Disease Control and Prevention, U.S. Department of Health and Human Services, Atlanta, Ga.

8. **Chernesky, M., M. Simieja, J. Schachter, J. Summersgill, L. Schindler, N. Solomon, K. Campbell, L. A. Campbell, A. Cappuccio, C. Gaydos, S. Chong, J. Moncada, J. Phillips, D. Jang, B. J. Wood, A. Petrich, M. Hammerschlag, M. Cerny, and J. Mahony.** 2002. Comparison of an industry-derived LCx *Chlamydia pneumoniae* PCR research kit to in-house assays performed in five laboratories. *J. Clin. Microbiol.* **40:**2357–2362.

9. **Dowell, S. F., R. W. Peeling, J. Boman, G. M. Carlone, B. S. Fields, J. Guarner, M. R. Hammerschlag, L. Jackson, C.-C. Kuo, M. Maass, T. O. Messmer, D. Talkington, M. L. Tondella, R. Zaki, P. Apfalter, C. Bandea, C. Black, L. A. Campbell, C. Cohen, C. Deal, I. Fong, C. Gaydos, M. Leionen, J. Mahony, S. O'Connor, J. M. Ossewaarde, J. Papp, P. Saikku, L. Schindler, A. Schuchat, V. Stevenes, D. Talkington, C. Taylor, M. L. Tondella, C. A. Van Benenden, S.-P. Wang, and E. Zell.** 2001. Standardizing *Chlamydia pneumoniae* assays: recommendations from the Centers for Disease Control and Prevention (USA), and the Laboratory Centre for Disease Control (Canada). *Clin. Infect. Dis.* **33:**492–502.

10. **Everett, K. D. E., R. M. Busy, and A. A. Andersen.** 1999. Emended description of the order *Chlamydiales*, proposal of *Parachlamydiaceae* fam. nov. and *Simkaniaceae* fam. nov., each containing one monotypic genus, revised taxonomy of the family *Chlamydiaceae*, including a new genus and five new species, and standards for the identification of organisms. *Int. J. Syst. Bacteriol.* **49:**415–440.

11. **Gaydos, C. A., M. Theodore, N. Dalesio, B. J. Wood, and T. C. Quinn.** 2004. Comparison of three nucleic acid amplification tests for detection of *Chlamydia trachomatis* in urine specimens. *J. Clin. Microbiol.* **42:**3041–3045.

12. **Gaydos, C. A., K. A. Crotchfelt, M. R. Howell, S. Kralian, P. Hauptman, and T. C. Quinn.** 1998. Molecular amplification assays to detect chlamydial infections in urine specimens from high school female students and to monitor the persistence of chlamydial DNA after therapy. *J. Infect. Dis.* **177:**417–424.

13. **Gaydos, C. A., M. R. Howell, J. C. Quinn, J. K. T. McKee, and J. C. Gaydos.** 2003. Sustained high prevalence of *Chlamydia trachomatis* infections in female army recruits. *Sex. Transm. Dis.* **30:**539–544.

14. **Gaydos, C. A., T. C. Quinn, D. Willis, A. Weissfeld, E. W. Hook, D. H. Martin, D. V. Ferrero, and J. Schachter.** 2003. Performance of the APTIMA Combo 2 assay for the multiplex detection of *Chlamydia trachomatis* and *Neisseria gonorrheae* in female urine and endocervical swab specimens. *J. Clin. Microbiol.* **41:**304–309.

15. **Girdner, J. L., A. P. Cullen, T. G. Salama, L. He, A. Lorincz, and T. C. Quinn.** 1999. Evaluation of the Digene hybrid capture II CT-ID test for the detection of *Chlamydia trachomatis* in endocervical specimens. *J. Clin. Microbiol.* **37:**1579–1581.

16. **Green, T. A., C. M. Black, and R. E. Johnson.** 1998. Evaluation of bias in diagnostic test sensitivity and specificity estimates computed by discrepant analysis. *J. Clin. Microbiol.* **36:**375–381.

17. **Hardick, J., N. Maldeis, M. Theodore, B. J. Wood, S. Yang, S. Lin, T. Quinn, and C. Gaydos.** 2004. Real-time PCR for *Chlamydia pneumoniae* utilizing the Roche Lightcycler and a 16S rRNA gene target. *J. Mol. Diagn.* **6:**132–136.

18. **Hermann, C., K. Graf, A. Groh, E. Straube, and T. Hartung.** 2002. Comparison of eleven commercial tests for *Chlamydia pneumoniae*-specific immunoglobulin G in asymptomatic healthy individuals. *J. Clin. Microbiol.* **40:**1603–1609.

19. **Howell, M. R., T. C. Quinn, and C. A. Gaydos.** 1998. Screening for *Chlamydia trachomatis* in asymptomatic women attending family planning clinics: a cost effectiveness analysis of three preventive strategies. *Ann. Intern. Med.* **128:**277–284.

20. **Hsieh, Y.-H., M. R. Howell, J. C. Gaydos, J. K. T. McKee, T. C. Quinn, and C. A. Gaydos.** 2003. Preference among female army recruits for use of self-administered vaginal swabs or urine to screen for *Chlamydia trachomatis* genital infections. *Sex. Transm. Dis.* **30:**769–773.

21. **Kuo, C. C., L. A. Jackson, L. A. Campbell, and J. T. Grayston.** 1995. *Chlamydia pneumoniae* (TWAR). *Clin. Microbiol. Rev.* **8:**451–461.

22. **Mahoney, J. B., and M. A. Chernesky.** 2003. Chlamydia and Chlamydophila, p. 991–1004. *In* P. R. Murray, E. J. Baron, J. H. Jorgensen, M. A. Pfaller, and R. H. Yolken (ed.), *Manual of Clinical Microbiology.* ASM Press, Washington, D.C.

23. **Martin, D. H., M. Nsuami, I. E. W. Hook, D. Ferrero, D. Willis, J. Schachter, A. Weissfeld, T. C. Quinn, and C. A. Gaydos.** 2004. Optimizing the use of nucleic acid amplification tests to define the infected patient standard in clinical trials of new diagnostic tests for *Chlamydia trachomatis* infections. *J. Clin. Microbiol.* **42:**4749–4758.

24. **Peeling, R. W., S.-P. Wang, J. T. Grayston, F. Blasi, J. Boman, A. Clad, H. Freidank, C. A. Gaydos, J. Gnarpe, T. Hagiwara, R. B. Jones, J. Orfila, K. Persson, M. Puolakkainen, P. Saikku, and J. Schachter.** 2000. *Chlamydia pneumoniae* serology: interlaboratory variation in microimmunofluorescence assay results. *J. Infect. Dis.* **181** (Suppl. 3):S426–S429.

25. **Rompalo, A. M., C. A. Gaydos, N. Shah, M. Tennant, K. A. Crotchfield, G. Madico, T. C. Quinn, R. Daniel, K. V. Shah, J. C. Gaydos, and J. K. T. McKee.** 2001. Evaluation of use of a single intravaginal swab to detect multiple sexually transmitted infections in active-duty military women. *Clin. Infect. Dis.* **33:**1455–1461.

26. **Schachter, J., W. M. McCormick, M. A. Chernesky, D. H. Martin, B. Van Der Pol, P. Rice, I. E. W. Hook,**

W. E. Stamm, T. C. Quinn, and J. M. Chow. 2003. Vaginal swabs are appropriate specimens for diagnosis of genital tract infection with *Chlamydia trachomatis*. *J. Clin. Microbiol.* **41:**3784–3789.

27. Schachter, J., R. S. Stephens, P. Timms, C. Kuo, P. M. Bavoil, S. Birkelund, J. Boman, H. Caldwell, L. A. Campbell, M. Chernesky, G. Christiansen, I. N. Clarke, C. Gaydos, J. T. Grayston, T. Hackstadt, R. Hsia, B. Kaltenboeck, M. Leinonnen, D. Ocjius, G. McClarty, J. Orfila, R. Peeling, M. Puolakkainen, T. C. Quinn, R. G. Rank, J. Raulston, G. L. Ridgeway, P. Saikku, W. E. Stamm, D. Taylor-Robinson, S. P. Wang, and P. B. Wyrick. 2001. Radical changes to chlamydial taxonomy are not necessary just yet. *Int. J. Syst. Evol. Microbiol.* **51:**249.

28. Smieja, M., J. Mahony, A. Petrich, J. Boman, and M. Chernesky. 2002. Association of circulating *Chlamydia pneumoniae* DNA with cardiovascular disease: a systematic review. *BMC Infect. Dis.* **2:**21–31.

29. Van Der Pol, B., D. Ferrero, L. Buck-Barrington, E. Hook III, C. Lenderman, T. C. Quinn, C. A. Gaydos, J. Moncada, G. Hall, M. J. Tuohy, and B. R. Jones. 2001. Multicenter evaluation of the BDProbeTec ET system for the detection of *Chlamydia trachomatis* and *Neisseria gonorrhoeae* in urine specimens, female endocervical swabs, and male urethral swabs. *J. Clin. Microbiol.* **39:**1008–1016.

30. Van Der Pol, B., T. C. Quinn, C. A. Gaydos, K. Crotchfelt, J. Schachter, J. Moncada, D. Jungkind, D. H. Martin, B. Turner, C. Peyton, and R. B. Jones. 2000. Evaluation of the AMPLICOR and automated COBAS AMPLICOR CT/NG tests for the detection of *Chlamydia trachomatis*. *J. Clin. Microbiol.* **38:**1105–1112.

31. Weisenfeld, H. C., D. L. B. Lowry, R. P. Heine, M. A. Krohn, H. Bittner, K. Kellinger, M. Schultz, and R. L. Sweet. 2001. Self-collection of vaginal swabs for the detection of Chlamydia, gonorrhea, and trichomoniasis: opportunity to encourage sexually transmitted disease testing among adolescents. *Sex. Transm. Dis.* **28:**321–325.

The *Rickettsiaceae, Anaplasmataceae, Bartonellaceae,* and *Coxiellaceae*

KARIM E. HECHEMY, YASUKO RIKIHISA, KEVIN MACALUSO,
ANDREW W. O. BURGESS, BURT E. ANDERSON, AND HERBERT A. THOMPSON

61

During the past two decades, significant changes have occurred in the rickettsial field, including the redefinition of the level of pathogenicity of some rickettsiae, the isolation of new species that have emerged as pathogens of old and new syndromes, and the reemergence of old pathogenic species. In addition, phylogenetic analyses of the rickettsiae by molecular taxonomic techniques have resulted in extensive changes in the taxonomy of the rickettsiae (12).

TAXONOMY

The order *Rickettsiales* (Fig. 1) consists of the family *Rickettsiaceae* and the family *Anaplasmataceae*. The family *Rickettsiaceae* contains the genus *Rickettsia* and the genus *Orientia*. Members of the family *Rickettsiaceae* are short rods or coccobacilli, and members of the family *Anaplasmataceae* are small pleomorphic cocci. All are obligate intracellular gram-negative bacteria.

The rickettsiae that cause diseases in humans belong to the families *Rickettsiaceae* and *Anaplasmataceae* (Fig. 1 and Table 1). All human pathogenic rickettsiae belong to the α1-group proteobacteria and are nonglycolytic. The family *Rickettsiaceae* includes two genera. The genus *Rickettsia* comprises the highly related typhus (TG) and spotted fever (SFG) groups and the genetically heterogeneous species *Orientia tsutsugamushi*, which includes several serovars.

The family *Anaplasmataceae* currently comprises five established genera, namely, *Ehrlichia, Anaplasma, Aegyptianella, Neorickettsia,* and *Wolbachia,* and two "*Candidatus*" genera, namely, "*Candidatus* Neoehrlichia" and "*Candidatus* Xenohaliotis." The genera *Bartonella* and *Coxiella* are now classified out of the order *Rickettsiales* and in the orders *Rhizobiales* (α-proteobacteria) and *Legionellales* (γ-proteobacteria), respectively. However, they are included in this chapter because of historical precedence (Fig. 1).

The family *Bartonellaceae* consists of two genera, one of which, *Bartonella,* includes human pathogens belonging to the α2-group proteobacteria. Nine species of the genus *Bartonella* have now been implicated in human disease. These include *Bartonella bacilliformis* (Oroya fever and verruga peruana), *Bartonella henselae* (cat scratch disease [CSD], bacillary angiomatosis [BA], bacillary peliosis [BP], and endocarditis), *Bartonella quintana* (BA, BP, endocarditis, and trench fever), *Bartonella clarridgeiae* (CSD), *Bartonella elizabethae, Bartonella vinsonii* subsp. *berkhoffii, B. vinsonii* subsp. *arupensis, Bartonella*

koehlerae (all causing endocarditis), and *Bartonella grahamii* (neuroretinitis) (10). The family *Coxiellaceae* includes one species, *Coxiella burnetii,* the agent of Q fever. It belongs to the γ group of proteobacteria and is glycolytic (46).

EPIDEMIOLOGY

The rickettsiae are endemic worldwide (Table 1). Rickettsiae are known or thought to be associated with invertebrates (arthropods and trematodes). Invertebrates are also the vectors that transmit the rickettsiae to humans and other vertebrates. Humans are accidental hosts to the rickettsiae, except for those that cause epidemic typhus and recrudescent typhus or Brill-Zinsser disease, which belong to the species *Rickettsia prowazekii.*

Some species of rickettsiae within a biogroup appear to be confined to certain geographic areas of the world. These species acquire some biologic, pathogenic, and genetic characteristics within their respective areas that make them different enough from each other within a biogroup to be classified as new species; e.g., the SFG member *Rickettsia japonica* is confined to Japan and *Rickettsia rickettsii* appears to be limited to the Western hemisphere. *Rickettsia felis,* a newly isolated rickettsia that causes an endemic typhus-like syndrome, has at present only been isolated in the Western hemisphere. *Rickettsia conorii* is primarily found in the Mediterranean basin and Africa, and *O. tsutsugamushi* is found in Southeast Asia, Japan, Korea, Northern Australia, and some island nations in the southwest Pacific, including the Philippines, New Guinea, and the Palau Archipelago.

In contrast, other species are ubiquitously found in various geographic areas of the world and appear to be biologically, genetically, and pathologically similar or nearly identical. Two examples are *C. burnetii* and *Rickettsia typhi,* which cause Q fever and endemic typhus, respectively. Q fever is found everywhere except New Zealand.

Epidemic typhus caused by *R. prowazekii* was found worldwide in the past. However, at present it appears to be confined to foci in areas of Africa, areas of the former Soviet Union, and South America. Members of the *Bartonella* genus implicated in CSD and in the new syndromes of BA and related extracutaneous manifestations are seen on both sides of the Atlantic. The syndrome of monocytic ehrlichiosis in humans (HME), which is caused by *Neorickettsia sennetsu* and was thought to be limited to Asia and Japan, has now

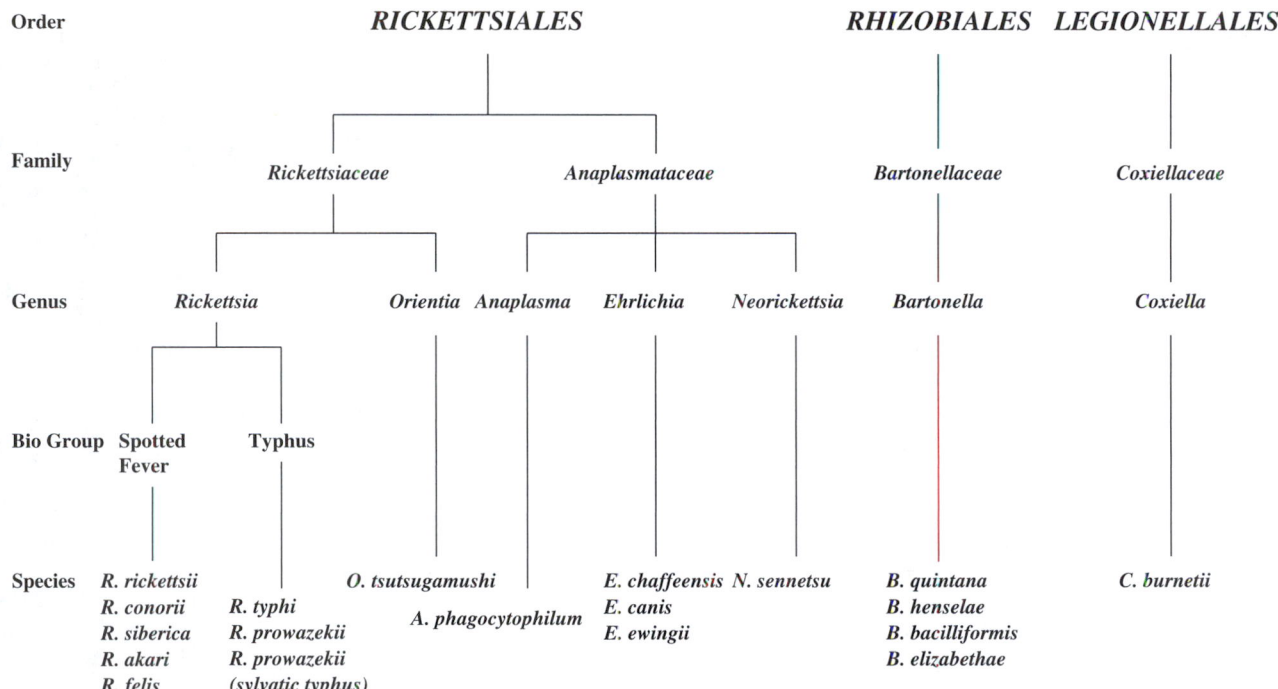

FIGURE 1 Taxonomy of human pathogens of the order *Rickettsiales*, with representative species from each genus and bacteria from genera that were formerly in the order *Rickettsiales* and were kept in this chapter for historical purposes.

been reported in other geographic regions. In the United States, the HME syndrome is caused by an ehrlichia species, *Ehrlichia chaffeensis*. In addition, a granulocytic ehrlichiosis which was reported for equines, ruminants, and canines is now diagnosed in humans (HGA). It is caused by *Anaplasma phagocytophilum*. *Ehrlichia ewingii*, once thought to infect only dogs, has recently been discovered to cause human granulocytic ehrlichiosis (HGE).

In the United States, Rocky Mountain spotted fever (RMSF), both types of endemic typhus caused by *R. typhi* and *R. felis*, HME, HGE, HGA, Q fever, CSD, and other diseases caused by *Bartonella* spp. are the most prevalent of the diseases described in this chapter. Most cases occur between May and September, except for *Bartonella* infections, which can occur year-round. Q fever is regional in occurrence and peaks slightly after the birthing seasons of ruminants (29). Between May and September, environmental conditions are optimal for tick activity, and human outdoor activities peak. However, a few cases have also been diagnosed during the winter months. Therefore, rickettsial diseases cannot be considered strictly seasonal.

In the United States, most RMSF cases occur east of the Rockies, with Oklahoma and the Carolinas leading the states. Ninety percent of endemic typhus cases in the United States are detected in the Southwest, especially in southern Texas, and in the West in southern California. A few endemic typhus cases have been reported from Virginia, North Carolina, Oklahoma, and California. Classic louse-borne epidemic typhus is not known to occur in the United States. However, a rickettsial organism closely resembling *R. prowazekii* was isolated from a flying squirrel.

Cases or outbreaks of Q fever are mainly associated with work-related exposures associated with carrier animals, e.g., sheep, cattle, and goats, especially during parturition. Also, patients with heart valve problems appear to be susceptible to

chronic infection with *C. burnetii*. *C. burnetii* is also known to be resistant to physical and chemical treatment. The importance of Q fever as a public health problem varies tremendously by country. In the United States, the disease was common in some states such as California, Texas, and the upper Midwestern states during the 1950s and 1960s; human infection is not reported at that frequency now. Although the possibilities of underreporting and misdiagnosis are often given as underlying reasons for the low frequency of Q fever in the United States, these are balanced by increased awareness of the disease due to its bioterrorism potential, the better availability of reliable tests and testing reagents, and the fact that the disease was made nationally notifiable in 1999. A relatively low frequency of sheep farming and sharply improved agricultural and mechanized dairy food production practices may have combined to make this disease comparatively less frequent in the United States, in spite of the fact that many, perhaps most, U.S. dairy herds show convincing serologic evidence of present or past infection (30).

It should be noted that *C. burnetii* is considered a biothreat (category B) agent with characteristics that place it high on the list of incapacitating agents (6). The organism's broad host range, ease of dispersal and survival, high environmental stability, and high infectivity rates for humans are major reasons for concern (45). The tendency of this organism to produce serious manifestations of persistent and chronic infections in humans adds further concern. In contrast to acute Q fever disease, the latter infections are difficult to manage and carry a significant fatality rate (29).

PATHOBIOLOGY

The pathobiology of the rickettsiae was reviewed in a monograph (3). The site of growth of all rickettsiae, except the members of the family *Bartonellaceae*, is intracellular in

TABLE 1 Representative types of pathogenic rickettsiae in humans

Species	Disease	Distribution	Agent of transmission	Target cells	Cellular location	LPS	C + G content (%)	Antigenic protein molecular mass(es) (kDa)	Plasmid
R. rickettsii	RMSF	Western hemisphere	Tick bite	Endothelium	Cytosol	Yes	32–33	190, 135	No
R. conorii	MSF	Middle East, Africa	Tick bite						
R. typhi	Endemic typhus	Worldwide	Infected flea feces						
R. prowazekii	Epidemic typhus	South America, Africa	Infected louse feces	Endothelium	Cytosol	Yes	29–30	135	No
	Recrudescent typhus	Worldwide	Reactivation of latent infection						
	Sylvatic typhus		Contact with flying squirrels						
O. tsutsugamushi	Scrub typhus	Asia	Chigger bite	Mononuclear phagocytes	Cytosol	No	28.5–30	70, 50, 63, 67	No
C. burnetii	Q fever	Worldwide	Inhalation of infected aerosol	Mononuclear phagocytes	Phagolysosome	Yes	43	28	Yes
N. sennetsu	Sennetsu ehrlichiosis	Japan, Malaysia	Metacercaria in fish	Mononuclear phagocytes	Early endosome	No		91, 70, 52, 44, 28, 20	No
E. chaffeensis	HME	United States	*Amblyomma americanum*	Mononuclear phagocytes	Early endosome	No		110, 64, 52, 42, 33, 28, 20	No
E. canis	HME	Venezuela	*Rhipicephacus sanguineus*	Mononuclear phagocytes	Early endosome			110, 64, 55, 42, 30	
A. phagocytophilum	HGE	United States	*Ixodes* ticks	Granulocytes	Nonlysosomal compartment			70, 55, 47, 44, 42	No
E. ewingii	HGE	United States	*Amblyomma americanum*	Granulocytes	Nonlysosomal compartment			74, 64, 47, 40	
B. quintana	Trench fever	Europe	Louse feces	Erythrocytes (extracellular)	Cytosol and epicellular	Yes	39–41	100, 75, 60, 35, 17	Yes
B. henselae	BA	United States, Europe				Yes			
	BA	United States, Europe	Cat fleas?						
B. elizabethae	Cat scratch fever	United States, Europe				Yes			
	Endocarditis?	United States							

the eukaryotic cell. However, there are differences in the intracellular sites of growth. Members of the SFG rickettsiae, e.g., *R. rickettsii*, grow in the cytoplasm and sometimes in the nucleus. In contrast, members of the TG, e.g., *R. typhi* and the organism causing scrub typhus, grow in the cytoplasm, while *C. burnetii* grows in the phagolysosomes of mononuclear phagocytes. Members of the family *Anaplasmataceae* replicate in the membrane-bound compartment that does not fuse with lysosomes. Except for members of *Wolbachia* and "*Candidatus* Xenohaliotis," members of the family *Anaplasmataceae* infect cells of hematopoietic and bone marrow origin of mammals or birds. Generally, wild animals are reservoirs of these bacterial infections and humans and domestic mammals or birds are infected by the bites of ticks infected with *Ehrlichia* or *Anaplasma* spp. or by the ingestion of trematodes infected with *Neorickettsia*. *Wolbachia* is so far known to infect only invertebrate cells. However, it can be found in the bloodstream of humans when released from filarial worms infesting the vertebrates. Among *Ehrlichia* species, so far *E. chaffeensis*, *E. ewingii*, and *Ehrlichia canis* have been isolated and/or detected in blood specimens from humans. For the genus *Anaplasma*, *A. phagocytophilum* is the only species, and for the genus *Neorickettsia*, *N. sennetsu* is the only species documented so far in humans.

No exotoxin has been reported to explain the pathogenic properties of the *Rickettsiaceae*, *Anaplasmataceae*, *Bartonellaceae*, and *Coxiellaceae*. The diseases caused by the rickettsiae are systemic illnesses exhibiting protean manifestations. The hallmark of the various diseases caused by the SFG and TG rickettsiae is the maculopapular rash; however, it is not found in every case. With SFG rickettsiae, it begins on the wrists and ankles and extends throughout the body. For scrub typhus and Mediterranean spotted fever (MSF), an eschar may develop at the site of the arthropod (mite or tick) bite. With TG rickettsiae, the rash is usually centrally distributed on the trunk and rarely involves the palms and soles. The internal lesions caused by the pathogen are a vasculitis localized in the endothelium and smooth muscles. Vascular permeability is increased, causing various degrees of hemorrhage, tissue edema, and peripheral circulatory failure. The extent of the internal vascular lesions is related to the degree of pathogenicity of a given species, e.g., for scrub typhus, vascular damage is not usually as severe as that seen with RMSF.

C. burnetii induces Q fever (29). Human Q fever manifests as two primary forms, an acute and a chronic from. About one-half of all human chronic infections are either mild or unrecognized. In these cases, only serologic analysis will portray evidence of a recent infection. The acute, recognized disease is often characterized by fever, headache, sweats, shaking chills, myalgia, and sometimes photophobia. In other cases, the presentation can be less constitutional, and the disease may cause pneumonia, hepatitis, and less commonly, neuritis or osteomyelitis. Interstitial pneumonia is often seen in patients with recognizable disease. For some patients, the course of events can lead to debilitating disease requiring a long period of recovery. In most cases, however, the disease is considered self-limiting, and recovery usually occurs in 10 to 20 days. Antibiotic (doxycycline) therapy can shorten the morbidity pattern.

The chronic or latent forms of the disease are of more concern. Endocarditis is the most common of these and is usually suspected only after most other diagnostic patterns and possible etiologic agents for infective endocarditis have been eliminated. The development of Q fever endocarditis usually occurs in those who have had the primary acute disease, either recognized or not, and who additionally have predisposing valvular,

vascular, or hemodynamic imperfections or deficiencies. Infective endocarditis in these patients can thus present years after the acute episode of the disease. Q fever endocarditis may or may not be characterized by nodules or vegetations on the endocardium. Thus, a lack of echocardiographic signals does not indicate a lack of infection or a lack of valvular immunopathology due to *C. burnetii*. A lingering chronic disease syndrome after acute Q fever has also been described and is termed "Q fatigue syndrome." Patients with this syndrome have indications of the organism in their bone marrow cells (presumably promonocytes) and do seem to get well (19). These patients are also characterized by a genetic proclivity to dysregulate normal cytokine shutdown after recovery from acute inflammatory episodes of Q fever (20).

Finally, the infection by *Coxiella* of human parturient tissues during pregnancy raises concerns that the proclivity of the organism to infect sheep and goat placental tissues and cow udder tissues may not be limited to ungulates. Indeed, there is increasing evidence and awareness of the dangers of exposure of pregnant human females to the organism (25). Infection of these tissues, as with defective valves, can occur long after acute disease. Unique among the rickettsiae, *C. burnetii* exhibits antigenic phase variation. It exists in two phases (I and II), which appear to be host influenced. Phase I exists in nature and changes to phase II after continuous subculturing in tissue or egg yolk sac cultures. This variation resembles the smooth-rough variation seen in other bacteria. Biochemical studies have suggested that this variation is due to changes in the sugar residue of the lipopolysaccharide (LPS). This phase variation is important in the preparation of diagnostic reagents and the interpretation of test results (29).

Human ehrlichiosis and anaplasmosis also exhibit nonspecific protean manifestations (11, 38), which are similar to those observed in patients with RMSF. However, only 20 to 30% of patients have a rash. The onset of illness is abrupt. Symptoms include fever, chills, headache, myalgia, anorexia, nausea or vomiting, and weight loss. Thrombocytopenia, leukopenia, and liver enzyme abnormality are often reported. A meningitis syndrome or an encephalitis or encephalopathy syndrome may occur with HME, and *E. chaffeensis* may be detected in the cerebrospinal fluid. Fatal seronegative infections have been reported for human immunodeficiency virus-infected patients, and secondary infections due to *Anaplasma*-induced immunosuppression may lead to severe disease and death. The patients also lack remarkable lesions such as cell lysis, tissue necrosis, abscess formation, or severe inflammatory reactions. The monocytes and granulocytes are the primary target cells for monocytic ehrlichiosis and granulocytic anaplasmosis, respectively. The replication site for the monocytic ehrlichia agents within the cell is the early endosome, where the bacteria are found.

Bartonellaceae bacteria grow preferentially on the surfaces of eukaryotic cells and sometimes intracellularly (35). The target cells are endothelial cells and erythrocytes. *Bartonella* spp. can be cultivated in cell-free culture on brain heart infusion agar and tryptic soy agar supplemented with 5% rabbit blood in a 5% CO_2 humidified atmosphere at 35°C. Original isolates take 9 to 15 days to grow. The bartonellas have a relatively simple pattern of three major fatty acids: octodecanoic, octodecenoic, and hexadecanoic. The clinical syndromes (35) associated with the *Bartonella* species are cutaneous BA, extracutaneous infection, BP of the liver and spleen, *Bartonella* bacteremic syndrome (fever and bacteremia), cat scratch fever, and trench fever. The histopathology of lymph nodes in CSD is characterized by granuloma, a nonspecific inflammatory infiltrate, and stellate abscesses. The organisms may be stained in sections with Warthy-Starry stain. In human immunodeficiency virus-infected patients with BA, multiple subcutaneous nodules that contain argyrophilic bacillary forms are present throughout the interstitium.

LABORATORY DIAGNOSIS

Serodiagnosis is presently the method of choice for the laboratory diagnosis of the diseases described in this chapter. However, serodiagnosis is confirmatory and retrospective. New molecular PCR-based and antigen capture techniques that have been developed for research purposes are being formatted for the laboratory diagnosis of these bacteria. In the coming years, it is expected that these molecular biological techniques will greatly enhance the ability of laboratories to identify and speciate rickettsial infections. Isolation of the bacteria causing the diseases described in this chapter from clinical specimens requires expertise and specialized facilities that are not readily available in the routine diagnostic laboratory. In addition, the time required for detection in culture of most of these organisms, as well as the danger associated with their handling, is beyond the capacity of most diagnostic facilities. For example, culturing *Bartonella* from clinical samples still remains difficult, with primary isolates typically appearing after 12 to 14 days, and sometimes up to 45 days, when blood agar is used (26). Therefore, isolation of the bacterium as a diagnostic tool is limited and is also retrospective. Isolation procedures have been described in the eighth edition of *Manual of Clinical Microbiology* (31).

In this chapter, we present some of the new techniques and review the classical serodiagnostic techniques. The details of the latter can be found in the sixth edition of *Manual of Clinical Laboratory Immunology* (39). It is expected that in the coming years, laboratory diagnoses of these bacteria will evolve significantly because of these new molecular techniques.

Serodiagnosis

Currently, the principal techniques used for the serodiagnosis of rickettsial diseases are probe-based immunoassays. Complement fixation using specific bacterial antigens and agglutination-based assays using whole bacteria or bacterial antigen extract-coated latex (latex agglutination [LA]) or red blood cell (indirect hemagglutination [IHA]) particles have been described previously (39). The LA test for the serodiagnosis of RMSF is available commercially by one manufacturer (Panbio). Note that serodiagnostic test results may not indicate the species within the group antigens that cause the infection without further laboratory studies and epidemiologic investigation.

Immunoprobes

Immunoprobe-based tests (39) include the indirect fluorescence assay (IFA) and its micromodification, the micro-IF or MIF test. The micro-IF test is still considered the gold standard. Other immunoprobe tests include immunoperoxidase assays (IPAs); enzyme-linked immunosorbent assays (ELISAs), in which the antigens are adsorbed either onto the well of a microtiter plate or onto nitrocellulose in a dot blot or slot blot configuration; and immunoblot assays (IBAs). IFAs and IPAs require the whole bacterium as the antigen. The remaining immunoprobe assays use either highly purified rickettsiae or an extract.

IFA

The rickettsia IFA and its modification, the micro-IF assay, are at present considered the gold standard. Both tests are relatively sensitive and specific. Also, the reagents for these tests are available commercially from several manufacturers. For the IFA, a suspension of one antigen is spread onto the slide. For the micro-IF test, several antigens are added as dots to a single well. This test has the added advantage of simultaneously detecting antibodies to up to nine rickettsial antigens with the same drop of serum in a single well containing bacterial antigen dots. Therefore, the micro-IF test economizes both time and reagents. More importantly, however, micro-IF is a more objective test modality when the cross-reactivity levels of the antibodies in a given serum are measured against a panel of antigens. It usually takes 7 to 9 days after the onset of the disease for sera to become significantly reactive, and they remain significantly reactive for years. As a result, IFA-based tests are suited for serodiagnostic purposes and seroepidemiologic studies. For step-by-step procedures and preparations of reagents, consult the references in reference 39. With the emergence of *Ehrlichia* and *Anaplasma* infections, it is suggested that a four-specific-antigen dot test be performed on submitted sera to rule out or rule in RMSF, typhus, ehrlichiosis, or *Anaplasma* infection. For the *Bartonella* spp., two or more antigens, as needed, e.g., *B. quintana* and *B. henselae* antigens, are placed on a slide. Usually, when testing for antibodies to *C. burnetii*, two dots are prepared, one containing *C. burnetii* phase I antigens and the other containing *C. burnetii* phase II antigens. For large numbers of sera, there may be a need to first screen the sera at a 1:64 dilution. Those that score reactive are then serially diluted and titrated to the end point of 2+ immunofluorescence. For the reading of *Bartonella* slides, the bacteria should be present mostly at the periphery and outside the eukaryotic cell, and few should be intracellularly located. For the reading of ehrlichia slides, try to find morulae (characteristic mulberry-like microcolonies of bacteria) (39) in the cytoplasm of cultured cells.

Because of the rising significance of Q fever as a biothreat agent, the IFA is described here with relatively more details. IFA can be done with impure or partially purified antigens. The specific measurement of immunoglobulin M (IgM), IgG, and IgA antibodies directed against either surface protein or LPS entities or both can be accomplished. Wild-type organisms found in human infections are in antigenic phase I, which means that they contain both a full-length (nontruncated) LPS and surface protein targets. The processing and presentation of these epitopes, however, are probably not simultaneous, and thus the IgM antibody response to phase II antigen is the first detectable serologic response to infection. This is followed by an IgM response to phase I antigen and then the IgG responses to both. Phase I and phase II antigens are available commercially from Focus Technologies, Cypress, Calif. (www.focustechnologies.com). Small quantities of reference reagents for IFA for use by public health laboratories are available from the Centers for Disease Control and Prevention. Direct requests to the Q Fever Laboratory, Viral and Rickettsial Zoonoses Branch, DVRD, MS G-13, 1600 Clifton Rd. NE, Atlanta, GA 30333, or telephone (404) 639-1075.

To reduce nonspecific fluorescence, the serum diluent is 1% albumin and 0.1 g of sodium azide in phosphate-buffered saline. The diluent of the secondary antibody probe is made by mixing heat-inactivated normal serum from the same species of animal used to prepare the antiserum to a final concentration of 1% in the dilution buffer. For step-by-step procedures and preparations of reagents, request the protocol from the Viral and Rickettsial Zoonoses Branch, Centers for Disease Control and Prevention. Studies are almost always done with a fluorescein isothiocyanate-conjugated goat anti-human polyvalent probe. By screening a serum batch at 1:16 and 1:256 dilutions, a group can be sorted into those giving negative results and those giving weak positive results. For individual human specimens of suspected acute or chronic disease, it is desirable to obtain IgG and IgM titers to both antigens. For IgG determinations, a goat anti-human IgG, gamma-chain-specific conjugated antibody is used in assays of unadsorbed antisera. For accurate IgM determinations, it is desirable to remove the IgG from the serum specimen by use of a recombinant protein G suspension available in kit form (Mini-Rapi-Sep-M). The resulting supernatant after centrifugation is a 1/8 dilution of the serum. The analysis for IgM is then performed with goat anti-human IgM (mu chain specific). The testing is done as for other IFAs. Serology remains the best confirmation method for Q fever.

IPA

The IPA was developed as an alternative to the IFA (reviewed in reference 39). The IPA uses an ordinary light microscope instead of a UV microscope. Claims have been made that the sensitivity and specificity of this methodology are similar to those obtained with the IFA. Tests for antibodies to *O. tsutsugamushi* and *Rickettsia israeli* have been the most studied with the IPA technology.

ELISA

The antigens used for ELISA must be purified antigens or extracts from purified antigens. Alternatively, ELISAs based on recombinant or recombinant truncated proteins are now being developed. The whole antigens used are sonicated (all rickettsiae), disrupted in French pressure cells (*Rickettsia*), lysed (*Ehrlichia* or *Anaplasma*) in distilled water, or chemically extracted (*Coxiella*) or are LPS-like material (SFG rickettsiae) or whole rickettsiae (genus *Bartonella*). Recently, attempts to use recombinant rickettsial antigens in the ELISA format were reported to be successful for *A. phagocytophilum* (Fig. 2) (44). In

general, the ELISA for rickettsiae is performed along previously described lines (39). The optimum antigen concentration in antigen mixtures used for ELISA is obtained by block titration. However, amounts of >2 μg of material per well should not be used to coat the wells. If the ELISA plates are prepared within the diagnostic laboratory, a buffer background control (no serum) at an optical density (OD) of 0.05 and a background control, a nonreactive serum with an OD of <0.2, should be obtained. Unless a commercial kit is used, each laboratory should establish an in-house standard of operation (39).

ELISA methods for *Coxiella* use yolk sac-grown, centrifugation gradient-purified phase I and II (separately) antigens, either whole or sonicated, or subcellular fractions thereof, at 1 to 2 μg per well. High-quality phase I and phase II (whole-cell-inactivated) antigens are not always available, and when available, are usually expensive. Presently, there is no widely used ELISA employing a recombinant protein.

Dot Blot and Slot Blot

Dot blot and slot blot tests (39) represent two configurations of antigens on membrane matrix supports and depend on how the antigen is applied. The antigens used are the same as those used in the ELISA. The matrices consist of either nitrocellulose or nylon sheets; the antigen can be applied in the dot or slot format, respectively. The steps are similar to those of the standard ELISA. The chromogen used for the last step should precipitate on the matrix upon development. A correlation of the immunodot assay and IFA (51), using *A. phagocytophilum*, is shown in Fig. 3. Such tests, when reactive, do indicate the presence of antibodies but do not differentiate between active or recent and past infections.

IBA

The interpretation of test results obtained with conventional serodiagnostic techniques, e.g., ELISA, IFA, and LA, is usually difficult when the titers of sera in the conventional assay are in the "gray zone" (relatively low positive results or results

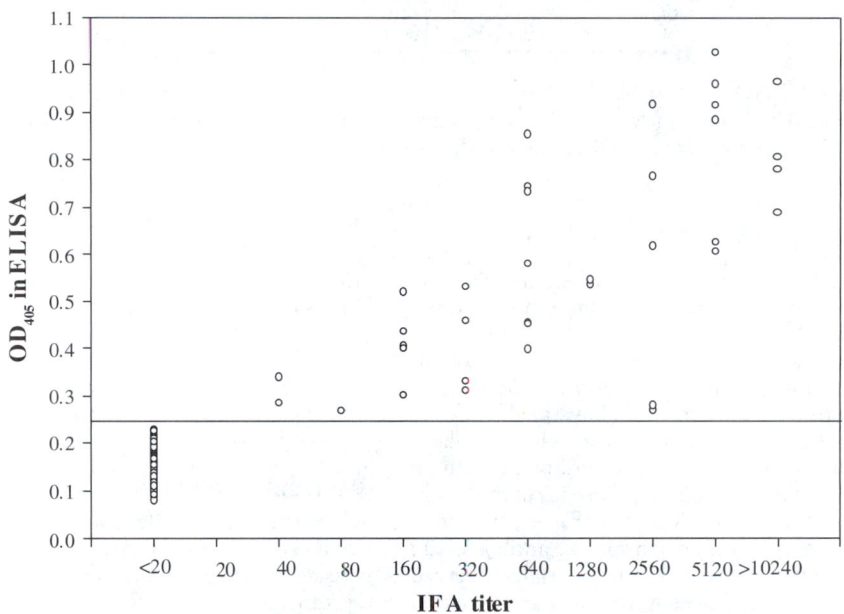

FIGURE 2 Correlation between IFA titers and ODs for ELISA with EK-rP44 as the antigen. Each circle represents one sample. The rho value calculated by Spearman's rank correlation was 0.740 ($P < 0.001$; $n = 181$). (Reprinted with permission from reference 44.)

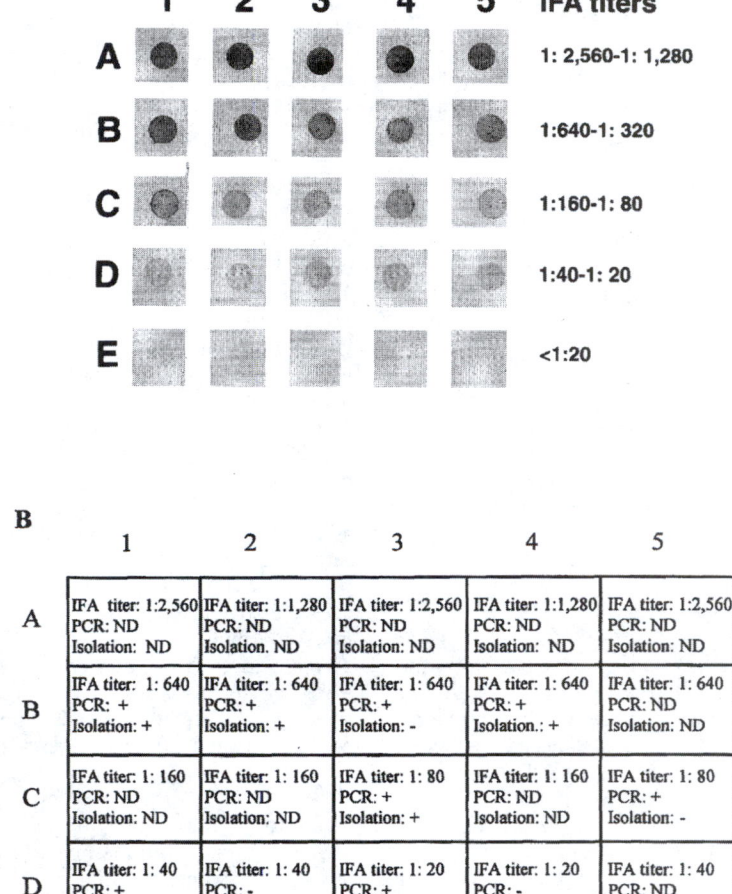

FIGURE 3 (A) Dot blot immunoassay of HGE patient sera with different IFA testing titers by use of 0.5 μg of affinity-purified recombinant P44 (rP44) antigen. The sera were diluted 1:1,000. (B) Layout of experiment. (Reprinted with permission from reference 51.)

at the minimum level of significance), when the titration results are irregular from one dilution to the other, or when there is no gradation in ODs when serum dilutions are tested. The IBA has become a necessary qualitative tool (39) for differentiating, for a significant number of events, true-positive from false-positive results. The IBA will allow the direct visualization of the antigen bands and hence help to make a determination from the antigen profile regarding the status of the test serum when whole antigens are used. Alternatively, when recombinant antigens are used (51) (Fig. 4), the direct visualization of the specific band when specific antibodies are present in the serum would confirm the test results observed with the conventional assays. Usually, the significant band(s) is determined by using sera from clinically well-defined cases. Bands for sera from patients with nonrickettsial disease that light up in the IBA for rickettsial antibodies should be noted. This reactivity is probably due to common epitopes among the rickettsial and certain nonrickettsial antigens, e.g., *Proteus* antigens. The "correct" banding pattern(s) would probably include a mixture of specific and nonspecific bands. Patterns of reactivity that include only nonspecific bands should not be considered positive. As with the dot blot and slot blot tests, reactive test results in the IBA do not differentiate between active or recent and past infections.

Molecular Diagnosis

Over the past decade, the development and refinement of PCR-based approaches to identify and differentiate rickettsiae have allowed for faster, more accurate diagnosis of rickettsial infections. Rickettsial DNA has been identified in host blood, serum, biopsy samples, and often, arthropod vectors (16) that have been collected from the patient or within the immediate surroundings of the patient. Through the amplification of portions of rickettsia-specific genes and the

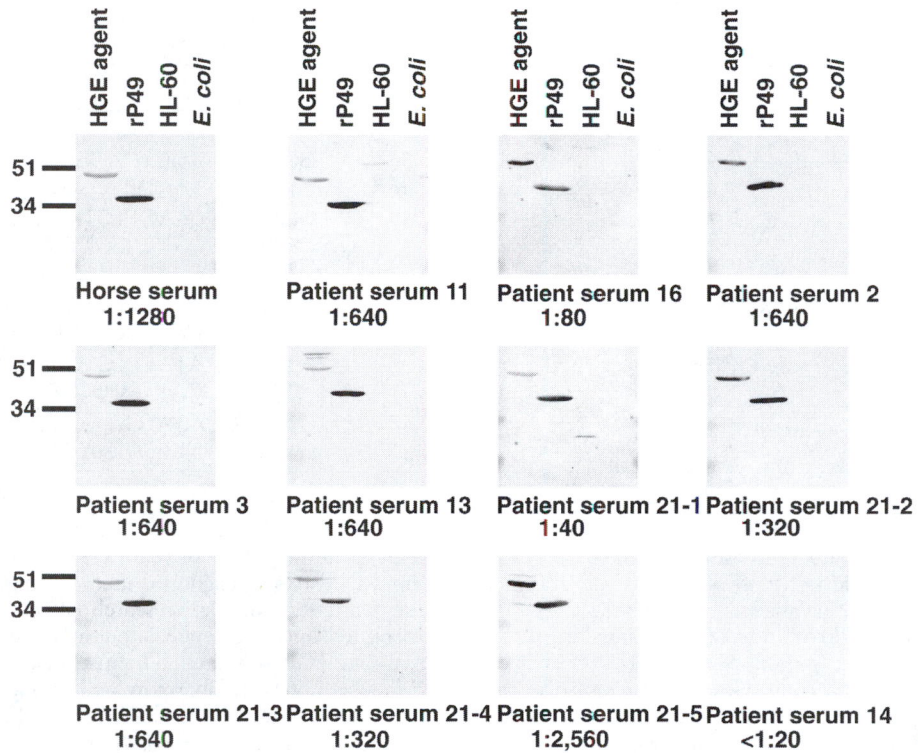

FIGURE 4 Western immunoblot analysis of anti-HGE (presently, anti-HGA) sera using purified HGE (presently, HGA) agent isolate 13 and rP44 antigen. The sera used for this study included a horse anti-HGE-agent serum; five convalescent-phase serum samples, from patients 2, 3, 11, 13, and 16; five serum samples collected at different times of illness over a 2-year period from patient 21, who was suspected of having persistent infection or reinfection; and negative control serum (IFA titer, <1:20). Samples subjected to sodium dodecyl sulfate-polyacrylamide gel electrophoresis consisted of 10 μg of purified whole-cell preparations of HGE agent strain 13, affinity-purified rP44, HL-60 cells, and *E. coli* BL21(DE30)/pLysS. These proteins were transferred to a nitrocellulose sheet and incubated with a 1:1,000 dilution of antisera. The number at the bottom of each panel represents the IFA test titer of the serum sample. The numbers on the left indicate molecular masses in kilodaltons based on broad-range prestained standards (Bio-Rad) (adapted and reprinted with permission from reference 51).

subsequent enzymatic digestion of amplicons, one is able to identify and determine the specific nature of the rickettsia in a matter of hours.

TG and SFG

Several options are available for the identification of rickettsiae from both the TG and SFG. While PCR sample preparation is of the user's preference, higher success rates for reactions are consistently observed when DNA is first isolated from the sample. The general philosophy and basic mechanics (e.g., sample preparation and salt, polymerase, and buffer concentrations) of PCR have been presented elsewhere in this volume and in reference 31. Therefore, only the details pertinent to rickettsial applications will be presented here.

Commonly used primer sets that amplify portions of genes that are unique to rickettsiae, as well as genes that are limited to SFG rickettsiae, are presented in Table 2. A screen for the presence or absence of rickettsial organisms is achieved by using genus-specific primers designed to amplify portions of genes encoding either citrate synthase or the 17-kDa genus-common antigen. A further analysis of positive samples for hypervariable portions of the genes encoding either the 120- or 190-kDa antigen common to the SFG rickettsiae can delin-

eate TG or SFG infection. Use a matched pair of primers and typical thermocycler conditions, including 35 cycles of denaturation (20 s at 95°C), annealing (30 s at 48°C), and extension (1 to 2 min at 60°C). A final extension period (7 min at 72°C) is typically added to allow for complete extension of the PCR amplicons (36). Appropriate positive and negative controls (genomic DNAs of previously characterized rickettsiae and water, respectively) should be used in place of the sample template with each reaction. PCR products should be resolved by electrophoresis on a 1% agarose gel. Amplicons matching the positive control should be considered positive. Initial reactions should determine rickettsial infection by the use of one of the genus-common primers, and subsequent PCRs should utilize one set of the SFG-specific primers listed in Table 2. A negative result with any of these three sets of primers would indicate the presence of TG rickettsiae. Exceptions exist, including *R. felis*, which will not be amplified by the SFG primers, although it is a member of the SFG rickettsiae. It is possible to separate *R. felis* from TG rickettsiae based on either sequencing or endonuclease digestion of the 17-kDa PCR product, as discussed below.

For a definitive identification of the rickettsial species, nucleotide sequence analysis of the amplicon from the

TABLE 2 Examples of PCR primer sets that allow for identification and differentiation of rickettsial species via RFLP analysis

Target gene or group	Primer	Reference	Nucleotide sequence (5'-3')
TG and SFG			
Citrate synthase gene	RpCS.877p	36	GGGGGCCTGCTCACGGCGG
	RpCS.1258n	36	ATTGCAAAAAGTACAGTGAACA
17-kDa antigen gene	Rr17.61p	49	GCTCTTGCAACTTCTATGTT
	Rr17.492n	49	CATTGTTCGTCAGGTTGGCG
SFG only			
190-kDa antigen (OmpA) gene	Rr190.70p	36	ATGGCGAATATTTCTCCAAAA
	Rr190.602n	36	AGTGCAGCATTCGCTCCCCCT
190-kDa antigen (OmpA) gene	Rr190.70p	36	ATGGCGAATATTTCTCCAAAA
	Rr190.701	40	AGTGCAGCATTCGCTCCCCCT
120-kDa antigen (OmpB) gene	Rr120	16	CTAGTGCAGATGCAAATG
			GTTTGAAATTGATAATTG

17-kDa protein- or citrate synthase-encoding gene can be used for the identification of most TG and some SFG rickettsiae. Likewise, nucleotide analysis of the amplicon from the gene encoding the 190-kDa antigen is the standard for the identification of every recognized species of SFG rickettsiae in the research laboratory setting. However, because the time and resources required to move from gel analysis to nucleotide sequence analysis are not feasible for many clinical laboratories, alternative analyses have been and are being developed. One commonly used technique involves enzymatic digestion of the original amplicon, which results in a unique digestion product for several of the TG and SFG rickettsiae. Another method is the use of real-time PCR, in which species-specific primers are used to identify the rickettsiae.

For all of the PCR-amplified products described above (encoding citrate synthase and the 17-, 120-, and 190-kDa antigens), restriction fragment length polymorphism (RFLP) analysis is a simple, cost-effective, and efficient method to aid in the specific identification of the rickettsiae. Currently, by utilizing the primers identified in Table 2 to generate a DNA template, the differentiation of rickettsiae can be achieved by using AluI for citrate synthase (15, 36) and the 17-kDa genus-common antigen (4, 49). For the 120-kDa SFG-specific antigen, digestion with RsaI (15) allows for the differentiation of several SFG rickettsiae. Based on the success of the 190.70n and 190.602p primer set (15, 16, 36), the most effective differentiation of SFG rickettsiae results from using the 190.70n (36) and 190.701 (40) primer set in combination with endonuclease digestion with RsaI, PstI, AluI, XbaI, and AvaII, which will allow for the differentiation of most of the recognized SFG rickettsiae (40).

Following the general PCR protocol described above, PCR products should be purified and an aliquot combined with 10 to 20 U of the endonuclease, the appropriate buffer, and water to a final volume of roughly 30 μl. The volume used for each component is dependent on the products used. The digestion reaction should be done according to the manufacturer's recommendations. Temperature requirements vary from 37 to 50°C, and digestion can be completed in as little as 1 h, or an overnight digestion may be suggested for best results. Due to the nature of the potential fragment sizes (~20 to ~650 bp) resulting from digestion, resolution of the digested products is best achieved by electrophoresis on an 8% polyacrylamide gel. The banding pattern can be compared to those available in the literature or to positive-control TG and/or SFG reactions carried out at the same time.

The development of real-time PCR-based diagnosis and rapid PCR-based diagnostic methods has been the focus of much attention in many research laboratories. The published literature concerning applications for rickettsial diagnosis using real-time PCR is limited. The instrumentation that has been developed for both laboratory and portable field applications was recently reviewed in the literature (24). Much real-time PCR development has focused on ensuring the specificity of the assay, identifying assay detection limits (quantitation), and determining the feasibility of utilizing different samples for template generation. Recent reports have assessed various aspects of real-time PCR for O. tsutsugamushi (22) and TG and SFG rickettsiae (14). Duplex assays for the detection of different species of Rickettsia are being developed. Similar to the PCR techniques described above, these real-time applications have been successful with infected tissue culture samples, animal tissues (blood and biopsies), and arthropod vectors.

Coxiella

The molecular identification of Coxiella species is performed with both conventional and real-time PCR methods, as summarized previously (46), and includes the use of an insertion sequence (IS1111), a superoxide dismutase gene (sod-1), an outer membrane protein gene (com-1), heat shock protein genes (htpAB), and other targets. A quantitative real-time assay has been published (5). Recently, a protein-based method for the detection of the small-cell variant protein A (ScvA) plus other protein markers comprising a Coxiella fingerprint via matrix-assisted laser desorption–time of flight (MALDI-TOF) mass spectrometry has been developed (43). The MALDI-TOF method may prove to be a powerful technique for strain and variant identification for this genus. This method works exceedingly well, with very high reproducibility, among protein samples possessing a highly basic character; with an average pI of 8.25, Coxiella contains more basic proteins than almost any other medically important genus (42).

Ehrlichia, Anaplasma, and Neorickettsia

There are two primary important facts to be aware of for the molecular diagnosis of members of the family Anaplasmataceae. Very few bacteria are generally present in blood or tissue specimens from infected humans or animals, e.g., one A. phagocytophilum genome equivalent per peripheral blood leukocyte of acutely infected horses (48). Also, enrichment or culture isolation of this group of bacteria is not practical, so testing is performed in the high background of the host cell DNA. For blood specimens from patients who had clinical signs and laboratory manifestation of HGA, 100% of culture isolation-positive specimens were PCR positive (21, 51). Also, in these studies 3 of 15 (20%) and 3 of 8 (38%) culture isolation-negative specimens were PCR positive, suggesting that PCR is more sensitive than culture isolation for the diagnosis of HGA. PCR diagnosis is more sensitive at the acute stage of infection with A. *phagocytophilum* and *E. chaffeensis* than serologic diagnosis (7, 51). However, patients who are negative by culture isolation or PCR at the acute stage seroconvert, or have a fourfold rise in IFA titers, during the convalescent stage (2, 21, 51). Thus, compared with IFA, PCR may give an overall lower clinical sensitivity. For determinations of the analytical sensitivity and specificity of the PCR test, the target specimens (human EDTA-anticoagulated blood) are spiked with serially diluted known amounts of *Anaplasma* or *Ehrlichia* DNA. The task force on consensus approach to *Anasplasmataceae* recommends that each laboratory establish its own assays and validate them with appropriate samples (47).

Single-step PCR, nested PCR, real-time PCR (27), reverse transcription-PCR, and PCR with reverse-line blot hybridization (41) are some methods employed, depending on the target gene and bacterial species being detected, to provide a sensitivity and specificity sufficient for each study purpose. As long as cross-contamination is carefully prevented, nested PCR is the most convenient and frequently used diagnostic method. The most commonly used target is the 16S rRNA gene. The *groEL* gene is another frequently used target gene. Since these genes are universally present in all bacteria, the primer sequence should be selected from bacterial species-specific regions. In the case of the 16S rRNA gene, this is near the 5′-end region. The PCR results should be unequivocal single distinct bands with the expected target size, as determined by alignment with a molecular size marker that is electrophoresed within the same gel. However, occasionally a nontarget band with a similar molecular size may be amplified from clinical specimens. The simplest way to deal with this nonspecific amplification is to sequence the nonspecific PCR product. By aligning the target and this newly obtained sequence, one can tailor new primers that selectively amplify the target sequence, but not the contaminant sequence, from given specimens. Since PCR sensitivity is affected by primer design and the PCR conditions, if a higher sensitivity is desired, these parameters should be experimentally optimized. From our experience, touch-down PCR may improve the sensitivity without requiring a change in the primer sequence for some specimens.

Other PCR targets used are repetitive-motif sequences that vary in the number of repeats among different isolates of *E. chaffeensis*. These are the variable-length PCR target gene, which has three to six 90-bp repeat units, and the 120-kDa antigen gene, which contains two to four 240-bp repeat units (33). A. *phagocytophilum* multigene family *p44* (*msp2*)-based nested PCR is approximately 50-fold more sensitive than 16S rRNA gene-based PCR due to the presence of a large number of *p44* paralogs in the genome (48). The ankyrin-rich genes (*ankA* and *epank1*) of A. *phagocytophilum* and the *omp-1* gene (*p28*) of *E. chaffeensis* are also sensitive species-specific PCR target genes.

For PCR testing, aseptically collected anticoagulated whole blood or buffy coat specimens are generally used; however, when whole blood has not been available, serum and plasma specimens have been used (28). When using serum or plasma specimens, one should keep in mind that negative results are not definitive but that positive results

are definitive. In addition to blood specimens, *E. chaffeensis* has been detected in human cerebrospinal fluids (13) and various other biopsy or postmortem human tissue specimens (9) by PCR and/or in situ hybridization. For paraffin-embedded or formalin-fixed specimens, a special precaution should be made to effectively recover and/or unmask the target DNA to reduce false-negative results.

Bartonella

The use of molecular techniques for the diagnosis of *Bartonella* infections is a rapidly expanding field. Presently, there is little consensus regarding the best test to use in the clinical laboratory. Furthermore, there are only a few comparative studies of clinical specimens regarding the sensitivity and specificity of the assays being used. Molecular techniques used for the diagnosis of *Bartonella* infections include PCR, RFLP analysis, and gene sequencing.

A PCR-RFLP method using the RNA polymerase beta-subunit gene, *rpoA*, amplifies an 825-bp region of the *rpoA* gene (37) from 13 *Bartonella* strains. Restriction enzyme analysis of the PCR fragment with ApoI, AluI, and AflIII can then differentiate the *Bartonella* strains. The application of this method to 94 lymph node samples or pus aspirates from patients suspected of having CSD resulted in 21 samples being positive for B. *henselae*.

PCR amplification targeting the riboflavin synthase gene (*ribC*) shows promise for use as a molecular diagnostic tool for CSD in the clinical laboratory (23). PCR using a unique primer pair highly homologous to segments of the *ribC* gene conserved among the *Bartonella* spp., but not to the corresponding segments in the genomes of unrelated bacteria, can amplify target DNAs from B. *henselae*, B. *quintana*, B. *bacilliformis*, B. *clarridgeiae*, B. *elizabethae*, and B. *vinsonii* subsp. *berkhoffii*. Species identification performed by restriction enzyme digestion with *TaqI* provides a unique pattern for each species. The primers appear to be specific for *Bartonella* since amplicons are not generated for a number of bacterial species, including *Afipia felis*. When used on 18 lymph node biopsies and 3 lymph node aspirates from patients with possible CSD, the assay detected B. *henselae* in 1 lymph node biopsy and all 3 lymph node aspirates (23).

PCR has also proven useful for the diagnosis of BA and BP. Unlike the localized infection of CSD, BA and BP are the result of disseminated infections caused by B. *henselae* and B. *quintana*. There are numerous case reports and case series showing the ability of PCR to detect *Bartonella* DNA in cutaneous tissues of BA patients and to identify the organism to the species level in other tissues such as bone and the brain (1). PCR can also be used to identify and determine the species of organisms obtained from cultures of tissues and blood from BA and BP patients. The latter would offer a minimally invasive approach to the diagnosis of BA and peliosis.

The molecular biology-based diagnosis of *Bartonella* endocarditis by the PCR-RFLP-based approach may lead to incorrect species identification. Since DNA sequencing is not commonly utilized in most clinical laboratories, the multigene PCR-RFLP approach should be used as a preliminary diagnostic step for patients with suspected *Bartonella* endocarditis. DNA sequencing should then follow for accurate species identification.

Real-time PCR is the most current molecular diagnostic tool for *Bartonella* infection. A real-time one-step nested PCR assay with a LightCycler instrument (LCN-PCR), using specimens of serum sampled early during the disease from 43 patients diagnosed as having *Bartonella* endocarditis, had a specificity of 100% and a sensitivity of 85.7% with serum stored for less than 1 year (50). The sensitivity gradually decreased as the length of serum storage increased. The sensitivity of this PCR method was higher than that of prolonged blood culturing but lower than that of PCR amplification from valvular biopsy specimens.

Another real-time PCR assay was recently used for the rapid detection and differentiation of *Bartonella* spp. involved in endocarditis and CSD in humans (8). The assay is based on the LightCycler instrument via fluorescence resonance energy transfer and probes hybridizing an internal 379-bp region of the *gltA* fragment amplified from genomic DNA. For the assay, PAC1 and PAC2 probes were selected to target the *gltA* gene, resulting in zero, two, or three mismatches for the different *Bartonella* species, which enabled species differentiation by melting point analysis. The assay appears to be reproducible and sensitive in that it was able to reproducibly detect up to 10 DNA copies at a concentration of one copy per reaction, on average. Species specificity was demonstrated by showing the lack of hybridization when purified DNAs from *R. prowazekii*, *R. rickettsii*, *Borrelia burgdorferi*, *C. burnetii*, and *Escherichia coli* were used in the LightCycler fluorescence resonance energy transfer assay. These organisms have the potential to result in a 379-bp PCR product from the *gltA* region as a consequence of the low-stringency annealing temperature (32). Due to its speed, sensitivity, specificity, and reproducibility, real-time PCR may be the molecular method of choice for diagnostic application to clinical samples. A summary of recent molecular methods used for the molecular diagnosis of bartonella diseases is presented in Table 3.

Interpretation of Test Results

Several aspects should be considered in the interpretation of test results for the rickettsial and other diseases described in this chapter. First, cross-reactivity within a biogroup will vary, depending on the technique used and on the host animal from which the antiserum is obtained. Human sera show extensive cross-reactivity within a biogroup. For example, cross-reactivity among the SFG or TG rickettsiae is so extensive that in most instances identification of the species within the biogroup cannot be accomplished by standard diagnostic techniques. Human antisera to the SFG rickettsiae *R. rickettsii* and *R. conorii* cannot be differentiated serologically (39). However, the geographic origin of the infection may indicate the infecting species. A reactive test result for either RMSF or MSF may be reported as reactive for SFG rickettsiae. It should be noted that for serodiagnostic purposes, identifying the species and determining the extent of cross-reactivity are not as important as they are for seroepidemiologic purposes. This is because the cure is the same, regardless of the specific rickettsial etiologic agent. In contrast to within-group cross-reactivity, cross-reactivity among groups (39) within a genus, e.g., among SFG and TG rickettsiae, may be present, but with the extent of the homologous titers being different enough from that of the heterologous titers to indicate the etiology of the rickettsial biogroup.

For scrub typhus rickettsiae, the various strains share cross-reacting epitopes that are observed in all of the various serologic procedures except the complement fixation test. The complement fixation test appears to be strain specific and therefore is contraindicated for use as a diagnostic screening procedure. For the *Ehrlichia* spp., there is apparently cross-reactivity within each of the three species, e.g., between *E. canis* and *E. chaffeensis*. In contrast, cross-reactivity among the genera of the *Anaplasmataceae*, e.g., between *E. chaffeensis* and *A. phagocytophilum*, appears at present to be minimal. Recently, a consensus statement was published for the diagnosis of human ehrlichioses (47). For

TABLE 3 Primers used for PCR

Primer name	Primer sequence (5′ to 3′)	Target organism	Target gene	PCR product size (bp)	PCR product analysis	Reference
BhCS.781p	GGGGACCAGCTCATGGTGG	*B. henselae*	*gltA* (citrate synthase)	379	Melting point analysis	8
BhCS.113n	AATGCAAAAAGAACAGTAAACA					32
PAC1	GCAAAAGATAAAAATGATTCTT-TCCG-fluorescein[a]					
PAC2	LCRed640-CTTATGGGTTTTGGT-CATCGAGT[a]					
91E	TCAAA(G,T)GAATTGACGGGGGC	Any bacterium	16S rRNA gene	492	Sequencing	17
13BS	GCCCGGGAACGTATTAC					
Zrib1F	CGGATATCGGTTGTGTTGAA	*Bartonella* species	*ribC* (riboflavin synthase)	NA	Sequencing	50
Zrib1R	CATCAATRTGACCAGAAACCA					
Zrib2F	GCATCAATTGCGTGTTCA					
Zrib2R	CCCATTTCATCACCCAAT					
BARTON-1	TAACCGATATTGGTTGTGTTGAAG	*Bartonella* species	*ribC* (riboflavin synthase)	585–588	RFLP with *Taq*I and *Ear*I	23
BARTON-2	TAAAGCTAGAAAGTCTGGCAACA-TAACG					
1400F	CGCATTGGCTTACTTCGTATG	*Bartonella* species	*rpoB* (RNA polymerase beta subunit)	825	RFLP with *Apo*I, *Alu*I, *Afl*III	37
2300R	GTAGACTGATTAGAACGCTG					

[a] Sequence of probe hybridizing an internal region of the *gltA* fragment during a real-time PCR assay.

Bartonella spp., cross-reactivity with human sera is relatively extensive. However, the homologous reactivity with a given serum is sometimes of a high enough amplitude that it can be differentiated from the heterologous reaction.

Next, for serodiagnosis, the definitive evidence of recent rickettsial infection is a minimum fourfold rise in titer between two or more serum specimens obtained at time intervals of between 7 and 21 days. Test results obtained with single serum specimens should be interpreted with caution. A negative or weakly reactive specimen taken within 2 weeks of the onset of disease may not necessarily indicate that the patient is negative for a given rickettsial disease. A second blood specimen drawn 1 or 2 weeks after the previous specimen should be requested. A positive serodiagnostic test result for one specimen usually establishes the presence of antibodies to the test antigen. It does not, however, indicate the presence of a disease state.

With the probe test, specific IgG to rickettsiae can remain positive and at a diagnostic level for years. Accordingly, a correlation of positive serologic results and an active disease condition is usually made if there is a significant increase in the antibody titer in sera between two paired serum specimens collected at ≥7-day intervals. Guidelines for the interpretation of test results are shown in reference 39. The titers stated are for reference purposes only. Laboratorians should be wary of serum samples in test runs that do not exhibit gradations in the intensity of the visual reaction (fluorescence, OD, or agglutination) as the serum dilutions reacting with the test antigen are close to the end point. Sera that exhibit gradations are probably true-positive samples. In contrast, test results for sera showing no gradation should be repeated or confirmed by a different methodology, e.g., the IBA. Such reactions might be due to nonspecific reactions, the explanation of which is at present unknown.

Agglutination-based assays (39) are best suited to detecting antibodies during active infection and are less suitable for past infections and serosurveys. This is because of the greater efficiency of specific IgM as an agglutinator than that of specific IgG. Therefore, a sample that scores reactive in such tests probably indicates an active infection or the presence of residual specific IgM. When comparing acute- and convalescent-phase sera, the paired sera should be run in the same assay to avoid interassay variation. For acute Q fever, phase II antibody titers are usually, but not always, higher than or equal to those from phase I determinations. The ratio is very dependent on when the specimens are drawn relative to the onset of symptoms. For chronic Q fever, the phase I titer for IgG is usually markedly higher than the phase II titer. An IFA titer of 1:16 or higher (class-specific or polyvalent immunoglobulins) plus signs and symptoms consistent with the disease comprises presumptive evidence of Q fever. A fourfold rise in titer is confirmatory. With only a single value, an IFA titer should be at least 1:64 to be considered positive. For surveillance studies, a value of 1:128 is considered a minimum value for a positive result.

PCR-based techniques are specific and efficient and have the potential to yield results from specimens obtained at the early stage of the disease and prior to antibiotic treatment. Subsequent analysis of infection after the clearance of rickettsiae associated with antibiotic treatment will result in negative PCR results. It should also be noted that conventional PCR may not be sensitive enough because of the relatively low number ($<10^4$ organisms/ml) (14) of these bacteria circulating in the blood of patients. Some of the more recent applications should be used to detect low levels of bacteria.

The usage of a broad-range PCR methodology can sometimes generate false-positive results due to the amplification of environmental contaminants or previously amplified products (amplicon carryover) that may be present in the clinical laboratory where PCR is routinely performed. These concerns regarding the validity of a positive result may hinder the wider usage of broad-range PCR for molecular diagnosis in the clinical laboratory. The substitution of dUTP for dTTP and the addition of uracil-N-glycosylase, both of which are compatible with direct sequencing, can be used to prevent carryover contamination (18). Simply dividing samples into multiple aliquots upon specimen arrival can serve as an important contamination control checkpoint for the subsequent procedures carried out in the laboratory (34). Confirmation of the results obtained with broad-range primers to amplify part of the 16S rRNA gene, followed by sequencing and a database search, can also be achieved by amplifying and sequencing a second genetic target, the heat shock protein gene *htrA*, specific for the identified organism (34). It should also be noted that PCR results may not be determinative in confirming the initial diagnosis for acute infections. This is because the time window for finding organisms in the blood for a successful PCR or culture test result is often narrow, probably the first 24 to 48 h after the onset of symptoms and prior to the administration of antibiotics.

Finally, the protean clinical manifestation of rickettsial diseases makes a definitive clinical diagnosis difficult without laboratory input. However, the correlation of test results with a clinical diagnosis may not always be possible because of the highly variable clinical presentation. It is recommended that diagnosticians consider the diagnosis of infection with one of the bacteria presented in this chapter if a patient presents with a high fever of unknown origin and without apparent clinical manifestations. In addition, it could be helpful to a clinician to obtain patient information pertaining to their travel to regions in which these diseases are endemic, outdoor activities, work environment (e.g., abattoirs for suspected Q fever), and other pertinent epidemiologic data. This could help diagnosticians in the clinical diagnosis of patients presenting with such protean manifestations. Because serodiagnosis is retrospective and until more molecular techniques are formatted for diagnostic use and are more accepted within the diagnostic community, it is suggested that physicians treat patients that they suspect of having one of the diseases described in this chapter before test results are available.

REFERENCES

1. **Agan, B. K., and M. J. Dolan.** 2002. Laboratory diagnosis of Bartonella infections. *Clin. Lab. Med.* **22:**937–962.
2. **Aguero-Rosenfeld, M. E., H. W. Horowitz, G. P. Wormser, D. F. Mckenna, J. Nowakowski, J. Munoz, and J. S. Dumler.** 1996. Human granulocytic ehrlichiosis: a case series from a medical center in New York State. *Ann. Intern. Med.* **125:**904–908.
3. **Anderson, B., H. Friedman, and M. Bendinelli.** 1997. *Rickettsial Infection and Immunity.* Plenum Press, New York, N.Y.
4. **Boostrom, A., M. S. Beier, J. A. Macaluso, K. R. Macaluso, D. Sprenger, J. Hayes, S. Radulovic, and A. F. Azad.** 2002. Geographic association of *Rickettsia felis*-infected opossums with human murine typhus, Texas. *Emerg. Infect. Dis.* **8:**549–554.
5. **Brennan, R. E., and J. E. Samuel.** 2003. Evaluation of *Coxiella burnetii* antibiotic resistance susceptibilities by real-time PCR assay. *J. Clin. Microbiol.* **41:**1553–1562.

6. **Centers for Disease Control and Prevention.** 2000. Recommendations and reports. Biological and chemical terrorism: strategic plan for preparedness and response. *Morb. Mortal. Wkly. Rep.* **49**(RR-4):1–14.

7. **Childs, J. E., J. W. Sumner, W. L. Nicholson, R. F. Massung, S. M. Standaert, and C. D. Paddock.** 1999. Outcome of diagnostic tests using samples from patients with culture-proven human monocytic ehrlichiosis: implications for surveillance. *J. Clin. Microbiol.* **37**:2997–3000.

8. **Ciervo, A., and L. Ciceroni.** 2004. Rapid detection and differentiation of Bartonella spp. by a single-run real-time PCR. *Mol. Cell. Probes* **18**:307–312.

9. **Dawson, J. E., C. D. Paddock, C. K. Warner, P. W. Greer, J. H. Bartlett, S. A. Ewing, U. G. Munderloh, and S. R. Zaki.** 2001. Tissue diagnosis of *Ehrlichia chaffeensis* in patients with fatal ehrlichiosis by use of immunohistochemistry, in situ hybridization, and polymerase chain reaction. *Am. J. Trop. Med. Hyg.* **65**:603–609.

10. **Dehio, C.** 2004. Molecular and cellular basis of Bartonella pathogenesis. *Annu. Rev. Microbiol.* **58**:365–390.

11. **Dumler, J. S., and J. S. Bakken.** 1995. Ehrlichial diseases of humans: emerging tick-borne infections. *Clin. Infect. Dis.* **20**:1102–1110.

12. **Dumler, J. S., A. F. Barbet, C. P. J. Bekker, G. A. Dasch, G. H. Palmer, S. C. Ray, Y. Rikihisa, and F. R. Rurangirwa.** 2001. Reorganization of genera in the families *Rickettsiaceae* and *Anaplasmataceae* in the order *Rickettsiales*: unification of some species of *Ehrlichia* with *Anaplasma*, *Cowdria* with *Ehrlichia* and *Ehrlichia* with *Neorickettsia*, descriptions of six new species combinations and designation of *Ehrlichia equi* and "HGE agent" as subjective synonyms of *Ehrlichia phagocytophila*. *Int. J. Syst. Evol. Microbiol.* **51**:2145–2165.

13. **Dunn, B. E., T. P. Monson, J. S. Dumler, C. C. Morris, A. B. Westbrook, J. L. Duncan, J. E. Dawson, K. G. Sims, and B. E. Anderson.** 1992. Identification of *Ehrlichia chaffeensis* morulae in cerebrospinal fluid mononuclear cells. *J. Clin. Microbiol.* **30**:2207–2210.

14. **Eremeeva, M. E., G. A. Dasch, and D. J. Silverman.** 2003. Evaluation of a PCR assay for quantitation of *Rickettsia rickettsii* and closely related spotted fever group rickettsiae. *J. Clin. Microbiol.* **41**:5466–5472.

15. **Eremeeva, M., X. Yu, and D. Raoult.** 1994. Differentiation among spotted fever group rickettsia species by analysis of restriction fragment length polymorphism of PCR-amplified DNA. *J. Clin. Microbiol.* **32**:803–810.

16. **Gage, K. L., R. D. Gilmore, R. H. Karstens, and T. G. Schwan.** 1992. Detection of *Rickettsia rickettsii* in saliva, hemolymph and triturated tissues of infected *Dermacentor andersoni* ticks by polymerase chain reaction. *Mol. Cell. Probes* **6**:333–341.

17. **Gauduchon, V., L. Chalabreysse, J. Etienne, M. Célard, Y. Benito, H. Lepidi, F. Thivolet-Béjui, and F. Vandenesch.** 2003. Molecular diagnosis of infective endocarditis by PCR amplification and direct sequencing of DNA from valve tissue. *J. Clin. Microbiol.* **41**:763–766.

18. **Goldenberger, D., T. Schmidheini, and M. Altwegg.** 1997. Detection of *Bartonella henselae* and *Bartonella quintana* by a simple and rapid procedure using broad-range PCR amplification and direct single-strand sequencing of part of the 16S rRNA gene. *Clin. Microbiol. Infect.* **3**:240–245.

19. **Harris, R. J., P. A. Storm, A. Lloyd, M. Arens, and B. P. Marmion.** 2000. Long-term persistence of *Coxiella burnetii* in the host after primary Q fever. *Epidemiol. Infect.* **124**:543–549.

20. **Helbig, K. J., S. L. Heatley, R. J. Harris, C. G. Mulligan, P. G. Bardy, and B. P. Marmion.** 2003. Variation in immune response genes and chronic Q fever. Concepts: preliminary test with post-Q fever fatigue syndrome. *Genes Immunity* **4**:82–85.

21. **Horowitz, H. W., M. E. Aguero-Rosenfeld, D. F. McKenna, D. Holmgren, T.-Z. Hsieh, S. A. Varde, S. J. Dumler, J. M. Wu, I. Schwartz, Y. Rikihisa, and G. P. Wormser.** 1998. Clinical and laboratory spectrum of culture-proven human granulocytic ehrlichiosis: comparison with culture-negative cases. *Clin. Infect. Dis.* **27**:1314–1317.

22. **Jiang, J., T. C. Chan, J. J. Temenak, G. A. Dasch, W. M. Ching, and A. L. Richards.** 2004. Development of a quantitative real-time polymerase chain reaction assay specific for *Orientia tsutsugamushi*. *Am. J. Trop. Med. Hyg.* **70**:351–356.

23. **Johnson, G., M. Ayers, S. C. McClure, S. E. Richardson, and R. Tellier.** 2003. Detection and identification of *Bartonella* species pathogenic for humans by PCR amplification targeting the riboflavin synthase gene (*ribC*). *J. Clin. Microbiol.* **41**:1069–1072.

24. **Kelly, D. J., A. L. Richards, J. Temenak, D. Strickman, and G. A. Dasch.** 2004. The past and present threat of rickettsial diseases to military medicine and international public health. *Clin. Infect. Dis.* **34**(Suppl. 4):S145–S169.

25. **Langley, J. M., T. J. Marrie, J. C. LeBlanc, A. Almudevar, L. Resch, and D. Raoult.** 2003. *Coxiella burnetii* seropositivity in parturient women is associated with adverse pregnancy outcomes. *Am. J. Obstet. Gynecol.* **189**:228–232.

26. **La Scola, B., and D. Raoult.** 1999. Culture of *Bartonella quintana* and *Bartonella henselae* from human samples: a 5-year experience (1993 to 1998). *J. Clin. Microbiol.* **37**:1899–1905.

27. **Loftis, A. D., R. F. Massung, and M. L. Levin.** 2003. Quantitative real-time PCR assay for detection of *Ehrlichia chaffeensis*. *J. Clin. Microbiol.* **41**:3870–3872.

28. **Massung, R. F., K. Slater, J. H. Owens, W. L. Nicholson, T. N. Mather, V. B. Solberg, and J. G. Olson.** 1998. Nested PCR assay for detection of granulocytic ehrlichiae. *J. Clin. Microbiol.* **36**:1090–1095.

29. **Maurin, M., and D. Raoult.** 1999. Q fever. *Clin. Microbiol. Rev.* **12**:518–553.

30. **McQuiston, J. H, and J. E. Childs.** 2002. Q fever in humans and animals in the United States. *Vector Borne Zoonotic Dis.* **2**:179–191.

31. **Murray, P. R., E. J. Baron, J. H. Jorgensen, M. A. Pfaller, and R. H. Yolken.** 2003. *Manual of Clinical Microbiology*, 8th ed. American Society for Microbiology, Washington, D.C.

32. **Norman, A. F., R. Regnery, P. Jameson, C. Greene, and D. C. Krause.** 1995. Differentiation of *Bartonella*-like isolates at the species level by PCR-restriction fragment length polymorphism in the citrate synthase gene. *J. Clin. Microbiol.* **33**:1797–1803.

33. **Paddock, C. D., J. W. Sumner, G. M. Shore, D. C. Bartley, R. C. Elie, J. G. McQuade, C. R. Martin, C. S. Goldsmith, and J. E. Childs.** 1997. Isolation and characterization of *Ehrlichia chaffeensis* strains from patients with fatal ehrlichiosis. *J. Clin. Microbiol.* **35**:2496–2502.

34. **Qin, X., and K. B. Urdahl.** 2001. PCR and sequencing of independent genetic targets for the diagnosis of culture negative bacterial endocarditis. *Diagn. Microbiol. Infect. Dis.* **40**:145–149.

35. **Regnery, R., and J. Tappero.** 1995. Unraveling mysteries associated with cat-scratch disease, bacillary angiomatosis, and related syndromes. *Emerg. Infect. Dis.* **1**:16–21.

36. **Regnery, R. L., C. L. Spruill, and B. D. Plikaytis.** 1991. Genotypic identification of rickettsiae and estimation of intraspecies sequence divergence for portions of two rickettsial genes. *J. Bacteriol.* **173**:1576–1589.

37. **Renesto, P., J. Gouvernet, M. Drancourt, V. Roux, and D. Raoult.** 2001. Use of *rpoB* gene analysis for detection and identification of *Bartonella* species. *J. Clin. Microbiol.* **39**:430–437.

38. **Rikihisa, Y.** 1999 Clinical and biological aspects of infections caused by *Ehrlichia chaffeensis. Microbes Infect.* **13:**367–376.

39. **Rose, N. R., R. G. Hamilton, and B. Detrick (ed.).** 2002. *Manual of Clinical Laboratory Immunology,* 6th ed. ASM Press, Washington, D.C.

40. **Roux, V., P.-E. Fournier, and D. Raoult.** 1996. Differentiation of spotted fever group rickettsiae by sequencing and analysis of restriction fragment length polymorphism of PCR-amplified DNA of the gene encoding the protein rOmpA. *J. Clin. Microbiol.* **34:**2058–2065.

41. **Schouls, L. M., I. Van De Pol, S. G. Rijpkema, and C. S. Schot.** 1999. Detection and identification of *Ehrlichia, Borrelia burgdorferi* sensu lato, and *Bartonella* species in Dutch *Ixodes ricinus* ticks. *J. Clin. Microbiol.* **37:**2215–2222.

42. **Seshadri, R., I. T. Paulsen, J. A. Eisen, T. D. Read, K. E. Nelson, W. C. Nelson, N. L. Ward, H. Tettelin, T. M. Davidsen, M. J. Beanan, R. T. Deboy, S. C. Daugherty, L. M. Brinkac, R. Madupu, R. J. Dodson, H. D. Khouri, K. H. Lee, H. A. Carty, D. Scanlan, R. A. Heinzen, H. A. Thompson, J. E. Samuel, C. M. Fraser, and J. F. Heidelberg.** 2003. Complete genome sequence of the Q-fever pathogen *Coxiella burnetii. Proc. Natl. Acad. Sci. USA* **100:**5455–5460.

43. **Shaw, E. I., H. Moura, A. R. Woolfit, M. Opsina, H. A. Thompson, and J. R. Barr.** 2004. Identification of biomarkers of whole *Coxiella burnetii* phase I by MALDI-TOF mass spectrometry. *Anal. Chem.* **76:**4017–4022.

44. **Tajima, T., N. Zhi, Q. Lin, Y. Rikihisa, H. W. Horowitz, J. Ralfalli, G. P. Wormser, and K. Hechemy.** 2000. Enzyme-linked immunosorbent assay using major outer membrane protein of the human granulocytic ehrlichiosis agent. *Clin. Diagn. Lab. Immunol.* **7:**652–657.

45. **Tigertt, W. D.** 1959. Studies on Q fever in man. Symposium on Q fever. *Med. Sci. Pub.* **6:**39–46.

46. **Waag, D., and H. A. Thompson.** 2004. Pathogenesis of and immunity to *Coxiella burnetii,* p. 185–207. *In* L. E. Lindler, F. K. Lebeda, and G. W. Korch (ed.), *Biological Weapons Defense: Infectious Disease and Counterbioterrorism.* Humana Press, Totowa, N.J.

47. **Walker, D. H., J. Bakken, P. Brouqui, J. Childs, L. Cullman, J. Dawson, J. S. Dumler, V. Fingerle, J. Goodman, P. Hogan, W. Hogrefe, J. Liz, L. A. Magnarelli, J. Markley, R. Massung, E. J. Masters, C. Murphy, J. Olano, C. Paddock, M. Petrovec, Y. Rikihisa, S. Standaert, G. P. Wormser, X.-Y. Yu, and T. A. Zupanic.** 2000. Consensus on diagnosis of human ehrlichioses. *ASM News* **66:**287–290.

48. **Wang, X., Y. Rikihisa, T. Lai, Y. Kumagai, N. Zhi, and S. M. Reed.** 2004. Rapid sequential changeover of expressed *p44* genes during the acute phase of *Anaplasma phagocytophilum* infection in horses. *Infect. Immun.* **72:** 6852–6859.

49. **Williams, S. G., J. B. Sacci, Jr., M. E. Schriefer, E. M. Andersen, K. K. Fujioka, F. J. Sorvillo, A. R. Barr, and A. F. Azad.** 1992. Typhus and typhus like rickettsiae associated with opossums and their fleas in Los Angeles County, California. *J. Clin. Microbiol.* **30:**1758–1762.

50. **Zeaiter, Z., P. E. Fournier, G. Greub, and D. Raoult.** 2003. Diagnosis of *Bartonella* endocarditis by a real-time nested PCR assay using serum. *J. Clin. Microbiol.* **41:**919–925.

51. **Zhi, N., N. Ohashi, Y. Rikihisa, H. W. Horowitz, G. P. Wormser, and K. Hechemy.** 1998. Cloning and expression of 44-kilodalton major outer membrane protein antigen gene of human granulocytic ehrlichiosis agent and application of the recombinant protein to serodiagnosis. *J. Clin. Microbiol.* **36:**1666–1673.

Serologic and Molecular Tools for Diagnosing *Bordetella pertussis* Infection

SCOTT A. HALPERIN

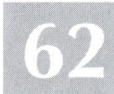

CLINICAL PRESENTATION AND EPIDEMIOLOGY OF INFECTIONS CAUSED BY *BORDETELLA PERTUSSIS*

B. pertussis is a gram-negative, pleomorphic coccobacillus for which humans are the only natural host. Infection by *B. pertussis* causes a prolonged coughing illness called pertussis or whooping cough. The spread of infection occurs person-to-person through the inhalation of infected respiratory droplets. After an incubation period of 7 to 10 days, symptoms of an upper respiratory infection develop, with rhinorrhea, lacrimation, malaise, low-grade fever, and a mild cough; this period is called the catarrhal stage and lasts from 1 to 2 weeks. With time, the cough becomes more frequent and severe, often occurring in bursts or fits (paroxysms), with multiple (5 to 10) coughs during a single expiration. During a cough, the infected individual may turn red in the face with bulging eyes, protruding tongue, and distended neck veins, all of which may progress to cyanosis. The coughing episode may terminate with a rapid in-drawing of air against a closed glottis, causing a "whooping" sound. Vomiting may also occur at the end of a paroxysmal cough, frequently associated with expulsion of a mucous plug. Paroxysms may be precipitated by eating, noise, or physical contact. Between episodes, the individual may look and feel healthy. Sleep disturbance and weight loss are common during the paroxysmal phase. Complications of pertussis typically appear during the paroxysmal phase and include pneumonia, pneumothorax, subconjunctival hemorrhage and other petechiae, inguinal and umbilical hernias, rib fractures, urinary incontinence, seizures, encephalopathy, and occasionally death (7). With time (2 to 4 weeks), the cough becomes less frequent and severe as the patient enters the convalescent stage. For up to a year, recurrent paroxysms can occur with any intercurrent upper respiratory infection.

Pertussis occurs at all ages, although most of the morbidity and virtually all of the mortality occur in young infants (27). As a result of universal childhood immunization, the incidence of pertussis has fallen by >95% in industrialized nations. However, the disease continues to occur in infants too young to have completed their three-dose primary immunization series. In the last decade, there has been a dramatic resurgence of pertussis, particularly in adolescents and adults, likely as the result of a waning of vaccine-induced immunity (23). In an effort to control adolescent pertussis and perhaps decrease the transmission of infection from adolescents to young infants, several countries have recently introduced a booster dose of pertussis vaccine in mid-adolescence (19).

DIAGNOSTIC METHODS TO DETECT *B. PERTUSSIS*

If all of the classical clinical symptoms of pertussis are present, clinical diagnosis is not difficult. However, symptoms may be atypical in young infants, adolescents, and adults, and the full classical clinical syndrome of pertussis may take weeks to develop. Laboratory confirmation of pertussis is therefore recommended. Detection of the etiologic agent is the optimal method of making a laboratory diagnosis; however, with *B. pertussis* infections, the nature of the infection and the natural history of the infection make this difficult. Table 1 and Fig. 1 summarize the diagnostic methods for the detection of *B. pertussis*.

Culture

The cornerstone of laboratory diagnosis of pertussis has been the culture of the causative organism from the nasopharynx. *B. pertussis* is most consistently found in the nasopharynx early in the clinical course, when the diagnosis is least likely to be considered. *B. pertussis* is present in the nasopharynx throughout the catarrhal stage and in the early paroxysmal stage; after a week or two of the paroxysmal stage, the organism can no longer be isolated from the nasopharynx, despite this being the period of maximal and classical symptomatology. The optimal specimen for culture is an aspirate of nasopharyngeal secretions (5), obtained by passing a fine, flexible plastic catheter attached to a 10-ml syringe through the nares into the nasopharynx and then withdrawing it while exerting gentle suction. A nasopharyngeal culture with a calcium alginate swab is also adequate (Dacron swabs are acceptable, but cotton swabs inhibit the growth of the organism and should not be used) and may be more acceptable to adults. Throat cultures are poor specimens for the recovery of *B. pertussis*, likely because the organism attaches to ciliated mucosal cells which are not present in the throat. Culture diagnosis has a high specificity; however, despite being the "gold standard," cell culture has a low sensitivity. *B. pertussis* is a fastidious, slow-growing organism that

TABLE 1 Characteristics of diagnostic tests for detection of *B. pertussis*[b]

Diagnostic test	Optimal use	Advantages	Disadvantages	Sensitivity	Specificity	Rapidity
Organism detection						
Culture	Diagnosis early in course of illness, particularly for young infants	No false-positive results, inexpensive, organism available for molecular epidemiology and antibiotic sensitivity (in rare cases, where indicated)	Moderately low sensitivity, requires special media and laboratory capability, specimen transport control is important	++	++++	++
PCR	Diagnosis early in course of illness	More sensitive than culture, less affected by prior treatment with antibiotics, positive for longer in clinical course than culture	Specificity affected by laboratory and environmental contamination, more expensive than culture, sophisticated equipment required	+++	+++	+++
DFA assay	Diagnosis early in course of illness	Rapid, inexpensive	Poor sensitivity and specificity, dependent on skill of operator and quality of reagents	+	+	++++
Serology						
Agglutinins	Population seroepidemiology studies	Easy to perform, correlates with population exposure to pertussis, long history of use	Poor correlation of titers with individual protection, no longer widely available	++	+++	+++, +[a]
CHO cell neutralization	Antibody to PT after immunization	Measures functional antibody	Labor-intensive, requires cell culture facilities, not widely available	+++	++++	+++, +[a]
IgG EIA						
PT	Diagnosis of infection or response to immunization	Specific for *B. pertussis*, most consistently immunogenic antigen, diagnosis late in clinical course, diagnosis of adolescents and adults	Cannot differentiate infection from immunization, young infants may have suboptimal immune response	+++	++++	+++, +[a]
FHA	Diagnosis of infection or response to immunization	Consistently immunogenic antigen, diagnosis late in clinical course, diagnosis of adolescents and adults	Cannot differentiate infection from immunization, cross-reacts with other *Bordetella* species and some other microorganisms	+++	+++	+++, +[a]
PRN	Diagnosis of infection or response to immunization	Diagnosis late in clinical course, diagnosis of adolescents and adults	Less consistently immunogenic antigen, cross-reacts with other *Bordetella* species, less standardized assay	++	+++	+++, +[a]
FIM	Diagnosis of infection or response to immunization (one vaccine)	Diagnosis late in clinical course, diagnosis of adolescents and adults	Less consistently immunogenic antigen, cross-reacts with other *Bordetella* species, less standardized assay	++	+++	+++, +[a]
IgA assays	Diagnosis of infection	Less likely to be positive after immunization	Less consistently positive	+	Depends on antigen	+++, +[a]

[a] +++ for single-serum diagnosis and + for paired serology.
[b] Adapted with permission from reference 4.

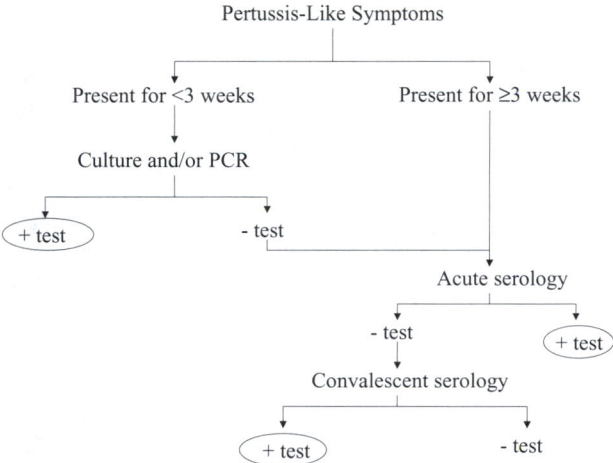

FIGURE 1 Algorithm for the laboratory diagnosis of pertussis.

requires special media (Bordet-Gengou or Regan-Lowe charcoal agar) and careful specimen handling (the organism is extremely sensitive to drying, so it must immediately be put on appropriate agar plates or into appropriate transport medium). The requirement for specialized and selective media means that the organism will not be isolated unless it is specifically sought. To further complicate matters, cultures are less likely to be positive from older individuals, previously immunized individuals, or those who have received an antimicrobial agent to which the organism is sensitive (18). *B. pertussis* is also slow growing, typically requiring 5 days of incubation before being identifiable, further decreasing the sensitivity of culture as a result of overgrowth of other, faster-growing organisms present in the nasopharynx. The incorporation of cephalexin into the growth medium is useful for the suppression of other organisms but may also inhibit the growth of some *B. pertussis* strains; therefore, culture is recommended to include both cephalexin-containing and cephalexin-free media. Despite these numerous methodological reasons for the decreased sensitivity of cell culture, the collection of specimens late in the clinical course, at a time when the microorganism is no longer present in the nasopharynx, is the major contributor to negative cultures from pertussis infections.

Once suspicious colonies with the appropriate morphology are detected on culture plates, the identification of *B. pertussis* is confirmed by biochemical tests, direct fluorescent antibody (DFA) staining, bacterial agglutination, or PCR (11).

DFA Staining

A more rapid method for the diagnosis of pertussis is to identify the organism directly in nasopharyngeal secretions, although the issue of the timing of specimen collection that limits the usefulness of culture also applies to DFA staining. Using fluorescein-labeled antibodies, one can directly observe *B. pertussis* in nasopharyngeal secretions, thereby providing almost immediate laboratory confirmation of the diagnosis. Although DFA reagents have been available commercially for decades, the test is fraught with problems of poor sensitivity and poor specificity and is highly dependent on the expertise of the technician performing the test (6). More specific reagents (monoclonal antibodies) have improved the specificity of the test but are not widely available (14). Because of the difficulties with the test, DFA staining should only be used in conjunction with culture;

some national surveillance systems do not accept DFA results as laboratory confirmation of pertussis infection.

PCR

More recently, molecular diagnostic techniques have been applied to the laboratory diagnosis of pertussis. The detection of *B. pertussis* by amplifying sections of the bacterial genome found in nasopharyngeal secretions has dramatically increased the sensitivity of bacterial detection methods. Various methods using different genomic sequences have been described; however, universally accepted target genes, amplification primers, and detection systems and a standardized methodology do not exist, and commercial kits are not widely available. PCR can be performed on nasopharyngeal aspirate specimens, although the secretions should be treated with a mucolytic agent and centrifuged to remove PCR-inhibiting substances and to concentrate the bacteria. Nasopharyngeal swabs can also be used; however, a DNA extraction method is required for specimens collected with calcium alginate swabs which is not required if Dacron swabs are employed (18, 26). Multiple target genes have been proposed, including repeated insertion sequences (3), the pertussis toxin (PT) promoter region (8), a DNA region upstream of the porin gene (10), and the adenylate cyclase toxin gene (1). Although the repeated insertion sequence intrinsically has greater sensitivity and is the most frequent target used, similar results can be obtained with all of the target genes by adjusting the number of amplification cycles. Most detection systems use ethidium bromide staining, although other methods (immunoblotting, Southern blotting, and dot blotting) have been described. With most reported methods, a sensitivity sufficient to detect <10 bacteria per reaction has been achieved. Recently, the most sensitive detection was achieved by using the insertion sequence in a real-time PCR format.

The ability to detect fewer organisms and the lesser importance of specimen handling because of the growth characteristics of the bacteria result in a far greater sensitivity of PCR. Also, the ability to detect nonviable organisms means that PCR likely remains positive for a longer time during the paroxysmal phase, when the organism is no longer cultivatable (although this increased duration has not been quantified). PCR is also less affected by antimicrobial effects than is cell culture, permitting laboratory diagnosis even after effective antibiotics have been initiated (2). With this increased sensitivity, however, there are more possibilities of cross-contamination leading to false-positive tests and decreased specificity. False-positive results can occur from contamination with other bacteria with similar genetic sequences, contamination with laboratory strains of *B. pertussis* or with other positive clinical specimens, or carryover from other specimens in the assay. Extreme care must be taken to avoid environmental contamination of specimens in the diagnostic laboratory with genomic DNA from previous specimens or bacterial cultures. Indeed, PCR is so sensitive that cross-contamination can occur from the presence of *B. pertussis* on surfaces and in the air of the specimen collection units (24). A strict separation of specimen processing areas and amplification and detection areas in the laboratory, the incorporation of known positive and negative controls into each assay, and the inclusion of blinded negative specimens improve the performance of PCR diagnosis. Real-time PCR methodology (9), which requires less specimen handling during the assay, and nested PCR techniques (21) have also decreased the risk of specimen contamination within the laboratory but do not affect the problems associated with specimen collection that are often outside the purview of laboratory quality control efforts. False-negative results may occur for many of the same reasons that affect the sensitivity of bacterial culture (collection of specimens late in the clinical course, prior antimicrobial use, inadequate specimen collection, or improper specimen handling or storage) as well as for reasons specific to PCR (presence of inhibitors such as blood in the specimen, insensitivity of the detection system, or presence of strain variants of *B. pertussis* with alterations in the target genetic sequence). Despite these limitations, PCR has consistently proven to have a superior sensitivity in the laboratory diagnosis of pertussis compared to that of bacterial culture.

SEROLOGIC METHODS FOR THE DIAGNOSIS OF *B. PERTUSSIS* INFECTIONS

Serologic methods for the diagnosis of pertussis have both advantages and disadvantages relative to organism detection methodologies. Since serology detects the host immune response to the infection, early acquisition of the specimen during the time when the organism is present in the nasopharynx is not required. In contrast to many infections for which one may have a falsely negative serologic test if specimens are obtained too early in the clinical course, with pertussis, by the time typical symptoms are present, the antibody response is usually well established. With pertussis, the difficulty with serology is demonstrating seroconversion because the timing of paired serology can more aptly be described as convalescent-late convalescent phase rather than the desired acute-phase–convalescent-phase pair. However, serologic assays have been the primary method of demonstrating the frequency of pertussis infections in adolescents and adults, for whom culture methods are less sensitive than for younger children. Indeed, in the United States, most cases of pertussis in adolescents and adults are reported from Massachusetts, one of the few jurisdictions that routinely performs serologic diagnostic testing for pertussis (28).

Pertussis Agglutinins

The measurement of pertussis agglutinins is one of the oldest assays used for determining antibody titers against *B. pertussis*. Widely used in the early and mid-20th century, particularly in the Medical Research Council clinical trials that demonstrated the efficacy of whole-cell pertussis vaccines, pertussis agglutinins correlated well with population immunity to pertussis but did not predict individual protection (16). The assay is currently performed as a microagglutination assay by vigorously mixing serial dilutions of patient sera with a standard concentration of whole phase I *B. pertussis* organisms in microtiter plates, incubating the mixtures overnight at 35°C, and observing them for bacterial agglutination. A negative agglutinin test appears as a thick button of cells at the bottom of the well, whereas complete (4+) agglutination appears as a sheet of cells covering the entire bottom of the well (13). Recently, agglutinin antibodies have been demonstrated to correlate best with antibodies against fimbriae (FIM), pertactin (PRN), and lipooligosaccharide (15). Agglutinins are no longer widely used and have no useful role in clinical diagnostic laboratories.

EIA

Enzyme-linked immunosorbent assays (EIAs) are the most widely used methodology for measuring antibodies against *B. pertussis*. A variety of solid-phase antigens have been used for EIA antibody detection, and assays have been described for immunoglobulin G (IgG), IgA, and IgM antibodies. The antigen(s) and antibody class(es) used affect both the sensitivity and specificity of the diagnostic test, so they must be selected carefully.

B. pertussis Antigens

EIAs have been developed with whole bacterial cells, PT, filamentous hemagglutinin (FHA), PRN (also referred to as the 69-kDa protein), FIM, lipooligosaccharide, and adenylate cyclase toxin. Commercially produced EIA kits have had limited availability; most have used sonicates of whole bacterial cells. Whole bacterial EIAs have the advantage of ease of antigen production (although a standardization of growth conditions is required to ensure consistent antigen expression by the bacteria) but are limited by cross-reactivity with related *Bordetella* species (most commonly *B. parapertussis*) and other unrelated bacteria (such as nonencapsulated *Haemophilus influenzae*).

PT is the most important pertussis antigen and is responsible for many of the biological activities of *B. pertussis*. PT is an A-B-type toxin with six subunits (S1 to S5). The B pentamer (made up of the S2, S3, two S4, and S5 subunits) is responsible for binding of the toxin to mammalian cells. The S1 protomer is the enzymatically active A subunit, which catalyzes the ADP-ribosylation of the membrane-bound regulatory protein G_i that normally inhibits adenylate cyclase, resulting in increased intracellular cyclic AMP. This results in the disruption of intracellular function, including decreased phagocytic activity and lymphocyte homing (resulting in lymphocytosis). PT is only produced by *B. pertussis*, making it a highly specific antigen (while *B. parapertussis* has the gene encoding PT, it is not expressed). PT is also included in all acellular pertussis vaccines currently manufactured worldwide and is an important protective antigen in the immune response to infection and immunization. Demonstration of an antibody rise to PT is diagnostic of pertussis (or of recent immunization), and the presence of antibodies against PT implies prior exposure to the organism or vaccine. Unfortunately, an antibody response to PT does not occur in all individuals after pertussis infection (young infants may not have an adequate response to PT) and may be diminished in previously immunized individuals. Thus, PT antibody assays are specific but by themselves are not of sufficient sensitivity for the reliable diagnosis of pertussis.

FHA is a component of the bacterial cell wall and plays an important role in binding to mucosal surfaces. FHA is a large, 220-kDa protein that forms filamentous structures on the bacterial cell surface. FHA has three distinct binding domains, including one that binds to sulfated sugars in the mucus of epithelial cells, an RGD domain that binds to integrins of macrophages and neutrophils, and a lactosylceramide binding site for attachment to macrophages and ciliated cells. EIAs with FHA are also widely used, typically in combination with PT assays. FHA is also a component of most acellular pertussis vaccines (with the exception being a monovalent PT vaccine), although whether or not FHA is a protective antigen is still controversial. Animal studies have been inconclusive; FHA has been demonstrated to induce protective antibodies in mice by some investigators, whereas others maintain that the protection induced was a result of trace contamination with PT. The presence of FHA antibody has not been correlated with protection in human studies. The antibody response to FHA is more consistent after infection, which increases the sensitivity of the test; however, all *Bordetella* species have FHA, so specificity is an issue. Indeed, anti-FHA antibodies have been demonstrated after infections caused by *H. influenzae* and *Mycoplasma pneumoniae*, suggesting that antibodies to unrelated antigens may cross-react with FHA.

PRN is another outer membrane adhesin protein that, like FHA, is mediated through an RGD sequence that promotes binding to the integrins of macrophages. PRN has a higher specificity for *B. pertussis* (although other *Bordetella* species produce related proteins). PRN is included in several widely used acellular pertussis vaccines and has been demonstrated to increase the efficacy of PT-FHA vaccines. PRN has also been correlated with protection after pertussis immunization. A PRN antibody response after infection may not occur as consistently as a response to PT (4). PRN-specific EIAs are not widely available and were shown to be associated with a greater degree of interlaboratory variability than either PT or FHA assays (12).

FIM are important hair-like surface antigens of *B. pertussis* that play a role in adherence to ciliated epithelial cells. Fimbrial antigens correlate best with agglutinogens, the components classically used to type *B. pertussis* isolates. Like the case for PRN, antibodies against FIM may occur less consistently than those against PT (4). FIM (types 2 and 3) are components of only one commercially available acellular pertussis vaccine, which limits access to supplies of the purified antigen for use in EIA (many of the purified antigens used in EIA are provided by the vaccine manufacturers). Thus, there is less information available on their use in diagnosis. Antibodies to FIM may cross-react with other bacterial species.

EIAs specific for other *B. pertussis* antigens, including the lipooligosaccharide and adenylate cyclase, have been described but are only available in a few research laboratories.

Antibody Class Assays

Although EIAs have been described for the detection of IgG, IgA, and IgM antibodies against *B. pertussis* antigens, IgG assays are the most frequently used as a diagnostic test, the best standardized, and the most widely available. IgG antibodies appear most consistently after infection or immunization; an antibody rise can typically be detected within 2 to 3 weeks after infection or primary immunization and as early as 1 week after a booster immunization. The antibody rise may be substantially slower in young infants. The rapidity of the antibody response may vary by antigen. PT and FHA antibodies are elicited most consistently, while PRN, FIM, and lipooligosaccharide antibodies are less predictable. PT antibodies appear somewhat later than antibodies against the surface antigens. IgG antibodies can be detected long after infection or immunization (decreasing over a 1- to 3-year period), so an elevated antibody titer may be the result of recent or remote infection or immunization (25). Although measurements of IgM might be useful for differentiating recent from remote infections, IgM assays have only occasionally been reported and are not well standardized. Little is known about the natural history of the IgM response after infection. To date, IgM assays have not provided any diagnostic utility.

Measuring the IgA response after pertussis infection has been proposed as a means of differentiating infection from immunization. IgA responses after infection occur less commonly (20 to 50%) than IgG responses (>90%) but are more frequent after infection than after immunization (18). IgA antibodies usually persist for up to a year after infection. The IgA response is even less predictable for young infants, and some IgA responses have been demonstrated after immunization with acellular pertussis vaccines, limiting the diagnostic specificity of the test (17). IgA serological diagnosis has not gained widespread acceptance to date but may be

increasingly useful, particularly for interpreting equivocal anti-PT antibody responses.

Combinations of assays (antigens or antibodies) have been used to increase the diagnostic sensitivity and specificity of tests (6). Using assays against two or more antigens and two or more antibody classes does increase the sensitivity of serological diagnosis but, depending on the antigen, may decrease the specificity if the antigen cross-reacts with antigens from other *Bordetella* species or other unrelated bacteria. Some investigators have used serological algorithms to minimize the loss of specificity, requiring a positive antibody response to two or more antigens that have cross-reactions (e.g., FHA and FIM) or a single antibody response to a unique *B. pertussis* antigen (e.g., PT), although the use of multiple antigens or antibody isotypes increases the cost of the diagnostic test (22). For all of these reasons, most clinical diagnostic laboratories offering serological diagnosis only use a PT or a PT-FHA IgG assay and limit the use of multiple antigens and antibody isotypes to seroepidemiological studies.

EIA Methodology

There is no universally accepted methodology for the performance of EIA for the detection of pertussis antibodies; however, most published assays are similar and follow basic EIA methodology. Purified pertussis antigen (PT, FHA, PRN, or FIM at 0.5 to 2 μg/ml) or whole bacterial cells are diluted in a neutral to alkaline coating buffer and bound to polystyrene EIA plates. After incubations of various durations (ranging from 1 to 2 h at 28 to 37°C to overnight at 4 to 28°C) and blocking of remaining binding sites with a blocking solution (typically containing a detergent such as Tween 20 and/or a high-protein solution such as bovine serum albumin or fetal calf serum), serum dilutions are added (typically starting at a dilution of 1:60 to 1:100 in phosphate-buffered saline at physiological pH) and incubated for a 1- to 3-h period at 28 to 37°C. After another series of washes with the blocking solution, a 1- to 16-h incubation is performed at 28 to 37°C with an enzyme-conjugated anti-human IgG (or IgA or IgM) antibody (e.g., alkaline phosphatase-conjugated goat anti-human IgG), after which a substrate is added; the enzyme-substrate combination results in a colorimetric change, which is read by a spectrophotometer at the substrate's optimal wavelength.

Antibody levels are typically quantified by assigning the test serum an EIA unitage by comparison to a simultaneously assayed standard serum that has been assigned an arbitrary antibody value. Standard sera for each of the pertussis antigens have been made available to diagnostic laboratories from the Pertussis Laboratory of the Center for Biologics Evaluation and Research of the U.S. Food and Drug Administration (FDA). Because of the limited supply of these standard sera, most pertussis serology laboratories have produced their own internal serum standards that are correlated with the FDA standard and then used with each assay. Various methods have been described to calculate the EIA unitage relative to the standard serum, but the reference-line method has been shown to be the most reproducible (20). With this method, the line generated by serial dilution of the test sample is assumed to have the same slope as the line generated by the reference serum, and the titer of the sample is calculated from the distance in dilution between the two lines (20).

The reproducibility of antibody titers measured by EIA is dependent on several factors. Variability can be attributed both to materials and to the operator. Intra-assay variability has been attributed to differences in binding characteristics of the EIA plates, to variability in binding related to the specimen's position on the plate (internal versus external wells), and to pipetting inaccuracies. Day-to-day (interassay) variability may be related to dilution differences and to variability in the reagents. Because of these variabilities, paired sera from an individual should be assayed together, preferably on the same EIA plate. To control for the inherent variability in EIA assays, pertussis serology laboratories should implement a quality control program to ensure that intra- and interassay variability is kept within acceptable limits. A positive control serum can be assayed on each plate, and the variability between assays can be expressed as the coefficient of variation (standard deviation divided by the mean and then multiplied by 100). Assays for which the control serum result falls outside a defined bound (such as ±2 standard deviations) should be rejected and repeated (20).

Antibody measurement by EIA is least accurate at low and high antibody concentrations, for which the antibody dilution curves are nonlinear. Low antibody levels are most difficult to measure accurately because the variability of the assay may be greater than the antibody level present. For each EIA, the coefficient of variation for the assay should be determined and should be <15%. A level of quantification should be determined which can then be used to determine the minimum level of detection (MLD) of the assay. Any antibody units with values lower than the MLD should be reported as less than the MLD.

Although EIA methodologies vary among laboratories providing serological diagnoses of pertussis, there have been efforts to explore whether results from various reference laboratories are comparable. Led by investigators at the FDA, 13 laboratories participated in an assessment of pertussis serological diagnosis by assaying a bank of test sera and comparing results. This study demonstrated that there was a good correlation for anti-PT IgG assays amongst the laboratories, a fair correlation for anti-FHA antibodies, and a relatively poor correlation for PRN and FIM antibodies (although the number of laboratories performing the last two assays was limited).

Other Serological Assays

Several other serological tests have been used to detect antibodies against *B. pertussis*, but none have gained wide acceptance or application. The most important of these is the measurement of neutralizing antibodies using the Chinese hamster ovary (CHO) cell neutralizing assay. CHO cells undergo a characteristic morphological change in the presence of PT that can be neutralized by anti-PT antibodies. The CHO assay quantifies these antibodies by assessing the ability of a serum to prevent the morphological change of a given, standardized quantity of PT. The CHO cell neutralizing titer is defined as the reciprocal of the last dilution that completely prevents the PT-induced morphological change. Proponents of the CHO cell neutralizing assay argue that the assay measures biologically active antibodies and thus might correlate better with protective antibodies. However, CHO titers have been shown to correlate well with the technically simpler to perform and easier to standardize anti-PT IgG EIA.

Use and Interpretation of Serological Tests for Pertussis

Serological tests for pertussis have important uses but also have several limitations. Measurements of antibodies have been used to evaluate the response to immunization (in clinical trials or after routine immunization) and for the diagnosis of natural infection. For the latter purpose, serology is most useful later in the course of illness, when bacterial or DNA detection assays may no longer be positive. Serology is also useful for older children, adolescents, and adults, for whom culture and PCR may be less consistently positive. Paired sera are the gold standard for serological diagnosis, demonstrating an antibody response after infection with *B. pertussis*. Fourfold increases in antibody levels have typically been used for pertussis agglutinins (and other assays that use serial dilutions), where a two-tube or -well change in titer is certain to be beyond the variability of the assay and to indicate a true increase in antibody. Fourfold dilutions are less defensible as a minimum indicator of an antibody increase in EIAs, for which test-to-test variability is measured by the coefficient of variation. With most well-performed EIAs, the coefficient of variation is sufficiently low (<15%) to allow a reliable differentiation of increases in antibodies of 50% or more; thus, a twofold increase in antibody level conservatively ensures that one is measuring a change in antibody level rather than assay variability. Despite this fact, however, fourfold responses are most often reported, most likely due to tradition.

Demonstrating a rise in antibody level is hindered by the late collection of the first specimen, by which time the antibody levels may have achieved the maximal levels after infection. In immunized individuals, the rapidity of the anamnestic antibody response may preclude the demonstration of an antibody rise. Single-serum criteria for the diagnosis of pertussis have been proposed, typically requiring an antibody level in excess of 3 standard deviations or the 99.99th percentile of a healthy age-matched population. These criteria have greatly increased the sensitivity of serological diagnosis, although, to retain a high specificity, requiring positive antibody titers against two or more antigens (except if against PT) is recommended. Single-serum diagnosis is becoming increasingly accepted as more age-specific reference values for IgG anti-PT antibodies become available. The interpretation of serological results for infants and young children must take into account any recent pertussis immunization, since acellular pertussis vaccines in current use contain two or more of these same antigens, therefore making differentiation between immunization and infection impossible. Serology testing is particularly useful for adolescents and adults, for whom culture is less sensitive and immunization is more remote. The recent implementation of adolescent booster doses of pertussis vaccine in a number of countries will further limit the use of serological diagnosis for these age groups unless assays are developed with consistently immunogenic and specific antigens that are not contained in the vaccines.

SUMMARY AND CONCLUSIONS

The laboratory diagnosis of pertussis continues to present challenges due to the fastidious nature of the organism, the natural history of the infection, whereby the organism is least likely to be present in the nasopharynx and thus detectable by culture or PCR when the clinical suspicion of pertussis is likely to be highest, the difficulty with demonstrating seroconversion because of the late collection of an acute-phase serum specimen, and the lack of a standardized, widely available assay specific for an antigen not included in acellular pertussis vaccines. Although molecular diagnosis (PCR) has revolutionized pertussis diagnosis by increasing the sensitivity of bacterial detection, the methodology is likely reaching its limits of improvement and is limited by the fact that the organism is no longer present in the host well before the clinical symptoms begin to resolve. Improvements in serological diagnosis have the greatest potential for improving the laboratory diagnosis of pertussis, particularly as the epidemiology shifts from young infants and children to adolescents and adults. The identification of a *B. pertussis*-specific antigen which consistently elicits an immune response but is not a vaccine candidate is a prerequisite for better serological diagnosis. The ability to differentiate recent from remote infections, perhaps through IgG and IgA assays, would make the test more interpretable. Standardization of the assay so that results from various laboratories can be compared is essential for the dissemination of such a diagnostic test.

I thank C. H. Wirsing von König, Annette Morris, Kevin Lynch, and Ann MacMillan for their thoughtful reviews of and comments on the manuscript.

REFERENCES

1. **Douglas, E., J. G. Coote, R. Parton, and W. McPheat.** 1993. Identification of *Bordetella pertussis* in nasopharyngeal swabs by PCR amplification of a region of the adenylate cyclase gene. *J. Med. Microbiol.* **38:**140–144.
2. **Edelman, K., S. Nikkari, O. Ruuskanen, Q. He, M. Viljanen, and J. Mertsola.** 1996. Detection of *Bordetella pertussis* by polymerase chain reaction and culture in the nasopharynx of erythromycin-treated infants with pertussis. *Pediatr. Infect. Dis. J.* **15:**54–57.
3. **Glare, E. M., J. C. Paton, R. R. Premier, A. J. Lawrence, and I. T. Nisbet.** 1990. Analysis of a repetitive DNA sequence from *Bordetella pertussis* and its application to the diagnosis of pertussis using the polymerase chain reaction. *J. Clin. Microbiol.* **28:**1982–1987.
4. **Hallander, H. O.** 1999. Microbiological and serological diagnosis of pertussis. *Clin. Infect. Dis.* **28**(Suppl. 2)**:** S99–S106.
5. **Hallander, H. O., E. Reizenstein, B. Renemar, G. Rasmusson, L. Mardin, and P. Olin.** 1993. Comparison of nasopharyngeal aspirates with swabs for culture of *Bordetella pertussis*. *J. Clin. Microbiol.* **31:**50–52.
6. **Halperin, S. A., R. Bortolussi, and A. J. Wort.** 1989. Evaluation of culture, immunofluorescence, and serology for the diagnosis of pertussis. *J. Clin. Microbiol.* **27:**752–757.
7. **Halperin, S. A., E. L. Wang, B. Law, E. Mills, R. Morris, P. Déry, M. Lebel, N. MacDonald, T. Jadavji, W. Vaudry, D. Scheifele, G. Delage, and P. Duclos.** 1999. Epidemiological features of pertussis in hospitalized patients in Canada, 1991–1997: report of the Immunization Monitoring Program—Active (IMPACT). *Clin. Infect. Dis.* **28:**1238–1243.
8. **Houard, S., C. Hackel, A. Herzog, and A. Bollen.** 1989. Specific identification of *Bordetella pertussis* by the polymerase chain reaction. *Res. Microbiol.* **140:**477–487.
9. **Kosters, K., M. Riffelmann, and C. H. Wirsing von König.** 2001. Evaluation of a real-time PCR assay for detection of *Bordetella pertussis* and *B. parapertussis* in clinical samples. *J. Med. Microbiol.* **50:**436–440.
10. **Li, Z., D. L. Jansen, T. M. Finn, S. A. Halperin, A. Kasina, S. P. O'Connor, T. Aoyama, C. R. Manclark, and M. J. Brennan.** 1994. Identification of *Bordetella pertussis* infection by shared-primer PCR. *J. Clin. Microbiol.* **32:**783–789.
11. **Loeffelholz, M. J.** 2003. *Bordetella*, p. 780–788. *In* P. R. Murray (ed.), *Manual of Clinical Microbiology*, 8th ed. ASM Press, Washington, D.C.
12. **Lynn, F., G. F. Reed, and B. Meade.** 1996. Collaborative study for the evaluation of enzyme-linked immunosorbent assays used to measure human antibodies to *Bordetella pertussis* antigens. *Clin. Diagn. Lab. Immunol.* **2:**689–700.
13. **Manclark, C. R., B. D. Meade, and D. G. Burstyn.** 1986. Serological response to *Bordetella pertussis*, p. 388–394. *In* N. R. Rose, H. Friedman, and J. L. Fahey (ed.), *Manual of Clinical Microbiology*, 3rd ed. American Society for Microbiology, Washington, D.C.
14. **McNicol, P., S. M. Giercke, M. Gray, D. Martin, B. Brodeur, M. S. Peppler, T. Williams, and G. Hammond.** 1995. Evaluation and validation of a monoclonal immunofluorescent reagent for direct detection of *Bordetella pertussis*. *J. Clin. Microbiol.* **33:**2868–2871.
15. **Meade, B. D., F. Lynn, G. F. Reed, C. M. Mink, A. Romani, A. Deforest, and M. A. Deloria.** 1994. Relationship between functional assays and enzyme immunoassays as measurements of responses to acellular and whole-cell pertussis vaccines. *Pediatrics* **96:**595–600.
16. **Medical Research Council.** 1956. Vaccination against whooping cough: relation between protection in children and results of laboratory tests. *Br. Med. J.* **2:**454–462.
17. **Mink, C. M., C. H. O'Brien, S. R. M. Wassilak, A. Deforest, and B. D. Meade.** 1994. Isotype and antigen specificity of pertussis agglutinins following whole-cell pertussis vaccination and infection with *Bordetella pertussis*. *Infect. Immun.* **62:**1118–1120.
18. **Müller, F. M. C., J. E. Hoppe, and C. H. W. von König.** 1997. Laboratory diagnosis of pertussis: state of the art in 1997. *J. Clin. Microbiol.* **35:**2435–2443.
19. **National Advisory Committee on Immunization.** 2003. Prevention of pertussis in adolescents and adults. *Can. Commun. Dis. Rep.* **29:**1–10.
20. **Reizenstein, E., H. O. Hallander, W. C. Blackwelder, I. Kuhn, M. Ljungman, and R. Möllby.** 1995. Comparison of five calculation methods for antibody ELISA procedures using pertussis serology as a model. *J. Immunol. Methods* **183:**279–290.
21. **Reizenstein, E., L. Lindberg, R. Möllby, and H. Hallander.** 1996. Validation of nested PCR in pertussis vaccine trial. *J. Clin. Microbiol.* **34:**810–815.
22. **Senzilet, L. D., S. A. Halperin, J. S. Spika, M. Alagaratnam, A. Morris, B. Smith, and the Sentinel Health Unit Surveillance System Pertussis Working Group.** 2001. Pertussis is a frequent cause of prolonged cough illness in adults and adolescents. *Clin. Infect. Dis.* **32:**1691–1697.
23. **Skowronski, D. M., G. De Serres, D. MacDonald, W. Wu, C. Shaw, J. Macnabb, S. Champagne, D. M. Patrick, and S. A. Halperin.** 2002. The changing age and seasonal profile of pertussis in Canada. *J. Infect. Dis.* **185:**1448–1453.
24. **Taranger, J., B. Trollfors, L. Lind, G. Zackrisson, and K. Beling-Holmquist.** 1994. Environmental contamination leading to false-positive polymerase chain reaction for pertussis. *Pediatr. Infect. Dis. J.* **13:**936–937.
25. **Tomoda, T., H. Ogura, and T. Kurashige.** 1994. The longevity of the immune response to filamentous hemagglutinin and pertussis toxin in patients with pertussis in a semiclosed community. *J. Infect. Dis.* **166:**908–910.
26. **Wadowsky, R. M., S. Laus, T. Libert, S. J. States, and G. D. Ehrlich.** 1994. Inhibition of PCR-based assay for *Bordetella pertussis* by using calcium alginate fiber and aluminum shaft components of a nasopharyngeal swab. *J. Clin. Microbiol.* **32:**1054–1057.
27. **Wortis, N., P. M. Strebel, M. Wharton, B. Bardenheier, and I. R. Hardy.** 1996. Pertussis deaths: report of 23 cases in the United States, 1992 and 1993. *Pediatrics* **97:**607–612.
28. **Yih, W. K., S. M. Lett, F. N. des Vignes, K. M. Carrison, P. L. Sipe, and C. D. Marchant.** 2000. The increasing incidence of pertussis in Massachusetts adolescents and adults, 1989–1998. *J. Infect. Dis.* **182:**1409–1416.

Bacillus anthracis Detection and Anthrax Diagnosis

ALEX R. HOFFMASTER AND TANJA POPOVIC

63

Anthrax is primarily a disease of herbivores, which acquire the disease by ingesting *Bacillus anthracis* spores from contaminated soil. Although anthrax is more common in parts of Central Asia and Africa, it still occurs sporadically in animals in parts of the United States, including the West, Midwest, and Southwest. There are three clinical forms of human anthrax, depending on the route of infection: cutaneous (acquired via skin abrasion), gastrointestinal (acquired via ingestion), and inhalation anthrax. While naturally acquired anthrax is rare in the United States, the fear of inhalation anthrax continues in this era of bioterrorism that became reality in 2001 when 22 people in the United States acquired anthrax from spores sent through the mail (16).

The genus *Bacillus* contains a wide range of endospore-forming species, of which very few are pathogens. *B. anthracis* and other members of the *B. cereus* group are exceptions to this general rule. *B. anthracis* is the etiologic agent of anthrax, *B. cereus* is most frequently associated with food poisoning but can cause a variety of serious infections, and *B. thuringiensis* is an insect pathogen but has also been implicated in some cases of gastroenteritis (20). These species have been shown to be phylogenetically very closely related by several methods (17, 29), resulting in some researchers suggesting that they be considered a single species (12). At least some of the differences in virulence between *B. anthracis* and most of its close relatives can be attributed to the presence of two virulence plasmids, pXO1 and pXO2. The pXO1 and pXO2 plasmids carry the genes which encode the anthrax toxins (lethal toxin and edema toxin) and the antiphagocytic poly-γ-D-glutamic acid capsule, respectively (23, 26). However, whether they are considered a single species or not, the need to rapidly differentiate them remains due to the different diseases they cause, potential bioterrorism use, and the implications for treatment.

Just a few years ago, anthrax was rarely encountered and few laboratories had the capacity to identify *B. anthracis* in the United States. Since the threat of bioterrorism and the development of the Laboratory Response Network (LRN), that situation has changed dramatically (22). Currently, there are LRN laboratories in every state that have the capacity to rapidly detect and identify *B. anthracis*. The number of methods, assays, and new instrumentation that are currently being used and described in the literature to detect *B. anthracis* is too exhaustive to be included in this review. This chapter will primarily focus on methods that are currently in use within LRN laboratories and on commercially available tests that have been approved by the U.S. Food and Drug Administration (FDA) and thus are widely available. This chapter includes four sections, covering culture, molecular, antigen, and antibody detection methods for the diagnosis of anthrax. Throughout the chapter, the methods are discussed relative to the Centers for Disease Control and Prevention (CDC) definitions of suspected and confirmed cases used during the 2001 anthrax outbreak. A confirmed case of anthrax was defined as a clinically compatible case that was laboratory confirmed by the isolation of *B. anthracis* from an affected tissue or by laboratory evidence based on at least two other supportive tests. A suspected case was defined as a clinically compatible illness without isolation of *B. anthracis* and with only a single supportive laboratory test or a clinically compatible case epidemiologically linked to a confirmed environmental exposure but without corroborative laboratory evidence (5). Supportive laboratory tests included the LRN PCR assay, immunohistochemical (IHC) staining of tissues, and anti-protective antigen (anti-PA) immunoglobulin G (IgG) detection by an enzyme-linked immunosorbent assay (ELISA) and are discussed later in the chapter.

CULTURE

Culturing *B. anthracis* from clinical specimens remains the standard for diagnosing anthrax. Biosafety level 2 practices are adequate for work with clinical materials and diagnostic quantities of infectious cultures. Biosafety level 3 practices and facilities are recommended for work involving larger quantities or concentrations of cultures and for activities with a high potential for aerosol production (1). *B. anthracis* may be present in blood, skin lesion exudates, cerebrospinal fluid, pleural fluid, sputum, and feces. If the *B. anthracis* infection has become systemic, it is generally easy to culture the organism from blood, with organisms reaching concentrations of 10^8 CFU/ml. Culturing *B. anthracis* from cutaneous lesions is more difficult, and growing the organism is not likely, regardless of the form of disease, once antimicrobial therapy has been initiated. The most common laboratory medium used for culturing and identification of *B. anthracis* is sheep blood agar. *B. anthracis* produces a characteristic ground-glass appearance and is nonhemolytic on this medium. Laboratories have also used polymyxin lysozyme

EDTA thallium acetate (PLET) semiselective medium when high levels of background contamination are expected (e.g., with environmental samples) (8, 18).

Despite the phylogenetic data suggesting that members of the *B. cereus* group may be considered a single species, *B. anthracis* can be readily distinguished from its close relatives by several phenotypic differences (20). *B. anthracis*, unlike *B. cereus* and *B. thuringiensis*, is not motile, is susceptible to penicillin, and is not hemolytic. Although exceptions to these phenotypes can occur, it is generally very easy to distinguish *B. anthracis* from *B. cereus* and *B. thuringiensis* based on these differences. In addition, susceptibility to lysis by a bacteriophage (gamma phage) has been used very successfully since the 1950s to help identify *B. anthracis* and is still in use today (3). *B. anthracis* is lysed (susceptible) by the gamma phage, while its close relatives are not. Resistant isolates of *B. anthracis* and susceptible isolates of *B. cereus* have been reported but are not common (10, 30). In addition, isolates can be tested by PCR and several of the antigen-based methods discussed later in this chapter. It is important that no single test can be used to rule out or identify *B. anthracis*.

Advantages and Disadvantages

All of these tests require an isolate of *B. anthracis* and require about 24 h to complete. However, they can easily be performed by most laboratories, with the possible exception of the gamma phage test, which is available at LRN reference laboratories. Once antimicrobial therapy has been initiated, it is very difficult to culture *B. anthracis* from patient specimens.

Specimen Collection and Transport

Isolates of *B. anthracis* or other *Bacillus* spp. can be transported on most common, nonselective laboratory media at room temperature. Clinical specimens such as swabs, stools, sputa, pleural fluid, and blood should be transported at 2 to 8°C. For cutaneous lesions in the vesicular stage, collect the vesicular fluid on a dry, sterile swab. For lesions in the eschar stage, lift an edge of the eschar and insert and rotate the swab without removing the eschar. Fresh tissue samples (e.g., not formalin fixed) should be sent frozen.

MOLECULAR DETECTION

PCR is another commonly used laboratory method for the detection of pathogens. In recent years, several different chemistries, assays, and instruments have become available for the performance of real-time PCR. These methods utilize fluorescent probes (primers labeled with fluorescent dyes) that allow the detection of amplicons by measuring fluorescence. Some of the common types of probes used include TaqMan (5′ exonuclease assay) probes, dual-hybridization probes, and molecular beacons (6, 21). The use of fluorescent primers as probes not only allows for real-time detection of the PCR products but also increases the specificity of the reaction since both the amplification primers and the fluorescent probes need to hybridize to the target in order to produce a signal.

Great efforts have been made to develop specific PCR assays for the detection of *B. anthracis*. The plasmids have generally proven to be reliable targets, particularly the toxin genes (*pagA*, *lef*, and *cya*) on pXO1 and the capsule operon (*capBCA*) on pXO2. However, false-positive amplification using primers specific for the *capB* gene has been reported previously (27), and recently pXO1 was identified in a *B. cereus* isolate (15). A commercial real-time PCR kit is available (Roche, Mannheim, Germany) that targets the toxin gene (*pagA*) and a capsule gene (*capB*) (2). However, this

section will focus on the LRN PCR assay used in the U.S. public health system.

LRN PCR

The LRN real-time PCR assay for the detection of *B. anthracis* is a 5′ exonuclease assay that includes three separate targets: one on the chromosome, one on pXO1, and one on pXO2 (14). This greatly reduces the risk of false-positive and false-negative results by not relying on a single target. This assay demonstrated 100% sensitivity and specificity when tested on a diverse set of 81 *B. anthracis* isolates and an extensive set of its close relatives (*n* = 56) (14). The limit of detection for this assay is approximately 5 to 10 spores based on PCRs performed directly on diluted spores. DNA extraction from the spores is not necessary since the spore surface is covered in DNA as a result of the sporulation process.

This assay was also used during the 2001 bioterrorism-associated anthrax outbreak to detect *B. anthracis* in environmental samples and clinical specimens to confirm anthrax diagnosis when the isolation of *B. anthracis* failed due to the initiation of antimicrobial drug treatment. The LRN PCR assay was particularly useful for detecting *B. anthracis* in pleural fluids of patients with inhalation anthrax but was also successfully used to detect *B. anthracis* in blood, serum, cerebrospinal fluid, lymph node tissue, lung tissue, sputum, pericardial fluid, and tissue from cutaneous lesions. Pleural fluid specimens were positive for all five inhalation anthrax patients from whom samples were received, despite the specimens having been taken after the initiation of antimicrobial therapy and consequently being culture negative (14).

Advantages and Disadvantages

The LRN real-time PCR assay is specific, sensitive, and rapid. Once the DNA has been extracted, the assays can be set up and results obtained in about 1 to 2 h. However, since PCR detects DNA from viable or nonviable cells, it is not useful for detecting *B. anthracis* contamination in the environment after decontamination since dead cells and spores will still be detected. In addition, the sensitivity greatly decreases if specimens are taken after the initiation of antimicrobial therapy.

Specimen Collection and Transport

As stated previously, isolates of *Bacillus* spp. for testing can be sent on most common, nonselective laboratory media at room temperature. Specimens such as swabs, stools, sputa, pleural fluid, and blood should be transported at 2 to 8°C and fresh tissue should be sent frozen.

ANTIGEN DETECTION

Several antibodies and antigen-based detection methods are in use for the detection and identification of *B. anthracis*. Regardless of the methodology, an antigen detection assay is limited by the affinity and specificity of the antibodies used, and in the case of clinical or environmental samples, the concentration of the antigen in the sample. Antibodies have been used successfully to detect the vegetative and spore forms of *B. anthracis*. This section will cover the following four methods: a direct fluorescent-antibody assay (DFA), time-resolved fluorescence (TRF) assays, an immunochromatographic assay, and IHC assays.

DFA

A two-component DFA using two different monoclonal IgM antibodies specific for a *B. anthracis* cell wall antigen (galactose–*N*-acetylglucosamine) and the *B. anthracis* capsule (poly-γ-D-glutamic acid) has been used successfully to identify vegetative cells of *B. anthracis* (7, 9, 10). Both antibodies are conjugated to fluorescein isothiocyanate, which when bound to *B. anthracis* allows for visualization of the fluorescent cells by using a UV microscope with a 40× or 100× objective. Although neither antibody is 100% specific for *B. anthracis*, when they are used in combination the assay is 100% specific to date (i.e., no isolates other than *B. anthracis* have been positive for both antigens) (7). In addition to being used directly on isolates, this assay successfully detected *B. anthracis* in pleural fluid, blood, lung tissue, and lymph node tissue collected during the 2001 bioterrorism-associated anthrax outbreak (7).

TRF Assays

In addition to the real-time PCR assay, some LRN laboratories have the capacity to detect spores or vegetative cells in samples by using a spore or vegetative cell-specific antibody in a dissociation-enhanced lanthanide fluoroimmunoassay (DELFIA; Perkin-Elmer). This type of assay is essentially comprised of noncompetitive sandwich ELISAs that utilize biotinylated capture antibodies and detector (secondary) antibodies labeled with a lanthanide chelate (europium) (24). Once the secondary antibody has been washed away, a low-pH (2 to 3) enhancement solution containing a β-diketone and Triton X-100 is added to the sample. The buffer interacts with the europium label to produce a highly fluorescent chelate suspended within a micelle, allowing for increased sensitivity and length of signal (24).

These assays can be used on various environmental and clinical specimens. Clinical specimens may include sera, nasopharyngeal swabs, bronchial or tracheal washings, or lesion exudates, but not whole blood. The *B. anthracis* TRF cell assay is specific for *B. anthracis* at concentrations of ≤10⁶ CFU/ml. The TRF spore assay utilizes an antibody that is specific for *B. anthracis* spores but also cross-reacts with *B. anthracis* vegetative cells. Both assays have a limit of detection of approximately 100 total spores or vegetative cells per reaction (LRN, unpublished data).

Immunochromatographic Methods

The development of lateral-flow immunochromatographic devices similar to many home pregnancy tests has remained an attractive concept due to their small size, speed, possible field use, and ease of operation. There are several varieties of tests, but typically a suspension of the sample (antigen) is added to a strip which rehydrates a monoclonal antibody labeled with colored beads or colloidal gold. The solution migrates via capillary action along the membrane, and if antigen is present, the labeled monoclonal antibody-antigen complex will be captured by a second antibody at the test line, resulting in a colored band that is easily visualized (24). Most attempts to utilize this type of technology for the detection of *B. anthracis* have suffered from low sensitivity, low specificity, or both.

The RedLine Alert test from Tetracore, Inc., is an immunochromatographic test utilizing an antibody specific for one of the *B. anthracis* S-layer proteins and has been approved by the FDA for use on nonhemolytic *Bacillus* colonies cultured on sheep blood agar plates. Restricting the test to nonhemolytic isolates reduces the risk of false-positive results that may be caused by hemolytic species such as *B. cereus* and *B. thuringiensis*. The test is easy to use, and results can be read within 15 min. The test was positive for a diverse set of *B. anthracis* isolates (143 of 145; 98.6% sensitive) and negative for all 49 nonhemolytic, non-*B. anthracis* isolates tested (manufacturer data); however, the identification of

B. anthracis with this test is considered presumptive, and the test should not be used as a stand-alone method.

IHC Assays

During the 2001 bioterrorism-associated anthrax outbreak, *B. anthracis*-specific IHC assays were among the supportive laboratory tests used to establish the diagnosis of anthrax when the culture of *B. anthracis* failed (11, 28). These assays were performed on 3-μm-thick sections of formalin-fixed, paraffin-embedded tissues and utilized antibodies specific for the *B. anthracis* cell wall and capsule as described for the DFA. A biotinylated anti-mouse IgM antibody, streptavidin-alkaline phosphatase complex, and naphthol-fast red substrate were used for the colorimetric detection of antigens within tissues. Analyses of specimens from inhalation anthrax patients revealed bacilli, bacillary fragments, and some granular antigen staining by use of the cell wall IHC assay, while the capsule IHC assay mostly detected bacterial granular antigens (11). IHC staining was attempted on tissues from the lymph nodes, lung, heart, liver, spleen, kidneys, conjunctiva, gastrointestinal tract, bronchial biopsies, pleural biopsies and pleural fluid cell blocks. Significantly, IHC staining of skin biopsies from 8 of 10 cutaneous cases tested was positive for both the capsule and cell wall antigens, making IHC staining particularly useful for establishing a diagnosis in these cases (28).

Advantages and Disadvantages

The DFA is 100% specific for *B. anthracis* when used on isolates, but this method will not detect strains cured of pXO2 since this plasmid is required for capsule production, and the cell wall-specific antibody has produced rare false-negative results (99% sensitive) (7). IHC assays have limitations similar to those of the DFA since the same antibodies are used. The LRN TRF assays are rapid and require minimal sample preparation; however, false-positive results can occur if a high level of innate europium is present in the samples. The RedLine Alert test is fast and easy to use but is intended for use on isolates only.

Specimen Collection and Transport

For IHC analysis of cutaneous lesions, a full-thickness punch biopsy fixed in 10% buffered formalin from a papule or vesicle lesion and including adjacent skin should be taken. Biopsies should also be taken from both the vesicle and eschar, if present (4, 28). Unlike fresh tissues (frozen), formalin-fixed samples can be sent at room temperature, while other specimens should be transported at 2 to 8°C.

SEROLOGY

Serology was the third approach, in addition to the LRN PCR and IHC assays, that was used to diagnose anthrax when the isolation of *B. anthracis* from patients failed. A quantitative anti-PA IgG ELISA was used during the 2001 outbreak to measure antibodies to the anthrax toxin protein, PA. Serology was only negative for a single patient with confirmed or suspected anthrax during the outbreak and was particularly useful for the diagnosis of cutaneous anthrax. In addition, quantitative ELISAs and the toxin neutralization assay (TNA) have also been used in vaccine-animal challenge studies to show that levels of anti-PA antibodies are a significant predictor of survival (19). Recently, a commercially available test was FDA approved to qualitatively measure anti-PA antibodies in human serum (QuickELISA Anthrax-PA kit).

Human Anti-PA IgG ELISA

The CDC has developed a quantitative ELISA for the detection of human IgG antibodies to PA, with a lower limit of quantification of 3.0 μg of anti-PA IgG/ml of serum (25). The assay has a 97.6% diagnostic sensitivity and 94.2% diagnostic specificity based on the analysis of specimens from confirmed anthrax cases and from anthrax vaccine adsorbed (AVA) vaccinees. A fourfold or higher rise from the baseline in the concentration of anti-PA IgG (acute- versus convalescent-phase serum sample) is considered reactive. Anti-PA IgG was detectable in 16 of 17 bioterrorism-associated patients with confirmed or suspected anthrax by 11 days after the onset of symptoms. Only a single patient with cutaneous anthrax failed to mount a detectable antibody response. In addition, serology was the only positive test for 3 of the 11 suspected or confirmed cutaneous anthrax cases.

A competitive inhibition anti-PA IgG ELISA can be used to enhance the diagnostic specificity to 100% (25). Briefly, one of two duplicate serum samples is treated with excess, purified recombinant PA (rPA). The sera are centrifuged to remove antibody-antigen complexes, and the supernatants are retested in the standard ELISA. A ≥ 85% suppression of reactivity in the competitive ELISA is used to discriminate between true-positive and false-positive results. For the analysis of the 2001 bioterrorism-related cases, the competitive ELISA was only used on serum samples that had an anti-PA IgG reactivity of ≥10 μg/ml and when paired sera were reactive but the anti-PA IgG concentration did not change over time.

TNA

Unlike the ELISA, the TNA is a measure of functional antibodies. This colorimetric assay measures the ability of antibodies to protect mouse macrophage cells (J774A.1) from anthrax lethal toxin cytotoxicity (13). Neutralization occurs when antibodies bind functional epitopes on PA, lethal factor (LF), or the PA receptor which inhibit toxin function. The ability of antibodies to neutralize lethal toxin activity and protect the cells is measured colorimetrically by use of a tetrazolium salt,

3-(4,5-dimethylthiazol-2-yl)-2,5-diphenyltetrazolium bromide (MTT). The degree of neutralization is reported as the serum dilution that effectively neutralizes 50% of the toxin-mediated cytotoxicity.

QuickELISA Anthrax-PA Kit

The FDA-approved QuickELISA Anthrax-PA kit from Immunetics (Boston, Mass.) has recently become available for the presumptive detection of anti-PA IgG and IgM antibodies in human serum. This assay is a qualitative detection assay for total antibodies against the PA protein. In principle, anti-PA antibodies present in serum bind strepavidin-rPA and horseradish peroxidase-rPA conjugates. The complex binds to biotin immobilized in the wells of a microtiter plate. The horseradish peroxidase-rPA-containing complex converts a chromogenic substrate containing tetramethylbenzidine, and the absorbance is measured. The assay exhibited > 99% specificity and 100% sensitivity when validated on sera from 19 individuals with anthrax, 49 individuals vaccinated with AVA, 583 healthy individuals, 205 sera from individuals with other infections, and 20 influenza vaccine recipients (manufacturer's data).

Advantages and Disadvantages

The major disadvantage of serology is the time required for seroconversion to occur after infection. Despite this, however, serology may be particularly useful for diagnosing cutaneous anthrax and for cases when the use of antimicrobial therapy results in negative cultures and PCR.

Specimen Collection and Transport

Sera should be transported frozen on dry ice.

SUMMARY

Numerous molecular and antigen-based methods are available for identifying B. anthracis and diagnosing anthrax. The advantages, disadvantages, and general availability of these tests are summarized in Table 1. Culturing of B. anthracis remains the definitive method for diagnosing anthrax, and

TABLE 1 Diagnostic tests for detection of B. anthracis

Test	Target	Availability	Advantages	Disadvantages
Culture	Spores or vegetative cells	LRN	Definitive identification of isolate and diagnosis	Isolation not likely after initiation of antimicrobial therapy
LRN PCR	Spores or vegetative cells	LRN	Rapid and 100% specific for use on isolates	Sensitivity decreases rapidly after initiation of antimicrobial therapy
DFA	Vegetative cells	LRN	100% specific for use on isolates	pXO2-cured strains will not be positively identified
TRF spore assay	Spores	LRN	Rapid, detects plasmid-cured strains	Samples with high innate europium levels can cause false-positive results
TRF cell assay	Vegetative cells	LRN	Rapid, detects plasmid-cured strains	Samples with high innate europium levels can cause false-positive results
IHC staining	Vegetative cells	CDC	Diagnosis of cutaneous anthrax cases	Not widely available
Immunochromatographic RedLine Alert test	Vegetative cells	Commercially available	Speed and ease of use	For use on isolates only
Serology ELISA TNA QuickELISA Anthrax-PA Kit	Immune response against toxin (PA)	CDC and commercially available	Diagnosis of cutaneous anthrax cases	Time to seroconversion

phenotypic, molecular, and antigen-based tests are available for the identification of isolates. It should be reiterated that no single phenotype or test should be used to rule out or positively identify *B. anthracis*. While culture is the standard, it is not always possible to isolate *B. anthracis*, particularly when specimens have been collected after the initiation of antimicrobial treatment. In these instances, the use of molecular, antigen-based, and antibody-based (serology) detection methods becomes even more important. If *B. anthracis* cannot be isolated, the CDC recommends that the diagnosis of anthrax be based on at least two supportive tests (5, 16). In recent years, there has been a rapid development and dissemination of assays for the detection of *B. anthracis* throughout the U.S. public health laboratory system. Current research interests and funding in this area will continue to yield novel technologies and new methods for the detection of *B. anthracis* and the diagnosis of anthrax in the future.

REFERENCES

1. **Anonymous.** 1999. Bacterial agents, p. 88–89. *In* J. Y. Richmond and R. W. McKinney (ed.), *Biosafety in Microbiological and Biomedical Laboratories*, 4th ed. U.S. Government Printing Office, Washington D.C.
2. **Bell, C. A., J. R. Uhl, T. L. Hadfield, J. C. David, R. F. Meyer, T. F. Smith, and F. R. Cockerill, III.** 2002. Detection of *Bacillus anthracis* DNA by LightCycler PCR. *J. Clin. Microbiol.* **40:**2897–2902.
3. **Brown, E. R., and W. B. Cherry.** 1955. Specific identification of *Bacillus anthracis* by means of a variant bacteriophage. *J. Infect. Dis.* **96:**34–39.
4. **Carucci, J. A., T. W. McGovern, S. A. Norton, C. R. Daniel, B. E. Elewski, S. Fallon-Friedlander, B. D. Lushniak, J. S. Taylor, K. Warschaw, and R. G. Wheeland.** 2002. Cutaneous anthrax management algorithm. *J. Am. Acad. Dermatol.* **47:**766–769.
5. **Centers for Disease Control and Prevention.** 2001. Update: Investigation of anthrax associated with intentional exposure and interim public health guidelines, October 2001. *Morb. Mortal. Wkly. Rep.* **50:**889–893.
6. **Cockerill, F. R., and T. F. Smith.** 2002. Rapid-cycle real-time PCR: a revolution for clinical microbiology. *ASM News* **68:**77–83.
7. **De, B. K., S. L. Bragg, G. N. Sanden, K. E. Wilson, L. A. Diem, C. K. Marston, A. R. Hoffmaster, G. A. Barnett, R. S. Weyant, T. G. Abshire, J. W. Ezzell, and T. Popovic.** 2002. Two-component direct fluorescent-antibody assay for rapid identification of *Bacillus anthracis*. *Emerg. Infect. Dis.* **8:**1060–1065.
8. **Dragon, D. C., R. P. Rennie, and B. T. Elkin.** 2001. Detection of anthrax spores in endemic regions of northern Canada. *J. Appl. Microbiol.* **91:**435–441.
9. **Ezzell, J. W., Jr., and T. G. Abshire.** 1988. Immunological analysis of cell-associated antigens of *Bacillus anthracis*. *Infect. Immun.* **56:**349–356.
10. **Ezzell, J. W., Jr., T. G. Abshire, S. F. Little, B. C. Lidgerding, and C. Brown.** 1990. Identification of *Bacillus anthracis* by using monoclonal antibody to cell wall galactose-N-acetylglucosamine polysaccharide. *J. Clin. Microbiol.* **28:**223–231.
11. **Guarner, J., J. A. Jernigan, W. J. Shieh, K. Tatti, L. M. Flannagan, D. S. Stephens, T. Popovic, D. A. Ashford, B. A. Perkins, and S. R. Zaki.** 2003. Pathology and pathogenesis of bioterrorism-related inhalational anthrax. *Am. J. Pathol.* **163:**701–709.
12. **Helgason, E., O. A. Okstad, D. A. Caugant, H. A. Johansen, A. Fouet, M. Mock, I. Hegna, and A.-B. Kolsto.** 2000. *Bacillus anthracis, Bacillus cereus,* and *Bacillus thuringiensis*—one species on the basis of genetic evidence. *Appl. Environ. Microbiol.* **66:**2627–2630.
13. **Hering, D., W. Thompson, J. Hewetson, S. Little, S. Norris, and J. Pace-Templeton.** 2004. Validation of the anthrax lethal toxin neutralization assay. *Biologicals* **32:**17–27.
14. **Hoffmaster, A. R., R. F. Meyer, M. D. Bower, C. K. Marston, R. S. Weyant, K. Thurman, S. L. Messenger, E. E. Minor, J. M. Winchell, M. V. Rassmussen, B. R. Newton, J. T. Parker, W. E. Morrill, N. McKinney, G. A. Barnett, J. J. Sejvar, J. A. Jernigan, B. A. Perkins, and T. Popovic.** 2002. Evaluation and validation of a real-time polymerase chain reaction assay for rapid identification of *Bacillus anthracis*. *Emerg. Infect. Dis.* **8:**1178–1182.
15. **Hoffmaster, A. R., J. Ravel, D. A. Rasko, G. D. Chapman, M. D. Chute, C. K. Marston, B. K. De, C. T. Sacchi, C. Fitzgerald, L. W. Mayer, M. C. Maiden, F. G. Priest, M. Barker, L. Jiang, R. Z. Cer, J. Rilstone, S. N. Peterson, R. S. Weyant, D. R. Galloway, T. D. Read, T. Popovic, and C. M. Fraser.** 2004. Identification of anthrax toxin genes in a *Bacillus cereus* associated with an illness resembling inhalation anthrax. *Proc. Natl. Acad. Sci. USA.* **101:**8449–8454.
16. **Jernigan, D. B., P. L. Raghunathan, B. P. Bell, R. Brechner, E. A. Bresnitz, J. C. Butler, M. Cetron, M. Cohen, T. Doyle, M. Fischer, C. Greene, K. S. Griffith, J. Guarner, J. L. Hadler, J. A. Hayslett, R. Meyer, L. R. Petersen, M. Phillips, R. Pinner, T. Popovic, C. P. Quinn, J. Reefhuis, D. Reissman, N. Rosenstein, A. Schuchat, W. J. Shieh, L. Siegal, D. L. Swerdlow, F. C. Tenover, M. Traeger, J. W. Ward, I. Weisfuse, S. Wiersma, K. Yeskey, S. Zaki, D. A. Ashford, B. A. Perkins, S. Ostroff, J. Hughes, D. Fleming, J. P. Koplan, J. L. Gerberding, and The National Anthrax Epidemiologic Investigation Team.** 2002. Investigation of bioterrorism-related anthrax, United States, 2001: epidemiologic findings. *Emerg. Infect. Dis.* **8:**1019–1028.
17. **Keim, P., A. Kalif, J. Schupp, K. Hill, S. E. Travis, K. Richmond, D. M. Adair, M. Hugh-Jones, C. R. Kuske, and P. Jackson.** 1997. Molecular evolution and diversity in *Bacillus anthracis* as detected by amplified fragment length polymorphism markers. *J. Bacteriol.* **179:**818–824.
18. **Knisely, R. F.** 1966. Selective medium for *Bacillus anthracis*. *J. Bacteriol.* **92:**784–786.
19. **Little, S. F., B. E. Ivins, P. F. Fellows, M. L. Pitt, S. L. Norris, and G. P. Andrews.** 2004. Defining a serological correlate of protection in rabbits for a recombinant anthrax vaccine. *Vaccine* **22:**422–430.
20. **Logan, N. A., and P. C. Turnbull.** 1999. *Bacillus* and recently derived genera, p. 357–369. *In* P. R. Murray, E. J. Baron, M. A. Pfaller, F. C. Tenover, and R. H. Yolken (ed.), *Manual of Clinical Microbiology*, 7th ed. ASM Press, Washington, D.C.
21. **McChlery, S. M., and S. C. Clarke.** 2003. The use of hydrolysis and hairpin probes in real-time PCR. *Mol. Biotechnol.* **25:**267–274.
22. **Morse, S. A., R. B. Kellogg, S. Perry, R. F. Meyer, D. Bray, D. Nichelson, and J. M. Miller.** 2003. Detecting biothreat agents: the laboratory response network. *ASM News* **69:**433–437.
23. **Okinaka, R. T., K. Cloud, O. Hampton, A. R. Hoffmaster, K. K. Hill, P. Keim, T. M. Koehler, G. Lamke, S. Kumano, J. Mahillon, D. Manter, Y. Martinez, D. Ricke, R. Svensson, and P. J. Jackson.** 1999. Sequence and organization of pXO1, the large *Bacillus anthracis* plasmid harboring the anthrax toxin genes. *J. Bacteriol.* **181:**6509–6515.
24. **Peruski, A. H., and L. F. Peruski, Jr.** 2003. Immunological methods for detection and identification of infectious disease and biological warfare agents. *Clin. Diagn. Lab. Immunol.* **10:**506–513.
25. **Quinn, C. P., V. A. Semenova, C. M. Elie, S. Romero-Steiner, C. Greene, H. Li, K. Stamey, E. Steward-Clark,**

D. S. Schmidt, E. Mothershed, J. Pruckler, S. Schwartz, R. F. Benson, L. O. Helsel, P. F. Holder, S. E. Johnson, M. Kellum, T. Messmer, W. L. Thacker, L. Besser, B. D. Plikaytis, T. H. Taylor, Jr., A. E. Freeman, K. J. Wallace, P. Dull, J. Sejvar, E. Bruce, R. Moreno, A. Schuchat, J. R. Lingappa, S. K. Martin, J. Walls, M. Bronsdon, G. M. Carlone, M. Bajani-Ari, D. A. Ashford, D. S. Stephens, and B. A. Perkins. 2002. Specific, sensitive, and quantitative enzyme-linked immunosorbent assay for human immunoglobulin G antibodies to anthrax toxin protective antigen. *Emerg. Infect. Dis.* **8:**1103–1110.

26. **Read, T. D., S. N. Peterson, N. Tourasse, L. W. Baillie, I. T. Paulsen, K. E. Nelson, H. Tettelin, D. E. Fouts, J. A. Eisen, S. R. Gill, E. K. Holtzapple, O. A. Okstad, E. Helgason, J. Rilstone, M. Wu, J. F. Kolonay, M. J. Beanan, R. J. Dodson, L. M. Brinkac, M. Gwinn, R. T. DeBoy, R. Madpu, S. C. Daugherty, A. S. Durkin, D. H. Haft, W. C. Nelson, J. D. Peterson, M. Pop, H. M. Khouri, D. Radune, J. L. Benton, Y. Mahamoud, L. Jiang, I. R. Hance, J. F. Weidman, K. J. Berry, R. D. Plaut, A. M. Wolf, K. L. Watkins, W. C. Nierman, A. Hazen,** R. Cline, C. Redmond, J. E. Thwaite, O. White, S. L. Salzberg, B. Thomason, A. M. Friedlander, T. M. Koehler, P. C. Hanna, A. B. Kolsto, and C. M. Fraser. 2003. The genome sequence of *Bacillus anthracis* Ames and comparison to closely related bacteria. *Nature* **423:**81–86.

27. **Reif, T. C., M. Johns, S. D. Pillai, and M. Carl.** 1994. Identification of capsule-forming *Bacillus anthracis* spores with PCR and a novel dual-probe hybridization format. *Appl. Environ. Microbiol.* **60:**1622–1625.

28. **Shieh, W. J., J. Guarner, C. Paddock, P. Greer, K. Tatti, M. Fischer, M. Layton, M. Philips, E. Bresnitz, C. P. Quinn, T. Popovic, B. A. Perkins, and S. R. Zaki.** 2003. The critical role of pathology in the investigation of bioterrorism-related cutaneous anthrax. *Am. J. Pathol.* **163:**1901–1910.

29. **Ticknor, L. O., A. B. Kolsto, K. K. Hill, P. Keim, M. T. Laker, M. Tonks, and P. J. Jackson.** 2001. Fluorescent amplified fragment length polymorphism analysis of Norwegian *Bacillus cereus* and *Bacillus thuringiensis* soil isolates. *Appl. Environ. Microbiol.* **67:**4863–4873.

30. **Turnbull, P. C.** 1999. Definitive identification of *Bacillus anthracis*—a review. *J. Appl. Microbiol.* **87:**237–240.

MYCOTIC AND PARASITIC DISEASES

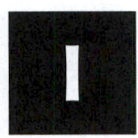

VOLUME EDITOR
ROBERT G. HAMILTON

SECTION EDITOR
THOMAS B. NUTMAN

Introduction

THOMAS B. NUTMAN

64

Combining the sections on clinical immunology of parasitic and fungal infections into one unit stems not so much from the similarity between parasites and fungi but rather from their not being part of either the infectious diseases or immunological mainstream. From a phylogenetic perspective, parasites (even the single-cell protozoa) differ from the fungi by a considerable evolutionary distance; interestingly, based on phylogenetic analyses, the differences between protozoan parasites and fungi are less significant than the differences between unicellular and multicellular parasites (Fig. 1).

Parasitic diseases are historically defined as infectious illnesses caused by unicellular protozoa or multicellular helminths distinct from viral, bacterial, or fungal etiologic agents. They are the special health care problem of tropical and subtropical countries, where their marked prevalence imposes a major medical and economic burden (5, 6). These infections afflict billions of people worldwide and are responsible for millions of deaths every year. The importance of parasitic illness has received recent additional emphasis as a result of the emergence of *Toxoplasma,* microsporidia, and *Cryptosporidium* as opportunistic pathogens in patients who are immunosuppressed.

Parasites encompass a heterogeneous group of organisms with extremely diverse biologies. Protozoa are usually a few micrometers in size, whereas worms are typically centimeters to meters in length. Tissue-dwelling protozoa are often intracellular parasites at some stage of infection, whereas helminths, being larger than most tissue cells, are almost always extracellular pathogens—the significant exception being *Trichinella spiralis,* which encysts within mammalian muscle cells. Protozoa usually replicate during infection of a single host; helminths do not reproduce without the assistance of intermediate hosts or passage through soil or water.

Both protozoan and helminth pathogens have complex life cycles, often with two or more developmental stages present in the host during infection (3). Because each stage of parasite development may be antigenically distinct, protozoan or helminth infections are often characterized by a series of discrete immune responses that develop at different times during the course of disease. Immune responses directed against a single stage may be circumvented by parasite differentiation. Each stage of parasite development may also entail a change in tissue tropism, introducing a compartmental feature to the immune responses. This temporal evolution of antigenic complexity and tissue tropism is unique to parasite immunology and further distinguishes this field from viral, fungal, and bacterial immunology.

Nevertheless, the immunology of fungal and parasitic infections converges at several levels. First, despite the enormous progress made in the biochemical purification and/or recombinant production of immunologically relevant antigens—some now based on parasite or yeast genomics—many of the diagnostic antigens used for either parasitic or fungal infections are crude (unfractionated) antigens that often contain epitopes (or whole antigens) that cross-react not only with organisms of different genera but also with those from unrelated species. Moreover, the diagnosis of mycotic infections cannot always be definitively addressed by culture or histology. Since the diagnosis of most parasitic infections has relied most commonly on the identification of the organism in appropriately collected specimens, those involved in the diagnosis of mycotic or parasitic infections have turned their attention to immunologic and molecular methods of diagnosis.

Traditionally, antibody-based diagnostic assays have suffered from a variety of difficulties that include: (i) the inability to distinguish between past infection and an active, current infection; (ii) poor specificity; (iii) reliance on changes in antibody isotypes or titers over the weeks or months following infection (retrospective diagnosis); and (iv) difficulty in their use in immunocompromised individuals. For many mycotic and parasitic infections, the limitations of standard serological assessments have been overcome by the use of antigen detection systems (see chapters 65 and 66) or methods of detecting microbial DNA (1, 2, 4) usually PCR.

Indeed, antigen detection methods have been extraordinarily useful in the diagnosis of fungal infections caused by *Aspergillus, Candida, Cryptococcus, Histoplasma,* and *Paracoccidioides* spp. and parasitic infections caused by *Entoamoeba, Giardia, Cryptosporidium, Wuchereria,* and *Trichomonas* spp. Many of these antigen detection systems have moved into the commercial arena and are available for clinical use. In contrast, PCR-based assays, although definitive in many instances, are not in widespread use. Nevertheless, PCR assays for the relatively rapid diagnosis of invasive *Candida* and *Aspergillus* spp. (see chapter 66) infections and for filarial and malarial organisms have moved beyond the laboratory bench and are offered in some clinical laboratories. Impediments to the widespread use of molecular diagnostics remain the lack of standardized methods for

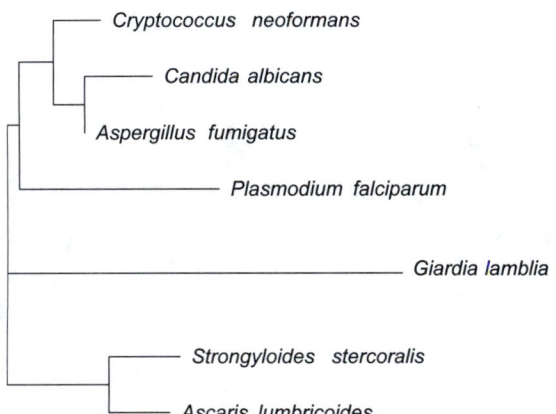

FIGURE 1 Phylogenetic dendrogram of selected pathogenic fungi and parasites based on 16S/18S ribosomal sequences.

sample preparation and difficulties extracting DNA from certain organisms and/or tissues.

Another area of progress in diagnostic mycology and parasitology is the use of immunohistochemistry to demonstrate particular organisms in tissue or body fluids. For example, the availability of fluorescently labeled antibodies for the detection of *Blastomyces dermatitidis, Coccidioides immitis, Histoplasma capsulatum, Pneumocystis carinii, Paracoccidioides basiliensis, Trichomonas vaginalis, Giardia lamblia,* and *Cryptosporidium parvum* among others has provided often rapid detection of organisms in appropriately collected specimens.

Continued efforts to improve the positive and negative predictive value of immunologic- and molecular-based assays remain the major goal of those interested in the accurate diagnosis of mycotic and parasitic infections. Although heralded as the new diagnostic gold standard, PCR-based assays are not yet in mainstream use. Notwithstanding the cost and issues related to quality control, the time required for sample preparation, PCR itself, and detection of the product suggests that other methods for clinical diagnosis of fungal and parasitic infections are needed, particularly rapid antigen detection systems.

REFERENCES

1. **Chen, S. C., C. L. Halliday, and W. Meyer.** 2002. A review of nucleic acid-based diagnostic tests for systemic mycoses with an emphasis on polymerase chain reaction-based assays. *Med. Mycol.* **40:**333–357.
2. **Iwen, P. C.** 2003. Molecular detection and typing of fungal pathogens. *Clin. Lab. Med.* **23:**781–799.
3. **Markell, E. K., and M. Voge.** 1976. *Medical Parasitology,* 4th ed. The W. B. Saunders Co., Philadelphia, Pa.
4. **McLintock, L. A., and B. L. Jones.** 2004. Advances in the molecular and serological diagnosis of invasive fungal infection in haemato-oncology patients. *Br. J. Haematol.* **126:**289–297.
5. **Stephenson, L. S., M. C. Latham, and E. A. Ottesen.** 2000. Malnutrition and parasitic helminth infections. *Parasitology* **121:**S23–238.
6. **Zaidi, A. K., S. Awasthi, and H. J. deSilva.** 2004. Burden of infectious diseases in South Asia. *Br. Med. J.* **328:** 811–815.

Molecular and Immunological Approaches to the Diagnosis of Parasitic Infections

MARIANNA WILSON, PETER M. SCHANTZ, AND THOMAS NUTMAN

65

The diagnosis of parasitic infections is definitively made by the identification of parasites in host tissue or excreta. Such identification is not generally possible for diseases such as toxoplasmosis or toxocariasis, in which parasites are located in deep tissue sites, and is not initially recommended for diseases such as cysticercosis or echinococcosis, for which invasive techniques with some risk to the patient are necessary to obtain material. The detection of antibodies can be very useful as an indicator that an individual has been infected with a specific parasite. A positive result for a person with no exposure to the parasite prior to recent travel in an area where disease is endemic may be interpreted as indicating recent infection. However, the detection of specific antibodies in a person who is native to an area where the parasite is endemic may reflect only a past infection unrelated to the current clinical status. In general, the detection of antibodies to parasitic diseases indicates only infection at some indeterminate time and not necessarily an acute or current infection. Levels of antibodies to parasites slowly decline after the patient is cured of the infection but generally last for at least 6 months to many years, depending on the infecting parasite, and thus are not generally reliable indicators of a successful cure.

The detection of specific immunoglobulin M (IgM) and IgA antibodies may be of value in determining the approximate time of initial infection with *Toxoplasma gondii*, but it is not recommended for any other parasitic disease. If infection with a parasite is suspected and blood film, stool, or urine examinations are either not indicated or negative, then the appropriate serology test for parasite-specific Ig or IgG antibodies should be requested. Tests for parasite-specific IgM, IgA, or IgE are generally not useful for diagnosis and should not be requested. If the parasite-specific Ig or IgG test is negative, then a positive IgM, IgA, or IgE result is generally a false-positive reaction and should not be considered when determining patient management.

The majority of parasitic immunodiagnostic procedures (Table 1) are performed in a few commercial laboratories, with reference testing available at the CDC. Although commercial kits for in vitro diagnostic use for some parasitic diseases are now available in the United States (Tables 2 to 4), the quality of these reagents is variable. Reagents for most parasitic diseases are classified as exempt from the U.S. FDA approval process; kits may be marketed in the United States without review, with the exceptions of *Toxoplasma* and *Trypanosoma* sp. serological reagents.

For most parasitic diseases, the antigen is generally the assay component which has the most influence on test sensitivity and specificity. Parasites generally have more than one life cycle stage, which may have both mutually shared antigens and stage-specific antigens. The matrix to which antigens are bound for use in a specific procedure also physically selects which antigen subset will be available for antibody binding. The decision of which parasite stage and antigen preparation will be used in a specific assay should not be made without an extensive review of the published literature. A determination of the sensitivity of a procedure should be made with specimens from patients in whom the specific parasite has been observed. Unfortunately, this is not possible for diseases such as toxoplasmosis, toxocariasis, or trichinosis because the parasites are sequestered in muscle or organ tissues and are generally not detectable. Specimens from well-defined clinical cases are acceptable for assay evaluations of these diseases, but they are usually difficult to obtain. The patient specimens should be characterized to suit the particular disease. The sensitivity of a procedure may be affected by the stage and type of the patient's disease. For example, patients who have undergone surgery for an echinococcal cyst in the liver almost always will have detectable antibodies, but they may be negative prior to surgery. A test evaluated with only postsurgery case specimens will have close to 100% sensitivity, but a test evaluated with presurgery case specimens will have a lower sensitivity which is more indicative of how efficient the assay is as an aid to establishing a diagnosis prior to surgery. Duplication of a published procedure does not necessarily mean that the results of several laboratories are identical without a comparable evaluation and, ideally, an exchange of reagents and sera. An organized, impartial proficiency program for parasitic serology assays other than those for *Babesia microti* and *Toxoplasma* does not exist to aid in determining comparability between tests and laboratories.

The diagnosis of human intestinal protozoa depends on microscopic detection of the various parasite stages in feces, duodenal fluid, or small intestine biopsy specimens. Since fecal examination is very labor-intensive and requires a skilled microscopist, both antibody tests and antigen detection tests have been investigated as alternatives. Antibody tests are of limited value except for invasive amebiasis due to

TABLE 1 Antibody and antigen detection tests for parasitic diseases

Disease	Antibody test(s)[a]	Antigen test(s)
Amebiasis	EIA	EIA, rapid
Angiostrongyliasis	EIA, IB	
Babesiosis	IFA	
Baylisascariasis	EIA	
Chagas' disease	EIA, IFA	
Cryptosporidiosis	EIA, IB	EIA, DFA, rapid
Cysticercosis	EIA, IB	
Echinococcosis	EIA, IB	
Fascioliasis	EIA	
Filariasis	EIA	Rapid
Giardiasis	IFA	EIA, DFA, rapid
Gnathostomiasis	IB	
Leishmaniasis	IFA, EIA	
Malaria	IFA	Rapid
Microsporidia		DFA, molecular
Paragonimiasis	EIA, IB	
Schistosomiasis	EIA, IB	
Strongyloidiasis	EIA	
Toxocariasis	EIA	
Toxoplasmosis	EIA, IFA	
Trichinellosis	EIA	
Trichomoniasis		DFA, rapid, molecular

[a] IB, immunoblot; rapid, rapid immunochromatographic test.

Entamoeba histolytica. The detection of parasite antigens is more indicative of a current infection and can be quickly performed by less skilled laboratory personnel than an experienced morphologist. Much work has been accomplished on the development of antigen detection systems, resulting in commercially available reagents for the intestinal parasites *Cryptosporidium parvum*, *E. histolytica*, *Giardia lamblia*, and *Trichomonas vaginalis.* In addition, rapid tests (dipstick-like) for antigen detection are available outside the United States for malaria and *Wuchereria bancrofti.*

Although molecular biology techniques show promise for improving the diagnosis of a variety of parasitic infections, they are generally research tools, with the exceptions of *B. microti* PCR, *Plasmodium* PCR, and *Toxoplasma* PCR, and probably will not be available for routine use in clinical diagnostic laboratories in the foreseeable future.

For detailed information on parasites and diagnostic procedures, go to DPDx (www.dpd.cdc.gov/dpdx), the Division of Parasitic Diseases, CDC, website for the laboratory diagnosis of parasitic diseases. For questions not addressed at the website, inquiries may be sent by e-mail through the website. For information and references regarding specific test procedures and protocols, the reader should contact the testing laboratories and the manufacturers of commercial kits.

Abbreviations. The following abbreviations are used in this chapter: **CDC,** Centers for Disease Control and Prevention; **CDC-EITB,** CDC enzyme-linked immunoelectrotransfer blot (immunoblot); **CSF,** cerebrospinal fluid; **DFA,** direct fluorescent antibody; **EIA,** enzyme immunoassay; **ES,** excretory-secretory; **FAST-ELISA,** Falcon Assay Screening Test (F.A.S.T.)–enzyme-linked immunosorbent assay; **FDA,** Food and Drug Administration; **IFA,** indirect fluorescent antibody; **IHA,** indirect hemagglutination assay; and **OLM,** ocular larva migrans.

SPECIMEN REQUIREMENTS

Specimens for Antibody Detection
For all antibody detection tests for parasitic diseases, sera or plasmas are acceptable specimens. For toxocariasis and toxoplasmosis, aqueous and vitreous eye fluids may be tested when accompanied by a serum specimen. For central nervous system infections such as cysticercosis or toxoplasmosis, CSF accompanied by a serum specimen may be tested. All specimens may be shipped at room temperature. In general, acute- and convalescent-phase specimens are not required; valid results generally can be obtained by testing only one specimen because many parasitic diseases are past the acute stage when initially considered.

Specimens for Antigen Detection
Fresh or preserved stool samples are acceptable for antigen detection testing with most kits, but please refer to the recommended collection procedure for each specific kit.

AFRICAN TRYPANOSOMIASIS
Immunodiagnostic tests for the detection of African sleeping sickness caused by infections with *Trypanosoma brucei rhodesiense* or *T. brucei gambiense* are not available without prior consultation with the CDC. If African trypanosomiasis is suspected, please call the Division of Parasitic Diseases, CDC, at (770) 488-7775 for information on diagnosis and clinical management.

TABLE 2 Antibody detection kits available commercially in the United States for parasitic diseases other than toxoplasmosis

Disease (organism)	Company[a]	Test[b]
Amebiasis (*Entamoeba histolytica*)	Chemicon	EIA
	IVD Research	EIA
Chagas' disease (*Trypanosoma cruzi*)	Chemicon	EIA
	Hemagen Diagnostics	EIA
	IVD Research	EIA
	InBios	EIA, rapid
Cysticercosis (larval *Taenia solium*)	Chemicon	EIA
	Immunetics	IB
	IVD Research	EIA
	InBios	EIA
Echinococcosis (*Echinococcus granulosus*)	Immunetics	IB
	IVD Research	EIA
Echinococcosis (*Echinococcus multilocularis*)	Bordier Affinity	EIA
Leishmaniasis, visceral (*Leishmania*)	Immunetics	IB
	InBios	Rapid
	IVD Research	EIA
Schistosomiasis (*Schistosoma*)	IVD Research	EIA
Strongyloidiasis (*Strongyloides stercoralis*)	IVD Research	EIA
Toxocariasis (*Toxocara canis*)	IVD Research	EIA
Trichinosis (*Trichinella spiralis*)	IVD Research	EIA

[a] Abbott Labs, Diagnostics Division, North Chicago, Ill.; Bordier Affinity Products, Chatanerie 2, CH-1023, Crissier, Switzerland; Chemicon, 28835 Single Oak Dr., Temecula, Calif.; Hemagen, 34-40 Bear Hill Rd., Waltham, Mass.; Immunetics, 380 Green St., Cambridge, Mass.; InBios, 562 1st Ave. South, Suite 600, Seattle, Wash.; IVD Research, 5909 Sea Lion Pl., Suite D, Carlsbad, Calif.

[b] IB, immunoblot; rapid, rapid immunochromatographic test.

TABLE 3 Commercially available kits for immunodetection of parasitic organisms or antigens

Organism and kit name	Manufacturer (distributor)[a]	Type of test[b]
Cryptosporidium parvum		
Cryptosporidium	IVD Research	EIA
Cryptosporidium	Novocastra	DFA
ProSpecT	Remel	EIA
Xpect	Remel	Rapid
Cryptosporidium	TechLab (Wampole)	EIA
Cryptosporidium parvum and *Giardia lamblia*		
ColorPAC	Becton Dickinson	Rapid
Crypto/Giardia	IVD Research	DFA, EIA
Merifluor	Meridian	DFA
ImmunoCardSTAT	Meridian	Rapid
ProSpecT	Remel	EIA
Xpect	Remel	Rapid
Cryptosporidium parvum, Giardia lamblia, and *Entamoeba histolytica*		
Triage	BioSite	Rapid
Entamoeba histolytica		
E. histolytica/E. dispar	IVD Research	EIA
ProSpecT	Remel	EIA
E. histolytica	TechLab (Wampole)	EIA
Giardia lamblia		
Giardia	Novocastra	DFA
ProSpecT	Remel	EIA
Giardia	TechLab (Wampole)	EIA
Trichomonas vaginalis		
Affirm VPIII	Becton Dickinson	NA
T.Vag.	Chemicon	DFA
OSOM Trichomonas	Genzyme	Rapid
XenoStrip-Tv	Xenotope	Rapid
Wuchereria bancrofti		
NOW Filariasis	Binax	Rapid

[a] Binax, 217 Read St., Portland, ME 04103; BioSite, 11030 Roselle St., San Diego, CA 92121; Becton Dickinson Diagnostic Systems, 7 Loveton Cir., Sparks, MD 21152; Chemicon, 28835 Single Oak Dr., Temecula, CA 92590; Genzyme Diagnostics, One Kendall Square, Cambridge, MA 02139; IVD Research, 5909 Sea Lion Place, Suite D, Carlsbad, CA 92008; Meridian Diagnostics, Inc., 3471 River Hills Dr., Cincinnati, OH 45244; Novocastra, 30 Ingold Rd., Burlingame, CA 94010; Remel, P.O. Box 14428, Lenexa, KS 66215; TechLab, VPI Research Park, 1861 Pratt Dr., Blacksburg, VA 24060; Wampole Laboratories, P.O. Box 1001, Cranbury, NJ 08512; Xenotope Diagnostics, 3463 Magic Dr., Suite 350, San Antonio, TX 78229.
[b] Rapid, rapid immunochromatographic test; NA, nucleic acid.

AMEBIASIS

EIA kits for *E. histolytica* antibody detection as well as for antigen detection are commercially available in the United States (Tables 2 and 3). Antibody detection is most useful for patients with extraintestinal disease, i.e., amebic liver abscess, for which organisms are not generally found upon stool examination. Antigen detection may be useful as an adjunct to microscopic diagnosis for detecting parasites and can distinguish between pathogenic and nonpathogenic *Entamoeba* infections (32).

Commercial EIA kits are available for routine serodiagnosis of amebiasis. The antigen consists of a crude soluble extract of axenically cultured organisms. The EIA detects antibodies specific for *E. histolytica* in approximately 95% of patients with extraintestinal amebiasis, 70% of patients with active intestinal infections, and 10% of asymptomatic persons who are passing cysts of *E. histolytica*. If antibodies are not detectable in patients with an acute presentation of suspected amebic liver abscess, a second specimen should be drawn 7 to 10 days later. If the second specimen does not show seroconversion, other agents should be considered. Detectable *E. histolytica*-specific antibodies may persist for years after successful treatment, so the presence of antibodies does not necessarily indicate acute or current infection. The specificity of the test is 95% or higher, and false-positive reactions rarely occur. Although the detection of IgM antibodies specific for *E. histolytica* has been reported, the test sensitivity is only about 64% for patients with current invasive disease. Several commercial EIA kits for antibody detection are available in the United States (Table 2).

Immunodetection of *E. histolytica* antigens in fecal specimens may be used to distinguish the morphologically identical pathogenic *E. histolytica* and nonpathogenic *Entamoeba dispar*. Fecal antigen assays employing monoclonal antibodies have improved sensitivities and specificities, resulting in the commercial availability of several EIA kits (Table 3). Organisms of both the pathogenic *E. histolytica* and the nonpathogenic *E. dispar* strains are morphologically identical. Detection of the galactose-inhibitable adherence protein, which appears to be necessary for pathogenesis, by tests for fecal antigen allows for the differentiation of pathogenic and nonpathogenic *Entamoeba* infections, thus avoiding unnecessary chemotherapy. A major drawback to this assay is that the test requires fresh stool samples instead of samples containing any fixative. Several EIA kits for antigen detection of the *E. histolytica*/*E. dispar* group are available in the United States, but only a TechLab kit is specific for *E. histolytica*.

TABLE 4 Toxoplasma kits available commercially in the United States

Company[a]	IgG kit(s)[b]	IgM kit(s)[b]
Abbott Labs	IMx, AxSYM	IMx, AxSYM
Bayer	Immuno1, Advia	Immuno1, Advia
Beckman	ACCESS	ACCESS
Biokit	LA	
bioMérieux	VIDAS	VIDAS
BioRad	EIA	EIA
Biotecx	EIA	EIA
Biotest	EIA	EIA
Diagnostic Products Corp.	Immulite	Immulite
Diamedix	EIA	EIA
DiaSorin	EIA	EIA
GenBio	EIA, IFA	EIA, IFA
Hemagen Diagnostics	EIA, IFA	EIA, IFA
MarDx	IB	IB
Meridian	EIA, IFA	EIA, IFA
Wampole Laboratories	EIA, IFA	EIA, IFA

[a] Abbott Labs, Diagnostics Division, North Chicago, IL 60064; Bayer Diagnostics, 511 Benedict Ave., Tarrytown, NY 10591; Beckman Coulter, 4300 N. Harbor Blvd., Fullerton, CA 92834; Biokit USA, 113 Hartwell Avenue, Lexington, MA 02173; bioMérieux, 595 Anglum Dr., Hazlewood, MO 63042; BioRad, 4000 Alfred Nobel Dr., Hercules, CA 94547; Biotecx Labs, 6023 S. Loop East, Houston, TX 77033; Biotest Diagnostics Corp., 66 Ford Rd., Suite 131, Denville, NJ 07834; Diagnostic Products Corp., 5700 W. 96th St., Los Angeles, CA 90045; Diamedix Corp., 2140 N. Miami Ave., Miami, FL 33127; DiaSorin, P. O. Box 285, Stillwater, MN 55082; GenBio, 15222 A. Avenue of Science, San Diego, CA 92128; Hemagen Diagnostics, 34-40 Bear Hill Rd., Waltham, MA 02154; MarDx, 5919 Farnsworth Court, Carlsbad, CA 92008; Meridian Diagnostics, 3471 River Hills Dr., Cincinnati, OH 45244; Wampole Laboratories, P.O. Box 1001, Cranbury, NJ 08512.
[b] ACCESS, Advia, AxSYM, Immulite, IMx, and VIDAS are automated assays.

The detection of *E. histolytica* and *E. dispar* DNA by PCR also allows for determinations of pathogenic versus nonpathogenic species. This assay is available in some state public health labs and the CDC. Contact information for each state lab is available at the Association of Public Health Laboratories website (www.aphl.org).

ANGIOSTRONGYLIASIS

Immunodiagnostic tests for the detection of antibodies to *Angiostrongylus* (*Angiostrongylus cantonensis*, which may cause eosinophilic meningitis, or *Angiostrongylus costaricensis*, the causative agent of abdominal angiostrongyliasis) are not currently available in the United States. If angiostrongylosis is suspected, please call the Division of Parasitic Diseases, CDC, at (770) 488-7775 for information on the availability of diagnostic testing and clinical management.

BABESIOSIS

Natural transmission of *B. microti* occurs primarily in the coastal areas of the northeastern United States and occasionally in Minnesota and Wisconsin. Rare human infections in California, Washington, Missouri, and Kentucky have occurred with *Babesia* sp. strains CA and WA1 and with *Babesia divergens*-like organisms which are antigenically and genotypically distinct from *B. microti* (8). Because the tick vector of *Babesia microti* also transmits the causative agents of Lyme disease and ehrlichiosis, dual and triple infections of *B. microti*, *Borrelia burgdorferi*, and *Ehrlichia* may occur.

The diagnosis of *Babesia* infection should be made by the observation of parasites in patients' blood films. However, antibody detection tests are useful for detecting infected individuals with very low levels of parasitemia, such as asymptomatic blood donors in transfusion-associated cases, for posttherapy diagnosis after parasitemia is no longer detectable, and for discrimination between *Plasmodium falciparum* and *B. microti* infection for patients whose blood film examinations are inconclusive and whose travel histories cannot exclude either parasite.

The IFA test using *B. microti* parasites as the antigen detects antibodies in 88 to 96% of patients with *B. microti* infections (15). IFA antigen slides are prepared by using washed, parasitized erythrocytes produced in hamsters. Patients' antibody levels generally rise to $\geq$1:1,024 during the first weeks of illness and decline gradually over 6 months to levels of 1:16 to 1:256, but antibodies may remain detectable at low levels for a year or more. The test specificity is 100% for patients with other tick-borne diseases or persons not exposed to the parasite. Cross-reactions may occur in serum specimens from patients with malaria infections, but generally, antibody levels are highest with the homologous antigen. The extent of antibody cross-reactivity between *Babesia* species appears variable. A negative antibody result with *B. microti* antigen for a patient exposed on the West Coast may be a false-negative reaction for a *Babesia* species other than *B. microti*. In those cases in which serology is negative but *Babesia* organisms are observed, identification to the species level may be accomplished by DNA sequence analysis of the organism (8). IFA tests for *Babesia* sp. strain WA1 and *B. divergens* are available from the CDC. IFA test kits are not available commercially, but one company offers *B. microti* IFA antigen slides for sale.

B. microti PCR assays are available in several commercial laboratories and at the CDC. PCR is at least as sensitive as microscopy, but the persistence of *Babesia* DNA is variable, ranging from 3 weeks posttherapy to 3 or more months in untreated patients. For the detection of *B. microti* infection in chronic carriers, such as asymptomatic infected blood donors, or in patients after therapy for *Babesia*, antibody detection by IFA is the initial test of choice because it is more sensitive than microscopy or nucleic acid detection in these situations.

BAYLISASCARIASIS

Immunodiagnostic tests for the detection of antibodies to *Baylisascaris* are available only at Purdue University. If infection with *Baylisascaris* is suspected, please call the Division of Parasitic Diseases, CDC, at (770) 488-7775 for information on the availability of diagnostic testing and clinical management.

CHAGAS' DISEASE

Infections with *Trypanosoma cruzi* are common in Central and South America. Many immigrants from areas where Chagas' disease is endemic currently reside in the United States and are potential sources of parasite transmission via infected blood. During the acute stage of illness, blood film examination generally reveals the presence of trypomastigotes. During the chronic stage of infection, parasites are rare or absent from the circulation. Immunodiagnosis is the method of choice for determining whether the patient is infected. Although differentiating between acute and chronic infections is very important in determining the necessity of therapy, serology cannot be used to do so. A positive antibody response indicates only infection at some unknown time, and not acute infection.

The IFA test and EIA are employed at the CDC. IFA antigen slides are prepared from a suspension of epimastigotes; crude soluble antigens of epimastigotes are used for EIA. Although the IFA test is sensitive, cross-reactivity occurs with sera from patients with leishmaniasis, a protozoan disease that occurs in the same geographical areas as *T. cruzi* infection. The sensitivity (93 to 98%) and specificity (99%, excluding leishmania patients) of EIAs that use crude antigens are similar to those of the IFA test. In the United States, the radioimmunoprecipitation assay has been used as a confirmatory test (17), but generally the results of a combination of tests are employed. A variety of cloned antigens have been investigated for use in diagnosis, but they are not yet available in the United States (34). Four EIA kits for antibody detection are available in the United States (Table 2).

CRYPTOSPORIDIOSIS

Tests for the detection of human antibodies specific for *C. parvum* are not currently recommended due to a lack of sensitivity and specificity. Both a plate EIA and an immunoblot assay for antibody detection have been reported, but their usefulness will probably be greatest for epidemiological studies and not as clinical diagnostic tools. Organism or antigen detection in stools is the current immunodiagnostic test of choice and provides equal or increased sensitivity over that of microscopy. Molecular tools are not recommended for clinical diagnosis but may be useful for isolate or strain identification for epidemiological purposes.

Table 3 lists 12 commercial products (3 DFA, 4 EIA, and 5 rapid tests) available in the United States for the immunodiagnosis of cryptosporidial infections. Several kits are combined tests for *Cryptosporidium*, *Giardia*, and *E. histolytica*. Factors such as ease of use, technical skill, and the time necessary to complete the test, single versus batch testing, and test cost must be considered when deciding on the test of choice for individual laboratories. The most sensitive (99%) and specific (100%) method is reported to be the DFA test, which identifies oocysts in concentrated or unconcentrated fecal samples by using a fluorescein isothiocyanate-labeled monoclonal antibody. A combined DFA test for the simultaneous detection of cryptosporidial oocysts and *Giardia* cysts is available.

Four commercial EIAs are available in the microplate format for the detection of cryptosporidial antigens in fresh or frozen stool samples and also in stool specimens preserved in formalin, merthiolate-iodine-formalin, or sodium acetate-acetic acid-formalin fixative. Concentrated or polyvinyl alcohol-treated samples are unsuitable for testing with antigen detection EIA kits. The kits are reportedly superior to microscopy (especially acid-fast staining) and show a high correlation with the monoclonal antibody-based DFA test. Kit sensitivities and specificities ranged from 93 to 100% when used in a clinical setting. Laboratories which use these EIA kits need to be aware of potential problems with false-positive results and take steps to monitor each kit's performance (3).

Five rapid immunochromatographic assays are available for the combined antigen detection of either *Cryptosporidium* and *Giardia* or *Cryptosporidium*, *Giardia*, and *E. histolytica*. These offer the advantages of a short test time and multiple results from one reaction device. Initial evaluations indicate a comparable sensitivity and specificity to those of previously available tests.

CYSTICERCOSIS (LARVAL *TAENIA SOLIUM*)

The CDC-EITB assay with purified *T. solium* antigens is the immunodiagnostic test of choice for confirming a clinical and radiologic presumptive diagnosis of neurocysticercosis (36). The CDC-EITB assay is based on the detection of antibodies to one or more of seven lentil lectin purified structural glycoprotein antigens from the larval cysts of *T. solium* in an immunoblot format. It is 99.9% specific and has a sensitivity superior to that of any other test yet evaluated. Serum specimens for 97% of 108 parasitologically confirmed cases of cysticercosis had detectable antibodies. No serum samples from 376 patients with other microbial infections contained antibodies that reacted with any of the *T. solium*-specific antigens. The most important factors identified as determining positive immunoblot reactions are the numbers and stage of development of cysticerci. Cumulative clinical experience has confirmed that for patients with multiple (more than two) lesions, the test has >95% sensitivity. Seropositivity for biopsy-confirmed patients with single, enhancing parenchymal cysts was <50%; for clinically defined patients with a single cyst but who were not biopsied, the sensitivity was 70%. Seropositivity in the sera and CSF of patients with multiple but only calcified cysts was 82 and 77%, respectively. Seropositivity in the sera and CSF of patients with intraventricular neurocysticercosis was 93% (single cyst) or 95% (two or more cysts). For all patients, regardless of clinical presentation, the immunoblot assay is 10% more sensitive for serum than for CSF specimens: consequently, there is no need to obtain CSF solely for use in the immunoblot assay.

The CDC-EITB assay is both more specific and more sensitive than the EIA systems with which it has been compared. Nonspecificity has been a major problem with most EIAs because of cross-reacting components in crude antigens derived from cysticerci; these components react with antibodies specific for other helminth infections, especially echinococcosis and filariasis. Most partially purified fractions evaluated in an EIA appear to have lower sensitivities than do crude antigens and do not necessarily achieve higher specificities. Assays employing crude antigens for the detection of antibody are not reliable for the identification of this disease; all positive results and any negative results strongly suspected of cysticercosis should be confirmed by immunoblot. Currently available antibody detection tests for cysticercosis do not distinguish between active and inactive infections and thus have not been useful for evaluating the outcomes and prognoses of medically treated patients. Both the CDC-EITB assay and an EIA are commercially available in the United States (Table 2).

ECHINOCOCCOSIS

Strategies for the diagnosis of echinococcosis were presented in a recent review (26). Immunodiagnostic tests can be very helpful for the diagnosis of echinococcal disease, and they should be used before invasive methods (19). However, the clinician must have some knowledge of the characteristics of the available tests and the patient and parasite factors associated with false results. False-positive reactions may occur in persons with other helminthic infections, cancer, and chronic immune disorders. Negative test results do not rule out echinococcosis because some cyst carriers do not have detectable antibodies. Whether the patient has detectable antibodies is dependent on the physical location, structural integrity, and vitality of the larval cyst. Cysts in the liver are more likely to elicit an antibody response than cysts in the lungs, and regardless of localization, antibody detection tests are least sensitive for patients with intact hyaline cysts. Cysts in the lungs, brain, and spleen are associated with decreased or nondetectable antibody levels, whereas those in bone appear to elicit a more detectable immune response. Fissuration or rupture of a cyst is followed by an abrupt stimulation of antibody production. A patient with senescent, calcified, or dead cysts is generally found to be seronegative.

Molecular tools are used primarily for isolate or strain identification for epidemiological purposes but not for clinical diagnosis.

Cystic Echinococcal Disease (*Echinococcus granulosus*)

IHA, IFA, and EIA are sensitive tests for detecting antibodies in sera of patients with cystic disease; sensitivity rates vary from 60 to 90%, depending on the characteristics of the cases. Crude hydatid cyst fluid is generally employed as the antigen. At present, the best available serologic diagnosis is obtained by using a combination of tests. EIA or IHA is used to screen all specimens; a positive reaction is confirmed by an immunoblot assay or any gel diffusion assay that demonstrates the presence of the echinococcal "Arc 5." Although these confirmatory assays give false-positive reactions with sera from 5 to 25% of persons with neurocysticercosis, the clinical and epidemiological presentation of neurocysticercosis patients should rarely be confused with that of cystic echinococcosis. One commercial EIA kit and one immunoblot kit for antibody detection are available in the United States (Table 2).

Circulating antigens have been detected in the sera of only about half of patients with cystic echinococcosis; however, these antigens may be detectable in the sera of many patients with negative or borderline antibody levels. Antigen assays might be useful as additional tests for those patients with no detectable *Echinococcus* antibodies, but such assays are not available in the United States.

Antibody responses have also been monitored as a way of evaluating the results of treatment, but with mixed results. Following successful radical surgery, antibody levels decline and sometimes disappear; antibodies rise again if secondary hydatid cysts develop. Tests for Arc 5 or IgE antibodies appear to reflect an antibody decline during the first 24 months postsurgery, whereas the IHA and other tests remain positive for at least 4 years. Chemotherapy has not been followed by consistent declines in antibody levels. Consequently, the usefulness of serology to monitor the course of disease is limited; imaging techniques provide a more accurate assessment of the patient's condition.

Alveolar Echinococcal Disease (*Echinococcus multilocularis*)

Most patients with alveolar echinococcal disease have detectable antibodies in tests using heterologous *E. granulosus* or homologous *Echinococcus multilocularis* antigens. With crude *Echinococcus* antigens, nonspecific reactions occur as described above. However, the affinity-purified *E. multilocularis* antigen (Em2) used for EIA allows the detection of positive antibody reactions in >95% of alveolar cases. Comparing the serologic reactivity to the Em2 antigen with that to antigens containing components of both *E. multilocularis* and *E. granulosus* permits the discrimination of patients with alveolar disease from those with cystic disease. The combined use of two purified *E. multilocularis* antigens (Em2 and the recombinant antigen II/3-10) in a single antibody detection assay allows for optimized sensitivity and specificity. These antigens are sold in a commercial EIA antibody detection kit in Europe, but not in the United States (Table 2). An *E. multilocularis* antigen prepared by isoelectric focusing and used for immunoblot and EIA was also sensitive for detecting alveolar disease and differentiating between cystic and alveolar disease (11). As with cystic echinococcosis, antibody detection tests are more useful for postoperative follow-up than for monitoring the effectiveness of chemotherapy.

FASCIOLIASIS

The acute manifestations of human fascioliasis may precede the appearance of eggs in the stool by several weeks; immunodiagnostic tests may be useful for an early indication of *Fasciola* infection as well as for confirmation of chronic fascioliasis when egg production is low or sporadic and for ruling out pseudofascioliasis associated with the ingestion of parasite eggs in sheep or calves' liver.

The current tests of choice for immunodiagnosis of human *Fasciola hepatica* infection are an IFA or EIA for antibody that uses ES antigens combined with the confirmation of positive results by immunoblot (9). Specific antibodies to *Fasciola* may be detectable within 2 to 4 weeks after infection, which is 5 to 7 weeks before eggs appear in the stool. The sensitivity of the FAST-ELISA was reported to be 95%, while the sensitivity of immunoblot using 12-, 17-, and 63-kDa antigens appeared to be 100%. However, cross-reactivity may occur in the FAST-ELISA with serum specimens from patients with schistosomiasis. Antibody levels decrease to normal 6 to 12 months after chemotherapeutic cure and can be used to predict the success of therapy. The IFA test with parasite sections as the antigen is still used extensively in Europe, but its sensitivity and specificity may not be optimal.

FILARIASIS

Among the eight filarial species that commonly infect humans, the four most likely to be pathogenic are three bloodborne filariae, *Brugia malayi*, *W. bancrofti*, and *Loa loa*, and the skin-dwelling organism *Onchocerca volvulus*. For each of these infections and for infections by other filariae (*Mansonella perstans*, *Mansonella ozzardi*, *Mansonella streptocerca*, and *Brugia timori*), demonstration of the parasite (microfilariae in the blood or skin or adult parasites in tissue samples) or of parasite DNA by PCR remains the "gold standard" for definitive diagnosis. Nevertheless, diagnosis can be elusive, not only because occult infections (low parasite burdens) occur but also because microfilariae (for most *Brugia* and *Wuchereria* organisms, at least) are nocturnally periodic.

Lymphatic Filariasis (*W. bancrofti* and *Brugia* spp.)

A definitive diagnosis of lymphatic filariasis can be made only by detection of the parasites and hence can be difficult. Adult worms localized in lymphatic vessels or nodes are largely inaccessible. Microfilariae can be found in blood, in hydrocele fluid, or (occasionally) in other body fluids. Such fluids can be examined microscopically, either directly or—for greater sensitivity—after concentration of the parasites by the passage of fluid through a polycarbonate cylindrical pore filter (pore size, 3 μm) or by the centrifugation of fluid fixed in 2% formalin (Knott's concentration technique). The timing of blood collection is critical and should be based on the periodicity of the microfilariae in the region of endemicity involved. Many infected individuals do not have microfilaremia, and a definitive diagnosis in such cases can be difficult. Assays for circulating antigens of *W. bancrofti* permit the diagnosis of microfilaremic and cryptic (amicrofilaremic) infections. Two tests are commercially available: one is an ELISA and the other is a rapid-format immunochromatographic card test (Table 3). Both assays have sensitivities that range from 96 to 100% and specificities that approach 100% (4, 35). There are currently no tests for circulating antigens in brugian filariasis.

PCR-based assays for DNAs of *W. bancrofti* and *B. malayi* in blood have been developed (38). Several studies indicate that this diagnostic method is of equivalent or greater sensitivity than parasitology-based methods, detecting patent infection in almost all infected subjects.

Immunologically based diagnostics which measure IgG responses against crude extracts of *Brugia* or *Dirofilaria* worms have traditionally suffered from poor specificities. Extensive cross-reactivity is found in the sera of individuals infected with closely related helminth parasites and even certain protozoal parasites. Furthermore, it is difficult to differentiate a previous infection or exposure to the parasite (aborted infection) from a current active infection; most residents of regions where filariasis is endemic are antibody positive. Nevertheless, such serologic assays for IgG antibodies have a definite place in diagnosis, as a negative assay result effectively excludes past or present infection. The prominent role of antifilarial antibodies of the IgG4 subclass in active filarial infection has led to the development of diagnostic serological assays based on antibodies of this subclass. Antifilarial IgG4-specific tests have an improved specificity (16), but positive results may still be seen for uninfected individuals living in areas of endemicity and for those infected with other filarial species (e.g., *O. volvulus*, *L. loa*, and *Mansonella* spp.).

In cases of suspected lymphatic filariasis, an examination of the scrotum or the female breast by the use of high-frequency ultrasound in conjunction with Doppler techniques may result in the identification of motile adult worms within dilated lymphatics. Worms may be visualized in the lymphatics of the spermatic cord in up to 80% of infected men.

Onchocerciasis

A definitive diagnosis of onchocerciasis depends on the detection of an adult worm in an excised nodule or, more commonly, of microfilariae in a skin snip or in the anterior chamber of the eye by use of a slit lamp. Skin snips are obtained with a corneal-scleral punch, which collects a blood-free skin biopsy sample extending to just below the epidermis, or by lifting of the skin with the tip of a needle and excision of a small (1 to 3 mm) piece with a sterile scalpel blade. The biopsy tissue is incubated in tissue culture medium or saline on a glass slide or flat-bottomed microtiter plate. After incubation for 2 to 4 h (or occasionally overnight for light infections), microfilariae emergent from the skin can be visualized by low-power microscopy.

Because the detection of parasites in the skin or eye is invasive and insensitive, immunodiagnostic assays have been sought. Antifilarial IgG antibody assays, while positive for individuals with onchocerciasis, suffer from the same lack of specificity and positive predictive value seen in the case of bloodborne filarial infections. The combined use of three groups of recombinant antigens provides sensitivities and specificities that approach 100% for the diagnosis of onchocerciasis (23). Although no recombinant antigen test is available commercially, an experimental rapid card test that detects IgG4 antibodies to the Ov-16 recombinant in serum or whole blood has been shown to have >90% sensitivity and specificity.

Antigen detection methods for use on serum or plasma samples or on urine are theoretically feasible, but prototypes have lacked both specificity and sensitivity. Assays using PCR to detect onchocercal DNA in skin snips are now in use in filariasis research laboratories and are highly sensitive and specific.

Loiasis

A definitive diagnosis of loiasis requires the detection of microfilariae in the peripheral blood or the isolation of the adult worm from the eye or from a subcutaneous biopsy specimen from a site of swelling developing after treatment. PCR-based assays for the detection of *L. loa* DNA in blood are now available in filariasis research laboratories and are highly sensitive and specific.

Antifilarial IgG and IgG4 may be useful for confirming the diagnosis of loiasis in visitors to areas of endemicity who have suggestive clinical symptoms or unexplained eosinophilia; however, currently available methods using crude antigen extracts from *Brugia* or *Dirofilaria* species do not differentiate between *L. loa* and other filarial pathogens. The utility of such testing in endemic populations is limited by the presence of antifilarial antibodies in up to 95% of individuals in some regions. Recently, a *Loa*-specific recombinant (L1-SXP-1) has been tested; IgG4 antibody-based assays have been found to be 98% specific but have a limited (56%) sensitivity (14).

GIARDIASIS

G. *lamblia* is the most common human intestinal protozoan pathogen in the United States and is an important cause of diarrhea in children and adults. Outbreaks of disease are common within day care centers as a result of person-to-person contact and may also occur in communities as a result of drinking water contaminated by infected human or animal feces. Infected persons often excrete cysts intermittently, so multiple stools collected over at least several days must sometimes be examined to detect the parasite. Tests for antibody detection in human *Giardia* infection are not currently recommended due to a lack of sensitivity and specificity. Molecular tools are most useful for isolate or strain identification and not for clinical diagnosis.

Table 3 lists 11 commercial products (3 DFA, 4 EIA, and 4 rapid tests) available in the United States for the immunodiagnosis of giardiasis. DFA assays may be purchased that employ a fluorescein isothiocyanate-labeled monoclonal antibody for the detection of *Giardia* cysts alone or in a combined kit for the simultaneous detection of *Giardia* cysts and *Cryptosporidium* oocysts. The sensitivity and specificity of these kits are both 100% compared to those of microscopy. They may be used for the quantitation of cysts and oocysts and thus may be useful for epidemiologic and control studies.

Four commercial EIAs are available in the microplate format for the detection of *Giardia* antigens in fresh or frozen stool samples and also in stool specimens preserved in formalin, merthiopate-iodine-formalin, or sodium acetate-acetic acid-formalin fixative. Concentrated or polyvinyl alcohol-treated samples are not suitable for testing with EIA kits. EIA kit sensitivity rates were recently reported as ranging from 94 to 100%, while specificity rates are all 100% (1, 7).

Four rapid immunochromatographic assays are available for the combined detection of either *Cryptosporidium* and *Giardia* or *Cryptosporidium*, *Giardia*, and *E. histolytica*. These offer the advantages of a short test time and multiple results from one reaction device. Initial evaluations indicate a comparable sensitivity and specificity to those of previously available tests.

GNATHOSTOMIASIS

Immunodiagnostic tests for the detection of antibodies to *Gnathostoma* are not currently available in the United States. If gnathostomiasis is suspected, please call the Division of Parasitic Diseases, CDC, at (770) 488-7775 for information on the availability of diagnostic testing and clinical management.

LEISHMANIASIS

IFA and EIA tests are used for the detection of antibodies to *Leishmania* (31). IFA slide antigens consist of cultured epimastigotes of various species, while EIA antigens are usually crude solubilized epimastigotes. These procedures can differentiate leishmaniasis from other clinically similar conditions but cannot determine the infecting species of *Leishmania*. Cross-reactions occur for patients with antibodies to *T. cruzi* (Chagas' disease), which is also endemic to some Central and South American countries where leishmaniasis occurs. If visceral leishmaniasis is suspected, antibody detection tests can be a useful adjunct to clinical findings because test sensitivities are >95%. However, the sensitivities of antibody tests for cutaneous leishmaniasis are poor: most patients do not develop a detectable circulating antibody response to the parasite, so diagnostic testing should include aspirate and tissue impression smears and parasite culture.

Although biochemical, immunologic, and molecular biology techniques have been used extensively in *Leishmania* research, molecular probes for the detection and identification of parasites are currently available only in research labs (24). If leishmaniasis is suspected, a consultation on diagnosis and therapy may be obtained by calling the Division of Parasitic Diseases, CDC, at (770) 488-7775.

MALARIA

The serodiagnosis of malaria is not recommended except for (i) screening blood donors involved in cases of transfusion-induced malaria when the donor's parasitemia may be below the detectable level of blood film examination and (ii) testing a patient with a febrile illness who is suspected of having malaria and from whom repeated blood smears are negative. IFA tests with organisms of the four human *Plasmodium* species for malarial antibody detection are 97% sensitive and 99% specific, but the presence of antibodies indicates that infection occurred at some time in the past and does not necessarily indicate a current infection (30). Determination of the infecting species by serology is usually not possible. One commercial EIA kit for antibody detection is available in Great Britain and has been evaluated for use in blood bank screening (13).

There are many rapid tests for the detection of *Plasmodium* antigens in blood or serum available outside the United States. A list of rapid tests may be found at the website of the World Health Organization at www.wpro.who.int/rdt/. Although these assays have been extensively evaluated and found useful in field trials, their use for individual patient diagnosis is not sufficiently sensitive or specific to warrant the replacement of conventional microscopic diagnosis in clinical laboratories in nonmalarious areas (20).

PCR is sometimes a more sensitive method than microscopy for the detection of acute *Plasmodium* infection (29) and is available in some state public health laboratories and at the CDC. If infection is suspected, submit blood smears for morphological examination and EDTA-anticoagulated blood for PCR. The blood smears should be examined first for the presence of parasites. If malarial parasites are observed and the species is determined, then the diagnosis is complete. However, if parasites are not observed or if parasites are observed but the infecting species cannot be determined morphologically, PCR can then be performed. *Plasmodium* DNA generally becomes nondetectable within a week of antimalarial chemotherapy. If a chronic infection is suspected or if the patient has been treated for malaria, serology is the most sensitive assay compared to PCR and blood film exam.

For more information about malaria and its diagnosis, please visit the CDC website (www.cdc.gov/malaria).

MICROSPORIDIA

Microsporidia are obligate intracellular parasites that have a variety of animal hosts. Gastrointestinal as well as systemic disease has been reported for humans, principally for patients with AIDS. Eight genera of microsporidia have been recognized in humans: *Enterocytozoon*, *Encephalitozoon*, *Vittaforma*, *Nosema*, *Pleistophora*, *Trachipleistophora*, *Brachiola*, and *Microsporidium*, a genus comprising all those organisms that are not yet classified. Polyclonal sera and monoclonal antibodies raised against the most frequently identified microsporidial pathogens in clinical specimens (*Enterocytozoon bieneusi*, *Encephalitozoon intestinalis*, *Encephalitozoon hellen*, and *Encephalitozoon cuniculi*) have been tested, and their use as diagnostic reagents has been proposed in several reports (6). Additionally, specific antibodies to microsporidia have been detected in humans, but the serologic diagnosis of microsporidial infections is of limited use. Molecular techniques used in assays for the detection of parasite DNA in patient specimens, including fecal samples, have been reported by several research groups. However, no reagents for the immunodetection of microsporidial parasites or soluble antigens are available commercially.

PARAGONIMIASIS

Pulmonary paragonimiasis is the most common presentation of patients infected with *Paragonimus* spp., although extrapulmonary (cerebral or abdominal) paragonimiasis may occur. The detection of eggs in sputa or feces of patients with paragonimiasis is often difficult; therefore, serodiagnosis may be helpful for confirming infections and for monitoring the results of individual chemotherapy. In the United States, the detection of antibodies to *Paragonimus westermani* has helped physicians differentiate paragonimiasis from tuberculosis in Indochinese immigrants.

EIA tests, in both plate and blot formats, have replaced the complement fixation test. The immunoblot assay for antibody detection performed with a crude antigen extract of *P. westermani* has been in use at the CDC since 1988 (27). Positive antibody reactions, based on a demonstration of reactivity with an 8-kDa antigen, were obtained with serum samples from 96% of patients with parasitologically confirmed *P. westermani* infection. The test specificity was ≥99%; of 210 serum specimens from patients with other parasitic and nonparasitic infections, only 1 serum sample from a patient with *Schistosoma haematobium* reacted. Antibody levels detected by EIA and immunoblot do decline after chemotheraputic cure, but not as rapidly as those detected by the complement fixation test. Most published literature deals with pulmonary paragonimiasis due to *P. westermani*, although in some geographic areas other *Paragonimus* species cause similar or distinct clinical manifestations of human infections. Cross-reactivity between species does occur, but at varying levels for different species.

SCHISTOSOMIASIS

Antibody detection can be useful to indicate schistosome infection in patients who have traveled in areas where schistosomiasis is endemic and for whom eggs cannot be demonstrated in fecal or urine specimens. Test sensitivity and specificity vary widely among the many tests reported for the serologic diagnosis of schistosomiasis and are dependent on both the type of antigen preparation used (crude, purified, adult worm, egg, or cercarial antigen) and the test procedure.

At the CDC, a combination of tests with purified adult worm antigens are used for antibody detection (2, 33). All serum specimens are initially tested by FAST-ELISA using *Schistosoma mansoni* adult microsomal antigen. A positive reaction indicates infection with a *Schistosoma* species. The sensitivity of the test for *S. mansoni* infection is 99%, that for *S. haematobium* infection is 95%, and that for *Schistosoma japonicum* infection is >50%. The specificity of this assay for detecting schistosome infection is 99%. Because test sensitivity with the *S. mansoni* adult microsomal antigen is reduced for species other than *S. mansoni*, immunoblots of the species appropriate to the patient's travel history are also tested to ensure antibody detection of *S. haematobium* and *S. japonicum* infections. Immunoblots with adult worm microsomal antigens are species specific, so a positive antibody reaction indicates the infecting species. The presence of antibody is indicative only of schistosome infection at some time and cannot be correlated with the clinical status, worm burden, egg production, or prognosis.

The detection of schistosome antigens in serum and urine, in addition to quantitative stool or urine exams, has been suggested as an indicator of cure after chemotherapy. Although these techniques may be useful for populations in areas of *Schistosoma* endemicity, test sensitivities for patients with low worm burdens and low egg output (<50 eggs/ml) are not adequate. Antigen detection tests are not available in the United States.

STRONGYLOIDIASIS

Immunodiagnostic tests for strongyloidiasis are indicated when the infection is suspected and the organism cannot be demonstrated by duodenal aspiration, string tests, or repeated examinations of stool. Antibody detection tests should use antigens derived from *Strongyloides stercoralis* filariform larvae for the highest sensitivity and specificity. Although IFA and IHA tests have been used, EIA is currently recommended because of its greater (95%) sensitivity. Immunocompromised persons with disseminated strongyloidiasis usually have detectable IgG antibodies despite their immunodepression (12). Cross-reactions in patients with filariasis and some other nematode infections may occur. Important test limitations are that (i) 5% of individuals infected with *Strongyloides* are seronegative and (ii) antibody test results cannot be used to differentiate between past and current infections. A positive test warrants continuing efforts to establish a parasitological diagnosis followed by antihelminthic treatment. Serologic monitoring may be useful for the follow-up of immunocompetent treated patients: antibody levels decrease markedly within 6 months after successful chemotherapy (18). The potential use of immunoblots for the immunodiagnosis of strongyloidiasis has been reported.

TOXOCARIASIS (LARVA MIGRANS)

Antibody detection tests are the only means of confirmation of a clinical diagnosis of visceral larva migrans, OLM, and covert toxocariasis, the most common clinical syndromes associated with *Toxocara* infections (5, 28). The currently recommended serologic test for toxocariasis is an EIA with larval-stage antigens extracted from embryonated eggs or released in vitro by cultured infective larvae. The latter, *Toxocara* ES antigens, are preferable to larval extracts because they are convenient to produce and because an absorption-purification step is not required to obtain maximum specificity.

Evaluation of the true sensitivities and specificities of serologic tests for toxocariasis in human populations is not possible because of the lack of parasitologic methods to detect *Toxocara* parasites. These inherent problems result in underestimations of sensitivity and specificity. Evaluation of the *Toxocara* EIA with groups of patients with presumptive diagnoses of visceral larva migrans or OLM indicated sensitivities of 78 and 73%, respectively, at antibody levels of ≥1:32. When the cutoff titer for OLM cases was lowered to 1:8, the sensitivity was increased to 90%. Further confirmation of the specificity of the serologic diagnosis of OLM can be obtained by testing aqueous or vitreous humor samples for antibodies. The specificity has been reported to be >90% at antibody levels of ≥1:32.

When interpreting serologic findings, clinicians must be aware that a detectable antibody level does not necessarily indicate a current clinical *Toxocara canis* infection. In most human populations, a small number of those tested have positive EIA antibody levels that apparently reflect the prevalence of asymptomatic toxocariasis. In the United States, 2.8% of nearly 9,000 persons tested showed such positive reactions, but the percentage varied significantly according to age, race, and socioeconomic status. A commercial EIA kit is available in the United States (Table 2).

TOXOPLASMOSIS

A Clinical and Laboratory Standards Institute (formerly NCCLS) guideline entitled *Clinical Use and Interpretation of Serologic Tests for Toxoplasma gondii* has been published as an aid for laboratorians and physicians in determining the status of patients potentially infected with *T. gondii* (22). *Toxoplasma* antibody detection tests are performed by a large number of laboratories with commercially available kits (Table 4). Comparisons of kits indicated that most perform comparably for detecting *Toxoplasma*-specific IgG antibodies but vary markedly for detecting *Toxoplasma*-specific IgM antibodies (37). Quantitative results obtained with kits from different companies must be compared as just positive or negative because of the lack of standardization of expression of results. The College of American Pathologists offers *Toxoplasma* antibody proficiency testing as part of the Virology Antibody Detection Survey. The participation of all laboratories that perform *Toxoplasma* antibody testing should be encouraged. The summary of data obtained by this program is not only an indication of individual laboratory performance but also an indication of kit performance. Laboratories with aberrant results should question the accuracy of the kit they use in addition to their technical performance.

An algorithm for the immunodiagnosis of toxoplasmosis is shown in Fig. 1. EIA or IFA tests for IgG and IgM antibodies are the tests most commonly used today. Persons should be initially tested for the presence of *Toxoplasma*-specific IgG antibodies to determine their immune status. A positive IgG titer indicates infection with the organism at some time. If more precise knowledge of the time of infection is necessary, then a person with a positive IgG titer should have an IgM test performed by an IgM-capture EIA. A negative IgM test essentially rules out infection in recent months. A positive IgM titer combined with a positive IgG titer may be suggestive of a recent infection. However, *Toxoplasma*-specific IgM antibodies may be detected by EIA for as long as 18 months after an acute acquired infection. If the patient is pregnant, an IgG avidity test should then be performed. A high-avidity result in the first 12 to 16 weeks of pregnancy (the time is dependent on the commercial test kit) essentially rules out an infection acquired during gestation. A low IgG avidity should not be interpreted as indicating recent infection, because some individuals have persistent low IgG avidity for many months after infection. A suspected recent infection in a pregnant woman should be confirmed prior to intervention by having samples tested at a toxoplasmosis reference laboratory such as the Toxoplasmosis Serology Lab, Palo Alto Medical Foundation, Palo Alto, Calif.

If a patient is tested initially for both *Toxoplasma*-specific IgM and IgG antibodies, the result will sometimes be a positive IgM titer but a negative IgG result. A positive IgM result with a negative IgG result in the same specimen should be viewed with great suspicion; the patient's blood should be redrawn 2 weeks after the first blood draw and tested together with the first specimen. If the first specimen was drawn very early after infection, the patient should have highly positive IgG and IgM antibodies in the second sample. If the IgG test is negative and the IgM test is positive for both specimens, the IgM result should be considered to be a false positive and the patient should be considered not infected.

Newborn infants suspected of congenital toxoplasmosis should be tested by both an IgM- and an IgA-capture EIA. The detection of *Toxoplasma*-specific IgA antibodies is more sensitive than IgM detection for congenitally infected babies. Although commercial kits for IgA detection are available in Europe, none are available yet in the United States.

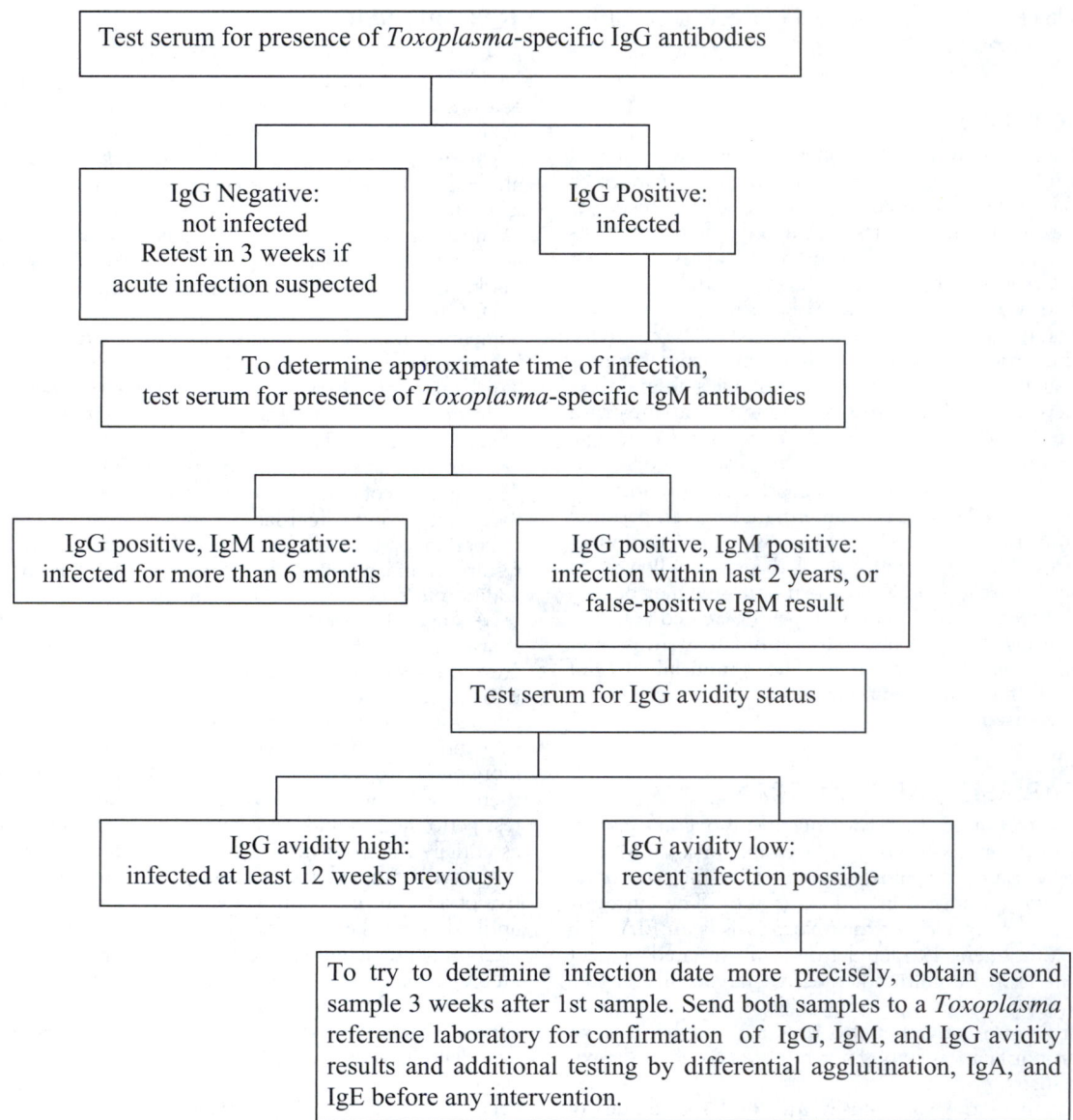

FIGURE 1   Algorithm for the serodiagnosis of toxoplasmosis in people older than 1 year of age.

The serological determination of active central nervous system toxoplasmosis in immunocompromised patients is not possible at this time. *Toxoplasma*-specific IgG antibody levels in AIDS patients are often low to moderate, but occasionally no specific IgG antibodies can be detected. Tests for IgM antibodies are generally negative. The detection of circulating antigen in AIDS patients has been evaluated, but the procedure lacks sensitivity.

TRICHINELLOSIS

Immunodiagnostic tests for trichinellosis currently available in the United States include EIAs for antibody detection. Antigen preparations may be crude antigens prepared from homogenates of *Trichinella spiralis* muscle larvae or ES products produced by cultured larvae (21). The TSL-1 group of larval secretory antigens is conserved in all species and isolates of *Trichinella* and thus can be used to detect infection in animals or people infected with any of the currently recognized types of *Trichinella*. Positive antibody reactions are detectable at some time during infection in serum samples from 80 to 100% of patients with clinically symptomatic trichinellosis. Antibody levels are often not detectable until 3 to 5 weeks postinfection, well after the onset of acute-stage illness. Antibody development is also affected by the infecting dose of larvae: the higher the infecting dose, the faster the patient's antibody response will develop. Multiple serum specimens should be drawn several weeks apart to demonstrate seroconversion in patients whose initial specimen was negative. IgG, IgM, and IgE antibodies are detectable in many patients; however, tests based on IgG antibodies are the most sensitive. Antibody levels peak in the second or third month postinfection and then decline slowly for several years.

In our experience at the CDC, the EIA with ES antigens detects antibodies earlier than the bentonite flocculation test in 25% of serum specimens from patients with acute infection, but the EIA also remains positive for longer periods after infection than the bentonite flocculation test and is reactive for a larger proportion of persons with no clinical evidence of trichinellosis. One commercial EIA kit for antibody detection is available in the United States (Table 2).

TRICHOMONIASIS

Trichomoniasis, an infection caused by *T. vaginalis*, is a common sexually transmitted disease. Diagnosis is made by the detection of trophozoites in vaginal secretions or urethral specimens by wet mount microscopic examination, culture, or the detection of parasite antigens or nucleic acids. The sensitivities of assays compared to that of culture were reported to be 60% for wet mounts, 86% for the DFA test, 80% for the Affirm VP test, 78.5% for the OSOM rapid test, and 78% for the XenoStrip rapid test (10, 25). A DFA test, a nucleic acid probe test, and two rapid antigen detection tests are available commercially (Table 3).

REFERENCES

1. **Aldeen, S. E., K. Carroll, A. Robison, M. Morrison, and D. Hale.** 1998. Comparison of nine commercially available enzyme-linked immunosorbent assays for detection of *Giardia lamblia* in fecal specimens. *J. Clin. Microbiol.* **36:**1338–1340.
2. **Al-Sherbiny, M. M., A. M. Osman, K. Hancock, A. M. Deelder, and V. C. W. Tsang.** 1999. Application of immunodiagnostic assays: detection of antibodies and circulating antigens in human schistosomiasis and correlation with clinical findings. *Am. J. Trop. Med. Hyg.* **60:**960–966.
3. **Centers for Disease Control and Prevention.** 2004. Manufacturer's recall of rapid cartridge assay kits on the basis of false-positive *Cryptosporidium* antigen tests—Colorado, 2004. *Morb. Mortal. Wkly. Rep.* **53:**198.
4. **Chanteau, S., J. P. Moulia-Pelat, P. Glaziou, M. L. Nguyen, P. Luquiaud, C. Plichart, P. M. Martin, and J. L. Cartel.** 1994. Og4C3 circulating antigen: a marker of infection and adult worm burden in *Wuchereria bancrofti* filariasis. *J. Infect. Dis.* **170:**247–250.
5. **Despommier, D.** 2003. Toxocariasis: clinical aspects, epidemiology, medical ecology, and molecular aspects. *Clin. Microbiol. Rev.* **16:**265–272.
6. **Garcia, L. S.** 2002. Laboratory identification of the microsporidia. *J. Clin. Microbiol.* **40:**1892–1901.
7. **Garcia, L. S., and R. Shimizu.** 1997. Evaluation of nine immunoassay kits (enzyme immunoassay and direct fluorescence) for detection of *Giardia lamblia* and *Cryptosporidium parvum* in human fecal specimens. *J. Clin. Microbiol.* **35:**1526–1529.
8. **Herwaldt, B. L., G. deBruyn, N. J. Pieniazek, M. J. Homer, K. H. Lofy, S. B. Slemenda, T. R. Fritsche, D. H. Persing, and A. P. Limaye.** 2004. *Babesia divergens*-like infection, Washington State. *Emerg. Infect. Dis.* **10:**622–629.
9. **Hillyer, G. V.** 1993. Serological diagnosis of *Fasciola hepatica*. *Parasitol. Dia* **17:**130–136.
10. **Huppert, J. S., B. E. Batteiger, P. Braslins, J. A. Feldman, M. M. Hobbs, H. Z. Sankey, A. C. Sena, and K. A. Wendel.** 2005. Use of an immunochromatographic assay for rapid detection of *Trichomonas vaginalis* in vaginal specimens. *J. Clin. Microbiol.* **43:**684–687.
11. **Ito, A., L. Ma, P. M. Schantz, B. Gottstein, Y.-H. Liu, J. J. Chai, S. K. Abdel-Hafez, N. Altintas, D. D. Joshi, M. W. Lightowlers, and Z. S. Pawlowski.** 1999. Differential serodiagnosis for cystic and alveolar echinococcosis using fractions of *Echinococcus granulosus* cyst fluid (antigen B) and *E. multilocularis* protoscolex (EM18). *Am. J. Trop. Med. Hyg.* **60:**188–192.
12. **Keiser, P. B., and T. B. Nutman.** 2004. *Strongyloides stercoralis* in the immunocompromised population. *Clin. Microbiol. Rev.* **17:**208–217.
13. **Kitchen, A. D., P. H. J. Lowe, K. Lalloo, and P. L. Chiodini.** 2004. Evaluation of a malarial antibody assay for use in the screening of blood and tissue products for clinical use. *Vox Sanguinis* **87:**150–155.
14. **Klion, A. D., A. Vijaykumar, T. Oei, B. Martin, and T. B. Nutman.** 2003. Serum immunoglobulin G4 antibodies to the recombinant antigen, L1-SXP-1, are highly specific for *Loa loa* infection. *J. Infect. Dis.* **187:**128–133.
15. **Krause, P. J.** 2003. Babesiosis diagnosis and treatment. *Vector-Borne Zoonotic Dis.* **3:**45–51.
16. **Lal, R. B., and E. A. Ottesen.** 1988. Enhanced diagnostic specificity in human filariasis by IgG4 antibody assessment. *J. Infect. Dis.* **158:**1034–1037.
17. **Leiby, D. A., S. Wendel, D. T. Takaoka, R. M. Fachini, L. C. Oliveira, and M. A. Tibbals.** 2000. Serologic testing for *Trypanosoma cruzi*: comparison of radioimmunoprecipitation assay with commercially available indirect immunofluorescence assay, indirect hemagglutination assay, and enzyme-linked immunosorbent assay kits. *J. Clin. Microbiol.* **38:**639–642.
18. **Loufty, M. R., M. Wilson, J. S. Keystone, and K. C. Kain.** 2002. Serology and eosinophil count in the diagnosis and management of strongyloidiasis in a non-endemic area. *Am. J. Trop. Med. Hyg.* **66:**749–752.
19. **McManus, D. P., W. Zhang, J. Li, and P. B. Bartley.** 2003. Echinococcosis. *Lancet* **362:**1295–1304.
20. **Moody, A.** 2002. Rapid diagnostic tests for malaria parasites. *Clin. Microbiol. Rev.* **15:**66–78.
21. **Murrell, K. D., and F. Brueschi.** 1994. Clinical trichinellosis. *Prog. Clin. Parasitol.* **4:**117–150.
22. **NCCLS.** 2004. Clinical use and interpretation of serologic tests for *Toxoplasma gondii*. Approved guideline. NCCLS, Wayne, Pa.
23. **Ramachandran, C. P.** 1993. Improved immunodiagnostic tests to monitor onchocerciasis control programmes—a multicenter effort. *Parasitol. Today* **9:**76–79.
24. **Schallig, H. D. F. H., and L. Oskam.** 2002. Molecular biological applications in the diagnosis and control of leishmaniasis and parasite identification. *Trop. Med. Int. Health* **7:**641–651.
25. **Schwebke, J. R., and D. Burgess.** 2004. Trichomoniasis. *Clin. Microbiol. Rev.* **17:**794–803.
26. **Siles-Lucas, M., and B. Gottstein.** 2001. Molecular tools for the diagnosis of cystic and alveolar echinococcosis. *Trop. Med. Int. Health* **6:**463–475.
27. **Slemenda, S. B., S. E. Maddison, E. C. Jong, and D. D. Moore.** 1988. Diagnosis of paragonimiasis by immunoblot. *Am. J. Trop. Med. Hyg.* **39:**469–471.
28. **Smith, J. V.** 1993. Antibody reactivity in human toxocariasis, p. 91–109. *In* J. W. Lewis and R. M. Maizels (ed.), *Toxocara and Toxocariasis: Clinical, Epidemiological, and Molecular Perspectives*. Institute of Biology and the British Society for Parasitology, London, United Kingdom.
29. **Snounou, G., S. Viriyakosol, X. P. Zhu, L. Pinheiro, V. E. do Rosario, S. Thaithong, and K. N. Brown.** 1993. High sensitivity detection of human malaria parasites by the use of nested polymerase chain reaction. *Mol. Biochem. Parasitol.* **61:**315–320.
30. **Sulzer, A. J., M. Wilson, and E. C. Hall.** 1969. Indirect fluorescent-antibody tests for parasitic diseases. V. An evaluation of a thick-smear antigen in the IFA test for malaria antibodies. *Am. J. Trop. Med. Hyg.* **18:**199–205.
31. **Sundar, S., and M. Rai.** 2002. Laboratory diagnosis of visceral leishmaniasis. *Clin. Diagn. Lab. Immunol.* **9:**951–958.
32. **Tanyuksel, M., and W. A. Petri, Jr.** 2003. Laboratory diagnosis of amebiasis. *Clin. Microbiol. Rev.* **16:**713–729.

33. **Tsang, V. C. W., and P. P. Wilkins.** 1997. Immunodiagnosis of schistosomiasis. *Immunol. Investig.* **26:**175–188.

34. **Umezawa, E. S., A. O. Luquetti, G. Levitus, C. Ponce, E. Ponce, D. Henriquez, S. Revollo, B. Espinoza, O. Sousa, B. Khan, and J. F. da Silveira.** 2004. Serodiagnosis of chronic and acute Chagas' disease with *Trypanosoma cruzi* recombinant proteins: results of a collaborative study in six Latin American countries. *J. Clin. Microbiol.* **42:**449–452.

35. **Weil, G. J., P. J. Lammie, and N. Weiss.** 1997. The ICT filariasis test: a rapid-format antigen test for diagnosis of bancroftian filariasis. *Parasitol. Today* **13:**401–404.

36. **Wilkins, P. P., M. Wilson, J. C. Allan, and V. C. W. Tsang.** 2002. *Taenia solium* cysticercosis: immunodiagnosis of neurocysticercosis and taeniasis, p. 329–341. *In* G. Singh and S. Prabhakar (ed.), *Taenia solium Cysticercosis: from Basic to Clinical Science.* CABI Publishing, New York, N.Y.

37. **Wilson, M., J. L. Jones, and J. M. McAuley.** 2003. *Toxoplasma,* p. 1970–1980. *In* P. R. Murray, E. J. Baron, M. A. Pfaller, J. H. Jorgensen, and R. H. Yolken (ed.), *Manual of Clinical Microbiology,* 8th ed. American Society for Microbiology, Washington, D.C.

38. **Zhong, M., J. Mccarthy, L. Bierwert, M. Lizotte-Waniewski, S. Chanteau, T. B. Nutman, E. A. Ottesen, and S. A. Williams.** 1996. A polymerase chain reaction assay for detection of the parasite *Wuchereria bancrofti* in human blood samples. *Am. J. Trop. Med. Hyg.* **54:**357–363.

Serological and Molecular Diagnosis of Fungal Infections

MARK D. LINDSLEY, DAVID W. WARNOCK, AND CHRISTINE J. MORRISON

66

Analysis of the signs and symptoms of disease, in conjunction with an evaluation of available epidemiologic information and the results of modern imaging procedures, can often provide a presumptive clinical diagnosis of a fungal infection. However, the clinical presentation of many mycotic diseases is nonspecific and a presumptive diagnosis must therefore be confirmed by appropriate laboratory tests. A definitive diagnosis of fungal disease is usually based upon the isolation of the etiologic agent in culture and/or microscopic demonstration of the organism in histopathologic or other clinical specimens. Unfortunately, these laboratory methods are insensitive and often unsuccessful, despite repeated sampling efforts. In the absence of positive microscopy or culture, immunologic and molecular tests offer alternative laboratory procedures to aid in the diagnosis of a mycotic disease. Advances in molecular diagnostic methods, and the commercial introduction of new antigen and antibody detection tests, hold promise for an earlier and more specific diagnosis than previously possible. Molecular and antigen detection tests are particularly valuable in the diagnosis of fungal infections in immunocompromised patients because such individuals often exhibit poor or variable antibody responses. In contrast, antibody detection tests are often helpful for the diagnosis of fungal infections in immunocompetent hosts. For example, when acute- and convalescent-phase serum specimens are tested, a fourfold rise in antibody titer can be diagnostic or prognostic for several fungal diseases in immunocompetent patients. Monitoring the results of serologic tests at regular intervals during infection can also reveal trends in disease progression or remission and may serve to guide antifungal therapy. In many cases, positive serologic test results lead to increased efforts to isolate and identify the suspected etiologic agent.

Despite recent advances in the production of purified antigens by biochemical and recombinant techniques, many antigens used in antibody detection tests possess cross-reactive epitopes that are shared among different fungal genera or which cross-react with entirely different classes of microorganisms. Other limitations of antibody detection tests include a requirement for the appropriate timing of serum collection so as to coincide with the occurrence of the antibody response. Negative antibody results do not exclude the presence of a mycotic infection, and sera that display low titers or demonstrate cross-reactivity among fungal antigens require the performance of additional laboratory tests to rule out infection. In such cases, an accurate serologic diagnosis relies on (i) the results of several serologic tests performed with a battery of antigens (including those from antigenically related genera), (ii) an examination of serial serum specimens to detect temporal changes in titer, and (iii) an analysis of the results of antigen detection tests, if such tests are available. In addition, knowledge of the clinical history of the patient and the therapy received is necessary for the correct interpretation of serologic test results.

Molecular biological tests, on the other hand, offer the promise of increased sensitivity compared to conventional diagnostic tests; i.e., nucleic acids, once extracted from clinical materials, can be amplified 10^6-fold or more using PCR or other DNA or RNA amplification technologies. In addition, in contrast to antibody detection, detection of fungal DNA is not dependent on a functioning immune system and may therefore allow a diagnosis early in the infectious episode, before an antibody response occurs. Another advantage of molecular diagnostic tests is the capacity to identify the infecting organism to the species level and to detect mixed as well as single-organism infections. However, whereas amplification technologies may provide greater test sensitivity and specificity for the above reasons, these advantages are counterbalanced by the concomitant increased risk of sample contamination resulting in false positivity and a loss of specificity. Moreover, the extraction of fungal DNA or RNA from clinical materials is not a straightforward or standardized process at present. The procedures used to remove inhibitors of the PCR assay may cause loss of target DNA, thereby reducing test sensitivity. Finally, although many DNA-based tests have been developed in single laboratories and are quite successful, confirmation of the usefulness of these technologies awaits multicenter clinical evaluation.

This chapter reviews the most extensively evaluated or routinely used tests for the serodiagnosis of mycotic infections. Commercially available antibody and antigen detection tests are listed in Tables 1 and 2. Specific details regarding the clinical indications for test application and the mechanics of test performance are presented in the body of the text. Experimental antigen and antibody detection tests and molecular biological tests are reviewed briefly in the text.

TABLE 1 Commercially available antibody detection tests for fungal diseases

Disease and test[a]	Specimen	Antigen	Interpretation	Sensitivity	Specificity	Source(s)[b] (reference[s])
Aspergillosis						
CF	Serum	Culture filtrate from A. fumigatus	Titer of ≥1:8 is strong evidence for Aspergillus infection; seroconversion or ≥4-fold increase in titer between acute- and convalescent-phase sera confirms diagnosis	Aspergilloma: 79% ABPA: 46% Invasive pulmonary or disseminated: 20%	95–100%	IMMY (6)
CIE	Serum	Cell homogenate from A. fumigatus; Culture filtrate from Aspergillus spp.[c]	≥1 line of identity indicates aspergilloma, ABPA or IA; 5–10 lines of identity are usually observed in cases of aspergilloma	ABPA: 70–90% Aspergilloma: 50%	100%	Bio-Rad (23, 158)
ID	Serum	Culture filtrate from Aspergillus spp.[c]	≥1 line of identity indicates aspergilloma, ABPA, or IA; ≥3 lines of identity is strong evidence for aspergilloma	ABPA: 50–61% Aspergilloma: 80–93%	97–100%	Gibson, IMMY, Meridian, Microgen (6, 19)
Blastomycosis						
CF	Serum	Purified A antigen	Titer of ≥1:8 is presumptive evidence of infection; titer of ≥1:32 is strongly presumptive evidence of recent infection Seroconversion or ≥4-fold increase in titer between acute- and convalescent-phase sera confirms diagnosis	Disseminated: 50% Localized: 33%	97–100%	IMMY (147)
ID	Serum	Purified A antigen	Presence of A band suggests recent infection	Disseminated: 85% Localized: 33%	100%	Gibson, IMMY, Meridian (147)
Candidiasis						
CIE	Serum	Culture filtrate from C. albicans	≥1 line of identity is positive for the presence of antibody; increase in line number correlates with progression of infection in immunocompetent patients	—[d]	—	Bio-Rad (24, 111)
		Cell homogenate from C. albicans		78–87%	75–97%	
EIA	Serum	Purified mannan from C. albicans	<5 AU[e] = negative; 5–<10 AU = intermediate; ≥10 AU = positive; >20 AU, dilute serum 1:4 and retest	C. albicans: 71–88% Other Candida spp.: 25–77%	63–94%	Bio-Rad (115)
ID	Serum	Culture filtrate and cell lysate of yeast-phase C. albicans	≥1 line of identity is positive for the presence of antibody; seroconversion or increase in number of lines suggests systemic infection; the greater the number of lines, the more severe the infection in immunocompetent patients	58–94%	94–98%	IMMY, Gibson (95)
IFA	Serum	Germ tubes of C. albicans	Titer of ≥1:640 suggests invasive candidiasis	76–96%	95–100%	Vircell (85, 98)
Coccidioidomycosis						
CF	Serum, CSF	Culture filtrate (coccidioidin)	Titer of ≥1:2, positive for acute pulmonary disease; titer of ≥1:16 suggests disseminated disease	75% (acute pulmonary disease); 98% (disseminated)	80–95%	IMMY, Meridian (107)

Test	Specimen	Antigen	Interpretation	%	%	Vendor (ref)
EIA	Serum, CSF	Mixture of purified TP and CF antigens to detect IgM or IgG, respectively	Absorbance values: <0.150 = negative; 0.150–<0.200 = indeterminate; ≥0.200 = positive	IgM only: 74% IgG only: 92% IgM and IgG: 97%	IgM only: 96% IgG only: 97% IgM and IgG: 94%	Meridian (92, 170)
IDCF	Serum, CSF	Culture filtrate (coccidioidin)	Band of identity with reference serum indicates active infection	77%	100%	IMMY, Meridian; Gibson (68)
IDTP	Serum	Heat-treated culture filtrate (coccidioidin 60°C for 30 min)	Band of identity with reference serum indicates active infection	75–91%	—	IMMY, Meridian (107)
LA	Serum	Heat-treated coccidioidin-coated latex particles	≥2+ agglutination is positive for the presence of antibody; must confirm with ID and/or CF	65–70%	93%	IMMY, Meridian (53)
Cryptococcosis						
TA	Serum	Suspension of weakly encapsulated *C. neoformans* yeast cells	Titer of ≥1:2 suggests recent or past infection; cross-reacts with blastomycosis and histoplasmosis	38–50%	89–95%	IMMY (105)
Histoplasmosis						
CF	Serum, CSF	Mycelial culture filtrate (histoplasmin)	Titer of ≥1:8 is presumptive evidence for infection; titer of ≥1:32 is strongly presumptive for infection	21%	81–99%	IMMY, Meridian (159)
	Serum, CSF	Yeast cell suspension	Titer of ≥1:8 is presumptive evidence for infection; titer of ≥1:32 is strongly presumptive for infection	82%	81–88%	
ID	Serum, CSF	Mycelial culture filtrate (histoplasmin)	M band alone indicates acute or chronic histoplasmosis (observed in 75% of patients); presence of both the H and M bands indicates acute histoplasmosis (observed in 20% of patients); positivity for H and/or M band using CSF indicates *Histoplasma* meningitis	65–100%	89–100%	IMMY, Meridian, Gibson (159)
LA	Serum	Mycelial culture filtrate (histoplasmin)	Titer of ≥1:16 is presumptive evidence of active or very recent infection	Acute: 97–100% Chronic: 46–96%	97% 97%	IMMY (36)
Paracoccidioidomycosis						
ID	Serum, CSF	Mycelial culture filtrate (contains gp43 and other antigens)	Band of identity with reference serum indicates active infection	94%	95–99%	IMMY (11, 22)
		Ag7		84%	99%	
Sporotrichosis						
LA	Serum	*Sporothrix* antigen	Titer of ≥1:8, presumptive evidence of sporotrichosis	Disseminated: 100%, Articular: 86–100%, Pulmonary: 73–87%, Cutaneous: 56–93%	100%	IMMY (10)

[a] For abbreviations, see beginning of chapter.
[b] Detailed vendor contact information is given at the end of the chapter. IMMY, Immunomycologics, Inc.
[c] Antigens from *A. fumigatus*, *A. flavus*, *A. nidulans*, *A. niger*, or *A. terreus* are tested separately.
[d] Insufficient data.
[e] Arbitrary units compared to a standard curve.

TABLE 2 Commercially available antigen detection tests for fungal diseases

Disease and/or test[a]	Specimen	Antigen detected[b]	Interpretation	Sensitivity	Specificity	Source(s)[b]
Aspergillosis						
EIA MAb (EB-A2)	Serum (boiled)	Galactomannan	EIA index: ≥0.5 units = positive; detection limit = 1 ng/ml	60–100%	78–99%	Bio-Rad (83, 91)
LA MAb (EB-A2)[c]	Serum (boiled)	Galactomannan	Any agglutination = positive; titrate positive sera; detection limit = 15 ng/ml	27–95%	86–100%	Bio-Rad (83, 149, 166)
Candidiasis						
EIA MAb (EB-CA1)	Serum (boiled)	α-(1,2)-Oligomannosides	<0.25 ng/ml = negative; ≥0.25 to <0.5 ng/ml = intermediate; ≥0.5 ng/ml = positive	Overall, 52%; C. albicans, 53–60%; other Candida spp., 20–70%	85–100%	Bio-Rad (129, 166)
LA MAb (EB-CA1)	Serum (boiled)	α-(1,2)-Oligomannosides	Any agglutination = positive; titrate positive sera Detection limit = 2.5 ng/ml	25–77%	99–100%	Bio-Rad (47, 129, 166)
LA PAb	Serum (not boiled)	Uncharacterized heat-labile C. albicans antigen	Titer of ≥1:4 suggests invasive candidiasis	Titer of 1:4, 48–81%; titer of 1:8, 2–59%; titer of 1:16, 59%	Titer of 1:4, 80–97%; titer of 1:8, 93–95%; titer of 1:16, 98%	Ramco (5, 96, 97)
Cryptococcosis						
EIA	Serum, CSF	Capsular polysaccharide antigen	Visual Definite yellow color = positive Spectrophotometric <0.100 OD = negative; ≥0.100–<0.150 = indeterminate; ≥0.150 = positive Detection limit = 0.63 ng/ml	96–100%	93–99%	Meridian (34)
LA PAb	Pronase-treated serum, CSF (boiled)	Capsular polysaccharide antigen	≥2+ agglutination = positive; titrate positive sera; titer of ≥1:8 strongly suggestive evidence for infection	93–100%	93–98%	IMMY, Wampole, Meridian (140)
LA MAb (E1)	Urine Pronase treated Serum, CSF, BAL fluid	Glucuronoxylomannan	Any agglutination = positive; titrate positive sera; detection limit = 50 ng/ml	Overall, 92%; urine, 93%; serum, 85%; CSF, 100%; BAL fluid, 100%	Overall, 98%; urine, 97%; serum, 100%; CSF, 100%; BAL fluid, 100%	Bio-Rad (142)
Panfungal[d]						
Modified Limulus amebocyte assay	Serum, BAL fluid	(1,3)-β-D-Glucan	≥60 pg/ml = positive (Associates of Cape Cod)	100%	90%	Associates of Cape Cod (108); Seikagaku Corp. (76)
	Plasma		≥20 pg/ml = positive (Seikagaku Corp.)	76–97%	100%	

[a]For abbreviations, see beginning of chapter and Table 1.
[b]Detailed vendor contact information at the end of the chapter.
[c]Clone name in parentheses.
[d]Detects species of Candida, Aspergillus, Pneumocystis, Fusarium, and Trichosporon asahii but not Zygomycetes or Cryptococcus spp.

Abbreviations. ABPA, allergic bronchopulmonary aspergillosis; **BAL,** bronchoalveolar lavage; **BDG,** (1,3)-β-D-glucan; **CDC,** Centers for Disease Control and Prevention; **CF,** complement fixation; **CIE,** counterimmunoelectrophoresis; **CNPA,** chronic necrotizing pulmonary aspergillosis; **CSF,** cerebrospinal fluid; **EIA,** enzyme immunoassay (fluid or solid phase); **ELISA,** enzyme-linked immunosorbent assay; **FDA,** Food and Drug Administration; **GM,** galactomannan; **HIV,** human immunodeficiency virus; **HPA,** *Histoplasma* polysaccharide antigen; **HSCT,** hematopoietic stem cell transplant; **IA,** invasive aspergillosis; **ID,** immunodiffusion in an agarose gel; **IDCF,** immunodiffusion variation to detect the CF F antigen in patients with coccidioidomycosis; **IDTP,** immunodiffusion variation to detect tube precipitin in coccidioidomycosis; **IFA,** immunofluorescent antibody; **Ig,** immunoglobulin; **ITS,** internal transcribed spacer region of the rRNA gene; **LA,** latex agglutination; **MAb,** monoclonal antibody; **OD,** optical density; **PAb,** polyclonal antibody; **PBS,** phosphate-buffered saline; **PCP,** *Pneumocystis* pneumonia; **QA,** quality assurance; **QC,** quality control; **rDNA,** DNA coding for the RNA gene; **SOT,** solid-organ transplant; **SRBCs,** sheep erythrocytes; **TA,** tube agglutinin; **TMB,** tetramethylbenzidine; **TP,** tube precipitin; **VBD,** vernal-buffered diluent; **WB,** Western blotting.

ASPERGILLOSIS

Background

Immunodiagnostic tests for aspergillosis consist of the detection of precipitating antibodies (precipitins) using ID (see Test 1 below) or CIE (Table 1) and the detection of serum GM antigen (see "Test 2. EIA To Detect *Aspergillus* Cell Wall GM" below and Table 2). The ID test is effective and specific for diagnosing aspergillosis in immunocompetent persons, and reagents can be purchased separately or as a complete kit (Immuno-Mycologics, Inc., Norman, Okla.; Gibson Laboratories, Lexington, Ky; and Bio-Rad Laboratories, Hercules, Calif.). The sensitivity of the CIE test equals that of the ID test, and its specificity is no greater. Therefore, the CIE test is not discussed further except to mention that the CIE test can be completed in a matter of hours rather than the days required for completion of the ID test. Reagents for the detection of anti-*Aspergillus fumigatus* antibodies by CF are available commercially, but test sensitivity has been reported to be low (29%) for tests using cell homogenate antigens and to be variable (20 to 79%) for tests employing culture filtrate antigens (Table 1). Few laboratories now use the CF test for the diagnosis of aspergillosis. A commercial monoclonal double-sandwich EIA to detect circulating serum GM antigen is effective in diagnosing IA in the immunocompromised host (Platelia *Aspergillus* EIA; Bio-Rad, Inc.), and it detects the disease earlier (approximately 1 week before clinical signs of infection) and is more sensitive than a commercial LA test, which uses the same MAb (Pastorex *Aspergillus*; Bio-Rad, Inc.); i.e., the LA test detects 15 ng of GM per ml, whereas the EIA detects 1 ng of GM per ml (see Test 2 below and Table 2) (122, 149). A murine MAb, WF-AF-1, directed against a cell wall fraction of *A. fumigatus*, is commercially available (DakoCytomation, Inc., Carpinteria, Calif.) for the immunohistochemical diagnosis of major *Aspergillus* species in tissues by IFA (59).

Clinical Indications and Diagnostic Rationale

Patients with ABPA, pulmonary aspergilloma (fungus ball), or CNPA and immunocompetent patients with obscure pulmonary or sinus infections should be tested for *Aspergillus* precipitins. ABPA should be considered in patients with asthma, transient pulmonary infiltrates, and peripheral eosinophilia. Pulmonary aspergilloma occurs when *A. fumigatus* or other *Aspergillus* species colonize preexisting cavities of tuberculosis, sarcoidosis, or bronchiectasis. The ID test to detect antibodies to *Aspergillus* species should be applied in such cases (see Test 1 below and Table 1). Antibody testing has been suggested by some to play a role in the diagnosis of IA in nonneutropenic, high-risk SOT recipients. The sensitivity of such testing may be low, however, requiring repeated testing to detect the antibody response.

Patients should be screened using the GM antigenemia test if they (i) display chest computed tomography or radiographic signs consistent with IA or (ii) develop an unexplained fever that fails to respond to broad-spectrum antibiotics while undergoing HSCT or SOT or while receiving immunosuppressive therapy for hematological malignancies. The commercial antigen detection test for IA detects circulating cell wall GM from medically important *Aspergillus* species (see Test 2 below and Table 2) (91).

Test 1. ID Test To Detect Antibodies to *Aspergillus* Species

Commercial kits for the ID test contain precast agar gels, antigens, and reference antisera. Vendors are listed in Table 1, and more detailed contact information is provided at the end of the chapter. The CDC Mycotic Diseases Branch uses the micro-ID test described below for aspergillosis, but most kits are marketed as macro-ID tests. Commercial antigens and antibodies should be used with the agar medium provided by the vendor.

Sample Requirements

A single serum specimen is usually sufficient for the diagnosis of aspergilloma, CNPA, or ABPA, particularly if multiple precipitin bands are detected. Precipitin bands are less frequent in patients with IA, and therefore absence of a precipitin band does not rule out IA. Precipitin-negative serum samples from patients with suspected IA should be retested after samples have been concentrated to one-fourth the original volume.

Materials and Reagents

Standardized and reproducible *A. fumigatus*, *A. flavus*, *A. niger*, and *A. terreus* antigens with either no or minimal C substance can be prepared from 5-week-old stationary Sabouraud dextrose broth cultures grown at 31°C. The culture filtrates are precipitated with cold acetone and concentrated to one-eighth of the original volume. The carbohydrate content of these antigens is determined by the anthrone test and adjusted with distilled water to contain 1,000 to 1,500 µg/ml (67). After standardization, all *Aspergillus* antigens should be examined for the presence of C substance by using serum known to contain C-reactive protein.

Stock Barbital Buffer (pH 8.6), 0.05 M, Made Up to 500 ml

Sodium diethylbarbiturate	5.16 g
Diethylbarbituric acid	0.92 g
Sodium acetate	2.05 g

Phenolized Medium

Noble agar (or equivalent)	1.00 g
Phenol, liquefied	0.25 ml

Stock barbital buffer (above) . . . . . .   25 ml
Distilled water . . . .   to 100 ml

Heat to boiling until the agar is completely dissolved.

Equipment

Plexiglas matrix (3-mm-diameter wells) with 17 patterns of seven wells each (Quality House, Cartersville, Ga.)

Plastic petri dish, 15 by 100 mm

Spatula, 1-mm tip (flattened)

Light box with indirect backlighting

Procedure

The micro-ID test is recommended to conserve test serum and reagents. In addition to the reference *Aspergillus* antigens and antisera, buffered phenolized agar is required. Care should be exercised when pipetting liquefied phenol.

1. Pipette 6.5 ml of agar into a petri dish (15 by 100 mm) and allow to harden.

2. Overlay the first agar layer with 3.5 ml of hot molten agar and immediately place the Plexiglas matrix on top of the liquid agar.

3. Plates may be used 30 min after the agar has solidified or may be stored in a humidified chamber at 4°C for up to 1 week.

4. Number each seven-well pattern on the bottom of the dish (not on the template).

5. Remove the excess agar from the wells down to the first agar layer with the pointed end of the spatula.

6. Place the reference serum in the top and bottom wells of each pattern and place patient's test sera in the four lateral wells (Fig. 1). Place the reference antigen in the center well of each pattern. All wells must be examined for air bubbles. If bubbles are observed, they should be broken by being gently pierced with toothpicks. Separate toothpicks should be employed for each different antigen and antibody solution. Incubate the reactants in a humidified chamber for 48 h at 25°C.

7. Remove the Plexiglas matrix by gently pressing the sides of the petri dish, and remove the agar overlay by gently sweeping the surface with a cotton swab. Wash the agar with distilled water to remove excess reactants. Cover the agar with distilled water, and examine the plate for lines of identity between test and reference wells.

QA/QC

Positive control sera must be included each time the test is performed. Three or more distinct precipitin lines ("bands") should be formed when *A. fumigatus* reference antiserum is allowed to react with *A. fumigatus* antigen. One or more distinct precipitin lines should be formed when *A. flavus, A. niger,* or *A. terreus* reference antiserum is allowed to react with the homologous antigen. The greatest number of aspergillosis cases may be detected by the use of *A. fumigatus, A. flavus, A. niger,* and *A. terreus* precipitinogens in separate ID tests performed at the same time. Some *Aspergillus* antigenic extracts contain C substance, and this can react with C-reactive protein in the serum of some patients with inflammatory disease. The resulting complex forms a precipitate, which may be erroneously interpreted as the presence of anti-*Aspergillus* antibodies. This false-positive reaction is easily eliminated if the test plates are soaked in 5% sodium citrate for 45 min before being read. In addition, C substance may produce lines of nonidentity with reference antisera.

Interpretation

Precipitins can be found in over 90% of patients with aspergillomas and in 70% of patients with ABPA or CNPA. Only serum samples that produce a line or lines of identity with reference serum from a patient with a proven case of human aspergillosis are considered positive in the ID test. Although one or two precipitins may occur when serum from patients with any clinical form of aspergillosis is used, the presence of three or more bands is usually associated with either aspergilloma or CNPA. Pulmonary fungus balls can also be produced by *Scedosporium apiospermum* (*Pseudallescheria boydii*) and by other fungi; noninfectious conditions or other abnormalities may also be misinterpreted as aspergillomas on chest radiographs. In such cases, the *Aspergillus* ID test is negative. However, the ID test may also be negative in some patients with aspergillosis who are receiving long-term antifungal or corticosteroid therapy.

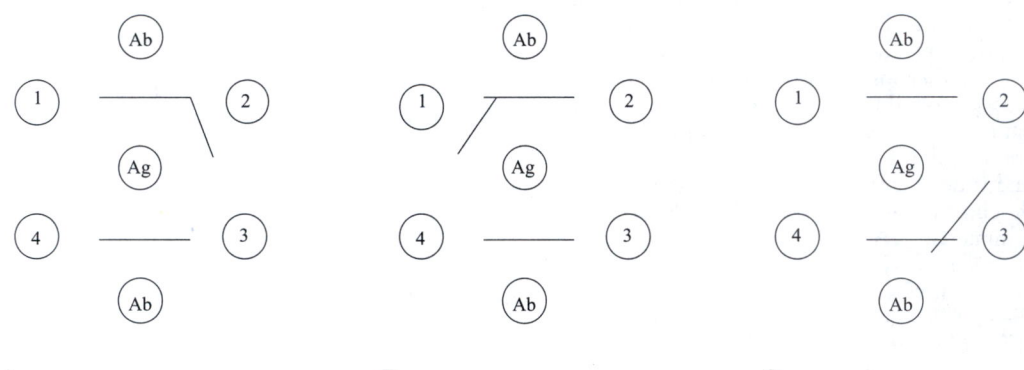

FIGURE 1 Examples of immunodiffusion results observed when a seven-well agar gel pattern is used. (A) Band of identity (patient 2); (B) band of partial identity (patient 1); (C) band of nonidentity (patient 3). Ag, reference antigen; Ab, reference antiserum; 1 to 4, patient test sera. A standard reference band is shown midway between the lower antiserum-containing wells and the central antigen-containing wells in all three panels.

Test 2. EIA To Detect *Aspergillus* Cell Wall GM

A commercial antigenemia detection test, the Platelia *Aspergillus* EIA, is a microtitration plate-based double antibody sandwich EIA (91) (Table 2). This assay uses a rat MAb, EB-A2, as both the capture and detector antibody for the $(1,5)$-β-D-galactofuranose residues of GM, an outer cell wall component found in the most clinically important species of *Aspergillus*.

Sample Requirements

Serum specimens should be collected serially during the infectious episode and may be collected at regular intervals before suspicion of infection if the test is to be used as a screening tool in high-risk patient populations such as in allogeneic HSCT recipients. Positive test results for two consecutively drawn serum samples is strong presumptive evidence of IA in the absence of factors that may contribute to false-positive results (see Interpretation, below); hence, multiple serum specimens, collected at least twice per week, are preferred. A 300-µl volume of patient serum is consumed each time the test is performed. Because the test may need to be repeated more than once and because some sample loss occurs during immune complex removal (precipitation of serum proteins during boiling in the presence of neutral disodium EDTA), at least 1 ml of patient serum is required for testing.

Materials and Reagents

Reagents provided in the kit include freeze-dried negative, positive, and cutoff (low-positive) control sera, EDTA solution, peroxidase-conjugated detector MAbs, wash solutions and buffers, H_2O_2, chromogen (TMB), stopping solution (1.5 N sulfuric acid), plate sealers, and microtiter plates precoated with capture anti-GM MAbs. Microtiter plates are composed of 12 eight-well strips so that the entire plate does not have to be used at one time. Strips are supplied in resealable pouches and should be used within 5 weeks of opening. Kits are stored at 2 to 8°C and should be brought to room temperature (18 to 25°C) before use.

Equipment

- Pipettes or multichannel pipettes, adjustable or fixed, to measure and dispense 50, 100, 300, and 1,000 µl
- 1.5-ml Eppendorf or similar polypropylene tubes with airtight stoppers, able to withstand boiling
- Centrifuge (for 1.5-ml polypropylene tubes) that can attain $10,000 \times g$
- Round, floating microcentrifuge rack for a 1-liter beaker
- Vortex agitator
- Boiling-water bath
- Incubator at 37 ± 1°C
- Manual or semiautomatic plate washer
- Microplate reader equipped with 450- and 620/630-nm filters

Procedure

A detailed stepwise procedure can be found in the package insert included with each kit. Briefly, GM is heat stable and is present in the circulation as soluble immune complexes. These complexes must be dissociated by boiling for 3 min in an EDTA solution provided in the kit. Samples are then centrifuged at $10,000 \times g$ for 10 min to remove precipitated serum proteins that could interfere with the test, and GM is recovered from the fluid phase. Peroxidase-conjugated detector antibodies are added to each test well of the microtiter plate that has been previously coated with EB-A2 capture MAbs by the manufacturer. Treated serum supernatants are then added, and plates are incubated for 90 min at 37°C before being washed five times. H_2O_2-TMB solution is added to each well, and the plates are incubated for 30 min in the dark at ambient temperature (18 to 25°C). Stopping solution is added, and the OD at 450 nm is determined within 30 min.

QA/QC

A negative control serum, a cutoff control serum (serving as a borderline-positive reaction), and a positive control serum containing 1 ng of GM per ml are included in each kit. A set of proficiency specimens can also be obtained from the manufacturer, and test values obtained in-house can be compared to those produced by the manufacturer. Results are expressed as an index (i.e., the ratio of the OD of the test sample to the OD of the mean cutoff control serum provided in the kit). OD values for the cutoff control serum must be ≥ 0.3 and ≤ 0.8; the index of the positive control serum must be greater than 2; and the index of the negative control serum must be less than 0.4.

Interpretation

As defined above, an index of ≥ 0.5 is considered a positive result and an index of <0.5 is considered a negative result. Positive results obtained with the Platelia *Aspergillus* EIA should be interpreted in conjunction with other diagnostic procedures including culture, histopathologic examination of biopsied tissues, and radiologic evidence of infection. For all positive patients, it is recommended that a second aliquot of the same sample be retested and a new sample, collected from the same patient, be tested in a follow-up procedure. In the absence of positive culture or histopathology, if tests for serum GM are repeatedly positive in patients at risk for IA, such results may be interpreted as a probable *Aspergillus* infection. On the other hand, negative test results do not rule out a diagnosis of IA. Even in cases of culture-proven or histopathologically proven IA, not every serum sample from each patient is expected to be positive.

Neonatal or pediatric serum samples have been reported to give a higher rate of false-positive results, and this may be related to the finding that the EB-A2 MAb used in the test reacts with components found in infant milk formulas and with the lipoteichoic acid of a common neonatal gut commensal, *Bifidobacterium bifidum*. False-positive test results may also occur in patients receiving piperacillin-tazobactam and amoxicillin-clavulanic acid antibiotics since these agents also react with the EB-A2 MAb in vitro. Positive test results in such individuals should be interpreted with caution and confirmed by other diagnostic means. Other fungal genera, including species of *Penicillium*, *Alternaria*, and *Paecilomyces*, have demonstrated reactivity with the EB-A2 MAb used in the Platelia *Aspergillus* test and could cause false-positive test results; however, these genera rarely cause invasive fungal disease. Other possible reasons for false-positive results have been suggested, including reactions with cyclophosphamide and/or adsorption of dietary GM through a damaged intestinal wall.

Reduced detection of GM may occur in patients with chronic granulomatous disease or Job's syndrome or in those with IA who are receiving antifungal therapy (150). Sera from such patients giving negative results should be retested. False-negative results have also been attributed to limited invasion of blood vessels by the organism or to especially high antibody titers in the host.

Experimental and Molecular Biological Approaches

Immunoblot analyses for the diagnosis of IA have been conducted to identify patient antibodies to a number of somatic or cell wall-derived proteins from *Aspergillus* species that range in molecular mass from 33 to 88 kDa (93). On the other hand, tests to detect immunoreactive protein antigens in patient serum and urine have also been described, including those to detect an 18-kDa ribonucleotoxin (3, 44) and one to detect an 88-kDa antigen, hypothesized to be analogous to the HSP90 heat shock protein of *Candida albicans* (14). In general, these antigen detection tests have not achieved the desired test sensitivity for an optimal diagnosis.

All nucleic acid detection tests for aspergillosis are experimental and limited to individual research laboratories. The most beneficial use of nucleic acid detection tests is for the early diagnosis of IA because this disease progresses rapidly and is associated with a high mortality rate (50 to 100%) in immunocompromised patients. Earlier detection of fungal DNA by PCR than by radiographic or culture methods was reported for a large series of patients (31). Fungal DNA extracted from whole blood was detected by PCR a median of 4 days before radiological signs were evident for 12 of 17 patients with hepatosplenic candidiasis or pulmonary aspergillosis. This method could also be used to monitor the response to antifungal therapy in patients with IA, since the number of PCR-positive samples declined in patients responding to therapy, in contrast to those who did not respond (31). This method was reported to have a sensitivity of 100% for patients with documented invasive infections when two or more blood samples were tested (31). Efficient sample preparation included a hot dilute alkali extraction step (0.05 M NaOH at 95°C for 10 min followed by neutralization with 1 M Tris-HCl [pH 7.0]) and the use of Zymolyase to digest fungal cells walls and release *Aspergillus* DNA (31).

BLASTOMYCOSIS

Background

Substantial improvement in the diagnosis of blastomycosis can be attributed to the use of a purified surface antigen of *Blastomyces dermatitidis* called the "A antigen" by one group of investigators (54) and WI-1 by another group (72); both are released from the yeast form of *B. dermatitidis* by autolysis and are recovered from culture filtrates. Immunologically, the A antigen and WI-1 are related in that antibodies directed against the WI-1 antigen recognize the A antigen and vice versa. The A antigen has a molecular mass of 135 kDa and is glycosylated, whereas the WI-1 antigen is a 120-kDa protein that is not glycosylated.

ID test kits and reagents to conduct the ID and CF tests are commercially available (Immuno-Mycologics, Inc.; Gibson Laboratories) for the detection of anti-*B. dermatitidis* antibodies. The A antigen is now incorporated into most commercially available kits and is also supplied as a reagent for in-house ID and CF testing. A positive reaction in an ID test using the purified A antigen is specific and diagnostic for blastomycosis. However, a negative ID test does not rule out a diagnosis of blastomycosis since this test has been reported to be negative in 10% of patients with disseminated infection and over 60% of patients with localized disease.

Initial CF assays for the diagnosis of blastomycosis used a crude yeast antigen which resulted in unsatisfactory sensitivity and specificity. With the incorporation of purified A antigen into the CF assay, the specificity improved markedly

from initial reports of 30 to 87% (73, 80, 148) to 97 to 100% (73, 148). However, the sensitivity still remains unsatisfactory for the diagnosis of disseminated infection (50%) or localized infection (33%) (73). Although the CF test is still in use, its sensitivity is poor and much reduced compared to the ID test, and it is therefore not discussed in further detail here. However, procedures for performing the CF test for the diagnosis of blastomycosis are the same as those for the diagnosis of histoplasmosis but *B. dermatitidis* A antigen is used instead of *H. capsulatum* antigens (see "Test 1. CF Test To Detect Antibodies to *H. capsulatum*" below).

Clinical Indications and Diagnostic Rationale

Antibody detection tests for blastomycosis should be performed with sera from patients showing signs of suspected acute pulmonary blastomycosis, especially if they reside in or have recently traveled to geographic areas where blastomycosis is endemic. Signs of acute pulmonary blastomycosis include a nonspecific respiratory infection characterized by fever, chills, productive cough, myalgia, arthralgia, pleuritic chest pain, and weight loss. Antibody detection tests should also be performed with sera from patients presenting with symptoms of chronic pulmonary blastomycosis, which are similar to those of tuberculosis and include productive cough, hemoptysis, night sweats, malaise, weight loss, and low-grade fever. Antibody detection can be helpful when lesions are present on the skin, a common site of dissemination, and for monitoring CSF specimens from patients with suspected blastomycotic meningitis.

Immunocompromised patients are predisposed to severe forms of the disease, which can relapse and are often associated with a high mortality rate. Up to 40% of AIDS patients with blastomycosis have central nervous system disease which manifests as either meningitis or brain lesions. Others have presented with a septic shock-like syndrome. Experimental antigen detection tests, should they prove to be sensitive and specific, would be helpful for the diagnosis of disseminated blastomycosis in immunocompromised patient populations whose antibody responses may be limited or variable.

Test 1. ID Test To Detect Antibodies to *B. dermatitidis*

Commercial kits for the ID test contain precast agar gels, antigens, and reference antisera. Vendors are listed in Table 1, and more detailed contact information is provided at the end of the chapter. Commercial kits use a precast, macro-ID gel template, whereas the CDC Mycotic Diseases Branch prefers using a micro-ID procedure and phenolized agar as described below.

Sample Requirements

A positive ID test result, giving a line of identity with the reference A precipitin band, is strong presumptive evidence of active or recent infection. Therefore, only a single serum sample is required if positive test results are obtained. However, because the reported sensitivity of the ID test is low, patients with negative serum reactions should have additional sera drawn 3 to 4 weeks after initial sampling to detect the development of an A precipitin band indicating seroconversion and recent infection.

Materials and Reagents

Antigens may be obtained from commercial sources (Table 1) or prepared from 1-week-old brain heart infusion broth (Difco Laboratories, Detroit, Mich.) cultures of yeast-form *B. dermatitidis* cells shaken at 150 rpm and 37°C. Culture filtrates are precipitated with acetone, and the precipitate is dissolved in a volume of phosphate-buffered saline (0.01 M PBS [pH 7.2]) equal to 1/10 the original filtrate volume.

Phenolized Medium

Sodium chloride	0.9 g
Noble agar (or equivalent)	1.0 g
Sodium citrate ($Na_3C_6H_5O_7 \cdot 2H_2O$) . .	0.4 g
Phenol, liquefied	0.25 ml
Glycine	7.5 g
Distilled water . . . . to 100 ml

Autoclave the mixture at a pressure of 15 lb/in² for 10 min. The final pH of the medium should be 6.3 to 6.4.

Equipment

The same equipment is used for the blastomycosis ID test as for the aspergillosis ID test.

Procedure

The same procedure is used as described for the aspergillosis ID test, except that serum samples are preincubated for 45 min at 25°C before antigen is added to wells of the ID plate. Reactants are incubated for 48 h at 25°C in a humidified chamber.

QA/QC

Positive control sera must be included each time the test is performed. The B. dermatitidis antiserum must react with the homologous reference antigen to form the specific A precipitin band. Only serum samples that produce lines of identity with the reference A precipitin band are considered positive for blastomycosis. Commercial kits most often provide reference antisera and antigens prediluted for optimal test performance. If in-house-produced reagents are being evaluated, it is important to cross-titrate reagents to determine the optimal working dilution. Optimal dilutions of serum and antigen are those that place the precipitin band midway between the serum and antigen wells.

Interpretation

The ID test performed using a B. dermatitidis yeast-form culture filtrate, containing the A antigen, is highly specific for blastomycosis. A positive reaction denotes a recent or current infection by B. dermatitidis. Positive reactions can therefore be the basis for immediate treatment of the patient without parallel testing for coccidioidomycosis or histoplasmosis. Negative test results, however, do not exclude a diagnosis of blastomycosis because the sensitivity of the ID test has been reported to range from 33% for localized infection to 88% for disseminated disease. In the absence of a positive A precipitin band or in cases where the CF test is positive for blastomycosis but the ID test is negative, patients should be examined extensively for culture or histologic evidence of infection by other endemic fungi as well as by B. dermatitidis (especially because the areas of endemicity for blastomycosis and histoplasmosis overlap and cross-reactivity can occur). In addition, sera should be drawn at 3-week intervals and examined by CF and ID tests with B. dermatitidis, C. immitis, and H. capsulatum antigens. Such testing will detect increases in CF titers to the causative organism, indicating infection by that organism, or the development of precipitin bands diagnostic for blastomycosis, histoplasmosis, or coccidioidomycosis. In established cases of blastomycosis, a decline in the number or the disappearance of precipitin lines is evidence for a favorable prognosis. The serologic response, however, is often not as rapid as the clinical response.

Experimental and Molecular Biological Approaches

More recently, a double-antibody sandwich EIA, employing rabbit polyclonal antibodies to detect an uncharacterized antigen from B. dermatitidis in urine, serum, CSF, BAL fluid, and other body fluids, has been developed. Test sensitivity was reported to be 89 and 100%, respectively, for the detection of urinary antigen in the disseminated and pulmonary forms of blastomycosis (28). Little or no cross-reactivity was observed when specimens obtained from healthy volunteers or from patients with aspergillosis, candidiasis, coccidioidomycosis, or cryptococcosis were used, but significant cross-reactivity occurred when specimens from patients with disseminated histoplasmosis (96%), paracoccidioidomycosis (100%), or penicilliosis marneffei (70%) were used (28). Because the areas of endemicity for blastomycosis and histoplasmosis overlap, additional tests are required to obtain a specific diagnosis. This test has not yet undergone adequate clinical evaluation and is available only as a fee-for-service test at a single reference laboratory.

A relatively small number of nucleic acid detection tests for blastomycosis have been published and are currently limited to individual research laboratories. Most studies have examined the use of molecular probes to detect B. dermatitidis DNA in paraffin-embedded tissues (7) or from pure cultures (86, 124). Using a gene encoding the WI-1 adhesin of B. dermatitidis as a target for nested PCR, Bialek et al. (7) detected B. dermatitidis DNA in 8 (62%) of 13 tissue samples from microscopically confirmed cases of canine blastomycosis but detected no PCR amplicons from microscopically negative biopsy specimens from dogs with blastomycosis or lymphosarcoma (negative controls). The deleterious effect of formalin on the target DNA during fixation of the tissues was hypothesized to be responsible for the low sensitivity of PCR detection (7).

CANDIDIASIS

Background

Tests for Candida antibodies have been extensively evaluated but remain of uncertain usefulness in the diagnosis of invasive forms of candidiasis. The clinical utility of these tests has been hampered by false-positive results in patients who are colonized with Candida species or who have superficial infections, as well as by false-negative results in immunocompromised patients who produce small or variable quantities of antibodies. On the other hand, in immunocompetent patients, a fourfold rise in the LA titer or seroconversion from no ID band to an ID band or an increase in the number of ID bands may be diagnostically helpful. Conversely, a fourfold decrease in LA titer may denote successful therapy. No LA test to detect anti-Candida antibodies is commercially available. ID kits are available from two commercial sources (Immuno-Mycologics, Inc.; Gibson Laboratories), and a CIE test is available from another (Bio-Rad Laboratories) (Table 1). CIE does not improve test sensitivity significantly compared to ID but can be completed in 90 min rather than in the several days required for the ID test. An EIA to detect antibodies to circulating mannoprotein, a major cell wall component of Candida species, is commercially available in some countries but not in the United States (Platelia Candida Antibody;

Bio-Rad Laboratories, Inc.). Clinical evaluations of the test in patients with invasive candidiasis demonstrated that the test specificity ranged from 63 to 94% but the test sensitivity ranged from 25 to 88%, depending on the identity of the infecting *Candida* species (the lowest sensitivity occurred for detecting *C. parapsilosis* infections, and the highest occurred for detecting *C. albicans* infections) (Table 1). An IFA test to detect antibodies directed to germ tube forms of *C. albicans* cells is also available commercially (Vircell Laboratories); the sensitivity and specificity ranged from 76 to 94% and 95 to 100%, respectively (98) (Table 1).

Because antibody detection tests have limited sensitivity for the diagnosis of invasive candidiasis in immunocompromised patients and because these patients may be in antigen excess, a variety of antigen detection assays have been developed. Among these are tests to detect heat-labile antigens by reverse passive LA (Cand-Tec test; Ramco Laboratories, Inc., Stafford, Tex.) and heat-stable *Candida* cell wall mannan by LA and EIA (the Pastorex *Candida* LA test and the Platelia *Candida* Ag EIA, respectively; Bio-Rad Laboratories, Inc.). The Cand-Tec test has been commercially available for many years. The nature of the antigen is unknown, but its susceptibility to heat (56°C), pronase, 2-mercaptoethanol, and sodium periodate treatment suggests that it may be a glycoprotein. Test sensitivity varied widely among studies (2 to 59%) whereas test specificity ranged from 93 to 95%, using a threshold titer of ≥1:8. A threshold titer of ≥1:4 resulted in a somewhat increased sensitivity (41 to 81%) and a specificity of 80 to 97% (5, 95, 96) (Table 2).

Both the Pastorex *Candida* LA test and the Platelia *Candida* Ag EIA use a rat EB-CA1 MAb directed against the α-1,2-oligomannosides of *Candida* mannan. The Pastorex *Candida* LA test employs agglutination of latex particles coated with this MAb to detect circulating *Candida* antigen, whereas the Platelia *Candida* Ag EIA uses the same MAb but employs it in a double-antibody sandwich EIA format (Table 2); neither of these tests is FDA approved at present. The range in reported sensitivity for the Pastorex *Candida* LA test is quite large (25 to 77%), although test specificity has been good (99 to 100%); in contrast, the Platelia *Candida* Ag EIA has an overall sensitivity of 52% and a specificity of 85 to 95%. Because the Platelia *Candida* Ag EIA gives superior test results compared to the Pastorex *Candida* LA test, only the EIA is described below.

Clinical Indications and Diagnostic Rationale

The LA and ID tests to detect antibodies to *Candida* species have been applied using sera from patients with acute disseminated candidiasis, chronic hepatosplenic candidiasis, or localized deep-organ candidiasis (e.g., endocarditis). Those most at risk for these infections include neutropenic cancer patients, HSCT and SOT recipients receiving immunosuppressive agents, and patients receiving critical care, particularly those in adult surgical and neonatal intensive care units. Patient serum containing antibodies that react with homogenate antigens of *C. albicans* in the ID test may produce one or several lines of identity. Systemic candidiasis should be suspected if serial serum specimens show an increase in titer or an increase in the number of reactive bands detected over time.

Serologic tests may also be employed to determine the potential clinical significance of *Candida* species recovered from various body sites. The detection of precipitins or the occurrence of fourfold changes in antibody titer in the LA test may be evidence of systemic candidiasis; however, such titers may also indicate colonization. The ID and LA tests for antibodies have a sensitivity of approximately 80% for confirmed cases of invasive candidiasis in immunocompetent hosts. The ID test is more specific than the LA test. In cases where candidiasis is suspected and ID reactions are negative for *C. albicans* antigens, the ID test should be performed with other *Candida* species antigens to rule out infections with those species. A decision to treat a patient with antifungal drugs must not be based on serologic data alone, however, but rather should be made after consideration of all available clinical and laboratory data.

Test 1. ID Test To Detect Antibodies to *C. albicans*

Commercial kits for the ID test contain precast agar gels, antigens, and reference antisera. Vendors are listed in Table 1, and more detailed contact information is provided at the end of the chapter. Commercial antigens and antibodies should be used with the agar medium provided by the vendor.

Sample Requirements

Results obtained with a single serum sample are difficult to interpret because a positive result may represent colonization rather than true systemic infection. Therefore, multiple sequential serum specimens, taken weekly or at least every 2 weeks, should be collected to detect seroconversion or an increase in the number of precipitin lines. The *Candida* ID test can also be performed in a semiquantitative manner by testing twofold serial dilutions of sera in normal saline or PBS in the same manner as undiluted sera (below) and recording the highest titer at which bands appear.

Materials and Reagents

Antigens for use in commercial *Candida* ID kits are crude or partially purified, uncharacterized components derived from culture filtrates and/or cell lysates of yeast-phase *C. albicans*. Reference antibodies are directed against the A serotype of *C. albicans* and form at least two precipitin lines against the reference *Candida* antigen.

Equipment

Humidified chamber
Light box with indirect backlighting

Procedure

1. Label ID plates with an identifying number and date.
2. Place plates on a dark background to facilitate well filling.
3. Place the reference serum in the top and bottom wells of the ID pattern, and place each patient's test serum in one of the four lateral wells. The closed plate may then be incubated at 25°C for 30 min to help intensify precipitin lines.
4. Place the reference antigen in the center well of each ID pattern.
5. Place closed plates on a level surface in a humidified chamber, and incubate at 25°C for 24 h.

QA/QC

A positive control serum, preferably containing three precipitin bands, should be included each time the ID test is performed. If bubbles occur during well-filling procedures, they must be broken by being gently pierced with toothpicks. Separate toothpicks should be used for each antigen and antibody solution.

Interpretation

Sera from candidiasis patients which react with homogenate antigens of *C. albicans* in the ID test may produce between one and seven precipitin bands. Systemic candidiasis should be suspected when serial serum specimens demonstrate seroconversion (i.e., when negative antibody test results become positive) or show temporal increases in the number of precipitins.

Test 2. EIA To Detect *Candida* Cell Wall Mannan

A commercial antigenemia detection test, the Platelia *Candida* Ag (Bio-Rad Laboratories), is a microtitration plate-based double-antibody sandwich EIA that can be conducted as either a quantitative (results are compared to a standard curve) or a semiquantitative (results are expressed as an index relative to the calibrator serum) test. This assay uses a rat MAb, EB-CA1, as both the capture and detector antibody for α-(1,2)-linked oligomannosides, outer cell wall components of most clinically important species of *Candida* (129).

Sample Requirements

The test can only be performed with serum samples collected into dry blood collection tubes (no additives or clot activators). Separated serum can be stored in a tightly closed tube at 2 to 8°C if the test is performed within 24 h or should be frozen at −20°C or colder for transport or if the test is not performed within 24 h. Serum can be submitted to a maximum of three freezing and thawing cycles, and frozen samples should be thoroughly mixed before being tested.

Serum specimens should be collected serially during the infectious episode. Sera may also be collected at regular intervals before suspicion of infection if the test is to be used as a screening tool in high-risk patient populations such as SOT recipients and critical-care patients. Mannan occurs in the serum in low nanogram-per-milliliter concentrations and is rapidly cleared from the circulation, necessitating frequent sampling of patients during periods of high risk. Therefore, the use of multiple serum specimens, collected at least twice per week, increases test sensitivity. A total of 300 μl of patient serum is consumed each time the test is performed. Because the test may need to be repeated more than once and because some sample loss occurs during immune complex removal (precipitation of serum proteins during boiling in the presence of neutral disodium EDTA), at least 1 ml of patient serum is required.

Materials and Reagents

Reagents provided in the kit include negative, positive, and calibrator sera, EDTA solution, peroxidase-conjugated detector MAbs, wash solutions and buffers, H_2O_2, chromogen (TMB), stopping solution (1.5 N sulfuric acid), plate sealers, and microtiter plates precoated with capture anti-mannan MAbs. Microtiter plates are composed of 12 eight-well strips so that the entire plate does not have to be used at one time. Strips are supplied in resealable pouches and should be used within 5 weeks of opening. Kits are stored at 2 to 8°C and should be brought to room temperature (18 to 25°C) before use.

Equipment and Procedure

The equipment and procedure for the Platelia *Candida* Ag EIA are the same as those for the Platelia *Aspergillus* Ag EIA (see "Test 2. EIA To Detect *Aspergillus* Cell Wall Galactomannan" above), except that a MAb directed against *Candida* mannan (EB-CA1) is used as the capture and detector antibody.

QA/QC

Strict compliance with the prescribed 100°C temperature for the boiling water bath is essential for success of the test. A negative control serum (no mannan), a calibrator serum (containing 2.0 ng of mannan per ml and the concentration from which to prepare a standard curve for the quantitative assay or from which to dilute to 0.5 ng for the qualitative assay), and positive control serum (containing between 0.5 and 1.5 ng of mannan) are included in each kit. Results are expressed in nanograms per milliliter extrapolated from the standard curve (quantitative assay) or as an index (semi-quantitative assay; i.e., the ratio of the OD of the test sample to the OD of the mean calibrator serum provided in the kit). In both test modes, OD values for the calibrator, for the four points comprising the standard curve (quantitative mode), and for the positive and negative controls must be within their designated ranges.

Interpretation

Serum samples with a mannan concentration of less than 0.25 ng/ml are considered to be negative, serum samples with a mannan concentration of between 0.25 and 0.5 ng/ml are considered to be intermediate, and serum samples with a mannan concentration greater than or equal to 0.5 ng/ml are considered to be positive. Range points used to plot the standard curve do not allow precise determination of mannan concentrations above 2.5 ng/ml, and strongly positive sera should be diluted 1:5 (vol/vol) with negative serum and retested. Positive results obtained with the Platelia *Candida* Ag test should be interpreted in conjunction with other diagnostic procedures including culture, histopathology of biopsied tissues, and radiographic evidence of infection. Negative test results do not rule out a diagnosis of invasive candidiasis. Even in cases of culture or histopathologically proven candidiasis, not every serum sample from each patient is expected to be positive.

The EB-CA1 MAb is specific for an α-linked mannopentaose common to all *Candida* species (135), but test sensitivity varies depending upon the *Candida* species being detected. For example, in a retrospective study conducted on 106 patients (366 sera) residing in various hospital wards (surgery, hematology, intensive care, burns, and others) and from whom *Candida* species were isolated from the blood or other sterile body sites, the overall sensitivity of the EIA was 52%. For infections by specific *Candida* species, however, sensitivities were 70% for *C. tropicalis*, 50 to 58% for *C. kefyr*, *C. albicans*, and *C. glabrata*, 38% for *C. parapsilosis*, and only 20% for *C. krusei*. The moderate sensitivity exhibited by the test does not provide an optimum negative predictive value for diagnosing invasive candidiasis. However, because the overall specificity of the EIA is so high (98%), a positive result obtained with samples from patients at risk suggests infection.

Experimental and Molecular Biological Approaches

Enolase, a 48-kDa cytoplasmic antigen of *C. albicans*, is a potentially useful diagnostic marker of invasive candidiasis. A clinical trial evaluating a commercial double-antibody liposomal immunoassay to detect enolase in cancer patients reported an overall sensitivity of 75% and a specificity of 96% (157). Unfortunately, this test is no longer available commercially.

An inducible, extracellularly secreted aspartyl proteinase (Sap), originally studied extensively as a virulence factor in the invasion and dissemination of *C. albicans* in animal models of infection (52, 79), has more recently been examined as a useful diagnostic marker of invasive candidiasis. An antibody detection assay and two antigen detection assays, employing a MAb specific for Sap, were compared in a retrospective analysis. The sensitivities and specificities, respectively, were 70 and 76% for the antibody detection assay and 94 and 92% for the antigen capture ELISA. The sensitivity and specificity of the inhibition ELISA to detect Sap antigen were greater than those of either the antibody detection test or the antigen capture test: 94 and 96%, respectively.

D-Arabinitol, a five-carbon polyol, is produced by the most medically important *Candida* spp. except for *C. krusei* and perhaps *C. glabrata* (18). Its production has been detected in serum or urine by gas-liquid chromatography, gas chromatography-mass spectrometry, and enzymatic fluorometric or enzymatic chromogenic assays (166). Serum creatinine levels, required to normalize results for the increased serum arabinitol concentrations observed during renal dysfunction, can be measured simultaneously with D-arabinitol by use of a centrifugal autoanalyzer (Roche). Patients with persistent candidemia had the highest D-arabinitol/creatinine levels (83% positive) compared to patients with transient candidemia (74%) or negative controls (14%) (166).

Commercial products are currently under development for the rapid extraction and recovery of *C. albicans* DNA from whole blood (MagNa Pure; Roche Molecular Biochemicals, Inc., Indianapolis, Ind.) (87) and for the identification of amplicons by real-time, quantitative PCR (Light Cycler *Candida* kit; Roche). Application of a commercial DNA extraction kit (MagNa Pure LC total nucleic acid Isolation kit; Roche) in conjunction with an automated DNA extraction system (MagNa Pure LC system; Roche) and a "real-time" PCR amplification and detection system (LightCycler) has been reported to detect as few as 1 CFU of *C. albicans* per ml of whole blood (87). This process could be completed in just 3 h. However, it was required that whole blood be treated to lyse and remove erythrocytes and that *C. albicans* cells in the specimen be disrupted by vortex mixing in the presence of glass beads before samples were added to the automated DNA extraction system (87). These additional steps make the application of this method for the extraction of *Candida* DNA too cumbersome for use in a clinical laboratory. However, amplicon detection by the real-time quantitative PCR system obviates the need for postamplification manipulation steps, making the LightCycler system more rapid than conventional PCR detection methods. This system has been adapted for use with species-specific primers, directed to target sequences from the 18S and 28S regions of rDNA, to detect and identify *C. albicans*, *C. glabrata*, *C. krusei*, *C. parapsilosis*, *C. tropicalis*, and *C. guilliermondii* (49) and to target sequences from the ITS regions and 18S rDNA region in *C. albicans*, *C. tropicalis*, and *C. krusei* (12). Multiplex real-time PCR and melting-curve analysis demonstrated the limit of test sensitivity to be 0.1 pg of fungal genomic DNA (12).

Other quantitative PCR methods have been described for the detection of *Candida* species, and one of these (TaqMan System; Perkin-Elmer Applied Biosystems, Inc.) takes advantage of the 5'-3' exonuclease activity of the *Taq* DNA polymerase to separate a quencher probe from a reporter probe, thereby producing a fluorescent signal proportional to the amount of target DNA amplified. Application of this system to sera obtained from pediatric hematology and oncology patients with culture-confirmed candidemia and clinically proven or suspected systemic candidiasis demonstrated a sensitivity of 100% for the detection of *C. albicans*, *C. glabrata*, *C. tropicalis*, and *C. parapsilosis* DNA (88).

Given the low sensitivity of antigen detection and the low specificity of antibody detection for the diagnosis of candidiasis, PCR-based diagnostic methods offer the promise of improved sensitivity and specificity. However, universally standardized methods for the extraction, purification, amplification, and detection of *Candida* species DNA require further development and evaluation.

COCCIDIOIDOMYCOSIS

Background

Tests to detect anti-*C. immitis* antibodies are of proven usefulness for the diagnosis and management of coccidioidomycosis. One of the original serologic methods for the diagnosis of this disease was the TP test which detects IgM antibodies reactive against a heat-stable, carbohydrate-containing component in coccidioidin (a filtrate of autolyzed *Coccidioides immitis* mycelial cultures). These antibodies can usually be detected within the first month of infection. Currently, the diagnosis of early acute disease can be established with similar results by using the same antigen but in an immunodiffusion test format (IDTP). An LA test, using particles adsorbed with heated coccidioidin, is a simple and rapid method to measure early antibody production corresponding to that detected by the TP or IDTP tests. The LA test is more sensitive than the TP or IDTP tests and can therefore be used as a rapid screening tool. However, the LA test is also associated with a false-positivity rate of greater than 5% (27, 53). This false-positivity rate is greater if sera have been diluted before testing. Therefore, the LA test can not be used as a quantitative test and results which are positive by this method must be confirmed by the IDTP test.

In contrast to the IDTP and LA tests, which detect early IgM antibody responses to coccidioidal infection, the CF test detects primarily IgG antibodies produced during the convalescent phase of disease or during chronic infections. The CF test measures the concentration of antibodies against a heat-labile protein antigen, found in coccidioidin, called the F antigen. This same antigen can be used to detect IgG antibodies in an immunodiffusion test format (IDCF). The CF procedure is the most widely used serologic test for the diagnosis of coccidioidomycosis, and reactive antibodies persist for longer periods than do those detected in the IDTP test. The CF test is diagnostic and prognostic: antibody titers rise in proportion to disease severity and subside in response to therapy. The IDCF test can also be conducted in a quantitative manner, using serially diluted serum. Whereas a single test by any of the above methods may provide an accurate diagnosis, performing both the IDCF and CF tests in parallel provides the highest sensitivity and specificity.

A commercial enzyme immunoassay, the Premier *Coccidioides* EIA (Meridian Diagnostics, Inc., Cincinnati, Ohio), is useful for the detection of anti-*Coccidioides* IgG and IgM antibodies in sera from patients with coccidioidomycosis (68). Microwells of an EIA plate are precoated by the manufacturer with a proprietary mixture of purified TP and CF antigens so that the detector antibodies employed can be used to differentiate between reactive IgM (early) and IgG (late) antibodies. Detection of both types of antibodies by the EIA gives the greatest sensitivity (97%) and specificity (94%), although confirmation of positive results by ID is recommended.

Clinical Indications and Diagnostic Rationale

Serologic tests should be considered whenever patients display signs and symptoms of coccidioidomycosis and have lived in or traveled to areas where *C. immitis* (California) or *C. posadasii* (Arizona, New Mexico, Utah, Texas, Mexico, and Central and South America) is endemic. Serum antibodies may be detected within 1 to 3 weeks after the onset of primary infection in a large percentage of cases. Detection of antibodies by the IDTP or LA tests is diagnostic but not prognostic since antibodies reactive in these tests are rarely detected 6 months after acute pulmonary infection. Reactive antibodies may reappear if the infection spreads or relapses or they may persist in disseminated cases. The CF test becomes positive later than the IDTP or LA tests and is most effective in monitoring disseminated disease. The CF titer rises in parallel with the severity of the infection (20, 107) and declines as the patient improves.

Test 1. IDTP and IDCF Tests To Detect Early and Late Antibodies to *Coccidioides* Species

The ID test format can be used to simultaneously detect IgM (IDTP) and IgG (IDCF) antibodies on a single plate. Both the IDTP and the IDCF tests are performed using a seven-well ID pattern formed in a gel or agar substrate. Positive control IDTP and IDCF sera are placed in independent wells and are tested against patient sera as well as against optimally diluted heated (for IDTP) or unheated (for IDCF) coccidioidin. Lines of identity between patient sera and positive reference sera, corresponding to reactive IgM (for IDTP) and IgG (for IDCF) antibodies, can then be observed for positive cases of early or late disease, respectively (107). Commercial sources for ID kits and reagents for use in ID tests are listed in Table 1.

Sample Requirements

Serum from symptomatic patients may give negative or indeterminate test results early in infection. Additional serum from such patients should be obtained 3 to 4 weeks later, and the tests should be repeated. CSF should be obtained and tested in parallel with serum specimens from patients presenting with signs and symptoms of meningitis. The sensitivity of the IDTP and IDCF tests can be increased by eightfold concentration of serum prior to testing. Serum can be concentrated by evaporation in vacuo (Speed-Vac; Savant Instruments, Inc., Holbrook, N.Y.) or by the use of centrifugal ultrafiltration devices (Centricon; Millipore, Billerica, Mass.). Concentration of test serum may be especially helpful to improve IDTP detection of low levels of IgM antibodies present early in infection and to improve IDCF detection of IgG antibodies in specimens from patients with chronic disease. Serum may demonstrate anticomplementary activity, making CF test results difficult to interpret; however, such sera can be successfully used in the ID test. In addition, the ID test is more specific than CF and may help resolve CF cross-reactivity issues often encountered among the endemic mycoses during CF testing.

Materials and Reagents

The antigens for both the IDTP and IDCF tests are filtrates of mycelial cultures of multiple or single isolates of *C. immitis*. Coccidioidin is prepared by a variety of procedures. In the most widely known procedure, filtrates are produced from cultures grown in synthetic asparagine-glycerol-salts medium originally devised for tuberculin production. The preparation of coccidioidin in this medium usually requires incubation for several weeks at room temperature. Coccidioidin antigens can also be prepared within 1 week by a toluene lysis technique (67). Heating coccidioidin at 60°C for 30 min destroys the F antigen responsible for the IDCF activity, but the heat-stable antigen responsible for the IDTP reactivity is retained (67).

Phenolized Medium

The same medium as that used for the blastomycosis ID test is used for the IDTP and IDCF tests (see "Test 1. ID Test To Detect Antibodies to *B. dermatitidis*" above). The final pH of the medium should be 6.3 to 6.4. The mixture is autoclaved at a pressure of 15 lb/in² for 10 min.

Equipment

The same equipment is used for the coccidioidomycosis ID test as for the aspergillosis ID test (see "Test 1. ID Test To Detect Antibodies to *Aspergillus* Species" above).

Procedure

The same procedure as that described for the aspergillosis ID test is used, except that the patient test sera and the corresponding reference sera must be incubated in test wells for 30 min at ambient temperature before the addition of the IDTP antigen to the center well of the ID test pattern. This preincubation interval provides time for the relatively large IgM antibody molecules (compared to IgG molecules) to adequately diffuse into the agar gel matrix. Antigen-antibody precipitin bands will then be located centrally between the antigen-containing and antibody-containing wells of the ID pattern.

QA/QC

Positive control sera must be included each time the test is performed. Patient serum must react with the homologous reference antigen to form a line of identity with the reference band in order to be considered positive for coccidioidomycosis. Occasionally, interference with test results occurs as a result of formation of a precipitation band resembling that of the IDTP reaction by sera from patients without coccidioidomycosis. The origin of this band is unknown but may be the result of reactions between coccidioidal antigens and C-reactive protein (or a related substance) in serum. Such bands can be dissolved by the addition of an aqueous solution of 1.5% EDTA, which leaves authentic IDTP bands unaffected.

Interpretation

IDTP

Observation of a band of identity in the IDTP assay indicates that the patient from whom the test serum was obtained is in the early stages of coccidioidomycosis. Of patients with coccidioidomycosis, 75% develop a detectable IDTP antibody response as early as 1 week after onset of symptoms; 91% are positive within 3 weeks. Negative test results, however, do not exclude a diagnosis of coccidioidomycosis. In the absence of a positive precipitin band, or in cases where the CF test is positive but the IDTP test is negative, patients should be examined extensively for culture or histopathologic evidence of infection by another endemic fungus as well as by *C. immitis*. In addition, sera should be drawn at 3-week intervals and examined by CF and ID tests with *B. dermatitidis*, *C. immitis*, and *H. capsulatum* antigens to detect increases in CF titer specific for infection by one of the endemic fungi or to detect the development of precipitin bands diagnostic for blastomycosis, histoplasmosis, or coccidioidomycosis. IDTP antibodies may not be detected in immunosuppressed patients with disseminated coccidioidomycosis (1). False-positive IDTP reactions have been reported to occur in 15% of sera obtained from cystic fibrosis patients in the absence of a positive culture for *C. immitis* (26). A positive IDTP test can also rarely indicate the presence of chronic pulmonary cavities. Although infrequent, a positive result using CSF in the IDTP test indicates the presence of acute meningitis. IDTP reactive antibodies may also occur in cases of disseminated coccidioidomycosis; 347 (48%) of 722 patients with disseminated infections demonstrated reactivity to this antigen, and in some cases, patient sera were reactive for up to several years (131). Persistence of IDTP reactive antibodies (along with positive CF titers) may therefore be an indication of disease severity.

IDCF

Observation of a band of identity in the IDCF assay is presumptive evidence that the patient from whom the test serum was obtained had recent or chronic coccidioidomycosis. IDCF reactive antibodies can usually be detected within 2 to 6 weeks after onset of symptoms. Cross-reactivity has been reported to occur when serum from patients infected with other fungi is used but not when serum from patients with cystic fibrosis is used. Occasionally, a band of nonidentity may be observed very close to the ID well containing the patient's serum. This band may represent the presence of reactive IgM antibodies; in such cases, the IDTP test should be performed. Serum or other body fluids may be tested unconcentrated and without prediffusion in ID wells, but the sensitivity of the qualitative test is improved and becomes greater than that of the CF test by concentration and prediffusion; concentration of CSF may result in the detection of IgG in CSF in the absence of meningitis. Although the IDCF test is generally not performed as a quantitative test, it can be used in this manner after serial dilution of patient serum to obtain an endpoint titer. Titers obtained by using the quantitative IDCF test are not identical to titers obtained from the CF test, but the observed trends are comparable (titers of each will rise or fall in parallel). Results using specimens collected longitudinally may show differences in the intensity of bands or in banding patterns which have prognostic value. On the other hand, IDCF reactive antibodies may not be detected in immunosuppressed patients with disseminated coccidioidomycosis (1).

Test 2. LA Test To Detect Antibodies to *Coccidioides* Species

The LA test is a qualitative slide agglutination assay using *C. immitis* TP antigen-coated latex particles to detect antibodies to *C. immitis*. Antibodies to *C. immitis* present in patient specimens bind to the antigen-coated latex particles, resulting in visible clumping (1+ to 4+ agglutination). Results are graded according to the level of agglutination observed for a particular dilution of serum. The assay measures predominantly IgM antibodies and therefore is used to diagnose early coccidioidomycosis. The assay is rapid and simple to perform, and no special equipment is needed. However, false-positive results can occur (>5%), making it necessary to confirm any positive results with the IDTP and/or CF tests (107). Commercial sources are listed in Table 1 and at the end of the chapter.

Sample Requirements

Blood should be collected into tubes that contain no anticoagulant since anticoagulant can interfere with test performance. Serum must be heat inactivated at 56°C for 30 min before being tested. The LA test should not be applied to CSF or to diluted sera, because false-positive reactions have

been reported. Test performance using pleural, joint, or ascitic fluid is unknown. Specimens can be held at 2 to 8°C for up to 72 h before being tested but must be placed at −20°C or colder for long-term storage. Specimens should not be stored in frost-free freezers because repeated freezing and thawing can affect test results.

Materials and Reagents

This test uses latex particles sensitized with coccidioidin that has been heated at 60°C for 30 min (TP antigen). All reagents including sensitized latex particles, positive control serum (from goats or rabbits immunized with *C. immitis*), and negative control serum (normal goat or human serum) can be obtained commercially from Immuno-Mycologics, Inc., or Meridian Diagnostics, Inc. Disposable glass slides with raised rings for the performance of the test are also supplied with the kits from Immuno-Mycologics, Inc.

Equipment

100- and 20-µl pipettes
Clinical rotator (optional)
Timer
Applicator sticks
Fluorescent or natural light source

Procedure

1. Add 25 µl of latex-positive control, negative control, and each undiluted specimen into separate rings on the glass slide.
2. Add 1 drop of optimally diluted sensitized latex particles into each ring.
3. Using separate applicator sticks, thoroughly mix the contents of each ring.
4. Rotate the slide by hand or place on a rotary shaker and rotate at 100 ± 25 rpm for 10 min at room temperature.
5. Immediately examine the slide, macroscopically, over a dark background, for signs of agglutination.

QA/QC

A positive and negative control must be run in parallel with test samples during the initial screening phase but are optional for the titration phase of the test. The LA test can not be used as a quantitative test because false-positive results have been reported with diluted sera. Additional QA/QC practices for the LA test include the following: (i) the latex-positive control must demonstrate 2+ or greater agglutination; (ii) the negative control must demonstrate less than 1+ agglutination; and (iii) periodically, the sensitivity of the latex reagent should be tested by titration of the positive control (i.e., the positive control should give an agglutination result of 1+ at a 1:4 dilution ± one dilution to be satisfactory for use). Agglutination is graded as follows: negative, a homogeneous suspension of particles with no visible clumping; 1+, fine granulation against a milky background; 2+, small but definite clumps against a slightly cloudy background; 3+, large and small clumps against a clear background; and 4+, large clumps against a clear or very clear background. Freezing of the latex particle suspension should be avoided since this can result in granularity leading to false-positive results. Materials should not be allowed to dry on the slide.

Interpretation

Agglutination of 2+ or greater is considered to be a positive test result indicating early or primary coccidioidomycosis, and agglutination of less than 2+ is defined as a negative result. The LA test is more sensitive than the IDTP test but is less specific; 5 to 10% false-positive rates have been reported. Therefore, a positive LA result with undiluted serum or CSF must be confirmed by ID and/or CF testing. The LA test, however, may yield a positive result earlier than the IDTP test. False-negative LA results may occur in specimens from immunocompromised patients. Also, 10 to 30% of individuals with culturally or serologically (CF or ID) positive results may demonstrate a negative or 1+ reaction in the LA test, limiting the test's negative predictive value. Such test negativity is thought to be related to the rapid rise and fall of IgM levels early in infection.

Test 3. CF Test To Detect Antibodies to *Coccidioides* Species

The CF assay, using unheated coccidioidin antigen, detects antibodies predominantly of the IgG subtype. Sera from approximately 98% of patients with disseminated infection are positive in the CF test within 2 to 6 weeks after onset of illness. The CF reactive antibodies typically disappear within 6 months after onset but can persist in disseminated or chronic infection. An advantage to the use of the CF test for the diagnosis of coccidioidomycosis is that it is a sensitive assay which provides quantitative results. Testing serial specimens to detect rising or falling antibody titers can reveal the progression or regression of illness and the response to antifungal therapy. The major disadvantage of the CF assay is that it is a laborious and time-consuming test that requires experienced personnel for optimum performance. No commercial CF test kit is available, but reagents for in-house use can be obtained from the vendors listed in Table 1.

Sample Requirements

The CF test may be performed with serum and CSF. Pleural, peritoneal, and joint fluids (in conjunction with serum) may also be tested when the corresponding anatomical sites are thought to be involved. Concentration of sera before performance of the CF test can be useful in the detection of chronic cases of coccidioidomycosis which might otherwise be missed.

Materials and Reagents

The antigen is prepared as described above for the IDCF test from cultures grown in synthetic asparagine-glycerol-salts medium (67). Because the CF antigen is destroyed by heating at 60°C for 30 min, this antigen should not be heated.

Equipment and Procedures

A microtitration version of the CF test is recommended when serum samples are tested for antibodies. Equipment and procedures for the CF test for the diagnosis of coccidioidomycosis are the same as those for histoplasmosis except that coccidioidin, prepared as described above for the IDCF test, is used instead of *H. capsulatum* antigens (see "Test 1. CF Test To Detect Antibodies to *H. capsulatum*" below). Also, unlike the *H. capsulatum* CF test, CF titers of <1:8 can be significant. Therefore, testing may begin using specimens diluted 1:2, or undiluted, if necessary.

QA/QC

Negative control serum and positive control serum from a human case of coccidioidomycosis (showing a *Coccidioides* CF titer of ≥1:32) should be included each time the CF test is performed. Anti-complementary activity in serum samples can occur (i.e., those showing <75% hemolysis in the serum

control without antigen), and results may be resolved by subsequent ID testing. However, the ID test may not be as sensitive as the CF test, particularly early in infection. Additional QA/QC measures are listed under "Test 1. CF Test To Detect Antibodies to *H. capsulatum*" below.

Interpretation

Sera demonstrating 30% or less hemolysis at a given dilution are considered to be positive at that titer. A CF titer to coccidioidin at any dilution should be considered presumptive evidence for *C. immitis* infection. Sera giving titers of 1:2 to 1:8 in the CF test that are also positive in the IDCF test reflect currently active or recent infection. CF titers of >1:16 generally indicate extrapulmonary dissemination, whereas titers of 1:2 or 1:4 usually indicate early, residual, or meningeal coccidioidomycosis. However, titers of 1:2 and 1:4 have also been obtained when sera from patients without coccidioidomycosis were used. The parallel use of the IDCF test and the CF test can therefore help confirm or refute the significance of low titers. Negative serologic test results do not exclude a diagnosis of coccidioidomycosis. Patients with clinical presentations consistent with coccidioidomycosis, whose sera give negative or low CF titers, should be retested at 3- to 4-week intervals; all sera collected from a given patient at all time points should then be tested in parallel to detect any increases in titer or to detect seroconversion. Approximately 5% of all CSF specimens from patients with coccidioidal meningitis are negative in the CF test. Sera from patients with chronic cavitary coccidioidomycosis may also frequently be negative.

Test 4. EIA To Detect Antibodies to *Coccidioides* Species

The Premier *Coccidioides* EIA (Meridian Diagnostics, Inc.) is a qualitative test to determine the presence of anti-*Coccidioides* IgG and IgM antibodies by using microtiter plates coated with a mixture of purified CF and TP antigens. Antibodies in serum or CSF are detected colorimetrically after addition of peroxidase-labeled, class-specific, anti-human IgM or IgG. The assay detects IgG and IgM antibodies separately, but maximum test sensitivity is achieved by using results from the detection of both IgG and IgM antibodies (Table 1). It is recommended that any positive result in the EIA be confirmed by the ID assay.

Sample Requirements

Serum and CSF are acceptable specimens for use in the Premier *Coccidioides* EIA, but this assay is not recommended for use with other clinical specimens. Heat-inactivated (56°C for 30 min) specimens may be used, but CSF containing blood is not acceptable. Specimens should be tested as soon as possible but may be stored at 2 to 8°C for up to 5 days and frozen at −20°C or colder for longer storage. It is recommended that specimens be divided into single-use aliquots before being frozen in order to avoid repeated freezing and thawing and that samples not be stored in a frost-free freezer.

Materials and Reagents

Reagents provided in the kit include positive control serum (prediluted positive human serum), sample diluent (buffered protein solution which also serves as the negative control), concentrated wash buffer, two enzyme conjugates (peroxidase-conjugated goat anti-human IgM and IgG), urea peroxide, chromogen (TMB), stopping solution (2 N sulfuric acid), and microtiter plates precoated with a mixture of CF and TP antigens. Microtiter plates are composed of 12 eight-well strips so that the entire plate does not have to be used at one time. Kits are stored at 2 to 8°C and should be brought to room temperature (22 to 25°C) before use.

Equipment

> Pipettes or multichannel pipettes, adjustable or fixed, to measure and dispense 10, 20, 100, and 200 µl
>
> 12- by 75-mm test tubes for the dilution of samples
>
> Timer
>
> Manual or semiautomatic plate washer
>
> Microplate reader equipped with a 450-nm filter

Procedure

A detailed stepwise procedure can be found in the package insert included with each kit. Briefly, specimens are diluted (serum, 1:441 [vol/vol]; CSF, 1:21 [vol/vol]) with the diluent provided in the kit before being added to the antigen-coated microtiter plate wells. Plates are incubated for 30 min at 22 to 25°C before being washed three times with buffer. Each of two peroxidase-conjugated detector antibodies is then added, in parallel, to separate wells of the microtiter plate (one conjugate detects IgM, and one detects IgG). Plates are incubated for an additional 30 min at 22 to 25°C and washed as above, and substrate solution is added to each well. Plates are then incubated for 5 min before addition of the stopping solution. Plates are read spectrophotometrically at 450 nm or at 450/630 nm, if a dual-wavelength plate reader is available.

QA/QC

Positive and negative controls must be included each time the test is performed and are included in the kit. Positive control samples should have a definite yellow color and absorbance values between ≥ 0.500 and ≤ 2.500 for each of the IgM and IgG conjugates. Negative control (sample diluent) values should be below 0.100 for both conjugates when samples are blanked on air (A_{450}) or below 0.050 when read on a dual-wavelength plate reader. If control sample results are outside of the required ranges, the assay should be repeated.

Interpretation

Absorbance values of ≥ 0.200 are considered positive, and values of <0.150 are considered negative. Specimens with absorbance values between 0.150 and 0.199 are defined as indeterminate, and testing must be repeated. A new specimen should be obtained from any patient whose original specimen gives repeatedly indeterminate results. Because the test uses a mixture of TP and CF antigens to coat microtiter plate wells, it does not distinguish between antibodies reactive to one antigen or the other. The kit may be used to detect reactive antibodies of a single class (IgG or IgM); however, optimum test sensitivity is obtained by using results for both Ig classes. Attempts to operate the Premier *Coccidioides* EIA as a quantitative test have not given results that correlate precisely with titers obtained by the conventional CF test. Nonetheless, the EIA has been used as a qualitative test in a series of evaluations and has been demonstrated to have an estimated sensitivity of 95 to 100%, a specificity of 96 to 99%, and positive and negative predictive values of >95% (68, 92, 170). The EIA, however, is not absolutely specific, since some sera from patients with blastomycosis or from patients with noncoccidioidal disease gave false-positive results. Therefore, positive EIA test

results should be confirmed by IDTP and IDCF assays. The standard CF test should be employed in cases where there is concern about possible extrapulmonary dissemination (61).

Experimental and Molecular Biological Approaches

The component of coccidioidin to which CF antibodies react is a 110-kDa protein that has been further identified as a chitinase (60, 171). Incorporating a recombinant form of the chitinase into an EIA format resulted in a test that was shown to be 96% sensitive and 100% specific for the detection of coccidioidal antibodies (61). A recombinant 190-amino-acid peptide was also examined in an EIA format and found to detect 95% of patients with coccidioidomycosis, with no cross-reactivity with serum from histoplasmosis or blastomycosis patients or from healthy subjects.

Galgiani et al. (35) isolated a 33-kDa immunoreactive protein from the walls of mature spherules which appeared to be different from the CF antigen. CSF from patients having suspected coccidioidal meningitis was tested for this antigen in an EIA test format. Of patients with meningitis, 72% yielded a positive result; in contrast, only 1.4% of patients without meningitis reacted positively.

Only a few studies describe the application of molecular methods to clinical materials for the diagnosis of coccidioidomycosis. Sandhu et al. (124) described the use of primers directed to the large (28S) rRNA subunit gene of *C. immitis* to produce PCR amplicons that could then be detected by a slot blot assay. All specimens had been demonstrated by smear or culture results to contain at least one species of fungus. An oligonucleotide probe was designed from *C. immitis* sequences within the 28S rRNA region. In a limited number of clinical specimens, this probe correctly identified *C. immitis* DNA that had been extracted and amplified from sputum or induced sputum but did not cross-react with amplicons derived from specimens containing other fungi (124).

Recently, based on single-nucleotide polymorphisms and differences in the size of microsatellites, the genus *Coccidioides* has been divided into two species: *C. immitis*, representing isolates found in California, and *C. posadasii*, representing isolates found outside of California (32). Accordingly, a nested PCR assay has since been developed to identify *C. posadasii* in paraffin-embedded tissues. The gene encoding Ag2/PRA, an immunoreactive proline-rich antigen specific for *Coccidioides* (9), was employed as the amplification target. All tissue specimens tested were microscopically positive for *Coccidioides* spherules, and all were also demonstrated to be PCR positive. In contrast, no PCR product was obtained from 20 human tissue samples shown to be positive by microscopy or by specific PCR assays for *H. capsulatum*, *P. brasiliensis*, or *B. dermatitidis*.

CRYPTOCOCCOSIS

Background

The *Cryptococcus* LA test to detect capsular polysaccharide in CSF and serum of patients infected with *C. neoformans* is one of the most reliable diagnostic tests in immunomycology. If more objective end points with equivalent sensitivity are desired, an EIA to detect serum and CSF antigen is also commercially available (see "Test 2. EIA To Detect *C. neoformans* Capsular Polysaccharide Antigen" below and Table 2). The EIA requires at least 1 h to perform, in contrast to the few minutes needed to complete the simpler LA test. Both the LA test and the EIA can be used to screen single test samples so that only positive specimens need to be subsequently subjected to titer determination. Unlike the LA test, for optimum sensitivity and specificity the EIA does not require serum to be heat inactivated or pretreated with pronase to remove immune complexes, nor does it require that CSF be boiled before testing (140, 142). Nonetheless, the LA test remains the most widely used procedure for detecting cryptococcal antigen because it is rapid, very specific, diagnostic, prognostic, and simple to perform. There are multiple commercial sources for LA tests to detect cryptococcal antigen, including those which adsorb latex particles with PAbs (Immuno-Mycologics, Inc., Meridian Diagnostics, and Wampole Laboratories, Inc., Cranbury, N.J.) or MAb (Bio-Rad Laboratories) (Table 2). Results and end-point titers vary among LA tests from different manufacturers, and reagents are not interchangeable. Similar sensitivities were reported for the MAb-based LA test (Pastorex Crypto Plus; Bio-Rad) compared to two PAb-based LA tests (CALAS, Meridian Biosciences, Inc.; Crypto-LA, Wampole Laboratories, Inc.) using sera obtained from patients with culture-confirmed cryptococcosis (142). Unlike the PAb-based tests, the MAb-based LA test is recommended for use with BAL fluid and urine specimens as well as with serum and CSF (142). A murine polyclonal antibody (DakoCytomation, Inc.), directed against the capsular glucuronoxylomannan of C. neoformans, is commercially available for the immunohistochemical staining of C. neoformans in tissues by IFA.

In addition to antigen detection tests, a TA test to detect antibodies to C. neoformans is commercially available (Immuno-Mycologics, Inc.; Table 1). Antibody detection is of value for the diagnosis of cryptococcosis during the early stages of the disease, before antibodies are neutralized by the large amount of capsular antigen released during evolution of infection. Antibodies may subsequently reappear after successful treatment, and it has been suggested that their detection is a favorable prognostic sign. However, cryptococcal antibody detection tests are generally less useful than those for antigen detection.

Clinical Indications and Diagnostic Rationale

Serologic tests to detect C. neoformans antigens are an indispensable tool for the rapid diagnosis of pulmonary, meningeal, or disseminated forms of cryptococcosis. The disease may be primary, but many cases are associated with HIV infection or other immunocompromising disorders. Serologic diagnosis for cryptococcosis should be considered for immunosuppressed patients with signs and symptoms of a subacute meningitis or meningoencephalitis. In HIV-infected persons, headache and fever are common but overt neurological symptoms and signs are unusual. In HIV-negative persons, headache is common but fever is often minimal or absent until late in the course of the infection.

Test 1. LA Test To Detect C. neoformans Capsular Polysaccharide Antigen

The LA test is a noncompetitive direct-binding slide agglutination test to detect C. neoformans antigens in clinical samples by employing latex particles adsorbed with rabbit polyclonal anti-C. neoformans antibodies (CALAS; Latex-Cryptococcus antigen test, Immuno-Mycologics; and Crypto-LA) or with mouse anti-glucuronoxylomannan MAb (Pastorex Crypto Plus; Bio-Rad Laboratories). These tests can be used to screen specimens for positivity, and

positive samples can subsequently be diluted serially to obtain an end-point titer (34, 140, 142).

Sample Requirements

Serum and CSF may be used in all commercial tests; serum, CSF, BAL fluid, and urine may be used in the Pastorex Crypto Plus test. Plasma may not be used. A minimum of 0.2 ml of serum or CSF is generally required to perform the test in a qualitative manner, and an additional 0.25 ml may be required to determine serum or CSF titers in a semiquantitative manner. Most kits recommend that sera be pretreated with pronase before being tested since this procedure has been demonstrated to increase the LA titer by 3 to 9 dilutions for 46 (81%) of 57 sera examined (41). Pronase is then inactivated with pronase inhibitor or by boiling. If no pronase pretreatment is recommended by the manufacturer (Wampole Laboratories), test sera should, at a minimum, be heat inactivated at 56°C for 30 min. Negative control sera (normal goat, rabbit, or human serum) should be heat inactivated each time the assay is performed. In contrast, antibody control serum (goat anti-rabbit serum, pronase control) should never be heated.

CSF should be heated in a boiling-water bath for 5 to 10 min as directed by the manufacturer. Pronase treatment of CSF is generally not recommended but was reported to increase LA titers by 2 to 3 dilutions in 14 (20%) of 70 CSF specimens tested (41). BAL fluids should be treated with pronase prior to assay. No anticoagulants should be used in the collection of blood or added to patient test samples prior to use or in preparation for storage. Specimens can be held at 2 to 8°C for up to 48 h before testing but must be placed at −20°C or colder for long-term storage. Specimens should not be stored in frost-free freezers because repeated freezing and thawing can affect test results.

Materials and Reagents

All reagents including sensitized latex particles, sample diluent, positive control serum, negative control serum, pronase reagents (pronase, pronase control, and, in some kits, pronase inhibitor), control latex particles, and glass slides with raised rings (or disposable reaction cards) are supplied with the test kits.

Equipment

Pipettes or multichannel pipettes to dispense 25, 100, and 200 μl

Clinical rotator capable of 140 rpm

Timer

Applicator sticks

12- by 75-mm borosilicate glass test tubes (nonsiliconized)

Water bath or heat block (56 and 100°C)

Fluorescent or natural light source

Procedure

The procedure for the cryptococcal LA test is essentially the same as that described for the Coccidioides LA test (see "Test 2. LA Test To Detect Antibodies to Coccidioides Species" above), except that (i) specimens are heat inactivated and/or pronase treated to remove immune complexes prior to use; (ii) end-point titer determinations for samples positive in the initial screening are conducted using serial twofold dilutions up to and including 1:1,024 (or higher, if testing determines that the specimen is still positive at the 1:1,024 dilution); and (iii) control latex particles, adsorbed with normal globulin, may be included in the kit.

QA/QC

QA/QC procedures are similar to those for the *Coccidioides* LA test. Latex particles should not be frozen since this can result in granularity, leading to false-positive results; excessive hand rotation during observation may also lead to misinterpretation of results. Different manufacturers' products can give different titers for the same clinical specimen. The reported range in end-point titers among different LA test kits varied from 6 dilutions above to 8 dilutions below those of the most sensitive kit examined, although high-titer results (≥1:256) were in better agreement than were low-titer results (140). Reagents must not be interchanged between kits from different companies or between different lots of kits from the same company.

False-negative reactions may occur as the result of immune complex formation or the presence of rheumatoid factor. Both of these interfering substances can be removed by performing a pronase treatment step or by boiling the specimen for 5 to 10 min before assay. Also, specimens containing a high concentration of cryptococcal antigen may display weak or no agglutination (prozone effect) and should be retested after dilution (1:10 and 1:100) in glycine-buffered saline. Rarely, false-negative results occur when sera from patients infected with acapsular or poorly encapsulated strains of *C. neoformans* are used. Such strains produce insufficient amounts of polysaccharide antigen to be detected and give false-negative results.

False-positive reactions have been reported to occur as the result of inadequate removal of detergent from the surface of the glass ring slides used for the LA test. Detergent can be removed by soaking slides in 10% bleach followed by thorough washing with distilled water. Rare false-positive results may be caused by the presence of contaminating hydroxyethyl starch, by nonspecific reactivity found in the serum of HIV-infected patients, and by cross-reactions with serum from patients infected with *Capnocytophaga animorsus* or *Trichosporon asahii*.

Periodically, the sensitivity of the latex particles coated with anti-cryptococcal globulin should be tested by titration against purified capsular polysaccharide antigen included in the kit. Pronase provided in the kit must be stored frozen in aliquots after initial reconstitution to eliminate exposure to repeated freezing and thawing and subsequent loss of enzyme activity. Also, at least once per month, an aliquot of frozen pronase should be examined for proteolytic activity by testing, in parallel, goat anti-rabbit globulin (PAb-based systems) or goat anti-mouse globulin (MAb-based systems) that have and have not been pronase treated before use. The untreated pronase control must demonstrate agglutination of 2+ or greater and the pronase-treated control must demonstrate agglutination of less than 1+ in the reaction.

Interpretation

The LA test to detect *C. neoformans* antigen has both diagnostic and prognostic value. A positive LA reaction at a titer of 1:4 or less using CSF, serum, or urine from an untreated patient is suggestive of cryptococcal infection, whereas titers of 1:8 or greater usually indicate active cryptococcosis (strong presumptive evidence). Antigen is detected in the CSF of over 90% of patients with untreated meningeal cryptococcosis. On the other hand, a negative serum antigen test result does not exclude a diagnosis of cryptococcosis, particularly if only a single specimen has been tested and the patient continues to have symptoms consistent with cryptococcal infection.

In HIV-negative patients, the antigen titer is usually proportional to the extent of infection, and increasing titers reflect progressive infection and a poor prognosis. Declining titers, on the other hand, generally indicate a favorable response to chemotherapy and progressive recovery; failure of the titer to fall during therapy suggests inadequate treatment. High initial titers of antigen (1:1,024 or greater) in the serum or CSF prior to treatment indicate a poor prognosis, and high titers at the end of treatment often predict later relapse. In contrast, HIV-positive patients may manifest elevated titers that decline very slowly even in the face of clinical improvement, whereas an unchanged or increased titer in the CSF of these patients is often associated with clinical and mycological failure to respond to treatment. Positive CSF antigen tests, despite no recovery of viable *C. neoformans* from the CSF, may indicate persistent release of capsular antigen from dead as well as from living cells or may indicate slow elimination of capsular antigen from the CSF rather than ongoing infection.

Test 2. EIA To Detect *C. neoformans* Capsular Polysaccharide Antigen

The Premier Cryptococcal Antigen test (Meridian Diagnostics, Inc.) is a double-antibody sandwich EIA for the detection of cryptococcal polysaccharide antigen in patient serum and CSF. Rabbit polyclonal anti-*C. neoformans* antibodies, adsorbed onto the surface of microtiter plate wells, are used to capture cryptococcal polysaccharide antigen found in the serum and CSF of patients with cryptococcosis. Peroxidase-labeled detector MAbs are applied, and plates are read visually or spectrophotometrically after the addition of peroxide and a colorimetric substrate. The EIA can be used as a screening test or as a semiquantitative test after titration of test samples to monitor the disease course and response to drug therapy. Its sensitivity has been reported to be equivalent to or somewhat better than that of the LA test produced by the same manufacturer, and it requires no pretreatment of specimens to remove complement, immune complexes, or rheumatoid factor (34, 140) (Table 2). The EIA is not subject to prozone effects and has also been reported to detect cryptococcal antigen earlier, and at lower concentrations, than does the LA test (34). LA titers and EIA titers are not equivalent but generally follow the same trend (i.e., both titers increase and decrease in parallel).

Sample Requirements

Serum and CSF samples may be tested, but urine may not be tested. Sample preparation of CSF and serum for the EIA consists only of centrifugation to remove any cells or other particulate matter. Pretreatment of specimens is not recommended by the manufacturer. However, samples that have previously been pronase or heat treated (56°C for 15 min) do not appear to be adversely affected and may be used in the screening assay. In contrast, pronase- or heat-treated samples should not be tested in the semiquantitative test mode since such treatment may alter EIA titration results. Therefore, it is recommended that all serial specimens from a given patient be pronase or heat treated in the same manner and that all samples be assayed in parallel when monitoring patients for disease changes or response to drug therapy; earlier specimens collected as part of these series should be aliquotted and frozen if stored for longer than 72 h at 2 to 8°C.

Materials and Reagents

All reagents are provided in the kit, including cryptococcal antigen (positive control), sample diluent (buffered protein solution which also serves as the negative control), concentrated wash buffer, enzyme conjugate (peroxidase-conjugated mouse anti-cryptococcal antigen-specific MAb), urea peroxide, chromogen (TMB), stopping solution (2 N sulfuric acid), and microtiter plates precoated with rabbit polyclonal antibodies specific for cryptococcal antigen. Microtiter plates are composed of 12 eight-well strips so that the entire plate does not have to be used at one time. Kits are stored at 2 to 8°C and should be brought to room temperature (20 to 30°C) before use.

Equipment

The equipment required to perform the EIA is the same as that for the Premier *Coccidioides* EIA (see "Test 4. EIA To Detect Antibodies to *Coccidioides* Species" above).

Procedure

The EIA can be performed in one of two modes: (i) as a screening assay, designed solely for the differentiation of positive from negative specimens, and (ii) as a semiquantitative assay to monitor relative changes in antigen levels in serum and CSF for the evaluation of patient progress and to monitor the efficacy of drug therapy. Whereas the screening assay examines a patient specimen at a single concentration (undiluted) at a single time point, the semiquantitative assay requires analysis of a series of specimens collected longitudinally, serially diluted to obtain an end-point titer for each. Values obtained using the screening assay may not be used to calculate an EIA titer. A detailed stepwise protocol can be found in the package insert included with each kit for both the screening assay and the semiquantitative assay.

Screening assay. Briefly, the screening assay is performed by placing the test specimen and positive and negative control samples into the bottom of separate microtiter plate wells, which are then incubated at ambient temperature for 10 min. The plates are washed between each step. Enzyme conjugate is added, and the plates are incubated again at ambient temperature for 10 min. Substrate is added, and the plates are incubated as above before addition of the stop solution and performance of visual or spectrophotometric reading at 450 nm (or 450/630 nm for dual-wavelength plate readers). Results are interpreted as follows. (i) For visual reading: negative, colorless well; positive, definite yellow color in well; (ii) for spectrophotometric reading with a single wavelength (OD_{450}): negative, <0.100; indeterminate, ≥0.100 and <0.150; positive, ≥0.150; and (iii) for spectrophotometric reading with a dual wavelength ($OD_{450/630}$): negative, <0.070; indeterminate, ≥0.070 and <0.100; positive, ≥0.100. Tests giving indeterminate results should be repeated; if the results are still indeterminate, a second specimen should be obtained and tested. Extremely strong reactions may produce a purple precipitate, but these samples are considered to be positive.

Semiquantitative assay. Five serial 1:5 dilutions of patient serum or CSF, beginning with a 1:2 dilution, are produced as follows: 1:2, 1:10, 1:50, 1:250, and 1:1,250 (further 1:5 dilutions may be carried out, if needed, to reach an end point). A positive antigen control and a negative control (reagent blank) are included on each test plate. Incubations with patient specimens and, after aspiration and washing, with conjugate are carried out for 10 min each at ambient temperature. Results are read spectrophotometrically at OD_{450} or $OD_{450/630}$. In instances where samples are read with a single-wavelength plate reader at OD_{450}, values for the negative control (sample diluent) must be subtracted from all OD_{450} values before calculation of the EIA titer. The results are analyzed as follows: (i) the highest OD_{450} value for a given sample that falls within the acceptable range (between 0.1 and 1.5) is identified, (ii) that serum dilution is multiplied by 10, and then (iii) the resulting number is multiplied by the OD value (e.g., if the test specimen gave an OD_{450} of 1.20 at the 1:50 dilution, the EIA titer would be $1.2 \times 50 \times 10 = 600$ or 1:600). These titers are not numerically equivalent to LA titers.

QA/QC

All reagents must be mixed gently and be at ambient temperature before use. Unused microwells must be placed back inside the foil ziplock pouch provided and sealed immediately to protect it from moisture. Inadequate plate washing may cause elevated background OD readings.

Interpretation

If the 1:2 dilution of the specimen yields an OD of <0.100, the assay should be repeated using undiluted samples. A positive test for undiluted serum is defined as one giving an OD_{450} of ≥0.15, provided that normal human serum gives a negative result when tested in parallel (undiluted). A negative result does not preclude a diagnosis of cryptococcosis, especially if only a single specimen has been tested and if the patient shows symptoms consistent with the disease. The sensitivity of the EIA was reported to be 93% for serum and 100% for CSF (140), whereas the specificity of the EIA was reported to be 97% (127).

Test 3. TA Test To Detect Antibodies to *C. neoformans*

A semiquantitative TA test is available commercially (YA-*Cryptococcus* antibody tube agglutination system; Immuno-Mycologics, Inc.) to detect anti-*C. neoformans* antibodies in the serum of patients with cryptococcosis. A standardized suspension of formalin-killed, small-capsule *C. neoformans* cells is mixed with an equal volume of serially diluted patient serum. The end-point titer is the highest serum dilution at which any agglutination is observed.

Sample Requirements

The test is performed only with serum. The specimen must not contain anticoagulants since these can interfere with the agglutination reaction. Sera should be heat inactivated at 56°C for 30 min before being tested. Specimens and reagents should not contain any particulate matter (except for the cryptococcal yeast antigen, which contains a suspension of *C. neoformans* yeast cells) and should show no signs of contamination. Specimens may be processed immediately, stored at 2 to 8°C for up to 48 h before being tested, or stored frozen at −20°C or below for longer periods.

Materials and Reagents

All reagents for the TA test are supplied by the manufacturer, including a standardized ($OD_{550} = 0.02$) suspension of formalin-killed *C. neoformans* yeast cells, specimen diluent (10× glycine buffer, pH 8.6, containing albumin), positive antibody control (lyophilized rabbit anti-*C. neoformans* antibodies), and a negative control (normal goat serum).

Equipment

Water bath (37 and 56°C)
Concave reading mirror

Procedure

1. Make twofold serial dilutions of the test serum (from 1:2 to 1:64) in 12- by 75-mm test tubes.

2. Place the mixture on a rotary shaker for 2 min.

3. Incubate mixtures at 37°C for 2 h, and then place in the refrigerator at 4°C for an additional 72 h, during which time readings are taken at 24-h intervals.

4. Examine tubes individually for agglutination by gentle tilting to allow the fluid to swirl the sedimented antigen (do not shake tubes).

5. Examine tubes for agglutination while tilting them over a concave mirror.

Reactions are graded as follows: negative, smooth suspension with no clumping; 1+, slight clumping; 2+, moderate clumping; 3+, moderate and large clumps; and 4+, large clumps.

QA/QC

Positive and negative controls must be included each time the test is performed and should be read first. The positive antibody control must give a 2+ reaction at a dilution of 1:4, and the negative control must not demonstrate any agglutination. If the control reagents do not perform properly, the test must be repeated. It is recommended that clean, disposable, borosilicate glass tubes be used for the test.

Interpretation

If no agglutination occurs at any serum dilution from 1:2 to 1:64, the result is negative. However, if agglutination occurs at any serum dilution, the test is reported as positive and the titer is reported as the highest specimen dilution with any degree of agglutination. A positive result (agglutination titers of 1:2 or greater) is presumptive evidence for recent or past infection with *C. neoformans* but may also indicate the presence of cross-reacting antibodies to *H. capsulatum* or *B. dermatitidis*. Titers of ≥1:16 are rarely observed. The presence of antibody in a single serum specimen is not diagnostic since most individuals are exposed to *C. neoformans* and become seropositive at an early age. In most instances, diagnosis using an antibody assay requires obtaining a second convalescent-phase serum sample 3 to 4 weeks after the first specimen in order to observe seroconversion or a fourfold or greater increase in serum titer. Antibodies may be detected early in disease or in localized infections. As disease progresses, capsular polysaccharide antigen is produced and released into body fluids, with concurrent complex formation or neutralization of antibody. Antibodies may reappear after successful treatment, and it has been suggested that their detection is a favorable prognostic sign. In immunocompetent patients, effective chemotherapy results in a decline in the antigen titer and antibodies may be detected. Therefore, concomitant use of antigen detection tests in addition to antibody detection tests is recommended for optimal detection of cryptococcal infection. Sera from approximately 50% of patients with active extrameningeal cryptococcosis are positive in the TA test, and the test has been reported to have a specificity of about 89%.

Experimental and Molecular Biological Approaches

A limited number of molecular biology-based tests to detect cryptococcal DNA in clinical specimens have been developed in an attempt to increase the sensitivity of diagnosis and to provide a tool for monitoring disease progression and therapeutic response. Initial studies conducted by Sandhu et al.

used the same methods as those described for the detection of *C. immitis* DNA (124). In this instance, *C. neoformans* DNA was extracted from tissue or CSF of patients with smear- or culture-confirmed cryptococcosis. A probe designed to detect the A serotype was found to correctly identify *C. neoformans* DNA in clinical specimens and did not cross-react with DNA extracted from specimens positive for *A. fumigatus*, *C. albicans*, or *C. immitis* (124).

Rappelli et al. (117) used primers directed to the ITS rRNA gene region to amplify *C. neoformans* DNA from the CSF of AIDS patients with acute cryptococcal meningitis. All 21 culture-confirmed cryptococcal meningitis cases (100%) were correctly identified by this test, and no PCR amplicons were obtained when CSF from 19 of 19 patients with viral or bacterial meningitis or cultures of other fungi known to cause meningitis was used. In addition, six specimens each of serum and CSF were collected from a single patient over a 5-month period to monitor the results of the PCR assay during anticryptococcal therapy. The nested PCR assay became negative at the time that India ink and culture results became negative (suggesting that the PCR assay may be useful for monitoring patient response to therapy.

A PCR method for the diagnosis of pulmonary cryptococcosis in HIV-negative patients was reported to detect four of five culture-positive specimens by using nested PCR primers (139). The sensitivity may have been reduced in this assay because PCR primers were directed to a single-copy gene target (*URA5*) rather than to a multicopy gene target. The specificity of the test, however, was 100% (10 of 10 culture-negative specimens were also PCR negative).

HISTOPLASMOSIS

Background

In the absence of culture or microscopic evidence of infection, the primary methods used to diagnose histoplasmosis are the CF, ID, and LA antibody detection tests and an EIA to detect *H. capsulatum* antigen. The CF microtitration procedure (105) yields information of both diagnostic and prognostic value. Over 90% of patients with culture-proven histoplasmosis are positive by the CF test if serum is collected and tested at 2- to 3-week intervals during infection. Therefore, the major advantage of the CF test is that it provides a quantitative measurement of the amount of antibody present in the test specimen. The titer for a given specimen can then be compared to the titer obtained by using a subsequent specimen to assess disease progression, or the efficacy of treatment, as measured by the respective increase or decrease in antibody titer. The major disadvantages of the CF test are as follows: (i) it is a relatively complex, labor-intensive assay that should be performed by only highly trained technical staff; (ii) accuracy depends on constant, complex quality control standardization or titration of test reagents (hemolysin, complement, sheep erythrocytes) each time a new lot of reagent is obtained; and (iii) specimens may possess anticomplementary activity (i.e., patient serum fixes or destroys complement in the absence of any added antigen), making test results indeterminate.

The CF assay for the diagnosis of histoplasmosis uses two different target preparations for the detection of anti-*H. capsulatum* antibodies: "histoplasmin," a soluble filtrate of mycelial-phase broth cultures (containing the H and M antigens), and *Histoplasma* yeast antigen, a suspension of merthiolate-killed, whole yeast-form cells. The CF assay is more sensitive (82% versus 21%) but less specific (88% versus

99%) when yeast cells rather than mycelial antigens are used. Antibodies to the yeast cells are usually the first to appear after infection and the last to disappear after the resolution of infection. However, antibodies produced during infection by other fungi, including those produced during infection by *C. immitis* or *B. dermatitidis*, as well as during some bacterial infections, such as tuberculosis, may react with the yeast antigen and give false-positive results (159). Antibodies to the yeast antigen usually appear within 4 weeks after exposure, whereas antibodies to the mycelial antigen occur later and have titers which are considerably lower.

The immunodominant antigens detected in the histoplasmosis ID test are referred to as the H and M antigens of *H. capsulatum* (45, 163). Precipitins against M antigen are the first to appear in acute pulmonary histoplasmosis and form the basis of an early presumptive diagnosis. H precipitins occur later and less frequently, and their presence is stronger evidence for recent infection. H bands rarely occur without the presence of an M band. Conversion from no bands to the presence of an M or H band is strong evidence for recent infection (seroconversion). Patients with extrapulmonary disseminated disease frequently exhibit H precipitins together with M precipitins. The ID test is generally less sensitive than the CF test, particularly early in infection, but is generally more specific. Because of this enhanced specificity, the ID test provides a more accurate diagnosis than the CF test, particularly in cases where sera display CF cross-reactivity to other fungal diseases. The ID test may also help to resolve the diagnosis in cases where the CF results are made uninterpretable by anticomplementary activity in the test sample.

The histoplasmosis LA test is a rapid, semiquantitative test that uses latex particles sensitized with histoplasmin for the detection of agglutinating antibodies against *H. capsulatum*. This assay measures predominantly the IgM subclass of antibodies and therefore is most useful in the early diagnosis of acute histoplasmosis. A positive LA test can be obtained as early as 2 to 3 weeks after exposure and has been reported to have an overall sensitivity (including both acute and chronic forms of the disease) of 62% and a specificity of 97% (48).

The HPA test is a colorimetric double-sandwich enzyme immunoassay that uses polyclonal rabbit antisera as both the capture and detector antibody (162). The antigen detected is poorly defined but is thought to be a polysaccharide based on its stability to heat (100°C for 30 min) and its reduced reactivity after passage through a concanavalin A affinity column (43, 119). Antigen can be detected very early in disease (during the first 2 weeks after the onset of symptoms), and then its level rapidly declines in self-limited disease. It can be detected for longer periods in cases of disseminated disease. The EIA has a reported sensitivity of 14, 75, and 92% for the detection of chronic pulmonary, acute pulmonary, and disseminated disease, respectively. Significant EIA cross-reactivity has been reported for the other endemic mycoses, particularly blastomycosis, paracoccidioidomycosis, and penicilliosis marneffei.

Clinical Indications and Diagnostic Rationale

Serologic tests for histoplasmosis should be applied to clinical specimens (serum, plasma, peritoneal fluid, CSF, or urine) from patients with respiratory illness, hepatosplenomegaly, signs of extrapulmonary systemic infection, or meningeal involvement. The patient's residence, travel, and occupation history is useful as a guide to the application of these tests. The CF test is very sensitive, but the current incorporation of unpurified antigens reduces test specificity. Cross-reactions may occur with sera from patients with blastomycosis,

coccidioidomycosis, and other mycoses. Sera from patients with leishmaniasis may cross-react in the CF test with *H. capsulatum* yeast-form antigens. It is generally recommended that both the ID as well as the CF test be applied to obtain maximum sensitivity and specificity. Use of the histoplasmosis ID and CF tests in parallel, with histoplasmin as the antigen, results in an overall sensitivity of approximately 85%. The CF and ID tests are also useful in diagnosing meningitis caused by *H. capsulatum* (99).

The histoplasmosis LA test is satisfactory for the detection of acute primary infections but may yield negative results for sera from persons with chronic histoplasmosis (48). It is particularly valuable in the detection of early disease. Because of the transitory nature of the agglutinins, the LA test cannot be considered a replacement for the CF test.

The EIA to detect HPA in urine and serum is useful for diagnosing disseminated histoplasmosis, particularly in AIDS patients (161). Antigen detection is less effective in diagnosing histoplasmosis in immunocompetent patients with self-limited disease or in cases of chronic pulmonary disease (162). Although less sensitive for the diagnosis of primary disease than disseminated disease, the test can be useful in the early stages of acute pulmonary disease (first 3 to 4 weeks after onset), permitting appropriate therapy to be initiated sooner. The use of urine as the test specimen has increased sensitivity (95%) compared to serum (85%) for the diagnosis of disseminated histoplasmosis. Recently, new procedures have been implemented which are reported by the manufacturer to give increased test sensitivity and specificity compared to the original test, primarily by the removal of human anti-rabbit IgG reactivity (www.miravistalabs.com). However, clinical evaluations to determine the overall test sensitivity and specificity after treatment to remove the antiglobulin activity have not yet been published.

Test 1. CF Test To Detect Antibodies to *H. capsulatum*

The standardized microadaptation of the CDC Laboratory Branch CF test with both *H. capsulatum* yeast-form and histoplasmin antigens is recommended for the determination of titer in sera from persons with suspected histoplasmosis. Because of the complexity of the procedure, only an abbreviated description of the CF test is outlined below. Readers are directed to a more detailed protocol (105) or a modified version, available from Immuno-Mycologics (www.immy.com), for use with their reagents. No commercial kits are available for the CF test, but antigens, antisera, and other reagents can be purchased individually from the commercial sources listed below and in Table 1. Detailed vendor information can be found at the end of this chapter.

Sample Requirements

Serum, peritoneal fluid, or CSF may be used in the CF test. Serum is most often tested in suspected cases of acute pulmonary histoplasmosis. CSF may be used to detect localized antibody production during *H. capsulatum* meningitis. Other body fluids are examined in cases of suspected disseminated disease. Acute-phase sera should be obtained after the onset of symptoms, and convalescent-phase sera should be collected 4 to 6 weeks later to identify changes in titer compared to the titer obtained for the acute-phase sera. Serum should be obtained from clotted blood collected into tubes without anticoagulants. Whereas excessively pigmented specimens must not be used, slightly pigmented specimens may be used because the color will be diluted out during the titer determination process and will therefore not interfere with test interpretation. Lipids should be removed with a 0.45- to 0.8-μm filter attached to a syringe (Millipore Corp.). CSF should be centrifuged before being tested, to remove any red or white blood cells. Sera and CSF are heated at 56°C for 30 min immediately prior to use to inactivate endogenous complement activity. Serum and CSF can be stored at 4°C for 72 h or stored for longer periods in frozen aliquots at −20°C or colder in a nondefrosting freezer. Repeated freezing and thawing of the samples, which can reduce reactivity, should be avoided.

Materials and Reagents

Two antigens are used in the CDC Laboratory Branch CF test: one is a suspension of merthiolate-killed, intact, yeast-form cells of *H. capsulatum*, and the second is a soluble, mycelial culture filtrate antigen, histoplasmin. Histoplasmin is produced by harvesting and filtering the supernatant from *H. capsulatum* cultures grown at 25°C for approximately 4 to 5 weeks in Smith's synthetic asparagine broth on a gyratory shaker at 150 rpm (78). The optimal dilution for each antigen is determined by a block titration against low- and high-titer positive human sera. These antigens may be purchased from Immuno-Mycologics, Inc., or from Meridian Diagnostics, Inc., in either prediluted or concentrated form. Other key materials, listed below, may be purchased from vendors that sell biological products (e.g., Cambrex Bio-Science, Walkersville, Md.; Rockland Immunochemicals, Inc., Gilbertsville, Pa.; TCS Biosciences Ltd., Buckingham, United Kingdom; and Colorado Serum Company, Denver, Colo.).

Equipment

pH meter

Centrifuge with microtiter plate carriers

Incubator (37°C)

Glass serologic tubes (15 by 125 and 12 by 75 mm)

Pipettes (1, 5, and 10 ml)

Water bath or heat block (37 and 56°C)

Refrigerator

Microtiter equipment

- 25- to 50-μl multichannel pipetter
- U-bottom polystyrene microtiter plates
- Reading mirror (concave, ×1.5 magnification)

Procedure

Reagent preparation and standardization

1. VBD. Dilute a 5× stock solution of VBD to 1× with 0.05% gelatin solution (see item 2 below) and use this throughout the test procedure as a reagent diluent. The pH of the 1× solution must be between 7.3 and 7.4; if it is not, prepare new 1× buffer from the 5× stock. Do not adjust the pH of the 1× buffer. If the pH of the 1× buffer is continually out of range, obtain new 5× buffer. Keep the VBD on ice during the assay. The shelf life of 1× VBD is 24 h at 4°C.

2. Gelatin solution. Make a 0.05% (wt/vol) solution of gelatin in deionized H₂O, and heat to 100°C; allow it to cool to room temperature, and use it to dilute 5× VBD to 1×. The shelf life of the solution is 7 days at 4°C.

3. SRBC, supplied in Alsever's solution. SRBCs must be washed three times with 1× VBD by gentle centrifugation on the day the CF test is to be performed (final working concentration, 2.8% [vol/vol] in 1× VBD). If after three consecutive washes red pigment remains, the SRBC are too old and too fragile for use. A fresh lot of SRBCs should be

obtained (SRBCs should be between 5 and 28 days old at the time of use). The shelf life of the stock SRBCs in Alsever's solution is 1 month, whereas the shelf life of washed and diluted SRBCs in 1× VBD is 24 h.

4. Hemolysin. Hemolysin (complement-fixing, anti-SRBC antibody) is used to "sensitize" (i.e., coat with antibody) the SRBCs, allowing them to be lysed in the presence of complement. To determine the optimal concentration of hemolysin for the sensitization of the SRBCs, serially dilute hemolysin in 1× VBD in 15- by 125-mm glass tubes (1:1,500, 1:2,000, 1:2,500, 1:3,000, 1:4,000, and 1:8,000) and titrate it against multiple dilutions of guinea pig complement (1:300, 1:350, 1:400 [see item 5 below]). After adding SRBCs and incubating them in a water bath at 37°C for 1 h, centrifuge tubes and determine the percent hemolysis in each tube by comparison to a standard curve (color standards) constructed from differing proportions of hemoglobin and 0.28% SRBCs (percent lysis = 0, 10, 20, 30, 40, 50, 60, 70, 80, 90, and 100). Plot the percent hemolysis against the hemolysin dilution, and identify the second dilution on the plateau of the graph. This hemolysin dilution is optimum to sensitize SRBCs for complement titration, antigen titration, and serum tests. Hemolysin must be titrated each time a new lot of SRBCs or hemolysin is obtained. The shelf life of the stock hemolysin (a 1:100 dilution of hemolysin in VBD containing 0.2% phenol) at 2 to 8°C is up to 1 year.

5. Guinea pig complement. Reconstitute guinea pig complement into single-use glass vials, and freeze at −70°C until ready to use. Storage in plastic vials will cause a reduction of complement activity over time. The complement must be subjected to titer determination before each use. Once determined, the optimal dilution must then sit on ice for 20 min and be used within 2 h. Titer determination must be done using sensitized, standardized SRBCs prepared as described in item 6 below. Serially dilute complement in 12- by 75-mm glass test tubes with VBD (1:200, 1:250, 1:300, 1:350, and 1:400) and add 0.20, 0.25, 0.30, and 0.40 ml of each complement dilution to 0.60, 0.55, 0.50, and 0.40 ml of VBD, respectively. Then add 0.20 ml of sensitized SRBCs to the tubes, shake the mixture, and incubate the tubes in a 37°C water bath for 30 min (shake again after 15 min and return the tubes to water bath). Remove the tubes, and centrifuge the cells. Determine the percent hemolysis compared to the color standards, and calculate the ratio of lysed to unlysed cells (lysis ratio = lysed/[100 − lysed], i.e., 10/[100 − 10] = 0.111). Using log-log graph paper, plot the volume of complement added to the tubes (0.20, 0.25, 0.30, and 0.40) against the lysis ratio. Two of the lysis ratio values must be less than 1, and two must be greater than 1. With a ruler, join the two points plotted for the two lowest volumes of complement and do the same for the two highest volumes. Draw a line connecting the midpoint of one line to the midpoint of the other line. From the point where this line intersects the vertical 1 line on the x axis, draw a horizontal line to the y axis on the left. This is the volume, in milliliters, that contains one 50% hemolytic unit of complement (1 CH₅₀ unit). Multiply this value by 5 to obtain the equivalent of 5 CH₅₀ units.

6. Sensitized SRBCs. Once the optimum concentration of hemolysin has been determined (see item 4 above), slowly add an equal volume of SRBCs with swirling. Incubate the mixture for 15 min in a 37°C water bath before use.

CF test

1. All reagents (hemolysin, complement, SRBCs, and VBD) must be optimally standardized as described above

before the test is used with patient samples or the positive control.

2. Using cold VBD, prepare a 1:8 dilution of the following samples in 12- by 75-mm glass test tubes: patient sample, positive control, and negative control. Samples may also be diluted 1:2 instead of 1:8 or may be diluted more than 1:8 during repeat testing to detect lower or higher antibody titers, respectively.

3. Heat the diluted sera for 30 min in a 56°C water bath, and cool to room temperature.

4. Label the microtiter plates as shown in Fig. 2.

5. Pipette 25 μl of cold VBD into the wells of rows B to H of columns 1 to 12 of the patient plate(s) (Fig. 2A) and columns 1 to 9 of the control plate (Fig. 2B).

6. Add 50 μl of heat-inactivated patient sera to wells 1 to 6 of row A for patient 1 and wells 7 to 12 of row A for patient 2. Add 50 μl of control sera to the appropriate wells in row A of the central plate that correspond to the appropriate antigen.

7. Using a multichannel pipette, serially pass 25 μl of serum sequentially from row A through row H, and mix. Remove 25 μl from the wells in row H, and discard (25 μl of serially diluted sera should remain in all wells).

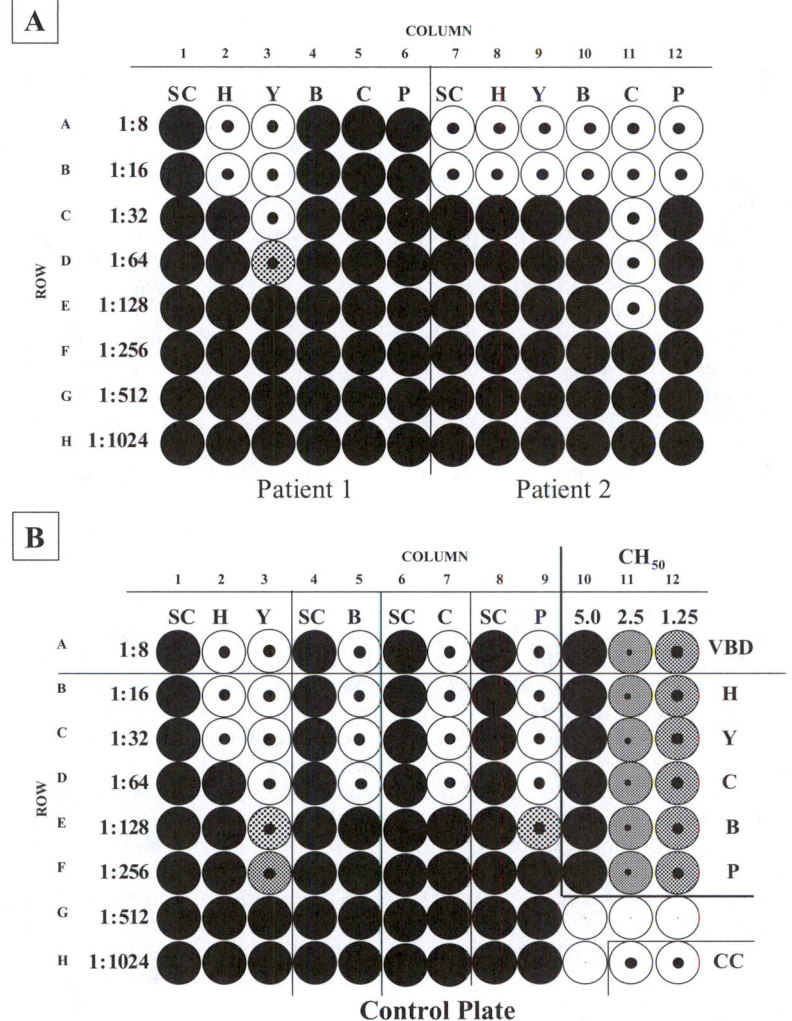

FIGURE 2   Diagram displaying organization of the microtiter plates and results for the complement fixation assay. Percent lysis: solid circles, 100% lysis; shaded circles, 30 to 90%; open circles, 0% lysis. SC, serum control wells receiving buffer in place of antigen; H, column receiving *Histoplasma* mycelial histoplasmin antigen; Y, column receiving *Histoplasma* yeast antigen; B, column receiving *Blastomyces* antigen; C, column receiving *Coccidioides* coccidioidin antigen; P, column receiving *Paracoccidioides* yeast antigen; CC, cell control. CH_{50}, amount of complement required for 50% lysis of SRBC. (A) Patient plate. Patient 1 demonstrates serum that is positive for *Histoplasma* antibodies with a 1:16 titer against mycelial histoplasmin antigen and a 1:64 titer against *Histoplasma* yeast antigen. Patient 2 displays serum that contains an anticomplementary titer of 1:16. However, because antibodies to coccidioidin are present at a titer that is >2 dilutions beyond the anticomplementary titer, the patient CF result is AC 1:16, *Coccidioides* 1:128. (B) Control plate. Percent lysis symbols as above. Columns 1 to 9 depict the reactivity of the control sera to specific fungal antigens. Columns 10 to 12, rows A to F, depict the results of the back titration of complement in CH_{50} units (5 through 1.25) in the presence of fungal antigens or the VBD buffer control. Columns 11 and 12, row H, depict the cell control wells that receive SRBC only.

8. Dilute fungal antigens to the appropriate concentration as determined by the antigen titration assay performed for that lot of antigen. Add 25 μl of diluted antigen to wells A through H of the appropriate columns as follows:

    a. *Histoplasma* mycelial antigen (histoplasmin) to columns 2 and 8 on patient plate(s) and column 2 of the control plate.

    b. *Histoplasma* yeast antigen to columns 3 and 9 on patient plate(s) and column 3 of the control plate.

    c. *Blastomyces* A antigen to columns 4 and 10 on patient plate(s) and column 5 of the control plate.

    d. *Coccidioides* culture filtrate antigen (coccidioidin) to columns 5 and 11 on the patient plate(s) and column 7 on the control plate.

    e. *Paracoccidioides* antigen in columns 6 and 12 on the patient plate(s) and column 9 on the control plate.

9. Add 25 μl of cold VBD to columns 1 and 7 on the patient plate(s) and columns 1, 4, 6, and 8 on the control plate to control for serum activity in the CF test.

10. Thaw guinea pig complement on ice, and dilute with cold VBD in a glass container to the concentration determined by the complement titration assay. Allow to stand on ice for at least 20 min, but use within 2 h.

11. Add 50 μl of diluted complement to all patient specimen wells and columns 1 to 9 of the control plate.

12. A complement "back titration" is performed with each assay to determine the accuracy of the complement titration/dilution. On the control plate, add 50 μl of cold VBD to rows A to F in columns 11 and 12.

13. Add 100 μl of diluted complement to wells A to F of column 10. Serially pass 50 μl of diluted complement from column 10 to column 11 and then to column 12. After gently mixing the content of the wells of column 12, remove 50 μl of diluted complement and discard.

14. Add 50 μl of cold VBD to wells 10 to 12 in row A. In wells 10 to 12 of rows B to F, add 25 μl of cold VBD.

15. Add 25 μl of diluted antigen from step 8 to the appropriate wells in rows B to F of columns 10 to 12.

16. Finally, add 100 μl of cold VBD to wells 11 and 12 of row H. All wells should now contain a total of 100 μl.

17. Mix the contents of the wells for 5 to 10 s on a vibrating microtiter plate shaker.

18. Place plates at 2 to 8°C for 15 to 18 h. Cover the plates to prevent evaporation (an unused plate can serve this function; plates can be placed in stacks of five to eight plates).

19. Add 25 μl of sensitized SRBCs (as described earlier) to all wells of the patient and control plates.

20. Mix the contents of the wells for 5 to 10 s on a vibrating microtiter plate shaker.

21. Cover the plates, and incubate them at 37°C for 30 min. Stack the plates no more than two high.

22. Centrifuge the plates for 5 min at 400 to 450 × g.

23. Read the plates for percent hemolysis compared to the color standard.

24. Wells that display ≤30% lysis are considered to be positive. The dilution at which the last well of serially diluted serum displays ≤30% lysis is the antibody titer for that sample. Serum control wells should display >70% lysis. Serum that displays ≤70% lysis in a serum control well is considered to be anticomplementary, and results cannot be interpreted for that dilution of the serum. (See Fig. 2A, patient 2.)

25. For a valid assay, control sera must display the titer recommended by the manufacturer (or the typical titer for laboratory-derived control sera) ± 1 dilution. Also, the complement back titration controls should display 95 to 100% lysis in column 10, 90 to 100% lysis in column 11, 30 to 50% lysis in the VBD control well (A of column 12), and 0 to 50% lysis in the antigen control wells (B to F of column 12). The cell control wells (H 11 to 12) should display no lysis (0%).

QA/QC

Negative control serum and positive control serum from human histoplasmosis patients demonstrating a CF titer of ≥1:32 with the homologous antigen should be tested each time the CF test is performed. Human positive-case serum is preferred for use as the positive control because the use of hyperimmune rabbit serum has, on occasion, given positive results with its homologous antigen in the absence of good reactivity to the same antigen by positive human case serum (84). Anticomplementary activity in serum samples can occur (i.e., those showing ≤70% hemolysis in the serum control wells without antigen) and may be resolved by subsequent ID testing. However, ID tests may not be as sensitive as the CF test. Also, all of the QC measures described in the text under the heading "Reagent preparation and standardization" above must be followed for optimal operation of the test.

Interpretation

CF tests can be valuable in the diagnosis of acute, chronic, disseminated, and meningeal histoplasmosis. Antibodies in primary pulmonary infections are generally demonstrable within 4 weeks after exposure to the fungus or, frequently, when symptoms appear. Antibodies to the yeast-form antigen are usually the first to appear (about 4 weeks after exposure) and the last to disappear after resolution of the infection. Antibodies to histoplasmin usually develop later in primary pulmonary cases, but titers are considerably lower than those obtained with the yeast-form antigen. In contrast, histoplasmin titers are usually higher when serum from patients with chronic histoplasmosis is used.

CF test results can be difficult to interpret because cross-reactions or nonspecific reactions with the yeast or histoplasmin antigens are often encountered. In such instances, titers usually range between 1:8 and 1:32 and occur mainly against the yeast-form antigen. Many serum samples from culture-proven cases of histoplasmosis, however, give titers in the same range. Consequently, titers of 1:8 and greater with either antigen are generally considered presumptive evidence of histoplasmosis. Titers above 1:32 or rising titers offer strong presumptive evidence of infection. The probability of infection increases in proportion to the CF titer.

On the other hand, one cannot rely solely on CF titers above 1:32 as a means of diagnosis because false-positive reactions of similar magnitude may occur in patients with other endemic mycoses. For example, in some situations, the first serologic response noted in a patient with histoplasmosis may be obtained only with *B. dermatitidis* antigen. Some patients with histoplasmosis may demonstrate antibodies against the antigens of *H. capsulatum*, *B. dermatitidis*, and *C. immitis* or may demonstrate antibodies to only some of these antigens or to none. Furthermore, a lack of immunologic response does not exclude histoplasmosis, particularly when only one specimen has been tested and when the clinical picture strongly suggests a pulmonary mycosis. For example, in cases of disseminated or terminal histoplasmosis, humoral antibody responses may or may not be positive. In contrast, the CF test is usually positive when CSF specimens obtained from patients with chronic meningitis are used; titers in such cases may range from 1:8 to 1:128.

Fourfold or greater increases or decreases in titer are significant indicators of disease progression or remission, respectively. However, culture, clinical, and other laboratory data should also be considered in assessing the patient's prognosis or making treatment decisions. Occasionally, in some patients, positive titers decline slowly and persist long after the patient has been cured. The significance of persistently elevated or fluctuating CF titers is unclear, as is the effect of antifungal treatment on antibody clearance.

Test 2. ID Test To Detect Antibodies to *H. capsulatum*

The ID procedure is recommended for the detection of *H. capsulatum* precipitins directed against the H and M glycoprotein antigens present in histoplasmin. Commercial kits use a macro-ID precast gel template, whereas the CDC Mycotic Diseases Branch prefers the use of a micro-ID procedure and phenolized agar as described under "Test 1. ID Test To Detect Antibodies to *B. dermatitidis*" earlier in this chapter. CIE for histoplasmosis can also be conducted, and its major advantages over ID are that test results are available within 2 h and the frequency to detect the H precipitin is somewhat increased.

Sample Requirements

Serum or CSF may be used in the ID test. Because the reported sensitivity of the ID test is low early in infection, patients with negative serum reactions during the acute phase of infection should have additional sera drawn 3 to 4 weeks later to detect the development of precipitin bands that would indicate seroconversion and recent infection. Concomitant evaluation of patient specimens by using the CF test is also recommended.

Materials and Reagents

Histoplasmosis ID reagents or kits may be purchased from Gibson Laboratories, Immuno-Mycologics, or Meridian Diagnostics. Commercial kits include mycelium-phase culture filtrates containing *H. capsulatum* H and M antigens, positive control sera containing antibodies directed against both the H and M antigens, and ID plates. For those who wish to make ID plates in-house, the recipe is as described earlier in this chapter (see "Test 1. ID Test To Detect Antibodies to *B. dermatitidis*" above). Histoplasmin may be produced in-house as described above for the CF test. However, the mycelium-phase filtrate antigen is concentrated 5- to 10-fold and titrated to determine the optimal dilution that demonstrates well-defined H and M bands on the ID plate when tested against serum from a patient with proven histoplasmosis. Control antisera containing H and M precipitins may also be prepared in animals by using precipitin arcs as immunogens.

Equipment and Procedure

The equipment and procedure for the histoplasmosis ID test are the same as those described for the blastomycosis ID test, except that histoplasmin, unknown sera, and control sera containing H and M precipitins are added to the ID plates simultaneously and no reagent requires preincubation in the agar gel. The ID plates are then incubated in a humidified chamber for 24 h at 25°C.

QA/QC

Positive control sera must be included each time the test is performed and must react with both the H and M antigens. If the reference bands are not visible in the agar, the assay must be repeated. Commercial kits most often provide reference antisera and antigens prediluted for optimal test performance.

If in-house-produced reagents are being evaluated, it is important to cross-titrate reagents to determine the optimal working dilutions. Optimal dilutions of serum and antigen are those that place the precipitin bands midway between the serum and antigen wells; the M precipitin band is closest to the antigen-containing well, and the H band is closest to the reference serum well.

Interpretation

The ID test is a useful screening procedure or adjunct to the CF test for the serologic diagnosis of histoplasmosis. In contrast to the CF test, the ID test is generally performed as a qualitative rather than a quantitative test. The ID assay is generally more specific but less sensitive than the CF test, so that when both assays are employed, the overall sensitivity and specificity to detect histoplasmosis is quite good (85%).

The M band is produced in the ID test by serum from patients with acute or chronic pulmonary histoplasmosis and is frequently the first to appear in patients with acute disease (4 to 8 weeks after exposure). The H band is produced in the ID test by serum from patients with active histoplasmosis and occurs less frequently later in infection. Antibodies to the H antigen are specific for active disease but occur in fewer than 20% of cases; they usually disappear within the first 6 months of infection and are seldom, if ever, found in the absence of M precipitins. The production of an M band in the ID test is considered presumptive evidence of *H. capsulatum* infection and may be attributed to active or previous disease. The demonstration of both the M and H precipitins in serum is highly suggestive of active histoplasmosis. The serum from about 70% of patients with proven histoplasmosis contains M precipitins, whereas sera from only 10% of patients with proven histoplasmosis demonstrate both the M and H precipitins. The detection of M and H precipitins in CSF specimens indicates meningeal histoplasmosis (99). Precipitins can frequently be detected in the CSF of patients with meningeal histoplasmosis at a time before *H. capsulatum* is detected by culture and when attempts to culture the microorganism fail.

Test 3. LA Test To Detect Antibodies to *H. capsulatum*

The LA test is useful for presumptive early detection of acute histoplasmosis. Commercially prepared histoplasmin-sensitized latex particles are available from Immuno-Mycologics, Inc. The LA test is a semiquantitative slide agglutination assay in which *H. capsulatum* antigen-coated latex particles are used to detect antibody to *H. capsulatum*. Antibody to *H. capsulatum* present in the patient's specimen binds to the antigen-coated latex particles, resulting in visible clumping. Results are graded according to the level of agglutination observed for a particular dilution of serum. The assay measures predominantly IgM antibodies and therefore is used to diagnose early stages of acute histoplasmosis. The assay is rapid and simple to perform, and no special equipment is needed.

Sample Requirements

Serum and CSF should be stored at 2 to 8°C if tested within 72 h after collection or at −20°C or colder in a nondefrosting freezer for longer periods. Repeated freezing and thawing of specimens must be avoided. Specimens should be heat inactivated at 56°C for 30 min and allowed to cool before use.

Materials and Reagents

The histoplasmosis LA test uses latex particles sensitized with histoplasmin antigen in a slide agglutination format to detect anti-*H. capsulatum* antibodies. All reagents including specimen diluent (concentrated glycine-buffered saline [pH 8.6] containing albumin), sensitized latex particles, positive control serum (from goats immunized with *H. capsulatum*), negative control serum (normal goat serum), and disposable glass slides with raised rings for the performance of the test can be obtained from Immuno-Mycologics, Inc.

Equipment and Procedure

The equipment and procedure for the histoplasmosis LA test are the same as those described for the *Coccidioides* LA test (see "Test 2. LA Test To Detect Antibodies to *Coccidioides*" above), except that the histoplasmosis LA test may be performed as a semiquantitative test. Specimens giving a 2+ or greater reaction during the initial screening phase of the test may be serially diluted twofold beginning with a 1:2 dilution to obtain an end-point titer.

QA/QC

Positive and negative control samples must be included each time the test is performed. The positive control must give a ≥2+ agglutination reaction, and the negative control must give a <1+ agglutination reaction. Unexpected reactions invalidate the test run, and all test runs with those specimens must be repeated. The sensitivity of the latex reagent should be tested periodically by titration against the positive control reagent. The sensitivity of the latex reagent is adequate if the positive control yields a result of 1+ at 1:4 ± 1 dilution. Agglutination is graded as follows: negative, a homogeneous suspension of particles with no visible clumping; 1+, fine granulation against a milky background; 2+, small but definite clumps against a slightly cloudy background; 3+, large and small clumps against a clear background; and 4+, large clumps against a clear or very clear background.

Interpretation

The LA test yields results in a matter of minutes and may be used with sera giving anticomplementary activity in the CF test. Although the LA test may be negative with sera from persons with chronic histoplasmosis or from immunosuppressed individuals, it is an excellent presumptive test aiding in the early diagnosis of acute histoplasmosis. A titer of 1:16 or greater is presumptive evidence of infection, and a titer of 1:32 or greater is considered strong presumptive evidence for active or very recent infection. Although a positive LA test result can be demonstrated as early as 2 to 3 weeks after infection by *H. capsulatum*, false-positive results can occur with other systemic mycoses. It is therefore recommended that results be confirmed by using the ID or other laboratory tests. Low-titer results from single specimens should especially be interpreted with caution. In such cases, the test should be performed with another specimen collected 4 to 6 weeks later.

Test 4. EIA To Detect *H. capsulatum* Polysaccharide Antigen

The *Histoplasma* polysaccharide antigen EIA (HPA test) is a microtitration plate-based double-antibody sandwich enzyme immunoassay to detect antigenuria and antigenemia in disseminated histoplasmosis. This test may also be useful in the diagnosis of early stages of acute pulmonary histoplasmosis. The major advantages of this test are that it is simple to perform, it does not require any major equipment, it can be very sensitive in cases of disseminated histoplasmosis where antibody responsiveness may be suboptimal, and it is quantitative without having to perform serial dilutions of the

specimen. No kit or reagents are commercially available for purchase, but this test is performed as a fee-for-service reference test (MiraVista Diagnostics, Indianapolis, Ind.; www.miravistalabs.com).

Sample Requirements

Preferred volumes for testing of urine, BAL fluid, serum, and CSF are 10, 10, 5, and 1 ml, respectively. Refrigeration, freezing, or specimen preservation is not required when shipped within the continental United States (see reference 120 for shipping information). To obtain maximum test sensitivity, it is recommended that both serum and urine specimens be tested in parallel. Treatment success or failure may be assessed by collecting specimens at least 14 days after initiation of treatment and testing the newly acquired sample in parallel with the last specimen that was positive before initiation of therapy. Serum samples are heated at 56°C for 1 h before being tested (to inactivate possible HIV), and urine is boiled for 5 min before use. Newly instituted procedures to remove test interference by human anti-rabbit immunoglobulins have been reported, but no details of the exact procedures employed have been described.

Materials and Reagents

The capture and detector antibodies are raised in rabbits against formalin-killed yeast forms of *H. capsulatum* in incomplete Freund adjuvant followed by multiple intravenous injections of live yeast forms. The percentage of high-responder rabbits producing antibody of suitable affinity for use in the EIA is low (i.e., < 5%), and the use of various immunization routes and schedules has not improved immune responsiveness.

Equipment

The equipment required to perform the HPA test is the same as that for the Premier *Coccidioides* EIA (see "Test 4. EIA To Detect Antibodies to *Coccidioides* Species" above), except that a boiling-water bath is also required.

Procedure

The EIA is conducted as described by Durkin et al. (29). Briefly, heat-treated samples are placed into wells of a microtiter plate coated with the polyclonal capture antibody. Biotinylated detector antibodies are then added, followed by peroxidase-labeled streptavidin. Each well is read after addition of and incubation with H_2O_2 and the colorimetric substrate (TMB) after the reaction is stopped using 1 M H_2SO_4. The substrate color change can then be read visually as a qualitative test result or on a spectrophotometer at OD_{450} as a quantitative test result. Because the exact nature of the antigen is not precisely known, there is no quantification of test results relative to a standard curve. Instead, EIA units (EU) are defined as the OD_{450} obtained for the patient sample divided by 1.5 times the mean of the OD_{450} of the negative control sample. Negative control samples (usually serum and urine) are obtained from normal subjects.

Interpretation

Specimens giving test results between 1 and 2 EU indicate a weak positive result corresponding to a diagnosis of probable histoplasmosis. In such cases, repeat testing is recommended. A test result of >2 to <10 EU corresponds to a moderate positive result, and a repeat test is necessary only if test results are inconsistent with clinical findings. Values of >10 EU reflect strongly positive results. The antigen concentration has been reported to subside in response to therapy and increase during relapses, but an increase of 0 to 1.9 EU indicates a stable condition. On the other hand, increases of 2 to 4 EU suggest possible treatment failures. In such cases, antigen testing should be repeated and cultures should be obtained. An increase of >4 EU corresponds to probable treatment failure, and more intense therapy is recommended (161).

The HPA test detected measurable antigen concentrations in urine from 50 (89%) of 56 patients with disseminated disease and 11 (37%) of 30 patients with self-limiting disease in a large outbreak in Indianapolis (29). In cases of disseminated or acute pulmonary histoplasmosis, the concentration of antigen is usually higher in urine than in serum when paired samples are tested. The HPA test has been reported to be positive in 21% of patients with chronic pulmonary histoplasmosis (164). Antigen has also been reported to be detected in the CSF of 25 to 50% of patients with *H. capsulatum* meningitis and in the BAL fluid of 70% of patients with diffuse pulmonary histoplasmosis. The test cross-reacts with antibodies from patients with blastomycosis, paracoccidioidomycosis, and penicilliosis marneffei but not from those with coccidioidomycosis; therefore, test results must be interpreted in light of the clinical presentation and the patient's history of travel to or residence in areas where these diseases are endemic and in conjunction with other laboratory results, including those for antibody detection and for culture.

It has been reported that false-positive results can occur when sera from SOT recipients who were treated with rabbit anti-thymocyte globulin are tested in the HPA assay (160). As a result, the HPA test was revised, in an unspecified manner, to reduce such false-positive results (www.miravistalabs.com).

Experimental and Molecular Biological Approaches

Attempts to replace the CF test with an EIA format have been frustrated because of cross-reactive carbohydrate moieties found on the immunodominant H and M antigens (65, 169). Periodate treatment of the M antigen before use in an immunoblot format, however, was reported to remove most of the cross-reactivity and increase the test specificity to 91% (43, 169). Recently, an ELISA for the early diagnosis of histoplasmosis was described in which purified native histoplasmin was compared to its deglycosylated counterpart (42). Deglycosylation resulted in an increase in test specificity from 93 to 96%; more surprisingly, the test sensitivity also increased from 57 to 92% (42). Other studies have employed monoclonal antibodies directed to an *H. capsulatum*-specific 70-kDa antigen in an attempt to improve test specificity (40). An inhibition EIA employing this antibody had 89 and 57% sensitivity for the detection of the acute and chronic forms of histoplasmosis, respectively, and a test specificity of 85% with serum from patients with chronic fungal or bacterial infections.

Aside from a few case reports in humans, a limited number of studies describe the application of molecular biological methods to clinical materials for the diagnosis of histoplasmosis. The most extensive study examined two nested PCR assays for the detection of *H. capsulatum* DNA in formalin-fixed, paraffin-embedded human tissue (8). Of the 29 samples that were described as positive for *H. capsulatum* by periodic acid-Schiff staining, 20 (69%) were PCR positive when a 100-kDa-like protein gene was used as the amplification target and 26 (90%) were positive when primers directed to the 18S rRNA gene were used. However, comparative DNA sequence analysis confirmed that only 20 of the latter 26 samples contained *H. capsulatum* DNA; the

remaining 6 samples were found to contain DNA from other fungi. Whereas the use of primers directed to the 100-kDa-like protein gene was 100% specific (33 samples negative by periodic acid-Schiff staining were also PCR negative), DNA sequence analysis demonstrated that 18 of the 33 histopathologically negative samples tested were falsely positive when primers directed to the 18S rRNA region were used. Although these data suggest that the application of primers directed to a single-copy *H. capsulatum* gene was more specific for the diagnosis of histoplasmosis than were broad-range fungal primers, another study successfully used similar broad-range fungal primers, also directed to the 18S rRNA gene (albeit to a different region of the gene), to amplify and detect *H. capsulatum* DNA from microscopically positive and culture-positive bone marrow (55). These researchers employed a LightCycler, real-time fluorescence PCR assay and melting-curve analysis along with DNA sequencing of the PCR products to confirm that the amplicons produced were derived from *H. capsulatum* DNA.

PARACOCCIDIOIDOMYCOSIS

Background

Serologic tests are useful for the rapid presumptive diagnosis of paracoccidioidomycosis, particularly for diagnosing cases of disseminated disease and for monitoring the response to treatment. The ID and CIE tests are simple to perform and are among the most specific procedures available (reported sensitivities, 84 to 94%; reported specificity, 99%). CF tests that use unpurified antigens have a similar sensitivity to the ID and CIE tests (87%) but are less specific (68%). Therefore, the CF test should be performed in conjunction with the ID test.

Clinical Indications and Diagnostic Rationale

Serologic tests for paracoccidioidomycosis should be performed on specimens from patients with symptoms of chronic disease or who present with ulcerative lesions of the mucosae (oral, nasal, or intestinal) or the skin. A history of travel to or residence in Latin America in conjunction with typical clinical signs should raise suspicion for paracoccidioidomycosis. The CF test detects antibodies in 80 to 96% of patients with paracoccidioidomycosis. CF antibodies are diagnostic, but the CF test results with *P. brasiliensis* yeast-form culture filtrate antigens are not always specific, and cross-reactions may occur when sera from patients with other endemic mycoses, particularly histoplasmosis, are used. These cross-reactions are infrequent and occur mainly at titers of 1:8 or below. Nonetheless, concomitant use of the CF and ID tests allows a correct serodiagnosis of paracoccidioidomycosis in over 98% of cases.

The ID test employing concentrated yeast-form culture filtrate antigens and reference sera is entirely specific and has a sensitivity of 94% when sera from patients with paracoccidioidomycosis are tested. The major diagnostic precipitin is a 43-kDa glycoprotein referred to as gp43 (also known as E_2 or A) and is found in 95 to 98% of patients with paracoccidioidomycosis (11, 113).

Test 1. CF Test To Detect Antibodies to *P. brasiliensis*

The standard microtitration CF test with *P. brasiliensis* yeast-form filtrate antigens is recommended for the determination of titers in sera from patients with suspected paracoccidioidomycosis. A detailed protocol for the CF test is available (105). No commercial kits are available for the paracoccidioidomycosis CF test.

Sample Requirements

The sample requirements are the same as those for the histoplasmosis CF test (see "Test 1. CF Test To Detect Antibodies to *H. capsulatum*" above).

Materials and Reagents

Culture filtrate antigens of *P. brasiliensis* are referred to as paracoccidioidin, an antigenic preparation that is suitable for use in the CF and ID tests. Paracoccidioidin is prepared by growing *P. brasiliensis* in a tryptic soy broth-dialyzate medium supplemented with glucose, ammonium sulfate, and vitamins (118). Yeast-form shake cultures of three stock isolates of *P. brasiliensis* are grown singly at 35°C in this medium for up to 4 weeks. References 13 and 21 give details about isolate selection. The culture filtrate from each isolate is dialyzed, concentrated 10-fold, and mixed in equal volumes with those from the other isolates. The optimal dilution for each antigen pool is determined by titration with low- and high-titer CF-positive sera from human paracoccidioidomycosis cases or by the use of ID tests with precipitin-positive sera. References 15 and 21 give details of the kinetics of *P. brasiliensis* antigen production during growth and discuss alternative growth media.

Equipment, Procedure, and QA/QC

The equipment, procedure, and QA/QC measures for the paracoccidioidomycosis CF test are the same as those described earlier in this chapter for the histoplasmosis CF test (see "Test 1. CF Test To Detect Antibodies to *H. capsulatum*").

Interpretation

CF titers of ≥1:8 are considered presumptive evidence of paracoccidioidomycosis. However, 85 to 95% of patients with active disease have titers of ≥1:32. Low CF titers are usually associated with localized disease or involvement of the mononuclear phagocyte system, whereas high titers are found in patients with pulmonary lesions or multifocal disease. Sera from young children with disseminated paracoccidioidomycosis are an exception and ordinarily show low or negative CF reactivity. The CF test has a sensitivity of 87% and a specificity of 68% (13). Serial CF determinations are prognostic in that a decreasing titer generally indicates effective therapy, whereas relapses are accompanied by increasing titers. High and fluctuating titers suggest a poor prognosis. Low levels of CF antibodies may persist long after the patient is cured.

Test 2. ID Test To Detect Antibodies to *P. brasiliensis*

The ID test for *P. brasiliensis* precipitins can be performed on a fee-for-service basis by Cerodex Laboratories, Inc., Washington, Okla., and commercial reagents are available from Immuno-Mycologics, Inc. No commercial kits are available for the performance of the paracoccidioidomycosis ID test.

Sample Requirements

The sample requirements for the paracoccidioidomycosis ID test are the same as those for the histoplasmosis ID test (see "Test 2. ID Test To Detect Antibodies to *H. capsulatum*" above).

Materials and Reagents

See the section on materials and reagents under the heading "Test 1. CF Test To Detect Antibodies to *P. brasiliensis*" (above) for a description of the antigen preparation used for the ID test. Commercial mycelium-phase *P. brasiliensis* culture filtrate antigens, containing gp43 and other antigens, are available from Immuno-Mycologics, Inc.

Interpretation

The ID test is valuable for the diagnosis of acute or chronic pulmonary infection and disseminated paracoccidioidomycosis. The CIE test gives similar results (13) and is not discussed further. The greatest number of precipitin bands has occurred when sera from patients with lung involvement or disseminated disease have been used; up to three precipitin bands have been observed (15). A major diagnostic precipitin is consistently found in the sera of patients with paracoccidioidomycosis, which reacts with a soluble, specific *P. brasiliensis* antigen. Band 1, which appears closest to the antigen-containing well, is thought to contain gp43 on the basis of immunochemical analysis. The precipitin that reacts with the gp43 antigen has been observed to occur in 95 to 99% of sera from patients with active paracoccidioidomycosis and can be found in patient serum for longer periods following infection than are the other two major serum precipitins; the latter disappear during a favorable response to treatment. The positive predictive value of a positive ID test result is 100%.

Experimental and Molecular Biological Approaches

An indirect EIA, measuring anti-gp43 IgG, has been described that provides a simpler test format than the CF test and, like the CF test, provides a quantitative measurement of antibody titer for therapeutic monitoring. The EIA was shown to be more sensitive than the CF test if the gp43 antigen was deglycosylated or if test sera were preadsorbed with mycelium-phase cells from *H. capsulatum* (13, 114). Variously purified and characterized antigens have been described in recent years in an attempt to discover antigens that would be without cross-reactivity, including 22- to 25-, 43-, 58-, and 87-kDa antigens. A 27-kDa antigen that appears to be free of cross-reacting epitopes has been described, and a 60-kDa heat shock protein has been cloned and characterized (57, 104).

Tests to detect antigens in serum, urine, CSF, and BAL fluid have also been described and may be particularly useful for the diagnosis of paracoccidioidomycosis in immunosuppressed patients and to monitor disease progression (39, 90, 94, 123). Paracoccidioidomycosis, in addition to its acute and chronic forms, has also been known to reactivate from quiescent endogenous foci. In such situations, the detection of antigenuria by immunoblotting may provide information not available by performing antibody tests alone. The occurrence of antigenuria in 11 (91.7%) of 12 patients tested in one study indicated that detection of antigenuria may be a promising diagnostic approach (123).

One study examined the detection of *P. brasiliensis* DNA from human clinical materials (38). In this study, a nested PCR assay was described in which primers directed to the gene encoding the gp43 antigen of *P. brasiliensis* were used. Sputa from 11 (100%) of 11 patients with proven chronic pulmonary paracoccidioidomycosis were positive in the PCR assay. Although no amplicons were produced when DNA from pure cultures of *C. albicans*, *H. capsulatum*, or *C. neoformans* was used as an amplification template, no clinical specimens from patients with other fungal diseases were tested and the clinical specificity of this test was not determined.

PENICILLIOSIS MARNEFFEI

Background

Disseminated infection with *Penicillium marneffei* is observed almost exclusively in immunocompromised patients who either live in or have traveled through southeast Asia.

Diagnosis of *P. marneffei* infections relies mainly on culture and/or histopathologic identification. Serologic procedures, which are still being evaluated, detect antibodies by ID and by IFA. More recently, antigen detection tests were developed to detect a 90-kDa cell wall mannoprotein (16). No commercial tests for the diagnosis of penicilliosis marneffei are currently available in the United States.

Clinical Indications and Diagnostic Rationale

Serologic tests for the diagnosis of *P. marneffei* infections should be considered for use with patients who have lived in or traveled to southeast Asia and who display symptoms of intermittent fever, marked weight loss, nonproductive cough, and debilitation. About 60 to 70% of patients present with multiple papular lesions, some of which show a central necrotic umbilication resembling molluscum contagiosum. Other presenting signs include hepatosplenomegaly, generalized lymphadenopathy, anemia, and thrombocytopenia. These symptoms may be confused with those of other fungal infections such as histoplasmosis or cryptococcosis as well as with those of tuberculosis.

Experimental and Molecular Biological Approaches

Detection of antibodies in suspected cases has relied on the ID test (128, 151) and on an IFA test (168). The ID test (69) detected antibody in only 2 of 17 HIV-positive patients with *P. marneffei* infection. More recently, an IFA test was developed that used germinating conidia and yeast-like forms as test antigens (168). Sera from 8 patients with confirmed *P. marneffei* cases had IgG titers of ≥1:160, whereas sera from 95 patients with other diseases and 78 healthy controls had titers of ≤1:40. A recombinant 90-kDa cell wall mannoprotein has been incorporated into an ELISA format to detect anti-*P. marneffei* antibodies. The ELISA was reported to detect 14 (82%) of 17 HIV-positive patients with penicilliosis marneffei with a test specificity of 100% when sera from patients with typhoid fever, tuberculosis, and normal healthy donors were used (16).

Antigenemia was detected using ID and LA tests (69), whereas antigenuria was detected in an EIA (25). The LA test was more sensitive (13 of 17 [77%]) than the ID assay (10 of 17 [59%]), whereas the antigenuria EIA was reported to have a sensitivity of 97% and a specificity of 98% (25). A sandwich EIA in which MAbs were used to detect *P. marneffei* soluble yeast exoantigen in sera had a reported test sensitivity of 72% and a specificity of 100% (106, 145).

One study described the application of a PCR method to the detection of *P. marneffei* DNA in clinical specimens (112). DNA was extracted from the blood of 19 AIDS patients, and amplicons of 331 and 251 bp, characteristic for *P. marneffei*, were detected by agarose gel electrophoresis and ethidium bromide staining. Of 19 blood cultures, 2 grew *P. marneffei*; both were PCR positive.

PNEUMOCYSTOSIS

Background

Until recently, the organisms responsible for pneumocystosis were referred to as *Pneumocystis carinii*. However, recent comparative DNA sequence analysis demonstrated that *Pneumocystis* organisms from different mammalian hosts were genetically quite dissimilar from one another. This finding resulted in a name change from *P. carinii* (which infects rats) to *P. jiroveci* for the organisms infecting humans (133). Until 1988 these organisms were widely thought to be protozoa, but comparative DNA sequence analysis demonstrated that *Pneumocystis* strains were phylogenetically more closely related to the fungi (30).

The laboratory diagnosis of pneumocystosis depends largely on the use of Gomori methenamine silver, Calcofluor white, Gram-Weigert, or toluidine blue-O staining of lung biopsy specimens, induced sputum, or BAL fluid specimens to detect the cyst form of the organism and the use of Giemsa stain to detect the trophozoite form or clusters of cysts containing intracystic bodies. Specific antipneumocystis MAbs have been developed that can detect not only the cyst form of the organism but also the significantly more abundant trophozoite form (37, 77). The sensitivity of the MAbs with either induced sputum or BAL fluid specimens has been reported to be similar to or somewhat greater than that of conventional staining methods.

Indirect and direct immunofluorescent assays employing MAbs have most commonly been used for the detection of *P. jiroveci* in induced sputum and in BAL fluid samples; however, less frequently, these reagents have also been used for tissue diagnosis (2, 74, 116). MAbs directed against *Pneumocystis* for use in direct or indirect staining procedures are available commercially from Axis-Shield Diagnostics (Dundee, United Kingdom), Bio-Rad Laboratories, Inc., Chemicon International, Inc. (Temecula, Calif.), and Meridian Diagnostics. Other immunologic methods including CIE, ELISA, Western blotting, and LA tests have also been developed experimentally and are discussed in more detail below. Finally, the increased sensitivity of molecular biology-based diagnostic methods may allow a minimally invasive procedure, such as oral washing (46), to be sufficient for diagnostic purposes.

Clinical Indications and Diagnostic Rationale

PCP is rare in immunocompetent adults but is a leading cause of illness and death in individuals with impaired immunity including malnourished or premature children, persons with AIDS, SOT recipients, and patients receiving long-term corticosteroid therapy. It is often described as interstitial plasma cell pneumonia; histopathologic studies of patients' lungs typically show alveolar interstitial thickening and the presence of a frothy eosinophilic exudate in the lumina. The clinical presentation in children is characterized by cyanosis, mild cough without fever, and, in severe disease, intercostal retractions. In contrast, adults with PCP frequently present with dyspnea, nonproductive cough, chest tightness, night sweats, and an inability to breathe deeply. Tachypnea and low-grade fever often occur, but hemoptysis is rarely present. Adults with CD4 counts below 200 per μl are at increased risk for PCP, and persons with AIDS have a more insidious progression than those who are immunosuppressed but HIV negative. Extrapulmonary pneumocystosis has been found in 1 to 3% of postmortem examinations of patients known to have pulmonary infections (100, 141) and most often involves the lymph nodes (44%) and the spleen, bone marrow, and liver (33%). Infection at multiple extrapulmonary sites is associated with a rapidly fatal outcome (100, 141).

The route of transmission of *P. jiroveci* is not understood, but seroprevalence studies have suggested that exposure occurs in early childhood. It was hypothesized that the strains acquired during first exposure persisted in the lungs in a dormant state throughout life and became active on subsequent immunosuppression of the host (133, 134). However, this hypothesis has recently been challenged, and it has been suggested that *P. jiroveci* organisms are frequently acquired and cleared by the immune system in immunocompetent hosts and do not persist (153).

Experimental and Molecular Biological Approaches

The serologic diagnosis of pneumocystosis has proven to be difficult because most humans become seropositive for *Pneumocystis* antibodies at an early age and are exposed to the organism multiple times throughout life. Therefore, the detection of serum antibodies may not correlate with true infection. In addition, conflicting results have been obtained primarily because different test methods have been used (CIE, LA, Western blotting, ELISA, indirect immunofluorescence), a variety of antigen sources have been employed (rat versus human), and the antigens used have been purified to different degrees (column purified or recombinant).

Other tests include the detection of antigens ranging from 35 to 45 kDa, as well as a 95-kDa major surface glycoprotein antigen, in BAL fluids (132). Western blot analysis demonstrated that the 35- to 45-kDa antigen was found in 88% of the BAL fluids tested whereas the 95-kDa antigen was detected in only 49% of the specimens. Yet another study demonstrated that levels of a panfungal antigen, (1,3)-β-D-glucan [see the section below on (1,3)-β-D-glucan], in plasma were found to parallel the clinical and radiographic improvement of a patient with PCP in a case report (143). Further evaluations of this test in larger studies are warranted.

Molecular diagnosis of pneumocystosis has primarily employed PCR primers directed to the multicopy gene family of the major surface glycoprotein of *P. jiroveci* (81) or to the mitochondrial rRNA gene (155). Both of these gene targets have been demonstrated to be sensitive and specific for the detection of *P. jiroveci* in BAL fluids (51, 154) and have been applied in single or nested PCR formats. Other target genes have included those for thymidylate synthase, heat shock protein 70, β-tubulin, dihydrofolate reductase, and the 5S, 18S, 28S, and ITS regions of rRNA. Most studies have indicated that PCR assays are more sensitive than conventional stains and are equal to or better than DFA or IFA tests for the diagnosis of pneumocystosis (110, 146). However, because 2 to 21% of individuals may be asymptomatic carriers of *P. jiroveci* (130), a positive PCR result in conjunction with a negative staining result may not represent active disease. To resolve this dilemma, researchers have investigated imposing cutoff values for PCR positivity (144) or the application of real-time quantitative PCR methods (33, 82) in an attempt to numerically differentiate the results for colonized patients from those of true cases.

The increased sensitivity of nucleic acid-based tests allows specimens that contain smaller numbers of organisms, and that are more easily obtained than BAL fluid or tissue, to be used for diagnostic purposes. For example, the use of oral wash fluids from patients suspected to have pneumocystosis has demonstrated test sensitivities and specificities of 89 and 94%, respectively; this compares to sensitivities and specificities of 100 and 91% that were obtained using BAL fluid during parallel testing (46). A diagnostic strategy may be to use less invasive procedures, such as oral washings, to obtain screening samples from patients presenting clinical signs consistent with the disease. The diagnostician would proceed to more invasive procedures only if the specimens obtained by less invasive means were negative.

Although respiratory samples such as induced sputum, BAL fluid, and oral and nasopharyngeal aspirates have most commonly been used to recover *P. jiroveci* DNA, other clinical specimens such as blood, serum, and peripheral blood mononuclear and polymorphonuclear cells have been tested with various degrees of success (4, 125, 137). In general,

PCR tests using blood-related specimens have given sensitivities of 41 to 86% and specificities of 100%. Tissues have also been used successfully in both PCR and in situ hybridization test formats (64, 75) but require invasive collection procedures. No commercial kits are currently available for PCR diagnosis of PCP in the clinical laboratory.

SPOROTRICHOSIS

Background

Serologic tests are sometimes helpful for the diagnosis of the extracutaneous or systemic forms of sporotrichosis. A slide agglutination test to detect anti-*Sporothrix schenckii* antibodies has been demonstrated to be the most useful method. This test has been reported to have sensitivities of 100, 86, 73, and 56% for disseminated, articular, pulmonary, and cutaneous disease, respectively, and a specificity of 100% (121). Antibodies are most probably directed toward a peptido-L-rhamno-D-mannan, localized in the outer layer of the *S. schenckii* cell wall. Comparable sensitivity for the detection of *S. schenckii* antibodies has not been reported for an ID test format.

Clinical Indications and Diagnostic Rationale

Serologic tests for sporotrichosis may be applied to sera from patients with skin lesions, subcutaneous nodules, bone and joint lesions, lymphadenopathy, or pulmonary disease and to CSF from patients with undiagnosed chronic meningitis. The disease should be suspected in individuals whose work brings them into contact with soil, plants, timber, plant materials, or sphagnum moss. Cutaneous sporotrichosis is more common in adults than in children, and extracutaneous disease is found more often in men older than 30 years. Although not common, disseminated infection is more likely to occur in immunosuppressed than immunocompetent individuals.

Test 1. LA Test To Detect Antibodies to *S. schenckii*

The LA test is a semiquantitative slide agglutination assay in which *S. schenckii* antigen-coated latex particles are used to detect antibody to *S. schenckii*. The assay is rapid and simple to perform and requires no special equipment. A commercial kit is available from Immuno-Mycologics, Inc.

Sample Requirements

Serum and CSF should be free of any particulates, and lipids should be removed using a 0.45- or 0.8-μm syringe filter. Specimens may be stored at 2 to 8°C if tested within 72 h after collection or at −20°C or colder in a nondefrosting freezer for longer periods. Repeated freezing and thawing of specimens should be avoided.

Materials and Reagents

All reagents including specimen diluent (concentrated glycine-buffered saline [pH 8.6] containing albumin), sensitized latex particles (sensitized with *S. schenckii* culture filtrate antigens), positive control serum (from rabbits immunized with *S. schenckii*), negative control serum (normal goat serum), and disposable glass slides with raised rings for the performance of the test can be obtained from Immuno-Mycologics, Inc. A properly standardized suspension of latex particles, which has an absorbance of 0.30 ± 0.02 after a 1:100 dilution, can be sensitized in-house with an equal volume of an optimal dilution of yeast-form *S. schenckii* culture filtrate antigens. The optimal quantity of culture filtrate antigen is the highest dilution that produces a clear 2+ agglutination reaction with the highest reactive dilution of rabbit anti-*S. schenckii* reference serum or serum from a human with sporotrichosis.

Equipment and Procedure

The equipment and procedure for the sporotrichosis LA test are the same as those for the coccidioidomycosis LA test (see "Test 2. LA Test To Detect Antibodies to *Coccidioides*" above), except that the sporotrichosis LA test may be performed as a semiquantitative test. Specimens giving a 2+ or greater reaction during the initial screening phase of the test may be serially diluted twofold, beginning with a 1:2 dilution to obtain an end-point titer.

QA/QC

QA/QC procedures for the sporotrichosis LA test are the same as those for the histoplasmosis LA test (see "Test 3. LA Test To Detect Antibodies to *H. capsulatum*" above).

Interpretation

LA titers of 1:8 or greater are considered presumptive evidence of sporotrichosis. False-positive reactions have, however, been noted at titers of 1:8 when sera from patients with nonfungal infections were used. Sera from patients with localized cutaneous, lymphocutaneous, or extracutaneous sporotrichosis may display titers ranging from 1:8 to 1:512. An increasing titer or a sustained high titer indicates pulmonary sporotrichosis. The test has limited prognostic value, since antibody levels may show little change during and after convalescence. Slide latex agglutinin titers of >1:8 with CSF are considered presumptive evidence of meningeal sporotrichosis.

Experimental and Molecular Biological Approaches

A CF test using culture supernatant antigen has been examined for the diagnosis of sporotrichosis, but whereas the specificity of the assay was good, and no cross-reactions with sera from patients infected with other fungi was observed, the assay lacked sensitivity (63). An enzyme immunoassay has also been described and used in a study of *S. schenckii* meningitis (126). A comparison between the LA test and EIA was performed with both serum and CSF from meningitis patients. Antibody titers were typically higher in the EIA (~100- to 1,000-fold higher) than in the LA test, and for a few cases, the EIA was more sensitive. Neither test became positive earlier in the course of disease than the other, although CSF specimens tested by the EIA remained positive for a longer period after disease onset than did those tested by the LA test (126).

S. schenckii DNA was detected in 11 of 12 tissues from various anatomical sites (including arm, hand, nose, foot, face, and neck) of patients with culture- or histopathology-proven sporotrichosis when a nested PCR assay and primers directed to the 18S rRNA gene were used. Negative PCR results were obtained with DNA extracts from common bacteria and fungi or from *S. schenckii*-negative skin specimens. The one culture-positive, PCR-negative specimen was shown to contain inhibitors of the PCR because purified *S. schenckii* DNA, artificially spiked into this sample, was not amplified (50).

ZYGOMYCOSIS

Background

The primary agents of zygomycosis in the order Mucorales include species of *Absidia*, *Apophysomyces*, *Cunninghamella*, *Mucor*, *Rhizopus*, *Rhizomucor*, and *Saksenaea*, and those in the order Entomophthorales include *Conidiobolus* and *Basidiobolus* (119, 156). In tissue, these organisms are difficult to differentiate and appear as sparsely septate, irregularly branched, broad, ribbon-like hyphae (17, 156). A murine MAb, WSSA-RA-1, directed against somatic antigens of *Rhizopus arrhizus*, has been reported to react specifically with *Absidia corymbifera*, *R. arrhizus*, and *Rhizomucor pusillus* when applied as an indirect immunofluorescent histopathology stain; this reagent is commercially available from DakoCytomation, Inc. (58). Although ID tests have been successfully used to detect antibodies in patients with active zygomycosis (65, 70), these methods have not been extensively evaluated.

Clinical Indications and Diagnostic Rationale

The major risk factors for zygomycosis are neutropenia, uncontrolled diabetes mellitus, other forms of metabolic acidosis, and burns. Other contributing factors include corticosteroid use and treatment with deferoxamine. Sera or CSF specimens from patients with diabetic ketoacidosis or evidence of rhinocerebral disease, those who are immunocompromised with renal disease, those with acute leukemia, or those who are debilitated and have signs of pulmonary or systemic infection should be tested for zygomycosis.

Experimental and Molecular Biological Approaches

Antibodies to *Rhizopus arrhizus* have been detected in the sera of patients with brain infections caused by this organism (62, 109). In addition, antibodies to *Absidia corymbifera* were found in the CSF and serum of a patient with culture-proven *Absidia* meningitis (89) and in the serum of a patient with histologically proven *A. corymbifera* brain abscess (109). There appears to be significant cross-reactivity among the major antigens of the genera *Rhizomucor*, *Absidia*, and *Rhizopus* as a result of the common peptido-L-fuco-D-mannan on their cell surfaces, confounding immunological differentiation of infections by these organisms (65, 165). Preliminary work using homogenized antigens from *Absidia corymbifera*, *Rhizomucor pusillus*, and *Rhizopus arrhizus* demonstrated a sensitivity of 70% and a specificity of 90% for these zygomycotic agents in an ID test format (65, 66). An EIA format was also evaluated and, using a 1:400 antigen titer as positive, was found to be 81% sensitive and 94% specific for zygomycosis (65, 70). This compared to an ID test for *Rhizopus arrhizus* that had a sensitivity of 66% and a specificity of 91% (70).

Experimental ID tests to detect antibodies to *Conidiobolus coronatus* and *Basidiobolus ranarum* in patients with subcutaneous or gastrointestinal infections have been developed using culture filtrate antigens from these organisms. The tests appear to be specific (66), but their sensitivity has not been determined. Studies of the molecular phylogeny of clinically important Zygomycetes have been conducted (152), but no molecular diagnostic tests using clinical materials have been developed to date.

PANFUNGAL DETECTION USING (1,3)-β-ᴅ-GLUCAN

The Fungitell test (Associates of Cape Cod, Inc., East Falmouth, Mass.) is a recently FDA-approved microtiter plate-based EIA for the detection of BDG in serum. BDG is a component of the cell wall of all fungi except the Zygomycetes, and only low levels of BDG are released from *C. neoformans* (101). BDG activates factor G, a coagulation enzyme found in *Limulus polyphemus* (horseshoe crab) amebocyte lysates. Although there are two *Limulus* amebocyte lysate coagulation pathways, one containing factors B and C and sensitive to activation by endotoxin and the other containing factor G and sensitive to BDG activation, the Fungitell test detects only the second, BDG-specific pathway. Once activated by BDG, the activated enzyme cleaves a chromogenic substrate (*t*-butyloxycarbonyl-Leu-Gly-Arg-*p*-nitroanilide) included in the test, releasing *p*-nitroanilide. The free *p*-nitroanilide can then be quantitated by its absorbance at 405 nm with respect to a glucan standard.

The test has been reported to detect low picogram quantities of BDG, and a serum BDG level of ≥60 pg/ml was chosen as the cutoff for positivity in a recent clinical evaluation of the test. Serial serum samples from 283 subjects with acute myeloid leukemia or myelodysplastic syndrome who were receiving antifungal prophylaxis were examined for the presence of BDG (103). For 100% of subjects with proven or probable invasive fungal infection, at least one serum sample was positive for BDG a median of 10 days before the clinical diagnosis of invasive fungal infection was established. Absence of a positive BDG result had a negative predictive value of 100%. Invasive fungal infections studied included aspergillosis, candidiasis, fusariosis, and trichosporonosis. The test specificity was reported to be 90% if a single test result was positive and greater than 96% if two or more sequential serum samples were positive.

Caveats in interpreting the results of BDG determinations are that plasma glucan activity increased in 36 of 45 patients with hematologic malignancies who were undergoing chemotherapy and who had no signs of invasive fungal disease (71). False-positive reactions have also been observed in patients after surgery or hemodialysis, possibly owing to extrinsic BDG present in surgical gauze or to the use of cellulosic membranes, such as cuprammonium rayon, which contain polysaccharides that are shed into the bloodstream during dialysis (102). Also, patients receiving parenteral infusions of plasma components, such as gamma globulin, which is filtered through cellulose membranes during manufacture, can give false-positive results (102). Recently, it was noted that the intramuscular administration of antitumor preparations containing BDG (lentinan and schizophyllan) can also produce false-positive results in the BDG test (56).

Although the BDG test cannot specifically identify the fungus responsible for infection, results can be obtained within 2 h. Such rapidity makes this test a very attractive screening tool to detect invasive infection by common as well as less common fungi, including those for which no other serologic test is available (167). Automation of this assay may make it more attractive for evaluation in prospective studies and for use in the clinical laboratory (138). Alternative colorimetric (Fungitec G Test MK; Seikagaku Kogyo Co., Ltd., Tokyo, Japan) (136) and turbidometric (Wako-WB003; Wako Pure Chemical Industries, Ltd., Tokyo, Japan) (71) forms of amebocyte lysate assays are available in Japan.

SUPPLIERS

Accurate Chemical & Scientific Corp., 300 Shames Drive, Westbury, NY 11590 (www.accuratechemical.com)

Associates of Cape Cod, 124 Bernard E. St. Jean Drive, East Falmouth, MA 02536 (www.acciusa.com)

Axis-Shield, Plc., Luna Place, Technology Park, Dundee, DD2 1XA, United Kingdom (www.axis-shield.com)

Bio-Rad Laboratories, Inc., 4000 Alfred Nobel Drive, Hercules, CA 94547 (www.biorad.com)

Chemicon International, Inc., 28820 Single Oak Drive, Temecula, CA 92590 (www.chemicon.com)

DakoCytomation California, Inc., 6392 Via Real, Carpinteria, CA 93013 (www.dakocytomation.us)

Gibson Laboratories, Inc., 1040 Manchester Street, Lexington KY 40508 (www.gibsonlabs.com)

Immuno-Mycologics, P.O. Box 1151, Norman OK 73070 (www.immy.com)

Meridian Diagnostics, Inc., 3471 River Hills Drive, Cincinnati, OH 45244 (www.meridiandiagnostics.com)

Microgen Bioproducts, Ltd., 1 Admiralty Way, Camberley, Surrey, GU15 3DT, United Kingdom (www.microgen-bioproducts.com)

Ramco Laboratories, Inc., 4100 Greenbriar Drive, Suite 200, Stafford, TX 77477 (www.ramcolab.com)

Remel Laboratories, Inc., 12076 Santa Fe Drive, Lenexa, KS 66215 (www.remelinc.com)

Vircell, S.L., Plaza Dominguez Ortiz, 1, 18320 Santa Fe, Granada, Spain (www.vircell.com)

Wampole, Inc., 2 Research Way, Princeton, NJ 08540 (www.wampolelabs.com)

Use of commercial sources is for identification purposes only and does not imply endorsement by the U.S. Department of Health and Human Services or CDC.

REFERENCES

1. **Abrams, D. I., M. Robia, W. Blumenfeld, J. Simonson, M. B. Cohen, and W. K. Hadley.** 1984. Disseminated coccidioidomycosis in AIDS. *N. Engl. J. Med.* **310**:986–987.

2. **Amin, M. B., E. Mezger, and R. J. Zarbo.** 1992. Detection of *Pneumocystis carinii.* Comparative study of monoclonal antibody and silver staining. *Am. J. Clin. Pathol.* **98**:13–18.

3. **Arruda, L. K., T. A. Platts-Mills, J. W. Fox, and M. D. Chapman.** 1990. *Aspergillus fumigatus* allergen I, a major IgE-binding protein, is a member of the mitogillin family of cytotoxins. *J. Exp. Med.* **172**:1529–1532.

4. **Atzori, C., F. Agostoni, E. Angeli, A. Mainini, G. Orlando, and A. Cargnel.** 1998. Combined use of blood and oropharyngeal samples for noninvasive diagnosis of *Pneumocystis carinii* pneumonia using the polymerase chain reaction. *Eur. J. Clin. Microbiol. Infect. Dis.* **17**:241–246.

5. **Bar, W., and H. Hecker.** 2002. Diagnosis of systemic *Candida* infections in patients of the intensive care unit. Significance of serum antigens and antibodies. *Mycoses* **45**:22–28.

6. **Bardana, E. J., Jr., J. D. Gerber, S. Craig, and F. D. Cianciulli.** 1975. The general and specific humoral immune response to pulmonary aspergillosis. *Am. Rev. Respir. Dis.* **112**:799–805.

7. **Bialek, R., A. C. Cirera, T. Herrmann, C. Aepinus, V. I. Shearn-Bochsler, and A. M. Legendre.** 2003. Nested PCR assays for detection of *Blastomyces dermatitidis* DNA in paraffin-embedded canine tissue. *J. Clin. Microbiol.* **41**:205–208.

8. **Bialek, R., A. Feucht, C. Aepinus, G. Just-Nubling, V. J. Robertson, J. Knobloch, and R. Hohle.** 2002. Evaluation of two nested PCR assays for detection of *Histoplasma capsulatum* DNA in human tissue. *J. Clin. Microbiol.* **40**:1644–1647.

9. **Bialek, R., J. Kern, T. Herrmann, R. Tijerina, L. Cecenas, U. Reischl, and G. M. Gonzalez.** 2004. PCR assays for identification of *Coccidioides posadasii* based on the nucleotide sequence of the antigen 2/proline-rich antigen. *J. Clin. Microbiol.* **42**:778–783.

10. **Blumer, S. O., L. Kaufman, W. Kaplan, D. W. McLaughlin, and D. E. Kraft.** 1973. Comparative evaluation of five serological methods for the diagnosis of sporotrichosis. *Appl. Microbiol.* **26:**4–8.

11. **Brummer, E., E. Castaneda, and A. Restrepo.** 1993. Paracoccidioidomycosis: an update. *Clin. Microbiol. Rev.* **6:**89–117.

12. **Bu, R., R. K. Sathiapalan, M. M. Ibrahim, I. Al-Mohsen, E. Almodavar, M. I. Gutierrez, and K. Bhatia.** 2005. Monochrome LightCycler PCR assay for detection and quantification of five common species of *Candida* and *Aspergillus. J. Med. Microbiol.* **54:**243–248.

13. **Bueno, J. P., M. J. Mendes-Giannini, G. M. Del Negro, C. M. Assis, C. K. Takiguti, and M. A. Shikanai-Yasuda.** 1997. IgG, IgM and IgA antibody response for the diagnosis and follow-up of paracoccidioidomycosis: comparison of counterimmunoelectrophoresis and complement fixation. *J. Med. Vet. Mycol.* **35:**213–217.

14. **Burnie, J. P., R. C. Matthews, I. Clark, and L. J. Milne.** 1989. Immunoblot fingerprinting *Aspergillus fumigatus. J. Immunol. Methods* **118:**179–186.

15. **Camargo, Z. P., C. Unterkircher, and L. R. Travassos.** 1989. Identification of antigenic polypeptides of *Paracoccidioides brasiliensis* by immunoblotting. *J. Med. Vet. Mycol.* **27:**407–412.

16. **Cao, L., D. L. Chen, C. Lee, C. M. Chan, K. M. Chan, N. Vanittanakom, D. N. Tsang, and K. Y. Yuen.** 1998. Detection of specific antibodies to an antigenic mannoprotein for diagnosis of *Penicillium marneffei* penicilliosis. *J. Clin. Microbiol.* **36:**3028–3031.

17. **Chandler, F. W., W. Kaplan, and L. Ajello.** 1980. *Color Atlas and Text of the Histopathology of Mycotic Diseases.* Year Book, Chicago, Ill.

18. **Christensson, B., G. Sigmundsdottir, and L. Larsson.** 1999. D-Arabinitol—a marker for invasive candidiasis. *Med. Mycol.* **37:**391–396.

19. **Coleman, R. M., and L. Kaufman.** 1972. Use of the immunodiffusion test in the serodiagnosis of aspergillosis. *Appl. Microbiol.* **23:**301–308.

20. **Cox, R. A., and D. M. Magee.** 1998. Protective immunity in coccidioidomycosis. *Res. Immunol.* **149:**417–428; discussion, 506–417.

21. **De Camargo, Z., C. Unterkircher, S. P. Campoy, and L. R. Travassos.** 1988. Production of *Paracoccidioides brasiliensis* exoantigens for immunodiffusion tests. *J. Clin. Microbiol.* **26:**2147–2151.

22. **De Camargo, Z. P., and M. F. de Franco.** 2000. Current knowledge on pathogenesis and immunodiagnosis of paracoccidioidomycosis. *Rev. Iberoam. Micol.* **17:**41–48.

23. **Dee, T. H.** 1975. Detection of *Aspergillus fumigatus* serum precipitins by counterimmunoelectrophoresis. *J. Clin. Microbiol.* **2:**482–485.

24. **Dee, T. H., G. M. Johnson, and C. S. Berger.** 1981. Sensitivity, specificity, and predictive value of anti-candida serum precipitin and agglutinin quantification: comparison of counterimmunoelectrophoresis and latex agglutination. *J. Clin. Microbiol.* **13:**750–753.

25. **Desakorn, V., M. D. Smith, A. L. Walsh, A. J. Simpson, D. Sahassananda, A. Rajanuwong, V. Wuthiekunan, P. Howe, B. J. Angus, P. Suntharasamai, and N. J. White.** 1999. Diagnosis of *Penicillium marneffei* infection by quantitation of urinary antigen by using an enzyme immunoassay. *J. Clin. Microbiol.* **37:**117–121.

26. **Dosanjh, A., J. Theodore, and D. Pappagianis.** 1998. Probable false positive coccidioidal serologic results in patients with cystic fibrosis. *Pediatr. Transplant.* **2:**313–317.

27. **Drutz, D. J., and A. Catanzaro.** 1978. Coccidioidomycosis. Part I. *Am. Rev. Respir. Dis.* **117:**559–585.

28. **Durkin, M., J. Witt, A. Lemonte, B. Wheat, and P. Connolly.** 2004. Antigen assay with the potential to aid in diagnosis of blastomycosis. *J. Clin. Microbiol.* **42:**4873–4875.

29. **Durkin, M. M., P. A. Connolly, and L. J. Wheat.** 1997. Comparison of radioimmunoassay and enzyme-linked immunoassay methods for detection of *Histoplasma capsulatum* var. *capsulatum* antigen. *J. Clin. Microbiol.* **35:**2252–2255.

30. **Edman, J. C., J. A. Kovacs, H. Masur, D. V. Santi, H. J. Elwood, and M. L. Sogin.** 1988. Ribosomal RNA sequence shows *Pneumocystis carinii* to be a member of the fungi. *Nature* **334:**519–522.

31. **Einsele, H., H. Hebart, G. Roller, J. Loffler, I. Rothenhofer, C. A. Muller, R. A. Bowden, J. van Burik, D. Engelhard, L. Kanz, and U. Schumacher.** 1997. Detection and identification of fungal pathogens in blood by using molecular probes. *J. Clin. Microbiol.* **35:**1353–1360.

32. **Fisher, M. C., T. J. White, and J. W. Taylor.** 1999. Primers for genotyping single nucleotide polymorphisms and microsatellites in the pathogenic fungus *Coccidioides immitis. Mol. Ecol.* **8:**1082–1084.

33. **Flori, P., B. Bellete, F. Durand, H. Raberin, C. Cazorla, J. Hafid, F. Lucht, and R. T. Sung.** 2004. Comparison between real-time PCR, conventional PCR and different staining techniques for diagnosing *Pneumocystis jiroveci* pneumonia from bronchoalveolar lavage specimens. *J. Med. Microbiol.* **53:**603–607.

34. **Gade, W., S. W. Hinnefeld, L. S. Babcock, P. Gilligan, W. Kelly, K. Wait, D. Greer, M. Pinilla, and R. L. Kaplan.** 1991. Comparison of the PREMIER cryptococcal antigen enzyme immunoassay and the latex agglutination assay for detection of cryptococcal antigens. *J. Clin. Microbiol.* **29:**1616–1619.

35. **Galgiani, J. N., T. Peng, M. L. Lewis, G. A. Cloud, D. Pappagianis, and The National Institute of Allergy and Infectious Diseases Mycoses Study Group.** 1996. Cerebrospinal fluid antibodies detected by ELISA against a 33-kDa antigen from spherules of *Coccidioides immitis* in patients with coccidioidal meningitis. *J. Infect. Dis.* **173:**499–502.

36. **Gerber, J. D., R. E. Riley, and R. Jones.** 1972. Evaluation of a microtiter latex agglutination test for histoplasmosis. *Appl. Microbiol.* **24:**191–197.

37. **Gill, V. J., G. Evans, F. Stock, J. E. Parrillo, H. Masur, and J. A. Kovacs.** 1987. Detection of *Pneumocystis carinii* by fluorescent-antibody stain using a combination of three monoclonal antibodies. *J. Clin. Microbiol.* **25:**1837–1840.

38. **Gomes, G. M., P. S. Cisalpino, C. P. Taborda, and Z. P. de Camargo.** 2000. PCR for diagnosis of paracoccidioidomycosis. *J. Clin. Microbiol.* **38:**3478–3480.

39. **Gomez, B. L., J. I. Figueroa, A. J. Hamilton, B. Ortiz, M. A. Robledo, R. J. Hay, and A. Restrepo.** 1997. Use of monoclonal antibodies in diagnosis of paracoccidioidomycosis: new strategies for detection of circulating antigens. *J. Clin. Microbiol.* **35:**3278–3283.

40. **Gomez, B. L., J. I. Figueroa, A. J. Hamilton, B. L. Ortiz, M. A. Robledo, A. Restrepo, and R. J. Hay.** 1997. Development of a novel antigen detection test for histoplasmosis. *J. Clin. Microbiol.* **35:**2618–2622.

41. **Gray, L. D., and G. D. Roberts.** 1988. Experience with the use of pronase to eliminate interference factors in the latex agglutination test for cryptococcal antigen. *J. Clin. Microbiol.* **26:**2450–2451.

42. **Guimaraes, A. J., C. V. Pizzini, H. L. De Matos Guedes, P. C. Albuquerque, J. M. Peralta, A. J. Hamilton, and R. M. Zancope-Oliveira.** 2004. ELISA for early diagnosis of histoplasmosis. *J. Med. Microbiol.* **53:**509–514.

43. **Hamilton, A. J.** 1998. Serodiagnosis of histoplasmosis, paracoccidioidomycosis and penicilliosis marneffei; current status and future trends. *Med. Mycol.* **36:**351–364.

44. **Haynes, K. A., J. P. Latge, and T. R. Rogers.** 1990. Detection of *Aspergillus* antigens associated with invasive infection. *J. Clin. Microbiol.* **28:**2040–2044.

45. **Heiner, D. C.** 1958. Diagnosis of histoplasmosis using precipitin reactions in agar gel. *Pediatrics* **22:**616–627.

46. **Helweg-Larsen, J., J. S. Jensen, T. Benfield, U. G. Svendsen, J. D. Lundgren, and B. Lundgren.** 1998. Diagnostic use of PCR for detection of *Pneumocystis carinii* in oral wash samples. *J. Clin. Microbiol.* **36:**2068–2072.

47. **Herent, P., D. Stynen, F. Hernando, J. Fruit, and D. Poulain.** 1992. Retrospective evaluation of two latex agglutination tests for detection of circulating antigens during invasive candidosis. *J. Clin. Microbiol.* **30:**2158–2164.

48. **Hill, G. B., and C. C. Campbell.** 1962. Commercially available histoplasmin sensitized latex particles in an agglutination test for histoplasmosis. *Mycopathologia* **18:**169–176.

49. **Hsu, M. C., K. W. Chen, H. J. Lo, Y. C. Chen, M. H. Liao, Y. H. Lin, and S. Y. Li.** 2003. Species identification of medically important fungi by use of real-time LightCycler PCR. *J. Med. Microbiol.* **52:**1071–1076.

50. **Hu, S., W. H. Chung, S. I. Hung, H. C. Ho, Z. W. Wang, C. H. Chen, S. C. Lu, T. T. Kuo, and H. S. Hong.** 2003. Detection of *Sporothrix schenckii* in clinical samples by a nested PCR assay. *J. Clin. Microbiol.* **41:**1414–1418.

51. **Huang, S. N., S. H. Fischer, E. O'Shaughnessy, V. J. Gill, H. Masur, and J. A. Kovacs.** 1999. Development of a PCR assay for diagnosis of *Pneumocystis carinii* pneumonia based on amplification of the multicopy major surface glycoprotein gene family. *Diagn. Microbiol. Infect. Dis.* **35:**27–32.

52. **Hube, B.** 1996. *Candida albicans* secreted aspartyl proteinases. *Curr. Top. Med. Mycol.* **7:**55–69.

53. **Huppert, M., E. T. Peterson, S. H. Sun, P. A. Chitjian, and W. J. Derrevere.** 1968. Evaluation of a latex particle agglutination test for coccidioidomycosis. *Am. J. Clin. Pathol.* **49:**96–102.

54. **Hurst, S. F., and L. Kaufman.** 1992. Western immunoblot analysis and serologic characterization of *Blastomyces dermatitidis* yeast form extracellular antigens. *J. Clin. Microbiol.* **30:**3043–3049.

55. **Imhof, A., C. Schaer, G. Schoedon, D. J. Schaer, R. B. Walter, A. Schaffner, and M. Schneemann.** 2003. Rapid detection of pathogenic fungi from clinical specimens using LightCycler real-time fluorescence PCR. *Eur. J. Clin. Microbiol. Infect. Dis.* **22:**558–560.

56. **Ishizuka, Y., H. Tsukada, and F. Gejyo.** 2004. Interference of (1 → 3)-beta-D-glucan administration in the measurement of plasma (1 → 3)-beta-D-glucan. *Intern. Med.* **43:**97–101.

57. **Izacc, S. M., F. J. Gomez, R. S. Jesuino, C. A. Fonseca, M. S. Felipe, G. S. Deepe, and C. M. Soares.** 2001. Molecular cloning, characterization and expression of the heat shock protein 60 gene from the human pathogenic fungus *Paracoccidioides brasiliensis. Med. Mycol.* **39:**445–455.

58. **Jensen, H. E., B. Aalbaek, P. Lind, and H. V. Krogh.** 1996. Immunohistochemical diagnosis of systemic bovine zygomycosis by murine monoclonal antibodies. *Vet. Pathol.* **33:**176–183.

59. **Jensen, H. E., B. Halbaek, P. Lind, H. V. Krogh, and P. L. Frandsen.** 1996. Development of murine monoclonal antibodies for the immunohistochemical diagnosis of systemic bovine aspergillosis. *J. Vet. Diagn. Investig.* **8:**68–75.

60. **Johnson, S. M., and D. Pappagianis.** 1992. The coccidioidal complement fixation and immunodiffusion-complement fixation antigen is a chitinase. *Infect. Immun.* **60:**2588–2592.

61. **Johnson, S. M., C. R. Zimmermann, and D. Pappagianis.** 1996. Use of a recombinant *Coccidioides immitis* complement fixation antigen-chitinase in conventional serological assays. *J. Clin. Microbiol.* **34:**3160–3164.

62. **Jones, K. W., and L. Kaufman.** 1978. Development and evaluation of an immunodiffusion test for diagnosis of systemic zygomycosis (mucormycosis): preliminary report. *J. Clin. Microbiol.* **7:**97–103.

63. **Jones, R. D., G. A. Sarosi, J. D. Parker, R. J. Weeks, and F. E. Tosh.** 1969. The complement-fixation test in extracutaneous sporotrichosis. *Ann. Intern. Med.* **71:**913–918.

64. **Kasolo, F., K. Lishimpi, C. Chintu, P. Mwaba, V. Mudenda, D. Maswahu, H. Terunuma, H. Fletcher, A. Nunn, S. Lucas, and A. Zumla.** 2002. Identification of *Pneumocystis carinii* DNA by polymerase chain reaction in necropsy lung samples from children dying of respiratory tract illnesses. *J. Pediatr.* **140:**367–369.

65. **Kaufman, L., J. A. Kovacs, and E. Reiss.** 1997. Clinical immunomycology, p. 585–604. *In* N. R. Rose, E. C. de Macario, J. D. Folds, H. C. Lane, and R. M. Nakamura (ed.), *Manual of Clinical Laboratory Immunology*, 5th ed. ASM Press, Washington, D.C.

66. **Kaufman, L., L. Mendoza, and P. G. Standard.** 1990. Immunodiffusion test for serodiagnosing subcutaneous zygomycosis. *J. Clin. Microbiol.* **28:**1887–1890.

67. **Kaufman, L., and E. Reiss.** 1992. Serodiagnosis of fungal diseases, p. 506–528. *In* N. R. Rose, E. V. de Macario, J. L. Fahey, H. Friedman, and G. M. Penn (ed.), *Manual of Clinical Laboratory Immunology*, 4th ed. American Society for Microbiology, Washington, D.C.

68. **Kaufman, L., A. S. Sekhon, N. Moledina, M. Jalbert, and D. Pappagianis.** 1995. Comparative evaluation of commercial Premier EIA and microimmunodiffusion and complement fixation tests for *Coccidioides immitis* antibodies. *J. Clin. Microbiol.* **33:**618–619.

69. **Kaufman, L., P. G. Standard, M. Jalbert, P. Kantipong, K. Limpakarnjanarat, and T. D. Mastro.** 1996. Diagnostic antigenemia tests for penicilliosis marneffei. *J. Clin. Microbiol.* **34:**2503–2505.

70. **Kaufman, L., L. F. Turner, and D. W. McLaughlin.** 1989. Indirect enzyme-linked immunosorbent assay for zygomycosis. *J. Clin. Microbiol.* **27:**1979–1982.

71. **Kawazu, M., Y. Kanda, Y. Nannya, K. Aoki, M. Kurokawa, S. Chiba, T. Motokura, H. Hirai, and S. Ogawa.** 2004. Prospective comparison of the diagnostic potential of real-time PCR, double-sandwich enzyme-linked immunosorbent assay for galactomannan, and a (1→3)-beta-D-glucan test in weekly screening for invasive aspergillosis in patients with hematological disorders. *J. Clin. Microbiol.* **42:**2733–2741.

72. **Klein, B. S., and J. M. Jones.** 1994. Purification and characterization of the major antigen WI-1 from *Blastomyces dermatitidis* yeasts and immunological comparison with A antigen. *Infect. Immun.* **62:**3890–3900.

73. **Klein, B. S., J. N. Kuritsky, W. A. Chappell, L. Kaufman, J. Green, S. F. Davies, J. E. Williams, and G. A. Sarosi.** 1986. Comparison of the enzyme immunoassay, immunodiffusion, and complement fixation tests in detecting antibody in human serum to the A antigen of *Blastomyces dermatitidis. Am. Rev. Respir. Dis.* **133:**144–148.

74. **Kobayashi, M., T. Moriki, Y. Uemura, N. Takehara, I. Kubonishi, H. Taguchi, and I. Miyoshi.** 1992. Immunohistochemical detection of *Pneumocystis carinii* in transbronchial lung biopsy specimens: antigen difference between human and rat *Pneumocystis carinii. Jpn. J. Clin. Oncol.* **22:**387–392.

75. **Kobayashi, M., T. Urata, T. Ikezoe, E. Hakoda, Y. Uemura, H. Sonobe, Y. Ohtsuki, T. Manabe, S. Miyagi, and I. Miyoshi.** 1996. Simple detection of the 5S ribosomal RNA of *Pneumocystis carinii* using in situ hybridisation. *J. Clin. Pathol.* **49:**712–716.

76. **Kondori, N., L. Edebo, and I. Mattsby-Baltzer.** 2004. Circulating beta (1-3) glucan and immunoglobulin G subclass antibodies to *Candida albicans* cell wall antigens in

patients with systemic candidiasis. *Clin. Diagn. Lab. Immunol.* **11:**344–350.

77. **Kovacs, J. A., V. Gill, J. C. Swan, F. Ognibene, J. Shelhamer, J. E. Parrillo, and H. Masur.** 1986. Prospective evaluation of a monoclonal antibody in diagnosis of *Pneumocystis carinii* pneumonia. *Lancet* **ii:**1–3.

78. **Kwon-Chung, J., and J. E. Bennett.** 1994. *Medical Mycology.* Lea & Febiger, Malvern, Pa.

79. **Kwon-Chung, K. J., D. Lehman, C. Good, and P. T. Magee.** 1985. Genetic evidence for role of extracellular proteinase in virulence of *Candida albicans. Infect. Immun.* **49:**571–575.

80. **Lambert, R. S., and R. B. George.** 1987. Evaluation of enzyme immunoassay as a rapid screening test for histoplasmosis and blastomycosis. *Am. Rev. Respir. Dis.* **136:**316–319.

81. **Larsen, H. H., L. Huang, J. A. Kovacs, K. Crothers, V. A. Silcott, A. Morris, J. R. Turner, C. B. Beard, H. Masur, and S. H. Fischer.** 2004. A prospective, blinded study of quantitative touch-down polymerase chain reaction using oral-wash samples for diagnosis of *Pneumocystis* pneumonia in HIV-infected patients. *J. Infect. Dis.* **189:**1679–1683.

82. **Larsen, H. H., H. Masur, J. A. Kovacs, V. J. Gill, V. A. Silcott, P. Kogulan, J. Maenza, M. Smith, D. R. Lucey, and S. H. Fischer.** 2002. Development and evaluation of a quantitative, touch-down, real-time PCR assay for diagnosing *Pneumocystis carinii* pneumonia. *J. Clin. Microbiol.* **40:**490–494.

83. **Latge, J. P.** 1999. *Aspergillus fumigatus* and aspergillosis. *Clin. Microbiol. Rev.* **12:**310–350.

84. **Leland, D. S., S. E. Zimmerman, E. B. Cunningham, K. A. Barth, and J. W. Smith.** 1991. Variability in commercial histoplasma complement fixation antigens. *J. Clin. Microbiol.* **29:**1723–1724.

85. **Linares, M. J., M. R. Javier, J. L. Villanueva, F. Solis, J. Torre-Cisneros, F. Rodriguez, J. M. Kindelan, and M. Casal.** 2001. Detection of antibodies to *Candida albicans* germ tubes in heroin addicts with systemic candidiasis. *Clin. Microbiol. Infect.* **7:**218–226.

86. **Lindsley, M. D., S. F. Hurst, N. J. Iqbal, and C. J. Morrison.** 2001. Rapid identification of dimorphic and yeast-like fungal pathogens using specific DNA probes. *J. Clin. Microbiol.* **39:**3505–3511.

87. **Loeffler, J., K. Schmidt, H. Hebart, U. Schumacher, and H. Einsele.** 2002. Automated extraction of genomic DNA from medically important yeast species and filamentous fungi by using the MagNA Pure LC system. *J. Clin. Microbiol.* **40:**2240–2243.

88. **Maaroufi, Y., N. Ahariz, M. Husson, and F. Crokaert.** 2004. Comparison of different methods of isolation of DNA of commonly encountered *Candida* species and its quantitation by using a real-time PCR-based assay. *J. Clin. Microbiol.* **42:**3159–3163.

89. **Mackenzie, D. W., J. F. Soothill, and J. H. Millar.** 1988. Meningitis caused by *Absidia corymbifera. J. Infect.* **17:**241–248.

90. **Marques da Silva, S. H., A. L. Colombo, M. H. Blotta, J. D. Lopes, F. Queiroz-Telles, and Z. Pires de Camargo.** 2003. Detection of circulating gp43 antigen in serum, cerebrospinal fluid, and bronchoalveolar lavage fluid of patients with paracoccidioidomycosis. *J. Clin. Microbiol.* **41:**3675–3680.

91. **Marr, K. A., S. A. Balajee, L. McLaughlin, M. Tabouret, C. Bentsen, and T. J. Walsh.** 2004. Detection of galactomannan antigenemia by enzyme immunoassay for the diagnosis of invasive aspergillosis: variables that affect performance. *J. Infect. Dis.* **190:**641–649.

92. **Martins, T. B., T. D. Jaskowski, C. L. Mouritsen, and H. R. Hill.** 1995. Comparison of commercially available enzyme immunoassay with traditional serological tests for detection of antibodies to *Coccidioides immitis. J. Clin. Microbiol.* **33:**940–943.

93. **Matthews, R. C., J. P. Burnie, and S. Tabaqchali.** 1987. Isolation of immunodominant antigens from sera of patients with systemic candidiasis and characterization of serological response to *Candida albicans. J. Clin. Microbiol.* **25:**230–237.

94. **Mendes-Giannini, M. J., J. P. Bueno, M. A. Shikanai-Yasuda, A. W. Ferreira, and A. Masuda.** 1989. Detection of the 43,000-molecular-weight glycoprotein in sera of patients with paracoccidioidomycosis. *J. Clin. Microbiol.* **27:**2842–2845.

95. **Merz, W. G., G. L. Evans, S. Shadomy, S. Anderson, L. Kaufman, P. J. Kozinn, D. W. Mackenzie, W. P. Protzman, and J. S. Remington.** 1977. Laboratory evaluation of serological tests for systemic candidiasis: a cooperative study. *J. Clin. Microbiol.* **5:**596–603.

96. **Misaki, H., H. Iwasaki, and T. Ueda.** 2003. A comparison of the specificity and sensitivity of two *Candida* antigen assay systems for the diagnosis of deep candidiasis in patients with hematologic diseases. *Med. Sci. Monit.* **9:**MT1–MT7.

97. **Mitsutake, K., T. Miyazaki, T. Tashiro, Y. Yamamoto, H. Kakeya, T. Otsubo, S. Kawamura, M. A. Hossain, T. Noda, Y. Hirakata, and S. Kohno.** 1996. Enolase antigen, mannan antigen, Cand-Tec antigen, and beta-glucan in patients with candidemia. *J. Clin. Microbiol.* **34:**1918–1921.

98. **Moragues, M. D., N. Ortiz, J. R. Iruretagoyena, J. C. Garcia-Ruiz, E. Amutio, A. Rojas, J. Mendoza, G. Quindos, and J. Ponton-San Emeterio.** 2004. Evaluacion de una nueva tecnica comercializada (*Candida albicans* IFA IgG) para el diagnostico de la candidiasis invasiva. *Enferm. Infecc. Microbiol. Clin.* **22:**83–88.

99. **Negroni, R., A. M. Robles, A. L. Arechavala, C. Iovannitti, S. Helou, and L. Kaufman.** 1995. Chronic meningoencephalitis due to *Histoplasma capsulatum.* Usefulness of serodiagnostic procedures in diagnosis. *Serodiagn. Immunother. Infect. Dis.* **7:**84–89.

100. **Ng, V. L., D. M. Yajko, and W. K. Hadley.** 1997. Extrapulmonary pneumocystosis. *Clin. Microbiol. Rev.* **10:**401–418.

101. **Obayashi, T., M. Yoshima, T. Mori, H. Goto, A. Yasuoka, H. Iwasaki, H. Teshima, S. Kohno, A. Horiuchi, and A. Ito.** 1995. Plasma (1→3)-beta-D-glucan measurement in diagnosis of invasive deep mycosis and fungal febrile episodes. *Lancet* **345:**17–20.

102. **Obayashi, T., M. Yoshida, H. Tamura, J. Aketagawa, S. Tanaka, and T. Kawai.** 1992. Determination of plasma (1→3)-beta-D-glucan: a new diagnostic aid to deep mycosis. *J. Med. Vet. Mycol.* **30:**275–280.

103. **Odabasi, Z., G. Mattiuzzi, E. Estey, H. Kantarjian, F. Saeki, R. J. Ridge, P. A. Ketchum, M. A. Finkelman, J. H. Rex, and L. Ostrosky-Zeichner.** 2004. Beta-D-glucan as a diagnostic adjunct for invasive fungal infections: validation, cutoff development, and performance in patients with acute myelogenous leukemia and myelodysplastic syndrome. *Clin. Infect. Dis.* **39:**199–205.

104. **Ortiz, B. L., A. M. Garcia, A. Restrepo, and J. G. McEwen.** 1996. Immunological characterization of a recombinant 27-kilodalton antigenic protein from *Paracoccidioides brasiliensis. Clin. Diag. Lab. Immunol.* **3:**239–241.

105. **Palmer, D. F., L. Kaufman, W. Kaplan, and J. J. Cavalaro.** 1977. *Serodiagnosis of Mycotic Diseases.* Charles C. Thomas, Springfield, Ill.

106. **Panichakul, T., R. Chawengkirttikul, S. C. Chaiyaroj, and S. Sirisinha.** 2002. Development of a monoclonal antibody-based enzyme-linked immunosorbent assay for the diagnosis of *Penicillium marneffei* infection. *Am. J. Trop. Med. Hyg.* **67:**443–447.

107. **Pappagianis, D., and B. L. Zimmer.** 1990. Serology of coccidioidomycosis. *Clin. Microbiol. Rev.* **3:**247–268.

108. **Pazos, C., J. Ponton, and A. Del Palacio.** 2005. Contribution of $(1 \rightarrow 3)$-beta-D-glucan chromogenic assay to diagnosis and therapeutic monitoring of invasive aspergillosis in neutropenic adult patients: a comparison with serial screening for circulating galactomannan. *J. Clin. Microbiol.* **43:**299–305.

109. **Pierce, P. F., Jr., S. L. Solomon, L. Kaufman, V. F. Garagusi, R. H. Parker, and L. Ajello.** 1982. Zygomycetes brain abscesses in narcotic addicts with serological diagnosis. *JAMA* **248:**2881–2882.

110. **Pinlaor, S., P. Mootsikapun, P. Pinlaor, A. Phunmanee, V. Pipitgool, P. Sithithaworn, W. Chumpia, and J. Sithithaworn.** 2004. PCR diagnosis of *Pneumocystis carinii* on sputum and bronchoalveolar lavage samples in immuno-compromised patients. *Parasitol. Res.* **94:**213–218.

111. **Porsius, J. C., H. J. van Vliet, J. H. van Zeijl, W. H. Goessens, and M. F. Michel.** 1990. Detection of an antibody response in immunocompetent patients with systemic candidiasis or *Candida albicans* colonisation. *Eur. J. Clin. Microbiol. Infect. Dis.* **9:**352–355.

112. **Prariyachatigul, C., A. Chaiprasert, K. Geenkajorn, R. Kappe, C. Chuchottaworn, S. Termsetjaroen, and S. Srimuang.** 2003. Development and evaluation of a one-tube seminested PCR assay for the detection and identification of *Penicillium marneffei*. *Mycoses* **46:**447–454.

113. **Puccia, R., S. Schenkman, P. A. Gorin, and L. R. Travassos.** 1986. Exocellular components of *Paracoccidioides brasiliensis*: identification of a specific antigen. *Infect. Immun.* **53:**199–206.

114. **Puccia, R., and L. R. Travassos.** 1991. 43-kilodalton glycoprotein from *Paracoccidioides brasiliensis*: immunochemical reactions with sera from patients with paracoccidioidomycosis, histoplasmosis, or Jorge Lobo's disease. *J. Clin. Microbiol.* **29:**1610–1615.

115. **Quindos, G., M. D. Moragues, and J. Ponton.** 2004. Is there a role for antibody testing in the diagnosis of invasive candidiasis? *Rev. Iberoam. Micol.* **21:**10–14.

116. **Radio, S. J., S. Hansen, J. Goldsmith, and J. Linder.** 1990. Immunohistochemistry of *Pneumocystis carinii* infection. *Mod. Pathol.* **3:**462–469.

117. **Rappelli, P., R. Are, G. Casu, P. L. Fiori, P. Cappuccinelli, and A. Aceti.** 1998. Development of a nested PCR for detection of *Cryptococcus neoformans* in cerebrospinal fluid. *J. Clin. Microbiol.* **36:**3438–3440.

118. **Restrepo-Moreno, A., and J. D. Schneidau, Jr.** 1967. Nature of the skin-reactive principle in culture filtrates prepared from *Paracoccidioides brasiliensis*. *J. Bacteriol.* **93:**1741–1748.

119. **Richardson, R. D., and D. W. Warnock.** 1997. *Fungal Infection. Diagnosis and Management*, 2nd ed. Blackwell Science, Malden, Mass.

120. **Richmond, J. Y., and R. W. Mickinney (ed.).** 1999. *Biosafety in Microbiological and Biomedical Laboratories*, 4th ed. U.S. Government Printing Office, Washington, D.C.

121. **Roberts, G. D., and H. W. Larsh.** 1971. The serologic diagnosis of extracutaneous sporotrichosis. *Am. J. Clin. Pathol.* **56:**597–600.

122. **Rohrlich, P., J. Sarfati, P. Mariani, M. Duval, A. Carol, C. Saint-Martin, E. Bingen, J. P. Latge, and E. Vilmer.** 1996. Prospective sandwich enzyme-linked immunosorbent assay for serum galactomannan: early predictive value and clinical use in invasive aspergillosis. *Pediatr. Infect. Dis. J.* **15:**232–237.

123. **Salina, M. A., M. A. Shikanai-Yasuda, R. P. Mendes, B. Barraviera, and M. J. Mendes Giannini.** 1998. Detection of circulating *Paracoccidioides brasiliensis* antigen in urine of paracoccidioidomycosis patients before and during treatment. *J. Clin. Microbiol.* **36:**1723–1728.

124. **Sandhu, G. S., B. C. Kline, L. Stockman, and G. D. Roberts.** 1995. Molecular probes for diagnosis of fungal infections. *J. Clin. Microbiol.* **33:**2913–2919. (Erratum **34:**1350, 1996.)

125. **Schluger, N., T. Godwin, K. Sepkowitz, D. Armstrong, E. Bernard, M. Rifkin, A. Cerami, and R. Bucala.** 1992. Application of DNA amplification to pneumocystosis: presence of serum *Pneumocystis carinii* DNA during human and experimentally induced *Pneumocystis carinii* pneumonia. *J. Exp. Med.* **176:**1327–1333.

126. **Scott, E. N., L. Kaufman, A. C. Brown, and H. G. Muchmore.** 1987. Serologic studies in the diagnosis and management of meningitis due to *Sporothrix schenckii*. *N. Engl. J. Med.* **317:**935–940.

127. **Sekhon, A. S., A. K. Garg, L. Kaufman, G. S. Kobayashi, Z. Hamir, M. Jalbert, and N. Moledina.** 1993. Evaluation of a commercial enzyme immunoassay for the detection of cryptococcal antigen. *Mycoses* **36:**31–34.

128. **Sekhon, A. S., J. S. Li, and A. K. Garg.** 1982. Penicillosis marneffei: serological and exoantigen studies. *Mycopathologia* **77:**51–57.

129. **Sendid, B., M. Tabouret, J. L. Poirot, D. Mathieu, J. Fruit, and D. Poulain.** 1999. New enzyme immunoassays for sensitive detection of circulating *Candida albicans* mannan and antimannan antibodies: useful combined test for diagnosis of systemic candidiasis. *J. Clin. Microbiol.* **37:**1510–1517.

130. **Sing, A., A. Roggenkamp, I. B. Autenrieth, and J. Heesemann.** 1999. *Pneumocystis carinii* carriage in immunocompetent patients with primary pulmonary disorders as detected by single or nested PCR. *J. Clin. Microbiol.* **37:**3409–3410.

131. **Smith, C. E., M. T. Saito, and S. A. Simons.** 1956. Pattern of 39,500 serologic tests in coccidioidomycosis. *JAMA* **160:**546–552.

132. **Smulian, A. G., M. J. Linke, M. T. Cushion, R. P. Baughman, P. T. Frame, M. N. Dohn, M. L. White, and P. D. Walzer.** 1994. Analysis of *Pneumocystis carinii* organism burden, viability and antigens in bronchoalveolar lavage fluid in AIDS patients with pneumocystosis: correlation with disease severity. *AIDS* **8:**1555–1562.

133. **Stringer, J. R., C. B. Beard, R. F. Miller, and A. E. Wakefield.** 2002. A new name (*Pneumocystis jiroveci*) for *Pneumocystis* from humans. *Emerg. Infect. Dis.* **8:** 891–896.

134. **Stringer, J. R., M. T. Cushion, and A. E. Wakefield.** 2001. New nomenclature for the genus *Pneumocystis*. *J. Eukaryot. Microbiol.* **48** (Suppl.)**:**184S–189S.

135. **Suzuki, S.** 1997. Immunochemical study on mannans of genus *Candida*. I. Structural investigation of antigenic factors 1, 4, 5, 6, 8, 9, 11, 13, 13b and 34. *Curr. Top. Med. Mycol.* **8:**57–70.

136. **Takesue, Y., M. Kakehashi, H. Ohge, Y. Imamura, Y. Murakami, M. Sasaki, M. Morifuji, Y. Yokoyama, M. Kouyama, T. Yokoyama, and T. Sueda.** 2004. Combined assessment of beta-D-glucan and degree of candida colonization before starting empiric therapy for candidiasis in surgical patients. *World J. Surg.* **28:**625–630.

137. **Tamburrini, E., P. Mencarini, E. Visconti, M. Zolfo, A. De Luca, A. Siracusano, E. Ortona, and A. E. Wakefield.** 1996. Detection of *Pneumocystis carinii* DNA in blood by PCR is not of value for diagnosis of *P. carinii* pneumonia. *J. Clin. Microbiol.* **34:**1586–1588.

138. **Tamura, H., Y. Arimoto, S. Tanaka, M. Yoshida, T. Obayashi, and T. Kawai.** 1994. Automated kinetic assay for endotoxin and $(1 \rightarrow 3)$-beta-D-glucan in human blood. *Clin. Chim. Acta* **226:**109–112.

139. **Tanaka, K., T. Miyazaki, S. Maesaki, K. Mitsutake, H. Kakeya, Y. Yamamoto, K. Yanagihara, M. A. Hossain,**

T. Tashiro, and S. Kohno. 1996. Detection of *Cryptococcus neoformans* gene in patients with pulmonary cryptococcosis. *J. Clin. Microbiol.* **34:**2826–2828.

140. Tanner, D. C., M. P. Weinstein, B. Fedorciw, K. L. Joho, J. J. Thorpe, and L. Reller. 1994. Comparison of commercial kits for detection of cryptococcal antigen. *J. Clin. Microbiol.* **32:**1680–1684.

141. Telzak, E. E., and D. Armstrong. 1994. Extrapulmonary infection and other unusual manifastations of *Pneumocystis carinii*, p. 361–380. *In* P. D. Walzer (ed.), *Pneumocystis carinii Pneumonia*, 2nd ed. Marcel Dekker, Inc., New York, N.Y.

142. Temstet, A., P. Roux, J. L. Poirot, O. Ronin, and F. Dromer. 1992. Evaluation of a monoclonal antibody-based latex agglutination test for diagnosis of cryptococcosis: comparison with two tests using polyclonal antibodies. *J. Clin. Microbiol.* **30:**2544–2550.

143. Teramoto, S., D. Sawaki, S. Okada, and Y. Ouchi. 2000. Markedly increased plasma $(1 \rightarrow 3)$-beta-D-glucan is a diagnostic and therapeutic indicator of *Pneumocystis carinii* pneumonia in a non-AIDS patient. *J. Med. Microbiol.* **49:**393–394.

144. Torres, J., M. Goldman, L. J. Wheat, X. Tang, M. S. Bartlett, J. W. Smith, S. D. Allen, and C. H. Lee. 2000. Diagnosis of *Pneumocystis carinii* pneumonia in human immunodeficiency virus-infected patients with polymerase chain reaction: a blinded comparison to standard methods. *Clin. Infect. Dis.* **30:**141–145.

145. Trewatcharegon, S., S. C. Chaiyaroj, P. Chongtrakool, and S. Sirisinha. 2000. Production and characterization of monoclonal antibodies reactive with the mycelial and yeast phases of *Penicillium marneffei*. *Med. Mycol.* **38:**91–96.

146. Tuncer, S., S. Erguven, S. Kocagoz, and S. Unal. 1998. Comparison of cytochemical staining, immunofluorescence and PCR for diagnosis of *Pneumocystis carinii* on sputum samples. *Scand. J. Infect. Dis.* **30:**125–128.

147. Turner, S., and L. Kaufman. 1986. Immunodiagnosis of blastomycosis. *Semin. Respir. Infect.* **1:**22–28.

148. Turner, S., L. Kaufman, and M. Jalbert. 1986. Diagnostic assessment of an enzyme-linked immunosorbent assay for human and canine blastomycosis. *J. Clin. Microbiol.* **23:**294–297.

149. Verweij, P. E., D. Stynen, A. J. Rijs, B. E. de Pauw, J. A. Hoogkamp-Korstanje, and J. F. Meis. 1995. Sandwich enzyme-linked immunosorbent assay compared with Pastorex latex agglutination test for diagnosing invasive aspergillosis in immunocompromised patients. *J. Clin. Microbiol.* **33:**1912–1914.

150. Verweij, P. E., C. M. Weemaes, J. H. Curfs, S. Bretagne, and J. F. Meis. 2000. Failure to detect circulating *Aspergillus* markers in a patient with chronic granulomatous disease and invasive aspergillosis. *J. Clin. Microbiol.* **38:**3900–3901.

151. Viviani, M. A., A. M. Tortorano, G. Rizzardini, T. Quirino, L. Kaufman, A. A. Padhye, and L. Ajello. 1993. Treatment and serological studies of an Italian case of penicilliosis marneffei contracted in Thailand by a drug addict infected with the human immunodeficiency virus. *Eur. J. Epidemiol.* **9:**79–85.

152. Voigt, K., E. Cigelnik, and K. O'Donnell. 1999. Phylogeny and PCR identification of clinically important Zygomycetes based on nuclear ribosomal-DNA sequence data. *J. Clin. Microbiol.* **37:**3957–3964.

153. Wakefield, A. E., A. R. Lindley, H. E. Ambrose, C. M. Denis, and R. F. Miller. 2003. Limited asymptomatic carriage of *Pneumocystis jiroveci* in human immunodeficiency virus-infected patients. *J. Infect. Dis.* **187:**901–908.

154. Wakefield, A. E., F. J. Pixley, S. Banerji, K. Sinclair, R. F. Miller, E. R. Moxon, and J. M. Hopkin. 1990. Amplification of mitochondrial ribosomal RNA sequences from *Pneumocystis carinii* DNA of rat and human origin. *Mol. Biochem. Parasitol.* **43:**69–76.

155. Wakefield, A. E., F. J. Pixley, S. Banerji, K. Sinclair, R. F. Miller, E. R. Moxon, and J. M. Hopkin. 1990. Detection of *Pneumocystis carinii* with DNA amplification. *Lancet* **336:**451–453.

156. Walsh, T. J., and S. J. Chanock. 1998. Diagnosis of invasive fungal infections: advances in nonculture systems. *Curr. Clin. Top. Infect. Dis.* **18:**101–153.

157. Walsh, T. J., J. W. Hathorn, J. D. Sobel, W. G. Merz, V. Sanchez, S. M. Maret, H. R. Buckley, M. A. Pfaller, R. Schaufele, and C. Sliva. 1991. Detection of circulating candida enolase by immunoassay in patients with cancer and invasive candidiasis. *N. Engl. J. Med.* **324:**1026–1031.

158. Warnock, D. W. 1977. Detection of *Aspergillus fumigatus* precipitins: a comparison of counter immunoelectrophoresis and double diffusion. *J. Clin. Pathol.* **30:**388–389.

159. Wheat, J., M. L. French, S. Kamel, and R. P. Tewari. 1986. Evaluation of cross-reactions in *Histoplasma capsulatum* serologic tests. *J. Clin. Microbiol.* **23:**493–499.

160. Wheat, L. J., P. Connolly, M. Durkin, B. K. Book, A. J. Tector, J. Fridell, and M. D. Pescovitz. 2004. False-positive *Histoplasma* antigenemia caused by antithymocyte globulin antibodies. *Transpl. Infect. Dis.* **6:**23–27.

161. Wheat, L. J., P. Connolly-Stringfield, R. Blair, K. Connolly, T. Garringer, B. P. Katz, and M. Gupta. 1992. Effect of successful treatment with amphotericin B on *Histoplasma capsulatum* variety *capsulatum* polysaccharide antigen levels in patients with AIDS and histoplasmosis. *Am. J. Med.* **92:**153–160.

162. Wheat, L. J., T. Garringer, E. Brizendine, and P. Connolly. 2002. Diagnosis of histoplasmosis by antigen detection based upon experience at the histoplasmosis reference laboratory. *Diagn. Microbiol. Infect. Dis.* **43:**29–37.

163. Wiggins, G. L., and J. H. Schubert. 1965. Relationship of histoplasmin agar-gell bands and complement fixation in histoplasmosis. *J. Bacteriol.* **89:**589–596.

164. Williams, B., M. Fojtasek, P. Connolly-Stringfield, and J. Wheat. 1994. Diagnosis of histoplasmosis by antigen detection during an outbreak in Indianapolis, Ind. *Arch. Pathol. Lab. Med.* **118:**1205–1208.

165. Wysong, D. R., and A. R. Waldorf. 1987. Electrophoretic and immunoblot analyses of *Rhizopus arrhizus* antigens. *J. Clin. Microbiol.* **25:**358–363.

166. Yeo, S. F., and B. Wong. 2002. Current status of nonculture methods for diagnosis of invasive fungal infections. *Clin. Microbiol. Rev.* **15:**465–484.

167. Yoshida, M., T. Obayashi, A. Iwama, M. Ito, S. Tsunoda, T. Suzuki, K. Muroi, M. Ohta, S. Sakamoto, and Y. Miura. 1997. Detection of plasma $(1 \rightarrow 3)$-beta-d-glucan in patients with *Fusarium*, *Trichosporon*, *Saccharomyces* and *Acremonium* fungaemias. *J. Med. Vet. Mycol.* **35:**371–374.

168. Yuen, K. Y., S. S. Wong, D. N. Tsang, and P. Y. Chau. 1994. Serodiagnosis of *Penicillium marneffei* infection. *Lancet* **344:**444–445.

169. Zancope-Oliveira, R. M., S. L. Bragg, E. Reiss, and J. M. Peralta. 1994. Immunochemical analysis of the H and M glycoproteins from *Histoplasma capsulatum*. *Clin. Diagn. Lab. Immunol.* **1:**563–568.

170. Zartarian, M., E. M. Peterson, and L. M. de la Maza. 1997. Detection of antibodies to *Coccidioides immitis* by enzyme immunoassay. *Am. J. Clin. Pathol.* **107:**148–153.

171. Zimmer, B. L., and D. Pappagianis. 1988. Characterization of a soluble protein of *Coccidioides immitis* with activity as an immunodiffusion-complement fixation antigen. *J. Clin. Microbiol.* **26:**2250–2256.

VIRAL DISEASES

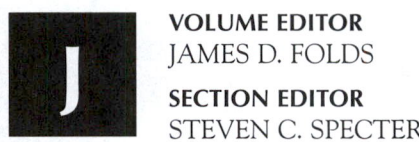

VOLUME EDITOR
JAMES D. FOLDS

SECTION EDITOR
STEVEN C. SPECTER

Introduction

STEVEN C. SPECTER

67

Viral diagnostics has continued to evolve significantly over the past 4 years since the publication of the 6th edition of the *Manual for Clinical Laboratory Immunology*. It is noteworthy that in the Introduction to the 6th edition Virology section there was an indication that increasing dependence would be placed on molecular diagnostic techniques in place of serologic detection of viruses. This is now reflected in the change of the title of the present 7th edition of this volume to *Manual of Molecular and Clinical Laboratory Immunology*.

The reliance on molecular techniques has expanded significantly; they have come into common usage for numerous virus infections. In addition, the number of viral agents recognized to have an etiologic role in human infections continues to expand. However, with all of this change taking place, protection of the blood supply, epidemiology, identification of the etiology of infectious diseases, and the monitoring of the progression of viral diseases in chronic infections continue to be the major reasons for performing laboratory diagnostic studies of viruses.

As we continue to develop new vaccines, antiviral drugs, more sophisticated technologies to detect viruses more rapidly, and better reagents, we have increased our reliance on the diagnostic laboratory. In addition, we have developed methods to combine cell culture diagnostics with direct detection systems, including antibodies, enzyme expression, and molecular methods, to combine viral isolation with identification. As a result we have succeeded in increasing sensitivity, specificity, and rapidity of diagnosis. More than any other advance, molecular diagnostic techniques have been increasingly applied in diagnostic virology and in several cases have become the "gold standard" for viral diagnosis. Furthermore, these molecular techniques can be applied quantitatively as well as qualitatively. As a result, they can be used to determine if there is a significant amount of virus in bodily fluids, determine whether there is a response to therapy, or use viral load as a prognostic indicator of disease progression.

The major pathogenic virus chapters have all been updated and there is considerable useful information on the latest developments in direct detection methods for viruses. This 7th edition has new chapters covering (i) rotavirus and noroviruses; (ii) Marburg, Ebola, and arenaviruses; (iii) coronaviruses including that causing severe acute respiratory distress syndrome, or SARS; (iv) poxviruses; and (v) prions and the transmissible spongiform encephalopathies they induce. In addition, the chapter on respiratory syncytial virus and parainfluenzaviruses has been expanded to include human metapneumovirus, which was not recognized as a human pathogen at last writing.

Rapid viral diagnosis, using a combination of direct detection, serology, cell culture, and molecular diagnostics, is now a reality for most virus diseases. This section provides an overview of the standards for viral diagnostics as well as the latest developments in the discipline.

Rapid Viral Diagnosis

MARIE LOUISE LANDRY

68

Over the past 3 decades, the populations at risk for serious or life-threatening viral infections have increased due to aggressive cancer chemotherapy, transplantation, the AIDS epidemic, and the survival of patients with chronic diseases. Antiviral therapies have become available but must be administered early in disease to be effective. Hence, a rapid diagnosis is essential. Viruses have also been recognized as serious pathogens in normal hosts. A rapid diagnosis can reduce costs of antibiotics, avert unnecessary and costly tests, prevent nosocomial transmission, and lead to shorter hospitalizations. The emergence of new viruses, such as severe acute respiratory syndrome (SARS) coronavirus and avian influenza virus, as well as threats of bioterrorism further underscores the importance of a rapid viral diagnosis.

In response to these needs, there has been an explosion in rapid viral diagnostic test development. Rapid diagnostic tests are now available that can provide results within 15 min of sample collection for some viruses and within hours for others, thus significantly shortening the time to diagnosis over conventional culture methods. Immunoassays provide the most rapid results, with some newer methods consisting of only one step and no reagent additions. Molecular amplification techniques have been significantly shortened by real-time detection and more rapid thermocycling. In addition, culture techniques using two cell cultures combined in one vial followed by pooled monoclonal antibody (MAb) staining facilitate rapid and efficient detection of multiple viruses.

Both the diagnostic techniques and the diagnostic approaches to specific viruses are described in detail in other parts of this manual. Therefore, this chapter will present an overview of rapid viral diagnosis, focusing on the advantages and limitations of common methods used, the factors involved in test selection, the validation and monitoring of test performance, and the critical importance of sample collection.

RAPID DIAGNOSTIC METHODS

The methods used for rapid viral diagnosis can be generally grouped according to the following strategies: (i) direct detection of viral proteins, nucleic acid, or particles in clinical specimens; (ii) biologic amplification of infectious virus in cell culture followed by detection of viral antigens in cultured cells; and (iii) detection of an immunoglobulin M (IgM) antibody response to viral infection. Advantages and limitations of these methods are listed in Table 1. With the exception of electron microscopy (EM), rapid tests detect only the specific agent(s) sought.

Direct Detection of Virus in Clinical Specimens

In general, the most rapid approach is to detect virus directly in clinical samples, rather than wait either for virus to grow in culture or for an antibody response to occur. The continuing improvements in sensitivity, specificity, reproducibility, and ease of use of direct methods have resulted in replacement of culture methods in many situations where only a specific virus is sought.

Viral Antigen

Rapid antigen tests remain the most commonly used of the rapid viral diagnostic methods, because of speed and cost. A number of simpler and more rapid tests have been developed in recent years, especially for influenza virus (13).

EIAs

Enzyme immunoassays (EIAs) detect both viral antigens expressed in infected cells and viral antigens in cell-free clinical samples. Therefore, EIAs can be used on respiratory samples and on samples such as serum and stool. Convenient commercial kits are available in a variety of formats. The methodology is well suited to automated, high-volume, batched-sample testing, with results determined by spectrophotometers and analyzed by computer. Alternatively, rapid membrane EIAs in single-sample cassettes with 15- to 30-min assay times can be used even in small laboratories or doctors' offices, and testing can be performed multiple times a day as needed.

However, with EIAs one cannot assess the quality of the sample and cannot distinguish nonspecific reactions unless a neutralization or blocking antibody test is done, which can greatly increase turnaround times. In serum, antibody present in the sample can bind antigen, rendering it undetectable; immune complex dissociation can improve sensitivity.

EIAs have been most successful in detecting viral antigens when high titers are present in clinical samples and have been especially useful for viruses that do not grow in routine cell cultures, such as rotavirus, hepatitis B virus (HBV), and enteric adenovirus. EIAs can provide same-day diagnosis and thus allow earlier intervention than culture methods for respiratory syncytial virus (RSV) and influenza

TABLE 1 Advantages and limitations of rapid viral diagnostic methods[a]

Rapid method	Common clinical applications	Time required	Advantages	Limitations[b]
Direct detection EIA Membrane	RSV, influenza virus, rotavirus	0.25–0.5 h	Simple format, minimal training required; can test single or multiple samples and run test multiple times a day; no major equipment	Relatively expensive per-test reagent; nonspecific reactions difficult to detect; single agent detected
Microwell, tube, or bead	RSV, rotavirus, HBV, HIV-1, influenza virus, HSV, adenovirus	2–4 h	Suitable for large test volumes, batching of samples; breakaway strips for smaller sample size; cheaper per-test reagent costs; objective endpoints, computerized data analysis, automated format	Sensitivity varies with virus and kit used; neutralization test needed to detect nonspecific reactions; multiple controls processed with each run; EIA reader and washer, multichannel pipette required
Latex agglutination	Rotavirus, enteric adenovirus	0.5 h	Simple format, no major equipment; suitable for single-sample testing	Subjective; weak positives difficult to read; nonspecific reactions; not as sensitive as EIA
Other rapid formats (IC, LFA, IGA, OIA, EVEA)[c]	Influenza virus, RSV, rotavirus	0.25–0.5 h	Simple format, some only one step; no major equipment; suitable for single-sample testing	Subjective; weak positives difficult to read; may have more false positives than EIA
Immunostaining: IF or IP	RSV, influenza virus, parainfluenza virus and adenovirus in respiratory cells; VZV and HSV in skin lesion smears; CMV in leukocytes	0.5–2 h	Can evaluate quality of sample, characteristic staining pattern and morphology; can detect a single positive cell, multiple pathogens in single sample, or quantitate CMV load in leukocytes; can test single or multiple samples; can run test multiple times a day	Requires significant expertise and training; endpoints subjective; needs good sample with adequate cells; requires fluorescence microscope with good-quality objectives for IF; cytocentrifuge desirable
Amplification techniques: PCR, NASBA, bDNA, hybrid capture	HIV-1 RNA and DNA, HBV, HCV, HTLV-1/2; herpes-, entero-, parvo-, adeno-, papilloma-, and polyomaviruses; respiratory viruses	3–9 h	Sensitivity generally exceeds that of culture; replaces hazardous, insensitive, and/or slow methods; potentially quantitative; high-quality, standardized commercial kits with EIA or real-time detection formats; multiplex formats can detect multiple agents, though sensitivity may decrease	Cross-contamination a problem, especially with PCR; amplification inhibitors may be present; reagents expensive; molecular expertise, meticulous technique, and quality control essential; in-house methods not standardized; extensive space (3 rooms) needed; expensive equipment requirements
EM (negative staining)	Gastroenteritis viruses	0.5–1 h	Open minded; can directly visualize virus and discover unsuspected or new viruses; can rapidly differentiate smallpox virus from VZV	Expensive equipment, extensive expertise needed; high viral titers required
Rapid culture[d] SVCC	CMV, VZV, HSV, respiratory viruses, adenoviruses, enteroviruses, HHV-6, and polyomavirus BK	16–48 h	Centrifugation enhances infectivity; characteristic staining pattern enhances specificity; can detect a single positive cell; can detect multiple viruses in one culture by combining two cell cultures in one shell vial and staining with pool of antibodies; detects replicating and not latent virus	Cell culture toxicity and contamination can reduce sensitivity; requires infectious virus; labor-intensive; need expertise in cell culture and IF; tissue culture facilities, centrifuge, and fluorescence microscope required
Immune response IgM antibody: capture EIA, IF	Parvovirus, EBV, arboviruses including West Nile virus, HBV, HAV, rubella, measles, CMV	2–4 h	Valuable when culture or antigen methods are not available or molecular methods are less sensitive; for parvovirus (fifth disease), HAV, HBV, and primary EBV, IgM antibodies detectable in almost all patients at clinical presentation	Compromised hosts and neonates may not have detectable antibodies; heterologous antibody rises can occur; appearance of IgM can be delayed until second week of illness; RF and IgG may interfere

[a]HIV-1, HIV type 1; HTLV-1/2, human T-cell leukemia virus type 1 or 2; HHV-6, human herpesvirus 6; bDNA, branched DNA.
[b]All rapid methods except EM are limited to the detection of suspected viruses; an unexpected or new virus will not be discovered.
[c]IC, immunochromatography; LFA, lateral flow assay; IGA, immunogold assay; OIA, optical immunoassay; EVEA, endogenous viral enzyme assay.
[d]Limited to viruses that grow in commonly available cell cultures.

viruses. Microtiter EIAs may be batched and not performed daily if sample numbers are insufficient. In contrast, membrane EIAs can be performed 24 h a day, whenever a rapid diagnosis is needed. Although readily implemented in laboratories without virology experience, EIAs may not be commercially available for the desired pathogen.

Agglutination

The advantages of agglutination assays include simplicity, speed, and lack of expensive equipment. However, the sensitivities are not as high as that of EIA (17). When the specimens contain large amounts of viral antigen, agglutination can be used with acceptable results. This would include rotavirus and enteric adenovirus in stools of infants with gastroenteritis. When antigen is present in great excess, however, a prozone reaction can occur, leading to a false-negative result. This can be detected by repeating the test at a higher sample dilution. The visual reading of agglutination is subjective, and reading borderline samples requires considerable expertise. In addition, some stools can agglutinate control beads. Nevertheless, this test can be used in smaller outpatient laboratories and in doctors' offices.

Other Rapid Antigen Formats

In recent years, a variety of other rapid test formats have become commercially available, especially for influenza A and B viruses and RSV (13). Whereas membrane EIAs usually involve a series of steps, including reagent additions, washes, and addition of stop reagent, newer rapid formats such as lateral flow immunochromatography require addition of one or no reagent and thus are very simple to perform. Optical immunoassays allow visualization of a physical change in molecular thin films, caused by antigen-antibody binding. One rapid influenza virus test utilizes an endogenous virus-encoded enzyme, influenza virus neuraminidase, to cleave a substrate and produce a colored product. Disadvantages include subjective interpretation, lack of automation, and lower sensitivity than immunofluorescence (IF) or culture methods.

IF

IF is a demanding technique that requires careful attention to detail throughout. Personnel training is significantly more rigorous for IF than for EIA. Since viral proteins are visualized in infected cells, IF is limited to samples that contain sufficient numbers of target cells. IF is commonly performed on cell smears from skin lesions, nasopharyngeal (NP) aspirates, tissue touch preparations, and peripheral blood leukocytes (PBLs). Advantages of IF include the opportunity to assess the quality of the sample, to discern specific from nonspecific staining patterns, to detect a single infected cell, and to test one sample for multiple viral pathogens. It can be applied to single or multiple samples, and per-test reagent costs are generally less than for other methods.

Recent improvements include shortening staining incubation time to as little as 20 min, using cytocentrifugation to enhance slide quality, and combining antibodies with different fluorochrome labels, such as fluorescein isothiocyanate and rhodamine B, to simultaneously detect and differentiate multiple viruses on the same slide. This approach has been used successfully to test for herpes simplex virus (HSV) and varicella-zoster virus (VZV) simultaneously in cell smears from skin lesions (1). In addition, a pool of MAbs to seven respiratory viruses can be used for detection of RSV, influenza viruses A and B, parainfluenza viruses 1, 2, and 3, and adenovirus in a single cell smear within 1 to 2 h of receipt of the sample, without compromising test sensitivity

(Color Plate 9) (7). Immunoperoxidase (IP) staining can be used in place of IF. IP slides are permanent and can be read with a light microscope; however, IP staining requires an extra step, the addition of a substrate.

The essential prerequisites for accurate IF testing are an experienced and well-trained microscopist, high-quality antibodies, a fluorescence microscope, and a sufficient and steady flow of samples to develop and maintain expertise. IF also works best in settings that allow education in sample collection and the ability to re-collect inadequate specimens. Established criteria for interpretation must be strictly followed, and results should be validated initially and intermittently thereafter by culture or other methods. MAbs have replaced polyclonal antibodies in most assays. However, low affinity and too narrow specificity of MAbs can be problems for clinical diagnosis, and a pool of two or more MAbs may be required. Antibodies should be selected specifically for the assay and sample type for which they will be used. For example, when cytomegalovirus (CMV) antigen is being detected in PBLs, a pool of MAbs to CMV matrix protein pp65 gives the best results (4). In contrast, early detection of CMV in shell vial centrifugation cultures requires an antibody to an immediate-early CMV protein. MAbs are now commercially available for most common viruses, allowing wide application of IF to clinical diagnosis.

IF staining is more sensitive than culture for detection of RSV in NP aspirates, VZV in skin lesions, and CMV in blood leukocytes. In addition, detection of CMV pp65 antigen in PBLs (Color Plate 10) allows direct quantitation of viral load in the blood, which correlates with clinical disease and can be used to monitor response to treatment. CMV antigenemia on PBLs can be as sensitive as CMV PCR on plasma and can be completed within 2 h (6). The sensitivity for other viruses or sample types is variable, ranging from 60 to 95% of that achieved by culture (7).

Viral Nucleic Acid

Amplification Methods

New developments in amplification methods continue to generate great interest in clinical laboratories due to their sensitivity and speed. In an age of SARS, avian influenza, and bioterrorism, the ability to inactivate virus prior to laboratory analysis is also very appealing. Nucleic acid amplification techniques biochemically amplify either a nucleic acid sequence or a detector molecule, resulting in a sensitivity that equals or exceeds those of culture methods. These methods have found their greatest initial application in the detection of viruses for which other methods are either too expensive, slow, or insensitive or simply unavailable, such as the detection of viruses in cerebrospinal fluid of patients with infections of the nervous system (e.g., enterovirus, HSV, and CMV); detection of human immunodeficiency virus (HIV), HBV, and hepatitis C virus (HCV) in blood; and detection of parvovirus B19 in immunocompromised hosts. In addition, amplification methods are amenable to quantification and thus have been extremely useful in monitoring viral load and response to therapy (e.g., HIV, HBV, HCV, and CMV). Furthermore, DNA is generally more stable than antigen or infectious virus, an important consideration when processing is delayed or samples are shipped to a distant reference laboratory.

To date, the most widely applied method is PCR. Initial PCR formats involved amplification of DNA in a thermal cycler followed by detection of the amplified product (amplicon) by gel electrophoresis, Southern blotting, or spot hybridization. Nested PCR methods provide increased sensitivity but are at high risk for cross-contamination. The development of commercial kits, enzyme-linked amplicon hybridization detection in microtiter plates, strict quality control guidelines, and strategies to prevent cross-contamination have all been important advances.

Recent emphasis has been on real-time detection methods that eliminate the need for a separate step to detect amplified products. Instead, an indicator or reporter is generated as amplification is occurring, and can be monitored in real time. Real-time assays are especially suitable for quantification of target. A high viral load may correlate with clinical disease, prognosis, and response to treatment, especially in compromised hosts. In addition, thermal cyclers with more rapid temperature cycling have been devised, such as LightCycler and Smartcycler, to shorten amplification time. Automated nucleic acid extraction instruments, commonly used in high-volume laboratories, result in both labor and time savings.

It is critical to note that in-house methods, including those used by reference laboratories, are not standardized. Sensitivity varies tremendously, due to different primers and probes, extraction methods, amplification protocols, detection methods, and platforms used, and cross-contamination remains a concern. Blind interlaboratory comparisons of PCR methods have found significant variation in both sensitivity and specificity among laboratories (10, 12). Thus, PCR results should be carefully monitored and performance characteristics should be clearly defined.

Signal amplification methods are also available in commercial kits and are widely used for genome detection and quantification. While slightly less sensitive than PCR, these methods do not suffer from amplicon carryover, are highly reproducible, and have a large dynamic range which facilitates quantification. Nucleic acid sequence-based amplification (NASBA) is very sensitive for RNA targets, and a basic kit that can be used in many applications is available (8). Since amplified product consists of single-stranded RNA transcripts, contamination of the environment is less of a problem than with DNA amplicons of PCR.

It should be kept in mind, however, that these highly sensitive methods are capable of detecting nonreplicating as well as replicating virus. Many of the viruses sought cause almost universal infection and persist in the host for life (e.g., herpesviruses and polyomaviruses). Thus, the clinical significance of a qualitative positive result, as well as the predictive value of a quantitative result, may be unclear and may vary among laboratories due to different methods employed.

Clinical use continues to increase, and in some large reference laboratories, amplification methods have essentially replaced cell culture (2). For the smaller laboratory, limitations include the need for molecular expertise and expensive equipment, extensive in-house validation required for all non-Food and Drug Administration-approved assays, and sufficient test volumes to make testing cost-effective. The costs of doing separate PCR assays for each virus in the differential can also be prohibitive. Development of multiplex assays, which detect multiple pathogens in a single assay, will help to reduce costs while broadening clinical utility (14).

Nucleic Acid Hybridization

Nucleic acid hybridization techniques without amplification are not widely used in diagnostic laboratories due to lack of sensitivity. However, in situ hybridization, which can provide cellular localization, remains a useful tool in pathology laboratories. Examples include the detection of the Epstein-Barr virus (EBV) genome in tumor tissue, human polyomavirus (JC) in brain tissue, or human papillomavirus in anogenital samples.

Viral Particles

EM

By use of EM, viral particles can be directly visualized. EM has received renewed attention recently due to concerns about the reintroduction of smallpox as a weapon of bioterrorism and due to the role of EM in the discovery of SARS coronavirus. Samples for EM can be processed within minutes by the negative staining technique. The limit of detection for negative staining is 10^7 to 10^8 virus particles/ml, but the sensitivity can be increased 100- to 1,000-fold by sample concentration with an airfuge. Addition of specific antibody aggregates virus particles, and the immune complexes thus formed can be directly visualized (immunoelectron microscopy). Antibody labeling with colloidal gold also enhances detection of virus. EM is a very labor-intensive and highly skilled procedure, and the basic equipment is very expensive to purchase and maintain. Nevertheless, it remains useful for the discovery and detection of a myriad of noncultivable gastroenteritis viruses and continues to be extremely useful for the detection and identification of unusual, unexpected, or new viruses.

Detection of Virus after Cell Culture Amplification

By this approach, the sensitivity of cell culture is combined with the speed of antigen detection. Isolation of virus by conventional methods involves infection of susceptible cell cultures followed by periodic examination of the cell monolayers for characteristic cytopathic effects (CPE). Depending upon the virus, the inoculum dose, and the cell system used, CPE may appear in less than 24 h to more than 3 weeks after infection. Early detection of viral proteins or nucleic acid, before CPE appears, shortens the time to reportable results. The greatest time savings are obtained for viruses with long replication cycles, and when antibodies to early replication proteins are available. A centrifugation step can be substituted for the standard stationary virus adsorption step to enhance virus infectivity and shorten time to detection.

Several formats for culture amplified rapid diagnosis have been used. Currently, the most common formats are: (i) inoculation of centrifugation cultures in shell vials or multiwell plates, followed by IP or IF staining at 1 to 2 days and microscopic examination; and (ii) inoculation of mixed cell cultures, either stationary or with centrifugation, followed by staining with pooled antibodies (Color Plate 11) (3, 9). The latter method reduces the number of cultures inoculated, read, and stained, while not sacrificing sensitivity for the spectrum of viruses detected. Mixed cell cultures, with corresponding pooled antibodies, are available for respiratory viruses, enteroviruses, and herpesviruses (i.e., HSV, VZV, and CMV).

Another approach to culture-amplified rapid diagnostic testing uses genetically altered cells. In one virus-inducible system, HSV infection activates a viral promoter which then triggers the production of beta-galactosidase (16). The addition of the substrate X-Gal (5-bromo-4-chloro-3-indolyl-β-D-galactopyranoside) results in a blue precipitate on infected cells. No antibodies, conjugates, or probes are needed.

Methods using microscopy and IF or IP have the ability to detect a single infected cell and to assess the morphology of the stained cell. Furthermore, nonspecific staining is less of a problem with cell culture monolayers than with clinical samples and training is more readily obtained. Both formats are helpful to laboratories lacking experience in discerning viral CPE. Multiple viruses can be detected by using a combined antibody pool to screen cultures, followed by separate antibodies to identify specific pathogens, or by using antibodies with different fluorochrome labels.

The optimal staining time after infection varies with the antibody, the virus, the inoculum dose (an unknown for clinical samples), and the susceptibility of the cell culture. One or 2 days' incubation will give a rapid turnaround but may miss low-titered samples. A longer incubation of 3 to 5 days may be necessary for maximum sensitivity, especially for adenovirus and VZV. In addition, samples may be toxic to the cell monolayers, reducing their ability to support viral replication.

Antibody Response

Rapid diagnostic techniques relying on the immune response have some basic limitations. Antibody develops in response to viral replication and therefore appears later. Thus, IgM is useful primarily when viral detection methods are not readily available or are too slow to give clinically useful results. Examples include arboviruses, rubella virus, and measles virus. IgM antibodies can usually be detected within 5 to 7 days of clinical symptoms but may require up to 2 weeks. For some virus infections, the clinical symptoms prompting medical attention are immune mediated; therefore, IgM is usually detectable at presentation (e.g., fifth disease due to parvovirus B19, EBV, hepatitis A virus [HAV], and HBV).

Limitations of IgM testing include weak or undetectable antibody responses in immunocompromised patients or neonates, heterologous IgM responses, interference by IgM class rheumatoid factor (RF), competition between IgG and IgM antibodies leading to false positives and false negatives, variability in test methods, failure to detect IgM due to timing of sample collection, persistence of IgM in some chronic or persistent viral infections, and frequent absence of IgM in reinfections or reactivations. For CMV, IgM antibody increases with age in seropositive individuals, presumably due to subclinical reactivation. Cross-reactions between anti-parvovirus, -rubella, and -measles IgM is a particular problem if a rash in pregnancy is being investigated. Hopefully, the use of synthetic peptides to replace virion antigen-based immunoassays will reduce interference by RF, nonspecific reactions, and cross-reactivity (15).

TEST SELECTION

Since each diagnostic method has advantages and limitations, test selection is ultimately a compromise that should be made with careful consideration of numerous factors. The sensitivity and specificity of a particular method will vary, depending upon the virus, the patient population, the sample type, and the laboratory setting. Nevertheless, the test selection process itself should be similar among laboratories and can be envisioned as a series of steps (Table 2).

The process should begin with a clear assessment and understanding of clinical needs. Therefore, the first step is to communicate with clinicians. Priorities should be established on the basis of knowledge of the patient populations served, the major viral pathogens in those populations, and in what settings intervention, either therapeutic or preventive, would be benefited by a laboratory diagnosis. In specific clinical situations, what test characteristics are most critical—sensitivity, specificity, or rapidity of results? Unfortunately, the most rapid method may not be the most sensitive.

The next step is to evaluate the methods available. For some viruses, the choices are currently limited. For others, there are several acceptable methods and numerous

TABLE 2 Guidelines for test selection

Step
Communicate and establish priorities together with clinicians according to:
Patient populations served
Major viral pathogens
Treatment and prevention strategies
Evaluate characteristics of available tests:
Commercial products vs in-house methods
Product literature, publications, experience of other laboratories
Personnel expertise and training requirements
Sensitivity, specificity, and turnaround time
Fit with laboratory workflow and hours of operation
Reagent cost, personnel time, reimbursement
Equipment and space required
Make test selection
Evaluate and validate test in-house
Educate clinicians in sample collection and test performance characteristics
Monitor test performance and periodically reevaluate
Communicate with clinicians for feedback

commercial products to choose from. Turnaround time, anticipated test volume, personnel expertise, fit with laboratory workflow, cost, equipment needed, etc., should be carefully considered.

In smaller hospital laboratories, testing may be limited to membrane EIAs or other rapid test formats suitable to small test volumes, and with less demanding training requirements. In laboratories serving large tertiary care hospitals, multiple methodologies are commonly available, including IF and nucleic acid amplification tests, and algorithms for test use should be in place. However, during hours when the virology laboratory is closed or has minimal staffing, EIA can be used in lieu of more technically demanding assays.

DIAGNOSTIC ALGORITHMS

While there is no consensus on the details of diagnostic algorithms for specific viruses, they must be developed in every laboratory, keeping in mind the limitations of each method and, most importantly, how results will be utilized clinically. A choice of tests accompanied by recommendations can be provided to the physician, or the diagnostic algorithm can be internal to the laboratory. The tests used will vary with the season, the clinical disease, age, risk factors, immune competence, and severity of illness. Diagnosis of RSV is given as an example in Fig. 1. In the normal child, if the rapid RSV antigen test is positive, detection of additional viruses does not appear to affect patient outcome and thus may not be justified. If the rapid test is negative but the purpose of the test is to cohort patients on admission to the hospital, a multiplex IF test could be done. Culture results available even 1 to 2 days later may be too late for infection control purposes, since many children will be ready for discharge by then. However, for a hospitalized patient, determining an accurate etiology may be important even if results are delayed.

Methods able to detect a spectrum of pathogens include IF, shell vial centrifugation culture (SVCC), conventional culture, and multiplex PCR. Laboratories capable of doing IF can screen for multiple respiratory pathogens in a single cell spot by using pooled MAbs and have results within 2 h of sample receipt (7). Alternatively, SVCC with pooled antibodies has

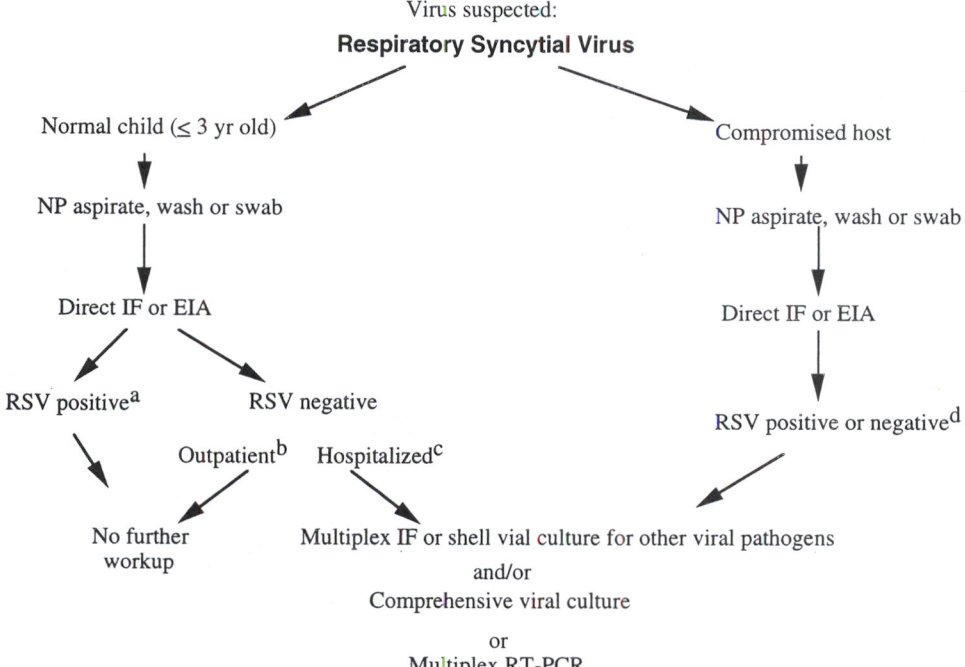

Virus suspected:
Respiratory Syncytial Virus

Normal child (≤ 3 yr old)

NP aspirate, wash or swab

Direct IF or EIA

RSV positive[a]　　　RSV negative

Outpatient[b]　Hospitalized[c]

No further workup

Multiplex IF or shell vial culture for other viral pathogens
and/or
Comprehensive viral culture

or
Multiplex RT-PCR

Compromised host

NP aspirate, wash or swab

Direct IF or EIA

RSV positive or negative[d]

FIGURE 1 Example of a diagnostic algorithm for RSV. (a) Coinfection with multiple viral pathogens does not appear to affect the outcome of RSV infection in the healthy child. (b) For the outpatient, no additional tests or a rapid influenza test may be indicated. (c) For the hospitalized child, either one or several tests can be done, depending upon the severity of illness, the resources available, and the need to cohort patients infected with other viral pathogens. (d) In compromised hosts, a comprehensive workup, including detection of mixed infections, is often indicated.

yielded acceptable results at 1 to 2 days for most common viruses (3, 9). Reports of multiplex PCRs have been published, but these PCRs are not widely available for clinical use. Since all methods miss a proportion of true positives, laboratories may employ multiple methods. To properly design a diagnostic algorithm, data on outcomes should be collected and analyzed to assess the benefits and the cost of each approach. It is apparent that appropriate testing requires clinical information. If this information is lacking, inadequate or superfluous laboratory testing can occur.

VALIDATION AND MONITORING OF TEST PERFORMANCE

Once a test is selected, it must be evaluated in the laboratory. It is important to establish how the test functions in the unique setting into which it will be introduced and to not rely on the manufacturer's claims in the package insert or publications from other institutions. If on initial evaluation the test does not function as anticipated, the reasons should be investigated (e.g., poor sample collection, improper test procedure, different patient population, lack of technical expertise, etc.) and corrective action should be taken or a more suitable method employed. Furthermore, each test offered by the laboratory should be monitored and periodically reevaluated to assess its performance and to determine whether it continues to serve the needs of patients and physicians. Test validation and monitoring are facilitated when more than one technique for a specific virus is in use in the laboratory. Use of two tests, such as IF and culture, in at least a proportion of patients facilitates training, serves as a cross-check, and increases expertise. For direct IF and in-house amplification methods in particular, the

pitfalls are many and careful monitoring of results is critical. Active seeking of both clinical correlation and feedback from clinicians is essential and should be ongoing.

THE IMPORTANCE OF SAMPLE COLLECTION

Poor specimens yield poor results, yet most physicians are unaware of the importance of or the factors involved in proper sample collection. The best samples contain high viral titers and/or numbers of infected target cells. Taking respiratory disease as an example, NP washes and NP aspirates give the highest yield of positive test results. NP swabs give variable results in inexperienced hands (5). Throat swabs (TS) have the lowest yield and are unacceptable for IF since they contain predominantly squamous and not ciliated epithelial cells. If TS are collected for culture or EIA, a combination of TS and NP swab in a single vial is recommended to improve results.

Samples should be collected early in illness, when virus titers are highest, using correct technique and swabs or tissues placed in transport medium appropriate for the tests to be performed. Body fluids should be submitted in sufficient volume for adequate testing. Transportation to the laboratory should be prompt, and samples for culture or IF should be kept on ice if a delay is anticipated. Alternatively, cells from lesions or NP swabs can be applied to slides and fixed in acetone immediately after collection. For CMV antigenemia, blood samples must be processed and leukocytes must be fixed within 6 h of collection for accurate quantitation; a decline in antigen-positive cells can be minimized by storage at 4°C. Nucleic acid amplification tests are also adversely affected by poor sample collection and handling, and requirements for samples for quantitative tests especially should be strictly followed.

Note that in published reports, individuals may have been trained in sample collection for the purpose of the study. The samples routinely submitted to clinical laboratories are collected by untrained persons and often yield inferior results. Since a significant percentage of samples submitted for IF can be inadequate or uninterpretable, IF may not be suitable for large reference laboratories where there is little control over sample collection or opportunity for re-collection.

For nucleic acid detection and quantitation methods, the sample types tested significantly impact the test sensitivity and viral load measurements. It has been shown that higher virus titers are found in plasma than in serum. For cell-associated viruses such as HIV and CMV, PBLs and whole blood contain more virus than does plasma alone.

Lastly, it has been shown that when physicians call the laboratory for advice prior to sample collection, the isolation rate doubles (11). Thus, unless clinicians are educated in sample collection procedures, the substantial effort expended on selecting the most sensitive test method will not yield the desired results.

SUMMARY AND CONCLUSIONS

The choices for rapid viral diagnosis continue to increase. A variety of test formats are available, from walk-away automated systems with computer-generated printouts to single-specimen membrane immunoassays read visually. Nucleic acid hybridization and amplification methods continue to evolve at a dazzling rate, with increasing automation in nucleic acid extraction, amplification, and detection, real-time reporting of amplification results, and faster time to result. Thus, viral diagnosis is no longer an esoteric discipline confined to a small number of university laboratories and state health departments but is becoming increasingly commonplace in community hospitals and even doctors' offices.

Since no method is 100% sensitive and specific and all rapid tests are limited in scope, test selection is ultimately a compromise that should be made with careful consideration of numerous factors. The number and types of techniques chosen will vary with the individual viruses, laboratory expertise, and clinical needs and will continue to change as both test methods and antiviral therapy evolve and improve. Laboratories must know the limitations of the tests offered—specifically, the performance of each test in their hands, with their transport system and their patient population—and communicate this information to clinicians. Once introduced, tests should be routinely monitored and periodically reevaluated.

To provide clinically relevant, cost-effective, and accurate information for patient management, it is important to go beyond the confines of the laboratory, to work with clinicians in establishing priorities, improving sample collection, and seeking clinical correlation and feedback.

REFERENCES

1. **Brumback, B. G., P. G. Farthing, and S. N. Castellino.** 1993. Simultaneous detection of and differentiation between herpes simplex and varicella-zoster viruses with two fluorescent probes in the same test system. *J. Clin. Microbiol.* **31:**3260–3263.
2. **Espy, M. J., P. N. Rys, A. D. Wold, J. R. Uhl, L. M. Sloan, G. D. Jenkins, D. M. Ilstrup, F. R. Cockerill III, R. Patel, J. E. Rosenblatt, and T. F. Smith.** 2001. Detection of herpes simplex virus DNA in genital and dermal specimens by LightCycler PCR after extraction using the IsoQuick, MagNA Pure, and BioRobot 9604 methods. *J. Clin. Microbiol.* **39:**2233–2236.
3. **Fong, C. K., M. K. Lee, and B. P. Griffith.** 2000. Evaluation of R-Mix FreshCells in shell vials for detection of respiratory viruses. *J. Clin. Microbiol.* **38:**4660–4662.
4. **Gerna, G., M. G. Revello, E. Percivalle, and F. Morini.** 1992. Comparison of different immunostaining techniques and monoclonal antibodies to the lower matrix phosphoprotein (pp65) for optimal quantitation of human cytomegalovirus antigenemia. *J. Clin. Microbiol.* **30:**1232–1237.
5. **Landry, M. L., S. Cohen, and D. Ferguson.** 2000. Impact of sample type on rapid detection of influenza virus A by cytospin-enhanced immunofluorescence and membrane enzyme-linked immunosorbent assay. *J. Clin. Microbiol.* **38:**429–430.
6. **Landry, M. L., and D. Ferguson.** 2000. 2-Hour cytomegalovirus pp65 antigenemia assay for rapid quantitation of cytomegalovirus in blood samples. *J. Clin. Microbiol.* **38:**427–428.
7. **Landry, M. L., and D. Ferguson.** 2000. SimulFluor respiratory screen for rapid detection of multiple respiratory viruses in clinical specimens by immunofluorescence staining. *J. Clin. Microbiol.* **38:**708–711.
8. **Landry, M. L., R. Garner, and D. Ferguson.** 2003. Rapid enterovirus RNA detection in clinical specimens by using nucleic acid sequence-based amplification. *J. Clin. Microbiol.* **41:**346–350.
9. **Navarro-Mari, J. M., S. Sanbonmatsu-Gamez, M. Perez-Ruiz, and M. De La Rosa-Fraile.** 1999. Rapid detection of respiratory viruses by shell vial assay using simultaneous culture of HEp-2, LLC-MK2, and MDCK cells in a single vial. *J. Clin. Microbiol.* **37:**2346–2347.
10. **Pembrey, L., M. L. Newell, P. A. Tovo, H. van Drimmelen, I. Quinti, G. Furlini, S. Galli, M. G. Meliconi, S. Burns, N. Hallam, A. Sonnerborg, G. Cilla, E. Serrano, P. Laccetti, G. Portella, S. Polywka, G. Icardi, B. Bruzzone, L. Balbo, and A. Alfarano.** 2003. Inter-laboratory comparison of HCV-RNA assay results: implications for multicentre research. *J. Med. Virol.* **69:**195–201.
11. **Ray, C. G., and L. L. Minnich.** 1987. Efficiency of immunofluorescence for rapid detection of common respiratory viruses. *J. Clin. Microbiol.* **25:**355–357.
12. **Schloss, L., A. M. van Loon, P. Cinque, G. Cleator, J. M. Echevarria, K. I. Falk, P. Klapper, J. Schirm, B. F. Vestergaard, H. Niesters, T. Popow-Kraupp, W. Quint, and A. Linde.** 2003. An international external quality assessment of nucleic acid amplification of herpes simplex virus. *J. Clin. Virol.* **28:**175–185.
13. **Storch, G. A.** 2003. Rapid diagnostic tests for influenza. *Curr. Opin. Pediatr.* **15:**77–84.
14. **Templeton, K. E., S. A. Scheltinga, M. F. C. Beersma, A. C. M. Kroes, and E. C. J. Claas.** 2004. Rapid and sensitive method using multiplex real-time PCR for diagnosis of infections by influenza A and influenza B viruses, respiratory syncytial virus, and parainfluenza viruses 1, 2, 3, and 4. *J. Clin. Microbiol.* **42:**1564–1569.
15. **Tranchand-Bunel, D., H. Gras-Masse, B. Bourez, L. Dedecker, and C. Auriault.** 1999. Evaluation of an Epstein-Barr virus (EBV) immunoglobulin M enzyme-linked immunosorbent assay using a synthetic convergent peptide library, or mixotope, for diagnosis of primary EBV infection. *J. Clin. Microbiol.* **37:**2366–2368.
16. **Turchek, B. M., and Y. T. Huang.** 1999. Evaluation of ELVIS HSV ID/Typing System for the detection and typing of herpes simplex virus from clinical specimens. *J. Clin. Virol.* **12:**65–69.
17. **Wilhelmi, I., J. Colomina, D. Martin-Rodrigo, E. Roman, and A. Sanchez-Fauquier.** 2001. New immunochromatographic method for rapid detection of rotaviruses in stool samples compared with standard enzyme immunoassay and latex agglutination techniques. *Eur. J. Clin. Microbiol. Infect. Dis.* **20:**741–743.

Enhanced Detection of Viruses in Cell Cultures

THOMAS F. SMITH

69

Prior to the mid-1980s, practical diagnosis of viral infections was based on the development of cytopathic effects (CPE) and the recognition of those changes in cell cultures. Several viruses such as herpes simplex virus (HSV), respiratory syncytial virus (RSV), influenza virus, and cytomegalovirus (CMV) were able to infect cells cultured in vitro, but the time for recognition of the CPE produced by these agents ranged from a few days to several weeks. With conventional tube cell culture techniques, diagnostic results of a CMV infection causing systemic disease in an organ transplant recipient or an AIDS patient may not have been available to the clinical service for several days.

The most significant step in the implementation of rapid cell culture techniques in the diagnostic virology laboratory has been the ability to develop epitope-specific monoclonal antibodies directed to select early antigens of viruses in the replication cycle (28, 59). Thus, rather than observing the development of CPE during a lengthy incubation period, monoclonal antibodies reacted with regulatory or structural components of viruses that were synthesized during the first few hours of infection in cell cultures; the presence of these early antigens could be recognized by using immunofluorescence or immunoperoxidase. Interestingly, cell culture (conventional tube and shell vial cell culture assays) has been the traditional "gold standard" for detection of virus infections in the clinical laboratory. These culture methods have been the benchmarks for comparison of automated commercially available platforms for performing nucleic acid amplification by PCR and other methods. In particular, real-time amplification of target nucleic acids provides more sensitive and rapid detection of viruses for support of clinical medical practices for the routine detection and quantitation of viruses from clinical specimens. Procedures previously implemented for the laboratory diagnosis of *Chlamydia trachomatis* infections by using shell vial cell cultures and low-speed centrifugation to enhance the efficiency of infection of this intracellular organism have been widely implemented for the detection of viruses by using specific monoclonal antibodies. More recently, the shell vial assay has been used for the rapid detection of rickettsiae and several other bacterial species (6, 23, 36, 37). The standard procedure, application for the detection of several viruses, and the technical variables that may affect the ability of the laboratory to provide sensitive and specific results with the shell vial assay are described in this chapter. Certainly, since the previous edition of this manual (57a) there has been significant incorporation of molecular methods into diagnostic virology laboratories. The transition of cell culture to routine nucleic acid-based methods is presented for consideration of future application in diagnostic virology laboratories.

GENERAL PRINCIPLES

Shell vials (1 dram [3.697 ml]) containing a circular coverslip are seeded with susceptible cells that develop into a monolayer. After removal of growth medium, specimen extracts are inoculated into 1-dram shell vials, which are then centrifuged at 700 × *g* (2,000 rpm) for 45 min. After addition of medium to the vials and overnight incubation (16 h at 36°C), cell monolayers on the coverslip are stained with a monoclonal antibody by the indirect immunofluorescence (preferably) or immunoperoxidase serologic technique (28, 59). The stained coverslips are then examined microscopically for specific stained foci. Detailed procedural steps, reagents, and equipment are provided in another American Society for Microbiology publication (76).

CELL CULTURES

Preparation of Shell Vial Cell Cultures
Monolayers on the surface of a 32-oz culture vial are removed and dispersed with a solution of trypsin-EDTA. The cells are resuspended in growth medium (~100 ml); 0.5 ml is dispensed into each shell vial to produce a monolayer in 1 to 3 days. Inoculation of preformed monolayers is preferable to simultaneous seeding and infecting of shell vials for the rapid detection of CMV infection (20).

Types
The choice of host cells used in the shell vial assay is based on the viruses to be isolated in a particular clinical setting, cost, and practicality. In the diagnostic laboratory, cell culture systems that provide the broadest range are usually chosen. Embryonic human diploid fibroblast (MRC-5) cells are optimal for the detection of CMV, HSV, varicella-zoster virus (VZV), and adenoviruses in shell vials, whereas mink lung, astrocytoma (U-373MG), and human lung carcinoma (A-549) cells have more restricted susceptibilities to infection by a wide range of viruses (8, 11, 39). MDCK cells can be used for primary detection of influenza virus type A (3). Generally,

617

cells that are diploid and are nearly confluent monolayers are optimal; neoplastic cell lines tend to produce multiple layers of cells, which makes a single virus-infected focus difficult to detect.

Age

Shell vial cell cultures ranging in age between 3 and 8 days should be used for inoculation of viral specimens. Monolayers exceeding this range are significantly less sensitive to CMV and are more fragile to toxic effects of certain specimens, particularly urine. Importantly, some commercially prepared shell vial cell cultures may be at least a week old when received at the clinical laboratory.

Specimens

Specimens from several sites are appropriate for inoculation into shell vial cell cultures for the diagnosis of herpesvirus (CMV, HSV, and VZV) and adenovirus. Detection of these viruses is optimal in MRC-5 human diploid fibroblast cells; however, HEp-2 cells (RSV), A-549 cells (RSV, influenza B virus, parainfluenza virus, and adenovirus), and primary rhesus monkey kidney or MDCK cells (influenza virus A and B and parainfluenza virus) should be used to detect these viruses in respiratory tract specimens (47, 61).

Urine

Urine is the best specimen for indication of CMV infection but does not provide definitive information about etiology because the virus is excreted commonly by asymptomatic patients, especially those who are immunosuppressed. Nevertheless, the predictive value for invasive disease with this specimen source is 40%. Because urine specimens do not have a high predictability for disease, continuous longitudinal monitoring of this source for CMV is not recommended. It is not necessary to adjust the pH of urine specimens to neutrality prior to inoculation to achieve maximal infection of shell vial cell cultures with CMV. The cellular fraction of urine (sediment after centrifugation) is the most productive specimen for detection of CMV from this specimen source (5).

BAL Fluid

Bronchoalveolar lavage (BAL) is an adaptation of routine bronchoscopic washing that involves wedging a fiberoptic bronchoscope into a subsegmented bronchus to sample cells in the lower respiratory tract. The technique is simple and obviates open lung biopsy, but it is invasive and patients are given atropine (subcutaneously), lidocaine is applied topically to the pharynx and upper airway, and supplemental oxygen is provided during the procedure (46). Most infectious CMV is associated with the cellular components of BAL specimens; however, there may be substantial amounts of virus in the cell-free fraction, particularly in specimens obtained from AIDS patients (14).

BAL specimens from bone marrow transplant patients yielded more positive results for CMV in the shell vial assay than did immunofluorescent antibody staining or cytologic identification of lung biopsy tissue. Nevertheless, CMV has been recovered from BAL specimens in the absence of disease and from patients simultaneously infected with other pathogenic organisms. Importantly, the specificity of BAL culture for CMV results varies greatly with the population being studied. A positive culture has greater clinical significance for solid-organ recipients than most other immunosuppressed patient groups.

Blood

Many viral infections have a viremic phase prior to the onset of clinical manifestations. In contrast, CMV viremia may persist for several days after a febrile episode in an immunocompromised patient. CMV infects leukocytes (lymphocytes, monocytes, and polymorphonuclear leukocytes [PMNs]); therefore, efficient recovery of this cellular fraction from anticoagulated blood specimens is necessary for maximum detection of this virus. For this purpose, HISTOPAQUE-1119 (Sigma Co., St. Louis, Mo.) separates these leukocytes from either EDTA-treated or heparinized blood specimens into a single diffuse band after centrifugation for approximately 20 min preparatory to inoculation into cell cultures. Generally, the greater the number of PMNs inoculated into shell vial cell cultures, the more likely that CMV viremia will be detected. For example, 96% of CMV strains were detected with an inoculum of 800,000 cells, compared to only 63% with an inoculum of 200,000 cells (58).

Detection of CMV in blood is considered a marker of systemic infection and correlates better with clinical disease and organ involvement than does the presence of the virus in urine or respiratory tract specimens (2). CMV accounts for over 90% of the viral isolates from blood cultures. Of 96 CMV strains recovered from blood specimens, 31 (32%) and 24 (25%) were detected exclusively in shell vial and conventional tube cell cultures, respectively (55). On the other hand, viremia with CMV may be transient or at least may not persist for more than a few hours even in immunocompromised patients (53). For example, of 46 CMV-viremic organ transplant patients who had repeat blood cultures performed after 1 to 3 days, only 40% were culture positive for the virus (53).

Although detection of CMV by PCR is more sensitive than the shell vial assay for early detection of the virus and preemptive therapy, the specificity of the shell vial technique (86%) is clearly superior to that of nucleic acid amplification (35%) for association with symptomatic infection (54).

Tissue

Lung tissue has been the single most productive source of viruses from these specimen types; however, BAL generally has replaced open lung biopsy as a technique for evaluation of lower respiratory tract disease due to CMV and other microorganisms (63).

Monoclonal Antibodies

Ideally, a monoclonal antibody directed to an immediate-early antigen product of replication is used for the immunologic detection of a virus infection. Indirect immunofluorescence assays are more sensitive but more labor-intensive than the use of direct labeled monoclonal antibodies to viral antigens. The ability of monoclonal antibodies to react with defined viral epitopes is extremely important for maximum sensitivity of the shell vial assay by immunologic techniques. For example, the 2H2.4 reagent is directed to a specific 72-kDa product of CMV synthesized in the first 3 h in the nucleus of the infected cell. In contrast, a monoclonal antibody reactive with a late product (2F3.0, 68 kDa; 48 to 72 h postinfection) detects structural antigens present in mature CMV particles rather than the regulatory and enzymatic products initially synthesized by the virus-infected cells.

Overall, characterization of the reactivity of monoclonal antibodies is most detailed for the herpesvirus group; however, specific reagents are commercially available for use in the shell vial assay for viruses causing respiratory tract disease.

Variables

Several technical steps of the shell vial assay must be followed to achieve maximum sensitivity for this cell culture detection system. In addition to the age of cells, condition of cell monolayers, and specificity of monoclonal antibodies for immediate-early or early viral antigens, other important variables include incubation temperature, number of shell vial cell cultures used per specimen, centrifugation, type of specimen (urine, blood, BAL fluid, tissue), quality of fluorescence equipment, chemical pretreatment of cell monolayers, and technical experience with the assay to subjectively evaluate specific results (Table 1).

Criteria for Diagnostic Results

Patterns of fluorescence after staining of infected cells are distinct and specific. Sometimes even a single focus (CMV), characterized by a dense immunofluorescence with prominent lobular staining in the nucleus, is sufficient to recognize a virus-infected cell. Both the smooth regularity of the nuclear membrane and the characteristic shape of the CMV-infected cell nuclei allow the specific recognition and distinction of this viral infection from background nonspecific debris that may fluoresce (Fig. 1).

Importantly, laboratory diagnosis can be achieved within 16 to 24 h postinoculation rather than several days after submission of the specimen to the laboratory. Even in laboratories that are not able to achieve maximum detection of virus by the shell vial assay, a significant number of results can be reported rapidly to the clinical service when the shell vial assay is used. Indeed, in 11 separate reports, the sensitivity of the shell vial assay ranged from 55 to 100% compared to eventual isolation of CMV in cell cultures (62). The shell vial assay is 90 to 100% sensitive for detecting VZV infections, whereas for viruses obtained from respiratory tract specimens (RSV, influenza A and B viruses, parainfluenza virus types 1, 2, and 3, adenovirus, and enterovirus), the sensitivity ranges from 60 to 94% compared with conventional tube cell culture (3, 25, 34, 35, 57, 75). Rapid detection of viral infections of the respiratory tract can reduce the time of hospitalization and patient care costs (4).

Mixed infections due to viruses can occur at frequencies that range from 7.6%, for mixed infections with RSV and CMV, rhinovirus, adenovirus, influenza and parainfluenza virus, echovirus, or HSV, to 35% for a simultaneous epidemic of parainfluenza virus and influenza virus (45). Each of these viruses can be specifically isolated and identified by CPE in tube cell cultures provided that susceptible cells are inoculated; eventual identification of each virus requires several days' time with this conventional technology. Generally, only infection with a single virus is recognized by rapid techniques like the shell vial assay, direct immunofluorescence of virus-infected cells, or enzyme immunoassay procedures, unless a mixture of monoclonal antibodies can be used as a single reagent (45). On the other hand, a monolayer stained with antibodies to CMV, for example, may be restained with antibodies to another virus. This procedure may be used in situations in which a rapid shell vial assay result is needed but inoculated, unstained cultures are not available.

QUALITY CONTROL

Cell Cultures

Cell cultures, especially from several commercial sources, may differ significantly in their susceptibility to virus infection. The laboratory should follow an appropriate quality control program extensively outlined in another American Society for Microbiology publication (73).

Positive Controls

Reference strains of viruses are used to inoculate shell vial cell cultures at a concentration designed to produce a countable number of fluorescent foci. The control cell cultures are processed (incubated and stained) in the same manner as specimens from patients.

Negative Controls

Uninoculated shell vial cell cultures are incubated and stained, using the same lot of cells used for the positive control and specimens from patients. No specific fluorescence patterns should be detectable in these controls.

COMPARISONS OF SHELL VIAL ASSAY WITH OTHER METHODS

Conventional Tube Cell Cultures

Performance characteristics of the shell vial assay compared with conventional tube cell cultures have generally been directly related to the effort expended by the laboratory to control the variables of the immunologic detection system used. Several comparisons have demonstrated that the shell vial assay is as sensitive as (for HSV and respiratory tract viruses [adenoviruses, parainfluenza virus types 1, 2, and 3, enterovirus, influenza A and B virus, measles virus, mumps virus, and RSV]) or even more sensitive than (for CMV) the recovery of these viruses in conventional tube cell cultures, which may require several days to weeks for recognition by CPE (25, 34, 35, 75). For some viruses (adenovirus and enterovirus), detection was more sensitive by the shell vial assay within 3 days after inoculation but conventional tube cell cultures ultimately yielded more viral isolates.

Acute respiratory tract infections caused by viruses are a significant cause of morbidity and mortality in all age groups but especially in immunocompromised patients and in individuals at increased risk for influenza virus-related complications (32). Importantly, influenza virus infections have been responsible for an average of approximately 36,000 deaths per year in the United States from 1990 to 1999 (68). Influenza virus vaccination is the primary method for preventing influenza and its severe complications as recommended by the Advisory Committee on Immunization Practices (32). However, antiviral drugs are an adjunct to influenza vaccine for controlling and preventing influenza; nevertheless, these agents are not a substitute for vaccination. Four licensed influenza antiviral agents are available in the United States: amantadine, rimantadine, zanamivir, and oseltamivir. Importantly, active influenza virus infections can now be treated in the early acute stage of disease. For example, oral administration of oseltamivir (Tamiflu) can be effective in patients identified with influenza virus infection within the initial 2 days of infection.

Rapid laboratory diagnosis of influenza virus infections by shell vial cell cultures will not be facilitative to guide specific therapy since recent publications indicate that the majority of isolates were identified only after 48 or 120 h postinoculation of R-mix (a mixed monolayer of human lung-derived cells [A-549] and mink lung-derived cells [Mv1Lu]) shell vial cell cultures (74). In another report, nearly all of the influenza virus infections were detected after 18 to 24 h postinoculation (17). These differences, including the lability of these viruses in transit to the laboratory, may be intrinsic to the variables inherent in cell culture methods (38, 64).

TABLE 1 Technical variables in the shell vial assay

Procedure step	Standard recommendations	Comments
Incubation temperature of virus-inoculated shell vial cultures	36°C	Incubation of inoculated cultures at 39 and 42°C does not increase the sensitivity compared with the standard 36°C
Time between inoculation and staining of shell vial cell cultures	Stain with monoclonal antibody to immediate-early antigen at 16–24 h	Time interval may be increased to 40 h to compensate for a suboptimal shell vial assay procedure, e.g., use of cell monolayers older than 8 days from time of preparation, use of one rather than two shell vial cell cultures, and staining with monoclonal antibodies with reactivity to late viral antigens
No. of cultures inoculated per specimen	Three shell vials should be inoculated with blood specimen; two shell vials are adequate for specimens from other sources	Inoculation of three shell vials versus two increases the rate of detection of CMV by 20%
Centrifugation	$700 \times g$ for 40 min	Both the rate and the efficiency of infection of host cells by viruses are significantly enhanced (10–20-fold) compared to shell vials not centrifuged after addition of the virus inoculum; the actual sensitivity of the shell vial assay for the detection of CMV infections increases from 40 to 100% with centrifugation; gravitational forces higher than recommended can cause cell damage and reduced sensitivity of the assay
Volume of inoculation and type of specimen	Urine, BAL fluid, and supernatant fraction of specimen (respiratory, dermal, tissue) extracts are inoculated into two shell vials (0.2 ml/vial); shell vial cell cultures must be used between 3 and 8 days after preparation to ensure maximum sensitivity to viruses	Higher volumes of inocula may produce more fluorescent foci than detected by using recommended amounts of specimen material; however, toxicity of cell monolayers can result from extra debris in larger specimen volumes
Peripheral blood leukocytes	Leukocytes are separated from anticoagulated blood specimens (10 ml) by HISTOPAQUE-1119 and suspended in 2 ml of medium; each of three shell vials receives 0.3 ml of inoculum	Shell vial coverslip cell cultures must be stained 16 h after inoculation with peripheral blood leukocytes to avoid toxicity of monolayers
Examination of infected cells	Fluorescence equipment with appropriate filters should be used to maximize detection of fluorescence with fluorescein isothiocyanate; the fluorescence pattern produced by a virus after immunostaining should be intracellular and produce consistent patterns compared to virus-infected controls	Xenon or mercury light sources are superior to halogen for the immunological detection of virus-infected cells
Detection label for monoclonal antibody (fluorescence, enzyme)	Commercial reagents are readily available for fluorescence detection of virus-infected cells	Sensitivity for detecting virus-specific antigens in infected cells is generally comparable to that of fluorescence or enzyme-labeled antibodies
Technical expertise	Shell vial assay should be standardized according to conditions demonstrated to be optimal; expertise with the assay is built by familiarization with the variables of the test; adequate time is needed to implement the test procedure according to specified procedures	Procedural changes in the laboratory should be implemented only after the results are compared to those of the standard shell vial assay
Chemical treatment of shell vial cell cultures	The role of routine use of 1% solutions of dimethyl sulfoxide and 10^{-5} M dexamethasone has not been consistently established	Effects of chemical treatment and shell vial cell cultures to enhance viral infection appear to be extremely variable in several reported publications; chemicals such as dimethyl sulfoxide and dexamethasone may be toxic to cell culture monolayers

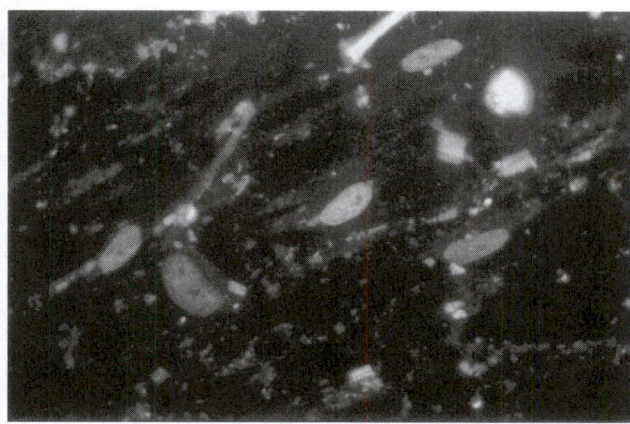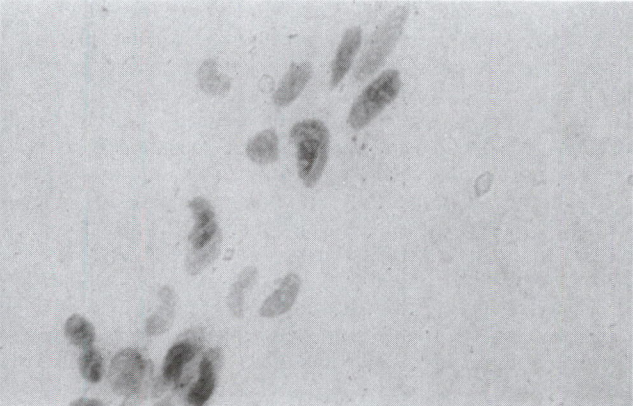

FIGURE 1 Detection of early antigens in the shell vial assay by immunofluorescence (left) and immunoperoxidase (right) stains. Magnification, ×400.

In addition, it was noted recently that R-mix cells can also be infected by severe acute respiratory syndrome coronavirus (SARS-CoV) in specimens from the respiratory tract which may be submitted to the laboratory from patients infected with this highly pathogenic and virulent virus. These findings indicate that further work is needed to enhance appropriate biosafety precautions for use of R-mix cells in diagnostic laboratories likely to process specimens containing SARS-CoV (27).

Antigenemia

The antigenemia test is a rapid (4- to 6-h) quantitative method for detecting CMV antigens in PMNs by using immunoperoxidase or immunofluorescence staining procedures. Importantly, pools of monoclonal antibodies must be directed to a 65-kDa lower matrix protein of the virus. Studies reporting the diagnostic utility of the antigenemia assay have been expanded to include solid-organ and bone marrow transplant patients and individuals with AIDS. In general, the performance characteristics of antigenemia parallel those reported for nucleic acid amplification techniques (PCR) (7, 56) (Table 2). Nevertheless, in most studies, real-time PCR assays detect the presence of CMV infection earlier and with greater sensitivity than do shell vial cell cultures (48) (Table 2). Note, however, that antigenemia and PCR are highly specific for CMV

infection, but these tests must be used in a quantitative fashion to predict and diagnose disease and to yield information for antiviral drug efficacy (10, 13, 41). Antigenemia assays are limited to blood specimens and have been restricted for general use by the cumbersome and nonstandardized technical aspects of sample processing (43). In contrast to nucleic acid amplification technology, automated instruments are not available for antigenemia testing. Lastly, quantification of CMV viremia is more accurate, precise, and measurable over a much wider dynamic range (29, 50). Typically, antigenemia values are reported in increments of 0, 1 to 10, 11 to 100, 101 to 1,000, and over 1,000 positive cells per 2×10^5 leukocytes. These values corresponded to median loads of 125, 1,593, 5,713, 16,825, and 5,425,000 copies/ml, respectively (40).

The test for antigenemia can be obtained in kit form, but the reagents and procedures are not generic. Similar to the shell vial assay, the results of the antigenemia test are influenced by technical variables, including the age of the blood specimen (optimal less than 4 h before processing), formalin fixation followed by permeabilization rather than methanol-acetone, avidity and specificity of monoclonal antibodies to the target pp65 antigen, number of PMNs stained, storage conditions of fixed slides, number of cells examined per slide (especially samples from neutropenic patients) and processing by cytospin preparation (neutropenic patients), quality of microscopic equipment, and technical experience of personnel in interpretation of specific results (9, 16, 26, 41, 42, 65, 77). The wide variability and the lack of standardization among laboratories restrict interpretation of the results of the antigenemia test to local use. The clinical role of this test is still evolving and is predicated on controlling important variables in the test. One of the biggest challenges for the laboratory processing the specimens for the antigenemia test is to stabilize the loss of antigen or viral (CMV) load during periods of specimen transport (12, 51). Importantly, specimens from patients with low-level antigenemia (fewer than five pp65-positive cells) may yield false-negative results if the blood samples are not processed within 4 h of collection.

PCR

Several advances in the performance of PCR and other nucleic acid amplification techniques have occurred in recent years. For example, in the past, conventional automated thermocycling instruments were programmed to perform 40 to 45 cycles of nucleic acid amplification that required 3 to 4 h; this was followed by gel electrophoresis of the PCR-amplified

TABLE 2 Sensitivity of detection of CMV DNA by real-time PCR compared to antigenemia results

Detection of DNA		Sensitivity			Reference
Earlier	Later	Higher	Lower	Same	
				X	44
X				X	66
				X	24
X		X			30
				X	31
X		X			49
X		X			77
X		X			33
		X			40
		X			50
X		X			16
X		X		X	52
X		X			29

products and Southern blotting with probe hybridization techniques. More recently, commercially available primers labeled with biotin or a fluorescent label have been incorporated into amplified products, which may be detected by colorimetric, fluorescent, or chemiluminescence methods (67). In addition, these detection methods have been incorporated into several automated platforms that yield quantitative CMV DNA, hepatitis C virus RNA, and human immunodeficiency virus type 1 RNA copy levels which may have application for disease prognosis and evaluation of antiviral efficacy (1, 7, 15, 18). For example, for eight liver transplant patients who developed relapsing CMV infection, the median levels of viral DNA were higher in pretreatment samples (leukocytes) than those in samples from individuals with resolved infection. Importantly, the relapsing group also had persistent detectable CMV DNA (median, 5,810 copies/10^6 leukocytes) after ganciclovir treatment, whereas CMV DNA was undetectable in the nonrelapsing group ($P < 0.0001$) (60).

The most significant innovations in PCR technology have been the availability of automated PCR instruments involving rapid thermocycling formats combined with the capability of quantitation and strain differentiation (e.g., HSV type 1 [HSV-1] and HSV-2) (22). The first system developed (LightCycler; Roche Molecular Biochemicals, Indianapolis, Ind.) combines rapid PCR thermocycling (45 cycles/30 to 40 min) with real-time (i.e., analysis of product after each cycle) specific probe detection and quantification of signal. Continuous monitoring of amplicon development by hybridization probes is based on the principle of fluorescence resonance energy transfer (FRET). Two hybridization probes, designed to anneal next to each other on the PCR amplicon, are used. A hybridization probe with a donor fluorophore, fluorescein, on the 3′ end is excited by an external light source and emits light. If the second probe, with an acceptor fluorophore, LC-Red 640, at the 5′ end, anneals next to the donor probe, the light from the fluorescein is absorbed. The acceptor fluorophore then emits light of a different wavelength which provides a signal that is proportional to the amount of specific PCR product, allowing specific detection and quantitation of the product.

In a prospective study of 200 genital and dermal specimens, we detected and confirmed 88 HSV strains by LightCycler, compared to only 69 by the shell vial cell culture assay. We found the LightCycler to be 100% specific and extremely sensitive in that 19 specimens (22%) were detected exclusively by LightCycler PCR (22).

Similarly, VZV was detected in only 23 (9.1%) of 253 dermal specimens by the shell vial cell culture assay, compared with 44 (17.4%) by LightCycler PCR (21). Collectively, these results (HSV and VZV) suggest that automated PCR such as the LightCycler system could replace cell culture for the detection of these viruses from genital and dermal sources because of the higher sensitivity, rapid results, and closed FRET detection system, which virtually eliminates the risk of crossover amplicon contamination for the routine laboratory.

Of seven studies that compared the detection of HSV DNA and VZV DNA by real-time PCR with shell vial cell culture (38,793 specimens), all demonstrated the superiority of the molecular amplification technology (Table 3). Similarly, real-time PCR was more sensitive for the detection

TABLE 3 Laboratory diagnosis of HSV and VZV infections by cell cultures and by real-time PCR

| Virus | Specimens | | Cells | Assay and sensitivity (%) | | Reference |
	Source	No.		Cell culture antibody-enhanced detection (shell vial)	Real-time PCR	
HSV	Genital	335	Human diploid fibroblasts	48.4	74.0	58
HSV	Genital, dermal, ocular	200	MRC-5	34.5	44	22
HSV	Genital, dermal, ocular	500	MRC-5	31.6	45	19
HSV	Genital, dermal, ocular, oral, BAL	668	Human embryonic fibroblasts	29.8	34.9	69
HSV	Various mucosal and dermal sites	36,471	Human diploid fibroblasts	2.98	12.1	71
VZV	Dermal	253	MRC-5	9.1	17.4	21
VZV	Dermal	366	Human embryonic fibroblasts	4.6	7.4	69
Influenza virus	Throat	233	MDCK (canine kidney cells)	24	60	72
Influenza virus types A and B	Combined nose and throat swabs or nasal washes	98	Tertiary monkey kidney cells (shell vial)	22.4	40.8	70
Influenza virus	Throat swabs, nasal washes, BAL, sputum, nasal swabs	557	R-mix (mink lung and A-549 cells)	9.2	16.5	Espy et al.[a]
RSV	Combined nose and throat swabs	168	Tertiary rhesus monkey kidney (shell vial)	2.4	4.9	70

[a]M. J. Espy, S. K. Schneider, P. A. Wright, S. Kidiyala, M. F. Jones, and T. F. Smith, Program Abstr. 20th Annual Clinical Virology Symposium, abstr. no. M51, 2004.

of influenza virus RNA than detection of this important pathogen by shell vial cell culture (Table 3).

The diagnostic laboratory may always find a use for cell cultures; however, the next level of test performance in the clinical laboratory will be formatted for the automated extraction and quantitation detection of target nucleic acids. Amplified nucleic acids will be monitored in real time by thermocycling instruments designed to be used in routine biosafety level 2 laboratories.

REFERENCES

1. **Anderson, J. C., J. Simonetti, D. G. Fisher, J. Williams, Y. Yamamura, N. Rodriguez, D. G. Sullivan, D. R. Gretch, B. McMahon, and K. J. Williams.** 2003. Comparison of different HCV viral load and genotyping assays. *J. Clin. Virol.* **28:**27–37.
2. **Badley, A. D., R. Patel, D. F. Portela, W. S. Harmsen, T. F. Smith, D. M. Ilstrup, J. L. Steers, R. H. Wiesner, and C. V. Paya.** 1996. Prognostic significance and risk factors of untreated cytomegalovirus viremia in liver transplant recipients. *J. Infect. Dis.* **173:**446–449.
3. **Bartholoma, N. Y., and B. A. Forbes.** 1989. Successful use of shell vial centrifugation and 16 to 18-hour immunofluorescent staining for the detection of influenza A and B in clinical specimens. *Am. J. Clin. Pathol.* **92:**487–490.
4. **Beekmann, S. E., H. D. Engler, A. S. Collins, J. Canosa, D. K. Henderson, and A. Freifeld.** 1996. Rapid identification of respiratory viruses: impact on isolation practices and transmission among immunocompromised pediatric patients. *Infect. Control Hosp. Epidemiol.* **17:**581–586.
5. **Bennion, D. W., L. J. Wright, R. A. Watt, A. A. Whiting, and J. F. Carlquist.** 1998. Optimal recovery of cytomegalovirus from urine as a function of specimen preparation. *Diagn. Microbiol. Infect. Dis.* **31:**337–342.
6. **Birg, M. L., B. La Scola, V. Roux, P. Brouqui, and D. Raoult.** 1999. Isolation of *Rickettsia prowazekii* from blood by shell vial cell culture. *J. Clin. Microbiol.* **37:**3722–3724.
7. **Blok, M. J., M. H. Christiaans, V. J. Goossens, J. P. van Hooff, P. Sillekens, J. M. Middeldorp, and C. A. Bruggeman.** 1999. Early detection of human cytomegalovirus infection after kidney transplantation by nucleic acid sequence-based amplification. *Transplantation* **67:**1274–1277.
8. **Boeckh, M., C. A. Gleaves, R. Bindra, and J. D. Meyers.** 1991. Comparison of MRC-5 and U-373MG astrocytoma cells for detection of cytomegalovirus in shell vial centrifugation cultures. *Eur. J. Clin. Microbiol. Infect. Dis.* **10:**569–572.
9. **Boeckh, M., P. M. Woogerd, T. Stevens-Ayers, C. G. Ray, and R. A. Bowden.** 1994. Factors influencing detection of quantitative cytomegalovirus antigenemia. *J. Clin. Microbiol.* **32:**832–834.
10. **Boivin, G., J. Handfield, E. Toma, G. Murray, R. Lalonde, V. J. Tevere, R. Sun, and M. G. Bergeron.** 1998. Evaluation of the AMPLICOR cytomegalovirus test with specimens from human immunodeficiency virus-infected subjects. *J. Clin. Microbiol.* **36:**2509–2513.
11. **Brinker, J. P., and G. V. Doern.** 1993. Comparison of MRC-5 and A-549 cells in conventional culture tubes and shell vial assays for the detection of varicella-zoster virus. *Diagn. Microbiol. Infect. Dis.* **17:**75–77.
12. **Bush, C. E., and J. A. Sluchak-Carlsen.** 1998. Evaluation of a leukocyte stabilization reagent for use in the cytomegalovirus pp65 antigenemia assay. *J. Clin. Microbiol.* **36:**3410–3411.
13. **Carton, J. A., A. Rodriguez-Guardado, S. Melon, J. A. Maradona, M. De Ona, and V. Asensi.** 1999. Cytomegalovirus antigenemia surveillance in the treatment of cytomegalovirus disease in AIDS patients. *J. Chemother.* **11:**195–202.
14. **Clarke, L. M., B. J. Daidone, R. Inghida, M. Kirwin, and M. F. Sierra.** 1992. Differential recovery of cytomegalovirus

from cellular and supernatant components of bronchoalveolar lavage specimens. *Am. J. Clin. Pathol.* **97:**313–317.
15. **Cook, L., K. W. Ng, A. Bagabag, L. Corey, and K. R. Jerome.** 2004. Use of the MagNA pure LC automated nucleic acid extraction system followed by real-time reverse transcription-PCR for ultrasensitive quantitation of hepatitis C virus RNA. *J. Clin. Microbiol.* **42:**4130–4136.
16. **Cortez, K. J., S. H. Fischer, G. A. Fahle, L. B. Calhoun, R. W. Childs, A. J. Barrett, and J. E. Bennett.** 2003. Clinical trial of quantitative real-time polymerase chain reaction for detection of cytomegalovirus in peripheral blood of allogeneic hematopoietic stem-cell transplant recipients. *J. Infect. Dis.* **188:**967–972.
17. **Dunn, J. J., R. D. Woolstenhulme, J. Langer, and K. C. Carroll.** 2004. Sensitivity of respiratory virus culture when screening with R-mix fresh cells. *J. Clin. Microbiol.* **42:**79–82.
18. **Elbeik, T., E. Charlebois, P. Nassos, J. Kahn, F. M. Hecht, D. Yajko, V. Ng, and K. Hadley.** 2000. Quantitative and cost comparison of ultrasensitive human immunodeficiency virus type 1 RNA viral load assays: Bayer bDNA Quantiplex versions 3.0 and 2.0 and Roche PCR Amplicor Monitor version 1.5. *J. Clin. Microbiol.* **38:**1113–1120.
19. **Espy, M. J., T. K. Ross, R. Teo, K. A. Svien, A. D. Wold, J. R. Uhl, and T. F. Smith.** 2000. Evaluation of LightCycler PCR for implementation of laboratory diagnosis of herpes simplex virus infections. *J. Clin. Microbiol.* **38:**3116–3118.
20. **Espy, M. J., and T. F. Smith.** 1987. Simultaneous seeding and infecting of shell vials for rapid detection of cytomegalovirus infection. *J. Clin. Microbiol.* **25:**940–941.
21. **Espy, M. J., R. Teo, T. K. Ross, K. A. Svien, A. D. Wold, J. R. Uhl, and T. F. Smith.** 2000. Diagnosis of varicella-zoster virus infections in the clinical laboratory by LightCycler PCR. *J. Clin. Microbiol.* **38:**3187–3189.
22. **Espy, M. J., J. R. Uhl, P. S. Mitchell, J. N. Thorvilson, K. A. Svien, A. D. Wold, and T. F. Smith.** 2000. Diagnosis of herpes simplex virus infections in the clinical laboratory by LightCycler PCR. *J. Clin. Microbiol.* **38:**795–799.
23. **Fournier, P. E., L. Bernabeu, B. Schubert, M. Mutillod, V. Roux, and D. Raoult.** 1998. Isolation of *Francisella tularensis* by centrifugation of shell vial cell culture from an inoculation eschar. *J. Clin. Microbiol.* **36:**2782–2783.
24. **Gault, E., Y. Michel, A. Dehee, C. Belabani, J. C. Nicolas, and A. Garbarg-Chenon.** 2001. Quantification of human cytomegalovirus DNA by real-time PCR. *J. Clin. Microbiol.* **39:**772–775.
25. **Germann, D., M. Gorgievski, A. Strohle, and L. Matter.** 1998. Detection of mumps virus in clinical specimens by rapid centrifugation culture and conventional tube cell culture. *J. Virol. Methods* **73:**59–64.
26. **Gerna, G., E. Percivalle, M. Torsellini, and M. G. Revello.** 1998. Standardization of the human cytomegalovirus antigenemia assay by means of in vitro-generated pp65-positive peripheral blood polymorphonuclear leukocytes. *J. Clin. Microbiol.* **36:**3585–3589.
27. **Gillim-Ross, L., J. Taylor, D. R. Scholl, J. Ridenour, P. S. Masters, and D. E. Wentworth.** 2004. Discovery of novel human and animal cells infected by the severe acute respiratory syndrome coronavirus by replication-specific multiplex reverse transcription-PCR. *J. Clin. Microbiol.* **42:**3196–3206.
28. **Gleaves, C. A., T. F. Smith, E. A. Shuster, and G. R. Pearson.** 1985. Comparison of standard tube and shell vial cell culture techniques for the detection of cytomegalovirus in clinical specimens. *J. Clin. Microbiol.* **21:**217–221.
29. **Gouarin, S., A. Vabret, E. Gault, J. Petitjean, A. Regeasse, B. Hurault de Ligny, and F. Freymuth.** 2004. Quantitative analysis of HCMV DNA load in whole blood

of renal transplant patients using real-time PCR assay. *J. Clin. Virol.* **29**:194–201.

30. **Griscelli, F., M. Barrois, S. Chauvin, S. Lastere, D. Bellet, and J. H. Bourhis.** 2001. Quantification of human cytomegalovirus DNA in bone marrow transplant recipients by real-time PCR. *J. Clin. Microbiol.* **39**:4362–4369.

31. **Guiver, M., A. J. Fox, K. Mutton, N. Mogulkoc, and J. Egan.** 2001. Evaluation of CMV viral load using TaqMan CMV quantitative PCR and comparison with CMV antigenemia in heart and lung transplant recipients. *Transplantation* **71**:1609–1615.

32. **Harper, S. A., K. Fukuda, T. M. Uyeki, N. J. Cox, and C. B. Bridges.** 2004. Prevention and control of influenza: recommendations of the Advisory Committee on Immunization Practices (ACIP). *MMWR Recomm. Rep.* **53**:1–40.

33. **Ikewaki, J., E. Ohtsuka, R. Kawano, M. Ogata, H. Kikuchi, and M. Nasu.** 2003. Real-time PCR assay compared to nested PCR and antigenemia assays for detecting cytomegalovirus reactivation in adult T-cell leukemia-lymphoma patients. *J. Clin. Microbiol.* **41**:4382–4387.

34. **Klespies, S. L., D. E. Cebula, C. L. Kelley, D. Galehouse, and C. C. Maurer.** 1996. Detection of enteroviruses from clinical specimens by spin amplification shell vial culture and monoclonal antibody assay. *J. Clin. Microbiol.* **34**:1465–1467.

35. **Kowalski, R. P., L. M. Karenchak, E. G. Romanowski, and Y. J. Gordon.** 1999. Evaluation of the shell vial technique for detection of ocular adenovirus. Community Ophthalmologists of Pittsburgh, Pennsylvania. *Ophthalmology* **106**:1324–1327.

36. **La Scola, B., G. Michel, and D. Raoult.** 1999. Isolation of *Legionella pneumophila* by centrifugation of shell vial cell cultures from multiple liver and lung abscesses. *J. Clin. Microbiol.* **37**:785–787.

37. **La Scola, B., and D. Raoult.** 1999. Culture of *Bartonella quintana* and *Bartonella henselae* from human samples: a 5-year experience (1993 to 1998). *J. Clin. Microbiol.* **37**:1899–1905.

38. **Leland, D. S., and D. Emanuel.** 1995. Laboratory diagnosis of viral infections of the lung. *Semin. Respir. Infect.* **10**:189–198.

39. **Leonardi, G. P., P. Costello, and P. Harris.** 1995. Use of continuous human lung cell culture for adenovirus isolation. *Intervirology* **38**:352–355.

40. **Li, H., J. S. Dummer, W. R. Estes, S. Meng, P. F. Wright, and Y. W. Tang.** 2003. Measurement of human cytomegalovirus loads by quantitative real-time PCR for monitoring clinical intervention in transplant recipients. *J. Clin. Microbiol.* **41**:187–191.

41. **Lipson, S. M., M. H. Kaplan, L. F. Tseng, and F. S. Mandel.** 1993. Use of the cytomegalovirus antigenemia (CMV-Ag) assay for the detection of CMV in the blood of AIDS patients. *Can. J. Microbiol.* **39**:1059–1065.

42. **Lipson, S. M., A. Toro, M. Lotlikar, M. E. Match, M. H. Kaplan, D. H. Shepp, and J. Gong.** 1997. Significance of leukocyte concentration in the performance of the quantitative cytomegalovirus (CMV) antigenemia assay. *Clin. Diagn. Virol.* **8**:151–158.

43. **Long, C. M., L. Drew, R. Miner, D. Jekic-McMullen, C. Impraim, and S. Y. Kao.** 1998. Detection of cytomegalovirus in plasma and cerebrospinal fluid specimens from human immunodeficiency virus-infected patients by the AMPLICOR CMV test. *J. Clin. Microbiol.* **36**:2434–2438.

44. **Machida, U., M. Kami, T. Fukui, Y. Kazuyama, M. Kinoshita, Y. Tanaka, Y. Kanda, S. Ogawa, H. Honda, S. Chiba, K. Mitani, Y. Muto, K. Osumi, S. Kimura, and H. Hirai.** 2000. Real-time automated PCR for early diagnosis and monitoring of cytomegalovirus infection after bone marrow transplantation. *J. Clin. Microbiol.* **38**:2536–2542.

45. **Maitreyi, R. S., S. Broor, S. K. Kabra, M. Ghosh, P. Seth, L. Dar, and A. K. Prasad.** 2000. Rapid detection of respiratory viruses by centrifugation enhanced cultures from children with acute lower respiratory tract infections. *J. Clin. Virol.* **16**:41–47.

46. **Martin, W. J., Jr., and T. F. Smith.** 1986. Rapid detection of cytomegalovirus in bronchoalveolar lavage specimens by a monoclonal antibody method. *J. Clin. Microbiol.* **23**:1006–1008.

47. **Matthey, S., D. Nicholson, S. Ruhs, B. Alden, M. Knock, K. Schultz, and A. Schmuecker.** 1992. Rapid detection of respiratory viruses by shell vial culture and direct staining by using pooled and individual monoclonal antibodies. *J. Clin. Microbiol.* **30**:540–544.

48. **Mazzulli, T., L. W. Drew, B. Yen-Lieberman, D. Jekic-McMullen, D. J. Kohn, C. Isada, G. Moussa, R. Chua, and S. Walmsley.** 1999. Multicenter comparison of the digene hybrid capture CMV DNA assay (version 2.0), the pp65 antigenemia assay, and cell culture for detection of cytomegalovirus viremia. *J. Clin. Microbiol.* **37**:958–963.

49. **Mori, T., S. Okamoto, R. Watanabe, T. Yajima, Y. Iwao, R. Yamazaki, T. Nakazato, N. Sato, T. Iguchi, H. Nagayama, N. Takayama, T. Hibi, and Y. Ikeda.** 2002. Dose-adjusted preemptive therapy for cytomegalovirus disease based on real-time polymerase chain reaction after allogeneic hematopoietic stem cell transplantation. *Bone Marrow Transplant.* **29**:777–782.

50. **Nitsche, A., O. Oswald, N. Steuer, J. Schetelig, A. Radonic, S. Thulke, and W. Siegert.** 2003. Quantitative real-time PCR compared with pp65 antigen detection for cytomegalovirus (CMV) in 1122 blood specimens from 77 patients after allogeneic stem cell transplantation: which test better predicts CMV disease development? *Clin. Chem.* **49**:1683–1685.

51. **Niubo, J., J. L. Perez, A. Carvajal, C. Ardanuy, and R. Martin.** 1994. Effect of delayed processing of blood samples on performance of cytomegalovirus antigenemia assay. *J. Clin. Microbiol.* **32**:1119–1120.

52. **Pang, A., M. F. Yuen, H. J. Yuan, C. L. Lai, and Y. L. Kwong.** 2004. Real-time quantification of hepatitis B virus core-promoter and pre-core mutants during hepatitis E antigen seroconversion. *J. Hepatol.* **40**:1008–1017.

53. **Patel, R., D. W. Klein, M. J. Espy, W. S. Harmsen, D. M. Ilstrup, C. V. Paya, and T. F. Smith.** 1995. Optimization of detection of cytomegalovirus viremia in transplantation recipients by shell vial assay. *J. Clin. Microbiol.* **33**:2984–2986.

54. **Patel, R., T. F. Smith, M. Espy, D. Portela, R. H. Wiesner, R. A. Krom, and C. V. Paya.** 1995. A prospective comparison of molecular diagnostic techniques for the early detection of cytomegalovirus in liver transplant recipients. *J. Infect. Dis.* **171**:1010–1014.

55. **Paya, C. V., A. D. Wold, and T. F. Smith.** 1988. Detection of cytomegalovirus from blood leukocytes separated by Sepracell-MN and Ficoll-Paque/Macrodex methods. *J. Clin. Microbiol.* **26**:2031–2033.

56. **Pellegrin, I., I. Garrigue, C. Binquet, G. Chene, D. Neau, P. Bonot, F. Bonnet, H. Fleury, and J. L. Pellegrin.** 1999. Evaluation of new quantitative assays for diagnosis and monitoring of cytomegalovirus disease in human immunodeficiency virus-positive patients. *J. Clin. Microbiol.* **37**:3124–3132.

57. **Perez, J. L., J. Niubo, D. Mariscal, F. Tubau, J. Salva, and R. Martin.** 1993. Evaluation of a monoclonal antibody for detection of varicella-zoster virus infections using a shell vial technique. *Eur. J. Clin. Microbiol. Infect. Dis.* **12**:875–879.

57a. Rose, N. R., R. G. Hamilton, and B. Detrick (ed.). 2002. *Manual of Clinical Laboratory Immunology*, 6th ed. ASM Press, Washington, D.C.

58. Ryncarz, A. J., J. Goddard, A. Wald, M. L. Huang, B. Roizman, and L. Corey. 1999. Development of a high-throughput quantitative assay for detecting herpes simplex virus DNA in clinical samples. *J. Clin. Microbiol.* 37:1941–1947.

59. Shuster, E. A., J. S. Beneke, G. E. Tegtmeier, G. R. Pearson, C. A. Gleaves, A. D. Wold, and T. F. Smith. 1985. Monoclonal antibody for rapid laboratory detection of cytomegalovirus infections: characterization and diagnostic application. *Mayo Clin. Proc.* 60:577–585.

60. Sia, I. G., J. A. Wilson, C. M. Groettum, M. J. Espy, T. F. Smith, and C. V. Paya. 2000. Cytomegalovirus (CMV) DNA load predicts relapsing CMV infection after solid organ transplantation. *J. Infect. Dis.* 181:717–720.

61. Smith, M. C., C. Creutz, and Y. T. Huang. 1991. Detection of respiratory syncytial virus in nasopharyngeal secretions by shell vial technique. *J. Clin. Microbiol.* 29:463–465.

62. Smith, T. F. 1994. Laboratory diagnosis of viral infections, p. 759–779. *In* B. J. Howard (ed.), *Clinical and Pathogenic Microbiology*. Mosby-Year Book, Inc., St. Louis, Mo.

63. Smith, T. F., A. D. Wold, M. J. Espy, and W. F. Marshall. 1993. New developments in the diagnosis of viral diseases. *Infect. Dis. Clin. N. Am.* 7:183–201.

64. St. George, K., N. M. Patel, R. A. Hartwig, D. R. Scholl, J. A. Jollick, Jr., L. M. Kauffmann, M. R. Evans, and C. R. Rinaldo, Jr. 2002. Rapid and sensitive detection of respiratory virus infections for directed antiviral treatment using R-Mix cultures. *J. Clin. Virol.* 24:107–115.

65. St. George, K., and C. R. Rinaldo, Jr. 1997. Comparison of commercially available antibody reagents for the cytomegalovirus pp65 antigenemia assay. *Clin. Diagn. Virol.* 7:147–152.

66. Tanaka, N., H. Kimura, K. Iida, Y. Saito, I. Tsuge, A. Yoshimi, T. Matsuyama, and T. Morishima. 2000. Quantitative analysis of cytomegalovirus load using a real-time PCR assay. *J. Med. Virol.* 60:455–462.

67. Tang, Y. W., P. S. Mitchell, M. J. Espy, T. F. Smith, and D. H. Persing. 1999. Molecular diagnosis of herpes simplex virus infections in the central nervous system. *J. Clin. Microbiol.* 37:2127–2136.

68. Thompson, W. W., D. K. Shay, E. Weintraub, L. Brammer, N. Cox, L. J. Anderson, and K. Fukuda. 2003. Mortality associated with influenza and respiratory syncytial virus in the United States. *JAMA* 289:179–186.

69. van Doornum, G. J., J. Guldemeester, A. D. Osterhaus, and H. G. Niesters. 2003. Diagnosing herpesvirus infections by real-time amplification and rapid culture. *J. Clin. Microbiol.* 41:576–580.

70. van Elden, L. J., A. M. van Loon, A. van der Beek, K. A. Hendriksen, A. I. Hoepelman, M. G. van Kraaij, P. Schipper, and M. Nijhuis. 2003. Applicability of a real-time quantitative PCR assay for diagnosis of respiratory syncytial virus infection in immunocompromised adults. *J. Clin. Microbiol.* 41:4378–4381.

71. Wald, A., M. L. Huang, D. Carrell, S. Selke, and L. Corey. 2003. Polymerase chain reaction for detection of herpes simplex virus (HSV) DNA on mucosal surfaces: comparison with HSV isolation in cell culture. *J. Infect. Dis.* 188:1345–1351.

72. Ward, C. L., M. H. Dempsey, C. J. Ring, R. E. Kempson, L. Zhang, D. Gor, B. W. Snowden, and M. Tisdale. 2004. Design and performance testing of quantitative real time PCR assays for influenza A and B viral load measurement. *J. Clin. Virol.* 29:179–188.

73. Warford, A. L. 1992. Quality control in clinical virology, p. 8.18.1–8.18.11. *In* H. D. Isenberg (ed.), *Clinical Microbiology Procedures Handbook*, vol. 2. American Society for Microbiology, Washington, D.C.

74. Weinberg, A., L. Brewster, J. Clark, and E. Simoes. 2004. Evaluation of R-Mix shell vials for the diagnosis of viral respiratory tract infections. *J. Clin. Virol.* 30:100–105.

75. Whistler, T., and N. Blackburn. 1997. A rapid culture assay for examining measles virus infections from urine specimens. *Clin. Diagn. Virol.* 7:193–200.

76. Wold, A. D. 1992. Shell vial assay for the rapid detection of viral infections, p. 8.6.1–8.6.10. *In* H. D. Isenberg (ed.), *Clinical Microbiology Procedures Handbook*, vol. 2. American Society for Microbiology, Washington, D.C.

77. Yakushiji, K., H. Gondo, K. Kamezaki, K. Shigematsu, S. Hayashi, M. Kuroiwa, S. Taniguchi, Y. Ohno, K. Takase, A. Numata, K. Aoki, K. Kato, K. Nagafuji, K. Shimoda, T. Okamura, N. Kinukawa, N. Kasuga, M. Sata, and M. Harada. 2002. Monitoring of cytomegalovirus reactivation after allogeneic stem cell transplantation: comparison of an antigenemia assay and quantitative real-time polymerase chain reaction. *Bone Marrow Transplant.* 29:599–606.

Herpes Simplex Virus

D. SCOTT SCHMID

70

Human infections with herpes simplex virus (HSV) type 1 (HSV-1) and HSV-2 are ubiquitous throughout the world. The clinical course of HSV infections is highly variable. Primary infection is subclinical or mild enough to be unrecognized in a majority of cases, whereas clinically apparent infection (1, 4, 35) may range from mild pharyngitis to severe generalized disease and sometimes death. The most frequent manifestation of primary HSV-1 infection is gingovostomatitis in young children, with pharyngitis occurring more commonly in adolescents. Conjunctivitis, keratitis, vesicular eruptions of the skin, herpes whitlow, and encephalitis occur much less frequently. HSV-2 is the most common cause of genital ulcer disease in the Western world, and in some demographic groups genital herpes is the most common sexually transmitted disease. The seroprevalence of HSV-2 has increased more than 30% in recent decades, and the majority of seropositive persons are unaware that they are infected (16). Other presentations of HSV-2 infection are aseptic meningitis and neonatal herpes. Infection in the newborn, which can also be caused by HSV-1, may be localized to the skin or may be generalized and may involve the central nervous system, eyes, skin, and other organs. Persons at risk for serious or prolonged active HSV infection are those with eczema, severe burns, or defective cell-mediated immunity, such as patients after organ transplantation or with AIDS.

Latent infection with both HSV-1 and HSV-2 is typically established after primary infection by viral colonization of the sensory neurons of either the trigeminal or the lumbosacrial ganglia (4, 35). Reactivation from either site may result in subclinical or clinical disease, both with viral shedding. Recurrent infection in the form of fever blisters or, rarely, ocular herpes occurs in up to 40% of the HSV-1-seropositive group (4, 35). Genital eruptions may recur in one-third to two-thirds of individuals infected with HSV-2 (4, 35). Because recurrent infections are frequently subclinical, they may result in unexpected virus spread and may be the source of neonatal infection (10, 24). It is important to understand that the initial clinically recognizable oral or genital HSV disease is not synonymous with primary infection. The term "primary infection" should be reserved for an HSV infection in a person who has not previously been infected with either HSV-1 or HSV-2. A previous oral HSV-1 infection does not protect a person against a genital HSV-2 infection; however, persons with prior HSV-1 infection who are subsequently infected with HSV-2 normally have a less severe clinical course (1, 35).

Infection with either type of HSV gives rise to humoral and cell-mediated immune responses that, while capable of neutralizing HSV and destroying virus-infected cells, do not eliminate latent infection or prevent recurrent disease. Humans produce antibody to the structural components of the virus, the envelope, capsid, and internal proteins, as well as soluble nonvirion antigens specified by the virus. A majority of persons in most population groups are HSV-1 seropositive by 20 years of age (1, 35). Consequently, evidence of antibody against HSV-1 or HSV-2 in a single serum sample by any serologic test, with the exceptions of an immunoglobulin M (IgM)-specific antibody assay (20, 22) and the avidity assay described below (19), provides no information about the time of onset of infection. Serologic diagnosis of active infection with either virus type depends on demonstration of a significant increase in antibody titer. The two HSV types share many epitopes that give rise to strongly cross-reacting antigens (4, 10), and a major portion of the antibody produced in response to a primary infection is to these shared antigens. Virus culture or type-specific serologic tests, some of which are now commercially available (6, 15, 17), must be performed to determine that an individual has been infected with HSV-1 or HSV-2 or both.

Primary infection with either HSV type is documented by testing for seroconversion in paired serum samples (consisting of an acute-phase serum sample collected as close as possible to the onset of illness and a convalescent-phase serum sample collected 10 days to 3 weeks later) by any of the common serologic tests. Detection of IgM in the absence of other evidence is proof of recent exposure (primary exposure, reactivation, or reexposure) but does not demonstrate a primary infection (20). One diagnostic method that can be used with a single serum sample is an IgG antibody avidity assay. The avidity assay (with 6 M urea) was found to distinguish primary HSV infections from nonprimary HSV infections for as long as 100 days after the onset of infection (19).

The immune response to recurrent infection or reinfection with either HSV type is much more complicated and depends on the number, frequency, and type of previous infections as well as the severity of the subsequent infection. After primary HSV infection, antibody levels may decline and then be boosted by subsequent recurrences or infection with the heterologous type. Patients who experience severe recurrences, particularly those associated with systemic or neurologic symptoms, may have a significant rise in antibody levels. On the other hand, most adults with recurrent localized HSV-1 or HSV-2 lesions show stable titers (1, 4) in the neutralization (NT) test, complement fixation (CF) test, and many enzyme immunoassays (EIAs) (20). Initial infection with HSV-2 in persons previously infected with HSV-1 (or vice versa) usually causes a significant rise in the level of antibodies to both the shared HSV antigens and the specific antigens of the infecting type.

The only human herpesvirus that shows significant cross-reactivity with HSV-1 and HSV-2 is varicella-zoster virus (VZV). Paired serum samples from patients with recent VZV infection who have preexisting HSV antibody may sometimes show a rise in the level of antibodies to HSV-1 and HSV-2 in nonspecific tests (1). A similar rise in the level of antibody to VZV may occur in patients with recent HSV infection who have prior antibody to VZV. This heterotypic anamnestic response has been observed by use of the CF test, the NT test, the indirect hemagglutination assay, and the immunofluorescence assay (IFA). Patients with atypical skin vesicles from whom a virus isolate was not obtained should have paired serum samples tested for antibodies against both HSV and VZV. Should a rise in the levels of antibodies to both viruses be found, cross-adsorption tests should be done to identify the cause of the current infection.

CLINICAL INDICATIONS

A presumptive clinical diagnosis of HSV infection can frequently be made from the appearance of cutaneous or mucosal lesions alone. The serologic results obtained after waiting to collect and test an appropriately timed convalescent-phase serum sample offer little guidance for therapy in the clinical management of most patients. The definitive diagnostic methods are virus isolation in cell culture (1) and direct detection in material from lesions (direct fluorescence assay and others, Tzanck smear, PCR). The direct detection methods are more rapid and, generally, considerably more sensitive than culture. Direct detection methods include (i) cytology for intranuclear inclusions and multinucleated giant cells (Giemsa; Tzanck smear); (ii) direct examination of specimens for viral antigens by either IFA, immunoperoxidase staining, or EIA; and (iii) detection of viral DNA in material from lesions, cerebrospinal fluid (CSF), and other tissues and fluids by PCR (12, 27, 30, 32). If possible, PCR results should be confirmed by virus isolation or by detection of antibodies in the CSF (11, 28, 35). Some patients with suspected viral encephalitis or other unusual clinical manifestations may have inconclusive initial diagnostic results, and serology could indicate recent HSV infection. When the etiology of encephalitis remains undiagnosed for 7 or more days after onset, CSF and serum should be tested in parallel for HSV antibody (13, 28). A CSF HSV antibody index of ≥ 2 (28) or an antibody titer in CSF that exceeds 6% of the titer in serum strongly suggests local production of antibody and recent central nervous system infection. Tests for HSV antibody may also be helpful in the diagnosis of HSV infection in immunosuppressed patients with prolonged fever of unknown etiology and infants with undiagnosed congenital disease. A recent case study revealed that HSV-1 and HSV-2 PCR testing should be considered as part of the rule-out diagnosis for suspected cases of bioterrorism-related smallpox (14, 18).

Procedures for determination of type-specific antibody to HSV are most useful in epidemiologic, clinicopathologic, and natural history studies (5, 16, 26, 32). They may also alert the physician to the need for prophylactic treatment of severely immunosuppressed patients. In addition, serologic confirmation of genital infection with HSV-2 permits the physician to discuss acyclovir therapy, the risk of recurrence, and ways to decrease the risk of HSV transmission to contacts. Moreover, an accurate diagnosis for persons with mild or unrecognized clinical manifestations also aids in infection control and in issues associated with pregnancy (11, 24). The prenatal detection of specific HSV-2 antibody indicates which women may be at risk of transmitting HSV to their infants at delivery, although the presence of IgG antibody does not indicate the time when active infection is present in the genital tract. Conversely, a negative result indicates that a woman may be at risk of acquiring HSV-2 during pregnancy, particularly if her partner is positive (11, 24).

Specimen Collection

Clinical specimens for HSV-1 or HSV-2 culture can be obtained by swabbing skin lesions that have been unroofed. Cotton or polyester swabs should be used. Culture may also be successfully performed with specimens of aspirated vesicular fluid or CSF. Direct detection methods require swabbing of the base of the lesion to ensure that infected epithelial cells are collected. In patients with disseminated HSV, peripheral blood mononuclear cells may be useful as specimens for either culture or PCR. For PCR or electron microscopy (EM) detection, scabs from crusted-over lesions are excellent specimens, but they are not useful for virus culture or direct detection methods. Specimens for PCR may be stored in a dry condition for extended periods at ambient temperature without substantial loss in specimen quality. In contrast, swabs collected for direct detection methods should be immersed in a small volume of isotonic transport medium and, ideally, tested within 24 h of collection. Virus isolation in cell culture is far more likely to succeed if specimens are inoculated immediately after collection.

VIRUS ISOLATION

Collected specimens are quite labile and must be transported to the laboratory and processed without delay. It is advisable to use several different HSV-susceptible cell lines, such as HEp-2, Vero-E6, and RD, to maximize the chance for successful culture. Inoculated cells should be checked daily for 7 days (incubated at 37°C, 5% CO_2) for the appearance of cytopathic effect. Positive wells should be used to reinoculate conventional tissue culture for additional confirmational testing.

EM

Suitable specimens for EM include dried smears of material from lesions (which can be resolubilized and placed on a copper grid), vesicular fluid, and scabs that have been ground in water. The chief limitations of this method are its relative insensitivity (the sensitivity is quite low compared with that of methods other than virus isolation) and the nonspecific result produced. EM is capable of identifying an agent as a member of the herpesvirus family on the basis of its distinctive morphology, but individual species cannot be discriminated on the basis of morphology. The method can be rendered specific by using type-specific monoclonal antibodies coupled to electron-dense particles.

DIRECT DETECTION METHODS

Tzanck (Giemsa) Smear

Smears of material from mucocutaneous lesions can be dried onto glass microscopic slides, stained with Giemsa reagent, and examined for the presence of cellular anomalies (syncytia, cytoplasmic ballooning, intranuclear inclusions). These anomalies are observed in all alphaherpesvirus infections and as such do not provide a specific diagnosis.

Direct Fluorescent-Antibody Assay

For the direct fluorescent-antibody assay, the same type of clinical specimen as for Tzanck smear is used, except the material is instead suspended in transport medium. Cellular matter is then pelleted by centrifugation, and the pellet is washed and resuspended in a small volume. Cell suspension is spotted onto glass slides, thoroughly air dried, fixed in ice-cold isopropyl alcohol, and stained with fluorescent antibodies specific for HSV-1 or HSV-2. If monoclonal antibody reagents are used in the protocol, it is preferable to use more than one type-specific antibody for each agent, since an individual epitope may be missing due to mutation in some circulating strains.

Variations on this method include the use of shell vial monolayers that are first inoculated with specimen and then examined with HSV-specific fluorescent antibody reagents. There is also a commercially available enzyme-linked virus-inducible system (ELVIS) that takes advantage of a genetically engineered reporter cell line. The cell line includes a hybrid gene that is induced by the HSV UL39 gene product to express bacterial β-galactosidase. Cells infected with HSV undergo a colorimetric change with the addition of substrate. Type specificity is determined by use of fluorescent antibodies.

SERODIAGNOSTIC TESTS

EIA, indirect hemagglutination assay, immunoblotting, IFA, and the NT test have had the widest application for serodiagnosis and serosurveys. Radioimmunoassays (4) are infrequently used because current EIA and immunoblotting procedures fulfill the same purpose and avoid the problem of using and disposing of radioisotopes. A latex agglutination assay is commercially available, but its use has not been widely reported.

Type-Specific Antibody Tests

The extensive cross-reactivity between HSV-1 and HSV-2 prevents accurate delineation of type-specific antibody with standard antigen preparations (1, 9, 10). Early efforts to devise type-specific serologic assays met with limited success, and none of these formats is currently regarded as reliable. The discovery of a type-specific protein, glycoprotein G (gG), and the crafting of assays using gG1 and gG2 have largely resolved the problem of discriminating antibodies to HSV-1 and HSV-2 (2, 9). A variety of protocols based on the use of gG have been developed over the years, including Western blotting (7, 25), monoclonal antibody blocking EIA (33), indirect IgG enzyme-linked immunosorbent assay (ELISA) (22), and capture ELISA (21), but until recently their use has been restricted to the research laboratory. Several commercial gG type-specific assays are now available; commercial methods using older technology, such as cross-absorption, are still marketed but do not adequately discriminate HSV-1 and HSV-2 antibodies.

Excellent reviews of the history of the development of type-specific and gG-based assays have been published by Bergström and Trybala (9) and Ashley (3). gC of HSV-1 was initially believed to be type specific but was later found to have epitopes that cross-react with HSV-2 antibodies (4, 26). Subsequently, gG1 and gG2 were discovered and shown to be type-specific targets for the human immune response by an immunodot EIA (26), immunoblot assays (4, 5, 32), and EIAs (22, 24). HSV-2-specific monoclonal antibodies have also been used to directly bind gG2 to microtitration plates and detect HSV-2 antibodies by EIA (1). Although the immune response to gG1 and gG2 is not immunodominant, sufficient antibodies to these proteins are made within a month postinfection (6) that gG assays can usually determine the type of HSV infection present.

Nonspecific Antibody Tests

A number of EIAs in which HSV antigen is noncovalently bound to a solid-phase support such as beads, disks, or microtitration plates have been described and are commercially available (4, 13, 22). These assays remain useful as a means for determining recent HSV infection (nonspecific) or recrudescence, by comparing paired acute-phase and convalescent-phase sera. The major advantages of the general EIA are its ability to objectively measure small concentrations of antibody, its use of reagents with long shelf lives, its ability to quickly screen large numbers of serum samples, and the availability of relatively simple instrumentation suitable for automation. However, since type-specific assays accomplish the same objectives, the role of nonspecific serologic methods in clinical practice is likely to diminish.

Immunoblotting

The immune response to HSV can be finely dissected by the immunoblot assay, which is thoroughly described by Ashley and colleagues (4, 5). Briefly, the antigenic proteins of HSV-1 and HSV-2 from infected cells are separated by sodium dodecyl sulfate-polyacrylamide gel electrophoresis (SDS-PAGE), transferred to nitrocellulose, and reacted with human sera. Bound antibody is detected with a peroxidase-conjugated anti-human IgG and a substrate with an insoluble colored product. In each test, one HSV-2 nitrocellulose strip is incubated with a monoclonal antibody that identifies the 92-kDa band of gG2 as a positive control. Sera with predominant reactivity on the HSV-1 strip and no reaction with the gG2 band on the HSV-2 strip have only HSV-1 antibodies. Sera with predominant reactivity on the HSV-2 strip, including the gG2 band, have HSV-2 antibodies. Sera with both profiles have antibodies to both viruses. Sera with atypical or equivocal results, without a clear 92-kDa gG2 band on the HSV-2 strip, are adsorbed separately with HSV-1 and HSV-2 antigens, and each aliquot is retested with both HSV strips.

The immunoblot assay described by Ashley et al. (5) is a highly sensitive and specific assay for HSV type-specific antibodies. Control sera with known reactivity for HSV-1 and HSV-2 are required. Since immunoblot assays include multiple HSV proteins that detect a range of both type-specific and type-common antibodies, they remain the standard by which other type-specific assays are evaluated (2, 9).

A modification of this approach using baculovirus-expressed gG1 and gG2 has also been described (22, 23). Abundant quantities of HSV gG1 and gG2 have been produced in insect cells by use of a baculovirus expression system (31). Insect cells infected with recombinant baculovirus expressing gG1 or gG2 are harvested and disrupted under conditions that release the proteins. The partially purified proteins are separated by SDS-PAGE, transferred to nitrocellulose, and incubated with test and control sera. This method has been extensively compared with other HSV antigen-specific methods and has high specificity and sensitivity (10, 31, 32). The availability of these type-specific recombinant or purified proteins from commercial sources (6, 15, 17) has now made possible large-scale testing of human sera in a variety of type-specific formats.

Immunodot EIA

Lee et al. (26) purified gG1 and gG2 antigens with immunoaffinity columns prepared with HSV type-specific murine monoclonal antibodies for an immunodot EIA performed on nitrocellulose disks in 96-well microtitration plates that required very little antigen. The assays are developed using an enzyme immunoaffinity colorimetric reaction. This is a high-throughput technique that has been instrumental in determining population-based seroprevalence rates for HSV-2 in the United States (16).

Monoclonal Antibody Blocking Assays

The monoclonal antibody blocking method was developed in the United Kingdom by the Central Public Health Laboratory, initially using a radioimmunoassay format. The protocol uses monoclonal type-specific antibody reagents directed against gG epitopes of HSV-1 and HSV-2. The method has been extensively validated against a number of alternative gG-based methods and performs with high sensitivity and specificity.

Several other gG-based methods that have performance standards comparable to those of the methods described above have been developed. With the advent of commercially available gG-based serological methods, these methods have rapidly become the standard of choice for performing HSV serology in both research laboratories and clinics. The assays are simple to perform and highly specific and have essentially the same sensitivities as procedures already in use.

Commercially Available Type-Specific Assays

An evaluation of three new commercial gG2-based EIAs has been made by testing serum samples from 25 persons with culture-confirmed infection with HSV-2 (13). The assays were based on recombinant gG2 produced by the baculovirus system or purified HSV-2 gG prepared from infected cell culture. The sensitivities and specificities and the level of concordance between the assays were high. However, caution was advised in the interpretation of low-positive results (possible false-positive results), and such samples might need another confirmatory test. Another report compared a rapid commercial assay, the POCkit-HSV-2 test (Diagnology, Belfast, United Kingdom), with the authors' immunoblot procedure and a gG2 type-specific EIA (Focus Technologies, Cincinnati, Ohio) (6). The sensitivity and specificity of the tests in comparison with the immunoblot results were in the 90 to 95% range. Timing in the collection of sera is important because it was shown that the median time for the POCkit-HSV-2 test and the immunoblot assay to become positive after the onset of symptoms was 13 days, and only 80% of the samples were positive at the end of 4 weeks.

Almost all of these methods that use HSV gG have shown good agreement when evaluated with specimens from cross-sectional studies (2). A current study with samples collected serially over a 2-year period from Thai military recruits found that the serologic status of some individuals determined by gG assays changed from positive to negative over time (32). The inaccuracy was found in four separate assays, and the variation was not confined to the same specimens with each assay. In some cases, the loss of positivity could be associated with weakly positive specimens. It is suggested that testing of cohort specimens from population-based studies in addition to clinical ones should be part of any assay evaluation scheme (32).

PCR Methods

Serological methods are not useful for detecting current HSV infection or viral shedding, and culture is relatively insensitive even when performed under optimal conditions. In the past decade, PCR has emerged as the method of choice for the direct detection of currently active HSV infection (30). HSV PCR on CSF has now supplanted brain biopsy as the method of choice for diagnosis of herpes encephalitis (34). The assays have been determined to be sufficiently specific and sensitive that a carefully performed test with a negative result excludes HSV as a diagnosis in encephalitis. A variety of different methods have been described, including single-agent methods (8, 30), multiplex methods (23, 27, 29), and real-time PCR (12). In studies directly contrasting the performance of PCR with culture, direct fluorescent-antibody assay, and other techniques, PCR is invariably more sensitive and at least comparably specific.

The most frequently used target genes for type-specific PCR are gD and gB, although reported methods have also targeted the thymidine kinase, gG, UL42, DNA polymerase, and ICP27 genes. The highly conserved DNA polymerase gene has been used most frequently for consensus PCR methods that amplify all recognized human herpesviruses.

As commercial PCR formats for clinical diagnosis have become more widely available, the use of PCR in clinical settings for routine diagnosis has become increasingly common. It is the most sensitive and specific method available for the detection of HSV in a wide variety of specimens. Since atypical HSV-1 and HSV-2 disease was, like varicella, historically misdiagnosed as smallpox prior to eradication, HSV PCR is also recommended as part of a testing panel to exclude smallpox used as a bioterrorist weapon.

It must also be kept in mind, however, that not all PCR methods are created equal. Direct comparisons of various formats have sometimes revealed substantial differences in the performance standards. In addition, care should be taken to ensure that substances potentially inhibitory to PCRs are eliminated during DNA purification.

REFERENCES

1. **Arvin, A. M., and C. G. Prober.** 1999. Herpes simplex viruses, p. 878–887. *In* P. R. Murphy, E. J. Baron, M. A. Pfaller, F. C. Tenover, and R. H. Yolken (ed.), *Manual of Clinical Microbiology*, 7th ed. American Society for Microbiology, Washington, D.C.
2. **Ashley, R. L.** 1998. Type-specific antibodies to HSV-1 and -2: review of methodology. *Herpes* **5:**33–38.
3. **Ashley, R. L.** 2001. Sorting out the new HSV type specific antibody tests. *Sex. Transm. Infect.* **77:**232–237.
4. **Ashley, R. L., and L. Corey.** 1989. Herpes simplex virus, p. 265–317. *In* N. J. Schmidt and R. W. Emmons (ed.), *Diagnostic Procedures for Viral, Rickettsial and Chlamydial Infections*, 6th ed. American Public Health Association, Washington, D.C.
5. **Ashley, R. L., J. Dalessio, J. Dragavon, L. A. Koutsky, F. Lee, A. J. Nahmias, C. E. Stevens, K. K. Holmes, and L. Corey.** 1993. Underestimation of HSV-2 seroprevalence in a high-risk population by microneutralization assay. *Sex. Transm. Dis.* **20:**230–235.
6. **Ashley, R. L., M. Eagleton, and N. Pheiffer.** 1999. Ability of a rapid serology test to detect seroconversion to herpes

simplex virus type 2 glycoprotein G soon after infection. *J. Clin. Microbiol.* **37:**1632–1633.

7. **Ashley, R. L., J. Militoni, F. Lee, A. Nahmias, and L. Corey.** 1988. Comparison of Western blot (immunoblot) and glycoprotein G-specific immunodot enzyme assay for detecting antibodies to herpes simplex virus types 1 and 2 in human sera. *J. Clin. Microbiol.* **26:**662–667.

8. **Athmanathan, S., S. B. Reddy, R. Nutheti, and G. N. Rao.** 2002. Comparison of an immortalized human corneal epithelial cell line with Vero cells in the isolation of herpes simplex virus-1 for the laboratory diagnosis of herpes simplex keratitis. *BMC Ophthalmol.* **2:**3.

9. **Bergström, T., and E. Trybala.** 1996. Antigenic differences between HSV-1 and HSV-2 glycoproteins and their importance for type-specific serology. *Intervirology* **39:**176–184.

10. **Berstein, M. T., and J. A. Stewart.** 1971. Method for typing antisera to herpesvirus hominis by indirect hemagglutination inhibition. *Appl. Microbiol.* **21:**680–684.

11. **Brown, Z. A., S. Selke, J. Zeh, J. Kopelman, A. Maslow, R. L. Ashley, D. H. Watts, S. Berry, M. Herd, and L. Corey.** 1997. The acquisition of herpes simplex virus during pregnancy. *N. Engl. J. Med.* **337:**509–515.

12. **Burrows, J., A. Nitsche, B. Bayly, E. Walker, G. Higgins, and T. Kok.** 2002. Detection and subtyping of herpes simplex virus in clinical samples by Light-Cycler PCR, enzyme immunoassay and cell culture. *BMC Microbiol.* **2:**12.

13. **Cremer, N. E., C. K. Cossen, C. V. Hanson, and G. R. Shell.** 1982. Evaluation and reporting of enzyme immunoassay determinations of antibody to herpes simplex virus in sera and cerebrospinal fluid. *J. Clin. Microbiol.* **15:**815–823.

14. **Damon, I., L. Rotz, J. Seward, and J. Hughes.** 2003. Comment on: Hanrahan, et al. 2003. A smallpox false alarm. *N. Engl. J. Med.* **348:**467–468. *N. Engl. J. Med.* **348:**468.

15. **Eis-Hübinger, A. M., M. Däumer, B. Matz, and K. E. Schneweis.** 1999. Evaluation of three glycoprotein G2-based enzyme immunoassays for detection of antibodies to herpes simplex virus type 2 in human sera. *J. Clin. Microbiol.* **37:**1242–1246.

16. **Fleming, D. T., G. W. McQuillan, R. E. Johnson, A. J. Nahmias, S. O. Aral, F. K. Lee, and M. E. St. Louis.** 1997. Herpes simplex virus type 2 in the United States, 1976 to 1994. *N. Engl. J. Med.* **337:**1105–1111.

17. **Groen, J., G. Van Dijk, H. G. M. Niesters, W. I. Van der Meijden, and A. D. M. E. Osterhaus.** 1998. Comparison of two enzyme-linked immunosorbent assays and one rapid immunoblot assay for detection of herpes simplex virus type-2-specific antibodies in serum. *J. Clin. Microbiol.* **36:**845–847.

18. **Hanrahan, J. A., M. Jakubowycz, and R. D. Bryan.** 2003. A smallpox false alarm. *N. Engl. J. Med.* **348:**467–468.

19. **Hashido, M., S. Inouye, and T. Kawana.** 1997. Differentiation of primary from nonprimary genital herpes infections by a herpes simplex virus-specific immunoglobulin G avidity test. *J. Clin. Microbiol.* **35:**1766–1768.

20. **Hashido, M., and T. Kawana.** 1997. Herpes simplex virus-specific IgM, IgA, and IgG subclass antibody responses in primary and nonprimary genital herpes patients. *Microbiol. Immunol.* **41:**415–420.

21. **Hashido, M., F. K. Lee, S. Inouye, and T. Kawana.** 1997. Detection of herpes simplex virus type-specific antibodies by an enzyme-linked immunosorbent assay based on glycoprotein G. *J. Med. Virol.* **53:**319–323.

22. **Ho, D. W. T., P. R. Field, E. Sjogren-Jansson, S. Jeansson, and A. L. Cunningham.** 1992. Indirect ELISA for the detection of HSV-2 specific IgG and IgM antibodies with glycoprotein G (gG-2). *J. Virol. Methods* **36:**249–264.

23. **Koenig, M., K. S. Reynolds, W. Aldous, and M. Hickman.** 2001. Comparison of Light-Cycler PCR, enzyme immunoassay, and tissue culture for detection of Herpes Simplex Virus. *Diagn. Microbiol. Infect. Dis.* **40:**107–110.

24. **Kulhanjian, J. A., V. Soroush, D. S. Au, R. N. Bronzan, L. L. Yasukawa, L. E. Weylman, A. M. Arvin, and C. G. Prober.** 1992. Identification of women at unsuspected risk of primary infection with herpes simplex virus type 2 during pregnancy. *N. Engl. J. Med.* **326:**916–920.

25. **Lee, F. K., R. M. Coleman, L. Pereira, P. D. Bailey, M. Tatsuno, and A. J. Nahmias.** 1985. Detection of herpes simplex virus type 2-specific antibody with glycoprotein G. *J. Clin. Microbiol.* **22:**641–644.

26. **Lee, F. K., L. Pereira, C. Griffin, E. Reid, and A. Nahmias.** 1986. A novel glycoprotein for detection of herpes simplex virus type 1-specific antibodies. *J. Virol. Methods* **14:**111–118.

27. **Markoulatos, P., A. Georgopoulou, C. Kotsovassilis, P. Karabogia-Karaphillides, and N. Spyrou.** 2000. Detection and typing of HSV-1, HSV-2, and VZV by a multiplex polymerase chain reaction. *J. Clin. Lab. Anal.* **14:**214–219.

28. **Monteyne, P., F. Albert, B. Weissbrich, E. Zardini, M. Ciardi, G. M. Cleator, and C. J. M. Sindic.** 1997. The detection of intrathecal synthesis of anti-herpes simplex IgG antibodies: comparison between an antigen-mediated immunoblotting technique and antibody index calculations. *J. Med. Virol.* **53:**324–331.

29. **Nicoll, S., A. Brass, and H. A. Cubie.** 2001. Detection of herpes viruses in clinical samples using real-time PCR. *J. Virol. Methods* **96:**25–31.

30. **O'Sullivan, C. E., A. J. Aksamit, J. R. Harrington, W. S. Harmsen, P. S. Mitchell, and R. Patel.** 2003. Clinical spectrum and laboratory characteristics associated with detection of herpes simplex virus DNA in cerebrospinal fluid. *Mayo Clin. Proc.* **78:**1347–1352.

31. **Sánchez-Martinez, D., D. S. Schmid, W. Whittington, D. Brown, W. C. Reeves, S. Chatterjee, R. J. Whitley, and P. E. Pellett.** 1991. Evaluation of a test based on baculovirus-expressed glycoprotein G for detection of herpes simplex virus type-specific antibodies. *J. Infect. Dis.* **164:**1196–1199.

32. **Schmid, D. S., D. R. Brown, R. Nisenbaum, R. L. Burke, D. Alexander, R. Ashley, P. E. Pellett, and W. C. Reeves.** 1999. Limits in the reliability of glycoprotein G-based type-specific serologic assays for herpes simplex virus types 1 and 2. *J. Clin. Microbiol.* **37:**376–379.

33. **Slomka, M. J., R. L. Ashley, F. M. Cowan, A. Cross, and D. W. Brown.** 1995. Monoclonal antibody blocking tests for the detection of HSV-1 and HSV-2 specific humoral responses: comparison with Western blot assay. *J. Virol. Methods* **55:**27–35.

34. **Tang, Y.-W., J. R. Hibbs, K. R. Tau, Q. Qian, H. A. Skarhus, T. F. Smith, and D. H. Persing.** 1999. Effective use of polymerase chain reaction for diagnosis of central nervous system infections. *Clin. Infect. Dis.* **29:**803–806.

35. **Whitley, R. J.** 1996. Herpes simplex viruses, p. 2299–2342. *In* B. N. Fields, D. M. Knipe, and P. M. Howley (ed.), *Fields Virology*, 3rd ed. Lippincott-Raven Publishers, Philadelphia, Pa.

Varicella-Zoster Virus

D. SCOTT SCHMID AND VLADIMIR LOPAREV

71

Varicella-zoster virus (VZV) is a highly contagious alphaherpesvirus that commonly causes two distinct clinical illnesses. Primary infection with VZV causes varicella, known more commonly as chickenpox, which is characterized by a generalized vesicular rash typically accompanied by fever and other nonspecific symptoms. VZV may reactivate decades after the primary infection to cause zoster, also called shingles, a dermatomally distributed vesicular rash. A number of zoster patients present with postherpetic neuralgia, characterized by severe pain that may persist for long periods after the rash has resolved. Some rare complications of zoster include encephalitis, conjunctivitis, keratitis and other eye disorders, Ramsey-Hunt syndrome, neurogenic bladder, and transverse myelitis. The majority of varicella cases are mild in nature and resolve without serious sequelae. On rare occasion, varicella may be complicated by bacterial infections, pneumonia, encephalitis, cerebellar ataxia, hepatitis, thrombocytopenia, and nephritis. Studies have shown that patients with recent varicella have a 40-fold greater risk of developing severe group A streptococcal disease. Populations at increased risk for serious VZV disease include immunocompromised adults and children, VZV-seronegative adults, pregnant women, and newborn infants. Prior to the introduction of varicella vaccine, complications of VZV infections resulted in approximately 100 deaths and 10,000 hospitalizations each year in the United States (1).

A live, attenuated varicella vaccine was approved for use in the United States in 1995 and is recommended for routine immunization of children and for susceptible adolescents and adults. Coverage for the vaccine in the United States is now estimated to be close to 90% for children, and a proportionate reduction in varicella incidence has been observed with evidence of herd immunity (9; J. Seward, personal communication). Vaccination occasionally produces a mild rash, and breakthrough infections by wild-type VZV strains sometimes occur in vaccinated patients, usually causing less severe disease than a typical primary infection.

When varicella was commonplace in the United States, laboratory testing to verify varicella was generally unnecessary, since both varicella and zoster could be readily diagnosed by a clinician. The dramatically reduced incidence of varicella, together with the increasingly common occurrence of modified disease, has made laboratory confirmation of VZV infection and discrimination of the vaccine strain from wild-type virus increasingly important.

The 90% reduction of varicella means physicians will be less likely to encounter cases of varicella and have an increased likelihood of encountering disease that does not meet the conventional case definition for varicella or zoster. Effective monitoring of the changing epidemiology of this virus will therefore hinge critically on the use of laboratory testing. In addition, laboratory services are essential for the identification of susceptible adults for the purposes of immunization of health care workers or individuals in other settings that carry high risk for exposure to varicella or zoster. The varicella vaccine is now recommended for the postexposure immunization of susceptible adults (3).

METHODS

Specimen Collection

Laboratory diagnosis of VZV infection requires the identification of the virus or one of its products in skin lesions, tissues, or fluids from the patient. Techniques include isolation of the virus in tissue culture, direct immunofluorescent staining of cells obtained from lesions, and detection of the virus genome by techniques based on PCR. Among these techniques, PCR-based detection methods are the most sensitive.

Specimens that are most commonly tested for VZV include smears or swabs of vesicular fluid, skin scrapings, crusts, cerebrospinal fluid, and various tissues obtained at autopsy. Vesicular lesions may be sampled by unroofing a vesicle with a sterile needle and then vigorously swabbing the base of the lesion with a sterile swab, applying enough pressure to collect epithelial cells without causing bleeding. Collection of infected epithelial cells from the base of the lesion is important because the majority of VZV virions are cell associated. It is best to use swabs made from synthetic materials, as it may be difficult to elute virus from cotton swabs, porous wooden sticks may absorb the extraction buffer, and substances in the wood may inhibit PCR. To avoid contamination, each swab must be placed directly into a separate tube and labeled. Vesicular fluid can also be collected onto a glass slide and air dried (again, taking care that specimens are placed in separate containers to avoid contamination). For virus isolation, vesicular fluid may be collected in sealed capillary tubes; however, VZV is extremely sensitive to heat and desiccation, making isolation difficult under the best circumstances. Ideally, vesicular fluid should be inoculated into cell culture immediately upon harvesting. Samples may be frozen at −80°C for several days prior to culture, but this procedure results in a significant loss of infectivity. Crusts are also outstanding specimens for PCR detection of VZV DNA; they may be collected in sterile tubes or plastic bags. Refrigeration is preferred for smears to be examined for viral antigen, but air-dried specimens for PCR can be kept at ambient temperature indefinitely.

Virus Isolation

VZV can be isolated from vesicular fluids of patients with zoster or varicella for a short period (1 to 3 days) following the onset of rash, but culture of VZV from respiratory secretions or biopsy specimens is rarely successful. Crusts do not contain infectious virus. Various cell cultures can be used to culture VZV from vesicular fluid, including human fetal diploid lung (HFDL) or kidney (HFDK) cells, human embryonic lung fibroblasts (MRC5 or WI 38), human melanoma (MeWo) cells, and human lung fibroblasts (HLFs). Our laboratory prefers the HLF and MeWo cell lines. Primary embryonic guinea pig cells will support VZV propagation but are generally less productive than human cells. Sufficient cell culture medium must be used to maintain the culture for 10 to 14 days without change. Several studies have shown that virus isolation, even under optimal conditions, is significantly less sensitive than direct immunodetection or PCR for the detection of VZV. VZV produces a distinctive specific cytopathic effect (CPE) in cell monolayers. Initially, in HLFs the CPE is characterized by discrete crescent-shaped foci of different sizes and consists of rounded and swollen cells. This may appear as early as day 3 or as late as day 14 after inoculation, but most appears between 4 and 7 days. If VZV-specific CPE has not appeared after a week to 14 days, it may be useful to passage the inoculated cultures. CPE may develop even if the amount of vesicular fluid in the capillary tube is barely discernible to the naked eye, if the specimens are obtained within the first 2 days of rash. Confirmation of VZV-specific CPE may be obtained if necessary by staining with fluorescein-labeled specific antibody.

The tendency of VZV to remain cell associated, together with its susceptibility to inactivation, renders virus isolation less sensitive than direct immunofluorescence or PCR. Preliminary identification of VZV can be made on the basis of characteristic CPE, which is usually more focal and progresses significantly more slowly than CPE from herpes simplex virus (HSV). However, the definitive identification of VZV requires additional testing with immunological assays or PCR. Specific identification of a VZV isolate can be made by demonstrating its ability to interact with reference serum from patients who have had a clinically diagnosed case of varicella or with VZV-specific monoclonal antibody. Human sera used for identification of VZV should be free of antibody against other human herpesviruses that may cross-react with VZV proteins due to structural homology (e.g., HSV type 1 [HSV-1] and HSV-2). VZV-specific monoclonal antibodies are commercially available and are the preferred reagent, since they significantly increase sensitivity and specificity of detection compared with human serum or polyclonal serum produced in animals. Specific VZV identification can be accomplished with direct or indirect immunofluorescent staining of infected cells.

Direct Examination of Material from Skin Lesions

Scrapings of vesicular lesions obtained with a scalpel blade can be examined for giant cells or intranuclear inclusions by staining with Giemsa reagent (Tzsank smear). Similar changes are seen with HSV; thus, the method is limited to identifying the presence of an alphaherpesvirus and is not species specific. Staining for examination for inclusions must be performed properly, using specific methods for this purpose, or specimens may yield false-negative results. It should be recognized that the presence of intranuclear inclusions or multinucleated giant cells is not specific for VZV. In contrast, direct fluorescence antibody (DFA) staining appears to have excellent sensitivity and specificity, although its performance is inferior to that of PCR. Staining of the scrapings with conjugated anti-VZV monoclonal antibodies can enable specific identification. A number of monoclonal antibodies are available for this purpose. Specimens must be collected with care; scraping of unroofed lesions must be sufficiently vigorous to ensure the collection of infected cells, but the specimen should contain as little blood as possible, since this can produce false-negative results. Crusts cannot be used for direct detection methods.

EM

Vesicular fluids, crusts that have been ground in water, or skin lesion sections can be examined by electron microscopy (EM). Good results can be obtained with air-dried smears of fluids prepared on glass microscope slides, which can be resolubilized and transferred to a grid. This method is useful only as an identification for herpesviruses; it does not facilitate the identification of VZV. The finding of virus with morphology characteristic of herpesviruses identifies the etiological agent as a member of this genus and serves to distinguish it from orthopoxviruses. However, this method does not provide a specific differentiation for VZV. In addition, this technique is relatively insensitive, capable of reliably detecting virions only at very high concentrations. It has been estimated that as much as 27% of DFA-positive specimens may give negative results by EM. VZV specificity can be conferred on EM by using VZV-specific immunoglobulin tagged with electron-dense materials.

Genetic Stability of VZV

A variety of techniques, including complete genomic sequencing, have been used to show the low degree of genetic variability among VZV isolates. However, at least three distinct VZV genotypes (European, Japanese, and Mosaic [M]) have been identified. Interestingly, the Japanese and European genotypes are dominant in countries with a temperate climate, although the Japanese strains are found almost exclusively in that country, whereas European strains are common to Europe, the United States, Canada, and other countries north or south of the 30th parallels (temperate/polar zones) (5). VZV strains of the M genotype are most common in countries with a tropical climate. Only about 0.1% of the nucleotides vary among individual strains of VZV, and the sequence diversity is distributed randomly throughout the genome. The attenuated vaccine strain (Oka) is derived from a Japanese genotype strain that has only about 40 base-pair differences from the parental strain. Vaccine preparations are now known to contain a number of subvariant strains, and only four of the vaccine markers (all in open reading frame 62 [ORF62]) are consistently maintained in all vaccine subvariants (unpublished observation). The mutations responsible for vaccine attenuation have not yet been determined, however. Genetic variability can have an effect on the performance of serological assays, particularly those involving the use of VZV-specific monoclonal antibodies.

PCR

PCR is the most accurate and sensitive method for VZV detection and differentiation. Taking into account that virus isolation is time-consuming and that viral DNA is much more stable than infectious virus, PCR is the preferred method for confirming the presence of VZV in a specimen. PCR is particularly useful to confirm mild VZV disease in vaccinees or in late stages of varicella when lesions contain no viable virus. Amplification and analysis of targeted VZV DNA regions is the method of choice for discriminating vaccine from wild-type VZV isolates. For routine laboratory diagnostic purposes, the best materials to use are vesicular fluids collected with capillaries or swabs, scrapings dried onto glass slides; or crusts from lesions. By this method, VZV DNA can be detected in various tissues, including lung, liver, kidney, skin and adrenal glands, trigeminal ganglia, and dorsal root ganglia. The viral genome can also be detected in peripheral mononuclear cells and, rarely, in cerebrospinal fluids, bronchoalveolar lavage, breast milk, oropharyngeal swabs, throat swabs, peripheral blood mononuclear cells, and nasal secretions. In some specific situations, VZV DNA can be found in the synovial fluid of patients with arthritis; intraocular fluids, corneal scrapings, and tear films of patients with retinal necrosis; temporal bone sections from patients who had herpes zoster oticus; and amniotic fluid, fetal tissues, and the placenta during neonatal varicella. We had experience of successful identification and typing of VZV strains from environmental swabs. A variety of PCR protocols have been used to detect VZV DNA. However, the current diagnostic convention combines specific VZV detection and wild-type and vaccine strain discrimination. Recently, it was documented that VZV vaccine preparations are heterogeneous, and more than 100 variant viruses carrying different arrays of vaccine-associated mutations exist. Identification of vaccine-specific single-nucleotide polymorphisms can be accomplished either by direct sequencing of a PCR product, by restriction fragment length polymorphism (RFLP), or by Förster resonance energy transfer (FRET)-based real-time PCR (4, 6). Recent studies indicate that while multiple polymorphisms were identified between vaccine and wild-type strains, detection of the sequence polymorphism at genome position 106262 is the most reliable method for discriminating the vaccine strain from wild-type VZV (4, 6). Perhaps the most important concern in the use of PCR is the quality of the template to be amplified. Care must be taken to optimize the purification of DNA from samples that may contain substances that inhibit PCRs. Most modern commercial kits designed for DNA purification from cells and tissues, used in accordance with the manufacturers' instructions, will provide good-quality DNA for immediate PCR amplification. Proper use of controls is an essential element of PCR protocols. Positive, negative, and blank (no virus DNA) controls allow inspection of the extraction, amplification, and product detection steps. In addition, as a universal control for the quality of sample processing, the amplification of human cellular genes (actin or globin) must be performed. This procedure is necessary in the case of negative PCR amplification with specific VZV primers to reduce the possibility of a false-negative result. Several primer sets that, when coupled with the step of restriction endonuclease digestion (RFLP), reliably discriminate between the vaccine strain and wild-type VZV have been identified. We have recently developed a number of PCR assays targeting single-nucleotide polymorphisms in ORF62 that more definitively discriminate vaccine strain than do markers described previously, such as those in ORF38 and ORF54 (4, 6). Recent advances in PCR technology, such as FRET-based approaches, have greatly shortened PCR cycling intervals and have made it possible to bypass the time-consuming endonuclease digestion step, greatly reducing the time required to obtain a strain discrimination result (as little as 3 h) and reducing the risk of contamination (6). We have now expanded the capability of PCR for use in the identification of wild-type VZV genotypes as well as multiple subvariants of VZV Oka, a tool that should prove invaluable to the monitoring of varicella vaccine impact (5).

Serologic Testing

Serologic testing is most often requested for determining susceptibility to VZV in outbreak settings, but on occasion it is needed for diagnosis. We have also used immunoglobulin G (IgG) enzyme-linked immunosorbent assay (ELISA) testing of acute- and convalescent-phase sera to support PCR evidence for breakthrough infection. Acute-phase serum should be obtained as soon as possible after the onset of illness, and the convalescent-phase serum should be obtained 4 to 6 weeks after onset. A variety of methods are available to determine whether there are significant rises in the level of VZV-specific serum immunoglobulin; however, all must be performed in an endpoint dilution format. Assay formats used for simple determination of VZV serostatus include ELISA, membrane fluorescence, and latex bead agglutination. Each of these test formats has limitations, which are discussed in greater detail below.

Rapid Serologic Tests

Rapid point-of-care assays for the detection of VZV antibodies have become commercially available in recent years. These include latex bead agglutination or flowthrough membrane-based enzyme immunoassay (EIA) methods. Serum, plasma, or whole blood can be tested. In general, these assays are designed to detect IgG antibodies; they have been reported to have good sensitivity and specificity, although none is as reliable as either glycoprotein-based ELISA (gpELISA) or fluorescent antibody to membrane antigen (FAMA) tests, particularly for detecting seroconversion in VZV-vaccinated persons. One recent study revealed that the latex bead agglutination test can be prone to false-positive results (2). Since one of the principal uses of these tests is to identify health care workers and other persons at high risk for susceptibility to VZV, a more specific commercial method is probably preferable for that purpose.

Western blotting

Western blotting of whole-cell lysates of VZV-infected cells permits a detailed analysis of antibody profiles and can be useful for the characterization of the antibody response to specific antigens. Western blotting is more cumbersome than most other approaches to antibody detection; in our hands, it has also been considerably less sensitive. In addition, Western blotting is limited to the detection of linear epitopes since the three-dimensional structure of antigens is destroyed by the sodium dodecyl sulfate used for high-performance gel electrophoresis. The resolving capacity of Western blotting is limited to the discrimination of only about 25 distinctive bands; as such, it may be difficult to distinguish between antigens of similar molecular sizes.

FAMA

FAMA is one of the most sensitive assays for the detection of VZV antibodies, when performed in an experienced laboratory.

It has been recognized for some time as one of the few tests sufficiently sensitive and specific to detect VZV antibodies in vaccinated individuals. In part, the enhanced sensitivity of this assay may be attributable to the fact that live, infected cells are used, thus preserving the conformational structure of the surface glycoprotein antigens. If cells are fixed, the antigenic structure is likely modified, and fixation generally results in decreased sensitivity. A modified FAMA assay in which cells are briefly fixed in 0.075% glutaraldehyde for 60 s at 0°C and stored at −70°C has been described (10). The FAMA assay can be used in various formats to detect any of the major classes of specific immunoglobulin. While this method can be quite powerful, optimal performance requires a long learning curve; the protocol requires live, virus-infected cells; and the method cannot be automated for large-scale screening.

gpELISA

Merck and Company developed a highly sensitive and specific ELISA method predicated on the use of a highly purified, high-concentration solution of VZV glycoproteins. It is the only method other than the FAMA test with performance standards adequate to reliably detect seroconversion to VZV vaccination. The method is not currently available commercially, although in recent years our laboratory has secured a supply of the antigen from the manufacturer. Direct comparison between the FAMA assay and gpELISA reveals that they have comparable levels of performance, and the ELISA method has the advantage of being easily performed. It is likely that this assay will become commercially available in the near future.

NT Tests

The presence of neutralizing antibodies in serum can be detected by using a neutralization (NT) assay based on reduction of plaque formation by titered VZV preparations pretreated with serum. Cell-free VZV is preferable for use in such assays and may be obtained from infected HLFs or MeWo cells after the development of visible CPE. The cells generally can be destroyed by sonication. Freeze-thawing procedures are not recommended because they inactivate the virus. Extracellular virus should be used immediately after preparation since it is susceptible to rapid inactivation, or preparations may be frozen at −70°C in calf serum or glycerol. VZV NT assays are rarely used in diagnostic laboratories today, and accompany early stages of vaccine licensing and vaccination efforts. NT methodology for VZV requires some improvement but will likely prove helpful for evaluating the duration of protective immunity among vaccinees. It will also be useful to identify the primary NT targets for VZV. There are no clear recommendations or standardized data for the evaluation of neutralizing antibody. Since it proved difficult to detect neutralizing antibody titers in vaccinated individuals, highly sensitive gpELISA and FAMA tests (both of which likely detect the principal neutralizing targets for VZV) were performed in parallel with, and in some instances completely supplanted the use of, NT tests during Oka vaccine efficacy trials.

Antibody Avidity

Measurement of IgM antibody in individuals with known recent exposure to VZV is inconsistent, and the detection of IgM may reflect either primary infection or reactivation. Evaluations of antibody avidity are straightforward to perform and can provide useful insights into the relative maturity of immunoglobulin responses to VZV. As such, they provide a useful adjunct tool for determining whether a person has a well-established, high-avidity antibody population specific for VZV. This parameter generally has not been investigated for VZV and could be particularly important for VZV vaccinees. It is conceivable that, as vaccination becomes nearly universal and natural reexposure to VZV becomes rare, fully mature immunoglobulin responses might not develop over time. Determination of antibody avidity is usually based on the separation of low- and high-avidity antibodies by using denaturing agents in immunoassays (EIA) or immunofluorescent assays. Several agents, such as guanidine hydrochloride, diethyleneamine, isothiocyanate, and urea, have been used for this purpose. Calculations of the avidity results have been approached in several ways. In general, avidity is expressed as percent ratio of antibody titers or EIA absorbance values with and without denaturation. Avidity results based on endpoint titration with and without denaturant are considered to be the "gold standard" for avidity determination.

INTERPRETATION

If results are required quickly, the preferred method is direct staining of cellular material from lesions, since it is sensitive, specific, and rapid. If, however, rapid turnaround is not an issue, PCR-based methods are more sensitive and informative, since they are agent specific and also can be designed to discriminate vaccine strain from wild-type isolates. That said, real-time FRET-based PCR and more rapid DNA extraction have made these methods comparable to DFA staining in the time required to obtain a result. Serologic testing is not a preferred method for confirming an acute infection. Significant rises in titer between acute-phase and convalent-phase sera are not always observed, and the determination of whether a titer found in such sera is consistent with an acute infection would depend on the test used.

For determination of susceptibility, a properly standardized and sensitive method is essential. As mentioned above, assay specificity trumps sensitivity as a consideration if the goal is to determine susceptibility to varicella in high-risk persons. Passively acquired antibody may also yield false-positive test results, and immunocompromised patients may have lower levels of antibody that may be difficult to detect in some immune patients if the test used is too insensitive.

ANALYTICAL SENSITIVITY AND SPECIFICITY, QUALITY CONTROL AND ASSURANCE, DATA ANALYSIS, PITFALLS, AND TROUBLESHOOTING

Serologic Testing

There have been several reports of inappropriate management of patients due to false-positive reactions (2, 7). While this is the greatest concern in settings where susceptible adults are at high risk of VZV exposure, it is also clear that the majority of VZV assays currently available fail to detect seroconversion in response to vaccination. In some public health organizations, this has led to unnecessary multiple vaccinations of the same individual. Suitable normal tissue control antigens in an ELISA are essential to reduce the risk of false-positive test results, although such controls are generally absent from commercially available assays. New methods are commonly validated by comparing performance with that of an established method that may itself be inaccurate. It is difficult to choose with certainty a set of negative sera that are ideal for this purpose. Sera from seronegative susceptible individuals who are known to have developed varicella can be used to standardize an assay, although, increasingly, vaccinees who fail to develop detectable antibody titers as determined by some methods and who might subsequently develop breakthrough disease might inadvertently be selected. Cord serum depleted of IgG can be used, but the elimination of IgG from these sera might also obscure nonspecific reactivity that could be present in normal serum specimens. A strategy that we adopted was to identify a set of sera that tested negative by a large panel of techniques, including FAMA tests, latex bead agglutination, immunoblotting, and several commercial and laboratory-based ELISAs. We developed a whole VZV-infected cell lysate-based ELISA that has become our preferred method. It should be emphasized that ELISAs vary considerably in their level of performance, and one should not assume that this method is generically better or worse than other methods. The means by which cutoff values for seropositivity (assessment of assay performance variability, selection of standardization sera, etc.) are established is crucial. More recently, we have been using lentil lectin-purified VZV glycoprotein preparations in the gpELISA format (8); this assay clearly has specificity and sensitivity comparable to those of the FAMA test, reliably detects vaccine seroconversion, and is far simpler and less subjective. Our current strategy is to first test with a whole-virus ELISA and then retest negative and equivocal specimens with the gpELISA.

None of the currently available serologic assays for VZV can reliably detect specific antibody in persons who have been vaccinated. This problem is most pronounced for measuring varicella vaccine seroconversion in adults. Among methods that are available only in selected laboratories, only the FAMA test and gpELISA are sufficiently sensitive and specific to reliably document VZV seroconversion in vaccinees. Unfortunately, FAMA testing cannot be recommended for routine use due to the technical difficulties in performance and interpretation. gpELISA is simple to perform but is not currently available commercially. Latex bead agglutination, which has been reported to perform similarly to the FAMA test, does not perform better than the whole VZV-infected cell ELISA in our hands. Efforts to develop more sensitive VZV serologic assay formats are currently being explored in our laboratory.

A number of studies have documented cases of individuals who develop detectable VZV-specific antibodies after immunization with varicella vaccine who subsequently developed varicella following exposure. This phenomenon should be borne in mind when serologic tests are used to identify adults who are protected from VZV infection in high-risk exposure environments. We recently documented cases of varicella in health care workers who were incorrectly identified as VZV seropositive by the latex bead agglutination method (2). It also should be recognized that immunocompromised patients may have received blood products that can result in transitory false-positive results.

IgM test results are difficult to interpret. IgM antibody capture assays are preferred, because they avoid the obfuscating effect of rheumatoid factor and because they are the most effective means for eliminating all of the IgG in serum specimens. IgM kits that rely on absorbants to remove IgG are commercially available, but they frequently do not remove all of the IgG from a specimen. In addition, extensive studies of sera from persons with documented recent exposures to VZV indicate that VZV IgM antibodies are inconsistently detectable in such persons.

Immunotherapy, Postexposure Prophylaxis in Pregnancy, and the Neonate

The fetuses of susceptible, pregnant women are at risk for severe, lifelong disabilities or death; fetuses of women infected during weeks 8 to 20 of gestation carry approximately a 2% risk of developing congenital varicella. Neonatal varicella contracted from the mother is often severe. VZV vaccination is contraindicated for women during pregnancy; however, administration of passive VZV immunoglobulin (VZIG) is recommended for seronegative pregnant women with possible VZV exposure, and administration to the infant is advisable if the mother develops varicella 5 days before to 2 days after delivery. A consensus reached at the 3rd Annual Meeting of the International Herpes Management Forum suggested that VZIG could reasonably be given as postexposure prophylaxis to neonates born to mothers who have varicella within 7 days before or after delivery. Despite VZIG prophylaxis, approximately two-thirds of infants exposed to maternal varicella around the time of delivery will become infected. Although in most cases the infection is mild, fatal outcomes have been reported for VZIG-treated infants whose mothers developed varicella rash in the period 4 days before to 2 days after delivery.

REMARKS AND CONCLUSIONS

Test selection must be made appropriate to the clinical circumstances for the individual patient; when appropriate and suitably reliable methods are limited and beyond the capacity of a laboratory, consideration should be given to providing specimens to a facility that is capable of performing the required method. The immunocompetence and history of a receipt of blood products need to be taken into account in the selection of serologic approaches to testing. The particular test selected may depend upon the interval between disease onset and the time required to obtain a test result. For example, the use of acute- and convalescent-phase serum testing is inappropriate in situations where evidence of recent exposure is needed quickly. If the circumstances require documentation of a vaccine adverse event, the use of conventional VZV PCR is not acceptable; RFLP or FRET PCR that specifically identifies the vaccine strain is required.

Immune status testing may be urgent if the patient is a candidate for postexposure varicella vaccination, as it must be administered within 72 h of exposure to be effective. The limitations of each method should be reflected in how the results are reported. Reporting of indeterminate results is of little use to the clinician attempting to use the results to manage a patient, but it is important to distinguish potentially false-negative results from those that are indeterminate. Seropositivity, whenever possible, should be equivalent to immunity. The specific methods selected will depend upon the experience of a particular laboratory.

REFERENCES

1. **Arao, Y., D. S. Schmid, P. E. Pellett, and N. Inoue.** 1999. Herpesviruses beyond HSV-1 and -2. *Clin. Microbiol. Newsl.* **21:**153–160.
2. **Behrman, A., D. S. Schmid, A. Crivaro, and B. Watson.** 2003. A cluster of primary varicella cases among healthcare workers with false-positive varicella-zoster virus titers. *Infect. Control Hosp. Epidem.* **24:**202–206.
3. **Galil, K., G. P. Mootrey, J. Seward, and M. Wharton.** 1999. Prevention of varicella: update recommendations of the Advisory Committee on Immunization Practices. *Morbid. Mortal. Wkly. Rep.* **48:**1–5.
4. **Loparev, V. N., T. Argaw, P. R. Krause, M. Takayama, and D. S. Schmid.** 2000. Improved identification and differentiation of varicella-zoster virus (VZV) wild-type strains and an attenuated varicella vaccine strain using a VZV open reading frame 62-based PCR. *J. Clin. Microbiol.* **38:**3156–3160.

5. **Loparev, V. N., A. Gonzalez, M. Deleon-Carnes, G. Tipples, H. Fickenscher, E. G. Torfason, and D. S. Schmid.** 2004. Three major genotypes of varicella-zoster virus: geographical clustering and strategies for genotyping. *J. Virol.* **78:**8349–8358.

6. **Loparev, V. N., K. McCaustland, B. P. Holloway, P. R. Krause, M. Takayama, and D. S. Schmid.** 2000. Rapid genotyping of varicella-zoster virus vaccine and wild-type strains with fluorophore-labeled hybridization probes. *J. Clin. Microbiol.* **38:**4315–4319.

7. **Martin, K., A. K. Junker, E. E. Thomas, M. I. Van Allen, and M. M. Friedman.** 1994. Occurrence of chickenpox during pregnancy in women seropositive for varicella-zoster virus. *J. Infect. Dis.* **170:**991–995.

8. **Provost, P. J., D. L. Krah, B. J. Kuter, D. H. Morton, T. L. Schofield, E. H. Wasmuth, C. J. White, W. J. Miller, and R. W. Ellis.** 1991. Antibody assays suitable for assessing immune responses to live varicella vaccine. *Vaccine* **9:**111–116.

9. **Seward, J. F., B. M. Watson, C. L. Peterson, L. Mascola, J. W. Pelosi, J. X. Zhang, T. J. Maupin, G. S. Goldman, L. J. Tabony, K. G. Brodovicz, A. O. Jumaan, and M. Wharton.** 2002. Varicella disease after introduction of varicella vaccine in the United States, 1995–2000. *JAMA* **287:**606–611.

10. **Zaia, J. A., and M. N. Oxman.** 1977. Antibody to varicella-zoster virus-induced membrane antigen: immunofluorescence assay using monodisperse glutaraldehyde-fixed target cells. *J. Infect. Dis.* **156:**519–530.

Epstein-Barr Virus

HAL B. JENSON

72

Epstein-Barr virus (EBV), a member of the *Herpesviridae* family, is a ubiquitous, worldwide infectious agent that is the cause of classic cases of infectious mononucleosis (13). Approximately 10% of cases of infectious mononucleosis-like illness are not caused by EBV. An important relationship between age, socioeconomic status, and disease exists with EBV infection. In developing countries and socioeconomically deprived areas of developed countries, most persons are infected with EBV during early childhood. Infection with EBV in socioeconomically advantaged areas of developed countries is delayed, with infection more frequently occurring during adolescence and young adulthood. Infection is symptomatic in one-half or more of older children and adults and is classically manifest as the syndrome of infectious mononucleosis that consists of the principal symptoms of fever, malaise, pharyngitis, and cervical lymphadenopathy. Primary EBV infection in infants and young children is usually asymptomatic, although the syndrome of infectious mononucleosis may be seen in these age groups.

EBV is generally acquired by oral transmission of virus in saliva. Following lytic replication in oropharyngeal epithelial cells with replication release of infectious virions from the cells, the virus selectively infects B lymphocytes in the peripheral blood and other reticuloendothelial tissues and establishes a lifelong latent, or quiescent, polyclonal infection of resting CD23$^-$ B7$^-$ B lymphocytes. EBV undergoes episodic reactivation of lytic replication with production of mature, infectious virions and intermittent shedding from the oropharynx even from asymptomatic persons. Reactivation is not typically accompanied by distinctive clinical symptoms. Virus is recoverable by culture at any given time from 12 to 33% of asymptomatic healthy seropositive adults and at significantly higher rates (49 to 82%) from immunocompromised persons, indicating greater levels of viral replication. Virus is detectable by PCR in oral secretions in up to 90% of healthy adults.

EBV has been linked with several human tumors including Hodgkin's disease, non-Hodgkin's lymphoma, nasopharyngeal carcinoma, some T-cell lymphomas, and leiomyosarcomas and B-cell lymphomas, especially in the central nervous system, in immunocompromised persons and organ transplant recipients (posttransplant lymphoproliferative disease) (2). Uncontrolled EBV replication in patients with human immunodeficiency virus (HIV) infection and AIDS in oral epithelium may develop into the lesion of oral hairy leukoplakia, and replication in the lungs appears to be the cause of lymphocytic interstitial pneumonitis that is observed in children. Fatal or severe systemic lymphoproliferative disease has occurred rarely in individuals who appear to be immunologically incapable of limiting the replication and dissemination of EBV-infected B cells. The X-linked lymphoproliferative (XLP) syndrome results from deletion or mutation of the *SH2D1A* gene (also known as DSHP or SAP), located in the chromosomal Xq25 region, which permits overwhelming and usually fatal infection upon primary EBV infection. The XLP protein may act as a blocker (inhibitor) or as a regulator (adaptor) of the critical events in T and NK cell signal transduction. Another, rare group of patients demonstrates chronic, progressive, and systemic involvement associated with an impaired immune response to EBV nuclear antigen 1 (EBNA-1).

Several laboratory methods have been applied to identify EBV infection by testing of clinical specimens, and many have developed into important diagnostic and research tools (Table 1). Serologic assays and viral culture have been used historically for diagnosis of EBV infection, but newer molecular methods provide greater insight into the presence and quantitation of lytic viral replication. The genomic origins of the targets used in molecular and serologic tests for the diagnosis of EBV infection have been well characterized (Table 2).

For serologic diagnosis, several distinct EBV-associated antigen systems and their corresponding antibodies have been characterized (5, 8, 18). These EBV antigen systems were initially described phenomenologically and can now be classified by the phase of the viral replicative cycle during which the target genes are expressed (Table 2). Only 10 viral genes are transcribed during latent infection, including the following: six EBV nuclear antigens, or proteins (EBNA-1, -2, -3A, -3B, -3C, and –LP [leader protein]), of which EBNA-1 is the principal constituent; three latent membrane proteins (LMP-1, -2A, and -2B); and two short EBV-encoded RNAs (EBER-1 and –2), which are not translated. LMP-1 and EBNA-2, in combination with the major histocompatibility complex antigens, constitute the lymphocyte-detected membrane antigen (MA), a cell surface antigen recognized by cytotoxic T cells. The early antigens (EAs) are produced during the initial stages of viral lytic replication prior to viral DNA synthesis. The EAs include two morphological components, diffuse (EA-D) and restricted (EA-R), which are distinguished on the basis of their distribution within the

TABLE 1 Tests used in the clinical diagnosis of EBV infection

Assay	Application (and comment)
Serologic tests	Identify acute infection (typically by positive heterophile antibody or positive anti-IgM-VCA)
	Identify remote infection ($\geq$3 months previously; typically by positive anti-EBNA)
	Identify relatively high levels of lytic replication (suggested by high VCA-IgG and high EA)
	Monitor disease status (especially EA-D and IgA antibody responses to VCA for nasopharyngeal carcinoma; serologic monitoring is less precise than monitoring quantitative EBV viral load by PCR and is also unreliable for immunocompromised persons)
Viral culture	Detect EBV in blood, body fluids, and tissues (requires 6–8 weeks and fresh human umbilical cord lymphocytes; much less sensitive than DNA PCR)
Virocyte assay	Semiquantitative EBV culture of infected circulating B lymphocytes
Electron microscopy	Detect whole virions in tissues (impractical for clinical diagnosis)
DNA PCR	
Qualitative	Detect EBV in blood, body fluids, and tissues (confounded by EBV in circulating lymphocytes in tissues)
Quantitative	Monitor viral load, implying lytic replication in blood or body fluids to follow disease status (by PCR amplification of EBER RNA or, alternatively, a DNA target)
Immunohistochemistry	Identify EBV protein expression in specific cell types in tissue samples (typically by identifying LMP-1 or, less frequently, EBNA-2)
	Identify lytic replication (by identifying BZLF1)
In situ hybridization	Identify EBV in specific cell types in tissue samples (using EBER probes)
Clonality assay	Distinguish monoclonal from oligoclonal and polyclonal cell infections
	Identify the presence of lytic replication (by the presence of a smaller ladder of terminal digestion fragments)

cells and by their differential denaturation by fixation procedures and proteolytic enzymes. EA-D and EA-R each comprise two different EBV proteins. The late antigens are produced after viral DNA synthesis and include the viral capsid antigens (VCAs), the structural proteins of the capsid. MAs are structural polypeptides of the virus expressed before and after viral DNA synthesis on the cell surface and also form part of the viral envelope.

HETEROPHILE ANTIBODY

The Paul-Bunnell heterophile antibody associated with acute infectious mononucleosis agglutinates sheep and horse erythrocytes, among others, and is adsorbed by beef erythrocytes but not guinea pig kidney cells (5). The latter adsorption property differentiates this response from other heterophile antibodies found in patients with serum sickness and rheumatic diseases and in some healthy individuals. The heterophile antibody response usually peaks during the second and third weeks of illness and is frequently detectable for several months after resolution of clinical symptoms (Fig. 1). The origin of the antigen is unknown, but it is not an EBV-encoded antigen. Heterophile antibody is primarily immunoglobulin M (IgM). There is no anamnestic response.

The most widely used method to detect Paul-Bunnell heterophile antibody is the qualitative, rapid slide test. The slide tests that use bovine or horse erythrocytes are more sensitive and detect heterophile antibody in 90% of cases of EBV-associated infectious mononucleosis in adults, with a false-positive rate of <10%. This method detects a heterophile response in about one-third of cases in children <4 years of age, although a greater proportion may have heterophile antibody detectable by the immune adherence hemagglutination procedure (18). Erroneous interpretations by the operator account for most of the false-positive results and some of the false-negative results. To improve accuracy, the package

directions must be followed very closely, positive and negative controls should be used with each test, and laboratory personnel need to gain experience with the test reactions. Heterophile antibody test kits utilizing sheep erythrocytes or those that lack a guinea pig kidney or beef absorption step (unless the method incorporates native and enzyme-treated erythrocytes for agglutination) should not be used.

Quantitative testing by the more cumbersome Paul-Bunnell-Davidsohn technique, or the simplified ox cell hemolysin technique, is performed rarely and usually for research purposes only. Other recently developed tests utilizing a variety of techniques, such as enzyme-linked immunosorbent assay (ELISA), immune adherence hemagglutination, and latex agglutination with purified forms of heterophile antigen, do not offer any significant or practical improvement over the rapid slide test (with the possible exception of the immune adherence method for testing of children <4 years of age).

Approximately 10% of cases of infectious mononucleosis-like illness are not caused by EBV and are uniformly not associated with a heterophile antibody response. Cytomegalovirus, *Toxoplasma gondii*, HIV, adenovirus, and possibly rubella virus have been identified as causative agents in some cases, although the majority of cases of heterophile-negative infectious mononucleosis remain of undetermined etiology. If the heterophile antibody test is negative and an EBV-associated disease is suspected, EBV-specific serologic testing is indicated to confirm the etiology. EBV-specific serologic testing is also useful in evaluating a positive heterophile antibody test associated with clinical or laboratory findings uncharacteristic of infectious mononucleosis.

EBV-SPECIFIC SEROLOGIC TESTS

The serologic profile of EBV-specific antibodies following infectious mononucleosis has been well documented (Fig. 1). The acute phase of infectious mononucleosis is characterized

TABLE 2 Genomic origins of EBV targets commonly used for diagnosis of EBV infection

Assay and antigen	EBV target		Use and interpretation
	Gene (protein mass)	Function	
Serology			
Latent antigens			
EBNA-1	BKRF1 (60–85 kDa)	DNA-binding protein to *oriP*, permitting episomal replication	Positive serology confirms EBV infection ≥3 months previously; remains positive for life
EBNA-2	BYRF1 (two alleles, EBNA-2A [85 kDa] and EBNA-2B [75 kDa], with 64% homology; EBNA-2B has a major internal deletion that removes a large portion of the polyproline stretch)	Transactivator; component of lymphocyte-derived membrane antigen	Positive serology with acute infection; may decline over time
Early antigens			
EA-D	BMRF1 (50 kDa)	DNA polymerase-associated processivity factor	Positive serology with acute infection; usually declines over time
	BSLF2/BMLF1 (60 kDa)	Transactivator/repressor	
EA-R	BORF2 (85 kDa)	Ribonucleotide reductase (large subunit)	Positive serology with acute infection; usually declines over time
	BHRF1 (17 kDa)	*bcl*-2 homolog (B-cell lymphoma/leukemia 2 proto-oncogene)	
Late antigens			
VCAs	BcLF1 (150 kDa, glycosylated; 135 kDa, unglycosylated)	Major capsid protein	Positive serology with acute infection; remains positive for life
Membrane antigens	BLLF1a/b (350/221 kDa, glycosylated; 135/100 kDa, unglycosylated)	Envelope glycoprotein and plasma membrane protein; ligand for cell attachment to CD21 (CR2)	
	BALF4 (125 kDa, glycosylated)	Membrane protein (gB); virus assembly	
Immunohistochemistry			
Latent antigens			
LMP-1	BNLF1 (58–63 kDa)	Morphological transformation	
EBNA-2	See EBNA-2 above		
Immediate early antigen			
BZLF1	BZLF1 (38 kDa)	Zta or ZEBRA; transcriptional activation of EBV early genes by binding to upstream Z-responsive elements	Positive result indicates viral replication
PCR and in situ hybridization	EBER-1 and EBER-2 (approximately 170 nucleotides)	Unknown	Best in situ hybridization target because of >10^6 copies/cell; not present in oral hairy leukoplakia
Clonality	Terminal repeats (not a gene)	Required for replication	Identifies monoclonal, oligoclonal, or polyclonal infection Identifies lytic replication, if present

by rapid IgM and IgG antibody responses to VCA and, in most cases, a lower IgG response to the EA complex. The IgM response to VCA is transient, lasting about 1 to 3 months. The IgG response to this antigen usually peaks during the acute illness, declines slightly over the next few weeks to months, and then persists at a relatively stable level for life. Anti-EA antibodies are usually present for several months but may persist for several years following resolution of the acute infection. Anti-EBNA antibodies typically appear much later, gradually emerging after 2 to 4 months, and

occasionally longer, following the onset of illness and lasting for life. Some immunocompromised patients demonstrate diminishing or undetectable levels of anti-EBNA antibodies.

EBV-specific antibody testing is useful in determining (i) susceptibility or immunity to primary EBV infection on an individual basis or as part of an epidemiologic study in a general population, (ii) the potential etiologic role of EBV in a heterophile antibody-negative infectious mononucleosis-like illness, (iii) the possible etiologic role of EBV in a variety of clinical syndromes that have occasionally been associated

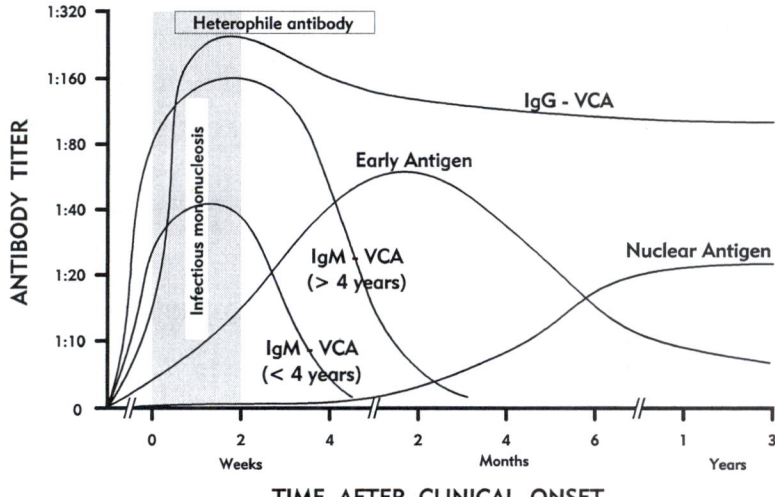

FIGURE 1 Schematic representation of the typical development of antibodies to various EBV antigens in patients with infectious mononucleosis, the prototype symptomatic primary EBV infection. The titers are geometric mean values expressed as reciprocals of the serum dilution. The minimum titers tested are 1:10 for VCA-IgG and EA, 1:8 for VCA-IgM, and 1:2.5 for EBNA. The IgM response to VCA is subdivided because of the significant differences noted according to age of the patient. (Adapted from references 8 and 18.)

with EBV infection, and (iv) the presence of EBV antigens in cells and tissues. In addition, serologic testing for IgA antibody responses to VCA and EA-D may be useful in the initial evaluation as well as the response to therapy for nasopharyngeal carcinoma.

The range of antibody responses can occasionally make it difficult to interpret an individual antibody profile (Table 3). The determination of IgM antibody to VCA (IgM-VCA) is the most valuable serologic procedure to diagnose acute EBV

infection; antibody panels that do not include IgM-VCA are not as dependable for detection of acute EBV infection. Properly performed, the IgM-VCA antibody test is quite reliable and specific. Very high titers of IgG-VCA alone do not necessarily indicate an acute infection. The vast majority of patients with infectious mononucleosis develop a transient antibody response to the EA-D component, although in some adult patients and especially in young children this response may be directed mainly against the EA-R component.

TABLE 3 Correlation of clinical status and characteristic serologic responses to EBV infection[a]

Clinical status	Heterophile antibody (qualitative only)	Characteristic antibody profile for:				
		EBV-specific antibody (negative reaction)				
		IgM-VCA (<1:8[b])	IgG-VCA (<1:10)	EA-D (<1:10)	EA-R (<1:10)	EBNA (<1:2.5)
Susceptible	−	−	−	−	−	−
Acute primary infection (infectious mononucleosis)	+	1:32 to 1:256	1:160 to 1:640	1:40 to 1:160	−[c]	− to 1:2.5
Recent primary infection (infectious mononucleosis)	±	− to 1:32	1:320 to 1:1,280	1:40 to 1:160	−[c]	1:5 to 1:10
Remote (past) infection	−	−	1:40 to 1:160	−[d]	− to 1:40	1:10 to 1:40
Reactivation in an immunosuppressed or immunocompromised individual	−	−	1:320 to 1:1,280	−[d]	1:80 to 1:320	− to 1:160
Burkitt's lymphoma	−	−	1:320 to 1:1,280	−[d]	1:80 to 1:320	1:10 to 1:80
Nasopharyngeal carcinoma	−	−	1:320 to 1:1,280	1:40 to 1:160	−[e]	1:20 to 1:160

[a]Adapted from numerous studies. Individual responses outside the characteristic range may occur. −, negative; +, positive; ±, positive or negative.
[b]Some laboratories report <1:10 as the lowest dilution tested.
[c]In young children and adults with asymptomatic infection and seroconversion, the anti-EA response may be mainly to the EA-R component.
[d]A minority of individuals will have the anti-EA response mainly to the EA-D component.
[e]A minority of individuals will have the anti-EA response mainly to the EA-R component.

The testing of a second, or convalescent-phase, serum sample 4 to 6 weeks after clinical onset is of limited assistance for diagnosing a preceding acute EBV infection, since <10% of cases have a significant antibody titer rise over this interval. A past, currently quiescent, EBV infection is characterized by the concurrent presence of moderate but stable titers of antibody to IgG-VCA and EBNA and absence of IgM-VCA. Antibodies to EA are often absent but, if present, are usually at a low level and are directed predominantly to the EA-R component. High titers of IgG-VCA and EA, considered to indicate enhanced EBV replication or reactivation, have been noted in individuals with Burkitt's lymphoma, nasopharyngeal carcinoma, or immunosuppressed or immunodeficient

states. The antibody response to EA is directed principally to the EA-R component in patients with Burkitt's lymphoma and immunosuppressed or immunodeficient individuals and to EA-D in patients with nasopharyngeal carcinoma. High levels of IgA-VCA and IgA-EA are also found in persons with nasopharyngeal carcinoma, including the early asymptomatic stages. In these patients, tumor activity and response to cancer therapy may be monitored by serial IgA-VCA and IgA-EA determinations.

The EBNA, EA, and VCA antigen systems are the most useful for clinical diagnostic purposes and are determined principally by indirect immunofluorescence assay (IFA) and ELISA (Table 4). ELISA-based tests using viral lysate proteins,

TABLE 4 Summary of methodologies of EBV antigen systems classically used for detecting EBV-specific antibodies

Antigen system	Type of test	Source of antigen[a]	Antigen-negative control	Result indicating positive test for antibody
Latent antigens				
EBNA	Anticomplement immunofluorescence	Acetone-methanol (1:1)-fixed cell smears of Raji cells	EBV genome-negative cell line (e.g., MOLT-4)	Indirect immunofluorescence of complement fixation (incubation with complement followed by FITC-conjugated anti-C3)
Early antigens				
EA-R, EA-D	Immunofluorescence	Acetone- or methanol-fixed cell smears of nonproducer cells (e.g., Raji) treated with halogenated pyrimidines (induction) or with virus concentrates of the HR_1K (P3-HR1) line (superinfection)	Nonproducer cell line (e.g. Raji), not induced or superinfected	Indirect immunofluorescence with FITC-conjugated anti-human IgG or IgA
Late antigens				
VCA	Immunofluorescence	Acetone-fixed cell smears of producer cell line (e.g, HR_1K [P3-HR1], B95-8) treated with TPA	EBV genome-negative cell line	Indirect immunofluorescence with FITC-conjugated antihuman IgM, IgG, or IgA
MA	Immunofluorescence	Living cells from Burkitt's lymphoma biopsies and some producer lymphoblastoid cell lines (shows MA on the cell membrane), or acetone-fixed cell smears of producer cell lines (e.g., HR_1K [P3-HR1], B95-8) treated with TPA (shows MA peripherally inside the cell due to fixation as well as on cell membrane)	EBV genome-negative cell line; autologous bone marrow	Blocking of immunofluorescence with FITC-conjugated reference human serum
VCA and MA	Serum neutralization assay	Concentrated extracellular fluid from the HR_1K (P3-HR1) cell line	Concentrated extracellular fluid from an EBV-negative cell line	Neutralization of EA production following superinfection of nonproducer cells or inhibition of colony formation by nonproducer cells (e.g., Raji)
	Serum neutralization assay of EBV transformation	Concentrated extracellular fluid from the B95-8 or Kaplan cell line	Concentrated extracellular fluid from a nonproducer cell line or from the HR_1K (P3-HR1) line (nontransforming)	Neutralization of transformation of primary human leukocytes into continuous cell lines

[a]Antigen is demonstrated by using either commercially available monoclonal antibodies to the antigen or reference human antisera empirically determined to contain antibodies against the specific antigen system.

recombinant proteins, or synthetic peptides are used in clinical laboratories most often. IFA methods are more specific but also more time-consuming and difficult to interpret, requiring experienced personnel. These methods are important for resolution of inconsistent results by other methodologies (e.g., ELISA) and testing for research purposes, and they remain the "gold standard" for evaluation of new tests. Neutralizing antibodies can be detected by the interference of biologic activity (e.g., neutralization of EBV transformation of primary human lymphocytes, or neutralization of induction of EA production in Raji cells following superinfection with the HR_1K EBV strain), although these are tedious assays to perform. Neutralizing antibodies correlate well with anti-VCA and anti-MA titers. Determination of complement-fixing antibodies against antigens extracted from EBV-positive lymphoblastoid cell lines is rarely performed.

Several antibody test kits utilizing immunofluorescence and ELISA kits to detect EBV-specific antibodies are commercially available. Many clinical laboratories prefer to use ELISA methods, although sufficient standardization of techniques and correlation of results among these kits have not been adequately performed. There is high concordance between commercial ELISA kits for intertest sensitivity (95 to 100%) and slightly less for intertest specificity (86 to 100%) (3). However, comparative testing of ELISA and IFA shows a sensitivity of ELISA of only approximately 71% for VCA-IgG, 95% for VCA-IgM, and 99% for anti-EBNA, with an overall specificity of 99%. Considerable investigation is ongoing with tests using purified or recombinant proteins.

IFA Testing for Antibodies to VCA

IgM-VCA

The detection of IgM-VCA alone is generally sufficient to diagnose acute EBV infection. This antibody response in almost all cases can be detected for 4 to 12 weeks after clinical onset of infectious mononucleosis. It is prudent to augment the IgM-VCA test with at least one other antibody determination, such as IgG-VCA or EBNA. IgM antibody to cytomegalovirus may be detected in sera of patients with EBV-associated infectious mononucleosis, but IgM-VCA antibody does not appear to be detectable with infectious mononucleosis-like illness caused by cytomegalovirus.

Because rheumatoid factor may produce a false-positive IgM reaction, it is essential to routinely utilize a method that removes or circumvents this factor, such as one involving an IgG-inactivating reagent (GullSORB; Meridian Diagnostics, Cincinnati, Ohio). An adsorption step to remove serum IgG and thus eliminate the false-positive reaction associated with rheumatoid factor also reduces the incubation time needed for a satisfactory reaction between VCA and the test serum. A less acceptable alternative is to test each IgM-VCA-positive serum undiluted for the presence of rheumatoid factor.

Protocol

1. Vigorously growing HR_1K cells at a concentration of 6×10^5 per ml are incubated with the phorbol ester 12-O-tetradecanoyl-phorbol-13-acetate (TPA) (20 ng/ml) for 5 days at 32°C. This increases the number of cells expressing VCA to approximately 30 to 50%.

2. Antigen smears are prepared using whole cells. Cells are washed twice for 5 min in filtered phosphate-buffered saline (PBS) and resuspended in PBS at a cell density adjusted to produce a confluent layer on a 5-mm-diameter spot (using 8- or 14-well slides) with 10 μl of cell suspension.

3. The cell smears are air dried and then fixed with cold acetone for 10 min. After fixation, the smears may be stored at −20°C for up to 6 months.

4. A 50-μl aliquot of GullSORB is pipetted into a microcentrifuge tube, and 5 μl of patient serum is added. Inactivation of IgG is instantaneous. A quick spin (30 s) removes the flocculent material. The supernatant is a 1:10 dilution of the serum.

5. Serial fourfold dilutions, from 1:10 to 1:160, of the IgG-free serum diluted with PBS are prepared in a microtiter plate.

6. Aliquots (20 μl) of serum dilutions are transferred onto the smears, which are then incubated in chambers humidified with moist gauze or paper for 90 min at 37°C. Cell smears must not be allowed to dry during or between incubations.

7. The smears are washed twice for 5 min in PBS, and liquid around the wells is removed by suction. The smears are then incubated for 30 min at 37°C with 20 μl of fluorescein isothiocyanate (FITC)-conjugated goat $F(ab')_2$ anti-human IgM (mu chain specific; BioSource International, Camarillo, Calif.) containing 0.004% Evans blue counterstain. The FITC-conjugated anti-human IgM is generally diluted 1:100 to 1:150 in PBS, predetermined by testing antiserum dilutions with each lot of slides and control sera.

8. The smears are washed twice for 5 min in PBS, rinsed in distilled water, and air dried; glycerol-PBS (9:1 [vol/vol], pH 8.5 to 9.0) is added; and a coverslip is placed for immunofluorescence reading. The highest dilution of serum showing immunofluorescence is the end point.

Controls

Known negative and low-titer and high-titer IgM-VCA-positive control sera should be employed with each assay. Satisfactory smears of induced HR_1K cells should contain at least 30 to 50% VCA-positive cells, which should be confirmed before serum testing by incubation with a monoclonal antibody to VCA (Advanced Biotechnologies, Columbia, Md.) and FITC-conjugated anti-mouse Ig (BioSource International).

IgG-VCA

IgG-VCA antibodies are determined as described for IgM-VCA antibodies, except that the serum absorption step to remove IgG is not performed, TPA stimulation to increase antigen production is not routinely used, and an FITC-conjugated anti-human IgG antibody is used. Acetone-fixed smears of HR_1K cells (after maintenance of cells at 32°C for 10 to 14 days without refeeding) are incubated with serial fourfold dilutions of test serum (from 1:10 to 1:2,560) at 37°C for 45 min. After being air dried, the smears are incubated with 20 μl of FITC-conjugated goat $F(ab')_2$ anti-human IgG (BioSource International), usually diluted 1:800, at 37°C for 45 min. Other washes and rinses are performed as in the IgM determination. Adequate cell smears should contain at least 10% fluorescing cells, which can be confirmed by reaction using commercial monoclonal antibody to VCA. Known negative and low-titer and high-titer IgG-VCA-positive control sera should be tested in parallel with each assay.

IgA-VCA

The IgA-VCA procedure is as described for IgG-VCA, except that IgG in the patient serum is removed by using GullSORB as for IgM-VCA, and an FITC-conjugated anti-IgA antibody (BioSource International) is used.

IFA Testing for Antibodies to EA

IgG-EA

Antigen for determination of EA antibodies is derived from normally nonproductive lymphoblastoid cell lines, usually Raji, induced either by the addition of halogenated pyrimidines such as 5-iododeoxyuridine (14) or by superinfection with the HR$_1$K EBV strain (10). The EA-R antigen shows staining restricted to the cytoplasm and is denatured by methanol or ethanol. The EA-D antigen is found in both the nucleus and the cytoplasm and is stable in methanol. Cells demonstrating EA-R antigen usually demonstrate EA-D antigen also, although the converse is not necessarily true. In cells demonstrating both antigens, the brilliant reactions to EA-D often obscure those to EA-R.

While some laboratories report separate titrations for antibodies to EA-D and EA-R components, many laboratories prefer the traditional reporting of a single interpretation that denotes the predominant reaction observed (anti-EA-D, anti-EA-R, or anti-EA-DR if a predominant reaction cannot be differentiated). A differential EA antibody response directed mainly against EA-D is characteristic of infectious mononucleosis and nasopharyngeal carcinoma, and a response directed against EA-R is characteristic of Burkitt's lymphoma and selected immunocompromised states. The basis for this is unclear. A significant antibody response to EA is found in current or recent infections or in diseases intimately associated with an enhanced replication or putative reactivation of EBV. Low levels of antibodies to EA-R may be found in a minority of the healthy general population with remote past EBV infection.

Protocol

1. Vigorously growing Raji cells at a concentration of 3×10^5 to 4×10^5 per ml are treated with 5-iododeoxyuridine (20 μg/ml; add 4 μl/ml of a stock solution of 5 mg/ml in 0.1 N NaOH) and hypoxanthine-aminopterin solution (14 and 0.4 μg/ml, respectively; 4 μl/ml of a stock solution of hypoxanthine [3.5 mg/ml] and aminopterin [0.1 mg/ml] in 0.1 N NaOH) for 24 h at 37°C. The cells are pelleted, washed with RPMI 1640 medium, and then incubated with hypoxanthine-thymidine solution (14 and 20 μg/ml, respectively; 4 μl/ml of a stock solution of hypoxanthine [3.5 mg/ml] and thymidine [5 mg/ml] in 0.1 N NaOH) for 24 h at 37°C to reverse the inhibitory effects of aminopterin. An alternative method for preparation of cells for EA is superinfection of Raji cells with the HR$_1$K EBV strain and incubation for 2 to 3 days (10).

2. Antigen smears are prepared with whole cells. The cells are washed twice for 5 min in PBS and resuspended in PBS at a cell density adjusted to produce a confluent layer on a 5-mm-diameter spot (using 8- or 14-well slides) with 10 μl of cell suspension.

3. The smears are air dried and then fixed with either prechilled acetone (4 min) or prechilled methanol (10 min). After fixation, the smears may be stored at −20°C for up to 6 months.

4. Serial fourfold dilutions from 1:10 to 1:160 of sera diluted with PBS are prepared in a microtiter plate.

5. Each dilution of test serum is reacted separately with an acetone- and a methanol-fixed cell smear according to the steps described for determination of IgG-VCA. Cells fixed with acetone contain both EA-D and EA-R; cells fixed with methanol contain only EA-D. There is no method to prepare cell antigen smears for EA-R alone.

6. The smears are washed twice for 5 min in PBS and then rinsed in distilled water. The smears are air dried, glycerol-PBS is added, and a coverslip is placed for immunofluorescence reading. The highest dilution of serum showing immunofluorescence is the end point.

Controls

Known negative and low-titer and high-titer IgG-EA-positive control sera should be tested in parallel with each assay. Satisfactory smears of Raji cells should contain at least 8 to 10% EA-positive cells, which should be confirmed by reaction with a monoclonal antibody to EA-D (Advanced Biotechnologies).

IgA-EA

The IgA-EA procedure is as described for IgG-EA, except that IgG in the patient serum is removed by using GullSORB as for IgM-VCA, and an FITC-conjugated anti-IgA antibody is used.

Anticomplement IFA Testing for Antibodies to EBNA

The EBNA antigen complex is composed of at least six EBV proteins (EBNA-1, EBNA-2, EBNA-3A, EBNA-3B, EBNA-3C, and leader protein), although EBNA-1 is the chief constituent. EBNA is found in all EBV-positive lymphoblastoid cell lines and biopsy tissues of various EBV-related malignancies. Modification of the anticomplement immunofluorescence method initially described by Reedman and Klein (16) is commonly used to detect antibodies to EBNA.

Protocol

1. Vigorously growing Raji cells are propagated for 48 h after splitting. Aliquots of 10 ml are pelleted and then fixed by adding 1 ml of cold acetone-methanol mixture (1:1), 1 drop at a time. The cells are pelleted and resuspended in cold acetone-methanol at a density to produce a thin, confluent layer on a 5-mm-diameter spot (using 8- or 14-well slides) with 10 μl of cell suspension. The cell suspension may be stored at 4°C for at least 8 weeks.

2. Stored, fixed Raji cells are mixed and then spotted on the wells of an 8- or 14-well slide. (Cell smears on slides cannot be stored.) The cell smears are air dried for at least 30 min.

3. Serum for anti-EBNA determinations must be heat inactivated (30 min at 56°C) to inactivate native complement. Serial fourfold dilutions from 1:2.5 to 1:160 of the serum with EBNA buffer (containing, per liter, 8 g of NaCl, 0.4 g of KCl, 0.2 g of MgSO$_4$·7H$_2$O, 0.185 g of CaCl$_2$·2H$_2$O, 1.8 g of Na$_2$HPO$_4$, and 0.6 g of KH$_2$PO$_4$) are prepared in a microtiter plate.

4. Aliquots (20 μl) of serum dilutions are transferred onto the smears, which are then incubated in chambers humidified with moist gauze or paper for 45 min at 37°C. Cell smears must not be allowed to dry during or between incubations.

5. The smears are rinsed in EBNA buffer and then incubated with 20 μl of diluted (usually 1:10 in EBNA buffer) guinea pig complement (GIBCO Laboratories, Grand Island, N.Y.) for 45 min at 37°C.

6. The smears are rinsed in EBNA buffer and then incubated for 45 min at 37°C with 20 μl of diluted (usually 1:100 to 1:150 in EBNA buffer) FITC-conjugated IgG fraction goat anti-guinea pig C3 (Cooper Biomedical, Malvern, Pa.) containing 0.002% Evans blue counterstain. Testing antiserum dilutions with each lot of slides and known sera

predetermines optimal dilutions of complement and FITC-conjugated anti-C3.

7. The smears are rinsed in EBNA buffer and then in distilled water. The smears are air dried, glycerol-PBS is added, and a coverslip is placed for immunofluorescence reading. The highest dilution of serum showing immunofluorescence is the end point.

Controls

False-positive anti-EBNA reactions are usually due to nonspecific antinuclear antibodies. To ascertain and eliminate this possibility, test serum is also reacted with cell smears of MOLT-4, an EBV-negative T-lymphoma cell line. Known negative and low-titer and high-titer EBNA-positive control sera should be tested in parallel with each assay.

NEUTRALIZING ANTIBODY

The presence of neutralizing antibodies in serum can be detected by using a neutralization assay based on interference of lymphocyte transformation (6). Cell-free B95-8 EBV is obtained from vigorously growing B95-8 cells after treatment with TPA (20 ng/ml) for 7 days at 32°C. The cells are pelleted, the supernatant is filtered through a 0.22-μm-pore-size filter, and the virus is concentrated by centrifugation at 40,000 × *g* for 2 h. Concentrated virus can be aliquoted and frozen at −70°C for at least 2 years. The titer (50% transforming dose [TD$_{50}$]/ml) is calculated according to the Reed and Muench method by transformation of human umbilical cord lymphocytes in 10-fold dilutions with at least three wells per dilution. Human umbilical cord lymphocytes are isolated by centrifugation of heparinized cord blood on Histopaque-1077 (Sigma, St. Louis, Mo.).

For the neutralization assay, concentrated B95-8 virus is diluted to $10^{2.3}$ to $10^{2.5}$ TD$_{50}$/0.1 ml, and aliquots (0.1 ml) of diluted virus are mixed with 0.1 ml of filtered, inactivated (56°C for 30 min) and diluted (1:5 through 1:3645) human serum and incubated at 37°C for 1 h. Fresh human umbilical cord lymphocytes are aliquoted at 1.5×10^5 cells in 0.15 ml of growth medium per well of a 96-well sterile tissue culture plate, and 0.02 ml of virus-serum mixture is added to each of triplicate wells at each serum dilution. The assay plate is incubated at 37°C and 5% CO_2 for 4 weeks with frequent changes (every 4 or 5 days) of one-half of the growth medium. Uninoculated cells, and virus without human serum, are included as controls with each assay. At the end of 4 weeks, the wells are scored as transformed or nontransformed and the 50% neutralizing endpoint titer is calculated by the Kärber method.

VIRUS ISOLATION

The transformation assay, used primarily for research purposes, can semiquantitatively assess the level of infectious EBV by measuring induction of lymphoproliferation or activation of B cells to Ig production. The number of virus-containing cells (virocytes) in a clinical specimen can be determined by the virocyte assay. Transforming EBV can generally be isolated from peripheral lymphocytes during acute infectious mononucleosis. Following acute infection, EBV is shed asymptomatically and intermittently in oropharyngeal secretions for life and occasionally can be isolated. Transforming virus is infrequently isolated from EBV-associated tumors or other pathologic lesions. Electron microscopy can be used to identify whole virions and confirm replicative viral infection but is impractical for clinical diagnosis.

Transformation Assay

Transforming virus may be found in either oral secretions or peripheral blood. For detection of transforming virus from the oral cavity, either saliva or a throat gargle with RPMI 1640 medium should be filtered through a 0.45-μm-pore-size filter (4). Samples are incubated in triplicate with aliquots of fresh human umbilical cord mononuclear cells (2×10^6 cells in 2 ml of RPMI 1640 medium supplemented with 20% fetal bovine serum). The cultures are observed for 6 weeks, with weekly changes of medium, for signs of cell transformation: proliferation and rapid growth, mitotic figures, large vacuoles and granular morphology, and cell aggregation. Transforming virus in peripheral blood is detected by isolating peripheral blood mononuclear cells from 10 to 30 ml of heparinized blood with Histopaque-1077, which are propagated in a medium containing cyclosporine (0.1 μg/ml), either alone or cocultivated with human umbilical cord leukocytes, and observing for signs of transformation. Cyclosporine is added to peripheral blood cultures to inhibit cytotoxic T cells that may cause regression of EBV-transformed B cells. The presence of EBV in transformed cultures can be confirmed by testing for the presence of EBNA, using an anticomplement IFA with a reference serum.

Virocyte Assay

An endpoint dilution assay is used to estimate the number of virus-containing cells (virocytes) in peripheral blood (17). Peripheral blood mononuclear cells, obtained as for the transformation assay, are serially diluted with RPMI-20 containing cyclosporine (0.1 μg/ml) to yield 2-ml volumes of 5×10^6, 5×10^5, 5×10^4, and 5×10^3/ml. Each dilution is dispensed in 0.1-ml volumes into a 96-well tissue culture plate (20 wells per dilution) containing 6×10^5 human umbilical cord lymphocytes per well. The plates are incubated for 8 weeks at 37°C with weekly changes of medium. The number of virocytes per 10^7 cells is calculated on the basis of the dilutions of cells showing signs of transformation.

IMMUNOHISTOCHEMICAL METHODS FOR ANTIGEN DETECTION

Detection of EBV antigens directly in body tissues by immunohistochemical procedures is widely done, but variability in assay interpretation justifies some caution in comparing results across studies. Tissue or tumor specimens or smears or touch preparations of specimens fixed in acetone may be tested by IFA. Monoclonal antibodies directed against components of EBNA-1, EBNA-2, LMP-1, EA, VCA, and BZLF1 are commercially available, although the commercial EBNA-1 monoclonal antibody has not proved satisfactory for direct antigen detection. Alternatively, characterized human reference serum may be used. LMP-1 immunostaining is most commonly used, primarily for evaluation of posttransplant lymphoproliferative disease, but is generally less sensitive than EBER in situ hybridization, especially for non-Hodgkin's lymphoma and carcinomas.

In contrast to latent antigens, it is unusual to detect replicative antigens (e.g., EA and VCA) in tissues with the exception of lesions of oral hairy leukoplakia, which is a purely lytic infection of oral epithelial cells that contain dense concentrations of VCA and EA. Some monoclonal antibodies are to minor EBV antigens, such as viral regulatory proteins (e.g., BLZF1) or minor structural components of the virus capsid. Testing for antibody responses against these minor EBV antigens is not necessary for the diagnostic evaluation of EBV infection but may be useful in defining the presence of lytic replication, or reactivation, of latent EBV.

Direct Detection of EBNA-2, LMP-1, and the BZLF1 Protein

Touch preparations of soft tissues (e.g., lymph node biopsies), cryostat sections of firm tissues, and smears of suspension cells (cultured cells or peripheral blood cells) are air dried on glass slides and fixed with cold acetone for 5 min or cold, freshly prepared acetone-methanol (1:1) for 2.5 min. The slides are air dried and stored at $-20°C$ until stained. Because the signal from these latent antigens is less intense than that from the replicative cycle antigens, signal amplification of the antigen-antibody reaction by use of streptavidin-biotin is necessary. Monoclonal antibodies to EBNA-2 or LMP-1 (Vector Laboratories, Burlingame, Calif.) or the BZLF1 protein (DakoCytomation, Carpinteria, Calif.) and mouse isotype control antibodies (Sigma) are diluted either 1:5 or 1:10 with PBS, and 10 to 20 µl of diluted monoclonal antibody is incubated with the smears in chambers humidified with moist gauze or paper for 1 h at 37°C. Cell smears must not be allowed to dry during or between incubations. After incubation, the slides are washed, the liquid around the smears is suctioned or blotted, and biotinylated anti-mouse IgG (Vector Laboratories) diluted 1:20 to 1:50 in PBS is added. The slides are incubated for 30 min at 37°C and washed in PBS, and 10 to 20 µl of streptavidin-fluorescein (Vector Laboratories) diluted 1:50 in PBS containing 0.001% Evans blue counterstain is added. The slides are mounted and viewed as described above. B95-8 cells (without TPA treatment) serve as positive control cells for EBNA-2 and LMP-1, and TPA-treated B95-8 cells serve as positive control cells for LMP-1 and BZLF1. Ramos cells are negative control cells for both assays.

Direct Detection of VCA and EA

Cryostat sections from biopsies, cultured cells from tumors, and smears of suspension cells (cultured cells or peripheral blood cells) are air dried on glass slides, fixed with cold acetone for 5 min, air dried, and stored at $-20°C$ until stained. The slides are thawed and air dried before staining. Monoclonal antibodies to gp350/220, VCA p160 and gp125, EA p50, and EA p85 and EA p17 (Advanced Biotechnologies) and mouse isotypes (Sigma) are diluted 1:100 (if the protein concentration of antibody is 1 mg/ml) or 1:200 (if the protein concentration of antibody is 2 mg/ml) with PBS, and 10 to 20 µl of diluted monoclonal antibody is incubated with the smears in chambers humidified with moist gauze or paper for 1 h at 37°C. Cell smears must not be allowed to dry during or between incubations. After incubation, the slides are washed and FITC-conjugated anti-mouse Ig (gamma and light chain specific; BioSource International) diluted 1:50 in PBS containing 0.001% Evans blue counterstain is added. The slides are incubated for 30 min, washed in PBS, mounted, and viewed as described above. Acetone-fixed smears of B95-8 or HR₁K cells treated with TPA serve as positive control cells for both VCA and EA assays. Acetone-fixed Ramos cells serve as negative control cells for each assay.

NUCLEIC ACID DETECTION

Nucleic acid hybridization is a very sensitive and specific method for detection of EBV DNA in clinical specimens and in certain circumstances has advantages over serologic methods. Direct detection of virus is more reliable than serologic

testing in immunosuppressed or immunocompromised patients who may not demonstrate a complete humoral response and in patients who have received immune globulin products, thereby precluding serologic diagnosis. The complete genome sequence of the B95-8 strain of EBV is known, although significant genomic diversity exists among EBV clinical isolates. Unlike culture of EBV by the transformation assay, nucleic acid hybridization will detect noninfectious (defective) as well as infectious virions, including nontransforming variants.

Southern blotting, dot blotting (also known as spot or slot blotting), PCR, and in situ hybridization for EBV DNA have been applied to peripheral blood cells, oropharyngeal secretions, cervical secretions, and fresh or frozen biopsy specimens, principally from lymphoproliferative lesions. Total intracellular DNA is prepared by standard methods. These techniques vary in sensitivity and specificity for identification of EBV DNA, and therefore the results of these tests for the establishment of the causal role of EBV for different syndromes and lesions must be interpreted within the limitations of each test. Approximations of the limits of sensitivity of these techniques for EBV detection are that Southern blotting can detect 10^5 EBV genomes, dot blotting can detect 10^4 genomes, conventional PCR can detect 10^1 to 10^3 EBV genomes, and real-time PCR can quantitate over a range between 10^2 and 10^7 genomes (11, 12). The specificity of dot hybridization, Southern blotting, and especially PCR for identifying EBV within selected cells of tissue specimens is diminished because of simultaneous detection of EBV genomes present in circulating lymphocytes. In situ hybridization is the most specific of these four molecular biological methods because it permits direct evaluation of individual cells (1, 9). Because of their complexity and lack of standardization, these tests currently are not used routinely or generally available for diagnostic testing for EBV infection, nor are they necessary in routine clinical situations.

Dot Blotting and Southern Blotting

Numerous radionucleotide probes derived from regions throughout the EBV genome have been successfully used in dot blotting and Southern blotting to demonstrate EBV in clinical specimens. Certain sequences, such as the large internal repeat (IR₁), have theoretical advantages for increased sensitivity because of multiple copies in each EBV genome. The sensitivity and specificity may vary for each nucleic acid probe, and therefore the limits must be established experimentally, using appropriate controls.

Dot blotting has been performed with either whole-cell lysates or purified intracellular DNA, although the former is less specific and is not recommended. Dot blotting may be more sensitive than Southern blotting but is very susceptible to false-positive results because of concentration of nonspecific hybridization within the area of the dot (7). Dot blotting uses total intracellular DNA and may be semiquantitated by using serial dilutions. Southern blotting uses total intracellular DNA digested with one or more restriction endonucleases followed by separation of restriction fragments by gel electrophoresis. Southern blotting is very specific, as restriction fragments can be distinguished from nonspecific hybridization. The precise pattern of hybridization is dependent upon the restriction endonuclease used to digest the sample DNA and the EBV probe used in the Southern blotting. Genomic variation, including large deletions, among different EBV isolates frequently results in restriction fragment length polymorphisms that may confound interpretation and lead to false-negative test results.

PCR

Similar to in situ hybridization, PCR is among the most sensitive methods available for detection of genomic EBV DNA (11, 12). Semiquantitative PCR assays, including quantitative competitive PCR, can be used to determine the EBV load in plasma, peripheral blood lymphocytes, or tissues. Demonstrating the presence of expected restriction endonuclease sites within the amplified fragment may increase the specificity. Real-time measurement of PCR products, using fluorescent TaqMan-based assays, provides better quantitation with excellent sensitivity, specificity, and reproducibility across a large dynamic range (11). The *Bam*HI W internal repeat, which is present in approximately six copies in various EBV strains, is often used as a target for DNA PCR (19), but is still less sensitive than targeting of EBER RNA, for which a commercial PCR amplification kit is available (BioSource International).

EBV viral load assays are more precise than monitoring serologic assays and are more reliable for immunocompromised persons. With acute infectious mononucleosis, mean EBV viral loads are 6×10^4 copies per ml (19). With posttransplant lymphoproliferative disease, EBV viral loads often exceed 10^6 copies per ml and may rise weeks to months before clinical manifestations, which suggests the need to monitor EBV viral loads routinely. EBV viral loads fall as immunosuppressive therapy is reduced to permit natural immunity to destroy EBV-infected cells. EBV viral load testing also shows promise for monitoring tumor burden and relapse in cases of nasopharyngeal carcinoma and Hodgkin's disease.

PCR has been used to characterize two different genotypes (EBNA-2A and EBNA-2B) of EBV based on EBNA-2 differences (ebnotypes). Diversity among EBV isolates has been utilized as a tool for studying the molecular epidemiology of EBV infection. Genomic variation is not randomly spread throughout the EBV genome; certain regions are highly conserved and may be preferable regions for Southern blot and PCR analysis. The occasional absence of a certain restriction endonuclease site in a clinical EBV isolate as determined by Southern blot or PCR analysis must be interpreted in the context of expected EBV genomic diversity. The sensitivity and specificity may vary for each set of PCR primers, so the limits must be established experimentally, using appropriate controls.

In Situ Hybridization

The EBER transcripts, EBER-1 and -2, are expressed in excess of 10^6 copies per cell in latently infected lymphocytes. They are separate but homologous genes that remain untranslated and are believed to function in controlling translation. They are the best target for EBV in situ hybridization because of their abundance (1, 9). These RNA polymerase III transcripts are approximately 170 nucleotides in length and have minimal homology with mammalian RNAs. Commercially available EBER oligonucleotide DNA probes, RNA probes (riboprobes), or peptide nucleic acid probes are labeled with biotin, digoxigenin, or fluorescein for detection (Fig. 2). In situ hybridization using nonisotopic EBER probes is more sensitive for detection of EBV than PCR is for detection of EBV DNA, provides cellular localization of EBV that demonstrates infected cells even when they are only a minor subpopulation, and can be applied to routinely processed paraffin-embedded tissue sections or cytology preparations. EBER transcripts are present in every EBV-associated infection with the exception of oral hairy leukoplakia, which is a purely lytic infection of oral epithelial cells. A hybridization control, often using a ubiquitous cellular transcript such as U6 RNA, must be performed to document that the RNA in the specimen is intact.

Clonality Assay

The EBV genome exists in two forms, circular (episomal) and linear. In latently infected cells, EBV is maintained only as

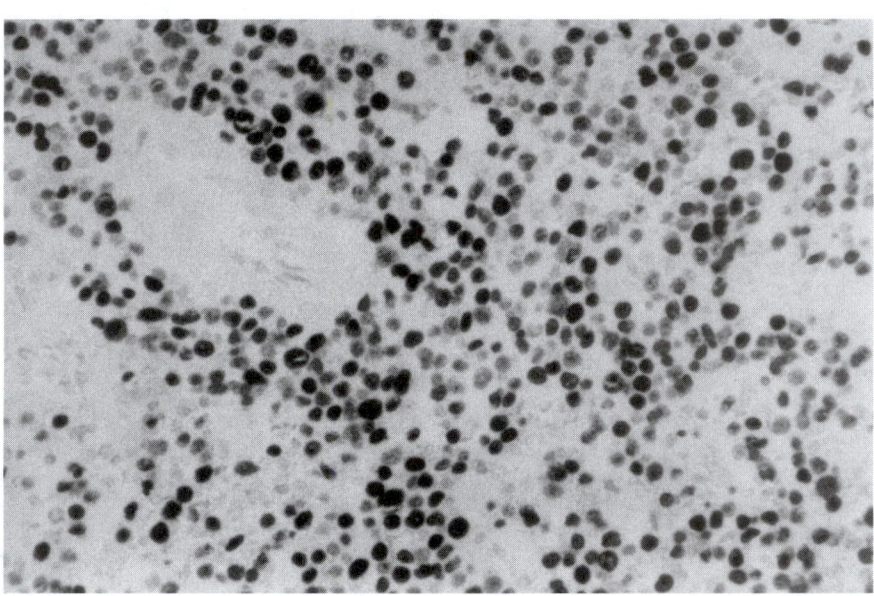

FIGURE 2 EBV in situ hybridization with a digoxigenin-labeled EBER-1 riboprobe in a lymphoproliferative tumor in a patient with an immunodeficiency. EBV is detected in the majority of lymphocytes. A blood vessel is present in the upper left portion. The slide is counterstained with methyl green. Magnification, ×400. Photograph courtesy of Margaret L. Gulley.

multiple episomal copies in the cell nucleus and replicates in a coordinated manner with cellular DNA synthesis. During lytic replication, which leads to cell death, EBV replicates with the formation of linear intermediates formed by the random cleavage between the variable number of terminal repeats of the EBV genome. The random cleavage produces linear EBV genomes containing different numbers of terminal repeats at the ends of the linear genomes. Upon malignant transformation, the same fused terminal repeat pattern is inherited by all progeny of the initial malignant cell.

The clonality assay is performed by digestion of EBV DNA with a restriction endonuclease (e.g., *Bam*HI) that does not cut the genome within the terminal repeats (15). The fragments containing the terminal repeats are detected in a Southern blot assay using specific probes (e.g., *Eco*RI I and *Xho*I a) for the two ends of the EBV genome. With monoclonal EBV infection, the fused termini of the episomes are present as a single size (usually 8 to 23 kbp) and appear as a single band. Multiple bands indicate oligoclonality or polyclonality, which suggests multiple EBV infection events in the cell population being assayed. In addition to confirming EBV infection and showing the clonality, a ladder of smaller terminal digestion fragments, if present, from linear genomes indicates active EBV replication.

REFERENCES

1. **Ambinder, R. F., and R. B. Mann.** 1994. Epstein-Barr-encoded RNA in situ hybridization. Diagnostic applications. *Hum. Pathol.* **25:**602–605.
2. **Baumforth, K. R., L. S. Young, K. J. Flavell, C. Constandinou, and P. G. Murray.** 1999. The Epstein-Barr virus and its association with human cancers. *Mol. Pathol.* **6:**307–322.
3. **Bruu, A. L., R. Hjetland, E. Holter, L. Mortensen, O. Natås, W. Petterson, A. G. Skar, T. Skarpaas, T. Tjade, and B. Åsjø.** 2000. Evaluation of 12 commercial tests for detection of Epstein-Barr virus-specific and heterophile antibodies. *Clin. Diagn. Lab. Immunol.* **7:**451–456.
4. **Chang, R. S., J. P. Lewis, and C. F. Abilgaard.** 1973. Prevalence of oropharyngeal excretors of leukocyte-transforming agents among a human population. *N. Engl. J. Med.* **289:**1325–1329.
5. **Davidsohn, I., and C. L. Lee.** 1969. The clinical serology of infectious mononucleosis, p. 177–200. *In* R. L. Carter and H. G. Penman (ed.), *Infectious Mononucleosis.* Blackwell Scientific Publications, Oxford, United Kingdom.
6. **de Schryver, A., G. Klein, J. Hewetson, G. Rocchi, W. Henle, G. Henle, D. J. Moss, and J. H. Pope.** 1974. Comparison of EBV neutralization tests based on abortive infection or transformation of lymphoid cells and their relation to membrane reactive antibodies (anti-MA). *Int. J. Cancer* **13:**353–362.
7. **Diaz-Mitoma, F., J. K. Preiksaitis, W. C. Leung, and D. L. J. Tyrrell.** 1987. DNA-DNA dot hybridization to detect Epstein-Barr virus in throat washings. *J. Infect. Dis.* **155:**297–303.
8. **Fleisher, G., W. Henle, G. Henle, E. T. Lennette, and R. J. Biggar.** 1979. Primary infection with Epstein-Barr virus in infants in the United States: clinical and serologic observations. *J. Infect. Dis.* **139:**553–558.
9. **Glaser, S. L., M. L. Gulley, M. J. Borowitz, F. E. Craig, R. B. Mann, S. L. Stewart, S. J. Shema, and R. F. Ambinder.** 2004. Inter- and intra-observer reliability of Epstein-Barr virus detection in Hodgkin lymphoma using histochemical procedures. *Leuk. Lymphoma* **45:**489–497.
10. **Henle, G., W. Henle, and G. Klein.** 1971. Demonstration of two distinct components in the early antigen complex of Epstein-Barr virus-infected cells. *Int. J. Cancer* **8:**272–282.
11. **Hubert, G. M. N., J. van Esser, E. Fries, K. C. Wolghers, J. Cornelissen, and A. D. M. E. Osterhaus.** 2000. Development of a real-time quantitative assay for detection of Epstein-Barr virus. *J. Clin. Microbiol.* **38:**712–715.
12. **Ikuta, K., Y. Satoh, Y. Hoshikawa, and T. Sairenji.** 2000. Detection of Epstein-Barr virus in salivas and throat washings in healthy adults and children. *Microbes Infect.* **2:**115–120.
13. **Jenson, H. B.** 2002. Infectious mononucleosis, p. 426–436. *In* H. B. Jenson and R. S. Baltimore (ed.), *Pediatric Infectious Diseases: Principles and Practice.* W. B. Saunders, Philadelphia, Pa.
14. **Long, C., J. G. Derge, and B. Hampar.** 1974. Procedure for activating Epstein-Barr virus early antigen in nonproducer cells by 5-iododeoxyuridine. *J. Natl. Cancer Inst.* **52:**1355–1357.
15. **Raab-Traub, N., and K. Flynn.** 1986. The structure of the termini of the Epstein-Barr virus as a marker of clonal cellular proliferation. *Cell* **47:**883–889.
16. **Reedman, B. M., and G. Klein.** 1973. Cellular localization of an Epstein-Barr virus (EBV)-associated complement-fixing antigen in producer and non-producer lymphoblastoid cell lines. *Int. J. Cancer* **11:**499–520.
17. **Rocchi, G., A. de Felici, G. Ragona, and A. Heinz.** 1977. Quantitative evaluation of Epstein-Barr-virus-infected mononuclear peripheral blood leukocytes in infectious mononucleosis. *N. Engl. J. Med.* **296:**132–134.
18. **Sumaya, C. V., and Y. Ench.** 1985. Epstein-Barr virus infectious mononucleosis in children. II. Heterophile antibody and viral-specific responses. *Pediatrics* **75:**1011–1019.
19. **Yamamoto, M., H. Kimura, T. Hiromaka, K. Hirai, S. Hasegawa, K. Kuzushima, M. Shibata, and T. Morishima.** 1995. Detection and quantification of virus DNA in plasma of patients with Epstein-Barr virus-associated diseases. *J. Clin. Microbiol.* **33:**1765–1768.

Cytomegalovirus

KIRSTEN ST. GEORGE, AKI HOJI, AND CHARLES R. RINALDO, JR.

73

Human cytomegalovirus (CMV) was first isolated independently in three laboratories in the mid-1950s (51). Initial infection with this ubiquitous *Betaherpesvirus* usually occurs early in life and is asymptomatic, after which the virus establishes a lifelong, latent infection. Transmission occurs during direct contact with body fluids such as occurs with breast-feeding, sexual contact, and the care of young children. Preschool-age children in close contact, either at home or in day care facilities, commonly acquire CMV from one another. Latent infections are periodically reactivated and usually result in asymptomatic shedding from various anatomical sites. CMV infection can, however, cause a spectrum of diseases, including congenital cytomegalic inclusion disease in the neonate, a serious but self-limiting mononucleosis syndrome in immunologically competent adults, and a broad range of potentially life-threatening illnesses in persons with impaired immune function. Congenital CMV infection is the major infectious cause of birth defects and a major cause of sensorineural hearing loss and mental retardation in developed countries. The most clinically significant diseases of the retina, gastrointestinal tract, liver, lungs, and central nervous system occur in immunosuppressed organ and tissue transplant recipients and in persons with severe immunodysfunction due to human immunodeficiency virus (HIV) infection. While the incidence of CMV disease in HIV-positive patients has decreased with the advent of combination antiretroviral therapy, CMV continues to be a major opportunistic pathogen in patients on antiretroviral therapy whose CD4+-T-cell counts remain low (49). In addition to its direct causation of disease, CMV infection in transplant recipients is also associated with an increased incidence of bacterial and fungal infections, organ rejection, and graft-versus-host disease (GVHD); accelerated cardiac allograft vasculopathy; increased hospital length of stay and cost of medical care; and decreased survival. Furthermore, people coinfected with CMV and either HIV or hepatitis C virus have more rapid progression of HIV disease or more severe cirrhosis, respectively (8).

CMV has a linear, double-stranded DNA genome of approximately 245 kb. It is surrounded by an icosahedral nucleocapsid, which in turn is bound by an amorphous tegument and a loose, host-derived lipid envelope. The genome is divided into unique short (US) and unique long (UL) regions, both of which are bounded by repeat sequences. These regions can be inverted, resulting in four isomers of CMV DNA found in equimolar amounts. There are more than 200 open reading frames, including virally encoded envelope glycoproteins; some of these have homology with prototype herpes simplex virus proteins, such as glycoproteins B and H (gB and gH). CMV viral particles have recently been shown to contain 71 virus-encoded proteins and more than 70 host cellular proteins, including cellular structural proteins, enzymes, and chaperones (54).

Replication of CMV begins with attachment to the host cell, followed by fusion of the viral envelope with the cell membrane and entry of the nucleocapsid into the cell cytoplasm. The viral DNA then moves from the nucleocapsid into the host nucleus, and a typical alpha-beta-gamma sequence of herpesvirus gene expression follows. The immediate-early (or alpha) gene proteins (primarily transactivators) appear in the infected cell first, followed by the early (or beta) gene proteins (primarily nonstructural) and, finally, the late (or gamma) gene proteins (primarily structural components of the progeny virions). The capsid is assembled, and CMV DNA is packaged into the capsids in the nucleus. The tegument is acquired in both the nucleus and the cytoplasm, and particles are enveloped by budding into the trans-Golgi network. Although CMV is considered to be a relatively slowly replicating virus, evidence suggests that the virus has an average doubling time of 1 day in peripheral blood.

CMV infection in vivo occurs in epithelial cells of the kidney, liver, bile ducts, salivary gland, gut, lung, and pancreas, as well as in endothelial cells. Furthermore, abortive CMV replication has been described to occur in polymorphonuclear leukocytes, monocytes, and T and B lymphocytes. Infected monocytes/macrophages and endothelial cells are important in latent and acute CMV infections, possibly providing transport of the agent to different organs. In contrast to its broad cellular tropism, CMV replication is highly species specific, both in vivo and in vitro.

The major immediate-early (MIE) promoter of CMV controls production of the immediate-early gene products. Activation of this promoter is essential for initiation of the replication cycle and for reactivation of CMV from the latent state. Interestingly, prostaglandins, tumor necrosis factor alpha, interleukin-1β (IL-1β), IL-6, and IL-10 all upregulate the MIE promoter (29). Since these are all products of activated macrophages, acute inflammation has been proposed as one potential trigger for CMV reactivation. Furthermore, MIE gene products have been shown to enhance IL-6 production, suggesting a role for CMV in the production of inflammatory states.

Monocytes, dendritic-like cells, and granulocyte-macrophage progenitor cells in the bone marrow and peripheral blood may be important sites of CMV latency. CMV reactivation can be induced in these cells by cocultivation with permissive cells, allogeneic stimulation, and cytokine treatment. Studies suggest that the percentage of cells latently infected is very low (0.004 to 0.01%) following natural infection (44).

Infection with one strain of CMV produces cross-reactive immunity to others, because of strong homology among all strains of CMV. However, immunity to one CMV strain does not always provide protection from superinfection by another strain, particularly in immunosuppressed hosts. Moreover, cell tropism and organ tropism may vary across different gB and other subtypes of the virus. This may relate to intragenic differences of gB types within a given isolate of CMV that result in variable immune specificity.

Cell-mediated immune responses play a major role in the control of CMV disease in an infected host. The presence of CMV-specific, major histocompatibility complex (MHC) class I-restricted CD8+ cytotoxic T-lymphocyte (CTL) responses correlates with recovery from acute CMV infection and avoidance of disease in bone marrow transplant recipients (38). Furthermore, CMV disease can be prevented in bone marrow transplant recipients by the transfusion of autologous, CMV-specific, CD8+ T-cell clones (56). CTL and MHC class II-restricted CD4+ helper T-cell responses have been reported for several nonstructural and structural proteins of CMV (26). The most prominent CD8+ T-cell responses are to the lower matrix tegument protein pp65, which is also the predominant protein in the virus particle. In contrast, there is no dominant viral protein specificity for CD4+ T-cell reactivity.

CMV may suppress immune function in numerous ways. Lymphocytes from patients with CMV mononucleosis show reduced responses to mitogens and viral antigens (39). Data suggest that CMV-infected monocytes produce both tumor necrosis factor alpha, which in turn induces release of arachidonic acid, and prostaglandin E_2, which suppresses T-cell function (35). Even more intriguing is the fact that several CMV proteins encoded in the US region of CMV down-regulate MHC class I and class II expression (19). US2 and US11 dislocate MHC class I heavy chains from the endoplasmic reticulum to the cytosol, US3 facilitates their retention in the endoplasmic reticulum, and US6 inhibits the transporter for antigen processing translocation of the peptides. CMV also inhibits MHC class II expression, with US2 causing degradation of two essential proteins in the MHC class II pathway. This inhibition reduces the presentation of CMV antigens and, by extension, recognition by CD8+ and CD4+ T cells in vitro, and it may be involved in virus escape from the cell-mediated immune responses in vivo.

Numerous interactions occur between CMV-encoded proteins and cell chemokines. At least three CMV genes, US27, US28, and UL33, encode proteins that have CC chemokine receptor homology. The US28 gene product, for example, can bind beta chemokines, an event that is followed by cell sequestration of the chemokines.

Thus, CMV infection has an intimate interrelationship with host immunity. Assessments of humoral and cellular immune responses to CMV are therefore central to our understanding of the pathogenesis of the virus, and to the development of suitable therapeutic and vaccine controls for CMV infection.

DIAGNOSIS AND TREATMENT

CMV can be cultured in vitro in diploid human fibroblasts through the use of both conventional and rapid centrifugation-enhanced (shell vial) methods. Classically, congenital CMV infection is diagnosed by the isolation of virus from urine or saliva within 3 weeks of birth. Direct antigen detection by immunostaining has been applied to tissue biopsy sections and to cell smears from bronchoalveolar lavage fluid, cerebrospinal fluid, and peripheral blood. The optimal reagents for staining of tissues and bronchoalveolar lavage cells target both early and late viral antigens. For the staining of leukocytes in cerebrospinal fluid, the pp65 antigen must be targeted; the assay is only useful for the diagnosis of polyradiculomyelopathy and not encephalitis. Optimal staining of peripheral blood leukocytes in the CMV antigenemia assay targets the pp65 protein, and this method has greatly increased the sensitivity of detection of infection (50). Additionally, the assay is quantitative and can be used to assess the likelihood of progression to disease and the response to antiviral therapy.

Molecular methods for the detection of viral nucleic acids have increasingly replaced many of the above-mentioned methods. The most frequently used diagnostic approach for CMV infection is currently molecular amplification and detection of either viral RNA or DNA in peripheral blood. For the detection of CMV DNA in tissues, hybridization reactions have been applied to biopsy sections and amplification reactions have been applied to tissue homogenates. The latter, however, have sometimes been found to be too sensitive for clinical utility. DNA detection by PCR or similar DNA amplification assays has proven to be the method of choice for determining virtually all CMV-related central nervous system diseases, whereas the detection of virus in throat and urine specimens by any method has generally been found to have little clinical utility, due to asymptomatic viral shedding and the consequent lack of disease association.

There is an extensive published literature on countless PCR and other DNA amplification methods for the detection of CMV nucleic acid in blood. These include qualitative and quantitative methods; commercial and in-house methods; and manual, semiautomated, and fully automated methods. Additionally, there has been extensive discussion as to the optimal blood compartment for disease specificity, whether serum or plasma, whole blood, or purified leukocytes. Furthermore, there have been some successful studies showing the clinical utility of the detection of viral RNA in blood; one such method is commercially available (12). Most workers in the field, however, consider quantitative assays for viral DNA in peripheral blood to be optimal for the diagnosis and prognosis of CMV infection. These provide the combination of high sensitivity of detection and of quantitation, factors which are valuable in the determination of likelihood of progression to symptomatic disease, and in the monitoring of response to antiviral therapy. In recent years, the use of real-time PCR assays has become increasingly popular, due to their advantages of rapid quantitative detection, long linear ranges, ease of automation, and sealed systems that minimize the risk of amplicon contamination. There are a variety of real-time chemistries and automated equipment available, as well as ever-increasing numbers of commercial reagents and kits.

Only three drugs are currently approved for the treatment of systemic CMV infection: ganciclovir, foscarnet, and cidofovir (17). Ganciclovir and cidofovir are nucleotide analogs, while foscarnet is a pyrophosphate analog. All are optimally administered intravenously and have considerable toxicity profiles. Oral ganciclovir, however, has a low bioavailability and is associated with an increased incidence of drug resistance. Fortunately, the valyl ester, valganciclovir, has much higher oral bioavailability, and its successful use is now widespread. Ganciclovir and valganciclovir remain the first drugs of choice and are usually administered prophylactically or preemptively to patients at high risk of disease. The antisense oligonucleotide fomivirsen is only approved for use as an intravitreal injection for CMV retinitis that is not responsive to ganciclovir or foscarnet. With the use of these drugs has come the emergence of resistant strains of CMV, particularly in HIV-positive patients under long prophylactic treatment regimens and in transplant recipients at high risk of severe CMV disease. Resistant strains are commonly virulent, and while some exhibit a decreased replication efficiency in vitro, their emergence in a patient is often associated with serious disease consequences (24).

ANTIBODY RESPONSES

The humoral response to CMV infection includes the production of immunoglobulin A (IgA), IgM, and IgG antibodies. IgM antibodies are the first to appear following a primary CMV infection and may be detectable for a prolonged period. Furthermore, their production can recur following reactivation of latent virus or reinfection with additional strains of CMV. Thus, detection of CMV IgM is not diagnostic of a primary or even a recent infection. IgG antibodies appear 6 to 8 weeks after primary infection and persist indefinitely, with fluctuations in titer believed to be due to reactivations of latent virus. More than 95% of the anti-CMV IgG in normal human serum is of subclass IgG1, and approximately 3% is IgG3. Most sera also have low levels of CMV-specific IgG2 and IgG4.

The CMV genome encodes approximately 65 glycoproteins with a wide variety of functions. gB (also known as UL55) was believed to be the most abundant protein in the CMV envelope; however, recent studies with the laboratory strain AD169 have found that gM (UL100) is in fact more abundant, with gH (UL75) being the next after gB (54). All clinical isolates of the virus express gB, and serological responses to gB can be detected in infected individuals. During primary CMV infection, the production of glycoprotein-specific antibodies is delayed relative to that of immunoglobulins directed against other CMV antigens. During reactivation or reinfection, however, antibody production is more synchronized, and most of the virus-neutralizing activity in the serum of naturally infected individuals is from antibodies against gB (10).

Antigenic domain 1 was the first antibody-binding site to be identified on gB (53). More than 50% of the gB-specific antibody response in serum is directed against antigenic domain 1, and studies with monoclonal antibodies (MAbs) and point mutations indicate various antigenic substructures within the domain (42). This is one of the most highly conserved regions of gB, suggesting a critical role in the structure or function of the protein. Antibodies to gH can also be detected following natural infection. Assays using full-length protein detect these CMV antibodies in 95% of seropositive persons, and in some individuals anti-gH comprises the majority of the virus-neutralizing activity of serum. Latency-associated transcripts have been identified, and antibodies to proteins encoded by them have been detected in the serum of blood donors.

CMV infections have been associated with autoimmune manifestations, including the production of autoantibodies.

For example, CD13-specific antibodies have been found in bone marrow transplant recipients following CMV disease or CMV viremia, presumably stemming from altered presentation to the immune system as part of the CMV virion. These CD13-specific autoantibodies are believed to play a role in chronic GVHD reactions (47). Likewise, the detection of antibodies to ganglioside GM2 in patients developing Guillain-Barré syndrome following CMV infection has suggested a role for these antibodies in the development of this condition.

Serological Assays

While the detection of IgG antibodies provides confirmation of previous exposure to CMV and implies the presence of latent virus, the presence of antibodies does not protect the individual from reactivation of the latent virus or superinfection with a different strain. The clinical utility of CMV IgG assays is therefore somewhat limited. There are instances in which the demonstration of seroconversion is appropriate, particularly in pregnant women. However, even here, additional data from tests of antibody avidity may help to clarify the prognosis (25). Serology is not generally recommended as a diagnostic methodology for immunocompromised patients, as they may be unable to mount a detectable humoral antibody response or may have circulating IgG antibodies resulting from transfusions or immunotherapy. The use of these antibody assays on intraocular eye fluids has been found to be unreliable for the diagnosis of CMV retinitis. Serological assays for CMV IgG are used extensively in blood banking to generate stocks of CMV-seronegative blood. These are important for reducing the risk of severe posttransfusion primary CMV infection in CMV-seronegative immunocompromised patients.

Transmission of CMV to the fetus in utero cannot be predicted by the presence of IgM antibodies in maternal serum, since not all primary infections result in a detectable IgM response and since IgM responses are often seen during reactivations. In fact, fewer than 10% of IgM-positive pregnant women subsequently deliver a congenitally infected infant (31). Likewise, IgM detection is not recommended for immunosuppressed patients and, since CMV IgM responses can be raised even in response to reactivations, the general utility is limited.

IgG Assays

The majority of commercially available assays for CMV IgG antibodies use either viral lysate preparations or semipurified viral proteins as antibody binding targets; the sensitivities of these assays do not vary widely. The most commonly used methods for the detection of IgG antibodies are indirect enzyme immunoassays (EIAs) with either a semiautomated or automated format. Semiautomated formats are generally microtiter-based systems with manual pipetting of reagents and plate-reading spectrophotometers. More highly automated robotic systems for microtiter plate assays are generally only found in very large laboratories. Microparticle systems have also become popular, as they lend themselves readily to smaller-scale automation. Antigen is bound to microparticles, which are suspended in liquid and flow through tubing systems on automated equipment. Antibody-antigen reactions take place on the surface of the microparticles, and the detecting antibody may be tagged with any one of a number of different compounds, to facilitate detection and quantitation. Care must be taken with these systems, however, to ensure homogeneous particle suspension prior to operation.

Another method for IgG detection, although now rarely used, is immunofluorescence. Antigen-containing cells are bound to the wells of a slide and are incubated with dilutions of patient serum. A second antibody tagged with a fluorescent label, usually fluorescein isothiocyanate, is then added, and the cell spot is viewed under fluorescence microscopy. A few laboratories still use complement fixation tests. The assay, which detects antibody via its ability to fix complement and thereby interfere with cell lysis, does not distinguish IgG from IgM, is time-consuming to perform, and does not lend itself readily to automation. Latex agglutination assays are also used in some laboratories as a rapid screening test for the presence of CMV antibodies, but they are less sensitive than EIAs.

IgM Assays

Assays for the detection of IgM antibodies show more variation in sensitivity than do those for IgG, depending on the antigen preparation used. In general, the necessity for detection of structural and nonstructural viral proteins, in order to achieve optimal sensitivity, renders those IgM assays that use viral lysates more sensitive than those that use semipurified viral protein preparations. However, certain pooled recombinant antigen preparations specifically designed for the purpose also have been found to be good and to avoid problems, such as patient antibody reactivity with cellular antigens, that may produce false-positive results.

As with IgG assays, the most common format for IgM detection is semiautomated EIA-based systems in microtiter plates, with microparticle-based systems also increasing in popularity. In contrast to the almost universal use of antigen coating on solid support to initially bind IgG antibodies, many IgM assays use IgM capture methods. In these systems, an anti-IgM antibody is bound to the solid support, either microtiter well or microparticle, to which any IgM antibody present in the serum will bind. CMV-specific IgM is then distinguished by the binding of CMV antigen to the immobilized IgM, with detection via a conjugated enzyme or other detector molecule. False-positive IgM results can occur with sera that contain high titers of IgG antibody, when an assay is used that relies on the absorption of IgG prior to the detection of IgM. IgM capture methods are not prone to the false-positivity problems caused by rheumatoid factor. The commercially available IgM assays are virtually universally qualitative, whereas many of the IgG assays are quantitative or semiquantitative.

Antibody Avidity

In organ transplant recipients, the delayed development of high-avidity antibody has been correlated with delayed viral clearance and a poor prognosis (32). Additionally, the measurement of antibody avidity has been found to be a powerful tool for distinguishing primary from nonprimary infections in pregnant women and for predicting CMV transmission to the fetus.

Antibody avidity assays are performed by the simple insertion of a chemical elution step in the EIA procedure. Following the incubation of serum with antigen, and prior to incubation with the conjugate, the strength of antibody binding, or avidity, is challenged by the addition of urea. The higher the antibody avidity, the greater the amount of IgG antibody that will remain bound to the antigen. Thus, by comparison of the test results with and without the urea incubation step, the percentage of antibody avidity is calculated.

Neutralization Assays

While antibody neutralization assays are now rarely used in diagnostic laboratories, they have been shown to assist in distinguishing primary from nonprimary infections. A microneutralization format has been shown to be helpful in predicting outcome in suspected maternal CMV infections during pregnancy (18).

T-LYMPHOCYTE RESPONSES

Blastogenesis (Proliferation)

CD4+ memory T helper cells from CMV-seropositive persons react to CMV antigens in vitro, when the antigens are presented as peptides in the context of MHC class II molecules by antigen-presenting cells (APCs). This clonal response is not evident in T cells from CMV-seronegative persons, although the distinction has become blurred, with reports of CMV DNA and virus in some CMV-seronegative persons. Recently, bacterial polysaccharides have been shown to be presented to CD4+ T cells by MHC class II molecules (15). This suggests that viral sugar moieties can be presented to T cells. Antigen-specific, activated CD4+ T cells provide "help" in the form of cytokines, such as IL-2 and gamma interferon (IFN-γ), that are produced after their antigen-specific interaction with APCs. These cytokines enhance activation and expansion of antiviral effector CD8+ CTLs. Activated CD4+ T cells also augment CD8+-T-cell activation by inducing maturation of APCs, in particular dendritic cells (DCs), through engagement of their CD40 ligand to CD40 on the surface of the APCs. The mature APCs express greater levels of T-cell ligands (MHC and costimulatory molecules) and cytokines (such as IL-12) that mediate activation and expansion of antigen-specific CD8+ T cells.

The conventional assay for CD4+-T-cell immunity is measurement of the turnover of cellular DNA, or blastogenesis. This is more commonly termed lymphocyte proliferation, since most (but not necessarily all) of the blasting cells undergo mitosis. Incorporation of [3H]thymidine into DNA is measured after 5 or 6 days of culture. The method is not commercially available in a kit format. We recommend a consensus lymphoproliferation assay protocol established in 2000 by the Immunology Research Agenda Committee of the Adult AIDS Clinical Trials Group (2). The assay requires in vitro stimulation and culture of the CD4+ T cells with viral antigen, so it is actually an assessment of the ability of precursor CD4+ T cells to replicate DNA and proliferate. Usually, nonreplicating CMV antigen is added to peripheral blood mononuclear cells (PBMCs) that contain the CD4+ T cells and the appropriate APCs (B cells, monocytes, and DCs) for processing of the CMV antigen. Laboratory strains of CMV are typically used as antigen (e.g., AD169, Davis, and Towne), since there is strong cross-antigenicity with clinical, wild-type isolates. Alternatively, recombinant CMV proteins (e.g., immediate-early protein, gB, and pp65) or predetermined MHC class II synthetic CMV peptides can be used to delineate CMV-specific CD4+-T-cell reactivity. Incorporation of [3H]thymidine into DNA is measured after 5 or 6 days of culture.

The results are reported as the difference in radioactivity between the antigen-stimulated cultures and the background control, or as a stimulation index (SI), which is the radioactivity in the antigen-treated cultures divided by that in the control culture. A positive result can be determined using as a lower limit the mean plus 3 standard deviations of the results for CMV-seronegative donors. A significant drawback to this test is that very low radioactive counts in the controls can result in artificially high SIs for biological responses that are relatively nonrobust. Moreover, the assay is only semiquantitative; i.e., it does not reveal the number of cells that duplicate their DNA or that proliferate in response to the antigens. Limiting-dilution assays have been developed to quantitate the number of proliferating, antigen-specific CD4[+] T cells, but these methods have not been widely adopted, due to their labor-intensive nature and technical difficulty.

The activation process described above does not distinguish T helper 1 (Th1) from T helper 2 (Th2) subpopulations of human CD4[+] T cells. These subtypes are primarily responsible for activation of antigen-specific CD8[+] CTLs and for B-cell antibody production, respectively. Another significant point concerning this assay is that the cells finally incorporating the thymidine label may include bystander, non-CMV antigen-specific T cells that have been activated by the secondary effects of cytokines that were initially produced by the CMV-specific CD4[+] T cells, such as IL-2. Finally, this assay is rarely used to assess blastogenesis of CD8[+] T cells; for such an application it would require CMV antigen processed by APCs through the MHC class I pathway.

In recent years, the intracellular fluorescent dye 5(6)-carboxyfluorescein diacetate succinimidyl-ester has been used to measure T-cell proliferation (5). As T cells labeled with this dye divide, the dye is successively diluted by half in each daughter cell. This therefore allows determination of the number of cells that have gone through cell divisions, by flow cytometry. The technique measures proliferation of CMV-specific CD4, as well as CD8, T cells. It is typically done in cell culture systems where fresh or frozen PBMCs are stimulated by the addition of either recombinant CMV proteins (e.g., pp65 produced by baculovirus), inactivated whole-virus preparations, or synthetic immunodominant CMV peptides (if the HLA type of the individual is known and if the peptide is available for the particular HLA type). The CMV proteins and virus will be processed through the exogenous MHC class II pathway by APCs in the PBMC cultures, and they will stimulate CMV-specific CD4[+] T cells. Stimulation of CMV-specific CD8[+] T cells can be done by the use of 8- to 10-mer MHC class I-restricted peptides. Moreover, this method, in combination with staining with CMV-specific MHC class I tetramers (see below), allows simultaneous detection of surface markers (immunophenotyping; see below) and of intracellular molecules that are either up- or down-regulated after antigen-specific stimulation. Thus, from a clinical standpoint, this method has a clear advantage over thymidine incorporation methods, in that it provides additional data for assessing whether CMV-specific T cells are functional or dysfunctional.

Healthy persons with latent CMV infection will have CD4[+] T-cell responses to whole CMV antigens and to some, but not always all, recombinant CMV proteins. In contrast, patients subject to immunosuppression, such as in HIV type 1 infection and during organ or tissue transplantation, will usually have low CD4[+] T-cell blastogenic responses to CMV antigens, depending on the duration and severity of their immunosuppression. This CMV-specific cellular immune dysfunction is in turn a determinant of their enhanced susceptibility to severe CMV-related disease.

Notably, there are no uniform standards that are widely available for these T-cell assays, leaving each laboratory to adopt internal, self-developed standards and controls. Also, because there are no proficiency testing services like those from the College of American Pathologists, laboratories are limited to proficiency panels provided to members of National Institutes of Health-sponsored programs, such as the AIDS Clinical Trials Group.

Cytokine Production

DCs and CD4[+] and CD8[+] T cells produce a group of cytokines before and after antigen-specific activation. These glycoproteins are a major factor in augmentation of effector T-cell responses to the virus and in helper function of the CD4[+] T cells. Cytokines predominantly produced by myeloid DCs are IL-12 and IL-15, which help to drive Th1 cell reactivity. Plasmacytoid DCs predominantly produce IFN-α, which can also enhance Th1 cell activity. Virus-specific T-cell-modulating activity by both types of DCs can be regulated through binding of natural ligands, such as lipopolysaccharides and CpG oligodeoxynucleotides, to toll-like receptors on the DCs (33).

Cytokines produced by Th1 cells, i.e., IFN-γ and IL-2, activate and expand the populations of antigen-specific effector CD8[+] CTLs. These cytokines also activate cells involved in innate immune responses, such as natural killer cells and macrophages. Lack of IL-12 production by DCs can lead to polarization of the T-cell response to Th2 cells instead of Th1 cells. Cytokines primarily produced by Th2 cells, such as IL-4 and IL-5, enhance B-cell antibody production. Thus, cytokine assays can, at least to some degree, distinguish Th1 from Th2 cells. A third set of CD4[+] T cells is T-regulatory (or Treg) cells, which are involved in maintaining tolerance by down-regulating effector T-cell responses. For CD8[+] T cells, there is a less well-documented division of CD8[+] type 1 and type 2 (Tc1 and Tc2) cells that produce cytokines similar to their T helper cell counterparts.

There exist a great number of commercially available EIAs for these cytokines. The test can be done on supernatants from cultures that have been stimulated as in the blastogenesis assay. The peak time for production of these cytokines is usually earlier than the peak blastogenic, or proliferative, response. For CD8[+] T cells, the major difference is the use of MHC class I-associated antigens by APCs. Since professional APCs do not support the CMV replication necessary for activation of CD8[+] T cells, stimulation of cytokines in CD8[+] T cells is done with APCs such as Epstein-Barr virus-immortalized B-lymphocyte cell lines (BLCLs) that have been infected with vectors such as vaccinia viruses expressing CMV proteins. Alternatively, PBMCs can be stimulated directly with synthetic CMV peptides representing predetermined MHC class I epitopes.

These assays have an advantage over the more quantitative tests in that they require relatively few PBMCs and are technically noncomplex. A significant drawback of these EIAs done on "bulk" culture supernatants, however, is that they are semiquantitative. That is, they do not distinguish whether differences in cytokine production are due to alterations in the amount of cytokine produced per cell or due to differing numbers of T cells. Moreover, they measure, to some extent, the levels of cytokines that have been induced through autocrine and paracrine loops by the CMV-specific CD4[+] or CD8[+] T cells that initially responded to the CMV MHC class II- or I-associated peptides, respectively, that are presented by the APCs. Thus, these assays do not unambiguously determine the numbers of CMV antigen-specific CD4[+] and CD8[+] T cells.

Single-cell EIA (ELISPOT) and intracellular flow cytometry assays of CMV-specific cytokine production by CD4[+] and CD8[+] T cells have steadily increased in usage in immunological research. These two assays are quantitative in that they delineate the number of CMV antigen-specific T cells that are producing the cytokines. Furthermore, if done within the first day of antigen stimulation, they essentially capture the CMV-specific memory T cells that are directly responding to MHC class I- or II-bound CMV peptides on the APCs.

For the ELISPOT assay, PBMCs, or enriched CD4+ or CD8+ T cells obtained by negative selection with magnetic beads coated with anti-HLA MAbs, are treated with HLA class I- or II-associated CMV antigens and seeded into commercially prepared microwells containing nitrocellulose membranes that have been impregnated with anticytokine MAb (27). Recently, large libraries of synthetic 15- to 20-mer peptides representing overlapping sequences of major immunogenic CMV proteins, e.g., pp65, have been used to generate anti-CMV CTLs for immunotherapy and for delineation of immunodominant epitopes (52). The 15- to 20-mer CMV peptides can be used in single or batched (up to 50 peptides each) formats. These libraries are a powerful approach in revealing new epitopes and changes in T-cell response to different viral epitopes. Such information is invaluable to the development of CMV vaccines, where it can be used to assess antigenic breadth. It is also notable that the once-strict definition of a specific HLA restriction for a single CMV epitope is now known to be much less rigid. This "degeneracy" is related to promiscuous binding of the peptide epitopes to several HLA class I molecules, which are termed supertype alleles (11).

The optimal time of incubation in the ELISPOT assay may vary according to the antigen preparation, ranging from 6 to 20 h. The dark spots are visible on the membranes for manual counting under a dissecting microscope, although computerized microscope readers are available (e.g., from Cell Technology, Columbia, Md.). Each spot theoretically represents cytokine produced from a single CD4+ or CD8+ T cell. The results are reported as the number of spot-forming cells. It should be noted that non-T cells can produce these cytokines, a fact which can complicate the results. However, if the CMV antigen is highly specific for activation of CD4+ or CD8+ T cells, there is less likelihood of cytokine production by the opposite T-cell subset or by the non-T cells in the preparation.

An alternative to the ELISPOT assay is intracellular staining of cells for cytokines and assessment by flow cytometry (55). The advantages of this method include relative ease and rapidity, less subjectivity in determining the results, and simultaneous determination of multiple cell surface and intracellular parameters of T-cell subpopulations. Thus, the numbers of CD4+ and CD8+ T cells producing cytokines can be directly assessed, without the need for laborious and expensive preenrichment of the cell subsets, as in the ELISPOT assay. However, intracellular staining is more costly, in that it requires flow cytometry for reading the assay, and it may require more PBMCs in cases where the number of positive cell "events" is relatively low.

Whole, anticoagulated blood or PBMCs are stimulated with either MHC class I or II CMV antigens. An inhibitor of protein secretion, such as brefeldin A or monensin, is added during the incubation to enhance the intracellular levels of the cytokines. The T cells are then labeled with anti-CD4 or anti-CD8 MAb and with anti-CD69 MAb (a type II membrane glycoprotein that is expressed on activated, but not resting, lymphocytes); these are each conjugated to different fluorescent dyes. Anti-CD28 MAb, which activates the CD28 molecule, which costimulates the T cells, can be added to enhance the CMV antigen-specific response. The PBMCs are permeabilized to allow intracellular entry of the fluorescence-conjugated anticytokine MAbs. The results, derived by flow cytometry, are expressed as the number of CD4+ or CD8+ T cells that are positive for the cytokine and CD69. Typical levels of T cells producing cytokines like IFN-γ or IL-2 in response to CMV antigens in healthy CMV-seropositive persons are 0.1 to 2.0%, so at least 50,000 cell events have to be read to obtain reliable results.

Cytotoxicity

CD8+ CTLs are the major effectors of host resistance to CMV infection. They are activated by engagement of their T-cell receptors and coreceptors by MHC class I-bound peptides and costimulatory receptors on APCs. Limited endogenous replication of CMV within APCs directly leads to processing of viral proteins through this pathway. DCs, however, may also engulf virus-infected apoptotic cells (e.g., CMV-infected endothelial cells) and may process viral proteins through the HLA class I pathway (termed "cross-priming") for activation of antiviral CD8+ CTLs. These CD8+-T-cell activation processes are enhanced by T helper cells, as described above. Lower numbers of CD4+ CTLs also are induced during CMV infection and are restricted by MHC class II molecules.

Once activated and expanded into effector cells, the CTLs make direct contact with the virus-infected target cells by the same T-cell receptor–MHC class I-restricted mechanism. The CTLs then mediate lysis, mainly by exocytosis of their granules, followed by perforin-dependent redistribution of CTL granzymes that activate the infected cell's apoptotic pathway. A second pathway of lysis that is not as prevalent in antiviral CTLs is engagement and oligomerization of Fas on the infected target cells by Fas ligand on the CTLs, with subsequent activation of the apoptotic pathway.

Anti-CMV CTL function cannot be reliably assayed directly from blood or tissues. Instead, CTLs are measured either by a bulk lysis procedure that is semiquantitative or by a quantitative limiting-dilution assay (40). These both require suitable stimulator cells expressing CMV peptides with the appropriate MHC class I molecules. For this, autologous fibroblasts previously grown from skin or tissue biopsy samples are infected with a laboratory strain of CMV. Alternatively, autologous BLCLs can be infected with viral vectors expressing CMV genes, such as vaccinia virus encoding CMV pp65. Such vectors are necessary, because BLCLs and other hematopoietic APCs are nonpermissive for full-cycle CMV replication. The vectors also allow differentiation of CMV protein-specific CTL responses. This system may stimulate CTLs specific for the Epstein-Barr virus that is used to transform the BLCLs, a response which must be differentiated from the CMV-specific T-cell response.

For the bulk lysis assay, PBMCs or enriched CD8+ T cells are stimulated with APCs loaded with either viral vectors expressing CMV proteins or synthetic CMV peptides representing known CD8+ T-cell epitopes and with IL-2. The IL-2 can instead be added after 2 to 3 days, so as to minimize nonspecific cell activation. Autologous or allogeneic, irradiated, uninfected cells are added as feeder cells to enhance cell viability and growth. Instead of feeder cells, which may introduce complicating factors such as alloreactivity, IL-7 can be added; this helps to maintain the viability of activated T cells. The cells are cultured for 10 days and then added to ^{51}Cr-labeled target cells at several effector/target cell ratios. Thus, the assay is, to a large degree, a measurement that is dependent on the in vitro proliferative capacity of the antigen-specific T cells.

The most convenient target cell systems are autologous cells that express CMV antigens in the context of HLA class I, such as the BLCLs loaded with synthetic peptides or infected with the CMV-vaccinia virus vectors. The percentage of lysis is calculated as follows: [(experimental cpm − spontaneous cpm)/(maximum cpm − spontaneous cpm)] × 100, where cpm is counts per minute. CMV-specific lysis is calculated as the lysis of the CMV antigen-expressing targets minus the lysis of the control targets. Data also can be calculated as lytic units per 10^7 cells; these units are derived from an exponential-regression analysis of the multiple effector/target cell ratios.

The limiting-dilution assay for anti-CMV CTLs is superior to the bulk lysis assay in that it quantitates the actual number of CD8$^+$ CTL precursors. This precursor frequency assay, however, is much more labor-intensive, and its use in the field has been declining in recent years. PBMCs are plated in two- or fourfold dilutions in 24 replicates. To each well are added irradiated allogeneic PBMCs as feeder cells, IL-2, and cells expressing HLA class I–associated CMV antigens. The cells are cultured as in the bulk lysis assay and on day 10 are split into replicate wells; cytotoxicity is then measured by the ^{51}Cr release assay. The fraction of nonresponding wells is the number of wells in which the ^{51}Cr release does not exceed the mean spontaneous release plus 10% of the incorporated ^{51}Cr, divided by the number of wells assayed. The precursor frequency is estimated by the maximum-likelihood method, using statistical programs that are described in the literature.

Flow cytometry-based assays for CTL function have slowly been accepted as replacements for the chromium release assay. These involve effector-to-target setups similar to those in the chromium release assays, but the target cells are stained with dyes such as 3,3'-dioctadecyloxacarocyanine, which labels green the cell membranes of viable cells. Target cells lysed by CTLs become permeable to counterstain dyes such as propidium iodide, which labels the accessible nuclei red (14). The assay is safer in that it does not use radioactive chromium, and it has been reported to be more sensitive and to have lower background than the chromium release assay. It is commercially available in a kit format from Molecular Probes (Eugene, Oreg.). Several other fluorescence-based assays of CTL function include measurements of apoptosis through assessment of caspase activity in the target cells (13). These proteases can be measured by caspase substrates having covalently bound and quenched dyes that fluoresce upon cleavage by the caspase. The reagents are commercially available from OncoImmunin (Gaithersburg, Md.). Prestaining of the targets with a nonspecific dye such as CellTracker Orange (Molecular Probes) can differentiate them from effector cells. Finally, the phenotype of the T cells mediating the lysis can be determined through costaining with MAbs to CD4 and CD8. The stained cells are assayed by multiparameter flow cytometry. This assay is thought to be more sensitive than other dye staining methods, because it measures early events in cell death, events that precede membrane disruption. Finally, new flow cytometric measures of CTL function include staining for CD107, a lysosomal-associated membrane glycoprotein that is exposed on the CTL surface during degranulation.

HLA Class I Tetramer Staining

In 1996, Altman and coworkers (4) reported that antiviral CD8$^+$ T cells could be directly labeled by staining with a soluble MHC class I tetramer with bound viral peptides. This tetramer staining method has several advantages over other assays for determination of antiviral CD8$^+$-T-cell numbers. First, it directly identifies virus-specific T cells without culturing them in vitro. To culture is to disturb: culture methods are fraught with pitfalls related to differential outgrowth of subpopulations of CD8$^+$ T cells, such as occurs due to apoptosis of activated T cells upon antigen-specific stimulation. Second, tetramer positivity correlates well with antiviral CTL and cytokine effector functions of CD8$^+$ T cells. Third, this method is a relatively objective and non-labor-intensive assay that is read on a flow cytometer. Drawbacks to the tetramer staining assay include, in some virus infections, a lack of correlation of tetramer-positive cells with functional activity, the

occurrence of nonspecific binding of the tetramers to other CD8$^+$ T cells, difficulty in preparing tetramers for certain CTL peptides, and restriction of the technique to known MHC class I epitopes. CMV-specific tetramers use immunodominant peptides such as pp65$_{495-503}$ (NLVPMVATV) (28). The method therefore potentially offers a powerful approach to assessment of numerous aspects of anti-CMV T-cell responses. In addition, HLA class II tetramers are in development and should be available in the near future for the measurement of anti-CMV CD4$^+$ T-cell responses (30).

T-Cell Phenotyping

Expression of certain molecules on the surface of T cells has been associated with their functional capacity. Sallusto and colleagues (41) first proposed two major subsets, termed central memory (CCR7$^+$ CD45RA$^+$) and effector memory (CCR7$^-$ CD45RA$^+$) T cells. This system was further refined by Appay and coworkers (6), who showed that expression of CD27 in combination with CD28 was related to distinct maturational stages. Naive T cells express both CD27 and CD28 (i.e., CD8$^+$ CD27$^+$ CD28$^+$). Conventional, early memory CD8$^+$ T cells maintain expression of CD27 and CD28 (i.e., CD8$^+$ CD27$^+$ CD28$^+$); they are poorly differentiated and weakly cytotoxic, but they can proliferate. As these memory CD8$^+$ T cells proliferate in response to antigen, they differentiate and lose expression of CD27 and CD28 (i.e., they become CD8$^+$ CD27$^-$ CD28$^-$), reflective of their more differentiated state. These cells have strong cytolytic function, due to high expression of the effector molecules perforin and granzymes, and they have been termed effector memory T cells. CD8$^+$ T cells specific for distinct antigens appear to be enriched in particular phenotypic subsets.

Such subsets can further be defined by expression of CD27 and CD28 or of CD27 and CD45RA. CMV-specific CD8$^+$ T cells are typically enriched in a CD27$^-$ CD28$^-$ (6) or CD27$^-$ CD45RA$^+$ (21) phenotypic compartment. This phenotypic subset is functionally equivalent to effector CD8$^+$ T cells, which have the capacity to lyse CMV-infected cells by releasing effector molecules such as granzymes and perforin. Interestingly, CMV-specific CD8$^+$ T cells from immunosuppressed individuals show a greater frequency and higher proportion of the CD27$^-$ CD45RA$^+$ effector subset than do latently infected healthy controls (21). A major factor that controls the size and phenotype of CMV-specific CD8$^+$ T cells appears to be up-regulation of CD70 upon antigenic stimulation (22). During CMV antigenic stimulation of the T cells, CD70 interacts with CD27 and leads to its down-regulation. Thus, development of the CMV-specific CD8$^+$ T-cell phenotypes is highly complex and is influenced by multiple factors present in the microenvironment in which they interact with virus-infected cells.

IMMUNOTHERAPY

Active Humoral Immunotherapy

Since primary CMV infection in pregnant women poses the greatest risk of congenital CMV in the infant, maternal immunization prior to pregnancy may protect newborns from this disease. In an effort to decrease the incidence of congenital CMV infection, it is suggested that recipients of a CMV vaccine include toddlers, preteen children, and young mothers. It should be noted that while preexisting immunity reduces the incidence of congenital CMV infection by 69% (20), such immunity does not significantly reduce the severity of outcome (23). However, the average incidence of congenital CMV infections in developed countries ranges from 0.5 to 2.0%, with approximately 10% of infected individuals being symptomatic at birth. Of those born without symptoms, 10 to 15% will progress to hearing loss or mental retardation (7, 16). CMV has been recognized as the leading infectious cause of fetal damage in the United States, Europe, and other developed areas of the world. For this reason, the Institute of Medicine in 1999 ranked the development of a CMV vaccine at the highest priority, based on the potential savings in economic costs, in years of life and disability, and in the human suffering that would be alleviated. Likewise, primary CMV infections in solid-organ transplant recipients carry the greatest risk of serious manifestations, and vaccination prior to transplantation may moderate the disease severity of subsequent infections.

Higher anti-CMV cell-mediated and humoral immune responses have been associated with a reduced risk of transmission to the fetus; however, the role of mucosal antibodies in protection is unknown. Circulating levels of anti-gB antibody have been shown to be inversely proportional to systemic viral load in HIV-infected patients (3), and high titers of glycoprotein-specific antibodies correlate with the absence of viral DNA in the blood of bone marrow transplant recipients (43). This suggests a role for antiglycoprotein antibodies in the prevention of CMV disease and in the modulation of its progression. However, for a vaccine, the relatively poor immunogenicity of CMV glycoproteins requires the addition of powerful adjuvants to purified gB proteins. Preliminary trials with one such mixture have shown promising results, but as many as four doses may be required to generate persistent neutralizing antibody responses.

Five types of candidate CMV vaccines have undergone preliminary trials in human subjects: (i) a classically attenuated CMV, (ii) a chimera between an attenuated CMV and wild-type virus, (iii) a nonreplicating canarypox vector with either a gB or pp65 antigen, (iv) recombinant envelope glycoprotein, and (v) a mixture of synthetic peptides including a T helper epitope and CD8+ T-cell epitopes (7). Other proposed vaccines include a DNA vaccine. Studies with live attenuated CMV Towne vaccine show that the majority of adult male, adult female, and pediatric recipients develop cell-mediated immune responses that persist for 6 months, as well as dose-dependent antibody titers comparable to those seen following natural infections. Importantly, seronegative recipients of seropositive kidneys who received this vaccine not only developed humoral and cellular immunity but also were protected from severe CMV disease. Combined-vaccine strategies have also been suggested, with recombinant canarypox live vaccine expressing CMV gB used to prime antibody responses prior to vaccination with the attenuated Towne vaccine (1). However, efficacy trials are still needed for those vaccines that have shown promise in phase I and II trials, and preliminary trials are still needed for the newer candidate vaccines.

Passive Humoral Immunotherapy

CMV immune globulin preparations have also been used in the prevention and treatment of CMV disease. Although results of clinical trials are variable, prophylactic CMV immune globulin appears overall to reduce the incidence of CMV disease and death in both bone marrow and solid-organ transplant recipients (46) and the incidence of acute GVHD in bone marrow transplant recipients (48). There have also been a number of encouraging studies with transplant recipients, using combinations of antiviral drugs and CMV immune globulin (34). In addition to reducing the incidence of CMV

disease, these combination therapies have also been shown to reduce the incidence or severity of CMV-exacerbated conditions, such as intimal thickening and coronary artery disease after cardiac transplantation (57), and fungal and parasitic superinfections following renal and liver transplantation (45). Unfortunately, however, the passive administration of anti-CMV antibodies postnatally is unlikely to modify the development or severity of congenital CMV sequelae (9).

Passive Cellular Immunotherapy

Adoptive immunotherapy has been proposed as an alternative to prophylactic treatments with antiviral drugs for the prevention of CMV disease in transplant recipients. Infusions of ex vivo-expanded CMV-specific, donor-derived CD8+ CTL clones and cell lines have been well tolerated, and they result in the in vivo expansion of CMV-specific CTLs. This immunotherapy is effective in reducing the incidence of CMV disease in high-risk bone marrow transplant recipients, although cytotoxic activity declines in patients who are deficient in CD4+ T helper cells (37, 56). An additional concern in this model is the choice of APCs. Autologous DCs are optimal in this regard, but they are difficult to obtain in large numbers. Nonhuman cell lines expressing a single HLA allele can also be effective APCs for generation of anti-CMV CTLs, but they are limited by single-allele specificity in the resulting effector T cells (36).

REFERENCES

1. Adler, S. P., S. A. Plotkin, E. Gonczol, M. Cadoz, C. Meric, J. B. Wang, P. Dellamonica, A. M. Best, J. Zahradnik, S. Pincus, K. Berencsi, W. I. Cox, and Z. Gyulai. 1999. A canarypox vector expressing cytomegalovirus (CMV) glycoprotein B primes for antibody responses to a live attenuated CMV vaccine (Towne). *J. Infect. Dis.* 180:843–846.
2. Adult AIDS Clinical Trials Group. 2005. Lymphoprolifer-ation assay protocol. *Immunology Consensus Protocols.* http://aactg.s-3.com/pub/download/labmanual/29-ALM-Lymphocyte-Proliferation-Assay.pdf.
3. Alberola, J., V. Dominguez, L. Cardenoso, J. Lopez-Aldeguer, M. Blanes, F. Estelles, C. Ricart, A. Pastor, R. Igual, and D. Navarro. 1998. Antibody response to human cytomegalovirus (HCMV) glycoprotein B (gB) in AIDS patients with HCMV end-organ disease. *J. Med. Virol.* 55:272–280.
4. Altman, J. D., P. A. Moss, P. J. Goulder, D. H. Barouch, M. G. Heyzer-Williams, J. I. Bell, A. J. McMichael, and M. M. Davis. 1996. Phenotypic analysis of antigen-specific T lymphocytes. *Science* 274:94–96.
5. Angulo, R., and D. A. Fulcher. 1998. Measurement of Candida-specific blastogenesis: comparison of carboxyfluorescein succinimidyl ester labelling of T cells, thymidine incorporation, and CD69 expression. *Cytometry* 34:143–151.
6. Appay, V., P. R. Dunbar, M. Callan, P. Klenerman, G. M. Gillespie, L. Papagno, G. S. Ogg, A. King, F. Lechner, C. A. Spina, S. Little, D. V. Havlir, D. D. Richman, N. Gruener, G. Pape, A. Waters, P. Easterbrook, M. Salio, V. Cerundolo, A. J. McMichael, and S. L. Rowland-Jones. 2002. Memory CD8+ T cells vary in differentiation phenotype in different persistent virus infections. *Nat. Med.* 8:379–385.
7. Arvin, A. M., P. Fast, M. Myers, S. Plotkin, and R. Rabinovich. 2004. Vaccine development to prevent cytomegalovirus disease: report from the National Vaccine Advisory Committee. *Clin. Infect. Dis.* 39:233–239.
8. Boeckh, M., and W. G. Nichols. 2003. Immunosuppressive effects of beta-herpesviruses. *Herpes* 1:12–16.
9. Boppana, S. B., J. Miller, and W. J. Britt. 1996. Transplacentally acquired antiviral antibodies and outcome

in congenital human cytomegalovirus infection. *Viral Immunol.* **9:**211–218.

10. Britt, W. J., L. Vugler, E. J. Butfiloski, and E. B. Stephens. 1990. Cell surface expression of human cytomegalovirus (HCMV) gp55-116 (gB): use of HCMV-recombinant vaccinia virus-infected cells in analysis of the human neutralizing antibody response. *J. Virol.* **64:**1079–1085.

11. Burrows, S. R., R. A. Elkington, J. J. Miles, K. J. Green, S. Walker, S. M. Haryana, D. J. Moss, H. Dunckley, J. M. Burrows, and R. Khanna. 2003. Promiscuous CTL recognition of viral epitopes on multiple human leukocyte antigens: biological validation of the proposed HLA A24 supertype. *J. Immunol.* **171:**1407–1412.

12. Caliendo, A. M., K. St. George, J. Allega, A. C. Bullotta, L. Gilbane, and C. R. Rinaldo. 2002. Distinguishing cytomegalovirus (CMV) infection and disease with CMV nucleic acid assays. *J. Clin. Microbiol.* **40:**1581–1586.

13. Chahroudi, A., G. Silvestri, and M. B. Feinberg. 2003. Measuring T cell-mediated cytotoxicity using fluorogenic caspase substrates. *Methods* **31:**120–126.

14. Chang, L., G. A. Gusewitch, D. B. Chritton, J. C. Folz, L. K. Lebeck, and S. L. Nehlsen-Cannarella. 1993. Rapid flow cytometric assay for the assessment of natural killer cell activity. *J. Immunol. Methods* **166:**45–54.

15. Cobb, B. A., Q. Wang, A. O. Tzianabos, and D. L. Kasper. 2004. Polysaccharide processing and presentation by the MHCII pathway. *Cell* **117:**677–687.

16. Collinet, P., D. Subtil, V. Houfflin-Debarge, N. Kacet, A. Dewilde, and F. Puech. 2004. Routine CMV screening during pregnancy. *Eur. J. Obstet. Gynecol. Reprod. Biol.* **114:**3–11.

17. De Clercq, E. 2004. Antiviral drugs in current clinical use. *J. Clin. Virol.* **30:**115–133.

18. Eggers, M., U. Bader, and G. Enders. 2000. Combination of microneutralization and avidity assays: improved diagnosis of recent primary human cytomegalovirus infection in single serum sample of second trimester pregnancy. *J. Med. Virol.* **60:**324–330.

19. Fortunato, E. A., A. K. McElroy, I. Sanchez, and D. H. Spector. 2000. Exploitation of cellular signaling and regulatory pathways by human cytomegalovirus. *Trends Microbiol.* **8:**111–119.

20. Fowler, K. B., S. Stagno, and R. F. Pass. 2003. Maternal immunity and prevention of congenital cytomegalovirus infection. *JAMA* **289:**1008–1011.

21. Gamadia, L. E., R. J. Rentenaar, P. A. Baars, E. B. Remmerswaal, S. Surachno, J. F. Weel, M. Toebes, T. N. Schumacher, I. J. Ten Berge, and R. A. van Lier. 2001. Differentiation of cytomegalovirus-specific CD8(+) T cells in healthy and immunosuppressed virus carriers. *Blood* **98:**754–761.

22. Gamadia, L. E., E. M. van Leeuwen, E. B. Remmerswaal, S. L. Yong, S. Surachno, P. M. Wertheim-van Dillen, I. J. Ten Berge, and R. A. van Lier. 2004. The size and phenotype of virus-specific T cell populations is determined by repetitive antigenic stimulation and environmental cytokines. *J. Immunol.* **172:**6107–6114.

23. Gaytant, M. A., E. A. Steegers, B. A. Semmekrot, H. M. Merkus, and J. M. Galama. 2002. Congenital cytomegalovirus infection: review of the epidemiology and outcome. *Obstet. Gynecol. Surv.* **57:**245–256.

24. Gilbert, C., J. Bestman-Smith, and G. Boivin. 2002. Resistance of herpesviruses to antiviral drugs: clinical impacts and molecular mechanisms. *Drug Resist. Update* **5:**88–114.

25. Grangeot-Keros, L., M. J. Mayaux, P. Lebon, F. Freymuth, G. Eugene, R. Stricker, and E. Dussaix. 1997. Value of cytomegalovirus (CMV) IgG avidity index for the diagnosis of primary CMV infection in pregnant women. *J. Infect. Dis.* **175:**944–946.

26. He, H., C. R. Rinaldo, Jr., and P. A. Morel. 1995. T cell proliferative responses to five human cytomegalovirus proteins in healthy seropositive individuals: implications for vaccine development. *J. Gen. Virol.* **76:**1603–1610.

27. Huang, X.-L., Z. Fan, C. Kalinyak, J. W. Mellors, and C. R. Rinaldo, Jr. 2000. CD8+ T-cell gamma interferon production specific for human immunodeficiency virus type 1 (HIV-1) in HIV-1-infected subjects. *Clin. Diagn. Lab. Immunol.* **7:**279–287.

28. Jin, X., M. A. Demoitie, S. M. Donahoe, G. S. Ogg, S. Bonhoeffer, W. M. Kakimoto, G. Gillespie, P. A. Moss, W. Dyer, M. G. Kurilla, S. R. Riddell, J. Downie, J. S. Sullivan, A. J. McMichael, C. Workman, and D. F. Nixon. 2000. High frequency of cytomegalovirus-specific cytotoxic T-effector cells in HLA-A*0201-positive subjects during multiple viral coinfections. *J. Infect. Dis.* **181:**165–175.

29. Kline, J. N., T. J. Waldschmidt, T. R. Businga, J. E. Lemish, J. V. Weinstock, P. S. Thorne, and A. M. Krieg. 1998. Modulation of airway inflammation by CpG oligodeoxynucleotides in a murine model of asthma. *J. Immunol.* **160:**2555–2559.

30. Lacey, S. F., D. J. Diamond, and J. A. Zaia. 2004. Assessment of cellular immunity to human cytomegalovirus in recipients of allogeneic stem cell transplants. *Biol. Blood Marrow Transplant.* **10:**433–447.

31. Lazzarotto, T., B. Guerra, P. Spezzacatena, S. Varani, L. Gabrielli, P. Pradelli, F. Rumpianesi, C. Banzi, L. Bovicelli, and M. P. Landini. 1998. Prenatal diagnosis of congenital cytomegalovirus infection. *J. Clin. Microbiol.* **36:**3540–3544.

32. Lazzarotto, T., S. Varani, P. Spezzacatena, P. Pradelli, L. Potena, A. Lombardi, V. Ghisetti, L. Gabrielli, D. A. Abate, C. Magelli, and M. P. Landini. 1998. Delayed acquisition of high-avidity anti-cytomegalovirus antibody is correlated with prolonged antigenemia in solid organ transplant recipients. *J. Infect. Dis.* **178:**1145–1149.

33. Lore, K., M. R. Betts, J. M. Brenchley, J. Kuruppu, S. Khojasteh, S. Perfetto, M. Roederer, R. A. Seder, and R. A. Koup. 2003. Toll-like receptor ligands modulate dendritic cells to augment cytomegalovirus- and HIV-1-specific T cell responses. *J. Immunol.* **171:**4320–4328.

34. Nicol, D. L., A. S. MacDonald, P. Belitsky, S. Lee, A. D. Cohen, H. Bitter-Suermann, J. Lowen, and A. Whalen. 1993. Reduction by combination prophylactic therapy with CMV hyperimmune globulin and acyclovir of the risk of primary CMV disease in renal transplant recipients. *Transplantation* **55:**841–846.

35. Nokta, M. A., M. I. Hassan, K. Loesch, and R. B. Pollard. 1996. Human cytomegalovirus-induced immunosuppression. Relationship to tumor necrosis factor-dependent release of arachidonic acid and prostaglandin E2 in human monocytes. *J. Clin. Investig.* **97:**2635–2641.

36. Papanicolaou, G. A., J. B. Latouche, C. Tan, J. Dupont, J. Stiles, E. G. Pamer, and M. Sadelain. 2003. Rapid expansion of cytomegalovirus-specific cytotoxic T lymphocytes by artificial antigen-presenting cells expressing a single HLA allele. *Blood* **102:**2498–2505.

37. Peggs, K. S., S. Verfuerth, A. Pizzey, N. Khan, M. Guiver, P. A. Moss, and S. Mackinnon. 2003. Adoptive cellular therapy for early cytomegalovirus infection after allogeneic stem-cell transplantation with virus-specific T-cell lines. *Lancet* **362:**1375–1377.

38. Quinnan, G. V., Jr., N. Kirmani, A. H. Rook, J. F. Manischewitz, L. Jackson, G. Moreschi, G. W. Santos, R. Saral, and W. H. Burns. 1982. Cytotoxic T cells in cytomegalovirus infection: HLA-restricted T-lymphocyte and non-T-lymphocyte cytotoxic responses correlate with recovery from cytomegalovirus infection in bone-marrow-transplant recipients. *N. Engl. J. Med.* **307:**7–13.

39. Rinaldo, C. R., Jr., W. P. Carney, B. S. Richter, P. H. Black, and M. S. Hirsch. 1980. Mechanisms of immunosuppression in cytomegaloviral mononucleosis. *J. Infect. Dis.* **141:**488–495.

40. Rinaldo, C. R., Jr., X.-L. Huang, Z. Fan, J. B. Margolick, L. Borowski, A. Hoji, C. Kalinyak, D. K. McMahon, S. A. Riddler, W. H. Hildebrand, R. B. Day, and J. W. Mellors. 2000. Anti-human immunodeficiency virus type 1 (HIV-1) CD8+ T-lymphocyte reactivity during combination antiretroviral therapy in HIV-1-infected patients with advanced immunodeficiency. *J. Virol.* **74:**4127–4138.

41. Sallusto, F., D. Lenig, R. Forster, M. Lipp, and A. Lanzavecchia. 1999. Two subsets of memory T lymphocytes with distinct homing potentials and effector functions. *Nature* **401:**708–712.

42. Schoppel, K., E. Hassfurther, W. Britt, M. Ohlin, C. A. Borrebaeck, and M. Mach. 1996. Antibodies specific for the antigenic domain 1 of glycoprotein B (gpUL55) of human cytomegalovirus bind to different substructures. *Virology* **216:**133–145.

43. Schoppel, K., C. Schmidt, H. Einsele, H. Hebart, and M. Mach. 1998. Kinetics of the antibody response against human cytomegalovirus-specific proteins in allogeneic bone marrow transplant recipients. *J. Infect. Dis.* **178:**1233–1243.

44. Slobedman, B., and E. S. Mocarski. 1999. Quantitative analysis of latent human cytomegalovirus. *J. Virol.* **73:**4806–4812.

45. Snydman, D. R. 2001. Historical overview of the use of cytomegalovirus hyperimmune globulin in organ transplantation. *Transplant. Infect. Dis.* **3**(Suppl. 2):6–13.

46. Snydman, D. R., B. G. Werner, B. Heinze-Lacey, V. P. Berardi, N. L. Tilney, R. L. Kirkman, E. L. Milford, S. I. Cho, H. L. Bush, Jr., A. S. Levey, et al. 1987. Use of cytomegalovirus immune globulin to prevent cytomegalovirus disease in renal-transplant recipients. *N. Engl. J. Med.* **317:**1049–1054.

47. Soderberg, C., S. Larsson, B. L. Rozell, S. Sumitran-Karuppan, P. Ljungman, and E. Moller. 1996. Cytomegalovirus-induced CD13-specific autoimmunity—a possible cause of chronic graft-vs-host disease. *Transplantation* **61:**600–609.

48. Sokos, D. R., M. Berger, and H. M. Lazarus. 2002. Intravenous immunoglobulin: appropriate indications and uses in hematopoietic stem cell transplantation. *Biol. Blood Marrow Transplant.* **8:**117–130.

49. Springer, K. L., and A. Weinberg. 2004. Cytomegalovirus infection in the era of HAART: fewer reactivations and more immunity. *J. Antimicrob. Chemother.* **54:**582–586.

50. St. George, K., and C. R. Rinaldo, Jr. 1999. Comparison of cytomegalovirus antigenemia and culture assays in patients on and off antiviral therapy. *J. Med. Virol.* **59:**91–97.

51. St. George, K., D. T. Rowe, and C. R. Rinaldo, Jr. 2000. Cytomegalovirus, varicella zoster virus and Epstein-Barr virus, p. 410–449. *In* S. C. Specter (ed.), *Clinical Virology Manual*, 3rd ed. ASM Press, Washington, D.C.

52. Trivedi, D., R. Y. Williams, R. J. O'Reilly, and G. Koehne. 2005. Generation of CMV-specific T lymphocytes using protein-spanning pools of pp65-derived overlapping pentadecapeptides for adoptive immunotherapy. *Blood* **105:**2793–2801.

53. Utz, U., W. Britt, L. Vugler, and M. Mach. 1989. Identification of a neutralizing epitope on glycoprotein gp58 of human cytomegalovirus. *J. Virol.* **63:**1995–2001.

54. Varnum, S. M., D. N. Streblow, M. E. Monroe, P. Smith, K. J. Auberry, L. Pasa-Tolic, D. Wang, D. G. Camp, K. Rodland, S. Wiley, W. Britt, T. Shenk, R. D. Smith, and J. A. Nelson. 2004. Identification of proteins in human cytomegalovirus (HCMV) particles: the HCMV proteome. *J. Virol.* **78:**10960–10966.

55. Waldrop, S. L., C. J. Pitcher, D. M. Peterson, V. C. Maino, and L. J. Picker. 1997. Determination of antigen-specific memory/effector CD4+ T cell frequencies by flow cytometry: evidence for a novel, antigen-specific homeostatic mechanism in HIV-associated immunodeficiency. *J. Clin. Investig.* **99:**1739–1750.

56. Walter, E. A., P. D. Greenberg, M. J. Gilbert, R. J. Finch, K. S. Watanabe, E. D. Thomas, and S. R. Riddell. 1995. Reconstitution of cellular immunity against cytomegalovirus in recipients of allogeneic bone marrow by transfer of T-cell clones from the donor. *N. Engl. J. Med.* **333:**1038–1044.

57. Weill, D. 2001. Role of cytomegalovirus in cardiac allograft vasculopathy. *Transplant. Infect. Dis.* **3**(Suppl. 2):44–48.

Human Herpesviruses 6, 7, and 8

RICHARD L. HODINKA

74

Herpesviruses 6, 7, and 8 are the most recently described members of the human herpesvirus family (Table 1). Like other herpesviruses, they have the ability to establish a latent or persistent infection following primary infection, and reactivation may occur in healthy and immunocompromised people in response to different stimuli. A variety of methods are available or under development for the laboratory diagnosis of each virus, including viral isolation in cell culture, demonstration of viral antigens or nucleic acids in body fluids or tissues, and serology for detection of virus-specific antibodies. This chapter focuses on the immunologic and molecular diagnosis and monitoring of infections with human herpesvirus 6 (HHV-6), HHV-7, and HHV-8 and provides information on the unique features of the epidemiology and biological and clinical characteristics of these viruses.

HHV-6

Introduction

HHV-6 is a lymphotropic virus which was discovered in 1986 in cultures of lymphocytes from patients with lymphoproliferative disorders and AIDS. Since that time, much has been learned about the biology, epidemiology, clinical features, and diagnosis of HHV-6, and a number of comprehensive reviews have been published (see references 4, 9, and 14 for examples of reviews).

HHV-6 is similar in morphology to other known human herpesviruses but is genetically and serologically distinct. The completed virion has a diameter of 160 to 200 nm and consists of an internal core containing double-stranded DNA of approximately 160 to 170 kb and an icosahedral nucleocapsid surrounded by a tegument and a protein-spiked envelope. The virus has a primary cell tropism for mature CD4$^+$ T lymphocytes but also infects CD8$^+$ T cells, natural killer (NK) cells, monocytes, macrophages, megakaryocytes, epithelial cells, endothelial cells, fibroblasts, and neural cells. CD46 has been identified as part of the cellular receptor for infection; this marker is expressed on the surfaces of many human cell types, leading to the broad cellular tropism of HHV-6. Viral replication occurs in the nucleus of the host cell, and the viral envelope is acquired during maturation within cytoplasmic vacuoles before budding of the completed virus from the host cell membrane.

The DNA genome of HHV-6 differs from that of other human herpesviruses by both restriction mapping and nucleic acid hybridization and is unique in that it has a significantly lower guanine-plus-cytosine content, 43 to 44%. Regions of sequence homology between HHV-6 and cytomegalovirus (CMV) have been identified, and HHV-6 is now classified with CMV among the betaherpesviruses. Genetic polymorphism among different isolates of HHV-6 exists, and evidence suggests that HHV-6 isolates form two distinct but very closely related groups (variants A and B) that differ in molecular, biological, and clinical properties. Most isolates of HHV-6 from patients with symptomatic primary infections have been of variant B. Variant A has been isolated or detected only rarely in children with primary HHV-6 infection, with the exception of African children with febrile illnesses. Both variants have been isolated from immunocompromised individuals, including AIDS patients, transplant recipients, and patients with leukemia; dual infections with both variants also have been described. Variant A is seen more frequently in patients with human immunodeficiency virus (HIV) infection, and it may be more neurotropic than variant B. Otherwise, an etiologic role for variant A in causing disease has not been clearly identified.

The HHV-6 genome has a coding capacity of approximately 80 to 100 proteins, although there has been little agreement about the actual number, size, and abundance of virus-specific proteins. More than 30 polypeptides ranging in size from 30 to 220 kDa, including six or seven glycoproteins, have been identified. A 101-kDa nucleocapsid protein was found to be highly reactive with human sera by Western immunoblotting and appears to be a specific marker for HHV-6 infection. A set of five monoclonal antibodies has been developed and used to identify nine proteins designated gp105 and gp82; gp116, gp64, and gp54; gp102; p41 and p110; and p135.

Similar to cases of CMV and Epstein-Barr virus (EBV) infection, infections with HHV-6 are common and often mild or inapparent; however, HHV-6 is now recognized as the causative agent of roseola (roseola infantum, exanthem subitum, sixth disease) in children aged 6 months to 3 years. The disease presents with an abrupt onset of fever (39 to 40°C) for 3 to 5 days, followed by the appearance of an erythematous, blanching, maculopapular, nonpruritic rash beginning on the face or trunk and spreading to other areas. The rash usually lasts for 1 to 3 days, and there is no subsequent

TABLE 1　Characteristics of HHV-6, HHV-7, and HHV-8

Characteristic	HHV-6	HHV-7	HHV-8
Family _Herpesviridae_			
Subfamily	Beta	Beta	Gamma
Genus	_Roseolovirus_	_Roseolovirus_	_Rhadinovirus_
Biological properties			
Genome (linear double-stranded DNA)	~159 kb; encodes 80–100 proteins	~145 kb; encodes at least 70 proteins	~165 kb; 97 genes identified
DNA relatedness (% homology)	CMV (66%)	HHV-6 (50–60%)	Herpesvirus saimiri (51%), EBV (39%)
Variants	HHV-6A, HHV-6B	Unknown	HHV-8 strains A, B, and C
Cell tropism in vitro	CD4+ T lymphocytes, NK cells, macrophages, CD8+T cells, megakaryocytes, neural and epithelial cells	CD4+ T lymphocytes	CD19+ B lymphocytes, spindle cells, endothelial cells
Virus interactions	EBV, CMV, HIV, parvovirus B19, human papillomaviruses	HHV-6, CMV, HIV	EBV, HIV
Epidemiology			
Distribution	Worldwide	Worldwide	Worldwide
Natural host	Human	Human	Human
Transmission	Oral secretions (HHV-6B only); possibly blood and urine; intrauterine and perinatal transmission suggested	Oral secretions; possibly blood and urine	Predominantly sexual contact; possibly oral secretions and blood; transplanted allograft
Seroprevalence	90% or greater	80–90%	0–25% in healthy American and European blood donors; higher in some African and Mediterranean populations; 75–95% of KS patients
Populations affected	Infants (0–3 yr), organ transplant recipients	Infants (1–5 yr)	Homosexual or bisexual HIV+ males or their sexual partners; Mediterranean males; Africans; organ transplant recipients
Incubation period	9–10 days	Unknown	Unknown
Attributable clinical illnesses	Exanthem subitum, infantile febrile illnesses, infectious mononucleosis-like illness in adults, malignancies, posttransplantation and central nervous system diseases, disseminated infections in AIDS	Exanthem subitum, infantile febrile illnesses, pityriasis rosea (?)	KS, primary effusion lymphomas, Castleman disease

desquamation or pigment changes. Recovery is usually rapid and without complications. Interestingly, most cases of acute primary HHV-6 infection in young children do not result in an illness recognizable as roseola. Studies have revealed that acute viremic HHV-6 infection accounts for 14% of febrile children younger than 2 years seen in an emergency room, most of whom have a nonspecific febrile illness without a rash. Other clinical manifestations of primary infection include rash without fever, intussusception, bulging of the anterior fontanelle, lymphadenopathy, hepatitis, an infectious mononucleosis-like syndrome, inflamed tympanic membranes, aseptic meningitis, meningoencephalitis, and encephalitis. Febrile seizures are a common complication of roseola; approximately one-third of all febrile seizures in childhood have been attributed to HHV-6 infection. Primary infection in adults is rare but may result in prolonged lymphadenopathy, hepatitis, or an illness resembling infectious

mononucleosis. Reactivated infection in healthy persons is asymptomatic. It remains to be established whether HHV-6 causes or contributes to disease in immunocompromised hosts, although reactivation in organ recipients following kidney, liver, bone marrow, or heart transplantation has been associated with isolated fever, hepatitis, leukopenia, delayed engraftment, neurologic dysfunction, skin rashes resembling graft-versus-host disease, bone marrow suppression, and interstitial pneumonitis (see references 7 and 10 for reviews). Evidence suggests that HHV-6 infection may contribute to disease progression with HIV type 1 (HIV-1) and may interact with other viruses, such as CMV, EBV, parvovirus B19, and human papillomaviruses, to affect their behavior and exacerbate disease. HHV-6 has also been associated with a number of other diseases in patients in whom elevated titers of HHV-6 antibody have been detected and from whom replicating virus was isolated and/or viral antigens or DNA was found. The role of the virus in most of these clinical settings, however, remains unproven and controversial.

HHV-6 is a ubiquitous virus, and humans are the only known natural host. The mode of transmission of the virus is poorly understood but presumably requires direct, personal contact. Virus has been identified in saliva, peripheral blood mononuclear cells (PBMC), cervical and vaginal secretions, urine, and various tissues, including skin, lymph nodes, liver, spleen, heart, lungs, kidneys, and brain. HHV-6B, but not HHV-6A, actively replicates in the salivary glands of children and adults, making oral secretions the most likely source of transmission for this variant. Intrauterine or perinatal transmission has been suggested. Congenital infections with HHV-6 have been described to occur in 1% of births; infected infants are asymptomatic at birth, in contrast to the acute febrile illnesses observed with primary postnatal infection (14). In this study, variant A was responsible for one-third of the congenital infections, whereas variant B was observed in all postnatal infections. The incidence of antibody to HHV-6 is high throughout the world, although variation in seroprevalence based on age and the serologic method employed has been reported. Newborn infants have titers of antibody to HHV-6 that are comparable to those in adults, suggesting passive transfer of transplacental maternal antibodies. With the loss of maternal antibody, the seroprevalence to HHV-6 decreases significantly by 4 to 6 months of age but subsequently rises to 90% at the end of the first year of life. By 3 years of age, almost 100% of individuals have antibody to HHV-6; immunity is maintained throughout childhood, adolescence, and early adulthood but may decline after 40 years of age and then rise to high titers following increased rates of reactivation in elderly persons. With the exception of HHV-7, no significant serologic cross-reactivity between different herpesviruses and HHV-6 has been detected.

Immunology of HHV-6 Infection

The host response to HHV-6 infection is thought to involve both humoral and cell-mediated immunity. Children with exanthem subitum develop an immunoglobulin M (IgM) response on day 4 of illness, and the response peaks between 7 and 14 days and declines over a period of 1 to 2 months. In addition, IgM antibodies to HHV-6 can persist for extended periods after a primary infection and can reappear in reactivated infections. IgG appears on day 7 of illness, peaks at approximately 4 weeks, and persists for long periods.

The role of cell-mediated immunity in HHV-6 infections is less well defined. However, the virus appears to have the ability to modulate or alter the expression of a number of cytokines and immune activation molecules. Increased levels of alpha interferon (IFN-α) have been found during the febrile phase of exanthem subitum, while an increase in NK cell activity has been observed during the exanthem period. In vitro infection of PBMC with HHV-6 decreases the expression of interleukin 2 (IL-2) and cell proliferation, upregulates NK cell cytotoxicity, and induces the synthesis of the soluble cytokines IFN-γ, IL-1β, tumor necrosis factor alpha, and IL-15. The virus can downregulate CD3, CD46, and CXCR4 expression and upregulate the chemokine receptor CCR7 in infected T cells and can stimulate IL-10 and IL-12 expression in monocytes and macrophages. Also, HHV-6 infection of transformed T-cell lines in vitro results in an enhanced susceptibility to apoptosis. The significance of these immunomodulating properties to the interaction of infected T cells with other components of the immune system and to the pathogenesis of the virus is unclear. Macrophages are infected with HHV-6 following primary

infection and may serve as a reservoir for reactivation of the virus.

Clinical Indications

Although a diagnosis of exanthem subitum in a child can be made on the basis of clinical presentation alone, laboratory confirmation is needed to detect atypical and more severe manifestations of HHV-6 infection and to more clearly define the role of HHV-6 in other childhood illnesses and in diseases of adults and immunocompromised persons.

Immunologic Diagnosis

Antigen Detection

Immunohistochemistry

Monoclonal antibodies suitable for the direct detection of HHV-6 antigens by immunofluorescence have been developed and employed with tissue samples (4). HHV-6 antigen has been demonstrated in biopsy material from allografts of kidney transplant patients, lung tissue from bone marrow transplant recipients with interstitial pneumonitis, cervical lymph nodes of patients with histiocytic necrotizing lymphadenitis and lymphoma, oligodendrocytes from patients with multiple sclerosis, abortive villous tissues from spontaneous abortions, patients with AIDS, and the salivary and bronchial glands of latently infected individuals. Productive infection of tissues with HHV-6 can be detecting by using monoclonal antibodies reactive against the structural protein p101 of variant B and the structural protein gp82 of variant A. Recently, an HHV-6 antigenemia assay similar to that described for detecting CMV has been developed to monitor active HHV-6 infection in liver and allogeneic stem cell transplant recipients (19, 34). This immunohistochemical method involves the cytocentrifugation of purified PBMC onto microscope slides followed by the detection of HHV-6-specific early and structural antigens by monoclonal antibodies and indirect immunoperoxidase staining. The significance of the results from immunohistochemical testing is still unclear, and the results must be further validated and correlated with clinical findings and data obtained from other laboratory tests.

EIA

A commercial antigen capture enzyme immunoassay (EIA) has been developed for the detection of HHV-6 antigens directly from clinical specimens (21). The assay is based on the gp116-gp64-gp54 antigen and is specific for HHV-6 variants A and B. The EIA has a sensitivity similar to that of viral culture from plasma obtained from children with exanthem subitum. Additional studies are needed to determine the utility of this EIA for rapid diagnosis of HHV-6 infection and for monitoring of HHV-6 activity in the immunocompromised host. The EIA has the advantages of being relatively simple and inexpensive to perform relative to culture or nucleic acid detection methods.

Viral Identification in Conventional Cell Culture

HHV-6 can be isolated from PBMC grown in primary culture or by cocultivation of these cells with stimulated cord blood cells (CBC) or donor PBMC (17). Saliva and other body fluids and tissues can be cocultured with activated donor cells for isolation of the virus as well. The optimal time for collection of specimens from children with roseola is during the febrile phase, before the development of rash. Infected PBMC show a specific cytopathic effect, with intracytoplasmic and intranuclear inclusion bodies appearing within 7 to 10 days. The cytopathic effect on primary isolation can be subtle and difficult to recognize, and virus production from infected cells should be confirmed by detection of viral antigens, in situ hybridization, or electron microscopy. Viral antigens can be detected by indirect immunofluorescence assay (IFA), anti-complement immunofluorescence (ACIF), or EIA with commercially available reagents or kits. IFA staining reveals a characteristic granular nuclear and cytoplasmic fluorescence in infected cells. The sensitivity and specificity of immunologic reagents for confirmation of viral growth have not been extensively studied, and it is recommended that appropriate antigen and antibody controls be used when attempting to identify infected cells. HHV-6 infects a number of established continuous T-cell lines, most notably HSB-2, MOLT-3, Sup-T1, J-Jhan, MT-4, and ET62, which are used mainly to grow virus following primary isolation. The two variants can be differentiated in culture by their growth in different cell lines; variant B strains of HHV-6 do not replicate in HSB-2 cells, and variant A strains do not replicate in MOLT-3 cells. The described culture methods are slow and labor-intensive and require a high level of technical expertise. Their routine use in clinical laboratories is limited.

Spin Amplification Shell Vial Assay

The human diploid lung fibroblast line MRC-5 has been reported to support primary virus isolation and has been used in a centrifugation-assisted shell vial amplification assay for the detection of the immediate-early antigen of HHV-6 from PBMC of patients (29). Panspecific polyclonal and monoclonal antibodies to the immediate-early antigen of variants A and B of HHV-6 and monoclonal antibodies specific to either variant A or B are commercially available; they stain the nucleus of infected MRC-5 cells as early as 12 h after infection and give maximum staining within 48 to 72 h of infection. In the assay, PBMC are obtained from heparinized whole blood by Ficoll-Hypaque density gradient centrifugation, washed once with Hanks' balanced salt solution, and resuspended in 1 ml of RPMI 1640 medium supplemented with 10% fetal bovine serum, 20 mM HEPES, and 2 µg of Polybrene per ml. MRC-5 cells are grown to confluency on 12-mm-diameter round coverslips in 1-dram (3.7-ml) vials and inoculated with 0.5 ml of specimen to each of two vials. After inoculation, the vials are centrifuged at $800 \times g$ for 45 min at 25°C, and then 1.5 ml of RPMI 1640 medium is added as described above. The cultures are incubated at 37°C for 48 to 72 h, fixed in cold (−20°C) acetone for 10 min, and stained by IFA. Uninfected and HHV-6-infected monolayers are included as negative and positive controls, respectively. The monolayers are counterstained with Evans blue. Coverslips are scanned at magnifications of ×200 to ×250 with a fluorescence microscope, and specific staining is confirmed at ×400 to ×630. Staining of immediate-early antigen occurs in the nucleus of an infected fibroblast and appears as a speckled or an even matte green fluorescence. The spin amplification shell vial assay has the important features of being more rapid and less labor-intensive than conventional culture, but the sensitivity and specificity of this assay remain to be defined. This test is currently not offered as a routine service in most clinical virology laboratories.

In general, positive culture results are most useful to diagnose primary infection but can be difficult to interpret for immunocompromised hosts and during reactivation of the virus, when the presence of the virus may be unrelated to the clinical presentation.

Antibody Detection

A number of tests have been developed for the serodiagnosis of HHV-6 infection, of which IFA, ACIF, EIA, and the neutralization (NT) test have been most commonly employed (see references 4 and 17 for reviews). The method that is chosen depends on the volume of specimens, turnaround time, cost, equipment needs, ease of performance, reagent availability, and levels of assay sensitivity and specificity. Overall, variation in the rates of seropositivity for HHV-6 appears to be related to the assay systems and the need for standardization of methods and reagents. The use of different cutoff values and serum dilutions and the method of preparing antigen substrates for individual assays can have a marked effect on the percentage of serum specimens that are determined to be positive for antibody to HHV-6. Overall, higher rates of seropositivity are observed when either NT or EIA is used than when the less sensitive method of IFA is used.

Collection and Storage of Specimens

Serum is the specimen of choice for most serologic assays, although plasma can normally be used as well. A total of 1 to 2 ml of serum should be collected from clotted blood. The serum should be refrigerated at 4°C shortly after collection and during transport to the laboratory. If an extended delay in transport or testing of a specimen is anticipated, the specimen should be frozen to at least −20°C. Freeze-thawing of specimens that have been frozen should be avoided. A single serum specimen is required to determine the immune status of an individual or to detect IgM-specific antibody. Paired serum specimens, collected 2 to 3 weeks apart, are required for the diagnosis of a current or recent HHV-6 infection when specimens for IgG antibody are examined. The acute-phase serum should be obtained as soon as possible after the onset of illness. The most useful results are obtained by submitting acute- and convalescent-phase sera together to be tested simultaneously.

Methods

IFA

The IFA is the most widely used method for detecting antibodies to HHV-6. Initially, IFAs were found to be both insensitive and nonspecific, in part because of the use of infected CBC as a source of antigen but also because of variations in the criteria used for positive results. With the preparation of HHV-6 antigen in continuous T-cell lines, such as HSB-2, MOLT-4, and J-Jhan, and following improvements in the definition of seropositivity, IFAs have become increasingly more sensitive and reliable.

In the IFA, HHV-6-infected cells are spotted onto wells of Teflon-coated slides, allowed to air dry completely, and then fixed in cold (−20°C) acetone for 10 min. Fixed slides can be used immediately or stored at 4°C for short periods or at −20 to −70°C for extended times. Serial dilutions of patient and positive and negative control sera are added to individual wells, and the slides are incubated at 37°C for 30 min in a humidified chamber. The slides are then washed two or three times in phosphate-buffered saline (PBS), and an appropriate dilution of fluorescein-labeled anti-human IgG or IgM is added to each well. The slides are again incubated at 37°C for 30 min in a humidified chamber, washed two or three times in PBS, counterstained with Evans blue, and air dried. Coverslips are mounted in buffered glycerol (pH 8.0), and the slides are examined at magnifications of ×200 to ×400 under a fluorescence microscope. The presence of HHV-6 antibodies in the serum is determined by the observation of positive fluorescence within infected cells. Antigen substrate slides can be purchased commercially, and some manufacturers provide kits that contain all the necessary reagents for staining, including diluted conjugated antibody, wash buffer, mounting fluid, control sera, and substrate slides. When testing for HHV-6-specific IgM antibodies, serum samples should be appropriately treated before the test, to decrease the incidence of false-positive results due to interfering rheumatoid factor or false-negative results caused by high levels of specific IgG antibodies blocking the binding of IgM to HHV-6 antigen.

ACIF

The ACIF test is an immunofluorescence assay that has been developed to reduce the nonspecific fluorescence observed when CBC are used in the IFA. It also has the added advantage of enhancing the fluorescent signal from positive cells. As with IFA, HHV-6-infected cells are spotted onto wells of Teflon-coated slides, allowed to air dry completely, and then fixed in cold ($-20°$C) acetone for 10 min. Sera are heat inactivated at $56°$C for 30 min, and serial dilutions are added to individual wells. The slides are incubated at $37°$C for 30 min in a humidified chamber and then washed two or three times in PBS. HHV-6-specific antibody bound to the infected cells is detected by incubating the slides with a source of complement at $37°$C for 30 min in a humidified chamber, washing the slides in PBS, and then incubating the slides with fluorescein-conjugated anticomplement antibodies for a final 30 min at $37°$C. The slides are washed, counterstained, air dried, mounted in buffered glycerol (pH 8.0), and examined at magnifications of $\times200$ to $\times400$ under a fluorescence microscope. The presence of nuclear and cytoplasmic fluorescence within infected cells indicates positivity for antibodies to HHV-6.

EIA

EIAs for the determination of HHV-6 antibodies have been developed. HHV-6-infected and uninfected HSB-2 cells are harvested by centrifugation and disrupted by one of several methods, such as sonication in glycine buffer (pH 9.5) for 30 s, solubilization in Tris-Triton X-100 buffer, or cycles of freezing and thawing. Polystyrene 96-well microtiter plates are then coated with optimal dilutions of antigen by overnight adsorption of the antigen at $4°$C. Coated plates can be stored at $-20°$C for extended periods. Prior to use, the plates are washed three times in PBS–0.05% Tween 20 and the wells are blocked for 30 min with PBS containing 1% bovine serum albumin. Diluted patient serum and controls are added to antigen wells of infected and uninfected cells, and the plates are incubated for 1 h at $37°$C. The plates are then washed three times with PBS-Tween 20, and bound antibody is detected by reaction with an enzyme-conjugated anti-human IgG or IgM antibody at $37°$C for 1 h. After washing is performed as described above, a substrate is added, and the plates are incubated for 30 to 45 min at room temperature. Following color development, the reaction is stopped and the absorbance of each well is read with a spectrophotometer. The results are calculated by subtracting the absorbance in wells containing uninfected cell antigen from the absorbance in wells containing infected cell antigen. The main advantages of the EIA are that it is rapid and more sensitive than the IFA and the results can be evaluated in an objective manner. In addition, the EIA is applicable to large numbers of specimens, and the potential for automation is excellent. Kits that detect HHV-6 IgG and IgM antibodies are now commercially available, although the performance of these reagents has not been fully examined. A μ-capture EIA has recently been developed to enhance the specificity for the detection of HHV-6-specific IgM antibody in human sera (22).

NT Assay

Neutralizing antibodies to HHV-6 are determined in the NT assay by mixing serial twofold dilutions of patient sera in microtiter plates with an equal volume of cell-free virus containing $10^{2.5}$ 50% tissue culture infective doses per 0.1 ml. After 1 h of incubation at $37°$C, 2×10^5 HSB-2 or MOLT-4 cells or CBC are added to each well, and the cultures are maintained for 7 days at $37°$C. The antibody titer is determined as the reciprocal of the highest dilution of serum that completely prohibits the observation of viral cytopathic effect or the detection of antigen by IFA. The NT assay has a sensitivity and a specificity that are comparable to those of EIA, but the method is cumbersome, labor-intensive, and less suited to a routine diagnostic laboratory.

Antibody Avidity Assay

An indirect immunofluorescence antibody avidity test has been used to distinguish primary from past infections with HHV-6 (35). Since the binding of an antibody increases with time after exposure to an antigen, a primary antibody response to HHV-6 infection would be of much lower avidity than an antibody response that had occurred in the more distant past or following viral reactivation. By using urea to denature proteins in serum samples treated prior to performing the immunofluorescence assay, low-avidity antibody-antigen reactions are preferentially disrupted and differentiated from high-avidity antibody-antigen reactions. This test has been successfully used to diagnose primary HHV-6 infection in children with rashes and to distinguish primary from secondary antibody responses in solid-organ transplant recipients.

Other Serologic Tests

Western immunoblots and radioimmunoprecipitation are other serologic assays that are used to measure antibody to HHV-6. These assays have been used mainly to identify and analyze the role of specific proteins in the immune response to HHV-6.

Molecular Diagnosis

The diagnosis of HHV-6 infection is increasingly being made by the amplification of viral DNA by PCR. Many in-house and some commercial qualitative assays have been developed, and the sensitivity and specificity of PCR for diagnosis of active HHV-6 infection are being evaluated. Multiplex conventional and real-time PCR assays for the simultaneous detection and differentiation of HHV-6 variants A and B and HHV-7 also have been described (16, 25). Amplification has been performed with a number of different primer pairs, including those from the immediate-early antigen 1 and 2, large tegument protein (U31), DNA polymerase, U22, U65-U66, and U67 regions of the HHV-6 genome. PCR has been used successfully to detect HHV-6 DNA in a variety of clinical specimens from solid-organ and bone marrow transplant recipients; children with roseola, acute febrile illnesses, encephalitis, and other clinical manifestations of primary HHV-6 infection; AIDS patients; and individuals with less common forms of HHV-6 infection. However, qualitative PCR for HHV-6 diagnosis cannot reliably distinguish between active disease and asymptomatic infection or latency, and HHV-6 DNA can often be detected in saliva and, to a lesser extent, in blood of healthy individuals. Measuring the level of HHV-6 DNA appears to be necessary to predict and diagnose HHV-6 disease, particularly in immunocompromised individuals such as transplant recipients with illnesses that may be associated with reactivation of the virus or that are possibly caused by another pathogen. Consequently, conventional (28) and real-time (13) quantitative PCR assays have been developed and used to monitor the levels of HHV-6 DNA in a variety of different body fluids and tissues of both healthy subjects and selected patient populations. Similar to the diagnostic paradigm for CMV, these assays may be useful to associate HHV-6 infection with disease, to predict and monitor disease progression, to assess the efficacy of antiviral drugs, and to facilitate our understanding of the natural history and pathogenesis of this virus. As with CMV, viremia is considered to be the best predictor of disease, and quantitative measures of HHV-6 DNA in PBMC, plasma, or serum have proven useful for the continued surveillance and management of transplant recipients. When testing transplant recipients, it is more important to monitor the relative changes in DNA levels from serial blood specimens collected over time, since absolute HHV-6 DNA levels or breakpoints for symptomatic disease have not been determined. It may also be important to monitor both plasma and PBMC fractions of blood, since it has been reported that both HHV-6 variants A and B are detected in plasma but only variant B can be found in PBMC of patients after bone marrow transplantation (23).

Reverse transcriptase PCR assays that qualitatively amplify specific HHV-6 mRNA transcripts that are expressed only during active infection have been used as a substitute for quantitative assays to assist in identifying patients at greatest risk for developing symptomatic infection (33). Alternatively, qualitative detection of HHV-6 in cell-free specimens such as serum or plasma can be diagnostically useful in supporting a causal relationship between active HHV-6 infection and disease (27).

Qualitative and Quantitative Real-Time TaqMan PCR

For the detection and quantitation of HHV-6 DNA by real-time TaqMan PCR in my laboratory, a total of 4 to 7 ml of EDTA-anticoagulated whole blood is collected. Leukocytes are isolated from 2.0 ml of whole blood using 6.0 ml of Puregene red blood cell lysis solution (Gentra Systems, Minneapolis, Minn.). The white blood cells are then pelleted by centrifugation for 2 min at $2,000 \times g$, washed once in 15 ml of PBS without Ca^{2+} or Mg^{2+}, and resuspended in 2.0 ml of PBS. The cells are counted using a hemocytometer, and the concentration of cells is adjusted to 2.0×10^6 cells/ml by dilution in PBS. The remainder of the whole blood is centrifuged at $500 \times g$ for 10 min to obtain plasma. Single-use aliquots of 250 μl of either cells or plasma are stored at $-70°C$.

The MagNA Pure LC instrument (Roche Diagnostics, Indianapolis, Ind.) and Total Nucleic Acid Isolation Kit (Roche Diagnostics) are used for the automated extraction and isolation of HHV-6 DNA from 200 μl of purified white blood cells or plasma. The samples are dissolved and simultaneously stabilized by incubation with a buffer containing denaturing agents and proteinase K. Nucleic acids released from the samples are bound to the surface of magnetic glass particles, and unbound substances are removed by several washes. The purified nucleic acids are then eluted in a low-salt buffer. Isolated total nucleic acids are diluted in a final volume of 66 μl of elution buffer and immediately processed for real-time PCR.

The primers used for the qualitative and quantitative HHV-6 DNA real-time PCR assays are from a portion of the HHV-6 DNA genome that carries the U65-U66 genes (13) and detect both variants; the generated DNA product is approximately 173 to 176 bp in length. To prepare standards for quantitative PCR, the 173- to 176-bp PCR product is produced using the High Fidelity PCR Master kit (Roche Applied Science, Indianapolis, Ind.) and is directly cloned into a pCRII-TOPO plasmid vector using the TOPO TA cloning kit (InVitrogen, Carlsbad, Calif.). The recombinant vector is then transformed into chemically competent cells of the DH5α-T1 strain of *Escherichia coli* using the rapid One Shot (InVitrogen) transformation procedure. Selected clones are amplified by overnight culture in LB broth containing 50 μg of ampicillin/ml and are then prescreened by PCR to confirm the size of the insert; the insert is also sequenced for verification. Plasmid DNA from the transformed clones is isolated in bulk using a Qiagen midi kit (Qiagen, Inc., Valencia, Calif.). The standards made from the plasmid are calibrated using a reference standard containing 1.4×10^{10} viral particles of HHV-6 strain U1102 variant A per ml (Advanced Biotechnologies, Inc., Columbia, Md.) as determined by electron microscopy. Serial 10-fold dilutions of this standard, ranging from 10^8 to 10^1 HHV-6 DNA copies per ml, are used to characterize the sensitivity, specificity, linearity, and precision of the quantitative assay. The standard curve is created automatically with software from an ABI Prism 7000 Sequence Detection System (Applied Biosystems, Foster City, Calif.) by plotting the threshold cycle (C_t) values against each standard of known concentration.

Both qualitative and quantitative HHV-6 DNA real-time PCR assays are performed in 50-μl volumes containing $1\times$ TaqMan Universal Master Mix (Applied Biosystems), 900 nM concentrations of forward and reverse primers, a 200 nM concentration of the fluorogenic probe labeled with FAM (6-carboxylfluorescein) at the 5′ end and TAMRA (tetramethylrhodamine) at the 3′ end, nuclease-free water with yeast tRNA (60 ng/ml; Roche Molecular Biochemicals, Indianapolis, Ind.), and 10 μl of islolated total nucleic acid. The mixtures are added to individual wells of 96-well reaction plates, and the plates are sealed with adhesive optical covers and then rotated on an orbital shaker for 30 s to thoroughly mix and remove air bubbles in the wells. The amplification and detection are completed using an ABI Prism 7000 Sequence Detection System. The thermal cycling parameters consist of 1 cycle for 2 min at 50°C, 1 cycle for 10 min at 95°C, and 45 two-step cycles of 15 s at 95°C and 60 s at 60°C. For the qualitative assay, one negative control (HHV-6-negative purified human white blood cells) and one positive control of HHV-6 strain Z-29 variant B at a concentration of 2×10^7 viral particles/ml (Advanced Biotechnologies, Inc.) are processed with each batch of clinical specimens from extraction of nucleic acids through the detection of amplified product. For the negative controls, cells are counted using a hemocytometer and the concentration of cells is adjusted to 2.0×10^6 cells/ml by dilution in PBS. Single-use aliquots of 250 μl of suspended material from each control are stored at $-70°C$. For the quantitative assay, the above controls are processed as well as a set of five standards ranging from 10^4 to 10^8 HHV-6 DNA copies/ml. Specimens and controls are tested singly for the qualitative assay and in triplicate when quantifying the amount of HHV-6 DNA. Specimens or controls are considered positive in the qualitative assay when the generated fluorescence signal at the C_t value exceeds a defined threshold limit. In the quantitative assay, the quantity of HHV-6 DNA in each specimen or control is determined from the generated standard curve. The quantitative real-time PCR can quantitate over a range of 140 to 140 million copies of HHV-6 DNA/ml at a 95% detection rate. Reliable results can be obtained below 140 copies/ml, but the detection rate diminishes as the DNA input drops below this value. A human albumin gene primer and probe set is used in separate PCRs as an internal positive control to ensure that samples contain nucleic acid and to exclude the presence of inhibitors.

Interpretation of Results

The ubiquitous distribution of HHV-6 throughout the world complicates the interpretation of laboratory studies, and a combination of methods may be required to confirm the relationship of HHV-6 infection with various diseases. Also, most diagnostic methods for HHV-6 are in the early stages of development; the sensitivity and specificity of each assay have not been systematically evaluated in controlled, prospective studies, and reagents have only recently been made available to diagnostic laboratories through commercial sources.

Serologic testing is most useful for diagnosing primary infections with HHV-6 in children with acute illnesses and for studies of the epidemiology, clinical pathology, and natural history of the virus. For interpretation of serologic tests, a history of seroconversion from a negative to a positive IgG antibody response to HHV-6 between acute- and convalescent-phase sera or the presence of IgM in a single serum sample during a primary infection helps establish HHV-6 as the causative agent. If a serum sample from early in an illness contains HHV-6 antibodies and a fourfold or greater rise in titer is demonstrated in a second specimen taken several weeks later, a diagnosis of recent infection due to reactivation or reinfection can be made. If acute- and convalescent-phase sera are both positive for HHV-6 antibody but the antibody titer is unchanged, the result is interpreted as HHV-6 infection at some time in the past. Screening a single serum specimen for IgG antibody to HHV-6 can also provide evidence of previous exposure to the virus and assists in identifying individuals at risk for HHV-6 infection.

The use of serologic techniques to establish the presence of active HHV-6 infection can be problematic; the detection of HHV-6-specific IgG or IgM antibodies may not always indicate primary infection, and in the setting of reactivation or latent infection, conventional serologic studies have a limited value in establishing an association with disease. Increased titers of IgG to HHV-6 may occur during infections with other herpesviruses, such as CMV, EBV, or HHV-7, and the relative importance of each virus in producing disease may be difficult to determine. Variations in the detection of HHV-6-specific antibodies have been observed and may be related to the methods and reagents used. The use of insensitive assays may inappropriately indicate that HHV-6 infection has been excluded or that a positive seroconversion had occurred when, in fact, this may represent an inability to detect low levels of antibody during reactivation. Assays should also be extensively evaluated for specificity to detect potential cross-reactivity with other herpesviruses. Results of serologic tests for IgM antibody should be interpreted with caution; IgM antibody can appear in both primary and reactivated HHV-6 infections and can persist for extended periods after a primary infection. Also, some children may not develop detectable IgM responses during primary infection. A recognized technical problem with HHV-6 IgM assays is the occurrence of false-positive and false-negative reactions due to high levels of competing rheumatoid factor and HHV-6-specific IgG.

The appropriate selection of methods for the diagnosis and monitoring of HHV-6 disease is a challenge. The lack of well-defined, commercially available reagents and standardized methods and controls has made the interpretation of laboratory results more difficult. Whenever possible, serologic diagnoses of HHV-6 infection should be confirmed by virus isolation or suitable direct detection methods. To implicate HHV-6 as the cause of certain diseases, it may also be necessary to use methods that measure active virus replication, since the qualitative detection of virus or viral DNA may simply indicate the presence of the virus in a latent state. A more accurate assessment of the involvement of HHV-6 in a given disease may be provided by the detection of cell-free viral DNA in serum or plasma by PCR, by qualitative amplification of specific HHV-6 mRNA transcripts, by detection of viral antigen expression in tissues or PBMC by immunohistochemistry or in situ hybridization, or by quantitative assessment of the viral load by DNA PCR.

HHV-7

Introduction

HHV-7 was first isolated in 1989 from PBMC of a healthy individual (12). In contrast to HHV-6, little is known about the prevalence, biology, and pathogenesis of this virus. HHV-7 is morphologically identical to other herpesviruses but, like HHV-6, is characterized by having a tropism for $CD4^+$ T lymphocytes, by causing infection early in life, and by being ubiquitous, with a seroprevalence rate of more than 85% in U.S. and European populations (see reference 1 for a review). Lower rates of seropositivity in Japan have been reported. After primary infection, HHV-7 can persist in the host in a latent state and reactivation can occur. Primary infection in children is thought to occur somewhat later in life than primary infection by HHV-6, usually after 24 months of age and by 5 years of age, although higher rates of seropositivity have been reported at a younger age (6). Salivary glands appear to be a main site of viral replication for HHV-7, and transmission is likely to occur from contact with respiratory secretions. Seroconversion to HHV-7 antibody positivity is a separate and distinct event from production of antibody to HHV-6. The virus can be grown in PBMC or CBC and shows a characteristic cytopathic effect of large, refractile cells indistinguishable from the cytopathic effect of HHV-6. A single continuous T-cell line (Sup-T1) can support the growth of HHV-7 with variable success. The virus is closely related to HHV-6 but has been shown to be genetically and immunologically distinct. Unlike for HHV-6, genetic variants have not been described for HHV-7. The DNA of HHV-7 has no homology to that of EBV, herpes simplex virus, or varicella-zoster virus and has limited homology to that of CMV. Therefore, HHV-7 has been classified as a member of the betaherpesviruses with HHV-6 and CMV. Western immunoblot analyses of viral proteins reveal different patterns for HHV-6- and HHV-7-infected cells, although monoclonal antibodies to HHV-6 can cross-react with HHV-7-infected cells. Several viral proteins have been identified for HHV-7, ranging in size from 30 to 136 kDa. The virus is frequently and consistently isolated from the saliva of infected individuals and can be detected in specimens such as peripheral blood, cervical secretions, and cerebrospinal fluid.

The clinical spectrum of disease caused by HHV-7 is poorly understood. HHV-7 has been associated with up to 10% of roseola cases and, as with HHV-6, is thought to be responsible for seizures and other neurologic events in children (see reference 20 for a review). The virus also has been isolated from two patients with a chronic viral syndrome and a child with a nonspecific febrile syndrome without rash. No viruses other than HHV-7 were isolated in these cases, and a seroconversion to HHV-7 but not HHV-6 positivity was documented. There is some evidence to suggest that HHV-7 also may play an etiologic role in pityriasis rosea. Little is known about disease caused by HHV-7 in immunocompromised patients, although reactivation of the virus in bone marrow and solid-organ transplant recipients is common (see reference 10 for a review). The glycoprotein CD4 is a critical component of the receptor on the surface of T lymphocytes for HHV-7; it has been shown that a selective and progressive downregulation of the expression of CD4 in HHV-7-infected T cells leads to a marked reciprocal interference of HIV infection. Infection of PBMC with HHV-7 enhances NK cell cytotoxicity by induction of IL-15. HHV-7 also may interact with other herpesviruses, leading to the reactivation of HHV-6 and CMV. Reactivation of HHV-7 has been reported to be a cofactor for the progression of CMV disease in renal transplant patients infected with CMV.

Immunologic and Molecular Diagnosis

The methods for laboratory diagnosis of HHV-7 are essentially identical to those for diagnosis of HHV-6 and currently include the direct examination of clinical specimens for viral antigens by immunohistochemistry (15) or viral nucleic acids by in situ hybridization and PCR (3, 28), virus identification in cell culture (12), and detection of antibodies against the virus (6). An HHV-7 antigenemia assay similar to that described above for HHV-6 has been developed for the detection of HHV-7 early and late antigens in PBMC isolated from recipients of liver and allogeneic stem cell transplants (19). The serodiagnosis of HHV-7 infection can be made by IFA, EIA, and Western immunoblot assays, using HHV-7-infected cells as an antigen source. Seroconversion to HHV-7 positivity, as determined by IFA, is independent of that to HHV-6 positivity and is diagnostic for primary infection. An antibody response to HHV-7 is induced only by HHV-7 infection, since neither seroconversion nor a significant rise in the titer of antibody to HHV-7 can be detected following primary infection with HHV-6. Conversely, seroconversion to HHV-7 positivity can cause a simultaneous rise in the titer of antibody to HHV-6. This is thought to be due to the ability of HHV-7 to induce a response of memory B cells against HHV-6 cross-reactive antigens or to be due to reactivation of HHV-6 during infection with HHV-7. HHV-6 antibodies are not protective against HHV-7 infection, since seroconversion to HHV-7 positivity can occur in the presence of high titers of antibody to HHV-6. The presence of antigenic cross-reactivity between HHV-6 and HHV-7 should be considered when performing serologic assays; it may be necessary to preadsorb patient sera to infected cells for specific determination of titers of antibody to each virus. An HHV-7 antibody avidity assay has recently been developed and validated and used in conjunction with the HHV-6 avidity test described above to detect and distinguish primary from past infections with either HHV-6 or HHV-7. In addition, dual primary HHV-6 and HHV-7 infections have been confirmed by using these assays.

Both conventional and real-time PCR assays have been described for the detection of HHV-7 DNA from clinical specimens. As with HHV-6, qualitative PCR assays are not able to differentiate active disease from asymptomatic infection or latency, and HHV-7 DNA is frequently found in saliva and PBMC of healthy individuals. To this end, PCR assays for quantitating HHV-7 DNA in infected individuals have been developed and are being evaluated for the ability

to correlate the viral load of HHV-7 with clinical disease and response to antiviral therapy, and to facilitate studies of the epidemiology of the virus (11, 28, 36).

The interpretation of laboratory results for HHV-7 is confounded by a paucity of commercially available reagents and, as with HHV-6, by the ubiquitous nature of this virus. In addition, caution is needed in interpreting the results of serologic studies because of the cross-reactivity of HHV-7 with HHV-6 and because of the ability of HHV-7 to reactivate other members of the herpesvirus family. With serologic evidence of dual infection, it may be difficult to determine the relative importance of each virus in causing disease. Virologic methods, including viral culture, rapid direct detection of antigens and/or nucleic acids, and serology, must be combined with a clinical assessment of the patient to provide a reliable determination of HHV-7 infection and to establish a clear relationship between infection and human disease. It may also be necessary to monitor viral load or other measures of active virus replication to help in our understanding of the natural history and pathogenesis of this virus.

HHV-8

Introduction

Using the molecular technique of representational difference analysis, HHV-8, also termed Kaposi's sarcoma (KS)-associated herpesvirus, was first identified by Chang et al. (5) in 1994 in more than 90% of KS tissues obtained from patients with AIDS. Subsequently, HHV-8 has been detected in patients with all forms of KS from all parts of the world, including AIDS-associated KS and classical KS in Mediterranean and Eastern European adults, HIV-1-negative African endemic KS of adults and children, and KS in persons with iatrogenic immunosuppression, most often organ transplant recipients (see references 2 and 26 for reviews). HHV-8 also has been detected in AIDS-related primary effusion lymphomas (formerly called body cavity-based lymphomas) and multicentric Castleman disease. In addition, HHV-8 has been implicated in the pathogenesis of other diseases, including multiple myeloma, sarcoidosis, angiosarcoma, non-KS skin lesions (including squamous and basal cell carcinomas) of immunocompromised patients, and multiple sclerosis. However, numerous follow-up studies using PCR-based and serologic assays have failed to corroborate the original findings, making it unlikely that HHV-8 is associated with these disorders. Little is known about primary HHV-8 infection in healthy individuals, and the diseases associated with this virus are thought to be more probably due to viral reactivation.

The biology, epidemiology, and pathogenesis of this virus are still not well understood (extensively reviewed in references 2 and 26). HHV-8 is classified as a gammaherpesvirus in the genus *Rhadinovirus* and has sequence homology to the simian virus herpesvirus saimiri and EBV. These viruses establish persistent, latent infection and are associated with immortalization and transformation of cells. The replicative form of the HHV-8 genome is approximately 165 kb in length, and 97 genes have been identified. Several genes have homology to human genes, such as those encoding cyclin D (a cell cycle inducer), various cytokines, and Bcl-2 (a blocker of apoptosis). Expression of these genes may help explain the association of HHV-8 with cell transformation and the development of tumors. Viral replication may be affected by interaction with other viruses such as HIV-1 and EBV, since body cavity lymphoma cells are frequently coinfected with EBV and tumors associated with HHV-8 are often seen in persons infected with HIV-1. It also has been demonstrated that HIV-1 can increase HHV-8 replication in a body cavity lymphoma cell line. Genetic diversity exists among viral isolates of HHV-8, resulting in the identification of strains A, B, and C; strain A has been found mainly in patients with AIDS-associated or classical KS, while strains B and C are seen more often among African patients. The virus has a cell tropism for $CD19^+$ B lymphocytes, the flat endothelial cells lining vascular spaces, and the perivascular spindle cells of KS lesions. Its distribution is worldwide, although it is not ubiquitous in most populations and there is considerable variation in its prevalence, which is related to the geographic and demographic distribution of KS. The precise modes of transmission are unknown. Based on the epidemiology of HHV-8, however, it is thought to be transmitted through sexual contact, predominantly among homosexual and bisexual HIV-1-positive males or their sexual partners. Likely sources of infection for sexual transmission are semen and possibly female genital secretions; HHV-8 DNA has been found in the semen of male AIDS patients and cervico-vaginal specimens from HHV-8-seropositive women. Although HHV-8 DNA has yet to be found in feces, sexual practices involving oral-anal contact may be a risk factor for homosexual transmission. HHV-8 also has been detected in oral secretions and PBMC of HIV-1-infected males and in the blood of an apparently healthy blood donor following multiple donations. Widespread horizontal transmission from oral secretions may be responsible for the high rate of HHV-8 infection in areas where KS is hyperendemic. However, the transmission of HHV-8 by blood or the respiratory route in populations at low risk for KS is likely to be uncommon. Transmission through organ transplantation has been documented and is of concern for this patient population.

Immunologic and Molecular Diagnosis

The laboratory diagnosis of HHV-8 infection is possible using molecular methods such as PCR or using serologic assays (see reference 32 for a review), although the clinical need for testing has not been defined. These methods have been used mainly to study the epidemiology of HHV-8 and to investigate the relationship between HHV-8 and the pathogenesis of various diseases. Assays are currently available only in research laboratories, and there are few commercial sources of reagents.

PCR is the primary method used for the direct detection of HHV-8 from tissues; body fluids such as serum, plasma, urine, saliva, bone marrow, and semen; and PBMC from infected individuals. The most widely used primers are those originally described by Chang et al. (5) and are specific for the highly conserved 233-bp region of the KS330Bam fragment (open reading frame [ORF] 26). Other useful primer sets have been evaluated and include those that amplify gene sequences of ORFs 8, 25, 37, 65, 72, 73, 75, K5, and K6. Quantitative conventional (8) and real-time (18, 31) PCR assays recently have been developed to measure the HHV-8 viral load in PBMC, plasma, or tissues of individuals with AIDS-associated KS, classical KS, AIDS-related primary effusion lymphomas, and multicentric Castleman disease and in organ transplant recipients. These assays may be useful to determine the exact mode(s) of transmission of the virus, to assist in the diagnosis of KS and other diseases associated with HHV-8 infection, to identify those individuals at highest risk of disease, to predict the progression to and development of KS, and to assess the efficacy of different therapeutic regimens. It has been shown that individuals with HHV-8-related diseases have more HHV-8 DNA in

either plasma or PBMC than do persons without disease, but the level of HHV-8 DNA in plasma is significantly higher than that in PBMC. Quantitation of HHV-8 in plasma, therefore, may be more accurate for evaluating the risk of HHV-8 disease progression and the efficacy of therapy.

Attempts to culture HHV-8 have met with great difficulty, and current methods are labor-intensive and impractical for diagnostic use. Nevertheless, $CD19^+$ B cells, the human papillomavirus-transformed endothelial cell line BB19, and the adenovirus-transformed human kidney epithelial cell line 293 have been used to grow virus from KS spindle cells, fluids from body cavity lymphomas, and filtered cell culture fluids from $CD19^+$ cells positive for HHV-8. However, continual replication in these cell lines has not been successful. Monoclonal antibodies specific to HHV-8 have been described and are currently being used to localize HHV-8 in infected cells and tissue by immunocytochemistry and flow cytometry. These antibodies are not widely available for diagnostic use.

Serologic testing for HHV-8 can be done by a variety of formats, including IFA, EIA, and immunoblot assays. Similar to serologic tests for EBV, these assays have been designed to detect antibody responses to HHV-8-specific antigens expressed during latency or lytic infection. Antigens currently used in HHV-8 serologic assays include purified viral particles, whole cells, or isolated nuclei prepared from HHV-8-infected cell lines derived from body cavity-based lymphomas, whole-cell lysates, recombinant viral proteins, and synthetic peptides.

IFAs for measuring HHV-8-specific antibody responses from patient sera are usually done with HHV-8-infected whole cells fixed onto slides as the substrate. The cell lines BC-1 and HBL-6, which are latently infected with HHV-8 and coinfected with EBV, were originally used to develop some of the first IFAs for the detection of HHV-8 antibodies against nonstructural latent antigens of the virus, particularly the latency-associated nuclear antigen (LANA). Antibody cross-reactivity is of primary concern with assays that use cells infected with both HHV-8 and EBV; cell lines such as BCP-1 and BCBL-1, which are infected with HHV-8 alone, are now being used in most whole-cell IFAs to minimize cross-reactions with antibodies to other herpesviruses. For measurement of antibodies to lytic antigens by IFA, HHV-8-infected cell lines are treated with phorbol esters or sodium butyrate. This results in the chemical induction of a lytic cycle of viral replication and the expression of lytic antigens that usually correspond to structural viral proteins. When using IFA, the presence of stippled immunofluorescence in the nuclei of uninduced cells is representative of an antibody response to LANA, while antibodies against HHV-8 lytic antigens are measured by observing fluorescence as diffuse cytoplasmic staining, spots in the nucleus, or localized to the membrane of the induced cells. A monoclonal antibody-enhanced IFA (mIFA) has been described and uses a mouse monoclonal antibody and induced or uninduced BCBL-1 cells for detecting antibodies to latent and lytic HHV-8 antigens. Although IFAs can be used to detect a range of antibody responses to various latent and lytic proteins of HHV-8, the procedures are labor-intensive and subjective, requiring considerable experience and critical evaluation to ensure reliable results. Extensive quality control is also needed to monitor the appropriate expression of lytic antigens in induced cells and to prepare the substrate slides.

EIAs have been developed that use whole viral lysates as antigens for detecting HHV-8 antibodies. The whole-virus EIA is designed to detect IgG antibodies to nonstructural and most structural HHV-8 antigens; it uses a viral lysate prepared from sucrose gradient-purified whole virions obtained from the cell line KS-1. More recently, recombinant proteins of the lytic viral capsid antigen from ORF 65 or peptides corresponding to a fragment of the minor capsid protein from ORF 26 have been used in the development of HHV-8 serologic EIAs.

Immunogenic latent (encoded by ORF 73 [LANA]) and lytic (encoded by ORFs 65, K8.1, K8.1A, and K8.1B) proteins have also been recombinantly expressed and used in immunoblot assays (37). Reactions to LANA on immunoblot assays are seen as a high-molecular-mass doublet of 226 and 234 kDa. The ORFs corresponding to K8.1 encode HHV-8-specific envelope glycoproteins of 35 to 40 kDa.

With most of the available serologic assays, HHV-8-specific antibodies have been detected in the majority of individuals with KS, AIDS-related primary effusion lymphomas, or multicentric Castleman disease. Among persons infected with HIV-1, the seroprevalence for HHV-8 is highest in HIV-1-infected homosexual males, indeterminate in intravenous drug users and persons infected through heterosexual contact, and lowest in hemophiliacs, women, and children. It also has been shown that seroconversion to HHV-8 positivity precedes the progression to KS and predicts the subsequent appearance of KS lesions in HIV-1-infected individuals. In the general population, the highest seroprevalence rates for HHV-8 are seen in sub-Saharan Africa and Mediterranean countries, while rates in northern European, North American, and southeast Asian countries are relatively low.

In several studies done to compare the various HHV-8 antibody assays (24, 30, 37), good assay correlation was obtained when testing sera from individuals with KS. The most significant discrepancies between assays were observed when determining the seroprevalence of HHV-8 in high-risk groups without KS or groups at minimal risk for HHV-8 infection, such as blood donors. While the different methods showed similar antibody trends within the various epidemiological and population groups, they did not always agree. Considerable variation in sensitivity and specificity was observed from one assay to another when testing individual serum specimens within defined panels of sera from different populations. This appears to be related to the choice of assays, the use of different serum dilutions and cutoff values, the selection and preparation of antigen(s) used, and the lack of standardized methods and reagents. In general, the mIFA using lytic antigens identifies the highest number of individuals with HHV-8-specific antibodies, while assays based on latent antigens or individual HHV-8 proteins and peptides are less sensitive. The specificity of the lytic mIFA has been questioned because this assay detects HHV-8 antibodies in a much higher percentage of healthy blood donors and the results have not been corroborated by other assays. However, it is still unknown whether the lytic mIFA is just more sensitive or truly detects cross-reactive antibodies. In general, nonspecific reactions have been found to occur when IFAs are performed with sera at dilutions of <1:40, particularly if the cells used as an antigen source were chemically induced. Dilutions as high as 1:100 or 1:160 have been recommended to avoid such reactions, but such dilutions also may lead to false-negative results. Single-antigen assays do not appear to detect all antibody responses to infection with HHV-8, but use of these tests has demonstrated that individuals may differ in their abilities to recognize different HHV-8 proteins and that different antibody profiles can develop during the course of HHV-8 infection (30). It is clear that no one assay is completely sensitive and specific, and that combinations of several assays or combination of several antigens in a single assay may be required to accurately determine the seropositivity to HHV-8, particularly in the general population (30). Zhu et al. (37) have recently shown that IFA positivity with both latent and lytic antigens followed by confirmation with an immunoblot assay using a panel of latent and lytic immunogenic recombinant antigens provides a reliable, sensitive, and specific measure of HHV-8 antibodies.

Until serologic assays are extensively evaluated and better standardized, their utility for diagnosing HHV-8 infection and for determining the immune status of an individual is limited and the interpretation of results is difficult. As with HHV-6 and HHV-7, it may be necessary to correlate serologic results with direct antigen and/or nucleic acid detection and to quantify the HHV-8 viral load to reliably detect infection and to establish a clear relationship between infection and human disease.

REFERENCES

1. **Ablashi, D. V., Z. N. Berneman, B. Kramarsky, J. Whitman, Jr., Y. Asano, and G. R. Pearson.** 1995. Human herpesvirus-7 (HHV-7): current status. *Clin. Diagn. Virol.* **4:**1–13.
2. **Ablashi, D. V., L. G. Chatlynne, J. E. Whitman, Jr., and E. Cesarman.** 2002. Spectrum of Kaposi's sarcoma-associated herpesvirus, or human herpesvirus 8, diseases. *Clin. Microbiol. Rev.* **15:**439–464.
3. **Berneman, Z. N., D. V. Ablashi, G. Li, M. Eger-Fletcher, M. S. Reitz, Jr., C. L. Hung, I. Brus, A. L. Komaroff, and R. C. Gallo.** 1992. Human herpesvirus 7 is a T-lymphotropic virus and is related to, but significantly different from, human herpesvirus 6 and human cytomegalovirus. *Proc. Natl. Acad. Sci. USA* **89:**10552–10556.
4. **Braun, D. K., G. Dominguez, and P. E. Pellett.** 1997. Human herpesvirus 6. *Clin. Microbiol. Rev.* **10:**521–567.
5. **Chang, Y., E. Cesarman, M. S. Pessin, F. Lee, J. Culpepper, D. M. Knowles, and P. S. Moore.** 1994. Identification of herpesvirus-like DNA sequences in AIDS-associated Kaposi's sarcoma. *Science* **266:**1865–1869.
6. **Clark, D. A., J. M. L. Freeland, P. L. K. Mackie, R. F. Jarrett, and D. E. Onions.** 1993. Prevalence of antibody to human herpesvirus 7 by age. *J. Infect. Dis.* **168:**252–253.
7. **Clark, D. A., and P. D. Griffiths.** 2003. Human herpesvirus 6: relevance of infection in the immunocompromised host. *Br. J. Haematol.* **120:**384–395.
8. **Curreli, F., M. A. Robles, A. E. Friedman-Kien, and O. Flore.** 2003. Detection and quantitation of Kaposi's sarcoma-associated herpesvirus (KSHV) by a single competitive-quantitative polymerase chain reaction. *J. Virol. Methods* **107:**261–267.
9. **Dockrell, D. H.** 2003. Human herpesvirus 6: molecular biology and clinical features. *J. Med. Microbiol.* **52:**5–18.
10. **Dockrell, D. H., and C. V. Paya.** 2001. Human herpesvirus-6 and -7 in transplantation. *Rev. Med. Virol.* **11:**23–36.
11. **Fernandez, C., D. Boutolleau, C. Manichanh, N. Mangeney, H. Agut, A. Gautheret-Dejean.** 2002. Quantitation of HHV-7 genome by real-time polymerase chain reaction assay using MGB probe technology. *J. Virol. Methods* **106:**11–16.
12. **Frenkel, N., E. C. Schirmer, L. S. Wyatt, G. Katsafanas, E. Roffman, R. M. Danovich, and C. H. June.** 1990. Isolation of a new herpesvirus from human CD4$^+$ T cells. *Proc. Natl. Acad. Sci. USA* **87:**748–752.
13. **Gautheret-Dejean, A., C. Manichanh, F. Thien-Ah-Koon, A. M. Fillet, N. Mangeney, M. Vidaud, N. Dhedin, J.-P. Vernant, and H. Agut.** 2002. Development of a real-time polymerase chain reaction assay for the diagnosis of human herpesvirus-6 infection and application to bone marrow transplant patients. *J. Virol. Methods* **100:**27–35.

14. Hall, C. B., M. T. Caserta, K. C. Schnabel, C. Boettrich, M. P. McDermott, G. K. Lofthus, J. A. Carnahan, and S. Dewhurst. 2004. Congenital infections with human herpesvirus 6 (HHV6) and human herpesvirus 7 (HHV7). *J. Pediatr.* **145:**472–477.

15. Kempf, W., B. Muller, R. Maurer, V. Adams, and G. C. Fiume. 2000. Increased expression of human herpesvirus 7 in lymphoid organs of AIDS patients. *J. Clin. Virol.* **16:**193–201.

16. Kidd, I. M., D. A. Clark, J. A. G. Bremner, D. Pillay, P. D. Griffiths, and V. C. Emery. 1998. A multiplex PCR assay for the simultaneous detection of human herpesvirus 6 and human herpesvirus 7, with typing of HHV-6 by enzyme cleavage of PCR products. *J. Virol. Methods* **70:**29–36.

17. Krueger, G. R. F., D. V. Ablashi, S. F. Josephs, S. Z. Salahuddin, U. Lembke, A. Ramon, and G. Bertram. 1991. Clinical indications and diagnostic techniques of human herpesvirus-6 (HHV-6) infection. *In Vivo* **5:**287–296.

18. Lallemand, F., N. Desire, W. Rozenbaum, J. C. Nicolas, and V. Marechal. 2000. Quantitative analysis of human herpesvirus 8 viral load using a real-time PCR assay. *J. Clin. Microbiol.* **38:**1404–1408.

19. Lautenschlager, I., M. Lappalainen, K. Linnavuori, J. Suni, and K. Hockerstedt. 2002. CMV infection is usually associated with concurrent HHV-6 and HHV-7 antigenemia in liver transplant patients. *J. Clin. Virol.* **25:**S57–S61.

20. Leach, C. T. 2000. Human herpesvirus-6 and -7 infections in children: agents of roseola and other syndromes. *Curr. Opin. Pediatr.* **12:**269–274.

21. Marsh, S., M. Kaplan, Y. Asano, D. Hoekzema, A. L. Komaroff, J. E. Whitman Jr., and D. V. Ablashi. 1996. Development and application of HHV-6 antigen capture assay for the detection of HHV-6 infections. *J. Virol. Methods* **61:**103–112.

22. Nielsen, L., and B. F. Vestergaard. 2002. A μ-capture immunoassay for detection of human herpes virus-6 (HHV-6) IgM antibodies in human serum. *J. Clin. Virol.* **25:**145–154.

23. Nitsche, A., C. W. Muller, A. Radonic, O. Landt, H. Ellerbrok, G. Pauli, and W. Siegert. 2001. Human herpesvirus 6A DNA is detected frequently in plasma but rarely in peripheral blood leukocytes of patients after bone marrow transplantation. *J. Infect. Dis.* **183:**130–133.

24. Rabkin, C. S., T. F. Schulz, D. Whitby, E. T. Lennette, L. I. Magpantay, L. Chatlynne, and R. J. Biggar for the HHV-8 Interlaboratory Collaborative Group. 1998. Interassay correlation of human herpesvirus 8 serologic tests. *J. Infect. Dis.* **178:**304–309.

25. Safronetz, D., A. Humar, and G. A. Tipples. 2003. Differentiation and quantitation of human herpesviruses 6A, 6B and 7 by real-time PCR. *J. Virol. Methods* **112:**99–105.

26. Sarid, R., S. J. Olsen, and P. S. Moore. 1999. Kaposi's sarcoma-associated herpesvirus: epidemiology, virology, and molecular virology. *Adv. Virus Res.* **52:**139–232.

27. Secchiero, P., D. R. Carrigan, Y. Asano, L. Benedetti, R. W. Crowley, A. L. Komaroff, R. C. Gallo, and P. Lusso. 1995. Detection of human herpesvirus 6 in plasma of children with primary infection and immunosuppressed patients by polymerase chain reaction. *J. Infect. Dis.* **171:**273–280.

28. Secchiero, P., D. Zella, R. W. Crowley, R. C. Gallo, and P. Lusso. 1995. Quantitative PCR for human herpesviruses 6 and 7. *J. Clin. Microbiol.* **33:**2124–2130.

29. Singh, N., and D. R. Carrigan. 1996. Human herpesvirus-6 in transplantation: an emerging pathogen. *Ann. Intern. Med.* **124:**1065–1071.

30. Spira, T. J., L. Lam, S. C. Dollard, Y. -X. Meng, C. P. Pau, J. B. Black, D. Burns, B. Cooper, M. Hamid, J. Huong, K. Kite-Powell, and P. E. Pellett. 2000. Comparison of serologic assays and PCR for diagnosis of human herpesvirus 8 infection. *J. Clin. Microbiol.* **38:**2174–2180.

31. Stamey, F. R., M. M. Patel, B. P. Holloway, and P. E. Pellett. 2001. Quantitative, fluorogenic probe PCR assay for detection of human herpesvirus 8 DNA in clinical specimens. *J. Clin. Microbiol.* **39:**3537–3540.

32. Tedeschi, R., J. Dillner, and P. Paoli. 2002. Laboratory diagnosis of human herpesvirus 8 infection in humans. *Eur. J. Microbiol. Infect. Dis.* **21:**831–844.

33. Van den Bosch, G., G. Locatelli, L. Geerts, G. Faga, M. Ieven, H. Goossens, D. Bottiger, B. Oberg, P. Lusso, and Z. N. Berneman. 2001. Development of reverse transcriptase PCR assays for detection of active human herpesvirus 6 infection. *J. Clin. Microbiol.* **39:**2308–2310.

34. Volin, L., I. Lautenschlager, E. Juvonen, A. Nihtinen, V. J. Anttila, and T. Ruutu. 2004. Human herpesvirus 6 antigenemia in allogeneic stem cell transplant recipients: impact on clinical course and association with other beta-herpesviruses. *Br. J. Haematol.* **126:**690–696.

35. Ward, K. N., D. J. Turner, X. Couto Parada, and A. D. Thiruchelvam. 2001. Use of immunoglobulin G antibody avidity for differentiation of primary human herpesvirus 6 and 7 infections. *J. Clin. Microbiol.* **39:**959–963.

36. Zerr, D. M., M.-L. Huang, L. Corey, M. Erickson, H. L. Parker, and L. M. Frenkel. 2000. Sensitive method for detection of human herpesviruses 6 and 7 in saliva collected in field studies. *J. Clin. Microbiol.* **38:**1981–1983.

37. Zhu, L., R. Wang, A. Sweat, E. Goldstein, R. Horvat, and B. Chandran. 1999. Comparison of human sera reactivities in immunoblots with recombinant human herpesvirus (HHV)-8 proteins associated with the latent (ORF 73) and lytic (ORFs 65, K8.1A, and K8.1B) replicative cycles and in immunofluorescence assays with HHV-8-infected BCBL-1 cells. *Virology* **256:**381–392.

Papillomaviruses and Polyomaviruses

KEERTI V. SHAH AND EUGENE O. MAJOR

75

Until recently, papillomaviruses and polyomaviruses were grouped together as papovaviruses, but they are now classified as two distinct families. The viruses of the two families are unrelated genetically and immunologically, and their genetic organizations and biology are quite dissimilar (12). Papillomaviruses infect only surface epithelia and are not transported to internal organs in the course of their infections. They are etiologically linked to a number of naturally occurring human and animal cancers. In contrast, polyomaviruses have a viremic phase during which they infect internal organs such as the kidneys and lymphoid cells.

PAPILLOMAVIRUSES

Papillomaviruses are widely distributed in nature and probably infect all higher vertebrates. They cannot be propagated in cell cultures. Therefore, rapid advances in our knowledge about papillomaviruses were possible only after molecular cloning became available in the 1970s. To date, over 100 human papillomaviruses (HPVs) have been characterized. Phylogenetic analyses of papillomaviruses reveal groupings that are consistent with the observed phenotypes, including species of origin, tissue tropism, and association with benign versus malignant lesions.

Papillomaviruses are nonenveloped viruses with a circular, covalently closed, double-stranded DNA genome of about 8,000 bp. All of the genomic information is carried on one strand. The genome is divided into an early region (E) that contains eight open reading frames (ORFs), a late region (L) that contains two ORFs, and a noncoding long control region in which the regulatory elements for viral DNA replication and transcription are located. The L1 and L2 genes code for, respectively, the major and minor capsid proteins of the virion. The E6 and E7 genes of high-risk HPV code for the transforming proteins that bind cellular tumor suppressor genes, p53 and Rb, respectively, and lead to dysregulation of the cell cycle and genetic instability. The E4 gene is expressed in the late stage of the virus cycle, even though it is located in the early region. The E1 gene is required for viral DNA replication, and the E2 gene modulates transcription of viral genes. No functions are known for the E3 and E8 ORFs.

HPVs are strictly epitheliotropic viruses that infect squamous epithelia of the skin and mucous membranes. Infection is initiated when the basal cells of the epithelium are exposed to infectious viral particles after minor trauma, e.g., during sexual intercourse or after skin abrasions. The expression of viral genes is tightly linked to the stages of cellular differentiation. In the basal and parabasal cells of the epithelium, only the early viral genes are expressed and the viral DNA is replicated in low copy numbers. In the upper, more differentiated layers of the epithelium, all viral genes are expressed, leading to extensive replication of viral DNA and the production of infectious viral particles. The presence of infectious virus in the most superficial cells of the infected epithelium, which are shed constantly, facilitates transmission. The relative lack of cells of the immune system in the epithelium, the site for the entire life cycle of HPV, probably accounts for the low immune responses seen in HPV infections.

HPVs fall naturally into two groups, mucosal HPVs and cutaneous HPVs. The genital tract is the main reservoir for mucosal HPVs, but two mucosal HPVs (types 13 and 32) exclusively infect the oral cavity. The clinical conditions associated with HPV infections are listed in Table 1.

Mucosal HPV

About 40 HPV types infect the genital tract. Genital HPV types are the most common sexually transmitted pathogens. In sexually active U.S. women, HPV prevalence, as measured by detection of viral sequences by PCR, may exceed 30%. HPV prevalence reaches its peak in young adults and declines in older age groups. Less than 10% of the women with HPV DNA in the genital tract have abnormal cervical cytology. Infections last for 1 to 2 years, and most individuals clear their infections completely. Immunodeficient women, e.g., women infected with the human immunodeficiency virus (HIV), have a high prevalence of HPV infections and of cervical cytological abnormalities.

Cervical Cancer

About 500,000 cases of cervical cancer occur annually worldwide. A large majority of these cases occur in developing countries, where cervical cancer is the most frequent malignancy among women. Epidemiologically, cervical cancer has long been known as having all the risk factors of a sexually transmitted disease. Studies over the past two decades have established that sexually transmitted HPV infections are etiologically linked to cervical cancer (3, 30) and that they initiate the multistep process that leads to cervical cancer (13). Invasive cervical cancer is preceded by

TABLE 1 Major clinical associations of HPV infections

Disease	Main HPV types	Mode of transmission
Mucosal HPV		
Anogenital warts	6, 11	Sexual contact
Juvenile-onset respiratory papillomas	6, 11	Mother to child, at birth
Cervical cancer	16, 18, 31, 45, and others	Sexual contact
Vulvar, penile and anal cancer	16 and others	Sexual contact
Focal epithelial hyperplasia (oral cavity)	13, 32	Nonsexual contact
Oropharynx cancer	16 and others	Unclear
Cutaneous HPV		
Cutaneous warts	1 to 4, 10, and others	Nonsexual contact
EV	5, 8, and others	Nonsexual contact
Skin cancers	EV-associated types and novel HPV types	Transmission and pathogenesis not clear

low-grade and high-grade squamous intraepithelial lesions (SIL), which are precursors of cervical cancer. The time interval between low-grade SIL and invasive cancer may span several decades. HPVs are found in a large majority of SIL and of cervical cancers. HPV infection precedes cervical SIL in prospective studies of cytologically negative women (13). Some HPV types, e.g., HPV-16 and HPV-18, are preferentially associated with invasive cancer, whereas some, e.g., HPV-6 and HPV-11, are almost never found in invasive cancers. In a large international study, HPV-16, HPV-18, HPV-45, and HPV-31 accounted for, respectively, 50, 14, 8, and 5% of cases of invasive cervical cancers (3). The viral genome is integrated into tumor cell DNA in a majority of women with cervical cancer but is present as free copies in women who are cytologically normal.

Laboratory studies strongly support the epidemiologic evidence in favor of the HPV etiology of cervical cancer (13). In phylogenetic analyses, high-risk and low-risk HPVs cluster in separate branches. The genomic DNAs of HPV-16 and HPV-18 can immortalize human keratinocytes and can produce lesions resembling high-grade SIL in organotypic cultures of cervical epithelium, but the genomic DNAs of HPV-6 and HPV-11 cannot do so.

In the United States, tens of millions of HPV infections occur annually, resulting in about 13,000 new cases of invasive cervical cancer. Most of the HPV infections, including infections with high-risk HPVs, are resolved on their own. The cervical SIL that may result from HPV infections can be detected in Pap smear screening programs and treated effectively. A history of inadequate Pap smear screening is the strongest risk factor for cervical cancer in the United States. In countries where cervical cancer incidence is high and effective Pap smear screening programs are not available, sexual promiscuity of the male population often accounts for the high rates of cervical cancer.

The evidence linking HPV with cervical cancer is as persuasive as that for any other human carcinogen. HPV infections account for 100% of cervical cancers and provide a unique example of a major human cancer that has a single etiology.

Cancers at Other Genital and Nongenital Sites

The high-risk HPV types, especially HPV-16, are etiologically linked to at least a proportion of anal, vaginal, and vulvar cancers. Among nongenital sites, HPV infections are linked to cancers of the oropharynx, especially tonsillar cancer (7).

Anogenital Warts (Condylomata)

Condylomata are benign tumors and are the best-known and most common clinical manifestation of genital HPV infections. It is estimated that in the United States, several million cases of condylomata occur annually. Infections with HPV-6 and HPV-11, types that are almost never associated with invasive cancer, are responsible for 90% of anogenital warts. Condylomata are transmitted to about 70% of sexual partners and have an incubation period of 3 weeks to 8 months.

RRP

Genital tract HPV-6 and HPV-11 are also responsible for recurrent respiratory papillomatosis (RRP), which may have onset in early childhood (juvenile-onset RRP) or in adult life (adult-onset RRP). Juvenile-onset RRP is most often caused by transmission of HPV-6 and HPV-11 at birth, during fetal passage through an infected birth canal. Cesarean delivery offers some protection against juvenile-onset RRP. Most cases of juvenile-onset RRP occur in the first 2 years of life. Patients with adult-onset RRP acquire HPV infection after birth.

Although infection of the genital tract with HPV-6 and HPV-11 is not uncommon, RRP is a rare disease, an indication that virus transmission from mother to child is inefficient. In the United States, the annual number of new cases of RRP is estimated to be about 1,000. Vocal cords in the larynx are the most frequent site of RRP. The tumors, although they are benign, may cause life-threatening respiratory obstruction.

HPV in the Oral Cavity

Two HPV types, HPV-13 and HPV-32, produce focal epithelial hyperplasia, a benign oral condition found frequently in some indigenous populations but only rarely in other groups. These types are not recovered from the genital tract. Genital HPVs, especially HPV-6 and HPV-11, may also infect the oral cavity, probably as a result of oral sex.

Cutaneous HPVs

Skin Warts

Skin warts are most prevalent in school-age children and young adults. They are transmitted by direct contact with infected tissue or by contact with virus-contaminated objects. There is a correlation between the site and morphology of a wart and the infecting HPV type. HPV-1 is strongly correlated with plantar warts, HPV-2 is correlated with common warts, and HPV-3 and -10 are correlated with flat warts. Skin warts almost never undergo malignant change.

Epidermodysplasia Verruciformis

Epidermodysplasia verruciformis (EV) is a very rare disease in which an extensive, lifelong, wart virus infection of the skin is never resolved (14). The disease is often familial. Clinically the warts are flat or are in the form of reddish-brown macular plaques. The disease generally has onset in infancy or childhood, with multiple, disseminated, wart-like lesions on the face, trunk and extremities, which tend to become confluent. In about one-third of the cases, malignant transformation occurs in the reddish-brown plaques in areas exposed to sunlight.

The flat warts of EV patients often have the same HPV types (e.g., HPV-3 and HPV-10) that are found in the flat warts of individuals without EV. However, the EV patients also harbor about 20 additional types (HPV-5, HPV-8, and other EV-associated HPV types) that are recovered predominantly from the macular plaques. The skin cancers of EV patients provide a model in which specific viral types (especially HPV-5 and HPV-8), host factors (genetic immunological defect), and environmental factors (sunlight) act together in the genesis of the malignant lesions.

Skin Cancers

Knowledge about HPVs in the skin is changing rapidly (22). With the use of highly sensitive assays, DNA sequences of many HPV types are easily recovered from plucked hairs of completely normal skin. Up to 50% of normal skin samples from immunocompetent individuals and nearly 100% of normal skin samples from immunodeficient individuals yield HPV sequences. HPV DNA is acquired early in life. The amount of viral DNA in the tissue is estimated to be very low, about one copy per hundreds of cells. The prevalence of HPV DNA is somewhat higher in nonmelanoma skin cancers than in normal skin. Most of the sequences belong to HPV types in the subgenus of EV-associated HPVs. Cutaneous HPVs have a weak transforming activity. Whether cutaneous HPVs contribute to the development of nonmelanoma skin cancers is unclear.

Role of Immunologic Assays

Diagnosis of Infections

Immunologic testing has played a relatively small role in diagnosis of HPV infections, but serologic assays are valuable in epidemiologic studies. Viral diagnosis is routinely made by nucleic acid hybridization tests, and most of the information acquired to date on HPV biology has been obtained on the basis of detection of HPV genomic sequences in tissues. Type-specific reagents are not commercially available for HPVs. Several factors have combined to limit the role of immunologic tests in viral diagnosis. (i) Because the viruses cannot be grown in culture, it has been difficult to develop immunologic reagents. (ii) As the cervical disease progresses from low-grade SIL to invasive cancer, synthesis of viral capsid proteins and of infectious particles is completely shut down. Therefore, serologic reagents that detect the capsid L1 and L2 proteins are of little value for the diagnosis of HPV types in cancer tissues. (iii) Other proteins of interest, e.g., the transforming E6 and E7 proteins, are expressed in such small amounts in affected tissues that their detection is very cumbersome.

As described below, assays have been developed for detection of antibodies to L1 proteins and to E6 and E7 proteins.

VLP Serology

Large numbers of sera have been tested for antibodies to HPV-16 in enzyme-linked immunosorbent assay (ELISA) with use of virus-like particles (VLPs) as the antigen (see Methods). A detectable antibody response occurs in a proportion of individuals with documented infection (Fig. 1). Antibody titers in positive sera are low. Higher rates of HPV seropositivity are associated with (i) persistent infection, (ii) infections that have a high viral burden, (iii) infection with HPV-related pathology, and (iv) residence in areas of high HPV endemicity.

Serology for HPV-16 E6 and E7 Proteins

Antibodies to the E6 and E7 proteins are markers of HPV-associated invasive cervical cancer (Fig. 2). These antibodies can be detected by ELISA with E6 and E7 peptides, by Western blot assays with E6 and E7 fusion proteins, and by radioimmunoprecipitation assays with in vitro-transcribed and -translated full-length E6 and E7 proteins. In a case-control study of cervical cancer, serum antibodies to E6 or E7 protein were detected in 63% of cases and 10% of controls. Elevated levels of antibodies to the E6 or E7 protein were found in 41% of cases but in only 0.5% of controls. The antibody response may reflect the tumor burden in invasive cervical cancer.

Cell-Mediated Immunity

It is very probable that a cell-mediated immune response to HPV is required for clearance of infection and for control of disease. Conditions that depress cell-mediated immunity (e.g., HIV infection, organ transplantation) exacerbate HPV-associated diseases. However, reagents to assess any measure of cell-mediated immune response to HPV infections are not yet routinely available.

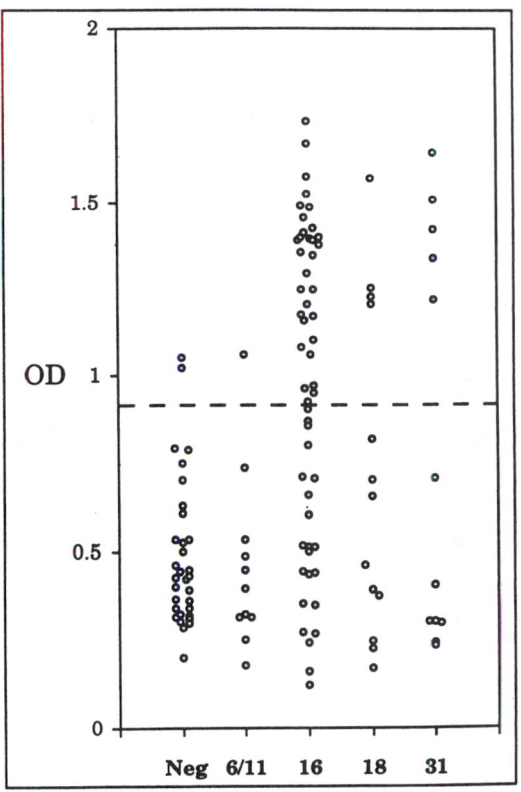

FIGURE 1 Reactivity of human sera to HPV-16 VLPs by HPV diagnosis of genital tract specimens. The dashed line at 0.89 represents the cutoff value. OD, optical density. (Reprinted from reference 16 with permission of the publisher.)

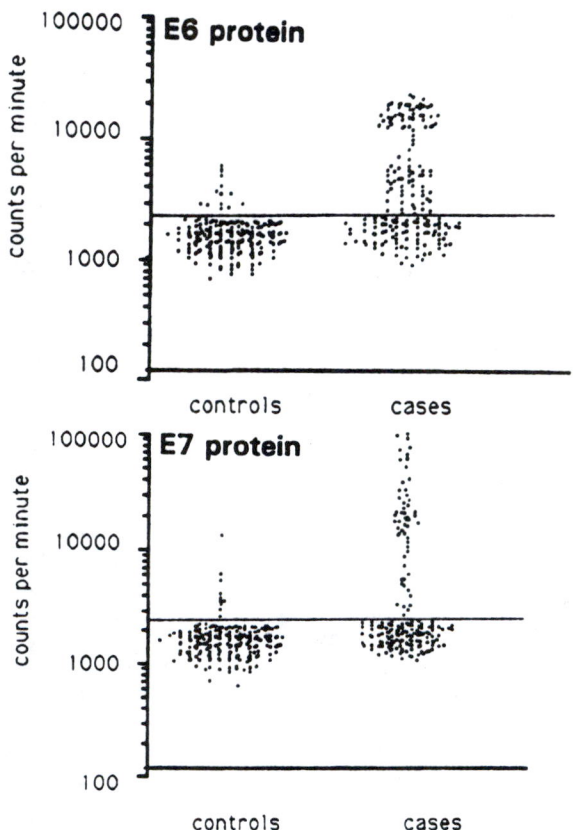

FIGURE 2 Distribution of counts per minute for serum reactivity to E6 and E7 proteins among cervical cancer cases and controls. Horizontal lines represent cutoff values for positivity. (Reprinted from reference 28 with permission of the publisher.)

HPV Vaccines

Attempts to develop prophylactic vaccines against HPV infections, employing the major capsid protein L1 as an antigen, have been remarkably successful in clinical trials. The L1 protein, when expressed by recombinant DNA technology, has the intrinsic ability to assemble into VLPs which are conformationally identical to authentic virions (27). Immunization of humans by intramuscular injection with VLPs results in a robust antibody response, with antibody titers far exceeding those resulting from natural infections. In a recent study, a vaccine based on HPV-16 VLPs administered as three intramuscular injections was tested in a placebo-controlled proof-of-principle trial in young U.S. women (17). The vaccine was found to prevent 100% of incident persistent HPV-16 infections and HPV-16-associated cervical intraepithelial neoplasia. The vaccine was genotype specific and it did not prevent cervical pathology due to types other than HPV-16. Studies in progress are examining the effectiveness of the vaccine in men and in HIV-infected individuals and are attempting to formulate vaccines that can be employed more easily in the developing world.

Methods

Detection of Viral Capsid Antigen

All HPV types have common antigenic determinants, some of which are located internal to the virion surface. Immunization of rabbits with detergent-disrupted virus capsids of an HPV, or of an animal papillomavirus, results in a broadly cross-reactive antiserum that can detect capsid antigens of any HPV in infected tissues. An antiserum prepared by immunization of rabbits with disrupted bovine papillomavirus capsids, and capable of detecting HPV capsid proteins, is commercially available (DAKO Corp., Carpinteria, Calif.).

The antigen can be detected by indirect fluorescent-antibody tests on frozen tissues or by an immunoperoxidase test on paraffin sections of formalin-fixed tissues. The specific staining is confined to the nuclei of infected epithelial cells. In positive tissues, the staining is most marked in the superficial layers of the epithelium, where viral capsids are synthesized. The proportion of cells in an infected tissue that contains the capsid antigen is highly variable; for example, capsid antigen is readily detected in plantar warts but may be present in only a very few cells in respiratory papillomas. Tissues that display viral cytopathic effect (koilocytosis) are likely to be capsid antigen positive, but the antigen is not detected in all koilocytotic cells in a tissue.

A positive test indicates productive infection with any of the HPVs. The infecting HPV type cannot be specifically diagnosed by the test because type-specific antisera are not available. A negative test does not imply that the lesion is not HPV associated. The test would be negative for capsid antigen in HPV-associated high-grade SIL and invasive cancers because viral particles are not synthesized in these lesions.

ELISA To Detect Antibody Response to HPV Infections

A serum antibody response to HPV infections can be detected with the use of antigens that maintain the conformational epitopes of native virions. HPV capsid proteins (L1) expressed in baculovirus or vaccinia virus have served satisfactorily as antigens. VLPs have been prepared for nearly all the medically important HPVs. This ELISA is not commercially available.

Conclusion

Although few immunologic tests for HPV are commercially available for use in clinical laboratories, this situation may change. Development of HPV-based vaccines against cervical cancer is a major goal of current research. Therefore, it is anticipated that standardized tests to measure HPV immune response will become available.

POLYOMAVIRUSES

Polyomaviruses consist of a double-stranded, circular DNA genome surrounded by a nonenveloped, icosahedral capsid that is approximately 45 nm in diameter, approximately 10 nm smaller than the papillomaviruses. The genomic organization of the polyomaviruses differs significantly from that of the papillomaviruses. This disparity, along with differences in biology, prompted the establishment of polyomaviruses into a separate family, *Polyomaviridae*. The genomic organization among the different polyomavirus family members is remarkably similar. The genome, which is approximately 5,000 bp, is functionally divided into an early region (2.4 kb), which is transcribed prior to DNA replication, and a late region (2.3 kb). Clockwise transcription from the origin of replication on one DNA strand yields the large, middle, and small T proteins for the mouse polyomavirus and the large and small T proteins for the primate polyomavirus. These early genes are necessary for subsequent transcription of the late region, which occurs in a counterclockwise direction and on the opposite strand of DNA. This late region codes for the structural proteins and the agnoprotein, which has been implicated in intracellular trafficking of viral proteins. In addition, there is a small noncoding region (0.4 kb) that contains the regulatory elements for viral replication and transcription. Structural differences in the regulatory region of the human polyomavirus JC virus (JCV) can be used as a basis for subtype classification. Furthermore, differences in transcription factor binding in this region have been strongly implicated in the regulation of the host range of these particular viruses (15, 19).

The polyomaviruses are broadly distributed in nature, with hosts including humans, rodents, birds, and rhesus macaques (Table 2). In humans, JCV is the etiologic agent for the fatal demyelinating disease progressive multifocal leukoencephalopathy (PML), while BK virus (BKV) infection is associated with urinary tract infections and nephropathy. Within the normal, healthy human population, JCV and BKV appear to circulate independently, with a vast majority of individuals exhibiting antibodies to these viruses. Initial infection and seroconversion appear to occur early in childhood and in the absence of any clinical symptoms. In the United States, approximately 50% of children develop antibodies to BKV by 3 years of age and antibodies to JCV by 12 to 14 years of age. Although the initial route of infection is unknown, it is likely that entry is via a commonly accessible route such as respiratory inhalation. The virus is then trafficked to the internal organs by viremia, where it can remain in a latent state. Both JCV and BKV are excreted in the urine during acute infections as well as after reactivation, which suggests that at least one site of latency is in kidney tissue. During periods of severe immune deficiency, reactivation of the virus eventually leads to pathology and clinical symptoms of the associated diseases. In the case of PML, it has been hypothesized that virus travels across the blood-brain barrier via circulating B lymphocytes (11), implicating lymphatic tissues as a site of latency as well.

Disease Associations

Progressive Multifocal Leukoencephalopathy

PML is the only demyelinating disease of the human central nervous system (CNS) for which the etiologic agent is a well-characterized virus, JCV. It was initially described in 1958 as a set of clinical symptoms and pathology in two patients with chronic lymphocytic leukemia (1), but it was not until 1971 that viral particles were isolated from the brain of a patient with non-Hodgkin's lymphoma who had died from PML (21). Early diagnosed cases were very few and were seen usually in conjunction with lymphoproliferative disorders. Presentation of clinical symptoms occurred later in life, in the fifth or sixth decade. However, since then, the disease has become much more common in association with HIV-1 infection and a rapidly growing population of immunosuppressed individuals. Although transplant recipients with acquired immunedeficiencies also comprise a small but significant percentage of PML patients, the number of PML cases with HIV-1 infection as the underlying immunosuppressive disorder is far greater than the combined total number of PML cases in all other patients. It has been estimated that 0.72% of all patients with AIDS have PML and that up to 5% will eventually develop the disease (2). PML is also an AIDS-defining illness in HIV-1-seropositive individuals, accounting for 1% of all diagnosed AIDS cases.

The clinical symptoms of PML have continued to evolve, particularly with the advent of highly active antiretroviral therapy in AIDS patients. Potent antiretroviral drugs have effectively reduced plasma HIV viral loads and increased CD4 cell counts, which could potentially lead to a decreased susceptibility to opportunistic infections such as PML. Studies have shown that in PML patients treated with highly active antiretroviral therapy, the course of PML may halt or go into remission in 50% of patients, with prolonged survival (5). The early signs of PML are sometimes difficult to diagnose, since they can present in a wide variety of neurological disturbances consistent with subcortical white matter involvement. Motor weakness, visual disturbances, and cognitive impairments are the three most common initial manifestations of PML, and they have been described as the classic "triad" of presenting symptoms (18). Diagnosis of PML currently tends to rely on a combination of radiographic findings and clinical history. The demonstration of viral particles or DNA from lesions within the brain had been the definitive evidence for PML but has now been replaced by JCV DNA levels in the cerebrospinal fluid (CSF).

TABLE 2 Polyomaviruses

Virus	Host species	Disease in natural host
BKV	Human	Acute hemorrhagic cystitis; acute respiratory tract disease; ureteral stenosis; nephropathy
JCV	Human	PML
SV40	Rhesus monkey	Natural infection of macaques; interstitial pneumonia; renal tubular necrosis; PML-like lesions in immunocompromised macaques
African green monkey polyomavirus (AGMPyV)	African green monkey	Natural infection; multiplies in B lymphoblasts
Baboon polyomavirus 2 (BPyV)	Baboon	Natural infection
Simian virus 12 (SV12)	Baboon	Natural infection; may persist in kidneys
Mouse polyomavirus (MPyV)	Mouse	Natural infection of wild mice; persists in kidneys; tumorigenesis
Murine pneumotropic virus (MPtV)	Mouse	Natural infection of mice; infects lung endothelium
Hamster polyomavavirus (HaPV)	Hamster	Subcutaneous tumorigenesis
Rabbit kidney vacuolating virus (RKV)	Rabbit	Natural infection of cottontail rabbits
Budgerigar fledgling disease virus (BFDV-1)	Parakeet	Highly infectious; multisystemic disease
Goose hemorrhagic polyomavirus (GHPV)	Goose	Hemorrhagic nephritis and enteritis
Bovine polyomavirus (BPyV)	Cattle	Natural infection of cattle; persists in kidneys

Infection appears to propagate by cell-to-cell contact, since viral particles are concentrated in cells at the periphery of the lesion. Furthermore, infected cells are often found near blood vessels in the brain, a finding that supports the theory of viral entry into the CNS via a hematogenous route, such as infected B lymphocytes (5). Within the lesioned area, lytically infected oligodendrocytes and reactive, enlarged astrocytes can be found, as well as macrophages that help to clear cellular debris. Neurons and axons are largely spared, since the virus rarely infects cells of neuronal lineage. However, there have been isolated reports of viral particles in cerebellar granule cells (6). Although the lytic infection of oligodendrocytes is the main event leading to the pathology of PML, it has been demonstrated that astrocytes and, more recently, human CNS progenitor cells in culture are also susceptible to JCV infection (19). The latter finding is of particular interest in regard to the pathogenesis of this disease. Since progenitor cells are responsible for repopulating various cell types in the brain, infection of this population of cells, as demonstrated in cell culture, could not only interfere with normal recovery after injury but also serve as a potential reservoir for virus during periods of latency.

Urinary Tract Diseases

The human polyomavirus BKV was first isolated in 1971 from the urine of a renal transplant recipient. Both of the human polyomaviruses, JCV and BKV, are excreted in the urine of healthy and immunocompromised individuals. Interestingly, there can also be an increased incidence of viruria in pregnant women, which may be indicative of the paradoxical immune suppression experienced by the body during pregnancy. Occasional cases of cystitis in healthy children have also been reported and have been associated with primary BKV infection. In both adult and pediatric patients with acquired immune deficiencies during the course of organ transplants, there is a particularly high risk of BKV reactivation and productive infection in the cells of the tubular epithelium, which could ultimately lead to allograft rejection. The incidence is indeed high enough to necessitate management of polyomavirus infections in transplant recipients, as well as potential screening of organ donors. Particularly in recent years, there has been a rapid increase in reported complications due to polyomavirus infections in renal and bone marrow transplant recipients. Because BKV remains latent in the kidneys, organ transplantation from seropositive donors to seronegative recipients may lead to BKV nephropathy in the setting of immunosuppressive regimens.

The hallmark of BKV nephropathy following transplantation has been considered to be the presence of "decoy" cells in the urine, which are infected cells with visible viral inclusion bodies that have been shed from the epithelium (9). However, urine analysis is best used as a screening process, since the definitive histologic signs of BKV nephropathy include viral inclusions or DNA in renal tubular cells and glomerular epithelial cells, as well as enlarged, irregular nuclei. Inflammatory infiltrates may be involved in persisting nephropathy, a condition that has been termed interstitial nephritis. End-stage disease is marked by fibrosis and tubular necrosis.

Human Malignancies

Much attention has been focused recently on the potential association between polyomavirus infection and the development of tumors in humans. Polyomaviruses are oncogenic in laboratory animals and can transform human cell lines. Indeed, "T" in simian virus 40 (SV40) large T was so named due to its transforming capability. During the period from 1955 through early 1963, millions of people worldwide were inadvertently exposed to SV40 via contaminated polio vaccines prepared using primary rhesus monkey cells. The accidental introduction of SV40 to humans and the demonstrated oncogenicity in human cells raised concerns about long-term effects of SV40 exposure (4). Similarly, DNA sequences from the human polyomaviruses JCV and BKV have been found in a variety of tumors, including those of the CNS (23). However, a recently completed study of the presence of JCV, BKV, and SV40 viral nucleotide sequences in a large sampling of human brain tumors did not reveal any association (25). As yet, a direct causal relationship has not yet been established (24), and the significance of these observations with respect to etiology remains mainly descriptive and unclear in relevance.

Detection of Viral Antigens

Immunostaining

Viral antigens can be identified in infected cells or tissues by use of antibody-based assays such as indirect immunofluorescence or immunoperoxidase staining. In the past, antisera made by immunizing rabbits with disrupted viral capsids and cross-reactive to JCV, BKV, and other polyomaviruses were utilized. However, there are now more specific polyclonal and monoclonal antibodies in existence that can identify either early or late proteins of specific polyomaviruses. In paraffin-embedded tissue or biopsy specimens, viral protein staining is usually confined to the nucleus.

ELISA of Urine Supernatants

JCV or BKV viral particles in urine specimens can be detected efficiently by a standard antigen capture ELISA protocol. Hyperimmune rabbit serum is used to coat the wells of microtiter plates as capture antibody. Urine supernatants are then added to the wells. Human sera having high titers to BKV or JCV are used as the detector antibody, and signal generation is obtained with an alkaline phosphatase-conjugated anti-human immunoglobulin G linked to an appropriate substrate. In this manner, relatively low levels of viruria can be rapidly detected to screen for potential reactivation in transplant recipients. However, PCR techniques have largely replaced ELISAs for the detection of viral nucleotide sequences in the urine and are increasingly directed toward the determination of viral copy numbers.

Hemagglutination Assay

The human polyomaviruses have the ability to agglutinate human type O erythrocytes (20). The antigen responsible for the hemagglutinating activity is located on the Vp1 capsid protein. Serial dilutions of samples are typically made in a microtiter plate in Alsever's solution, after which purified human type O erythrocytes are added to the wells. After a 6- to 12-h incubation at 4°C, an approximate virus titer in hemagglutination units can be read as the reciprocal of the highest dilution of sample that results in hemagglutination.

Detection of Viral DNA Sequences

In Situ DNA Hybridization

A definitive diagnosis of PML requires the demonstration of JCV virions or DNA in biopsy specimens taken from lesions in the brain or the presence of JCV DNA in the CSF. The most specific and reliable assay for detecting replicating viral DNA is in situ DNA hybridization using a JCV-specific, biotinylated DNA probe (10). After overnight hybridization, the probe is detected using a streptavidin-biotin-horseradish peroxidase signal-generating system and diaminobenzidine. If viral DNA is present, the nuclei stain light to dark brown. Unlike immunofluorescent staining, which uses cross-reactive antibodies, in situ DNA hybridization can be performed using very specific probes that can selectively identify JCV, BKV, or SV40. Furthermore, since the sensitivity of this assay is in the range of approximately 100 genome copies, a positive result is indicative of replicating viral DNA and active infection.

PCR Analysis

Polyomavirus DNA sequences can be detected from a number of tissues and fluids by PCR, which makes it a very powerful tool in helping to diagnose infection and pathogenesis of associated diseases. Specific primers can be designed to selectively amplify viral DNA from each of the polyomaviruses. Of more recent interest is the concept of quantifying viral copy numbers from CSF as a potential marker for disease progression in PML patients. Similarly, rising BKV copy numbers in the urine could be an indicator of reactivation in transplant recipients. To this end, real-time quantitative PCR protocols have been established for the human polyomaviruses by using serial dilutions of plasmid containing whole viral genomes to generate the standard curve (26). This technique is very sensitive and efficient and can detect down to one viral copy with reproducibility. In terms of clinical use, the presence of polyomavirus DNA sequences in CSF or urine provides support for a differential diagnosis.

Serology

Hemagglutination Inhibition Assay

To determine antibody titers against the human polyomaviruses, a hemagglutination inhibition assay can be performed using viral antigen to coat the wells of microtiter plates and then adding serial dilutions of human serum. Human type O erythrocytes are then used for hemagglutination. An antibody titer can be read as the reciprocal of the highest dilution that inhibits hemagglutination. Polyomavirus VLPs have been developed by self-assembly of purified Vp1 proteins. For assay purposes, VLPs have replaced the use of infected-cell culture supernatants as the source of antigen (29). Hemagglutination inhibition assays were heavily employed in the past in early serological studies to examine the worldwide distribution of these viruses.

ELISA

A more rapid and reproducible measurement of antibody titers is obtained by ELISA (8). Just as in hemagglutination inhibition, the polyomavirus VLP of interest is used to coat microtiter plate wells and serial dilutions of sera are layered on top. Labeled anti-human secondary antibodies are added to detect the antipolyomavirus antibodies bound to the antigen. Colorimetric detection and readings at specified wavelengths are then used to determine end-point dilutions. Alternatively, readings can be compared to a standard curve. Using either BKV or JCV VLPs, it has been demonstrated that antibodies against these viruses are very specific and do not cross-react. Furthermore, titers to JCV and BKV generally demonstrate a reciprocal relationship, indicating that individuals most probably experienced independent infections by the two viruses.

Conclusion

Immunologic assays are generally not helpful in diagnosing disease, since seroconversion occurs very early in life and persists throughout adulthood. High antibody titers to JCV have not been associated with an increased incidence of PML, although there is some evidence that a link may exist between BKV antibody titers in renal transplant donors and recipients and the risk for allograft rejection. Furthermore, serological data do not show a correlation of JCV and BKV antibody titers with an increased incidence of tumor formation in humans. Diagnostic testing at present relies heavily on DNA-based technologies such as in situ DNA hybridization and quantitative PCR.

REFERENCES

1. **Astrom, K. E., E. L. Mancall, and E. P. Richardson, Jr.** 1958. Progressive multifocal leuko-encephalopathy; a hitherto unrecognized complication of chronic lymphatic leukaemia and Hodgkin's disease. *Brain* **81:**93–111.
2. **Berger, J. R.** 2000. Progressive multifocal leukoencephalopathy. *Curr. Treat. Options Neurol.* **2:**361–368.
3. **Bosch, F. X., M. M. Manos, N. Munoz, M. Sherman, A. M. Jansen, J. Peto, M. H. Schiffman, V. Moreno, R. Kurman, and K. V. Shah, and the International Biological Study on Cervical Cancer Study Group.** 1995. Prevalence of human papillomavirus in cervical cancer: a worldwide perspective. *J. Natl. Cancer Inst.* **87:**796–802.
4. **Dang-Tan, T., S. M. Mahmud, R. Puntoni, and E. L. Franco.** 2004. Polio vaccines, simian virus 40, and human cancer: the epidemiologic evidence for a causal association. *Oncogene* **23:**6535–6540.
5. **De Luca, A., M. L. Giancola, A. Ammassari, S. Grisetti, M. G. Paglia, M. Gentile, A. Cingolani, R. Murri, G. Liuzzi, A. D. Monforte, and A. Antinori.** 2000. The effect of potent antiretroviral therapy and JC virus load in cerebrospinal fluid on clinical outcome of patients with AIDS-associated progressive multifocal leukoencephalopathy. *J. Infect. Dis.* **182:**1077–1083.
6. **Du Pasquier, R. A., S. Corey, D. H. Margolin, K. Williams, L. A. Pfister, U. De Girolami, J. J. Mac Key, C. Wuthrich, J. T. Joseph, and I. J. Koralnik.** 2003. Productive infection of cerebellar granule cell neurons by JC virus in an HIV+ individual. *Neurology* **61:**775–782.
7. **Gillison, M. L., W. M. Koch, R. B. Capone, M. D. Spafford, W. H. Westra, L. Wu, M. L. Zahurak, R. W. Daniel, M. Viglione, D. E. Symer, K. V. Shah, and D. Sidransky.** 2000. Evidence for a causal association between human papillomavirus and a subset of head and neck cancers. *J. Natl. Cancer Inst.* **92:**709–720.
8. **Hamilton, R. S., M. Gravell, and E. O. Major.** 2000. Comparison of antibody titers determined by hemagglutination inhibition and enzyme immunoassay for JC virus and BK virus. *J. Clin. Microbiol.* **38:**105–109.
9. **Hirsch, H. H., W. Knowles, M. Dickenmann, J. Passweg, T. Klimkait, M. J. Mihatsch, and J. Steiger.** 2002. Prospective study of polyomavirus type BK replication and nephropathy in renal-transplant recipients. *N. Engl. J. Med.* **347:**488–496.
10. **Houff, S. A., D. Katz, C. V. Kufta, and E. O. Major.** 1989. A rapid method for in situ hybridization for viral DNA in brain biopsies from patients with AIDS. *AIDS* **3:**843–845.
11. **Houff, S. A., E. O. Major, D. A. Katz, C. V. Kufta, J. L. Sever, S. Pittaluga, J. R. Roberts, J. Gitt, N. Saini, and W. Lux.** 1988. Involvement of JC virus-infected mononuclear cells from the bone marrow and spleen in the pathogenesis of progressive multifocal leukoencephalopathy. *N. Engl. J. Med.* **318:**301–305.

12. **Howley, P. M., and D. R. Lowy.** 2001. Papillomaviruses and their replication, p. 2197–2229. *In* D. M. Knipe and P. M. Howley (ed.), *Fields Virology*, 4th ed. Lippincott Williams & Wilkins, Philadelphia, Pa.

13. **International Agency for Research on Cancer.** 1995. *IARC Monograph on the Evaluation of Carcinogenic Risks to Humans*, vol. 64. *Human Papillomaviruses*. International Agency for Research on Cancer, Lyon, France.

14. **Jablonska, S., and S. Majewski.** 1972. Epidermodysplasia verruciformis: immunological and clinical aspects, p. 157–175. *In* H. zur Hausen (ed.), *Human Pathogenic Papillomaviruses*. Springer Verlag KG, Heidelberg, Germany.

15. **Khalili, K., J. Rappaport, and G. Khoury.** 1988. Nuclear factors in human brain cells bind specifically to the JCV regulatory region. *EMBO J.* **7:**1205–1210.

16. **Kirnbauer, R., N. L. Hubbert, C. M. Wheeler, T. M. Becker, D. R. Lowy, and J. T. Schiller.** 1994. A virus-like particle enzyme-linked immunosorbent assay detects serum antibodies in a majority of women infected with human papillomavirus type 16. *J. Natl. Cancer Inst.* **86:**494–499.

17. **Koutsky, L. A., K. A. Ault, C. M. Wheeler, D. R. Brown, E. Barr, F. B. Alvarez, L. M. Chiacchierini, and K. U. Jansen.** 2002. A controlled trial of a human papillomavirus type 16 vaccine. *N. Engl. J. Med.* **347:**1645–1651.

18. **Major, E. O., K. Amemiya, C. S. Tornatore, S. A. Houff, and J. R. Berger.** 1992. Pathogenesis and molecular biology of progressive multifocal leukoencephalopathy, the JC virus-induced demyelinating disease of the human brain. *Clin. Microbiol. Rev.* **5:**49–73.

19. **Messam, C. A., J. Hou, R. M. Gronostajski, and E. O. Major.** 2003. Lineage pathway of human brain progenitor cells identified by JC virus susceptibility. *Ann. Neurol.* **53:**636–646.

20. **Padgett, B., and D. Walker.** 1976. New human papovaviruses. *Prog. Med. Virol.* **22:**1–35.

21. **Padgett, B. L., D. L. Walker, G. M. Zu Rhein, R. J. Eckroade, and B. H. Dessel.** 1971. Cultivation of papova-like virus from human brain with progressive multifocal leukoencephalopathy. *Lancet* **i:**1257–1260.

22. **Pfister, H.** 2003. Human papillomavirus and skin cancer. *J. Natl. Cancer Inst. Monogr.* **31:**52–56.

23. **Reiss, K., and K. Khalili.** 2003. Viruses and cancer: lessons from the human polyomavirus, JCV. *Oncogene* **22:**6517–6523.

24. **Rollison, D. E., K. J. Helzlsouer, A. J. Alberg, S. Hoffman, J. Hou, R. Daniel, K. V. Shah, and E. O. Major.** 2003. Serum antibodies to JC virus, BK virus, simian virus 40, and the risk of incident adult astrocytic brain tumors. *Cancer Epidemiol. Biomarkers Prev.* **12:**460–463.

25. **Rollison, D. E. M., U. Utaipat, C. Ryschkewitsch, J. Hou, P. Goldthwaite, R. Daniel, K. J. Helzlsouer, P. C. Burger, K. V. Shah, and E. O. Major.** 2004. An investigation of human brain tumors for the presence of polyomavirus genome sequences by two independent laboratories. *Int. J. Cancer* **121:**217–221.

26. **Ryschkewitsch, C. F., P. N. Jensen, J. Hou, G. Fahle, S. Fischer, and E. O. Major.** 2005. Comparison of PCR-Southern hybridization and quantitative real time PCR for the detection of JC and BK viral nucleotide sequences in urine and cerebrospinal fluid. *J. Virol. Methods* **121:**217–221.

27. **Schiller, J. T., and D. R. Lowy.** 2004. Preventive human papillomavirus vaccines, p. 325–343. *In* T. Rohan and K. V. Shah (ed.), *Cervical Cancer: from Etiology to Prevention*. Kluwer Academic Publishers, Dordrecht, The Netherlands.

28. **Sun, Y., J. Eluf-Neto, F. X. Bosch, N. Muñoz, M. Booth, J. M. Walboomers, K. V. Shah, and R. P. Viscidi.** 1994. Human papillomavirus-related serological markers of invasive cervical carcinoma in Brazil. *Cancer Epidemiol. Biomarkers Prev.* **3:**341–347.

29. **Viscidi, R. P., D. E. Rollison, E. Viscidi, B. Clayman, E. Rubalcaba, R. Daniel, E. O. Major, and K. V. Shah.** 2003. Serological cross-reactivities between antibodies to simian virus 40, BK virus, and JC virus assessed by virus-like-particle-based enzyme immunoassays. *Clin. Diagn. Lab. Immunol.* **10:**278–285.

30. **Walboomers, J. M. M., M. V. Jacobs, M. M. Manos, F. X. Bosch, J. A. Kummer, K. V. Shah, P. J. F. Snijders, J. Peto, C. J. L. M. Meijer, and N. Muñoz.** 1999. Human papillomavirus is a necessary cause of invasive cervical cancer worldwide. *J. Pathol.* **189:**12–19.

Adenoviruses

LETA K. CRAWFORD-MIKSZA

76

The accidental discovery in 1953 of "spontaneous" cytopathic degeneration in cell cultures of human adenoid tissue led to the discovery of a new family of viruses. The original name proposed for this phenomenon was "adenoid degeneration agent" (36). Observation of this type of cytopathology in cell cultures inoculated with specimens from a number of clinical syndromes quickly followed, leading to the designation adenoidal-pharyngeal-conjunctival agents in 1954 (25), replaced by the less cumbersome adenovirus (Ad) within 2 years. Since then, it has become clear that Ads are ubiquitous microorganisms, isolated from every mammalian, marsupial, bird, and reptile species that has been studied, yet they are host specific, even among primates. They share a nonenveloped, icosahedral capsid structure and a linear double-stranded DNA genome of approximately 36 kbp. There are three capsid proteins on the surface of the virus. The icosahedral faces are covered with 240 hexon capsomers, each composed of a trimer of the hexon protein. The 12 vertex capsomers are composed of the penton base, containing five copies of the penton protein, and the protruding fiber attachment complex with one or two fibers, each carrying a trimer of the fiber protein (49). Ads are classified into serotypes with immunological reagents that delineate (i) type-specific neutralization, defined by epitopes on the hexon protein, and (ii) type-specific hemagglutination-inhibition (HI), defined by epitopes on the fiber attachment protein (46). To date, the human adenoviruses (HAds) number 51 serotypes that are subdivided into six species (A through F) on the basis of fiber protein characteristics, DNA homology, and biological properties (15, 23, 40). Among adults, transmission occurs by respiratory droplet, but among young children fecal-oral spread predominates. Even in overt respiratory disease, HAds are shed in stools in greater numbers for a longer period than from the respiratory tract, and asymptomatic persistent shedding of virus for weeks to months is common (17).

Within the viral genome, the hexon capsid protein contains regions with both the greatest degree of conservation and the highest degree of mutability. The hexon protein elicits two types of immunological response in HAd infection. Type-specific neutralizing antibody is directed against epitopes on the exposed surfaces of the hexon that are unique to each serotype (12), and nonneutralizing, broadly cross-reactive antibody that is directed against conserved genus-specific regions of this protein is shared by all known HAds.

Early studies showed that neutralizing antibody appeared within 2 weeks of primary infection, at relatively low titers of 8 to 80, and then declined to undetectable levels over a 2-year period if reexposure did not occur (25). Seroprevalence of any given serotype therefore depends on the levels of that virus circulating in the community. Seroprevalence of endemic serotypes associated with respiratory infections, such as HAd type 2 (HAd2) and HAd7a, has been found in 25 to 100% of the populations studied, consistent with continuous reexposure, while antibodies to the serotypes involved in sporadic outbreaks of keratoconjunctivitis were found in 0 to 6% (44). The presence of neutralizing antibody does not affect persistence or protect against subsequent colonization with the same serotype but does protect against development of clinical disease (17). The level of nonneutralizing cross-reactive antibody also rises and declines within the same time frame, but there is a low-level anamnestic boost with each subsequent HAd infection (20). The levels of nonspecific indicators of inflammation, C-reactive protein and interleukin-6, are also substantially elevated during HAd infection (3, 26).

Apart from their role as human pathogens, there is currently enormous interest in the development of Ads as vectors for both gene delivery and chemotherapeutic agents. The majority of these are recombinant, engineered, replication-deficient variants of HAd5. This intense focus on Ad biology has resulted in a large and detailed body of information on the interactions between virus and host cell that may soon have therapeutic applications for clinical infections.

Laboratory diagnosis of HAd infections can be accomplished by three standard approaches. The first approach, isolation of the agent in cell culture followed by confirmation with a group-specific immunofluorescent reagent, is the usual method employed in most clinical settings. With the exception of the enteric serotypes HAd40 and -41, HAds are regarded as relatively easy to culture in several human heteroploid cell lines derived from carcinomas of the respiratory tract (HEp-2, A549, or KB). Diploid lung fibroblasts, used by most clinical virology laboratories for culture of cytomegalovirus and herpes simplex viruses, are also sensitive to most HAds but may be slower to display typical cytopathology. Serotype identification can be accomplished with neutralization tests in cell culture employing standardized immune serum pools, type-specific antisera, or molecular techniques. Although culture of an agent from a specimen collected from the site of pathology may constitute the definitive diagnosis, it may require 1 to 2 weeks, even with the improvements of shell vial culture and monoclonal antibodies for detection.

The second approach, using rapid methods of detection involving direct detection of viral antigens or nucleic acid in clinical materials, has improved the speed of diagnosis. Since the number and efficacies of antiviral chemotherapeutics are increasing, this is of direct benefit to the patient. At present, the only readily available methods of diagnosing gastroenteritis caused by HAd40 or -41 are direct detection of viral antigens in stool specimens by antigen capture, latex agglutination, or electron microscopy.

The third approach to diagnosis is through serologic tests. Serologic tests for HAd infections detect anti-HAd immunoglobulin M (IgM) in an acute-phase specimen and measure rises in group- or type-specific antibodies in paired serum specimens. Detection of IgM is now one of the earliest laboratory indicators of infection, often preceding culture results. Serologic diagnosis is particularly important when viral culture is delayed or not available and for confirmation of an etiologic relationship when a virus is isolated from a peripheral site. Virus isolation, identification, and antigen detection methods are discussed elsewhere (43). This chapter concentrates on serologic methods for diagnosis of HAd infections and recent advances in molecular detection of viral nucleic acid.

The most widely used methods for measuring HAd cross-reactive, genus-specific antibodies of both the IgG and the IgM classes are enzyme immunoassay (EIA) and indirect immunofluorescence (IIF) assay (also called indirect fluorescent-antibody assay). Complement fixation (CF), once used extensively, is the most standardized serologic test for diagnosis of HAd infection. However, by comparison with EIA and IIF, CF is cumbersome and much less sensitive, and its use is now limited to reference laboratories that still maintain CF capability for antigens for which there is no other suitable method. The EIA and IIF methods appear to have equivalent sensitivities, so the choice of one versus the other is more a matter of convenience, depending on the format and equipment being used for other serologies in the laboratory and personnel expertise. Laboratories may elect to use one method routinely and use the other as confirmation for problem specimens that are difficult to interpret, for example, when antinuclear antibody, rheumatoid factor, or other nonspecific reactions are present.

For some cases, in which an HAd is isolated from a peripheral site not directly involved in pathology, it is desirable to confirm an etiologic relationship by documenting a rise in the titer of type-specific neutralizing antibody between acute- and convalescent-phase specimens with that isolate. This can be accomplished by serum neutralization (SN) or HI tests. SN tests are also used extensively in serosurveys for the presence of neutralizing antibody to a specific serotype in defined populations, such as military recruits tested for serostatus to HAd4 and HAd7a (30), or to quantify preexisting antibody in those who are candidates to receive an adenoviral vector as a chemotherapeutic or gene transfer agent.

Specimen requirements for HAd serodiagnosis are standard: collection of whole blood that is allowed to clot and then separated. Care must be taken to collect the acute-phase specimen in the first few days of illness in order to detect the presence of IgM and avoid the anamnestic rise in group-specific antibody. Convalescent-phase specimens can be collected within 2 to 4 weeks after onset.

CLINICAL FEATURES

HAds are associated with a broad spectrum of clinical pathology (Table 1). Severity of infection may vary from asymptomatic subclinical infection to fulminant disseminated disease, but the individual contributions of viral virulence factors and host factors to pathogenesis are, as yet, poorly understood. In recent years, HAds have emerged as significant pathogens in fatal outbreaks in Malaysia, the United States, Israel, Japan, Korea, and Argentina, which may reflect an increase in the pathogenic potential of the strains involved (9, 48). While there are at least 51 human serotypes, the majority of clinical disease manifestations involve approximately one-fourth of them.

TABLE 1 Illnesses commonly associated with HAd infections

Disease(s)	Population at risk	Associated serotype(s)[a]
Acute febrile pharyngitis	Infants, young children	1, 2, 3, 5, 6, 7, and 7a
Pharyngoconjunctival fever	School-age children	3, 7, and 14
ARD	Military recruits, residential communities	4, 7, and 7a (3, 11, and 21)[b]
Pertussis-like syndrome	Infants, young children	5
Pneumonia	Any age group	1, 2, 3, 4, 5, 7, 7a, and 21
Epidemic keratoconjunctivitis	Any age group	8, 19, and 37 (3)
Acute hemorrhagic cystitis	Infants, young children, immunocompromised individuals	11 and 21 (7)
Gastroenteritis	Infants, young children	40 and 41
Intussusception	Infants, young children	Species C
Meningitis, encephalitis	Infants, young children	3, 5, 6, 7, 7a, and 12
Myocarditis, pericarditis	Infants, young children	1, 2, 3, 7, 7a, and 21
Disseminated disease, multiple organ involvement	Immunocompromised individuals	All, including many species D

[a]We have included the serotype designations for HAd7 and -7a. Early serology (36a) and recent genetic evidence (14) indicate that they are distinct strains, but most of the literature does not distinguish between them. Available sequence data for HAd7 genotypes determined by restriction enzyme profiles as 7b and 7d denote that they are of the 7a serotype (14).

[b]Serotypes in parentheses are less frequently associated with the syndrome.

Respiratory Diseases

The greatest numbers of clinical HAd infections involve the respiratory tract. It has been estimated that HAd infections account for 7% of all respiratory disease in children, including pneumonia, pneumonitis, bronchiolitis, croup, pharyngitis, bronchitis, and upper respiratory infections (8). HAds are responsible for serious and sometimes fatal outbreaks of acute respiratory disease (ARD) in closed residential communities, such as military barracks, orphanages, summer camps, chronic care facilities, and schools (10). Historically, epidemics of ARD in military personnel were the most significant cause of morbidity, hospitalizations, and work-time loss in new recruits and trainees until introduction of vaccines for HAd4 and HAd7a in the early 1970s. In 1996, the manufacturer of the vaccines discontinued production, and stocks of the vaccines were exhausted in 1998. Multiple military training centers have since experienced large outbreaks of HAd-induced ARD, and many more outbreaks are anticipated before a new vaccine can be produced and approved (19). Progression of HAd respiratory infections to pneumonia occurs in both adults and children and can be fatal even among immunocompetent individuals.

Diseases of the Eye

HAds are the etiologic agent of 20% of acute conjunctivitis in children (18) and 5% of epithelial keratitis in adults and children (11). Species D serotypes HAd8, -19, and -37 are well documented in numerous outbreaks of epidemic keratoconjunctivitis in adults and children in both community and institutional settings, including nosocomial infections in ophthalmology clinics.

Gastroenteritis

HAds account for 3 to 10% of pediatric gastroenteritis worldwide (6). The enteric HAds, HAd40 and HAd41, account for the majority of outbreaks, but many other serotypes have been associated with sporadic cases in children and adults, as well as gastrointestinal symptoms concomitant with respiratory disease.

Myocarditis and Pericarditis

A growing number of reports have linked HAds and acute myocarditis, with and without pericarditis, in infants and young children (31); sudden infant death associated with myocarditis (41); and idiopathic left ventricular dysfunction in adults (32). For the most part, diagnosis has been made by inference from throat or rectal cultures because isolation from heart tissue has not been productive. The difficulty in establishing a causal relationship through peripheral site culture has been resolved by the recent molecular characterization of HAds directly from heart tissue.

Infections in Immunocompromised Individuals

The rapid expansion of transplantation procedures and the longer survival times of persons with AIDS have contributed to an increasing population whose immune systems have been compromised by disease, chemotherapy, or genetics and who are particularly susceptible to viruses that establish latent and persistent infections. A wide range of pathology involving almost every organ system has been associated with HAd infection in this population, including fulminant hepatitis, encephalitis, cystitis, nephritis, and renal failure. HAds account for approximately 10% of the chronic diarrhea and colitis that are among the earliest manifestations of human immunodeficiency virus (HIV) infection (27). Since the introduction of effective chemotherapeutics for herpesviruses, HAds have emerged as one of the most significant causes of fatal infections in organ and bone marrow transplant patients, particularly allogeneic bone marrow and stem cell transplant recipients (27). HAd infection is also a significant risk factor for decreased survival time in persons with AIDS (37). This has led to recognition of the need for rapid and quantitative molecular assays to monitor adenoviral load during antiviral therapy, similar to those used for HIV (21, 22, 28).

In addition to the major disease syndromes, HAds have been linked to sporadic cases of more unusual presentations, including toxic shock-like syndrome, meningoencephalitis with and without flaccid paralysis, Reye's syndrome, venereal disease, hemorrhagic fever-like syndrome, and intussusception and mesenteric lymphadenopathy in young children. As with myocarditis, molecular detection of an HAd genome in the affected organs is moving us closer to establishing an etiologic relationship.

HAd serology is rarely requested alone but is usually requested as part of the differential diagnosis for the syndromes listed above. A respiratory agent battery may include HAd, influenza viruses A and B, *Mycoplasma pneumoniae*, respiratory syncytial virus, and *Chlamydia pneumoniae*. HAd serology may also be included in panels for conjunctivitis, gastroenteritis, meningitis, childhood rashes, myocarditis, and lymphadenopathy.

TEST PROCEDURES

EIA

EIA is now one of the most automated tests in the clinical laboratory and, for the most part, uses the 96-well microplate format, automated plate washers, and readers that define experimental parameters and interpret results. It is adaptable to any number of antigens, with a variety of anti-immunoglobulin enzyme conjugates and substrates. A recent innovation is the use of single-row microwell strips, or modules, that obviate the need for a whole 96-well plate, conserving antigen, reagents, and operator time. The availability of commercially prepared HAd antigen for EIA is currently unpredictable, but antigen can be prepared in-house if there are cell culture facilities.

EIA for both IgG and IgM detects genus-specific cross-reactive antibody so that, theoretically, any serotype may be used as an antigen. It is common practice to use one of the low-numbered endemic serotypes that grow to high titers in any of the cell cultures described above, i.e., HAd2, -3, -4, -5, or -7a. Flasks of cells that have just reached confluence are changed to maintenance medium of 98% Eagle's minimal essential medium in Hanks' balanced salt solution with 2% fetal bovine serum. A virus inoculum that induces a 4+ cytopathic effect in 3 to 5 days is used. Cells and fluids are harvested, subjected to three freeze-thaw cycles, and clarified of cell debris by centrifugation at $1,000 \times g$ for 10 min at 4°C. Whole virus is recovered by ultracentrifugation of the supernatant at $40,000 \times g$ for 4 h. The virus pellet is resuspended and disrupted in a small amount of solubilizing alkaline buffer (pH 9.0) containing 10 mM Tris, 0.14 M NaCl, 4 mM EDTA, 0.1% sodium desoxycholate, and 0.1% NP-40. Viral lysate is titrated and then diluted in 5 mM phosphate-buffered saline (PBS) (pH 7.2 to 7.4), usually diluted 1:50 to 1:200. This working dilution of antigen is used to coat 96-well plates or strip wells by evaporation to dryness at 37°C. Plates and strips specifically treated for antigen absorption are commercially available. Stored in airtight plastic bags with desiccant at 4°C, this antigen is stable for 1 year.

Uninfected cell cultures are treated exactly the same for use as negative cell controls.

The commercial conjugates for EIA that are currently available are anti-human immunoglobulins labeled with one of two types of enzyme, either horseradish peroxidase or alkaline phosphatase. The choices of substrate, stop solution, and detection wavelength are determined by the enzyme used. Substrate and stop solutions are commercially available as well. For horseradish peroxidase, the substrate may be o-phenylenediamine or tetramethylbenzidene with hydrogen peroxide, the reaction may be stopped with acid (1 N HCl or 2 M phosphoric acid), and the results may be read at A_{492} or A_{450}, respectively. For alkaline phosphatase, the substrate is usually p-nitrophenyl phosphate for EIA applications, the reaction is stopped with alkaline solutions (50 mM trisodium phosphate, pH 12.6), and the results are read at A_{405}. The optimal dilution of conjugate should be determined in each laboratory according to the manufacturer's guidelines.

Specimens to be tested for IgM are first treated with a commercially available anti-human IgG according to the manufacturer's recommendations. The wash buffer is 5 mM PBS (pH 7.2 to 7.4) with 0.05% Tween 20. The diluent for both sera and conjugates is wash buffer with 1% casein blocking agent. Sodium azide (0.01%) may be added to the wash and diluent buffers as a preservative. Plates or strip wells are removed from 4°C storage and washed three times, drained, and blotted. Serial dilutions of test sera, beginning at 1:200, are added to antigen and control wells, and the plates are incubated at 37°C for 1 h in a moist chamber or sealed. After the plates are washed five times, drained, and blotted, diluted anti-IgG or -IgM conjugates are added and the plates are incubated at 37°C for 1 h. The plates are washed five times, substrate is added, and the plates are incubated for 15 to 30 min. Stop solution is added, and the plates are read in an automated plate reader at the required wavelength. Each EIA run should contain negative cell controls, reagent controls, and positive-control sera. The optical density of the substrate solution alone should be <0.6 U, and for other negative controls it should be <1.0 U.

IIF

IIF detects genus-specific, cross-reactive anti-HAd antibodies of both the IgG and the IgM classes, depending on the conjugates used. It provides a good alternative to EIA when relatively few samples are being tested or when results are needed as quickly as possible. It does require a good-quality epifluorescence microscope and experienced laboratory personnel. Antigen slides with HAd grown in cell culture, normal cell controls, anti-human immunoglobulins conjugated with fluorescein isothiocyanate with counterstain, and control sera are currently available commercially from several sources. Optimal working dilutions of conjugates must be determined with each new lot according to the manufacturer's guidelines. It is also possible to prepare antigen slides in-house, if desired. Preprinted glass slides with 8, 10, or 12 wells are used. As in the case of EIA, the choice of HAd serotype is not critical, and the same viruses and cells listed above may be used. Cell culture flasks are infected with an inoculum that produces cytopathic effect in 50 to 75% of the cells (2+ to 3+) in 2 to 3 days. Uninfected cell cultures are maintained at the same time. Infected and uninfected cells are harvested by gentle trypsinization and resuspended in a small volume of PBS. Uninfected cells are pooled with infected cells at a 1:2 ratio so that an optimal 25 to 30% of cells will stain with control sera. Uninfected cells are used to make cell control spots on the same or separate glass slides. Infected and uninfected cell suspensions are dotted onto printed slides, allowed to air dry, and fixed in cold fresh acetone for 10 min. Stored at −70°C, they are stable for >1 year. Each new lot of antigen must be validated with the conjugates for sensitivity and specificity.

Specimens tested for anti-HAd IgM are absorbed with anti-IgG as described above. Test sera are diluted fourfold in PBS (pH 7.2 to 7.4), beginning at 1:8 for IgG determinations and 1:10 for absorbed sera for IgM determinations. A 1:8 or 1:10 dilution of each test serum is added to a negative control well, and PBS alone is added to infected and uninfected wells as a conjugate control. Slides are incubated in a moist chamber at 35 to 37°C for 20 min. Sera are decanted, and the slides are washed in fresh PBS for 5 min. Working dilution of conjugate is added, and the slides are incubated and washed as described above and then allowed to air dry. A preservative mounting medium of 10% polyvinyl alcohol (crystalline, type II)–20% glycerol in 50 mM Tris buffer (pH 8.5) is applied, and a coverslip is applied. The slides are examined for the degree and location of fluorescence. HAd antigen is located primarily in the nucleus, where viral replication takes place, but also may be seen in the cytoplasm. The degree of fluorescence is calibrated as for any other immunofluorescent procedure, from 1+ to 4+, with 1+ as the cutoff for positivity. When paired sera are tested and the rise in titer is greater than fourfold, no further testing is required. However, if endpoints fall relatively close together, the test may need to be repeated with serial twofold dilutions bracketing the endpoints.

SN

Rarely, a type-specific immune response must be determined, and SN is the test of choice. Several microplate formats that facilitate the use of multichannel pipettors, plate washers, and even automated plate readers have been described (13, 24). In a clinical setting, the virus used is usually the patient isolate or stock virus culture of the serotype of interest. There are a few species D serotypes that do not grow to high enough titers to be tested in a microplate format and require testing in a tube format, but they are not often encountered. A colorimetric microneutralization procedure using a spectrophotometer capable of reading an A_{550} is the simplest and most automated of the microtiter formats (13). The tube format is described elsewhere (43).

HI

HAds are able to hemagglutinate several types of mammalian erythrocytes in vitro. They were originally grouped by their hemagglutination properties, which are based on fiber protein characteristics (Table 2). The immune response to HAd infection includes type-specific antibody directed against the fiber protein, which inhibits hemagglutination. HI was originally used to serotype an HAd isolate with standardized antisera and was evaluated as a diagnostic test for serologic diagnosis of HAd infection. Its utility as a diagnostic test is limited by the requirements for the patient's own virus isolate, fresh sources of rat and rhesus erythrocytes, and pretreatment of test sera to remove nonspecific inhibitors of hemagglutination. While it is still the means to characterize the fiber protein for new and untypeable HAd strains, even this has been complicated by the increasing emergence of naturally occurring recombinant HAd strains that express the hexon protein of one serotype and fiber protein of another. A description of the test is given in a previous edition of this manual (15a).

TABLE 2 Ad serotypes grouped into species by hemagglutination and DNA homology

Species	Serotype(s)	Hemagglutination pattern
A	12, 18, and 31	Rat, incomplete[a]
B	B1 (3, 7, 7a, 16, 21, and 50) and B2 (11, 14, 34, and 35)	Rhesus, complete
C	1, 2, 5, and 6	Rat, incomplete[a]
D	8–10, 13, 15, 17, 19, 20, 22–30, 32, 33, 36–39, 42–49, and 51	Rat, complete
E	4	Rat, incomplete[a]
F	40 and 41	Rat, incomplete[a]

[a]Requires the presence of 1% heterotypic antiserum in diluent for complete agglutination.

MOLECULAR TECHNIQUES FOR DIAGNOSIS

Detection of viral nucleic acid in clinical materials is the most rapidly expanding diagnostic methodology in medicine, overtaking culture as the "gold standard" for diagnosis of infectious disease. Several different strategies have been developed for both target and signal amplification and incorporated into commercially prepared kits and detection systems for a variety of microorganisms. Of these, PCR amplification of viral nucleic acid has demonstrated the greatest versatility and applicability. The obvious advantages of PCR include speed and increased sensitivity in situations in which virus isolation is unproductive or impossible. Outcome studies have documented the clinical and financial advantages of rapid diagnosis (5, 35). The disadvantages include the lack of a viable isolate to characterize biologically, the limited information available from conserved regions when consensus primers are used, and the problems associated with PCR contamination. Despite these difficulties, PCR is the most thoroughly studied and most widely used amplification tool today. The refinements of real-time PCR, multiplexing, and nested protocols have only increased its utility.

PCR

Nucleic Acid Extraction

Nucleic acid extraction is the limiting step in all amplification protocols. In a clinical setting, the identity of the microbial agent of infection is rarely known prior to testing, so that DNA and RNA viruses, as well as bacteria, yeasts, and parasites, may be part of the differential diagnosis. For this reason, we recommend an extraction procedure that isolates total nucleic acid, so that both PCR and reverse transcriptase-mediated PCR may be performed from the same extract. The all-purpose extraction method of Boom et al. (7), in which guanidinium isothiocyanate (GuSCN) is used with silica adsorbent, has been used successfully for bacteria and RNA and DNA viruses. Briefly, 100 μl of body fluids or 100 mg of tissue is dissolved for 20 min in 0.9 ml of lysis buffer (5 M GuSCN in 50 mM Tris-HCl [pH 6.4]–20 mM EDTA–1.5% [vol/vol] Triton X-100), with disposable microtube pestles used for homogenization if necessary. Large fragments of debris are removed by centrifugation. Powdered silica is added to adsorb nucleic acid, which is then washed sequentially in wash buffer (lysis buffer without EDTA or Triton X-100), 70% ethanol, and acetone to dry, and finally eluted in 100 μl of RNase-free 10 mM Tris (pH 7.5).

Automated nucleic acid extraction machines, using this or other chemistry, are available from several vendors, as are numerous commercially available cartridges, columns, and reagents, which work well with some clinical specimens but not others, especially tissue.

Formalin-fixed, paraffin-embedded tissues present different but not insurmountable extraction problems. Several protocols have been described elsewhere (1, 45). Again, we recommend a procedure that extracts total nucleic acid for the reasons given above. In our laboratory, we have adapted a method for extraction that provides total nucleic acid using phenol-chloroform-isoamyl alcohol at pH 8.0 (42).

Amplification

A number of PCR protocols have been devised for HAd amplification, and many target conserved genes in one of two ways. Conservation among Ads is a relative term: while protein sequence may be conserved in a given region, DNA sequence may be extremely degenerate, and therefore the primers used must contain some level of degeneracy. The hexon gene carries regions of maximum protein conservation, and several assays target short sequences within these regions with degenerate consensus primers (4). The drawback is that the serotype or genotype cannot be deduced from these amplicons, merely the presence or absence of HAd. Other assays target regions of type specificity with type-specific primers when a limited number of serotypes are suspected, as in gastroenteritis outbreaks or ARD in military recruits (14). Real-time PCR assays use this approach because real-time assays cannot tolerate degeneracy in primers or probes (16). The drawback of this approach is the limitation in detectable serotypes, which is not optimal for community-acquired infections or infections in the immunocompromised. More recently, nested PCR protocols that increase the sensitivity of detection as well as increase the size of the amplicon so that further characterization is possible by restriction fragment length polymorphism analysis or sequencing have been described (2, 29, 38, 39). Our laboratory and others now routinely use a nested protocol to amplify six of the type-specific hypervariable regions of the hexon protein so that serotype identification is possible by sequencing (2, 39). Others use multiplex formats to determine species, if not serotype (33, 47). Appropriate controls are critical for PCR. As in all laboratory tests, there is an element of risk for cross-contamination of specimens and reagents, but this appears to be even greater with molecular biology-based techniques. There should be sufficient negative controls to rule out PCR contamination and internal controls to assess the quality of nucleic acid present.

The choice of any given format for a laboratory depends on a number of considerations, particularly the patient population to which it will be applied. Military hospitals do not have the same needs as a tertiary-care teaching hospital with a large transplant population. Logistics within the laboratory itself, in terms of equipment, trained personnel, and cost-benefit analysis, play an equally important role.

INTERPRETATION

The classical fourfold or greater rise in titer of either group- or type-specific antibody between acute-phase and convalescent-phase specimens is considered diagnostic of HAd infections. The difficulty with this is that after 2 to 4 weeks postonset the clinical relevance may be lost. There are also difficulties in documenting a fourfold rise when the acute-phase specimen is not collected early enough. The increased sensitivity of EIA and IIF for the detection of genus-specific antibody, compared with that of CF, usually means that there is some level of antibody in the population due to constant exposure to endemic serotypes. The heterotypic anamnestic rise that occurs early in infection may obscure a fourfold rise in titer of antibody to the infecting serotype when the acute-phase specimen is not collected in the first few days.

The presence or absence of IgM may be determined in the acute phase and therefore be more clinically relevant. IgM determinations by EIA or IIF are well standardized procedures for a number of infectious agents. However, the clinical significance of IgM in HAd infection has not been well studied. Most of the serologic surveys that defined the immunological response to HAd infection predate our ability to distinguish the IgM component. This is certainly a subject that requires further study.

However, serologic tests for HAd infections are only one part of the total laboratory diagnostic workup that may include culture and antigen or nucleic acid detection. Each of these approaches confirms and validates the others, and diagnosis is rarely made by just one approach. A recent comparison of six methods for ARD diagnosis showed that traditional viral culture, PCR, and serology had almost equivalent sensitivities but that each of these three methods detected a slightly different segment of the cohort (34). It is therefore desirable to augment serologic diagnosis with one or more additional approaches.

The significance of a PCR result, i.e., the presence or absence of the viral genome in a given specimen, should be interpreted in the same way that a positive or negative culture result is interpreted. HAds are capable of persistent and latent infection, and various factors must be taken into account, including the site from which the specimen is taken (peripheral versus site of pathology), the timing and integrity of specimen collection, the sensitivity of the assay employed, and consistency with clinical presentation. The possibility of PCR contamination must also be evaluated. As with interpretation of serological test results, it is better to have the corroboration of additional methods of diagnosis if possible.

REFERENCES

1. **Akhtar, N., J. Ni, C. Langston, G. J. Demmler, and J. A. Towbin.** 1996. PCR diagnosis of viral pneumonitis from fixed-lung tissue in children. *Biochem. Mol. Med.* **58:**66–76.
2. **Allard, A., B. Albinson, and G. Wadell.** 2001. Rapid typing of human adenoviruses by a general PCR combined with restriction endonuclease analysis. *J. Clin. Microbiol.* **39:**498–505.
3. **Appenzeller, C., R. A. Ammann, A. Duppenthaler, M. Gorgievski-Hrisobo, and C. Aebi.** 2002. Serum C-reactive protein in children with adenovirus infection. *Swiss Med. Wkly.* **132:**345–350.
4. **Avellon, A., P. Perez, J. C. Aguilar, R. O. de Lejarazu, and J. E. Echevarria.** 2001. Rapid and sensitive diagnosis of human adenovirus infections by a generic polymerase chain reaction. *J. Virol. Methods* **92:**113–120.
5. **Barenfanger, J., C. Drake, N. Leon, T. Miller, and T. Troutt.** 2000. Clinical and financial benefits of rapid detection of respiratory viruses: an outcomes study. *J. Clin. Microbiol.* **38:**2824–2828.
6. **Bon, F. P. F., M. Dauvergne, D. Tenenbaum, H. Planson, A. M. Petion, P. Pothier, and E. Kohli.** 1999. Prevalence of group A rotavirus, human calicivirus, astrovirus, and adenovirus type 40 and 41 infections among children with acute gastroenteritis in Dijon, France. *J. Clin. Microbiol.* **37:**3055–3058.
7. **Boom, R., C. J. A. Sol, M. M. M. Salimans, C. L. Jansen, P. M. E. Wertheim-van Dillen, and J. van der Noordaa.** 1990. Rapid and simple method for purification of nucleic acids. *J. Clin. Microbiol.* **28:**495–503.
8. **Brandt, C. D., H. W. Kim, A. J. Vargosko, B. C. Jeffries, J. O. Arrobio, B. Rindge, R. H. Parrott, and R. M. Chanock.** 1969. Infections in 18,000 infants and children in a controlled study of respiratory tract disease. I. Adenovirus pathogenicity in relation to serologic type and illness syndrome. *Am. J. Epidemiol.* **90:**484–500.
9. **Cardosa, M. J., S. Krishnan, P. H. Tio, D. Perera, S. C. Wong.** 1999. Isolation of subgenus B adenovirus during a fatal outbreak of enterovirus 71-associated hand, foot and mouth disease in Sibu, Sarawak. *Lancet* **354:**987–991.
10. **Centers for Disease Control.** 1998. Civilian outbreak of adenovirus acute respiratory disease—South Dakota, 1997. *Morb. Mortal. Wkly. Rep.* **47:**567–570.
11. **Chodosh, J., D. Miller, W. G. Stroop, and S. C. Pflugfelder.** 1995. Adenovirus epithelial keratitis. *Cornea* **14:**167–174.
12. **Crawford-Miksza, L. K., and D. P. Schnurr.** 1996. Analysis of 15 adenovirus hexon proteins reveals the location and structure of seven hypervariable regions containing serotype-specific residues. *J. Virol.* **70:**1836–1844.
13. **Crawford-Miksza, L. K., and D. P. Schnurr.** 1994. Quantitative colorimetric microneutralization assay for characterization of adenoviruses. *J. Clin. Microbiol.* **32:**2331–2334.
14. **Crawford-Miksza, L. K., R. N. Nang, and D. P. Schnurr.** 1999. Strain variation in adenovirus serotypes 4 and 7a causing acute respiratory disease. *J. Clin. Microbiol.* **37:**1107–1112.
15. **De Jong, J. C., A. G. Wermendol, M. W. Verweij-Uijterwaal, K. W. Slaterus, P. Wertheim-Van Dillen, G. J. J. Van Doornum, S. H. Khoo, and J. C. Hierholzer.** 1999. Adenoviruses from human immunodeficiency virus-infected individuals, including two strains that represent new candidate serotypes Ad50 and Ad51 of species B1 and D, respectively. *J. Clin. Microbiol.* **37:**3940–3945.
15a. **Erdman, D. D., and J. E. Hierholzer.** 1997. Adenoviruses, p. 661–666. *In* N. R. Rose, E. Conway de Macario, J. D. Folds, H. C. Lane, and R. M. Nakamura (ed.), *Manual of Clinical Laboratory Immunology*, 5th ed. ASM Press, Washington, D.C.
16. **Faix, D. J., H.-S. H. Houng, J. C. Gaydos, S.-K. S. Liu, J. T. Connors, X. Brown, L. V. Asher, D. W. Vaughn, and L. N. Binn.** 2004. Evaluation of a rapid quantitative diagnostic test for adenovirus type 4. *Clin. Infect. Dis.* **38:**391–397.
17. **Fox, J. P., and C. E. Hall.** 1980. *Viruses in Families*, p. 294–334. PSG Publishing, Littleton, Mass.
18. **Gigliotti, F., W. T. Williams, F. G. Hayden, and J. O. Hendley.** 1981. Etiology of acute conjunctivitis in children. *J. Pediatr.* **98:**531–536.
19. **Gray, G. C., J. D. Callahan, A. W. Hawksworth, C. A. Fisher, and J. C. Gaydos.** 1999. Respiratory diseases among U.S. military personnel: countering emerging threats. *Emerg. Infect. Dis.* **5:**379–387.
20. **Grayston, T. J., C. G. Loosli, P. B. Johnston, M. E. Smith, and R. L. Woolridge.** 1956. Neutralizing and complement fixing antibody response to adenovirus infection. *J. Infect. Dis.* **99:**199–206.
21. **Gu, Z., S. W. Belzer, C. S. Gibson, M. J. Bankowski, and R. T. Hayden.** 2003. Multiplexed real-time PCR for quantitative detection of human adenovirus. *J. Clin. Microbiol.* **41:**4631–4641.
22. **Heim, A., C. Ebnet, G. Harste, and P. Pring-Akerblom.** 2003. Rapid and quantitative detection of human adenovirus DNA by real-time PCR. *J. Med. Virol.* **70:**228–239.
23. **Hierholzer, J. C., R. Wigand, L. J. Anderson, T. Adrian, and J. W. M. Gold.** 1988. Adenoviruses from patients with AIDS: a plethora of serotypes and a description of five new serotypes of subgenus D (43–47). *J. Infect. Dis.* **158:**804–813.

24. **Hierholzer, J. C., and P. G. Bingham.** 1978. Vero microcultures for adenovirus neutralization tests. *J. Clin. Microbiol.* **7:**499–506.
25. **Huebner, R. J., W. P. Rowe, T. G. Ward, R. H. Parrott, and J. A. Bell.** 1954. Adenoidal-pharyngeal-conjunctival agents: a newly recognized group of common viruses of the respiratory system. *N. Engl. J. Med.* **251:**1077–1086.
26. **Kawasaki, Y., M. Hosoya, M. Katayose, and H. Suzuki.** 2002. Correlation between serum interleukin 6 and C-reactive protein concentrations in patients with adenoviral respiratory infection. *Pediatr. Infect. Dis. J.* **21:**370–374.
27. **Kojaoghlanian, T., P. Flomenberg, and M. S. Horwitz.** 2003. The impact of adenovirus infection on the immunocompromised host. *Rev. Med. Virol.* **13:**155–171.
28. **Leruez-Ville, M., V. Minard, F. Lacaille, A. Buzyn, E. Abachin, S. Blanche, F. Freymuth, and C. Rouzioux.** 2004. Real-time blood plasma polymerase chain reaction for management of disseminated adenovirus infection. *Clin. Infect. Dis.* **38:**45–52.
29. **Li, Q.-G., A. Henningsson, P. Juto, F. Elgh, and G. Wadell.** 1999. Use of restriction fragment analysis and sequencing of a serotype-specific region to type adenovirus isolates. *J. Clin. Microbiol.* **37:**844–847.
30. **Ludwig, S. L., J. F. Brundage, P. W. Kelley, R. N. Nang, C. Towle, D. P. Schnurr, L. K. Crawford-Miksza, and J. C. Gaydos.** 1998. Prevalence of antibodies to adenovirus serotypes 4 and 7 among unimmunized US army trainees: results of a retrospective nationwide seroprevalence study. *J. Infect. Dis.* **178:**1776–1778.
31. **Martin, A. B., S. Webber, F. J. Fricker, R. Jaffe, G. Demmler, D. Kearney, Y.-H. Zhang, J. Bodurtha, B. Gelb, J. Ni, J. T. Bricker, and J. A. Towbin.** 1994. Acute myocarditis: rapid diagnosis by PCR in children. *Circulation* **90:**330–339.
32. **Pauschinger, M., N. E. Bowles, F. J. Fuentes-Garcia, V. Pham, U. Kuehl, P. L. Schwimmbeck, H.-P. Schultheiss, and J. A. Towbin.** 1999. Detection of adenoviral genome in the myocardium of adult patients with idiopathic left ventricular dysfunction. *Circulation* **99:**1348–1354.
33. **Pehler-Harrington, K., M. Khanna, C. R. Waters, and K. J. Henrickson.** 2004. Rapid detection and identification of human adenovirus species by Adenoplex, a multiplex PCR-enzyme hybridization assay. *J. Clin. Microbiol.* **42:**4072–4076.
34. **Raty, R., M. Kleemola, K. Melen, M. Stenvik, and I. Julkunen.** 1999. Efficacy of PCR and other diagnostic methods for the detection of respiratory adenoviral infections. *J. Med. Virol.* **59:**66–72.
35. **Rocholl, C., K. Gerber, J. Daly, A. T. Pavia, and C. L. Byington.** 2004. Adenoviral infections in children: the impact of rapid diagnosis. *Pediatrics* **113:**e51–e56.
36. **Rowe, W. P., R. J. Huebner, L. K. Gilmore, R. H. Parrott, and T. J. Ward.** 1953. Isolation of a cytopathogenic agent from human adenoids undergoing spontaneous degeneration in tissue culture. *Proc. Soc. Exp. Biol. Med.* **84:**570–573.
36a.**Rowe, W. P., R. J. Huebner, L. K. Gilmore, R. H. Parrott, and T. J. Ward.** 1957. Serotype composition of the adenovirus group. *Proc. Soc. Exp. Biol. Med.* **97:**465–470.
37. **Sabin, C. A., G. S. Clewley, J. R. Deayton, A. Mocroft, M. A. Johnson, C. A. Lee, J. E. McLaughlin, and P. D. Griffiths.** 1999. Shorter survival in HIV-positive patients with diarrhoea who excrete adenovirus from the GI tract. *J. Med. Virol.* **58:**280–285.
38. **Saitoh-Inagawa, W., A. Oshima, K. Aoki, N. Itoh, K. Isobe, E. Uchio, S. Ohno, H. Nakajima, K. Hata, and H. Ishiko.** 1996. Rapid diagnosis of adenoviral conjunctivitis by PCR and restriction fragment length polymorphism analysis. *J. Clin. Microbiol.* **34:**2113–2116.
39. **Sarantis, H., G. Johnson, M. Brown, M. Petric, and R. Tellier.** 2004. Comprehensive detection and serotyping of human adenoviruses by PCR and sequencing. *J. Clin. Microbiol.* **42:**3963–3969.
40. **Schnurr, D. P., and M. E. Dondero.** 1993. Two new candidate adenovirus serotypes. *Intervirology* **36:**79–83.
41. **Shimizu, C., C. Rimbaud, G. Cheron, C. Rouzioux, G. M. Lozinski, A. Rao, G. Stanway, H. F. Krous, and J. C. Burns.** 1995. Molecular identification of viruses in sudden infant death associated with myocarditis and pericarditis. *Pediatr. Infect. Dis. J.* **14:**584–588.
42. **Shimizu, H., D. P. Schnurr, and J. C. Burns.** 1994. Comparison of methods to detect enteroviral genome in frozen and fixed myocardium by polymerase chain reaction. *Lab. Investig.* **71:**612–616.
43. **Swanson, P. D., G. Wadell, A. Allard, and J. C. Hierholzer.** 2003. Adenoviruses, p. 1404–1417. *In* P. R. Murray, E. J. Baron, J. H. Jorgensen, M. A. Pfaller, and R. H. Yolken (ed.), *Manual of Clinical Microbiology*, 8th ed. ASM Press, Washington, D.C.
44. **Tai, F.-H., and J. T. Grayston.** 1962. Adenovirus neutralizing antibodies in persons on Taiwan. *Proc. Soc. Exp. Biol. Med.* **109:**881–884.
45. **Turner, P. C., A. S. Bailey, R. J. Cooper, and D. J. Morris.** 1993. The polymerase chain reaction for detecting adenovirus DNA in formalin-fixed, paraffin-embedded tissue obtained *post mortem*. *J. Infect.* **27:**43–46.
46. **Willcox, N., and V. Mautner.** 1976. Antigenic determinants of adenovirus capsids. *J. Immunol.* **116:**19–24.
47. **Xu, W., M. C. McDonough, and D. D. Erdman.** 2000. Species-specific identification of human adenoviruses by a multiplex PCR assay. *J. Clin. Microbiol.* **38:**4114–4120.
48. **Yamadera, S., K. Yamashita, M. Akatsuka, N. Kato, and S. Inouye.** 1998. Trend of adenovirus type 7 infection, an emerging disease in Japan. *Jpn. J. Med. Sci. Biol.* **51:**43–51.
49. **Yeh, H.-Y., N. Pieniazek, D. Pieniazek, H. Gelderblom, and R. B. Luftig.** 1994. Human adenovirus type 41 contains two fibers. *Virus Res.* **33:**179–198.

Parvovirus B19

STANLEY J. NAIDES

77

Autonomous parvoviruses capable of helper virus-independent replication have been isolated from many animal species. Human parvovirus-like particles were first isolated from stools of a patient with enteritis, but their classification remains controversial. The human serum parvovirus B19 was accidentally discovered in 1975 in healthy donor blood used in the development of hepatitis B virus surface antigen diagnostic tests. To date, three genotypes have been described: types 1 (B19), 2 (A6/K71), and 3 (V9). Genotype-specific disease variation has not been reported (8, 19). Clinical disease was historically attributed to B19 before recognition of the A6/K71 and V9 genotypes. The most frequent clinical presentation of B19 infection is erythema infectiosum, or fifth disease, a common childhood exanthem. Application of sensitive molecular biological and immunological methods to viral diagnosis has allowed recognition of the ever-expanding spectrum of clinical presentation (28).

BIOLOGICAL, CLINICAL, AND EPIDEMIOLOGICAL FEATURES

Physicobiochemical Characteristics

B19 and its variants are members of the *Erythrovirus* genus, subfamily *Parvovirinae*, family *Parvoviridae*; the genus contains members of the family that infect mammalian hosts and are autonomous in their ability to replicate in host erythroid precursors. Parvovirus B19 is the smallest (18 to 26 nm in diameter) DNA virus known to infect humans. It forms nonenveloped icosahedral virions. The single-stranded genome contains approximately 5,600 nucleotides (37). B19 encapsidates a single copy of genome. Progeny virus populations are represented by equal numbers of virions containing positive- or negative-sense DNA.

B19 employs a simple coding strategy. A single strong promoter at map unit 6 initiates transcription for both a left-handed nonstructural protein region and a right-handed structural protein region (5). The nonstructural protein, NS1, is approximately 74,000 Da and is encoded between nucleotides 435 and 2448. NS1 is a helicase that provides the "nickase" activity for reduction of replicative DNA forms to progeny virus DNA that can be packaged into the virion and may also play a role in the assembly of viral DNA into mature capsids during viral replication. Recently, studies have shown that NS1 causes apoptosis in its erythroid precursor cell target as well as in nonpermissive cells, e.g., hepatocytes (26, 36).

Both structural proteins, VP1 and VP2, are encoded in the same open reading frame by nucleotides at positions 2444 to 4786 and 3125 to 4786 and are 84,000 and 58,000 Da, respectively. VP2 transcription is initiated at an alternate start site at nucleotide 3125 (6).

Pathogenesis and Pathology

Experiments on healthy volunteers provided a detailed picture of the natural history of B19 infection in the normal host. When B19 viremic plasma was inoculated into the nostrils of previously seronegative individuals, B19 was first detected in recipient serum by day 6 postinoculation. Viremia lasted up to 7 days, with the peak occurring on days 8 and 9 postinoculation. During this period, B19 DNA appeared in nasal and oropharyngeal secretions but virus was not detected in urine or stool. Approximately 11 days postinoculation, high-titer anti-B19 immunoglobulin M (IgM) antibody developed, followed by the appearance of anti-B19 IgG antibody. Volunteers with a significant level of preexistent anti-B19 antibody did not show any evidence of viremia or anti-B19 IgM response. During the viremic phase, some of the subjects had a flu-like illness with malaise, myalgia, and transient fever. Coincident with the onset of viremia, reticulocytosis was absent and remained so for up to 10 days. Viremia was cleared with the onset of the anti-B19 IgM antibody response, which was associated with the second phase of clinical illness, characterized by rash, arthralgia, and arthritis (2). The cell receptors for B19 were reported to be neutral glycosphingolipids, including globoside, which are widely distributed in various cell types (12, 13). $\alpha_5\beta_1$-Integrins may serve as coreceptors (43).

During natural infection, the incubation period may vary from 6 to 18 days, with a maximum of 28 days. By the time most patients present, usually with rash, polyarthralgia, and/or polyarthritis, an anti-B19 IgM response has begun and the patients are not infectious. An exception is the patient with aplastic crisis, who typically presents during the viremic phase. Usually, anti-B19 IgM is present for up to 2 to 3 months postinfection, after which its level may wane. Specific IgG response to B19 is long-lived. Approximately 50% of the adult population have anti-B19 IgG antibodies (14).

Clinical Manifestations

The clinical spectrum of parvovirus B19 infection may be classified by common (Table 1) and uncommon (Table 2) manifestations.

Nearly half of infected children and adults have subclinical or asymptomatic infection. Erythema infectiosum, or fifth disease of childhood, is the best-known manifestation of B19 infection. Children aged 4 to 7 years are typically infected as they enter school, but children as young as 1 year of age and adolescents may present with fifth disease. Prodromal symptoms are often mild. The majority of the children have the hallmark rash characterized by bright red "slapped cheeks." The rash may also appear on the torso and extremities. It may recur after sun exposure, hot bath, or physical activity. Usually the exanthem is a lacy, reticular, "fish net," or blotchy macular or maculopapular eruption, but occasionally it is vesicular or hemorrhagic. Other symptoms usually are mild and include sore throat, headache, fever, cough, anorexia, vomiting, diarrhea, and arthralgia. Children presenting with rash usually have serum anti-B19 IgM antibody present at presentation. Uncommon dermatological manifestations include vesiculopustular eruption, purpura with or without thrombocytopenia, and a "socks-and-gloves" erythema. Erythema infectiosum may also be encountered in adults in whom the rash tends to be more subtle and the bright red slapped-cheeks symptom is often absent; the flu-like symptoms tend to be more severe in adults.

Approximately 10% of children with erythema infectiosum have associated arthritis and arthralgia. In adults, the polyarthralgia and joint swelling tend to be more prominent (27, 31). The arthropathy typically appears as an acute, moderately severe, symmetric, peripheral polyarthritis. The joints most frequently affected include the metacarpophalangeal joints, proximal interphalangeal joints, knees, wrists, and ankles. The duration of these symptoms is usually brief (approximately 10 days), but one-third of patients continue to have persistent joint symptoms 2 to 3 months after onset of the disease. About half of patients who have chronic parvovirus arthropathy meet the criteria of the American Rheumatism Association for a diagnosis of rheumatoid arthritis (31). Patients may have transient expression of autoantibodies, usually in low to moderate titer, including rheumatoid factor, anti-DNA, antilymphocyte, antinuclear, anticardiolipin, and antiphospholipid antibodies (25). Initial studies of major histocompatibility predisposition suggested an association between chronic B19 arthropathy and HLA DR4, but subsequent studies by the same authors failed to substantiate this association (22, 44). The pathogenesis of B19 arthropathy has not been fully elucidated. In patients with chronic B19 arthropathy, B19 DNA may be found in bone marrow aspirates and in synovial biopsy specimens, suggesting B19 viral persistence in apparently immunocompetent individuals (15, 27). B19 DNA has been detected

TABLE 1 Common clinical manifestations of parvovirus B19 infection

Asymptomatic infection
Aplastic crisis
Erythema infectiosum (fifth disease)
Hydrops fetalis
Arthropathy, acute and/or chronic
Chronic or recurrent bone marrow suppression in
  immunocompromised individuals

TABLE 2 Less common clinical manifestations of parvovirus B19 infection

Skin
  Vesiculopustular eruption
  Henoch-Schönlein purpura
  Thrombotic thrombocytopenic purpura
  Socks-and-gloves syndrome

Hematological
  Anemia
  Thrombocytopenia
  Leukopenia
  Benign acute lymphadenopathy
  Hemophagocytic syndrome

Vasculitis
  Polyarteritis nodosa
  Wegener's granulomatosis

Liver
  Hepatocellular enzyme elevations
  Non-A, non-B, non-C, non-E, non-G fulminant liver failure

Nervous system
  Paresthesias
  Meningitis
  Sensorineural hearing loss

in the normal synovium of young adults by using sensitive PCR techniques (38). One group reported B19 DNA and capsid protein in rheumatoid synovium (40). Coculture of B19-positive rheumatoid synovium with normal cells increased tumor necrosis factor alpha production, a finding typical of rheumatoid arthritis. The group suggested that B19 may be a causative agent of rheumatoid arthritis, a provocative suggestion that remains to be confirmed (41). Transgenic mice expressing B19 nonstructural protein, NS1, are prone to developing polyarthritis (42).

Fetal parvovirus B19 infection presents as fetal or congenital anemia, hydrops fetalis, spontaneous abortion, or stillbirth. In some cases, fetal infection is asymptomatic and self-limited. During B19 infection in utero, virus infects fetal erythroid progenitor cells, causing maturation arrest and severe anemia. The resulting hypoxia causes high-output cardiac failure with fluid accumulation in body cavities and generalized edema of the fetus. B19 may also infect the fetal liver, spleen, kidneys, heart, lungs, thymus, adrenal glands, skeletal muscle, eyes, and placental tissue (27).

Individuals with inherited or acquired conditions causing a decrease in reticulocyte production or abnormal destruction of erythrocytes may develop aplastic crisis during an acute B19 infection. These predisposing conditions include iron deficiency; congenital dyserythropoietic anemia; α- and β-thalassemias; hereditary spherocytosis, stomatocytosis, or elliptocytosis; deficiencies in the production of erythrocyte enzymes such as glucose-6-phosphate dehydrogenase, pyruvate kinase, pyrimidine-5'-nucleotidase; sickle cell disease; chronic autoimmune hemolytic anemia; antibody-mediated autoimmune hemolytic anemia; paroxysmal nocturnal hemoglobinuria; virus-associated hemophagocytosis; and blood loss. In healthy individuals, B19 causes transiently decreased reticulocyte production, but this is not usually clinically evident (29).

Chronic or recurrent bone marrow suppression with anemia, thrombocytopenia, and/or leukopenia has been found in patients with immune compromise including Nezelof's syndrome; those who had undergone prior chemotherapy for lymphoproliferative disorders including acute lymphocytic leukemia, chronic myeloid leukemia, Burkitt's lymphoma, acute lymphoblastic lymphoma, myelodysplastic syndrome, astrocytoma, and Wilms' tumor; those with human immunodeficiency virus infection and AIDS; and those who were receiving immunosuppressive therapy for bone marrow or organ transplantation. In immunocompetent hosts, anti-B19 IgM and acute-phase IgG antibody recognize antigenic determinants on VP2 and may last for 2 months or more. Convalescent-phase anti-B19 IgG antibody recognizes determinants on VP1 (23). VP1 differs from VP2 by containing unique N-terminal determinants absent from the shorter VP2 (37). Patients with congenital or acquired immunodeficiencies fail to produce convalescent-phase IgG antibodies to VP1, and their serum is unable to neutralize B19 in vitro (29). Since IgG seroprevalence in the adult population is approximately 50%, it was not surprising that neutralizing activity to B19 was detected in commercially available pooled immunoglobulin. Administration of commercial immunoglobulin with anti-B19 activity to patients with immunodeficiency who have chronic B19 infection and cytopenias is effective in clearing B19 infection and allowing bone marrow recovery (16).

Recently, several uncommon manifestations of B19 infection have been described, including idiopathic thrombocytopenia purpura, transient erythroblastopenia of childhood, Diamond-Blackfan anemia, encephalitis, aseptic meningitis, brachial plexus neuropathy, paresthesias, neuralgic amyotrophy, and motor weakness. Unusual rheumatologic presentations attributed to B19 infection include systematic vasculitis, Henoch-Schönlein purpura, Kawasaki's disease, polyarteritis nodosa, adult Still's disease, fibromyalgia, and systemic lupus erythematosus. Parvovirus B19 has also been associated with acute fulminant liver failure, myocarditis, mononucleosis-like syndrome, Koplik's spots, and pneumonia (21, 24, 29, 36, 39, 40).

Epidemiology

Parvovirus B19, genotype 1, has a worldwide distribution. Genotypes 2 and 3 tend to be found in Europe and Africa (8, 19). B19 infection occurs in all age groups throughout the year in epidemics or as sporadic cases. The peak incidence is seasonal, occurring predominantly in late winter and early spring. Serological studies show that B19 has usually infected 2 to 15% of children under the age of 5 years, 15 to 60% of school age children (5 to 19 years old), and 30 to 60% of adults. A total of 20% of children and 26% of adults found to be seropositive had experienced a previous asymptomatic infection. The highest rates of natural infection (50 to 60%) were observed during outbreaks of erythema infectiosum or B19-induced aplastic crisis (3, 9).

Natural transmission of B19 occurs mostly via respiratory secretions or vertically from mother to fetus. Recently, transmission via transfusion of blood and blood products was reported. The frequency of contamination of blood obtained from single donors usually ranges from 1 in 30,000 to 1 in 50,000 donations. However, the frequency of contamination of pooled clotting-factor concentrates can be much higher (45).

LABORATORY DIAGNOSIS

Cell Culture

A major limitation in studies of B19 has been the absence of appropriate cell lines permissive for the virus. Attempts to detect B19 virus in standard cell cultures have not been successful. Several investigators use cell cultures of erythroid origin for B19 propagation. B19 infection of primary cell cultures of erythroid precursors derived from human fetal liver and bone marrow or of human megakaryocytic leukemic cell lines has been successful. However, cultivation of B19 in these cell cultures is not routine, and the viral yield tends to be low. Attempts to use animals, including anthropoid primates, for modeling B19 infection have been unsuccessful.

Electron Microscopy

Standard electron microscopy methods of negative staining allow the examination of a liquid sample dried on an electron microscopy grid that had been previously coated with a thin layer of plastic, followed by staining with phosphotungstic acid or uranyl acetate. Electron-dense material accumulates around viral particles, giving a bas relief appearance or negative-contrast image (Fig. 1).

Specific viral identification may be confirmed by immunoaggregation with polyclonal or monoclonal anti-B19 antibodies (immunoelectron microscopy [IEM]), or by immunogold labeling. However, successful IEM requires the absence of excess endogenous anti-B19 antibody in the sample. In serum samples, "bare" virions are present only in the very early stages of infection before specific antibody develops. IEM may be useful when used with nonserum body fluids or tissues in which anti-B19 antibody is not present in high titer. After incubation of the sample with specific antiserum or anti-B19 monoclonal antibody, centrifugation, and negative staining, the aggregated virions can be seen by electron microscopic examination.

Combined pseudoreplica-immunochemical staining may be more useful, even in the presence of endogenous anti-B19 antibody, since even a few antigenic sites may be adequate to allow the labeling of B19 by specific anti-B19 monoclonal antibodies. Virus can be detected in various body fluids by this method (32). In the pseudoreplica technique, a sample is absorbed into an agarose block, leaving viral particles on the surface. The agarose is then overlaid with a plastic film, which, after hardening, is floated off of the agarose, inverted, applied to a support grid, and negatively stained. Combined pseudoreplica-immunochemical staining uses second-stage gold-conjugated labeling antibodies to detect first-stage anti-B19 monoclonal antibody before negative staining. Examination of viral particles with specific colloidal-gold-conjugated antibodies permits species identification. Otherwise, it may be difficult to discriminate B19 virions from other nonenveloped icosahedral viruses of a similar size, such as enteroviruses, on the basis of morphology alone. B19 may be present as "full" particles with the contrast stain excluded, or stain may enter the capsid, giving the appearance of an "empty" shell (Fig. 1). Although these methods have high specificity, they require special equipment and experienced examiners and are labor-intensive, rendering them suboptimal for routine diagnosis (32).

Immunoassays

Immunofluorescence assay, radioimmunoassay (RIA), and enzyme-linked immunosorbent assay (ELISA) have been used to detect both B19 antigen and specific anti-B19 antibody. The indirect immunofluorescence assay was successfully applied to the cellular localization of B19 antigen in tissue and cell culture samples but has not found wide clinical application. Several RIA and ELISA systems were developed for detecting B19 antigen and anti-B19 IgM and IgG antibody. They can be divided into two major groups. The

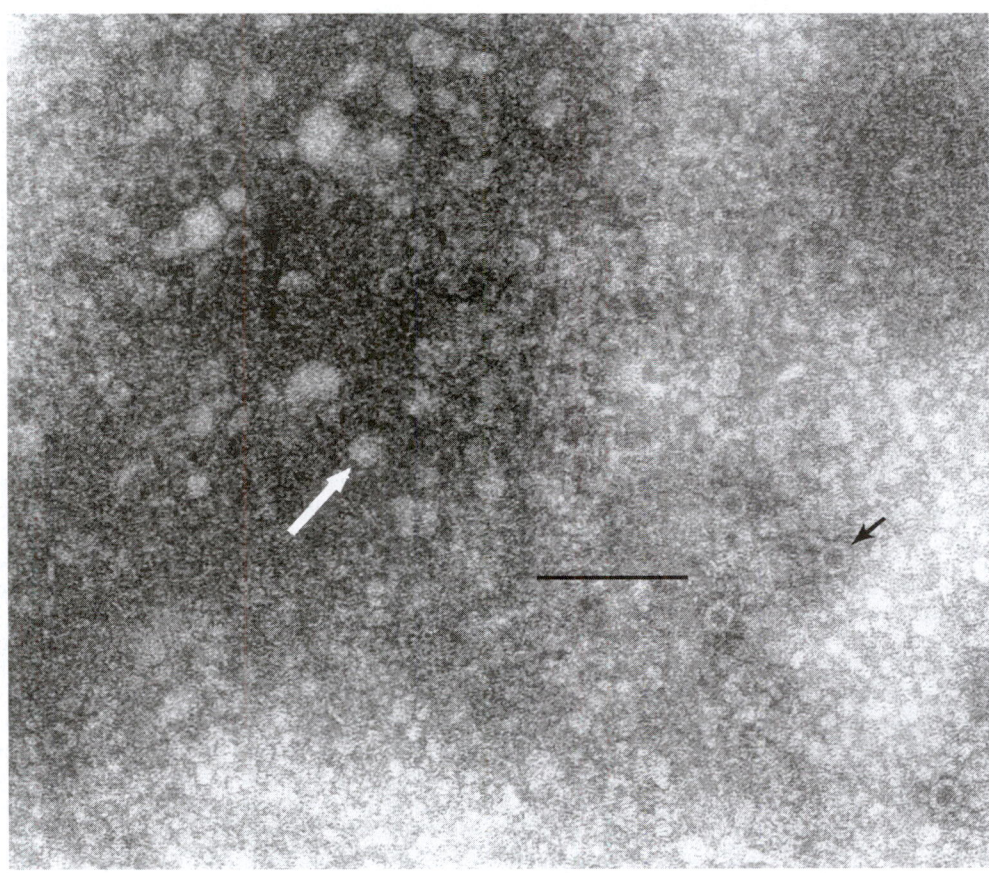

FIGURE 1 Electron micrograph of serum from a patient with sickle cell disease and aplastic crisis, showing full (white arrow) and empty (black arrow) nonenveloped, icosahedral viral particles measuring ~23 nm in diameter, visualized by negative staining with uranyl acetate. Bar, 100 nm (original magnification, × 196,000). Reprinted from reference 31 with permission of the publisher.

first system developed consisted of tests using native virus from viremic patients as an antigen source (Fig. 2A) (11). Briefly, for antibody capture RIA or ELISA to detect anti-B19 IgM or anti-B19 IgG, microtiter plates (solid phase) are coated with anti-human IgM (μ-chain specific) or anti-human IgG (γ-chain specific) antibody diluted in carbonate-bicarbonate buffer during an overnight incubation. After the plates have been washed with phosphate-buffered saline

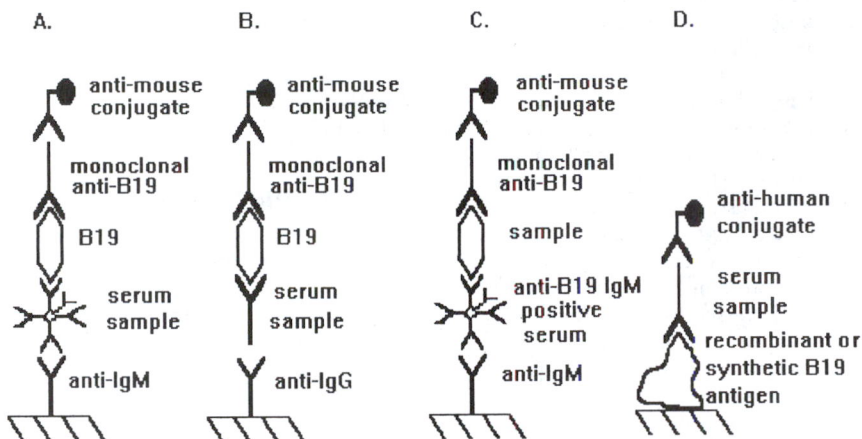

FIGURE 2 ELISA-based tests showing antibody capture ELISA for anti-B19 IgM antibody (A), antibody capture ELISA for anti-B19 IgG antibody (B), antigen capture ELISA for B19 virus (C), and recombinant or synthetic B19 antigen-based ELISA for detection of B19 antibody (D).

containing a low concentration of nonionic detergent to prevent nonspecific aggregation, the serum to be tested for antibody is added; if the RIA or ELISA is used for detection of antigen, a defined serum with high-titer anti-B19 IgM is added instead. After incubation and washing with buffer, a high-titer B19 viremic serum without endogenous anti-B19 specific antibodies is added as an antigen source; if the RIA or ELISA is used for detection of antigen, the serum to be tested for virus is added instead. In the antibody capture assay, an antigen-negative control serum may be added to parallel wells at the antigen step to detect nonspecific reagent cross-reactivity. Detection of such cross-reactivity may be necessary to avoid false-positive results for patients presenting with autoantibodies such as rheumatoid factor (30). In the antigen capture assay, parallel wells with an anti-B19 IgM negative control capture serum and parallel wells with appropriate virus negative control sample (e.g., normal serum, body fluid, and cell lysate) must be added to detect nonspecific reagent cross-reactivity.

After overnight incubation and washing with buffer, monoclonal antibody with anti-B19 activity is added. After nonadherent anti-B19 murine monoclonal antibody is washed off, anti-mouse class-specific antibody labeled with ^{125}I (RIA) or peroxidase (ELISA) is added. After incubation and washing, radioactivity is counted or color developer in the presence of H_2O_2 is added to each well. The reaction is stopped with 2 M H_2SO_4. We considered an antibody capture assay positive when the absorbance of the sample incubated with the virus was greater than 3 standard deviations above the mean value of background controls (i.e., all serum samples in an assay incubated with nonviremic serum at the antigen step) and the difference between the mean of test well values and the mean of background well values for a given sample was greater than 3 standard deviations of the mean of the background wells for all sera tested (4).

Identification of a stock of high-titer viremic serum without endogenous anti-B19 antibody for use as antigen in immunoassays (Fig. 2A and B) may require significant effort. B19 virus in a panel of candidate antigen sources may be detected by screening antigen capture RIA or ELISA (Fig. 2C) and confirmed by direct DNA hybridization. Alternatively, PCR with B19-specific primers followed by hybridization of the amplified product with B19-specific probes may be used. Antigen detection by ELISA is usually not as sensitive as direct DNA hybridization or PCR amplification (1), but it is useful in screening for high-titer viremic sera. Candidate antigen sources then need to be screened by an antibody capture assay to eliminate those with endogenous antibody.

To overcome the problem of limited access to antigen for diagnostic testing, a second group of solid-phase immunoassays were developed based on recombinant protein or synthetic peptides representing B19 antigenic structures (Fig. 2D). Initially, Chinese hamster ovary cells were transfected with a plasmid containing the B19 nucleotide sequence allowing the expression of both VP1 and VP2 viral proteins that self-assembled into empty capsids (20). These proteins were subsequently expressed using bacterial or baculovirus vectors and form the basis of commercially available diagnostic kits. Several groups have synthesized peptides based on published B19 DNA sequences for use as antigen in immunoassays. For antibody assays, synthetic protein or peptide with B19 antigenic activity is absorbed onto the solid phase. Recent comparison of several commercial kits to each other and to indirect antibody capture ELISA addressed their sensitivity and specificity (7, 34, 35).

Antibodies to genotypes 1 and 3 may be detected equally well by using ELISAs targeting B19 or V9, respectively (17).

Methods for Detection of B19 Nucleic Acid

B19 DNA may be detected by hybridization with cDNA probes, riboprobes (synthetic RNA), or synthetic oligonucleotide probes. Hybridization may be performed directly on tissue or cells by in situ hybridization allowing localization of viral DNA. Disrupted virus-containing sample or extracted DNA may be blotted onto a nitrocellulose or nylon membrane before being hybridized with B19-specific probe. Recently, numerous modifications of this basic approach have been used to detect B19 in body fluids, blood products, tissue, and cell culture extracts. Nonradioactive labels for probes may be used for safety and long shelf life. B19 DNA has been detected in serum by using a digoxigenin-labeled RNA probe to hybridize with target DNA, followed by capture of the hybrid onto a solid phase (microtiter wells) previously coated with a second anti-B19 oligonucleotide probe to an unhybridized portion of the B19 target DNA; an alkaline phosphatase-conjugated anti-digoxigenin antibody and chemiluminescent substrate allow the detection of B19 DNA on a scintillation counter.

PCR-based technologies offer exquisite sensitivity and the ability to detect B19 DNA in different types of clinical specimens. Various oligonucleotide primers directed against sequences in both the nonstructural and viral capsid protein genes have been used (10). PCR is more sensitive than traditional dot blot hybridization; the use of an internal radiolabeled probe to detect amplification product by Southern analysis is still more sensitive than dot blot hybridization. Many investigators have now reported the use of PCR to detect B19 in fetal and adult tissues, body fluids, blood products, and cell cultures. However, PCR detection of B19 DNA in clinical samples is not problem free. The most common problem is the presence in clinical samples of inhibitors of *Taq* polymerase (18). Different approaches to avoid this problem have been used, including controlled heating of the sample, detergent extraction of DNA, and the use of a second round of amplification with nested primers. In antigen capture or immunoadherence PCR, virus is adhered to PCR tubes precoated with anti-B19 monoclonal antibody, and after incubation and washing, the PCR mixture (containing primers, deoxynucleoside triphosphates, and *Taq* polymerase) is added, virions are disrupted by heating, and viral DNA is amplified. This approach avoids nonspecific inhibition and provides high sensitivity and specificity (21, 24). PCR primers may be chosen to preferentially amplify genotypes 2 and 3, although the practical impact of differentiating B19 (genotype 1) from genotypes 2 (K71/A6) or 3 (V9) has not been defined (19, 33).

DISEASE PREVENTION AND THERAPY

Parvovirus B19 infection is widespread in the community. It is therefore difficult to prevent exposure and to control the spread of infection. Community and household contacts are frequently asymptomatic. Hospital exposures may occur. However, isolation of viremic patients may decrease the level of exposure (29).

Specific antiviral therapy has not been identified. In general, patient management is symptomatic and supportive. Patients with acute aplastic crisis may require blood transfusion. Adults with chronic B19 arthropathy are managed with nonsteroidal anti-inflammatory drugs (31). Fetal transfusion in utero may be required to support the fetus during

B19 infection complicated by severe anemia; fetuses transfused in utero and surviving the aplastic crisis have been born without apparent long-term sequelae (29). Immunocompromised patients who lack neutralizing anti-B19 antibodies and who present with manifestations of persistent B19 infection benefit from commercial intravenous immunoglobulin (16). Intramuscular immunoglobulin for prophylaxis following B19 exposure has not yet been adequately evaluated. Specific antiviral chemotherapy for parvovirus B19 has not been demonstrated.

REFERENCES

1. **Anderson, L. J., R. A. Tsou, T. L. Chorba, H. Wulff, P. Tattersall, and P. P. Mortimer.** 1986. Detection of antibodies and antigens of human parvovirus B19 by enzyme-linked immunosorbent assay. *J. Clin. Microbiol.* **24:**522–526.
2. **Anderson, M. J., P. G. Higgins, L. R. Davis, J. S. Willman, S. E. Jones, I. M. Kidd, J. R. Pattison, and D. A. Tyrrell.** 1985. Experimental parvoviral infection in humans. *J. Infect. Dis.* **152:**257–265.
3. **Anonymous.** 1989. Leads from the MMWR. Risks associated with human parvovirus B19 infection. *JAMA* **261:**1406–1408.
4. **Bell, L. M., S. J. Naides, P. Stoffman, R. L. Hodinka, and S. A. Plotkin.** 1989. Human parvovirus B19 infection among hospital staff members after contact with infected patients. *N. Engl. J. Med.* **321:**485–491.
5. **Blundell, M. C., C. Beard, and C. R. Astell.** 1987. In vitro identification of a B19 parvovirus promoter. *Virology* **157:**534–538.
6. **Brunstein, J., M. Soderlund-Venermo, and K. Hedman.** 2000. Identification of a novel RNA splicing pattern as a basis of restricted cell tropism of erythrovirus B19. *Virology* **274:**284–291.
7. **Bruu, A.-L., and S. A. Nordbo.** 1995. Evaluation of five commercial tests for detection of immunoglobulin M antibodies to human parvovirus B19. *J. Clin. Microbiol.* **33:**1363–1365.
8. **Candotti, D., N. Etiz, A. Parsyan, and J. P. Allain.** 2004. Identification and characterization of persistent human erythrovirus infection in blood donor samples. *J. Virol.* **78:**12169–12178.
9. **Chorba, T., P. Coccia, R. C. Holman, P. Tattersall, L. J. Anderson, J. Sudman, N. S. Young, E. Kurczynski, U. M. Saarinen, and R. Moir.** 1986. The role of parvovirus B19 in aplastic crisis and erythema infectiosum (fifth disease). *J. Infect. Dis.* **154:**383–393.
10. **Clewley, J. P., and B. J. Cohen.** 1995. Investigation of human parvovirus B19 infection using PCR, p. 205–215. *In* J. P. Clewley (ed.), *The Polymerase Chain Reaction (PCR) for Human Viral Diagnosis.* CRC Press, Inc., Boca Raton, Fla.
11. **Cohen, B. J., P. P. Mortimer, and M. S. Pereira.** 1983. Diagnostic assays with monoclonal antibodies for the human serum parvovirus-like virus (SPLV). *J. Hyg.* **91:**113–130.
12. **Cooling, L. L., D. S. Zhang, S. J. Naides, and T. A. Koerner.** 2003. Glycosphingolipid expression in acute non-lymphocytic leukemia: common expression of shiga toxin and parvovirus B19 receptors on early myeloblasts. *Blood* **101:**711–721.
13. **Cooling, L. L. W., T. A. Koerner, and S. J. Naides.** 1995. Multiple glycosphingolipids determine the tissue tropism of parvovirus B19. *J. Infect. Dis.* **172:**1198–1205.
14. **Eis-Hubinger, A. M., J. Oldenburg, H. H. Brackmann, B. Matz, and K. E. Schneweis.** 1996. The prevalence of antibody to parvovirus B19 in hemophiliacs and in the general population. *Zentbl. Bakteriol.* **284:**232–240.
15. **Foto, F., K. G. Saag, L. L. Scharosch, E. J. Howard, and S. J. Naides.** 1993. Parvovirus B19-specific DNA in bone marrow from B19 arthropathy patients. Evidence for B19 viral persistence. *J. Infect. Dis.* **167:**744–748.
16. **Frickhofen, N., J. L. Abkowitz, M. Safford, J. M. Berry, J. Antunez de Mayolo, A. Astrow, R. Cohen, I. Halperin, L. King, D. Mintzer, B. Cohen, and N. S. Young.** 1990. Persistent B19 parvovirus infection in patients infected with human immunodeficiency virus type 1 (HIV-1): a treatable cause of anemia in AIDS. *Ann. Intern. Med.* **113:**926–933.
17. **Heegaard, E. D., K. Qvortrup, and J. Christensen.** 2002. Baculovirus expression of erythrovirus V9 capsids and screening by ELISA: Serologic cross-reactivity with erythrovirus B19. *J. Med. Virol.* **66:**246–252.
18. **Hicks, K. E., S. Beard, B. J. Cohen, and J. P. Clewley.** 1995. A simple and sensitive DNA hybridization assay used for the routine diagnosis of human parvovirus B19 infection. *J. Clin. Microbiol.* **33:**2473–2475.
19. **Hokynar, K., P. Norja, H. Laitinen, P. Palomaki, A. Garbarg-Chenon, A. Ranki, K. Hedman, and M. Soderlund-Venermo.** 2004. Detection and differentiation of human parvovirus variants by commercial quantitative real-time PCR tests. *J. Clin. Microbiol.* **42:**2013–2019.
20. **Kajigaya, S., T. Shimada, S. Fujita, and N. S. Young.** 1989. A genetically engineered cell line that produces empty capsids of B19 (human) parvovirus. *Proc. Natl. Acad. Sci. USA* **86:**7601–7605.
21. **Karetnyi, Y. V., P. R. Beck, R. S. Markin, A. N. Langnas, and S. J. Naides.** 1999. Human parvovirus B19 infection in acute fulminant liver failure. *Arch. Virol.* **144:**1713–1724.
22. **Klouda, P. T., S. A. Corbin, B. A. Bradley, B. J. Cohen, and A. D. Woolf.** 1986. HLA and acute arthritis following human parvovirus infection. *Tissue Antigens* **28:**318–319.
23. **Kurtzman, G. J., B. J. Cohen, A. M. Field, R. Oseas, R. M. Blaese, and N. S. Young.** 1989. Immune response to B19 parvovirus and an antibody defect in persistent viral infection. *J. Clin. Investig.* **84:**1114–1123.
24. **Langnas, A. N., R. S. Markin, M. S. Cattral, and S. J. Naides.** 1995. Parvovirus B19 as a possible causative agent of fulminant liver failure and associated aplastic anemia. *Hepatology* **22:**1661–1665.
25. **Meyer, O.** 2003. Parvovirus B19 and autoimmune diseases. *Joint Bone Spine* **70:**6–11.
26. **Moffatt, S., N. Yaegashi, K. Tada, N. Tanaka, and K. Sugamura.** 1998. Human parvovirus B19 nonstructural (NS1) protein induces apoptosis in erythroid lineage cells. *J. Virol.* **72:**3018–3028.
27. **Naides, S. J.** 1998. Rheumatic manifestations of parvovirus B19 infection. *Rheum. Dis. Clin. North Am.* **24:**375–401.
28. **Naides, S. J.** 1999. Infection with parvovirus B19. *Curr. Infect. Dis. Rep.* **1:**273–278.
29. **Naides, S. J.** 2000. Parvoviruses, p. 487–500. *In* S. Specter, R. L. Hodinka, and S. A. Young (ed.), *Clinical Virology Manual.* ASM Press, Washington, D.C.
30. **Naides, S. J., and E. H. Field.** 1988. Transient rheumatoid factor positivity in acute human parvovirus B19 infection. *Arch. Intern. Med.* **148:**2587–2589.
31. **Naides, S. J., L. L. Scharosch, F. Foto, and E. J. Howard.** 1990. Rheumatologic manifestations of human parvovirus B19 infection in adults. Initial two-year clinical experience. *Arthritis Rheum.* **33:**1297–1309.
32. **Naides, S. J., and C. P. Weiner.** 1989. Antenatal diagnosis and palliative treatment of non-immune hydrops fetalis secondary to fetal parvovirus B19 infection. *Prenat. Diagn.* **9:**105–114.
33. **Nguyen, Q. T., S. Wong, E. D. Heegaard, and K. E. Brown.** 2002. Identification and characterization of a second novel human erythrovirus variant, A6. *Virology* **301:**374–380.
34. **Patou, G., and U. Ayliffe.** 1991. Evaluation of commercial enzyme linked immunosorbent assay for detection of B19 parvovirus IgM and IgG. *J. Clin. Pathol.* **44:**831–834.

35. **Pickering, J. W., B. Forghani, G. R. Shell, and L. Wu.** 1998. Comparative evaluation of three recombinant antigen-based enzyme immunoassays for detection of IgM and IgG antibodies to human parvovirus B19. *Clin. Diagn. Virol.* **9:**57–63.
36. **Poole, B. D., Y. V. Karetnyi, and S. J. Naides.** 2004. Parvovirus B19-induced apoptosis of hepatocytes. *J. Virol.* **78:**7775–7783.
37. **Shade, R. O., M. C. Blundell, S. F. Cotmore, P. Tattersall, and C. R. Astell.** 1986. Nucleotide sequence and genome organization of human parvovirus B19 isolated from the serum of a child during aplastic crisis. *J. Virol.* **58:**921–936.
38. **Soderlund-Venermo, M., K. Hokynar, J. Nieminen, H. Rautakorpi, and K. Hedman.** 2002. Persistence of human parvovirus B19 in human tissues. *Pathol. Biol.* (Paris) **50:**307–316.
39. **Sokal, E. M., M. Melchior, C. Cornu, A. T. Vandenbroucke, J. P. Buts, B. J. Cohen, and G. Burtonboy.** 1998. Acute parvovirus B19 infection associated with fulminant hepatitis of favourable prognosis in young children. *Lancet* **352:**1739–1741.
40. **Stahl, H. D., B. Seidl, B. Hubner, S. Altrichter, R. Pfeiffer, B. Pustowoit, U. G. Liebert, J. Hofmann, G. Salis-Soglio, and F. Emmrich.** 2000. High incidence of parvovirus B19 DNA in synovial tissue of patients with undifferentiated mono- and oligoarthritis. *Clin. Rheumatol.* **19:**281–286.
41. **Takahashi, Y., C. Murai, S. Shibata, Y. Munakata, T. Ishii, K. Ishii, T. Saitoh, T. Sawai, K. Sugamura, and T. Sasaki.** 1998. Human parvovirus B19 as a causative agent for rheumatoid arthritis. *Proc. Natl. Acad. Sci. USA* **95:**8227–8232.
42. **Takasawa, N., Y. Munakata, K. K. Ishii, Y. Takahashi, M. Takahashi, Y. Fu, T. Ishii, H. Fujii, T. Saito, H. Takano, T. Noda, M. Suzuki, M. Nose, S. Zolla-Patzner, and T. Sasaki.** 2004. Human parvovirus B19 transgenic mice become susceptible to polyarthritis. *J. Immunol.* **173:**4675–4683.
43. **Weigel-Kelley, K. A., M. C. Yoder, and A. Srivastava.** 2003. Alpha5beta1 integrin as a cellular coreceptor for human parvovirus B19: requirement of functional activation of beta one integrin for viral entry. *Blood* **102:**3927–3933.
44. **Woolf, A. D., G. V. Campion, P. T. Klouda, A. Chiswick, B. J. Cohen, and P. A. Dieppe.** 1987. HLA and the manifestations of human parvovirus B19 infection. *Arthritis Rheum.* **30:**S52.
45. **Wu, C. G., B. Mason, J. Jong, D. Erdman, L. McKernan, M. Oakley, M. Soucie, B. Evatt, and M. Y. Yu.** 2005. Parvovirus B19 transmission by a high-purity factor VIII concentrate. *Transfusion* **45:**1003–1010.

Influenza Viruses

JACQUELINE M. KATZ, ALEXANDER I. KLIMOV,
STEPHEN E. LINDSTROM, AND NANCY J. COX

78

Epidemics caused by influenza viruses may be identified by their explosive onset in a given population, their seasonal characteristics in regions of temperate climate, the respiratory and systemic symptoms associated with illness, and the high attack rate among susceptible individuals. Based on these distinct features, influenza epidemics have been tracked through history, well before the first isolation of the virus in 1933 and the availability of laboratory methods for their identification.

The influenza virus types A, B, and C belong to the family *Orthomyxoviridae*. Antigenic properties of the two major structural internal proteins of influenza viruses, the matrix protein (M1) and the nucleoprotein (NP), allow for differentiation between the virus types. Orthomyxoviruses are enveloped and pleomorphic to spherical, with a diameter of approximately 80 to 120 nm, and contain a segmented RNA of negative sense. Influenza A viruses are further classified into subtypes according to the antigenic characteristics of their two major surface glycoproteins, the hemagglutinin (HA) and the neuraminidase (NA). Sixteen distinct HA and 9 NA subtypes have been identified thus far (14, 27, 46). At present, only influenza A viruses bearing the H1 or H3 HA and N1 or N2 NA cocirculate with influenza B viruses in the human population. All subtypes of influenza A viruses are maintained in wild aquatic birds, the reservoir from which certain subtypes have (i) infrequently crossed species to establish stable lineages in humans, swine, and horses; (ii) more frequently crossed species to circulate widely in domestic poultry; and (iii) been transmitted sporadically to aquatic or other mammalian species. Influenza B viruses have also been isolated from seals (34). In recent years, wholly avian influenza viruses of the H5, H9, and H7 subtypes have been transmitted directly from domestic poultry to humans and caused a spectrum of illness, from mild to severe and fatal disease (7, 27, 35, 43).

The nomenclature of influenza viruses includes the type, the geographic location where the virus was isolated, a laboratory identification number, and the year of isolation, followed by the subtype, e.g., A/New Caledonia/20/99 (H1N1). The species is included for viruses of animal origin, e.g., A/Seal/Massachusetts/133/82 (H4N5).

CLINICAL ASPECTS

Influenza epidemics are caused by influenza A and/or B viruses almost every year. Influenza C viruses usually cause mild to inapparent disease, primarily in children. Therefore, routine diagnosis of influenza C is not commonly undertaken. Influenza epidemics are often associated with excess morbidity and mortality, although the latter is to some extent dependent on the virus type and the age of the affected population (39).

Influenza viruses replicate predominantly in the ciliated columnar epithelium of the respiratory tract. Early in infection, large amounts of virus are shed into respiratory secretions which when expelled through sneezing and coughing can be transmitted to close contacts. Spread by direct contact with contaminated hands or surfaces is also possible. An incubation period of 1 to 4 days is typical but may extend to 7 days. The typical clinical picture of influenza virus infection is sudden onset of fever of >38°C of 3 to 4 days' duration and is often associated with headache, myalgia, and malaise as well as respiratory symptoms, including sore throat, cough, rhinorrhea, nasal congestion, and/or tracheobronchitis. However, there is a great deal of variation in the clinical presentation of laboratory-confirmed cases, which may depend on the age of the patients. Fever and cough are the most common symptoms in all age groups and are often the only clinical manifestations in the elderly, whereas vomiting and diarrhea occur more often in children than in adults (1, 9, 33). Data from epidemiological studies indicate that influenza A viruses of the H3N2 subtype cause more severe illness than influenza B viruses, which in turn are more severe than H1N1 infections. While all age groups are affected by influenza A infections, influenza B viruses predominantly cause illness in children. Certain chronic medical conditions, such as diabetes, asthma, chronic heart and lung diseases, and immunosuppression, predispose individuals to severe complications from influenza. The incidences of influenza-related hospitalizations and deaths are highest among those over 64 years of age. Complications from influenza often present as lower respiratory tract problems. Complications requiring hospitalization include primary viral or, more commonly, secondary bacterial pneumonia with fatal outcome. Otitis media is a common complication of influenza virus infection seen in young children. A large proportion of influenza patients have abnormal electrocardiograms, yet myocarditis and arrhythmia with fatal outcome are relatively rare events (32).

Relatively little is known about the epidemiology and the clinical significance of influenza C viruses. These viruses cause upper respiratory infection predominantly in children, adolescents, and young adults, and they occasionally have been associated with outbreaks, but they show no particular seasonality. Fever and cough are the predominant symptoms, but in rare instances, influenza C virus has been isolated from patients with lower respiratory tract infections (32). The focus of this chapter is diagnosis of influenza A and B viruses since these types are the major human pathogens.

INFLUENZA VIRUS GENE PRODUCTS AND REPLICATION

The replication and molecular biology of influenza viruses have been extensively reviewed elsewhere (19, 28) and are summarized only briefly here. Influenza A and B viruses possess eight segments of negative-sense RNA which encode at least 10 proteins. Contact between the virus and cell surface is mediated by the HA, which binds to terminal residues of *N*-acetylneuraminic (sialic) acid linked to cell surface glycoproteins or glycolipids. The virus enters the cell through receptor-mediated endocytosis via clathrin-coated pits. In the reduced pH of the endosome, the HA molecule undergoes structural changes that promote the fusion of the HA with the endosomal membrane. The low pH of the late endosome activates the transmembrane M2 ion channel protein, allowing a flow of H$^+$ to the inner part of the virion, which leads to the dissociation of the M1 protein, the major structural protein of the virus, from the ribonucleoprotein (RNP) complexes. The RNP complex, which is composed of three polymerase proteins surrounded by the NP, is released into the cytoplasm and is rapidly transported into the nucleus. In the nucleus of the host cell, viral RNAs are transcribed into mRNAs, from which viral proteins are synthesized, and into complementary RNAs, which serve as templates for the synthesis of viral progeny RNA segments. The three viral polymerases, PA, PB1, and PB2, catalyze this process. PA is involved in viral RNA replication, while PB1 and PB2 are essential for mRNA synthesis. The nonstructural protein (NS1) inhibits processing of host mRNA, thus allowing the preferential translation of viral mRNA in the cytoplasm, using the host cell's ribosomal machinery. Newly synthesized viral polymerases, NP, and nuclear export protein are transported to the nucleus and complexed with viral RNA segments to form RNPs that under the influence of M1 and nuclear export protein are exported to the cytoplasm. The viral membrane proteins, i.e., the HA and NA of influenza A and B viruses, as well as the transmembrane proteins M2 of influenza A and the NB and BM2 proteins of influenza B, undergo posttranslational modifications in the endoplasmic reticulum and, after transport through the Golgi complex, are inserted into specific areas of the cellular membrane. The M1 protein lines the inner leaflet of the plasma membrane and associates the RNP with the transmembrane proteins. Finally the assembled virions bud from the membrane of the host cell. The NA cleaves sialic acid moieties on the host cell membrane to facilitate release of the HA and the mature virus particles into the extracellular space.

INFLUENZA VIRUS VARIATION

The virus-encoded RNA polymerases do not exhibit proofreading activities. Therefore, point mutations in the viral genome occur at a frequency of approximately one per 10^4 nucleotides. Such point mutations may lead to the emergence of variant viruses that are antigenically distinct from previously circulating strains of the same subtype. Amino acid changes in the globular distal part of the HA molecule are of particular importance, because neutralizing antibodies to antigenic sites

in this region provide protection from reinfection with identical or closely related virus strains. Thus, amino acid changes in the HA and NA surface glycoproteins frequently give rise to new epidemic strains to which immunity acquired through previous infection with a homologous type or subtype or by vaccination offers only limited protection. Such new antigenic variants are responsible for the almost yearly epidemics of influenza A and B. Genetic reassortment, i.e., the exchange of gene segments between two viruses, provides an additional evolutionary pathway for influenza A viruses. During simultaneous infection of a host cell with two viruses of different subtypes, gene segments from the two parent viruses can reassort, producing progeny containing segments from both viruses. A virus that has acquired a novel HA from the reservoir of influenza viruses circulating among wild aquatic birds, with or without a novel NA, may be able to infect individuals lacking immunity to the novel HA. If the virus also has the ability to spread from human to human, it may give rise to a pandemic, i.e., a global epidemic caused by a virus in a susceptible population (46).

In the 20th century, pandemics occurred after the appearance of the H1N1 subtype during the "Spanish Flu" in 1918, the emergence of the H2N2 subtype during the "Asian" pandemic in 1957, and the H3N2 viruses during the "Hong Kong" pandemic in 1968. The viruses that caused the last two pandemics were reassortant viruses that had acquired a novel HA and one or two other genes from an avian influenza virus along with the ability to be transmitted efficiently from human to human. Since swine are susceptible to both avian and human influenza viruses, they have been proposed to be an intermediate mammalian host in which reassortment may take place. However, it is now established that influenza A viruses from other species may also be transmitted directly to humans, and so it is also possible that a reassortant virus with pandemic potential may arise in humans without the need for an intermediate host.

IMMUNITY TO INFLUENZA VIRUSES

Strain-specific virus-neutralizing antibody directed against the HA is the primary immune mediator of protection against infection and clinical illness, while antibody directed against the NA may reduce the severity of disease through enhancing viral clearance (16). Antibodies to NP and M1 are of diagnostic importance. Significant rises in antibody directed against the abundant internal structural proteins NP and M1 can be detected after primary infection and reinfection with viruses of the homologous type and are of diagnostic significance. Antibodies to the transmembrane M2 protein may also be produced after repeated influenza virus infections. Antibody to the ectodomain of the protein has been shown to play a role in viral clearance in mice, but the contribution of anti-M2 antibodies to viral clearance in human influenza infection is unknown. CD4$^+$ and CD8$^+$ T cells also play an important role in immunity to influenza and, in contrast to the strain-specific response of antibodies, tend to be more cross-reactive among subtypes, recognizing more conserved epitopes on the surface proteins and/or internal viral proteins. CD4$^+$ T cells provide help for the antibody response and the induction of CD8$^+$ T cells, whereas CD8$^+$ T cells have been associated with accelerated clearance of virus and recovery from infection (41). The ability to recognize a given T-cell epitope is dependent on the HLA phenotype of an individual.

Upon primary infection with influenza viruses, strain-specific immunoglobulin M (IgM), IgG, and IgA antibodies to the HA are detected in serum and in respiratory secretions.

As seen in infections with other viruses, IgM and IgA serum antibodies peak approximately 2 weeks after onset of symptoms and then decline, whereas anti-HA IgG antibodies reach maximum levels a few weeks after infection and persist for many years. The durability of the IgG response to influenza was demonstrated during the 1977 reemergence of H1N1 viruses, when individuals with immunologic memory of H1N1 strains circulating before 1957 were to a large extent protected against reinfection. Antibodies to NA generally reach detectable levels in serum only after repeated infections with related strains. In primed individuals, infection with related viruses results in serum IgG and IgA and mucosal (nasal) IgA antibodies in most cases. Antibody-secreting cells of all three immunoglobulin classes may be detected in local lymphatic tissues and peripheral blood as early as 2 days after vaccination of primed individuals (4, 11). The level of the IgM response in primed individuals is most likely dependent on the antigenic relatedness of the infecting virus to previously encountered influenza viruses.

A number of cytokines and chemokines, such as interleukins 6 and 10, tumor necrosis factor alpha, and gamma interferon, can be detected in nasal washes of individuals experimentally infected with influenza viruses. The levels and kinetics of production of some of these cytokines can be correlated with those of clinical symptoms of influenza virus infection (15).

INFLUENZA SURVEILLANCE

Because of the major medical and socioeconomic impact of influenza and because of the constant threat of the emergence of new epidemic or pandemic strains, the World Health Organization established an international network for the global surveillance of influenza as one of its first activities in 1947 (18). The primary goals of this network are to monitor influenza activity worldwide, to identify new epidemic or pandemic strains in a timely manner, to make recommendations for the formulation of the annually updated vaccine, and to make new virus strains available for vaccine production.

PREVENTION AND CONTROL OF INFLUENZA

Vaccination is the primary means to reduce the impact of influenza viruses and the disease they cause. In the United States, annual immunization with influenza vaccine is recommended for individuals and their caregivers who are at increased risk for influenza-related complications (6). Inactivated intramuscular vaccines are licensed for individuals aged >6 months, while live attenuated cold-adapted intranasal vaccines are currently licensed for individuals 5 to 49 years of age (6). Due to the rapid evolution of influenza viruses, the composition of the vaccine has to be updated annually. The response to influenza vaccines is dependent on age, risk status, and immune status of an individual. Influenza vaccine is 70 to 90% effective in preventing influenza illness in younger, healthy adults when the vaccine strain is well matched antigenically with the circulating virus (6).

In addition to vaccine, antiviral agents can be used for prevention and treatment of influenza virus infections. In the United States, amantadine and rimantadine have been licensed for prophylactic and therapeutic use for several years. The prophylactic efficacy of these two compounds is comparable to that of vaccination. Their selective action against influenza A viruses, their side effects (particularly in the case of amantadine), and the rapid emergence of drug-resistant viruses in treated individuals have each contributed to the limited use of these compounds. Drug-resistant viruses can be spread to close contacts and can cause typical influenza (20). Recently a high proportion of amantadine- or rimantadine-resistant viruses were found in several countries (3, 38).

Another class of antivirals against influenza, the NA inhibitors zanamivir and oseltamivir, have been licensed for therapeutic use (17, 21, 22). One major advantage of these two drugs is their activity against both influenza A and influenza B. In clinical studies, NA inhibitors have been shown to reduce complications from influenza (8, 24). Viruses resistant to both zanamivir and oseltamivir were generated in vitro (20, 31). However, no resistant mutants have been isolated so far from immunocompetent patients treated with zanamivir. It was shown that resistant mutants can be isolated from approximately 1% of adults and from 5 to 18% of pediatric patients treated with oseltamivir (26, 36). However, the infectivity of mutant viruses tested has generally been compromised (23, 31).

DIAGNOSIS OF INFLUENZA VIRUS INFECTIONS

Identification of the illness-causing agent, assistance in the selection of optimal treatment, genetic and antigenic characterization of an influenza virus isolate, determination of vaccine immungenicity and efficacy, screening for drug-resistant isolates, providing epidemiological data, and contributing clinical isolates for the selection of vaccine strains are some of the functions performed by laboratories engaged in influenza virus diagnosis. Virus cultivation in cell culture or embryonated hens' eggs, detection of viral antigens or nucleic acids in clinical specimens, or measuring virus-specific antibodies in serum and other specimens are the techniques commonly applied. The reliability and the clinical impact of laboratory diagnosis are greatly influenced by the quality of the clinical specimens and the timing of the specimens' collection, the conditions for transport from the patient to the laboratory, the selection of appropriate methods and reagents, the expertise of the laboratory staff, and quality assurance of the laboratory services.

Specimens for the isolation of viruses or for the direct detection of viral antigens or nucleic acids should be taken early during the course of illness, i.e., during the first 4 days after onset of symptoms. Nose and throat swabs (collected by using a cotton applicator and placed in a suitable transport medium), nasopharyngeal aspirates, and nasal washes are all suitable specimens. The primary goal when collecting such samples should be to obtain as many virus-infected epithelial cells as possible. To avoid inactivation of virus, the specimen should be shipped to the laboratory without delay, preferably refrigerated. If the elapsed time between specimen collection and processing in the laboratory exceeds 72 h, the specimen should be stored frozen at temperatures well below $-40°C$. Paired serum samples collected during the acute phase and 2 to 4 weeks later are required for a serological diagnosis of influenza.

Point-of Care Tests

Although virus isolation is still considered the "gold standard" for diagnosis of influenza, results of virus culturing become available only in several days. The availability of NA inhibitors (see above) stimulated development of rapid diagnostic tests that can be used at the point of care, allowing physicians to prescribe available drugs in a timely manner and reduce unnecessary use of antibiotics (2).

TABLE 1 Rapid diagnostic tests for influenza

Test	CLIA[a] waived	Antigen detected[b]	Specimen type[c,d]	Specimen storage[c]
Directigen Flu A (Becton Dickinson)	No	A	NP wash/aspirate/swab, throat swab	2–8°C, 72 h
Directigen Flu A+B (Becton Dickinson)	No	A+B	NP wash/aspirate/swab, nasal wash, throat swab, BAL	2–8°C, 72 h
Flu OIA (Thermo Electron)	No	A/B	Nasal aspirate/swab, throat swab, sputum	2–8°C, 24 h
Flu OIA A/B (Thermo Electron)	No	A+B	Nasal aspirate/swab, throat swab, sputum	2–8°C, 24 h
Xpect Flu A & B (Remel)	No	A+B	Nasal wash/swab, throat swab	2–8°C, 72 h, or −20°C, 6 mo
NOW Influenza A & B (Binax)	No	A+B	Nasal wash/aspirate, NP swab	2–8°C, 24 h
QuickVue Influenza (Quidel)	Yes	A/B	Nasal wash/aspirate/swab	2–8°C, 8 h, or 15–30°C, 8 h
QuickVue Influenza A+B (Quidel)	Yes	A+B	Nasal wash/aspirate/swab	2–8°C, 8 h, or 15–30°C, 8 h
SAS Influenza A, SAS Influenza B	No	A+B	NP wash/aspirate	4–8°C, 24 h
Clearview Flu A/B (Wampole)	No	A+B	Nasal wash/swab, throat swab	2–8°C, 72 h, or −20°C, 6 mo
ZstatFlu (ZymTx)	Yes	A/B	Throat swab	0–40°C, 24 h

[a]CLIA, Clinical Laboratory Improvement Amendments.
[b]A+B, test differentiates between influenza A and B viruses; A/B, test does not differentiate between A and B viruses.
[c]Per manufacturer test inserts.
[d]NP, nasopharyngeal; BAL, bronchoalveolar lavage.

Most of the point-of-care tests are based on immunoassay detection of viral antigens in clinical samples, while one of them detects virus NA activity (Table 1). These tests require minimal expertise and can be completed within only 10 to 30 min. They are widely available now, although more sensitive and less expensive tests are highly desired. More than 10 rapid diagnostic tests are licensed in the United States (http://www.cdc.gov/flu). Directigen A can identify influenza A only, while some other tests do not distinguish between influenza A or B (Flu OIA, Quick Vue Influenza, and ZstatFlu). Certain tests were designed to differentiate between these two types of influenza (Directigen Flu A+B, Flu OIA A/B, NOW Influenza A & B, QuickVue Influenza A+B, SAS Influenza A and Influenza B, Clearview Flu A/B, and Xpect Flu A & B). Nasopharyngeal washes, nasopharyngeal swabs, nasal aspirates, and nasal swabs are the most common specimens used, although bronchial lavage fluid, throat swabs, and sputum are also mentioned as appropriate specimens in inserts accompanying some rapid diagnostic tests.

Appropriate use of rapid diagnostic tests requires a clear understanding of the predictive value of the tests, which depends on their sensitivity and specificity as well as on the level of influenza activity in the tested population (Table 2). Sensitivity is defined as the percentage of true influenza cases among true-positive (TP) plus false-negative (FN) test results, while specificity is the percentage of true-negative (TN) influenza cases among TN plus FP test results. Variable sensitivity and specificity have been demonstrated for the different rapid diagnostic tests. For example, compared with those of viral culture, the median sensitivity and the median specificity for the Directigen Flu A + B test were shown to be 89.8% (86.6 to 100%) and 98.7% (95.5 to 100%), respectively, in detecting influenza A viruses and 87.5% (62.5 to 88.9%) and 96.8% (88.1 to 100%), respectively, in detecting influenza B viruses (44). Recent study of more than 4,000 respiratory samples revealed that the sensitivity of the Directigen Flu A+B test was 43 to 45% for detection of both influenza A and B viruses in patients with respiratory

symptoms, while the test specificity was more than 99% (5). The median sensitivity and the median specificity of the ZstatFlu test were 68.8% (48.1 to 96%) and 83% (62.7 to 92.4%), respectively, in several studies combined (44).

The positive predictive value (PPV) of a test is equal to the percentage of the value obtained by the equation TP/(TP + FP). The negative predictive value (NPV) of a test is defined as the percentage of the value obtained by the equation TN/(TN + FN). PPV and NPV are important characteristics of a rapid test, since even highly sensitive and specific tests can have low PPVs and high NPVs if the prevalence of influenza in the community is low and, therefore, FP results are most likely to be obtained. When the activity of influenza in the community is low, it is important to confirm positive test results by virus culture or other methods (immunofluorescence or PCR). Accordingly, FN results are more likely during the influenza season.

Rapid diagnostic tests are becoming widely used by many clinics and physicians. However, the accuracy of currently available tests is less than optimal, and these tests have the further limitation of not providing virus isolates for further characterization.

Direct Detection Using FA

The detection by fluorescent antibody (FA) staining of viral antigens in exfoliated epithelial cells of the respiratory tract is a sensitive method that can produce results within 2 to 3 h.

TABLE 2 Sensitivity, specificity, and predictive values of tests[a]

Test result	Disease	
	Present	Absent
Positive	TP	FP
Negative	FN	TN

[a]Determined as described in the text.

Specific monoclonal antibodies for some of the clinically most relevant respiratory viruses can be purchased from several suppliers.

For a successful application of this technique it is essential that the specimen is processed in the laboratory within hours after collection. Briefly, epithelial cells are freed from contaminating mucus, fixed on microscope slides, stained by FA staining methods, and, finally, identified by fluorescence microscopy. Adequate controls, i.e., cell culture-grown preparations, known positive clinical specimens, and monoclonal antibodies with different specificities, should be included in each test run.

1. Dilute the specimen 1:2 to 1:5 in phosphate-buffered saline (PBS), pH 7.4, containing 10 mM dithiothreitol to partly solubilize mucus. Transfer the specimen to a centrifuge tube, add half the volume of 45% Percoll, mix gently with a pipette, and centrifuge at $700 \times g$ for 5 min. Carefully remove the supernatant and resuspend the cell pellet in 3 ml of PBS by gentle pipetting. Underlay the suspension with a 1- to 2-ml cushion of 20% Percoll, and centrifuge at $700 \times g$ for 5 min. Remove the supernatant and resuspend the cells in 0.1 to 1.0 ml of PBS. Add a drop of cell suspension (20 to 50 μl) to marked areas on clean microscope slides. Make an appropriate number of spots for the identification of influenza A and B and eventually other viruses. (Note: The optimal cell density should be determined using microscopic examination; dilute cells sufficiently to avoid overlapping of cells.) Allow slides to dry completely in a fume hood or in a laminar-flow hood and then fix using cold acetone for 5 min.

2. Apply 20 to 50 μl of appropriately diluted monoclonal antibody to each cell spot, place the slide in a moist chamber, and incubate at 37°C for 30 min. Rinse slide thoroughly with washing solution. Add 20 to 50 μl of fluorescein isothiocyanate-conjugated antibodies to mouse immunoglobulins (monoclonal antibodies) to each spot, place the slide in a moist chamber, and incubate at 37°C for 30 min. Rinse the slide thoroughly with washing solution. Drain excess washing solution, tap the slide dry on soft tissue, add mounting medium, and place a coverslip over the cells.

3. Examine the slide by fluorescence microscope at a magnification of ×250 to ×400. Virus-positive cells are identified by intracellular appearance of bright, apple-green fluorescence. A cell spot stained with a virus-negative (control) monoclonal antibody should not contain any fluorescing cells.

With optimal specimens, adequate handling, high-quality reagents, and experienced laboratory personnel, this technique reaches a sensitivity of 80 to 90% compared to standard virus isolation. However, the speed by which a result is obtained outweighs in many cases the reduced sensitivity.

Virus Isolation

Virus isolation in embryonated hens' eggs or in cell cultures continues to be the gold standard in the laboratory diagnosis of influenza virus infections. Days to weeks are required to obtain a conclusive result by virus isolation; therefore, this technique has limited utility in a clinical setting. Yet virus isolation is an invaluable method, because it provides an isolate for antigenic and genetic characterization, which is of utmost importance for the surveillance of influenza and for vaccine production. The continuous line of Madin-Darby canine kidney cells (MDCK) is the cell line of choice for the cultivation of influenza viruses. Trypsin, preferably 1-tosylamide-2-phenylethyl chloromethyl ketone-treated trypsin, at a concentration of 2 μg/ml must be added to the cell culture medium to allow for a continued replication of

influenza viruses in these cells. Primary monkey kidney cells have a wider virus spectrum than MDCK cells, and they do not require addition of trypsin to the medium. However, high cost and occasional contamination with endogenous viruses limit their use in many laboratories. Identification of influenza viruses must be done by hemadsorption, HA titration, or FA staining (25).

Rapid culture, i.e., a combination of virus isolation with detection of viral antigens in the cultured cells by immunoperoxidase staining before changes in the cell morphology can be identified, combines the sensitivity of standard virus isolation with the speed of some culture-independent methods. Protocols have been designed for a type- and subtype-specific identification of influenza viruses 16 to 24 h after inoculation (49).

RT-PCR

Reverse transcriptase PCR (RT-PCR) offers a rapid and highly sensitive method for the identification of influenza and other respiratory viruses in clinical specimens (10, 47). Although this method does not produce an isolate for further analysis, genetic variation of epidemic strains can be identified by nucleic acid sequencing, and with appropriate selection of primers, amino acid changes in the antigenic sites on the HA can be identified.

RT-PCR can be used for the detection of influenza viruses in original respiratory samples from patients, or for the characterization of viruses grown in tissue culture or embryonated eggs. Isolated virus RNA is first reverse transcribed into a cDNA copy using RT. The cDNA is then subjected to a repeated thermal cyclic reaction causing template denaturation (95°C), primer annealing (45 to 60°C), and product extension (72°C). RT-PCR requires an RNA template, a pair of oligonucleotides (or forward and reverse primers) that are complementary to the template, four deoxyribonucleoside triphosphates RT, and a thermostable DNA polymerase, such as *Taq* or *Tth*, that is not inactivated at 95°C. Since products of one round of amplification serve as templates for the next, each cycle of PCR doubles the amount of copied DNA. One-step RT-PCR reagent kits that combine reverse transcription and PCR reagents in one tube are available as well. Because it is not necessary to open the reaction tube to add PCR reagents following the reverse transcription reaction, one-step RT-PCR makes the amplification procedure simpler and less susceptible to contamination.

Nested or seminested RT-PCRs can significantly increase the sensitivity and specificity of PCR by further amplification of DNA using another set of forward and/or reverse primers. These secondary primers are complementary to regions located within the DNA copy amplified during the first round of PCR. The sensitivity of nested PCR in detection of influenza A(H1N1), A(H3N2), and B viruses can be as high as one to four target gene copies per reaction (45).

Recently, PCR strategies have been designed that utilize fluorescent probes for detection and/or quantitation of amplified DNA in real time (30). The most common real-time PCR strategy utilizes a dually labeled oligonucleotide probe (e.g., Taqman probe) that is labeled with a fluorescent dye, or fluorophore, and a quencher dye. Because the probe binds to the specific target and does not bind to nonspecific products, fluorescence is only observed if the desired DNA is amplified. A number of other real-time formats for detection of specific targets have been designed. Nevertheless, the sensitivity and specificity of real-time PCR as well as conventional RT-PCR depend on the quality of clinical samples and their storage

(42) as well as on the quality of the oligonucleotide primers and probes used for amplification.

Because of genetic diversity among influenza viruses, it is possible to design PCR primers and probes that will specifically detect only one influenza type or subtype. On the other hand, the M gene is the most conserved influenza virus gene and is widely used as a target for the detection of all influenza A type viruses. Specific primers that amplify the HA and NA genes are used for detection of influenza A virus subtypes. In addition, a number of protocols have been designed for the detection of influenza B viruses based on their NS genes (13, 29, 40, 45).

In order to avoid contamination and to protect the integrity of the sample RNA, it is important to comply with certain conditions during PCR performance:

- Work surfaces, pipettes, and centrifuges should be cleaned routinely to minimize the risk of contamination from DNA or RNA as well as RNase. Gloves should be used and changed as needed.
- All reagents should be kept on ice during assay setup.
- Negative ("water") controls and viral RNA-positive controls should be included in each run.
- Viral RNA controls should be added as the final step after all reagents, primers, and sample RNAs are sealed.
- When original clinical materials are used for detection of influenza virus genes, a primer and probe set to a host gene mRNA such as the human RNase P gene can be used as a positive control (12). Amplification of this RNA by conventional or real-time RT-PCR serves to validate the quality of the clinical sample. Failure to detect RNase P RNA in any of the clinical samples may be the result of an insufficient number of human cells in the sample, of improper extraction (loss) of RNA from clinical materials, or of the presence of RT-PCR inhibitors in a clinical specimen.
- Excessive amounts of RNA or DNA in the specimen may result in FN results. If a high level of nucleic acid is suspected, the sample may be tested at several dilutions to verify the negative results.

Serological Detection of Infection

Serodiagnosis of influenza virus infection can be established by a >4-fold increase of antibody titers between serum samples collected during the acute and convalescent phases of the illness. Acute-phase sera should be collected as soon as possible but no more than 7 days from the onset of illness. The convalescent-phase sera should be collected 2 to 3 weeks after the acute-phase sera. Because of the possibility of detection of antibody induced by prior infection or vaccination with influenza, single serum samples generally cannot be used for serodiagnosis of recent influenza virus infection, regardless of the type of assay to be used. Due to the need for paired sera, serodiagnosis of infection is necessarily retrospective in nature and is therefore not useful for patient management. Nevertheless, serodiagnosis may be useful to determine the etiology of a respiratory illness when virus isolation has not been successful or possible. The gold standard for serodiagnosis of infection or response to vaccination with human influenza viruses is the hemagglutination inhibition (HAI) assay (25). The microneutralization test is an alternative method for the detection of strain-specific antibodies to influenza viruses and in some cases may be more sensitive than the HAI test (37). This is particularly important for the detection of antibodies to avian influenza viruses in human sera, for

which the microneutralization assay should be used due to the fact that the HAI test is not sensitive enough to detect these antibodies. Although rarely used, the complement fixation test can be performed using unconcentrated virus in tissue culture supernatants or allantoic fluid, and it predominantly detects antibodies directed against the influenza virus NP and thus does not allow for a subtype- or strain-specific diagnosis. Although the complement fixation test is less specific than tests mentioned below, it may be useful during periods when antigens prepared from currently circulating viruses are not yet available. Enzyme immunoassays are typically performed to measure virus-specific IgG, IgM, or IgA antibodies in paired samples, e.g., acute- and convalescent-phase sera or pre- and postvaccination serum or respiratory samples. Such immunoassays perform optimally when concentrated and/or purified preparations of viral antigen are used to detect antibodies.

HAI Test

The HAI test is the standard method for characterizing the antigenic properties of influenza virus isolates, for serodiagnosis of influenza virus infections as well as for seroepidemiological studies detecting human influenza virus infection (25, 48). The HAI test measures strain-specific antibodies (Table 3); thus, the identity of the infecting strain can be established or the response to single components of the trivalent vaccine can be precisely determined. The quality of results obtained by the HAI test can be influenced by several factors. First, inhibitors present in some sera must be removed before testing. Treatment of sera with receptor-destroying enzyme from *Vibrio cholerae* is the usual method of choice, but trypsin-periodate treatment with heat may also effectively remove inhibitors from sera. Second, the source and quality of the red blood cells, which may be turkey, guinea pig, or human type O red blood cells, can greatly influence the test result. Third, the growth substrate of the antigen and the treatment of the antigen may also influence the test results. Because of the instability of the HA, the working dilution of antigen must be precisely determined and titered each time the HAI assay is performed. Well-characterized standard positive and negative reference sera must be included in each test (47). A detailed protocol is available on the World Health Organization website (http://www.who.org).

Microneutralization Test

The microneutralization test is a highly sensitive assay applicable to the identification of virus-specific antibody in human sera. The neutralization test has several additional advantages for detecting antibody to influenza virus. First, the assay primarily detects antibodies to the influenza virus HA and thus can identify functional, strain-specific antibodies in human serum. Second, since infectious virus is used, the assay can be developed quickly upon recognition of a novel virus and is available before suitable purified viral proteins become available for use in other assays. The microneutralization test is a sensitive and specific assay for detecting virus-specific antibody to avian influenza A viruses in human serum. The microneutralization test could detect H5-specific antibody in human serum at titers that could not be detected by the HAI assay, the traditional test used for the detection of antibodies to human influenza A and B viruses (37).

The microneutralization test has been designed to be a more rapid neutralization test in that it can yield results within 2 days, compared with other neutralization assays that take 3 to 4 days. The neutralization test is performed in two stages. The first is a virus-antibody reaction step in which serially diluted serum is preincubated with a standardized

TABLE 3 Antigenic drift of H3N2 viruses between 1968 and 2004 as demonstrated by their cross-reactivities in HAI tests using postinfection ferret sera

Strain designation	Cross-reactivity (HAI titer) of serum to:															
	HK68	ENG72	VIC75	TEX77	BAN79	PHI82	MIS85	SHN87	BEI89	BEI92	JHB94	NAN95	SYD97	PAN99	WYO3	NY04
A/Hong Kong/1/68 (HK68)	2,560	1,280	5	5	5	5	10	10	5	5	5	5	5	5	5	5
A/England/42/72 (ENG72)	320	1,280	80	20	5	5	5	5	5	5	5	5	5	5	5	5
A/Victoria/3/75 (VIC75)	5	80	320	40	10	20	10	5	5	5	5	5	5	5	5	5
A/Texas/1/77 (TEX77)	5	80	160	1,280	160	320	320	10	5	5	5	5	5	5	5	5
A/Bangkok/1/79 (BAN79)	5	5	80	640	640	640	640	20	5	5	5	5	5	5	5	5
A/Philippines/2/82 (PHI82)	5	5	10	40	40	320	160	10	5	5	5	5	5	5	5	5
A/Mississippi/1/85 (MIS85)	5	5	40	160	80	640	640	40	20	20	5	5	5	5	5	5
A/Shanghai/11/87 (SHN87)	5	5	5	5	5	5	80	320	160	40	10	10	10	5	5	5
A/Beijing/353/89 (BEI89)	5	5	5	5	5	5	5	160	320	640	20	5	5	5	5	5
A/Beijing/32/92 (BEI92)	5	5	5	5	5	5	10	20	80	160	160	40	5	5	5	5
A/Johannesburg/33/94 (JHB94)	5	5	5	5	5	5	5	10	20	20	640	40	5	5	5	5
A/Nanchang/933/95 (NAN95)	5	5	5	5	5	5	5	10	5	5	40	1,280	40	20	5	5
A/Sydney/5/97 (SYD97)	5	5	5	5	5	5	5	5	5	5	5	40	640	160	40	5
A/Panama/2007/99 (PAN99)	5	5	5	5	5	5	5	5	5	5	5	40	160	640	320	40
A/Wyoming/3/2003 (WYO3)	5	5	5	5	5	5	5	5	5	5	5	5	40	160	1,280	320
A/New York/55/2004 (NY04)	5	5	5	5	5	5	5	5	5	5	5	5	5	40	320	640

amount of virus and then inoculated into MDCK cell culture. After an overnight incubation, the cells are fixed and the presence of influenza A virus NP in infected cells is detected by enzyme-linked immunosorbent assay. The absence of infectivity constitutes a positive neutralization reaction and indicates the presence of virus-specific antibodies capable of neutralizing virus infectivity in human or animal sera prior to the addition of MDCK cells. As with other serological assays, well-characterized standard positive and negative reference sera must be included in each test. A protocol for a microneutralization test-enzyme immunoassay has been described previously (37). A detailed protocol for this assay will soon be available on the World Health Organization website (http://www.who.org).

CONCLUSIONS

Although influenza is often identified by its clinical presentation, multicenter studies using well-trained clinicians have shown that clinical diagnosis of influenza has an accuracy of 50 to 75% (21). Laboratory diagnostic services are therefore essential for several reasons. Early during the influenza season, the presence of influenza viruses in the community should be verified and the antigenic match between the circulating epidemic strains and the vaccine viruses should be determined. Laboratory diagnosis should be considered for atypical cases presenting during the influenza season and in cases where treatment with antiviral agents may be of benefit for the patient. In these instances, a rapid method such as detection of viral antigens in clinical specimens is the method of choice. Virus isolation and detection of virus antigens or nucleic acids in clinical specimens become more difficult a few days after onset of illness, when the amount of virus shed by the patient typically is decreasing. If a laboratory diagnosis is required during this stage, serological methods may provide the answer. It is often during the late part of an epidemic that new antigenic variants emerge. These variants are of particular interest because they may possess antigenic characteristics that will be predominant in viruses of the following season. For this reason, it is desirable to collect a representative number of isolates for antigenic characterization at the end of the season. Virus isolation should also be attempted when suspected cases occur outside the typical influenza season. With the availability of effective drugs for the prevention and treatment of influenza, the need for rapid diagnostic services is increasing. Some of these tests can be performed in a doctor's office or on a hospital ward, and they are of great importance for the appropriate use of antiviral medications and antibiotics. However, specialized laboratories must continue to use more sophisticated techniques such as virus isolation, RT-PCR, and serological methods in order to monitor the antigenic and genetic characteristics of influenza viruses circulating worldwide.

REFERENCES

1. **Betts, R. F.** 1995. Influenza virus, p. 1546–1567. *In* G. L. Mandell, J. E. Bennett, and R. Dolin (ed.), *Principles and Practice of Infectious Diseases.* Churchill Livingstone Inc., New York, N.Y.

2. **Bonner, A. B., K. W. Monroe, L. I. Talley, A. E. Klasner, and D. W. Kimberlin.** 2003. Impact of the rapid diagnosis of influenza on physician decision-making and patient management: results of a randomized, prospective, controlled trial. *Pediatrics* **112:**363–367.

3. **Bright, B. A., M. J. Medina, X. Xu, G. Perez-Oronoz, T. R. Wallis, L. Povinelli, N. J. Cox, and A. I. Klimov.** Increasing incidence of adamantane resistance among

influenza A(H3N2) viruses, isolated globally from 1994 to 2004: a cause for concern. *Lancet* **366:**1175–1181.

4. **Brockstad, K. A., R. J. Cox, J. Olofsson, R. Johsson, and L. R. Haaheim.** 1995. Parenteral influenza vaccination induces a rapid systemic and local immune response. *J. Infect. Dis.* **171:**198–203.

5. **Cazacu, A. C., S. E. Chung, J. Greer, and G. J. Demmler.** 2004. Comparison of the Directigen Flu A+B membrane enzyme immunoassay with viral culture for rapid detection of influenza A and B viruses in respiratory specimens. *J. Clin. Microbiol.* **42:**3707–3710.

6. **Centers for Disease Control and Prevention.** 2004. Prevention and control of influenza. Recommendations of the Advisory Committee on Immunization Practices (ACIP). *Morb. Mortal. Wkly. Rep.* **53:**1–39.

7. **Claas, E. C. J., A. D. M. E. Osterhaus, R. van Beek, J. C. De Jong, G. F. Rimmelzwaan, D. A. Senne, S. Krauss, K. F. Shortridge, and R. G. Webster.** 1998. Human influenza A H5N1 virus related to a highly pathogenic avian influenza virus. *Lancet* **351:**472–477.

8. **Cooper, N. J., A. J. Sutton, K. R. Abrams, A. Wailoo, D. Turner, and K. G. Nicholson.** 2003. Effectiveness of neuraminidase inhibitors in treatment and prevention of influenza A and B: systematic review and meta-analyses of randomized controlled trials. *Br. Med. J.* **326:**1235–1239.

9. **Cox, N. J., and K. Subbarao.** 1999. Influenza. *Lancet* **354:**1277–1282.

10. **Ellis, J. S., D. M. Fleming, and M. C. Zambon.** 1997. Multiplex reverse transcription-PCR for surveillance of influenza A and B viruses in England and Wales in 1995 and 1996. *J. Clin. Microbiol.* **35:**2076–2082.

11. **El-Madhun, A. S., R. J. Cox, A. Soreide, J. Olofsson, and L. R. Haaheim.** 1998. Systemic and mucosal immune responses in young children and adults after parenteral influenza vaccination. *J. Infect. Dis.* **178:**933–939.

12. **Emery, S. L., D. D. Erdman, M. D. Bowen, B. R. Newton, J. M. Winchell, R. F. Meyer, S. Tong, B. T. Cook, B. P. Holloway, K. A. McCaustland, P. A. Rota, B. Bankamp, L. E. Lowe, T. G. Ksiazek, W. J. Bellini, and L. J. Anderson.** 2004. Real-time reverse transcription-polymerase chain reaction assay for SARS-associated coronavirus. *Emerg. Infect. Dis.* **10:**311–316.

13. **Fouchier, R. A., T. M. Bestebroer, S. Herfst, L. Van Der Kemp, G. F. Rimmelzwaan, and A. D. M. E. Osterhaus.** 2000. Detection of influenza A viruses from different species by PCR amplification of conserved sequences in the matrix gene. *J. Clin. Microbiol.* **38:**4096–4101.

14. **Fouchier, R. A., V. Munster, A. Wallensten, T. M. Bestebroer, S. Herfst, D. Smith, G. F. Rimmelzwaan, B. Olsen, and A. D. Osterhaus.** 2005. Characterization of a novel influenza A virus hemagglutinin subtype (H16) obtained from black-headed gulls. *J. Virol.* **79:**2814–2822.

15. **Fritz, R. S., F. G. Hayden, D. P. Calfee, L. M. R. Cass, A. W. Peng, W. G. Alvord, W. Strober, and S. E. Straus.** 1999. Nasal cytokine and chemokine responses in experimental influenza A virus infection: results of a placebo-controlled trial of intravenous zanamivir treatment. *J. Infect. Dis.* **180:**586–593.

16. **Gerhard, W.** 2001. The role of the antibody response to influenza virus infection. *Curr. Top. Microbiol. Immunol.* **260:**171–190.

17. **Gubareva, L. V., L. Kaiser, and F. G. Hayden.** 2000. Influenza virus neuraminidase inhibitors. *Lancet* **355:**827–835.

18. **Hampson, A. W.** 1997. Surveillance for pandemic influenza. *J. Infect. Dis.* **176:**S8–S13.

19. **Hay, A. J.** 1998. The virus genome and its replication, pp. 43–53. *In* K. G. Nicholson, R. G. Webster, and A. J. Hay (ed.), *Textbook of Influenza.* Blackwell Science Ltd., Oxford, United Kingdom.

20. **Hayden, F. G., R. B. Belshe, R. D. Clover, A. J. Hay, M. G. Oakes, and W. Soo.** 1989. Emergence and apparent transmission of rimantadine-resistant influenza A virus in families. *N. Engl. J. Med.* **321:**1696–1702.

21. **Hayden, F. G., A. D. M. E. Osterhaus, J. J. Treanor, D. M. Fleming, F. Y. Aoki, K. G. Nicholson, A. M. Bohnen, H. M. Hirst, O. Keene, and K. Wightman.** 1997. Efficacy and safety of the neuraminidase inhibitor zanamivir in the treatment of influenza virus infections. *N. Engl. J. Med.* **337:**874–880.

22. **Hayden, F. G., J. J. Treanor, R. S. Fritz, M. Lobo, R. F. Betts, M. Miller, N. Kinnersley, R. G. Mills, P. Ward, and S. E. Straus.** 1999. Use of the oral neuraminidase inhibitor oseltamivir in experimental human influenza. *JAMA* **282:**1240–1246.

23. **Herlocher, M. L., J. Carr, J. Ives, S. Elias, R. Truscon, N. Roberts, and A. S. Monto.** 2002. Influenza virus carrying an R292K mutation in the neuraminidase gene is not transmitted in ferrets. *Antivir. Res.* **54:**99–111.

24. **Kaiser, L., C. Wat, T. Mills, P. Mahoney, P. Ward, and F. Hayden.** 2003. Impact of oseltamivir treatment on influenza-related lower respiratory tract complications and hospitalizations. *Arch. Intern. Med.* **163:**1667–1672.

25. **Kendal, A. P., J. J. Skehel, and M. S. Pereira.** 1982. *Concepts and Procedures for Laboratory-Based Influenza Surveillance.* Centers for Disease Control, Atlanta, Ga.

26. **Kiso, M., K. Mitamura, Y. Sakai-Tagawa, K. Shiraishi, C. Kawakami, K. Kimura, F. G. Hayden, N. Sugaya, and Y. Kawaoka.** 2004. Resistant influenza A viruses in children treated with oseltamivir: descriptive study. *Lancet* **364:**759–765.

27. **Koopmans, M., B. Wilbrink, M. Conyn, G. Natrop, H. van der Nat, H. Vennema, A. Meijer, J. van Steenbergen, R. Fouchier, A. Osterhaus, and A. Bosman.** 2004. Transmission of H7N7 avian influenza A virus to human beings during a large outbreak in commercial poultry farms in the Netherlands. *Lancet* **363:**587–593.

28. **Lamb, R. A., and R. M. Krug.** 1996. Orthomyxoviridae: the viruses and their replication, pp. 1353–1395. *In* B. N. Fields, D. M. Knipe, and P. M. Howley (ed.), *Fields Virology,* 3rd ed. Lippincott-Raven, Philadelphia, Pa.

29. **Lee, M. S., P. C. Chang, J. H. Shien, M. C. Cheng, and H. K. Shieh.** 2001. Identification and subtyping of avian influenza viruses by reverse transcription-PCR. *J. Virol. Methods* **97:**13–22.

30. **Mackay, I. M., K. E. Arden, and A. Nitsche.** 2002. Real-time PCR in virology. *Nucleic Acids Res.* **30:**1291–1305.

31. **McKimm-Breschkin, J. L.** 2000. Resistance of influenza viruses to neuraminidase inhibitors—a review. *Antivir. Res.* **47:**1–17.

32. **Moriuchi, H., N. Katsushima, H. Nishimura, K. Nakamura, and Y. Numazaki.** 1991. Community-acquired influenza C virus infection in children. *J. Pediatr.* **118:**235–238.

33. **Nicholson, K. G.** 1998. Human influenza, pp. 219–264. *In* K. G. Nicholson, R. G. Webster, and A. J. Hay (ed.), *Textbook of Influenza.* Blackwell Science Ltd., Oxford, United Kingdom.

34. **Osterhaus, A. D., G. F. Rimmelzwaan, B. E. Martina, T. M. Bestebroer, and R. A. Fouchier.** 2000. Influenza B virus in seals. *Science* **288:**1051–1053.

35. **Peiris, M., K. Y. Yuen, C. W. Leung, K. H. Chan, P. L. Ip, R. W. Lai, W. K. Orr, and K. F. Shortridge.** 1999. Human infection with influenza H9N2. *Lancet* **354:**916–917.

36. **Roberts, N.** 2001. Treatment of influenza with neuraminidase inhibitors: virological implications. *Philos. Trans. R. Soc.* **356:**1895–1897.

37. **Rowe, T., R. A. Abernathy, J. Hu-Primmer, W. W. Thompson, X. Lu, W. Lim, K. Fukuda, N. J. Cox, and J. M. Katz.** 1999. Detection of antibody to avian influenza

A(H5N1) virus in human serum by using a combination of serologic assays. *J. Clin. Microbiol.* **37:**937–943.

38. **Shiraishi, K., K. Mitamura, Y. Sakai-Tagawa, H. Goto, N. Sugaya, and Y. Kawaoka.** 2003. High frequency of resistant viruses harboring different mutations in amantadine-treated children with influenza. *J. Infect. Dis.* **188:**57–61.

39. **Simonsen, L., K. Fukuda, L. B. Schonberger, and N. J. Cox.** 2000. The impact of influenza epidemics on hospitalization. *J. Infect. Dis.* **181:**831–837.

40. **Spackman, E., D. A. Senne, T. J. Myers, L. L. Bulaga, L. P. Garber, M. L. Perdue, K. Lohman, L. T. Daum, and D. L. Suarez.** 2002. Development of a real-time reverse transcriptase PCR assay for type A influenza virus and the avian H5 and H7 hemagglutinin subtypes. *J. Clin. Microbiol.* **40:**3256–3260.

41. **Stevenson, P. G., and P. C. Doherty.** 1998. Cell-mediated immune response to influenza virus, pp. 278–287. *In* K. G. Nicholson, R. G. Webster, and A. J. Hay (ed.), *Textbook of Influenza.* Blackwell Science Ltd., Oxford, United Kingdom.

42. **Stone, B., J. Burrows, S. Schepetiuk, G. Higgins, A. Hampson, R. Shaw, and T. W. Kok.** 2004. Rapid detection and simultaneous subtype differentiation of influenza A viruses by real time PCR. *J. Virol. Methods* **117:**103–112.

43. **Subbarao, K., A. Klimov, J. Katz, H. Regnery, W. Lim, H. Hall, M. Perdue, D. Swayne, C. Bender, J. Huang, M. Hemphill, T. Rowe, M. Shaw, X. Xu, K. Fukuda, and N. Cox.** 1998. Characterization of an avian influenza A (H5N1) virus isolated from a child with a fatal respiratory illness. *Science* **279:**393–396.

44. **Uyeki, T.** 2003. Influenza diagnosis and treatment in children. A review of studies on clinically useful tests and antiviral treatment for influenza. *Pediatr. Infect. Dis. J.* **22:**164–177.

45. **Van Elden, L. J. R., M. Nihuis, P. Shipper, R. Schuurman, and A. M. van Loon.** 2001. Simultaneous detection of influenza viruses A and B using real-time quantitative PCR. *J. Clin. Microbiol.* **39:**196–200.

46. **Webster, R. G., W. J. Bean, O. T. Gorman, T. M. Chambers, and Y. Kawaoka.** 1992. Evolution and ecology of influenza A viruses. *Microbiol. Rev.* **56:**152–179.

47. **Weinberg, G. A., D. D. Erdman, K. M. Edwards, C. B. Hall, F. J. Walker, M. R. Griffin, B. Schwartz, and the New Vaccine Surveillance Network Study Group.** 2004. Superiority of reverse-transcription polymerase chain reaction to conventional viral culture in the diagnosis of acute respiratory tract infections in children. *J. Infect. Dis.* **189:**706–710.

48. **Wood, J. M., R. E. Gaines-Das, J. Taylor, and P. Chakraverty.** 1994. Comparison of influenza serological techniques by international collaborative study. *Vaccine* **12:**167–174.

49. **Ziegler, T., H. Hall, A. Sanchez-Fauquier, W. C. Gamble, and N. J. Cox.** 1995. Type- and subtype-specific detection of influenza viruses in clinical specimens by rapid culture assay. *J. Clin. Microbiol.* **33:**318–321.

Respiratory Syncytial Virus, Human Metapneumovirus, and the Parainfluenza Viruses

PEDRO A. PIEDRA AND GUY BOIVIN

79

Respiratory syncytial virus (RSV), human metapneumovirus (HMPV), and the parainfluenza viruses (PIVs) are the major viral causes of acute respiratory tract disease in infants and children (32, 37). RSV is the single most important cause of bronchiolitis and pneumonia among young children. It is the major virus associated with hospitalization for acute lower respiratory tract disease in children younger than 5 years of age. Most of the hospitalizations occur in children younger than 12 months of age (32). HMPV is a recently recognized paramyxovirus that causes respiratory tract disease similar to that due to RSV (20, 37). It appears to be the second most common cause of bronchiolitis and pneumonia among young children. HMPV is often detected in children with underlying chronic conditions. Coinfection with RSV and HMPV may cause a more severe illness than infection with RSV or HMPV alone (19). PIVs regularly cause pneumonia, bronchiolitis, and croup among infants and children. Like RSV and HMPV, PIVs are associated mostly with acute upper respiratory tract illnesses in children. Among adults, RSV and PIVs cause a modest number of community-acquired pneumonias, especially in immunocompromised and elderly persons (9, 18). HMPV appears also to be a cause of community-acquired pneumonias in elderly adults (37). Limited information is available on the impact of HMPV in the immunocompromised host. RSV has been documented to cause outbreaks among elderly persons in semiclosed institutions, such as nursing homes, and is associated with high attack rates of pneumonia and significant case fatality rates (14). Nosocomial RSV, HMPV, and PIV infections occur among infants, children, and adults.

RSV, HMPV, and PIVs belong to the *Paramyxoviridae* family of respiratory viruses. The *Pneumovirnae* subfamily contains the *Pneumovirus* and *Metapneumovirus* genera. RSV is a pneumovirus that comprises two subgroups, A and B; HMPV is a metapneumovirus that also consists of two subgroups, A and B. The PIVs, members of the paramyxovirus group, include four serotypes, 1, 2, 3, and 4A and 4B. RSV, HMPV, and PIV are transmitted mainly by direct contact and uncommonly by aerosols. Epidemics of RSV and HMPV occur annually in the fall, winter, and spring in temperate climates. RSV epidemics last for approximately 20 weeks starting in October or November and ending in March or April. There are geographic differences with respect to the onset, peak, and end of the RSV epidemics. In the United States, RSV outbreak arrives earlier in the southern and midwestern states than in the northern and western states. Subgroups A and B circulate together in epidemics; however, subgroup A occurs about three times as often as subgroup B and may cause somewhat more severe illness. HMPV subgroups A and B cocirculate during the outbreak. The severity of HMPV disease has yet to be associated with a particular subgroup. PIVs exhibit differing epidemiological patterns: PIV type 3 occurs endemically with outbreaks in early spring, PIV type 2 occurs sporadically, and PIV type 1 occurs mainly in epidemics during the fall of alternate years.

Rapid diagnosis of RSV infection is very important because of the availability of effective treatment modalities for children with serious infections and for reduction of nosocomial infection. These are ribavirin, an established anti-RSV drug, and a new humanized monoclonal antibody for prophylaxis, designated palivizumab (32). Although ribavirin is an approved drug for the treatment of RSV disease, its use remains controversial because of its expense and limited benefit in shortening the duration of hospitalization. A potential long-term benefit of ribavirin treatment of RSV illness in children free of underlying disease may be a reduction in the frequency of reactive airway disease later in life (11). Ribavirin administered as an aerosol provides some therapeutic benefit in the treatment of RSV infection in infants with underlying cardiopulmonary diseases. Its current use is restricted primarily to children and adults who are immunocompromised. Palivizumab is directed against the fusion (F) protein of RSV and is effective in the prevention of hospital-related RSV infections in preterm infants, children with bronchopulmonary dysplasia, and children with hemodynamically unstable congenital heart disease (16, 21, 36). Vaccines for RSV, HMPV, and PIV remain in the developmental stage despite substantial research and clinical testing of various candidate vaccines.

LABORATORY DIAGNOSTIC TESTS

Rapid laboratory diagnosis of RSV, HMPV, and PIV infections, using sensitive and specific procedures that are cost-effective, can lead to a decrease in diagnostic evaluation tests, avoids indiscriminate use of antibiotics, reduces the number of nosocomial infections, and allows a rational use for specific anti-RSV treatment measures. A number of major approaches to the laboratory diagnosis of these virus infections are available: (i) tissue culture for virus isolation from respiratory secretions of the upper and lower respiratory tract, (ii) rapid detection of viral antigen in respiratory secretions or middle ear effusions (in otitis media), (iii) viral RNA detection in respiratory secretions, and (iv) determination of specific antibody responses by serological assays.

Common Diagnostic Tests in a Hospital Laboratory

RSV and PIV infections can be rapidly diagnosed by the demonstration of viral antigen in exfoliated respiratory tract epithelial cells present in respiratory tract secretions, including nasal wash specimens. The "gold standard" for the diagnosis of RSV and PIV infection is virus isolation from respiratory tract specimens; however, this requires several days until virus growth in tissue cultures can be identified, often after the acute phase of illness subsides. Also, attention to transport and processing of the specimen is required because of virus lability. A shell vial technique reduces the time for virus isolation and identification to 24 to 48 h. Most hospital laboratories are not able to isolate HMPV in tissue culture because frequently the optimal cell line is not used, serum-free medium containing trypsin is needed, and the detection of viral cytopathic effect (CPE) requires a long incubation. Reverse transcription-PCR (RT-PCR) is currently the preferred test for the detection of HMPV (8, 37).

RSV and PIV infection can be rapidly diagnosed by demonstrating viral antigens in exfoliated respiratory tract mucosal cells. Several sensitive and specific assays have been described for identifying viruses in exfoliated cells, including immunofluoresence (IF), enzyme linked immunosorbent assay (ELISA), time-resolved fluoroimmunoassay, and RT-PCR (6, 7, 24, 35, 40). These procedures employ monoclonal antibodies directed against one of the major structural proteins of the virus or DNA primers to cDNA of the specific viruses. Diagnostic kits based on ELISA procedures contain all reagents and provide "self-contained" reasonably sensitive and specific assays for routine diagnosis in the hospital laboratory. Antigen detection diagnostic kits are routinely used for RSV. IF for identifying RSV and PIV antigens in exfoliated cells is used in some hospital laboratories, but this test requires well-trained technicians. In general, antigen tests are not very sensitive or useful in testing adults because the reduced viral loads in adults are frequently below the lower limits of detection of the tests. Commercial reagents for HMPV are currently not available. Multiplex PCR or RT-PCR is used in some hospital laboratories as the preferred method for rapid detection of common childhood respiratory viruses including RSV, HMPV, and PIVs. With the emphasis on the rapidity of diagnostic information and cost, procedures such as the antigen detection diagnostic kits and IF are often preferred in the hospital laboratory.

Common Serologic Tests in a Research Laboratory

Serologic assays are infrequently used in the hospital laboratory for the detection of RSV, HMPV and PIVs; however, these assays are frequently used for research purposes. They include the detection of RSV-specific immunoglobulin A (IgA), IgG, and IgM antibody in secretions, breast milk, and serum and the detection of diagnostic (fourfold) antibody rises between acute-phase and convalescent-phase serum specimens ("paired" serums). The Western blot (WB) test is useful in identifying RSV infection, in particular, in persons who have received an investigational RSV subunit vaccine (33). Antibody to RSV, HMPV, and PIV can be assayed by ELISA, virus neutralization (NT), direct or indirect IF, complement fixation (CF), and, for PIV, hemagglutination inhibition (HI). ELISA is a sensitive and specific procedure and

is the mainstay of serologic procedures for the diagnosis of RSV, HMPV, and PIV. A shortcoming of ELISA is that it measures the amount of binding antibody, which does not always correlate with protection against disease. NT assays such as the microneutralization and plaque reduction assays are similar to ELISA in sensitivity and specificity. The advantage of an NT assay is that it measures the neutralizing-antibody activity of serum, which is a better correlate of immunity than is binding antibody (34). NT assays, however, are more labor-intensive and require longer for completion.

The levels of antibody to RSV, HMPV, and PIV in large groups of infants, children, and adults can be measured in epidemiologic surveys by ELISA, including immunoglobulin-specific ELISA, as well as IF and NT tests that detect serum IgG antibody (or "protective" antibody) and reflect the immune status. Since HI antibody to PIV correlates well with the level of NT antibody, HI provides a sensitive, reliable, and rapid method for the survey of type-specific PIV antibody. The NT tests provide an excellent means of detecting protective antibody to RSV, HMPV, and PIV, but these procedures are labor-intensive and are generally performed only in research laboratories. Immunoglobulin-specific ELISA provides a highly specific and sensitive method of measuring individual serum IgA, IgG, and IgM responses. Infants younger than 6 months respond less than half the time with a brisk and high-titer IgG or NT antibody response because they all possess maternal antibody to RSV, HMPV, and PIV and because of their immature immunological systems (4, 18). In this age group, determination of antibody responses to infection with RSV, HMPV, and PIV should include several different assays to increase the likelihood of detecting an antibody response (5).

A site-specific ELISA employing as antigen one or more synthetic peptides of the reactive site of the large glycoprotein (G) and F protein of RSV provides an additional means of detecting antibody to RSV, mainly in research studies (2). A single peptide comprising 15 amino acids (peptide 12) of the G protein of RSV selectively reacts with monoclonal antibodies generated against the G protein. Use of peptides from subgroup A and B strains of RSV provides a means of measuring subgroup-specific antibody responses. This approach does not appear to be as sensitive as ELISA procedures employing whole virus antigen (3).

CLINICAL INDICATIONS FOR SEROLOGIC STUDIES

The choice of an assay for measuring antibody to RSV, HMPV, and PIV depends on several factors, including the objective of the test, information needed concerning current or past infection, the immunological status and age of the person being tested, and the sensitivity, specificity, rapidity, and complexity of the test employed. ELISA, HI, IF, NT, and WB procedures provide highly specific and especially reliable means for the determination of antibody to RSV, HMPV, and PIV. The HI test applies only to PIVs. The IgM ELISAs give serologic evidence of an acute infection even if only a single specimen of respiratory tract secretions or a single serum specimen, obtained soon after the onset of illness, is used. The WB test for RSV also provides serologic evidence of a recent infection even if a single serum specimen is used (33). It is likely that a WB profile for recent infection also can be developed for HMPV and PIVs. ELISA seems the best assay for antibody detection in the hospital diagnostic laboratory because it is highly sensitive, specific, and easy to use and provides the most practical method for detecting antibody to RSV, HMPV, and PIV in persons of all ages, including infants and children younger than 6 months.

Paired serum specimens can be used for the diagnosis of RSV, HMPV, and PIV infection in patients with an acute illness; a wait of usually 18 to 21 days, but preferably not later than 35 days, is necessary before the convalescent-phase (second) serum specimen can be collected. This approach does not seem practical for acutely ill patients, because by this time the patient has recovered. Recent infection is signaled by detection of a fourfold or greater rise in antibody level in the convalescent-phase serum compared to the acute-phase serum. A diagnostic rise in antibody titer that is temporally associated with illness provides serologic evidence that the illness resulted from infection with that virus. However, when mitigating circumstances exist, the convalescent-phase serum can be obtained earlier, between 10 and 17 days after the acute-phase serum is collected. Importantly, use of a convalescent-phase serum specimen drawn too soon after the acute-phase serum specimen or an acute-phase serum drawn too late after onset of disease diminishes the opportunity of detecting a diagnostic antibody rise.

INTERPRETATION

The detection of a high level of RSV IgM or PIV IgM in a single specimen of respiratory secretions or serum or a fourfold or greater increase in antibody titer during convalescence indicates acute infection. Most infants, children, and adults infected with RSV, HMPV, or PIV develop IgA-, IgM-, and IgG-specific ELISA antibody. Site-directed ELISAs employing synthetic peptides of subgroups A and B of RSV as antigen (which allow the detection of antibody responses to linear epitopes) also detect subgroup-specific diagnostic rises in titer during RSV infection. WB test using sucrose gradient-purified RSV antigen detects RSV infection with similar sensitivity and specificity to those of ELISA and NT. HI tests provide similar sensitivity for infections with the serotypes of PIV. Although much less sensitive than either ELISA or the HI test, CF detects diagnostic rises in titer of paired serum specimens in less than half of infections among adults.

At birth all children possess maternal neutralizing antibody to RSV that wanes during the first 6 months of life; the presence of maternal antibody precludes the detection of antibody responses to RSV by most techniques (5). The WB test can detect most RSV infections because it measures not only responses to the surface G and F glycoproteins but also to the internal viral proteins (nucleoprotein [NP], phosphoprotein [P], and matrix protein [M]). The ELISA procedure can detect fourfold or greater rises in the titer of antibody to RSV in 50% of infected children in this age group. The ELISA that measures IgA anti-RSV antibody is more sensitive than the ELISA that measures IgG anti-RSV antibody in infants younger than 6 months of age. The NT test, WB assay, and ELISA are equally efficient in detecting antibody responses to RSV infection in children older than 6 months. CF fails to detect antibody responses in children younger than 6 months (5).

Heterotypic antibody responses detected by HI and CF tests frequently occur in patients with PIV infections. Increases in the PIV antibody titer occur after mumps virus infections. It is difficult to identify the infecting PIV serotype based solely on serologic procedures. The serotype may be identified by virus isolation with subsequent serotyping of the isolate by hemadsorption inhibition (HadI) or HI or by demonstration of antigen in exfoliated nasal epithelium by IF with a panel of monospecific antibodies or by RT-PCR.

REAGENTS

Selected Vendors for Reagents

Immunological, RT-PCR and tissue culture reagents can be purchased readily from many sources. Selected commercial sources include the following.

BioWhittaker, Inc. (www.biowhittaker.com), 8830 Biggs Ford Rd., Walkersville, MD 21793; 1-800-638-8174

DAKO Corp. (www.dakousa.com), 6392 Via Real, Carpinteria, CA 93103; 1-800-235-5673

GIBCO BRL Life Technologies (www.lifetech.com), 3175 Stanley Rd., Grand Island, NY 14072-0068; 1-800-828-6686

ICN Biomedicals, Inc. (www.icnbiomed.com), 3300 Hyland Ave., Costa Mesa, CA 92626; 1-800-854-0530

Intracel Corporation (www.intracel.com), 93 Monocacy Blvd A-8, Frederick, MD 21701; 1-877-289-5476

Labsystems, Inc. (www.labsystems.fi), P.O. Box 3655, Boston, MA 02241-3635; 1-800-522-7763

Midland Certified Reagent Company (www.mcrc.com), 3112-A West Cuthbert Ave., Midland, TX 79701-5511; 1-800-247-8766

PGC Scientifics (www.pgcscientifics.com), 7311 Governors Way, Frederick, MD 21704; 1-800-424-3300

Promega Corp. (www.promega.com), 2800 Woods Hollow Road, Madison, WI 53711; 1-800-356-9526

Qiagen Inc. (www1.qiagen.com), 27220 Turnberry Lane, Valencia, CA 91355; 1-800-426-8157

Chemicals and other reagents can be purchased from the following suppliers.

Amersham (www.apbiotech.com), 800 Centennial Ave., P.O. Box 1327, Piscataway, NJ 08855-1327; 1-800-526-3593

Bio-Rad Laboratories (www.discover.bio-rad.com), 2000 Alfred Nobel Dr., Hercules, CA 94547; 1-800-424-6723

Fisher Scientific (www.fishersci.com), 2000 Park Lane, Pittsburgh, PA 15275; 1-800-766-7000

Sigma-Aldrich Corp. (www.sigma-aldrich.com), 3050 Spruce St., St. Louis, MO 63103; 1-800-521-8956

VWR Scientific (www.vwrsp.com), P.O. Box 626, Bridgeport, NJ 08014; 1-800-932-5000

TEST PROCEDURES

Tissue Culture Cell Methods for Isolation of RSV, HMPV, and PIVs

Isolation of RSV and PIVs by tissue culture technique has been the gold standard by which all other diagnostic tests are compared. The isolation of current wild-type virus strains is important for molecular epidemiology, evaluation of antiviral drugs, identification of escape mutants to antiviral therapy and immune prophylaxis, selection of viral strain for vaccine development, production of antigens or virus strains for serologic assays, use in evaluation of disease pathogenesis, correlates of immunity, development of vaccine with animal models, development of human virus challenge pools, and evaluation of diagnostic tests. These are just some examples of how current wild-type virus strains benefit research and the practice of medicine. To optimize the isolation of RSV, HMPV, and PIVs, a good-quality specimen (nasal wash is preferred over throat swab or nose swab), timely transport of a specimen on ice to the laboratory, and use of cell lines permissive to RSV, HMPV, and PIVs are required. A transport medium such as 40% sucrose in Eagle minimal essential medium (EMEM) or 15% plant glycerol (Fisher Scientific, catalogue no. G-33-500) in Iscove's medium (BioWhittaker, Inc., catalog no. 12-722Q) stabilizes RSV, HMPV, and PIVs and improves the recovery of virus during prolonged transportation of the specimen. The nasal wash specimen is combined with the transport medium in a 1:1 ratio. Normally 2 ml of nasal wash is added to 2 ml of transport medium. Transport media should not contain fetal bovine proteins, an important issue for vaccine development. A disadvantage for sucrose-containing transport media is that at concentrations above 5%, sucrose is toxic to the cell monolayer and a final sucrose concentration of 15% or greater is required to stabilize RSV. Nasopharyngeal aspirates can be sent undiluted to the laboratory if they are transported rapidly on ice and processed within 4 h of collection.

A cell culture tube is the conventional cell culture method for growing respiratory viruses. It is a simple and inexpensive procedure, but RSV and PIV can take 3 to 14 days to grow, depending on the concentration of viable virus in the specimen. A shell vial method can identify RSV or PIV in 24 to 48 h but is more complicated and expensive and at times less sensitive. The shell vial method uses low-speed centrifugation to inoculate the specimen onto the cell monolayer which is growing on a glass coverslip. At 24 to 48 h, the monolayer is fixed and an IF assay is used to detect RSV or PIVs. Antibody against HMPV is not currently commercially available. A hospital or diagnostic laboratory is able to isolate and easily identify RSV and PIVs; however, HMPV is not isolated unless special growth conditions are used. The procedure described in this section has been published previously (18, 33, 41), but more detail is included here.

Materials

A HEp-2 cell culture tube (BioWhittaker, Inc., catalog no. 71-136D) is used for isolation of RSV; an LLC-MK2 cell culture tube (a monkey kidney cell line; BioWhittaker, Inc., catalog no. 71-197D) is used for isolation of HMPV; and a rhesus monkey kidney (Rh MK) cell culture tube (BioWhittaker, Inc., catalog no. 70-103D) is used for isolation of PIVs. These cell lines are most permissive to the above-mentioned viruses; however, any of the viruses can at times be isolated from most cell lines. The cell culture tubes, EMEM, antibiotics, antifungal, and trypsin are commercially available.

Identification of RSV or PIV Antigens in Epithelial Cells Shed in Nasal Secretions

Rapid diagnosis of either RSV or PIV infection can be confirmed in a few minutes to a few hours by demonstration of viral antigen in exfoliated cells in respiratory secretions or nasal wash specimens. In the past decade, a number of ELISA-based commercial tests have been developed for this purpose, each of reasonably high sensitivity and specificity for use in diagnosis of children, as an alternative to the more tedious IF procedures for detecting virus in exfoliated cells. They use proprietary reagents formulated on a matrix (e.g., a tablet or membrane) that forms the substrate on which an aliquot of respiratory secretions is layered. The matrix develops a color reaction when the secretions contain a sufficient amount of virus to react in a positive manner. Several direct enzyme immunoassays for RSV are available (DAKO Directigen RSV; Abbott TestPack RSV). The choice of commercial kit depends on the sensitivity and specificity and the rapidity of the color reaction (29, 40). Also, several IF kits have been developed to simplify this procedure, including a monoclonal antibody-based IF test (Imagen RSV; DAKO) to facilitate the detection of viral antigen in exfoliated cells (15, 22). IF kits are available that incorporate monoclonal antibodies to several respiratory viruses, including RSV and PIV, and provide a rapid screening procedure to identify these infections in clinical samples of respiratory secretions (22).

RT-PCR for Detection of Viral RNA Sequences of RSV, HMPV, and PIVs

RT-PCR is a technique for in vitro amplification of specific viral RNA sequences. It can identify infections missed by cell culture, IF assays, and rapid diagnostic test kits. It is ideally suited for the detection of viruses that are difficult to isolate by cell culture. RT-PCR is currently the best available method for detecting HMPV and frequently enhances the ability to diagnose infection, particularly in adults (4). RT-PCR can be applied to the detection of viral nucleic acid in cell culture harvest of specimens positive for CPE or Had, clinical samples of respiratory secretions and middle ear effusions, and other sites of virus infection. RT-PCR is being increasingly used in some hospital laboratories. There is growing interest in its use as a screening procedure for detecting viral RNA of several respiratory viruses simultaneously in clinical specimens (multiplex RT-PCR), for detecting viruses that are difficult to cultivate, and for detecting viruses for which commercial diagnostic reagents are lacking. It is highly sensitive and specific. A limitation of RT-PCR is the expense and meticulous attention required to prevent carryover contamination. Prevention of carryover contamination requires a separate room for sample preparation, a separate area for RT-PCR setup, and a separate room for post-PCR analysis. In addition, there is the need for traffic control from clean or pre-PCR to dirty or post-PCR areas. Use of dedicated lab coats and plugged pipette tips also helps reduce carryover contamination.

RT-PCR is divided into three major procedures: nucleic acid extraction, cDNA synthesis and amplification, and detection of cDNA product. An additional procedure for the confirmation of the virus-specific amplicon by Southern hybridization can be performed and is often desirable for research. Significant advancements have been made in facilitating the use of RT-PCR assays in hospital and research laboratories. Commercially available reagents and kits such as the viral RNA extraction kits (Q1Amp viral RNA mini kit; Qiagen Inc., Valencia, Calif.), the One Step Qiagen kit (Qiagen Inc.) for cDNA synthesis and amplification, primers, and the affordability of thermocyclers have made it feasible for RT-PCR to become a common and invaluable laboratory assay. The development of real-time PCR utilizing a LightCycler platform, a combined thermocycler and fluorimeter, has added to the speed, reproducibility, specificity, and sensitivity of the assay compared to conventional RT-PCR (25). An additional benefit of real-time PCR is the use of a single closed reaction vessel for nucleic acid amplification and detection, thus reducing the risk for environmental contamination from the amplicons.

RT-PCR is used for specific detection of RSV, HMPV, and PIV genomes in clinical specimens (1, 4, 7, 10, 13, 29). Advances in the technical aspects of this technique now allow both RT and PCR to be carried out in the same tube.

The amplified DNA PCR products are analyzed by agarose gel electrophoresis, in which DNA of known size is visualized by ethidium bromide staining of the gel when viewed under UV light (and photographed for a permanent copy) or by hybridization with a specific probe (Southern hybridization). Alternatively, fluorescent adjacent or TaqMan probes are used in the real-time PCR format. Depending on the virus, different genes are targets of amplification. The genes encoding the NP, F (note that G is very variable and mainly used for epidemiological studies), and SH proteins of RSV, the NP, L, F, and M proteins of HMPV, and the M and hemagglutinin-neuraminidase (HN) genes of PIV are often targeted for amplification. Selection of amplification primers aims at the sequences of the conserved regions of these genes and is based on analyses of these known sequences from several strains of the virus as available in published databases such as GenBank (10). The success of the amplification depends on the quality of the primer sets and on whether more than one set, called nested primers, are needed for amplification. Various RT-PCR procedures including real-time PCR for detection of RSV, HMPV, and PIV, using different primers and genes, have been developed and provide a starting point for applying this procedure to the diagnosis of RSV, HMPV, and PIV in clinical specimens (1, 4, 7, 8, 10, 13, 15, 17, 28, 29). Antigenic and genetic heterogeneities exist within the two major antigenic groups of RSV and HMPV and can be differentiated by PCR-based assays and restriction fragment analysis. Methods for the rapid analysis of samples of RSV using PCR followed by restriction mapping have been described (6). Clinical samples or tissue culture-grown RSV and HMPV can readily be divided into subgroups and then further classified into lineages. These methods enable the examination of large numbers of isolates by molecular biology-based techniques, thereby facilitating research into the molecular epidemiology of the virus. A description of a conventional RT-PCR procedure used in our laboratory for the identification of HMPV from infected LLC-MK2 cell culture can be found in reference 4.

A partial list of primers for RSV, HMPV, and PIVs is given in Table 1. Most of the primers listed are for HMPV because RT-PCR is currently the principal method for the detection of HMPV. In general, primers targeting the L, N, and F genes of HMPV provide the greatest sensitivity for detecting clinical HMPV isolates. Each set of primers listed below will require different thermocycling times according to its reference. It is important to use quality control procedures to ensure the accuracy of the RT-PCR test and to reduce carryover contamination.

COMMON SEROLOGIC TESTS

There are a number of substrates that work well for ELISA. Appropriate substrates for individual enzymes are available from several commercial sources. 5-AS forms a vivid purple color when acted upon by peroxidase, but other substrates of horseradish peroxidase can be used equally well.

ELISA for Measurement of RSV Antibodies

Several ELISA procedures for whole virus or viral proteins have been devised for the measurement of binding antibodies to RSV in serum, breast milk, and respiratory tract specimens from persons of all ages (12, 26, 27, 33, 34, 38, 39). Examples of some of these procedures can be found in the above references.

IF Test for Determination of RSV Antibodies

IF procedures for determination of RSV antibodies in human serum have been used for at least two decades. The procedure is easy to perform but not easily adapted to the evaluation of large numbers of specimens (23).

WB Test for Detection of Antibodies to Surface and Internal RSV Proteins

WB analysis has been used to help discriminate immune responses associated with subunit RSV vaccine from those associated with natural RSV infection (33). The WB assay is used to detect antibody binding to internal and surface

TABLE 1 Primers for HMPV, RSV, and PIV RT-PCR

Virus	Target	Primer name	Primer sequence	Reference
HMPV	F	F1F	5′-CTT TGG ACT TAA TGA CAG ATG	31
		F1R	5′-GTC TTC CTG TGC TAA CTT TG	
HMPV	L	L-1	5′-GTT GCC ATA GAG AAT CCT GTT A	8
		L-2	5′-CAT TCA GAC TGT TGC TTA CCC A	
HMPV	NP	N-1	5′-ATG GAC AAG TGA AAA TGT C	8
		N-3	5′-GCA TTT CCG AGA ACA ACA C	
HMPV	F	F-1	5′-ATG TCT TGG AAA GTG GTG	8
		F-2	5′-TCT TCT TAC CAT TGC AG	
HMPV	NP	01.2	5′-AAC CGT GTA CTA AGT GAT GCA CTC	25
		02.2	5′-CAT TGT TTG ACC GGC CCC ATA A	
HMPV	NP	N3F	5′-GTC TCT TCA AGG GAT TCA CC	4
			5′-ATT ATT GGT GTG TCT GGT GC	
RSV	F	F-F	5′-ATT GGC ATT AAG CCT ACA AAG CA	4
		F-R	5′-CTT GAC TTT GCT AAG AGC CAT CT	
PIV-1	M	PF526	5′-ATT TCT GGA GAT GTC CCG TAG GAG AAC	4
		PR678	5′-CAC ATC CTT GAG TGA TTA AGT TTG ATG A	
PIV-2	M	P2 –F	5′-CAT GTA CTA TAC TGA TGG TGG	4
		P2 -R	5′-GTT AGT AAC TTA AAT AGG GTA AC	
PIV-3	M	P3HN1	5′-CTC GAG GTT GTC AGG ATA TAG	4
		P3HN2	5′-CTT TGG GAG TTG AAC ACA GTT	

proteins of RSV. The antigen used is sucrose-purified RSV. Color development of bands with molecular masses 76, 50, 42, 35, and 28 kDa corresponded to RSV proteins G, F_1, NP, P, and M, respectively. The identities of the RSV proteins are confirmed using purified monoclonal antibodies to the proteins. Significant antibody detection occurs if there is an increase in the intensity of a preexisting band or the identification of one or more new bands that correspond to RSV proteins.

HI Test for Determination of PIV Antibody

Antigen consisting of untreated virus harvested from cell culture can be prepared by low-multiplicity infection of rhesus monkey kidney cells and harvesting of the virus at maximal hemagglutination activity. A sample of culture medium is tested daily for the presence of viral antigen and virus is harvested on the day of high-titer antigen, usually after 5 days of incubation. The untreated virus is then frozen in small aliquots at $-70°C$, incorporating bovine serum albumin (BSA) at a final concentration of 0.5% for antigen stabilization. A 0.1-ml volume of a 10% suspension of sterile BSA is added to each 1.9 ml of virus antigen, and the solution is adjusted to pH 7 with 1 or 2 drops of 1 N NaOH.

Treatment of Cell Culture-Grown Virus with Tween 80 and Ether Increases the Hemagglutinin Titer

Tween 80 at a final concentration of 0.01% is added to the virus harvested from cell culture. Ether is added to increase the total volume by one-third. Hemagglutination antigens can be purchased from commercial sources also (e.g., BioWhittaker, Inc.). For the microtiter procedure, U-well plastic disposable plates are preferred, since the hemagglutination patterns in U-shaped wells are interpreted readily. Initially, antigen lots must be titrated, and a dilution of antigen containing 1 hemagglutinin unit per unit volume should be determined. Antigen is used at 4 U per unit volume in the HI test.

NT Test for Determination of RSV Antibody

Neutralizing antibody to RSV can be measured by plaque reduction, by tube NT procedures, or in microtiter plates. The plaque reduction and microneutralization assays provide an especially sensitive measurement of neutralizing antibody to RSV subgroups A and B. The use and interpretation of these assays are facilitated by techniques which produce either large, clear plaques (1 to 2 mm in diameter [plaque reduction assay]) or tissue destruction (microneutralization assay) in susceptible cell monolayers (HEp-2 or Vero cells). The sensitivity of HEp-2 cells for replication of RSV varies with the source of the cells, and several lines may have to be tested before a sensitive one is detected. Several plaque reduction and microneutralization procedures for RSV neutralizing-antibody measurement have been described, each with slight but modest variations in test procedures. The microneutralization procedure provides end points in 6 to 7 days (33, 34). The microneutralization assay is performed on HEp-2 cells in 96-well tissue culture plates. Plaque-purified RSV is frequently used. Serial twofold dilutions of heat-inactivated sera are made in duplicate, often starting at 3 $\log_2$ dilution. The last serum dilution at which a $\geq$50% reduction in viral CPE is observed is defined as the neutralizing-antibody titer.

HMPV Microneutralization Protocol

HMPV microneutralization is similar to the RSV microneutralization assay except for some key points. A 48-well microtiter plate works best for this assay. The medium consists of EMEM with trypsin, glutamine, and antibiotics but without fetal calf serum (as described earlier in Tissue Culture Cell Methods). A complete cell monolayer of LLC-MK2 cells rather than trypsinized cells is used for the assay. Serial twofold dilutions of heat-inactivated sera are incubated with HMPV before being transferred onto wells with complete LLC-MK2 monolayers (41).

Measurement of NT Antibody for PIV

For the measurement of the level of antibodies to the four PIVs, individual tests must be carried out with the specific virus type as the test virus in the NT test. Since PIVs do not usually produce CPE in cell culture but do exhibit hemadsorption, the end point of the NT procedure is the demonstration of HadI.

REFERENCES

1. **Aguilar, J. C., M. P. Perez-Brena, M. L. Garcia, N. Cruz, D. D. Erdman, and J. E. Echevarria.** 2000. Detection and identification of human parainfluenza viruses 1, 2, 3, and 4 in clinical samples of pediatric patients by multiplex reverse transcription-PCR. *J. Clin. Microbiol.* **38:**1191–1195.
2. **Akerlind-Stopner, B., G. Utter, M. A. Mufson, C. Orvell, R. A. Lerner, and E. Norrby.** 1990. A subgroup-specific antigenic site in the G protein of respiratory syncytial virus forms a disulfide-bonded loop. *J. Virol.* **64:**5143–5148.
3. **Akerlind-Stopner, B., G. Utter, E. Norrby, and M. A. Mufson.** 1995. Evaluation of subgroup-specific peptides of the G protein of respiratory syncytial virus for characterization of the immune response. *J. Med. Virol.* **47:**120–125.
4. **Beckham, J. D., A. Cadena, J. Lin, P. A. Piedra, W. P. Glezen, S. B. Greenberg, and R. L. Atmar.** 2005. Respiratory viral infections in patients with chronic, obstructive pulmonary disease. *J. Infect.* **50:**322–330.
5. **Brandenburg, A. H., J. Groen, H. A. van Steensel-Moll, E. C. Claas, P. H. Rothbarth, H. J. Neijens, and A. D. Osterhaus.** 1997. Respiratory syncytial virus specific serum antibodies in infants under six months of age: limited serological response upon infection. *J. Med. Virol.* **52:**97–104.
6. **Cane, P. A., and C. R. Pringle.** 1995. Molecular epidemiology of respiratory syncytial virus: a review of the use of reverse transcription-polymerase chain reaction in the analysis of genetic variability. *Electrophoresis* **16:**329–333.
7. **Corne, J. M., S. Green, G. Sanderson, E. O. Caul, and S. L. Johnston.** 1999. A multiplex RT-PCR for the detection of parainfluenza viruses 1–3 in clinical samples. *J. Virol. Methods* **82:**9–18.
8. **Côté, S., Y. Abed, and G. Boivin.** 2003. Comparative evaluation of real-time PCR assays for the detection of the human metapneumovirus. *J. Clin. Microbiol.* **41:**3631–3635.
9. **Dowell, S. F., L. J. Anderson, H. E. Gary, Jr., D. D. Erdman, J. F. Plouffe, T. M. File, Jr., B. J. Marston, and R. F. Breiman.** 1996. Respiratory syncytial virus is an important cause of community-acquired lower respiratory infection among hospitalized adults. *J. Infect. Dis.* **174:**456–462.
10. **Echevarria, J. E., D. D. Erdman, E. M. Swierkosz, B. P. Holloway, and L. J. Anderson.** 1998. Simultaneous detection and identification of human parainfluenza viruses 1, 2, and 3 from clinical samples by multiplex PCR. *J. Clin. Microbiol.* **36:**1388–1391.
11. **Edell, D., E. Bruce, K. Hale, and V. Khoshoo.** 1998. Reduced long-term respiratory morbidity after treatment of respiratory syncytial virus bronchiolitis with ribavirin in previously healthy infants: a preliminary report. *Pediatr. Pulmonol.* **25:**154–158.
12. **Erdman, D. D., and L. J. Anderson.** 1990. Monoclonal antibody-based capture enzyme immunoassays for specific serum immunoglobulin G (IgG), IgA, and IgM antibodies to respiratory syncytial virus. *J. Clin. Microbiol.* **28:**2744–2749.

13. **Eugene-Ruellan, G., F. Freymuth, C. Bahloul, H. Badrane, A. Vabret, and N. Tordo.** 1998. Detection of respiratory syncytial virus A and B and parainfluenzavirus 3 sequences in respiratory tracts of infants by a single PCR with primers targeted to the l-polymerase gene and differential hybridization. *J. Clin. Microbiol.* **36:**796–801.

14. **Falsey, A. R., and E. E. Walsh.** 2000. Respiratory syncytial virus infection in adults. *Clin. Microbiol. Rev.* **13:**371–384.

15. **Fan, J., and K. J. Henrickson.** 1996. Rapid diagnosis of human parainfluenza virus type 1 infection by quantitative reverse transcription-PCR-enzyme hybridization assay. *J. Clin. Microbiol.* **34:**1914–1917.

16. **Feltes, T. F., A. K. Cabalka, H. C. Meissner, F. M. Piazza, D. A. Carlin, F. H. Top, E. M. Connor, H. M. Sondheimer, and the Cardiac Synagis Study Group.** 2003. Palivizumab prophylaxis reduces hospitalization due to respiratory syncytial virus in young children with hemodynamically significant congenital heart disease. *J. Pediatr.* **143:**532–540.

17. **Freymuth, F., A. Vabret, F. Galateau-Salle, J. Ferey, G. Eugene, J. Petitjean, E. Gennetay, J. Brouard, M. Jokik, J. F. Duhamel, and B. Guillois.** 1997. Detection of respiratory syncytial virus, parainfluenzavirus 3, adenovirus and rhinovirus sequences in respiratory tract of infants by polymerase chain reaction and hybridization. *Clin. Diagn. Virol.* **8:**31–40.

18. **Glezen, W. P., S. B. Greenberg, R. L. Atmar, P. A. Piedra, and R. B. Couch.** 2000. Impact of respiratory virus infections on persons with chronic underlying conditions. *JAMA* **283:**499–505.

19. **Greensill, J., P. S. McNamara, W. Dove, B. Flanagan, R. L. Smyth, and C. A. Hart.** 2003. Human metapneumovirus in severe respiratory syncytial virus bronchiolitis. *Emerg. Infect. Dis.* **9:**372–375.

20. **Hamelin, M. E., A. Abed, and G. Boivin.** 2004. Human metapneumovirus: a new player among respiratory viruses. *Clin. Infect. Dis.* **38:**983–990.

21. **IMpact-RSV Study Group.** 1998. Palivizumab, a humanized respiratory syncytial virus monoclonal antibody, reduces hospitalization from respiratory syncytial virus infection in high-risk infants. *Pediatrics* **102:**531–537.

22. **Irmen, K. E., and J. J. Kelleher.** 2000. Use of monoclonal antibodies for rapid diagnosis of respiratory viruses in a community hospital. *Clin. Diagn. Lab. Immunol.* **7:**396–403.

23. **Kerr, M. H., and J. Y. Paton.** 1999. Surfactant protein levels in severe respiratory syncytial virus infection. *Am. J. Respir. Crit. Care Med.* **159:**1115–1118.

24. **Landry, M. L., and D. Ferguson.** 2000. SimulFluor respiratory screen for rapid detection of multiple respiratory viruses in clinical specimens by immunofluorescence staining. *J. Clin. Microbiol.* **38:**708–711.

25. **Mackay, I. M., K. C. Jacob, D. Woolhouse, K. Waller, M. W. Syrmis, D. M. Whiley, D. J. Siebert, M. Nissen, and T. P. Sloots.** 2003. Molecular assays for the detection of human metapneumovirus. *J. Clin. Microbiol.* **41:**100–105.

26. **Meddens, M. J., P. Herbrink, J. Lindeman, and W. C. van Dijk.** 1990. Serodiagnosis of respiratory syncytial virus (RSV) infection in children as measured by detection of RSV-specific immunoglobulins G, M, and A with enzyme-linked immunosorbent assay. *J. Clin. Microbiol.* **28:**152–155.

27. **Mufson, M. A., R. B. Belshe, C. Orvell, and E. Norrby.** 1987. Subgroup characteristics of respiratory syncytial virus strains recovered from children with two consecutive infections. *J. Clin. Microbiol.* **25:**1535–1539.

28. **Osiowy, C.** 1998. Direct detection of respiratory syncytial virus, parainfluenza virus, and adenovirus in clinical respiratory specimens by a multiplex reverse transcription-PCR assay. *J. Clin. Microbiol.* **36:**3149–3154.

29. **Paton, A. W., J. C. Paton, A. J. Lawrence, P. N. Goldwater, and R. J. Harris.** 1992. Rapid detection of respiratory syncytial virus in nasopharyngeal aspirates by reverse transcription and polymerase chain reaction amplification. *J. Clin. Microbiol.* **30:**901–904.

30. **Pedersden, K. A., E. C. Sadasiv, P. W. Chang, and V. J. Yates.** 1990. Detection of antibody to avian viruses in human populations. *Epidemiol. Infect.* **104:**519–525.

31. **Peret, T. C. T., G. Boivin, Y. Li, M. Couillard, C. Humphrey, A. D. M. E. Osterhaus, D. D. Erdman, and L. J. Anderson.** 2002. Characterization of human metapneumoviruses isolated from patients in North America. *J. Infect. Dis.* **185:**1660–1663.

32. **Piedra, P. A., J. A. Englund, and W. P. Glezen.** 2002. Respiratory syncytial virus and parainfluenza viruses, p. 763–790. *In* D. D. Richman, R. J. Whitley, and F. G. Hayden (ed.), *Clinical Virology*, 2nd ed. ASM Press, Washington, D.C.

33. **Piedra, P. A., S. G. Cron, A. Jewell, N. Hamblett, R. McBride, M. A. Palacio, R. Ginsberg, C. M. Oermann, P. W. Hiatt, and Purified Fusion Protein Vaccine Study Group.** 2003. Immunogenicity of a new purified fusion protein vaccine to respiratory syncytial virus: a multi-center trial in children with cystic fibrosis. *Vaccine* **21:**2448–2460.

34. **Piedra, P. A., A. M. Jewell, S. G. Cron, R. L. Atmar, and W. P. Glezen.** 2003. Correlates of immunity to respiratory syncytial virus (RSV) associated-hospitalization: establishment of minimum protective threshold levels of serum neutralizing antibodies. *Vaccine* **21:**3479–3482.

35. **Pitkaranta, A., J. Jero, E. Arruda, A. Virolainen, and F. G. Hayden.** 1998. Polymerase chain reaction-based detection of rhinovirus, respiratory syncytial virus, and coronavirus in otitis media with effusion. *J. Pediatr.* **133:**390–394.

36. **Scott, L. J., and H. M. Lamb.** 1999. Palivizumab. *Drugs* **58:**305–311.

37. **van den Hoogen, B. G., A. D. M. E. Osterhaus, and R. A. M. Fouchier.** 2004. Clinical impact and diagnosis of human metapneumovirus infection. *Pediatr. Infect. Dis. J.* **23:**S25–S32.

38. **van Wyke Coelingh, K. L., C. C. Winter, E. L. Tierney, S. L. Hall, W. T. London, H. W. Kim, R. M. Chanock, and B. R. Murphy.** 1990. Antibody responses of humans and nonhuman primates to individual antigenic sites of the hemagglutinin-neuraminidase and fusion glycoproteins after primary infection or reinfection with parainfluenza type 3 virus. *J. Virol.* **64:**3833–3843.

39. **Welliver, R. C., T. N. Kaul, T. I. Putnam, M. Sun, K. Riddlesberger, and P. L. Ogra.** 1980. The antibody response to primary and secondary infection with respiratory syncytial virus: kinetics of class-specific responses. *J. Pediatr.* **96:**808–813.

40. **Wren, C. G., B. J. Bate, H. B. Masters, and B. A. Lauer.** 1990. Detection of respiratory syncytial virus antigen in nasal washings by Abbott TestPack enzyme immunoassay. *J. Clin. Microbiol.* **28:**1395–1397.

41. **Wyde, P. R., S. N. Chetty, A. M. Jewell, G. Boivin, and P. A. Piedra.** 2003. Comparison of the inhibition of human metapneumovirus and respiratory syncytial virus by ribavirin and immune serum globulin in vitro. *Antiviral Res.* **60:**51–59.

Measles and Mumps

DIANE S. LELAND

80

Measles virus, also called rubeola, and mumps virus are both RNA viruses of the family *Paramyxoviridae*, subfamily *Paramyxovirinae*; measles virus is in the *Morbillivirus* genus, and mumps virus is in the *Rubulavirus* genus. These viruses cause classic 7-day measles and mumps, respectively. Both were included among the expected illnesses of childhood in the United States prior to the introduction of vaccination programs in the late 1960s. Measles epidemics involving 500,000 to 700,000 cases occurred every 2 years (4), and approximately 150,000 cases of mumps were reported annually (7). Measles continues to be a major concern globally, ranking as the fifth leading cause of mortality worldwide for children younger than 5 years. Of 777,000 childhood deaths attributed to measles in 2000, most occurred in Africa (58%) and Southeast Asia (26%) (9).

In measles virus infection, after 1 to 2 weeks of incubation, fever, rhinorrhea, cough, and conjunctivitis appear, followed by a maculopapular rash and Koplik spots (1- to 3-mm-diameter red spots with a bluish-white speck in the center located on the buccal mucosa—pathognomonic for measles). The rash usually lasts 7 days, and recovery is rapid and complete. The complications of measles may include otitis media, lower respiratory infections, confusion, and seizures. Subacute sclerosing panencephalitis (SSPE) is believed to be a persistent measles infection of the central nervous system. Onset is 4 to 7 years after the initial measles episode and is characterized by personality changes, mental deterioration, involuntary movements, and muscular rigidity, invariably ending in death (4).

Mumps, which is clinically inapparent in 25 to 30% of cases, is typically mild and characterized by slightly elevated temperature and enlargement of one or both parotid glands. Complications of mumps include meningoencephalitis (up to 15% of cases) and, in postpubertal individuals, orchitis (20 to 30% of males) and oophoritis (7% of females) (7). Mumps remains common throughout much of the world.

The epidemiology of both measles and mumps, along with that of rubella virus (3-day or German measles), changed dramatically with the aggressive vaccination programs implemented in the United States in the 1960s. The number of measles and mumps cases in the United States decreased rapidly throughout the 1970s and 1980s. In 1986 to 1987, there was a brief resurgence of mumps cases that peaked at 8,000 to 12,000 cases. A similar resurgence in the number of measles cases occurred in 1989 to 1991, peaking

at nearly 30,000 cases. Resurgences were attributed to susceptible populations of children under 5 years of age residing in urban settings and to an accumulation of underimmunized children born between 1967 and 1977 (4).

Following the resurgences mentioned above, a two-dose schedule was implemented for the combination measles, mumps, and rubella (MMR) vaccine in the United States. The first dose is given between 12 and 15 months, and the second dose is given between 4 and 6 or 11 to 13 years. The protective value of the second dose of vaccine is reflected in the current low numbers of measles and mumps cases. The United States experienced a record low of 44 confirmed cases of measles in 2002. Eighteen of these cases were internationally imported; 15 additional cases resulted from exposure to the imported cases, and 3 additional cases were caused by measles viruses with genotypes consistent with imported sources (8). SSPE has been largely eliminated in countries like the United States in which measles has been reduced to low levels for more than a decade. Only 231 mumps cases were reported in the United States in 2002 (8), but isolated outbreaks continue to occur.

Transplacental transfer of antibodies traditionally provided protection from measles and mumps infections for infants for 6 months or longer after birth. Currently, the level of transplacental antibody is lower at birth and infants are more susceptible because the level of protection is lower in infants born to mothers whose measles and mumps immunity is vaccine induced. By 6 months of age, only 18% of infants born to vaccinated mothers were shown to have protective levels of measles antibodies; this is in contrast to the 50% of infants born to naturally infected mothers (24). Premature infants (<32 weeks gestation and weighing <1,000 g) may demonstrate seronegativity of 45% for measles and 55% for mumps, with further deterioration of immunity over the next 3 months, resulting in seronegativity of 94% for measles and 100% for mumps (13).

Interestingly, despite the lower levels of measles-specific antibody following vaccination compared to those after natural infection, antibody in vaccinated individuals has been shown to persist (12). Measles antibody has been detected in two-dose MMR vaccine recipients 26 to 33 years after vaccine administration, with 92% of these individuals showing antibody at protective levels.

With the decrease in incidence of both measles and mumps, the demand for diagnostic services has changed.

Although previously diagnosed on clinical grounds alone, both infections are now so rare that they are not readily recognized by physicians. Likewise, they may occur in underimmunized individuals or in immunocompromised individuals, in whom typical clinical signs and symptoms are absent. Due to the low incidence of measles in the United States, the clinical case definition, which included generalized maculopapular rash, fever, and either a cough, coryza, or conjunctivitis, currently has a low positive predictive value. Serological (or other laboratory-defined) confirmation is essential to ensure an accurate diagnosis (16).

DIAGNOSTIC STRATEGIES

Although both measles virus and mumps virus can be isolated in cell culture, isolation may be difficult due to the need to collect specimens very early in the infection process and to the slow proliferation and weak to absent production of cytopathogenic effect by these viruses in traditional tube cell cultures. Newer modified cell culture techniques involving detection of viral antigen in shell vial cultures have improved the sensitivity and speed of measles and mumps virus isolation. However, for both viruses, cell lines optimal for virus isolation and the specialized reagents needed for confirmation may not be kept on hand at many diagnostic laboratories. Virus isolation, although desirable because of the yield of a viral product that can be used in additional studies such as genotyping, may be unsuccessful even in confirmed cases.

Molecular techniques, which do not rely on the presence of viable virus, can be used to detect viral RNA directly in clinical samples. Molecular testing by reverse transcriptase PCR (RT-PCR) may yield positive results in instances when virus culture is unsuccessful. Measles virus RNA has been detected in many types of clinical samples at various time intervals. Measles virus RNA has been detected in throat samples of 93% of patients during the period of 5 days before until 12 days after onset of symptoms, and 88% of patients may secrete measles virus RNA in their urine until 5 weeks after onset of symptoms (25). In a study of nearly 30 measles virus-infected patients, measles virus RNA was detected by RT-PCR within 3 days of appearance of the rash in plasma of 100% of the patients and in nasopharyngeal samples and peripheral blood mononuclear cells of 96% of the patients (20). Shedding of measles virus RNA in urine, nasopharyngeal samples, and peripheral blood mononuclear cells has been documented for 30 to 60 days after the onset of rash, with shedding more frequently prolonged in human immunodeficiency virus-infected children (21). Likewise, mumps virus RNA has been detected by RT-PCR in oral fluids, cerebrospinal fluid (CSF) (22), saliva or throat specimens, and urine specimens (1). Molecular methods are more expensive than virus isolation but may provide a viable approach for confirming the presence of measles or mumps virus.

The serologic approach, relying on detection of antibodies for confirmation of infection, has long been the most accessible and reliable diagnostic tool for confirming measles and mumps virus infections. In natural infection by both measles and mumps viruses, the antibody response upon infection is predictable and consistent. Immunoglobulin M (IgM) is detectable initially within 3 to 4 days of appearance of clinical symptoms and persists for 8 to 12 weeks. IgG is detectable within 7 to 10 days of the onset of symptoms, is maintained at high levels for years, and remains detectable for life. After vaccination, measles virus-specific IgM positivity

rates have been reported as follows: 2% at 1 week, 61% at 2 weeks, 79% at 3 weeks, and 60% at 4 weeks. IgM may persist for 8 weeks or longer. After vaccination, measles IgG positivity rates are as follows: 0% at 1 week, 14% at 2 weeks, 81% at 3 weeks, and 85% at 4 weeks (15).

Although antibodies against various viral proteins are produced, protection is most closely correlated with antibodies to the measles virus hemagglutinin (H) protein and the mumps virus hemagglutinin-neuraminidase (HN) protein. Most assays use whole virus or viral extract antigens that will detect antibodies of various specificities, but most detect antibodies against the measles H and mumps HN proteins effectively.

The most widely used methods in measles and/or mumps antibody detection are enzyme immunoassay (EIA) and indirect immunofluorescence assay (IFA). Complement fixation (CF), hemagglutination inhibition (HI), neutralization (NT), and plaque reduction neutralization (PRN) are seldom used in diagnostic laboratories but may be available at reference or research facilities. A brief description of each of these methods is presented later in this chapter. EIAs and IFAs can be designed to detect either IgG or IgM, and PRN can be modified to allow a comparison of IgM and IgG levels, as well as to measure the total (IgG and IgM) response. The other methods detect total response and do not distinguish between IgG and IgM. Commercial kits for EIA and IFA are readily available, and testing is not difficult to perform. The other assays are more complicated, requiring a variety of reagents and considerable expertise on the part of the technologist.

Acute infection or vaccination with either measles or mumps virus is confirmed when virus-specific IgM, regardless of level, is detected in a sample collected 4 days to 6 weeks after the virus exposure or onset of symptoms. EIA, IFA, and PRN are suitable methods for detecting IgM, but these assays may be available only at reference or state health laboratories. Acute infections can also be confirmed with IgG-specific EIA and IFA or by total antibody detection by CF, HI, NT, or PRN, if the antibody level in the second of two samples collected 2 weeks apart can be shown to be significantly higher than that of the first sample. With assays performed in serial twofold dilutions, a fourfold increase in antibody level between acute- and convalescent-phase samples confirms infection. For methods such as EIA that are not performed with serial dilutions, the manufacturer must provide guidelines for defining significant differences in antibody level. No standardized interpretation is available.

The laboratory confirmation of SSPE is less straightforward. Measles virus often cannot be isolated, due to its defective nature, and antibodies are detectable but in abnormally high quantities. A comparison of levels of antibody in serum and CSF shows greater elevations in the CSF than in the serum (5).

Most measles and mumps antibody testing in the United States is conducted to determine the immune status of health care workers or to assess vaccine effectiveness. Commercially available EIAs and IFAs have shown acceptable sensitivity and specificity for this purpose. EIA endpoints, however, are usually set to maximize confidence in positive results, causing these methods to yield false-negative results in low-titered immunity (5). In situations where very low levels of antibody are suspected, the NT and HI assays for measles and mumps antibodies and the PRN assay (for measles) may need to be requested.

TECHNOLOGY

Molecular Methods

Reagents and procedures for molecular methods for measles and mumps virus RNA detection are not well standardized, so protocols for these assays will not be presented here. RT-PCR, which is described elsewhere in this volume, is the approach of choice and has been applied for detection of measles and mumps virus RNA in infected cell cultures as well as in clinical samples. Simple detection as well as genotyping may be accomplished with this approach. Various gene targets on the viruses, primer and probe compositions, amplification methods, and visualization protocols have been employed. Sources cited below present procedural details for RT-PCR as reported in individual studies.

A one-step RT-PCR for measles virus RNA performed directly on plasma, nasopharyngeal samples, and peripheral blood mononuclear cells has been described elsewhere (20). A new multiplex nested RT-PCR has been shown to simultaneously detect and identify measles and rubella viruses, along with human parvovirus B19, in using pharyngeal exudates, CSF, and serum (18). As a result of the current lack of standardization, comparison of various in-house RT-PCR assays for measles virus RNA has shown that laboratories could differ in sensitivity by as much as 1,000-fold in their ability to detect measles virus (2).

A nested RT-PCR assay has been used to detect mumps virus RNA (1). RT-PCR has also been applied after enrichment of viral template RNAs by overnight culture of the virus in Vero cells and the substitution of polyacrylamide gel analysis for agarose gel electrophoresis (6). These modifications enhanced sensitivity, providing for detection of 1 to 20 infectious units of virus or an equivalent of 1 to 10 pg of mumps virus-specific plasmid DNA. A TaqMan-based one-step real-time RT-PCR for detection and quantification of mumps virus RNA was able to quantify concentrations of a mumps virus gene ranging from 10^1 to 10^8 copies per reaction (17).

Serologic Methods

(Note: the basic principles underlying many of the following assays are described elsewhere in this volume.)

The specimen collection guidelines are similar for most serologic assays: collect whole blood, separate serum, store the serum in the refrigerator (2 to 8°C) for up to 48 h, and freeze the serum (−20°C) if testing will be performed after 48 h. For most methods, heat inactivation of the serum (incubation at 56°C for 30 min) is not required. Some methods specify that heat-inactivated samples cannot be used. In general, contaminated, hemolyzed, lipemic, or icteric specimens should not be used.

An alternative to serum collected by venipuncture is whole blood obtained by fingerstick or heel prick, spotted on Whatman filter paper, air dried, sealed in air-tight packets, and stored at 2 to 8°C. Venous blood collected by venipuncture may also be spotted on filter paper and stored. Following elution and dilution of the dried blood sample, commercial EIAs may be used to test the sample. Results of EIA testing for measles (3, 10, 11, 14, 19) and mumps (11) virus IgG and IgM from dried blood spots have shown excellent correlation with those of fresh serum or plasma testing. Storage of blood spots for up to 24 months without significant change in antibody testing results has been demonstrated, although storage for 6 months or less is recommended (23). Prior to testing, the dried blood is eluted from the filter paper by using phosphate-buffered saline (PBS) with Tween 20 at room temperature for 30 min. The eluted sample is then diluted in PBS containing 5% fat-free milk powder before being tested by EIA (11).

EIA

Most diagnostic laboratories use commercially supplied measles and mumps antibody EIA systems. Protocols provided and validated by the manufacturer must be followed without modification if results are to be of the expected quality. The typical configuration involves an antigen-coated solid phase (often microwells). The antigen may be an extract of cells infected with virus (often Edmonston strain for measles and Enders strain for mumps) or a recombinant protein. Testing is performed either manually or with an automated system. All controls are supplied by the manufacturer to ensure accuracy and reproducibility. Most EIAs detect only IgG, but IgM-specific EIAs are available. These may include an "IgM capture" step featuring microwells coated with antibodies against human IgM. In the first step of the assay, the patient's serum is added to the antibody-coated microwell, and any IgM present in the sample is bound, or captured. In subsequent steps, reagents are added to confirm that the captured IgM is indeed specific for the virus. Most large reference laboratories list measles- and mumps-specific IgM testing in their menus.

IFA

IFA is used for both measles and mumps antibody detection. Written procedures, along with proper reagents and controls, are included with each commercial product, and manufacturers' guidelines must be followed. Like the EIAs, most IFAs are designed to detect IgG antibodies, but they can be used for IgM detection. Usually, IgM-specific IFA testing is preceded by an IgM separation step (column separation or addition of anti-IgG) to separate IgM from IgG.

CF

CF depends on the binding of antibodies to the viral antigen to make antigen-antibody complexes that bind complement. CF is a lengthy and cumbersome method of antibody detection. Few diagnostic laboratories currently use this method for measles or mumps antibody determinations because the EIAs and IFAs are more sensitive and so much easier to perform.

NT

Virus NT measures the capacity of serum antibody to neutralize live virus, thus preventing it from infecting susceptible cell cultures. NT testing requires laboratory facilities suitable for management of live, infectious viruses and cell cultures. The virus must be quantitated prior to the start of the assay, and cell cultures are observed to determine the result. This method is sometimes considered the reference method against which other assays should be compared because neutralizing antibodies considered protective for infection are measured.

HI

An overview of the HI test for measles and mumps antibodies is presented below. A detailed procedure is available in previous editions of this manual (23a, 23b).

Antigens

Commercially purchased measles and mumps virus hemagglutinating antigens are used. Antigen suspensions must be treated to break up antigenic particles and titrated to determine a challenge dose of 2 50% hemagglutinating units.

Erythrocytes

For measles virus antibody testing, use African green, Patas, or rhesus monkey erythrocytes. For mumps virus antibody testing, use chick, goose, or monkey cells.

Specimen Preparation

Serum, plasma, or CSF may be used. Nonspecific inhibitors of agglutination must be removed from serum or plasma by treatment with saturated ammonium sulfate, and nonspecific agglutinins must also be removed by mixing inhibitor-free sample with packed erythrocytes. CSF is usually free of nonspecific inhibitors and agglutinins.

Performance of the Test

A U-bottom microwell plate may be used to prepare serial twofold dilutions from 1:2 to 1:2,048 for each sample for the measles virus test and from 1:10 to 1:640 for the mumps virus test. Add prepared, titrated hemagglutinating antigen to serum dilutions, incubate the mixture, and add a 0.5% erythrocyte suspension to all wells. Allow erythrocytes to settle. Read for hemagglutination.

IgG and IgM titers can be determined separately in a series of three titrations. The first is carried out as described above. The second titration uses serum that has been extracted with *Staphylococcus aureus* protein A, and the third titration is conducted on sera that have been further treated for 30 min with 0.2 volume of 1 M 2-mercaptoethanol. The IgG level is the difference between the arithmetic titers of the first two tests, and the IgM level is the difference between those of the second and third tests. IgG3 and IgA remain in the third test.

PRN (Measles Only)

An overview of the PRN test is presented below. A detailed procedure is available in previous editions of this manual (23a, 23b).

Challenge Virus

Use a line of virus that has been through a plaque passage fewer than five cycles previously.

Cell Cultures

Use Vero cells grown to confluence in 24-well (16-mm-diameter) plates.

Performance of the Test

Mix portions of serial dilutions of inactivated serum with an equal volume of virus containing 125 PFU. Incubate the mixtures for 1 h at 37°C. Use this mixture to inoculate cell cultures drained of their medium. Incubate the cultures for 1 h at 37°C. Replace the inoculum with agarose overlay. Incubate for 4 to 7 days (with timing determined by plaque formation). Remove the overlay, stain the cells with neutral red diluted in cell culture medium, and count the plaques. A 50% reduction in plaque count, relative to controls, is considered the endpoint.

INTERPRETATION

Measles

The presence of measles virus RNA in clinical samples is evidence for current or very recent infection or vaccination. The interpretation of measles serologic testing results is gen-erally uncomplicated, with the presence of IgM indicating current or recent experience with the virus, either through infection or vaccination. However, interpretation of a positive IgM result from a person with suspected measles can be difficult if the person has recently received measles vaccine. Because measles virus-specific IgM may appear as early as 8 days after vaccination and persists for at least 8 weeks after primary vaccination, IgM-positive results obtained during this time should not be assumed to confirm infection (15). IgM is not produced routinely upon revaccination of previously immunized persons but may be detected following clinical measles in these individuals (4). An absence of IgM does not rule out measles virus infection. Samples collected within 72 h after onset of rash may not yet contain detectable IgM, and IgM may not be produced in infection of those previously immunized (4).

A significant increase in IgG level between acute- and convalescent-phase samples is also indicative of infection or vaccination but may be seen in individuals with a history of natural infection or vaccination when they are again exposed to the virus. Failure to detect a significant increase between acute- and convalescent-phase samples in infection may occur if the samples are collected too long after the onset of symptoms.

Mumps

As with measles virus infection, the presence of mumps virus RNA in clinical samples is evidence for current or very recent infection or vaccination. However, the interpretation of mumps antibody testing results is less straightforward than that of measles. Mumps IgM may be detected, along with significant increases in IgG, in patients infected with related viruses, such as the paramyxoviruses. In general, cross-reactivity with related viruses can be ruled out by testing for these antibodies in parallel with mumps antibody testing. The greatest increase in antibody level should identify the true infection. Virus isolation is the most accurate method for resolving this issue. Interpretation of mumps serology, like that of measles, can be obscured in patients who were previously vaccinated. Various therapeutic treatment regimens such as chemotherapy may result in a decrease in seropositivity for measles and mumps.

Interpretation and Applications of Laboratory Results in Diseases of Low Prevalence

Even assays of high specificity will have a low positive predictive value in populations with low prevalence (<1%) of infection, making a high percentage of positive results false positives (3). This precautionary note fits well with the current status of measles and mumps infections in the United States, suggesting that a single positive laboratory value should be carefully scrutinized. Thorough clinical histories and confirmatory laboratory testing are warranted in order to differentiate true-positive from false-positive laboratory findings. For example, a single positive measles IgM result should be supported or confirmed with follow-up measles IgG testing to demonstrate serconversion from negative to positive or a significant increase in IgG titer. Also, in this case, detection of measles virus RNA in clinical samples would give the necessary confirmation and would do so more quickly than monitoring of the IgG level.

REFERENCES

1. **Afzal, M. A., J. Buchanan, J. A. Dias, M. Cordeiro, M. L. Bentley, C. A. Shorrock, and P. D. Minor.** 1997. RT-PCR

based diagnosis and molecular characterisation of mumps viruses derived from clinical specimens collected during the 1996 mumps outbreak in Portugal. *J. Med. Virol.* **52:**349–353.

2. **Afzal, M. A., A. D. Osterhaus, S. L. Cosby, L. Jin, J. Beeler, K. Takeuchi, and H. Kawashima.** 2003. Comparative evaluation of measles virus-specific RT-PCR methods through an international collaborative study. *J. Med. Virol.* **70:** 171–176.

3. **Bellini, W. J., and R. F. Helfand.** 2003. The challenges and strategies for laboratory diagnosis of measles in an international setting. *J. Infect. Dis.* **187**(Suppl. 1)**:**S283–S290.

4. **Bellini, W. J., and P. A. Rota.** 1999. Measles (rubeola) virus, p. 603–621. *In* E. H. Lennette and T. F. Smith (ed.), *Laboratory Diagnosis of Viral Infections*, 3rd ed. Marcel Dekker, Inc., New York, N.Y.

5. **Black, F. L.** 1997. Measles and mumps, p. 688–692. *In* N. R. Rose, E. C. de Macario, J. D. Folds, H. C. Lane, and R. M. Nakamura (ed.), *Manual of Clinical Laboratory Immunology*, 5th ed. ASM Press, Washington, D.C.

6. **Boriskin, Y. S., J. C. Booth, and A. Yamada.** 1993. Rapid detection of mumps virus by the polymerase chain reaction. *J. Virol. Methods* **42:**23–32.

7. **Centers for Disease Control.** 1989. Mumps prevention. *Morb. Mortal. Wkly. Rep.* **38:**388–391.

8. **Centers for Disease Control and Prevention.** 2004. Summary of notifiable diseases, US, 2002. [Online.] http://www.cdc.gov/mmwr/summary.html.

9. **Centers for Disease Control and Prevention.** 2003. Update: global measles control and mortality reduction—worldwide, 1991–2001. *Morb. Mortal. Wkly. Rep.* **52:**471–475.

10. **Chakravarti, A., D. Rawat, and S. Yadav.** 2003. Whole blood samples as an alternative to serum for detection of immunity to measles virus by ELISA. *Diagn. Microbiol. Infect. Dis.* **47:**563–567.

11. **Condorelli, F., G. Scalia, A. Stivala, R. Gallo, A. Marino, C. M. Battaglini, and A. Castro.** 1994. Detection of immunoglobulin G to measles virus, rubella virus, and mumps virus in serum samples and in microquantities of whole blood dried on filter paper. *J. Virol. Methods* **49:**25–36.

12. **Dine, M. S., S. S. Hutchins, A. Thomas, I. Williams, W. J. Bellini, and S. C. Redd.** 2004. Persistence of vaccine-induced antibody to measles 26–33 years after vaccination. *J. Infect. Dis.* **189**(Suppl. 1)**:**S123–S130.

13. **Glick, C., S. Feldman, M. R. Norris, and J. Butler.** 1998. Measles, mumps, and rubella serology in premature infants weighing less than 1,000 grams. *South. Med. J.* **91:**159–160.

14. **Helfand, R. F., H. L. Keyserling, I. Williams, A. Murray, J. Mei, C. Moscatiello, J. Icenogle, and W. J. Bellini.** 2001. Comparative detection of measles and rubella IgM and IgG derived from filter paper blood and serum samples. *J. Med. Virol.* **65:**751–757.

15. **Helfand, R. F., S. Kebede, H. E. Gary, Jr., H. Beyene, and W. J. Bellini.** 1999. Timing of development of measles-specific immunoglobulin M and G after

primary measles vaccination. *Clin. Diagn. Lab. Immunol.* **6:**178–180.

16. **Hutchins, S. S., M. J. Papania, R. Amler, E. F. Maes, M. Grabowsky, K. Bromberg, V. Glasglow, T. Speed, W. J. Bellini, and W. A. Orenstein.** 2004. Evaluation of the measles clinical case definition. *J. Infect. Dis.* **198**(Suppl. 1)**:**S153–S159.

17. **Kubar, A., M. Yapar, B. Besirbellioglu, I. Y. Avci, and C. Guney.** 2004. Rapid and quantitative detection of mumps virus RNA by one-step real-time RT-PCR. *Diagn. Microbiol. Infect. Dis.* **49:**83–88.

18. **Mosquera, M., F. de Ory, M. Moreno, and J. E. Echevarria.** 2002. Simultaneous detection of measles virus, rubella virus, and parvovirus B19 by using multiplex PCR. *J. Clin. Microbiol.* **40:**111–116.

19. **Mubarak, H. S., S. Yukel, O. M. Mustafa, S. A. Ibrahim, A. D. Osterhaus, and R. L. de Swart.** 2004. Surveillance of measles in the Sudan using filter paper blood samples. *J. Med. Virol.* **73:**624–630.

20. **Nakayama, T., T. Mori, S. Yamaguchi, S. Sonoda, S. Asamura, R. Yamashita, Y. Takeuchi, and T. Urano.** 1995. Detection of measles virus genome directly from clinical samples by reverse transcriptase-polymerase chain reaction and genetic variability. *Virus Res.* **35:**1–16.

21. **Permar, S. R., W. J. Moss, J. J. Ryon, M. Monze, F. Cutts, T. C. Quinn, and D. E. Griffin.** 2001. Prolonged measles virus shedding in human immunodeficiency virus-infected children, detected by reverse transcriptase-polymerase chain reaction. *J. Infect. Dis.* **183:**532–538.

22. **Poggio, G. P., C. Rodriguez, D. Cisterna, M. C. Freire, and J. Cello.** 2000. Nested PCR for rapid detection of mumps virus in cerebrospinal fluid from patients with neurological diseases. *J. Clin. Microbiol.* **38:**274–278.

23. **Riddell, M. A., J. A. Leydon, M. G. Catton, and H. A. Kelly.** 2002. Detection of measles virus-specific immunoglobulin M in dried venous blood samples by using a commercial enzyme immunoassay. *J. Clin. Microbiol.* **40:**5–9.

23a. **Rose, N. R., E. Conway de Macario, J. D. Folds, H. C. Lane, and R. M. Nakamura (ed.).** 1997. *Manual of Clinical Laboratory Immunology*, 5th ed. ASM Press, Washington, D.C.

23b. **Rose, N. R., R. G. Hamilton, and B. Detrick (ed.).** 2002. *Manual of Clinical Laboratory Immunology*, 6th ed. ASM Press, Washington, D.C.

24. **Szenborn, L., A. Tischer, J. Pejcz, Z. Rudkowski, and M. Wojcik.** 2003. Passive acquired immunity against measles in infants born to naturally infected and vaccinated mothers. *Med. Sci. Monitor* **9:**CR541–CR546.

25. **van Binnendijk, R. S., S. van den Hof, H. van den Kerkhof, R. H. Kohl, F. Woonink, G. A. Berbers, M. A. Conyn-van Spaendonck, and T. G. Kimman.** 2003. Evaluation of serological and virological tests in the diagnosis of clinical and subclinical measles virus infections during an outbreak of measles in The Netherlands. *J. Infect. Dis.* **188:**898–903.

Rubella Virus

JAMES B. MAHONY

81

For most virology laboratories in North America, rubella virus has all but dropped off the radar screen, with few diagnostic requests. This is in part due to the World Health Organization's effort to reduce congenital rubella syndrome (CRS) from its current level of over 100,000 cases annually via the introduction of mass vaccination programs in resource-poor countries. Live attenuated vaccines, introduced in the late 1960s, are currently in use in roughly half of the countries in the world. National immunization programs for rubella have increased from 78 countries in 1996 to 123 by the end of 2002 (2). Despite the introduction of new vaccination programs, rubella outbreaks continue to occur in many countries around the world, and babies diagnosed with CRS have recently been reported in Italy, Greece, China, Australia, and Japan (17). Recent surveys of rubella virus antibody titers in women of child-bearing age (20) indicate that vaccination programs are not reaching all populations and that the risk of CRS remains. A recent case of a congenitally infected baby born to a vaccinated woman with detectable rubella antibody has raised concern about the efficacy of the measles, mumps, and rubella (MMR) vaccine (22). The efficacy and safety of the MMR vaccination have been under intense scrutiny over the past 2 years, with links between MMR vaccine and autism (15). In the wake of recent discussions about the safety of live vaccines in patients with DiGeorge syndrome/velocardiofacial syndrome (14), novel approaches to immunization have been initiated, including the development of a recombinant rubella virus E1 glycoprotein vaccine.

Rubella virus is a single-stranded RNA virus with 9,762 nucleotides and is classified as a member of the *Togaviridae* family. Rubella virus possesses three major structural proteins: two envelope glycoproteins, E1 and E2 (58 and 42 to 47 kDa, respectively), and a nucleocapsid protein, C (33 kDa). Morphologically, rubella virus is spherical (diameter, 60 to 70 nm) and possesses a dense nucleoprotein core surrounded by a lipid bilayer that contains glycoproteins E1 and E2. Rubella virus is destroyed by proteinases and lipid solvents but is relatively resistant to freezing and thawing or sonication. Viral RNA and protein are synthesized in the cytoplasm and combine to form nucleoprotein cores, which are then assembled into mature virions at marginal cytoplasmic membranes by joining with viral glycoproteins previously compartmentalized in the Golgi network. Although this mechanism of virus replication is similar to that of other togaviruses, rubella virus is unique and immunologically distinct from all other togaviruses. Rubella virus is antigenically stable, and antigenic variation has so far not been an issue for vaccination or serological diagnosis; the significance of the possible emergence of new international subgenotypes of rubella virus is unknown (24). Rubella virus is found only in human populations and as far as we know has no counterpart in the animal kingdom. It is for this reason that rubella virus has been placed as the only member in the separate genus *Rubivirus*.

Postnatal rubella (German measles) is transmitted chiefly through direct or droplet contact from nasopharyngeal secretions. The peak incidence of infection is in the late winter and early spring. Subclinical infection is common. The period of maximum communicability appears to be a few days before and 5 to 7 days after onset of the rash. Volunteer studies indicate the presence of rubella virus in nasopharyngeal secretions from 7 days before to 14 days after the onset of the rash. Infants with congenital rubella may continue to shed virus in nasopharyngeal secretions and urine for 1 year or more and may transmit infection to susceptible contacts. Virus can be isolated from the nasopharynx at 6 months of age in approximately 10 to 20% of these patients.

Prior to the widespread use of rubella virus vaccine, rubella was an epidemic disease with 6- to 9-year cycles; the majority of cases occurred in children. Currently, in North America, the incidence of rubella has declined by more than 99% in comparison with the prevaccine era. In North America, the risk of acquiring rubella has declined sharply in all age groups, with a greater percentage of the cases now occurring in young, unvaccinated adults. Recent serological surveys in the developed world have indicated that 10 to 20% of young adults are susceptible to rubella. This degree of susceptibility in young adults is due predominantly to underutilization of vaccine in this population, not to waning immunity in immunized persons. In developing countries where mass vaccination programs have not been initiated, significantly larger proportions of the population are susceptible to rubella virus infection. For this reason, most infections seen in North America occur in immigrants from countries where immunization has not reached.

The incubation period for postnatal rubella ranges from 10 to 21 days, averaging 16 to 18 days. It is usually a mild disease characterized by an erythematous maculopapular discrete rash, postauricular and suboccipital lymphadenopathy, and slight fever. Some 25 to 50% of infections are asymptomatic.

Transient polyarthralgia and polyarthritis that occasionally occur in children are extremely common in older individuals. Encephalitis and thrombocytopenia are rare complications.

Antibodies to the virus appear as the rash fades (Fig. 1), and initially, both immunoglobulin G (IgG) and IgM antibodies can be detected. Antibodies of the IgM class generally do not persist beyond 4 to 5 weeks after onset of illness (13), while IgG antibodies usually persist for life. Reinfection with the virus can occur, but it is almost always asymptomatic and can be detected by a rise in IgG antibodies. The risk of fetal damage resulting from reinfection during pregnancy is low, but a recent case of CRS in a woman who seroconverted following vaccination has been reported (22). The attenuated virus vaccines induce production of IgM and IgG antibodies similar to that observed with natural infections except that the titers are generally lower. Reinfection rates with wild-type virus are greater among vaccinees than among persons previously infected under natural conditions.

LABORATORY DIAGNOSIS

Clinical laboratories are called upon to diagnose rubella virus infections and to perform rubella immunity screening. Because virus isolation procedures are slow and expensive and host antibody responses are rapid and specific, serological procedures are usually performed for disease diagnosis (the exception would be virus isolation from a congenitally infected newborn). Reliable and sensitive laboratory technology has been developed for the measurement of rubella antibodies of the IgM and IgG classes. These serological tests are used to diagnose congenital rubella and postnatal rubella infections (usually in children or young adults) and to determine the immune status for rubella. In the past, various techniques have been used to measure rubella antibodies, including hemagglutination inhibition (HI), passive hemagglutination (PHA), hemolysis in gel, latex agglutination (LA), enzyme immunoassay (EIA), fluorescence immunoassay, radioimmunoassay, complement fixation (CF), and a variety of rubella virus-specific IgM antibody assays. However, laboratories now generally use commercially available EIAs for IgG and IgM detection. An international standard serum is now available,

and an antibody concentration of 10 IU/ml is generally accepted as the level conferring immunity.

Investigation of rubella virus infection in pregnancy presents a special challenge demanding a rapid and accurate diagnosis. If the patient develops clinical signs, a serum specimen should be collected immediately and tested for the presence of rubella virus-specific IgM by EIA (1, 3). Alternatively, it may be paired with a second serum sample collected 5 days later. The two samples should be investigated in parallel in the same test on the same day. A fourfold or greater rise in HI, CF, or neutralization antibodies, together with clinical symptoms, is diagnostic for recent infection, as is a significant change in optical densities or binding ratios in a solid-phase immunoassay (SPIA). A seroconversion in any patient indicates recent rubella virus infection. Patients without clinical symptoms but with diagnostic serology pose a special problem. They may have a primary infection or reinfection with an anamnestic antibody boost. The absence of late-rising PHA or CF antibodies in the first serum sample in this type of patient would provide evidence that the infection was primary (Fig. 1). Measurement of rubella IgG avidity by EIA may also help to differentiate primary infection from reinfection. The third type of case involves the patient whose serum samples are collected several days after the infection, when all serological tests are in plateau (Fig. 1); in this situation, testing for IgM may be helpful. If time is available, a third serum sample collected several weeks later and run in parallel with the others may demonstrate a fourfold decline in titer, which would be diagnostic. Serological examination of the suspected contacts may also be helpful in this situation.

Investigation of a suspected case of congenital rubella could include several approaches. One approach is to demonstrate rubella virus-specific IgM antibody in the infant's serum, which would be diagnostic of congenital rubella. A second approach is to perform serial serum antibody titrations (HI or SPIA) during the first 6 months of life; a persistence of a high titer in the infant during this time (Fig. 2) is highly suggestive of congenital rubella. A third approach is to perform immunoblotting and peptide EIA on sera collected during the neonatal period, looking for

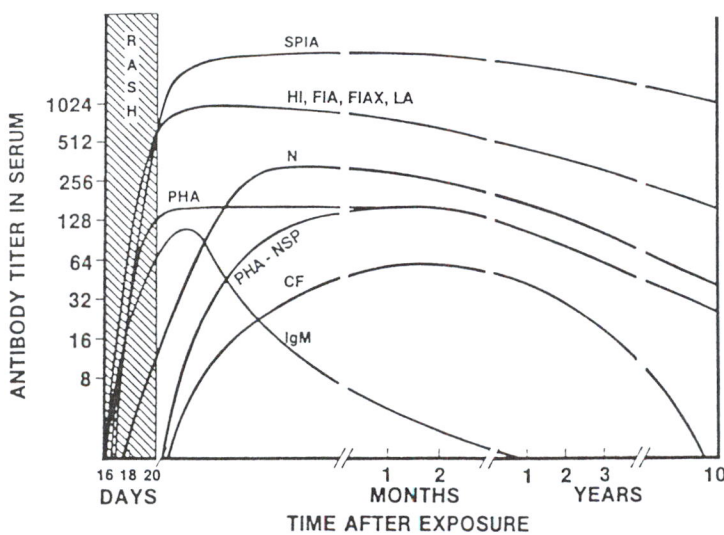

FIGURE 1 Antibody response after rubella virus infection. FIA, fluorescence immunoassay (FIAX); N, neutralization; NSP, nonstructural protein.

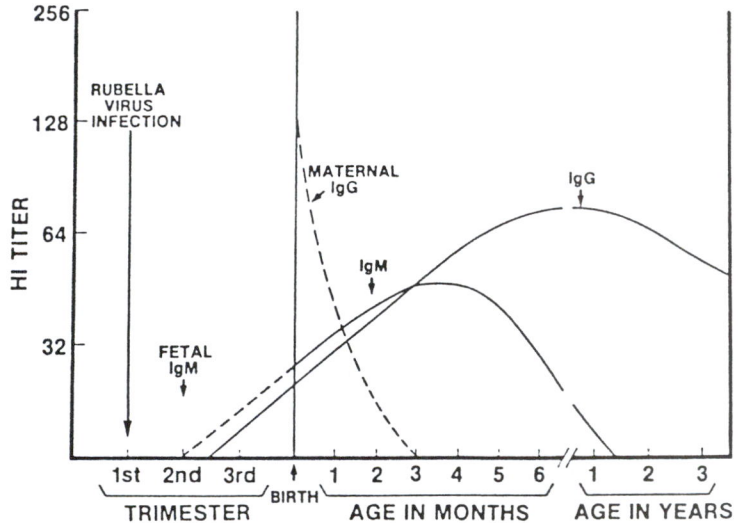

FIGURE 2 Antibody responses in an infant congenitally infected with rubella virus.

reduced bands for E1 and E2 proteins (10). Nonserological approaches for diagnosis include virus isolation and nucleic acid detection by PCR.

TESTING PROCEDURES

Specimens
For details of procedures for the collection and storage of serum, urine, nasopharyngeal, throat, or cerebrospinal fluid specimens, see reference 8. Testing of oral fluid samples as an alternative to serum offers many advantages. These specimens have been positive for rubella virus-specific IgM or rubella virus RNA in a large proportion of CRS cases (10).

PHA
PHA is a rapid, inexpensive way of screening for rubella immunity. PHA antibody in response to nonstructural proteins (Fig. 1) parallels CF and neutralization responses after infection, whereas PHA to structural protein is more closely aligned with HI and SPIA. Both antibodies remain measurable for years after infection or immunization and indicate immunity. PHA employs human type O erythrocytes, stabilized with formaldehyde-pyruvic aldehyde and sensitized with rubella virus antigen. The erythrocytes agglutinate in the presence of specific rubella antibody. In the test, phosphate buffer is added to V-bottom microwells. Specimens, as well as positive and negative controls, are added and then mixed before the addition of the sensitized cells. A row of erythrocytes without rubella antigen is used as a control and allows more objective scoring of results. A button of erythrocytes signifies the absence of antibody (susceptibility to rubella), whereas disperse settling of erythrocytes indicates a positive reaction (immunity to rubella).

Radial Hemolysis
Radial hemolysis can be used to screen large numbers of serum samples by preparing plates in advance and storing them at 4°C. We have successfully used the method of Russell et al. (18). Freshly drawn sheep erythrocytes are washed with dextrose-gelatin-Veronal buffer, treated with 2.5 mg of trypsin (Difco, Detroit, Mich.) per ml in dextrose-gelatin-Veronal for

1 h at room temperature, and sensitized with rubella HA antigen (Flow Laboratories, McLean, Va.) (240 hemagglutination units [HAU] per ml) in HEPES-saline-albumin-gelatin buffer (HSAG; pH 6.2) for 1 h at 4°C. Sensitized erythrocytes (0.15 ml of a 50% suspension) are mixed with 0.4 ml of guinea pig complement (Behringwerke, Marburg, Germany) and added to 10 ml of 0.8% agarose preheated to 43°C, and the mixture is poured into a square petri dish (100 by 15 mm). The plates can be stored at 4°C and used for up to 14 days. Prepoured radial hemolysis plates are available from Orion Diagnostics, Helsinki, Finland. Sera are inactivated at 56°C for 30 min, pipetted into 3-mm-diameter wells punched in the agarose, and allowed to diffuse overnight at 4°C in a humidified atmosphere. The plates are then incubated for 2 h at 37°C. Plates with incomplete hemolysis are flooded with 4 ml of guinea pig complement (diluted 1:3) and reincubated. All sera are also tested in control plates containing unsensitized erythrocytes to monitor nonspecific hemolysis. Zones of hemolysis in control plates range from 3.5 to 5 mm in diameter. Zone diameters of >5 mm on antigen-containing test plates indicate immunity.

LA
Rapid LA tests are used predominantly for immunity screening. The tests incorporate antigen-coated latex particles and may be performed on a card or in a tray. Agglutination lends itself to processing small numbers of specimens.

EIA
EIA kits are commercially available from a number of North American and European suppliers and have been developed for rubella virus-specific IgG and IgM antibody. All of the commercially available EIAs are solid-phase capture assays using either microplate wells, beads, or filters and measure antibodies to envelope and/or capsid proteins. Most are performed in a couple of hours and are low in cost. Automation is built into some EIAs, whereas others are manual. Most of the tests are quantitative or semiquantitative and incorporate both positive and negative controls. At the present time, we are using a microparticle EIA which is automated for detection of IgG or IgM on the solid phase. The antibodies are detected by use of anti-human IgG or IgM antibody

coupled to alkaline phosphatase followed by methylumbel-liferyl phosphate substrate (1). The assay is performed with IMX or AXSYM analyzers (Abbott Laboratories, North Chicago, Ill.), providing test results in 1 h.

HI

Although different laboratories use modifications of the standard rubella HI test, the following is a description of the test that we have consistently found to give good results. The test is conveniently performed in disposable plastic or vinyl V-bottom microtiter plates. The rubella HA antigen is titrated each time the test is performed. Serial twofold dilutions of the antigen are made in 0.025 ml of HSAG (pH 6.2) to which 0.05 ml of a 0.25% washed suspension of pigeon erythrocytes is added. Control cups containing no antigen are included. The plates are sealed and placed at 4°C for 1 h, after which they are placed at room temperature for 15 min before the results are read. The highest dilution that produces a pattern of complete hemagglutination is considered 1 HAU; 4 HAU is used in the HI test. Before the HI test is performed, nonspecific inhibitors of hemagglutination and nonspecific agglutinins must be removed from sera. Test serum (0.1 ml) is added to 0.1 ml of HSAG and 0.6 ml of a 25% suspension of kaolin. The suspension is mixed and allowed to sit at room temperature for 20 min with frequent agitation. The kaolin is pelleted in a clinical centrifuge, and the supernatant fluid is transferred to a clean tube containing 0.05 ml of a 50% suspension of pigeon erythrocytes. After 60 min of incubation at 4°C the erythrocytes are centrifuged, and the supernatant fluid is removed and heated at 56°C for 30 min. This final sample, which represents a dilution of 1:8, is now ready to be incorporated into the test. Alternatively, nonspecific inhibitors may be removed by precipitation with heparin and manganous chloride. The serum sample is diluted 1:4 with 0.15 M NaCl. To each 0.8 ml of diluted serum is added 0.03 ml of sodium heparin (200 U) and 0.04 ml of 1 M manganous chloride. The sample is held at 4°C for 20 min, and the precipitate which forms is pelleted by centrifugation. The supernatant fluid is then absorbed with pigeon erythrocytes as described above.

Known positive and negative control sera are treated similarly. Further serial twofold dilutions of each serum are made in 0.025-ml volumes of HSAG. An area of the plate is reserved for duplication of the first three dilutions of each serum. These receive HSAG in place of antigen and serve as serum controls. To each other dilution of serum is added 4 HAU of antigen in a volume of 0.025 ml. The antigen is back-titrated in a separate section of the plate by doubling dilutions in 0.025 ml of HSAG to represent 4, 2, 1, and 0.5 HAU. The plates are incubated for 1 h at room temperature, after which 0.05 ml of a 0.25% suspension of pigeon erythrocytes is added to each well and the plates are mixed on a plate vibrator. The hemagglutination pattern is read after 1 h at 4°C. The reciprocal of the highest dilution of serum which completely inhibits hemagglutination is taken as the endpoint or rubella titer.

Since the original description of the HI test for rubella (21), several modifications have been introduced. These include the choice of indicator erythrocytes (5), optimal pH of reagents (6), methods for removal of nonspecific inhibitors from sera (7), methods for preparation of the antigen (19), and duration of incubation of antigen with the sera (16). The widely used commercial HI tests available in the 1980s and 1990s, including Rubindex (Ortho Diagnostics, Raritan, N.J.) and Rubatech (Abbott), are no longer available in North America.

CF

The CF test is performed by a standard technique (23).

IFA

The indirect fluorescent-antibody (IFA) test for rubella antibody, first described in 1964, used chronically infected LLC-MK$_2$ cell cultures as the solid-phase antigen. Other acutely infected cell systems or even purified rubella antigens have since been used for the rubella IFA test. For the classic IFA test, acutely infected cells are grown either on Leighton tube coverslips or in culture flasks, and they are then trypsinized and deposited on slides as cell smears. The cytoplasm of cells infected with rubella virus contains rubella antigens. These antigens are used to detect specific antibodies by the indirect method in which an anti-human globulin conjugated with fluorescein isothiocyanate is employed. The technique is rapid and relatively inexpensive and allows detection of IgG and IgM antibodies; however, IFA test results are read visually with a fluorescence microscope and are open to subjective interpretation.

A soluble rubella antigen immobilized on an opaque plastic surface has also been used in an IFA test. In the FIAX test, the antigen-sensitized surface is allowed to react in a two-step procedure with the serum and the fluorescein-labeled conjugate, and the resulting fluorescence signal is measured objectively in a fluorometer. The intensity of the fluorescence signal correlates with the titer of rubella antibody. The sensitivity and specificity of this assay method correlate well with those of the HI test.

Other assays for detecting rubella antibody include mixed hemadsorption and time-resolved fluoroimmunoassay. These tests have their own characteristics and have not gained widespread usage.

Rubella IgM Assays

Commercial EIAs are available for testing whole sera for rubella virus-specific IgM. These EIAs usually employ a pretreatment step or use anti-IgM capture antibody on the solid phase to isolate IgM from IgG and Fab antibody fragments in the indicator reagent to eliminate rheumatoid factor false-positive results. They possess a high level of sensitivity and specificity (3, 4).

Rubella virus-specific IgM antibodies can be separated from IgG by sucrose density gradient fractionation and then detected by HI, EIA, or IFA test. Density gradient centrifugation entails diluting the test serum 1:3 in phosphate-buffered saline and adsorbing it with pigeon erythrocytes. After removal of the erythrocytes, the serum is placed on a discontinuous sucrose gradient that is constructed by layering sucrose solutions in phosphate-buffered saline in a 5-ml cellulose nitrate tube (37, 33, 28, 24, 18, and 12% [wt/vol], as determined by refractometer readings). Before the test serum is layered, the gradient is allowed to equilibrate by overnight diffusions at 4°C. The specimen is carefully laid on top, and the tube is centrifuged for 16 to 18 h at 150,000 × g. The bottom of the tube is carefully punctured with a needle-type fraction collector, and 10 to 12 fractions are collected (0.3 ml per fraction; about 20 drops). Fractions 2 to 4 usually contain IgM; fractions 6 to 9 contain IgG, and the top two fractions contain nonspecific inhibitors of hemagglutination. Alternatively, other immunoglobulin separation techniques such as gel filtration, staphylococcal protein A absorption, quaternary aminoethyl-Sephadex chromatography, and 2-mercaptoethanol destruction have been used with variable success. Density gradient centrifugation for IgM purification has been replaced with affinity chromatography using immobilized IgG.

Virus Isolation

Few laboratories have the techniques or expertise to culture rubella virus, and when virus detection is clinically important, laboratories may want to consider detection of rubella virus RNA by PCR. A wide variety of cell types are susceptible to infection by rubella virus. For primary isolation from clinical specimens, primary African green monkey kidney (AGMK), Vero, or RK-13 cell cultures are commonly used (21). Rubella virus is detected by interference with the cytopathic effects (CPE) of a challenge virus. For virus isolation in AGMK cells, four tubes containing cell monolayers are drained of medium; 0.2 ml of the specimen is used to inoculate each tube and allowed to absorb for 1 h at 35 to 36°C for 10 days. Uninoculated AGMK cell cultures serve as controls. At the end of the incubation period, the tubes are examined for any CPE. If none is found, two inoculated and two control tubes are challenged with 100 to 1,000 50% tissue culture infectious doses ($TCID_{50}$) of a challenge virus. The challenge viruses most commonly used for rubella virus isolation in AGMK cells are echovirus 11 and coxsackievirus A9. Challenged tubes are read 3 to 4 days after challenge. The presence of rubella virus is indicated by little or no CPE in the inoculated tubes and complete destruction of the control cells infected with challenge virus in the absence of rubella virus. Confirmation of the presence of rubella virus requires specific neutralization of the interference with rubella antibody.

Specimens with low concentrations of rubella virus may produce little or partial interference in the culture tubes initially inoculated. The culture fluids may have to be passaged to demonstrate the virus. Fluid from the cultures that were not challenged should be used to inoculate an additional four tubes of AGMK cells. Additional control tubes are also included. These tubes should be incubated for a further 7 to 8 days. Two inoculated tubes and two control tubes are then challenged with echovirus 11 and observed for CPE. The absence of rubella virus interference with the echovirus cytopathogenicity on passage of fluid from tubes that did not demonstrate interference initially confirms the absence of rubella virus in the original tube. If virus is not found after such a passage, it is rarely found by further passages.

Some laboratories use RK-13 or Vero cells for isolation of rubella virus. In these cell systems, rubella virus produces CPE; however, the CPE is not always clear on primary isolation, and cell culture fluids may need to be passaged several times for full detection of virus. These cell systems, however, do offer the advantage of direct neutralization for identification of an isolate. An indirect immunofluorescence staining method has also been shown to be specific and sensitive for identifying rubella virus isolates in these cells.

Fresh unfrozen tissue specimens may be of particular value in attempts to isolate virus from fetal tissues and organs. A convenient method is to explant minced tissue fragments with growth medium and allow sufficient time for the outgrowth of cells. When the cells have formed monolayers, the extracellular fluids can be harvested and tested for the presence of an interfering agent, as described above. This is a more sensitive method for rubella virus isolation than the method in which tissue extracts or homogenates of ground tissue are used.

Rubella virus can be neutralized specifically with rubella antiserum prepared in rabbits. Such antisera are available from several commercial sources. Immune rabbit serum is diluted to contain 4 U of neutralizing antibody. A normal preimmune (rubella antibody-free) rabbit serum is diluted similarly for the control titration. The media from the two companion, unchallenged cultures containing the interfering agent are pooled, and serial 10-fold dilutions are made in maintenance medium (undiluted to 10^{-6}); 0.1-ml samples of each dilution are used to inoculate three culture tubes. The 10^{-1}, 10^{-2}, and 10^{-3} dilutions are also combined with an equal volume of the prediluted rubella antiserum and of the prediluted normal rabbit serum. After 1 h of incubation at 35°C, 0.2 ml of each of the mixtures is used to inoculate three tubes of AGMK cells. The tubes are incubated at 35 to 36°C for 7 to 8 days, challenged with echovirus 11, and observed for the development of enterovirus CPE. Destruction of the AGMK monolayers inoculated with the isolate dilution containing between 10 and 100 $TCID_{50}$ plus the immune rabbit serum, but not of those with the normal rabbit serum, indicates that the isolate is rubella virus.

Nucleic Acid Detection

PCR has been used to detect rubella virus RNA in amniotic fluid specimens or from biopsies of chorionic villi from the fetus in utero (9, 16). Reverse transcriptase PCR first uses reverse transcriptase to make a cDNA copy of genomic RNA and then PCR amplification using rubella virus-specific oligonucleotides in either a one- or a two-step reaction. The product is detected by Southern blotting. Compared to those of rubella IgM antibody for diagnosing congenital rubella, the sensitivity and specificity of PCR in a recent study were 95 and 100%, respectively (9).

Lymphocyte Transformation Assay

A rubella-specific lymphocyte transformation assay, using cryopreserved mononuclear cells, has been developed (12). A negative rubella-specific lymphocyte transformation response in a seropositive child 3 years of age or younger was highly suggestive of congenitally acquired rubella.

MATERIALS AND REAGENTS

Erythrocytes for PHA are sensitized with rubella antigen by the standard tannic acid treatment. The reagents come standardized in a kit (Rubacell; Abbott).

HA antigen is prepared by infecting monolayers of BHK-21 cells in 32-oz (960-ml) bottles with 5 to 10 ml of rubella virus stock containing 10^4 or more $TCID_{50}$/ml. After the virus has adsorbed for 2 h at 37°C, the monolayers are covered with Eagle's medium containing 2% fetal bovine serum that has previously been adsorbed with kaolin (to remove nonspecific agglutinins). The medium is changed after 24 h, and then HA antigen is harvested after 5 and 7 days of incubation. High-titered antigen can be extracted from the monolayers by extracting the cell-associated antigen with alkaline buffers. The cell-associated antigen preparations have CF activity and can be used as the antigen source in the CF test. We have found that good-quality CF and HI antigens in lyophilized form can be purchased from commercial sources such as BioWhittaker Inc. (Walkerville, Md.) and Ortho Diagnostics.

Red blood cells for HI are prepared by collecting blood from a wing vein of a pigeon into modified Alsever's solution. The erythrocytes are washed three times in HSAG buffer, and the packed cells are suspended in an equal volume of HSAG to make a 50% suspension; part of this suspension is used to absorb nonspecific agglutinins from the test sera. A 10% working suspension is made in HSAG, from which the 0.25% suspension to be used in the test is prepared.

Acid-washed kaolin powder to be used in an HI test can be purchased from most scientific supply companies. A 25-g amount of kaolin is washed with Tris buffer until a pH of 7.0 or greater is achieved. The Tris buffer is made by mixing 12.1 g of Trizma base (Sigma Chemical Co., St. Louis, Mo.), 80 ml of 1 N HCl, and 0.85 g of NaCl and bringing the volume to 1 liter. This solution is then further diluted 1:10 in distilled water for washing the kaolin. After the final wash in Tris buffer, the kaolin pellet is suspended in 100 ml of Tris-bovine albumin buffer (Tris-BSA). This buffer is made by adding to 96.67 ml of Tris buffer the following ingredients: 0.33 ml of a 35% sterile solution of BSA (Nutritional Biochemicals Corp., Cleveland, Ohio), 1 ml of a 0.5% $MgCl_2 \cdot 6H_2O$ solution, 1 ml of an 8% NaN_3 solution, and 1 ml of a 0.5% $CaCl_2$ solution.

HSAG is made from three different stock solutions: (i) 5×HEPES-saline, (ii) 2×BSA, and (iii) 100×gelatin. HEPES-saline is made by adding 29.8 g of HEPES powder, 40.95 g of NaCl, and 0.74 g of $CaCl_2 \cdot 2H_2O$ to 1 liter of water and adjusting the pH to 6.2. BSA is made by adding 20 g of BSA powder to 1 liter of water. Gelatin is made by adding 25 mg of gelatin to 2 liters of water. All solutions are filtered. A working solution of HSAG is made by adding 200 ml of HEPES-saline to 500 ml of BSA solution and 100 ml of gelatin stock solution. The volume is made up to 1 liter by adding 200 ml of sterile distilled water. The pH of the working solution should be 6.25. The solution can be stored for 2 months if it remains sterile. HSAG may be purchased from several commercial sources (Flow Laboratories; GIBCO Laboratories, Grand Island, N.Y.; or M. A. Bioproducts).

QUALITY CONTROL AND INTERPRETATION

Confirmation of clinical rubella requires the demonstration of a fourfold rise in antibody titers in paired sera, the presence of rubella virus-specific IgM, or the detection of rubella virus RNA by PCR in the case of congenital rubella. There is considerable variability in the antibody titers maintained during life, and a firm diagnosis cannot be made on the absolute titer of a single serum sample. Because of day-to-day variations in the results of tests, paired sera must be tested in parallel. Differences in titers of paired sera tested on different days may reflect test-to-test variation and not a true change in antibody concentration. This observation is especially important when paired sera are collected from pregnant women who have not experienced clinical illness. Judgments regarding therapy should be withheld until the sera have been retested in parallel on the same day. False-positive IgM results are more likely to occur with indirect assays than capture IgM assays and might also occur with rheumatoid factor-positive sera or with sera containing cross-reacting IgM antibody. For this reason, a second IgM assay using a different format should be done to confirm maternal rubella during the first trimester, before patients make a decision to terminate the pregnancy in jurisdictions where it is legal.

EIA titers should be converted to HI antibody equivalence since the latter expressed as international units has been routinely used to determine immunity. Currently, advisory groups suggest that between 10 and 15 IU represents immunity to rubella in the majority of cases, where a dilution of 1:8 in the HI test is equivalent to 15 IU.

PHA or radial-hemolysis tests are used to detect "late" antibody indicative of a convalescent phase or immunity. When these tests are negative and sera test positive by tests that pick up "early" rubella antibody (EIA and HI), the combination of a negative late antibody and positive early antibody result indicates a recent infection. Sera giving this pattern of antibody results are invariably rubella IgM antibody positive.

Patients without detectable antibodies are usually susceptible to infection by rubella virus; however, a small percentage of adults may not have detectable antibodies and yet are immune. Neutralizing antibodies at low dilutions can usually be detected in the sera of these patients. The lack of serological responses to rubella virus vaccine in women who do not have detectable antibodies is often due to low levels of neutralizing antibodies. With the HI test described here, the first dilution in the test is 1:8. A patient's serum that is positive only at 1:8 should be retitrated to rule out a possible false-positive reaction.

REFERENCES

1. **Abbott, G. G., J. W. Safford, R. G. MacDonald, M. C. Craine, and R. R. Applegren.** 1990. Development of automated immunoassays for immune status screening and serodiagnosis of rubella virus infection. *J. Virol. Methods* **27:**227–240.
2. **Banatvala, J. E., and D. W. G. Brown.** 2004. Rubella. *Lancet* **363:**1127–1137.
3. **Best, J., S. Palmer, P. Morgan-Capner, and J. Hodgson.** 1984. A comparison of Rubazyme-M and MACRIA for the detection of rubella-specific IgM. *J. Virol. Methods* **8:**99–109.
4. **Chernesky, M. A., L. Wyman, J. B. Mahony, S. Castriciano, J. T. Unger, J. W. Safford, and P. S. Metzel.** 1984. Clinical evaluation of the sensitivity and specificity of a commercially available enzyme immunoassay for detection of rubella virus-specific immunoglobulin M. *J. Clin. Microbiol.* **20:**400–404.
5. **Gupta, J. D., and J. D. Harley.** 1970. Use of formalinized sheep erythrocytes in the rubella hemagglutination-inhibition test. *Appl. Microbiol.* **20:**843–844.
6. **Gupta, J. D., and V. J. Peterson.** 1971. Use of a new buffer system with formalinized sheep erythrocytes in the rubella hemagglutination-inhibition test. *Appl. Microbiol.* **21:**749–750.
7. **Jin, L., A. Vyse, and D. W. Brown.** 2002. The role of RT-PCR assay or oral fluid for diagnosis and surveillance of measles, mumps, and rubella. *Bull. W. H. O.* **80:**76–77.
8. **Liebhaber, H.** 1970. Measurement of rubella antibody by hemagglutination inhibition. II. Characteristics of an improved HAI test employing a new method for removal of non-immunoglobulin HA inhibitors from serum. *J. Immunol.* **104:**826–834.
9. **Mace, M., D. Cointe, C. Six, D. Levy-Bruhl, I. Parent du Chatelet, D. Ingrand, and L. Grangeot-Keros.** 2004. Diagnostic value of reverse transcriptase PCR of amniotic fluid for prenatal diagnosis of congenital rubella infection in pregnant women with confirmed primary rubella infection. *J. Clin. Microbiol.* **42:**4818–4820.
10. **Meitsch, K., G. Enders, J. S. Wolinsky, R. F. Faber, and B. Pustowoit.** 1997. The role of rubella-immunoblot and rubella-peptide-EIA for the diagnosis of the congenital rubella syndrome during the prenatal and newborn periods. *J. Med. Virol.* **51:**280–283.
11. **Miller, J. M., and H. T. Holmes.** 1999. Specimen collection, transport and storage, p. 33–63. *In* P. R. Murray, E. J. Baron, M. A. Pfaller, F. C. Tenover, and R. H. Yolken (ed.), *Manual of Clinical Microbiology*, 7th ed. ASM Press, Washington, D.C.
12. **O'Shea, S., J. Best, and J. E. Banatvala.** 1992. A lymphocyte transformation assay for the diagnosis of congenital rubella. *J. Virol. Methods* **37:**139–148.
13. **Pattison, J. R., D. S. Dane, and J. E. Mace.** 1975. Persistence of specific IgM after natural infection with rubella virus. *Lancet* **i:**185–187.

14. **Perez, E. E., A. Bokszczanin, D. McDonald-McGinn, E. H. Zackai, and K. E. Sullivan.** 2003. Safety of live viral vaccines in patients with chromosome 22q11.2 deletion syndrome (DiGeorge syndrome/velocardiofacial syndrome). *Pediatrics* **112:**e325.

15. **Purssell, E.** 2004. Exploring the evidence surrounding the debate on MMR and autism. *Br. J. Nurs.* **13:**834–838.

16. **Revello, M. G., F. Baldanti, A. Sarasini, M. Zavattoni, M. Torsellini, and G. Gerna.** 1997. Prenatal diagnosis of rubella virus infection by direct detection and semiquantitation of viral RNA in clinical samples by reverse transcription-PCR. *J. Clin. Microbiol.* **35:**708–713.

17. **Robertson, S. E., D. A. Featherstone, M. Gacic-Dodo, and B. S. Hersh.** 2003. Rubella and congenital rubella syndrome: global update. *Rev. Panam. Salud. Publica* **14:**306–315.

18. **Russell, S. M., S. R. Benjamin, M. Briggs, M. Jenkins, P. P. Mortimer, and S. B. Payne.** 1978. Evaluation of the single radial hemolysis (SRH) technique for rubella antibody measurement. *J. Clin. Pathol.* **31:**521–526.

19. **Schmidt, N. J., and E. H. Lennette.** 1966. Rubella complement fixing antigens derived from the fluid and cellular phases of infected BHK-21 cells: extraction of cell-associated antigen with alkaline buffers. *J. Immunol.* **97:**815–821.

20. **Sheridan, E., C. Aitken, D. Jeffries, M. Hird, and P. Thayalasekaran.** 2002. Congenital rubella syndrome: a risk in immigrant populations. *Lancet* **359:**674–675.

21. **Stewart, G. L., P. D. Parkman, H. E. Hopps, R. D. Douglas, J. P. Hamilton, and H. M. Meyer, Jr.** 1967. Rubellavirus hemagglutination-inhibition test. *N. Engl. J. Med.* **276:**554–557.

22. **Uchida, M., S. Katow, and S. Furukawa.** 2003. Congenital rubella syndrome due to infection after maternal antibody conversion with vaccine. *Jpn. J. Infect. Dis.* **56:**68–69.

23. **U.S. Public Health Service.** 1965. Standardized diagnostic complement fixation method and adaptation to Micro Test. U.S. Public Health monograph 74. U.S. Public Health Service, Washington, D.C.

24. **Zheng, D. P., T. K. Frey, J. Icenogle, S. Katow, E. S. Abernathy, K.-J. Song, W.-B. Xu, V. Yarulin, R. G. Desjatskova, Y. Aboudy, G. Enders, and M. Croxson.** 2003. Global distribution of rubella virus genotypes. *Emerg. Infect. Dis.* **9:**1523–1530.

Enteroviruses

DAVID SCHNURR

82

Poliovirus, the prototype for the enterovirus group, is of current and historic interest as the agent of paralytic poliomyelitis. Polio has been known for centuries and occurred in epidemic fashion until the development and application of poliovirus vaccines starting in the 1950s. A goal of the World Health Organization (WHO) was the complete eradication of naturally transmitted poliovirus by the year 2000 (references 15 and 16 and this manual provide an excellent review of the enteroviruses). While eradication has not been achieved, transmission of wild-type poliovirus has been restricted to a few areas in the world, and complete eradication remains the goal. However, recent complications involving the spread of wild-type poliovirus have provided new challenges (18).

The search for other agents causing poliomyelitis-like syndromes resulted in the discovery of the group A and B coxsackieviruses from human specimens cultured in mice. The use of cell cultures for viral isolation resulted in the discovery of a number of related viruses, named the echoviruses (for enteric cytopathogenic human orphan virus). Poliovirus, coxsackie A and B viruses, and echoviruses make up the *Enterovirus* genus. Current taxonomy based on sequence analysis divides the human enteroviruses into five species, poliovirus and human enteroviruses A to D, containing 65 serotypes (6).

More recently, the application of molecular techniques has contributed to enterovirus diagnostics and taxonomy. Application of molecular methods, especially PCR, has resulted in more rapid and sensitive diagnostic assays and molecular biology-based taxonomy.

THE AGENTS

The *Enterovirus* genus belongs to the family of *Picornaviridae*, viruses with a single-stranded, positive-sense RNA genome. The virions are unenveloped, 28 to 30 nm in diameter, and composed of 60 subunits, named protomers, each composed of the four viral proteins. The genus was created in 1957 in order to group together agents with similar properties that inhabit the alimentary tract. The enteroviruses are currently composed of 65 serotypes: poliovirus types 1 to 3, 23 serotypes of group A coxsackieviruses, 6 serotypes of group B coxsackieviruses, 29 serotypes of echoviruses, and enteroviruses 68 to 71. These are classified into five species: poliovirus (3 serotypes) and human enteroviruses A

(12 serotypes), B (37 serotypes), C (11 serotypes), and D (2 serotypes) (6).

The 5′ end of the genome is untranslated and highly conserved. These conserved sequences are the targets for primers of the PCR, which recognizes all or almost all of the enteroviruses, and thus provide for group detection and identification. Enterovirus-specific PCR primers do not amplify the RNA of echovirus 22 or 23, now classified as members of the genus *Parechovirus*.

The enteroviruses are extremely stable in the environment. They retain viability indefinitely at −70°C and for years at −20°C and are not inactivated by ether or chloroform. Infectivity is lost when they are heated at 50°C for 2 min or more. Virions are protected from heat inactivation by addition of divalent cations. UV light, formaldehyde treatment, or sodium hypochlorite (0.3 to 0.5 ppm of chlorine) treatment inactivates infectivity.

Serotypes are defined by the lack of cross protection with hyperimmune serum in the neutralization assay. Type-specific determinants reside on the surface of the virion and have been defined by use of monoclonal antibodies (MAbs) (16). Taxonomy based on the nucleotide sequences of the structural proteins correlates closely with the results of typing with hyperimmune sera (12).

Heating or UV light converts the infectious N particle to the noninfectious H form. The conversion exposes epitopes, which cross-react among enteroviruses. MAbs, which react with all human enteroviruses and presumably react with these epitopes, have been described elsewhere (23, 25).

Various types of antigenic variants occur among the enteroviruses. MAbs have been used to show the range of antigenic variants within a serotype (23). A prime strain is an antigenic variant not neutralized by antiserum to the parental virus, while antiserum to a prime strain neutralizes the prime strain virus and parental virus alike.

CLINICAL INDICATIONS

Enteroviral infections range from asymptomatic to severe and sometimes cause fatal diseases. Certain serotypes are more likely to be involved in a given syndrome than others, but there is considerable overlap between the syndromes caused by the various enteroviruses.

The central nervous system is a major target for enteroviral infections. Paralytic poliomyelitis, due to poliovirus types 1 to 3, is among the most serious of all the enteroviral syndromes. The incidence has decreased sharply due to the use of the poliovirus vaccine and concerted efforts to vaccinate as many susceptible persons as possible. Enhanced surveillance has been maintained in order to ensure that all new cases are detected. Poliomyelitis-like disease is occasionally associated with vaccine virus reverting to virulence in immunocompromised persons or infection by other enteroviruses, particularly enterovirus 71. Enterovirus 71 has been described as the cause of brain stem encephalitis with up to 10% mortality in Taiwanese children (22). A more frequent but less severe disease is aseptic meningitis, for which enteroviruses are the major cause. Rapid diagnosis of enterovirus infection by PCR has direct, important benefits, reducing antibiotic treatment and allowing for earlier discharge of children from the hospital. Chronic enteroviral meningoencephalitis in agammaglobulinemic patients is a rare disease caused by persistent infection of the central nervous system, usually by an echovirus or occasionally by a group A or B coxsackievirus.

Coxsackie A virus infections frequently result in skin rashes or respiratory infections. Herpangina, characterized by fever, mouth lesions, and sore throat, is caused by several of the coxsackie A viruses. Coxsackie A16 virus and enterovirus 71 are the most common causes of hand, foot, and mouth disease and a syndrome that can occur in large epidemics (2). A number of coxsackie A serotypes are also associated with respiratory infections, especially in children.

Coxsackievirus A24 and enterovirus 70 are associated with epidemic conjunctivitis and acute hemorrhagic fever. Enterovirus 70 infections can also result in severe neurologic complications. The coxsackie B viruses cause viral myocarditis and pancreatitis and are important agents in the etiology of neonatal disease.

Echovirus infections result in a variety of syndromes. Large outbreaks of echovirus 30-associated aseptic meningitis occur periodically, most recently in 1991 to 1993 and again in the late 1990s (13).

LABORATORY DIAGNOSIS

Enterovirus infections are protean in their expression, ranging from asymptomatic to presenting a wide range of symptoms and syndromes. A definitive diagnosis depends on laboratory detection of infection. Although particular serotypes are associated with certain syndromes, an etiologic association cannot be established on clinical grounds alone. Laboratory diagnosis is done by isolation and identification of the agent, serology, or direct detection. In many situations, direct detection by PCR is the method of choice because it is rapid and sensitive.

For best results, specimens for viral culture or direct detection should be collected as early in the course of the illness as possible. Specimens that should be collected include a respiratory sample, a stool or rectal swab, and cerebrospinal fluid (CSF) for aseptic meningitis.

Isolation and Identification

Culture of the agent from host material in cell culture or newborn mice has been the standard for diagnosis of enteroviral infection. Although no one cell type supports growth of all enteroviruses, all members of the group, except for coxsackie A viruses 1, 19, and 22, can be grown in cell cultures. All of the group A and B coxsackieviruses can be grown in mice.

Since no single cell type supports the replication of all the enteroviruses, more than one cell type should be inoculated for optimal recovery. A human fetal diploid line such as WI-38 or MRC-5, primary monkey kidney cells, and BGMK and RD are cell lines sensitive to a variety of enteroviruses. The range of viruses that will grow in any cell type can be enhanced or selected by introducing specific cell surface molecules that act as viral receptors by genetic engineering. For instance, cells expressing CD155 are targeted to polioviruses (3), and BGMK cells expressing decay-accelerating factor are reported to be sensitive to a broader range of serotypes than the parental BGMK cells (4). Another innovation designed to broaden the sensitivity of cell culture has been to combine two cell types, such as engineered BGMK and CaCo cells, in a single culture (4).

Enterovirus growth in cell culture is recognized by observation of the characteristic cytopathic effect (CPE). Depending on the dose of the inoculum, cell type inoculated, and the strain of virus, CPE may take up to several days to develop. The shell vial technique is a method for making the results of cell culture isolation available in 24 to 72 h (20). Inoculated cultures are stained with group-reactive MAbs, frequently allowing detection of virus before CPE has developed.

Although a presumptive identification of an enterovirus can be made, based on knowledge of host symptoms, the specimen, type and progression of CPE, and the cell type in which the virus grows, confirmation that the isolate is an enterovirus requires a specific immunological or molecular test.

MAbs which react with most or all enteroviruses (group-reactive MAbs) may be used in indirect immunofluorescence assays for confirmation. The MAb described by Yousef et al. (25) has high specificity and low sensitivity, while the MAbs described by Yagi et al. (23) are more sensitive but less specific. Confirmation that an enterovirus has been grown in culture can also be achieved by PCR amplification of the viral genome from the tissue culture fluids.

Another approach to confirm that an isolate is an enterovirus is neutralization with type-specific immune sera. This technique confirms that the isolate is an enterovirus and identifies the serotype in the same test. For most purposes, identification of an isolate as an enterovirus without knowing the serotype is sufficient. However, for enterovirus epidemiology and practical questions such as tracing the circulation of poliovirus, serotyping is of importance.

On the basis of epidemiological information, a particular serotype may be targeted by attempting to neutralize the isolate with one or a few specific immune sera. However, because of the large number of serotypes and the inability to reliably associate particular serotypes with a given syndrome or symptoms, pools of immune sera have been used for typing. The widely used Lim-Benesch Melnick (LBM) immune serum pools are available from the WHO. Typing results are subject to error (21), perhaps because with the LBM pools the serotype is determined by neutralization with one, two, or three of the pools. Confirmation of the pool results by neutralization with a single, type-specific immune serum provides for the most reliable serotyping. More rapid and economical typing may be done by indirect immunofluorescent staining using type-specific MAbs, which are commercially available for the most frequently isolated serotypes (17).

Confirmation that an isolate is an enterovirus can be done by enterovirus-specific PCR (see the PCR discussion below ["Direct Detection"]). A real-time PCR assay which can reliably differentiate between entero- and rhinoviruses has been described elsewhere (5).

Due to a variety of factors associated with serotyping, including antigenic variation and drift, viral aggregation, expense, and the time required to complete the characterization, there is a great interest and need for development and application of molecular methods for typing enteroviruses (1, 7, 8, 11, 12). Molecular methods such as restriction fragment length polymorphism of PCR amplicons and nucleotide sequencing of different regions of the genome have been evaluated for their use in typing. The type as determined by sequencing from the VP1 region correlates almost exactly with the type determined serologically (12). Even isolates that cannot be serotyped by using standard WHO and Centers for Disease Control and Prevention immune sera were typed by VP1 sequence data, and the type as indicated by sequencing was confirmed by neutralization with type-specific immune sera (11).

Enterovirus isolates that were not typeable by sequencing of the VP1 region were further characterized by sequencing of the remainder of the genome. On the basis of molecular and biologic data, these untypeable enteroviruses are now proposed as new enterovirus serotypes (14).

Serology

Serology has not been used extensively for diagnosis of enteroviral infections because the serotype-specific nature of the neutralization assay makes it difficult to select which virus should be used as the target in the test. Neutralization tests on a single serum are generally not useful because many individuals have antibody from previous infections. However, a fourfold rise in neutralizing titer between acute- and convalescent-phase sera is of value when there is interest in only a few serotypes, as in the case of paralytic poliomyelitis. Use of a single antigen is also possible when epidemic outbreaks with a particular serotype occur, such as with enterovirus 71 in Taiwan (2) or echovirus 30 (13). Broadly cross-reactive immunoglobulin M (IgM) antibodies detected by enzyme-linked immunosorbent assay are useful in detecting recent infection. The IgM assay can be group or serotype specific, depending on the treatment of the antigen. Heating exposes cross-reactive antigens, while capture with type-specific antibodies results in preservation of type specificity. Reactivity in the IgM assay depends on the selection of the test antigen and the individual host response.

Direct Detection

Direct detection of a virus in clinical material provides the most rapid and therefore clinically most useful information. Nucleic acid amplification by PCR is sensitive and specific and is the method of choice for direct detection of enteroviruses. Highly conserved, panenterovirus, group-reactive sequences located in the 5′ noncoding region of the genome are targets for primers and probes for detection of enterovirus RNA. Enteroviruses from various specimens have been successfully amplified and detected by use of these primers and probes. The 5′ end of the genome contains sufficient sequence homology with rhinoviruses that cross-reactivity between the enteroviruses and rhinoviruses occurs. Depending on the specimen and goals of the assay, this cross-reactivity can be used as a screen for both entero- and rhinoviruses (5), or enterovirus-specific primers may be used (10).

A variety of specimens such as blood, respiratory, stool, CSF, and paraffin-embedded or fresh myocardial tissue samples have been successfully used as the source of enterovirus RNA for molecular detection. Molecular testing of CSF for enterovirus has been especially beneficial in reducing hospital stay and antibiotic use in pediatric patients with neurologic symptoms. Detection of the viral genome in the CSF is positive evidence of invasion, is more sensitive than culture, and provides results in a clinically useful time frame.

The specimen should be collected as early in the acute phase of illness as possible and transported to the laboratory for processing within 48 h or frozen at −70°C until tested. Care must be taken not to cross contaminate specimens. Guanidine thiocyanate-based RNA extraction methods work well with specimens likely to yield enteroviruses, and false negatives are reported not to be a problem with this method (9). The RNA is copied into cDNA by reverse transcription (RT) using *T*th polymerase (19) or reverse transcriptase. The *T*th enzyme has both RT and thermostable DNA polymerase activity in a single molecule. When an RT enzyme is used, the thermostable DNA polymerase must be added separately to the reaction mix.

PCR results in a many-fold increase of amplicons, doubling in number for each round of amplification. The basic principle of PCR technology has remained relatively unchanged, while methods for detection of the amplified product have evolved.

The products of the PCR can be detected and sized by electrophoresis and staining of the gel with ethidium bromide. The size of amplicons is estimated by comparing the positions of nucleic acid bands in the stained gel with those of known molecular weight standards. If a band is of the expected size for the enterovirus amplicon, that is presumptive evidence that the amplicon is enterovirus specific. However, the size of the amplicon does not guarantee specificity; hybridization of the amplicon with an oligonucleotide probe complimentary to the amplified sequence provides confirmation that the amplicon is enterovirus specific. The hybridization reaction can be done following Southern blotting from the gel, by plate or liquid hybridization. Southern blotting of the PCR products onto a solid-phase surface is followed by hybridization to a probe labeled with a radioactive element, biotin, or some other tracer molecule. For plate hybridization, the probe is bound to the plate and the products of the PCR are hybridized to the bound probe. Plate and blot hybridization can be measured by enzyme immunoassay using primers labeled with biotin (19) that are incorporated into the amplicon during amplification or by use of a MAb that reacts with the double-stranded DNA probe and amplicon hybrid (24). The enzyme is conjugated to avidin, which binds strongly to biotin or to an antibody directed against the species type of the primary antibody.

More recently, real-time detection methods have reduced the time for obtaining a diagnosis (5, 10). Real-time formats provide results in hours from the setup of the assay.

Standards for reporting results on human specimens are set by the Clinical Laboratory Improvement Amendments (CLIA) and can be found in the *Federal Register* 1992 and 24 January 2003 issues. PCR methods for enterovirus detection are home brew assays and therefore require a verification protocol that addresses criteria set by the CLIA regulations. This protocol must be completed and documented before the assay results can be reported. The criteria are accuracy, precision, sensitivity, specificity, reportable range of test results, and normal values. Determination of sensitivity and specificity for clinical specimens is difficult because culture, the "gold standard" for enterovirus detection, is less sensitive than molecular methods. Establishing the sensitivity and specificity for an assay that is more sensitive than the gold standard is a special problem. One approach to resolve discrepant results between molecular methods and culture is to sequence amplification products from PCR-positive, culture-negative specimens. Knowledge of the amplicon sequence can be used to determine if it was copied from an enterovirus template. Sequence analysis also provides information on the similarity of the amplicon to positive-control RNA that is used in the assay. The amplicons should be of enteroviral origin but should differ from each other and from the positive-control nucleic acid. One caveat is that the sequences may be very similar or perhaps identical in cases where outbreaks with a single serotype of closely related strains occurs. Clinical diagnosis of enteroviral infection can be used to establish sensitivity in cases where the PCR is positive and there is strong epidemiological evidence of an enterovirus infection in the absence of positive viral culture.

A reportable assay must include the proper controls. For each assay, there must be a positive and negative control. For specimens for which the extract may inhibit the PCR and as a positive control for the extraction, a PCR for an RNA that should be present, that is, a housekeeping gene, should also be included. The housekeeping gene is not required if it can be demonstrated that the particular specimen type does not contain inhibitory substances.

Proficiency testing is an important quality control issue and is required by CLIA. Proficiency testing for molecular detection of enterovirus is not available through the regular providers of proficiency panels in the United States. Options are to share specimens between laboratories or to set up an internal proficiency testing program within a laboratory. There is a European source for enterovirus proficiency test specimens through Quality Control for Molecular Diagnostics (http://www.qcmd.org).

One current difficulty with PCR is that virtually all tests are developed for use at individual laboratories. Until reagents and protocols are standardized and proficiency testing is made available, it is difficult to compare results between laboratories, and the sensitivity and specificity of any given test must be carefully evaluated. Although work remains to be done, for many purposes nucleic acid amplification methods are rapidly becoming the tests of choice for enterovirus detection.

INTERPRETATION

Isolation and identification remain an important standard for enterovirus diagnosis. However, because of their sensitivity and rapid turnaround, nucleic acid amplification methods are becoming more prominent and are preferable for testing where results may yield clinically useful information. If an enterovirus is identified, the significance of the detection depends on the known association of the agent with the syndrome and the site from which the virus was detected. For example, a positive result for CSF is more significant than a positive test for a stool or respiratory specimen in evaluating the etiology of aseptic meningitis.

Direct detection, especially in aseptic meningitis, is a valuable diagnostic aid allowing the discontinuation of antibiotic therapy and hospital discharge for children. Direct detection by PCR or other sensitive methods is likely to be the highest priority for clinical diagnostic virology laboratories.

The role of enteroviruses, especially group B coxsackieviruses, in the etiology of myocarditis is a question that has been extensively investigated. A viral isolate from the heart is highly significant compared to one from the stool. There have been a number of studies using PCR to detect enteroviral RNA in myocardial tissue of humans. Persistence of enteroviral RNA in the absence of infectious virus does occur. However, the significance of this persistence has not been adequately explained. In any situation, failure to detect a virus does not rule out a viral etiology.

A fourfold or greater rise in neutralizing antibody titer is the strongest serologic evidence for recent infection. The presence of enterovirus-specific IgM is evidence of a recent infection but does not establish proof of etiology. A high titer of neutralizing antibody in a single serum is of questionable significance.

Enterovirus infections will remain an important clinical entity, and diagnostic tools and their applications for these agents will continue to evolve. The use of molecular methods, particularly PCR, is an important advance that will contribute greatly to more rapid and sensitive diagnostics for enteroviruses.

REFERENCES

1. **Caro, V., S. Guillot, F. Delpeyroux, and R. Crainic.** 2001. Molecular strategy for "serotyping" of human enteroviurses. *J. Gen. Virol.* **82:**79–91.
2. **Ho, M., E. Chen, K. Hsu, S. Twu, K. Chen, S. Tsai, J. Wang, and S. Shih.** 1999. An epidemic of enterovirus 71 infection in Taiwan. *N. Engl. J. Med.* **341:**929–942.
3. **Hovi, T., and M. Stenvik.** 1994. Selective isolation of poliovirus in a recombinant murine cell line expressing the human poliovirus receptor gene. *J. Clin. Microbiol.* **32:**1366–1368.
4. **Huang, Y. T., P. Yam, H. Yan, and Y. Sun.** 2002. Engineered BGMK cells for sensitive and rapid detection of enteroviruses. *J. Clin. Microbiol.* **40:**366–371.
5. **Kares, S., M. Lonnrot, P. Vuorinen, S. Oikarinen, S. Taurianen, and H. Hyoty.** 2004. Real-time PCR for rapid diagnosis of entero- and rhinovirus infections using LightCycler. *J. Clin. Virol.* **29:**99–104.
6. **King, A. M. Q., F. Brown, P. Christian, T. Hovi, T. Hyypia, N. J. Knowles, S. M. Lemon, P. D. Minor, A. C. Palmenberg, T. Skern, and G. Stanway.** 2000. *Picornaviridae*, p. 657–678. *In* M. H. V. Van Regenmortel, C. M. Fauquet, D. H. L. Bishop, E. B. Carstens, M. K. Estes, S. M. Lemon, J. Maniloff, M. A. Mayo, D. J. McGeoch, C. R. Pringle, and R. B. Wickner (ed.), *Virus Taxonomy. Seventh Report of the International Committee on Taxonomy of Viruses.* Academic Press, San Diego, Calif.
7. **Kubo, N., I. Hobuhiro, and Y. Seto.** 2002. Molecular classification of enteroviruses not identified by neutralization tests. *Emerg. Infect. Dis.* **8:**298–304.
8. **Manzara, S., M. Muscillo, G. La Rosa, C. Marianelli, P. Cattani, and G. Fadda.** 2002. Molecular identification and typing of enteroviruses isolated from clinical specimens. *J. Clin. Microbiol.* **40:**4554–4560.
9. **Muir, P., A. Ras, P. E. Klapper, G. M. Cleator, K. Korn, C. Aepinus, A. Fomsgaard, P. Palmer, A. Samuelsson, A. Tenorio, B. Weissbrich, and A. M. van Loon.** 1999. Multicenter quality assessment of PCR methods for detection of enteroviruses. *J. Clin. Microbiol.* **37:**1409–1414.
10. **Nijhuis, M., N. van Maarseveen, R. Schuurman, S. Verkuijlen, M. de Vos, K. Hendriksen, and A. M. van Loon.** 2002. Rapid and sensitive detection of all members of the genus *Enterovirus* in different clinical specimens by real-time PCR. *J. Clin. Microbiol.* **40:**3666–3670.
11. **Oberste, S. M., K. Maher, M. R. Flemister, G. Marchetti, D. R. Kilpatrick, and M. A. Pallansch.** 2000. Comparison of classic and molecular approaches for the identification of untypeable enteroviruses. *J. Clin. Microbiol.* **38:**1170–1174.
12. **Oberste, S. M., K. Maher, D. R. Kilpatrick, M. R. Flemister, B. A. Brown, and M. A. Pallansch.** 1999. Typing of human enteroviruses by partial sequencing of VP1. *J. Clin. Microbiol.* **37:**1288–1293.

13. **Oberste, M. S., K. Maher, M. L. Kennett, J. J. Campell, M. S. Carpenter, D. Schnurr, and M. A. Pallansch.** 1999. Molecular epidemiology and genetic diversity of echovirus type 30 (E30): genotypes correlate with temporal dynamics of E30 isolation. *J. Clin. Microbiol.* **37:**3928–3933.

14. **Oberste, S. M., D. Schnurr, K. Maher, S. al-Busaidy, and M. A. Pallansch.** 2001. Molecular identification of new picornaviruses and characterization of a proposed enterovirus 73 prototype. *J. Gen. Virol.* **82:**409–416.

15. **Pallansch, M. A., and R. P. Roos.** 2001. Enteroviruses: polioviruses, coxsackieviruses, echoviruses, and newer enteroviruses, p. 723–774. *In* D. M. Knipe and P. M. Howley (ed.) *Fields Virology.* Lippincott Williams & Wilkins, Philadelphia, Pa.

16. **Racaniello, V. R.** 2001. Picornaviridae: the viruses and their replication, p. 685–722. *In* D. M. Knipe and P. M. Howley (ed.). *Fields Virology.* Lippincott Williams & Wilkins, Philadelphia, Pa.

17. **Rigonan, A.S., L. Mann, and T. Chromaitree.** 1998. Use of monoclonal antibodies to identify serotypes of enterovirus isolates. *J. Clin. Microbiol.* **36:**1877–1881.

18. **Roberts, L.** 2004. Polio. The final assault. *Science* **303:**1960–1968.

19. **Rotbart, H. A., M. H. Sawyer, S. Fast, C. Lewinski, N. Murphy, E. F. Keyser, J. Spadoro, S. Kao, and M. Loeffelholz.** 1994. Diagnosis of enteroviral meningitis by using PCR with a colorimetric microwell detection assay. *J. Clin. Microbiol.* **32:**2590–2592.

20. **Van Doornum, G. J. J., and J. C. De Jong.** 1998. Rapid shell vial culture technique for detection of enteroviruses and adenoviruses in fecal specimens: comparison with conventional virus isolation method. *J. Clin. Microbiol.* **36:**2865–2868.

21. **Van Loon, A. M., C. C. Gleator, and A. Ras.** 1999. External quality assessment of enterovirus detection and typing. *Bull. W. H. O.* **77:**217–223.

22. **Wang, S., C. Liu, H. Tsent, J. Wang, C. Huang, Y. Chen, Y. Yang, S. Lin, and T. Yeh.** 1999. Clinical spectrum of enterovirus 71 infection in children in southern Taiwan, with an emphasis on neurological complications. *Clin. Infect. Dis.* **29:**184–190.

23. **Yagi, S., D. Schnurr, and J. Lin.** 1992. Spectrum of monoclonal antibodies to coxsackievirus B-3 includes type- and group-specific antibodies. *J. Clin. Microbiol.* **30:**2498–2501.

24. **Young, P. P., R. S. Buller, and G. A. Storch.** 2000. Evaluation of a commercial DNA enzyme immunoassay for detection of enterovirus reverse transcription-PCR products amplified from cerebrospinal fluid specimens. *J. Clin. Microbiol.* **38:**4260–4261.

25. **Yousef, G. E., I. N. Brown, and J. F. Mowbray.** 1987. Derivation and biochemical characterization of an enterovirus group specific monoclonal antibody. *Intervirology* **28:**163–170.

Viral Hepatitis

MAURO BENDINELLI, MAURO PISTELLO, GIULIA FREER,
MARIALINDA VATTERONI, AND FABRIZIO MAGGI

83

In recent decades, the importance of viruses as causative agents of liver parenchymal inflammation has been fully appreciated, with the discovery of five major hepatitis-inducing viruses and the development of sensitive diagnostic tools for each of them. In addition, two more viruses with still uncertain liver tropism and pathogenicity have been identified in patients suffering from hepatitis of unknown origin (Table 1). By convention, hepatitis is labeled acute when it lasts less than 6 months and chronic when it persists longer. In spite of extensive use of vaccines against hepatitis A and B in many countries and despite considerable underreporting, acute or chronic viral hepatitis still ranks among the most frequent reportable infectious diseases throughout the world. In particular, hepatitis B virus (HBV) and hepatitis C virus (HCV) are known to infect several hundred million people worldwide. Diagnostic laboratories are therefore frequently confronted with the need to confirm clinical diagnosis of acute or chronic hepatitis, identify the causative virus, and evaluate disease progression and therapy outcome.

Diagnosis of hepatitis and assessment of its severity rely largely on the biochemical analysis of liver integrity and function (Table 2). Aspartate-aminotransferase and especially alanine-aminotransferase (ALT) are of utmost importance, since their levels in serum are highly sensitive indicators of hepatocellular damage and provide simple means of monitoring liver inflammation. Liver endoscopy and especially liver biopsy (when indicated) are essential for accurate determination of the stage and outcome of chronic hepatitis and for deciding the optimal therapeutic strategy. However, clinical features and biochemical, imaging, and histopathological changes are of little help in differentiating the responsible virus. Thus, etiological diagnosis of acute and chronic hepatitis depends extensively on laboratory tests that are specific for each individual virus and are generally used in a stepwise fashion (see below). A feature common to all hepatitis-inducing viruses is that they are poorly cultivable in vitro, if at all, and, with the exception of hepatitis E virus (HEV), they do not infect small laboratory animals. Laboratory diagnosis has therefore always relied on the use of immunoassays that measure viral antigens or antibodies. The more recently introduced molecular tests that detect and quantify viral genomes complement the information obtained immunologically and, due to rapid turnaround times and the availability of user-friendly commercial kits, have acquired a key position in both the diagnosis and the follow-up of viral hepatitis. On the other hand, in the near future, molecular assays are likely to prove useful also in assessing host factors predictive of hepatitis virus infection outcome. Polymorphisms in human cytokine genes or their promoter sequences are beginning to be associated with infectious disease severity and may ultimately become criteria for optimizing therapeutic regimens for individual patients.

HEPATITIS-INDUCING VIRUSES

The vast majority of acute forms of hepatitis are the result of primary infection by the hepatitis viruses designated A to E (Table 1). These viruses differ greatly both genetically and structurally but have in common marked hepatotropism and the ability to trigger variable degrees of liver damage. Primary infection is often nonsymptomatic or accompanied by mild influenza-like manifestations and minimal aberrations of biochemical liver tests. When symptoms of liver damage are clinically evident, these symptoms are essentially uncharacteristic of the causative virus and range from those associated with mild, anicteric or icteric hepatitis (low-grade fever, malaise, anorexia, blunting of taste, nausea, easy fatiguability, and myalgia) to those associated with rare but frequently fatal fulminant hepatitis.

A major difference between A and E hepatitis and the other forms of viral hepatitis is that, whereas hepatitis A and E are constantly self-limiting and resolve in very few weeks or months, variable proportions of HBV, HCV, and hepatitis D virus (HDV) infections do not resolve but tend to persist for protracted periods, frequently for the life span of the infected patient. The clinical consequences of chronic infection by HBV, HCV, and HDV vary greatly both in pattern and severity; thus, patients may remain relatively asymptomatic for extended periods or indefinitely (healthy carriers) or present jaundice and other liver inflammation symptoms of varying severity, with either a stable or a remittent course. Eventually, after variable but generally long intervals, chronicity may result in progressive hepatic failure (decompensated hepatitis) and cirrhosis. Chronically infected patients also are at highly increased risk (20- to 300-fold, depending on the specific populations considered) of developing hepatocellular carcinoma (HCC), and they may suffer from a number of extrahepatic manifestations, including arthralgias, glomerulonephritis, the vasculitis known as

TABLE 1 Viruses discussed in this chapter

Virus	Type of infection	Main route(s) of transmission
Viruses with marked hepatotropism		
HAV	Self-limiting	Oral-fecal
HBV	Self-limiting or persistent	Parenteral
HCV	Self-limiting or persistent	Parenteral
HDV	Self-limiting or persistent	Parenteral
HEV	Self-limiting	Oral-fecal
Viruses with uncertain hepatotropism[a]		
GBV-C or HGV	Self-limiting or persistent	Parenteral
TTV	Self-limiting or persistent	Oral-fecal/parenteral/ respiratory/others

[a]The existence of the putative hepatitis F virus has never been confirmed.

polyarteritis nodosa (especially HBV), and cryoglobulinemia (especially HCV). The proposed association with other diseases, such as Sjögren's syndrome and porphyria cutanea tarda, is much less well established.

Acute hepatitis can also be observed during the course of systemic infections by many other viruses that are not primarily hepatotropic but occasionally produce clinically significant liver damage. These include Epstein-Barr virus, cytomegalovirus, and, less frequently, certain adenoviruses and enteroviruses, parvovirus B19, yellow fever virus, and others. In these infections, liver involvement is usually a minor component of overall pathobiology, and the coexistence of symptoms other than those of hepatitis is an important guide for etiologic diagnosis. The laboratory tests used for diagnosis are discussed in the specific chapters dealing with these viruses.

In addition to the above forms, a relatively small number of cases of acute and chronic hepatitis that cannot be ascribed to any currently known virus also occur. The search for agents that might be responsible for these cryptogenetic forms by modern molecular approaches has led to the discovery of other candidate hepatitis-inducing viruses (Table 1). GB virus type C (GBV-C, also called hepatitis G virus [HGV]) and torquetenovirus (TTV), the prototype of the novel genus *Anellovirus*, are widespread, but their hepatopathogenic potential is much less pronounced than originally proposed or may even be nonexistent. These viruses are considered here because they were discovered in hepatitis patients and because for some of them the ability to injure the liver, alone or in association with other agents, is still under scrutiny.

TABLE 2 Serum parameters useful for the biochemical evaluation of liver necrosis and function

Test	Information provided
ALT and aspartate-aminotransferase	Degree of hepatocellular injury and necrosis
γ-Glutamyl transferase	Marker of cholestasis
Alkaline phosphastase	Confirmation of cholestasis
Direct bilirubin	Degree of cholestasis
Albumin, cholinesterase, total cholesterol, prothrombin time, etc.	Degree of damage to liver protein synthetic activity
Ferritin	Degree of damage to liver storage activity
Immunoglobulin profile	Immune system activation

The mechanisms by which viruses damage the liver are only partially understood, but, at least in the viral systems most thoroughly investigated, data converge to indicate that tissue injury is mainly mediated by the host's immune attack on viral antigen-expressing hepatocytes, while the direct effects produced by viral replication itself are of marginal importance, if any. Indeed, when cell-mediated immune responses are feeble, as typically occurs in individuals infected perinatally or those undergoing immunosuppressive treatments, the manifestations of hepatitis B and C are usually less severe than when the immune system is mature and uncompromised. Conversely, in patients chronically infected with HBV or HCV, abrupt withdrawal of immunosuppressive treatments is often followed by worsening of the clinical and biochemical picture, although viral replication declines. On the other hand, chronic HBV and HCV infections of immunocompromised individuals, primarily those who are coinfected with human immunodeficiency virus type 1 (HIV-1), are particularly difficult to treat with some success.

HCC develops in 2 to 4% of chronic hepatitis patients, mostly those with a background of liver cirrhosis. It is generally accepted that the extensive cell death and regeneration that occur in the chronically infected liver, together with the resulting persistent inflammation, are major driving forces in tumorigenesis; however, the fine mechanisms of hepatocyte transformation remain unclear. The HCCs developed in patients chronically infected with HBV almost universally carry, integrated in their cells, fragments of the viral genome. The role played by these fragments, however, remains essentially unresolved. The pathogenetic mechanisms of the extrahepatic manifestations associated with hepatitis viruses are also poorly understood.

HBV, HCV, and HDV produce long-lasting viremias and are frequently transmitted parenterally through infected blood (blood-borne hepatitis) or sexually. In contrast, hepatitis A and E viruses, which are abundantly excreted with the feces and can be found only briefly in blood, follow epidemiological patterns typical of classical infections transmitted via the oral-fecal route. Most epidemiological features of GBV-C and anelloviruses are still poorly defined, but current evidence indicates that the usual route of transmission is parenteral for HGV and enteric or respiratory for anelloviruses. HBV and HCV infections observed in neonates are generally acquired during parturition or postnatally.

The viruses considered in this chapter are examined separately because of their distinctive properties. For each virus, a concise summary of the most relevant biopathological features is provided, and the approaches used for diagnosis and follow-up are discussed. Regarding the latter aspect, special emphasis is given to the methods that are most widely used, have entered the clinical laboratory most recently, or have only been proposed but appear suitable for routine use in the near future. For assays that are no longer in common usage, the reader is referred to previous editions of this manual. The procedures for commercial assays are accurately described in the manufacturers' accompanying leaflets and should be strictly followed, while those for in-house methods are too varied to be detailed here. Guidelines for the correct selection of tests in different clinical situations are given at the end of the chapter.

HAV

Hepatitis A virus (HAV) is a 27- to 32-nm, nonenveloped icosahedral virus with a linear, single-stranded, positive-sense RNA genome. The RNA is approximately 7.5 kb in length and encompasses a single open reading frame (ORF), two untranslated regions (UTRs) at the 5′ and 3′ ends, and a poly(A) tail. The 5′-UTR contains an extensive secondary structure required for cap-independent translation and is covalently linked to a 2.4-kDa protein (VPg protein). The ORF is translated into a whole polyprotein that is sequentially cleaved, mostly by a viral protease, into precursor and then mature structural (VP) and nonstructural (NS) proteins. Three capsid proteins (VP1, VP2, and VP3) are found in mature virions, while a small VP4 protein is released during morphogenesis. End products also include the protease, an RNA-dependent RNA polymerase, and other NS proteins. Several of these features are common to the *Enterovirus* genus within the family *Picornaviridae*. However, the genomic organization of HAV is partially different, and the degree of genetic homology to enteroviruses is very low. Also, HAV does not react with enterovirus-specific monoclonal antibodies, is not cytopathic in culture, and is highly resistant to physicochemical agents. For these and other reasons, HAV is classified in a picornavirus genus of its own, *Hepatovirus*. Although the degree of heterogeneity is high (at least nine variants between genotypes and subtypes and three antigenic variants have been distinguished), only one serotype is known (8). Adaptation of wild-type HAV to culture conditions is slow and troublesome, but some laboratory strains grow readily in primate cells. The main protective antigenic site is conformational and contributed to by both VP1 and VP3. Therefore, a significant neutralizing antibody response is elicited only by whole-virus preparations, while disrupted virions and recombinant proteins have not been proven effective in inducing protective immunity (17).

Exposure to HAV is usually enteric. The virus invades the liver, possibly following a phase of gastrointestinal amplification, and replicates extensively in hepatocytes, from where it is shed into the bloodstream and bile. Viremia, which was traditionally considered more short-lived, has been shown to start roughly 15 days before peak liver enzyme levels and to last between a month and a year (5). Fecal shedding is also significantly longer than previously believed. The antibody response is considered a key element in elimination of infectious HAV in both blood and feces, while cell-mediated mechanisms are probably most important in pathogenesis and clearance of virus from the liver. An immunoglobulin M (IgM) antibody response is invariably detected, usually in concomitance with the disappearance of viral antigen from the bloodstream. Anti-HAV IgG follows and persists for years, conferring lifelong protection (Fig. 1).

HAV infection is clinically silent in over 90% of children under 5 years old and in 70 to 80% of adults. Overt forms range in severity from a mild, short-lived anicteric illness to more protracted severe icteric hepatitis. Fatal liver failure is rare and usually occurs in patients with preexisting chronic hepatitis B or C or other forms of liver damage. Signs and symptoms, often preceded by a nonspecific prodromic phase, develop after an incubation period of 10 to 50 days and are typical of acute liver inflammation. Biochemical and clinical abnormalities usually resolve in 4 to 6 weeks, albeit liver enzymes may take longer to normalize. HAV does not cause chronic disease, but some patients may experience generally mild relapses weeks after recovery from the primary disease.

Primates are the only hosts. HAV is transmitted mainly through person-to-person contact by the fecal-oral route and, due to its remarkable resistance in the environment, may give rise to massive water- and food-borne epidemic dissemination. In developing countries, 10-year-old children are almost invariably anti-HAV positive. In industrialized countries, the circulation of HAV has been declining for several decades, leading to increased proportions of susceptible adolescents and adults. However, HAV remains the most common cause of hepatitis in the United States and elsewhere. In industrialized countries, epidemics still occur from time to time, and clinical severity increases with age, leading to the paradoxical effect of greater morbidity and

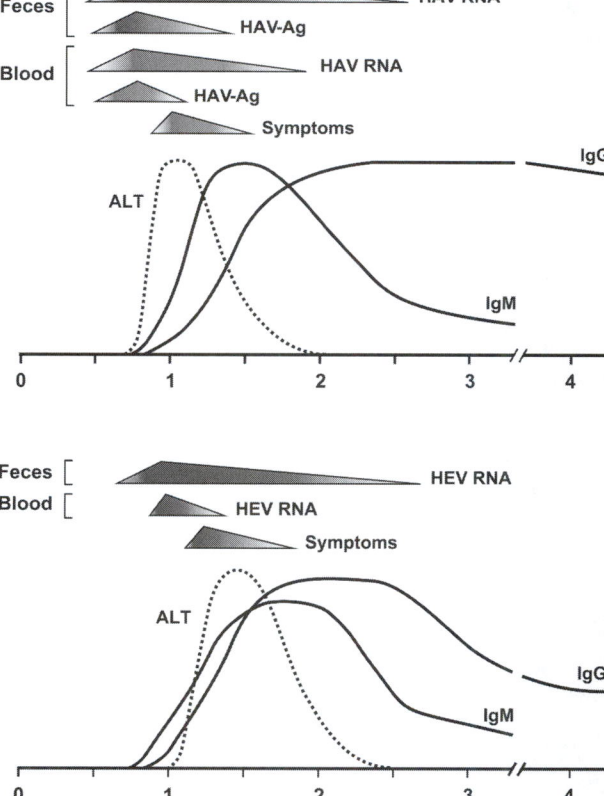

Months post-exposure

FIGURE 1 Typical course of immunovirological events and manifestations of liver damage in symptomatic infection by the enterically transmitted HAV (top) and HEV (bottom). Both viruses produce many more inapparent than symptomatic infections, but the immunovirological events are similar to the ones depicted. Neither virus produces chronic infections.

mortality in older age groups and increasing economic costs (14). Small outbreaks take place primarily among infants in preschool day care centers and their contacts and among people living in poor neighborhoods, while sporadic cases are generally traced to the consumption of raw bivalve shellfish and to travel to countries with poor sanitation. Parenteral transmission is suspected in hemophiliacs and injecting drug users (IDUs). Tissue culturing of some HAV strains has greatly facilitated the development of inactivated and attenuated vaccines, but only the former have been licensed and extensively employed, either alone or in combination with anti-HBV vaccine. Administration of immune serum globulins to contacts and targeted vaccination campaigns are highly effective at reducing infection severity and incidence, respectively.

Assay Systems for HAV

An algorithm for use and interpretation of laboratory tests for HAV infection is provided in Fig. 2.

Testing for Antiviral Antibody

The first choice for diagnosis of ongoing HAV infection is to search for anti-HAV IgM. This marker is almost invariably present from onset of clinical symptoms and remains detectable for 3 to 6 months in approximately 80 to 90% of patients and for up to 1 year in the remaining patients (Fig. 1). Commercial tests are generally both sensitive and specific. Currently, testing is generally carried out by enzyme immunoassays (EIAs). The most convenient and widely used tests are in the solid-phase antibody capture format, using μ-chain-specific antibody to bind any IgM present in the test serum, the addition of HAV grown in culture and purified to trace specific IgM, and an enzyme-conjugated anti-HAV IgG to reveal bound antigen.

Because there is virtually no temporal lag between the appearance of anti-HAV IgM, IgG, and IgA, comparison of the titers of these classes of antibody has no diagnostic value. Total anti-HAV antibody (both IgG and IgM) is measured to determine whether individuals have been exposed to HAV, either by natural infection or vaccination, and to assess the need for or the efficacy of immunoprophylaxis in contacts and in persons at risk of infection because of their profession, travel to areas of high endemicity, or contact with infected persons. Commercial kits generally use solid-phase competitive inhibition EIAs with purified HAV as the test antigen. While the original anti-HAV assays were designed for use with serum, other types of specimen, such as urine, have been investigated because they are more convenient for diagnostic and epidemiological purposes. Appositely modified EIAs have been proposed. Results can be expressed as international units (IU) for comparison with appropriate reference standards. Discrimination between past infection and past vaccination is rarely necessary but can be achieved by testing sera for antibodies to NS proteins, which are not elicited by the inactivated vaccines currently in use. The use of HAV neutralization tests is restricted to the biologic control of vaccine manufacturing.

Testing for Viral Antigen

Direct detection of the infectious agent has an ancillary role in the laboratory diagnosis of hepatitis A due to the reliability and ease of anti-HAV IgM testing. Even now, although sensitive and easy genome amplification assays are available, the greatest utility of virus detection lies in the identification of individuals who spread the virus in the course of outbreaks and the infection fomites. In clinical settings, detection of HAV antigen is generally carried out by EIA methods.

Testing for Viral RNA

Viral RNA is tested for mainly by reverse transcriptase PCR (RT-PCR). Studies have demonstrated that real-time RT-PCR detects HAV in serum for up to >1 year after clinical onset, with peaks in the order of magnitude of 10^5 viral copies/ml at the time of diagnosis (5). Stool samples are found HAV RNA positive for months, i.e., for much longer periods than detectable by the most sensitive immunoassays (Fig. 1). However, only stool samples containing detectable

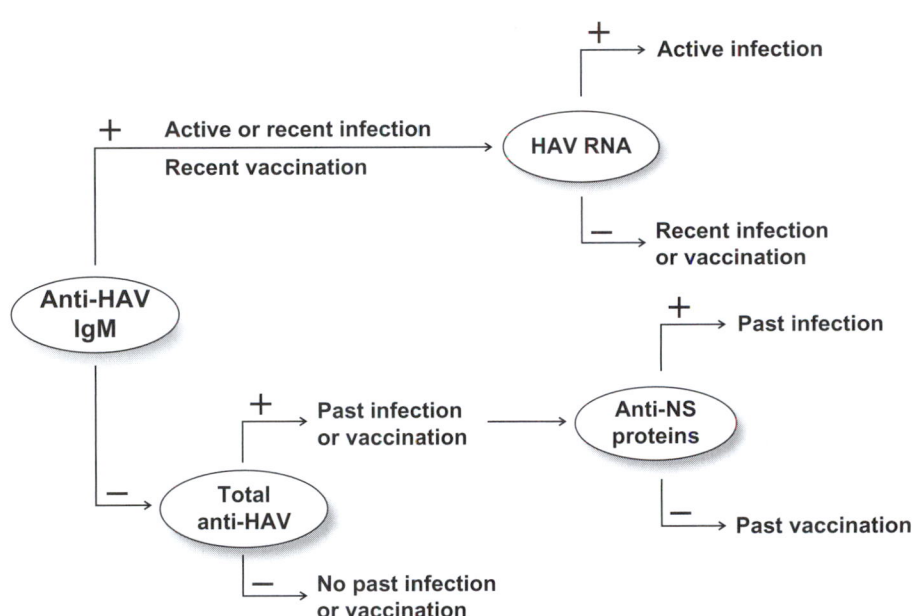

FIGURE 2 Algorithm for use and interpretation of laboratory tests for HAV infection. HAV RNA detection is usually carried out with stool samples.

HAV antigen proved infectious when used to inoculate primates (33). RT-PCR detection of HAV RNA in serum before seroconversion has been recommended for early diagnosis of hepatitis A during outbreaks (9). RT-PCR is also particularly suitable for detecting virus in wastewater and shellfish, where its concentration can be particularly low. In addition, molecular techniques can be designed to permit subsequent evaluation of the genetic relatedness of different clinical or environmental isolates, which can be epidemiologically useful.

HBV

HBV is classified within the family *Hepadnaviridae*, together with related viruses of animals. Virions are double-shelled particles, 40 to 42 nm in diameter, with a tight outer lipoprotein envelope that contains three forms of a virus-encoded glycoprotein (designated surface antigen [HBsAg]). Inside the envelope is the 27-nm icosahedral capsid, or core, composed of approximately 200 copies of a single phosphoprotein (core antigen [HBcAg]). This encloses a relaxed-circular, partially duplex DNA genome of 3.2 kb and the polymerase, which performs the synthesis of viral DNA as well as other functions. Among the smallest of all known animal virus genomes, the HBV genome has four extensively overlapping primary ORFs: the *S* gene, coding for the HBsAg proteins; the *C* gene, coding for the HBcAg and hepatitis B e antigen (HBeAg); the *P* gene, coding for the DNA polymerase; and the *X* gene, coding for a multifunctional regulatory protein with transactivating properties essential for replication. The virus is relatively heat stable but is rapidly destroyed by acids and lipid solvents.

The only cells that have proved susceptible to HBV infection in vitro are primary hepatocytes of humans and chimpanzees (the only susceptible species); all attempts to grow the virus in more readily available systems have failed. Mice transgenic for all or part of the viral genome are therefore used extensively to explore aspects of HBV molecular biology and pathogenesis. In vivo, the virus replicates predominantly in hepatocytes, although some viral DNA is also found at extrahepatic sites, including kidney, pancreas, and mononuclear cells. A key feature of HBV replication is that the genome is synthesized via an RNA intermediate. Following cell entry through a still-undefined receptor(s), the partially double-stranded DNA genome is released from the core, transported to the nucleus, and converted into a covalently closed circular DNA molecule which serves as a template for the synthesis of genomic and subgenomic RNAs by host RNA polymerase II. Assembly takes place in the cytosol; here, genomic RNA and viral proteins encoded by the subgenomic RNAs associate to form the nucleocapsid. After encapsidation, genomic RNA is reverse-transcribed into a strand of DNA, which is then transformed into the partially duplex molecule found in mature virions. Subsequently, the nucleocapsids acquire the envelope by budding through intracellular membranes at sites where viral glycoproteins have accumulated and are released extracellularly, with no evident direct cytopathology. However, in the context of laboratory diagnosis, the most noteworthy features of HBV replication are as follows. (i) Virion release by hepatocytes is sustained and long-lasting. (ii) The envelope glycoproteins are produced in great excess relative to what is needed for virion morphogenesis and are released as spherical and tubular subvirion aggregates as well as intact virions; in the bloodstream, the former typically outnumber virions by 3 to 5 orders of magnitude, thus representing a large part of the HBsAg. (iii) A fraction of C gene products is not incorporated into virions but reaches the Golgi apparatus, where it is cleaved to form HBeAg by cellular proteases; HBeAg is then released as such by infected cells and circulates freely in blood, where it is detectable as a distinct antigen.

HBV has been classified into immunotypes and genotypes, based on distinctive antigenic determinants in the HBsAg and genetic relatedness, respectively. One antigenic determinant (designated *a*) is cross-reactive among all immunotypes, whereas the others tend to be present in one of two allelic forms (e.g., *d-y* and *w-r*). This results in different antigenic formulas, of which the most frequent worldwide are *adw*, *adr*, and *ayw*. Due to the presence of an important cross-protective moiety in the universal *a* determinant, however, there is only a single serotype of HBV, and the usefulness of immunotypes is solely epidemiological. Of the eight genotypes currently recognized, genotype A is pandemic, whereas the others are more geographically restricted (genotypes B and C prevail in Asia, genotype D prevails in southern Europe, E in Africa, F in the Americas, and G in the United States and France, and genotype H has been recently identified in Central America). In recent studies, Caucasian patients infected with genotype A were found to be more likely to resolve the infection than Caucasian genotype D patients, and Asians with genotype B developed milder forms of hepatitis and responded better to therapies than Asian genotype C patients (15, 53). Certainly more important for laboratory diagnosis and disease management, however, are the so-called HBeAg-minus core or precore mutants of the virus, which are unable to express HBeAg due to a stop codon in the C gene, and the drug-resistant variants that are commonly found in patients undergoing therapy (see below). The clinical significance, if any, of mutations increasingly found in the S gene of HBV isolates obtained from vaccinated children is still unclear.

Most primary HBV infections evolve with moderately altered liver enzymes but no appreciable symptoms. Clinically evident acute hepatitis is observed only in <5% of perinatal HBV infections and in 20 to 30% of adult infections. Symptoms of acute hepatitis B develop after a longer incubation period (usually 1.5 to 3 months) and tend to be more severe and longer-lasting than in other forms of acute viral hepatitis (Fig. 3). Acute-phase HBV-infected patients normally contain large numbers of virions in their blood (10^9 per ml or greater), although viremia usually undergoes a slight decline when the symptoms of acute hepatitis develop, most likely as a result of the mounting immune responses. The viral components detectable in viremic blood include HBsAg (present both as whole virions and subvirion aggregates), HBeAg, HBV DNA, and the virion-associated DNA polymerase. HBcAg instead usually remains hidden within intact virions or complexed with antibodies. Serologically, during this stage the host's immune response is revealed only by the presence of antibodies to the internal capsid protein (anti-HBc).

In the absence of complications, clinical resolution of acute hepatitis B occurs within 2 to 6 months from onset and is generally paralleled by the clearance of viral antigen and DNA from blood and followed by the development of antibodies to HBsAg (anti-HBs). Anti-HBs possess virus-neutralizing activity and confer lifelong immunity. Recovery, however, is believed to be mediated mainly by cytokines and cytotoxic T lymphocytes. Self-limited HBV infections are characterized by a progressive decline of viremia (Fig. 3). For example, a >40% reduction of HBsAg concentration is

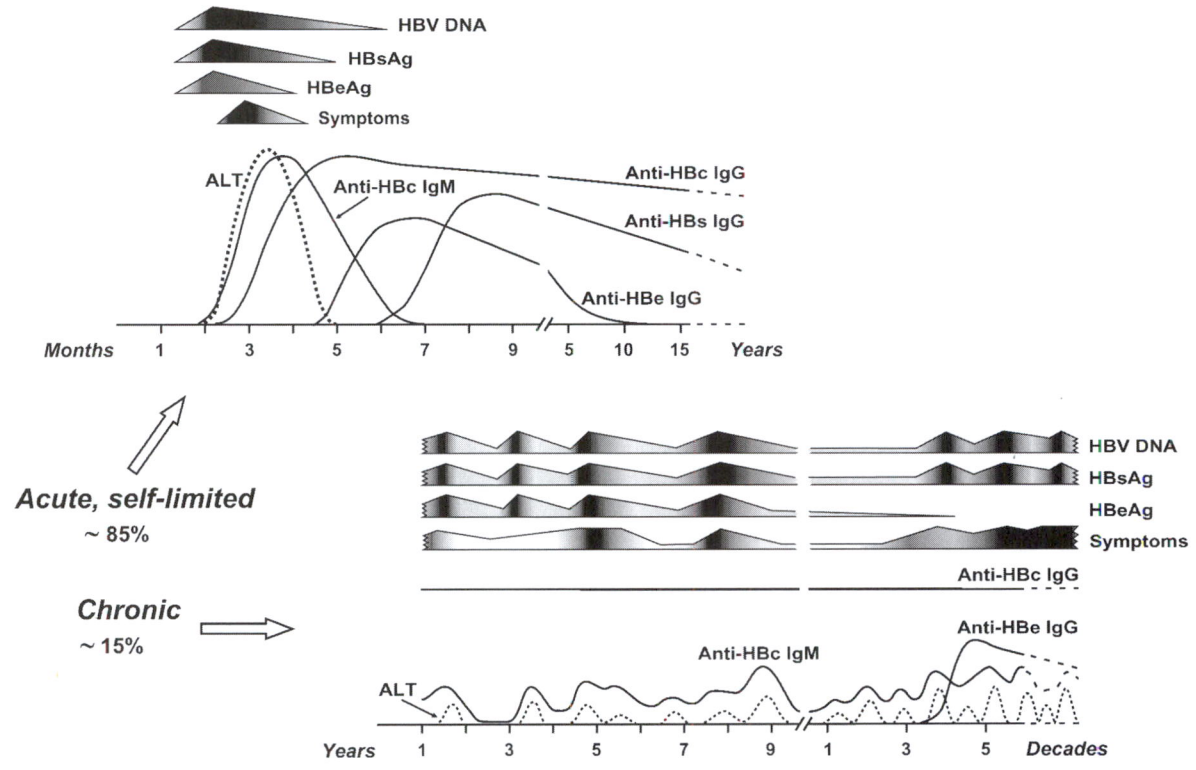

FIGURE 3 Typical course of immunovirological events and manifestations of liver damage in symptomatic acute, self-limiting, and chronic HBV infection. The proportion of infections that chronicize is indicated as 15% but in fact varies widely, depending on the patient's age and other variables (see text). The initial, acute phases are essentially the same, regardless of whether the infection resolves or becomes chronic. The vast majority of HBV infections do not produce overt disease or do so after many years of persistence; however, the immunovirological events are similar to the ones depicted.

considered suggestive of a favorable prognosis. Importantly, resolution of infection is usually preceded by the disappearance of HBeAg from blood and appearance of detectable antibodies to this antigen (anti-HBe). Concomitantly or subsequently to these changes, hepatic histology, biochemical parameters, and clinical conditions normalize. Thus, by all classical criteria, both acute hepatitis B and the underlying infection are resolved.

Recently, however, sensitive genome amplification assays (typically, nested PCR) have revealed that 30 to 80% of patients who have apparently resolved an acute hepatitis B infection may continue to harbor low levels of HBV DNA in the serum, blood mononuclear cells, and liver for years. This condition, which is often referred to as occult HBV infection and is especially frequent in patients coinfected with HCV and HIV-1, needs to be better understood because it is not even known whether the viral DNA detected is full-length genomes and whether it is enclosed within potentially infectious virions. Helping to obscure the picture, a similar status has been observed also in individuals lacking any other marker of ongoing or past HBV infection, including anti-HBc (2).

As mentioned above, a proportion of acutely infected individuals, regardless of whether they are symptomatic or not (in fact, the forms of hepatitis with mild or no symptoms have an increased tendency to persist), fail to clear the virus, do not develop readily detectable anti-HBs, and progress to chronicity. Of several variables which affect the frequency of

this occurrence, the patient's age is by far the most important. Indeed, perinatal infections become chronic in more than 90% of cases, compared with 15 to 30% of cases in childhood and fewer than 5% in adulthood. The behavior of infection markers is clearly distinct from the one described for self-limiting transient infections. The picture is dominated by the persistence of variably high levels of HBsAg and other markers of viremia in serum usually for life, while clinical manifestations vary from alternating periods of remission (chronic hepatitis B) to no symptoms at all (healthy HBV carriers). Chronic viremia may remain essentially stable over time but more often fluctuates somewhat, with peaks in concomitance with elevated levels of ALT and of anti-HBc IgM and a deteriorated clinical picture (Fig. 3). It has been calculated that chronically infected patients release as many as 10^{11} or more virions per day in the bloodstream and that the daily turnover of circulating virions is about 50% (35). At any rate, with passing years, the levels of infectious virus in blood tend to slowly decline, as revealed by decreasing concentrations of HBeAg and HBV DNA. Ultimately, generally after many years of persistence, HBeAg becomes undetectable, and this is generally followed by seroconversion to anti-HBe. Nonetheless, HBsAg and HBV DNA continue to be readily detectable in the circulation (Fig. 3).

During chronic hepatitis B, liver damage accumulates and in approximately 20% of cases ultimately leads to cirrhosis. In turn, cirrhosis determines a 100-fold or more increased risk of developing HCC. Importantly, chronically infected individuals with no detectable HBeAg have a mild disease course, exhibit a relatively low risk for progression to cirrhosis and HCC, and transmit the virus with reduced efficiency. However, it is imperative to consider that, particularly in Asia and southern Europe, failure to demonstrate HBeAg can not only represent an indicator of low infection activity but also be the consequence of active infection by HBeAg-minus variants of the virus.

Spontaneous resolution of persistent HBV infection is rare, occurring annually in less than 1% of subjects. The few cases of chronic infection which do eventually completely resolve exhibit an evolution of infection markers similar to the one discussed for resolution of self-limiting acute infections, albeit much slower in pace. Recently, these similarities have been seen to include the long-term detectability of minute amounts of viral DNA in plasma and liver by sensitive amplification methods, in spite of consistently negative HBsAg tests (2, 15, 44).

The prevalence rates of chronic HBV infection vary widely throughout the world, from as high as 25% in certain areas of sub-Saharan Africa, China, and Southeast Asia to as low as 0.1 to 0.5% in western Europe and North America. Niches of especially high endemicity, however, can be found within specific ethnic, behavioral, and professional groups of any geographical region. Infected humans shed HBV with body fluids, including saliva, urine, semen, vaginal and menstrual fluids, tears, and breast milk. Vertical transmission from infected mothers to babies during parturition or postnatally is a major mechanism of virus diffusion especially in areas where HBV is hyperendemic, where intrafamilial spread with no other apparent form of exposure also occurs and seems to be especially important for young children. Sexual transmission is also frequent, as shown by high rates of infection among sexually active young adults living in areas of low endemicity, with peaks among male homosexuals. However, IDUs show the highest rates of infection in these areas. Recognized fomites include toilet articles and contaminated medical instruments. Transmission by blood transfusions and clotting factor replacement therapy is currently uncommon as a result of donor screening, virucidal treatment of blood derivatives, and other measures. Several intervention strategies have been implemented to limit HBV dissemination, but vaccination of newborns with recombinant HBsAg is by far the most powerful and is used extensively in many parts of the world. Indeed, increasing implementation of vaccination is rapidly modifying HBV epidemiology in many countries.

Natural and recombinant alpha interferon (IFN-α) and, more recently, its pegylated form pegIFN-α have shown limited utility for treatment of chronic HBV infection. The recent advent of nucleoside or nucleotide analogs that target the viral polymerase has, however, started a new therapeutic era. Lamivudine and adefovir dipivoxil have proved efficacious and generally well tolerated and have consequently been elevated to the rank of first-line therapies. Several other antiviral compounds currently under scrutiny are showing promise and might become therapeutically available in the near future. Current treatments often lead to sustained improvement of clinical symptoms, ALT level normalization, and reduction or clearance of viremia. However, total eradication of infection is infrequent. In any case, due to the rapid emergence of resistant P gene mutants, most patients relapse after withdrawal of therapy. Liver transplantation remains the only treatment for decompensated cirrhosis and HCC. Unfortunately, recurrence of

HBV infection in the grafted liver is common and shows a particularly aggressive course, in spite of recent pharmacological attempts. For more comprehensive reviews of HBV pathobiology, consult references 11, 15, 24, and 44.

Assay Systems for HBV

Customarily, the laboratory diagnosis of HBV infection has been carried out by using commercial immunoassays that detect the viral antigens or the corresponding antibodies and provide most of the information needed at relatively low cost. The kits currently used to this purpose exploit various principles and formats (including dipsticks), are generally characterized by good to excellent specificity and sensitivity, and have often been automated to deal with large numbers of samples. HBV DNA detection and quantitation, however, are being increasingly used for assessment and management of hepatitis B. Commercially available molecular assays also have different formats and are generally reliable, standardized, and simple to use or automated but remain relatively expensive. Criteria for use and interpretation of HBV test systems are provided in Fig. 4 and Table 3.

Testing for HBsAg

HBsAg becomes detectable in serum 2 to 10 weeks after initiation of infection (i.e., 2 to 6 weeks before ALT abnormalities and 2 to 5 weeks before clinical onset) and reaches peak concentrations of 50 to 300 μg per ml in the late incubation or early acute phase. The capture EIAs and other immunoassays currently in use for HBsAg detection and quantitation have a lower limit of sensitivity in the range of 0.1 to 2 ng of HBsAg per ml of serum, corresponding to roughly 3×10^7 viral particles. Given this high sensitivity, a negative test implies that no active HBV replication is ongoing or, more rarely, that the virus produced is too scarce for consistent HBsAg detectability, as occasionally is observed during acute infections accompanied with massive liver necrosis (fulminant hepatitis) and in neonatal infections. Mutations in the a determinant may also affect the performance of HBsAg immunoassays. Importantly, since sporadic false positives do occur (due to accidental contamination, insufficient washing of microwells or beads, or the presence of anticoagulants in test samples), a first positive HBsAg result should always be confirmed with the same test or a different type of test, such as specific inhibition with unlabeled anti-HBs or, more conveniently, by assaying for other markers of infection. Before molecular assays became routine, the customary confirmatory marker was total anti-HBc. Since anti-HBc is the first antibody to appear and the most persistent, a positive HBsAg test in the absence of a corroborating positive anti-HBc test always had to be interpreted with great caution. Currently, testing for HBV DNA should be considered the confirmation method of choice.

By itself, a confirmed positive HBsAg test proves that an HBV infection is ongoing but does not distinguish between acute self-limiting infection, acute infection with no tendency to resolve, and chronic infection with moderate or exuberant virus replication. Accurate investigation of the patient is required to distinguish among these possibilities, including direct measurement of viremia levels, testing for HBeAg, and testing for the presence and concentration of anti-HBc IgM, anti-HBe, and anti-HBs.

Testing for Viral DNA

Since the tests currently in use may have detection limits as low as 10^2 viral genomes per ml, to date, HBV DNAemia is the most accurate marker of ongoing HBV replication.

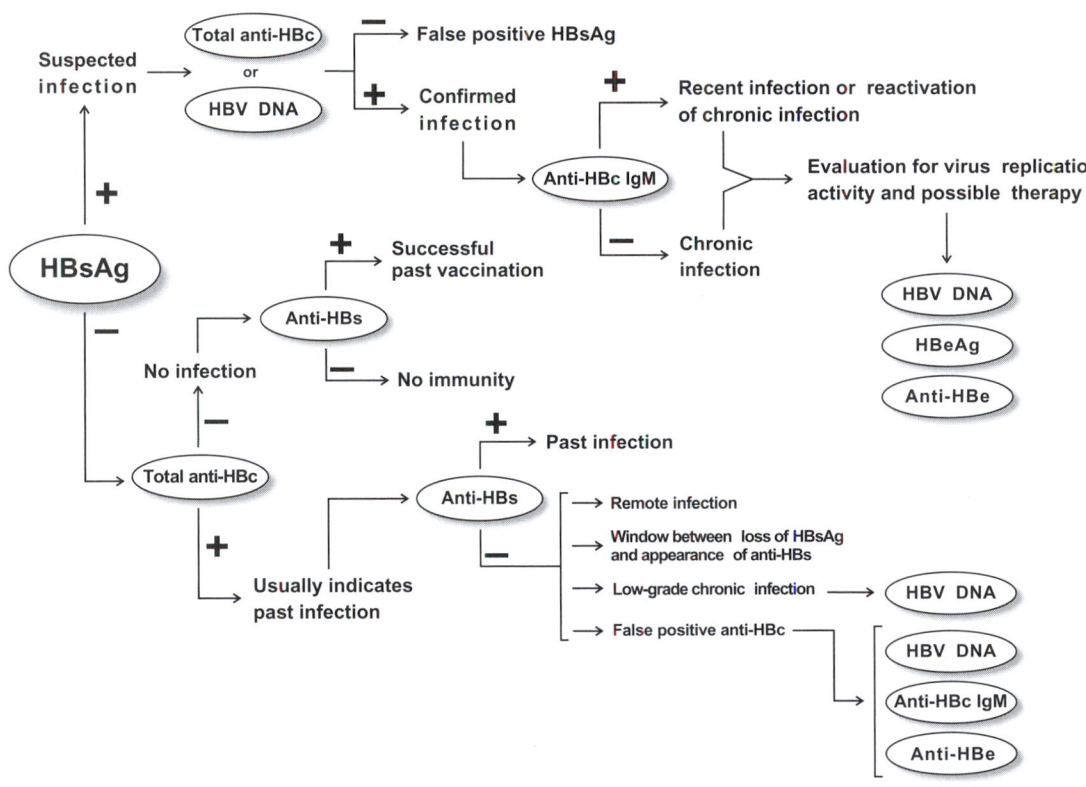

FIGURE 4 Algorithm for use and interpretation of laboratory tests for HBV infection. See also Table 3.

Determination of HBV DNA also circumvents the problem of demonstrating and staging infections sustained by genetic variants of HBV, such as the HBeAg-minus mutants.

HBV DNA assays usually target the C gene and can be both qualitative and quantitative. However, the qualitative tests are being rapidly replaced by quantitative methods that perform equally well and are of greater utility in the follow-up of patients, especially when the patients are undergoing antiviral treatments. The commercially available tests have different sensitivities and linear ranges, but their precision

TABLE 3 Interpretation of immunovirological profiles for HBV

Genome (HBV DNA)	Antigens		Antibodies				Interpretation
	HBsAg	HBeAg[a]	Anti-HBe	Anti-HBc IgM	Anti-HBc IgG	Anti-HBs	
							Acute infection
+	+	+	−	−	−	−	Very early stages
+	+	+	−	+	−	−	Early stages
+	+	+	−	−	+	−	Late stages
−	−	−	+	±	+	+	Resolution
							Chronic infection
+	+	±	−	−	+	−	Typical profile
+	+	±	±	+	+	−	Reactivation
−	−	−	+	−	+	+	Resolution
+	−	−	−	−	±	±	Occult infection
−	−	−	±	−	±	±	Remote infection
−	−	−	−	−	−	+	Past vaccination
−	+	−	−	−	−	−	Likely false positive
−	−	−	−	−	+	−	False positive, passively acquired antibody, resolved infection with loss of detectable anti-HBs
−	−	−	−	−	−	−	No infection

[a]In infections by HBeAg-minus virus variants, HBeAg may test negative and anti-HBe may test positive in spite of active HBV replication.

and reproducibility characteristics are generally good. Among the assays, the so-called real-time methods, which quantify the viral nucleic acids in test samples by measuring the amplicons while they form during the exponential phase of amplification, have reached the diagnostic laboratory only recently but thanks to their excellent characteristics (linearity of up to 7 logs versus the 3 to 4 logs of conventional PCR assay, sensitivity up to 50 to 100 copies/ml, high throughputs, cost-effectiveness) are setting a new standard for quantitative assays. A plethora of in-house single-round and nested quantitative PCR assays have also been described, with reported sensitivities ranging from 5 to 10 viral particles/ml (nested PCR) to 600 copies/ml (single-round PCR), but many suffer from small linearity ranges and other limitations. Additional innovative technologies, such as DNA chips and other microarray technologies, have the potential to simultaneously quantitate the virus and characterize its genetic features but have yet to reach the clinical virology laboratory.

The wide array and decreasing costs of available quantitation methods have led to consideration of periodic measurement of HBV DNA as the key parameter for the management of HBV patients. However, uncertainties still exist with regard to what levels of HBV DNAemia can be associated with a lack of clinically significant liver damage and what levels instead demand antiviral intervention (7, 22). Recently, a viremia of 10^5 HBV DNA copies per ml of serum was proposed as the cutoff level for distinguishing healthy carriers from chronic hepatitis patients (20), but further studies are clearly warranted.

Testing for Anti-HBc

Typically, anti-HBc IgM develops at the same time as ALT changes in acute infection (i.e., 1 to 2 weeks after HBsAg) and rapidly reaches considerable titers. The presence of high-titer anti-HBc IgM is therefore diagnostic for acute or recent HBV infection and, together with HBV DNA, may be the only marker present in neonatal infections or when the amount of HBsAg produced remains under the threshold of test sensitivity, as occasionally occurs in fulminant hepatitis. In the subsequent 4 to 6 months, IgM predominates but then slowly declines and is overwhelmed by increasing titers of anti-HBc IgG. In self-limiting infections, anti-HBc IgM becomes undetectable in a few months, although low titers are sometimes found for up to 2 years. In chronic low-grade infections, anti-HBc IgM is either undetectable or low in titer but usually reappears or increases (>10 IU/ml) when viral replication exacerbates, thus representing an indicator of infection activity. Tests for total anti-HBc (IgM and IgG) remain positive after complete eradication of infection, and the antibodies persist for life in >90% patients.

Testing for HBeAg, Anti-HBe, and Anti-HBs

As mentioned above, HBeAg appears in blood at the same time as HBsAg and is detectable whenever the virus is actively replicating. Conversely, disappearance of HBeAg is indicative of reduced viral replication. Note, however, that anti-HBe can coexist with active virus replication in patients infected by HBeAg-minus variants. For example, in patients undergoing antiviral treatment, the emergence of an HBeAg-minus mutant should always be suspected when elevated ALT levels persist despite HBeAg clearance.

In acute infection, conversion from HBeAg positivity to anti-HBe positivity is prognostic for resolution since it is usually followed by the disappearance of HBsAg (but, as discussed above, not always of HBV DNA) from serum and by the appearance of anti-HBs within weeks or months. In chronic infection, loss of HBeAg and acquisition of anti-HBe tend to be associated with biochemical and histological improvement.

Anti-HBs become measurable just before or, more typically, a few weeks after HBsAg clearance and, being virus neutralizing, are a marker for complete clinical recovery and acquired immunity. Anti-HBs are usually permanent but, many years after infection resolution, they have a somewhat higher tendency than anti-HBc to become undetectable.

Determining Viral Genotype or Immunotype

HBV can be immunotyped with monoclonal antibodies and genotyped by characterization of amplified segments of the viral DNA by sequence analysis, restriction pattern analysis, or inverse hybridization. To date, HBV typing has generally remained restricted to epidemiological studies. If confirmed, the recent indications that HBV genotype might affect disease severity and responsiveness to therapies (15) might render HBV genotyping a routine laboratory test, similar to what already occurs with HCV. Although no standard HBV genotyping method has yet been established, sequence analysis will most likely become the method of reference, in analogy to what happens with other viruses.

Testing for HBeAg-Minus and Drug-Resistant Mutants

As discussed above, some HBV mutants are of clinical interest. Determination of whether HBV has evolved clinically significant mutations is becoming increasingly important. Patients with undetectable HBeAg but high HBV DNA levels and severe liver damage can carry mutants altered in the precore or core region of the C gene of the virus that are unable or impaired in the ability to produce HBeAg. These mutants can be identified by sequencing the region of the viral genome involved (the most frequent has a stop codon at codon 28 of the precore region). Less cumbersome methods have also been proposed but still need to be properly evaluated.

Breakthroughs in the response of HBV to therapies are often the result of the emergence of mutations in the target site of the drug being used. For example, during long-term therapy with lamivudine, the frequency of lamivudine-resistant mutants has been seen to rise from between 15 and 30% in the first year to 60% or more by the fourth year of treatment. As there are no phenotypic resistance assays available, HBV drug resistance is monitored by genotypic analysis. Most lamivudine-resistant mutants have an exchange of the methionine at codon 552 within the YMDD amino acid motif of the catalytic site of the DNA polymerase to either valine or isoleucine, which narrows the active site pocket and blocks drug binding. Direct sequencing of selected regions of ORF *P* (approximately 600 nucleotides) is the method of choice; however, more rapid assays similar in principle to the ones developed for HIV-1 drug resistance analysis have been developed and are commercially available.

HCV

HCV, the major agent of parenterally transmitted non-A, non-B hepatitis, remained elusive until the late 1980s, when its genome was molecularly cloned from experimentally infected chimpanzees. The genome is a linear molecule of single-stranded, positive-sense RNA approximately 9.5 kb in length. It contains one large ORF and two relatively short

UTRs at the 5′ and 3′ ends that play essential roles in genome expression and replication. The ORF is translated into a large polyprotein precursor of approximately 3,000 amino acids which is cleaved post- and cotranslationally into a dozen mature proteins. Of these, three are essentially structural (the capsid, or C, protein and the envelope glycoproteins E1 and E2) while the others (p7, NS2, NS3, NS4A and -B, and NS5A and -B) have enzyme activity (an RNA-dependent RNA polymerase, two proteases, and a helicase) and other poorly defined functions. Recent studies have shown that p7 has ion channel activity. A new protein with undetermined functions (protein F) encoded by an ORF overlapping the C region has also been identified. The virion, which has proved hard to visualize, is round, 55 to 65 nm in diameter, and consists of a 30- to 35-nm icosahedral nucleocapsid formed by numerous copies of the C protein and an outer lipoprotein envelope with small projections containing the E1 and E2 glycoproteins. Its infectivity is relatively unstable. On the basis of genomic organization and other criteria, HCV is classified within the family *Flaviviridae*, genus *Hepacivirus*.

Diversity among HCV isolates is minimal in the 5′-UTR and maximal in the E2 glycoprotein, where a stretch of 31 amino acids (hypervariable region 1) has been proposed to function as a decoy for immune escape, similarly to the V3 loop of HIV. Analyses have distinguished six major genotypes, designated 1 through 6, each one divided into subtypes designated by lowercase letters. A few recombinants have been reported from Russia and Peru (subtypes 2k/1b and 1a/1b, respectively). As discussed below, it is generally accepted that the infecting genotype of HCV may influence the likelihood of a patient's response to therapies. The impact of genetic heterogeneity in cross-protective immunity and pathogenic potential is instead poorly understood, although evidence has recently been obtained for multiply exposed IDUs and experimentally infected chimpanzees for the existence of at least some intra- and intergenotype protection (16) and of limited between-genotype differences in disease progression (29).

Dissection of HCV-host cell interactions lags far behind, mainly due to the lack of suitable tissue culture systems, while information about the dynamics of infection in the organism is derived mainly from posttransfusion hepatitis and chimpanzees. HCV shows a distinct tropism for hepatocytes but also replicates in lymphoid cells, circulating plasmocytoid dendritic cells, and other cell types, although much less productively. In typical primary infections, the virus becomes detectable in blood within 1 to 3 weeks and peaks a few weeks later; then it gradually declines over the following months. Just before and shortly after seroconversion, the load of HCV in plasma can fluctuate extensively and drop to very low levels. In this phase, spontaneous clearance of primary infection has been observed in a proportion of cases that has varied between 15 and 50% in different reports and appears to be most frequent in female and young patients (25). However, in the majority of subjects, the infection becomes persistent. Modulation and clearance (when it occurs) of acute-phase viremia are believed to result from the host's immune response, which is vigorous but tends to be slower than in most other systemic viral infections. In particular, the window period between the appearance of virus in plasma and that of antiviral antibodies (anti-HCV) usually lasts 7 to 9 weeks and, occasionally, as long as 9 months (Fig. 5). However, there are no established immunological or virological markers that can be used to reliably predict whether acute HCV infection will be cleared or become chronic, although an association of certain major histocompatibility complex class II alleles with infection outcome has been reported.

In untreated chronically infected patients, the number of virions produced and cleared per day is on the order of 10^{10} to 10^{12}; the levels of circulating HCV remain essentially stable or slowly increase over time, with fluctuations that do not usually exceed 1 log_{10}, hardly ever falling below the level of detection. For these patients, concentrations and spectra of anti-HCV are approximately the same as observed in advanced acute infection (Fig. 5). Complete spontaneous resolutions of chronic infections have hardly been reported. On the contrary, recently, by use of very sensitive detection methods, HCV RNA has been detected in the blood of patients who have apparently undergone a well-documented spontaneous or therapy-induced resolution of infection. Reportedly, the peripheral blood mononuclear cells of these patients also harbor the negative, replicative strand of the viral genome, suggesting that HCV can be even more difficult to eradicate than previously believed (30). Also, a recent report has suggested that hard-to-detect (occult) HCV infection might be responsible for abnormal liver function in patients with no anti-HCV antibodies and no other known causes of hepatitis (6).

More than 70% of acute infections are symptom-free or present with nonspecific manifestations. When clinical hepatitis is present, it develops after an incubation period of 4 to 20 weeks and is generally mild and brief. Fulminant hepatic failure is very rare. ALT concentrations may exhibit different elevation patterns (single or multiple peaks, plateaus, etc.) but infrequently exceed 1,000 IU/liter, generally reflecting moderate liver damage, and usually progressively normalize within a few weeks. As a matter of fact, because acute infections are so inconspicuous, they frequently go undiagnosed, and many people are discovered to be HCV infected during chronicity as a fortuitous finding of blood testing for unrelated reasons. In accord with the concept that acute liver damage by HCV is essentially immune system mediated, self-limited infections appear to be more frequent among symptomatic than asymptomatic patients (42).

The clinical importance of HCV is due mainly to its long-term persistence and to the consequent accumulation of hepatocellular damage, which progresses more slowly but possibly more severely than during chronic hepatitis B. In about a third of chronic infections, ALT levels remain normal for prolonged periods. Most patients start to show intermittently or persistently elevated levels of ALT and progressively deteriorated liver functions after 2 or 3 decades of infection, and up to 20% go on to develop cirrhosis. HCC can develop in 10% of cirrhotic livers. Male gender, old age at the time of infection, alcohol intake, elevated ALT levels, and coinfection with HBV and/or HIV-1 are all factors that negatively affect prognosis (12, 54).

Humans are the only known natural reservoir for HCV. About 3% of the world population is estimated to be infected, with prevalence rates ranging around 2% in North America and western Europe and >10% in some Asian and African countries. Because many infected people may be clinically healthy and unaware of their infections, apparent prevalence is likely to increase in future years. The National Institutes of Health has estimated that the prevalence of chronic infection in the United States will keep increasing at least until the year 2015 (25). Thanks to much-improved blood screening, the risk of acquiring HCV infection as a result of blood transfusions or treatments with blood derivatives is currently extremely low. Nevertheless, iatrogenic

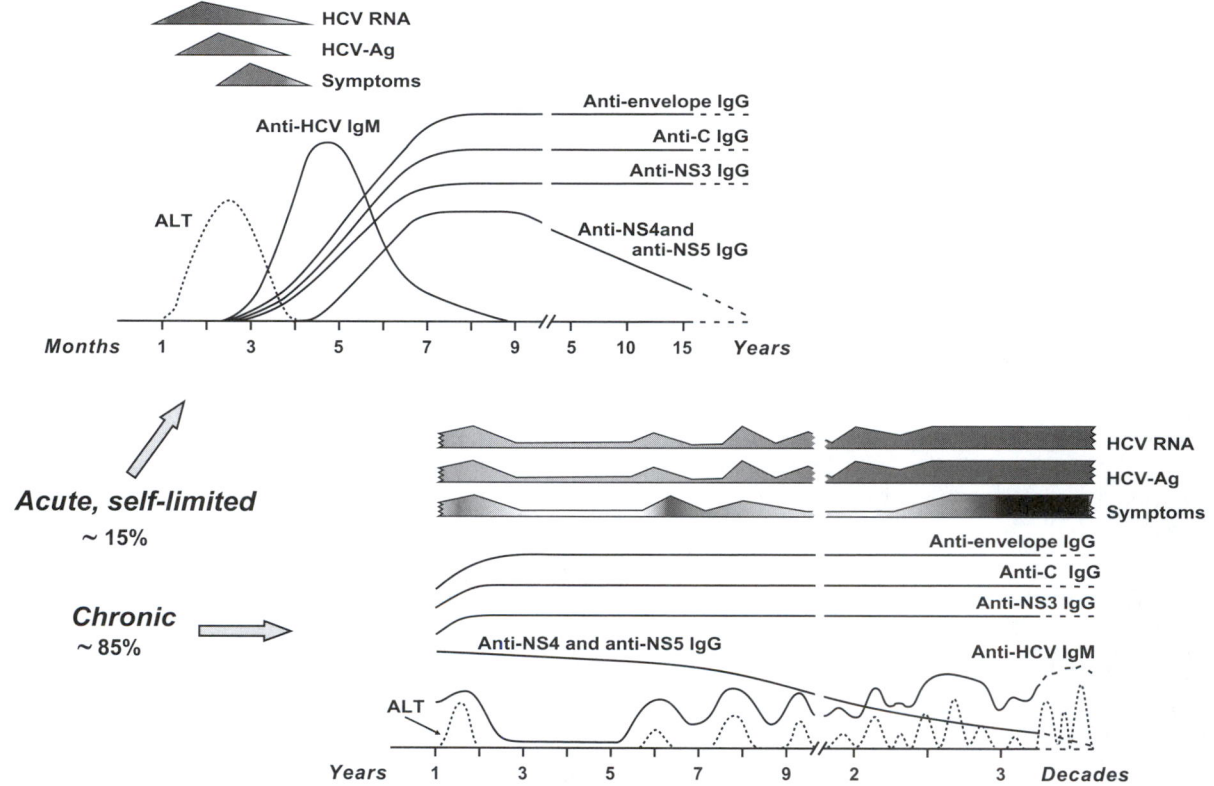

FIGURE 5 Typical course of immunovirological events and manifestations of liver damage in symptomatic, acute self-limiting and chronic HCV infection. The initial, acute phases are essentially the same, regardless of whether infection resolves or becomes chronic. HCV has a greater tendency to persist than HBV. The vast majority of both acute and chronic infections do not produce overt disease or do so after many years of persistence; however, the immunovirological events are similar to the ones depicted.

transmission is still observed in dialysis units, and there are also sporadic reports of HCV transmission from infected health care personnel to patients. In low-prevalence developed countries, intravenous drug abuse accounts for most new infections. Tattooing, acupuncture, body piercing, and any practice that may cause exposure to contaminated blood also contribute to dissemination. Mother-to-baby and sexual transmission are relatively ineffective, unless conditions that favor high viral loads, such as concurrent HIV-1 infection, coexist. Transmission to household contacts is infrequent, and there is no evidence for insect vectors. A significant proportion of HCV infections, designated community acquired or sporadic, occur apparently in the total absence of risk factors. Surveys have shown that HCV subtype 1a is predominant in North America, subtype 1b is predominant in western Europe and Japan, and types 4 and 5 are predominant in Africa, while type 6 appears to be restricted to Southeast Asia. Subtype 2c, previously considered a rare genotype, was found to be the second most frequent genotype in Italian patients with community-acquired infection (31). Differences in genotype distribution have also been observed, depending on the mode of infection.

Primary and secondary prevention activities are similar to those for HBV, except that no vaccine is available. Attempts to develop vaccines against HCV are under way but are encountering considerable hurdles. The efficacy of postexposure prophylaxis with immunoglobulins is probably only marginal. Treatment has improved significantly in recent years, and currently pegIFN-α in combination with ribavirin is the standard of care for chronically infected patients. This combination therapy produces sustained virological responses in a much higher proportion of cases than monotherapy with IFN-α alone: up to 80% in infections by genotype 2 and 3 HCV and around 50% in infections by the other genotypes. A variety of other compounds, mostly targeting the viral enzymes, are being evaluated for possible clinical use, and hopefully some will became therapeutically exploitable in the near future. At least 25% of liver transplants worldwide are carried out in patients with HCV cirrhosis and HCC. Nearly all recipients relapse with hepatitis C in the grafted organ: this is usually a very precocious event, which leads to severe hepatitis and cirrhosis in up to 30% of patients (26).

Assay Systems for HCV

The first approach to diagnosis of HCV infection is detection of anti-HCV IgG (Fig. 6). In the context of first diagnosis, testing for the presence of virus in blood by either nucleic acid or antigen is useful for (i) identifying patients and blood or tissue donors who are still in the preserological phase (as discussed above, with HCV the window period is particularly extended), (ii) resolving indeterminate serological results, (iii) recognizing the relatively few patients who still possess anti-HCV but have spontaneously resolved the infection, and (iv) sorting vertically infected newborns from those who have merely received transplacental anti-HCV

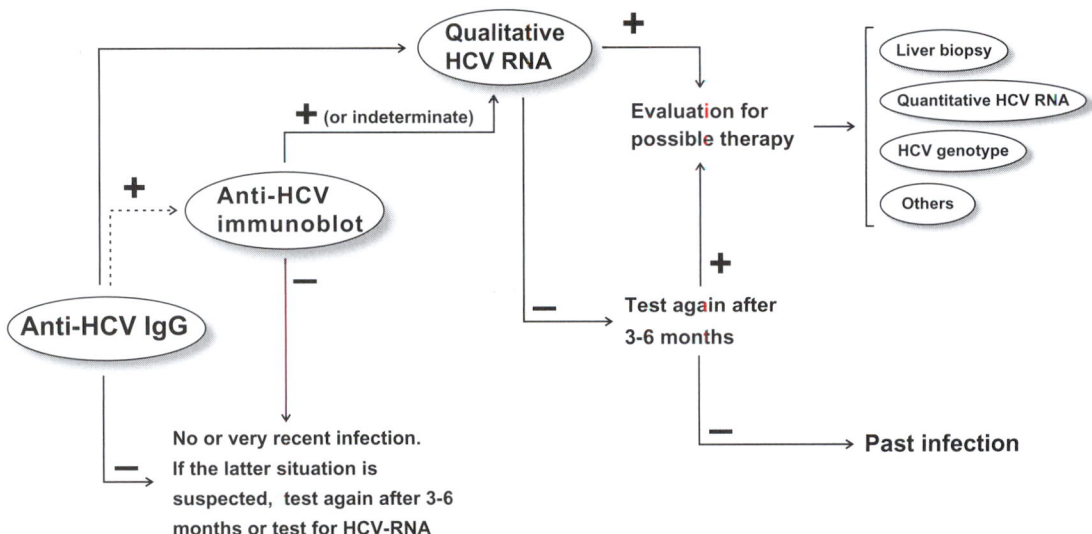

FIGURE 6 Algorithm for use and interpretation of laboratory tests for HCV infection. Under selected circumstances, HCV-Ag detection and measurement can be used in place of HCV RNA detection. Immunoblotting as a means to confirm positive EIA results is currently skipped by many laboratories, which proceed directly to HCV RNA detection and use confirmation by immunoblotting only for the patients who test HCV RNA negative.

from their mothers. On the other hand, detection and especially quantitation of viremia are invaluable for correct clinical management of infected patients, since they provide an evaluation of HCV replicative activity in the liver (which should not be equated with severity of liver damage; see below).

Testing for Antiviral Antibodies

Commercial kits for anti-HCV IgG screening have been redesigned several times to shorten the duration of the window period and to augment sensitivity and specificity, thus meeting the needs of blood banks as well as of diagnostic laboratories. The ones in use at present (third generation) have reduced the window period by 4 to 6 weeks and consist of EIAs and other immunoassays using optimized combinations of recombinant and synthetic antigens representing conserved domains of the C, NS3, NS4, and NS5 proteins. Their specificity is generally excellent. The very few false-positive results observed have been attributed to hypergammaglobulinemia, aged serum samples, and rheumatoid factors or have remained unexplained.

For patients at high risk of infection with increased ALT levels and high anti-HCV reactivity, supplemental anti-HCV testing can be skipped, since correlation between a positive screening test and infection is essentially 100%, and it is less costly to proceed directly to testing for viremia (Fig. 6). In all other circumstances and especially when ALT levels are normal, certain laboratories validate positive results with a second immunoassay, possibly different from the one used for screening, while others prefer to proceed directly to testing for viremia. Serological validation is most often carried out by immunoblotting, which permits a dissection of antibodies directed to different viral determinants. Sera that react with products derived from at least two viral genes are considered positive and indeterminate when reactive with a single protein; reactivity to the carrier polypeptide fused to recombinant antigens (usually human superoxide dismutase)

shows that the positivity might be nonspecific. Indeterminate immunoblot results may be indicative of false positivity, especially for low-risk individuals, but they are frequent also for HCV-infected immunocompromised patients, whose reactivity is often restricted to C and NS3 antigens. It should also be kept in mind that IgG antibodies tend to be produced later in response to NS4 and NS5 than to other viral proteins and to wane earlier following spontaneous or posttreatment resolution of infection; therefore, absence of reactivity to envelope, C, and NS3 proteins may be indicative of recent infection, in patients still seroconverting, or of a resolved infection. Since the avidity of anti-HCV IgG increases significantly with duration of infection, tests that measure this parameter can help to sort out recent from remote infection, but they have not become routine.

The first anti-HCV antibody detected in infected patients is usually IgM. This class of antibody, however, cannot be used as a marker of acute-phase infection because it is also found in 50 to 70% of chronic infections. In the latter, the detection of anti-HCV IgM is frequently discontinuous, and some investigators consider this marker an indicator of increased virus activity, since it correlates nicely with ALT and viremia levels (Fig. 5). Unfortunately, the sensitivity and specificity of currently available commercial kits for anti-HCV IgM are far from perfect. Thus, even the optimized anti-HCV assays in use at present provide no reliable clues to discriminate resolved from ongoing infection and to evaluate the extent of viral replication. As mentioned above, this can be achieved by testing and measuring viremia.

Testing for Viral RNA

Detection and measurement of HCV RNA in plasma or serum are most frequently carried out with commercial assays that exploit RT-PCR and other gene amplification techniques similar to those discussed for HBV. The sensitivity, specificity, and hands-on requirements of most current commercial assays are highly satisfactory; the lower detection limits are as low as 25 to 50 IU per ml, and intra- and interassay variabilities are small. Due to the wide genetic variability of HCV, correct selection of the genome segment targeted by amplification methods is critical. The preferred target is the 5′-UTR, but even in this highly conserved region only some segments are sufficiently homogeneous to permit an equal efficiency with all viral genotypes. This explains why early commercial quantitative kits underestimated the titers of certain HCV genotypes by approximately 1 log, a shortcoming virtually eliminated in current versions. The availability of automated devices for nucleic acid extraction, detection, and quantitation has markedly increased throughputs and reduced (although not eliminated) the risks of specimen contamination. False negatives are usually the result of carelessness in the preanalytical phase.

Qualitative nucleic acid-based tests are most useful in assessing the safety of blood donations but prove useful also when a suspicion of active infection based on serological grounds needs to be confirmed. In this case, it is advisable to retest negative patients several times at intervals of several weeks in order to identify the ones who might have intermittent viremia, as is frequently observed in the course of spontaneous resolution or antiviral therapy.

Quantification of HCV RNA in serum or plasma probably has its greatest utility in aiding in the decision of whether and when to start treating patients and in monitoring their responsiveness to antivirals, but, given that the costs and accuracies of the test methods are similar, they are also increasingly used as an alternative to simple HCV RNA detection. Viral loads may reach peaks of 10^7 IU per ml or more during primary infection but in untreated chronic infections usually range around 10^5 to 10^6 IU per ml, with considerable variations in individual patients. A positive correlation between HCV RNA levels in plasma and viral replication in the liver has been documented, but it is generally recognized that viral loads are of limited relevance for prognosis at the level of single patients. Despite partially different dynamic ranges and analytical sensitivities, most current commercial tests quantify HCV with similar efficiencies. The introduction of IU to express viral loads has greatly facilitated the comparison of results obtained with different methods, but it is nevertheless recommended that individual patients be monitored for viremia level by consistent use of the same assay throughout their follow-up. This is especially important if the patient is undergoing treatment (23).

Testing for Viral Antigen

Immunoassays for direct demonstration and quantitation of HCV antigen in serum have become commercially available more recently than genome-targeted molecular methods. The assays currently on the market target the core antigen and generally use classical EIAs. They are highly specific and perform equally well regardless of the infecting HCV genotype, with a lower limit of sensitivity of 1.5 pg (reportedly, 1 pg of HCV antigen corresponds to 8,000 to 8,500 IU of HCV RNA per ml, as detected by molecular methods). Reports have argued that, despite its low sensitivity, HCV antigenemia quantitation could be a relatively inexpensive alternative to molecular assays as a means of monitoring the efficiency of antiviral treatments. However, it is important to note that the test becomes positive a few days after the appearance of HCV RNA and is rather insensitive when the viral load is <10,000 IU/ml (45).

Determining Viral Genotype

The major indication for HCV genotyping is the need to obtain all the information for customizing treatment protocols. In fact, it is generally accepted that successful treatment of genotype 1 and 4 HCV infection with combined pegIFN-α and ribavirin therapy requires higher doses of ribavirin (1,000 to 1,200 mg daily versus 800 mg) and longer durations (48 versus 24 weeks) than treatment of infection by other genotypes (42). Sequence analysis of the viral genome is the "gold standard" for any genotype determination, and in the case of HCV sequencing, carefully selected short segments of the 5′-UTR, NS5B, or E1 are sufficient for practical purposes. In particular, analysis within the 5′-UTR permits an accurate definition of genotype, while assignment to subtypes is generally achieved by analyzing the NS5B region. Sequencing of the HVR1 and NS5B regions is indicated solely to trace epidemiological linkages when suspected transmission events need to be confirmed.

Automated sequencers have become increasingly available in recent years, yet genome sequencing is still expensive, time-consuming, and feasible only in laboratories with skilled expertise. Alternative easier-to-perform methods include type- or subtype-specific RT-PCR, restriction fragment length polymorphism analysis of RT-PCR amplicons obtained from informative domains of the viral genome, and other techniques. A frequently used commercial test exploits the ability of 5′-UTR amplicons to hybridize to type-specific probes immobilized on nitrocellulose strips (line probe assay). Assessment of the reactivity of a patient's antiviral antibodies against genotype-specific synthetic peptides deduced from the C and NS4 regions of the genome (improperly called "serotyping") does not distinguish subtypes and is less accurate. A commercial direct-sequencing kit targeting the 5′-UTR and NS5B regions and incorporating all the machinery needed to achieve a report—from RNA extraction to the database of reference strains—is also announced. It is likely, however, that genotyping will soon be based on real-time techniques capable of differentiating types and subtypes by melting curve analysis or hybridization with type-specific probes labeled with different fluorescent dyes.

Viral Quasispecies Analysis

Similarly to many other viruses, HCV is present in infected hosts in the form of a variably complex mix of genetic variants, generally known as quasispecies. Several investigations have addressed the issue of whether the complexity and diversity of the viral quasispecies may represent useful parameters in decision making about the management of HCV-infected patients, but no firm conclusions have been reached. In any case, the methods currently in use for quasispecies analysis (cloning followed by sequencing, single-strand polymorphism analysis, etc.) are too laborious for routine use.

HDV OR DELTA VIRUS

HDV is a satellite infectious agent that was first identified while an unusual antigen (delta antigen, or HDAg) found in certain HBV-infected patients was investigated and was subsequently found to resemble certain subviral agents of plants. HDV derives its outer envelope protein from HBV, and hence it grows only in HBV-infected hosts. The virion, a slightly pleomorphic 36-nm-diameter sphere, consists of (i) the above-mentioned external envelope composed of HBsAg and lipids; (ii) a circular, negative-sense single-stranded RNA of approximately 1.7 kb, which is the smallest genome of any known animal virus; and (iii) a poorly defined capsid made of numerous copies of HDAg, the only known protein it encodes. The single-stranded RNA forms a rod-shaped imperfect duplex due to pairing of roughly 70% of its nucleotides and has well-characterized ribozyme activities. Self-cleavage and self-ligation are essential for processing the RNA intermediates generated by a rolling-circle mechanism of replication that uses cellular RNA polymerases. In virions and infected cells, the HDAg is present in two isoforms (small, or S-HDAg, of 195 amino acids, and large, or L-HDAg, which has 19 more terminal amino acids), which result from differential posttranscriptional RNA editing and have distinct regulatory functions during viral replication. Being unique among animal viruses, HDV is classified as the only member of the free-standing genus *Deltavirus*.

Unlike for HBV, extrahepatic replication of HDV has never been detected. Experimentally, HDV replicates only in HBV-infected chimpanzees (with more severe consequences than other human hepatitis viruses), in mice engrafted with HBV-infected primary human hepatocytes, and in eastern woodchucks infected by the respective hepadnavirus. Cells exposed to HDV alone can replicate the viral genome in the absence of any HBV gene product but with no production of complete virions and, with the exception of a subtle growth disadvantage, no consequences for the cells (46). Thus, there is no practical cell culture system for in vivo isolation.

HDV infection may occur either as coinfection in patients who are concomitantly infected with HBV or as superinfection of already HBV-infected patients, and the course and consequences of infection differ considerably in the two situations (Fig. 7). In coinfection, HDV replication is slowed by the scarce HBsAg available and generally peaks at low levels 1 week after HBV and evokes feeble immune responses. On the other hand, the dynamics of HBV replication and HBV-specific immune responses are scarcely affected relative to those of single HBV infection. Both viruses are generally cleared in a few months, and only 1 to 3% of coinfections become chronic. Clinical manifestations, when present, are indistinguishable from those caused by HBV alone except that they tend to be more severe and biphasic. The natural history of the few coinfection cases that fail to resolve is also similar to that of chronic hepatitis B alone, but bouts of HDV replication may occur. These are usually associated with transient reductions of HBV viremia due to competition for HBsAg.

During superinfection, because HBsAg is already abundant in hepatocytes, HDV replication is more prompt and florid than in coinfection and causes a more profound suppression of preexisting HBV viremia. Immune responses to HDV also mount rapidly but, in spite of persistent high titers of anti-HDV antibodies (anti-HDs), over 70% of superinfected patients continue to circulate HDV indefinitely, although at lower levels than in earlier stages (Fig. 7). In

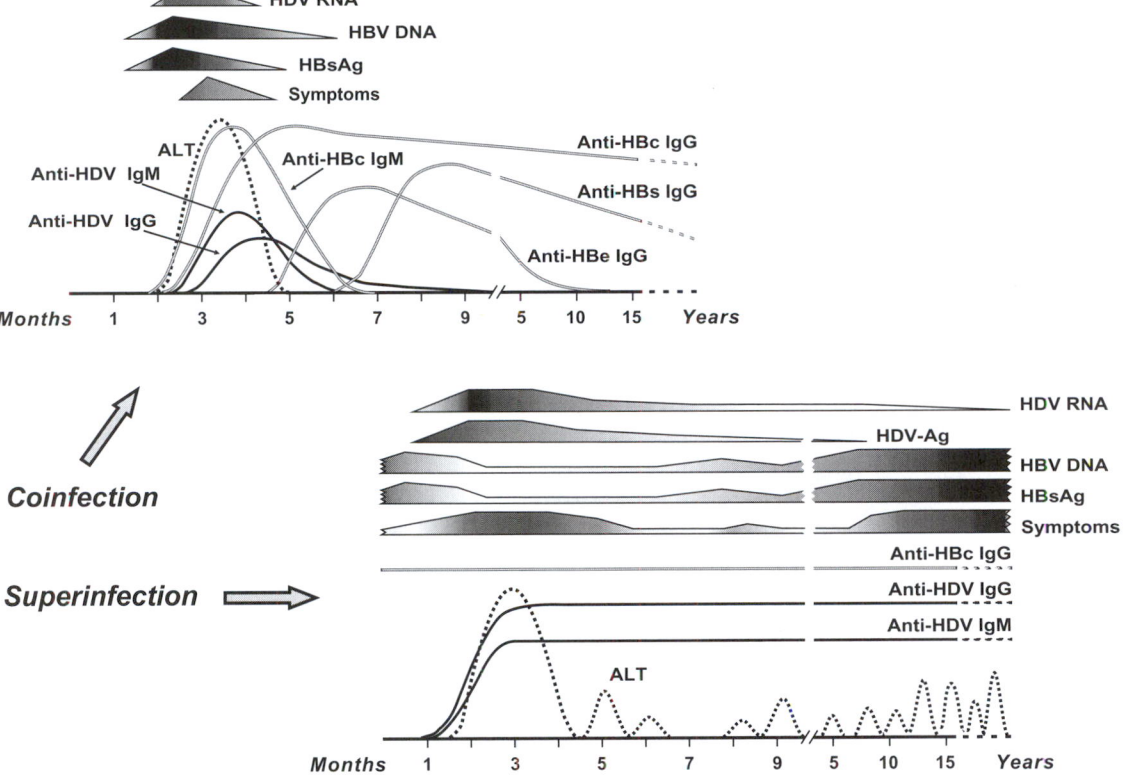

FIGURE 7 Typical course of immunovirological events and manifestations of liver damage in symptomatic HDV infection. In concomitant infection (coinfection) of naive individuals with HBV and HDV, HBV markers are affected very little by concurrent HDV replication, and HDV markers may escape detection due to their transient nature. In superinfection of individuals already infected with HBV, HDV replication is particularly florid and may produce transient reductions or undetectability of HBV DNA and HBsAg (see text).

patients who eventually succeed in resolving HDV infection, anti-HD IgG usually persists for the remainder of life. The acute phase of superinfection often, though not invariably, causes exacerbation of liver damage and a significant rate of fulminant hepatitis. The manifestations and outcome of chronic dual infection are also usually severe, with accelerated evolution toward cirrhosis, liver decompensation, and HCC.

Roughly 20 million people are believed to be HDV infected worldwide. The prevalence of HDV is uneven, however, ranging from 0.5 to 2% of HBV-infected individuals in North America and northern Europe, where HDV is virtually confined to IDUs, to 20 to 60% in South America and central and east Asia. The fact that the nucleotide sequences of different isolates may vary by 30% or more has led to distinguishing of three unevenly distributed HDV genotypes and two subtypes: type I is present worldwide, type II is present in Japan and Taiwan, and type III is present in northern South America, where acute infection is associated with particularly severe disease. Although HDV transmission routes are poorly understood, it is generally accepted that they are the same as for HBV.

As may be obvious in the light of HDV dependence on HBV, anti-HBV therapies (especially IFN-α) have been seen to significantly improve the long-term clinical outcome and survival of patients with chronic hepatitis D, even if they already have cirrhosis before treatment is initiated. Most importantly, HDV endemicity has considerably decreased where HBV vaccination is extensively used. Nevertheless, HDV is still an important cause of severe and fulminant hepatitis in developing countries (for recent reviews, see references 40 and 43).

Assay Systems for HDV

The possible coexistence of HDV infection is an important consideration in the management of hepatitis B, especially in areas of high HDV endemicity and in IDUs worldwide. In particular, it should be suspected in all cases of fulminant hepatitis B and in individuals with chronic HBV infections that undergo a sudden deterioration of symptoms which remains unexplained on the basis of parameters of HBV infection and other possible hepatotoxic events or do not improve as a result of lamivudine treatment. Traditionally, diagnosis used to rely mainly on assays for anti-HD, but HDV RNA detection methods have now become of great importance. Figure 8 provides a scheme for using and interpreting these tests.

Testing for Viral RNA

Detection of HDV RNA in the serum of HBV-infected patients is a particularly useful marker, as it indicates ongoing active HDV replication and is almost invariably positive in all types of HDV infection (13). Currently, HDV RNA is assayed mostly by RT-PCR assays, which especially in the real-time format have shown high sensitivity (lower detection limit, 10^2 to 10^3 genomes/ml) and specificity. HDV RNA quantitation is especially useful for patient follow-up in the course of therapy and often correlates with extent of liver injury (51). Liver biopsy can be complemented with the demonstration of HDV RNA located primarily in the nuclei of hepatocytes.

Testing for Viral Antigen

Although the presence of HDAg in serum is also a marker of ongoing active HDV replication, its clinical utility is very limited, as it is readily detectable only during the acute stages of superinfection, when HDV replicates extensively and reaches titers of up to 10^{11} infectious doses/ml of serum in 2 weeks (often causing a transient reduction of HBV viremia down to undetectable HBsAg). In contrast, most individuals with coinfections and chronic infections test HDAg negative because virus replication is moderate and/or the patients' anti-HDs interfere with HDAg detection in current assays (Fig. 7). Western blotting suffers less from the latter limitation and has the additional advantage of allowing separate visualization of S-HDAg and L-HDAg, but it is labor-intensive and commercially unavailable. In the past, immunohistological identification of HDAg in liver biopsy specimens has also been widely used.

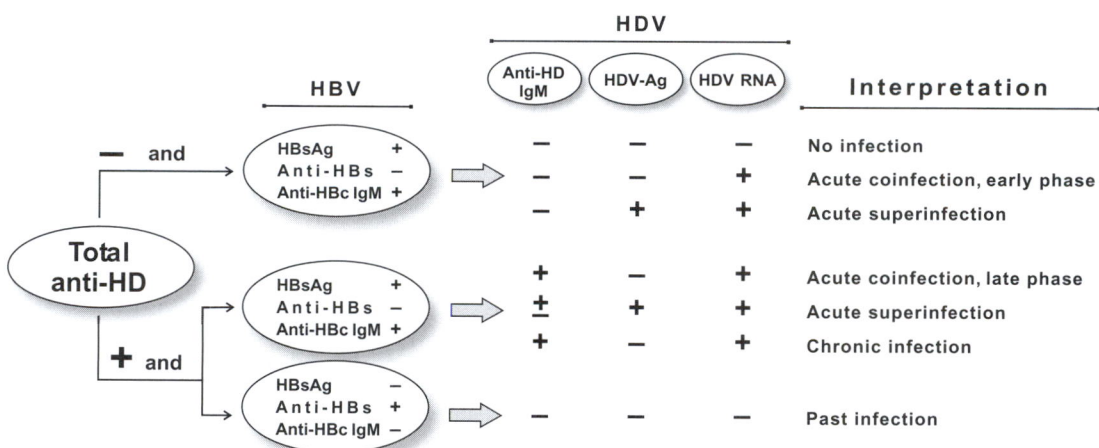

FIGURE 8 Algorithm for use and interpretation of laboratory tests for HDV infection. A prerequisite for HDV testing is that the patient is infected with HBV. In regions of high HDV endemicity, HDV testing should be carried out every second or third year or whenever there is an unexplained aggravation of hepatitis. In regions of low endemicity, HDV testing should essentially be limited to IDUs or people returning from areas of endemicity.

Testing for Antiviral Antibodies

Assays for anti-HD use ex vivo-derived or recombinant HDAg. However, it is important to note that anti-HDs can be missed in self-limited coinfection because they develop late, remain low in titer, are mostly IgM, and persist briefly. In chronic infection, the presence of anti-HD IgM and high titers of total anti-HD are indicators of poor prognosis, though the correlation is far from absolute (13). Finding high titers of anti-HBc IgM is also useful in defining management and prognosis, since they indicate recent HBV infection and thus ongoing coinfection.

Determining Viral Genotype

HDV typing can be carried out by restriction fragment length polymorphism analysis or sequencing of selected amplicons, but currently its utility is limited to epidemiological surveys (50).

HEV

Hepatitis E, a major form of enterically transmitted hepatitis, is widespread in many developing countries but is currently considered an emerging threat also for other areas. HEV is nonenveloped, spherical, and roughly 30 to 34 nm in diameter. The genome is a capped, positive-sense, single-stranded, linear RNA of approximately 7.2 kb and is organized into three potential ORFs, two terminal short UTRs, and a poly(A) tail at the 3′ end. ORF1 has motifs characteristic for RNA-dependent RNA polymerase, RNA helicase, and other enzymes; ORF2 encodes the putative capsid protein; and ORF3 overlaps with the other ORFs and encodes a small immunogenic, cytoskeleton-associated phosphoprotein of unknown functions. HEV was classified within the family Caliciviridae until recently, but it is currently considered a genus of its own, the hepatitis E-like viruses. Several isolates have been entirely sequenced and, albeit phylogenetic analysis is still incomplete, at least three genotypes have been recognized: types I (Burma strain; Asia and Africa), II (Mexico), and III (United States). Genetic heterogeneity observed among different isolates is moderate except in a segment of ORF1. Only one serotype appears to exist, on the basis of serological cross-reactivity and cross-protection studies in experimental animals. HEV was definitively identified by inoculation into nonhuman primates soon after HCV was recognized as the principal cause of parenteral non-A, non-B hepatitis and was subsequently shown to infect other mammals as well. However, to date, HEV has not been reproducibly propagated in simple cell culture systems. Evidence indicates that HEV is a labile virus; therefore, storage of infected fecal extracts in liquid nitrogen is recommended for preservation (for a comprehensive review, see reference 49).

In several hepatitis E outbreaks, young adults 15 to 40 years of age were most at risk of developing overt illness. Lower disease rates for younger individuals were attributed to subclinical infection. The disease has an incubation period that ranges from 15 to 60 days (average, 40 days) and resembles hepatitis A but tends to be more severe (Fig. 1). In different epidemics, fatalities due to fulminant liver failure have usually been around 0.5 to 2% in hospitalized patients and are observed almost exclusively among third-trimester pregnant women and/or their unborn babies.

Antibodies are already present at clinical onset and peak by 1 month. Antiviral IgM is detected in >90% of patients and persists for at least 3 months in half of them, while IgG declines more gradually (Fig. 1). Anti-HEV antibody has been

detected as long as 14 years after infection in roughly half of the patients. Reports of patients who have become seronegative much earlier may be due to improper choice of the antigens used in the assays for anti-HEV detection. Viremia and fecal excretion are short-lived and generally over soon after biochemical resolution of hepatitis in most patients (1).

HEV is present primarily in the Indian subcontinent, central and Southeast Asia, the Middle East, Mexico, and other developing countries with inadequate environmental sanitation, where it causes >50% of all cases of acute hepatitis. It is usually transmitted by fecally contaminated drinking water, and extensive waterborne epidemics are not infrequent. In highly developed countries, the infection is mostly imported by immigrants and travelers (and possibly infected animals as well) and shows little or no tendency to spread to contacts; however, cases with no risk factors in the medical history also occur. In such areas, anti-HEV is found in roughly 2% of healthy blood donors, but a certain number of false-positive results cannot be excluded. Chronic infection has never been detected in humans. Sporadic infection may be responsible for virus survival during interepidemic periods, but a role of nonhuman reservoirs is also very likely, since HEV or HEV-like agents are widespread in rodents, pigs, and other animals. Additional evidence indicating that HEV infection might be a zoonosis derives from sequence comparison of human and animal virus isolates (47). At the time of writing, no commercial vaccine against HEV infection is available; however, vaccination with recombinant HEV capsid protein has conferred protection in rhesus macaques, and a promising phase II clinical trial of this vaccine is ongoing in Nepal (34).

Assay Systems for HEV

Testing for Antiviral Antibodies

Detection of anti-HEV IgM is a well-recognized marker of recent infection and the most convenient one for diagnosis during the acute phase. Anti-HEV IgG antibodies are measured to discriminate remote from recent infections (Fig. 9). Since HEV cannot be cultivated or purified in large quantities, serology relies essentially on immunoassays using

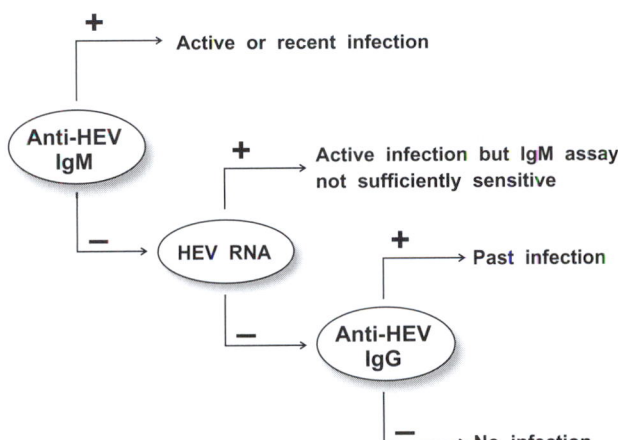

FIGURE 9 Algorithm for use and interpretation of laboratory tests for HEV infection. HEV RNA assays should be performed only when there are solid reasons for suspecting HEV infection (see text), on stool samples collected within 2 to 3 weeks from clinical onset.

recombinant or synthetic ORF2 and/or ORF3 peptides of variable length (49). Recent comparisons have indicated that ORF2-based serological assays are more reliable than ORF3-based ones, possibly because the former contain epitopes more conserved among viral isolates. Thanks to considerable improvements, currently available commercial kits perform significantly better than previous ones (52). Western blotting has been used in small-scale studies to validate serological results.

Testing for Viral RNA

Because viremia frequently subsides before symptoms arise, feces (possibly collected within 1 week of symptoms) is a more appropriate specimen than blood for direct demonstration of the virus. RT-PCR assays using primers targeted to conserved segments of ORF1 or ORF2 generally perform well and detect the full range of clinical isolates. However, a negative result does not exclude infection, and the detection of anti-HEV IgM should be considered more informative.

GBV-C OR HGV

In the mid-1990s, two independent groups characterized two novel viral agents in the blood of patients with cryptogenetic hepatitis by the use of molecular approaches similar to the ones used for identifying HCV (18, 39). The viruses were called GBV-C and HGV, but sequence data soon showed that they were different isolates of the same species. The virion is an enveloped sphere, 40 to 60 nm in diameter. The genome is single-stranded, positive-sense linear 9.4-kb RNA, consisting of a single, long ORF and two UTRs located at the 5' and 3' termini. The ORF encodes a large polyprotein that is posttranslationally cleaved into mature structural proteins (namely, envelope glycoproteins E1 and E2) and NS proteins (NS2 to NS5, with motifs typical of an RNA-dependent RNA polymerase, two proteases, and a helicase). Notably, location of the gene for the nucleocapsid or C protein is still debated. It might be within the genomic RNA, possibly in a reading frame different from that of the major ORF, or within negative-sense RNA where a second ORF with no known functions has been described. Apart from this, the genomic organization of GBV-C is similar to that of HCV and other flaviviruses. The degree of nucleotide homology with HCV, however, is low (<30%). Overall genetic diversity among isolates is limited, but at least five major genotypes, some of which are further divided into subtypes, have been demonstrated and have different geographic distributions.

The immunobiology and pathogenic potential of GBV-C are poorly understood. Most acute infections resolve within a few weeks, but approximately 25% persist. In self-limiting infection, the disappearance of viremia is preceded by the development of antibodies to the E2 protein (anti-E2). In infections that become chronic, anti-E2 instead remains undetectable, and the virus continues to circulate in blood for many months or years, apparently bound to low-density lipoproteins but not to antibody. While this strongly suggests that anti-E2 is important for virus eradication, antibodies to the nucleocapsid protein have no apparent role in virus clearance.

To date, an unequivocal demonstration that GBV-C is implicated in any pathology is lacking. There are numerous reports of acute and chronic GBV-C infections in individuals with no evidence of hepatitis or other disease. In the few patients infected with GBV-C alone with otherwise unexplained elevated ALT levels, biochemical alterations were usually modest and temporally unrelated to GBV-C viremia fluctuations. Sites of GBV-C replication and persistence are poorly defined, but the liver does not appear to be a major one. Even in HBV- and HCV-infected patients, concomitant GBV-C infection did not seem to affect the severity of liver damage or outcome of therapy. However, the possibility that GBV-C may occasionally induce hepatitis, similarly to other viruses which may occasionally become hepatotropic, cannot be totally excluded. Interestingly, recent reports have indicated that HIV-1 patients coinfected with GBV-C by several years have lower HIV loads, progress to AIDS more slowly, and tend to survive longer than singly HIV-1-infected patients, suggesting that GBV-C might inhibit HIV-1 replication through mechanisms that remain to be elucidated (48).

Epidemiological surveys have shown that 2 to 20% of healthy people worldwide have antibodies against GBV-C, with the lowest rates found in Asia and North America and the highest rates found in Africa and South America. The prevalence rates of viremia are lower, varying between 1 and 4% in the general populations of different countries but with peaks of 25 to 75% in IDUs and other subjects at risk for parenteral infection in general. The high frequency of GBV-C infection in HCV- and HBV-infected patients (10 to 19%) demonstrates that these infections disseminate through similar routes. Mother-to-child transmission has been documented, while sexual transmission is considered likely (for a comprehensive review, see reference 41).

Assay Systems for GBV-C

Because there is growing consensus that GBV-C is an orphan virus in search of a disease, diagnostic tests are performed almost exclusively for research purposes. Nonetheless, laboratory diagnosis of infection may still be indicated for those forms of acute or chronic hepatitis that appear to be viral in origin but in which no other known virus can be implicated.

Testing for Viral RNA

Methods for isolating GBV-C in tissue culture and for detecting GBV-C antigen are currently unavailable. The diagnosis of active GBV-C infection is therefore carried out by molecular methods. Serum is the specimen of choice, although saliva, semen, and numerous tissues including liver, bone marrow, spleen, and white blood cells have been shown to contain small concentrations of virus. Conversion from detectable to undetectable viral RNA, especially if this occurs in concomitance with the development of anti-E2, shows a strong correlation with recovery from infection. However, intermittent viremia has also been observed in persistently infected individuals. RT-PCR assays that target the 5'UTR are preferable, since those targeting the coding regions NS3 and NS5 lead to some false-negative results, apparently due to a low level of homology. Use of the latter should be limited to confirmation of results for samples that have had a positive reaction by use of the 5'-UTR. More standardization is clearly needed. Several RT-PCR kits are commercially available and appear to have comparable sensitivities. Quantitative assays exploiting real-time or competitive PCR and genotyping methods using restriction fragment length polymorphism analysis, genotype-specific primers, or sequencing have also been described but at this time have no demonstrated clinical utility.

Testing for Antiviral Antibodies

Several distinct strongly reactive epitopes have been detected in the NS proteins. Since they appear to be conformation sensitive, the procedure used for their production is critical for antigenicity. The only antibody detection approach fairly well validated to date is EIA using E2 protein expressed in CHO cells as a test antigen (commercial kits available). On the basis of the evidence discussed above, anti-E2 is considered a marker of clearance of infection. However, considerable uncertainty still exists about the correct interpretation of test results for individual patients. This is due to the facts that the assay can remain negative for months after exposure to the virus and that anti-E2-positive individuals may undergo reactivations of the infecting virus as well as reinfections with a different GBV-C genotype. Moreover, despite considerable improvements, current tests still yield a significant proportion of false-positive and false-negative results. Testing for NS3 antibodies has been proposed but has not yet been fully validated as a means of improving the reliability of GBV-C serology. Confirmatory tests proposed include a line probe assay based on recombinant structural and NS proteins, a radioimmunoprecipitation assay using E2 protein expressed in BHK-21 cells, and a sandwich EIA using E2 protein expressed in CHO cells, but all of these tests must be validated, and at least some are clearly impractical for routine use. Anti-E2 IgG lasts for >3 years at fairly constant titers, while attempts to develop reliable specific IgM assays have been frustrating so far. Thus, no serologic test that may provide information on the duration of GBV-C infection is available.

TTV AND OTHER ANELLOVIRUSES

The free-standing genus *Anellovirus* was created recently to accommodate a large group of viruses that are often highly divergent from each other in sequence but have in common a remarkably small circular single-stranded DNA genome of negative polarity. Torquetenovirus (from the Latin torques, necklace, and tenuis, thin) (TTV), the prototype of the group, was first identified in 1997 in the serum of a patient with cryptogenetic posttransfusion hepatitis (27). Subsequent studies revealed the existence of numerous clearly related additional viruses, some of which were classified in the separate species mini-torquetenovirus (TTMV), due to their even smaller genome. SEN virus (SENV), thus named for the HIV-positive patient in whose blood it was first identified, was initially considered an independent entity but is now classified within the 5 genogroups and over 30 genotypes in which TTV is currently subdivided as a result of its extreme genetic diversity.

TTV has not yet been visualized with certainty by electron microscopy or grown in tissue culture. As determined by examining infected plasma, the viral particle has a diameter of 30 to 50 nm, is nonenveloped, and appears to be very stable in the environment. About two-thirds of the 3.8-kb genome is made up of a large ORF (ORF1, coding capacity for approximately 770 amino acids) and several partially or totally overlapping smaller ones. The rest (UTR) of the viral genome is noncoding and contains various regulatory elements probably involved in replication. Although the natural history of infection is poorly understood, it is well documented that TTV is extremely prevalent worldwide (80% or more of healthy subjects are viremic at titers ranging from 10^3 to 10^8 DNA copies per ml), frequently if not invariably establishes chronic productive infections, and shows replication dynamics as active as those of other chronic viremia-producing viruses, such as HBV, HCV, and HIV. Cases of seemingly self-limited acute infection have also been described; however, it is unclear whether they reflect true virus eradication. On the other hand, mixed infections by multiple TTV genogroups

and genotypes are quite common, thus suggesting that immune responses are inefficient at eradicating the virus and provide no significant cross-protection. Transmission is believed to occur by the oral-fecal route and parenterally and transplacentally, but the upper respiratory tract also is an important route by which abundant virus can be shed into the environment. The discovery that TTV viremia is so widespread among the general population rendered early data on its high prevalence in hepatitis patients meaningless. Also, reports that infection with certain TTV genotypes, such as SENV, may be specifically associated with self-limited non-A non-E hepatitis have not been clearly substantiated (37). To date, therefore, TTV does not appear to be a significant agent of hepatitis and should actually be considered a virus in search of a disease since no other clinical involvement has been demonstrated with reasonable certainty (3). Interestingly, the loads of TTV in nasal samples of infants hospitalized for acute respiratory infections were recently seen to correlate with disease severity. Indications that TTV might be immunomodulatory in young children have also been reported (19).

Assay Systems for TTV

As long as the pathological implications of TTV remain undefined, diagnosis of infection will be of uncertain clinical utility.

Testing for Viral DNA

Because of the lack of sensitive in vitro culture systems and viral antigen detection methods, the only described approach for demonstrating TTV is by PCR amplification. The virus can be easily detected in serum and other specimens such as stools, saliva, nasopharyngeal and genital fluids, and breast milk. Due to the great genetic diversity of TTV, "universal" PCR methods are targeted to a small, highly conserved segment of the UTR. Use of these methods has greatly increased the rates of TTV-positive samples and revealed viremia titers 10- to 100-fold higher than those determined by ORF1-based PCR assays. None of the PCR protocols proposed, however, has been validated for detection of the entire spectrum of TTV variants. Typing of TTV has most frequently been carried out by sequencing of ORF1 segments; however, genogroup-specific PCR assays have recently been designed for appropriately selected UTR or ORF1 regions. PCR primers have also been designed for selective detection of SENV or other TTV genotypes and are targeted mainly to the ORF1. Quantitative assays based on microwell hybridization of amplicons obtained with primers specific for SENV isolates have also been described.

Testing for Antiviral Antibody

To date, there are no validated immunoassays of practical use in the clinical laboratory. The only reports on the presence of anti-TTV antibody in infected patients involved PCR-assisted immunoprecipitation of whole virus extracted from fecal samples, Western blotting with a truncated ORF1 recombinant protein, and an EIA against ORF1 synthetic peptides. These and other studies have shown that anti-TTV IgG is present in most viremic and nonviremic subjects and that a large proportion of the TTV found in blood is immunocomplexed.

CHOOSING TESTS ACCORDING TO DIAGNOSTIC PURPOSE

The sections above have described the complete range of diagnostic tests available for each virus discussed. However, testing should be modulated depending on the information sought, the characteristics of the specific patient under scrutiny (e.g., age, clinical features, risk factors, etc.), and epidemiological circumstances. This planning avoids needless costs in terms of reagents, equipment, technical time, and expertise. The following considerations are meant to assist in choosing the optimal testing protocol in different situations.

Etiologic Diagnosis of Hepatitis

The existence of risk factors for parenteral transmission (e.g., abuse of injecting drugs, transfusions of blood or blood derivatives, recent major surgery, promiscuous sex life, etc.) should immediately raise the suspicion that acute hepatitis is due to HBV or HCV. By contrast, a history of risky behavior for enteric transmission (e.g., recent visit of unvaccinated individuals to areas of HAV endemicity, ingestion of raw bivalve shellfish, etc.) should orient the clinician toward hepatitis A or E diagnosis. The diagnostician should also keep in mind that hepatitis A and E tend to occur in outbreaks of variable size, while hepatitis B and C are usually sporadic. Clinical presentation may also provide some guidance. Abrupt initiation of symptoms with a fever of >38.5°C and a sharp elevation of ALT levels above 1,000 IU/liter are usually indicative of HAV infection. In contrast, insidious onset of symptoms and moderately elevated ALT levels are more typical of hepatitis B and C. Cholestasis is especially prominent in hepatitis E.

In practice, however, in order to shorten diagnostic times and recognize possible mixed infections—which are not uncommon, especially in IDUs and other high-risk groups—clinicians investigating the origin of a recently diagnosed hepatitis usually request simultaneous testing for HAV, HBV, and HCV. A standard protocol for diagnosing acute viral hepatitis includes determination of anti-HAV IgM, HBsAg, anti-HBc IgM, and anti-HCV. A single testing for anti-HAV IgM and HBsAg is usually sufficient to confirm or exclude infection by HAV or HBV, respectively. As discussed in the appropriate section, anti-HAV IgM is a reliable marker of recent infection. If HBsAg is found in serum, it is customary to proceed to test for total anti-HBc, which is confirmatory for diagnosis, and for anti-HBc IgM, which is present at high titers in acute infection and in exacerbated chronic infection. It is also worth recalling that testing for anti-HBc IgM is usually enough to identify the few cases of fulminant or neonatal HBV hepatitis that test HBsAg negative (see above). In any case, testing for HBV DNA will help solve any diagnostic doubt that might persist. The presence of anti-HCV is evidence of active infection in approximately 80% of cases and warrants further assessment. In contrast, the absence of anti-HCV does not exclude acute hepatitis C because 30 to 50% of patients are not reactive at clinical onset. It is thus necessary to further assay seronegative patients for HCV RNA, which circulates in blood well before any biochemical or clinical change, and/or retest these patients for anti-HCV after 3 months or more. The possibility that antiviral antibodies are passively acquired should also be considered when dealing with neonates or persons treated with serum immunoglobulins. Outside areas of endemicity, testing for HDV should be reserved for HBV-infected patients who have traveled to such areas or who abuse injecting drugs. Testing for HEV should be limited primarily to patients living in or recently arrived from areas where the virus is endemic and, in the absence of such risk factors, when all other causes of hepatitis have been excluded. Finally, if all of the above viruses have been ruled out, the patient may be assayed for viremia by HGV or TTV

and other anelloviruses, although the clinical significance of positive tests remains generally unclear.

Follow-Up of Hepatitis after Etiology Has Been Established

Accurate follow-up of patients infected by hepatitis viruses that may give persistent infection (HBV, HCV, and HDV) is important. Because primary infection is often clinically silent, the ex novo appearance of symptoms of hepatitis may result from recrudescence of unrecognized chronic infection as well as from primary infection. Distinguishing between these possibilities requires additional tests, as schematically indicated in Table 3 and Fig. 4, 6, and 8. Moreover, the ALT levels of patients with HBV, HCV, and HDV infection should be monitored at relatively close intervals. Parameters that provide a direct evaluation of virus replication are also of great utility, but, unless the clinical picture undergoes significant changes, they can be examined at longer intervals. Because the liver is by far the major body site of HBV and HCV replication, viremia levels are a dependable measure of virus replication within this organ, although not of liver damage progression. Measurement of HBsAg in paired serum samples obtained 4 to 6 weeks apart can help in distinguishing acute HBV infections that have no tendency for recovery, because in this case antigenemia shows no appreciable decline. The presence of circulating HBeAg is also an important marker of vigorous HBV replication, while its disappearance followed by the development of anti-HBe usually precedes, by weeks or months, the disappearance of HBsAg and the development of anti-HBs, which are hallmarks of resolution. Anti-HBc IgM levels are useful for diagnosis of reactivation of chronic infection, as well as acute infections. Currently, however, quantification of HBV DNA levels in blood circulation is commonly used, since this test provides the most direct and accurate indication of HBV replicative activity and also detects the HBeAg-minus mutants that persist despite the presence of anti-HBe. Also, patients with persistently high HBV DNA loads should be carefully monitored for HCC. HBV-infected individuals who abuse illicit drugs or live in areas where HDV is highly prevalent should also be tested for markers of superinfection by HDV every 2 to 3 years and, in any case, whenever symptoms deteriorate abruptly or persist in spite of HBeAg unreactivity. HDV superinfection is an important element in decisions about patient management.

Hepatitis C has much less propensity to spontaneously resolve than hepatitis B. Serology is of little or no value for staging HCV infection because current anti-HCV IgM assays perform poorly, and the humoral profiles show very slow, if any, change in the course of persistence, even after virus clearance. Follow-up is carried out by periodically measuring HCV RNA or, less frequently, HCV antigen loads. Over 95% of viremic patients test positive for HCV antigen at levels that generally but not invariably correlate with the viral loads determined by molecular assays (38, 45). HCV viremia values vary extensively for individual patients but, except in the acute phase of infection, tend to remain stable over time. Direct visualization of necroinflammatory liver changes is currently irreplaceable for prognosis and management of chronic hepatitis. Biopsy should preferably be carried out during periods of relatively low hepatitis activity.

Predicting and Evaluating the Outcome of Antiviral Therapy

As discussed above, the options currently available for treatment of viral hepatitis are limited. In particular, although numerous new drugs are under evaluation or development, there are no antiviral drugs approved for hepatitis A and E, and those that can be used to contain and possibly eradicate HBV and HCV are still few. The decisions regarding antiviral therapy of chronic hepatitis B and C are generally made on clinical, histopathological, and immunovirological grounds and should be carefully weighed against side effects and cost. The goals are a sustained virological response (virus undetectable in blood) or at least a sustained biochemical response (normalization of ALT levels for >12 months) and improved histopathology. Once the decision to initiate therapy is made, the dynamic changes of viremia during treatment are an important guide, together with parameters of disease progression such as ALT levels, in deciding whether the therapy should be continued, discontinued, or adjusted.

Treatment of chronic hepatitis B has improved greatly in recent years, thanks to the development of new antiviral drugs which, alone or in combination with IFN-α, effectively inhibit HBV replication and improve disease status and prognosis. The best noninvasive approach for monitoring the response of chronic HBV infection to therapy is measurement of the markers of virus activity, including HBsAg, HBeAg, and HBV DNA, as well as ALT values at intervals. Initially, the response to therapy in terms of viral load is generally very sustained, but relapses are almost the rule due to the selection of drug-resistant virus mutants. How drug-resistant HBV mutants can be identified has been described in a previous section. Since HDV replicates only if HBV is also present, treatments that cure HBV also eradicate HDV. Evidence, however, indicates that concurrent infections by two or more hepatitis viruses are difficult to treat. Also extremely difficult to treat are HBV and HCV infections in HIV-1-positive patients. These dual or triple infections have recently emerged as major causes of morbidity and mortality, with liver damage that progresses more rapidly than in singly infected individuals, and they may significantly decrease tolerance to highly active antiretroviral therapy (28, 36).

With regard to chronic hepatitis C, there is wide consensus that all patients with persistently elevated ALT levels, high viremia levels, and portal and bridging liver fibrosis should be treated because their risk of developing cirrhosis is prominent. It is also generally agreed that patients with consistently normal levels of ALT and patients with advanced cirrhosis should be managed on an individual basis or in the context of clinical trials. A decrease of liver fibrosis in some treated HCV-infected patients has recently been described (32). Features that correlate with poor response of chronic hepatitis C to therapy include the following: viral genotypes 1 and 4; high viremia loads; highly complex viral quasispecies; and, in Asian type 1b isolates, the amino acid composition of a specific segment of the NS5A protein as well as patients' old age, male gender, African-American ethnicity, and presence of advanced liver fibrosis (54). Thus, therapeutic strategies and regimens need to be customized on the basis of numerous variables, among which the viral ones are of utmost importance (10). Current guidelines suggest that genotype 1 or 4 HCV-infected patients should be administered a 48-week course of pegIFN-α and ribavirin, whereas patients infected by genotype 2 or 3 should be treated for 24 weeks only and with lower dosages of ribavirin. Pretreatment viral burdens are also very relevant: baseline viral loads higher than 800,000 IU per ml have been seen to correlate with reduced rates of sustained responses, especially in genotype 1 HCV-infected subjects. The early effects of treatment on viral load are considered useful for predicting

the eventual response to therapy and adjusting the therapeutic protocol accordingly, since a sustained virological response is most likely in patients whose plasma HCV RNA drops to undetectable levels or shows a 2-$\log_{10}$ decrease by 12 weeks of treatment (early responders). Contrariwise, HCV RNA titers above 450,000 and 30,000 IU per ml at 4 and 12 weeks of therapy, respectively, have been reported to correlate with failure to undergo a sustained virological response (4). In this context, measuring the level of HCV antigen in blood has also shown utility: a negative antigenemia by 1 month of therapy was reported to be highly predictive of favorable response (21). With the therapies in use at present, many HCV-infected patients who initially appear to respond well relapse, as documented by the return to abnormal ALT levels and high virus levels in serum. The causes of hepatitis C relapses are poorly understood.

Guidelines for treatment of acute hepatitis C are still poorly defined. It has been suggested that therapy should begin as early as possible for asymptomatic patients but start only 2 to 4 months after acute onset for those with symptoms, since they are more likely to clear the infection spontaneously (42).

Evaluation of Immune Status

Evaluation of immune status is generally needed to decide whether persons scheduled for vaccination are already immune as a result of past infection and to evaluate the immunizing effect of vaccination. For HAV, total anti-HAV is the test of choice. For hepatitis B, anti-HBs is usually sufficient, and total anti-HBc may be used to discriminate previous infection from vaccination. A low level of anti-HBs alone in the absence of a history of vaccination might be a false-positive result.

Epidemiological Surveys

Because evaluation of the prevalence rates of viruses in selected populations or groups requires the examination of large numbers of samples, a compromise between the sensitivity/specificity and the cost of a test(s) is usually sought. Total anti-HAV persists long after infection or vaccination; thus, serosurveys are of limited value in the determination of the extent of actual HAV circulation in a population at the time of testing. Examination of sewage samples for the presence of HAV by molecular methods is more informative and relatively simple. This method is proving useful also for monitoring HEV infection in areas of endemicity, while serosurveys are of value for surveillance of HEV penetration in areas of low or no endemicity. Anti-HCV positivity rates provide a valid estimate of actual HCV prevalence because approximately 80% of seropositive individuals are also virus carriers. Similarly, tests for HBsAg provide an accurate estimate of HBV carrier prevalence. Sensitive molecular assays have shown that a number of patients continue to harbor minute copy numbers of HBV DNA long after HBsAg is no longer detectable, but the significance of these subjects in epidemiology is unknown. Because antibody detection tests for GBV-C and anelloviruses are under validation or not yet available, respectively, epidemiological investigations for these viruses have used molecular assays. In general, these are more expensive than immunoassays but can be designed in such a way as to provide information also about prevailing virus genotypes.

Screening of Blood, Tissue, and Organ Donors

In most countries, donor screening for hepatitis viruses is still limited to testing of sera for HBsAg and anti-HCV.

A small number of cases of HCV infection still occur in recipients, due to the fact that anti-HCV tests do not reveal donors in the window period. Since these cases can be further reduced by tests that detect HCV RNA, the blood banks of several countries have introduced them in their routine. The so-called surrogate markers for non-A, non-B hepatitis, such as ALT and anti-HBc, have lost impact after the development of HCV tests, but they still help to exclude risky donors. Testing of donors for other blood-borne viruses, including GBV-C and TTV and other anelloviruses, is instead generally viewed as an additional burden, totally unproductive in terms of blood and organ supply safety.

This work was supported in part by the Ministero della Università e Ricerca Scientifica, Rome, and the University of Pisa and the Azienda Ospedaliero-Universitaria Pisana, Pisa, Italy.

REFERENCES

1. **Aggarwal, R., D. Kini, S. Sofat, S. R. Naik, and K. Krawczynski.** 2000. Duration of viremia and fecal excretion in acute hepatitis. *Lancet* **356:**1081–1082.
2. **Allain, J. P.** 2004. Occult hepatitis B infection. *Transfus. Clin. Biol.* **11:**18–25.
3. **Bendinelli, M., M. Pistello, F. Maggi, C. Fornai, G. Freer, and M. L. Vatteroni.** 2001. Molecular properties, biology, and clinical implications of TT virus, a recently identified widespread infectious agent of humans. *Clin. Microbiol. Rev.* **14:**98–113.
4. **Berg, T., C. Sarrazin, E. Herrmann, H. Hinrichsen, T. Gerlach, R. Zachoval, B. Wiedenmann, U. Hopf, and S. Zeuzem.** 2003. Prediction of treatment outcome in patients with chronic hepatitis C: significance of baseline parameters and viral dynamic during therapy. *Hepatology* **37:**600–609.
5. **Bower, W. A., O. V. Nainan, X. Han, and H. S. Margolis.** 2000. Duration of viremia in hepatitis A virus infection. *J. Infect. Dis.* **182:**12–17.
6. **Castillo, I., M. Pardo, J. Bartolomé, N. Ortiz-Movilla, E. Rodriguez-Inigo, S. de Lucas, C. Salas, J. A. Jimenez-Heffernan, A. Pérez-Mota, J. Graus, J. M. Lopez-Alcorocho, and V. Carreno.** 2004. Occult hepatitis C virus infection in patients in whom the etiology of persistently abnormal results of liver-function tests is unknown. *J. Infect. Dis.* **189:**7–14.
7. **Chu, C. J., M. Hussain, and A. S. F. Lok.** 2002. Quantitative serum HBV DNA levels during different stages of chronic hepatitis B infection. *Hepatology* **36:**1408–1415.
8. **Costa-Mattioli, M., A. Di Napoli, V. Ferrè, S. Billaudel, R. Perez-Bercoff, and J. Cristina.** 2003. Genetic variability of hepatitis A. *J. Gen. Virol.* **84:**3191–3201.
9. **de Paula, V. S., L. M. Villar, L. M. Morais, L. L. Lewis-Ximenez, C. Niel, and A. M. Gaspar.** 2004. Detection of hepatitis A virus RNA in serum during the window period of infection. *J. Clin. Virol.* **29:**254–259.
10. **Fried, M. W.** 2004. Viral factors affecting the outcome of therapy for chronic hepatitis C. *Rev. Gastroenterol. Disord.* **4:**S8–S13.
11. **Ganem, D., and A. M. Prince.** 2004. Hepatitis B infection—natural history and clinical consequences. *N. Engl. J. Med.* **350:**1118–1129.
12. **Hoofnagle, J. H.** 2002. Course and outcome of hepatitis C. *Hepatology* **36:**S21–S29.
13. **Huang, Y. H., J. C. Wu, W. Y. Sheng, T. I. Huo, F. Y. Chang, and S. D. Lee.** 1998. Diagnostic value of anti-hepatitis D virus (HDV) antibodies revisited: a study of total and IgM anti-HDV compared with detection of HDV-RNA by polymerase chain reaction. *J. Gastroenterol. Hepatol.* **13:**57–61.
14. **Jenson, H. B.** 2004. The changing picture of hepatitis A in the United States. *Curr. Opin. Pediatr.* **16:**89–93.
15. **Lai, C. L., V. Ratziu, M.-F. Yuen, and T. Poynard.** 2003. Viral hepatitis B. *Lancet* **362:**2089–2094.
16. **Lanford, R. E., B. Guerra, D. Chavez, C. Bigger, K. M. Brasky, X. H. Wang, S. C. Ray, and D. Thomas.** 2004. Cross-genotype immunity to hepatitis C virus. *J. Virol.* **78:**1575–1581.
17. **Lewis, J. A.** 1999. Hepatitis A vaccines, p. 317–375. *In* S. Specter (ed.), *Viral Hepatitis: Diagnosis, Therapy, and Prevention.* Humana Press Inc., Totowa, N.J.
18. **Linnen, J., J. Wages, Jr., Z. Y. Zhang-Keck, K. E. Fry, K. Z. Krawczynski, H. Alter, E. Koonin, M. Gallagher, M. Alter, S. Hadziyannis, P. Karayiannis, K. Fung, Y. Nakatsuji, J. W. K. Shih, L. Young, M. Piatak, Jr., C. Hoover, J. Fernandez, S. Chen, J. C. Zou, T. Morris, K. C. Hyams, S. Ismay, J. D. Lifson, G. Hess, S. H. K. Foung, H. Thomas, D. Bradley, H. Margolis, and J. P. Kim.** 1996. Molecular cloning and disease association of hepatitis G virus: a transfusion-transmissible agent. *Science* **271:**505–508.
19. **Maggi, F., M. Pifferi, E. Tempestini, C. Fornai, L. Lanini, E. Andreoli, M. L. Vatteroni, S. Presciuttini, A. Pietrobelli, A. Boner, M. Pistello, and M. Bendinelli.** 2003. TT virus loads and lymphocyte subpopulations in children with acute respiratory diseases. *J. Virol.* **77:**9081–9083.
20. **Martinot-Peignoux, M., N. Boyer, M. Colombat, R. Akremi, B. N. Pham, S. Ollivier, C. Castelnau, D. Valla, C. Degott, and P. Marcellin.** 2002. Serum hepatitis B virus DNA levels and liver histology in inactive HBsAg carriers. *J. Hepatol.* **36:**543–546.
21. **Maynard, M., P. Pradat, P. Berthillon, G. Picchio, N. Voirin, M. Martinot, P. Marcelin, and C. Trepo.** 2003. Clinical relevance of total core antigen testing for hepatitis C monitoring and for predicting patients' response to therapy. *J. Viral Hepat.* **10:**318–323.
22. **Mommeja-Martin, H., E. Mondou, M. R. Blum, and F. Rousseau.** 2003. Serum HBV DNA as a marker of efficacy during therapy for chronic HBV infection: analysis and review of the literature. *Hepatology* **37:**1309–1319.
23. **Morishima, C., M. Chung, K. W. Ng, D. J. Brambilla, and D. R. Gretch.** 2004. Strengths and limitations of commercial test for hepatitis C virus RNA quantification. *J. Clin. Microbiol.* **42:**421–425.
24. **Nakamoto, Y., and S. Kaneko.** 2003. Mechanisms of viral hepatitis induced liver injury. *Curr. Mol. Med.* **3:**537–544.
25. **National Institutes of Health.** 2002. NIH consensus statement on management of hepatitis C. *NIH Consens. State Sci. Statements* Jun 10–12 **19:**1–46. [Online.] http://www.consensus.nih.gov/.
26. **Neumann, U. P., T. Berg, M. Bahra, G. Puhl, O. Guckelberger, J. M. Langrehr, and P. Neuhaus.** 2004. Long-term outcome of liver transplants for chronic hepatitis C: a 10-year follow-up. *Transplantation* **77:**226–231.
27. **Nishizawa, T., H. Okamoto, K. Konishi, H. Yoshizawa, Y. Miyakawa, and M. Mayumi.** 1997. A novel DNA virus (TTV) associated with elevated transaminase levels in posttransfusion hepatitis of unknown etiology. *Biochem. Biophys. Res. Commun.* **241:**92–97.
28. **Nunez, M., M. Puoti, N. Camino, and V. Soriano.** 2003. Treatment of chronic hepatitis B in the human immunodeficiency virus-infected patient: present and future. *Clin. Infect. Dis.* **37:**1678–1685.
29. **Pawlotsky, J.-M.** 2004. Pathophysiology of hepatitis C infection and related liver disease. *Trends Microbiol.* **12:**96–102.
30. **Pham, N. Q., S. A. MacParland, P. M. Mulrooney, H. Cooksley, N. V. Naumov, and T. I. Michalak.** 2004. Hepatitis C virus persistence after spontaneous or treatment-induced resolution of hepatitis C. *J. Virol.* **78:**5867–5874.

31. **Pistello, M., F. Maggi, C. Fornai, A. Leonildi, A. Morrica, M. L. Vatteroni, and M. Bendinelli.** 1999. Classification of hepatitis C virus type 2 isolates by phylogenetic analysis of core and NS5 region. *J. Clin. Microbiol.* **37:**2116–2117.

32. **Pol, S., F. Carnet, B. Nalpas, J.-L. Lagneau, H. Fontaine, J. Serpaggi, L. Serfaty, P. Bedossa, and C. Brechot.** 2004. Reversibility of hepatitis C virus-related cirrhosis. *Hum. Pathol.* **35:**107–112.

33. **Polish, L. B., B. H. Robertson, B. Khanna, K. Krawczynski, J. Spelbring, F. Olson, and C. N. Shapiro.** 1999. Excretion of hepatitis A virus (HAV) in adults: comparison of immunologic and molecular detection methods and relationship between HAV positivity and infectivity in tamarins. *J. Clin. Microbiol.* **37:**3615–3617.

34. **Purcell, R. H., H. Nguyen, M. Shapiro, R. E. Engle, S. Govindarajan, W. C. Blackwelder, D. C. Wong, J. P. Prieels, and S. U. Emerson.** 2003. Pre-clinical immunogenicity and efficacy trial of a recombinant hepatitis E vaccine. *Vaccine* **2:**2607–2615.

35. **Ribeiro, R. M., A. Lo, and A. S. Perelson.** 2002. Dynamics of hepatitis B virus infection. *Microbes Infect.* **4:**829–835.

36. **Rockstroh, J. K., and U. Spengler.** 2004. HIV and hepatitis C virus co-infection. *Lancet Infect. Dis.* **4:**437–444.

37. **Sagir, A., O. Kirschberg, T. Heintges, A. Erhardt, and D. Haussinger.** 2004. SEN virus infection. *Rev. Med. Virol.* **14:**141–148.

38. **Schuttler, C. G., C. Thomas, T. Discher, G. Friese, J. Lohmeyer, R. Schuster, S. Schaefer, and W. H. Gerlich.** 2004. Variable ratio of hepatitis C virus RNA to viral core antigen in patient sera. *J. Clin. Microbiol.* **45:**1977–1981.

39. **Simons, J. N., T. P. Leary, G. J. Dawson, T. J. Pilot-Matias, A. S. Muerhoff, G. G. Schlauder, S. M. Desai, and I. K. Mushahwar.** 1995. Isolation of novel virus-like sequences associated with human hepatitis. *Nat. Med.* **1:**564–569.

40. **Smedile, A., and G. Verme.** 1999. Hepatitis D virus. Biology, pathogenesis, epidemiology, clinical description, and therapy, p. 129–150. *In* S. Specter (ed.), *Viral Hepatitis: Diagnosis, Therapy, and Prevention.* Humana Press Inc., Totowa, N.J.

41. **Stapleton, J. T.** 2003. GB virus type C/hepatitis G virus. *Semin. Liver Dis.* **23:**137–148.

42. **Strader, D. B., T. Wright, D. L. Thomas, and L. B. Seeff.** 2004. Diagnosis, management, and treatment of hepatitis C. *Hepatology* **39:**1147–1171.

43. **Taylor, J. M.** 2003. Replication of human hepatitis delta virus: recent developments. *Trends Microbiol.* **11:**185–190.

44. **Torbenson, M., and D. L. Thomas.** 2002. Occult hepatitis B. *Lancet Infect. Dis.* **2:**479–486.

45. **Veillon, P., C. Payan, G. Picchio, M. Maniez–Montreuil, P. Guntz, and F. Lunel.** 2003. Comparative evaluation of the total hepatitis C virus core antigen, branched-DNA, and Amplicor Monitor assays in determining viremia for patients with chronic hepatitis C during interferon plus ribavirin combination therapy. *J. Clin. Microbiol.* **41:**3212–3220.

46. **Wang, D., J. Pearlberg, Y. T. Liu, and D. Ganem.** 2001. Deleterious effects of hepatitis delta virus replication on host cell proliferation. *J. Virol.* **75:**3600–3604.

47. **Wang, Y. C., H. Y. Zhang, N. S. Xia, G. Peng, H. Y. Lan, H. Zhuang, Y. H. Zhu, S. W. Li, K. G. Tian, W. J. Gu, J. X. Lin, X. Wu, H. M. Li, and T. J. Harrison.** 2002. Prevalence, isolation, and partial sequence analysis of hepatitis E virus from domestic animals in China. *J. Med. Virol.* **67:**516–521.

48. **Williams, C. F., D. Klinzman, T. E. Yamashita, J. Xiang, P. M. Polgreen, C. Rinaldo, C. Liu, J. Phair, J. B. Margolick, D. Zdunek, G. Hess, and J. T. Stapleton.** 2004. Persistent GB virus C infection and survival in HIV-infected men. *N. Engl. J. Med.* **350:**981–990.

49. **Worm, H. C., W. H. M. van der Poel, and G. Brandstaetter.** 2002. Hepatitis E: an overview. *Microbes Infect.* **4:**657–666.

50. **Wu, J. C., I. A. Huang, Y. H. Huang, J. Y. Chen, and I. J. Sheen.** 1999. Mixed genotypes infection with hepatitis D virus. *J. Med. Virol.* **57:**64–67.

51. **Yamashiro, T., K. Nagayama, N. Enomoto, H. Watanabe, T. Miyagi, H. Nakasone, H. Sakugawa, and M. Watanabe.** 2004. Quantitation of the level of hepatitis delta virus RNA in serum, by real-time polymerase chain reaction and its possible correlation with the clinical stage of liver disease. *J. Infect. Dis.* **189:**1151–1157.

52. **Yu, C., R. E. Eagle, J. P. Bryan, S. U. Emerson, and R. H. Purcell.** 2003. Detection of immunoglobulin M antibodies to hepatitis E virus by class capture enzyme immunoassay. *Clin. Diagn. Lab. Immunol.* **10:**579–586.

53. **Yuen, M. F., E. Sablon, H. J. Yuan, D. K. L. Wong, C. K. Hui, B. C. Y. Wong, A. O. O. Chan, and C. L. Lai.** 2003. Significance of hepatitis B genotype in acute exacerbation, HBeAg seroconversion, cirrhosis-related complications and hepatocellular carcinoma. *Hepatology* **37:**562–567.

54. **Zeuzem, S.** 2004. Heterogeneous virologic response rates to interferon-based therapy in patients with chronic hepatitis C: who responds less well? *Ann. Intern. Med.* **140:**346–355.

Rotaviruses and Noroviruses

NINGGUO FENG AND SUZANNE M. MATSUI

84

ROTAVIRUS

Group A rotavirus, a member of the family *Reoviridae*, is a major cause of infectious gastroenteritis in infants and young children throughout the world. This pathogen alone accounts for 20 to 70% of hospitalizations due to diarrhea and 400,000 to 500,000 deaths per year in developing countries (34). The impact of rotavirus diarrhea is also substantial in industrialized countries, where nearly all children experience a rotavirus infection by the time they are 5 years old. In the United States each year, rotavirus diarrhea results in 500,000 physician visits and 50,000 hospitalizations (33, 39). Given the magnitude of the global public health problem associated with rotavirus infection and the observation that natural infection ameliorates the rate and severity of reinfection, strategies to develop effective vaccines have been pursued intensively.

Rotavirus was first identified by electron microscopy (EM) of duodenal biopsy specimens from children with diarrhea (2). Viral particles were found to be 70 nm in diameter, with a distinctive appearance. Ultrastructural analysis by electron cryomicroscopy disclosed that the viral capsid is formed by three concentric protein layers with external spikes. Within the innermost layer is the viral genome, composed of 11 segments of double-stranded RNA. The antigenic capsid proteins important for rotavirus detection are VP6 (encoded by gene segment 6), the middle-layer protein that specifies the subgroup; VP7 (encoded by gene segment 7, 8, or 9, depending on the strain), the glycoprotein that forms the lunar-like surface of the outer capsid shell and determines G serotype; and VP4 (encoded by gene segment 4), the protease-sensitive spike protein of the outer capsid that determines the P serotype (reviewed in reference 8).

The ability to detect rotavirus infection is essential in epidemiologic surveys, vaccine studies, and investigations of outbreaks of gastroenteritis. A variety of methods are available to facilitate the diagnosis of rotavirus infection, from imaging the virus directly to detecting viral antigens immunologically to detecting viral nucleic acid. EM is a highly sensitive and specific method that allows direct visualization of the virus and has the potential to identify other enteric viruses within a sample as well, but it requires expert operators and specialized equipment that are not readily available in all settings and cannot process large numbers of samples rapidly. Diagnostic methods based on immunologic

detection of rotavirus antigens have been developed to circumvent some of these problems (46). Enzyme immunoassay (EIA), in particular, has been used extensively to establish the incidence and prevalence of rotavirus infection and to define antigenic characteristics of the virus. The simplicity and high sensitivity and specificity of the assay, along with its ability to handle large numbers of samples efficiently, are distinct advantages of EIA.

EIA

Two EIA formats have been developed to detect rotavirus antigen. In the direct assay (Fig. 1), the anti-rotavirus antibody is labeled with enzyme. The capture antibody (Ab_1 in Fig. 1) and rotavirus antibody conjugated with an enzyme (Ab–Enzyme) may be derived from the same host. Once the Ab–Enzyme is produced and its characteristics are defined, the assay can be performed rapidly and without difficulty. In the indirect assay (Fig. 2), an unlabeled antiviral antibody is bound to a solid phase and enzyme-labeled antiglobulin is used to quantify the amount of antigen bound (Fig. 2). The capture antibody (Ab_1 in Fig. 2) and the detector antibody (Ab_2) must be derived from two different animal species. This format is well suited to a laboratory that performs a number of different EIAs, since a single, commercially available enzyme-labeled immunoglobulin can be used for any EIA. In addition, the relatively higher degree of sensitivity attainable with the indirect EIA is advantageous in evaluating samples from large epidemiological surveys.

Modification of the EIA by incorporating a high-affinity marker-antimarker combination yields rapid and reproducible results (46). One strategy is to label the liquid-phase antibody with biotin and then allow it to react with avidin. In EIA systems, the assay can be completed by reaction with avidin that has been covalently coupled to an enzyme or complexed with biotin-substituted enzyme. The latter format yields signal-to-noise ratios that are superior to those encountered when enzyme-linked avidin derivatives are used. If avidin directly labeled with enzyme is used, avidin derived from avidin-producing strains of streptomycetes or egg white avidin which has been modified to minimize the extent of nonspecific reactions is preferable to unmodified egg white avidin.

A distinct advantage of the biotin EIA method is that virtually all of the immunological and enzymatic activities

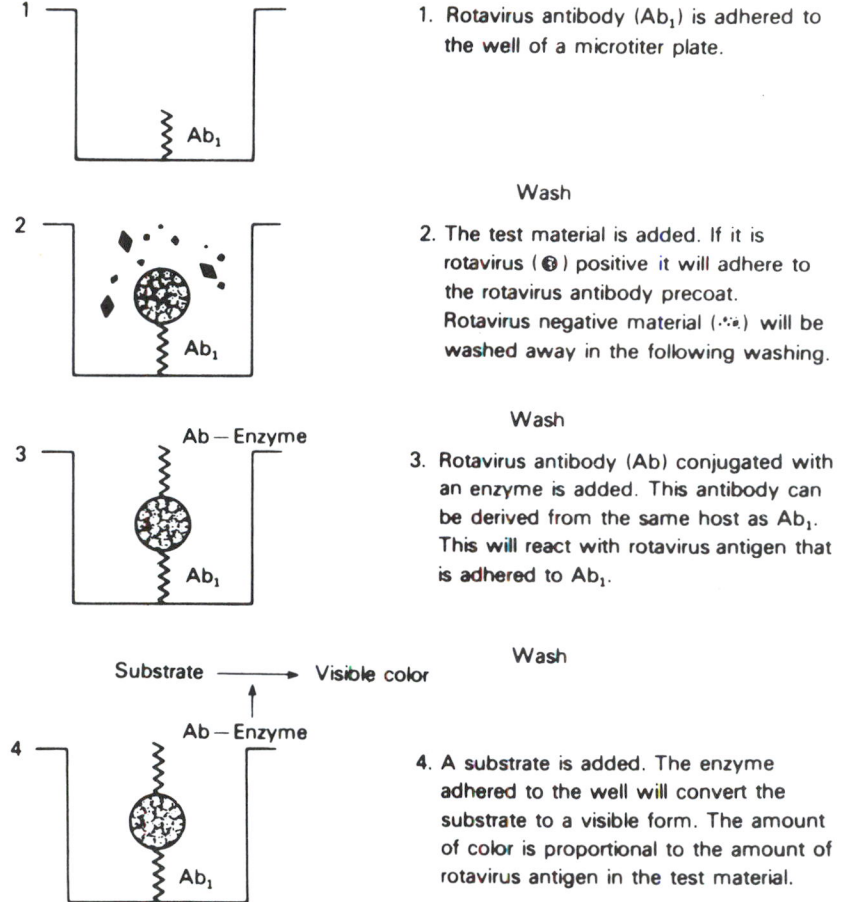

1. Rotavirus antibody (Ab₁) is adhered to the well of a microtiter plate.

Wash

2. The test material is added. If it is rotavirus (❸) positive it will adhere to the rotavirus antibody precoat. Rotavirus negative material (⠒⠒) will be washed away in the following washing.

Wash

3. Rotavirus antibody (Ab) conjugated with an enzyme is added. This antibody can be derived from the same host as Ab₁. This will react with rotavirus antigen that is adhered to Ab₁.

Wash

4. A substrate is added. The enzyme adhered to the well will convert the substrate to a visible form. The amount of color is proportional to the amount of rotavirus antigen in the test material.

FIGURE 1 Direct EIA for antigen measurement. Reproduced from reference 24 with permission.

of the reagents are maintained throughout the immunoassay procedure, since the enzyme is not directly linked to immunoglobulin. In addition, the fact that a single molecule of avidin can react with up to four molecules of biotin offers the potential for increased sensitivity due to magnification at the level of avidin-biotin interactions. On the other hand, since avidin-biotin systems do not utilize anti-immunoglobulins, they are less subject to nonspecific interactions with other anti-immunoglobulin materials often present in clinical specimens. EIA systems that use biotin are often more specific than equivalent systems that involve unlabeled antibodies and enzyme-labeled immunoglobulins.

The EIA can also be designed to detect rotavirus antibody in one of two ways. In the binding assay, rotavirus antigen is bound to the solid phase either directly or through an antibody. Dilutions of test specimen are added, and the amount of bound immunoglubulins is determined by the addition of the appropriate enzyme-labeled anti-immunoglobulin and, after incubation, the appropriate substrate. By using class-specific anti-immunoglobulins, immunoglobulin G (IgG), IgM, and IgA can be specifically quantified. In practice, the ability to measure anti-rotavirus IgM levels in serum can be greatly improved by first removing serum IgG with staphylococcal protein A or streptococcal protein G or by ion-exchange chromatography (47). Alternatively, IgM (an indicator of recent infection) can be measured by a reverse-capture system, in which IgM is bound to a solid phase by means of anti-human IgM and then IgM directed at

rotavirus is quantified by the addition of rotavirus antigen and labeled anti-rotavirus antibody. The measurement of anti-rotavirus IgA is important in the measurement of anti-rotavirus antibody in human body secretions such as intestinal fluids and milk (49). One problem with the binding method is that a different antiglobulin is required for each species of animal in which antibody is to be measured. When antibody from a number of animal species is to be tested, a blocking assay can be used. Such assays simply involve the mixing of the test specimen with a known amount of rotaviral antigen and, after a suitable incubation period, the measurement of antigen not neutralized by the serum. Such blocking tests are simple to perform and use the same reagents as do the antigen detection tests. However, they do not provide information about the immunoglobulin subclass of the rotavirus antibody.

General Considerations

Solid Phase

All of the EIAs described above require the initial binding of a reactant to a solid phase. The most widely used and versatile is the microtiter plate, from which results can be obtained rapidly with a microplate spectrophotometer. In preparation for screening a large number of samples, a large number of plates can be coated at once. If the coated plates are carefully sealed with plastic film and stored at 4°C in a moist chamber, they display minimal loss of activity for up to 4 months of storage.

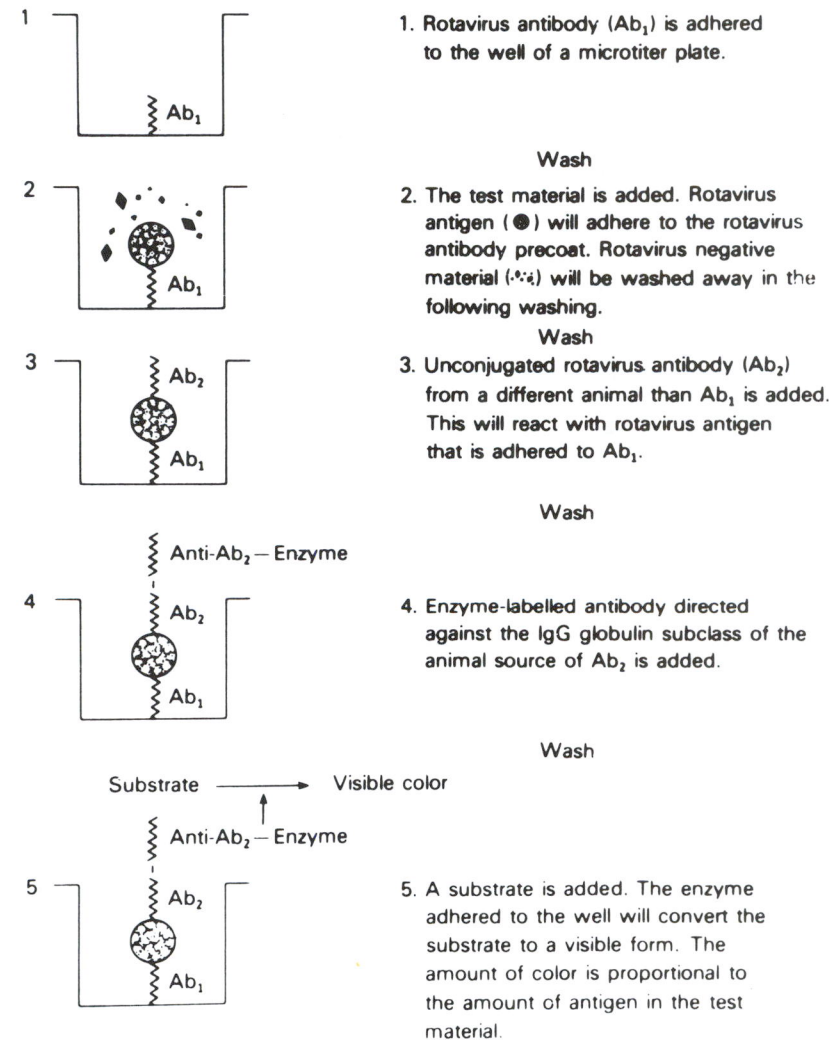

1. Rotavirus antibody (Ab₁) is adhered to the well of a microtiter plate.

Wash

2. The test material is added. Rotavirus antigen (●) will adhere to the rotavirus antibody precoat. Rotavirus negative material (⋅⋅) will be washed away in the following washing.

Wash

3. Unconjugated rotavirus antibody (Ab₂) from a different animal than Ab₁ is added. This will react with rotavirus antigen that is adhered to Ab₁.

Wash

4. Enzyme-labelled antibody directed against the IgG globulin subclass of the animal source of Ab₂ is added.

Wash

5. A substrate is added. The enzyme adhered to the well will convert the substrate to a visible form. The amount of color is proportional to the amount of antigen in the test material.

FIGURE 2   Indirect EIA for rotavirus antigen measurement. Reproduced from reference 24 with permission.

Washing

Washing facilitates the separation of reactants bound to the solid phase from unreacted reagents that could yield false-positive results. This is best accomplished by adding a nonionic detergent such as Tween 20 to the wash fluid and washing with at least 200 μl of wash fluid in each well. To avoid incomplete removal of reactants and sporadic mixing of reagents between wells, aspiration of wash fluid with a suction device (e.g., a suction manifold or a Pasteur pipette attached to a vacuum) is recommended over simple inversion of the microtiter plate.

Enzymes

Although a number of enzymes can form active conjugates with immunoglobulin, most EIAs use either peroxidase or alkaline phosphatase. Conjugates prepared with either enzyme can be used for rotavirus EIAs, and the choice of enzyme depends on the particular needs of the investigator. Peroxidase has the advantage of being relatively inexpensive and having substrates which form a dark color and thus are easy to read visually. Peroxidase conjugates are stable at 4°C,

but their action is largely destroyed by bacteriostatic agents such as sodium azide. Sodium azide is commonly added to fecal specimens to deter bacterial overgrowth, but it should not be used in the steps immediately preceding and during the use of the peroxidase. Alkaline phosphatase, on the other hand, is not sensitive to bacteriostatic agents and thus is more stable under field conditions. In addition, the reaction between alkaline phosphatase and the substrate can be completely stopped by raising the pH above 12, and alkaline phosphatase has a large number of substrates (see below). Both alkaline phosphatase- and peroxidase-conjugated anti-immunoglubulin antibodies are available from a number of commercial sources; alkaline phosphatase is somewhat more expensive than peroxidase. An overview of enzyme-antibody conjugates is found elsewhere in this manual (chapter 2).

Substrates

The simplest substrates for use in EIAs are those which yield a visible product on interaction with the bound enzyme. The amount of color can be estimated visually or quantified with a spectrophotometer. There are a number of such substrates available, including p-nitrophenyl phosphate for alkaline phosphatase and o-phenylenediamine, 5-aminosalicylic acid, and diaminobenzidine (in conjunction with peroxide) for peroxidase.

Reagents

The sensitivity of EIAs makes it necessary to use highly specific reagents to minimize undesired cross-reactivity. Specific reagents are best prepared from rotavirus strains that have been adapted to tissue culture systems. While numerous strains can be used, the simian strain SA11 is well suited for use in immunoassay systems since it can be grown to high titer in a number of different tissue culture cell lines. Antigen obtained from tissue culture cells should be purified by multiple sedimentation on sucrose and cesium chloride gradients, using standard ultracentrifugation techniques, before being used to immunize animals; this avoids the problem of nonspecific interactions due to the generation of antibodies to nonviral tissue culture components. Antigens cloned and expressed in recombinant forms or synthetic peptides may also serve as antigens for solid-phase immunoassays (25). However, care should be taken to exclude the possibility of reaction to vector-derived proteins or to cross-reacting peptides; the use of molecular sources of antigen does not remove the need for performance of careful control reactions to ensure assay specificity.

Purified antigen can be used to immunize a variety of laboratory animals, most commonly mice, guinea pigs, rabbits, goats, and sheep. Antiserum is collected from the animals by bleeding at multiple intervals after immunization and is monitored by the immunoassays described above. Rotavirus reagents are also available from commercial and nonprofit sources. Reagents obtained from these sources should be carefully evaluated for sensitivity and specificity prior to use. Rotavirus antigen can also be used to prepare monoclonal antibodies by means of mouse immunization and standard hybridoma techniques. The availability of enzyme-labeled anti-immunoglobulins which have been affinity purified to remove nonspecific reactivity has greatly improved the specificity and reduced the background activity of indirect immunoassays. The use of highly specific anti-immunoglobulins is recommended in all assay formats.

It should be noted that although there are antigenic differences among human and animal rotaviruses, all group A rotaviruses share sufficient common antigenic determinants to allow detection by reagents to one strain. On the other hand, if highly specific or monoclonal reagents are used, quantitative determinations can be performed to determine the subgroup and serotype of rotavirus isolates by the comparison of homotypic and heterotypic reactions (26). Different reagents may be required to detect rotaviruses that do not share the rotavirus common antigen. Since reagents vary in potency according to their source and method of preparation, optimal dilutions for use in the EIA should be determined by titration.

Nonspecific Reactions

Positive reactions that are not due to the presence of rotavirus antigen or antibody can occur by a variety of mechanisms. Nonspecific interactions among the antisera can cause high background in the absence of any added specimen. This problem can be overcome by the use of purified reagents as described above and, in the indirect assay, by the use of enzyme-labeled conjugates prepared from antiglobulins of high specificity. In addition, some stool specimens

contain material that can react nonspecifically with an animal immunoglobulin. These specimens can be identified by the fact that they react with wells coated with normal serum as well as with those coated with specific anti-rotavirus serum; the exact nature of this cross-reacting material is not known. Nonspecific activity is detected by processing each specimen in wells coated with serum that does not contain antibody to rotavirus as well as in wells coated with anti-rotavirus antiserum. Specific rotavirus activity is defined as the difference between the activity in the specimen processed in wells coated with the anti-rotavirus serum and that in the same specimen processed in wells coated with the nonimmune serum (Fig. 3).

Buffers

The buffers used in the rotavirus assays are similar to those used in other solid-phase immunoassay systems. Animal proteins are often added to such buffers to reduce nonspecific activity. Care should be taken that the "normal" animal proteins used in rotavirus assays are free of rotavirus antibodies. Particular care should be observed in the use of proteins derived from bovine sources, since most cows contain endogenous antibodies to rotavirus proteins. Thus, blocking agents, such as neonatal calf serum, bovine serum albumin, and cows' milk, should be screened for antibodies to rotavirus proteins before they are used in rotavirus assays. The blocking assay described below is particularly suited for these measurements since it can be used to measure antibody levels in any animal species.

Commercial Assay Kits

EIA and latex agglutination kits are available commercially for the detection of group A rotavirus antigen in fecal samples. Most EIA kits are designed with polyclonal and/or monoclonal antibodies that are specific for group A rotavirus proteins, primarily VP6. At least 90 min is required to complete the test, and the results are read in a spectrophotometer. Sensitivity and specificity are generally high, averaging well over 90 and 95%, respectively. In the latex agglutination test, latex beads coated with rotavirus-specific antibody interact with rotavirus antigens in the samples. Although results can be obtained more quickly (20 min), the test is substantially less sensitive and slightly less specific than EIA in a head-to-head comparison (44).

Immunochromatography is a newer technique that is both rapid (10 min) and simple. The fecal sample, introduced at the bottom port of the device, mixes with gold particles that have an anti-rotavirus monoclonal antibody coating and is allowed to migrate along a nitrocellulose membrane for 10 min at room temperature. In the capture area, the migrating sample interacts with control (goat anti-mouse antibody) and test (anti-rotavirus polyclonal capture antibody) lines. A positive result is indicated by a red-purple line in the test area, indicating complex formation between the immunogold-labeled sample and the capture antibody. Immunochromatographic tests have performed with sensitivity, specificity, and positive and negative predictive values comparable to those of commercial EIAs (6, 44). Choosing a kit or format will depend largely on the specific needs of the laboratory, the setting in which the test is to be performed (e.g., field versus research laboratory), budgetary issues, and the availability of technical expertise and equipment.

Nucleic Acid Amplification

Rotavirus nucleic acid can also be detected in clinical samples by reverse transcription-PCR (RT-PCR) and nucleic

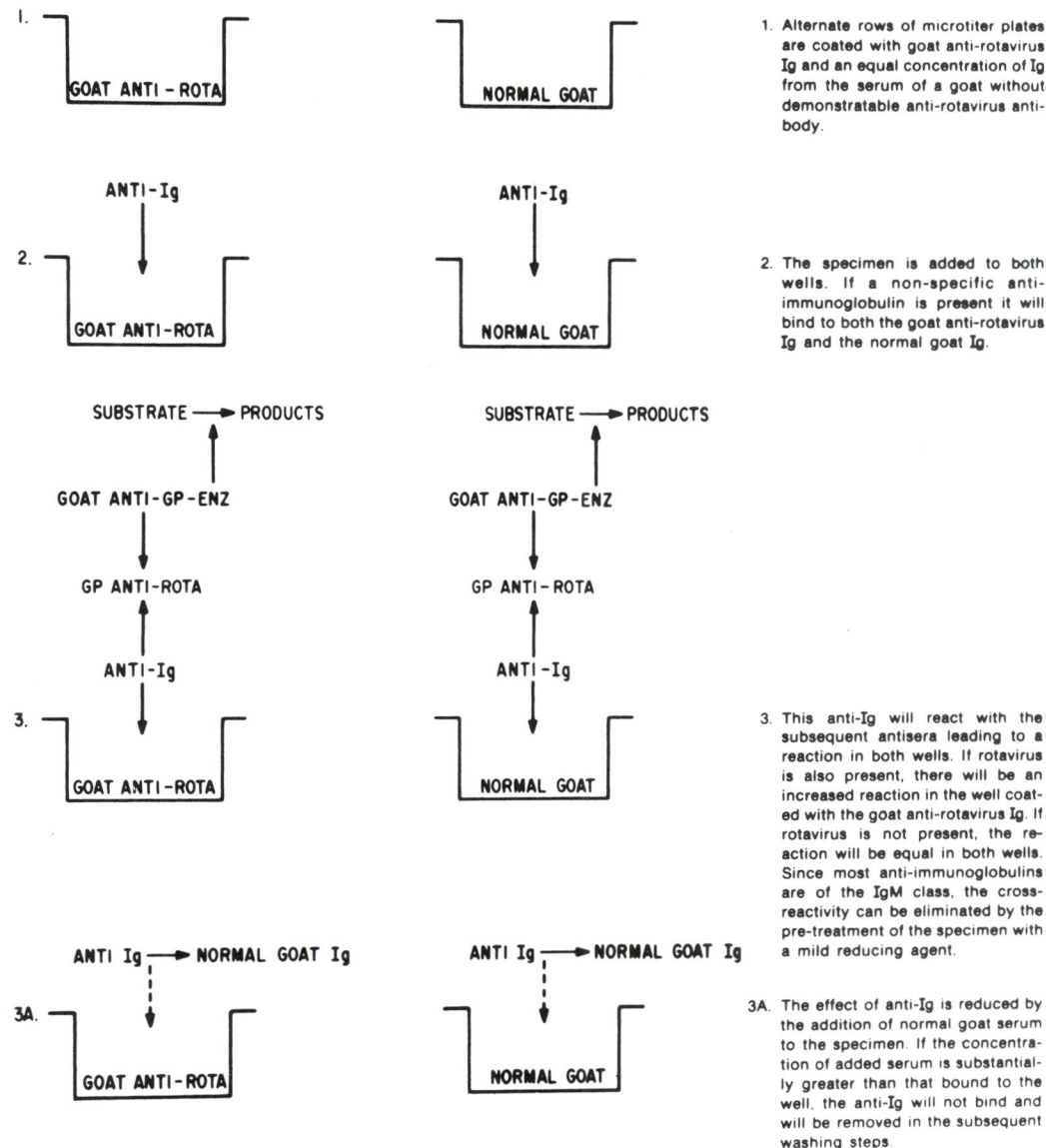

1. Alternate rows of microtiter plates are coated with goat anti-rotavirus Ig and an equal concentration of Ig from the serum of a goat without demonstratable anti-rotavirus antibody.

2. The specimen is added to both wells. If a non-specific anti-immunoglobulin is present it will bind to both the goat anti-rotavirus Ig and the normal goat Ig.

3. This anti-Ig will react with the subsequent antisera leading to a reaction in both wells. If rotavirus is also present, there will be an increased reaction in the well coated with the goat anti-rotavirus Ig. If rotavirus is not present, the reaction will be equal in both wells. Since most anti-immunoglobulins are of the IgM class, the cross-reactivity can be eliminated by the pre-treatment of the specimen with a mild reducing agent.

3A. The effect of anti-Ig is reduced by the addition of normal goat serum to the specimen. If the concentration of added serum is substantially greater than that bound to the well, the anti-Ig will not bind and will be removed in the subsequent washing steps.

FIGURE 3 Cross-reactivity due to anti-immunoglobulin.

acid hybridization techniques. PCR has the greatest potential in terms of assay sensitivity and specificity; RT-PCR is estimated to be 100 to 1,000 times more sensitive than immunoassays. This technique is especially useful in identifying rotavirus nucleic acid in body fluids and environmental samples in which small quantities of virus may be present (4) and for discerning genotypes of the G and P serotypes. The principles of PCR are discussed in detail elsewhere in this manual (chapter 5).

Numerous oligonucleotide primer pairs and reaction conditions have been devised for the detection of rotavirus group-specific and species-specific genomic regions. Oligonucleotide primers derived from conserved regions of the gene encoding the group-reactive antigen VP6 can detect all available strains of group A rotavirus (48). Comparative evaluations have indicated that PCR assays involving these primers can detect rotaviruses in tissue culture and fecal samples at levels below those detectable by immunoassay methods (41). The application of this assay in clinical studies can, under certain circumstances, result in the detection of rotavirus RNA before antigens are shed in the stool in sufficient quantity to allow for immunoassay detection (43). In addition, PCR has been applied to the detection of rotavirus RNA on fomites and other environmental samples (42).

The inherent high level of sensitivity of PCR also can present a number of potential problems of which the investigator must be aware. False-positive results may occur from contamination and sample carryover. It is also theoretically possible that the assay system will not clearly differentiate between rotavirus gastroenteritis and an asymptomatic carrier state associated with the passage of low levels of rotavirus RNA. Although fecal samples can contain substances that inhibit the enzymatic reactions used in the conversion of RNA to cDNA by reverse transcription and the amplification of the cDNA by PCR, sufficiently inhibitor-free rotavirus RNA can be extracted from fecal specimens using commercial RNA extraction kits.

EIA for Determining Serotype

Two outer capsid proteins, VP4 and VP7, are the determinants of rotavirus serotype. The VP4 serotype is designated P type to indicate the sensitivity of VP4 to proteases such as trypsin. Trypsin cleavage of VP4 is necessary for rotavirus infectivity. The VP7 serotype is designated G type for the VP7 glycoprotein. Antibodies directed against VP4 and VP7 neutralize rotaviruses both in vitro and in vivo in a serotype-specific manner. Antiserum prepared against virus of one serotype tends to neutralize homotypic rotaviruses more efficiently than it neutralizes heterotypic viruses. A number of human and animal studies have shown that protection induced either by natural infection or immunization may also be serotype specific (reviewed in reference 22). As a consequence, recent epidemiological surveys have included determination of serotype in the analysis to monitor the spectrum of rotavirus strains in different populations and the emergence of new serotypes. This information is critical for developing an effective rotavirus vaccine.

Rotavirus serotypes were initially defined by cross-neutralization using hyperimmune serum against purified rotaviruses (reviewed in reference 9). Reference antisera generated from viruses with established serotype were used to type field isolates. It has been shown that this type of assay identifies VP7 serotypes to the exclusion of VP4 serotypes. This viral cross-neutralization assay is most suitable for viruses adapted to growth in tissue culture. Stool samples, anal swipes, and other clinical samples obtained directly from patients cannot be used in this assay. For these samples, EIA based on serotype-specific monoclonal antibodies to different G types is used to determine the VP7 or G serotype. Ten different VP7 serotypes have been identified from human isolates. G serotypes 1, 2, 3, and 4 are the most common serotypes associated with virulent rotavirus strains that cause diarrheal disease in humans, while other emerging serotypes, including 5, 6, 8, 9, and 10, have been isolated in different areas of the world. In recent years, some of the rarer viral serotypes have appeared more frequently in humans (16). For example, serotype 9 rotavirus has been reported to be the dominant epidemic strain in diverse populations in Asia, and serotype 8 is the dominant epidemic strain in Africa. It is not certain whether vaccines that include only serotype 1 (GSK's Rotarix [G1, P1A[8], currently in trials]) or serotypes 1 to 4 (previously licensed vaccine; Wyeth's RotaShield [G1-4] and Merck's RotaTeq [WC-3-based pentavalent bovine-human reassortments, currently in trials]) will protect vaccinated infants broadly against the strains not specifically included in the vaccine formulation (11). Therefore, it is of utmost importance that monitoring systems be in place to detect changes in rotavirus serotype and emergence of new serotypes. Commonly used VP7 serotyping monoclonal antibodies and their serotype specificity are listed in Table 1.

VP4 serotyping is substantially more difficult. Hyperimmune serum from animals immunized with purified rotavirus has low titer against VP4. It cannot be used directly to determine VP4 serotype because of interference from the predominant VP7 neutralizing antibody. Several modified methods have been devised to determine the VP4 serotype, including cross-neutralization using hyperimmune serum against reassortant viruses that have identical VP4 to the test virus but a different VP7 (15) or hyperimmune serum generated against recombinant VP4 expressed in the baculovirus system (12). Seven P types have been identified from human rotaviruses. P1A, P1B, and P2 are the most common. P1A and P1B are associated with the most virulent human rotaviruses that cause diarrhea.

TABLE 1 Reference viruses and a partial list of VP7 monoclonal antibodies for G serotyping

G serotype	Reference viruses	Monoclonal antibodies
1	Wa, Ku, RV-4, K8	5E8, RV4-1, KU-4, RV4-2
2	DS-1, RV-5, S2	IC10, S2-2G10, RV5-3
3	P, YO, RV-3, SA11	YO-1E2, 159, RV3-1
4	ST-3, VA70, HOSO	ST-2G7, ST3-1
5	TFR41, OSH	5B8
6	UK	UK7/IC3
7		
8	69M, B37	B37:1
9	F45, WI61, Au32	F45:8, WI61:3

Determining the VP4 serotype using monoclonal antibodies is also very difficult. Most of the anti-VP4 monoclonal antibodies that have been isolated are cross-reactive. Only a small number of monoclonal antibodies are available to detect a limited number of human and animal rotavirus P serotypes. Table 2 lists several monoclonal antibodies that have been used in EIA to determine the P types of common human rotaviruses.

An alternative to EIA-based rotavirus serotyping is rotavirus genotyping which uses RT-PCR (10) or RNA-RNA hybridization with type-specific probes (32) to compare the nucleic sequences that define VP7 or VP4 genotypes. VP7 genotype designation is identical to serotype, but VP4 genotype designation is different from serotype; the genotype is indicated in brackets. In theory, the genotype is not a direct reflection of the serotype that is defined by a specific neutralization activity. However, several of the P or G genotypes that have been identified match perfectly with the P or G serotype determined separately (examples are given in Table 2). Genotyping based on RT-PCR has been used frequently in recent epidemiological studies. A detailed discussion of rotavirus genotyping is beyond the scope of this chapter (see references 9 and 10 for more details).

Protocols for EIA

Antigen Assays

Assays to detect rotavirus antigen are performed by using the direct (Fig. 1) or indirect (Fig. 2) format. Viral antigen is most likely to be detected if fecal specimens are collected between the first and fourth day of rotavirus illness (22).

Interpretation of results. Calculate a rotavirus-specific activity by subtracting the mean activity of the specimen in wells coated with the rotavirus-negative serum from the mean activity in the wells coated with the anti-rotavirus serum. To ensure accurate quantification, specimens giving readings of greater than 1.2 optical density (OD) units should be diluted 1:10 and retested. Calculate the mean and standard deviation of the rotavirus-specific activity of the

TABLE 2 Reference viruses and a partial list of VP4 monoclonal antibodies for P serotyping

P serotype [P genotype]	Reference viruses	Monoclonal antibodies
1A[8]	Wa, Ku, YO, F45, RV-4	F45:4, 1A10
1B[4]	DS-1, RV-5, S2	RV-5:2
2[6]	ST-3, RV-3, M37	ST-3:3, HS6, HS11

negative controls. A specimen is considered positive if its mean activity is greater than 2 standard deviations above the mean activity of the negative controls. Alternatively, a specimen may be considered positive if its activity is greater than that of the weakly positive control.

If qualitative visual determinations are used, a specimen is considered positive if its color in the goat anti-rotavirus wells is more intense than its color in the normal goat immunoglobulin wells and the color of the weakly positive control in the goat anti-rotavirus wells. Note that if the β-lactamase starch-iodine system is used, a positive reaction is manifested by a decrease in color.

Antibody Assays

Binding Test for Antibody Measurement: Antiglobulin Method

To measure antibody binding, microtiter plate wells coated with purified rotavirus are contrasted with wells coated with control antigen. If purified antigen is not available, wells can be coated first with anti-rotavirus antibody and then with unpurified rotavirus. Fourfold dilutions of test samples (to a final dilution of at least 1:2,560 for serum or 1:256 for other specimens) are assayed.

Interpretation of results. For each dilution, calculate a rotavirus-specific antibody activity by subtracting the activity in wells treated with the control antigen from the activity in wells treated with the viral antigen. A dilution is considered to contain antibody if the rotavirus-specific antibody activity is equal to or greater than the rotavirus-specific antibody activity of the positive control specimen at its end point. The antibody can be more accurately quantified by extrapolating from a standard curve generated by using specimens of known specific antibody concentrations. Antibody concentrations can also be calculated from computer programs that have been developed for this purpose (35).

Measurements of IgM or IgA in serum are more accurate if excess IgG is first removed. The immunoglobulins can be separated by physicochemical or immunological methods (28).

Blocking Assay for Antibody Determination

In general, the blocking assay is used less commonly than the binding assay. The presence of antibody in a dilution is manifested by a reduction in the activity of antigen as a result of virus neutralization.

Interpretation of results. A dilution of the specimen is considered to contain antibody if it yields a value that is less than or equal to that of the positive control specimen at its end point. Alternatively, a predetermined reduction of activity, such as a fixed percentage (at least 20%) or 2 standard deviations below that in wells in which negative control serum was added, can be used to calculate the end points. If visual determinations are used, wells that have less color visibly than wells to which negative control serum has been added are considered positive for antibody.

EIA To Determine VP7 G Serotype

To prepare for the VP7 serotype EIA, hyperimmune serum against one reference rotavirus representing each of the G types should be procured. Since the conformational integrity of VP7 is dependent on binding Ca^{2+}, we recommend that all buffers used in the EIA contain Ca^{2+}. Wells are coated with hyperimmune sera against rotavirus G types 1 to 9 or with rotavirus-negative serum from the same species that

was used to produce the hyperimmune serum. A partial list of serotyping monoclonal antibodies for G types 1 to 6, 8, and 9 is shown in Table 1. The concentration of each of the monoclonal antibodies should be adjusted before use in the assay, such that comparable OD readings to those of the reference virus are achieved. If serotyping monoclonal antibodies are used to coat the wells initially, hyperimmune serum against rotavirus may be used as the detector antibody.

Interpretation of results. The serotype of a test virus is determined if OD of virus from one serotype monoclonal antibody is greater than or equal to two times the OD from antibodies of other serotypes (positive OD/negative OD ≥ 2.0).

EIA To Determine VP4 P Serotype

The protocol for the EIA to determine the VP4 serotype is similar to that for the VP7 serotyping EIA described above, except that VP4 serotyping antibodies (listed in Table 2) are used. In addition, it has been shown that the sensitivity of VP4 serotyping increases if the hyperimmune serum used to coat the plates matches the G type of the test virus. Thus, G typing should precede P typing. Sensitivity of VP4 serotyping is compromised if the fecal samples are repeatedly frozen and thawed.

NOROVIRUS

It is estimated that ingestion of contaminated food accounts for about 76 million cases of gastroenteritis and leads to hospitalization in over 300,000 cases each year in the United States (30). Of the known pathogens, viruses as a group are thought to account for at least two-thirds of these illnesses, with the largest number of cases (23 million estimated) attributable to noroviruses. Although food-borne gastroenteritis is not associated significantly with mortality, its economic impact may be considerable since ill individuals may require medical attention or days off from school or work owing to symptoms which include vomiting and/or watery diarrhea that can lead to dehydration, abdominal cramps, low-grade fever, myalgia, and headache. While the symptoms usually resolve within 1 to 3 days, virus may be shed in feces for up to 2 weeks afterward.

Norovirus, a genus of the family *Caliciviridae*, comprises a genetically diverse but related group of small, nonenveloped, plus-strand RNA viruses. In the literature prior to 2002, they were more commonly referred to as Norwalk-like viruses (after the outbreak in Norwalk, Ohio, that led to the discovery of these agents) and small round structured viruses (after their ultrastructural features).

Immunological methods have played a key role in the detection and study of the human caliciviruses, beginning with the discovery of Norwalk virus in 1972 by Albert Kapikian and coworkers (23). For this seminal work, immunoelectron microscopy (IEM) was applied to fecal extracts from a patient with a secondary case in the 1968 outbreak of gastroenteritis at a school in Norwalk, Ohio, and resulted in the visualization of the 27-nm viral agent thereafter known as Norwalk virus. Subsequently, IEM was instrumental in determining the biophysical characteristics of Norwalk virus, tracking the course of viral shedding in ill individuals, and identifying other viruses that infect the gastrointestinal tract and liver. Solid-phase immunoassays were also developed, but their widespread use was curtailed by virtue of their dependence on limited supplies of native viral antigen.

Standard virological techniques were not readily applicable to the study of Norwalk virus and other related human caliciviruses, given that these viruses could not be propagated in cell culture or studied in a laboratory animal model (7). (The very recent description of a mouse model that supports infection by a mouse norovirus holds promise for future studies [45].) In the early 1990s, reports of cloning the Norwalk virus genome (17, 18, 29) opened new avenues of investigation and presented fresh opportunities to develop reliable diagnostic tests. Knowledge of the viral genomic sequence enabled the application of RT-PCR to detect viral nucleic acid in a variety of samples (summarized in reference 40). Data acquired over the years have allowed the classification of the noroviruses into four genogroups (GI, GII, GIII, and GIV) that can be divided into 20 or more genetic clusters. Human infections are most commonly caused by GI and GII noroviruses, representing 15 or more genotypes (reviewed in reference 13).

Expression of Norwalk virus capsid sequence in the baculovirus system was another important milestone, since it yielded large numbers of noninfectious virus-like particles (VLPs) that were easily purified from cell culture supernatant fluids (19) and had antigenic features comparable to those of wild-type virus. Subsequently, VLPs of other noroviruses have been produced (listed in reference 5). The VLPs have been used directly as antigens in EIAs to measure antibody response and as immunogens to develop serological reagents that can be used to detect viral antigen in clinical samples (reviewed in reference 20).

EIA To Detect Antigen

For antigen detetion EIAs, highly purified norovirus VLPs were used initially to immunize laboratory animals to produce polyclonal antibodies. The antibodies from one animal species (e.g., mouse) were then used to coat the EIA plate and serve as capture antibody, while the antibodies from a second animal species (e.g., rabbit) were used as the detector antibody in a sandwich EIA format. In general, the rabbit polyclonal antibodies showed high specificity for the genetic subgroup of the immunizing VLPs. More recently, mouse monoclonal antibodies that are reactive with a wider variety of noroviruses (GI and GII) have been identified. Two commercial EIAs for the detection of norovirus antigen in fecal samples, using these more broadly reactive monoclonal antibodies, have been marketed in Europe and Asia but are not currently available in the United States.

It is not clear whether these EIAs are sensitive enough to be recommended as a screening test for norovirus infection. A study from the United Kingdom (36) compared the Dako IDEIA assay and EM with RT-PCR detection of noroviurses. Compared with RT-PCR, the sensitivity and specificity of the EIA were 55.5 and 98.3%, respectively, versus 23.9 and 99.2%, respectively, for EM. To facilitate identification of the cause of a norovirus-like outbreak, six or more samples from an outbreak needed to be tested to improve the sensitivity and specificity of the EIA to 71.4 and 100%, respectively. Although these investigators suggest that this EIA may be used as a preliminary screening tool, they recommend using RT-PCR to examine samples from outbreaks that test negative by EIA and to further characterize the viral strains identified by EIA.

In a separate study, the Dako IDEIA NLV assay from the United Kingdom was compared to the Denko SRSV (II)-AD assay from Japan (5). The Dako kit demonstrated low sensitivity overall (less than 30% for six genogroup II subgroups) and high specificity (100%). The Denko kit, by contrast, had higher sensitivity, achieving a sensitivity of greater than 70% for 10 of the 14 subgroups, but lower specificity (69%). In addition, the Dako kit could distinguish between GI and GII noroviruses while the Denko kit exhibited nonspecific cross-reactivity of GI and GII noroviruses, as well as sapoviruses. As a result, these investigators were unable to recommend either of these EIA-based kits as practical alternatives to RT-PCR for the detection of noroviruses.

EIA To Detect Antibody

In contrast to EIAs that detect norovirus antigen, which tend to be more highly strain specific (estimated >95% identity in the RNA polymerase region), EIAs developed for detection of norovirus antibody have the distinct feature of being more broadly reactive, such that the presence of antibody does not necessarily indicate the individual has been infected with the specific virus represented by the VLP in the assay. It has been estimated that 70% identity to the test strain in the region of the RNA polymerase is sufficient to cause the antibody detection EIA to be positive. Although antibody to a heterologous strain of norovirus can be detected by this type of assay, homologous or more genetically closely related strains display more frequent and vigorous responses (reviewed in reference 20).

An EIA designed to measure salivary antibodies to Norwalk virus and a related outbreak strain has been reported (31). Wells of microtiter plates were coated with recombinant Norwalk virus antigen and blocked. Saliva samples were then added, and IgG- or IgA-specific antibodies were detected by a colorimetric reaction. Use of this approach to determine the cause of an outbreak has some clear advantages, including the ability to quickly and noninvasively acquire the saliva from affected individuals. It is not possible, however, to make the diagnosis on the basis of a single sample, since many people have anti-Norwalk virus salivary IgA and IgG. Two samples are required, one on day 4 (or as early in the infection as possible) and the other on about day 14, and a fourfold increase in antibody titer between the samples must be demonstrated. Compared to the antigen detection EIA tested previously by Richards et al. (36) (see above), a slightly higher sensitivity (78%) and nearly equivalent specificity (95 to 100%) were achieved. Potential applications of this test include its use in studies of epidemic and endemic infection, as well as host immune response, particularly in groups of individuals for whom it may be difficult to obtain adequate clinical material for testing.

Nucleic Acid Detection

Since the cloning of the Norwalk virus genome, methods to detect norovirus nucleic acid in clinical samples by using RT-PCR have been developed and used widely to diagnose norovirus infection. Amplicons derived by these methods can be verified by hybridization with specific probes or sequencing. Although highly sensitive, RT-PCR has been difficult to standardize for widespread use for a number of reasons (40).

First, by nature of the infection, detection of norovirus nucleic acid is performed with stool samples which contain inhibitors to RT-PCR. Although methods to minimize the presence of these compounds have been developed, they require additional time to perform, necessitate extra handling of the sample (which may reduce the amount of antigen/nucleic acid available in the final sample), and add to the cost of the test. In addition, these methods are not standardized and vary from laboratory to laboratory (40). Assaying other materials, such as prepared food or raw shellfish through which infection may be transmitted, may require different methods to extract the virus or its nucleic acid from these matrices (27).

Second, significant sequence diversity among the multitude of norovirus strains has made it difficult to design primers that detect all strains of norovirus. As the sequences of more norovirus strain genomes have been elucidated, the ability to select primers that are more broadly reactive and useful for detecting currently circulating strains has improved. In general, primers capable of identifying a wider range of noroviruses are based on a conserved area of open reading frame 1 (ORF1) that encodes the viral RNA polymerase. Primers targeting sequences of the 2C helicase, the 5′ end of the capsid, or ORF3 tend to be more strain specific.

Third, the RT-PCR methods used most extensively to date are neither the simplest nor the fastest. Contamination of the sample is always a concern in carrying out highly sensitive tests that require multiple steps and sample manipulation. In addition, verifying the specificity of the amplicon necessitates additional analysis, including probe hybridization and variations of this technique, as well as sequencing the product.

Recent efforts have attempted to address some of these problems. A promising strategy has been the application of real-time RT-PCR, a quantitative test that permits both amplification of viral nucleic acid and detection of virus-specific amplicons, using intercalating dyes or fluorescent probes or primers. Two fluorescence techniques, in single-tube formats, are increasingly studied to detect noroviruses in clinical samples, water, and shellfish: SYBR green dye incorporation into amplicons (1, 37, 38) and the TaqMan fluorogenic detection system (14, 21).

The TaqMan assay uses virus-specific primer sets and fluorogenic probes that identify GI and GII sequences (14). The fluorogenic probes are labeled with a fluorescent reporter and quencher dye. After the probe hybridizes with the norovirus target sequence, the 5′-3′ nuclease activity of *Taq* polymerase cleaves the TaqMan probe during amplification, thus separating the quencher dye from the reporter. The increase in fluorescence intensity of the reporter is proportional to the starting copy number of the target nucleic acid and enables the quantitation of norovirus RNA when compared to a standard curve. Besides the high sensitivity of this test, other benefits of this one-tube method include the potential to screen large numbers of samples expeditiously, lower chance of sample contamination, and no need to confirm the validity of the product by additional tests. For this approach to yield reliable results, however, the probe must bind to the amplicon of interest, which presents a challenge to probe designers, given the great diversity in sequence among noroviruses. Kageyama et al. (21) sought to minimize the potential probe-binding problem by amplifying with degenerate primers (one set for genogroup I and a second set for genogroup II) a highly conserved region of the norovirus genome that spanned the junction between ORF1 and ORF2.

The strategy involving SYBR green detection, rather than TaqMan probes, has the advantage that the fluorescent dye is incorporated into amplicons and does not rely on a probe binding to a norovirus sequence that may not be sufficiently complementary. Richards et al. (37) recently were able to detect noroviruses from five genetic clusters of genogroup I and eight genetic clusters of genogroup II, which represents most of the known circulating strains of human noroviruses. They designed two sets of degenerate primers (for genogroups I and II, respectively) based on sequences from the RNA-dependent RNA polymerase region for use in a one-step, hot-start real-time RT-PCR. The highly degenerate primers necessitated increasing the time for denaturation, annealing, and extension, as well as low temperatures for optimal annealing and extension, compared

to standard RT-PCR. SYBR green is also known to intercalate into primer-dimers, as well as the amplicons of interest. To ensure proper interpretation of their test results, the authors imposed a 6-s optical read step at 77°C (after the normal 60°C extension step) for each PCR cycle to fully melt primer-dimers and other undesired products that had lower melting temperatures than the norovirus amplicon, thereby reducing the fluorescence from the nonspecific products.

Developing the optimal molecular detection assay for the highly diverse noroviruses continues to be a challenge that is being pursued by scientists throughout the world. For the present, in the United States, diagnostic testing for noroviruses is limited largely to public health and research laboratories. The Centers for Disease Control and Prevention has provided primers and reagents to state and local laboratories to facilitate their efforts in investigating outbreaks of gastroenteritis (3). The Centers for Disease Control and Prevention also maintains CaliciNet, a database of norovirus sequences from outbreaks, to facilitate the study of relationships between outbreaks and to gain more insight into the norovirus strains in circulation.

We acknowledge Robert H. Yolken, the author of this chapter in a previous edition of this manual.

REFERENCES

1. **Beuret, C.** 2004. Simultaneous detection of enteric viruses by multiplex real-time RT-PCR. *J. Virol. Methods* **115:**1–8.
2. **Bishop, R. F., G. P. Davidson, I. H. Holmes, and B. J. Ruck.** 1973. Virus particles in epithelial cells of duodenal mucosa from children with acute nonbacterial gastroenteritis. *Lancet* **i:**1281–1283.
3. **Bresee, J. S., M.-A. Widdowson, S. S. Monroe, and R. I. Glass.** 2002. Foodborne viral gastroenteritis: challenges and opportunities. *Clin. Infect. Dis.* **35:**748–753.
4. **Buesa, J., J. Colomina, J. Raga, A. Villanueva, and J. Prat.** 1996. Evaluation of reverse transcription and polymerase chain reaction (RT/PCR) for the detection of rotaviruses: applications of the assay. *Res. Virol.* **147:**353–361.
5. **Burton-MacLeod, J. A., E. M. Kane, R. S. Beard, L. A. Hadley, R. I. Glass, and T. Ando.** 2004. Evaluation and comparison of two commercial enzyme-linked immunosorbent assay kits for detection of antigenically diverse human noroviruses in stool samples. *J. Clin. Microbiol.* **42:**2587–2595.
6. **Dennehy, P. H., M. Hartin, S. M. Nelson, and S. F. Reising.** 1999. Evaluation of the ImmunoCardSTAT! Rotavirus assay for detection of group A rotavirus in fecal specimens. *J. Clin. Microbiol.* **37:**1977–1979.
7. **Duizer, E., K. J. Schwab, F. H. Neill, R. L. Atmar, M. P. G. Koopmans, and M. K. Estes.** 2004. Laboratory efforts to cultivate noroviruses. *J. Gen. Virol.* **85:**79–87.
8. **Estes, M. K.** 2001. Rotaviruses and their replication, p. 1747–1785. *In* D. M. Knipe, P. M. Howley, D. E. Griffin, R. A. Lamb, M. A. Martin, B. Roizman, and S. E. Straus (ed.), *Fields Virology*, 4th ed. Lippincott Williams & Wilkins, Baltimore, Md.
9. **Fischer, T. K., and J. R. Gentsch.** 2004. Rotavirus typing methods and algorithms. *Rev. Med. Virol.* **14:**71–82.
10. **Gentsch, J. R., R. I. Glass, P. Woods, V. Gouvea, M. Gorziglia, J. Flores, B. K. Das, and M. K. Bhan.** 1992. Identification of group A rotavirus gene 4 types by polymerase chain reaction. *J. Clin. Microbiol.* **30:**1365–1373.
11. **Glass, R. I., J. S. Bresee, U. D. Parashar, B. Jiang, and J. Gentsch.** 2004. The future of rotavirus vaccines: a major setback leads to new opportunities. *Lancet* **363:**1547–1550.
12. **Gorziglia, M., G. Larralde, A. Z. Kapikian, and R. M. Chanock.** 1990. Antigenic relationships among human

rotaviruses as determined by outer capsid protein VP4. *Proc. Natl. Acad. Sci. USA* **87:**7155–7159.

13. **Green, K. Y., R. M. Chanock, and A. Z. Kapikian.** 2001. Human caliciviruses, p. 841–874. *In* D. M. Knipe, P. M. Howley, D. E. Griffin, R. A. Lamb, M. A. Martin, B. Roizman, and S. E. Straus (ed.), *Fields Virology*, 4th ed. Lippincott, Williams & Wilkins, Baltimore, Md.

14. **Hohne, M., and E. Schreier.** 2004. Detection and characterization of norovirus outbreaks in Germany: application of a one-tube RT-PCR using a fluorogenic real-time detection system. *J. Med. Virol.* **72:**312–319.

15. **Hoshino, Y., and A. Z. Kapikian.** 1994. Rotavirus antigens. *Curr. Top. Microbiol. Immunol.* **185:**179–227.

16. **Hoshino, Y., and A. Z. Kapikian.** 2000. Rotavirus serotypes: classification and importance in epidemiology, immunity, and vaccine development. *J. Health Popul. Nutr.* **18:**5–14.

17. **Jiang, X., D. Y. Graham, K. Wang, and M. K. Estes.** 1990. Norwalk virus genome: cloning and characterization. *Science* **250:**1580–1583.

18. **Jiang, X., M. Wang, K. Wang, and M. K. Estes.** 1993. Sequence and genomic organization of Norwalk virus. *Virology* **195:**51–61.

19. **Jiang, X., M. Wang, D. Y. Graham, and M. K. Estes.** 1992. Expression, self-assembly, and antigenicity of the Norwalk virus capsid protein. *J. Virol.* **66:**6527–6532.

20. **Jiang, X., N. Wilton, W. M. Zhong, T. Farkas, T. W. Huang, E. Barrett, M. Guerrero, G. Ruiz-Palacios, K. Y. Green, J. Green, A. D. Hale, M. K. Estes, L. K. Pickering, and D. O. Matson.** 2000. Diagnosis of human caliciviruses by use of enzyme immunoassays. *J. Infect. Dis.* **181**(Suppl. 2)**:**S349–S359.

21. **Kageyama, T., S. Kojima, M. Shinohara, K. Uchida, S. Fukushi, F. B. Hoshino, N. Takeda, K. Katayama.** 2003. Broadly reactive and highly sensitive assay for Norwalk-like viruses based on real-time quantitative reverse transcription-PCR. *J. Clin. Microbiol.* **41:**1548–1557.

22. **Kapikian, A. Z., Y. Hoshino, and R. M. Chanock.** 2001. Rotaviruses, p. 1787–1833. *In* D. M. Knipe, P. M. Howley, D. E. Griffin, R. A. Lamb, M. A. Martin, B. Roizman, and S. E. Straus (ed.), *Fields Virology*, 4th ed. Lippincott, Williams & Wilkins, Baltimore, Md.

23. **Kapikian, A. Z., R. G. Wyatt, R. Dolin, T. S. Thornhill, A. R. Kalica, and R. M. Chanock.** 1972. Visualization by immune electron microscopy of a 27 nm particle associated with acute infectious nonbacterial gastroenteritis. *J. Virol.* **10:**1075–1081.

24. **Kapikian, A. Z., R. H. Yolken, H. B. Greenberg, R. G. Wyatt, A. R. Kalica, R. M. Chanock, and H. W. Kim.** 1979. Gastroenteritis viruses, p. 927–995. *In* E. H. Lennette and N. Schmidt (ed.), *Diagnostic Procedures for Viral, Rickettsial and Chlamydial Infections*, 5th ed. American Public Health Association, New York, N.Y.

25. **Larralde, G., and J. Flores.** 1990. Identification of gene 4 alleles among human rotaviruses by polymerase chain reaction-derived probes. *Virology* **179:**469–473.

26. **Linhares, A. C., Y. B. Gabbay, J. Mascarenhas, R. B. Freitas, T. H. Flewett, and G. M. Beards.** 1988. Epidemiology of rotavirus subgroups and serotypes in Belem Brazil: a three year study. *Ann. Inst. Pasteur Paris* **139:**88–99.

27. **Loisy, F., R. L. Atmar, P. Guillon, P. Le Cann, M. Pommepuy, and F. S. Le Guyader.** 2005. Real-time RT-PCR for norovirus screening in shellfish. *J. Virol. Methods* **123:**1–7.

28. **Martins, T. B., T. D. Jaskowski, C. L. Mouritsen, and H. R. Hill.** 1995. An evaluation of the effectiveness of three immunoglobulin G (IgG) removal procedures for routine IgM serological testing. *Clin. Diagn. Lab. Immunol.* **2:**98–103.

29. **Matsui, S. M., J. P. Kim, H. B. Greemberg, W. Su, Q. Sun, P. C. Johnson, H. L. DuPont, L. S. Oshiro, and G. R. Reyes.** 1991. The isolation and characterization of a Norwalk virus-specific cDNA. *J. Clin. Investig.* **87:**1456–1461.

30. **Mead, P. S., L. Slutsker, V. Dietz, L. F. McCaig, J. S. Bresee, C. Shapiro, P. M. Griffin, and R. V. Tauxe.** 1999. Food-related illness and death in the United States. *Emerg. Infect. Dis.* **5:**607–625.

31. **Moe, C. L., A. Sair, L. Lindesmith, M. K. Estes, and L.-A. Jaykus.** 2004. Diagnosis of Norwalk virus infection by indirect enzyme immunoassay detection of salivary antibodies to recombinant Norwalk virus antigen. *Clin. Diagn. Lab. Immunol.* **11:**1028–1034.

32. **Nakagomi, O., H. Oyamada, and T. Nakagomi.** 1989. Use of alkaline Northern blot hybridization for the identification of genetic relatedness of the fourth gene of rotaviruses. *Mol. Cell. Probes* **3:**263–271.

33. **Parashar, U. D., R. C. Holman, M. J. Clarke, J. S. Bresee, and R. I. Glass.** 1998. Hospitalization associated with rotavirus diarrhea in the United States, 1993 through 1995: surveillance based on the new ICD-9-CM rotavirus specific diagnostic code. *J. Infect. Dis.* **177:**7–13.

34. **Parashar, U. D., E. G. Hummelman, J. S. Bresee, M. A. Miller, and R. I. Glass.** 2003. Global illness and deaths caused by rotavirus disease in children. *Emerg. Infect. Dis.* **9:**565–572.

35. **Peterman, J. H., and J. E. Butler.** 1989. Computer analysis for enzyme immunoassays. *BioTechniques* **7:**601–605.

36. **Richards, A. F., B. Lopman, A. Gunn, A. Curry, D. Ellis, H. Cotterill, S. Ratcliffe, M. Jenkins, H. Appleton, C. I. Gallimore, J. J. Gray, and D. W. Brown.** 2003. Evaluation of a commercial ELISA for detecting Norwalk-like virus antigen in feces. *J. Clin. Virol.* **26:**109–115.

37. **Richards, G. P., M. A. Watson, R. L. Fankhauser, and S. S. Monroe.** 2004. Genogroup I and II noroviruses detected in stool samples by real-time reverse transcription-PCR using highly degenerate universal primers. *Appl. Environ. Microbiol.* **70:**7179–7184.

38. **Richards, G. P., M. A. Watson, and D. H. Kingsley.** 2004. A SYBR green, real-time RT-PCR method to detect and quantitate Norwalk virus in stools. *J. Virol. Methods* **116:**63–70.

39. **Tucker, A. W., A. C. Haddix, J. S. Bresee, R. C. Holman, U. D. Parashar, and R. I. Glass.** 1998. Cost-effectiveness analysis of a rotavirus immunization program for the United States. *JAMA* **279:**1371–1376.

40. **Vinjé, J., H. Vennema, L. Maunula, C.-H. von Bonsdorff, M. Hoehne, E. Schreier, A. Richards, J. Green, D. Brown, S. S. Beard, S. S. Monroe, E. de Bruin, L. Svensson, and M. P. G. Koopmans.** 2003. International collaborative study to compare reverse transcriptase PCR assays for detection and genotyping of noroviruses. *J. Clin. Microbiol.* **41:**1423–1433.

41. **Wilde, J., J. Eiden, and R. Yolken.** 1990. Removal of inhibitory substances from human fecal specimens for detection of group A rotaviruses by reverse transcriptase and polymerase chain reactions. *J. Clin. Microbiol.* **28:**1300–1307.

42. **Wilde, J., R. Van, L. Pickering, J. Eiden, and R. Yolken.** 1992. Detection of rotaviruses in the day care environment by reverse transcriptase polymerase chain reaction. *J. Infect. Dis.* **166:**507–511.

43. **Wilde, J., R. Yolken, R. Willoughby, and J. Eiden.** 1991. Improved detection of rotavirus shedding by polymerase chain reaction. *Lancet* **337:**323–326.

44. **Wilhelmi, I., J. Colomina, D. Martin-Rodrigo, E. Roman, and A. Sanchez-Fauquier.** 2001. New immunochromatographic method for rapid detection of rotaviruses in stool

samples compared with standard enzyme immunoassay and latex agglutination techniques. *Eur. J. Clin. Microbiol. Infect. Dis.* **20:**741–743.

45. **Wobus, C. E., S. M. Karst, L. B. Thackray, K.-O. Chang, S. V. Sosnovtsev, G. Belliot, A. Krug, J. M. Mackenzie, K. Y. Green, and H. W. Virgin IV.** 2004. Replication of *Norovirus* in cell culture reveals a tropism for dendritic cells and macrophages. *PLoS Biol.* **2:**e432.

46. **Yolken, R. H.** 1990. Immunoassays for diagnosis of infectious diseases. *Methods Enzymol.* **184:**529–537.

47. **Yolken, R. H.** 1990. Laboratory diagnosis of viral infections, p. 141–181. *In* G. J. Galasso, R. J. Whitley, and

T. C. Merigan (ed.), *Antiviral Agents and Viral Diseases of Man*, 3rd ed. Raven Press, New York, N.Y.

48. **Yolken, R. H.** 1997. Enzyme immunoassays for detection of rotavirus antigen and antibody, p. 719–728. *In* N. R. Rose, E. Conway de Macario, J. D. Folds, H. C. Lane, and R. M. Nakamura (ed.), *Manual of Clinical Laboratory Immunology*, 5th ed. ASM Press, Washington, D.C.

49. **Yolken, R. H., R. G. Wyatt, L. Mata, J. J. Urrutia, B. Garcia, R. M. Chanock, and A. Z. Kapikian.** 1978. Secretory antibody directed against rotavirus in human milk—measurement by means of enzyme-linked immunosorbent assay. *J. Pediatr.* **93:**916–921.

Arboviruses

ROBERT S. LANCIOTTI AND JOHN T. ROEHRIG

85

The arthropod-borne viruses (arboviruses) represent a diverse amalgam of more than 500 animal viruses that are grouped together because of their ability to replicate in both vertebrates and arthropods. While more than 150 arboviruses are known to cause human illness or infection, the list of the most medically important viruses is considerably shorter (Table 1) (8, 17, 27). Because of the vast number of agents that potentially should be considered in a differential diagnosis, the use of epidemiologic, ecologic, and clinical data to guide the choice and interpretation of clinical laboratory diagnostic tests is essential. Most arboviruses are transmitted seasonally in specific geographic locations or ecological habitats. The patient's history of travel, activities, and potential exposures to arthropods or habitats associated with arbovirus transmission provides vital data for selection of appropriate antigens and relevant diagnostic approaches. Knowledge of the patient's immunizations against yellow fever (YF), Japanese encephalitis (JE), or tick-borne encephalitis (TBE) viruses is also important for the proper interpretation of serological results. Although the laboratory diagnosis of arboviral infections still relies chiefly on serology, other approaches that directly detect viral antigen or genomic material and not antibodies are now routine.

METHODS

Antibody Detection

IgM ELISA

Assays that detect virus-elicited immunoglobulin M (IgM) are useful because they detect antibodies produced within days of a primary viral infection. IgM antibody capture enzyme-linked immunosorbent assay (MAC-ELISA) is the preferred approach to IgM detection because it is simple, sensitive, and applicable to serum and cerebrospinal fluid (CSF) samples. False-positive reactions due to rheumatoid factor also are minimized (2, 22). While most ELISAs are based on a 96-well microplate format, assays are being developed and adapted to microsphere-based systems. These new systems require very small volumes of test specimens and permit antigen multiplexing, resulting in a considerable savings of time and money (30, 31).

IgM from serum or CSF is first captured onto the solid phase with μ-chain-specific antispecies antibody. IgM antibodies of all reactivities are thus concentrated, but during an acute infection, IgM antibodies directed at the etiologic agent are the principal circulating species. Virus antigen is next added, and if virus-specific IgM is present, viral antigen is bound to the plate. A variety of antigen sources such as virus-infected mouse brain, lysed cells, cell culture supernatant, or recombinant antigen can be employed. The bound antigen can be detected by a variety of means; however, the most practical approach is to use an enzyme-labeled antiviral monoclonal antibody. Since the reactivity of the patient's IgM with the test antigen in part defines the specificity of the assay, broadly reactive labeled antibodies can be used as detectors for most of the medically important arboviruses, e.g., monoclonal antibodies reactive against flavivirus group (6B6C-1), alphavirus group (2A2C-3), and California serogroup (10G5.4) (Table 2) (7).

Approximately 75% of patients with flavivirus encephalitis (e.g., JE or St. Louis encephalitis [SLE]) have detectable IgM in serum or CSF in the first 4 days of illness, and nearly 100% of samples are reactive by 7 days. Similar levels of sensitivity have been reported for patients with LaCrosse (LAC) encephalitis or alphavirus encephalitis and in patients with dengue (DEN) or YF. For patients with central nervous system (CNS) infections, greater sensitivity and specificity are obtained by also testing CSF.

The specificity of the MAC-ELISA is similar to that of the complement fixation (CF) test, and heterologous antibodies to related viruses may interfere with interpretation, particularly in patients with previous related infections. To improve diagnostic specificity, ratios of absorbances to related viruses can be calculated, yielding indices that are better discriminators than the individual absorbances alone. For example, antibodies to DEN and JE viruses cross-react in hemagglutination inhibition (HI) tests and ELISAs, but patients with the respective infections can be identified by calculating ratios of ELISA absorbances to the two viruses. Similarly, ratios of absorbances in IgM and IgG capture tests have a high predictive value in discriminating recent from previous infections with these viruses (5).

Although levels of IgM antibodies generally decline after 2 to 4 weeks and are absent after 90 to 120 days, IgM persists for a year or more after infection in some patients. This phenomenon has been reported for patients with JE, SLE, West Nile (WN) encephalitis, Murray Valley encephalitis (MVE), LAC encephalitis, and Sindbis and Ross River (RR) virus

TABLE 1 Characteristics of selected medically important arbovirus disease

Disease	Viral agent	Arthropod vector or source	Clinical syndrome(s)	Geographic distribution	Risk factor(s)	Case-fatality ratio (%)
EEE	Alphavirus	Mosquito	CNS infection	Eastern United States, Central and South America	Advanced age	30
JE	Flavivirus	Mosquito	CNS infection	Asian rice-growing areas	Exposure to rural areas	15–30
LAC encephalitis	Bunyavirus	Mosquito	CNS infection	East-central United States (children)	Males > females; agricultural occupations	<1
Rocio encephalitis	Flavivirus	Mosquito	CNS infection	Sao Paulo state, Brazil	Males > females; agricultural occupations	5
SLE	Flavivirus	Mosquito	CNS infection	North, Central, and South America	Advanced age	7
TBE	Flavivirus	Tick	CNS infection	Europe, Asia	Forest exposure	1–10
Powassan encephalitis	Flavivirus	Tick, mosquito	CNS infection	Canada, United States, Russia, China	Forest exposure	10
WEE	Alphavirus	Mosquito	CNS infection	Western United States, South America, Canada, Mexico	Males > females; extremes of age	5
CTF	Coltivirus	Tick	Febrile grippe	Rocky Mountain states, South Dakota, California, western Canada	Exposure to areas >5,000 ft (ca. 1,500 m) in elevation	<1
DEN	Flavivirus	Mosquito	Febrile grippe and rash; hemorrhagic fever	Tropical locations worldwide	Urban, peridomestic exposure	5
WN fever	Flavivirus	Mosquito	Febrile grippe and rash; encephalitis	United States, Africa, Europe, Asia	Advanced age	<1
Oropouche fever	Bunyavirus	Midge	Febrile grippe	Central and South America	Agricultural occupation	<1
Phlebotomus fever	Phlebovirus	Phlebotomine fly	Febrile grippe	Europe, Africa, Asia	Peridomestic exposure	<1
Chikungunya	Alphavirus	Mosquito	Febrile polyarthropathy and rash; rarely hemorrhagic fever	Africa, Asia	Urban, peridomestic exposure	<1
Mayaro fever	Alphavirus	Mosquito	Febrile polyarthropathy and rash	Central, South America	Males > females; forest exposure	<1
RR arthropathy	Alphavirus	Mosquito	Febrile polyarthropathy and rash	Australia, Pacific	Females > males	<1
Sindbis virus fever	Alphavirus	Mosquito	Febrile polyarthropathy and rash	Africa, Europe, Asia	Woodland exposure	<1
Crimean-Congo hemorrhagic fever	Nairovirus	Tick, infected blood	Hemorrhagic fever	Africa, Europe, Asia	Animal husbandry; agricultural and medical occupations	10–50
Rift Valley fever	Phlebovirus	Mosquito, infected blood	Febrile grippe; hemorrhagic fever	Africa, Middle East	Animal husbandry; butchering	<1
YF	Flavivirus	Mosquito	Febrile grippe; hemorrhagic fever	South America, West and Central Africa	Forest or rural exposure	15

TABLE 2 Selected arbovirus monoclonal antibodies for serologic and antigen detection assays[a]

Antibody[b]	Prepared against:	Reactivity	Use
6B6C-1	SLE virus (MSI-7)	Flavivirus group	As HRP[c] conjugate in antigen capture and IgM capture ELISAs
4G2	DEN virus 2 (New Guinea C)	Flavivirus group	Viral identification by IF or ELISA; ELISA capture antibody
6B4A-10	JE virus (Nakayama)	JE-SLE-WN-MVE complex	Capture antibody in antigen capture ELISA
JE314H52	JE virus (Nakayama)	JE virus specific	Viral identification by IF or ELISA
6B5A-2	SLE virus (MSI-7)	SLE virus specific	Viral identification by IF and neutralization
4A4C-4	SLE virus (MSI-7)	SLE virus specific	Capture antibody in antigen capture ELISA
4B6C-2	MVE virus (original)	MVE virus specific	Viral identification by IF or ELISA
D2-1F-3	DEN virus 1 (Hawaii)	DEN virus 1 specific	Viral identification by IF or ELISA
3H5-1-21	DEN virus 2 (New Guinea C)	DEN virus 2 specific	Viral identification by IF or ELISA
D6-8A1-12	DEN virus 3 (H87)	DEN virus 3 specific	Viral identification by IF or ELISA
1H10-6-7	DEN virus 4 (H-241)	DEN virus 4 specific	Viral identification by IF or ELISA
5E-3	YF virus (17D)	YF virus specific	Capture antibody in antigen capture ELISA
117	YF virus (Asibi)	YF wild-type virus specific	Viral identification by IF
864	YF virus (17D)	YF vaccine virus specific	Identification of vaccine strains by IF
4D9	TBE virus	Tick-borne flavivirus complex	Viral identification by IF or ELISA
H5.46	WN virus	WN virus specific	Viral identification by IF or ELISA
2A2C-3	WEE virus (McMillan)	Alphavirus group	As HRP conjugate in antigen and IgM capture ELISAs
2A3D-5	WEE virus (McMillan)	WEE complex	Capture antibody for WEE and HJ antigen capture ELISA
2B1C-6	WEE virus (McMillan)	WEE virus specific	Viral identification by IF or ELISA; as HRP conjugate in antigen capture ELISA
1B5C-3	EEE virus (NJ 60)	EEE North American virus specific	Viral identification by IF or ELISA; as HRP conjugate in antigen capture ELISA
1C1J-4	EEE virus (BeAn 5122)	EEE South American virus specific	Viral identification by IF or ELISA
1B1C-4	EEE virus (BeAn 5122)	EEE complex specific	Viral identification by IF or ELISA
2D4-1	Highlands J virus (B230)	Highlands J virus specific	Viral identification by IF or ELISA; as HRP conjugate in antigen capture ELISA
1A2B-10	VEE virus (E2 peptide)	VEE complex	Viral identification by IF or ELISA
5B4D-6	VEE virus (TC-83)	TC-83 (vaccine) specific	Viral identification by IF or ELISA
1A3A-5	VEE virus (IC)	Epizootic VEE virus	Viral identification by IF or ELISA
1A1B-9	VEE virus (IE)	Enzootic VEE virus	Viral identification by IF or ELISA
807-18	LAC virus (original)	LAC virus specific	Viral identification by HI, neutralization, or ELISA
10G5.4	LAC virus (original)	California serogroup reactive	Viral identification by ELISA

[a]Adapted from reference 19.
[b]Antibodies and/or conjugates are available from the Centers for Disease Control and Prevention.
[c]HRP, horseradish peroxidase.

polyarthropathy, and it is common in patients with YF or after YF vaccination. This observation is of diagnostic importance, because in areas where the diseases are endemic, IgM from infection during a previous transmission season could be mistaken as evidence of recent infection. For this reason, demonstration of IgM in a single serum sample alone does not necessarily indicate a recent infection. Virus-specific IgM in CSF has been detected 50 to 180 days after onset of acute JE, indicating continuing intrathecal production of antibody and the possibility of persistent CNS infection. However, these appear to be unusual cases, and in most circumstances, detection of arbovirus-specific IgM in CSF is a reliable indication of recent infection.

A practical problem in implementing the MAC-ELISA is the unavailability of positive-control sera containing IgM for all the antigens of interest. Although reactive human sera for many of the common arbovirus infections are available from the Centers for Disease Control and Prevention and other laboratories, human positive-control sera for less prevalent infections are unavailable. These laboratories can provide testing panels of serum for quality control of test

performance. Unlike the HI, CF, and neutralization tests described below, in which mouse immune fluids can be used as controls, the MAC-ELISA incorporates a species-specific capture antibody and requires reactive human samples. MAC-ELISAs for agents of arbovirus encephalitis are offered by commercial reference laboratories, and a kit for TBE diagnosis is available in Europe. Commercial dot blot kits for DEN and JE are available in Asia, but their sensitivity and specificity require further characterization.

MAC-ELISAs also have been developed to detect eastern equine encephalitis (EEE), western equine encephalitis (WEE), and Venezuelan equine encephalitis (VEE) virus antibodies in horses; EEE, SLE, WEE, and WN virus antibodies in birds; and JE virus antibody in pigs. The test formats are identical to the procedure described above for human sera, except that commercially available anti-horse, anti-chicken, and anti-pig IgM, respectively, replaces the anti-human capture antibody. Horses immunized with inactive EEE, WEE, and VEE vaccines produce HI and neutralizing antibodies that cannot be readily distinguished from naturally acquired antibodies; however, IgM antibodies to the viruses are usually detectable only after natural infection. The MAC-ELISA is sensitive when serum samples are obtained within 1 week of the onset of illness, and it is now the procedure of choice in the laboratory diagnosis of arbovirus encephalitis in horses.

Sparrows and other passerine birds are the principal amplifying hosts for SLE, WN, and WEE viruses. Serologic surveillance of wild birds and sentinel chickens is a means by which state and local health agencies monitor the risk of epidemic arbovirus transmission. Likewise, in certain areas of Asia, seroconversions in pigs are monitored in JE surveillance programs. IgM antibodies to SLE and WEE viruses in sparrows rise and fall to undetectable levels within 2 weeks of infection, and the MAC-ELISA (using commercially available anti-chicken IgM) is useful only in monitoring recent infections among sparrows. HI and/or neutralizing antibodies are still valuable indicators of more remote infections.

IgG ELISA

IgG ELISA has replaced the HI test for the diagnosis of some infections because the procedure is less cumbersome and titration curves for the two procedures are similar. Various indirect procedures to measure the levels of IgG antibodies to arboviruses differ chiefly in the procedures for antigen preparation and methods for their attachment to the solid phase. Conventional mouse brain antigens extracted with sucrose and acetone generally do not have adequate potency as antigens unless they are first captured and concentrated onto the solid phase with antibody (mouse monoclonal or polyclonal ascitic fluid) (6). Dot ELISAs, in which antigens are adsorbed to nitrocellulose or other membranes, also have been used successfully. The sensitivities of IgG ELISAs generally are similar to or greater than those of HI tests, and their specificities correspondingly are equal or lower.

IF Test

Indirect immunofluorescence (IF) tests for IgG and IgM antibodies are described in chapter 48. The procedures for arbovirus diagnosis generally use virus-infected Vero or other cells fixed onto slides in monovalent or polyvalent preparations. Commercially available spot slides with SLE, WEE, EEE, and LAC virus-infected cells make it possible to screen a serum sample simultaneously against the principal arbovirus agents of encephalitis in the United States. A similar polyvalent slide is available to screen patients with suspected viral hemorrhagic fever for antibodies against Crimean-Congo and Rift Valley fever (RVF) viruses, two strains of Ebola virus, and Lassa and Marburg viruses in a single CRE$_2$LM (derived from the names of the viruses) slide. Virus-specific IgM and IgG antibodies in CSF also can be measured by IF, although the titers generally are lower than in serum. With all indirect tests for IgM, the confounding effects of IgM rheumatoid factors should be controlled.

Indirect IF, HI, and neutralization tests have similar sensitivities, but IF is less sensitive than ELISA. The indirect IF test for antibodies to most arboviruses is as specific as or less specific than the HI test. Indirect IF cannot be relied upon to distinguish infections among the flaviviruses, among the alphaviruses, or among viruses in bunyavirus serogroups. However, the broad reactivity of IF can be exploited in screening tests and in epidemiologic studies.

HI and CF Tests

Classical serodiagnosis of arbovirus infections relied on the HI and CF tests. These technically demanding assays rely on the availability of goose or other erthrocytes and have largely been abandoned in favor of the more readily standardizable IgM and IgG ELISAs exept in the largest diagnostic reference laboratories (1). The major advantage of both the HI and the CF test is that species-specific positive-control reagents are not necessary. Consequently, more readily available, experimentally derived antiviral antibodies from mice, rabbits, or goats can be used in these tests.

HI antibodies are long-lived, and for this reason HI has often been used as a screening test, especially in serosurveys. After infection, HI antibodies rise within the first week, peak by the third week, and decline to low levels that may persist for years or decades. HI antibodies arising from a primary infection are relatively specific; however, with second and repeated flavivirus infections (superinfection), such as with DEN, YF, or JE virus, the antibody response broadens and heterologous reactions preclude differentiation of the most recent infection from previous infections. Patients with repeated exposures to flaviviruses routinely develop heterologous antibodies to agents to which they have never been exposed. Often, these heterologous reactions have titers that are equal to or higher than those of the presumed homologous reaction. More specific assays, described below, are required to differentiate these cross-reactions.

The CF test provides a level of specificity intermediate between those of HI and neutralization tests (1). CF antibody levels usually are late to rise, and in some patients they are not detectable until 6 weeks after infection. In up to one-third of proven SLE patients, no CF antibodies can be detected. Because of its insensitivity, the CF test should not be used alone as a diagnostic procedure. The test remains useful for viruses that do not hemagglutinate, such as Colorado tick fever (CTF) virus. The kinetics of the rise and fall (half-life of 2 years) of CF antibody levels can be exploited to identify infections that have occurred relatively recently, in the period after which IgM antibodies have disappeared. The test also is relatively specific in differentiating natural from vaccine-induced immunity to YF virus. Immunized patients generally do not produce detectable CF antibodies to YF virus unless they have had previous flavivirus infections.

Neutralization Test

The serum neutralization test is the most virus-specific test for serologic diagnosis and is used to confirm other serologic testing results (1). The serum dilution-plaque reduction neutralization test performed in cell culture is the standard method; however, animal, especially mouse, protection tests follow the same principle. Dilutions of heat-inactivated serum are added to equal volumes of a viral preparation, known to contain a predetermined viral input dose from previous infectivity titrations. The resulting mixtures of serum, beginning at a 1:10 final dilution, and virus (100 plaques for 35-mm-diameter wells and 25 plaques for 16-mm-diameter wells) are incubated either overnight at 4°C or for 1 h at 37°C for viral neutralization to proceed. The resulting mixtures are used to inoculate confluent cell monolayers and overlaid with a nutrient semisolid or solid medium (methylcellulose, agarose, gum tragacanth, or agar can be used); after a suitable interval (e.g., 2 to 7 days, depending on the virus), when plaques have formed, a vital stain is added to differentiate infected nonviable cells, which appear as unstained plaques, from the uninfected stained monolayer. Neutral red in agar or as a liquid solution is conventionally used, but when removable semisolid overlays are used, a permanent record of the test can be made by fixing the monolayer and staining it with amido black or crystal violet.

Numerous variations of the procedure have been described, including (i) the use of DEAE-dextran or other cationic polymers to reduce electrostatic charges on agar that interfere with virus-cell interactions and (ii) the addition of complement or normal human or animal serum to serum-virus mixtures to increase the sensitivity of neutralization.

The last serum dilution that significantly reduces the input dose of virus is the end point (80 to 90% reduction of the plaque count in the virus control). End points in animal protection assays are calculated by the Reed-Muench or Karber method, and six animals per serum dilution should be the minimum number used.

For viruses that do not produce cytopathic effects, fluorescent focus reduction assays or their equivalent, using enzyme-labeled conjugates, can be used to measure viral neutralization. Similarly, the in situ ELISA technique described above can be applied to automate large-scale tests if 96-well cell culture panels are used.

Neutralizing-antibody levels generally rise within days of the onset of illness, peak in the second week, and decline slowly to moderate or low levels, where they persist for years and often a lifetime. The sensitivity of the test is high, usually equal to that of HI or IF tests, but, most importantly, no other approach is as virus specific.

An alternative approach to measuring the neutralizing power of a serum is the constant serum-varying virus dilution test, resulting in a log neutralization index. This procedure has fallen into disuse because it is somewhat less specific than the serum dilution method and large quantities of serum are needed.

Antigen Detection

Certain arboviruses produce a viremia of sufficient magnitude and duration that the viruses can be isolated from blood during the acute phase of illness, e.g., 0 to 5 days after onset. Epidemiologically, this is significant because during the period of viremia, the viruses may be transmitted from person to person by biting vectors. Examples of these viruses include the agents of YF, DEN, chikungunya, sandfly, RR, and Oropouche fevers. The viremia in CTF is unique because it can extend for weeks or months and infection has been transmitted by transfusion.

While VEE virus can be recovered from the throat of one-fourth of patients, person-to-person spread has not been conclusively proven. SLE virus and certain hantaviruses can be detected in urine (see below). Many encephalitogenic arboviruses can be recovered from CSF obtained during the acute phase of illness, and, rarely, SLE, JE, WEE, and EEE viruses have been recovered from blood. The virus of TBE commonly contaminates milk of infected sheep, cows, and goats, but its occurrence in human milk has not been reported.

Antigen Capture ELISA

Antigen capture ELISA has been used to directly detect antigens of YF, DEN, sandfly fever, Rift Valley fever, Sindbis, and chikungunya viruses directly in blood. In some cases, viral antigens complexed with antibody must first be dissociated by use of a reducing agent, e.g., dithiothreitol. Generally, an overnight incubation of antigen maximizes sensitivity, which approaches 10^3 PFU/0.1 ml. The sensitivity of antigen capture ELISA for YF virus is similar to that of viral isolation from cell cultures, mosquitoes, or mice and is accomplished 3 to 7 days more quickly.

Antigen capture ELISA also has proved useful in epidemiologic surveillance of arbovirus infection rates in vector mosquitoes. A single infected mosquito in a pool can be detected rapidly and cheaply by the direct detection of antigen, allowing greater flexibility and time to implement emergency vector control measures. This approach has been applied to SLE, WN, EEE, and LAC viruses (28). The SLE and EEE virus tests have been converted to a commercial dipstick format. Other arbovirus antigens have been detected directly in sandflies and ticks.

Immunohistochemical Staining

Certain arbovirus infections can be rapidly diagnosed by direct detection of virus-infected cells by IF or other histochemical techniques (see chapter 45 for a general discussion of these procedures). The various causes of potentially fatal viral hemorrhagic fever, including DEN virus, cannot be reliably differentiated on a clinical basis, and immunohistochemical examination of liver tissues is a means by which a specific diagnosis can be reached. When liver biopsy specimens from patients with suspected YF are available, ordinary histopathological examination should be supplemented with more specific immunohistochemical techniques such as indirect IF. Similarly, IF and immunoperoxidase staining of brain biopsy or autopsy specimens have been helpful in differentiating arbovirus infections such as WEE, EEE, and LAC virus infections from other causes of encephalitis.

In disseminated infections such as YF and DEN, viral antigen has been demonstrated in various sites, including myocardium and kidney (YF) and bone marrow, spleen, lymph nodes, and dermal mononuclear cells (DEN) (3).

The CTF virus is unusual because it infects erythrocyte precursors and infected erythrocytes can be detected in peripheral blood for the life of the infected cells. Examination of peripheral blood smears by IF is the most rapid approach to diagnosis and is more sensitive than serology. For patients with RR virus polyarthropathy, IF viral antigen has been found in monocytes and macrophages of synovial exudates, and it has been possible to rapidly identify infected patients by examining fluid from inflamed joints. Peripheral blood mononuclear cells are a principal replicative site for DEN virus and other flaviviruses. DEN and JE virus-infected mononuclear cells have been detected in peripheral blood by IF, and JE virus-infected cells have been found in CSF, making a specific diagnosis possible within hours of a diagnostic lumbar puncture. SLE virus-infected cells have been detected by IF in urinary sediment of some patients, and free viral particles were visualized by electron microscopy; however, virus was not recovered from urine. Patients with suspected viruria had urinary incontinence and other symptoms possibly associated with myelitis.

IF is the simplest approach to identifying viral isolates recovered from clinical samples. The source of the isolate, the rapidity and characteristics of viral growth in cell culture, and mortality patterns and average survival time in mice may provide clues to its identity; e.g., alphaviruses kill suckling mice and produce plaques in cell culture within 1 to 5 days. The basic approach to viral identification is to prepare spot slides with an infected cell culture suspension. After being dried, the slides are fixed in acetone and stained by the indirect method with a series of mouse ascitic grouping fluids, containing antibodies to various groups of arboviruses (National Institutes of Health grouping fluids) or broadly cross-reactive monoclonal antibodies (Table 2). A positive reaction to a single grouping fluid is followed by further IF and neutralization tests with monospecific ascitic fluids or monoclonal antibodies until the virus is identified (4, 20, 21, 23, 24). Inoculated cell cultures that do not show cytopathic effects still should be tested by the aforementioned method because arboviruses may not be lytic in every cell line. Alternatively, frozen brain sections of intracerebrally inoculated suckling mice or squashes of intrathoracically inoculated mosquitoes can be stained by the same procedure. Morphologic characteristics of the isolate should be confirmed by electron microscopy, but definitive antigenic classification requires the production of a homologous antibody (immune mouse ascitic fluid) and cross-serologic tests, especially cross-neutralization tests, with antigenically related agents.

In situ ELISA combines the sensitivity of cell culture systems for viral isolation with the rapidity of ELISA to identify the amplified isolates. Virus in clinical specimens is amplified briefly by growth in cell culture in 96-well panels; after fixation, the resulting amplified cell-associated antigens are detected directly by ELISA in the same vessel. Infected cell cultures can be identified within 24 to 72 h after inoculation, depending on the titer of the inoculum and viral growth characteristics. The approach is especially useful for mass screening, such as for inhibitory effects of candidate antiviral drugs and for viruses that do not produce cytopathic effects. If a long-working-distance objective is available, the monolayer also can be examined microscopically for infected foci.

Detection of Viral Genomic Sequences

In Situ Hybridization

A general outline of the procedure for in situ hybridization is given in chapter 46. In situ hybridization has been used to identify genomic sequences of LAC virus and other bunyaviruses, SIN virus, and DEN virus in mosquitoes; bluetongue virus in sandflies; and DEN and YF virus genomic sequences in formalin-fixed, paraffin-embedded liver tissue (18).

The principal advantage of in situ hybridization over immunohistochemical detection of viral proteins is the greater stability of viral RNA than of viral protein antigens in fixed, embedded specimens. Paraffin-embedded liver samples that had been stored at ambient temperatures for 23 years still had detectable viral RNA when viral antigens were undetectable by immunohistochemical stains. Non-isotope-labeled probes, such as biotin, have been used for the detection of DEN virus in human tissues.

NAATs for the Detection of Arboviruses

A variety of nucleic acid amplification platforms have been successfully utilized for the detection of arboviruses, including standard reverse transcriptase PCR (RT-PCR) (with agarose gel analysis), real-time RT-PCR using fluorescent probes, and nucleic acid sequence-based amplification (NASBA). Each of these technologies will be described below; however, several important issues common to each approach will be presented first. In general, the sensitivity of any of the nucleic acid amplification tests (NAATs) in identifying arboviruses has been shown to be equal to or greater than that of the most sensitive viral isolation procedures (either in cultured cells or in neonatal mice) while providing equal specificity in identifying specific viruses. The dynamics of in vivo viral replication and tissue tropisms must be carefully considered so that the utility of a NAAT to a particular arbovirus can be properly applied and interpreted. For example, the encephalitic flaviviruses (i.e., WN, SLE, and JE viruses) demonstrate a short viremia which is low or absent at the time of clinical presentation of CNS symptoms. With

these viruses, the detection of virus in serum by NAAT (or any method) is typically unproductive and a negative result is not informative. Detection of virus in CSF obtained from meningitis or encephalitis patients is often better. In one study of WN encephalitis patients, virus was detected by a real-time RT-PCR in 14% of acute-phase serum specimens and 57% of CSF specimens (14). In contrast, the DEN viruses often achieve a much higher viremia of longer duration which can be detected by virus isolation or NAAT methods; as a result, NAATs are a good choice for detecting and serotyping the DEN viruses. In general, the alphaviruses demonstrate replication kinetics similar to those of the flaviviruses and are not commonly detected in acute-phase serum and/or CSF specimens, although detection is generally greater than with the flaviviruses. In contrast, NAATs have been highly successful in detecting arboviruses from tissues obtained from fatal human cases when the appropriate tissue target is known and assayed (i.e., brain tissue for WN virus, LAC or EEE virus cases, liver tissue from YF cases, etc.).

The use of NAATs for the detection of arboviruses in surveillance protocols is highly successful, in particular the testing of field-collected mosquitoes. In this application, NAATs have often demonstrated superior sensitivity compared to virus isolation or antigen detection assays. With the addition of automation, these NAAT approaches have been used to test hundreds of mosquito specimens in a single day (26). NAATs have also been successfully utilized in environmental surveillance by detecting arboviruses from tissues obtained from field-collected vertebrate hosts. Detection of WN virus in field-collected dead birds and detection of EEE virus from fatal equine cases are typical applications of this technology.

RNA Extraction and Purification

Most arboviruses have a single-stranded RNA genome, and as a result the sensitivity and specificity of all amplification strategies depend upon the efficient extraction and purification of the target RNA template. In the past, RNA extraction protocols were developed primarily in-house and suffered from inconsistency due to RNA degradation during purification; however, a variety of highly efficient RNA extraction and purification protocols which allow for more rapid, consistent, and high-volume sample processing are now commercially available. Most of these utilize a chaotropic lysis buffer for efficient solubilization and stabilization of RNA from a variety of sources, followed by binding to silica, subsequent washing, and then elution in a low-salt solution. This approach also has been automated, and hundreds of samples can be processed within a single day. The use of a chaotropic lysis buffer has also enabled the efficient extraction of intact RNA from a variety of sources, including serum or plasma, whole blood, CSF, tissues, and homogenized ticks or mosquitoes. The last are particularly useful for environmental surveillance of arboviruses.

Testing Algorithms and Interpretation

Sound testing algorithms for NAATs are necessary to ensure that results have a high degree of confidence. The most desirable testing algorithm is one in which the amplification assays are complemented by another virus detection assay, such as an alternate NAAT, virus isolation, antigen capture ELISA, or direct IF assay. At a minimum, NAAT-positive results should be confirmed by retesting using the same technology with an additional primer set. NAAT assays must also incorporate the appropriate controls to ensure against false-positive or false-negative results. At a minimum, clinical samples should be tested in duplicate. Positive controls included in each assay should contain various levels of target RNA (high, medium, low, etc.) to evaluate the sensitivity of each test in comparison with previous tests. An internal positive control also can be very useful when specimens that may contain inhibitors of RT-PCR (i.e., blood, mosquito lysates, etc.) are tested. In all amplification-based technologies, it is essential that proper laboratory procedures be followed that prevent cross contamination of nascent samples with amplified DNA (amplicon) from previous tests, resulting in the generation of false-positive results. In general, there should be complete physical separation of pre- and postamplification laboratory space and equipment. Of particular importance is the use of several no-template (negative) controls spaced randomly throughout the assay to monitor for amplicon contamination.

RT-PCR

Standard RT-PCR-based assays (compared to the real-time assays described below) to detect arbovirus genomic sequences have been developed for a number of agents (9). These assays use either virus-specific primers or consensus primers that are designed to amplify genetically related viruses. These "first-generation" assays typically involve RT-PCR amplification followed by agarose gel electrophoresis with DNA visualization by staining with ethidium bromide to characterize the amplified DNA by molecular weight. Obtaining a DNA fragment of the predicted size is considered by some to be diagnostic. However, note that in some instances nonspecific amplification can generate DNA products with mobility on agarose gels similar or identical to that of the predicted fragment, which would lead to a false-positive interpretation of results. Greater specificity can be achieved by using sequence-specific approaches for detecting and confirming the identity of the amplified DNA, including hybridization with virus-specific probes (e.g., Southern blot, dot blot, or microtiter plate hybridization), PCR amplification with additional primers internal to the original primers (nested or seminested PCR), restriction endonuclease digestion of the DNA product, or nucleic acid sequence analysis. When consensus primers are utilized, a sequence-specific detection method such as one of those described above must be employed to specifically identify the resulting DNA, since by the design of the assay all related viruses would all be amplified. Consensus RT-PCR assays have been described for alphaviruses, flaviviruses, and the California and Bunyamwera serogroup bunyaviruses (10, 13, 19, 25). Virus-specific assays include assays for the DEN viruses; the YF, JE, WEE, EEE, SLE, MVE, Powassan, TBE, and WN viruses; the California serogroup viruses; and the RR and Ockelbo and CTF viruses.

Real-Time 5'-Exonuclease Fluorogenic Assays (TaqMan)

TaqMan RT-PCR assays combine RT-PCR amplification with fluorescently labeled virus-specific probes able to detect amplified DNA during the amplification reaction. These assays offer numerous advantages over standard RT-PCR, namely, increased sensitivity and specificity, quantitation of initial target RNA, high throughput, and rapid turnaround of results. The increased specificity of the TaqMan assay compared to that of standard RT-PCR is due to the use of the virus-specific internal probe during the amplification. The hybridization of this probe to the target sequence is detectable by the increase in fluorescence in real time. This sequence-specific detection

obviates the need for any postamplification characterization of the amplified DNA. As a result, amplified DNA is not manipulated in the laboratory as occurs with standard RT-PCR, thus greatly reducing the likelihood of amplicon contamination. Real-time fluorogenic assays also offer the advantage of the ability to detect multiple targets at the same time in the same amplification reaction (multiplexing). This can be accomplished by using multiple oligonucleotide probes (up to four in some instruments) each labeled with fluorescent reporter dyes with discrete emission spectra. Several TaqMan assays for the detection of arboviruses have been described, including assays for WN, SLE, TBE, DEN, EEE, WEE, and LAC viruses (11, 14, 16, 29).

NASBA

Another amplification technology which has successfully been used for the detection and identification of arboviruses is NASBA. This approach shows some similarities to RT-PCR at the initial stages. However, there are several significant differences; namely, the reaction is isothermic (41°C); the enzymes utilized are RT, RNase H, and T7 RNA polymerase; and the final amplification product is single-stranded RNA. Amplified RNA can be detected in a sequence-specific manner either by utilizing an electrochemiluminescence probe detection format or by using a fluorescently labeled molecular beacon probe in real time. These approaches have been successfully employed for the detection of a number of arboviruses, including WN, SLE, EEE, WEE, LAC, and DEN viruses (11, 15, 32).

SELECTION AND SEQUENCE OF TESTS

The laboratory diagnosis of an arbovirus infection presents a unique set of problems because of the large number of arbovirus agents that must be considered in a differential diagnosis. The approach is simplified by first considering the viruses according to the clinical illness they produce, e.g., viruses that produce principally CNS infection, hemorrhagic fever, polyarthritis, or nonspecific febrile illnesses with or without a rash (Table 1). The geographic distribution of certain arboviruses may be restricted to certain countries or regions, and the choice of antigens to be included in a diagnostic battery can be reduced further by including only those that are relevant to the patient's history of travel and exposure. If the patient gives a history of exposure to a specific vector, the choice of antigens can be narrowed further; e.g., if the patient reports an attached tick or tick exposure, antigens of tick-borne viruses should be emphasized.

When brain or liver specimens are available from patients with encephalitis or hemorrhagic fever, respectively, the tissues should be submitted for viral isolation and detection of viral genome or antigens. The tissue should be divided, and portions should be fixed in buffered formalin for histochemical staining and frozen in liquid N_2 on dry ice or in a mechanical freezer at −70°C for viral isolation or molecular detection. If sufficient quantities are available, tissues in 10% (wt/vol) suspensions should be used to inoculate cell cultures and to intracerebrally inoculate suckling mice for viral isolation. While areas of the cerebral cortex have served as good sources of virus and antigen for many arboviruses, recent experience with WN virus suggested that more virus and antigen can be obtained from the brain stem and spinal cord. This observation is supported by the flaccid paralysis demonstrated by WN virus-infected patients.

Although a probable diagnosis sometimes can be made serologically from a single serum specimen, paired sera should always be used when possible. In patients with a CNS infection, an accompanying CSF sample should be requested routinely. The MAC-ELISA is more sensitive when CSF samples are tested, and IgM can often be demonstrated in CSF slightly earlier than in acute-phase serum. MAC-ELISA is now the serologic test of first choice in the laboratory diagnosis of arbovirus infections because of its sensitivity and the possibility that a presumptive diagnosis can be made in an early stage of infection.

The conventional sequence of serologic testing, which is still a valid and sensitive approach, is to test paired sera to quantify a change in antibody titer. Often, an elevated titer in an acute-phase serum sample is sufficient information upon which to make a presumptive diagnosis. If heterologous reactions are present, the sera are tested subsequently by neutralization to better elucidate the cause of infection.

INTERPRETATION OF RESULTS

Serologic test results should be interpreted in the context of the clinical and epidemiologic features of the case. Heterologous antibodies from previous infections or from immunizations (namely, to YF) may interfere with the correct interpretation of a result, especially if serum specimens are tested by a single screening assay. For example, anti-SLE virus antibody may be present in people who previously were infected with DEN virus during travel or residence in tropical countries of South or Central America or Asia. Unless changes in antibody titer or specific IgM antibody levels are demonstrable or more specific tests are done, it may be difficult to differentiate these reactions. Epidemiologically and clinically, fourfold changes in serum antibody titer or the presence of virus-specific IgM in CSF confirms a recent infection.

Until the introduction of WN virus into the United States, the incidence of arbovirus infections had been low and the diseases occurred in certain geographic locations or episodically. Seroprevalence remains low, except in areas where WN virus outbreaks have been documented or where LAC virus is transmitted in an endemic pattern. Therefore, the discovery of specific arbovirus antibodies in a single serum specimen of an ill patient is likely to be associated with a recent infection. The recent introduction of WN virus into the United States has also complicated the serodiagnosis of SLE virus infections in regions where these viruses may cocirculate (12). Seroprevalence to EEE virus is the lowest among all the domestic arboviruses, and the positive predictive value of a single seroreactive serum sample for other arboviruses depends on the clinical and epidemiological circumstances of the case. For example, the majority of SLE virus infections are asymptomatic or result in mild symptoms of headache and fever. The probability of SLE in seroreactive patients without frank signs of CNS infection normally is low, but in an epidemic, seroreactions in patients with less distinctive symptoms, such as acute fever and headache, may have a high predictive value.

The interpretation of ELISA results is not standardized, and the significance of raw absorbance values has been determined by methods established in individual laboratories. Thorough evaluations of the operating characteristics of arbovirus ELISAs have been hampered by the large number of agents for which assays must be established and the scarcity of positive human specimens for rare infections. A frequently used standard for a positive absorbance value is 3 standard errors above the mean absorbance of a sample of known negative sera. An alternative approach is to calculate the ratio of the sample absorbances with test (positive) and control (negative) antibodies (positive-to-negative ratio). With the diagnosis of RR and JE virus infections, a binding index, in which the sample absorbance is expressed in units in relation to the absorbance of a known positive sample, has also been used.

The isolation and identification of an arbovirus or its antigen or viral genomic sequences in a clinical sample generally are specific evidence of a recent infection. With few exceptions, arboviruses cause acute self-limited infections without persistence or latency. Certain flavivirus infections, however, cause subacute or persistent CNS infection. A progressive degenerative infection of the brain stem and cervical spinal cord leading to paralysis and atrophy of the shoulder girdle and upper arm after infection with viruses of the tick-borne flavivirus complex has been described, and in a small proportion of patients with JE, clearance from the CNS is delayed for several months after the onset of acute illness. Experimental infection of monkeys with WN virus, another flavivirus, also results in persistent CNS infection. IgM antibodies to YF virus remain detectable in a large proportion of patients for years or decades following infection or immunization, leading to the suspicion that this flavivirus persists in some individuals. Infections with certain viruses of the *Bunyaviridae* family also are followed by persistent silent infections in animals, of which the clearest examples are the lifelong infections of rodents with Hantaan, Seoul, and Prospect Hill viruses and other hantaviruses. There is no evidence, however, of persistent bunyavirus infections in humans.

CONCLUSIONS

Arbovirus infections in the wealthy countries of the world are usually rare events. As a result, funding for research on arborviruses had fallen dramatically, resulting in only small advances and improvements in the diagnosis of arboviral infections. Two events which have shifted these priorities have occurred in recent years. One is the renewed emphasis on preparedness for bioterrorist events. Three of these arboviruses (VEE, EEE, and WEE viruses) have been classified as possible biological threats. This designation has renewed interest in rapid and sensitive diagnosis of alphaviruses. The second event was the introduction of WN virus into the Western Hemisphere for the first time, reminding us of the ease with which new and emerging infections can travel great distances. As mentioned above, the introduction of a second mosquito-borne flaviviral encephalitis virus into the United States resets the diagnostic algorithms. It will be imperative for the diagnostic virologist to keep close watch for new, faster, and more sensitive diagnostic methods which will undoubtedly result from this new level of recognition of this group of viral pathogens.

REFERENCES

1. **Beaty, B. J., C. H. Calisher, and R. W. Shope.** 1989. Arboviruses, p. 797–856. *In* N. J. Schmidt and R. W. Emmons (ed.), *Diagnostic Procedures for Viral, Rickettsial and Chlamydial Infections*, 6th ed. American Public Health Association, Washington, D.C.
2. **Burke, D. S., A. Nisalak, M. A. Ussery, T. Laorakpongse, and S. Chantavibul.** 1985. Kinetics of IgM and IgG responses to Japanese encephalitis virus in human serum and cerebrospinal fluid. *J. Infect. Dis.* **151:**1093–1099.
3. **De Brito, T., S. A. Siqueira, R. T. Santos, E. S. Nassar, T. L. Coimbra, and V. A. Alves.** 1992. Human fatal yellow fever. Immunohistochemical detection of viral antigens in the liver, kidney and heart. *Pathol. Res. Pract.* **188:**177–181.

4. **Hunt, A. R., and J. T. Roehrig.** 1985. Biochemical and biological characteristics of epitopes on the E1 glycoprotein of western equine encephalitis virus. *Virology* **142:**334–346.

5. **Innis, B. L., A. Nisalak, S. Nimmannitya, S. Kusalerdchariya, V. Chongswasdi, S. Suntayakorn, P. Puttisri, and C. H. Hoke.** 1989. An enzyme-linked immunosorbent assay to characterize dengue infections where dengue and Japanese encephalitis co-circulate. *Am. J. Trop. Med. Hyg.* **40:**418–427.

6. **Johnson, A. J., D. M. Martin, N. Karabatsos, and J. T. Roehrig.** 2000. Detection of anti-arboviral IgG by using a monoclonal antibody-based capture ELISA. *J. Clin. Microbiol.* **38:**1827–1831.

7. **Johnson, A. J., D. A. Martin, N. Karabatsos, and J. T. Roehrig.** 2000. Detection of anti-arboviral immunoglobulin G by using a monoclonal antibody-based capture enzyme-linked immunosorbent assay. *J. Clin. Microbiol.* **38:**1827–1831.

8. **Karabatsos, N.** 1985. *International Catalogue of Arboviruses.* American Society for Tropical Medicine and Hygiene, San Antonio, Tex.

9. **Kuno, G.** 1998. Universal diagnostic RT-PCR protocol for arboviruses. *J. Virol. Methods* **72:**27–41.

10. **Kuno, G., C. J. Mitchell, G. J. Chang, and G. C. Smith.** 1996. Detecting bunyaviruses of the Bunyamwera and California serogroups by a PCR technique. *J. Clin. Microbiol.* **34:**1184–1188.

11. **Lambert, A. J., D. A. Martin, and R. S. Lanciotti.** 2003. Detection of North American eastern and western equine encephalitis viruses by nucleic acid amplification assays. *J. Clin. Microbiol.* **41:**379–385.

12. **Lanciotti, R. S., J. T. Roehrig, V. Deubel, J. Smith, M. Parker, K. Steele, B. Crise, K. E. Volpe, M. B. Crabtree, J. Scherret, R. Hall, J. MacKenzie, C. B. Cropp, B. Panigrahy, E. Ostlund, B. Schmitt, M. Malkinson, C. Banet, J. Weissman, N. Komar, and H. Savage.** 1999. Origin of the West Nile virus responsible for an outbreak of encephalitis in the northeastern U.S. *Science* **286:**2333–2337.

13. **Lanciotti, R. S., C. H. Calisher, D. J. Gubler, G. J. Chang, and A. V. Vorndam.** 1992. Rapid detection and typing of dengue viruses from clinical samples by using reverse transcriptase polymerase chain reaction. *J. Clin. Microbiol.* **30:**545–551.

14. **Lanciotti, R. S., A. J. Kerst, R. S. Nasci, M. S. Godsey, C. J. Mitchell, H. M. Savage, N. Komar, N. A. Panella, B. C. Allen, K. E. Volpe, B. S. Davis, and J. T. Roehrig.** 2000. Rapid detection of West Nile virus from human clinical specimens, field-collected mosquitoes, and avian samples by a TaqMan reverse transcriptase-PCR assay. *J. Clin. Microbiol.* **38:**4066–4071.

15. **Lanciotti, R. S., and A. J. Kerst.** 2001. Nucleic acid sequence-based amplification assays for rapid detection of West Nile and St. Louis encephalitis viruses. *J. Clin. Microbiol.* **39:**4506–4513.

16. **Laue, T., P. Emmerich, and H. Schmitz.** 1999. Detection of dengue virus RNA in patients after primary or secondary dengue infection by using the TaqMan automated amplification system. *J. Clin. Microbiol.* **37:**2543–2547.

17. **Monath, T. P.** 1988. *Arboviruses: Epidemiology and Ecology,* vol. 1. CRC Press, Boca Raton, Fla.

18. **Monath, T. P., M. E. Ballinger, B. R. Miller, and J. J. Salaun.** 1989. Detection of yellow fever viral RNA by nucleic acid hybridization and viral antigen by immunocytochemistry in fixed human liver. *Am. J. Trop. Med. Hyg.* **40:**663–668.

19. **Pfeffer, M., B. Proebster, R. M. Kinney, and O. R. Kaaden.** 1997. Genus-specific detection of alphaviruses by a seminested reverse transcription-polymerase chain reaction. *Am. J. Trop. Med. Hyg.* **57:**709–718.

20. **Roehrig, J. T.** 1986. The use of monoclonal antibodies in studies of the structural proteins of alphaviruses and flaviviruses, p. 251–278. *In* S. Schlesinger and M. J. Schlesinger (ed.), *The Viruses: The Togaviridae and Flaviviridae.* Plenum Press, New York, N.Y.

21. **Roehrig, J. T., and R. A. Bolin.** 1997. Monoclonal antibodies capable of distinguishing epizootic from enzootic varieties of subtype 1 Venezuelan equine encephalitis viruses in a rapid indirect immunofluorescence assay. *J. Clin. Microbiol.* **35:**1887–1890.

22. **Roehrig, J. T., T. M. Brown, A. J. Johnson, N. Karabatsos, D. M. Martin, C. J. Mitchell, and R. Nasci.** 1998. Alphaviruses, p. 7–18. *In* J. R. Stephenson and A. Warnes (ed.), *Methods in Molecular Biology: Diagnostic Virology Protocols.* Humana Press, Totowa, N.J.

23. **Roehrig, J. T., A. R. Hunt, G. J. Chang, B. Sheik, R. A. Bolin, T. F. Tsai, and D. W. Trent.** 1990. Identification of monoclonal antibodies capable of differentiating antigenic varieties of eastern equine encephalitis viruses. *Am. J. Trop. Med. Hyg.* **42:**394–398.

24. **Roehrig, J. T., J. H. Mathews, and D. W. Trent.** 1983. Identification of epitopes on the E glycoprotein of Saint Louis encephalitis virus using monoclonal antibodies. *Virology* **128:**118–126.

25. **Scaramozzino, N., J.-M. Crance, A. Jouan, D. A. DeBriel, F. Stoll, and D. Garin.** 2001. Comparison of *Flavivirus* universal primer pairs and development of a rapid, highly sensitive heminested reverse transcription-PCR assay for detection of flaviviruses targeted to a conserved region of the NS5 gene sequences. *J. Clin. Microbiol.* **39:**1922–1927.

26. **Shi, P. Y., E. B. Kauffman, P. Ren, A. Felton, J. H. Tai, A. P. Dupuis II, S. A. Jones, A. Ngo, D. C. Nicholas, J. Maffei, G. D. Ebel, K. A. Bernard, and L. D. Kramer.** 2001. High-throughput detection of West Nile virus RNA. *J. Clin. Microbiol.* **39:**1264–1271.

27. **Tsai, T. F.** 1995. Arboviruses, p. 980–996. *In* P. R. Murray, E. J. Baron, M. A. Pfaller, F. C. Tenover, and R. H. Yolken (ed.), *Manual of Clinical Microbiology,* 6th ed. American Society for Microbiology, Washington, D.C.

28. **Tsai, T. F., R. A. Bolin, M. Montoya, R. E. Bailey, D. B. Francy, M. Jozan, and J. T. Roehrig.** 1987. Detection of St. Louis encephalitis virus antigen in mosquitoes by capture enzyme immunoassay. *J. Clin. Microbiol.* **25:**370–376.

29. **Wicki, R., P. Sauter, C. Mettler, A. Natsch, T. Enzler, N. Pusterla, P. Kuhnert, G. Egli, M. Bernasconi, R. Lienhard, H. Lutz, and C. M. Leutenegger.** 2000. Swiss Army Survey in Switzerland to determine the prevalence of *Francisella tularensis,* members of the Ehrlichia phagocytophila genogroup, Borrelia burgdorferi sensu lato, and tick-borne encephalitis virus in ticks. *Eur. J. Clin. Microbiol. Infect. Dis.* **19:**427–432.

30. **Wong, S. J., R. H. Boyle, V. L. Demarest, A. N. Woodmansee, L. D. Kramer, H. Li, M. Drebot, R. A. Koski, E. Fikrig, D. A. Martin, and P. Y. Shi.** 2003. Immunoassay targeting nonstructural protein 5 to differentiate West Nile virus infection from dengue and St. Louis encephalitis virus infection and from flavivirus vaccination. *J. Clin. Microbiol.* **41:**4217–4223.

31. **Wong, S. A., V. L. Demarest, R. H. Boyle, T. Wang, M. Ledizet, K. Kar, L. D. Kramer, E. Fikrig, and R. A. Koski.** 2004. Detection of human anti-flavivirus antibodies with a West Nile virus recombinant antigen microsphere immunoassay. *J. Clin. Microbiol.* **42:**65–72.

32. **Wu, S. J., E. M. Lee, R. Putvatana, R. N. Shurtliff, K. R. Porter, W. Suharyono, D. M. Watts, C. C. King, G. S. Murphy, C. G. Hayes, and J. R. Romano.** 2001. Detection of dengue viral RNA using a nucleic acid sequence-based amplification assay. *J. Clin. Microbiol.* **39:**2794–2798.

Hantavirus Infections

BRIAN HJELLE AND STEPHEN A. YOUNG

86

The genus *Hantavirus* is composed of plus-strand RNA viruses within the family *Bunyaviridae* (22, 23). The members of the genus *Hantavirus* have a tripartite single-stranded RNA genome, an enveloped virion containing two viral transmembrane glycoproteins, and a helical nucleocapsid. The individual hantaviruses each cause persistent infections of one or a small number of closely related rodent species that serve as the primary natural reservoir(s). The genomic RNA segments are named according to their size: the mRNA from the large segment, L, encodes an RNA-dependent RNA polymerase and endonuclease (200 kDa); the mRNA from the middle (M) segment encodes the precursor (GPC) for the two glycoproteins, G1 (72 kDa) and G2 (56 kDa); and the mRNA from the small (S) genomic segment encodes the nucleocapsid protein (50 kDa).

OLD WORLD HANTAVIRUSES

The genus is named for the prototypical virus species, Hantaan virus (HTNV). The disease caused by Hantaan virus, now called hemorrhagic fever with renal syndrome (HFRS), came to the attention of western medicine during the Korean war, when soldiers presented with symptoms of fever, hemorrhage, hypotension, and renal failure (6). The rodent associated with Korean hemorrhagic fever was identified when Lee and his coworkers showed that human convalescent-phase sera react with antigen in the lungs of a particular species of field mice, *Apodemus agrarius* (18). Because the mice were captured in the Hantaan river basin of Korea, the prototype virus was called Hantaan virus. Serial propagation of Hantaan virus in *A. agrarius* resulted in the first continuous source of viral antigen for laboratory testing, but the virus was later adapted to cell culture. The isolation of HTNV was followed shortly thereafter by the isolation of two other common causes of milder forms of HFRS: the European Puumala virus (PUUV) followed by the commensal rat-borne Seoul virus (SEOV), which, despite its worldwide distribution, causes disease almost exclusively in Eastern Asia (22).

Over the ensuing few years, investigators from several continents isolated additional viruses that antigenically, morphologically and genetically resembled the pathogenic strains but were known solely from their presence among field rodents. The identification of those distinctive molecular and morphologic features enabled investigators to recognize that a number of different isolates collectively could be grouped under a single genus of the family *Bunyaviridae* (23). Since then, investigators have recognized that hantaviruses fall into three major clades (groups of viruses sharing a common ancestor), based on their serologic, genetic, and epidemiologic features (22). All of the viral groups except for the shrew-borne Thottapalayam virus are carried by rodents of the family *Muridae*, but members of each clade are carried by rodents of a different subfamily: *Sigmodontinae*, *Murinae*, and *Arvicolinae*. These three groups include the New World clade, which encompasses all of the viruses that have been linked to hantavirus cardiopulmonary syndrome (HCPS or HPS) and which is associated with rodents of the subfamily *Sigmodontinae*; the Old World clade, including HTNV, which is carried by rodents of the subfamily *Murinae*; and the clade carried by voles of the subfamily *Arvicolinae*, which are indigenous to both the Old World and New World.

NEW WORLD HANTAVIRUSES

Serological surveys in the United States revealed the presence of HTNV or related virus enzootic in domestic rats as well as several autochthonous rodent species (27). Several viruses were isolated that were serologically distinct from HTNV but grouped with Seoul virus. In the early 1980s, the prototypical indigenous North American hantavirus, Prospect Hill virus (PHV), was isolated from the lung tissue of a vole, *Microtus pennsylvanicus* (P. W. Lee, H. L. Amyx, D. C. Gajdusek, R. T. Yanagihara, D. Goldgaber, and C. J. Gibbs, Jr., Letter, *Lancet* **ii**: 1405, 1982). During the 1980s, investigators detected numerous patients from the United States with evidence of past exposure to one or another hantavirus through serological surveys of healthy blood donors, but the results were difficult to interpret with the information that was available at that time (27). Attempts to identify autochthonous cases of HFRS in the New World went largely unrewarded, although a few cases caused by SEOV were eventually detected among residents of inner-city Baltimore and possible cases were also identified in coastal Brazil.

Clinicians and medical investigators reported a cluster of cases of an unexplained and frequently fatal acute illness in the southwestern United States in the spring of 1993 (20). The disease, HCPS, evolves in three stages: the prodromal, cardiorespiratory, and convalescent phases (19). Patients in the prodromal phase of HCPS most frequently report symptoms of fever, chills, myalgias, nausea and vomiting. The prodromal phase, which usually lasts 3 to 6 days, is followed by a pulmonary phase during which the patient experiences shortness of breath and cough. Laboratory findings either at presentation or during disease progression include elevated lactate dehydrogenase and aspartate aminotransferase levels in serum, metabolic acidosis, prolonged partial thromboplastin time, hemoconcentration, leukocytosis with a specific pattern of atypical lymphocytes (immunoblasts), and highly immature granulocytes, often including myelocytes or promyelocytes in the peripheral smear (16, 19). Many patients with HCPS require intubation and mechanical ventilation to treat progressive hypoxemia due to noncardiogenic pulmonary edema. During the intubation, providers sometimes must remove impressive amounts of a flaxen proteinaceous fluid by endotracheal suctioning, as much as 1 liter per h. A significant number of patients have unmanageable hypotension that results in death.

In the midst of the original outbreak in 1993, after extensive local efforts to identify a pathogen were unsuccessful, the Centers for Disease Control and Prevention (CDC) in Atlanta tested serum samples from HCPS patients for specific antibodies against known hantaviruses, using an immunoglobulin M (IgM) capture enzyme immunoassay (EIA) and an IgG EIA. The antigen source for these assays consisted of lysates of Vero E6 cells that had been infected with HTNV, SEOV, Puumala, or Prospect Hill viruses. The low-titer and rather mixed patterns of reactivity to these four viral antigens suggested that the patients had become infected with a previously unrecognized hantavirus (20). This initial impression was confirmed when the cDNA of a newly recognized hantavirus, now called Sin Nombre virus (SNV), was amplified from the tissues of several patients by reverse transcription-PCR (RT-PCR) with consensus primers (10, 20).

Armed with genetic and serologic evidence that a new hantavirus was circulating in the Four Corners region of the United States, investigators conducted intensive trapping in the vicinity of case households in an attempt to identify a rodent reservoir for SNV. The most frequently captured rodent was *Peromyscus maniculatus* (the deer mouse), and deer mice were the most frequently serologically positive rodent captured during the initial investigation (20). The nucleotide sequence of the amplimer obtained from the lung tissue of a deer mouse captured at a case-patient's residence was nearly identical to that of the amplimer obtained from the tissues of the patient obtained at necropsy, lending further support to the hypothesis that the patient had contracted the virus from a deer mouse. This suspicion was abundantly confirmed through further investigation (13). It was not for another 5 to 6 months that virologists at CDC and the U.S. Army Medical Research Institute of Infectious Diseases first isolated SNV from the tissues of wild infected deer mice by serial passages in laboratory *P. maniculatus* and/or by direct inoculation of Vero E6 cells.

Originally, because the primary focus of the disease was the lung, the disease was termed hantavirus pulmonary syndrome (HPS). More recently, as investigators came to realize that most deaths due to SNV infection occur from declining cardiac output rather than from noncardiogenic pulmonary edema, many publications have referred to the syndrome as hantavirus cardiopulmonary syndrome (HCPS).

Several cases of HCPS that occurred outside the range of *P. maniculatus* have been investigated, leading to the recognition of three other etiologic agents in North America. These investigations revealed four known or presumed cases of HCPS due to Bayou virus that occurred in Louisiana and eastern Texas (8, 24). Investigators later determined that the predominant carrier rodent for Bayou hantavirus is the rice

rat *Oryzomys palustris* (24; N. Torrez-Martinez and B. Hjelle, Letter, *Lancet* **346**:780–781, 1995). In another case, a patient from Dade County, Fla., contracted HCPS, and while the pathogen was never conclusively identified at the molecular level, the presence of a novel SNV-like agent called Black Creek Canal virus (BCCV) in nearby cotton rats (*Sigmodon hispidus*) led investigators to conclude that BCCV was the etiologic agent (15). Two hantavirus infections that were both traced to exposures in Shelter Island, N.Y., in the mid-1990s led to fatal cases of HCPS in patients from Rhode Island and New York. The etiologic virus, now called New York virus (NYV or sometimes NY-1V), is a distinctive SNV-like pathogen that is carried by island populations of white-footed mice, *P. leucopus* (11; J. W. Song, L. J. Baek, D. J. Gajdusek, R. Yanagihara, I. Gavrilovskaya, B. J. Luft, E. R. Mackow, and B. Hjelle, Letter, *Lancet* **344**:1637, 1994).

The four species of rodents that carry the viruses that are implicated in causing HCPS in the United States have a host range that encompasses the contiguous United States and a large part of Canada and Mexico. As of 1 September 2004, 49 cases of HCPS had been confirmed in Canada, with most cases occurring in the three westernmost provinces (H. Artsob, personal communication). Although most Central American countries and Mexico have reported no cases, Panama has recognized endemic cases of hantavirus infection since 2000, with a collective total of 64 cases as of November 2004 (25; J. M. Pascale, personal communication). The etiologic agent, Choclo virus, is distinct from known North and South American hantaviruses, and the associated disease is unusually mild, causing relatively little cardiac depression and an overall case fatality ratio of 15%.

The proposed existence of hantaviruses indigenous to South America was confirmed by the description of Rio Mamoré virus in pygmy rice rats (*Oligoryzomys microtis*) in early 1996 (B. Hjelle, N. Torrez-Martinez, and F. T. Koster, Letter, *Lancet* **347**:57, 1996). Subsequent surveillance for HCPS-like diseases in South America resulted in the identification of both HCPS epidemics and sporadic cases. HCPS has been detected in Argentina, Bolivia, Brazil, Chile, Paraguay, and Uruguay. One prototypical etiologic agent of HCPS, Andes virus, is phylogenetically rather more closely related to Bayou virus and BCCV than it is to SNV, and it causes a form of HCPS with increased renal involvement, similar to that described for Bayou virus and BCCV. At the molecular level, Andes virus is closely allied to and may be synonymous with forms with designations such as Oran, Bermejo, Castelo dos Sonhos, Araraquara, Lechiguanas, and Juquitiba viruses. Andes virus is the only hantavirus for which person-to-person transmission of HCPS has been described, with the first examples occurring during an outbreak in Argentina in 1996 (21). Additional subsequent examples of interpersonal transmission of Andes virus have certainly occurred but as of yet have not been reported in the peer-reviewed literature; at present it appears that sexual contacts may be at substantially increased risk of disease relative to nonsexual contacts (M. Ferres, personal communication). However, the great majority of cases in South America are sporadic cases associated with exposure to infected rodents. Collectively approximately 600 cases have been recorded in Argentina, 400 have been recorded in Chile, 350 have been recorded in Brazil, and 20 have been recorded in each of Uruguay and Bolivia since HCPS was first recognized in South America.

In 1997, investigators reported 23 laboratory-confirmed cases of a rather less severe form of HCPS in Paraguay that were linked to Laguna Negra virus, a Rio Mamoré-like virus carried by the vesper mouse (*Calomys laucha*). Serological testing of the population during this outbreak revealed a high hantavirus antibody prevalence in the indigenous population. Although the indigenous Indians constituted a majority of the antibody-positive population, the population with Mennonite ancestry constituted the majority of confirmed HCPS cases (26). It is thought that all or nearly all of the approximately 75 cases of HCPS occurring in Paraguay were caused by Laguna Negra virus, which is closely allied to the *Oligoryzomys*-borne Rio Mamoré virus. A list of pathogenic New World hantaviruses and their primary rodent vector, disease, and geographic distribution is presented in Table 1.

CLINICAL INDICATIONS

The CDC established clinical and postmortem screening criteria for HCPS in persons with respiratory disease of unknown origin: (i) a febrile illness ($>101°F$ [$>38.3°C$]) occurring in a previously healthy person, characterized by an unexplained adult respiratory distress syndrome; (ii) bilateral interstitial pulmonary infiltrates developing within 1 week of hospitalization with respiratory compromise requiring supplemental oxygen; or (iii) an unexplained respiratory illness resulting in death in conjunction with an autopsy examination demonstrating noncardiogenic pulmonary edema without an identifiable cause of death. For the diagnosis of HCPS to be confirmed, one or more of the following diagnostic markers must be positive: (i) presence of hantavirus-specific IgM or rising titers of IgG, (ii) presence of hantavirus RNA by RT-PCR, and (iii) positive immunohistochemistry for hantavirus antigen.

In practice, HCPS in its more fulminant forms presents in a very stereotypical manner, with a constellation of clinical abnormalities that has scant overlap with other disease entities (19). The clinical diagnosis of HCPS during the prodromal phase of illness is more problematic, because the clinical characteristics are so nonspecific that it is difficult to make a diagnosis on initial presentation. Other conditions that can mimic HCPS depend on the geographic region. In North America those conditions might include influenza or community-acquired pneumonia in many areas and septicemic plague in the southwestern United States, but in Latin America such conditions as dengue fever or leptospirosis may present with symptoms similar to early HCPS. Laboratory findings that may help confirm hantavirus infection progressing to hypoxemia/pulmonary edema are (i) low albumin levels in serum (<3.5 g/dl) or a decreasing albumin level in serum, (ii) thrombocytopenia ($<150,000$ platelets/μl) or a decreasing platelet count, and (iii) presence of circulating immunoblasts (16). While unfortunately it is uncommon for HCPS to be suspected during the prodromal phase of illness, serological tests or RT-PCR for viral RNA with peripheral blood mononuclear cell (PBMC) or blood clot RNA as the template are generally positive in all but the smallest fraction of very earliest cases (9, 12).

SPECIMENS

The specimen requirement for serological testing is blood drawn into a serum collection tube (red top) that contains no additive but is silicone coated. For ideal diagnostic purposes, the sample should be drawn at or immediately following admission, a second specimen should be drawn just before the samples are shipped for testing, and a third should be drawn 3 weeks after the first sample. For autopsy samples, heart blood should be collected in a red-top tube. The blood should be centrifuged, and the serum should be aliquoted. The aliquot used for testing can be stored at 4°C for 24 h but should be frozen at $-70°C$ if more than 24 h will elapse before testing can be performed. The sample may be shipped either frozen or on ice pack, and such samples are not considered to be "etiologic agents" for purposes of shipment even if the patient is already known to have HCPS.

CDC HANTAVIRUS EIA

Reagents

The CDC supplies state and public health laboratories with reagents needed to perform anti-SNV IgG and IgM EIA assays (5). The IgG EIA antigen is affinity-purified SNV nucleocapsid fusion protein expressed in *Escherichia coli*, and control antigen is affinity-purified protein expressed from the vector in which the SNV nucleoprotein gene was inserted in the opposite orientation and the fusion was expressed in *E. coli* (7). The IgM EIA antigen is a gamma-irradiated lysate prepared from SNV-infected Vero E6 cells in serum diluent, and the control antigen is a gamma-irradiated lysate prepared

TABLE 1 Pathogenic New World hantaviruses and their suspected rodent hosts

Virus	Rodent host	Disease	Geographic distribution
Sin Nombre virus	*Peromyscus maniculatus*	HCPS	United States except Gulf Coast, Canada except far north
New York virus	*Peromyscus leucopus*	HCPS	Shelter Island, Long Island, N.Y. (*P. leucopus* is more widespread, but through most of its range it is a minor carrier of SNV)
Bayou virus	*Oryzomus palustris*	HCPS	Southern United States
Black Creek Canal virus	*Sigmodon hispidus* (eastern form)	HCPS	Florida
Andes virus (including variant forms such as Oran, Juquitiba, Araraquara, Pergamino Lechiguanas, Hu39641, and Bermejo viruses)	*Oligoryzomys longicaudatus* (*Oligoryzomys chacoensis* for Bermejo virus)	HCPS	Argentina, Brazil, and Chile
Laguna Negra virus	*Calomys laucha*	HCPS	Paraguay and Bolivia
Choclo virus	*Oligoryzomys fulvescens*	HCPS	Panama

from uninfected Vero E6 cells in the serum diluent. Additional reagents required for these assays include human sera positive for SNV IgG and IgM, human sera negative for SNV, and hyperimmune mouse ascitic fluid containing antibodies directed against the SNV nucleocapsid antigen (17).

IgM Test Procedure

The IgM EIA is an immune capture procedure in which specific and nonspecific human IgM is first captured using an anti-human mu chain. The wells of microtiter plates are precoated overnight with the anti-human mu chain antibody. The coated plates may be prepared weekly. The titer of each serum sample is determined in duplicate in fourfold dilutions starting at 1:100 and ending at 1:6,400. The bound anti-mu antibody captures IgM antibodies of all specificities. The plate is then washed, SNV-infected cell lysate is added to rows A through D, and lysates from the uninfected cells are added to rows E through H. The antigen binds any plate-bound anti-hantavirus-specific IgM. Bound antigen is detected in a three-step process. The first step involves incubation with an anti-SNV nucleocapsid hyperimmune mouse ascitic fluid, which sandwiches N antigen that was captured by the IgM. The second detection reagent is a horseradish peroxidase-conjugated anti-mouse IgG (heavy and light chains), and the final reagent is 2,2-azinobis (3-ethylbenzthiazolinesulfonic acid) (ABTS)–peroxide substrate. The optical density (OD) of the color reaction is read spectrophometrically.

Interpretation of IgM Test Results

Quality control measures used in each run are an IgM-positive sample run in duplicate and an IgM-negative sample run in duplicate, along with up to four samples in duplicate. The results are interpreted by subtracting the OD value of each serum dilution well without SNV antigen from the OD value of the corresponding serum dilution well that contains SNV antigen. A dilution is considered to be positive if the corrected OD value is greater than 0.1. The test is reported as positive if any dilution above 1:100 is positive. A sample that is positive only at the 1:100 dilution is not reported as positive, but the test is repeated. Quality assurance for acceptable test variation can be judged by summing the OD values of the controls in each assay and monitoring the summation over time for fluctuations in the signals.

The sensitivity and specificity of this assay are high but must be viewed with caution. There is no "gold standard" to which any HCPS serological assay can be compared. As of September 2004, the CDC listed a cumulative total of only 379 cases in the United States (http://www.cdc.gov/ncidod/diseases/hanta/hps/noframes/caseinfo.htm). Therefore, the total number of positive samples is limited, meaning that only tests with excellent specificity will have acceptable predictive value when positive. Samples collected early in the course of illness have occasionally had specific IgM that was missed by EIA, but fortunately many or most such samples can be detected by a strip immunoblot assay (SIA). Few non-HCPS patient samples have been positive for anti-SNV IgM; therefore, the specificity appears to be close to 100% and the sensitivity appears to be in the upper 90% range.

IgG Test Procedure

The IgG test is also performed in a microtiter format but is different in that the antigen preparation, the affinity-purified nucleoprotein fusion expressed in *E. coli*, is itself used to coat rows A through D. Rows E through H are coated with affinity-purified control fusion antigen expressed in *E. coli*. The

dilution scheme used for the IgG assay is identical to the IgM assay, and horseradish peroxidase-conjugated mouse anti-human IgG (heavy and light chain) is used for detection.

Interpretation of IgG Test Results

The OD value of the serum dilutions with antigen is corrected by subtracting the OD obtained from the no-antigen control well with the corresponding dilution of serum. The serum dilution is considered positive for anti-hantavirus IgG if the corrected OD value is greater than 0.2. In the IgG assay, any dilution with an OD over 0.2 is interpreted as a positive result. The sensitivity of this assay is close to 100% in samples collected late in the course of illness but is about 60% in samples collected very early in the disease process. The specificity is high, but precise numbers are not available.

COMMERCIAL HANTAVIRUS EIA

Hantavirus IgM EIA and hantavirus IgG EIA are also available commercially from Focus Diagnostics (Los Angeles, Calif.) as research use only (RUO) kits. Information regarding these kits can be obtained at the Focus Diagnostics web site (http://www.focustechnologies.com/focus/0-home/index.asp).

Reagents

Hantavirus N antigens are coated onto 12 eight-well polystyrene microwells. The antigen is a cocktail of baculovirus-expressed recombinant N proteins, derived from HNTV, SEOV, PUUV, Dobrava virus, and SNV.

Procedure for Anti-Hantavirus IgM Test

Each specimen or control serum is diluted 1:101 in IgM sample diluent. The sample diluent contains anti-human IgG and binds IgG in the samples. After incubation, the IgM conjugate is added to all of the wells, followed by substrate reagent. After 10 min, the reaction is stopped by the addition of 100 μl of stop reagent. The OD of each well is measured at 450 nm.

Procedure for Anti-Hantavirus IgG Test

Samples (100 μl) of each specimen as well as the control samples and calibrator are diluted 1:2 in sample diluent, after microwell pretreatment. The remainder of the procedure is identical to the IgM procedure.

Test Interpretation and Quality Control

The index value for all samples and controls is calculated by dividing the OD of each sample or control by the mean OD value of the cutoff calibrators. The index values of the controls should be as follows: high-positive control OD, >3.0; low-positive control OD, 1.5 to 3.0; negative control OD, <0.8. The index values of the samples are interpreted as follows: a positive sample has an index value of >1.10, a negative sample has an index value of <0.9, and samples with equivocal results have index values of ≥0.90 to ≤1.10.

SIA

Reagents

SIA is performed at the Genetics and Cytometry Division of TriCore Reference Laboratories (Albuquerque, N.M.). It is a descendent of the first specific test for anti-SNV antibodies (Western blot), developed during the 1993 outbreak of HCPS in the Four Corners region of the United States (34). The test was refined to increase its specificity over tests that used intact viral antigen preparations after epitope-mapping studies using serum samples from SNV HCPS case-patients were incorporated into its design. The original Western blot assay used in the epitope-mapping studies was soon replaced by the first (Chiron) SIA, which used purified recombinant viral antigens that are attached to a membrane via vacuum rather than by electrophoresis (27). The Chiron SIA was supplanted by a version of the SIA that detected and distinguished anti-hantavirus antibodies of both IgG and IgM class. To make SIA test strips, investigators apply each of several antigens and control materials in separate lanes to the membrane by using a vacuum manifold, and the membrane is then cut into 1.6-mm wide strips lengthwise using a paper shredder. Affinity-purified full-length SNV N protein from *E. coli* is used to coat one band, while another band is coated with an *E. coli*-derived phage MS2 coat protein fused to an immunodominant 31-amino-acid epitope of the SNV G1 antigen. Two other bands consisting of high and low concentrations of human serum IgM or IgG are also coated onto the membrane to serve as controls to demonstrate the proper functions of the anti-human IgM and IgG antibody conjugates, respectively, as well as for the proper function of the substrates and developer solutions.

Test Procedure

The patient's serum is first diluted 1:200 into a blocking reagent that contains a 5% lysate of *E. coli* cells in which an empty pET vector (Novagen) has been induced. The mixture is incubated for 1 h or more to allow the preadsorption of any antibody that recognizes *E. coli* protein(s). Investigators apply N antigen (typically 2.4 μg/membrane), G1 fusion antigen (typically 3 μg/membrane), and the serum equivalent of 0.3 and 0.05 μl of human IgG or IgM onto each membrane before the membrane is shredded into about 40 strips for storage at 4°C. Each assay strip is a section of nitrocellulose containing, from top to bottom, Coomassie brilliant blue for strip orientation, "high-intensity" (3+) human IgM or IgG preparation, RecN T7 His$_6$ fusion protein, MS2-G1 His$_6$ fusion protein, and "low-intensity" (1+) human IgM or IgG preparation. In addition to the strip for the sample, a weak-IgM SNV-positive human serum sample and a negative human serum sample are assayed in each run. The blot is added to the serum/blocking reagent after the 1- to 4-h preadsorption interval and rocked in the reagent for 4 h or overnight at room temperature. The strips are incubated with alkaline phosphatase-conjugated goat anti-human IgG or alkaline phosphatase-conjugated goat anti-human IgM and then placed in substrate buffer with alkaline phosphatase substrate, leading to color deposition over the bands. The investigator stops the reaction with an excess of water.

Test Interpretation

The investigator considers the intensity of the color of each reactive band in the positive-control serum blot to determine whether an unknown sample is positive or negative. The criteria used in a positive test for acute HCPS are a positive IgM reaction to the nucleocapsid antigen with or without a positive IgM G1 glycoprotein and the IgG positive for both N and G1.

This assay has been used to evaluate sera from well over 200 patients who were acutely ill with HCPS. With one exception, which was also negative in the CDC EIA, the IgM assay has always been positive for the nucleoprotein fusion, including the Florida case where the hantavirus was BCCV. The IgG assay is positive in about 95% of cases. In fewer than 0.1% of cases, the IgM assay gives a false-positive result, but such false reactions typically are easily identified

by considering a combination of clinical history or the (generally unchanging) results of serial SIAs, performed using serum samples collected over 2 days or more.

MOLECULAR BIOLOGY-BASED DIAGNOSIS OF HANTAVIRUS INFECTION

Two molecular biology-based diagnostic methods, both based on RT-PCR, are in common use: nested RT-PCR for detection and/or sequencing and TaqMan quantitative RT-PCR (qRT-PCR) for detection and/or quantitation of hantavirus genomes. Neither method is approved by the U.S. Food and Drug Administration, and neither method is in use in any commercial or government laboratory except for confirmatory or investigational usage. An almost unlimited number of different potential variants of both methods are available, for example involving many different published primer combinations. A representative procedure for each method is described below.

Nested RT-PCR

Because the concentration of hantavirus RNA in any particular sample can be quite low, one cannot reliably detect hantavirus genomes without conducting a second round of nested PCR (12). To conduct second-round PCR, the investigator uses primers that are internal to those used in the first round. The high abundance of inner-round PCR product lends itself to downstream manipulations of the amplimer such as cloning or sequencing.

Because the S genome is the most abundant, we recommend using primers in the S genome for routine diagnostic work. The existence of a second open reading frame is useful diagnostically because its consistent presence in SNV imposes an additional constraint on sequence variability in that part of the genome. Because SNV can vary by nearly 20% in nucleotide sequence across geographic space while encoding virtually identical proteins, it is sometimes advantageous to choose primers spanned by the S genome's overlapping open reading frames to help ensure that the template will be adequately complementary to the primers.

Reagents

To control temperatures during the RT and amplification reactions, use a Peltier-based or equivalent 96-well thermal cycler such as the ABI model 9700 GeneAmp unit. The protocol calls for four SNV-specific primers (two for the outer RT-PCR and two for the inner PCR), four nucleoside triphosphates (20 mM each; Pharmacia), 5×RT-PCR buffer (Boehringer Mannheim) for the outer reaction, 10×PCR buffer II (with 15 mM MgCl$_2$) for the inner reaction, 0.2-ml thin-walled snap-cap test tubes for PCR (Fisher), β-mercaptoethanol (Sigma), avian myeloblastosis virus reverse transcriptase (Boehringer Mannheim), and AmpliTaq (Roche) (12). Before storage, the following primers are diluted in aliquots to 100 μM and stored frozen:

Har S 167+: 5′ AGC ACA TTA CAG AGC AGA CGG GC (outer RT-PCR)

Har S 190+: 5′ AGC TGT GTC TGC ATT GGA GA (inner PCR)

Har S 401−: 5′ TAG AAT GTA GAG TCC GAT GGA (inner PCR)

Har S 423−: 5′ GGA TAA TCG GTA ATG CAA AAC T (outer RT-PCR)

All manipulations of all reagents should be carried out exclusively with plugged pipette tips. Great caution must be taken to separate pre-PCR from nesting from post-PCR steps, including use of separate pipetters, pipette tips, and bench spaces or hoods.

Test Procedure

The most commonly used nested RT-PCR protocols are those using one-tube systems for the first-step (outer) RT and PCR procedures. The term "one-tube" indicates that all of the reagents needed for both the RT and amplification reactions are placed into the same tube initially and the tube is neither transferred nor opened until it is time to perform the nesting reaction. There is some loss of sensitivity, negligible for most diagnostic applications, relative to separately preparing a cDNA reverse transcript and later utilizing that cDNA for PCR, but because a one-tube system does not require that low-abundance cDNA templates are manipulated, it also greatly reduces the chances of PCR contamination.

RNA preparations should be made from human serum or plasma by using kits designed to prepare RNA from substances with a low abundance of nucleic acids, such as the Qiagen viral RNA miniprep kit. When using tissues or cultured cells as the source of viral RNA, the investigator should use kits intended for samples containing significant amounts of RNA, such as the Qiagen RNeasy kit or the BioChemika Ultra RNA isolation kit (Sigma), as recommended by the manufacturer. The equivalent of about 5 to 25 μl of plasma should be used for each RT-PCR. If one is using RNA prepared from tissues, PBMC, or cultured cell lysates, one should use 0.1 to 0.5 μg of RNA per RT-PCR. The final concentration of RNA should be adjusted so that those quantities can be delivered in 5 μl. At minimum, a positive-control RNA, a negative-control RNA and a negative-control water sample are subjected to RT-PCR.

The investigator prepares for the assay by preparing a cocktail or master mix of reagents in advance, using a sufficient volume to conduct two or three more assays than are needed, to compensate for mechanical losses due to pipetting. The reagents are added to the master mix in the following order: water to take the final volume of each tube to 50 μl, 5× Boehringer RT buffer, 3.5 μl of 25 mM MgCl$_2$, 0.5 μl of β-mercaptoethanol, 0.5 μl of 20 mM each deoxynucleoside triphosphate mix, 0.25 μl of 100 μM each outer primer, 5 U of reverse transcriptase, and 2.5 U of AmpliTaq polymerase. The investigator then adds 45 μl of master mix to each 200-μl thin-walled PCR tube, followed by 5 μl of RNA. After brief trituration of the contents with the pipette the PCR tube is placed into the thermal cycler that is programmed to expose the sample to an RT step (1 h at 42°C) followed by 30 cycles at 95°C (10 s), 55°C (10 s), and 72°C (15 s), followed by a single extension step of 72°C for 10 min and then reduction to "soak" temperature at 4°C until the sample can be processed for the nesting step.

For the nesting reaction, the investigator prepares a cocktail as above but containing enough water to bring the final volume to 50 μl, 10× PCR buffer II (Roche), 0.5 μl of 20 mM deoxynucleoside triphosphate mix, 0.25 μl of each 100 μM inner primer, and 0.5 μl of AmpliTaq polymerase per tube, with enough volume to prepare two or three extra tubes. After returning all of the stock buffers, enzymes, and reagents to the freezers, the investigator distributes 48 μl of the cocktail into each 0.2-ml snap-cap thin-walled PCR tube and then transfers 2 μl of the outer product into the new tube. The reaction is allowed to proceed through amplification as described in the previous step, except that no RT step is included. The outer product is stored at 4°C until the assay has come to a satisfactory ending, in case there is a failure of the nesting reaction.

After the second round of amplification, the investigator adds 5 μl of 10× loading buffer to each tube, runs the entirety of each 50-μl PCR product on a 1.5% submarine agarose gel for 1.5 h at 100 V in Tris acetate-EDTA (TAE) buffer, and stains the gel with ethidium bromide to visualize the PCR product under UV light. Using the S-genomic primers listed above, the investigator should expect a 211-bp PCR product to arise from positive samples. In many cases the product of nested RT-PCR is of sufficient abundance that it can be subjected to sequencing or cloning.

Interpretation of Test Results

Viral RNA is present in samples from patients with SNV infection only during the acute phases of infection, specifically the prodrome phases and early in the cardiorespiratory phase. In later phases of illness, viral RNA becomes increasingly less abundant until it is undetectable, usually within 7–12 days after hospitalization. With serum samples as the source of RNA, an investigator using nested PCR can detect viral genetic material in about 70% of acute-phase samples. The fraction of positive samples approaches 100% when one uses PBMC RNA templates collected within 1 to 5 days of hospitalization, and similar sensitivities are encountered when using lung or kidney samples collected at necropsy (10, 12). A smaller fraction of serum samples are positive when Andes virus is the etiologic agent.

Because RT-PCR assays are positive only transiently in the course of SNV infection, RT-PCR and qRT-PCR will probably remain relegated to secondary or confirmatory assays relative to serologic assays. They are of use primarily for molecular epidemiology, such as identification of the emergence of new virus genotypes or serotypes in a region (nested RT-PCR) or for studies of pathogenesis (qRT-PCR) (see below).

TaqMan Quantitative RT-PCR

Compared to nested RT-PCR, qRT-PCR has somewhat diminished sensitivity, at about 3,000 to 5,000 RNA copies/μl of blood compared to ~2 to 5 copies/μl, but despite this limitation the sensitivity of qRT-PCR in detection of viral genomes in patient samples is more modestly reduced at 50 to 60% compared with ~70% for nested RT-PCR.

qRT-PCR (TaqMan) assays are conducted with instruments such as the ABI model 7000 sequence detection system. One-tube systems are not available or are not reliable. While it is possible to conduct qRT-PCR assays by using random hexamer primers, for hantavirus assays one must appose the positive effects of hexamers (priming of the reverse transcriptase enzyme) against their negative effects (inhibition of the subsequent PCR amplification). There is no concentration at which hexamers can be added that isolate the positive effects at the expense of the negative effects. Furthermore, in some cases the primers used in PCR are less efficient in priming the RT step than in priming the *Taq* polymerase; for that reason, it is recommended that primers used in the RT step should lie external to those used in PCR (2).

Primers with melting temperatures well suited for qRT-PCR can be predicted by using programs such as PrimerExpress (ABI). Two systems for qRT-PCR have been promulgated in the real-time RT-PCR literature: those that detect the increase in abundance of a product that is detected through intercalation of a dye, SYBR green, and those that detect the production of a product by virtue of the associated degradation of a probe that lies between the primers on an amplimer (TaqMan). This chapter discusses only the latter method, since it has performed with reasonable sensitivity and specificity in the detection of SNV RNA in our laboratory and we have not similarly evaluated intercalating dyes (1–3).

To use TaqMan RT-PCR, one begins by producing a cDNA product without further amplification using RT, and then continues by conducting PCR in the presence of an excessive amount of a single-stranded DNA oligodeoxynucleotide probe that lies internal to the primers used for PCR The probe, labeled with both fluor and quencher moieties, competes for hybridization to one strand of the amplimer, but in the course of PCR it is increasingly degraded as the concentration of amplimer increases. The probe is degraded because, as *Taq* polymerase encounters it in hybridization to a strand of the amplimer, it uses an endonuclease activity to break the probe into shorter fragments, thus liberating the reporter fluor from the quencher. The sequence detection system instrument continuously (in real time) interrogates each tube by using light and simultaneously monitors the intensity of light of the wavelength emitted in response by the fluor. After the intensity of the emission wavelength exceeds a predetermined threshold level, the sample is called positive for hantavirus RNA and the number of amplification cycles required to reach that threshold level is recorded. The positive reaction is always scored during the phase of exponential amplification, which helps ensure that the inverse log-linear relationship between the threshold cycle value (minimum number of cycles needed to score the sample as positive) and the input copy number remains close.

An investigator can establish a parallel standard curve using a template molecule of known concentration and thus determine the absolute quantity of S segment RNA in a sample. While it is possible to determine the absolute number of copies of hantavirus RNA in a sample and express that number relative to the quantity of total RNA in the assay tube or the volume of serum used, such a determination is beyond the scope of this chapter and is not necessary to render a diagnosis of hantavirus infection.

Procedure for the TaqMan Assay

The investigator uses the two-step TaqMan Gold RT-PCR protocol as recommended by the manufacturer (ABI), subjecting each sample to triplicate testing. For the RT, 5 μl of template RNA derived from a 140-μl plasma sample is mixed with the S-segment coordinate-167 sense primer 5′ AGCACATTACA-GAGCAGACGGGC in a volume of 100 μl at 25°C for 10 min, 48°C for 30 min, and 95°C for 5 min. Then 5 μl of cDNA is removed for subsequent PCR. The S-segment primers used for the PCR step are the coordinate-179 sense primer 5′ GCA-GACGGGCAGCTGTG and the coordinate-245 antisense primer 5′ AGATCAGCCAGTTCCCGCT. The fluorescent probe, labeled with fluor FAM and quencher TAMRA (Perkin-Elmer Applied Biosystems) is a positive-sense oligonucleotide at coordinate 198 of the S genome, 5′ (FAM) TGCATTGGA-GACCAAACTCGGAGAACTT (TAMRA) 3′. All oligonucleotides are used at a final concentration of 200 nM. After an initial step in which the reaction is heated for 10 min at 95°C, PCR is conducted through 40 repetitions of 95°C for 10 s, 50°C for 10 s, and 72°C for 30 s. A standard curve containing dilutions ranging from 50 to 5×10^7 copies of template can be used optionally on each 96-well plate, should exact quantitation be desired. If not, a single low-copy-number template representing 5 or 50 copies of template can be used as the positive control and a no-RNA sample and an uninfected-human-serum RNA preparation control can be used as the negative control sample.

REFERENCES

1. **Botten, J., K. Mirowsky, D. Kusewitt, M. Bharadwaj, J. Yee, R. Ricci, R. M. Feddersen, and B. Hjelle.** 2000. Experimental infection model for Sin Nombre hantavirus in the deer mouse (*Peromyscus maniculatus*). *Proc. Natl. Acad. Sci. USA* **97:**10578–10583.

2. **Botten, J., K. Mirowsky, D. Kusewitt, C. Ye, K. Gottlieb, J. Prescott, and B. Hjelle.** 2003. Persistent Sin Nombre virus infection in the deer mouse (*Peromyscus maniculatus*) model: sites of replication and strand specific expression. *J. Virol.* **77:**1540–1550.

3. **Botten, J., K. Mirowsky, C. Ye, K. Gottlieb, M. Saavedra, L. Ponce, and B. Hjelle.** 2002. Shedding and intracage transmission of Sin Nombre hantavirus in the deer mouse (*Peromyscus maniculatus*) model. *J. Virol.* **76:**7587–7594.

4. **Centers for Disease Control and Prevention.** 1994. Laboratory management of agents associated with hantavirus pulmonary syndrome: interim biosafety guidelines. *Morb. Mortal. Wkly. Rep.* **43:**1–7.

5. **Centers for Disease Control and Prevention.** 1994. Hantavirus pulmonary syndrome—United States, 1993. *Morb. Mortal. Wkly. Rep.* **43:**45–48. (Erratum, **43:**127.)

6 **Earle, D. P.** 1954. Analysis of sequential physiologic derangements in epidemic hemorrhagic fever. *Am. J. Med.* **16:**690–709.

7. **Feldmann, H., A. Sanchez, S. Morzunov, C. F. Spiropoulou, P. E. Rollin, T. G. Ksiazek, C. J. Peters, and S. T. Nichol.** 1993. Utilization of autopsy RNA for the synthesis of the nucleocapsid antigen of a newly recognized virus associated with hantavirus pulmonary syndrome. *Virus Res.* **30:**351–367.

8. **Hjelle, B., D. Goade, N. Torrez-Martinez, M. Lang-Williams, J. Kim, R. L. Harris, and J. A. Rawlings.** 1996. Hantavirus pulmonary syndrome, renal insufficiency, and myositis associated with infection by Bayou hantavirus. *Clin. Infect. Dis.* **23:**495–500.

9. **Hjelle, B., S. Jenison, N. Torrez-Martinez, B. Herring, S. Quan, A. Polito, S. Pichuantes, T. Yamada, C. Morris, F. Elgh, H. W. Lee, H. Artsob, and R. Dinello.** 1997. Rapid and specific detection of Sin Nombre virus antibodies in patients with hantavirus pulmonary syndrome by a strip immunoblot assay suitable for field diagnosis. *J. Clin. Microbiol.* **35:**600–608.

10. **Hjelle, B., S. Jenison, N. Torrez-Martinez, T. Yamada, K. Nolte, R. Zumwalt, K. MacInnes, and G. Myers.** 1994. A novel hantavirus associated with an outbreak of fatal respiratory disease in the southwestern United States: evolutionary relationships to known hantaviruses. *J. Virol.* **68:**592–596.

11. **Hjelle, B., S. W. Lee, W. Song, N. Torrez-Martinez, J. W. Song, R. Yanagihara, I. Gavrilovskaya, and E. R. Mackow.** 1995. Molecular linkage of hantavirus pulmonary syndrome to the white-footed mouse, *Peromyscus leucopus*: genetic characterization of the M genome of New York virus. *J. Virol.* **69:**8137–8141.

12. **Hjelle, B., C. F. Spiropoulou, N. Torrez-Martinez, S. Morzunov, C. J. Peters, and S. T. Nichol.** 1994. Detection of Muerto Canyon virus RNA in peripheral blood mononuclear cells from patients with hantavirus pulmonary syndrome. *J. Infect. Dis.* **170:**1013–1017.

13. **Hjelle, B., N. Torrez-Martinez, F. T. Koster, M. Jay, M. S. Ascher, T. Brown, P. Reynolds, P. Ettestad, R. E. Voorhees, J. Sarisky, R. E. Enscore, L. Sands, D. G. Mosley, C. Kioski, R. T. Bryan, and C. M. Sewell.** 1996. Epidemiologic linkage of rodent and human hantavirus genomic sequences in case investigations of hantavirus pulmonary syndrome. *J. Infect. Dis.* **173:**781–786.

14. **Jenison, S., T. Yamada, C. Morris, B. Anderson, N. Torrez-Martinez, N. Keller, and B. Hjelle.** 1994. Characterization of human antibody responses to Four Corners hantavirus infections among patients with hantavirus pulmonary syndrome. *J. Virol.* **68:**3000–3006.

15. **Khan, A. S., M. Gaviria, P. E. Rollin, W. G. Hlady, T. G. Ksiazek, L. R. Armstrong, R. Greenman, E. Ravkov, M. Kolber, H. Anapol, E. D. Sfakianaki, S. T. Nichol,**

C. J. Peters, and R. F. Khabbaz. 1996. Hantavirus pulmonary syndrome in Florida: association with the newly identified Black Creek Canal virus. *Am. J. Med.* **100**:46–48.

16. Koster, F., K. Foucar, B. Hjelle, A. Scott, Y. Y. Chong, R. Larson, and M. McCabe. 2001. Rapid presumptive diagnosis of hantavirus cardiopulmonary syndrome by peripheral blood smear review. *Am. J. Clin. Pathol.* **116:** 665–672.

17. Ksiazek, T. G., C. J. Peters, P. E. Rollin, S. Zaki, S. Nichol, C. Spiropoulou, S. Morzunov, H. Feldmann, A. Sanchez, and A. S. Khan. 1995. Identification of a new North American hantavirus that causes acute pulmonary insufficiency. *Am. J. Trop. Med. Hyg.* **52:**117–123.

18. Lee, H. W., P. W. Lee, and K. M. Johnson. 1978. Isolation of the etiologic agent of Korean hemorrhagic fever. *J. Infect. Dis.* **137:**298–308.

19. Mertz, G. J., B. L. Hjelle, and R. T. Bryan. 1997. Hantavirus infection. *Adv. Intern. Med.* **42:**369–421.

20. Nichol, S. T., C. F. Spiropoulou, S. Morzunov, P. E. Rollin, T. G. Ksiazek, H. Feldmann, A. Sanchez, J. Childs, S. Zaki, and C. J. Peters. 1993. Genetic identification of a hantavirus associated with an outbreak of acute respiratory illness. *Science* **262:**914–917.

21. Padula, P. J., A. Edelstein, S. D. Miguel, N. M. Lopez, C. M. Rossi, and R. D. Rabinovich. 1998. Hantavirus pulmonary syndrome outbreak in Argentina: molecular evidence for person-to-person transmission of Andes virus. *Virology* **241:**323–330.

22. Schmaljohn, C., and B. Hjelle. 1997. Hantaviruses: a global disease problem. *Emerg. Infect. Dis.* **3:**95–104.

23. Schmaljohn, C. S., S. E. Hasty, J. M. Dalrymple, J. W. Leduc, H. W. Lee, C. H. von Bonsdorff, M. Brummer-Korvenkontio, A. Vaheri, T. F. Tsai, and H. L. Regnery. 1985. Antigenic and genetic properties of viruses linked to hemorrhagic fever with renal syndrome. *Science* **227:**1041–1044.

24. Torrez-Martinez, N., M. Bharadwaj, D. Goade, J. Delury, P. Moran, B. Hicks, B. Nix, J. L. Davis, and B. Hjelle. 1998. Bayou virus-associated hantavirus pulmonary syndrome in Eastern Texas: identification of the rice rat, *Oryzomys palustris*, as reservoir host. *Emerg. Infect. Dis.* **4:**105–111.

25. Vincent, M. J., E. Quiroz, F. Gracia, A. J. Sanchez, T. G. Ksiazek, P. T. Kitsutani, L. A. Ruedas, D. S. Tinnin, L. Caceres, A. Garcia, P. E. Rollin, J. N. Mills, C. J. Peters, and S. T. Nichol. 2000. Hantavirus pulmonary syndrome in Panama: identification of novel hantaviruses and their likely reservoirs. *Virology* **277:**14–19.

26. Williams, R. J., R. T. Bryan, J. N. Mills, R. E. Palma, I. Vera, F. De Velasquez, E. Baez, W. E. Schmidt, R. E. Figueroa, C. J. Peters, S. R. Zaki, A. S. Khan, and T. G. Ksiazek. 1997. An outbreak of hantavirus pulmonary syndrome in western Paraguay. *Am. J. Trop. Med. Hyg.* **57:**274–282.

27. Yanagihara, R. 1990. Hantavirus infection in the United States: epizootiology and epidemiology. *Rev. Infect. Dis.* **12:**449–457.

Filoviruses and Arenaviruses

JAMES E. STRONG, ALLEN GROLLA, PETER B. JAHRLING,
AND HEINZ FELDMANN

87

Emerging viral infections have recently captured the interest and concern of the general public. This concern stems in part from the revelation that exotic viral disease agents, such as the viral hemorrhagic fever (VHF) viruses, are significant human pathogens with the potential for introduction into populations of the industrialized world either through international travel or through potential bioterrorism (4, 13). It is feared that the highly virulent nature of some of these infections, coupled with a potential for aerogenic transmission to a susceptible population and with inadequate diagnostic and therapeutic strategies, could result in a major epidemic.

The VHF-causing filoviruses and arenaviruses have been a particular focus of discussion, given their high lethality and, in the case of Ebola virus (EBOV) and Lassa virus (LAS), previously demonstrated introductions into countries where they are not endemic. They are classified as biosafety level 4 (BSL-4) and have been deemed to be category A bioterrorism agents (http://www.bt.cdc.gov/Agent/Agentlist.asp). Although exotic to many parts of the world, filoviruses and arenaviruses are important public health problems in parts of Africa and South America. Patients with these infections frequently present with similar, nonspecific clinical signs resembling malaria, typhoid, and pharyngitis. Early diagnosis is critical to timely implementation of specialized patient isolation and clinical management procedures and limited therapeutic intervention with, for example, hyperimmune globulin (South American arenaviruses) and ribavirin (arenaviruses).

The need for sensitive, specific viral diagnostics and for having procedures in place to handle such agents is essential for the correct identification and containment of outbreaks of VHFs. Travel histories have historically been important in deciphering etiologies. Events occurring since 11 September 2001, including the anthrax scare, have raised the possibility of potential bioterrorism including utilizing these VHFs in countries where they are not endemic. Outbreak management in rural African or South American hospitals, in cases of natural epidemics, has its own challenges. Clinicians here must always keep a high index of suspicion and rely on the clinical and epidemiological information available to set in motion a train of events including the cautious collection of appropriate samples for sophisticated virologic investigations. The World Health Organization (http://who.int/csr/don/en/) and several other organizations, such as ProMed, provide up-to-date information on outbreaks including those from VHFs. The mobilization of adequate logistics to permit the collection, transport, and processing of clinical specimens and other laboratory samples presents numerous difficulties in remote areas of rural Africa and South America. These technical and logistic questions remain of paramount importance to the physician practicing in remote rural populations as well as to those responsible for epidemiological surveillance and public health in countries at risk.

Since the procedures for initial isolation, clinical management, and virologic diagnoses of patients with suspected arenavirus and filovirus infections are similar, these taxonomically distinct viruses are discussed together in this chapter.

VIRAL AGENTS

Arenaviridae

The family *Arenaviridae* comprises at least 23 viral species within the single genus *Arenavirus* (Table 1). All arenaviruses share a unique morphology when observed in thin section by electron microscopy (EM). They are round to pleomorphic and range in size from 50 to 300 nm (mean, 110 to 130 nm) (Fig. 1A). The genome consists of two single-stranded, negative-sense RNA segments, designated large (L) and small (S). Each segment encodes two different proteins in two nonoverlapping reading frames of opposite polarities (ambisense coding strategy) separated by an intergenic noncoding region with the potential to form hairpin structures. The L segment encodes the viral RNA-dependent RNA polymerase (L) and the zinc binding protein (Z); the S segment encodes the nucleoprotein (NP) and the glycoprotein precursor that is posttranslationally cleaved into GP-1 and GP-2 (5, 32).

Both serology and phylogenetic analyses divide the arenaviruses into two complexes. The first group includes the Old World complex with *Lymphocytic choriomeningitis virus* (LCMV) and the Lassa viruses, including a number of apparently benign LAS-like strains from Mozambique, Zimbabwe, and the Central African Republic. All of these have been isolated from rodents of the family Muridae (Table 1). The second group includes the Tacaribe or New World complex with the four South American VHF-causing arenaviruses *Junin* (Argentine HF) (JUN), *Machupo* (Bolivian HF) (MAC), *Guanarito* (Venezuelan HF) (GTO) and *Sabia*

TABLE 1 Characteristics of arenaviruses

Classification	Acronym	Geographic distribution	Reservoir species	Human disease	Year discovered
New World					
Junin	JUN	Argentina	*Calomys musculinus*	Argentinian hemorrhagic fever	1958
Machupo	MAC	Bolivia	*Calomys callosus, C. laucha*	Bolivian hemorrhagic fever	1963
Sabia	SAB	Brazil	?	Brazilian hemorrhagic fever	1993
Guanarito	GTO	Venezuela	*Sigmodon alstoni, Zygodontomys brevicauda*	Venezuelan hemorrhagic fever	1989
Tacaribe	TCR	Trinidad	*Artibeus* spp. (bats)	Unknown	1956
Cupixi	CPX	Brazil	*Oryzomys gaeldi, O. megacephalis*	Unknown	1998
Amapari	AMA	Brazil	*Oryzomys capito, Neacomys guianae*	Unknown	1964
Whitewater Arroyo	WWA	New Mexico, California	*Netoma albigula*	Adult respiratory distress syndrome	1996
Tamiami	TAM	United States	*Sigmodon hispidus*	Unknown	1970
Bear Canyon	BCN	California	*Peromyscus californicus*	Unknown	2002
Pichinde	PIC	Colombia	*Oryzomys albigularis*	Unknown	1967
Pirital	PIR	Venezuela	*Sigmodon alstoni*	Unknown	1997
Flexal	FLE	Brazil	*Oryzomys* spp.	Unknown	1975
Parana	PAR	Paraguay	*Oryzomys buccinatus*	Unknown	1965
Allpahuayo	ALL	Peru	*Oecomys bicolour, O. paricola*	Unknown	2001
Oliveros	OLV	Argentina	*Bolomys obscurus*	Unknown	1996
Latino	LAT	Bolivia	*Callomys callosus*	Unknown	1965
Pampa	PAM	Argentina	*Bolomys* spp.	Unknown	1997
Old World					
Lassa	LAS	Nigeria, Ivory Coast, Guinea, Sierra Leone	*Mastomys* spp.	Lassa fever	1969
Lymphocytic choriomeningitis	LCM	Europe, Americas	*Mus musculus, M. domesticus*	Meningitis/encephalitis and congenital defects	1933
Mopeia	MOP	Mozambique	*Praomys* spp., *Mastomys natelensis*	Unknown	1977
Mobala	MOB	Zimbawa, Central African Republic	*Praomys* spp., *Mastomys natelensis*	Unknown	1983
Ippy	Ippy	Central African Republic	*Arvicanthus* spp.	Unknown	1970

A

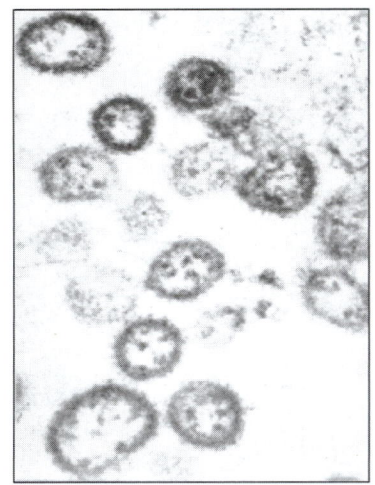
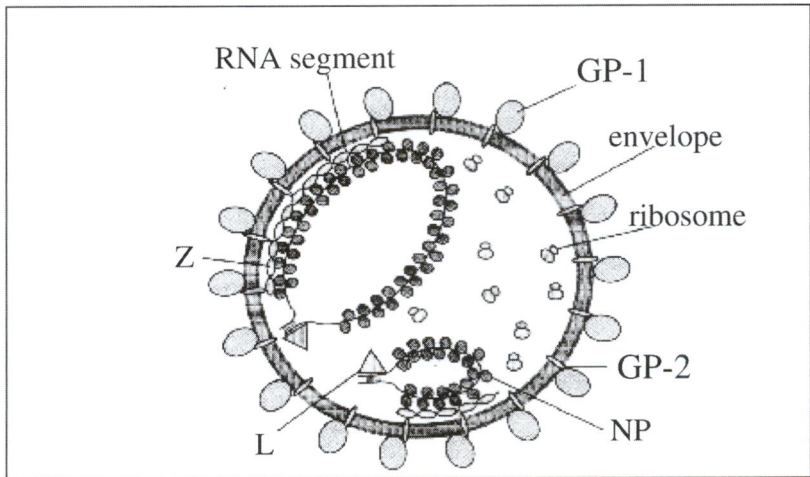

B

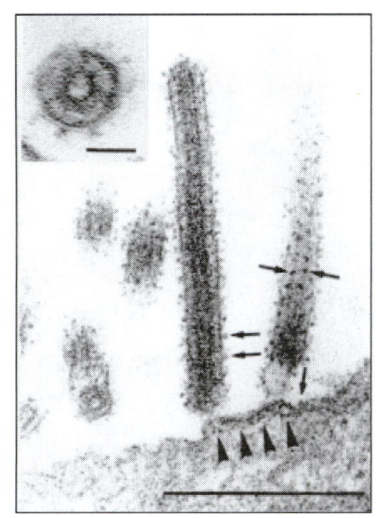
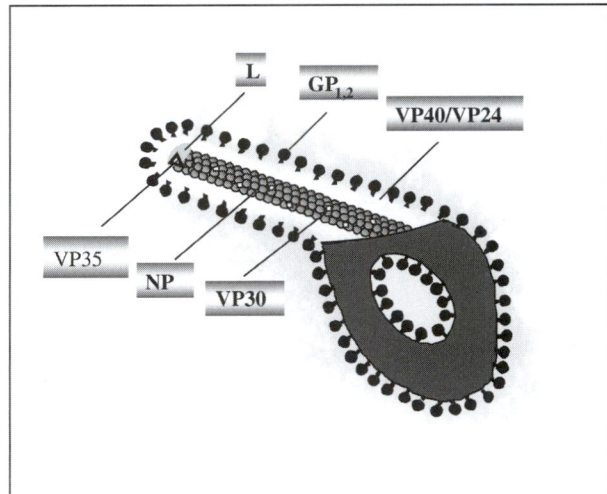

FIGURE 1 Morphology of virus particles. (A) Arenaviruses. Arenaviruses are round to pleomorphic enveloped particles with a bisegmented, single-stranded, negative-sense RNA genome. Two proteins are involved in nucleocapsid formation: RNA-dependent RNA polymerase (L) and nucleoprotein (NP). The glycoproteins (GP-1 and GP-2) form the spikes on the virion surface. The Z protein functions as the matrix protein. Ribosomes are usually incorporated during particle maturation. (B) Filoviruses. Filoviruses are filamentous enveloped particles with a nonsegmented, single-stranded, negative-sense RNA genome. Four proteins are involved in nucleocapsid formation: RNA-dependent RNA polymerase (L), nucleoprotein (NP), virion structural protein 30 (VP30), and VP35. The glycoprotein (GP$_{1,2}$) forms the spikes on the virion surface (arrows in electron micrograph). VP40 functions as the matrix protein; VP24 is membrane associated.

(Brazilian HF) (SAB) viruses. All New World complex viruses have been isolated from rodents of the family Cricetidae, or, in the case of *Tacaribe virus*, from bats (Table 1). The Old and New World complexes are distantly related; only when very high-titer antisera are used can cross-reactions be observed. The use of monoclonal antibodies with specificities for structural proteins of arenaviruses suggests that the nucleoprotein is the group-reactive determinant while the envelope glycoproteins (GP-1 and GP-2) are responsible for type specificity (6, 32).

All arenaviruses are maintained in nature by establishing chronic viremia in their reservoir host (almost exclusively rodents) and are transmitted to humans through contaminated animal excreta or occasionally bites. Person-to-person transmission (secondary infection) also occurs with LAS and less frequently with the South American VHF-causing arenaviruses (5, 32).

LAS is the etiologic agent of Lassa fever, a West African VHF (Table 1). The original outbreaks described were hospital associated, occurring first in Nigeria in 1969 and later in Liberia, Sierra Leone, and the Republic of Guinea. Different percentages (8 to 52%) of the population of this area are seropositive. LAS is now recognized to persist in endemic foci, and the true incidence of human Lassa fever is thought to be thousands to tens of thousands per year. Among hospitalized patients with Lassa fever, the mortality rate is currently estimated to be 15 to 20%. Overall mortality, including subclinical cases identified serologically, is substantially lower, perhaps less than 1%. Arenaviruses serologically related to yet distinct from LAS have been isolated from rodents in Mozambique (Mopeia virus), Zimbabwe and the Central African Republic (Mobala virus, Ippy virus). These viruses have not been associated with naturally occurring human disease and may, in fact, elicit protective immunity against virulent LAS infection.

JUN, the causative agent of Argentine HF (AHF) (Table 1), was first isolated in 1958, although the disease had been recognized since 1943 in Argentina, where it has been associated with annual outbreaks primarily among agricultural workers. From 1958 to the present, annual fluctuations in AHF cases range from 100 to 3,500, with several hundred cases occurring in most years. Since the recent introduction of a live attenuated vaccine for JUN in Argentina, the annual incidence of disease now numbers 10 to 100 cases. The mortality rate for patients with laboratory-confirmed AHF who do not receive specific immune plasma therapy is reported to be 14 to 17%. The vesper mouse, *Calomys musculinus*, is considered the primary reservoir because it was the most commonly trapped rodent in the area of endemic infection and because persistent viremia and virus shedding via saliva have been shown both in naturally infected and laboratory-infected animals (5, 6).

MAC, the etiologic agent of Bolivian HF (BHF) (Table 1), was first isolated in 1963, although reports of sporadic outbreaks began in 1959 and a series of devastating epidemics occurred from 1962 to 1964; these involved more than 1,000 patients and had an 18% mortality rate. Another severe outbreak occurred in Cochabamba, Bolivia, in 1971 and was associated entirely with nosocomial spread from an index case apparently infected in the region of endemicity. Following a long quiescence, Machupo virus reemerged in Bolivia in 1994, in association with a small outbreak. The reservoir of MAC is the rodent *Calomys callosus*, and the infection most often affects agricultural workers during spring and summer (5, 6).

GTO was first recognized in association with an outbreak of HF thought initially to be dengue fever in Venezuela in 1989 (Table 1). During 3 years of epidemiologic surveillance, from September 1989 to December 1991, 88 cases of VHF were documented, with a fatality rate of 34%. The Venezuelan virus was first discovered in a zone in which tropical forest was removed to permit the establishment of small farms and ranches. Apparently, a local rodent species that carries the virus found the cleared areas hospitable and multiplied in proportion to the increased food supplies available in fields and houses. Since then, only sporadic cases have emerged, causing a lower percentage of deaths. All cases were in rural areas, and the cotton rat, *Sigmodon alstoni*, is the major host and natural reservoir of GTO. As with the other arenaviruses, transmission from rodents to humans is thought to relate primarily to contact with food, water, or air contaminated with rodent urine. Person-to-person transmission is uncommon (5, 6).

SAB was isolated from a patient with a fatal case of VHF thought initially to be yellow fever in Brazil in 1993 (Table 1). During characterization of this virus, a laboratory technician became infected, probably via the aerosol route; he eventually recovered. This virus once again infected a virologist in 1994. The emergence of both GTO and SAB and the initial confusion with other viral fevers including dengue and yellow fever illustrate the importance of developing specific, definitive diagnostic tools for these agents (5, 6).

Filoviridae

Marburg virus (MARV) and EBOV are classified in the order *Mononegavirales*, family *Filoviridae*. The family *Filoviridae* consists of the genera *Marburgvirus* and *Ebolavirus*. The *Ebolavirus* genus is subdivided into three distinct African species, *Ivory Coast ebolavirus* (ICEBOV), *Sudan ebolavirus* (SEBOV), and *Zaire ebolavirus* (ZEBOV), and a single Asian species, *Reston ebolavirus* (REBOV). Serologically, MARV and EBOV strains are distinct. EBOV species have some epitopes in common, responsible for the serological cross-reactivity observed in broadly reactive tests (9).

Filovirus particles are bacilliform but can also appear as branched, circular, U-shaped, 6-shaped, and long filamentous forms (Fig. 1B). They have a uniform diameter of approximately 80 nm but vary greatly in length. Negatively contrasted particles, regardless of serotype or host cell, contain an electron-dense central axis (19 to 25 nm in diameter) surrounded by an outer helical layer (45 to 50 nm in diameter) with cross-striations at 5-nm intervals. This central core is formed by the ribonucleoprotein complex, which is surrounded by a lipid envelope derived from the host cell plasma membrane. Spikes of approximately 7 nm in diameter and spaced at about 5- to 10-nm intervals are seen as globular structures on the surface of virions (9, 33).

Virus particles contain a nonsegmented single-stranded negative-sense linear RNA genome that does not contain a poly(A) tail and is noninfectious. Virions are made of seven structural proteins with presumed identical functions for the different viruses. Four proteins make up the ribonucleoprotein complex (NP, virion protein 35 [VP35], VP30, and L), together with the viral RNA, while the remaining three proteins are membrane associated (glycoprotein [$GP_{1,2}$], VP40, and VP24). The single type I transmembrane glycoprotein ($GP_{1,2}$) is inserted in the envelope as a homotrimer and functions in receptor binding and fusion; VP40 has been identified and characterized as the matrix protein, but the function of VP24 is unknown. EBOV expresses a nonstructural soluble glycoprotein (sGP) as the primary gene product of the glycoprotein gene, which is efficiently secreted from infected cells; its functions remain unknown (9, 33).

MARV and the species ICEBOV, SEBOV, and ZEBOV are indigenous to Central Africa in an area approximately between the 10th parallel north and south of the equator as indicated by the locations of known outbreaks and seroepidemiologic studies (Fig. 2). The geographic range of EBOV may extend to other regions in Africa, for which adequate serosurveys are lacking. In 1994 ICEBOV was isolated in West Africa during an outbreak of HF among wild chimpanzees in the Tai Forest. Before that, the identification of REBOV suggested for the first time the presence of a filovirus in Asia that may be associated with wild nonhuman primates (8, 33). Since 1995, reports have been accumulating of EBOV infection in great apes (chimpanzees and gorillas) in Gabon and the Republic of Congo, in which 80% of the world's population of these great apes are found. It is predicted that in some regions the gorilla population is threatened by extinction. Understanding the maintenance strategy of filoviruses in nature is essential to prediction of their emergence and to their control.

Many outbreaks have been traced to index cases, in which an infected person probably came into contact with an as yet unidentified reservoir. It is likely that monkeys do not serve as reservoir hosts since their pathogenicity is similar to our own. However, nonhuman primates may serve as the intermediate host of some outbreaks, such as has been demonstrated in the Republic of Congo. The reservoirs are

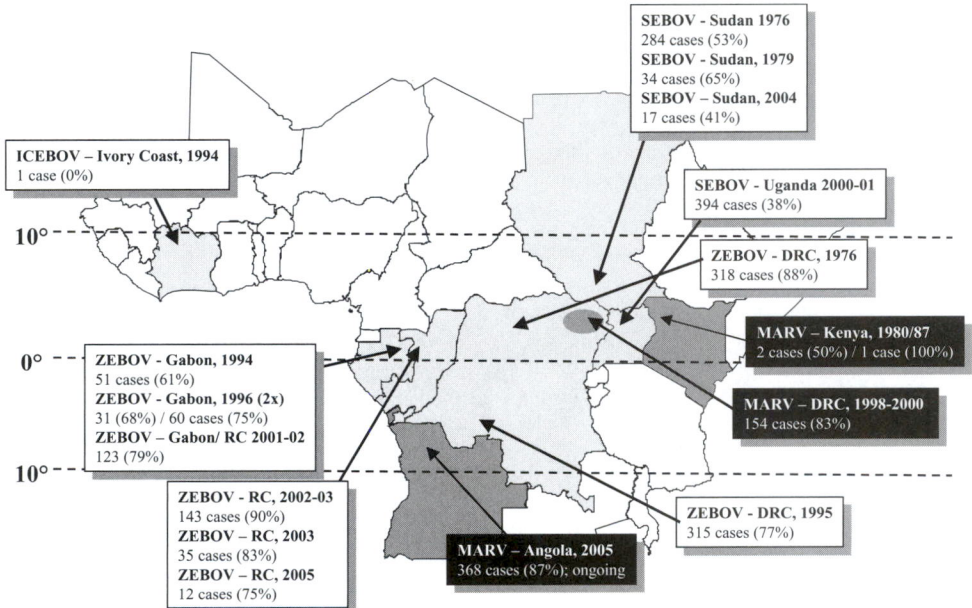

FIGURE 2 Filovirus outbreaks in Central Africa. Reported outbreaks of HF caused by MARV (dark gray) and EBOV (light gray) in the affected countries are indicated with the corresponding year, case numbers, and percentage lethality. DRC, Democratic Republic of the Congo; ICEBOV, Ivory Coast ebolavirus; RC, Republic of the Congo; SEBOV, Sudan ebolavirus; ZEBOV, Zaire ebolavirus.

likely to be other mammals, birds, or invertebrate species including mosquitoes and ticks. Bat species are currently the most favored candidate due to some epidemiologic links and experimental studies demonstrating replication of EBOV in bats. From the index case, transmission among humans is principally due to direct contact, such as among family members but also from infected patients to nurses, doctors, and other health care workers (8, 10, 33).

CLINICAL ASPECTS

Arenaviruses
Initial symptoms of the VHF-causing arenaviruses are rather nonspecific and follow an incubation period of 2 to 16 days. Patients experience an insidious or sudden onset of progressive fever (that may be biphasic), chills, malaise, generalized myalgias and arthralgias, headache, anorexia, and cough. Most patients have a severe sore throat and may have epigastric pain, vomiting, and diarrhea. Typical physical findings are not distinctive; they include nonspecific conjunctival injection, facial and truncal flushing, petechiae, purpura, ecchymoses, icterus, epistaxis, gastrointestinal and genitourinary bleeding, and lymphadenopathy. Severe illness is associated with hypotension and shock, relative bradycardia, pneumonitis, pleural and pericardial effusions, hemorrhage, encephalopathy, seizures, coma, and occasionally death.

For LAS infection, fever and myalgia develop insidiously between 3 and 16 days after exposure and increase in severity during the following week. Lassa fever patients usually come to the hospital within 5 to 7 days of onset, with sore throat, severe lower back pain, and conjunctivitis. Pneumonitis and pleural and pericardial effusions with friction rub frequently occur. A maculopapular rash may develop, but although Lassa fever is grouped with the hemorrhagic fevers, frank hemorrhage is seen only in a small proportion of the

more severe cases. Death, due to sudden cardiovascular collapse as a consequence of hepatic, pulmonary, and myocardial damage, occurs in the second or third week in approximately 15 to 20% of hospitalized patients. Although few Lassa fever patients develop central nervous system (CNS) signs, tinnitus or deafness may develop as recovery begins. Lassa fever is a particularly severe disease among pregnant women, for whom mortality rates are somewhat higher. Swollen-baby syndrome describes severe Lassa fever in infants and toddlers, with anasarca, abdominal distension, and spontaneous bleeding, but pediatric disease otherwise is no different from that observed in older patients. Clinical laboratory studies are usually not helpful for Lassa fever; specific virological diagnosis is required (5, 30).

The clinical pictures for AHF (JUN) and BHF (MAC) are well characterized; for VHF caused by GTO and SAB, less information is available. However, all these infections are sufficiently similar to each other to be discussed as a single entity, South American HF. Incubation periods range from 7 to 14 days, and very few subclinical cases are thought to occur. Following a gradual onset of fever, anorexia, and malaise over several days, constitutional signs involving gastrointestinal, cardiovascular, and CNS symptoms become apparent by the time patients present to the hospital. On initial examination, AHF and BHF patients are febrile, acutely ill, and mildly hypotensive. They frequently complain of back pain, epigastric pain, headache, retro-orbital pain, photophobia, dizziness, constipation or diarrhea, and coughing. Vascular phenomena, including flushing of the face, neck, and chest, as well as bleeding from the gums, are common. Enanthema are almost invariably present; petechiae or tiny vesicles spread over erythematous palate and fauces. Neurologic involvement, ranging from mild irritability and lethargy to abnormalities in gait, tremors of the upper extremities, and, in severely ill patients, coma, delirium, and convulsions, occurs in more than half of the patients. During the second week of illness, clinical improvement may begin, or complications may develop. The latter include extensive petechial hemorrhages, oozing from puncture wounds, melena, and hematemesis. These manifestations of capillary damage and thrombocytopenia do not result in life-threatening blood loss. However, hypotension and shock, complicated by gross hemorrhaging, may develop, often in combination with serious neurologic signs in the 15% of patients who die. Survivors begin to show improvement by the third week. Recovery is slow; weakness, fatigue, and mental difficulties may last for weeks. In contrast to Lassa fever, clinical laboratory studies are frequently useful. Total white blood cell counts usually fall to 1,000 to 2,000 cells/mm³, although the differential remains normal. Platelet counts fall precipitously, usually to 25,000 to 100,000/mm³, and occasionally lower. Routine clotting parameters are usually normal or slightly deranged, but in severe cases, evidence of disseminated intravascular coagulation (DIC) is apparent (6, 30, 36).

Filoviruses

MARV and EBOV infections are clinically similar. MARV HF manifests after an incubation period of 5 to 10 days, with a sudden onset of marked fever, chills, headache, and myalgia. Patients may develop a maculopapular rash, most prominent on the trunk (chest, back, or stomach) on the fifth day after onset of symptoms. Nausea, vomiting, chest pain, sore throat, abdominal pain, and diarrhea may then appear. Symptoms become increasingly severe and may include jaundice, pancreatitis, severe weight loss, delirium, shock, liver failure, massive hemorrhaging, and multiorgan dysfunction. The hemorrhaging may be the result of a combination of DIC and hepatic failure. Uveitis has occurred following MARV infection, after a 2-month asymptomatic period, and may persist for several weeks. MARV has been cultured from the anterior chamber of the eye following such infection (29, 33).

Human infections with ZEBOV, SEBOV, and ICEBOV follow similar courses and typically include incubation periods of 2 to 8 days in primary cases to slightly longer in secondary cases. Cases with longer incubation periods of 19 and 21 days have been observed. The onset of clinical symptoms is often sudden, and clinical findings depend on the stage of disease at which patients present. Early in the disease, symptoms include pharyngitis, severe headache, arthralgias or myalgias, fever, anorexia, and asthenia, followed by gastrointestinal symptoms, including abdominal pain, nausea and vomiting, and diarrhea later in the course. There may be mucous membrane involvement including conjunctivitis with effusions, odynophagia or dysphagia. Chemical hepatitis without clinical jaundice is usual, and multiple organ systems become involved. A characteristic maculopapular rash develops over the trunk. Petechiae, mucous membrane hemorrhages, and bleeding from multiple sites along the gastrointestinal tract are occasionally accompanied by uncontrollable bleeding from venipuncture sites. Although the mechanism is unclear, hiccups have been noted in fatal cases of ZEBOV in both the 1976 and the 1995 outbreaks in the Democratic Republic of Congo. Terminally ill patients often are normothermic, obtunded, anuric, tachypneic, and in shock. Late in the disease, patients often develop an expressionless hippocratic face—"the mask of death." Myocarditis and pulmonary edema also are seen in the later stages of the disease. Development of shock occurs soon before death, often 6 to 16 days after onset of illness (29, 33).

Early nonvirologic laboratory studies are nonspecific and often unavailable in an outbreak setting. These include thrombocytopenia and leukopenia with pronounced lymphopenia. After several days, neutrophilia occurs and may be associated with elevations in aspartate aminotransferase and alanine aminotransferase levels. Hyperbillirubinemia can occur. Prothrombin and partial thromboplastin times are prolonged, with the notable presence of fibrin split products, particularly in MARV disease. Platelet counts decline to 50,000 to 100,000/mm³ during the hemorrhagic phase. Later in the clinical course, elevated blood urea nitrogen and serum creatinine levels occur in association with the onset of anuria. Also, secondary bacterial infections may occur later in the course, with associated elevation of the white blood cell counts. Metabolic acidosis with compensatory hyperventilation can develop in terminally ill patients.

COLLECTION AND PREPARATION OF CLINICAL SAMPLES

Special precautions and equipment are required for the safe handling of diagnostic specimens obtained from patients suspected of being infected with arenaviruses and filoviruses (www.who.int/entity/csr/resources/publications/biosafety/WHO_CDS_CSR_LYO_2004_11/en [*Laboratory Biosafety Manual*], http://www.cdc.gov/od/ohs/biosfty/biosfty.htm [*Biosafety in Microbiology and Biomedical Laboratories*]). Current recommendations are that samples from such infected patients be manipulated only at the maximum biological containment level, BSL-4. In the field, personnel caring for patients and obtaining diagnostic specimens should wear disposable caps, gowns, shoe covers, surgical gloves, and masks; full-face respirators equipped with high-efficiency particulate air (HEPA) filters are preferable. Suggestions for reducing the risk of handling patient samples prior to shipment to a BSL-4 laboratory are detailed elsewhere (28; see also the websites given above). For transport of infectious material, specimens should be packaged in accordance with international regulations (International Air Transport Association [IATA] [http://www.thecompliancecenter.com/forms.htm]) and forwarded, after consultation, to a specialized national or international reference laboratory that maintains diagnostic capability for these agents. With a few exceptions, these are BSL-4 facilities; Table 2 lists laboratories that are organized in the International High Security Laboratory Network (IHSLN).

For virus isolation, serum or plasma (or, less ideally, whole blood) obtained during the acute, febrile stage of illness should be frozen on dry ice or in liquid nitrogen vapor. Storage at higher temperature may be unavoidable in some circumstances but leads to rapid loss in infectivity. Throat washings and urine specimens should also be collected and mixed with a buffered diluent containing protein (e.g., 10% fetal bovine serum or normal rabbit serum) before being frozen. Specimens collected for viral isolation are also suitable for testing by antigen capture enzyme-linked immunosorbent assay (ELISA); maintenance at −20°C for periods up to several weeks is adequate for antigen preservation. Impression smears of infected tissues may be fixed by immersion in cold acetone and stored frozen for viral antigen staining by direct immunofluorescence assay (DFA). Formaldehyde-fixed tissues and paraffin-embedded blocks are also suitable for immunohistochemical (IHC) identification of viral antigens. Blood obtained in early convalescence for serodiagnosis may be infectious despite the presence of antibodies and should be handled accordingly. Maintenance of samples at −20°C or below is sufficient to preserve antibody titers and antigenicity, but lower

TABLE 2 International High Security Laboratory Network (IHSLN) list of members

Country	Institution
Australia	Victorian Infectious Diseases Reference Laboratory, 10 Wreckyn Street, North Melbourne 3051, Victoria
Canada	Special Pathogens Program, National Microbiology Laboratory, Public Health Agency of Canada, 1015 Arlington Street, Winnipeg, MB R3E 3R2
	National Centre for Foreign Animal Diseases, Canadian Food Inspection Agency, 1015 Arlington Street, Winnipeg, MB R3E 3R2
France	Centre de Recherche Merieux-Pasteur a Lyon, Laboratoire P4, 21 Avenue Tony Garnire, 69365 Lyon Cedex 07
Gabon	Centre International de Recherches Medicales de Franceville, BP 769, Franceville
Germany	Bernhard-Nocht Institute of Tropical Medicine, Department of Virology, Bernhard-Nocht-Str. 74, D-20359 Hamburg Institute of Virology, Philipps-University, Robert-Koch-Str. 17, D-35-37 Marburg
Japan	Special Pathogens Laboratory, National Institute of Infectious Disease, Gakuen 4-7-1, Musashimurayama, Tokyo 208-0011
Russia	State Research Center of Virology & Biotechnology (SRCVB) "Vector," Koltsovo, Novosibirsk region, 630559
South Africa	National Institute for Communicable Diseases, Special Pathogens Unit, Private Bag x4, Sandringham, 2131
Sweden	Swedish Institute for Infectious Disease Control, Centre for Microbiological Preparedness, Tomtebodavagen 12B, Solna, SE-171-82
United Kingdom	Centre for Applied Microbiology Research, 11 Sherfield, Winterbourne Dauntsey, Salisbury, SP4 0JG
	PHLS Central Public Health Laboratory, 61 Colindale Avenue, Colindale, London, NW9 6HF
United States	Special Pathogens Branch, Centers for Disease Control and Prevention, 1600 Clifton Rd., Atlanta, GA 30333
	US Army Medical Research Institute for Infectious Diseases, 1425 Porter Street, Fort Detrick, MD 21702-5011
	Southwest Foundation for Biomedical Research, 7620 NW Loop 410, San Antonio, TX 78227
	University of Texas Medical Branch, 301 University Boulevard, Galveston, TX 77555-0609
	Georgia State University, Herpes B Virus Resource Laboratory, 50 Decatur Street, Atlanta, GA 30302-4118 (herpes B only)

temperatures are required to preserve infectivity. Citrate and oxalate should be avoided as anticoagulants because of interference with the indirect immunofluorescence assay (IFA) and nonspecific cytopathic effect in Vero and MA-104 cells used for virus isolation. Heparin seems to be the best anticoagulant for antibody and antigen detection systems, and EDTA is the best for PCR diagnostics.

LAS is frequently isolated from acute-phase sera and throat washings for several weeks following onset of clinical signs, but it is only occasionally isolated from urine. Sera obtained as late as 15 days after onset have yielded LAS. JUN is usually recoverable from serum for 3 to 10 days after onset and is often recoverable from throat washings for a similar period but is rarely recovered from urine. MAC is recovered from only one of five acute-phase sera and even less frequently from throat washings or urine. MARV and EBOV are usually recoverable from acute-phase sera; various specimens including throat washings, urine, soft tissue effusates, semen, and anterior eye fluid have yielded these viruses, even when the specimens are obtained late in convalescence (Fig. 3). LAS, MAC, JUN, MARV, and EBOV are all readily isolated from spleen, lymph nodes, liver, and kidneys obtained at autopsy but rarely, if ever, are recovered from brain or other CNS tissues. Notably, LAS is usually isolated from the placentas of infected pregnant women.

All arenaviruses and filoviruses are readily inactivated by ethyl ether, chloroform, sodium deoxycholate, and acid media (pH less than 5). β-Propiolactone and gamma irradiation (on dry ice) are both reported to inactivate viral infectivity while preserving reactivity in standard serologic and antigen detection tests. RNA extraction medium containing guanidinium isothiocyanate in general inactivates viral infectivity but has only been experimentally proven for some commercially available extraction buffers (unpublished data). It should be noted that arenaviruses and particularly filoviruses can be stable at room temperature for several hours to days. In the field, infectivity of samples may be greatly reduced, if not totally inactivated, by the addition of sodium dodecyl sulfate (SDS) and Triton-X-100 (0.1% SDS; 0.1% Triton X-100) and treatment with heat (60°C for 30 min). Treated specimens may subsequently be safely used in serologic or antigen detection assays.

DIAGNOSTIC PROCEDURES

The differential diagnosis of HF, especially in individual patients, presents considerable difficulties. Although the VHF-causing viruses are the most worrisome infectious agents in regard to public health and case patient management, bacterial, fungal, and protozoal infections must also be considered. Severe sepsis syndromes with DIC and shock diatheses caused by any infectious agents also should be included in the differential diagnosis. Complicating matters is the possibility of noninfectious entities (including acute leukemia, lupus erythematosus, thrombocytopenia of various etiologies, and hemolytic-uremic syndromes) as well as combinations of these infectious and noninfectious entities.

Laboratory diagnosis can be achieved in two ways, measurement of host-specific immune responses to the infection and detection of viral antigen and/or genomic RNA (Table 3). Because of the presence of high titers of infectious virus in blood and tissues even during early stages, antigen and nucleic acid detection plays the most important role in early detection of VHF infections caused by arenaviruses and filoviruses. Here the assays of choice would be the antigen capture ELISA and reverse transcription-PCR (RT-PCR).

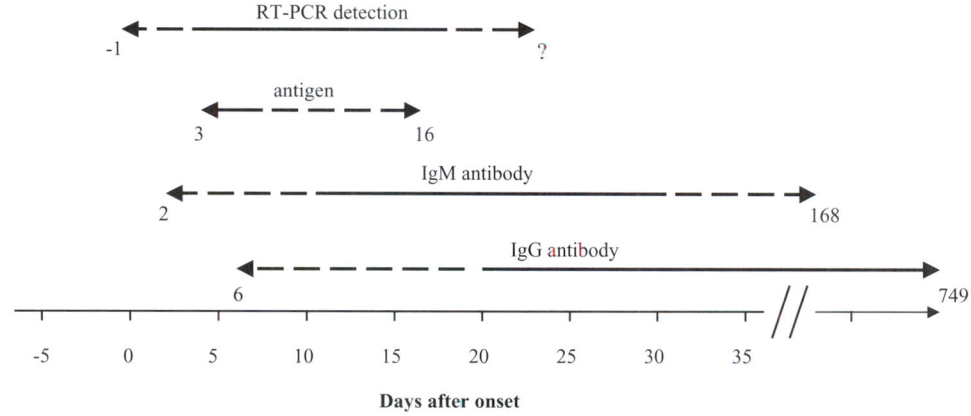

FIGURE 3 Time line for diagnostic sampling. The scheme demonstrates an approximate time line for sampling and testing of EBOV-infected patients. The numbers indicate days after onset of symptoms.

With the development of more sensitive tests, such as the immunoglobulin M (IgM) capture ELISA and the direct IgG test, antibody detection has become more valuable in early diagnosis but is still considered second line for acute diagnostics (Fig. 3). Electron microscopy has been particularly useful in the diagnosis of filovirus infections in the past but can also be applied for arenaviruses. IHC on formalin-fixed material and paraffin-embedded tissues as well as DFA on impression smears of tissues can be used for viral antigen detection. Virus isolation from serum and/or other clinical material should always be attempted in tissue culture (e.g., Vero or MA-104 cells). However, most filoviruses and arenaviruses do not cause extensive cytopathic effect on primary isolation. Isolation attempts in animals frequently fail due to a lack of

susceptibility of the most commonly used small-animal models and are thus less valuable.

In the following sections, the current commonly used diagnostic procedure are discussed under the headings of "Detection of Viral Antigen and Nucleic Acid" and "Detection of Virus-Specific Antibodies." Furthermore, a few additional procedures are discussed. Figure 4 presents an outline of the important steps from clinical to laboratory-confirmed diagnosis.

Detection of Viral Antigen and Nucleic Acid

Antigen Capture ELISA

The development of antigen capture ELISAs for quantitative detection of viral antigen in clinical specimens has facilitated

TABLE 3 Laboratory diagnosis

Test	Target	Source	Remarks
Detection of viral antigen/nucleic acid			
Antigen capture enzyme-linked immunosorbent assay	Viral antigen	Blood, serum, tissues	Rapid and sensitive, but requires special equipment
Reverse transcription-PCR (RT-PCR)	Viral nucleic acid	Blood, serum, tissues	Rapid and sensitive, but requires expensive and special equipment
Direct fluorescence assay (DFA)	Viral antigen	Tissues (e.g., liver)	Rapid and easy, but prone to subjective interpretation
Immunohistochemistry (IHC)	Viral antigen	Tissues (e.g., skin, liver)	Inactivated material, but requires time
Detection of virus-specific antibodies			
Enzyme-linked immunosorbent assay (ELISA)	Antiviral antibodies	Serum	Specific and sensitive, but initial response is slower than indirect immunofluorescence assay
Indirect immunofluorescence assay (IFA)	Antiviral antibodies	Serum	Simple to perform, but prone to nonspecific positives and subjective interpretation
Neutralization test (NT)	Antiviral antibodies (neutralizing activity)	Serum	Specific, but requires time
Additional diagnostic procedures			
Virus isolation	Viral particle	Blood, tissues	Virus available for studies, but requires time and biocontainment
Electron microscopy (EM)	Viral particle	Blood, tissues	Unique morphology (immunostaining possible), but insensitive and requires expensive equipment

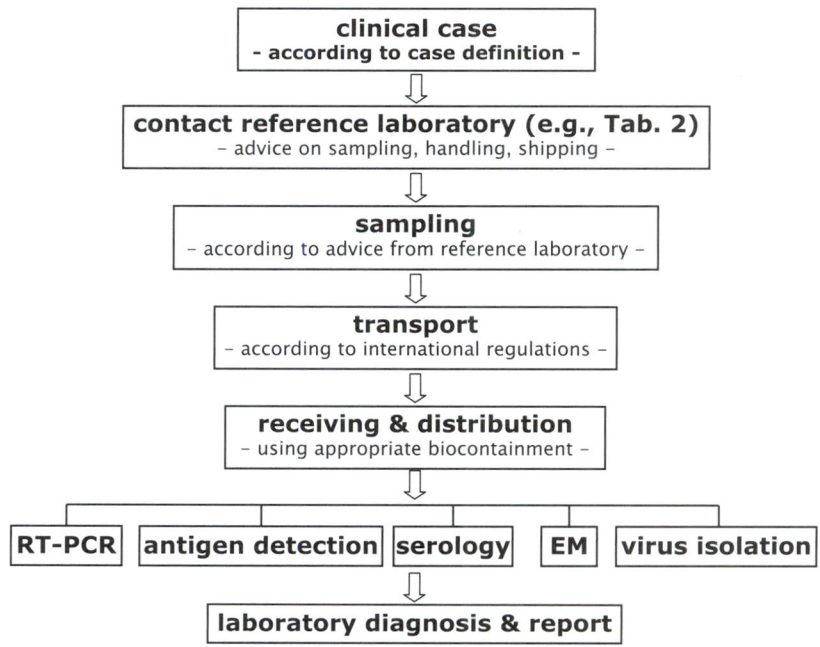

FIGURE 4   Diagnostic flowchart. For further information, see the text.

the early detection and identification of these agents and is both sensitive and specific (3, 16, 20, 23, 26). These tests reliably detect antigens in samples inactivated by either β-propiolactone or gamma irradiation; thus, they can be conducted safely without elaborate BSL-4 facilities. The threshold sensitivities for these assays are approximately 1.3×10^2 to 3.2×10^2 PFU/ml; therefore, they are sufficiently sensitive to detect antigen in most acute-phase VHF viremias, as well as virus concentrations in late-phase throat wash and urine samples. The antigen capture ELISA developed for EBOV serves as a generic model for antigen capture ELISAs for both arenavirus and filovirus groups (20). The assay is a double-sandwich capture ELISA. Plates are coated overnight with a mixture of monoclonal antibodies and washed, and unknowns are added in fourfold dilutions. Following incubation and wash steps, polyclonal antibodies (mainly rabbit serum) against the virus to be tested are added, and the plates are incubated and washed; an anti-species antibody (e.g., anti-rabbit IgG) is then added. Color development, by the horseradish peroxidase-ABTS [2,2'-azino-di-(3-ethylbenzthiazoline sulfonate)] system, is proportional to the quantity of viral antigen captured on the plate.

A few researchers have developed and compared antigen capture ELISAs by using monoclonal versus polyclonal antibodies against various EBOV proteins. The antigen capture ELISA developed by Ksiazek et al. (20) uses a pool of five mouse monoclonal antibodies for coating. Others use NP or VP40 and/or GP-secific specific monoclonal antibodies (23, 26). Most published antigen capture ELISAs use polyclonal rabbit serum for detection. Polyclonal antisera often show higher sensitivity and avidity than do monoclonal antibodies. On the other hand, monoclonal antibodies may have the advantages of higher specificity and availability in unlimited amounts of the same quality.

In the REBOV epizootic setting, very close concordance was obtained between conventional isolation and the antigen capture ELISA techniques. The suitability of this test for use with clinical materials from human patients with ZEBOV was also validated during the 1995 Zaire outbreak. Similar formats have been devised and tested for LAS and JUN. For LAS, good correlation with viral isolation was found for serum samples collected in West Africa, provided that the infectious virus titers exceeded 1.3×10^2 PFU/ml. Substitution of monoclonal antibody of high avidity and appropriate specificities for polyclonal sera generally increases the sensitivities and specificities of these antigen capture ELISAs. However, monoclonal antibodies with broad cross-reactivities are potentially useful for the development of a general pan-arenavirus detector system.

RT-PCR

Nucleic acid detection assays based on PCR have been developed as very useful tools for rapid, definitive diagnosis of most VHF infections. The procedures for performing this assay vary and are sometimes performed through the use of commercially available kits. The process starts with an RNA purification step. Most commonly, total RNA is extracted from clinical specimens with commercially available RNA extraction kits on the basis of denaturation using a monophasic solution of guanidine thiocyanate, thus inactivating the infectious material. At this stage, the specimen can be removed from biocontainment and processed in a standard molecular diagnostic setting under BSL-2 conditions.

The RT and amplification steps are ideally performed in a one-tube system to simplify handling and avoid cross-contamination. Several commercial kits are available and perform more or less equally well in amplification. Alternate PCRs can be set up by designing primer sets against specific areas of the viral gene of interest. The presence of amplification products of the appropriate size when run on agarose gels confirms the presence of RNA from the original sample. It is strongly recommended that a positive PCR result be confirmed by determination of the amplicon DNA sequence and amplification of a second target gene. The sequence information can be used for further phylogenetic analyses.

More recently, real-time PCR methods for rapid nucleic acid detection have been developed which allow for online evaluation. The systems also can be used for quantitation, which becomes important for the evaluation of treatment protocols. Several methods are available at present to monitor the amplification process. A sequence-specific fluorogenic probe(s) can be incorporated into the amplified products and detected through 5′ nuclease action or fluorescence resonance energy transfer, or fluorescent dyes (SYBR Green I) can intercalate into the amplified double-stranded DNA nonspecifically. This method requires a further "melt curve analysis" to verify the identity of the amplified products. In general, these methods eliminate the need for agarose gels and thus limit the potential for contamination.

There are many assays available, and specific details can be obtained from the appropriate publications (see references 7, 22, 34, and 35). Assays can be set up for the detection of a group of viruses such as the Old World or New World arenaviruses or members of a genus such as *Ebolavirus* or *Marburgvirus*. Many assays target the nucleoprotein gene (thought to be the most abundant viral RNA species in infected cells) or polymerase gene (thought to be the most highly conserved genome region). For virus-specific assays, the glycoprotein gene, the most variable genome region, is preferred. Figures 5 and 6 provide examples of real-time RT-PCR analysis for filoviruses and arenaviruses based on methods developed in our laboratory (unpublished data).

Amplification of DNA is prone to several drawbacks, notably the serious potential of cross-contamination and, thus, false-positive results. Several of the conventional RT-PCR assays include a second-round amplification (nested PCR), which can increase the sensitivity and specificity of the amplification reaction but is particularly prone to template contamination due to the inherent need for opening first-round reactions, exposing the environment to amplification products prior to the last amplification step. Because of this potential, most researchers advocate the use of a second independent RT-PCR targeting a different region of the genome, an independent extraction of RNA, or a confirmatory test based on a different technique such as the antigen capture ELISA. Another potential problem with PCR-based diagnostics is the considerable genetic variability of these viruses, which must be accounted for when designing oligonucleotide primers and probes. This problem is enhanced when multiple primer-probe combinations are necessary for real-time assays and a failure of one component to properly hybridize gives a false-negative result. The use of novel agents and strains also provides a situation where PCR-based techniques may fail due to the specificity inherent in the reaction, a situation that has arisen in the past and promises to arise again.

A side-by-side comparison of standard single-round and nested RT-PCR and real-time RT-PCR (34) demonstrated that the real-time RT-PCR detection systems might be more sensitive than standard RT-PCR. The threshold for detection by standard single-round RT-PCR was approximately 10^5 genomic-sense RNA copies per ml. Nested RT-PCR assays from the Gulu Sudan EBOV outbreak demonstrated a threshold of detection of approximately 10^4 copies per ml. The one-step real-time RT-PCR method demonstrated a sensitivity of detection to the level of approximately 10^3 copies per ml. The sensitivity of PCR can be much higher than that of antigen detection (antigen capture ELISA) or virus isolation. However, it must be remembered that the volume of clinical sample which is actually tested in the RT-PCR analysis is quite small, usually between 1 and 10 μl (our

standard is approximately 3 μl of serum or blood); thus, the concentration of infectious virions in the clinical material must exceed 500/ml to expect a positive RT-PCR signal.

An RT-PCR has also been evaluated by using sera from two small series of Lassa fever patients from West Africa (35). The sensitivity by RT-PCR relative to conventional viral isolation was 82%, and the specificity was 68%. The RT-PCR assay was positive for more of the disease course than was isolation, perhaps a reflection of the early antibodies associated with acute Lassa fever. These results predict good success with detection of LAS in tissue samples obtained at autopsy, although this has not been field tested. Likewise, various strategies for RT-PCR have been devised to detect JUN and MAC RNA in clinical materials (22). RT-PCR strategies also exist for GTO but remain to be field tested. The sensitivity of the JUN RT-PCR is reported to be 1 infected cell in a population of 10^4 (22).

DFA

To process infected cells for DFA examination and presumptive identification, inoculated cell monolayers are dispersed by trypsinization, diluted in phosphate-buffered saline containing 10% calf serum, washed, and resuspended in phosphate-buffered saline to a final concentration of 10^6 cells/ml. Small drops (10 to 20 μl) of cell suspensions are placed onto circular areas of specially prepared epoxy-coated microscope slides, cleaned previously by immersion in ethanol followed by polishing to remove residual oily deposits. These "spotslides" are air dried, fixed in acetone at room temperature for 10 min, and either stained immediately or stored frozen at −70°C until used. Note that although acetone fixation greatly reduces the amount of infectious intracellular virus, spotslides prepared in this manner should still be considered infectious and handled accordingly. Spotslides are usually rendered noninfectious by gamma radiation, with no diminution in fluorescent-antigen intensity reported; this treatment is recommended if the appropriate equipment is available. Alternatively, infected cells may be biologically inactivated with β-propiolactone.

For DFA tests, specific immune globulin, prepared by ethanol or ammonium sulfate precipitation of immune sera followed by conjugation with fluorescein, is diluted to a working concentration predetermined by box titration and flooded onto the infected cells, which are incubated at room temperature in a moist chamber. After incubation, the slides are washed, dipped in water to remove salts, dried by evaporation, and mounted under coverslips. Specific viral fluorescence is characterized as intense, punctuate to granular aggregates confined to the cytoplasm of infected cells. In addition, specific MARV and EBOV fluorescence may include large, bizarrely shaped aggregates up to 10 μm across. Nonspecific fluorescence is rarely a problem in DFA procedures for these viruses.

DFA can also be applied to impression smears from biopsy or autopsy material (e.g., liver, spleen, or kidney tissue) obtained from infected individuals. A suspension of the material is prepared in PBS and applied to microscope slides that are subsequently air dried and acetone fixed. DFA also has been used successfully to detect MARV antigen on dried, citrated human blood smears and on impression smears from blood, tissues, nasal turbinates, and even urine from REBOV-infected macaques (31). In addition, the approach has been successfully applied to JUN-infected cells in peripheral blood and urinary sediment.

Detection of MARV, EBOV, and LAS antigens by DFA is usually considered sufficient for a definitive diagnosis.

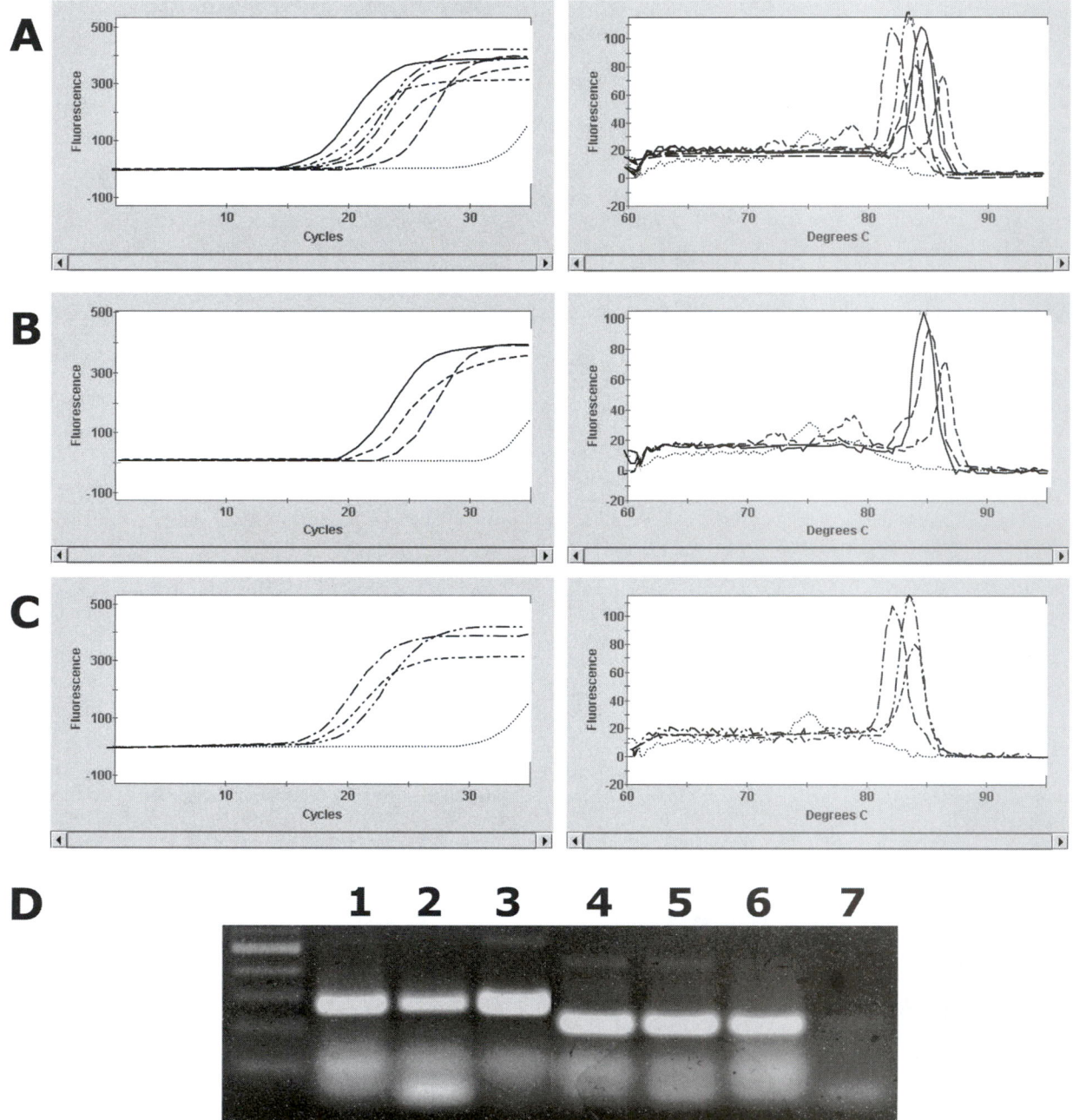

FIGURE 5 Real-time RT-PCR detection of filoviruses. (A) Amplification curves and melting point analysis of *Zaire ebolavirus* (ZEBOV) (long dash, D-1), *Sudan ebolavirus* (SEBOV) (dash, D-2), *Ivory Coast ebolavirus* (ICEBOV) (solid, D-3), *Marburgvirus* (MARV) strain Musoke (dash dot, D-4), MARV strain Ravin (long dash dot, D-5), MARV strain Ozolin (long dash dot dot, D-6), and a control (round dot, D-7). (B and C) Separate amplification curves and melting point analyses for the EBOV species (ZEBOV, SEBOV, and ICEBOV) and MARV strains, respectively. (D) Agarose gel electrophoresis of the amplification products of the real-time filovirus RT-PCR with a 100-bp DNA ladder. Viral RNA was extracted from tissue culture supernatants by using a Qiagen viral RNA kit followed by real-time RT-PCR with a Lightcycler RNA SYBR Green I kit with 0.2 µM each primer and cycling parameters of RT reaction at 50°C for 20 min, denaturation at 94°C for 120 s, and amplification of 40 cycles at 95°C for 15 s, 50°C for 30 s, and 72°C for 30 s. Primers target the EBOV (EVSP5 [5′ ACATCTTTCTTTCTTTG GGTAAT] and EVSP3 [5′ CAGT TCTCAGC-CCATTCACCAGCTT]) and MARV (MVSP5 [5′AAAGTTGCTGAT TCCCCTTTGGA] and MVSP3 [5′ GCATGAGG GTTTTGACCTTGAAT]) glycoprotein genes and produce 273- and 223-bp amplification products, respectively. Melting-point analysis was done by heating the amplification products from 60 to 95°C at 0.2°C/s while monitoring the samples for loss of fluorescence, indicating the point at which double-stranded DNA melts and the intercalating dye loses fluorescence. The first derivative of the melting curve is shown here for ease of interpretation. The presence of peaks at appropriate melting temperatures distinguishes authentic product from nonspecific products and primer-dimers as seen for the control (round dot).

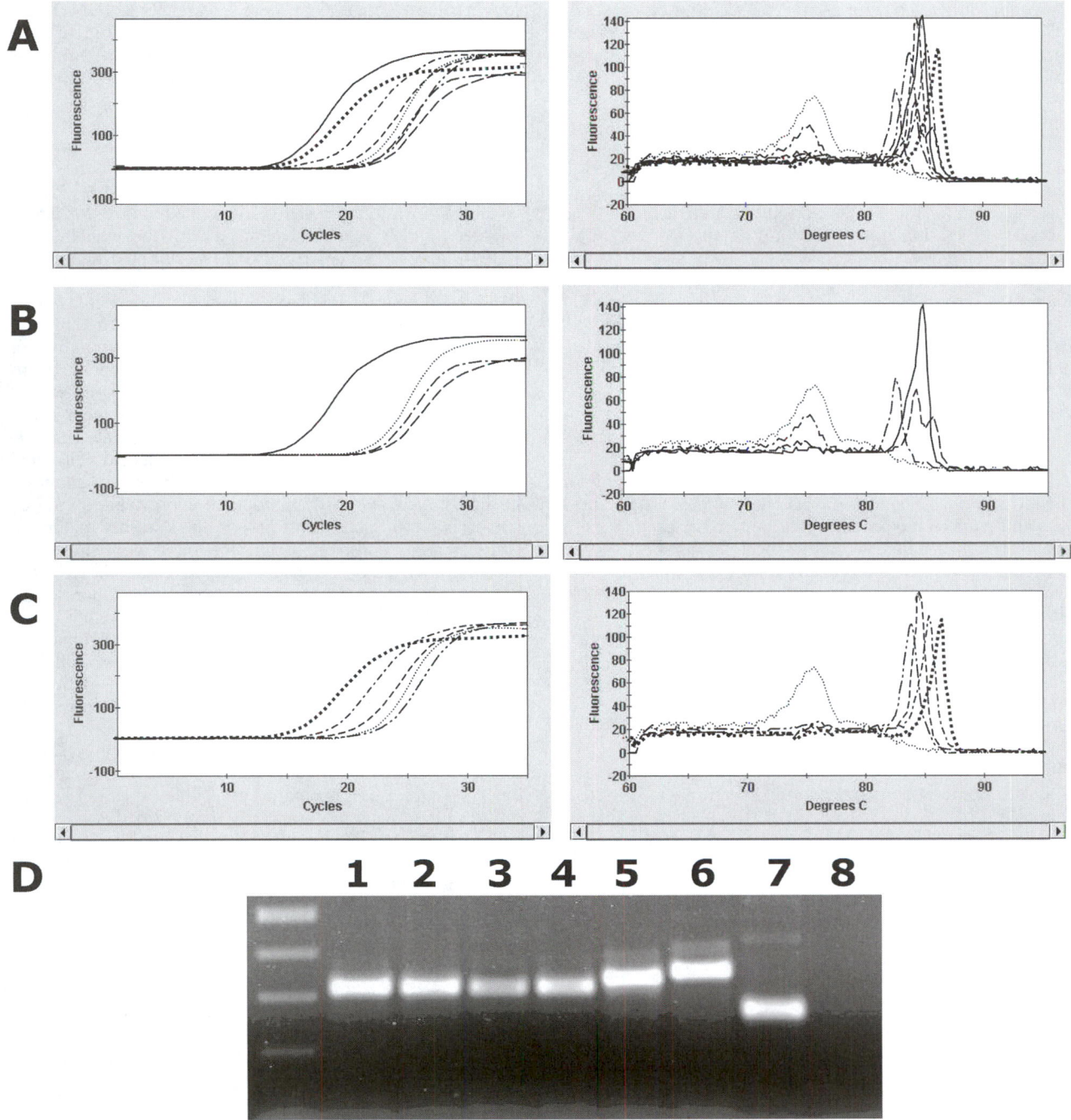

FIGURE 6 Real-time RT-PCR detection of arenaviruses. (A) Amplification curves and melting-point analysis of Machupo (MAC) (dash, D-1), Junin (JUN) (square dot, D-2), Sabia (SAB) (dash dot, D-3), Guanarito (GTO) (long dash dot, D-4), Lassa (LAS), strain Josiah (solid, D-5), LAS strain Pinneo (long dash, D-6), *Lymphocytic choriomeningitis* virus (LCMV) (long dash dot, D-7), and a control (round dot, D-8). (B and C) Separate amplification curves and melting point analysis for the New World complex species (MAC, JUN, GTO, and SAB) and the Old World complex species (LAS and LCMV), respectively. (D) Agarose gel electrophoresis of the amplification products of the arenavirus real-time RT-PCR with a 100-bp DNA ladder. RNA was extracted from tissue culture supernatants by using a Qiagen viral RNA kit followed by real-time RT-PCR with a Lightcycler RNA SYBR Green I kit with 0.2 μM each primer and cycling parameters of RT reaction at 50°C for 20 min, denaturation at 94°C for 120 s, and amplification of 40 cycles at 95°C for 15 s, 50°C for 30 s, and 72°C for 30 s. Primers target the NP gene for New World arenaviruses (NWA5 [5′ TTTGAAGC-CTTTCTCATCATG] and NWA3 [5′ TGGCCTTACATTGGTTC(CA)AG(AG)TC]) and the GPC gene of the Old World arenaviruses (OWA5 [5′ ACCGGGGATCCTAGGCATTT] and OWA3 [5′ ATATAATGATGACTGTTGTTCTTTGTCA]) and produce amplification products of 288 and ~250 to 345 bp, respectively. Melting-point analysis was achieved by heating the amplification products from 60 to 95°C at 0.2°C/s while monitoring the samples for loss of fluorescence, indicating the point at which double-stranded DNA melts and the intercalating dye loses fluorescence. The first derivative of the melting curve is shown here for ease of interpretation. The presence of peaks at appropriate melting temperatures distinguishes authentic product from nonspecific products and primer-dimers as seen for the mock infection (round dots).

Detection of antigen from South American arenaviruses by DFA constitutes a presumptive diagnosis since these viruses can be reliably distinguished from each other only by neutralization tests (NTs).

IHC

The development of IHC techniques for detection of filovirus and arenavirus antigens in formalin-fixed tissues has recently advanced to the point that results are far more satisfactory than for DFA examination of frozen, acetone-fixed sections. Obtaining frozen sections for diagnosis is rarely worth the biohazard incurred, especially since the threshold sensitivity for detection exceeds 6 $\log_{10}$ PFU/g. For filoviruses, paraffin blocks of tissues are sectioned and mounted on silane-coated slides. They are deparaffinized, hydrated, digested with protease, and stained for the presence of viral antigens with cocktails of monoclonal antibodies. Biotinylated anti-mouse antiserum is then added, and the reaction product is developed with a streptavidin-alkaline phosphatase system. Substitution of other chromogens can further increase sensitivity while reducing background. These techniques are expected to prove especially useful for the retrospective diagnosis of viral infections in archived tissues and paraffin blocks. However, systematic examinations of archived materials have not yet been reported.

Remarkable success was reported in application of IHC to detect viral antigens in formalin-fixed skin biopsy specimens obtained from EBOV patients (37). This tool facilitates a definitive diagnosis of patients when liquid nitrogen or dry ice is not available and simplifies submission of the samples to a reference laboratory, since fixation inactivates the virus.

Detection of Virus-Specific Antibodies

ELISA

The current method of choice for diagnostic antibody detection is ELISA (3, 11, 17, 21, 24, 27). The best-evaluated assays use infected cell lysates as antigen. Normally, for IgG detection, infected cells are treated with Triton X-100 followed by inactivation using gamma irradiation. This antigen is coated onto 96-well plates overnight. The plates are washed, and serum or plasma is applied to the wells in a serial fourfold dilution normally starting at 1:100. This is followed by washing and addition of a species-specific secondary antibody mostly coupled with horseradish peroxidase. Color development is measured by the horseradish peroxidase-ABTS system. In parallel, each sample is run against a negative control antigen (uninfected cell lysate prepared using the same method).

For IgM detection, many laboratories use a capture format (21, 27). Microtiter plates are coated with anti-human IgM, washed, and incubated with a serial fourfold dilution of the clinical specimen (serum or plasma) normally starting at 1:100. In the next step, viral antigen is applied after being prepared by sonication and gamma irradiation of infected cells. Subsequently, the antigen is detected using a polyclonal antiserum following the IgG protocol.

ELISAs have been developed using recombinant-expressed viral proteins as antigens for detection of virus-specific antibodies. These assays thereby abrogate the need for BSL-4 infections to establish antigen supplies. Stably expressing cell lines, bacterial recombinant-expressed as well as recombinant baculovirus-expressed viral proteins, have been used for the detection of EBOV and LAS antigens (1, 2, 11, 14, 17). The sensitivity and specificity of the EBOV recombinant ELISAs compared to those of the

immunofluorescence assay were 92 and 99%, respectively. Similar results were shown for the nucleocapsid of LAS expressed from a baculovirus system as well as from the recombinant bacterium-expressed LAS nucleocapsid.

IFA

IFA is currently the most simple method for documenting recent filovirus and arenavirus infections in the field. Preparation of spotslides using infected Vero or MA-104 cells is identical to the procedure described above for DFA. Uninfected cells are often admixed with the virus-infected cells to aid discrimination between specific and nonspecific fluorescence. Although monovalent spotslides are usually desired and are prepared with cells optimally infected with a single virus, polyvalent spotslides can also be prepared by mixing cells infected with different viruses selected from these or other taxonomic groups which have similar geographic distributions (19). Test sera are diluted serially, usually in twofold increments, starting at 1:4 or 1:10. Prozones may occur in low dilutions. Thus, for screening procedures, sera are commonly tested at both 1:10 and 1:80 dilutions. Infected cells (and uninfected control cells) are incubated with serum dilutions, washed, reincubated with appropriate fluorescein-conjugated anti-globulin (or specific anti-IgM or -IgG), washed, mounted, and observed. End-point determination is very subjective. Most experienced observers consider the end point to be the highest dilution producing typical cytoplasmic fluorescence clearly positive relative to uninfected cells. Although it is possible to obtain reproducible end points within individual laboratories, discrepancies in titers determined by different laboratories are common and probably relate to variations in interpretation, epi-illumination intensity, filtration systems, and fluorescein conjugates.

Previous investigations of the seroprevalence of EBOV relied on inactivated infected cells as the source of antigen for IFA, requiring the preparation of slides in BSL-4 laboratories. Others have more recently developed IFA to detect IgG based on cell lines stably expressing viral proteins such as REBOV nucleoprotein or cell lines infected with a recombinant baculovirus expressing an appropriate antigen (15). If this proves reliable in the future, antigen production would be independent on BSL-4 facilities.

Despite the simplicity of the assay, IFA, particularly for the detection of filovirus-specific immune responses, has often been not very reliable, probably because of cross-reactivities with other viruses. For example, significant proportions of human and nonhuman primate sera have been shown to react with filovirus and arenavirus antigens without an apparent history of such exposure.

NT

Neutralization tests (NT) are considered definitive for arenavirus identification but are rarely necessary since, with the exceptions of JUN, MAC, and perhaps LAS and the LAS-like viruses (Mopeia and Mobala viruses), these viruses may be readily distinguished on the basis of IFA, ELISA, or other less frequently used antibody detection tests such as immunoblot assay or radioimmunoprecipitation (not described here). NT depends on inhibition of viral replication by a specific immune serum; the format is determined in part by the availability of tools to measure infectivity or viral antigens (e.g. plaques, DFA, ELISA, or in vivo infectivity). The most generally applied NT is a plaque reduction neutralization test (PRNT) using Vero cells and the serum dilution-constant virus format. The serum dilution calculated (by probit analysis) to reduce the control number of plaques by

50% (PRNT-50) is usually taken as the end point, although in some laboratories the highest serum dilution producing 80% reduction (PRNT-80) is used. The PRNT-80 test is commonly used to distinguish JUN from MAC. For LAS, neutralizing-antibody activity is rapidly lost on dilution; for this reason, the constant serum dilution-varying virus format is preferred. The same principles apply to neutralization of MARV and EBOV, for which NTs have been notoriously imprecise. Neutralization of Old World arenaviruses is also markedly enhanced by addition of complement; thus, 10% fresh guinea pig serum is routinely added to the diluent. Plaque reduction is further enhanced by addition of either anti-immunoglobulin or protein A. PRNTs in various formats have largely replaced animal protection tests for measurement of neutralizing antibodies to these viruses.

Acute-phase sera from Lassa fever patients frequently contain both infectious virus and IFA and complement fixation antibodies. In survivors, neutralizing antibodies to LAS virus first appear very late in convalescence (6 weeks or later), long after viremia has disappeared. Neutralizing antibodies against JUN and MAC become detectable 3 to 4 weeks after onset, soon after the termination of viremia. For MARV and EBOV, as for LAS, neutralizing antibodies evolve late; while neutralizing antibodies are thought to be important in protection against reinfection, their role in resolution of acute infections is less firmly established (18).

Additional Diagnostic Procedures

Virus Isolation

The ultimate goal of diagnostic efforts should always be the isolation of the infectious agent in either tissue culture or animal models. The method of choice for isolation of pathogenic filoviruses and arenaviruses is the inoculation of appropriate cell cultures, usually Vero cells (especially clone E6), MA-104 cells, or SW-13 cells, followed by examination of inoculated cells at intervals for the presence of viral antigens by using an immunological staining method such as DFA or immunoperoxidase assays. This approach has been successfully applied to routine primary isolations from field-collected materials. Isolation of some filoviruses, such as SEBOV, by Vero cell inoculation is less reliable since several blind passages might be required. SW-13 and MA-104 cells are reported to be more sensitive and preferable for primary isolations of filoviruses. Other cell lines, including human diploid lung (MRC-5) and BHK-21 cells, have been substituted for Vero cells with reasonable success. Although MAC and JUN were historically isolated by inoculation of newborn hamsters and mice, respectively, Vero cells are approximately as sensitive and are far less cumbersome to manage in BSL-4 containment. Furthermore, Vero cells permit isolation and identification, usually within 1 to 5 days, a significant advantage over the use of animals, which can require a 7- to 20-day incubation period for illness to develop. For primary isolation of other arenaviruses, and for MARV and EBOV, animal inoculations are still used when cell cultures are not available. Guinea pigs are the species of choice for these studies, particularly for filoviruses that initially do not grow well in tissue culture. Often several passages within these animals are required to produce uniformly fatal disease.

EM

MARV and EBOV have been successfully visualized directly by EM of both heparinized blood and urine obtained during the febrile period, as well as tissue culture supernatant fluids following isolation attempts from human material (Fig. 1B).

The concentrations of virus in tissues, blood, and often urine of febrile patients are sufficiently high, and the morphology is sufficiently distinct, to permit a preliminary diagnosis of filovirus infection even when the isolate had been previously unknown, such as with REBOV. Filovirus particles and intracellular inclusions can be used in the diagnosis of suspected VHF cases since these are morphologically distinct features associated with filovirus infections and even have serotype-specific features (12). The materials are processed by immediate fixation with 0.5% glutaraldehyde followed by low-speed centrifugation. Virions are sedimented at $12,000 \times g$ for 15 min, resuspended in 1/100 original sample volumes, and placed on Formvar-carbon coated EM grids, which are then negatively stained with 1% phosphotungstic acid for 30 s and examined.

For confirmation, immune EM (IEM) techniques are used. Monoclonal or polyclonal antibodies have been successfully applied to recent filovirus isolates. These IEM techniques also work well for diagnosis of arenavirus infections, although the morphology of the virions is less striking (Fig. 1A).

For filoviruses, ultrathin sections of cell pellets prepared from peripheral blood leukocytes by Hypaque-Ficoll gradients frequently reveal clusters of virus associated with monocytes. Ultrathin sections of formalin-fixed tissues, most often liver, spleen, or kidney, have frequently revealed typical filovirus and arenavirus particles (Fig. 1). This approach is successful because infectious virus concentrations are frequently very high. Thin-section EM finds utility in retrospective examination of archived tissues.

EVALUATION AND INTERPRETATION OF RESULTS

Early laboratory diagnosis of arenavirus and filovirus infection is most desirable because of the implications for case patient management and public health interventions. Specific antiviral treatment is limited, but specific immune plasma (South American arenaviruses) and the antiviral drug ribavirin (arenaviruses) are most effective when treatment is started soon after onset.

Despite all the achievements in laboratory diagnostics in the past decades, it should be kept in mind that the diagnosis of arenavirus and filovirus infections initially has to be based on clinical assessment (Fig. 4). For this purpose, contingency plans should be developed; these are still missing in many countries, particularly developing countries. Since clinical microbiology and public health laboratories are not generally equipped for diagnosis of VHF caused by arenaviruses and filoviruses, it is necessary that samples be sent to national and/or international reference laboratories capable of performing the required assays (Table 2). In addition, many nations encounter difficulties in sample transport, which can cause substantial delays in laboratory response. Once samples are received, the laboratory response is fairly reasonable and results can be expected within 24 to 48 h.

Of the available techniques for diagnosis, antigen capture ELISA and RT-PCR are currently the most useful for making a diagnosis in an acute clinical setting. RT-PCR assays seem to be favored by many investigators because BSL-4 biocontainment is not necessary after proper inactivation and because of sensitivity, specificity, and rapidity of the technique. However, the diagnosis of index cases of outbreaks or of single imported cases should not be based solely on RT-PCR because of the problem of cross-contamination and, thus, false-positive results. Confirmation by an independent assay such as antigen capture ELISA should always be attempted. If confirmatory techniques and biocontainment (virus isolation) are not available, RT-PCR on an independent target gene and/or independent sample should be the minimum confirmation. In such cases it might be useful to seek confirmation through another reference laboratory.

Serology can be useful for confirmation, but it should be kept in mind that negative serology is not exclusive since patients, particularly filovirus-infected individuals, often die without mounting a proper humoral immune response. Currently, IgM capture ELISA and IgG ELISA are the assays of choice for serology because of their sensitivity, specificity, and reliability. For all the arenavirus and filovirus pathogens, a rising IgM or IgG titer constitutes a strong presumptive diagnosis. However, a single positive result should be confirmed by using a follow-up sample preferentially taken a week later. Decreasing IgM and/or increasing IgG titers (fourfold) in successive paired sera are highly suggestive of a recent infection.

EM can be used as a confirmatory diagnostic procedure but is far less sensitive than any other assay. Virus isolation should be achieved, although its utility as a diagnostic procedure is restricted by time and biosafety concerns. For nonoutbreak surveillance, IHC on formalin-fixed biopsy or autopsy material is available for some of the agents (e.g., filoviruses) and has several advantages including its simplicity and specificity and the lack of any need for enhanced biocontainment.

QUALITY ASSURANCE

Since filoviruses and the VHF-causing arenaviruses have been designated category A bioterrorism agents, procedures for rapid diagnoses have been recently implemented by many countries to enable rapid, sensitive, and efficient detection of these special pathogens. PCR technologies are most widely utilized for this testing (see reference 7), but because of the restricted availability of virologic and clinical material, the evaluation and standardization of test procedures are difficult. Recently, external agencies have been designated to provide external quality assurance of the levels of PCR diagnostic proficiency of responsible laboratories in Europe and Canada through the European Network for Imported Viral Diseases (ENIVD) (25). A total of 28 laboratories from 17 countries were invited to participate in the study. For these, the cumulative fraction of positively testing results for all virus-containing samples (including filoviruses, LAS, and orthopoxviruses) ranged between 70 and 78%. If the samples contained low levels of virus, the detection rates plummeted to between 40 and 46%. Although most laboratories in this study showed reasonable abilities to detect category A agents, a small but significant fraction of laboratories demonstrated rather poor sensitivities. Thus, continued and extended quality assurance studies are required to maximize the robustness of these testing procedures.

FUTURE DEVELOPMENTS

Because of the constant threat posed by emerging infectious diseases and the limitations of existing approaches used to identify new pathogens, there is a great demand for new technological methods for VHF diagnostics. These advances include improved immunologic reagents matched with improved laboratory technologies that are more readily available, more portable, less cumbersome, and less expensive. These have ranged from automated analyzers and microarrays that facilitate the analysis of large numbers of samples to self-contained, disposable miniaturized devices that enable immunoassays to be performed in a field setting. Together, these novel reagents and new technologies are likely to transform diagnostic medicine over the next decade and will probably have large impacts in the field of VHFs.

Outbreaks of filovirus and arenavirus infections often occur in remote, isolated communities that do not have ready access to sophisticated medical resources. This often means that cases must be managed based solely on clinical presentation and contact history, with little or no timely diagnostic support. Patients with unrelated fevers may not be recognized as infected and may risk potential exposure to a more lethal virus. The development of truly portable real-time thermocyclers and simple immunological assays for use in the field has made the provision of a field diagnostic laboratory a reasonable undertaking. Teams developed for rapid response to bioterrorism events are readily adaptable for outbreak response and can prove to be a valuable tool in managing these events.

Since it is not possible to relocate an entire laboratory to remote settings, it is necessary to bring the equipment essential to provide a safe work environment while completing the necessary testing. The initial and most important task is to protect the workers from the virus. Ideally this can be accomplished by using a portable class III biosafety cabinet, if time and logistics permit. This allows safe handling of samples until the infectious agents are inactivated or packaged appropriately for shipping. Although portable, this unit is often too large to travel as checked baggage on commercial flights and would need to be shipped cargo or by charter. Alternatively, personal protective equipment similar to that used by the isolation ward medical staff can be used to protect workers while handling infectious material. Inactivated samples can be used directly in diagnostic assays, as is the case with serological assays, or nucleic acids can be isolated for molecular biology-based assays by using a suitable commercial kit. Real-time PCR-based assays run on machines designed to be portable are well suited to these environments and can be extremely sensitive and provide results in a very short time. In addition to confirming the presence of a virus in patient samples, real-time tests provide a quantitative assay that may be of use when viral-load determination is necessary, as in trials of antivirals or other treatment regimens. Tests for other agents that may be confounding and mistaken originally as the causative agent (e.g., *Plasmodium* spp.) should also be included in the reagent inventory. Logistical issues must be addressed; these include the fact that in truly remote locations a source of reliable electrical power can be difficult to obtain. The provision of a generator with surge protection may be needed and is best obtained locally if rapid response is necessary. Ensuring that the team has all the necessary equipment and reagents can be a significant challenge. In our experience, it is possible to equip a team of two persons for rapid response to an outbreak situation by using six suitcase-sized cases with enough reagents for 500 assays.

An immunofiltration assay for the direct detection of EBOV antigen (which will most probably also be applicable for other VHF agents) in sera and other body fluids will soon be available in column format (unpublished data). These assays have a number of features that make them suitable for rapid tests that can be used in a field or outbreak setting. Refrigeration is not required for any component, nor is there any need for electrical power sources other than a battery-driven photometer. A simple protocol consisting of rehydration of the column and sequential loading of the sample followed by addition of test reagents and substrate provides a colormetric determination in approximately 30 min. Antibody detection assays based on this system are also under development (unpublished data). This method should be applicable to most arenaviruses and filoviruses and should lend itself very well to field applications.

We thank many colleagues in the field for fruitful and stimulating discussion. Work on arenaviruses and filoviruses in Winnipeg was supported over the years by grants from the following agencies: Canadian Institute of Health Research (CIHR), Deutsche Forschungsgemeinschaft (DFG), and Health Canada/Public Health Agency of Canada.

REFERENCES

1. Barber, G. N., J. C. Clegg, and J. Chamberlain. 1987. Expression of Lassa virus nucleocapsid protein segments in bacteria: purification of high-level expression products and their application in antibody detection. *Gene* **56:**137–144.

2. Barber, G. N., J. C. Clegg, and G. Lloyd. 1990. Expression of the Lassa virus nucleocapsid protein in insect cells infected with a recombinant baculovirus: application to diagnostic assays for Lassa virus infection. *J. Gen. Virol.* **71:**19–28.

3. Bausch, D. G., P. E. Rollin, A. H. Demby, M. Coulibaly, J. Kanu, A. S. Conteh, K. D. Wagoner, L. K. McMullan, M. D. Bowen, C. J. Peters, and T. G. Ksiazek. 2000. Diagnosis and clinical virology of Lassa fever as evaluated by enzyme-linked immunosorbent assay, indirect fluorescent-antibody test, and virus isolation. *J. Clin. Microbiol.* **38:**2670–2677.

4. Borio, L., T. Inglesby, C. J. Peters, A. L. Schmaljohn, J. M. Hughes, P. B. Jahrling, T. Ksiazek, K. M. Johnson, A. Meyerhoff, T. O'Toole, M. S. Ascher, J. Bartlett, J. G. Breman, E. M. Eitzen, Jr., M. Hamburg, J. Hauer, D. A. Henderson, R. T. Johnson, G. Kwik, M. Layton, S. Lillibridge, G. J. Nabel, M. T. Osterholm, T. M. Perl, P. Russell, K. Tonat, and the Working Group on Civilian Biodefense. 2002. Hemorrhagic fever viruses as biological weapons: medical and public health management. *JAMA* **287:**2391–2405.

5. Buchmeier, M. J., M. D. Bowen, and C. J. Peters. 2001. *Arenaviridae*: the viruses and their replication, p. 1635–1668. *In* B. N. Fields and D. M. Knipe (ed.), *Virology*, 4th ed. Raven Press, Philidelphia, Pa.

6. Charrel, R. N., and X. de Lamballerie. 2003. Arenaviruses other than Lassa virus. *Antiviral Res.* **57:**89–100.

7. Drosten, C., S. Göttig, S. Schilling, M. Asper, M. Panning, H. Schmitz, and S. Günther. 2002. Rapid detection and quantification of RNA of Ebola and Marburg viruses, Lassa virus, Crimean-Congo hemorrhagic fever virus, Rift Valley fever virus, Dengue virus, and yellow fever virus by real-time reverse transcription-PCR. *J. Clin. Microbiol.* **40:**2323–2330.

8. Feldmann, H., S. Jones, H. D. Klenk, and H. J. Schnittler. 2003. Ebola virus: from discovery to vaccine. *Nat. Rev. Immunol.* **3:**677–685.

9. Feldmann, H., T. W. Geisbert, P. B. Jahrling, H. D. Klenk, S. V. Netesov, C. J. Peters, A. Sanchez, R. Swanepoel, and V. E. Volchkov. 2004. Filoviridae, p. 645–653. *In* C. M. Fauquet, M. A. Mayo, J. Maniloff, U. Desselberger, and L. A. Ball (ed.), *Virus Taxonomy, VIIIth Report of the ICTV.* Elsevier/Academic Press, London, United Kingdom.

10. Feldmann, H., V. Wahl-Jensen, S. M. Jones, and U. Stroeher. 2004. Ebola virus ecology: a continuing mystery. *Trends Microbiol.* **12:**433–437.

11. Garcia Franco, S., A. M. Ambrosio, M. R. Feuillade, and J. I. Maiztegui. 1988. Evaluation of an enzyme-linked immunosorbent assay for quantitation of antibodies to Junin virus in human sera. *J. Virol. Methods* **19:**299–305.

12. Geisbert, T. W., and P. B. Jahrling. 1995. Differentiation of filoviruses by electron microscopy. *Virus Res.* **39:**129–150.

13. Geisbert, T. W., and P. B. Jahrling. 2004. Exotic emerging viral diseases: progress and challenges. *Nat. Med.* **10:**S110–S121.

14. Groen, J., B. G. van den Hoogen, C. P. Burghoorn-Maas, A. R. Fooks, J. Burton, C. J. Clegg, H. Zeller, and A. D. Osterhaus. 2003. Serological reactivity of baculovirus-expressed Ebola virus VP35 and nucleoproteins. *Microbes Infect.* **5:**379–385.

15. Ikegami, T., M. Saijo, M. Niikura, M. E. Miranda, A. B. Calaor, M. Hernandez, D. L. Manalo, I. Kurane, Y. Yoshikawa, and S. Morikawa. 2002. Development of an immunofluorescence method for the detection of antibodies to Ebola virus subtype Reston by the use of recombinant nucleoprotein-expressing HeLa cells. *Microbiol. Immunol.* **46:**33–38.

16. Ikegami, T., M. Niikura, M. Saijo, M. E. Miranda, A. B. Calaor, M. Hernandez, L. P. Acosta, D. L. Manalo, I. Kurane, Y. Yoshikawa, and S. Morikawa. 2003. Antigen capture enzyme-linked immunosorbent assay for specific detection of Reston Ebola virus nucleoprotein. *Clin. Diagn. Lab. Immunol.* **10:**552–557.

17. Ikegami, T., M. Saijo, M. Niikura, M. E. Miranda, A. B. Calaor, M. Hernandez, D. L. Manalo, I. Kurane, Y. Yoshikawa, and S. Morikawa. 2003. Immunoglobulin G enzyme-linked immunosorbent assay using truncated nucleoproteins of Reston Ebola virus. *Epidemiol. Infect.* **130:**533–539.

18. Jahrling, P. B., T. W. Geisbert, N. K. Jaax, M. A. Hanes, T. G. Ksiazek, and C. J. Peters. 1996. Experimental infection of cynomolgus macaques with Ebola-Reston filoviruses from the 1989–1990 U.S. epizootic. *Arch. Virol. Suppl.* **11:**115–134.

19. Johnson, K. M. L., L. Elliott, and D. L. Heymann. 1981. Preparation of polyvalent viral immunofluorescent intracellular antigens and use in human serosurveys. *J. Clin. Microbiol.* **14:**527–529.

20. Ksiazek, T. G., P. E. Rollin, P. B. Jahrling, E. Johnson, D. W. Dalgard, and C. J. Peters. 1992. Enzyme immunosorbent assay for Ebola virus antigens in tissues of infected primates. *J. Clin. Microbiol.* **30:**947–950.

21. Ksiazek, T. G., C. P. West, P. E. Rollin, P. B. Jahrling, and C. J. Peters. 1999. ELISA for the detection of antibodies to Ebola viruses. *J. Infect. Dis.* **179:**S192–S198.

22. Lozana, M. E., P. D. Ghiringhelli, V. Romanowski, and O. Grau. 1993. A simple nucleic acid amplification assay for the rapid detection of Junin virus in whole blood samples. *Virus Res.* **27:**37–53.

23. Lucht, A., R. Grunow, C. Otterbein, P. Moller, H. Feldmann, and S. Becker. 2004. Production of monoclonal antibodies and development of an antigen capture ELISA directed against the envelope glycoprotein GP of Ebola virus. *Med. Microbiol. Immunol.* **193:**181–187.

24. Morales, M. A., G. E. Calderon, L. M. Riera, A. M. Ambrosio, D. A. Enria, and M. S. Sabattini. 2002. Evaluation of an enzyme-linked immunosorbent assay for detection of antibodies to Junin virus in rodents. *J. Virol. Methods* **103:**57–66.

25. Niedrig, M., H. Schmitz, S. Becker, S. Gunther, J. ter Meulen, H. Meyer, H. Ellerbrok, A. Nitsche, H. R. Gelderblom, and C. Drosten. 2004. First international quality assurance study on the rapid detection of viral agents of bioterrorism. *J. Clin. Microbiol.* **42:**1753–1755.

26. Niikura, M., T. Ikegami, M. Saijo, I. Kurane, M. E. Miranda, and S. Morikawa. 2001. Detection of Ebola viral antigen by enzyme-linked immunosorbent assay using a novel monoclonal antibody to nucleoprotein. *J. Clin. Microbiol.* **39:**3267–3271.

27. **Niklasson, B. S., P. B. Jahrling, and C. J. Peters.** 1984. Detection of Lassa virus antigens and Lassa-specific IgG and IgM by enzyme-linked immunosorbent assay. *J. Clin. Microbiol.* **20:**239–244.

28. **Peters, C. J., P. B. Jahrling, and A. Khan.** 1996. Patients infected with high-hazard viruses: scientific basis for infection control. *Arch. Virol. Suppl.* **11:**141–168.

29. **Peters, C. J., and J. W. LeDuc.** 1999. An introduction to Ebola: the virus and the disease. *J. Infect. Dis.* **179:**S1–S288.

30. **Peters, C. J.** 2002. Human infection with arenaviruses in the Americas. *Curr. Top. Microbiol. Immunol.* **262:**65–74.

31. **Rollin, P. E., T. G. Ksiazek, P. B. Jahrling, M. Haines, and C. J. Peters.** 1990. Direct detection of Ebola-like viruses by immunofluorescence (IF) in impression smears from macaque tissues. *Lancet* **336:**1591.

32. **Salvato, M. S., J. C. S. Clegg, M. J. Buchmeier, R. N. Charrel, J. P. Gonzalez, I. S. Lukashevich, C. J. Peters, R. Rico-Hesse, and V. Romanowski.** 2004. *Arenaviridae,* p. 725–733. *In* C. M. Fauquet, M. A. Mayo, J. Maniloff, U. Desselberger, and L. A. Ball (ed.), *Virus Taxonomy, VIIIth Report of the ICTV.* Elsevier/Academic Press, London, United Kingdom.

33. **Sanchez, A., A. Khan, S. Zaki, G. Nabel, T. Ksiazek, and C. J. Peters.** 2001. "Filoviridae" Marburg and Ebola viruses, p. 1279–1304. *In* D. M. Knipe and P. M. Howley (ed.), *Fields Virology,* 4th ed., vol. 1. Lippincott Williams & Wilkins, Philadelphia, Pa.

34. **Towner, J. S., P. E. Rollin, D. G. Bausch, A. Sanchez, S. M. Crary, M. Vincent, W. F. Lee, C. F. Spiropoulou, T. G. Ksiazek, M. Lukwiya, F. Kaducu, R. Downing, and S. T. Nichol.** 2004. Rapid diagnosis of Ebola hemorrhagic fever by reverse transcription-PCR in an outbreak setting and assessment of patient viral load as a predictor of outcome. *J. Virol.* **78:**4330–4341.

35. **Trappier, S. G., A. L. Conaty, B. B. Farrar, D. D. Auperin, J. B. McCormick, and S. P. Fisher-Hoch.** 1993. Evaluation of the polymerase chain reaction for diagnosis of Lassa virus infection. *Am. J. Trop. Med. Hyg.* **49:**214–221.

36. **Vainrub, B., and R. Salas.** 1994. Latin American hemorrhagic fever. *Infect. Dis. Clin. North Am.* **8:**47–59.

37. **Zaki, S. R., W. J. Shieh, P. W. Greer, C. S. Goldsmith, T. Ferebee, J. Katshitshi, F. K. Tshioko, M. A. Bwaka, R. Swanepoel, P. Calain, A. S. Khan, E. Lloyd, P. E. Rollin, T. G. Ksiazek, C. J. Peters, and Commission de Lutte contre les Epidemies a Kikwit.** 1999. A novel immunohistochemical assay for the detection of Ebola virus in skin: implications for diagnosis, spread, and surveillance of Ebola hemorrhagic fever. *J. Infect. Dis.* **179:**S36–S47.

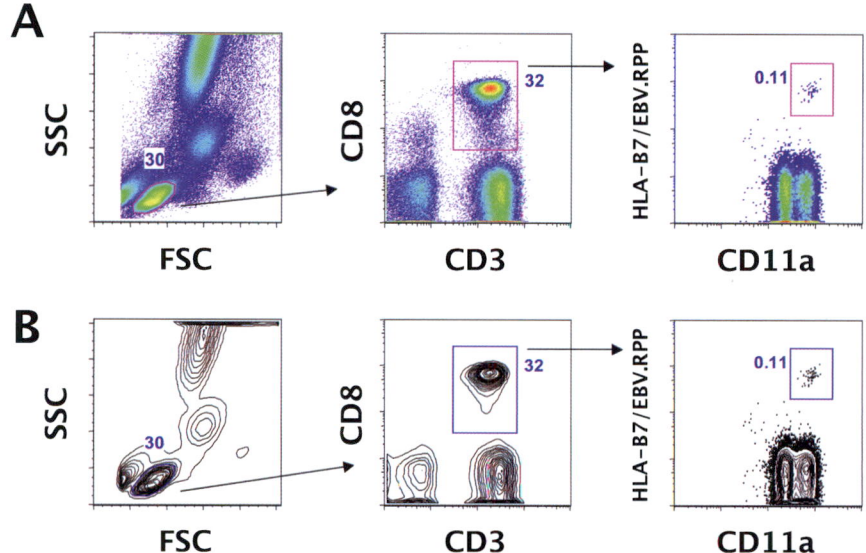

COLOR PLATE 1 (chapter 23) A standard approach to analyzing flow cytometry data from tetramer-stained whole blood. Whole blood from an individual who was HLA-B7[+] and seropositive for EBV was stained with anti-CD3, anti-CD8, anti-CD11a, and an HLA tetramer composed of the HLA-B*0701 heavy chain and a well-characterized B7-restricted CD8[+] T-cell epitope from EBV (RPP, for the first three amino acids in its peptide sequence). The same hierarchical gating procedure is shown in panels A and B. (A) Data displayed in pseudo-color dot plot format; (B) contour plot format, with the show-outliers option turned on for the third panel to show the low-frequency tetramer-positive population.

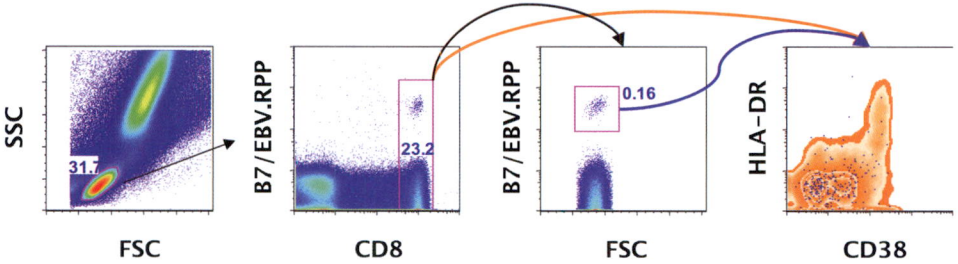

COLOR PLATE 2 (chapter 23) Use of overlay plots to show the phenotype of a tetramer-positive population with two markers. In this example, whole blood from the same donor as in Color Plate 1 was stained with anti-CD8, anti-CD38, anti-HLA-DR, and the B7/EBV.RPP tetramer. After gating on lymphocytes and CD8[hi] cells (two left-hand panels), CD8[hi] cells are plotted as forward scatter versus tetramer, and a gate on the tetramer-positive cells is set. Finally, an overlay plot is created where all CD8[+] cells are shown in orange (as a zebra-plot format), while the tetramer-positive cells are presented as an overlay of blue dots.

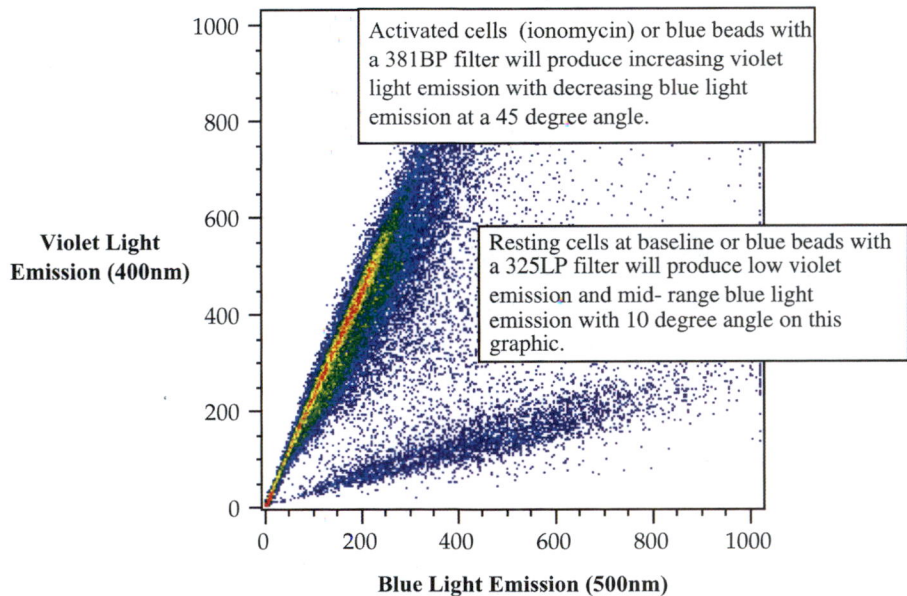

COLOR PLATE 3 (chapter 36)   Blue light emission versus violet light emission as measured by INDO-1-loaded cells or control blue beads. Control positions of blue beads used in the alignment and UV detection of the calcium method can produce either a 45° angle or a 10° angle depending on the light filters used. The expected positions of simulated (free calcium release) and resting cells at baseline are indicated.

The text within the plot reads:

Activated cells (ionomycin) or blue beads with a 381BP filter will produce increasing violet light emission with decreasing blue light emission at a 45 degree angle.

Resting cells at baseline or blue beads with a 325LP filter will produce low violet emission and mid-range blue light emission with 10 degree angle on this graphic.

The y-axis is labeled "Violet Light Emission (400nm)" and the x-axis is labeled "Blue Light Emission (500nm)".

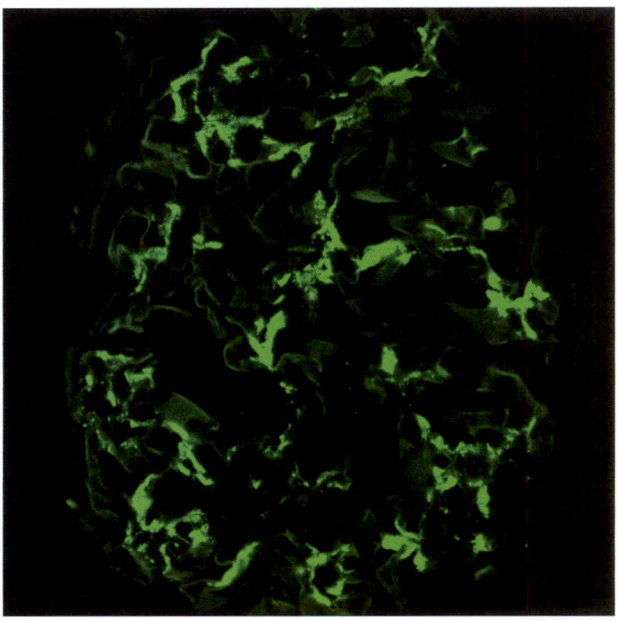

COLOR PLATE 4 (chapter 48)   Direct immunofluorescence of a frozen section from a renal biopsy specimen from a patient with IgA nephropathy, stained with FITC–rabbit anti-human IgA and showing diffuse granular staining in the glomerular mesangium.

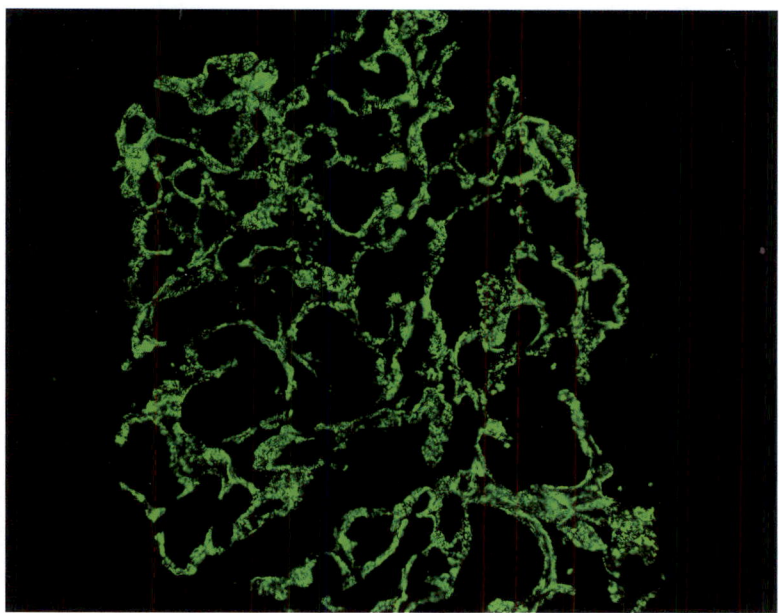

COLOR PLATE 5 (chapter 48)   Direct immunofluorescence of a frozen section from a renal biopsy specimen from a patient with membranous glomerulonephritis, stained with FITC–rabbit anti-human IgG and showing diffuse granular deposits of IgG along the glomerular basement membrane.

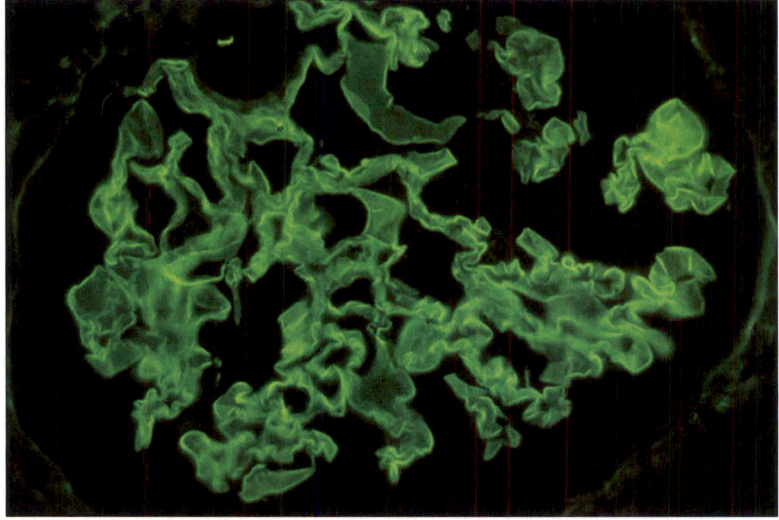

COLOR PLATE 6 (chapter 48)   Direct immunofluorescence of a frozen section from a renal biopsy specimen from a patient with anti-GBM disease, stained with FITC–rabbit anti-human IgG and showing diffuse linear staining along the glomerular basement membrane.

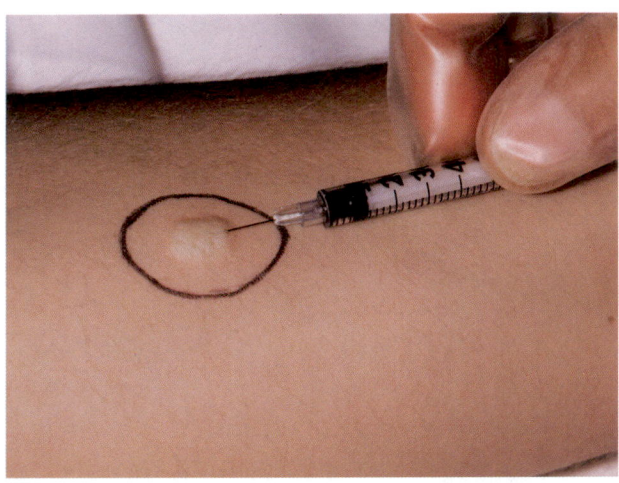

COLOR PLATE 7 (chapter 58) Mantoux test. Intradermal injection of tuberculin raises a weal with a characteristic peau d'orange appearance.

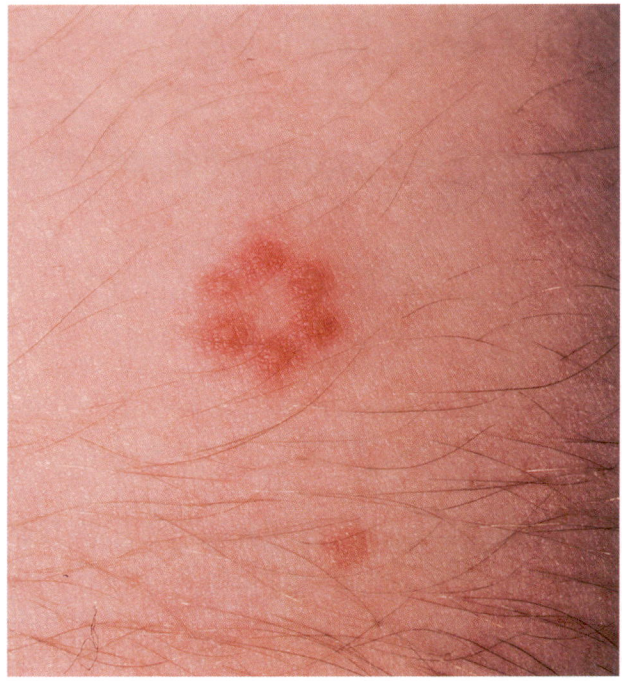

COLOR PLATE 8 (chapter 58) Multipuncture Heaf test. This grade 1 reaction is commonly seen in healthy subjects who have received BCG vaccination.

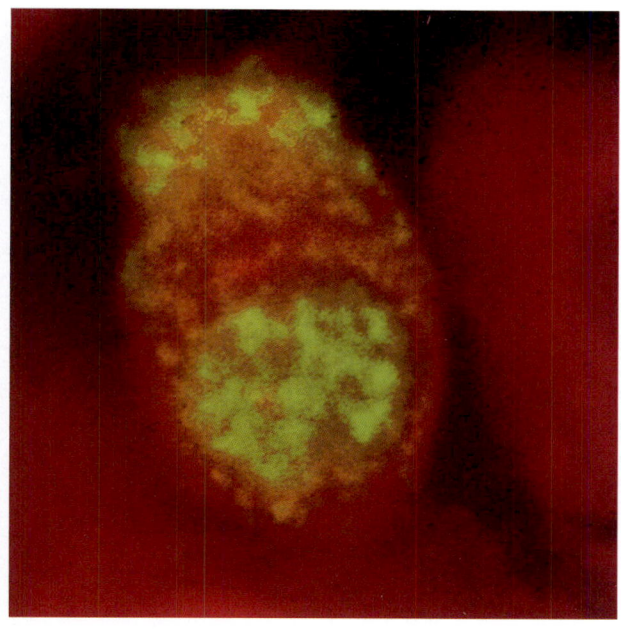

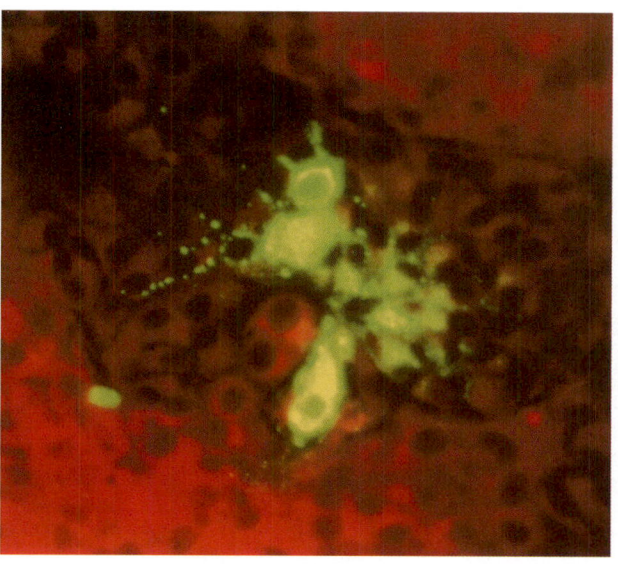

COLOR PLATE 9 (chapter 68) Detection of influenza A virus in columnar respiratory epithelial cell by using a respiratory screen reagent. (Immunofluorescent staining; magnification, ×400.)

COLOR PLATE 10 (chapter 68) Detection of influenza A virus infection in R-mix cells by immunofluorescent staining at 24 h postinfection. (Courtesy Caroline Fong; magnification, ×200.)

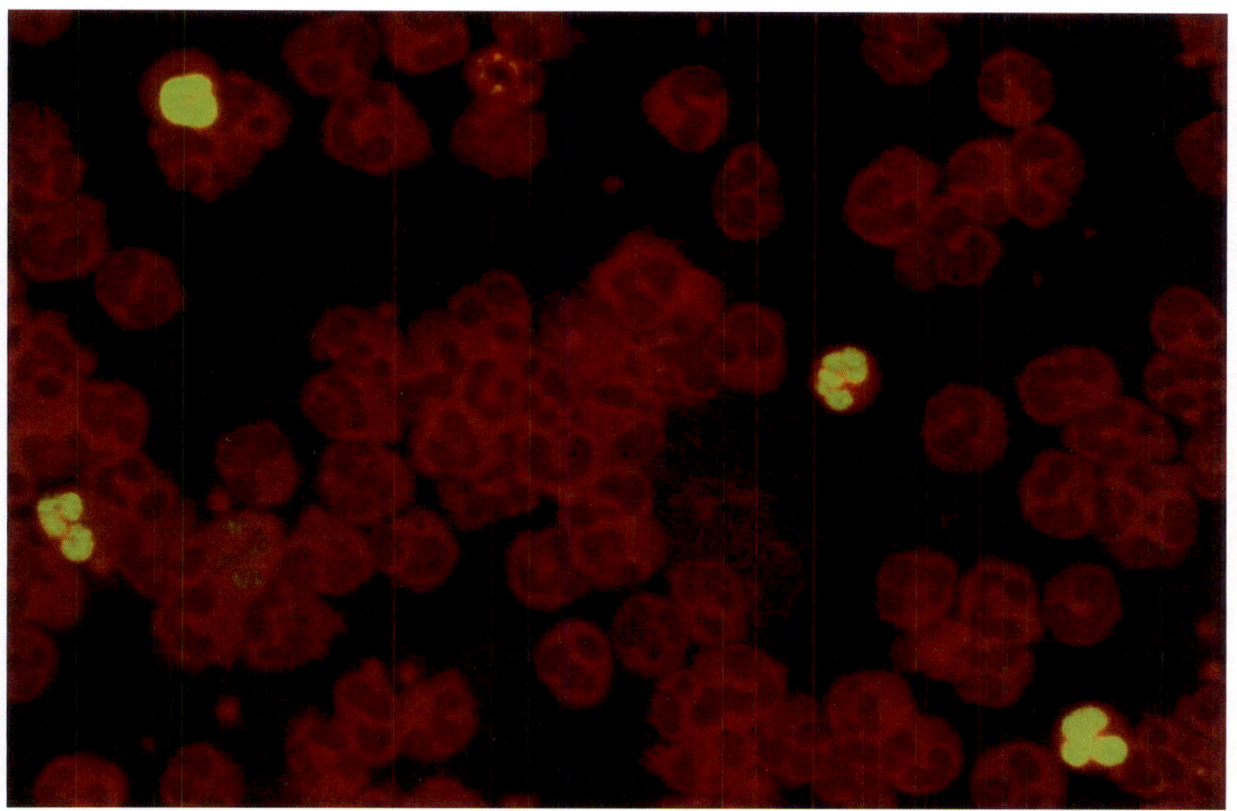

COLOR PLATE 11 (chapter 68) Detection of CMV pp65 antigen in PBL nuclei by immunofluorescent staining. (Magnification, ×400.)

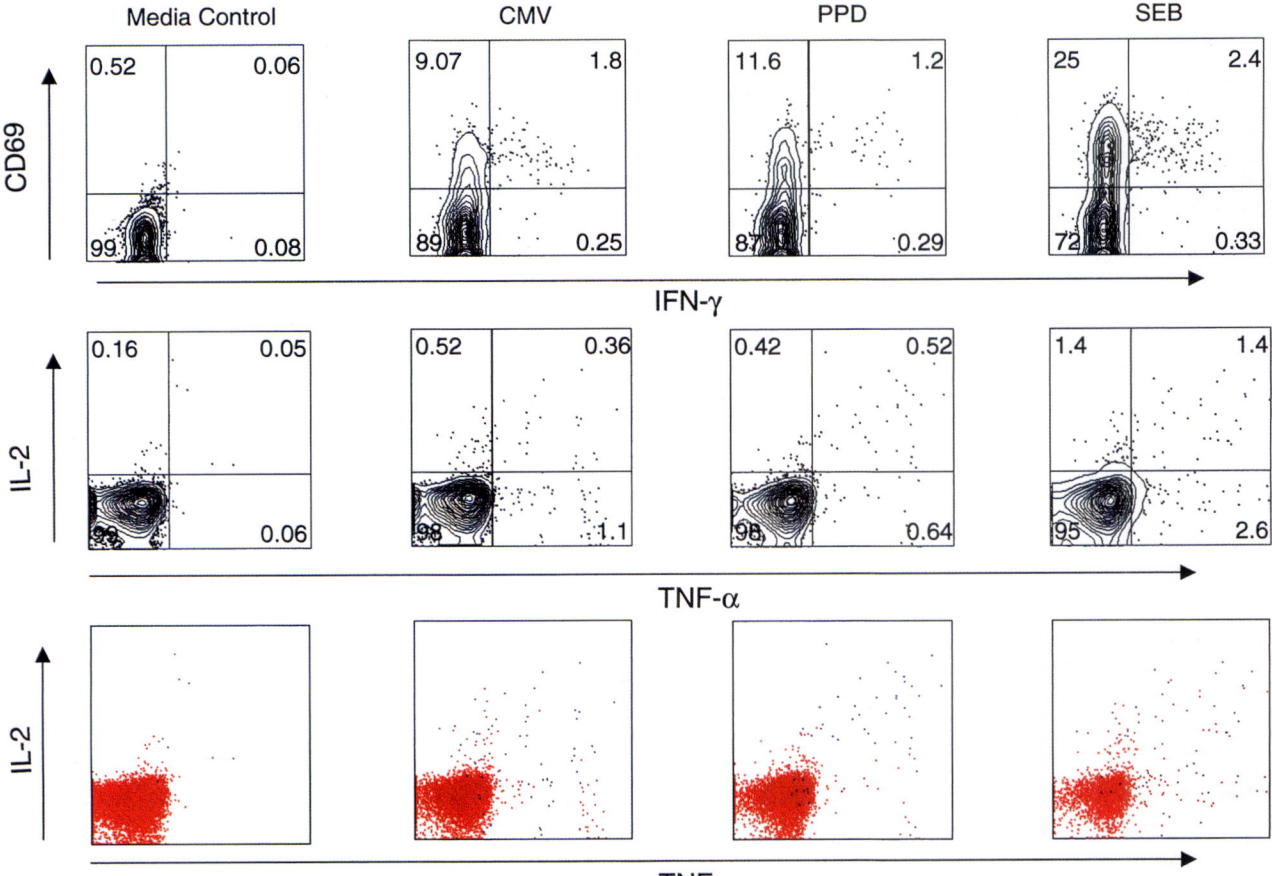

COLOR PLATE 12 (chapter 97) Whole blood from an individual with untreated latent *Mycobacterium tuberculosis* infection was analyzed to determine the frequency of immediate cytokine-producing *M. tuberculosis*-specific CD4[+] T cells. Whole blood was stimulated with PPD for 20 h, the final 4 h in the presence of brefeldin A. CD4[+] T cells were analyzed on a flow cytometer (gating strategies not shown) for expression of various intracellular cytokines after stimulation with medium control, CMV, PPD, and SEB antigens (as shown across the top panel). In the first row of dot plots, with CD4[+] T cells expressing both CD69 (a marker of short-term activation) and IFN-γ, it is shown that 1.2% of CD4[+] T cells express both markers after stimulation with PPD antigen. By subtracting the 0.06% background frequency measured after stimulation with medium control antigen, the proportion of *M. tuberculosis* (really PPD)-specific CD4[+] T cells is 1.14%. In the second row of dot plots, parallel tubes demonstrate the frequency of CD4[+] T cells expressing both TNF-α and IL-2 under the same conditions. In the third row of dot plots, the events (cells) enumerated in the second row are visualized but color coded (gating strategy not shown) to indicate cells expressing all three cytokines of interest (i.e., the blue dots indicate CD4[+] T cells expressing IFN-γ, with TNF-α and/or IL-2 or neither, while the red dots indicate expression of TNF-α and/or IL-2 or neither).

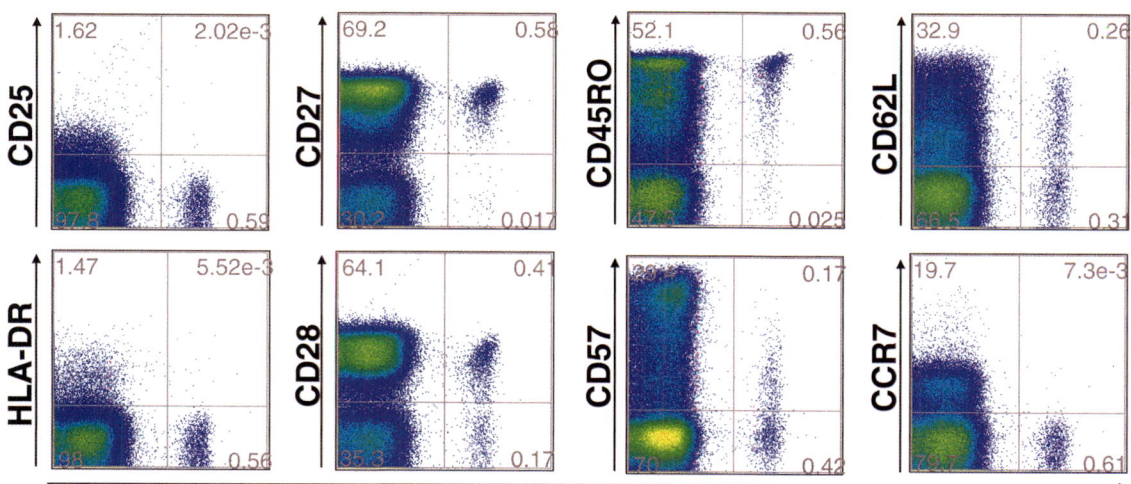

B57-p24 Tetramer

COLOR PLATE 13 (chapter 97) PBMCs from an HIV-infected long-term nonprogressor were surface labeled with MAb to cell surface molecules and an HLA class I tetramer (HLA57 tetramer loaded with a peptide from the p24 protein). Cell frequencies from each of four quadrants from each of the eight dot plots representing the surface molecules tested are on the y axis (CD25, HLA-DR, CD27, CD28, CD45RO, CD57, CD62L, and CCR7), while tetramer staining is shown on the x axis. The data show that the frequency of antigen-specific CD8$^+$ T cells in this individual was ~0.59% of all CD3$^+$ T cells (gating strategy not shown). In addition, the data show that these antigen-specific cells found in the peripheral blood were nearly all CD25$^-$, HLADR$^-$, CD45RO$^+$, CCR7$^-$, and heterogenous for the other markers measured. These data illustrate how HLA tetramers can help tease apart antigen-specific T-cell responses, particularly if immunophenotyping (shown here) is coupled with functional assays (e.g., CFSE proliferation assays and/or intracellular cytokine responses).

Rabies Virus

D. CRAIG HOOPER

88

Rabies virus, the type species of the genus *Lyssavirus* of the family *Rhabdoviridae*, order *Mononegavirales*, is the causative agent of rabies, an invariably lethal neurological disease of a wide variety of animals and humans. The virus is endemic throughout much of the world as an extensive range of variants, each associated with a particular wildlife or domestic animal host species but with the capacity to infect secondary targets, including humans. In developing countries, the major carrier of viruses causing human rabies is the dog. However, significant reservoirs of rabies viruses exist throughout much of the world in foxes, coyotes, skunks, raccoons, various bat species, and a variety of other mammals. Rabies virus can be transmitted from these natural host species to humans either directly or by intermediate animals that are not normally associated with rabies, such as cats, rabbits, etc. Moreover, transplantation of organs from rabies virus-infected individuals has led to the lethal infection of the recipients.

The rabies virion is a characteristically bullet-shaped, enveloped particle of, on average, 75 by 180 nm (26). Projections of glycoprotein (G), the primary target of neutralizing antibodies, are dispersed evenly over the surface, and a helical nucleocapsid contains a single-stranded negative-sense RNA genome encoding five proteins: the nucleoprotein (N), the phosphoprotein (NS), the polymerase (L), the matrix protein (M), and the viral glycoprotein. Since distinct rabies virus strains are endemic in different reservoir species in diverse geographical regions, antigenic or gene sequence analysis of a particular virus isolate can determine its origin and help understanding of the etiology of an infection, which is important in developing risk management strategies. Variability between different virus isolates is extensive for G protein at both sequence and antigenic levels, while N is more conserved. Thus, N-protein-specific antibodies have greater utility for the general detection of rabies virus infection by direct immunofluorescence or immunohistochemical analysis of tissue biopsies or corneal impressions. Identification of a particular virus isolate is commonly accomplished by assessing G-protein nucleic acid structure.

In the absence of treatment, progression to clinical rabies in humans is dependent upon the location and severity of the exposure, the virus strain involved, and, likely, the immune status of the host. For attacks by infected animals, historical evidence suggests that the highest mortality occurs with patients bitten on the head and face (at least 40 to 80%), with diminishing mortality as the bite site becomes more distant from the central nervous system (CNS). Generally, the initial signs of disease appear 2 to 6 weeks after exposure, but there have been occasional cases that developed a number of years after exposure. Clinical rabies becomes apparent initially in nonspecific symptoms which may include general malaise, chills, fever, headache, photophobia, anorexia, sore throat, cough, and musculoskeletal pain. In the case of a bite, there is often itching, burning, numbness, or paresthesia around the site. This prodromal period generally lasts from 2 to 10 days and precedes the acute neurologic phase in which patients manifest signs of neurological dysfunction such as anxiety, agitation, paralysis, or episodes of delirium. A variable proportion of patients exhibit the classical pathognomonic sign of rabies, hydrophobia. Disease progression is variable but usually proceeds through coma to death from respiratory arrest by approximately 30 to 60 days after infection. Survival may be prolonged somewhat by respiratory assistance, but death invariably occurs due to other complications.

Recognition of potential exposure is the most important criterion for successful postexposure prophylaxis, which entails the passive administration of rabies virus-neutralizing antibodies and immunization with a potent vaccine and must be commenced as soon as practical after exposure. Such intervention invariably fails if begun after the appearance of clinical signs of rabies. When potential exposure is due to the bite, or contact with saliva through broken skin or mucosal surfaces, of an animal that might have rabies, the decision to administer postexposure prophylaxis can be based on testing of the animal, if it is available, for the virus. If the animal cannot be located, the decision to intervene is the standard of care since, unlike their predecessors, modern vaccines are safe, efficacious, and readily administered. As a consequence of the widespread use of postexposure prophylaxis when contact with rabies virus is suspected, human mortality from rabies virus infection in the United States is primarily the result of cases where exposure was not recognized. These cases are often initially classified as encephalitis of unknown origin and only correctly identified as rabies either in the terminal stages of the disease or postmortem. In the United States, cases of cryptic rabies, where exposure was unknown, have most often been caused by virus strains associated with several different bat species, including the silver-haired and Mexican free-tailed bats. In several instances, there has been a confirmed or anecdotal reference to contact between the victim and a bat; however, the mode of transmission, which may be by an unnoticed bite or scratch or across a mucosal surface, is unknown.

The failure to diagnose rabies can be significant, as an infected individual presents a risk of infection to others. For example, in 2004, the kidneys, liver, and a segment of the iliac artery were transplanted from a donor who had died of undiagnosed rabies, resulting in the death of all four recipients from rabies and the need to administer postexposure prophylaxis to hundreds of contacts (4, 5). Since most rabies viruses replicate largely in the CNS, rabies in animals or humans has been most often confirmed by the histological identification of Negri bodies (intraneuronal cytoplasmic inclusions of rabies virus nucleocapsid [RNP]) in the brain tissue of victims or suckling mice that had been injected with suspect brain material. However, Negri bodies are not always present in rabies virus-infected brain tissue or may be confused with other viral inclusion bodies. Thus, immunohistochemical techniques using nucleoprotein-specific antibodies have supplanted simple histology in testing of tissue specimens for evidence of rabies. Detection of rabies virus nucleoprotein in histological specimens, such as brain tissue and peripheral nerve biopsies as well as corneal imprints, using fluorescein-conjugated antibody remains the accepted method for the diagnosis of rabies virus infection.

Fluorescein isothiocyanate (FITC)-conjugated monoclonal antinucleoprotein antibodies are also the basis of the rapid fluorescent focus inhibition test (RFFIT), the in vitro neutralization test commonly used to monitor vaccine efficacy or the immune status of humans or animals that have been immunized against the virus. Enzyme-linked immunosorbent assay (ELISA) techniques can also be used for the general screening of virus-specific antigen-antibody interactions when information about neutralizing capacity is unnecessary. While epitope-specific antibodies have been used for the identification and characterization of individual rabies virus isolates, technologies based on the reverse transcriptase (RT)-dependent PCR (RT-PCR) technology are now more widely utilized for these purposes. For example, real-time quantitative RT-PCR is well suited for the detection and characterization of viral genome or mRNA in relatively small tissue samples of variable quality. The existence of cryptic rabies and proof that transmission of the disease between humans can occur by organ transplantation indicate that screening of potential donors with encephalitis of unknown origin for rabies is prudent. This can be accomplished by the analysis of tissue biopsies for either rabies virus antigens or nucleic acids and serology, as many victims of clinical rabies exhibit high serum or cerebrospinal fluid (CSF) titers of rabies virus-specific antibodies prior to their death.

TECHNOLOGY

The control of human rabies is dependent upon determination of whether the animal vector responsible for a potential exposure is rabid. Thus, animals that have bitten an individual and are known reservoirs or secondary vectors of rabies virus are routinely tested for either the presence of the virus or evidence of previous immunization against rabies. Cases of fatal human rabies, most often due to infection with bat rabies virus variants, occur when exposure has gone unnoticed. Due to the nonspecificity of the clinical signs of rabies, these cases are generally undiagnosed during the course of the disease and rabies infection is confirmed only postmortem. Although little can be done once clinical disease has become evident, the diagnosis of rabies is important for management purposes. Immunological technologies are the accepted standards for the assessment of rabies virus infection as well as antiviral-immune status. However, molecular approaches to assessing rabies virus infection are becoming increasingly popular due to their sensitivity, utility for specimens of poor quality, and specificity.

As noted in Table 1, a considerable variety of laboratory, or "fixed," rabies virus strains are available for use in the various assays. Challenge virus standard (CVS) strain 11 (CVS-11) and Evelyn-Rokitnicki-Abelseth (ERA) are commonly used for in vitro assays and may be readily produced in cultures of baby hamster kidney (BHK) cells. Viruses obtained from infected wildlife, termed "street" rabies viruses, often

TABLE 1 Selected laboratory (fixed) strains of rabies virus

Virus designation (abbreviation)	Origin
Challenge virus standard (CVS)	Thought to be derived from the original Pasteur rabies virus isolate passaged in rabbit brain and then mouse brain; a number of variants exist in different laboratories (e.g., CVS-11, passaged in cell culture; CVS-24, passaged in mouse brain)
Evelyn-Rokitnicki-Abelseth (ERA)	Derived from SAD by passage in mouse brain
Flury Low egg passage (LEP) High egg passage (HEP)	Isolated from a human with rabies by mouse brain inoculation and then passaged in chick brain and chicken embryo
Kelev	Isolated from a rabid dog by mouse brain inoculation and then passaged in chicken embryo
Louis Pasteur Virus (PAST)	Isolated from a rabid cow infected by dog bite, passaged in rabbit brain and then primary hamster kidney cell culture
Pasteur Virus (PV)	Believed to be derived from the original Pasteur rabies virus isolate passaged in rabbit brain and then cell culture
Pitman Moore (PM)	Thought to be derived from a rabbit brain-passaged isolate from the original Pasteur rabies virus, adapted to cell culture
Street Alabama-Dufferin (SAD)	Isolated from a rabid dog by mouse brain inoculation and then passaged in chicken embryo and cell culture

replicate poorly in BHK cells but can often be cultured in mouse neuroblastoma (NA) cells. Alternatively, these viruses can be expanded in the suckling (1- to 3-day-old) mouse brain. Where desired, rabies virus may be purified by zonal centrifugation in a sucrose density gradient (21).

Fluorescent-Antibody Detection of Rabies Virus Antigen

A variety of different antibody-based tests have been developed to provide specificity and improve the sensitivity of the assessment of specimens for rabies virus antigen. The direct fluorescent-antibody (DFA) test, for detection of viral antigen in brain tissue sections, impressions, or smears (brain stem and cerebellum are preferred) by use of FITC-conjugated rabies virus nucleoprotein-specific antibodies, is the minimum standard for the diagnosis of rabies virus infection in the United States (7, 24). A detailed protocol for the postmortem diagnosis of rabies in animals by DFA that includes sample preparation and details of the test procedure as well as a list of reagent suppliers can be found on the Centers for Disease Control and Prevention (CDC) website (www.cdc.gov/ncidod/dvrd/rabies). DFA testing is also used to analyze ante- and postmortem samples (neural tissue biopsy, skin biopsy, saliva, corneal impressions) from humans suspected of having died of rabies, as a firm diagnosis can have important implications for postexposure prophylaxis of the patient's contacts. Sample preparation from field specimens and clinical isolates for DFA analysis has been extensively detailed elsewhere (19).

The DFA test is more sensitive and specific than the histochemical visualization of Negri bodies in CNS tissues and can be readily applied to tissue impressions and smears, as well as to fixed and frozen material of variable quality. This allows a specific diagnosis to be made earlier in the infection, providing that appropriate samples are available. The fluorescein-conjugated N-specific monoclonal antibodies capable of detecting all known rabies virus variants that are used for DFA tests are commercially available. N-specific antibodies are employed for such general screening since N antigenic determinants are more highly conserved among rabies virus isolates than those of the G protein. However, characterization of a rabies virus variant that has infected an individual will identify the originating reservoir species, which is critical to understanding the etiology of an infection. Panels of monoclonal anti-N and anti-G antibodies have been widely used in DFA tests to differentiate rabies virus variants on the basis of their expression of unique patterns of antigenic epitopes (e.g., reference 22) (Table 2). Immunohistochemical approaches using peroxidase- and alkaline phosphatase-conjugated N-specific antibodies have also been described as being reliable for studies of formalin-fixed, paraffin-embedded tissues (e.g., see references 8 and 22).

ELISA-Based Tests for Detection of Rabies Virus Antigen

The dependence of the DFA test on fluorescence microscopy has led to the development of several ELISA-based methods for the detection and quantification of rabies virus antigens that may be more suited for use in the field. The rapid rabies enzyme immunodiagnosis (RREID) and its variants are essentially ELISAs in which rabies virus antigens are detected by a substrate reaction, the product of which, under optimal conditions, is visible to the naked eye. In RREID, plates coated with anti-N antibodies are used to trap RNP from specimen preparations, which is then detected with enzyme-conjugated anti-N antibodies and conventional ELISA methods. The use of biotinylated N-specific antibodies and peroxidase-streptavidin can reduce the requirement for labeled antibody (15). Both the sensitivity and the specificity of RREID are considered to be somewhat lower than those of the DFA test with appropriately prepared samples. However, sample quality may be less critical than for the DFA test and positive results may be visualized without microscopy in dot ELISA (10) and RREID. Moreover, ELISA-based assays are more readily amenable to quantitation of antigen content than is DFA analysis (11).

Titration of Rabies Virus by the Fluorescent Focus Assay

The presence of infectious rabies virus in a particular sample is generally confirmed by determining whether the virus replicates in the brains of 1- to 3-day-old suckling mice. However, many rabies virus variants also replicate in cultures of mouse NA cells (NA C1300). Methods for the isolation of rabies virus in cell culture and by mouse inoculation are detailed elsewhere (19). As rabies virus infection is generally nonlytic, titration of the virus is generally performed with a fluorescent focus test in which foci of virus-infected cells in culture are enumerated by use of fluorescein-conjugated

TABLE 2 Antigenic variation among diverse North American rabies virus isolates

| Rabies virus isolate | Monoclonal antibody reaction pattern at antigenic sites[a]: | | | | | | | | |
| | Nucleocapsid specific | | | Glycoprotein specific | | | | | |
	NS I	N I	N III	I	II A	II B	II C	III A	III B
Bat type									
BT-I	a			h	ij	kl	m	o	qsuvxy
BT-II	a		c	h	ij		nm	op	qrsuvwxyαβ
BT-IV	a		c	h	ij		m		vwyβ
BT-VI	a	b	e	h	ij		m		svwxyβ
Fox type F-I	a					k	n	p	qtvz
Arctic fox type F-II			dg		j		m		wxyβ
Skunk type									
S-I						j	m		wyβ
S-II	a		cfg		j				tvyβ
Raccoon type R-I	a				ij		m		vwxyβ

[a]Letters denote monoclonal antibodies of unique specificities. The absence of a letter indicates that the monoclonal antibody failed to bind nucleocapsid (NC-specific antibodies) or neutralize virus (G-specific antibodies) of the indicated isolate. Adapted from the work of Rupprecht et al. (16).

rabies antigen-specific antibodies. BHK cells [BHK-21(C-13); ATCC CCL 10] are suitable targets for fixed laboratory strains of rabies virus such as CVS and ERA, but street virus isolates often infect these cells poorly. NA cells, known to be susceptible to infection by all street virus isolates tested so far, are appropriate for both virus titration and tests of antibody neutralization when street virus isolates are employed. Briefly, 10-fold dilutions of virus are made in medium (10 μl in 90 μl) and added (90 μl) to 30 μl of BHK or NA cells in suspension (approximately 2.5×10^6 cells per ml). The mixtures are transferred to the wells of flat-bottom 96-well microtiter plates (or, alternatively, 10-μl portions are transferred to the wells of Terasaki plates) which are then incubated for 24 to 48 h at 34°C, washed once with phosphate-buffered saline, and fixed with ice-cold 80% acetone for 20 to 30 min. The acetone is then removed, the plates are dried, and the cell monolayers are stained with fluorescein-labeled antirabies virus antibodies. N-protein-specific antibodies are preferred because the antigenic structure of N is more conserved than that of G and because certain rabies virus strains express relatively low levels of G protein. The results of the assay, with each initially infecting virion being represented by a focus of fluorescent infected cells, are read with a fluorescence microscope. The rabies virus titer is then reported in focus-forming units.

Titration of Rabies Virus-Specific Neutralizing Antibody

The level of protective immunity exhibited by a vaccinated individual or animal is determined by quantifying the titer of rabies virus-neutralizing antibody. For humans vaccinated against rabies due to an occupational risk of exposure, World Health Organization (WHO) guidelines recommend that effectiveness of immunization as well as the persistence of immunity be assessed by virus neutralization at 6-month intervals and that a booster vaccination be administered if the neutralizing titer drops below 0.5 IU/ml (24). As noted above, virus titers are normally determined by enumerating foci originating from single infecting virions in vitro, visualized with fluorescein-conjugated antibodies to N. Consequently, the most widely used virus neutralization assay is the RFFIT, which is based on antibody-mediated reduction in the titer of fixed, tissue culture-adapted virus (e.g., CVS or ERA) infecting susceptible cell lines (e.g., BHK, BSR, or NA cells) (25). Through the use of appropriate target cells, the RFFIT can be employed to assess antibody neutralizing activity for fixed and street strains of rabies virus. There are many variations and adaptations of this technique in practice, and a representative microculture protocol is presented here. Sera to be tested are inactivated at 56°C for 30 min prior to their use. Test serum or antibody preparations are serially diluted (e.g., threefold starting at 1:5) in medium in the wells of a microtiter plate to give a final volume of 50 μl. Rabies virus (e.g., CVS-11) is diluted so that 30 μl contains sufficient virus to give 50 to 70% infection of 30 μl of a suspension (2.5×10^6 per ml) (note that cell monolayers are not suitable for rabies virus neutralization tests) of BHK or NA cells (e.g., 5 to 10 focus-forming units per cell) and added to the serum dilutions (and a control row of medium alone) in an equal volume, and the mixture is incubated at 37°C for 60 min. Then 30 μl of BHK or NA cell suspension (1×10^6 to 2×10^6 cells per ml) is added to each well, the contents are mixed, and the cells are cultured in 96-well flat-bottom microtiter plates (alternatively, 10-μl portions can be transferred to Terasaki plates). The plates are incubated overnight at 37°C, washed once with phosphate-buffered saline, and

then fixed and stained as described for the fluorescent focus assay above. The numbers of infected cells are read by using a fluorescence microscope. The virus-neutralizing antibody titer is defined as the highest antibody dilution which gives a 50% reduction in infected cells. A standard antirabies serum (e.g., WHO reference serum) with a virus-neutralizing titer of at least 2 IU per ml should be included in each test so that the assays can be standardized.

To take into account variables in the assay such as the percent control infection obtained and the reference serum titer, the RFFIT results may be calculated as follows.

1. Determine the average percentage of infected cells in the control (virus plus cells without serum) wells (C).

2. Determine the dilution of reference serum that causes C/2 percent infected cells in the wells containing virus plus cells plus reference serum dilutions. Determine the percentage of infection in wells containing the next higher dilution of serum (A) as well as the percentage of infection in wells containing the next higher concentration of serum (B). The 50% dilution point of the reference serum is calculated as: dilution of serum giving $A - \{[(C/2 - B)/(A - B)] \times$ (dilution of serum giving B − dilution of serum giving A)}. This number represents the dilution of reference serum that contains 2 IU (S).

3. Calculate the 50% dilution point in the test serum, using the same formula and substituting the test values of A and B, and their respective dilutions (the result of this calculation = T).

4. The titer of the test serum can now be expressed in international units by using the following relationship: titer of test serum (IU) = $2 \times S \times (1/T)$.

The fluorescent-antibody virus neutralization (FAVN) test, based on the fluorescence principle used in the RFITT but with an endpoint titer determined by the absence of fluorescence, has also been described (6). No significant differences in specificity or sensitivity between the RFFIT and FAVN were detected in comprehensive comparisons (3, 14), and the assessment of fluorescence in both assays has been automated (14), which is highly advantageous in the screening of large numbers of serum samples.

Analysis of Rabies Virus Antigen-Specific Antibody in ELISA

ELISA or radioimmunoassay can be used for the general assessment of rabies virus-specific antibody titers, particularly when a neutralization test is either unavailable or less appropriate. For example, the majority of antibodies specific for rabies virus N protein fail to neutralize, yet are readily detectable by ELISA. Since rabies virus N protein is more highly conserved among different isolates of the virus than rabies virus G protein, and a significant segment of the humoral response to rabies virus is directed against N, detection of rabies antibodies by ELISA may have particular utility where there may be significant antigenic differences between the virus that elicited the antibody and those available in the laboratory. Another situation in which ELISA for rabies virus-specific antibodies may also be more advantageous than a neutralization test is for the screening of serum and CSF from individuals with encephalitis of undiagnosed origin. Late in the disease process, individuals infected with rabies virus often produce some rabies virus-specific antibodies. ELISA can be used to detect these antibodies regardless of whether they are neutralizing. Moreover, ELISA is more suited for automated screening than neutralization tests. Increasing titers of rabies virus-specific antibodies in consecutive serum samples or the appearance of such antibodies in CSF is indicative of an active infection.

ELISA for rabies virus-specific antibody is straightforward (see part I of this manual, "General Methods"). Briefly, ELISA plates (e.g., Immunolon 4 [Dynatech, Chantilly, Va.]) can be readily coated with purified inactivated (β-propriolactone) virus (to detect G- and N-specific antibodies), isolated virus RNP (to detect N-specific antibodies), or recombinant-expressed G and N. As an alternative to directly coating plates with rabies antigens, plates can be sensitized with rabies antigen-specific antibodies to specifically trap the antigens from crude preparations containing the virus (e.g., infected suckling mouse brain). After incubation, bound virus-, G-, or N-specific antibodies can be detected by using secondary peroxidase- or alkaline phosphatase-conjugated antibodies and conventional methods. Commercial ELISA kits for the detection of rabies virus-specific antibodies are available.

RT-PCR for Rabies Virus mRNA

RT-PCR has been found to be a sensitive way of detecting evidence of rabies virus infection in tissue from experimentally infected animals as well as in human autopsy material, including fresh, snap-frozen, formalin-fixed, and paraffin-embedded material (e.g., see references 9, 12, 18, and 23). RNA purified from these specimens by conventional technology, or in situ, can be subjected to RT-PCR or nested RT-PCR if greater sensitivity is required. A number of different procedures for RT-PCR detection and characterization of rabies virus RNA using a variety of oligonucleotide primers and probes specific for conserved or strain-specific sequences have been developed (1, 9, 12, 13, 17, 18, 23). For general RT-PCR screening of infection, primers derived from the nucleoprotein gene sequence, such as sense 10g (5'-CTA-CAATGGATGCCGAC3') (position 66, near the initial methionine codon of N) and antisense 304 (5'-TTGACG-AAGATCTTGCTCAT3') (position 1533, close to the initial methionine residue of the NS protein), are appropriate for amplifying rabies virus RNA from a range of street virus isolates (19). This pair of primers will amplify a fragment of 1.4 kb. When nested PCR is desired for increased sensitivity, a second PCR can be performed with primer 113 (5'GTAGGATGCTATATGGG3') (genomic sequence around position 900). If the above primers fail to detect rabies virus-specific sequences and analysis of β-actin RNA reveals that a specimen is of poor quality, the RT reaction can be performed with primer RabNfor [5'TTGT(AG)GA(TC)CAATATGAGTACAA3'] and the

PCR can be performed with primers RabNfor and RabNbat1.1 (5'TTCCATAGCTGGTCCAGTCA3'). These primers amplify a fragment of about 200 nucleotides of RNA from a large variety of rabies virus strains, including a silver-haired bat rabies virus, and are more likely to successfully amplify partially degraded RNA. PCR amplification of viral mRNA can also be performed but has proven to be more problematic for diagnostic use with specimen material. RT-PCR analysis using strain-specific primers of sequences from the remnant Ψ pseudogene found between the G and L cistrons (18) or the N gene (13) are particularly useful in discriminating between different rabies virus isolates, as is sequence analysis of RT-PCR products (e.g., see reference 1).

Real-time, quantitative RT-PCR (Q-RT-PCR) is well suited for the analysis of samples for rabies virus genome or mRNA. In addition to its specificity and sensitivity, this technology is based upon the replication of only a relatively short stretch of RNA (120 to 150 nucleotides) and therefore has utility for a wide variety of samples of varying quality, including archived paraffin tissue sections. The quality of a sample and the success of extracting usable RNA are controlled by examining the levels of expression of a housekeeping gene, such as the gene for ribosomal protein L13a or glyceraldehyde-3-phosphate dehydrogenase (GAPDH), at the same time as rabies virus RNA. Because of the extensive variability between rabies virus strains, as in other technologies the choice of primers and probes for Q-RT-PCR is of paramount importance. The specificity is such that primer and probe sets for the N mRNA of laboratory strains of the virus, such as CVS, fail to detect similar mRNA from a street rabies virus variant derived from the silver-haired bat (Table 3). In the latter case, a unique primer-probe set was necessary. To accurately assess the level of rabies virus infection of a tissue sample as well as provide a positive control for the Q-RT-PCR, a synthetic DNA template for the PCR is advantageous. With this approach, the number of copies of the rabies virus mRNA in a sample can be determined and normalized to the quality of tissue studied as established by the level of expression of a housekeeping gene.

Rabies Vaccine Potency Tests

While the potency of a rabies vaccine may partly be inferred by assessing the level of total or neutralizing rabies virus-specific antibody elicited by vaccination, the National Institutes of Health potency test is the best means of evaluating vaccine efficacy. In this test, groups of 4- to 6-week-old outbred mice are given a range of doses of vaccine intraperitoneally and then challenged intracerebrally 14 days later

TABLE 3 Primer and probe sets for quantitative PCR of rabies N-protein mRNA

Primer and probe set[a]	Rabies virus strain[b]	
	CVS	SHBRV
Forward: 5'-CAC-TTC-CGT-TCA-CTA-GGC-TTG-A-3' Reverse: 5'-GAC-CCA-TGT-AGC-ATC-CAA-CAA-3' Probe: 5'-**FAM**-TGA-ACA-CAT-GAC-CGA-CAG-CAT-TCG-A-**BHQ**-3'	+ + +	−
Forward: 5'-TGT-GCG-CTA-ACT-GGA-GTA-CCA-3' Reverse: 5'-GTG-CCT-ACC-CTA-ATT-GCT-GAA-3' Probe: 5'-**FAM**-CCG-AAC-TTC-AGA-TTC-CTA-GCT-GGA-ACC-**BHQ**-3'	−	+ + +

[a]Primers and probes were designed from the N mRNA sequences of CVS (NCBI accession no. AF406696) and SHBRV-18 (NCBI accession no. AY705373). FAM, carboxyfluorescein; BHQ, Black Hole Quencher.
[b]Q-RT-PCR was performed with a Bio-Rad iCycler on samples of mouse brain infected with CVS-24, CVS-N2c, CVS-F3, and a silver-haired bat rabies virus (SHBRV) isolate obtained from a human rabies case.

with 5 to 50 50% lethal doses of rabies CVS so that all unvaccinated mice die. While this is the accepted method for testing a vaccine, the extensive antigenic differences between CVS and wildlife rabies virus strains suggest that assessment of protection against diverse virus isolates may be appropriate under certain cirucumstances.

QUALITY ASSURANCE AND CONTROL

The variable spread of rabies virus into different areas of the CNS, the existence of extensive antigenic diversity in rabies virus isolates, particularly in the G protein, and methodological variability between different laboratories present significant concerns in the diagnosis of rabies virus infection. Nevertheless, all of the immunological and molecular rabies virus detection approaches have sensitivity which is limited by the nature and quality of the sample, the quality of the specialized reagents necessary, and expertise with the technology. For instance, a major concern when monoclonal antibodies are employed for DFA detection of rabies virus infection is that the antibodies utilized can detect the full range of antigenically disparate rabies virus strains. In this case, N-specific antibodies are more appropriate than those specific for G because of the more conserved antigenic structure of the former. Recommended standardized reagents and DFA methods for the detection of rabies antigen are detailed on the CDC rabies website (www.edc.gov/ncidod/dvrd/rabies) and elsewhere (17). These recommendations should be followed to minimize technical failures in the diagnosis of infection. False-positive results, which are not uncommon when immunofluorescent approaches are used, are best minimized by the use of commercially available monoclonal antibody preparations (e.g., FITC-anti-rabies monoclonal globulin [Fujirebio Diagnostics, Inc.; catalog no. 800-092]). Proper sample handling and storage are important, and positive-control tissues should always be utilized. A positive DFA reaction should be considered definitive; however, a negative DFA result only implies that the particular tissue sample does not contain virus antigen. A negative result is considered conclusive only if the studies include a complete cross section of the brainstem and cerebellum or hippocampus and have been performed with fluorescein-conjugated anti-rabies virus antibodies from two different sources. Due to the procedures involved, laboratories performing the DFA test for rabies in the United States should participate in the national rabies virus proficiency testing program, available through the Wisconsin State Laboratory of Hygiene (details may be found on their website, www.slh.wisc.edu/pt). Bench training and consultation on the basic aspects of rabies training are available in the United States through a variety of state public health laboratories and the CDC. RT-PCR using primers specific for conserved regions of rabies virus N RNA is gaining acceptance for rabies diagnosis in laboratories where the technology is available because of the sensitivity of this technique, its utility for samples that are not suitable for immunohistological approaches, and the ability to use sequence analysis of the products to identify different rabies virus strains. A duplex RT-PCR protocol using rRNA as an internal control to assess sample degradation may reduce the probability of false-negative results (20). However, similar to the importance of choosing the right antibodies for the DFA test, the selection of primers is critical. For quantitative RT-PCR, both primers and probes must be appropriate. This may limit the utility of RT-PCR technology for general screening purposes unless reagents that can detect all possible rabies virus isolates are available. Due to sensitivity of RT-PCR-based technologies, false positives can be a major concern, particularly if the work is performed in laboratories where the virus is being grown or processed. Controls to ensure that the RT-PCR reagents, laboratory supplies, and environment are not contaminated with rabies virus RNA are essential.

The assessment of rabies virus-specific neutralizing antibody titers by fluorescent focus inhibition tests like the RFFIT requires technical expertise. With variability in the quality of the cell culture, the percentage of cells infected by the assay virus in the absence of antibody, and changes in the appearance of the fluorescent signal when different assay viruses are used, individual assays give results which can be difficult to interpret and must be equilibrated by using antibody standards. The FAVN test shows particular promise in having accuracy which is similar to that of RFFIT yet requiring less expertise to read. On the other hand, ELISA-based technologies are relatively straightforward technically but cannot discriminate between neutralizing and nonneutralizing antibodies. Thus, ELISA has limited value in assessing protective immunity. However, quantitation by ELISA of rabies virus N produced in culture by cells incubated with rabies virus in the presence and absence of antiserum can be used to provide an estimate of antibody neutralizing activity, but these and similar assays in which virus replication is assessed by RT-PCR have not been generally accepted. For all of these approaches, note that antigenic disparity between the fixed assay virus and the infecting or vaccine strain that elicited the antibody may be a concern and the proper controls should always be utilized.

INTERPRETATION

Rabies continues to be an all too common disease of wildlife throughout much of the world. Reducing animal reservoirs of rabies by vaccination has proven effective in various animal species. Vaccination of potential intermediary vectors of rabies virus, such as cats, can also limit human exposure to the virus. Nevertheless, the thousands of animals submitted for testing that are found to be positive for rabies virus each year in the United States necessitate the administration of postexposure prophylaxis to human contacts at a rate of up to 40,000 times a year. These measures, which limited annual fatal human cases of rabies in the United States to an average of fewer than 6 per year in the late 1990s, are dependent upon prompt confirmation of rabies infection in a suspect animal. Routine evaluation of the levels of rabies virus-neutralizing antibody in the sera of individuals immunized against rabies because of a risk of exposure through the nature of their employment or travel to areas of the world with endemic dog rabies is also recommended.

The apparent emergence of cases of human rabies without known exposure, associated predominantly with bat-borne rabies virus strains, has led to the suggestion that rabies virus infection may be a more common cause of lethal encephalitis of unknown origin than is currently thought. The failure to correctly diagnose rabies as a cause of fatal encephalitis has recently led to the death from rabies of a number of individuals who received organ transplants contaminated with the virus. At the least, this indicates that more vigorous attempts should be made to rule out rabies virus infection as a cause of encephalitis progressing to coma. Thus, techniques for the rapid detection of rabies virus antigens, for the identification of rabies virus strains, and for the assessment of immunity to the virus continue to have considerable value. A confirmed elevation in serum rabies virus-specific antibody titer has diagnostic value, but the appearance of rabies virus-specific antibody in CSF is more conclusive of an infection, as such antibodies are never seen in CSF following immunization. However, negative results for the presence of rabies virus-specific antibody in CSF and serum from an infected individual are not uncommon. The detection of rabies virus antigen in various histological specimens or RT-PCR detection of rabies virus-specific RNA sequences is more reliable. With proper care being taken to control for false-positive reactions, a confirmed positive result from a single sample is taken as definitive. Negative results are considered less meaningful since viral replication may be limited to sites which have not been sampled.

The U.S. Department of Health and Human Services, Public Health Service, CDC, and National Institutes of Health recommend Biosafety Level 2 practices and facilities for all activities with materials infected or potentially infected with rabies virus. Immunization is recommended for individuals whose occupations or other activities may predispose them to exposure to rabies virus. It is noteworthy in this regard that antigenic cross-reactivity between rabies virus G and human immunodeficiency virus type 1 (HIV-1) gp120 has been described, and sera from rabies-immune individuals have occasionally cross-reacted against HIV-1 gp120 in ELISA (2).

REFERENCES

1. **Arai, Y. T., K. Yamada, Y. Kameoka, T. Horimoto, K. Yamamoto, S. Yabe, M. Nakayama, and M. Tashiro.** 1997. Nucleoprotein gene analysis of fixed and street rabies virus variants using RT-PCR. *Arch. Virol.* **142:**1787–1796.
2. **Bracci, L., S. K. Ballas, A. Spreafico, and P. Neri.** 1997. Molecular mimicry between the rabies virus glycoprotein and human immunodeficiency virus-1 GP120: cross-reacting antibodies induced by rabies vaccination. *Blood* **90:**3623–3628.
3. **Briggs, D. J., J. S. Smith, F. L. Mueller, J. Schwenke, R. D. Davis, C. R. Gordon, K. Schweitzer, L. A. Orciari, P. A. Yager, and C. E. Rupprecht.** 1998. A comparison of two serological methods for detecting the immune response after rabies vaccination in dogs and cats being exported to rabies-free areas. *Biologicals* **26:**347–355.
4. **Centers for Disease Control and Prevention.** 2004. Investigation of rabies infections in organ donor and transplant recipients—Alabama, Arkansas, Oklahoma, and Texas, 2004. *Morb. Mortal. Wkly. Rep.* **53:**586–589.
5. **Centers for Disease Control and Prevention.** 2004. Update: investigation of rabies infections in organ donor and transplant recipients—Alabama, Arkansas, Oklahoma, and Texas, 2004. *Morb. Mortal. Wkly. Rep.* **53:**615–616.
6. **Cliquet, F., M. Aubert, and L. Sagné.** 1998. Development of a fluorescent antibody virus neutralisation test (FAVN test) for the quantitation of rabies-neutralising antibody. *J. Immunol. Methods* **212:**79–87.
7. **Dean, D. J., and M. K. Abelseth.** 1973. The fluorescent antibody test. *WHO Monogr. Ser.* **23:**73–84.
8. **Hamir, A. N., G. Moser, T. Wampler, A. Hattel, B. Dietzschold, and C. E. Rupprecht.** 1996. Use of a single anti-nucleocapsid monoclonal antibody to detect rabies antigen in formalin-fixed, paraffin-embedded tissues. *Vet. Rec.* **138:**114–115.
9. **Heaton, P. R., L. M. McElhinney, and J. P. Lowings.** 1999. Detection and identification of rabies and rabies-related viruses using rapid-cycle PCR. *J. Virol. Methods* **81:**63–69.
10. **Jayakumar, R., G. Thirumurugan, K. Nachimuthu, and V. D. Padmanaban.** 1995. Detection of rabies virus antigen in animals by avidin-biotin dot ELISA. *Zentbl. Bakteriol.* **285:**82–85.
11. **Katayama, S., M. Yamanaka, S. Ota, and Y. Shimizu.** 1999. A new quantitative method for rabies virus by detection of nucleoprotein in virion using ELISA. *J. Vet. Med. Sci.* **61:**411–416.
12. **Kulonen, K., M. Fekadu, S. Whitfield, and C. K. Warner.** 1999. An evaluation of immunofluorescence and PCR methods for detection of rabies in archival carnoy-fixed, paraffin-embedded brain tissue. *J. Vet. Med.* **46:**151–155.
13. **Nadin-Davis, S., W. Huang, and A. I. Wandeler.** 1996. The design of strain-specific polymerase chain reactions for discrimination of the raccoon rabies virus strain from indigenous rabies viruses of Ontario. *J. Virol. Methods* **57:**1–14.
14. **Péharpré, D., F. Cliquet, E. Sagné, C. Renders, F. Costy, and M. Aubert.** 1999. Comparison of visual microscopic and computer-automated fluorescence detection of rabies virus neutralizing antibodies. *J. Vet. Diagn. Investig.* **11:**330–333.
15. **Perrin, P., C. Gontier, E. Lecocq, and H. Bourhy.** 1992. A modified rapid enzyme immunoassay for the detection of rabies and rabies-related viruses: RREID-lyssa. *Biologicals* **20:**51–58.
16. **Rupprecht, C. E., B. Dietzschold, W. H. Wunner, and H. Koprowski.** 1991. Antigenic relationships of Lyssaviruses, p. 69–100. *In* G. M. Baer (ed.), *The Natural History of Rabies*, 2nd ed. CRC Press, Boca Raton, Fla.
17. **Sabouraud, A., J. S. Smith, L. A. Orciari, C. de Mattos, C. de Mattos, and R. Rohde.** 1999. Typing of rabies virus isolates by DNA enzyme immunoassay. *J. Clin. Virol.* **12:**9–19.
18. **Sacramento, D., H. Bourhy, and N. Tordo.** 1991. PCR technique as an alternative method for diagnosis and molecular epidemiology of rabies virus. *Mol. Cell. Probes* **6:**229–240.
19. **Smith, J.** 1999. Rabies virus, p. 1099–1106. *In* P. R. Murray (ed.), *Manual of Clinical Microbiology*, 7th ed. ASM Press, Washington, D.C.
20. **Smith, J., L. M. McElhinney, P. R. Heaton, E. M. Black, and J. P. Lowings.** 2000. Assessment of template quality by the incorporation of an internal control into a RT-PCR for the detection of rabies and rabies-related viruses. *J. Virol. Methods* **84:**107–115.
21. **Sokol, F.** 1973. Purification of rabies virus and isolation of its components. *WHO Monogr. Ser.* **23:**165–178.
22. **Warner, C., M. Fekadu, S. Whitfield, and J. Shaddock.** 1999. Use of anti-glycoprotein monoclonal antibodies to characterize rabies virus in formalin-fixed tissues. *J. Virol. Methods* **77:**69–74.
23. **Warner, C. K., S. G. Whitfield, M. Fekadu, and H. Ho.** 1997. Procedures for reproducible detection of rabies virus antigen mRNA and genome in situ in formalin-fixed tissues. *J. Virol. Methods* **67:**5–12.
24. **WHO Expert Committee on Rabies.** 1992. WHO Expert Committee on Rabies, 8th report. *WHO Technical Report Series no. 824.* WHO, Geneva, Switzerland.
25. **Wiktor, T. J., R. I. Macfarlan, C. M. Foggin, and H. Koprowski.** 1984. Antigenic analysis of rabies and Mokola virus from Zimbabwe using monoclonal antibodies. *Dev. Biol. Stand.* **57:**199–211.
26. **Wunner, W. H.** 1991. The chemical composition and molecular structure of rabies viruses, p. 31–67. *In* G. M. Baer (ed.), *The Natural History of Rabies*, 2nd ed. CRC Press, Boca Raton, Fla.

Human T-Cell Lymphotropic Virus Types 1 and 2

SUSAN B. NYLAND, THOMAS P. LOUGHRAN, AND KENNETH E. UGEN

89

VIRAL CHARACTERISTICS

The human T-cell leukemia virus type 1 (HTLV-1) is a member of the family *Retroviridae*, consisting of enveloped, single-stranded, positive-polarity RNA (two copies make the virus diploid) viruses using RNA-dependent DNA polymerase (reverse transcriptase, [RT]). It is classified as an oncovirus. Although the virus has proliferative capabilities similar to true type C oncogenic retroviruses, it does not appear to express a defined "conventional" viral oncogene, and thus it is unique within the oncovirus subfamily. HTLV-1 is transmitted by parenteral, vertical, and sexual routes, in descending order of efficiency. Its seroprevalence varies according to geographical region. Historically, regions of endemic infection have included Japan, South America, Central Africa, and the Caribbean basin, with a seropositivity range of 3 to 30%. More recently, HTLV-1 infection has become more common in the southeastern United States and in injecting drug users (IDU) worldwide. In the general U.S. population, the seropositivity level is about 0.06%, while in the southern United States, it ranges from 0.5 to 2% in the non-IDU population and around 20% in the IDU population (16). HTLV-2 has 66% homology to HTLV-1, and although it transforms cells similarly to HTLV-1 in vitro, it is less able to do so in vivo and hence is considered the less pathogenic of the two retroviruses. HTLV-2 is endemic to several Amerindian tribes, and it is estimated that 2 to 30% of some tribal populations are carriers of this retrovirus. From 3 to 18% of IDU in the United States and Europe are also infected with the virus (9, 16). Recent in vitro data relevant to HTLV and human immunodeficiency virus (HIV) seropositivity in IDU suggest that morphine/heroin exposure at levels relevant to heroin addiction enhanced HTLV infection in cells coinfected with HIV and HTLV, perhaps increasing the likelihood of disease development in coinfected IDU (17).

HTLV-1 was reported in 1980 by Bernard Poiesz and Robert Gallo as the first retrovirus shown to be pathogenic to humans (19). HTLV-1 preferentially infects CD4$^+$ lymphocytes, with rare infections noted in dendritic cells, CD8$^+$ T lymphocytes, and null (CD4$^-$ CD8$^-$) T lymphocytes. HTLV-2 exhibits expanded tropism and infects macrophages in addition to all of the cell types mentioned above. In the later stages of HTLV-1 diseases, viral proteins can be detected in a variety of affected tissues; however, the virus itself has not been identified in other tissue cells. The virus is transmitted predominantly by direct contact with infected cells; therefore, whole packed blood is infectious while cell-free serum is not. HTLV-1 is extremely difficult to isolate, and cell-free clones typically exhibit titers so low that infection can be detected only by PCR techniques. This cell-dependent quality has made the virus somewhat more difficult to study than its lentiviral cousin, HIV. With the exception of the glucose transporter GLUT-1 (13), receptors used by the virus for attachment remain unconfirmed. Cell adhesion molecules may also play an important role in infection (1).

Once the virus is in the host cell, the HTLV RNA genome is reverse transcribed into proviral DNA, which is then integrated into the host DNA. When the host cell is activated, cellular transcription factors initiate the synthesis of new viral mRNA. Translation of the viral mRNA produces the 40-kDa Tax protein as well as other viral proteins. Tax focuses the cellular transcriptional machinery by dominating the interactions with cell transcription factors, such as NF-κB and cyclic AMP response element binding proteins (3). The enhancer activity induced by Tax is located in the viral long terminal repeat sequences of the proviral DNA. The long terminal repeat contains a 21-bp repeat sequence, which is a Tax response element that functions as a viral cyclic AMP response element. Thus, more viral proteins are produced and eventually processed into progeny for cell-to-cell transmission.

In addition to virus production, the promiscuous interactions of Tax with host transcription factors contribute to a constitutively activated state of the infected cell. Secreted Tax acts in a similar fashion on noninfected bystanders. Two cytokines associated with activation, interleukin 2 (IL-2) and IL-6, are abundantly present in HTLV-1-infected cell cultures (5, 7). IL-2 is considered an essential cytokine for the initiation of cell-mediated immune responses and is necessary for the proliferation of T lymphocytes. IL-6 is best known for its role in inflammatory immune responses. Thus, the constantly activated state is thought to be responsible for the diseases associated with HTLV infection.

DISEASES ASSOCIATED WITH HTLV INFECTION

As can be surmised from the description of some mechanisms of pathogenesis, the diseases associated with HTLV infection have inflammatory and/or proliferative attributes. HTLV-1 and HTLV-2 diseases are usually classified as malignant or nonmalignant clinical presentations. Nonneoplastic disease states may be due to an oligoclonal proliferation of infected cells, while the proliferation of only a few infected clones is thought to lead to the development of neoplasia. It has been postulated that all HTLV infections begin with oligoclonal proliferation (4). With time and other unknown factors, a few dominant infected clones evolve; therefore, the progression of nonmalignant disease may be related to the risk of developing a malignancy.

Nonneoplastic Diseases Due to Infection with HTLV-1

HAM/TSP

HTLV-associated myelopathy/tropical spastic paraparesis (HAM/TSP) is probably the best-known nonmalignant syndrome attributed to HTLV infection. Although HAM/TSP is attributed mostly to the effects of HTLV-1 infection contracted after the onset of adulthood, spinal cord lesions from a few patients have demonstrated evidence of HTLV-2 infection (9). The lifetime risk of developing HAM/TSP in seropositive carriers is currently estimated to be 2%. HAM/TSP is characterized by a set of progressive neurological disorders that include incontinence with constipation, hyperreflexia, hypoesthesias, Babinski reflex, clonus, ataxia, and weakness of the lower extremities. Activated immune cells are thought to contribute to the inflammatory process in the central nervous system during HAM (12, 18) by direct and indirect pathways. The diagnosis of HAM/TSP is based on clinical presentation, lack of documented history of other known causes of paraparesis, and the presence of antibodies against HTLV-1 in the blood or cerebrospinal fluid. HAM patients are treated symptomatically, with danazol for incontinence and with corticosteroids and benzodiazepines.

HU

HTLV uveitis (HU) presents clinically as an intraocular inflammation in one or both eyes, accompanied by visual impairment. HU can occur with or without HAM, and the lifetime risk to HTLV-1 carriers is approximately 2.5%, somewhat higher than the risk of developing HAM. Concurrent Graves' disease may also be observed. An examination of the eye reveals iritis, retinal vasculitis with the presence of gray-white bodies, a nontransparent vitreous humor, decreased tear breakup time, and keratoconjunctivitis. The development of HU in HTLV-1 carriers is attributed to the infiltration of infected, activated T lymphocytes and their secreted cytokines. A high level of viral antigen can be found in ocular fluids, as well as relatively elevated levels of IL-6 (15). HU patients typically have a greater viral load than asymptomatic carriers. Diagnosis of uveitis is based on clinical presentation and the presence of antibodies to HTLV-1 as well as the confirmation of proviral DNA by PCR. Because uveitis can be caused by other infectious agents, infections such as syphilis, tuberculosis, toxoplasmosis, or cytomegalovirus infection need to be ruled out (14). HU responds well to topical treatment with corticosteroids.

HTLV-1-Associated ID

HTLV-1-associated infective dermatitis (ID) is manifested primarily in children who have acquired HTLV-1 by vertical transmission (11). Clinically overt symptoms include severe eczema on the head, neck, and groin, with a clear nasal discharge. The affected areas of the head include the scalp, ears, nose, and eyelid margins. Cultures of skin biopsy specimens usually demonstrate that colonization by *Staphylococcus aureus* or beta-hemolytic streptococcal species has occurred, and testing of biopsy material reveals the presence of HTLV-1 proviral DNA. Elevated CD4$^+$ and CD8$^+$ T-cell counts, found in dermal exudates as well as in peripheral blood, contribute to an increased susceptibility to bacterial infection, due to nonspecific activation of B cells via activated T-cell-secreted cytokines. The combination of apparent dermatitis with nasal discharge and antibodies to HTLV-1 is necessary for the diagnosis of ID (11). Additional symptoms may include anemia, lymphadenitis, and abnormally high serum globulin. Long-term antibiotic therapy is required for treatment of ID, since recurrence is common when antibiotics are withdrawn.

HTLV-1-Associated Sicca Syndrome

HTLV-1-associated sicca syndrome, resembling Sjögren's syndrome, can be observed in some HAM/TSP patients as well as in otherwise asymptomatic carriers. Sjögren's syndrome is an autoimmune disorder complete with the expression of anticentromere antibodies, while the antibodies expressed with sicca syndrome are to HTLV-1 (2). Clinical presentation includes dry eyes and dry mouth frequently accompanied by recurrent fever and myelopathy. Lymphocyte infiltration, as well as viral Tax, is evident in the salivary glands (2). Diagnosis is dependent on clinical presentation with detection of HTLV-1 infection. Sicca syndrome can be due to a variety of infectious agents and chemical agents; therefore, other possible causes should be ruled out. Treatment includes topical and oral steroids and artificial tears.

Nonneoplastic Diseases Due to Infection by HTLV-2

HTLV-2 infection is associated with a progressive ataxia similar to HAM/TSP in some patients (8); however, the risk of developing this symptom in HTLV-2 carriers has not been determined. The role of HTLV-2 infection in subclinical neurological sequelae and greater susceptibility to infectious disease overall has been recently reported (16). A positive history of recurrent bladder and kidney infections, minor fungal infections, and pneumonia may indicate HTLV-2 infection. Confirmation of infection is determined by the presence of antibodies and proviral DNA.

Neoplastic Diseases Due to Infection by HTLV-1

HTLV-1 infection acquired prior to the onset of adulthood carries a higher risk of neoplastic disease than does infection acquired later in life. Adult T-cell leukemia/lymphoma (ATL) appears in about 3 to 5% of HTLV-1 carriers decades after infection (6, 20). Skin lesions constitute the most common initial clinical presentation of disease and can appear as papules, nodules, infiltrated plaques, tumors, or erythroderma. A general diagnosis of ATL is made on the basis of clinical presentation, hematological examination, and presence of antibodies to HTLV-1 and by the molecular confirmation of proviral DNA. The immune system may fail to respond to HTLV-1 due to the production of defective virus particles in neoplastic cells. If so, antibody levels may be insufficient for detection. The diagnosis is completed by a determination of (i) smoldering, (ii) chronic, (iii) lymphoma, or (iv) acute ATL, based on additional criteria. These four subtypes of ATL have been designated by the Lymphoma Study Group of Japan (20).

In smoldering-type ATL, the patient has a normal to slightly elevated lymphocyte count, with about 5% abnormal lymphocytes. Serum lactate dehydrogenase (LDH) levels are elevated to about 1.5 times the normal value. There is usually a positive history of HAM/TSP. About half of these patients will progress to acute ATL. The median survival time after diagnosis is approximately 4 years.

Lymphocytosis with 5 to 10% abnormal T cells is evident in chronic-type ATL. These consist of small cells with cerebriform nuclei and basophilic cytoplasms together with large cells containing convoluted, multilobed nuclei. The larger cells are called flower cells and are considered characteristic of ATL. From 5 to 20% of the abnormal leukocytes may consist of flower cells, which can be viewed by Giemsa staining. The serum LDH level is about twice the normal level. As with smoldering-ATL patients, about half of the chronic ATL patients will progress to acute ATL. At that time, hypercalcemia is present. Unlike patients with other ATL subtypes, chronic ATL patients may present with concomitant HAM/TSP. The median survival time after diagnosis is 3 to 4 years.

In contrast to chronic ATL, lymphocytosis is not evident during lymphoma-type ATL. Blood histology reveals 1% or fewer abnormal lymphocytes in the patient's peripheral blood. The serum LDH level is elevated. Most patients present clinically with a generalized lymphadenopathy, and approximately half have hypercalcemia. Hepatomegaly and splenomegaly may also be present, indicating extensive organ involvement. Histologically, lymphoma-type ATL may mimic Hodgkin's disease. The abnormal cells are observed as a pleiomorphic T-cell lymphoma, with a large and bilobed Reed-Sternberg-like morphology. The median survival time after diagnosis of lymphoma-type ATL is less than 1 year.

The acute-type ATL is the most common subtype of ATL. More than 10% of the peripheral blood consists of abnormal lymphocytes. Giemsa stains of blood smears reveal a pleiomorphic T-cell lymphoma similar to chronic ATL, with 5 to >70% of the abnormal cells identified as ATL flower cells. Generalized lymphadenopathy, hypercalcemia, and skin lesions are common to the clinical picture. An additional manifestation of the skin resembling a mycosis fungoides-like rash is likely to emerge. The patient may exhibit uveitis or retinitis, with a somewhat extensive involvement of the liver and spleen. Acute ATL is rapidly fatal, with a median survival of only 6 months after diagnosis.

The treatment of ATL consists of chemotherapy, alpha interferon, and zidovudine. Relapses are common, and when they occur, treatment is generally ineffective. About 9 of 10 ATL patients have ATL cells that overexpress multidrug resistance genes (10), and this is thought to contribute to the resistance of ATL to chemotherapy. The main cause of death is disease progression combined with hypercalcemia and septicemia (20).

DETECTION OF HTLV INFECTION

The detection of HTLV-1 and -2 relies on the presence of serum or plasma antibodies and proviral DNA. Enzyme-linked immunosorbent assays (ELISAs), Western immunoblots, and radioimmunoprecipitation assays (RIPAs) are used to confirm repeatedly reactive or inconclusive findings. In serum samples, antibodies against the core antigen proteins appear first, followed by antibodies to the viral envelope and finally by anti-Tax antibodies. Patients who have a combination of relevant symptoms and risk factors should be monitored even if their serum is nonreactive in diagnostic ELISAs, due to the previously described antibody suppression that sometimes occurs during infection. The detection process is illustrated and summarized in Fig. 1.

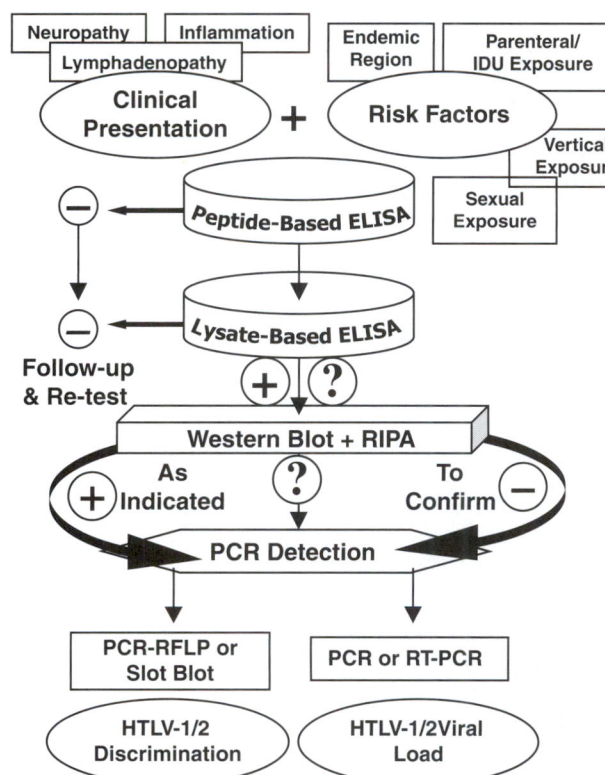

FIGURE 1 Flowchart for HTLV-1 and -2 detection and discrimination. For patients with combined clinical presentation and risk factors, detection of HTLV-1 and -2 infection begins with ELISA testing. When both ELISA results are negative (−), it is recommended that follow-up include documentation of other possible causes for the clinical presentation, as well as additional testing if other causes are ruled out. Repeatedly reactive (+) results must be confirmed by Western blot analysis and then analyzed by PCR if indicated. Indeterminate (?) or reactive ELISA results that are nonreactive on Western blotting should be confirmed by RIPA. Repeatedly indeterminate results can be clarified by PCR-related methods. RFLP, restriction fragment length polymorphism.

ELISA kits approved for diagnostic use in the United States are evaluated by the Food and Drug Administration Center for Biologics Evaluation and Research (FDA/CBER). According to the current CBER website, updated in March 2004 (www.fda.gov/cber/products/testkits/htm), only two approved kits are available, although other testing kits are listed elsewhere on the site. These two kits are the Abbott HTLV-1/2 ELISA (Abbott Laboratories, Diagnostics Division) and the Vironostika HTLV-1/2 MicroElisa system (marketed by Ortho at Johnson & Johnson). Abbott Laboratories recently introduced a chemiluminescent version of its diagnostic ELISA, called the Prism chLIA, which is not yet on the CBER-approved list. Briefly, recombinant HTLV-1 and -2 gag and env antigens are immobilized onto microtiter plates. A blocking agent is added to decrease nonspecific reactions. Samples containing antibodies are reacted with the immobilized antigens. The nonreactive portion of the sample is removed, while the reactive (antibody) portion remains tightly bound to the antigen. An enzyme-conjugated secondary antibody is reacted with sample and standard control antibodies and is detected colorimetrically (or with chemiluminescence if the Prism test is used). A more detailed description of the ELISA technique is provided in chapter 3 of this volume. A positive result usually has a colorimetric value of at least 2 standard deviations greater than negative controls. Certified ELISAs involving the use of recombinant proteins or peptides are developed to reduce the number of indeterminate results or values that are between the cutoff values of the negative and positive controls. Indeterminate results can occur when the patient is undergoing seroconversion, usually very early in the infection. A retest later for such patients usually resolves this type of indeterminate finding. Certain autoimmune diseases may mimic some of the symptoms of HTLV infection, and the sera of such patients may also yield indeterminate results in the ELISA format. Patients with rheumatoid factor or antinuclear antibodies are examples of noninfected individuals who may have indeterminate results for HTLV-1 and -2 serum antibodies.

Indeterminate blood can be sent to a clinical reference laboratory. Specialty Laboratories (www.specialtylabs.com), Laboratory Corporation of America (LabCorp; www.labcorp.com), the Molecular Infectious Disease Laboratory (MIDL) division of the Genetics and IVF Institute (www.givf.com/midl), and Quest Diagnostics Laboratories (www.questdiagnostics.com) were among the reference laboratories found online with resources for confirming HTLV-1 and -2 infections. These laboratories perform several types of Western immunoblot assays with or without RIPA. The criterion for a positive Western blot assay is the detection of antibodies to a series of core antigens (gag) and envelope glycoproteins. When a sample exhibits reactivity to only one set of viral proteins or lacks reactivity to HTLV gag p24 and env proteins, it is still considered indeterminate (14). There must be no band development in order for the results to be considered seronegative.

Inconclusive ELISA and Western immunoblot findings can be further tested by RIPA, which is more sensitive to smaller amounts of serum antibody, before PCR analyses are performed. Quest Diagnostics Laboratories, LabCorp, and MIDL also have specialized facilities to perform real-time PCR analyses of genomic DNA from EDTA-treated whole blood. PCR targets typically include conserved regions of *gag* and *pol*. This technique is also useful for differentiating between HTLV-1 and HTLV-2, as well as for detecting proviral DNA in tumor tissue, exudates, and skin biopsy specimens. In addition, the use of PCR allows a determination of the viral load, which may correlate with disease progression. The following PCR-related methods of virus detection and differentiation are described in chapter 5 of this volume.

A slot blot is the combination of PCR with probe hybridization techniques. Standard primer pair sets are available for this purpose from Synthetic Genetics (San Diego, Calif.) and Roche Diagnostics. For example, genomic DNA is extracted from the sample and primer pairs for HTLV-1 and -2 *pol* genes are used to amplify a conserved region of proviral DNA. After PCR amplification, the reaction products are isolated by electrophoresis and then transferred to a nylon membrane. The subsequent hybridization with labeled HTLV-1 and -2 *pol*-specific probes to detect differently sized amplimers allows a classification of immunologically indeterminate samples (22).

Because of the genomic differences between HTLV-1 and HTLV-2, the detection of restriction fragment length polymorphisms on agarose gels after PCR amplification products have been digested is a useful alternative to the blot technique (21). The interpretation of PCR-restriction fragment length polymorphism findings is based on the comparison to the banding patterns of known standards.

The development of recombinant RT has greatly reduced the cost and uncertainty of viral-load quantification by RT-PCR. In this technique, viral RNA is reverse transcribed using RT. The resultant cDNA is then amplified by PCR and compared to amplified standards containing known amounts of target cDNA. The preferred specimen for this type of clinical test is usually EDTA-treated plasma.

Although PCR-related methods are not approved by the Food and Drug Administration and are not routinely used for screening, they have proved to be reliable and sensitive tools for the detection and discrimination of HTLV-1 and -2 from previously indeterminate samples. Thus, the ability to use or at least understand these techniques can serve to confirm and to further clarify differential diagnoses of HTLV-associated diseases.

REMARKS ON PREVENTION AND TREATMENT OF INFECTION

HTLV-1- and HTLV-2-seropositive patients should be counseled about prevention of transmission. Patients are advised to use condoms during sexual intercourse and are prohibited from donating blood or blood products. HTLV-positive female patients of childbearing age should refrain from breast-feeding. This will prevent about 90% of the incidences of vertical transmission (from 30% with breast-feeding to 3% without breast-feeding). Intimate contacts and children of patients are at risk for acquiring infection. Accordingly, testing for the corresponding virus would be appropriate for these individuals. Because of the role played by vertical transmission, parents of patients who are not suspected of acquiring the disease by parenteral or sexual routes might also prove to be seropositive. Casual household and social contacts are not at risk.

Currently, there are no antiviral drugs designed specifically for HTLV-1 or HTLV-2. Because of the differences between lentiviruses and oncoviruses, most anti-HIV drugs, including the protease and nonnucleoside RT inhibitors, are generally ineffective against the leukemia viruses. The use of zidovudine, a nucleoside analogue, in combination chemotherapy protocols appears to offer only a transient benefit to patients. Several highly conserved regions found in the genomes of both viruses make them likely candidates for successful vaccine prophylaxis (1, 14). In fact, the more genetically conserved nature of HTLV-1 and -2 compared to HIV-1 makes a vaccine against HTLV-1 and -2 more logistically feasible than is a vaccine to HIV-1. However, the development of such vaccines has been slow, and ongoing research is relatively scarce. Consequently, the treatment of HTLV-seropositive patients is directed at the amelioration of HTLV-associated disease symptoms.

REFERENCES

1. Agadjanyan, M. G., K. E. Ugen, B. Wang, W. V. Williams, and D. B. Weiner. 1994. Identification of an 80-kilodalton membrane glycoprotein important for human T-cell leukemia virus type I and type II syncytium formation and infection. *J. Virol.* **68:**485–493.
2. Beby-Defaux, A., F. Frugier, A. Bourgoin, D. Moynet, C. Hajjar, S. Sainte-Foie, B. Guillemain, and G. Agius. 1999. Nucleotide sequence analysis of human T-cell lymphotropic virus type I pX and LTR regions from patients with sicca syndrome. *J. Med. Virol.* **59:**245–255.
3. Brady, J. N. 1996. Biology of HTLV-I: host cell interactions, p. 79–112. *In* P. Hollsberg and D. A. Hafler (ed.), *Human T-Cell Lymphotropic Virus Type I.* John Wiley & Sons, Inc., New York, N.Y.

4. **Carrington, C. V. F., and T. F. Schulz.** 1996. Virology of HTLV-I infection, p. 113–139. *In* P. Hollsberg and D. A. Hafler (ed.), *Human T-Cell Lymphotropic Virus Type I.* John Wiley & Sons, Inc., New York, N.Y.

5. **Cereseto, A., J. C. Mulloy, and G. Franchini.** 1996. Insights on the pathogenicity of human T-lymphotropic/leukemia virus types I and II. *J. Acquir. Immune Defic. Syndr. Hum. Retrovirol.* **13**(Suppl. 1):S69–S75.

6. **Gessain, A.** 1996. Epidemiology of HTLV-I and associated diseases, p. 33–65. *In* P. Hollsberg and D. A. Hafler (ed.), *Human T-Cell Lymphotropic Virus Type* I. John Wiley & Sons, Inc., New York, N.Y.

7. **Good, L., S. B. Maggirwar, and S. C. Sun.** 1996. Activation of the IL-2 gene promoter by HTLV-I Tax involves induction of NF-AT complexes bound to the CD28-responsive element. *EMBO J.* **15**:3744–3750.

8. **Hall, W. W., R. Ishak, S. W. Zhu, P. Novoa, N. Eiraku, H. Takahashi, C. Ferreira Mda, V. Azevedo, M. O. Ishak, C. Ferreira Oda, C. Monken, and T. Kurata.** 1996. Human T lymphotropic virus type II (HTLV-II): epidemiology, molecular properties, and clinical features of infection. *J. Acquir. Immune Defic. Syndr. Hum. Retrovirol.* **13**(Suppl. 1):S204–S214.

9. **Hall, W. W., T. Kubo, S. Ijichi, H. Takahashi, and S. W. Zhu.** 1994. Human T cell leukemia/lymphoma virus, type II (HTLV-II): emergence of an important newly recognized pathogen. *Semin. Virol.* **5**:165–178.

10. **Ikeda, K., M. Oka, Y. Yamada, H. Soda, M. Fukuda, A. Kinoshita, K. Tsukamoto, Y. Noguchi, H. Isomoto, F. Takeshima, K. Murase, S. Kamihira, M. Tomonaga, and S. Kohno.** 1999. Adult T-cell leukemia cells overexpress the multidrug-resistance protein (MRP) and lung-resistance protein (LRP) genes. *Int. J. Cancer* **82**:599–604.

11. **La Grenade, L., A. Manns, V. Fletcher, D. Derm, C. Carberry, B. Hanchard, E. M. Maloney, B. Cranston, N. P. Williams, R. Wilks, E. C. Kang, and W. A. Blattner.** 1998. Clinical, pathologic, and immunologic features of human T-lymphotropic virus type I-associated infective dermatitis in children. *Arch. Dermatol.* **134**:439–444.

12. **Levin, M. C., S. M. Lee, F. Kalume, Y. Morcos, F. C. Dohan, Jr., K. A. Hasty, J. C. Callaway, J. Zunt, D. Desiderio, and J. M. Stuart.** 2002. Autoimmunity due to molecular mimicry as a cause of neurological disease. *Nat. Med.* **8**:509–513.

13. **Manel, N., F. J. Kim, S. Kinet, N. Taylor, M. Sitbon, and J. L. Battini.** 2003. The ubiquitous glucose transporter GLUT-1 is a receptor for HTLV. *Cell* **115**:449–459.

14. **Manns, A., M. Hisada, and L. La Grenade.** 1999. Human T-lymphotropic virus type I infection. *Lancet* **353**:1951–1958.

15. **Muller, K., M. Zak, S. Nielsen, F. K. Pedersen, P. de Nully, and K. Bendtzen.** 1997. Interleukin-1 receptor antagonist in neonates, children and adults, and in patients with pauci- and polyarticular onset juvenile chronic arthritis. *Clin. Exp. Rheumatol.* **15**:439–444.

16. **Murphy, E. L., S. A. Glynn, J. Fridey, J. W. Smith, R. A. Sacher, C. C. Nass, H. E. Ownby, D. J. Wright, and G. J. Nemo.** 1999. Increased incidence of infectious diseases during prospective follow-up of human T-lymphotropic virus type II- and I-infected blood donors. Retrovirus Epidemiology Donor Study. *Arch. Intern. Med.* **159**:1485–1491.

17. **Nyland, S. B., C. Cao, Y. Bai, T. P. Loughran, and K. E. Ugen.** 2003. Modulation of infection and type 1 cytokine expression parameters by morphine during in vitro coinfection with human T-cell leukemia virus type I and HIV-1. *J. Acquir. Immune Defic. Syndr.* **32**:406–416.

18. **Osame, M.** 2002. Pathological mechanisms of human T-cell lymphotropic virus type I-associated myelopathy (HAM/TSP). *J. Neurovirol.* **8**:359–364.

19. **Poiesz, B. J., F. W. Ruscetti, A. F. Gazdar, P. A. Bunn, J. D. Minna, and R. C. Gallo.** 1980. Detection and isolation of type C retrovirus particles from fresh and cultured lymphocytes of a patient with cutaneous T-cell lymphoma. *Proc. Natl. Acad. Sci. USA* **77**:7415–7419.

20. **Pombo De Oliveira, M. S., P. Loureiro, A. Bittencourt, C. Chiattone, D. Borducchi, S. M. De Carvalho, H. S. Barbosa, M. Rios, A. Sill, F. Cleghorn, W. Blattner, and The Brazilian ATLL Study Group.** 1999. Geographic diversity of adult T-cell leukemia/lymphoma in Brazil. *Int. J. Cancer* **83**:291–298.

21. **Tuke, P. W., P. Luton, and J. A. Garson.** 1992. Differential diagnosis of HTLV-I and HTLV-II infections by restriction enzyme analysis of 'nested' PCR products. *J. Virol. Methods* **40**:163–173.

22. **Vandamme, A. M., K. Van Laethem, H. F. Liu, M. Van Brussel, E. Delaporte, C. M. de Castro Costa, C. Fleischer, G. Taylor, U. Bertazzoni, J. Desmyter, and P. Goubau.** 1997. Use of a generic polymerase chain reaction assay detecting human T-lymphotropic virus (HTLV) types I, II and divergent simian strains in the evaluation of individuals with indeterminate HTLV serology. *J. Med. Virol.* **52**:1–7.

Coronavirus Including Severe Acute Respiratory Syndrome (SARS)

JAMES B. MAHONY AND CHENGSHENG ZHANG

90

Coronavirus, a genus within the family *Coronaviridae*, contains a number of enveloped viruses that infect both animals and humans. Coronaviruses possess a positive-strand RNA genome, 27 to 32 kb in size, which is the largest known genome among all RNA viruses. The genomic RNA is capped and polyadenylated and comprises several genes encoding both structural and nonstructural proteins. The genome organization of coronaviruses has the characteristic order 5′-replicase, spike (S), envelope (E), membrane (M), nucleocapsid (N)-3′ (11). The G+C content ranges from a low of 32% for coronavirus HKU1 (CoV-HKU1) to a high of 41% for severe acute respiratory syndrome (SARS)-associated coronavirus (SARS-CoV). In addition to the S, E, M, and N structural proteins, the genome also encodes a chymotrypsin-like protease, replicase (polymerase), helicase, and hemagglutinin-esterase. For the replicase gene, a frameshift interrupts the protein coding regions and separates open reading frames (ORFs) 1a and 1b. Both the 5′ and the 3′ ends contain short untranslated regions. The RNA genome is translated as a polyprotein which is subsequently cleaved by the chymotrypsin-like protease activity. The S gene encodes the spike glycoprotein, which binds to the host cell receptor (ACE-2 in the case of SARS-CoV and aminopeptidase N or CD13 for HCoV-229E) and leads to membrane fusion and viral entry.

Coronaviruses have been identified in mice, rats, chickens, turkeys, swine, dogs, cats, rabbits, horses, cattle, and humans and cause a variety of severe diseases, including gastroenteritis and respiratory tract diseases. Up until 2002, there were only two known human coronaviruses (HCoVs), HCoV-OC43 and HCoV-229E. On the basis of genotypic and serological characterization, coronaviruses have been divided into three distinct groups, with HCoV-229E in group 1 and HCoV-OC43 in group 2 (11). Since 2002, three additional HCoVs have been discovered, bringing the total number of HCoVs to five. In 2002, SARS emerged from mainland China and SARS-CoV was identified as the causative agent (16). On the basis of genome analysis, SARS-CoV was originally assigned to a fourth CoV group but more recently has been recognized as a distant relative to the group 2 coronaviruses and has been considered as a group 2 subgroup (14). In 2004, a novel group 1 HCoV associated with respiratory tract infections, HCoV-NL63, was discovered in The Netherlands and its genome was sequenced (24). In 2005, the fifth HCoV, a group 2 HCoV, was discovered in patients with pneumonia in Hong Kong and its genome was sequenced (25).

HCoV-OC43 and -229E were identified in the mid-1960s as a cause of mild self-limited upper respiratory infection and were subsequently shown to cause about one-third of "common cold"-like illnesses in adults. Overall, they account for between 5 and 30% of respiratory tract infections, and outbreaks may occur at 3- to 4-year intervals (23). Like infections caused by other respiratory viruses, HCoV-OC43 and -229E infections can present with a variety of signs and symptoms ranging from a self-limiting common cold including cough, runny nose, and fever to a lower respiratory tract infection with bronchiolitis or pneumonia. HCoV-OC43 and -229E have been associated with respiratory tract infection in a variety of settings, including nosocomial infections in high-risk immunocompromised children, hospitalized elderly patients with noninfluenza severe respiratory tract infection and pneumonia, and newborns, children, and hospital staff (4, 17, 22). In one recent prospective study of 501 patients in France, HCoV-OC43 was found in 6% of patients compared with 6.1% for respiratory syncytial virus, 7.8% for influenza virus, 6.4% for rhinovirus, 1% for parainfluenzavirus 2, 2% for adenovirus, and 1% for enterovirus (22). Symptoms included fever (59%), rhinitis (37%), pharyngitis (30%), laryngitis (3%), otitis (13%), bronchitis (17%), bronchiolitis (10%), and pneumonia (7%). Like other respiratory viruses, HCoV-OC43 and -229E are spread by large-droplet infection. Of concern to infection control practitioners is a recent finding that HCoV-229E can survive for up to 3 h when dried on solid surfaces and for up to 6 days in saline solution at room temperature.

SARS first appeared as a potentially fatal cause of pneumonia in Guangdong Province of China in November 2002. The first human case was identified on 16 November, and within 6 months SARS spread to 29 countries, infecting 8,098 people and killing 774 individuals (26). The last known case in this outbreak occurred 15 July 2003 in Taiwan. This outbreak had a profound effect on public health and economies worldwide, with an estimated $100 billion lost from global economies. SARS has arguably been the most significant event in medical virology since the emergence of human immunodeficiency virus and AIDS in the early 1980s.

SARS-CoV is believed to be zoonotic in origin, having crossed into humans most likely from animal hosts in the wild-game markets in Guangdong Province. Many of the first infected individuals in November and December 2002 had contact with the live-game trade. The disease was first called "infectious atypical pneumonia" because it caused clusters of disease in families and health care workers. The etiologic agent of SARS was identified as a new coronavirus by Peiris and coworkers at the University of Hong Kong (16), and the viral genome was fully sequenced in a record time of 3 weeks first by workers at the University of British Columbia, Vancouver, Canada (14). Genomic analysis revealed that SARS-CoV was a new coronavirus not previously found in humans. The absence of antibody in healthy humans suggested that SARS-CoV had recently emerged in the human population and that animal-to-human interspecies transmission was the most probable explanation for its emergence. Specimens collected from apparently healthy animals in the wild-game animal markets in China indicated that a number of animals, including the Himalayan palm civet cat and raccoon dogs, yielded a SARS-CoV-like virus with more than 99% nucleotide homology to human SARS-CoV. Many animal handlers with no previous history of a SARS-like illness had serum antibodies to SARS-CoV. Taken together with the fact that a number of SARS cases had an epidemiological link to wild-game animals, it is very likely that the wet markets in Guangdong provided the interface for transmission to humans. The early transmissions to humans were probably inefficient, causing little disease or human-to-human transmission. The animal SARS-CoV-like virus probably adapted in humans for efficient human-to-human transmission, and SARS-CoV emerged. There is evidence that the SARS-CoV evolved towards greater "fitness" during the SARS outbreak, since human viruses isolated late in the outbreak showed a 29-nucleotide deletion in ORF 8 that was absent from both human viruses isolated early in the outbreak and animal viruses (8). Similarly, the gene encoding the spike protein that mediates viral entry shows high rates of nonsynonymous mutations in early isolates that are absent in later isolates, probably reflecting the ongoing adaptations to the new host.

The major route of transmission in humans is droplet infection, aerosolization, and fomites. Deposition of droplets onto the respiratory epithelium probably initiates infection. Whether infection can occur through the oral or conjunctival epithelium remains unknown, but SARS-CoV has been detected in tears. Although exposure to the animal SARS-like virus may have caused asymptomatic infection, once the virus adapted to the human host, asymptomatic infection seemed to be a rare event. Despite the rapid spread of SARS worldwide, the average number of secondary infections caused by any one case is low (2.2 to 3.7) compared with influenza (5 to 25), and household transmission of SARS is relatively inefficient (6). Superspreading events in which a few infected individuals disproportionately contribute to transmission (e.g., a difficult intubation in the intensive care unit resulting in infection of a number of house staff) were characteristic of the outbreak. The factors associated with superspreading events are not well understood but may include coinfection with other viruses, host factors such as immunosuppression, and/or environmental factors.

At the beginning of the SARS outbreak, nosocomial infections played an important role. The first major outbreak in Hong Kong occurred in the Prince of Wales Hospital around 10 March 2003, resulting in 138 SARS cases, 69% of which were hospital workers. By the end of the outbreak there were 1,755 SARS cases in Hong Kong, 339 of which were workers in 16 hospitals. The attack rates for hospital workers varied widely during the outbreak. The overall attack rate for workers in the 16 hospitals in Hong Kong was 1.2%. In Canada, the first large outbreak occurred also in a community hospital, affecting 128 patients, of which 37% were hospital staff. In the

Canadian outbreak, the attack rates among nurses ranged from 10.3 to 60%, depending on which department they were serving. The number of infected staff was strongly correlated with the number of admitted SARS patients, the length and type of exposure, and the use of personal protective equipment such as gloves and masks. Later in the outbreak it was shown that personal protective equipment significantly decreased nosocomial infections and played a significant role in outbreak management. These and other studies indicated that the transmission of SARS is driven by exposure.

The natural history of SARS-CoV has been documented in several studies. The initial symptoms are unremarkable and common to all upper respiratory tract viral infections. A few days of cough and low-grade fever progresses rapidly to a full-blown pneumonia requiring hospitalization and often mechanical ventilation. Fever, malaise, lymphopenia, elevated liver enzymes, and infiltrates and consolidation on chest X ray are usually present. Quantitative PCR studies have shown that the viral load is high in the lower respiratory tract but low in the upper respiratory tract. Viral load in the upper respiratory tract and feces is low during the first 4 days and peaks at around day 10 of illness (19). This is in marked contrast to other respiratory viral infections such as influenza that peak soon after the onset of symptoms. This unusual feature of SARS-CoV infection explains its low transmissibility early in the illness and perhaps explains why outbreaks in some countries were limited to only a few cases. More importantly, it explains the poor sensitivity of early reverse transcriptase PCR (RT-PCR) tests on nasopharyngeal (NP) specimens collected early in the illness.

Although the main clinical symptoms are those of severe respiratory tract disease, the virus also infects other organs. About a quarter of SARS patients had a watery diarrhea, and virus can be cultured from the feces and urine as well as the respiratory tract. Virus can also be detected in serum, plasma, and peripheral blood leukocytes by RT-PCR; however, the viremia may be short-lived. Patients have a pronounced peripheral T-cell lymphocytopenia with reduced CD4 and CD8 cell counts, with one-third of individuals having a CD4 count of <200 cells/mm^2. Infected individuals with high viral loads in serum have a poor prognosis. Between days 10 and 15 of illness, high viral loads in NP aspirates (NPA), feces, and serum are independent predictors of adverse clinical outcome. SARS-CoV is invariably found in the lungs of individuals dying of SARS, but the viral load is usually higher in those dying earlier in the course of illness (<21 days). About one-quarter of patients with SARS require management in intensive care units, and the overall fatality rate is ~11%. Disease severity and mortality are correlated with age, with the highest mortality rates (52%) for those >65 years of age and the lowest rate for the 0- to 24-year-old group. Children who acquire SARS seldom require intensive care or mechanical ventilation (10). Although SARS-CoV can be found for months in the feces of an infected individual, there is no evidence that the virus persists following resolution of the illness.

The fourth human coronavirus, HCoV-NL63, was first discovered in The Netherlands in a 7-month-old boy who presented with coryza, conjunctivitis, and fever and who had chest X-ray findings consistent with bronchiolitis (24). The virus grew in tertiary monkey kidney cells, which distinguished it from HCoV-OC43 and -229E. Sequencing of the genome indicated that the virus was not a recombinant virus but genetically distinct from all other HCoVs. After the first case, NL63 was detected in five additional children and three adults, two of whom were immunocompromised. NL63 has also been detected in 2% of prospectively studied patients with respiratory tract infections in Brisbane, Australia. Fourchier et al. independently reported a novel group 1 HCoV with a 27,555-nucleotide genome with 34% G+C (5). This virus was first isolated in 1988 from an 8-month-old with pneumonia in monkey kidney cells and is most likely the same virus as NL63. RT-PCR assays and primers based on the first isolate were able to detect this virus in 4 of 139 specimens collected from pediatric patients with upper respiratory infections between 2000 and 2002, indicating that this virus has been circulating in The Netherlands for a number of years.

The fifth HCoV, HCoV-HKU1, was discovered in January 2004 in Hong Kong in a 71-year-old man returning from Shenzhen, China. He presented with fever and a productive cough with purulent sputum and had a chest radiograph showing patchy infiltrates. All attempts to grow a virus from NP specimens failed, but coronavirus RNA was detected in the NPA by RT-PCR using *pol* gene consensus primers (25). Quantitative PCR indicated high titers of virus (10^{-6}) present in the NPA during the first week of illness, with decreasing titers in the second week and undetectable levels of virus in the third and fourth weeks. The virus was absent from urine or stool specimens. A recombinant nucleocapsid protein-based enzyme-linked immunosorbent assay (ELISA) indicated seroconversion in the first week of infection, with both immunoglobulin M (IgM) and IgG antibody detectable. A second case was subsequently identified, a 35-year-old woman with pneumonia with unknown etiology. The recent discovery over the past 2 years of two new group 1 and 2 HCoVs from the upper respiratory tract of symptomatic patients suggests that additional as yet unidentified HCoVs may await discovery.

LABORATORY DIAGNOSIS

Infections due to HCoV-OC43 and -229E are best diagnosed by detection of viral RNA in NP specimens using a nucleic acid amplification technique such as RT-PCR. RT-PCR is more sensitive than both virus isolation and immunofluorescence staining of NP specimens. Individual coronaviruses can be detected by one of two approaches: type-specific primers can be used to amplify single HCoV types (20, 23), or consensus primers targeting conserved regions of the *pol* gene can be used to amplify all five HCoVs and the amplified RNA can be digested with specific restriction enzymes or sequenced to determine the type of HCoV present (1, 23). The diagnosis of SARS, however, presents a bigger challenge.

Isolation of SARS-CoV in cell culture followed by determination of its partial genome sequence led to the first generation of RT-PCR assays for diagnosing SARS. The first PCR assays targeted the ORF 1b *pol* gene, the first part of the genome to be sequenced. Early serological tests used SARS-CoV-infected cells and ELISAs employing crude cell lysates containing SARS-CoV antigens. Virus culture was less sensitive than RT-PCR, labor-intensive, and too slow for clinical management and required a biosafety level 3 (BSL3) laboratory. Although these tests, when used together with multiple specimens, proved useful for identifying patients at the beginning of the outbreak, they proved less satisfactory for diagnosing new cases in the first few days after onset of symptoms.

The first-generation RT-PCR assays proved more useful after the first week of illness, with only 40 to 60% of specimens testing positive in the first few days of the disease (2, 21). NP specimens had the highest positivity rates in the second week of illness, peaking at about day 10. The poor sensitivity of RT-PCR with NP specimens prompted the examination of other specimens, leading to the discovery of

virus in fecal and urine specimens. Replication of SARS-CoV in the gastrointestinal tract was confirmed by electron microscopy and RT-PCR testing of biopsy and postmortem specimens. These findings indicated that the virus rapidly disseminates from the NP to other tissues and suggested that the virus could be transmitted by the fecal route. The use of quantitative PCR assays on respiratory specimens and testing of serial specimens showed that unlike for other respiratory viral infections, the viral load and rates of positivity of SARS-CoV in the upper respiratory tract increased steadily and peaked at around day 10 after disease onset (15). Whereas viral RNA could be detected for several weeks or even months in stool specimens, virus culture was positive only during the first 2 to 3 weeks of illness. It is possible that virus replication continues for weeks but that virus is complexed with antibody and is no longer infective or transmissible. This is consistent with epidemiological findings.

In addition to being found in respiratory tract specimens, viral RNA is detected in stool, blood, cerebrospinal fluid, urine, and tears. Of these nonrespiratory specimens, stool specimens have the highest positivity rates and highest viral loads, suggesting that fecal specimens are a good alternative to respiratory tract specimens for identification of SARS patients. The low RT-PCR positivity rates for NP specimens early in the course of disease prompted examination of other approaches to increase the sensitivity of viral RNA detection. Real-time nested-PCR strategies are useful for detecting low levels of SARS-CoV in the early stage of illness, but nested PCR doubles the cost and workload and carries with it the potential for false positives due to carryover contamination. Quantitative one-step RT-PCR in a sealed reaction vessel not only reduces the chance of false positives but adds valuable viral load information. Quantitative PCR also revealed that viral loads were highest in lower respiratory tract specimens (bronchoalveolar lavage, sputum, endotracheal aspirates) and higher in NP specimens than in throat swabs (3). Fecal specimens have a high viral load at the end of the first week of illness and are the specimen of choice during the second week of disease.

Other approaches to increasing the sensitivity of PCR include testing multiple serial specimens or enhancing RNA extraction. This approach, although not comprehensively evaluated for SARS-CoV, has proven useful for detecting other microorganisms when present in low levels in clinical specimens. Targeting the nucleocapsid gene for RT-PCR should enhance the sensitivity of PCR for diagnosis, since subgenomic RNA transcripts contain nucleocapsid gene sequences following discontinuous transcription. This, however, turned out not to be the case for SARS-CoV, as RT-PCR assays targeting the nucleocapsid gene failed to be more sensitive than *pol* gene assays and subsequent studies showed that most of the viral RNA in clinical specimens was genomic RNA. The availability of nucleocapsid RT-PCR assays, however, did provide a confirmatory assay for positive specimens early in the epidemic (13). Another approach to improving sensitivity involves extraction of a larger volume of the clinical specimen and using more RNA in the PCR assay. By extracting a larger portion of NPA specimens, the sensitivity of RT-PCR was increased from about 50 to 80% for specimens collected from days 1 to 3 of disease onset while retaining 100% specificity (18). In this particular study, there was no increase in amplification inhibitors during RNA purification, but this should be controlled for by the use of an amplification control in the PCR to rule out false negatives due to PCR inhibition. Testing of serum or plasma for viral RNA was disappointing at first, but subsequent studies have shown 50 and

78% positivity rates for serum and plasma, respectively, during the first week of illness. A second study confirmed these results for plasma, with a 79% positivity rate during the first 3 days of illness (7). The demonstration of SARS-CoV RNA in peripheral leukocytes may provide another alternative for early diagnosis. Efforts aimed at optimizing RNA extraction from a larger volume of specimens such as stool or plasma should raise the sensitivity of RT-PCR for these nonrespiratory specimens for identifying SARS patients. Real-time PCR assays that provide viral loads may also be useful for identifying patients at increased risk for worse outcomes in terms of survival and requirement for intensive care and assisted ventilation. Recent studies confirmed that a high viral load in NPA specimens was associated with the need for intensive care and was an independent predictor of mortality. Thus, quantitative PCR assays may provide useful prognostic information for clinical management, including the use of antiviral therapy.

The serodiagnosis is currently the "gold standard" for confirmation of a diagnosis of SARS. The first tests were immunofluorescence assays (IFAs) using virus-infected cells spotted onto microscope slides and ELISAs using extracts from virus-infected cells to coat microtiter well plates. Both methods proved useful in diagnosing SARS, but soon after their deployment it became clear that serology had a major limitation for diagnosis. Seroconversion following infection with SARS-CoV usually occurred in weeks 2 and 3 of illness, and a few patients seroconverted as late as 28 days postinfection. Thus, serology is not useful for the early diagnosis of SARS. SARS-CoV IgM appears after IgG antibody and therefore does not assist in the serodiagnosis. IgA antibody appears about the same time as IgG and persists in serum for 1 to 2 months. IgM antibody persists for about 11 weeks and is then undetectable, whereas IgG persists for months and perhaps years. The whole-cell IFA is about 92% sensitive and 96% specific, with about 4% of serum specimens from healthy individuals giving a positive result. ELISAs using crude antigens showed sensitivity and specificity similar to those of the IFA. Early IFAs and ELISAs required the cultivation of virus in a BSL3 laboratory, and this limitation resulted in the development of serological assays utilizing recombinant proteins. Western blot (WB) assays using whole virus cell lysates show the presence of a predominant N-protein band (often a doublet or triplet around 36 to 48 kDa), a spike antibody band at 150 kDa, and less predominant antibody bands at 80, 60, 32, and 24 kDa (12). Recombinant spike and nucleocapsid proteins have quickly replaced viral lysates in ELISAs and WB and immunodot assays and provide a safe, low-cost alternative for serodiagnosis. The nucleocapsid protein has been shown to be the immunodominant protein of SARS-CoV and an excellent antigen for use in the ELISA. The recombinant N-protein ELISA has an improved sensitivity and specificity compared with those of the whole cell lysate assay and can measure IgG, IgA, and IgM class antibodies by use of specific conjugates. In one study, the N-protein ELISA had a sensitivity of 94.3% and a specificity of 95.3% when evaluated with 106 SARS patient serum samples and 149 blood donor control serum samples (24a), and in another study it performed with a sensitivity and specificity of 100%. Other laboratories have compared the use of the recombinant N protein in a WB, immunodot assay, and ELISA and found sensitivities and specificities in the same range (94 to 96% and 96 to 98%, respectively). Although the spike protein is an important viral protein and elicits neutralizing antibody, it has not been used as widely in serological tests. Further evaluations with larger numbers of serum specimens will be required to determine the true performance of these research tests.

The gold standard test for detecting SARS-CoV antibody is the neutralization (NT) test. The performance of all new serological tests should be evaluated by comparing them with the NT test. Because this test measures neutralizing antibody by reacting serum with live virus, the test can be performed only in a BSL3 laboratory and is therefore limited to only a few laboratories. For this reason, the kinetics for the appearance of NT antibody and the role of IgM and IgA class antibodies in virus NT are poorly understood. The recent development of SARS-CoV pseudotype virions and their use in NT and virus entry assays provide a novel method for assessing neutralizing antibody in SARS patients' sera that is safe (doesn't require BSL3 containment) and cost-effective (9). This assay can easily be automated for high-throughput capacity for the large-scale screening of neutralizing antibody for vaccine trials.

TESTING PROCEDURES

Specimens
For details of procedures for the collection and storage of specimens for detection of HCoVs, see *Manual of Clinical Microbiology*, 8th edition (4a).

Virus Isolation
Cell culture has proven unreliable for primary isolation of HCoV, and some strains grow in cell culture only after adaptation. HCoV-OC43 and -229E can be isolated in human embryonic lung cells (L132) or MRC-5 cells. HCoV-NL63 and HCoV-HKU1 can be isolated in tertiary monkey kidney (*Cynomolgus* monkey) or LLC-MK2 cells. Cytopathic effect may take 7 to 10 days to appear and may vary in appearance from a ground-glass refractive appearance to cell rounding and detachment, depending on the host cell. SARS-CoV can be isolated in Vero E6 cells, although this must not be attempted outside a BSL3 laboratory.

Antigen Detection
HCoV antigens can be detected in cells prepared from NP specimens by standard methods and stained with coronavirus-specific monoclonal antibodies and a fluorescence-labeled anti-mouse IgG conjugate (20).

Antibody Detection
Serum antibody to SARS-CoV can be detected by immunofluorescence staining of fixed SARS-CoV-infected Vero E6 cells. Replicate cell monolayers on glass coverslips in 1-dram shell vials are infected with SARS-CoV at a multiplicity of infection (MOI) of 1. After 24 h, the monolayers are fixed and permeabilized with cold 100% methanol and the cells are rehydrated in phosphate-buffered saline (PBS) containing 5% bovine serum albumin. Serum samples are heat inactivated at 56°C for 30 min, serial dilutions are prepared in PBS containing 0.05% Tween 20 (PBS-T) and incubated on cell monolayers for 1 h at 37°C and the cells are washed three times with PBS-T. Fluorescent anti-human IgG conjugates (either Alexa 488 from Molecular Probes, Eugene, Oreg., or fluorescein isothiocyanate from Sigma, St. Louis, Mo.) are diluted according to the manufacturer's instructions and added, and the mixtures are incubated for 1 h at room temperature. The cells are washed with PBS-T and deionized water and viewed using a fluorescence microscope. A SARS IFA antibody kit is commercially available from Euroimmune GmbH (Luebeck, Germany).

WB

SARS-CoV-infected cell lysates are generated by infecting Vero E6 cells with SARS-CoV (Tor2 or Urbani strain) at an MOI of 1 to 5 for 24 h and then lysing the cells in NP-40 lysis buffer. The lysates are heated to 65°C for 1 h, and sodium dodecyl sulfate (SDS) is added to a final concentration of 2%. (Inactivation of virus should be confirmed by cell culture inoculation.) For WB analysis, 20 μl of lysate is electrophoresed on SDS–10% polyacrylamide gels. Proteins are transblotted to nitrocellulose (Nytran from Schleicher & Schuell), and the membranes are blocked with 5% nonfat dried milk in TBS-T buffer (50 mM Tris [pH 7.6], 150 mM NaCl, containing 0.5% Tween 20) for 1 h at room temperature. A serum dilution of 1:500 in blocking buffer is incubated with the membrane for 1 h at room temperature, and the membranes are washed three times for 15 min each with TBS-T. Bound antibody is detected by enhanced chemiluminescence using goat anti-human IgG, IgM, or IgA antibody-horseradish peroxidase conjugate diluted 1:2,000 in blocking buffer (1 h, room temperature) and ECL substrate (Amersham) according to the manufacturer's instructions.

ELISA

Viral antigens, either recombinant nucleocapsid or spike protein or viral lysates, are bound to wells of Immunlon II microtiter plates by dilution of protein (0.05 to 1.0 μg/0.1 ml) in carbonate buffer (pH 9.6) and adsorption overnight at 4°C. The plates are blocked with PBS containing 5% skim milk powder. The assay is performed essentially as described by Leung et al. (12). Briefly, 100 μl of serum diluted 1:500 in PBS-T is added to the wells, and the mixture is incubated for 1 h at room temperature. The plates are washed, incubated with a 1:2,000 dilution of horseradish peroxidase-conjugated goat anti-human IgG conjugate (Sigma) for 30 min at room temperature, washed, and incubated with tetramethylbenzidine substrate for 15 min at room temperature. The plates are read in a Dynatech reader at 450 nm. Cutoffs are established as the mean plus 3 standard deviations of 20 negative sera. ELISA kits are commercially available from Beijing Genomics Institute (Beijing, China).

Nucleic Acid Detection

HCoV RNA can be detected by RT-PCR, nucleic acid sequence-based amplification (NASBA), and loop-mediated isothermal (LAMP) amplification techniques. For RT-PCR, conventional heat block or real-time assays using a one- or two-step format have been used to detect HCoV-OC43 and HCoV-229E (1, 20, 23) and SARS-CoV (2, 3, 7, 13, 15, 18). For a two-step assay, cDNA is prepared by using 5 μl of sample RNA in a 20-μl reaction volume containing Moloney murine leukemia virus RT with 50 μM random hexamer primers, and then 4 μl of the RT reaction mixture is used in a 50-μl conventional thermal cycler or 20-μl LightCycler PCR assay. Oligonucleotide primers can target either conserved or unique regions of the *nuc* or *pol* genes (Table 1). For conventional assays, the products are analyzed by agarose gel electrophoresis with ethidium bromide staining. Real-time assays in either the LightCycler or ABI 7500/7700/7900 instruments acquire the signal in "real time" during amplification using either SYBRGreen dye or Taqman or fluorescent resonance energy transfer probes and do not require post-run analysis. Forty cycles of amplification is usually sufficient to detect a single RNA copy; 50-cycle reactions do not usually add sensitivity and often make it difficult to distinguish weak positives from background. Positive and negative controls should be included in every run, and internal amplification controls (spiked RNA) are useful for detecting amplification inhibitors in specimens.

Commercially available tests have recently appeared and include the RealArt HPA CoV RT-PCR assay from Artus GmbH (Hamburg, Germany), the SARS Coronavirus NP and POL MultiCode-RTx kits from EraGen Biosciences (Madison, Wis.), and the LightCycler SARS-CoV kit from Roche Diagnostics (Branchburg, N.J.). Meaningful evaluations of these commercial assays have not yet appeared, since their true performance has not yet been determined.

QUALITY CONTROL AND INTERPRETATION

Caution must be exercised when antibody results are interpreted for diagnosis of SARS because of the late seroconversion following infection. A negative antibody result in a patient with pneumonia and an epidemiological link to a known SARS patient cannot be used to rule out SARS due to the possibility of a late seroconversion. A negative antibody result for a sample collected on or after 28 days following onset of illness can, however, rule out SARS since most SARS patients seroconvert by this time. If an in-house, recombinant protein-based ELISA is used (e.g., rN protein), performance must be determined in advance since any given recombinant protein may yield different sensitivities and specificities when used in different formats in different

TABLE 1 RT-PCR assays for detection of HCoV

Virus	Gene	Primers	Format[a]	Amplicon (bp)	Reference
OC43	*nuc*	5′-CCC AAG CAA ACT GCT ACC TCT CAG-3′ 5′-GTA GAC TCC GTC AAT ATC GGT GCC-3′	2-step CB	305	20
229E	*nuc*	E7 5′-TCT GCC AAG AGT CTT GCT CG-3′ E9 5′-AGC ATA GCA GCT GTT GAC GG-3′ Hybrid probe 5′-biotin GGA AGT GCA GGT GTT GTGGC	1-step CB	214	23
SARS-CoV	*pol* ORF lb	5′-ATG AAT TAC CAA GTC AAT GGT TAC-3′ 5′-CAT AAC CAG TCG GTA CAG CTA-3′	LC (SYBRGreen)	190	3
	nuc	5′-TGA ATA CAC CCA AAG ACC AC-3′ 5′-TGA TGA GGA GCG AGA AGA-G-3′ 5′-6FAM-CCT AAT AAC AAT GCT GCC ACC GT-TAMRA-3′	LC (TaqMan)	149	13

[a]CB, conventional heat block assay; LC, LightCycler assay.

laboratories. Commercially available antibody assays are just now appearing and will require careful evaluation prior to their use. IgM antibody testing has not proven useful for SARS since IgM antibody may actually appear later than IgG antibody. A positive antibody test alone cannot be used to diagnose SARS due to the potential cross-reactivity of antibody to other HCoVs such as OC43 and 229E. Any positive antibody test should therefore be confirmed with an NT antibody test. A single confirmed antibody test in the absence of another positive test such as RT-PCR should also be viewed with caution since the positive predictive values of IFA and ELISA are not 100%.

A negative RT-PCR test on an NP specimen from a suspected SARS patient does not rule out SARS, since SARS-CoV is present in low levels in the upper respiratory tract in the first week of infection. Since the level of viral RNA in the NP and stool rises in the second week of illness, a follow-up NP and/or fecal specimen should be collected and tested by PCR. Negative PCR results for specimens from the upper tract could trigger sampling from the lower tract, where the titers of virus are higher, although collection of these invasive specimens is associated with an increased risk of nosocomial transmission. Detection of SARS-CoV in plasma or peripheral leukocytes should be considered, since this approach provides sensitivities of around 80% during the first week of illness. The use of multiple and serial respiratory tract and fecal specimens will improve the sensitivity of PCR for making a diagnosis, especially when a larger volume of the sample is extracted and a larger proportion of the sample RNA is used for amplification. A positive RT-PCR result should be confirmed by testing a different specimen with an independent molecular test targeting a different gene and also confirmed by an independent reference laboratory. The first commercially available PCR assays for SARS are only 65 to 75% sensitive and should not be used alone without sending parallel specimens to an experienced reference laboratory for testing. Recognizing that the first human infections were caused by a zootic virus that adapted to its new human host and that we face the continuing possibility for the introduction of new variants of animal SARS-associated viruses (which may cause milder disease with low levels of replicating virus), greater vigilance will be required to make a diagnosis of infection with SARS-associated animal coronaviruses.

REFERENCES

1. **Adachi, D., G. Johnson, R. Draker, M. Ayers, T. Mazzulli, P. J. Talbot, and R. Tellier.** 2004. Comprehensive detection and identification of human coronaviruses, including SARS-associated coronavirus, with a single RT-PCR assay. *J. Virol. Methods* **122:**29–36.
2. **Chan, K. H., L. L. M. Poon, V. C. C. Cheng, et al.** 2003. Detection of SARS coronavirus (ScoV) by RT-PCR, culture, and serology in patients with severe acute respiratory syndrome (SARS). *Emerg. Infect. Dis.* **10:**194–199.
3. **Drosten, C., L. L. Chiu, M. Panning, H. N. Leong, W. Preiser, J. S. Tam, S. Gunther, S. Kramme, P. Emmerich, W. L. Ng, H. Schmitz, and E. S. Koay.** 2004. Evaluation of advanced reverse transcription–PCR assays and an alternative PCR target region for detection of severe acute respiratory syndrome-associated coronavirus. *J. Clin. Microbiol.* **42:**2043–2047.
4. **Falsey, A. R., E. E. Walsh, and F. G. Hayden.** 2002. Rhinovirus and coronavirus infection-associated hospitalization: among older adults. *J. Infect. Dis.* **185:**1338–1341.
4a. **Forman, M. S., and A. Valsamakis.** 2003. Specimen collection, transport, and processing: virology, p. 1227–1241.

In P. R. Murray et al. (ed.), *Manual of Clinical Microbiology*, 8th ed. ASM Press, Washington, D.C.
5. **Fourchier, R. A. M., N. G. Hartwig, T. M. Bestebroer, B. Niemeyer, J. C. de Jong, J. H. Simon, and A. D. M. E. Osterhaus.** 2004. A previously undescribed coronavirus associated with respiratory disease in humans. *Proc. Natl. Acad. Sci. USA* **101:**6212–6216.
6. **Goh, D. L., B. W. Lee, K. S. Chia, B. H. Heng, M. Chen, S. Ma, and C. C. Tan.** 2004. Secondary household transmission of SARS, Singapore. *Emerg. Infect. Dis.* **10:**232–234.
7. **Grant, P. R., J. A. Garson, R. S. Tedder, P. K. Chan, J. S. Tam, and J. J. Sung.** 2003. Detection of SARS coronavirus in plasma by real-time PCR. *N. Engl. J. Med.* **349:**2468–2469.
8. **Guan, Y., B. J. Zeng, Y. Q. He, X. L. Liu, Z. X. Zhuang, C. L. Cheung, S. W. Luo, P. H. Li, L. J. Zhang, Y. J. Guan, K. M. Butt, K. L. Wong, K. W. Chan, W. Lim, K. F. Shortridge, K. Y. Yuen, J. S. Peiris, and L. L. Poon.** 2003. Isolation and characterization of viruses related to the SARS coronavirus from animals in Southern China. *Science* **302:**276–278.
9. **Han, P., H. G. Kim, Y. B. Kim, L. L. M. Poon, and M. W. Cho.** 2004. Development of a safe neutralization assay for SARS-CoV and characterization of S-glycoprotein. *Virology* **326:**140–149.
10. **Hon, K. L., et al.** 2004. Clinical presentation and outcome of severe acute respiratory syndrome in children. *Lancet* **361:**1701–1703.
11. **Lai, M. M., and D. Cavanagh.** 1997. The molecular biology of coronaviruses. *Adv. Virus Res.* **48:**1–100.
12. **Leung, D. T. M., F. C. H. Tam, C. H. Ma, P. K. S. Chan, J. L. K. Cheung, H. Niu, J. S. L. Tam, and P. L. Lim.** 2004. Antibody response of patients with severe acute respiratory syndrome (SARS) targets the viral nucleocapsid. *J. Infect. Dis.* **190:**379–386.
13. **Mahony, J. B., A. Petrich, L. Louie, X. Song, S. Chong, M. Smieja, M. Chernesky, M. Loeb, and S. Richardson.** 2004. Performance and cost evaluation of one commercial and six in-house conventional and real-time reverse transcriptase PCR assays for detection of severe acute respiratory syndrome coronavirus. *J. Clin. Microbiol.* **42:**1471–1476.
14. **Marra, M. A., S. J. Jones, C. R. Astell, R. A. Holt, A. Brooks-Wilson, Y. S. Butterfield, J. Khattra, J. K. Asano, S. A. Barber, S. Y. Chan, et al.** 2003. The genome sequence of the SARS-associated coronavirus. *Science* **300:**1399–1404.
15. **Peiris, J. S., C. M. Chu, V. C. Cheng, et al.** 2003. Clinical progression and viral load in a community outbreak of coronavirus-associated SARS pneumonia: a prospective study. *Lancet* **361:**1767–1772.
16. **Peiris, J. S. M., S. T. Lai, L. L. Poon, Y. Guan, L. Y. Yam, W. Lim, J. Nicholls, W. K. Yee, W. W. Yan, M. T. Cheung, V. C. Cheng, K. H. Chan, D. N. Tsang, R. W. Yung, T. K. Ng, K. Y. Yuen, and SARS Study Group.** 2003. Coronavirus as a possible cause of severe acute respiratory syndrome. *Lancet* **361:**1319–1325.
17. **Pene, F., A. Merlat, A. Vabret, F. Rozenberg, A. Buzyn, F. Dreyfus, A. Cariou, F. Freymuth, and P. Lebon.** 2003. Coronavirus 229E-related pneumonia in immunocompromised patients. *Clin. Infect. Dis.* **37:**929–932.
18. **Poon, L. L. M., B. M. Wong, K. H. Chan, C. S. Leung, K. Y. Yuen, Y. Guan, and J. S. Peiris.** 2004. A one step quantitative RT-PCR for detection of SARS coronavirus with an internal control for PCR inhibitors. *J. Clin. Virol.* **30:**214–217.
19. **Poutanen, S. M., D. E. Low, B. Henry, S. Finkelstein, D. Rose, K. Green, et al.** 2003. Identification of severe acute respiratory syndrome in Canada. *N. Engl. J. Med.* **348:**1995–2005.

20. Sizun, J., N. Arbour, and P. J. Talbot. 1998. Comparison of immunofluorescence with monoclonal antibodies and RT-PCR for the detection of human coronaviruses 229E and OC43 in cell culture. *J. Virol. Methods* **72:**145–152.

21. Tang, P., M. Louie, S. Richardson, M. Smieja, A. E. Simor, F. Jamieson, M. Fearon, S. M. Poutanen, T. Mazzulli, R. Tellier, J. Mahony, M. Loeb, A. Petrich, M. Chernesky, A. McGeer, D. E. Low, E. Phillips, S. Jones, N. Bastien, Y. Li, D. Dick, A. Grolla, L. Fernando, T. F. Booth, B. Henry, A. R. Rachlis, L. M. Matukas, D. B. Rose, R. Lovinsky, S. Walmsley, W. L. Gold, and S. Krajden. 2004. Interpretation of diagnostic laboratory tests for severe acute respiratory syndrome; the Toronto experience. *Can. Med. Assoc. J.* **170:**47–54.

22. Vabret, A., T. Mourez, S. Gouarin, J. Petitjean, and F. Freymuth. 2003. An outbreak of coronavirus OC43 respiratory infection in Normandy, France. *Clin. Infect. Dis.* **36:**985–989.

23. Vallet, S., A. Gagneur, P. J. Talbot, M. Legrand, J. Sizun, and B. Picard. 2004. Detection of human coronavirus 229E in nasal specimens in large scale studies using an RT-PCR hybridization assay. *Mol. Cell. Probes* **18:**75–80.

24. Van der Hoek, L., K. Pyrc, M. F. Jebbink, W. Vermeulen-Oost, R. J. M. Berkhout, K. C. Wolthers, P. M. E. Wertheim-van Dillen, J. Kaandorp, J. Spaargaren, and B. Berkhout. 2004. Identification of a new human coronavirus. *Nat. Med.* **10:**368–373.

24a. Woo, P. C., S. K. Lan, B. H. Wong, H. W. Tsai, A. M. Fung, K. H. Chan, V. K. Tam, J. S. Peiris, and K. Y. Yuen. 2004. Detection of specific antibodies to severe acute respiratory syndrome (SARS) coronavirus nucleocapsid protein for serodiagnosis of SARS coronavirus pneumonia. *J. Clin. Microbiol.* **42:**2306–2309.

25. Woo, P. C. Y., S. K. P. Lau, C.-M. Chu, K.-H. Chan, H.-W. Tsoi, Y. Hwang, B. H. L. Wong, R. W. S. Poon, J. J. Cai, W.-K. Luk, L. L. M. Poon, S. S. Y. Wong, Y. Guan, J. S. M. Peiris, and K.-Y. Yuen. 2005. Characterization and complete genome sequence of a novel coronavirus, coronavirus HKU1, from patients with pneumonia. *J. Virol.* **79:**884–895.

26. World Health Organization. Summary of probable SARS cases with onset of illness from 1 November 2002 to 31 July 2003. http://www.who.int/cst/sars/country/talbe2004_04_21/en/.

Poxviruses

KEVIN L. KAREM AND INGER K. DAMON

91

Poxviruses are large double-stranded DNA viruses that have a wide range of susceptible host species. The family *Poxviridae* includes two subfamilies: *Chordopoxvirinae* and *Entomopoxvirinae*, which infect vertebrate and insect hosts, respectively, and replicate in their cytoplasm (13). The complexity of these viruses relies on the large genome which encodes most proteins required for viral replication and maturation, and their ability to modify and evade host responses to the benefit of the virus. This chapter limits discussion to the diagnostic capabilities for the subfamily *Chordopoxvirinae*, which contains viruses capable of infecting humans (Table 1). Among the *Chordopoxvirinae* are two agents that are specific for humans, variola virus (a member of the OPXs and the etiologic agent of smallpox) and molluscum contagiosum virus, a benign exanthem of the genus *Molluscipoxvirus* (7).

Within the *Chordopoxvirinae*, the genus considered most relevant to human disease is OPX. The OPXs are highly homologous, morphologically similar viruses that, with the exception of variola virus, have a broad animal host range. This genus also includes monkeypox, vaccinia, cowpox, and camelpox viruses and several other lesser known species. Other genera with species that cause any human illness are the *Yatapoxvirus* (tanapox virus and occasionally yaba monkey tumor virus [YMTV]), *Parapoxvirus* (orf, pseudocowpox; see below), and *Molluscipoxvirus* (the sole member is molluscum contagiosum virus). The poxvirus of the greatest historical significance is variola virus, the agent of smallpox and the single greatest killer of humans of all infectious diseases known. Observed since at least Egyptian times, variola major was endemic worldwide and has caused high morbidity and mortality on at least six continents (14). The eradication program of the mid to late 20th century resulted in the eradication of naturally occurring smallpox cases worldwide, with the ultimate isolation and consolidation of stocks of variola viruses in two locations worldwide (14). However, historical use of variola virus as a bioweapon and knowledge of active research into the use of variola virus as a bioweapon have heightened the awareness of the possibility that nonsanctioned stocks may exist and that rogue states or terrorists may intentionally release variola virus. Diagnostic capabilities for smallpox are therefore of utmost importance globally and have evolved significantly over the past decade.

More recent events since the eradication of smallpox have increased interest in and need for diagnostic capabilities for other OPXs. Disease caused by monkeypox was recognized in primates as early as 1958 and has been the cause of ongoing human disease in central Africa since the 1980s. Monkeypox is of increased interest since its importation into the United States in 2003 and has increased concerns of zoonotic transmission of poxviruses. The emergence of human monkeypox highlights the importance of improving and maintaining diagnostic capacities not only for variola virus but also for other poxviruses.

This chapter addresses molecular and immunological diagnostic issues for detection of viral infections associated with four genera of the *Chordopoxvirinae* that cause human disease and their public health significance (Table 1). Diagnostic methods are similar for these viruses and are addressed cumulatively. A description of specific viruses and associated diseases is presented based on genus.

GENUS OPX

Variola Virus

The primary challenge presented by smallpox for clinicians is identifying, quickly and with confidence, a disease that has been extinct for over 25 years. To facilitate the detection of variola in patients, clinical awareness has been promoted to assist a medical community that has never observed this disease except in textbooks. Humans are the only known reservoir for variola, a fact that played in favor of the eradication campaign since vaccination of a single species (humans) could facilitate extinction. Clinical illness associated with variola virus infection has been described extensively and reviewed recently (5). Airborne exposure is the mode of infection from human to human via respiratory droplets. Following exposure, upper and lower respiratory pathways are infected followed by regional lymph nodes, with subsequent viremia in most cases. The incubation period lasts from 7 to 17 days, during which the patient is not contagious. In ordinary smallpox (historically 90% of disease presentations) a prodromal stage follows, in which first symptoms appear. These symptoms include fever, malaise, head and body aches, and sometimes vomiting. Notable is a high fever, usually in the range of 101 to 104°F. During the prodromal stage patients are typically too sick to perform daily duties and are essentially incapacitated. The prodrome lasts 2 to 4 days, and during this period the patient may be contagious. Following the prodrome is the rash onset stage of

TABLE 1 Subfamily *Chordopoxvirinae*

Genus	Disease in humans	Virus	Disease (host[s])
Avipoxvirus	No	Fowlpox	Fowlpox (chickens, turkeys)
		Canarypox	Canarypox (pet bird species)
Capripoxvirus	No	Goatpox	Goatpox (goat, sheep)
		Sheeppox	Sheeppox (goat, sheep)
		Lumpy skin	Lumpy skin disease (cattle, buffalo)
Leporipoxvirus	No	Myxoma	Myxomatosis (rabbits)
Molluscipoxvirus	Yes	Molluscum	Molluscum contagiosum (humans)
OPX	Yes	Variola	Smallpox (humans)
		Monkeypox	Monkeypox (humans, monkeys, rodents)
		Vaccinia	Vaccine adverse events (humans)
		Rabbitpox	Rabbitpox (colonized rabbits)
		Buffalopox	Buffalopox (buffalo, cattle, humans)
		Cowpox	Cowpox (cattle, felines, rodents, humans)
		Taterapox	Taterapox (gerbils)
		Camelpox	Camelpox (camels)
		Ectromelia	Mousepox (mice)
		Volepox	Volepox (California voles, mice)
		Raccoonpox	Raccoonpox (North American raccoons, unknown)
		Skunkpox	Skunkpox (North American skunks, unknown)
Parapoxvirus	Yes	Orf	Orf (sheep, goats, cattle, humans)
		Pseudocow, paravaccinia	Milker's nodules (cattle, humans)
		Bovine papular stomatitis	Bovine papular stomatitis (cattle, humans)
Suipoxvirus	No	Swinepox	Swinepox (domestic swine)
Yatapoxvirus	Yes	Tanapox	Tanapox (primates, humans)
		YMTV	YMTV (primates)

illness. The rash emerges between day 7 and day 17 postexposure, on average day 10 to 12, as an exanthem consisting of small red spots on the oral mucosa, including the tongue, and shortly thereafter as an exanthem consisting of macules on the epidermis. The exanthem develops into sores that break open and spread large amounts of the virus into the mouth and throat, largely accounting for the contagious nature of the disease. The exanthem appears on the skin of the face and spreads to the arms and legs and then the feet and hands, including the soles and palms. The rash typically spreads to all parts of the body within 24 h (Fig. 1). Concurrently, the fever typically falls as the rash spreads to distal extremities. The rash develops through macular to papular to vesicular and then pustular stages. By the third to fourth day of the rash the lesions become raised bumps filled with a thick opaque fluid with a depression in the center that looks like a belly button (this is a major distinguishing characteristic of smallpox). The fever typically rises again at this time and remains high until scabs form over all of the lesions. Pustules develop soon after and become firm to the touch. During this pustule stage the patient remains contagious. After 5 or 6 days after rash onset, the pustules begin to form a crust and then to scab. Over the next 5 days scabs form over the sores while the patient remains contagious. Scabs then resolve and begin to fall off, leaving pitted scar areas over the next 6 days or so. Upon complete resolution and falling off of scabs, the patient is no longer contagious. At this stage the lesions are healed, leaving significant scarring.

Recently the use of clinical algorithms designed to differentiate smallpox from other febrile vesiculo-pustular rash illnesses has been promoted (17, 48). These algorithms use the historic classic features of ordinary smallpox described previously and contrast them with similar symptoms in other febrile vesiculo-pustular rash illnesses. A primary focus of the algorithm is the discrimination of varicella virus and other herpesvirus infections; historically, infections caused by these pathogens were most often confused with smallpox.

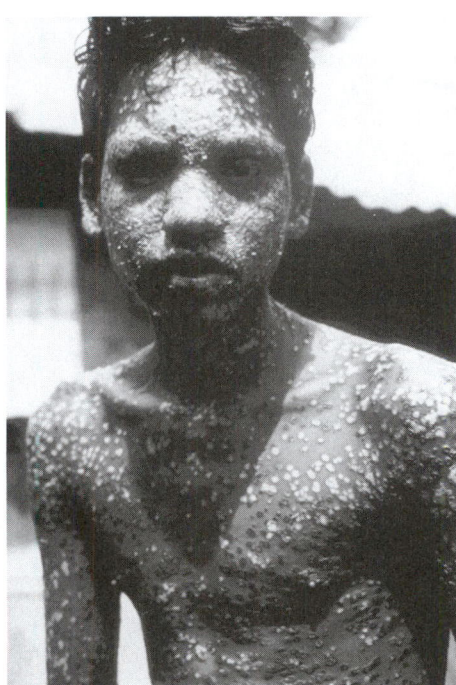

FIGURE 1 This photograph is of a Bangladeshi boy with smallpox, revealing the distribution of maculopapular lesions. (Source: CDC Public Health Image Library, James Hicks, 1973.)

Treatments for smallpox infection are limited and are largely supportive, using traditional methods of giving fluids and rest for viral infections. Advances in supportive care and improvements in intensive care strategies would likely enhance treatment efficacies should smallpox recur. Experimentally, several compounds are effective in vitro, such as cidofovir, but may have toxicities in vivo. Alterations in cidofovir structurally have remedied the toxicity to some degree in animal models and in vitro; however, approval of any compounds to treat poxviruses by the Food and Drug Administration remains elusive. Vaccinia immunoglobulin (VIG) is another therapy that is effective at neutralizing OPX infections and is typically used to treat adverse reactions to smallpox vaccination (see below). VIG is a polyclonal serum pool from vaccinia virus recipients that works effectively to neutralize virus in vivo and subsequently limit infection and halt adverse vaccine reactions. There are no data that currently support the use of VIG as a therapy for smallpox.

Vaccination against smallpox using the closely related live OPX vaccinia virus was used effectively to eradicate variola in the mid to late 20th century. Use of vaccinia virus was and continues to be considered prudent for protection of military and medical public health responder personnel against bioterrorism threats. Further discussion of vaccinia virus and variants is presented below.

Monkeypox Virus

Monkeypox was first recognized in primate colonies in the late 1950s to early 1960s as a disease resembling smallpox infections in humans. However, it was not until the 1970s that human disease associated with monkeypox was recognized (Fig. 2). During the eradication campaign against smallpox, human monkeypox was observed in central and western Africa. With the eradication of smallpox and with the emergence of monkeypox in central and western Africa, the World Health Organization conducted a surveillance program in the Democratic Republic of the Congo (DRC) from 1981 to 1986 that was aimed at determining the risk of

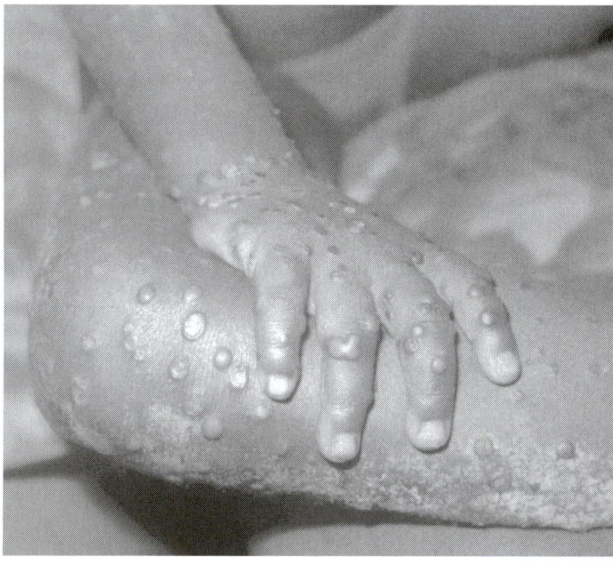

FIGURE 2 Close-up photograph of monkeypox lesions on the arm and leg of a 4-year-old female child in Liberia. (Source: CDC Public Health Image Library, 1971.)

monkeypox becoming a smallpox-like epidemic and its potential to pose a threat to the eradication program. Results indicated a high level of zoonotic infections, with a substantially lower human-to-human secondary attack rate (7.5%) than that of smallpox (60%). Ecological studies indicated an association with squirrels of the *Funisciurus* and *Heliosciurus* species. With a low secondary attack rate and primarily zoonotic transmission, the threat to the eradication of smallpox-like disease globally was considered remote. Few cases were reported until 1996, when suspected cases of monkeypox were reported from the DRC during a period of civil unrest (18). In addition to difficulties caused by civil unrest, cocirculation of chickenpox became a clinical presentation confounding to accurate diagnosis of monkeypox. Interest in monkeypox has remained high due to its clinical presentation being similar to that of smallpox, its genomic similarity to variola virus, and ongoing disease in central Africa since 1996. Awareness of the potential for monkeypox to emerge as a human disease outside of Africa occurred with the export of the virus, along with exotic animals intended for pet trade, to the United States in 2003. Importation of these African species included several suspected hosts/reservoirs of monkeypox and triggered an outbreak of monkeypox in six states in the Midwestern United States (15, 44). Outbreak investigations identified potential sources of the initial transmission from African species (Gambian rats and dormice) to native prairie dogs of North America. All subsequent human case-patients had contact with infected prairie dogs (Fig. 3). Monkeypox isolates from prairie dogs and humans were most closely related to a west African strain of monkeypox based on single-gene phylogenetics (29, 44). Differences in the severity of human disease were noted between the U.S. outbreak and a concurrent outbreak in the DRC (26). Genetic analysis of the U.S. isolate compared to a central African isolate (Zaire) reveals genomic differences (phylogenetic clades) which may hold the key to differences observed in clinical presentation, transmissibility, and virulence (29). Further analysis of strain differences may provide additional insight into the pathogenesis of monkeypox and identify targets for treatment or vaccines.

Treatment of monkeypox infection is similar to that of other OPX infections, including supportive medical care and antibiotic use to prevent secondary bacterial infection of lesion sites. Literature from the active surveillance efforts in the DRC in the 1980s demonstrated a protective benefit against disease acquisition and against disease severity (21). Prior vaccinia virus vaccination does not always prevent infection, and prevention may be related to the temporal interval since vaccination or to other unidentified host factors. During the U.S. outbreak in 2003, many confirmed case-patients were recipients of smallpox vaccine during childhood.

Vaccinia Virus

The origins of vaccinia virus remain obscure. Edward Jenner's vaccine evolved through a complex series of experiments to propagate the vaccine for use in faraway lands. Techniques used have been implicated in the development of a novel OPX with characteristics differing from those of other related viruses, such as cowpox and variola virus. Although vaccinia virus has been shown to be able to infect a wide variety of animal species, the natural reservoir and origin for vaccinia (as we know it) remains a mystery (1).

The eradication of smallpox was achieved by vaccination with vaccinia virus using intradermal inoculation resulting in a localized infection, or "take" (Fig. 4). The virus causes a

Inoculation Lesions

Disseminated Lesions

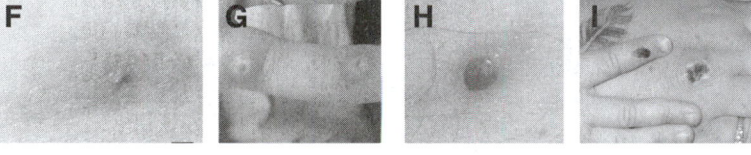

FIGURE 3 Monkeypox lesions from the 2003 U.S. outbreak, showing primary inoculation reactions (A, B, and C), examples of smallpox-like (D) and umbilicated varicella-like (E) disseminated monkeypox lesions, and morphologic appearance of disseminated lesions over time (F, G, H, and I). Panel A shows a primary inoculation reaction at the site of a prairie dog bite, panel B shows a prairie dog scratch, and panel C shows a preexisting cat scratch. Panel F shows a disseminated lesion less than 24 h after its appearance, panel G shows lesions after 6 days, panel H shows a lesion after 96 h, and panel I shows a lesion after more than 9 days. (Reproduced from reference 44 with permission.)

vesicular-pustular lesion followed by scab formation. A successful take is considered an indication of protective vaccination. However, vaccination is not without risk. Clinical disease or adverse outcomes may result from vaccination. Persons with immunosuppression or skin conditions such as eczema are at higher risk of adverse events from vaccinia virus exposure. Eczema vaccinatum, severe skin dissemination of vaccinia virus, may result from vaccination of persons with eczema or of contacts of vaccine recipients who have eczema. Progressive vaccinia, or vaccinia necrosum, may also occur in vaccine recipients. This potentially fatal illness is characterized by progressive necrosis in the area of vaccination, often with metastatic lesions. In the past, it was estimated that progressive vaccinia occurred in approximately 1 to 2 per million primary vaccinations, and it was almost always fatal before the introduction of VIG and antiviral agents. Nearly all instances have been in people with defined cell-mediated immune defects (T-cell deficiency). Progressive vaccinia was considered rare during the eradication campaign, but with concern over wide use of immunosuppressive drugs

and a larger immunocompromised population, rates may increase in today's population. Treatment of infection with vaccinia virus includes supportive care and may include antibiotics for control of secondary bacterial infections. Steroid use is contraindicated since immunosuppression and viral growth may ensue. Laboratory workers are susceptible to infection, and vaccination is recommended but not required in all facilities. Adverse events associated with vaccinia may be treated with VIG.

Cowpox Virus

Cowpox is endemic in parts of Europe and Asia, and disease associated with this zoonotic virus is typically associated with agricultural exposure. Despite its name, cowpox is not enzootic in cattle. With a host range from rodents to domestic cats, the reservoir for this virus is thought to include both European rodent species and domestic cats. Zoonotic disease has been observed in a variety of captive species in European zoos, such as cheetahs, lions, anteaters, rhinoceroses, elephants, and okapis, with transmission on occasion to animal

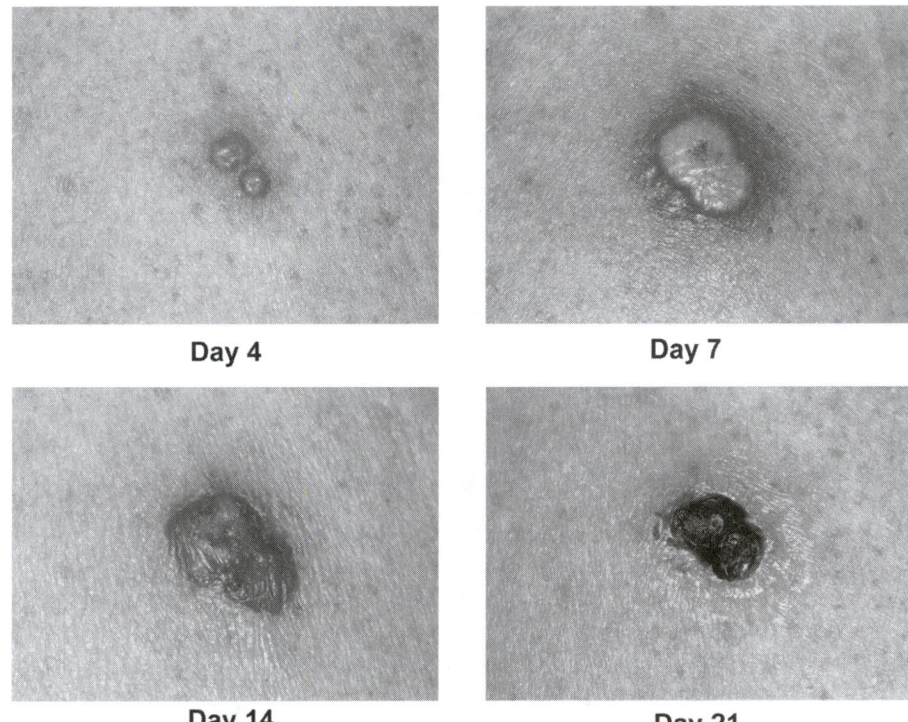

Day 4

Day 7

Day 14

Day 21

FIGURE 4 Major (primary) reaction—expected vaccine site reaction and progression following primary smallpox vaccination or revaccination after a prolonged period between vaccinations. Vaccinia virus vaccination results in a take under normal circumstances. A take is used as a measure of vaccine efficacy. The inoculation site becomes pustular around day 4 and then vesicular by day 7 and begins to scab around day 14. (Source: CDC [http://www.cdc.gov].)

handlers (2, 3, 41). Disease in humans is typically limited to the fingers following direct contact with infected animals, particularly cats. Redness and swelling occur, followed by papule and vesicular development in 4 to 5 days. Lesions are commonly painful, with erythema and edema at the vesicle and pustular stages. Resolution of lesions occurs from 2 to 4 weeks, with illness taking 6 to 8 weeks for complete recovery. Scarring is usually permanent. At greater risk are those with immunocompromised conditions.

Person-to-person transmission has not been reported, suggesting low infectivity for humans. Control of this disease is mainly through careful handling of infected animals and care of lesions once they appear. Management is supportive, with antibiotics to control secondary infections. Acyclovir has no activity against poxviruses. Steroids are contraindicated.

GENUS *PARAPOXVIRUS*

Parapoxviruses are structurally distinct from other *Chordopoxvirinae* and commonly cause agricultural disease of sheep, goats, and cattle that may be transmitted by direct contact to humans. Parapoxvirus commonly causes pustular skin and oral (mouth) lesions in sheep and goats that upon direct contact can be transmitted to humans and that are most often referred to as "contagious pustular dermatitis" or "orf." In cattle, the parapoxvirus-caused diseases most likely to be encountered by humans are pseudocowpox or paravaccinia (in dairy cattle, which causes milker's nodule in humans) or bovine papular stomatitis in calves and beef cattle. In humans, milker's nodule occurs as a reddened hemispheric

papule that matures to a purplish, smooth, firm nodule varying up to 2 cm in diameter; the lesions usually are not painful and can persist for about 6 weeks. Disease in livestock can have high morbidity, causing severe oral lesions and subsequent weight loss. In humans, lesions are typically limited to the fingers, hands, and arms and occur through direct contact with infected animals and transmission to existing cuts or scratches. Self-limiting illness follows, with local inflammation and the potential for secondary infections of open lesions. Lymphadenopathy and malaise are uncommon. Clinical presentation may cause difficulties if severe or prolonged lesions are observed. Large granulomatous or papillomatous lesions may be misdiagnosed as malignancies and result in inappropriate treatment, such as amputation (22).

Virions within the lesions are usually detectable by electron microscopic (EM) analysis, providing rapid and efficient diagnosis. The virus can be grown in cell culture, but this is not routinely done due to poor growth in transformed cell lines. Some molecular techniques are available, but widespread use is not yet apparent.

Interestingly, prior exposure is not thought to confer protection from subsequent exposure. Theories for reinfection with orf include heterologous but related viruses that do not provide cross-protective immunity or distinct ability to evade host immunity. The immune response to naturally occurring infection in humans has been studied, and a short-lived cell-mediated response and humoral response have been noted (53, 54). Treatment for orf infections is limited to control to prevent spread of the virus to other humans or animals. A vaccine is available for sheep but is fully virulent and can cause human infections. Use of vaccine is recommended annually to prevent outbreaks in livestock and more frequently for control in affected areas.

GENUS *MOLLUSCIPOXVIRUS*

Molluscipoxvirus is a distinct genus within the *Chordopoxvirinae* that contains only one known virus, molluscum contagiosum virus (Table 1). Molluscum contagiosum virus, like variola virus, is specific for humans. Infection causes a benign skin rash illness and has no known systemic phase. In children, the rash is distributed on the face, trunk, and limbs and is transmitted by direct contact. In adults, the lesions are found in the lower abdominal and pubic region, genitalia, and inner thighs and are transmitted through sexual contact. The appearance of the rash is typically sufficient for clinical diagnosis. Virions can be observed by EM using slide preparations of lesion material. Lack of inflammation and failure to isolate virus by cell culture or other means is a hallmark of molluscum contagiosum.

Infection with molluscum contagiosum virus is benign and self-limiting. Treatment may be implemented for cosmetic reasons to ease scarring, particularly from facial lesions. Treatments have included the use of chemicals such as phenolic compounds, silver nitrate, and trichloroacetic and glacial acetic acids. Curettage and cryotherapy also have been used as a physical intervention. Trauma may induce viral clearance, presumably due to the release of immune factors that provide higher antiviral immunity.

Prevention is based on personal hygiene and improvements in living conditions. The suggestion that molluscum may contribute to or be a marker for more serious conditions has been made (40). No vaccine is available.

GENUS *YATAPOXVIRUS*

Tanapox

Tanapoxvirus was first recognized in humans in 1957 in the River Tana region of Kenya. Particular interest occurred during the smallpox eradication campaign, and descriptions of human cases were documented in Zaire (DRC) in the 1980s (10, 20). Infection occurs on the skin, with epidermal hyperplasia and little dermal involvement. A prodromal illness of fever and malaise may occur but is short in duration. Macular lesion development progresses to a nodular (raised) stage that becomes umbilicated. Lesions are large (~10 mm) and typically become ulcerated. Erythema, edema, and lymphadenopathy are commonly associated with infection. Most cases present with only one lesion, and distribution may occur anywhere on the body, with the head usually being spared.

Illnesses associated with tanapox have been reported outside of Africa, and travel to or from regions of endemicity should be considered in diagnosis of rash illness with clinical presentation consistent with yatapox (9). The virus is restricted to Africa and particularly Kenya and the DRC. Simian species are the likely reservoir, and human-to-human transmission does not occur naturally. Transmission from primates to humans is thought to occur due to overcrowding during natural disasters, such as flooding, and civil unrest. Treatment is limited to supportive care, and vaccination is not available.

YMTV

YMTV has occurred in human primate-animal handlers (46). YMTV produces epidermal histiocytomas, tumor-like masses of histiocytic polygonal mononuclear cell infiltrates that advance to suppurative inflammatory sites. Only rare, anecdotal reports of human disease exist.

DIAGNOSTICS

Introduction to Laboratory Diagnosis

The basis for diagnosis of any poxviruses can be attributed historically to smallpox. Clinical presentation of smallpox was distinctive and usually sufficient for diagnostic recognition in order to implement public health control measures. However, in the presence of other rash illnesses, such as chickenpox and syphilis, to name a few, the diagnosis based purely on clinical presentation was often confusing. The oldest laboratory tests for poxviruses relied on visual inspection of lesion samples by light microscopy for the presence of poxviruses. More recently, EM has been utilized for the detection of poxviruses in lesion or cultured material. EM is rapid and efficient and may discriminate at the genus level for the parapoxviruses (8). Serological tests in use since the mid-1900s detect poxvirus antibodies, although discrimination among species within a genus using serology has remained difficult. Testing for serum antibodies or viral antigen has provided evidence of poxvirus exposure and has been used as a surveillance tool for the past half century. However, definitive molecular and immunology laboratory diagnostic capabilities arose only in conjunction with the eradication of smallpox in 1978. For the past several decades, poxvirus diagnosis was primarily related to vaccinia virus research as a vaccine vector and public health studies using serology and PCR testing during monkeypox outbreaks in central Africa, or isolated occurrences of cowpox, vaccinia virus-like infections, or other anecdotal poxvirus infections. Recent advances, driven by concerns of bioterrorism and a renewed vaccination campaign, have greatly improved diagnostic capabilities for a variety of poxviruses.

Physical Features of the *Poxviridae*

Poxviruses are among the largest viruses known and are brick shaped or ovoid, with an outer membrane surrounding a core that contains the double-stranded DNA genome. The genome contains 200 to 300 kb, with a G+C content of approximately 35% in OPX and yatapox virus and around 60% in parapoxviruses and molluscum virus. The size of viruses ranges from around 170 to 200 nm by 200 to 300 nm for OPXs, molluscum virus, and yatapox virus, while parapox virus is more ovoid, at 140 to 170 nm by 220 to 310 nm. The discrimination of parapoxviruses from other poxviruses is possible using EM, due to the subtle differences in physical appearance which are reviewed below.

VIRUS ISOLATION AND IDENTIFICATION

OPXs typically result in rash skin lesions that contain high levels of viral particles. During clinical disease, specimens such as rash exudates, crusts or scrapings, and vesicular fluids are suitable for growth and isolation in cell culture. Currently at the Centers for Disease Control and Prevention (CDC), identification of cytopathic effect in cell culture is followed by passage in cell culture and confirmation of viral species by PCR. Isolates are then anonymized and stored for development of diagnostic reagents, such as DNA for molecular testing and antigen for serological tests. Specimens of poxvirus rash lesions or viral cultures from such lesions are suitable for diagnosis by EM (Fig. 5). EM analysis provides

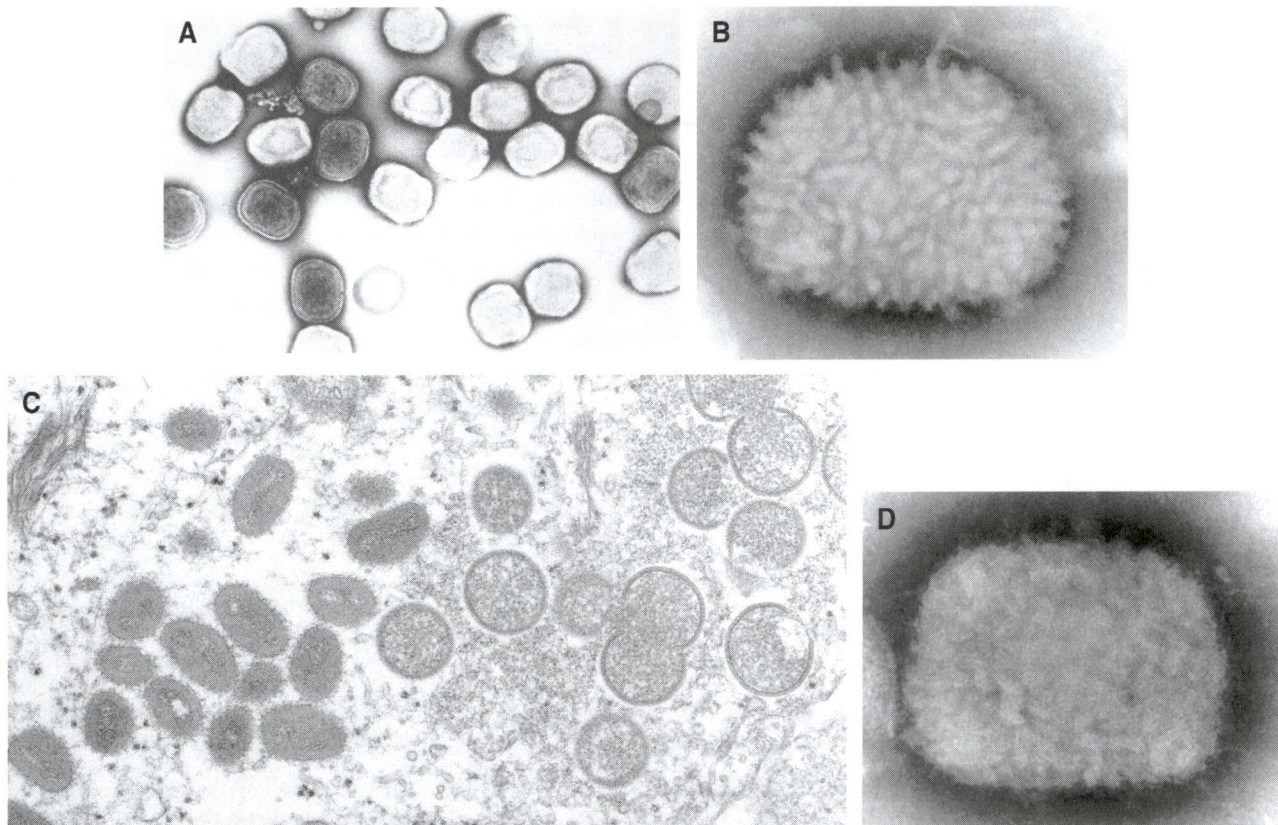

FIGURE 5 EM of vaccinia virus (A and B) and monkeypox virus (C and D) from clinical lesions collected during the 2003 U.S. outbreak. Bar equals 100 nm. (Source: CDC [vaccinia, Cynthia Goldsmith and Yasou Ichihashi; monkeypox, Cynthia Goldsmith and Christopher D. Paddock].)

the most rapid and characteristically clear distinction of poxviruses over other exanthems. Despite its utility, EM cannot distinguish between viruses within the genus OPX with any reliability. This genus includes most of the viruses of highest risk to human public health, such as variola, vaccinia, monkeypox, and cowpox viruses. Only members of the genus *Parapoxvirus* can be differentiated by EM; their distinctive morphology of a cross-hatched appearance (caused by tubule formations) and an ovoid shape (Fig. 6) allows discrimination from other poxviruses that are brick shaped

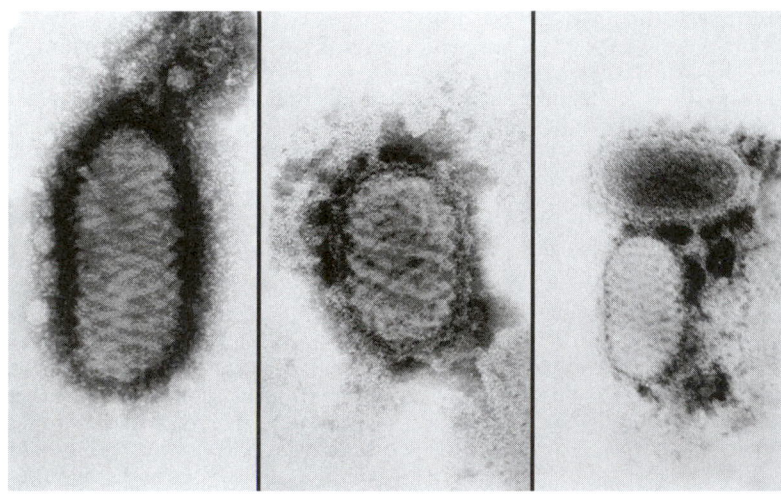

FIGURE 6 EM of parapoxvirus (orf) from a human lesion. Bar equals 100 nm. (Source: CDC [Cynthia Goldsmith and Fred A. Murphy].)

(Fig. 5). Differential diagnosis of rash illnesses associated with exanthematous viruses (e.g., varicella) other than *Poxviridae* is easily performed using EM. Tissues or rash-derived biopsy samples may also be subjected to immunohistochemistry for detection of OPX antigen.

Specimen Collection

For serological testing, serum or plasma is optimal with refrigeration of samples at a minimum and freezing of samples for storage longer than a few days prior to testing. Samples may be kept refrigerated for short periods while transporting or testing with sufficient results. For neutralization testing, heat inactivation of serum at 56°C for 20 to 30 min is recommended to avoid complement-mediated activity of the serum that may be independent of pure neutralizing capabilities.

Poxviruses will remain infective at ambient temperatures, particularly if kept dry. If specimens cannot be tested immediately, infectivity is retained during transportation at ambient temperatures by mail courier without the need for special transport medium. Vesicle fluid should be smeared on a slide and air dried. On receipt, the material can be reconstituted in buffer and used for EM, PCR, and viral isolation. Scrapings from molluscum and parapox lesions can be treated similarly. The infectivity of virus in dried crusts is retained for long periods. Virus may be extracted from such material by freeze-thawing and ultrasonic treatment. However, if the differential diagnosis includes pathogens less resistant than poxviruses, greater care should be taken and appropriate transport medium, etc., should be used.

Serology Introduction

Detection of humoral antibody responses by serology is an indirect approach to diagnosis and has been a hallmark for laboratory diagnosis of viral infections. In the absence of suitable viral samples for PCR, culture, or EM testing, serology may be the only method for diagnosing poxvirus infections. For this reason, serological tests have historically provided a standard for disease monitoring and surveillance. Characterization of the detection of humoral immune induction against smallpox provided a complement to the time line of disease progression as a measure of host response (4, 14). However, serological testing does not reliably or reproducibly provide information regarding the "type" or strain of OPX in question. This is the major limitation of serological tests to date. We review various serology methods and discuss recent advances that provide diagnostic capacity. Methods of antibody detection historically have included agar precipitation (Ouchterlony), immunofluorescence, complement fixation, hemagglutination inhibition (HI), plaque reduction neutralization testing (PRNT), and enzyme-linked immunosorbent assays (ELISAs). The most pragmatic serology tests are reviewed and include HI, PRNT, and ELISA, with methods described for PRNT and ELISA.

HI

HI exploits the fact that OPXs contain a hemagglutination protein that binds to avian or sheep red blood cells (RBCs), causing agglutination of the RBCs and forming a "shield" as compared to negative or inhibition (button or pellet) at the bottom of the well. Mixture of OPX antigen with patient serum prior to the addition of RBCs allows one to test for the presence of anti-OPX antibodies. Binding of specific antibody (if present) to the antigen prevents binding of the OPX antigen to the RBCs and subsequent agglutination of RBCs

in solution. HI has been used and is currently used for detection of virus-specific antibodies in studies for a number of viruses. For OPXs, HI has been successfully used for serological surveys of exposure to OPX, but it lacks specificity to differentiate between member species of these closely related viruses. Most often, chicken RBCs are used for agglutination, with approximately 50% of chickens having RBCs that can be agglutinated by vaccinia virus (37). HI antibody is detected 4 to 7 days after infection with OPXs. Testing of paired serum is vital to the diagnostic potential of HI tests. A rise or fall in titer is indicative of poxvirus infection. Since the advent of ELISA, the use of HI for OPX antibody detection has decreased.

PRNTs

PRNTs provide significant information regarding not only the presence of virus-specific antibodies but also their ability to neutralize viral particles in vitro. Neutralization of virus is considered to provide some evidence of a protective immune response due to prevention of viral infection of cell culture in vitro and passive transfer protection in animal models.

Virus particles form plaques in cell culture monolayers by adhering to and infecting cells and subsequently adjacent cells, forming a visible hole. The presence of anti-OPX antibodies in serum results in inhibition of plaque formation and thus plaque reduction that can be visually monitored and quantified (Fig. 7). It should be noted that a strong correlation is observed between ELISA reactivity and virus neutralization in studies of smallpox vaccination efficacy. Despite being labor-intensive and difficult to validate and transfer, the PRNT remains a vital laboratory test for determination of smallpox vaccine efficacy.

Recently, several novel neutralization tests have been developed that reduce labor and increase sensitivity and reproducibility by utilizing fluorescence or enzymatic colorimetric signals as a readout for the presence of virus. These assays may provide standardization of serum neutralization as a method for testing vaccine efficacy (11, 31). Use of gene expression as a readout prevents the need to count plaques and provides a format with potential for performing high-throughput testing in 96- or 384-well plates. The methods for performing these tests are described elsewhere and are not included here (11, 31). A traditional neutralization protocol is described below.

PRNT Method

Serum samples to be tested for neutralization should be heat inactivated to prevent complement-mediated activity of antibody. Serial twofold dilutions of test samples are prepared and incubated with an equal volume of vaccinia virus at a concentration of 100 PFU/ml and incubated at 35°C with 6% CO_2 for 3 h, with gentle rocking or vortexing every 15 min. Six-well titer plates are prepared to have confluent monolayers of adherent cells. For each well of the six-well plates, 1 ml of serum and antibody mixture is added. For every sample, duplicate wells should be used. Plates are incubated for 1 h, with rocking every 15 min, at 37°C with 6% CO_2. The inoculum is then removed from each well, 2 ml of fresh medium (2% protein) is added to each well, and plates are incubated at 35°C with 6% CO_2 for 2 days. After incubation, 1 ml of crystal violet stain solution (0.2% crystal violet, 4.5% formaldehyde, and 7.5% ethanol in phosphate-buffered saline [PBS]) is added to each well for 20 min at room temperature. Plates are then rinsed with water and allowed to air dry. Plaques are then counted and test serum

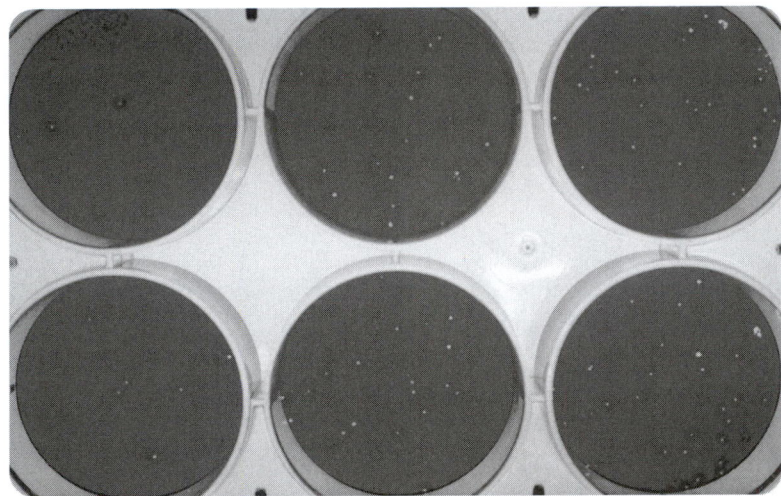

FIGURE 7 PRNT using control sera positive for plaque reduction. Sera were tested at 20-, 40-, and 80-fold dilutions. Plaque counts are the lowest in the 20-fold dilution wells (far left) and increase with higher dilutions. (Source: CDC [Poxvirus Program, Kevin L. Karem].)

wells are compared to virus-only control wells to determine the percentage of plaque reduction. Significant plaque reduction is typically considered to be equal to or greater than 50%.

ELISA

Three types of ELISA are routinely run at the CDC and represent some advances in the assays as well as analysis of the efficacy of the assays to perform during an OPX outbreak (19, 23, 47). All are indirect ELISAs and detect anti-OPX antibodies by an indirect conjugate reaction or by detection using enzyme-linked secondary antibodies against human immunoglobulin or non-species-specific immunoglobulin.

In the absence of viral samples for PCR or culture testing, active infection is difficult to determine and diagnosis is limited except for the use of serology. Efficacy of diagnosis by serology relies heavily on the collection of paired or multiple serum collections from an individual to compare the levels of antibody over time. A rise or fall in antibody levels is indicative of viral infection. More recently, the development of an OPX-specific immunoglobulin M (IgM) ELISA allowed the detection of recent exposure (or vaccination) against OPX by exploiting the biology of IgM production as a marker for acute-phase immune responses. During the monkeypox outbreak of 2003, IgM ELISA provided diagnostic support for evaluation of OPX infection, and evidence of the time line of infection correlated to illness onset. During this investigation, IgM ELISA provided 92% sensitivity in detection of cases confirmed by PCR (23). Together with epidemiology and clinical history, the IgM test may provide support of diagnosis of OPX infection even in the absence of material sufficient for viral isolation or detection (culture, EM, or PCR).

ELISA Methods

IgG ELISA. For the IgG ELISA, microtiter plates (Immulon II) are coated with 100 μl of vaccinia virus (purified vaccinia virus; Wyeth, Madison, N.J.) at 1.2×10^5 PFU/well in carbonate buffer overnight at 4°C. Plates are then blocked for 30 min at room temperature with assay diluent (PBS plus 0.05% Tween 20 [PBST], 5% skim milk, 2% bovine serum albumin, and 2% goat serum) followed by washing three times with PBST. Test samples are then added at dilutions of 1:100 for serum and incubated for 1 h at 37°C. Plates are washed and goat anti-human IgG-horseradish peroxidase conjugate (Kirkegaard & Perry [KPL], Gaithersburg, Md.) is added at a 1:2,000 dilution for 1 h at 37°C. Plates are washed, tetramethyl benzidine (TMB) one-component substrate is added, and development is allowed to proceed for 5 to 15 min. Plate reactions are stopped by addition of stop solution (KPL) and read at 450 nm on an optical density reader (Molecular Devices Corporation, Sunnyvale, Calif.). Values reported represent the average of duplicate wells of each sample. Known positive and negative sera from smallpox vaccine recipients are used as assay controls. On each day that assays are performed, cutoff values for ELISA are determined based on the mean plus 3 standard deviations of five negative control sera.

IgM ELISA. For the IgM ELISA, microtiter plates (Immulon II) are coated with 100 μl of a 1:800 dilution of goat anti-human IgM (KPL) diluted in PBS (pH 7.4) and incubated for 1 h at 37°C. Plates are then washed five times with PBST (PBS plus 0.1% Tween 20) and blocked for 30 min at room temperature with assay diluent solution (PBST, 0.5% gelatin, 2% bovine serum albumin, 5% skim milk, and 2% normal goat serum). Plates are washed and patient serum samples are added at a 1:50 dilution in assay diluent. Patient samples are incubated on the plates for 1 h at 37°C, followed by washing. Antigen (purified vaccinia virus; Wyeth) is then added at a concentration of 6.15×10^5 PFU/well (in diluent), and the plates are incubated for 1 h at 37°C. Plates are washed, and anti-OPX antiserum (concentration to be determined) is added for 1 h at 37°C. Plates are washed and conjugate (KPL) is added at 37°C for 30 min. Plates are washed and TMB one-component substrate is added for 5 to 20 min of development (KPL). Reactions are stopped by addition of stop solution (KPL) and read at 450 nm on an optical density reader. Values reported represent the average of duplicate wells of each sample. Positive and negative control sera are used as assay controls.

Molecular (Nucleic Acid) Testing

With the increasing knowledge of pox viral genomic nucleic acid sequence information, a number of methods have been developed to discriminate viruses based on nucleic acid testing. Early methods involved restriction fragment length polymorphism (RFLP) comparison of whole genomes; the preferred methods today involve PCR methodologies, as well as "chip-based" hybridization detection methods.

Single-gene PCR, followed by RFLP analysis of the amplicon, permits species identification of OPX. A number of methods have been published (30, 32, 35, 45, 49). One PCR assay targets the gene for hemagglutinin (HA) because this locus is unique for the genus OPX. Other published PCR methods target the gene for the A-type inclusion body protein (34), and another targets the gene for the B cytokine response modifier (CrmB), one of several different tumor necrosis factor receptor homologs produced by OPXs (30). In these assays, PCR is done by using primers anticipated to amplify a segment of DNA that would be present in any OPX, the amplicon is digested with an appropriate restriction endonuclease, and gel electrophoresis separation of digest fragments is used to discriminate species by comparing the fragment profiles with reference virus RFLP profiles.

Other strategies are based on the amplification of a region of nucleic acid unique for a specific species or genus of poxvirus. Such strategies have been developed for parapoxvirus and tanapox virus identification (9, 50, 51). Nucleic acid sequencing of the amplicon, regardless of whether it is predicted to be specific for one species, and its comparison to sequence databases can also provide diagnostic confirmatory information (52). The use of a multiplex format (42, 43) approach also has been described for the detection of the OPX variola virus in specimens. Another multiplex OPX assay targets the essential DNA polymerase gene (9).

Real-time PCR strategies, which can provide quantitative and qualitative information, as well as chip-based diagnostic methods have been developed for the OPXs (24, 25, 39). Most recently, such assays have demonstrated utility in detection of monkeypox during the 2003 U.S. outbreak (24, 27, 28, 38). Such assays also have been developed to specifically detect variola virus as part of bioterrorism response efforts (39). Within the United States, member laboratories of the Laboratory Response Network (a consortium of state and federal microbiology laboratories) have the capacity to test for OPXs in specimens using real-time PCR methods. Additional capacity is contained within the World Health Organization Collaborating Center for Smallpox and other Poxviruses within the Poxvirus Program of the CDC in Atlanta, Ga.

As mentioned previously, detailed nucleic acid diagnostic detection methods of poxvirus identification have been published, in addition to a recent detailed review of molecular PCR methods (32). Some commonly used methods employed by the World Health Organization reference center at the CDC include single-gene OPX HA and A-type inclusion (ATI) amplification, followed by RFLP analysis for species identification. These methods work well for clinical specimens anticipated to have large quantities of viral material, as found in rash-derived specimens. More recently, methods using real-time PCR detection also have been used. These methods are more sensitive and were used for rapid analysis of specimens during the U.S. monkeypox outbreak (28, 39).

Detailed Single-Gene PCR RFLP Methods

Perhaps the best-described locus for PCR-based detection of OPX is the HA gene. Species-generic primer amplification using EACP1 and -2 or NACP1 and -2 primers allows a positive signal to detect an Old World (Eurasian) or New World (North American) OPX species, respectively (45). Subsequent restriction digestion of the HA PCR product with TaqI or RsaI allows species-specific identification. EACP1 and -2 are used to detect the Old World OPXs vaccinia, cowpox, monkeypox, and variola viruses as well as ectromelia, camelpox, and gerbilpox viruses (not known to infect humans), via amplification of an ~950-nucleotide (nt) fragment. The methods for amplification are detailed elsewhere (45), and recent optimizations are described briefly here.

Materials (PCR for HA)

Primers: EACP1 at 250 ng/µl (forward, ATG ACA CGA TTG CCA ATA C), EACP2 at 250 ng/µl (reverse, CTA GAC TTT GTT TTC TG)

Sample nucleic acid at 50 ng per reaction

Positive controls: 5-µl volume containing 100 ng of vaccinia, variola, or monkeypox virus DNA

Negative control: nontemplate control (5 µl of H_2O). Other negative controls could include a cell culture lysate or non-OPX DNA (e.g., varicella virus).

PCR tubes or plate with caps and a programmable thermocycler

Add master mix (buffer, deoxynucleoside triphosphates, primer, polymerase, and H_2O) to each tube or well. Add test sample or control to each well, bringing the final volume to 50 µl. Cap each tube or well and place on the thermocycler. Denature the reactions for 2 min at 92°C. Perform 10 cycles as follows: 92°C for 10 s, 55°C for 30 s, and 72°C for 30 s. Then perform 20 cycles as follows: 92°C for 10 s, 55°C for 30 s, and 72°C for 35 s. Continue elongation at 72°C for 2 min, followed by a hold at 4°C. The total time for the PCR is approximately 90 min. The PCR product can be visualized by agarose gel electrophoresis.

RFLP of HA PCR Product

If a PCR product is observed by agarose gel electrophoresis, then restriction enzyme digestion will permit species determination of the OPX based on product fragments. TaqI restriction enzyme is used to digest the PCR fragment, and the resulting fragments are analyzed by agarose gel electrophoresis. Digestion with TaqI yields fragments of 452, 295, 105, and 97 nt (vaccinia virus); 303, 289, 115, 96, and 91 nt (cowpox virus); 536 and 406 nt (variola virus); and 451, 220, 105, 91, and 75 nt (monkeypox virus). NACP1 and -2 primers are used to specifically detect the New World OPXs (45) raccoonpox, volepox, and skunkpox viruses, which are not documented to be human pathogens.

PCR for A-Type Inclusion Protein

Amplification of the A-type inclusion protein is another method used to differentiate OPXs. Primer pairs ATI-low-1 and ATI-up-1 are used to amplify 1,500- to 1,700-bp fragments from vaccinia, cowpox, variola, or monkeypox virus, and amplicon identity can be confirmed with BglII or XbaI RFLP.

Materials (PCR for HA)

Primers: ATI-up used at 250 ng/µl (forward, AAT ACA AGG AGG ATC T), ATI-up used at 250 ng/µl (reverse, (CTT AAC TTT TTC TTT CTC)

Sample nucleic acid at 50 ng per reaction

Positive controls: 5-μl volume containing 100 ng of vaccinia, variola, or monkeypox virus DNA

Negative control: nontemplate control (5 μl of H₂O). Other negative controls could include a cell culture lysate or non-OPX DNA (e.g., varicella virus).

PCR tubes or plate with caps and a programmable thermocycler

Add master mix (buffer, deoxynucleotide triphosphates, primer, polymerase, and H₂O) to each tube or well. Add test sample or control to each well, bringing the final volume to 50 μl. Cap each tube or well and place on the thermocycler. Denature the reactions for 2 min at 92°C. Perform 10 cycles as follows: 92°C for 10 s, 40°C for 30 s, and 72°C for 45 s. Then perform 15 cycles as follows: 92°C for 10 s, 40°C for 30 s, and 72°C for 50 s. Continue elongation at 72°C for 2 min, followed by a hold at 4°C. The total time for the PCR is approximately 90 min. The PCR product can be visualized by agarose gel electrophoresis.

RFLP of A-Type Inclusion PCR Product

If a PCR product is observed by agarose gel electrophoresis, then restriction enzyme digestion will permit species determination of the OPX based on product fragments. BglII restriction enzyme is used to digest the PCR fragment, and the resulting fragments are analyzed by agarose gel electrophoresis. Digestion with BglII yields six fragments of 470, 444, 291, 165, 154, and 72 bp for vaccinia virus; six fragments of 522, 466, 293, 165, 154, and 72 bp for cowpox virus; and six fragments of 475, 470, 180, 165, 154, and 64 bp for monkeypox virus.

An RFLP using XbaI enzyme can also be used. XbaI has also been used to discriminate vaccinia, monkeypox, variola, and cowpox virus DNA. After XbaI digestion, variola virus generates two fragments sized at 154 and 1,018 nt. Vaccinia, cowpox, and monkeypox viruses all yield five fragments after XbaI digestion. Monkeypox species can be classified into Zairian and non-Zairian isolates based on the restriction profile.

With advances in genomic sequencing and analysis, there is an increased recognition that one genetic locus may not sufficiently identify a poxvirus as a member of a particular species (6, 16, 33, 36, 52). The use of testing strategies which discriminate genus and species based on the characterization of multiple genetic loci, in concert with protein-based diagnostics, will enhance the ability to accurately identify poxviruses as members of a particular genus and species. Use of existing molecular and immune diagnostic testing has allowed detection and diagnosis of OPX infections related to vaccine adverse events as well as outbreaks of naturally occurring viruses, such as monkeypox. Continued efforts to incorporate laboratory research advances into diagnostic testing regimens are expected to facilitate more efficient and specific tests for species of viruses within the genus OPX.

REFERENCES

1. **Baxby, D.** 1981. *Jenner's Smallpox Vaccine: the Riddle of Vaccinia Virus and Its Origin.* Heinemann Educational Books, London, England.
2. **Baxby, D., and M. Bennett.** 1997. Poxvirus zoonoses. *J. Med. Microbiol.* **46:**17–20.
3. **Baxby, D., and M. Bennett.** 1997. Cowpox: a re-evaluation of the risks of human infection based on new epidemiological information. *Arch. Virol.* **13:**1–12.
4. **Breman, J. G., J. Bernadou, and J. H. Nakano.** 1977. Poxvirus in West Africa nonhuman primates: serological survey results. *Bull. W. H. O.* **55:**605–612.
5. **Breman, J. G., and D. A. Henderson.** 2002. Diagnosis and management of smallpox. *N. Engl. J. Med.* **346:**1300–1308.
6. **Damaso, C. R., J. J. Esposito, R. C. Condit, and N. Moussatche.** 2000. An emergent poxvirus from humans and cattle in Rio de Janeiro State: Cantagalo virus may derive from Brazilian smallpox vaccine. *Virology* **277:**439–449.
7. **Damon, I. K., and J. Esposito.** 2003. Poxviruses that infect humans, p. 1583–1591. *In* P. R. Murray, F. C. Tenover, E. J. Baron, et al. (ed.), *Manual of Clinical Microbiology,* 8th ed. ASM Press, Washington, D.C.
8. **Damon, I. K., P. Jahrling, and J. LeDuc.** 2004. Poxviruses, p. 491–507. *In* A. J. Zuckerman, J. E. Banatvala, J. R. Pattison, P. Griffiths, and B. Schoub (ed.), *Principles and Practice of Clinical Virology,* 5th ed. John Wiley, Chichester, England.
9. **Dhar, D., A. E. Werchniak, Y. Li, J. B. Brennick, C. S. Goldsmith, R. Kline, I. Damon, and S. N. Klaus.** 2004. Tanapox infection in a college student. *N. Engl. J. Med.* **350:**361–366.
10. **Downie, A. W., C. H. Taylor-Robinson, A. E. Caunt, G. S. Nelson, P. E. Manson-Bahr, and T. C. Matthews.** 1971. Tanapox: a new disease caused by a pox virus. *Br. Med. J.* **1:**363–368.
11. **Earl, P. L., J. L. Americo, and B. Moss.** 2003. Development and use of a vaccinia virus neutralization assay based on flow cytometric detection of green fluorescent protein. *J. Virol.* **77:**10684–10688.
12. **Esposito, J., and J. H. Nakano.** 1992. Human poxviruses, p. 643. *In* E. H. Lennette (ed.), *Laboratory Diagnosis of Viral Infections,* 2nd ed. Marcel Dekker, Inc., New York, N.Y.
13. **Esposito, J. J., and F. Fenner.** 2001. Poxviruses, p. 2885–2921. *In* D. M. Knipe and P. M. Howley (ed.), *Fields Virology,* 4th ed. Lippincott Williams and Wilkins, Philadelphia, Pa.
14. **Fenner, F., D. A. Henderson, I. Arita, Z. Jezek, and I. Ladnyi.** 1988. *Smallpox and Its Eradication.* World Health Organization, Geneva, Switzerland.
15. **Guarner, J., B. J. Johnson, C. D. Paddock, W. Shieh, C. S. Goldsmith, M. G. Reynolds, I. K. Damon, R. L. Regnery, S. R. Zaki, and the Veterinary Monkeypox Virus Working Group.** 2004. Monkeypox transmission and pathogenesis in prairie dogs. *Emerg. Infect. Dis.* **10:**426.
16. **Gubser, C., H. Hue, P. Kellam, and G. L. Smith.** 2004. Poxvirus genomics: a phylogenetic analysis. *J. Gen. Virol.* **85:**105–117.
17. **Hanrahan, J. A., M. Jakubowycz, B. R. Davis, I. Damon, L. Rotz, J. Seward, and J. Hughes.** 2003. A smallpox false alarm. *N. Engl. J. Med.* **348:**467–468.
18. **Hutin, Y. J., R. J. Williams, P. Malfait, R. Pebody, V. N. Loparev, S. L. Ropp, M. Rodriguez, J. C. Knight, F. K. Tshioko, A. S. Khan, M. V. Szczeniowski, and J. J. Esposito.** 2001. Outbreak of human monkeypox, Democratic Republic of Congo, 1996 to 1997. *Emerg. Infect. Dis.* **7:**434–438.
19. **Hutson, C. L., K. Lee, J. Abel, D. Carroll, J. Montgomery, V. Olson, Y. Li, W. Davidson, C. Hughes, M. Dillon, P. Spurlock, M. Reynolds, Z. Braden, K. Karem, I. Damon, and R. Regnery.** Unpublished data.
20. **Jezek, Z., I. Arita, M. Szczeniowski, K. M. Paluku, K. Ruti, and J. H. Nakano.** 1985. Human tanapox in Zaire: clinical and epidemiological observations on cases confirmed by laboratory studies. *Bull. W. H. O.* **63:**1027–1035.
21. **Jezek, Z., and F. Fenner.** 1988. Human monkeypox. *Monogr. Virol.* **17:**1–140.
22. **Johannesen, J. V., H. K. Krogh, I. Solberg, A. Dalen, H. van Wijngaarden, and B. Johansen.** 1975. Human orf. *J. Cutan. Pathol.* **2:**265–283.
23. **Karem, K. L., M. Reynolds, Z. Braden, G. Lou, N. Bernard, J. Patton, and I. K. Damon.** 2005.

Characterization of acute-phase humoral immunity to monkeypox: use of immunoglobulin M enzyme-linked immunosorbent assay for detection of monkeypox infection during the 2003 North American outbreak. *Clin. Diagn. Lab. Immunol.* **12:**867–872.

24. **Kulesh, D. A., B. M. Loveless, D. Norwood, J. Garrison, C. A. Whitehouse, C. Hartmann, E. Mucker, D. Miller, L. P. Wasieloski, Jr., J. Huggins, G. Huhn, L. L. Miser, C. Imig, M. Martinez, T. Larsen, C. A. Rossi, and G. V. Ludwig.** 2004. Monkeypox virus detection in rodents using real-time 3′-minor groove binder TaqMan assays on the Roche LightCycler. *Lab. Investig.* **84:**1200–1208.

25. **Lapa, S., M. Mikheev, S. Shcheklkunov, V. Mikhailovich, A. Sobolev, V. Blinov, I. Babkin, A. Guskov, E. Sokunova, A. Zasedatelev, L. Sandakhchiev, and A. Mirzabekov.** 2002. Species level identification of orthopoxvirus with an oligonucleotide microchip. *J. Clin. Microbiol.* **40:**753–757.

26. **Learned, L. A., M. G. Reynolds, D. W. Wassa, Y. Li, V. A. Olson, K. Karem, L. L. Stempora, Z. H. Braden, R. Kline, A. Likos, F. Libama, H. Moudzeo, J. D. Bolanda, P. Tarangonia, P. Boumandoki, P. Formenty, J. M. Harvey, and I. K. Damon.** 2005. Extended interhuman transmission of monkeypox in a hospital community in the Republic of the Congo, 2003. *Am. J. Trop. Med. Hyg.* **73:**428–434.

27. **Li, Y., V. A. Olson, T. Laue, M. T. Laker, I. V. Babkin, C. Drosten, S. N. Shchelkunov, M. Niedrig, I. K. Damon, and H. Meyer.** 2004. Real-time PCR system for detection of orthopoxviruses and simultaneous identification of smallpox virus. *J. Clin. Microbiol.* **42:**1940–1946.

28. **Li, Y., V. A. Olson, T. Laue, M. T. Laker, and I. K. Damon.** Unpublished data.

29. **Likos, A. M., S. A. Sammons, V. A. Olson, A. M. Frace, Y. Li, M. Olsen-Rasmussen, W. Davidson, R. Galloway, M. L. Khristoval, M. G. Reynolds, H. Zhao, D. S. Carroll, A. Curns, P. Formenty, J. J. Esposito, R. L. Regnery, and I. K. Damon.** 2005. A tale of two clades: monkeypox viruses. *J. Gen. Virol.* **86:**2261–2672.

30. **Loparev, V. N., R. F. Massung, J. J. Esposito, and H. Meyer.** 2001. Detection and differentiation of Old World orthopoxviruses: restriction fragment length polymorphism of the *crmB* gene region. *J. Clin. Microbiol.* **39:**94–100.

31. **Manischewitz, J., L. R. King, N. A. Bleckwenn, J. Shiloach, R. Taffs, M. Merchlinsky, N. Eller, M. G. Mikolajczyk, D. J. Clanton, T. Monath, R. A. Weltzin, D. E. Scott, and H. Golding.** 2003. Development of a novel vaccinia-neutralization assay based on reporter-gene expression. *J. Infect. Dis.* **188:**440–448.

32. **Meyer, H., I. K. Damon, and J. J. Esposito.** 2004. Orthopoxvirus diagnostics. *Methods Mol. Biol.* **269:**119–134.

33. **Meyer, H., H. Neubauer, and M. Pfeffer.** 2002. Amplification of variola virus-specific sequences in German cowpox isolates. *J. Vet. Med. B* **49:**17–19.

34. **Meyer, H., S. L. Ropp, and J. J. Esposito.** 1997. Gene for A-type inclusion body protein is useful for a polymerase chain reaction assay to differentiate orthopoxviruses. *J. Virol. Methods* **64:**217–221.

35. **Meyer, H., S. L. Ropp, and J. J. Esposito.** 1998. Poxviruses, p. 199–212. *In* J. R. Stephenson and L. Warnes (ed.), *Diagnostic Virology Protocols* (*Methods in Molecular Medicine*). Humana Press, Totowa, N.J.

36. **Meyer, H., A. Totmenin, E. Gavrilova, and S. Shchelkunov.** 2004. Variola and camelpox virus-specific sequences are part of a single large open reading frame identified in two German cowpox virus strains. *Virus Res.* **108:**39–43.

37. **Nakano, J. H.** 1979. Poxviruses, p. 257. *In* E. H. Lennette and N. J. Schmidt (ed.), *Diagnostic Procedures for Viral, Rickettsial and Chlamydial Infections*, 5th ed. American Public Health Association, Washington, D.C.

38. **Neubauer, H., U. Reischl, S. Ropp, J. J. Esposito, H. Wolf, and H. Meyer.** 1998. Specific detection of monkeypox virus by polymerase chain reaction. *J. Virol. Methods* **74:**201–207.

39. **Olson, V. A., T. Laue, M. T. Laker, I. V. Babkin, C. Drosten, S. N. Shchelkunov, M. Niedrig, I. K. Damon, and H. Meyer.** 2004. Real-time PCR system for detection of orthopoxviruses and simultaneous identification of smallpox virus. *J. Clin. Microbiol.* **42:**1940–1946.

40. **Oriel, J. D.** 1987. The increase in molluscum contagiosum. *Br. Med. J.* **294:**74.

41. **Pilaski, J., and A. Rösen-Wolff.** 1988. Poxvirus infection in zoo-kept mammals, p. 84–100. *In* G. Darai (ed.), *Virus Diseases in Laboratory and Captive Animals*. Martinus Nijhoff, Boston, Mass.

42. **Pulford, D., H. Meyer, G. Brightwell, I. Damon, R. Kline, and D. Ulaeto.** 2004. Amplification refractory mutation system PCR assays for the detection of variola and Orthopoxvirus. *J. Virol. Methods* **117:**81–90.

43. **Pulford, D. J., H. Meyer, and D. Ulaeto.** 2002. Orthologs of the vaccinia A13L and A36R virion membrane protein genes display diversity in species of the genus orthopoxvirus. *Arch. Virol.* **147:**995–1015.

44. **Reed, K. D., J. W. Melski, M. B. Graham, R. L. Regnery, M. J. Sotir, M. V. Wegner, J. J. Kazmierczak, E. J. Stratman, Y. Li, J. A. Fairley, G. R. Swain, V. A. Olson, E. K. Sargent, S. C. Kehl, M. A. Frace, R. Kline, S. L. Foldy, J. P. Davis, and I. K. Damon.** 2004. The detection of monkeypox in humans in the Western Hemisphere. *N. Engl. J. Med.* **350:**342–350.

45. **Ropp, S. L., Q. Jin, J. C. Knight, R. F. Massung, and J. J. Esposito.** 1995. PCR strategy for identification and differentiation of smallpox and other orthopoxviruses. *J. Clin. Microbiol.* **33:**2069–2076.

46. **Rouhandeh, H.** 1988. Yaba virus, p. 1–15. *In* G. Darai (ed.), *Virus Diseases in Laboratory and Captive Animals*. Martinus Nijhoff, Boston, Mass.

47. **Sejvar, J. J., Y. Chowdary, M. Schomogyi, J. Stevens, J. Patel, K. L. Karem, M. Fischer, M. Kuehnert, S. R. Zaki, C. D. Paddock, J. Guarner, W. Shieh, J. L. Patton, N. Bernard, Y. Li, V. A. Olson, R. L. Kline, V. N. Loparev, D. S. Schmid, B. Beard, R. L. Regnery, and I. K. Damon.** 2004. Human monkeypox infection: a family cluster in the Midwestern United States. *J. Infect. Dis.* **190:**1833–1840.

48. **Seward, J. F., K. Galil, I. Damon, S. A. Norton, L. Rotz, S. Schmid, R. Harpaz, J. Cono, M. Marin, S. Hutchins, S. S. Chaves, and M. M. McCauley.** 2004. Development and experience with an algorithm to evaluate suspected smallpox cases in the United States, 2002–2004. *Clin. Infect. Dis.* **39:**1477–1483.

49. **Stemmler, M., H. Neubauer, and H. Meyer.** 2001. Comparison of closely related orthopoxvirus isolates by random amplified polymorphic DNA and restriction fragment length polymorphism analysis. *J. Vet. Med. B* **48:**647.

50. **Stich, A., H. Meyer, B. Kohler, and K. Fleischer.** 2002. Tanapox: first report in a European traveller and identification by PCR. *Trans. R. Soc. Trop. Med. Hyg.* **96:**178–179.

51. **Torfason, E. G., and S. Gunadottir.** 2002. Polymerase chain reaction for the laboratory diagnosis of orf virus infections. *J. Clin. Virol.* **24:**79–84.

52. **Trindade, G. S., G. da Fonseca Flavio, J. T. Marques, S. Diniz, J. A. Leite, S. De Bodt, Y. Van der Peer, C. A. Bonjardim, P. C. Ferreira, and E. G. Kroon.** 2004. Belo Horizonte virus: a vaccinia-like virus lacking the A-type inclusion body gene isolated from infected mice. *J. Gen. Virol.* **85:**2015–2021.

53. **Yirrell, D. L., and J. P. Vestey.** 1994. Human orf infections. *J. Eur. Acad. Dermatol. Venereol.* **3:**451–459.

54. **Yirrell, D. L., J. P. Vestey, and M. Norval.** 1994. Immune responses of patients to orf virus infection. *Br. J. Dermatol.* **130:**438–443.

Prion Diagnostics

STEPHEN DEALLER

92

INTRODUCTION

Transmissible spongiform encephalopathies (TSEs) (3, 5, 10) are a group of pathological animal conditions in which an infectious agent gives rise, after logarithmic growth in the brain, to cerebral damage but to little sign of inflammation. No antibodies are produced to the agent in the body, and TSEs were not realized to be infective until around the middle of the last century. Transmission experiments showed that they had extremely long incubation periods, often 20% of the normal life expectancy of the animal, that the infectious agent was similar in size to a virus, and that it could be filtered out using 100-nm-pore-size filters. The rapid expansion in research due to the epidemic rise of bovine spongiform encephalopathy (BSE) in the United Kingdom has widened the understanding of these TSEs, and the importance that they may have for other conditions that may be infective in similar ways (e.g., Alzheimer's disease and Parkinson's disease) has become clear.

It is now widely accepted that the infectious agent is largely proteinaceous and that the increase in infectivity during the incubation period is due to the alteration of a normal protein found in the body, the prion protein labeled PrP^c, to an abnormal (disease-associated) form called PrP^d that is not destroyed adequately by body enzymes, and that this abnormal form will cause the further alteration of PrP^c to PrP^d and build up within tissues. There is still argument as to the mode of infectivity of the agent, but it can be stated that PrP^c is required for infection to take place and that without it further infectivity is not found.

The protein infectious form is called the prion, which is resistant to irradiation, UV light, a wide range of enzymes (including powerful peptidases), antiseptic chemicals, heat, and antiviral agents. PrP^c is found throughout the animal kingdom. It has a series of well-preserved segments and two heparin binding sites, and it has retained a section normally associated with Cu^{2+} ions. It is hydrophobic in nature and tends to form into crystalloids within the tissues in which it is present. The natural forms of prion disease are shown in Table 1. Various forms and strains of prion disease are seen for different species; these vary by incubation period, brain and peripheral tissue distribution, chemical glycoform nature of the PrP^d that is produced, and different ranges of further species (usually about 50%) that may be infected by the strain experimentally.

The prion is derived from the normal (PrP^c) form of the protein, which is found throughout the body except on red cells, but to a much greater degree on various leukocytes, and brain cells. As such it may infect the body not only through the brain but also through peripheral tissues, which themselves become infectious. However, because of cellular turnover, the quantity of prions present in these tissues remains low and it is only in the brain where late in the disease PrP^d builds up to such a degree that stimulation is seen of microglia and their release of cytokine peptides along with other inflammatory intermediates. These processes result in progressive neurocytic apoptosis, leading to death of the animal.

Diagnostics for TSEs have become important following the realization that several of them may infect humans (or should be assumed to do so) and that, because of modern agricultural and medicinal techniques, large numbers of people may be put at risk (see below). Also, prophylactic agents and progress in potential methods of treatment for Creutzfeldt-Jakob disease (CJD) patients suggest that diagnostics may be necessary to permit the therapeutics to be used early in a symptomatic phase.

BSE, Variant CJD (v-CJD), and Blood Transfusion (3): the Worries that Made Rapid and Effective Diagnostics Worthwhile (2)

BSE was first diagnosed in 1987 and was quickly realized to be rapidly rising in the United Kingdom's bovine population. Epidemiology showed that the condition was spread through the feeding of infective material made from the carcass of one infected bovine to another, and this practice was stopped in the United Kingdom in 1988. Unfortunately, as cattle die generally at around 3 to 6 years due to BSE but are commonly slaughtered much earlier, most of the infected animals were eaten presymptomatically. Ultimately, it was possible to say that over a million infected cattle were present in the United Kingdom, probably at a peak around 1991, that the peak of animals dying of BSE was in 1993, that over 95% of cattle in the United Kingdom were from infected herds by 1995, and that in that country everyone had eaten, on average, approximately 50 meals made from the tissues of infected cattle by 1996. The recurrent denial by the United Kingdom's Ministry of Agriculture Fisheries and Food (MAFF) that there was any risk to humans because BSE was simply scrapie in cattle (and hence would have the same infective range among other

TABLE 1 Natural forms of prion disease

Natural TSE	Natural host(s)	Incubation period	Age of infection	World distribution
Scrapie	Sheep and goats	2 yr	<6 mo	Widespread except in Australia and New Zealand
Sporadic CJD	Humans	? >30 yr	Unknown. Familial forms seen in less than 50%.	Worldwide
GSS	Humans	30–50 yr	Familial condition	Worldwide
FFI	Humans	40 yr	Familial condition	Worldwide
Kuru	Humans	6–>40 yr	Neonate to adult	Papua New Guinea
v-CJD	Humans	?5–?40 yr	Unclear, possibly teenage or younger	United Kingdom, France, Canada, United States
BSE	Bovines (+ other animals fed BSE in error)	3–10 yr	<7 mo	United Kingdom and countries importing cattle from the United Kingdom
CWD	Deer and elk	?2–10 yr	Various points in life	United States, Canada
TME	Mink	<2 yr	<6 mo	United States, Russia, Finland

species) during this period was followed by evidence that BSE infected cats (considered immune to scrapie) and monkeys but not hamsters (common research tool for scrapie infection). The government of the United Kingdom also decided not to fund research into the field adequately; it said that if it did fund aspects including diagnostic or treatment research, then the people in that country would question the MAFF's statement that BSE was of no risk to humans and stop eating beef. However, in 1990, under pressure from the scientific society, the MAFF banned the availability in food of a progressive range of central nervous system (CNS) and lymphoid tissues that were expected to carry the highest titer of infectivity. Also, all cattle with symptoms of BSE automatically became the property of the MAFF, and therefore no tissues were available for research to any group outside the control of the government of the United Kingdom.

The incubation period of a TSE is considered to be much longer when TSE is passed from one species to another; when the dose is low or given orally, as may have been the case in BSE in human food, it was thought to be longer. Also, the incubation period rises in proportion to the normal life expectancy of the recipient animal. BSE was considered to have infected the cattle shortly after birth (within the first 7 months), and the peak incidence was at 5 years of age. Bovines have a natural life expectancy of 20 to 30 years, and humans have one of 70 years, i.e., between two and four times longer. Hence, if it was passed from other humans we might expect a human incubation period of 10 to 20 years, but because it was passed from cattle at a low dose and by mouth, this was expected to be between 20 and 40 years. As such, a peak of clinical disease in humans transferred from cattle was calculated to be 2010 to 2030.

In March 1996, v-CJD was reported for young people in the United Kingdom and was realized to be BSE in humans. The disease could be passed back to animals to produce the same tissue distribution of prion infection as seen when BSE was inoculated into them with the same type of glycosylation (see below) in the prion proteins that were extracted from humans, and from the animals with BSE; this was not true for any known form of CJD.

The initial cases of v-CJD were worrying in that it was not at all clear how the first case could appear so early without representing the beginning of a very large epidemic in the United Kingdom. It was this factor and the realization that BSE must have been exported by the United Kingdom

to countries all around the world that caused major research progress and political action. As of this writing, only 146 cases of v-CJD have been reported in the United Kingdom, the case numbers are no longer rising, and all but one are of a single PrP genotype. The reason for this is unclear. Unfortunately, there have been now two cases of v-CJD derived from blood transfusion, one of which was of a different, more common PrP genotype, and it is realized that a further epidemic of v-CJD in that genotype must be expected as a result of oral transmission of BSE.

It is because of these factors that diagnostic techniques in cattle to remove asymptomatic BSE-infected bovines from the human diet were required urgently, human diagnostic techniques were needed in that v-CJD did not have classical electroencephalogram (EEG) changes or its initial clinical symptoms, and blood testing systems were needed to avoid the transmission of v-CJD in blood and other medical practices.

CWD

Chronic wasting disease (CWD) (2, 19) was originally reported at Fort Collins, Colo., in captive mule deer in the late 1960s, but case numbers have expanded in deer and elk in the Rocky Mountains and are spreading both northward and eastward. This slow spread of what now appears to be an epidemic disease becoming endemic raises several problems in that there is no proof that the disease is not infectious to humans, and there is no clear mechanism of natural transmission. A widespread attempt has been made to monitor its growth by the testing of all slaughtered and fallen (i.e., found dead) deer and elk using a rapid testing method, and the eating of nervous tissue from these animals has been warned against by officials in specific states.

METHODS

A wide range of tests, international guidances, and local protocols are available that use basic methods (12, 14, 15, 23, 20).

Diagnostics for Prion Disease Using Transmission of the Condition to Other Animals

In the past, using transmission of prion disease to other animals was looked on as the only reliable method for diagnostics, and the minimum quantity of tissue that was found to transmit the disease to another animal of the same species by inoculation directly into the brain was said to contain

TABLE 2 Dose of infection required to transmit the disease when inoculated into various sites

Tissue into which inoculum is injected	Dose required for transmission (IU)
Brain	1
Blood	5–>10
Peritoneum	>400
Given orally	>10^4 (lower possibly in neonates)

1 infection unit (IU). The reason for this technique was that the transmission from one species to another was commonly found to require 10^4 times the quantity of tissue (the "species barrier"), and when inoculated into peripheral tissues a much larger amount might be needed; see Table 2.

When prions are inoculated into the brain a short incubation period is seen, and this still represents the most sensitive method for measuring prion infectivity. The method is unfortunately inaccurate, expensive, and ethically complex. In addition, simply because such small amounts (generally less than 3 mg) of tissue can be inoculated into mice, approximately 2 orders of magnitude of the sensitivity is lost, with a minimum of 300 IU per g required for infection to be transmitted.

Attempts were made to pass the species barrier and permit mice to be used to measure human tissue infectivity with CJD using the transgenic development of the human PrP gene in the mouse embryo. This process has proved inadequate, but progress is being made (13).

It should be noted that once a prion disease has been passed between species, the further transmission from the recipient animal to another of the same species is markedly more sensitive (i.e., the species barrier is lost or reduced). As a result, many scientific studies are carried out using human prions from CJD that have been transferred into mice. A problem with this method is that, having been transmitted between species, the range of further animals that the prion will infect changes, and the distribution of disease in the animal body also changes.

Tissue infectivity varies during the incubation period. Following peripheral inoculation of prions into the body, infectivity is found in peripheral tissues starting at a concentration that is dependent on the dose that was inoculated but dropping over a short period to a generally unmeasurable level. Following this, lymphoid tissue and reticuloendothelial tissues become infectious and rise relatively early in the incubation period to reach a plateau at a relatively low level compared with the final infectivity of brain tissue. After half the incubation period the infectivity is also found in the CNS, building up in a logarithmic manner until the death of the animal.

Quantification of infectivity in tissues may be carried out by comparing the incubation period in the animals into which a tissue inoculum has been passed with a standard range or by inoculation of a series of logarithmic dilutions of the tissue into the brains of animals, generally five for each dilution, of the same species. The cost of the large numbers of animals needed and the difficulty of carrying this out have meant that these methods are used only when disease quantity must be certain. Therefore, they are commonly used to confirm the sensitivity of other test systems.

EM

Several methods are claimed to show tubulofilamentous particles present in brain (22) that are specific to TSEs and start to appear in the tissues at around half the incubation period

of the disease. However, it now seems that they do not contain immunoreactive PrP (17) and hence probably show an early brain secondary pathological process. The buildup of PrP^d in the brain can be shown at a later point using immunogold electron microscopy (EM) staining of 65-nm sections etched in sodium periodate for 60 min, immunogold labeled to detect PrP using specific PrP monoclonal antibodies (see below), and with grids counterstained using uranyl acetate and lead citrate (11).

Scrapie-associated fibrils (SAF) can be demonstrated in brain tissue diagnosed by histopathology. This tissue is homogenized and pretreated or not with proteinase inhibitors or with dimethyl sulfoxide acting as a precipitant. SAF also can be extracted efficiently by adding a 10% solution of Sarkosyl to the homogenate and can be enriched by differential centrifugation and buffer extraction. Following centrifugation, this material can be stored at 4 or −70°C before EM is performed at a later date (9, 28; WHO Infection Control Guidelines for Transmissible Spongiform Encephalopathies, 1999 [http://www.who.int/emc-documents/tse/docs/whocdscsraph 2003.pdf]). The SAF appear under EM as long, thin, crystalloid structures that can be stained using an immunogold anti-PrP technique and are copurified with infectivity. The original hypothesis that SAF are actually the infective particles is now considered unlikely but rather that they represent the coagulation of hydrophobic PrP^d.

Histopathological Methods

Standard staining methods can be used for the demonstration of specific histopathological changes (8) in the brain, e.g., hematoxylin and eosin stains. However, tissue can be decontaminated in 96% formic acid for 1 h prior to processing in paraffin wax. A problem with this technique is that, as with BSE, where approximately 15% of cases were misdiagnosed, the spongiform changes appear late in the incubation period; although this is unlikely to be a problem with humans dying of CJD, it cannot be reliable with slaughtered animals that are killed when symptoms start. Also, the development of Congo red-stained amyloid as PrP plaques is seen in only 10% of the cases, particularly in the cerebellum in CJD, and occurs late in disease. Many samples of the brain must be taken to be sure that spongiform changes are not present, as some parts of the brain may have no changes. In CJD, spongiform change is relatively reliable in various layers of the cerebral cortex; fine vacuole-like holes appear in the neuropil as vacuoles 20 to 200 μm in diameter but become confluent at times to create larger ones, substantially distorting the cytoarchitecture. Similar vacuoles in the cytoplasm of larger cortical neurons may be seen. Cortical involvement is usually accompanied by spongiform change in the cerebellar cortex and basal ganglia. Microvacuolar change may be seen in the cerebellum. In clinical cases involving patients who die after long periods of symptomatic disease, neuronal loss may be severe and a status spongiosus appears where collapse of the cytoarchitecture appears in the cortex, leaving a distorted edge of gliotic tissues. The neurons also die in the basal ganglia, and there is a dramatic drop in granular and Purkinje cell populations. Gliosis involving astrocytes and microglia is present throughout areas associated with neuronal loss, and microglia also increase around PrP amyloid plaques. For further images and comparisons with other neurological pathology, see http://www.cjd.ed.ac.uk/path.htm; however, it should be remembered that there is a poor relationship between the course of disease and pathology distribution.

Immunostaining for PrP in brain and tonsils is of particular value in that an excess of PrP amyloid plaques would create a certain diagnosis. Ultrastructural and immunocytochemical studies of both human and animal prion diseases have demonstrated that microglial cells are intimately involved in PrP plaque formation and may play a role in the processing of PrP into an amyloid structure (8, 10). The appearance of PrP by immunostaining in the human tonsils or those of deer is also important in that PrP is found in early clinical cases of v-CJD and CWD (24), whereas this is not true with other forms of TSE. Third-eyelid tissue biopsy in CWD is an effective and relatively simple confirmatory test (3).

EEG Changes

A gradual loss of normal EEG patterns is seen in sporadic CJD, and in 60 to 80% of cases, generalized bi- or triphasic periodic sharp wave complexes appear with a frequency of around one or two per second. With clinical signs similar to those of sporadic CJD, this would be a useful confirmation of the diagnosis. Initially, EEG changes may be unilateral, as may periodic complexes. Unfortunately, this pattern is not universally found, and many other dementia-causing illnesses may show some similar signs. The point during the clinical progression of the disease at which this periodic pattern is found may vary and indeed may not be until very late; hence, weekly EEG tests may be needed, often an unrealistic requirement. This periodic pattern appears less frequently in genetic or human growth hormone-related CJD. It is not seen in v-CJD, which even in itself may be help to separate a case of sporadic CJD from v-CJD in an older patient.

MRI Scanning

It has been noted late in the clinical period of v-CJD that a reliable, symmetrical high-intensity signal is observable in the pulvinar by high-intensity MRI scanning (4). This is not seen in other forms of human disease, although magnetic resonance imaging (MRI) sequences, only as diffusion-weighted images of the cortex, showed unequivocal pathology in CJD, and clear atrophy was only seen late in disease with a long clinical period.

Rapid Specific Diagnostic Techniques (28, 29)

Brain Samples

It was realized that cattle incubating BSE were still reaching human food supplies in Europe and that the prions would not be destroyed by cooking processes. Consequently, several technical methods were developed that would indicate PrP^d in the brain of the slaughtered animal in a manner that would permit the carcass, kept overnight, to be destroyed the next day, when the result was ready, and not reach the human diet. Several companies are now selling assessed and licensed methods for testing tissue derived from the base of the brain and obtained as a sample through the foramen magnum. Homogenized samples of around 100 mg or less are resuspended and tested using enzyme-linked immunosorbent assay systems. The company tests involved have approximately the same sensitivity and specificity, but certain types might be considered of advantage in specific conditions; see Table 3.

At the time of this writing, no testing of bovine tissue in the United States has been requested, but this is required in Canada, Europe, and Japan. Also, the Organisation International Epizoites has made it clear that the United States has a high chance of developing BSE, and therefore testing systems should be considered. All of these methods have the same problem in that they cannot ensure that the animal being slaughtered is not infected with BSE but simply does not carry enough of the PrP^d in its brain to be indicated. The tests are expected to become positive probably some time between 50 and 75% of the clinical incubation period.

Confirmation is required for all carcasses that have a positive test for BSE. This is carried out by repetition of the first test (with another method if possible) and sending of samples to the government laboratory of the individual country. In the United States, confirmation is currently being carried out by the Animal and Plant Health Inspection Service (APHIS) in Iowa (http://www.aphis.usda.gov/oa/pubs/ pub_ahbse.html).

Confirmation by Western blotting is carried out using a proteinase K-treated sample of brain tissue suspended in buffer and electrophoresed. The blotting shows a series of bands generally between 27 and 30 kDa representing three forms of the PrP^d that carry both glycosyl chains, only one of them, or none. Full confirmation must be done by inoculation of the bovine tissues into another animal, but this is now rarely used.

Specific diagnostic methods for the testing of sheep and cattle have been decided and directed at an international level (e.g., Organisation International Epizoites Laboratory Manual [http://www.oie.int/eng/normes/mmanual/A_00064.htm and http://www.oie.int/eng/normes/mmanual/A_154.html]); methods that are commercially available for animal testing must be licensed by the Food and Drug Administration and specifically

TABLE 3 Comparison of licensed rapid brain tissue tests for PrP^d that are used commercially for the testing of asymptomatic cattle for BSE[a]

Company source of test	Speed of test	Complexity of test	Specificity	Cost	Experience in veterinary use
Enfer (Abbott, Abbott Park, Ill.)	Slow	Complex because of proteinase K step	++	Medium	Medium
Bio-Rad (Hercules, Calif.)	Slow	Complex because of proteinase K step	++	Relatively high because of equipment	Very high
Idexx (Westbrook, Maine)	Rapid	Simple because Seprion ligand used	++	Relatively low because complex equipment not needed	Medium (large amounts in CWD)
InPro (San Francisco, Calif.)	Slow	Complex	+++	Computerized equipment needed	Low
Prionics (Zurich, Switzerland)	Slow	Relatively simple because specific anti-PrP^d used	+++ because Western blot also available for confirmation	Relatively high because of antibody cost	High

[a]Data from references 20 and 29. Poor-comparison-related assessments have been carried out. All have high false-negative rates due to low levels of prions present in early stages of disease.

handled. Standard methods are also available from the European Commission in this respect. In the United States, currently the Department of Agriculture through APHIS is testing groups of cattle: nonambulatory cattle; cattle exhibiting signs of a CNS disorder; cattle exhibiting other signs that may be associated with BSE, such as emaciation or injury; and dead cattle. These groups of cattle are calculated to give a good indication as to the prevalence of BSE in the United States.

Blood Samples

No rapid technique is currently commercially available for detecting PrP^d in blood. However, several methods are currently well advanced in development. For further information on these, contact Microsens Biotechnology (London, United Kingdom; http://www.microsens.co.uk) or BioMerieux (http://www.biomerieux-usa.com).

Urine Samples

It was realized that a PrP^d form was in fact being excreted from much of the tissues of the body in some way because there was little local damage. The turnover of infected cells in the body and gut wall suggested that prions may be present in both urine and feces but in extremely small amounts. Complex testing systems have shown the presence of altered forms of PrP^d in the urine (28), and this result has been confirmed by other scientists but the systems are not available commercially.

Nonspecific Diagnostic Techniques (6, 7, 16, 18, 21, 25–27)

Late in the incubation period of prion disease, the pathological processes in the brain and elsewhere cause local release of cytokines and alterations in the relative quantities of proteins in the cerebrospinal fluid (CSF) and blood. The major problem for all of these tests is that the findings may also be found in other conditions that may cause symptoms similar to those of CJD. However, they may be of use in following the progress of the patient's illness, and potentially the value of treatment.

Also, because the tests in blood and the vasovagal response test are so easily carried out, they may be used to help in diagnosis in clinically ill patients. For test types, see Table 4.

Genetic PrP Changes Associated with Prion Disease and Glycoside Changes Found in Some Clinical Strains

In humans the prion protein with 253 amino acids is encoded on the short arm of chromosome 20 from its specific gene (PRNP), and small changes in amino acids of the PrP^c are seen between mammals. Small but specific changes are seen in familial forms of the disease, Gerstmann-Sträussler-Scheinker syndrome (GSS) and fatal familial insomnia (FFI). No changes are seen in the forms in which infection is considered to have taken place. However, the incubation period may be altered according to the structure (see the Weizmann Library [http://bioinfo.weizmann.ac.il/cards-bin/carddisp?PRNP]).

In humans there is a specific polymorphic mutation at codon 129 giving rise to either a valine or methionine at the peptide site and both a wide change in the incubation period and clinical symptoms of CJD results.

Glycosylation changes (1, 3) in the ratio of PrP^d carrying two, one, or zero glycosyl chains have been reported for different strains of CJD, v-CJD, transmissible mink encephalopathy (TME), and scrapie. If this is required for full diagnosis or investigation of epidemic outbreaks of disease, then CJD researchers (Gambetti et al.) should be contacted at Case Western University, Cleveland, Ohio. The importance of this glycoform research data is realized as a change in some sheep scrapie, which has now been suggested to be BSE transmission to sheep.

ANALYTICAL SENSITIVITY AND SPECIFIC DIFFICULTIES CURRENTLY ENCOUNTERED WITH PRION DIAGNOSTIC ASSAYS: QUALITY CONTROL

The growth of academic groups in the field of prion research has led to a tendency for each of them to be large enough to

TABLE 4 Nonspecific tests for TSE also used to follow disease progression[a]

Change reported[b]	Tissue source	Change seen	Availability of test
14-3-3 protein (6)	CSF	Increased in CJD but not all TSEs	Neuropathology, Case Western Reserve University, or CJD Surveillance Unit, Edinburgh, Scotland
GFAP, protein S-100B, NSE, MBP (6, 24)	CSF	GFAP is more available than the others by ELISA[c]; all of these proteins are associated with brain damage and gliosis.	Neurological research groups
FABP (7)	Blood and CSF	May be increased in TSE conditions; further research required	Research groups
PrP or IFN-γ, or LR or LRP (21)	Blood	Altered in clinical conditions of TSE as a range of changes	Research groups (Proteome Sciences)
EDRF (18)	Blood	Low in scrapie and possibly other TSEs	Not commercially available. Research at Roslin Institute, Edinburgh, Scotland.
R spectra for plasma (26)	Blood	Plasma from BSE asymptomatic cattle shown to have changes in IR spectra	Roche Inc. (the test is currently unavailable)
Vasovagal reflex (25)		Loss of heart rate changes with breathing during progression of TSE	Tsens Ltd.

[a]Data from references 20, 21 to 26, and WHO Infection Control Guidelines for Transmissible Spongiform Encephalitis, 1999 (http://www.who.int/emc-documents/tse/docs/whocdscsraph 2003. pdf).

[b]GFAP, glial fibrillary acidic protein; NSE, neuron-specific enolase; MBP, myelin basic protein; FABP, fatty acid binding protein; IFN-γ, gamma interferon; LR, laminin receptor; LRP, LR precursor; EDRF, erythroid differentiation-related factor; IR, infrared.

[c]ELISA, enzyme-linked immunosorbent assay.

declare that their own methods are adequate. As a result, the lack of standard testing systems has been a major problem for any new quantitative or qualitative assay system. Because of the rapid growth in BSE in Europe, there has been political pressure for specific tissues to be available from international standards laboratories, but complex difficulties have given rise to a severe shortfall for many tissue samples. It has become necessary for central laboratories that hold them to limit their distribution and to question the validity of testing procedures. Also, human tissues have been exceptionally difficult for research groups to gain access to because of ethics procedures that are enforced, and as a result postmortem tissues of known dilution may be all that are available.

Currently, the Veterinary Laboratories Agency (D. E. Bunce, TSE Office, New Haw, Addlestone, Surrey, United Kingdom KT15 3NB; phone, UK-1932-357875; e-mail address, d.e.bunce@vla.maff.gsi.gov.uk) is making an attempt to have available samples of BSE- and scrapie-infected tissue. For CJD, samples might be available from the National Institute of Biological Standards and Controls (20) (NIBSC, Blanche Lane, South Mimms, Potters Bar, United Kingdom); for reagents and samples, contact the TSE Resource Centre (Institute for Animal Health, Compton, Newbury, Berkshire, United Kingdom RG20 7NN; phone, UK-1635-577294; e-mail address, tse.rc@bbsrc.ac.uk; URL, http://www.iah. bbsrc.ac.uk/tse-rc). Currently in the United States, small tissue samples can be requested from the academic research groups at the National Institutes of Health (NIH) (P. Brown) and Wyoming State University (E. Williams).

Quality control for prion testing systems is exceptionally difficult in that standard reagents containing known amounts of infectivity require complex quantitative assays. Consequently, they are expensive and infectious and must be stored under specific conditions. Currently they are used mainly for research and for the assessment of rapid diagnostic techniques. The nonspecific systems either use reagents that are commonly available through standard suppliers (e.g., Sigma), or must use reagents that are not available easily, and hence the tests are carried out only in centralized laboratories where reliable comparisons between the results of separate patient samples can be carried out (e.g., 14-3-3 protein).

Precautions for Working with Potentially Prion-Infected Material

One of the major problems with TSE diagnostics is that certain procedures should be carried out using specific methods and precautions to prevent risk of infection to any staff or cross-contamination (e.g., WHO Infection Control Guidelines for Transmissible Spongiform Encephalopathies, 1999 [http://www.who.int/emc-documents/tse/docs/whocdscsraph2003.pdf], and the Advisory Committee on Dangerous Pathogens 2002 Transmissible Spongiform Encephalopathy Agents: Safe Working and the Prevention of Infection [http://www.advisorybodies.doh.gov.uk/acdp/tseguidance/index. htm]).

Some methods require specific biohazard containment facilities and the reliable and audited use of specific policies. However, methods involving bovine tissues and the rapid techniques are not currently required in the United States except in research laboratories.

Examples of precautions are shown in Table 5. Notably, the Centers for Disease Control and Prevention (CDC) and NIH would recommend some aspects of dealing with prion-infected tissue at biosafety level 2 and some at level 3. The CDC or NIH should be contacted before laboratory testing is developed. Currently in the United States cattle are not considered infected with BSE until a test is shown to be positive. However, samples being taken for testing from symptomatic cattle and sent to APHIS should be transferred as infectious material.

DISCUSSION AND INTERPRETATION

The development of many diagnostic systems and methods has meant that many groups have difficulty knowing which would be of most value for individual patients despite the appearance of national and international guidelines (10, 14, 20, 23). In animals, the tests that are performed depend to a large degree on official direction at the time (20, 23). An attempt is made in Table 6 to list the diagnostic actions that are considered useful with clinical syndromes that fit the pattern of the individual disease. Note that some methods described earlier cannot be used clinically and are only of value in research.

TABLE 5 Precautions for working with high- and low-infectivity tissues from patients with known or suspected TSEs[a]

1. Whenever possible and where available, specimens should be examined in a laboratory or center accustomed to handling high- and low-infectivity tissues; in particular, high-infectivity tissue specimens should be examined by experienced personnel in a TSE laboratory.
2. Samples should be labeled "Biohazard."
3. Single-use protective clothing is preferred as follows:
    Liquid-repellent gowns over plastic apron
    Gloves (cut-resistant gloves are preferred for brain cutting)
    Mask
    Visor or goggles
4. Use disposable equipment wherever possible.
5. All disposable instruments that have been in contact with high-infectivity tissues should be clearly identified and disposed of by incineration.
6. Use disposable nonpermeable material to prevent contamination of the work surface. This covering and all washings, waste material, and protective clothing should be destroyed and disposed of by incineration.
7. Fixatives and waste fluids must be decontaminated by a decontamination method described in another section of the WHO advisory document or adsorbed onto materials such as sawdust and disposed of by incineration as a hazardous material.
8. Laboratories handling large numbers of samples are advised to adopt more stringent measures because of the possibility of increased residual contamination, e.g., restricted-access laboratory facilities, the use of dedicated microtomes and processing labware, and decontamination of all wastes before transport out of the facility for incineration.

[a]Data from reference 20.

TABLE 6 Value of specific tests in the diagnosis of TSEs[a]

Clinical syndrome	EEG	MRI	Brain biopsy	Tonsillar biopsy	Genetic analysis	Rapid brain sample test	Nonspecific CSF test
Sporadic CJD	+	+	May be unhelpful	−	−	−	14-3-3 test only
Familial CJD, GSS, or FFI	+++ in FFI	+	−	−	++	−	−
v-CJD	++ no specific changes	Pulvinar sign	May be unhelpful	++	+	−	14-3-3 test negative
Kuru	+	+	+	−	−	−	−
TME	−	−	+	−	−	Only positive with some test methods	−
Scrapie	−	−	+	−	+ used to decrease scrapie in flock	Only positive with some test methods	−
CWD	−	−	Confirmatory tests needed if new area of United States affected	−	−	++	−
BSE	−	−	Western blotting and animal transfer experiments to confirm rapid-test positives in United States	−	−	Currently not required by U.S. government as screening of cattle for human food	−

[a]Data from references 1, 10, 20, and 23. EEG changes are not reliable, so false-negative results may be seen in sporadic CJD but positive results are useful in diagnosis. MRI tests in human disease must always be carried out to rule out other disease. Histopathological testing of postmortem human samples, including immunological staining, should be used to confirm the diagnosis. Histopathological testing of samples from BSE, scrapie, and CWD cases may produce false-negative results without further testing (e.g., Western blot for PrPd). Asymptomatic infected animals may have negative rapid screening tests. Genetic analysis of v-CJD and scrapie is useful only in that some genotypes are more likely to have the disease than others but cannot be diagnostic. Symptomatic kuru is largely clinically diagnostic, and the tests suggested here are used only when a possible case is seen outside Papua New Guinea. Nonspecific vasovagal tests should be considered if available but mainly to follow the progression of the disease. EM of brain biopsy material is helpful in diagnosis, but its availability is exceedingly limited. It must be realized that certainty in antemortem diagnosis is commonly difficult to achieve. +, may be of value; ++, useful for diagnosis; −, not considered worthwhile.

REMARKS AND CONCLUSIONS

The change over the past 15 years from TSE being the subject of research carried out in a few laboratories to its being a major international problem with testing and assessing taking place widely shows how agricultural practices may spread an illness widely and potentially create major risks. The crushing effect of this on specific industries and hospital practices has been widespread and has been at an immense cost (considered to be over $10 billion) to mainly the European population. However, it is now realized how similar TSEs are to Alzheimer's and Parkinson's diseases. Potential diagnostics, animal models, and treatment systems may be derived from the study of TSEs, so a clear benefit may be gained for these more common afflictions.

Currently over 20 million cattle are being tested annually for BSE in Europe, and blood transfusion risks may demand that a similar number of blood donations also be tested for the foreseeable future. The development of potential clinical treatment for CJD would make the testing of large numbers of older people useful, and the gradual growth in Alzheimer's disease as the demographics of the populations grow older would mean that any test for this would become valuable. As a result, we should expect progress from commercial and academic groups despite the extreme difficulty in diagnostics and treatment.

At the time of this writing, the U.S. Department of Agriculture has not permitted the widespread testing of asymptomatic cattle for BSE in the United States and does not have CDC laboratory guidance on it. However, it should not be surprising if animal and human testing in the United States does expand.

REFERENCES

1. **Atkinson, P. H.** 2004. Glycosylation of prion strains in transmissible spongiform encephalopathies. *Aust. Vet. J.* **82:**292–299.
2. **Belay, E. D., R. A. Maddox, E. S. Williams, M. W. Miller, P. Gambetti, and L. B. Schonberger.** 2004. Chronic wasting disease and potential transmission to humans. *Emerg. Infect. Dis.* **10:**977–984.
3. **Bender, S., J. Alverson, L. M. Herrmann, and K. I. O'Rourke.** 2004. Histamine as an aid to biopsy of third eyelid lymphoid tissue in sheep. *Vet. Rec.* **154:**662–663.
4. **Collie, D. A., D. M. Summers, R. J. Sellar, J. W. Ironside, S. Cooper, M. Zeidler, R. Knight, and R. G. Will.** 2003. Diagnosing variant Creutzfeldt-Jakob disease with the pulvinar sign: MR imaging findings in 86 neuropathologically confirmed cases. *Am. J. Neuroradiol.* **24:**1560–1569.
5. **Collins, S. J., V. A. Masters, and C. L. Lawson.** 2004. Transmissible spongiform encephalopathies. *Lancet* **363:**51–61.
6. **Green, A. J.** 2002. Use of 14-3-3 in the diagnosis of Creutzfeldt-Jakob disease. *Biochem. Soc. Trans.* **30:**382–386.
7. **Guillaume, E., C. Zimmermann, P. R. Burkhard, D. F. Hochstrasser, and J. C. Sanchez.** 2003. A potential cerebrospinal fluid and plasmatic marker for the diagnosis of Creutzfeldt-Jakob disease (FABP). *Proteomics* **3:**1495–1499.
8. **Head, M. W., D. Ritchie, N. Smith, V. McLoughlin, W. Nailon, S. Samad, S. Masson, M. Bishop, L. McCardle, and J. W. Ironside.** 2004. Peripheral tissue involvement in sporadic, iatrogenic, and variant Creutzfeldt-Jakob disease: an immunohistochemical, quantitative, and biochemical study. *Am. J. Pathol.* **164:**143–153.
9. **Hilmert, H., and H. Diringer.** 1984. A rapid and efficient method to enrich SAF-protein from scrapie brains of hamsters. *Biosci. Rep.* **4:**165–170.
10. **Ironside, J. W., and M. W. Head.** 2004. Neuropathology and molecular biology of variant Creutzfeldt-Jakob disease. *Curr. Top. Microbiol. Immunol.* **284:**133–159.
11. **Jeffrey, M., C. M. Goodsir, M. E. Bruce, P. A. McBride, and J. R. Fraser.** 1997. In vivo toxicity of prion protein in murine scrapie: ultrastructural and immunogold studies. *Neuropathol. Appl. Neurobiol.* **23:**93–101.
12. **Knight, R., M. Brazier, and S. J. Collins.** 2004. Human prion diseases: cause, clinical and diagnostic aspects. *Contrib. Microbiol.* **11:**72–97.
13. **Korth, C., K. Kaneko, D. Groth, N. Heye, G. Telling, J. Mastrianni, P. Parchi, P. Gambetti, R. Will, J. Ironside, C. Heinrich, P. Tremblay, S. J. DeArmond, and S. B. Prusiner.** 2003. Abbreviated incubation times for human prions in mice expressing a chimeric mouse-human prion protein transgene. *Proc. Natl. Acad. Sci. USA* **100:**4784–4789.
14. **Kovac, G. G., T. Voigtlander, E. Gelpi, and H. Budka.** 2004. Rationale for diagnosing human prion disease. *W. J. Biol. Psychiatry* **5:**83–91.
15. **Kubler, E., B. Oesch, and A. J. Raeber.** 2003. Diagnosis of prion diseases. *Br. Med. Bull.* **66:**267–279.
16. **Lamers, K. J., P. Vos, M. M. Verbeek, F. Rosmalen, W. J. van Geel, and B. G. van Engelen.** 2003. Protein S-100B, neuron-specific enolase (NSE), myelin basic protein (MBP) and glial fibrillary acidic protein (GFAP) in cerebrospinal fluid (CSF) and blood of neurological patients. *Brain Res. Bull.* **61:**261–264.
17. **Liberski, P. P., and M. Jeffrey.** 2000. Tubulovesicular structures: what are they really? *Microsc. Res. Tech.* **50:**46–57.
18. **Miele, G., J. Manson, and M. Clinton.** 2001. A novel erythroid-specific marker of transmissible spongiform encephalopathies. *Nat. Med.* **7:**361–364.
19. **Miller, M. W., and E. S. Williams.** 2004. Chronic wasting disease of cervids. *Curr. Top. Microbiol. Immunol.* **284:**193–214.
20. **Minor, P., J. Newham, N. Jones, C. Bergeron, L. Gregori, D. Asher, F. van Engelenburg, T. Stroebel, M. Vey, G. Barnard, M. Head, and the WHO Working Group on International Reference Materials for the Diagnosis and Study of Transmissible Spongiform Encephalopathies.** 2004. Standards for the assay of Creutzfeldt-Jakob disease specimens. *J. Gen. Virol.* **85:**1777–1784.
21. **Nagra, R. M., M. P. Heyes, and C. A. Wiley.** 1994. Viral load and its relationship to quinolinic acid, TNF alpha, and IL-6 levels in the CNS of retroviral infected mice. *Mol. Chem. Neuropathol.* **22:**143–160.
22. **Narang, H. K.** 1992. Scrapie-associated tubulofilamentous particles in human Creutzfeldt-Jakob disease. *Res. Virol.* **143:**387–395.
23. **O'Rourke, K. I., D. Zhuang, A. Lyda, G. Gomez, E. S. Williams, W. Tuo, and M. W. Miller.** 2003. Abundant PrP(CWD) in tonsil from mule deer with preclinical chronic wasting disease. *J. Vet. Diagn. Investig.* **15:**320–323.
24. **Petzold, A., G. Keir, A. J. Green, G. Giovannoni, and E. J. Thompson.** 2004. An ELISA for glial fibrillary acidic protein. *J. Immunol. Methods* **287:**169–177.
25. **Pomfrett, C. J., D. G. Glover, B. G. Bollen, and B. J. Pollard.** 2004. Perturbation of heart rate variability in cattle fed BSE-infected material. *Vet. Rec.* **154:**687–691.
26. **Schmitt, J., M. Beekes, A. Brauer, T. Udelhoven, P. Lasch, and D. Naumann.** 2002. Identification of scrapie infection from blood serum by Fourier transform infrared spectroscopy. *Anal. Chem.* **74:**3865–3868.
27. **Shaked, G. M., Y. Shaked, Z. Kariv-Inbal, M. Halimi, I. Avraham, and R. Gabizon.** 2001. A protease-resistant

prion protein isoform is present in urine of animals and humans affected with prion diseases. *J. Biol. Chem.* **276:**31479–31482.

28. **Stack, M. J., A. M. Aldrich, A. D. Kitching, and A. C. Scott.** 1995. Comparative study of electron microscopical techniques for the detection of scrapie-associated fibrils. *Res. Vet. Sci.* **59:**247–254.

29. **Wu, D., and C. P. Stowell.** 2003. Prion diseases: recent developments toward diagnostic tests. *Am. J. Clin. Pathol.* **120**(Suppl.)**:**S46–S52.

HUMAN IMMUNODEFICIENCY VIRUS

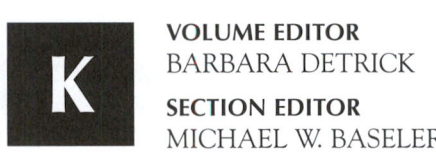

VOLUME EDITOR
BARBARA DETRICK
SECTION EDITOR
MICHAEL W. BASELER

Introduction

MICHAEL W. BASELER

93

No single disease has had such an impact on the diagnostic immunology laboratory as human immunodeficiency virus (HIV) infection and its sequelae. The laboratory evaluation of patients with HIV infection has evolved from basic flow cytometry to detailed molecular analysis of viral quasispecies and quantitation of tetramer-positive T cells. As the number of HIV infections worldwide continues to increase, the need for laboratory capabilities for the monitoring of these patients has increased as well. This need is even greater given recent advances in treatment strategies that will hopefully turn this disease into a chronic manageable illness. This section deals with the laboratory immunologic and virologic perspectives. In the chapter "Principles and Procedures of Human Immunodeficiency Virus Serodiagnosis," Dewar et al. review the current assay systems available for the serodiagnosis of HIV. These assay systems include standard enzyme-linked immunosorbent assays, the currently available rapid assay systems, and Western blot confirmatory analysis, as well as the recently Food and Drug Administration-approved home testing kits. This chapter also discusses point-of-care testing, which is critical in resource-poor settings such as developing nations, where more than 95% of all new infections are emerging.

In the chapter "General Immunologic Evaluation of Patients with Human Immunodeficiency Virus Infection," Stevens et al. discuss how to evaluate the cellular immune response in patients with HIV. Functional assays and the state of the art in immunophenotyping with flow cytometry are emphasized. Singe-platform immunophenotyping versus dual-platform immunophenotyping is also highlighted within this chapter. With the advent of better therapeutic interventions, the ability to monitor patients' immune systems over long periods becomes critical.

Along with the need to monitor cellular immune function in patients with HIV, it is equally critical to monitor viral load and drug resistance. Elbeik et al., in the chapter "Quantitation of Viremia and Determination of Drug Resistance in Patients with Human Immunodeficiency Virus Infection," outline the state-of-the-art procedures for monitoring viral load and drug resistance with time. The measurement of drug resistance is critical in managing patients with HIV in light of the multiple therapeutic modalities that are currently available.

For the more research-oriented laboratories, Hengel et al., in the chapter "Measurement of T-Cell-Specific Immunity in Patients with Human Immunodeficiency Virus Infection," discuss state-of-the-art research tools that are able to more specifically define the pathologic effects of HIV infection on T-cell-specific immunity. These advanced methods are very complementary to the more broadly characterizing methods described by Stevens et al.

The HIV epidemic has provided the standard clinical immunology laboratory with a unique opportunity and an important challenge. The close relationship between immunologic status, as determined by CD4 T-lymphocyte quantitation, and stage of disease has made immunologic monitoring an important part of the clinical management of HIV-infected patients. The combination of CD4 count and HIV RNA level provides the clinician with important information that has led to marked improvements in patient care. From determining a patient's relative risk of developing an opportunistic infection to monitoring immunologic responses to candidate vaccines, the clinical immunology lab plays a major role in the area of HIV.

Principles and Procedures of Human Immunodeficiency Virus Serodiagnosis

ROBIN DEWAR, HELENE HIGHBARGER, RICHARD DAVEY, AND JULIA METCALF

94

The first published reports of AIDS appeared in 1981, and the causative agent, human immunodeficiency virus type 1 (HIV-1), was identified in 1983 to 1984. Over the next two decades, HIV-1 infection and AIDS became one of the leading causes of illness and death worldwide. The Joint United Nations Program on HIV/AIDS (UNAIDS) reported in July 2004 that as of the end of 2003, an estimated 37.8 million people worldwide—35.7 million adults and 2.1 million children younger than 15 years—were living with HIV/AIDS. Approximately two-thirds of these people (25.0 million) live in sub-Saharan Africa; another 20% (7.4 million) live in Asia and the Pacific. More than 20 million people with HIV/AIDS have died since the first AIDS cases were identified in 1981 (41). In 2003 alone, HIV/AIDS-associated illnesses caused the deaths of approximately 2.9 million people worldwide, including an estimated 490,000 children younger than 15 years (41). In 2000, the Centers for Disease Control and Prevention (CDC) estimated that 850,000 to 950,000 U.S. residents are living with HIV infection, one-quarter of whom are unaware of their infection (16). As of the end of 2002, an estimated 385,000 people in the United States were living with AIDS and an estimated 500,000 people with AIDS in the United States had died (8). An estimated 4.8 million new HIV infections occurred worldwide during 2003, that is, about 14,000 infections each day. More than 95% of these new infections occurred in developing countries (41), while approximately 40,000 new HIV infections occur each year in the United States (7).

An important early impetus for the development and testing of serologic methods to detect HIV infection was the need to guarantee the safety of the blood supply. A quick review of the statistics above makes clear the need for the continued development of serologic methods, including point-of-care testing, that are useful especially in resource-poor settings.

ANTIBODY DETECTION ASSAYS

Screening Tests

The standard screening tests for HIV infection involve detection of HIV-specific antibodies. Early in 1985, routine testing of donated blood by a rapid solid-phase approach became available through the development, testing, and licensure of the first enzyme-linked immunosorbent assay (ELISA) kit. By 1987 a total of eight different commercial ELISAs had been licensed by the Food and Drug Administration (FDA), and the HIV-1 ELISA was rapidly established as a primary diagnostic screening tool (21). Test sites that were established nationwide in government-sponsored clinics to allow for confidential or anonymous testing of at-risk individuals were soon supplemented by wide-scale availability of these assays through other means, such as hospital-based or commercial laboratories. Since the first screening ELISAs and Western blot (immunoblot) assays came onto the market in 1985, technology has evolved to include novel assays based on a variety of immunologic principles (Table 1). The present-day assays have improved sensitivity and specificity, can better resolve indeterminate results, and help to identify infections in newborns. Some of these newer assays include augmented Western blot assays, class-specific antibody capture assays, particle agglutinations, substrate amplification procedures, tests that can differentiate antibody isotypes, rapid assays (requiring just minutes to perform), and tests that can simultaneously detect HIV-1 (including subtype O [for "other"]), HIV-2, human T-cell lymphotropic virus type 1 (HTLV-1), HTLV-2, and HIV antigen (44, 47).

Infection with HIV results in the induction of a humoral antibody response specific to viral proteins. Most exposed individuals will develop antibody against the virus within a few weeks to a few months after viral infection. There is only a single case report of a previously healthy individual who failed to produce antibodies following HIV infection. Wide-scale serologic testing of infected individuals has revealed that the major antigens against which antibodies are produced are also fairly consistent within the population, although the exact timing of appearance and the relative intensity of individual antibody responses may vary from person to person. The genome of HIV-1 is known to code for three structural polyproteins and seven regulatory proteins. The structural proteins of HIV-1 (Fig. 1) are the targets for the majority of the circulating antibodies directed against the virus and are as follows.

- Envelope (*env*) proteins: the surface glycoprotein (gp120), the transmembrane glycoprotein (gp41), and their precursor glycoprotein (gp160)
- Polymerase (*pol*) proteins: the reverse transcriptase (p66), the endonuclease-integrase (p31), and the protease (p10)
- Core (*gag*) proteins: the matrix protein (p18), the internal capsid protein (p24), the nucleocapsid protein (p7), and their precursor protein (p55)

TABLE 1 Commercial kits for HIV testing[a]

Assay	Commercial name	Company
Screening assays		
ELISA for HIV-1	HIVAB HIV-1 EIA	Abbott Laboratories
	HIV1 rLAV EIA	Genetic Systems (Bio-Rad)
	Vironostika HIV-1 Plus O Microelisa	bioMerieux
	HIVAB HIV-1 EIA	Abbott Laboratories
	HIV-1 Urine EIA	Calypte Biomedical
ELISA for HIV-1 and HIV-2	HIVAB HIV-1/HIV-2 (rDNA) EIA	Abbott Laboratories
	HIV1/HIV2 Plus O EIA	Bio-Rad Laboratories
	Abbott HIV-1/HIV-2 3rd Generation Plus	Abbott Laboratories
Rapid tests	OraQuick Rapid HIV-1 Antibody Test	OraSure Technologies, Inc.
	Determine HIV-1/2/O	Abbott Laboratories
	Reveal Rapid HIV-1 Antibody Test	MedMira Laboratories, Inc.
	Serodia HIV-1/2	Fujirebio
p24 antigen assay	HIV-1 p24 Antigen Assay	Coulter Corporation
	HIVAG-1 Monoclonal	Abbott Laboratories
	HIV-1 p24 Core Profile ELISA	DuPont
Combination assays	Enzymun-Test HIV Combi	Boehringer Mannheim
	VIDAS HIV DUO Plus	bioMerieux
	AxSYM HIV Ag-Ab Combo	Abbott Laboratories
Confirmatory assays		
Western blot assay	Bio-Rad New LAV Blot 1	Bio-Rad Laboratories
	HIV-1 Western Blot	Calypte/Cambridge Biotech
	OraSure HIV-1 Western Blot	OraSure Technologies, Inc.
	Bio-Rad Genetic Systems HIV-1	Bio-Rad Laboratories
	HIV-2 Western Blot	Genelabs Diagnostics
	HIV-1 Urine Western Blot	Calypte/Cambridge Biotech
IFA	Fluorognost HIV-1 IFA	Waldheim Pharmazeutika
	Virgo IFA	Pharmacia
Line immunoassay	RIBA HIV-1/HIV-2 SIA	Chiron Corporation
	INNO-LIA HIV Confirmation	Innogenetics

[a]Partial listing; see also references 4 and 11.

Within a few weeks (usually between 4 and 8 weeks, although a duration as short as 8 days has been described) after exposure to the virus, infected individuals may experience a brief period of constitutional illness (fever, fatigue, myalgia, rash, gastrointestinal complaints, and, rarely, neurological symptoms) that has been likened to a mononucleosis-like viral illness. This period lasts anywhere from a few days to a few weeks and has been shown to be accompanied by a burst of active viral replication in the host, as documented by high levels of circulating virus and viral p24 antigen in plasma. With subsidence of the acute symptomatology, increasing levels of virus-specific antibody begin to appear and can be quantified by a variety of serologic detection methods (Table 1). Antibodies against p24 and against the viral envelope proteins (gp160 and gp41 in particular) are among the first detectable HIV-1-specific immunoglobulins produced during this period of acute seroconversion (Fig. 2) (1). Of note, the ELISA appears to be especially sensitive to the early detection of anti-p24 antibody, whereas certain other tests, such as the radioimmunoprecipitation assay (RIPA), may show early reactivity due to antibody directed against the higher-molecular-weight antigens, such as gp160. The ELISA is the standard screening test for HIV-1 infection. Individuals with indeterminate or positive ELISA results should undergo confirmation testing (generally by Western blotting [immunoblotting]) to determine if the reactivity is primarily directed to HIV-1 infection or secondarily directed to cross-reacting antibodies (11, 15). A commonly accepted algorithm for the sequential application of the serologic tests in the evaluation of sera from patients with potential HIV exposure is shown in Fig. 3.

ELISAs

ELISAs and enzyme immunoassays for the detection of a serologic response to HIV-1 infection were developed in a series of stages. The first generation of enzyme immunoassays that were licensed as diagnostic kits and many of those still used today are based on the use of viral lysate antigens derived from viruses that are grown in human T-lymphocyte lines. The presence of traces of host cell components, in which the virions were propagated, in these lysates may lead to false-positive results. The basis for a majority of these assay kits is a solid-phase indirect-antibody detector system (use of microtiter plate wells is most common, although polystyrene or latex beads are used by some manufacturers). The relative amounts of each of the major structural and expressed proteins of HIV-1 may differ significantly between the various commercial preparations. Both the external envelope glycoprotein (i.e., gp120 and its precursor, gp160) and the Gag-derived products (p24 and p18 antigen in particular) are generally well represented in the bound material. Using known positive and negative samples, which are run with each test as controls, a standard curve for the colorimetric

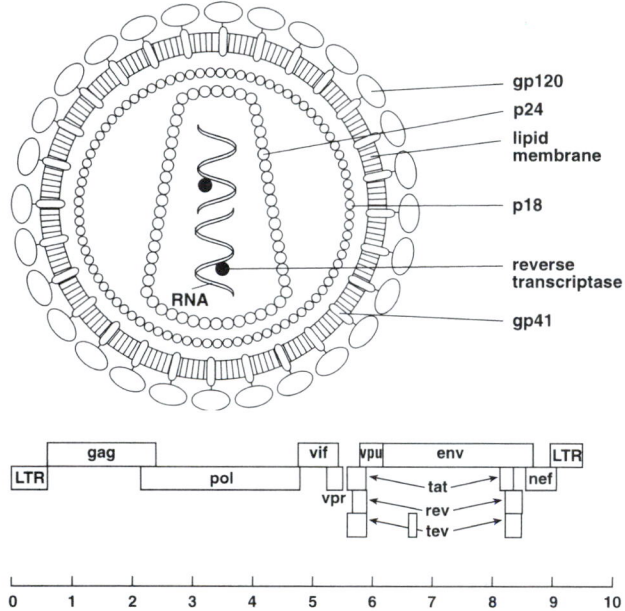

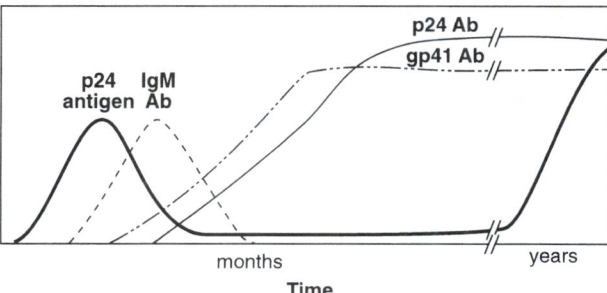

FIGURE 2 Hypothetical time course for the appearance of p24 antigen and HIV-1 antibodies (Ab) in serum during HIV-1 infection.

FIGURE 1 Diagrams of HIV-I virion structure (A) and the HIV-1 viral genome (B).

reaction is generated, and the optical density (OD) values of test samples are compared against this. A cutoff value for the lowest OD still regarded as consistent with a positive determination can be calculated on the basis of a statistical comparison of the intensity of a panel of positive control samples with that of a panel of negative sera. Whereas test sera with OD values well above the cutoff point are recorded as unequivocally positive, the scoring of samples with OD readings skirting the cutoff range can be more problematic. Sera with positive or indeterminate results should be further evaluated by a confirmatory test (Western blotting).

A significant advance in the efforts to optimize the sensitivity and specificity of existing solid-phase immunoassays came via the introduction of viral antigens produced through recombinant DNA technology and/or synthetic antigens to

supplement or replace the crude mixtures of proteins derived from lysates. Not only can the recombinant antigens be produced with considerably more purity and in larger amounts than proteins derived from viral lysates, but also they can be bound to solid-phase surfaces with much tighter control over protein ratios and concentrations. These second-generation assays, which were introduced in the late 1980s, combine both HIV-1- and HIV-2-specific antigens. Combination assays allow screening for multiple retroviral agents simultaneously. A potential drawback of such recombinant proteins is that they may afford a more limited repertoire of antigenic sites. This appeared to have clinical significance in the failure of several of the commercial preparations used in Europe and Africa to detect infection with the subtype O strain of HIV-1 (see below). Thus, despite the use of recombinant and synthetic antigens, some of these anti-HIV ELISAs may yield a relatively poor sensitivity and/or specificity when difficult serum samples are tested. The recombinant antigens may also differ somewhat from native proteins by virtue of altered patterns of glycosylation. Nonetheless, the avidity between these antigens and anti-HIV-1 antibodies still appears to be quite high. In addition to diagnostic utility in the screening of individuals and blood products, these newer-generation immunoassays have proven especially valuable in the research setting. Immunoassays enriched in external envelope antigen such as gp160, for

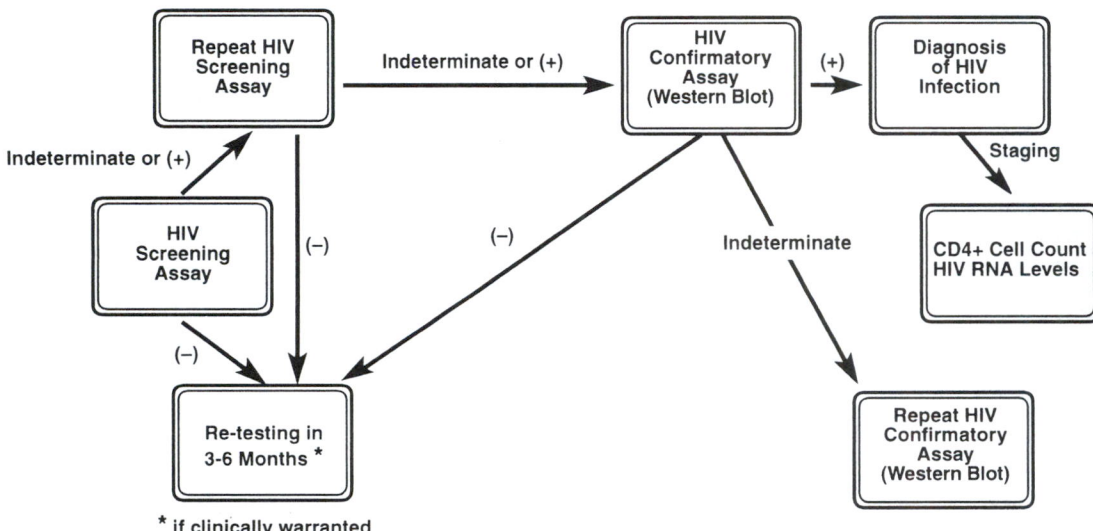

FIGURE 3 Algorithm for the correct use and sequence of serologic testing in the diagnosis of HIV infection.

example, are useful in the detection of anti-envelope antibody responses in individuals immunized with candidate anti-HIV-1 vaccines, particularly those employing either recombinant gp160 or gp120 protein as an immunogen. These assays have provided significantly enhanced sensitivity to early antibody responses over that afforded by a more conventional ELISA.

Most ELISA (see chapter 39) kits utilize enzyme-tagged anti-human immunoglobulin G (IgG) as the probe to detect the presence of bound HIV-1-specific antibody within a test well. Another refinement that may help to improve the sensitivity of existing immunoassays, leading to earlier detection of seroconversion, involves either the addition or the substitution of enzyme-labeled anti-human IgM for anti-human IgG at this stage of the assay. With some kits, care must be taken to minimize the use of heat-inactivated sera, as a higher rate of false positivity has been reported when sera are treated in this fashion prior to testing.

In the third-generation ELISA, specific recombinant antigens conjugated with enzyme are used to detect the antigen-antibody complex (antigen sandwich ELISA). Briefly, human serum or plasma is diluted in a specimen diluent and incubated with a polystyrene bead coated with recombinant HIV-1 *env* and *gag* and HIV-2 *env* proteins; specific antibody present in the sample reacts with the antigens on the coated bead. After removal of the unbound materials by washing of the bead, specific immunoglobulins bound to the solid phase are detected by incubating the bead-antigen antibody complex with a solution containing HIV-1 *env* and *gag* and HIV-2 *env* recombinant proteins labeled with horseradish peroxidase, which is then detected by incubation with *o*-phenylenediamine substrate solution. This format was developed to allow the simultaneous detection of IgG and IgM (which are present during the early stages of HIV infection) and even IgA antibodies to HIV-1 and HIV-2.

Interpretation of ELISA Results

As noted above, serum from an individual infected with HIV-1 should be positive by commercial HIV-1 ELISA within a few months of exposure. Because these assays are enriched both in Gag-derived proteins and envelope glycoproteins, antigens against which the humoral response in the host is characteristically brisk, the ELISA is usually quite sensitive for detection of early seroconversion. Given the uniformly high sensitivity of most commercial preparations, a negative ELISA reading at an appropriate interval following exposure strongly mitigates against the likelihood of infection in the majority of cases. In general, barring procedural errors in the performance of the assay, there is usually no reason to require that a screening ELISA with a negative result be immediately repeated under these circumstances. A common exception to this guideline is if the interval between testing and presumed exposure is unknown and there is the possibility that the original test was performed relatively early after a possible infection. In this situation, it may be advisable to repeat the test on a new sample within a few months of the initial assay.

Another circumstance under which repeat ELISA testing may be warranted is if the initial results showed borderline reactivity according to the internal OD standards generated within each test kit. OD readings falling slightly under (e.g., less than 1 standard deviation below) the cutoff value may simply reflect high background signals from true seronegative sera or, alternatively, could represent the initial stages of reactivity in serum from an individual undergoing incipient seroconversion. Since the immunoassay is not capable of

differentiating these two possibilities, all of the following have been used as a means of attempting to resolve this diagnostic uncertainty: repeating the test on a fresh specimen, repeating the test with the same sera but using a different commercial assay, and using a combination of these two approaches. In those situations where borderline reactivity persists despite repetitive testing, a minimal recommendation would be to repeat the ELISA within a few weeks. Failure of the OD value to rise substantially over time is suggestive that the low level of reactivity does not represent true infection. In this setting, it is prudent to perform a Western blot assay and a direct measurement of HIV RNA to help rule out an unusual serologic response to true infection.

Highly divergent strains of HIV-1 grouped provisionally as subtype O were isolated from certain patients from Cameroon and other regions of west-central Africa. Initial screening with several of the commercial ELISA kits commonly used in Europe and Africa failed to detect antibody reactivity in some of these patients (29, 36, 39). Those kits employing synthetic peptides or recombinant antigens were particularly prone to this defect. One of the nine tests, which was based on synthetic peptides, was insensitive against serum specimens from all nine infected persons, and four other tests were each unreactive against at least one of four different specimens (29). Assays based on whole-virus lysates performed better. While a retrospective study in the United States did not document any serum samples with peptide reactivity consistent with HIV-1 group O infection (33), manufacturers in the Unites States and abroad have revised their test kit antigens to enhance detection of antibodies against subtype O (3). Whether there might exist other, as-yet-uncharacterized strains of HIV-1 that could also fail to show reactivity on current commercial assays is not known.

Unlike the situation in parts of West Africa and India, documented cases of HIV-2 infection remain generally rare in the United States. The majority of cases identified to date have involved individuals who have imported the infection into this country from elsewhere, e.g., recent immigrants, U.S. servicemen and -women who were deployed overseas, or expatriates with exposure to endemic diseases (e.g., Peace Corps workers). Nonetheless, over the past 1 to 2 years, most major manufacturers of commercial ELISA kits have incorporated HIV-2 antigens in their preparations in order to enhance the sensitivity of these assays for both major types of HIV. It has now become the standard practice in blood banks to screen donated blood samples with one of the new HIV-1-HIV-2 combination ELISAs.

Cautionary Remarks

Since the ELISA was originally designed primarily as a screening assay, it was optimized to have a very high sensitivity and thus will give false-positive reactions. Because of the availability of backup or confirmatory assays to validate positive findings as well as the potentially serious consequences of undiagnosed infections, this reduction in the number of false negatives at the expense of a slightly higher rate of false positives is a reasonable trade-off. Thus, the ELISA, while an excellent test for screening, should not be used for making a diagnosis of HIV-1 infection without a positive confirmatory test. In large-scale testing of individuals with high-risk behavior for HIV-1 acquisition, most of the commercially marketed ELISA preparations have been shown to have a sensitivity of at least 99.5% and a specificity of more than 99.8%. However, the positive predictive value of the standard HIV-1 ELISA may fluctuate widely depending upon the population being screened. In an investigation to study the sensitivity and specificity of 13 current anti-HIV-1/HIV-2 enzyme immunoassays for the detection of anti-HIV antibodies in human serum or plasma, a panel of 454 well-characterized specimens was tested. Observed sensitivities ranged from 96.9 to 100%, and observed specificities ranged from 89.9 to 100% (30). The false-positivity rate in low-risk populations is substantially higher than that in high-risk populations, an observation that must be taken into account in the interpretation of preliminary test results. In a large study by the American Red Cross of a low-risk pool of volunteer blood donors, only 13% of those individuals with a repeatedly reactive HIV-1 ELISA were confirmed to be HIV-1 infected on the basis of a confirmatory Western blot (21). Such data have obvious implications for wide-scale screening of donated blood products, for which the majority of positive ELISA reactions may be expected to be false-positive readings. In contrast, the rate of false-negative results with conventional ELISAs remains quite low, with such results generally occurring no more often than once in every 40,000 samples (43). As continued refinements in solid-phase technology lead to development of even more sensitive probes, this rate should continue to drop further.

As with any assay capable of processing large numbers of test sera at any one time, ELISA methodology is subject to a number of technical drawbacks that may diminish the significance of any single positive result. These range from procedural errors in the handling of samples, such as mislabeling of specimens, to deficiencies in the manual or automated performance of sample processing, such as well-to-well carry-over during pipetting and resultant contamination of neighboring wells. A false-positive result can also be caused by inadequate washing of the specimen or incorrect dilution of the sample or of any one of the assay reagents. Usually such false-positive reactions are corrected either by repeating the assay or by testing with another manufacturer's ELISA kit. Apart from these purely technical considerations, the causes of false-positive ELISA results may be both varied and obscure. In some cases, however, certain common elements that may provide an explanation for these findings have been identified. Chief among these is the presence of cross-reactive antibodies against certain common human leukocyte antigens (HLA-DR and other class II antigens in particular) present in some patients' sera as a result of exposure to fetal leukocytes during pregnancy or by blood transfusion. These antibodies presumably recognize and bind to cellular contaminants that are present in the viral lysates used in these kits. The use of the CEM cell line to propagate virus in tissue culture has been reported to reduce or eliminate this particular cause of cross-reactivity. Newer test kits incorporate the use of recombinant or synthetic peptide antigens and offer improvements in test performance (47).

Other causes of false-positive ELISA readings that have been identified include the presence of autoreactive antibodies (e.g., antinuclear or antimitochondrial antibodies), heat inactivation of sera prior to testing, repetitive freeze-thaw cycles prior to assaying, severe hepatic disease, passive immunoglobulin administration (isolated cases of transient seroconversion have been reported for patients receiving passive IgG injections), recent exposure to certain vaccine preparations (e.g., influenza vaccine), renal transplantation, Stevens-Johnson syndrome, alcoholic hepatitis, history of multiple pregnancies, Epstein-Barr virus infections, and certain malignancies (12). The commercial ELISA cannot distinguish positive results due to antibody response to candidate HIV vaccines from those due to seroconversion as a result of HIV infection. Cross-reactivity of sera from patients with HIV-2 also occurs. In contrast, cross-reactivity in the HIV-1 ELISA generally does not occur with sera from patients with HTLV-1 infection. The causes of false-negative ELISA findings are also varied and, in addition to improper handling of reagents in individual test kits, include performance of the assay too early in the period after HIV-1 exposure (i.e., prior to seroconversion, the window period), immunosuppressive therapy, and replacement transfusion, as well as conditions that cause B-cell dysfunction and defective antibody synthesis, such as severe hypogammaglobulinemia. Powder from disposable gloves worn by technicians performing the test has been shown to absorb macromolecules such as immunoglobulins that could cause an otherwise positive sample to give a negative reaction (12).

Rapid Assays

The technical complexity and expense associated with some of the more conventional anti-HIV-1 antibody detection methods fostered a search for simplified, less costly methods of serologic screening, particularly those that could be more suitable for use under field conditions in developing nations or medically disadvantaged regions where HIV infection is endemic. These tests do not require any specialized instrumentation and are developed as a cost-effective alternative to conventional ELISA and Western blot tests. These newer tests may also offer some practical advantages in developed nations as well by providing results in a very short period, thus increasing the likelihood that patients will wait to receive their results. Some of these tests are extremely rapid (ranging from 2 to 10 min), easy to perform, stable at room temperature, and with sensitivities comparable to those of commercially available ELISAs (4, 5). Rapid and sensitive assays for HIV may also prove to be useful in organ donation centers, emergency departments, and physicians' offices. In general, tests that work on whole blood will also work on serum or plasma, but approval from the FDA requires medium-specific proof of efficacy.

SUDS HIV-1 Test

The SUDS HIV-1 test (Murex Inc., Norcross, Ga.), the first rapid test to obtain FDA approval, utilizes a microfiltration enzyme immunoassay procedure. The solid-phase capture reagent is a mixture of latex particles coated with HIV-1 p24 and gp41 synthetic peptides. The test device is a small plastic cartridge designed to filter, concentrate, and adsorb all liquid reagents added during the test, including the specimen. The test is performed at room temperature. Human serum or plasma is incubated in a sample cup with reaction diluent and the capture reagent. The mixture is transferred into the test cartridge, where the latex particles coated with antigens and any bound HIV-1 antibodies are trapped by a fiberglass filter. Following the addition of a wash reagent to remove unbound materials, an enzyme-labeled anti-human immunoglobulin is added to detect the presence of bound antibodies. Following a second incubation and washing, the substrate solution is added to develop the color reaction. A sample is considered reactive if any blue color is observed in the center circle in the bottom of the cartridge. A portion of the fiberglass filter that does not contain the capture reagent should remain white to indicate that the wash steps were performed correctly. The whole procedure takes approximately 10 min. This test is shown to have 99.9% sensitivity and 99.6% specificity. The requirement for reagent refrigeration, multiple procedural steps, and lack of an internal control make the SUDS test less well suited for point-of-care testing.

OraQuick Rapid HIV-1/2 Antibody Test

The OraQuick Rapid HIV-1/2 antibody test (OraSure Technologies, Inc., Bethlehem, Pa.) has FDA approval for the detection of antibodies to HIV-1 and HIV-2 in finger stick whole-blood and venipuncture samples. It is a qualitative immunoassay composed of a single-use test device and a single-use vial containing a premeasured amount of a buffered developer solution. The test utilizes a lateral-flow immunoassay procedure, and the plastic housing of the device holds an assay test strip that provides the matrix for the immunochromatography of the specimen and the platform for indication of the test result. The assay contains synthetic peptides representing the HIV envelope region and a goat anti-human IgG test assay control immobilized onto a nitrocellulose membrane in the test (T) zone and the control (C) zone, respectively. A finger stick whole-blood or venipuncture whole-blood specimen is collected and transferred to the vial of developer solution, followed by the insertion of the test device. The developer solution facilitates the flow of the specimen into the device and onto the test strip. As the diluted specimen flows through the device, it rehydrates the protein A colloidal gold colorimetric reagent contained in the device. As the specimen migrates up the strip, it encounters the T zone. A positive result is indicated by a reddish purple line in the T zone. The intensity of the line color is not directly proportional to the amount of antibody present in the specimen. Further up the assay strip, the sample encounters the C zone. This built-in procedural control validates that a specimen was added to the vial and that the fluid has migrated adequately through the test device. A reddish purplish line will appear in the C zone if the test was performed properly, regardless of the result in the T zone. The test must be interpreted at least 20 min but not more than 40 min after the test device was placed in the solution containing the specimen. This test is shown to have 99.6% sensitivity and 100% specificity.

Reveal Rapid HIV-1 Test

The Reveal Rapid HIV-1 antibody test (MedMira Laboratories, Halifax, Nova Scotia, Canada) is an FDA-approved, qualitative immunoassay to detect antibodies to HIV-1 in serum or plasma specimens. The test is composed of a single-use cartridge containing an immunoreactive test membrane coated with synthetic peptides corresponding to conserved regions of HIV structural proteins. This functions to capture anti-HIV-1 antibodies present in serum or plasma when a drop of specimen is added. Following the application of the sample, the membrane is washed to remove any nonspecifically bound antibodies. Captured anti-HIV-1 antibodies are visualized through a reaction with a protein A-colloidal gold conjugate, followed by a second washing step to clarify the test result. The test results must be read immediately following the second washing step. A sample is considered reactive when a distinctive red dot is produced on the test membrane, regardless of intensity. This test is shown to have 99.8% sensitivity and 99.1% specificity.

Uni-Gold Recombigen HIV Test

The Uni-Gold Recombigen HIV (Trinity Biotech PLC, Bray, County Wicklow, Ireland) is an immunochromatographic rapid test that has FDA approval for the detection of antibodies to HIV-1 in plasma, serum, and whole blood (venipuncture). The test employs genetically engineered recombinant proteins representing the immunodominant regions of the envelope proteins of HIV-1. The recombinant proteins are immobilized at the test region of a nitrocellulose strip. These proteins are also linked to colloidal gold and impregnated below the test region of the device. A narrow band of the nitrocellulose membrane is also sensitized as a control region for procedure performance. One drop of sample is added to the sample port using a pipette provided with the kit, followed by the addition of wash solution. The test must be read after 10 min of incubation. A sample is considered to be reactive if a visible pink-red band forms in the test region of the device. The control line should always appear as a pink-red line in the control region of the device to indicate that the test device is functioning properly. This test is shown to have 100% sensitivity and 99.7% specificity.

Abbott Determine HIV-1/2 Test

The Abbott Determine HIV-1/2 (Abbott Laboratories, Abbott Park, Ill.) is an immunochromatographic test for the qualitative detection of antibodies to HIV in serum, plasma, and whole blood. While this test is not approved by the FDA, it is widely employed worldwide as the rapid test of choice. Fifty microliters of sample is added to the sample pad of the test strip. If the sample is whole blood (from either venipuncture or finger stick), a drop of chase buffer must be added to the sample pad. As the sample migrates through the conjugate pad, it reconstitutes and mixes with the selenium colloidal-antigen conjugate. This mixture continues to migrate through the solid phase to the immobilized recombinant antigens and synthetic peptides in the patient window site. A sample is considered reactive if a red line forms in the patient window. For the test to be considered valid, a red line must also show up in the control window. This test is shown to have 100% sensitivity and 99.8% specificity.

Cautionary Remarks

All reactive rapid HIV test results require confirmatory testing. CDC protocols recommend that (i) either a Western blot or indirect immunofluorescence assay (IFA) be performed even if a subsequent ELISA screening test is negative, and (ii) persons with negative or indeterminate confirmatory test results receive follow-up testing 4 weeks after the initial positive rapid test result (6).

Confirmatory Tests

HIV-1 Western Blot

In low-risk populations, the frequency of false-positive ELISA readings is relatively high. All reactive ELISA samples must be tested by one of the confirmatory assays to determine the actual presence of specific anti-HIV antibodies. Among several confirmatory assays, HIV-1-specific (or HIV-2-specific) Western blotting is the most popular test in the United States and elsewhere. While the algorithm shown in Fig. 3 should be followed on samples from all individuals, it is particularly true for individuals without risk factors for HIV-1 or HIV-2 exposure, for whom the majority of positive ELISA results will be false positives. A positive Western blotting result not only confirms the presence of antibodies reactive with HIV in the infected individual but also permits identification of the specific viral components to which that individual has raised a detectable humoral response. By performing serial dilutions of the test sample, it can also be used to grade the intensity of the individual components of that response qualitatively and, in some cases, quantitatively over time.

Use of the commercially available Western blot kits requires a minimal amount of sample handling, and they can now be completed within a few hours. By comparison with

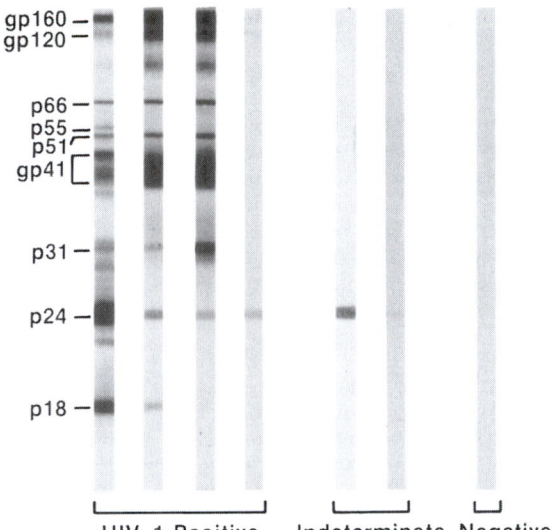

FIGURE 4 Illustration of various patterns of positive HIV-1 Western blots, showing antibody banding at the major viral proteins that can be identified using this technique. For comparison, a negative Western blot and two examples of indeterminate Western blots are also shown.

control sera as well as with internal reference standards usually provided with each kit, results can be scored visually in terms of the pattern and number of antibody bands present. Recognized viral antigens produce bands at p18, p24, p31, gp41, p51, p55, p66, gp120, and gp160 (numbers refer to apparent molecular masses, in kilodaltons). Alternatively, densitometry techniques permit quantitation of bands. Such quantitation is useful in evaluating the humoral response to candidate AIDS vaccines in noninfected seronegative recipients following primary and booster immunizations.

When used to confirm seroreactivity in a patient with presumed HIV infection, Western blotting will generally reveal variable degrees of antibody reactivity with *env*, *gag*, and *pol* gene products of HIV-1 (Fig. 4). The specific pattern of banding may vary from individual to individual, and the intensity may fluctuate according to both the relative amounts of specific anti-HIV-1 antibody circulating at any given time and the particular commercial preparation being used. As noted previously, most commercial Western blot preparations are especially sensitive for the detection of anti-p24 antibody, and its appearance on immunoblotting may occur relatively early in the period after exposure, occasionally serving to herald the process of seroconversion. The appearance of detectable levels of antibody against *pol* and *env* gene products may be delayed until somewhat later, although this lag period is usually sufficiently brief such that its impact on serodiagnosis is minor. Antibodies against other gene products of HIV-1, such as *nef* or other regulatory elements, are generally not detected by conventional immunoblotting techniques.

Interpretation of Western Blotting Results

Since official FDA licensure of the first commercial Western blot preparation in April 1987, a number of different manufacturers' preparations have been introduced on the market. However, the correct interpretation or scoring of a Western blotting result for HIV has not been universally established. Even today, not all laboratories agree upon a common algorithm for the grading of immunoblot banding patterns. Occasionally this has led to some confusion in the reporting of test results, particularly when separate laboratories using different criteria have been asked to perform confirmatory assays on the same specimens.

Depending upon the rigor of the definition applied, it is generally agreed that a negative Western blotting result means that either (i) no bands are present at any location or (ii) at least no bands corresponding to the molecular weights of known viral proteins can be detected. The presence of bands at locations not corresponding to known viral antigens is a fairly common finding and is presumed to reflect contaminants within the preparation to which some degree of antibody binding occurs. The molecular weights of these so-called aberrant bands may vary from manufacturer to manufacturer and even, occasionally, from lot to lot in kits produced by the same manufacturer.

Cautionary Remarks

The definition of what should constitute a positive Western blotting result has been considerably more difficult to codify, particularly since there has been some disagreement among investigators as to whether appropriate stringency of the definition should require the presence of antibody against any two versus all three of the major viral gene products. Antibody against a protein (or proteins) from all three groups has always been accepted as unequivocal evidence of a positive finding, and the Biotech-DuPont kit was licensed with the manufacturer's recommendation that reactivity with all three gene products be present in order for a positive determination to be made. This was also the position adopted by the American Red Cross at that time. Since then, however, convincing evidence has been presented that antibody against only two of the three major groups may also be equally diagnostic of true seroreactivity to HIV-1. In 1988, for example, the Consortium for Retrovirology Serology Standardization recommended that positive scoring of a Western blot be made on the basis of the following pattern: anti-p24 or anti-p31 occurring in the presence of either anti-gp41 or anti-gp160/anti-gp120. Other groups, in contrast, suggested that the presence or absence of antibody against *pol* gene products such as p31 not be included within this definition.

While this controversy still continues to some degree today, the majority of laboratories have accepted the 1989 recommendations of the Association of State and Territorial Public Health Laboratory Directors and the CDC. According to these criteria, a Western blot can be considered positive if it contains two of the three key bands considered by the Association to be of diagnostic significance, namely, p24, gp41, and gp120/gp160.

By definition, Western blotting results that cannot be classified as either negative or positive are grouped into the category known as indeterminate findings. Bands present may correspond to the molecular weights of known HIV-1 proteins as well as to those of contaminating cellular proteins on the nitrocellulose paper. Reactivity at the p24 and/or p55 band is particularly common in Western blots falling into the indeterminate category, regardless of whether one is surveying patients whose histories might classify them as being at high or low risk for HIV-1 infection. However, the vast majority of indeterminate Western blotting results occur for patients with no other evidence of HIV-1 infection, and it is presumed that this limited antibody recognition represents reactivity by antibodies with various contaminants of the immunoblot preparation. For example, reactivity with class I and II HLA antigens, present as cellular contaminants within the viral lysate, appears to account for a significant percentage of false-positive banding. Other causes of false-positive or indeterminate Western blotting results for HIV include the presence of antibodies to mitochondrial, nuclear, and T-cell leukocyte antigens; anticarbohydrate antibodies; globulins produced during polyclonal gammopathy; a high concentration of bilirubin in serum; and passively acquired antibodies (12). As in ELISA, some of the anti-HIV-1 subtype O specimens fail to show the complete array of HIV-1 bands and may be interpreted as indeterminate or even negative when tested using HIV-1 Western blot kits (20). Immunoblot assays utilizing recombinant-derived viral antigens or synthetic peptides corresponding to the conserved regions among different subtypes rather than viral lysates may reduce the incidence of indeterminate reactivity, although this remains to be confirmed in large-scale testing.

If clinically warranted (e.g., in the setting of a recent history of possible HIV exposure), the finding of an indeterminate Western blot pattern in the presence of a positive HIV-1 ELISA should prompt one first to repeat the Western blotting, using either the same or, if available, a fresh serum specimen. If the repeat assay result is still indeterminate, one should then consider retesting the patient within a few weeks, inasmuch as it is possible that the patient was first tested early in the process of seroconversion and that, upon serial examination, follow-up studies may reveal the full pattern of antibody reactivity. As several studies have confirmed, however, the likelihood that an indeterminate Western blotting finding represents incipient seroconversion remains low for most patients. Rather, upon serial testing, the vast majority of indeterminate findings will remain indeterminate (with either identical or different patterns of banding), revert to full seronegativity, or vacillate between the two categories. Thus, as with the ELISA, failure of the Western blot to evolve from an indeterminate to a positive test within a few months strongly mitigates against the possibility that the patient is HIV infected. Nonetheless, plagued by the anxiety generated during this period of diagnostic uncertainty, many physicians and patients understandably will opt to consult other diagnostic procedures, such as the p24 antigen capture or HIV RNA and proviral DNA assays, in an attempt to rule out more conclusively the possibility of early HIV infection.

It is particularly important to note that Western blotting is an inappropriate initial screening test for HIV infection. Among homosexual or bisexual men testing negative for HIV-1 both by ELISA and by PCR, it has been found that 20 to 30% may still show one or more bands on Western blotting. Moreover, during evaluations performed every 1 to 3 months over the course of 1 year or more, 70% of an HIV-1 ELISA-negative, PCR-negative cohort of homosexual men with an initial indeterminate Western blotting result continued to show one or more bands on serial immunoblots (13). Other studies using low-risk populations have noted similar findings. Given this high frequency of indeterminate reactivity—the overwhelming preponderance of which will be nonspecific binding—Western blotting is not appropriate for use as a primary screening tool in the population at large. Rather, its strength is as a confirmatory assay in the setting of a positive or indeterminate HIV-1 ELISA or other initial screening test result.

As mentioned above, the majority of commercial ELISA test kits in widespread use in the United States now react with antibodies against either HIV-1 or HIV-2. Given the preponderance of infection with HIV-1 in this country, a repeatedly reactive ELISA should generally first prompt use of a specific HIV-1 Western blot test as a confirmatory assay. If HIV-2 infection is suspected on epidemiologic grounds or the HIV-1 Western blot shows an atypical pattern of banding suggestive of HIV-2 cross-reactivity, then the next level of evaluation should be to perform an HIV-2 ELISA, and if the result is positive or indeterminate, to go on to HIV-2 immunoblotting. Currently, there are no HIV-2 immunoblot kits licensed by the FDA. Nonetheless, at least one company (Genelabs Diagnostics, Singapore, Singapore) manufactures a kit that is commercially available for research purposes. A positive result for HIV-2 is scored when bands are seen at *env* proteins (gp125 or gp36) and either *gag* protein (p26) or *pol* proteins (p68 or p31 or p56 or p53).

While estimates for the sensitivity and specificity of the HIV-1 Western blot test vary somewhat depending upon the manufacturer, comparative surveys have shown that most preparations afford a sensitivity of at least 96%. When the Western blot is used properly as a confirmatory test in sequence with an initial positive screening assay, the combination of these two tests should have a positive predictive value greater than 99% for both low- and high-risk populations.

IFA

IFA is performed in some laboratories for screening and/or as a substitute for conventional immunoblotting as a confirmatory assay. IFA is rapid and relatively simple to perform. However, IFA requires the use of an expensive fluorescence microscope. The assay uses immortalized human T cells that express HIV-1 antigens on their surface. The cells are fixed to the surface of an IFA glass slide with methanol-acetic acid. Fixed, uninfected T cells are provided as a control. To perform the assay, a serum or plasma specimen is diluted, and aliquots are placed in the infected and uninfected cell wells of the IFA slide and incubated in a humidified chamber for a defined period of time (Fig. 5). If HIV-1 antibodies are present in the sample, they will bind to HIV-1 viral antigens present on the infected cell surface. Unbound material is removed by aspiration and washing. Antibody to human immunoglobulin conjugated with a fluorescent dye such as fluorescein isothiocyanate is added to the infected and uninfected cell wells of the IFA slide and again incubated as described above. Unbound material is removed by aspiration and washing. A glass coverslip is mounted to the IFA slide, and the slide is viewed under a microscope with UV light. If antibodies to HIV-1 are present in the specimen, a characteristic pattern of fluorescence will become visible under UV light. The interpretation of this fluorescence is evaluated by comparing and differentiating the pattern and intensity of fluorescence in the uninfected and infected cell wells for

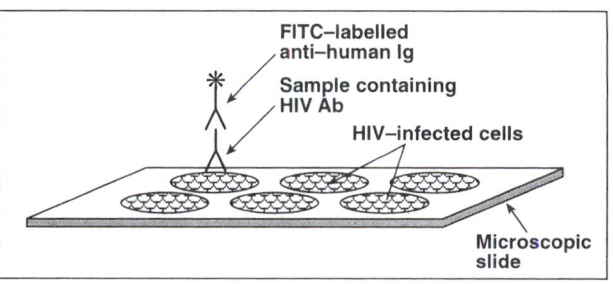

FIGURE 5 The principle of the IFA test. FITC, fluorescein isothiocyanate; Ab, antibody.

each sample. With use of the proper technique, background staining should be minimal. As with any of the standard antibody detection methods, proper quality control requires that serum from a known seropositive individual also be included as a positive control.

In addition to the relative ease with which it can be performed, the IFA offers the advantage of generally turning positive earlier in the course of infection than either a conventional ELISA or Western blot test. Time to development of a positive IFA result after an acute seroconversion to HIV-1 can be further reduced by substituting fluorescein isothiocyanate-labeled anti-human IgM as the developing conjugate. Most authors agree that, in clinical use, the sensitivity and specificity of the IFA are equivalent to those of Western blotting (22), although occasionally there can be some variability in appropriate scoring of samples due to inexperience with the technique. Manufacturers of a commercially available IFA (Fluorognost HIV-1 IFA; Waldheim Pharmaceutika, Vienna, Austria) estimate a sensitivity of 99.7%. IFA has also been employed for screening and confirming HIV-2 infections and to discriminate between HIV-1 and HIV-2 infections. It has been shown to be as sensitive as the ELISA in screening, and it is superior to Western blotting in discriminating HIV-1 and HIV-2 infection (27).

A sample result is considered indeterminate when fluorescence is observed in both infected and uninfected cells. Indeterminate IFA results are expected to occur with a slightly higher frequency in specimens from patients with certain autoimmune diseases (such as systemic lupus erythematosus) and certain viral infections such as hepatitis, cytomegalovirus, and Epstein Barr virus. Hyperlipemic or extremely icteric specimens and samples heavily contaminated with bacteria may show atypical background fluorescence.

Cautionary Remarks

The intensity of the fluorescence observed in the IFA does not bear a strict correlation to antibody titer. One of the limitations of the IFA in the research setting is that, unlike Western blotting, it does not permit precise delineation of specific patterns of antibody reactivity. The assay requires highly skilled, well-trained laboratory personnel to read and interpret the results. In addition, the test becomes cumbersome to perform if many samples are tested at one time.

RIPA

RIPA was first used as an alternative test to detect HIV antibodies in the mid-1980s and is still reserved as a research tool, since it involves a somewhat rigorous procedure requiring the use of radioactively labeled antigens. RIPA has the advantage of using minimally denatured antigens, provides appropriate conditions for identification of the large viral glycoproteins, and is sometimes preferred as a confirmatory assay over conventional Western blotting. However, its use is largely restricted to laboratories that have the facilities and expertise to propagate HIV-1 in continuous cell culture (9, 34).

Cautionary Remarks

Several aspects of the standard RIPA preclude its use by many clinical laboratories. The need to maintain viral stocks and active cell culture lines, the requirement for storing and handling of radioactive tracer materials, the time and technical expertise required to perform the assay properly, and the overall expense of this test have all contributed to making the RIPA substantially less attractive than Western blotting for routine use. For this reason, most assays of this type

are performed in research laboratories where the skills and materials required are more readily accessible. Nonetheless, occasionally there are circumstances in which the clinician may find the RIPA helpful, such as for detecting low levels of antibody positivity or aiding in the evaluation of individuals with indeterminate Western blot results.

Line Immunoassays

The line immunoassay, a variant of the Western blot test, involves application of recombinant proteins or synthetic peptides in a band pattern on plastic-backed nitrocellulose strips and testing in a manner similar to that for the Western blot assay. In this assay, optimal concentrations of antigens can be applied, enabling easier reading and interpretation. It also eliminates or minimizes the problem of indeterminate or atypical bands that are a problem in conventional Western blotting. Antigens from HIV-1 (including group O) and HIV-2 can also be combined and added for use as a combination assay (17, 26, 46); two such kits are the RIBA HIV-1/HIV-2 SIA (Chiron Corporation, Emeryville, Calif.) and the INNO-LIA HIV Confirmation (Innogenetics, Ghent, Belgium).

Home Test Kit

Using the FDA-approved home test kit Home Access Express Test (marketed by Home Access Health Corp., Hoffman Estates, Ill.), a person begins the testing process by reading a pretest counseling booklet about HIV and AIDS. Using a lancet, the person takes a finger stick blood sample and places it on a designated area of a test card precoded with a unique identification number. The test card is mailed in a protective envelope to a certified laboratory for testing. The results can be obtained over the telephone when the user keys in a special personal identification number.

Urine and Saliva Tests

Although difficult to collect and process, serum or plasma is regularly used for HIV antibody testing. Assays that use other body fluids such as saliva, oral mucosal transudates, and urine have recently been developed. Use of these alternate body fluids has obvious advantages: collection of these fluids is easy and less expensive and requires no invasive procedures. In addition, since these body fluids contain very low concentrations of virus, they are less biohazardous than serum. HIV antibodies are known to be present in body fluids from infected individuals and can be detected with routine screening and confirmatory tests (2, 10, 14, 45). The sensitivity and specificity of different assays for saliva samples are in the range of 97.3 to 100% and 99.4 to 100%, respectively (18, 24, 45). Since secretory IgA and IgG isotypes of antibodies are found in saliva, conjugates incorporating anti-human IgA and anti-human IgG enhance their detection. Test kits for detecting HIV-1 antibodies in urine and oral fluid have been recently approved by the FDA. The tests to detect HIV antibodies in urine (Calypte HIV-1 Urine EIA and the Cambridge Biotech HIV-1 Urine Western Blot) are marketed by Calypte/Cambridge Biomedical Corporation, Berkeley, Calif. Since neither urine test is as accurate as blood tests, they were approved as supplemental diagnostic tests but not as substitutes for the standard blood test to screen donors at blood banks. The two procedures in combination do, however, provide a full algorithm for HIV-1 antibody testing using urine only. The FDA has recently approved the use of the OraQuick Rapid HIV-1/2 antibody assay (OraSure Technologies, Inc.) as a Clinical Laboratory Improvement Amendments-waived test for the detection of antibodies to HIV-1 in saliva samples. To perform the test, the person being tested for HIV-1 takes the device, which has an exposed absorbent pad at one end, and places the pad above the teeth and against the outer gum. The person then gently swabs completely around the outer gums, both upper and lower, one time around. The tester then takes the device and completes the assay in the same manner as if using a blood sample (see above). In a recent multicenter clinical trial, blood and saliva samples were collected from 3,750 subjects. The results of this study showed that saliva testing is a highly accurate alternative to blood testing, providing correct results in 99.97% of cases.

VIRAL ANTIGEN DETECTION ASSAYS

The major core protein of HIV-1 is p24 (Fig. 1). The assay to detect the p24 antigen has been used for many years in the prognostic staging and management of infected individuals (32) and is licensed in the United States as part of routine blood donor screening. Most commercial HIV-1 antigen capture assays are solid-phase techniques designed to provide a quantitative measure of the level of viral p24 antigen present within serum or other body fluids. Viral p24 protein circulates in the bloodstream of an infected individual during the early viremic phase prior to seroconversion and again during advanced stages of infection (Fig. 2). Failure to detect p24 antigen between seroconversion and advanced infection has been ascribed to the formation of immune complexes, which lowers the amount of free antigen. Earlier generations of the conventional p24 antigen capture assay detected only the free p24 antigen. Recent modified versions detect both bound and free antigen.

While the levels of p24 antigen in serum may vary from individual to individual, it is known that in many patients this antigen can be detected relatively early in the period after exposure to HIV-1 and will often precede the process of seroconversion by several weeks (19, 40). This rise in measurable p24 antigen level presumably correlates with the burst in viral replication, detectable by other methods such as measurements of HIV-1 RNA or plasma viremia, that has been shown to occur shortly after primary infection. p24 antigen usually drops below the threshold of detection by conventional methods, as anti-p24 antibody is formed during seroconversion and may remain undetectable during the subsequent years of asymptomatic infection. Thereafter, depending upon an individual's immune status as reflected in the dynamic equilibrium with levels of anti-p24 antibody, it may again become detectable as the infection proceeds to a more advanced stage.

Because only 20 to 30% of individuals with asymptomatic HIV-1 infection will have levels of p24 antigen in serum detectable by standard methodology, this assay compares unfavorably to either the conventional ELISA as a diagnostic tool for HIV-1 infection or the HIV-1 RNA assays for monitoring the levels of viral activity within the known infected host. Its main use today is as a routine diagnostic tool for HIV infection in blood donors who have not yet developed antibodies. It has been chosen for this role because of its ease of performance and low cost. It is estimated that somewhere between 6 and 20 HIV-1-infected donors will be eliminated from the donor pool each year as a result of routine p24 antigen testing. With regard to its role as an indicator of viral replication, it is well established that conventional antiretroviral therapy with a nucleoside analog such as zidovudine can at least temporarily reduce the serum p24 antigen level in antigenemic patients, presumably reflecting an overall inhibition of the level of viral activity within the treated patient. On the basis of these data, the p24 antigen test was used as a surrogate marker of antiviral efficacy in a number of clinical trials of antiretroviral agents.

With respect to its role in prognostic stratification, it has been shown that patients with detectable p24 antigen in serum as a group may progress more rapidly to the development of AIDS-defining illnesses than a similar group of patients lacking this serum marker (28, 35). In a 1988 study of a cohort from San Francisco, Calif., it was found that over a 3-year period, p24-antigenemic patients developed AIDS-defining conditions at a rate that was more than three times higher than that within a similar cohort of p24 antigen-negative individuals (31).

The serum p24 antigen capture assay is a solid-phase immunoassay that has been available since 1986; it is commercially marketed by several different manufacturers, including Abbott Laboratories and Coulter Corporation. While specific reagents differ among various manufacturers, the assay is generally performed as follows. Test or control sera are allowed to react with monoclonal or polyclonal anti-HIV-1 antibody (reactive to p24 antigen) bound either to the bottom of a microtiter well or used to coat polystyrene beads. After appropriate incubation and washing, the well or beads are incubated with goat or rabbit anti-HIV-1 p24 antibody which will, in turn, bind in proportionate amounts to any p24 antigen captured on the solid phase. Washing is followed by the addition of an enzyme-tagged anti-goat (or anti-rabbit) immunoglobulin that, in the presence of an appropriate substrate, will produce a colorimetric reaction whose intensity can be measured spectrophotometrically. Using dilutions of a serum with a known concentration of p24 antigen as a positive control, one can generate a standard curve of OD versus concentration, against which the absorbance values of test sera can be compared quantitatively. Most commercially available kits define their lower limits of p24 antigen detection as being in the range of 50 pg/ml, although the actual linear portion of the standard curve will often permit reliable measurements as low as 10 to 20 pg/ml. Of note, as a confirmation of the specificity of the assay, positive test sera can also be retested in the presence of human sera containing a known high concentration of anti-HIV-1 antibody. With most kits, a reduction in the test serum's OD of 50% or greater by this neutralization procedure is confirmatory of the specificity of the p24 measurement.

As mentioned, a major limitation of the overall utility of the earlier forms of the p24 antigen capture assay was that they were capable of detecting only free p24 antigen and not antigen complexed with anti-p24 antibody. A significant improvement in the sensitivity of this test was achieved through incorporation of methods to dissociate such immune complexes prior to assay. In particular, it was found that heating (37) or lowering the pH (23, 32, 42) of samples markedly increased the level of p24 antigen detectable in sera from both asymptomatic and advanced HIV-1-infected patients. One method that has been developed involves the addition of dilute hydrochloric acid to samples and subsequent neutralization with alkali (32). An alternative method involves acidification with a mild organic acid such as glycine (pH 1.85) followed by neutralization with alkaline Tris buffer (pH 8.6) (23, 42). It offers the potential advantage of being less likely to denature epitopes on p24 antigen prior to measurement. In one of these studies (42), a 300% increase in the number of p24-reactive samples and a 3- to 12-fold increase in the quantity of antigen were observed when samples were pretreated with 1.5 M glycine buffer.

COMBINATION ASSAYS

Fourth-generation assays, which allow the simultaneous detection of HIV antigen and antibody, have been recently developed. Such tests include the Enzymun-Test HIV Combi manufactured by Boehringer Mannheim (Penzberg, Germany), the VIDAS HIV DUO manufactured by bioMerieux (Marcy l'Etoile, France), and the AxSYM HIV Ag-Ab Combo manufactured by Abbott Laboratories (Abbott Diagnostika GmbH & Co. KG, Wiesbaden, Germany) (38, 44). Fourth-generation assays may permit an earlier diagnosis of HIV infection than third-generation assays through the detection of p24 antigen.

HIV Combi is an enzyme immunoassay for the simultaneous detection of HIV antigen and IgG and IgM antibodies to HIV-1 (including subtype O) and HIV-2. In the first reaction step, the sample is incubated with biotinylated and digoxigenin-labeled HIV antigens (synthetic peptides gp41 and gp36 and recombinant reverse transcriptase) and biotinylated and digoxigenin-labeled monoclonal anti-p24 antibody. After washing, o-phenylenediamine-conjugated antidigoxigenin antibody is added. After a final wash, HIV antigen and/or antibody is detected by the addition of diammonium 2,2′-azinobis(3-ethylbenzthiazoline-6-sulfonate) (ABTS) substrate. The minimum volume of sample required is 400 μl, and the total test time is 4 h. All of the assay steps are performed automatically by the Enzymun system (ES 300 or ES 600/700). At the end of the assay, results are automatically calculated by the Enzymun system in relation to the cutoff (0.14 × extinction of positive calibrator + 1.0 × extinction of the negative calibrator). Samples with an index value (extinction of the sample/cutoff) of >1 are considered positive.

VIDAS HIV DUO is an IFA for the simultaneous detection of p24 antigen and IgG antibodies to HIV-1 (including subtype O) and HIV-2. The first reaction step, which is for the detection of anti-HIV-1 and anti-HIV-2 IgG, is performed in the lower part of a solid phase receptacle (SPR), which is coated with synthetic peptides (gp41 and gp36). Anti-human IgG labeled with alkaline phosphatase is used as the conjugate. The second reaction, for the detection of p24, is performed in the upper part of the SPR, which is coated with monoclonal anti-p24 antibodies. During incubation, p24 is released through viral lysis and binds to the monoclonal antibodies on the SPR and also to the biotinylated anti-p24 antibodies. The antibody-antigen-antibody complex binds to alkaline phosphatase-labeled streptavidin. The final detection step is the same for both reactions. The substrate (4-methylumbelliferyl phosphate) is catalyzed by the conjugate into a fluorescent product (4-methylumbelliferone). A sample volume of 200 μl is required, and the total test time is 1.5 h. All of the assay steps are performed automatically in the VIDAS instrument. The test value is calculated by dividing the patient reference value by the reference value of the standard. A test value of >0.35 is considered positive.

AxSYM Combo is a three-step process that combines microparticle, fluorescence, and enzyme-linked immunoassay technologies in an automated, random-access system. After specimens are loaded into the instrument, AxSYM mixes serum or plasma specimens with a detergent-enriched, buffered specimen diluent formulated to disrupt HIV for optimal p24 exposure and to decrease or eliminate nonspecific or interfering reactions of undesirable plasma or serum components with the microparticles. In the second step, antibody (anti-gp41) and/or antigen (p24 core antigen) sandwiches are formed by automated addition of biotinylated

probes (biotinylated recombinant transmembrane proteins, biotinylated peptides derived from the immunodominant regions of gp41, and biotinylated monoclonal [anti-p24] antibodies) to microparticle-bound immune complexes. In the third step, biotinylated probes bound to the solid phase via sandwich formation are reacted with an antibiotin rabbit antibody complexed with alkaline phosphatase (conjugate) presented in a diluent formulated to enhance the formation of biotin-antibiotin immune complexes and to limit nonspecific binding of the conjugate. AxSYM detects the formation of antibody (anti-gp41) and antigen (p24 core protein) immune complexes by automated addition of 4-methylumbelliferyl phosphate, which is a fluorescent substrate for alkaline phosphatase. As 4-methylumbelliferyl phosphate is converted to methylumbelliferone by alkaline phosphatase, AxSYM detects and quantifies the fluorescent signal. The signal is proportional to the amount of antibody (anti-gp41) or antigen (p24 core protein) contained in the original plasma or serum sample.

The AxSYM Combo assay delivers specimen results as a ratio of the specimen signal (in rate units) to the cutoff value. Ratios of ≥1 are considered reactive and indicate the presence of anti-HIV immunoglobulin and/or p24.

QUALITY ASSURANCE PROGRAM

An overall program of quality assurance, including quality control and proficiency testing, is required to ensure the accuracy of laboratory results. Such a program consists of written policies and procedures that the laboratory has implemented to ensure that its performance is acceptable to its clients and licensing agencies.

CONCLUSIONS

Serologic assays to detect antibodies to HIV are the most widely used means of laboratory diagnosis of HIV infection (11). Most HIV testing algorithms include an ELISA as the screening component and Western blotting as the confirmatory method (25). The ELISA is used for screening because of its high sensitivity for detecting antibody, and the Western blot assay is used for confirmation because of its high specificity. Several problems related to the laboratory diagnosis of HIV infection still exist; these include the need for detection of early infection, the resolution of indeterminate results, the need for detection of infection in the newborn, and the need for less expensive confirmatory strategies. The estimated risk of transmitting HIV by transfusion of screened blood in the United States is very small, primarily because all blood donations are tested with a combination antibody test for HIV-1 and HIV-2 and are examined for the presence of p24 antigen. The use of rapid tests in point-of-care settings should have significant positive public health benefits within the United States and globally.

REFERENCES

1. **Allain, J. P., Y. Lourian, D. A. Paul, and D. Senn.** 1986. Serological markers in early stages of human immunodeficiency virus infection in hemophiliacs. *Lancet* **ii:**1233–1236.
2. **Archibald, D. W., J. P. Johnson, P. Nair, L. S. Alger, C. A. Hebert, E. Davis, and S. E. Hines.** 1990. Detection of salivary immunoglobulin A antibodies to HIV-1 in infants and children. *AIDS* **4:**417–420.
3. **Bachmann, P., J. Beyer, S. Brust, W. Engelhardt, L. G. Gurtler, K. O. Habermehl, A. Karakassopoulos, U. Michl, A. Muhlbacher, M. Stoffler-Meilicke, and R. Thorstensson.**

1995. Multicentre study of diagnostic evaluation of an assay for simultaneous detection of antibodies to HIV-1, HIV-2 and HIV-1 subtype O (HIV-O). *Infection* **23:**322–333.

4. **Branson, B. M.** 2003 Point-of-care rapid tests for HIV antibodies. *J. Lab. Med.* **27:**288–295.

5. **Carlson, J. R., J. L. Yee, E. J. Watson-Williams, M. B. Jennings, S. C. Mertens, M. B. Gardner, J. Ghrayeb, and R. J. Biggar.** 1987. Rapid, easy, and economical screening tests for antibodies to human immunodeficiency virus. *Lancet* **i:**361–362.

6. **Centers for Disease Control and Prevention.** 2004. Protocols for confirmation of reactive rapid HIV tests. *Morb. Mortal. Wkly. Rep.* **53:**221–222.

7. **Centers for Disease Control and Prevention.** 2001. HIV and AIDS—United States, 1981–2001. *Morb. Mortal. Wkly. Rep.* **50:**430–434.

8. **Centers for Disease Control and Prevention.** 2002. *HIV/AIDS Surveillance Report*, vol. 14, p. 1–40. Centers for Disease Control and Prevention, Atlanta, Ga.

9. **Chiodi, F., U. Bredberg-Raden, G. Biberfeld, B. Bottiger, J. Albert, B. Asjo, E. M. Fenyo, and E. Norrby.** 1987. Radioimmunoprecipitation and Western blotting with sera of human immunodeficiency virus infected patients: a comparative study. *AIDS Res. Hum. Retrovir.* **3:**165–176.

10. **Connell, J. A., J. V. Parry, P. P. Mortimer, R. J. Duncan, K. A. McLean, A. M. Johnson, M. H. Hambling, J. Barbara, and C. P. Farrington.** 1990. Preliminary report: accurate assays for anti-HIV in urine. *Lancet* **335:**1366–1369.

11. **Constantine, N. T.** 1993. Serologic tests for the retroviruses: approaching a decade of evolution. *AIDS* **7:**1–13.

12. **Cordes, R. J., and M. E. Ryan.** 1995. Pitfalls in HIV testing, application and limitation of current tests. *Postgrad. Med.* **98:**177–180.

13. **Davey, R. T., Jr., L. R. Deyton, J. A. Metcalf, M. Easter, J. A. Kovacs, M. B. Vasudevachari, M. Psallidopoulos, L. M. Thompson III, J. Falloon, M. A. Polis, H. Masur, and H. C. Lane.** 1992. Indeterminate Western blot patterns in a cohort of individuals at high risk for human immunodeficiency virus (HIV-1) exposure. *J. Clin. Immunol.* **12:**185–192.

14. **Desai, S., H. Bates, and F. J. Michalski.** 1991. Detection of antibody to HIV-1 in urine. *Lancet* **337:**183–184.

15. **Farzadegan, H.** 1994. HIV antibodies and serology. *Clin. Lab. Med.* **14:**257–269.

16. **Fleming, P. L., R. H. Byers, P. A. Sweeney, D. Daniels, J. M. Karon, and R. S. Janssen.** 2002. HIV prevalence in the United States, 2000, abstr. 11. *Programs Abstr. 9th Conf. Retrovir. Opportunistic Infect.*

17. **Fransen, K., D. E. Potlet, M. Peeters, I. van Kerckhoven, G. Beelaert, G. Vercauteren, P. Piot, and G. van der Groen.** 1991. Evaluation of a line immunoassay for simultaneous confirmation of antibodies to HIV-1 and HIV-2. *Eur. J. Clin. Microbiol. Infect. Dis.* **10:**939–946.

18. **Frerichs, R. R., N. Silarug, N. Eskes, P. Pagcharoenpol, A. Rodklai, S. Thangsupachai, and C. Wongba.** 1994. Saliva-based HIV-antibody testing in Thailand. *AIDS* **8:**885–894.

19. **Goudsmit, J., J. M. Lange, W. J. A. Krone, M. B. M. Teunissen, L. G. Epstein, S. A. Danner, H. van den Berg, C. Breederveld, L. Smit, M. Bakker, F. de Wolf, R. A. Coutinho, and J. van der Noordaa.** 1987. Pathogenesis of HIV and its implications for serodiagnosis and monitoring of antiviral therapy. *J. Virol. Methods* **17:**19–34.

20. **Gurtler, L. G., L. Zekeng, F. Simon, J. Eberle, J. M. Tsague, L. Kaptue, S. Brust, and S. Knapp.** 1995. Reactivity of five anti-HIV-1 subtype O specimens with six different anti-HIV screening ELISAs and three immunoblots. *J. Virol. Methods* **51:**177–184.

21. **Houn, H. Y., A. A. Pappas, and E. M. Walker, Jr.** 1987. Status of current clinical tests for human immunodeficiency virus (HIV): applications and limitations. *Ann. Clin. Lab. Sci.* **17:**279–285.

22. **Iltis, J. P., N. M. Patel, S. R. Lee, S. L. Barmat, and W. C. Wallen.** 1990. Comparative evaluation of an immunofluorescent antibody test, enzyme immunoassay and Western blot for the detection of HIV-1 antibody. *Intervirology* **31:**122–128.

23. **Kestens, L., G. Hoofd, P. L. Gigase, R. Deleys, and G. van der Groen.** 1991. HIV antigen detection in circulating immune complexes. *J. Virol. Methods* **31:**67–76.

24. **King, A., S. A. Marion, D. Cook, M. Rekart, P. J. Middleton, M. V. O'Shaughnessy, and J. S. G. Montaner.** 1995. Accuracy of a saliva test for HIV antibody. *J. Acquir. Immune Defic. Syndr.* **9:**172–175.

25. **King, R., S. Frey, R. Beisha, P. Van de Perre, E. Karita, and S. Allen.** 1993. The presence or absence of gp120/gp160 bands on indeterminate Western blots: predictive value for HIV seroconversion. *AIDS* **7:**437–438.

26. **Kline, R. L., D. McNairn, M. Holodniy, L. Mole, D. Margolis, W. Blattner, and T. C. Quinn.** 1996. Evaluation of Chiron HIV-1/HIV-2 recombinant immunoblot assay. *J. Clin. Microbiol.* **34:**2650–2653.

27. **Kvinesdal, B. B., C. M. Nielsen, A.-G. Poulsen, and N. Hojlyng.** 1989. Immunofluorescence assay for detection of antibodies to human immunodeficiency virus type 2. *J. Clin. Microbiol.* **27:**2502–2504.

28. **Lange, J. M., D. A. Paul, H. G. Huisman, F. de Wolf, H. van den Berg, R. A. Coutinho, S. A. Danner, J. van der Noordaa, and J. Goudsmit.** 1986. Persistent HIV antigenaemia and decline of HIV core antibodies associated with transition to AIDS. *Br. Med. J.* **293:**1459–1462.

29. **Loussert-Ajaka, I., T. D. Ly, M. L. Chaix, D. Ingrand, S. Saragosti, A. M. Courouce, F. Brun-Vezinet, and F. Simon.** 1994. HIV-1/HIV-2 seronegativity in HIV-1 subtype O infected patients. *Lancet* **343:**1393–1394.

30. **McAlpine, L., J. Gandhi, J. V. Parry, and P. P. Mortimer.** 1994. Thirteen current anti-HIV-1/HIV-2 enzyme immunoassays: how accurate are they? *J. Med. Virol.* **42:**115–118.

31. **Moss, A. R., P. Bacchetti, D. Osmonap, W. Krampf, R. E. Chaisson, D. Stites, J. Wilber, J. P. Allain, and J. Carlson.** 1988. Seropositivity for HIV and the development of AIDS or AIDS related condition: three year follow up of the San Francisco General Hospital cohort. *Br. Med. J.* **296:**745–750.

32. **Nishanian, P., K. R. Huskins, S. Stehn, R. Detels, and J. L. Fahey.** 1990. A simple method for improved assay demonstrates that HIV p24 antigen is present as immune complexes in most sera from HIV-infected individuals. *J. Infect. Dis.* **162:**21–28.

33. **Pau, C. P., D. J. Hu, C. Spruill, C. Schable, E. M. Lackritz, M. Kai, J. R. George, M. A. Rayfield, T. J. Dondero, A. E. Williams, M. P. Busch, A. E. Brown, F. E. McCutchan, and G. Schochetman.** 1996. Surveillance for human immunodeficiency virus type I group O infections in the United States. *Transfusion* **36:**398–400.

34. **Pinter, A., and W. J. Honnen.** 1988. A sensitive radioimmunoprecipitation assay for human immunodeficiency virus (HIV). *J. Immunol. Methods* **112:**235–241.

35. **Portera, M., F. Vitale, R. La Licata, D. R. Alesi, G. Lupo, F. Bonura, N. Romano, and G. Di Cuonzo.** 1990. Free and antibody-complexed antigen and antibody profile in apparently healthy HIV seropositive individuals and in AIDS patients. *J. Med. Virol.* **30:**30–35.

36. **Schable, C., L. Zekeng, C. P. Pau, D. Hu, L. Kaptue, L. Gurder, T. Dondero, J. M. Tsague, G. Schochetman, H. Jaffe, and J. R. George.** 1994. Sensitivity of United States HIV antibody tests for detection of HIV-1 group O infections. *Lancet* **344:**1333–1334.

37. **Schupbach, J., and J. Boni.** 1992. Quantitative and sensitive detection of immune-complexed and free HIV antigen after boiling of serum. *J. Virol. Methods* **43:** 247–256.

38. **Sickinger, E., M. Stieler, B. Kaufman, H.-P. Kapprell, D. West, A. Sandridge, S. Devare, G. Schochetman, J. C. Hunt, and D. Daghfal.** 2004. Multicenter evaluation of a new, automated enzyme-linked immunoassay for detection of human immunodeficiency virus-specific antibodies and antigen. *J. Clin. Microbiol.* **42:**21–22.

39. **Simon, F., T. D. Ly, A. Baillou-Beaufils, V. Fauveau, J. De Saint-Martin, I. Loussert-Ajaka, M. L. Chaix, S. Saragosti, A. M. Courouce, et al.** 1994. Sensitivity of screening kits for anti-HI-1 subtype O antibodies. *AIDS* **8:**1628–1629.

40. **Stramer, S., J. S. Heller, R. W. Coombs, J. V. Parry, D. D. Ho, and J. P. Allain.** 1989. Markers of HIV infection prior to IgG antibody seropositivity. *JAMA* **262:**64–69.

41. **UNAIDS.** 2004. *Report on the Global AIDS Epidemic, July, 2004.* UNAIDS, Joint United Nations Programme on HIV/AIDS, Geneva, Switzerland.

42. **Vasudevachari, M. B., N. P. Salzman, D. P. Woll, T. C. Mast, K. W. Uffelman, G. Toedter, D. Hofheinz, J. A. Metcalf, and H. C. Lane.** 1993. Clinical utility of an enhanced human immunodeficiency virus type 1 p24 antigen capture assay. *J. Clin. Immunol.* **13:**185–192.

43. **Ward, J. W., S. D. Holmberg, J. R. Allen, D. L. Cohn, S. E. Critchley, S. H. Kleinman, B. A. Lenes, O. Ravenholt, J. R. Davis, M. G. Quinn, and H. W. Jaffe.** 1988. Transmission of human immunodeficiency virus (HIV) by blood transfusions screened as negative for HIV antibody. *N. Engl. J. Med.* **318:**473–478.

44. **Weber, B., E. H. M. Fall, A. Berger, and H. W. Doerr.** 1998. Reduction of diagnostic window by new fourth-generation human immunodeficiency virus screening assays. *J. Clin. Microbiol.* **36:**2235–2239.

45. **Wesley, W. E., S. F. Paparello, C. F. Decker, J. M. Sheffield, and F. H. Lowe-Bey.** 1995. A modified ELISA and Western blot accurately determine anti-human immunodeficiency virus type I antibodies in oral fluids obtained with a special collecting device. *J. Infect. Dis.* **171:**1406.

46. **Zaaijer, H. L., G. A. van Rixel, J. N. Kromosoeto, D. R. Balgobind-Ramdas, H. T. Cuypers, and P. N. Lelie.** 1998. Validation of a new immunoblot assay (LiaTek HIV III) for confirmation of human immunodeficiency virus infection. *Transfusion* **38:**776–781.

47. **Zhang, X., N. T. Constantine, J. Bansal, J. D. Callahan, and V. C. Marsiglia.** 1992. Evaluation of a new generation synthetic peptide combination assay for detection of antibodies to HIV-1, HIV-2, HTLV-I and HTLV-II simultaneously. *J. Med. Virol.* **38:**49–53.

General Immunologic Evaluation of Patients with Human Immunodeficiency Virus Infection

RANDY A. STEVENS, RICHARD A. LEMPICKI, VEN NATARAJAN,
JEANETTE HIGGINS, JOSEPH W. ADELSBERGER, AND JULIA A. METCALF

95

AIDS was first recognized in 1981 as a new clinical entity and has since become a devastating, worldwide epidemic. It is estimated that by the end of 2003, roughly 37.8 million people worldwide were living with human immunodeficiency virus (HIV) and that during 2003, approximately 14,000 new infections occurred each day (26). Since AIDS was first identified, more than 20 million people with HIV/AIDS have died, and in 2003 alone, HIV infection was responsible for the death of nearly 3 million people worldwide (26). Throughout the globe, numerous clinical trials are currently being conducted to examine preventive HIV vaccines, as well as treatments for both HIV infection and its associated infections and cancers. Because of this epidemic and the need to discover new and more effective therapies for HIV/AIDS, the clinical immunology laboratory plays a critical role in the evaluation and monitoring of patients with HIV infection.

The hallmark of HIV infection is the destruction of $CD4^+$ T lymphocytes and the concomitant destruction of the immune system. A variety of quantitative and functional immunologic abnormalities have been described to occur in individuals infected with HIV (13, 16, 17). These abnormalities affect virtually every compartment of the cellular and humoral immune systems and include (i) decreased percentage and absolute number of helper/inducer T lymphocytes ($CD4^+$ T cells), (ii) decreased proliferative responses of lymphocytes to mitogens and antigens, (iii) increased rates of peripheral T-cell turnover, (iv) decreased thymic function, (v) hypergammaglobulinemia, (vi) decreased cytotoxic lymphocyte and natural killer (NK) cell activity, and (vii) abnormalities in serum components, including elevated levels of β_2-microglobulin, neopterin, and soluble immune complexes.

When evaluating the immunologic status of individuals with HIV infection, or when developing strategies for clinical monitoring of therapeutic trials, immunologic monitoring should be conducted in a manner appropriate for the evaluation of any patient population that is suspected of having multiple defects in cell-mediated immunity. Basic testing should include immunophenotypic analysis of T-lymphocyte subpopulations ($CD3^+$, $CD4^+$, and $CD8^+$ cells) by flow cytometry, with particular attention to both the percentage and absolute number of $CD4^+$ T cells. Where appropriate, additional testing may include further phenotypic analysis of peripheral blood mononuclear cells (PBMCs), to include markers for monocytes; NK cells; B cells; T-cell activation markers, such as HLA-DR, CD38, and CD25; markers of naive and memory lymphocytes, such as CD45RO, CD45RA, CD62L, and CD27; and HIV coreceptors, such as CC-CKR5 and CXCR4. Routine assessment of immune function may include the measurement of proliferative responses of T lymphocytes to antigens and mitogens, as well as measurement of NK cell cytotoxicity and T-cell-mediated cytotoxicity. Lymphocyte turnover rates may be measured by intracellular staining for the nuclear antigen Ki67 or by ex vivo labeling of cells with the thymidine analog bromodeoxyuridine (BrdU). Most recently, techniques have been developed to study cell turnover in vivo using deuterium or BrdU to label proliferating cells. Thymic function may be assessed by the quantitation of T-cell receptor rearrangement excision circles (TRECs).

The intent of this chapter is to provide proven methods for the routine immunologic monitoring of the cellular immune status of patients with HIV infection. Since a majority of immunologic assays are performed with PBMCs, procedures for the isolation and cryopreservation of PBMCs are also discussed. The section describing each procedure is prefaced with an explanation of the rationale behind the described assay, quality control measures necessary for standardization of testing, and practical advice on pitfalls to avoid. In-depth theoretical discussions of each of the major types of monitoring procedures such as flow cytometry, lymphocyte proliferation assays (LPAs), and the quantification of TRECs are provided elsewhere in this manual.

CELL PREPARATION

When monitoring the immunologic status of patients with HIV infection, isolation of lymphoid cells is often required for performing several immunologic procedures, such as lymphocyte immunophenotyping and measurement of lymphocyte function. Lymphoid cells are most commonly obtained from peripheral whole blood, but they may also be collected from other lymph tissue, such as lymph node and tonsil. Described below is a procedure whereby PBMCs can be easily isolated from whole blood, leukapheresis packs, or lymphoid tissue preparations by use of Ficoll-Hypaque density gradient centrifugation. Alternatively, whole-blood mononuclear cells may be isolated using a Percoll gradient or by using BD Vacutainer CPT cell preparation tubes, which are available from Becton Dickinson (http://www.bd.com/). The CPT tube combines a blood collection tube, anticoagulant, Ficoll-Hypaque density fluid, and a polyester gel, which facilitates the separation of the mononuclear cells. The advantage of the CPT tube method is that blood collection and separation occur in one tube, thereby reducing the risk of specimen contamination and reducing the time and materials needed to process the specimens. Disadvantages of CPT tubes are that recovery of PBMCs may be less than with the Ficoll method described below, and multiple CPT tubes are needed to process large volumes of blood, since each tube holds only 9 ml of blood. Once the PBMCs have been obtained, they can be further purified into various leukocyte subsets using flow cytometry cell sorting or by using immunomagnetic separation technologies that are available from Dynal, Inc. (http://www.dynal.no/) and Miltenyi Biotec (http://www.miltenyibiotec.com/).

Human peripheral blood is obtained by venipuncture into vacuum tubes or syringes containing preservative-free sodium heparin (20 U/ml of blood). Alternatively, cells obtained by leukapheresis may be used. Following phlebotomy, the heparinized blood or leukapheresis sample can be stored for up to 24 h at room temperature before further processing. PBMCs are then obtained from the whole blood or leukapheresis sample by Ficoll-Hypaque density gradient centrifugation. This procedure is accomplished by carefully layering whole blood diluted 1:2 with sterile phosphate-buffered saline (PBS) over Ficoll-Hypaque, which is commercially available from several manufacturers. After a short centrifugation at room temperature, mononuclear cells are harvested from the interface between the Ficoll-Hypaque and plasma layers. The amount of diluted whole blood layered on top of the Ficoll-Hypaque should not exceed two to three times the volume of the Ficoll-Hypaque. For small amounts of whole blood (≤5 ml), the procedure can be carried out in 15-ml conical polypropylene centrifuge tubes. Larger volumes of whole blood should be separated in 50-ml conical centrifuge tubes. The use of polystyrene or polycarbonate tubes to purify and wash the PBMCs should be avoided because of undesired cell adhesion to these types of plastics.

The separation of PBMCs by this technique is straightforward, but consistent and reproducible separations can be accomplished only through close attention to procedural detail. The end result of this procedure will be a clean population of PBMCs virtually free of erythrocyte (RBC), granulocyte, and platelet contamination. Occasionally, the PBMC layer will be contaminated with RBCs due to low mean corpuscular hemoglobin content, or contaminated with granulocytes due to degranulation of the granulocytes. This is especially true with end-stage AIDS patients or acutely ill patients. In these cases, it is not possible to remove the contaminating cells by reprocessing the sample. If RBC contamination is a problem, the cells can be removed by hypotonic or ammonium chloride lysis. It is not practical to attempt to remove contaminating granulocytes, since they do not interfere appreciably in functional assays and can be easily discriminated during phenotypic analysis using flow cytometry.

Equipment

Low-speed centrifuge
Hemacytometer or automated cell counter
50- or 15-ml sterile polypropylene conical centrifuge tubes
Disposable sterile pipettes

Reagents

1× PBS without Ca^{2+} or Mg^{2+}
Ficoll-Hypaque solution (density, 1.077 g/ml)
Cell culture medium, such as RPMI 1640 medium without L-glutamine, 2% 1 M HEPES buffer, 1% 200 mM L-glutamine, 50 μg gentamicin per ml, and 10% fetal calf serum (FCS)

Procedure

1. Bring PBS to room temperature.
2. Dilute fresh, heparinized whole blood with equal parts PBS, and place the samples into 50-ml conical tubes.
3. Add 15 ml of Ficoll-Hypaque to another 50-ml conical tube.
4. Carefully layer 30 ml of diluted blood on top of the Ficoll-Hypaque by hooking the lip of the Ficoll-Hypaque tube onto the lip of the diluted whole blood tube and gently transferring the whole blood into the Ficoll-Hypaque tube. Note: Allow the blood mixture to flow gently onto the top of the Ficoll surface without breaking the surface plane of the Ficoll. Do not allow the Ficoll to mix with the diluted blood. This method takes practice to master but can dramatically reduce preparation time over the alternative method of underlayering the diluted blood with Ficoll-Hypaque by using a pipette.
5. Centrifuge the samples for 10 min at 1,640 × g and 20°C.
6. Remove the cloudy layer of cells at the plasma–Ficoll-Hypaque interface with a disposable sterile pipette. Avoid aspiration of the Ficoll solution located below the cell layer.
7. Resuspend cells in 50 ml of PBS, and centrifuge them for 10 min at 840 × g and 20°C.
8. Wash the cell pellet twice with PBS for 10 min at 470 × g and 20°C.
9. Resuspend the cells in an appropriate cell culture medium, such as RPMI 1640 medium without L-glutamine, 2% 1 M HEPES buffer, 1% 200 mM L-glutamine, 50 μg of gentamicin per ml, and 10% FCS. Perform a cell count using a hemacytometer or automated cell counter and adjust the cell concentration as needed. Cell viability should be determined either by the standard trypan blue staining method or by the flow cytometry-based propidium iodide staining method. Cells may be used immediately for experimentation, stored as pry pellets, or cryopreserved as viable cell suspensions (see cryopreservation procedure below).

IMMUNE CELL PHENOTYPING BY FLOW CYTOMETRY

HIV infection and AIDS are characterized by a significant and progressive destruction of $CD4^+$ T lymphocytes that results in a state of profound immunodeficiency and exposes the host to opportunistic pathogens and disease. In addition to the steady decline of $CD4^+$ T lymphocytes during infection, there is a concomitant increase in $CD8^+$ T lymphocytes as part of the normal immune response to viral infection. Measurement of the percentage and absolute number of $CD4^+$ T lymphocytes is the most useful laboratory test for determining the immunologic status of patients with HIV infection, making decisions regarding antiretroviral therapy, and determining when to initiate prophylaxis for opportunistic pathogens. For example, patients should be started on regimens for *Pneumocystis carinii* pneumonia prophylaxis once their absolute CD4 count is <200 cells/μl or their CD4 level is <14% (3). Patients with CD4 counts of >200 but <250 cells/μl may be considered for treatment as well (3). Antiretroviral medications have vastly improved the morbidity and mortality of HIV-infected patients, and current treatment guidelines recommend delaying antiretroviral treatment until CD4 counts are ≤350 cells/μl (4). In addition to the prognostic value of monitoring the percentage and absolute number of CD4+ lymphocytes, these parameters have been recommended by the American College of Physicians and the Institute of Medicine as surrogate markers in the analysis of clinical trials involving HIV/AIDS patients.

Currently, there are two accepted methods for the identification and enumeration of CD4+ T cells obtained from peripheral whole blood. In 1997, the Centers for Disease Control and Prevention (CDC) issued revised guidelines for performing CD4+-T-cell determinations in persons with HIV infection (2). This method involves a dual-platform process in which the absolute CD4 cell count is calculated by multiplying together three independent measurements: the CD4 percentage, which is measured by three- or four-color flow cytometry, and the white blood cell (WBC) count and percentage of lymphocytes, which are measured by conventional hematology. In 2003, the CDC issued guidelines for performing CD4+-T-cell determinations by a single-platform technology (5). With single-platform technology, absolute cell counts are measured solely on a flow cytometer and are derived by performing standard three- or four-color flow cytometry and simultaneously counting fluorospheres, which have been added to the blood at a known concentration, thus eliminating the need for a separate hematology instrument. Two suppliers of single-platform fluorospheres are Beckman Coulter (http://www.beckman.com) and BD Biosciences (http://www.bdbiosciences.com). There are advantages and disadvantages associated with both the single- and dual-platform methodologies, so each laboratory must determine which method best suits their needs and capabilities. A major disadvantage of the dual-platform method is that errors in each of the three independent measurements (WBCs, percent lymphocytes, and percent CD4 cells) are multiplied when the absolute count is calculated. The age of blood must also be considered when deciding which method to use. For the single-platform method, blood is stable for up to 72 h after draw, whereas for the dual-platform method, flow cytometry should not be performed on blood that is more than 30 h old and hematology must be performed within the time specified by the manufacturer of the hematology instrument used (often 8 h from the time of blood draw). This can be a major consideration when there is a need to have blood collected off-site and shipped to the testing laboratory. Compared to the single-platform method, the dual-platform method can also be quite expensive, since this method involves the purchase and maintenance of both a flow cytometer and a hematology analyzer. The major disadvantage of the single-platform method involves the need for precise pipetting, compared to the dual-platform method, because accurate results rely on the precise addition of a known number of fluorospheres to fixed volumes of blood and monoclonal antibodies (22, 24). Therefore, quality assessment becomes even more imperative with single-platform methodologies.

When performing immunophenotypic determinations by flow cytometry, peripheral whole blood is first stained with fluorescently labeled monoclonal antibodies which are specific for cell surface antigens. Next, RBCs are removed from the cell suspension by lysis and the remaining WBCs are fixed using a commercial lysing/fixing reagent. The resulting cell preparation is then suitable for analysis on a flow cytometer. Whole blood for immunophenotyping should be drawn by venipuncture into containers with either EDTA or sodium heparin anticoagulant, and the specimens should be processed as soon as possible (2, 5). If single-platform technology is used, whole blood can be stored at room temperature for up to 72 h, whereas with dual-platform technology, whole blood must be processed within 30 h.

Table 1 lists suggested three- and four-color panels of monoclonal antibodies that may be used for the basic monitoring of patients with AIDS (5). Using the panels listed in this table, one can enumerate CD4+ and CD8+ T cells and ensure the quality of the results. For each of these basic panels, lymphocytes are identified using a CD45 fluorescence and side-scatter gating strategy. Lymphocytes stain brightly for CD45 and have low light-scatter properties. When appropriate, additional testing may include further phenotypic analysis of PBMCs to include T-cell activation markers such as HLA-DR, CD25, CD38, and Ki67. One may also wish to characterize CD4+ and CD8+ T lymphocytes as naive or memory by using markers such as CD45RA, CD45RO, CD62L, and CD27. Companies that provide monoclonal antibodies for the immunophenotyping of patients include the following: Beckman Coulter, BD Biosciences, Biosource (http://www.biosource.com), Caltag (http://www.caltag.com), Dako Cytomation (http://www.dakocytomation.com), Molecular Probes (http://www.probes.com), and R & D Systems (http://www.rdlabs.com). Additional suppliers can be found at http://www.antibodyresource.com. It should be

TABLE 1 Suggested monoclonal antibody panels for lymphocyte immunophenotyping of patients with HIV infection

Panel[a]	Monoclonal antibodies	Specificity
Three color	CD3 × CD4 × CD45	CD3+ T cells and CD3+ CD4+ T cells
	CD3 × CD8 × CD45	CD3+ T cells and CD3+ CD8+ T cells
	CD3 × CD19 × CD45	CD3+ T cells and CD19+ B cells
	CD3 × CD16/56 × CD45	CD3+ T cells and NK cells
	CD27 × CD45RO × CD4	Memory and naive CD4 cells
	CD27 × CD45RO × CD8	Memory and naive CD8 cells
Four color	CD3 × CD8 × CD45 × CD4	CD3+, CD3+ CD4+, and CD3+ CD8+ T cells
	CD3 × CD16/56 × CD45 × CD19	CD3+ T cells, NK cells, and CD19+ B cells
	CD27 × CD45RO × CD3 × CD4	Memory and naive CD4 cells
	CD27 × CD45RO × CD3 × CD8	Memory and naive CD8 cells

[a]Lymphocytes are gated using CD45 and side scatter.

noted that monoclonal antibodies are supplied in various concentrations and are available in unconjugated form or conjugated to one of the following fluorochromes: fluorescein isothiocyanate (FITC), R-phycoerythrin (R-PE), BD Cy-Chrome (also known as PE-Cy5), peridinin chlorophyll protein (PerCP), PerCP-Cy 5.5, allophycocyanin (APC), and APC-Cy7. Each laboratory must determine the optimal concentration of each antibody and select the appropriate fluorochromes for its needs and applications.

Once the whole blood has been stained with the appropriate immunofluorescent antibodies, the specimens are analyzed on a flow cytometer. The two major manufacturers of clinical flow cytometers are Beckman Coulter and BD Biosciences. Prior to analysis of samples with a flow cytometer, it is imperative that the instrument be standardized and calibrated in order to provide accurate and reproducible data on a consistent basis. Detailed guidelines for the quality control and quality assurance of flow cytometric immunophenotyping in clinical laboratories have been published by the National Committee for Clinical Laboratory Standards (21). Every clinical laboratory involved in immunophenotyping of lymphocytes must develop a rigid set of protocols for the quality control and quality assurance of its flow cytometry. Such protocols should include daily calibration of the flow cytometer by using standardized immunofluorescent particles, which are available from several manufacturers. These standardized immunofluorescent particles should be used daily to verify that the optical alignment of the flow cytometer meets the manufacturer's specifications, and to calibrate the immunofluorescence and forward and right-angle light scatter properties that are appropriate for the fluorochrome-labeled cells (5). Fluorescence resolution and spectral-overlap compensation should be performed on a daily basis in accordance with National Committee for Clinical Laboratory Standards guidelines (21).

Quality control of the staining procedure is also necessary. For this purpose, laboratories should use a commercially available standardized preserved lymphocyte preparation, such as Status Flow (R & D systems), CD-Chex Plus (Streck [http://www.streck.com]), or BD Multi-Check (BD Biosciences) to serve as a positive control. The preserved lymphocytes should be stained with the same monoclonal antibodies as used in the basic immunophenotyping panel. The use of these cells will allow the clinical laboratory to determine inter- and intra-assay variation as well as provide long-term control for assay drift. The values obtained from a standardized lymphocyte panel should always fall within 2 standard deviations of a predetermined mean value for each phenotypic marker in the panel. The mean percentage of the values for any set of standardized lymphocytes should be calculated on the basis of at least 20 separate determinations made by using a completely calibrated flow cytometer. If the daily-standardized lymphocytes fall outside these specifications, then the results obtained for the patients' lymphocytes should be closely examined for accuracy and the determination should be repeated if appropriate. In addition to the use of standardized lymphocytes, fresh blood from healthy donors may be used as a positive control. However, it is not always possible to obtain fresh donors on any given day; therefore, the standardized lymphocytes offer the advantage of providing a calibrated control that can be analyzed with each set of specimens. When one is analyzing any cell population with a flow cytometer, it is important to collect between 5,000 and 10,000 cells during the analysis. The collection of this number of cells will effectively eliminate any

variability due to poor sampling numbers and provide good statistical power. Additionally, to ensure the satisfactory performance of CD4$^+$-T-cell measurements, clinical laboratories must participate in a performance evaluation program and demonstrate an acceptable level of performance (5). Performance evaluation programs for flow cytometry are offered by the DAIDS IQA Program (http://aactg.s-3.com), the College of American Pathologists Proficiency Testing Program (http://www.cap.org), and the Model Performance Evaluation Program (http://www.phppo.cdc.gov/MPEP/). If the dual-platform method is used for performing CD4$^+$-T-cell determinations, then the laboratory must also participate in a proficiency testing program for hematology, such as the College of American Pathologists program. Additionally, laboratories within the United States that perform CD4$^+$-T-cell determinations should be certified under the Clinical Laboratory Improvement Amendments (see http://www.cms.hhs.gov/clia).

In addition to reporting the percentage of positives for each of the lymphocyte populations in the standard immunophenotyping panel, one also reports the absolute number of these cells. As mentioned previously, absolute counts may be obtained with either the dual- or single-platform approach. If using the dual-platform approach to report absolute lymphocyte numbers, one must obtain a WBC and differential lymphocyte count on the patient sample. Once the percentages of lymphocytes are obtained from the differential, one can calculate the absolute number of cells in any subpopulation of lymphocytes by using the following formula: percentage of lymphocytes from differential × WBC × percentage of specific subpopulation obtained from appropriately calibrated flow cytometer = absolute number. Differential lymphocyte counts can be obtained from an automated hematology analyzer, or they can be performed by the manual method. Automated differential cell counting offers the advantage of being able to examine and count large numbers of cells (up to 10,000 lymphocytes), lending great statistical power. However, for patients who have AIDS, approximately 25 to 30% of the automated differentials may be flagged by the hematology instrument as containing unreadable cells. In these cases, an experienced hematology technician will be required to manually perform a visual evaluation of that slide. A manual differential count has the disadvantage of being a labor-intensive operation that does not offer the statistical power of the automated cell counters. However, a well-trained staff of hematology technicians can provide reliable and accurate differential cell counting from day to day and can also provide the clinicians with valuable information concerning unusual morphology of WBCs due to drug-induced changes or infection with HIV.

When using the single-platform method to provide absolute cell counts, most manufacturers of fluorospheres provide software that will automatically report calculated cell counts. If the program does not automatically calculate the values, then use the following formula: absolute cell count = (number of lymphocytes in bright CD45 region/number of fluorospheres in fluorosphere region) × (number of fluorospheres added/volume of blood added) (5).

In summary, immunophenotyping of patients with HIV infection can provide the most clinically relevant information as to the immunologic status of these patients. In light of the complex nature of the instrumentation required to perform immunophenotyping and the multiple steps necessary to prepare the cells for immunophenotyping, every laboratory must develop rigid quality assessment programs. Only through careful monitoring of immunophenotyping will it be possible to determine the efficacy of any experimental therapy. Described below is a dual-platform procedure for staining whole blood for immune cell phenotyping by flow cytometry, using Optilyse C lysing reagent. If using an alternative lysing reagent, follow the manufacturer's instructions.

Monoclonal Antibody Staining Procedure for Flow Cytometry (Three-Color)

Equipment

> Low-speed refrigerated centrifuge and carriers for 12- by 75-mm tubes
>
> Vortex mixer
>
> Polystyrene or polypropylene tubes (12 by 75 mm)

Reagents

> Optilyse C lysing buffer
>
> PBS
>
> Monoclonal antibodies

Procedure

1. Collect blood into EDTA anticoagulant. Mix blood thoroughly for a minimum of 1 to 2 min. Blood collected in acid-citrate-dextrose or heparin is also acceptable for this procedure; however, if one wishes to perform hematological testing and immunophenotyping from the same tube of blood, then EDTA is the preferred anticoagulant.

2. Label tubes (polypropylene or polystyrene, 12 by 75 mm) with sample identification and monoclonal antibody name.

3. To each tube add the appropriate fluorescently labeled monoclonal antibody at the manufacturer's recommended amount.

4. Carefully add 100 μl of patient blood to the bottom of each tube. When adding blood to the tubes, avoid making air bubbles and avoid getting blood on the inner sides of the tube. Excess blood on the inner side of a tube should be removed with a cotton swab. Specimens with WBC counts of ≤3,000/μl require double volumes of blood (200 μl).

5. Gently vortex all tubes and incubate them for 15 min at room temperature, in the dark (cover tube rack with aluminum foil).

6. Add 500 μl of Optilyse C lysing solution to each tube, and then immediately vortex each tube briefly. Allow lysing solution to incubate at room temperature in the dark (cover tube rack with aluminum foil) for at least 10 min. (Cells may be incubated in the lysing solution for up to 2 h without adversely affecting the results.)

7. Add 2 ml of PBS to each tube, vortex each tube immediately after the addition of the PBS, and centrifuge each tube at 250 to 300 × g for 5 min at room temperature. Resuspend the cell pellet by gently vortexing.

8. Wash the cells again with 2 ml of PBS; centrifuge at 300 × g for 5 min at room temperature.

9. Resuspend the cells in 400 μl of PBS and store at 4°C in the dark until analysis is performed.

10. Perform analysis on a flow cytometer within 24 h.

LPA

HIV infection results in a severe immunodeficiency which can be characterized by a selective depletion of the helper/inducer subset of T lymphocytes (CD4+). Some of the functional defects related to the loss of CD4+ T cells include decreases in in vitro lymphocyte proliferative responses to polyclonal mitogens, soluble antigens, and alloantigens. Consequently, the measurement of lymphocyte proliferative responses can be a very useful tool for determining the functional capacity of lymphocytes and for monitoring immunologic responses to therapy. During the course of HIV infection, the earliest proliferative dysfunction that appears is the inability of CD4+ T cells to recognize and proliferate in response to soluble recall antigens such as tetanus toxoid (TT), diphtheria toxin, *Candida albicans*, or purified protein derivative. Response to TT is the easiest of these antigens to monitor because a majority of the population has been previously exposed to this common immunogen. As the disease state progresses, the next proliferative response that disappears is the response to class II alloantigens, expressed on donor mononuclear cells in a mixed lymphocyte culture (MLC). During end-stage disease, a decline in proliferative responses to polyclonal mitogens such as phytohemagglutinin (PHA), pokeweed mitogen (PWM), and concanavalin A (ConA) can be seen. The order of loss of responsiveness in most patients is PWM, ConA, and finally PHA. Therefore, when one is monitoring proliferation of lymphocytes from AIDS patients, a basic panel of stimuli may include TT, MLC, PWM, PHA, and ConA. While lymphocyte proliferative responses are rather easy to monitor, it is not clear if these parameters have any clinical utility over the measurement of CD4 counts.

Additional monitoring of lymphocyte proliferation may be appropriate in the setting of certain therapeutic interventions. For example, when one is monitoring a trial in which a biological response modifier such as interleukin-2 (IL-2) is being administered, it is important to measure spontaneous proliferation of freshly isolated PBMCs. This assay consists of the in vitro assessment of the proliferative state of PBMCs in the absence of mitogen or antigen, and it can be used in lieu of cell cycle analysis to determine the relative fraction of cells synthesizing DNA in vivo. Similarly, if one is monitoring an HIV vaccine trial, the purified immunogen may be used as an in vitro proliferative stimulus in order to measure HIV-specific T-lymphocyte responses evoked by the vaccine. In such assays, an irrelevant protein which has been expressed in the same system as used to manufacture the vaccine should be included as a background control. Titration of the immunogen against a positive control cell population (cells known to respond to the immunogen) will help to determine the dose of immunogen necessary to achieve maximum proliferation. If a suitable human positive control is not available, PBMCs from other species, such as chimpanzees, immunized with the immunogen may be used for dose titration. Finally, cellular immune responses to HIV type 1 (HIV-1) may be detected by measuring proliferative responses to HIV-1-associated proteins and glycoproteins such as HIV-1 p24 antigen or HIV-1 envelope glycoprotein 120.

The measurement of lymphocyte proliferation involves the in vitro culture of PBMCs in the absence or presence of a stimulus. At the end of a specified incubation period, a radiolabeled DNA precursor (usually tritiated thymidine) is added, and the amount of radioactivity incorporated into the DNA of dividing cells is measured. Although the principle of this assay is straightforward, careful consideration must be given to standardization and quality control in order to minimize significant day-to-day variability. The best positive controls for this assay are cryopreserved PBMCs from at least three healthy donors who have been preselected for a defined level of proliferative activity. The positive control cells may be obtained by leukapheresis and cryopreserved in aliquots containing 5 million to 10 million cells. The positive control cells should be tested with each assay, and their activity may be used to monitor assay variability and to determine if the assay is working well. Each laboratory must also determine the optimal conditions for measuring proliferation. Each lot of antigen or mitogen should be titrated against normal PBMCs to achieve the correct concentration for maximum stimulation. It is also necessary to determine the optimal culture incubation times for each antigen or mitogen. Optimal polyclonal mitogen stimulation usually occurs in 2 to 4 days, while optimal antigen stimulation may take 5 to 7 days. An exception to this rule is PWM, for which the peak proliferative response is seen at day 6. Another variable, which should not be underestimated, is the choice of serum to be used in the assay medium. Not all lots of serum support cell growth equally; therefore, several lots should be tested to find one which gives low spontaneous background proliferation and supports optimal growth in the presence of mitogens or antigens. Pooled human AB serum from HIV-seronegative donors (final concentration, 15%) is recommended due to low backgrounds and high levels of stimulation.

As in all immunologic testing, quality control is an important part of the assay procedure. All pipetting devices should be calibrated to ensure accurate and consistent dilution of mitogens and antigens. All equipment, such as the incubator, cell harvester, and scintillation counter, should be calibrated periodically. All reagents and cultures must be kept sterile, since culture times range from 2 to 7 days. The use of laminar-flow hoods during all technical procedures is recommended to decrease the probability of bacterial or fungal contamination. The LPA may be performed with PBMCs that have been isolated from either heparin- or acid-citrate-dextrose-anticoagulated blood. EDTA is not a suitable anticoagulant for LPA. In order to minimize the effects of blood storage conditions on LPA, blood must be held at room temperature and PBMCs should be isolated within 30 h of venipuncture. Cells should be plated in the assay as soon as possible. Although cryopreserved PBMCs may be tested with the assay, freshly isolated PBMCs are often the best choice because cells from some HIV-infected patients do not survive cryopreservation well.

The data generated by LPAs can be expressed in various ways. Although the method of data expression is left to the discretion of each laboratory, the three most commonly used methods are net counts per minute (cpm), stimulation index, and relative proliferation index.

Net cpm = cpm of stimulated culture − cpm of unstimulated culture

Stimulation index = cpm of stimulated culture/cpm of unstimulated culture

Relative proliferation index = net cpm of patient sample/mean net cpm of a panel of at least three healthy donors that have been tested simultaneously in the assay

Equipment

96-well U-bottom microtiter plates
Humidified incubator with 5% CO_2
Cell harvester (Harvester 96 Mach 3M, Tomtec)
Scintillation fluid (Betaplate Scint, LKB Wallac)
Scintillation counter (Microbeta Trilux, LKB Wallac)
Mechanical pipettes
96-well filtermats (LKB Wallac)

Filtermat sample bags (LKB Wallac)
Heat sealer (LKB Wallac)

Reagents

Serumless medium: RPMI 1640 medium without L-glutamine, 2% 1 M HEPES buffer, 1% 200 mM L-glutamine, 50 μg of gentamicin per ml

30% human AB medium: serumless medium supplemented with 30% heat-inactivated human AB serum

[methyl-³H]thymidine, specific activity of 6.7 Ci/mmol (NEN Research Products)

Dulbecco's PBS without Ca^{2+} or Mg^{2+}, pH 7.4

Mitogen and Antigen Preparation

PHA (Murex; catalog no. HA16): Make a 1:100 dilution of stock PHA (2 mg/ml) with 30% human AB medium (final concentration, 20 μg/ml). Use 20 μl per well (final concentration, 2 μg/ml).

ConA (Sigma; catalog no. C-2010): Make a 1:2 and a 1:4 dilution of ConA stock (2 mg/ml) with 30% human AB medium (final concentrations, 1 and 0.5 mg/ml). Use 20 μl per well (final concentrations, 100 and 50 μg/ml).

MLC: Obtain PBMCs from six healthy donors by the Ficoll-Hypaque method. Cryopreserve cells from each donor in aliquots of 5×10^6 cells per ml, using a controlled-rate freezer, and irradiate them in the frozen state with 7,500 rads from a ^{137}Cs irradiator. On the day of assay, thaw one aliquot of each normal sample and pool the aliquots. Adjust the cell concentration to 10^6 cells per ml with 30% human AB medium. Use 50 μl (total of 50,000 cells) per well.

TT (Calbiochem; catalog no. 582231): Reconstitute 25 μg of TT with 2.5 ml of 30% human AB medium (final concentration, 10 μg/ml). Use 20 μl per well (final concentration, 1 μg/ml).

PWM (Sigma; catalog no. L-9379): Make a 1:80 dilution of stock PWM with 30% human AB medium. Use 20 μl per well (final dilution of 1:800).

Recombinant HIV-1 MN envelope glycoprotein 120 (catalog no. 1021; Immunodiagnostics, Inc.): Make a 1:10 and a 1:2 dilution of gp120 stock (100 μg/ml) with 30% human AB medium (final concentrations, 10 and 50 μg/ml). Use 20 μl per well (final concentrations, 1 and 5 μg/ml).

Recombinant HIV-1 NY5 p24 viral protein (Protein Sciences Corp.; catalog no. 2004): Make a 1:2 dilution of p24 stock (100 μg/ml) with 30% human AB medium (final concentration, 50 μg/ml). Use 20 μl per well (final concentration, 5 μg/ml).

Procedure

1. Isolate PBMCs by the Ficoll-Hypaque method, and adjust the concentration to 10^6 cells per ml in serumless medium.

2. Plate three control wells per patient per stimulus. Control wells contain mononuclear cells with no stimulus: 100 μl of cells (10^6/ml) in serumless medium and 100 μl of 30% human AB medium.

3. Plate three stimulated wells per patient per stimulus. Stimulus wells contain mononuclear cells and a stimulus.
    a. For PHA, ConA, TT, PWM, p24, or gp120: 100 μl of cells (10^6/ml) in serumless medium, 80 μl of 30% human AB medium, and 20 μl of appropriate mitogen or antigen.

b. For MLC: 100 μl of cells (10^6/ml) in serumless medium, 50 μl of 30% human AB medium, and 50 μl of MLC.

4. For spontaneous blastogenesis, plate six wells per patient. Each well contains the following: 100 μl of cells (10^6/ml) in serumless medium and 100 μl of 30% human AB medium.

5. Place 200 μl of PBS into all empty wells (this prevents fluid loss from sample wells due to evaporation).

6. Keep plates sterile and incubate them at 37°C in a humidified, 5% CO_2 incubator. Incubation times are as follows: 0 h for spontaneous blastogenesis; 3 days for PHA and ConA; 5 days for p24, gp120, and MLC; and 6 days for TT and PWM.

7. Pulse each well with 0.4 μCi of [^{3}H]thymidine in 20 μl of serumless medium at the end of the specified incubation period.

8. Incubate the plates for an additional 4 h at 37°C in a humidified, 5% CO_2 incubator.

9. Harvest cells onto fiberglass filtermats with a cell harvester (LKB Wallac) or equivalent. Allow the filtermats to air dry. Add scintillation fluid to each filtermat, and count cells in a liquid scintillation counter for 1 min.

10. Determine the mean, standard deviation, and standard error of the mean for each triplicate. Note: Since incubation times vary with mitogen, PHA and ConA may be put on the same 96-well plate (3 days), whereas MLC, p24, and gp120 must be run on a plate with appropriate controls (5 days); TT and PWM can be put on the same plate (6 days).

EVALUATION OF CELL TURNOVER

Much debate exists over the mechanisms by which HIV-1 infection disrupts CD4 T-cell homeostasis. Numerous procedures for measuring cell turnover rates have been employed to further our understanding of T-cell dynamics during HIV-1 infection, including assessing the impact of highly active antiretroviral therapy and IL-2 immunotherapy. Some of the methods introduced in such studies include ex vivo [^{3}H]thymidine incorporation (16), telomere terminal restriction fragment length (7), T-cell rearrangement excision circles (6), Ki67 staining (23), ex vivo and in vivo BrdU incorporation (15, 18), and in vivo incorporation of deuterated glucose or deuterated water (10, 11).

In recent years investigators have focused on more direct measures of cell turnover by directly quantitating the fraction of cycling cells. One such ex vivo method includes flow cytometric analysis of the expression of the nuclear protein Ki67 (8). Ki67 expression increases in late G_1 phase of the cell cycle and remains elevated throughout mitosis (8). Antisense experiments indicate that Ki67 expression may be important for cellular proliferation and survival (12, 16). Importantly, Ki67 is not expressed in resting cells (1), thereby making this molecule a reasonable marker of cell cycle progression. One of the main advantages of Ki67 detection is that it can be used on cryopreserved cells; however, one potential disadvantage is that cells blocked in cell cycle progression or cells in a preactivated nondividing state may be positive for Ki67. Another ex vivo method of measuring cell turnover is BrdU incorporation. BrdU is a thymidine analog taken up by cells through the nucleotide salvage pathway, converted into BrdUTP, and incorporated into the DNA of dividing cells. Monoclonal antibodies are available to detect DNA-incorporated BrdU by flow cytometry. The one main disadvantage of the ex vivo BrdU labeling method

is that it must be done on freshly isolated cells. The Ki67 detection and ex vivo BrdU labeling methods provide a rapid and relatively inexpensive "snapshot" of the level of dividing cells in the blood or lymph nodes.

In vivo kinetic studies are extremely informative; however, they are significantly more expensive to conduct since they require the use of large amounts of labeling reagent, a clinical infrastructure, and long-term longitudinal follow-up (months to years) to obtain sufficient data points during the labeling and delabeling phases of the study. The main advantage of kinetic studies is that mathematical modeling can simultaneously determine the values of numerous biological parameters, including the portion of actively dividing cells, cell proliferation and death rates, the fraction of newly added cells, and the effects of cellular trafficking. The biological assumptions underlying the various models are controversial, and thus investigators partaking in such studies should consult with a mathematician. In vivo infusions of BrdU, deuterated glucose, or deuterated water are currently the methods of choice for in vivo labeling studies. Deuterated glucose is taken up by cells and converted de novo to deuterated deoxynucleoside triphosphates (dNTPs) via the pentose phosphate pathway, followed by incorporation into the DNA of dividing cells. Differences among the conclusions of a number of published papers describing in vivo labeling kinetics in patients with HIV-1 infection are mostly due to the differences in the assumptions and design of the mathematical models as opposed to the results of the raw kinetic data; i.e., there are relatively consistent findings in the raw labeling-delabeling kinetics. Despite these shortcomings, mathematical modeling is allowing for the generation of testable hypotheses that should address some of the model assumptions.

The following sections describe optimized protocols for ex vivo and in vivo BrdU incorporation, Ki67 staining, and in vivo labeling with deuterated glucose. Representative data from cross-sectional and longitudinal studies comparing these methods are presented and show that the different techniques are well correlated.

In Vivo Labeling of Lymphocytes with Deuterated Glucose

In Vivo Cell Labeling and Isolation

For the method described below, all subjects participated in an Institutional Review Board-approved clinical protocol and all subjects provided written informed consent. Deuterated glucose (Isotec, Inc., Miamisburg, Ohio, or Cambridge Isotope Laboratories, Inc., Andover, Mass.) was administered to subjects by continuous intravenous infusion over 5 days at a dose of 60 g per day. Subjects underwent a one- or two-pass lymphapheresis, and PBMCs were obtained following Ficoll-Hypaque gradient centrifugation. PBMCs were further separated by flow cytometric sorting into lymphocyte subsets by following manufacturer's recommended instructions with the monoclonal antibodies CD3 FITC, CD4 PE (BD Immunocytometry Systems, San Jose, Calif.), and CD8 Cy-Chrome (BD Biosciences Pharmingen, San Diego, Calif.). Cell sorting was performed using an amorphous forward light scatter and 90° light scatter gate and a linear gate on CD3 FITC$^+$ fluorescence to identify T lymphocytes. T lymphocytes were further divided into CD4 and CD8 subsets based on amorphous gates for CD4 PE$^+$ fluorescence and CD8 Cy-Chrome$^+$ fluorescence. CD4 and CD8 T-cell purity was documented by flow cytometry to be >99.0%.

Genomic DNA Isolation and Hydrolysis

Genomic DNA was isolated from the 0.5 million to 4 million frozen pelleted cells using the Puregene kit (Gentra Systems, Minneapolis, Minn.) and pelleted DNA hydrated overnight with 25 μl of deionized water. In preparation for DNA hydrolysis, phosphodiesterase I (PDE I) (Worthington Biochemical Corp., Lakewood, N.J.) is reconstituted to 0.05 U/μl with PDE I storage buffer (100 mM Tris-HCl [pH 8.8], 100 mM NaCl, 15 mM MgCl$_2$, 50% glycerol) and stored at -20°C for no more than 3 months. The 25 μl of rehydrated genomic DNA was hydrolyzed to free deoxyribonucleosides by adding 25 μl of hydrolysis solution (30 U of DNase I [Invitrogen, Frederick, Md.], 0.1 U of reconstituted PDE I, 25 U of bacterial alkaline phosphatase [Invitrogen], 10 mM freshly added dithiothreitol, 100 mM NaCl, 40 mM Tris-HCl [pH 8.0], 20 mM MgCl$_2$) and incubating overnight at 37°C. Digestates were stored at -20°C until analysis. Prior to analysis, the digestate was cleaned up by reversed-phase solid-phase extraction, using an Oasis HLB (30 mg) 96-well extraction plate (Waters Corp., Milford, Mass.) prepared as follows: 1 ml of methanol was aspirated through each well under vacuum, followed by 1 ml of deionized water. To each well were pipetted 300 μl of 100 mM phosphate buffer (pH 7.0) and 50 μl of the DNA digestate. The sample solution was aspirated through the sorbent bed, followed by 0.5 ml of deionized water, and allowed to dry by aspirating air. Aspirating 0.5 ml of methanol effects elution of the deoxyribonucleosides. The eluate was collected, split into two equal volumes, and evaporated to dryness using a vacuum centrifuge (model RC10.10; Jouan, Winchester, Va.). For micro-column high-performance liquid chromatography/mass spectrometry (μHPLC/MS) analysis the residue was reconstituted in 50 μl of deionized water, followed by agitation for 1 min on a vortex mixer, and then transferred to a 96-V-shaped-well polypropylene microtiter plate and analyzed by μHPLC/MS.

Quantitation of Deuterated-dA Enrichment in Genomic DNA by HPLCEIS/MS

All μHPLC-electrospray ionization (ESI)/MS experiments were carried out using Agilent Technology 1110 series instrumentation. The μHPLC system was connected on-line to an MSD/Trap equipped with an ESI source, and with Hewlett-Packard (Palo Alto, Calif.) Vectra PC running Chemstation software for data acquisition and instrument control. Chromatography was carried out using a glass-lined stainless steel (SGE, Austin, Tex.) microanalytical column (100 mm long by 0.5 mm [internal diameter]) packed in-house with Luna C$_{18}$, 5 μM particles (Phenomenex, Torrance, Calif.). A sample volume of 1 μl was injected and eluted using a 15-μl/min mobile phase gradient beginning at 3% (vol/vol) acetonitrile and 97% 5 mM ammonium acetate, pH 5.0, for 1 min and increased linearly to 40% (vol/vol) acetonitrile over 6 min and held for 3 min, after which initial conditions were restored. EIS/MS data were acquired in positive-ion mode using the following ion source conditions: drying gas temperature, 250°C at a flow of 7 liters/min; nebulizer pressure, 15 lb/in^2; and capillary voltage, $-3,000$ V. The ion trap settings used were as follows: accumulation time, 100 ms; ion charge control target, 30,000; and scan range, m/z 248 to 258. Extracted ion chromatograms were generated for m/z 252 and 254, corresponding to the protonated molecular ions $(M + H)^+$ of deoxyadenosine (dA) and deuterated dA, respectively. Quantitation was performed using a standard calibration curve. The ratio of the peak area of deuterated dA (m/z 252) to that of the total

dA pool (m/z 252 + 254) was determined and compared to a concentration-independent calibration curve generated by mixtures of deuterated dA (Cambridge Isotope Laboratories, Inc.) and dA (Sigma, St. Louis, Mo.) of known composition from 0 to 10% enrichment.

Extraction and Processing of Serum Glucose

Glucose was extracted from 200 μl of serum by the addition of 800 μl of methanol, incubation for 1 h and centrifugation at 16,000 × g for 15 min. The supernatant containing the extracted glucose was stored at -20°C until analysis. Glucose extracts were dried using a vacuum concentrator or dry nitrogen gas and resuspended in 200 μl of 11% aldolnitrile. The samples were transferred to 1-ml glass autosampler vials, and the solution was evaporated to dryness at 50°C under a stream of nitrogen gas. The dried sample is derivatized by adding 150 μl of 2% hydroxylamine HCl in dry pyridine (2% [wt/wt]). The vials are sealed and heated at 90°C for 1 h. The aldolnitrile penta-acetate derivative of glucose was synthesized by adding 50 μl of acetic anhydride. The vials were sealed and heated at 60°C for 1 h. The solvents in the resulting solution were evaporated under a stream of nitrogen gas at 50°C, and 100 μl of acetonitrile was added to the dry reaction mixture and vortexed for 30 s.

Technical notes: Deuterium will be incorporated into all four dNTPs through the de novo-synthesized pathway and incorporated into genomic DNA of dividing cells; however, deuterated dA is the easiest to detect. As a result of dNTPs being synthesized through pathways that do not include glucose as a precursor, only a maximum of 60% of the dA in the genomic DNA will become enriched with deuterated dA; thus, raw enrichment values must be correct by a factor of 1.67. An additional adjustment must be made for the dilution of deuterated glucose by endogenous blood glucose. This is accomplished by daily measurements of deuterated-glucose enrichment levels in serum during the infusion (see procedure below) and multiplying serum deuterated-glucose enrichment values by the average daily dilution factor.

Quantitation of Deuterated Glucose in Serum by GC/MS

Derivatized glucose samples were analyzed using an HP 5790 (Hewlett-Packard) gas chromatograph (GC) interfaced to a VG 70-250HF (VG Analytical, Ltd., Manchester, United Kingdom) mass spectrometer. One microliter of the sample was injected onto a 60-m, 0.32-mm (inside diameter), 15-μm-film DB-17ht (J & W Scientific, Folsom, Calif.) fused silica capillary column via splitless injection. Helium at a flow rate of 1 ml/min was used as the carrier gas. Injector, transfer line, and ion source temperatures were 260, 270, and 220°C, respectively. The GC oven was programmed for 140°C with a 1-min hold followed by a ramp of 15°C per min to 280°C, with a 5-min hold at 280°C. The mass spectrometer is operated in the electron ionization selected ion recording mode. It is set to monitor the fragment ions at m/z 217 and 219. Dwell times on each ion are 50 ms, with a 10-ms interchannel delay. Other MS experimental parameters are as follows: resolution, 1,000; trap current, 100 μA; electron multiplier, 2.5 to 3.0 kV; and electron energy, 70 eV. Quantitation was performed using a standard calibration curve. The ratio of the peak area of deuterated glucose (m/z 219) to that of the total glucose pool (m/z 217 + 219) was determined and compared to a concentration-independent calibration curve generated by mixtures of deuterated glucose (Cambridge Isotope Laboratories, Inc.) and glucose (Sigma) of known composition from 0 to 50% enrichment.

In Vivo BrdU Labeling of Dividing Lymphocytes

Patients and BrdU Infusion

For the method described below, HIV-infected subjects who were infused with BrdU were participants in an Institutional Review Board-approved clinical protocol, and all subjects provided written informed consent. Subjects who were pregnant or breast-feeding or receiving 5-fluorouracil were excluded from participation. While BrdU has been used in cancer patients as a marker for rates of cell turnover without any observed toxicities, it has been shown to be teratogenic in animal models. For this reason, the risk/benefit ratio precludes the infusion of BrdU in healthy volunteers. Participants in the study were counseled to practice effective contraception. BrdU (NEOMARK-BU) was supplied by NeoPharm through the National Cancer Institute and infused at a dose of 200 mg/m^2 over 30 min.

Cell Staining and Flow Cytometry

Ten milliliters of whole blood was collected into an EDTA-containing tube at various times following BrdU administration. Lymph node biopsy samples were collected from some subjects, teased to release lymphocytes and pushed through a mesh screen to obtain a single cell suspension, and then processed as for whole blood. Two 1-ml aliquots from each tube were used for three-color flow cytometric staining with monoclonal antibodies anti-BrdU FITC and anti-CD45RO PE (BD Immunocytometry Systems) crossed with either anti-CD4 PC5 or anti-CD8 PC5 (Beckman Coulter). Nonspecific antibody binding sites were blocked by adding 100 μl of 25-mg/ml immunoglobulin G (ChemiCon International, Inc., Temecula, Calif.) and incubating the mixtures for 10 min. Each cell surface-staining fluorescent antibody was added to the appropriate tube and incubated for 15 min. RBCs were lysed by incubation with 5 ml of Optilyse C lysing solution (Immunotech, Westbrook, Maine) for 10 min. Cells were washed twice with PBS and then fixed and permeabilized by incubation with 1 ml of 1% para formaldehyde plus 1% Tween 20 for 15 min at 37°C. Cells were washed with PBS and incubated with 300 μl of DNase I solution (100 U of DNase I [Roche Applied Science, Indianapolis, Ind.], PBS, 4.2 mM MgCl$_2$ [pH 5.0]) for 30 min at 37°C. The reaction was terminated by the addition of 1 ml of DNase I stopping solution (1% bovine serum albumin [BSA], 0.5% Tween 20, PBS). Cells were washed with PBS and incubated with 100 μl of 25-mg/ml mouse immunoglobulin G for 10 min. Precleared anti-BrdU was added to each tube and incubated for 30 min, followed by two washes with 3 ml of PBS. Cells were resuspended in 500 μl of PBS and analyzed on a Coulter XL flow cytometer. A total of 20,000 to 50,000 gated events were collected for most samples; a minimum of 5,000 gated events were collected when the gated cell count was low.

Technical notes: The DNA in the cells must be digested in order for the anti-BrdU antibody to bind to the incorporated BrdU in the DNA structure. The action of DNase is time, temperature, and pH dependent and should be optimized in each laboratory setting. The BrdU-negative gate is determined by using a sample of blood drawn before the infusion of BrdU. The positive staining of in vivo-labeled BrdU cells is not well separated from the BrdU-negative cells, and thus it takes a skilled, experienced operator to set the gates. This procedure has an impact on the light scatter properties of the cells, and care must be taken to exclude monocytes and granulocytes from analysis due to their autofluoresence properties. This autofluoresence may appear as positive BrdU staining. BrdU labeling peaks at approximately day 1 after infusion with lymph node T cells and at days 3 to 5 in peripheral blood T cells.

Ex Vivo BrdU Labeling of Dividing Cells in Whole Blood

Cell Labeling

Ten milliliters of whole blood was collected into an EDTA-containing tube and 4.5 ml was aliquoted into two 15-ml tubes. Ten microliters of BrdU (Sigma) at 3 μg/ml was added to one tube of blood, with the other tube serving as a BrdU-negative control. Samples were incubated at 37°C and 5% CO$_2$ for 4 h. Cell staining and flow cytometry were performed as described in "In Vivo BrdU Labeling of Dividing Lymphocytes."

Technical notes: Comments are the same as for in vivo BrdU labeling except that the BrdU-positive cells are determined by setting the gate based on the "without BrdU" sample.

Detection of Dividing Cells by Ki67 Staining

Cell Staining

Ki67 can be detected in lymphocytes of either freshly isolated whole blood or cryopreserved PBMCs. For each sample four tubes are prepared for cell surface phenotyping and Ki67 analysis: (i) CD3 FITC/isotype PE/CD4 PE-Cy5, (ii) CD3 FITC/Ki67 PE/CD4 PE-Cy5, (iii) CD3/isotype PE/CD8 PE-Cy5, and (iv) CD3/isotype PE/CD8 PE-Cy5. CD3 FITC, isotype PE, CD4 PE-Cy5, and CD8 PE-Cy5 were purchased from BD Biosciences Pharmingen. Cell surface staining was performed by incubating the appropriate antibodies with 1 ml of whole-blood cells or 1 ml of PBMCs (one million to five million cells) for 15 min. RBCs were lysed with 5 ml of Optilyse C lysing solution (Immunotech) for 10 min. Cells were washed twice with PBS and then fixed and permeabilized by incubation with 1 ml of 1% paraformaldehyde plus 1% Tween 20 for 15 min at 37°C. Cells were washed twice in PBS, resuspended in 1 ml of Ki67 staining buffer (anti-Ki67 PE or isotype PE antibody, PBS with 1% BSA and 0.5% Tween 20), and incubated for 30 min. Cells were washed twice and resuspended in 600 μl of PBS and analyzed on a Coulter XL flow cytometer.

Technical notes: Gating for Ki67-positive cells is accomplished by setting the region on the isotype control to less than 1% positive.

Comparison of Ex Vivo and In Vivo T-Cell Labeling Methods

An important question that should be addressed before drawing conclusions based on T-cell turnover data derived from whole blood is whether blood, a compartment that only contains about 2% of the total body T cells, is representative of major body compartments harboring the majority of T cells. To evaluate this, ex vivo BrdU incorporation was measured in CD4 and CD8 T cells in paired samples of freshly drawn blood and freshly isolated lymph nodes from 14 HIV-infected subjects (Fig. 1A). There was good correlation between the proliferation rates of the T cells in the blood and lymph nodes, implying that the measures in the blood are representative of division rates in the peripheral tissue.

Ex vivo BrdU incorporation in T cells was compared to Ki67 staining in a cross-sectional study of 56 blood samples that were isolated from healthy controls and HIV-infected subjects (Fig. 1B). Significant correlations existed between ex vivo BrdU incorporation rates and Ki67 positivity in both CD4 and CD8 T cells, although the level of Ki67 was significantly lower in CD8 cells than it was in CD4 cells. Ex vivo BrdU incorporation was also compared to Ki67 staining in a longitudinal study of three HIV-infected subjects (Fig. 1C). High within-subject correlations were seen for CD4 T cells. These results show that Ki67 and ex vivo BrdU incorporation measure similar changes in proliferation rates and thus are qualitatively comparable despite yielding different absolute numbers. The difference in absolute numbers is due to BrdU being incorporated only into those cells going through S phase, while Ki67 is expressed in cells in late G_1, S, and G_2/M phases of the cell cycle whether the cell is actively dividing or not.

Two studies showed that ex vivo BrdU incorporation and Ki67 staining correlated with in vivo BrdU labeling levels. In the first study, ex vivo BrdU incorporation levels in CD4 and CD8 T cells determined in 14 subjects just before a 30-min BrdU administration were shown to correlate with peak in vivo BrdU incorporation levels (Fig. 2A); BrdU peaks in lymph node and blood T cells around day 1 and days 3 to 5, respectively, and is in approximately equal levels in both compartments after about 1 day (15). In a second study of six subjects infused with BrdU, levels of Ki67 staining in T cells were found to correlate with the in vivo incorporation of BrdU in T cells (Fig. 2B). Ex vivo BrdU incorporation and Ki67 measures are comparable to each other and to in vivo BrdU labeling, giving confidence that these methods measure similar biological events.

Comparison of in vivo deuterated-glucose labeling and in vivo BrdU incorporation showed high correlation between these methods. Figure 3 shows the results of a double-label infusion in which a subject was given deuterated glucose for 5 days, followed by a 30-min infusion of BrdU on day 5. Samples were collected longitudinally for 16 months. Deuterated-dA enrichment in genomic DNA of CD4 cells and in vivo BrdU incorporation levels in CD4 cells were determined. Decay rates of the two labels in CD4 T cells were similar (Fig. 3A) and are highly correlated (Fig. 3B).

Summary

A number of methods have been developed to measure T-cell turnover rates in HIV-infected subjects. Protocols for two ex vivo methods, BrdU incorporation and Ki67 staining, and two in vivo methods, BrdU incorporation and deuterated-glucose labeling, are described and shown to yield data that are well correlated. The main differences in studies of cell turnover in subjects with HIV infection come in the design and interpretation of in vivo kinetic models, despite the studies yielding similar raw kinetic data. Additional creative studies are required to test the various conclusions drawn from the in vivo modeling studies.

QUANTITATION OF THYMIC FUNCTION

During maturation in the thymus, T cells undergo rearrangement of their T-cell receptor genes. The antigen recognition domains of the T-cell receptor are generated by site-specific somatic DNA recombination events. During the generation of a coding T-cell receptor chain chromosomal DNA, intervening DNA sequences are excised as episomal circles. These episomes, TRECs, are stable and persist in newly matured T cells; they do not replicate and are diluted out during mitosis of these cells or lost when these cells die. Quantitation of TRECs present in naive T cells is considered to be an accurate measure of thymic function.

A.

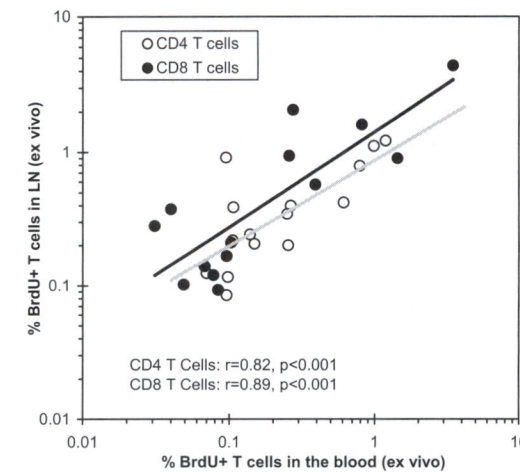

B.

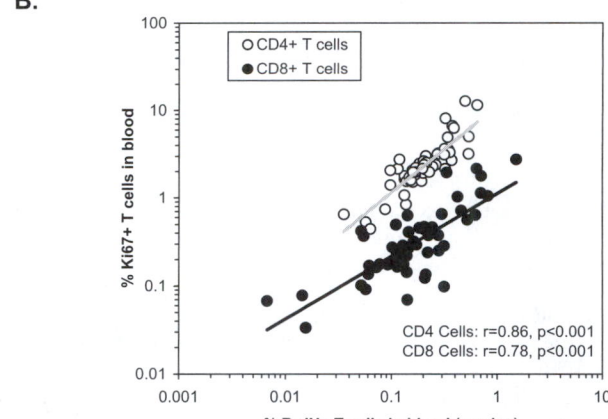

C.

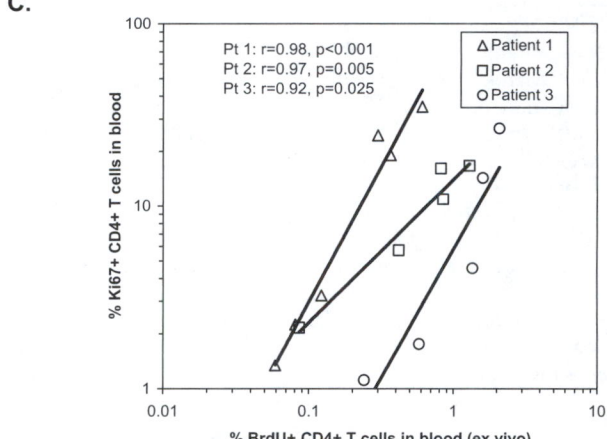

FIGURE 1 Ex vivo methods of cell turnover are well correlated. (A) Ex vivo BrdU incorporation levels for CD4 and CD8 T cells correlated in paired samples from freshly isolated blood and lymph node suspensions from 14 subjects infected with HIV-1; (B) ex vivo BrdU incorporation correlated with Ki67 staining using the same blood samples from 56 individuals that were either healthy controls or infected with HIV; (C) ex vivo BrdU incorporation correlated with Ki67 staining in CD4 T cells from longitudinal blood samples taken once every day or two from three HIV-infected subjects.

A.

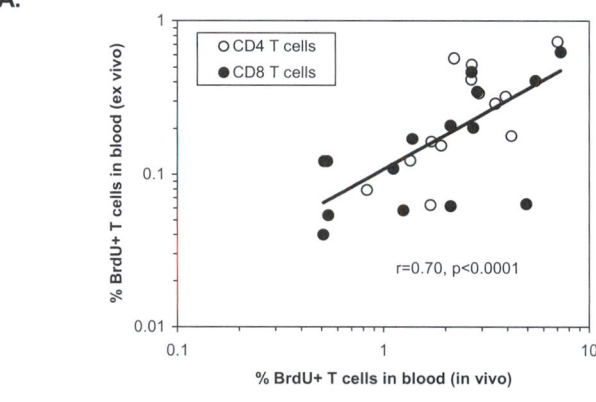

B.

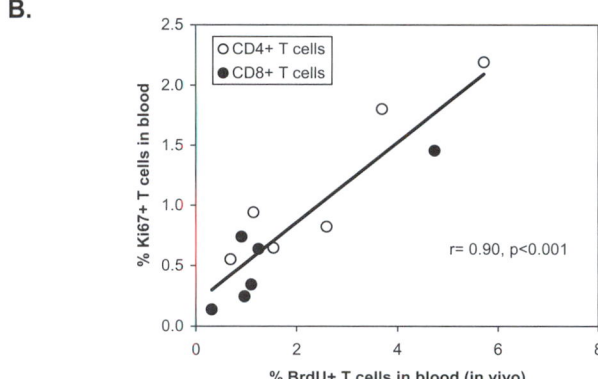

FIGURE 2 Ex vivo BrdU incorporation and Ki67 staining methods correlated with in vivo BrdU labeling. (A) Ex vivo BrdU incorporation levels in CD4 and CD8 T cells determined for 14 HIV-infected subjects just before a 30-min in vivo BrdU administration were shown to correlate with peak in vivo BrdU incorporation levels; (B) Ki67 T-cell staining levels were found to correlate with the in vivo BrdU T-cell incorporation levels in six HIV-infected subjects infused with BrdU.

The natural course of HIV-1 infection involves depletion of $CD4^+$ T cells and a continuous demand for production of $CD4^+$ T cells. Even though the thymus may shrink with age, recent data suggest that the thymus is still functionally active in adults. A desirable consequence of successful treatment of HIV infection is the restoration of thymic function. Therefore, laboratories interested in immune reconstitution during HIV treatment may find it helpful to use TRECs as a marker to assess thymic function (20).

TRECs in PBMCs and purified $CD4^+$ and $CD8^+$ cells may be quantitated by real-time PCR, based on the Taqman principle (http://www.appliedbiosystems.com/support/apptech/#rt_pcr) (9). Real-time PCR measures the amount of DNA present in the sample by PCR amplification as it occurs using a fluorescently labeled probe (Taqman probe). A probe, labeled with a fluorescent reporter dye at the 5′ end and a quencher dye at the 3′ end, is added to the PCR mixture along with the primers. The probe is designed to bind internally to PCR primers. When the probe is intact, the emission intensity of the fluorescent dye is reduced by the quencher dye. During PCR, while extending the primer, the DNA polymerase digests the probe and the fluorescent dye is

A.

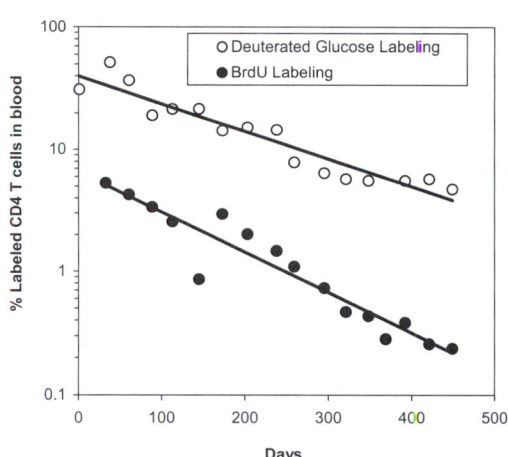

B.

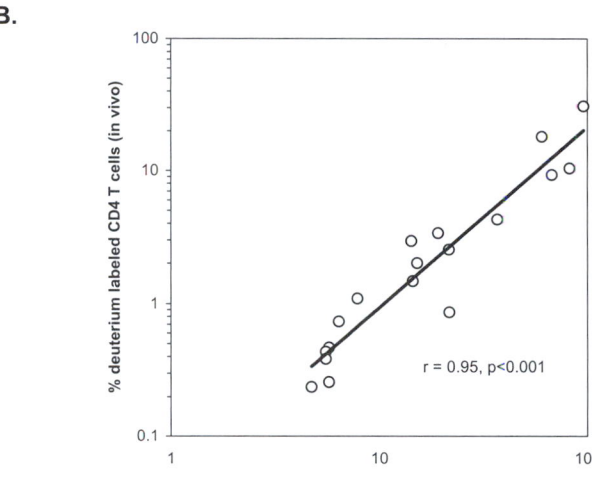

FIGURE 3 In vivo BrdU incorporation correlates with in vivo deuterated-glucose labeling in a double-labeling study. A 30-min infusion of BrdU and a 5-day continuous infusion of deuterated glucose were administered to an HIV-infected subject. (A) Samples were assayed for label incorporation and decay in CD4 T cells over a 1.5-year period; (B) in vivo BrdU incorporation and decay were highly correlated with incorporation and decay levels of deuterated glucose.

released from the quencher dye. The intensity of the fluorescence is proportional to the amount of DNA present in the sample. The cycle at which the fluorescence intensity is statistically significant at a point above the baseline value is designated as the threshold cycle. The level of TRECs in experimental samples is derived from a standard curve generated by plotting the log concentration of the standard against the threshold cycle (Fig. 4).

Equipment

Real-time PCR system (ABI Prism 7700 sequence detector)
Heat blocks at 65 and 95°C
Low-speed centrifuge
0.2-ml PCR tubes

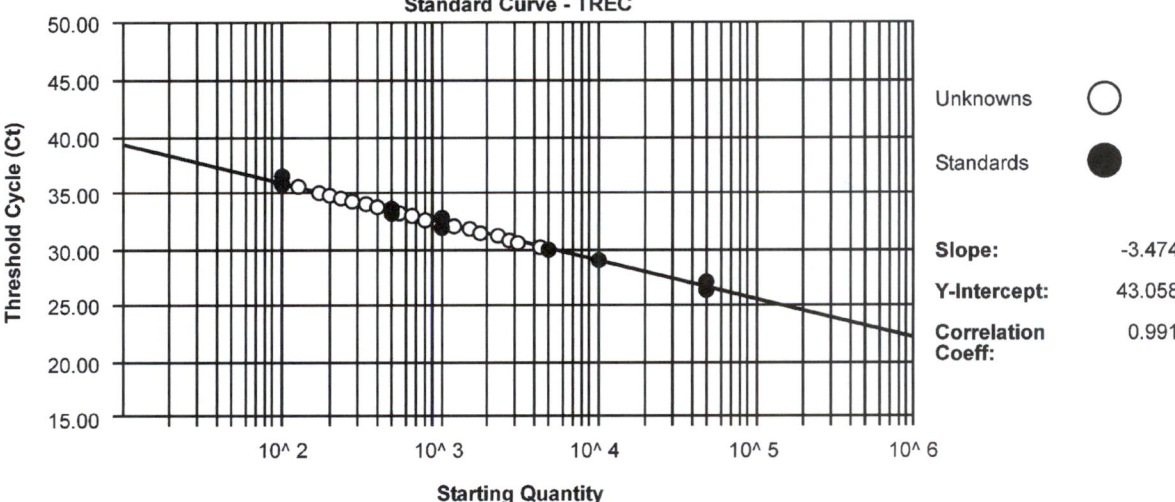

FIGURE 4 Quantitation of TRECs in patient samples. Shown is a standard curve plotting log starting TREC copy number versus threshold cycle. The amounts of TREC in unknown samples were calculated from the standard curve by using ABI Prism 7700 software.

Reagents

Lysis buffer A: 10 mM Tris-HCl (pH 8.0), 100 mM KCl, and 2.5 mM MgCl$_2$

Lysis buffer B: 10 mM Tris-HCl (pH 8.0), 2.5 mM MgCl$_2$, 1% NP-40, and 1% Tween 20

Proteinase K (catalog no. 1964372; Roche Applied Science). Add proteinase K to a final concentration of 20 mg/ml to buffer B just before using buffer B.

Platinum Taq polymerase, 10× PCR buffer, 50 mM MgCl$_2$ (Invitrogen kit; catalog no. 10966-026), and 10 mM concentration of dNTP mixture (catalog no. 18427-013; Invitrogen).

Passive reference dye Blue 636 (Megabases Inc.)

PCR primers and probe: Primers and probe can be purchased from a number of vendors.

  Reverse primer: 5′-GCCAGCTGCAGGGGTTTAGG-3′

  Forward primer: 5′-CACATCCCTTTCAACCAT-GCT-3′

  Probe: 5′–6-carboxyfluorescein (6-FAM)–ACACCT-CTGGTTTTTGTAAAGGTGCCCACT-3′ carboxy-tetramethylrhodamine (TAMRA)

Jurkat cell line (American Type Culture Collection): Maintain in RPMI 1640 medium.

Plasmid standard: SJ plasmid that contains TREC sequence is used as a standard in PCR (19). This plasmid is diluted to 1 pg/μl (280,000 copies/μl) in water and stored as aliquots at −20°C. The plasmid is further diluted with Jurkat cell lysate for inclusions in PCR as a standard.

Lysis of patient and Jurkat cells:

  (i) Suspend the cells in lysis buffer A (250 μl per million cells) and add an equal volume of lysis buffer B.

  (ii) Mix equal volumes of lysis buffer A and B to use as a negative control.

  (iii) Incubate at 65°C for 1.0 h in a heat block.

  (iv) Incubate at 95°C for 15 min. The samples are ready to use for PCR or can be stored at 4°C. Long-term storage should be at −20°C.

PCR master mix (one reaction)

10× Platinum Taq buffer	10 μl
50 mM MgCl$_2$	7 μl
10 mM concentration each of dATP, dGTP, dTTP, and dCTP	2 μl
25 pmol of forward primer per μl	2 μl
25 pmol of reverse primer per μl	2 μl
7.5 pmol of probe per μl	2 μl
10 pmol of internal reference dye Blue 636 per μl ..	0.25 μl
5 U of Platinum Taq per μl	0.25 μl
water	24.5 μl

Master mix without Taq polymerase can be prepared in a large volume and stored in 1-ml aliquots at −20°C. Prior to using in PCR, thaw an aliquot and add Taq polymerase.

Procedure

1. Prepare dilutions of the plasmid (SJ) standard containing 100, 500, 1,000, 5,000, 10,000 and 50,000 copies of TREC in 50 μl of Jurkat cell lysate.

2. Add the following components to a 0.2-ml PCR tube.
   a. Master mix (50 μl)
   b. Patient sample or Jurkat cell lysate containing the standard plasmid (50 μl)

3. Set up patient samples in duplicate and the standard plasmid in triplicate. Also set up no-template controls without any input DNA by adding 50 μl of lysis buffer.

4. Using the ABI Prism 7700 software, enter the sample, standard, and no-template control information and load the plate with the corresponding tubes.

5. Perform the PCR with the following cycling conditions: 95°C for 5 min followed by 40 cycles at 95°C for 30 s and 60°C for 1 min.

6. Analyze the data with the ABI Prism 7700 (sequence detection) software and determine the TREC values in patient samples.

7. An example of TREC quantitation is shown in Fig. 4. If the sample has fewer than 100 copies of TREC per 50,000 cells, the amount of patient DNA sample added per reaction should be increased by purifying the DNA instead of using the cell lysate.

CRYOPRESERVATION AND THAWING OF PBMCs

The cryopreservation of PBMCs plays a significant role in the modern clinical research laboratory. For evaluating the cellular functions and immunophenotypes of patients, particularly during longitudinal studies, in which it is not possible to use fresh cells, cells from each time point can be cryopreserved and then assayed in batch at the completion of the study. The use of cryopreserved cells in this manner can significantly reduce the cost of performing assays and help to minimize assay variability. However, cryopreservation of patient samples can also affect the functions of some cells. The exact effect of cryopreservation on the tests of interest should be determined ahead of time. Another use of cryopreservation is to provide a consistent source of positive control donor cells for use in the standardization of LPAs, NK cell assays, and immunophenotyping of cells.

There are two basic methods for the cryopreservation of WBCs. In the first method, WBCs are mixed with medium containing serum and a cryoprotectant, such as dimethyl sulfoxide (DMSO). The cells are then immediately placed in a slow-freeze container (such as the "Mr. Frosty" Freezing Container, available from Nalgene [http://nalgenelab. nalgenunc.com/default.asp]), and stored in a $-70°C$ freezer for 4 to 24 h. Upon freezing, the cells are transferred to a $-135°C$ vapor-phase liquid-nitrogen freezer for long-term storage. Because of the variable rate of cooling that is inherent with this process, some laboratories may not achieve maximal cell recovery and cell viability with this method. The best method for cryopreserving WBCs is the controlled-rate method described below (25). Briefly, this method uses a controlled-rate freezing apparatus (such as a Cryomed Freezer, available from Thermo Electron Corp. [http://thermo.com/]) to gradually cool the cells at a controlled rate. Once the cells reach $-90°C$, they are transferred to vapor-phase liquid nitrogen for storage. The major advantage of using a controlled-rate freezing apparatus is that the device is programmed to compensate for the release of latent heat that occurs during the crystallization process, thereby improving cell viability. This method should consistently yields cell recoveries of >80% and cell viabilities of >85%. Cells frozen in this manner can be stored for years in liquid nitrogen and remain viable, although some functional activities may be compromised.

Several important factors must be considered when attempting to cryopreserve cells. The cryoprotectant DMSO must be added to the cells very slowly to allow the DMSO to penetrate the cells. The final concentration of DMSO should not exceed 7.5%. The cell-freezing medium should contain a final concentration of 10% FCS as an added protectant. Once the DMSO has been added, the cells should be kept at 4°C prior to freezing in order to avoid DMSO toxicity. After all samples are prepared for freezing, they must be immediately transferred to the controlled-rate freezer. After freezing, the cells must be quickly transferred to vapor-phase liquid nitrogen to minimize warming of the cells.

To recover the best possible functional activity of cryopreserved cells, a precise thawing method such as the one outlined below must be used. It is generally recognized that cryopreserved cells are initially more sensitive to mechanical stress than are fresh cells. Therefore, care must be taken to avoid rigorous pipetting and centrifuging of the cells during the thawing procedure. The most critical step in the procedure involves the dilution of DMSO from the cell suspension. A careful dropwise dilution of the DMSO with warm medium containing 20% serum is necessary to allow for

osmotic equilibrium of the cells. The cells should then be washed to completely remove the DMSO. Careful handling of these cells should result in maximum immunologic activity.

Since the freeze-thaw process may cause physiological and morphological changes to some cells, one should always assess the viability of cryopreserved PBMCs before using them in immunologic assays. Cell viability can easily be determined by the standard trypan blue dye exclusion method. Alternatively, one can use flow cytometry to simultaneously measure apoptosis and cell viability (14). In this method, cells are stained in combination with annexin V and propidium iodide. Nonapoptotic cells are negative for both annexin V and propidium iodide, apoptotic cells are positive for annexin V and negative for propidium iodide, and necrotic cells are positive for both propidium iodide and annexin V. To assess the validity of the cryopreservation procedure, PBMCs should be obtained from a healthy donor each day and included as a control each time patient specimens are frozen. Cell viability and recovery should be determined for each control. The viability of frozen cells obtained from healthy individuals should exceed 90%, and cell recovery should exceed 80%. If these parameters are not met, then all phases of the cryopreservation process should be evaluated for error.

Equipment

Low-speed centrifuge

37°C water bath

Controlled-rate freezing system (Thermo Electron Corp.)

Liquid-nitrogen freezer

2-ml polypropylene cryovials

15-ml round-bottom plastic tubes

Reagents

Freezing medium (RPMI 1640 plus 20% FCS, RPMI 1640 plus 15% DMSO, or RPMI 1640 plus 10% FCS plus 7.5% DMSO)

Thawing medium (RPMI 1640 plus 20% FCS)

Procedure for Preparing PBMCs for Cryopreservation

1. Separate PBMCs from heparinized peripheral blood by the Ficoll-Hypaque method.

2. Resuspend PBMCs in room temperature RPMI 1640 plus 20% FCS in half the desired final freezing volume (usually 0.5 ml).

3. Add dropwise an equal volume (0.5 ml) of 4°C RPMI 1640 plus 15% DMSO, giving a final freezing solution of RPMI 1640 plus 10% FCS plus 7.5% DMSO.

4. Transfer the cell suspension to a sterile cryovial and place it in a cryovial rack that is on ice in order to maintain vials at 4°C.

5. Prepare one control cryovial to regulate the controlled-rate freezer, using the same volume and concentrations as for the final freezing solution (usually 1 ml of complete RPMI 1640 plus 10% FCS plus 7.5% DMSO). Place the freezer thermocouple probe inside this cryovial.

6. Transfer cryovials immediately to the controlled-rate freezer and freeze them as follows.

Cryopreservation Procedure

The controlled-rate freezer should be precooled to a starting temperature of 4°C. Once the sample vials have been placed into the freezing chamber, the sample temperature and chamber temperature must be allowed to equilibrate to 4°C.

After equilibration, the freezing procedure must follow a defined set of rate kinetics. From the starting temperature of 4°C, the samples should be cooled to −4°C at a rate of −1°C/min. To compensate for the heat of fusion released during the crystallization process, the samples must then be supercooled to −42°C and allowed to warm to −9°C. From this point, the samples must be cooled to −35°C at a rate of −1°C/min and then cooled to −90°C at a rate of −5°C/min. After the samples have reached −90°C, they should be immediately transferred to vapor-phase liquid-nitrogen storage.

Procedure for Thawing Cryopreserved PBMCs

1. Remove cells from the freezer and immediately thaw them by gently shaking the vial in a 37°C water bath.

2. Remove the vial from the water bath just before the last ice crystal has melted.

3. Gently transfer the cell suspension to a 15-ml round-bottom plastic tube at room temperature.

4. Immediately add 2 drops of RPMI 1640 plus 20% FCS which is 1/20 the original volume (1 ml) to the cell suspension and mix gently (to start diluting DMSO).

5. Repeat the addition, doubling the number of drops each time, until the DMSO concentration is 3%. (For an initial volume of 1.0 ml, this occurs after five additions, when the total volume is 2.5 ml.)

6. Add 7.5 ml of medium to achieve a final 1:10 dilution of the sample.

7. Centrifuge the cell suspension for 10 min at no more than 200 × g.

8. Pour off the supernatant. Resuspend the cells gently in the appropriate medium; count and measure the viability of the cells.

Notes: (i) Do not thaw more than three vials at one time. (ii) Do not mix, vortex, or pipette the cells vigorously, since cells that have been frozen are initially more sensitive to mechanical stress than are fresh cells. (iii) Viability is usually >90%.

REFERENCES

1. **Bruno, S., and Z. Darzynkiewicz.** 1992. Cell cycle dependent expression and stability of the nuclear protein detected by Ki-67 antibody in HL-60 cells. *Cell Prolif.* **25:**31–40.

2. **Centers for Disease Control and Prevention.** 1997. 1997 revised guidelines for the performance of CD4+ T-cell determination in persons infected with human immunodeficiency virus (HIV). *Morb. Mortal. Wkly. Rep.* **46**(RR-2):1–29.

3. **Centers for Disease Control and Prevention.** 2002. Guidelines for preventing opportunistic infections among HIV-infected persons—2002. *Morb. Mortal. Wkly. Rep.* **51** (RR-8):1–46.

4. **Centers for Disease Control and Prevention.** 2002. Guidelines for using antiretroviral agents among HIV-infected adults and adolescents. *Morb. Mortal. Wkly. Rep.* **51**(RR-7):1–71.

5. **Centers for Disease Control and Prevention.** 2003. 2003 guidelines for performing single-platform absolute CD4+ T-cell determinations with CD45 gating for persons infected with human immunodeficiency virus (HIV). *Morb. Mortal. Wkly. Rep.* **52**(RR-2):1–13.

6. **Douek, D. C., R. D. McFarland, P. H. Keiser, E. A. Gage, J. M. Massey, B. F. Haynes, M. A. Polis, A. T. Haase, M. B. Feinberg, J. L. Sullivan, B. D. Jamieson, J. A. Zack, L. J. Picker, and R. A. Koup.** 1998. Changes in thymic function with age and during the treatment of HIV infection. *Nature* **396:**690–695.

7. **Effros, R. B., R. Allsopp, C. P. Chiu, M. A. Hausner, K. Hirji, L. Wang, C. B. Harley, B. Villeponteau, M. D. West, and J. V. Giorgi.** 1996. Shortened telomeres in the expanded CD28− CD8+ cell subset in HIV disease implicate replicative senescence in HIV pathogenesis. *AIDS* **10:**17–22.

8. **Gerdes, J., H. Lemke, H. Baisch, H. H. Wacker, U. Schwab, and H. Stein.** 1984. Cell cycle analysis of a cell proliferation-associated human nuclear antigen defined by the monoclonal antibody Ki-67. *J. Immunol.* **133:**1710–1715.

9. **Heid, C. A., J. Stevens, K. J. Livak, and P. M. Williams.** 1996. Real time quantitative PCR. *Genome Res.* **6:**986–994.

10. **Hellerstein, M., M. B. Hanley, D. Cesar, S. Siler, C. Papageorgopoulos, E. Wieder, D. Schmidt, R. Hoh, R. Neese, D. Macallan, S. Deeks, and J. M. McCune.** 1999. Directly measured kinetics of circulating T lymphocytes in normal and HIV-1-infected humans. *Nat. Med.* **5:**83–89.

11. **Hellerstein, M. K., R. A. Hoh, M. B. Hanley, D. Cesar, D. Lee, R. A. Neese, and J. M. McCune.** 2003. Subpopulations of long-lived and short-lived T cells in advanced HIV-1 infection. *J. Clin. Investig.* **112:**956–966.

12. **Kausch, I., A. Lingnau, E. Endl, K. Sellmann, I. Deinert, T. L. Ratliff, D. Jocham, G. Sczakiel, J. Gerdes, and A. Bohle.** 2003. Antisense treatment against Ki-67 mRNA inhibits proliferation and tumor growth in vitro and in vivo. *Int. J. Cancer* **105:**710–716.

13. **Koenig, S., and A. S. Fauci.** 1988. AIDS: immunopathogenesis and immune response to the human immunodeficiency virus, p. 61–77. *In* V. T. DeVita, Jr., S. Hellman, and S. A. Rosenberg (ed.), *AIDS: Etiology, Diagnosis, Treatment, and Prevention*, 2nd ed. J. B. Lippincott Co., Philadelphia, Pa.

14. **Koopman, G., C. P. M. Reutelingsperger, G. A. M. Kuijten, R. M. J. Keehnen, S. T. Pals, and M. H. J. van Oers.** 1994. Annexin V for flow cytometric detection of phosphatidylserine expression on B cells undergoing apoptosis. *Blood* **84:**1415–1420.

15. **Kovacs, J. A., R. A. Lempicki, I. A. Sidorov, J. W. Adelsberger, B. Herpin, J. A. Metcalf, I. Sereti, M. A. Polis, R. T. Davey, J. Tavel, J. Falloon, R. Stevens, L. Lambert, R. Dewar, D. J. Schwartzentruber, M. R. Anver, M. W. Baseler, H. Masur, D. S. Dimitrov, and H. C. Lane.** 2001. Identification of dynamically distinct subpopulations of T lymphocytes that are differentially affected by HIV. *J. Exp. Med.* **194:**1731–1741.

16. **Lane, H. C., J. M. Depper, W. C. Green, G. Whalen, T. A. Waldmann, and A. S. Fauci.** 1985. Qualitative analysis of immune function in patients with acquired immunodeficiency syndrome: evidence for a selective defect in soluble antigen recognition. *N. Engl. J. Med.* **313:**79–84.

17. **Lane, H. C., and A. S. Fauci.** 1985. Immunologic abnormalities in the acquired immunodeficiency syndrome. *Annu. Rev. Immunol.* **3:**477–500.

18. **Lempicki, R. A., J. A. Kovacs, M. W. Baseler, J. W. Adelsberger, R. L. Dewar, V. Natarajan, M. C. Bosche, J. A. Metcalf, R. A. Stevens, L. A. Lambert, W. G. Alvord, M. A. Polis, R. T. Davey, D. S. Dimitrov, and H. C. Lane.** 2000. Impact of HIV-1 infection and highly active antiretroviral therapy on the kinetics of CD4+ and CD8+ T cell turnover in HIV-infected patients. *Proc. Natl. Acad. Sci. USA* **97:**13778–13783.

19. **McFarland, R. D., D. C. Douek, R. A. Koup, and L. J. Picker.** 2000. Identification of a human recent thymic emigrant phenotype. *Proc. Natl. Acad. Sci. USA* **97:** 4215–4220.

20. **Natarajan, V., R. A. Lempicki, I. Sereti, Y. Badralmaa, J. W. Adelsberger, J. A. Metcalf, D. A. Prieto, R. Stevens, M. W. Baseler, J. A. Kovacs, and H. C. Lane.** 2002. Increased peripheral expansion of naive CD4+ T cells in

vivo after IL-2 treatment of patients with HIV infection. *Proc. Natl. Acad. Sci. USA* **99:**10712–10717.

21. **National Committee for Clinical Laboratory Standards.** 1989. *Clinical Applications for Flow Cytometry: Quality Assurance and Immunophenotyping of Peripheral Blood Lymphocytes; Proposed Guideline.* NCCLS document H42-P. National Committee for Clinical Laboratory Standards, Villanova, Pa.

22. **Reimann, K. A., M. R. G. O'Gorman, J. Spritzler, C. L. Wilkening, D. E. Sabath, K. Helm, D. E. Campbell, and The NIAID DAIDS New Technologies Evaluation Group.** 2000. A multisite comparison of CD4 and CD8 T lymphocyte counting by single vs. multiple platform methodologies: evaluation of Beckman Coulter Flow-Count Fluorospheres and tetraONE System. *Clin. Diagn. Lab. Immunol.* **7:**344–351.

23. **Sachsenberg, N., A. S. Perelson, S. Yerly, G. A. Schockmel, D. Leduc, B. Hirschel, and L. Perrin.** 1998.

Turnover of CD4(+) and CD8(+) T lymphocytes in HIV-1 infection as measured by Ki-67 antigen. *J. Exp. Med.* **187:**1295–1303.

24. **Schnizlein-Bick, C. T., J. Spritzler, C. L. Wilkening, J. K. A. Nicholson, M. R. G. O'Gorman, Site Investigators, and The NIAID DAIDS New Technologies Evaluation Group.** 2000. Evaluation of TruCount absolute-count tubes for determining CD4 and CD8 cell numbers in human immunodeficiency virus-positive adults. *Clin. Diagn. Lab. Immunol.* **7:**336–343.

25. **Strong, D. M., J. R. Ortaldo, F. Pandolfi, A. Maluish, and R. B. Herberman.** 1982. Cryopreservation of human mononuclear cells for quality control in clinical immunology. I. Correlations in recovery of K- and NK-cell functions, surface markers and morphology. *J. Clin. Immunol.* **2:**216–221.

26. **UNAIDS.** 2004. *2004 Report on the Global AIDS Epidemic: 4th Global Report.* UNAIDS, Geneva, Switzerland.

Quantitation of Viremia and Determination of Drug Resistance in Patients with Human Immunodeficiency Virus Infection

TAREK ELBEIK, HELENE HIGHBARGER, ROBIN DEWAR, VEN NATARAJAN, HIROMI IMAMICHI, AND TOMOZUMI IMAMICHI

96

In the current environment of human immunodeficiency virus type 1 (HIV-1) treatments under highly active antiretroviral therapy (HAART), not only an increase in the number of CD4+ T lymphocytes but also a decrease in the level of plasma viremia (7, 13, 20, 41, 44) is expected; thus, it is essential to be able to quickly and accurately assess viral load. Several methods for quantitation of HIV-1 RNA in human plasma are outlined here. These are the Bayer Corporation Quantiplex HIV-1 RNA assay (branched-DNA [bDNA] assay), the Amplicor Roche Monitor assay, and the internally controlled virion PCR (ICVPCR). Although the different procedures may show good correlation and agreement, there is variability between assays not only within one subtype but also in the ability to quantify different HIV-1 subtypes. With some geographic regions experiencing an increased mixture of subtypes, intra-assay variability makes it preferable that patients be tested with the same assay throughout treatment (6, 31, 35).

Although the use of HAART has resulted in a decrease in virus replication in plasma to less than 50 copies/ml for prolonged periods in many patients with HIV-1 infection (27, 29), many lines of evidence have demonstrated that complete suppression of viral replication may not be possible with current HAART regimens (8, 12, 16, 21, 23, 28, 40, 48, 54, 55, 56). The persistence of low levels of ongoing viral replication may eventually lead to resistance. Continuous low-level viral replication, noncompliance issues, and gradual deterioration of the immune system have all contributed to the emergence of drug-resistant HIV-1 (32). HIV drug resistance presents another challenge for clinicians (5).

Until recently, the accepted approach to treating infected individuals with drug-resistant HIV-1 was thorough treatment history and viral load data. While initial resistance assays measured replication of the patient's viral isolate in culture with the presence of drug, these assays were highly labor-intensive, poorly reproducible, prone to variability, and insensitive; they required at least a month for results; and they were very expensive (36). Nonetheless, the demand for HIV-1 drug resistance assays increased as the numbers of patients failing HAART increased. As a result, commercially available HIV-1 resistance assays, incorporating innovative molecular technologies to overcome the handicaps of the earlier assays, have been introduced to address the needs of the treating clinician and the infected individual. We outline several commercially available resistance tests as well as a cloning-microculturing technique for measuring drug resistance.

HIV-1 RNA ASSAYS

Sample Collection and Processing

The HIV-1 RNA assays are performed on stored ($-70°C$) acid-citrate-dextrose- or EDTA-treated plasma. These anticoagulants show the least interference with amplification and detection (15). Plasma separation is achieved by centrifugation of whole blood at $500 \times g$ for 15 min.

HIV-1 RNA Quantitation Using bDNA

HIV-1 RNA is quantitated in plasma by bDNA signal amplification-based hybridization using the Quantiplex HIV-RNA assay kit in conjunction with the Quantiplex System 340 instrument according to the manufacturer's instructions (Bayer Corporation, Norwood, Mass. [formerly Chiron Diagnostics, Emeryville, Calif.]). These instructions are outlined below (Fig. 1). Virus is concentrated from 1-ml plasma specimens by centrifugation in a bench top microcentrifuge (Heraeus centrifuge model 17RS, rotor 3753) at $23,500 \times g$ for 1 h. The virus pellet is resuspended in a buffer containing proteinase K, capture probes, lithium laurel sulfate, and target probes complementary to the HIV *pol* gene and incubated at 63°C for 2 h. The extract is then spun, vortexed, transferred to microwells coated with capture probe, and placed in the automated Quantiplex 340 instrument. The RNA-probe complex is captured onto the surface of the microwell during a 63°C overnight incubation (16 to 18 h) via hybridization of the solid-phase capture probe with a subset of the target probes. The next day the wells are washed automatically and preamplifier molecules (added manually) are hybridized to the immobilized target-probe complex during a 30-min 63°C incubation, followed by another wash and 30-min 63°C hybridization of the bDNA amplifier molecules to the immobilized preamplifier complex. After another wash, multiple copies of alkaline phosphatase-labeled probes hybridize to each bDNA molecule during a 45-min 63°C incubation. The complex is then washed a final time and incubated for 30 min at 37°C with a chemiluminescent substrate (dioxetane), after which light emission is measured and analyzed by the Quantiplex System 340 and 340 Data Management System. The light emission is directly proportional to the amount of HIV RNA present in the plasma specimen. The concentration of RNA in each specimen is expressed as HIV-1 RNA copies per milliliter, determined from a standard curve, using β-propiolactone-treated virus in six known concentrations

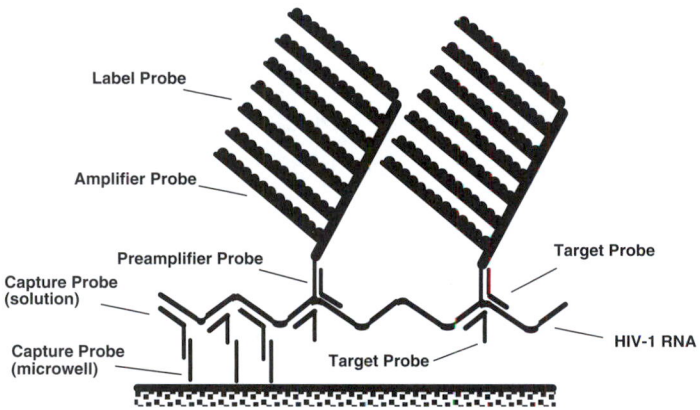

FIGURE 1 Principle of the bDNA assay.

with a dynamic range of 50 to 500,000 RNA copies per ml of plasma. The bDNA assay is capable of detecting all HIV-1 subtypes, including subtype O.

Amplicor Roche Monitor Assay

The Roche Monitor assay is an in vitro nucleic acid amplification test for the quantitation of HIV-1 virus RNA present in most bodily fluids, including plasma, serum, and breast milk. The kit is supplied by Roche Diagnostic Systems, Indianapolis, Ind. The test can be used with either the standard or ultrasensitive specimen processing procedure. When the standard specimen processing procedure is used, the test can quantitate HIV-1 RNA over the range of 400 to 750,000 copies/ml. When the ultrasensitive specimen processing procedure is used, the test can quantitate HIV-1 RNA over the range of 50 to 75,000 copies per ml. There are two plates per kit, and 10 patient samples can be assayed per plate in addition to a positive and negative control. Before this assay can be purchased from Roche Diagnostic Systems, two things are required by Roche—first, that someone be trained in the use of the assay by a Roche Diagnostic Systems representative and, second, that the laboratory successfully perform a qualification assay set for certification.

The standard Roche Monitor assay procedure requires 200 μl of plasma, while the ultrasensitive assay procedure requires 500 μl of plasma. RNA is extracted by using guanidium thiocyanate and isopropanol. The use of an internal quantitation standard (IQS) monitors the efficiency of extraction and amplification and eliminates the need for a standard curve. The IQS RNA transcript has the same *gag* primer binding sites for SK-462 and SK-431 as the HIV-1 virus target RNA and the same size and base composition as the HIV-1 virus target but possesses a non-HIV-1 probe region. The amplification efficiency is monitored internally in each sample since the amplification efficiency of the IQS will be equivalent to that of the HIV-1 target RNA. The IQS is noncompetitive and does not interfere with the amplification of the HIV-1 RNA; it yields a quantitative value over a 4-log dynamic range (45).

To minimize the possibility of cross-contamination of samples with amplicon, target DNA, or target RNA, the assay process is performed in four physically distinct locations with the flow being one way. The areas are reagent preparation, sample preparation, amplification, and detection-analysis. In addition, the use of uridine instead of thymidine in the amplification reaction has allowed the use of uracil-N-glycosylase (42) to help minimize the possibility of uridine-containing amplicon carryover from specimens previously amplified. The following procedure describes the use of the quantitative HIV-1 RNA Amplicor Roche Monitor assay, including reagent preparation, processing of whole-blood specimens, amplification, and detection-analysis by enzyme-linked immunosorbent assay.

Reagent Preparation

1. Add 100 μl of manganese solution containing pink dye to one tube of master mix. The master mix and manganese solution are provided in single-use vials, sufficient for 12 tests, and up to three runs can be done simultaneously with one positive and negative control.

2. Pipette 50 μl of working master mix to each PCR tube. Amplification must begin within 4 h of preparation of the working master mix.

3. Prepare 70% ethanol using diethylpyrocarbonate-treated water, and aliquot 100% isopropanol.

4. For each batch of 12 samples, prepare the working lysis reagent by adding the indicated volume (varies by lot) of HIV quantitation standard RNA (QS RNA) to one bottle of the lysis reagent. Vortex well.

Standard Assay Specimen Preparation

1. Dispense 600 μl of working lysis reagent into each 1.5-ml Sarstedt screw-cap conical tube.

2. Thaw plasma specimens at room temperature. Vortex each sample for 5 s, and then add 200 μl of plasma or control to each labeled tube containing the working lysis reagent.

3. Vortex for 5 s and incubate the tubes for 10 min at room temperature.

4. Add 800 μl of 100% isopropanol to each tube. Re-cap the tubes, and mix contents thoroughly by inverting the tubes 5 to 10 times and vortexing for 5 s.

5. Centrifuge samples at $16,000 \times g$ with the Heraeus centrifuge for 15 min at room temperature. Remove the samples from the rotor immediately, and proceed. Do not let the samples sit following centrifugation, or you will lose the pellets.

6. Beginning with the control tubes, carefully draw off the supernatant without disturbing the pellet by using a fine-tip disposable pipette. The pellet may not be obviously visible or at best will appear translucent. If the pellet is disturbed, you may repeat the centrifugation.

7. Add 1.0 ml of 70% ethanol to each tube, vortex for 5 s, and repeat steps 5 and 6.

8. Add 400 μl of specimen diluent to each pellet, and vortex vigorously for 10 s to resuspend the pellet, which contains the extracted RNA. RNAs should be amplified or frozen immediately. For short-term storage, −20°C is adequate; however, for long periods, −80°C is preferred.

9. Pipette 50 μl of the RNA prepared from controls and patient specimens into the appropriate MicroAmp tubes.

Ultrasensitive Assay Specimen Preparation

1. Thaw plasma specimens at room temperature, and then add 500 μl of each patient specimen to the appropriately labeled 1.5-ml Sarstedt screw-cap conical tube.

2. For each negative and positive control, add 500 μl of normal human plasma to each appropriately labeled tube.

3. Centrifuge specimen and control tubes containing normal human plasma at $23,600 \times g$ at 2 to 8°C for 60 min.

4. Remove as much liquid as possible without disturbing the pellet. Withdraw the supernatant slowly, allowing the liquid to drain completely off the sides of the tube. *Do not use vacuum aspiration.*

5. Dispense 600 μl of ultrasensitive assay working lysis reagent into each tube.

6. For each negative and positive control, add 12.5 μl of HIV-1 (−) C, HIV-1 L (+) C, and HIV-1 H (+) C to the appropriately labeled tubes.

7. Cap and vortex each sample for 5 s following addition of lysis reagent.

8. Incubate the tubes for 10 min at room temperature.

9. Add 600 μl of 100% isopropanol to each tube. Re-cap the tubes, and mix contents thoroughly by inverting 5 to 10 times and vortexing for 5 s.

10. Centrifuge samples at $16,000 \times g$ with the Heraeus centrifuge for 15 min at room temperature.

11. Beginning with the control tubes, carefully draw off the supernatant without disturbing the pellet by using a fine-tip disposable pipette. The pellet may not be obviously visible or at best will appear translucent. If the pellet is disturbed, you may repeat the centrifugation.

12. Add 1.0 ml of 70% ethanol to each tube, vortex for 5 s, and repeat steps 10 and 11.

13. Add 100 μl of specimen diluent to each pellet, and vortex vigorously for 10 s to resuspend the pellet, which contains the extracted RNA.

14. Pipette 50 μl of the RNA prepared from controls and patient specimens into the appropriate MicroAmp tubes, and move to the amplification and detection area.

PCR Amplification

1. Place the MicroAmp reaction tray in a Perkin-Elmer thermocycler (model 9600), and run the following program.

Hold:	2 min at 50°C
Hold:	30 min at 60°C
Cycle (4 cycles):	10 s at 95°C, 10 s at 55°C, and 10 s at 72°C
Cycle (26 cycles):	10 s at 90°C, 10 s at 60°C, and 10 s at 72°C
Hold:	15 min at 72°C

2. After amplification, immediately pipette 100 μl of the Monitor denaturation solution to each PCR tube, and mix by pipetting up and down five times. The denatured amplification reaction products should be held for no more than 2 h at room temperature before proceeding to detection. If detection of the amplicon cannot be performed within 2 h, store the denatured amplification reaction products at 4°C. Under these conditions the denatured amplicon is stable for up to 1 week.

Detection and Analysis

1. Remove the appropriate number of both target and QS microwell strips, and place them into a microwell frame.

2. Pipette 100 μl of HIV Monitor hybridization solution into each well of the microwell plate (MWP). Rows A to F of the HIV Monitor MWP are coated with the HIV-specific oligonucleotide probe; rows G and H are coated with the QS-specific oligonucleotide probe.

3. Add 25 μl of denatured amplification reaction product from the first row of the amplification tray into the first row of HIV wells. Mix by pipetting up and down five times, and then transfer 25 μl to the next row of wells. Repeat this procedure four more times, so as to generate five fivefold dilutions (neat, 1:5, 1:25, 1:125, 1:625, and 1:3,125) in rows A through F. Remove and discard 25 μl from row F after mixing.

4. Add 25 μl of the same amplicon from the first row of the amplification tray into the first row of the IQS wells (row G). Mix by pipetting up and down five times, and then transfer 25 μl of this dilution to the next row (row H) of wells (1:25). Remove and discard 25 μl from row H after mixing. Incubate for 1 h at 37°C.

5. Wash each MWP five times with working wash solution.

6. Add 100 μl of avidin-horseradish peroxidase conjugate to each well, and incubate for 15 min at 37°C. Wash the MWP as described in step 5.

7. Add 100 μl of working substrate to each well.

8. Allow color to develop for 10 min at room temperature (20 to 25°C) in the dark (lab drawer).

9. Add 100 μl of stop solution to each well.

10. Start the data capture and analysis program using either an Excel or Lotus spreadsheet supplied for this purpose by Roche Molecular Systems. Measure the optical density (OD) at 450 nm on the plate reader.

11. The actual HIV copy number per milliliter of sample is calculated in the following manner. First determine the OD value and sample amplicon dilution that yields an OD value next above a 0.2-OD cutoff. Also determine the OD value and QS amplicon dilution that yields an OD value next above a 0.3-OD cutoff. Subtract a standard empirically determined background OD value of 0.07 from each of the assay OD values, and multiply each of the resulting OD values by their respective dilution factor. Divide the resulting calculated sample value by the value calculated for the QS internal standard. This value represents the efficiency of the amplification of the sample relative to the input QS. This value is multiplied by the number of initial input QS RNA copies, and the result is the total HIV-1 RNA copies in 25 μl of starting plasma. This value (copies per PCR) is multiplied by 40 (if performing a standard assay) or by 4 (if performing an ultrasensitive assay) to get the number of PCR copies per milliliter of plasma. The Roche Amplicor Monitor assay has a 4-log dynamic range and detects from 400 to 750,000 HIV RNA copies per ml with the standard sample preparation procedure and from 50 to 75,000 HIV RNA copies per ml with the ultrasensitive sample preparation procedure. Roche Amplicor version 1.5 is currently marketed outside of the United States for the detection of non-B subtypes of HIV-1.

QUANTITATION OF HIV-1 RNA BY INTERNALLY CONTROLLED PCR

PCR has been used to quantitate levels of RNA and DNA from a variety of samples. With clinical specimens, the presence of inhibitors of PCR and small variations in amplification efficiency between different samples make it difficult to accurately estimate the amount of the specific sequence present in the starting material (3, 10). To avoid these problems, an internally controlled competitive PCR procedure can be used (25). In this method, various known amounts of an internal standard that shares the same primers as the target RNA but that contains either a deletion or an insertion are added to equal aliquots of the sample containing the unknown target sequence. The internal standard and the target sequence compete equally for primer binding and amplification in the PCR. Variables such as the efficiency of amplification and the number of cycles will have the same effect on both templates. Equal amounts of products will be formed when the initial concentrations of the templates are equal. Experimentally, the ratio of products formed can be determined, and the equivalence point can be calculated. This method has been successfully employed to quantify the amount of HIV-1 RNAs in clinical samples (9, 52). This method, however, does not control for the variable loss of RNA during purification steps. It has been estimated that, on average, 36% of the RNA sample can be lost due to the extraction procedures used (44).

An alternative method for measuring the HIV-1 RNA in patients' plasma or sera uses an infectious mutant virus as an internal control (49). The mutant virus, VX-46, has a 25-bp insert in a conserved region between the primer binding and major splice donor sites. To utilize this virus as an internal control, different dilutions of this virus are added to aliquots of the plasma or serum sample to be measured, and RNA is isolated and reverse transcribed to cDNA. PCR is performed with primers selected to include the sequences on either side of the insert contained in the externally added virus. The DNA product from the control virus is 25 bp longer than that from the virus present in plasma. The amount of viral RNA present in a plasma sample is calculated after the PCR-amplified products are separated by gel electrophoresis. This ICVPCR assay eliminates errors introduced by variable recovery during the RNA purification step, and thus the accuracy of the assay is enhanced. This method can also be applied to other DNA or RNA viruses.

Oligodeoxyribonucleotide Primer and Probe Sequences

Primer designation	Sequence $5' \rightarrow 3'$
ICVPCR-9 (reverse transcription-primer)	TCCCTGCTTGCCCATACTA
ICVPCR-16 (+strand)	ATCTCTCGACGCAGGACT
ICVPCR-17 (−strand)	GCTCTCGCACCCATCTCT
ICVPCR-18 (probe)	ACTAGCGGAGGCTAGAAGGA

RNA Isolation and cDNA Synthesis

Sample (200 μl) is mixed with 400 μl of 6.0 M guanidium thiocyanate, 60 μl of 2.0 M sodium acetate (pH 4.0), and 600 μl of phenol-chloroform-isoamyl alcohol (25:24:1). The samples are mixed after each addition, incubated on ice for 20 min, and centrifuged at room temperature for 20 min. The aqueous phase is aspirated and mixed with 10 μg of carrier RNA (Sigma Chemical Co., St. Louis, Mo.) and precipitated with an equal volume of isopropanol. Prepare guanidium thiocyanate in 42 mM sodium citrate buffer,

pH 4.0, containing 0.83% sodium lauroylsarcosine and 0.2 mM β-mercaptoethanol.

RNA recovered by centrifugation is washed with cold 70% ethanol and dissolved in 8 μl of water and is used for cDNA synthesis in a 20-μl reaction mixture with a cDNA cycle kit obtained from Invitrogen Corporation (San Diego, Calif.) using ICVPCR-9 as the primer for reverse transcription.

PCR Amplification

cDNA (5 μl) is used in a reaction mixture containing 10 mM Tris-HCl (pH 8.3), 50 mM KCl, 1.5 mM MgCl$_2$, 0.001% gelatin, 0.2 mM deoxynucleoside triphosphates (dNTPs), 25 pmol each of primers ICVPCR-16 and -17, and 2.5 U of AmpliTaq DNA polymerase (Perkin-Elmer) in a final volume of 50 μl. Amplification is carried out in a Perkin-Elmer thermocycler (model 9600) with the following PCR cycle program: 1 cycle at 94°C for 60 s, 55°C for 10 s, and 72°C for 30 s; 30 cycles at 94°C for 15 s, 55°C for 30 s, and 72°C for 60 s; and a final incubation at 72°C for 10 min.

Analysis of the PCR Product by Liquid Hybridization

Liquid hybridization is carried out as described in reference 17a, with oligonucleotide ICVPCR-18 as a probe. Hybridized PCR products are analyzed on 10% polyacrylamide gels. The amount of radioactivity present in each band is quantitated with a Bio-Image analyzer (37). We use Fuji Medical Systems (Stamford, Conn.) BAS1000.

Estimation of RNA Present in a VX-46 Virus Preparation

The amount of RNA in a VX-46 virus preparation is estimated using a competitor plasmid (pA1) containing the pNL4.3 nucleotide sequences (GenBank accession no. M19921) from positions 501 to 1448. cDNA from VX-46 virus is PCR amplified in the presence of different amounts of plasmid pA1. The PCR product is hybridized with ICVPCR-18 labeled at the 5′ end with ^{32}P and then is separated in an acrylamide gel. The primers selected should generate 123- and 148-bp DNA PCR products from the wild-type and mutant viral sequences, respectively. The amounts of radioactivity in the specific bands are determined, and the ratios between the amounts of radioactivity present in wild-type and mutant DNA bands are plotted against the amount of input wild-type competitor plasmid DNA. The copy number of the mutant viral RNA is calculated from the plot for the ratio of 1 between the amount of radioactivity present in wild-type and mutant DNA bands.

ICVPCR To Determine the Level of HIV-1 RNA in Plasma

By using this standardized VX-46 virus as the competitor during the RNA isolation, the amount of HIV-1 viral RNA in patients' plasma can be estimated. Aliquots (100 μl) of serial dilutions of the mutant virus, VX-46, that span the estimated range are added to 100 μl of patient plasma or serum. Commonly, about four dilutions are sufficient to determine the equivalence point between the mutant and sample viral RNAs in PCR. If the equivalence point cannot be determined by these dilutions, the amount of the added mutant virus is adjusted.

RNA extracted from the samples containing patient serum and the added mutant virus is used for cDNA synthesis and for PCR, and the PCR products are analyzed as described above. The amount of radioactivity present in each band is estimated, and the ratio of radioactivity present in mutant

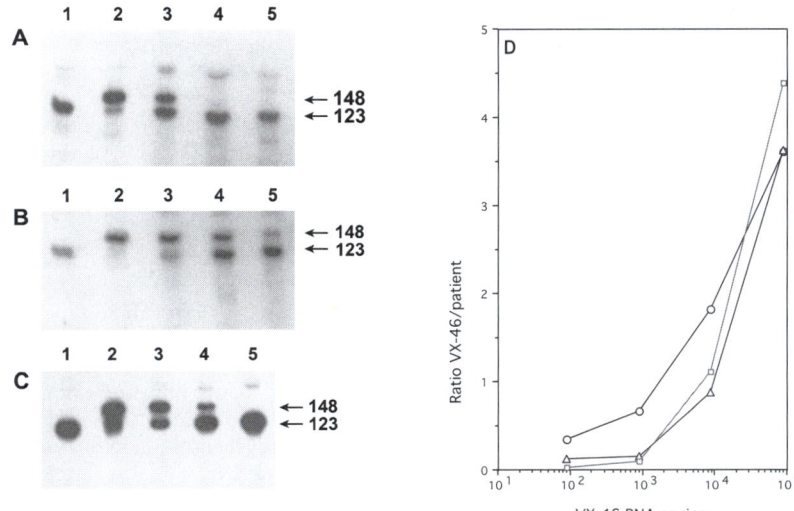

FIGURE 2 ICVPCR for the estimation of HIV-1 RNA in patient plasma. (A, B, and C) Different dilutions of mutant virus (VX-46) containing 0 pg (lane 1), 30 pg (lane 2), 3 pg (lane 3), 0.3 pg (lane 4), and 0.03 pg (lane 5) of p24 antigen were added to 100 μl aliquots of patients' plasma. RNA isolation, cDNA synthesis, and PCR were carried out as described in the text. The sizes of DNA products from the mutant (148) and wild type (123) are shown on the right. Each panel is for plasma from one of three different patients. (D) Estimation of HIV-1 RNA in patients' plasma. Patient 1 (triangles) had 10,000 copies, patient 2 (squares) had 7,600 copies, and patient 3 (circles) had 16,000 copies of RNA in 100 μl of plasma.

DNA bands to that in the wild-type (patient) DNA bands is plotted against the input mutant viral RNA. The amount of viral RNA present in the patient sample is calculated from the plot for the ratio of 1 between the amount of radioactivity present in patient and mutant DNA bands (Fig. 2).

The mutant virion can play the roles of both a control for the RNA extraction procedure and a source of competitive RNA template in the PCR. Any inhibitors present in the sample that will affect the cDNA synthesis and/or PCR will affect equally the product formed from the RNA present in the sample as well as the mutant viral RNA, thereby increasing the accuracy of the PCR quantitation. This method also could provide a guide for determining if an inhibitor of reverse transcriptase PCR (RT-PCR) is present in the sample, thus suggesting the use of a procedure to remove the inhibitor.

RESISTANCE TESTING

Technologies Used for HIV-1 Genotypic and Phenotypic Resistance Assays

Resistance assays are divided into two groups—genotypic and phenotypic—and are directed toward the analysis of the protease (*pro*) and the RT (*rt*) genes. However, several research groups are utilizing these assays to evaluate mutations within the group specific antigen (*gag*) gene and correlation to drug resistance (13, 19, 24, 47, 57).

The genotypic assays provide sequencing information that can be used to identify known resistance codons. The phenotypic assay, a function-based system, derives resistance data from the expression of the patient's viral isolate in the presence of drug in vitro. Also included under phenotypic assays is the virtual phenotype (extrapolates a phenotypic result through comparison of the genotype to matched genotype-phenotype resistance profiles) and replication capacity

(a component of viral fitness). Finally, online services available to analyze HIV-1 sequences for genotypic drug resistance are addressed.

Genotypic Resistance

There are currently three commercially available systems that are in use: GeneSeq (ViroLogic, South San Francisco, Calif.), TRUGENE (Bayer HealthCare LLC, Tarrytown, N.Y.) (38), and ViroSeq (Celera Diagnostics, Alameda, Calif.) (11). GeneSeq is a service provided by ViroLogic and is not available in a kit format, while TRUGENE and ViroSeq are obtainable in a kit format and available for setup in clinical and research laboratories.

TRUGENE and ViroSeq involve similar technical steps that require a highly adept group of technologists for successful operation. TRUGENE and ViroSeq are approved for use on HIV-1 subtype B; however, several groups demonstrate reduced performance, by 25 to 50%, on non-B subtypes, including failed RT-PCR or partial bidirectional sequences (2, 18, 22, 35, 43). In comparative studies, ViroSeq performs better than TRUGENE on non-B subtypes (2, 22); however, use of prototype primers improves the performance of TRUGENE (35).

GeneSeq HIV

ViroLogic offers the in-house HIV-1 genotypic drug resistance assay GeneSeq HIV. A patient plasma sample with ≥500 copies of HIV-1 RNA/ml is submitted to ViroLogic or one of the approved laboratories for in-house testing. GeneSeq HIV utilizes dideoxy sequencing technology (see "ViroSeq" below), and the resulting patient genotype is analyzed with ViroLogic's algorithm to determine the patient HIV-1 drug resistance profile. The subtype is also reported; however, there are no peer-reviewed publications on the performance characteristics of GeneSeq HIV on non-B subtypes. Additional information on GeneSeq HIV can be obtained from the ViroLogic website (http://www.virologic.com).

TRUGENE

TRUGENE has been cleared by the Food and Drug Administration for in vitro diagnostic use with the OpenGene DNA sequencing system. TRUGENE provides all components required to genotype the HIV-1 *pro* and *rt* genes for drug resistance, including those for RT-PCR and sequencing of a total of 30 genotyping reactions (four clinical samples and one positive and one negative control per reaction plate, or a total of 23 clinical samples and seven controls when run in batch). It does not, however, contain reagents necessary for HIV-1 RNA extraction and purification, which must be purchased separately. It is recommended to process six samples in one batch (four clinical samples and one positive and one negative control) for each RT-PCR set. The lower limit of detection for TRUGENE is 1,000 copies of HIV-1 RNA per ml and has been approved for diagnostic sensitivity only to HIV-1 subtype B.

Long-Read Tower and MicroGene Clipper sequencers, computer, Gel Toaster gel units, disposable MicroCel acrylamide gel cassettes, and sequencing software are purchased separately from Bayer HealthCare LLC. All other hardware (thermal cyclers and microcentrifuges) and disposables (reaction tubes, 96-well plates, aerosolized tips, etc.) are purchased by the operator. Bayer HealthCare LLC does not provide an HIV-1 RNA extraction kit; however, various extraction methods produce HIV-1 RNA samples compatible with the TRUGENE HIV-1 genotyping kit (see "Extraction and Purification of HIV-1 RNA" below).

Three physically defined areas are recommended for this procedure: area 1, RNA preparation; area 2, reagent preparation; and area 3, sequencing and detection. A unidirectional flow from area 1 to area 2 to area 3 is required; i.e., one cannot backtrack from area 3 to area 2 or area 1 in the same day.

All technical procedures require strict adherence to techniques for working with RNA: aerosolized tips; cleaning down of all surfaces with 10% bleach followed by 70% ethanol, and frequent use of clean, powder-free gloves and lab coats; and ensuring that all disposables and reagents are RNase free. The negative control is a Tris-HCl buffered solution containing wheat germ tRNA. The positive control contains noninfectious HIV-1$_{BH10S}$ transcripts diluted in a negative control. While RNA is extracted and purified from the clinical plasma samples using any one of the recommended techniques (see below), neither positive nor negative controls are subjected to RNA extraction.

Extraction and purification of HIV-1 RNA. Purified HIV-1 RNA from plasma with a viral load of ≥1,000 copies of HIV-1 RNA per ml can be obtained by the following approved extraction procedures using the Qiagen QIAamp Viral RNA minikit, Qiagen Ultra HIV-1 RNA extraction method, Roche Amplicor HIV-1 Monitor test, Roche Amplicor HIV-1 Monitor with ultrasensitive specimen preparation, or Organon-Teknika NASBA NucliSens HIV-1 QT nucleic acid solution reagents.

Adaptations of each method, if needed, are listed in the Bayer HealthCare LLC TRUGENE package insert, and limits of recovery for each extraction method are listed in the corresponding manufacturer product package insert. The extracted HIV-1 RNA should be immediately placed on wet ice and either used the same day or frozen at −70°C for future use (i.e., for next-day setup).

RT-PCR amplification. A two-step single-tube RT-PCR is used to amplify a 1.3-kb sequence of the *pro* and *rt* regions (*pro* codon 1 through *rt* codon 333). Master mix I (primers and deoxynucleotides) for six samples is prepared in a 0.5-ml sterile RNase-free tube on wet ice (42.0 μl of RT-PCR primers, 10.5 μl of dNTP solution, 7.0 μl of dithiothreitol [DTT] solution, and 3.5 μl of RNase inhibitor), vortexed for 5 s, and microcentrifuged for 5 s. Aliquots (9.0 μl) of master mix I are dispensed into six 0.2-ml individual (not strip) prelabeled thin-wall PCR tubes and stored on wet ice. Master mix II (enzymes and buffer) is similarly prepared in a 0.5-ml sterile RNase-free tube on wet ice (70 μl of RT-PCR buffer, 3.5 μl of RNase inhibitor, 7.0 μl of reverse transcriptase enzyme, and 17.5 μl of DNA polymerase), vortexed for 7 to 10 s, and microcentrifuged for 7 to 10 s. Master mix II is held in wet ice but must be used within 15 min. Both master mixes I and II, as well as the samples and controls, are transferred, on wet ice, to a dead-air box in area 3, and the thermal cycler is prewarmed to 90°C. While maintaining the thin-walled PCR tubes containing master mix I on wet ice, 17.0 μl of each sample, including both positive and negative controls, is added to its corresponding tube and simultaneously mixed using the pipette. The tubes are capped and transferred to the thermal cycler, and cycling is commenced at 90°C for 2 min, followed by 50°C for 60 min. After 5 min at 50°C, the tubes are uncapped, 14.0 μl of master mix II is added, and the tubes are re-capped. Program the thermal cycler prior to setting up the RT reaction as follows.

One cycle of:	90°C for 2 min (tubes paced in thermal cycler), 50°C for 60 min (add master mix II after 5 min at 50°C), and 94°C for 2 min
20 cycles of:	94°C for 30 s, 57°C for 30 s, and 68°C for 2 min
17 cycles of:	94°C for 30 s, 60°C for 30 s, and 68°C for 2.5 min
One cycle of:	68°C for 7 min and hold at 4°C (for a maximum of 24 h, or similarly in the fridge at 2 to 8°C for 24 h)

Sequencing reaction (CLIP). Four sets of primers—two sets within *pro* (protease and P2 primer pairs) and two sets within *rt* (RT-beginning and RT-end)—are used for the sequencing reaction. Each primer set generates a bidirectional sequence of the identical region, thus allowing for cross-checking during sequence analysis.

A 96-well sequencing tray (or 96-well plate containing 0.2-ml thin-walled 12-well strip tubes) is used for a total of six samples (four primer sets per sample, with a total of 16 reactions per sample). Bayer HealthCare LLC recommends that the positive and negative controls be included in each run. The sequencing tray is labeled vertically (plate orientation with columns of 12 wells and rows of 8 wells) with the reaction primers' designations so that the first 4 wells of row 1 are for protease and the remaining four wells (wells 5 to 8) of row 1 are for RT-beginning. The first four wells of row 2 are for RT-middle, and the remaining four wells (wells 5 to 8) of row 2 are for P2. Hence, each sample (or control) tested will occupy two rows of 16 wells. Using a 100-μl repeat pipettor, 7 μl of CLIP terminator mix (A, C, G, and T; columns 1 and 5, 2 and 6, 3 and 7, and 4 and 8, respectively) is added to the respective well for each primer.

CLIP master mix is prepared with 474 μl of DNase-free water, 120 μl of CLIP buffer, and 22.5 μl of CLIP enzyme; gently vortexed for 7 to 10 s; and placed on ice. An aliquot of 95 μl of CLIP master mix is transferred to each of six 0.5-ml microcentrifuge tubes. Tubes containing the CLIP master mix and the plate containing CLIP terminator mix are held on ice in area 3.

An aliquot of 5 μl of RT-PCR product from the samples or the negative or positive control is transferred to the corresponding tube containing CLIP master mix. Each tube is vortexed for 5 s, microcentrifuged for 5 s, and transferred to ice. An aliquot of 5 μl from each tube is transferred to the appropriate well in the 96-well plate, capped, and placed in a preheated thermal cycler set at 94°C. The cycling conditions are as follows.

One cycle of:	94°C for 5 min
30 cycles of:	94°C for 20 s, 56°C for 20 s, and 70°C for 1.5 min
One cycle of:	70°C for 5 min
4°C hold	

All reactions are terminated with the addition of 14 μl of stop loading dye to each well of the 96-well plate. The plate is vortexed gently for 7 to 10 s to ensure proper mixing. The plate is either placed on ice prior to electrophoresis or stored overnight at 2 to 8°C.

Electrophoresis and data analysis. Acrylamide gels are prepared using kit products. One SureFill cartridge (containing a 6% acrylamide gel) is brought to room temperature. During this time the Long-Read Tower power is turned on, including the computer workstation. From the GeneObjects software, select "Create New Run." In the "Preference" menu, set the following parameters: heterozygosity to partial (20%), peak distance at 7 to 10, automatic basecalling and automatic save assay, and save run. In "Run Information," set the appropriate database and then the Long-Read Tower, and select "Connect." In "Sequencer Control," select the following parameters: gel temperature, 60°C; gel voltage, 2,000 V; laser power, 50%; run clock (sampling interval), 0.5 s; and run clock (run duration), 50 min.

Press "Go" and select "Prerun." Insert splash guard into the bottom of the fill fixture unit. Attach the SureFill 6% sequencing gel cartridge to the Gel Toaster polymerization unit, making sure that there are no air bubbles in the connection tube. Insert the Softplug comb into the MicroCel 500 cassette, secure with clips provided, and place a strip of Scotch tape (not shiny tape, as it will prevent polymerization) across the plate, just below the comb, to prevent acrylamide from seeping onto the glass plate. The assembled cassette is placed in the Gel Toaster polymerization unit, and the cassette is filled with acrylamide. The Gel Toaster polymerization unit is turned on for 3 min to photopolymerize the acrylamide, after which the Softplug comb and the Scotch tape are removed. Make sure there are no bubbles in the gel; generate a new gel if bubbles are detected. The cassette is placed in the Long-Read Tower with 1× Tris-borate-EDTA in the upper and lower chambers. The gel is prerun for 5 to 10 min, but no longer than 10 min, prior to loading the samples. The prerun is completed when the "Run" and "Prerun" lights on the Long-Read Tower are illuminated.

During prerun, the samples (one sample or control of 16 reactions per gel) are denatured in the 96-well plate using a thermal cycler for 1 min at 85 to 95°C and immediately transferred to wet ice. Immediately prior to loading samples, the residual urea and air bubbles are removed from the MicroCel wells by flushing with 1× Tris-borate-EDTA using a transfer pipette or a syringe. A 1.5-μl aliquot of each denatured sample is transferred to the MicroCel wells using an eight-cylinder expandable multichannel pipettor. The reaction aliquots are added in the same manner as with the plate format; the first eight reaction aliquots include protease and RT-beginning of sample 1, row 1, the second eight reaction aliquots include RT-middle and P2 of sample 1, row 2, and so on. The condensation cover is placed on the upper buffer chamber, the door is closed, and pressing "Go" commences the sequencer and data collection.

Upon completion of the sequencing run, the data are assessed for quality. Acceptable data include strong signal, low background, and even peaks. Differences in nucleotide sequence of the sample are compared to the reference sequence of HIV-1$_{LAV-1}$. The final sequence result is based upon RT-beginning, RT-middle, and either protease or P2 but not both (the better signal generated by either protease or P2 should be used). The software translates all known mutations identified from the sample to the corresponding drug resistance profile. Novel mutations are also identified. Additional information is available at http://www.trugene.com.

ViroSeq

ViroSeq has been cleared by the Food and Drug Administration for in vitro diagnostic use with ViroSeq HIV-1 Genotyping System Software version 2.6 on the following platform: ABI Prism 377 DNA sequencer (no longer manufactured), ABI Prism 3100 genetic analyzer, ABI Prism 3100-*Avant* genetic analyzer, or ABI Prism 3700 DNA analyzer.

ViroSeq consists of four modules, including the sample preparation module, RT-PCR module, sequencing module, and 8E5 control module, for a total of 48 genotyping reactions. This translates into 46 clinical samples, one negative control, and one positive control if the entire kit is used in one go; otherwise, split into separate batches (up to four), each requiring one positive and one negative control. To optimize work flow and operating efficiency, it is recommended that operators configure test batches in multiples of 12.

The lower limit of detection for ViroSeq is 2,000 copies of HIV-1 RNA per ml, is intended for use on samples with a viral load between 2,000 and 750,000 copies/ml, and has been approved for diagnostic sensitivity only to HIV-1 subtype B. The entire HIV-1 *pro* region from codons 1 to 99 and two-thirds of *rt* from codons 1 to 335 are genotyped.

ViroSeq kits are purchased from Abbott Diagnostics, while platforms and sequencing software, as well as certain disposables and specialty reagents (96-well plates, polymer, BigDye Terminator version 1.1 sequencing standard, and Hi-Di formamide), are purchased directly from Applied Biosystems or through Abbott. The assay should be performed in three physically defined areas as described above.

Procedure. ViroSeq is based on six major processes: sample preparation, reverse transcription, PCR, sequencing, sequence detection, and software analysis. All technical procedures require strict adherence to techniques for working with RNA—aerosolized tips, cleaning down of all surfaces with 10% bleach followed by 70% ethanol, and frequent use of clean gloves and lab coats; all disposables and reagents must be RNase free. The negative control is human plasma free of HIV-1 RNA and nonreactive for antibodies to HIV-1 and -2, hepatitis C virus, human T-cell lymphotropic virus type 1, and HBsAG. The positive control contains in vitro-cultured defective HIV-1$_{8E5}$ diluted in negative control to a concentration between 50,000 and 100,000 copies of HIV-1 RNA/ml. Negative and positive controls and clinical samples are processed in the identical manner, from RNA extraction to sequencing reactions.

Sample preparation (extraction and purification of HIV-1 RNA). Purified HIV-1 RNA from patient EDTA-treated plasma with a viral load of ≥2,000 copies of HIV-1 RNA per ml is generated using the HIV sample prep module provided. Plasma samples are thawed at room temperature, mixed thoroughly using a vortex, and pulse-centrifuged for 3 to 5 s. A 500-μl aliquot of patient plasma is transferred to a 1.5-ml Sarstedt microcentrifuge tube. The positive control includes a 50-μl kit positive control mixed with a 450-μl kit negative control, and the negative control includes a 500-μl kit negative control. Using a black indelible marker, place an orientation mark on one side of the tube, and place the tube in the rotor so that the orientation mark faces outward (this is where the subsequent pellet will align). Centrifuge at 21,000 to 25,000 ×g at 2 to 8°C for 1 h. During centrifugation, prepare 70% ethanol (maintain at 4°C), and thaw the viral lysis buffer and RNA diluent at room temperature. Briefly vortex the thawed viral lysis buffer and RNA diluent; store the RNA diluent on wet ice. Upon completion of centrifugation, aspirate the clarified plasma with a fine-tip transfer pipette opposite the orientation mark; avoid disturbing the viral pellet. Add 600 μl of viral lysis buffer to the pellet, vortex for 3 to 5 s, pulse-centrifuge for 1 to 2 s, and incubate at room temperature for 10 min, followed by the addition of 600 μl of isopropanol. Vortex the tube for 3 to 5 s, and, with the orientation mark facing outward, centrifuge at 12,500 to 15,000 ×g for 15 min. Remove the supernatant using a fine-tip transfer pipette opposite the orientation mark. Aspiration must be performed in one motion without any backflow that would otherwise dislodge the pellet. Add 1 ml of 70% ethanol, vortex for 3 to 5 s, and, with the orientation mark facing outward, centrifuge at 12,500 to 15,000 ×g for 5 min. Aspirate the ethanol using a fine-tip transfer pipette (opposite the orientation mark). Pulse-spin the tube at 2000 ×g (orientation mark facing outward) for 1 to 2 s to collect residual ethanol at the bottom of the tube, and remove the residual ethanol with a new fine-tip transfer pipette (opposite the orientation mark). Air dry the pellet, with the cap removed, for 1 to 5 min to ensure that all residual ethanol is removed; otherwise, the traces will inhibit RT-PCR. Based upon the sample's viral load, resuspend the RNA pellet in 50 μl of RNA diluent if the viral load is unknown or less than 15,000 copies of HIV-1 RNA per ml, or in 100 μl of RNA diluent if the viral load is greater than 15,000 copies of HIV-1 RNA per ml. The positive control and negative control are resuspended in 50 μl of RNA diluent. Vortex for 10 s, and then pulse-centrifuge at 2,000 × g for 1 to 2 s. Hold on ice for immediate continuation to reserve transcription, or transfer to −65 to −80°C for storage.

RT-PCR amplification. A two-step one-tube RT-PCR is used to amplify a 1.8-kb sequence of *pro* and *rt* (*pro* codon 1 through *rt* codon 333). Only GeneAmp 9600 or 9700 thermal cyclers are recommended by the manufacturer. The HIV RT mix and DTT solution are thawed at room temperature, vortexed, and transferred to ice. The RNase inhibitor and murine leukemia virus RT are held in a −20°C cooler. RT master mix for one sample (one reaction) is prepared in an RNase-DNase-free 1.5-ml microcentrifuge tube on ice. Aliquots of 8 μl of HIV RT mix, 1 μl of RNase inhibitor, 1 μl of murine leukemia virus RT, and 0.4 μl of DTT are combined, vortexed for 2 to 3 s, and pulse-centrifuged at 2,000 ×g for 1 to 2 s. The RT master mix must be kept at room temperature prior to being added to the reaction tubes; however, it must not be kept at room temperature for more than 30 min. Always prepare additional volumes for one or two extra reactions.

Add 10 μl of purified RNA to a thin-walled 200-μl MicroAmp reaction tube, and transfer directly to the thermal cycler for one cycle of 65°C for 30 s to relax the RNA secondary structure and increase RT binding sites. Only after the second cycle of 45°C for 5 min are the tubes removed and 10 μl of RT master mix is added to each sample, the reaction tubes are capped, and then they are returned to the thermal cycler. Program the thermal cycler prior to setting up the RT reaction as follows.

One cycle of :	65°C for 30 s (to relax RNA secondary structure)
One cycle of:	42°C for 5 min (cools for optimum enzyme activity)
One cycle to:	Manually pause the thermal cycler for the maximum permitted time of 10 min. Remove tubes and add 10 μl of RT master mix to each reaction and return to thermal cycler. This step must be completed within 10 min
One cycle of:	42°C for 60 min (reverse transcription)
One cycle of:	99°C for 5 min (inactivates murine leukemia virus RT)
Hold:	4°C (at least 10 min, but no greater than 18 h, until proceeding to the PCR step)

The reserve transcription product can be used immediately for PCR or stored at −15 to −25°C but for no longer than 2 weeks.

PCR master mix for one sample (one reaction) is prepared in an RNase-DNase-free 1.5-ml microcentrifuge tube on ice (29.5 μl of HIV PCR mix, 0.5 μl of AmpliTaq Gold DNA polymerase, and 1 μl of AmpErase UNG), vortexed for 3 to 5 s, and pulse-centrifuged at 2,000 ×g for 1 to 2 s. Always prepare an additional volume for one extra reaction. An aliquot of 30 μl of PCR master mix is added to the RT reaction tube, and the tube is capped and pulse-centrifuged at 2,000 ×g for 5 to 10 s. Thermal cycler conditions are as follows.

One cycle of:	50°C for 10 min
One cycle of:	93°C for 12 min
40 cycles of:	93°C for 20 s, 64°C for 45 s, and 66°C for 3 min
One cycle of:	72°C for 10 min
Hold:	4°C for up to, but no longer than, 24 h (if the PCR product cannot be sequenced within 24 h, store at −15 to −25°C)

The PCR product is purified using a YM-100 microconcentrator, supplied with the kit, as follows. Insert the YM-100 spin column, reservoir facing up, into the YM 1.5-ml collection tube. Add 300 μl of sterile, deionized water to the reservoir, followed by the addition of the entire 50-μl PCR product. Cap the YM-100 microconcentrator, and centrifuge in a fixed-angle rotor at 450 to 550 ×g for 15 min. Following centrifugation, remove the cap, add 35 μl of sterile, deionized water to the reservoir, and transfer the YM-100 microconcentrator to a new 1.5-ml collection tube with the reservoir facing down. Centrifuge in a fixed-angle rotor at 450 to 550 ×g for 5 min. The purified PCR product (35 to 60 μl) in the 1.5-ml collection tube is either used immediately or stored at −15 to −25°C, but for no longer than 2 weeks.

Prior to the sequencing reaction, the purified PCR product is quantified by agarose gel electrophoresis. A 1.0% agarose gel containing 0.5 μg of ethidium bromide per ml is used. An aliquot of 5 μl of PCR product and 5 μl of agarose gel loading buffer is mixed in a microcentrifuge tube, vortexed, and pulse-centrifuged at 2,000 × g for 1 to 2 s, and the entire 10 μl is loaded onto the gel. Two aliquots, one of 3 μl and the other of 6 μl, of DNA mass ladder solution (with 5 μl of loading buffer) are loaded into the exterior flanking wells of the gel. The products are resolved at 10 V per cm until the bromophenol blue has migrated 5 cm into the gel. The image is recorded by photography under UV illumination. A dilution scheme is called for, based on the intensity of the PCR product compared to the mass ladder, as follows:

If the mass of the 1.8 kbp product band is:	Then:
Greater than 100 ng	1:10 dilution with double-distilled water
60 to 100 ng	1:4 dilution with double-distilled water
40 to 60 ng	1:2 dilution with double-distilled water
20 to 40 ng	Bring to 60 μl with double-distilled water
Less than 20 ng	Not suitable for sequencing

Once adjusted to the correct concentration, the diluted sample is vortexed for 3 to 5 s and pulse-centrifuged at 2,000 × g for 1 to 2 s; the sample is now ready for sequencing.

Sequencing reaction. Seven primers, four forward and three reverse, provide double coverage of the entire region spanning *pro* codon 1 to *rt* codon 320.

Once the product has been adjusted to the appropriate concentration, the sequencing reaction is prepared. Use the MicroAmp optical 96-well reaction plate (provided with the kit) or MicroAmp reaction tubes or MicroAmp eight-strip reaction tubes in a MicroAmp tray. For the MicroAmp optical 96-well reaction plate, label the first seven rows (from top to bottom) with the letter corresponding to the primer: A, B, C, D, F, G, or H. Label the columns across 1 to 12. In the last row, label columns 1 through 7 with A, B, C, D, F, G, and H, respectively. Thaw the HIV sequence master mix (A, B, C, D, F, G, and H) tubes at room temperature. Add 12 μl of each HIV SEQ mix to the row corresponding to the HIV SEQ letter (i.e., HIV SEQ mix A to row A, HIV SEQ mix B to row B, etc.). For the last row, add each HIV SEQ mix to each corresponding well (A through H). Next, add 8 μl of the clinical sample PCR product to each of the seven wells in its designated column. The wells are capped with the MicroAmp optical 96-well reaction plate cover and centrifuged at low speed for 5 to 10 s. The plate is transferred to a GeneAmp 9600 or 9700 thermal cycler with the following setup: 25 cycles of 96°C for 10 s, 50°C for 5 s, and 60°C for 4 min and hold at 4°C. Sequenced samples may be stored for no more than 3 days at −15 to −25°C.

Three methods are recommended to purify the sequence reaction, including isopropanol (similar to the procedure used by Roche Amplicor HIV-1 Monitor to precipitate the HIV-1 RNA), ethanol-sodium acetate, and the CENTRI•SEP 96 plate. This section deals with purification by the CENTRI•SEP 96 plate.

Equilibrate the CENTRI•SEP 96 plate to room temperature for 2 h. Remove the lower adhesive foil sealing, place the plate on a MicroAmp optical 96-well reaction plate embedded in a 96-well base, remove the upper adhesive foil sealing, and tape the plates and base together. Without letting the plate dry, immediately transfer it to a swinging rotor and centrifuge

at 700 × g for 2 min to pack the columns. Replace the MicroAmp optical 96-well reaction plate with a Princeton 96-well collection plate, place the CENTRI•SEP 96 plate on top of the Princeton 96-well collection plate, and tape the plate to the 96-well base. Using a multichannel pipettor, transfer the entire sequence reaction volume of approximately 20 μl from each well to the corresponding wells on the CENTRI•SEP 96 plate, being sure to maintain the exact orientation. Immediately transfer to a swinging rotor and centrifuge at 700 × g for 2 min. Transfer the Princeton 96-well collection plate containing the purified sequence reaction product (approximately 20 μl) to a Speed-Vac and dry. The desiccated product can be kept by sealing the plate with ThermaSeal and storing at −15 to −25°C in the dark, but samples need to be analyzed within 1 week.

Automated sequence detection. The HIV-1 genotyping system can be run on a multitude of automated sequence detection platforms, including the ABI Prism 3100 genetic analyzer, ABI Prism 3100-*Avant* genetic analyzer, and ABI Prism 3700 DNA analyzer. The ABI Prism 377 DNA sequencer, an acrylamide gel-based system, is also approved for use but is no longer manufactured; details on use of this platform have been previously described (17).

To perform the analysis on an ABI Prism 3100 genetic analyzer, power on the platform and the computer workstation. Ensure a constant green light status (located next to the on/off button) on the platform before proceeding; the green light must not be blinking. To prepare for sequence collection, select "Start > Applied Biosystems > 3100 Data Collection." A window will pop up with plate record identifiers and an impression for both plates. At this point the ABI Prism 3100 genetic analyzer will require final preparation for loading. Reagents required include POP-6 polymer, a 50-cm 16-capillary array, and 10× genetic analysis buffer with EDTA, diluted to 1× with deionized water. Inspect the level of POP-6 polymer in the ABI Prism 3100 genetic analyzer and add as needed (polymer must be changed every 7 days). Ensure that both the anode and cathode reservoirs are filled to the "fill line" with freshly prepared 1× genetic analysis buffer with EDTA. Water reservoirs must be filled to the fill line with deionized water. Inspect the channels in the polymer block for bubbles, and expel by pushing down on the syringe. Once the ABI Prism 3100 genetic analyzer is prepared, the "Collection Software, v.1.1" is activated on the computer workstation as follows. In "Preferences," select "Data Analysis and Extraction," and then make the following selections: select "Enable AutoAnalysis" On, clear "Extract to Sequence Collector," select "By Run," and then specify the format for the sample file name prefix: "Sample Name," "Well Position," or "<none>." End by selecting "OK." To continue, select "Plate View" and then "New," and under the "Tools Bar," select "Plate Editor." In the plate editor dialog box, name the plate (do not use space bar in naming plate), specify the application and the plate type, select "OK" to complete the application, and close the plate editor dialog box. Under "Application," select "Sequencing," and under "Plate Type," select "96-well," and then select "Finish." At this point the plate editor spreadsheet opens which allows naming of each sample. A specific naming convention is used and should be adhered to: it is patient identification, underscore, and primer; for example, patient 41/288_A to patient 41/288_H.

The following settings are set for each sample in the spreadsheet (note: when the appropriate setting is selected for the first sample, select the column heading to highlight the entire column and from the "Edit" menu select the "Fill Down" command): Dye Set, E; Mobility File, DT3100POP6{BD}v2.mob;

Comments, enter your comments; BioLIMS Project, N/A; Project Name, 3100-Project; Run Module 1, StdSeq50_POP6-DefaultModule; and Analysis Mode 1, BC-3100POP-6SR_SeqOffFtOff.saz.

To prepare the samples for analysis, bring those stored at −15 to −25°C to room temperature; otherwise proceed directly with those samples that have just been desiccated. In the Princeton 96-well collection plate, resuspend each dried sample by adding 20 μl of Hi-Di formamide, and then vortex for 10 to 15 s. Centrifuge the Princeton 96-well collection plate at $2,000 \times g$ for 20 to 30 s. Heat denaturing is not required, and the plate is now ready to load onto the ABI Prism 3100 genetic analyzer. Attach the ABI Prism 3100 genetic analyzer 96-well septa to the plate, and insert the plate in the "snap" on the ABI Prism 3100 genetic analyzer retainer and base. Load the framed plate onto the ABI Prism 3100 genetic analyzer, orienting the plate so that the A1 well is in the upper right corner, and verify that the plate position indicator is yellow. From the "Pending Plate Records" table, select the entered plate name in "Plate Record," and then select the corresponding plate on the position indicator (either A or B); the position indicator will turn from yellow to green and the plate name under "Pending Plate Record" will automatically transfer to either the A or B row under "Linked Plate Records." The plate is now linked to the plate record. Select the "Run View" tab to view the run schedule, and select each run to verify that the appropriate wells have been highlighted; if a well is not highlighted, it will not be analyzed. To start the run, click the green "Run Instrument Button" (green arrow). The software will automatically check the available space in the database and drive D and will advise accordingly; if the database or drive D is full, make more space and then click "Run Instrument." Once the instrument is running, select the "Status View" tab to confirm the electric current parameters. Should there be no indication of current, the most likely cause is a bubble in the polymer. Cancel the run, clear the bubble from the polymer, and restart the instrument.

When the run is complete, Sequence Analysis Software version 3.7 is launched and all the files (completed sequences from the run) are transferred from the run folder to the Sample Manager. The following settings are selected for each sample: Basecaller, Basecaller_3100SR; Spacing: Defined by Instrument; Basecaller Setting, HIV580; Peak 1 Location, Set by software, Start Point, Set by software; DyeSet/Primer, DT3100POP6{BD}v2.0; and Factura Setting, none (this function is not used with the ViroSeq assay).

Select the "A" (analyze) check box for each sample, clear the "P" (print) and "F" (Factura) columns, and then click "Start." Confirm analysis by checking the column A status color. If it is green, then the sample was analyzed; however, if it is red, then the sample was not analyzed (review the settings and reanalyze the data).

After proper sequence analysis, the data are ready to be used by HIV-1 Genotyping System Software version 2.6. This software incorporates and aligns all seven primer sequences of a sample into a single project with one consensus sequence. The sample consensus sequence is then compared to a reference sequence of HIV-1$_{HXB-2}$. The software performs automatic basecalling, and several options are selected to review the data. Manual editing is performed at "positions of interest," which include all resistance mutations found in the sample. The user resolves mixed-base positions in the same manner. Once editing is complete, a genotyping report is generated that contains a list of all the known resistance mutations found in *pro* and *rt* (compared with the Los Alamos National Laboratories reference database) as well as a separate list of all

novel mutations. Additional information is available at http://www.celeradiagnostics.com.

Phenotypic Resistance

There are two commercially available phenotypic assays, the Antivirogram assay (Virco, Mechelen, Belgium) and the PhenoSense HIV assay (ViroLogic); however, the patient plasma sample is sent to the manufacturer or to a recommended reference laboratory (access websites below for information) for testing.

Phenotypic assays are not available in a kit format because of their technical complexity. The technically challenging aspect is derived, in part, from generating a viral construct of a vector containing the patient's viral *pro* and *rt* insert. Viral constructs are necessary, because it is generally quite difficult to directly isolate and propagate patient-derived plasma virus, except from those infected individuals with progressive disease and high viral loads (14, 39). Therefore, complicated manual and robotic procedures that rely upon strict quality control and monitoring are required for the successful outcome of each analysis.

Comparative analysis demonstrates that Antivirogram and PhenoSense HIV generate essentially concordant results on matched clinical samples (53). However, similar to genotypic assays, Antivirogram performance is less efficient, by approximately 25%, with certain non-B subtypes (33); to date there are no peer-reviewed publications for PhenoSense HIV on non-B subtype performance.

Antivirogram

The Antivirogram assay is available for the quantitative measurement of HIV-1 phenotypic resistance from patient plasma samples. Briefly, purified HIV-1 RNA is derived from patient plasma by concentration of virus through high-speed centrifugation, viral lysis, and nucleic acid purification. The patient's HIV-1 *rt* and *pro* region is amplified as one continuous 2.2-kbp fragment by nested RT-PCR. The PCR-amplified fragment is cotransfected into MT-4 cells (CD4+ T-lymphocyte cell line) with a provirus-deleted plasmid pGEMT3ΔPRT (HXB2 viral backbone, of which the majority of *pro* and *rt* has been deleted). Chimeric virus is generated through homologous recombination, harvested after 7 to 8 days in culture, and titrated. Drug susceptibility is determined using a highly sensitive reporter-based assay system that specifically measures ongoing viral replication at the single-cell level. Resistance is reported as the 50% inhibitory concentration (IC$_{50}$) of the patient's chimeric virus compared with the control, recombinant HIV-1$_{IIIB/LAI}$. Generally, patient plasma samples with a viral load as low as 500 copies of HIV-1 RNA per ml can be analyzed; however, the highest sensitivity is obtained in plasma samples with a viral load of ≥1,000 copies of HIV-1 RNA per ml. The assay generally takes 18 laboratory working days to generate results (30). Additional information is available at http://www.vircolab.com/index.jhtml?product=none.

PhenoSense HIV

The PhenoSense HIV assay is available for phenotypic evaluation of patient plasma samples (51). Virus is concentrated from patient plasma by high-speed centrifugation, the virus pellet is lysed and viral RNA is purified using standard procedures. A 1.5-kbp fragment from the patient's HIV-1 RNA encompassing the entire *pro* (amino acids 1 to 99) coding region and a large portion of the *rt* (amino acids 1 to 305) coding region is amplified by RT-PCR. Using conventional molecular cloning procedures, the amplified 1.5-kbp fragments are inserted into a modified infectious, replication-defective molecular clone, HIV_{NL4-3}, to generate resistance test vectors (RTVs). RTVs contain a luciferase expression cassette inserted in a deleted region of the envelope gene. RTVs are prepared as libraries (or pools) containing many different variants of the 1.5-kbp patient insert, thus preserving the heterogeneity of the patient's quasispecies. The replication-defective patient's RTV DNA is cotransfected with amphotropic murine leukemia virus envelope expression vector DNA into human embryonic kidney 293 cells. The amphotropic murine leukemia virus envelope expression vector provides envelope proteins in *trans* to support the assembly of infectious pseudotyped HIV-1 particles. This methodology allows for only a single replication cycle format and thus avoids in vitro selection of virus populations through multiple rounds of replication.

To evaluate susceptibility to protease inhibitors, transfected cells are propagated in the presence of serial dilutions of protease inhibitors, and progeny virus is harvested and used to infect fresh 293 target cells in the absence of drugs. To evaluate susceptibility to RT inhibitors, virus is harvested from transfected cells propagated in the absence of drugs and used to infect 293 target cells in the presence of serial dilutions of RT inhibitors. Infection is measured by quantitating luciferase expression in target cells 48 to 72 h after virus inoculation. The percent inhibition of luciferase activity (i.e., infection) at each drug concentration is determined by dividing the luciferase activity produced in the presence of drug by the luciferase activity produced in the absence of drug. The IC_{50} is extrapolated from the data by plotting percent inhibition versus drug concentration. The fold change in patient HIV-1 drug susceptibility is determined by comparing the patient virus IC_{50} with the IC_{50} for a drug-susceptible reference virus that is run in parallel. Additionally, ViroLogic has ascertained the biological cutoff of drug susceptibility for several wild-type viruses with a variety of drugs and, by utilizing the natural variation of wild-type drug susceptibility, has calculated a more accurate fold change over baseline susceptibility to determine the clinical cutoff (resistance) for patient viral isolates (50). The performance characteristics of the assay have been validated for HIV-1 group M, subtype B. Patient plasma samples with viral loads of ≥500 copies of HIV-1 RNA per ml can be evaluated, and the assay reproducibly detects ≥2.5-fold changes in susceptibility.

The assay is performed in ViroLogic's licensed clinical reference laboratory, and results are reported within 2 weeks from the date of sample receipt. The replication capacity may also be evaluated as part of PhenoSense HIV (see "Replication Capacity" below). Additional information is available at http://www.virologic.com.

PhenoSense GT

ViroLogic offers a comprehensive analysis package, PhenoSense GT, whereby the same patient plasma sample is assayed for phenotypic and genotypic drug resistance, HIV-1 subtype (from sequence analysis), and replication capacity (a component of viral fitness); phenotypic analysis is performed on the sample and is not derived from a database as described below for Virco's *Virtual*Phenotype. The sample is tested by PhenoSense HIV (see above) and GeneSeq HIV (see above) for phenotypic and genotypic resistance, respectively, and replication capacity is tested as described below. Additional information is available at http://www.virologic.com.

Virtual Phenotype

Virtual phenotype refers to the procedure whereby the phenotype is extrapolated from the genotype using shared sequence data. This is achieved from large databases containing data correlating the genotype to the phenotype from patient samples. Hence, these databases allow the entry of genotypic sequence data, which are compared with sequence data of phenotyped samples, and a virtual phenotype is then constructed based upon the best available match. However, the association may not be 100% across the sequence; the level of correlation is indicated on a virtual-phenotype report. A virtual phenotype can be interpreted as long as the genotypic sequence is continuous. Although this is a less expensive means of obtaining a phenotype, it still remains a "virtual" interpretation, because it is an extrapolation of data with the best possible fit and thus may not represent the exact phenotypic characteristics of that patient's isolate.

To generate a *Virtual*Phenotype, the HIV-1 plasma isolate is submitted to Virco and genotyped utilizing their in-house procedure, VircoGEN II, which makes use of dideoxy sequencing technology, similar to that described for ViroSeq (see above). Briefly, amplification of the target sequence is accomplished by nested PCR, generating a 2.2-kbp product encompassing the *pro* and *rt* coding sequences. Sequencing primers, developed by Virco, allow for sequence analysis of the entire *pro* gene and up to codon 400 of the *rt* gene. The sequence is then analyzed against databanks to generate the *Virtual*Phenotype report. Additional information is available at http://www.vircolab.com/index.jhtml?product=none.

Replication Capacity

Replication capacity (ViroLogic) (4) is an outcome of PhenoSense HIV where the pseudotyped patient HIV-1 particle replication is expressed as a percentage of pseudotyped wild-type HIV-1 particle replication (see "PhenoSense HIV" above). Knowledge of replication capacity can be used to aid in treatment assessment (4). ViroLogic offers the replication capacity assay as part of the PhenoSense HIV and PhenoSense GT products. Additional information is available from http://www.virologic.com.

Online Services

Online options are available to the testing laboratory and clinician for the evaluation of HIV-1 drug resistance. Specifically, once a sequence has been derived from a clinical sample, the user may elect to either submit the sequence online for a third party to analyze and generate reports or directly analyze the sequence online. VircoNET (Virco) and Virodec-HIV (F. Hoffmann-La Roche Ltd., Basel, Switzerland) are examples of these services.

The benefits of using online services vary depending on the product options available. From the clinical laboratory director's standpoint, these online services permit utilization of any available technology to generate the sequence data for genotypic resistance analysis. For example, the laboratory may elect to use ViroSeq or TRUGENE to generate the sequence or may consider other options, such as a potentially less costly homebrew assay, with the appropriate quality assurance and quality control programs. Ultimately, cost model analysis may be used to determine the most cost-effective package.

From the perspective of the clinician or researcher, data can be analyzed using up-to-date algorithms and with different reference stains (see "Virodec-HIV" below).

VircoNET

The HIV-1 sequence (obtained by either TRUGENE, ViroSeq, or homebrew) is submitted to Virco's online service to VircoNET to obtain a *Virtual*Phenotype. A result is provided within 2 working days. Additional information is available at http://www.vircogen.com.index.jhtml?product=none.

Virodec-HIV

Virodec-HIV (F. Hoffmann-La Roche Ltd.) is a browser-based service for analysis of complex data, utilizing the IDNS (Integrated Database Network System) technology. While its backbone structure includes database and web functionalities, customized disease-specific modules are offered to customers for complex diseases such as HIV. Virodec-HIV allows the user to enter disease-relevant and virus sequence data from HIV-1 *rt* and *pro*, as well as *gag* and envelope (*env*) genes, for resistance analysis and a patient report; a charge is levied for the service, and various pricing models are available to suit the needs of the user.

The platform can function online through access with the Internet and a web browser, or it can be stand-alone, or within an intranet infrastructure, with upgrades and updates accessible through connection with the Internet. To maintain security, data are encrypted for transmission. Numerous algorithms can be incorporated for analyzing data and generating drug resistance reports. The service is provided with the Stanford algorithm; however, the user can incorporate additional algorithms. The drug resistance report includes a list of HIV-1 antiretroviral drugs, their corresponding generic names, mutations detected, score and range, and interpretation of result. Planned upgrades of the service allow this information to be uploaded into the accompanying patient data management form, which also includes the clinical condition and treatment regimen of the patient. Multiple chronological entries for the same patient provide the option of a longitudinal data record that is presented in both numeric and graphic format.

The Virodec-HIV service can be made available online to permit network communications to other users using a secure pass code system. Databases can be generated for this purpose to allow other investigators to access and share and compare information; however, only the database creator can alter or add information. The data are shared only by authorized access.

From the clinician and researcher standpoint, Virodec-HIV provides options to custom analyze data, to recognize genetic profiles of both B and non-B subtype clinical isolates (using the clade finder in the Virodec program), to reanalyze data as technology advances by using up-to-date reference strains and algorithms, to consolidate clinical information, and to share data with other team members for, as an example, consultations or manuscript preparation.

For the realization of the Virodec product line, F. Hoffmann-La Roche Ltd. collaborates closely with SmartGene GmbH, Zug, Switzerland, and integrates the SmartGene IDNS technology in its offering.

Procedure. Sequence data may be generated using one of the commercial assays (ViroSeq or TRUGENE, for example) or one of several available homebrew assays.

To access the software, turn on the computer workstation and, using name and password, log into the "Specimen Management" window. Enter patient identification, date of birth, sample date, sample label, laboratory label, sample specimen, and comments. Select the "Application" tab to access the three applications, including "Reference Sequences" (blue box), "Sample Sequences" (red box), and "Clipboard(s)" (gray box).

The "Reference Sequences" function contains HIV reference sequences (B and non-B subtypes) that are used for alignment with the clinical specimen sequence for determination of mutations, which could be resistance relevant. The reference sequences are continually kept up-to-date by Virodec support staff. The user cannot edit the reference database; however, the user may elect to generate a customized reference database, which in turn can be edited only by the user.

The "Sample Sequences" function is where the patient sample sequence and additional disease-relevant data are entered, generating a database that can be shared with other authorized users. Entered sequences and sample data sets are also accessed in this section and can be reanalyzed as needed.

The "Clipboard(s)" function permits the user to input and analyze data from different samples sequenced over a period of time. This allows for longitudinal analysis of same or related patient samples (i.e., source and recipient patients) or samples from patients on the same regimen, as well as contamination check for samples run in the same or successive batches; the flexibility of the system allows for numerous analyses.

Sequence analysis. Using the "Sample Sequences" function, select "Add Record in Virodec HIV Samples" tab. A proofreading window opens where the sequence can be either uploaded or copy pasted. The Virodec proofreading module automatically executes alignment and orientation of the sequence. Uploading the electropherogram assists in detecting and correcting ambiguities and aids in verification of the sequence. The consensus sequence is selected and compared against the patient sequence; *rt*, *pro*, *gag*, and *env* are included in the consensus sequence. The software identifies codons conferring resistance and can be executed using either the manual or automated system. Virodec accounts for insertions and deletions. The sequence can also be subtyped (select "Subtype Analysis" tab), and can be compared to other isolates with similar sequences (select "Search Sequence Similarity in a Sample Database" in "Sample Sequences" function). A drug resistance report is generated utilizing the preferred algorithm available on Virodec.

Patient management. Soon-to-be-available features of the Virodec software will allow the patient genotypic report to be incorporated into the "Patient Data Management" screen that includes numerous options to record disease states, clinical conditions, and treatment regimen. Integration of these data allows for a graphic display of results and permits the user to generate longitudinal records for each patient. Additional information is available at http://www.virodec.com.

Cloning and Microculturing Technique

As described above, both commercially phenotypic assays are now available in a kit format. In the assays, HIV protease and RT genes are inserted into replication-defective molecular clones to generate chimeric clones (see above). However, the produced recombinant chimeric clones occasionally possess a low level of replication competence due to lack of mutations in the *gag* (p7/p1/p6) cleavage site (57). To obtain accurate drug resistance profiles, it is often necessary to construct chimeric clones containing mutations in the *gag* cleavage site with high replication competence. From this point of view, a modified molecular clone, pNL4.3PFB (Fig. 3), has been designed to obtain the chimeric recombinant viruses containing mutations in the cleavage sites (34).

PCR Amplification

A 1,685-bp fragment of the HIV-1 genome containing the *gag* (p7/p1/p6) regions, the protease gene, and part of the RT gene is amplified by PCR as described above with the following primer pairs: forward primer (nucleotides [nt] 1881 to 1904) 5′-GAAGCAATGAGCCAAGTAACAAAT-3′

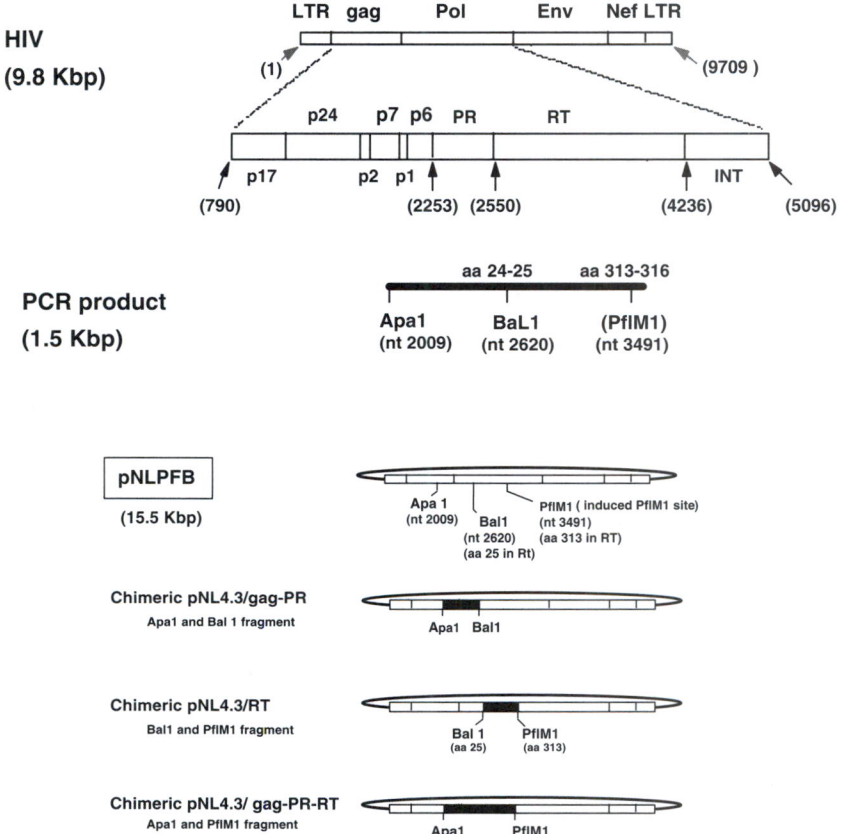

FIGURE 3 Structure of chimeric HIV. The PCR-amplified products are digested with restriction enzymes depending on the drug to be tested. To investigate drug resistance to protease inhibitor, RT inhibitor, or a combination of protease inhibitor and RT inhibitor, the products are digested with *Apa*1 plus *Bal*1, *Bal*1 plus *Pfl*M1, or *Apa*1 plus *Pfl*M1. The digested products are ligated into pNLPFB backbone. LTR, long terminal repeat; aa, amino acid; PR, protease.

and reverse primer (nt 3543 to 3566) 5′-GATATGTC-CATTGGCCTTGCCCCT-3′. A nested PCR is then carried out with the following primer pairs: forward primer (nt 1965 to 1988) 5′-TTCAATTGTGGCAAAGAAGGGCA-3′ and reverse primer (nt 3482 to 3505) 5′-ATAATACACTC-CATGTACTGGTTC-3′. The reaction mixtures (50 μl) containing 1× Expand High Fidelity buffer, oligonucleotide pairs (400 nM), dNTPs (200 nM), and 1.75 U of Expand High Fidelity PCR System enzyme mix, are subjected to 25 cycles of 95°C for 30 s, 55°C for 30 s, and 72°C for 2 min, with the final extension at 72°C for 7 min. The PCR products are purified with the QIAquick spin PCR purification kit (Qiagen).

Cloning and Sequencing

The purified PCR products are ligated into the pCRII vector (Invitrogen), and the ligation products are used to transform *Escherichia coli* TOP10F competent cells (Invitrogen). Positive colonies are identified and the presence of a 1.6-kbp insert is confirmed by restriction enzyme digestion with *Eco*RI. Plasmid DNAs containing the PCR fragments are purified with the S.N.A.P. Miniprep kit (Invitrogen). Sequencing reactions are performed with the BigDye Terminator Cycle Sequence kit (Applied Biosystems, Foster City, Calif.), and the reaction products are resolved by electrophoresis on 6.0%

polyacrylamide gels and analyzed with an Applied Biosystems 377 automated sequencing system. The nucleotide sequences of the *gag* (p7/p1/p6) regions, the protease gene, and the RT gene are translated and aligned with the Sequence Navigator (Applied Biosystems). Changes in the RT regions are compared with the HIV-1 clade B consensus sequence as a reference (46).

Construction of Molecular Chimeric Clones

The plasmid (pNL4.3PFB is available through the National Institute of Allergy and Infectious Diseases) contains one *Bal*1 site at nt 2622 and one *Pfl*M1 site at nt 3492 in the *rt* gene (Fig. 3). These two restriction enzyme sites are then utilized to construct a series of chimeric infectious clones of HIV-1. To obtain virus-containing *gag-pro-rt*, the clones are digested with *Apa*1 and *Pfl*M1. The fragments from *Apa*1 and *Pfl*M1 digestion are used to replace the corresponding fragment of pNL4.3PFB (Fig. 3). DNA sequencing is used to ascertain that each of the chimeric NLPFB and mutated NL4.3PFB variants possesses the intended mutations.

Transfections, Infections, and Generation of Viral Stocks

Transfections are performed with TranSit LT1 (Panvera) as previously described (26, 34, 57). Briefly, 3.5×10^5 RD cells in 35-mm culture dishes are used for each transfection with 2 µg of the molecular clones in 5 ml of EMEM-10. After 24 h of transfection, 10^6 fresh MT-2 cells are added to the dishes and incubated at 37°C for another 24 h. The MT-4 cells thus infected are collected, washed, and cultured at 37°C for 3 days in 5 ml of RPMI-10. Cell-free culture supernatants are obtained and stored at −80°C until used as viral stocks. Nucleotide sequencing of the stocks is performed to confirm that each stock has the intended mutation(s) in the *rt* gene. The 50% tissue culture infectious dose (TCID$_{50}$) of each stock is determined as previously described (34, 57). Cultures of MT-4 cells and serial fourfold dilutions of the appropriate recombinant HIV stock are set up in triplicate. The tissue culture plates are incubated at 37°C for 7 days, after which culture supernatants are collected and p24 antigen assays are performed (p24 antigen capture kit; Beckman Coulter, Miami, Fla.). Using a cutoff value for p24 of <50 pg/ml, TCID$_{50}$s are calculated for each stock by the Spearman-Karber method (1).

Drug Resistance Assays

MT-4 cells (4×10^6) are incubated with 2,500 TCID$_{50}$s of HIV-1 for 2 h at 37°C, washed twice, and resuspended at a density of 0.2×10^6 cells/ml in RPMI-10. An aliquot of the suspension (0.2 ml) is added to each well of a 96-well flat-bottom plate in the presence or absence of various concentrations of anti-HIV-1 drugs, such as protease inhibitors or RT inhibitors, for 7 days at 37°C. HIV replication is monitored by measurement of p24 amount in culture supernatant with the p24 antigen capture kit (Beckman Coulter). Each assay is performed in quadruplicate. Sensitivities are reported as the concentrations of the drugs that inhibited p24 production by 50% (34).

REFERENCES

1. **AIDS Clinical Trials Group.** 2004. *Virology Manual for HIV Laboratories.* [Online.] Division of AIDS, National Institute of Allergy and Infectious Diseases, Bethesda, Md. http://www.niaid.nih.gov./daids/vir_manual.
2. **Beddows, S., S. Galpin, S. H. Kazmi, A. Ashraf, A. Johargy, A. J. Frater, N. White, R. Braganza, J. Clarke, M. McClure, and J. N. Weber.** 2003. Performance of two commercially available sequence-based HIV-1 genotyping systems for the detection of drug resistance against HIV type 1 group M subtypes. *J. Med. Virol.* **70:**337–342.
3. **Beutler, E., T. Gelbart, and W. Kuhl.** 1990. Interferences of heparin with the polymerase chain reaction. *BioTechniques* **9:**166.
4. **Buckheit, R. W., Jr.** 2004. Understanding HIV resistance, fitness, replication capacity and compensation: targeting viral fitness as a therapeutic strategy. *Exp. Opin. Investig. Drugs* **13:**933–958.
5. **Carpenter, C. C. J., D. A. Cooper, M. A. Fischl, J. M. Gatell, B. G. Gazzard, S. M. Hammer, M. S. Hirsch, D. M. Jacobsen, D. A. Katzenstein, J. S. Montner, D. D. Richman, M. S. Saag, M. Schechter, R. T. Schooley, M. A. Thompson, S. Vella, P. G. Yeni, and P. A. Volberding.** 2000. Antiretroviral therapy in adults: updated recommendations of the International AIDS Society— USA panel. *JAMA* **283:**381–390.
6. **Chew, C. B., B. L. Herring, F. Zheng, C. Browne, N. K. Saksena, A. L. Cunningham, and D. E. Dwyer.** 1999. Comparison of three commercial assays for the quantification of HIV-1 RNA in plasma from individuals infected with different HIV-1 subtypes. *J. Clin. Virol.* **14:**87–94.
7. **Chun, T. W., D. Engel, S. B. Mizell, L. A. Ehler, and A. S. Fauci.** 1998. Induction of HIV-1 replication in

latently infected CD4+ T cells using a combination of cytokines. *J. Exp. Med.* **188:**83–91.
8. **Chun, T. W., L. Stuyver, S. B. Mizell, L. A. Ehler, J. A. M. Mican, M. Baseler, A. L. Lloyd, M. A. Nowak, and A. S. Fauci.** 1997. Presence of an inducible HIV-1 latent reservoir during highly active antiretroviral therapy. *Proc. Natl. Acad. Sci. USA* **94:**13193–13197.
9. **Clementi, M., S. Menzo, P. Bagnarelli, A. Manzin, A. Valenza, and P. E. Varaldo.** 1993. Quantitative PCR and RT-PCR in virology. *PCR Methods Applic.* **2:**191–196.
10. **Coutlee, F., P. Saint-Antoine, C. Olivier, A. Kessous-Elbaz, H. Voyer, F. Berrada, P. Begin, L. Giroux, and R. Viscidi.** 1991. Discordance between primer pairs in the polymerase chain reaction for detection of human immunodeficiency virus type 1: a role for Taq polymerase inhibitors. *J. Infect. Dis.* **164:**817–818.
11. **Cunningham, S., B. Ank, D. Lewis, W. Lu, M. Wantman, J. A. Dileanis, J. B. Jackson, P. Palumbo, P. Krogstad, and S. H. Eshleman.** 2001. Performance of the Applied Biosystems ViroSeq human immunodeficiency virus type 1 (HIV-1) genotyping system for sequence-based analysis of HIV-1 in pediatric plasma samples. *J. Clin. Microbiol.* **39:**1254–1257.
12. **d'Arminio Monforte, A., L. Testa, F. Adorni, E. Chiesa, T. Bini, G. C. Moscatelli, C. Abeli, S. Rusconi, S. Sollima, C. Balotta, M. Musicco, M. Galli, and M. Moroni.** 1998. Clinical outcome and predictive factors of failure of highly active antiretroviral therapy in antiretroviral-experienced patients in advanced stages of HIV-1 infection. *AIDS* **12:**1631–1637.
13. **Dauber, D. S., R. Ziermann, N. Parkin, D. J. Maly, S. Mahrus, J. L. Harris, J. A. Ellman, C. Petropoulos, and C. S. Craik.** 2002. Altered substrate specificity of drug-resistant human immunodeficiency virus type 1 protease. *J. Virol.* **76:**1359–1368.
14. **Dewar, R. L., H. C. Highbarger, M. D. Sarmiento, E. S. Lawton, M. B. Vasudevachari, J. A. Kovacs, R. T. Davey, R. E. Walker, H. C. Lane, and N. P. Salzman.** 1992. Isolation of HIV-1 from plasma of infected individuals; an analysis of experimental conditions affecting successful virus propagation. *J. Acquir. Immune Defic. Syndr.* **5:**822–828.
15. **Dickover, R. E., S. A. Herman, K. Saddiq, D. Wafer, M. Dillon, and Y. J. Bryson.** 1998. Optimization of specimen-handling procedures for accurate quantitation of levels of human immunodeficiency virus RNA in plasma by reverse transcriptase PCR. *J. Clin. Microbiol.* **36:**1070–1073.
16. **Dornadula, G., H. Zhang, B. VanUitert, J. Stern, L. Livornese, Jr., M. J. Ingerman, J. Witek, R. J. Kedanis, J. Natkin, J. DeSimone, and R. J. Pomerantz.** 1999. Residual HIV-1 RNA in blood plasma of patients taking suppressive highly active antiretroviral therapy. *JAMA* **282:**1627–1632.
17. **Elbeik, T., T. W. Chun, H. Imamichi, T. Imamichi, V. Natarajan, D. Waters, R. L. Dewar, and H. Highbarger.** 2002. Quantitation of viremia and determination of drug resistance in patients with human immunodeficiency virus infection, p. 772–789. *In* N. R. Rose, R. G. Hamilton, and B. Detrick (ed.), *Manual of Clinical Laboratory Immunology*, 6th ed., ASM Press, Washington, D.C.
17a. **Elbeik, T., R. L. Dewar, and V. Natarajan.** 1997. Isolation and detection of human immunodeficiency virus, p. 781–787. *In* N. R. Rose, E. Conway de Macario, J. D. Folds, H. C. Lane, and R. M. Nakamura (ed.), *Manual of Clinical Laboratory Immunology*, 5th ed. ASM Press, Washington, D.C.
18. **Eshleman, S. H., J. Hackett, Jr., P. Swanson, S. P. Cunningham, B. Drews, C. Brennan, S. G. Devare, L. Zekeng, L. Kaptue, and N. Marlowe.** 2004. Performance of the Celera Diagnostics ViroSeq HIV-1 Genotyping System for sequence-based analysis of diverse human immunodeficiency virus type 1 strains. *J. Clin. Microbiol.* **42:**2711–2717.

19. Feher, A., I. T. Weber, P. Bagossi, P. Boross, B. Mahalingam, J. M. Louis, T. D. Copeland, I. Y. Torshin, R. W. Harrison, and J. Tozser. 2002. Effect of sequence polymorphism and drug resistance on two HIV-1 Gag processing sites. *Eur. J. Biochem.* **269:**4114–4120.

20. Ferrando, S., W. van Gorp, M. McElhiney, K. Goggin, M. Sewell, and J. Rabkin. 1998. Highly active antiretroviral treatment in HIV infection: benefits for neuropsychological function. *AIDS* **12:**F65–F70.

21. Finzi, D., M. Hermankova, T. Pierson, L. M. Carruth, C. Buck, R. E. Chaisson, T. C. Quinn, K. Chadwick, J. Margolick, R. Brookmeyer, J. Gallant, M. Markowitz, D. D. Ho, D. D. Richman, and R. F. Siliciano. 1997. Identification of a reservoir for HIV-1 in patients on highly active antiretroviral therapy. *Science* **278:**1295–1300.

22. Fontaine, E., C. Riva, M. Peeters, J. C. Schmit, E. Delaporte, K. Van Laethem, K. Van Vaerenbergh, J. Snoeck, E. Van Wijngaerden, E. De Clercq, M. Van Ranst, and A. M. Vandamme. 2001. Evaluation of two commercial kits for the detection of genotypic drug resistance on a panel of HIV type 1 subtypes A through J. *J. Acquir. Immune Defic. Syndr.* **28:**254–258.

23. Furtado, M. R., D. S. Callaway, J. P. Phair, K. J. Kunstman, J. L. Stanton, C. A. Macken, A. S. Perelson, and S. M. Wolinsky. 1999. Persistence of HIV-1 transcription in peripheral-blood mononuclear cells in patients receiving potent antiretroviral therapy. *N. Engl. J. Med.* **340:**1614–1622.

24. Gatanaga, H., Y. Suzuki, H. Tsang, K. Yoshimura, M. F. Kavlick, K. Nagashima, R. J. Gorelick, S. Mardy, C. Tang, M. F. Summers, and H. Mitsuya. 2002. Amino acid substitutions in Gag protein at non-cleavage sites are indispensable for the development of a high multitude of HIV-1 resistance against protease inhibitors. *J. Biol. Chem.* **277:**5952–5961.

25. Gilliland, G., S. Perrin, K. Blanchard, and H. F. Bunn. 1990. Analysis of cytokine mRNA and DNA: detection and quantitation of competitive polymerase chain reaction. *Proc. Natl. Acad. Sci. USA* **87:**2725–2729.

26. Gonzales, M. J., E. Johnson, K. M. Dupnik, T. Imamichi, and R. W. Shafer. 2003. Colinearity of reverse transcriptase inhibitor resistance mutations detected by population-based sequencing. *J. Acquir. Immune Defic. Syndr.* **34:**398–402.

27. Gulick, R. M., J. W. Mellors, D. Havlir, J. J. Eron, C. Gonzalez, D. McMahon, D. D. Richman, F. T. Valentine, L. Jonas, A. Meibohm, E. A. Emini, and J. A. Chodakewitz. 1997. Treatment with indinavir, zidovudine, and lamivudine in adults with human immunodeficiency virus infection and prior antiretroviral therapy. *N. Engl. J. Med.* **337:**734–739.

28. Gunthard, H. F., S. W. Frost, A. J. Leigh-Brown, C. C. Ignacio, K. Kee, A. S. Perelson, C. A. Spina, D. V. Halvir, M. Hezareh, D. J. Looney, D. D. Richman, and J. K. Wong. 1999. Evolution of envelope sequences of human immunodeficiency virus type 1 in cellular reservoirs in the setting of potent antiviral therapy. *J. Virol.* **73:**9404–9412.

29. Hammer, S. M., K. E. Squires, M. D. Hughes, J. M. Grimes, L. M. Demeter, J. S. Currier, J. J. Eron, Jr., J. E. Feinberg, H. H. Balfour, Jr., L. R. Deyton, J. A. Chodakewitz, and M. A. Fischl For the AIDS Clinical Trial Group 320 Study Team. 1997. A controlled trial of two nucleotide analogues plus indinavir in persons with human immunodeficiency virus infection and CD4 cell counts of 200 per cubic millimeter or less. *N. Engl. J. Med.* **337:**725–733.

30. Hertogs, K., M.-P. De Bethune, V. Miller, T. Ivenes, P. Schel, A. Van Cauwenberge, C. Van Den Eynde, V. Van Gerwen, H. Azijn, M. Van Houtte, F. Peeters, S. Staszewski, M. Conant, S. Bloor, S. Kemp, B. Larder, and R. Pausels. 1998. A rapid method for simultaneous detection of phenotypic resistance to inhibitors of protease and reverse transcriptase in recombinant human immunodeficiency virus type 1 isolates from patients treated with antiretroviral drugs. *Antimicrob. Agents Chemother.* **42:**269–276.

31. Highbarger, H., W. G. Alvord, M. K. Jiang, A. Shah, J. Metcalf, H. C. Lane, and R. Dewar. 1999. Comparison of the Quantiplex version 3.0 assay and a sensitized Amplicor Monitor assay for measurement of human immunodeficiency virus type 1 RNA levels in plasma samples. *J. Clin. Microbiol.* **37:**3612–3614.

32. Hirschel, B., and M. Opravil. 1999. The year in review: antiretroviral treatment. *AIDS* **13**(Suppl. A):S177–S187.

33. Holguin, A., K. Hertogs, and V. Soriano. 2003. Performance of drug resistance assays in testing HIV-1 non-B subtypes. *Clin. Microbiol. Infect.* **9:**323–326.

34. Imamichi, T., S. C. Berg, H. Imamichi, J. C. Lopez, J. A. Metcalf, J. Falloon, and H. C. Lane. 2000. Relative replication fitness of a high-level 3'-azido-3'-deoxythymidine-resistant variant of human immunodeficiency virus type 1 possessing an amino acid deletion at codon 67 and a novel substitution (Thr→Gly) at codon 69. *J. Virol.* **74:**10958–10964.

35. Jagodzinski, L. L., D. L. Wiggins, J. L. McManis, S. Emery, J. Overbaugh, M. Robb, S. Bodrug, and N. L. Michael. 2000. Use of calibrated viral load standards for group M subtypes of human immunodeficiency virus type 1 to assess the performance of viral RNA quantitation tests. *J. Clin. Microbiol.* **38:**1247–1249.

36. Japour, A. J., D. L. Mayers, V. A. Johnson, D. R. Kuritzkes, L. A. Beckett, J.-M. Arduino, J. Lane, R. J. Black, P. S. Reichelderfer, R. T. D'Aquila, C. S. Crumpacker, The RV-43 Study Group, and the AIDS Clinical Trials Group Virology Committee Resistance Working Group. 1993. Standardized peripheral blood mononuclear cell culture assay for determination of drug susceptibilities of clinical human immunodeficiency virus type 1 isolates. *Antimicrob. Agents Chemother.* **37:**1095–1101.

37. Johnston, R. F., S. C. Pickett, and D. L. Barker. 1990. Autoradiography using storage phosphor technology. *Electrophoresis* **11:**355–360.

38. Kuritzkes, D. R., R. M. Grant, P. Feorino, M. Griswold, M. Hoover, R. Young, S. Day, R. M. Lloyd, Jr., C. Reid, G. F. Morgan, and D. L. Winslow. 2003. Performance characteristics of the TRUGENE HIV-1 genotyping kit and the Opengene DNA sequencing system. *J. Clin. Microbiol.* **41:**1594–1599.

39. Lathey, J. L., S. A. Fiscus, S. Rasheed, J. C. Kappes, B. P. Griffith, T. Elbeik, S. A. Spector, and P. S. Reichelderfer. 1994. Optimization of quantitative culture assay for human immunodeficiency virus from plasma. Plasma Viremia Group Laboratories of the AIDS Clinical Trials Group (National Institute of Allergy and Infectious Diseases). *J. Clin. Microbiol.* **32:**3064–3067.

40. Lewin, S. R., M. Vesanen, L. Kostrikis, A. Hurley, M. Duran, L. Zhang, D. D. Ho, and M. Markowitz. 1999. Use of real-time PCR and molecular beacons to detect virus replication in human immunodeficiency virus type 1-infected individuals on prolonged effective antiretroviral therapy. *J. Virol.* **73:**6099–6103.

41. Li, T. S., R. Tubiana, C. Katlama, V. Calvez, H. Ait Mohand, and B. Autran. 1998. Long-lasting recovery in CD4 T-cell function and viral-load reduction after highly active antiretroviral therapy in advanced HIV-1 disease. *Lancet* **351:**1682–1686.

42. Longo, M. C., M. S. Berninger, and J. L. Hartley. 1990. Use of uracil DNA glycosylase to control carry-over contamination in polymerase chain reaction. *Gene* **93:**125–128.

43. Maes, B., Y. Schrooten, J. Snoeck, I. Derdelinckx, M. Van Ranst, A. M. Vandamme, and K. Van Laethem. 2004. Performance of ViroSeq HIV-1 genotyping system in

routine practice at a Belgian clinical laboratory. *J. Virol. Methods* **119:**45–49.

44. **Menzo, S., P. Bagnarelli, M. Giacca, A. Manzin, P. E. Varaldo, and M. Clementi.** 1992. Absolute quantitation of viremia in human immunodeficiency virus infection by competitive reverse transcription and polymerase chain reaction. *J. Clin. Microbiol.* **30:**1752–1757.

45. **Mulder, J., N. McKinney, C. Christopherson, J. Sninsky, L. Greenfield, and S. Kwok.** 1994. Rapid and simple PCR assay for quantitation of human immunodeficiency virus type 1 RNA in plasma: application to acute retroviral infection. *J. Clin. Microbiol.* **32:**292–300.

46. **Myers, G., B. T. Korber, S. Wain-Hobson, R. Smith, and G. N. Pavlakas.** 1995. *Human Retroviruses and AIDS: a Compilation and Analysis of Nucleic Acid and Amino Acid Sequences.* [Online.] Theoretical Biology and Biophysics Group T-10, Los Alamos National Laboratory, Los Alamos, N.Mex. http://hiv-web.lanl.gov.

47. **Myint, L., M. Matsuda, Z. Matsuda, Y. Yokomaku, T. Chiba, A. Okano, K. Yamada, and W. Sugiura.** 2004. Gag non-cleavage site mutations contribute to full recovery of viral fitness in protease inhibitor-resistant human immunodeficiency virus type 1. *Antimicrob. Agents Chemother.* **48:**444–452.

48. **Natarajan, V., M. Bosche, J. A. Metcalf, D. J. Ward, H. C. Lane, and J. A. Kovacs.** 1999. HIV-1 replication in patients with undetectable plasma virus receiving HAART. *Lancet* **353:**119–120.

49. **Natarajan, V., R. J. Plishka, E. W. Scott, H. C. Lane, and N. P. Salzman.** 1994. An internally controlled virion PCR (ICVPCR) for the measurement of HIV-1 RNA in plasma. *PCR Methods Applic.* **3:**346–350.

50. **Parkin, N. T., N. S. Hellmann, J. M. Whitcomb, L. Kiss, C. C. Chappey, and C. J. Petropoulos.** 2004. Natural variation of drug susceptibility in wild-type human immunodeficiency virus type 1. *Antimicrob. Agents Chemother.* **48:**437–443.

51. **Petropoulos, C. J., N. T. Parkin, K. L. Limoli, Y. S. Lie, T. Wrin, W. Huang, H. Tian, D. Smith, G. A. Winslow, D. J. Capon, and J. M. Whitcomb.** 2000. A novel phenotypic drug susceptibility assay for human immunodeficiency virus type 1. *Antimicrob. Agents Chemother.* **44:**920–928.

52. **Piatak, M. M., Jr., S. Saag, L. C. Yang, S. J. Clark, J. C. Kappes, K.-C. Luk, B. H. Hahn, G. M. Shaw, and J. D. Lifson.** 1993. High levels of HIV-1 in plasma during all stages of infection determined by competitive PCR. *Science* **259:**1749–1754.

53. **Qari, S. H., R. Respess, H. Weinstock, E. M. Beltrami, K. Hertogs, B. A. Larder, C. J. Petropoulos, N. Hellmann, and W. Heneine.** 2002. Comparative analysis of two commercial phenotypic assays for drug susceptibility testing of human immunodeficiency virus type 1. *J. Clin. Microbiol.* **40:**31–35.

54. **Sharkey, M. E., I. Teo, T. Greenough, N. Sharova, K. Luzuriaga, J. L. Sullivan, R. P. Bucy, L. G. Kostrikis, A. Haase, C. Veryard, R. E. Davaro, S. H. Cheeseman, J. S. Daly, C. Bova, R. T. Ellison III, B. Mady, K. K. Lai, G. Moyle, M. Nelson, B. Gazzard, S. Shaunak, and M. Stevenson.** 2000. Persistence of episomal HIV-1 infection intermediates in patients on highly active anti-retroviral therapy. *Nat. Med.* **6:**76–81.

55. **Wong, J. K., M. Hezareh, H. F. Gunthard, D. V. Havlir, C. C. Ignacio, C. A. Spina, and D. D. Richman.** 1997. Recovery of replication-competent HIV despite prolonged suppression of plasma viremia. *Science* **278:**1291–1295.

56. **Zhang, L., B. Ramratnam, K. Tenner-Racz, H. Yuxian, M. Vesanen, S. Lewin, A. Talal, P. Racz, A. S. Perelson, B. T. Korber, M. Markowitz, and D. D. Ho.** 1999. Quantifying residual HIV-1 replication in patients receiving combination antiretroviral therapy. *N. Engl. J. Med.* **340:**1605–1613.

57. **Zhang, Y.-M., H. Imamichi, T. Imamichi, H. C. Lane, J. Falloon, M. B. Vasudevachari, and N. P. Salzman.** 1997. Drug resistance during indinavir therapy is caused by mutations in the protease gene and in its Gag substrate cleavage sites. *J. Virol.* **71:**6662–6670.

Measurement of T-Cell-Specific Immunity in Patients with Human Immunodeficiency Virus Infection

RICHARD L. HENGEL, TOMOZUMI IMAMICHI, AND STEPHEN A. MIGUELES

97

BACKGROUND

Despite more than 20 years of intensive research, the precise mechanism of human immunodeficiency virus (HIV) pathogenesis remains unknown. Nowhere is this shortcoming more frustrating than in the field of HIV vaccine development, where empirical rather than rational vaccines continue to be necessary until we have a better understanding of how HIV causes disease. Until then, intensive research must continue, building on what is already known.

Most people with untreated HIV infection develop clinical immunodeficiency. For those without access to treatment, the median time to life-threatening opportunistic infection or malignancy averages about 10 years (13). For those fortunate enough to have access to treatment, new anti-HIV drugs can prevent this eventuality, perhaps indefinitely. However, even these individuals may suffer subtle immunodeficiency before meeting current criteria to start treatment. Clinically, such immunodeficiency can manifest by an increased susceptibility to diseases like thrush or tuberculosis.

Fortunately, while we do not yet know how HIV causes disease, we do have significant insights into correlates of the disease and, in particular, how HIV disease correlates with heightened levels of HIV replication, CD4+-T-cell depletion, immune activation, and cellular turnover. Earlier in the HIV epidemic, similar correlations with disease and functional assays of immune function included impaired responses to immunization, and functional measures of T-cell responsiveness to recall antigen (9). More recently, more sophisticated assays of T-cell function have been developed, mostly owing to improvements in multiparameter flow cytometry and to improvements in T-cell isolation techniques. These new assays promise to further help refine insights into HIV pathogenesis by dissecting the intricate interactions of antigen-specific cell function from immune activation and CD4+-T-cell lymphopenia. Many of these assays are now capable of more specifically measuring the human immune response directly, and many may soon be ready for clinical application. Examples could include helping physicians decide about the need for revaccination or the need for prophylaxis for latent tuberculosis infection in developed countries where widespread treatment is not yet feasible.

While the ultimate mechanism of HIV pathogenesis remains elusive, one fortunate consequence of two decades of HIV research has been the development and optimization of new tools to investigate the human immune response, both in health and in disease. In this chapter we outline both old and new tools used in evaluating patients with HIV disease. Some of these are used in clinical settings, some in the research setting. However, it seems only a matter of time before most or all of the research tools ultimately make their way into clinical use.

TCR REPERTOIRE ANALYSIS

An individual's T-cell repertoire is determined when T cells traffic through the thymus. A T-cell receptor (TCR) that binds with too much or too little avidity for a self-peptide presented within a self-major histocompatibility complex molecule will cause the death of that T cell. Only T-cell clones with just the right amount of binding affinity will survive to populate the peripheral circulation and make up an individual's T-cell repertoire. Theoretically, an individual's T-cell repertoire is capable of responding to all the different antigenic epitopes on earth. Such immense diversity is possible not through germ line genetic diversity alone, but through the miracle of genetic recombination, additional genetic diversity is generated within the T cell itself (4). This occurs when clusters of gene segments responsible for encoding the subunits that make up the TCR undergo combinatorial joining prior to T-cell repertoire determination. Because this random combinatorial joining generates random and different gene lengths for any given T-cell clone, measuring the diversity of these gene lengths can therefore indirectly measure T-cell clonal diversity. In this section we outline the so-called Vβ spectratyping analysis (also known as the "immunoscope" technique), which measures gene length diversity within the CDR3 region of the Vβ gene cluster (12). Overall T-cell clonal diversity is then measured by enumerating the relative frequency of clones having the same CDR3 gene length. The greater the number of CDR3 gene lengths found, the greater the T-cell clonal diversity within the T-cell repertoire. Applications of this technique are shown in Fig. 1 and 2. In Fig. 1, CD4 T-cell clonal diversity increases over time following treatment of late-stage HIV infection. Rather than comparing T-cell clonal diversity over time, Fig. 2 shows how clonal diversity varies for the same individual at a single time point, comparing CD4 T-cell subsets, in this case comparing clonal diversity within central memory to effector memory CD4 T cells.

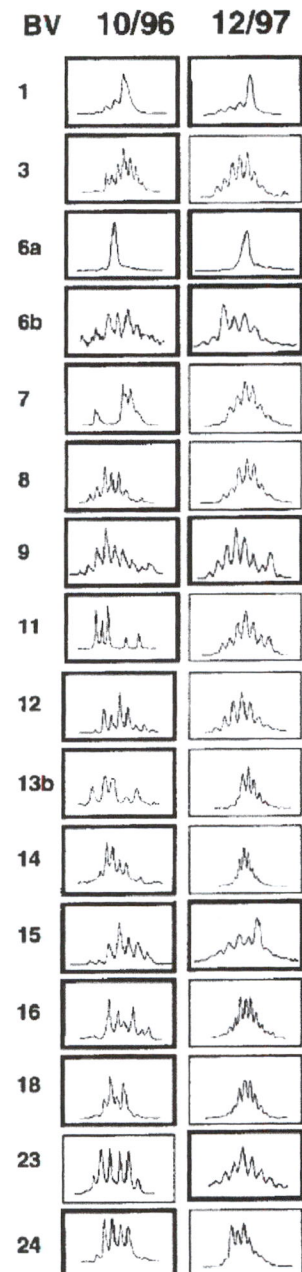

BV 10/96 12/97

1
3
6a
6b
7
8
9
11
12
13b
14
15
16
18
23
24

FIGURE 1 As recently reported by Gea-Banacloche et al., PBMCs were separated into CD4⁺ T-cell fractions and then compared at two different time points for the same HIV-infected individual starting treatment for HIV infection. Such an analysis is typical of how the CDR3 sizing assay is applied to HIV-infected patients. The Vβ family is indicated along the y axis, while CDR3 sizing analysis is indicated along the x axis (each peak corresponding to the relative frequency of PCR products of the same size). Abnormal patterns are identified by bolded boxes around the frequency distribution graphs. Comparisons between the early and late time periods indicate an improvement in the Vβ repertoire (i.e., less skewing), presumably because of this individual's HIV treatment regimen (5).

Equipment

PCR hood with UV light
PCR GeneAmp 9700 (PE Applied Biosystems)
High-speed centrifuge
RNEasy kit (Qiagen)
Vortex machine
GeneScan 500 XL TAMRA (PE Applied Biosystems)
Heat block

Materials and Reagents

RNase-free tubes
Diethyl pyrocarbonate (DEPC) water
Pipettors and pipette tips
Trizol
Isopropanol
Ethanol
Chloroform
β-Mercaptoethanol
DEPC water
25 mM MgCl₂
Fam Cβ
Deoxynucleoside triphosphate (dNTP) mixture
AmpliTaq Gold
RNAlater (Ambion)
RNase OUT RNase inhibitor

Procedure

Step 1: Extraction and Quantitation of RNA

RNA extractions should be performed in a PCR hood, making sure to run the UV light for sufficient time before beginning in order to avoid any cross-contamination. Two methods, chemical (phenol) and nonchemical (column), are available to isolate RNA from cells.

A. Phenol method
1. Using the Trizol reagent (*not* Trizol LS—the LS is intended for liquid samples, whereas the reagent can be applied directly to the cell pellet), add 1 ml to each sample, making sure to keep them on ice until the Trizol is added.
2. Resuspend the pellet by repeat pipetting until no clumps of cells are visible.
3. Incubate the tubes at room temperature for 5 min to ensure complete lysis of the cells.
4. Add 200 μl of chloroform to each tube and shake them vigorously for 30 60 s, and then let stand for 10 to 15 min, ensuring that the supernatant is relatively cleared.
5. Spin samples at 4°C at maximum speed for 15 min.
6. Remove the supernatant (should be around 600 μl) to a clean RNase-free tube, making sure not to pick up any protein or organic material.
7. Add 3 μl of microcarrier to each sample and flick well to mix (do not vortex), then add 1 volume (usually around 600 μl) of isopropanol to the tubes, mix by inverting or flicking, and incubate at room temperature for 10 min.
8. Centrifuge samples at 4°C and at maximum speed for 20 to 30 min, placing the notches on the lids to the outside to orient the tubes so that the pellet is

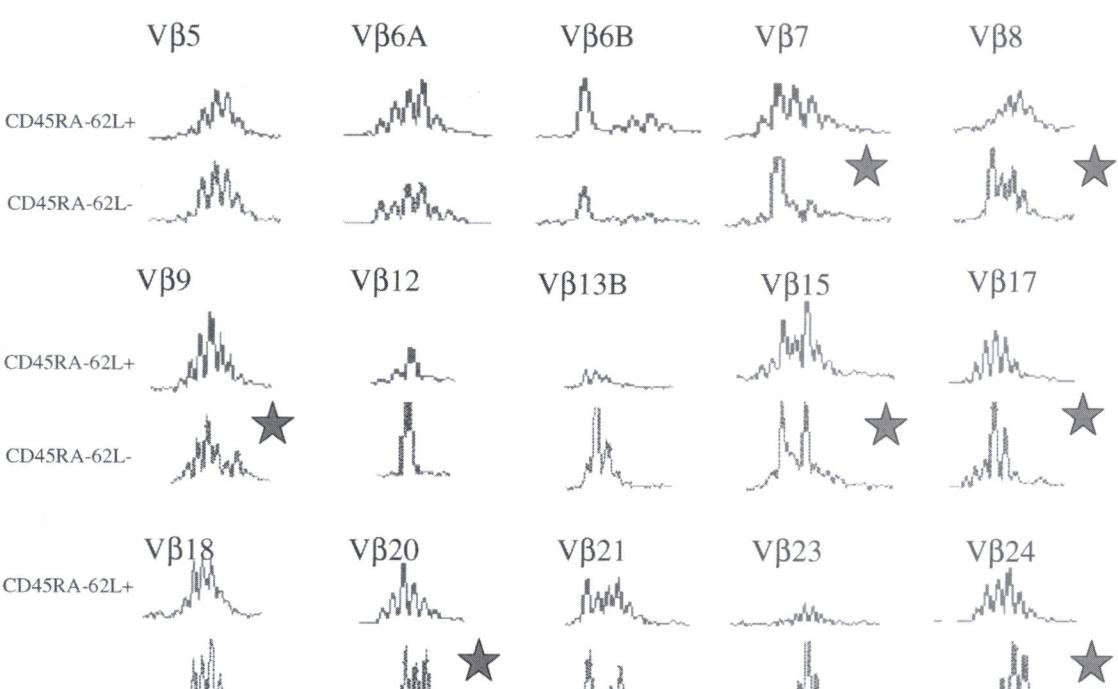

FIGURE 2 PBMCs from an HIV-seronegative individual were separated into CD4$^+$ CD45RA$^-$ and then into CD62L$^+$ and CD62L$^-$ fractions using magnetic beads to determine whether T-cell repertoire differences observed in later-stage HIV-seropositive individuals might be because these individuals have decreased ratios of central to effector memory (as well as naive to memory) CD4$^+$ T cells accompanying their advancing HIV infection. CDR3 gene length analysis was performed on the separated subsets, and while abnormal patterns were found among both subsets, further exaggeration was found among CD62L$^-$ effector memory subsets (as indicated with adjacent stars), suggesting some support for the hypothesis that a decreased Vβ repertoire in late-stage HIV infection may be due to a combination of a relative decrease in naive and central memory and a reciprocal increase in effector memory CD4$^+$ T cells.

easily found (it will be translucent and have a gel-like consistency).

9. Remove most of the isopropanol, being careful not to discard the pellet.

10. Wash twice with chilled 70% ethanol, mixing each time by inversion and spinning at 4°C and full speed for 5 min. (The pellet will whiten and become more rigid so that all of the liquid can be removed after the second wash.)

11. Uncap tubes and dry for 3 to 5 min in a desiccator, being careful to minimize the exposure of the pellets to air outside of the hood.

12. Pellets can be stored at −70°C until needed.

13. Working in a hood, add 10 μl of DEPC water to each pellet.

14. Dissolve the pellets by placing the tubes in a 70°C heating block for 3 to 5 min, flicking them every minute.

15. After the pellets are dissolved, immediately place tubes on ice.

16. Make appropriate dilutions in DEPC water for the spectrophotometer nucleotide-RNA program that is used, and measure the samples (usually about 1 μg/μl with the optical density at 260 to 280 nm at about 1.8 to 2.0).

B. Column method. The nonchemical method extracts RNA using the RNEasy kit (Qiagen) with QIAShredder spin column (Qiagen).

1. Add 600 μl of RNAlater (Ambion) onto a pellet of 5 million to 10 million cells in a 1.5-ml RNase-free tube. Samples can be stored at −80°C without resuspension.

2. If samples are frozen, thaw the pellet for about 10 min at 37 to 42°C in a prewarmed heat block to ensure that there are no crystals. Vortex well, and pipette up and down to ensure a monosuspension of cells.

3. Add 600 μl of phosphate-buffered saline (PBS) to sample, mix well, and spin for 5 min at maximum speed at 4°C.

4. Draw off the supernatant as completely as possible without losing any cells.

5. Add RTL with β-mercaptoethanol and follow protocol from the kit.

6. Elute RNA from spin column in 20 μl of kit-provided water into an RNase-free tube preloaded with 1 μl of RNase OUT RNase inhibitor (kit provided).

7. Take optical density in Tris-EDTA (TE) at 260 and 280 nm.

Step 2: First-strand synthesis (Reverse Transcription)

Take 3.5 to 5 μg of the RNA sample for use in the Superscript first-strand synthesis system for reverse transcription-PCR (Invitrogen). The protocol can be followed exactly as it is written in the kit instructions. If the RNA concentration is low, the first-strand synthesis is performed in twice the usual volume: e.g., 20 μl rather than 10 μl. Each reaction to set up cDNA synthesis is performed in a Sarstedt screw-cap 1.5-ml microcentrifuge tube.

Step 3: PCR Amplification of the Vβ Subfamilies (2, 3)

All primers (Table 1) should be aliquoted for single use only and not repeatedly freeze-thawed.

1. Remove all primers and reagents from the freezer to thaw. After being pulse-vortexed and spun down, all tubes should be kept on ice.

2. With the rack of tubes in a cold block, add 5 μl of each V β primer (5 μM) in sequential order to the tubes for each sample. For these purposes, Vβ 1 to Vβ 24 are used. Vβ 6A is substituted for Vβ 10, and Vβ 13B is substituted for Vβ 19. Equal amounts of Vβ 6.1, 6.2, and 6.3 primers are mixed and used as Vβ 6. Equal amounts of Vβ 12.1 and 12.2 are mixed to use as Vβ 12.

TABLE 1 PCR primers for Vβ CDR3 sizing analysis

Vβ family	Primer sequence (5′→3′)[a]
Fam-labeled Cβ	ACACAGCGACCTCGGGTGGG
Unlabeled Cβ	CGTGCTGCTCCTTGAGGGGCTGCG
Tet-labeled Cα	ATCATAAATTCGGGTAGGATCC
Unlabeled Cα	GAACCCTGACCCTGCCGTGTACC
Vβ 1	CCGCACAACAGTTCCCTGACTTGC
Vβ 2	CACAACTATGTTTTGGTATCGTC
Vβ 3	CGCTTCTCCCTGATTCTGGAGTCC
Vβ 4	TTCCCATCAGCCGCCCAAACCTAA
Vβ 5	GATCAAAACGAGAGGACAGC
Vβ 6A	GATCCAATTTCAGGTCATACTG
Vβ 6.1	CAGGGCCCAGAGTTTCTGAC
Vβ 6.2	CAGGGGCCAGAGTTTCTGAC
Vβ 6.3	CAGGGCTCAGAGGTTCTGAC
Vβ 7	CCTGAATGCCCCAACAGCTCT
Vβ 8	GGTACAGACAGACCATGATGC
Vβ 9	TTCCCTGGAGCTTGGTGACTCTGC
Vβ 11	GTCAACAGTCTCCAGAATAAGG
Vβ 12.1	TCCCCCTCACTCTGGAGTC
Vβ 12.2	TCCTCCTCACTCTGGAGTC
Vβ 13A	GGTATCGACAAGACCCAGGCA
Vβ 13B	AGGCTCATCCATTATTCAAATAC
Vβ 14	GGGCTGGGCTTAAGGCAGATCTAC
Vβ 15	CAGGCACAGGCTAAATTCTCCCTG
Vβ 16	GCCTGCAGAACTGGAGGATTCTGG
Vβ 17	TCCTCTCACTGTGACATCGGCCCA
Vβ 18	CTGCTGAATTTCCCAAAGAGGGCC
Vβ 20	TGCCCCAGACTCTCTCAGCCTCCA
Vβ 21	GGAGTAGACTCCACTCTCAAG
Vβ 22	GATCCGGTCCACAAAGCTGG
Vβ 23	ATTCTGAACTGAACATGAGCTCCT
Vβ 24	GACATCCGCTCACCAGGCCTG

[a]Concentration of each reconstituted Vβ primer is 5 μM in TE. Concentrations of Fam-labeled Cβ, unlabeled Cβ, Tet-labeled Cα, and unlabeled Cα primers are 100 μM in TE.

3. On ice or a cold block, prepare a master mix for each cDNA sample that will be used, making enough for 27 tubes each.

DEPC water	943 μl
10× PCR buffer for TaqGold (Applied Biosystems, Roche)	135 μl
25 mM MgCl₂ (Applied Biosystems, Roche)	81 μl
10 mM dNTP mixture (Roche Applied Science)	27 μl
cDNA (3.5 to 5.0 μg)	15 μl
AmpliTaq Gold (Applied Biosystems, Roche)	7 μl

4. Vortex and spin down the mix after adding the Taq, and then add 45 μl to each tube, making sure not to cross-contaminate the primers.

5. Place the tubes in a PE Applied Biosystems GeneAmp PCR system 9700 and run the reaction for 40 cycles using the following program.

Hold:	10 min at 95°C
Cycle (40 cycles):	25 s at 94°C, 45 s at 60°C, and 45 s at 72°C
Hold	5 min at 72°C

6. In order to label the products, a "runoff" reaction must be set up and run for seven cycles. One master mix can be made for every sample. The following is the mix for 27 tubes (one sample) and can be multiplied to accommodate more samples.

DEPC water	154.0 μl
10× PCR buffer	27.5 μl
25 mM MgCl₂	33.0 μl
10 mM dNTP mixture	5.5 μl
Fam Cβ (10 μM)	2.75 μl
AmpliTaq Gold	1.0 μl

7. Add 8 μl of the runoff mix to each tube of a new tray of empty tubes, and transfer 2 μl of product obtained during the first 40 cycles to the appropriate corresponding new tube.

Step 4: Gel Loading Preparation

1. In order to load labeled PCR product, a molecular size marker (GeneScan 500 XL TAMRA; PE Applied Biosystems) needs to be added in loading dye. The following is a master mixture of loading dye.

Deionized formide (Sigma)	75 μl
TAM 500	15 μl
Loading dye	15 μl

2. Add 3.5 μl of the master mix to the PCR tube.
3. Add 2.5 μl of PCR product.
4. Denature and quench immediately before loading the gel. This involves incubation at 90°C for 2 min followed by 4°C.
5. Run 1.5 μl of loading sample on a 6% DNA sequencing gel. The gel size is 36 cm, with 2-mm spacers. Run for 3 h. The plate should be scanned and prerun for 10 to 20 min using 1× Tris-borate-EDTA buffer. Urea should be blown out of the wells before loading the samples (there is no need to skip lanes as is done with the sequencing gels). Before beginning data collection, set up and save sample

sheet within GeneScan analysis and be sure to select the "settings" within "GeneScan Collection."

Step 5: Cα Relative Quantitation of Vβ Subfamilies

1. Follow steps 1 to 3 above, using the following master mix:

```
DEPC water............................. 938 μl
10× PCR buffer ......................... 135 μl
25 mM MgCl₂ ...........................  81 μl
10 mM dNTP mixture ....................  27 μl
Fam Cβ primer (100 μM) ................   7 μl
3′ Tet Cα (100 μM).....................   7 μl
5′ unlabeled Cα (100 μM)...............   7 μl
cDNA (2.5 to 5.0 μg) ..................   6 μl
AmpliTaq Gold..........................   7 μl
```

2. Follow the same steps as above, only run the sample for 25 to 27 cycles. This ensures that the PCRs will not go to saturation and that amounts of product will be proportional to the individual amounts of starting template.

3. In a fresh tray of tubes, add 18 μl of the 20% EDTA-blue dextran in formamide mixture to each tube. Two microliters of each reaction product can be directly added to the corresponding tubes of loading mix.

4. Follow the denaturation and loading steps above.

Quality Control and Quality Assurance

1. Adequate cell numbers to yield an adequate amount of total RNA are critical to generating reliable and reproducible results. Obtain ~10^7 cells to yield 5 μg of total RNA (3 μg minimum). Monitor T-cell purity and ensure that it exceeds 95%.

2. Vortex samples well for consistent results.

3. Use dry heat blocks rather than water baths to avoid RNase contamination.

4. Do not use powdered gloves.

5. Use only RNase-DNase-free screw-cap tubes and micropipette tips.

6. Aliquot all primers for single use (do not refreeze-thaw).

7. Use cold blocks to keep reaction tubes cold while setting up the PCR.

8. After 40 PCR cycles, run 5 μl of PCR mix in a 1% agarose gel to confirm PCR product reaction. The expected molecular size of the PCR product is ~300 bp.

Interpretation

1. Decreases in CDR3 gene length diversity can be associated with the relative loss of a diverse number of antigen-specific T-cell clones (polyclonal contraction), the relative gain of a limited number of antigen-specific T-cell clones (oligoclonal expansion), or both phenomena at the same time. Therefore, while Vβ spectratyping analysis provides insight into the breadth of the T-cell repertoire, it does not address how such a limited (or "skewed") repertoire might have come about in the first place.

2. Similarly, while CDR3 gene length diversity should correlate with gene sequence diversity, direct sequencing of the genes is necessary to absolutely confirm this correlation.

3. While limited repertoires are often obvious by visual inspection of the pattern of CDR3 length distributions, subtle differences are often found. Distinguishing whether these subtle differences are significant can be challenging. Several groups have attempted to apply statistical techniques to

quantifying differences between samples, but caution should be exercised when visual inspection alone does not convey obvious differences in comparator CDR3 length distribution patterns (5).

INTRACELLULAR CYTOKINE ANALYSIS

The ability of T cells to rapidly secrete cytokines following stimulation by their cognate antigen is an important hallmark of the memory T-cell response. This response can help enumerate the frequency of antigen-specific T cells in the peripheral blood. Application of this technique is shown in Color Plate 12, where the frequency of cytomegalovirus (CMV)-specific and purified protein derivative (PPD)-specific CD4 T cells, as defined by gamma interferon (IFN-γ), interleutin 2 (IL-2), or tumor necrosis factor alpha (TNF-α) production, is enumerated for one individual at a single time point. In this section we outline two popular methods to detect cytokine-secreting antigen-specific T cells using multiparameter flow cytometry. One method uses whole blood, which is more convenient and perhaps more physiological than other methods (15). The second method uses peripheral blood mononuclear cells (PBMCs). It is capable of using cells from a variety of clinical samples and may have less background noise than other methods (14). As both methods only enumerate antigen-specific cells that are capable of rapidly secreting cytokines (and certainly only those expressing the cytokines measured), antigen-specific T cells not having these characteristics are not enumerated using these assays.

Whole-Blood Method

Equipment

Centrifuge
Three- or four-color flow cytometer
Vortex mixer
Incubator (5% CO_2 at 37°C)
37°C water bath

Materials and Reagents

15-ml conical polypropylene tubes
12- by 75-mm polystyrene tubes
Pipettor and pipette tips
Micropipettor and micropipette tips
FACSLyse *or equivalent*
FACSPerm 2 *or equivalent*
Brefeldin A
Dimethyl sulfoxide (DMSO)
Paraformaldehyde (PFA)
PBS (without Ca^{2+} or Mg^{2+})
Staphylococcus enterotoxin B (SEB)

Procedure

Step 1: Material and Reagent Preparation

1. Brefeldin A (catalog no. B-7651; Sigma-Aldrich, St. Louis, Mo.) is supplied as a powder and when dissolved in DMSO (catalog no. D8779; Sigma-Aldrich) can be frozen in small aliquots (e.g., 60 μl) at a concentration of 10 mg/ml for up to 1 year. Just prior to use, dilute a thawed aliquot 1:50 using PBS (or medium) to make up a 1-μg/μl

working solution (e.g., add 50 μl of thawed aliquot to 2.5 ml of PBS). Store at 4°C for use the same day. Do not refreeze.

2. Prepare 4% PFA solution in a fume hood by adding 40 g of crystalline PFA (catalog no.150146; ICN Biomedicals, Inc., Aurora, Ohio), 13.4 g of $Na_2HPO_4 \cdot 7H_2O$ (molecular weight [MW], 268) and 6.9 g of $NaH_2PO_4 \cdot H_2O$ (MW, 138) to 900 ml of distilled H_2O in a measuring cylinder, then placing the cylinder on a hotplate/stirrer, heating to 60 to 70°C, and stirring moderately. In solution, the PFA will become clear (do not overheat or spill solution, which is a potential carcinogen). After cooling, add enough distilled H_2O to total 1,000 ml. Adjust to pH 7.0. Aliquot into 5- to 15-ml tubes and freeze at −20°C (good for at least 3 months). Prior to use, thaw and prepare 1% solution by diluting with PBS (good for 2 weeks at 4°C).

3. Prepare FACSLyse and FACSPerm 2 solutions (catalog no. 349202 and 340973; Becton Dickinson Immunocytometry Systems, San Jose, Calif.) according to the manufacturer's recommendations. Both are supplied premixed as 10× solutions and use deionized water as diluent (*do not* use PBS or other buffers).

4. Prepare intracellular cytokine staining wash buffer using PBS with 0.5% (wt/vol) bovine serum albumin (BSA) and 0.5% (wt/vol) sodium azide (NaN_3). Store at 4°C for up to 2 weeks.

5. Purified SEB is supplied as a lyophilized powder (catalog no. BT-202; Toxin Technology, Sarasota, Fla.) and is dissolved in pure water and then stored at a working concentration of 1 mg/ml at 4°C for up to 3 months.

6. Peptides or antigens are supplied from various vendors or researchers, either as lyophilized powders or as solutions, and are usually resuspended in solution and then frozen in small aliquots for later use. Specifics depend on the antigen and supplier.

Step 2: Antigenic Stimulation

1. Label 15-ml polypropylene tubes (activated lymphocytes are less likely to adhere to polypropylene than polystyrene) for each stimulation condition desired. Include both positive and negative control conditions.

2. Use only well-mixed sodium heparin-anticoagulated whole blood which has been stored at room temperature for less than 12 h (blood should be used as soon as possible). Other anticoagulants (e.g., EDTA, acid-citrate-dextrose, and lithium heparin) are not suitable, as they may interfere with cytokine secretion by chelating cations. Reject samples which are obviously hemolyzed or have been exposed to extremes of heat or cold.

3. The amount of blood needed per stimulation condition is determined by how many flow cytometry tubes will be analyzed per stimulation condition, how many cells are present in whole blood, and the cell number target for flow cytometry acquisition (e.g., 10,000 $CD4^+$-T-cell events). Blood volumes are typically 0.5 to 2 ml per stimulation condition.

4. Add CD28 and CD49d (catalog no. 347690; Becton Dickinson Immunocytometry Systems) at a final concentration of 10 μl/ml of whole blood in each of the 5-ml stimulation tubes (CD28 and CD49d are used for costimulation and alone do not trigger cytokine secretion from T cells).

5. Add the appropriate concentration of stimulating peptide, antigen, or superantigen/mitogen to each of the labeled stimulation tubes (these should be pretitrated for optimal responses, but final concentrations of antigen preparations are often ~10 μg per ml of blood). To negative control tubes

add 10 μl of RPMI 1640, and to positive control tubes add 10 μg of SEB per ml of blood (i.e., 10 μl of 1-μg/μl working solution per ml of blood).

6. Aliquot the appropriate amount of blood into each 15-ml tube.

7. Incubate between 6 and 24 h at 37°C and 5% CO_2. Incubation times can be adjusted depending on the antigen(s) used or scheduling issues, but once chosen, incubation times must remain constant for relevant comparisons (6).

8. Four hours prior to completion of the incubation (i.e., after 2 to 20 h of incubation), add brefeldin A for a final concentration of 10 μg per ml of whole blood.

Step 3: Cell Preparation for Flow Cytometric Analysis

1. Label 12- by 75-mm polystyrene tubes (include compensation control tubes).

2. Add monoclonal antibody (MAb)-fluorochrome conjugates to stain the desired cell surface epitope (e.g., CD3 or CD4) for analysis in each flow cytometry tube (7, 8).

3. After vortexing each 15-ml stimulation tube on high for 10 s, remove the desired amount of blood and add it to the corresponding flow cytometry tube(s). Usually either 100 or 200 μl of stimulated blood is added to each flow cytometry tube. If more blood is needed (e.g., for individuals with few $CD4^+$ T cells in late-stage HIV disease), prepare additional parallel tubes (rather than additional blood per tube). In this case, cells from such parallel tubes can be recombined after processing but prior to acquisition on the flow cytometer (some researchers add EDTA at a final concentration of 2 mM just prior to this step to help decrease the number of adherent activated cells from the sides of tubes).

4. Remove blood splattered on the sides of tubes with cotton swabs wetted with deionized water (unstained blood can spuriously alter cell frequencies).

5. Vortex gently and incubate at room temperature for 15 min in the dark.

6. Add 2 ml of 1× FACSLyse (3 ml for tubes with 200 μl of blood) to the blood-MAb mixture. Vortex gently and incubate at room temperature for 10 min in the dark.

7. Centrifuge at 400 × g for 5 min. Remove supernatant without disturbing the cell pellet.

8. Add 500 μl of 1× FACSPerm. Vortex gently and incubate at room temperature for 10 min in the dark. Add 2 ml of wash buffer and centrifuge at 500 × g for 5 min. Remove supernatant without disturbing the cell pellet.

9. Add MAb for each intracellular epitope of interest to the appropriate flow cytometry tubes (e.g., IFN-γ, TNF-α, or IL-2). Vortex gently and incubate at room temperature for 30 min in the dark. Add 2 ml of wash buffer and centrifuge at 500 × g for 5 min. Remove supernatant without disturbing the cell pellet.

10. Add 200 μl of 1% PFA working solution to pellet and vortex. Analyze on the flow cytometer or store at 4°C with wax and foil covers for analysis up to 24 h later.

Quality Control and Quality Assurance

1. Volumes of blood and not cell numbers determine volumes of MAb-fluorochrome conjugates.

2. Pretiter fluorochrome-antibody conjugates to determine optimal antibody concentration.

3. Particular care and practice in removing supernatants are necessary to avoid losing cells. This is particularly true when cells are permeabilized, as their densities decrease and

they are suspended in supernatants with higher protein concentrations. Under these conditions, many investigators prefer decanting to aspirating the pellet. When decanting, do not tip twice.

4. Remove blood splatters from the tube walls with deionized water on cotton tip swabs to prevent this unstained blood from subsequently being enumerated during analysis.

5. The standard staining volume of whole blood is 100 μl but a maximum of 200 μl per tube if the patient is lymphopenic or if large numbers of cells are needed to acquire the target number of >50 positive events.

Interpretation

Blood volume is determined by the needs of each experiment. For example, an experiment to determine IFN-γ, IL-2, and TNF-α expression from activated (CD69$^+$) CD3$^+$ CD4$^+$ T cells on a four-color flow cytometer would require three flow cytometry tubes. Alternatively, when using newer multiparameter (i.e., six- or nine-color) flow cytometers, the same experiment can be performed using a single tube. Beyond the convenience of not having to separate whole blood, and having fewer steps than other methods, another possible reason to choose the whole-blood method is that autologous plasma proteins and innate immune cells may be important contributors to the acquired cellular immune response, thus theoretically making this method more physiological than others.

Saponin-Based Method

Equipment
The equipment is the same as for the whole-blood method.

Materials and Reagents

5-ml V-bottom tubes

4-ml V-bottom tubes (catalog no. 57.477; Sarstedt, Newton, N.C.).

Corning U-bottom tissue culture tubes

15-ml conical polypropylene tubes

Pipettor and pipette tips

Micropipettor and micropipette tips

Brefeldin A (Sigma)

PFA

DNase I (20,000 U, 50 to 375 U/μl; Invitrogen, Cambridge, United Kingdom)

RPMI 1640

PBS

Saponin (Sigma)

Nonfat dried milk

BSA

Autologous Epstein-Barr virus (EBV)-transformed cell lines (lymphoblastoid B-cell lines [EBV-LCL])

Vaccinia virus constructs (e.g., vTFnef and vVK1) for option 1 (see below)

Procedure

Step 1: Reagent Preparation

1. Brefeldin A (10 mg/ml in DMSO) and PFA (4% at pH 7.0) are prepared as outlined for the whole-blood method, except that PFA is not diluted in PBS prior to use and is used at 4% after thawing.

2. Complete medium (CM) is prepared using RPMI 1640 with 10% fetal calf serum and 2% glutamine. Store at 4°C for 1 week.

3. DNase is supplied at between 50 and 375 IU/μl (Invitrogen) and used in aliquots between 1.5 and 4 μl per tube, depending on needs.

4. Intracellular cytokine staining wash buffer is prepared using sterile PBS with 0.1% (wt/vol) BSA and 0.1% (wt/vol) NaN₃. Store at 4°C for up to 2 weeks.

5. Cell culture freezing medium-DMSO (catalog no. 11101-011; Gibco) may be used to cryopreserve stimulated cells for future use.

6. For blocking and staining procedure:

a. PBS-S solution is prepared using PBS with 0.2% saponin.

b. PBS-S–5% milk solution is prepared using PBS-S with 5% nonfat dried milk. Store at 4°C for 2 to 6 months.

c. PBS-BSA is prepared using 0.1% BSA.

7. Peptides and antigens are supplied from various vendors or researchers, either as lyophilized powders or as solutions, and are usually resuspended in solution and then frozen in small aliquots for later use. Specifics depend on the antigen and supplier.

Step 2: PBMC Isolation

1. Isolate PBMCs by the Ficoll-Hypaque method, washing cells twice with Hanks' balanced salt solution with Ca^{2+} and Mg^{2+} or RPMI 1640. Count cells during the washing.

2. Resuspend PBMCs in CM and leave at room temperature.

3. If frozen PBMCs are to be used, results are improved by incubating them overnight in CM at a concentration of approximately 10^6/ml.

4. Plate PBMCs at $4 \times 10^6/2$ ml in a U-bottom tissue culture tube, using prewarmed medium.

Step 3: Antigenic Stimulation of CD4$^+$ T Cells

1. Add anti-CD28 to a final concentration of 1 μg/ml.

2. Add antigen (e.g., p24 or p55). It is very important to try proteins from different manufacturers initially, as there may be significant differences in the results. Typically ≈10 μg/ml is used.

Step 4: Antigenic Stimulation of CD8$^+$ T Cells

1. Option 1: EBV-transformed vaccinia virus-infected stimulator cells (5). In this case, a large diversity of HIV antigens will be presented.

a. Autologous EBV-LCL are infected overnight with the desired vaccinia virus constructs (e.g., vTFnef and vVK1) for an optimal duration of 12 to 16 h prior to being mixed with effectors.

b. Aliquot 2.5×10^6 EBV-transformed B cells for each target cell type to be prepared in 15-ml conical tubes.

c. Centrifuge at $400 \times g$ for 10 min.

d. Aspirate the supernatant and leave the cell pellet.

e. Add 150 μl of CM containing 2.5×10^6 to 10×10^6 (each virus has to be titrated to find out which infection ratio is best) PFU of the desired recombinant vaccinia virus.

f. Vortex gently.

g. Incubate in the 15-ml conical tubes with loosened caps in a 5% CO_2 incubator at 37°C for 90 min. Vortex gently at 30 and 60 min.

h. Wash twice with 10 ml of CM, centrifuging each time at $400 \times g$ for 10 min.

i. Resuspend in 1.25 ml of RPMI 1640 medium with 20% fetal bovine serum and transfer to a culture flask.

j. Incubate overnight (16 h) at 37°C in a 5% CO_2 atmosphere.

k. On the following day, add 200 µl of the vaccinia virus-infected EBV-LCL to the 2 ml of effector PBMCs in the U-bottom tubes, for a final PBMC/EBV-LCL ratio of 10:1. The results are usually consistent within ratios of 1:1 to 100:1.

2. Option 2: peptide pulsing (11). In this case, the EBV-LCL, instead of being infected with HIV-vaccinia virus constructs, are incubated for 1 h with the peptides of interest at 37°C in the U-bottom stimulation tubes. Effector PBMCs are then added with the peptide-pulsed EBV-LCL. The peptides (typically previously synthesized fragments from different HIV proteins) will occupy the groove of the HLA class I molecules on the EBV-LCL and in this fashion will be presented to the PBMCs.

3. Option 3: Direct peptide pulsing, for a final peptide concentration of 1 to 10 µM or approximately 2 to 10 µg of peptide/10^6 cells/ml.

4. Option 4: Polyclonal stimulation followed by electronic gating on cellular subsets of interest.

Step 5: Cell Incubation

1. Cap tubes and spin at $400 \times g$ for 5 min.
2. Incubate in 5% CO_2 at 37°C for 2 h.
3. Warm up brefeldin A at 37°C for 5 min, and vortex until dissolved (5 to 10 min). Dilute 1:50 in CM and vortex.
4. Add 100 µl of the brefeldin solution/tube (final concentration, 10 µg/ml). Mix gently without disrupting the pellet.
5. Incubate for 4 to 8 h in 5% CO_2 at 37°C. Depending on the cytokine that is going to be determined, different incubation times will be needed. Six hours total (4 h after adding brefeldin) gives adequate results for IL-2, TNF-α, and IFN-γ, but it is too short for IL-10 and IL-16 (these two may need 24 h).

Step 6: Cell Fixation (Adapted from Reference 14)

1. Add approximately 500 U of DNase to each tube. Gently vortex. Incubate for 5 min at 37°C. (This step is needed only when the stimulus used is polyclonal, e.g., phorbol esters plus calcium ionophore or soluble MAbs targeting the TCR-CD3 complex, as the intense cellular activation originates significant cell death with release of DNA.)
2. Remove cells with a pipette.
3. Place cells in a 4-ml V-bottom tube.
4. Place 4% PFA in a 37°C water bath to warm. Cool centrifuge to 4°C.
5. Spin down ($400 \times g$ for 10 min) and aspirate supernatant.
6. Break up the pellet by knocking the tubes against a white "pincushion" test tube rack.
7. Resuspend with 1 ml of cold PBS. Spin down ($400 \times g$ for 10 min).
8. Remove PFA from water bath and set on counter at room temperature.
9. Remove PBS from the tubes by aspiration.

Note: At this point, the cells have been washed twice and have not been fixed yet. If separate surface staining is required, it may be performed here. Most surface antibodies

will work on fixed cells, but occasionally they will not. Staining with HLA tetrameric complexes is suboptimal on fixed cells, so it is mandatory to perform surface staining with tetramers at this point. Regarding tetramer use, staining at 4°C for 30 min typically provides good results, with bright fluorescence of tetramer-labeled cells, although each tetramer should be tried at 4°C, room temperature, and 37°C for 15 to 60 min to optimize the signal-to-noise ratio. The higher the temperature, the less time used for staining. All conditions should work, but depending on the HLA-peptide combination, one temperature may be better than the other (17). The tetramer staining is performed as a MAb staining: the tetramer is added to PBS–0.1% BSA, typically 1:5 to 1:50 (1 to 10 µl of tetramer in 50 µl of PBS-BSA). Other MAbs can be added to the solution so a "master mix" for surface staining is prepared. The cell pellet to be stained is resuspended in the tetramer solution (or master mix) and incubated for 20 to 30 min (see above regarding need for different temperature-time combinations). After the surface staining, continue the protocol as follows.

10. Break up the pellet by knocking the tube.
11. Add 0.5 ml of 4% PFA to each tube. Incubate for 5 min.
12. Vortex each tube for ≈3 to 5 s three or four times over the 5 min of incubation (essential to avoid clumping).
13. After 5 min, add 2 ml of ice-cold 0.1% BSA–PBS azide.
14. Cap tubes and vortex to mix.
15. Centrifuge at ≈$1,200 \times g$ (3,000 rpm) for 5 min. Remove supernatant by aspiration.

At this point, the cells have been fixed. If desired, it is possible to proceed to permeabilization and intracellular staining immediately. Alternatively, the fixed cells may be frozen in DMSO for future use. Fixed and frozen cells stored at -80°C are equivalent to freshly analyzed cells for at least a year. Therefore, if desired, resuspend each tube in 1 ml of cell culture freezing medium-DMSO. Aliquot each tube or tube equivalent into one cryovial and freeze at -80°C.

Step 7: Cell Permeabilization, Blocking, and Intracellular Staining

1. If not freezing the cells for future use, proceed directly to step 6. If cells were cryopreserved, thaw frozen cells and continue to step 2.
2. Transfer to 4-ml V-bottom tubes.
3. Add 1 ml of PBS-BSA.
4. Spin down at $1,200 \times g$ (~3,000 rpm) for 5 min at 4°C.
5. Aspirate supernatant. Watch for pellet.
6. Add 50 µl of PBS-S–5% milk per each ≈1×10^6 to 2×10^6 cells, 50 µl minimum in order to permeabilize and block the fixed cells. Excess protein minimizes nonspecific binding to permeabilized cells.
7. Leave for 1 h or overnight on ice in the cold room.
8. For intracellular staining, make a master mix with your MAbs of choice in PBS-S–5% milk. The mixture of antibodies should be spun down at maximum speed for 10 min to decrease background. (It must be emphasized that each staining protocol has to be optimized according to the reagents used. We have had excellent results with the following mix for four-color staining to study IFN-γ-producing CD8 T cells: CD3 fluorescein isothiocyanate, 10 µl; CD8 PerCP, 10 µl; CD69 phycoerythrin [Beckon Dickinson], 20 µl; IFN-γ allophycocyanin [Pharmingen], 2.5 µl; and

PBS-S–5% milk, 7.5 μl. Staining was done in a 50-μl total volume per sample.)

9. Aliquot cells into 4-ml V-bottom tubes, ≈2 × 10⁶ to 10 × 10⁶ cells/tube. Use PBS-S to resuspend for aliquoting.

10. Spin down samples. Aspirate supernatant, avoiding the pellet.

11. Add diluted MAb (after centrifuging the master mix) to cells in a 50-μl volume, resuspending the cells in the process.

12. Incubate for 30 min at 4°C.

13. Add 1 ml of PBS-S to each tube and vortex.

14. Spin down samples. Aspirate supernatant, avoiding the cell pellet.

15. Break up the pellet by knocking tube.

16. Add 1 ml of PBS-S to each tube and vortex.

17. Spin down samples. Aspirate supernatant, again avoiding the pellet.

18. Repeat above starting with step 8, if staining with secondary MAbs. If finished, resuspend in 150 to 300 μl of PBS-BSA for flow cytometric analysis.

Quality Control and Quality Assurance

1. Results obtained with cryopreserved PBMCs that have been rested overnight are comparable to results obtained with rested fresh PBMCs. Using PBMCs immediately post-Ficoll gives significantly lower frequencies of antigen-specific T cells.

2. MAbs should be titered out before use for optimal signal-to-noise ratios.

3. MAb master mixes that will be used for intracellular staining should be diluted in PBS-S–5% milk and centrifuged prior to being mixed with cells in an effort to minimize nonspecific background staining.

4. HLA class I tetrameric complexes can be combined in a master mix containing a CD8 MAb and others for surface labeling of stimulated cells prior to fixation and intracellular staining.

5. We have successfully stained up to 15 × 10⁷ PBMCs with a single aliquot of tetramer before aliquoting the cells into other tubes for staining of other markers or prior to fixation, permeabilization, and intracellular cytokine staining.

6. Be careful to minimize light exposure of all fluorochrome-conjugated reagents during the preparation of the master mixes, at the time of staining, upon completion of staining, and in handling during the analysis.

Interpretation

This sensitive, highly quantitative, and highly reproducible method affords one the ability to study the frequencies of cytokine-secreting antigen-specific T cells using a technique characterized by very low background. The major drawbacks relate to the inconveniences of isolating PBMCs by leukapheresis and sodium diatrizoate density centrifugation. However, once PBMCs are available, one has the capability to examine multiple parameters of individual cell subsets and make conclusions about frequency, phenotype, and function. Compared with older techniques, such as limiting-dilution analysis, considerably higher frequencies of antigen-specific T cells have been measured in this manner. Although this has not been established, the methods outlined herein are probably superior to ELISPOT assays, which are limited by spatial constraints and numbers of antigen-presenting cells (APC) and typically yield results that are 10 to 100 times lower than the magnitudes detected by intracellular cytokine analysis.

DETECTION OF ANTIGEN-SPECIFIC T CELLS USING HLA TETRAMERS

HLA tetramer technology revolutionized the investigation of antigen-specific T-cell clones (1). Unlike other assays and technologies, HLA tetramers can enumerate T-cell clones regardless of their functional behavior, such as proliferation, killing, or cytokine production. An example of the application of this technique is shown in Color Plate 13, where tetramer staining is combined with cell surface immunophenotype markers to better characterize these antigen-specific cells in one HIV-infected individual at one time point. The technology can also be coupled with assays measuring these functional responses, such as the intracellular cytokine production, saponin-based method, as outlined above, or the lymphocyte proliferation assays (LPAs), outlined later in this chapter. Combined analysis of antigen-specific T-cell responses using these assays allows the teasing apart of complex T-cell immunological responses, as may occur in HIV-infected patients. In this section we outline the basic method for staining with HLA class I tetramers.

Technology

The technology is the same as for intracellular cytokine production, saponin-based method.

Materials and Reagents

Same as for intracellular cytokine production, saponin-based method

HLA tetramers

Procedure

Step 1: Prepare Cells

1. PBMCs: <100 × 10⁶ cells in 50 to 100 μl (10⁶ cells/100 μl)

2. Whole blood: 200 μl

Note: Following stimulation with peptides or polyclonal activators (e.g., phorbol esters plus calcium ionophore or soluble MAbs directed against subunits of the TCR-CD3 complex), cells can be washed, resuspended in medium at a concentration of 10⁶/ml, and rested for 1 h at 37°C to preserve the fluorescence intensity of tetramer staining.

Step 2: Prepare HLA Class I Tetramers

1. Use 5 to 10 μl per test. See "Saponin-Based Method, Procedure, Step 6 (Cell Fixation)," item 9 note.

2. MAbs directed against CD8 subunits and other surface markers may be included in a master mix.

3. Centrifuge at 16,000 × g for 20 min at 4°C to decrease nonspecific staining.

Note: Minimize exposure of this reagent to light during storage or incubation.

4. Incubate cells with tetramer at 4°C (or room temperature) for 30 min. See "Saponin-Based Method, Procedure, Step 6 (Cell Fixation)," item 9 note.

5. Wash with PBS twice, aspirating the supernatant after each wash.

6. Cells may be analyzed immediately or fixed, permeabilized, and stained for intracellular cytokines and other proteins per standard protocols.

7. If cells are not going to be analyzed immediately following step 5, store at 4°C in the dark and analyze within 24 to 48 h.

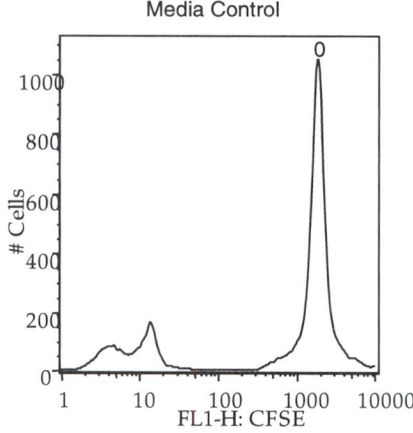
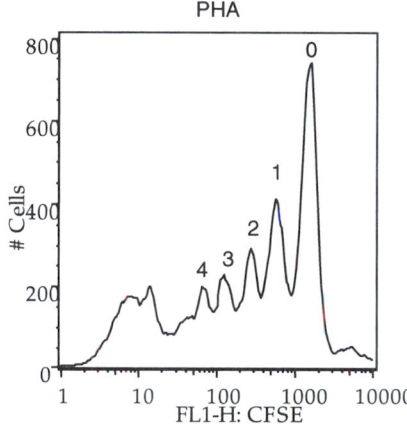

FIGURE 3 PBMCs were separated into CD4+ T cells using magnetic beads and then labeled with CFSE to track cell division over 5 days following stimulation with either medium control or phytohemagglutinin (PHA), as indicated in the two dot plots. Arbitrary cell number is indicated on the y axis, while CFSE fluorescence intensity (measured in FL-1 on the flow cytometer) is shown on the x axis. A single CFSE bright peak (0) is shown under the medium control conditions, indicating that no cell division has occurred (the dim peak is from non-CFSE-labeled irradiated PBMCs that were added into these and parallel tubes for presentation of other antigens in the experiment). Conversely, the PHA-stimulated condition shows four cell (1 to 4) divisions beyond the peak of undivided cells (0), in addition to the dim peak of unlabeled irradiated PBMCs.

Quality Control and Quality Assurance

Quality control and quality assurance are the same as for intracellular cytokine production, saponin-based method.

Interpretation

While HLA tetramer technology is a very powerful tool to investigate immunological responses in the setting of HIV infection, its major drawback reflects its high degree of specificity. In other words, when enumerating an antigen-specific T-cell clone, only T cells specific for a particular epitope loaded onto a particular HLA molecule are enumerated. Given that T-cell responses to any given pathogen may include dozens (if not hundreds) of antigenic epitopes, and HLA haplotypes can vary significantly between individuals, HLA tetramer technology is highly inductive, making interindividual comparisons difficult.

LYMPHOCYTE PROLIFERATION

The ability of lymphocytes to expand exponentially after encountering their cognate antigen is a critical attribute that allows the acquired immune response to contain otherwise lethal pathogenic challenges. For decades, immunologists have measured this response using the LPA. This assay, coupled with limiting-dilution analysis, was one of the first methods used to quantitate antigen-specific T-cells. However, because the assay does not enumerate cells with low proliferative potential, quantitation of antigen-specific T-cell precursor frequencies has been supplanted by flow cytometric techniques, such as HLA tetramer and intracellular cytokine expression assays. Nevertheless, the ability to measure proliferation in response to cognate antigen(s) remains an important functional characteristic of antigen-specific T cells.

The standard LPA uses tritiated-thymidine pulse-labeling of cellular DNA within PBMCs at the peak of proliferation in tissue culture as a surrogate measure of the precursor frequency of antigen-specific cells. Cells dividing during the period of pulse-labeling (usually 6 h) incorporate the tritiated thymidine in the daughter DNA strands. Subsequently, cells are harvested, and quantitation of radioactivity measured from each tissue culture well correlates with the magnitude of cellular expansion during the period of labeling. This assay is outlined in chapter 95.

In this section, we outline another popular method to measure lymphocyte proliferation using a membrane-tracking fluorescent dye that spontaneously and irreversibly binds to cells (10). Once labeled, the fluorescent dye is divided equally among any subsequent daughter cells. This decay of fluorescence per generation of daughter cells is conveniently resolved using the log scale of one of the fluorescence detectors of a multiparameter flow cytometer (see Fig. 3). Simultaneous measurement of T-cell surface immunophenotype, using the other fluorescence detectors on the flow cytometer, allows determination of which T-cell subsets are proliferating, as shown in Fig. 4.

5- and 6-Carboxyfluorescein Diacetate Succinimidyl Ester (CFSE) Cell Division Assay

Equipment

    Centrifuge
    Three- or four-color flow cytometer
    Vortex mixer
    Incubator (5% CO_2 at 37°C)
    37°C water bath

Materials and Reagents

    15- and 50-ml conical polypropylene tubes
    12- by 75-mm polystyrene tubes
    Pipettor and pipette tips
    Micropipettor and micropipette tips
    1× PBS (without Ca^{2+} or Mg^{2+})
    RPMI 1640

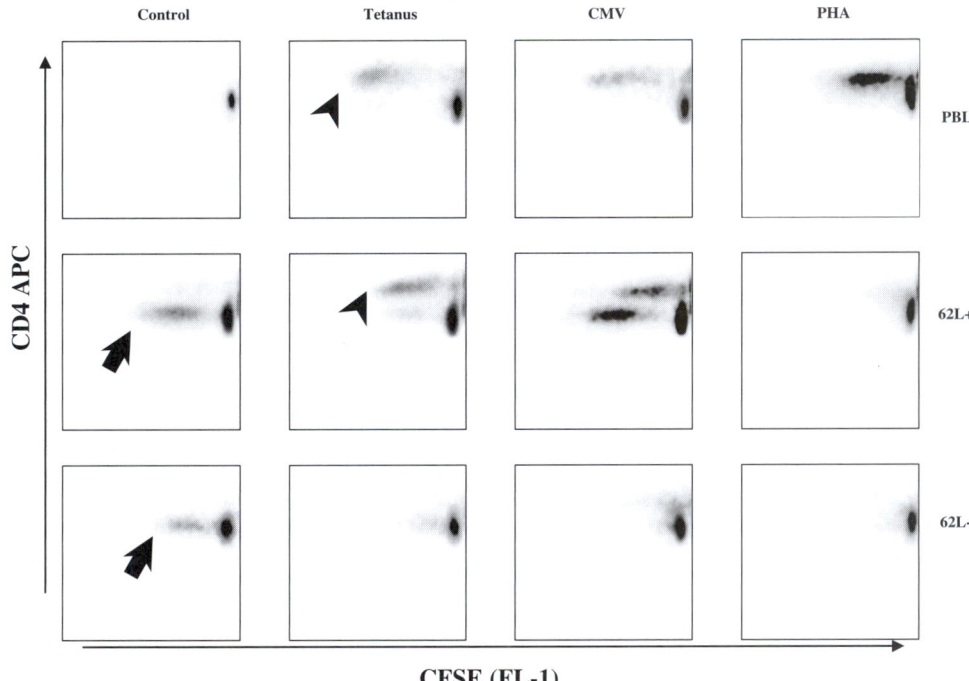

FIGURE 4 PBMCs were either set aside, irradiated, or separated into CD4$^+$ CD62L$^+$ or CD4$^+$ CD62L$^-$ T cells. PBMCs (unirradiated) and separated CD4$^+$ T-cell subsets were then stimulated with medium control, tetanus toxoid, CMV, or phytohemagglutinin (PHA) (as shown across the top of all dot plots) for 2 days in the presence of irradiated PBMCs as APC. Cells were then harvested and labeled with CFSE and placed back into medium for an additional 6 days. Cells were harvested again and then labeled with MAb for surface markers (CD3 and CD4) and analyzed on a flow cytometer to track cell division. The arrowheads identify tetanus toxoid-specific cell division (bright for CD4) found in PBMCs that corresponded to division found in CD4$^+$ CD62L$^+$ T cells but not CD4$^+$ CD62L$^-$ T cells, while the arrows identify homeostatic cell division (dim for CD4) that is mostly confined to CD4$^+$ CD62L$^+$ T cells. Proliferation measured by CFSE cell division was confirmed with standard tritiated-thymidine LPA results at 5 days (results not shown). Separated PHA stimulations do not show proliferation, likely as these cells lost CFSE signal (death or >8 divisions) by day 8 of stimulation.

Human AB serum

L-Glutamine (200 mM solution)

HEPES (1 M solution)

Gentamicin

DNase I (20,000 U, 50 to 375 U/μl; Invitrogen, Cambridge, United Kingdom)

EDTA

CFSE

Antibody-fluorochrome conjugates for immunophenotyping

Antigen, peptides, or mitogens for cell stimulation

Procedure

Step 1: Reagent Preparation

1. Prepare wash buffer as PBS with 0.1% (wt/vol) BSA. Store at 4°C for up to 2 weeks.

2. Prepare culture medium as RPMI 1640, 10% (vol/vol) human AB serum (heat inactivated for 30 min at 55°C), 2 mM L-glutamine, 10 mM HEPES, and 50 μg of gentamicin per ml. Sterile filter through a 0.22-μm-pore-size polyethersulfone filter and store for up to 2 weeks at 4°C.

3. CFSE (catalog no. C1157; Molecular Probes, Eugene, Oreg.) is supplied as 25 mg of lyophilized powder (MW, 557). Dissolve 25 mg in DMSO to a final concentration of 5 mM (i.e., 2.785 mg/ml) and freeze in 50-μl aliquots at −80°C under desiccating conditions for up to 1 year.

4. DNase is supplied at between 50 and 375 IU/μl (Invitrogen) and used in aliquots between 1.5 and 4 ml per tube, depending on needs.

Step 2: Cell Labeling

1. Isolate cells of interest using density gradient centrifugation (see chapter 95).

2. Wash cells once in room temperature PBS.

3. Count and aliquot 15×10^6 to 30×10^6 cells into 15-ml conical polypropylene tubes for CFSE labeling.

4. Pellet and resuspend in 1 ml of PBS per 15-ml conical tube.

5. Prepare CFSE by thawing one vial of stock 5 mM CFSE in a 37°C water bath, diluting 4,000 times by first adding 50 μl of stock solution to 50 ml of room temperature PBS and then adding 12.5 ml of this solution to 37.5 ml of PBS (it is wise to optimize the assay to your particular cells and antigens by first testing several different CFSE concentrations). Shield from light prior to cell labeling.

6. Mix an equal volume of cell suspension with diluted CFSE solution (i.e., at 1:1). Vortex immediately and periodically (e.g., 10 times, each lasting for a few seconds) during 7 min of incubation at room temperature.

7. Quench cell staining reaction by adding 2 ml of 4°C heat-inactivated human AB serum. Vortex immediately and let sit for 1 min (the high protein content of the medium binds excess CFSE in this and subsequent wash steps).

8. Wash cells two additional times in culture medium containing heat-inactivated human AB serum.

9. Plate cells in U-bottomed plates (e.g., 1-ml-deep 96-well tissue culture plates, catalog no. P9626-S; PGC Scientifics, Frederick, Md.) in one-half the desired final tissue culture volume at twice the desired final concentration (e.g., 0.5 ml of suspension containing 4×10^6-cells/ml).

10. If using $CD4^+$ T cells previously isolated by either fluorescence-activated cell sorting or magnetic bead separation, consider adding irradiated autologous monocytes or PBMCs as APC. These should be added in one-quarter the desired final tissue culture volume at four times the desired final concentration. Ideally, the APC concentration should be previously determined in an APC titration (dose-response curve) experiment. Typically, irradiated PBMCs are plated at a final concentration of $\sim 0.5 \times 10^6$ cells/ml.

11. Add antigen or peptide (or mitogen) to each tissue culture well in the appropriate remaining volume (i.e., in one-half the desired final tissue culture volume at twice the desired final concentration if using irradiated APC or in one-half the desired final tissue culture volume at twice the desired final concentration if not using irradiated APC).

12. Incubate the cells at 37°C and 5% CO_2 for the appropriate duration (between 5 and 8 days, usually 6 days). However, time course experiments will help determine the optimal harvest day for your particular antigens and cells.

13. On the day of harvest, add approximately 500 U of DNase to each tube. Gently vortex. Incubate for 5 min at 37°C. (This step is needed after prolonged cellular activation and turnover result in significant cell death with release of DNA.)

14. Label surface and intracellular epitopes using the saponin-based intracellular cytokine detection method outlined above (many investigators insist that dead-cell exclusion methods be used, in which case labeling with propridium iodide, 7-amino-actinomycin D (7-AAD), or TOPRO-3 to subsequently exclude positively labeled dead cells should be done prior to cell permeabilization [16]).

Step 3: Cell Analysis

1. If a dead-cell exclusion dye is used, then exclude these cells from subsequent analysis. Propidium iodide can be used to exclude brightly staining cells from FL-2 and still use another fluorochrome in the same channel, but compensation between FL-2 and FL-1 can be difficult depending on CFSE fluorescence intensity (see below). 7-AAD and TOPRO-3 can exclude positively staining dead cells from FL-3 and FL-4, respectively, but use of these agents precludes use of another fluorochrome in the same channels. Ultimately, the choice of a dead-cell exclusion dye is dependent on the particular applications, and a single approach is impossible to recommend.

2. When using CFSE, compensation between FL-2 and FL-1 can be difficult in the extreme (e.g., FL-2–FL-1 can be upwards of 90%). Make certain to have the appropriate compensation controls (i.e., single-color control tubes with CFSE, FL-2, FL-3, and FL-4 reagents). Difficulties in compensation

can be addressed by either avoiding FL-2 altogether, using a bright FL-2 fluorochrome, decreasing the photomultiplier tube voltage in FL-1, or decreasing the CFSE labeling concentration to 5 mM or less (leading to diminished sensitivity for later cell divisions).

Quality Control and Quality Assurance

1. Wash buffer should be kept on wet ice to keep it cold for use in the quenching step.

2. Always pretiter MAb concentrations prior to routine use to determine the minimal amount of antibody necessary for saturation and maximal fluorescence intensity.

3. Always pretiter antigens used in stimulation experiments for maximal optimal response at the minimal antigen concentration on the day of interest.

4. Always perform a time course experiment to determine the optimal cell harvest time for the cells and antigens used in the particular application.

5. Make certain to pretitrate out the optimal CFSE staining concentration prior to use in your particular application.

Interpretation

Using membrane dye dilution methods to track cell division on a multiparameter flow cytometer is an extremely powerful tool to investigate which cells within PBMCs respond to antigen, how they differentiate over time, and what their surface immunophenotype is as they go through successive rounds of cell division. However, it is always important to remember that the technique does not analyze cells that disappear from the culture system, thus increasing representation of cells that remain. Thus, care should be taken in making conclusions about cells that did not proliferate in an assay that only measures cells that did proliferate after about 6 days in tissue culture.

REFERENCES

1. **Altman, J. D., P. A. Moss, P. J. Goulder, D. H. Barouch, M. G. McHeyzer-Williams, J. I. Bell, A. J. McMichael, and M. M. Davis.** 1996. Phenotypic analysis of antigen-specific T lymphocytes. *Science* **274:**94–96.

2. **Arden, B., S. P. Clark, D. Kabelitz, and T. W. Mak.** 1995. Human T-cell receptor variable gene segment families. *Immunogenetics* **42:**455–500.

3. **Connors, M., J. A. Kovacs, S. Krevat, J. C. Gea-Banacloche, M. C. Sneller, M. Flanigan, J. A. Metcalf, R. E. Walker, J. Falloon, M. Baseler, I. Feuerstein, H. Masur, and H. C. Lane.** 1997. HIV infection induces changes in CD4+ T-cell phenotype and depletions within the CD4+ T-cell repertoire that are not immediately restored by antiviral or immune-based therapies. *Nat. Med.* **3:**533–540.

4. **Davis, M. M., and P. J. Bjorkman.** 1988. T-cell antigen receptor genes and T-cell recognition. *Nature* **334:** 395–402.

5. **Gea-Bancloche, J. C., L. Martino, J. M. Mican, C. W. Hallahan, M. Baseler, R. Stevens, L. Lambert, M. Polis, H. C. Lane, and M. Connors.** 2000. Longitudinal changes in CD4+ T cell antigen receptor diversity and naive/memory cell phenotype during 9 to 26 months of antiretroviral therapy of HIV-infected patients. *AIDS Res. Hum. Retrovir.* **16:**1877–1886.

6. **Hengel, R. L., M. C. Allende, R. L. Dewar, J. A. Metcalf, J. M. Mican, and H. C. Lane.** 2002. Increasing CD4+ T cells specific for tuberculosis correlate with improved clinical immunity after highly active antiretroviral therapy. *AIDS Res. Hum. Retrovir.* **18:**969–975.

7. **Hengel, R. L., B. M. Jones, M. S. Kennedy, M. R. Hubbard, and J. S. McDougal.** 1999. Lymphocyte kinetics

and precursor frequency-dependent recovery of CD4(+)CD45RA(+)CD62L(+) naive T cells following triple-drug therapy for HIV type 1 infection. *AIDS Res. Hum. Retrovir.* **15:**435–443.

8. **Hengel, R. L., and J. K. Nicholson.** 2001. An update on the use of flow cytometry in HIV infection and AIDS. *Clin. Lab. Med.* **21:**841–856.

9. **Lane, H. C., J. M. Depper, W. C. Greene, G. Whalen, T. A. Waldmann, and A. S. Fauci.** 1985. Qualitative analysis of immune function in patients with the acquired immunodeficiency syndrome. Evidence for a selective defect in soluble antigen recognition. *N. Engl. J. Med.* **313:**79–84.

10. **Lyons, A. B., and C. R. Parish.** 1994. Determination of lymphocyte division by flow cytometry. *J. Immunol. Methods* **171:**131–137.

11. **Migueles, S. A., M. S. Sabbaghian, W. L. Shupert, M. P. Bettinotti, F. M. Marincola, L. Martino, C. W. Hallahan, S. M. Selig, D. Schwartz, J. Sullivan, and M. Connors.** 2000. HLA B*5701 is highly associated with restriction of virus replication in a subgroup of HIV-infected long term nonprogressors. *Proc. Natl. Acad. Sci. USA* **97:**2709–2714.

12. **Pannetier, C., J.-P. Levraud, A. Lim, J. Even, and P. Kourlisky.** 1997. The immunoscope approach for the analysis of T-cell repertoires, p. 287–325. *In* J. Oksenberg (ed.), *The Human Antigen T-Cell Receptor: Selected Protocols and Applications.* R. G. Landes, Austin, Tex.

13. **Porter, K., A. Babiker, K. Bhaskaran, J. Darbyshire, P. Pezzotti, and A. S. Walker.** 2003. Determinants of survival following HIV-1 seroconversion after the introduction of HAART. *Lancet* **362:**1267–1274.

14. **Prussin, C., and D. D. Metcalfe.** 1995. Detection of intra-cytoplasmic cytokine using flow cytometry and directly conjugated anti-cytokine antibodies. *J. Immunol. Methods* **188:**117–128.

15. **Waldrop, S. L., C. J. Pitcher, D. M. Peterson, V. C. Maino, and L. J. Picker.** 1997. Determination of antigen-specific memory/effector CD4+ T cell frequencies by flow cytometry: evidence for a novel, antigen-specific homeostatic mechanism in HIV-associated immunodeficiency. *J. Clin. Investig.* **99:**1739–1750.

16. **Wells, A. D., H. Gudmundsdottir, and L. A. Turka.** 1997. Following the fate of individual T cells throughout activation and clonal expansion. Signals from T cell receptor and CD28 differentially regulate the induction and duration of a proliferative response. *J. Clin. Investig.* **100:**3173–3183.

17. **Whelan, J. A., P. R. Dunbar, D. A. Price, M. A. Purbhoo, F. Lechner, G. S. Ogg, G. Griffiths, R. E. Phillips, V. Cerundolo, and A. K. Sewell.** 1999. Specificity of CTL interactions with peptide-MHC class I tetrameric complexes is temperature dependent. *J. Immunol.* **163:**4342–4348.

IMMUNODEFICIENCY DISEASES

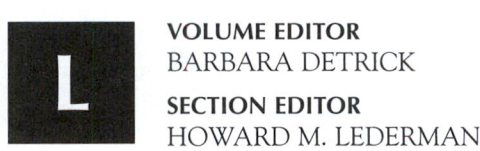

VOLUME EDITOR
BARBARA DETRICK

SECTION EDITOR
HOWARD M. LEDERMAN

The Primary Immunodeficiency Diseases

HOWARD M. LEDERMAN

98

Patients with primary immunodeficiency diseases most often are recognized because of their increased susceptibility to infection (chronic or recurrent infections without other explanation, infection with an organism of low virulence, or infection of unusual severity). However, these patients may also present with autoimmune or inflammatory disorders (e.g., hemolytic anemia, inflammatory bowel disease, vasculitis, or systemic lupus erythematosus) or with part of a syndrome complex (Table 1).

SYMPTOMS OFTEN CAN GUIDE THE LABORATORY EVALUATION

The type of pathogen and the location of the infection may give valuable insight into the nature of the immunologic defect. For example, individuals with antibody deficiencies are unusually susceptible to encapsulated bacteria and enteroviruses, which cause infections along mucosal surfaces. Individuals with defects in cell-mediated immunity can have problems with almost any microorganism, including opportunistic pathogens. Individuals with complement deficiencies most often present with bacteremia, septic arthritis, and meningitis, caused by encapsulated bacteria. And finally, phagocytic disorders are characterized by bacterial and fungal infections of the skin and abscesses in the reticuloendothelial system (lymph nodes, spleen, and liver).

Autoimmune and inflammatory diseases are more commonly seen in particular primary immunodeficiency diseases, most notably common variable immunodeficiency, selective immunoglobulin A (IgA) deficiency, chronic mucocutaneous candidiasis, and deficiencies of early components of the classical complement pathway (C1 to C4).

When immunodeficiency is part of a constellation of signs and symptoms in a syndrome complex, the diagnosis of immunodeficiency may be made before there are any clinical manifestations of that deficiency. For instance, children with DiGeorge syndrome are most often first identified because of the neonatal presentation of congenital heart disease and/or hypocalcemic tetany. This should lead to T-lymphocyte evaluation prior to the onset of opportunistic infections. Similarly, a diagnosis of Wiskott-Aldrich syndrome can often be made in young boys with eczema and thrombocytopenia even prior to the onset of infections.

LABORATORY EVALUATION

Although immune system dysfunction can be suspected by the clinician after careful review of the history and physical exam, specific diagnoses are rarely evident without the use of the laboratory. However, the types of infections and other symptoms should help to focus the laboratory workup on specific compartments of the immune system (Table 2).

TABLE 1 Examples of immunodeficiency syndromes

Syndrome	Usual clinical presentation(s)	Immunologic abnormality
DiGeorge syndrome	Congenital heart disease, hypoparathyroidism, abnormal facies	Thymic hypoplasia
Wiskott-Aldrich syndrome	Thrombocytopenia, eczema	Variable B- and T-lymphocyte dysfunction
Ataxia-telangiectasia	Ataxia, telangiectasia	Variable B- and T-lymphocyte dysfunction
Ivemark syndrome	Congenital heart disease, bilateral three-lobed lungs	Asplenia
Polyendocrinopathy syndrome	Endocrine organ dysfunction	Chronic mucocutaneous candidiasis

TABLE 2 Patterns of illness associated with primary immunodeficiency

Disorder	Illnesses	
	Infection	Other
Antibody	Sinopulmonary (pyogenic bacteria) Gastrointestinal (enterovirus, giardiasis)	Autoimmune disease (autoantibodies, inflammatory bowel disease)
Cell-mediated immunity	Pneumonia (pyogenic bacteria, *Pneumocystis jerovici*, and viruses) Gastrointestinal (viruses) Skin, mucous membranes (fungi)	
Complement	Sepsis and other blood-borne infections (streptococci, pneumococci, and neisseriae)	Autoimmune disease (systemic lupus erythematosus, glomerulonephritis)
Phagocytosis	Skin, reticuloendothelial system, abscesses (*Staphylococcus*, enteric bacteria, fungi, and mycobacteria)	

Screening tests that should be performed for almost all patients include a complete blood count with differential and quantitative measurement of serum immunoglobulins. Other tests should be guided by the clinical features of the patient (Table 3). Finally, whenever primary immunodeficiency is suspected, consideration must also be given to secondary causes of immunodeficiency, including human immunodeficiency virus infection, therapy with anti-inflammatory medications (e.g., corticosteroids), and other underlying illnesses (e.g., lymphoreticular neoplasms and viral infections, such as infectious mononucleosis). Details about the selection and performance of specific laboratory tests are discussed in the following chapters, organized by immunologic compartment: antibody, cell-mediated immunity (severe combined immunodeficiency), complement, and phagocytes.

TABLE 3 Screening tests for primary immunodeficiency

Suspected abnormality	Diagnostic test(s)
Antibody	Quantitative immunoglobulins (IgG, IgA, and IgM) Antibody response to immunization
Cell-mediated immunity	Lymphocyte count T-lymphocyte enumeration (CD4 and CD8) HIV[a] serology Delayed-type-hypersensitivity tests
Complement	Total hemolytic complement
Phagocytosis	Neutrophil count Nitroblue tetrazolium dye test or equivalent

[a]HIV, human immunodeficiency virus.

SUGGESTED READING

1. **Bonilla, F. A., and R. S. Geha.** 2003. Primary immunodeficiency diseases. *J. Allergy Clin. Immunol.* **111:**S571–S581.

2. **Chapel, H., R. Geha, and F. Rosin for the IUIS PID Classification Committee.** 2003. Primary immunodeficiency diseases: an update. *Clin. Exp. Immunol.* **132:**9–15.

3. **Folds, J. D., and J. L. Schmitz.** 2003. Clinical and laboratory assessment of immunity. *J. Allergy Clin. Immunol.* **111:**S702–S711.

4. **Stiehm, E. R., H. D. Ochs, and J. A. Winkelstein.** 2004. Immunodeficiency disorders: general considerations, p. 289–355. *In* E. R. Stiehm, H. D. Ochs, and J. A. Winkelstein (ed.), *Immunologic Disorders in Infants and Children,* 5th ed. Elsevier Saunders, Philadelphia, Pa.

Approach to the Diagnosis of Severe Combined Immunodeficiency

CHAIM M. ROIFMAN

99

Severe combined immunodeficiency (SCID) includes a genetically heterogeneous group of disorders that present with a distinct clinical and immunological phenotype. The phenotype is related to the profound T-cell defect which is common to all types of SCID. Central to the adaptive immune system, T cells protect the host from intracellular pathogens by mediating cytolytic activity and releasing Th1 cytokines. In addition, through release of soluble mediations such as interleukin 4 (IL-4) and IL-10 and interactions with antigen-presenting cells and B cells, T cells regulate the production of antibody against protein antigens (3). Consequently, severe defects in T-cell function result in a combined cellular and humoral immunodeficiency leading to increased susceptibility to viral, fungal, and microbial infections in infancy (21). SCID is caused by a variety of genetic aberrations in genes which appear to be critical for the normal development and expansion of the T-cell repertoire, or in genes whose products are responsible for effective elimination of metabolites which are toxic to T-cell precursors (Table 1 and Fig. 1).

In addition to T-cell deficiency, some aberrations, such as mutations in IL-2 receptor (IL-2R) gamma and its downstream signaling partner JAK-3, prevent the normal development of NK cells. Other forms of SCID, such as recombination-activating gene (RAG) deficiency, may block the maturation of B cells as well as T cells. Nevertheless, a profound selective deficiency in the T-cell lineage such as in CD3δ deficiency is sufficient to produce a full phenotype of SCID with extreme susceptibility to microbes of even low pathogenicity (Table 1).

MOLECULAR BASIS OF SCID

T⁻ B⁻ SCID

RAG Deficiency

Patients who lack circulating T lymphocytes as well as B lymphocytes are most frequently found to have mutations in one of the RAGs RAG1 and RAG2 (35). The corresponding enzymes play a critical role in the complex process of assembling the V(D) and J segments which together form the variable parts of immunoglobulin and T-cell receptor (TCR) protein chains. In the absence of effective recombination, the development of a full repertoire of T cells or B cells is greatly limited, hence the reduced number of circulating T cells and B cells in patients with abnormal RAG1 or RAG2 activity.

Missense mutations limiting, but not completely abolishing, the function of RAG1 or RAG2 were implicated as a cause of Omenn's syndrome, which is characterized by erythroderma, lymphadenopathy, hepatosplenomegaly, eosinophilia, and high immunoglobulin E levels (9, 22, 40, 41, 43).

ARTEMIS Deficiency

An essentially identical phenotype of complete absence of circulating T cells and B cells results from mutations which render the ARTEMIS enzyme inactive (19). Similar to the case with RAG1 or RAG2, partial activity of ARTEMIS may result in an Omenn's syndrome phenotype (11).

ADA Deficiency

Markedly reduced T-cell and B-cell numbers are also typical of adenosine deaminase (ADA) deficiency. This enzyme mediates conversion of adenosine into inosine and of deoxyadenosine into deoxyinosine (14). In ADA deficiency the injury to early lymphocyte precursors is caused by the intracellular accumulation of deoxyadenosine and its phosphorylated metabolites. Partial enzymatic deficiency of ADA may result in a delayed and/or milder clinical presentation (24).

Reticular Dysgenesis

Reticular dysgenesis, an exceedingly rare type of SCID, is caused by a defect in early lymphoid and myeloid precursors (10). Patients present with profound neutropenia and lymphopenia. The thymus gland is barely detectable by ultrasound and appears to be completely dysplastic when assessed by histology and immunohistochemistry.

T⁻ B⁺ (NK⁻) SCID

XL-SCID

The most common type of SCID is inherited as an X-linked trait. This disease is caused by a mutation in the gene that encodes the IL-2R common gamma chain (γc) located at Xq12-13.1 (20). Together with the IL-2Rα and -β chains, the γc forms the high-affinity receptor for IL-2, which is required for clonal expansion of T cells. The γc chain is also an essential partner to other receptors, including those for IL-4, IL-7, IL-9, IL-15, and IL-21. The typical immunotype of XL-SCID is an absence of circulating T cells and NK cells and normal numbers of B cells. This can be easily explained by a lack of

TABLE 1 Genetic and immunological features of SCID[a]

Phenotype and disease	Genetic features (gene/inheritance)	Circulating white blood cells				Thymus
		T cells	B cells	NK cells	Neutrophils	Imaging/histology
T⁻ B⁻						
RAG deficiency	RAG1, RAG2/AR	↓	↓	N	N	Small/dysplastic
ARTEMIS deficiency	ARTEMIS/AR	↓	↓	N	N	Small
Reticular dysgenesis	UK/AR	↓	↓	↓	↓	Small/dysplastic
ADA deficiency	ADA/AR	↓	↓	↓N	N	Small/dysplastic
T⁻ B⁺ (NK⁻)						
X-linked SCID	γc/XL	↓	N	↓	N	Small/dysplastic
JAK-3 deficiency	JAK-3/AR	↓	N	↓	N	Small/dysplastic
T⁻ B⁺ (NK⁺)						
IL-7Rα deficiency	IL-7R/AR	↓	N	N	N	Small/dysplastic
CD3δ deficiency	CD3δ AR	↓	N	N	N	N size, no HC
CD45 deficiency	CD45/AR	↓	N	N	N	UK
CD25 deficiency	IL2-Rα/AR	↓	N	N	N	N size, no HC, no CM
PNP deficiency	PNP/AR	↓	N	N	N	Small/poor HC
CHH	RMRP/AR	↓	N	N	N	Dysplastic but leaky
T⁺ B⁺ (NK⁺)						
ZAP-70 deficiency	ZAP-70/AR	N (CD8↓)	N	N	N	N size, N HC, N CM
HLA class II deficiency	CIITA, RFXANK, RFX5, RFXAP/AR	N↓ (CD4↓)	N	N	N	UK
Multiple cytokine defects	UK/AR	N	N	N	N	UK
Variable						
Omenn's syndrome	RAG1/RAG2/AR	N↓↑ (clonal)	↓	N	N	Small/dysplastic
	ARTEMIS/AR	↓	↓	N	N	Small
	UK/AR	N↓↑ (clonal)	N	N	N	UK
Atypical X-linked SCID	γc/XL	N	N	N	N	N HC, N CM

[a]HC, Hassall's corpuscles; CM, corticomedullary distinction; UK, unknown; N, normal; AR, autosomal recessive; XL, X-linked; RMRP, RNase mitochondrial RNA processing.

activity of IL-7R and IL-15R, respectively. Rarely, atypical cases of XL-SCID may have near normal to normal numbers of circulating T cells and NK cells (Table 1) (26, 37).

JAK-3 Deficiency

Phenotypically identical to XL-SCID but inherited in an autosomal recessive fashion are cases of SCID caused by mutations in the JAK-3 gene, which is located at chromosome 19 (16, 34). This tyrosine kinase mediates signal transduction stemming from the γc chain and IL-2R (23, 33).

T⁻ B⁺ (NK⁺)

IL-7Rα Deficiency

IL-7R is essential for the development of T cells in humans (25). It is therefore not surprising that mutations in this receptor result in the absence of circulating T cells with preserved development of B and NK cells (27, 32). IL-7R consists of two subunits, the γc chain and IL-7Rα, which is specific for IL-7R. The receptor is expressed very early in lymphoid precursor cells, including some CD34⁺ stem cells, hence the block of T-cell development at an early stage (double negative) and the resultant small and dysplastic thymus (Fig. 1 and Table 1).

CD3δ Deficiency

CD3δ subunits are the signaling molecules of the TCR. While deficiencies of CD3γ result in mild to moderate cellular deficiency (1), mutations in CD3δ cause a complete arrest in the transition from double-negative to double-positive thymocytes (7). Patients would therefore have no circulating αβ TCR- or γδ TCR-positive cells. B-cell and NK-cell numbers are normal. The thymus in these patients appears normal in size, but it contains mainly immature double-negative thymocytes and lacks Hassall's corpuscles (30). A similar phenotype has been recently identified in a case with complete CD3ε deficiency (8).

CD45 Deficiency

CD45 deficiency results in a similar phenotype, including a complete lack of circulating T cells with normal B cells and NK cells. The CD45 protein is a phosphatase that modulates TCR/CD3 signaling (15, 39).

IL-2Rα (CD25) Deficiency

IL-2Rα deficiency in humans is fascinating. It results in inefficient negative selection in the thymus that leads to expansion of autoreactive clones which infiltrate multiple tissues (29). Indeed, the thymus in such patients is densely populated with thymocytes. However, Hassall's corpuscles and corticomedullary distinctions are lacking. The number of circulating T cells is reduced, but B-cell and NK-cell numbers are normal (29, 36).

PNP Deficiency

Purine nucleoside phosphorylase (PNP) deficiency, similar to ADA deficiency, results in an accumulation of toxic phosphorylated metabolites. These block ribonucleotide reductase, which is essential for DNA synthesis. Along the purine metabolism pathway, PNP converts guanosine into guanine and deoxyguanosine into deoxyguanine (6). Accumulating deoxyguanosine metabolites are selectively toxic to T-cell

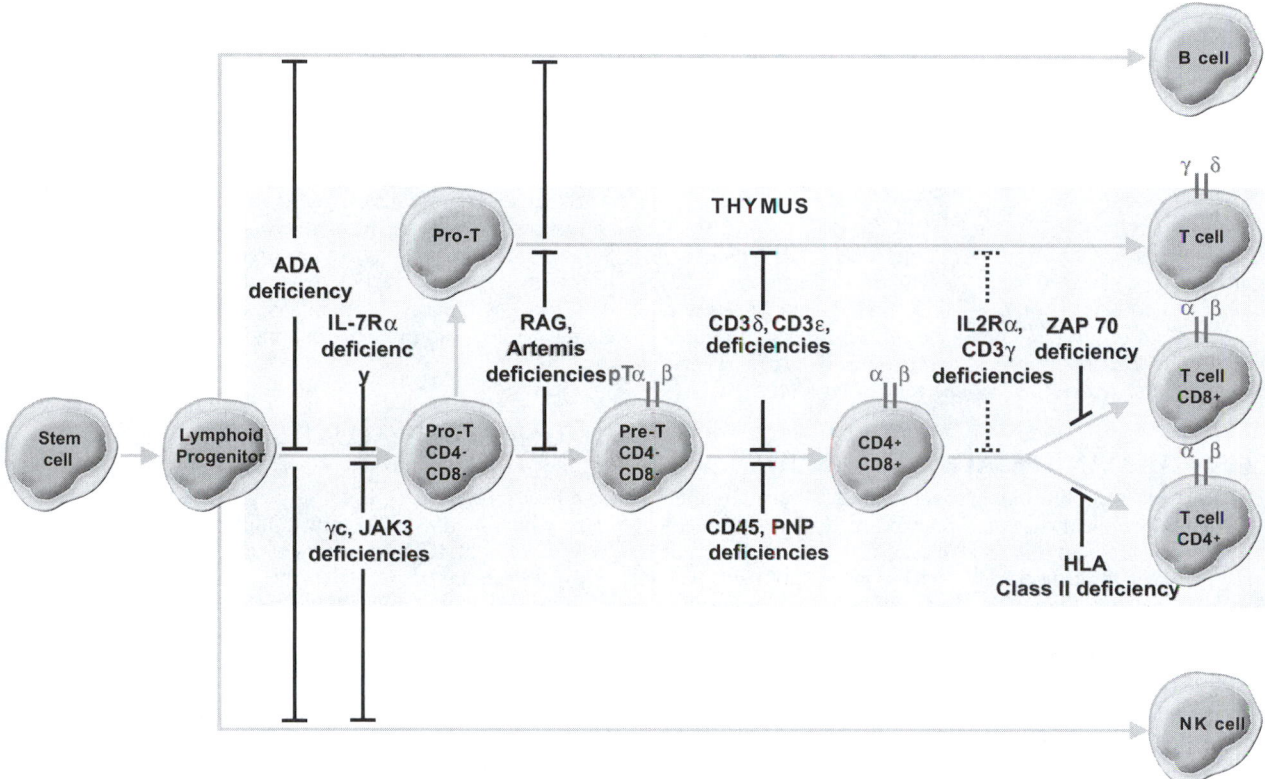

FIGURE 1 Simplified scheme of the block in T-cell, NK-cell, and B-cell development caused by aberrations in genes which cause SCID. The symbol "⊥" represents complete block, while the symbol "⊥" represents partial block. Stem cells which originate in the bone marrow mature into putative lymphoid progenitor cells which either populate the thymus gland and become T-lineage precursors or develop into NK or B cells. The TCR complex consists of the α and β or γ and δ variant chains, paired as mutually exclusive heterodimers in association with the invariant chains CD3 γ, δ, ε, and ζ. After rearrangements of the δ and then γ genes, some thymocytes develop into a distinct population of γδ TCR⁺ T cells. Precursors of the αβ T-cell lineage undergo three major stages of maturation, defined by the expression of CD4 and CD8. The earliest precursors are designated double negative, expressing neither CD4 nor CD8. They progress to a stage of dual expression of CD4 and CD8 (double positive) before committing to the expression of either CD4 or CD8 alone (single positive) and leaving the thymus. A rearrangement of TCRβ occurs at the double-negative stage and precedes the rearrangement of TCRα. Transition from the double-negative stage to CD4⁺ CD8⁺ double positivity requires the surface expression of TCRβ and precursor TCRα (pTα) forming the pre-TCR, whereas the maturation from double-positive to single-positive CD4 or CD8 cells is dependent on the surface expression of the αβ TCR complex.

precursors. Patients with PNP deficiency present with progressive T-cell lymphopenia and eventually a SCID phenotype within the first few years of life (6, 13).

CHH

Patients with cartilage-hair hypoplasia (CHH) may, rarely, present with a SCID phenotype. Typically, these patients have metaphyseal dysplasia, fine hair, and immunodeficiency. Mutations in the RNA component of MRP have been identified in these patients (28). Most patients with CHH have a milder phenotype with moderate T-cell dysfunction and, infrequently, humoral deficiency.

T⁺ B⁺ (NK⁺)

ZAP-70 Deficiency

Patients with ZAP-70 deficiency present clinically with a typical SCID phenotype, yet unusually, these patients have normal numbers of circulating T cells, B cells, and NK cells (31). Flow

cytometry analysis reveals a complete or near complete absence of circulating CD8⁺ T cells (31). Circulating CD4⁺ cells, although normal in number, fail to respond to mitogens. ZAP-70 is an intracellular protein tyrosine kinase which is required for T-cell activation following ligation of the TCR. The deficiency underscores the critical role of ZAP-70 in the maturation of CD8⁺ T cells in the thymus and in the clonal expansion (mitogenic and antigenic responses) of peripheral lymphocytes (2, 12).

HLA Class II Deficiency

Patients with HLA class II deficiency can present with a SCID phenotype, although frequently patients may present later than 1 year of age and survive beyond infancy with only antimicrobial treatment. The immunological basis for the deficiency lies with the inability of T cells to recognize antigens in the context of self-HLA class II molecules expressed by antigen-presenting cells (17). In addition, development of CD4⁺ T cells is hampered by the lack of expression of major histocompatibility complex class II molecules on thymic epithelial cells, hence the reduction in circulating CD4+ T cells in these patients.

The disease is caused by mutations not in the genes which encode HLA class II molecules but, rather, in genes that encode transcription factors which control HLA class II gene expression (Table 1) (17, 18, 38, 42).

Cytokine Deficiencies (IL-2 Deficiency)

IL-2 deficiency is a functional defect of T cells which are unable to produce normal levels of endogenous IL-2. Defective production of IL-4, IL-5, and gamma interferon has also been observed. The exact pathogenesis and molecular defect remain unknown. Exogenous IL-2 can reverse the defect in vitro and to some extent in vivo (4, 5).

CLINICAL MANIFESTATIONS OF SCID

All forms of SCID present in a remarkably similar manner. Patients with typical cases are referred to tertiary-care centers between the ages of 4 to 12 months because of recurrent and persistent viral, bacterial, and fungal infections as well as failure to thrive (Table 2). Most commonly, patients suffer from chronic protracted diarrhea and interstitial pneumonitis. Viruses such as rotavirus and adenovirus readily grow in their stool cultures. Bronchial secretions or lung biopsy specimens frequently harbor *Pneumocystis carinii*, parainfluenza virus, or cytomegalovirus. Persistent oral thrush which responds poorly to topical anti-fungal medications is also a common feature. Other frequent clinical manifestations include increased liver enzymes and disseminated cytomegalovirus. Lack of palpable lymph nodes and a small to undetectable thymus shadow, as evaluated by radiography or ultrasound, are also very common in SCID.

Skin rashes may also be prominent in SCID. A maculopapular rash has been recognized in ZAP-70 deficiency, and it may be a manifestation of graft-versus-host disease due to maternal engraftment. Although maternally derived T cells are frequently found in SCID patients with profound lymphopenia, clinical symptoms of graft-versus-host disease are less common.

Some forms of SCID may present with additional typical features. Severe universal erythroderma and alopecia, which

TABLE 2 Clinical presentation of SCID

Feature	Patients
Common nonspecific	
Pneumonitis	All
Chronic protracted diarrhea	All
Failure to thrive	All
Oral thrush	All
Family history (consanguinity)	All
Early presentation (4–12 mo)	Typical cases
Specific	
Erythroderma	Omenn's syndrome
Lymphadenopathy	Omenn's, CD25 deficiency
Hepatosplenomegaly	Omenn's, CD25 deficiency
Short limbs	CHH, Omenn's syndrome
Neurological disorders and hepatic dysfunction	ADA deficiency
Gait abnormalities	PNP deficiency

is associated with lymphadenopathy, hepatosplenomegaly, and eosinophilia, are typical of Omenn's syndrome and are likely caused by expanded autoreactive T-cell clones (Table 2).

Hepatic dysfunction and neurological manifestations, including cortical atrophy and cognitive abnormalities, are detected in ADA deficiency, while ataxia is common in PNP deficiency.

Skeletal abnormalities such as metaphyseal dysplasia causing short limb dwarfism are typical of CHH and may also be associated with Omenn's syndrome. Cupping and flaring of the ribs are seen in ADA deficiency. Hematological disorders such as hemolytic anemia are common in PNP deficiency, while profound neutropenia is a hallmark of reticular dysgenesis.

DIAGNOSTIC EVALUATION OF SCID

The most basic and informative laboratory test which can be used as a screen for SCID at all health care levels is a complete white blood cell count. Lymphopenia is observed in most cases of SCID, and counts of fewer than 2,000 lymphocytes/μl should prompt further investigation. Neutropenia in addition to lymphopenia should raise the possibility of reticular dysgenesis, while hemolytic anemia might point to PNP deficiency (Fig. 2).

However, a significant proportion of SCID patients have normal or near normal number of circulating lymphocytes (Omenn's syndrome, major histocompatibility complex class II deficiency, and ZAP-70 deficiency). Flow cytometry analysis will help decipher these cases and will aid in pinpointing the molecular defect by providing insight into the number of B cells and NK cells. It is therefore recommended that all infants with a putative diagnosis of SCID have their lymphocyte subsets analyzed. The markers to be tested include CD3, CD2, CD4, and CD8 for T cells; CD19 or CD20 for B cells; and CD16 or CD56 for NK cells. HLA class II should also be tested. In most cases this analysis should be sufficient to define which gene defect should be analyzed (Fig. 2)

Evaluation of T-cell function in vitro is helpful when flow cytometry is normal or inconclusive. Mitogenic responses to phytohemagglutinin and anti-CD3 antibody in the presence or absence of exogenous IL-2 can help in the diagnosis of atypical cases of XL-SCID, multiple cytokine deficiency, or Omenn's syndrome. Assessment of the T-cell repertoire can identify oligoclonality in Omenn's syndrome. This can be performed by determination of the relative expression of various Vβ families using PCR or flow cytometry (Fig. 2).

In cases where the diagnosis of SCID is suspected from the clinical presentation but cannot be ascertained using standard investigations, a thymus biopsy can be helpful. The lack of Hassall's corpuscles and the loss of corticomedullary distinction are indicative of a primary immunodeficiency. In contrast, depletion of thymocytes in the presence of normal Hassall's corpuscles suggests changes secondary to stress or treatment with corticosteroids. Analysis of a thymus biopsy not only helps in distinguishing primary from secondary immunodeficiency but also can help identify novel genetic aberrations leading to SCID, as demonstrated in the discoveries of ZAP-70 deficiency, CD3δ deficiency, and IL-2Rα deficiency.

In cases of extreme lymphopenia, ADA and PNP enzymatic activity in red cells can establish the diagnosis of these conditions.

Finally, since the genes responsible for many forms of SCID have already been identified, it is important to perform mutation analysis. In addition to providing definitive diagnosis, it

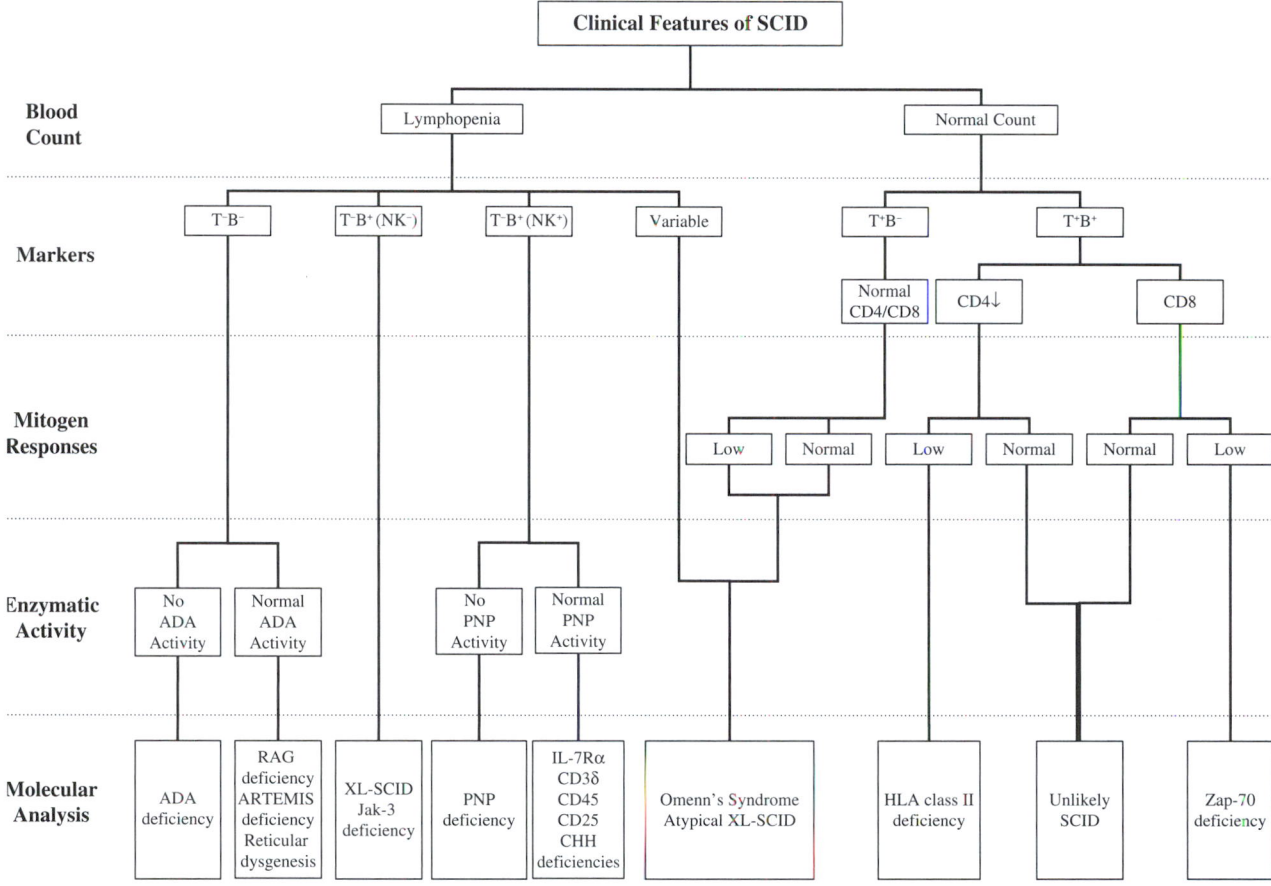

FIGURE 2 Step-by-step laboratory evaluation of patients who present within the first year of life with typical manifestations of SCID (see Table 2) and after secondary causes, such as human immunodeficiency virus infection and medications, have been excluded.

allows for appropriate genetic counseling and future consideration of prenatal diagnosis and gene therapy.

REFERENCES

1. Alarcon, B., J. R. Regueiro, A. Arnaiz-Villena, and C. Terhorst. 1988. Familial defect in the surface expression of the T-cell receptor-CD3 complex. *N. Engl. J. Med.* **319:**1203–1208.

2. Arpaia, E., M. Shahar, H. Dadi, A. Cohen, and C. M. Roifman. 1994. Defective T cell receptor signaling and CD8+ thymic selection in humans lacking Zap-70 kinase. *Cell* **76:**947–958.

3. Benoist, C., and D. Mathis. 1999. T-lymphocyte differentiation and biology, p. 367–409. *In* W. E. Paul (ed.), *Fundamental Immunology*, 4th ed. Lippincott-Raven Publishers, Philadelphia, Pa.

4. Castigli, E., R. Pahwa, R. A. Good, R. S. Geha, and T. A. Chatila. 1993. Molecular basis of a multiple lymphokine deficiency in a patient with severe combined immunodeficiency. *Proc. Natl. Acad. Sci. USA* **90:**4728–4731.

5. Chatila, T., E. Castigli, R. Pahwa, S. Pahwa, N. Chirmule, N. Oyaizu, R. A. Good, and R. S. Geha. 1990. Primary combined immunodeficiency resulting from defective transcription of multiple T-cell lymphokine genes. *Proc. Natl. Acad. Sci. USA* **87:**10033–10037.

6. Cohen, A., D. Doyle, D. W. Martin, Jr., and A. J. Ammann. 1976. Abnormal purine metabolism and purine overproduction in a patient deficient in purine nucleoside phosphorylase. *N. Engl. J. Med.* **295:**1449–1454.

7. Dadi, H. K., A. J. Simon, and C. M. Roifman. 2003. Effect of CD3δ deficiency on maturation of α/β and γ/δ T-cell lineages in severe combined immunodeficiency. *N. Engl. J. Med.* **349:**1821–1828.

8. de Saint Basile, G., F. Geissmann, E. Flori, B. Uring-Lambert, C. Soudais, M. Cavazzana-Calvo, A. Durandy, N. Jabado, A. Fischer, and F. Le Deist. 2004. Severe combined immunodeficiency caused by deficiency in either the δ or the ε subunit of CD3. *J. Clin. Investig.* **114:**1512–1517.

9. de Saint Basile, G., F. Le Deist, J. P. de Villartay, N. Cerf-Bensussan, O. Journet, N. Brousse, C. Griscelli, and A. Fischer. 1991. Restricted heterogeneity of T lymphocytes in combined immunodeficiency with hypereosinophilia (Omenn's syndrome). *J. Clin. Investig.* **87:**1352–1359.

10. de Vaal, O. M., and V. Seynhaeve. 1959. Reticular dysgenesis. *Lancet* **ii:**1123–1124.

11. Ege, M., Y. Ma, B. Manfras, K. Kalwak, H. Lu, M. R. Lieber, K. Schwarz, and U. Pannicke. 2005. Omenn syndrome due to ARTEMIS mutations. *Blood* **105:**4179–4186.

12. Elder, M. E., D. Lin, J. Clever, A. C. Chan, T. J. Hope, A. Weiss, and T. G. Parslow. 1994. Human severe combined immunodeficiency due to a defect in ZAP-70, a T cell tyrosine kinase. *Science* **264:**1596–1599.

13. Grunebaum, E., J. Zhang, and C. M. Roifman. 2004. Novel mutations and hot spots in patients with purine

nucleoside phosphorylase deficiency. *Nucleosides Nucleotides Nucleic Acids* **23**:1411–1415.

14. **Hershfield, M. S.** 2000. Immunodeficiency caused by adenosine deaminase deficiency. *Immunol. Allergy Clin. N. Am., T Cell Immunodeficiencies* **20**:161–175.

15. **Kung, C., J. T. Pingel, M. Heikinheimo, T. Klemola, K. Varkila, L. I. Yoo, K. Vuopala, M. Poyhonen, M. Uhari, M. Rogers, S. H. Speck, T. Chatila, and M. L. Thomas.** 2000. Mutations in the tyrosine phosphatase CD45 gene in a child with severe combined immunodeficiency disease. *Nat. Med.* **6**:343–345.

16. **Macchi, P., A. Villa, S. Giliani, M. G. Sacco, A. Frattini, F. Porta, A. G. Ugazio, J. A. Johnston, F. Candotti, J. J. O'Shea, et al.** 1995. Mutations of Jak-3 gene in patients with autosomal severe combined immune deficiency (SCID). *Nature* **377**:65–68.

17. **Mach, B., V. Steimle, and W. Reith.** 1994. MHC class II-deficient combined immunodeficiency: a disease of gene regulation. *Immunol. Rev.* **138**:207–221.

18. **Masternak, K., E. Barras, M. Zufferey, B. Conrad, G. Corthals, R. Aebersold, J. C. Sanchez, D. F. Hochstrasser, B. Mach, and W. Reith.** 1998. A gene encoding a novel RFX-associated transactivator is mutated in the majority of MHC class II deficiency patients. *Nat. Genet.* **20**:273–277.

19. **Moshous, D., I. Callebaut, R. de Chasseval, B. Corneo, M. Cavazzana-Calvo, F. Le Deist, I. Tezcan, O. Sanal, Y. Bertrand, N. Philippe, A. Fischer, and J. P. de Villartay.** 2001. Artemis, a novel DNA double-strand break repair/V(D)J recombination protein, is mutated in human severe combined immune deficiency. *Cell* **105**:177–186.

20. **Noguchi, M., H. Yi, H. M. Rosenblatt, A. H. Filipovich, S. Adelstein, W. S. Modi, O. W. McBride, and W. J. Leonard.** 1993. Interleukin-2 receptor gamma chain mutation results in X-linked severe combined immunodeficiency in humans. *Cell* **73**:147–157.

21. **Notarangelo, L. D.** 2003. T cell immunodeficiencies, p. 99–107. *In* D. Y. M. Leung, H. A. Sampson, R. S. Geha, and S. J. Szefler (ed.), *Pediatric Allergy Principles and Practice.* Mosby Inc., St. Louis, Mo.

22. **Omenn, G. S.** 1965. Familial reticuloendotheliosis with eosinophilia. *N. Engl. J. Med.* **273**:427–432.

23. **O'Shea, J. J., L. D. Notarangelo, J. A. Johnston, and F. Candotti.** 1997. Advances in the understanding of cytokine signal transduction: the role of Jaks and STATs in immunoregulation and the pathogenesis of immunodeficiency. *J. Clin. Immunol.* **17**:431–447.

24. **Ozsahin, H., F. X. Arredondo-Vega, I. Santisteban, H. Fuhrer, P. Tuchschmid, W. Jochum, A. Aguzzi, H. M. Lederman, A. Fleischman, J. A. Winkelstein, R. A. Seger, and M. S. Hershfield.** 1997. Adenosine deaminase deficiency in adults. *Blood* **89**:2849–2855.

25. **Peschon, J. J., P. J. Morissey, K. H. Grabstein, F. J. Ramsdell, E. Maraskovsky, B. C. Gliniak, L. S. Park, S. F. Ziegler, D. E. Williams, C. B. Ware, J. D. Meyer, and B. L. Davison.** 1994. Early lymphocyte expansion is severely impaired in interleukin 7 receptor-deficient mice. *J. Exp. Med.* **180**:1955–1960.

26. **Puck, J. M.** 1996. IL2RGbase: a database of γc-chain defects causing human X-SCID. *Immunol. Today* **17**:507–511.

27. **Puel, A., S. Ziegler, R. H. Buckley, and W. J. Leonard.** 1998. Defective IL7R expression in T−B+NK+ severe combined immunodeficiency. *Nat. Genet.* **20**:394–397.

28. **Ridanpää, M., H. van Eenennaam, K. Pelin, R. Chadwick, C. Johnson, B. Yuan, W. vanVenrooij, G. Pruijn, R. Salmela, S. Rockas, O. Makitie, I. Kaitila, and A. de la Chapelle.** 2001. Mutations in the RNA component of RNase MRP cause a pleiotropic human disease, cartilage-hair hypoplasia. *Cell* **104**:195–203.

29. **Roifman, C. M.** 2000. Human IL-2 receptor alpha chain deficiency. *Pediatr. Res.* **48**:6–11.

30. **Roifman, C. M.** 2005. Studies of patients' thymi aid in the discovery and characterization of immunodeficiency in humans. *Immunol. Rev.* **203**:143–155.

31. **Roifman, C. M., D. Hummel, H. Martinez-Valdez, P. Thorner, P. J. Doherty, S. Pan, F. Cohen, and A. Cohen.** 1989. Depletion of CD8+ cells in human thymic medulla results in selective immune deficiency. *J. Exp. Med.* **170**:2177–2182.

32. **Roifman, C. M., J. Zhang, D. Chitayat, and N. Sharfe.** 2000. A partial deficiency of interleukin-7Rα is sufficient to abrogate T-cell development and cause severe combined immunodeficiency. *Blood* **96**:2803–2807.

33. **Russell, S. M., J. A. Johnston, M. Noguchi, M. Kawamura, C. M. Bacon, M. Friedmann, M. Berg, D. W. McVicar, B. A. Witthuhn, O. Silvennoinen, et al.** 1994. Interaction of IL-2Rβ and γc chains with Jak1 and Jak3: implications for XSCID and XCID. *Science* **266**:1042–1045.

34. **Russell, S. M., N. Tayebi, H. Nakajima, M. C. Riedy, J. L. Roberts, M. J. Aman, T. S. Migone, M. Noguchi, M. L. Markert, R. H. Buckley, J. J. O'Shea, and W. J. Leonard.** 1995. Mutation of Jak3 in a patient with SCID: essential role of Jak3 in lymphoid development. *Science* **270**:797–800.

35. **Schwarz, K., G. H. Gauss, L. Ludwig, U. Pannicke, Z. Li, D. Lindner, W. Friedrich, R. A. Seger, T. E. Hansen-Hagge, S. Desiderio, M. R. Lieber, and C. R. Bartram.** 1996. RAG mutations in human B cell-negative SCID. *Science* **274**:97–99.

36. **Sharfe, N., H. K. Dadi, M. Shahar, and C. M. Roifman.** 1997. Human immune disorder arising from mutation of the chain of the interleukin-2 receptor. *Proc. Natl. Acad. Sci. USA* **94**:3168–3171.

37. **Somech, R., and C. M. Roifman.** 2005. Mutation analysis should be performed to rule out γc deficiency in children with functional SCID despite apparently normal immunity. *J. Pediatr.* **147**:555–557.

38. **Steimle, V., L. A. Otten, M. Zufferey, and B. Mach.** 1993. Complementation cloning of an MHC class II transactivator mutated in hereditary MHC class II deficiency (or bare lymphocyte syndrome). *Cell* **75**:135–146.

39. **Tchilian, E. Z., D. L. Wallace, R. S. Wells, D. R. Flower, G. Morgan, and P. C. Beverley.** 2001. A deletion in the gene encoding the CD45 antigen in a patient with SCID. *J. Immunol.* **166**:1308–1313.

40. **Villa, A., S. Santagata, F. Bozzi, S. Giliani, A. Frattini, L. Imberti, L. B. Gatta, H. D. Ochs, K. Schwarz, L. D. Notarangelo, P. Vezzoni, and E. Spanopoulou.** 1998. Partial V(D)J recombination activity leads to Omenn syndrome. *Cell* **93**:885–896.

41. **Villa, A., C. Sobacchi, L. D. Notarangelo, F. Bozzi, M. Abinun, T. G. Abrahamsen, P. D. Arkwright, M. Baniyash, E. G. Brooks, M. E. Conley, P. Cortes, M. Duse, A. Fasth, A. M. Filipovich, A. J. Infante, A. Jones, E. Mazzolari, S. M. Muller, S. Pasic, G. Rechavi, M. G. Sacco, S. Santagata, M. L. Schroeder, R. Seger, D. Strina, A. Ugazio, J. Valiaho, M. Vihinen, L. B. Vogler, H. Ochs, P. Vezzoni, W. Friedrich, and K. Schwarz.** 2001. V(D)J recombination defects in lymphocytes due to RAG mutations: a severe immunodeficiency with a spectrum of clinical presentations. *Blood* **97**:81–88.

42. **Villard, J., B. Lisowska-Grospierre, P. van den Elsen, A. Fischer, W. Reith, and B. Mach.** 1997. Mutation of RFXAP, a regulator of MHC class II genes, in primary MHC class II deficiency. *N. Engl. J. Med.* **337**:748–753.

43. **Zhang, J., L. Quintal, A. Atkinson, B. Williams, E. Grunebaum, and C. M. Roifman.** 2005. Novel RAG1 mutation in a case of severe combined immunodeficiency. *Pediatrics* **116**:445–449.

Investigation of Signal Transduction Defects

MELISSA E. ELDER

100

Several forms of severe combined immunodeficiency syndrome (SCID) and other inherited T- and B-cell defects have been shown to result from mutations in signaling molecules required to transduce antigen receptor-binding events to intracellular biochemical pathways. Activation of these signaling pathways synergistically results in transcription of specific genes encoding lymphocyte functions such as cytolysis, cytokine secretion, isotype switching, cell differentiation, and proliferation. In the following discussion, antigen-receptor signal transduction pathways for both T cells and B cells are reviewed and methods to evaluate these pathways in children with inherited immune deficiencies are described.

T-CELL SIGNAL TRANSDUCTION PATHWAY

The T-cell receptor (TCR) is a multisubunit complex consisting of a disulfide-linked α/β heterodimer noncovalently associated with the CD3γ, -δ, and -ε chains and a ζζ homodimer (22, 24, 33). The polymorphic α/β chains are responsible for recognition of peptide bound to a self-major histocompatibility complex molecule; these chains lack signaling capability. In contrast, the ζ and CD3 proteins contain conserved immunoreceptor tyrosine-based activation motifs (ITAMs) within their extensive cytoplasmic domains that are able to transduce extracellular antigen-binding events to intracellular signaling pathways through associations with cytoplasmic protein tyrosine kinases (PTKs) (22, 24, 33). PTKs known to associate with ITAMs include the Src family kinases Lck and Fyn and the Syk family kinases ZAP-70 and Syk (22, 33). Activation of Lck and ZAP-70 is absolutely required for normal TCR signaling, lymphocyte development, and differentiation (5, 9, 18, 22, 24, 33). PTK activation is a rapid and critical event that leads to phosphorylation of numerous downstream molecules, including phospholipase C-γ1, the adaptor molecules LAT (linker of activated T cells) and SLP-76 (Src homology 2 domain-containing leukocyte protein of 76 kDa), and the Tec family of PTKs (22, 24, 25, 27, 34). These tyrosine phosphorylation reactions are required for mobilization of intracellular free calcium ($[Ca^{2+}]_i$) and activation of the Ras, mitogen-activated protein kinase (MAPK), and phosphatidylinositol-3 kinase pathways, and they culminate in T-cell activation and initiation of T-cell-specific responses (22, 25).

One of the best-characterized PTKs is Lck, which is associated with the cytoplasmic domains of CD4 and CD8 (5, 33).

Lck substrates include the ITAMs of ζ and CD3, as well as ZAP-70 (22, 24, 33). Recruitment of ZAP-70 to the TCR and its subsequent phosphorylation and activation largely by Lck are essential for all downstream signaling events (5, 9, 18, 22, 24). Activated ZAP-70 phosphorylates the adaptor molecules SLP-76 and LAT, thereby triggering distal pathways that bring about T-cell activation (22, 25, 33). Syk is a related PTK family member with structural homology to ZAP-70. Although essential for normal B-cell receptor (BCR) signaling, Syk is not essential for normal TCR signaling unless ZAP-70 is deficient.

The hematopoietic lineage-specific leukocyte common antigen, CD45, is a transmembrane protein tyrosine phosphatase that dephosphorylates Src family PTKs and is a positive regulator of Lck in TCR signal transduction (11, 22). CD45 is critical to both TCR and BCR signal transduction, and its deficiency results in SCID in humans characterized by few peripheral T cells but normal B-cell numbers (13, 29).

ZAP-70 Deficiency

ZAP-70 deficiency was the first described TCR-associated PTK defect in humans (2, 5, 9). It is a rare form of autosomal recessive SCID characterized by normal numbers of CD3+ T cells, abundant nonfunctional CD4+ T cells, and an absence of CD8+ T cells in the circulation. Most affected patients have mutations within the kinase domain of ZAP-70 that abrogate both protein expression and enzymatic function; however, mutations in other protein domains have been identified (2, 5, 9, 10, 16, 20, 31). The presence of peripheral CD4+ T cells in ZAP-70-deficient patients contrasts with their absence in ZAP-70 knockout mice, which are blocked at the CD4+ CD8+ stage of thymocyte differentiation (18).

The diagnosis of ZAP-70 deficiency is suggested by a clinical phenotype of SCID with normal numbers of CD3+ T cells and absent CD8+ T cells in the peripheral blood. Moreover, markedly defective T-cell proliferation in response to TCR-mediated stimuli (mitogens and alloantigen) in vitro is observed, in contrast to preserved proliferation in response to phorbol myristic acetate (PMA) plus ionomycin (10). Markedly defective cytoplasmic protein tyrosine phosphorylation and $[Ca^{2+}]_i$ mobilization after TCR stimulation are seen (10). However, immunoblot analysis of ZAP-70 protein and DNA sequencing are required to confirm inheritance of two mutant ZAP-70 alleles in patients with SCID characterized by a paucity of circulating CD8[+] T cells.

CD3 Deficiency

T-cell signaling abnormalities that are not associated with mutations in PTKs have also been identified in patients with SCID and primary T-cell immune deficiencies. These include abnormal cell surface expression of the TCR resulting from defects in the CD3 subunits ε, γ, and δ (6–8, 28). A diagnosis of CD3ε or -γ deficiency may be suggested by flow cytometry (fluorescence-activated cell sorter [FACS] analysis), since affected children have decreased numbers of peripheral T cells that weakly express TCRα/β and CD3. Mutations in CD3γ result in defective T-cell immunity, but affected patients do not require hematopoietic stem cell transplantation (1). The phenotype of CD3ε deficiency appears to be dependent on the level of residual CD3ε expression: an absence of CD3ε causes T[−] B[+] NK[+] SCID, while partial CD3ε expression results in decreased T-cell numbers but only mild immune deficiency (1, 7, 28). In contrast, defective CD3δ expression results in SCID characterized by complete arrest of thymocyte development prior to development of CD4[+] CD8[+] thymocytes (7). Like for other forms of SCID or T-cell immune deficiency, gene sequencing is required to confirm CD3 deficiency.

CD45 Deficiency

The hematopoietic lineage-specific protein tyrosine phosphatase, CD45, is a positive regulator of Src family PTKs involved in T- and B-cell antigen-receptor signaling, and Lck in particular (11, 22). Mutations that result in the absence of CD45 expression on leukocytes are associated with the development of T[−] B[+] NK[−] SCID (3, 13, 30). NK cells and CD3[+] T cells expressing an α/β TCR are markedly reduced in the peripheral blood of affected infants (3, 13, 30). In contrast, γ/δ T cells develop normally. Despite elevated numbers of circulating B cells, serum immunoglobulin levels decrease with age and antibody responses are defective.

Defects of the IL-2 Signaling Pathway

Mutations in the γ chain (γc) common to the receptors for interleukin 2 (IL-2), IL-4, IL-7, IL-9, IL-15, and IL-21 are found in boys with X-linked recessive SCID (SCID-X1) (3, 19, 26). Although not involved in antigen-receptor signaling, the γc molecule is essential for the intracellular transmission of cytokine signals and is required for T-cell development (21, 26). The absence of γc-containing cytokine receptor complexes results in early arrest of T- and NK-cell development and production of immature B cells that exhibit defective isotype switching (3, 19, 26). Approximately 45% of SCID cases in the United States are due to mutations in γc (3, 26).

Most SCID-X1 T cells fail to express CD132 (γc) as determined by flow cytometry. However, because most SCID-X1 families have unique mutations, sequencing of the coding regions of the *IL2RG* gene should be performed in order to confirm deleterious mutations (3, 26). Sequencing of maternal DNA can also be informative, but many boys with SCID-X1 have spontaneously arising mutations without evidence of an inherited mutant maternal X chromosome either by DNA sequencing or by nonrandom pattern of X chromosome inactivation (3, 8).

Females, as well as some males, with the typical SCID-X1 phenotype do not have mutations in γc. These patients instead have autosomal recessive SCID due to mutations in

the cytoplasmic tyrosine kinase JAK3 (3, 8, 14, 21). JAK3 activation is required for transduction of ligand-binding signals from γc-containing cytokine receptors, and its deficiency results in T[−] B[+] NK[−] SCID indistinguishable from SCID-X1 (3, 14, 21). In contrast, mutations in the α chain of the IL-7 receptor (IL-7Rα) arrest human thymocyte development at the CD4[−] CD8[−] stage but do not affect NK-cell development (3, 21). The T[−] B[+] NK[+] phenotype of IL-7Rα-deficient SCID emphasizes the critical and nonredundant role of IL-7 in T-cell development, differentiation, and survival (21). Most JAK3 and IL-7Rα mutations abolish mRNA or protein expression, and molecular methods are required to confirm these diagnoses (3, 21).

B-CELL SIGNAL TRANSDUCTION PATHWAY

The BCR is composed of a membrane immunoglobulin molecule noncovalently associated with a disulfide-linked heterodimer of immunoglobulin α and β chains (CD79) (12, 33). Similar to CD3, CD79 functions to transduce extracellular binding events to intracellular signaling pathways through binding of nonreceptor-associated PTKs, culminating in specific B-cell responses such as antibody production, isotype switching, cellular differentiation, and proliferation (12, 27, 33). Additional components of the BCR signaling complex include CD72, CD5, CD21/CD19/CD81, and the negatively regulated immunoreceptor tyrosine-based inhibitory motif-containing coreceptors FcγRIIb and CD22 (12, 33).

Similar to T-cell signaling, ligand engagement of the BCR is associated with rapid activation of Syk; the Src family PTKs Lyn, Fyn, Blk, and Lck; and the Tec family PTK Bruton's tyrosine kinase (Btk) (12, 33). Similar to TCR signal transduction, PTK activation results in phosphorylation of downstream cytoplasmic signaling molecules, which include phospholipase C-γ2, BLNK (B-cell linker protein), and Vav1 (12, 23, 27, 33). Phosphorylation of these downstream substrates results in [Ca^{2+}]$_i$ flux and activation of the Ras, MAPK, phosphatidylinositol-3 kinase, and NF-κB pathways, which are required for B-cell activation, development, and induction of B-cell effector functions (12, 27, 33).

Syk binds ITAMs within CD79 via its tandem Src homology 2 domains and is absolutely required for normal B-cell function (12, 27, 33). Btk is activated in response to BCR stimulation and is expressed in early B-lineage cells, but not in terminally differentiated plasma cells. Mutations in Btk result in abnormal B-cell differentiation and development of X-linked agammaglobulinemia (XLA) in humans (3, 32). BLNK (SLP-65) is an adaptor molecule similar to SLP-76 and LAT in T cells that is required for NF-κB activation and B-cell survival (29). Mutations in BLNK result in arrest of B-cell development and absence of B cells in the peripheral blood in affected humans (17, 23, 29).

XLA

In boys with XLA, mutations in Btk result in a nearly complete block in development at an early pre-B-cell stage (3, 32). Residual B-cell development can occur, but usually <2% B cells are detected in the peripheral blood. These B cells are unable to respond to BCR engagement. A diagnosis of XLA is suggested by the absence of peripheral B cells, but confirmation of diagnosis requires sequencing of the coding portions of the *XLA* gene. Immunoblot or FACS analysis of Btk expression is difficult when peripheral blood mononuclear cells (PBMC) are used, since the number of B cells is insufficient for protein assays. However, analysis of

Btk protein expression using bone marrow-derived pre-B cells or Epstein-Barr virus (EBV)-transformed lymphoblastoid lines is possible. Unfortunately, generation of EBV-transformed lines from Btk-deficient bone marrow is technically difficult and often unsuccessful.

BLNK Deficiency

Similar to XLA, mutations in BLNK result in an absence of peripheral B cells (3, 17, 23, 29). This diagnosis should be considered in females without detectable B cells or in boys with few B cells who do not have mutations in Btk. BLNK protein expression can be evaluated on marrow-derived EBV-transformed pre-B-cell lines, but DNA sequence analysis is required to make a diagnosis of BLNK deficiency.

METHODS

Flow Cytometry

FACS analysis for cell surface expression of the TCR or BCR, CD40L, CD69, and cytokine or coreceptor molecules is discussed in chapters 18 and 19 of this volume. Since CD69 expression is dependent on activation of the Ras/MAPK pathway, the absence of CD69 on stimulated T or B cells may suggest a proximal signal transduction defect (10). Moreover, intracellular cytokine expression using FACS analysis may be useful in characterizing the scope of T-cell defects.

TCL and BCL

Because insufficient numbers of lymphocytes are available from children with primary immune deficiencies, generation of cultured cell lines is useful as a source of DNA and RNA for molecular studies. T-cell lines (TCL) may be generated using human T-cell lymphotropic virus type 1 (HTLV-1) or herpesvirus saimiri (HVS) transformation, while B-cell lines (BCL) are generally produced by EBV transformation. Unfortunately, HTLV-1 and EBV may affect cell signaling (14); alterations in cellular function appear to be less problematic when HVS is used (4).

Lymphocyte Proliferative Assays

T-cell proliferation in response to PMA plus ionomycin in vitro may be used to screen for proximal signaling defects in patients with SCID or T-cell immune deficiencies in whom SCID-X1, enzyme abnormalities (such as adenosine deaminase deficiency), or defects in recombination (RAG-1/RAG-2 deficiency or Omenn syndrome) have been eliminated.

1. Suspend PBMC or peripheral blood T cells that have been positively selected using CD3$^+$ magnetic beads (Miltenyi Biotec, Auburn, Calif.) in complete RPMI medium (RPMI 1640 plus 10% fetal calf serum, 100 μg of penicillin per ml, 100 U of streptomycin per ml, and 2 mM L-glutamine) at a concentration of 10^6 cells/ml.

2. Incubate 10^5 cells in 200 μl of complete RPMI medium at 37°C for 72 h in flat-bottomed 96-well plates with 50 ng of anti-CD3 monoclonal antibody (MAb) (Caltag Laboratories, Burlingame, Calif.) per ml or 0.5 ng of PMA (Sigma-Aldrich, St. Louis, Mo.) per ml plus 1 μM ionomycin (Calbiochem, San Diego, Calif.).

3. Pulse wells with 0.96 μCi of [^{3}H]thymidine per well for 6 h, harvest, and count in a scintillation counter.

[Ca^{2+}]$_i$ Flux

If T-cell or B-cell proliferation in response to antigen receptor-mediated stimulation is not seen, measurements of [Ca^{2+}]$_i$ mobilization may be indicated in order to localize a putative signaling defect. [Ca^{2+}]$_i$ flux assays may be done either by fluorimetry or by FACS analysis. Fluorimetric methods require more cells but do not require concomitant cell staining with potentially stimulatory MAbs. This assay is best done using fresh PBMC, but bone marrow-derived lymphocytes, BCL, or TCL rested overnight in medium without IL-2 or mitogen may also be used.

1. Rest TCL in complete RPMI medium for 16 to 24 h before analysis.

2. Suspend PBMC or bone marrow-derived lymphocytes (preferably enriched for T or B cells via magnetic bead selection) or TCL or BCL at 2 × 10^7 cells/ml in complete RPMI medium and load with 3 μM Indo-1 (Molecular Probes Invitrogen, Eugene, Oreg.) for 20 min at 37°C. Dilute cell suspension to 2 × 10^6 cells/ml with complete RPMI medium and incubate for 20 min at 37°C.

3. Wash cells three times in calcium buffer (Hanks balanced salt solution plus 1% bovine serum albumin, 1 mM CaCl$_2$, and 0.5 mM MgCl$_2$), resuspend at 5 × 10^6 cells/ml in calcium buffer, and keep on ice until use.

4. Warm 400 μl of cell suspension at 37°C for 2 min in a cuvette before analysis. Measure absorbance at an excitation wavelength of 355 nm and emission wavelengths of 400 and 500 nm using a fluorescence spectrophotometer (Hitachi High Technologies America, San Jose, Calif.). Maximal fluorescence is determined after cell lysis with 5 μl of 10% Triton X-100 detergent; minimal fluorescence is determined after addition of 50 μl of 1 M Tris base and 15 μl of 0.4 M EGTA.

5. Recordings are made before and after cells are stimulated by the addition of TCR or BCR cross-linkers. For T-cell analysis, add 2 μl of biotinylated anti-CD3 MAb (BD Pharmingen, San Diego, Calif.) plus 5 μg of streptavidin (Sigma-Aldrich) per ml; immunoglobulin M (IgM) MAb to TCR may be used instead if available. For B-cell analysis, add 10 to 40 μg of anti-IgM F(ab')$_2$ antibody (Southern Biotechnology Associates, Birmingham, Ala.) per ml. To ensure proper loading of Indo-1, add 1 μl of 1 mM ionomycin to nonresponding cell suspensions after 5 min.

Protein Tyrosine Phosphorylation Assay

Analysis of tyrosine phosphoproteins is indicated if a defect in proximal antigen receptor signaling is suggested by defective lymphocyte proliferation or [Ca^{2+}]$_i$ mobilization in response to TCR stimulation. This method may also be used to evaluate BCR signaling in children with primary B-cell immune deficiencies, especially in patients of either sex who have severe hypogammaglobulinemia but normal numbers of peripheral B cells. Males without circulating B cells likely have XLA; methods to detect XLA are described in chapter 101 of this volume. However, rare patients without peripheral B cells have mutations in signaling molecules, such as BLNK, as described previously.

1. Incubate 100 μl of 2 × 10^6 TCL or CD3-enriched PBMC for 20 min on ice with 2 μl each of biotinylated anti-CD3 MAb plus biotinylated anti-CD4 MAb or phosphate-buffered saline alone. Wash cells, resuspend in 100 μl of phosphate-buffered saline, and cross-link with 5 μg of avidin per ml for 4 min at 37°C. For analysis of B-cell signaling events, 100 μl of 2 × 10^6 EBV-transformed BCL, CD2-depleted PBMC, or CD19-enriched PBMC or bone marrow cells may be stimulated with 10 to 40 μg of anti-IgM F(ab')$_2$ antibody per ml.

2. Lyse cells in 45 μl of Nonidet P-40 (NP-40) buffer (1% NP-40 plus 10 mM Tris) [pH 7.6], 150 mM NaCl, 0.5 mM

EDTA, 10 mM NaF, 1 mM phenylmethylsulfonyl fluoride, 1 μg of pepstatin A per ml, 10 μg of leupeptin per ml, 1 μg of aprotinin per ml, and 1 mM Na$_3$VO$_4$) for 30 min at 4°C. Centrifuge cells at 12,000 × g at 4°C for 10 min, collect supernatants, and mix with 15 μl of 4× sample buffer dye (2% sodium dodecyl sulfate [SDS], 5% 2-mercaptoethanol, 250 mM Tris, 10% glycerol, and 1 mg of bromophenol blue per ml, pH 6.8). Boil at 90°C for 5 min prior to separation by SDS–12% polyacrylamide gel electrophoresis under reducing conditions.

3. Electrophoretically transfer separated protein bands to Immobilon-P membranes (Millipore Corporation, Billerica, Mass.), block in blotting buffer (Tris-buffered saline plus 0.1% Tween) plus 3% bovine serum albumin, and incubate at room temperature for 1 h in blotting buffer with 4G10 (antiphosphotyrosine MAb; Upstate Biotechnology, Waltham, Mass.).

4. Wash filters three times in blotting buffer, and incubate with horseradish peroxidase-conjugated goat anti-mouse MAb (Southern Biotechnology Associates) for 1 h at room temperature. Phosphoproteins are assayed using an enhanced chemiluminescence detection system (ECL; Amersham Biosciences, Piscataway, N.J.).

Immunoblot Analysis

If abnormal protein tyrosine phosphorylation is demonstrated, the expression of specific PTKs known to be involved in T- or B-cell signal transduction may be evaluated by immunoblotting using PBMC, T- or B-cell-enriched PBMC or cultured lines, or marrow-derived lymphocytes. For analysis of specific PTKs or other signaling proteins, separate PBMC, TCL, or BCL extracts by SDS-polyacrylamide gel electrophoresis as described above and analyze for protein expression using the enhanced chemiluminescence system.

IL-2 Production

Distal TCR signal transduction events, as well as the IL-2 pathway, may be analyzed by measurement of IL-2 production in response to TCR-mediated stimuli. Abnormal IL-2 production may lead to evaluation of other molecules that are beyond the scope of this chapter. Analysis of IL-2 production is performed as follows. Stimulate 2 × 10^5 PBMC in complete RPMI medium with 50 ng of anti-CD3 per ml plus 0.5 to 5 μg of anti-CD28 MAb (BD Biosciences) per ml or 0.5 ng of PMA per ml plus 1 mM ionomycin at 37°C for 24 h in flat-bottomed 96-well plates. Collect supernatants and quantitate IL-2 levels using standardized immunoassay kits (BioSource International, Camarillo, Calif.).

ANALYTICAL SENSITIVITY AND SPECIFICITY, QUALITY CONTROL AND ASSURANCE, DATA ANALYSIS, PITFALLS, AND TROUBLESHOOTING

In vitro T-cell proliferative studies are useful in the screening of immunodeficient patients for proximal signal transduction defects. Restoration of T-cell proliferation by PMA and ionomycin indicates a possible defect in a TCR-associated PTK; lack of stimulation by these second messengers suggests a defect in a T-cell signaling event distal to activation of Ras and [Ca^{2+}]$_i$ flux, respectively. Results of proliferative assays for patients must be compared to those for healthy individuals of similar age. Immunoblot and kinase assays may be informative in documenting PTK defects, but they

may be adversely affected by viability and quantity of cells available for study and specificity of antibodies used. Protease inhibitors and sodium orthovanadate must be included in the protein lysis buffer in order to control inadvertent protein degradation and phosphatase activity. Therefore, protein techniques require controls in order to assess the quality of the results. [Ca^{2+}]$_i$ assays may be affected by temperature and improper loading of the calcium-sensitive dye; nonresponding cells should be incubated with ionomycin to ensure that cells were properly loaded. Finally, TCL and BCL may be the only source of patient cells; therefore, analysis of signal transduction defects using transformed lines may be complicated by the effects of HTLV-1 and EBV, and possibly HVS, on lymphocyte signaling pathways.

INTERPRETATION

The described methods are valuable both to screen and to diagnose signaling defects in patients with inherited T- or B-cell immune deficiencies. However, inherited immune defects, other than those characterized as XLA, X-linked hyper-IgM syndrome, SCID-X1, and adenosine deaminase deficiency, are very rare, occurring in fewer than 1 in 10^6 children.

REMARKS AND CONCLUSIONS

Signaling pathways resulting in abnormal T- or B-cell activation and development of immune deficiency are the focus of much investigation at present. Although better understood, the roles of Tec family PTKs, adaptor molecules, and downstream signaling proteins in lymphocyte activation in humans remain to be well characterized. Knockouts or mutations in many signaling molecules have been evaluated in inbred-mouse models but have not been diagnosed in immunodeficient humans. This likely is due to the limited quantities of patient cells available for analysis and current management techniques that lead to fairly rapid stem cell transplantation prior to genetic diagnosis.

REFERENCES

1. **Arnaiz-Villena, A., M. Timon, A. Corell, P. Perez-Aciego, J. M. Martin-Villa, and J. R. Regueiro.** 1992. Primary immunodeficiency caused by mutations in the gene encoding the CD3-γ subunit of the T-lymphocyte receptor. *N. Engl. J. Med.* **327:**529–533.
2. **Arpaia, E., M. Shahar, H. Dadi, A. Cohen, and C. M. Roifman.** 1994. Defective T cell receptor signaling and CD8$^+$ thymic selection in humans lacking ZAP-70 kinase. *Cell* **76:**947–958.
3. **Buckley, R. H.** 2004. Molecular defects in human severe combined immunodeficiency and approaches to immune reconstitution. *Annu. Rev. Immunol.* **22:**625–655.
4. **Cabanillas, J. A., R. Cambronero, A. Pacheco-Castro, M. C. Garcia-Rodriguez, J. M. Martin-Fernandez, G. Fontan, and J. R. Regueiro.** 2002. Characterization of Herpesvirus saimiri-transformed T lymphocytes from common variable immunodeficiency patients. *Clin. Exp. Immunol.* **127:**366–373.
5. **Chan, A. C., T. A. Kadlecek, M. E. Elder, A. H. Filipovich, W.-L. Kuo, M. Iwashima, T. G. Parslow, and A. Weiss.** 1994. ZAP-70 deficiency in an autosomal recessive form of severe combined immunodeficiency. *Science* **264:**1599–1601.
6. **Dadi, H. K., A. J. Simon, and C. M. Roifman.** 2003. Effect of CD3δ deficiency on maturation of α/β and γ/δ

T cell lineages in severe combined immunodeficiency. *N. Engl. J. Med.* **349:**1821–1828.

7. de Saint Basile, G., F. Geissmann, E. Flori, B. Lambert, C. Soudais, M. Cavazzana-Colvo, A. Durandy, N. Jabado, A. Fischer, and F. Le Diest. 2004. Severe combined immunodeficiency caused by deficiency in either the δ or the ε subunit of CD3. *J. Clin. Investig.* **114:**1512–1517.

8. Elder, M. E. 2000. T-cell immunodeficiencies. *Pediatr. Clin. N. Am.* **47:**1253–1274.

9. Elder, M. E., D. Lin, J. Clever, A. C. Chan, T. J. Hope, A. Weiss, and T. G. Parslow. 1994. Human severe combined immunodeficiency due to a defect in ZAP-70, a T cell tyrosine kinase. *Science* **264:**1596–1599.

10. Elder, M. E., S. Skoda-Smith, T. A. Kadlecek, F. L. Wang, J. Wu, and A. Weiss. 2001. Distinct T cell developmental consequences in humans and mice expressing identical mutations in the DLAARN motif of ZAP-70. *J. Immunol.* **166:**656–661.

11. Hermiston, M. L., Z. Xu, and A. Weiss. 2003. CD45: a critical regulator of signaling thresholds in immune cells. *Annu. Rev. Immunol.* **21:**107–137.

12. Kelly, M. E., and A. C. Chan. 2000. Regulation of B cell function by linker proteins. *Curr. Opin. Immunol.* **12:**267–275.

13. Kung, C., J. T. Pingel, M. Heikinheimo, T. Klemola, K. Varkila, L. I. Yoo, K. Vuopala, M. Poyhonen, M. Uhari, M. Rogers, S. H. Speck, T. Chatila, and M. L. Thomas. 2000. Mutations in the tyrosine phosphatase CD45 gene in a child with severe combined immunodeficiency. *Nat. Med.* **6:**343–345.

14. Levitsky, V., and M. G. Masucci. 2002. Manipulation of immune responses by Epstein-Barr virus. *Virus Res.* **88:**71–86.

15. Macchi, P., A. Villa, S. Gillani, M. G. Sacco, A. Frattini, F. Porta, A. G. Ugazio, J. A. Johnston, F. Candotti, J. J. O'Shea, P. Vezzoni, and L. D. Notarangelo. 1995. Mutations of Jak-3 gene in patients with autosomal severe combined immune deficiency (SCID). *Nature* **377:**65–68.

16. Matsuda, S., T. Suzuki-Fujimoto, A. Minowa, H. Ueno, K. Katamura, and S. Koyasu. 1999. Temperature-sensitive ZAP70 mutants degrading through a proteasome-independent pathway. *J. Biol. Chem.* **274:**34515–34518.

17. Minegishi, Y., J. Rohrer, E. Coustan-Smith, H. M. Lederman, R. Pappu, D. Campana, A. C. Chan, and M. E. Conley. 1999. An essential role for BLNK in human B cell development. *Science* **286:**1954–1957.

18. Negishi, I., N. Motoyama, K.-I. Nakayama, K. Nakayama, S. Senju, S. Hatakeyama, Q. Zhang, A. C. Chan, and D. Y. Loh. 1995. Essential role for ZAP-70 in both positive and negative selection of thymocytes. *Nature* **376:**435–438.

19. Noguchi, M., H. Yi, H. M. Rosenblatt, A. H. Filipovich, S. Adelstein, W. S. Modi, O. W. McBride, and W. J. Leonard. 1993. Interleukin-2 receptor γ chain mutation results in X-linked severe combined immunodeficiency in humans. *Cell* **73:**147–157.

20. Noraz, N., K. Schwarz, M. Steinberg, V. Dardalhon, C. Rebouissou, R. Hipskind, W. Friedrich, H. Yssel, K. Bacon, and N. Taylor. 2000. Alternative antigen receptor (TCR) signaling in T cells derived from ZAP-70-deficient patients expressing high levels of Syk. *J. Biol. Chem.* **275:**15832–15838.

21. O'Shea, J. J., M. Husa, D. Li, S. R. Hofmann, W. Watford, J. L. Roberts, R. H. Buckley, P. Changelian, and F. Candotti. 2004. Jak3 and the pathogenesis of severe combined immunodeficiency. *Mol. Immunol.* **41:**727–737.

22. Palacios, E. H., and A. Weiss. 2004. Function of the Src-family kinases, Lck and Fyn, in T-cell development and activation. *Oncogene* **23:**7990–8000.

23. Pappu, R., A. M. Cheng, B. Li, Q. Gong, C. Chiu, N. Griffin, M. White, B. P. Sleckman, and A. C. Chan. 1999. Requirement for B cell linker protein (BLNK) in B cell development. *Science* **286:**1949–1954.

24. Qian, D., and A. Weiss. 1997. T cell antigen receptor signal transduction. *Curr. Opin. Cell Biol.* **9:**205–212.

25. Rudd, C. E. 1999. Adaptors and molecular scaffolds in immune cell signaling. *Cell* **96:**5–8.

26. Schmalstieg, F. C., and A. S. Goldman. 2002. Immune consequences of mutations in the human common γ-chain gene. *Mol. Genet. Metab.* **76:**163–171.

27. Sieomi, L., S. Kliche, J. Lindquist, and B. Schraven. 2004. Adaptors and linkers in T and B cells. *Curr. Opin. Immunol.* **16:**304–313.

28. Soudais, C., J. P. Villartay, F. Le Diest, A. Fischer, and B. Lisowska-Grospierre. 1993. Independent mutations of the human CD3-ε gene resulting in a T cell receptor/CD3 complex immunodeficiency. *Nat. Genet.* **3:**77–81.

29. Tan, J. E., S. C. Wong, S. K. Gan, S. Xu, and K. P. Lam. 2001. The adaptor protein BLNK is required for B-cell antigen receptor-induced activation of NF-κB and cell cycle entry and survival of B lymphocytes. *J. Biol. Chem.* **276:**20055–20063.

30. Tchilian, E. Z., D. L. Wallace, R. S. Wells, D. R. Flower, G. Morgan, and P. C. Beverley. 2001. A deletion in the gene encoding the CD45 antigen in a patient with SCID. *J. Immunol.* **166:**1308–1313.

31. Toyabe, S.-I., A. Watanabe, W. Harada, T. Karasawa, and M. Uchiyama. 2001. Specific immunoglobulin E responses in ZAP-70-deficient patients are mediated by Syk-dependent T-cell receptor signaling. *Immunology* **103:**164–171.

32. Tsukada, S., D. C. Saffran, D. J. Rawlings, O. Parolini, R. C. Allen, I. Klisak, R. S. Sparkes, H. Kubagawa, T. Mohandas, S. Quan, J. W. Belmont, M. D. Cooper, M. E. Conley, and O. N. Witte. 1993. Deficient expression of a B cell cytoplasmic tyrosine kinase in human X-linked agammaglobulinemia. *Cell* **72:**279–290.

33. Weiss, A., and A. L. DeFranco. 1999. Signal transduction by T and B lymphocyte antigen receptors, p. 66–81. *In* H. D. Ochs, C. I. E. Smith, and J. M. Puck (ed.), *Primary Immunodeficiency Diseases: a Molecular and Genetic Approach.* Oxford University Press, New York, N.Y.

34. Zhang, W., J. Sloan-Lancaster, J. Kitchen, R. P. Trible, and L. E. Samelson. 1998. LAT: the ZAP-70 tyrosine kinase substrate that links T cell receptor to cellular activation. *Cell* **92:**83–92.

Primary Antibody Deficiency Diseases

MARY ELLEN CONLEY

101

Antibody deficiencies are a heterogeneous group of disorders that share an unusual susceptibility to recurrent or persistent infections with encapsulated bacteria, particularly *Streptococcus pneumoniae* and *Haemophilus influenzae*. The types of infections seen in affected patients are ones that are typical for these organisms. Young children with antibody deficiencies usually have a cough, recurrent otitis, and purulent nasal discharge (5). Adults are likely to have a cough, sinusitis, and recurrent pneumonias (7). Dramatic infections, like meningitis, cellulitis, empyema, or epiglottitis, are not uncommon and are often the findings that lead to an evaluation of the immune system. Additional types of infections or medical complications are more specific to particular antibody deficiencies. For example, approximately 50% of patients with X-linked hyper-immunoglobulin M (hyper-IgM) syndrome (CD40 ligand deficiency) have *Pneumocystis jiroveci* (formerly called *Pneumocystis carinii*) pneumonia in the first year of life (37). *Pneumocystis* pneumonia is seen in other antibody deficiencies, but it is quite rare.

Although all patients with antibody deficiencies are treated with gamma globulin replacement, a specific diagnosis permits a better understanding of potential complications, a more accurate prediction of prognosis, and more informative genetic counseling. Several of the antibody deficiencies that present in early childhood are inherited in an X-linked manner. These disorders, which include X-linked agammaglobulinemia (XLA) (Btk deficiency), X-linked hyper-IgM syndrome (CD40 ligand deficiency), ectodermal dysplasia with immunodeficiency (NEMO deficiency), X-linked severe combined immunodeficiency (cytokine common gamma chain deficiency), and X-linked lymphoproliferative syndrome (SAP deficiency), are seen almost exclusively in males. It is essential to take a detailed family history that goes back at least three generations in the maternal lineage; however, it is important to remember that only about 50% of affected males have a positive family history of disease. This is because these disorders are maintained in the population by new mutations.

In recent years several rare autosomal recessive disorders that result in antibody deficiency have been reported. These disorders, which include defects in μ heavy chain (18), CD79 (20), λ5 (part of the surrogate light chain) (21), BLNK (23), CD40 (9), activation-induced cytidine deaminase (AID) (31), uracil DNA glycolase (UNG), ICOS (12), CD19, TACI, and BAFF receptor, are more likely to occur in consanguineous or isolated populations. In taking a family history, it is useful to know if grandparents or great-grandparents came from the same small village. Most patients are homozygous for their mutations, and most mutations are relatively specific to particular geographic regions. For example, in North America AID deficiency is more common in Lumbee Indians from North Carolina and French Canadians from eastern Quebec (22).

IgA deficiency and common variable immunodeficiency (CVID) are usually considered multifactorial disorders (7). That is, they are not inherited in a simple Mendelian pattern; instead, multiple susceptibility genes and environmental factors combine to cause disease. Affected patients may have a family history of autoimmune disease or abnormalities of immunoglobulin production, but the pattern of inheritance usually does not conform to an autosomal recessive or dominant pattern. CVID should be considered a diagnosis of exclusion. Particularly in young children, it is important to rule out single gene defects of the immune system. Occasionally, adults present with delayed recognition of single gene defects that are more commonly diagnosed in childhood.

Some antibody deficiencies are part of a more broadly expressed systemic disorder or part of an immunodeficiency that affects T cells and/or NK cells as well as B cells. For example, patients with ataxia telangiectasia often have IgA, IgE, and IgG2 deficiency (25). These patients may present for medical attention with recurrent infections and mild cerebral palsy. Patients with severe combined immunodeficiency may have infections that suggest antibody deficiency, but the T-cell deficiency must be recognized to institute appropriate therapy. Defects in activation markers expressed on T cells, for example, CD40 ligand or ICOS, result in antibody deficiency, although, strictly speaking, the B-cell lineage is normal.

AN APPROACH TO EVALUATION OF PATIENTS WITH SUSPECTED ANTIBODY DEFICIENCY

The possibility of immunodeficiency should be considered in any patient who is hospitalized for a major infection requiring intravenous therapy. This does not mean that laboratory studies should be performed for every patient, but a careful family history should be taken and a record of the number and nature of past infections should be obtained. If the infection results in admission to an intensive care unit or the history is suggestive of immunodeficiency (for example, a relative died of infection or the patient has received multiple courses of antibiotics), a complete blood count with differential, quantitative serum IgG, IgM, and IgA, and total hemolytic complement should be performed. Further evaluation depends on the type of infection seen in the patient and the index of suspicion. If the infection strongly suggests an antibody deficiency, for example, *H. influenzae* epiglottitis in an immunized patient, or if the screening evaluation demonstrates low serum IgM or IgG, titers of antibody to vaccine antigens should be obtained. It is useful to test for antibodies to both T-cell-independent antigens, like antiblood group substances (isohemagglutinins) and antipneumococcal antibodies, and T-cell-dependent antigens, like anti-tetanus toxoid or anti-measles virus antibodies. Patients who have low serum immunoglobulins and poor titers of antibody to vaccine antigens should be analyzed for lymphocyte cell surface markers to determine the number and percentage of T cells and B cells.

Dramatic infections frequently elicit an evaluation of the immune system. Patients with repeated infections who are treated on an outpatient basis may not be evaluated for immunodeficiency for many, many years, and these patients may develop bronchiectasis before they are recognized to have an antibody deficiency. Children, particularly boys, who have had 10 or more courses of antibiotics for otitis, sinusitis, or pneumonia in a 2-year period should have serum immunoglobulins measured. The same is true for adults, males or females, who have had five or more courses of antibiotics in a 2-year period.

Most patients with antibody deficiencies have very low concentrations of serum IgG and IgA (less than 10% of normal adult values). The IgM level is more variable. If an individual has concentrations of serum immunoglobulins that fall just below the normal range, it is important to measure titers of antibody to vaccine antigens. Some patients with low normal concentrations of serum immunoglobulins make antibodies to some, but not all, pneumococcal serotypes. It is often difficult to know how to interpret these results. Most investigators feel that these patients may respond to chronic prophylactic antibiotics and good medical follow-up. For the purposes of this discussion, patients with antibody deficiencies are divided into those with defects in early B-cell development, that is, patients with less than 2% B cells in the peripheral circulation, and those with late defects in B-cell development, i.e., patients with more than 2% B cells in the blood.

DEFECTS IN EARLY B-CELL DEVELOPMENT

XLA

XLA accounts for approximately 85% of patients with defects in early B-cell development (6). Most patients with XLA develop recurrent or persistent infections in the first 4 to 8 months of life, and the majority are recognized to have immunodeficiency at less than 3 years of age (5). Almost all patients have recurrent otitis, many have pneumonias, and some have sepsis, meningitis, arthritis, or cellulitis. Pyoderma, neutropenia, and pseudomonas or staphylococcal disease may be seen at presentation but are rarely seen after gamma globulin replacement therapy is started. In addition to their susceptibility to encapsulated bacteria, patients with XLA are also vulnerable to giardia (17), mycoplasma (10), and enteroviral (19) infections, including vaccine-associated

polio. Currently, patients are treated with gamma globulin replacement and aggressive use of antibiotics.

The protein responsible for XLA, Btk, is a cytoplasmic tyrosine kinase encoded in 19 exons spread over 37 kb in the mid-portion of the long arm of the X chromosome (34). Btk is expressed in all hematopoietic cells except T cells and plasma cells, but the consequences of Btk deficiency are limited to the B-cell lineage. Cross-linking of the pre-B-cell or B-cell antigen receptor results in phosphorylation and activation of Btk. In turn, Btk phosphorylates the lipid kinase phospholipase-Cγ2; this results in a sustained calcium flux, cell proliferation, and differentiation (29). In patients with XLA, B-cell differentiation is blocked at the pro-B-cell to pre-B-cell transition, the stage at which the pre-B-cell receptor is first expressed. However, the block is leaky, and almost all patients with XLA do have a small number of pre-B-cells in the bone marrow and B cells in the peripheral circulation.

Laboratory studies for the majority of patients with XLA reveal very low concentrations of serum IgM, IgG, IgA, and IgE, but most patients do have some serum IgG and approximately 10% of patients have a serum IgG or IgM concentration that is normal or near normal (28). The IgM falls to low levels after gamma globulin therapy is started. With very rare exceptions, titers of antibody to all vaccine antigens are negative. The most consistent laboratory feature in patients with XLA is the marked reduction in the number of B cells in the peripheral circulation. The threshold for detection for B cells in most clinical laboratories is 1%. Patients who have less than 1% B cells are reported as having 0%. The mean percentage of B cells in patients with XLA is 0.1% (3), and I have not seen any patients with XLA (over 200 evaluated) who had more than 1.5% CD19$^+$ cells. The B cells that are present have a distinctive phenotype with very high intensity expression of surface IgM and variable expression of CD19 (see below). Bone marrow studies demonstrate normal numbers of CD34$^+$ CD19$^+$ surface IgM$^-$ (sIgM$^-$) pro-B cells but very few CD34$^-$ CD19$^+$ sIgM$^-$ pre-B cells (24). Because Btk is expressed in platelets and myeloid cells, as well as B-lineage cells, immunofluorescence studies which evaluate Btk in monocytes or platelets or Western blot studies are useful screening tests (11); however, the reagents to perform these tests reliably are not commercially available. Further, 10 to 15% of patients with XLA have mutations in Btk that result in normal amounts of Btk protein in these cells. Definitive diagnosis of XLA requires mutation detection. The mutations in Btk are highly variable, and no single mutation accounts for more than 3% of all mutations (4). Over 90% of mutations in Btk are single base pair substitutions or the insertion or deletion of less than 10 bp within the coding sequence or flanking splice sites. These mutations are easily detected by single-strand conformation polymorphism (SSCP) analysis.

Autosomal Recessive Agammaglobulinemia

Approximately 7 to 10% of patients with early onset of infections, profound hypogammaglobulinemia, and an absence of B cells are girls. One must assume that there is an equal number of boys with disease that is not X linked. The clinical presentation of these patients is identical to that seen in patients with XLA; however, as a group, these patients tend to have more severe complications, and they are recognized to have immunodeficiency at a younger age (less than 2 years of age).

Defects in μ heavy chain account for about one-third of the patients with autosomal recessive agammaglobulinemia (18). These patients do not have a leaky defect, and their serum immunoglobulins are generally below the level of detection in clinical laboratories. If the laboratory reports detectable concentrations of serum immunoglobulins in these patients, it is because the laboratory has difficulty measuring very low concentrations, not because the patient is making serum immunoglobulins. Bone marrow studies show normal numbers of pro-B cells but no pre-B cells. Two types of mutations account for half of the pathological alterations in the μ heavy-chain gene. These are large deletions that remove all of the μ constant region as well as the D and J genes and a recurrent single base pair substitution at the alternative splice site in exon 4 of the constant-region gene (18). A PCR-based test for these mutations is described below.

Mutations in other components of the B-cell and pre-B-cell signaling pathway can also cause autosomal recessive agammaglobulinemia. Small numbers of patients with defects in Igα (CD79a), Igβ (CD79b), λ5, and BLNK have been seen. The clinical and laboratory findings in these patients are indistinguishable from those in patients with mutations in Btk or μ heavy chain. The bone marrow in these patients demonstrates a complete block at the pro-B-cell to pre-B-cell transition, and patients have normal numbers of pro-B cells but less than 10% of the normal number of pre-B cells. The most efficient way to make the diagnosis in patients with these rare autosomal recessive disorders is mutation detection.

Differential Diagnosis

There are patients with less than 2% circulating B cells who do not have defects in one of the genes listed above. Several groups have described patients with intrauterine growth retardation and/or microcephaly who have agammaglobulinemia and an absence of B cells (1, 30, 35). The causative defects in these patients are unknown. Some children with myelodysplasia come to medical attention because of recurrent infections and an absence of B cells. Bone marrow studies for these patients show markedly reduced numbers of pro-B cells as well as pre-B-cells (33). A small percentage of adults with late onset of recurrent infections and clinical and laboratory features consistent with CVID do not have B cells and do not have defects in one of the known genes associated with defects in early B-cell development (7). Some patients with Good's syndrome, that is, thymoma with immunodeficiency, have less than 2% B cells in the peripheral circulation. These patients also have decreased numbers of pro-B cells as well as pre-B cells.

LATE DEFECTS IN B-CELL DEVELOPMENT

X-Linked Hyper-IgM Syndrome (CD40 Ligand Deficiency)

Hyper-IgM syndrome is a term used to describe a group of disorders characterized by normal or elevated serum IgM with low concentrations of IgG and IgA and normal numbers of B cells. Approximately 60% of patients with early onset of infections and the laboratory features of hyper-IgM syndrome have defects in CD40 ligand (16), a member of the tumor necrosis factor family encoded in five exons on the long arm of the X chromosome. CD40 ligand is expressed transiently on the surface of activated T cells, particularly CD4+ T cells. Its cognate receptor, CD40, is expressed on B cells, monocytes, and dendritic cells. Activated endothelial and epithelial cells may also express CD40. Stimulation of B cells through CD40 results in cell

activation, short- and long-term cell proliferation, and, in the presence of cytokines, isotype switching. Cross-linking of CD40 on monocytes and dendritic cells results in cell activation and production of multiple cytokines, particularly interleukin 12. The cytokines feed back to T cells and further enhance T-cell activation.

The clinical spectrum of disease in patients with CD40 ligand deficiency is very broad. As noted above, many patients present with *Pneumocystis* pneumonia in the first year of life. Neutropenia, oral ulcers, and severe diarrhea are common in these patients. In addition to the increased susceptibility to encapsulated bacteria, patients with CD40 ligand deficiency are more vulnerable to cytomegalovirus, *Cryptococcus*, and *Cryptosporidium* infection and histoplasmosis. Carcinomas affecting the liver, pancreas, biliary tree, and associated neuroectodermal endocrine cells have been reported, particularly for patients with chronic gastrointestinal infections (13). Rare patients are relatively asymptomatic until they develop persistent anemia secondary to parvovirus B19 infection as young adults.

Flow cytometric analysis of activated T cells can be used as a screening evaluation to diagnose CD40 ligand deficiency; however, this assay has several drawbacks. T cells must be activated before analysis, and a control for T-cell activation, for example, CD69 or CD25, should be used. Some mutations in CD40 ligand permit normal cell surface expression of CD40 ligand; therefore, the presence of CD40 ligand on the cell surface does not rule out the diagnosis. Because the gene for CD40 ligand is small, mutation detection is often an easier and more definitive method of making the diagnosis of CD40 ligand deficiency.

Autosomal Recessive Hyper-IgM Syndrome

A small number of patients with mutations in CD40 have been reported (9). These patients have a clinical phenotype that is identical to that seen in patients with defects in CD40 ligand. Thus far, all of the reported patients have had mutations in CD40 that result in a failure to express CD40 on the cell surface. As a result, cell surface staining of B cells is a good first step in evaluating a patient suspected of having defects. If the index of suspicion is high, mutation detection might be appropriate even if staining for CD40 was normal. The gene for CD40 is encoded in nine exons on chromosome 20q13.2.

Two additional autosomal recessive forms of hyper-IgM syndrome have been identified. AID (31) and UNG (14) are required for normal isotype switching and somatic hypermutation. B cells activated with CD40 ligand and cytokines, in the context of the germinal center, transiently express the enzyme AID, which deaminates cytidine at target sites within the immunoglobulin variable-region genes and switch regions. The resulting uracil is then removed by UNG, leaving the site vulnerable to cleavage or mismatched repair.

Patients with defects in AID or UNG have a disease that is less severe than that seen in most patients with defects in CD40 ligand or CD40. Like all patients with antibody deficiencies, patients with defects in AID or UNG have recurrent upper and lower respiratory tract infections. Many have lymphoid hyperplasia, and patients with AID deficiency have increased incidences of autoimmune or inflammatory disorders. However, patients with AID or UNG deficiency do not have the opportunistic infections seen in patients who are deficient in CD40 and CD40 ligand, and their antibody deficiency is not as severe as that seen in patients with XLA or other defects in early B-cell development. The genes for both AID and UNG are relatively small; the AID gene consists of five exons spanning 11 kb on chromosome 12p13, and the UNG gene consists of seven exons spanning 13 kb on chromosome 12q23. Mutation detection is the most practical way of making a definitive diagnosis.

Differential Diagnosis of Hyper-IgM Syndrome

Some adults with CVID have normal or mildly elevated concentrations of serum IgM with low concentrations of serum IgG and IgA. If these individuals did not have recurrent infections as children, it is unlikely that they have defects in the genes listed above. Males with mutations in the X chromosome encoded gene for NEMO (NF-κB essential modulator) may have elevated IgM with low IgG and IgA levels (8). These patients generally have mild ectodermal dysplasia, with sparse hair, conical incisors, and inadequate sweating. Response to encapsulated bacterial infection is particularly poor in patients with defects in NEMO, and these patients may continue to have problems with infection even after gamma globulin replacement is initiated.

CVID

CVID is a term used to describe patients with low concentrations of serum immunoglobulins, particularly IgG and IgA, poor antibody response to vaccine antigens, and no known cause of immunodeficiency (7). It should be considered a diagnosis of exclusion. Low concentrations of serum immunoglobulins may be seen after the use of certain drugs or in association with leukemia or lymphoma. As noted above, single gene defects of the immune system may have features in common with CVID. One should be particularly cautious in giving the diagnosis of CVID to a child with the onset of symptoms at less than 10 years of age, siblings who appear to have CVID, or debilitated patients with immunodeficiency.

The typical patient with CVID has the onset of disease in the second, third, or fourth decade of life. Most patients have had several pneumonias before they are recognized to have immunodeficiency. Autoimmune or inflammatory disorders, particularly autoimmune thrombocytopenia, hemolytic anemia, inflammatory bowel disease, and arthritis, are seen in 20 to 30% of patients and may precede the onset of recurrent infections. Laboratory studies in patients with CVID are quite variable. T cells may be abnormal in number or function, and there may be a reversal of the normal CD4/CD8 ratio. Proliferation in response to mitogens may be decreased. Although the majority of patients with CVID have normal numbers and percentages of B cells, approximately 10% have less than 2% CD19+ B cells.

Recent studies suggest that analysis of B-cell phenotype may be useful in identifying patients with CVID who have more severe disease. In the healthy individual, 10 to 40% of CD19+ cells express the memory marker CD27. The CD27-positive cells can be divided into IgM memory cells which express CD27, IgD, and IgM and "switch memory B cells" which express CD27 but not IgD or IgM. Patients lacking switch memory B cells tend to have lower concentrations of serum immunoglobulins and a higher incidence of lymphadenopathy and splenomegaly (2, 15, 27, 36).

METHODS

Flow Cytometry

Either whole blood or density gradient-separated mononuclear cells can be used to examine lymphocyte cell surface markers. Blood that has been anticoagulated with heparin or EDTA can be used for up to 24 h after the blood has been drawn. Most laboratories use directly labeled monoclonal antibodies to CD19 or CD20 to assess the percentage of B cells in the peripheral circulation. Either marker is satisfactory. To examine memory B cells, cells are stained with antibodies to CD19, surface IgD, and CD27. Directly labeled polyclonal goat antibodies to surface IgD are used. Isotype controls are essential. To decrease background staining, it is helpful to add unlabeled rabbit IgG. The principles of cell surface staining are the same for all staining reagents. B-cell staining in patients with possible XLA is used as an example.

Materials and Reagents

5-ml snap-top tubes (no. 352052; Falcon)

Staining buffer: phosphate-buffered saline with 0.2% sodium azide and 0.2% bovine serum albumin

Fix buffer: phosphate-buffered saline with 0.5% paraformaldehyde (make fresh at least every 2 weeks and filter before use)

Phycoerythrin (PE) CD19 (no. 349209; BD Pharmingen)

Fluorescein isothiocyanate (FITC)–goat anti-human IgM (no. 2020-02; Southern Biotech)

FITC-CD3 (no. 349201; BD Pharmingen)

Rabbit IgG (for blocking) (no. 090310; DAKO)

Isotype controls: PE-mouse IgG1 (no. 349043; BD Pharmingen), FITC-mouse IgG1 (no. 349041; BD Pharmingen), and FITC-goat IgG (no. 0109-02; Southern Biotech)

At least 3×10^6 cells from a control and the patient

Procedure

1. Resuspend cells to a concentration of $10^6/100$ μl.
2. Place 50 μl of cells from the control and the patient into each of five tubes on ice.
3. Add 50 μl of rabbit IgG to each tube. Vortex gently.
4. Add staining reagents in a volume of less than 50 μl. The reagents listed below are used neat except for the FITC–goat anti-human IgM and its isotype control (goat IgG), which are used at a 1:40 dilution. For consistent staining, always add the antibodies in the same order.

> Tube 1: 40 μl of staining buffer (no stain control)
> Tube 2: 20 μl each of FITC-mouse IgG1 and PE-mouse IgG1 (isotype controls for tube 4)
> Tube 3: 20 μl each of FITC-goat IgG and PE-mouse IgG1 (isotype controls for tube 5)
> Tube 4: 20 μl of FITC-CD3 and PE-CD19
> Tube 5: 20 μl of FITC–anti-human IgM and PE-CD19

5. Vortex each tube gently and incubate for 15 min on ice in the dark.
6. Wash by adding 1 ml of staining buffer per tube and vortex gently. Then add an additional 2 ml of staining buffer.
7. Centrifuge the tubes at 1,300 rpm in a Beckman CPKR centrifuge for 3 min at 4°C.
8. Carefully aspirate the supernatant and wash again as in step 6 and centrifuge as in step 7.
9. Resuspend the pellet in 200 to 500 μl of fix buffer. Cells may be analyzed immediately or stored in the dark and cold for analysis within 4 days.

Because the number of B cells in patients with XLA is very low, low background fluorescence in the isotype control tubes is essential. Cells that are in less than optimal condition will autofluoresce, making accurate analysis very difficult. To determine the number and phenotype of B cells in patients with suspected XLA, at least 175,000 to 300,000 events should be analyzed (Fig. 1).

Mutation Detection

A variety of techniques can be used to provide mutation detection. The size of the gene, the variability of the mutations, and the structure and GC content of a gene will influence the choice of technique. In evaluating any gene, it is important to keep in mind that not all alterations represent mutations. Some genes are highly polymorphic. Premature stop codons, frameshift mutations, and base pair substitutions within the invariant regions of the splice consensus sequences are clearly mutations. Amino acid substitutions may represent mutations; alternatively, they may represent uncommon polymorphic variants. If the amino acid substitution is not seen in 200 chromosomes from individuals of the same ethnic background as the patient, the substitution is probably a mutation. There are base pair substitutions within the coding sequence that do not change the amino acid sequence but still cause disease. Some of these base pair alterations affect splicing, while others may act as regulatory regions. Functional assays may be required to demonstrate that a base pair or amino acid substitution is the cause of disease. The advantages and disadvantages of some techniques are listed below.

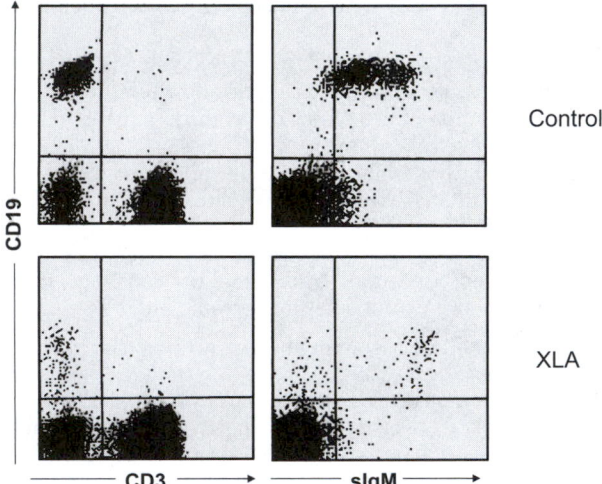

FIGURE 1 Fluorescence-activated cell sorter analysis of B cells from a patient with XLA. Density gradient-separated peripheral blood mononuclear cells from a control (top panels) and a patient with XLA (bottom panels) were stained with PE-CD19 and either FITC-CD3 (left panels) or FITC–polyclonal anti-human IgM (right panels). The dot plot shows approximately 20,000 gated events from the control sample and 200,000 events from the patient sample. The control sample contains 7.3% CD19+ cells, and the patient sample contains 0.07% CD19+ cells. Note that the intensity of CD19 staining is homogeneous in the control sample but variable in the patient sample. Additionally, the majority of the B cells from the patient are very brightly stained for surface IgM, whereas those from the control are variable in surface IgM expression.

PCR Protocol for Mutation-Specific Assay

A simple PCR-based assay can be used to detect up to 60% of the mutations in μ heavy chain. Approximately 30 to 40% of mutations in μ heavy chain are large deletions that remove all of the coding regions for the D, J, and constant segments. Failure to amplify any part of this region suggests a deletion. Another 20 to 30% of mutations in μ heavy chain consist of a recurrent single base pair substitution found at the −1 position of the alternative splice site in exon 4. This G-to-A substitution in codon 433 results in the loss of an MspI restriction site. PCR amplification of the 3′ end of exon 4 of μ heavy chain, followed by MspI digestion and gel electrophoresis, will detect both deletions and the base pair substitution in codon 433.

Materials and Reagents

0.5-ml microcentrifuge tubes

Sterile water

DNA polymerase (Qiagen kit 201205—contains polymerase, 10× buffer, and Q buffer)

Primers at 10 mM concentration: sense primer, 5′-CAACAGGGTCACCGAGAGG-3′; antisense primer, 5′-GCACTCAGGACCAGTATC-3′

Deoxynucleoside triphosphates (dNTPs) at 1 mM (no. 27-2035-01; Amersham/Pharmacia)

DNA from controls and patients at a concentration of 100 ng/μl

MspI (no. R0106L; New England Biolabs)

Agarose (no. 15510-027; Life Technologies)

Ethidium bromide (E-1510; Sigma)

Gel electrophoresis apparatus

Procedure

1. PCR is very vulnerable to contamination. Before the assay is begun, the work area should be wiped down with 10% bleach. If possible, the PCR should not be done in a room where DNA is extracted, purified, stored, or analyzed. Some PCR machines require that the sample be overlaid with mineral oil. Know your machine!

2. Program the PCR machine to the following conditions: 95°C for 5 min, followed by 30 cycles of 95°C for 30 s, 56°C for 30 s, and 72°C for 30 s, with a final extension at 72°C for 5 min. Set the machine to hold at 95°C. Remove reagents from freezer and place on ice to thaw.

3. Roll up sleeves and put on fresh gloves.

4. Label two Eppendorf tubes for each control, each patient sample, and a negative control. One will be for the undigested DNA and the other will be for the digested DNA.

5. Place 2 μl (200 ng) of control or patient DNA into the tube for the undigested DNA. Place 2 μl of water into the negative control tube.

6. Prepare the PCR mixture for the total number of samples plus the negative control plus one extra sample (to make sure that you do not run out of reaction mixture). Keep all reagents on ice at all times. Add the following items, per sample, in the following order:

Water	23.75 μl
Q buffer	10 μl
10× buffer	5 μl
Sense primer	4 μl
Antisense primer	4 μl
dNTP	1 μl
Qiagen Taq	0.25 μl

7. Mix the above reagents well, and then distribute 48 μl into each DNA containing tube. Mix well with the DNA by pipetting up and down several times. Discard the tip between samples.

8. Place the samples in the PCR machine and begin to cycle.

9. At the end of the PCR, remove the tubes and take 25 μl from each tube and place it in the paired empty tube. This tube will be used for the digested DNA.

10. Add 1 μl of MspI along with 2.5 μl of appropriate 10× buffer (NEB2) into each tube labeled for digestion and incubate for 1 h at 37°C.

11. Run the paired samples on a 3% agarose gel.

12. Stain the gel with ethidium bromide, and examine and photograph.

If the patient sample shows no amplification product, the patient may have a deletion. However, it important to make sure that the patient DNA is intact by amplifying a segment from a different part of the genome. DNA from a normal individual will be completely digested by MspI and will demonstrate a 214-bp segment. If the patient has a base pair substitution in codon 433, the DNA will not be digested and the DNA exposed to MspI will be the same size as the undigested DNA.

SSCP

SSCP is a screening technique that is often used to analyze large genes with highly variable mutations. In SSCP assays, PCR is used to amplify a small segment of DNA. The PCR product is heat denatured to separate the two strands of DNA, and then the DNA is electrophoresed through a non-denaturing gel. A commercially available gel, MDE gel, is particularly useful for SSCP. The fact that the gel is non-denaturing allows the strands of DNA to form secondary structures which influence their migration through the gel (26, 32). Even single base pair substitutions change the secondary structure and therefore the migration. The ideal length of the PCR product for SSCP is 110 to 280 bp. For many genes, this length fits well with the size of exons plus flanking splice sites. If many samples are analyzed together, it is easier to identify subtle variations. The gel is run on a sequencing apparatus and is transferred to a filter, like a sequencing gel.

Materials and Reagents

As above for PCR-based mutation specific assay, with the following additions:

Primers specific for the reaction at 10 mM
[^{32}P]dCTP (no. BLU513H; Du Pont NEN)
MDE gel solution (no. 50620; Cambrex Bioscience)
Stop solution (no. 70724; USB)

Procedure

As above for PCR-based mutation-specific assay, with the following change: total volume is 25 μl rather than 50 μl.

1. Same as above.

2. Same as above. PCR conditions may vary depending on the reaction.

3. Same as above.

4. Label an Eppendorf tube for each control, each patient sample, and a negative control.

5. Place 1 μl (100 ng) of control or patient DNA into each tube. Place 1 μl of water into the negative control tube.

6. Prepare the PCR mixture for the total number of samples plus the negative control plus one extra sample (to make sure that you do not run out of reaction mixture). Keep all reagents on ice at all times. Add the following items, per sample, in the following order:

Water . . . . 11.25 μl
Q buffer . . . .   5 μl
10× buffer. . . . .   2.5 μl
Sense primer. . . . .   2 μl
Antisense primer. . . . .   2 μl
dNTP . . . .   1 μl

7. After adding the dNTPs to the reaction mixture, transfer the reaction mixture and the tubes containing the template DNA to an area behind a radioactive shield and add 0.3 μl of [^{32}P]dCTP per sample and 0.25 μl of DNA polymerase per sample to the reaction mixture.

8. Mix the above reagents well, and then distribute 24 μl of reaction mixture into each DNA-containing tube. Mix well with the DNA by pipetting up and down several times. Discard the tip between samples.

9. Place the samples in the PCR machine and begin to cycle.

10. Prepare the MDE gel according to instructions. It will take 30 min for the gel to set.

11. At the end of the PCR, transfer 3 μl of PCR product to 8 μl of stop solution.

12. Denature all of the samples at 95°C for 5 min, and then leave on ice for 1 min prior to loading onto the gel.

13. The gel should be run in the cold (4°C) at 3 W for 4 h. Longer PCR products may require a longer run time.

An example of an SSCP gel is shown in Fig. 2. I have used SSCP to screen for mutations in Btk, CD40 ligand, ICOS, and AID.

Direct Sequencing

Direct sequencing is used to analyze small genes or genes that are not easily evaluated by screening techniques. Essential regions of the gene are amplified by PCR, the PCR product is gel purified, and the primers used to amplify the segment, or primers that recognize sites within the product, are used to sequence the segment on an automated sequencer. The PCR product must be quite clean, and the template-to-primer ratio must be appropriate to allow sequencing. Generally, 600 to 800 bp of sequence can be obtained from a single run. I have found that direct sequencing is more efficient than SSCP analysis to identify alterations in the exons encoding the constant region of μ heavy chain. The four exons of the μ heavy-chain constant region are too large (approximately 300 bp) to examine in a single SSCP reaction, and together the four exons are only 2.2 kb in length.

No single technique will identify all mutations. Although sequencing of cDNA may be a useful first screen, this approach often misses splice site defects and defects within regulatory regions. Direct sequencing of critical regions of the gene may miss base pair alterations within introns that create splice sites and pseudoexons. These mutations are found by sequencing cDNA. SSCP screening will miss duplications and inversions that are most easily detected by Southern blot analysis.

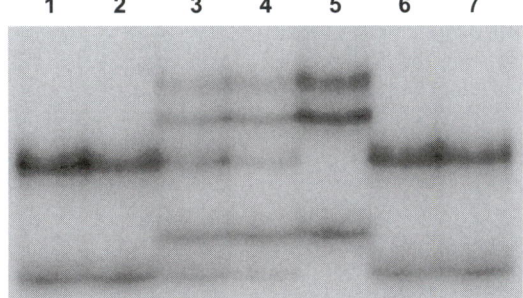

FIGURE 2 SSCP analysis of DNA from a patient with XLA and his family members. Exon 17 of Btk was amplified using primers that flank the coding sequence and splice sites. The PCR products were denatured in heat and then allowed to renature as they migrated through an electrophoresis gel. Lanes 1, 2, 6, and 7 contain DNA from controls. The DNA sample in lane 5 is from a patient with XLA. DNA samples from the patient's mother and sister are in lanes 3 and 4, respectively.

SUMMARY

Evaluation of patients with suspected antibody deficiency should proceed in a stepwise fashion. A detailed history of past infections, a careful family history, and a physical examination that focuses on sites typically involved in antibody deficiencies should come before any laboratory tests. The extent of the preliminary evaluation should depend on the index of suspicion. A screening evaluation may include only quantitative serum immunoglobulins and isohemagglutinins, or it may include additional tests such as titers of antibody to vaccine antigens and lymphocyte cell surface markers. For patients with defects in early B-cell development of unknown etiology, a bone marrow aspirate may be useful to document the numbers of pro-B cells and pre-B cells. A gene-specific diagnostic test should be performed if genetic counseling is desired and preliminary tests support the diagnosis.

REFERENCES

1. **Adderson, E. E., D. H. Viskochil, J. C. Carey, A. O. Shigeoka, J. C. Christenson, J. F. Bohnsack, and H. R. Hill.** 2000. Growth failure, intracranial calcifications, acquired pancytopenia, and unusual humoral immunodeficiency: a genetic syndrome? *Am. J. Med. Genet.* **95:**17–20.
2. **Brouet, J. C., A. Chedeville, J. P. Fermand, and B. Royer.** 2000. Study of the B-cell memory compartment in common variable immunodeficiency. *Eur. J. Immunol.* **30:**2516–2520.
3. **Conley, M. E.** 1985. B cells in patients with X-linked agammaglobulinemia. *J. Immunol.* **134:**3070–3074.
4. **Conley, M. E., A. Broides, V. Hernandez-Trujillo, V. Howard, H. Kanegane, T. Miyawaki, and S. A. Shurtleff.** 2005. Genetic analysis of patients with defects in early B-cell development. *Immunol. Rev.* **203:**216–234.
5. **Conley, M. E., and V. Howard.** 2002. Clinical findings leading to the diagnosis of X-linked agammaglobulinemia. *J. Pediatr.* **141:**566–571.
6. **Conley, M. E., D. Mathias, J. Treadaway, Y. Minegishi, and J. Rohrer.** 1998. Mutations in Btk in patients with presumed X-linked agammaglobulinemia. *Am. J. Hum. Genet.* **62:**1034–1043.
7. **Cunningham-Rundles, C., and C. Bodian.** 1999. Common variable immunodeficiency: clinical and immunological features of 248 patients. *Clin. Immunol.* **92:**34–48.
8. **Doffinger, R., A. Smahi, C. Bessia, F. Geissmann, J. Feinberg, A. Durandy, C. Bodemer, S. Kenwrick, S. Dupuis-Girod, S. Blanche, P. Wood, S. H. Rabia, D. J. Headon, P. A. Overbeek, F. Le Deist, S. M. Holland, K. Belani, D. S. Kumararatne, A. Fischer, R. Shapiro, M. E. Conley, E. Reimund, H. Kalhoff, M. Abinun, A. Munnich, A. Israel, G. Courtois, and J. L. Casanova.** 2001. X-linked anhidrotic ectodermal dysplasia with immunodeficiency is caused by impaired NF-kappaB signaling. *Nat. Genet.* **27:**277–285.
9. **Ferrari, S., S. Giliani, A. Insalaco, A. Al Ghonaium, A. R. Soresina, M. Loubser, M. A. Avanzini, M. Marconi, R. Badolato, A. G. Ugazio, Y. Levy, N. Catalan, A. Durandy, A. Tbakhi, L. D. Notarangelo, and A. Plebani.** 2001. Mutations of CD40 gene cause an autosomal recessive form of immunodeficiency with hyper IgM. *Proc. Natl. Acad. Sci. USA* **98:**12614–12619.
10. **Furr, P. M., D. Taylor-Robinson, and A. D. Webster.** 1994. Mycoplasmas and ureaplasmas in patients with hypogammaglobulinaemia and their role in arthritis: microbiological observations over twenty years. *Ann. Rheum. Dis.* **53:**183–187.
11. **Futatani, T., T. Miyawaki, S. Tsukada, S. Hashimoto, T. Kunikata, S. Arai, M. Kurimoto, Y. Niida, H. Matsuoka, Y. Sakiyama, T. Iwata, S. Tsuchiya, O. Tatsuzawa, K. Yoshizaki, and T. Kishimoto.** 1998. Deficient expression of Bruton's tyrosine kinase in monocytes from X-linked agammaglobulinemia as evaluated by a flow cytometric analysis and its clinical application to carrier detection. *Blood* **91:**595–602.
12. **Grimbacher, B., A. Hutloff, M. Schlesier, E. Glocker, K. Warnatz, R. Drager, H. Eibel, B. Fischer, A. A. Schaffer, H. W. Mages, R. A. Kroczek, and H. H. Peter.** 2003. Homozygous loss of ICOS is associated with adult-onset common variable immunodeficiency. *Nat. Immunol.* **4:**261–268.
13. **Hayward, A. R., J. Levy, F. Facchetti, L. Notarangelo, H. D. Ochs, A. Etzioni, J. Y. Bonnefoy, M. Cosyns, and A. Weinberg.** 1997. Cholangiopathy and tumors of the pancreas, liver, and biliary tree in boys with X-linked immunodeficiency with hyper-IgM. *J. Immunol.* **158:**977–983.
14. **Imai, K., G. Slupphaug, W. I. Lee, P. Revy, S. Nonoyama, N. Catalan, L. Yel, M. Forveille, B. Kavli, H. E. Krokan, H. D. Ochs, A. Fischer, and A. Durandy.** 2003. Human uracil-DNA glycosylase deficiency associated with profoundly impaired immunoglobulin class-switch recombination. *Nat. Immunol.* **4:**1023–1028.
15. **Jacquot, S., L. Macon-Lemaitre, E. Paris, T. Kobata, Y. Tanaka, C. Morimoto, S. F. Schlossman, and F. Tron.** 2001. B-cell co-receptors regulating T cell-dependent antibody production in common variable immunodeficiency: CD27 pathway defects identify subsets of severely immunocompromised patients. *Int. Immunol.* **13:**871–876.
16. **Lee, W. I., T. R. Torgerson, M. J. Schumacher, L. Yel, Q. Zhu, and H. D. Ochs.** 2005. Molecular analysis of a large cohort of patients with the hyper immunoglobulin M (IgM) syndrome. *Blood* **105:**1881–1890.
17. **LoGalbo, P. R., H. A. Sampson, and R. H. Buckley.** 1982. Symptomatic giardiasis in three patients with X-linked agammaglobulinemia. *J. Pediatr.* **101:**78–80.
18. **Lopez, G. E., A. S. Porpiglia, M. B. Hogan, N. Matamoros, S. Krasovec, C. Pignata, C. I. Smith, L. Hammarstrom, J. Bjorkander, B. H. Belohradsky, G. F. Casariego, M. C. Garcia Rodriguez, and M. E. Conley.** 2002. Clinical and molecular analysis of patients with defects in mu heavy chain gene. *J. Clin. Investig.* **110:**1029–1035.
19. **McKinney, R. E., Jr., S. L. Katz, and C. M. Wilfert.** 1987. Chronic enteroviral meningoencephalitis in agammaglobulinemic patients. *Rev. Infect. Dis.* **9:**334–356.

20. Minegishi, Y., E. Coustan-Smith, L. Rapalus, F. Ersoy, D. Campana, and M. E. Conley. 1999. Mutations in Igα (CD79a) result in a complete block in B cell development. *J. Clin. Investig.* **104:**1115–1121.

21. Minegishi, Y., E. Coustan-Smith, Y.-H. Wang, M. D. Cooper, D. Campana, and M. E. Conley. 1998. Mutations in the human λ5/14.1 gene result in B-cell deficiency and agammaglobulinemia. *J. Exp. Med.* **187:**71–77.

22. Minegishi, Y., A. Lavoie, C. Cunningham-Rundles, P. M. Bedard, J. Hebert, L. Cote, K. Dan, D. Sedlak, R. H. Buckley, A. Fischer, A. Durandy, and M. E. Conley. 2000. Mutations in activation-induced cytidine deaminase in patients with hyper IgM syndrome. *Clin. Immunol.* **97:**203–210.

23. Minegishi, Y., J. Rohrer, E. Coustan-Smith, H. M. Lederman, R. Pappu, D. Campana, A. C. Chan, and M. E. Conley. 1999. An essential role for BLNK in human B cell development. *Science* **286:**1954–1957.

24. Noordzij, J. G., S. Bruin-Versteeg, W. M. Comans-Bitter, N. G. Hartwig, R. W. Hendriks, R. de Groot, and J. J. van Dongen. 2002. Composition of precursor B-cell compartment in bone marrow from patients with X-linked agammaglobulinemia compared with healthy children. *Pediatr. Res.* **51:**159–168.

25. Nowak-Wegrzyn, A., T. O. Crawford, J. A. Winkelstein, K. A. Carson, and H. M. Lederman. 2004. Immunodeficiency and infections in ataxia-telangiectasia. *J. Pediatr.* **144:**505–511.

26. Orita, M., Y. Suzuki, T. Sekiya, and K. Hayashi. 1989. Rapid and sensitive detection of point mutations and DNA polymorphisms using the polymerase chain reaction. *Genomics* **5:**874–879.

27. Piqueras, B., C. Lavenu-Bombled, L. Galicier, F. Bergeron-van der Cruyssen, L. Mouthon, S. Chevret, P. Debre, C. Schmitt, and E. Oksenhendler. 2003. Common variable immunodeficiency patient classification based on impaired B cell memory differentiation correlates with clinical aspects. *J. Clin. Immunol.* **23:**385–400.

28. Plebani, A., A. Soresina, R. Rondelli, G. Amato, C. Azzari, F. Cardinale, G. Cazzola, R. Consolini, D. De Mattia, G. Dell'Erba, M. Duse, M. Fiorini, S. Martino, B. Martire, M. Masi, V. Monafo, V. Moschese, L. Notarangelo, P. Orlandi, P. Panei, A. Pession, M. Pietrogrande, C. Pignata, I. Quinti, V. Ragno, P. Rossi, A. Sciotto, A. Stabile, A. Ugazio, and the Italian Pediatric Group for XLA-AIEOP. 2002. Clinical, immunological, and molecular analysis in a large cohort of patients with X-linked agammaglobulinemia: an Italian multicenter study. *Clin. Immunol.* **104:**221–230.

29. Rawlings, D. J. 1999. Bruton's tyrosine kinase controls a sustained calcium signal essential for B lineage development and function. *Clin. Immunol.* **91:**243–253.

30. Revy, P., M. Busslinger, K. Tashiro, F. Arenzana, P. Pillet, A. Fischer, and A. Durandy. 2000. A syndrome involving intrauterine growth retardation, microcephaly, cerebellar hypoplasia, B lymphocyte deficiency, and progressive pancytopenia. *Pediatrics* **105:**E39.

31. Revy, P., T. Muto, Y. Levy, F. Geissmann, A. Plebani, O. Sanal, N. Catalan, M. Forveille, R. Dufourcq-Lagelouse, A. Gennery, I. Tezcan, F. Ersoy, H. Kayserili, A. Ugazio, N. Brousse, M. Muramatsu, L. Notarangelo, K. Kinoshita, T. Honjo, A. Fischer, and A. Durandy. 2000. Activation-induced cytidine deaminase (AID) deficiency causes the autosomal recessive form of the hyper-IgM syndrome (HIGM2). *Cell* **102:**565–575.

32. Sheffield, V. C., J. S. Beck, A. E. Kwitek, D. W. Sandstrom, and E. M. Stone. 1993. The sensitivity of single-strand conformation polymorphism analysis for the detection of single base substitutions. *Genomics* **16:**325–332.

33. Srivannaboon, K., M. E. Conley, E. Coustan-Smith, and W. C. Wang. 2001. Hypogammaglobulinemia and reduced numbers of B cells in children with myelodysplastic syndrome. *J. Pediatr. Hematol. Oncol.* **23:**122–125.

34. Tsukada, S., D. C. Saffran, D. J. Rawlings, O. Parolini, R. C. Allen, I. Klisak, R. S. Sparkes, H. Kubagawa, T. Mohandas, S. Quan, J. W. Belmont, M. D. Cooper, M. E. Conley, and O. N. Witte. 1993. Deficient expression of a B-cell cytoplasmic tyrosine kinase in human X-linked agammaglobulinemia. *Cell* **72:**279–290.

35. Verloes, A., M. F. Dresse, H. Keutgen, C. Asplund, and C. I. Smith. 2001. Microphthalmia, facial anomalies, microcephaly, thumb and hallux hypoplasia, and agammaglobulinemia. *Am. J. Med. Genet.* **101:**209–212.

36. Warnatz, K., A. Denz, R. Drager, M. Braun, C. Groth, G. Wolff-Vorbeck, H. Eibel, M. Schlesier, and H. H. Peter. 2002. Severe deficiency of switched memory B-cells (CD27(+)IgM(−)IgD(−)) in subgroups of patients with common variable immunodeficiency: a new approach to classify a heterogeneous disease. *Blood* **99:**1544–1551.

37. Winkelstein, J. A., M. C. Marino, H. Ochs, R. Fuleihan, P. R. Scholl, R. Geha, E. R. Stiehm, and M. E. Conley. 2003. The X-linked hyper-IgM syndrome: clinical and immunologic features of 79 patients. *Medicine* (Baltimore) **82:**373–384.

Hereditary and Acquired Complement Deficiencies

PATRICIA C. GICLAS

102

Complement comprises an interactive system of more than 30 plasma and cell membrane-associated recognition molecules, enzymes, cofactors, control proteins, and receptors. It plays an important role in the host's response to infection by coating microbial surfaces with complement fragments that enhance uptake and killing by phagocytes. As a major effector arm of the innate immune system, complement serves as a link between many of the activities of acquired immunity and other defense mechanisms, with ties to diverse cell signal responses in an ever-increasing number of tissues.

Activation of the complement enzyme cascade produces peptide fragments that exhibit inflammatory properties, including chemotactic activity and the ability to regulate local blood flow and vascular permeability. Complement also has a host of "housekeeping" activities, such as clearance of immune complexes, effete and apoptotic cells, and cellular debris. Deficiencies or mutations in complement components, whether inherited or acquired, predispose an individual to infections, autoimmune diseases, impaired immune responses, and diverse conditions such as fetal loss, renal disease, vasculitis, allergic reactions, angioedema (AE), and age-related macular degeneration. The discussion that follows touches on examples of these and other complement-related functions that go awry when one or more of the proteins in the system is missing or functions abnormally. The reader is referred to Fig. 1 for a review of these pathways and the proteins involved.

A previous chapter published in the fifth edition of this manual (39) describes a process by which the appropriate laboratory methods can be used to determine which component(s) is deficient and whether the deficiency is hereditary or acquired. In general, starting with basic screening tests, such as CH50 and AH50 or their equivalents for total classical and alternative pathway function, will help pinpoint the pathway involved and limit the number of tests required. A test for lectin pathway (LP) function will further narrow the search. Since all three initiating pathways (classical pathway [CP], alternative pathway [AP], and LP) share the same terminal pathway, a missing component unique to any of the early steps will affect only the pathway involved, while a missing component in the terminal pathway will affect all of the others. As with other complement tests, care must be taken in specimen collection, handling, and shipping. It is strongly advised to contact the laboratory to which the specimen will be sent for instructions for specific assays. More labs

are now offering genotyping for complement components, so the collection of specimens for DNA from the patient and family is recommended as well.

DEFICIENCIES OF THE CP: C1q, C1r, C1s, C2, AND C4

The CP is activated when the C1 complex ($C1qC1r_2C1s_2$) binds to an appropriate activator through the latter's interaction with C1q. Although often this may be an immune complex or aggregate of immunoglobulin G (IgG) (IgG3 > IgG1 > IgG2) or IgM, many other substances can serve as activators of the CP. Once bound, the C1 complex undergoes a relaxation of the constraint on C1r and C1s and the esterase activities of these subcomponents can then be expressed. The substrate of C1r is C1s, and the substrates of C1s are C4 and C2. The activities of these two enzymes are very rapidly controlled in normal plasma by C1-esterase inhibitor (C1-Inh).

The CP is critical for the clearance of immune complexes, and it also participates in the removal of apoptotic cells. The phenotype of C1q and other early CP component deficiencies is closely linked to diseases in which these processes are impaired, such as systemic lupus erythematosus (SLE), and rheumatologic disorders such as anaphylactoid purpura, vasculitis, and membranoproliferative glomerulonephritis (30). The incidences of SLE in patients with known C1q, C4, or C2 deficiency are roughly 90, 75, and 15%, respectively, while partial C4 deficiency (C4A) is also implicated in 15%. SLE patients with C1q or C4 deficiencies have characteristic features such as earlier age of onset, prominent photosensitivity, lower frequency of renal disease, variable antinuclear antibody titers, and a nearly equal male-to-female ratio. In addition to SLE and other immune complex diseases, CP deficiencies also lead to recurrent pyogenic infections with streptococcal, staphylococcal, and other common encapsulated bacteria but less likely *Neisseria*, and should not be overlooked in the workup for immune dysfunction. The CH50 or equivalent assays are the best screens for these deficiencies, since the absence of any one of the CP proteins will block CP activity (38).

The gene for human C1q is located on chromosome 1, at 1p34-1p36.3 (82). The protein is related to the collectin family, possessing both collagen-like and globular structure. There are six each of three different polypeptide chains in the intact 460-kDa molecule. These chains are combined to

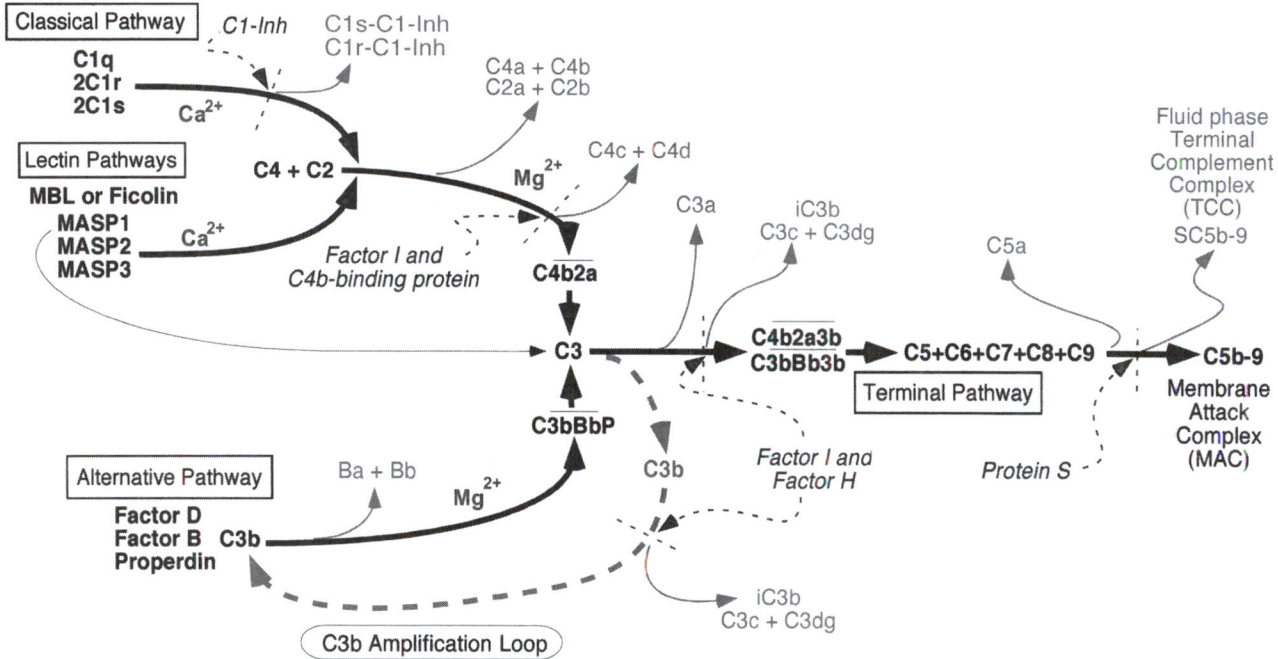

FIGURE 1 CP, LP, and AP of the human complement system, showing the control steps and where some of the biologically active split products are produced.

form six triple-chain helices that make up the collagen-like "stalk" of the molecule, and then they branch away at a flexible hinge region into six smaller stalks ending in globular heads. The molecule has been described as a bunch of six tulips, based on electron microscopic photographs.

The primary synthesis of C1q is by cells of monocyte/macrophage lineage, with follicular dendritic cells as a secondary site. C1q deficiency is an autosomal recessive condition, with deficient patients having little or no detectable protein or C1q function in the circulation. Mutations have been identified in the genes for each of the three chains. Almost all patients with documented C1q deficiency have developed SLE-like disease, and linkage studies demonstrate that the C1q gene is close to that for other proposed SLE susceptibility genes on chromosome 1 in humans (91).

The genes for C1r and C1s are located on chromosome 12, at 12p13, where the two genes lie in tandem (60). C1r and C1s are synthesized as single-chain proenzyme molecules that associate in a tail-to-tail fashion, with two C1r-C1s pairs in a calcium-dependent complex with each C1q. Each proenzyme is activated by cleavage of a single bond to produce two disulfide-linked peptides, the smaller of which has esterase activity. C1r has very limited trypsin-like activity, with C1r autoactivation followed by cleavage of C1s. C1s has trypsin-like activity against C4 and C2, each of which it cleaves into two fragments: C4a and C4b, and C2a and C2b.

C1r and C1s are synthesized primarily in the liver by hepatocytes, but monocytes, macrophages, epithelial and endothelial cells, and some cells of the central nervous system provide secondary synthesis sites. Deficiencies of C1r and C1s are rare and may be partial or combined. They predispose the patient to recurrent pyogenic infections as well as immune complex disease (65).

The proteins C4 and C2 are both required for formation of the C3 convertase enzyme of the CP (C4b2a). The absence of either protein leads to a complete block of CP

activity and is associated with recurrent infections and immune complex disease as described above. In spite of this, many patients with C2 deficiency remain asymptomatic for long periods, if not for life. The genes for C4 and C2, along with those for factor B (BF), are present in the major histocompatibility complex (MHC) on chromosome 6 in the group known as class III MHC genes (5).

C4 is produced primarily by hepatocytes but can also be made by many other cells. It is synthesized as a single chain that undergoes posttranslational modification to three chains that are disulfide linked. The alpha chain contains an internal thioester linkage that forms a covalent bond with nearby substances when the C4a is clipped off during activation. This bond provides a means for attachment of C4b to the nearest protein or carbohydrate group when activation occurs and results in long-lasting deposition of C4b and its breakdown fragment, C4d, on the activator.

Human C4 exists in two forms, C4A and C4B, coded for by different genes and present in equal amounts (two alleles of C4A and two of C4B) in approximately 75% of the population (104). The differences between the two forms of C4 are in a few amino acids near the thioester group and affect the ability of the C4b fragment to bind to proteins (C4A) or carbohydrate residues on cell surfaces (C4B). Standard assays for C4 do not distinguish between these forms. Variation in C4 gene number is not uncommon, and the gene number can range from none to eight or more copies, giving this protein a wide range of concentrations in the general population (103, 104). Most of the partial C4 deficiencies are without consequence, but some individuals have a total deficiency of one haplotype. C4A deficiency is increased (8 to 12%) in Caucasian lupus patients compared to control individuals (1 to 3%) due to the decreased binding of C4A to protein antigens and antibodies and consequent difficulty with immune complex clearance. An increased incidence of C4B null alleles was recently reported for patients with Henoch-Schönlein purpura (86). Close to 100 different polymorphisms in the C4 protein make it one of the most variable proteins in the circulation.

C2 is synthesized by hepatocytes, monocytes, macrophages, fibroblasts, astroglioma cells, and alveolar type II cells. It is produced as a single-chain proenzyme that expresses its esterase activity only after it has been cleaved. This activity is very weak in the fluid phase but becomes efficient when the C2a fragment is bound to C4b on a surface. C2-deficient patients have increased susceptibility to infections, particularly streptococcal pneumonia, as well as the previously mentioned association with immune complex diseases. In Caucasian patients with rheumatologic disorders such as SLE, the incidence of C2 deficiency approaches 1/100, as opposed to the general population, where incidence is estimated to be 1/10,000 (4, 54). There are two forms of C2 deficiency. Type I deficiency, which affects over 90% of patients, results from a complete lack of synthesis, while type II C2 deficiency results from a secretion defect. The former deficiency is characterized by little or no detectable protein in the circulation, and the latter is characterized by up to 10% of normal levels and function.

DEFICIENCIES OF THE LP: MBL, FICOLINS, AND MASPs

Mannose-binding lectin (MBL) has also been known as mannose-binding protein, mannan-binding protein, or core-specific lectin. Similar in structure to C1q, it is made up of trimers of single polypeptide subunits, two to six of which combine to form oligomers. MBL is a pattern recognition lectin that binds with high affinity to the mannose, peptidoglycan, and N-acetylglucosamine residues that are found on the surfaces of bacteria, yeasts, and fungi (92). Like C1q, it is associated with several serine proteases, or MASPs (MBL-associated serine proteases), that become active when binding of the MBL occurs (62). In addition to activating complement, MBL may be able to act directly as an opsonin by interacting directly with cell surface receptors.

The gene for MBL is found on chromosome 10, at 10q11.2-q21, with another gene that encodes a truncated protein at 10q22.2-22.3 (42, 79). There is a wide range of serum concentrations of MBL, due in part to the presence of gene variants that produce different amounts of the protein. Approximately 5 to 10% of individuals studied to date are MBL deficient (16). Because complement activation by the LP is antibody and C1 independent, it is thought to play an important role in innate immunity during infancy before the adaptive immune responses are mature (93). Deficiency of MBL has been linked to an increased frequency of pyogenic infections and sepsis, particularly in neonates and young children. It has been implicated as a risk factor in ischemia-reperfusion injury, Behçets disease, cystic fibrosis, severe acute respiratory syndrome, and several other respiratory infections (14, 36, 46, 51, 52). There is a two- to threefold increase in MBL deficiency in lupus patients who tend to have more frequent and severe infections, and worse outcomes are observed in rheumatoid arthritis patients with MBL deficiency. Autoantibodies that reacted with MBL were found in a Japanese study of patients with SLE, but the significance of these antibodies was not evident from the disease characteristics of the patients (87).

The ficolins are a group of proteins that are similar to C1q and MBL, with a collagen-like region and a C-terminal fibrinogen domain that is thought to be the ligand-binding site for N-acetylglucosamine (61, 62). There are several forms of ficolins that have been described: ficolin-L and ficolin-H are found in the circulation, while ficolin-M is a secretory protein that is found in the cytoplasm of neutrophils, monocytes, and type II alveolar epithelial cells. All forms have similar opsonizing capacities for pathogens and are associated with the MASP enzymes found with MBL. Although the ficolins were first described as opsonins in 1996, little is known of the prevalence or phenotype of ficolin deficiencies.

The four MASP proteins, MASP-1, MASP-2, MASP-3, and Map19, are encoded by two genes (81). Structurally they are similar to C1r and C1s, with a serine protease domain in the B chain. MASP-1 and MASP-3 are alternative splice products of one gene (MASP1/3) that have the same A chain but different B chains. A different gene encodes MASP-2 and Map19, the latter of which has only the first two domains of MASP-2 plus an additional four amino acids. MASP-2 is responsible for the cleavage of C4 and C2, making it analogous to C1s in function. Although there have been mutations found in the genes for the MASP proteins, the mutations in MBL that prevent the assembly of the complete complex are the major known cause of functional deficiency of these proteins (85, 93).

DEFICIENCIES OF THE CP AND LP CONTROL PROTEINS: C1-Inh AND C4BP

The active enzyme forms of C1r and C1s are regulated solely by C1-Inh, a member of the SERPIN family of serine protease inhibitors. C1-Inh also contributes to the control of other enzymes, including coagulation factors XIa, XIIa, plasmin, and plasma kallikrein. When the enzyme and inhibitor interact, the enzyme cleaves a "bait-sequence" on the inhibitor and the resulting change in conformation forms a tight complex, rendering the enzyme inactive. The complexes formed in these reactions are cleared from the circulation by cells of the reticuloendothelial system. C1-Inh deficiency can be of hereditary origin (HAE) or acquired (AAE) through clearance of inhibitor-enzyme complexes or through action of autoantibodies that react with the inhibitor and result in its inappropriate cleavage. Symptoms are similar regardless of the origin of the deficiency, so careful evaluation is required to distinguish between HAE and AAE. The kinin-like biochemical mediator(s) of AE, not yet definitively identified, could arise from defective regulation of either the complement or coagulation pathways. The argument for bradykinin is strengthened by current studies in an animal model and success with treatment of patients using a kallikrein inhibitor (20, 45).

C1-Inh is inherited in an autosomal codominant pattern in which each allele produces approximately half of the protein in the circulation, although increased catabolism often causes decreases of the normal gene product to below the predicted 50% level. To date, no patient homozygous for deficiency of C1-Inh (both alleles defective) has been reported, and the heterozygous state determines the phenotype (32). Patients with C1-Inh deficiency suffer various degrees of intermittent AE characterized by nonpainful, nonpruritic, and nonerythematous subcutaneous and submucosal swelling that spontaneously subsides within 72 h (21, 32). Swelling may arise sporadically and spontaneously, or it may be triggered by mild trauma or psychological stress. It is not accompanied by urticaria and is not responsive to antihistamines, steroids, or beta agonists. Symptoms usually begin in adolescence and range in severity from mild edema of the extremities to life-threatening laryngeal edema.

Edema of the bowel wall results in severe colicky abdominal pain, nausea, and vomiting that can be distinguished from acute abdominal syndromes by the absence of fever, peritoneal signs, and elevated white blood cell count. Angiotensin inhibitors may increase attack frequency (33). There are several new drugs being developed that may help control AE, including recombinant human C1-Inh, human C1-Inh purified by new methods, and kallikrein antagonists.

Genetic defects in C1-Inh range from single nucleotide polymorphisms that may alter the function of the protein produced to inappropriate stop codons resulting in large deletions and no protein production. Since each patient has one normal allele and one abnormal allele, he or she will have variable amounts of C1-Inh protein in the circulation, from very low to elevated, depending upon the particular mutation in the affected gene. In the majority of patients, low levels of C1-Inh are indicative of the defect, but final diagnosis of HAE should be based on the functional activity of C1-Inh protein in conjunction with decreased levels of C4, the clinical presentation, and family history. Spontaneous mutations in C1-Inh genes have been documented in about 20% of cases, so the lack of family history does not rule out the defect (12, 18, 22). The prevalence of C1-Inh deficiency is 1/10,000 in Caucasian populations. MASP-1 and MASP-2 are controlled in a 1:1 manner by C1-Inh, in the same way that C1r and C1s are controlled. The control of MASP-3 is not known at this time.

The two forms of HAE behave the same clinically. Type I HAE (80% of patients) is defined by a reduction of C1-Inh to less than half of normal antigenic and functional levels. Type II patients have normal or elevated antigenic C1-Inh levels but synthesize a dysfunctional protein with reduced or absent C1-Inh function. Recent studies have identified a third type in which the patients, all women, have clinical findings consistent with HAE but normal C1-Inh level and function (9, 11). The underlying estrogen-dependent defect has not been identified.

As in HAE, two forms of acquired AE have been described. In type I AAE, patients with B-cell lymphoproliferative diseases produce circulating anti-idiotype antibodies. The immune complexes produced by these antibodies cause a persistent activation of the CP, resulting in profound C1-Inh consumption as the enzyme-inhibitor complexes are cleared (13, 64). In this form of AAE, the C1q level is decreased, whereas in the hereditary forms it is not. In type II AAE, inactivation of C1-Inh is caused by autoantibodies to the C1-Inh protein (53). In type II AAE, the C1-Inh level can be normal by immunoassay, but the protein is dysfunctional. The autoantibody can be detected by enzyme-linked immunosorbent assay, and a cleaved form of the C1-Inh molecule can be detected by Western blotting.

The fluid-phase control of C4aC2b, the C3 convertase of the CP and LP, is accomplished through the combined effects of C4b-binding protein (C4BP) and factor I (FI). Also known as proline-rich protein, human C4BP is a member of the family known as regulators of complement activation (RCA). Characterized by multiple short consensus repeat motifs, also referred to as complement control protein (CCP) units, the RCA proteins bind C3b and C4b fragments and possess various control properties that are critical for regulation of complement activity. These small globular CCP units are typically connected in linear fashion like beads on a string. They occur in all of the RCA and many other complement proteins in various numbers.

C4BP has several isomers made up of two types of subunits: six or seven alpha chains and zero or one beta chain.

These are connected at a central joining region and radiate outward, giving the molecule a spider-like appearance (19). The alpha chains bind to C4b and accelerate the dissociation of C4bC2a to form free C2a and C4b-C4BP. C2a is unable to bind to newly formed C4b and becomes inactivated, while C4b undergoes degradation by FI (with C4BP as a cofactor) to form C4c and C4d (34). C3 convertase activity by the CP enzyme is short-lived due to the efficiency of C4BP. For this reason, activation of the CP does not produce a large amount of C3 fragments and activation often stops at this point in the cascade unless the AP is activated. In the absence of C1-Inh, it is the control of C4bC2a activity by C4BP and FI that accounts for the stability of C3 in HAE patients in spite of decreased C4 and C2 (41). The beta chain has a binding site for the anticoagulant protein S and may play a role in control of coagulation.

C4BP is synthesized in the liver by hepatocytes. The genes for the C4BP alpha and beta chains are located in the RCA gene cluster on chromosome 1, at 1q32. Circulating concentrations of C4BP vary according to genetic determinants as well as fluctuations due to consumption during disease states. Deficiencies of C4BP are very rare and would logically be associated with uncontrolled activation of C3 through the CP. The only documented case was a patient with an atypical form of Behçet's disease and AE (90).

DEFICIENCIES OF THE AP: FD, Bf, AND PROPERDIN (P)

Factor D (FD) is the smallest of the complement proteins and is the only serine protease of the system that does not require enzymatic cleavage in order to become active. Instead, its enzyme activity is a function of its conformational state, and it can flip between the active and inactive forms depending on its proximity to its substrate: C3b-bound Bf (94). Like other complement proteins, it is synthesized by cells of monocyte/macrophage lineage, but its major source of synthesis is adipose tissue (101). FD is the only initiating enzyme for the AP. It binds to and cleaves Bf only when the Bf is bound to C3b. The resulting complex, C3bBb, is the AP C3 convertase.

FD is synthesized by a gene located on chromosome 19. One family with FD deficiency has been described to date. In five generations of family members, the propositus was a 23-year-old woman who presented with meningococcemia from *Neisseria meningitidis*, three relatives had FD deficiency with no health problems, and a deceased family member had a history of meningitis in his twenties and died from pneumonia and meningitis caused by *Streptococcus pneumoniae* at age 81 (8). Complement studies for the patient and family members included C3 and C4 levels and CH50 (normal in all). The AH50 was <10% of normal in homozygous deficient individuals but was normal in all others, including those heterozygous for the deficiency. When FD was analyzed, it was found to be slightly elevated in those members who were homozygous for the wild-type FD gene, about half the normal level in those heterozygous for the mutation, and undetectable in the four patients homozygous for the mutation.

In addition to its participation in the AP of complement, FD plays a role in fatty acid metabolism, and the $C3a_{desArg}$ fragment produced by FD-mediated cleavage of C3 has been identified as the autocrine mediator of hyperapobetalipoproteinemia (57, 101). It is tempting to speculate that this involvement with lipid metabolism may be impaired or dysregulated somehow in those rare patients with partial lipodystrophy who have increased cleavage of C3 due to the presence of autoantibodies to the C3bBb complex (C3 nephritic factors).

Bf has been known variably as glycine-rich beta glycoprotein, properdin factor B, C3 proactivator, C3 convertase, C5 convertase, and EC 3.4.21.47. The gene for Bf is in the MHC complex on chromosome 6, at 6p21.1-6p21.3, 3′ to the C2 gene (15). It is synthesized primarily in the liver, with additional protein produced by cells of monocyte/macrophage lineage, fibroblasts, endothelial cells, and alveolar type II epithelial cells. Secreted as a single polypeptide chain proenzyme, Bf is activated only when it is bound to C3b and cleaved by FD. Its activity is specific for C3 and C5, but it requires C3b as a cofactor to cleave the former and an additional C3b to cleave the latter. The hydrolyzed form of C3 known as C3•H₂O can serve as the first ligand for Bf binding.

Bf is an acute-phase protein and increases during inflammation. There are two polymorphic forms of Bf, BF*F and BF*S, based on their electrophoretic mobilities on immunoelectrophoresis. The amount of Bf in the circulation is higher in individuals homozygous for the former and lower in individuals homozygous for the latter, with heterozygous individuals intermediate (66). There has only been one unconfirmed report of a Bf deficiency in humans and none in animals except Bf gene knockout mice. The latter do not appear to have problems in specific-pathogen-free conditions.

P is a unique protein that acts as a stabilizer for the AP C3 convertase and makes possible the amplification loop that very efficiently cleaves C3 when the AP is activated. P is a single-chain linear molecule with no enzyme activity, but it forms head-to-tail polymers, about half of which are trimers, with dimers and tetramers making up the remainder. P binds to C3b with increasing avidity depending on the number of C3b molecules in a cluster, and its affinity increases when Bb is present (26, 27).

P is the only complement protein that is X-linked, with its gene at Xp11.3-Xp11.23 (40). The protein is synthesized by monocytes, granulocytic cells, and T cells. Three types of P deficiency have been described. Type I deficiency is associated with fulminant meningococcal infections, and the patients had little or no P detectable in the circulation (83). Partial P deficiency found in another family with neisserial septicemia was characterized by about 10% of normal levels of P in the serum (84). Several dysfunctional mutant forms of the protein have been identified that result in decreased AP function, making this type III deficiency (100). P deficiency increases the susceptibility to bacterial infections, including *Neisseria* infections. Carriers of a defective or absent P gene cannot be reliably identified from the protein's level in the circulation, and genetic typing is necessary to provide evidence of the carrier state (59).

CONTROL PROTEINS OF THE AP: CFH AND FI

The amplification, or feedback, loop of the AP makes it one of the most efficient enzyme systems in the circulation (28). As long as P can stabilize the C3 convertase (C3bBbP), C3 cleavage continues unchecked. This leads to deposits of C3 clusters on the surface of cells, where the C3bBb is bound, and greatly enhances opsonization and other inflammatory cell interactions with the C3-coated particles due to the increased avidity provided by multiple closely spaced C3 fragments for C3 receptor interaction. The two major controls of the fluid-phase activation of the AP are factor H (CFH) and FI. The former is a member of the RCA family,

described above for C4BP, and the latter is a serine protease with specificity for C3b and C4b.

CFH is synthesized as a single chain with 20 complement control protein modules. The gene for CFH is located in the RCA cluster of genes on chromosome 1, at 1q32 (48). CFH is produced primarily in the liver, but like other complement components, it can also be made by monocytes, macrophages, fibroblasts, endothelial cells, and myoblasts. There are several variant forms of CFH, referred to as FH-like or FH-related proteins, that differ in size and function from CFH. In humans, these different forms of CFH appear to represent products of alternative splicing of the CFH gene, rather than separate genes (25).

CFH has multiple binding sites that interact with C3b, heparin, chondroitin sulfate and other polyanions, bacterial surface components, DNA, and endothelial cells. Its mode of action as a control protein is to bind to C3b and displace the Bb enzyme component of the C3 convertase. If additional C3b fragments are bound to or near the convertase, the avidity of this binding is increased. Once Bb has been removed, FI can use CFH as a cofactor in cleaving C3b to form iC3b, C3d,g, and C3c, thus preventing the C3b from interacting with B to form a new convertase. The fragments iC3b and C3d,g can interact with CR3 receptors on phagocytic cells and with CR2 receptors on B cells and dendritic cells, respectively (96, 97). In addition to its function as a fluid-phase control protein, CFH has been reported to have chemotactic activity for monocytes (69, 73). It also functions as an adhesion protein for neutrophils, possibly through the RGD sequence in the fourth CCP module. CFH binds to many cell types, including endothelial cells, through its polyanion binding regions and can serve as a cell surface control protein in this capacity.

CFH deficiency involves compromise of the complement regulatory action, which can be severe in patients that lack CFH protein completely. These patients have varied presentations, including recurrent infections, membranoproliferative glomerulonephritis, SLE, and atypical hemolytic-uremic syndrome (aHUS) (6, 67, 71). Initial lab results may identify them as C3 deficient, since without functional CFH, the C3 in their circulation is diminished or absent. More subtle deficiencies stem from point mutation in the CFH gene and result in decreased ability of the CFH to control complement on cell surfaces, particularly in the kidney (aHUS) and in the eye (age-related macular degeneration [AMD]) (24, 43, 44, 58, 77, 78). In the latter case, the mutated protein has not yet been characterized functionally but the gene defect was strongly associated with the susceptibility to AMD. An acquired form of aHUS was reported for a patient with anti-CFH autoantibodies (23).

Another disease-related property of CFH is the prevalence of bacterial or viral binding surface proteins that have evolved to bind it and thus wrap the microbe in a protective coating that prevents complement activation on their surfaces. Among the microbes that use this scheme to escape complement attack are strains of *Borrelia*, *Streptococcus*, *Yersinia*, and *Neisseria* (10, 17, 49, 63, 70, 76). This method of acquiring serum resistance also includes binding of other regulatory proteins (C4BP and membrane cofactor protein [MCP]) as well as RCA-like proteins encoded by the microbial DNA and expressed on the surface.

FI, also known in the literature as C3b-inactivator and KAF (conglutinogen-activating factor), is a single-chain serine protease that cleaves two sites on the α chains of both C4b and C3b: one on either side of the thioester bond region. This stops further participation of these molecules in complement activation and creates first iC4b or iC3b, followed by the final breakdown fragments C4c and C4d, and C3c and C3d,g. FI requires C4BP (for C4b cleavage) or CFH (for C3b cleavage) for cofactor activity in the fluid phase. On cell surfaces, the complement receptors CR1 and CR3 and MCP can fill this role as cofactors. FI is synthesized by hepatocytes, monocytes, fibroblasts, endothelial cells, myoblasts, glial cells, and Raji cells. The gene for FI is on chromosome 4, at 4q25. FI deficiency was first identified in a patient with little or no C3 in the circulation (1, 2). FI deficiencies, like those of CFH, are characterized by low or absent C3 in the circulation. FI deficiency is associated with recurrent severe pyogenic infections, vasculitis, glomerulonephritis, and aHUS (34, 37, 95).

DEFICIENCIES OF THE TERMINAL PATHWAY (LATE) COMPONENTS: C3, C5, C6, C7, C8, AND C9

Because C3 occupies the central position where the three initiating pathways merge with the terminal pathway, it is critical in the functioning of the system as a whole. C3 is an acute-phase reactant, increasing as much as twofold during inflammation. This increase may mask decreases due to activation, making it difficult to determine what is actually happening in vivo. Cleavage of C3 during complement activation produces a sequence of fragments, most of which have biological activities associated with opsonization, phagocytosis, immune adherence, effects on local vasodilation, smooth muscle contraction, and induction of mediator release, including histamine, from inflammatory cells. The absence of C3, either due to an inherited defect or an acquired condition, renders the individual highly susceptible to bacterial infections, membranoproliferative glomerulonephritis, and immune complex-mediated diseases such as lupus. The internal thioester bond in C3 is like that described earlier for C4 and leads to permanent attachment of the C3b and C3d fragments to the surface of the activating particle or molecule.

Most of the C3 in the circulation comes from hepatocytes, but many other cells can produce C3 and contribute to the local supply. The gene for human C3 is located on chromosome 19, at 19p13.3-p13.2 (102). Inheritance follows an autosomal recessive pattern in which the C3 protein is undetectable in the homozygous state and is approximately half the normal level in heterozygous individuals. The acquired forms of C3 deficiency can be profound and have been mistaken for genetic C3 deficiency on occasion. The usual causes of acquired C3 deficiency are secondary to deficiencies of FI or CFH, or the presence of autoantibodies to either of the C3 convertases, C3 or C4 nephritic factors, resulting in uncontrolled C3 cleavage in the circulation. In these cases, C3 fragments (iC3b, C3c, or C3a) can usually be detected in the circulation, and incubation of the patient's serum with normal serum or with purified C3 leads to C3 cleavage in the normal serum.

C5 is structurally similar to C3 but lacks the internal thioester bond that characterizes C3 and C4. When cleaved during activation, C5 also gives rise to similar fragments, but their activities are different from those for C3 and C4: C5b participates in the initiation and formation of the lytic complex (C5b-9) that inserts into the membrane of the target cells, and C5a is one of the most potent chemoattractants for neutrophils and other inflammatory cells. As an anaphylatoxin, C5a induces changes in vascular permeability, smooth muscle contraction, cell activation, upregulation of adherence molecules, and release of enzymes, mediators such as histamine, and cytokines.

Like C3, C5 is produced mainly in the liver but can also be synthesized by cells in the lung, spleen, and intestine, as well as by monocytes, macrophages, and alveolar type II cells. The gene for C5 is located on the ninth chromosome, at 9q33. Homozygous deficiency of C5 is associated with severe infections, often from *N. meningitidis* or *Neisseria gonorrhoeae*. C5-deficient individuals lack bactericidal activity and are unable to mobilize their neutrophils and other inflammatory cells to respond to bacterial infections. Other presentations have included discoid lupus and Sjögren's syndrome (3, 80). Several strains of mice have spontaneously occurring C5 deficiency.

C6 and C7 are similar proteins that are encoded by genes on the fifth chromosome, at 5p12-14. Another complement gene, C9, is close to this locus as well. Unlike the previously discussed complement proteins up through C5 in the activation pathways, none of the late components (C6, C7, C8, and C9) is cleaved during activation, but all are integral proteins in the formation of the membrane attack complex (MAC) or the terminal complement complex. C6 binds to a neoepitope exposed on C5b, forming the C5b-6 complex that is rapidly expanded to C5b-6-7 by the addition of C7. The final complex formation occurs on a membrane surface when C8 binds and C9 polymerizes to form the membranolytic complement lesion, C5b-9, on the cell surface, leading to osmotic lysis of the cell.

Deficiencies of C6 and C7 are associated with recurrent severe neisserial infections as well as infections caused by other pyogenic bacteria, although there have been reports of lupus in individuals with these deficiencies as well. A number of cases of combined deficiency of C6 and C7 have been reported, as well as the influence of one gene upon the synthesis rate of the other, leading to decreased production of one of the proteins from an otherwise normal gene. Subtotal deficiencies of both proteins were accompanied in one patient by a lower-molecular-weight form of C6 that was associated with a defect in the 5′ splice donor site of intron 15 of the C6 gene. The same patient had low C7 as well, with the C7 protein containing an Arg→Ser substitution that altered the protein's isoelectric point. Patients with complete deficiency of C6 or C7 lack measurable protein and have little or no hemolytic activity in the CH50 or AH50 assays. Subtotal deficiencies of C6 or C7 are similar, although loss of hemolytic function is not complete (29).

C8 is a complex protein made up of three nonidentical polypeptide chains: a disulfide-linked α-γ pair and a noncovalently linked β chain. Each one of the chains is coded for by a separate gene and the protein is assembled intracellularly, although there is evidence from deficiencies that C8α-γ and C8β may be produced and secreted independently. The intact molecule is required for function in the lysis of the target cell (88).

The genes for the C8 subunits are located on the first (C8α and C8β at 1p32) and ninth (C8γ at 9q34.4) chromosomes. The three chains of C8 are interesting in that C8α and C8β are similar to C6, C7, and C9 in their structure, while C8γ is more closely related to the lipocalin family of proteins that bind and transport small hydrophobic ligands (56). Because C8 deficiency is due to decreased or a lack of synthesis of only part of the complex molecule (C8α chain or C8β chain), the part of the molecule that is produced is recognized by the antisera used for measuring C8 levels in serum, giving, in effect, a false-positive result. This makes it necessary to use caution in diagnosing C8 deficiency from protein levels alone, and a functional test should be done as well. C8 deficiency, like that of other MAC proteins, is characterized by recurrent infections, most often caused by neisserial species. C8 is synthesized primarily by hepatocytes, although it can also be produced by cells of monocyte/macrophage lineage, astrocytes, oligodendrocytes, fibroblasts, and endothelial cells.

As the MAC is assembled on the cell surface, the C5 to C8 proteins are joined by C9, the final protein in the terminal complement pathway. The C9 protein unfolds to form polymers that penetrate the membrane and create perturbations that lead to osmotic lysis of the target cells. Estimates of the number of C9 molecules required to form a lytic pore range from 6 to 18 (68). C9 is produced primarily by hepatocytes and secondarily by monocytes, glial cells, fibroblasts, and other local cells at sites of inflammation. It is an acute-phase protein and is coded for by a gene at 5p13, close to the genes for C5 and C6.

Many cases of C9 deficiency have been reported, and the remarkable thing is the lack of strong association of disease phenotypes with this complement deficiency. Although there have been scattered reports of neisserial infections, most C9-deficient patients appear to be healthy. This is most likely because C9 is not absolutely required for lysis of the target cell. C9 is the most common complement component deficiency in Japan and perhaps in other Asian populations as well (35, 50, 55).

CONTROL PROTEINS OF THE TERMINAL PATHWAY: S-PROTEIN, CLUSTERIN, AND CD59

Protection of host cells from "bystander lysis" caused by insertion of fluid-phase C5b-9 (MAC) complexes is accomplished by several mechanisms. Two proteins, S-protein (vitronectin) and clusterin (SP 40,40 or apolipoprotein J), act as solubilizing factors to bind the MAC and block its hydrophobic insertion into the membranes of nearby cells. These proteins can bind to C5b-7 and C5b-8 in the fluid phase, preventing membrane interaction and C9 polymerization, although at least one C9 molecule is associated with the final SC5b-9 complexes detected in the circulation. This complex is relatively long-lived and may serve as a marker for complement activation when most other complement fragments (C3a, C5a, etc.) have been cleared from the circulation. No deficiency of either of these proteins has been identified to date.

CD59 is a membrane-bound glycoprotein that inhibits the polymerization of C9 and the lytic activity of the MAC. It is expressed on a wide variety of cell types, including erythrocytes. Because it is species specific, it is the primary cell surface protector against lysis mediated by homologous complement. CD59 is linked to the cell membrane by a glycophosphatidylinositol anchor that is variably lost from cells in patients with paroxysmal nocturnal hemoglobinuria; CD59 loss provides one of the mechanisms for hemolysis in these patients.

THERAPY FOR COMPLEMENT DEFICIENCIES

Treatment of patients with complement deficiencies has been limited to treatment of infection and autoimmunity. At this point in time the use of recombinant components for a completely deficient patient is possible, but the hurdles of economics and potential of immune responses to the recombinant proteins make this tactic unlikely to succeed. Blood

transfusion to replace C2 was tried with some success in two SLE patients and several HUS patients with CFH deficiency (6, 7). Purified plasma C1-Inh has been successful at the time of attacks, but other possible drugs are currently in the pipeline, including recombinant C1-Inh and a specific inhibitor of the bradykinin receptor BK2.

Recombinant or monoclonal antibody complement inhibitors have been used in ischemia-reperfusion injury, cardiopulmonary bypass surgery, and autoimmune disorders. Soluble CR1 acts against the C3 and C5 convertases of both the AP and CP (74, 75, 105, 106), and a humanized anti-C5 monoclonal antibody that prevents cleavage of C5 to C5a and C5b has been effective in animal models and clinical trials (31, 89, 98, 99). In paroxysmal nocturnal hemoglobinuria, however, complement inhibition by one of the C5 inhibitors led to a prompt reversal of the hemolytic process (72). Given this beginning, it seems only a matter of time until most patients with complement deficiencies can be helped by compounds that will reverse the acute symptoms as well as provide long-term prevention of the often devastating diseases associated with malfunction of this important immune pathway.

REFERENCES

1. **Abramson, N., C. A. Alper, P. J. Lachmann, F. S. Rosen, and J. H. Jandl.** 1971. Deficiency of C3 inactivator in man. *J. Immunol.* **107:**19–27.

2. **Alper, C. A., N. Abramson, R. B. Johnston, Jr., J. H. Jandl, and F. S. Rosen.** 1970. Studies in vivo and in vitro on an abnormality in the metabolism of C3 in a patient with increased susceptibility to infection. *J. Clin. Investig.* **49:**1975–1985.

3. **Asghar, S. S., G. T. Venneker, M. van Meegen, M. M. Meinardi, R. F. Hulsmans, and L. P. de Waal.** 1991. Hereditary deficiency of C5 in association with discoid lupus erythematosus. *J. Am. Acad. Dermatol.* **24**(Part 2): 376–378.

4. **Atkinson, J. P.** 1989. Complement deficiency: predisposing factor to autoimmune syndromes. *Clin. Exp. Rheumatol.* **7:**95–101.

5. **Atkinson, J. P., and P. M. Schneider.** 1999. Genetic susceptibility and class III complement genes, p. 91–104. *In* R. G. Lahita (ed.), *Systemic Lupus Erythematosus.* Academic Press, San Diego, Calif.

6. **Ault, B. H.** 2000. Factor H and the pathogenesis of renal diseases. *Pediatr. Nephrol.* **14:**1045–1053.

7. **Bala Subramanian, V., M. K. Liszewski, and J. P. Atkinson.** 2000. The complement system and autoimmunity. *In* R. G. Lahita, N. Chiorazzi, and W. Reeves (ed.), *Textbook of Autoimmune Diseases.* Lippincott-Raven, Philadelphia, Pa.

8. **Biesma, D. H., A. J. Hannema, H. van Velzen-Blad, L. Mulder, R. van Zwieten, I. Kluijt, and D. Roos.** 2001. A family with complement factor D deficiency. *J. Clin. Investig.* **108:**233–240.

9. **Binkley, K. E., and A. E. Davis III.** 2003. Estrogen-dependent inherited angioedema. *Transfus. Apher. Sci.* **29:**215–219.

10. **Blackmore, T. K., V. A. Fischetti, T. A. Sadlon, H. M. Ward, and D. L. Gordon.** 1998. M protein of the group A *Streptococcus* binds to the seventh short consensus repeat of human complement factor H. *Infect. Immun.* **66:**1427–1431.

11. **Bork, K., S. E. Barnstedt, P. Koch, and H. Taupe.** 2000. Hereditary angioedema with normal C1-inhibitor activity in women. *Lancet* **356:**1440–1441.

12. **Bowen, B., J. J. Hawk, and S. Sibunka.** 2001. A review of the reported defects in the human C1 esterase inhibitor

gene producing hereditary angioedema including four new mutations. *Clin. Immunol.* **87:**157–163.

13. **Caldwell, J. R., S. Ruddy, P. H. Schur, and K. F. Austen.** 1972. Acquired C1 inhibitor deficiency in lymphosarcoma. *Clin. Immunol. Immunopathol.* **1:**39–52.

14. **Carlsson, M., A. G. Sjoholm, L. Eriksson, S. Thiel, J. C. Jensenius, M. Segelmark, and L. Truedsson.** 2005. Deficiency of the mannan-binding lectin pathway of complement and poor outcome in cystic fibrosis: bacterial colonization may be decisive for a relationship. *Clin. Exp. Immunol.* **139:**306–313.

15. **Carroll, M. C., R. D. Campbell, D. R. Bentley, and R. R. Porter.** 1984. A molecular map of the human major histocompatibility complex class III region linking complement genes C4, C2 and factor B. *Nature* **307:**237–241.

16. **Casanova, J. L., and L. Abel.** 2004. Human mannose-binding lectin in immunity: friend, foe, or both? *J. Exp. Med.* **199:**1295–1299.

17. **China, B., M. P. Sory, B. T. N'Guyen, M. De Bruyere, and G. R. Cornelis.** 1993. Role of the YadA protein in prevention of opsonization of *Yersinia enterocolitica* by C3b molecules. *Infect. Immun.* **61:**3129–3136.

18. **Cicardi, M., and A. Agostoni.** 1996. Hereditary angioedema. *N. Engl. J. Med.* **334:**1666–1667.

19. **Dahlback, B., C. A. Smith, and H. J. Muller-Eberhard.** 1983. Visualization of human C4b-binding protein and its complexes with vitamin K-dependent protein S and complement protein C4b. *Proc. Natl. Acad. Sci. USA* **80:**3461–3465.

20. **Davis, A. E.** 2003. The pathogenesis of hereditary angioedema. *Transfus. Apher. Sci.* **29:**195–203.

21. **Davis, A. E. I.** 1998. C1 inhibitor gene and hereditary angioedema, p. 229–444. *In* J. E. Volanakis and M. M. Frank (ed.), *The Human Complement System in Health and Disease.* Marcel Dekker, New York, N.Y.

22. **Donaldson, V. H., and J. J. Bissler.** 1992. C1 inhibitors and their genes: an update. *J. Lab. Clin. Med.* **119:**330–333.

23. **Dragon-Durey, M. A., C. Loirat, S. Cloarec, M. A. Macher, J. Blouin, H. Nivet, L. Weiss, W. H. Fridman, and V. Fremeaux-Bacchi.** 2005. Anti-factor H autoantibodies associated with atypical hemolytic uremic syndrome. *J. Am. Soc. Nephrol.* **16:**555–563.

24. **Edwards, A. O., R. Ritter III, K. J. Abel, A. Manning, C. Panhuysen, and L. A. Farrer.** 2005. Complement factor H polymorphism and age-related macular degeneration. *Science* **308:**421–424.

25. **Estaller, C., W. Schwaeble, M. Dierich, and E. H. Weiss.** 1991. Human complement factor H: two factor H proteins are derived from alternatively spliced transcripts. *Eur. J. Immunol.* **21:**799–802.

26. **Farries, T. C., P. J. Lachmann, and R. A. Harrison.** 1988. Analysis of the interaction between properdin and factor B, components of the alternative-pathway C3 convertase of complement. *Biochem. J.* **253:**667–675.

27. **Farries, T. C., P. J. Lachmann, and R. A. Harrison.** 1988. Analysis of the interactions between properdin, the third component of complement (C3), and its physiological activation products. *Biochem. J.* **252:**47–54.

28. **Fearon, D. T.** 1979. Activation of the alternative complement pathway. *Crit. Rev. Immunol.* **1:**1–32. (Review.)

29. **Fernie, B. A., R. Wurzner, A. Orren, B. P. Morgan, P. C. Potter, A. E. Platonov, I. V. Vershinina, G. A. Shipulin, P. J. Lachmann, and M. J. Hobart.** 1996. Molecular bases of combined subtotal deficiencies of C6 and C7: their effects in combination with other C6 and C7 deficiencies. *J. Immunol.* **157:**3648–3657.

30. **Figueroa, J. E., and P. Densen.** 1991. Infectious diseases associated with complement deficiencies. *Clin. Microbiol. Rev.* **4:**359–395.

31. **Fitch, J. C., S. Rollins, L. Matis, B. Alford, S. Aranki, C. D. Collard, M. Dewar, J. Elefteriades, R. Hines, G. Kopf, P. Kraker, L. Li, R. O'Hara, C. Rinder, H. Rinder, R. Shaw, B. Smith, G. Stahl, and S. K. Shernan.** 1999. Pharmacology and biological efficacy of a recombinant, humanized, single-chain antibody C5 complement inhibitor in patients undergoing coronary artery bypass graft surgery with cardiopulmonary bypass. *Circulation* **100:**2499–2506.

32. **Frank, M. M.** 1993. Hereditary angioedema, p. 229–243. *In* K. Whaley, M. M. Loos, and J. M. Weiler (ed.), *Complement in Health and Disease.* Kluwer Academic, Dordrecht, The Netherlands.

33. **Frank, M. M., F. Gelfand, and J. P. Atkinson.** 1976. Hereditary angioedema: clinical syndrome and its management. *Ann. Intern. Med.* **84:**580–593.

34. **Fujita, T., I. Gigli, and V. Nussenzweig.** 1978. Human C4-binding protein. II. Role in proteolysis of C4b by C3b-inactivator. *J. Exp. Med.* **148:**1044–1051.

35. **Fukumori, Y., K. Yoshimura, S. Ohnoki, H. Yamaguchi, Y. Akagaki, and S. Inai.** 1989. A high incidence of C9 deficiency among healthy blood donors in Osaka, Japan. *Int. Immunol.* **1:**85–89.

36. **Gadjeva, M., S. R. Paludan, S. Thiel, V. Slavov, M. Ruseva, K. Eriksson, G. B. Lowhagen, L. Shi, K. Takahashi, A. Ezekowitz, and J. C. Jensenius.** 2004. Mannan-binding lectin modulates the response to HSV-2 infection. *Clin. Exp. Immunol.* **138:**304–311.

37. **Genel, F., A. G. Sjoholm, L. Skattum, and L. Truedsson.** 2005. Complement factor I deficiency associated with recurrent infections, vasculitis and immune complex glomerulonephritis. *Scand. J. Infect. Dis.* **37:**615–618.

38. **Giclas, P. C.** 2002. Choosing complement tests: differentiating between hereditary and acquired deficiency, p. 111–116. *In* N. R. Rose, R. G. Hamilton, and B. Detrick (ed.), *Manual of Clinical Laboratory Immunology,* 6th ed. ASM Press, Washington, D.C.

39. **Giclas, P. C.** 1997. Complement tests, p. 181–186. *In* N. R. Rose, E. Conway de Macario, J. D. Folds, H. C. Lane, and R. M. Nakamura (ed.), *Manual of Clinical Laboratory Immunology,* 5th ed. ASM Press, Washington, D.C.

40. **Goundis, D., S. M. Holt, Y. Boyd, and K. B. Reid.** 1989. Localization of the properdin structural locus to Xp11.23-Xp21.1. *Genomics* **5:**56–60.

41. **Gronski, P., L. Bodenbender, E. J. Kanzy, and F. R. Seiler.** 1988. C4-binding protein prevents spontaneous cleavage of C3 in sera of patients with hereditary angioedema. *Complement* **5:**1–12.

42. **Guo, N., T. Mogues, S. Weremowicz, C. C. Morton, and K. N. Sastry.** 1998. The human ortholog of rhesus mannose-binding protein-A gene is an expressed pseudogene that localizes to chromosome 10. *Mamm. Genome* **9:**246–249.

43. **Hageman, G. S., D. H. Anderson, L. V. Johnson, L. S. Hancox, A. J. Taiber, L. I. Hardisty, J. L. Hageman, H. A. Stockman, J. D. Borchardt, K. M. Gehrs, R. J. Smith, G. Silvestri, S. R. Russell, C. C. Klaver, I. Barbazetto, S. Chang, L. A. Yannuzzi, G. R. Barile, J. C. Merriam, R. T. Smith, A. K. Olsh, J. Bergeron, J. Zernant, J. E. Merriam, B. Gold, M. Dean, and R. Allikmets.** 2005. A common haplotype in the complement regulatory gene factor H (HF1/CFH) predisposes individuals to age-related macular degeneration. *Proc. Natl. Acad. Sci. USA* **102:**7227–7232.

44. **Haines, J. L., M. A. Hauser, S. Schmidt, W. K. Scott, L. M. Olson, P. Gallins, K. L. Spencer, S. Y. Kwan, M. Noureddine, J. R. Gilbert, N. Schnetz-Boutaud, A. Agarwal, E. A. Postel, and M. A. Pericak-Vance.** 2005. Complement factor H variant increases the risk of age-related macular degeneration. *Science* **308:**419–421.

45. **Han, E. D., R. C. MacFarlane, A. N. Mulligan, J. Scafidi, and A. E. Davis III.** 2002. Increased vascular permeability

in C1 inhibitor-deficient mice mediated by the bradykinin type 2 receptor. *J. Clin. Investig.* **109:**1057–1063.

46. **Hart, M. L., K. A. Ceonzo, L. A. Shaffer, K. Takahashi, R. P. Rother, W. R. Reenstra, J. A. Buras, and G. L. Stahl.** 2005. Gastrointestinal ischemia-reperfusion injury is lectin complement pathway dependent without involving C1q. *J. Immunol.* **174:**6373–6380.

47. **Hellwage, J., S. Kuhn, and P. F. Zipfel.** 1997. The human complement regulatory factor-H-like protein 1, which represents a truncated form of factor H, displays cell-attachment activity. *Biochem. J.* **326**(Part 2):321–327.

48. **Hing, S., A. J. Day, S. J. Linton, J. Ripoche, R. B. Sim, K. B. Reid, and E. Solomon.** 1988. Assignment of complement components C4 binding protein (C4BP) and factor H (FH) to human chromosome 1q, using cDNA probes. *Ann. Hum. Genet.* **52**(Part 2):117–122.

49. **Horstmann, R. D., H. J. Sievertsen, J. Knobloch, and V. A. Fischetti.** 1988. Antiphagocytic activity of streptococcal M protein: selective binding of complement control protein factor H. *Proc. Natl. Acad. Sci. USA* **85:**1657–1661.

50. **Inai, S., H. Kitamura, S. Hiramatsu, and K. Nagaki.** 1979. Deficiency of the ninth component of complement in man. *J. Clin. Lab. Immunol.* **2:**85–87.

51. **Inanc, N., G. Mumcu, E. Birtas, Y. Elbir, S. Yavuz, T. Ergun, I. Fresko, and H. Direskeneli.** 2005. Serum mannose-binding lectin levels are decreased in Behcet's disease and associated with disease severity. *J. Rheumatol.* **32:**287–291.

52. **Ip, W. K., K. H. Chan, H. K. Law, G. H. Tso, E. K. Kong, W. H. Wong, Y. F. To, R. W. Yung, E. Y. Chow, K. L. Au, E. Y. Chan, W. Lim, J. C. Jensenius, M. W. Turner, J. S. Peiris, and Y. L. Lau.** 2005. Mannose-binding lectin in severe acute respiratory syndrome coronavirus infection. *J. Infect. Dis.* **191:**1697–1704.

53. **Jackson, J., R. B. Sim, A. Whelan, and C. Feighery.** 1986. An IgG autoantibody which inactivates C1-inhibitor. *Nature* **323:**722–724.

54. **Johnson, C. A., P. Densen, R. A. Wetsel, F. S. Cole, N. E. Goeken, and H. R. Colten.** 1992. Molecular heterogeneity of C2 deficiency. *N. Engl. J. Med.* **326:**871–874.

55. **Kang, H. J., H. S. Kim, Y. K. Lee, and H. C. Cho.** 2005. High incidence of complement C9 deficiency in Koreans. *Ann. Clin. Lab. Sci.* **35:**144–148.

56. **Kaufman, K. M., and J. M. Sodetz.** 1994. Genomic structure of the human complement protein C8 gamma: homology to the lipocalin gene family. *Biochemistry* **33:**5162–5166.

57. **Kildsgaard, J., E. Zsigmond, L. Chan, and R. A. Wetsel.** 1999. A critical evaluation of the putative role of C3adesArg (ASP) in lipid metabolism and hyperapobetalipoproteinemia. *Mol. Immunol.* **36:**869–876.

58. **Klein, R. J., C. Zeiss, E. Y. Chew, J. Y. Tsai, R. S. Sackler, C. Haynes, A. K. Henning, J. P. SanGiovanni, S. M. Mane, S. T. Mayne, M. B. Bracken, F. L. Ferris, J. Ott, C. Barnstable, and J. Hoh.** 2005. Complement factor H polymorphism in age-related macular degeneration. *Science* **308:**385–389.

59. **Kolble, K., A. J. Cant, A. C. Fay, K. Whaley, M. Schlesinger, and K. B. Reid.** 1993. Carrier detection in families with properdin deficiency by microsatellite haplotyping. *J. Clin. Investig.* **91:**99–102.

60. **Kusumoto, H., S. Hirosawa, J. P. Salier, F. S. Hagen, and K. Kurachi.** 1988. Human genes for complement components C1r and C1s in a close tail-to-tail arrangement. *Proc. Natl. Acad. Sci. USA* **85:**7307–7311.

61. **Lu, J., C. Teh, U. Kishore, and K. B. Reid.** 2002. Collectins and ficolins: sugar pattern recognition molecules of the mammalian innate immune system. *Biochim. Biophys. Acta* **1572:**387–400.

62. **Matsushita, M., Y. Endo, and T. Fujita.** 2000. Cutting edge: complement-activating complex of ficolin and mannose-binding lectin-associated serine protease. *J. Immunol.* **164:**2281–2284.

63. **McDowell, J. V., J. Wolfgang, E. Tran, M. S. Metts, D. Hamilton, and R. T. Marconi.** 2003. Comprehensive analysis of the factor H binding capabilities of *Borrelia* species associated with Lyme disease: delineation of two distinct classes of factor H binding proteins. *Infect. Immun.* **71:**3597–3602.

64. **Melamed, J., C. A. Alper, M. Cicardi, and F. S. Rosen.** 1986. The metabolism of C1 inhibitor and C1q in patients with acquired C1-inhibitor deficiency. *J. Allergy Clin. Immunol.* **77:**322–326.

65. **Morgan, B. P., and M. J. Walport.** 1991. Complement deficiency and disease. *Immunol. Today* **12:**301–306.

66. **Mortensen, J. P., and L. U. Lamm.** 1981. Quantitative differences between complement factor-B phenotypes. *Immunology* **42:**505–511.

67. **Moseley, H. L., and K. Whaley.** 1980. Control of complement activation in membranous and membranoproliferative glomerulonephritis. *Kidney Int.* **17:**535–544.

68. **Muller-Eberhard, H. J.** 1985. The killer molecule of complement. *J. Investig. Dermatol.* **85**(1 Suppl.):47s–52s. (Review.)

69. **Nabil, K., B. Rihn, M. C. Jaurand, J. M. Vignaud, J. Ripoche, Y. Martinet, and N. Martinet.** 1997. Identification of human complement factor H as a chemotactic protein for monocytes. *Biochem. J.* **326** (Part 2):377–383.

70. **Neeleman, C., S. P. Geelen, P. C. Aerts, M. R. Daha, T. E. Mollnes, J. J. Roord, G. Posthuma, H. van Dijk, and A. Fleer.** 1999. Resistance to both complement activation and phagocytosis in type 3 pneumococci is mediated by the binding of complement regulatory protein factor H. *Infect. Immun.* **67:**4517–4524.

71. **Nielsen, H. E., K. C. Christensen, C. Koch, B. S. Thomsen, N. H. Heegaard, and J. Tranum-Jensen.** 1989. Hereditary, complete deficiency of complement factor H associated with recurrent meningococcal disease. *Scand. J. Immunol.* **30:**711–718.

72. **Ninomiya, H., Y. Kawashima, and T. Nagasawa.** 2000. Inhibition of complement-mediated haemolysis in paroxysmal nocturnal haemoglobinuria by heparin or low-molecular weight heparin. *Br. J. Haematol.* **109:**875–881.

73. **Ohtsuka, H., T. Imamura, M. Matsushita, S. Tanase, H. Okada, M. Ogawa, and T. Kambara.** 1993. Thrombin generates monocyte chemotactic activity from complement factor H. *Immunology* **80:**140–145.

74. **Perry, G. J.** 1998. Phase I safety trial of soluble complement receptor type (TP 10) on acute myocardial infarction. *J. Am. Coll. Cardiol.* **31:**411A.

75. **Quigg, R. J.** 2002. Use of complement inhibitors in tissue injury. *Trends Mol. Med.* **8:**430–436.

76. **Ram, S., A. K. Sharma, S. D. Simpson, S. Gulati, D. P. McQuillen, M. K. Pangburn, and P. A. Rice.** 1998. A novel sialic acid binding site on factor H mediates serum resistance of sialylated *Neisseria gonorrhoeae. J. Exp. Med.* **187:**743–752.

77. **Richards, A., J. A. Goodship, and T. H. Goodship.** 2002. The genetics and pathogenesis of haemolytic uremic syndrome and thrombotic thrombocytopenic purpura. *Curr. Opin. Nephrol. Hypertens.* **11:**431–435.

78. **Richards, A., E. J. Kemp, M. K. Liszewski, J. A. Goodship, A. K. Lampe, R. Decorte, M. H. Muslumanoglu, S. Kavukcu, G. Filler, Y. Pirson, L. S. Wen, J. P. Atkinson, and T. H. Goodship.** 2003. Mutations in human complement regulator, membrane cofactor protein (CD46), predispose to development of familial hemolytic uremic syndrome. *Proc. Natl. Acad. Sci. USA* **100:**12966–12971.

79. Sastry, K., G. S. Herman, L. Day, E. Deignan, G. Bruns, C. C. Morton, and R. A. Ezekowitz. 1989. The human mannose-binding protein gene. Exon structure reveals its evolutionary relationship to a human pulmonary surfactant gene and localization to chromosome 10. *J. Exp. Med.* **170:**1175–1189.

80. Schoonbrood, T. H., A. Hannema, C. A. Fijen, H. M. Markusse, and A. H. Swaak. 1995. C5 deficiency in a patient with primary Sjogren's syndrome. *J. Rheumatol.* **22:**1389–1390.

81. Schwaeble, W., M. R. Dahl, S. Thiel, C. Stover, and J. C. Jensenius. 2002. The mannan-binding lectin-associated serine proteases (MASPs) and MAp19: four components of the lectin pathway activation complex encoded by two genes. *Immunobiology* **205:**455–466.

82. Sellar, G. C., C. Cockburn, and K. B. Reid. 1992. Localization of the gene cluster encoding the A, B, and C chains of human C1q to 1p34.1-1p36.3. *Immunogenetics* **35:**214–216.

83. Sjoholm, A. G., J. H. Braconier, and C. Soderstrom. 1982. Properdin deficiency in a family with fulminant meningococcal infections. *Clin. Exp. Immunol.* **50:**291–297.

84. Sjoholm, A. G., C. Soderstrom, and L. A. Nilsson. 1988. A second variant of properdin deficiency: the detection of properdin at low concentrations in affected males. *Complement* **5:**130–140.

85. Sorensen, R., S. Thiel, and J. C. Jensenius. 2005. Mannan-binding-lectin-associated serine proteases, characteristics and disease associations. *Springer Semin. Immunopathol.* **27:**299–319.

86. Stefansson Thors, V., R. Kolka, S. L. Sigurdardottir, V. O. Edvardsson, G. Arason, and A. Haraldsson. 2005. Increased frequency of C4B*Q0 alleles in patients with Henoch-Schonlein purpura. *Scand. J. Immunol.* **61:**274–278.

87. Takahashi, R., A. Tsutsumi, K. Ohtani, D. Goto, I. Matsumoto, S. Ito, N. Wakamiya, and T. Sumida. 2004. Anti-mannose binding lectin antibodies in sera of Japanese patients with systemic lupus erythematosus. *Clin. Exp. Immunol.* **136:**585–590.

88. Tedesco, F., P. Densen, M. A. Villa, B. H. Petersen, and G. Sirchia. 1983. Two types of dysfunctional eighth component of complement (C8) molecules in C8 deficiency in man. Reconstitution of normal C8 from the mixture of two abnormal C8 molecules. *J. Clin. Investig.* **71:**183–191.

89. Thomas, T. C., S. A. Rollins, R. P. Rother, M. A. Giannoni, S. L. Hartman, E. A. Elliot, S. H. Nye, L. A. Matis, S. P. Squinto, and M. J. Evans. 1996. Inhibition of complement activity by humanized anti-C5 antibody and single-chain Fv. *Mol. Immunol.* **33:**1389–1401.

90. Trapp, R. G., M. Fletcher, J. Forristal, and C. D. West. 1987. C4 binding protein deficiency in a patient with atypical Behcet's disease. *J. Rheumatol.* **14:**135–138.

91. Tsao, B. P. 2000. Lupus susceptibility genes on human chromosome 1. *Int. Rev. Immunol.* **19:**319–334.

92. Turner, M. W. 1996. Mannose-binding lectin: the pluripotent molecule of the innate immune system. *Immunol. Today* **17:**532–540.

93. Turner, M. W. 2003. The role of mannose-binding lectin in health and disease. *Mol. Immunol.* **40:**423–429.

94. Volanakis, J. E., and S. V. Narayana. 1996. Complement factor D, a novel serine protease. *Protein Sci.* **5:**553–564. (Review.)

95. Vyse, T. J., B. J. Morley, I. Bartok, E. L. Theodoridis, K. A. Davies, A. D. Webster, and M. J. Walport. 1996. The molecular basis of hereditary complement factor I deficiency. *J. Clin. Investig.* **97:**925–933.

96. Walport, M. J. 2001. Complement: first of two parts. *N. Engl. J. Med.* **344:**1058–1066.

97. Walport, M. J. 2001. Complement: second of two parts. *N. Engl. J. Med.* **344:**1140–1144.

98. Wang, Y., Q. Hu, J. A. Madri, S. A. Rollins, A. Chodera, and L. A. Matis. 1996. Amelioration of lupus-like autoimmune disease in NZB-WF1 mice after treatment with a blocking monoclonal antibody specific for complement component C5. *Proc. Natl. Acad. Sci. USA* **93:**8563–8568.

99. Wang, Y., S. A. Rollins, J. A. Madri, and L. A. Matis. 1995. Anti-C5 monoclonal antibody therapy prevents collagen-induced arthritis and ameliorates established disease. *Proc. Natl. Acad. Sci. USA* **92:**8955–8959.

100. Westberg, J., G. N. Fredrikson, L. Truedsson, A. G. Sjoholm, and M. Uhlen. 1995. Sequence-based analysis of properdin deficiency: identification of point mutations in two phenotypic forms of an X-linked immunodeficiency. *Genomics* **29:**1–8.

101. White, R. T., D. Damm, N. Hancock, B. S. Rosen, B. B. Lowell, P. Usher, J. S. Flier, and B. M. Spiegelman. 1992. Human adipsin is identical to complement factor D and is expressed at high levels in adipose tissue. *J. Biol. Chem.* **267:**9210–9213.

102. Whitehead, A. S., E. Solomon, S. Chambers, W. F. Bodmer, S. Povey, and G. Fey. 1982. Assignment of the structural gene for the third component of human complement to chromosome 19. *Proc. Natl. Acad. Sci. USA* **79:**5021–5025.

103. Yang, Y., E. K. Chung, B. Zhou, C. A. Blanchong, C. Y. Yu, G. Fust, M. Kovacs, A. Vatay, C. Szalai, I. Karadi, and L. Varga. 2003. Diversity in intrinsic strengths of the human complement system: serum C4 protein concentrations correlate with C4 gene size and polygenic variations, hemolytic activities, and body mass index. *J. Immunol.* **171:**2734–2745.

104. Yu, C. Y., C. A. Blanchong, E. K. Chung, K. L. Rupert, Y. Yang, Z. Yang, B. Zhou, and J. M. Moulds. 2002. Molecular genetic analysis of human complement components C4A and C4B, p. 117–131. *In* N. R. Rose, R. G. Hamilton, and B. Detrick (ed.), *Manual of Clinical Laboratory Immunology*, 6th ed. ASM Press, Washington, D.C.

105. Zamora, M. R., R. D. Davis, S. H. Keshavjee, L. Schulman, J. Levin, U. Ryan, and G. A. Patterson. 1999. Complement inhibition attenuates human lung transplant reperfusion injury: a multicenter trial. *Chest* **116**(1 Suppl.):4S.

106. Zimmerman, J. L., R. P. Dellinger, R. C. Straube, and J. L. Levin. 2000. Phase I trial of the recombinant soluble complement receptor 1 in acute lung injury and acute respiratory distress syndrome. *Crit. Care Med.* **28:**3149–3154.

Neutropenia and Neutrophil Defects

STEVEN M. HOLLAND

103

Concern about the neutrophil status of a patient is usually raised on the basis of the frequency, severity, distribution, or specific infectious agent(s) involved in one or more episodes that are, or are thought to be, infectious. The clinical presentations of patients with neutrophil disorders usually share a few common features: gingivitis, periodontal disease, and oral ulceration. Cutaneous infections with *Staphylococcus aureus* are often recurrent and can be severe. In neutrophil disorders characterized by inadequate inflammation (neutropenia, leukocyte adhesion deficiency [LAD], Chédiak-Higashi syndrome, and specific granule deficiency), infections can extend locally and subcutaneously with little reaction until marked destruction has taken place. Clinically relevant neutrophil abnormalities fall into several broad categories: neutropenia, abnormalities of neutrophil adherence and locomotion, abnormalities of neutrophil granule formation or content, and abnormalities of killing. With the widespread use of therapies which modulate the immune system either by design (e.g., steroids and monoclonal antibodies) or incidentally (e.g., cytotoxic chemotherapy), the most common causes of immunodeficiency are iatrogenic. The recognition, characterization, identification, and cloning of disease-related genes and, in some cases, genetic correction of immune defects are moving rapidly. As specific and genetic treatments become available, making the correct diagnosis early takes on greater therapeutic importance (reviewed in reference 6).

The clinical history should include type, location, microbiology, severity, and frequency of infections; family history with specific questioning as to consanguinity; and physical examination of the oral mucosa and any lesions or scars. Complete peripheral blood count with differential and examination of the peripheral smear are necessary initial studies to determine whether the patient has a quantitative, qualitative, or combined abnormality of neutrophils.

NEUTROPENIA

The normal neutrophil count in peripheral blood is about 4,000/mm³, with a large variation among racial and ethnic groups, especially certain West Indian and African blacks and Yemeni Jews, who may have much lower neutrophil counts. Neutropenia is determined by the presence of fewer than 1,500 neutrophils/mm³. Increased risk of infections does not occur until the absolute neutrophil count (the sum of mature and band form neutrophils) falls below 1,000/mm³; risk of serious infections occurs below 500 neutrophils/mm³. Since about 90% of the body's neutrophils are kept in reserve in the bone marrow, neutropenias with impaired marrow stores are associated with greater infection risk than neutropenias with normal marrow stores. Thus, acute neutropenias associated with lack of marrow reserves, such as those induced by cancer chemotherapy, are usually associated with greater infectious complications than chronic neutropenias.

There are three basic mechanisms by which neutropenia can occur: decreased neutrophil production, increased neutrophil destruction, or abnormal neutrophil trafficking (either defective release of neutrophils from the bone marrow or an abnormal increase in the marginated or tissue pools). Recently, an autosomal dominant disorder with mild neutropenia due to neutrophil retention in the bone marrow (myelokathexis) has been molecularly characterized. The syndrome of warts, hypogammaglobulinemia, infections, and myelokathexis (WHIM) is due to mutations in the chemokine receptor CXCR4 which lead to retention of mature neutrophils on their marrow-expressed ligand stromal cell-derived factor 1 (SDF1; CXCL12). Major causes of intrinsic, acquired, and apparent neutropenia are listed in Table 1. An acquired cause of neutrophil destruction is antineutrophil antibodies. These antibodies can be detected in the clinical laboratory by either immunofluorescence or agglutination, procedures which are readily available in most laboratories.

Methods of neutrophil preparation and isolation are reviewed in chapter 31 of this volume.

Antineutrophil Antibodies

Principle

Antineutrophil antibodies may cause neutrophils to be more susceptible to complement-mediated lysis, enhance neutrophil sequestration via Fc receptors on tissue macrophages, or affect the maturation and development of myeloid precursors. Detection of these antibodies in a flow cytometer relies upon demonstration of specific binding of patient immunoglobulin G (IgG) and IgM to neutrophils (2, 3, 9). Many of these antibodies are directed against FcγRIII (CD16). Techniques which are not dependent on flow cytometry are more difficult to interpret.

TABLE 1 Causes of neutropenia[a]

Disease	Clinical features	Mechanism	Diagnosis	Treatment
Intrinsic				
Severe chronic neutropenia (Kostmann syndrome)	Neutropenia (<200 PMN/mm³) at birth; recurrent, severe infections, autosomal dominant and recessive	Mutations in neutrophil elastase (CLA2) and GFI1	Bone marrow aspiration shows maturation defect at promyelocyte/myelocyte stage	G-CSF
Myelokathexis	Neutropenia; hypogammaglobulinemia, warts; familial cases reported	Mutations in CXCR4	Bone marrow aspiration, no evidence of peripheral destruction, abnormal marrow release on steroid challenge	G-CSF
Shwachman-Diamond syndrome	Moderate to severe neutropenia, anemia, growth retardation, exocrine pancreatic insufficiency, bone abnormalities; some patients may develop aplastic anemia or malignancy	Mutations in SDBS	Demonstration of fatty infiltration of the pancreas	G-CSF
Cyclic neutropenia (cyclic hematopoiesis)	Severe neutropenia ca. every 21 days for about 4–5 days; fever, cutaneous, oral infections; autosomal dominant, spontaneous, and acquired forms	Mutations in neutrophil elastase (ELA2)	Serial blood counts (6 wk) at least every 3 days; mutation detection	G-CSF
Benign chronic neutropenia	Infantile severe neutropenia (<200 PMN/mm³) without serious infections; can last for years	Unknown	Bone marrow aspiration shows normal morphology and development of myeloid series	None
Chédiak-Higashi syndrome	Mild to moderate neutropenia, partial oculocutaneous albinism, recurrent cutaneous, pulmonary infections; fatal lymphoproliferative syndrome in some cases; autosomal recessive	Mutations in LYST	Demonstration of giant primary granules in peripheral blood neutrophils and in other lysosome-containing cells	Supportive; bone marrow transplantation
Reticular dysgenesis	Neonatal neutropenia, hypogammaglobulinemia, thymic abnormalities, lymphopenia; usually fatal	Unknown	Absent myeloid development in bone marrow; other lines may be normal	Supportive
Acquired				
Cytotoxic chemotherapy	Severity of neutropenia depends on dose and specific agent, commonly profound; neutropenia onset variable after treatment; fevers, oral ulcers, bacteremia (e.g., cyclophosphamide)	Reduction of dividing cells	Clinical history	Supportive; G- or GM-CSF in some cases
Drug induced				
Immune	Requires sensitization of neutrophils to antibody (e.g., β-lactams); antibodies may cross placenta	Peripheral destruction of neutrophils	Demonstration of antineutrophil antibodies	Discontinuation of drug, supportive, G-CSF in some cases
Nonimmune	Dose-related or idiopathic reaction to drug, may cause profound neutropenia (e.g., chloramphenicol or clozapine)	Suppression of bone marrow precursors	Clinical history	Supportive; G-CSF in some cases

(Continued on next page)

TABLE 1 (*Continued*)

Disease	Clinical features	Mechanism	Diagnosis	Treatment
Isoimmune	Neonatal neutropenia due to maternal alloimmunization; lasts for several weeks; may be moderate to severe; predominantly cutaneous infections	Antibody-mediated peripheral destruction of neutrophils; against FcγRIII (CD16) epitopes	Clinical history, demonstration of antineutrophil antibodies	Supportive; G-CSF in some cases
Autoimmune	Antibody-mediated neutropenia during collagen vascular diseases (e.g., rheumatoid arthritis with splenomegaly, Felty syndrome; systemic lupus erythematosus)	Sequestration, peripheral destruction of neutrophils	Clinical history, demonstration of antineutrophil antibodies	Treatment of underlying disease; splenectomy in Felty syndrome; steroids in some cases; G-CSF in some cases
Splenomegaly	Mild to moderate neutropenia with moderate to massive splenomegaly due to mechanical (e.g., portal hypertension), infectious (e.g., chronic malaria), or neoplastic causes; often accompanied by anemia and thrombocytopenia	Sequestration with or without destruction of neutrophils	Clinical history and exam, normal bone marrow examination	Treatment of underlying disease; no specific therapy usually required
LGL induced	Moderate to severe acquired cyclic neutropenia; onset usually in adulthood	Clonal proliferation of T cells; probably acts on stem cells	LGL, serial blood sampling, demonstration of LGL proliferation	Treatment of underlying disease; supportive; G-CSF, steroids, or immunosuppression in some cases
Nutritional deficiency	Mild to severe neutropenia associated with vitamin B₁₂, folate, or copper deficiency; protein-energy malnutrition (marasmus)	Ineffective myelopoiesis	Clinical history, determination of specific nutrient levels	Treatment of underlying disease; supportive
AIDS	Moderate to severe neutropenia in AIDS; pyomyositis and aspergillosis seen	HIV related; treatment related (e.g., zidovudine and ganciclovir)	Demonstration of HIV infection; drug history	Discontinuation of drug if possible; G-CSF
Apparent				
Severe infections	Mild neutropenia seen early in severe infections; resolves relatively rapidly	Increase in marginated tissue neutrophil pools	Demonstration of acute infection (e.g., gram-negative sepsis)	Treatment of underlying infection
Hemodialysis	Mild to moderate neutropenia seen during hemodialysis; resolves off dialyzer	C5a-induced stiffening of neutrophils leads to transient trapping in lung	Clinical history, no evidence of acute infection	None

^aG-CSF, granulocyte colony-stimulating factor; GM-CSF, granulocyte-macrophage colony-stimulating factor; HIV, human immunodeficiency virus; LGL, large granular lymphocyte; LYST, lysosomal transporter; PMN, polymorphonuclear leukocytes.

Specimen Collection

Patient serum, stored at −70°C, 1 ml

Pooled normal sera from several donors, stored at −70°C, 200-μl aliquots

Isolated neutrophils from three healthy donors, prepared as described above (≥10⁷ neutrophils per serum sample to be assayed)

Reagents and Equipment

Phosphate-buffered saline, pH 7.2 (PBS), 1×

Bovine serum albumin (BSA), 0.22% (1 ml of 22% BSA plus 99 ml of PBS; make fresh; stable for 1 week at 4°C)

Paraformaldehyde, 4% stock solution (2 g of paraformaldehyde in 45 ml of 0.85% normal saline; warm to 70°C with dropwise addition of 1 N NaOH solution, adjust final pH to 7.2 with dropwise addition of 1 N HCl, bring volume to 50 ml, and store in the dark at 4°C) and 1% working solution (1 volume of 4% stock solution in 3 volumes of PBS; can be stored for 1 week at 4°C)

Fluorescein isothiocyanate-conjugated goat anti-human IgG and IgM, diluted 1:10 with PBS

Microcentrifuge

Flow cytometer

Procedure

1. Label triplicate pairs of microcentrifuge tubes for each serum sample to be assayed (i.e., assays for antineutrophil IgG and IgM with each of three normal donor neutrophil preparations).

2. Dilute the patient and control sera 1:1 with PBS.

3. Resuspend the healthy-donor neutrophils in PBS and sediment at $300 \times g$ for 7 min.

4. Remove and discard the supernatants and resuspend in 2 ml of 1% paraformaldehyde; allow this to stand for 5 min at room temperature.

5. Resuspend in 20 ml of PBS and sediment at $300 \times g$ for 7 min.

6. Resuspend treated cells in PBS to 3×10^7 neutrophils/ml.

7. Transfer 50 μl of each diluted serum sample to the appropriate microcentrifuge tube.

8. Add 50 μl of the neutrophil suspension to the appropriate microcentrifuge tube and incubate at 4°C for 30 min.

9. Wash twice with ice-cold 0.22% BSA, sedimenting the cells for 10 s in a microcentrifuge.

10. Remove and discard the supernatants, add 50 μl of the diluted conjugated anti-human IgG or IgM to the appropriate tube, and incubate at 4°C for 30 min.

11. Wash once with ice-cold 0.22% BSA, sedimenting the cells for 10 s in a microcentrifuge.

12. Remove and discard the supernatants; resuspend the pellets in 1 ml of PBS and transfer to tubes appropriate for analysis in the flow cytometer (usually 12 by 75 mm).

Interpretation

Patient sera are examined for a distinct shift in the peak fluorescence relative to that of the control samples run the same day. Modest and great shifts of fluorescence should be noted through both the histograms and the determinations of channel fluorescence. Increased binding of IgG or IgM over the normal control sera is considered abnormal and is reported. The report should be descriptive, including the antibody subclass implicated and the number of normal donors (out of the day's controls) to which it bound.

NEUTROPHIL DYSFUNCTION

The determination of a qualitative defect of neutrophil function is more complex than the simple determination of neutropenia, since it requires the demonstration of a dysfunctional phenotype. Methods for diagnosis of these abnormalities range from inspection of the peripheral blood smear to fluorescence-activated cell sorting (FACS). Some of these diseases simultaneously affect several limbs of neutrophil function, making prior determination of the single best diagnostic test in a given case important. The clinical history, peripheral blood neutrophil count, and inspection of the peripheral smear readily indicate the direction of further evaluation of a possible neutrophil functional abnormality.

The major classes of neutrophil defects highlight the major neutrophil functions: adhesion, chemotaxis, phagocytosis, degranulation, and killing (Table 2). General features which suggest clinically relevant neutrophil disorders include recurrent, severe infections, often requiring intravenous antibiotics, hospitalization, or surgery. Cutaneous and oral infections are common. The microbiology of specific infectious episodes may be quite informative: infections with *Burkholderia* (*Pseudomonas*) *cepacia*, *Serratia marcescens*, *Chromobacterium violaceum*, *Nocardia* species, *Aspergillus* species, or *Paecilomyces* species, or hepatic abscesses with *S. aureus*, suggest the diagnosis of chronic granulomatous disease (CGD) (8). Since patients with CGD are most susceptible to infections with catalase-producing organisms, severe infections with organisms which do not produce catalase (e.g., streptococci) would suggest abnormalities outside the superoxide-generating pathway.

Adhesion Disorders

The normal neutrophil exits the bone marrow and remains in the circulation for about 7 h before entering the tissue, the intestinal lumen, or the oral cavity. During its time in the peripheral circulation it is frequently "rolling" along and sampling the endothelium for evidence of infection or tissue damage. The low-affinity rolling of the neutrophil along the postcapillary endothelium is mediated by interacting glycoproteins on the endothelial surface (endothelial [E]-selectin and platelet [P]-selectin) and the neutrophil surface (sialyl-Lewisˣ, CD15s). When the neutrophil encounters endothelium activated by chemokines or other stimuli, it adheres to specific molecules (intercellular adhesion molecules [ICAM] 1 and 2) by way of the heterodimeric leukocyte integrins (leukocyte functional antigen 1 [LFA-1] and Mac-1 or complement receptor 3 [CR3]) which contain CD18 as their common β chain. Disorders in both of these critical pathways have been described as LAD. LAD type 1 (LAD1) is due to loss of leukocyte integrin function secondary to CD18 deficiency (6); LAD2 is due to loss of neutrophil selectin binding due to loss of CD15s (3). Both diseases lead to profound impairment of the ability of neutrophils to exit the circulation to sites of infection. One of the CD18-containing molecules (CD18/CD11b, Mac-1, or CR3) also serves as the receptor for the cleaved, inactivated third component of complement (C3bi). Therefore, the absence of CD18-containing leukocyte integrins leads to the inability of neutrophils to perform complement-mediated phagocytosis as well. The cellular signal from CD18 ligation leads to adherence and movement toward the ligand. Rac2 is the G protein that tethers CD18 to cytoskeletal actin. In Rac2 deficiency, CD18 expression is intact, but adherence is reduced and the clinical presentation is like that of LAD1.

TABLE 2 Neutrophil defects[a]

Disease	Clinical features	Mechanism	Diagnosis	Treatment
Adhesion disorders				
LAD1	Neutrophilia (>15,000 PMN/mm³), delayed umbilical stump separation; recurrent, severe infections; autosomal recessive	Defective leukocyte integrin expression; neutrophils unable to exit circulation to sites of infection	FACS analysis for CD18 and the integrins it constitutes: LFA-1 (CD18/CD11a), Mac-1/CR3 (CD18/CD11b), p150,95 (CD18/CD11c); abnormal complement-mediated phagocytosis; impaired chemotaxis	Supportive; bone marrow transplantation where possible
LAD2	Neutrophilia, short stature, abnormal facies, mental retardation, recurrent infections; autosomal recessive	Defective neutrophil selectin ligand (CD15s)	FACS analysis for sialyl-Lewis^x (CD15s) on neutrophils	Supportive
Rac2 deficiency	Neutrophilia, recurrent infections	Rac2 defect	Defective adhesion; defective chemotaxis; absence of Rac2 on immunoblot	Supportive; bone marrow transplantation probably indicated
Granule disorders				
Chédiak-Higashi syndrome	Mild to moderate neutropenia, partial oculocutaneous albinism, recurrent cutaneous or pulmonary infections, fatal lymphoproliferative syndrome in some cases; autosomal recessive	LYST defect	Demonstration of giant primary granules in peripheral blood neutrophils and in other lysosome-containing cells; delayed staphylococcal killing	Supportive; bone marrow transplantation
Specific granule deficiency	Recurrent infections, poor inflammatory response; rare; autosomal recessive	C/EBPε mutation; absence of neutrophil secondary granules and defensins	Absent secondary granules; bi- and trilobed neutrophil nuclei; absence of neutrophil lactoferrin defensins; impaired chemotaxis	Supportive; bone marrow transplantation probably indicated
Chemotactic disorders				
Actin dysfunction	Recurrent infections, poor inflammatory response; rare; autosomal recessive	Defective actin polymerization	Impaired chemotaxis and staphylococcal killing; absence of 47-kDa protein	Supportive; bone marrow transplantation
Oxidative metabolism disorders				
MPO deficiency	No clinical phenotype except in diabetics, in whom severe Candida infections occur; most common neutrophil abnormality; autosomal recessive	Abnormalities in MPO gene	Absence of peroxidase staining of peripheral blood neutrophils; impaired candidacidal activity	No treatment needed in most cases
CGD	Recurrent life-threatening infections with catalase-positive organisms; tissue granuloma formation; X-linked and autosomal recessive forms	Defective superoxide formation	Impaired superoxide production: abnormal NBT test, chemiluminescence, DHR oxidation, or cytochrome c reduction; impaired staphylococcal killing	Supportive; antibiotic and gamma interferon prophylaxis indicated; bone marrow transplantation possibly indicated

[a]PMN, polymorphonuclear leukocytes; LYST, lysosomal transport.

Diagnosis of LAD1 should be made by FACS staining for CD18 and its associated alpha chains, CD11a, CD11b, and CD11c. The functional assays below can help to suggest the diagnosis. LAD2 is rarer and clinically distinct; it can be definitively diagnosed by FACS staining for sialyl-Lewis^x (CD15s). The diagnosis of Rac2 deficiency requires specialized research laboratory resources.

Neutrophil Adherence to Nylon Wool

Principle

Normal neutrophils adhere to several synthetic surfaces, including glass, plastic, and nylon wool, in addition to the endothelium. This adherence is impaired in LAD1 and by aspirin, ethanol, and prednisone.

Specimen collection

Heparinized blood is used, 5 ml each from the patient and three healthy subjects.

Reagents and equipment

Analytical balance

Apparatus for counting leukocytes and performing differential counts

Scrubbed nylon fiber (3 denier, 4 cm, type 200; Fenwal Labs, Morton Grove, Ill.)

Tuberculin syringes, 1 ml, without needle (three per sample)

Small collecting tubes (polypropylene preferred)

Procedure

1. Weigh out 40 mg of nylon wool/column to be used.
2. Using the plunger, pack each column with the 40 mg of nylon wool to the 0.4-ml mark on the syringe.
3. Aliquot and reserve 1 ml of blood from each sample for total leukocyte and differential counts ("precolumn" sample).
4. Place the packed syringes in a rack with their tips inside but not touching the sides or bottom of the small tubes.
5. Add 1.0 ml of heparinized blood to the column and allow it to filter by gravity for 10 min at room temperature.
6. Discard the columns.
7. Perform complete and differential leukocyte counts of the pre- and postcolumn samples.

Interpretation

The percent neutrophils adherent to the nylon wool is calculated as follows: 100% − ([cells per milliliter postcolumn/cells per milliliter precolumn] × 100) = percent cells adherent. Normally, 68% ± 7% neutrophils adhere in this assay. Adherence of a significantly lower percentage of neutrophils is suggestive of an adherence defect. Neutrophil adherence to plastic or glass requires more specialized techniques and is described elsewhere (5).

Flow Cytometric Determination of LAD

FACS analysis (chapter 31) of peripheral blood or isolated neutrophils is required for definitive diagnosis of LAD1 or LAD2. In LAD1, levels of CD18 are profoundly reduced on neutrophils and monocytes, leading to low levels of the associated molecules CD11a, CD11b, and CD11c (method given in chapter 31). Levels of CD18 expression below 0.5% of normal are seen in the "severe" phenotype and are associated with more devastating disease and earlier mortality in the absence of bone marrow transplantation. Levels of CD18 expression between 0.5 and 10% of normal are

associated with the "moderate" phenotype of LAD1 and are associated with a better rate of survival. The display of CD18/CD11 complexes, which are stored in secondary granules, is upregulated by neutrophil activation.

Demonstration of sialyl-Lewis^x (CD15s) deficiency on neutrophils confirms the diagnosis of LAD2. These patients also have the relatively rare Bombay (Hh) blood type, another manifestation of the underlying genetic defect in fucosylation caused by mutations in the GDP-fucosyl transferase. This disease is also now named congenital disorder of glycosylation II c. Rac2 deficiency should be suspected in cases in which surface display of CD18 and CD15s is normal but adherence is impaired, as is superoxide production (7).

Granule Disorders

In the normal course of neutrophil ontogeny, the large (about 0.8 μm in diameter) azurophilic or primary granules, containing myeloperoxidase (MPO), lysozyme, β-glucuronidase, and defensins, among others, appear at the promyelocyte stage; the smaller (about 0.5 μm in diameter) specific or secondary granules, containing lactoferrin, vitamin B$_{12}$-binding protein, cytochrome b_{558}, and CR3, among others, appear during the myelocyte stage.

In Chédiak-Higashi syndrome, neutrophil primary granulogenesis is initially normal, but the primary granules readily fuse to each other and subsequently to some secondary granules as well, resulting in giant primary granules that are easily appreciated under the light microscope. Chédiak-Higashi syndrome is due to autosomal recessive mutations in the gene lysosomal transporter (LYST or CHS1). Neutrophils from Chédiak-Higashi syndrome patients show delayed bactericidal activity against *S. aureus*. Other clinical features include partial oculocutaneous albinism, irregular melanization of hair, peripheral neuropathy later in life, and an eventual lymphoma-like "accelerated phase" in most patients.

In specific granule deficiency, the secondary granules are rare or absent, as are secondary granule proteins, such as lactoferrin. One form of secondary (specific) granule deficiency is due to an autosomal recessive mutation in the CCAAT/enhancer binding protein C/EBPε. Since lactoferrin is present in other secretions, it appears to be a tissue-specific phenomenon. Defensins, a primary granule product, are also low to absent, because the defect is in a transcription factor important in neutrophil ontogeny and granule protein expression. Careful inspection of the peripheral smear suggests the diagnosis, as these neutrophils are larger and paler than normal. The diagnosis is confirmed by electron microscopy, showing an absence of secondary granules, or demonstration of the absence of lactoferrin in patient neutrophils by direct immunofluorescence or enzyme-linked immunosorbent assay. Methods for the detection of lactoferrin and other secondary and primary granule proteins are detailed elsewhere (4).

Chemotaxis

The neutrophil's ability to locomote up a chemoattractant gradient is chemotaxis, whereas the stimulation of shape change and random locomotion induced by a uniform concentration of a chemoattractant is chemokinesis. These properties are critical for the neutrophil response to infection. Disorders involving chemotaxis are found in only a few diseases; secondary causes of depressed chemotaxis are more common (e.g., aspirin, prednisone, and ethanol). Actin dysfunction, Chédiak-Higashi syndrome, LAD1, Rac2 deficiency, secondary granule deficiency, and Job's syndrome (intermittently) all show decreased chemotaxis, although the mechanisms are quite disparate. In none of these disorders is the demonstration of a chemotactic defect diagnostic. The several assays of chemotaxis all require fresh neutrophils and an experienced laboratory. The sensitive techniques (Boyden chamber migration or the multiwell chamber) require highly specialized equipment, radioactivity, or both (4). In view of the complexity of the current chemotactic assays and their extremely limited diagnostic value, I recommend that for cases in which chemotactic determination appears to be appropriate, specialty reference or research laboratories be contacted. Chemotaxis assays are discussed in reference 5.

Oxidative Metabolism Disorders

The neutrophil, eosinophil, and macrophage use the NADPH oxidase enzyme complex to augment molecular oxygen by one electron yielding superoxide (O_2^-). This in turn is converted to hydrogen peroxide (H_2O_2) by superoxide dismutase. H_2O_2 is combined with halide (X^-) by MPO to produce hypohalous acid (HOX); in the neutrophil, which uses chloride for its halide, this is bleach (HOCl). Defects in the proximal portion of this pathway, at the level of the NADPH oxidase, lead to life-threatening infections in CGD; defects in the latter portion of the pathway caused by MPO deficiency are clinically quite inapparent and lead to infectious problems only when coupled to other diseases, such as diabetes mellitus.

CGD is a genetic disorder estimated to occur in about 1/250,000 persons and is characterized by severe, recurrent life-threatening infections with catalase-producing bacteria and fungi and tissue granuloma formation (8). Four separate genotypes (one X-linked, gp91^{phox}; three autosomal recessive, p22^{phox}, p47^{phox}, and p67^{phox}) can give rise to the phenotype of CGD, but there are slight differences in clinical phenotype and obvious differences in genetic transmission and associated counseling. Since all of the relevant genes have been cloned and characterized, a definitive molecular diagnosis can be made. Molecular diagnoses can be performed by reference and commercial laboratories. All patients with CGD should be referred for definitive characterization of their CGD, at least to the protein level.

Several methods are available for diagnosis of CGD. Nitroblue tetrazolium (NBT) reduction and dihydrorhodamine (DHR) oxidation are the simplest tests available and are discussed here. Chemiluminescence and staphylococcal killing are also discussed since they not only are used in the demonstration of CGD functional defects but also occasionally may help in diagnosis. Superoxide production, hydrogen peroxide production, and cytochrome *c* reduction are other techniques which bear on the integrity of oxidative metabolism covered elsewhere in this text (chapter 31).

NBT Test

Principle

Superoxide produced by neutrophils reduces NBT from a soluble yellow dye to blue-black formazan, which is readily apparent as a cytoplasmic precipitate. Neutrophils unable to produce superoxide fail to reduce NBT and are therefore free of precipitate. Because this assay is read by light microscopy, individual cells reducing or not reducing NBT can be recognized. Mothers of patients with X-linked CGD show mosaicism of peripheral blood neutrophil NBT reduction since X chromosome inactivation (lyonization) occurs randomly in hematopoietic precursors.

Interpretation

More than 95% of normal neutrophils will reduce NBT, showing orange nuclei with clumps of blue-black precipitate in the cytoplasm. In a patient with CGD, there is usually no NBT reduction. Since X chromosome inactivation is thought to be random in females, there should be two populations of neutrophils in the peripheral blood of X-linked carriers, NBT reducing (normal) and non-NBT reducing (CGD). This mosaic pattern can range anywhere from 0.001 to 97% of neutrophils, although most carriers will fall within about 20 to 80% NBT reducing. At the extremes of lyonization, these X-linked carriers are indistinguishable from CGD patients or healthy subjects, respectively. It is best to report the results as percent NBT-reducing neutrophils to avoid the confusion surrounding the terms positive and negative in this setting. The drug D-penicillamine can act as a superoxide-generating source when oxidized and therefore can cause unreliable NBT results.

The X-linked form of CGD is the most common (about 65% of cases). One can often rapidly determine whether a male patient is X-linked or autosomal recessive by analysis of the mother's blood at the time of the initial NBT test. In this way genotype can be approximated at the same time as phenotype in most cases.

There are several reports of patients with variant forms of X-linked CGD in whom a dysfunctional gp91^{phox} protein is normally expressed. These patients may have apparently normal NBT reduction. In cases in which the clinical suspicion is high, testing by DHR oxidation, quantitative superoxide generation, or bactericidal activity should be pursued.

DHR Oxidation

Principle

DHR 123 is oxidized to rhodamine 123 by H_2O_2 and O_2^-, with the emission of bright fluorescence upon stimulation by blue light (488 nm). This dye is freely able to permeate cells and can be used in whole blood to determine whether granulocytes produce H_2O_2 and O_2^-, upon stimulation with phorbol myristate acetate (PMA), a potent stimulus of NADPH oxidase activity.

This technique is simple, sensitive, and quantitative and can be performed on whole blood shipped overnight. PMA-stimulated and unstimulated samples are run simultaneously (1).

Specimen Collection

Collect 1 ml of heparin-anticoagulated peripheral blood in plastic, endotoxin-free tubes.

Reagents and Equipment

Lysis buffer (store at room temperature)

Ammonium chloride	4.15 g
Sodium bicarbonate	0.84 g
0.5 M EDTA, pH 8.0	1 ml
Distilled water	500 ml

Suspension buffer (store at room temperature)

Hanks' balanced salt solution (HBSS) (without Ca^{2+}, Mg^{2+}, or phenol red)	500 ml
Albumin (human fraction V)	0.5 g
0.5 M EDTA, pH 8.0	1 ml

Catalase stock solution (1,400 U/μl)

Catalase (C40; Sigma) .... 28 mg
Suspension buffer .... 400 μl

Store 10-μl aliquots at −70°C.

Catalase working solution: Dilute 10 μl of stock with
130 μl of suspension buffer immediately before use.
Use 5 μl for each 500-μl tube (final concentration,
1,000 U/ml).
PMA stock (2 μg/μl)

PMA (P8139; Sigma) .... 1 mg
Dimethyl sulfoxide (DMSO) (D2650; Sigma) ... 500 μl

Store 10-μl aliquots at −70°C.

PMA working solution (1:1000 dilution): 2 μl of PMA
stock solution combined in 1,998 μl of suspension
buffer immediately before use. Add 100 μl to tubes for
a final concentration 400 ng/ml.
DHR stock (29 mM)

DHR 123 (catalog no. D-632; Molecular
Probes, Eugene, Oreg.) .... 10 mg
DMSO .... 1 ml

Store 25-μl aliquots at −70°C. Add 1.8 μl of stock to
each reaction tube.

Procedure

1. Add 4 ml of prewarmed, 37°C lysis buffer to polypropylene tubes.
2. Add 100 to 300 μl of whole blood to each of two tubes
for each sample to be assayed, mix by inversion, and let
stand for 5 min at room temperature.
3. Centrifuge at 800 × g at room temperature for 5 min to
pellet leukocytes.
4. Discard supernatant and blot tubes.
5. Resuspend the leukocyte pellet in 4 ml of suspension
buffer and centrifuge as described above.
6. Discard supernatant, blot tubes, and resuspend in
400 μl of suspension buffer.
7. Add 5 μl of the catalase working solution.
8. Add 1.8 μl of DHR 123 stock solution and incubate
for 5 min in a 37°C shaking water bath.
9. Add 100 μl of PMA working solution to one tube and
100 μl of suspension buffer to the other (unstimulated) tube.
10. Incubate for 15 min in a 37°C shaking water bath.
11. Analyze by flow cytometry, collecting forward and
side scatter as well as FL2.

Interpretation

Histograms are compared for unstimulated and PMA-
stimulated tubes. In normal neutrophils, PMA-stimulated
DHR oxidation yields between 50- and 200-fold more mean
channel fluorescence than unstimulated DHR oxidation.
CGD neutrophils usually show less than 10-fold augmentation
of DHR oxidation by PMA. X-linked carriers show two distinct populations of neutrophils, those which oxidize normally
in the presence of PMA and those which do not. This technique is sensitive to at least 0.01% normal cells among 99.99%
CGD cells and is therefore able to identify highly lyonized carriers (1). Given the general availability of FACS machines and

the ease, sensitivity, and reproducibility of this assay, this test
should be widely applied for the diagnosis of CGD.

Chemiluminescence

Principle

In the normal neutrophil, stimulation of the NADPH
oxidase leads to the generation of H_2O_2, which couples with
hypochlorite (OCL^-) to produce singlet oxygen ($^1O_2$),
water, and chloride (Cl^-). Singlet oxygen is molecular oxygen with an electron lifted to a higher orbit with inversion of
spin. The return of this electron to its ground state is associated with light emission which can be measured as chemiluminescence with several different reagents (5).

Specimen Collection

Isolated neutrophils, $2 × 10^4$/ml, are used.

Reagents and Equipment

Chemiluminometer or fluorometer with only one photomultiplier tube, or beta counter that can be shifted to
only one photomultiplier tube, since the coincidence
sum cannot be used.
Use the ^3H channel; background is usually 25,000 to
50,000 cpm.
Glass 20-ml scintillation vials (keep in the dark) or
microtiter plates
37°C incubator with rotator
Luminol stock solution (A8511; Sigma) (275 μM in
DMSO stored at room temperature in the dark; the
final concentration for the assay is 1 μM) or lucigenin
stock solution (M8010; Sigma) (6.88 μM in distilled
water stored at room temperature in the dark; the
final concentration for the assay is 25 μM)
PMA stock solution (P8139; Sigma) (200 μg/ml in
DMSO, aliquot and store at −70°C)
Zymosan stock solution (Z4250)

Zymosan .... 500 mg
PBS .... 50 ml

Boil for 1 h and then cool. Centrifuge at 500 × g for 10 min
and discard supernatant. Resuspend pellet in 10 ml of
PBS and keep at 4°C in the dark.
Opsonized zymosan: On the day of use, suspend 1 part
zymosan stock in 9 parts pooled human serum. Rotate
for 15 min at 37°C. Centrifuge at 500 × g for 10 min
and discard supernatant. Resuspend to 1.25 mg/ml in
$HBSS^+$ HBSS (with Ca^{2+} and Mg^{2+}).

Procedure

1. To each vial add 400 μl of opsonized zymosan or 55 μl
of PMA, 20 μl of luminol solution, and $HBSS^+$ to 4.5 ml.
2. Place scintillation vials in counter in the dark for at
least 20 min before adding the cells.
3. Arrange control vials:
        HBSS plus luminol
        HBSS plus luminol plus zymosan or PMA
        HBSS plus luminol plus cells
4. Record the background chemiluminescence of the vials.
5. At 1 min intervals, add 1 ml of cells to each vial
sequentially, swirling each vial for 30 s before replacing the
vial in the counter.

6. Count vials sequentially for 1-min periods continuously for 1 h.

7. Plot the counts per minute versus time.

Interpretation

The normal range of chemiluminescence values is 300,000 to 600,000 cpm, with peak values between 8 and 12 min. Chemiluminescence is not entirely specific for singlet oxygen, but it is a sensitive technique for detecting abnormalities in oxidative metabolism. Very low chemiluminescence is consistent with CGD. Heterozygotes can be detected as intermediate between normal subjects and CGD patients. If performed with opsonized zymosan instead of PMA, this assay can detect abnormalities of phagocytosis, such as in LAD1, in which the receptor for C3bi (CR3 or CD18/CD11b) is deficient.

The assay given here is adaptable to laboratories without highly specialized equipment. These procedures are now routinely performed in many laboratories in microtiter plates on specialized chemiluminometers. Recently, an enhancer of chemiluminescence has been marketed (Diogenes, order no. CL-202; National Diagnostics, Atlanta, Ga.) which allows ≥100-fold amplification of the chemiluminescent signal using essentially the same protocol. For experiments using B cells, cells, or cell lines which produce small amounts of superoxide, or very low numbers of neutrophils, the Diogenes system should be considered.

MPO

MPO is the enzyme that makes pus green and catalyzes the conversion of hydrogen peroxide to bleach in the neutrophil. Deficiency of MPO is the most common neutrophil disorder, occurring in about 1/2,000 persons. Despite the important role of MPO in the neutrophil, clinical disease from MPO deficiency is quite rare and has been reported mostly for diabetics with disseminated *Candida* infections. MPO is an important marker of myeloid maturation, appearing at the promyelocyte stage of development. This procedure will stain peroxidase-containing granules in neutrophils, eosinophils, and monocytes.

Specimen Collection

Cytocentrifuged neutrophils on glass slides are preferred, but peripheral blood can be used.

Reagents and Equipment

Fixative, 10% formyl ethanol

Ethanol (absolute)	90 ml
Formaldehyde (37%)	10 ml

Stain, pH 5.8 to 6.5

Ethanol (30%)	100 ml
Benzidine hydrochloride (carcinogen)	0.3 g
Zinc sulfate · 7H$_2$O (3.6%)	1.0 ml
Sodium acetate	1.0 g
Hydrogen peroxide (30%)	70 µl
Safranin O	0.2 g

Mix reagents well in the order listed. The benzidine hydrochloride may leave a slight residue, which will not dissolve. A precipitate forms on the addition of the zinc sulfate, which will dissolve with addition of the remaining reagents. Filter and store capped at room temperature. This solution is good for 6 months.

Procedure

1. Fix the slide in formyl ethanol for 60 s.

2. Rinse slide thoroughly to remove residual formyl ethanol, since this can inactivate the benzidine hydrochloride stain.

3. Place the slide in the stain for 45 s.

4. Rinse thoroughly, and allow to air dry.

Interpretation

Neutrophils show a blue cytoplasm with discrete blue granules, monocytes stain more weakly but still display discrete granules, and eosinophils stain most intensely, often tinged brown-black or green-black. Lymphocytes, basophils, and platelets do not stain. Cells from patients with MPO deficiency do not stain.

This research was supported by the Intramural Research Program of the National Institute of Allergy and Infectious Diseases, National Institutes of Health.

REFERENCES

1. **Anderson-Cohen, M., S. M. Holland, D. B. Kuhns, T. A. Fleisher, L. Ding, S. Brenner, H. L. Malech, and J. Roesler.** 2003. Severe phenotype of chronic granulomatous disease presenting in a female with a de novo mutation in gp91-phox and a nonfamilial, extremely skewed X chromosome inactivation. *Clin. Immunol.* **109:**308–317.

2. **Berliner, N., M. Horwitz, and T. P. Loughran, Jr.** 2004. Congenital and acquired neutropenia. *Hematology* (Am. Soc. Hematol. Educ. Progr.) **2004:**63–79.

3. **Bruin, M., A. Dassen, D. Pajkrt, L. Buddelmeyer, T. Kuijpers, and M. de Haas.** 2005. Primary autoimmune neutropenia in children: a study of neutrophil antibodies and clinical course. *Vox Sang.* **88:**52–59.

4. **Metcalf, J. A., J. I. Gallin, W. M. Nauseef, and R. K. Root.** 1986. *Laboratory Manual of Neutrophil Function.* Raven Press, New York, N.Y.

5. **Poznansky, M. C., D. T. Scadden, and A. D. Luster.** 2002. Chemokine and chemokine receptor analysis, p. 357–367. In N. R. Rose, R. G. Hamilton, and B. Detrick (ed.), *Manual of Clinical Laboratory Immunology*, 6th ed. ASM Press, Washington, D.C.

6. **Rosenzweig, S. D., and S. M. Holland.** 2004. Phagocyte immunodeficiencies and their infections. *J. Allergy Clin. Immunol.* **113:**620–626.

7. **Rosenzweig, S. D., G. Uzel, and S. M. Holland.** 2004. Phagocyte disorders. In E. R. Stiehm, H. D. Ochs, and J. Winkelstein (ed.), *Immunologic Disorders in Infants and Children*, 5th ed. Elsevier, Amsterdam, The Netherlands.

8. **Segal, B. H., T. L. Leto, J. I. Gallin, H. L. Malech, and S. M. Holland.** 2000. Genetic, biochemical, and clinical features of chronic granulomatous disease. *Medicine* (Baltimore) **79:**170–200.

9. **Stroncek, D. F.** 1997. Neutrophil antibodies. *Curr. Opin. Hematol.* **4:**455–458.

ALLERGIC DISEASES

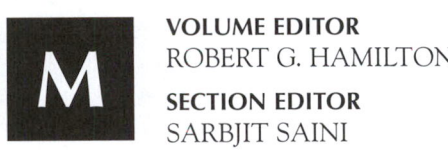

VOLUME EDITOR
ROBERT G. HAMILTON

SECTION EDITOR
SARBJIT SAINI

Introduction

SARBJIT SAINI

104

In 1968, immunoglobulin E (IgE) was identified as the reagin in human serum (1). This single event initiated an explosion in research that has culminated in the detection and quantitation of a number of analytes that aid in the diagnosis and management of human allergic disease. Section M covers the important topics of the allergen, in vivo and in vitro confirmatory IgE antibody testing, mediators and markers of allergic inflammation, and application of the analytical measurements to food allergy and hypereosinophilic syndromes. While accurate detection of IgE antibody in the skin is important for confirmation, it is the clinical history that drives the diagnosis of human allergic disease. The temporal association between an allergen exposure and the occurrence of an allergic symptom leads an allergist to suspect that an individual has an allergic disorder. Only after this inference has been made should confirmatory testing for IgE antibody be performed to support the working diagnosis of allergic disease.

Chapter 105, by deVore and Slater, examines assays that are used in the quantification and standardization of allergens that are glycoproteins which elicit allergic reactions in susceptible individuals. Presently, only 19 of the hundreds of allergen extracts used clinically are standardized. Chapter 105 describes (i) characterization of an allergen extract's total protein in protein nitrogen units per milliliter by the Kjeldahl method, (ii) assignment of bioequivalent allergen units using the in vivo method of intradermal dilution for 50-mm sum of erythema, and (iii) in vitro immunoassays that assess allergen potency by direct binding or inhibition of the binding of IgE from pooled allergic sera to reference allergens. Finally, research-based assays, such as basophil histamine release and basophil surface activation marker assays by flow cytometry, are discussed within the context of allergen characterization.

Chapter 106, by Damin and Peebles, examines in vivo confirmatory assays for the detection of allergen-specific IgE antibody in patients suspected of having allergic disease. The authors provide a detailed account of the rationale, reagent requirements, and procedures for prick/puncture and intradermal skin testing. In vivo provocation procedures are then discussed with a particular focus on intranasal challenge, whole-lung antigen challenge, and methacholine and histamine challenges. Chapter 106 concludes that of the in vivo diagnostic methods available, skin testing has a high degree of sensitivity and specificity for identifying the allergen specificities that cause allergic symptoms. However, caution should be exercised that the presence of a positive skin test does not necessarily indicate that a specific allergen causes symptoms specific for a certain organ system. In some cases, provocation testing may better define whether allergen exposure or nonspecific hyperreactivity is involved in the observed allergic symptoms.

Chapter 107, by Hamilton, examines the diagnostic analytes that are measured in the diagnostic allergy clinical and research laboratory to aid in the diagnosis and management of human allergic disease. Clinically used and research assays for total and allergen-specific IgE and allergen-specific IgG antibody measurements are discussed in detail. Presently, no molecular biology methods are used clinically, except for the generation of recombinant allergenic molecules that are used as reagents in antibody assays.

Chapter 108, by Schroeder and Saini, overviews mediators and markers of inflammation that are associated with immediate-type hypersensitivity reactions. More specifically, the chapter examines the design, performance, and interpretation of immunologic or flow cytometry-based assays for the measurement of mediators (histamine and leukotriene C_4), basophil cytokine secretion (interleukins 4 and 13), and basophil activation-linked surface markers (CD63, CD69, and CD203c). The performance, utility, and quality control of assays for the quantification of mast cell tryptase, eosinophil major basic protein, and eosinophil cationic protein are overviewed. Newer specimens and analytes are discussed, including the exhale condensates and nitric oxide measurements for assessing inflammation during allergic reactions.

Immediate-type hypersensitivity reactions to foods affect about 6% of children younger than 3 years. Chapter 109, by Fleischer and Wood, discusses diagnostic tests that are useful in the workup of food allergy. The diagnostic sensitivity and specificity are examined for prick/puncture and intradermal skin tests with commercially available extracts and fresh foods, atopic patch testing, elimination diets, oral food challenges, and in vitro assays for food allergen-specific IgE antibody. Since the last edition of this manual, the kilo-international unit-per-liter levels of chicken egg-, cow's milk-, soy-, wheat-, and peanut-specific IgE antibodies in serum as measured by third-generation assays have reached general acceptance as a useful predictor of the likelihood of a reaction following consumption of one of these foods.

Finally, the authors discuss the literature that indicates the lack of diagnostic utility of food-specific IgG antibodies, total serum IgE levels, basophil histamine release, and serum tryptase concentrations.

Once parasitic infections, neoplasms, drug hypersensitivity reactions, and immunodysregulatory disorders associated with secondary eosinophilia have been excluded, subtyping of hypereosinophilic syndromes can be facilitated by laboratory analyses. In chapter 110, Klion overviews the clinical features, pathogenesis, and variants of hypereosinophilic syndromes. Subtype identification is accomplished by detecting

fusion tyrosine kinase using nested reverse transcriptase PCR or fluorescent in situ hybridization. Finally, this chapter discusses the controversies surrounding the diagnosis of hypereosinophilic syndrome.

REFERENCE

1. **Bennich, H. H., K. Ishizaka, S. G. Johansson, D. S. Rowe, D. R. Stanworth, and W. D. Terry.** 1968. Immunoglobulin E: a new class of human immunoglobulin. *Immunology* **3:**323–324.

Quantification and Standardization of Allergens

NICOLETTE C. deVORE AND JAY E. SLATER

105

Allergic reactions and allergic diseases are the most common human disorders of immune regulation. Diseases may include localized responses in the skin and various portions of the airway, or systemic responses characterized by extensive skin involvement, severe airway compromise, or cardiovascular collapse. Mechanisms include mast cell or basophil activation by the cross-linking of allergen-specific homocytotropic immunoglobulin E (IgE), cellular infiltration following mast cell or basophil mediator release, complement activation, the deposition of immune complexes in susceptible tissues, and the infiltration of activated T lymphocytes. The degree of impairment from allergic disease varies widely, with most reactions posing minor inconvenience but with rare episodes requiring intensive—and sometimes unsuccessful—interventions to prevent death.

While the treatment of allergic diseases often includes highly effective and specific pharmacotherapy, for many allergic disorders allergen avoidance and allergen immunotherapy remain the best and safest options. Specific allergen diagnosis—a prerequisite for effective avoidance or immunotherapy—may be achieved by controlled in vivo allergen challenge (skin testing or, less often, ocular or respiratory challenge) (see chapter 106, this volume) or by in vitro methods (such as radioallergosorbent testing [RAST], basophil histamine release, or lymphocyte stimulation). Specific allergen immunotherapy or desensitization is achieved by the graded administration of the identified allergens to achieve at least a temporary reduction in allergic response, either through receptor saturation, antibody depletion, the formation of blocking antibodies, or T-cell tolerance (currently the most favored hypothesis). Remarkably, the purity of the allergen being tested is not essential for diagnostic or therapeutic efficacy; in fact, purity has not been achieved for any commercially available allergen preparations. However, for each of these evaluations or treatments it is critical that the allergen used be correctly identified and that it be present in sufficient bioactive form to achieve the expected diagnostic or therapeutic performance. Thus, for the successful use of allergens in allergy diagnosis or immunotherapy, it is important that we be able to identify and measure the allergen being used.

Allergens are molecules that elicit allergic reactions in susceptible individuals. Typically, allergens are naturally occurring proteins or glycoproteins derived from plants or animals, but biomolecules derived from single-cell organisms (such as molds), synthetic compounds, metals, and small molecules may elicit significant allergic reactions as well. In this chapter, we limit our discussion to natural or recombinant proteins or glycoproteins used in the diagnosis and/or treatment of IgE-mediated allergic disease.

Allergen extracts are manufactured and sold worldwide for the diagnosis and treatment of IgE-mediated allergic disease. These are crude extracts of natural animal or plant source materials and are complex mixtures of natural biomaterials. Each extract contains proteins, carbohydrates, enzymes, and pigments, of which the allergens—presumably the active ingredients—may constitute only a small proportion (48).

All current U.S. allergenic products were licensed prior to the efficacy requirements that were established for biologics in 1972. The safety, efficacy, and labeling of these products were evaluated by a review panel in the 1970s, which considered all of the products available at that time and made separate recommendations for the diagnosis and therapy indications of these products (7a). Although some allergenic products were removed from the market following the panel's deliberations, most were deemed presumptively safe and effective for therapy and/or diagnosis.

Traditionally, allergen extracts have been labeled either with a designation of extraction ratio (weight per volume) or with a protein unit designation which is determined by the Kjeldahl method (protein nitrogen units per milliliter). However, there is little correlation between these two designations and biological measures of allergen potency (2, 3). In the absence of a concerted effort to maintain product consistency, lot-to-lot variations in allergen content may be considerable. Product consistency may be enhanced by the inherent nature of the raw materials; for example, pollen and pure mite extracts (34) generally have greater lot-to-lot consistency than mold, house dust, and insect extracts (28). In addition, manufacturers can increase the consistency of their products by controlled collection, storage, and processing of the raw materials; by reproducible and optimized extraction and manufacturing techniques; and by expiration dates based on real-time stability data. However, consistency can be ensured only by measuring the potency of each lot of extract and by marketing only those lots whose potency falls within an acceptable range. When such additional tests and specifications are applied to similar products from more than one manufacturer, those products are said to be standardized.

The Food and Drug Administration (FDA) allergen standardization regulation [21 CFR 680.3(e)] mandates that when an appropriate potency test exists, manufacturers must test each lot of an allergen extract for potency prior to distribution. In practice, the FDA has provided manufacturers with a U.S. reference standard to which each new lot of allergen extract may be compared. The purpose of allergen standardization is to ensure that the extracts are well characterized in terms of allergen content and that variation between lots is minimized even among different manufacturers (49). Since standardized allergenic extracts are compared to a single, national potency standard, patients and their physicians can switch from one manufacturer's product to another with minimized risk of adverse reaction.

Currently, there are 19 standardized allergen extracts available from manufacturers in the United States (Table 1). For each of these products, there is a U.S. standard of potency to which each lot is compared prior to release for sale to the public. The potency measures and the assays used to determine these measures are specified in the approved product license applications of each manufacturer for each product.

OVERVIEW OF IN VIVO ASSESSMENTS OF ALLERGEN POTENCY

Allergen standardization in the United States comprises two important components: the selection of a reference preparation

TABLE 1 Allergenic extracts currently standardized in the United States

Allergen extract	Current lot release tests	Labeled unitage	Current standard (date placed in service)	Method(s) to establish equivalence to previous standard
Dust mites				
Dermatophagoides farinae	Competition ELISA, protein	AU/ml (equivalent to BAU/ml)	E8-Df (2000)	Competition ELISA
Dermatophagoides pteronyssinus	Competition ELISA, protein		E7-Dp (1999)	Competition ELISA
Cat (*Felis domesticus*)				
Pelt	Fel d 1 (RID), IEF, protein	BAU/ml	E3-cat pelt (1996)	RID, IEF
Hair	Fel d 1 (RID), IEF, protein	5–9.9 Fel d 1 U/ml = 5,000 BAU/ml; 10–19.9 Fel d 1 U/ml = 10,000 BAU/ml	E4-cat hair (2001); C10-cat (calibration set, 2001)	RID, IEF
Grasses				
Bermuda grass (*Cynodon dactylon*)	Competition ELISA, IEF, protein[a]	BAU/ml	E6-Ber (2004)	Competition ELISA
Red top grass (*Agrostis alba*)			E5-Rt (1999)	
June (Kentucky blue) grass (*Poa pratensis*)			E5-Jkb (1998)	
Perennial ryegrass (*Lolium perenne*)			E12-Rye (1995)	
Orchard grass (*Dactylis glomerata*)			E5-Or (1999)	
Timothy grass (*Phleum pratense*)			E8-Ti (2004)	
Meadow fescue grass (*Festuca elatior*)			E5-Mf (1999)	
Sweet vernal grass (*Anthoxanthum odoratum*)			E6-Sv (2000)	
Short ragweed (*Ambrosia artemisiifolia*)	Amb a 1 (RID)	Amb a 1 U	E15-Ras; C14-Ras (calibration set, 2004)	RID
Hymenoptera				
Yellow hornet (*Vespa* spp.)	Hyaluronidase and phospholipase activity[b]	μg of protein	V2-HB	
Wasp (*Polistes* spp.)				
Honeybee (*Apis mellifera*)				
White-faced hornet (*Vespa* spp.)				
Yellow jacket (*Vespula* spp.)				
Mixed vespid (*Vespa* + *Vespula* spp.)				

[a]The current lot release tests are the same for all grasses listed.
[b]The current lot release tests are the same for all Hymenoptera listed.

of allergenic extract and the selection of the procedures to compare manufactured products with the reference extract (37, 38, 40). In the United States, the use of a biological model of allergen standardization has permitted the assignment of bioequivalent allergen units (BAU) for most standardized allergens (38). Once a specific unitage is assigned to a reference, then all allergenic extracts from the same allergenic source can be assigned units based on the relative potency (RP) with respect to the reference, using the established quantitative in vitro potency method (41).

In theory, standardizing an allergenic extract might involve purifying each allergen in the extract and establishing with precision the importance of these allergens. However, most allergenic extracts are complex mixtures of several relevant allergens of as yet uncertain immunodominance. In addition, an individual allergen in a particular lot may be less "allergenic" due to instability or denaturation. The choice of the best potency test depends on the extract to be standardized. In the absence of data supporting the safety of potency designations based on single-allergen content, a measure of overall allergenicity may be a better predictor of safe dosing. For two allergenic extracts (short ragweed and cat hair), data have supported the use of single-allergen determinations (Amb a 1 and Fel d 1, respectively); for cat pelt and hymenopteran venoms, the presence of two allergens (Fel d 1 and albumin for cat pelt; hyaluronidase and phospholipase A2 for hymenopteran venoms) is verified for each lot; for dust mites and grass pollens, overall allergenicity is determined.

For initial overall allergenicity assessment, The Center for Biologics Evaluation and Research (CBER) has developed a method using erythema size following serial intradermal testing of highly allergic individuals. Intradermal testing was chosen over prick-puncture testing to achieve greater dosing accuracy; erythema size was chosen over wheal size to achieve greater accuracy in reaction measurements (41). This method, called $ID_{50}EAL$ (intradermal dilution for 50-mm sum of erythema determines the BAU), can be used to compare the allergenicities of extracts, regardless of source. Subsequent comparisons of extracts from the same source material are made by a variant analysis called the parallel line bioassay. Both of these methods are described in CBER's "Methods of the Allergenic Products Testing Laboratory" (1994, FDA Docket 94N-0012).

In the $ID_{50}EAL$ method, allergenic extracts are evaluated in subjects maximally reactive to the respective reference concentrates. Each subject is tested with serial threefold dilutions of the reference extract. After 15 min, the sum of the longest and midpoint orthogonal diameters of erythema (ΣE) is determined at each dilution, and the log dose producing a 50-mm ΣE response (D_{50}) is calculated (41) (Fig. 1).

Extracts that produce similar D_{50}s can be considered bioequivalent and are assigned similar units (BAU). Because the modal D_{50} of a series of extracts was 14 (a 3^{-14} or 1:4.8 million dilution), extracts with a mean D_{50} of 14 were arbitrarily assigned the value of 100,000 BAU/ml (38). Thus, the formula for the determination of potency from the D_{50} is:

$$\text{Potency} = 3^{-(14 - \text{mean } D_{50})} \times 100,000 \text{ BAU/ml}$$

By a similar technique and analysis, bioequivalent doses of test extracts from the same source as the reference extract can be determined by the parallel line bioassay (44). The inverse ratio of the doses of test extract required to produce identical D_{50}s to a reference extract is the RP of that extract. This analysis requires that the log dose-response curves of the test extract and the reference extract be parallel; if the two dose-response lines are not parallel, then the ratio of skin test doses for identical responses (and the RP) will vary with the dose. In this situation, which strongly suggests compositional differences between the two extracts, the distance between the two lines is different at each dose and a meaningful RP cannot be determined (36, 37) (Fig. 2).

In the original 1994 protocol, the mean D_{50} for 15 highly allergic individuals was used to determine the D_{50} for the extract. In a recent reanalysis of the statistical considerations underlying such potency studies, Rabin et al. (30) applied the following formula for the number of study subjects, n, that would be required:

$$n = 2 \left(\frac{\sigma}{\delta} \right)^2 (z_{1-\alpha} + z_{1-\beta/2})^2$$

where σ is the standard deviation of the measurement, δ is the acceptable difference in D_{50}s of two equivalent products, and the z values are the critical values from the cumulative normal distribution table for a significance level α and a

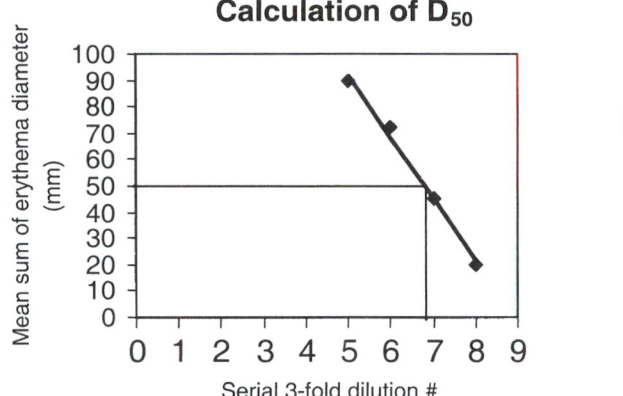

Calculation of D_{50}

$y = -23.7x + 210.8$

$D_{50} = \dfrac{50 - \text{intercept}}{\text{slope}}$

$D_{50} = \dfrac{50 - 210.8}{-23.7}$

$D_{50} = 6.78$

FIGURE 1 Sample calculation of D_{50}. Serial threefold dilutions of test material were injected, and the ΣE responses were plotted against the negative log dilutions. The D_{50} is determined from the best-fit line by using the formula $D_{50} = (50 - \text{intercept})/\text{slope}$. The calculated D_{50} of 6.78 corresponds to a value of $3^{-(14 - 6.78)} \times 100,000 \text{ BAU/ml} = 35.9 \text{ BAU/ml}$.

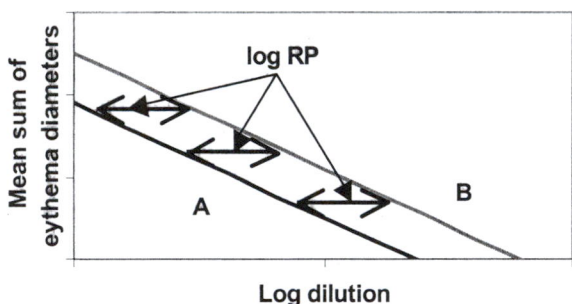
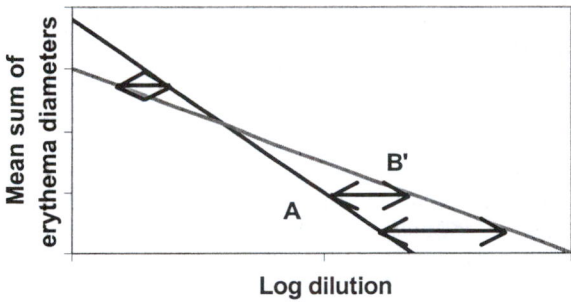

FIGURE 2— Hypothetical parallel line bioassay curves. (Left) The bioassay curves are parallel, and the difference of log dilutions resulting in the same diameters is constant at all diameters. The log RP of test sample B compared to reference A is represented by the difference. (Right) The curves are not parallel, and the differences vary with the strength of the reaction. Thus, the log RP of B′ compared to A cannot be calculated.

power of $1 - \beta$ (31). From this formula, n is a function of the squares of σ and δ. The value of n will depend on the particular allergen to be tested, but, for typical values of σ and δ, n will usually be larger than 15.

In Europe, the Committee for Proprietary Medicinal Products issued a Note for Guidance on Allergen Products that was revised in 1996 (http://www.emea.eu.int/pdfs/human/bwp/024396en.pdf). The European system for standardizing allergens and determining allergenic extract potency is different from the system used in the United States, as follows.

1. Manufacturers ensure batch-to-batch consistency by using an in-house standard. The in-house standard may be characterized by a number of physicochemical and immunologic assays, with demonstration of the presence of individual allergens preferred.

2. There are no external reference standards to ensure consistency among manufacturers.

3. Potency may be determined by any validated measure of in vitro IgE binding or other immunoassay. The potency of the in-house standard may also be tested by a skin test technique.

4. An in vivo method by which European products may be tested is called the Nordic technique (21). This skin test method differs from the CBER $ID_{50}EAL$ method in its use of prick skin tests, its focus on wheal size rather than erythema, its choice of study subjects, and its use of a histamine dose-response curve to determine unitage. The method very likely provides a reasonable estimate of extract potency. In theory, the comparison of the skin test reactivity of all allergens to a single standard (histamine dihydrochloride, 10 mg/ml) allows the assignment of universal unitage without the development or maintenance of specific allergen reference standards. However, the Note for Guidance does not prescribe the specifics of the skin test technique to be used, and manufacturers are free to modify it as needed as long as the test is validated. Thus, as applied in Europe, this method cannot provide a level of standardization among the different manufacturers that market products in the European Union.

$ID_{50}EAL$ Test

Study Sequence

1. Identify three or four testing sites to achieve geographic and ethnic diversity of study populations.

2. Recruit 6 to 10 subjects per tester for proficiency testing (subjects need not be atopic). In order to generate useful data, the $ID_{50}EAL$ and parallel line bioassay methods must be performed by individuals proficient in the accurate and reproducible delivery of intradermal skin test doses and the precise measurement of the skin test responses. Hence, a proficiency program has been developed to qualify personnel. This program (not described in detail here) involves puncture skin testing with histamine base (0.1 mg/ml) and intradermal testing with eight serial threefold dilutions of histamine. The tester then analyzes the data and compares the results with normative data. Thus, the proficiency program examines the tester's ability to prepare accurate dilutions, administer the skin tests with precision, and record and analyze the data properly.

3. Recruit 10 to 20 study subjects for initial allergen skin testing.

4. Skin test subjects and analyze skin test data. Analysis will include determination of σ for intradermal testing.

5. On the basis of the initial data, determine the final study size.

6. Recruit study subjects, skin test the subjects, and analyze skin test data.

7. Prepare final study report.

Selection of Subjects

Select individuals within the target age range with a history of allergic disease relevant to the allergen being tested, who have puncture sum of erythema diameter responses (ΣE) to the allergen concentrate of at least 30 mm. Exclude individuals with asthma whose peak flow is <75% of the flow predicted at the time of testing, whose skin coloring or skin condition would preclude the measurement of erythema responses, who are dermographic, or who are currently using antihistamines, tricyclic antidepressants, monoamine oxidase inhibitors, and beta-blockers.

Dilution of Allergens for Skin Testing

Starting with the undiluted or reconstituted lyophilized extract, prepare serial threefold dilutions, using sterile technique, down to a dilution of 3^{-17}. For convenience, label the dilution by the $-\log_3$ doses: undiluted extract is labeled 0, and the 3^{-17} dose is labeled 17.

Preparation of Subjects

Skin tests may be placed on the back or the glabrous skin of the volar surface of the arms, avoiding a 1-in. area above and below the antecubital fossa and a 1-in. area above the wrist. For consistency, the back should be used for final titrations.

Injection Technique

The volume of solution to be injected is 0.05 ml. Insert the needle of a 27-gauge 0.5-ml syringe at a 30° angle, bevel down. A distinct injection bleb should be observed. Injections in which gross leakage of extract around the needle, an indistinct bleb, or a subcutaneous injection occurs should be repeated at a different site.

Measurement of Skin Tests

THIS IS A TIME-DEPENDENT ASSAY. Exactly 15 min following injection, the wheal and erythema margins are outlined with a fine, roller-tip pen with washable ink. In order to make a permanent record of the skin test reaction, transparent surgical tape is placed on the skin over the skin test outline. Lifting of the tape from the skin results in transfer of the outline to the tape. The tape is then placed in a notebook for future reference.

The size of the skin response is obtained by measuring and recording the longest diameter of erythema and the orthogonal erythema diameter measured at one-half the longest erythema diameter (Fig. 3). The sum of the longest and orthogonal erythema diameters (ΣEs) (or wheal [ΣW]) constitutes the skin response at that site. Measurements are made from the inner edge of the skin test outlines.

Skin Test Procedure

The dose-response line for each product is generated by using four serial threefold dilutions with graded erythema responses which bracket a ΣE of 50 mm and include the end point where ΣE = 0 or ΣE $\sim$ ΣW. The skin response (ΣE) should fall within the limits of $\geq$0 to $\leq$125 mm. Each more concentrated dilution should produce a graded erythema response. The four dilutions selected should span a wide range of ΣEs (for example, from 0 to 20 mm to 80 to 125 mm) and bracket a ΣE of 50 mm.

Inject the test and reference extracts, beginning with dilution 15. The expected change in ΣE going from one dilution to the next dilution is about 20 mm. Therefore, if dilution 15 is negative, proceeding to dilution 12 would not be expected to exceed a ΣE response of 60 mm. Similarly, if dilution 12 is negative, proceed to dilution 9. Do not inject reference extract dilutions more concentrated than no. 5 unless the extract is known to be of low potency. Apply each dilution singly for each product and reference. Always include an intradermal diluent control test.

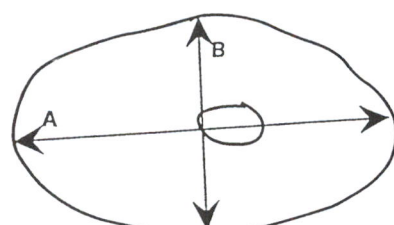

FIGURE 3 Diameters are measured from the inner margins of the penned outline. Longest (A) plus midpoint orthogonal (B) diameters and summed diameters (A + B) are recorded.

OVERVIEW OF IN VITRO ASSAYS OF ALLERGEN POTENCY

Although skin testing is an essential component of the allergen standardization program, it is not intended for routine use in the testing of manufactured lots of extracts prior to release. In vitro potency assays that accurately predict the in vivo activity of extracts have been developed (36). Once an in vivo assay has been utilized to assign unitage to a reference extract, then an appropriate surrogate in vitro assay can be used to assign units to test extracts from the same sources. These methods can be based on quantitation of the total protein content (Hymenoptera venoms), the specific allergen content within the allergenic extract (short ragweed and cat hair), or the inhibition of binding of IgE from pooled allergic sera to reference allergen (grasses and mites) (31). For the Hymenoptera venom allergens, the potency determination is also based on the content of the known principal allergens within the extract, hyaluronidase and phospholipase, which is determined by enzyme activity (Table 1).

The potency units for short ragweed extracts were originally assigned on the basis of their Amb a 1 content. Subsequent data suggested that 1 U of Amb a 1 is equivalent to 1 µg of Amb a 1, and 350 Amb a 1 U/ml is equivalent to 100,000 BAU/ml. However, the original unitage has been retained. Grass pollen extracts are labeled in BAU per milliliter, based on $ID_{50}EAL$ testing. In some cases, the assignment of potency units to standardized allergenic extracts in the United States has changed as better bioequivalence data have become available (41). Cat pelt extracts were originally standardized on the basis of their Fel d 1 content, with arbitrary unitage (AU per milliliter) tied to the Fel d 1 determinations. Subsequent $ID_{50}EAL$ testing suggested that the 100,000-AU/ml cat pelt extracts, which contained 10 to 19.9 Fel d 1 U/ml, should be relabeled as 10,000 BAU/ml (22). In addition, 20% of individuals allergic to cat were found to have antibody to non-Fel d 1 proteins (43), and the identification of a cat albumin band on isoelectric focusing (IEF) gels was added as a requirement for cat pelt extracts. Dust mite extracts were originally standardized (in AU per milliliter) on the basis of RAST inhibition assays. Subsequent $ID_{50}EAL$ testing indicated that the arbitrary unitage was statistically bioequivalent to BAU per milliliter (22, 42); in this case, the original unitage was retained (39).

TESTS FOR INDIVIDUAL ALLERGENS

Individual allergens may be measured and detected by various approaches using monospecific antisera or antibodies. Assay designs using these antisera include the radial immunodiffusion (RID) assay, crossed immunoelectrophoresis/crossed radioimmunoelectrophoresis (CIE/CRIE), and enzyme-linked immunosorbent assay (ELISA) variants (direct, two-site, and competition). Each of the assays utilizes monospecific antisera or antibodies to detect and quantify the specified allergen. The RID assay is currently applied to two standardized allergenic extracts, short ragweed and cat hair, in which the immunodominant allergens (Amb a 1 and Fel d 1, respectively) have been identified and defined. Sheep antisera are used for the RID performed at CBER/FDA, but polyclonal and monoclonal antibodies from several species have been used with success for many of these assays. Specifications for the antibodies vary with the assay system. For example, antibodies for the RID assay must form a discrete precipitin ring, the two antibodies for the two-site ELISA must recognize different epitopes on the allergen molecule, and, in all cases, the epitope(s) recognized must be present on the allergen and reflective of its bioactivity.

Antibodies

Monospecific antisera that recognize the allergen of interest may be purchased or, alternatively, obtained by inoculating an animal with the appropriate amounts of recombinant or purified allergen. Monoclonal antibodies or recombinant antibodies (such as scFv or Fabs) can also be generated for these assays.

Sandwich ELISA

Antibody sandwich ELISAs are two- to fivefold more sensitive than ELISAs in which the antigen is bound directly to the plate (10). The capture antibody is diluted to 0.2 to 10 μg/ml in phosphate-buffered saline (PBS) and allowed to bind to 96-well polystyrene plates overnight at 4°C. The plates are washed, blocked, and washed again. A standard antigen dilution series is prepared by serial 1:3 dilutions of the antigen in blocking buffer and typically falls in the range of 0.1 to 1,000 ng/ml. A few serial dilutions of the test antigen should also be prepared so that the concentration falls in the range of 1 to 100 ng/ml. Incubate the plates for 3 to 4 h at room temperature and then wash them. Incubate in 50 μl of specific secondary antibody-enzyme conjugate. Develop the reaction in the appropriate solution, and read the results in a plate reader (Laboratory of Immunobiochemistry—Standard Operating Procedures 7, revised November 1998). To analyze these data, construct a graph using the values obtained from the standard antigen dilution and interpolate.

RID Assay

In this assay, used by CBER and most U.S. allergen manufacturers to measure the allergen content of short ragweed and cat allergen extracts, monospecific antiserum is added to an agar solution, which is allowed to solidify. Wells are then cut into the agar, and test allergen is placed in the wells. As the specific allergen diffuses out into the agar a precipitin ring forms, which delineates the equivalence zone for antigen-antibody binding. The radius of the precipitin ring can then be measured. Since the antibody concentration in the agar is constant, the antigen concentration decreases with increasing distance from the well and is proportional to the log of the concentration of the applied test allergen in comparison to the reference extract (Laboratory of Immunobiochemistry—Standard Operating Procedures 5 and 6, revised November 1993).

1. Prepare a solution consisting of 1% Noble agar (Difco) and 1% sodium azide in water. Heat in a boiling water bath until the solution is clear. Allow the temperature to equilibrate in a 55°C water bath.

2. Once the solution has cooled to 55°C, add 0.2 ml of monospecific antiserum to 2 ml of agar solution. Mix thoroughly but gently and pour onto a microscope slide that has been precoated with 0.01% Noble agar. Allow the agar to solidify at room temperature.

3. After the agar has hardened, place the slide on a sheet of graph paper that contains a template with five evenly spaced dots, approximately 1.5 mm apart. Cut wells into the agar over each dot with a gel cutter, and carefully pipette 8 μl of allergen test solutions into each well. Incubate the slides in a sealed humidified chamber at room temperature for 72 h.

4. Fix the slides by soaking them in 10% acetic acid for 2 min and then rinsing them briefly in deionized water. The diameters of the precipitin rings can be measured to the nearest 0.1 mm with a calibrating viewer (Transidyne General Corp., Ann Arbor, Mich.).

5. After the diameters of the precipitin rings are measured, the reference standard data are graphed on a semilog scale. The average ring size of the unknown can then be used to determine the amount of allergen by interpolation.

Troubleshooting the RID Assay

Before this assay is performed on an unknown, a dose-response curve should be made to determine the antiserum concentration at which the ring diameter plateaus. If multiple RID assays are going to be compared, person-to-person variability should be established by direct comparison of an identical test profile. Likely sources of person-to-person variability may include (i) pipetting errors leading to spillover of samples applied to the wells and (ii) measurement errors with the calibrating viewer.

CIE/CRIE

In CIE, allergen extract is typically separated by electrophoresis on a 1% agarose gel, and a narrow strip of gel containing the separated antigen is then transferred to a clean glass plate. The remaining area of the plate is then filled with agarose containing polyspecific antisera against the antigen. A second electrophoresis is performed at right angles to the first one (hence the name "crossed" electrophoresis). Immune complexes form precipitin arcs that can be visualized by Coomassie blue staining (45, 46).

In CRIE, the unstained CIE preparation is incubated in the presence of appropriately diluted patient sera containing specific IgE, which is detected by overnight incubation in ^{125}I-labeled anti-IgE (20).

Enzyme Activity Assays

Hymenoptera venoms contain multiple glycoprotein enzymes, the most important of which are hyaluronidase and phospholipases A1 and A2. Venom allergenic extracts are standardized by enzymatic assays, which estimate hyaluronidase and phospholipase content on the basis of their enzymatic activity. In these assays, an agar solution is prepared with the appropriate enzymatic substrate and test samples are then added to cut wells. As the enzyme present in the sample diffuses into the agar, it digests the substrate, forming clearing zones around the wells. The radius of the clear zones is then measured and calculated as the log of the concentration of the enzyme present in the sample (Laboratory of Immunobiochemistry—Standard Operating Procedures 1 and 2, revised January 1995).

TESTS OF OVERALL POTENCY

The potency of standardized allergen extracts for which the immunodominant components have not been identified with certainty may be estimated by assays for IgE-antigen binding that compare the overall IgE binding properties of test and reference extracts, using pooled allergic sera. Initially, a RAST inhibition assay was used for this purpose; CBER adopted the competition ELISA as its standard assay because of its greater precision and convenience. After the wells of the polystyrene microtiter plate are coated with the reference allergen and the wells are blocked with bovine serum albumin, a mixture of the extract to be tested and a reference serum pool is added to the wells. The greater the amount of immunoreactive allergen in the mix, the less free

IgE antibody will be available from the serum pool to bind to the immobilized allergen on the plate. The concentration of the allergens in the extract is determined by comparison to the reference allergen extract. However, since this assay does not explicitly measure a specific allergen, the allergen concentration is expressed as RP, with the reference extract assigned an arbitrary RP of 1.0. Early studies showed an excellent correlation between RP assigned by titration skin testing and RP determined by RAST inhibition assay (38); subsequent studies showed the competition ELISA to be equivalent as well (18).

Method Summary—Inhibition Immunoassays

The inhibition immunoassays for the determination of overall allergen potency share basic design features.

1. Known allergens are bound to a solid-phase support.
2. The solid support is then exposed to serum containing IgE antibodies from an allergic individual, mixed with dilutions of unknown competing allergen.
3. IgE binds to the allergens on the solid phase, forming antigen-allergen complexes. The competing (soluble) unknown allergen reduces the binding of specific IgE to the solid-phase allergen.
4. The unbound IgE is washed away. Labeled anti-IgE is allowed to bind to the antigen-IgE complexes. After a final wash, the label remaining bound to the antigen-allergen complex is related to the quantity of the IgE antibody present in the serum of the patient.
5. The results are then plotted, and the 50% binding value determined is proportional to the potency of the extract. In addition to finding the 50% binding value, the slopes of different extracts can be compared; extracts with similar slopes have similar antigen compositions. The RP may then be determined as illustrated in Fig. 2.

RAST

RAST was first described in 1967 (47). In this assay, intended to determine the presence of specific IgE in a serum sample, allergen is bound to cyanogen bromide-activated paper disks, which are then incubated with patient serum. After unbound antibody is washed away, ^{125}I-radiolabeled anti-IgE is used to detect the bound IgE. Following the approach outlined above, the RAST inhibition assay is used to establish the overall allergen content of an unknown extract.

CAP

Pharmacia introduced the CAP system as an alternative to the paper-based RAST in 1990. Instead of paper disks, a sponge cellulose material is used to bind the allergen; the secondary antibody is an anti-human IgE–β-galactosidase conjugate; and the substrate is 4-methylumbelliferyl-β-D-galactoside, cleavage of which by the β-galactosidase generates a detectable fluorogen. The CAP system has been shown to have increased sensitivity for some allergens (hymenopteran venoms [11, 15], cat [5, 7, 15], *Dermatophagoides pteronyssinus* [5, 7, 15], and *Alternaria* [5, 7]), while other studies have not shown a significant improvement in sensitivity (24, 27). This assay can be used to measure overall allergen content in a similar way to RAST.

Overview of ELISA Inhibition, or Competition ELISA

In this assay, the one used by CBER and most U.S. allergen manufacturers to determine the RP of standardized grass pollen and dust mite allergenic extracts, serial dilutions of an extract to be tested are placed in a well that has been precoated with a known amount of reference extract. Optimal concentrations of the reference extract and the detecting antibody conjugate must be determined by checkerboard titration for each new set of reagents.

The detecting antibody is a critical component of the assay. It is essential that the antibodies used reflect the broadest range of allergens considered relevant to the overall allergenicity of the allergenic extract being tested, and the antibodies should be evaluated by Western blotting or a comparable technique. IgE is biologically relevant for allergic disease, but each batch of IgE-containing sera is likely to vary in the specificity of the IgE, and—since most atopic donors are multiallergic—may well include IgE molecules that recognize irrelevant allergens as well. Such extraneous IgE will only interfere in the assay to the degree that the coating allergen contains cognate irrelevant allergens. Human sera containing IgE antibodies should be collected from as many allergic individuals as possible, with a minimum of 6, but preferably 10 to 20 (Laboratory of Immunobiochemistry—Standard Operating Procedure 13, revised October 1998). Other polyspecific antisera can also be utilized for these assays and are discussed above.

ELISA Inhibition Procedure (Laboratory of Immunobiochemistry—Standard Operating Procedure 7, revised November 1998)

1. Coat the microplate wells with 100 µl of the reference extract per well and allow binding at 4°C overnight. Wash the plates in 0.05% Tween in PBS (PBS-T).
2. Block at room temperature for 1.5 h in blocking buffer (1% bovine serum albumin in PBS-T), and wash in PBS-T.
3. Into duplicate wells, pipette 1:3 serial dilutions of the reference extract. Into the remaining wells, pipette 1:3 serial dilutions of the test extracts in duplicate.
4. Immediately add 50 µl of the detecting antibody at the appropriate concentration.
5. Incubate the plate overnight at 4°C.
6. Wash the plate with PBS-T, develop, and read results as appropriate.
7. The results are plotted with the values of the optical density along the y axis and the log of the dilution factor along the x axis. The 50% binding value that is determined is proportional to the potency of the extract; the RP is estimated by comparing the x intercepts of the test and reference extracts. The slopes of the different extracts can also be compared; extracts with identical slopes as determined by the t test are presumed to have similar antigen compositions.

Histamine Release

Basophil histamine release is an in vitro surrogate for skin testing and, as with other assays based upon interactions between allergen and specific IgE, the release of histamine from sensitized human basophils may be used to measure the allergen content of an unknown solution. Histamine release assays have been performed on heparinized whole blood (12, 26), crude leukocyte preparations (17), purified basophils (8, 13, 35), cell lines (4, 19), and rabbit leukocytes (33). The drawbacks of this assay are that histamine release assays with whole or fractionated blood require large amounts of recently drawn blood, and specialized cell lines are not readily available. In addition, basophils from 20% or more of skin test-positive patients do not release histamine in vitro (1), even in the presence of cross-linking anti-IgE. However, the same individuals' serum IgE may still be used in histamine release experiments by passively sensitizing basophils from other donors with the heterologous IgE (16). In all variants of this assay, released histamine may be quantified by radioimmunoassay or fluorimetry (32). Although this technique and its variants have been used to assess allergen potency (9, 14, 29), it does not appear to have any advantage over other assays that depend upon specific allergen-antibody interactions.

Flow Cytometry

In the past decade, the discovery of basophil activation markers CD63, CD45, CD69, and CD203c have led to a flow cytometric approach that assesses the in vitro activation of basophils. Most commonly, basophil activation markers CD63 and CD203c are used (6). CD63 is weakly expressed on the surface of basophils in both allergic and nonallergic patients. When FcεRI-bound IgE encounters an allergen, granules containing large quantities of CD63 fuse with the plasma membrane, resulting in a large increase in CD63 on the surface of basophils. However, CD63 is expressed not only by basophils, but also by mast cells, macrophages, and platelets (23, 25). Therefore, when CD63 is used in a flow cytometric analysis, a separate antibody that recognizes IgE must also be used. CD203c is a basophil-specific marker that is not expressed on other blood leukocytes and is upregulated in the presence of IgE cross-linking in a manner similar to that of CD63. Because CD203c is a basophil-specific marker, a second antibody is not required for specificity.

IDENTITY TESTING

The identity of an allergen extract may be verified by visualizing the separated allergen proteins on the basis of their size and isoelectric points (48). The IEF assay is an important safety test in the lot release of grass pollen and cat allergen extracts. The patterns produced by the crude allergen mixtures are reproducible enough to consistently indicate the presence of known allergens, to identify possible contaminants present in the extracts, and to check lot-to-lot variation in the extracts (50). In addition, IEF is used to verify the presence of cat albumin in cat pelt extracts.

Method Summary: Identity Testing

IEF

Polyacrylamide gels (PAGplates), wicks, applicators, cellophane preserving sheets, and the Multiphor II electrophoresis unit are available from Pharmacia-LKB. No specific buffer is required for IEF, but salt concentrations of >50 mM should be avoided as they will cause band distortions.

1. Place the polyacrylamide gel (PAGplate, pH 3.5 to 9.5) on the electrophoresis unit, using the screen print as a guide. The Multiphor II unit serves to both apply the electric current to the gel and keep the gel cool during the run.

2. Soak one electrode wick with anode buffer (1 M H_3PO_4) and one with freshly made cathode buffer (1 M NaOH). Remove excess moisture with tissue paper and place the damp electrode wicks along the length of the gel, being sure to position the strips along the appropriate ends of the gel.

3. For sample application, place dry IEF/SDS sample applicator strips on the cathode end of the gel. Apply 5 to 20 µl of the sample to the applicator. If a greater volume of sample is required, then up to five applicator strips may be stacked vertically and 20 µl of the sample can be loaded per strip. (Note that for cat pelt 0.6 to 0.8 Fel d 1 U must be used, and more may be needed for cat hair extracts.) When larger proteins are being focused, the sample applicator should be placed near, but not at, the expected pI.

4. For each sample, a reference extract and a pI marker should also be run from the cathode end of the gel. To monitor progress visually, 20 µl of a 1% solution of methyl green (MP Biomedicals) in deionized water will separate into three colored bands as the gradient is established when the sample is placed just to the left of the anode. For best results, the gel should be run for 60 to 75 min with a maximum voltage of 500 V, maximum current of 50 mA, and power of 30 W. Maintain the temperature at 8 to 10°C.

5. After the gel has been run, the gel is immediately fixed for 15 to 30 min in 7.5% sulfosalicylic acid–12.5% trichloroacetic acid, washed with destain (7% acetic acid–10% methanol), and stained for 1 to 3 h in 0.05% Coomassie brilliant blue R250 in 10% acetic acid–50% methanol. Destain over a period of 16 to 24 h with several exchanges of destain until the background is clear.

6. An image of the gel may be captured by using a densitometer (Molecular Dynamics) and saved as a TIF. Alternatively, the gel may be photographed with high-contrast film and a yellow filter. To preserve the gel, incubate it in preserving solution (10% glycerol in destain) for 1 h at room temperature. Then place the gel on a glass plate and cover with a cellophane preserving sheet that has been soaked in the preserving solution. Allow the gel and cellophane to dry for 24 to 48 h and store away from bright light.

7. The pI of the sample proteins can be determined by interpolation on a calibration curve utilizing the IEF marker that was resolved along with the sample.

REFERENCES

1. **Asero, R., M. Lorini, S. U. Chong, T. Zuberbier, and A. Tedeschi.** 2004. Assessment of histamine-releasing activity of sera from patients with chronic urticaria showing positive autologous skin test on human basophils and mast cells. *Clin. Exp. Allergy* **34:**1111–1114.
2. **Baer, H., H. Godfrey, C. J. Maloney, P. S. Norman, and L. M. Lichtenstein.** 1970. The potency and antigen E content of commercially prepared ragweed extracts. *J. Allergy* **45:**347–354.
3. **Baer, H., C. J. Maloney, P. S. Norman, and D. G. Marsh.** 1974. The potency and group I antigen content of six commercially prepared grass pollen extracts. *J. Allergy Clin. Immunol.* **54:**157–164.
4. **Barsumian, E. L., C. Isersky, M. G. Petrino, and R. P. Siraganian.** 1981. IgE-induced histamine release from rat basophilic leukemia cell lines: isolation of releasing and nonreleasing clones. *Eur. J. Immunol.* **11:**317–323.
5. **Bousquet, J., P. Chanez, I. Chanal, and F. B. Michel.** 1990. Comparison between RAST and Pharmacia CAP system: a new automated specific IgE assay. *J. Allergy Clin. Immunol.* **85:**1039–1043.
6. **Ebo, D. G., M. M. Hagendorens, C. H. Bridts, A. J. Schuerwegh, L. S. De Clerck, and W. J. Stevens.** 2004. In vitro allergy diagnosis: should we follow the flow? *Clin. Exp. Allergy* **34:**332–339.
7. **Ewan, P. W., and D. Coote.** 1990. Evaluation of a capsulated hydrophilic carrier polymer (the ImmunoCAP) for measurement of specific IgE antibodies. *Allergy* **45:**22–29.
7a.**Federal Register.** 1985. Biological products; allergenic extracts; implementation of efficacy review, proposed rule. *Fed. Regist.* **50:**3082.

8. **Gibbs, B. F., T. Noll, F. H. Falcone, H. Haas, E. Vollmer, I. Vollrath, H. H. Wolff, and U. Amon.** 1997. A three-step procedure for the purification of human basophils from buffy coat blood. *Inflamm. Res.* **46:**137–142.

9. **Hoffmann, A., L. Vogel, S. Scheurer, S. Vieths, and D. Haustein.** 1997. Potency determination of allergenic extracts using mediator release of rat basophil leukemia cells. *Arb. Paul Ehrlich Inst. Bundesamt Sera Impfstoffe Frankf. A M.* **91:**203–208.

10. **Hornbeck, P.** 2004. Induction of immune response, p. 2.1.2–2.1.20. *In* J. E. Coligan, D. H. Margulies, E. M. Sherach, and B. Bierer (ed.), *Current Protocols in Immunology.* John Wiley & Sons, Inc., New York, N.Y.

11. **Jeep, S., E. Kirchhof, A. O'Connor, and G. Kunkel.** 1992. Comparison of the Phadebas RAST with the Pharmacia CAP system for insect venom. *Allergy* **47:**212–217.

12. **Katz, G., and S. Cohen.** 1941. Experimental evidence of histamine release in allergy. *JAMA* **117:**1782.

13. **Kepley, C., S. Craig, and L. Schwartz.** 1994. Purification of human basophils by density and size alone. *J. Immunol. Methods* **175:**1–9.

14. **Kordash, T. R., L. L. Freshwater, and M. J. Amend.** 1995. Standardization of allergenic extracts by basophil histamine release. *Ann. Allergy Asthma Immunol.* **75:**101–106.

15. **Leimgruber, A., J. P. Lantin, and P. C. Frei.** 1993. Comparison of two in vitro assays, RAST and CAP, when applied to the diagnosis of anaphylactic reactions to honeybee or yellow jacket venoms. Correlation with history and skin tests. *Allergy* **48:**415–420.

16. **Levy, D. A., and A. G. Osler.** 1966. Studies on the mechanisms of hypersensitivity phenomena. XIV. Passive sensitization in vitro of human leukocytes to ragweed pollen antigen. *J. Immunol.* **97:**203–212.

17. **Lichtenstein, L. M., and A. G. Osler.** 1964. Studies on the mechanisms of hypersensitivity phenomena. IX. Histamine release from human leukocytes by ragweed pollen antigen. *J. Exp. Med.* **120:**507–530.

18. **Lin, Y., and C. A. Miller.** 1997. Standardization of allergenic extracts: an update on CBER's standardization program. *Arb. Paul Ehrlich Inst. Bundesamt Sera Impfstoffe Frankf. A M.* **91:**127–130.

19. **Lowe, J., P. Jardieu, K. VanGorp, and D. T. Fei.** 1995. Allergen-induced histamine release in rat mast cells transfected with the alpha subunits of Fc epsilon RI. *J. Immunol. Methods* **184:**113–122.

20. **Lowenstein, H.** 1978. Quantitative immunoelectrophoretic methods as a tool for the analysis and isolation of allergens. *Prog. Allergy* **25:**1–62.

21. **Malling, H. J.** 1997. Skin prick testing in biological standardization of allergenic products. *Arb. Paul Ehrlich Inst. Bundesamt Sera Impfstoffe Frankf. A M.* **91:**157–163.

22. **Matthews, J., and P. C. Turkeltaub.** 1992. The assignment of biological allergy units (AU) to standardized cat extracts. *J. Allergy Clin. Immunol.* **89:**151.

23. **Metzelaar, M. J., H. J. Schuurman, H. F. Heijnen, J. J. Sixma, and H. K. Nieuwenhuis.** 1991. Biochemical and immunohistochemical characteristics of CD62 and CD63 monoclonal antibodies. Expression of GMP-140 and LIMP-CD63 (CD63 antigen) in human lymphoid tissues. *Virchows Arch. B Cell Pathol. Incl. Mol. Pathol.* **61:**269–277.

24. **Nalebuff, D. J., R. G. Fadal, and B. C. May.** 1993. A comparative study of the diagnostic characteristics of the modified RAST and Pharmacia CAP System. *Otolaryngol. Head Neck Surg.* **109:**601–605.

25. **Nieuwenhuis, H. K., J. J. van Oosterhout, E. Rozemuller, F. van Iwaarden, and J. J. Sixma.** 1987. Studies with a monoclonal antibody against activated platelets: evidence that a secreted 53,000-molecular weight lysosome-like granule protein is exposed on the surface of activated platelets in the circulation. *Blood* **70:**838–845.

26. **Noah, J. W., and A. Brand.** 1954. Release of histamine in the blood of ragweed sensitive individuals. *J. Allergy* **25:**210–214.

27. **Pastorello, E. A., C. Incorvaia, V. Pravettoni, A. Marelli, L. Farioli, and M. Ghezzi.** 1992. Clinical evaluation of CAP System and RAST in the measurement of specific IgE. *Allergy* **47:**463–466.

28. **Patterson, M. L., and J. E. Slater.** 2002. Characterization and comparison of commercially available German and American cockroach allergen extracts. *Clin. Exp. Allergy* **32:**721–727.

29. **Poulsen, L. K., M. H. Pedersen, M. Platzer, N. Madsen, E. Sten, C. Bindslev-Jensen, C. G. Dircks, and P. S. Skov.** 2003. Immunochemical and biological quantification of peanut extract. *Arb. Paul Ehrlich Inst. Bundesamt Sera Impfstoffe Frankf. A M.* **94:**97–105.

30. **Rabin, R. L., J. E. Slater, P. Lachenbruch, and R. W. Pastor.** 2003. Sample size considerations for establishing clinical bioequivalence of allergen formulations. *Arb. Paul Ehrlich Inst. Bundesamt Sera Impfstoffe Frankf. A M.* **94:**24–33.

31. **Schuirmann, D. J.** 1987. A comparison of the two one-sided tests procedure and the power approach for assessing the equivalence of average bioavailability. *J. Pharmacokinet. Biopharm.* **15:**657–680.

32. **Siraganian, R. P., and M. J. Brodsky.** 1976. Automated histamine analysis for in vitro allergy testing. I. A method utilizing allergen-induced histamine release from whole blood. *J. Allergy Clin. Immunol.* **57:**525–540.

33. **Siraganian, R. P., and A. G. Osler.** 1970. Antigenic release of histamine from rabbit leukocytes. *J. Immunol.* **104:**1340–1347.

34. **Slater, J. E., and R. W. Pastor.** 2000. The determination of equivalent doses of standardized allergen vaccines. *J. Allergy Clin. Immunol.* **105:**468–474.

35. **Tanimoto, Y., K. Takahashi, M. Takata, N. Kawata, and I. Kimura.** 1992. Purification of human blood basophils using negative selection by flow cytometry. *Clin. Exp. Allergy* **22:**1015–1019.

36. **Turkeltaub, P. C.** 1986. In vivo methods of standardization. *Clin. Rev. Allergy* **4:**371–387.

37. **Turkeltaub, P. C.** 1988. Assignment of bioequivalent allergy units based on biological standardization methods. *Arb. Paul Ehrlich Inst. Bundesamt Sera Impfstoffe Frankf. A M.* **82:**19–40.

38. **Turkeltaub, P. C.** 1989. Biological standardization of allergenic extracts. *Allergol. Immunopathol.* (Madrid) **17:**53–65.

39. **Turkeltaub, P. C.** 1994. Use of skin testing for evaluation of potency, composition, and stability of allergenic products. *Arb. Paul Ehrlich Inst. Bundesamt Sera Impfstoffe Frankf. A M.* **87:**79–87.

40. **Turkeltaub, P. C.** 1997. Biological standardization. *Arb. Paul Ehrlich Inst. Bundesamt Sera Impfstoffe Frankf. A M.* **91:**145–156.

41. **Turkeltaub, P. C.** 1999. Allergen vaccine unitage based on biological standardization: clinical significance, p. 321–340. *In* R. Lockey and S. C. Bukantz (ed.), *Allergens and Allergen Immunotherapy,* vol. 12. Marcel Dekker, Inc., New York, N.Y.

42. **Turkeltaub, P. C., M. C. Anderson, and H. Baer.** 1987. Relative potency (RP), compositional differences (CD), and assignment of allergy units (AU) to mite extracts (Dp and Df) assayed by parallel line skin test (PLST). *J. Allergy Clin. Immunol.* **79:**235.

43. **Turkeltaub, P. C., and P. J. Gergen.** 1992. Epidemiology of allergic disease and allergen skin test reactivity in the US population: data from the second National Health and Nutrition Examination Survey (1976–1980)-NHANES II. *Arb. Paul Ehrlich Inst. Bundesamt Sera Impfstoffe Frankf. A M.* **85:**59–80.

44. **Turkeltaub, P. C., S. C. Rastogi, H. Baer, M. C. Anderson, and P. S. Norman.** 1982. A standardized quantitative skin-test assay of allergen potency and stability: studies on the allergen dose-response curve and effect of wheal, erythema, and patient selection on assay results. *J. Allergy Clin. Immunol.* **70:**343–352.

45. **Weeke, B.** 1973. A manual of quantitative immunoelectrophoresis. Methods and applications. 1. General remarks on principles, equipment, reagents and procedures. *Scand. J. Immunol. Suppl.* **1:**15–35.

46. **Weeke, B.** 1973. Crossed immunoelectrophoresis. *Scand. J. Immunol. Suppl.* **1:**47–56.

47. **Wide, L., H. Bennich, and S. G. Johansson.** 1967. Diagnosis of allergy by an in-vitro test for allergen antibodies. *Lancet* **ii:**1105–1107.

48. **Yunginger, J. W.** 1983. Allergenic extracts: characterization, standardization and prospects for the future. *Pediatr. Clin. N. Am.* **30:**795–805.

49. **Yunginger, J. W.** 1998. Allergens: recent advances. *Pediatr. Clin. N. Am.* **35:**981–993.

50. **Yunginger, J. W., C. R. Adolphson, and M. C. Swanson.** 2002. Standardization of allergens, p. 868–874. *In* R. G. Hamilton, N. R. Rose, and B. Detrick (ed.), *Manual of Clinical Laboratory Immunology*, 6th ed. ASM Press, Washington, D.C.

In Vivo Diagnostic Allergy Testing

DEREK A. DAMIN AND R. STOKES PEEBLES, JR.

106

In recent decades, understanding of atopic diseases has increased exponentially. Pollens, fungi, animal dander, insects, and foods have been implicated in such diseases as allergic rhinitis, extrinsic asthma, atopic dermatitis, and anaphylaxis. Phenotypic association has been replaced with a profound understanding of biomolecular pathways, signaling molecules, and receptors. Despite marked advancements in the understanding of the pathophysiology of allergic disease, the simple idea of challenging subjects with antigenic material to reproduce a biological response remains fundamental in investigation.

Prick-puncture and intradermal skin testing are the most commonly used methods for the diagnosis of immediate hypersensitivity in allergic disease, while airway challenges may be used in the evaluation of rhinitis and asthma. This chapter describes the technique and utility of in vivo skin testing, intranasal allergen challenge, and specific and nonspecific lower airway challenge testing. These tools provide clinically useful information in the evaluation of the atopic patient.

SKIN TESTING

Overview

Allergen skin testing is considered to be the most convenient, least expensive, and most specific screening method in the diagnosis of allergic diseases. The first skin test recorded was in 1865, when Charles H. Blackley placed pollen grains on abraded skin (3). The prick skin test was first documented in the early 1920s, but scarification was the method of choice until the 1970s (13). Prick testing reemerged as the most common method when studies revealed increased false-positive and -negative results with scarification. During the 1980s, further studies elucidated the correlation of skin test reactivity with allergic symptoms to specific allergens. In recent years, major advancements have been made in allergen reagent standardization and national organizations have appealed for universal reporting methods to aid testing interpretation of an increasingly mobile population (see chapter 105, this volume).

Skin test positivity is an indication of individual immunoglobulin E (IgE) production. Allergen-specific IgE produced by plasma cells binds to specific receptors on the surface of mast cells and basophils. After introduction of allergen into the skin either by prick-puncture or by needle injection, the allergen may cross-link the allergen-specific IgE on the mast cell and/or basophil surface, resulting in cellular degranulation and mediator release. These mediators, including histamine, leukotrienes, and others, produce the sharply demarcated area of edema and even larger area of erythema characteristically referred to as the "wheal and flare" response. Demonstrable results are produced within minutes, and marked reactivity can be impressive.

Alternative Assessments

Serum assays allowing direct measurement of allergen-specific IgE antibodies are described in chapter 107. Skin testing is more economical per test than in vitro IgE assays, but in vitro testing should be utilized for patients with extensive dermatitis or dermatographism or for patients who cannot withhold interfering medications or refuse testing. Sensitivity for in vivo and in vitro testing varies, depending on the antigen being tested. Wood and colleagues compared predictive values of skin tests and radio allergosorbent tests (RASTs) in the diagnosis of cat allergy (33). Depending on the outcome measured, sensitivity for prick testing ranged from 79 to 97% while that of the RAST ranged from 69 to 91% (33). More comparative studies are needed for individual antigens, but sensitivity for in vivo testing is usually 10 to 25% greater than that for in vitro testing. In the diagnosis of food allergy, threshold in vitro values that have 95% positive and 90% negative predictive values have been derived (36).

An alternative to skin testing to assess the potential role of allergy in clinical symptoms is to assess basophil mediator release. This topic is reviewed extensively in chapter 108.

Clinical Indications

Allergen skin testing is indicated for the further evaluation of symptoms suspected of being mediated by allergen-specific IgE antibodies. In the evaluation of rhinitis, asthma, and conjunctivitis, aeroallergen assessment is performed with extracts of clinical relevance to the geographical area where testing is performed or symptoms are experienced. Assessment of foods is often indicated in the evaluation of eczema and systemic reactions suggestive of anaphylaxis. In the evaluation of stinging-insect hypersensitivity, purified venoms and whole-body extracts are used in the evaluation of systemic reactions to insects of the order Hymenoptera. Although much less defined, skin testing with nonirritating concentrations of medications is used when medication hypersensitivity is being assessed.

In the evaluation of aeroallergens and stinging-insect hypersensitivity, proper allergen identification is essential in accurate immunotherapy prescription and administration. Identification of food allergens is necessary for appropriate avoidance. In vivo testing is also essential in identifying medications that should be avoided or to which desensitization should be initiated.

Aeroallergen Assessment

Aeroallergen assessment is routinely performed by the prick-puncture method and has excellent positive predictive value. The use of intracutaneous or "intradermal" skin testing in aeroallergen assessment is less supported. Nelson and colleagues found a poor correlation between timothy grass intradermal positivity and symptom provocation (22, 33). However, intracutaneous testing may detect relevant sensitivity in some populations when prick-puncture testing is negative but sensitivity is strongly suggested on the basis of exposure and symptomatic history.

Food Allergy Assessment

A vast amount of information exists on the evaluation of food allergy (see chapter 109). General principles that relate to in vivo examination are discussed here. Food allergens are implicated in approximately 30 to 40% of children with eczema (28). The "gold standard" of diagnosis is the double-blind placebo-controlled food challenge (DBPCFC). However, DBPCFC is limited by the risk of systemic reaction. Prick-puncture testing, therefore, is often the initial choice for evaluation. Intradermal testing is not routinely performed in the evaluation of food allergy secondary to high false-positive and low false-negative rates compared to DBPCFC (26). Negative skin prick testing essentially rules out allergy to that food with >95% negative predictive accuracy (27). In the diagnosis of eczema in which a food is the etiologic agent, 80 to 90% is accounted for by allergies to milk, egg, wheat, soy, peanut, tree nuts, fish, and shellfish. One caveat of testing, however, is false-negative results with manufactured extracts from fruits and vegetables due to the lack of relevant antigens. Freshly prepared extracts should be used for definitive exclusion (24).

Stinging-Insect Assessment

The diagnosis and treatment of stinging-insect hypersensitivity remain controversial. For in vivo testing, intradermal injection is required for definitive diagnosis when prick-puncture testing is negative. Initially, prick-puncture testing is started at 1.0 μg/ml. If negative, the protocol proceeds with intracutaneous testing started at 0.01 μg/ml and injections are advanced in single logarithmic increases to 1.0 μg/ml. In vitro IgE assays have additional utility in the diagnosis of hymenopteran sensitivity. Ten percent of skin test-negative patients being evaluated for insect allergy will have increased serum-specific IgE antibodies detected. Currently, a combination of in vivo and in vitro testing is used for patients with a history of systemic reaction to provide maximum sensitivity for detecting at-risk individuals (10).

Medication Adverse Reaction Assessment

Skin testing can be utilized as a diagnostic tool when the adverse reaction to a medication is suspicious of an IgE-mediated mechanism. Skin testing for allergy to medications is not well defined, and more studies are needed to establish reproducible parameters for individual medications. Also, in many instances, the relevant antigen is not the parent compound and therefore not commercially available for testing.

It is important that interpreters realize that the antigenic epitope responsible for the reaction may be a metabolized product of the parent compound. Currently, the only group of medications for which the predictive values have been elucidated is beta-lactam antibiotics. If tested to the major (benzyl penicilloyl polylysine) and minor (benzylpenicillin, benzylpenilloate, and benzyl penicilloate) determinants of penicillin, negative testing confers a 97 to 99% negative predictive value. If positive, there is approximately a 60% chance of immediate reaction with subsequent exposure (31). False-negative testing is possible if major or minor determinants are tested alone. Several obstacles exist for appropriate testing. First, the only commercially available, major determinant skin test reagent (PREPEN; Bayer) has been plagued by manufacturing shortages. Second, minor determinant mixtures are generally available only at major medical centers through complex preparative methods.

If skin testing is performed for other medications, control subjects should be tested to rule out an irritant response, and the results should be interpreted cautiously, given the lack of predetermined validity. A commonly used method for testing various medications is to determine the threshold dilution titration by preparing serial dilutions of the original concentration for testing. Prick-puncture testing is performed with the original concentration along with appropriate controls. If negative, intradermal testing is performed with a 1:1,000 dilution and increased until a positive reaction develops or the original concentration is tolerated.

Procedures

Several preparatory measures are required for successful testing outcomes. All interfering medications must be discontinued in order to achieve interpretable results. It is advised that narrow-spectrum antihistamines be discontinued 24 to 72 h before testing, hydroxyzine 96 h prior to testing, broad-spectrum antihistamines 4 to 7 days before testing, and tricyclic antidepressants 7 to 14 days before testing (1, 2). Testing should not be done on areas of active dermatitis and should be done with caution in patients with dermatographism because of difficulties in interpretation. Testing can be performed on pregnant patients but is not advisable unless the information gained from testing is deemed to outweigh the risk of adverse effects on the fetus if a systemic reaction is encountered. Although prick-puncture and intradermal skin testing are exceptionally safe, rare systemic reactions have occurred. In a 5,063-subject cohort of patients in a sexually transmitted disease clinic who were being screened for penicillin allergy, mild anaphylaxis occurred in 1 patient and 11 others experienced systemic pruritus or urticaria, for an overall incidence of adverse reactions to skin tests of 1.2% (9). Therefore, a supervising physician and resuscitation materials should be on hand in case of systemic reaction. First-line treatment for a systemic reaction is 0.3 ml of 1:1,000 aqueous epinephrine for adults and 0.01 ml/kg of body weight (up to 0.3 ml) for children, administered intramuscularly (29). Other resuscitative materials should include antihistamines, corticosteroids, oxygen, and normal saline for volume replacement. Patients with life-threatening reactions should be transported to the nearest emergency department. The risk of systemic reaction is higher with intracutaneous testing. A practical approach is to use prick-puncture testing for screening and intradermal testing for confirming equivocal or negative percutaneous testing results (32).

The number of individual extracts tested is dependent on many variables, including the condition for which testing is required, geographical area, age, and knowledge of antigen cross-reactivity. Special consideration should be given to infants and very young children. In this population, few tests are needed and relevant antigens are usually limited to constant environmental exposures, including foods, dust mites, and animal dander.

Testing sites are cleansed with 70% isopropyl alcohol and marked for identification. Using barrier precautions, allergen extracts of known composition are introduced into the skin, usually on the volar aspect of the arm or the upper back. Either site is appropriate, but the back is associated with clinically significant higher sensitivity, whereas the arm affords tourniquet application if systemic reaction is encountered (19). Individual tests should have sufficient spacing, usually 2.5 cm, and should not be placed within 5 cm of the wrist or 3 cm of the antecubital fossa. False-positive results from adjacent reactions are unlikely to be caused when there is at least 2 cm between individual test sites (19).

Controls

Positive and negative controls must be applied in the absence of interfering medications. Histamine as a positive control must be read at 15 min to achieve peak reactivity. For prick-puncture testing in the United States, a concentration of 2.7 mg of histamine phosphate per ml (1 mg/ml equivalent of histamine base) is used, whereas a 100-fold dilution is used for intradermal testing. A negative control must be performed with the same diluent used for the extracts (2).

Prick-Puncture Tests

Several devices and techniques can be used in performing the prick-puncture test. The purpose is to introduce a small quantity of allergen into the skin after interruption of the epidermal barrier. Disposable lancets on single- or multitipped devices as well as various needles can be used for the prick-puncture technique. Lancets are usually 1 mm long with a plastic rim to prevent excessive penetration. Variables involved in testing include the device being used, the angle and depth of penetration, and the force applied by the applicator. Testers should be aware of trauma associated with different devices and their influence on interpretability (20, 21). Proper application should not cause excessive trauma or bleeding at the site. Single- and multitipped devices often simultaneously place a drop of allergen extract while puncturing the skin. If such devices are not used, a drop of extract is placed on the skin and the needle or lancet is used to prick through the extract.

Intradermal Tests

Intradermal testing is usually performed on the volar aspect of the arm to allow application of a tourniquet in the event of a systemic reaction. The concentration used is usually 100- to 1,000-fold more dilute than the concentration used in the prick-puncture method. As in the previous method, the skin test site is cleansed and marked for individual allergen identification. Using a 27-gauge tuberculin needle, 0.01 to 0.05 ml of diluted extract is introduced into the skin. With the skin held taut, the needle is inserted bevel down at a 45° angle to the skin. After initial insertion, the syringe is lowered parallel to the skin and advanced only sufficiently to provide an intradermal injection. A small wheal about 3 mm in diameter is usually formed. A new needle is used for each injection.

Interpretation

Quality interpretation can depend on many variables, including skin color, testing site, skin reactivity, and reader skill. Tests should be read 15 to 20 min after application. Reporting in a standardized manner as recommended by the American College of Allergy, Asthma and Immunology and the American Academy of Allergy, Asthma and Immunology should include the following information: subject name and date of birth, longest diameter of wheal and flare in millimeters, device used, time, date, reader, and extracts tested. A semiquantitative manner of reporting using 1+, 2+, etc., is not advised. Marked interphysician variability has been noted to occur with semiquantitative reading of prick-puncture tests, with the exception of the extreme positive result (16). If semiquantitative scores are reported, the grading system should be included in the report. The goal is to include a sufficient amount of information in the report to eliminate the need for repeat testing if interpreted by another physician or provider. A wheal diameter of 3 mm greater than that of the diluent control is considered positive and representative of the presence of IgE antibodies with prick-puncture testing. A wheal diameter of 8 mm greater than the diluent control is considered positive for intradermal testing. Accurate interpretation is enhanced when erythema is considered (32). Readers must be proficient to maximize intra- and interpatient validity. Prick-puncture testing is usually considered more specific and less sensitive than intracutaneous testing. Interpretation is dependent on clinical correlation and an understanding of testing limitations, since the presence of IgE antibodies does not always imply symptom culpability.

Reagents

Reconstitution, Stability, and Storage

A vast number of commercial extracts are available from companies that collect and purify allergens, but the number of standardized antigens available is a very small percentage (see chapter 105). Reproducible and precise extract constitution through standardization has been a major advancement in the utility of allergy skin testing. Extract standardization is important in providing test reliability and minimizing lot-to-lot variability. Concentration assignment in bioequivalence allergy units is a method of reporting potency based on a skin test bioassay reducing lot-to-lot variability. Standardized extracts exist for short ragweed, cat hair, grass pollens, dust mites, and hymenopteran venoms. Until universal standardization, many allergen extracts will continue to be supplied in weight per volume and may have significant variation in lot-to-lot concentration (17).

It is important to understand extract thermal stability, compatibility, and cross-reactivity when storing and mixing different reagents for testing or injectable immunotherapy. Allergen extract potency deteriorates with time, dilution, and increased temperature. Several studies have demonstrated extract degradation with higher temperatures, fungal and insect protease activity, and percent glycerin of diluent (11, 18). Protease activity from fungal and insect extracts can have degradative effects on other antigens. An understanding of protease degradation and unnecessary inclusion of redundant cross-reactive extracts is required when mixing extracts for injectable therapy. Glycerinated extracts protect unstable allergens from denaturation, inhibit protease degradation, and increase thermal stability. Diluted extracts need to be remixed every 2 to 3 months in buffered saline or normal saline diluent and every 6 months in 10% glycerin or human serum albumin diluent. Allergen extracts should be stored at 4°C (11).

Recombinant Allergens

Many recombinant allergens have been generated for basic and clinical investigation. Further investigation is needed for recombinant allergens to be licensed for human use in the United States and become useful for skin testing. One problem with recombinant allergens is that allergenicity does not equal immunogenicity, and antigen epitopes may be excluded when single recombinant allergens, versus their natural counterparts, are used. They do, however, afford the opportunity of having greater purity and stability as well as improved delivery since protease degradation can be avoided. Diagnostic products may be ineffective for immunotherapy, and immunotherapy products may be ineffective for diagnosis. Diagnostic and therapeutic uses will have to be defined as each allergen is approved (30).

AIRWAY CHALLENGES

Although antigens that elicit IgE-mediated reactions can be identified in an individual by either skin or serologic testing, there may be variability in the nature and the intensity of challenged organs in that subject. For example, a dose of inhaled ragweed might cause intense immediate rhinitis symptoms in a patient who also has allergic asthma; however, even much larger doses of ragweed may cause minimal or no asthmatic symptoms. Similarly, the same subject might have a greater skin test reaction to ragweed than to timothy grass, yet small doses of inhaled timothy grass cause intense bronchoconstriction while the ragweed at even greater concentrations has no effect on pulmonary symptoms. The benefit of using organ-specific antigen challenges is that allergens that precipitate clinical symptoms can be identified. In this section, we will focus on both upper (intranasal) and lower (bronchial) airway challenges that are used to diagnose rhinitis and asthma. In addition, we will briefly mention the rationale and procedures for the bronchial methacholine and histamine challenges as diagnostic tools, since they are often used to assess the presence of asthma.

Clinical Indications

Airway challenges, either intranasal or bronchial, can be used to determine whether a single allergen may be responsible for symptoms of either rhinitis or asthma or both conditions. In general, most allergists use a combination of patient-reported rhinitis symptoms and positive skin tests to identify the most likely culprit of allergic nasal symptoms. Intranasal challenges are more often used to determine the effect of antiallergic drugs in an experimental setting. Bronchial challenge is more often used to measure airway reactivity in the diagnosis of asthma but also has been utilized to determine the effectiveness of pharmacologic agents.

Two bronchial challenge models that have been developed to mimic allergic asthma are the whole-lung and segmental antigen challenges. Segmental challenge involves installation of antigen solution through a bronchoscope into a subsegment of the lung. Since it may be performed only by those trained in bronchoscopy and is used almost exclusively for research investigation, it will not be discussed further in this chapter. Whole-lung antigen challenge can be used both as a diagnostic and as a research tool and is useful in determining relevant environmental asthmatic stimuli for a patient who cannot define exacerbating factors. In addition to its diagnostic application, whole-lung antigen challenge is also used to determine the effects of treatment methods to block allergic physiologic changes and asthmatic symptoms.

Both intranasal and whole-lung antigen challenges initiate allergic reactions and may precipitate bronchoconstriction. Therefore, these techniques should be used with caution under the supervision of a physician or similarly trained health care professional who can treat allergic emergencies. Equipment to treat such emergencies should be ready when these challenges are being performed. Several contraindications to performing either intranasal or whole-lung antigen challenge must be observed to protect the subject. Neither should be performed during asthmatic exacerbations, since such a condition might significantly worsen as a result of the challenge. Also, the results of whole-lung antigen challenge may be misinterpreted during asthma flares, as increases in nonspecific bronchial reactivity occur during exacerbations. In general, it is not recommended that whole-lung antigen challenge be performed if the forced expiratory volume in 1 s (FEV_1) is <60% of predicted values (5). Other health problems such as underlying heart disease must be considered, since whole-lung antigen challenge may result in prolonged bronchoconstriction and potentially hypoxia.

Test Procedures

Intranasal Challenge

Several methods have been developed to test the effect of antigen exposure on the nasal mucosal surface in allergic reactions. First, a specific antigen is identified by a combination of history consistent of allergic symptoms upon exposure to the antigen and positive skin testing, followed by intranasal challenge with that antigen. The two most commonly used methods of intranasal challenge include instillation of antigen into the nares either by spray pump (14) or by nebulizer (8). Symptoms of rhinorrhea and nasal congestion can be scored, the sneezes can be counted, and measurements of nasal patency may be made by rhinometry. These outcomes can be determined at various time points, including baseline before the subject starts the challenge protocol, subsequent to administration of the vehicle in which the antigen is dissolved, and after each dose of antigen. Antigen doses are usually increased at log or half-log intervals, starting at very low antigen concentrations (approximately 0.0001 allergy units for ragweed, for instance) (14). The period between the administrations of consecutive doses of antigen may vary, depending on the challenge protocol, but most frequently the interval is either 5 or 10 min. Completion of the challenge protocol may be determined by a preordained level of symptoms or physiologic changes or by administration of a defined number of individual antigen concentrations. Another outcome which may be measured during intranasal challenges is nasal secretion weight, in which paper disks are placed on the nasal mucosa, removed after a defined period, and then weighed, or alternatively the weight and/or number of paper tissues into which a subject has blown his or her nose is determined (8). Other possible end points include the number of inflammatory cells and mediators measured in the nasal secretions. Some investigators use nasal lavage with 2.5 ml of saline after antigen challenge to collect nasal secretions for determination of inflammatory parameters (14). In such cases, a nasal decongestant such as oxymetazalone may be used as a pretreatment before antigen instillation to ensure nasal patency, as this agent has been shown not to alter allergen-induced inflammation in the nose (15).

Since there is no standardized protocol for intranasal challenge and different investigators have used a wide variety of methods and doses of antigen instillation, there are few reports concerning the reproducibility of intranasal challenge. Doyle and colleagues, using a three-antigen dose protocol administered by nebulizer, found a high degree of correlation when the challenges were performed out of the specific allergen season (8). In this study, ragweed challenge resulted in highly correlated intraindividual responses for the outcomes of sneeze count and secretion weight, while there was moderate correlation in rhinorrhea and congestion symptom scores. Some authors recommend that individuals be challenged no more frequently than once every 2 weeks to minimize the "priming effect," in which an exposure to allergen augments the response to subsequent exposure to the same allergen (14).

Whole-Lung Antigen Challenge

Skin test titration is first performed to determine the concentration of antigen that will be used. The procedure defined earlier in this chapter for a threshold dilution titration with a 10-fold dilution series is initiated. The lowest concentration of this dilution series is given intradermally, and after 15 min the wheal is measured. The concentration given intradermally is then increased at 15-min intervals until a wheal response of 10 mm is obtained. One log higher than this concentration will be used to initiate the inhaled challenge.

The choice of an apparatus to deliver aerosolized solutions is important for ensuring delivery of test doses reproducibly (25). Technical factors that may vary include the preparation and storage of test solutions, generation and inhalation of the aerosol to be delivered, and reporting methods. Factors that affect aerosol delivery from a nebulizer apparatus include output, particle size, and whether the aerosol is delivered continuously or intermittently. Additionally, there may be intrasubject variability in the lung volume at the start of the inhalation, the inspiratory volume and flow rate, and the time that each breath after aerosol inhalation is held. The solutions to be inhaled should be obtained sterile from the manufacturer or sterile filtered before use.

The particle size generated from the nebulizer is critical to ensure consistent delivery of the solution to be aerosolized. Particles of >5 μm tend to be deposited in the mouthpiece apparatus, oropharynx, and upper airway, while particles smaller than 1 μm can be lost through exhalation. The inspiratory flow rate through the nebulizer should be consistent, in the range of 0.13 ml/min, by keeping the flow through the nebulizer at 7 to 9 liters/min.

The Wright and DeVilbiss nebulizers are widely used. The Wright nebulizer generates an aerosol that is inhaled by tidal breathing for 2 min for each dose. It generates an output of 0.13 ml/min, with a particle size of 1.3 μm aerodynamic mass median diameter. With this apparatus, the speed of inhalation and the volume of aerosol inspired are not regulated, and there is no breath holding after each inhalation (25). In our experiments, we have used a DeVilbiss no. 646 nebulizer attached to a solenoid tuning circuit and compressed air source. Two milliliters of the solution to be inhaled is added to the nebulizer well. During a slow, deep inspiration, the solenoid is then activated, delivering compressed air at 10 lb/in^2 for 0.6 s to the nebulizer. An electronic metronome and breath counter is integrated with the solenoid timing device to assist the subject in performing a 3-s inhalation and a 3-s breath hold. This system delivers a mean volume of 0.051 ml of solution, with a standard error of 0.007 ml. The mass median diameter of the droplets is 1.6 μm, with a geometric deviation of 3.14 μm (25). When either the Wright or the DeVilbiss nebulizer device is regulated by a dosimeter, the reproducibility of results in the same subject is similar.

At the start of the procedure, baseline pulmonary function testing is performed and the FEV_1 is recorded. Next, the subject takes five breaths of sterile 10% phosphate-buffered saline solution used as a diluent via the nebulizer. Spirometry is performed 3 min later. If the FEV_1 decreases by more than 10%, the study should be terminated since the specificity of the antigen challenge cannot be evaluated. Five breaths of the initial antigen concentration are then inhaled, and the FEV_1 is measured 10 min later. Five breaths of half-log-increasing concentrations of antigen are inhaled at 10-min intervals until either a >20% decrease in FEV_1 or the maximum dose is achieved.

The maximal dose of antigen to be employed must be carefully considered and may vary for each antigen. High concentrations of antigen solution will cause allergic subjects with rhinitis to have asthma symptoms, even though they may have never experienced such symptoms before. If a whole-lung antigen challenge is to determine a cause-and-effect relationship between an antigen and asthma symptoms, then the use of too high a dose may give false-positive data.

After a 20% fall in FEV_1 has been observed (Fig. 1), the bronchoconstriction can be immediately reversed with a bronchodilator, or hourly pulmonary function measurements can be made to determine whether the subject experiences an asthmatic late-phase reaction. The presence of a late-phase reaction is defined as an FEV_1 measurement 4 to 8 h after the whole-lung antigen challenge that is <15% of the saline control FEV_1 measurement. Approximately 30 to 40% of subjects who have at least a 20% immediate decrease in FEV_1 with whole-lung antigen challenge experience a late-phase reaction. The physiologic mechanisms behind late-phase reactions are unclear. The three factors that are thought to contribute to the allergen-induced late-phase reaction are smooth muscle constriction, airway swelling as a result of increased vascular permeability, and increased mucus production causing airflow obstruction.

Several medications have been shown to affect either the immediate or the late-phase response or both. To avoid a confounding effect of these medications on whole-lung antigen challenge, patients should be instructed to abstain from the following medications for the times listed below based on recent American Thoracic Society (ATS) guidelines (5):

8 h, inhaled short-acting beta-agonists and inhaled cromolyn

24 h, oral beta-agonists, short-acting anticholinergic agents, and leukotriene-modifying agents

48 h, long-acting theophylline preparations, long-acting beta-agonists, long-acting anticholinergics, and inhaled nedocromil

72 h, classical antihistamines

5 days, nonsedating antihistamines

2 weeks, inhaled corticosteroids and nasal steroids

4 weeks, oral corticosteroids

Note: the ATS guidelines do not recommend routinely withholding oral or inhaled corticosteroids if needed for symptom control. However, if these agents are to be withheld to answer either a research or a clinical question, they should be discontinued for the periods listed above, as their anti-inflammatory effect may decrease bronchial responsiveness.

Methacholine and Histamine Challenges

Methacholine and histamine challenges are used to assess nonspecific bronchial reactivity (5). Although neither test is specific for asthma, both tests are commonly used in the evaluation of patients who describe asthmatic symptoms and who have not been observed during an exacerbation. The

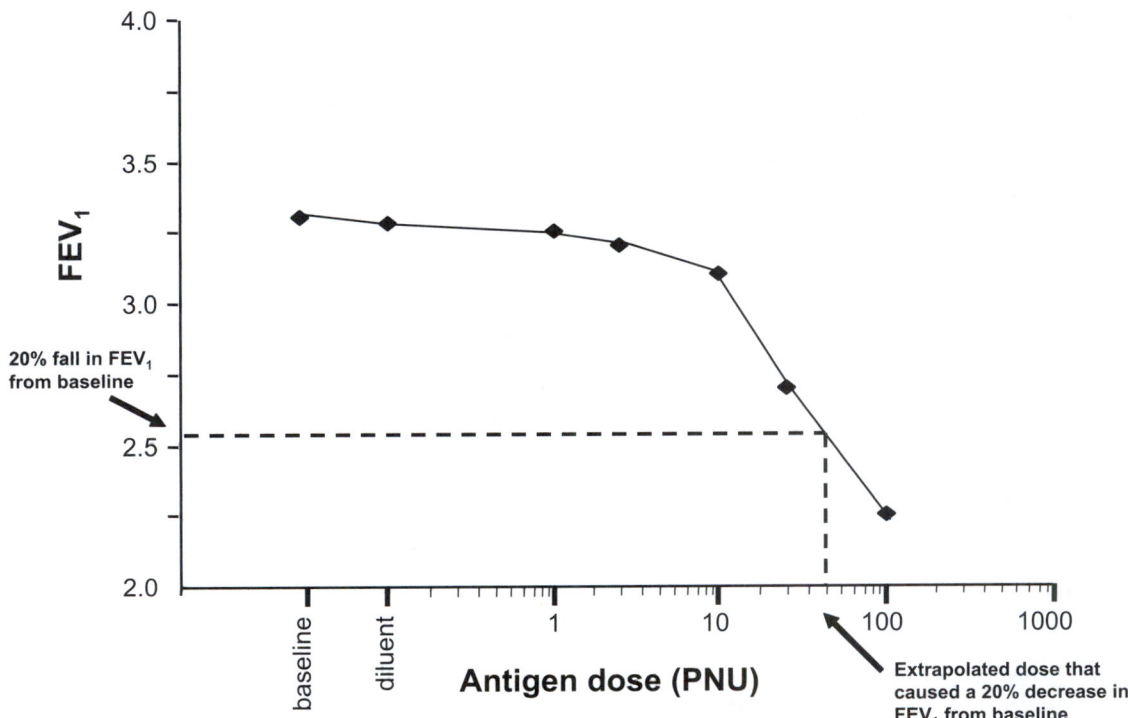

FIGURE 1 Graph of the change of FEV_1 that occurs in an allergic asthmatic subject during a typical whole-lung challenge to which the subject is sensitive. Protein nitrogen units (PNU) are one measure of allergen quantity.

contraindications for methacholine and histamine challenges are essentially the same as for whole-lung antigen challenge.

Methacholine directly interacts with muscarinic receptors to produce smooth muscle contraction. The peak of methacholine effect occurs within 1 to 4 min after inhalation, and the duration of activity is between 1 and 2 h. There is no tachyphylaxis (decreasing response when doses are repeated) associated with methacholine challenges, although there can be diurnal variation (up to 1 to 2 doubling doses) in effecting a 20% fall in FEV_1 during challenges. Methacholine is very safe when administered properly. Rare patients will experience flushing with administration of higher concentrations, but there are no clear predictors as to who will be affected. Methacholine is stable in solution for up to 3 months and is relatively inexpensive.

Histamine has the same onset of action as methacholine, but the duration of activity, 10 to 30 min, is much shorter (34). Histamine can cause bronchoconstriction by stimulating sensory nerves that elicit vagally mediated reflex bronchoconstriction. In addition, histamine can cause airway constriction by binding to histamine receptors on bronchial smooth muscle (34). Tachyphylaxis is reported to occur with histamine challenge and can last up to 6 h. The degree of diurnal variation that occurs with histamine challenge is similar to that for methacholine. Although histamine challenge is safe when administered properly, it is associated with greater side effects, i.e., flushing, headache, and tachycardia. Histamine is stable for 1 to 3 months in solution and is also inexpensive.

Both methacholine and histamine inhalational challenges are similar to antigen challenge in that baseline pulmonary function tests are recorded and then saline challenge

is done to assess nonspecific bronchial reactivity. If the fall in FEV_1 after saline challenge is less than 10% of the baseline, the methacholine or histamine challenge can be started. The ATS has issued recommended guidelines for methacholine challenge protocol for both the 2-min tidal breathing and the five-dose dosimeter methods (5). When the 2-min tidal breathing method is employed, twofold concentration increases are recommended according to the following schedule: 0.03, 0.06, 0.125, 0.25, 0.50, 1, 2, 4, 8, and 16 mg/ml. When the five-dose dosimeter method is used, the doses of methacholine are 0.06, 0.25, 1, 4, and 16 mg/ml. A recent report revealed that when these ATS protocols were used in a study population of stable asthma patients in a crossover manner, there was no intrasubject difference between the provocative concentration that causes a drop in FEV_1 of 20% from the saline control value (PC_{20}) obtained by either method on randomized study days (35). Histamine can be administered with the same dosing schedule protocol outlined for methacholine.

Some investigators suggest that adenosine or hypertonic saline challenges might be a useful adjunct to methacholine in epidemiologic studies. This argument is based on the hypothesis that inhalation of adenosine or hypertonic saline induces the release of inflammatory mediators from mast cells and eosinophils, which in turn causes bronchoconstriction, whereas methacholine principally acts on cholinergic nerve endings to effect airway obstruction (6, 7). Currently, there are no ATS guidelines for adenosine challenges.

Data Analysis

Values for whole-lung antigen, methacholine, and histamine challenges are calculated similarly, and the major end point is usually the PC_{20} (5). Generally, the PC_{20} is expressed as a noncumulative measurement in milligrams per milliliter. A few groups express results as the provocative dose (PD_{20}) that is usually reported as a cumulative dose, in terms of either micromoles or "breath units." The number of breath units is determined by the following formula: breath units = concentration (micrograms per milliliter) × breath number (23). The results of any of the challenges described are determined by a dose-response curve, using a semilogarithmic scale. The dose (either cumulative or noncumulative) of the challenge substance is plotted on the logarithmic abscissa, while the FEV_1 responses as a percentage of the saline control inhalation are plotted on the linear ordinate. The line of best fit for the values obtained is determined, and the PC_{20} or PD_{20} is calculated by interpolating from the final two concentrations or doses the point at which the FEV_1 is 20% decreased from that of the saline control.

Interpretation

Whole-lung allergen challenge is considered to be the definitive method to test the specificity of a particular antigen to cause bronchial reactions. False-positive reactions can occur when the antigen is given in high enough concentrations to cause asthma symptoms in allergic rhinitis patients or normal subjects who previously have never experienced asthma. The reproducibility of whole-lung allergen challenge from day to day is less than twofold in concentration and is improved if the prechallenge FEV_1 is within 10% on the two challenges.

The diagnostic sensitivity of methacholine and histamine challenges for asthma has been studied by several investigators, but the results have varied because of a lack of uniform diagnostic criteria for asthma. The concentrations for methacholine and histamine that are regarded as positive for bronchial reactivity (FEV_1 fall of >20%) are both 8 mg/ml. Two studies have reported widely accepted values for the sensitivity of methacholine and histamine challenges. Hopp et al. reported that the sensitivity of an 8-mg/ml concentration of methacholine for diagnosing asthmatic subjects was 85%, while the specificity was 95% (12). Cockroft and his colleagues reported that the sensitivity of a PC_{20} for histamine of 8 mg/ml or less was 100%, while the specificity was 93% for the diagnosis of asthma (4). Currently, the ATS categorizes bronchial responsiveness thus (5) for the indicated PC_{20} (in milligrams per milliliter):

>16, normal bronchial responsiveness
4–16, borderline bronchial responsiveness
1–4, mild bronchial responsiveness
<1, moderate to severe bronchial responsiveness

The reproducibility of inhalational challenges is dependent not only on the technique, but also on the health of the subject. Subjects should not be studied during asthmatic exacerbations, for two reasons. First, natural allergen exposures such as animals or seasonal pollens increase nonspecific bronchial reactivity and fail to provide a clear answer. Second, an allergen reactivity priming effect may potentiate so that lower doses may result in excessive responses and diminish the safety of the procedure. Active upper respiratory tract infections can also increase nonspecific reactivity. Patients should be free of symptoms from colds, bronchitis, and sinus infections for at least 2 weeks before challenge. Persons exposed to oxidizing pollutants, smokers, and cystic fibrosis patients may also have increased reactivity based on methacholine and histamine challenges.

CONCLUSION

Challenge procedures can be extremely useful in the investigation of allergy. Skin testing has a high degree of sensitivity and specificity for determining antigens that cause allergic symptoms. However, positive skin tests do not necessarily indicate that a specific allergen causes symptoms specific for a certain organ system. Provocation testing can help define both relevant allergens that cause asthma symptoms and nonspecific bronchial hyperreactivity to pharmacologic agents. These tests have predictive profiles that make them useful diagnostic tools and can be safe when performed properly and under close supervision by experienced health care personnel.

This work was supported by the American Academy of Allergy, Asthma, and Immunology ERT Award, grant NIH 1 RO1 HL 069949, and grant NIH 1 RO1 AI 054660.

REFERENCES

1. **Almind, M., A. Dirksen, N. H. Nielsen, and U. G. Svendsen.** 1988. Duration of the inhibitory activity on histamine-induced skin weals of sedative and non-sedative antihistamines. *Allergy* **43:**593–596.
2. **Bernstein, I. L., and W. W. Storms.** 1995. Practice parameters for allergy diagnostic testing. Joint Task Force on Practice Parameters for the Diagnosis and Treatment of Asthma. The American Academy of Allergy, Asthma and Immunology and the American College of Allergy, Asthma and Immunology. *Ann. Allergy Asthma Immunol.* **75:**543–625.
3. **Blackley, C. H.** 1873. Experimental researches on the causes and nature of Catarrhus Aestivus (hay fever or hay-asthma). Balliere, Tindall and Cox, London, England.
4. **Cockcroft, D. W., R. E. Ruffin, P. A. Frith, A. Cartier, E. F. Juniper, J. Dolovich, and F. E. Hargreave.** 1979. Determinants of allergen-induced asthma: dose of allergen, circulating IgE antibody concentration, and bronchial responsiveness to inhaled histamine. *Am. Rev. Respir. Dis.* **120:**1053–1058.
5. **Crapo, R. O., R. Casaburi, A. L. Coates, P. L. Enright, J. L. Hankinson, C. G. Irvin, N. R. MacIntyre, R. T. McKay, J. S. Wanger, S. D. Anderson, D. W. Cockcroft, J. E. Fish, and P. J. Sterk.** 2000. Guidelines for methacholine and exercise challenge testing—1999. *Am. J. Respir. Crit. Care Med.* **161:**309–329.
6. **De Meer, G., D. J. J. Heederik, B. Brunekreef, and D. S. Postma.** 2001. Repeatability of bronchial hyperresponsiveness to adenosine-5'-monophosphate (AMP) by a short dosimeter protocol. *Thorax* **56:**362–365.
7. **De Meer, G., G. B. Marks, and D. S. Postma.** 2004. Direct or indirect stimuli for bronchial challenge testing: what is the relevance for asthma epidemiology? *Clin. Exp. Allergy* **34:**9–16.
8. **Doyle, W. J., D. P. Skoner, J. T. Seroky, and P. Fireman.** 1995. Reproducibility of the effects of intranasal ragweed challenges in allergic subjects. *Ann. Allergy Asthma Immunol.* **74:**171–176.
9. **Gadde, J., M. Spence, B. Wheeler, and N. F. Adkinson, Jr.** 1993. Clinical experience with penicillin skin testing in a large inner-city STD clinic. *JAMA* **270:**2456–2463.
10. **Golden, D. B., J. M. Tracy, T. M. Freeman, and D. R. Hoffman; Insect Committee of the American Academy of Allergy, Asthma and Immunology.** 2003. Negative venom skin test results in patients with histories of systemic reaction to a sting. *J. Allergy Clin. Immunol.* **112:**495–498.
11. **Grier, T., D. Hazelhurst, E. Duncan, and R. Esch.** 2001. Stability, compatibility, and cross-reactivity of allergens: immunochemical reactivities and practical considerations. Presented at ACAAI Annual Meeting, 16 to 20 November 2001, Orlando, Fla.

12. Hopp, R. J., A. K. Bewtra, N. M. Nair, and R. G. Townley. 1984. Specificity and sensitivity of methacholine inhalation challenge in normal and asthmatic children. *J. Allergy Clin. Immunol.* **74:**154–158.

13. Lewis, T., and R. T. Grant. 1924. Vascular reactions of the skin to injury. Part II. The liberation of a histamine-like substance in injured skin, the underlying cause of factitious urticaria and of wheals produced by burning; and observations upon the nervous control of certain skin reactions. *Heart* **11:**209–265.

14. Lin, H., K. M. Boesel, D. T. Griffith, C. Prussin, B. Foster, F. A. Romero, R. Townley, and T. B. Casale. 2004. Omalizumab rapidly decreases nasal allergic response and FcepsilonRI on basophils. *J. Allergy Clin. Immunol.* **113:**297–302.

15. Majchel, A. M., F. Baroody, A. Kagey-Sobotka, L. M. Lichtenstein, and R. M. Naclerio. 1993. Effect of oxymetazoline on the early response to nasal challenge with antigen. *J. Allergy Clin. Immunol.* **92:**767–770.

16. McCann, W. A., and D. R. Ownby. 2002. The reproducibility of the allergy skin test scoring and interpretation by board-certified/board-eligible allergists. *Ann. Allergy Asthma Immunol.* **89:**368–371.

17. Nelson, H. S. 2004. Preparing and mixing allergen vaccines. *Clin. Allergy Immunol.* **18:**457–479.

18. Nelson, H. S., D. Ikle, and A. Buchmeier. 1996. Studies of allergen extract stability: the effects of dilution and mixing. *J. Allergy Clin. Immunol.* **98:**382–388.

19. Nelson, H. S., J. Knoetzer, and B. Bucher. 1996. Effect of distance between sites and region of the body on results of skin prick tests. *J. Allergy Clin. Immunol.* **97:**596–601.

20. Nelson, H. S., C. Kolehmainen, J. Lahr, J. Murphy, and A. Buchmeier. 2004. A comparison of multiheaded devices for allergy skin testing. *J. Allergy Clin. Immunol.* **113:**1218–1219.

21. Nelson, H. S., J. Lahr, A. Buchmeier, and D. McCormick. 1998. Evaluation of devices for skin prick testing. *J. Allergy Clin. Immunol.* **101:**153–156.

22. Nelson, H. S., J. Oppenheimer, A. Buchmeier, T. R. Kordash, and L. L. Freshwater. 1996. An assessment of the role of intradermal skin testing in the diagnosis of clinically relevant allergy to timothy grass. *J. Allergy Clin. Immunol.* **97:**1193–1201.

23. Peebles, R. S., Jr., E. M. Wagner, M. C. Liu, D. Proud, R. G. Hamilton, and A. Togias. 2001. Allergen-induced changes in airway responsiveness are not related to indices of airway edema. *J. Allergy Clin. Immunol.* **107:**805–811.

24. Rosen, J. P., J. E. Selcow, L. M. Mendelson, M. P. Grodofsky, J. M. Factor, and H. A. Sampson. 1994. Skin testing with natural foods in patients suspected of having food allergies: is it a necessity? *J. Allergy Clin. Immunol.* **93:**1068–1070.

25. Ryan, G., M. B. Dolovich, R. S. Roberts, P. A. Frith, E. F. Juniper, F. E. Hargreave, and M. T. Newhouse. 1981. Standardization of inhalation provocation tests: two techniques of aerosol generation and inhalation compared. *Am. Rev. Respir. Dis.* **123:**195–199.

26. Sampson, H. A. 1988. Comparative study of commercial food antigen extracts for the diagnosis of food hypersensitivity. *J. Allergy Clin. Immunol.* **2:**718–726.

27. Sampson, H. A. 2004. Update on food allergy. *J. Allergy Clin. Immunol.* **113:**805–819.

28. Sicherer, S. H., and H. A. Sampson. 1999. Food hypersensitivity and atopic dermatitis: pathophysiology, epidemiology, diagnosis, and management. *J. Allergy Clin. Immunol.* **104:**S114–S122.

29. Simons, F. E., X. Gu, and K. J. Simons. 2001. Epinephrine absorption in adults: intramuscular versus subcutaneous injection. *J. Allergy Clin. Immunol.* **108:**871–873.

30. Slater, J. E. 2004. Recombinant allergens in the US. *Methods* **32:**209–211.

31. Sogn, D. D., R. Evans III, G. M. Shepherd, T. B. Casale, J. Condemi, P. A. Greenberger, P. F. Kohler, A. Saxon, R. J. Summers, P. P. VanArsdel, J. G. Massicot, W. C. Blackwelder, and B. B. Levine. 1992. Results of the National Institute of Allergy and Infectious Diseases Collaborative Clinical Trial to test the predictive value of skin testing with major and minor penicillin derivatives in hospitalized adults. *Arch. Intern. Med.* **152:**1025–1032.

32. Turkeltaub, P. C. 2000. Percutaneous and intracutaneous diagnostic tests of IgE-mediated diseases (immediate hypersensitivity). *Clin. Allergy Immunol.* **15:**53–87.

33. Wood, R. A., W. Phipatanakul, R. G. Hamilton, and P. A. Eggleston. 1999. A comparison of skin prick tests, intradermal skin tests, and RASTs in the diagnosis of cat allergy. *J. Allergy Clin. Immunol.* **103:**773–779.

34. Woolcock, A. J., K. Yan, and C. Salome. 1983. Methods for assessing bronchial reactivity. *Eur. J. Respir. Dis.* **64**(Suppl. 128)**:**181–194.

35. Wubbel, C., M. J. Asmus, G. Stevens, S. E. Chesrown, and L. Hendeles. 2004. Methacholine challenge testing: comparison of the two American Thoracic Society-recommended methods. *Chest* **125:**453–458.

36. Yuninger, J. W., S. Ahlstedt, P. A. Eggleston, H. A. Homburger, H. S. Nelson, D. R. Ownby, T. A. Platts-Mills, H. A. Sampson, S. H. Sicherer, A. M. Weinstein, P. B. Williams, R. A. Wood, and R. S. Zeiger. 2000. Quantitative IgE antibody assays in allergic diseases. *J. Allergy Clin. Immunol.* **105:**1077–1084.

Immunological Methods in the Diagnostic Allergy Clinical and Research Laboratory

ROBERT G. HAMILTON

107

Almost 40 years have passed since immunoglobulin E (IgE) was identified as the reagin or serum antibody that sensitizes skin and mediates immediate-type hypersensitivity reactions in humans (2, 6). Since this pivotal event, the diagnostic allergy laboratory has provided the clinician with an array of analytical measurements that aid in the diagnosis, management, and study of the epidemiology of IgE-mediated diseases. Table 1 summarizes the analytes that are currently measured in diagnostic allergy laboratories. Total and allergen-specific IgE antibodies are the primary analytes measured to support the diagnosis of human allergic disease (Table 2). Mast cell tryptase, eosinophil cationic protein, IgG antivenom, cotenine (a metabolite of nicotine and indicator of passive smoke exposure), and the levels of indoor aeroallergens in surface dust are less frequently measured to aid in allergic disease diagnosis or management. The goal of this chapter is to overview clinically used and research methods for the quantification of total and allergen-specific IgE antibodies and allergen-specific IgG antibodies. The performance of immunoassays for these analytes has continued to improve with the availability of new solid-phase matrices, conjugate labeling technology, standardized reference reagents, and data processing methods. Methods for the measurement of the other analytes listed in Table 1 are discussed elsewhere (7, 13) and are not discussed further here.

ANALYTES RELEVANT TO ALLERGIC DISEASE

Immediate-type hypersensitivity or allergic disease manifests as a spectrum of symptoms involving respiratory responses (asthma or rhinitis), skin reactions (urticaria and dermatitis), gastrointestinal symptoms, or life-threatening anaphylactic shock. These symptoms are produced as a result of the reexposure of a previously sensitized (IgE antibody-positive) individual to one or many sensitizing allergens. These allergens are ubiquitous proteins that are released from pollens of grasses, weeds, and trees or antigenic proteins released from mites, rodents, domestic animals, insects, and mold spores and present in some drugs and generally well-tolerated foods.

IgE mediates allergic reactions by binding onto high-affinity Fcε receptors on mast cells and basophils and initiating the release of vasoactive mediators following allergen binding and cell surface IgE antibody cross-linking (18). Total serum IgE has been used clinically as a diagnostic analyte, since a moderately elevated total serum IgE level reinforces the clinical

diagnosis of atopic disorders, including allergic rhinitis, allergic asthma, and atopic dermatitis. Moreover, high IgE levels are commonly observed in parasite infections and are necessary in the definitive diagnosis of bronchopulmonary aspergillosis and hypergammaglobulinemia E syndrome (Table 2). Serial total serum IgE levels can confirm an expected seasonal boost in serum IgE that is commonly seen after environmental exposure to the allergen to which the patient has become sensitized. However, the wide overlap in total serum IgE levels among atopic and nonatopic individuals diminishes their general diagnostic utility. Thus, the clinician must refrain from discounting allergy when total IgE levels are low or from automatically inferring an allergic etiology when the total serum IgE is high.

Allergen-specific IgE antibody is the primary analyte used to support the definitive diagnosis of IgE-mediated allergic disease (Table 2). IgE antibody can be detected in vivo using puncture or intradermal skin tests that provoke IgE-mediated skin mast cell release and elicitation of a wheal and erythema. The skin test is extensively discussed in chapter 106 and is not further discussed here. Some generalized skin conditions, such as eczema, dermatographism, psoriasis, and urticaria, make skin testing problematic. Moreover, skin testing of children under 10 years can be difficult. There are also occasions when skin reactivity has been suppressed by prolonged use of antihistamines and other medications that cannot be stopped prior to skin testing. In all of these cases, analysis of a serum specimen for allergen-specific IgE antibody may be preferred over skin testing in the diagnostic workup of a suspected allergic patient (12, 16).

Antigen-specific IgG antibody levels in serum can sometimes serve to document exposure of an individual to a potent antigen. However, IgG antibody that is specific for allergenic substances is not generally assayed because there has been no clear clinical indication for these measurements. The exception is Hymenoptera venom hypersensitivity, where IgG antibody levels may serve as an indicator of the effectiveness of various antigen doses used to induce a specific immune response during venom immunotherapy (5) (Table 2). IgG antibody has been used to monitor venom-allergic patients when maintenance venom immunotherapy doses are first achieved (after 3 to 6 months) for comparison with pretreatment levels to assess the adequacy of the humoral immune response. The venom-specific IgG level can also serve as a baseline for future immunological monitoring

TABLE 1 Analytes measured in the diagnostic allergy laboratory

Analyte
Diagnosis
Allergen-specific IgE (individual allergen specificities and multiallergen screens)
Total serum IgE, and free serum IgE for patients on anti-IgE (omalizumab) therapy
Mast cell tryptase (alpha and beta tryptase); indicator for mast cell-mediated anaphylaxis
Management
Eosinophil cationic protein
IgG antivenom (monitoring Hymenoptera venom patients on immunotherapy)
Environmental testing
Cotinine (monitoring secondhand smoke exposure)
Indoor aeroallergen quantification
Dust mite: *Dermatophagoides pteronyssinus* group 1 allergen (Der p 1)
Dust mite: *Dermatophagoides farinae* group 1 allergen (Der f 1)
Cat: *Felis domesticus* group 1 allergen (Fel d 1)
Dog: *Canis familiaris* group 1 allergen (Can f 1)
German cockroach: *Blatella germanica* group 1 and 2 allergens (Bla g 1 and 2)
Mouse: *Mus musculus* group 1 allergen (Mus m 1)
Rat: *Rattus norvegicus* group 1 allergen (Rat n 1)
Bacterial endotoxin
Viable mold spore analysis

and at 12- to 18-month intervals to monitor the efficacy of the maintenance immunotherapy regimen. Comparison with previous levels can be useful as a periodic guide to plan modifications in venom immunotherapy, such as increasing the maintenance injection interval, changing the dose, or discontinuing some or all venoms. IgG antibody levels can be used to assist in the evaluation of clinical problems such as adverse reactions to venom injections during venom treatment or an inadvertent field sting. Finally, levels of specific IgG antibody to venom and other model antigens, such as ragweed, are used in research studies to document humoral immune responses to an antigen to which the individual has been accidentally or intentionally exposed.

TOTAL SERUM IgE

Historically, total human serum IgE has been measured by several assays, including competitive-binding liquid-phase immunoprecipitation (double-antibody or labeled-antigen) assays, competitive-binding solid-phase labeled-antigen immunoassays, noncompetitive solid-phase two-site (sandwich) immunometric (labeled-antibody) assays, and nephelometric assays. Of these assays, the two-site immunometric assay has become the most widely used clinical and research assay for the quantification of total serum IgE. The first reported noncompetitive solid-phase two-site immunometric assay used polyclonal anti-human IgE covalently bound to a solid phase (paper disks) to bind IgE from unknown and calibrated reference and control sera. Following a buffer wash, radiolabeled anti-IgE was added to detect bound IgE. The amount of radiolabeled anti-IgE bound was directly related to the IgE content in the original serum. The assay displayed excellent sensitivity (as low as 0.2 ng of IgE per ml) and precision (coefficients of variation [CV] of ≤5%), and it was minimally affected by nonspecific serum factors as a result of the washing step. Reliable commercial sources of polyclonal and monoclonal anti-IgE are now available. Clinical laboratories perform one of several Food and Drug Administration (FDA)-cleared immunometric assays, such as the Pharmacia ImmunoCAP, Diagnostic Products Corporation Immulite 2000, Bayer ADVIA Centaur, Beckman Access/2, or Behring Nephelometer, for measuring total serum IgE. Since their performance has been extensively discussed elsewhere (13), it is not further discussed here.

Occasionally, researchers need to measure total serum IgE using an inexpensive and flexible assay that can accommodate unusual specimens other than serum. One monoclonal antibody-based noncompetitive solid-phase two-site immunoenzymetric assay (IEMA) is described here as the procedure of choice for research investigations of total serum IgE. This assay is a 1-day microtiter plate-based enzyme immunoassay (EIA) that uses monoclonal anti-human IgE adsorbed onto plastic wells to bind IgE and a different labeled monoclonal anti-human IgE to detect bound IgE (11). The use of a murine IgM monoclonal anti-human IgE Fc capture antibody and biotinylated murine IgG monoclonal anti-human IgE Fc detection antibody optimizes both assay sensitivity and specificity.

Reagents

Mouse IgM-k anti-human IgE Fc (clone HP6061; EMD Biosciences, La Jolla, Calif.) should be obtained in purified form at 2 mg/ml in phosphate-buffered saline (PBS) with no added protein. Mouse IgG2a-k anti-human IgE Fc (clone HP6029; EMD Biosciences) should be obtained in biotinylated form at 1 mg/ml in PBS containing 10 mg of bovine serum albumin (BSA) per ml. Buffers and other reagents required for the assay include PBS, PBS–0.05% Tween 20 (PBS-Tween), PBS–1% BSA, streptavidin-horseradish peroxidase (streptavidin-HRP), 1 mM 2,2'-azino-di-(3-ethylbenzthiazoline sulfonic acid) (ABTS) substrate in 70 mM citrate phosphate buffer, and 2 mM sodium azide. These buffers are prepared using endotoxin-free water and chemicals obtained from Sigma Chemical Company (St. Louis, Mo.).

Specimen Requirements

The IEMA is designed to measure the level of IgE protein in human serum. Heparinized or cation-chelated plasma may be used, although fibrin formation can reduce pipetting accuracy. This assay can also be used to measure IgE levels in tear fluid, bronchial alveolar lavage fluid, saliva, nasal washings, and peripheral blood cell culture supernatants.

TABLE 2 Clinical conditions in which serological determinations may be useful in differential diagnosis

Clinical condition	Total serum IgE	Allergen-specific IgE	Allergen-specific IgG
Atopic disorders: allergic rhinitis, allergic asthma, atopic dermatitis	Moderately elevated levels positively reinforce clinical diagnosis; however, low or normal IgE level is not incompatible with diagnosis.	Positive allergen-specific IgE antibody level supports the diagnosis of IgE-mediated atopic disorders.	In the absence of allergen immunotherapy, the level of allergen-specific IgG antibody can be low or undetectable.
Intrinsic (nonallergic) asthma	Normal or low levels suggest that IgE mechanisms play only a minor role in the pathogenesis of asthma.	Negative IgE antibody levels support the diagnosis of intrinsic asthma.	Not useful in the definitive diagnosis of intrinsic asthma
ABPA[a]	Normal serum IgE levels virtually exclude diagnosis.	Positive *Aspergillus*-specific IgE antibody is required for definitive diagnosis of ABPA.	Precipitating IgG antibodies are required for definitive diagnosis of ABPA.
Wiskott-Aldrich syndrome	Elevated levels are commonly found in patients who exhibit eczema.		
Hypergammaglobulinemia E syndrome (elevated IgE, increased susceptibility to infection and dermatitis)	Very high serum IgE levels are necessary for definitive diagnosis of hyper-IgE syndrome.		
Parasitism	Many parasitic infections produce extreme elevations in serum IgE; a very high IgE level in the absence of other explanations strongly suggests the possibility of parasitism.	The presence of parasite-specific IgE antibodies confirms the diagnosis of parasitism.	Parasite-specific IgG antibodies confirm a present or recent parasite infection.
Eosinophilia	A normal IgE level makes the diagnosis of parasitism less likely as a cause of eosinophilia; eosinophilia with normal serum IgE is a common feature of nonallergic asthma.		
Allergen immunotherapy	Same as for atopic disorders (above)	Specific IgE antibodies are not helpful in monitoring patients on immunotherapy or assessing its clinical efficacy.	Used in Hymenoptera venom immunotherapy to confirm adequate immunotherapy dosages and assess relative risk for reactions upon resting

[a]ABPA, allergic bronchopulmonary aspergillosis.

Use of specimens other than serum and plasma requires the analysis of an appropriate non-IgE-containing "negative" control to define the magnitude of the nonspecific binding produced by matrix proteins that can vary widely. The antigenic properties of IgE protein are maintained almost indefinitely when serum is stored frozen at −20 or −70°C. Transportation of serum specimens at ambient temperatures for more than several days is not generally recommended without packaging in insulated mailers.

IEMA Procedure

The IEMA has been designed to balance good performance with a reasonable turnaround time.

1. Plastic 96-well microtiter plates are coated for 1 h at room temperature (RT; ~23°C) and then overnight at 4°C with mouse IgM monoclonal anti-human IgE Fc (clone HP6061, 100 μl/well) which has been diluted in PBS to 10 μg/ml just prior to use. Plates are covered with Parafilm between each step to minimize evaporation and dust contamination.

2. Each plate is washed once with PBS-Tween using a 12-channel handheld Corning washing system or a comparable washing device, and 0.3 ml of PBS–1% BSA is added to each well to block unreacted sites.

3. After a second wash (four times) with PBS-Tween, 0.1 ml of reference, control, or test serum is added to its respective well. The standard curve is composed of 8 to 10 twofold dilutions in duplicate of a reference serum, beginning with a concentration of 100 kIU/liter (1 IU of IgE = 2.4 ng). Test sera are initially screened undiluted in duplicate and reanalyzed at several dilutions up to 1:100 if they exceed the top point of the dose-response curve. A buffer blank is analyzed to control for nonspecific binding. Each plate is pipetted within 15 min without interruption. The plates are then incubated for 2 h at RT. Two or three dilutions of high, medium, and low IgE serum controls are analyzed in different regions of the plate to demonstrate that the assay is in control.

4. Following a PBS-Tween buffer wash (four times), biotin-conjugated mouse IgG anti-human IgE Fc (clone HP6029) is added (0.1 ml per well, 1 μg/ml in PBS–1% BSA) with a multichannel pipette and the plates are incubated for 1 h at RT.

5. The plates are washed four times with PBS-Tween buffer, streptavidin-HRP (avidin HRP; Sigma S5512) is

added with a multichannel pipette (0.1 ml per well, 1 μg/ml in PBS–1% BSA), and the plates are incubated for 1 h at RT.

6. Plates are washed four times and 0.1 ml of substrate is added. Three substrates have been successfully used in this assay: 1,3-benzenediamine (also known as *o*-phenlyenediamine) (free base; Sigma P2903), ABTS (Sigma A1888), and 3,3',5,5'-tetramethylbenzidine (Sigma T5525). For routine analysis of human sera, 1 mM ABTS is prepared in 70 mM citrate-phosphate buffer. Immediately prior to use, 1 μl of 30% hydrogen peroxide is added per ml of ABTS required. The substrate is immediately pipetted into the plate (0.1 ml/well) using a multichannel pipette.

7. The peroxidase enzymatic reaction is stopped by adding 0.1 ml of 2 mM sodium azide per well when the top point on the standard curve reaches an optical density of 1.5 to 2.0 (usually within 5 to 15 min). The plate is read on a microtiter plate reader at 410 nm, and optical densities of the unknown sera are interpolated from the standard curve in kilo-international units per liter traceable to the World Health Organization total serum IgE reference preparation using an interpolation program.

Standardization

The World Health Organization international reference standard for human IgE or the U.S. IgE reference serum preparation can be used as a primary standard from which secondary standard serum pools can be cross-calibrated for IgE content by the value transfer technique (e.g., 3 to 5 dilutions in 10 assays). Alternatively, commercially available precalibrated IgE standards can be used (e.g., Pharmacia). Once a secondary working standard has been reproducibly cross-calibrated, it can be used in routine assays with periodic reevaluation against the primary reference preparation to ensure quality control. Nonparallelism may be observed in the high-end range of the IEMA possibly because of an atypical nonspecific binding when sera containing >2,000 kIU/liter are used as reference sera.

Working Range, Sensitivity, Reproducibility, and Parallelism

The minimal detectable concentration and working range of the IEMA are dependent on the dilution and affinity of the capture and detection antibodies and duration of the serum, conjugate, and substrate incubations. One practical goal in assay design is to achieve a clinically useful assay working range (e.g., 1 to 200 IU/ml added) while minimizing nonspecific binding effects and reagent use. A sensitivity of 0.5 IU/ml (1.2 μg/liter) can be achieved with this total IgE IEMA. Agreement among replicates is usually excellent (CV, <5%), and an interexperimental reproducibility of <15% (CV) can be achieved. Finally, parallelism is assessed by analyzing test sera at two or more dilutions and computing an interdilutional CV following correction for serum dilution. Interdilutional CV of <15% are achievable with most test sera.

Quality Control

The total serum IgE IEMA can be quality controlled by inclusion of two or three well-studied sera within each assay. The three quality control sera should have low (<10 IU/ml), moderate (100 to 250 IU/ml), and high (>1,000 IU/ml) levels of IgE, respectively.

Because total serum IgE is a regulated analyte as defined by the amended Clinical Laboratory Improvement Act of 1988, licensed clinical laboratories providing this analytical measurement must demonstrate proficiency in an external proficiency survey such as the Diagnostic Allergy (SE) survey conducted by the College of American Pathologists. In the SE survey, five challenge sera are sent to each participating laboratory during each of three cycles per year (15 challenges per year) and each is tested for total serum IgE and allergen-specific IgE antibody. The total serum IgE levels range from <10 to >10,000 IU/ml to test the laboratory's ability to accurately measure a wide spectrum of IgE levels in serum.

Interpretation

Total serum IgE levels are age dependent. The level of IgE in cord serum is usually less than 2 IU/ml since IgE does not cross the placental barrier in significant amounts. Mean serum IgE levels progressively increase in healthy children until 10 to 15 years of age (1). Atopic infants have an earlier and steeper rise in serum IgE levels during the early years of life than do nonatopic controls. An age-dependent decline in total serum IgE typically occurs from the second to eighth decade of life. Individuals with total serum IgE levels above the upper 95% confidence limit (12, 13) (Table 2) often have atopic disorders such as allergic rhinitis, extrinsic or allergic asthma, and atopic dermatitis. However, the overlap between atopic and nonatopic populations is considerable. In one study of adults with allergic asthma, the mean serum IgE level was 1,589 ng/ml (range, 55 to 12,750 ng/ml). Only about one-half of these asthmatic patients had serum IgE levels above the upper 95% confidence limit for nonatopic individuals of the same age. In another study, high levels of serum IgE (mean, 978 kIU/liter; range, 1.3 to 65,208 kIU/liter) were observed in approximately 90% of patients with atopic dermatitis.

Modification of Total IgE IEMA for Free IgE Quantification in Serum

In 2003, omalizumab, a recombinant humanized IgG1 monoclonal anti-human IgE Fc (Xolair), was licensed for therapeutic use in the United States to treat persistent allergic asthma. Omalizumab binds circulating IgE, blocking its binding to alpha chain of FcεR1 receptors and down regulating the FcεR1 receptor number on mast cells and basophils (18). Reduced cell-bound IgE can result in a concomitant reduction in mediator release and reduced allergy symptoms. Comparison of the total and free IgE levels in serum before and 1 to 3 months after treatment can serve as one measure of an effective omalizumab dose administration (14). A modification of the total serum IEMA described above allows the quantification of the level of "free" or non-omalizumab-bound IgE in serum. In this assay, IgE is captured from serum with monoclonal anti-human IgE (clone HP6061) and detected with biotin-labeled FcεR1α. In the absence of omalizumab, working ranges of the free and total IgE IEMAs were comparable (10 to 1,000 kIU/liter), with excellent precision, reproducibility, and parallelism. Pre-omalizumab administration total and free IgE levels by IEMA are highly correlated, and in vitro reduction of free IgE (>90%) has been observed with omalizumab/IgE molar ratios of 2 to 20 (14).

ALLERGEN-SPECIFIC IgE ANTIBODY

Historically, the first-generation assay for allergen-specific IgE antibody in human serum was the radioallergosorbent test (19). In this assay, an allergen-coated solid phase (paper disks) was incubated with human serum, during which time specific antibody of all immunoglobulin classes (if present) bound. The solid phase was then washed, and radiolabeled anti-human IgE antibody detected bound IgE. The quantity of bound radioactivity directly correlated with the quantity of specific IgE antibody in the original serum. IgE antibody results were compared to a calibrated standard reference serum, and insolubilized allergen and radiolabeled anti-IgE antibody were used in molar excess.

Clinical Allergen-Specific IgE Antibody Assays

Over the past ~40 years, there have been major improvements in the design and performance of allergen-specific IgE assays. FDA-cleared commercially available semiautomated and automated allergen-specific IgE antibody assays have been developed. An overview of these commercial IgE antibody assays is presented the sixth edition of this manual (4) and elsewhere (12, 13, 17). These assays have in common an allergen-containing reagent (typically a solid-phase allergosorbent); a panel of reference, control, and test human sera; and a labeled anti-human IgE reagent. The Pharmacia ImmunoCAP system and the Diagnostic Products Corporation Immulite 2000 have achieved the highest degree of quantification and automation. Tighter precision around the positive/negative threshold and a more rapid, robust chemistry have been achieved with automation. With automation comes the need to analyze quality control sera with IgE antibody levels across the measured dose-response curve range. The quality control sera containing different specificities of IgE antibody should be randomly sprinkled through the assay run to investigate the quality of the whole assay analysis. Daily monitoring of results from these positive control sera in the form of Levey-Jennings plots verifies that the instrument is performing all of its serum and reagent addition, incubation, washing, and data analysis steps accurately.

Analyte-Specific Reagents

In the United States, the FDA regulates the sale of in vitro diagnostic products under regulation 21 CFR 809. This includes allergen-specific IgE antibody assay reagents that are intended for human use. One component of the IgE antibody assay reagent is the allergen extract, which is often a complex protein mixture. Presently, only 19 of the hundreds of allergen specificities of clinical interest have been standardized (see chapter 105). Some allergen extracts that have been insolubilized on allergosorbents for use in allergen-specific IgE assays have not yet been cleared by the FDA. These can be provided to clinical laboratories under an "analyte-specific reagent" classification. These allergosorbents can be used by laboratories that are qualified to perform high-complexity testing; however, a disclaimer must be included in the report indicating that a measurement was performed with an analyte-specific reagent.

Research Allergen-Specific IgE Assays

Researchers sometimes have need of a versatile immunoassay to measure allergen-specific IgE antibody. A number of polymers have been used for allergen insolubilization, including carbohydrate matrices (Sephadex, agarose, and cellulose) and polystyrene test tubes and 96-well microtiter plates. Each of these polymers differs with respect to its allergen-binding capacity, nonspecific binding properties, stability, and ease of washing. The use of a solid phase with the highest allergen-binding capacity is needed when maximum sensitivity is required, or when sera from hyperimmunized patients with high levels of allergen-specific IgG antibodies are to be studied for the presence of IgE antibody. For suitably equipped

clinical laboratories with adequate facilities for centrifugation, aspiration, and pipetting, one of the carbohydrate particle matrices is preferred because of its high antigen-binding capacity. Alternatively, polystyrene solid phases (plastic microtiter plates) are quite satisfactory with some allergens (e.g., purified proteins). Plastic solid phases, however, can display selectivity and variable and limited binding capacity that make them less than ideal for use in IgE antibody immunoassays involving crude mixtures with multiple protein antigens.

One research assay has been effectively used for the measurement of IgE antibody specific for crude allergen mixtures. It is a noncompetitive radioallergosorbent test that uses an agarose carbohydrate solid phase to which allergenic protein is covalently coupled to bind specific antibody. Radiolabeled anti-human IgE is then used to detect bound IgE. This assay has been described in detail in the fifth edition of this manual (11) and is not discussed further here. An alternative is the microtiter plate-based EIA for the detection of IgE antibody to a purified allergen such as Amb a 1, the group 1 allergen in short ragweed. This EIA format is described in detail below for IgG anti-Amb a 1 detection in human serum. A modification of this assay format, using more concentrated serum (neat to 1:5) and a biotin-conjugated murine anti-human IgE detection antibody (e.g., HP6061-biotin; EMD Biosciences), allows the IgG antibody assay format to detect Amb a 1-specific IgE antibody in human serum.

Specimen Requirements

The commercially available third-generation assays for allergen-specific IgE antibody and the research-based microtiter plate-based EIA are designed to measure levels of IgE antibody in human serum. While heparinized or cation-chelated plasma can be used with good results, fibrin formation may cause high interassay variation and increased levels of nonspecific binding in the assay. Serum is best stored at −20 or −80°C until used. Allowing blood samples to clot and retract overnight at 4°C before centrifugation and storage has no detectable effect on the measurement of serum IgE antibody levels.

Standardization

The National Committee on Clinical Laboratory Standards has prepared a guideline that extensively examines the issue of standardization of IgE antibody assays (17). Several approaches have been used by researchers to standardize IgE antibody-containing reference sera (3). One approach involves elution of a portion of the specific IgE bound to the allergen-solid phase followed by measurement of the quantity and proportion of IgE eluted. This approach allows standardization of reference and test sera in weight/volume terms, usually in nanograms per milliliter. Another approach involves the total depletion of specific antibody by immunoabsorption and subsequent measurement of the reduction of total IgE protein observed with a total serum IgE assay. This approach is useful only when the IgE antibodies of interest comprise a significant fraction of the total serum IgE. In both cases, it is necessary to only standardize the reference serum. The quantity of IgE antibody in the test sera may then be estimated by homologous interpolation from a standard curve that has been constructed with multiple dilutions of the reference serum that contains defined levels of IgE antibody of the same allergen specificity. This outcome allows comparison of IgE antibody results in different allergen systems, each with its own calibrated reference serum, and it facilitates interlaboratory standardization.

From a practical point of view, preparing separate calibrated IgE antibody-containing reference sera for each of the hundreds of allergen specificities of clinical importance is not possible. An alternative generic strategy for calibrating IgE antibody assays has been adopted which uses heterologous interpolation from a total serum IgE reference curve that is run in parallel with the IgE antibody assay (3, 17). This approach requires that the total serum IgE (heterologous) curve is diluted out in parallel with control and test sera analyzed in the IgE antibody portion of the assay. Parallelism ensures reproducible estimates of IgE antibody when sera are analyzed at different dilutions. With heterologous interpolation, IgE antibody from any of hundreds of different allergen specificities can be interpolated from a single total serum IgE dilution curve that is traceable to defined levels of IgE (in kilo-international units per liter) in a primary standard.

Quality Control

The most important region of the IgE antibody assay dose-response curve from a clinical point of view is the minimal detectable dose. Positive thresholds can differ according to the blank subtraction and reporting methods used (17). Therefore, each allergen-specific IgE antibody assay should contain one or more positive and negative serum controls for each allergosorbent in addition to a reference serum dilution curve. All samples should be analyzed in duplicate to identify and minimize procedural errors. Since the quality of each antibody measurement depends on parallelism between the dilution curves of the reference serum and test sera under study, 2 or 3 dilutions of IgE antibody-positive test serum should be analyzed to confirm parallelism.

Clinical laboratories performing allergen-specific IgE antibody assays are required by federal licensing requirements to participate in an external proficiency testing program. The College of American Pathologists conducts the SE survey, which sends five sera in each of three cycles per year to participating laboratories. Each serum is analyzed for total serum IgE and IgE antibody to five allergen specificities that cycle among the weeds, grasses, trees, pet epidermal, mold, occupational allergen, and food allergen groups. Results are submitted to the survey's coordinating center, and performance of a participating laboratory is examined in relation to that of its peer laboratories using the same assay. Since IgE antibody is still a nonregulated analyte, participation in a national proficiency survey is required for licensure but the individualized laboratory performance is not formally graded.

Interpretation

The presence of allergen-specific IgE antibody in serum indicates that the individual is sensitized to that allergen and has an increased probability of experiencing allergic symptoms that are associated with IgE-mediated disease. Moreover, the relative quantity of IgE antibody in serum may but does not always correlate with the risk of severity of these symptoms. The association between antibody quantity and allergic symptoms can be confounded by many variables, including antibody affinity, the presence of IgG blocking antibodies, and, most importantly, the relative biochemical sensitivity or "releasability" of the subject's IgE-laden effector cells. Thus, IgE antibody is necessary but not sufficient for expression of allergic disease. For many food, drug, and insect allergies, only about half of those individuals with IgE antibody will react clinically when challenged. IgE results must therefore be carefully integrated with other clinical information for proper diagnostic interpretation.

Quantitative results (in kilo-international units per liter) from commercial IgE antibody assays have allowed investigators to study whether the quantity of serum IgE antibody has any predictive utility in defining clinical sensitivity. Several groups have shown that the quantity of specific IgE antibody in serum to peanut, egg white, cow's milk, and fish can accurately define a patient's current clinical sensitivity as determined diagnostically with double-blind placebo-controlled food challenges. The probability distribution for a positive food challenge as a function of food-specific IgE antibody in serum using the Pharmacia CAP assay has been published for five foods (13). Using probability curves, it has been possible to define IgE thresholds for provocative testing below which there is >95% probability that the challenge will be negative. Alternatively, upper limits define IgE levels above which a positive challenge test is >95% likely, thereby avoiding the need for this cumbersome, expensive, and sometimes uncomfortable clinical procedure.

IgE antibody serology has recently become a diagnostic test complementary to the skin test for those patients who experience a systemic reaction following a hymenopteran venom sting in the face of a negative intradermal skin test. The American Academy of Allergy, Asthma and Immunology practice parameters were modified in 2003 to recommend IgE antivenom serology in cases where a positive clinical history is not confirmed by intradermal venom skin testing.

Multiallergen Screen

In cases where the clinical indication for allergic disease is weak, a single qualitative screening assay for IgE antibody to multiple allergen specificities can support the absence of allergic disease. In the multiallergen screen, a panel of up to 15 allergen specificities representing those primarily involved in aeroallergen-induced allergic disease are coupled to a single allergosorbent. The IgE antibody results from these screening assays can be highly predictive of individual IgE antibody results obtained by a panel of separate skin tests or in vitro IgE antibody tests. Screening assays provide a positive or negative result. If negative, it may be the single best test for confirming the absence of significant atopic disease in individuals who are suspected of having an intrinsic or non-IgE-mediated disease process. The negative predictive value of this single test is higher than total serum IgE or any single specific IgE antibody measurement for identifying nonatopic individuals. Such a test can minimize the need for multiple in vivo or in vitro allergen-specific IgE measurements in patients with a questionable clinical history for allergic disease.

ALLERGEN-SPECIFIC SERUM IgG ANTIBODY

The levels of specific IgG antibodies are generally low or nondetectable in an unimmunized individual who has been naturally exposed to clinically important antigens (e.g., aeroallergens from weeds, grass, and tree pollens and dust mite, mold, and animal epidermal antigens). The analytical sensitivity and specificity of an IgG antibody assay used to assess these sera therefore become important because nanogram-per-milliliter levels of specific IgG must be measured in the presence of milligram-per-milliliter levels of nonspecific IgG. In contrast, individuals who have received injections of an antigen, either by accidental exposure (e.g., bee sting or drug injection) or by active allergen immunotherapy, can produce high microgram-per-milliliter levels of specific IgG. At these levels, nonspecific binding and assay sensitivity become less critical and assay parallelism, precision, and accuracy and human antibody standards become the focus of assay design.

An early research assay that measured antigen-specific IgG in human serum employed a reaction between a radio-labeled antigen mixture and antibody-containing serum. IgG was then selectively precipitated from other antibody isotypes in serum with a polyclonal anti-human IgG reagent. This assay, called the radioimmunoprecipitation or double-antibody assay, has remained a research tool for the measurement of IgG antibody specific to purified antigens. However, it is difficult to uniformly radioiodinate or enzyme label complex mixtures of protein antigens that vary widely in isoelectric point and molecular weight. Nonparallelism and differential plateauing (variable maximum binding) can result with the double-antibody assay when a labeled protein mixture is used, indicating that the assay will not perform in a uniform, quantitative manner with all human sera. To address this problem with complex antigen mixtures, a non-competitive solid-phase radioimmunoassay (SPRIA) was developed based on the assay design described above for IgE antibody except that it uses staphylococcal protein A or protein G to detect bound IgG antibody. This assay is still in use today to assess Hymenoptera venom-specific IgG (8). Since there are naturally occurring IgG antibodies for carbohydrates present in the agarose solid-phase matrix that interfere in this assay, all sera analyzed in this assay are routinely preadsorbed with uncoupled agarose (10). The generic SPRIA for IgG antibody specific for complex protein mixtures has been discussed in detail in the fifth edition of this manual (11; see also references 8 and 9) and is not discussed further here.

A versatile nonisotopic monoclonal antibody-based EIA for the detection of IgG antibodies specific for purified allergens such as ragweed group 1 allergen (Amb a 1) is presented. Although a crude aqueous extract can be used as an antigen source, it contains many irrelevant proteins that readily adsorb onto plastic surfaces. In doing so, these occupy limited sites on the plastic surface that can be used to bind more relevant antigens. Because the microtiter plate well has a limited surface area for binding proteins, well-characterized purified antigens are recommended for use with the microtiter plate-based EIAs. The assay uses documented murine monoclonal antibodies that bind to the Fc regions of all four subclasses of human IgG and are purified and biotinylated or HRP conjugated (clone HP6043; EMD Biosciences Corporation). The biotinylated monoclonal anti-human IgG PAN reagent can be used with an avidin-enzyme preparation to maximize the working range of the assay while minimizing nonspecific binding.

Specimen Requirements

The antigen-specific IgG EIAs are designed to measure the level of specific IgG antibody in human serum. Heparinized or cation-chelated plasma can be used with good results, but fibrin formation may cause high interassay variation and increased levels of nonspecific binding in the assay. The serum is best stored at −20°C until used. Allowing blood samples to clot and retract overnight at 4°C before centrifugation and storage has no detectable effect on the measurement of serum IgG antibody levels. While serum is desired, plasma and other body fluids (e.g., bronchial alveolar lavage fluid, tears, and nasal secretions) can be tested if the appropriate negative controls are analyzed in the same assay to identify the level of nonspecific binding.

Assay Procedure

1. Flat-bottom 96-well microtiter plates are coated for 1 h at RT and then overnight at 4°C with purified antigen (e.g., Amb a 1 or Der p 1; 0.1 ml per well) which has been diluted in endotoxin-free PBS to a final concentration of 10 µg/ml just prior to use. Since these proteins bind by means of adsorption, caution must be exercised so as not to lose antigen on plastic tubes, pipettes, and reservoirs used for dispensing it into the microtiter plate. A variety of plastic microtiter plates (e.g., Costar or Nunc) have been successfully used as solid phases. The plates are covered with Parafilm between each step to minimize evaporation and dust contamination.

2. Each plate is washed once with PBS–0.5% Tween 20 using a 12-channel handheld Corning washing system or equivalent, and 0.3 ml of PBS–1% BSA is added to each well to block unreacted sites on the microtiter plate wells (1 h at RT).

3. After a second wash (four times) with PBS-Tween, 0.1-ml volumes of antigen-specific IgG-containing reference, control, and test sera (diluted at least 1:50 in PBS–1% BSA) are added to their respective wells. The standard curve is composed of 8 to 10 twofold dilutions in duplicate of a reference serum, beginning with a concentration of 1,000 ng of IgG antibody per ml. Test sera are initially screened at a 1:50 dilution in duplicate and reanalyzed at several dilutions up to 1:10,000 if they exceed the top point of the dose-response curve.

Soluble antigen can be added at this step to confirm assay specificity by competitive inhibition (see chapter 105). A buffer blank and a negative control serum are analyzed to control for nonspecific binding. The 1:50 negative serum control consistently produces an optical density above that of the buffer blank. The plates are incubated for 2 h at RT or overnight at 4°C. Two or three dilutions of high, medium, and low IgG anti–Amb a 1 serum controls are analyzed in different regions of the plate to ensure that the assay is in control.

4. Following a PBS-Tween buffer wash (four times), HRP-conjugated mouse anti-human IgG Fc (HP6043-HRP; EMD Biosciences Corporation) is added (0.1 ml per well, 1 µg/ml in PBS–1% BSA) with a multichannel pipette and the mixture is incubated for 1 h at RT.

5. Plates are washed four times for the last time and developed with ABTS substrate as described above for the total and free serum IgE EIAs. The enzyme reaction is stopped with the addition of 0.1 ml of 2 mM sodium azide when the top point on the standard curve reaches an A_{410} of 1.5 to 2.0 (usually in 5 to 15 min). The plate is read on a microtiter plate reader at 410 nm, and optical densities of unknown sera are interpolated from a standard curve into estimates of antibody concentration using a computer data processing program.

Standardization

Reference serum dose-response curves are plotted using optical density as the response variable and then used to interpolate test serum results. Nonspecific binding produced by the negative control serum should be subtracted from the replicate means for all points on the reference curve as well as each test serum.

Working Range, Sensitivity, Reproducibility, and Parallelism

The SPRIA and EIA are capable of measuring nanogram quantities of IgG antibody. The working range of the agarose-based

SPRIA spans from 10 to 2,000 ng of specific IgG per ml. While the theoretical sensitivity of the EIA is 1 ng of IgG per ml, the observed sensitivity typically ranges from 5 to 15 ng/ml, which is comparable to that of the SPRIA. Both the sensitivity and working range of these assays are dependent on the density of the antigen on the solid phase; the dilution and affinity of the detection antibody; the duration of the serum, conjugate, and substrate incubations; and the relative amount of specific antibody of other isotypes (e.g., IgE, IgA, and IgM) that compete for available solid-phase antigen epitopes. Parallelism between the reference and test serum dilution curves remains good over the working range of both assays, with interdilutional CV typically of <20%. The CV for within-experiment replicates averages typically 5%, and the CV for results between assays when all reagents remain constant should be 10 to 15%.

Quality Assurance

The most important region of the IgG SPRIA and EIA dose-response curves from a clinical point of view is the low portion of the working range. The minimum detectable concentration of the assay varies as a function of the negative serum subtraction and reporting methods used. Therefore, each assay should contain one or more positive and negative serum controls for each allergosorbent used in the assay, in addition to the reference serum dilution curve. All samples should be analyzed in duplicate to identify and minimize systematic (procedural) and random errors. At present, there are no external proficiency surveys for assays that monitor allergen-specific human IgG antibodies.

Interpretation

An IgG antibody measurement is commonly performed to document an exposure of an individual to an immunizing dose of antigen. In some cases, it can serve as an indicator of the effectiveness of various antigen doses used to induce a specific IgG antibody response in immunotherapy. In research applications, specific IgG antibody levels are used to quantitatively monitor the humoral immune response to an antigen to which a patient has been accidentally or intentionally exposed.

In the 1930s, allergen-specific IgG antibodies were identified as "blocking antibodies" that could block transfer of reaginic activity in the Prausnitz-Küstner reaction and basophil leukocyte histamine release assays. Presently, the only cited clinical application for IgG antibody measurements in the field of allergy is their use in the evaluation of hymenopteran venom-allergic patients who are initiating venom immunotherapy or who have been receiving maintenance injections for a number of years. In a 1992 study (5), 211 insect sting challenges were performed in 109 patients over a 4-year period to investigate the clinical significance of venom-specific IgG levels measured by the protein A SPRIA. In individuals on immunotherapy for less than 4 years, systemic symptoms occurred in only 1.6% of individuals with venom-specific IgG levels greater than 3.5 μg/ml but in 16% of individuals with levels lower than 3.5 μg/ml. The venom-specific IgG level had no predictive value for risk in patients who received therapy for more than 4 years. This study concluded that venom-specific IgG levels of <3.5 μg/ml are associated with an increased risk of allergic reactions upon a resting during the first 4 years of immunotherapy with yellow jacket or mixed vespid venoms. The observations described in other published studies of IgG antibody levels in patients receiving ragweed, grass, and dust mite immunotherapy have remained research observations that relate the antigen exposure to IgG (humoral) immune responses.

CONCLUDING THOUGHTS

In summary, the diagnostic allergy laboratory uses a number of immunoassay methods to measure IgE and IgG antibodies that aid the clinician in the diagnosis and management of individuals with allergic disease. At present, there are no molecular biology techniques explicitly used by allergy laboratories to facilitate the diagnosis of allergic disease. Recombinant-DNA technology to date has only been used in the generation of allergenic proteins that have become incorporated as reagents in some research-based microarray assays for IgE antibody (15). As more is learned about genetic polymorphisms that predispose individuals to allergic disease, molecular biology methods may also be employed in the diagnostic allergy laboratory of the future.

REFERENCES

1. **Barbee, R. A., M. Halomen, M. Lebowitz, and B. Burrows.** 1981. Distribution of IgE in a community population sample: correlations with age, sex and allergen skin test reactivity. *J. Allergy Clin. Immunol.* **68:**106–111.
2. **Bennich, H. H., K. Ishizaka, S. G. O. Johansson, D. S. Rowe, D. R. Stanworth, and W. D. Terry.** 1968. Immunoglobulin E: a new class of human immunoglobulin. *Immunology* **3:**323–324.
3. **Butler, J. E., and R. G. Hamilton.** 1981. Quantitation of specific antibodies: methods of expression, standards, solid phase considerations and specific applications, p. 173–198. In J. E. Butler (ed.), *Immunochemistry of Solid Phase Immunoassays.* CRC Press, Boca Raton, Fla.
4. **Dolen, W. K.** 2002. The diagnostic allergy laboratory, p. 883–890. In N. R. Rose, R. G. Hamilton, and B. Detrick (ed.), *Manual of Clinical Laboratory Immunology*, 6th ed. ASM Press, Washington, D.C.
5. **Golden, D. B. K., I. D. Lawrence, R. G. Hamilton, A. Kagey Sobotka, M. D. Valentine, and L. M. Lichtenstein.** 1992. Clinical correlation of the venom-specific IgG antibody level during maintenance venom immunotherapy. *J. Allergy Clin. Immunol.* **90:**386–393.
6. **Hamilton, R. G.** 2005. Science behind the discovery of IgE. *J. Allergy Clin. Immunol.* **115:**648–652.
7. **Hamilton, R. G.** 2005. Assessment of indoor allergen exposure. *Curr. Allergy Asthma Rep.* **5:**394–401.
8. **Hamilton, R. G., and N. F. Adkinson, Jr.** 1979. Solid phase radioimmunoassay for quantitation of antigen-specific IgG in human serum with I-125 protein A from *Staphylococcus aureus. J. Immunol.* **122:**1073–1079.
9. **Hamilton, R. G., and N. F. Adkinson, Jr.** 1980. Quantitation of antigen-specific IgG in human serum. I. Standardization by a *Staphylococcus aureus* solid phase radioimmunoassay elution technique. *J. Immunol.* **124:**2966–2971.
10. **Hamilton, R. G., and N. F. Adkinson, Jr.** 1985. Naturally-occurring carbohydrate antibodies: interference in solid phase immunoassays. *J. Immunol. Methods* **77:**95–108.
11. **Hamilton, R. G., and N. F. Adkinson, Jr.** 1997. Immunological tests for diagnosis and management of human allergic disease: total and allergen specific IgE and allergen specific IgG, p. 881–892. In N. R. Rose, E. C. de Macario, J. D. Folds, H. C. Lane, and R. M. Nakamura (ed.), *Manual of Clinical Laboratory Immunology*, 5th ed. ASM Press, Washington, D.C.
12. **Hamilton, R. G., and N. F. Adkinson, Jr.** 2003. Clinical laboratory assessment of IgE-dependent hypersensitivity. *J. Allergy Clin. Immunol.* **111:**687–701. (Review.)
13. **Hamilton, R. G., and N. F. Adkinson, Jr.** 2004. In vitro assays for IgE mediated sensitivities. *J. Allergy Clin. Immunol.* **114:**213–225. (Review.)
14. **Hamilton, R. G., G. V. Marcotte, and S. S. Saini.** 2005. Immunological methods for quantifying free and total

serum IgE levels in allergy patients receiving Omalizumab (Xolair) therapy. *J. Immunol. Methods* **303**:81–91.

15. **Hiller, R., S. Laffer, C. Harwanegg, et al.** 2002. Microarrayed allergen molecules: diagnostic gatekeepers for allergy treatment. *FASEB J.* **16**:414–416.

16. **Huss, K., N. F. Adkinson, P. Eggleston, C. Dawson, M. Van Natta, and R. G. Hamilton.** 2001. House dust mite and cockroach exposure are strong risk factors for positive allergy skin tests in the Childhood Asthma Management Program. *J. Allergy Clin. Immunol.* **107**:48–54.

17. **Matsson, P., and R. G. Hamilton.** 1997. *Evaluation Methods And Analytical Performance Characteristics of Immunological Assays for Human IgE Antibody of Defined Allergen Specificities: Guideline.* National Committee for Clinical Laboratory Standards, document 1/LA20-A. NCCLS, Wayne, Pa.

18. **Saini, S. S., D. W. MacGlashan, S. A. Sterbinsky, A. Togias, D. C. Adelman, L. M. Lichtenstein, and B. S. Bochner.** 1999. Down-regulation of human basophil IgE and Fc epsilon RI alpha surface densities and mediator release by anti-IgE infusions is reversible *in vitro* and *in vivo*. *J. Immunol.* **162**:5624.

19. **Wide, L., H. H. Bennich, and S. G. O. Johannson.** 1967. Diagnosis by an *in vitro* test for allergen antibodies. *Lancet* **ii**:1105–1107.

Assay Methods for Measurement of Mediators and Markers of Allergic Inflammation

JOHN T. SCHROEDER AND SARBJIT SAINI

108

With the discovery of immunoglobulin E (IgE) as the source of reaginic activity in serum, the release of histamine from leukocyte suspensions challenged with a specific antigen has been used as a reliable in vitro correlate of immediate hypersensitivity (5). Indeed, much of the knowledge obtained during the past 40 years concerning the detection and treatment of allergic disease has come from in vitro studies investigating the parameters, mechanisms, and pharmacologic control of the inflammatory mediators released from basophils and mast cells. Both of these cell types express the high-affinity receptor for IgE (FcεR1) and are responsible for the anaphylactic release of mediators in response to an allergen. However, basophils, by virtue of their accessibility and the fact that they are the sole source of histamine among the leukocytes in blood, continue to facilitate these studies to a greater extent than tissue-derived mast cells. Thus, an antigen (or anti-IgE antibody) that has the ability to bind and cross-link IgE-receptor complexes when simply added to a suspension of washed leukocytes in the presence of calcium is sufficient to trigger a complex cascade of signals within basophils, resulting in the release of preformed histamine and newly generated mediators.

Although histamine remains the most commonly measured mediator released following this IgE-mediated reaction, it is now well established that other mediators are also released from basophils and are important markers of allergic inflammation (see Fig. 1). The lipid mediator leukotriene C$_4$ (LTC4), which is derived from the metabolism of arachidonic acid, is secreted at concentrations nearly 100-fold lower (on a molar basis) than those of histamine. However, since LTC4 is some 100 to 6,000 times more potent in contracting smooth muscle than is histamine, it may be responsible for more of the symptoms of asthma and, therefore, has gained considerable attention in recent years. Clinical studies with antihistamines have not shown benefit for the treatment of asthma, but leukotriene receptor antagonists have shown efficacy, which supports the importance of LTC4 as a bronchoconstrictive agent. Cytokines represent a third class of mediators released from cells expressing FcεR1, but unlike histamine and LTC4, they are generated de novo (13). In particular, human basophils secrete high levels of interleukin-4 (IL-4) and IL-13—arguably the two most important cytokines in allergic disease given the primary role of these cytokines in regulating IgE synthesis from B cells. The importance of this response has only recently been appreciated,

with evidence that basophils in IL-4-transgenic mice are, indeed, a major source of this cytokine (9, 20). Therefore, it has been the objective of this chapter during the last two editions of this manual to focus on the laboratory procedures commonly performed for measuring the release of these inflammatory mediators, both in vitro and in biological fluids. However, rather than concentrating on those procedures that have changed little during the course of three decades, this chapter will focus on more recent approaches for measuring these mediators and will refer to previous editions when specific details are deemed necessary. In particular, this chapter will highlight the growing interest in the use of flow cytometry assays to monitor activation-linked markers (e.g., CD63, CD69, and CD203c) on basophils and the applicability of such assays as surrogate indicators of mediator release. Emphasis will also be given to those mediators that are not necessarily produced by basophils but that are commonly found in lavage fluids taken from sites of allergic inflammation. In particular, an update of the assays used for the detection of tryptase (a mast cell product) and major basic protein (MBP; a product of eosinophils) will be included in this discussion. Novel approaches regarding the potential use of exhalation condensates and measurements of nitric oxide (NO) in assessing the overall inflammation occurring during allergic reactions will be reviewed. Finally, although several technical advances have made these detection assays more applicable for clinical use, it is important that some of these methods remain time-consuming and are presently useful only in specialized clinical situations or for research purposes.

HISTAMINE

Laboratory Assays

While commercial assays for measuring histamine (see below) are becoming increasingly popular as a result of their not requiring specialized equipment, the automated fluorometric technique remains perhaps the most rapid, accurate, and sensitive way to measure histamine, particularly when there is a need for high throughput. Since the original development of this technique by Siraganian in the mid-1970s (19), it has become possible to analyze, with more modern machines, as many as 45 to 60 samples per hour. The procedure is based on the extraction of histamine and its coupling with ophthalaldehyde (OPT) at a highly alkaline pH to form a fluorescent product. Samples tested must be relatively free of protein and other interfering compounds, such as histidine. The machine achieves this extraction and coupling by first extracting histamine into *n*-butanol from a salt-saturated, alkalinized solution. In addition, before the condensation step with OPT, histamine is back extracted into an aqueous solution of diluted HCl by adding heptane. The histamine-OPT complex is stable at an acid pH, which increases the fluorescence intensity of the compound. The automated technique requires a sample volume of 0.6 to 1.0 ml and is capable of detecting histamine levels in the range of 0.5 to >100 ng/ml. Although the automated methodology for histamine measurement is preferable, similar results can be obtained manually with minor loss of sensitivity and precision. The assay is linear from 0.5 to 1,000 ng/ml. The advantage of automated fluorometry over other systems is its ability to rapidly process, with reproducibility and ease, a large quantity of samples. This is the method of choice, however, only when samples are obtained from studies using low-protein-concentration buffer systems such as that involving the in vitro release of histamine from basophil or mast cell cultures. It has also been useful for determining levels of histamine released at sites of experimental allergen challenge in the nose, lung, and skin by assaying fluids from lavages performed with normal saline. Fluorometric measurement of histamine in whole blood and in serum at concentrations greater than 10% requires extensive acid precipitation and/or dialysis to remove protein, cumbersome manipulations that lead to a loss of assay sensitivity.

The radioenzymatic assay (REA) has the advantage of detecting very low levels of histamine, with a sensitivity of approximately 10 pg/ml. Importantly, unlike the fluorometric method, the REA is not subject to interference from high protein levels, which makes it an excellent protocol for measuring plasma histamine levels. The assay involves the transfer of ^{3}H- or ^{14}C-labeled methyl groups from S-adenosylmethionine to histamine by using the enzyme histamine N-methyltransferase, which is commonly derived from crude extracts of rat kidney (Pel-Freez, Rogers, Ark.). The product, radiolabled methylhistamine, is extracted from the reaction mixture by using a solvent such as chloroform or toluene. This compound is then recovered into an aqueous solution by using NaOH saturated with NaCl. In addition to the standard curve generated with each assay, internal standards are often incorporated into the protocol by adding a trace amount of histamine (labeled with a second isotope or simply left unlabeled) to the unknown sample. The ratio of the counts obtained for the "spiked" sample to those obtained for the internal standard itself is proportional to the amount of histamine in the original sample. The REA has a narrower working range (50 pg/ml to 20 ng/ml) but is more sensitive than the fluorometric assay. The REA also has the advantage of requiring a small sample size (0.02 ml). However, since the assay is performed manually, it is relatively time-consuming and lacks the reproducibility achieved with the automated fluorometric system. Presently, one must also establish this assay in-house, since greater appeal of the enzyme-linked immunosorbent assay (ELISA) and the enzyme immunoassay (see below) have diminished the commercial availability of the REA.

The standards used in both the fluorometric assay and the REA are made from stock solutions prepared by accurately weighing an appropriate amount of histamine dihydrochloride (see Appendix). Standard solutions used for the fluorometric assay are stable at 4°C when the stock solution

is diluted in water containing 2% $HClO_4$. The standards used in the REA are prepared fresh by diluting the stock in the diluent best representing the samples to be tested but in the absence of $HClO_4$, which interferes with the histamine N-methyltransferase used in the assay.

Commercial Histamine Assays

An enzyme immunoassay and an ELISA are offered by Cayman Chemicals and Immuno-Biological Laboratories, respectively, for the detection of histamine in a variety of biological specimens, including culture supernatant, urine, and plasma. As the REA, these assays have the advantage of needing relatively small sample volumes (e.g., 0.050 to 0.100 ml), are less bothered by high-protein contamination than automated fluorometry, and are cost-effective for low-throughput needs. On the other hand, their use remains somewhat limited and they should be evaluated for sensitivity and specificity prior to application.

Clinical Indications for Measuring In Vitro Histamine Release from Basophils

Measuring the release of histamine from basophil leukocytes in vitro continues to serve as a valuable test for evaluating IgE-mediated reactions. In fact, the indications for the use of this method are, at this time, more extensive than those for any other test described in this chapter. Yet because the parameters involved in the histamine release assay have been extensively described in previous editions of this book, they will be only briefly mentioned here. Some of its more common uses are outlined below.

Evaluation of Allergic Status

It was noted some 40 years ago that there is good correlation between the level of histamine released from basophils in response to allergens (e.g., antigen E, or Amb a I, and Fel d1, etc.) and the severity of clinical symptoms suffered by individuals who are allergic to these allergens (7). In fact, studies show that allergen sensitivity is related to the levels of specific IgE in serum, with very low concentrations of an allergen often causing histamine release from basophils in vitro when allergen-specific IgE antibody levels are high. As a result, the release of histamine from basophils in vitro can serve as a dependable and precise indicator of the allergic status of an individual, with few false positives compared to skin-testing techniques. However, a caveat is that the presence of allergen-specific IgE is not sufficient and must be combined with the clinical history to indicate the presence of disease given the widespread prevalence of IgE specific to insect venoms, latex, and food allergens. Also, since many dilutions of an antigen can be readily tested for reactivity, the histamine release assay can be more quantitative than skin testing, which often relies on a somewhat less precise endpoint. Most important, basophil analyses can be performed safely using "crude" allergens and products not yet approved for in vivo use. However, any clinical applicability is limited to a positive assay result, since in vitro histamine release from basophils does not necessarily predict a negative skin test reaction. Due to the complexities of the assay, direct measures of specific IgE rather than histamine release are more commonly used in clinical practice (see chapter 107, this volume).

Demonstration of IgE Antibody Activity

Measuring the release of histamine from normal donor leukocyte suspensions passively sensitized with IgE is a useful technique for detecting allergen-specific antibody in the sera (or plasma) of patients presenting with clinical symptoms (6). In fact, the histamine release assay has some advantages over the more commonly used radioallergosorbent test (RAST) in the detection of allergen-specific IgE. First, it gives a quick and precise assessment of whether serum contains biologically active IgE. The RAST, although more easily standardized, simply quantifies the amount of allergen-specific IgE that is in serum. Second, very little antigen is required to induce histamine release from passively sensitized basophils. In contrast, the RAST requires relatively large quantities of pure allergen in order to successfully couple the allergen to an insoluble matrix for subsequent binding of allergen-specific IgE. Third, the basophil histamine release assay is excellent for studies investigating, by direct analysis and after passive sensitization, whether a patient has become sensitized to an uncommon allergen for which a RAST is not available. Naturally, a disadvantage of these assays is their requirement for a fair amount of fresh leukocytes from a nonallergic subject whose cells can withstand the rigors of passive sensitization (see below) and retain responsiveness. In this respect, the histamine release assay is at a disadvantage to the RAST, which is technically far less challenging. In addition, there is the potential for serum to contain priming factors (homologous restriction factor and IL-3, etc.) that can trigger the recipient basophils in a nonspecific fashion, even though proof of this has yet to emerge.

Quality Control of Prepared Allergens

It is often desirable to check the quality of allergens, whether commercially prepared or made in-house, by testing their ability to induce histamine release from leukocytes obtained from allergic donors. This is becoming particularly useful for immunotherapy studies for which modified allergens can be evaluated for biological activity or cross-reactivity prior to testing in vivo.

Alternative for Skin Testing

In some instances, it is desirable to avoid skin testing and to use the in vitro basophil histamine release assay as an alternative approach for evaluating allergic status. However, given the prevalence of RAST, this particular indication is rarely practiced.

Test Procedures

Induction of Histamine Release from Washed Human Leukocytes: General Method

While there are presently many variations of the protocol originally described for inducing histamine release from basophils in vitro, these relate primarily to the method used for histamine analysis. Otherwise, little has changed during the past 40 years since its first description. The reader is therefore directed to previous editions of this book for specific details, as this section will emphasize only certain aspects of the assay. Also, the techniques described herein are, for the most part, used when histamine is analyzed by automated fluorometry.

Blood is drawn into a plastic syringe, preferably by using a butterfly infusion set with the needle size reflecting the desired volume required for the assay. Usually 1 ml of blood per reaction tube will provide total histamine levels of approximately 20 ng, with some variation occurring among donors. Dextran sedimentation remains the method of choice for preparing washed leukocytes for histamine release, as it requires little technical expertise and is the least

manipulative toward the cells. These issues are necessary to consider when both preparation time and retention of cell function are of greatest importance. In this instance, whole blood is immediately transferred into disposable 50-ml polypropylene centrifuge tubes (catalog no. 25330; Corning Incorporated, Corning, N.Y.) each containing 12.5 ml of dextran, 5.0 ml of 0.1 M EDTA, and 375 mg of dextrose, which allows proper mixing for up to 20 ml of blood. After sitting for 60 to 90 min at room temperature (23 to 25°C), the leukocyte-rich plasma layer is carefully removed and centrifuged and the cell pellet is washed two to three times in PIPES [piperazine-N,N'-bis(2-ethanesulfonic acid)]-albumin-glucose (PAG) buffer (see Appendix) to remove platelets. It is sometimes useful to do one or more washes in PAG containing EDTA (~4 mM), since this reagent chelates calcium and prevents platelet clumping. However, it is important that the final wash be done in the absence of EDTA, since histamine release requires calcium and residual EDTA may prevent the reaction cascade. After the final wash, the cell pellet is resuspended in PAG buffer containing 1 mM $CaCl_2$ and 1 mM $MgCl_2$ (PAGCM) to a volume sufficient to allow the addition of the required amount of cells to each reaction tube as per the protocol. Histamine release can be induced in almost any variety of test tube, but total reaction volumes usually range from 0.1 to 1.0 ml. The washed leukocytes in PAGCM and the reaction tubes are then warmed separately in a 37°C water bath before mixing with one another. The total histamine content (called "completes") is obtained by the lysis of cells in a duplicate set of reaction tubes using perchloric acid at a final concentration of 1.6%. The amount of histamine released spontaneously (usually less than 5% of the total) is determined by incubating cells in buffer alone. Reactions are allowed to proceed at 37°C for 30 to 45 min, at which time buffer is added to a 1-ml total volume, the cells are centrifuged, and the cell-free supernatants are decanted into 2-ml autoanalyzer cups (Sarstedt, Inc., Princeton, N.J.; catalog no. 73.641) and stored at 4°C in plastic racks (Elkay Products Inc., Shrewsbury, Mass.). To prevent evaporation, samples should be frozen at −20°C if histamine cannot be analyzed within 2 weeks.

Any samples requiring added protein during the reaction may require acid precipitation in order to prevent interference with histamine measurements using the automated fluorometric technique. In such instances, much of the protein can be precipitated prior to analysis by adding perchloric acid to the cell-free supernatant at a final concentration of 1.6%, incubating overnight at 4°C, and recentrifuging prior to analysis. Alternatively, histamine can be measured using either the REA or ELISA.

Inhibition of Histamine Release from Basophils

As a modification of the standard assay, the inhibition of histamine release from basophils can be useful in testing whether a patient's serum contains an antigen-neutralizing blocking antibody. This assay has been used to monitor patients receiving allergen immunotherapy, since this treatment causes an increase in allergen-specific IgG antibodies (1). However, the assay has largely been replaced by radioimmunoassays (RIAs) and REAs, which both directly measure specific IgG antibody. In brief, the protocol involves the use of a reference donor (or donors) whose basophils are known to release high levels (>70%) of histamine in response to an antigen. The patient's serum or normal (type AB) serum (at ~10% final concentration) is then mixed with a dose of an antigen that will cause approximately half of the maximal histamine release from the reference cells. After preincubating for up to 60 min at 37°C, washed leukocytes are added for an additional 45-min incubation, with the cell-free supernatants then collected for histamine analysis as described above.

Although its clinical utility is somewhat limited, the inhibition of in vitro histamine release is often used to determine the effectiveness of pharmacologic agents. This test also involves a modification of the standard release assay but differs slightly from that used in measuring IgG antibodies. In brief, washed leukocytes are mixed with PAGCM alone or with several concentrations of the drug diluted in buffer. Final drug concentrations of 10^{-4} M to 10^{-6} M are useful for initial screening. After preincubation (usually for 10 to 15 min) at 37°C, several concentrations of an antigen (or anti-IgE antibody) are added for an additional 45 min for the induction of histamine release. Once again, it is best to use stimulus concentrations that normally cause approximately half of the maximal histamine release. In addition to the usual controls (completes and blanks), it is important to include cells incubated with the drugs alone to assess any lytic effects of the drugs, as well as drugs diluted in buffer (no cells) to control for fluorescent compounds if the OPT-based assay is used.

Passive Sensitization of Basophils

The basophils isolated from some donors express sufficient numbers of unoccupied IgE FcεR1 sites to enable these cells to be passively sensitized with IgE antibody from an unrelated source. Thus, the serum or plasma of an allergic individual can be tested for antigen-reactive IgE antibodies by sensitizing the basophils of a nonallergic donor and inducing histamine release from these cells by using the antigen in question. The success of studies using this technique requires the use of nonallergic donors whose basophils normally release well in response to IgE-dependent stimulation and whose cells have naturally unoccupied IgE FcεR1 sites that can be passively sensitized with IgE antibody. Since only an estimated 1 out of 20 nonallergic individuals has basophils that meet these criteria, lactic acid is often used to remove endogenous basophil-bound IgE, thereby increasing one's ability to passively sensitize cells. In fact, the details of performing this procedure are outlined elsewhere (11) and are also described in previous editions of this chapter. As a result, it seems appropriate to note here only a few considerations, since the reader can refer to the above-mentioned references for specific information. First, these assays are best done using mixed leukocytes prepared by sedimentation and must use cells from a donor whose basophils respond to IgE-mediated stimulation. The lactic acid solution (pH 3.9) works best when fresh and can be used either at room temperature (25°C) or on ice (4°C) for up to 5 min. Cells are then immediately washed to remove unbound IgE before passive sensitization (30 min at 37°C) with an appropriate dilution of patient serum in PAG containing 10 U of heparin/ml and 4 mM EDTA. An important negative control includes acid-treated cells sensitized with an equal amount of irrelevant IgE in control serum. It is also important to leave a portion of cells untreated with acid solution in order to control for any effect this treatment may have on basophil responsiveness. After washing twice in PAG buffer, the leukocytes are tested for histamine release by using identical test conditions. The antigen-induced release of histamine by leukocytes passively sensitized with the patient's serum, but not with control serum, indicates positivity. Of course, non-passively sensitized cells should not react with the antigen, while cells subjected to all conditions of passive

sensitization should still respond to anti-IgE used as a positive control.

LIPID MEDIATORS

LTC4

The secretion of LTC4 by basophils and mast cells is also rapid, nearly paralleling the release of histamine, and is essentially complete by 30 min after activation. IL-3 has been shown to enhance the levels of LTC4 generated by basophils in response to IgE-dependent activation by nearly 100-fold, and following IL-3 priming, release of LTC4 occurs with stimulation by C5a, a secretagogue that alone does not normally cause the release of this mediator. Essentially no release of prostaglandins from basophils occurs in response to activation, indicating that cyclooxygenase enzyme activity is not prominent in these cells. However, all human mast cells studied to date do produce prostaglandin D_2 (PGD2) and lung and mucosal cells secrete levels of LTC4 nearly identical to those secreted by basophils but usually only in response to IgE-dependent stimuli.

The assays for LTC4 are, most commonly, competitive RIAs. Briefly, ^{3}H labeling is added to all sample tubes and to unlabeled LTC4 standards. This step is followed by the addition of a limiting quantity of anti-LTC4 antibody (usually polyclonal in origin) sufficient to bind all of the ^{3}H-labeled LTC4. The standards or unknowns containing LTC4 compete with radiolabeled LTC4 for antibody binding sites, and the antigen-antibody complexes formed in this reaction are then precipitated and removed by activated charcoal, thus leaving unbound ^{3}H-labeled LTC4. As the levels of sample LTC4 increase, less radioactive label is bound to the antibody, leading to higher remaining radioactivity. The levels of LTC4 are then measured by comparing the radioactivity in the unknown samples to that in the standard curve. With most RIAs, picogram quantities of LTC4 can be accurately measured with a range of <10 pg/ml to 100 ng/ml. RIAs are quite reliable for use with buffer systems. However, the signal-to-noise ratio for serum and other biological fluids (e.g., nasal and bronchial lavage and skin blister fluids) makes the measurement of LTC4 difficult and less quantitative. The ^{3}H-labeled LTC4 standards used in this assay were prepared from commercially available stock solutions (New England Nuclear Corp.).

ELISA kits that measure LTC4 using a competitive immunoassay approach are also commercially available (Assay Designs and Cayman Chemicals) and have the advantage of being free of radioactive isotopes. These assays are also generally quite sensitive (~50 pg/ml), showing only slight cross-reactivity with LTD4 and LTE4.

Clinical Indications

Evaluation of Allergic Status

LTC4 is generated from several cell types, including monocytes and eosinophils. However, the formation and secretion of this mediator from washed leukocytes can serve as an in vitro test of allergic status, since the basophil is the only cell in these preparations that responds to IgE-mediated stimulation. In practice, however, since histamine is released in parallel with LTC4 and the assays for it are less cumbersome and more reliable, histamine is more often used as an index of allergen sensitivity. Nonetheless, measurements of LTC4 in biological specimens may be useful in assessing the inhibitory actions of the 5-lipoxygenase inhibitors, which do not affect histamine release.

Test Procedures

Washed leukocytes are prepared from peripheral blood using dextran sedimentation as described above for histamine release from basophils; LTC4 and histamine release are assessed simultaneously. However, the reactions are done in a total volume of 0.1 ml in PAGCM buffer. PAG buffer (0.2 ml) is added to all tubes at the end of the reaction, and after centrifugation, a portion of the supernatant (0.1 ml) is carefully removed for LTC4 analysis. An additional 0.5 to 0.8 ml of PAG buffer is then added to the reaction tubes, and following recentrifugation, the supernatant is obtained for histamine analysis by automated fluorometry as described above. By measuring the release of these two mediators from the same aliquot of cells, the LTC4 levels can be normalized to the amount of histamine released (i.e., picograms of LTC4 per nanograms of histamine).

CYTOKINE GENERATION BY BASOPHILS

Much effort during the past 30 years has been directed at understanding the stimuli, activation and desensitization mechanisms, and pharmacologic control of histamine release and LTC4 generation by basophils. During the past decade, there has emerged solid evidence that human basophils are the predominant source of IL-4 (and likely IL-13) among the cells circulating in blood and they appear to constitute a significant source of these cytokines among the cells infiltrating allergic lesions (10, 14). Both IL-4 and IL-13 promote IgE production from B lymphocytes and activate the endothelium for the selective adherence and transendothelial migration of eosinophils. IL-4 is also the only cytokine known to direct the conversion of Th1 lymphocytes into the Th2 phenotype, with concomitant changes in cytokine profiles. The parameters important for the generation of these cytokines in basophils indicate that both proteins, much like histamine, are important correlates of immediate hypersensitivity (15). In fact, both IL-4 and IL-13 are secreted following IgE cross-linking, and the concentration of a stimulus required for optimal release is nearly 10-fold less than that necessary for histamine release. This is particularly true for cells stimulated by anti-IgE antibody, but it is also found with activation by an antigen. IL-4 protein levels peak after 4 to 6 h of activation, with IL-13 secretion being somewhat slower, beginning at ~4 h and peaking after some 20 h of incubation (Fig. 1). The generation of both cytokines is inhibited by the addition of cycloheximide, suggesting that their production occurs de novo and that neither is stored and released during degranulation or produced minutes following stimulation, as is true for histamine and LTC4.

Clinical Indications for Measuring In Vitro Basophil IL-4 and IL-13 Secretion

At the time the previous edition of this book was published, the clinical indications for measuring IL-4 and IL-13 appeared to be the same as those described for measuring histamine release from basophils. This remains true in that these cytokines show increased sensitivity to IgE-mediated stimulation and are somewhat specific for this type of activation: IgE-independent secretagogues, including C5a and N-formyl-methionyl-leucyl phenylalanine (FMLP), which are potent stimuli for histamine release, do not normally induce IL-4 and IL-13. However, in recent studies comparing cells from allergic and nonallergic subjects, greater levels of IL-13

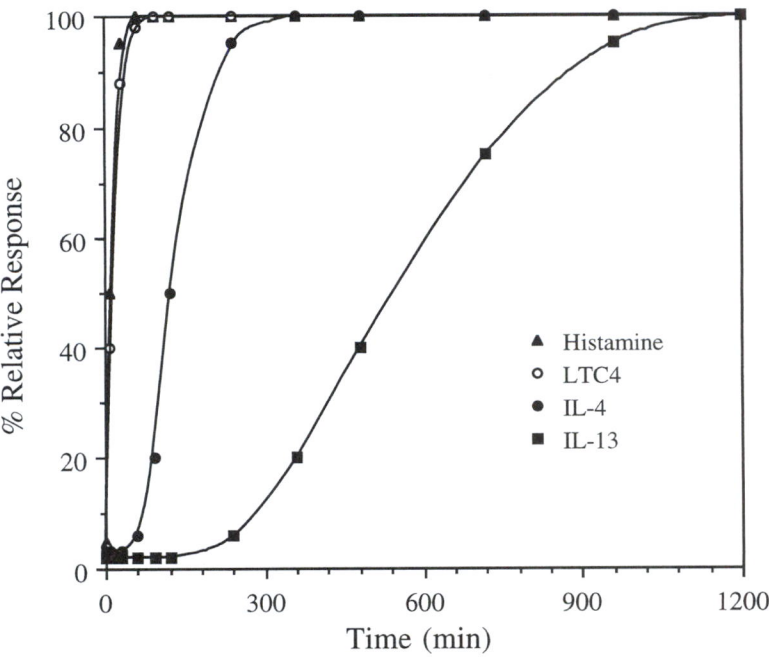

FIGURE 1 Diagrammatic representation of the time course for histamine, LTC4, and IL-4 and IL-13 protein release by human basophils following IgE-dependent activation. Both preformed histamine and newly generated LTC4 are released within minutes after stimulation. The generation of IL-4 and IL-13 is thought to occur de novo, with protein detectable only after 1 to 2 h for IL-4 and after 4 h for IL-13, following stimulation.

were secreted by cells of the latter group in response to specific non-IgE-dependent stimuli. For instance, it has been found that cells from allergic subjects secrete three to seven times more IL-13 following direct stimulation with IL-3 and/or nerve growth factor than cells from nonallergic subjects (18). Moreover, there is recent evidence that IL-13 is spontaneously produced in vitro from basophils of allergic subjects repeatedly exposed to allergen via nasal challenge (12). Overall, these findings suggest a novel indication for measuring basophil secretion of cytokines (particularly IL-13), since these cytokines are observed in the absence of mediator (histamine) release, and may also be indicative of underlying systemic Th2-like responses occurring as a result of allergen exposure. Nonetheless, the clinical applicability of measuring IL-4 and IL-13 remains less than that of measuring histamine, since measuring IL-4 and IL-13 is time-consuming and requires multiple assay systems.

IL-4 and IL-13 Protein: Methods of Cytokine Detection

As that of many other cytokines, the measurement of IL-4 and IL-13 protein most often employs an ELISA. Many sources of commercial kits now exist, and some assays have sensitivities of 1 pg/ml to 1 ng/ml. Alternatively, the development of in-house ELISAs is economically desirable if the appropriately matched antibody pairs for the cytokine of interest are available. With respect to IL-4 and IL-13, several companies now offer such antibody combinations for use in developing in-house assays. Since there are protocols described elsewhere in this manual that are devoted to ELISA design, specific details will not be belabored here other than to make some general comments. First, when quantifying IL-4 and IL-13 protein by ELISA (as with any protein ELISA), there are potential problems that may arise with interassay variation. This is particularly true since many assays, including commercially available kits, are supplied with standards that are likely to give different results among assays. It is important, therefore, to calibrate in-house standards against a variety of other available standards, ideally those set by World Health Organization specifications. In addition, it is important to store IL-4 and IL-13 stock solutions in working aliquots frozen at −20°C or below, since protein degradation may occur at 4°C or with repeated freezing and thawing.

While ELISAs detect secreted protein, it has become increasingly popular to monitor cytokine generation at the single-cell level by using multicolor flow cytometry. The technique requires the inclusion of a protein transport inhibitor, such as brefeldin A or monensin, which is added to cell cultures during stimulation to prevent the secretion of cytokines from activated cells. Intracellular cytokines are subsequently detected in paraformaldehyde-fixed, detergent-permeabilized cells using fluorescence-conjugated antibodies. With the use of a two-color staining protocol, it was recently shown that basophils account for most of the IL-4 and IL-13 produced in peripheral blood mononuclear cell suspensions following in vitro stimulation with an allergen (3). While multicolor flow cytometry has significant potential as an analytical technique for monitoring cytokine generation in specific cell types, particularly those found in low frequencies, its success depends on antibodies that are compatible with fixation and permeabilization. Fixation with paraformaldehyde (4%) is usually necessary to maintain cell integrity for permeabilization with detergent (e.g., saponin, 0.1%), which allows intracellular access by fluorescence-conjugated antibodies. These procedures, however, can

often affect antigenic binding sites, making cytokines unrecognizable by antibodies (particularly those monoclonal in nature) that would ordinarily detect native protein. When antibodies do stain, it is important to establish specificity by performing neutralization experiments with unlabeled antibody. In fact, there are presently many commercially available anticytokine monoclonal antibodies directly conjugated with a variety of fluorochromes that have been subjected to such testing and appear to be suitable for multicolor flow cytometry.

Preparation of Basophil Suspensions for Cytokine and/or Mediator Release

Enriched Suspensions

Basophil-enriched suspensions are prepared by density centrifugation on isotonic Percoll gradients to allow simultaneous assessment of cytokine secretion and histamine release (15). For IL-4 and IL-13 production, 5 ml of blood per reaction tube, approximately five times the amount required for histamine release, is anticoagulated with 10 mM EDTA. The plasma layer, obtained following centrifugation ($300 \times g$; 15 min; 24°C), is aspirated without disturbing the leukocyte interface (buffy coat). The buffy coat interface is then removed and transferred into a tube containing an equal volume of PAG-EDTA buffer (approximately 20 ml of buffy coat per 50 ml of whole blood). Diluted buffy coat (20 ml) is then layered onto gradients consisting of 12.5 ml of 55% isotonic Percoll (approximate density, 1.072 g/ml) underlaid with 12.5 ml of 61% isotonic Percoll ($d \approx 1.082$ g/ml), as illustrated in Fig. 2. Note that an alternative to performing this "double Percoll" approach is the simple use of the 61% Percoll solution for a "single Percoll" protocol. While this typically results in a basophil purity of less than 3%, it adequately removes excessive red cells, producing a leukocyte suspension suitable for investigating cytokine expression by flow cytometry. In any case, the gradients are centrifuged ($700 \times g$; 20 min; 24°C). The cells banding at the 55% Percoll interface and penetrating the top half of this layer are removed and discarded. Basophils are present in the fraction consisting of the lower half of the 55% Percoll layer, the 61% interface, and the upper half of this layer. These leukocytes are immediately transferred into clean tubes containing 35 ml of PAG-EDTA buffer and centrifuged ($150 \times g$; 10 min; 24°C). After combining and transferring the cells into 15-ml polypropylene tubes, the cells are washed twice in cold PAG (6 to 10 ml per wash). The mean percentage of basophils found in these fractions ranges from 5 to 50% (using the double Percoll approach), as determined by cell counts in Spiers-Levy chambers using alcian blue (4).

Mixed Leukocyte Preparations

Yet another alternative is simply to use washed leukocytes obtained from dextran sedimentation. In fact, the availability of ultrasensitive ELISAs allows the measurement of IgE-mediated IL-4 secretion by using the same preparation technique and number of basophils (~20,000) as those used for histamine release. Note, however, that this protocol does not allow the simultaneous analysis of the histamine released into the culture supernatant, since the entire supernatant volume is needed for the IL-4 measurement. Furthermore, it is important not to culture the total number of cells at an excessively high density (~20×10^6 cells/ml), which is thought to decrease somewhat the ability to detect any cytokine secreted. Rather than depending on ELISA methodology for detecting secreted protein, protocols for

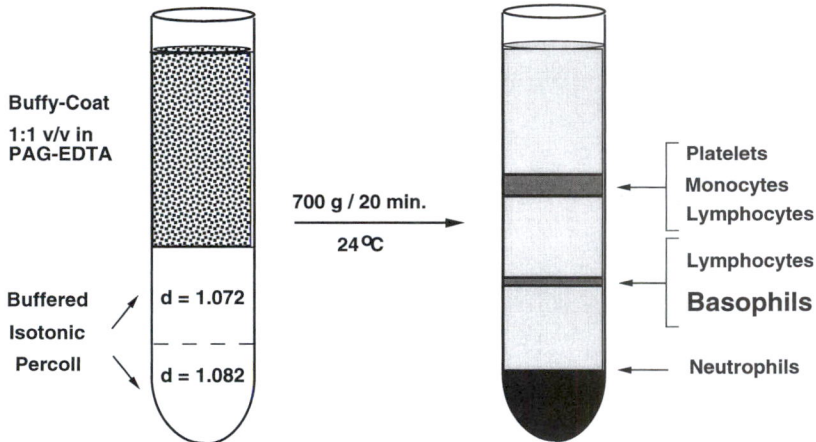

FIGURE 2 Diagrammatic representation of preparation of peripheral blood basophils by discontinuous Percoll density centrifugation. Leukocyte interface cells (buffy coat) are prepared from whole blood by centrifugation. Diluted buffy-coat cell suspensions are layered onto buffered isotonic gradients consisting of two Percoll densities (d) of 1.072 and 1.082 g/ml. Following centrifugation ($700 \times g$, 20 min, at 24°C), basophils band on the 1.082-g/ml Percoll interface and range from 5 to 50% purity. v/v, vol/vol.

detecting intracellular cytokines may be more appropriate when cells prepared in this manner are used. The rationale is that any cytokine retained in the cell, and under conditions of chemical fixation, is more likely to be absorbed or metabolized by contaminating cells in crowded cell cultures.

Culture Procedure

For cytokine protein secretion from basophils, leukocytes obtained directly or from Percoll gradients are resuspended in a culture medium such as Iscove's modified Dulbecco's medium, pH 7.4, supplemented with 5% heat-inactivated (56°C for 30 min) fetal bovine serum, nonessential amino acids, and 5 μg of gentamicin per ml (C-IMDM). For simultaneous analysis of histamine release and IL-4 protein secretion, basophil-enriched suspensions are prepared on Percoll gradients, and 100,000 to 200,000 basophils, accurately enumerated by counting of alcian blue-stained cells, are added per well in a 96-well microtiter plate. The cells are added in 125 μl of C-IMDM and are brought to 37°C in a CO_2 incubator (5% CO_2), after which 125 μl of C-IMDM with or without a stimulus (e.g., a specific antigen) at 37°C is added for a 4-h incubation. The cultures are then centrifuged, and the cell-free supernatants are collected for analysis. A portion of the supernatant is obtained for histamine measurement by carefully removing the upper 25 to 50 μl of supernatant and adding this to 1 ml of PAG buffer containing 1.6% $HClO_4$. After precipitation of protein overnight at 4°C, the histamine in the samples is measured by automated fluorometry or by other methods. Histamine release is reported as a percentage of the total histamine, which is measured by taking a portion of the starting leukocyte suspension, containing a number of basophils proportional to the amount of supernatant used for analysis, for direct lysis in 1 ml of acid solution. The supernatant remaining is then collected for IL-4 protein analysis by ELISA.

As noted, the conditions necessary for IgE-dependent secretion of IL-13 are essentially the same as those important for secretion of IL-4, with the only difference being that detection of the former cytokine requires an 8- to 20-h incubation.

Thus, the protocol described above for IL-4 also applies to IL-13 secretion with the exception that longer incubation times are required.

NOVEL NON-IgE STIMULI OF BASOPHILS

Recently, there has been great interest in the role innate immunity plays in directing the course of acquired immunity, including that associated with allergic disease. At the core of this attention are the Toll-like receptors (TLRs), their expression on various immune cells (particularly antigen-presenting cells), and the cellular responses resulting from the binding of their putative ligands. For instance, basophils are now reported to express several of the 11 known TLRs, including TLR1, 2, 4, 6, 8, 9, and 10. There is also mounting evidence that specific ligands for these receptors can either augment or suppress both mediator release and cytokine secretion by these basophils (and mast cells). For example, TLR2 ligands (such as the peptidoglycan derived from the cell wall of gram-positive bacteria) will directly induce IL-4 and IL-13 from basophils and are capable of augmenting IgE-dependent secretion of all mediator classes (histamine, LTC4, and cytokines) as well as IgE-independent secretion of IL-13 (2). While the significance of these findings pertains more, at this time, to the pathogenesis of allergic disease itself, they do raise potential issues with regard to the tests described above. For instance, it is not uncommon for allergen preparations to be contaminated with microbial products (e.g., endotoxin), and such contamination may become even more of a problem as recombinant allergens are developed for use in skin testing and immunotherapy. Thus, it is reasonable to believe that products containing endotoxin could affect basophil function as well as any interpretations arising from assay results.

BASOPHIL SURFACE ACTIVATION MARKERS

Several groups have reported the use of select surface markers readily measured by flow cytometry as another means to detect basophil activation, particularly via the IgE receptor.

Specifically, CD63, CD69, and CD203c have been put forward as surface markers that are sensitive to basophil activation after exposure to an allergen (CD63 and CD203c), exposure to IL-3 (CD69), or exposure to other degranulation stimuli such as FMLP and ionophores. The use of these activation markers as part of diagnostic evaluation of the presence of allergic reaction-specific IgE, such as in the case of venom allergy, has been reported, and limited evidence suggests specificity in the pattern and degree of basophil activation. However, several questions remain as to the specificity of these markers for diagnostic testing with specific allergens. As apparent from basophil histamine release assays, a broad range of allergen doses must be utilized to allow the use of these tests across a given population. Access to sufficient blood basophils for each individual allergen to be tested must be considered, as well as the potential that nearly 1 in 20 subjects may have nonresponding basophils, which may hamper the ability to interpret the results. In addition, there is some controversy about the preferred surface marker or the use of a panel of all three markers and the potential for the kinetics for each individual marker to shift. Given the number of issues, the application of these markers as an in vitro diagnostic tool remains to be seen.

Although it is accepted that CD69 is the marker on basophils that is most sensitive to prolonged IL-3 exposure, several additional factors must be considered. The use of whole blood for assay of these surface markers is quite popular; however, the conditions used for the lysis of contaminating red cells may also deliver an activation stimulus to the basophils. Other isolation strategies such as Percoll isolation may be desirable, but negative selection procedures for highly purified basophil preparation may evoke nonspecific basophil activation due to prolonged handling of basophils. In addition, controls to monitor for false signals from other cell types that bear CD69 and CD63, such as adherent platelets, must be considered in assays. Although some studies have shown expression of activation markers in parallel with histamine release from basophils, at least one study has shown discordance between the elevation of activation marker expression and basophil histamine release in response to a polyclonal anti-IgE stimulus (8). Thus, the potential for these surface markers to become an adjunct or surrogate to other diagnostic tests such as mediator detection awaits the development of rigorous standards and procedures.

NON-BASOPHIL-SECRETED MEDIATORS AND MARKERS

Tryptase

Tryptase is a neutral protease with trypsin-like substrate specificity that is found in relatively large quantities in mast cells ($\sim$10 pg per lung mast cell and up to 135 pg per skin mast cell), where it is most commonly stored in the secretory granules as an active enzyme complexed to, and stabilized by, heparin. Although several forms have been described (I, IIβ, III, α, and transmembrane tryptase) and all are found in mast cells, only the β and, less frequently, α species are clinically relevant. Since negligible amounts are found in basophils (0.04 pg per cell), tryptase is considered to be a specific marker of mast cell activation. Although tryptase is generally accepted as a mediator of immediate hypersensitivity, its biological role is not known. However, several in vitro activities of tryptase, such as its ability to sensitize smooth muscle to histamine and to stimulate fibroblast proliferation, have suggested a direct role for this enzyme in conditions ranging from asthma to wound healing.

Clinical Indications: Assessment of In Vivo Mast Cell Activation

Unlike that of histamine release from basophils, measurement of tryptase release as a routine in vitro correlate of immediate hypersensitivity is not practical, since this requires preparation of tissue mast cells from human subjects. However, the ability to readily detect tryptase in many types of biological specimens, such as serum, bronchial lavage fluid, nasal lavage fluid, skin blister fluid, and tears, has made this enzyme a valuable marker of in vivo mast cell activation. Thus, in conjunction with histamine measurements, the detection of tryptase is useful in determining the involvement of mast cells in immediate allergic responses occurring in many different reaction sites. Like histamine, β-tryptase is released from mast cells within 15 min following in vitro degranulation and is the predominant form detected in the serum 1 to 2 h following anaphylaxis. However, since α-tryptase is spontaneously secreted from mast cells and often elevated in mastocytosis patients during mast cell burden, quantifying ratios of α and β forms in serum provides the best indication of mast cell activation (16).

Test Procedures for Detection of Tryptase

Several laboratories have developed antibodies against purified human pulmonary mast cell tryptase, enabling the specific detection of this protein in a variety of biological fluids. The measurements are most often performed by ELISA, utilizing an anti-lung tryptase antibody as the primary antibody and biotinylated secondary antibodies in a two-site immunoenzymatic assay, much like that described above for IL-4 protein measurements. Polyclonal antibodies are also useful for detecting tryptase by RIA, although nonspecific binding and protein interference are often problematic. Human lung mast cell tryptase is often used as a source of standards in both the ELISA and RIA techniques and requires extensive purification protocols. While at least one company (Promega) offers recombinant tryptase, its usefulness as a standard has not been fully determined. It is now possible to measure tryptase using the commercially available ImmunoCAP assay (Pharmacia, Uppsala, Sweden), which is designed as a sandwich immunoassay involving a cellulose-derivative solid-phase component. The assay is reported to be suitable for serum or nasal lavage specimens collected between 15 min and 3 h after mast cell activation.

PGD2

Cyclooxygenase enzyme activity is prevalent in mast cells, since the proinflammatory mediator PGD2 is released from these cells ($\sim$60 ng/10^6 cells) upon activation. In contrast, as mentioned above, basophils do not produce PGD2, making this prostanoid a specific marker of IgE-mediated mast cell activation. PGD2 is also a proinflammatory mediator, capable of causing bronchoconstriction, dilation, and increased permeability of the microvasculature. Recent studies indicate that PGD2 is an important chemoattractant, selectively recruiting cells expressing its receptor, CRTH2, including basophils and Th2 cells. Unlike assays for LTC4, PGD2 assays should be performed as quickly as possible, especially when skin mast cells are involved, since this mediator is susceptible to degradation even when stored at $-20°$C. PGD2 is most often measured using a competitive RIA, either a commercially available or an in-house assay.

Because of the technical problems observed, especially with high-protein-concentration fluids, some laboratories have developed gas chromatographic technology, which is considered the method of choice for detection of prostanoids in biologic fluids. The addition of tetradeuterated standards overcomes problems of differential degradation, and chromatography of samples using Sep-Pak columns removes interfering proteins and other substances in biologic matrices. PGD2 is not regularly analyzed as a mediator of allergic inflammation, since tryptase is more readily detected in the same biological specimens and is generally accepted as a more specific marker of mast cell activation (see below).

MBP and ECP

No cell type shows more striking infiltration into allergic lesions than the eosinophil. In fact, patients with mild to moderate asthma often have blood eosinophilia that correlates with the severity of disease, and activated eosinophils have been demonstrated to be present in bronchial biopsy specimens and in the lavage fluids taken from reaction sites in the lung. Eosinophils contain many granule-associated proteins that are thought to be responsible for much of the tissue destruction occurring in diseases such as asthma. In particular, both MBP and eosinophil cationic protein (ECP) account for a large portion of the protein found in the cytoplasmic granules of eosinophils, and both are released upon activation. Both are rich in arginine residues, making them very basic proteins that are highly toxic to host cells, particularly those of the tracheal epithelium. MBP is also known to activate basophils, mast cells, and neutrophils, causing mediator release from these cells, which can contribute to the overall response. MBP is found at relatively high concentrations in eosinophils, averaging nearly 5 $\mu g/10^6$ cells in normal donors. Although low levels of this protein are found in basophils (<1 $\mu g/10^6$ cells), this is thought to be an artifact, resulting from internalization of MBP by these cells.

Clinical Indications: Assessment of Eosinophil Activation

Since MBP and ECP are often detected in a variety of biological specimens, including serum, sputum, and lavage fluid collected from a variety of reaction sites, they are becoming recognized as important in vivo correlates of eosinophil activation. In fact, increased levels of these proteins in these biological specimens show a strong correlation with the severity of clinical symptoms in asthma and rhinitis, particularly as they relate to decreased airway function. In vitro studies investigating the release of MBP and ECP from highly enriched eosinophil suspensions prepared from peripheral blood have also been useful in elucidating the mechanisms of eosinophil activation.

Test Procedures for Detecting MBP and ECP

MBP is most commonly measured by competitive RIA using polyclonal anti-MBP antibody and radiolabeled MBP. The technique, therefore, is similar to the procedure outlined above for the RIA used in the measurement of LTC4 but remains specialized in that antibodies to MBP are usually made in-house. At least one company (HyTest, Oy, Finland) now offers a rabbit polyclonal antibody reportedly suitable for the detection of human pro-MBP by either ELISA or Western blotting. Serum ECP levels can now be determined using the commercially available ImmunoCAP assay (Pharmacia) much as noted for measuring tryptase. However, the success of the assay is very much dependent on specimen preparation, as collection tubes, coagulation time,

and temperature will all affect the levels measured in serum samples.

NO

Many studies show that increased levels of exhaled NO are associated with airway inflammation, particularly that transpiring in allergic disease (17). Several nitric oxide synthases (NOS) have a role in the production of NO from many substrate species found in the lung (e.g., O_2, NADPH, and L-arginine). Endothelial cell membrane-associated NOS (type III) is constitutively expressed and is primarily responsible for NO generated in response to shear stresses in the systemic and pulmonary circulation. Neuronal NOS (type I) has a role in neurotransmission and is also constitutively expressed. Thus, both the type I and III forms mediate physiologic functions. In contrast, inducible NOS (iNOS, or type II) is the form associated with inflammation, and although it is expressed in many cell types, its expression is markedly increased in the bronchial epithelia of asthmatics. Allergen challenge, in fact, will induce epithelial expression of iNOS, resulting in increased production of NO. More recently, it has been shown that IL-1, tumor necrosis factor alpha, and IL-4, when combined with gamma interferon, can upregulate iNOS expression in epithelial cell lines, suggesting a role for proinflammatory cytokines in regulating exhaled NO levels. NO is quite unstable and rapidly autooxidizes into a variety of metabolites, including nitrite (NO_2^-), nitrate (NO_3^-), peroxynitrite ($OONO^-$), and nitrothiols. These nitrogen oxides have been shown to modulate many different effects, ranging from bronchodilation to immune defense, including chemotaxis and apoptosis.

Clinical Indications: Assessment of Allergic Airway Disease

Measurements of exhaled NO are noninvasive and can be performed on children as well as adults. This convenience, along with evidence that increased levels of NO correlate with methacholine responsiveness and with sputum eosinophilia, has sparked interest in this mediator as a sensitive marker of ongoing allergic inflammation in the lower airways. Evidence shows, in fact, that exhaled NO can be used as a parameter to discriminate asthmatics from nonasthmatics and to monitor the therapeutic efficacy of certain anti-inflammatory drugs (e.g., corticosteroids) that inhibit iNOS activity and thus reduce NO levels. However, underlying viral infections, acute allograft lung rejection, and collagen diseases with lung involvement have been shown to increase levels of exhaled NO. Thus, there are some instances that warrant caution against oversimplification in interpreting levels of exhaled NO. At this time, further evaluation is required in assessing the utility of nasal NO measurements in the diagnosis of upper airway inflammation, such as that associated with allergic rhinitis.

Measurement of Exhaled NO

Exhaled NO is most commonly measured by chemiluminescence, in which sample NO is drawn into a reaction cell and reacted with ozone, resulting in the emission of light that is detected by a photomultiplier tube. Values are reported as parts per billion, with some instruments sensitive to parts per trillion. On-line and off-line measurements can be performed. For off-line measurements, specimens are collected into special receptacles (e.g., Mylar balloons and Tedlar bags), which allow the convenience of sampling at home or at sites distant from the analyzer. Patients inhale to total lung capacity, and the exhalant is then collected while mouth pressure, expiratory resistance, and expiratory flow rate are monitored. The same parameters of fixed pressure and resistance are monitored during on-line measurements in which NO profiles are simultaneously displayed, allowing the collection of reproducible tracings. For adults, an NO plateau of 3 to 6 s should be obtained, whereas a 2-s plateau is sufficient for children of less than 12 years old. The most precise measurements are obtained when subjects inhale air from a source containing <5 ppb of NO, since surrounding NO levels may be higher than endogenous levels. Measurements should be performed before spirometry so as not to decrease the levels of exhaled NO. Other factors that lower NO levels and which need to be controlled for include smoking, the use of glucocorticoids, and bronchoconstriction. In contrast, bronchodilators increase NO levels; thus, their use should be well documented. As noted above, exhaled NO levels also increase in certain infections; thus, measurements should be postponed until recovery is evident.

QUALITY ASSURANCE

Since none of the assays described above are regulated by the Clinical Laboratory Improvement Act of 1988, interlaboratory proficiency surveys are presently not available. However, there are certain critical steps that can be taken to ensure the validity of the analytical measurements. The first deals with the tests performed to detect in vitro correlates of immediate hypersensitivity (i.e., histamine, LTC4 and IL-4 and IL-13 protein release from basophils). When the allergic status of an individual is evaluated, it is important to include controls to ensure basophil reactivity, especially when the challenging allergen does not induce the release of the mediator in question. For histamine and LTC4 release, this inclusion is most commonly achieved by stimulating basophils with anti-IgE antibody and/or with FMLP, which are both quite effective in inducing the release of these mediators from basophils obtained from most donors. For IL-4 and IL-13 protein, anti-IgE antibody alone is usually sufficient to induce the secretion of the cytokine from most donors' basophils. However, as noted above, a calcium ionophore (ionomycin or A23187) has been shown to be a potent and relatively specific stimulus for the secretion of both cytokines by basophils. The lack of reactivity with these stimuli could indicate that calcium is missing from the reaction buffer or that the temperature is not 37°C (e.g., it is above 40°C). It is also important that IL-3 pretreatment (15 min) will often enhance the IgE-mediated release of all of the above-listed mediators and may be employed when basophils show marginal release in response to an antigen alone. In contrast, false-positive histamine release may occur as a result of cell lysis due to solvents found in allergen preparations. In this instance, it is important to include controls showing that, in the absence of allergen, the solvents cause no additional release above the spontaneous release (blanks). Similarly, in studies investigating substances that inhibit mediator release, it is important to show that final concentrations of the solvent (e.g., dimethyl sulfoxide) have no effect on secretion.

There are several other factors to consider when performing assays that are used to directly measure mediators and markers of allergic inflammation. The first deals with the general use of standards for these assays. Stock solutions should always be prepared using established methodology to prevent interassay variability. It is also important to store stock solutions in small aliquots to avoid repeated freezing and thawing

that may result in loss of activity. Since the type of buffer used and the amount of protein present have a profound effect in all of the assays described above, it is also extremely important that the standards be prepared in diluent identical to, or closely resembling, that found in the test samples. For example, when culture supernatants are tested for IL-4 or IL-13 protein, it is important that the standards be diluted in medium identical to that used in the cultures, since medium containing serum may produce different background levels compared to buffer containing little to no protein. Finally, data analysis for these assays is greatly facilitated by the use of computer application programs, which are often commercially available from equipment manufacturers. They are especially helpful for histamine measurements determined by automated fluorometry, in which many samples can be assayed at a given time and the data can be saved and stored for later access and rapid analysis.

SUMMARY

It is now possible to measure a number of inflammatory mediators released from cells participating in allergic disease. Measurement of the release of preformed histamine from peripheral blood basophils challenged with a specific antigen is among several tests available, and histamine release remains a valuable in vitro correlate of immediate hypersensitivity reactions. However, other mediators that have a role in allergic inflammation, such as LTC4 and IL-4, are also generated by basophils upon IgE-dependent activation, and in vitro assays have recently been developed to measure these products. These assays, combined with those available for the detection of several other mediators occurring in biological fluids, have produced data that have significantly added to our understanding of the parameters, mechanisms, and pharmacologic control of allergic inflammation.

APPENDIX

Special reagents and equipment

RFA 300 rapid flow analyzer for histamine measurement by fluorometry (Astoria-Pacific International, Clackamas, Oreg.)

Filtered reagents for fluorometry

Phosphoric acid (0.73 M)

30% NaCl

5 N NaOH

1 N NaOH containing 1 mM EDTA

0.1 N HCl

Brij-saline-EDTA: 0.17 M NaCl, 1.5 mM EDTA, 0.015% Brij 35 (Perstorp Analytical, Silver Spring, Md.)

Heptane

Butanol

OPT solution: 50 mg of OPT (Sigma, St. Louis, Mo.) recrystallized in ligroine solvent (Eastman Kodak Co., Rochester, N.Y.), 1 ml of spectranalyzed methanol (Fisher Scientific, Pittsburgh, Pa.), and 99 ml of borate buffer (0.5 M)

Histamine standards (for fluorometry)

Histamine dihydrochloride (molecular weight, 184.1)

Histamine (molecular weight, 111.0)

Make a 1-mg/ml solution of histamine.

Note that 1 mg of histamine equals 1.66 mg of histamine dihydrochloride.

Dilute the 1-mg/ml solution 1/1,000 in 2% $HClO_4$ to give a 1-μg/ml stock and store at $-20°C$ in 6-ml aliquots. Six milliliters of 1-μg/ml histamine added to 294 ml of 2% $HClO_4$ yields 20 ng/ml; 50 ml of 20-ng/ml standard added to 50 ml of 2% $HClO_4$ yields 10 ng/ml.

10× PIPES buffer, pH 7.4: 250 mM PIPES (Sigma Chemical Co.), 1.10 M NaCl, 50 mM KCl

PAG buffer: 10% 10× PIPES, 0.003% human serum albumin (Calbiochem-Behring Corp., La Jolla, Calif.), 0.1% D-glucose

PAG-EDTA buffer: PAG containing 4 mM EDTA

PAGCM buffer: PAG containing 1 mM $CaCl_2$ and 1 mM $MgCl_2$

Isotonic Percoll: 9 parts Percoll (Pharmacia, Piscataway, N.J.) plus 1 part 10× PIPES

Lactic acid buffer (pH 3.9): 90.1 mg of lactic acid (Calbiochem-Behring Corp.), 817.6 mg of NaCl, 37.28 mg of KCl, 100 ml of distilled water

This work was supported in part by NIH grant AI42221.

REFERENCES

1. **Alberse, R., R. van der Gaag, and J. van Leeuwen.** 1983. Serologic aspects of IgG$_4$ antibodies. 1. Prolonged immunization results in an IgG$_4$-restricted response. *J. Immunol.* **130:**722–726.

2. **Bieneman, A., K. Chichester, Y.-H. Chen, and J. Schroeder.** 2005. Toll-like receptor 2 ligands activate human basophils for both IgE-dependent and IgE-independent secretion. *J. Allergy Clin. Immunol.* **115:**295–301.

3. **Devouassoux, G., G. Foster, L. M. Scott, D. D. Metcalfe, and C. Prussin.** 1999. Frequency and characterization of antigen-specific IL-4- and IL-13-producing basophils and T cells in peripheral blood of healthy and asthmatic subjects. *J. Allergy Clin. Immunol.* **104:**811–819.

4. **Gilbert, H. S., and L. Ornstein.** 1975. Basophil counting with a new staining method using alcian blue. *Blood* **46:**279–286.

5. **Ishizaka, T., R. DeBernardo, H. Tomioka, L. M. Lichtenstein, and K. Ishizaka.** 1972. Identification of basophil granulocytes as a site of allergic histamine release. *J. Immunol.* **108:**1000–1008.

6. **Levy, D., and A. Osler.** 1966. Studies on the mechanisms of hypersensitivity phenomena. XIV. Passive sensitization in vitro of human leukocytes to ragweed pollen antigen. *J. Immunol.* **97:**203–212.

7. **Lichtenstein, L. M., P. Norman, and W. Winkenwerder.** 1968. Clinical and in vitro studies on the role of immunotherapy in ragweed hay fever. *Am. J. Med.* **44:**514–524.

8. **MacGlashan, D. W., Jr.** 1995. Graded changes in the response of individual human basophils to stimulation: distributional behavior of events temporally coincident with degranulation. *J. Leukoc. Biol.* **58:**177–188.

9. **Min, B., M. Prout, J. Hu-Li, J. Zhu, D. Jankovic, E. Morgan, J. Urban, Jr., A. Dvorak, F. Finkelman, G. LeGros, and W. E. Paul.** 2004. Basophils produce IL-4 and accumulate in tissues after infection with a Th2-inducing parasite. *J. Exp. Med.* **200:**507–517.

10. **Nouri-Aria, K., A.-M. Irani, M. Jacobson, F. O'Brien, E. Varga, S. Till, S. Durham, and L. Schwartz.** 2001. Basophil recruitment and IL-4 production during human allergen-induced late asthma. *J. Allergy Clin. Immunol.* **108:**205–211.

11. **Pruzansky, J. J., L. C. Grammer, R. Patterson, and M. Roberts.** 1983. Dissociation of IgE from receptors on human basophils. I. Enhanced passive sensitization for histamine release. *J. Immunol.* **131:**1949.

12. **Saini, S., D. Bloom, A. Bieneman, K. Vasagar, A. Togias, and J. Schroeder.** 2004. Systemic effects of allergen exposure on blood basophil IL-13 secretion and FcεR1β expression. *J. Allergy Clin. Immunol.* **114:**768–774.

13. **Schroeder, J. T., D. W. MacGlashan, and L. M. Lichtenstein.** 2001. Human basophils: mediator release and cytokine production. *Adv. Immunol.* **77:**93–122.

14. **Schroeder, J. T., L. M. Lichtenstein, E. Roche, H. Xiao, and M. C. Liu.** 2001. IL-4 production by human basophils found in the lung following segmental allergen challenge. *J. Allergy Clin. Immunol.* **107:**265–271.

15. **Schroeder, J. T., D. W. MacGlashan, Jr., A. Kagey-Sobotka, J. M. White, and L. M. Lichtenstein.** 1994. IgE-dependent IL-4 secretion by human basophils: the relationship between cytokine production and histamine release in mixed leukocyte cultures. *J. Immunol.* **153:**1808–1818.

16. **Schwartz, L., D. Metcalfe, J. Miller, H. Earl, and T. Sullivan.** 1987. Tryptase levels as an indicator of mast cell activation in systemic anaphylaxis and mastocytosis. *N. Engl. J. Med.* **316:**1622–1626.

17. **Silkoff, P. E., R. A. Robbins, B. Gaston, J. O. N. Lundberg, and R. G. Townley.** 2000. Endogenous nitric oxide in allergic airway disease. *J. Allergy Clin. Immunol.* **105:**438–448.

18. **Sin, A., E. Roche, A. Togias, L. Lichtenstein, and J. Schroeder.** 2001. Nerve growth factor or IL-3 induces more IL-13 production from basophils of allergic subjects than from basophils of nonallergic subjects. *J. Allergy Clin. Immunol.* **108:**387–393.

19. **Siraganian, R. P.** 1974. An automated continuous-flow system for the extraction and fluorometric analysis of histamine. *Anal. Biochem.* **57:**383–394.

20. **Voehringer, D., K. Shinkai, and R. Locksley.** 2004. Type 2 immunity reflects orchestrated recruitment of cells committed to IL-4 production. *Immunity* **20:**267–277.

Tests for Immunological Reactions to Foods

DAVID M. FLEISCHER AND ROBERT A. WOOD

109

Food allergy is defined as an adverse immunological response to food. Food allergic disorders can be divided into those that are immunoglobulin E (IgE) mediated and those that are non-IgE mediated. Disorders with acute onset of symptoms, defined typically as occurring within 2 h after ingestion, are usually mediated by IgE antibodies, while subacute and chronic food allergic disorders may be cell mediated (primarily T cell) or of mixed origin with both cell-mediated and IgE-associated mechanisms, and they usually affect the gastrointestinal tract. In Table 1, a number of IgE-, cell-, and mixed IgE- and cell-mediated disorders are listed.

The diagnosis of food allergy must first begin with a careful medical history, as the information gathered will be used to guide the best mode of diagnosis, or it could lead to dismissal of the problem by history alone. In fact, it is well documented in several studies in which double-blind, placebo-controlled food challenges (DBPCFCs) were used to diagnose food allergy that only about 40% of patient histories of suspected food-induced allergic reactions can be verified (4). In cases of acute reactions such as anaphylaxis and urticaria after the ingestion of an isolated food, the medical history has a much higher predictive value than in chronic disorders such as atopic dermatitis and allergic eosinophilic gastroenteritis (AEG) (32). The history should focus on the food(s) and quantity of food suspected of provoking the reaction, the type of symptoms attributed to food ingestion (acute versus chronic), the timing between ingestion and onset of symptoms, patterns of reactivity, the most recent reaction, and whether other associated activities play a role in inducing symptoms (e.g., exercise or alcohol ingestion). When gathering the history, one must also be aware of other foods eaten at the same time, potentially contaminated foods that may have been packaged on nondedicated lines, and hidden sources of ingredients.

Once a symptom history is established (see Table 2 for signs and symptoms of food-induced allergic reactions), the search for a food-related etiology needs to be put in context with the prevalence that food allergy is implicated as the causative factor. For example, food-allergic reactions account for about 20% of acute urticaria, <10% of chronic urticaria, and about 35% of moderate to severe atopic dermatitis in children, but food allergy is not a common cause of atopic dermatitis in adults (32). While food allergy may affect up to 5% of children with asthma and 1 to 2% of children with allergic rhinitis, it is not a common cause (<1%)

of isolated upper or lower respiratory disease in either children or adults (40). Also, the prevalence of food hypersensitivities is greatest in the first few years of life, affecting about 6% of children <3 years of age and then decreasing to a steady prevalence of 1 to 2% by late childhood through adulthood (35). Furthermore, although any food could theoretically cause an allergic reaction, a small number of foods account for about 90% of verified food reactions: milk, egg, soy, wheat, peanut, tree nuts, and fish for children and peanuts, tree nuts, fish, and shellfish for adults. Finally, the physician should realize that the majority of food allergy is outgrown, usually as a child. In fact, about 85% of children lose their sensitivity to the most allergenic foods (milk, egg, soy, wheat) within the first 3 to 5 years of life (41). However, sensitivity to peanut, tree nuts, fish, and shellfish is rarely lost and thus persists into adulthood; for example, only about 20% of children achieve tolerance to peanut. Some of the tests to be discussed in this chapter not only aid in the diagnosis of food allergies, but also are useful in monitoring the natural history of patients' food allergies over time, from diagnosis to oral tolerance.

Once a thorough history has been obtained, the physical examination should focus on detecting other atopic features, which are more commonly found in patients with IgE-mediated allergic reactions. After completing the history and physical, the physician should first determine whether the patient's findings implicate a food-induced disorder based on the information gathered, and then determine whether an IgE-mediated or non-IgE-mediated mechanism is most likely responsible. Typically, the clinical presentations of allergic reactions listed in Table 2, such as urticaria, angioedema, and wheezing, have a rapid onset in IgE-mediated disorders, whereas other presentations such as vomiting, diarrhea, and bloody stools may not develop for hours to days after ingestion of the allergen in non-IgE-mediated disorders. For disorders with mixed IgE- and cell-mediated mechanisms, clinical features may be variable in onset. Once food allergy has been identified as the likely cause of symptoms, confirmation of the diagnosis and identification of the implicated food(s) can begin. There are a number of tools that aid in the diagnosis of food allergy, some of which are more commonly used, and they vary in their ability to provide an accurate diagnosis. In general, laboratory tests are more useful in delineating the specific foods responsible for IgE-mediated reactions, whereas they are of limited value in non-IgE-mediated

TABLE 1 Food allergy disorders

IgE mediated
  Gastrointestinal: oral allergy syndrome, gastrointestinal
    anaphylaxis
  Cutaneous: urticaria, angioedema, morbilloform rashes and
    flushing
  Respiratory: acute rhinoconjunctivitis, wheezing
  Generalized: anaphylactic shock

Mixed IgE and cell mediated
  Gastrointestinal: allergic eosinophilic esophagitis/AEG
  Cutaneous: atopic dermatitis
  Respiratory: asthma

Cell mediated
  Gastrointestinal: food protein-induced enterocolitis, proctocoli-
    tis, and enteropathy syndromes; celiac disease
  Cutaneous: contact dermatitis, dermatitis herpetiformis
  Respiratory: food-induced pulmonary hemosiderosis (Heiner
    syndrome)

disorders. Available studies include in vivo tests such as skin prick and intradermal testing, oral food challenges (OFCs), elimination diets, and patch testing and in vitro tests such as quantification of food-specific IgE and basophil histamine release (BHR). The utility of these and other test modalities will be discussed in detail.

IN VIVO TESTS

Skin Prick Testing

Skin prick tests (SPTs) are commonly used to screen patients with suspected IgE-mediated food reactions. While the patient is off antihistamines for an appropriate amount of time (short acting, 72 h; long acting, 7 days), a device such as a bifurcated needle, lancet, plastic probe, or the tip of a small-gauge needle is used to puncture the skin through a glyceri-nated food extract (1:10 or 1:20, wt/vol) into the epidermis. Positive (histamine) controls are used to show that the skin response is not blocked, and negative (saline-glycerine) con-trols are used to show that there is not dermatographism or other potential causes for false-positive results such as irritant and contact reactions from the diluent used to preserve aller-gen extracts or poor technique of the tester. Food skin testing with large panels of foods is generally not advised because there could be many irrelevant positive results, but should rather be limited to the most common food allergens and foods that are suspected of provoking symptoms gathered on history (5). If food-specific antibody is present, mast cells with the same food-specific IgE bound to their surface degranulate and release mediators that result in a local wheal-and-flare reaction within 15 to 20 min.

SPTs are generally considered positive if there is a mean wheal diameter of ≥3 mm, after subtraction of the negative control wheal. The mean diameter of the wheal is calculated by measuring the greatest diameter of the wheal and the largest diameter perpendicular to it and then averaging the sum of these diameters. When an SPT is positive, it indi-cates the possible association between the food tested and the patient's reactivity to that food because the positive pre-dictive accuracies of SPTs are <50% compared to those of DBPCFCs. On the other hand, negative responses virtually exclude the possibility of an IgE-mediated reaction because

their negative predictive value exceeds 95% (32). Therefore, negative SPTs are an excellent means of excluding IgE-mediated food allergies, although they are not perfect (31), and positive SPTs are only suggestive of the presence of symptomatic allergy. However, a positive SPT may be con-sidered diagnostic in patients who have experienced a sys-temic anaphylactic reaction to an isolated food (32).

Several key studies have looked at the performance char-acteristics of SPTs in predicting true food allergy at different wheal cutoffs compared to the outcome of DBPCFCs. Sampson (31), in a study of 87 patients (median age, 7.9 years) who all had atopic dermatitis and underwent DBPCFCs to rule out food hypersensitivities after SPTs, reported that a 3-mm wheal had a 96% sensitivity in identi-fying children with cow's milk allergy, 98% with egg allergy, and 90% with peanut allergy, with corresponding specifi-cities of 51, 53, and 29%, respectively. Sporik et al. (43) showed corresponding sensitivities for a 3-mm wheal of 74% for cow's milk, 84% for egg, and 96% for peanut, with respective specificities of 79, 70, and 71% from 535 chal-lenges in 467 children (median age, 3 years). For each food, Sporik et al. (43) were also able to identify a SPT wheal diameter at and above which negative food challenges did not occur, thus in theory reducing the need for formal food challenges if the wheal size equaled or exceeded these val-ues: 8 mm for cow's milk, 7 mm for egg, and 8 mm for peanut in a group of children with a median age of 3 years. For chil-dren 2 years of age or younger, the SPT wheal diameter cut-offs were lower: 6 mm for cow's milk, 5 mm for egg, and 4 mm for peanut. Finally, Eigenmann and Sampson (13) reevaluated SPTs in the diagnosis of food allergy in a group of children (median age, 4.6 years) with a history of atopic dermatitis. They used as cutoffs wheal sizes at the upper 95% confidence interval for food-tolerant patients; these were 5 mm for cow's milk, 4 mm for egg, and 6 mm for peanut. The corresponding sensitivities were 89% for cow's milk,

TABLE 2 Signs and symptoms of food-induced allergic reactions

Skin
  Urticaria/angioedema
  Flushing
  Erythematous, pruritic rash
  Atopic dermatitis

Gastrointestinal
  Pruritus and/or swelling of the lips, tongue, or oral mucosa
  Nausea
  Abdominal pain or colic
  Vomiting or reflux
  Diarrhea

Respiratory
  Nasal congestion
  Rhinorrhea
  Pruritus/sneezing
  Laryngeal edema, staccato cough, and/or dysphonia
  Wheezing/repetitive cough

Cardiovascular
  Hypotension/shock
  Dizziness

Other
  Feeling of "impending doom"

98% for egg, and 63% for peanut, and the specificities were 68, 61, and 71%, respectively.

When the test is appropriately performed, SPT results have been shown to be highly reproducible (31). The accuracy of SPTs does vary, however, depending on which food antigen is being studied, the quality of the food extract, and the technical skills of the tester. There are a number of other variables that have to be considered when interpreting SPTs. First, children <1 year old may have negative SPT responses but still have IgE-mediated disease, and infants <2 years old may have smaller wheals, which is presumably due to lower levels of food-specific IgE and skin reactivity. Second, skin testing on areas of the skin that have been treated frequently with topical steroids or in patients on long-term, high-dose systemic corticosteroid therapy may result in reduced wheal size. Third, histamine control wheals <5 mm in diameter may indicate the presence of antihistamines, other interfering medications, or decreased skin reactivity that results in decreased wheal size and possible false-negative test responses (32).

SPTs have several advantages: they are quick, patients can see the reaction of a positive test result on the skin, and they are relatively inexpensive compared with serologic methods for allergy investigation (each SPT on average costs less than one-half as much as measuring the food-specific IgE level in serum). They are also safe: no lethal reactions have been reported after SPTs (11). However, SPTs are often not helpful in determining if a patient who was allergic to a particular food has achieved tolerance to that food, as skin tests often remain significantly positive for years following attainment of clinical tolerance determined by OFC (40).

Intradermal Skin Testing

In 1978, Bock et al. (5) performed DBPCFCs on 76 children aged 5 months to 15 years who exhibited a wheal of 3.0 mm or greater in response to an SPT with one or more of 14 foods, regardless of whether or not they reported a history of an adverse reaction to that food. SPTs with 1:20 (wt/vol) food extracts identified all subjects who exhibited adverse reactions during their challenges. In addition, intradermal skin tests (ISTs) were performed with 1:1,000 (wt/vol) extracts. For each of the 14 foods, between 19 and 39 additional patients (mean, 26) who were negative by SPT had a 3.0 mm or greater wheal in response to intradermal testing. Using peanut as an example, 26 patients were identified by SPT, 12 of whom failed DBPCFCs, and an additional 28 patients, all of whom had negative DBPCFCs, were identified by positive intradermal tests. As a result of this study, it was shown that ISTs with food extracts had no positive advantage over SPTs, and it was concluded that the increased sensitivity of ISTs would lead to even more false-positive tests than seen with the prick technique (34). Furthermore, fatalities after intradermal testing for food allergies have been reported (32). In 1929, a 5-month-old infant died after intradermal injection of ovomucoid. Between 1964 and 1984, sufficient information was available to analyze six fatalities from skin testing. Of these six, two were children aged 10 and 11, both with asthma, who received either ISTs without prior SPTs or ISTs with food extracts (45).

FFSPTs

Fresh food skin prick tests (FFSPTs) are not commonly performed, since the indications for doing so are limited. Some commercially prepared extracts frequently lack the labile proteins that are responsible for IgE-mediated sensitivity to many fruits and vegetables (e.g., apples, oranges, bananas, pears, melons, potato, carrots, and celery), as is seen in patients with oral allergy syndrome (OAS), because the proteins are degraded or lose allergenicity during extract preparation (23). OAS, or pollen-food allergy syndrome, is a condition in which patients develop pruritus, tingling, and angioedema, usually localized to the lips and mouth, due to certain plant proteins in fresh fruits and vegetables cross-reacting with airborne allergens, such as ragweed, birch, and mugwort pollens. Negative SPTs with commercially available extracts that contradict a convincing history of a food-induced allergic reaction should be repeated with the fresh food before conclusion that food-specific IgE is absent (13). Rosen et al. (30) also suggested that patients be tested with the food in the form that caused the reaction (e.g., raw or cooked). FFSPTs are usually done in one of two manners, depending on the type of food. In the prick-plus-prick technique, the needle or lancet device is first embedded in the fresh food and is then immediately used to prick the patient's skin, whereas foods with a harder consistency, such as peanut, are often ground first and diluted in buffered saline.

Several studies have been performed with various combinations of comparisons of FFSPTs with commercial extracts, food-specific-IgE levels, and/or food challenges. In a study by Ortolani et al. (23), 100 patients with OAS and 32 nonallergic control subjects were enrolled. Patients had FFSPTs, commercial extract SPTs, and Phadebas radioallergosorbent tests (RASTs), and 14 patients with OAS underwent open OFCs. The results showed that with FFSPTs there was better sensitivity to foods such as carrot, celery, cherry, apple, and potato, but that sensitivity was better with commercial extract SPTs for peanut, almond, banana, and pea. Rosen et al. (30) confirmed the superiority of fresh extracts in a study of 22 patients, including 9 children. Fourteen of the 22 patients presented with anaphylactic reactions, and the remaining 8 presented with OAS. For 18 of the 22 patients, the foods presumed to be the offending allergens were not limited solely to fruits or vegetables, but included fish, crustaceans, mollusks, milk, egg, peanut, and tree nuts. All of the patients demonstrated a negative response to SPTs with commercial extracts but positive responses to SPTs with natural food extracts, although no food challenges were performed to confirm that these foods were the ones that caused the symptoms. Rance et al. (27), using commercial extracts and fresh foods, compared SPT results for milk, egg, and peanut to the results obtained with labial and/or oral challenge. They found that the overall correlations between positive SPT ($\geq$3 mm) and positive challenges with commercial extracts were 58.8 and 91.7% with fresh foods. They also observed that challenges were positive for 40.5% of subjects with negative commercial SPTs, while only 7.4% of challenges were positive for subjects with negative FFSPTs.

One must be careful, however, in extrapolating these data to the allergic population as a whole. One must also be careful when performing FFSPTs, as safety is an issue with this type of skin testing as well. Two cases of anaphylactic reactions in adults were reported after FFSPTs (11). Devenney and Falth-Magnusson (11) reported six cases of generalized reactions requiring treatment with antihistamine and/or epinephrine in six infants <6 months of age when FFSPTs were used.

Atopy Patch Testing

Atopy patch tests (APTs) have been proposed as a mode of diagnosis of non-IgE-mediated food allergy and for identification of allergens in delayed-onset clinical reactions. APTs are performed epicutaneously, usually on a patient's back. Instead of using type IV allergens such as metals or perfumes, typical immediate-type allergens such as foods are used. A small amount of a food is placed on filter paper, which is then applied to uninvolved skin and covered by an aluminum cup. The application sites are checked after 15 to 20 min for immediate reactions and then are usually kept occluded for 48 h. Results are usually read 20 min after removal of the cups and again 24 h later for the final evaluation. Final reactions are then scored; a type of scoring system used is 1+ for erythema and slight infiltration, 2+ for erythema and papules, and 3+ for erythema and vesicles. Irritant reactions, which have been described as sharply defined, brownish erythema, blistering, and a lack of clear infiltration, are not regarded as positive (28).

Although the exact pathomechanism of the APT is not known, it has been proposed that when the allergen that is applied to the skin under occlusion and penetrates the epidermis, it is captured by IgE molecules which are bound to IgE receptors on Langerhans cells. Allergen-specific T cells are then activated, possibly by IgE-mediated antigen presentation by these Langerhans cells, and initiate an eczematous reaction, which immunocytochemically resembles that seen in atopic dermatitis. APT reactions are therefore associated with the T-lymphocyte-mediated allergen-specific immune response (44). The patch test reaction to aeroallergens seems to be specific for sensitized patients with atopic dermatitis, as it does not occur in healthy volunteers or in patients suffering from asthma or rhinitis (10).

The outcome of APTs in different studies shows large variations due to differences in patient selection and, more importantly, differences in method. At this time, there are large disparities in the type and concentrations of allergens used and in the duration of application and reading time (10). Nonspecific irritation is a common finding in standard patch testing and therefore requires a good deal of skill in differentiating it from a positive reaction (35). These facts make interpretation of studies somewhat difficult due to reliability issues, but a number of investigators have examined the use of the APTs in addition to SPTs for the diagnosis of non-IgE-mediated food allergy, primarily in patients with atopic dermatitis (20), but also in patients with allergic eosinophilic esophagitis.

Roehr et al. (28) studied 173 challenges in 98 patients with atopic dermatitis and used APTs, SPTs, and food-specific IgE levels with cow's milk, egg, soy, and wheat to see if the combination of a positive APT result plus a positive food-specific-IgE level, a positive SPT, or both would make DBPCFCs unnecessary. Patients were observed for 48 h on an inpatient basis after challenges to document late-phase reactions (>2 h postchallenge) of eczema exacerbations, which were counted as positive challenges if they occurred either alone or in combination with early reactions. Positive APT results alone correlated with high positive predictive values (PPVs) for cow's milk (95%), hen's egg (94%), and wheat (94%) compared to positive DBPCFCs, but with only a 50% PPV for soy (only four children reacted to soy). Combination of the APT with proof of specific IgE for cow's milk (≥0.35 kU of antibody [kU_A] per liter) and for egg (≥17.5 kU_A/liter) increased the PPVs to 100%, thus making DBPCFCs superfluous. Addition of SPTs to the other two tests did not further improve results. Spergel et al. (42) studied 26 patients with biopsy-proven eosinophilic esophagitis and performed both SPTs and APTs. Allergies to a total of 68 foods were identified by SPTs in 19 patients and to 67 foods by APTs in 21 patients, and specific foods were

eliminated from patients' diets on the basis of those results. Eighteen patients reported complete resolution of symptoms on the restricted diet, and six reported partial improvement. Posttreatment biopsies also showed decreased numbers of eosinophils per high-powered field, and in some patients, symptoms returned when foods that were positive on patch testing were reintroduced.

Elimination Diets

The purpose of an elimination diet is to determine whether a patient's symptoms will resolve when foods are restricted from the diet. Once certain foods are suspected of being responsible for a food-induced allergic disorder, an elimination diet is started as an attempt to support the diagnosis. If a patient's symptoms persist despite a very strict avoidance diet, it is unlikely that the food accounts for the patient's complaints (6). There are three types of elimination diets: elimination of one or more suspect foods, elimination of all but a defined group of allowed foods that are rarely antigenic (oligo-antigenic diet), and an elemental diet consisting of a hydrolyzed or amino acid-based formula (40). The type of diet chosen depends upon the clinical presentation being evaluated and the results of IgE antibody tests.

Elimination of one or more foods in the first diet type may be the obvious course of action and therapeutic in the case of an acute reaction to a food and the presence of a positive test for IgE to that food. It may also be especially helpful in evaluating infants who are on a very limited diet. In the oligo-antigenic diet, a large number of foods suspected to cause a chronic problem are removed, and the patient is given a list of allowed foods. This type of diet is useful for evaluation of chronic disorders such as atopic dermatitis in children or chronic urticaria. The foods eliminated usually are those that are common causes of food-allergic reactions. In the most extreme diet, the elemental diet, a hydrolyzed (Nutramigen, Alimentum) or amino acid-based (Neocate, EleCare) formula provides all the nutrition. The elemental diet provides the most definitive trial, but it can be difficult to undertake and maintain, especially in patients beyond infancy. This diet may be necessary when the other two diets mentioned above have failed but the suspicion for food-related illness remains high. It may also be necesssary in disorders such as AEG, which is often associated with multiple food allergies. If a patient's symptoms do not disappear on an elemental diet, then it is very unlikely that ingested substances are the problem (6, 40). The length of trial is dependent on the type of symptoms, but 1 to 6 weeks is the usual range required.

If symptoms resolve on an elimination diet, some form of food challenge is generally warranted, especially in chronic disorders such as atopic dermatitis. One must be careful when a food to which the patient is sensitized is removed from the diet during a chronic disorder because reintroduction could induce severe reactions (41). Suspect foods should not be reintroduced at home except under the direction of a physician. With gastrointestinal allergies such as AEG, endoscopy and biopsy after 6 to 8 weeks on an elimination diet showing resolution of pathology will confirm that the implicated foods were likely responsible for the disorder (32).

With any of these diets, specific information needs to be reviewed carefully to ensure adherence, as it is common for patients to make errors. For example, eliminating egg from someone's diet means reading labels for key words such as ovalbumin, lysozyme, and globulin. Contamination of the food being eliminated and hidden ingredients can be issues that hinder strict avoidance. Organizations such as the Food Allergy and Anaphylaxis Network (http://www.foodallergy. org) may provide assistance for patients. When multiple foods are eliminated from the diet, it may be necessary to consult the aid of a nutritionist to maintain a balanced diet.

OFCs

OFCs are performed by feeding suspected foods in gradually increasing amounts over hours or days under the supervision of a physician. OFCs can be done openly, where both the physician and the patient know the food being challenged; single-blind, where only the physican knows; or double-blind, placebo-controlled, where neither patient nor physician knows the content of the challenge. Open food challenges are best performed when it is not very likely that symptoms will develop and when there is little psychologic play that could bias results (40). The DBPCFC is considered to be the "gold standard" for the diagnosis of food allergy, and it is the least prone to bias and confounding factors (38, 40). OFCs can be used to assess any kind of adverse response to foods. When several foods are under consideration, tests for IgE are positive, and elimination resulted in resolution of symptoms, the OFCs for each food may allow expansion of the diet. For acute anaphylactic reactions in which there is no specific IgE for the suspected food found, an OFC would be indicated to safely reintroduce the food in case of a false-negative skin test or RAST. If an elimination diet did not alleviate symptoms and suspicion is still high for a food-related cause, then the OFC may be needed to resolve the issue. For those who have been previously diagnosed with an IgE-mediated food allergy, the OFC can also be used to determine whether the patients have outgrown their clinical reactivity. Finally, for non-IgE-mediated reactions, OFCs are often the only means of diagnosis (41).

To optimize challenge conditions, the suspected food should be eliminated from the diet for 1 to 2 weeks (and up to 8 to 12 weeks in some gastrointestinal disorders), potentially interfering medications should be withdrawn (antihistamines, β-agonists), symptoms of chronic diseases such as asthma and atopic dermatitis should be adequately controlled, fresh or dehydrated foods should be used, and challenge vehicles should not contain fat, which can interfere with protein absorption. The OFC should be administered in the fasting state in a graded fashion, starting with a dose that is unlikely to produce symptoms (25 to 500 mg of lyophilized food). Some physicians start with a labial food challenge as an added precaution before actual ingestion, whereby a small amount of the challenge food is placed on the lower lip for 2 min and then the patient is observed for some time; if this test is negative, then an OFC follows. In suspected IgE-mediated reactions, if there is no reaction with the starting dose, then the dose is doubled every 15 to 60 min (the interval time may need to be increased for more delayed reactions) until 8 to 10 g of dried food, 60 to 100 g of the wet food, or 100 ml of liquid has been consumed (32, 40). Once the challenge is finished, patients should generally be observed for up to 2 h. Once the patient has tolerated one of the above amounts in the challenge, then clinical reactivity has generally been ruled out, since a negative challenge has a high negative-predictive value (33). However, for blinded challenges, all negative challenges should be confirmed by an open feeding of the suspected food made in its commonly prepared state and served in normal meal-size quantities under medical supervision to exclude the rare false-negative challenge response (6).

In suspected non-IgE-mediated food allergies such as AEG and food protein-induced enterocolitis syndrome (FPIES), since there are no specific laboratory tests for these illnesses, the OFC may be the only way to identify causative foods. OFCs for FPIES may require up to 0.3 to 0.6 g of food/kg of body weight given in two doses, and patients need to be observed for 2 to 6 h for possible profuse vomiting and diarrhea (intravenous access is usually placed prior to challenge as a precaution). For AEG, patients may require several feedings over a 1- to 3-day period. In most IgE-mediated disorders, further challenges can be conducted every 1 or 2 days, or even on the same day 4 h apart for each part of the DBPCFC. Most non-IgE-mediated disorders, however, require a longer interval of 3 to 5 days between challenges (32, 40).

The decision to perform OFCs should not be taken lightly, as severe anaphylactic reactions can occur, and the challenges are time-consuming, cost-intensive, and stressful to the patient and families. To aid in making the decision of when to challenge, some information has already been presented regarding the use of SPT wheal size cutoffs and the likelihood of true allergy based upon DBPCFCs; other tools that help determine whether to challenge a patient will be mentioned when food-specific-IgE levels are discussed later in this chapter. Recent and severe anaphylaxis after an isolated ingestion with a positive test for specific IgE to the causal food is an example of a relative contraindication to challenge, as this is a convincing history and would not warrant further investigation (41). Because of the risk of anaphylaxis, the physician must be comfortable with a potential severe reaction and be prepared to treat it with emergency medications and equipment. Patients must be examined before the challenge begins, as well as frequently during the OFC for objective signs of a reaction, and challenges need to be terminated promptly when a reaction becomes apparent. As a general rule, challenges should not be done at home (41); when the skin test is negative, though, and the history of a reaction to that food is doubtful, the food may be replaced at home with a 99% expectation that the food will be tolerated (6). However, reintroduction of foods should never be done at home if there is even the slightest chance of severe symptoms developing.

As with any diagnostic test, there can be false-positive and false-negative results. From two university centers in the United States, the average false-positive rate for the DBPCFC was reported to be 0.7%, and the false-negative rate was 3.2% (33). Caffarelli and Petroccione (8) reported that 5 patients of 193 (3%) challenged by DBPCFCs had passed a DBPCFC and then reacted the next day to an open feeding of the same food at home. Occasionally, an open challenge is positive in the face of a negative blinded challenge. Several possibilities explain this phenomenon. First, the patient's threshold response may have been higher than was achieved during the blind challenge. This possibility could be tested in a blind challenge with greater amounts of food. Second, the allergenicity of the food may have been different because of the way it was prepared; this is rarely confirmed because the open consumption of the food after the blinded challenge usually eliminates the notion that cooking, digestion, and other factors may have altered the food. Third, the reaction may have been due to psychological factors (6).

IN VITRO TESTING

Quantification of Food-Specific IgE

Another way to identify food-specific IgE that is more widely available to the general practitioner is the RAST. In this type of test, the allergen in question is bound to a solid matrix and exposed to the patient's serum. If there is specific IgE for that allergen in the patient's serum, it binds to the protein matrix. After a buffer wash to remove unbound serum proteins, bound human IgE antibodies are detected with a radiolabeled anti-human IgE Fc. Different manufacturers use various substrates, and results can be reported as classes (class 1 to 5 or 6), percentages, counts, or arbitrary units of concentration (kU_A/liter) (41).

The first-generation RAST results compared with clinically diagnosed food allergy showed false-positive rates of 3 to 40% and false-negative rates of 3 to 48%, depending largely on how the diagnosis of food hypersensitivity was made and on the antigens used in the RAST (36). Much of this disparity had to do with relying on patient history in making the diagnosis, which, as stated previously, is confirmed only about 40% of the time by DBPCFCs. Using DBPCFCs and eight common food antigens, Sampson and Albergo (36) studied 40 patients with atopic dermatitis and compared SPT and Phadebas RAST results with the challenge results. They found that the sensitivities and specificities of the SPTs and RASTs were similar if a Phadebas RAST score of 3+ or higher was considered positive. RASTs are generally considered less sensitive than SPTs, but the development of the second-generation RAST, the CAP System FEIA (Pharmacia-Upjohn Diagnostics, Uppsala, Sweden), improved the allergosorbent's overall antibody-binding capacity, which led to more rapid assay kinetics and an enhanced assay sensitivity. The Pharmacia CAP System also uses standardized allergens and is calibrated against the World Health Organization IgE standard (38) (for more quality control issues, please refer to chapter 107).

The development of the CAP System allowed better quantitation of food-specific IgE antibodies (on a scale from <0.35 kU_A/liter, or negative, to the upper limit of >100 kU_A/liter), which have been shown in key studies to be more predictive of symptomatic IgE-mediated food hypersensitivity. These studies of children provided support that certain concentrations of food-specific IgE were associated with a high likelihood of reactions, or true allergy. Because sensitivity and specificity are inherent properties of a test and predictive values reflect the inherent properties of the test plus the prevalence of disease in the population under investigation, an alternative approach used in the studies mentioned below to minimize the effect of disease prevalence has been the use of the 90 or 95% specificity values to establish diagnostic decision points (34).

In a retrospective study of 196 children and adolescents (mean age, 5.2 years) with atopic dermatitis, Sampson and Ho (38) compared the levels of food-specific IgE with the results of DBPCFCs and found that concentrations of 6 kU_A/liter or greater for egg, 32 kU_A/liter or greater for cow's milk, 15 kU_A/liter or greater for peanut, and 20 kU_A/liter or greater for codfish were 95% predictive of an allergic reaction. Therefore, a patient with a food-specific-IgE level greater than the 95% PPV could be considered reactive and an OFC would not be warranted. If, however, the level of food-specific IgE was less than the 95% PPV, a patient may be reactive but would need an OFC to confirm the diagnosis. There are caveats with this study that affect its use in the general population: first, all patients had atopic dermatitis, and these patients tend to have higher IgE levels; and second, this group of patients had a much higher prevalence of food allergy than is seen in most populations. Because of these factors, Sampson performed a prospective study of 100 children (median age, 3.8 years) not selected for atopic

dermatitis (only 61% had this disorder), with similar results, except the 95% PPV cutoff was lower for milk at 15 kU_A/liter (34).

Different results were obtained in studies of younger infants and children with different clinical histories. Garcia-Ara et al. (14) showed that an even lower concentration of food-specific IgE to milk had a high predictive capability, although their study was of a much younger patient population of 170 infants (mean age, 4.8 months) without atopic dermatitis or gastrointestinal allergy. They determined the 95% PPV cutoff to be >5 kU_A/liter but recommended 2.5 kU_A/liter or greater as the cutoff to not challenge because it still had a high probability of a positive challenge (90%) without a significant reduction in sensitivity. Finally, Osterballe and Bindslev-Jensen (24) determined the 95% PPV for egg to be 1.5 kU_A/liter in a population of 56 children with atopic dermatitis and a median age of 2.2 years, while Boyano et al. (7), in a population of 81 children under 2 years of age (43% with atopic dermatitis), determined that an OFC was unnecessary to establish the diagnosis of egg allergy if the egg white-specific IgE was ≥0.35 kU_A/liter and the patient had a history of immediate hypersensitivity to egg.

The use of food-specific-IgE concentrations can also be helpful in monitoring allergen-specific IgE values on an annual basis as part of a routine follow-up of food-allergic patients to assess their ongoing sensitivity because they provide numerical values that can be monitored from an initial reference point. Moreover, food-specific-IgE values have been pivotal in determining other cutoff points below which patients should undergo OFCs because they might have lost their clinical reactivity. To define guidelines of when an IgE level is low enough to warrant challenges, Perry et al. (26) retrospectively reviewed the levels of food-specific IgE for five major foods at the time of open OFCs with the results of 604 challenges carried out in 391 patients. Challenges were performed when oral tolerance was suspected due to the lack of any reaction to the suspect food within the previous year and, for most patients, when the food-specific-IgE level was <0.35 kU_A/liter or approached one-fourth of the previously established 95% PPVs for milk, egg, and peanut or one-fourth of the 50 and 75% PPVs for soy and wheat, respectively. For analysis, patients were divided into two groups as follows, based on their reaction history: group 1, patients who clearly had a history of an allergic reaction or had previously failed a challenge to that food; and group 2, patients who were avoiding the suspect food solely on the basis of a positive test for food-specific IgE or who had an unclear history of reaction, such as worsening atopic dermatitis.

Perry et al. (26) found that when looking for a food-specific-IgE level at which 50% of patients would be expected to pass OFCs, which has been a reasonable and acceptable pass rate with both physicians and parents given the risk, expense, and time that each challenge entails, clear values were found for milk, egg, and peanut. The proposed cutoff level for milk-specific IgE was 2 kU_A/liter, below which 53% of patients passed their challenge, and for egg-specific IgE the cutoff was also 2 kU_A/liter, below which 60% of patients passed their challenge both with and without a clear history of reaction. For peanut, they recommended that patients with a clear history of reaction be challenged when the peanut-specific-IgE level is <2 kU_A/liter, whereas a cutoff level of 5 kU_A/liter should be used for those patients with no clear history of ingestion. Firm recommendations could not be provided for soy and wheat, a problem seen with results in other studies as well (34, 38). However, they generally recommended that if the level of wheat-specific IgE is <10 kU_A/liter or the level of soy-specific IgE is <5 kU$_A$/liter, challenges should be considered, although higher levels may be appropriate for some patients, depending on the clinical history.

There are several important points regarding food-specific-IgE levels that need to be mentioned. The level of food-specific IgE, like the size of the SPT, does not usefully correlate with the severity or type of reaction a patient will have, but especially high concentrations are associated with a very high likelihood of reactions occurring (34). Also, it is preferable to obtain food-specific-IgE levels instead of performing SPTs in certain clinical situations: in patients with significant dermatographism for whom there could be many false-positive tests, in patients with severe skin disease and limited area for testing, in patients who cannot discontinue taking antihistamines, and in patients with intense sensitivity to certain foods for whom SPTs could be dangerous (38).

Quantification of Food-Specific IgG

Food-specific IgG or IgG4 antibodies can be measured by immunoassay. The levels of IgG subclasses other than IgG4 rise in response to long-term exposure in both symptomatic and asymptomatic conditions (1). They are generally elevated in patients with food allergy affecting the gastrointestinal tract, but their specificities typically reflect the type of foods ingested and are not indicative of food-related pathogenesis (38). Roger et al. (29) measured egg-specific IgG4 and IgE antibodies in 104 patients and found that while IgG4 levels may be high in food-allergic patients, detection of IgG4 had little diagnostic value in childhood allergy to egg as determined by OFCs. In addition, food-specific IgG4 was a frequent finding in patients who tolerated egg. Bjorksten et al. (3), studying 47 children with cow's milk allergy, found no relationship between the presence of milk-specific IgG4 antibodies and the results of OFCs, nor was there a relationship between the presence of IgG4 and IgE antibodies against milk. Finally, Morgan et al. (19) looked at the relationship among shrimp-specific IgG subclass antibodies and results of DBPCFCs in their study with 31 patients with a history of immediate adverse reactions to shrimp and 20 control subjects who were shrimp tolerant. None of the shrimp-specific IgG subclass responses was predictive of a positive response to DBPCFC, and therefore they were not diagnostic of shrimp intolerance. In summary, food-specific IgG antibodies play no role in the diagnosis of food hypersensitivity reactions.

Total IgE

IgE concentrations in serum are highly age dependent, rising gradually through childhood until they peak between ages 10 and 15 and then steadily decline throughout adulthood. Klink et al. (17) analyzed serum IgE levels in 2,657 subjects grouped into skin test-positive or skin test-negative rhinitic, asthmatic, or asymptomatic individuals. They found that although serum IgE concentrations tend to be higher in allergic children and adults than in nonallergic individuals, the range of IgE in all groups was extremely wide. There is usually a large overlap in the ranges of IgE between atopic and nonatopic populations, resulting in no single level of IgE that clearly distinguishes the different groups at a level of precision that is clinically meaningful. This large overlap greatly limits the diagnostic sensitivity of total serum IgE as a screening test for allergy (17).

There are many conditions that can be associated with greatly elevated total IgE levels, but probably the most common and the one associated with food allergy in 30% of children is atopic dermatitis. High serum IgE levels, with a mean of 978 IU/ml (range, 1.3 to 65,208), have been observed in patients with atopic dermatitis (15). Total serum IgE levels are related to the probability of an individual having detectable allergen-specific IgE. In a large adult study population, patients with total serum IgE levels in the highest quintile (>66 IU/ml) were 37 times more likely to have one or more allergen-specific IgE antibodies (25). Because of this, patients with high IgE levels, especially those with atopic dermatitis, can have many false-positive food-specific antibodies if their total IgE level is greatly elevated, thus making the diagnosis of true food allergy in these patients more difficult. In summary, total serum IgE levels are not useful diagnostic tests for food allergy.

BHR

BHR has been proposed as an in vitro correlate to in vivo allergic responses (12). BHR as a method of diagnosing food allergy was reported by Nolte (21) to correlate well with SPTs, RASTs, and open food challenges but did not correlate with histamine release from intestinal mast cells obtained by duodenal biopsy in children. Another study by Sampson comparing BHR, SPTs, and DBPCFCs, however, showed that the BHR assay was no more effective in predicting clinical sensitivity than SPTs (38).

The clinical use of BHR is complicated by several factors. It is not a widely available test, blood needs to be processed within a certain amount of time for cells to be viable, and there are no standardized methods for performing BHR. About 8 to 20% of patients in a normal population fail to show BHR upon immunological activation of their basophils (21). Increased spontaneous release of up to 35% of the total basophil histamine associated with mononuclear cell-derived production of basophil-releasing factors has been reported for patients with atopic dermatitis and food allergy documented by DBPCFC (37), although the use of whole blood now in these assays reportedly overcomes this problem of spontaneous histamine release. Also, there are functional differences between mast cells and basophils that cause the BHR tests to be a controversial means for diagnosing food allergy. BHR assays are now used primarily in research settings.

Serum Tryptase

An increased level of serum tryptase, a neutral protease found almost exclusively in mast cells, has been found to be an excellent marker of mast cell activation in anaphylactic reactions. Basophils, the only other cell type in which tryptase has been found, contain 100 to 1,000 times less tryptase than mast cells (22). Tryptase level elevations are believed to begin at 1 h after mast cell stimulation (18), and the half-life of tryptase in the circulation is approximately 2 h (22).

An increase in serum tryptase in food-induced anaphylaxis, however, is rarely seen and therefore is not a reliable marker of food-related allergic reactions. The short half-life of serum tryptase, its quick rise in relation to onset of reaction, and the required special processing in a limited number of specialty laboratories make it even less useful as a diagnostic test for food allergy. The absence of a substantial increase in mast cell tryptase in food-induced reactions suggests that other mediators from mast cells may play a more central role or that basophils, which contain significantly less tryptase, may play a more important role in these reactions. It is also possible that other cells such as macrophages, monocytes, and endothelial cells become activated through FcεII receptors or by cytokines and mediators released early in the allergic reaction to foods (39).

Future Directions: Specific Epitope Analysis

While it has been shown that measurement of food-specific IgE concentrations in the serum and SPT wheal diameter is helpful in determining possible patient clinical reactivity, many patients still require OFCs because their food-specific-IgE levels or wheal diameters fall below the 95% PPV diagnostic decision levels or because they may have lost their clinical reactivity. Recent technological advances have enabled investigators to map allergenic epitopes of many major food allergens, including milk, egg, and peanut, and determine specifically where a patient's IgE antibodies bind to those proteins. As a result, it was discovered that conformational and sequential (or linear) epitopes might be responsible for allergic reactions. Researchers also found that individuals who possess IgE antibodies to sequential epitopes react to the allergenic food in any form, whether extensively cooked or partially hydrolyzed, while patients with IgE antibodies to conformational epitopes appear to tolerate small amounts of the food after extensive cooking or partial hydrolysis because the tertiary structure of the allergenic protein is altered and the conformational epitopes are destroyed (35).

Additionally, in several studies of egg- and milk-allergic patients (9, 16), it was shown that certain patients with IgE antibodies to sequential epitopes have a propensity to have persistent allergy, while patients with IgE antibodies primarily to conformational epitopes tend to have clinical tolerance. Therefore, screening for antibodies to those epitopes may prove useful in identifying children who will not outgrow their allergy and thus will possibly be candidates for immunotherapy when it becomes available (9). Further analysis of epitope binding in peanut-allergic patients demonstrated that there are differences in peanut allergenic epitope recognition patterns between patients with symptomatic peanut allergy and those who are sensitized but clinically tolerant. Therefore, the addition of epitope-specific IgE determinations might prove to be a more valuable tool for diagnosing symptomatic peanut allergy than quantitative IgE antibodies to the whole protein and may be particularly useful for patients with peanut-specific-IgE levels below the diagnostic decision levels (2). It has also been demonstrated that patients with peanut allergy and IgE antibodies to many epitopes, called broad epitope diversity, tend to have more severe allergic reactions than those who have IgE binding to relatively few epitopes (35). The clinical use of epitope-specific IgE antibodies as diagnostic tools requires further research.

CONCLUSIONS

The diagnosis of immunological reactions to foods must begin with a thorough history and physical, as this provides the basis for making decisions of what testing, if any, needs to be done to confirm the history. A number of valid diagnostic tools exist for diagnosing IgE-mediated food reactions, both in vivo methods such as skin testing and food challenges and in vitro methods including measurement of food-specific-IgE concentrations in serum. Both methods of testing have their advantages and limitations, depending on the clinical situation, but for non-IgE-mediated food reactions, elimination diets and OFCs may be the only means of diagnosis for this group of disorders. Tests that have not proven helpful in food allergy diagnosis include quantification of food-specific IgG, total serum IgE levels, BHR, and serum tryptase concentrations. Tests

that need further study but show some promise include the APT, which may aid in the diagnosis of non-IgE-mediated disorders and delayed reactions to foods. The identification of epitopes to which IgE binding correlates with a high risk of clinical reactions might not only prove useful in enhancing the diagnostic value of SPTs and RASTs, but also provide a means of determining the clinical course of food allergy. Regardless of the test chosen, the DBPCFC still remains the gold standard for diagnosing food allergy. Finally, important features of the studies mentioned in this chapter for the described tests that need to be appreciated by clinicians are (i) that the data generated may be particular to the study population and test material and (ii) that the age and clinical disease of the patients are important variables. Clinicians must therefore be careful in applying the results in these published studies to their own individual clinical situations.

REFERENCES

1. **AAAI Board of Directors.** 1995. Measurement of specific and nonspecific IgG$_4$ levels as diagnostic and prognostic tests for clinical allergy. *J. Allergy Clin. Immunol.* **95:**652–654.
2. **Beyer, K., L. Ellman-Grunther, K.-M. Jarvinen, R. A. Wood, J. Hourihane, and H. A. Sampson.** 2003. Measurement of peptide-specific IgE as an additional tool in identifying patients with clinical reactivity to peanuts. *J. Allergy Clin. Immunol.* **112:**202–207.
3. **Bjorksten, B., S. Ahlstedt, F. Bjorksten, B. Carlsson, S. V. Fallstrom, K. Juntunen, M. Kajosaari, and A. Kober.** 1983. Immunoglobulin E and immunoglobulin G4 antibodies to cow's milk in children with cow's milk allergy. *Allergy* **38:**119–124.
4. **Bock, S. A., and F. M. Atkins.** 1990. Patterns of food hypersensitivity during sixteen years of double-blind, placebo-controlled food challenges. *J. Pediatr.* **117:**561–567.
5. **Bock, S. A., W. Y. Lee, L. Remigio, A. Holst, and C. D. May.** 1978. Appraisal of skin tests with food extracts for diagnosis of food hypersensitivity. *Clin. Allergy* **8:**559–564.
6. **Bock, S. A., H. A. Sampson, F. A. Atkins, R. S. Zeiger, S. Lehrer, M. Sachs, R. K. Bush, and D. D. Metcalfe.** 1988. Double-blind, placebo-controlled food challenge (DBPCFC) as an office procedure: a manual. *J. Allergy Clin. Immunol.* **82:**986–997.
7. **Boyano, M. T., C. Garcia-Ara, J. M. Diaz-Pena, F. M. Munoz, S. G. Garcia, and M. M. Esteban.** 2001. Validity of specific IgE antibodies in children with egg allergy. *Clin. Exp. Allergy* **31:**1464–1469.
8. **Caffarelli, C., and T. Petroccione.** 2001. False-negative food challenges in children with suspected food allergy. *Lancet* **358:**1871–1872.
9. **Chatchatee, P., K.-M. Jarvinen, L. Bardina, K. Beyer, and H. A. Sampson.** 2001. Identification of IgE- and IgG-binding epitopes on α$_{s1}$-casein: difference in patients with persistent and transient cow's milk allergy. *J. Allergy Clin. Immunol.* **107:**379–383.
10. **De Bruin-Weller, M.S., E. F. Knol, and C. A. F. M. Bruijnzeel-Koomen.** 1999. Atopy patch testing—a diagnostic tool? *Allergy* **54:**784–791.
11. **Devenney, I., and K. Falth-Magnusson.** 2000. Skin prick tests may give generalized allergic reactions in infants. *Ann. Allergy Asthma Immunol.* **85:**457–460.
12. **Du Buske, L. M.** 1993. Introduction: basophil histamine release and the diagnosis of food allergy. *Allergy Proc.* **14:**243–249.
13. **Eigenmann, P. A., and H. A. Sampson.** 1998. Interpreting skin prick tests in the evaluation of food allergy in children. *Pediatr. Allergy Immunol.* **9:**186–191.

14. Garcia-Ara, C., M. T. Boyano, J. M. Diaz-Pena, F. Martin-Munoz, M. Reche-Frutos, and M. Martin-Esteban. 2001. Specific IgE levels in the diagnosis of immediate hypersensitivity to cow's milk protein in the infant. *J. Allergy Clin. Immunol.* **107:**185–190.

15. Hamilton, R. G. 2003. Laboratory tests for allergic and immunodeficiency disease, p. 611–630. *In* N. F. Adkinson, Jr., J. W. Yunginger, W. B. Busse, B. S. Bochner, S. T. Holgate, and F. E. R. Simons (ed.), *Middleton's Allergy: Principles & Practice*, 6th ed. Mosby, Inc., Philadelphia, Pa.

16. Jarvinen, K.-M., K. Beyer, L. Villa, P. Chatchatee, P. L. Busse, and H. A. Sampson. 2002. B-cell epitopes as a screening instrument for persistent cow's milk allergy. *J. Allergy Clin. Immunol.* **110:**293–297.

17. Klink, M., M. G. Cline, M. Halonen, and B. Burrows. 1990. Problems in defining normal limits for serum IgE. *J. Allergy Clin. Immunol.* **85:**440–444.

18. Lin, R. Y., L. B. Schwartz, A. Curry, G. R. Pesola, R. J. Knight, H. S. Lee, L. Bakalchuk, C. Tenenbaum, and R. E. Westfal. 2000. Histamine and tryptase levels in patients with acute allergic reactions: an emergency department-based study. *J. Allergy Clin. Immunol.* **106:**65–71.

19. Morgan, J. E., C. B. Daul, and S. B. Lehrer. 1990. The relationships among shrimp-specific IgG subclass antibodies and immediate adverse reactions to shrimp challenge. *J. Allergy Clin. Immunol.* **86:**387–392.

20. Niggemann, B., S. Reibel, and U. Wahn. 2000. The atopy patch (APT)—a useful tool for the diagnosis of food allergy in children with atopic dermatitis. *Allergy* **55:**281–285.

21. Nolte, H. 1993. The clinical utility of basophil histamine release. *Allergy Proc.* **14:**251–254.

22. Ohtsuka, T., S. Matsumaru, K. Uchida, M. Onobori, T. Matsumoto, K. Kuwahata, and M. Arita. 1993. Time course of plasma histamine and tryptase following food challenges in children with suspected food allergy. *Ann. Allergy* **71:**139–146.

23. Ortolani, C., M. Ispano, E. A. Pastorello, R. Ansaloni, and G. C. Magri. 1989. Comparison of results of skin prick tests (with fresh foods and commercial food extracts) and RAST in 100 patients with oral allergy syndrome. *J. Allergy Clin. Immunol.* **83:**683–690.

24. Osterballe, M., and C. Bindslev-Jensen. 2003. Threshold levels in food challenge and specific IgE in patients with egg allergy: is there a relationship? *J. Allergy Clin. Immunol.* **112:**196–201.

25. Ownby, D. R. 2003. Clinical significance of immunoglobulin E, p. 1087–1103. *In* N. F. Adkinson, Jr., J. W. Yunginger, W. B. Busse, B. S. Bochner, S. T. Holgate, and F. E. R. Simons (ed.), *Middleton's Allergy: Principles & Practice*, 6th ed. Mosby, Inc., Philadelphia, Pa.

26. Perry, T. T., E. C. Matsui, M. K. Conover-Walker, and R. A. Wood. 2004. The relationship of allergen-specific IgE levels and oral food challenge outcome. *J. Allergy Clin. Immunol.* **114:**144–149.

27. Rance, F., A. Juchet, F. Bremont, and G. Dutau. 1997. Correlations between prick skin tests using commercial extracts and fresh food, specific IgE, and food challenges. *Allergy* **52:**1031–1035.

28. Roehr, C. C., S. Reibel, M. Ziegert, C. Sommerfeld, U. Wahn, and B. Niggemann. 2001. Atopy patch tests, together with determination of specific IgE levels, reduce the need for oral food challenges in children with atopic dermatitis. *J. Allergy Clin. Immunol.* **107:**548–553.

29. Roger, A., M. Pena, J. Botey, J. L. Eseverri, and A. Marin. 1994. The value of specific IgG4 determination in childhood allergy to egg in relation to specific IgE and the provocation test. *J. Invest. Allergol. Clin. Immunol.* **4:**87–90.

30. Rosen, J. P., J. E. Selcow, L. M. Mendelson, M. P. Grodofsky, J. M. Factor, and H. A. Sampson. 1994. Skin testing with natural foods in patients suspected of having food allergies: is it a necessity? *J. Allergy Clin. Immunol.* **93:**1068–1070.

31. Sampson, H. A. 1988. Comparative study of commercial food antigen extracts for the diagnosis of food hypersensitivity. *J. Allergy Clin. Immunol.* **82:**718–726.

32. Sampson, H. A. 1999. Food allergy. Part 2. Diagnosis and management. *J. Allergy Clin. Immunol.* **103:**981–989.

33. Sampson, H. A. 2001. Use of food-challenge tests in children. *Lancet* **358:**1832–1833.

34. Sampson, H. A. 2001. Utility of food-specific IgE concentrations in predicting symptomatic food allergy. *J. Allergy Clin. Immunol.* **107:**891–896.

35. Sampson, H. A. 2004. Update in food allergy. *J. Allergy Clin. Immunol.* **113:**805–819.

36. Sampson, H. A., and R. Albergo. 1984. Comparisons of results of skin tests, RAST, and double-blind, placebo-controlled food challenges in children with atopic dermatitis. *J. Allergy Clin. Immunol.* **74:**26–33.

37. Sampson, H. A., K. R. Broadbent, and J. Bernhisel-Broadbent. 1989. Spontaneous release of histamine from basophils and histamine-releasing factor in patients with atopic dermatitis and food hypersensitivity. *N. Engl. J. Med.* **321:**228–232.

38. Sampson, H. A., and D. G. Ho. 1997. Relationship between food-specific IgE concentrations and the risk of positive food challenges in children and adolescents. *J. Allergy Clin. Immunol.* **100:**444–451.

39. Sampson, H. A., L. Mendelson, and J. P. Rosen. 1992. Fatal and near-fatal anaphylactic reactions to food in children and adolescents. *N. Engl. J. Med.* **327:**380–384.

40. Sicherer, S. H. 1999. Food allergy: when and how to perform oral food challenges. *Pediatr. Allergy Immunol.* **10:**226–234.

41. Sicherer, S. H. 2002. Food allergy. *Lancet* **360:**701–710.

42. Spergel, J. M., J. L. Beausoleil, M. Mascarenhas, and C. A. Liacouras. 2002. The use of prick skin tests and patch tests to identify causative foods in eosinophilic esophagitis. *J. Allergy Clin. Immunol.* **109:**363–368.

43. Sporik, R., D. J. Hill, and C. S. Hosking. 2000. Specificity of allergen skin testing in predicting positive open food challenges to milk, egg and peanut in children. *Clin. Exp. Allergy* **30:**1540–1546.

44. Stromberg, L. 2002. Diagnostic accuracy of the atopy patch test and the skin-prick test for the diagnosis of food allergy in young children with atopic eczema/dermatitis syndrome. *Acta Paediatr.* **91:**1044–1049.

45. Zacharisen, M. C. 2000. Allergy skin testing infants: a safe or risky procedure? *Ann. Allergy Asthma Immunol.* **85:**429–430.

Diagnosis of Hypereosinophilic Syndromes

AMY D. KLION

110

HYPEREOSINOPHILIC SYNDROMES

Whereas mild to moderate eosinophilia has been reported in as many as 0.1% of North American outpatients (5) and may be due to seasonal allergies, asthma, or other common conditions, marked eosinophilia ($>1,500/mm^3$) is relatively infrequent and should always prompt a diagnostic evaluation. The differential diagnosis of marked eosinophilia is broad and includes secondary causes of eosinophilia (Table 1), such as hypersensitivity reactions, helminth infection, and neoplastic and inflammatory disorders, as well as several disorders for which eosinophilia is thought to be the primary etiology. In many cases, a thorough diagnostic evaluation will reveal a secondary cause of the eosinophilia, and appropriate treatment can be instituted. In other instances, a well-defined, single organ-restricted, primary eosinophil disorder, such as eosinophilic esophagitis, eosinophilic fasciitis, or eosinophilia cystitis, is identified. Once secondary causes and alternative diagnoses have been excluded, however, a systemic primary eosinophil disorder should be considered. The diagnostic evaluation of this small subgroup of eosinophilic patients will be the focus of this chapter.

Historical Definition

The term hypereosinophilic syndromes (HES) was first used in 1968 by Hardy and Anderson to describe three patients with marked peripheral eosinophilia, hepatosplenomegaly, and cardiac and/or pulmonary symptoms (16). Diagnostic criteria for HES were proposed in 1975 by Chusid et al. and include idiopathic hypereosinophilia ($>1,500$ eosinophils/mm^3) of >6 months' duration with signs and symptoms of eosinophil-mediated or unexplained end organ damage (7). Whereas this definition is extremely useful as a first step in identifying patients with systemic hypereosinophilic syndromes, as more sophisticated diagnostic testing becomes available and subgroups of patients with HES of known causes are described, the "idiopathic" nature of HES has been called into question. Furthermore, the availability of effective treatment for HES often leads to the resolution of eosinophilia before the requisite 6 months have elapsed. Finally, the classification of eosinophilic syndromes of unknown cause with distinctive clinical patterns, such as episodic angioedema and eosinophilia and chronic eosinophilic pneumonia, which are not excluded by this definition, remains unresolved (see below).

Clinical Features

Using Chusid's criteria, several characteristic features of HES have been described (7, 11). Although some of these, such as the male predominance (9:1), are likely due to skewing by a single HES subtype (see below), some general conclusions can be drawn.

HES typically occurs between the ages of 20 and 50, but may present in childhood or advanced age. The clinical manifestations of HES are extremely varied, ranging from nonspecific complaints, such as fatigue, myalgias, and rhinitis, to severe end organ damage, including endomyocardial fibrosis, restrictive pulmonary disease, and neuropathy (11, 42). Furthermore, some patients may remain asymptomatic for decades despite markedly elevated eosinophil counts. Although data from a number of published case series suggest that cardiac, neurologic, and dermatologic manifestations are most common (11, 42), any organ can be affected. A description of the many and varied end organ manifestations of HES is beyond the scope of this chapter but can be found in some excellent reviews (1, 42). Notably, increased susceptibility to infection is not a feature of HES; thus, a history of recurrent infection should prompt an investigation for secondary causes of eosinophilia, including malignancy and immunodeficiencies.

Pathogenesis

Bone marrow eosinophils are increased in number in all forms of HES and may reflect a primary myeloproliferative process (as in Fip1-like 1/platelet-derived growth factor alpha (F/P)-associated HES) or a response to eosinophilopoietic cytokines produced by nonmyeloid cells. Regardless of the mechanism of increased eosinophil production, increased numbers of activated eosinophils released into the peripheral blood and tissues are thought to play a primary role in the tissue damage observed in this disorder through the local release of a variety of inflammatory mediators, including cationic proteins, leukotrienes, and cytokines.

RECENT DEFINITION OF SUBTYPES

Although it has long been appreciated that HES are a heterogeneous group of disorders (11, 40), it is only recently that advances in molecular and immunologic techniques have begun to delineate the precise pathogenesis of HES in some groups of patients. Of these defined groups, the most

TABLE 1 Secondary causes of marked eosinophilia[a]

Cause
Allergic disorders
Asthma and/or atopic disease (rare)
Allergic bronchopulmonary aspergillosis
Drug hypersensitivity reactions
Infectious diseases
Helminth infection
Ectoparasite infestations (scabies and myiasis)
Protozoal infection (rarely in isosporiasis and sarcocystis)
Fungal infection (especially coccidiomycosis)
HIV infection
Neoplasms
Leukemia, lymphoma, or adenocarcinoma
Hypoadrenalism
Diseases associated with immunodysregulation
Sarcoidosis, inflammatory bowel disease, or connective tissue disorders
Other
Cholesterol embolization, radiation exposure

[a]This list is not exhaustive.

common appear to be a clonal myeloproliferative disorder associated with the constitutive activation of platelet-derived growth factor receptor alpha (PDGFRA) (9, 15) and a lymphocytic variant characterized by the presence of a clonal population of lymphocytes (35, 39). An autosomal dominant familial form of HES mapped to chromosome 5q31-33 has also been described, although the exact nature of the molecular abnormality remains to be elucidated (24, 31). Finally, additional subgroups of HES with distinctive clinical manifestations await characterization at the molecular and immunologic levels.

Imatinib-Responsive HES

Imatinib is a tyrosine kinase inhibitor with potent activity against ABL, ARG, BCR-ABL, KIT, and PDGFRA and -B. Following the report of a clinical response to imatinib in a single patient with HES (36), several small clinical trials were initiated to explore the utility of imatinib for the treatment of HES (2, 13, 22). This led to the identification of F/P, a fusion tyrosine kinase associated with the majority of cases of imatinib-responsive HES (9, 15). Although patients with F/P-associated HES occasionally have cytogenetic abnormalities (9, 26), in the vast majority of cases the *FIP1L1-PDGFRA* fusion gene is created by a small interstitial deletion in chromosome 4, del(4)(q12q12), that is undetectable by standard cytogenetics (9, 15). The breakpoints in *FIP1L1* are variable but are typically located in a 40-kb region spanning introns 7 to 10 of *FIP1L1*. In contrast, the breakpoints in *PDGFRA* appear to be restricted to a region of exon 12 that contains the WW-like region of the juxtamembrane domain (9). Disruption of this WW-like domain has been shown to cause constitutive kinase activation in members of the PDGFR family of tyrosine kinases, including PDGFRA (17).

Clinical, hematologic, and molecular responses are rapidly achieved with imatinib treatment in the setting of the F/P mutation and appear to be sustained (23), although the long-term efficacy of this drug for the treatment of HES remains to be proven. A resistance mutation (T674I) in F/P that is homologous to the well-described T315I mutation in BCR-ABL seen in patients with imatinib-resistant chronic myelogenous leukemia has been described for a single patient with HES who relapsed during therapy (9), further confirming the etiologic role of the fusion gene in this disorder.

Imatinib-responsive patients with HES in whom the F/P mutation cannot be demonstrated have been reported in several studies (12, 41). Clinical and hematologic responses in these patients are generally slower and incomplete and require higher doses of imatinib than responses in patients with F/P-associated disease. Although molecular abnormalities have been described for a few of these patients, the basis of the response remains uncharacterized in most instances.

Lymphocytic Variant HES

Despite isolated reports of clonal populations of T cells in patients with HES as early as 1994 (6, 8), it was not until 1999 that a distinct subgroup of patients with lymphocyte-driven HES was first described (39). Hypereosinophilia in these patients appears to occur in response to the production of eosinophilopoietic cytokines, particularly interleukin 5 (IL-5), by clonal populations of phenotypically abnormal activated T lymphocytes. Although the levels of IL-5 in the serum are often normal for patients with the lymphocytic variant, an increased production of IL-5 by stimulated peripheral blood mononuclear cells and/or phenotypically abnormal T-cell populations can be demonstrated in most patients with the lymphocytic variant of HES, consistent with this hypothesis (34, 35). Other evidence of Th2 activation in patients with this variant include elevations of immunoglobulin E (IgE) and thymus and activation-regulated chemokine (TARC) in serum (10). Cytogenetic abnormalities are occasionally present in patients with the lymphocytic variant, although no consistent pattern has been delineated (34).

Familial Eosinophilia

The occurrence of marked eosinophilia in multiple members of the same family is rare, with only a few reports in the literature to date (24). Autosomal dominant transmission appears to be the most common form of transmission. In one such family, the gene responsible for the eosinophilia has been mapped to chromosome 5q31-33 (31). Despite marked eosinophilia (2,000 to 6,000/mm³) from birth, a minority of family members with familial eosinophilia develop eosinophil-mediated end organ damage (21). This paucity of clinical manifestations is associated with a relative lack of eosinophil activation compared to that in patients with non-familial HES. Whether the sudden disease progression in a small number of these patients after a lifetime of asymptomatic eosinophilia represents a second mutation remains unknown at this time.

Other

Several other HES of unknown etiology have distinctive clinical patterns that appear to set them apart. One of the most intriguing of these is episodic angioedema and eosinophilia (Gleich's syndrome) (14). Gleich's syndrome is characterized by episodic, but pronounced, eosinophilia and angioedema. In most cases, the episodes occur monthly and last for 7 to 11 days. Cyclical increases in eosinophilopoietic cytokines, most often IL-5, can be demonstrated preceding the rise in peripheral eosinophil counts (14). Although some patients with this syndrome ultimately progress to HES and/or develop clonal populations of lymphocytes (25), the unique clinical presentation is suggestive of a common and distinct etiology for this clinical subgroup of patients.

A second, less well-defined clinical subgroup of patients presents with marked eosinophilia and clinical features highly suggestive of Churg-Strauss syndrome, including a long history of asthma, paranasal sinus abnormalities, and recurrent pulmonary infiltrates, without demonstrable vasculitis. Although some of these patients likely have occult Churg-Strauss vasculitis, in some cases biopsies of affected tissues repeatedly fail to show evidence of vasculitis, and antineutrophil cytoplasmic antibodies are undetectable in serum. The pathologic basis of end organ damage in this subgroup of patients remains to be elucidated.

Primary eosinophilic disorders affecting a single organ, such as eosinophilic gastroenteritis, eosinophilic fasciitis, and chronic eosinophilic pneumonia, may be associated with peripheral eosinophilia of >1,500/mm^3. When this occurs, it can be difficult to determine whether the patient has HES with single organ involvement or a distinct primary eosinophilic disorder. A more useful classification system for these patients awaits advances in our understanding of the etiology of single-organ-restricted disease, particularly the mechanisms of eosinophil homing to specific sites, such as the gastrointestinal tract and the lungs.

IMPORTANCE OF SUBTYPES

Subtype identification has profound implications for the patient with respect to the clinical manifestations, prognosis, and treatment of HES. This is best illustrated by the differences between F/P-associated HES and the lymphocytic variant (see below).

Clinical Manifestations

Current data suggest that 10 to 20% of HES cases that meet Chusid et al.'s classic definition have F/P-associated disease (27). Most of these cases belong to a distinct clinical subgroup characterized by extreme male predominance, pathologic evidence of eosinophil-related tissue damage and tissue fibrosis, elevated serum tryptase levels, splenomegaly, anemia, thrombocytopenia, and bone marrow hypercellularity with reticulin fibrosis and increased atypical mast cells (see below) (22). Interestingly, some clinical manifestations, such as endomyocardial fibrosis, restrictive lung disease, and mucosal ulcerations, appear to occur predominantly, if not exclusively, in patients with F/P-associated disease. Leukemic transformation is rare, but it does occur in this subgroup (12, 41).

The F/P mutation has also been described for a subset of eosinophilic patients presenting with clinical features of systemic mastocytosis that are indistinguishable from those of c-kit mutation-driven systemic mast cell disease (27). It is extremely important to distinguish these patients from those with c-kit mutation-driven disease, as 816V, the most common c-kit mutation associated with systemic mastocytosis, is resistant to imatinib.

Interestingly, the clinical presentation of patients with symptomatic familial eosinophilia shares many features with F/P-associated HES, with the exception of male predominance. Endomyocardial fibrosis and neurologic involvement are the most common clinical manifestations, and the response to conventional therapies, including steroids, alpha interferon, and hydroxyurea, is limited. Data on the presence of the F/P mutation and/or imatinib responsiveness are not available at this time. The clinical manifestations of patients with HES and features of myeloproliferative disease, but no evidence of the F/P mutation, have not been systematically examined.

The lymphocytic variant of HES appears to be equally distributed between men and women. Although the clinical manifestations of this subgroup of patients can be extremely varied, tissue fibrosis, including endomyocardial fibrosis, is uncommon. In addition, patients with the lymphocytic variant of HES share several clinical characteristics, the most striking of which is the predominance of dermatologic manifestations, including pruritus, urticaria, angioedema, and erythroderma (34). Gastrointestinal symptoms and obstructive pulmonary disease are also extremely common. Many patients have a history of atopic disease, and elevated IgE and IgG levels are common, but not restricted, to this subgroup of patients with HES. The prevalence of this subtype of HES is unknown, since the largest series reported in the literature to date recruited patients predominantly from dermatology clinics.

Prognosis

The prognosis of HES varies considerably depending on the underlying cause and is poorest for patients with the *FIP1L1/PDGFRA* fusion (22, 41). The dismal survival rates reported in the literature (29) likely reflect the high morbidity and mortality from cardiac and neurologic complications in this subgroup. Although imatinib treatment results in dramatic improvement in most of the clinical manifestations of F/P-associated HES, cardiac involvement appears to be relatively refractory to treatment (23). A report of the reversal of cardiac abnormalities with imatinib treatment in a single patient with the F/P mutation and recent-onset cardiac involvement underscores the importance of early identification of patients with F/P-associated disease (33).

In contrast to F/P-associated HES, severe end organ damage is uncommon in the lymphocytic variant of HES (39). Despite the relatively low mortality rate for this subgroup, the morbidity, due both to the underlying disease and to secondary effects of treatment, is significant. Furthermore, progression to T-cell lymphoma appears to be most common in this subgroup of patients and should be suspected in the setting of increasing numbers of aberrant T cells and/or the development of lymphadenopathy (34, 35). Two features that appear to be associated with an increased likelihood of progression to lymphoma are the CD3$^-$ CD4$^+$ surface phenotype and the presence of cytogenetic abnormalities.

Therapy

Finally, and perhaps most importantly, the identification of the HES subtype has profound implications for therapy. Whereas conventional first-line therapy for HES in most patients should continue to be steroids, patients with F/P-associated HES are typically resistant to steroids and should receive targeted therapy with imatinib mesylate. Although imatinib resistance has been reported in several patients with a documented F/P fusion (9), the incidence of resistance remains extremely low. The utility of imatinib therapy in patients without the F/P mutation remains to be determined, although some patients have demonstrated a response. It should be noted that imatinib therapy is not without risk, as life-threatening complications have occurred in patients with eosinophilic cardiac disease (30, 32). Troponin levels in serum have been proposed as a pretreatment marker for the development of this complication (30).

Imatinib does not appear to be useful for treating patients with the lymphocytic variant of HES (26) and should not be used as first-line therapy for these patients. Historically, steroids have been used successfully in the majority of cases to control clinical symptoms, and significant decreases in clonal populations in response to steroid therapy have been described (35). In patients with steroid-refractory disease or who are intolerant of the side effects of steroid treatment, a number of immunomodulatory agents with effects on Th2 cytokine production and T-cell proliferation, including alpha interferon, cyclosporine, and intravenous immunoglobulin, have been shown to have a therapeutic effect. Although stable responses have been achieved with relatively low doses of alpha interferon over prolonged periods of time, in vitro data demonstrating an inhibition of apoptosis of clonal $CD3^-$ $CD4^+$ T cells (37) suggest that interferon monotherapy should be avoided for this subgroup of patients (34). New agents, such as antibody to IL-5, that directly target eosinophilipoietic cytokines remain to be assessed.

DIAGNOSTIC ALGORITHM

The first step in the diagnosis of HES is to exclude other disorders associated with marked peripheral eosinophilia. These include parasitic infections, drug hypersensitivity reactions, neoplasms, and immunodysregulatory disorders associated with secondary eosinophilia (Table 1). Once it is established that the patient has eosinophilia of >1,500/mm^3 of unknown cause, it is important to determine if the patient has one of the identifiable subtypes of HES, as these have prognostic and therapeutic implications as discussed above (Table 2).

Exclusion of Other Disorders

It is beyond the scope of this chapter to provide a comprehensive diagnostic approach to eosinophil-associated disorders. Nevertheless, several general principles apply.

TABLE 2 Evaluation of patients with presumed HES

Test or measurement
Complete blood count with differential[a]
Bone marrow aspirate and biopsy (with staining for reticulin and tryptase)
Conventional cytogenetics
Assessment of end organ pathology
Echocardiogram
Pulmonary function tests
Skin or gastrointestinal biopsies, if indicated
Chest and abdomen computed tomography scan
Subtype differentiation: myeloproliferative disease
Examination of peripheral smear for myeloid precursors or dysplasia
Tryptase level in serum
Vitamin B$_{12}$ level in serum
Testing for *FIP1L1/PDGFRA* fusion (by RT-PCR or FISH)
Subtype differentiation: lymphoproliferative disease
Serum immunoglobulins, including IgE
Lymphocyte phenotyping[b]
TCR and B-cell-receptor gene rearrangement analysis
TARC level in serum
Assessment of T-cell cytokine profile, if reliable assays are available

[a]This should be performed every 3 days for 1 month in the absence of steroid treatment (if possible) for patients presenting with angioedema to exclude episodic angioedema and eosinophilia.

[b]Antibodies specific for the following additional markers should be included if routine phenotyping is normal and the lymphocytic variant is suspected: CD2, CD5, CD6, CD7, CD8, CD25, CD27, CD45RO, TCRα/β, TCRγ/δ, HLA-DR, and CD95.

First, a thorough clinical history and physical examination is essential and should include a detailed travel history, medication and dietary history (including the use of dietary and herbal supplements), past medical history (including risk factors for human immunodeficiency virus [HIV] infections), and family history. It should be noted that HES occurs in countries where helminth infections are common, and some helminth infections associated with marked eosinophilia, including strongyloidiasis, occur worldwide. Second, whenever possible, all medications and supplements should be discontinued for a minimum of 1 month (or longer, depending on the half-life of the particular agent). Finally, if routine laboratory results (including HIV testing) and diagnostic testing do not lead to an alternative diagnosis, computed tomography of the chest, abdomen, and pelvis, as well as a bone marrow examination, should be performed in all patients to exclude occult malignancy before a diagnosis of HES is confirmed.

Hematologic malignancies that may present with marked eosinophilia include T-cell lymphoma, chronic myelomonocytic leukemia, and pre-B-cell acute lymphocytic leukemia. If a bone marrow aspirate is not possible due to myelofibrosis or other reasons, lymphocyte clonality should be assessed by PCR analysis of T-cell receptor (TCR) and immunoglobulin heavy chain gene usage, as the diagnosis may be obscured upon biopsy by the presence of markedly increased numbers of eosinophils and eosinophil precursors (32). Chronic eosinophilic leukemia (CEL), defined by the World Health Organization as HES with evidence of clonality on the basis of chromosome abnormalities or X-inactivation studies (4), represents a special situation for several reasons. First, although the presence of F/P is indicative of eosinophil clonality (and thus of CEL), in most cases it is not detectable by standard cytogenetic analysis. Since the clinical presentation of HES with clonal eosinophilia overlaps with other forms of HES, it seems arbitrary to call those cases for which testing for F/P is available and positive CEL and to call the rest HES. Second, F/P is the causative mutation in some, but not all, cases of HES in which clonal eosinophilia can be demonstrated (41). For the purposes of this chapter, therefore, HES with the F/P mutation is referred to as F/P-associated HES rather than CEL.

Subtype Identification

The "gold standard" for the diagnosis of F/P-associated HES is detection of the fusion tyrosine kinase by nested reverse transcription-PCR (RT-PCR) or fluorescence in situ hybridization (FISH). If these tests are not available, a number of clinical and laboratory features may be helpful in identifying the patients most likely to have imatinib-responsive HES. Notably, some clinical manifestations, such as mucosal ulcerations, appear to occur exclusively in patients with F/P-associated HES. Since patients with familial eosinophilia may present with clinical features indistinguishable from those of F/P-associated HES, it is important to elicit a family history of eosinophilia from all patients with suspected HES.

The identification of a population of phenotypically abnormal circulating lymphocytes by flow cytometry is considered the hallmark of the lymphocytic variant of HES. In the majority of cases, T-cell clonality can also be demonstrated by an analysis of TCR rearrangement patterns. Although one or both of these features may be considered sufficient to make a diagnosis of the lymphocytic variant of HES for the purposes of clinical management, it is important to recognize that neither clonality nor an abnormal surface phenotype is synonymous with an increased secretion of eosinophilopoietic cytokines, the pathologic basis for this subtype of HES.

For patients whose primary complaint is swelling and/or weight gain, it is useful to measure eosinophil counts every 3 days for several weeks off therapy in order to identify episodic angioedema and eosinophilia. Often, the periodicity is missed because of intermittent steroid use and the measurement of eosinophil counts only when symptoms are present. Clonal T-cell populations have been described for this subgroup of patients and should be assessed by flow cytometry and TCR rearrangement analysis.

In general, IL-5 levels in serum are not useful for the differentiation between primary and secondary disorders of eosinophilia or between the various HES subtypes. Furthermore, they do not appear to predict a therapeutic response to imatinib mesylate (22), or interestingly, to anti-IL-5 antibody therapy (20).

SPECIALIZED DIAGNOSTIC TESTS

Myeloproliferative HES

The F/P fusion can be detected in peripheral blood or bone marrow mononuclear cells by using either nested RT-PCR or FISH. Although published data to date suggest that these methods have comparable sensitivities for the detection of the *FIP1L1/PDGFRA* fusion gene (41), FISH has the theoretical advantage of being able to detect cases with variant *FIP1L1* breakpoints, translocations, or alternative *PDGFRA* fusion partners that appear negative by nested RT-PCR. On the other hand, FISH is more technically challenging, and the high autofluorescence of eosinophil granules makes an exact quantification of the number of positive cells difficult. If neither of these tests is available, surrogate markers for F/P-associated HES can be used, as described below.

Nested RT-PCR for *FIP1L1/PDGFRA*

Following total RNA isolation from peripheral blood mononuclear cells by standard methods, first-strand cDNA is synthesized from 2 μg of total RNA by the use of random hexamer primers. The fusion of *FIP1L1* to *PDGFRA* is detected by nested PCR. The first PCR amplifies 2 μl of cDNA in a 50-μl reaction mix; using primers FIP1L1-F1 (5′-ACCTGGTGCTGATCTTTCTGAT) and PDGFRA-R1 (5′-TGAGAGCTTGTTTTTCACTGGA) and the following cycle conditions: 3 min at 95°C followed by 35 cycles of 95°C for 30 s, 58°C for 30 s, and 72°C for 1 min and a final extension at 72°C for 4 min. The product is then diluted 1/100, and 1 μl is used in a second PCR with primers FIP1L1-F2 (5′-AAAGAGGATACGAATGGGACTTG) and PDGFRA-R2 (5′-GGGACCGGCTTAATCCATAG) and the same cycle conditions. Multiple bands are often present upon gel electrophoresis and represent splice variants (9, 22). The EOL-1 cell line (ACC386; available from the Deutsche Sammlung von Mikroorganismen und Zellkulturen [http://www.dsmz.de]) has been shown to possess the F/P mutation (15) and is useful as a positive control. RT-PCR for a housekeeping gene, such as the glyceraldehyde-3-phosphate dehydrogenase gene, should also be performed as a control for the amount and quality of the RNA template.

FISH

Slides for FISH are prepared by standard methods. BAC clones 120K16 (mapped centromeric of *FIP1L1*), 3H20 (mapped between *FIP1L1* and *PDGFRA*), and 24O10 (mapped telomeric of *PDGFRA*), can be obtained from the RPCI11 Roswell Park Cancer Institute library (http://www.chori.org/BACPAC) for three-color labeling by nick translation. Following hybridization, interphase nuclei are examined for the presence or absence of the 3H20 signal, which is lost as a result of the interstitial deletion in cells with the *FIP1L1/PDGFRA* fusion gene (9).

One-color FISH with a probe for the cysteine-rich hydrophobic domain 2 (*CHIC2*) locus situated between *FIP1L1* and *PDGFRA* on chromosome 4q has been suggested as a surrogate for detection of the fusion gene to identify patients with the F/P fusion gene (28). Although it is less cumbersome, this method is not useful for the detection of F/P fusion genes in which there is a translocation. A two-color modification of this approach has recently been reported by the same authors (27) and appears to be comparable to the three-color strategy outlined above.

Other (Bone Marrow Features and Level of Tryptase in Serum)

In addition to the assays described above, several clinical and laboratory features are supportive of a diagnosis of F/P-positive HES (22) and may serve as surrogates if formal testing for the mutation is not available. These include male gender, elevated tryptase levels in serum, splenomegaly, clinical evidence of fibrotic end organ involvement, bone marrow features of myeloproliferative disease (including hypercellularity and reticulin fibrosis), increased and spindle-shaped bone marrow mast cells, anemia, thrombocytopenia, and elevated vitamin B_{12} levels in serum. Although none of these features is by itself diagnostic of the *FIP1L1/PDGFRA* fusion gene, the presence of an elevated tryptase level in serum and four or more of the above clinical features has correlated with the presence of the fusion gene in all of the patients evaluated at our center to date. Measurements of tryptase levels in serum are performed by several commercial laboratories. Enzyme-linked immunosorbent assay (ELISA) kits are also available from a number of sources.

Lymphoproliferative HES

The diagnosis of the lymphocytic variant of HES is based on the identification of a clonal population of phenotypically abnormal T cells in the peripheral blood by flow cytometry (see chapter 18, this volume). The sensitivity of this assay depends to a large degree on the number of antibodies used and the ability of the laboratory to detect subtle changes in the surface phenotype. Although T-cell clonality is not always present in cases with a demonstrable population of aberrant lymphocytes and is not essential for the diagnosis of the lymphocytic variant, identification of a clonal population of T cells by TCR rearrangement analysis is strongly supportive of this diagnosis. Other diagnostic tests that may be helpful in establishing the diagnosis include the measurement of TARC levels in serum and the assessment of the lymphocyte production of eosinophilopoietic cytokines.

Lymphocyte Phenotype

Although the most common aberrant phenotype of the lymphocytic variant of HES appears to be $CD3^- CD4^+$, several other surface phenotypes have been described, including $CD3^+ CD4^- CD8^-$ and $CD2^- CD3^+$ (39). In many cases, the aberrant population may be identifiable only by markers that are not included in routine panels (such as CD5, CD6, CD7, CD27, and CD95) or by slight alterations in staining intensity. Therefore, if the lymphocytic variant is suspected and routine lymphocyte phenotyping is normal, surface staining for additional markers, including CD5, CD6, CD7, and CD27, should be considered. Activation markers, such as CD25 and HLA-DR, are commonly increased on the surfaces of aberrant T cells, providing additional markers.

Other (TCR Rearrangement Analysis, Measurement of TARC Levels, and Cytokine Assays)

T-cell clonality can be assessed in peripheral blood or bone marrow samples by PCR evaluation of TCR usage and has been reported to be present in approximately 75% of patients with the lymphocytic variant of HES, as defined by flow cytometry. When present, the demonstration of clonality may be helpful, although false-negative results may occur when the clonal population is very small or involves clonal deletion of TCR chain genes (35). In addition, restricted (or oligoclonal) patterns of TCR usage are common in all forms of HES, necessitating a very strict interpretation of banding results.

TARC is a CC chemokine thought to be involved in Th2-mediated immune responses. TARC levels in serum can be measured reliably by using several commercially available ELISA kits and are markedly elevated (>1,000 pg/ml) in patients with lymphocytic HES (10). TARC levels in serum are also markedly elevated in patients with cutaneous T-cell lymphoma (18), a disorder that may overlap with HES in clinical presentation, and rarely in patients with atopic dermatitis (38) or helminth infection (19). Thus, although TARC levels in serum may be a useful surrogate marker for T-cell clonality in HES, the presence of elevated levels should not replace a thorough diagnostic evaluation.

The ultimate proof of lymphocyte-driven HES is the documentation of an increased production of eosinophilopoietic cytokines by circulating lymphocytes. Enhanced levels of IL-3, IL-5, and/or granulocyte-macrophage colony-stimulating factor have been detected by ELISA in supernatants from in vitro cultures of peripheral blood mononuclear cells or purified T cells from patients with the lymphocytic variant of HES (35, 39). Increased percentages of lymphocytes positive for eosinophilopoietic cytokines have also been demonstrated by intracellular flow cytometry in these patients. Although these assays are not routinely available in clinical laboratories at this time, they may be helpful, particularly in situations where an abnormal surface phenotype is not detected by more standard methods.

CONTROVERSIES

Several controversies currently exist surrounding the diagnosis of HES and its classification into subtypes. These include (i) the classification of patients with marked eosinophilia and no evidence of end organ damage, (ii) the distinction between HES and other organ-specific eosinophilic disorders of unknown etiology (e.g., eosinophilic gastroenteritis or chronic eosinophilic pneumonia) in patients with concomitant peripheral eosinophilia, and (iii) the diagnostic classification of patients with the *FIP1L1/PDGFRA* fusion gene (chronic eosinophilic leukemia versus myeloproliferative HES versus systemic mastocytosis with eosinophilia) (3). As the number of chemotherapeutic agents with specific molecular and immunologic targets continues to grow, the resolution of these issues will become increasingly important for the appropriate management of patients with primary eosinophilic disorders.

REFERENCES

1. Assa'ad, A. H., R. L. Spicer, D. P. Nelson, N. Zimmerman, and M. E. Rothenberg. 2000. Hypereosinophilic syndromes. *Chem. Immunol.* **76:**208–229.
2. Ault, P., J. Cortes, C. Coller, E. S. Kaled, and H. Kantarjian. 2002. Response of idiopathic hypereosinophilic syndrome to treatment with imatinib mesylate. *Leuk. Res.* **26:**881–884.
3. Bain, B. 2004. Eosinophilic leukemia and idiopathic hypereosinophilic syndrome are mutually exclusive diagnoses. *Blood* **104:**3836.
4. Bain, B., R. Pierre, M. Imbert, J. W. Vardiman, R. D. Brunning, and G. Flandrin. 2001. Chronic eosinophilic leukemia and the hypereosinophilic syndrome, p. 29–31. *In* E. S. Jaffe, N. L. Harris, H. Stein, and J. W. Vardiman (ed.), *World Health Organization Classification of Tumors: Pathology and Genetics of Tumors of Haematopoietic and Lymphoid Tissues.* IARC Press, Lyon, France.
5. Brigden, M., and C. Graydon. 1997. Eosinophilia detected by automated blood cell counting in ambulatory North American outpatients. Incidence and clinical significance. *Arch. Pathol. Lab. Med.* **121:**963–967.
6. Brugnoni, D., P. Airò, G. Rossi, A. Bettinardi, H. U. Simon, L. Garza, C. Tosoni, R. Cattaneo, K. Blaser, and A. Tucci. 1996. A case of hypereosinophilic syndrome is associated with the expansion of a CD3−CD4+ T-cell population able to secrete large amounts of interleukin-5. *Blood* **87:**1416–1422.
7. Chusid, M. J., D. C. Dale, B. C. West, and S. M. Wolff. 1975. The hypereosinophilic syndrome: analysis of fourteen cases with review of the literature. *Medicine* **54:**1–27.
8. Cogan, E., L. Schandene, A. Crusiaux, P. Cochaux, T. Velu, and M. Goldman. 1994. Brief report: clonal proliferation of type 2 helper T cells in a man with the hypereosinophilic syndrome. *N. Engl. J. Med.* **330:**535–538.
9. Cools, J., D. J. DeAngelo, J. Gotlib, E. H. Stover, R. D. Legare, J. Cortes, J. Kutok, J. Clark, I. Galinski, J. D. Griffin, N. C. P. Cross, A. Tefferi, J. Malone, R. Alam, S. L. Shrier, J. Schmid, M. Rose, P. Vandenberghe, G. Verhoef, M. Boogaerts, I. Wlodarska, H. Kantarjian, P. Marynen, S. Coutre, R. Stone, and D. G. Gilliland. 2003. A tyrosine kinase created by the fusion of the PDGFRA and FIP1L1 genes as a therapeutic target of imatinib in idiopathic hypereosinophilic syndrome. *N. Engl. J. Med.* **348:**1201–1214.
10. de Lavareille, A., F. Roufosse, P. Schmid-Grendelmeier, A. Roumier, L. Schandené, E. Cogan, and H. Simon. 2002. High serum thymus and activation-regulated chemokine levels in the lymphocytic variant of the hypereosinophilic syndrome. *J. Allergy Clin. Immunol.* **110:**476–479.
11. Fauci, A. S., J. B. Harley, W. C. Roberts, V. J. Ferrans, H. R. Gralnick, and B. H. Bjornson. 1982. The idiopathic hypereosinophilic syndrome. Clinical, pathophysiologic, and therapeutic considerations. *Ann. Intern. Med.* **97:**78–92.
12. Gilliland, G., J. Cools, E. H. Stover, I. Wlodarska, and P. Marynen. 2004. FIP1L1-PDGFRa in hypereosinophilic syndrome and mastocytosis. *Hematol. J.* **5:**S133–S137.
13. Gleich, G. J., K. M. Leiferman, and A. Pardanani. 2002. Treatment of hypereosinophilic syndrome with imatinib mesilate. *Lancet* **359:**1577–1578.
14. Gleich, G. J., A. L. Schroeter, J. P. Marcoux, M. I. Sachs, E. J. O'Connell, and P. F. Kohler. 1984. Episodic angioedema associated with eosinophilia. *N. Engl. J. Med.* **310:**1621–1626.
15. Griffin, J. H., J. Leung, R. J. Bruner, M. A. Caligiuri, and R. Briesewitz. 2003. Discovery of a fusion kinase in EOL-1 cells and idiopathic hypereosinophilic syndrome. *Proc. Natl. Acad. Sci. USA* **100:**7830–7835.

16. **Hardy, W. R., and R. E. Anderson.** 1968. The hypereosinophilic syndromes. *Ann. Intern. Med.* **68:**1220–1229.

17. **Irusta, P. M., and D. DiMaio.** 1998. A single amino acid substitution in a WW-like domain of diverse members of the PDGF receptor subfamily of tyrosine kinases causes constitutive receptor activation. *EMBO J.* **17:**6912–6923.

18. **Kakinuma, T., M. Sugaya, K. Nakamura, F. Kaneko, M. Wakugawa, K. Matsushima, and K. Tamaki.** 2003. Thymus and activation-regulated chemokine (TARC/CCL17) in mycosis fungoides: serum TARC levels reflect the disease activity of mycosis fungoides. *J. Am. Acad. Dermatol.* **48:**23–30.

19. **Katoh, S., N. Matsumoto, K. Matsumoto, M. Tokojima, J. Ashitani, F. Nakamura-Uchiyama, K. Matsushima, S. Matsukura, and Y. Nawa.** 2004. A possible role of TARC in antigen-specific Th2-dominant responses in patients with paragonimiasis westermani. *Int. Arch. Allergy Immunol.* **134:**248–252.

20. **Klion, A. D., M. A. Law, P. Noel, Y. Kim, T. P. Haverty, and T. B. Nutman.** 2004. Safety and efficacy of the monoclonal anti-interleukin-5 antibody SCH55700 in the treatment of patients with hypereosinophilic syndrome. *Blood* **103:**2939–2941.

21. **Klion, A. D., M. A. Law, W. Riemenschneider, M. L. McMaster, M. R. Brown, M. Horne, B. Karp, M. Robinson, V. Sachdev, E. Tucker, M. Turner, and T. B. Nutman.** 2004. Familial eosinophilia: a benign disorder? *Blood* **103:**4040–4055.

22. **Klion, A. D., P. Noel, C. Akin, J. Cools, M. A. Law, G. Gilliland, D. D. Metcalfe, and T. B. Nutman.** 2003. Elevated serum tryptase levels identify a subset of patients with a myeloproliferative variant of idiopathic hypereosinophilic syndrome associated with tissue fibrosis and poor prognosis. *Blood* **101:**4660–4665.

23. **Klion, A. D., J. Robyn, C. Akin, P. Noel, M. Brown, M. A. Law, D. D. Metcalfe, C. Dunbar, and T. B. Nutman.** 2003. Molecular remission and reversal of myelofibrosis in response to imatinib mesylate treatment in patients with the myeloproliferative variant of hypereosinophilic syndrome. *Blood* **103:**473–478.

24. **Lin, A. Y., T. B. Nutman, D. Kaslow, J. J. Mulvihill, L. Fontaine, B. J. White, T. Knutsen, K. S. Theil, P. K. Raghuprasad, A. M. Goldstein, and M. A. Tucker.** 1998. Familial eosinophilia: clinical and laboratory results of a U.S. kindred. *Am. J. Med. Genet.* **76:**229–237.

25. **Morgan, S. J., H. M. Prince, D. A. Westerman, C. McCormack, and I. Glaspole.** 2003. Clonal T-helper lymphocytes and elevated IL-5 levels in episodic angioedema and eosinophilia (Gleich's syndrome). *Leuk. Lymphoma* **4:**1623–1625.

26. **Musto, P., G. Perla, M. M. Minervini, and A. M. Carella.** 2004. Imatinib-mesylate for all patients with hypereosinophilic syndrome? *Leuk. Res.* **28:**773–774.

27. **Pardanani, A., S. R. Brockman, S. F. Paternoster, H. C. Flynn, R. P. Ketterling, T. L. Lasho, C. Ho, C. Li, G. W. Dewald, and A. Tefferi.** 2004. FIP1L1-PDGFRA fusion: prevalence and clinicopathologic correlates in 89 consecutive patients with moderate to severe eosinophilia. *Blood* **104:**3038–3045.

28. **Pardanani, A., R. P. Ketterling, S. R. Brockman, H. C. Flynn, S. F. Paternoster, B. M. Shearer, T. L. Reeder, C. Li, J. Cools, D. G. Gilliland, G. W. Dewald, and A. Tefferi.** 2003. CHIC2 deletion, a surrogate for *FIP1L1-PDGFRA* fusion, occurs in systemic mastocytosis associated with eosinophilia and predicts response to imatinib therapy. *Blood* **102:**3093–3096.

29. **Parrillo, J. E., A. S. Fauci, and S. M. Wolff.** 1978. Therapy of the hypereosinophilic syndrome. *Ann Intern Med.* **89:**167–172.

30. **Pitini, V., C. Arrigo, D. Azzarello, G. La Gattuta, C. Amata, M. Righi, and S. Coglitore.** 2003. Serum concentration of cardiac troponin T in patients with hypereosinophilic syndrome treated with imatinib is predictive of adverse outcomes. *Blood* **102:**3456–3457.

31. **Rioux, J. D., V. A. Stone, M. J. Daly, M. Cargill, T. Green, H. Nguyen, T. Nutman, P. A. Zimmerman, M. A. Tucker, T. Hudson, A. M. Goldstein, E. Lander, and A. Y. Lin.** 1998. Familial eosinophilia maps to the cytokine gene cluster on human chromosomal region 5q31-q33. *Am. J. Hum. Genet.* **63:**1086–1094.

32. **Robyn, J., P. Noel, I. Wlodarska, M. Choksi, P. O'Neal, D. Arthur, C. Dunbar, T. Nutman, and A. Klion.** 2004. Imatinib-responsive hypereosinophilia in a patient with B cell ALL. *Leuk. Lymphoma* **45:**2497–2501.

33. **Rotoli, B., L. Catalano, M. Galderisi, L. Luciano, G. Pollio, A. Guerriero, A. D'Errico, C. Mecucci, R. La Starza, F. Frigeri, R. Di Francia, and A. Pinto.** 2004. Rapid reversion of Loeffler's endocarditis by imatinib in early stage clonal hypereosinophilic syndrome. *Leuk. Lymphoma* **45:**2503–2507.

34. **Roufosse, F., E. Cogan, and M. Goldman.** 2004. Recent advances in the pathogenesis and management of hypereosinophilic syndromes. *Allergy* **59:**673–689.

35. **Roufosse, F., L. Schandene, C. Sibille, K. Willard-Gallo, B. Kennes, A. Efira, M. Goldman, and E. Cogan.** 2000. Clonal Th2 lymphocytes in patients with the idiopathic hypereosinophilic syndrome. *Br. J. Haematol.* **109:**540–548.

36. **Schaller, J. L., and G. A. Burkland.** 2001. Case report: rapid and complete control of idiopathic hypereosinophilia with imatinib mesylate. *Med. Gen. Med.* **3:**9.

37. **Schandene, L., F. Roufosse, A. de Lavareille, P. Stordeur, A. Efira, B. Kennes, E. Cogan, and M. Goldman.** 2000. Interferon alpha prevents spontaneous apoptosis of clonal Th2 cells associated with chronic hypereosinophilia. *Blood* **96:**4285–4292.

38. **Shimada, Y., K. Takehara, and S. Sato.** 2004. Both Th2 and Th1 chemokines (TARC/CCL17, MDC/CCL22, and Mig/CXCL9) are elevated in sera from patients with atopic dermatitis. *J. Dermatol. Sci.* **34:**201–208.

39. **Simon, H. U., S. G. Plotz, R. Dummer, and K. Blaser.** 1999. Abnormal clones of T cells producing interleukin-5 in idiopathic eosinophilia. *N. Engl. J. Med.* **341:**1112–1120.

40. **Spry, C. J., J. Davies, P. C. Tai, E. G. Olsen, C. M. Oakley, and J. F. Goodwin.** 1983. Clinical features of fifteen patients with the hypereosinophilic syndrome. *Q. J. Med.* **52:**1–22.

41. **Vandenberghe, P., I. Wlodarska, L. Michaux, P. Zachee, M. Boogaerts, D. Vanstraelen, M. C. Herregods, A. Van Hoof, D. Selleslag, F. Roufosse, M. Maerevoet, G. Verhoef, J. Cools, D. G. Gilliland, A. Hagemeijer, and P. Marynen.** 2004. Clinical and molecular features of FIP1L1-PDGFRA(+) chronic eosinophilic leukemias. *Leukemia* **18:**734–742.

42. **Weller, P. F., and G. J. Bubley.** 1994. The idiopathic hypereosinophilic syndrome. *Blood* **83:**2759–2779.

SYSTEMIC AUTOIMMUNE DISEASES

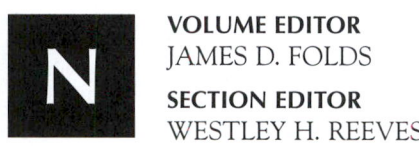

VOLUME EDITOR
JAMES D. FOLDS

SECTION EDITOR
WESTLEY H. REEVES

Introduction

WESTLEY H. REEVES

111

Systemic autoimmune diseases are often associated with the production of autoantibodies that recognize a diverse array of cytoplasmic and nuclear antigens. These autoantibodies are used as adjuncts in the diagnosis of autoimmune disease, for monitoring disease activity and severity, and for predicting the outcome of autoimmune disease. As the diagnosis of systemic autoimmune disease is not always straightforward, the widespread use of autoantibody testing has significantly improved our ability to diagnosis complex autoimmune disorders. However, autoantibody test results, particularly those based on enzyme-linked immunosorbent assays (ELISAs), must be interpreted with caution due to the occasional occurrence of false-positive results. It is important to interpret the results of autoantibody tests in light of both the clinical context and the methodology employed. In some cases, confirmatory testing, analogous to the use of Western blot to verify positive ELISA test results for HIV infection, is warranted.

Conversely, it is important to understand that positive autoantibody tests can be harbingers of autoimmune disease in otherwise healthy individuals, especially in the case of disease-specific autoantibodies, which may appear months, years, or even decades before the onset of clinical symptoms. The detection of disease-specific autoantibodies in asymptomatic individuals may permit early diagnosis and preventative treatment. Good examples are antimitochondrial antibodies in primary biliary cirrhosis, anti-Sm, RNP, Ro(SSA), and double-stranded DNA autoantibodies in systemic lupus erythematosus (SLE), and specific autoantibodies associated with rheumatoid arthritis, polymyositis, and scleroderma, all of which may appear prior to the onset of clinical manifestations. Thus, in the case of an unexpectedly positive autoantibody test, it is important to consider two possibilities: (i) that the test result is a false positive, or (ii) that the autoantibody is present, perhaps as the initial manifestation of an autoimmune disorder.

Autoantibody testing is an evolving field. Older tests, such as double immunodiffusion in gels and agglutination assays, are highly specific but less sensitive than more recent ELISA and addressable bead assays. The older tests also are frequently less amenable to automation, which has led to their rapid abandonment in favor of other tests. The past 15 years has seen a rapid shift from double immunodiffusion and agglutination assays to the ELISA format. Newer technologies are on the horizon, including fluorescence-based assays employing addressable beads, which permit screening for multiple specificities in a single assay.

The chapters in this section reflect both the evolving technology and the need for reliable confirmatory tests, which frequently are older or more labor-intensive assays that are not readily available. Bradwell et al. review the importance of a classical screening test, the fluorescent antinuclear antibody assay, in the serodiagnosis of systemic autoimmune disease. Although automated (ELISA) testing is available, it has not yet replaced the more labor-intensive fluorescence-based assay, and is unlikely to do so in the near future. In the following chapter, Reeves et al. discuss the clinical application of double immunodiffusion, radioimmunoprecipitation, and Western blotting, relatively specific immunological tests that are generally available only in specialized or referral laboratories. With the exception of Western blot and other solid-phase assays, these tests are probably too labor-intensive for general screening, but they can be invaluable in confirming the significance (or lack thereof) when a screening test yields an unexpectedly positive result. The chapter by Chan et al. deals with the mainstream autoantibody assays employing solid-phase antigens, both natural and recombinant. The newly developing technology of addressable laser bead assays for detecting autoantibodies against multiple antigens is reviewed along with future prospects for this exciting new approach.

The following four chapters deal with autoantibody testing relevant to particular diseases or syndromes. Tran and Pisetsky review the approach for detecting anti-DNA antibodies, a specificity pathognomonic for SLE. The importance of distinguishing antibodies against double-stranded DNA (disease specific) from those against single-stranded DNA (not specific) is detailed, as well as an approach to the interpretation of anti-DNA test results. Narain et al. discuss the classical rheumatoid factor assays used to screen for rheumatoid arthritis, along with newer assays for autoantibodies against citrulline-modified proteins that appear to be more specific for rheumatoid arthritis than rheumatoid factor. Schmitz covers the various antibodies associated with the antiphospholipid antibody syndrome and tests to detect and evaluate them. Finally, Wiik discusses the clinical use of antineutrophil cytoplasmic antibody testing in the diagnosis of vasculitis syndromes and the newer tests that detect autoantibodies against specific neutrophil proteins.

The identification of a wide variety of disease-specific autoantibodies over the past 30 years and the increasing sophistication of autoantibody testing have greatly facilitated the diagnosis of systemic autoimmune disease. Automation of autoantibody testing is a more recent development, raising hope that in the future, screening for these biological markers may be useful not only for confirming a clinical diagnosis, but also for establishing a diagnosis during the preclinical phase of the illness, when it may be more amenable to therapy.

Immunofluorescent Antinuclear Antibody Tests

ARTHUR R. BRADWELL, RICHARD G. HUGHES, AND ABID R. KARIM

112

BACKGROUND

Detection and identification of antinuclear autoantibodies (ANAs) are essential for the assessment of systemic and organ-specific autoimmune diseases. The initial screening test is usually done by immunofluorescence on HEp-2 cells followed by identification of individual antibodies with specific assays. Over 40 years, this test has proved remarkably robust and, with a few minor changes, it has retained its important position in most laboratories. It combines the detection of a wide range of autoantibodies with good sensitivity, reproducibility, economy, and ease of use. Such is its dominance that it is the most commonly performed autoantibody test worldwide and the most frequently performed test in clinical immunology laboratories. Competitors in the form of enzyme immunoassays (EIAs) have been available since the early 1990s, but to date they have not upset the hegemony of this enduring immunofluorescent assay (IFA). This chapter reviews the history and the method for ANA testing on HEp-2 cells and its utility in a laboratory setting. Further details can be obtained from the extensive reviews and monographs on the subject which, in particular, show details of the numerous patterns produced by the various autoantibodies on HEp-2 cells (3, 5, 13, 15, 26).

Antinuclear antibody tests have their origin in the "L.E." cell phenomenon, which was the observation that neutrophils from patients with systemic lupus erythematosus (SLE) ingested other leukocytes. This was first demonstrated in 1948 by Hargraves et al. (10) while working at the Mayo Clinic and became widely used as a diagnostic test for SLE but was rather insensitive and difficult to standardize. Lee et al. (14) then showed that the L.E. phenomenon was caused by a gamma globulin protein on the leukocytes, which was thought to be an antibody. In 1957, Holborow et al. (11) (Canadian Red Cross Memorial Hospital, Taplow, United Kingdom) used the fluorescence-labeled antibody technique, developed by Coons and Kaplan (6), to demonstrate that the sera of patients positive for L.E. cells contained antibodies that produced homogeneous nuclear fluorescence on human tissues.

It was soon apparent that different patterns occurred, and in 1961, Beck (2) (National Institute for Medical Research, London, United Kingdom) used rat liver sections to demonstrate homogeneous, speckled, and nucleolar staining of nuclei by sera from patients with a variety of different rheumatic diseases. He also showed that washing the cells in saline caused alterations in the patterns, which was the precursor of extractable nuclear antigen (ENA) tests. The use of human cell lines subsequently became popular, and the work of Tan (20) (Scripps Clinic, La Jolla, Calif.) and others with ENAs and HEp-2 cells led to a huge increase in the number of antigens and patterns recognized in the 1970s and 1980s. Widespread commercial production of HEp-2 cells and the development of national quality control schemes ensured that the test entered worldwide routine laboratory usage. While rodent tissues proved useful in their day, poor sensitivity and variable quality have been conspicuous problems (1, 8), so for the detection of ANAs they have now been replaced by HEp-2 cells in almost all laboratories.

HEp-2 cells, originally considered to originate from a human laryngeal carcinoma, are now known to have been established from a HeLa cell contamination (HEp-2 cells: CCL-23, American Type Culture Collection; depositor, A. E. Moore). This was shown by several techniques, including isoenzyme analysis and DNA fingerprinting. The cells are grown as monolayers on microscope slides. These slides provide a sensitive substrate, and their advantages over rodent tissues include the following:

1. They have increased sensitivity because of greater antigen expression.
2. Human origin ensures better specificity.
3. Cell division rates are higher, so cell cycle-dependent antibodies are easily identified.
4. The cells are grown in monolayers so that all nuclei are visible.
5. The nuclei are much larger, so complex nuclear details can be seen.
6. Antigen distribution is uniform.
7. There is no obscuring intercellular matrix.
8. They are widely available as a standardized immortal cell line.

HEp-2 cells allow recognition of over 30 different nuclear and cytoplasmic patterns that are given by upwards of 50 different autoantibodies. Some patterns, such as centromere patterns, are antigen specific, but most can be attributed to several different autoantibodies. For this

TABLE 1 HEp-2 cell patterns, autoantigens, and disease associations[a]

HEp-2 cell pattern		Antigen target(s)	Disease association(s)
Nucleus	Homogeneous	dsDNA, histones	SLE, drug-induced lupus (histones)
	Nuclear membranous	Lamins A, B1, B2, and C	Mixed chronic autoimmune disorders and chronic fatigue syndrome
	Nuclear membrane pores	gp210 and nucleoporin	PBC and polymyositis
	Nuclear matrix	hnRNP	MCTD, RA, SLE, and scleroderma
	Coarse nuclear speckles	Sm, U1-snRNP, U2-snRNP, U4/U6-snRNP	MCTD, SLE, scleroderma-polymyositis, Raynaud's phenomenon, Sjögren's syndrome, and systemic sclerosis
	Fine nuclear speckles	SSA/Ro, SSB/La, RNA Ku, polymerases I and II, Ki, and Mi-2	SLE, Sjögren's syndrome, scleroderma, myositis, and MCTD
	Few nuclear dots (1–6)	p80-coilin	PBC and chronic active hepatitis
	Multiple nuclear dots (≈10)	Sp-100, PML, and NDP53	PBC, Sjögren's syndrome, and occasionally SLE
	Homogeneous or fine speckled nuclei	Scl-70 (topoisomerase I)	Systemic sclerosis; may also be present in Raynaud's phenomenon and SLE
Nucleolus	Homogeneous	Pm-Scl	Myositis-scleroderma overlap; less frequent in systemic sclerosis and myositis
		Th/To (7-2 RNA and 8-2 RNA)	Systemic sclerosis, Raynaud's phenomenon, SLE, polymyositis and RA
	Clumpy	Fibrillarin (in snoRNP)	Systemic sclerosis
	Dense speckled	RNA helicase II	Systemic sclerosis, SLE, undifferentiated connective tissue disease, and watermelon stomach disease
	Speckled with mitotic dots	RNA polymerase I	Mainly in systemic sclerosis; also SLE, RA, and MCTD
		NOR-90/hUBF	Scleroderma, Raynaud's phenomenon, SLE, RA, and malignancies
Cell cycle related	Centromere, 40–80 discrete nuclear speckles	Centromere (CENP-A, B, C, D)	CREST
	Nuclear pleomorphic pattern (PCNA)	DNA-polymerase associated protein (cyclin)	SLE
	Mitotic spindle (pole-pole) and cytoplasmic fibers	Tubulin	Nonspecific
	1–2 perinuclear cytoplasmic dots, located at spindle poles in mitosis	Centriole/centrosome proteins	Raynaud's phenomenon, scleroderma, Sjögren's syndrome, and CREST
	Spindle poles and fibers in close proximity to poles with fine speckled nuclei	NuMA-1/MSA-1 (210 kDa)	Nonspecific; reported in SLE, Sjögren's syndrome, MCTD, and polyarthritis
	Spindle poles and fibers (pole-pole), midbody and intercellular bridge	NuMA-2, HsEg5	SLE and Sjögren's syndrome
	Cleavage furrow and midbody, staining of chromatin in metaphase and speckled nuclei in interphase	MSA-2, Unknown antigen	Systemic sclerosis and Raynaud's phenomenon
	Speckles along spindle poles. Fine, dense nuclear speckling in some interphase cells	MSA-3, unknown antigen	Unknown
	G$_2$ granular nuclei and nuclear rim. Kinetochores, cleavage furrow, and either side of the midbody	CENP-F/Na (367 kDa)	Neoplasms (breast and lung cancer)

(Continued on next page)

TABLE 1 (*Continued*)

HEp-2 cell pattern		Antigen target(s)	Disease association(s)
Cytoplasmic staining	Fine speckled staining concentrated around the nucleus	Jo-1 (histyl-tRNA synthetase) and other amino-acyl-tRNA synthetases	Polymyositis, dermatomyositis, associated with interstitial pulmonary diseases
	Granular filamentous cytoplasmic staining	Mitochondrial (frequently M2, PDC E2 antigen)	PBC; less frequent in scleroderma, CREST, SLE, and Sjögren's syndrome
	Fine, dense granular to homogeneous cytoplasm, with nucleolar staining	Ribosome P phosphoproteins (PO, P1, P2), 28S rRNA, S10, Ja, L12, L5/5S	SLE (associated with neuropsychiatric symptoms)
	Fine speckled to granular cytoplasmic staining	Signal recognition particle (SRP); 54-kDa protein is major antigen	Polymyositis, dermatomyositis
	Large irregular cytoplasmic speckles	Lysosomal; antigens are poorly characterized	SLE
	Fine, uniform cytoplasmic speckles	Peroxisomal; antigens are unknown	Nonspecific
	Speckled granular staining adjacent to one part of the nucleus	Golgi complex, golgins (-67, -95, -97, -160, and -245) and macrogolgin/giantin	SLE, Sjögren's syndrome, and other rheumatic diseases
Cytoplasmic fibers	Fine fibers running the length of the cell	Actin	Chronic active hepatitis; also seen in PBC and connective tissue diseases
	Reticular pattern throughout the cytoplasm. Cytoplasmic speckles in mitosis	Cytokeratin 8, 18, and 19	Nonspecific
	Stress fibers running the length of the cells	Tropomyosin	Nonspecific
	Fine whorled fibers	Vimentin	Nonspecific
	Short fibers adjacent to nuclear and cytoplasmic membranes	Vinculin	Nonspecific
	Fine cytoplasmic filaments with cytoplasmic speckles in mitosis	Desmin	Nonspecific
	Short filaments from the cytoplasmic membrane	Cytoplasmic anchoring proteins, e.g., paxillin and zyxin	Unknown, although reported in early systemic sclerosis

*ᵃ*Abbreviations: CENP, centromere protein; CREST, syndrome of calcinosis, Raynaud's phenomenon, esophageal dismotility, sclerodactyly, and telangiectasia; MCTD, mixed connective tissue diseases/overlap syndromes; MSA, mitotic spindle apparatus; PBC, primary biliary cirrhosis; RA, rheumatoid arthritis; SLE, systemic lupus erythematosus.

reason and because patients' sera frequently contain several autoantibodies, specific tests are usually performed. Nevertheless, the broad specificity and sensitivity of HEp-2 cells are ideal for an initial screening assay (Table 1), so HEp-2 cells are unlikely to disappear from the clinical laboratory for many years to come.

TECHNOLOGY

The immunofluorescent HEp-2 test is used for several purposes:

- as a general screen to identify patients with ANAs
- to link autoantibody patterns with individual diseases for guidance on specific tests
- to help monitor patients during treatment
- to screen out patients who have negative tests

To meet this broad range of requirements, the test needs a variety of characteristics. It must be sufficiently sensitive to detect a whole range of autoantibodies, yet sufficiently specific that healthy individuals are not falsely identified as positive. Since modest levels of autoantibodies are common in elderly people, normal ranges must be carefully selected. As regards the use of HEp-2 for identifying individual autoantibodies, some patterns such as centromere are antigen

specific (Table 1), but for most, specificity should be confirmed against individual proteins.

Monitoring of autoantibodies is normally achieved with specific tests such as anti-double-stranded DNA (anti-dsDNA) assays for SLE. However, the low cost and broad specificity of HEp-2 assays allow them to be used in parallel with specific tests during the management of patients.

The immunofluorescence patterns seen on HEp-2 cells depend upon their stage in the cell cycle. Since most autoantibodies are directed against interphase antigens, most HEp-2 cells should be at this stage of development (Fig. 1). Autoantibodies directed against antigens in the cytoplasm of HEp-2 cells are frequently observed, and some of them are important diagnostically. They can be classified into either speckled or fibrous patterns. Autoantibodies with a speckled appearance bind to targets such as histidyl-tRNA synthetase (e.g., Jo-1), signal recognition particles, mitochondria, lysosomes, and peroxisomes. The cytoplasmic fibers are of many types, and low-titer antibodies to these proteins are found in healthy people, so disease specificity is low. Several autoantibodies produce characteristic patterns on cells that are in division. The following is a brief outline of the various phases of HEp-2 cells during their reproductive cycle and should assist in understanding of autoantibody patterns.

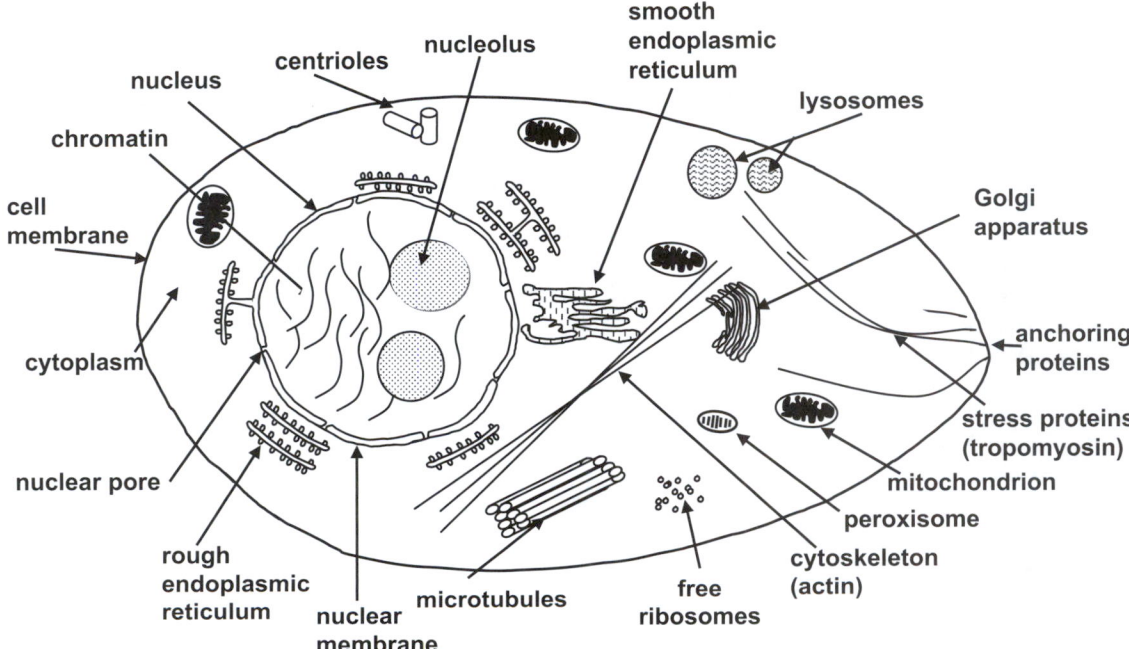

FIGURE 1 Diagrammatic representation of HEp-2 cell antigens during interphase.

The Cell during Interphase

In interphase, the chromosomes form a fibrillar network of chromatin, more or less uniformly distributed throughout the nucleoplasm and delimited by the nuclear membrane. Only the nucleoli are well differentiated. Cytoplasmic organelles and fibrous structures are most visible at this stage and tend to largely disappear or change their appearance during mitosis. Interphase is subdivided into three successive periods: G_1, S, and G_2 (G = gap, S = synthesis). The G_1 phase is preparatory to the biosynthesis and doubling of DNA which occur during S phase. Once the cell reaches the G_2 phase, DNA synthesis is complete and the pairs of chromatids remain joined at the centromere. In the M phase (M = mitosis), the DNA per cell drops to one-half as the cell divides. There are numerous autoantigens in the nucleus, some associated with the chromosomes such as dsDNA and histones, and many associated with ribosomes, polymerases, and nucleoli (Table 1).

The Nuclear Envelope

The nuclear envelope is the membrane that maintains the integrity of the nucleoplasm during interphase. There are three distinct layers, comprising the nuclear lamina and the inner and outer nuclear membranes. The membranes are interrupted by the nuclear pore complexes, and the outer nuclear membrane is continuous with the endoplasmic reticulum with attached ribosomes. The transcriptionally active euchromatin is found in the vicinity of the nuclear pore complexes, whereas the heterochromatin is found adjacent to the nuclear lamina, which in turn is attached to the inner nuclear membrane. Autoantibodies against lamins A, B1, B2, and C are found and are seen as linear nuclear membranous staining, while antibodies directed against the nuclear pore complexes show granular nuclear membrane staining.

The Cell during Division

Mitosis takes place during 10 to 15% of the cell cycle and is divided into four successive phases: prophase, metaphase, anaphase, and telophase.

During prophase, DNA condensation gives rise to the appearance of individual chromosomes while the nucleolar contents are distributed throughout the nucleoplasm. Meanwhile, the mitotic spindle forms around the nucleus and terminates at the polar centrioles (or centrosomes). During mid-prophase, the nuclear membrane disrupts and then disappears. The chromosomes are attached to the mitotic spindle by microtubules (tubulin) which originate from the kinetochores and attach to the chromosome centromeres. Metaphase is characterized by the localization of condensed chromosomes at the equator of the spindle apparatus through the action of microtubules. In anaphase, each pair of chromatids splits at the centromere and the chromatids migrate separately to each pole of the spindle. Microtubules disappear at the end of anaphase as the chromatids reach opposite poles of the mitotic spindle. In telophase, the nuclear membrane re-forms around each of the two daughter nuclei. The nucleoli reappear, and the chromosomes become decondensed in the newly formed nuclei.

Mitosis is followed by cytoplasmic division or cytokinesis, which proceeds at the midbody region of the dividing cell. During this process, the cytoplasmic membrane invaginates around the middle of the cell at right angles to the mitotic spindle and between the two daughter nuclei. As membrane invagination proceeds, the midbody is progressively constricted and finally disappears as the two daughter cells separate.

Important autoantibodies are found against most of the cell cycle-related structures that have been mentioned, such as the centromeres, proliferating cell nuclear antigen, mitotic spindle proteins, and centriole proteins. The pattern on HEp-2 cells is usually sufficient to identify most of these autoantibodies (Table 1).

What Is the Best Fluorescent Conjugate for the Autoantibodies?

The species of animals commonly used for the fluorescein-conjugated antibody are goat, sheep, and rabbit. Affinity-purified antibodies are preferable because they produce the least background staining, although immunoglobulin fractions are widely used and quite satisfactory. Antibodies are conjugated with fluorescein at a fluorescein/protein molar ratio of approximately 3. This applies to all animal species, although some individual monoclonal antibodies may perform better with a higher fluorescein content.

There is considerable variation in laboratory usage for the fine specificity of the conjugated antibody. Immunoglobulin G (IgG) ANAs are undoubtedly the most important in terms of diagnosis and monitoring of rheumatic diseases and must always be measured. IgM ANAs may coexist with IgG but are usually of secondary importance, except perhaps in pediatric SLE. If IgM antibodies dominate, they indicate a milder or nonspecific disease with a better prognosis and less renal or other organ damage. IgA ANAs correlate with IgG antibodies and offer little additional information and so are generally ignored (4).

The majority of laboratories use a non-affinity-purified, fluorescein-conjugated second antibody directed against IgG, -A, and -M heavy chains (or anti-IgG heavy and light chains). This detects IgG, IgM, and IgA antibodies but with a bias towards IgG, and the results are reported without identification of the antibody class. Many laboratories use a second antibody directed against IgG heavy chains alone, thereby ignoring IgM antibodies on the basis that they are rarely of clinical importance.

Alternative Technology

ANA EIA screens, available since the early 1990s, are viable alternatives to ANA detection on HEp-2 cells. Given the subjectivity of IFA interpretation and the high number of negative samples, an EIA method for ANA screening has considerable potential. Assay conditions of EIAs are optimized for performance; however, the sensitivity of the ANA EIA screen ultimately depends on the choice of antigens, and for every antigen used the cost increases.

The antigens of choice are the major markers for the autoimmune diseases of interest, such as SLE, Sjögren's syndrome, mixed connective tissue disease, scleroderma, and the syndrome of calcinosis, Raynaud's phenomenon, esophageal dismotility, sclerodactyly, and telangiectasia. The antigens are from either purified or recombinant sources. Since the antigens on the plate are known, one can further identify the specificity of positive samples by using single EIAs (25). This approach will detect the majority of ANAs, but a proportion of ANA samples will be missed. These may be of limited clinical importance, as the specificities will be towards minor antigens that have little known significance. An alternative approach is to include nuclear and/or nucleolar extracts to supplement the specific antigens. This may increase the number of positive ANA samples detected, but a number of these will be difficult to characterize as the antigen targets may be unknown or of little clinical consequence.

In one study (13), five EIA kits were compared with HEp-2 cells for 600 patient samples and 200 blood donor samples. Overall, agreement with IFA was approximately 90% (range, 87 to 96%), the sensitivity of EIA was 90% of that of IFA (range, 70 to 96%), and the specificity was 95% (range, 81 to 98%), the figures being dependent upon the cutoff selection for sensitivity and specificity. None of the EIAs was 100% sensitive, having failed to demonstrate a few atypical as well as classical HEp-2 patterns, and some kits produced rather discordant results. Other studies comparing HEp-2 cells with EIA for ANA detection have produced similar results (7) and rather poor detection rates for antibodies against dsDNA and Sm in some EIAs (24). Also,

low-affinity autoantibodies are more readily detected in the "capacity" EIAs, so discordance between results tends to be worse at low antibody concentrations. Correlation between the results for the two techniques is, perhaps, remarkably good, considering their differences.

More recently, ANA screens have become available as multianalyte immunoassays based on multibead arrays, which can be read by use of flow cytometers. The bead arrays are interpreted with the new generation of flow cytometers, e.g., the Luminex system (Luminex Corporation) and the FACSarray (BD Biosciences). Such systems allow for the screening of samples while at the same time providing semiquantitative results on individual specificities for positive samples. Protein microarrays also have potential as multiplex platforms for ANA detection (9). The results of these are read by using fluorescence imaging systems, and they use the technology from DNA microarray analysis. Multiplex platforms are limited, like the EIA ANA screens, by their dependence on the antigens of choice present in the assay, and development difficulties are compounded by the tight performance criteria required for each individual specificity. Due to the infancy of multiplex systems, it is difficult to predict their impact on the preeminence of the HEp-2 immunofluorescent ANA screen.

ASSAY PROCEDURES

Sample Requirements

Ideally, serum samples that have been collected within the previous few hours should be used. Storage at 4°C is sufficient for samples analyzed up to a week after collection, while for longer periods (months or years) storage at −20°C is preferable. Frequent thawing and freezing of the sample may lead to a decrease of antibody activity, while long-term storage may lead to lyophilization, resulting in an increase in titer. Addition of sodium azide (100 μg/ml) is recommended.

Serum dilution is an important issue. The first studies of immunofluorescence detection of ANA on rat liver sections used patients' sera diluted 1:10. With the use of HEp-2 cells, improved microscope lenses, and better-labeled second antibodies, 1:10 dilutions would produce a huge false-positive rate from normal samples, so now it is common practice to screen at a 1:80 dilution on HEp-2 cells. Since the frequency of ANAs varies with age, it can be argued that for children a 1:40 dilution would be reasonable while 1:160 might be preferable for patients >65 years of age. However, some low-titer autoantibodies may be clinically significant. One study (22) recommended that samples should be tested at both 1:40 and 1:160 dilutions and that information should be supplied to the clinicians about the numbers of healthy individuals, of the same age and sex, who have positive results at those dilutions (see quality control section below).

Materials and Reagents

Production of HEp-2 Cells

HEp-2 cells can be grown in the laboratory, but slides are normally purchased in kits that contain all the necessary reagents. For those who wish to prepare their own slides, the following is a brief description of the important steps in their preparation (12).

1. Cells are maintained in long-term storage in liquid nitrogen.
2. Short-term growth is maintained in flasks in which the cells become adherent and confluent.

3. For the production of HEp-2 slides, the cells are dissociated, checked for bacterial contamination, counted, and added to incubation flasks for rapid growth over 1 to 2 days.

4. The cells are dissociated from the flasks, separated by being passed through a fine needle, counted, and added to slide wells that have been carefully cleaned.

5. Slides are incubated for approximately 24 h in a humid CO_2 incubator at 37°C.

6. Slides are removed and drained prior to fixation. Fixation procedures vary considerably and commercial manufacturers have optimized their procedures, both to preserve the antigens and to render the membranes permeable. However, a reasonable guide would be to use a mixture of cooled (−20 to +4°C) acetone (80 to 90%) and methanol (10 to 20%) for 20 min. It is important to assess the fixation procedure for the preservation of antigens; in particular, sensitivity for the SS-A antigen may be affected.

7. The fixative is drained off, and the slides are dried with warm air.

8. Each slide is sealed in a foil bag with a desiccant such as silica gel and stored at 4°C.

9. For quality control, the slides are stained and checked by using a panel of sera for morphology, mitotic figures (>4 per field of view at 400× magnification), negative staining (background), weak and strong positive staining, different staining patterns, and titration characteristics of common autoantibodies.

10. Several slides are stored for long-term assessment of stability.

Fluorescent Conjugated Antibodies

The specificity and type of antibody have been discussed above, and these reagents are normally purchased. Affinity-purified, anti-human IgG (heavy and light chain) fluorescein isothiocyanate is widely used. In commercial kits, the reagent is normally supplied prediluted and matched for optimal reactivity and sensitivity with the HEp-2 cells. Undiluted antibodies must be assessed at a working dilution against a variety of different sera.

Commercial preparations tend to use derivatives of fluorescein, and for the purposes of IFA on HEp-2 cells they are amply sensitive. However, the fluorescein fluorophores are pH sensitive and susceptible to photobleaching. There are other fluorophores available that overcome these drawbacks to a certain extent. For example, the Alexa fluor dyes (Molecular Probes) give increased signals when used for immunofluorescence, although the limited benefit of detecting low concentrations of autoantibodies may not justify the associated increase in cost.

Equipment and Instrumentation

The HEp-2 cells should be observed by using an epifluorescence microscope fitted with filters appropriate for fluorescein detection. A 40× objective (dry or water immersion), along with a 10× magnification eyepiece (giving a final 400× magnification), allows easy identification of all common patterns.

Test Procedure for Immunofluorescence ANA Detection

1. Prepare phosphate-buffered saline (PBS) (pH 7.2 to 7.4) with 0.1 g of sodium azide per liter. Tween 20 (0.5 g/liter), bovine serum albumin (20 g/liter) or dilute HEp-2 medium can be added to the PBS to reduce nonspecific binding of serum globulins to the HEp-2 cells.

2. Sample dilutions:

a. Screening. We recommend diluting samples 1:80 when screening, by adding 10 μl of serum to 790 μl of PBS buffer. See "Sample Requirements" (above) for discussion of recommended screening dilutions.

b. Titration. Make serial dilutions of positive samples in PBS buffer (e.g., 1:80, 1:160, 1:320, etc.).

3. HEp-2 slides. Allow the slides to reach room temperature over 30 min prior to removal from their pouches. Label slides appropriately, place them in the humid chamber, and add 1 drop of each positive and negative control serum to separate wells. Add 25 μl of the diluted patients' samples to the remaining wells. Care should be taken to ensure that there is no crossover of serum samples into neighboring wells, particularly in the case of 24-well slides.

4. Incubate the slides in a humid chamber at room temperature for 30 min, ensuring that no wells dry out.

5. Remove the slides from the humid chamber and rinse thoroughly but gently with PBS. Do not squirt PBS directly onto the wells. Place the slides in a rack, immerse them in PBS, and agitate or stir for 10 min.

6. Shake off the excess PBS and blot around the wells. Immediately return the slides to the humid chamber and add a drop of fluorescein-conjugated antibody to each well. Do not leave the wells uncovered for more than 15 s, since drying out will change the results. It is important to optimize the second antibody if it is not supplied prediluted and no recommendations are provided. "Checkerboard" titrations can be used to determine the appropriate secondary-antibody concentration (19).

7. Incubate the slides for 20 min in a humid chamber at room temperature in the dark.

8. Wash again as in step 5. Counterstain as required by adding 2 or 3 drops of 1% Evans Blue per 100 ml of PBS prior to washing or immersion (not recommended if the microscopist is color-blind).

9. Remove one slide at a time from the PBS wash. Quickly dry around the wells and add a drop of mounting medium to each well (e.g., 90% glycerol in PBS, pH 8.6). {Note: chemicals should be added to the mounting medium to improve retention of fluorescence upon illumination. DABCO (1,4-diazabicyclo [2,2,2]-octane, Sigma-Aldrich Company, Ltd.), 2.5 g per 100 ml of mounting medium, is frequently used.} Carefully add a coverslip, ensuring that there are no trapped air bubbles.

10. Finished slides should be viewed as soon as possible, but they may be stored at 2 to 8°C in the dark for many days with little loss of fluorescence activity.

11. The intensity and patterns of fluorescence are assessed and recorded. A serum specimen is considered to be positive when the observed fluorescence is significant compared with that of the controls. The intensity can be expressed according to a scale of values compatible with the guidelines established for reference sera (18) as 1+ to 4+ or as negative. A semiquantitative evaluation can be obtained by performing serial dilutions of the test serum to endpoint fluorescence.

12. The procedure can be semiautomated; this saves on labor and is particularly beneficial in laboratories that have a high throughput of samples. Instruments are available which can perform dilutions and run IFAs up to the point of but not including the mounting of the coverslips. Other instruments which can perform the dilutions alone are available.

Enzyme Immunohistochemical Staining

Autoantibody patterns on HEp-2 cells can also be demonstrated by using enzyme-conjugated second antibodies.

The immunoperoxidase technique produces excellent, permanent staining. Advantages are that HEp-2 cells can be interpreted with conventional light microscopy, there is a permanent record, and the slides can be sent to different laboratories for quality control purposes. However, the technique is slightly less sensitive and the extra technical steps are time-consuming, so the procedure is not widely used.

QUALITY ASSURANCE AND QUALITY CONTROL IMPLEMENTATION

In 1980, the Arthritis Foundation in the United States, in collaboration with the Centers for Disease Control and Prevention (CDC), Atlanta, Ga., established a committee on antinuclear antibody serology with the purpose of producing a repository of ANA reference sera. Aliquots (0.5 ml) from large plasmapheresis donations of defined specificity were dispensed into borosilicate ampoules, freeze-dried, and sealed under reduced pressure. The standard requirements for establishing reference reagents, such as measurements of mean dry weight, water content, and stability, were met, and data were provided with each ampoule. The reagents were assessed before and after processing in several laboratories, and in 1982 five reference reagents were made available to laboratories as primary standards (23).

It was subsequently agreed by various international bodies that standardization of ANAs should be extended to other autoantibodies. In 1988 (21), in conjunction with the International Union of Immunological Societies and the World Health Organization, the reference sera at the CDC were expanded to 10 different specificities, and in 1997, these sera were further characterized by immunofluorescence and Western blotting (18) (Table 2). These various standards are satisfactory for the common autoantibodies and provide an important basis for HEp-2 cell usage. For rarer antibodies, appropriate sera should be exchanged to standardize interlaboratory practice.

Quality Control

Known positive and negative control sera must be tested with each group of slides. Prototype sera are available from many commercial sources and from the CDC (see above). It is important to use not only samples that produce typical patterns but also weak samples that test the sensitivity limits of each batch of slides.

Each laboratory should determine the border between positive and negative results. Approximately 200 serum samples from healthy local controls, equally distributed over age and sex, and 100 serum samples from local patients with definite SLE and other relevant diseases should be assessed.

Quality Assurance

There are several national, international, and commercial quality assurance schemes, of which two are indicated below. These schemes are widely used and cover the common autoantibodies. Samples are issued several times a year and a consensus report is produced so that individual laboratories can compare their performance with that of other participants.

A scheme for autoimmune serology is available from The College of American Pathologists, 325 Waukegan Road, Northfield, IL 60093-2750.

The United Kingdom National External Quality Assessment Schemes for Autoimmune Serology are available from the Department of Immunology, P.O. Box 894, Sheffield S5 7YT, United Kingdom.

PITFALLS AND TROUBLESHOOTING

Because HEp-2 cells for ANA tests are so widely used, laboratories have gained huge experience, and the results are generally satisfactory. The largest variation in results reported to quality control schemes relates to differences in fluorescence intensity of the samples. As shown in Table 2, even expert laboratories vary in their opinion. Samples regarded as 4 + (1:2,560) in one laboratory may be considered only 1 + (1:160) in another. Such variation is accounted for more by differences in the fluorescent conjugates and quality of microscopes (and age of the mercury vapor bulb) than differences in HEp-2 preparations. Generally, the use of a widely distributed commercial kit will ensure a high-quality substrate and give good consensus on quality control schemes. Nevertheless, individual HEp-2 batches do vary, so each batch should be assessed against a standard set of control sera. When problems are encountered it is sensible to make some simple checks, such as the production and expiration dates of the slides and conjugates and the recommended storage conditions (Table 3). The age of the bulb in the microscope should also be checked. Odd results should be reported to the manufacturer in order to

TABLE 2 Arthritis Foundation/CDC antinuclear antibody reference sera[a]

Serum	Designated specificity	IF[b] result at 1:160 or recommended Western blot dilution
AF/CDC1	Homogeneous ANA (anti-dsDNA)	2+ to 4+
AF/CDC3	Speckled-pattern ANA	2+ to 4+
AF/CDC6	Nucleolar-pattern ANA (antifibrillarin)	1+ to 3+
AF/CDC8	Centromere pattern ANA	1+ to 4+
AF/CDC2	SS-B (La) and speckled-pattern ANA	1:200
AF/CDC4	Anti-U1-snRNP	1:100
AF/CDC5	Anti-Sm (U1, U2, U5, U4/6 snRNPs)	1:2,000
AF/CDC7	SS-A (Ro)	Negative (IF +ve only)
AF/CDC9	Anti-Scl-70	1:100
AF/CDC10	Anti-Jo-1	1:100

[a]These sera are available from the Centers for Disease Control and Prevention, Atlanta, GA 30333, or CLB, Plesmanlaan 125, 1066 Cx, P.O. Box 9190, 1006 AD, Amsterdam, The Netherlands.
[b]IF, immunofluorescence; +ve, positive.

TABLE 3 Troubleshooting guide for ANA testing on HEp-2 cells

Problem	Possible reason or solution
Weak positive sera are negative or difficult to interpret	Conjugate too weak; too much Evans Blue
Excessive staining of negative cells	Conjugate too strong
Poor morphology	Slides not allowed to warm up from refrigerator or allowed to dry out during procedure
Neighboring wells positive with similar patterns	Samples splashed over several wells, particularly on 24-well slides. Ensure careful pipetting.
Mechanical damage to cells	Use care with pipettes and washing procedures and when adding coverslips
Speckles on slide and cells destroyed	Infected sample. Use new sample or heat to 65°C to destroy bacterial enzymes, filter, and reapply
Immunofluorescence fades too quickly	Use antifading agent such as DABCO
Slides stick to the microscope	Too much mounting medium
Bubbles under coverslip	Gently wash off the coverslip and carefully remount
Fluorescent film over the cells	Drying of substrate wells between reagent additions or nonspecific binding of conjugate to proteins. Add blocking agent to buffers.
Weak nucleolar staining	Samples diluted in water or glassware dirty. Use cleaner procedures and dilute samples in PBS.
Insufficient mitotic figures, cells overconfluent or too sparse	Change batch of HEp-2 cells

determine whether other users have experienced similar problems or whether the unusual results are specific to the individual laboratory.

TEST VALIDATION

The ANA immunofluorescent HEp-2 test is intended to be used for screening and titration of circulating antinuclear antibodies. The results of the test serve as an aid in the diagnosis of SLE, Sjögren's syndrome, rheumatoid arthritis, and other connective tissue disorders. The test has a class II performance standard classification from the Food and Drug Administration (FDA), requiring 510(k) submission. The submission must include performance criteria, which include precision, sensitivity, and specificity data. For a list of commercial suppliers of FDA-approved HEp-2 immunofluorescent ANA tests, either refer to the FDA website (http://www.fda.gov) or contact individual suppliers. All ANA immunofluorescent HEp-2 tests must conform to the standards already mentioned above ("Quality Assurance and Quality Control Implementation").

COST ASSESSMENT—COMMERCIAL KITS OR IN-HOUSE MANUFACTURE?

ANA tests were traditionally performed on rodent tissues that had been prepared by laboratory staff. Since animals and cryostats are readily available in most pathology laboratories, it is natural that these practices should have persisted. HEp-2 cells, in contrast, are less easily handled, and specialist knowledge is required to prepare slides in a satisfactory condition. In contrast and from a commercial point of view, HEp-2 production can be scaled up to produce batches of much larger size and better uniformity than rodent tissue sections. This has led to a proliferation of commercial suppliers of HEp-2 cells.

The actual costs of running these tests depend in some degree upon the number of tests performed. Based on a reasonable throughput, 100 or so samples per day, where 25% of the samples are positive, one would estimate about 3.5 h of labor (3 h of setup and 1/2 h of interpretation). An estimated figure would therefore be $1.90 per test (reagent cost [$1.45] + labor cost [$0.45]); notably, this does not include capital equipment investments such as microscopes, etc.

Inevitably, HEp-2 production techniques vary, and there are no standard publications or international agreement on optimal culture techniques, ideal fixatives, drying procedures, etc. Commercial HEp-2 cells therefore differ in their performance characteristics, so care should be taken when choosing a product (8). There will also be batch-to-batch variation from both in-house and commercial suppliers. It is therefore common practice to test and then reserve batches that are particularly satisfactory. This leads to minimal variation of the HEp-2 cells with time and confidence in their performance.

Much of the discussion about the quality variations has focused on preservation of the SS-A antigens. Normally, HEp-2 cells contain abundant SS-A antigen, but the antigen is destroyed by some chemical fixatives. A multicenter European study (1) clearly showed that some HEp-2 cell preparations did not contain adequate amounts of SS-A and could produce negative or confusing results with SS-A-positive sera. HEp-2 cells that contained satisfactory amounts of SS-A produced results that correlated well with very sensitive EIAs and Western blot assays. Care must therefore be exercised when preparing the cells or when selecting commercial products.

The commercial HEp-2 cells known as HEp-2000 have been genetically modified to produce extra SS-A, which allows the autoantibodies to be specifically identified by the initial screening test. However, other commercial kits containing conventionally produced HEp-2 cells express adequate amounts of SS-A, and even use of HEp-2000 cells may miss some SS-A autoantibodies compared with EIA techniques (17).

INTERPRETATION

Autoantibodies occur in both physiological and pathological conditions. In general, high titers (>1:160) are significant disease indicators, but low or absent titers do not exclude disease. Circulating autoantibodies may be absent or not detected because of poor target antigens or unsatisfactory assay technique or even because the disease is so active that antigens released into the circulation have adsorbed all the antibodies. In contrast, low-titer antibodies may be found in healthy people, relatives of patients with autoimmune conditions, and a variety of diseases, such as chronic inflammation and cancer, which have no autoimmune basis. Autoantibodies may also appear months or years before overt manifestations of an autoimmune disorder. Autoantibodies also increase in prevalence with age, particularly in women, without necessarily being harmful. Interpretation must be made with reference to the individual's medical history, age, and existing conditions (Table 4). While ANA tests are diagnostically important, results must be interpreted in the context of the clinical information. Of equal importance are awareness of the limitations of the tests and quality control of the substrates and reagents.

Recognizing autoantibody patterns on HEp-2 cells is relatively straightforward (Fig. 2), but assessing fluorescence intensity and its clinical significance requires considerable experience. The ability to make decisions on fluorescence intensity can be gained only with practice and by regularly viewing batches of normal, or allegedly normal, sera in order to obtain the picture of a "negative" background. Interpretation of staining is partly subjective, so there may be considerable variation in the reported results from day to day and between different observers. Should discrepancies arise, particularly between past and present specimens, it is important to identify the previous sample and compare it directly with the current one. When there is doubt about a sample, the physician should be involved and the final judgment should be made in the context of the patient's clinical problems.

Reporting practices vary, but the following is a guide to commonly used protocols.

1. HEp-2 slides for ANA testing are run at the screening concentration and are scored from weak to strong positive by experienced personnel. They are reported as +/− (weak), + (positive), 2+ (strong positive), and 3+ and 4+ (very strong positive), which correspond to titrations of approximately 1:80 (+/−), 1:160 to 1:320 (+), 1:640 (2+), 1:1,280 (3+), or 1:2,560 (4+). All positive samples from new patients should be titrated. Follow-up samples are frequently titrated or skilled personnel may judge the titer from the fluorescence intensity since this approach may be clinically sufficient and is less costly.

2. All slides should be stored for a minimum of 28 days. It is good practice for results to be transcribed onto computer-generated worksheets by the person reading the slides so that mistakes are minimized. When results have been verified, with particular reference to the age, sex, and diagnosis of the patient, they are authorized for reporting. The clinical immunologist adds appropriate comments and signs the result form for dispatch. Comments should include something to the effect of "Titers of 1:80 are of limited importance for patients over 50 years of age." If a query arises, the appropriate test may be readily located by diary date, slide number, and well number and the sample can be checked.

Comments on interpretation:

1. ANA patterns are only indicative of the autoantibody, and precise determination of their specificity must be assessed by other techniques, such as immunodiffusion, immunoblotting, and EIA. Samples negative by HEp-2 can confidently be reported as such. Occasional samples will demonstrate low-titer autoantibodies by EIAs that are negative as determined by use of HEp-2 cells, but that depends upon the cutoff level of sensitivity for either assay.

2. Mixed patterns occur when patients' sera contain more than one antibody. For example, when U1-snRNP antibodies are associated with dsDNA antibodies in the serum of SLE patients, a homogeneous nuclear pattern will be observed and the chromosomal region of mitotic cells will be strongly positive. However, after serial dilution the typical speckled pattern for U1-snRNP antibodies may appear. Different serum dilutions therefore produce different fluorescence patterns, so an autoantibody titer should be assessed only by a serial dilution of the sample.

3. Mitotic figures are important for the identification of centromere antibodies and others that bind to antigens involved with cell division. The specificity of centromere antibodies can be established directly from the HEp-2 pattern after examining a few mitotic figures.

4. Unexpected or rare HEp-2 patterns can be reported to the physicians even if they do not apparently relate to the patient's stated diagnosis. The clinicians can choose to ignore the results, or it can be indicated that the autoantibodies are of no known significance. These results can be reviewed from time to time to assess their clinical and laboratory importance.

TABLE 4 Diseases associated with ANA-positive sera

Disease, condition, or group	% ANA positive
Chronic discoid lupus	5–50
Chronic infections	10–50
Dermatomyositis, polymyositis	30–40
Drug-associated SLE-like syndromes	<50
Felty's syndrome	95–100
Healthy population	<5
Healthy relatives of SLE patients	25
Juvenile arthritis	15–30
Lupoid hepatitis	95–100
Neonatal lupus syndrome	>90
Neoplastic diseases	10–30
Normal old age	<30
Polyarteritis nodosa	15–25
Pregnancy	5–10
Primary biliary cirrhosis	95–100
Rheumatoid arthritis	<95
Rheumatic fever	>5
Sjögren's syndrome	<95
SLE	95–100
Systemic sclerosis (scleroderma)	>90

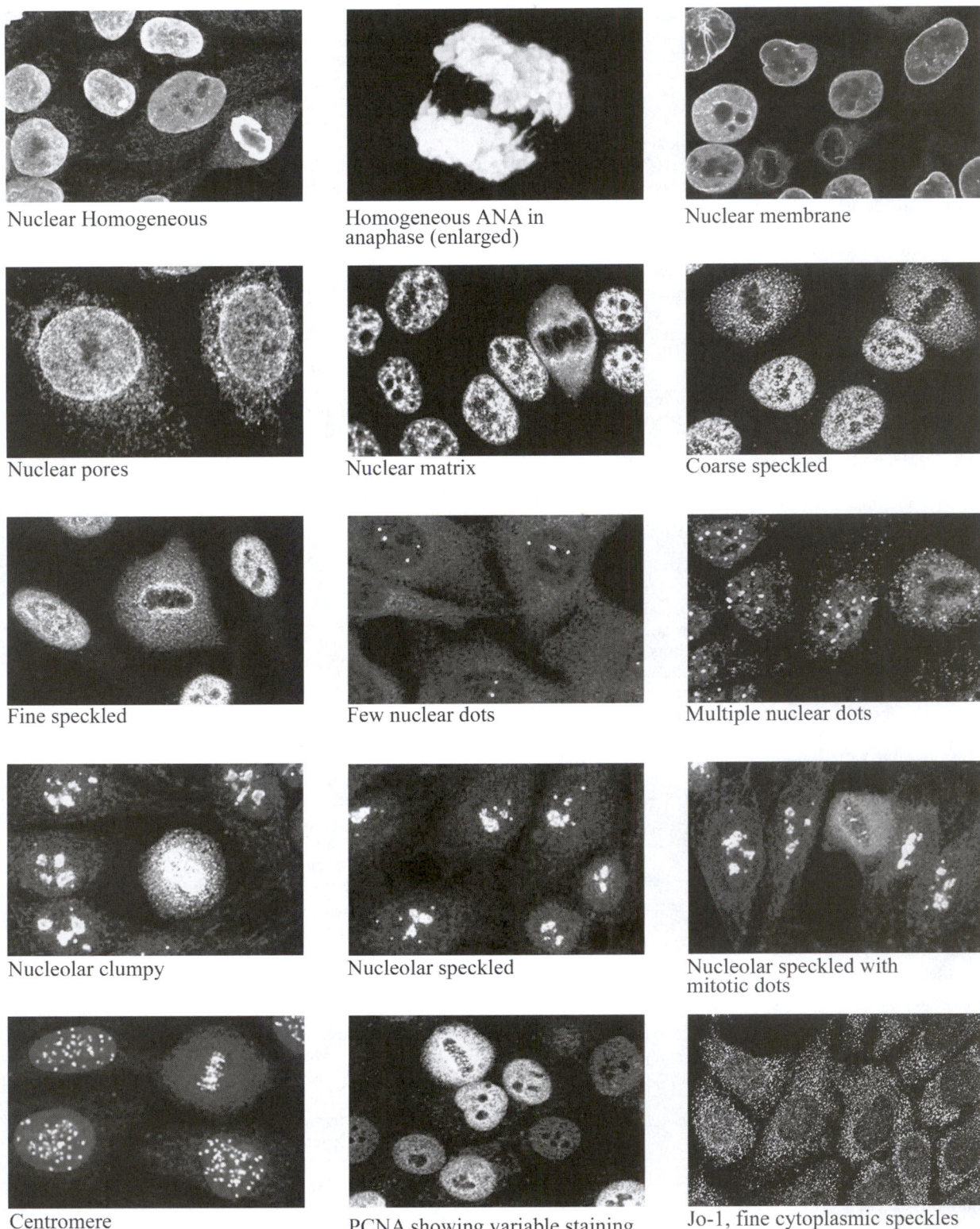

Nuclear Homogeneous

Homogeneous ANA in anaphase (enlarged)

Nuclear membrane

Nuclear pores

Nuclear matrix

Coarse speckled

Fine speckled

Few nuclear dots

Multiple nuclear dots

Nucleolar clumpy

Nucleolar speckled

Nucleolar speckled with mitotic dots

Centromere

PCNA showing variable staining of interphase nuclei

Jo-1, fine cytoplasmic speckles

FIGURE 2   Common autoantibody patterns on HEp-2 cells.

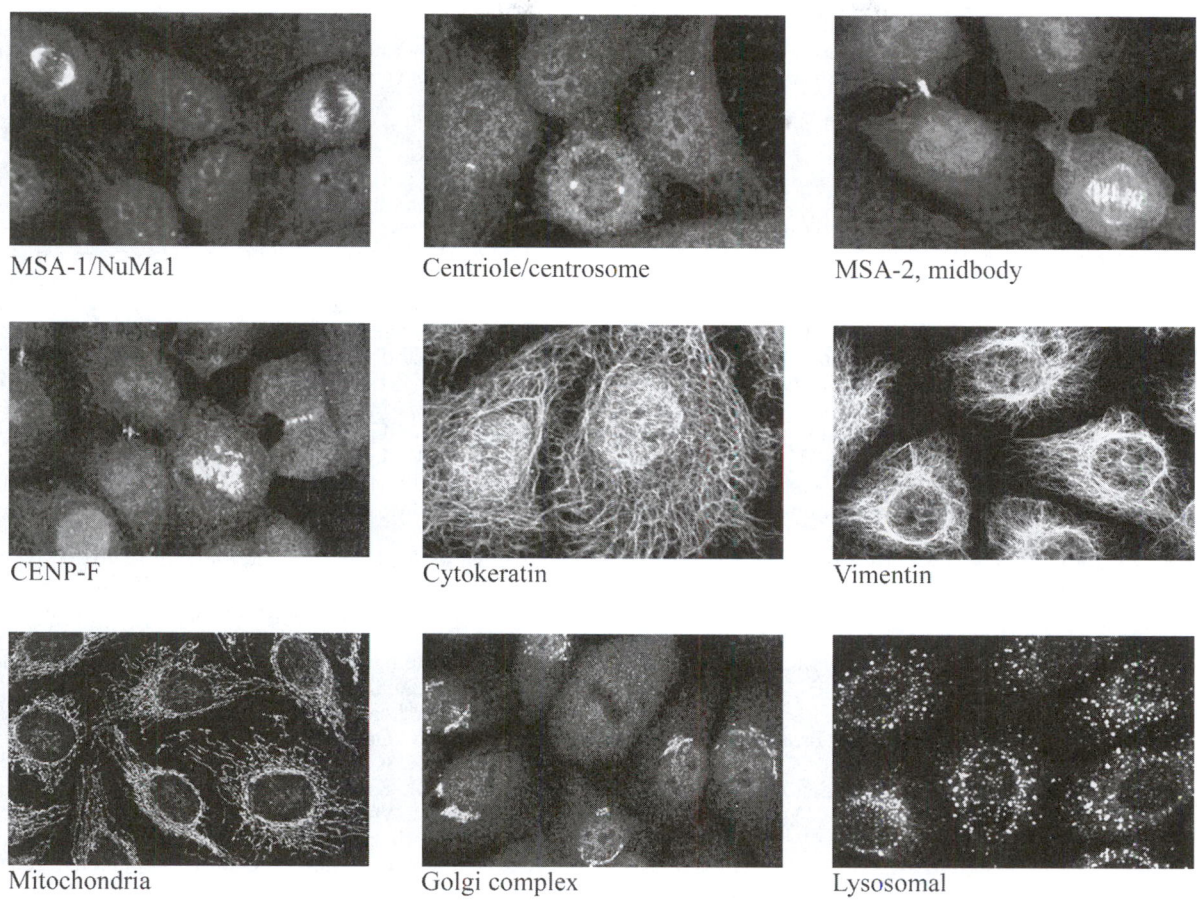

MSA-1/NuMa1   Centriole/centrosome   MSA-2, midbody

CENP-F   Cytokeratin   Vimentin

Mitochondria   Golgi complex   Lysosomal

FIGURE 2   (*Continued*)

Specific immunoassays are used to analyze HEp-2-positive sera in more detail. The following is a brief description of the different methods, but details should be sought elsewhere.

1. Immunodiffusion and countercurrent immunoelectrophoresis (CIE). These are the simplest and most specific but least sensitive methods of ENA identification. An initial screening assay uses a polyvalent antigen extract that contains all common ENAs. The test is inexpensive, and negative samples (70 to 80%) are easily screened out. Positive sera are then further tested against well-characterized, monospecific antibodies by a similar procedure. A mask for sample application on CIE gels increases the sensitivity and precision of the assay.

2. Immunoblotting. The Western blot assay is an essential tool for the detailed characterization of many autoantibodies. Molecular mass markers and positive and negative controls are run together in each assay. These provide the necessary comparison bands alongside those of the patient sera. However, the assay is relatively expensive in comparison with EIAs. Furthermore, the antigens are displayed as linear polypeptides, which distorts conformational epitopes, so the results are not always accurate. For example, the international SS-A (anti-Ro) material AF/CDC7 is negative by Western blot although positive on HEp-2 cells (Table 2). This has also been observed with other antigens, such as PM-Scl (16).

3. EIAs. These are widely used for quantifying samples with antibodies against dsDNA and ENAs, and more recently, some laboratories use them when screening for ANAs. The dsDNA and ENA EIAs are very sensitive assays, and monitoring patients with quantitative measurements for autoantibodies against dsDNA and some ENAs is useful (e.g., Jo-1). In the case of anti-dsDNA autoantibodies, there is a clear relationship between disease activity and antibody titer. However, many autoantibodies do not fluctuate with disease activity, so accurate quantitation is not always necessary.

REFERENCES

1. Abuaf, N., G. Chyderiotis, L. Grangeot-Keros, A.-M. Rouquette, G. Servais, R.-J. van de Stadt, and R. Stokes. 1998. Étude européenne, multicentrique: comparison de la sensibilité des lames de cellules HEp-2 avec des sérums contenent des anticorps anti-SSA/Ro. *Option/Bio* **220:**(Suppl.)7–13.
2. Beck, J. S. 1961. Variations in the morphological patterns of autoimmune nuclear fluorescence. *Lancet* **1:**1203–1205.
3. Bradwell, A. R., R. G. Hughes, and E. L. Harden. 2003. *Atlas of HEp-2 Patterns*, 2nd ed. The Binding Site Ltd., Birmingham, United Kingdom.
4. Bradwell, A. R., R. P. Stokes, and G. P. Mead. 1999. *Advanced Atlas of Autoantibody Patterns*. The Binding Site Ltd., Birmingham, United Kingdom.
5. Conrad, K., W. Schlosler, F. Hiepe, and M. J. Fritzler. 2002. *Autoantibodies in Systemic Autoimmune Disease. A Diagnostic Reference*, vol. 2. Pabst Science Publishers, Berlin, Germany.

6. **Coons, A. H., and M. H. Kaplan.** 1950. Localization of antigen in tissue cells. II. Improvements in a method for the detection of antigen by means of fluorescent antibody. *J. Exp. Med.* **91**:1–13.

7. **Emlen, W., and L. O'Neill.** 1997. Clinical significance of antinuclear antibodies: comparison of detection with immunofluorescence and enzyme-linked immunosorbent assays. *Arthritis Rheum.* **40**:1612–1618.

8. **Feltkamp, T. E. W.** 1996. Antinuclear antibody determination in a routine laboratory. *Ann. Rheum. Dis.* **55**:723–727.

9. **Feng, Y., X. Ke, R. Ma, Y. Chen, G. Hu, and F. Liu.** 2004. Parallel detection of autoantibodies with microarrays in rheumatoid diseases. *Clin. Chem.* **50**:416–422.

10. **Hargraves, M. M., H., Richmond, and R. Morton.** 1948. Presentation of 2 bone marrow elements; "tart" cell and "L.E." cell. *Proc. Mayo Clin.* **23**:25–28.

11. **Holborow, E. J., D. M. Weir, and G. D. Johnson.** 1957. A serum factor in lupus erythematosus with affinity for tissue nuclei. *Br. Med. J.* **2**:732–734.

12. **Humbel, R. L.** 1994. Detection of antinuclear antibodies by immunofluorescence, p. 1–16. *In* W. J. Van Venrooij and R. N. Maini (ed.), *Manual of Biological Markers of Disease*, vol. A2. Kluwer Academic Publishers, Dordrecht, The Netherlands.

13. **Jaskowski, T. D., C. M. S. Schroder, T. B. Martins, C. L. Mouritsen, C. M. Litwin, and H. R. Hill.** 1996. Screening for antinuclear antibodies by enzyme immunoassay. *Am. J. Clin. Pathol.* **105**:468–473.

14. **Lee, S. L., S. R. Michael, and I. L. Vural.** 1951. The L.E. (Lupus Erythematosus) cell. *Am. J. Med.* **10**:446–451.

15. **Mimori, T., M. Kanai, and Y. Ishihara.** 1999. *Atlas of Antinuclear Antibodies.* Medical and Biological Laboratories Co., Ltd., Nagoya, Japan.

16. **Odis, C. V., and I. N. Targoff.** 1996. PM-Scl autoantibodies, p. 642–650. *In* J. B. Peter and Y. Shoenfeld. (ed.), *Autoantibodies.* Elsevier Science B.V., Amsterdam, The Netherlands.

17. **Pollock, W., and T. Ban-Hock** 1999. Routine immunofluorescence detection of Ro/SS-A autoantibody using HEp-2 cells transfected with human 60 kDa Ro/SS-A. *J. Clin. Pathol.* **52**:684–687.

18. **Smolen, J. S., B. Butcher, M. J. Fritzler, T. Gordon, J. Hardin, J. R. Kalden, R. Lahita, R. N. Maini, W. Reeves, M. Reichlin, N. Rothfield, Y. Rakasaki, W. J. van Venrooij, and E. M. Tan.** 1997. Reference sera for antinuclear antibodies. II. Further definition of antibody specificities in international antinuclear antibody reference sera by immunofluorescence and Western blotting. *Arthritis Rheum.* **40**:413–418.

19. **Storch, W. B.** 2000. *Immunofluorescence in Clinical Immunology* (English edition). Birkhäuser Verlag, Basel, Switzerland.

20. **Tan, E. M.** 1982. Antibodies to nuclear antigens (ANA): their immunobiology and medicine. *Adv. Immunol.* **33**:167–240.

21. **Tan, E. M., T. E. W. Feltkamp, D. Alarcon-Segovia, R. L. Dawkins, H. Homma, J. R. Kalden, P. H. Lambert, A. Lange, R. N. Maini, F. C. McDuffie, J. S. McDougal, R. Norberg, and M. Wilson.** 1988. Reference reagents for antinuclear antibodies. *Arthritis Rheum.* **31**:1331.

22. **Tan, E. M., T. E. W. Feltkamp, J. S. Smolen, B. Butcher, R. Dawkins, M. J. Fritzler, T. Gordon, J. A. Hardin, J. R. Kalden, R. G. Lahita, R. N. Maini, J. S. McDougal, N. F. Rothfield, R. J. Smeenk, Y. Takasaki, A. Wiik, M. R. Wilson, and J. A. Koziol.** 1997. Range of antinuclear antibodies in "healthy" individuals. *Arthritis Rheum.* **40**:1601–1611.

23. **Tan, E. M., M. J. Fritzler, J. S. McDougal, F. C. McDuffie, R. M. Nakamura, M. Reichlin, C. B. Reimer, G. C. Sharp, P. H. Schur, M. R. Wilson, and R. J. Winchester.** 1982. Reference sera for antinuclear antibodies. I. Antibodies to native DNA, Sm, nuclear RNP and SS-B/La. *Arthritis Rheum.* **25**:1003–1005.

24. **Tan, E. M., J. Smolen, J. S. McDougal, B. T. Butcher, D. Conn, R. Dawkins, M. J. Fritzler, T. Gordon, J. A. Hardin, J. R. Kalden, R. G. Lahita, R. N. Maini, N. A. Rothfield, R. Smeenk, Y. Takasaki, W. J. van Venrooij, A. Wiik, M. Wilson, and J. A. Koziol.** 1999. A critical evaluation of enzyme immunoassays for detection of antinuclear autoantibodies of defined specificities. *Arthritis Rheum.* **42**:455–464.

25. **Tan, E. M., J. Smolen, J. S. McDougal, M. J. Fritzler, T. Gordon, J. A. Hardin, J. R. Kalden, R. G. Lahita, R. N. Maini, W. H. Reeves, N. F. Rothfield, Y. Takasaki, A. Wiik, M. Wilson, and J. A. Kozoil.** 2002. A critical evaluation of enzyme immunoassay kits for detection of antinuclear autoantibodies of defined specificities. II. Potential for quantitation of antibody content. *J. Rheum.* **29**:68–74.

26. **Von Muhlen, C. A., and E. M. Tan.** 1995. Autoantibodies in the diagnosis of systemic rheumatic diseases. *Semin. Arthritis Rheum.* **24**:323–358.

Detection of Autoantibodies against Proteins and Ribonucleoproteins by Double Immunodiffusion and Immunoprecipitation

WESTLEY H. REEVES, MINORU SATOH, ROBERT LYONS, CODY NICHOLS, AND SONALI NARAIN

113

INTRODUCTION AND BACKGROUND

Antinuclear antibodies (ANA) are markers for systemic autoimmune disease but also can be seen at low titers in healthy individuals (20). Thus, there has been considerable interest in identifying ANA subsets with greater diagnostic specificity for particular diseases. Autoantibodies specific for systemic lupus erythematosus (SLE), systemic sclerosis (SSc), polymyositis or dermatomyositis (PM/DM), and other systemic autoimmune disorders have been identified (Table 1) and are of considerable importance as diagnostic markers. The prevalence of some of the more useful autoantibody markers for various diseases is summarized in Table 2.

SLE

Several autoantibodies are produced uniquely in SLE. Anti-double-stranded DNA (anti-dsDNA) antibodies are found in ~70% of SLE patients' sera at some point during their disease and are 95% specific. Levels of anti-dsDNA antibodies may vary reciprocally with complement levels, serving as a marker of disease activity. Anti-Sm antibodies are produced by 7 to 25% of lupus patients, depending on ethnic origin, and, like anti-dsDNA, are virtually pathognomonic of SLE (12). Unlike anti-DNA antibodies, the levels of anti-Sm antibodies generally do not correlate with disease activity. Anti-nRNP antibodies, which recognize proteins associated with the Sm antigen, are not disease specific (Table 1). They are present at high levels in mixed connective tissue disease (MCTD) (12). The frequency of anti-nRNP antibodies in SLE is 20 to 40%. All but a few sera containing anti-Sm antibodies contain anti-nRNP autoantibodies as well. However, anti-nRNP antibodies frequently occur without anti-Sm.

Antiribosomal antibodies which recognize the P0, P1, and P2 antigens (Table 1) are found in about 15% of SLE patients (5). They also are highly specific for SLE. Anti-proliferating cell nuclear antigen (anti-PCNA) (2 to 5% of patients) antibodies are specific for SLE as well.

Sicca Syndrome and Sjögren's Syndrome

Anti-Ro (SS-A) and anti-La (SS-B) autoantibodies are associated with Sjögren's syndrome as well as other systemic autoimmune diseases when they are accompanied by sicca symptoms (e.g., SLE). Anti-Ro (SS-A) antibodies are found in 10 to 50% of serum samples from SLE patients and 60 to 80%

of primary Sjögren's syndrome sera (24). They recognize two antigens, one of 60 kDa (Ro60) and the other of 52 kDa (Ro52) (see below and Table 1). Anti-La (SS-B) autoantibodies are produced by 10 to 20% of SLE patients and at a somewhat higher frequency in Sjögren's syndrome. Anti-La is virtually always associated with anti-Ro, whereas anti-Ro antibodies frequently are detected in the absence of anti-La.

Congenital Complete Heart Block

Cardiac conduction abnormalities in neonates are strongly associated with maternal antibody against the Ro (especially Ro52) and La antigens (2). Screening for these autoantibodies in pregnant women with systemic autoimmune disease is important. Since these autoantibodies may be present in asymptomatic individuals, screening also is carried out in mothers of children with congenital cardiac conduction abnormalities.

SSc

A nucleolar pattern on fluorescent ANA testing is common in SSc. Nucleolar antigens recognized by SSc-specific autoantibodies include fibrillarin, the To/Th ribonucleoprotein, and RNA polymerases I and III (RNAP I/III) (10 to 20% of patients [Table 1]) (9, 15). The nucleoplasmic and nucleolar enzyme topoisomerase I (topo I) (Scl-70) also is an important marker found in ~15% of patients. Anti-topo I and RNAP I/III both are associated with a poor prognosis and with proximal scleroderma rather than just sclerodactyly. Autoantibodies against RNAP II also are present in SSc but are not disease specific. When present along with anti-topo I, antibodies against the phosphorylated form of RNAP II predict a poor outcome (17). Antifibrillarin (5 to 8% of patients) and anti-To/Th (5%) antibodies also are diagnostically useful specificities (Table 1).

PM/DM

Autoantibodies to a set of cytoplasmic antigens, many of which are aminoacyl tRNA synthetases, are diagnostic markers for PM/DM (Table 1). These antibodies are rare in the absence of myositis. The most common is anti-histidyl-tRNA synthetase (anti-Jo-1), which is produced by 20% or more of adult myositis patients (Table 1) (22). Other tRNA synthetases recognized by PM/DM sera include threonyl (anti-PL-7; 3% of patients), alanyl (anti-PL-12; 3 to 8% of patients), isoleucyl (anti-OJ; 2% of patients), glycyl (anti-EJ; 2% of patients), and

TABLE 1 Some non-DNA/chromatin autoantibodies useful in the diagnosis of systemic autoimmune disease

Disease(s)	Autoantibody	Protein component(s)	RNA component(s)
SLE	Sm	B′/B (29/28 kDa), D1/2/3 (16 kDa), E/F/G (12, 11, 10 kDa)	U1, U2, U4–U6, U5
	Ribosomal P	P0, P1, P2 (38, 19, 17 kDa)	rRNA
	PCNA	36 kDa	None
MCTD and others	RNP	70K (70 kDa), A (33 kDa), C (23 kDa)	U1
Sicca syndrome	Ro (SS-A)	Ro60 (60 kDa), Ro52 (52 kDa)	hY1, hY3, hY4, hY5
	La (SS-B)	48 kDa	8-2, 7-2, 7SL, 5S, hY1, hY3, hY4, hY5, tRNAs
SLE, MCTD, PM, SSC	Ku	Ku80 (80 kDa); Ku70 (70 kDa)	None
SLE, SSC	RNAP II	240 (IIO), 220 (IIA), 140 (IIB) kDa	None
PM/DM	Various tRNA synthetases	His (50 kDa), Thr (80 kDa), Ala (110 kDa), Ile (150 kDa), Gly (75 kDa), Leu (130 kDa), Asp (65 kDa)	Corresponding tRNAs
	SRP	72, 68, 54, 19, 14, 9 kDa	7SL
SSc	Topoisomerase I	100 kDa	None
	Fibrillarin	34 kDa	U3
	RNAP I/III	RNAP I: 190 (IA), 126 (IB) kDa; RNAP III: 155 (IIIA), 138 (IIIB) kDa	None
	To/Th	40 kDa (not readily visualized)	7-2, 8-2

asparaginyl (Table 1). For unclear reasons, only one antisynthetase autoantibody is usually detected in an individual patient. All of these autoantibodies are associated with myositis, interstitial lung disease, Raynaud's phenomenon, mechanic's hands (roughened skin over the fingertips), arthritis, and fever, a constellation known as antisynthetase autoantibody syndrome. Autoantibodies to the signal recognition particle (SRP) also are myositis specific (4% of patients) and may be a marker for severe disease.

Conclusions

Autoantibodies recognize a diverse array of nuclear and cytoplasmic antigens. Some of these autoantibodies are clinically useful markers for subsets of systemic autoimmune disease, such as SLE, SSc, or PM/DM. Others are useful because they point to organ involvement, e.g., lacrimal or salivary gland involvement with anti-Ro (SS-A) or anti-La (SS-B), though they are not disease specific. Finally, other autoantibodies are useful prognostically (e.g., anti-topo I or anti-RNAP I/III in SSc and anti-SRP in PM). Despite the importance of these autoantibodies as clinical markers, diagnostic tests for them often are less than optimal. This chapter deals with how to detect them reliably in a clinical or research setting. It is hoped that newer tests based on recombinant autoantigens will eventually take the place of some of the more technically difficult tests described below.

DID IN AGAROSE GELS (OUCHTERLONY)

Double immunodiffusion (DID) (Ouchterlony method) is a classic immunoassay to detect interactions of antigens and antibodies. Anti-Sm was the first lupus-specific autoantibody

TABLE 2 Prevalence of some non-DNA/chromatin autoantibodies by disease

Autoantibody	Prevalence in disease subset (%)			
	SLE (n = 288)	Sjögren's (n = 50)	PM/DM (n = 30)	Scleroderma (n = 42)
Sm	10	0	0	0
RNP	39	6	0	12
Ribosomal P	2	0	0	0
PCNA	0.3	0	0	0
Ro60 (SS-A)	33	58	13	12
Ro52[a]	28	36	49	15
La (SS-B)	11	28	7	0
Jo-1[b]	1	ND[c]	22	0
Alanyl tRNA synthetase[b]	0	ND	6	ND
Ku	2	0	0	2
RNAPI/III	0	0	0	21
RNAP II	5	2	0	7
Scl-70 (topo I)	0.3	0	0	7

[a] Recombinant antigen ELISA (SLE, n = 265; Sjögren's, n = 50; PM/DM, n = 35; scleroderma, n = 40).
[b] Recombinant antigen ELISA (SLE, n = 74; PM/DM, n = 51; scleroderma, n = 36).
[c] ND, not done.

system to be defined as a precipitin line (21). Additional precipitating autoantibodies were defined by using sera from patients with systemic rheumatic diseases, including anti-nRNP, anti-Ro (SS-A), anti-La (SS-B), anti-topo I (Scl-70), and Jo-1 (12). Antigens, such as rabbit thymus extract (RTE) or human lymphocyte extract, are added to wells punched in an agarose gel. Serum samples are placed in adjacent wells. Antigenic proteins or protein complexes in the cell extract and antibodies in the serum diffuse toward one another in the gel and form insoluble antigen-antibody complexes when the antigen-to-antibody ratio is near equivalence. Formation of insoluble immune complexes in the gel is seen as a white precipitin line.

Technology and Instrumentation

Instrumentation for the DID assay is simple, consisting of a suitable agarose gel and apparatus for punching holes in the gel, viewing the precipitin lines, and documenting the pattern photographically. The following equipment is needed: a magnetic stirrer and hot plate, a light box with black background, and a gel puncher (commercial suppliers are becoming scarce; as an alternative, a gel puncher can be made with straws or similar materials by assembling short-cut pieces with Super Glue [Fig. 1]).

The agarose gel is prepared by heating 0.6% (wt/vol) agarose in phosphate-buffered saline (PBS) with 0.02% NaN_3 and stirring the mixture on a heating plate until clear. Boiling should be avoided. A microwave oven can be used initially to shorten the heating time. A 100-mm-diameter petri dish is placed on a level surface, and 15 ml of agarose gel solution is added per plate (the amount of gel differs depending on the size of the wells and amount of extract or serum). The lid is replaced after the gel cools, and the plate is stored overnight to several weeks at 4°C in a humidified chamber or else sealed with Parafilm.

Just before use, wells are made in the agarose with a homemade gel puncher by pushing straight down gently until the bottom of the plate is reached. Pieces of gel in the wells are aspirated by use of vacuum suction and a Pasteur pipette. If the vacuum is too strong, it may damage the gel. Pieces of gel should be picked up from inside the wells by making a circular movement with the pipette. Appropriate dilutions of antigens, serum samples, and reference sera are prepared (see below) with PBS, and 40 μl is added slowly to

each well to avoid overflow. The petri dishes should be left undisturbed in a humid chamber (wet gauze or paper towels in a tightly capped plastic box work well).

Several sources of antigens can be used, including commercial extracts (e.g., RTE) and extracts of human cell lines. To prepare RTE, rabbit thymus acetone powder is stirred at a concentration of 0.2 g/ml in PBS in a flask or beaker at 4°C overnight and then centrifuged at 9,000 × g for 30 min at 4°C in a microcentrifuge. The supernatant is collected, and small aliquots are frozen at −80°C until use.

K562 (human erythroleukemia) cells grown in log-phase culture (the medium is RPMI 1640 with 10% fetal bovine serum, penicillin-streptomycin, and L-glutamine) are a convenient source of human cellular proteins. They are collected by centrifugation, washed once with PBS, counted, and pelleted at 800 × g for 10 min. After the PBS is aspirated, the cell pellet is frozen (−80°C) for future use. To prepare extract, 100 μl of PBS is added per 10^8 cells to either frozen cells or a freshly prepared cell pellet. The cells are sonicated on ice to disrupt them (Branson sonifier, 30% output setting 3, for 50 s). The lysate is centrifuged at 9,000 × g for 30 min at 4°C (microcentrifuge). The supernatant is collected and aliquots are frozen at −80°C.

Other antigens can be used, including calf thymus acetone powder (Pel-Freez), fresh calf thymus extract, Wil-2 cell extract, human spleen extract, etc. Antibodies that can be detected with RTE, calf thymus extract, or K562 cell extract are summarized in Table 2.

Assays

Sera stored at 4°C with NaN_3 or frozen at −80 or −20°C can be used. The following materials and reagents are needed:

PBS (0.15 M NaCl–20 mM sodium phosphate, pH 7.2)

Agarose (SeaKem ME; FMC Bioproducts, Rockland, Maine [catalog no. 50010])

10% NaN_3 in distilled water

Plastic petri dish (diameter, 100 mm for four sets of seven wells)

Rabbit thymus acetone powder, calf thymus acetone powder (Pel-Freez), or cell pellet (human lymphocytes, spleen cells, K562, HeLa, or other cells)

Serum samples from patients with systemic rheumatic diseases frequently form more than one precipitin line, and the optimal dilution to form precipitin lines may vary (Fig. 2B). Even if the sample forms only one precipitin line, some sera contain autoantibodies at such a high titer that the precipitin line can be seen only with highly diluted samples. Therefore, it is essential to test serially diluted serum first to see whether precipitin lines are formed. Sera are undiluted (1:1) or diluted with PBS 1:4, 1:16, 1:64, 1:256, and 1:1,024. The diluted samples are used to identify an appropriate dilution for each precipitin line prior to comparison with reference sera. For this purpose, antigen can be placed in the center well with serially diluted serum samples set around it in clockwise order (Fig. 2B).

The precipitin lines should be sketched, and the appropriate dilution and titer for each precipitin line should be determined. At the optimal dilution, a precipitin line should form about halfway between the antigen and antibody wells. Sometimes, a dilution at which two or more precipitin lines are clearly separated may need to be used (Fig. 2C and D). It is easier to interpret the results if the precipitin lines are not too close to the antigen or serum wells.

Dilutions of the reference sera are determined as described above for the test samples. The appearance of precipitin lines

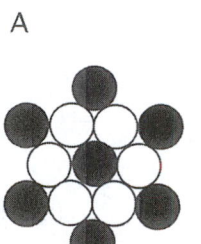
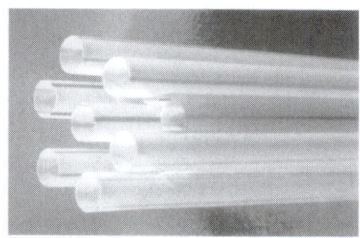

FIGURE 1 Homemade gel puncher for DID. A design for assembling a simple "cookie cutter" punch for agarose gels out of drinking straws is shown. (A) Arrangement of the straws. Seven straws (black) are used to punch holes in the gel, and six additional straws (white) are used as spacers and recessed so that they do not contact the agarose gel. (B) Assembled hole puncher. Straws are assembled as shown in the diagram, using Super Glue. Note the recessed spacer straws that maintain the proper distance between holes.

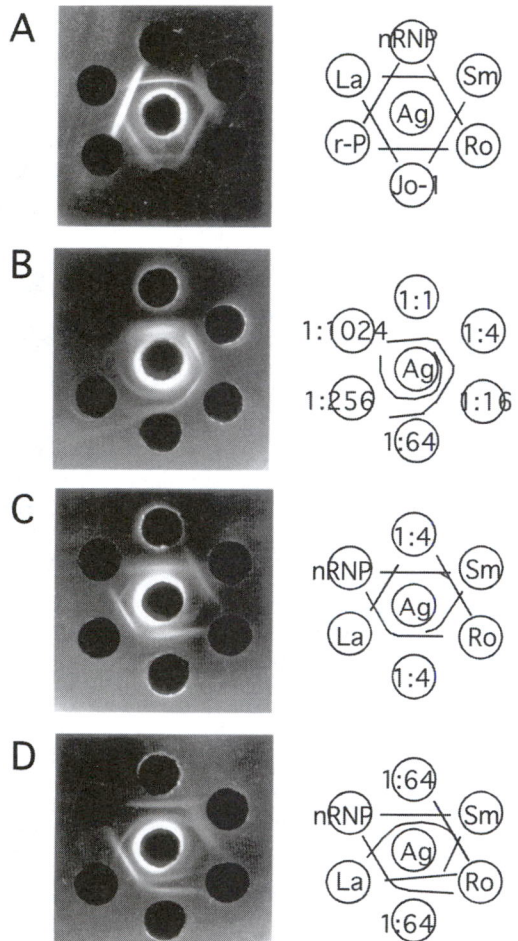

FIGURE 2 DID in agarose gels. A photograph of the assay is shown on the left, and an interpretation is diagrammed on the right. (A) Appearance of precipitin lines when properly diluted reference sera with the following specificities are used: anti-nRNP, anti-Sm (note line of partial identity with anti-nRNP), anti-Ro, anti-Jo-1, anti-ribosomal P (r-P), and anti-La. (B) Determining the optimal serum dilution. Test serum was diluted 1:1, 1:4, 1:16, 1:64, 1:256, and 1:1,024 with PBS. The optimal dilution for precipitin line 1 is 1:4; optimal dilution for line 2 is 1:64. (C and D) DID using dilutions of 1:4 (C) and 1:64 (D) of the serum shown in panel B. Precipitin line 1 is identified as anti-La (C). Precipitin line 2 is identified as anti-nRNP (D).

when properly diluted reference sera are used is illustrated in Fig. 2A. When a test sample does not form precipitin lines, it is considered negative by DID and not tested further. When the sample forms one or more precipitin lines, a second assay must be carried out. The arrangement of samples with unknown precipitin lines, reference sera, and antigens will differ depending on the situation. Examples are shown in Fig. 3. If the sample has unknown precipitin lines that need to be tested for several different specificities, the arrangements in Fig. 3A and B are convenient. If the sample forms precipitin lines with different antigens (e.g., one line with RTE and another with human lymphocyte extract), Fig. 3B may be useful. If several samples (u1 to u4) need to be tested for a single specificity, the arrangements in Fig. 3C and D can be used. If the antigen is valuable, the arrangement in

Fig. 3A or C will help to minimize the amount used. If the serum sample is limited, the arrangement in Fig. 3B will be useful. Figure 3C or D (especially the latter) should be useful when the amount of reference serum is limited.

Attention should be given to which specificities will be tested. Information from the fluorescent ANA test and/or suspected diagnosis can be used to focus attention on particular antigens for more efficient screening of unknown precipitin lines. For example, if the clinical diagnosis is SLE, a panel of lupus-related reference sera such as anti-Sm and ribosomal P should be tested initially rather than scleroderma or myositis reference sera (Table 1). Similarly, there are autoantibodies associated with certain symptoms such as Raynaud's phenomenon (anti-nRNP) or sicca (Ro/SS-A, La/SS-B) (Table 1). Consideration of the clinical diagnosis or clinical manifestations will help to identify precipitin lines more efficiently and less expensively. Similarly, the ANA pattern (e.g., nuclear or cytoplasmic) can be used to narrow the list of diagnostic possibilities, avoiding unnecessary testing. In many cases, sera positive for ANA may be screened for a set of common autoantibodies such as anti-nRNP, -Sm, -Ro, and -La. If they are negative, additional specificities can be tested on the basis of clinical information or ANA pattern. However, there are pitfalls to this approach. First, a cytoplasmic pattern may not be reported consistently by the laboratory. Second, when cytoplasmic staining is brighter than nuclear staining, ANA can be reported as negative because it is often difficult to tell whether there is coexisting (but weaker) nuclear staining.

Quality Assurance, Quality Control, and Test Validation

Normal human serum can be used as a negative control. Positive reference sera are available from the Centers for

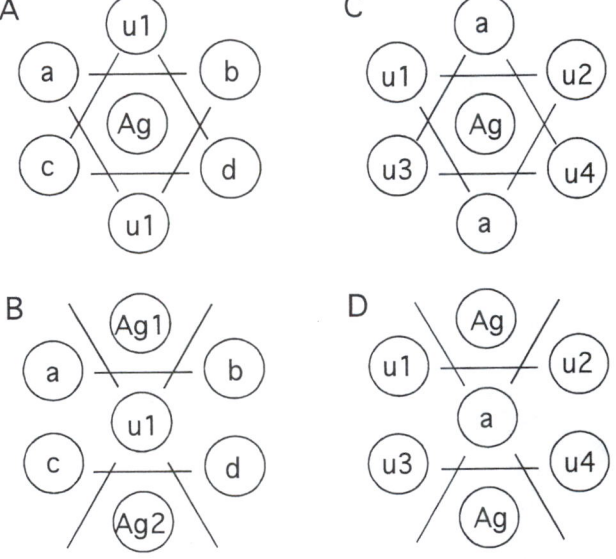

FIGURE 3 Typical arrangements of sera and antigens for DID. (A and B) Arrangements for testing an unknown precipitin line for several specificities. Panel A illustrates the use of a single antigen; Panel B illustrates use of two different test antigens (e.g., RTE and human lymphocyte extract). (C and D) Arrangements for testing several sera for a single autoantibody specificity when reference serum is precious. Ag1 and Ag2, antigens; u1 to u4, sera with unknown specificities; a to d, reference sera.

Disease Control and Prevention (CDC) and commercially. It often is convenient to develop a set of in-house standards monospecific for individual precipitin lines. In-house reference sera should form a single strong precipitin line that fuses with the precipitin line formed by the CDC reference serum. Once good sera are found, try to obtain 20 to 30 ml or more of each in order to maintain a stock that can be used over a period of several years.

It is best to make a large amount of antigen and freeze small aliquots at −80°C. When a new lot of antigen is prepared, it must be tested for all antibody systems that normally form precipitin lines. The titer of each reference serum with each antigen should be recorded. This is the highest serum dilution at which a precipitin line can be seen clearly. It is ideal to standardize (by diluting, if necessary) the antigen with a panel of reference sera. Adjustment of the antigen concentration so that the titers are ±1 dilution will assure lot-to-lot reproducibility. Only freshly thawed antigens should be used, and they should not be refrozen.

Antigens in cell extracts can be heavily degraded. Antigens in acetone powder are more denatured than the same antigens in calf thymus extract or lymphocyte extract. Antibodies that preferentially recognize native molecules may not bind denatured antigens in acetone powder but may recognize the more native molecules in a cell extract. Although detergents such as Nonidet P-40 (NP-40) and Tween 20 extract proteins efficiently and are used to prepare extracts for other immunoassays, they cause artifacts in DID and should not be used.

The advantage of DID is its simplicity. DID is highly specific when autoantibodies produce precipitin lines that are strong and sharp and when only a single precipitin line exists. Although all specificities may not be identified on initial screening, autoantibodies to various antigens can be detected by a single test without purifying the target antigens.

A major disadvantage of DID is the difficulty in interpreting weak precipitin lines when multiple lines, especially strong and diffuse lines, coexist in the same sample. If there is only one precipitin line, the chance of misinterpretation is low. Autoantibodies that form sharp, strong precipitin lines, such as anti-nRNP and anti-La (SS-B), are easy to interpret. On the other hand, weak and faint lines, such as anti-Ro (SS-A) and anti-Ku, can be misinterpreted, especially in the presence of another strong or diffuse line. Other disadvantages include the large amounts of sera and antigens used and the fact that the reaction takes several days. Although DID is useful for many autoantibody systems, some autoantibodies, such as antifibrillarin, anti-RNA polymerases, and anti-7-2 RNP, do not produce precipitin lines and are undetectable by DID.

Although DID has been used for over 30 years to detect autoantibodies such as anti-Sm and anti-nRNP, the precise mechanism of formation of precipitin lines is not completely understood. For example, it is not known which component of the U snRNP is responsible for the precipitin lines. There is no clear explanation why the anti-nRNP precipitin line disappears when cell extract is pretreated with RNase.

Cost Assessment

Over 30 years after the initial reports, and despite the introduction of more sophisticated techniques, DID remains a standard method for detecting many clinically useful autoantibody systems because of its simplicity and reliability. However, it is labor-intensive and has gradually fallen out of common use in favor of enzyme-linked immunosorbent assays (ELISAs) and other techniques that are more amenable to automation. Because of the difficulty in automating DID, this assay is relatively expensive. Despite its cost, the false-positive rate is significantly lower than that seen with ELISAs (S. Narain et al., unpublished data). Thus, the DID assay is highly cost-effective, since the expense (both monetary and psychological) of a false-positive test can be considerable.

Interpretation

The result is interpreted visually by examining the precipitin lines after 1, 2, 3, and 5 days. The observer should sketch the precipitin lines and judge if they fuse (identity = positive), cross (nonidentity = negative), or partially fuse (partial identity, some common part of the two antibody-antigen systems) with the lines formed by reference sera. The gels are washed carefully with PBS, avoiding bubbles, especially under the agarose gel. Afterward, PBS is added to a level 1 to 2 mm above the gel, 2 to 3 drops of 10% NaN$_3$ are added, and the gel can be stored at 4°C. The gel is photographed on a dark background for documentation.

Generally, the sensitivity of DID is good, and the results correlate well with more sensitive and specific methods, such as radioimmunoprecipitation (henceforth referred to as immunoprecipitation). DID remains one of the methods of choice for detecting common autoantibodies in clinical practice. In particular, commercial ELISAs for anti-Sm are unreliable, and no simple alternative to DID is available at present. The passive hemagglutination assay (11) is a good alternative but has fallen out of use.

Since the titers often are not reported and the significance of changing titers has not been emphasized, DID usually is not considered a quantitative assay. However, it can be made semiquantitative by determining the highest dilution of serum that forms a clear precipitin line.

Clear fusion of two precipitin lines is highly specific for identity. Conversely, if the precipitin lines formed by the sample and the reference serum cross, it indicates nonidentity. Partial fusion between anti-nRNP and anti-Sm precipitin lines is observed, but specificity should be verified by using monospecific anti-nRNP and anti-Sm reference sera.

Remarks and Conclusions

DID is a classic method to detect autoantibodies found in sera from patients with systemic rheumatic diseases. Positive results usually are very reliable. However, at times, false-negative or -positive results can occur due to multiple specificities, technical difficulties, or low sensitivity. Nevertheless, DID is a useful test, especially in view of the lack of good alternatives for detecting certain autoantibodies, such as anti-Sm.

IMMUNOPRECIPITATION: PROTEINS

Gel diffusion and ELISA, unlike Western blot assays (see below), allow the detection of autoantibodies to native antigenic determinants, but the composition of the antigenic particles and fine specificities of the autoantibodies cannot readily be determined. Western blotting, although useful for defining fine specificities, is of limited value for detecting antibodies against conformational epitopes. For this reason, immunoprecipitation of radiolabeled cell extracts has become an important research tool for examining antibody specificities. For the detection of a number of clinically important specificities, immunoprecipitation should be considered the "gold standard" against which other techniques are measured (Table 3).

TABLE 3 Gold standards for autoantibody testing (non-DNA/chromatin antigens)[a]

Autoantibody	Gold standard	Other good alternatives
Sm	R-IPP, DID	P-IPP
RNP	R-IPP, P-IPP, DID	
Ro60 (SS-A)	P-IPP	R-IPP, EIA, DID
Ro52	WB	EIA
La (SS-B)	R-IPP, DID	P-IPP, ELISA, WB
Ribosomal P	P-IPP	DID; P-peptide EIA
Ku	P-IPP	DID, EIA
Jo-1 (histidyl tRNA synthetase)	R-IPP	DID, recombinant antigen EIA
PL-7 (threonyl tRNA synthetase)	P-IPP, R-IPP	DID
SRP	P-IPP, R-IPP	
RNAP I, II, III	P-IPP	
Topoisomerase I	DID	WB, P-IPP
Fibrillarin	R-IPP	WB, P-IPP
To/Th	R-IPP	

[a] P-IPP, protein immunoprecipitation; R-IPP, RNA immunoprecipitation; WB, Western blot; EIA, enzyme immunoassay.

Technology and Instrumentation

Radiolabeled antigens are allowed to form immune complexes with autoantibodies and purified onto protein A-Sepharose beads. After the immune complexes are dissociated from the beads, the radiolabeled proteins are separated by sodium dodecyl sulfate (SDS)-polyacrylamide gel electrophoresis and detected by autoradiography (16). A similar approach can be used to analyze the nucleic acid components of small ribonucleoprotein particles (see below) (8). Required apparatus includes an electrophoresis power supply, vertical electrophoresis apparatus (e.g., models from CBS Scientific, Del Mar, Calif.), tabletop centrifuge, CO_2 incubator, cell sonicator (Branson), and microcentrifuge.

The following materials and reagents are needed:

Phenylmethylsulfonyl fluoride (PMSF) (Sigma no. P7626): 50 mM in absolute ethanol stored at $-20°C$ ($=100\times$ stock)

Aprotinin (Sigma, catalog no. A6279): 24 trypsin inhibitor units (TIU) in double-distilled H_2O ($=100\times$ stock)

Protein A-Sepharose CL4B (PAS) (Pharmacia no. 17-0780-01). Prepare the PAS as follows:

1. Add H_2O to 1.5 g of dry PAS in a 15-ml centrifuge tube and incubate with intermittent inversion for 20 to 30 min at room temperature to swell the beads.
2. Centrifuge for 1 min in a tabletop centrifuge ($800 \times g$).
3. Wash the beads three times with H_2O and centrifuge to pellet the beads.
4. To the packed beads, add an equal volume of H_2O. Add 2 M Tris-HCl (pH 8.0) to a final concentration of 20 mM (1:100). Add NaN_3 to a final concentration of 0.1%. The beads can be stored at 4°C in this buffer.

0.5 M NaCl NET/NP-40 buffer: 50 mM Tris-HCl (pH 7.5), 0.5 M NaCl, 2 mM EDTA, 0.3% NP-40

NET buffer: 50 mM Tris-HCl (pH 7.5), 0.15 M NaCl, 2 mM EDTA

3× sample buffer: mix 0.5 M Tris-HCl (pH 6.8) (6.0 ml), 1% bromophenol blue (0.6 ml), 2-mercaptoethanol (3.0 ml), 25% SDS (4.8 ml), and glycerol (6.0 ml). This mixture can be stored at $-20°C$.

Sterile Dulbecco's PBS (D-PBS): NaCl (160 g), Na_2HPO_4 (dibasic; 23 g), KCl (8 g), KH_2PO_4 (monobasic; 4 g).

Add double-distilled water (Milli-Q filtered) to 20 liters, and adjust conductivity to 15,000 to 16,000 and pH to 7.4.

D-PBS-dialyzed fetal bovine serum: 50 ml of fetal bovine serum (Gibco-BRL or HyClone) is dialyzed for 3 days at 4°C against D-PBS (500 ml). Change the D-PBS twice daily.

[35S]Methionine-cysteine (Dupont/New England Nuclear, NEG 072): upon receipt, the isotope should be snap-frozen in small aliquots sufficient for one labeling reaction and stored at $-80°C$.

Methionine- and cysteine-free RPM1 1640 (Cellgro, Fisher catalog no. 17-104-CI)

Penicillin (10,000 IU/ml)-streptomycin (10,000 μg/ml) ($=100\times$ Pen-Strep; Gibco BRL, catalog no. 15140-031)

L-Glutamine, 200 mM ($=100\times$; Gibco BRL, catalog no. 25030-081)

Fetal bovine serum (Gibco BRL, catalog no. 26140-079)

35S-labeling medium: 39 ml of methionine and cysteine-free media, 4.5 ml of D-PBS-dialyzed fetal bovine serum, 0.45 ml L-glutamine, 45 μl of Pen-Strep, 1.35 ml of regular RPMI (for 10^8 cells)

Assays

Radiolabeled cell extract is prepared from K562 cells (ATCC CCL-243). The cells are thawed 2 to 3 days before use and grown at a density of 0.5×10^6 to 1.5×10^6/ml in RPMI 1640 plus L-glutamine (1:100), penicillin-streptomycin (1:100), and 10% fetal bovine serum in 750-ml tissue culture flasks (Corning, catalog no. 430199) at 37°C in a 5% CO_2 atmosphere. Cells should be in the mid-log phase of growth and should be visually inspected before labeling. Rapidly growing cells are labeled more efficiently than slowly growing ones. *Note: K562 cells grow in small nonadherent or weakly adherent clusters when healthy. If they are not healthy, they will start to adhere to the flask and differentiate. Cells that have begun to differentiate are deficient in some antigens, such as topoisomerase I (Scl-70).*

The night before use, collect the cells by centrifugation ($600 \times g$ for 5 min in a tabletop centrifuge), resuspend them in 20 ml of sterile D-PBS, and count them. The cells should be adjusted to 10^8 cells per 45 ml of 35S-labeling medium (recipe above) in a 250-ml flask. Add 2 mCi of freshly thawed

[^{35}S]methionine-cysteine, and incubate the cells for 12 to 16 h at 37°C in a 5% CO_2 atmosphere. The following day, the cells are collected by centrifugation (1,000 rpm, 5 min). *Note: the level of RNAP II decreases after 16 h, so it is important not to label for too long.* After labeling, there should be ~1.8×10^8 cells and the medium should have turned yellow. Collect the cells in a centrifuge tube, rinse the empty flask with D-PBS, and combine. Make aliquots of 2×10^7 cells in 15-ml polypropylene centrifuge tubes. Spin the tubes at $800 \times g$ in a tabletop centrifuge (5 min) and aspirate the supernatant. Freeze tubes with their cell pellets at −70°C. *Be sure to use polypropylene centrifuge tubes (e.g., Corning no. 430052) so they will not crack when frozen.*

Immunoprecipitation is carried out with serum that has been centrifuged ($9,000 \times g$ for 5 min) to remove insoluble materials. Frozen serum samples (−20°C) should be recentrifuged before analysis. Serum samples also may be stored for 10 to 15 years at 4°C after addition of sodium azide (NaN$_3$; final concentration, 0.05%). The procedure is as follows. In a 1.5-ml microcentrifuge tube combine 40 μl of 50% PAS slurry in Tris-HCl (pH 8.0), 8 μl of human serum, and 500 μl of 0.5 M NaCl NET/NP-40. Rotate the tube end-over-end at 4°C for 1 to 2 h or at room temperature for 1 to 3 h. *Avoid vortexing the beads at any stage of the procedure.* During this incubation, prepare cell extract from radiolabeled K562 cells (see above). For a standard reaction, we use extract from 2×10^6 radiolabeled cells per sample. Add 2 ml of 0.5 M NaCl NET/NP-40 plus 1:100 (20 μl) PMSF plus 1:100 (20 μl) aprotinin to the pellet (final cell concentration, 10^7/ml). *Do not put PMSF directly on the cell pellet because the ethanol will denature the proteins.* Sonicate the cells for 1 min (duty cycle 30%, output 3). Place on ice for 1 min and then sonicate again for 1 min. Transfer the cell lysate to microcentrifuge tubes and centrifuge at $9,000 \times g$ for 30 min at 4°C. Carefully collect the lysate (avoid disturbing the small pellet). Combine all of the lysate into one tube before dispensing. Extract from 2×10^7 cells is sufficient for 12 immunoprecipitations. *Note: when using frozen cells, do not thaw the cell pellet at 37°C. Once the cells are thawed, they are disrupted and protein degradation commences. Also, avoid excessive heating of the cell suspension during sonication. The extract may become hot enough to denature proteins if not chilled on ice.*

Pellet the serum-coated PAS beads by microcentrifuging for 3 s. Aspirate the supernatant by using a drawn-out Pasteur pipette attached to a vacuum. Add 1 ml of 0.5 M NaCl NET/NP-40 and microcentrifuge for 3 s. Aspirate the supernatant. *Carefully remove any air bubbles on the surface of the samples first, since they may cause high background.* To each PAS pellet, add 150 to 160 μl of cell extract. Rotate end-over-end for 1 h at 4°C. Microcentrifuge for 3 s and aspirate the supernatant. Wash the beads three times with 1 ml of 0.5 M NaCl NET/NP-40 and then once with 1 ml of NET. Carefully aspirate the supernatant. Add 50 μl of 1× sample buffer to each pellet. Samples may be kept at −80°C for at least 1 month (keep in mind that the half-life of ^{35}S is ~60 days). To analyze, boil the samples for 3 min, pellet the beads, and load 15 to 20 μl of supernatant per lane of an SDS–12.5% polyacrylamide gel. For large proteins (>100 kDa), resolution may be enhanced by using a 10 or 8% polyacrylamide gel. It usually takes 3 to 5 h for the tracking dye to reach the bottom of the gel at a constant voltage of 100 to 130 V.

Note: if performing immunoprecipitations with antibodies that do not bind protein A (e.g., human immunoglobulin γ3 [IgG3] or mouse IgG1), it will be necessary to use protein G-Sepharose.

The proteins associated with the immunoprecipitates are analyzed by SDS-polyacrylamide gel electrophoresis and fluorography. Reagents are as follows:

25% SDS (Fisher or Bio-Rad). *Note: filter this solution and all other stock solutions through a 0.45-μm bottle top filter.*

Coomassie blue stain: Coomassie brilliant blue R-250 (Bio-Rad, catalog no. 161-0400) (5 g), methanol (1,200 ml), glacial acetic acid (400 ml); add distilled water to 4,000 ml

Destaining solution: 2 liters of glacial acetic acid, 7 liters of methanol, 11 liters of distilled water

2, 5-Diphenyloxazole (PPO) (Fisher, catalog no. D144-100), 20% (wt/vol) in dimethyl sulfoxide (DMSO). *Note: PPO is carcinogenic.*

Glycerol

BioMax MR film (Eastman Kodak, catalog no. 870-1302)

30% acrylamide–0.8% bisacrylamide stock: 30% (wt/vol) acrylamide (Fisher, catalog no. BP170-500) plus 0.8% bisacrylamide (Bio-Rad, catalog no. 160-0201) (wt/vol) in water (ratio, 37.5:1); filter through a 0.45-μm bottle top filter.

5× Tris-glycine (for running buffer): 120 g of Tris base plus 576 g of glycine; add distilled water to 4 liters (no need to adjust pH; can be stored at room temperature).

The procedure for preparing gels is as follows. *Note: precast minigels may be substituted for homemade ones. They can be purchased from Bio-Rad or other vendors. If casting your own gels, keep in mind that acrylamide is a neurotoxin and suspected carcinogen.* Gel plates, spacers, and rubber gaskets are washed thoroughly with detergent and water (e.g., PCC-54, Pierce, Rockford, Ill.), rinsed carefully, and wiped dry with ethanol. Gel plates should be assembled and clamped together, starting at the bottom and working your way up the sides.

A 12.5% resolving gel is made by combining distilled water (15.6 ml), 2 M Tris HCl (pH 8.8) (7.5 ml), 30% acrylamide–0.8% bisacrylamide (16.6 ml), and 25% SDS (160 μl). *Immediately before use (wearing gloves)* add 10% ammonium persulfate (200 μl) and TEMED (N, N, N′, N′-tetra methylenediamine) (20 μl; Bio-Rad) to start polymerization. Mix gently, avoiding bubbles. Carefully pour between the glass gel plates, again avoiding bubbles. Using a Pipetteman, gently layer 70% ethanol above the resolving gel (~3- to 5-mm-thick layer) to exclude air from the gel as it polymerizes. The gel should polymerize in about 1 h. Pour off the ethanol, and rinse the top of the gel with water. Use a filter paper strip to carefully remove water droplets between the plates. *It is critical to use fresh ammonium persulfate and TEMED for polymerizing the gel. Both reagents should be stored at 4°C. Prepare 10% ammonium persulfate fresh. Do not use TEMED older than 1 year.*

Stacking gel is made by combining distilled water (12.2 ml), 0.5 M Tris HCl (pH 6.8) (5 ml), 30% acrylamide–0.8% bisacrylamide (2.6 ml), and 25% SDS (80 μl). *Immediately before use (wearing gloves)* add 10% ammonium persulfate (100 μl) and TEMED (20 μl) to start polymerization. Mix gently, avoiding bubbles. Carefully pour between the glass gel plates up to the top, avoiding bubbles. Carefully insert the comb at the top of the gel. Clamp the top. *This prevents gel bits from adhering to the wells after the comb is removed.* Stacking gel should polymerize in about 45 min at room temperature.

The gel is run as follows.

1. Make 1 liter of running buffer: 200 ml of 5× Tris-glycine plus distilled water to make 1,000 ml; add 4 ml of 25% SDS and mix well.

2. Boil samples, including molecular weight standards, for 3 min in a water bath immediately before loading the gel.

3. Carefully remove the comb and bottom spacer from the SDS-polyacrylamide gel.

4. Clamp the gel to the gel apparatus and add running buffer to the top and bottom chambers to cover the top and bottom of the gel.

5. Remove bubbles from the bottom of the gel, using a syringe with a bent (90°) 18-gauge needle.

6. Gently wash out wells with running buffer, using a Hamilton syringe.

7. Add 20 μl (or desired volume) of boiled sample per well.

8. Attach leads to the electrodes of the gel apparatus (proteins treated with SDS are negatively charged and will migrate toward the cathode).

9. Attach to power supply and run at 100 V until the blue tracking dye reaches the resolving gel. At this time, the voltage may be increased to 120 V.

10. Run the gel until the blue tracking dye reaches the bottom of the gel (do not run the dye off the gel).

11. Turn off the power, remove the electrodes, and unclamp the gel from the gel apparatus. Carefully pry the plates apart, leaving the gel adherent to one of the plates. Using a pizza cutter, cut off the stacking gel and diagonally cut off a small piece of the gel from the upper right-hand corner to aid in orienting the gel.

12. Stain the gel for 20 min with Coomassie blue solution. Destain and fix the gel with several changes of destaining solution.

After staining and fixation, the gel is fluorographed as follows.

1. Place the gel in a Tupperware (polyethylene or polypropylene but not polystyrene) container and remove as much of the destaining solution as possible. Immerse the gel in 100 to 200 ml of DMSO, cover the container, and rotate gently on a shaker for 30 min. Discard DMSO.

2. Transfer to 100 to 200 ml of fresh DMSO, cover, and rotate for 30 min. After use, this DMSO solution is removed and can be saved for use as the first DMSO wash for another gel.

3. Add 100 to 200 ml of 20% (wt/vol) PPO in DMSO, cover, and rotate gently for 60 min. Save the DMSO-PPO mixture. It can be reused for several gels, although the effectiveness gradually diminishes. The solution can be "recharged" by adding additional PPO. *Note: PPO is a carcinogen, and DMSO can penetrate standard laboratory gloves. Wear heavy rubber gloves (e.g., Playtex) and handle DMSO-PPO solution carefully.*

4. Wash the gel with several changes of water to rehydrate (at least 30 min, until the smell of DMSO is no longer apparent). The PPO will precipitate in the gel. Add glycerol to the final wash to a concentration of ~3%. Remove the gel, which will have turned white and opaque, place on 3MM paper (Whatman) and dry with a vacuum gel dryer. Wash out the tray with ethanol to remove traces of PPO (which is insoluble in water). We use a Bio-Rad gel dryer (model 583) at 60°C with the timer set to 3 h. After 1.5 h, the gel is removed. Vent the gel dryer, and remove the gel and attached 3MM paper.

5. Tape dried gels to a used piece of X-ray film. If it is sticky, dust the gel lightly with talc to prevent sticking. Place this in a cassette and (in the darkroom) place in direct contact with BioMax MR film. *This film is coated on one side, and the coated side must contact the gel.* Expose the gel to film in the cassette for 3 days or more at −70°C before developing.

Quality Assurance, Quality Control, and Test Validation

It is important to include a sample of normal human serum as a negative control. Whenever possible, it is advisable to use a known positive control serum (reference serum). Expression of individual antigens may vary, depending on the cell line used.

Molecular weight standards (Sigma, catalog no. SDS-7 [low molecular weight] or SDS-6H [high molecular weight]) are analyzed in an adjacent lane of the gel and detected by Coomassie blue staining. Migration of molecular weight standards and immunoglobulin heavy and light chains (~50 and 25 kDa, respectively) can be examined to assess the quality of separation. By using reference or prototype sera and normal human serum, the technical adequacy of the gel can be assessed. Multiple weak bands with normal human serum may indicate problems with washing.

Immunoprecipitation is a highly sensitive and specific technique for detecting a variety of autoantibodies. However, clinical application of this approach is greatly limited because it is labor-intensive and technically demanding and requires the use of radioisotopes. Nevertheless, the immunoprecipitation technique is extremely useful for validating other assays, such as ELISAs.

Cost Assessment

The protein immunoprecipitation technique is demanding and labor-intensive. However, these drawbacks are offset by the considerable information on multiple autoantibody systems gained from a single assay.

Interpretation

The major autoantibodies that can be evaluated by these techniques are summarized below.

Anti-Sm and Anti-nRNP

Anti-Sm and anti-nRNP antibodies recognize different subsets of the protein components of the U1 snRNP particle. This is an RNA-protein complex consisting of proteins U1-70K (70 kDa), A (33 kDa), B′/B (29 and 28 kDa, respectively), C (23 kDa), D1/2/3 (16 kDa), E (12 kDa), F (11 kDa), and G (10 kDa). The proteins are associated with a single U1 small nuclear RNA molecule (12). Proteins B′/B, D, E, F, and G assemble into a stable Sm core particle, which is reactive with anti-Sm, but not anti-nRNP, antibodies. The Sm core particle is a component of several additional snRNPs, each with a unique uridine-rich (U) RNA species as well as unique proteins. These include the U2, U4/U6, and U5 snRNPs, as well as other less abundant U snRNPs (12). Anti-Sm, but not anti-nRNP, antibodies immunoprecipitate the unique 200- to 205-kDa proteins of the U5 snRNP, which are associated with the Sm core particle (Fig. 4). Although autoantibodies specific for these proteins have been reported, they are unusual. Thus, immunoprecipitation of the U5 200- to 205-kDa doublet by a serum that immunoprecipitates the A to G proteins provides evidence for the presence of anti-Sm autoantibodies, a diagnostic marker for SLE (12). Anti-nRNP antibodies are not disease specific and are of limited utility in diagnosing SLE or in predicting its course. Different fine specificities of anti-nRNP and anti-Sm antibodies can be distinguished if immunoprecipitation is carried out after the U1 snRNP is dissociated into its components by use of MgCl$_2$ or RNase (18, 19).

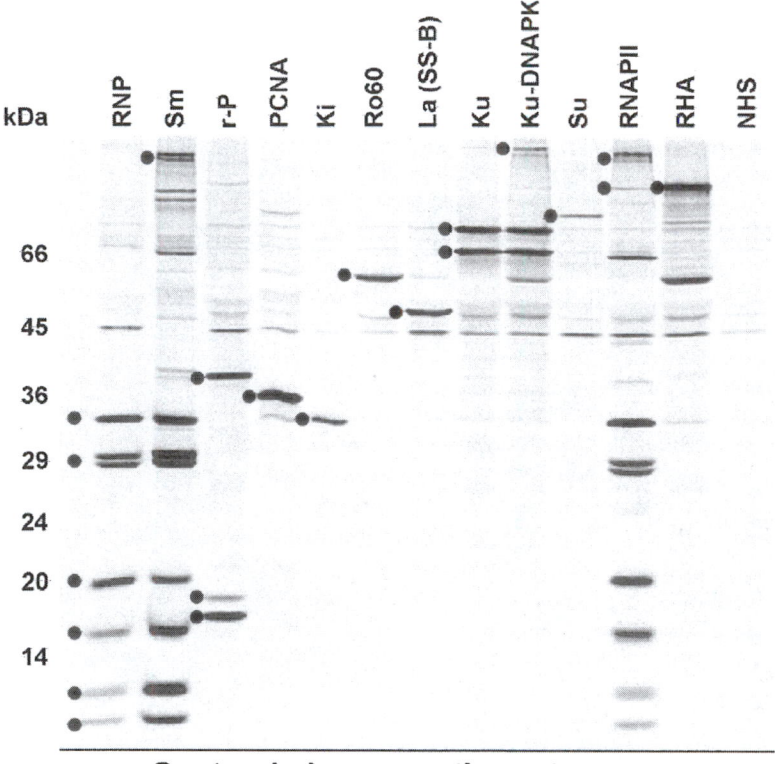

Systemic lupus erythematosus

FIGURE 4 Protein immunoprecipitation for analyzing SLE sera. Sera were tested according to the protocol in the text, and immunoprecipitated proteins were resolved on a 12.5% gel. Sera containing the following autoantibodies were tested: anti-nRNP (RNP), anti-Sm, anti-ribosomal P (r-P), anti-PCNA, anti-Ki, anti-Ro60, anti-La (SS-B), anti-Ku, anti-Ku plus anti-DNA-PK$_{cs}$ (Ku-DNAPK) anti-Su, anti-RNAP II, anti-RNA helicase A (RHA), and normal human serum (NHS). Positions of molecular weight standards are shown on the left (in kilodaltons). Protein components of the antigens are indicated (dots).

Anti-Ro (SS-A) and Anti-La (SS-B)

Sera containing anti-Ro (SS-A) autoantibodies may recognize two proteins: a 60-kDa protein (Ro60) that binds to the stem of four small RNAs designated hY1, hY3, hY4, and hY5 (3) and a 52-kDa protein (Ro52) (12) reactive with many, but not all, anti-Ro (SS-A) sera. It is controversial whether or not Ro52 interacts with Ro60 or the Y RNAs. Anti-Ro52 autoantibodies can immunoprecipitate the protein (12), but they are not reliably detected by that means, and many sera immunoprecipitate Ro60 but not Ro52. Anti-Ro60 autoantibodies are readily detected by protein immunoprecipitation (Fig. 4).

La (SS-B) antigen is a 47-kDa protein associated transiently with the precursors of several small RNAs synthesized by RNAP III (12). It can be detected readily by protein immunoprecipitation (Fig. 4), but the band often is distorted because it migrates near the immunoglobulin heavy chain ("heavy chain artifact"). Anti-La (SS-B) autoantibodies are virtually always associated with anti-Ro (SS-A) (24).

Anti-ribosomal P

Anti-ribosomal P antibodies recognize three proteins of ∼38, 19, and 17 kDa (P0, P1, and P2) that are components of the large (60S) ribosomal subunit (Fig. 4). These autoantibodies recognize mainly a conserved epitope contained on the C-terminal 22 amino acids of P0, P1, and P2 (4). Antibodies to the ribosomal P0, P1, and P2 antigens are highly specific for the diagnosis of SLE (12). Anti-P antibodies have been linked with neuropsychiatric lupus, especially psychosis, and their levels may be useful in predicting a relapse of lupus psychosis (12). Despite controversy regarding their relevance to neuropsychiatric lupus, the specificity for SLE is widely accepted. Immunoprecipitation is probably the standard test for this specificity, but DID, ELISA, and immunoblotting also are reliable (1, 23). There appear to be some sera that are positive by ELISA but negative by immunoprecipitation, however.

Anti-PCNA

PCNA is a 36-kDa protein recognized by autoantibodies found in about 2 to 5% of SLE sera (12). These antibodies, though unusual, are highly specific for SLE (6, 10). Immunoprecipitation is probably the most reliable way to detect these autoantibodies (Fig. 4), but DID also is suitable.

Anti-Ku

Ku antigen is a heterodimer of ∼80- and 70-kDa subunits (p80 and p70, respectively) that binds to termini of dsDNA (12). These proteins associate with an ∼460-kDa DNA-dependent protein kinase (DNA-PK catalytic subunit [DNA-PK$_{cs}$]). Autoantibodies are produced against both of the Ku subunits as well as DNA-PK$_{cs}$. A subset of autoantibodies recognizes epitopes formed by the assembly of these proteins into a particle, which can be detected only by techniques that preserve the quaternary structure of the Ku/DNA-PK antigen. Immunoprecipitation is the gold standard for detecting autoantibodies against Ku/DNA-PK (Fig. 4 and Table 3). Antibodies that recognize specifically the DNA-PK$_{cs}$ protein must be detected following dissociation from Ku, e.g., by exposure to 0.5 to 1.5 M NaCl. Autoantibodies against Ku antigen are found in several diseases, including PM-SSc overlap syndrome, SLE, MCTD, and SSc.

Anti-tRNA Synthetases

Autoantibodies against aminoacyl tRNA synthetases are diagnostic markers for PM/DM and the antisynthetase autoantibody syndrome (see above). The most common is anti-histidyl-tRNA synthetase (anti-Jo-1), but many others have been reported, including threonyl (anti-PL-7), alanyl (anti-PL-12), isoleucyl (anti-OJ), glycyl (anti-EJ), and asparaginyl (anti-KS) tRNA synthetases. The antisynthetase autoantibodies immunoprecipitate proteins of characteristic molecular weights (Table 1) as well as the corresponding tRNA molecule (7, 22). Both the proteins and the tRNAs have distinctive mobilities on electrophoresis (Fig. 5). Recombinant antigen-based ELISAs,

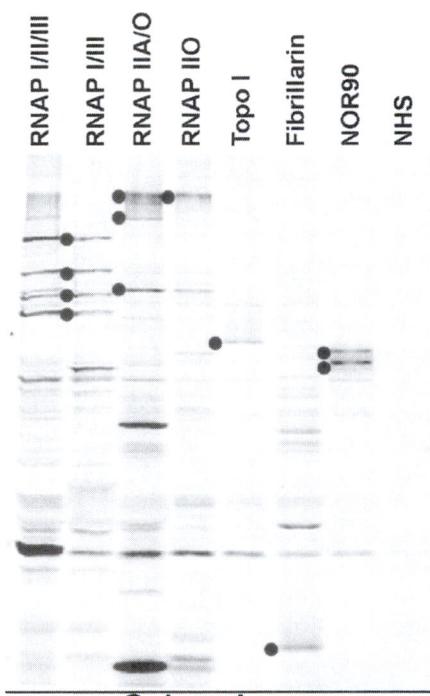

Scleroderma

FIGURE 6 Protein immunoprecipitation for analyzing scleroderma sera. Sera were tested according to the protocol in the text, and immunoprecipitated proteins were resolved on an SDS–8% polyacrylamide gel. Sera containing the following autoantibodies were tested: anti-RNAP I, II, and III (RNAP I/II/III); anti-RNAP I and III (RNAP I/III); anti-RNAP II, unphosphorylated and phosphorylated forms (RNAP IIA/O); anti-RNAP II, phosphorylated form (RNAP IIO); anti-topo I (100 kDa); antifibrillarin (34 kDa); and anti-NOR90 (doublet ~95 kDa). Protein components of the antigens are indicated (dots).

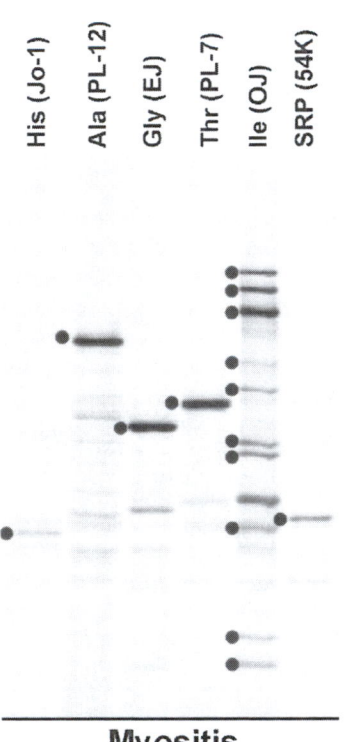

Myositis

FIGURE 5 Protein immunoprecipitation for analyzing myositis (PM/DM) sera. Sera were tested according to the protocol in the text, and immunoprecipitated proteins were resolved on an SDS–8% polyacrylamide gel. Sera containing the following autoantibodies were tested: anti-histidyl tRNA synthetase (Jo-1, 50 kDa), anti-alanyl tRNA synthetase (PL-12, 110 kDa), anti-glycyl tRNA synthetase (EJ, 75 kDa), anti-threonyl tRNA synthetase (PL-7, 80 kDa), anti-isoleucyl tRNA synthetase (OJ, 150 kDa and multiprotein complex), and anti-signal recognition particle (SRP, 54-kDa protein and multiprotein complex). Protein components of the antigens are indicated (dots).

DID (histidyl, threonyl), and Western blotting (e.g., glycyl) also may be useful.

Anti-SRP

Autoantibodies against SRP are myositis specific and recognize an RNA-protein complex consisting of a single molecule of 7SL RNA and proteins of 72, 68, 54, 19, 14, and 9 kDa (13). The major antigenic determinants are located on the 54-kDa protein. Immunoprecipitation is the only technique at present for detecting anti-SRP (Fig. 5).

Anti-topo I (Scl-70)

Autoantibodies against topo I are highly associated with diffuse scleroderma and portend a poor outcome (15). The antigen is a 100-kDa nuclear protein that is not RNA associated. Although the autoantibodies are reliably detected by DID using calf thymus extract, Western blotting or immunoprecipitation (Fig. 6) is also helpful.

Antifibrillarin (U3 RNP)

Fibrillarin is a 34-kDa nucleolar protein associated with the U3 small nucleolar RNA species. Autoantibodies to this protein are highly specific for scleroderma and produce a nucleolar immunofluorescence pattern on ANA testing (15). Screening can be carried out by immunofluorescence ("clumpy" anti-nucleolar staining). Immunoprecipitation probably should be regarded as the gold standard (Fig. 6 and Table 3).

Anti-RNAP I, II, and III

RNAP I and III are multiprotein complexes that synthesize rRNA and a class of small cellular RNAs, respectively. RNAP I is located in the nucleolus, and autoantibodies against it are associated with a nucleolar ANA pattern. The largest subunits of RNAP I are 190 and 126 kDa, whereas the large subunits of RNAP III are 155 and 138 kDa. Autoantibodies against these proteins are highly associated with scleroderma and with a poor prognosis (14). Although RNAP I, II, and III have different large subunits, some of the smaller subunits are shared. Thus, some sera with anti-RNAP antibodies immunoprecipitate all three enzymes (Fig. 6).

RNAP II is a multiprotein complex consisting of 8 to 12 proteins that synthesizes mRNA. The C-terminal domain of the largest subunit is phosphorylated in the transcriptionally active form of the enzyme. The two largest subunits (220 and 140 kDa) are the main proteins recognized by autoantibodies, though the smaller subunits may be targeted as well. Unlike anti-RNAP I and III, anti-RNAP II autoantibodies are found in 10% of SLE sera as well as in scleroderma (16). A significant number of sera having autoantibodies specific for RNAP II recognize only the phosphorylated form (RNAP IIO, 240 kDa) of the largest subunit (Fig. 6). In scleroderma, anti-RNAP IIO antibodies may be associated with anti-topoisomerase I antibodies and with more severe disease (17). At present, the only reliable assay for anti-RNAP I, II, or III is immunoprecipitation.

IMMUNOPRECIPITATION: SMALL RNAs

The same general procedure used for analyzing proteins recognized by autoantibodies can be adapted for analyzing the RNA components of these antigens. The following is a description of the modifications necessary to analyze these RNAs. *Note: this procedure generates highly radioactive cells and liquid and/or solid waste. It is essential to use adequate protection against the strong β radiation produced and to dispose of radioactive waste properly.*

Technology and Instrumentation

See "Immunoprecipitation: Proteins" (above).

Assays

K562 cells are labeled with [^{32}P]orthophosphate, which is incorporated into nucleic acids. The cells are labeled in RPMI 1640–10% fetal bovine serum (cells must be actively dividing for good labeling). Cells are washed twice with D-PBS and resuspended at 10^6/ml in low phosphate minimal essential medium (MEM) (phosphate-free MEM, Joklik modification, Gibco formula 81-5165) plus 10% normal saline-dialyzed (*not D-PBS-dialyzed*) fetal bovine serum. Add 1:100 L-glutamine and 1:100 penicillin-streptomycin plus 1.5% regular (i.e., phosphate-containing) MEM (10 mM HEPES [Cellgro; Fisher catalog no. 25-060-CI], pH 7.4, can be added to increase the buffering capacity of the medium). We typically label 2×10^7 to 4×10^7 cells in 20 to 40 ml of medium. Add 25 μCi of [^{32}P]orthophosphate (NEX-053 [Du Pont/New England Nuclear], carrier free in water) per ml of culture medium. For a typical experiment, 500 to 1,000 μCi is added to 20 to 30 ml of culture. Incubate at 37°C overnight (shield the culture flask with Lucite or incubate in a water bath to protect against strong β radiation).

After labeling, the cells are centrifuged at $600 \times g$ in a tabletop centrifuge (use appropriate shielding). Supernatant is removed to ^{32}P waste, and the cells are washed once with ice-cold D-PBS. Cells are resuspended at 10^7/ml in ice-cold hypotonic lysis buffer (10 mM Tris [pH 7.5], 10 mM KCl, 1 mM EDTA) containing 0.5 mM PMSF (add PMSF fresh from a $100 \times$ stock in ethanol) and incubated for 10 min on ice. The cells are then disrupted with 12 strokes with a tight-fitting Dounce homogenizer (*to avoid generating radioactive aerosols, we do not sonicate the cells*), and NaCl is added to a final concentration of 0.2 M. Extract is then microcentrifuged ($9,000 \times g$) for 10 min at 4°C, and the supernatant is collected into clean tubes before being spun again and saved. Fresh extract is used for immunoprecipitation.

Immunoprecipitation is carried out as described for protein immunoprecipitation. For each immunoprecipitation, use 1.5×10^6 cell equivalents of extract, 8 to 10 μl of serum, and 40 μl of 50% PAS slurry in water. Incubation is carried out for 30 to 45 minutes at 4°C. Washing is the same as for protein immunoprecipitation. RNA is then isolated from the immunoprecipitates. (*Note: precautions must be taken to prevent RNases [e.g., from the hands] from degrading the isolated RNA. Use only autoclaved glassware, microcentrifuge tubes, buffers, etc., and wear gloves at all stages of isolation procedure.*) The procedure is as follows.

1. Resuspend the washed beads in 200 μl of NET.
2. Extract by vortexing with 400 μl of phenol-chloroform-isoamyl alcohol (24:24:1). Save the aqueous phase into clean, RNase-free (autoclaved) 1.5-ml microcentrifuge tubes.
3. Optional: repeat step 2.
4. Extract once with 400 μl of chloroform-isoamyl alcohol (24:1), saving the aqueous phase.
5. Add 10 μl of 5 M NaCl to each tube (final NaCl concentration, 0.25 M).
6. Add 500 μl of ethanol (=2.5 volumes).
7. Store overnight at −20°C.
8. Incubate the tubes at −70°C for 30 min.
9. Thaw and centrifuge at 4°C for 20 to 30 min in a microcentrifuge ($9,000 \times g$). Orient the hinges of the caps upward so that you know the location of the invisible pellet.
10. Carefully aspirate the ethanol with a drawn-out Pasteur pipette.
11. Add 20 μl of RNA gel sample buffer (recipe below) to each tube.

The RNA is analyzed by polyacrylamide gel electrophoresis in the presence of urea:

1. Gel solution (100 ml): 7% acrylamide (23.3 ml of 30% acrylamide–0.8% bisacrylamide stock), 7 M urea (42.4 g of "Ultra Pure" urea from Schwarz/Mann, catalog no. 821519), $1 \times$ Tris-borate-EDTA (TBE: 20 ml of $5 \times$ TBE stock), 60 μl of TEMED. To polymerize, add 400 μl of freshly made 10% ammonium persulfate. Pour the gel between long glass plates (40 cm or more).
2. $5 \times$ TBE (1 liter): 54 g of Trizma base (Sigma), 27.5 g of boric acid, 50 ml of 0.2 M EDTA (pH 8.0); add distilled water to make 1 liter.
3. Electrophoresis buffer: $1 \times$ TBE.
4. Sample buffer for RNA gels (500 μl): 100 μl of $5 \times$ TBE, 100 μl of 0.1% bromophenol blue solution in distilled water, 100 μl of 1% xylene cyanol solution in distilled water, 0.212 g of urea; add distilled water to make 500 μl.

This is not a stacking gel system. The gel is run as follows. Clean out the wells using a syringe to gently dislodge acrylamide gel fragments. Prerun the gel at 400 to 500 V for 15 to 30 min. The plates should become warm but not so hot that you cannot touch them. After prerunning the gel, clean out the wells again. Carefully load the samples, and run the gel at 400 to 500 V constant voltage until the bromphenol blue tracking dye is about two-thirds of the way to the bottom of the plates. After electrophoresis, fix the gel on one of the glass plates for 20 to 30 min in 5% glacial acetic acid–water. Carefully transfer onto 3MM paper (place paper on top of the gel and glass plate and flip over). Dry gel under vacuum and then expose to XAR5 film (Eastman Kodak; overnight exposure at −80°C using intensifier screens).

Quality Assurance, Quality Control, and Test Validation

See "Immunoprecipitation: Proteins" (above).

Cost Assessment

See "Immunoprecipitation: Proteins" (above).

Interpretation

Anti-Sm and anti-nRNP sera immunoprecipitate distinctive subsets of small RNAs, as shown by analysis of the ^{32}P-labeled RNAs (8). Both anti-nRNP and anti-Sm sera immunoprecipitate U1 RNA, whereas the U2, U4, U5, and U6 small RNAs are immunoprecipitated only by anti-Sm, providing a useful means for unequivocally distinguishing the two specificities. Anti-Ro60 antibodies can be detected by immunoprecipitation of the hY1, hY3, hY4, and hY5 RNAs. Anti-La (SS-B) autoantibodies also can be detected by immunoprecipitation of 5S, 7SL, 7-2, 8-2, tRNA, and other small RNAs.

REFERENCES

1. **Arnett, F. C., J. D. Reveille, H. M. Moutsopoulos, L. Georgescu, and K. B. Elkon.** 1996. Ribosomal P autoantibodies in systemic lupus erythematosus. *Arthritis Rheum.* **39:**1833–1839.
2. **Buyon, J. P.** 1993. Congenital complete heart block. *Lupus* **2:**291–295.
3. **Chan, E. K. L., and J. P. Buyon.** 1994. The SS-A/Ro antigen, p. B4.1;1–18. *In* W. J. van Venrooij and R. N. Maini (ed.), *Manual of Biological Markers of Disease.* Kluwer Academic Publishers, Dordrecht, The Netherlands.
4. **Elkon, K., S. Skelly, A. Parnassa, A. Moller, W. Danho, H. Weissbach, and N. Brot.** 1986. Identification and chemical synthesis of a ribosomal protein antigenic determinant in systemic lupus erythematosus. *Proc. Natl. Acad. Sci. USA* **83:**7419–7423.
5. **Elkon, K. B., E. Bonfa, and N. Brot.** 1992. Antiribosomal antibodies in systemic lupus erythematosus. *Rheum. Dis. Clin. N. Am.* **18:**377–390.
6. **Fritzler, M. J., G. A. McCarty, J. P. Ryan, and T. D. Kinsella.** 1983. Clinical features of patients with antibodies directed against proliferating cell nuclear antigen. *Arthritis Rheum.* **26:**140–145.
7. **Hirakata, M., A. Suwa, S. Nagai, M. A. Kron, E. P. Trieu, T. Mimori, M. Akizuki, and I. N. Targoff.** 1999. Anti-KS: identification of autoantibodies to asparaginyl-transfer RNA synthetase associated with interstitial lung disease. *J. Immunol.* **162:**2315–2320.
8. **Lerner, M. R., and J. A. Steitz.** 1979. Antibodies to small nuclear RNAs complexed with proteins are produced by patients with systemic lupus erythematosus. *Proc. Natl. Acad. Sci. USA* **76:**5495–5499.
9. **Medsger, T. A.** 1993. Systemic sclerosis (scleroderma), localized forms of scleroderma, and calcinosis, p. 1253–1292.

In D. J. McCarty and W. J. Koopman (ed.), *Arthritis and Allied Conditions.* Lea & Febiger, Philadelphia, Pa.
10. **Miyachi, K., M. J. Fritzler, and E. M. Tan.** 1978. Autoantibody to a nuclear antigen in proliferating cells. *J. Immunol.* **121:**2228–2234.
11. **Nakamura, R. M., C. L. Peebles, and E. M. Tan.** 1978. Microhemagglutination test for detection of antibodies to nuclear Sm and ribonucleoprotein antigens in systemic lupus erythematosus and related diseases. *Am. J. Clin. Pathol.* **70:**800–807.
12. **Reeves, W. H., S. Narain, and M. Satoh.** 2004. Autoantibodies in systemic lupus erythematosus, p. 1497–1521. *In* W. J. Koopman and L. W. Moreland (ed.), *Arthritis and Allied Conditions.* Lippincott Williams & Wilkins, Baltimore, Md.
13. **Reeves, W. H., S. K. Nigam, and G. Blobel.** 1986. Human autoantibodies reactive with the signal recognition particle. *Proc. Natl. Acad. Sci. USA* **83:**9507–9511.
14. **Reimer, G., K. M. Rose, U. Scheer, and E. M. Tan.** 1987. Autoantibody to RNA polymerase I in scleroderma sera. *J. Clin. Invest.* **79:**65–72.
15. **Rothfield, N. F.** 1992. Autoantibodies in scleroderma. *Rheum. Dis. Clin. N. Am.* **18:**483–498.
16. **Satoh, M., A. K. Ajmani, T. Ogasawara, J. J. Langdon, M. Hirakata, J. Wang, and W. H. Reeves.** 1994. Autoantibodies to RNA polymerase II are common in systemic lupus erythematosus and overlap syndrome. Specific recognition of the phosphorylated (IIO) form by a subset of human sera. *J. Clin. Invest.* **94:**1981–1989.
17. **Satoh, M., M. Kuwana, T. Ogasawara, A. K. Ajmani, J. J. Langdon, D. Kimpel, J. Wang, and W. H. Reeves.** 1994. Association of autoantibodies to topoisomerase I and the phosphorylated (IIO) form of RNA polymerase II in Japanese scleroderma patients. *J. Immunol.* **153:**5838–5848.
18. **Satoh, M., J. J. Langdon, K. J. Hamilton, H. B. Richards, D. Panka, R. A. Eisenberg, and W. H. Reeves.** 1996. Distinctive immune response patterns of human and murine autoimmune sera to U1 small nuclear ribonucleoprotein C protein. *J. Clin. Invest.* **97:**2619–2626.
19. **Satoh, M., H. B. Richards, K. J. Hamilton, and W. H. Reeves.** 1997. Human anti-nRNP autoimmune sera contain a novel subset of autoantibodies that stabilizes the molecular interaction of U1RNP-C protein with the Sm core proteins. *J. Immunol.* **158:**5017–5025.
20. **Tan, E. M., T. E. Feltkamp, J. S. Smolen, B. Butcher, R. Dawkins, M. J. Fritzler, T. Gordon, J. A. Hardin, J. R. Kalden, R. G. Lahita, R. N. Maini, J. S. McDougal, N. F. Rothfield, R. J. Smeenk, Y. Takasaki, A. Wiik, M. R. Wilson, and J. A. Koziol.** 1997. Range of antinuclear antibodies in "healthy" individuals. *Arthritis Rheum.* **40:**1601–1611.
21. **Tan, E. M., and H. G. Kunkel.** 1966. Characteristics of a soluble nuclear antigen precipitating with sera of patients with systemic lupus erythematosus. *J. Immunol.* **96:**464–471.
22. **Targoff, I. N.** 1992. Autoantibodies in polymyositis. *Rheum. Dis. Clin. N. Am.* **18:**455–482.
23. **van Dam, A., H. Nossent, J. de Jong, J. Meilof, E. J. ter Borg, T. Swaak, and R. Smeenk.** 1991. Diagnostic value of antibodies against ribosomal phosphoproteins. A cross sectional and longitudinal study. *J. Rheumatol.* **18:**1026–1034.
24. **Wasicek, C. A., and M. Reichlin.** 1982. Clinical and serological differences between systemic lupus erythematosus patients with autoantibodies to Ro versus patients with antibodies to Ro and La. *J. Clin. Invest.* **69:**835–843.

Detection of Autoantibodies by Using Immobilized Natural and Recombinant Autoantigens

EDWARD K. L. CHAN, RUFUS W. BURLINGAME, AND MARVIN J. FRITZLER

114

Autoantibodies directed against intracellular antigens are characteristic features of a number of human autoimmune diseases and certain malignancies (5, 12, 50–52). Studies in systemic rheumatic diseases have provided strong evidence that autoantibodies are maintained by antigen-driven responses (42, 52, 56) and that autoantibodies can be reporters from the immune system revealing the identity of antigens involved in the disease pathogenesis (51). Historically, autoantibody detection and analysis have relied on a number of different technologies, such as hemagglutination and particle aggregation, immunodiffusion (ID), indirect immunofluorescence (IIF), complement fixation, counterimmunoelectrophoresis (CIE), Western and dot blotting, immunoprecipitation (IP), enzyme-linked immunosorbent assay (ELISA), and functional assays that demonstrate inhibition of the catalytic or other functional activity of the antigen of interest. These conventional technologies have limitations because they tend to be labor-intensive and time-consuming, are limited in throughput, are semiquantitative, and are not adaptable to leading-edge research. ID has been used for more than 50 years and is still used in clinical laboratories because it is inexpensive and specific, but it lacks sensitivity and can take up to 48 h before precipitin lines are interpretable. Western blot is costly and time-consuming, and not all autoantibodies are detected by this technique. For example, in the SS-A/Ro system it has been observed that IP techniques are required to identify some sera that contain antibodies reacting only with the "native" SS-A/Ro particle (2). IP protocols that use extracts from [^{35}S]methionine-labeled cells are not suitable for the detection of all autoantibodies, such as antibodies to the 52-kDa SS-A/Ro protein (6). ELISA techniques have rapidly advanced, but highly specific, sensitive, and reliable assays that use highly purified or recombinant proteins can be expensive and are limited by intermanufacturer and interlaboratory variation (53). Some laboratories continue to use CIE for the detection of certain autoantibodies, such as SS-A/Ro, because this technique was found to be the most reliable method for the detection of these autoantibodies (33, 35). However, ID and CIE generally favor high-titer sera and often cannot discriminate multiple autoantibody responses that are characteristic of sera from patients with systemic rheumatic disease.

Despite the advantages of IP, CIE, and ELISA, IIF remains the least expensive and, perhaps, the screening assay of choice for many autoantibodies (1, 60). HEp-2 cells are currently the most commonly used cell substrate in diagnostic autoantibody tests for systemic rheumatic diseases. However, the use of IIF on HEp-2 cells to detect autoantibodies can be limited by a lack of specificity and sensitivity when the antigen in question is of low abundance, or when epitopes are hidden or lost through cell fixation. These factors have resulted in variability of commercial HEp-2 cell substrates (17). In addition to variation in kits produced by various manufacturers, significant lot-to-lot variation in kits from single manufacturers has also been noted, and variations in different batches from the same manufacturer have also been observed. Another limitation of current IIF substrates is that there is significant variation in the sensitivity of different commercially available substrates to detect different antibodies. This limitation can be compounded by sera that contain multiple autoantibodies, for which it is necessary to use other techniques to definitively identify as many autoantibodies as possible in a single serum sample.

Human sera contain autoantibodies that are notably heterogeneous with respect to antigen and epitope specificity and polyclonality of the B-cell response that leads to their formation. For example, it is not uncommon to see sera that show a complex pattern of IIF staining that might include reactivity with the nuclear envelope, mitochondrial antibodies, and homogeneous staining of interphase nuclei. Further analyses of these sera with a variety of techniques confirm that there is reactivity with a variety of antigens, which might include chromatin, SS-A/Ro, pyruvate dehydrogenase complex (PDC; also called M2 antigen), nuclear pore complex antigens (39), and p97/valosin-containing protein (VCP) (36). Of interest, autoantibodies directed to the last autoantigen VCP are not associated with a distinctive IIF staining pattern and are not detected by Western blotting when denaturing agents are utilized (37). Complex sera like those referenced here point to the need for multiplexed autoantigen arrays to provide an accurate picture of the autoantibody profile of any patient.

With the use of expression cloning and autoantibodies as probes to screen λ phage cDNA libraries, the identities of many autoantigens have been determined and validated. A logical strategy is to take advantage of the availability of recombinant autoantigens, generated from the cDNA in *Escherichia coli* or other appropriate expression systems, as substrates for immunoassays such as ELISA and multiplex assays. This chapter focuses on the methodology in purification of recombinant autoantigens used in the authors' laboratories and recent advances in multiplex immunoassays that are suitable for autoantibody detection.

ANTIGEN TECHNOLOGY

A rapid expansion of new technologies developed by basic and applied immunology is making a significant impact on a broad spectrum of biomedical investigation (13, 43). The identification of biomarkers of disease onset, progression, and response to therapy is now made possible with the application of a variety of reagents in a number of novel platforms (7, 20, 23, 57). Polyclonal, monoclonal, and single-component antibodies have become valuable tools in basic research and diagnostic technologies, and more recently they have become a very successful approach for therapeutics in oncology, a broad spectrum of systemic rheumatic diseases, a variety of autoimmune conditions, and cell and organ transplantation. Accompanying these developments has been the appearance of a broad spectrum of DNA, RNA, and protein arrays. Protein arrays in particular are gaining acceptance as an approach to multiplexed detection of autoantibodies in biological fluids and the detection of changes in cell physiology after various physiological triggers and therapeutic interventions (43). To capitalize on these advances, there has been a need for the parallel development of new technology platforms to produce and utilize the arrays in clinical settings. These have included new adaptations of the fluorescence-activated cell sorter, which is now a standard device in most clinical immunology centers (55). In addition, devices that produce protein arrays by binding analytes of interest on solid-phase substrates have become a necessary technology of research-intensive institutions. Some of these emerging technologies include addressable laser beads, microfluidics and laboratory-on-a-chip platforms, and nanotechnology (13, 22, 54, 58, 61).

Purification of Natural and Recombinant Autoantigens

One requirement in the development of a successful immunoassay for the detection of autoantibodies is that the antigen must be recognized efficiently. Many recombinant autoantigens generated in E. coli can be used successfully for functional as well as immunological assays. In the analysis of systemic rheumatic diseases, recombinant human SS-B/La antigen is an excellent example, since most human anti-SS-B/La-positive sera recognize multiple epitopes, most of which are readily expressed in recombinant forms. However, some recombinant autoantigens are found to be not suitable at all. For example, SmD1 antigen generated in E. coli is not suitable for ELISA, while the same antigen expressed from a baculovirus system is (40). Recombinant antigens derived from the E. coli expression system that are not suitable for the detection of autoantibodies may lack posttranslational modifications required directly or indirectly for the reactivity of the epitope(s). There is a subgroup of autoantigens derived from E. coli expression systems that are not completely nonreactive but are clearly not optimal as substrates for autoantibody detection. A member of this subgroup includes the 60-kDa SS-A/Ro antigen. Only a low percentage of anti-SS-A/Ro-positive sera are reactive to the recombinant protein generated from E. coli compared to the native affinity-purified bovine 60-kDa protein. It is not clear why the native preparation is more immunoreactive than the one derived from E. coli, but probable explanations are that the native

antigen has a conformation, a posttranslational modification, or a cofactor that the protein made in E. coli lacks. Another instance where a cloned antigen does not have as much reactivity as the native proteins is U1 RNP. In this case, the increased reactivity with the native antigen is caused by antibodies in patients with mixed connective tissue disease that only react with the quaternary structure found in the RNA-multiprotein complex but not in the individual components.

Use of Natural Autoantigens

There remain many reasons that autoantigens are purified from natural rather than recombinant sources. Historical uses and costs are some of the issues that lead to the use of bovine chromatin preparations as substrates for the detection of antichromatin antibodies. Classical biochemical purification is still used for the purification of large quantities of different chromatin fractions as well as subunits that are useful for detecting a clinically relevant subset of antibodies (3). Additionally, it has been demonstrated that some diagnostically important antibodies react with epitopes present on the native histone-DNA complex found in chromatin. These epitopes are absent in purified histones and DNA (4). The antigen tissue transglutaminase, recognized by sera from people with celiac disease, is easily isolated by biochemical techniques from red blood cells and other tissue sources. To obtain native autoantigens that are in relatively low abundance in animal tissue, affinity column purification using well-defined human autoantibodies coupled to solid-phase matrices is routinely used. Because it is possible to obtain the large quantities of tissue that are needed at a relatively low cost, bovine spleen and thymus are often the starting material for native antigens. Examples in this category include all of the extractable nuclear antigens, such as Sm, RNP, 60-kDa SS-A/Ro, SS-B/La, Scl-70, and Jo-1.

Use of Peptide Antigens

Patients with autoimmune diseases make a wide spectrum of autoantibodies to specific antigens, and some of these antibodies will react with peptides from the antigen. Usually, the peptides are not as reactive as the whole protein in immunoassays, and thus they are not clinically useful. However, in a few instances, antibodies against peptides have been shown to be at least as clinically useful as antibodies against the corresponding native protein. In particular, the C-terminal 22 amino acids of ribosomal P proteins are the immunodominant peptide in certain patients with systemic lupus erythematosus (SLE) (9), as is a dimethylated peptide from SmD3 antigen (32). Citrullinated peptides derived from filaggrin and other sources are very reactive with sera from patients with rheumatoid arthritis (RA) (45).

Construction of Recombinant Proteins

The strategy in the design of recombinant constructs is beyond the scope of this chapter; however, some key aspects related to the production of recombinant autoantigens are discussed briefly below. The construction of recombinant proteins to be used in the detection of autoantibodies should take into consideration the suitability of the construct design and the ease of purification of resulting proteins. Earlier attempts in the production of recombinant proteins were faced with lengthy biochemical purification protocols to remove unwanted E. coli proteins. More importantly, most of these protocols have to be adjusted for each individual recombinant protein with distinct biochemical characteristics. Currently it is preferable to design recombinant proteins with an affinity tag that can be utilized for subsequent purification using a one-step solid-phase affinity chromatography protocol that can be shared among most recombinant proteins largely independent of their biochemical properties. The preferred affinity tag should be short, like the six-histidine tag that can be attached to the N terminus or C terminus of the recombinant protein using vectors such as pET28 (Novagen/EMD Biosciences, Inc., San Diego, Calif.) or pDEST17 (Invitrogen, Carlsbad, Calif.). The glutathione S-transferase (GST) fusion proteins, although used by many investigators for the expression of autoantigens, may not be suitable for general use, since anti-GST antibodies have been reported in some patients with autoimmune hepatitis (24).

In most designed recombinant autoantigens, full-length constructs are preferred so as to ensure that all the epitopes are well represented. When the autoantigen is a large protein, such as the Golgi complex protein giantin, which has a molecular mass of ~350 kDa, it is technically difficult to produce the complete protein in E. coli or even in a mammalian expression system. Thus, overlapping fragments of giantin that can be used alone or as a mixture for the detection of autoantibodies were produced (38).

Purification of Recombinant Proteins

As discussed above, the purification of recombinant proteins depends on the strategy and requirements. It is beyond the scope of this chapter to discuss purification of different types of recombinant proteins, and thus the following discussion represents two key modifications or improvements in overcoming problems encountered during the production of six-histidine-tagged recombinant proteins for use in the detection of autoantibodies. The first concern is the purity of the preparation to ensure that there are no false-positive results caused by antibodies that bind to E. coli protein contaminants. A modification of the established purification protocol for six-histidine-tagged proteins has been used to achieve a higher degree of purity by repeating the affinity purification step (41). Preliminary studies showed that twice-purified recombinant proteins had lower background reactivity with normal human sera than once-purified preparations. This two-time affinity purification protocol has been used in several studies (38, 62). In brief, six-histidine-tagged recombinant proteins are purified from E. coli lysates under denaturing conditions as described in the Qiagen manual The QIAexpressionist (41) and are eluted from a nickel affinity column using buffer E (8 M urea, 100 mM NaH$_2$PO$_4$, and 10 mM Tris Cl, pH 4.5). Fractions are pooled, the pH is adjusted to 8.0 with 1 N NaOH, and the nickel column is regenerated by washing in 2 volumes of buffer A (6 M guanidine hydrochloride, 100 mM NaH$_2$PO$_4$, and 10 mM TrisCl, pH 8.0). The second purification simply utilizes the pooled fraction and the regenerated affinity column identical to that in the first purification.

Use of Rosetta Bacteria for the Production of Large Recombinant Proteins

The second improvement addresses the low yield of recombinant protein in E. coli, especially when the recombinant protein to be produced has a high molecular mass. Most recombinant autoantigens up to ~70 kDa have been successfully produced in standard E. coli strain BL21(DE3) or JM109(DE3). Examples include SS-B/La and SS-A/Ro proteins of 52 and 60 kDa. Problems are often encountered when proteins of ~100 kDa or higher are generated in these E. coli strains. Figure 1 illustrates the problem encountered when the Golgi autoantigen p115 (115 kDa) was expressed in JM109(DE3) and the major products were only about

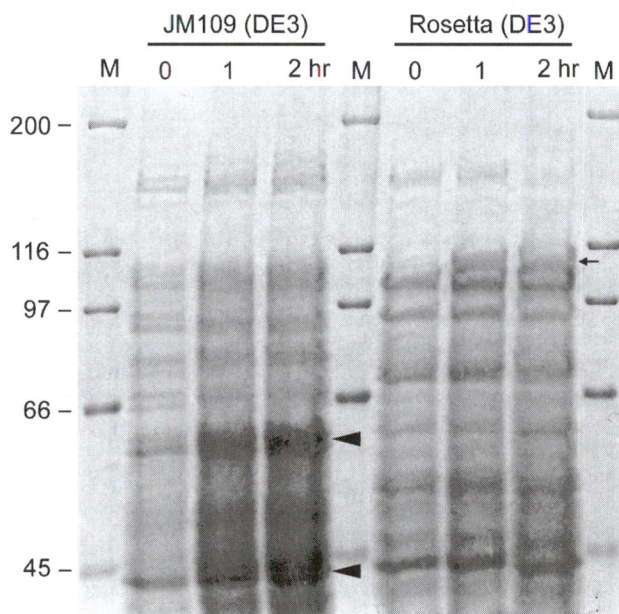

FIGURE 1 Enhanced expression of recombinant proteins is illustrated by the effect on the bacterial host. A construct, pET-p115, was transformed into either bacterial strain JM109(DE3) or Rosetta(DE3), and recombinant proteins were produced with the transformed bacteria using the same culture medium (2YT) and conditions. To cultured bacteria was added 1 mM isopropyl-β-D-thiogalactopyranoside (IPTG) at time zero, and cells were harvested as pellets after 1 or 2 h, solubilized in gel sample buffer, and analyzed by sodium dodecyl sulfate-polyacrylamide gel electrophoresis using a 5% acrylamide gel. Proteins were detected by Coomassie brilliant blue G-250 stain. Note that the recombinant JM109(DE3) culture generated major products of ~60 kDa (arrowhead) plus other lower-molecular-mass products, whereas the Rosetta culture yielded major products (arrow) corresponding to the native protein.

60 kDa. Similarly low-molecular-mass products were obtained with the BL21(DE3) bacteria. However, the expression was improved significantly using a new strain known as Rosetta(DE3), and a protein band corresponding to 115 kDa was generated (Fig. 1). Rosetta host strains from Novagen/EMD Biosciences, Inc., are E. coli BL21 derivatives engineered to increase the expression of eukaryotic proteins that contain codons rarely used in E. coli. These strains contain tRNA genes for AGG, AGA, AUA, CUA, CCC, and GGA in a chloramphenicol-resistant plasmid and thus provide for "universal" translation which is otherwise limited by the codon usage of E. coli. Our experience is that the use of the Rosetta cells has made a significant positive impact on the production of recombinant human autoantigens in E. coli.

ADVANCES IN ASSAYS

Newer autoantibody assay systems include cells transfected with cDNAs of antigens of interest (16, 25, 26), "LINE" assays (34), solid-phase antigen arrays (46), and addressable laser bead arrays (ALBA) where relevant native or recombinant antigens are bound to a solid-phase matrix or to laser-reactive beads. These new advances are only the beginning of a rapid succession of newer technologies such as microfluidics, lab-on-a-chip platforms, and nanotechnology (58). Comparison of performance and costs of some of these technologies to those of conventional assays suggest that they are reliable, highly sensitive, and cost-effective. Clinical analyses suggest that gains in accuracy and repeatability obtained in these new technologies may be clouded by a need to reevaluate current paradigms of the diagnostic and prognostic specificity of autoantibodies. One of the challenges of adapting new technologies will be to differentiate natural autoantibodies from those that are related to pathogenesis. Each assay has limitations in terms of determining the sensitivity, specificity, and positive predictive value for the detection of autoantibodies. The balance of this chapter focuses on addressable laser bead technology and recent experience with it in a clinical laboratory setting with addressable laser bead immunoassays (ALBIA).

ALBA and ALBIA

ALBA represent an application of array and flow technologies that has already entered the market and has demonstrated flexibility in a variety of genomic, proteomic, and immunoassay applications (8). Although there are several applications of this technology, much experience has centered on the Luminex 100 platform (Luminex Corp., Austin, Tex.), which incorporates laser-based flow technology that can analyze reactants in a microtiter plate format. A key component of this technology is the ability to differentiate up to 100 classes of microspheres based on various amounts of laser-reactive dyes embedded in each class, called 100 different colors for simplicity. This platform has been developed to measure antibodies in biological fluids (18, 44), screen supernatants for monoclonal antibodies of interest (21, 47), quantitate cytokines in cell extracts and biological fluids (27), detect bacterial pathogens, perform HLA typing, detect single nucleotide polymorphisms, track cell signaling responses, and monitor gene expression. The robust application of numerous technologies in this platform suggests that a future use may be to profile patients in a variety of diagnostic and therapeutic settings (8).

ALBA and ALBIA that utilized the Luminex (Labmap) platform in research and clinical laboratory settings have been evaluated in a number of studies. In practice, an antigen of interest is chemically coupled to a specific colored microsphere. Other antigens are coupled to microspheres of different colors. After the coupling and stabilizing reactions, the antigen-coupled spheres are combined into a single microtiter well to provide a single assay that has the ability to detect multiple antibodies in a single specimen. The test samples (sera or other biological fluids) and a fluorochrome-coupled secondary antibody are added to the wells, and after an incubation time, they are analyzed. The principles of the assay are similar to those of flow cytometry with one laser identifying the specific antigen-coupled bead passing through the path and a second laser determining the presence and quantity of secondary antibody bound to the bead. The data are displayed in a number of formats but are expressed as a quantitative analysis of multiple analytes and the relative amount of antibody bound to the antigen. We have found the development of our in-house assays to be easier, more efficient, and more economical than earlier technologies such as Western blotting, IP, or ELISA. Research applications have included the development of assays to detect monoclonal antibodies and autoantibodies directed to a number of autoantigens, including early endosome antigen 1 (48, 49), GW182 (10, 11), translocated promoter region (39), and VCP (36).

TABLE 1 Reactivity of sera from 100 PBC patients in ALBIA

Antigen	% Reactivity		
	PBC (n = 100)	IBD[a] (n = 50)	Healthy (n = 100)
Chromatin	12	2	2
SLA	0	0	0
M2/PDC	72	0	0
LKM	0	0	0
p97/VCP	18	0	0

[a] IBD, inflammatory bowel disease.

In addition, a research kit used to detect antibodies to liver kidney microsomal antigen (LKM), M2 (PDC), soluble liver antigen (SLA), and chromatin (QUANTA Plex liver panel; INOVA Diagnostics Inc., San Diego, Calif.) was evaluated in the setting of autoimmune liver diseases. In a separate ALBIA, beads that were coupled to p97/VCP were also prepared (36). In a study of 25 sera from primary biliary cirrhosis (PBC) patients, 19 (76%) reacted with the M2 (PDC) antigen, 5 (20%) reacted with VCP, 2 (8%) reacted with chromatin, and none reacted with LKM or SLA (Table 1). Only one serum sample reacted with chromatin in the inflammatory bowel disease control group. In the same PBC cohort, 84% had a positive antimitochondrial antibody test as measured by IIF on rodent liver substrates. The apparent lack of sensitivity of the ALBIA is likely due to antimitochondrial antibody directed to other mitochondrial autoantigens that were not included in the ALBIA PDC antigen source (15, 28).

In a clinical service laboratory setting an autoantigen panel (QUANTA Plex; INOVA Diagnostics, Inc.) based on ALBIA was evaluated and compared to the routine diagnostic protocol, which analyzed 870 sequential unselected sera received over a 6-month period (13). In this study, the sera were submitted primarily by clinicians who were considering a diagnosis of systemic rheumatic disease. The conventional serological algorithm used IIF on HEp-2 cell substrates (HEp-2000; ImmunoConcepts, Inc.) to screen all sera. Antibodies to SS-A/Ro can be detected in this IIF assay because this substrate includes cells that are transfected with, and overexpress, the 60-kDa SS-A/Ro autoantigen (14, 25). Sera that were found to be positive in this IIF assay were then evaluated by ID for antibodies to Sm, U1-RNP, SS-A/Ro, SS-B/La, Scl-70 (topoisomerase I), and other saline-soluble autoantigens. Antibodies to double-stranded DNA (dsDNA) were detected by IIF on *Crithidia luciliae* substrate (ImmunoConcepts). This comparison showed that ALBIA agreed with the conventional test result 92% of the time. An exception was a lack of high correlation of anti-dsDNA measured by the *Crithidia* assay and the ALBIA. Because of this, anti-DNA is no longer included in this profile.

When the results of the ALBIA were compared to those of the conventional assay, it was noted that, on average, 25% of sera exhibited a positive result that was not detected by conventional autoantibody testing. The accuracy and validity of the ALBIA result could be confirmed by other techniques, such as IP and immunoblotting. This observed increased sensitivity of ALBIA was studied in various serological cohorts. The results of one such study are shown in Table 2; in that study were included 30 highly characterized sera that were previously shown to react with ribosomal P in at least one commercial ELISA (Euroimmun, Pharmacia,

TABLE 2 Comparison of ELISA and ALBIA detection of anti-ribosomal P autoantibodies in 30 sera

Serum no.	Value for test from indicated vendor[a]			
	Euroimmun, ratio (cutoff, >1)	MBL, U/ml (cutoff, 11.6)	INOVA, U (cutoff, 20)	QUANTA Plex, ratio (cutoff, >1)
1	9.1	219	202	15
2	5.6	144	164	8
3	7.9	124	200	14
4	2.2	24	185	11
5	4.4	76	140	17
6	5.1	63	178	8
7	6.8	111	165	12
8	7.7	169	197	25
9	8.9	246	212	13
10	7.5	187	198	12
11	8.9	69	87	8
12	2.8	72	139	6
13	6.6	125	184	13
14	6.3	130	181	12
15	5.2	116	173	14
16	3.4	87	148	5
17	6.0	136	164	10
18	5.3	118	155	20
19	5.8	100	150	3
20	7.8	170	206	17
21	7.1	146	199	16
22	1.0	11	20	1.5
23	2.1	19	39	4
24	7.4	155	204	10
25	3.9	76	54	10
26	7.6	143	192	9
27	7.2	148	203	23
28	9.1	239	219	27
29	3.2	38	75	2
30	1.6	55	66	2

[a] Data extracted from reference 31 and rounded to the nearest whole number.

MBL) (30, 31). Comparison of the data show excellent agreement of ALBIA with the ELISAs, including those that utilize the C22 terminal ribosomal P peptide (31).

Unselected sera from various disease cohorts were also studied to determine if the frequency of autoantibodies as detected by the ALBIA was consistent with the published frequency of autoantibodies (Table 3). This study showed that the frequency of various autoantibodies in SLE, systemic sclerosis (SSc), Sjögren's syndrome (SjS), and RA was in keeping with published reports. Interesting exceptions included antibodies to Scl-70 (topoisomerase I), which were found in 8% of sera from SLE patients, and antibodies to

TABLE 3 Frequency of autoantibodies detected by INOVA QUANTA Plex assay in cohorts of patients with systemic rheumatic diseases, those with multiple sclerosis, and controls[a]

Antigen	SLE (n = 200)	SSc (n = 100)	SjS (n = 100)	RA (n = 200)	IBD (n = 50)	MS (n = 100)	Healthy (n = 50)
Chromatin	60	20	20	8	2	4	0
dsDNA	48	0	0	2	0	0	0
U1 RNP	24	10	0	4	0	8	0
Sm	18	4[b]	0	0	0	1	0
Scl-70	6	24	0	0	0	4	0
SS-A/Ro	34	24	35	0	0	5	0
SS-B/La	8	5	20	2	0	10	0
Jo-1	0	3	15	0	0	4	0
Rib-P	16	2	0	0.5	0	5	0

[a] Abbreviations: IBD, inflammatory bowel disease; MS, multiple sclerosis.
[b] Low positive.

TABLE 4 Advantages, challenges, and opportunities relating to new array technologies

Advantages	Challenges and opportunities
Multiple autoantibodies detected in single assay	New clinical correlations and paradigms based on autoantibody and epitope profiling
Personnel costs	Costs of maintenance contracts and budgeting for laser replacement
Rapid test performance and automated test reporting	Medical centers not equipped or configured to accept digital reports can jeopardize rapid turnaround times.
Small sample volumes	Adoption of new technologies that do not require conventional venipuncture
High correlation with other immunoassays, particularly ELISA	Low correlation with ID
Ease of establishing new assays	Research and development required to provide broader spectrum of autoantigens (nucleolar, paraneoplastic, phospholipids)
Equipment and technology can be used for variety of relevant assays: cytokine, SNP, HLA, gene activation, cell activation, drug discovery	Emergence of other microarray and nanotechnology platforms will complicate standardization.

Jo-1 (histidyl-tRNA synthetase), which were found in 15% of sera from SjS patients and 4% of sera from SSc patients. It was noted that the reactivity of sera from SLE patients with Scl-70 was in the borderline region of positivity. Similar observations were made with anti-Sm, which was found in 5% of sera from SSc patients, but all of these demonstrated a measurement of mean fluorescence units that was just above the cutoff. Follow-up testing of these sera found that none bound the SmD3 peptide, which is highly specific for SLE (29, 32). The observation that some sera from SLE patients bind Scl-70 is interesting in light of other reports that anti-Scl-70 antibodies were found in sera from SLE patients (19). Likewise, the finding of anti-Jo-1 antibodies in sera from SjS and SSc patients was surprising but may be related to more recent observations that sera with anti-Jo-1 antibodies are occasionally found to contain antibodies to the 52-kDa SS-A/Ro autoantigen (59). Of note, none of the sera from healthy or inflammatory bowel disease controls were positive for any of the antigens used in the INOVA QUANTA Plex ALBIA.

Early studies of ALBIA kits are showing a high level (>90%) of agreement with antinuclear antibody and conventional ELISA techniques. For example, in a study of 37 sera from SjS patients that compared a conventional ELISA to an ALBIA kit (Athena Multi-Lyte ANA Test System), a 99% concordance between the two assays was found (18).

Taken together, there are advantages and challenges that come with the adoption of the ALBA platform to detect autoantibodies (Table 4). The capacity of one assay to analyze and detect a complex array of autoantibodies in a single small serum sample (>10 μl) with speed and precision is a significant advantage. There are now several ALBIA kits on the market that detect eight or more autoantibodies relevant to systemic rheumatic diseases. In some kits, the secondary antibody is added but no subsequent washing of beads is required. In addition, test reports can be automatically generated through standard database management software. These factors combine to generate test results very rapidly, since analysis of multiple antibodies in a single well typically takes less than 2 min. In our laboratory, the turnaround time from receipt of the serum sample to generation of the laboratory report using the conventional technologies was 4 to 5 days. By comparison, the turnaround time using ALBIA is 1 to 2 days. This marked improvement is predicated on a laboratory algorithm that tests samples daily, as opposed to batch runs of ~90 sera. Last, although we have not performed detailed cost analyses, there is little additional cost because the throughput has been effectively

doubled and this throughput was managed with the same staff complement as with the conventional protocols. In fact, the staff now has more time for quality assurance and research projects that were formerly delegated to other staff. The tradeoff for these apparent cost savings is countered by more expensive maintenance contracts, upgrades to software, and a budget allocation for replacement of lasers.

A major challenge and opportunity in the adoption of multiplexed autoantibody analyses is the breadth of autoantibody profiles provided in the laboratory reports. This increased amount of information presents a significant challenge to clinicians who are accustomed to dealing with one or two autoantibody results for any given patient. It is likely that with autoantibody profiling, a new wave of clinical studies and clinical correlations based on more complete autoantibody profiles will emerge. The clinical picture may be enhanced by extending the breadth of this technology to epitope mapping and epitope spreading as an approach to monitoring disease progression or remission. Last, history has taught us that standardization of the new multiplexed platforms will be the most significant challenge. The utilization of international reference sera for standardization of secondary antibodies to establish controls and cutoff values will be very important. At present, because the ALBA equipment and hardware are based primarily on the Luminex platform and accompanying software, diversity of this hardware is not a significant issue.

This work was supported in part by Canadian Institutes for Health Research grant MOP-38034 and National Institutes of Health grants AI47859 and AI39645. M.J.F holds the Arthritis Society Chair at the University of Calgary.

REFERENCES

1. **Bizzaro, N., and A. Wiik.** 2004. Appropriateness in antinuclear antibody testing: from clinical request to strategic laboratory practice. *Clin. Exp. Rheumatol.* **22:**349–355.
2. **Boire, G., F.-J. Lopez-Longo, S. Lapointe, and H. A. Menard.** 1991. Sera from patients with autoimmune disease recognize conformational determinants on the 60-kd Ro/SS-A protein. *Arthritis Rheum.* **34:**722–730.
3. **Burlingame, R. W., M. L. Boey, G. Starkebaum, and R. L. Rubin.** 1994. The central role of chromatin in autoimmune responses to histones and DNA in systemic lupus erythematosus. *J. Clin. Investig.* **94:**184–192.
4. **Burlingame, R. W., and R. L. Rubin.** 1990. Subnucleosome structures as substrates in enzyme-linked immunosorbent assays. *J. Immunol. Methods* **134:**187–199.

5. **Chan, E. K. L., and L. E. C. Andrade.** 1992. Antinuclear antibodies in Sjögren's syndrome. *Rheum. Dis. Clin. N. Am.* **18**:551–570.

6. **Chan, E. K. L., and J. P. Buyon.** 1994. The SS-A/Ro antigen, p. 1–18. *In* W. J. van Venrooij and R. N. Maini (ed.), *Manual of Biological Markers of Disease.* Kluwer Academic Publishers, Dordrecht, The Netherlands.

7. **Chan-Hui, P. Y., K. Stephens, R. A. Warnock, and S. Singh.** 2004. Applications of eTag trademark assay platform to systems biology approaches in molecular oncology and toxicology studies. *Clin. Immunol.* **111**:162–174.

8. **Earley, M. C., R. F. Vogt, Jr., H. M. Shapiro, F. F. Mandy, K. L. Kellar, R. Bellisario, K. A. Pass, G. E. Marti, C. C. Stewart, and W. H. Hannon.** 2002. Report from a workshop on multianalyte microsphere assays. *Cytometry* **50**:239–242.

9. **Elkon, K., S. Skelly, A. Parnassa, W. Moller, W. Danho, H. Weissbach, and N. Brot.** 1986. Identification and chemical synthesis of a ribosomal protein antigenic determinant in systemic lupus erythematosus. *Proc. Natl. Acad. Sci. USA* **83**:7419–7423.

10. **Eystathioy, T., E. K. L. Chan, M. Mahler, L. M. Luft, M. L. Fritzler, and M. J. Fritzler.** 2003. A panel of monoclonal antibodies to cytoplasmic GW bodies and the mRNA binding protein GW182. *Hybrid. Hybrid.* **22**:79–86.

11. **Eystathioy, T., E. K. L. Chan, K. Takeuchi, M. Mahler, L. M. Luft, D. W. Zochodne, and M. J. Fritzler.** 2003. Clinical and serological associations of autoantibodies to GW bodies and a novel cytoplasmic autoantigen GW182. *J. Mol. Med.* **81**:811–818.

12. **Fritzler, M. J.** 1993. Autoantibodies in scleroderma. *J. Dermatol.* **20**:257–268.

13. **Fritzler, M. J.** 2002. New technologies in the detection of autoantibodies, p. 50–63. *In* K. Conrad, M. J. Fritzler, M. Meurer, U. Sack, and Y. Shoenfeld (ed.), *Autoantigens, Autoantibodies, Autoimmunity.* Pabst Scientific Publishers, Lengerich, Germany.

14. **Fritzler, M. J., C. Hanson, J. Miller, and T. Eystathioy.** 2002. Specificity of autoantibodies to SS-A/Ro on a transfected and overexpressed human 60 kDa Ro autoantigen substrate. *J. Clin. Lab. Anal.* **16**:103–108.

15. **Fritzler, M. J., and M. P. Manns.** 2002. Anti-mitochondrial antibodies. *Clin. Appl. Immunol. Rev.* **3**:87–113.

16. **Fritzler, M. J., and B. J. Miller.** 1995. Detection of autoantibodies to SS-A/Ro by indirect immunofluorescence using a transfected and overexpressed human 60 kD Ro autoantigen in HEp-2 cells. *J. Clin. Lab. Anal.* **9**:218–224.

17. **Fritzler, M. J., A. Wiik, M. L. Fritzler, and S. G. Barr.** 2003. The use and abuse of commercial kits used to detect autoantibodies. *Arthritis Res. Ther.* **5**:192–201.

18. **Gilburd, B., M. Abu-Shakra, Y. Shoenfeld, A. Giordano, E. B. Bocci, F. delle Monache, and R. Gerli.** 2004. Autoantibodies profile in the sera of patients with Sjogren's syndrome: the ANA evaluation—a homogeneous, multiplexed system. *Clin. Dev. Immunol.* **11**:53–56.

19. **Gussin, H. A., G. P. Ignat, J. Varga, and M. Teodorescu.** 2001. Anti-topoisomerase I (anti-Scl-70) antibodies in patients with systemic lupus erythematosus. *Arthritis Rheum.* **44**:376–383.

20. **Illei, G. G., E. Tackey, L. Lapteva, and P. E. Lipsky.** 2004. Biomarkers in systemic lupus erythematosus. I. General overview of biomarkers and their applicability. *Arthritis Rheum.* **50**:1709–1720.

21. **Jia, X. C., R. Raya, L. Zhang, O. Foord, W. L. Walker, M. L. Gallo, M. Haak-Frendscho, L. L. Green, and C. G. Davis.** 2004. A novel method of multiplexed competitive antibody binding for the characterization of monoclonal antibodies. *J. Immunol. Methods* **288**:91–98.

22. **Joos, T. O., D. Stoll, and M. F. Templin.** 2002. Miniaturised multiplexed immunoassays. *Curr. Opin. Chem. Biol.* **6**:76–80.

23. **Kantor, A. B., W. Wang, H. Lin, H. Govindarajan, M. Anderle, A. Perrone, and C. Becker.** 2004. Biomarker discovery by comprehensive phenotyping for autoimmune diseases. *Clin. Immunol.* **111**:186–195.

24. **Kato, T., H. Miyakawa, and M. Ishibashi.** 2004. Frequency and significance of anti-glutathione S-transferase autoantibody (anti-GST A1-1) in autoimmune hepatitis. *J. Autoimmun.* **22**:211–216.

25. **Keech, C. L., S. Howarth, T. Coates, M. Rischmueller, J. McCluskey, and T. P. Gordon.** 1996. Rapid and sensitive detection of anti-Ro (SS-A) antibodies by indirect immunofluorescence of 60kDa Ro HEp-2 transfectants. *Pathology* **28**:54–57.

26. **Keech, C. L., J. McCluskey, and T. P. Gordon.** 1994. Transfection and overexpression of the human 60-kDa Ro/SS-A autoantigen in HEp-2 cells. *Clin. Immunol. Immunopathol.* **73**:146–151.

27. **Kellar, K. L., R. R. Kalwar, K. A. Dubois, D. Crouse, W. D. Chafin, and B. E. Kane.** 2001. Multiplexed fluorescent bead-based immunoassays for quantitation of human cytokines in serum and culture supernatants. *Cytometry* **45**:27–36.

28. **MacKay, I. R., S. Whittingham, S. Fida, M. Myers, N. Ikuno, M. E. Gershwin, and M. J. Rowley.** 2000. The peculiar autoimmunity of primary biliary cirrhosis. *Immunol. Rev.* **174**:226–237.

29. **Mahler, M., M. J. Fritzler, and M. Bluthner.** 2005. Identification of a SmD3 epitope with a single symmetrical dimethylation of an arginine residue as a specific target of a subpopulation of anti-Sm antibodies. *Arthritis Res. Ther.* **7**:R19–R29.

30. **Mahler, M., K. Kessenbrock, J. Raats, and M. J. Fritzler.** 2004. Technical and clinical evaluation of anti-ribosomal P protein immunoassays. *J. Clin. Lab. Anal.* **18**:215–223.

31. **Mahler, M., K. Kessenbrock, J. Raats, R. Williams, M. J. Fritzler, and M. Bluthner.** 2003. Characterization of the human autoimmune response to the major C-terminal epitope of the ribosomal P proteins. *J. Mol. Med.* **81**:194–204.

32. **Mahler, M., L. M. Stinton, and M. J. Fritzler.** 2005. Improved serological differentiation between systemic lupus erythematosus and mixed connective tissue disease by use of an SmD3 peptide-based immunoassay. *Clin. Diagn. Lab. Immunol* **12**:107–113.

33. **Manoussakis, M. N., K. G. Kistis, X. Liu, V. Aidinis, A. Guialis, and H. M. Moutsopoulos.** 1993. Detection of anti-Ro(SSA) antibodies in autoimmune diseases: comparison of five methods. *Br. J. Rheumatol.* **32**:449–455.

34. **Meheus, L., W. J. van Venrooij, A. Wiik, P. J. Charles, A. G. Tzioufas, O. Meyer, G. Steiner, D. Gianola, S. Bombardieri, A. Union, S. De Keyser, E. Veys, and F. De Keyser.** 1999. Multicenter validation of recombinant, natural and synthetic antigens used in a single multiparameter assay for the detection of specific anti-nuclear autoantibodies in connective tissue disorders. *Clin. Exp. Rheumatol.* **17**:205–214.

35. **Meilof, J. F., I. Bantjes, J. De Jong, A. P. Van Dam, and R. J. Smeenk.** 1990. The detection of anti-Ro/SS-A and anti-La/SS-B antibodies. A comparison of counterimmunoelectrophoresis with immunoblot, ELISA, and RNA-precipitation assays. *J. Immunol. Methods* **133**:215–226.

36. **Miyachi, K., Y. Hirano, T. Horigome, T. Mimori, H. Miyakawa, Y. Onozuka, M. Shibata, M. Hirakata, A. Suwa, H. Hosaka, S. Matsushima, T. Komatsu, H. Matsushima, R. W. Hankins, and M. J. Fritzler.** 2004. Autoantibodies from primary biliary cirrhosis patients with anti-p95c antibodies bind to recombinant p97/VCP and inhibit in vitro nuclear envelope assembly. *Clin. Exp. Immunol.* **136**:568–573.

37. **Miyachi, K., H. Matsushima, R. W. Hankins, M. Hirakata, T. Mimori, H. Hosaka, Y. Amagasaki,**

H. Miyakawa, M. Kako, M. Shibata, Y. Onozuka, and U. Ueno. 1998. A novel antibody directed against a three-dimensional configuration of a 95-kDa protein in patients with autoimmune hepatic diseases. *Scand. J. Immunol.* **47:**63–68.

38. **Nozawa, K., M. J. Fritzler, C. A. von Mühlen, and E. K. L. Chan.** 2004. Giantin is the major Golgi autoantigen in human anti-Golgi complex sera. *Arthritis Res. Ther.* **6:**R95–R102.

39. **Ou, Y., P. Enarson, J. B. Rattner, S. G. Barr, and M. J. Fritzler.** 2004. The nuclear pore complex protein Tpr is a common autoantigen in sera that demonstrate nuclear envelope staining by indirect immunofluorescence. *Clin. Exp. Immunol.* **136:**379–387.

40. **Ou, Y., D. Sun, G. C. Sharp, and S. O. Hoch.** 1997. Screening of SLE sera using purified recombinant Sm-D1 protein from a baculovirus expression system. *Clin. Immunol. Immunopathol.* **83:**310–317.

41. **Qiagen.** 2003. *The QIAexpressionist. A Handbook for High-Level Expression and Purification of 6xHis-Tagged Proteins*, 5th ed. http://www1.qiagen.com/literature/handbooks/PDF/Protein/Expression/QXP_QIAexpressionist/1024473_QXPHB_0603.pdf.

42. **Radic, M. Z., and M. Weigert.** 1994. Genetic and structural evidence for antigen selection of anti-DNA antibodies. *Annu. Rev. Immunol.* **12:**487–520.

43. **Robinson, W. H., C. DiGennaro, W. Hueber, B. B. Haab, M. Kamachi, E. J. Dean, S. Fournel, D. Fong, M. C. Genovese, H. E. de Vegvar, K. Skriner, D. L. Hirschberg, R. I. Morris, S. Muller, G. J. Pruijn, W. J. van Venrooij, J. S. Smolen, P. O. Brown, L. Steinman, and P. J. Utz.** 2002. Autoantigen microarrays for multiplex characterization of autoantibody responses. *Nat. Med.* **8:**295–301.

44. **Rouquette, A. M., C. Desgruelles, and P. Laroche.** 2003. Evaluation of the new multiplexed immunoassay, FIDIS, for simultaneous quantitative determination of antinuclear antibodies and comparison with conventional methods. *Am. J. Clin. Pathol.* **120:**676–681.

45. **Schellekens, G. A., H. Visser, B. A. de Jong, F. H. Van Den Hoogen, J. M. Hazes, F. C. Breedveld, and W. J. van Venrooij.** 2000. The diagnostic properties of rheumatoid arthritis antibodies recognizing a cyclic citrullinated peptide. *Arthritis Rheum.* **43:**155–163.

46. **Scussel-Lonzetti, L., F. Joyal, J. P. Raynauld, A. Roussin, E. Rich, J. R. Goulet, Y. Raymond, and J. L. Senecal.** 2002. Predicting mortality in systemic sclerosis: analysis of a cohort of 309 French Canadian patients with emphasis on features at diagnosis as predictive factors for survival. *Medicine* (Baltimore) **81:**154–167.

47. **Seideman, J., and D. Peritt.** 2002. A novel monoclonal antibody screening method using the Luminex-100 microsphere system. *J. Immunol. Methods* **267:**165–171.

48. **Selak, S., and M. J. Fritzler.** 2004. Altered neurological function in mice immunized with early endosome antigen 1. *BMC Neurosci.* **5:**2.

49. **Selak, S., M. Mahler, K. Miyachi, M. L. Fritzler, and M. J. Fritzler.** 2003. Identification of the B-cell epitopes of the early endosome antigen 1 (EEA1). *Clin. Immunol.* **109:**154–164.

50. **Tan, E. M.** 1991. Autoantibodies in pathology and cell biology. *Cell* **67:**841–842.

51. **Tan, E. M.** 1989. Antinuclear antibodies: diagnostic markers for autoimmune diseases and probes for cell biology. *Adv. Immunol.* **44:**93–151.

52. **Tan, E. M., E. K. L. Chan, K. F. Sullivan, and R. L. Rubin.** 1988. Antinuclear antibodies (ANAs): diagnostically specific immune markers and clues toward the understanding of systemic autoimmunity. *Clin. Immunol. Immunopathol.* **47:**121–141.

53. **Tan, E. M., J. S. Smolen, J. S. McDougal, M. J. Fritzler, T. Gordon, J. A. Hardin, J. R. Kalden, R. G. Lahita, R. N. Maini, W. H. Reeves, N. F. Rothfield, Y. Takasaki, A. Wiik, M. Wilson, and J. A. Koziol.** 2002. A critical evaluation of enzyme immunoassay kits for detection of antinuclear autoantibodies of defined specificities. II. Potential for quantitation of antibody content. *J. Rheumatol.* **29:**68–74.

54. **Templin, M. F., D. Stoll, J. Bachmann, and T. O. Joos.** 2004. Protein microarrays and multiplexed sandwich immunoassays: what beats the beads? *Comb. Chem. High Throughput Screen.* **7:**223–229.

55. **Thiel, A., A. Scheffold, and A. Radbruch.** 2004. Antigen-specific cytometry—new tools arrived! *Clin. Immunol.* **111:**155–161.

56. **Tillman, D. M., N. T. Jou, R. J. Hill, and T. N. Marion.** 1992. Both IgM and IgG anti-DNA antibodies are the products of clonally selective B cell stimulation in (NZB × NZW)F1 mice. *J. Exp. Med.* **176:**761–779.

57. **Utz, P. J.** 2004. Multiplexed assays for identification of biomarkers and surrogate markers in systemic lupus erythematosus. *Lupus* **13:**304–311.

58. **Utz, P. J.** 2004. "Hot technologies" for clinical immunology research. *Clin. Immunol.* **111:**153–154.

59. **Venables, P. J.** 1997. Antibodies to Jo-1 and Ro-52: why do they go together? *Clin. Exp. Immunol.* **109:**403–405.

60. **Wiik, A. S., T. P. Gordon, A. F. Kavanaugh, R. G. Lahita, W. Reeves, W. J. van Venrooij, M. R. Wilson, and M. Fritzler.** 2004. Cutting edge diagnostics in rheumatology: the role of patients, clinicians, and laboratory scientists in optimizing the use of autoimmune serology. *Arthritis Rheum.* **51:**291–298.

61. **Xue, Q., A. Wainright, S. Gangakhedkar, and I. Gibbons.** 2001. Multiplexed enzyme assays in capillary electrophoretic single-use microfluidic devices. *Electrophoresis* **22:**4000–4007.

62. **Zhang, J. Y., C. A. Casiano, X. X. Peng, J. A. Koziol, E. K. L. Chan, and E. M. Tan.** 2003. Enhancement of antibody detection in cancer using panel of recombinant tumor-associated antigens. *Cancer Epidemiol. Biomark. Prev.* **12:**136–143.

Detection of Anti-DNA Antibodies

TRINH T. TRAN AND DAVID S. PISETSKY

115

Antibodies to DNA (anti-DNA) are prototypic autoantibodies found prominently in the sera of patients with systemic lupus erythematosus (SLE). This generalized autoimmune disease is characterized by multisystem involvement in association with abundant autoantibody production. Of these autoantibodies, those directed to components of the cell nucleus (antinuclear antibodies, or ANA) occur almost invariably in patients, with anti-DNA as a major ANA specificity, serving as a serological marker of diagnostic and prognostic significance. As established by the American College of Rheumatology, anti-DNA also represents a criterion in the classification of patients for SLE. The close association of anti-DNA with SLE has suggested that anti-DNA antibodies can signal critical events in SLE pathogenesis as well as guide patient evaluation in the clinical setting (10, 22).

As a macromolecule with a nonrepeating structure, DNA presents a potentially large array of antigenic determinants related to its sequence, conformation, and backbone structure. In its simplest form, however, DNA can be categorized antigenically as single-stranded DNA (ssDNA) or double-stranded DNA (dsDNA); dsDNA is also sometimes denoted native DNA. For this categorization, natural DNA of mammalian or bacterial origin serves as the antigen. While DNAs from various species likely differ in antigenic structure, anti-DNA antibodies in SLE sera appear to bind epitopes expressed widely on DNA, independent of its origin (15). Other antigenic forms of DNA can be prepared by using synthetic or cloned DNA, but these antigens have not produced assays that are either more sensitive or more specific than those using natural DNA.

In addition to reactivity to antigenic sites on DNA, anti-DNA antibodies can be differentiated in terms of their isotype, avidity, and pathogenicity. In general, anti-DNA immunoglobulin G (IgG) is linked more closely to disease than IgM antibodies. Indeed, IgM anti-DNA antibodies can appear in the sera of even healthy individuals, where they are designated natural autoantibodies (4, 9). Among IgG antibodies, anti-dsDNA antibodies are more specific to SLE than anti-ssDNA antibodies. Anti-ssDNA, which occurs more frequently in SLE patients than anti-dsDNA, nevertheless occurs in the sera of patients with other autoimmune and inflammatory diseases as well as in healthy subjects (6). Many antibodies cross-react with both dsDNA and ssDNA, however, making these distinctions operational. In patients with SLE, anti-dsDNA is present in approximately 40% of patients, whereas anti-ssDNA is present in approximately 70% of patients at some point.

Although expressed pathologically, anti-DNA antibodies nevertheless differ in their ability to mediate inflammation and tissue damage, in particular glomerulonephritis. Antibodies promoting nephritis are denoted as pathogenic or nephritogenic. Since nephritis in SLE results at least in part from immune complex deposition, pathogenic antibodies likely display properties that allow the formation of complexes that deposit in the kidney. These properties include avidity, fine specificity, and the ability to fix complement (18, 21). Assays of anti-DNA based on these properties have not been developed, although ultimately, the assessment of pathogenicity involves the transfer of disease by antibodies in an animal model. Such an assessment is useful only in the research setting.

While the precise properties conferring pathogenicity are not well defined, for many patients the presence of high-avidity anti-dsDNA antibodies of the IgG isotype correlates well with the disease activity of lupus nephritis. Furthermore, the levels of these antibodies frequently vary significantly over time, with levels rising as nephritis intensifies and falling with effective therapy. These correlations are not invariable, however, and nephritis can occur in the absence of anti-DNA levels. This finding suggests that antibodies binding antigens other than DNA are pathogenic or that the assay used for anti-DNA determination misses the relevant antibody population (18). In this regard, anti-DNA levels may not correlate with other clinical manifestations of SLE or overall disease activity.

In the clinical setting, testing of anti-DNA antibodies has two distinct purposes. The first is diagnosis. For the evaluation of patients with complex, multisystem disease, anti-DNA assays are commonly performed in conjunction with testing for other ANA to assess the likelihood of SLE. Depending on the assay used, ANA positivity, while essentially ubiquitous in SLE and a criterion for classification, occurs in many other conditions, including rheumatoid arthritis and Sjögren's syndrome. Anti-DNA thus provides a more specific marker of diagnosis, and along with anti-Sm, another ANA linked to SLE, points to the diagnosis (7, 16). Since anti-DNA occurs in only some patients and since the levels vary strikingly, its use diagnostically has limitations. In this regard, anti-DNA expression can occur years prior to clinical manifestations, suggesting that for some patients, this specificity may have predictive value as well (1, 2).

The second purpose of anti-DNA testing relates to disease activity. Since anti-DNA antibodies appear to be a major cause of SLE renal disease, the correlations between levels of these antibodies and nephritis are the clearest and most demonstrable by the use of various assay approaches (25). For some patients, anti-DNA testing has less value as an activity marker, in which case testing of complement levels (a measure of complement consumption during immune complex deposition) can provide adjunctive information. Clinically, for each patient, it is useful to establish the best serological or laboratory correlate of disease activity and not to rely exclusively on any one test. Since the "gold standard" for active lupus remains elusive, there is inherent uncertainty in this assessment (23).

While the role of anti-DNA in immune complex renal disease may underlie the correlation with disease activity, anti-DNA antibodies may have other functions that contribute to this association. As shown in studies of the human and murine systems, DNA–anti-DNA immune complexes have immunomodulatory effects and can promote B-cell activation and the production of cytokines such as interferon (19, 27). This action may be related to the ability of immune complexes to deliver DNA to internal sites in cells, where it can stimulate Toll-like receptor 9 (5, 17). Since the DNA in the complexes is needed for immune activity, an assay of antibodies alone may not reveal the potential for immune stimulation. In this regard, antibodies to DNA are a subset of antibodies to nucleosomes, the form of DNA in the nucleus, with many of these antibodies potentially able to stimulate the immune system as long as the nucleic acid component is present in the complex. This feature of anti-DNA function could suggest the basis of a more general correlation of anti-DNA with SLE in terms of both diagnosis and activity.

Despite their lower frequency in patient sera, anti-dsDNA antibodies are more specific for SLE than anti-ssDNA antibodies. Most clinical laboratories now perform tests that specifically detect anti-dsDNA antibodies, although anti-ssDNA can provide useful information for assessing disease activity; anti-ssDNA assays are also easier to perform. Currently, the methods available for anti-DNA include the radioimmunoassay (RIA), the *Crithidia luciliae* immunofluorescence (CLIF) assay, and the enzyme-linked immunosorbent assay (ELISA). Their advantages and disadvantages are discussed below (14, 16).

TECHNOLOGY

Farr Assay

The most commonly used RIA for anti-DNA measurement is the Farr assay. In this assay, a radiolabeled source of dsDNA is incubated with serum to form immune complexes, which are precipitated from solution with ammonium sulfate at 50% saturation. The quantity of anti-dsDNA antibodies is represented as the amount of radioactivity in the precipitate. A circular bacteriophage DNA or a circular plasmid DNA is used to ensure double strandedness.

The Farr assay measures high-affinity anti-DNA antibodies which do not dissociate under the high salt conditions of ammonium sulfate saturation. Given the properties of the antibodies detected, the Farr assay is specific for SLE. The results are reproducible, with high titer values in combination with other features of SLE signifying diagnosis;

moreover; the titers measured in the Farr assay can correlate with disease activity. The Farr assay, however, does not discriminate between IgM and IgG anti-dsDNA antibodies and may also detect immune complexes with proteins other than antibodies. The assay is currently used infrequently because of the cumbersome nature and risks associated with radioactivity.

Other RIA approaches are available. Thus, the precipitation of bound radioactive DNA can be accomplished by using polyethylene glycol rather than ammonium sulfate to bring down immune complexes. Alternatively, the complexes can be separated from free radioactive DNA by filtration on nitrocellulose. In this variation of the assay, the immune complexes are soluble, with binding of antibody to the filter as the basis for the physical separation of the complexes.

CLIF Assay

The *Crithidia luciliae* immunofluorescence (CLIF) assay measures the binding of antibodies to the kinetoplast of the hemoflagellate *C. luciliae*. This kinetoplast contains a piece of circular dsDNA that is not associated with histone proteins. For assay purposes, the parasite is fixed to a microscope slide and incubated with serum, and a fluorescently labeled secondary anti-Ig reagent is added. There is no contamination by ssDNA in this assay, leading to its high specificity. Different anti-dsDNA antibody isotypes can be detected by using separate anti-Ig reagents. Although this assay has a sensitivity similar to that of the Farr assay, quantitation is more difficult and the titers correlate less closely with disease activity for lupus nephritis.

ELISA

An ELISA measures the binding of antibodies to an antigen adhered to a surface, with bound antibodies measured colorimetrically from the product of the enzyme of the anti-Ig conjugate. For this assay, a plastic microtiter plate is coated with purified dsDNA, often from calf thymus, and serum dilutions are then added to the wells. Anti-dsDNA antibodies in the serum are detected by the use of an enzyme-labeled anti-Ig reagent followed by the addition of a substrate for color development. This technique is easy to perform and allows testing of many samples at one time.

In general, an ELISA is more sensitive than the Farr or CLIF assay since it detects both high- and low-avidity antibodies. Since the specificity of the anti-Ig conjugate can be varied, different isotypes can also be readily measured. In contrast to the case of the Farr or CLIF assay, the DNA source for an ELISA is more likely to be contaminated by ssDNA. This assay can also be limited by nonspecific binding of immune complexes or other immunoglobulins to the plates. In addition, the interaction of dsDNA with the plastic surface may not be reproducibly uniform, leading to the use of binding agents such as positively charged proteins to increase DNA adherence. A modification of this assay can also involve the use of biotinylated DNA to bind streptavidin-coated plates to provide more sensitive and reproducible measurements and reduce nonspecific binding (13).

Other Assays

Some other, older techniques that have been used by clinical laboratories in the past for the detection of anti-DNA antibodies include immunodiffusion, hemagglutination, and complement fixation. These are now surpassed by the assays described above.

Newer tests have been developed and described in the literature. These include the fluorometric PicoGreen assay and microarrays (3, 12). These tests have been used for research purposes only and have not been characterized sufficiently to allow their general use in clinical laboratories. The following are brief descriptions of these techniques.

Fluorometric PicoGreen Assay

The flurometric PicoGreen assay is similar to the Farr assay in principle but has the advantage of not using radiolabeled DNA. For this assay, a source of dsDNA is added to serum. After ammonium sulfate precipitation, the DNA bound in the immune complexes is detected by means of a fluorescent dye, PicoGreen, which binds specifically to dsDNA and allows the detection of DNA in the nanogram-to-picogram range. Nonspecific binding of other DNA binding proteins may lead to false-positive results for anti-DNA antibodies. The sensitivity and specificity of this assay for SLE have not been defined (3).

Microarrays

The new technology of microarrays allows the detection of several antibodies in a single experiment. In the array format, nucleic acids or protein antigens are immobilized as microspots in rows or columns on a solid chip, which is then exposed to serum. Antibodies binding to their immobilized counterparts are detected by fluorescence, radioactive labeling, chemiluminescence, mass spectrometry, or electrochemical methods.

Placing autoantigens in different concentrations on a single array allows the measurement of multiple autoantibodies from a minimal amount of serum in a single test. The titer can be defined as the lowest antigen concentration at which a product can be detected. Alternatively, titer determination can be achieved by incubation of a fixed antigen concentration with a series of serum dilutions. While both approaches should yield similar results, the determination of the titer will depend on the array format, the spot size, the amount of the antigen immobilized within the spots, and the detection system.

Parallel detection and quantification of several autoimmune diseases can be performed with the microarray assay. In addition, microarrays enable the identification of the specificity as well as the isotype and require only small amounts of samples. Microarrays will likely be a valuable technique in the future, given their flexibility and adaptability to a wide range of autoimmune diseases (12).

Measurement of Avidity and Isotype

Although high-avidity anti-dsDNA antibodies of certain IgG isotypes are both pathologic and pathogenic, clinical assessments of anti-DNA avidities and isotypes have not been done routinely. For research purposes, usual measurements of avidity have been performed by competitive inhibition in binding assays (28). More recently, surface plasmon resonance (or the BIAcore assay) has enabled a more precise detection and calculation of the antibody-antigen affinity and kinetics. In this assay, the purified dsDNA is immobilized on a streptavidin-coated sensor chip. Samples containing different concentrations of purified IgG are then flowed over the chip at a defined flow rate. The interaction between the antibody and the DNA is measured in real time and is shown by a sensorgram, from which the affinity can be derived as the ratio between the association and the dissociation rate constants (20, 24).

Assay Selection

The ELISA is now the most widely used technique for detecting anti-dsDNA antibodies. Very few clinical laboratories are still performing the Farr assay or the CLIF assay. As the number of commercially available ELISA kits for measuring anti-dsDNA has increased, most clinical laboratories would consider cost and efficiency in selection. It is important to choose an assay that has the highest sensitivity and specificity. Often, the benefit of having a sensitive assay is offset by a low specificity, and some laboratories may use a combination of two or three techniques to increase the diagnostic value of the test result. For example, a positive result by an ELISA can be confirmed by a more specific test for SLE such as the Farr RIA or CLIF assay. The application of other tests should be done in consultation with a clinician and should reflect the needs for patient evaluation (11).

The Medical Devices Agency performs critical evaluations of in vitro diagnostic kits on behalf of the UK Department of Health. The reports provided by the Medical Devices Agency can assist with decisions regarding the choice of commercially available kits to meet laboratory requirements. These reports are accessible at www.medical-devices.gov.uk. For use in clinical laboratories in the United States, these kits must be FDA approved, and the list of approved kits can be found at the research section of www.FDA.gov.

METHODOLOGY

Anti-DNA assays are currently available as kits from several manufacturers. Some details of these assays, however, are proprietary. Detailed descriptions of the procedures can be obtained from the manufacturer. Presented here are short outlines for the Farr, CLIF, and ELISA assays as adapted from kits. While information from kits from Inova Diagnostics, Inc. (www.inovadx.com) has been used in this discussion, the principles are general. Reference to these kits does not imply any preference or superiority.

Farr Assay

An anti-DNA kit is available from Inova Diagnostics, Inc.

Materials

Radioactive iodinated DNA (^{125}I-dsDNA) (recombinant dsDNA is preferable to avoid contamination with ssDNA)

Anti-DNA calibrators prepared from a World Health Organization standard anti-dsDNA pool

Ammonium sulfate precipitating solution

Anti-DNA controls

Patient serum

Plain 12- by 75-mm polypropylene tubes

All materials are stored at 2 to 8°C.

Procedure

1. Pipette 25 µl of each calibrator, control, and patient serum sample into duplicate tubes.
2. Add 200 µl of ^{125}I-DNA and mix.
3. Incubate samples at 37°C for 2 h.
4. Add 1.0 ml of cold ammonium sulfate precipitating solution.
5. Centrifuge at 2,000 × g for 15 min in the cold.
6. Decant the supernatant.

7. Count in a gamma counter.

8. Determine anti-DNA concentrations from the calibration curve.

CLIF Assay

The Nova Lite dsDNA kit available from Inova Diagnostics, Inc., is an indirect immunofluorescent antibody test employing the hemoflagellate *C. luciliae* as a substrate.

Materials

The following reagents are included in the kit.

  C. luciliae slides (dsDNA)
  Goat anti-human IgG conjugated with fluorescein isothiocyanate
  dsDNA-positive serum
  Immunofluorescence assay system negative control

Procedure

1. Prepare 1× phosphate-buffered saline (PBS).

2. Dilute serum samples in PBS, with 1:10 as the initial dilution.

3. For titration, prepare serial dilutions of all positive samples with PBS (1:20, 1:40, 1:80, ...).

4. Place substrate slides in a moist chamber, and add 1 drop (30 to 50 μl) of positive and negative controls and diluted patient sample to wells.

5. Incubate slides for 30 min.

6. Wash with PBS.

7. Add fluorescent conjugate and incubate the slide for an additional 30 min.

8. Examine under a fluorescence microscope.

Quality Control

dsDNA-positive and immunofluorescence assay system–negative controls should be run on every slide to ensure proper assay performance.

Results

The specific staining of the kinetoplast can be visualized using a fluorescence microscope with a 495-nm exciter and 515-nm barrier filter. A sample is considered positive if specific kinetoplast staining or kinetoplast-plus-nuclear staining is more intense than that of the negative control. Staining of other structures such as the flagellum, body, or nucleus without kinetoplast staining is considered negative. All positive samples should be titrated to the endpoint. Since the results are obtained from titrations, there are potential errors that propagate from inaccurate dilutions. In addition, the range of the assay is more limited since the smallest difference in values is twofold.

ELISA

Materials

The following materials are included in the kit.

  Polystyrene microtiter plates coated with a purified calf thymus dsDNA antigen (pretreated with S1 nuclease enzyme to remove single-stranded regions)
  Positive and negative controls
  Anti-dsDNA calibrator containing antibodies to dsDNA
  Horseradish peroxidase (HRP)–goat anti-human IgG conjugate
  Tetramethyl benzidine dihydrochloride chromogen
  HRP stop solution

Procedure

1. Prepare a 1:100 dilution of each patient sample.

2. Add 100 μl of the prediluted anti-dsDNA calibrator, anti-dsDNA positive and negative controls, and diluted patient samples to the wells.

3. Incubate for 30 min at room temperature.

4. Wash three times.

5. Add HRP-IgG conjugate to each well; incubate wells at room temperature for 30 min.

6. Wash.

7. Add tetramethyl benzidine dihydrochloride chromogen and incubate in the dark.

8. Add HRP stop solution.

9. Read the absorbance (optical density [OD]) of each well on a plate reader at 450 nm within 1 h of stopping the reaction.

Quality Control

The anti-dsDNA ELISA calibrator and anti-dsDNA positive and negative controls should be run with every batch of samples, with calculated positive control and negative control values (international units per milliliter or WHO units per milliliter) falling within the range specified for the lot number. In addition, the absorbance of the dsDNA positive control must be greater than the absorbance of the calibrator, which must be greater than the absorbance of the dsDNA negative control. The positive control must have an absorbance of >1.0, and the negative control's absorbance should not be over 0.2. The dsDNA ELISA calibrator absorbance must be more than twice that of the negative control or over 0.25. The assay must be repeated if the quality control criteria are not met.

Calculation of Results

Sample value (units)

$$= \frac{\text{sample OD} \times \text{dsDNA calibrator (units)}}{\text{dsDNA ELISA calibrator OD}}$$

Results

As a solid-phase assay, the ELISA likely detects a broader array of anti-DNA specificities, including lower-avidity species, than a fluid-phase assay, especially the Farr assay. Furthermore, depending on the antigen preparation and the type of microtiter plate used, reproducibility can be variable. As a result, some ELISAs involve the use of a positively charged protein such as protamine sulfate or methylated bovine serum albumin to promote more consistent binding of the DNA. The impact of such an agent on the array of anti-DNA specificities detected is not known.

Fluorometric Anti-DNA Assay

Materials

The following reagents are needed for this assay.

  Patient serum
  Positive and negative anti-DNA controls
  Purified calf thymus dsDNA
  PicoGreen (purchased from Molecular Probes, Inc., Eugene, Oreg.) diluted 1:200 in TEN buffer (10 mM Tris, 1 mM EDTA, 100 mM NaCl [pH 8.8])

100% saturated ammonium sulfate solution
Black 96-well microtiter plates (Costar, Corning, N.Y.)

Procedure

1. Mix serum diluted 1:20 with a solution of dsDNA (1:1) in 100 μl in a microtiter plate.
2. Incubate for 1 h.
3. Add 100 μl of 100% ammonium sulfate solution and incubate for 1 h at 4°C.
4. Centrifuge for 10 min at 3,000 × g and wash four times with 50% ammonium sulfate.
5. Dissolve precipitate in 100 μl of TEN buffer.
6. Add 100 μl of PicoGreen.
7. Measure fluorescence by using a microplate fluorescence reader (excitation wavelength of 485 nm and emission wavelength of 535 nm).
8. Calculate the DNA concentration by using a standard curve of dsDNA.

Quality Control

This assay has been successfully performed with sera from murine models of SLE. There is less experience with human samples. Since PicoGreen binds only dsDNA, it is important that the DNA used as the antigen as well as the standard DNA used for calibration is highly purified and lacks significant contamination with ssDNA. Digestion with S1 nuclease can be used to ensure the purity of the dsDNA used. Standard positive and negative sera can be used to assess the assay performance and to ensure appropriate quantitative assessments.

QUALITY CONTROL AND TEST VALIDATION

Currently, assays for anti-DNA involve kits that have been extensively tested by their respective manufacturers and approved for diagnostic use. Many clinical laboratories routinely verify their tests by using a panel of well-defined sera for which patient diagnoses are well verified and previous test results are known. As new tests are introduced or laboratories implement new technology, validation is important. Given the range of anti-DNA antibody specificities and avidities, differences in test performance will often occur. Thus, a patient whose serum showed anti-DNA positivity with one assay may be negative in another, and vice versa. Clinicians must therefore be informed of any changes in the testing and back-up assays provided, especially for patients for whom anti-DNA testing is important for management.

COST ASSESSMENT

Measurements of anti-DNA levels are indicated for the evaluation of patients for whom the diagnosis of SLE is considered. Depending on considerations of cost and patient convenience, this test can be performed concurrently with an ANA test or after a positive ANA test is obtained. In this regard, some patients will have a positive anti-DNA test in the absence of a positive ANA test, but the significance of this result is unclear.

Anti-DNA tests can also be performed as a part of routine patient management to assess disease activity, especially nephritis. For those patients whose anti-DNA levels have been correlated with disease activity, more frequent testing may be indicated to predict flare-ups. For those patients with manifestations of SLE other than nephritis or for whom correlations with anti-DNA have not been observed, repeat testing has less value. The predictive value of anti-DNA testing has been a source of investigation and controversy, with some studies even showing that a fall, rather than a rise, in the anti-DNA level predates renal disease activity (8). Pending studies to more fully validate the marker function of anti-DNA for selective use in patients are indicated to avoid confusion and to promote more cost-effective utilization.

INTERPRETATION

Each laboratory should develop its own normal range based on its techniques, controls, equipment, and patient population. Depending on the technique used, the result of anti-dsDNA measurements can be reported as being negative, equivocal, or positive, with results of quantitative assays provided as titers or numerical values. A positive result usually indicates the presence of anti-dsDNA antibodies and supports the diagnosis of SLE. In contrast, a negative anti-dsDNA result does not exclude the diagnosis of SLE since only some patients with SLE express this specificity and since levels vary with disease activity. Samples with equivocal results should be retested with the same technique at another time or with another technique to define the antibody status.

For diagnostic purposes, a positive test result for the CLIF assay or Farr assay may be more useful than that obtained by ELISA. Studies have suggested that the relative specificities of these tests for SLE differ, although interpretation of these data is dependent on the patient and control populations selected for analysis. In general, the CLIF assay appears to be more specific for SLE (7, 16, 26). Data on newer assays such as microarrays are not yet available.

For patients with SLE and glomerulonephritis, the changes in anti-dsDNA levels over time can provide valuable information on both disease activity and the response to treatment. Since anti-dsDNA antibodies are associated with renal disease in many patients, a rise in anti-dsDNA antibody levels may predict an exacerbation or relapse (25). This pattern may not always occur in SLE patients, with the frequency of testing also affecting the apparent fluctuation of the response and the relationship to disease activity.

In the clinical setting, the interpretation of the results needs to be individualized based on the history of the patient and preceding serological events. In this regard, some SLE patients may show persistent elevations of anti-dsDNA levels but nevertheless lack evidence of active renal disease. These patients may produce nonpathogenic antibodies or lack antigens to form immune complexes (18). The predictive value of anti-dsDNA antibodies is increased when used in combination with supportive evidence of a high likelihood of SLE based on patient history, physical examination, and other laboratory tests such as complement levels.

Since the sensitivity and specificity for diagnosing SLE increase with the detection of more than one specific autoantibody, microarrays and other multiplex assays will likely play an increasing role in patient evaluation. Pending the refinement of such approaches, the ELISA will likely remain the preferable assay used for the purpose of disease activity monitoring.

REFERENCES

1. **Arbuckle, M. R., J. A. James, K. F. Kohlhase, M. V. Rubertone, G. J. Dennis, and J. B. Harley.** 2001. Development of anti-dsDNA autoantibodies prior to clinical diagnosis of systemic lupus erythematosus. *Scand. J. Immunol.* **54:**211–219.

2. **Arbuckle, M. R., M. T. McCain, M. V. Rubertone, R. H. Scofield, G. J. Dennis, J. A. James, and J. B. Harley.** 2001. Development of autoantibodies before the clinical onset of systemic lupus erythematosus. *N. Engl. J. Med.* **349:**1526–1533.

3. **Bjorkman, L., C. F. Reich III, and D. S. Pisetsky.** 2003. The use of fluorometric assays to assess the immune response to DNA in murine systemic lupus erythematosus. *Scand. J. Immunol.* **57:**525–533.

4. **Bootsma, H., P. E. Spronk, E. J. ter Borg, E. J. Hummel, G. de Boer, P. C. Limburg, and C. G. Kallenberg.** 1997. The predictive value of fluctuations in IgM and IgG class anti-dsDNA antibodies for relapses in systemic lupus erythematosus. *Ann. Rheum. Dis.* **56:**661–666.

5. **Boule, M. W., C. Broughton, F. Mackay, S. Akira, A. Marshak-Rothstein, and I. R. Rifkin.** 2004. Toll-like receptor 9-dependent and -independent dendritic cell activation by chromatin-immunoglobulin G complexes. *J. Exp. Med.* **199:**1631–1640.

6. **Carson, D. A.** 1991. The specificity of anti-DNA antibodies in systemic lupus erythematosus. *J. Immunol.* **146:**1–2.

7. **Egner, W.** 2000. The use of laboratory tests in the diagnosis of SLE. *J. Clin. Pathol.* **53:**424–432.

8. **El Hachmi, M., M. Jadoul, C. Lefebvre, G. Depresseux, and F. A. Houssiau.** 2003. Relapses of lupus nephritis: incidence, risk factors, serology and impact on outcome. *Lupus* **12:**692–696.

9. **Forger, F., T. Matthias, M. Oppermann, H. Becker, and H. Helmke.** 2004. Clinical significance of anti-dsDNA antibody isotypes: IgG/IgM ratio of anti-dsDNA antibodies as a prognostic marker for lupus nephritis. *Lupus* **13:**36–44.

10. **Hahn, B. H.** 1998. Mechanism of disease: antibodies to DNA. *N. Engl. J. Med.* **338:**1359–1368.

11. **Haugbro, J., J. C. Nossent, T. Winkler, Y. Figenschau, and O. P. Rekvig.** 2004. Anti-dsDNA antibodies and disease classification in antinuclear antibody positive patients: the role of analytical diversity. *Ann. Rheum. Dis.* **63:**386–394.

12. **Hueber, W., P. J. Utzl, L. Steinman, and W. L. Robinson.** 2002. Autoantibody profiling for the study and treatment of autoimmune disease. *Arthritis Rheum.* **4:**290–295.

13. **Hylkema, M. N., H. Huygen, C. Kramers, T. J. V. D. Wall, J. de Jong, M. C. J. van Bruggen, A. J. G. Swaak, J. H. M. Berden, and R. J. T. Smeenk.** 1994. Clinical evaluation of a modified ELISA, using photobiotinylated DNA, for the detection of anti-DNA antibodies. *J. Immunol. Methods* **170:**93–102.

14. **Isenberg, D., and R. Smeenk.** 2002. Clinical laboratory assays for measuring anti-dsDNA antibodies. Where are we now? *Lupus* **11:**797–800.

15. **Karounos, D. G., J. P. Grudier, and D. S. Pisetsky.** 1988. Spontaneous expression of antibodies to DNA of various species origin in sera of normal subjects and patients with systemic lupus erythematosus. *J. Immunol.* **83:**125–139.

16. **Kavanaugh, A. F., D. H. Solomon, and the American College of Rheumatology Ad Hoc Committee on Immunologic Testing Guidelines.** 2002. Guidelines for immunologic laboratory testing in the rheumatic diseases: anti-DNA antibody tests. *Arthritis Rheum.* **47:**546–555.

17. **Leadbetter, E. A., I. R. Rifkin, A. M. Hohlbaum, B. C. Beaudette, M. J. Shlomchik, and A. Marshak-Rothstein.** 2002. Chromatin-IgG complexes activate B cells by dual engagement of IgM and Toll-like receptors. *Nature* **416:**603–607.

18. **Lefkowith, J. B., and G. S. Gilkeson.** 1996. Nephritogenic autoantibodies in lupus: current concepts and continuing controversies. *Arthritis Rheum.* **39:**894–903.

19. **Lovgren, T., M. L. Eloranta, U. Bave, G. V. Alm, and L. Ronnblom.** 2004. Induction of interferon-alpha production in plasmacytoid dendritic cells by immune complexes containing nucleic acid released by necrotic or late apoptotic cells and lupus IgG. *Arthritis Rheum.* **50:**1861–1872.

20. **Malmqvist, M.** 1993. Surface plasmon resonance for the detection and measurement of antibody-antigen affinity and kinetics. *Curr. Opin. Immunol.* **5:**282–286.

21. **Mohan, C., and S. K. Datta.** 1995. Lupus: key pathogenic mechanisms and contributing factors. *Clin. Immunol. Immunopathol.* **77:**209–220.

22. **Rekvig, O. P., K. Andreassen, and U. Moens.** 1998. Antibodies to DNA—towards an understanding of their origin and pathophysiological impact in systemic lupus erythematosus. *Scand. J. Rheumatol.* **27:**1–6.

23. **Reveille, J. D.** 2004. Predictive value of autoantibodies for activity of systemic lupus erythematosus. *Lupus* **13:**290–297.

24. **Sem, D. S., P. A. Mcneeley, and M. D. Linnik.** 1999. Antibody affinities and relative titers in polyclonal populations: surface plasmon resonance analysis of anti-DNA antibodies. *Arch. Biochem. Biophys.* **372:**62–68.

25. **ter Borg, E. J., G. Horst, E. J. Hummel, P. C. Limburg, and C. G. Kallenberg.** 1990. Measurement of increases in anti-double-stranded DNA antibody levels as a predictor of disease exacerbation in systemic lupus erythematosus. A long-term, prospective study. *Arthritis Rheum.* **33:**634–643.

26. **Tzioufas, G. A., C. Terzoglou, E. D. Stavropoulos, S. Athanasiadou, and H. M. Moutsopoulos.** 1990. Determination of anti-ds-DNA antibodies by three different methods: comparison of sensitivity, specificity and correlation with lupus activity index (LAI). *Clin. Rheumatol.* **9:**186–192.

27. **Vallin, H., A. Perers, G. V. Alm, and L. Ronnblom.** 1999. Anti-double-stranded DNA antibodies and immunostimulatory plasmid DNA in combination mimic the endogenous IFN-alpha inducer in systemic lupus erythematosus. *J. Immunol.* **163:**6306–6313.

28. **Villalta, D., P. B. Romelli, C. Savina, N. Bizzaro, R. Tozzoli, E. Tonutti, A. Ghirardello, and A. Doria.** 2003. Anti-dsDNA antibody avidity determination by a simple reliable ELISA method for SLE diagnosis and monitoring. *Lupus* **12:**31–36.

Autoantibody Testing in Rheumatoid Arthritis

SONALI NARAIN, MEGHAVI KOSBOTH, AND PAULETTE HAHN

116

Rheumatoid arthritis (RA) is a chronic, systemic, inflammatory disorder thought to affect 0.5 to 1% of the global population, predominantly women, although most studies have been carried out in North America and northern Europe. Clinical and pathogenic effects characterized by chronic inflammation and synovial proliferation result in destruction of joints, with subsequent disability and increased morbidity. Extra-articular manifestations of RA may involve most organ systems. Pulmonary, ocular, and cardiovascular involvement is common. Thus, the complications of RA are not limited to the joints and "classic" extra-articular sites. Early diagnosis of RA may help avoid these complications, resulting in decreased disability, morbidity, and mortality.

RA is thought to result from multiple poorly defined factors, including both genetic and environmental risk factors as well as age, gender, and ethnicity. Environmental associations may include hormonal effects, smoking, infections, diet, and socioeconomic factors (4). There tends to be a bimodal age distribution in the development of RA. The peak of disease onset is in the fifth decade of life.

Twin and family studies suggest an association of RA with both HLA and non-HLA genetic factors. An association with HLA-DR4 has been recognized for more than 20 years, and more recent data suggest a stronger association with particular DR4 alleles, such as DRB1*0401, DRB1*0404, DRB1*0405, and DRB1*0408. The presence of the "shared epitope" confers an even higher relative risk of the disease and is associated with a higher likelihood of developing erosive disease requiring more aggressive therapy (139).

Infectious factors in the development of RA have been proposed. It may be that infection serves as an environmental trigger in a genetically susceptible individual. Viral infections and increased titers of antibody against Epstein-Barr virus and other viruses have been found in patients with RA, yet a causal relationship remains to be established (79). Recently there has been a proposed association of elevated immunoglobulin M (IgM) and IgA antibodies to *Proteus mirabilis* and IgM to *Escherichia coli* with rheumatoid factor (RF) positivity. It may be that genetically susceptible patients with chronic clinical or subclinical infections may have onset of synovitis. The mechanism is not known.

In 1987 the American College of Rheumatology established criteria for the diagnosis of RA (8, 69). Although the criteria are useful to diagnose established RA, they are of limited utility for recognizing early disease. With new developments in the therapy of RA and evidence that therapy is most effective when started early in the disease process, it becomes increasingly important to develop criteria that will permit the accurate diagnosis of disease prior to the onset of radiographic changes. The challenge will be to distinguish early RA from other inflammatory arthritides, such as spondyloarthropathies or infectious arthritis.

RF

RF is an antibody directed against the Fc portion of human IgG. RF-IgG immune complexes can deposit in tissues, activate the classical complement pathway, and lead to tissue damage (78, 110, 145). Although RF may be IgG, IgM, IgA, or IgE, IgM RF is the species most commonly measured in clinical assays. It was initially described by Waaler (138) in 1940, when he noted that sera from some RA patients caused agglutination of sheep erythrocytes coated with rabbit antibodies. Subsequently, IgM RF was used as a diagnostic test for RA (30). The sensitivity of RF in the diagnosis of RA is 75%. However, chronic infections, such as bacterial endocarditis, may cause the production of RF (74, 142). Recently, Newkirk et al. suggested an association between RF-positive RA and anti-*P. mirabilis* IgM and IgA antibodies and anti-*E. coli* IgM antibodies in patients with recent onset of synovitis (80). However, although an attractive hypothesis, it remains unclear that infections are involved in the pathogenesis of RA.

RF-positive patients tend to have more severe disease, with extra-articular involvement (nodulosis, ulcers, vasculitis, and neuropathy) and increased mortality (37, 50, 119, 126). In addition, there is some evidence to suggest that when RA is successfully treated, the RF titer tends to fall and that loss of RF positivity confers improved prognosis (86, 92). The presence of RF in the blood is one of the diagnostic criteria used for RA. However, it is important to keep in mind that its specificity for the disease is low. RF can be seen in infections such as tuberculosis, leprosy, osteomyelitis, syphilis, bacterial endocarditis, infectious mononucleosis, and hepatitis C (66). In addition, RF is found in many patients with other systemic autoimmune diseases, such as primary Sjögren's syndrome, systemic lupus erythematosus, vasculitis, and idiopathic pulmonary fibrosis. Some patients with B-cell malignancies, such as Waldenström's macroglobulinemia, non-Hodgkin's

TABLE 1 Comparison of features of RF assays

Assay	Antigen	Equipment expense	Reagent expense	Automation	Interlaboratory precision	Result	Interferences	Class detected	Sensitivity
Sheep cell agglutination	Rabbit IgG	Low	Low	No	Low	Titer or IU[a]	C1q, anti-rabbit IgG, anti-sheep erythrocytes	IgM	Low
Latex fixation agglutination	Human IgG	Low	Low	No	Low	Titer or IU	C1q, fibrin?	IgM	Medium
Nephelometry	Human or other IgG	High	Moderate	Yes	High	IU	Fibrin? Cryoglobulins? Other immune complexes if assay is polymer enhanced	IgM	High
ELISA	Variable	Moderate to high	Moderate	Variable	Moderate	IU	Nonspecific plastic binders, heterophilic anti-immunoglobulins	IgM, IgA, IgG (with modification)	High

[a]IU, International Units.

lymphoma, or chronic lymphocytic leukemia, have monoclonal gammopathies with RF activity. However, RF can be present in the absence of disease states. It has been suggested that smoking is associated with chronically elevated RF in the absence of rheumatic disease, and the presence of RF and antibodies to nuclear antigens is associated with cardiovascular disease even in patients without RA (3, 49, 114).

Antigenic Specificity of RF

The antigen detected by RF is the Fc portion of the IgG molecule. There is some evidence that the recognition of human isotype IgG3 by RF is different from recognition of other IgG subclasses (92). Many RFs bind in domain C_v2 or C_v3 of IgG and often require both for binding, suggesting the presence of a conformational epitope requiring both domains for successful binding (15, 98). X-ray crystallography of the C_v2-C_v3 binding site indicates that up to half of the RFs bind conformational determinants on the Fc surface, while some IgM RF Fab fragments bind antigen unusually at the edge of the usual antigen binding via linear polypeptide determinants scattered in the C_v2 and C_v3 regions (22, 105, 107, 143).

Genetic studies of RF revealed that many monoclonal RFs are encoded by a limited number of germ line genes that are preferentially expressed in early development (101). However, RF produced in the synovial tissue of patients with RA is different. Synovial tissue RF is produced by genes encoding immunoglobulin V region that have undergone genetic mutation, while monoclonal RFs from patients with B-cell malignancies are derived from V-region genes similar to unmutated germ line genes (87, 88). This somatic mutation and evidence of class switch from IgM to IgG and other Ig subfamilies suggest that RF production in RA patients is a T-cell-driven process (60).

Assays for RF

The presence of RF can be detected by a variety of techniques (Table 1), such as agglutination of IgG-sensitized sheep erythrocytes, bentonite or latex particles coated with human IgG, radioimmunoassay, indirect immunofluoresence, enzyme-linked immunoadsorbent assay (ELISA), and laser nephelometry (54, 61, 63, 85, 93, 138). The antigen source for most RF assays is usually gamma globulin pools from humans, rabbits, or cattle (18). IgG fractions from various species differ in their abilities to be bound by RF, resulting in variability of reported results. Rabbit IgG is most commonly used as the antigen source due to its lower sensitivity but higher specificity compared to those of human IgG.

Agglutination Assays

Agglutination methods have been used for many years to detect RF. The classical Waaler-Rose test uses sheep erythrocytes coated with rabbit IgG. If RF is present, the erythrocytes agglutinate (96, 138). This technique is most sensitive for IgM RF since IgM antibodies are more efficient in agglutination reactions. Commercial reagents use stabilized preparations of sensitized sheep cells to allow adequate shelf life. The latex agglutination and bentonite flocculation methods employ particles coated nonspecifically with human or rabbit gamma globulin. When mixed with serum samples containing RF, they agglutinate or flocculate. The agglutination assays described originally were performed in test tubes with agglutination prompted by temperature-controlled incubation and centrifugation of cells or particles. Semiquantitative analysis to determine the antibody content of a serum involves doubling dilutions of the serum and determination of an endpoint (the last doubling dilution at which agglutination can be visualized). The reciprocal of this dilution is known as the antibody titer. Results are typically expressed as titers or international units. Interlaboratory coefficient of variation has been reported as 30 to 50% based on a U.S. College of Pathologists voluntary survey. The latex agglutination test is sensitive, but it can result in a fairly high number of false positives (77). Nonspecific agglutination of latex particles by sera from healthy individuals is not uncommon (9). A potential drawback to the manual and visual agglutination techniques is that they are dependent on the skill and consistency of the technologist performing the assay and require a subjective determination of final titer.

ELISA

ELISA is used to determine RF by measuring the amount of immunoglobulin that binds to target antigen (IgG or its fragments) adsorbed to a solid phase, usually a polystyrene microtiter plate (1, 48, 82). This method can determine the immunoglobulin class of the antibody by using class-specific antibodies as reagents for human immunoglobulin binding. Microwells are coated with purified antigen (human IgG) followed by blocking of the unreacted sites to reduce nonspecific binding. Controls, calibrators, and patient serum samples are incubated in the antigen-coated wells, allowing RF present in the patient's serum to bind, forming antigen-antibody complexes. Unbound serum proteins are removed by washing the microwells. Enzyme-conjugated anti-human IgM (or IgG for IgG RF) is added to the wells. The enzyme conjugate binds to the antigen-antibody complex, and excess conjugate is washed away. Addition of specific substrate begins a hydrolytic reaction with the bound enzyme conjugate, causing color development. The intensity of the color change is proportional to the amount of IgM (or IgG) RF antibody bound to the wells, which is read using a spectrophotometer. The net absorbance is calculated by subtracting the absorbance value of the specimen blank from the value for the coated microwell. A calibration standard assayed with each plate is used to calculate IgM (or IgG) RF activity. The results are expressed in international units per milliliter. The use of IgG from different species would yield different results (35). Another pitfall may be nonspecific binding of patient sera to the plastic wells. This is overcome by subtracting the optical density from wells that are blocked but not coated with antigen.

Radioimmunoassay

Radioimmunoassays for RF were used in the past but are no longer in widespread use due to the problems of dealing with radioactivity.

Nephelometry

Laser and rate nephelometry have recently been adapted for the determination of RF activity in serum. In this method, mixing antigen and antibody under antibody excess conditions results in the formation of antigen-antibody complexes whose concentration is determined by light dispersion. When a beam of light is passed through tubes containing a fixed amount of antibody and variable concentrations of antigen, the concentration of immune complexes formed in the tube determines the extent of light scatter. The amount of light scattered is measured at angles varying from 0 to 90°. Since the antibody concentration remains constant, the light scattered is proportional to the concentration of antigen

in the mixture. Target antigen is heat-aggregated or chemically cross-linked human IgG. In latex-enhanced models, human or rabbit IgG is used to coat latex particles as in agglutination assays, with the nephelometer providing more automated and objective quantification of agglutination. Individual nephelometric assay kits come with complete instructions, which are dependent on instrumentation and software particular to the nephelometer and should be followed accordingly. Intralaboratory coefficient of variation of nephelometric methods has been reported to be fairly low, at 2% (84, 94). The nephelometric technique is considered superior because of its ability to detect changes in absolute levels at earlier stages and its low interassay coefficient of variation, 11% (93). In general, there is greater precision with ELISA and nephelometric assays, allowing greater confidence in interpreting a low-positive result.

Quality Assurance/Quality Control Implementation

Nephelometric assays and ELISAs use calibrators measured against standard sera established by the World Health Organization (6) or the Centers for Disease Control and Prevention (112) to promote uniformity in IgM RF quantification (55, 111). However, the World Health Organization standard does not contain IgG or IgA standard and therefore cannot be used for IgG or IgA RF (122). Quality control for nephelometric and ELISA values should include the multirule Shewart chart/Westgard rules for accepting or rejecting an assay (141). Control sera should be run with each assay and ideally should detect one negative serum and at least two positive sera: one at a low positive cutoff and the other at a high positive cutoff. Agglutination assays dependent on dilution titers should calculate the between-run geometric mean and standard deviation of quality control specimens (111) and use the Westgard rules to accept or reject a given run. Alternatively, the given value plus or minus one tube dilution may be an acceptable quality control. RF assays that report quantitative results such as titers or units need quantitative quality control measures for controls as well. Each lot of reagents should be evaluated to ensure equivalent results with previous reagents. It is advisable to evaluate plasma or serum without RF activity, since different reagent lots vary in their likelihood of having false-positive results in the presence of fibrin or fibrinogen (FBG).

The percentage of positive results found in normal sera within a given laboratory should be monitored and compared to a normal reference population periodically. Standardization between methods is often suboptimal; therefore, results in a given laboratory should be verified with a reference method and/or proficiency surveys to ensure reliable results.

Factors That Interfere with RF Measurements

Several factors can interfere with the measurement of RF. Agglutination and nephelometric assays can give false-positive results if a patient's serum has highly elevated levels of C1q, which binds and cross-links IgG (15, 16). This becomes important in inflammatory disorders since C1q is an acute-phase reactant. This can be avoided by heating the serum to 56°C for 15 to 30 min, since C1q is heat labile. Other approaches to complement inhibition can be employed, such as adding polyvinyl sulfonate to the reaction mixture (16, 22). The presence of fibrin or FBG in plasma or incompletely clotted serum can interfere with or induce agglutination or aggregation in nephelometric and agglutination assays, leading to false-positive or false-negative results. Nephelometric techniques that use polyethylene glycol or similar polymers to accelerate immune complex formation may give false-positive results from polymer-enhanced delayed aggregation of fibrin, lipoproteins, cryoglobulins, or other immune complexes (128, 140). This can be avoided by subtracting background light scatter with specimens that are allowed to react for an equivalent amount of time as the nephelometric measurement but in the absence of aggregated IgG target antigen or by eliminating the use of polymer. Since RFs are frequently enriched in cryoprecipitates, they may be lost if the cryoprecipitate separates from the remainder of the serum or if the cryoprecipitate in cooled serum is not dissolved prior to assay, rendering a false-negative or diminished level of RF (98). Histidine-rich glycoprotein, a plasma protein, inhibits formation and enhances solubilization of insoluble immune complexes formed by RF, presumably due to competitive binding to the IgG (33). Some small molecules, such as aspartame, have been described as inhibitors of RF activity (87); due to its rapid metabolism, however, aspartame concentrations in serum are not likely to be high enough to influence RF detection in humans.

ELISA and sandwich immunoassays for measurement of RF may yield false results due to the presence of heterophilic anti-immunoglobulin antibodies. These are naturally occurring antibodies reacting with immunoglobulins from other species. They can react with intact IgG or F(ab) or F(ab')$_2$ fragments of IgG from one or more species. About 15% of the heterophile antibodies recognize the Fc portion of IgG and can be considered analytically true-positive versus the other 85%, which recognize the F(ab')$_2$ fragments and are not RF. Their detection would be considered a false-positive result. These antibodies were present at low titers in up to 40% of sera from a healthy population when using sandwich assays based on monoclonal murine antibodies (17). Interference by heterophile antibodies may be eliminated by using rabbit F(ab) or F(ab')$_2$ fragments (38).

RF can interfere with other immunoassays (62), especially those depending on the binding of two antibodies for detecting an antigen. Recent studies have reported a false-positive elevation of serum troponin in patients with seropositive RA (23, 52, 53) and sera from patients with systemic lupus erythematosus can give false-positive reactions in cytokine assays due to the presence of RF (148). In general, RFs are more likely to bind rabbit IgG than goat or mouse IgG, so this interference may be less frequent in assays employing murine monoclonal antibodies.

Measurement of RF Isotypes

The measurement of RF isotypes is challenging due to various confounders. RF activity within immunoglobulin subtypes is typically quantified by sandwich radioimmunoassays or enzyme immunoassays. The solid-phase antigen is usually IgG or purified Fc (component a) and the source of RF antibody is diluted serum (component b), detected by labeled or unlabeled appropriate subclass-specific detection antibodies (component c). If molecule c is unlabeled, an additional labeled antibody (component d) that reacts with antibodies of the detection antibody species is used. Since components a to d are all IgG molecules or immunoglobulin fragments, they can potentially be bound by RF. For this reason, measurement of RF may require modifications. Designers of an assay must verify that the detecting antibody components (components c and d) do not react directly with the target antigen (component a). They must also ensure that the RF being measured (component b) does not lead to false results because of RF recognition of antigenic determinants on the detecting antibody components (components

c and d). Various pairs of antigen and detecting antibodies or their fragments may be employed to ensure specificity of assay results. For example, intact rabbit IgG or the Fc fragment can be used as the target antigen (a), with F(ab')$_2$ fragments of anti-human IgG as the detection antibody (c). If RFs reacting specifically with human IgG are to be measured, then the detecting antibody (c) can be F(ab')$_2$ fragments of antibodies to the Fd region [heavy-chain region of the F(ab) fragment] of the IgG, so that the IgG in the RF (b) can be measured without cross-reactions of c with anti-a or b with anti-c. Papain digestion of serum has been advocated to allow accurate quantification of IgG RF (56). Another potential problem with measuring IgG RF is that it can self-associate (70), since both antigen and antibody are IgG. In addition, non-RF serum IgG may bind IgM or IgA RF and give falsely elevated titers of IgG RF.

In general, all RF isotypes occur together in the same patient and the titers of the different isotypes correlate with each other. Some studies suggest that agglutination assays may detect IgA RF in addition to IgM RF (28, 123). Recent studies suggest that IgA may have a role in predicting disease outcome, especially in combination with anti-cyclin citrullinated peptide (anti-CCP) antibodies (11, 65). When agglutination assays are compared with isotype-specific RF assays, they are found to perform similarly in predicting the long-term course of RA (113). However, all RF isotypes have been reported for subjects who do not develop RA, and smoking is associated with a higher positivity rate for IgG RF and IgA RF in patients without evidence of arthritis (49).

Clinical Interpretation

RFs are marker antibodies for RA, and among the seven American College of Rheumatology criteria, RF is the only serologic test (8). It does not establish the diagnosis of RA but serves a factor contributing to the diagnosis. Elderly individuals, especially females, may have low titers of RF in the absence of RA (19, 67); thus, clinical interpretation should consider the patient's age and gender. A positive RF test has a sensitivity of 60 to 80% in RA and a specificity of 75 to 93% in a clinical rheumatic disease population (Table 2) (144). The concentration of serum RF may change over time, and in patients with RA, RF levels may correlate with the degree of inflammation and disease activity. Fluctuations in RF activity can be measured sufficiently precisely only by using nephelometry or ELISA rather than agglutination titers (40, 84, 93). Measurements of disease activity such as erythrocyte sedimentation rate (ESR) and C-reactive protein (CRP) are also very useful when used together with RF in the evaluation of patients with inflammatory arthritis (63). Subjects without RA are more likely than RA patients to have transient serum RFs that do not persist on long-term follow-up (36). Substantial variations in RF titer with reversal of seropositivity and seronegativity have been observed. Most patients are RF positive within 6 months of onset of symptoms, but the RF test may turn positive a year or more before the onset of disease (44). The functional avidity of RF changes over time (97). Persistently high levels of RF have been shown to be associated with more severe radiographic joint destruction over a 3-year follow-up period (83). Patients with monoclonal gammopathies due to B-cell malignancies may have serum RF activity. Those with mixed cryoglobulinemia have serum RF that precipitates in the cryoglobulin. Conversely, in patients with Sjögren's syndrome, loss of RF activity has been a marker suggestive of the development of lymphoma. According to Bayes' theorem, the clinical utility of

TABLE 2 Comparison of the sensitivities and specificities of RF isotypes and anti-CCP combinations

Reference	Anti-CCP + IgM RF		Anti-CCP + IgA RF	
	Sensitivity (%)	Specificity (%)	Sensitivity (%)	Specificity (%)
14	33	99.6		
45	33.3	97.5		
64	56.9	91.1		
11	48	96	44	98
116	79.3	80.7	73.6	88.4
34	90	81		

a diagnostic test depends substantially on the pretest probability of having the disease, and this is true for RF detection (102, 103).

ANTIBODIES TO CCPs

The relatively low specificity of RF and the fact that high concentrations of IgM RF are detected not only in RA but also in other conditions with polyclonal stimuli to B cells (39) create a need for improved laboratory markers with a higher disease-related specificity and sensitivity. A variety of antibodies, not very specific to RA, are seen in the sera of patients with RA, such as anti-RA-33, anticalpastatin, anti-collagen type II, anti-glucose-6-phosphate isomerase, antifibronectin, antineutrophil cytoplasmic antibodies, and antinuclear antibody, while other antibodies demonstrate a high specificity, such as anti-BiP, anti-Sa, and anti-citrullinated protein antibodies (APF, AKA, antifilaggrin, and anti-CCP) (135).

Anti-perinuclear factor (APF) antibodies, first described in 1964, showed an acceptable sensitivity and a much higher specificity than RF (42). In 1979, another group of RA-specific antibodies, antikeratin antibodies (AKA), was shown to have a specificity comparable to that of APF (43), and could be demonstrated to precede the onset of RA (59). These tests, however, were never implemented in routine practice, as they were inconvenient, laborious, and difficult to standardize. It was later discovered that APF and AKA target the antigen identified as the epithelial protein filaggrin (filament-aggregating protein), yielding a high specificity (99%) in patients with RA, with the sensitivity and specificity depending on the method of filaggrin purification

and the difficulty in obtaining antigen preparations with reproducible citrulline content (39).

Importance of Protein Citrullination

In 1998, Schellekens et al. (99) showed that citrulline is a major constituent of the antigenic determinants recognized by antibodies frequently found in sera from patients with RA. This family of autoantibodies includes the APF, AKA, antifilaggrin antibodies, anti-CCP antibodies, and anti-Sa antibodies. All recognize epitopes containing citrulline. Citrulline is a nonstandard amino acid that is not incorporated into proteins during translation (131). However, it is generated by posttranslational modification (deimination, citrullination) of protein-bound arginine by peptidylarginine deiminase (PAD) enzymes (Fig. 1), first described in 1977 (95).

Four related isoforms of PAD exist in mammals and other vertebrates (137). All isoforms can citrullinate most proteins with accessible arginine residues in vitro, although certain proteins are citrullinated more rapidly than others by individual PADs (137). Amino acids flanking the arginine residue influence its susceptibility to citrullination. PAD2 is the most widely expressed type of PAD, with its expression regulated at the transcriptional and the translational level. Two natural substrates for PAD2 are known: myelin basic protein in the central nervous system and vimentin in skeletal muscle and macrophages. Macrophages express PAD2, but the cytosolic Ca^{2+} concentration is too low for enzyme activity (132). Human PAD5 is a homolog of mouse and rat PAD4 and is mainly expressed in granulocytes and monocytes, detectable in a variety of tissues. It is the only isoform residing in the cell nucleus.

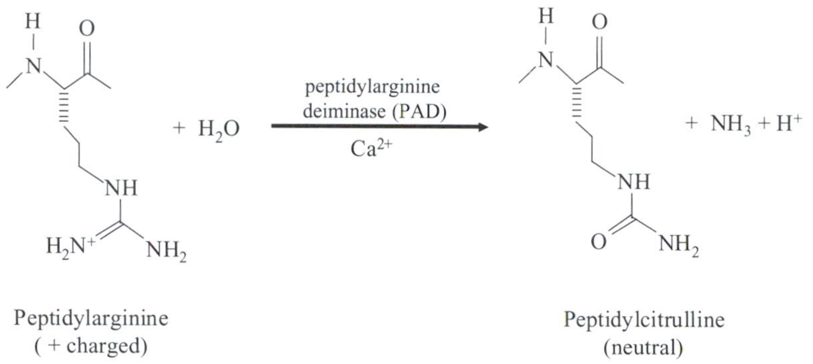

FIGURE 1 Citrullination (deimination) of peptidylarginine to peptidylcitrulline by PAD.

FBG, one of the targets of citrullination, is a glycoprotein found in blood plasma at concentrations of ~3 mg/ml, increasing to >7 mg/ml during inflammation. FBG or fibrin deposits in the inflamed joints may play an important role in RA (106). Deimination of FBG is mediated by PAD (108). The production of antibodies to deiminated FBG in humans may be a specific marker for RA, as antibodies to deiminated human FBG appear before the onset of joint symptoms, indicating that these antibodies may be of predictive value (108, 131).

Vimentin is citrullinated in dying human macrophages (132), which are abundant in the rheumatoid synovium. The Sa antigen, recently identified as citrullinated vimentin (130), has also been detected in rheumatoid pannus (26). Granulocytes, present in the inflamed synovium (especially the synovial fluid), have a life span of only about 3 days. They die in large numbers at inflammatory sites, triggering histone citrullination. The three proteins considered to be candidate autoantigens in RA are citrullinated fibrin, citrullinated histone, and citrullinated vimentin (134).

Oxygen metabolism is in disequilibrium in inflamed rheumatoid synovium, leading to hypoxia and synovial microinfarctions. Plaques of extravascular fibrin can be found at these sites. The inflamed synovium also contains many PAD2-expressing macrophages and sometimes PAD4-containing granulocytes. During cell death, the loss of the integrity of the plasma membrane causes an influx of calcium from the extracellular space and subsequent activation of intracellular PAD (134). Alternately, when cells are dying, as in RA synovium, due to oxidative stress, intracellular PAD enzymes might leak out and become activated in the presence of extracellular Ca^{2+}, inducing the citrullination of extracellular proteins such as fibrin (131). The calcium influx in the dying macrophages has also been hypothesized to lead to the production of citrullinated vimentin in the inflamed synovium (132).

The subclass distribution of anti-CCP antibodies (predominantly IgG1) (21, 136) is consistent with a T-cell-dependent antibody response and HLA involvement, and the antibodies are thought to be produced by local plasma cells (71). Anti-CCP-producing B cells have also been detected in the synovial fluid of RA patients (133). The initial events leading to their production are unknown, though it is believed that in principle any stress leading to death of PAD-expressing cells may suffice to initiate abnormal protein citrullination. In a susceptible individual (125) and in the appropriate environment (73) the citrullinated proteins may stimulate an immune response.

Two explanations have been offered for the high specificity of autoantibodies against citrullinated antigens for RA. First, there may be an RA-specific overexpression of citrullinated antigens in the synovium, leading to an immune response. This is supported by studies showing genetic polymorphisms of the PAD4 gene (108) and the association of a PAD4 haplotype with susceptibility to RA. This could lead to increased PAD4 enzyme expression, increased protein citrullination, and a higher chance of developing anti-CCP antibodies (108, 125). Second, the presence of citrullinated proteins is perhaps a common phenomenon in any inflamed (synovial) tissue but RA patients show an abnormal humoral response to them. This possibility is supported by studies that show the presence of citrullinated proteins in the synovium in RA patients and in deposits of extravascular fibrin (21, 72). Furthermore, citrullinated proteins have also been detected not only in RA patients but also in individuals with osteoarthritis or reactive arthritis (104, 134).

Assays for Antibodies to Citrullinated Proteins

The citrulline moiety is so important for antigenicity that essentially every citrullinated peptide or protein is recognized by autoantibodies in sera from RA patients, albeit with different sensitivities and specificities (124). The oxygen group of peptidylcitrulline is specifically recognized by autoantibodies in RA (99). The CCPs have a three-dimensional design optimally structured for recognition of the antigenic group by the heterogeneous population of RA autoantibodies. Using a single CCP as antigen in an ELISA, the sensitivity was ~68%, with a specificity of more than ~97% (118, 124). To improve the anti-CCP test, peptides from libraries of citrullinated peptides were tested with RA sera to select the most reactive species (24, 41, 117). Selected cyclic peptides have been synthesized and utilized for a second-generation anti-CCP assay, distributed worldwide as the CCP2 test (136).

Studies have compared the sensitivities and specificities of the commercially available second-generation anti-CCP antibody tests. The CCP2 ELISA provides the best combination of sensitivity and specificity for detecting RA, with little difference among various assays (27, 31, 34). The anti-CCP test has a sensitivity comparable to that of the IgM RF test but a much higher specificity (Table 3).

At present, there are five distributors of CCP2 ELISA kits: Euro-Diagnostica, Arnhem, The Netherlands (Immunoscan RA); Axis-Shield Diagnostics Ltd., Dundee, United Kingdom (Diastat Anti-CCP); Inova Diagnostics Inc., San Diego, Calif. (QUANTA Lite CCP IgG ELISA); EUROIMMUN Medizinische Labordiagnostika AG, Lübeck, Germany; and Pharmacia Diagnostics AB, Uppsala, Sweden (ELIA CCP). The ELIA CCP is a fully automated testing system for CCP antibodies that is somewhat easier to use and gives reliable results: a sensitivity of 80% and a specificity of 97% (39). At this time, only ELIA anti-CCP and QUANTA Lite CCP IgG ELISA are approved by the Food and Drug Administration.

Further research has led to the development of the third-generation anti-CCP antibody test (CCP3) that has shown comparable specificity to but increased sensitivity over previous anti-CCP assays. Two linear peptides, CCP3A (67% sensitivity) and CCP3B (55% sensitivity), are used (G.J. Pruijn et al., unpublished data). Though the CCP3B peptide has lower sensitivity, it reacts with sera from RA patients nonreactive in the CCP2 assay, leading to the conclusion that a combination of peptides (CCP2-CCP3) is required for optimal sensitivity.

Additionally, a new semiquantitative ELISA kit (INOVA Diagnostics) more sensitive than the CCP2 ELISA (QUANTA Lite CCP IgG ELISA; INOVA) has been developed, with a sensitivity of 74%, versus 69% for the old kit, and a specificity of 96%, versus 98% for the old kit, with agreement between the two assays of 96%. The new assay has an interassay variability of 2.9% and an intra-assay coefficient of variation ranging between 3.4 and 5.5% (R.W. Burlingame et al., unpublished data). However, this kit is not yet available commercially.

Quality Assurance/Quality Control Implementation

The test is performed on serum or citrated plasma specimens. Samples must be stored for a maximum of 48 h at 4 to 8°C but can be frozen at −20°C for prolonged storage. Repeat freeze-thaw cycles should be avoided. Frozen specimens must be thawed and mixed well prior to testing. Preservatives such as sodium azide at 0.1% will not affect sample results. Adequate maintenance and calibration of the plate reader should be performed according to the manufacturer's

TABLE 3 Sensitivities and specificities of anti-CCP and IgM RF antibody measurements in sera of patients with RA[a]

Reference	Anti-CCP		IgM RF	
	Sensitivity (%)	Specificity (%)	Sensitivity (%)	Specificity (%)
100	68	98	54	91
32	50	90	66	87
14	41	98	62	84
12	68	96	75	74
45	43	98	50	93
124	82	98		
126a	79	97		
64	66	90	72	80
108a	88	89	70	82
147	47	97	59	
97a	47	93	41	
84a	80	98		
7a	81	92		
27	65	96	60	70
31a	71	95	91	31
116	64	97	66	82
146	77	97	74	77
7	88	81		
109	67.5	99.3	66.3	82.1

[a]Although there is consensus among different studies about the specificity of anti-CCP, there is considerable variation in the diagnostic sensitivity. This variation can be attributed to the different serum dilutions tested or, more probably, to the different cutoff values (12). Furthermore, the observed differences in the sensitivity and specificity most likely are the consequence of the patient selection for the different cohorts used.

instructions. The ELISA kits are accompanied by detailed instructions and include calibrators and negative and positive control samples. Positive and negative controls should be run in all assays. Additional quality controls for ELISA values should include reference to National Committee for Clinical Laboratory Standards (NCCLS) document C24-A or the usual multirule Shewart chart/Westgard rules for accepting or rejecting an assay. The commercially available anti-CCP ELISAs have low analytical error. The dilution test, if performed in accordance with the NCCLS, shows a high grade of analytical reliability (109). Interassay and intra-assay coefficients of variation for different manufacturers' anti-CCP tests are comparable, ranging between 2.6 and 13.6% (interassay) and 3 and 17% (intra-assay).

Calculations and interpretation of test results are described by each manufacturer, and hence the cutoff values vary depending upon the kit used for the assay. The cutoff values established by the manufacturer are based on specific populations and may not necessarily reflect the literature. Reference ranges and appropriate cutoff points should all be evaluated for the specific populations serviced by the user. Overall, the anti-CCP has good discriminative ability. If a patient with RA and a control were to be selected at random, the RA patient would be 10 times more likely to have a higher anti-CCP antibody concentration (12).

Anti-CCP Test in Early RA

About 35 to 40% of RF-negative RA patients are positive for anti-CCP (116, 124). The diagnostic advantage of anti-CCP for RF-negative patients is even more convincing in early disease; RA patients with disease duration of less than 1 year who were CCP positive tested negative for IgG RF, IgM RF, and IgA RF (116).

The anti-CCP test predicts which patients with early arthritis would receive a clinical diagnosis of RA with a sensitivity of 55.4% and specificity of 96.7% (45). An evaluation of anti-CCP and RF behavior in RA patients in relation to the duration of the disease showed that in patients with early arthritis (diagnosis <1 year before the study), the correlation with anti-CCP was highly significant (14). A number of studies suggest that anti-CCP and IgA RF are the best predictors of future development of RA, especially in ambiguous cases or RF-negative RA (2, 81, 89, 90, 115). Additionally, anti-CCP antibodies are useful in predicting the development of RA in patients with undifferentiated arthritis (120).

Progression of RA

Preliminary studies have demonstrated that anti-CCP antibodies also have prognostic significance, as patients with antibodies develop significantly more severe radiographic damage (58, 75, 121). Anti-CCP is associated with a higher probability of radiographic signs of joint damage, while RF is associated with higher functional disability (11). Anti-CCP also is a good predictor of disease activity (116) and is better than RF in predicting disease activity over 3 years after the onset of RA (51). ESR, CRP, DAS28, and physician's global assessment were consistently higher in the anti-CCP-positive group than in the anti-CCP-negative group.

Visser et al. (129) assessed a clinical prediction model in early RA patients for three arthritis outcomes: self-limiting, persistent nonerosive, and persistent erosive arthritis. Anti-CCP was more strongly associated with erosive arthritis and severe joint destruction than RF. Anti-CCP antibodies predicted progression of the Larsen score over 2 years better than RF, and the presence of both antibodies (anti-CCP and RF) did not increase the predictive ability

(29, 127). Longitudinal studies to assess the utility of anti-CCP antibody in predicting the outcome of very early synovitis (≤3 months' duration) also show that anti-CCP antibodies are one of the significant independent predictors of persistence (91).

Fluctuation of Anti-CCP Levels

Anti-CCP antibody levels can change substantially in RA patients (7); most show elevated levels at the first visit, followed by a decrease in the majority of cases and fluctuation over time. Moreover, the change in anti-CCP levels parallels disease activity (severity of arthritis and deterioration of laboratory parameters such as ESR and CRP) (11, 46, 58, 124). A decline in anti-CCP levels in RA patients receiving therapy with other disease-modifying antirheumatic drugs has been reported (76). Though an earlier study reported that anti-CCP antibody levels decrease following infliximab (tumor necrosis factor alpha) therapy in RA patients, recent studies have indicated that its levels are relatively stable and not modulated by therapeutic interventions (5, 20, 25). It also has been hypothesized that the fluctuation in the anti-CCP levels may simply reflect the natural history of the autoantibody production over a course of time and that the level may peak early in the disease process, irrespective of therapeutic interventions, before declining and reaching baseline (76).

Combined Use of Anti-CCP and RF

Earlier studies have reported that if both RF and anti-CCP antibodies are required to be present, sensitivity decreases without a substantial increase in specificity relative to that of anti-CCP alone. However, more recent studies suggest that by evaluating the presence of either autoantibody (RF or anti-CCP), sensitivity for RA is increased without substantially altering the specificity (34, 64). These data are summarized in Table 2.

Genetic Associations of Anti-CCP Antibody

The HLA-DRB1 locus is associated with RA, especially in individuals with compound heterozygosity for shared-epitope genes (47). In addition, HLA-DRB1*0401, DRB1*1001, DQB1*0302, and DQB1*0501 are associated with the presence of anti-CCP antibodies and with more severe disease and a higher rate of joint damage (120). Studies combining the serologic (RF, anti-CCP antibodies) and genetic (SE, defined as DRB1*0404 and DRB1*0401) factors suggest that the presence of both SE and anti-CCP antibodies is strongly predictive of risk for future development of RA (11, 13). The results do not support the notion that the SE is a direct risk factor for the production of anti-CCP antibodies, but rather suggest synergy between the SE and the presence of anti-CCP (or RF).

In a study of early RA, a significant association between anti-CCP antibodies and expression of DRB1*0404 or DRB1*0101 was reported (32), suggesting that SE-positive individuals may have more sustained T- and B-cell responses to citrullinated antigens than noncarriers. These data support the hypothesis that in individuals carrying one or two SE genes, a T-cell-dependent immune response to citrullinated peptides may contribute to the pathogenesis of RA. An alternative explanation is that HLA antigens do not predispose to the autoimmune disease per se but rather fail to provide protection (13). A recent report presented numerous single nucleotide polymorphisms in PAD4, several of which are strongly associated with RA (108). Carriers of the susceptible haplotype had antibodies against citrullinated proteins significantly more often than noncarriers (108).

Association of Anti-CCP Antibodies with Other Conditions

Anti-CCP antibodies can be detected in patients with juvenile idiopathic arthritis, but generally at low levels and less commonly than in adults with RA (10). In patients with juvenile idiopathic arthritis, the presence of anti-CCP antibodies does not correlate statistically with the presence of RF, except in patients with RF-positive polyarthritis (68). Anti-CCP antibodies also help to differentiate hepatitis C virus-related arthropathy from RA (5). Anti-CCP antibody levels are not elevated in nonarthritic patients with chronic hepatitis C virus. Anti-CCP may be positive in patients with psoriatic arthritis (PsA), and its presence in PsA patients is associated with more severe disease. The association of the prevalence of anti-CCP with radiographic erosions in PsA suggests some phenotypic overlap of PsA with RA (57). The mechanism is unclear, although it is possible that the antibodies, by sustaining the inflammatory response, are directly involved in joint damage.

REFERENCES

1. **Aggarwal, A., S. Dabadghao, S. Naik, and R. Misra.** 1994. Serum IgM rheumatoid factor by enzyme-linked immunosorbent assay (ELISA) delineates a subset of patients with deforming joint disease in seronegative juvenile rheumatoid arthritis. *Rheumatol. Int.* **14:**135–138.

2. **Aho, K., T. Palosuo, M. Heliovaara, P. Knekt, P. Alha, and R. von Essen.** 2000. Antifilaggrin antibodies within "normal" range predict rheumatoid arthritis in a linear fashion. *J. Rheumatol.* **27:**2743–2746.

3. **Aho, K., J. T. Salonen, and P. Puska.** 1982. Autoantibodies predicting death due to cardiovascular disease. *Cardiology* **69:**125–129.

4. **Alamanos, Y., and A. A. Drosos.** 2005. Epidemiology of adult rheumatoid arthritis. *Autoimmun. Rev.* **4:**130–136.

5. **Alessandri, C., M. Bombardieri, N. Papa, M. Cinquini, L. Magrini, A. Tincani, and G. Valesini.** 2004. Decrease of anti-cyclic citrullinated peptide antibodies and rheumatoid factor following anti-TNFalpha therapy (infliximab) in rheumatoid arthritis is associated with clinical improvement. *Ann. Rheum. Dis.* **63:**1218–1221.

6. **Anderson, S. G., M. W. Bentzon, V. Houba, and P. Krag.** 1970. International reference preparation of rheumatoid arthritis serum. *Bull. W. H. O.* **42:**311–318.

7. **Aotsuka, S., M. Okawa-Takatsuji, K. Nagatani, C. Nagashio, T. Kano, K. Nakajima, K. Ito, and A. Mimori.** 2005. A retrospective study of the fluctuation in serum levels of anti-cyclic citrullinated peptide antibody in patients with rheumatoid arthritis. *Clin. Exp. Rheumatol.* **23:**475–481.

7a. **Araki, C., N. Hayashi, M. Moriyama, S. Morinobu, M. Mukai, M. Koshiba, S. Kawano, and S. Kumagai.** 2004. Usefulness of anti-cyclic citrullinated peptide antibodies (anti-CCP) for the diagnosis of rheumatoid arthritis. *Rinsho Byori* **52:**966–972. (In Japanese.)

8. **Arnett, F. C., S. M. Edworthy, D. A. Bloch, D. J. McShane, J. F. Fries, N. S. Cooper, L. A. Healey, S. R. Kaplan, M. H. Liang, H. S. Luthra, et al.** 1988. The American Rheumatism Association 1987 revised criteria for the classification of rheumatoid arthritis. *Arthritis Rheum.* **31:**315–324.

9. **Ash, K. O.** 1980. Reference intervals (normal ranges): a challenge to laboratorians. *Am. J. Med. Technol.* **46:**504–511.

10. **Avcin, T., R. Cimaz, F. Falcini, F. Zulian, G. Martini, G. Simonini, V. Porenta-Besic, G. Cecchini, M. O. Borghi, and P. L. Meroni.** 2002. Prevalence and clinical significance of anti-cyclic citrullinated peptide antibodies

in juvenile idiopathic arthritis. *Ann. Rheum. Dis.* **61:** 608–611.

11. Bas, S., S. Genevay, O. Meyer, and C. Gabay. 2003. Anticyclic citrullinated peptide antibodies, IgM and IgA rheumatoid factors in the diagnosis and prognosis of rheumatoid arthritis. *Rheumatology* (Oxford) **42:**677–680.

12. Bas, S., T. V. Perneger, M. Seitz, J. M. Tiercy, P. Roux-Lombard, and P. A. Guerne. 2002. Diagnostic tests for rheumatoid arthritis: comparison of anti-cyclic citrullinated peptide antibodies, anti-keratin antibodies and IgM rheumatoid factors. *Rheumatology* (Oxford) **41:**809–814.

13. Berglin, E., L. Padyukov, U. Sundin, G. Hallmans, H. Stenlund, W. J. Van Venrooij, L. Klareskog, and S. R. Dahlqvist. 2004. A combination of autoantibodies to cyclic citrullinated peptide (CCP) and HLA-DRB1 locus antigens is strongly associated with future onset of rheumatoid arthritis. *Arthritis Res. Ther.* **6:**R303–R308.

14. Bizzaro, N., G. Mazzanti, E. Tonutti, D. Villalta, and R. Tozzoli. 2001. Diagnostic accuracy of the anti-citrulline antibody assay for rheumatoid arthritis. *Clin. Chem.* **47:**1089–1093.

15. Bonagura, V. R., S. E. Artandi, A. Davidson, I. Randen, N. Agostino, K. Thompson, J. B. Natvig, and S. L. Morrison. 1993. Mapping studies reveal unique epitopes on IgG recognized by rheumatoid arthritis-derived monoclonal rheumatoid factors. *J. Immunol.* **151:**3840–3852.

16. Borque, L., A. Rus, and R. Ruiz. 1991. Automated turbidimetry of rheumatoid factor without heat inactivation of serum. *Eur. J. Clin. Chem. Clin. Biochem.* **29:**521–527.

17. Boscato, L. M., and M. C. Stuart. 1988. Heterophilic antibodies: a problem for all immunoassays. *Clin. Chem.* **34:**27–33.

18. Butler, V. P., Jr., and J. H. Vaughan. 1964. Hemagglutination by rheumatoid factor of cells coated with animal gamma globulins. *Proc. Soc. Exp. Biol. Med.* **116:**585–593.

19. Cammarata, R., G. P. Rodnan, and R. H. Fennell. 1967. Serum anti-gamma-globulin and antinuclear factors in the aged. *JAMA* **199:**455–458.

20. Caramaschi, P., D. Biasi, E. Tonolli, S. Pieropan, N. Martinelli, A. Carletto, A. Volpe, and L. M. Bambara. 2005. Antibodies against cyclic citrullinated peptides in patients affected by rheumatoid arthritis before and after infliximab treatment. *Rheumatol. Int.* **26:**58–62.

21. Chapuy-Regaud, S., L. Nogueira, C. Clavel, M. Sebbag, C. Vincent, and G. Serre. 2005. IgG subclass distribution of the rheumatoid arthritis-specific autoantibodies to citrullinated fibrin. *Clin. Exp. Immunol.* **139:**542–550.

22. Corper, A. L., M. K. Sohi, V. R. Bonagura, M. Steinitz, R. Jefferis, A. Feinstein, D. Beale, M. J. Taussig, and B. J. Sutton. 1997. Structure of human IgM rheumatoid factor Fab bound to its autoantigen IgG Fc reveals a novel topology of antibody-antigen interaction. *Nat. Struct. Biol.* **4:**374–381.

23. Dasgupta, A., S. K. Banerjee, and P. Datta. 1999. False-positive troponin I in the MEIA due to the presence of rheumatoid factors in serum. Elimination of this interference by using a polyclonal antisera against rheumatoid factors. *Am. J. Clin. Pathol.* **112:**753–756.

24. de Koster, H. S., R. Amons, W. E. Benckhuijsen, M. Feijlbrief, G. A. Schellekens, and J. W. Drijfhout. 1995. The use of dedicated peptide libraries permits the discovery of high affinity binding peptides. *J. Immunol. Methods* **187:**179–188.

25. De Rycke, L., X. Verhelst, E. Kruithof, F. Van den Bosch, I. E. Hoffman, E. M. Veys, and F. De Keyser. 2005. Rheumatoid factor, but not anti-cyclic citrullinated peptide antibodies, is modulated by infliximab treatment in rheumatoid arthritis. *Ann. Rheum. Dis.* **64:**299–302.

26. Despres, N., G. Boire, F. J. Lopez-Longo, and H. A. Menard. 1994. The Sa system: a novel antigen-antibody system specific for rheumatoid arthritis. *J. Rheumatol.* **21:**1027–1033.

27. Dubucquoi, S., E. Solau-Gervais, D. Lefranc, L. Marguerie, J. Sibilia, J. Goetz, V. Dutoit, A. L. Fauchais, E. Hachulla, R. M. Flipo, and L. Prin. 2004. Evaluation of anti-citrullinated filaggrin antibodies as hallmarks for the diagnosis of rheumatic diseases. *Ann. Rheum. Dis.* **63:**415–419.

28. Elkon, K. B., D. L. Delacroix, A. E. Gharavi, J. P. Vaerman, and G. R. Hughes. 1982. Immunoglobulin A and polymeric IgA rheumatoid factors in systemic sicca syndrome: partial characterization. *J. Immunol.* **129:**576–581.

29. Forslind, K., M. Ahlmen, K. Eberhardt, I. Hafstrom, and B. Svensson. 2004. Prediction of radiological outcome in early rheumatoid arthritis in clinical practice: role of antibodies to citrullinated peptides (anti-CCP). *Ann. Rheum. Dis.* **63:**1090–1095.

30. Fraser, K. J. 1988. The Waaler-Rose test: anatomy of the eponym. *Semin. Arthritis Rheum.* **18:**61–71.

31. Garcia-Berrocal, B., C. Gonzalez, M. Perez, J. A. Navajo, I. Moreta, C. Davila, and J. M. Gonzalez-Buitrago. 2005. Anti-cyclic citrullinated peptide autoantibodies in IgM rheumatoid factor-positive patients. *Clin. Chim. Acta* **354:**123–130.

31a. Girelli, F., F. G. Foschi, E. Bedeschi, V. Calderoni, G. F. Stefanini, and M. G. Martinelli. 2004. Is anticyclic citrullinated peptide a useful laboratory test for the diagnosis of rheumatoid arthritis? *Allerg. Immunol.* (Paris) **36:**127–130.

32. Goldbach-Mansky, R., J. Lee, A. McCoy, J. Hoxworth, C. Yarboro, J. S. Smolen, G. Steiner, A. Rosen, C. Zhang, H. A. Menard, Z. J. Zhou, T. Palosuo, W. J. Van Venrooij, R. L. Wilder, J. H. Klippel, H. R. Schumacher, Jr., and H. S. El-Gabalawy. 2000. Rheumatoid arthritis associated autoantibodies in patients with synovitis of recent onset. *Arthritis Res.* **2:**236–243.

33. Gorgani, N. N., J. G. Altin, and C. R. Parish. 1999. Histidine-rich glycoprotein prevents the formation of insoluble immune complexes by rheumatoid factor. *Immunology* **98:**456–463.

34. Greiner, A., H. Plischke, H. Kellner, and R. Gruber. 2005. Association of anti-cyclic citrullinated peptide antibodies, anti-citrullin antibodies, and IgM and IgA rheumatoid factors with serological parameters of disease activity in rheumatoid arthritis. *Ann. N. Y. Acad. Sci.* **1050:**295–303.

35. Grunnet, N., and G. T. Espersen. 1988. Comparative studies on RF-IgA and RF-IgM ELISA—human or rabbit IgG as antigen? *Scand. J. Rheumatol. Suppl.* **75:**36–39.

36. Halldorsdottir, H. D., T. Jonsson, J. Thorsteinsson, and H. Valdimarsson. 2000. A prospective study on the incidence of rheumatoid arthritis among people with persistent increase of rheumatoid factor. *Ann. Rheum. Dis.* **59:**149–151.

37. Heliovaara, M., K. Aho, P. Knekt, A. Aromaa, J. Maatela, and A. Reunanen. 1995. Rheumatoid factor, chronic arthritis and mortality. *Ann. Rheum. Dis.* **54:**811–814.

38. Hennig, C., L. Rink, U. Fagin, W. J. Jabs, and H. Kirchner. 2000. The influence of naturally occurring heterophilic anti-immunoglobulin antibodies on direct measurement of serum proteins using sandwich ELISAs. *J. Immunol. Methods* **235:**71–80.

39. Herold, M., V. Boeser, E. Russe, and W. Klotz. 2005. Anti-CCP: history and its usefulness. *Clin. Dev. Immunol.* **12:**131–135.

40. Hicks, M. J., M. Heick, P. Finley, E. P. Gall, L. Minnich, and R. J. Williams. 1982. Rheumatoid factor activity by rate nephelometry correlated with clinical activity in rheumatoid arthritis. *Am. J. Clin. Pathol.* **78:**342–345.

41. Hiemstra, H. S., W. E. Benckhuijsen, R. Amons, W. Rapp, and J. W. Drijfhout. 1998. A new hybrid resin for stepwise screening of peptide libraries combined with single bead Edman sequencing. *J. Pept. Sci.* **4:**282–288.

42. Hoet, R. M., A. M. Boerbooms, M. Arends, D. J. Ruiter, and W. J. van Venrooij. 1991. Antiperinuclear factor, a marker autoantibody for rheumatoid arthritis: colocalisation of the perinuclear factor and profilaggrin. *Ann. Rheum. Dis.* **50:**611–618.

43. Hoet, R. M., and W. J. Van Venrooij. 1992. *The Perinuclear Factor and Antikeratin Antibodies in Rheumatoid Arthritis.* Springer Verlag, Berlin, Germany.

44. Jacoby, R. K., M. I. Jayson, and J. A. Cosh. 1973. Onset, early stages, and prognosis of rheumatoid arthritis: a clinical study of 100 patients with 11-year follow-up. *Br. Med. J.* **2:**96–100.

45. Jansen, A. L., I. van der Horst-Bruinsma, D. van Schaardenburg, R. J. van de Stadt, M. H. de Koning, and B. A. Dijkmans. 2002. Rheumatoid factor and antibodies to cyclic citrullinated peptide differentiate rheumatoid arthritis from undifferentiated polyarthritis in patients with early arthritis. *J. Rheumatol.* **29:**2074–2076.

46. Jansen, L. M., D. van Schaardenburg, I. van der Horst-Bruinsma, R. J. van der Stadt, M. H. de Koning, and B. A. Dijkmans. 2003. The predictive value of anti-cyclic citrullinated peptide antibodies in early arthritis. *J. Rheumatol.* **30:**1691–1695.

47. Jawaheer, D., and P. K. Gregersen. 2002. Rheumatoid arthritis. The genetic components. *Rheum. Dis. Clin. N. Am.* **28:**1–15.

48. Jonsson, T., J. A. Arnason, and H. Valdimarsson. 1986. Enzyme-linked immunosorbent assay (ELISA) screening test for detection of rheumatoid factor. *Rheumatol. Int.* **6:**199–204.

49. Jonsson, T., J. Thorsteinsson, and H. Valdimarsson. 1998. Does smoking stimulate rheumatoid factor production in non-rheumatic individuals? *APMIS* **106:**970–974.

50. Jonsson, T., and H. Valdimarsson. 1993. Is measurement of rheumatoid factor isotypes clinically useful? *Ann. Rheum. Dis.* **52:**161–164.

51. Kastbom, A., G. Strandberg, A. Lindroos, and T. Skogh. 2004. Anti-CCP antibody test predicts the disease course during 3 years in early rheumatoid arthritis (the Swedish TIRA project). *Ann. Rheum. Dis.* **63:**1085–1089.

52. Katwa, G., G. Komatireddy, and S. E. Walker. 2001. False positive elevation of cardiac troponin I in seropositive rheumatoid arthritis. *J. Rheumatol.* **28:**2750–2751.

53. Kenny, P. R., and D. R. Finger. 2005. Falsely elevated cardiac troponin-I in patients with seropositive rheumatoid arthritis. *J. Rheumatol.* **32:**1258–1261.

54. Keshgegian, A. A., C. W. Straub, E. F. Loos, and B. K. Grenoble. 1994. Rheumatoid factor measured with the QM300 nephelometer: clinical sensitivity and specificity. *Clin. Chem.* **40:**943.

55. Klein, F., M. B. Janssens, L. K. van Romunde, and G. A. Eilers. 1990. Comparative study of test kits for measurement of rheumatoid factors by the latex fixation test. *Ann. Rheum. Dis.* **49:**801–804.

56. Kleveland, G., T. Egeland, and T. Lea. 1988. Quantitation of rheumatoid factors (RF) of IgM, IgA and IgG isotypes by a simple and sensitive ELISA. Discrimination between false and true IgG-RF. *Scand. J. Rheumatol. Suppl.* **75:**15–24.

57. Korendowych, E., P. Owen, J. Ravindran, C. Carmichael, and N. McHugh. 2005. The clinical and genetic associations of anti-cyclic citrullinated peptide antibodies in psoriatic arthritis. *Rheumatology* (Oxford) **44:**1056–1060.

58. Kroot, E. J., B. A. de Jong, M. A. van Leeuwen, H. Swinkels, F. H. van den Hoogen, M. van't Hof, L. B. van de Putte, M. H. van Rijswijk, W. J. van Venrooij, and P. L. van Riel. 2000. The prognostic value of anti-cyclic citrullinated peptide antibody in patients with recent-onset rheumatoid arthritis. *Arthritis Rheum.* **43:**1831–1835.

59. Kurki, P., K. Aho, T. Palosuo, and M. Heliovaara. 1992. Immunopathology of rheumatoid arthritis. Antikeratin antibodies precede the clinical disease. *Arthritis Rheum.* **35:**914–917.

60. Kyburz, D., M. Corr, D. C. Brinson, A. Von Damm, H. Tighe, and D. A. Carson. 1999. Human rheumatoid factor production is dependent on CD40 signaling and autoantigen. *J. Immunol.* **163:**3116–3122.

61. Larkin, J. G., R. D. Sturrock, and W. H. Stimson. 1986. A rapid enzyme immunoassay for the detection of IgM rheumatoid factor—a comparison of "sero-negative" and "sero-positive" rheumatoid patients. *J. Clin. Lab. Immunol.* **20:**207–209.

62. Larsson, A., and J. Sjoquist. 1988. False-positive results in latex agglutination tests caused by rheumatoid factor. *Clin. Chem.* **34:**767–768.

63. Lawrence, R. C., C. G. Helmick, F. C. Arnett, R. A. Deyo, D. T. Felson, E. H. Giannini, S. P. Heyse, R. Hirsch, M. C. Hochberg, G. G. Hunder, M. H. Liang, S. R. Pillemer, V. D. Steen, and F. Wolfe. 1998. Estimates of the prevalence of arthritis and selected musculoskeletal disorders in the United States. *Arthritis Rheum.* **41:**778–799.

64. Lee, D. M., and P. H. Schur. 2003. Clinical utility of the anti-CCP assay in patients with rheumatic diseases. *Ann. Rheum. Dis.* **62:**870–874.

65. Lindqvist, E., K. Eberhardt, K. Bendtzen, D. Heinegard, and T. Saxne. 2005. Prognostic laboratory markers of joint damage in rheumatoid arthritis. *Ann. Rheum. Dis.* **64:**196–201.

66. Linker, J. B., III, and R. C. Williams, Jr. 1986. Tests for detection of rheumatoid factors, p. 759–761. *In* N. R. Rose, H. Friedman, and J. L. Fahey (ed.), *Manual of Clinical Laboratory Immunology*, 3rd ed. American Society for Microbiology, Washington, D.C.

67. Litwin, S. D., and J. M. Singer. 1965. Studies of the incidence and significance of anti-gamma globulin factors in the aging. *Arthritis Rheum.* **8:**538–550.

68. Low, J. M., A. K. Chauhan, D. A. Kietz, U. Daud, P. H. Pepmueller, and T. L. Moore. 2004. Determination of anti-cyclic citrullinated peptide antibodies in the sera of patients with juvenile idiopathic arthritis. *J. Rheumatol.* **31:**1829–1833.

69. Lunt, M., D. P. Symmons, and A. J. Silman. 2005. An evaluation of the decision tree format of the American College of Rheumatology 1987 classification criteria for rheumatoid arthritis: performance over five years in a primary care-based prospective study. *Arthritis Rheum.* **52:**2277–2283.

70. Mannik, M., and F. A. Nardella. 1985. IgG rheumatoid factors and self-association of these antibodies. *Clin. Rheum. Dis.* **11:**551–572.

71. Masson-Bessiere, C., M. Sebbag, J. J. Durieux, L. Nogueira, C. Vincent, E. Girbal-Neuhauser, R. Durroux, A. Cantagrel, and G. Serre. 2000. In the rheumatoid pannus, anti-filaggrin autoantibodies are produced by local plasma cells and constitute a higher proportion of IgG than in synovial fluid and serum. *Clin. Exp. Immunol.* **119:**544–552.

72. Masson-Bessiere, C., M. Sebbag, E. Girbal-Neuhauser, L. Nogueira, C. Vincent, T. Senshu, and G. Serre. 2001. The major synovial targets of the rheumatoid arthritis-specific antifilaggrin autoantibodies are deiminated forms of the alpha- and beta-chains of fibrin. *J. Immunol.* **166:**4177–4184.

73. Matzinger, P. 2002. The danger model: a renewed sense of self. *Science* **296:**301–305.

74. Messner, R. P., T. Laxdal, P. G. Quie, and R. C. Williams, Jr. 1968. Rheumatoid factors in subacute bacterial

endocarditis—bacterium, duration of disease or genetic predisposition? *Ann. Intern. Med.* **68:**746–756.

75. **Meyer, O., B. Combe, A. Elias, K. Benali, J. Clot, J. Sany, and J. F. Eliaou.** 1997. Autoantibodies predicting the outcome of rheumatoid arthritis: evaluation in two subsets of patients according to severity of radiographic damage. *Ann. Rheum. Dis.* **56:**682–685.

76. **Mikuls, T. R., J. R. O'Dell, J. A. Stoner, L. A. Parrish, W. P. Arend, J. M. Norris, and V. M. Holers.** 2004. Association of rheumatoid arthritis treatment response and disease duration with declines in serum levels of IgM rheumatoid factor and anti-cyclic citrullinated peptide antibody. *Arthritis Rheum.* **50:**3776–3782.

77. **National Committee for Clinical Laboratory Standards.** 1985. *User Comparison of Quantitative Clinical Laboratory Methods Using Patient Samples; Proposed Guideline.* NCCLS document EP9-P. National Committee for Clinical Laboratory Standards, Villanova, Pa.

78. **Nemazee, D. A.** 1985. Immune complexes can trigger specific, T cell-dependent, autoanti-IgG antibody production in mice. *J. Exp. Med.* **161:**242–256.

79. **Newkirk, M. M., K. N. Duffy, A. Paleckova, E. Ivaskova, A. Galianova, J. Seeman, K. Vojtechovsky, and C. Dostal.** 1995. Herpes viruses in multicase families with rheumatoid arthritis. *J. Rheumatol.* **22:** 2055–2061.

80. **Newkirk, M. M., R. Goldbach-Mansky, B. W. Senior, J. Klippel, H. R. Schumacher, Jr., and H. S. El-Gabalawy.** 2005. Elevated levels of IgM and IgA antibodies to *Proteus mirabilis* and IgM antibodies to *Escherichia coli* are associated with early rheumatoid factor (RF)-positive rheumatoid arthritis. *Rheumatology* **44:**1433–1441.

81. **Nielen, M. M., D. van Schaardenburg, H. W. Reesink, R. J. van de Stadt, I. E. van der Horst-Bruinsma, M. H. de Koning, M. R. Habibuw, J. P. Vandenbroucke, and B. A. Dijkmans.** 2004. Specific autoantibodies precede the symptoms of rheumatoid arthritis: a study of serial measurements in blood donors. *Arthritis Rheum.* **50:**380–386.

82. **Oka, H., S. Hirohata, T. Inoue, S. Iwamoto, and T. Miyamoto.** 1990. Quantitative determination of IgM-rheumatoid factor by enzyme immunoassay—standardization using a serum from a rheumatoid arthritis patient. *Clin. Chim. Acta* **188:**147–159.

83. **Paimela, L., T. Palosuo, M. Leirisalo-Repo, T. Helve, and K. Aho.** 1995. Prognostic value of quantitative measurement of rheumatoid factor in early rheumatoid arthritis. *Br. J. Rheumatol.* **34:**1146–1150.

84. **Painter, P. C., J. M. Lyon, J. H. Evans, W. W. Powers, R. L. Whittaker, and M. J. Decker.** 1982. Performance of a new rate-nephelometric assay for rheumatoid factor, and its correlation with tube-titer results for human sera and synovial fluid. *Clin. Chem.* **28:**2214–2218.

84a. **Pinheiro, G. C., M. A. Scheinberg, M. Aparecida da Silva, and S. Maciel.** 2003. Anti-cyclic citrullinated peptide antibodies in advanced rheumatoid arthritis. *Ann. Intern. Med.* **139:**234–235.

85. **Plotz, C. M., and J. M. Singer.** 1956. The latex fixation test. I. Application to the serologic diagnosis of rheumatoid arthritis. *Am. J. Med.* **21:**888–892.

86. **Pope, R. M., J. Lessard, and E. Nunnery.** 1986. Differential effects of therapeutic regimens on specific classes of rheumatoid factor. *Ann. Rheum. Dis.* **45:**183–189.

87. **Ramsland, P. A., B. F. Movafagh, M. Reichlin, and A. B. Edmundson.** 1999. Interference of rheumatoid factor activity by aspartame, a dipeptide methyl ester. *J. Mol. Recognit.* **12:**249–257.

88. **Randen, I., K. M. Thompson, V. Pascual, K. Victor, D. Beale, J. Coadwell, O. Forre, J. D. Capra, and J. B. Natvig.** 1992. Rheumatoid factor V genes from patients

with rheumatoid arthritis are diverse and show evidence of an antigen-driven response. *Immunol. Rev.* **128:**49–71.

89. **Rantapaa-Dahlqvist, S.** 2005. Diagnostic and prognostic significance of autoantibodies in early rheumatoid arthritis. *Scand. J. Rheumatol.* **34:**83–96.

90. **Rantapaa-Dahlqvist, S., B. A. de Jong, E. Berglin, G. Hallmans, G. Wadell, H. Stenlund, U. Sundin, and W. J. van Venrooij.** 2003. Antibodies against cyclic citrullinated peptide and IgA rheumatoid factor predict the development of rheumatoid arthritis. *Arthritis Rheum.* **48:**2741–2749.

91. **Raza, K., M. Breese, P. Nightingale, K. Kumar, T. Potter, D. M. Carruthers, D. Situnayake, C. Gordon, C. D. Buckley, M. Salmon, and G. D. Kitas.** 2005. Predictive value of antibodies to cyclic citrullinated peptide in patients with very early inflammatory arthritis. *J. Rheumatol.* **32:**231–238.

92. **Reilly, P. A., J. A. Cosh, P. J. Maddison, J. J. Rasker, and A. J. Silman.** 1990. Mortality and survival in rheumatoid arthritis: a 25 year prospective study of 100 patients. *Ann. Rheum. Dis.* **49:**363–369.

93. **Roberts-Thomson, P. J., R. McEvoy, T. Langhans, and J. Bradley.** 1985. Routine quantification of rheumatoid factor by rate nephelometry. *Ann. Rheum. Dis.* **44:**379–383.

94. **Roberts-Thomson, P. J., R. M. Wernick, and M. Ziff.** 1982. Quantitation of rheumatoid factor by laser nephelometry. *Rheumatol. Int.* **2:**17–20.

95. **Rogers, G. E., H. W. Harding, and I. J. Llewellyn-Smith.** 1977. The origin of citrulline-containing proteins in the hair follicle and the chemical nature of trichohyalin, an intracellular precursor. *Biochim. Biophys. Acta* **495:**159–175.

96. **Rose, H. M., C. Ragan, E. Pearce, and M. O. Lipman.** 1949. Differential agglutination of normal and sensitized sheep erythrocytes by sera of patients with rheumatoid arthritis. *Proc. Soc. Exp. Biol. Med.* **68:**1–11.

97. **Saraux, A., B. Bendaoud, M. Dueymes, P. Le Goff, and P. Youinou.** 1997. The functional affinity of IgM rheumatoid factor is related to the disease duration in patients with rheumatoid arthritis. *Ann. Rheum. Dis.* **56:**126–129.

97a. **Saraux, A., J. M. Berthelot, V. Devauchelle, B. Bendaoud, G. Chales, C. Le Henaff, J. B. Thorel, S. Hoang, S. Jousse, D. Baron, P. Le Goff, and P. Youinou.** 2003. Value of antibodies to citrulline-containing peptides for diagnosing early rheumatoid arthritis. *J. Rheumatol.* **30:**2535–2539.

98. **Sasso, E.** 2000. The rheumatoid factor response in the etiology of mixed cryoglobulins associated with Hep C virus infection. *Ann. Med. Interne* **151:**41–45.

99. **Schellekens, G. A., B. A. de Jong, F. H. van den Hoogen, L. B. van de Putte, and W. J. van Venrooij.** 1998. Citrulline is an essential constituent of antigenic determinants recognized by rheumatoid arthritis-specific autoantibodies. *J. Clin. Investig.* **101:**273–281.

100. **Schellekens, G. A., H. Visser, B. A. de Jong, F. H. van den Hoogen, J. M. Hazes, F. C. Breedveld, and W. J. van Venrooij.** 2000. The diagnostic properties of rheumatoid arthritis antibodies recognizing a cyclic citrullinated peptide. *Arthritis Rheum.* **43:**155–163.

101. **Schrohenloher, R. E., S. L. J. Bridges, and W. J. Koopman.** 1999. *Rheumatoid Factor.* The Williams & Wilkins Co., Baltimore, Md.

102. **Shmerling, R. H., and T. L. Delbanco.** 1992. How useful is the rheumatoid factor? An analysis of sensitivity, specificity, and predictive value. *Arch. Intern. Med.* **152:**2417–2420.

103. **Shmerling, R. H., and T. L. Delbanco.** 1991. The rheumatoid factor: an analysis of clinical utility. *Am. J. Med.* **91:**528–534.

104. **Smeets, T. J., E. R. Vossenaar, W. J. van Venrooij, and P. P. Tak.** 2002. Is expression of intracellular citrullinated proteins in synovial tissue specific for rheumatoid

arthritis? Comment on the article by Baeten et al. *Arthritis Rheum.* **46**:2824–2826. (Author reply, **46**: 2826–2827.)

105. **Sohi, M. K., B. J. Sutton, A. L. Corper, T. Wan, R. N. Maini, C. Brown, T. Rijnders, D. Beale, A. Feinstein, A. S. Humphreys, et al.** 1994. Crystallization and preliminary X-ray analysis of the Fab fragment of a human monoclonal IgM rheumatoid factor (2A2). *J. Mol. Biol.* **242**:706–708.

106. **Sonderstrup, G.** 2003. Development of humanized mice as a model of inflammatory arthritis. *Springer Semin. Immunopathol.* **25**:35–45.

107. **Sutton, B., A. Corper, V. Bonagura, and M. Taussig.** 2000. The structure and origin of rheumatoid factors. *Immunol. Today* **21**:177–183.

108. **Suzuki, A., R. Yamada, X. Chang, S. Tokuhiro, T. Sawada, M. Suzuki, M. Nagasaki, M. Nakayama-Hamada, R. Kawaida, M. Ono, M. Ohtsuki, H. Furukawa, S. Yoshino, M. Yukioka, S. Tohma, T. Matsubara, S. Wakitani, R. Teshima, Y. Nishioka, A. Sekine, A. Iida, A. Takahashi, T. Tsunoda, Y. Nakamura, and K. Yamamoto.** 2003. Functional haplotypes of PADI4, encoding citrullinating enzyme peptidylarginine deiminase 4, are associated with rheumatoid arthritis. *Nat. Genet.* **34**:395–402.

108a. **Suzuki, K., T. Sawada, A. Murakami, T. Matsui, S. Tohma, K. Nakazono, M. Takemura, Y. Takasaki, T. Mimori, and K. Yamamoto.** 2003. High diagnostic performance of ELISA detection of antibodies to citrullinated antigens in rheumatoid arthritis. *Scand. J. Rheumatol.* **32**:197–204.

109. **Tampoia, M., V. Brescia, A. Fontana, P. Maggiolini, G. Lapadula, and N. Pansini.** 2005. Anti-cyclic citrullinated peptide autoantibodies measured by an automated enzyme immunoassay: analytical performance and clinical correlations. *Clin. Chim. Acta* **355**:137–144.

110. **Tarkowski, A., C. Czerkinsky, and L. A. Nilsson.** 1985. Simultaneous induction of rheumatoid factor- and antigen-specific antibody-secreting cells during the secondary immune response in man. *Clin. Exp. Immunol.* **61**:379–387.

111. **Taylor, R. N., K. M. Fulford, and W. L. Jones.** 1977. Reduction of variation in results of rheumatoid factor tests by use of a serum reference preparation. *J. Clin. Microbiol.* **5**:42–45.

112. **Taylor, R. N., A. Y. Huong, K. M. Fulford, V. A. Przybyszewski, and T. L. Hearn.** 1979. *Quality Control for Immunologic Tests.* HEW publication no. (CDC) 79-8376. U.S. Department of Health, Education and Welfare, Atlanta, Ga.

113. **Tuomi, T., K. Aho, T. Palosuo, R. Kaarela, R. von Essen, H. Isomaki, M. Leirisalo-Repo, and S. Sarna.** 1988. Significance of rheumatoid factors in an eight-year longitudinal study on arthritis. *Rheumatol. Int.* **8**:21–26.

114. **Tuomi, T., M. Heliovaara, T. Palosuo, and K. Aho.** 1990. Smoking, lung function, and rheumatoid factors. *Ann. Rheum. Dis.* **49**:753–756.

115. **Vallbracht, I., and K. Helmke.** 2005. Additional diagnostic and clinical value of anti-cyclic citrullinated peptide antibodies compared with rheumatoid factor isotypes in rheumatoid arthritis. *Autoimmun. Rev.* **4**:389–394.

116. **Vallbracht, I., J. Rieber, M. Oppermann, F. Forger, U. Siebert, and K. Helmke.** 2004. Diagnostic and clinical value of anti-cyclic citrullinated peptide antibodies compared with rheumatoid factor isotypes in rheumatoid arthritis. *Ann. Rheum. Dis.* **63**:1079–1084.

117. **van Boekel, M. A., B. de Jong, J. W. Drijfhout, M. H. de Koning, J. van Delft, and W. J. Van Venrooij.** 2000. *Selection of Diagnostic Marker Peptides for Autoimmune Diseases Using Synthetic Peptide Libraries.* Pabst Science, Lengerich, Germany.

118. **van Boekel, M. A., E. R. Vossenaar, F. H. van den Hoogen, and W. J. van Venrooij.** 2002. Autoantibody systems in rheumatoid arthritis: specificity, sensitivity and diagnostic value. *Arthritis Res.* **4**:87–93.

119. **Van der Heijde, D., P. L. Van Riel, M. H. Van Rijiswijk, and L. B. Van de Putte.** 1988. Influence of prognostic features in the final outcome in rheumatoid arthritis. A review of literature. *Semin. Arthritis Rheum.* **17**:284–292.

120. **van Gaalen, F. A., S. P. Linn-Rasker, W. J. van Venrooij, B. A. de Jong, F. C. Breedveld, C. L. Verweij, R. E. Toes, and T. W. Huizinga.** 2004. Autoantibodies to cyclic citrullinated peptides predict progression to rheumatoid arthritis in patients with undifferentiated arthritis: a prospective cohort study. *Arthritis Rheum.* **50**:709–715.

121. **van Jaarsveld, C. H., E. J. ter Borg, J. W. Jacobs, G. A. Schellekens, F. H. Gmelig-Meyling, C. van Booma-Frankfort, B. A. de Jong, W. J. van Venrooij, and J. W. Bijlsma.** 1999. The prognostic value of the antiperinuclear factor, anti-citrullinated peptide antibodies and rheumatoid factor in early rheumatoid arthritis. *Clin. Exp. Rheumatol.* **17**:689–697.

122. **van Leeuwen, M. A., J. Westra, P. C. Limburg, H. J. de Jong, J. Marrink, and M. H. van Rijswijk.** 1988. Quantitation of IgM, IgA and IgG rheumatoid factors by ELISA in rheumatoid arthritis and other rheumatic disorders. *Scand. J. Rheumatol. Suppl.* **75**:25–31.

123. **van Snick, J. L., and P. L. Masson.** 1980. Incidence and specificities of IgA and IgM anti-AgG autoantibodies in various mouse strains and colonies. *J. Exp. Med.* **151**:45–55.

124. **van Venrooij, W. J., J. M. Hazes, and H. Visser.** 2002. Anticitrullinated protein/peptide antibody and its role in the diagnosis and prognosis of early rheumatoid arthritis. *Neth. J. Med.* **60**:383–388.

125. **van Venrooij, W. J., E. R. Vossenaar, and A. J. Zendman.** 2004. Anti-CCP antibodies: the new rheumatoid factor in the serology of rheumatoid arthritis. *Autoimmun. Rev.* **3**(Suppl. 1):S17–S19.

126. **van Zeben, D., J. M. Hazes, A. H. Zwinderman, A. Cats, E. A. van der Voort, and F. C. Breedveld.** 1992. Clinical significance of rheumatoid factors in early rheumatoid arthritis: results of a follow up study. *Ann. Rheum. Dis.* **51**:1029–1035.

126a. **Vasishta, A.** 2002. Diagnosing early-onset rheumatoid arthritis: the role of anti-CCP antibodies. *Am. Clin. Lab.* **21**:34–36.

127. **Vencovsky, J., S. Machacek, L. Sedova, J. Kafkova, J. Gatterova, V. Pesakova, and S. Ruzickova.** 2003. Autoantibodies can be prognostic markers of an erosive disease in early rheumatoid arthritis. *Ann. Rheum. Dis.* **62**:427–430.

128. **Virella, G., W. A. Hipp, J. F. John, Jr., B. Kahaleh, M. Ford, and H. H. Fudenberg.** 1979. Nephelometric detection of soluble immune complexes: methodology and clinical applications. *Int. Arch. Allergy Appl. Immunol.* **58**:402–410.

129. **Visser, H., L. B. Gelinck, A. H. Kampfraath, F. C. Breedveld, and J. M. Hazes.** 1996. Diagnostic and prognostic characteristics of the enzyme linked immunosorbent rheumatoid factor assays in rheumatoid arthritis. *Ann. Rheum. Dis.* **55**:157–161.

130. **Vossenaar, E. R., N. Despres, E. Lapointe, A. van der Heijden, M. Lora, T. Senshu, W. J. van Venrooij, and H. A. Menard.** 2004. Rheumatoid arthritis specific anti-Sa antibodies target citrullinated vimentin. *Arthritis Res. Ther.* **6**:R142–R150.

131. **Vossenaar, E. R., S. Nijenhuis, M. M. Helsen, A. van der Heijden, T. Senshu, W. B. van den Berg, W. J. van Venrooij, and L. A. Joosten.** 2003. Citrullination of synovial proteins in murine models of rheumatoid arthritis. *Arthritis Rheum.* **48:**2489–2500.

132. **Vossenaar, E. R., T. R. Radstake, A. van der Heijden, M. A. van Mansum, C. Dieteren, D. J. de Rooij, P. Barrera, A. J. Zendman, and W. J. van Venrooij.** 2004. Expression and activity of citrullinating peptidylarginine deiminase enzymes in monocytes and macrophages. *Ann. Rheum. Dis.* **63:**373–381.

133. **Vossenaar, E. R., T. J. Smeets, M. C. Kraan, J. M. Raats, W. J. van Venrooij, and P. P. Tak.** 2004. The presence of citrullinated proteins is not specific for rheumatoid synovial tissue. *Arthritis Rheum.* **50:**3485–3494.

134. **Vossenaar, E. R., and W. J. van Venrooij.** 2004. Citrullinated proteins: sparks that may ignite the fire in rheumatoid arthritis. *Arthritis Res. Ther.* **6:**107–111.

135. **Vossenaar, E. R., and W. J. van Venrooij.** 2004. Anti-CCP antibodies, a highly specific marker for (early) rheumatoid arthritis. *Clin. Appl. Immunol. Rev.* **4:** 239–262.

136. **Vossenaar, E. R., A. J. Zendman, and W. J. Van Venrooij.** 2004. Citrullination, a possible functional link between susceptibility genes and rheumatoid arthritis. *Arthritis Res. Ther.* **6:**1–5.

137. **Vossenaar, E. R., A. J. Zendman, W. J. van Venrooij, and G. J. Pruijn.** 2003. PAD, a growing family of citrullinating enzymes: genes, features and involvement in disease. *Bioessays* **25:**1106–1118.

138. **Waaler, E.** 1940. On the occurrence of a factor in human serum activating the specific agglutination of sheep red blood cell corpuscles. *Acta Pathol. Microbiol. Scand.* **17:**172–173.

139. **Wagner, U., S. Kaltenhauser, H. Sauer, S. Arnold, W. Seidel, H. Hantzschel, J. R. Kalden, and R. Wassmuth.** 1997. HLA markers and prediction of clinical course and outcome in rheumatoid arthritis. *Arthritis Rheum.* **40:**341–351.

140. **Wener, M. H., and P. R. Daum.** 1992. Nephelometry measurement of C4 concentration is influenced by ethylene glycol. *Clin. Chem.* **38:**1076S.

141. **Westgard, J. O., and P. L. Barry.** 1986. *Cost-Effective Quality Control: Managing the Quality and Productivity of Analytical Processes.* AACC Press, Washington, D.C.

142. **Williams, R. C., Jr., and H. G. Kunkel.** 1962. Rheumatoid factor, complement, and conglutinin aberrations in patients with subacute bacterial endocarditis. *J. Clin. Investig.* **41:**666–675.

143. **Williams, R. C., Jr., and C. C. Malone.** 1994. Rheumatoid-factor-reactive sites on CH2 established by analysis of overlapping peptides of primary sequence. *Scand. J. Immunol.* **40:**443–456.

144. **Wolfe, F., M. A. Cathey, and F. K. Roberts.** 1991. The latex test revisited. Rheumatoid factor testing in 8,287 rheumatic disease patients. *Arthritis Rheum.* **34:**951–960.

145. **Wong, A., T. P. Kenny, R. Ermel, and D. L. Robbins.** 1994. IgG3 reactive rheumatoid factor in rheumatoid arthritis: etiologic and pathogenic considerations. *Autoimmunity* **19:**199–210.

146. **Zendman, A. J., E. R. Vossenaar, and W. J. van Venrooij.** 2004. Autoantibodies to citrullinated (poly) peptides: a key diagnostic and prognostic marker for rheumatoid arthritis. *Autoimmunity* **37:**295–299.

147. **Zeng, X., M. Ai, X. Tian, X. Gan, Y. Shi, O. Song, and F. Tang.** 2003. Diagnostic value of anti-cyclic citrullinated peptide antibody in patients with rheumatoid arthritis. *J. Rheumatol.* **30:**1451–1455.

148. **Zhuang, H., S. Narain, E. Sobel, P. Y. Lee, D. C. Nacionales, K. M. Kelly, H. B. Richards, M. Segal, C. Stewart, M. Satoh, and W. H. Reeves.** Association of anti-nucleoprotein autoantibodies with upregulation of type I interferon-inducible gene transcripts and dendritic cell maturation in systemic lupus erythematosus. *Clin. Immunol.*, in press.

Laboratory Testing for Antibodies Associated with Antiphospholipid Antibody Syndrome

JOHN L. SCHMITZ

117

Testing for the presence of antiphospholipid antibodies (aPL) is typically performed for patients with vascular thrombosis and/or recurrent fetal morbidity—clinical features of aPL syndrome (APS), a disease of autoimmune nature. aPL are a heterogeneous group of antibodies that are present not only in patients with APS but also in patients in other disease states, recipients of certain drugs, and some healthy individuals. Various characteristics such as target antigen, isotype, and titer distinguish presumed pathogenic from nonpathogenic aPL. Adding to the complexity of this antibody system is the fact that several distinct types of assays are used to detect their presence and a variety of both home brew and kit-based enzyme-linked immunosorbent assay (ELISA) systems are in use, which have contributed significant variability in test performance, results, and interpretation. Nonetheless, detection of aPL is considered clinically useful. Of the several types of aPL described, lupus anticoagulant (LA) antibodies and anticardiolipin antibodies (aCL) are the types most clearly associated with APS, the latter being the focus of this chapter.

BACKGROUND ON aPL

The earliest described aPL were attributed not to an autoimmune disease but rather to an infectious disease, syphilis. The Wasserman test, a complement fixation assay that detected nontreponemal antibody, employed extracts from the livers of syphilitic newborns (73) that provided the phospholipid cardiolipin as the antigen. Subsequently cardiolipin was identified as the antigenic component of the serologic tests for syphilis (54). The Venereal Disease Research Laboratory (VDRL) and rapid plasma reagin tests were then developed, both employing purified cardiolipin combined with cholesterol and lecithin as the antigen. In the early 1980s investigators recognized an association between systemic lupus erythematosus (SLE) patients and LA-mediated thrombosis which was mediated by antibodies to phospholipids (55). A number of SLE patients also had a biological false-positive serologic test for syphilis, thus indicating a possible similarity between these two phenomena. Limitations of the LA and VDRL tests led to the development of the more sensitive radioimmunoassay (RIA) (35) for detection of aPL using cardiolipin as the test antigen. The RIA was subsequently modified to an ELISA format (28), the most common technique employed for the direct detection of aPL. The recognition of APS and the association with aPL

has led to diagnostic application of this test, a disease classification system dependent upon detection of these antibodies, and international efforts at assay standardization.

APS

Classification of patients with APS considers both clinical and laboratory criteria (Table 1). Vascular thrombosis and/or pregnancy complications in conjunction with a persistent presence of moderate to high levels of anticardiolipin immunoglobulin M (IgM) or IgG antibodies or LA antibodies establishes a definite diagnosis (74). The syndrome is classified as primary APS when not associated with another disease and accounts for over 50% of cases (12). Secondary APS is most frequently diagnosed in patients with SLE, lupus-like syndromes, Sjögren's syndrome, rheumatoid arthritis, systemic sclerosis, systemic vasculitis, and dermatomyositis (12).

Virtually any organ system can be affected in APS; however, the frequency of specific manifestations may vary with gender, age, type of associated aPL, and the presence of SLE. Recurrence is common in APS. The most frequent features associated with APS are venous thrombosis, thrombocytopenia, livedo reticularis, stroke, superficial thrombophlebitis, pulmonary embolism, fetal loss, transient ischemic attack, and hemolytic anemia (12, 40). In addition to the cerebrovascular system, manifestations are described to occur in the pulmonary, cardiovascular, renal, ocular, cutaneous, endocrine, gastrointestinal, and hematologic systems. APS in the background of SLE does not have a distinctly different array of clinical or laboratory manifestations. A small fraction of cases (<1%) may exhibit catastrophic APS resulting from widespread thrombosis in multiple organ systems leading to organ failure and a mortality rate of near 50% (4).

Fetal morbidity associated with APS typically occurs after 10 weeks of gestation (20, 40). Criteria for APS-associated fetal morbidity include three or more losses prior to the 10th week of gestation, one or more losses after the 10th week, or one or more premature deliveries at or before the 34th week because of preeclampsia, eclampsia, or placental insufficiency with the exclusion of other causes.

ANTIBODIES ASSOCIATED WITH APS

aPL are a heterogeneous group of antibodies in terms of target antigen and isotype (61). The first category of aPL,

TABLE 1 Summary of the criteria for classification of APS[a]

Clinical criteria

    1. Vascular thrombosis, including one or more episodes of arterial, venous, or small-vessel thrombosis in any tissue or organ

    2. Pregnancy morbidity, including one or more fetal deaths beyond the 10th week of gestation; one or more premature births of a morphologically normal neonate at or before the 34th week of gestation because of severe preeclampsia, eclampsia, or placental insufficiency; three or more consecutive spontaneous abortions before the 10th week of gestation with the exclusion of parental anatomic, hormonal, and chromosomal causes

Laboratory criteria

    1. Detection of aCL of IgG and/or IgM isotype at medium or high titer on two or more occasions at least 6 weeks apart as measured by a β2GPI-dependent assay

    2. Detection of LA or two or more occasions at least 6 weeks apart following established guidelines[b]

    [a]This table is adapted from reference 74. Definite APS is present when at least one clinical criterion and one laboratory criterion are present.
    [b]These guidelines can be found in reference 9.

LA antibodies, are detected with certain phospholipid-dependent coagulation assays. These may be the sole aPL found in APS patients or may be found in association with a second category of aPL that are detected with ELISAs. Included in this second group of aPL are those that bind directly to the phospholipid molecule (infection associated but not APS associated), those that bind to phospholipid-serum protein complexes, and those that bind directly to serum protein cofactors in the absence of phospholipid. The last two types of ELISA-detected aPL can both be found in patients with APS with or without LA. The aCL assay is the most common ELISA-based aPL assay in use to date, although other assays employing different antigens are being evaluated and in some cases used clinically (see below).

LAs

LAs are antibodies that are prothrombotic in vivo but display anticoagulant properties in vitro (i.e., they prolong certain coagulation tests). The antibodies detected in these LA assays are directed to serum proteins, including beta 2-glycoprotein I (β2GPI) and prothrombin (2, 65). Compared to other aPL tests, the LA test is considered less sensitive but more specific for APS (21, 50). However, there are patients with APS who exhibit only LA (55). The advantages of LA assays relative to aCL assays include increased specificity and a resulting higher predictive value (21, 27). A consensus approach has been developed for detection of LA (8) that defines the characteristics of APS-associated LA as (i) prolonging phospholipid-dependent clotting time assays (including activated partial thromboplastin time, dilute prothrombin time, dilute Russell's viper venom time, and Kaolin clotting time); (ii) not correctable by addition of normal plasma at a 1:1 ratio; (iii) phospholipid dependence confirmed by correction upon addition of phospholipids; and (iv) not due to inhibitors. Testing for LA is not addressed further in this chapter.

PHOSPHOLIPID-BINDING ANTIBODIES DETECTED WITH THE aCL ELISA

Antibodies associated with APS that are detected in aCL ELISAs were originally thought to bind to the phospholipid molecule. However, it was determined that binding was dependent upon the serum proteins. The protein identified as mediating this effect was β2GPI (26, 46). Not all aCL-reactive sera require β2GPI for binding. In particular, patients with certain infections were shown to have cofactor-independent aCL. aCL have been found in patients with a variety of infectious diseases, including human immunodeficiency virus (1, 14, 17, 43), malaria (22, 66), leprosy (18, 32), hepatitis C virus (39), and human T-cell lymphotropic virus type 1 (23, 75), although their reported prevalences vary (41). These infection-associated aPL do not require serum cofactors to enhance binding and are not usually associated with thrombotic events (61). Infection-associated aPL are more commonly of the IgM isotype, have less avid binding, and are generally transient, declining with resolution of infection. Although not typical, some patients with infections do have detectable cofactor-specific antibodies. Both prothrombin and β2GPI antibodies have been detected in patients with several infectious diseases (41).

AUTOIMMUNE aPL

An appreciation of the presence of aPL in SLE patients, and their association with thrombosis, led to the development of an RIA for detection of aCL antibodies (35) and subsequently an ELISA-based format (28). aCL associated with APS are most frequently IgG antibodies and of moderate to high levels in the blood (28, 34, 51). In contrast to aCL detected in patients with infections, the autoimmune aCL are typically cofactor (β2GPI) dependent. β2GPI enhancement of aCL binding is the result of the negatively charged phospholipids promoting higher density coating of the ELISA plate by β2GPI. The higher density of β2GPI enhances detection of these typically low-avidity antibodies. The use of "high binding" ELISA plates can replace the need for phospholipid in promoting high-density coating of plates (62).

    aCL may consist of one or more isotypes of antibody. Various combinations of IgG, IgM, and IgA aPL may be present in an individual with APS. IgG antibodies are the most prevalent and clinically relevant isotype (12, 28, 40, 48), although IgM and IgA isotypes have been associated with APS. The prevalence of aCL-specific isotypes may vary by ethnicity (15, 48). A small fraction of patients have solely IgM aCL (12). While these have been shown to be associated with APS in some cases, as discussed above, IgM isotype aCL are often associated with infection. IgA aCL have a variable prevalence in various patient groups (63); however, studies indicate that IgA aCL are the predominant isotype in African-American APS patients (15). Like other aCL isotypes, IgA aCL appear to be cofactor dependent in their binding to phospholipids, but further studies are needed to establish a clear clinical association, as studies are conflicting (63).

COFACTOR-SPECIFIC AND OTHER TESTS FOR aPL

Alternative tests have been developed to enhance the specificity of aPL testing due to concerns with the specificity of the aCL test and the recognition that aCL binding is actually cofactor targeted. Some of these alternate tests are in use, while for others further study is necessary to determine their utility. The best known and most used of these is the test for β2GPI-specific antibodies (70). This test utilizes purified β2GPI and is performed as a standard ELISA with high-binding ELISA plates to facilitate greater binding of antigen to the plate, which is a requirement for detection of characteristically low-affinity aPL antibodies (62). β2GPI-binding antibodies may consist of IgG, IgM, or IgA isotypes. Positive results in this test are associated with several manifestations of APS (13, 38, 44, 52). In addition, this may be the only positive test for certain APS patients (50).

Another ELISA-based alternative to aCL testing is the APhL test (APL Diagnostics, Louisville, Ky.), which employs a mixture of negatively charged phospholipids designed to enhance specificity for APS. Published studies indicate that this test is as sensitive for APS as the aCL assays but with improved specificity (16, 47). The improved specificity of this test was demonstrated by comparison with several aCL tests, a β2GPI test, and a flow cytometry-based test (57). The sensitivities of all tests were 90% or greater. The specificities, however, varied extensively, from 37 to 100%, with the APhL test giving the best specificity.

Several other test systems for aPL have been reported in the literature. Other anionic phospholipid antibody specificities may be found in patients, including antibodies to phosphatidylserine, phosphatidylethanolamine, and phosphatidylinositol (10). In addition, other cofactor-specific assays have been developed, including prothrombin (3, 7) and protein-C and protein-S (53) tests. None of these tests are considered first-line assays for APS at this time, however.

ASSAYS FOR DETECTION OF aPL

Home brew as well as a variety of commercially available ELISA-based aCL assays are in use (29). Commercially available kits include tests for IgG, IgM, and IgA aCL that can be reported qualitatively or quantitatively. A significant effort has been put into the characterization of these tests due to the recognition of significant variability between commercial and home brew tests as well as between laboratories. International consensus conferences have focused on optimizing performance of these tests. Proficiency testing surveys are available from such organizations as the College of American Pathologists.

Quantitative aCL assays typically report results in IgG aPL (GPL) and IgM aPL (MPL) units, which are equivalent to the activity of 1 μg of standard antibody preparation. Negative and low, moderate, and high positive ranges have been defined for these units (36). However, the cutoffs for a positive result vary by manufacturer. As discussed below, cutoff levels should be validated in each laboratory performing aPL testing.

STANDARDIZATION OF aPL TESTING

Appreciation of the utility of aCL and the resultant availability of a variety of commercially available ELISA kits as well as home brew tests has proven problematic as evidenced by publications that have documented significant variability between different commercially available kits and home brew tests (5, 19, 24, 25, 58, 76). Wong et al. (76) reported an assessment of intra- and interassay variability in nine laboratories employing one home brew and eight commercial and IgG aCL assays. The mean intra-assay variability (coefficient of variation [CV]) on three samples ranged from 3.6 to 32.4%, and the mean interassay variability ranged from 8.8 to 18.6%. Six of nine labs had an interassay CV of <20%. Qualitative agreement (positive versus negative) was suboptimal. Summary data from a proficiency testing program (24) demonstrated that 90% or greater consensus was achieved in only 42% of cases during a 1-year period. In an evaluation of 10 commercial tests and one home brew test using 62 sera, the rate of positive results varied by kit from 18 to 64% (5). Based on clinical criteria, the sensitivities of the kits ranged from 65 to 90% and specificities ranged from 33 to 77%.

Because of the importance of these tests and the significant variation in performance, international workshops have been held to evaluate aCL testing parameters (33, 36, 37, 57). The first of these workshops established methods and units of measure and identified standards for aCL testing (36). GPL and MPL units were established that were equivalent to 1 μg of affinity-purified antibody per ml. In the second workshop, improvements in between-laboratory agreement were determined to be better if a semiquantitative aCL measure (reported as negative, low positive, moderate, and high positive) was used (33).

Several groups have identified and published what are felt to be important aspects of aPL testing and have recommended specific consensus guidelines for the use and performance of aPL tests (31, 67, 77). The guidelines that provide the most extensive recommendations suggest the following minimally acceptable practices for aPL testing (77): test for IgG with or without IgM; serum is the preferred sample; and controls and calibrators should be run with the goal of achieving an interassay CV of <20%. Other guidelines (67) urge running samples in duplicate, in-house cutoff determination based on 50 to 100 healthy age- and sex-matched controls, percentile-based cutoffs, and the use of external controls.

As with aCL tests, β2GPI testing appears to be susceptible to significant variability (60). Several factors may affect the performance of β2GPI tests, including the source of β2GPI, the type of ELISA tray, blocking buffer, sample integrity, secondary-antibody used, and lack of standards, as well as variability in cutoff levels used (6).

INDICATIONS FOR aPL TESTING

Indications for aPL testing have been discussed by Greaves (30) and Triplett (68). Although sensitive, aPL is not indicated as a screening test for APS due to its low specificity. As discussed previously, aPL can be found in a variety of conditions not associated with thrombosis or pregnancy morbidity as well as in apparently healthy individuals. Derksen and de Groot (20) suggest that aPL testing is indicated in patients with SLE and/or the clinical criteria associated with APS. Because pathological aPL are persistently detected, positive results should be confirmed by repeat testing after 6 weeks.

aPL testing may also be indicated in other clinical situations. For example, the presence of aPL may, in part, influence decisions regarding oral contraception or use of estrogen (13a). The accurate and precise determination of aPL is important not only diagnostically but also because it may guide therapeutic decisions such as prophylaxis (1a) or duration of therapy (44a).

Given the variety of tests available, which should be performed? Though not all studies are consistent, the consensus is that LA and IgG aCL tests are sufficient for most cases of APS (49). Additional testing for IgA aCL may be warranted in patients with negative IgG and IgM aCL tests, as IgA may be the sole isotype present in some instances and in certain ethnic groups. Testing for IgG, IgM, and IgA β2GPI-specific antibodies (56) has been recommended because of their greater specificity. In addition, they may be the sole aPL present in some patients (59). Multiple tests for aPL should be used since no one is sufficiently sensitive to identify all patients. Alternative phospholipids and/or cofactor antibodies may be detected in patients with APS.

INTERPRETATION OF RESULTS

The interpretation of aPL tests should take into consideration patient characteristics such as age, drugs, infection, and the presence of autoimmune disease as well as the isotype and titer of the aPL. The aCL test is sensitive and as such may be positive for individuals with no history of thromboses or adverse pregnancy outcomes. Surveys of healthy blood donors demonstrated positivity rates for IgM and IgG aCL of 9.4 and 6.5%, respectively (71). However, this rate may vary depending upon the cutoff level used (42), and the tests are often negative upon repetition (71). The prevalence of aPL may be increased in the elderly (71). aPL may be present in patients with autoimmune diseases (11, 64), patients taking certain drugs (45, 69), and patients with a variety of infectious diseases as discussed previously.

aCL antibodies are found in more than 80 to 90% of patients with APS (55). In general, the higher the antibody level, the more likely that the clinical event(s) is due to APS (28, 40). An incidental- or low-titer aCL test usually has no clinical significance (20). β2GPI-specific antibodies may be present with aCL or may be the sole antibody found in 2 to 10% of APS patients (59). Occasional patients with APS do not have aCL, LA, or β2GPI antibodies. In these cases testing for reactivity to other phospholipids may identify the presence of an aPL (see above). Clinically significant aCL are also persistent (i.e., detected on two separate occasions), a characteristic that is addressed in the APS classification scheme.

REAGENTS

A detailed method for a home brew aCL ELISA test can be found in the previous version of this chapter (29). Commercially available aCL kits are available from the following companies:

1. The Binding Site
   San Diego, CA 92121
2. DL Diagnostika
   Hamburg, Germany
3. Corgenix
   Denver, CO 80234
4. Diamedix
   Miami, FL 33127
5. DiaSorin
   Stillwater, MN 55082
6. Hemagen-Virgo
   Columbia, MD 21045
7. Hycor Biomedical
   Garden Grove, CA 92841
8. IMMCO Diagnostics
   Buffalo, NY 14228
9. Immuno Concepts
   Sacramento, CA 95827
10. INOVA Diagnostics, Inc.
    San Diego, CA 92131
11. Louisville APL Diagnostics
    Louisville, KY 40202
12. MBL International
    Woburn, MA 01801
13. Pharmacia Diagnostics
    Uppsala, Sweden
14. TheraTest
    Lombard, IL 60148
15. Trinity Biotech
    Berkeley Heights, NJ 07922
16. Wampole
    Princeton, NJ 08540

REFERENCES

1. **Abuaf, N., S. Laperche, B. Rajoely, R. Carsique, A. Deschamps, A. M. Rouquette, C. Barthet, Z. Khaled, C. Marbot, N. Saab, J. Rozen, P. M. Girard, and W. Rozenbaum.** 1997. Autoantibodies to phospholipids and to the coagulation proteins in AIDS. *Thromb. Haemost.* **77:**856–861.
1a.**Alarcón-Segovia, D., M. C. Boffa, W. Branch, R. Cevera, D. Gharavi, M. Kharmashta, Y. Shoenfeld, W. Wilson, and R. Roubey.** 2003. Prophylaxis of the antiphospholipid syndrome: a consensus report. *Lupus* **12:**499–503.
2. **Arnout, J., C. Wittevrongel, M. Vanrusselt, M. Hoylaerts, and J. Vermylen.** 1998. Beta-2-glycoprotein I dependent lupus anticoagulants form stable bivalent antibody beta-2-glycoprotein I complexes on phospholipid surfaces. *Thromb. Haemost.* **79:**79–86.
3. **Arvieux, J., L. Darnige, C. Caron, G. Reber, J. C. Bensa, and M. G. Colomb.** 1995. Development of an ELISA for autoantibodies to prothrombin showing their prevalence in patients with lupus anticoagulants. *Thromb. Haemost.* **74:**1120–1125.
4. **Asherson, R., R. Cervera, J. C. Piette, J. Font, J. T. Lie, A. Burcoglu, K. Lim, F. J. Munoz-Rodriguez, R. A. Levy, F. Boue, J. Rossert, and M. Ingelmo.** 1998. Catastrophic antiphospholipid syndrome: clinical and laboratory features of 50 patients. *Medicine* (Baltimore) **77:**195–207.
5. **Audrain, M. A., F. Colonna, F. Morio, M. A. Hamidou, and J. Y. Muller.** 2004. Comparison of different kits in the detection of autoantibodies to cardiolipin and beta2glycoprotein 1. *Rheumatology* (Oxford) **43:**181–185.
6. **Bas de Laat, H., R. H. Derksen, and P. G. de Groot.** 2004. Beta2-glycoprotein I, the playmaker of the antiphospholipid syndrome. *Clin. Immunol.* **112:**161–168.
7. **Bevers, E. M., M. Galli, T. Barbui, P. Comfurius, and R. F. Zwaal.** 1991. Lupus anticoagulant IgG's (LA) are not directed to phospholipids only, but to a complex of lipid-bound human prothrombin. *Thromb. Haemost.* **66:**629–632.
8. **Brandt, J. T., L. K. Barna, and D. A. Triplett.** 1995. Laboratory identification of lupus anticoagulants: results of the Second International Workshop for Identification of Lupus Anticoagulants. On behalf of the Subcommittee on Lupus Anticoagulants/Antiphospholipid Antibodies of the ISTH. *Thromb. Haemost.* **74:**1597–1603.
9. **Brandt, J. T., D. A. Triplett, B. Alving, and I. Scharrer.** 1995. Criteria for the diagnosis of lupus anticoagulants: an

update. On behalf of the Subcommittee on Lupus Anticoagulant/Antiphospholipid Antibody of the Scientific and Standardisation Committee of the ISTH. *Thromb. Haemost.* **74:**1185–1190.

10. Carreras, L., R. Forastiero, and M. Martinuzzo. 2000. Which are the best biological markers of the antiphospholipid syndrome? *J. Autoimmun.* **15:**163–172.

11. Cervera, R., and R. A. Asherson. 2003. Clinical and epidemiological aspects in the antiphospholipid syndrome. *Immunobiology* **207:**5–11.

12. Cervera, R., J. C. Piette, J. Font, M. Khamashta, Y. Shoenfeld, M. T. Camps, S. Jacobsen, G. Lakos, A. Tincani, I. Kontopoulou-Griva, M. Galeazzi, P. Meroni, R. Derksen, P. G. de Groot, E. Gromnica-Ihle, M. Baleva, M. Mosca, S. Bombardieri, F. Houssiau, J. C. Gris, I. Quere, E. Hachulla, C. Vasconcelos, B. Roch, A. Fernandez Nebro, M. C. Boffa, G. Hughes, and M. Ingelmo. 2002. Antiphospholipid syndrome: clinical and immunologic manifestations and patterns of disease expression in a cohort of 1000 patients. *Arthritis Rheum.* **46:**1019–1027.

13. Chamley, L. W. 1997. Antiphospholipid antibodies or not? The role of beta 2 glycoprotein 1 in autoantibody-mediated pregnancy loss. *J. Reprod. Immunol.* **36:**123–142.

13a. Chandramouli, N. B., and G. M. Rodgers. 2001. Management of thrombosis in women with antiphospholipid syndrome. *Clin. Obstet. Gynecol.* **44:**36–47.

14. Constans, J., V. Guerin, A. Couchouron, M. Seigneur, A. Ryman, A. D. Blann, J. Amiral, A. Amara, E. Peuchant, J. F. Moreau, I. Pellegrin, J. L. Pellegrin, H. Fleury, B. Leng, and C. Conri. 1998. Autoantibodies directed against phospholipids or human beta 2-glycoprotein I in HIV-seropositive patients: relationship with endothelial activation and antimalonic dialdehyde antibodies. *Eur. J. Clin. Investig.* **28:**115–122.

15. Cucurull, E., A. E. Gharavi, E. Diri, E. Mendez, D. Kapoor, and L. R. Espinoza. 1999. IgA anticardiolipin and anti-beta2-glycoprotein I are the most prevalent isotypes in African American patients with systemic lupus erythematosus. *Am. J. Med. Sci.* **318:**55–60.

16. Day, H. M., P. Thiagarajan, C. Ahn, J. D. Reveille, K. F. Tinker, and F. C. Arnett. 1998. Autoantibodies to beta2-glycoprotein I in systemic lupus erythematosus and primary antiphospholipid antibody syndrome: clinical correlations in comparison with other antiphospholipid antibody tests. *J. Rheumatol.* **25:**667–674.

17. de Larranaga, G. F., R. R. Forastiero, L. O. Carreras, and B. S. Alonso. 1999. Different types of antiphospholipid antibodies in AIDS: a comparison with syphilis and the antiphospholipid syndrome. *Thromb. Res.* **96:**19–25.

18. de Larranaga, G. F., R. R. Forastiero, M. E. Martinuzzo, L. O. Carreras, G. Tsariktsian, M. M. Sturno, and B. S. Alonso. 2000. High prevalence of antiphospholipid antibodies in leprosy: evaluation of antigen reactivity. *Lupus* **9:**594–600.

19. de Moerloose, P., G. Reber, and J. J. Vogel. 1990. Anticardiolipin antibody determination: comparison of three ELISA assays. *Clin. Exp. Rheumatol.* **8:**575–577.

20. Derksen, R. H., and P. G. de Groot. 2004. Clinical consequences of antiphospholipid antibodies. *Neth. J. Med.* **62:**273–278.

21. Derksen, R. H., P. Hasselaar, L. Blokzijl, F. H. Gmelig Meyling, and P. G. De Groot. 1988. Coagulation screen is more specific than the anticardiolipin antibody ELISA in defining a thrombotic subset of lupus patients. *Ann. Rheum. Dis.* **47:**364–371.

22. Facer, C. A., and G. Agiostratidou. 1994. High levels of anti-phospholipid antibodies in uncomplicated and severe *Plasmodium falciparum* and in *P. vivax* malaria. *Clin. Exp. Immunol.* **95:**304–309.

23. Faghiri, Z., W. A. Wilson, F. Taheri, E. N. Barton, O. S. Morgan, and A. E. Gharavi. 1999. Antibodies to cardiolipin and beta2-glycoprotein-1 in HTLV-1-associated myelopathy/tropical spastic paraparesis. *Lupus* **8:**210–214.

24. Favaloro, E. J., and R. Silvestrini. 2002. Assessing the usefulness of anticardiolipin antibody assays: a cautious approach is suggested by high variation and limited consensus in multilaboratory testing. *Am. J. Clin. Pathol.* **118:**548–557.

25. Favaloro, E. J., R. C. Wong, R. Silvestrini, R. McEvoy, S. Jovanovich, and P. Roberts-Thomson. 2005. A multilaboratory peer assessment quality assurance program-based evaluation of anticardiolipin antibody, and beta2-glycoprotein I antibody testing. *Semin. Thromb. Hemost.* **31:**73–84.

26. Galli, M., P. Comfurius, C. Maassen, H. C. Hemker, M. H. De Baets, P. J. Van Breda-Vriesman, T. Barbui, R. F. Zwaal, and E. M. Bevers. 1990. Anticardiolipin antibodies (ACA) directed not to cardiolipin but to a plasma cofactor. *Lancet* **335:**1544–1547.

27. Galli, M., D. Luciani, G. Bertolini, and T. Barbui. 2003. Lupus anticoagulants are stronger risk factors for thrombosis than anticardiolipin antibodies in the antiphospholipid syndrome: a systematic review of the literature. *Blood* **101:**1827–1832.

28. Gharavi, A., E. N. Harris, R. Asherson, and G. Hughes. 1987. Anticardiolipin antibodies: isotype distribution and phospholipid specificity. *Ann. Rheum. Dis.* **46:**1–6.

29. Gharavi, A. E., and M. D. Lockshin. 2002. Antiphospholipid antibody tests, p. 973–980. *In* N. R. Rose, R. G. Hamilton, and B. Detrick (ed.), *Manual of Clinical Laboratory Immunology*, 6th ed. ASM Press, Washington, D.C.

30. Greaves, M. 2000. Antiphospholipid syndrome: state of the art with emphasis on laboratory evaluation. *Haemostasis* **30**(Suppl. 2):16–25.

31. Greaves, M., H. Cohen, S. J. MacHin, and I. Mackie. 2000. Guidelines on the investigation and management of the antiphospholipid syndrome. *Br. J. Haematol.* **109:**704–715.

32. Guedes Barbosa, L. S., B. Gilbrut, Y. Shoenfeld, and M. A. Scheinberg. 1996. Autoantibodies in leprosy sera. *Clin. Rheumatol.* **15:**26–28.

33. Harris, E. N. 1990. Special report. The second international anti-cardiolipin standardization workshop/the Kingston anti-phospholipid antibody study (KAPS) group. *Am. J. Clin. Pathol.* **94:**476–484.

34. Harris, E. N., J. K. Chan, R. Asherson, V. R. Aber, A. Gharavi, and G. Hughes. 1986. Thrombosis, recurrent fetal loss, and thrombocytopenia: predictive value of the anticardiolipin antibody test. *Arch. Intern. Med.* **146:**2153–2156.

35. Harris, E. N., A. Gharavi, M. L. Boey, B. M. Patel, C. Mackworth-Young, S. Loizou, and G. Hughes. 1983. Anticardiolipin antibodies: detection by radioimmunoassay and association with thrombosis in systemic lupus erythematosus. *Lancet* **ii:**1211–1214.

36. Harris, E. N., A. Gharavi, S. P. Patel, and G. Hughes. 1987. Evaluation of the anti-cardiolipin antibody test: report of an international workshop held 4 April 1986. *Clin. Exp. Immunol.* **68:**215–222.

37. Harris, E. N., S. Pierangeli, and D. Birch. 1994. Anticardiolipin wet workshop report. Fifth International Symposium on antiphospholipid antibodies. *Am. J. Clin. Pathol.* **101:**616–624.

38. Katano, K., A. Aoki, H. Sasa, M. Ogasawara, E. Matsuura, and Y. Yagami. 1996. Beta 2-glycoprotein I-dependent anticardiolipin antibodies as a predictor of adverse pregnancy outcomes in healthy pregnant women. *Hum. Reprod.* **11:**509–512.

39. Leroy, V., J. Arvieux, M. C. Jacob, M. Maynard-Muet, M. Baud, and J. P. Zarski. 1998. Prevalence and significance of anticardiolipin, anti-beta2 glycoprotein I and

anti-prothrombin antibodies in chronic hepatitis C. *Br. J. Haematol.* **101:**468–474.

40. **Levine, J. S., D. W. Branch, and J. Rauch.** 2002. The antiphospholipid syndrome. *N. Engl. J. Med.* **346:**752–763.

41. **Loizou, S., S. Singh, E. Wypkema, and R. A. Asherson.** 2003. Anticardiolipin, anti-beta(2)-glycoprotein I and antiprothrombin antibodies in black South African patients with infectious disease. *Ann. Rheum. Dis.* **62:**1106–1111.

42. **Love, P. E., and S. A. Santoro.** 1990. Antiphospholipid antibodies: anticardiolipin and the lupus anticoagulant in systemic lupus erythematosus (SLE) and in non-SLE disorders. Prevalence and clinical significance. *Ann. Intern. Med.* **112:**682–698.

43. **Maclean, C., P. J. Flegg, and D. C. Kilpatrick.** 1990. Anticardiolipin antibodies and HIV infection. *Clin. Exp. Immunol.* **81:**263–266.

44. **Martinuzzo, M. E., R. R. Forastiero, and L. O. Carreras.** 1995. Anti beta 2 glycoprotein I antibodies: detection and association with thrombosis. *Br. J. Haematol.* **89:**397–402.

44a. **McCrae, K. R.** 1996. Antiphospholipid antibody associated thrombosis: a consensus for treatment? *Lupus* **5:**560–570.

45. **McNeil, H. P., and S. A. Krilis.** 1991. Antiphospholipid antibodies. *Aust. N. Z. J. Med.* **21:**463–475.

46. **McNeil, H. P., R. J. Simpson, C. N. Chesterman, and S. Krilis.** 1990. Anti-phospholipid antibodies are directed against a complex antigen that includes a lipid-binding inhibitor of coagulation: beta2-glycoprotein I (apolipoprotein H). *Proc. Natl. Acad. Sci. USA* **87:**4120–4124.

47. **Merkel, P. A., Y. Chang, S. S. Pierangeli, E. N. Harris, and R. P. Polisson.** 1999. Comparison between the standard anticardiolipin antibody test and a new phospholipid test in patients with connective tissue diseases. *J. Rheumatol.* **26:**591–596.

48. **Molina, J. F., S. Gutierrez-Urena, J. Molina, O. Uribe, S. Richards, C. De Ceulaer, C. Garcia, W. A. Wilson, A. E. Gharavi, and L. R. Espinoza.** 1997. Variability of anticardiolipin antibody isotype distribution in 3 geographic populations of patients with systemic lupus erythematosus. *J. Rheumatol.* **24:**291–296.

49. **Musial, J., J. Swadzba, A. Motyl, and T. Iwaniec.** 2003. Clinical significance of antiphospholipid protein antibodies. Receiver operating characteristics plot analysis. *J. Rheumatol.* **30:**723–730.

50. **Nash, M. J., R. S. Camilleri, S. Kunka, I. J. Mackie, S. J. Machin, and H. Cohen.** 2004. The anticardiolipin assay is required for sensitive screening for antiphospholipid antibodies. *J. Thromb. Haemost.* **2:**1077–1081.

51. **Neville, C., J. Rauch, J. Kassis, E. R. Chang, L. Joseph, M. Le Comte, and P. R. Fortin.** 2003. Thromboembolic risk in patients with high titre anticardiolipin and multiple antiphospholipid antibodies. *Thromb. Haemost.* **90:**108–115.

52. **Ogasawara, M., K. Aoki, E. Matsuura, H. Sasa, and Y. Yagami.** 1996. Anti beta 2glycoprotein I antibodies and lupus anticoagulant in patients with recurrent pregnancy loss: prevalence and clinical significance. *Lupus* **5:**587–592.

53. **Oosting, J. D., R. H. Derksen, I. W. Bobbink, T. M. Hackeng, B. N. Bouma, and P. G. de Groot.** 1993. Antiphospholipid antibodies directed against a combination of phospholipids with prothrombin, protein C, or protein S: an explanation for their pathogenic mechanism? *Blood* **81:**2618–2625.

54. **Pangborn, M. C.** 1941. A new serologically active phospholipid from beef heart. *Proc. Soc. Exp. Biol. Med.* **48:**484–486.

55. **Pierangeli, S. S., A. E. Gharavi, and E. N. Harris.** 2001. Testing for antiphospholipid antibodies: problems and solutions. *Clin. Obstet. Gynecol.* **44:**48–57; quiz, 58–59.

56. **Pierangeli, S. S., and E. N. Harris.** 2005. Clinical laboratory testing for the antiphospholipid syndrome. *Clin. Chim. Acta* **357:**17–33.

57. **Pierangeli, S. S., M. Stewart, L. K. Silva, and E. N. Harris.** 1998. An antiphospholipid wet workshop: 7th International Symposium on Antiphospholipid Antibodies. *J. Rheumatol.* **25:**156–160.

58. **Reber, G., J. Arvieux, E. Comby, D. Degenne, P. de Moerloose, M. Sanmarco, and G. Potron.** 1995. Multicenter evaluation of nine commercial kits for the quantitation of anticardiolipin antibodies. The Working Group on Methodologies in Haemostasis from the GEHT (Groupe d'Etudes sur l'Hemostase et la Thrombose). *Thromb. Haemost.* **73:**444–452.

59. **Reber, G., and P. de Moerloose.** 2004. Anti-beta2-glycoprotein I antibodies—when and how should they be measured? *Thromb. Res.* **114:**527–531.

60. **Reber, G., I. Schousboe, A. Tincani, M. Sanmarco, T. Kveder, P. de Moerloose, M. C. Boffa, and J. Arvieux.** 2002. Inter-laboratory variability of anti-beta2-glycoprotein I measurement. A collaborative study in the frame of the European Forum on Antiphospholipid Antibodies Standardization Group. *Thromb. Haemost.* **88:**66–73.

61. **Roubey, R. A.** 1994. Autoantibodies to phospholipid-binding plasma proteins: a new view of lupus anticoagulants and other "antiphospholipid" autoantibodies. *Blood* **84:**2854–2867.

62. **Roubey, R. A., R. A. Eisenberg, M. F. Harper, and J. B. Winfield.** 1995. "Anticardiolipin" autoantibodies recognize beta 2-glycoprotein I in the absence of phospholipid. Importance of Ag density and bivalent binding. *J. Immunol.* **154:**954–960.

63. **Samarkos, M., R. A. Asherson, and S. Loizou.** 2001. The clinical significance of IgA antiphospholipid antibodies. *J. Rheumatol.* **28:**694–697.

64. **Sebastiani, G. D., M. Galeazzi, A. Tincani, J. C. Piette, J. Font, F. Allegri, A. Mathieu, J. Smolen, E. de Ramon Garrido, A. Fernandez-Nebro, A. Jedryka-Goral, C. Papasteriades, G. Morozzi, F. Bellisai, O. De Pita, and R. Marcolongo.** 1999. Anticardiolipin and anti-beta2GPI antibodies in a large series of European patients with systemic lupus erythematosus. Prevalence and clinical associations. European Concerted Action on the Immunogenetics of SLE. *Scand. J. Rheumatol.* **28:**344–351.

65. **Simmelink, M. J., D. A. Horbach, R. H. Derksen, J. C. Meijers, E. M. Bevers, G. M. Willems, and P. G. De Groot.** 2001. Complexes of anti-prothrombin antibodies and prothrombin cause lupus anticoagulant activity by competing with the binding of clotting factors for catalytic phospholipid surfaces. *Br. J. Haematol.* **113:**621–629.

66. **Soni, P. N., C. C. De Bruyn, J. Duursma, B. L. Sharp, and D. J. Pudifin.** 1993. Are anticardiolipin antibodies responsible for some of the complications of severe acute Plasmodium falciparum malaria? *S. Afr. Med. J.* **83:**660–662.

67. **Tincani, A., F. Allegri, G. Balestrieri, G. Reber, M. Sanmarco, P. Meroni, and M. C. Boffa.** 2004. Minimal requirements for antiphospholipid antibodies ELISAs proposed by the European Forum on antiphospholipid antibodies. *Thromb. Res.* **114:**553–558.

68. **Triplett, D. A.** 2002. Antiphospholipid antibodies. *Arch. Pathol. Lab. Med.* **126:**1424–1429.

69. **Triplett, D. A.** 1998. Many faces of lupus anticoagulants. *Lupus* **7**(Suppl. 2):S18–S22.

70. **Viard, J. P., Z. Amoura, and J. F. Bach.** 1992. Association of anti-beta 2 glycoprotein I antibodies with lupus-type circulating anticoagulant and thrombosis in systemic lupus erythematosus. *Am. J. Med.* **93:**181–186.

71. **Vila, P., M. C. Hernandez, M. F. Lopez-Fernandez, and J. Batlle.** 1994. Prevalence, follow-up and clinical significance of the anticardiolipin antibodies in normal subjects. *Thromb. Haemost.* **72:**209–213.

72. **Wahl, D. G., E. De Maistre, F. Guillemin, V. Regnault, C. Perret-Guillaume, and T. Lecompte.** 1998. Antibodies against phospholipids and beta 2-glycoprotein I increase the

risk of recurrent venous thromboembolism in patients without systemic lupus erythematosus. *Q. J. Med.* **91:**125–130.

73. **Wassermann, A., A. Neisser, and C. Bruck.** 1906. Eine serodiagnostiche Reaction bei Syphilis. *Dtsch. Med. Wochenschr.* **32:**745–746.

74. **Wilson, W., A. Gharavi, T. Koike, M. Lockshin, D. W. Branch, J. C. Piette, R. Brey, R. Derksen, E. N. Harris, G. Hughes, D. A. Triplett, and M. Khamashta.** 1999. International consensus statement on preliminary classification criteria for definite antiphospholipid syndrome. *Arthritis Rheum.* **42:**1309–1311.

75. **Wilson, W. A., C. Morgan Ost, E. N. Barton, M. Smikle, B. Hanchard, W. A. Blattner, S. Doggett, and A. E. Gharavi.** 1995. IgA antiphospholipid antibodies in HTLV-1-associated tropical spastic paraparesis. *Lupus* **4:**138–141.

76. **Wong, R., E. Favaloro, W. Pollock, R. Wilson, M. Hendle, S. Adelstein, K. Baumgart, P. Homes, S. Smith, R. Steele, A. Sturgess, and D. Gillis.** 2004. A multi-centre evaluation of the intra-assay and inter-assay variation of commercial and in-house anti-cardiolipin antibody assays. *Pathology* **36:**182–192.

77. **Wong, R. C., D. Gillis, S. Adelstein, K. Baumgart, E. J. Favaloro, M. J. Hendle, P. Homes, W. Pollock, S. Smith, R. H. Steele, A. Sturgess, and R. J. Wilson.** 2004. Consensus guidelines on anti-cardiolipin antibody testing and reporting. *Pathology* **36:**63–68.

Antineutrophil Cytoplasm Antibodies (ANCAs) and Strategy for Diagnosing ANCA-Associated Vasculitides

ALLAN WIIK

118

BACKGROUND

The initial organ involved in vasculitis, and therefore the type of vasculitis, may vary extensively. Hence, the physician who initially sees a patient may be a generalist or any one of a great number of subspecialists. For the nephrologist, dermatologist, and rheumatologist in a secondary- or tertiary-care center, the level of awareness of systemic vasculitis may be high because such conditions are not uncommonly seen, but for primary-care doctors and specialists, these diseases are rare and may easily be misdiagnosed or may be left undiagnosed. Since this chapter concentrates on vasculitides which are associated with presence of antineutrophil cytoplasm antibodies (ANCAs), it focuses only on idiopathic small-vessel vasculitides (SVV), but it will also mention some of the clinical conditions where other types of neutrophil-specific autoantibodies (NSA) are commonly produced.

The diagnosis of a primary vasculitic condition must rest on sound clinical judgment of more or less characteristic constellations of symptoms and features, with some being indicative of vasculitis and others reflecting just a general inflammatory condition (arthralgias, fever, fatigue, loss of appetite, hypersedimentation, etc.). It is of paramount importance to put emphasis on the latter signs so that the systemic nature of the vasculitic condition can be recognized and so that the clinician can start looking for involvement of those organs most commonly affected by vasculitis, like the kidneys, the lungs, and the upper airways. The clinical spectrum of manifestations must generally be supported by defined histopathological findings in biopsy specimens from affected organs to provide a histologic "gold standard" for diagnosis. Unfortunately, this does not always work, as many biopsy specimens, e.g., nasal biopsy specimens, are frequently dominated by nonspecific inflammation.

In patients with focal necrotizing SVV involving venules, capillaries, and/or arterioles, neutrophilic granulocytes are assumed to be instrumental in causing the vessel damage and inducing ANCA production. It is thus not unexpected that ANCAs may occur in patients with SVV, but the very pronounced B-cell reactivity toward only one of two azurophil granule components, proteinase 3 (PR3) or myeloperoxidase (MPO), is unique for SVV and quite different from the B-cell reactivities for other neutrophil-dominated inflammatory conditions, e.g., rheumatoid synovitis, ulcerative colitis, chronic hepatitis, and primary sclerosing cholangitis (8), in which NSA are less strongly expressed and target very

different neutrophil antigens. Already at the first visit the doctor thus needs to set a tentative diagnosis so that the order for autoantibody tests is as rational as possible and the results of laboratory tests, including ANCA screening, can be put into a proper diagnostic context in order to avoid incorrect interpretation of the results. Also, laboratories should take care that clinically significant levels of PR3-ANCA and MPO-ANCA combined with NSA detected by indirect immunofluorescence (IIF) are reported in a different way than NSA seen only by IIF or by a whole-cell enzyme-linked immunosorbent assay (ELISA). This being said, strongly positive results for NSA by IIF combined with clearly positive results for PR3- or MPO-ANCAs obtained by using clinically validated assay techniques strongly support a diagnosis of necrotizing SVV, such as Wegener's granulomatosis (WG), microscopic polyangiitis (MPA), or Churg-Strauss syndrome (CSS), or the clinically limited forms of any of these, e.g., "renal limited" focal necrotizing glomerulonephritis or "upper airway-limited" WG (4).

Although this chapter focuses on the methodologies used to detect ANCAs, it also stresses important aspects of setting clinically validated assay cutoff values, controlling laboratory performance quality, knowing frequent pitfalls, and how to exercise troubleshooting. It also mentions possibilities for reporting laboratory data with due consideration toward differential diagnostics, potential clinical utility, and interpretation. The narrow definition of ANCAs includes only antibodies to cytoplasmic constituents of neutrophils and monocytes, but today most groups in the world call all autoantibodies to these cells ANCAs, although the cellular targets are mostly unknown. This chapter will try to make a case for naming autoantibodies to neutrophils which are detectable only by IIF "NSA" to avoid clinical misinterpretation, false diagnosis, and wrong therapy.

MAIN CLINICAL INDICATIONS FOR ANCA TESTING

ANCA testing is mainly indicated for patients with a tentative or a definite diagnosis of primary SVV, i.e., SVV in the absence of a recognized immunoinflammatory rheumatic disease, chronic infection, drug-related condition, or malignancy. In the nomenclature for primary vasculitides, several names were previously used for a single disease or one name was used for separate conditions. This inconsistency has tentatively been dealt with by an expert-driven proposal to use a simple, nonoverlapping nomenclature for vasculitides with accompanying short definitions (5) as a common means of scientific communication and nosologic standardization. According to this nomenclature, ANCA testing is mainly indicated for patients with suspected primary SVV, such as WG, MPA, CSS, and oligotypic forms of these conditions. In all other types of primary vasculitides, ANCAs sensu strictu are not commonly found.

Classical cytoplasmic ANCAs (C-ANCAs) (Fig. 1) prevail in patients with WG (70 to 85% of the patients, depending on the population studied), whereas perinuclear ANCAs (P-ANCAs) (Fig. 2) prevail in patients with MPA, CSS, and renal-limited SVV (60 to 80% of the patients, depending on the population studied). A positive IIF result for NSA needs to be substantiated by a positive result for PR3-ANCA or MPO-ANCA to support the diagnosis of ANCA-associated vasculitis (AAV). If true ANCAs (ELISA-positive, IIF-positive ANCAs) are found in a patient with arterial involvement and with features of polyarteritis nodosa (e.g., radiological artery aneurysms) or giant-cell arteritis (e.g., temporal artery inflammation), AAV is highly likely to coexist (2). A careful clinical search for SVV in such patients is mandatory since therapy for vasculitis in small or large arteries (mainly corticosteroids) is different from that for necrotizing SVV, in which both corticosteroids and immunosuppressive treatment are most frequently necessary. According to the Chapel Hill consensus proposal, the SVV diagnosis then becomes the main diagnosis (5). If ANCAs are found in a patient with seemingly skin-limited vasculitis, a systemic SVV should be suspected and looked for, especially if constitutional signs of disease and inflammation are present. The same is true if a patient has had long-standing purulent or hemorrhagic rhinitis, otitis, or laryngitis.

ANCAs directed toward neutrophil elastase (EL) and MPO (and sometimes other azurophil granule constituents) commonly develop in patients who develop signs of arthritis, skin exanthem, or vasculitis during prolonged drug treatment, e.g., with tetracyclines, propylthiouracil, penicillamine, quinidine, hydralazine, and other drugs. A small number of P-ANCA- and EL-ANCA-positive patients may have primary SVV that has not been provoked by drugs, but such patients are rare. In patients with an established diagnosis of SVV, it is generally advised that the level of the particular ANCA harbored by the patient be monitored for several reasons: (i) the level of ANCA is commonly higher in a patient with signs of active vasculitis than in a patient in remission;

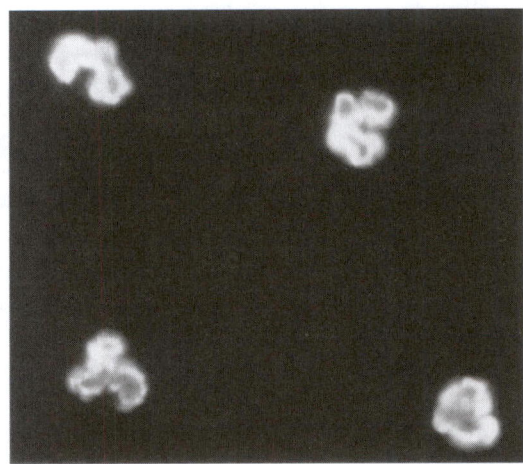

FIGURE 2 Typical P-ANCA pattern seen on ethanol-fixed neutrophils by MPO-ANCA-containing sera, here stained for IgG.

(ii) in more than half of WG patients, a steep rise in the PR3-ANCA level over a short time heralds disease exacerbation or extension; (iii) patients who become ANCA negative during a clinical remission get clearly fewer exacerbations of the disease than patients who remain positive, despite a lack of overt disease activity, most probably due to persistent presence of smoldering disease; and (iv) patients who are getting an infection may have symptoms like those of patients who have an exacerbation, but ANCA levels generally do not rise during infections. There may be exceptions to this notion, since infections with *Staphylococcus aureus* have been found to cause exacerbations in some patients with WG. In the clinical follow-up of patients with AAV, intervals between ANCA tests can be determined only on clinical grounds, such as if the patient has shown a tendency to get frequent disease exacerbations, or if critical-organ damage has already been inflicted by the disease (e.g., decreased renal or lung function). It can also be taken into consideration whether the patient has shown successful response to previous remission-inducing treatment or has shown little response to conventional therapies. It is highly recommended that ANCA levels in AAV patients be judged by very experienced vasculitis specialists. A high persistent level of PR3-ANCA or MPO-ANCA usually does not herald disease exacerbation or reflect active disease, whereas a sudden rise is a clear warning sign.

ANCA ANTIGENS

The two main antigens targeted by vasculitis-associated ANCAs are PR3 and MPO, both being enzymes located in the azurophil granules of neutrophils and in homologous granules of monocytes. PR3 is a single-chain, 229-amino-acid serine protease with four disulfide bridges and two potential glycosylation sites. It migrates as a triple band around 29 kDa in sodium dodecyl sulfate-polyacrylamide gel electrophoresis. This apparent heterogeneity is due to the existence of differently glycosylated subspecies. PR3 is most likely identical to neutrophil proteinase 4, myeloblastin, and azurophil granule protein 7 mentioned in earlier literature, and it is partly homologous to neutrophil EL and cathepsin G as well as to the antimicrobial proteins heparin-binding protein/bacterial-permeability-increasing protein (BPI) and azurocidin, which

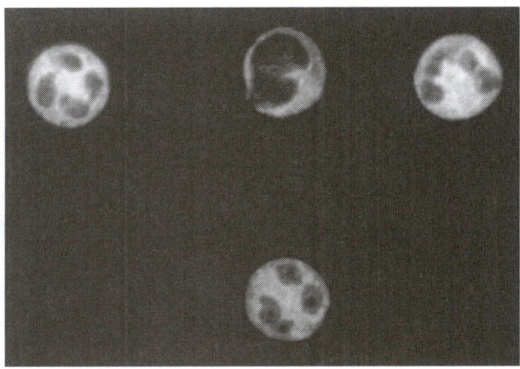

FIGURE 1 Typical C-ANCA pattern seen on ethanol-fixed neutrophils and monocytes by PR3-ANCA-containing sera, here stained for IgG.

are not enzymes. PR3-ANCA mainly recognizes conformational epitopes on PR3, but linear epitopes have also been described.

MPO, the second major ANCA antigen, is important for defense against microorganisms, its main function being the catalysis of the production of hypochloric acid, which is an important microbicidal agent in the phagolysosome. The concurrent production of highly reactive oxygen radicals can cause oxidative changes both in the cells themselves and in surrounding tissues. MPO is a heterodimer consisting of two light chains and two heavy chains. It contains two heme groups and has at least four potential glycosylation sites. The molecule is very cationic, with a pI of >11 and a molecular mass of about 140 kDa. MPO-ANCA associated with SVV mainly recognizes conformational epitopes.

When IIF is used with ethanol-fixed leukocytes, PR3-ANCA produces a granular cytoplasmic staining pattern (C-ANCA) (Fig. 1), whereas MPO-ANCA typically gives rise to an artifactual perinuclear or nuclear staining pattern (P-ANCA) due to the redistribution of MPO onto the polymorphonuclear leukocyte (PMN) nucleus and even neighboring cell nuclei after ethanol fixation (Fig. 2) (see below). Many groups have produced recombinant PR3 in the hope of eliminating the need for repeated purification of PR3 from normal neutrophils and to obtain pure PR3 preparations in sufficient amounts. However, only a few of these recombinants have been found to be useful for routine ANCA testing. To acquire full enzymatic activity and have the optimal conformation for ANCA reactivity, recombinant PR3 needs to have both the signal peptide and the proenzyme dipeptide cleaved off, processes which take place in myeloid precursor cells when PR3 leaves the endoplasmic reticulum and enters into the azurophil granules (12). Also, pure MPO has been prepared by recombinant synthesis technology and has been successfully used for MPO-ANCA determination.

METHODS USED TO DETECT ANCA

IIF

Human leukocytes were introduced as a convenient substrate for autoantibody demonstration soon after the IIF technique had been described as a screening method in serology (see chapter 112, this volume). In the mid-1960s autoantibodies that appeared to specifically recognize nuclear components of neutrophils were found by this technique in the sera of patients with rheumatoid arthritis, and a technique was developed to easily identify these so-called "granulocyte-specific" antinuclear antibodies (ANAs). The same technique was later adopted as a sensitive and reliable method for the detection of ANCAs (14), and its use has led to comparable recognition of C-ANCAs and P-ANCAs in multicenter studies of patients with primary vasculitides (3).

Slide Preparation

A 10-ml volume of blood is drawn into a syringe, and the blood is immediately transferred to a conical flask for defibrination with 10 glass beads (10 mm in diameter). Just after the clot has formed, the defibrinated blood is transferred into a polypropylene tube and thoroughly mixed with 250 IU of heparin. Aliquots of 2 ml are layered onto 5-ml dextran-sodium diatrizoate gradients (50 ml of 32.8% sodium diatrizoate [Nycomed] and 100 ml of 6% dextran T500 in distilled H_2O [Pharmacia]) in 10-ml polypropylene tubes, and these are left at room temperature for 45 min for

sedimentation of erythrocytes. The leukocyte-containing plasma layers are combined in a 10-ml tube.

The cells are pelleted at $200 \times g$ for 10 min and are resuspended in 1% human serum albumin in phosphate-buffered saline (PBS [pH 7.4]; 8.0 g of NaCl, 200 mg of KCl, 1.44 g of $Na_2HPO_4 \cdot 2H_2O$, 200 mg of KH_2PO_4, and distilled H_2O to 1,000 ml) and centrifuged again as described above to wash away plasma constituents. The cells are then resuspended in human serum albumin plus PBS and are pelleted by centrifugation at $200 \times g$. The last centrifugation is best done in a conical tube, so that the cells are concentrated in a small space in the bottom to allow removal of practically all washing medium, leaving only 150 to 200 µl of fluid over the pellet. The cells are then resuspended by tapping the tube, and a fine-tipped Pasteur pipette that has been drawn over a gas flame is used as a capillary pipette to deposit 1-mm-diameter droplets on carefully defatted objective slides. These droplets must be smeared immediately with a ground-edged glass slide. Deposition of leukocytes on the slides may also be done by cytocentrifugation of a leukocyte suspension onto glass slides. After air drying, the slides are fixed in cold (4°C) 99% ethanol for 5 min, a selected area is encircled with a glass marker, and the slides are ready for use as a substrate for the IIF technique. If not used directly, the slides should be wrapped in an airtight container and stored at −20°C for use within a week.

Staining

Negative control serum, C-ANCA- and P-ANCA-positive control sera, and patient sera diluted in PBS to the agreed cutoff dilution (usually 1:20 to 1:40) are added as a drop on the encircled smear area, the controls on the first three slides. Some laboratories will use the fourth slide for a sensitivity control, i.e., a weakly positive IIF reaction that needs to be detectable in each routine run. Incubation at room temperature for 30 min takes place in a humid chamber, and the smears are washed in PBS and left totally immersed in PBS for 10 min. The washing procedure is repeated, and the excess PBS around the circle is removed, leaving a minute drop of PBS in the circle to avoid drying of the specimen. A fluorescein isothiocyanate-labeled immunoglobulin G (IgG) fraction of antiserum to human Fcγ chains is added at an appropriate dilution (usually 1:25 to 1:100) and left for incubation in the humid chamber as described above, and the washing steps are then repeated. After removal of the surrounding PBS, a 2:1 glycerol-PBS mixture is then applied to each smear and a cover glass is mounted. The preparations are now ready for fluorescence microscopy, which is best done in an epi-illumination microscope at a magnification of × 400 with an objective having a high numerical aperture to allow optimal excitation of the fluorochrome.

Annotations

It is important to avoid leukocyte activation during isolation and washing of the cells, and diligent handling of the cells is therefore mandatory. Each step must be followed immediately by the next step to avoid activation artifacts and leakage of antigens out of the cells until the slides have been fixed in ethanol. Do not use paraformaldehyde fixation even in combination with a permeabilizing agent (ethanol or acetone), since such fixation destroys the reactivities of many antigens and the fixation procedure often gives unpredictable results from batch to batch of cell preparations. Extra hands must help with the smearing of the cells to avoid drying of the small suspension droplet on the slide.

Use fluorescein isothiocyanate conjugates with a low mean fluorescein/protein molar ratio, around 2.5, since higher ratios will cause nonspecific staining of neutrophils and eosinophils. *Whole buffy coat must be used to ensure the presence of a satisfactory concentration of lymphocytes on the final slides, since these cells serve as important controls for both C-ANCAs and P-ANCAs (see below).* ANCA levels may be estimated by twofold titration or reactivity judged from the strength of the fluorescence staining (weak, intermediate, or strong).

Interpretation and Controls for Non-Organ-Specific Autoantibodies

A granular cytoplasmic fluorescence which is more intense in the vicinity of the nucleus than in the periphery of the neutrophils is characteristic for C-ANCA. Monocytes are more uniformly stained in the cytoplasm (Fig. 1). Lymphocytes and eosinophils should show no fluorescence. If non-organ-specific anticytoplasmic antibodies (such as anti-Jo-1 or anti-ribosomal ribonucleoprotein antibodies) are present, it may be difficult to demonstrate C-ANCAs on leukocytes. Titration of such samples on the buffy coat substrate by using isolated human lymphocytes from the same donor as a separate control substrate may help provide a solution to the problem if a clearly higher titer of ANCAs is found. HEp-2 cells are less well suited for such titer comparisons, although HEp-2 cells may be excellent for demonstration of some anticytoplasmic antibodies (6). The C-ANCA pattern is most commonly produced by autoantibodies to PR3. C-ANCA-positive sera should be further tested by ELISA for two reasons: PR3-ANCA is are very narrowly linked to WG and to, in a minority of patients, other types of SVV, whereas C-ANCAs that are not directed to PR3 may be seen in patients with infection-related vasculitis (directed to BPI) or patients without vasculitis. In addition, in rare cases MPO-ANCA may give a classical C-ANCA pattern (9).

P-ANCAs related to SVV are seen as a perinuclear or a nuclear fluorescence on neutrophils and monocytes (Fig. 2). This staining pattern is an artifact caused by the ethanol fixation, which partially dissolves the lipid membranes of the cells, making the various intracellular compartments accessible to the autoantibodies. Cationic proteins of the cytoplasm, however, can now freely redistribute onto the anionically charged nucleus of the same cell or a closely adjacent cell (Fig. 3), and antibodies attaching to the adjacent cell nuclei will show an ANA-like pattern. Since neutrophils contain a number of cationic components (e.g., MPO, EL, cathepsin G, lysozyme, azurocidin, and lactoferrin), autoantibodies to each of these will mostly be seen as P-ANCA or atypical ANCA reactivity.

To eliminate false interpretation, inclusion of control cells, like lymphocytes, is therefore mandatory to discriminate P-ANCAs from homogeneous or peripheral non-organ-specific ANAs. Lymphocytes from the buffy coat donor are very reliable for this purpose if they are present in sufficient numbers in the smear or if they are separated from neutrophils being deposited in a separate field on the slide. ANAs that give rise to a homogeneous or peripheral nuclear reactivity will then be seen to be reactive with neutrophils, eosinophils, and lymphocytes (Fig. 4), whereas P-ANCAs will selectively stain neutrophil and monocyte nuclei and sometimes a lymphocyte lying just adjacent to a neutrophil, but the majority of lymphocytes as well as eosinophils will be negative (Fig. 3). If non-organ-specific ANAs and P-ANCAs are found in the same serum sample, twofold titration of the sample can be done; a clearly higher P-ANCA level (at least 2 dilution steps) indicates

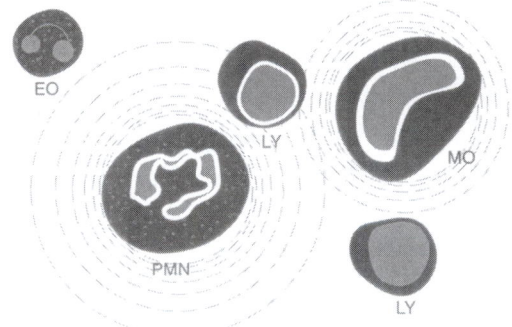

FIGURE 3 Diagram showing typical peripheral staining of neutrophil (PMN) and monocyte (MO) nuclei and the nucleus of an adjacent lymphocyte (LY), while a more distantly located lymphocyte and an eosinophil (EO) are not stained. The artifactual ANA-like pattern on positive cells is due to redistribution of soluble, diffusible molecules (such as the cationic MPO) onto the anionic nuclei located close by, here symbolized by the circles around the PMN and monocyte.

the presence of both autoantibodies. P-ANCAs are detected at 1:20 dilution on blood neutrophils whereas ANAs are detected at 1:160 dilution on HEp-2 cells. Therefore, titers cannot be directly compared. If the ANAs are very characteristic and distinguishable on the lymphocyte nuclei (e.g., nucleolar patterns, nuclear dot patterns, or centromere patterns), P-ANCAs are separable from such ANAs already at the screening dilution and titration is not necessary.

To summarize, in patients with primary vasculitides, P-ANCA reactivity is ordinarily due to autoantibodies to MPO. P-ANCA-positive sera must be studied for MPO-ANCA by ELISA, since strong MPO-ANCA activity is very characteristic of primary SVV or a drug-induced syndrome, whereas weak or absent MPO-ANCA activity in the presence of P-ANCA is more characteristic of another chronic inflammatory disease, e.g., rheumatoid arthritis, ulcerative colitis, chronic active hepatitis, primary sclerosing cholangitis, or systemic lupus erythematosus (8), altogether diseases that are much more frequent than AAV and thus recognized by finding NSA and not ANCA.

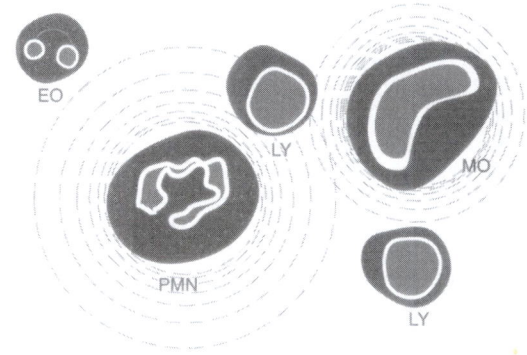

FIGURE 4 Diagram showing typical peripheral staining of all leukocyte nuclei by serum containing anti-double-stranded DNA. Diffusion of soluble and freely diffusible molecules such as MPO is symbolized by the circles around the PMN and the monocyte (MO). LY, lymphocyte; EO, eosinophil. Note that all cell nuclei in the field are positive.

Attempts at Standardizing Direct ELISA Techniques

Since data from the First and the Second International Workshops on ANCAs clearly indicated that results obtained by solid-phase techniques were not comparable, a collaborative study among seven European laboratories was organized in 1991. The aim was to study the available solid-phase methods for quantifying ANCA and to standardize the most promising techniques. These methods could then be used to evaluate their clinical utility in large populations of patients with primary SVV by using critical disease control patients with secondary vasculitides as well as healthy donor controls, including data from 14 different vasculitis centers all over Europe.

It quickly became apparent that PR3 and MPO were the main neutrophil autoantigens in primary vasculitides and that purified PR3 and MPO were superior to various mixed extracts from neutrophils or azurophil granules, probably due to the scarcity of the important antigens in such crude extracts. MPO could be obtained either from commercial sources or by simple purification methods, so the second part of the study concentrated on isolation of PR3 in four laboratories which all used different purification methods. Purity was judged by sodium dodecyl sulfate-polyacrylamide gel electrophoresis, immunoblotting, and direct ELISA techniques with specific antibodies to possible contaminants. The PR3 preparations were then applied in direct ELISAs by using the assay procedures recommended by the laboratory that delivered the preparation and a series of well-characterized but coded ANCA-positive sera (3).

After six rounds of testing in which assay conditions were gradually more strictly defined, the variability among all participating centers had reached a level of <20%. There was no significant difference among the three different PR3 preparations used regarding intracenter or intercenter variability. One preparation of MPO was used by all groups for direct ELISA with the assay specifications from Copenhagen, Denmark. Whereas PR3 is stable, it was found that MPO is very unstable if it is used to coat plates to be sent from one center to another, but if it is used for coating locally just before use, it was found to be suitable and gave reproducible results. The direct ELISAs detailed below reflect the assay conditions recommended from Copenhagen in the study described above. PR3 can now be obtained from several commercial sources, can be isolated by published methods (3), or can be obtained as recombinant PR3 (10, 12). An international reference preparation for C-ANCAs was established in 1988, but new International Union of Immunological Societies standards are being developed for MPO-ANCA and PR3-ANCA for distribution through the Centers for Disease Control and Prevention in Atlanta, Ga.

Direct PR3-ANCA ELISA

1. The wells of high-level-of-binding microtiter plates (Maxisorb; Nunc) are coated with 100 ml of PR3 (0.5 mg/ml) in 0.05 M sodium carbonate buffer (pH 9.6) containing 0.01% Triton X-100. The plates are incubated overnight at 4°C.

2. The plates are washed three times in 0.15 M NaCl containing 0.05% Tween 20, each time leaving the washing solution in the wells for 1 min before removal.

3. A negative control serum sample, a PR3-ANCA-positive serum sample with an intermediate level of antibody (or three standard serum samples with different antibody levels), and the patient sera are diluted 1:50 in

20°C incubation buffer (0.05 M Tris, 0.15 M NaCl, 0.05% Tween 20, and 0.2% bovine serum albumin).

4. These samples are added to duplicate wells (100 μl per well), and the plates are incubated for 1 h at room temperature.

5. The wells are washed three times with washing solution as described above.

6. Alkaline phosphatase-conjugated goat anti-human IgG (Sigma) diluted 4,000 times in incubation buffer (Tris-bovine serum albumin) is added to each well (100 μl per well), and the plate is incubated at room temperature for 30 min.

7. The wells are again washed three times with washing solution as described above.

8. To each well is added 100 μl of substrate consisting of 1 mg of para-nitrophenyl phosphate disodium per ml in 1 M diethanolamine buffer (pH 9.8) (97 ml of diethanolamine, 700 ml of distilled H_2O [the pH is adjusted to 9.8 with 5 M HCl–0.101 g of $MgCl_2 \cdot 6H_2O$; distilled H_2O is added to 1 liter]), and the plate is incubated at room temperature for 30 min. This buffer will keep for 4 weeks if 2 ml of NaN_3 is added to prevent bacterial growth.

9. The optical densities at 405 nm are measured in an ELISA reader.

10. The values relative to the values on the standard curve are calculated in arbitrary units.

Direct MPO-ANCA ELISA

1. Microwells of high-level-of-binding microtiter plates (Maxisorb; Nunc) are coated with 100 μl (1 μg/ml) of purified MPO in cold 0.05 M sodium carbonate buffer (pH 9.6) containing 0.01% Triton X-100, and the plates are incubated overnight at 4°C to be used the next day. Coated microplates may be stored under nitrogen in the dark for several months.

2. The procedure is continued with MPO-ANCA controls and the procedures described above in steps 2 through 10 for the PR3-ANCA ELISA.

Interpretation of Direct ELISA Results

When a decision as to the cutoff levels for PR3-ANCA and MPO-ANCA ELISAs must be made, it is advised that testing be done not only with sera from healthy donors but also with sera from patients with various forms of chronic or long-standing immunoinflammatory diseases, which in practical clinical work may pose differential diagnostic problems. The most important disease controls are those of vasculitis related to infections, rheumatoid arthritis, or other systemic rheumatic diseases. The diagnostic specificity toward disease controls should be >95%, and that toward healthy controls should be 100%. Such high degrees of specificity will eliminate most positive results in the gray area, albeit at the expense of a slightly lower nosographic sensitivity. Note that cutoff values for commercial ELISAs should be set locally in just the same way, since the diagnostic value of the results must be evaluated for local control patients with the ethnic composition and the differential diagnostic spectrum prevailing in the individual center.

Pitfalls and Troubleshooting

Since sera studied for ANCAs by ELISA may contain "sticky IgG" (probably immune complexes, conformationally altered IgG, or high levels of IgG), many laboratories will prefer to run all sera also in control wells that have been left uncoated in parallel with wells coated with autoantigen. If high background values are seen in uncoated wells, the problem must be taken into account when results are reported, although no general formula on how to do that can be given. The background problem seems to arise especially when sera from pediatric patients and patients with systemic lupus erythematosus are studied by using wells with a blocking agent, e.g., bovine serum albumin, ovalbumin, or gelatin. In such patients, levels of antibodies to blocking agents such as bovine serum albumin or ovalbumin are higher than those in healthy controls, and human serum albumin in the incubation buffer or on the solid phase may thus be preferred, if a blocking agent is used at all. Low-avidity antibodies to MPO can actually be present in sera from patients with systemic lupus erythematosus, and the conditions in the ELISA may be adjusted to eliminate weak MPO reactivity by increasing the ionic strength or the concentration of Tween 20 in the incubation buffer. These variables of method refinement need to be looked at locally whether in-house or commercial ELISAs are used. Since only one ANCA specificity is ordinarily present in a given serum sample, positivity for two ANCAs should arouse suspicion of false assay positivity.

Other Methods Used To Detect ANCA

Radioimmunoprecipitation and immunoblotting have been used previously to detect ANCAs, but these techniques are not practical for use in a routine serology setting. Monoclonal mouse antibodies to PR3, MPO, and EL have been used to capture the respective antigens from cell extracts, and the captured antigen has then been used as the target in an ELISA (1). This type of assay should ideally use capture antibodies recognizing epitopes that are rarely or never seen by human antibodies. Although promising results have been obtained by use of such assays (11, 13), the clinical applicability must be tested in multicenter studies.

A quantitative immunoprecipitation method based on binding of [^{3}H]diisopropyl fluorophosphate ([^{3}H]DFP) to PR3 and EL was recently introduced (7) for PR3-ANCA (and EL-ANCA) quantitation, and preliminary results indicating that this assay will reflect the presence of ANCAs directed solely to conformationally preserved enzymes look promising. In this respect, both the capture PR3-ANCA ELISA and the [^{3}H]DFP quantitative immunoprecipitation assay may better reflect the particular types of PR3-ANCA being produced in patients with active vasculitis (7, 13).

REFERENCES

1. Goldschmeding, R., E. C. van der Schoot, D. Ten Bokkel Huinink, C. E. Hack, M. E. van den Ende, C. G. M. Kallenberg, and A. E. G. K. von dem Borne. 1989. Wegener's granulomatosis autoantibodies identify a novel diisopropyl-fluorophosphate binding protein in the lyso-somes of normal human neutrophils. *J. Clin. Investig.* **84:**1577–1587.

2. Guillevin, L., F. Lhote, J. Amouroux, R. Gherardi, P. Callard, and P. Casassus. 1996. Antineutrophil cytoplasmic antibodies, abnormal angiograms and pathological findings in polyarteritis nodosa and Churg-Strauss syndrome: indications for the classification of vasculitides of the polyarteritis nodosa group. *Br. J. Rheumatol.* **35:**958–964.

3. Hagen, E. C., K. Andrassy, E. Csernok, M. R. Daha, G. Gaskin, W. L. Gross, B. Hansen, Z. Heigl, J. Hermans, D. Jayne, C. G. M. Kallenberg, P. Lesavre, C. M. Lockwood, J. Lüdemann, F. Mascart-Lemone, E. Mirapeix, C. D. Pusey, N. Rasmussen, R. A. Sinico, A. Tzioufas, J. Wieslander, A. Wiik, and F. J. van der Woude. 1996. Development of solid phase assays for the detection of antineutrophil cytoplasmic antibodies (ANCA). A report on the second phase of an international cooperative study on the standardization of ANCA assays. *J. Immunol. Methods* **196:**1–15.

4. Hagen, E. C., M. Daha, J. Hermans, K. de Groot, R. A. Sinico, C. D. Pusey, P. Lesavre, J. Liidemann, N. Rasmussen, A. Wiik, and F. J. van der Woude. 1998. Diagnostic value of standardized assays for anti-neutrophil cytoplasmic antibodies in idiopathic vasculitis. *Kidney Int.* **53:**743–753.

5. Jennette, J. C., R. J. Falk, K. Andrassy, P. A. Bacon, J. Churg, W. L. Gross, E. C. Hagen, G. S. Hoffman, G. G. Hunder, C. G. M. Kallenberg, R. T. McCluskey, R. A. Sinico, A. J. Rees, L. A. van Es, R. Waldherr, and A. Wiik. 1994. Nomenclature of systemic vasculitides: the proposal of an international consensus conference. *Arthritis Rheum.* **37:**187–192.

6. La Cour, B. B., A. Wiik, M. Høier-Madsen, and B. Baslund. 1995. Clinical correlates and substrate specificities of antibodies exhibiting neutrophil nuclear reactivity. A methodological study. *J. Immunol. Methods* **187:**287–295.

7. Lucena-Fernandez, F., G. Dalpé, P. Dagenais, C. Richard, R. Calvert, G. Boire, and H. A. Menard. 1995. Detection of antineutrophil cytoplasmic antibodies by immunoprecipitation. *Clin. Investig. Med.* **18:**153–162.

8. Savige, J., D. Gillis, E. Benson, D. Davies, V. Esnault, R. J. Falk, E. C. Hagen, D. Jayne, J. C. Jennette, B. Paspaliaris, W. Pollock, C. Pusey, C. O. Savage, R. Silvestrini, F. van der Woude, J. Wieslander, and A. Wiik for the International Group for Consensus Statement on Testing and Reporting of Antineutrophil Cytoplasmic Antibodies. 1999. International consensus statement on testing and reporting of antineutrophil cytoplasmic antibodies (ANCA). *Am. J. Clin. Pathol.* **111:**507–513.

9. Segelmark, M., B. Baslund, and J. Wieslander. 1994. Some patients with anti-myeloperoxidase antibodies have a c-ANCA pattern. *Clin. Exp. Immunol.* **96:**458–465.

10. Specks, D., D. N. Fass, M. P. Fautsch, A. M. Himmel, and M. A. Viss. 1996. Recombinant human proteinase 3, the Wegener's autoantigen, expressed in HMC-l cells is enzymatically active and recognized by c-ANCA. *FEBS Lett.* **390:**265–270.

11. Sun, J., D. N. Fass, J. A. Hudson, M. A. Viss, J. Wieslander, H. A. Homburger, and D. Specks. 1998. Capture-ELISA based on recombinant proteinase 3 (PR3) is sensitive for PR3-ANCA testing and allows detection of PR3 and PR3-ANCA/PR3 immune complexes. *J. Immunol. Methods* **211:**111–123.

12. Sun, J., D. N. Fass, M. A. Viss, A. M. Hummel, H. Tang, H. A. Homburger, and D. Specks. 1998. A proportion of proteinase 3-specific anti-neutrophil cytoplasmic antibodies only react with proteinase 3 after cleavage of its N-terminal activation peptide. *Clin. Exp. Immunol.* **114:**320–326.

13. Westman, K. W. A., D. Selga, P. Bygren, M. Segelmark, B. Baslund, A. Wiik, and J. Wieslander. 1998. Clinical evaluation of a capture ELISA for detection of proteinase 3 antineutrophil cytoplasmic antibody. *Kidney Int.* **53:**1230–1236.

14. Wiik, A. 1989. Delineation of a standard procedure for indirect immunofluorescence detection of ANCA. *Acta Pathol. Microbiol. Immunol. Scand.* **97**(Suppl. 6):12–13.

ORGAN-LOCALIZED AUTOIMMUNE DISEASES

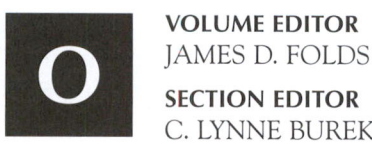

VOLUME EDITOR
JAMES D. FOLDS

SECTION EDITOR
C. LYNNE BUREK

Introduction

C. LYNNE BUREK

119

Autoimmunity is common, while autoimmune disease is not. It is not clear how or why a benign autoimmune response becomes "malignant," thereby leading to pathogenic changes of a target organ. Few autoimmune diseases fulfill the strict criteria by which the autoimmune response is directly related to pathogenesis. However, many findings, either cellular or humoral, can provide circumstantial evidence that autoimmunity is strongly associated with a particular disease. Often, the humoral responses that we detect in the laboratory are best considered to be markers rather than causes of disease. They are useful for diagnosis or prognosis, for excluding other conditions, for classifying disease, or for monitoring therapy. However, whenever we test for autoimmune disease by evaluating autoantibodies, we must consider that individuals without evidence of disease may also exhibit these autoantibodies. Therefore, all results must be evaluated in context with the entire clinical picture; autoantibodies are never the sole criteria for disease.

Autoimmune disease can be divided into two types. The first type, the systemic diseases, are conditions in which the whole body may be involved. They include such disorders as systemic lupus erythematosus and rheumatoid arthritis. The second category consists of the organ-specific autoimmunities. These conditions generally involve one particular organ of the body. In earlier editions of this manual, the section covering organ-specific autoimmunity was small and was combined within the overall section on autoimmune diseases. In the 5th edition, organ-specific autoimmune diseases warranted their own section. In the 6th edition, the section was expanded approximately 25%. In this edition, topics have been expanded to include molecular methods of diagnosis. In certain chapters, such as the one on endocrinopathies, some things have changed only a little. Like in the previous edition, the endocrinopathy chapter contains collected descriptions of the various procedures currently used to detect circulating autoantibodies in patients with immune-mediated endocrine disease, i.e., thyroiditis, Graves' disease, insulin-dependent diabetes mellitus, Addison's disease, and pernicious anemia. However, certain of the neurological autoimmunities and the section on hemolytic anemia will be found only in the 6th edition. Since the number of organ-specific diseases that display diagnostically important autoantibodies is ever expanding, we have included a new section on autoimmune uveitis. The test strategies change once individual antigens are identified. More and more of the assays are now based on enzyme-linked immunosorbent assay using purified antigens or recombinant antigens. However, there is still a role for the "older" assays, such as indirect immunofluorescence, that can be used for screening tests and for identification of antibodies for which the precise antigen is not yet known. Certain new assays use immunoblots of tissue extracts or digested purified antigens. These assays have promise for screening several antigens or epitopes simultaneously.

As antigens are identified, more and more commercial sources are producing reagents for assays in the form of Food and Drug Administration-approved kits. However, manufacturers often use different processes to obtain components (e.g., native antigens versus recombinant peptides). There is no standardization among the assays. The result is that different antibody specificities may be recognized, which is one reason not all kits give identical results. The role of the clinical laboratory is changing from one in which new assays are developed to one of evaluating the new technologies. Yet our goal of helping the patient remains the same.

Endocrinopathies

C. L. BUREK, P. E. BIGAZZI, N. R. ROSE, M. ZAKARIJA, J. M. McKENZIE,
L. YU, J. WANG, AND G. S. EISENBARTH

120

In this chapter, we have collected descriptions of the various procedures currently used to detect circulating autoantibodies in patients with endocrine disease, i.e., thryoiditis, Graves' disease, insulin-dependent diabetes mellitus, Addison's disease, and pernicious anemia.

AUTOANTIBODIES IN CHRONIC THYROIDITIS, ADDISON'S DISEASE, AND PERNICIOUS ANEMIA

(This section was written by C. L. Burek, P. E. Bigazzi, and N. R. Rose.)

General Method for Indirect IF Test for Antibodies

The general method of indirect immunofluorescence (IF) is the screening test used most frequently to detect tissue- or organ-specific autoantibodies. The procedure is essentially the same for all of the autoantibodies, except for the selection of an appropriate tissue that contains the antigen of interest.

Materials

Phosphate-buffered saline (PBS), pH 7.2

Rabbit or goat antiserum to human immunoglobulins conjugated to fluorescein isothiocyanate (FITC conjugate). Most conjugates are commercial preparations and include information by the company on their characteristics, i.e., immunologic analysis of conjugate to show its specificity; antibody, protein, and fluorescein concentrations; and fluorescein-to-protein ratio. When a commercial conjugate is obtained, the lot number should be recorded, and the optimal dilution should be checked by testing several dilutions in a chessboard titration. The same lot should then be used as long as possible.

Buffered glycerol. Mix 9 volumes of glycerol with 1 volume of phosphate buffer (pH 7.2).

Cryostat-cut frozen sections (4 μm thick) of the appropriate tissue on a glass slide

Coverslips

Procedure

1. Prepare 1:10 dilutions in PBS of all sera to be tested (unknown and positive and negative controls). Sera may be screened at 1:10 dilutions or titrated in serial twofold dilutions until the endpoint is reached.

2. Incubate diluted sera with cryostat-cut sections of tissue in a humid chamber at room temperature for 30 min.

3. Wash the slides in PBS for 30 min at room temperature. Effective washing can be performed by gently stirring with a magnetic stirrer and changing the wash solution three times.

4. Incubate sections with the appropriate dilution of FITC conjugate in a humid chamber at room temperature for 30 min.

5. Wash again for 30 min as described in step 3.

6. Mount the coverslip with buffered glycerol, and read with a UV microscope.

Antibodies to Thyroid-Specific Antigens

Sera from patients with chronic thyroiditis (Hashimoto's disease) may contain several types of antibody to thyroid antigens. Antibodies to thyroglobulin or to cytoplasmic antigens of the thyroid epithelial cell are most commonly detected by routine diagnostic procedures; antibodies to the second colloid antigen (called CA2) and to antigens of the thyroid cell surface are less frequently observed and are not of clinical value. In addition to being found in chronic thyroiditis patients, these antibodies may be found in patients with other thyroid disorders, such as primary myxedema, hyperthyroidism, colloid goiter, nodular goiter, and thyroid tumors (3). Thyroid antibodies have also been observed in sera of patients with pernicious anemia, adrenal insufficiency, diabetes mellitus, and other conditions. Screening for thyroid autoantibodies in pregnant women appears to be an effective way to identify individuals who may develop postpartum thyroiditis (8). Finally, antithyroid antibodies are seen in a certain proportion of healthy subjects, as discussed below (3).

Antibodies to Thyroglobulin

Thyroglobulin antibodies can be demonstrated by several procedures, such as precipitation in agar, indirect IF, passive hemagglutination of cells coated with thyroglobulin, radioimmunoassay, and enzyme-linked immunosorbent assay (ELISA) (3). Precipitation in agar is simple to perform but of low sensitivity, detecting only antibodies present in relatively large amounts. Passive hemagglutination tests with the use of tanned erythrocytes (tanned-cell hemagglutination [TCH]) or chromic chloride-treated erythrocytes (chromic chloride hemagglutination [CCH]) are very sensitive and thus detect antibodies to thyroglobulin in patients with a variety of conditions other than thyroiditis, a possible disadvantage from the diagnostic point of view. Commercial hemagglutination kits for thyroglobulin antibodies are less sensitive than the TCH test described below (5). The frequency of thyroglobulin autoantibodies is dependent upon the assay used for evaluation (discussed elsewhere in depth [5]). Indirect IF is less sensitive but reportedly can detect nonagglutinating antibodies that are missed by hemagglutination procedures (3). ELISA procedures for thyroglobulin antibodies are also highly sensitive and demonstrate both agglutinating and nonagglutinating antibodies. Commercial ELISA kits for thyroglobulin autoantibodies are also available and are very sensitive. Indirect IF can also detect antibodies to CA2, which are undetectable by hemagglutination.

TCH Test for Antibodies to Thyroglobulin

Erythrocytes treated with tannic acid are capable of adsorbing protein antigens on their surfaces. When added to serial dilutions of patient serum, these erythrocytes will react with the appropriate antibody, if present, with a visible agglutination reaction. Tanned erythrocytes coated with thyroid extract or purified thyroglobulin are used to detect antibodies to thyroglobulin. The method is highly sensitive but requires fresh erythrocytes and reagents for best results. The procedure, which is described in detail in the previous editions of this manual, has generally been replaced by the CCH test.

CCH Test for Antibodies to Thyroglobulin

Chromic chloride can be used to couple thyroglobulin to erythrocytes, providing a simpler alternative to the tannic acid method (3). The CCH and TCH tests appear to be comparable in sensitivity and specificity. The method of microtitration is given.

Materials

Patient serum (heat inactivated at 56°C for 30 min)

Saline solution (8.5 g of NaCl in 1 liter of double distilled water). Phosphate ions must be avoided, since they interfere with the coupling of antigens to erythrocytes.

Normal rabbit serum (NRS) diluent (heat-inactivated NRS diluted 1:100 in saline)

Chromic chloride solution

1. Stock
   0.125 g of $CrCl_3 \cdot 6H_2O$
   10 ml of saline
2. Wash solution
   0.1 ml of stock
   100 ml of saline
3. Coating solution (0.1% solution made up fresh)
   0.8 ml of stock solution
   9.2 ml of saline

Human thyroglobulin. In a 50-ml tube, mix 0.1 ml of human thyroid extract (prepared by mincing thyroid tissue in PBS, incubating it overnight in the cold, and then centrifuging it at $64,000 \times g$ for 45 min) with 5.0 ml of saline solution. Purified thyroglobulin can be prepared by precipitation with 1.60 to 1.70 M ammonium sulfate followed by filtration through Sephadex G-400. The first peak should be separated and concentrated. Thyroglobulin can be lyophilized or stored frozen. It is used as a 200-μg/ml solution. Do not repeatedly freeze and thaw thyroglobulin.

Human group O erythrocytes. Collect 10 ml of human group O erythrocytes in 3.8% sodium citrate. Use for up to 10 days.

Inactivated test sera; positive and negative control sera
Plates, pipettes, diluters, and tube

Procedure

1. Wash human group O erythrocytes three times with the chromic chloride wash solution. Pack. Centrifuge at $200 \times g$ for 10 min. Remove fluid by aspiration.
2. Pipette 0.2 ml of packed erythrocytes into a 12-ml centrifuge tube.
3. In the centrifuge tube, combine 0.2 ml of packed erythrocytes, 0.2 ml of $CrCl_3$ coating solution, and 0.2 ml of diluted thyroglobulin (or 1:200 NRS for control cells). Mix, and incubate for 4 min at room temperature.
4. Add 10 ml of saline to stop the reaction. Centrifuge as before.
5. Wash the mixture twice in NRS diluent.
6. After the last wash, suspend the erythrocytes in 19.8 ml of NRS diluent to make a 1% suspension.
7. With NRS diluent, prepare 1:5 dilutions of sera to be tested, including control sera.
8. With a pipette dropper, place 0.025 ml of NRS diluent into each of wells 1 through 12.
9. With a 0.025-ml microtitration diluter, take a loopful of 1:5 serum dilution and place it in the first well. Mix and transfer a loopful to the next well, and so on until well 9.
10. With a 0.025-ml microtitration diluter, take a loopful of 1:5 serum dilution and place it in well 11. Mix, and transfer a loopful to well 12. (Alternatively, the dilutions can be made using a multichannel pipette with a 0.025-ml volume.)
11. Repeat these steps for all sera to be tested, including positive and negative control sera.
12. Add 0.025 ml of antigen-coated erythrocytes to wells 1 through 10. Add 0.025 ml of control cells to each of wells 11 and 12.
13. Gently shake the plate to mix.
14. Incubate the plates at room temperature until the cells settle (usually 1 h), and then incubate the plates overnight at 4°C. To avoid evaporation, stack the plates on top of one another, and cover the top plate with plastic or another empty plate.
15. Read the patterns of sedimentation on the bottom of the wells. Strong agglutination usually gives an even mat over the bottom of the well. Weaker reactions give ragged doughnut-shaped patterns, whereas the absence of agglutination gives a smooth, doughnut-shaped, compact button of cells in the center of the well. The reciprocal of the last serum dilution to give a positive reaction is considered to be the titer.

Interpretation of Hemagglutination Test Results

At present, the TCH or CCH test is most commonly used for the detection of antibodies against thyroglobulin. The prevalence of these antibodies detectable by the TCH test is approximately 90% in patients with chronic thyroiditis, 75% in patients with myxedema, and 40% in patients with Graves' disease or thyroid tumors. Approximately 30% of patients with chronic thyroiditis have CCH titers ranging from 1×10^3 to 2.5×10^6. Such high titers are found in only about 10% of patients with Graves' disease. Low titers of thyroglobulin antibodies may be found in juveniles with autoimmune thyroiditis. Low titers of thyroglobulin antibodies may also be found in healthy individuals. The prevalence of such antibodies in subjects without overt thyroid disease is higher in women than men. The incidence also increases with age: 18% of women over 40 years old have antibodies to thyroglobulin.

Indirect IF Test for Antibodies to Thyroglobulin

Indirect IF performed on sections of human or monkey thyroid can demonstrate antibodies to thyroglobulin, CA2, and microsomes of thyroid epithelial cells, and antinuclear antibodies. Tests for these antibodies may be performed on unfixed sections, but in most laboratories, IF for antibodies to thyroglobulin and CA2 is performed on methanol-fixed (56°C methanol for 3 min) or acetone-treated sections. The pattern of staining that is obtained when methanol-fixed sections are used with thyroglobulin antibodies is characteristic and has a floccular "puffy" appearance (3). The less commonly observed CA2 pattern has been described as diffuse, with a "ground glass" appearance. This test is rarely performed for thyroglobulin antibodies.

Interpretation of IF Test Results

The same considerations apply for results of the IF test as for results of the hemagglutination tests except that the sensitivity of IF seems to be lower.

ELISA for Antibodies to Thyroglobulin

ELISA is increasingly used for the measurement of antibodies to thyroglobulin.

Materials

Prepare human thyroglobulin as for the CCH test (see above).

Procedure

1. Dilute thyroglobulin to a concentration of 1 μg/ml in carbonate-bicarbonate buffer (1.56 g of Na_2CO_3 plus 2.93 g of $NaHCO_3$ made up to 1 liter with distilled water and adjusted to pH 9.6). Add the diluent (200 μl) to each well of an Immulon II ELISA plate (Dynatech), and incubate the plate in a humid chamber overnight at 4°C to allow passive adsorption of the thyroglobulin to the surface.
2. Remove unreacted material by washing the plate three times with PBS-Tween (0.15 M PBS [pH 7.4] containing 0.05% Tween 20). Shake the plate dry before adding the next reagent.
3. Dilute the test serum or plasma specimens 1:100 in PBS-Tween, and add 200-μl samples to wells in the plate, permitting duplicate tests on each sample. Incubate the plates for 4 h at 37°C in a humid chamber.
4. Repeat the washing as described in step 2.
5. Add conjugate (200 μl), consisting of goat anti-human globulin labeled with alkaline phosphatase standardized and diluted in PBS-Tween, to each well, and incubate the plate overnight at 4°C.
6. Repeat the washing as described in step 2.
7. Add to each well 200 μl of the enzyme substrate (p-nitrophenyl phosphate [1 mg/ml] in 10% diethanolamine buffer [97 ml of diethanolamine and 800 ml of H_2O with 1 M HCl added to yield a pH of 9.8, made up to 1 liter with H_2O]), and incubate the plate for 20 min at room temperature.
8. Add NaOH (50 μl of 3 M NaOH) to each well to stop the enzyme substrate reactions.
9. Read at A_{405} in an ELISA reader.

Chessboard Titrations

It is necessary to determine the optimal concentration of thyroglobulin for coating the plates and the optimal dilution of the serum or plasma to be used in the tests. These determinations are made by a chessboard titration of positive and negative sera on plates coated with various concentrations of thyroglobulin. A coating solution containing 1 μg of thyroglobulin per ml generally gives the best separation of values between the reference positive and negative sera to be used in subsequent tests.

Interpretation of ELISA Results

The overall correlation of ELISA and CCH titers is presented in Fig. 1. Of samples for which CCH was negative, 95% gave ELISA values below 1.4. Values over 1.4 were considered positive. Only three of the CCH-negative individuals had values significantly greater than 1.4. All were hospital patients. One person (ELISA value of 4.0) had sustained a traumatic injury to the thyroid; the other two patients (ELISA values of 2.2 and 2.4) had antibodies to the microsomal fraction of the thyroid as measured by indirect IF. Values for Fig. 1 were based on an ELISA that used polyvinyl plates. While protein adsorption appears to be higher for polyvinyl, it is impractical for current ELISA readers. Therefore, Immulon II plates have been substituted. Optical density values are much lower with Immulon plates but still show their relative reactivity as on the polyvinyl plates. Many (45%) of the sera with very low (2, 4, or 8) CCH titers had ELISA values under 1.4, as did 22% of the sera with low (16, 32, 64, or 128) CCH titers. All sera with medium (256 to 2,048) or high (4,096 to 16,384) CCH titers were positive by ELISA values and CCH titers (Fig. 1). The Spearman rank correlation is 0.82 (P < 0.001). It is apparent that ELISA readily detects antibody to thyroglobulin in those sera that have medium to high CCH titers but is not very efficient at discriminating between negatives and those samples with low CCH titers. The reason for this lack is not clear; possibly the

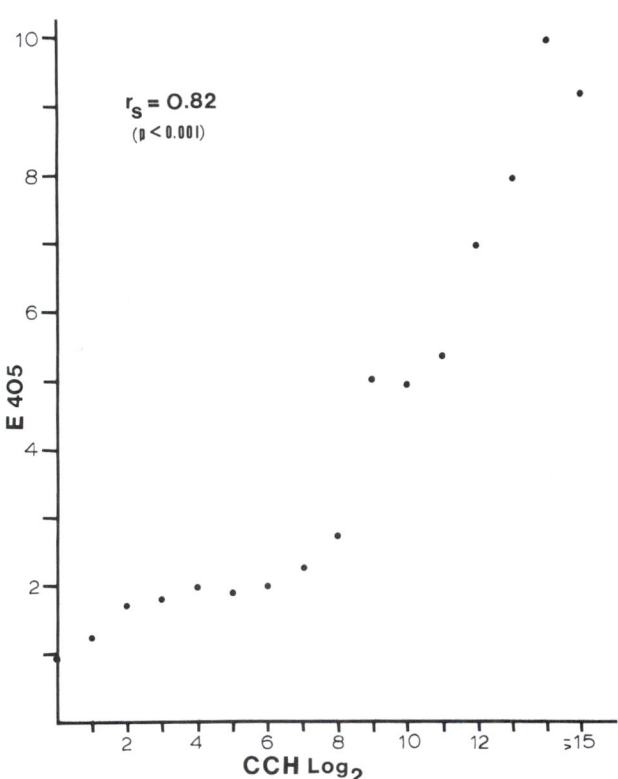

FIGURE 1 Overall correlation between the CCH test and ELISA. Each dot represents the mean ELISA value for the group of sera with the individual CCH titers.

ELISA is less sensitive than CCH to particular subclasses of antibody to thyroglobulin. Recent evidence shows that the antigenic specificity of autoantibodies to thyroglobulin in patients with thyroiditis is different from that in people with antibody but no disease. The naturally occurring antibodies from healthy individuals are directed primarily to sites on the molecule that are shared among species (i.e., conserved), whereas those found primarily in patients are directed to human-specific regions (4). In the future, a test for thyroglobulin autoantibodies specific for those individuals with disease may be of more value in diagnosis.

Antibodies to TPO
The microsomal antigen of the thyroid epithelial cell has been identified as thyroid peroxidase (TPO) (6). The most commonly used tests for determining TPO antibodies are indirect IF and commercially available hemagglutination assays or ELISAs. Preparations of isolated thyroid microsomes are often contaminated with thyroglobulin. Therefore, the commercially prepared tanned-cell kit uses a special diluent containing thyroglobulin to block any antibody that may inadvertently react. Special attention must be paid to any serum that contains high titers of thyroglobulin autoantibodies. There may be insufficient thyroglobulin to remove all traces of the antithyroglobulin antibody, and the serum will give a false-positive result. Serum titers obtained by the indirect IF procedure may reach 1,200 or higher. Titers of TPO antibody obtained by TCH may reach well over 25,000. ELISAs using either purified microsomes or recombinant TPO are also available in commercial kits. These ELISAs are also very sensitive (9). However, those kits that use recombinant antigens may be less sensitive, as the posttranslational modification of the antigens may be lacking. The antibodies to TPO belong predominantly to the immunoglobulin G (IgG) class and, when detected by indirect IF, stain the cytoplasm of thyroid cells (Fig. 2). The nucleus is unstained. This

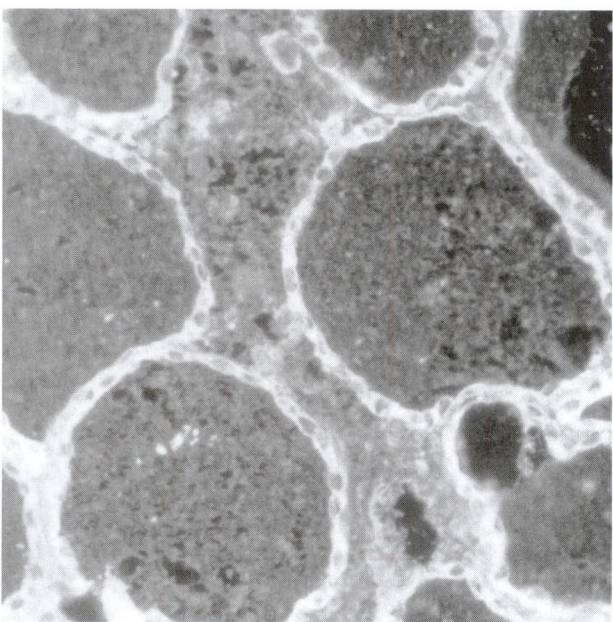

FIGURE 2 Indirect IF for antibodies to thyroid microsomes with an unfixed, air-dried section of monkey thyroid. Only the cytoplasm of the thyroid epithelial cells is stained. (Magnification, ×80.)

pattern of staining must be distinguished from the much coarser granular cytoplasmic staining obtained with mitochondrial antibodies. For better differentiation, sera should be tested on both thyroid and kidney sections.

Indirect IF Test for Antibodies to TPO

Materials and Procedure
The reagents and procedures described above for the general indirect IF test are used. Frozen sections of primate tissue (unfixed and air dried) are used as the tissue substrate.

Interpretation of Test Results
The indirect IF test for antibodies to TPO is positive for approximately 90% of patients with chronic thyroiditis. It is also positive for 64% of patients with primary hypothyroidism, 50% of patients with thyrotoxicosis, 10% of patients with simple goiters, and 17% of patients with thyroid tumor (3, 9).

Antibodies to Adrenal Antigens
Patients with idiopathic Addison's disease have circulating antibodies to adrenal antigens. Such antibodies have been detected by a variety of procedures (3), but the method most commonly used is indirect IF. Antibodies detected by IF stain the cytoplasm of cells of the adrenal cortex and are directed to an antigen associated with the microsomes of these cells. The antibodies belong predominantly to the IgG class and, in general, have rather low titers (not higher than 100). Recent studies suggest that different steroidogenic enzymes of the cytochrome P-450 family may be the target autoantigens of autoimmune Addison's disease. Sera from patients with autoimmune Addison's disease contain autoantibodies to 21-hydroxylase (21-OH) or 17-α-hydroxylase (1, 2, 11). A sensitive radioimmunoassay using the 21-OH antigen has been developed, but the usage is limited (2). Patients with autoimmune polyendocrine syndrome type I (Addison's disease plus hypoparathyroidism and chronic mucocutaneous candidiasis) have circulating autoantibodies to the P-450 cholesterol side chain cleavage enzyme. It is still uncertain whether these autoantigens are expressed on the surfaces of adrenal cells or are otherwise accessible to adrenal antibodies in vivo.

Indirect IF Test for Antibodies to Adrenal Antigens

Materials and Procedure
The reagents and procedures previously described for the general indirect IF test are used. Frozen sections of primate adrenal tissue are used as a substrate. These sections are available commercially from certain vendors that deal with autoimmune test kits. Positive and negative control sera can also be purchased commercially.

Interpretation of Test Results
Antibodies to adrenocortical cells are detected in the serum of 38 to 60% of patients with idiopathic Addison's disease (2, 3). The antibodies are present in 7 to 18% of patients with tuberculous Addison's disease and in 1% of healthy subjects. The presence of antibodies to adrenocortical cells is a good indication that the disease is idiopathic and not of a tubercular or other nature. Different patterns of staining have been observed: most sera stain the whole cortex, with a brighter fluorescence in the glomerulosa zone (Fig. 3 and 4), but a few sera stain only the fasciculata and reticularis zone, not the glomerulosa zone. The latter pattern has been reported with sera that also stain the interstitial cells of the testis and the theca interna cells of the ovary.

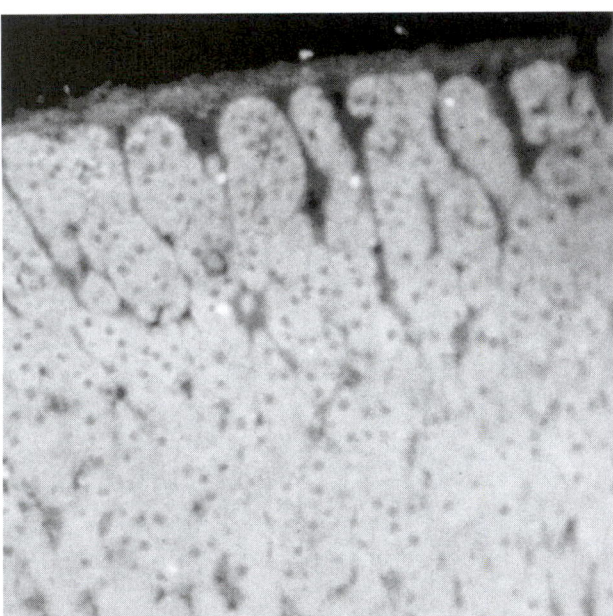

FIGURE 3 Indirect IF for antibodies to adrenal cortex, with an unfixed, air-dried section of monkey adrenal cortex. All layers of the adrenal cortex are stained. (Magnification, ×32.)

Antibodies to Antigens of Ovary, Testis, and Placenta

Antibodies staining the cytoplasm of cells of the theca interna, interstitial cells and corpus luteum cells of the ovary, interstitial cells of the testis, and trophoblast of the placenta have been detected in the sera of patients with Addison's disease and of patients with premature ovarian failure (2, 3). The antigens involved have not been very well characterized,

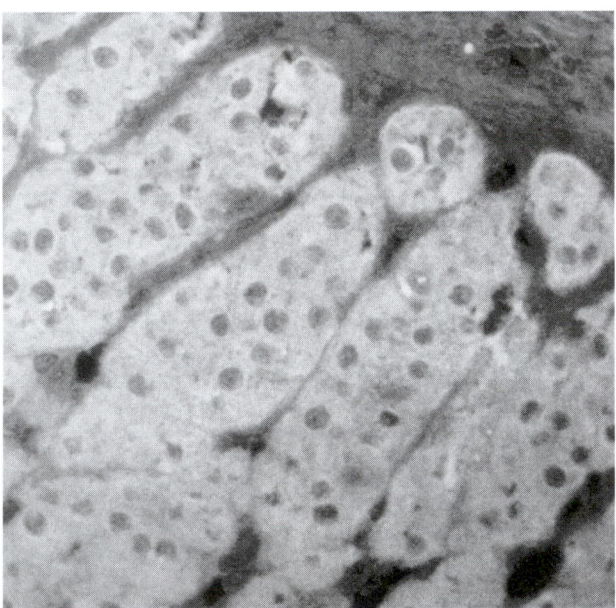

FIGURE 4 Same as Fig. 3 but at a higher magnification. Only the cytoplasm of the adrenal cells is stained. (Magnification, ×80.)

and the test itself is at present more of research than of diagnostic interest (see chapter 126).

Antibodies to Parathyroid Antigens

Sera from patients with idiopathic hypoparathyroidism (IHP) contain antibodies to antigens of parathyroid cells. Such antibodies have been detected by indirect IF on sections of normal human parathyroid tissue obtained at autopsy (3). They are directed not against parathyroid hormone but against cytoplasmic antigens of parathyroid cells.

Indirect IF Tests for Antibodies to Parathyroid Antigens

Materials and Procedure

The reagents and procedures are the same as those used for the other IF tests. The test is performed with unfixed cytostat sections of primate parathyroid as the substrate.

Interpretation of Test Results

Antibodies to parathyroid cells are found in the serum of approximately 38% of patients with IHP, 26% of patients with idiopathic Addison's disease, 12% of patients with chronic thyroiditis, and 6% of controls. Since approximately 60% of patients with IHP do not have demonstrable parathyroid antibodies, a negative test obviously does not exclude IHP. On the other hand, a positive test, while indicating IHP, is not necessarily diagnostic, since the patient may have adrenal insufficiency or thyroiditis or a combination of these disorders.

Antibodies to Gastric Parietal Cells

Circulating autoantibodies to intracytoplasmic antigens of gastric parietal cells (parietal cell antibodies), to the Bl2 binding site of intrinsic factor, and to the intrinsic factor Blt complex occur with high frequency in patients with autoimmune gastritis leading to end-stage disease of pernicious anemia (10). Antibodies to intrinsic factor may be detected by several radioassay procedures. However, these methods are not yet regularly performed in most hospitals. Parietal cell antibodies are detected primarily by indirect IF. Parietal cell antibodies, when detected by indirect IF, bind to the cytoplasm of parietal cells of the gastric fundal mucosa of humans and various animals, like monkeys, rats, and guinea pigs (Fig. 5). As noted above, the pattern of staining resembles that seen with mitochondrial antibodies; therefore, a control test on kidney should be performed. The autoantigens to which gastric parietal cell antibodies are directed have been identified as the alpha- and beta-subunits of the gastric H/K ATPase, the enzyme responsible for acid secretion in the stomach (7).

Indirect IF Test for Antibodies to Gastric Parietal Cells

Materials and Procedure

The materials used are the same as those described previously for other IF tests. Unfixed sections of rat stomach (gastric mucosa) are used as the substrate. Unfixed rat kidney sections are used as controls for staining because of mitochondrial antibodies.

Interpretation of Test Results

Parietal cell antibodies are found in about 90% of patients with pernicious anemia (10). These antibodies are also present in patients with a number of other conditions,

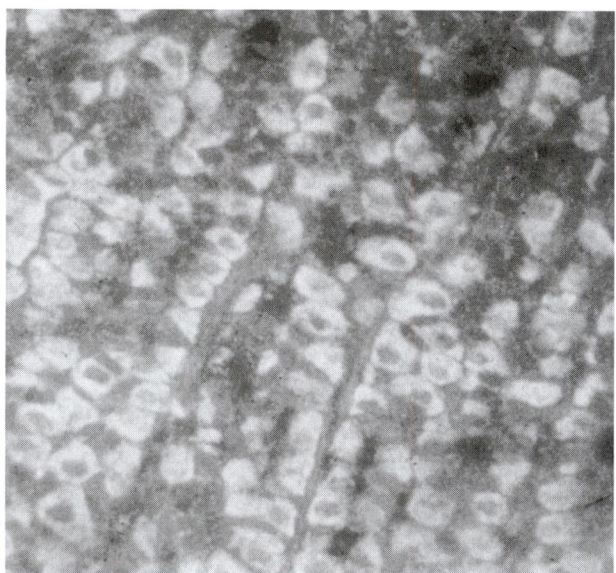

FIGURE 5 Indirect IF for antibodies to parietal cells of the gastric mucosa, with an unfixed, air-dried section of rat stomach. The cytoplasm of most cells is stained. (Magnification, ×100.)

such as chronic thyroiditis (33%), Sjögren's sicca syndrome (15%), atrophic gastritis (60%), and gastric ulcer (22%). Antibodies to parietal cells have been reported for about 20 to 30% of patients with *Helicobacter pylori*-associated gastritis, although the titers may be lower than in autoimmune gastritis (10). Whether *H. pylori* is an environmental agent triggering the autoimmune condition is still not known. The antibodies are also found in the healthy population, with an incidence that varies according to age, i.e., from 2% in subjects younger than 20 years to 16% in subjects older than 60 years. They are more common in women than in men. It is also not known whether these antibodies are a biomarker of latent disease, as the interval between autoimmune gastritis with parietal cell antibodies and pernicious anemia may be as long as 20 to 30 years (10). As of yet, no longitudinal studies have addressed this issue.

HYPERTHYROIDISM OF GRAVES' DISEASE AND ANTIBODIES TO THE THYROTROPIN RECEPTOR

(This section was written by M. Zakarija and J. M. McKenzie.)

Thyroid function and growth are under control of the pituitary hormone thyrotropin (TSH), with thyroid hormones exerting negative feedback control of TSH secretion. Binding of TSH to its receptor (TSH-R), a member of a subfamily of G protein-coupled receptors for polypeptide hormones, follicle-stimulating hormone, luteinizing hormone, and TSH, initiates metabolic events in the gland mainly by activating a cyclic AMP (cAMP) cascade and, to a minor degree, phospholipase C (for a review, see reference 22). The major structural difference between TSH-R and receptors for follicle-stimulating hormone and luteinizing hormone is a 50-amino-acid insertion in the extracellular domain, the cleavage of which leaves an extracellular A subunit and a transmembrane B subunit, linked by disulfide bonds. Further degradation of B subunit, with the dissolution of disulfide

bonds, releases the A subunit, at least from cultured cells. This may have implications for the induction of autoimmunity to the TSH-R (18). In Graves' disease, hyperactivity and enlargement of the thyroid are due to an antibody that mimics the action of TSH on its receptor (for reviews, see references 15 and 16). From the initial discovery of this activity (16), named long-acting thyroid stimulator, and its identification as an IgG, through gradual development of better assay techniques accompanied by numerous acronyms, the present name—thyroid-stimulating antibody (TSAb)—has been agreed upon. That TSAb truly stimulates human thyroid in vivo was established by the finding of neonatal hyperthyroidism due to transplacental passage of the antibody from mother to fetus.

In contrast to the agonist action of TSAb, another antibody (also an IgG), thyroid-blocking antibody (TBAb), was found to act as an antagonist by inhibiting TSH binding and action. TBAb is a probable cause of hypothyroidism in some patients with atrophic thyroiditis and is responsible for transient hypothyroidism in neonates of mothers who have this antibody (16). The final proof that TSAb and TBAb interact with the TSH-R came from work with the cloned receptor (14, 16, 17, 22), and the term TSH-R antibodies (TRAb) encompasses both antibodies.

Current Assays for TSH-R Antibodies

In the last decade, FRTL5 cells (a cloned Fisher rat thyroid cell line) have been the most uniform and widely used preparation for the stimulation-type assay of TSAb. These cells depend on TSH for function and growth and are propagated in a well-defined medium that includes TSH. After withdrawal of TSH for several days, metabolically quiescent cells become sensitive to both TSH and TSAb. More recently, Chinese hamster ovary cells transfected with the recombinant human TSH-R (CHO–TSH-R) have become the preparation of choice because they express the homologous receptor for TSAb and are easier and cheaper to maintain in culture. The assay entails incubation of cells with either purified IgG or polyethylene glycol-precipitated immunoglobulins from patients' sera. The endpoint of the assay is the concentration of cAMP in the cells (Fig. 6) when the incubation medium is isotonic Hanks' balanced

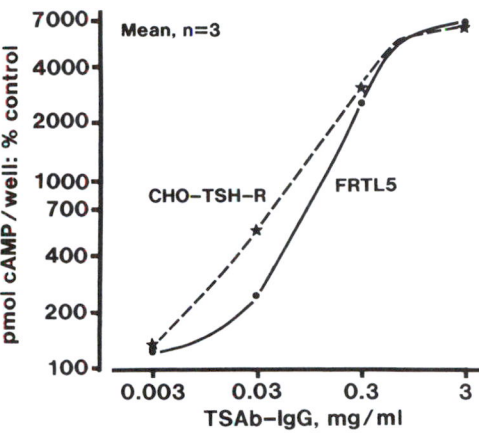

FIGURE 6 TSAb-induced cAMP accumulation in FRTL5 and CHO–TSH-R cells incubated in isotonic medium. Cells were incubated for 2 h in the absence (control) or presence of the indicated concentrations of TSAb (purified IgG), and cAMP was measured in cell extracts.

salt solution (pH 7.4) buffered with HEPES and supplemented with 3-isobutyl-1-methylxanthine (blocker of cAMP phosphodiesterase). Improved sensitivity to TSAb is achieved with the use of a low-salt solution (Hanks' balanced salt solution devoid of NaCl), in which case cAMP released into the medium is measured. With this method, detection of TSAb in patients with Graves' disease reaches almost 100%. Results are usually expressed as percent increase in cAMP over that in the control wells (cells incubated with normal IgG), and values of >130 to 150% are considered positive.

The ability of TSAb to displace ^{125}I-TSH from the TSH-R is the basis of another technique, called the TSH binding inhibition (TBI) assay (Fig. 7). Commercially available kits use solubilized porcine thyroid cell membranes as a source of the receptor. The attraction of this assay is the ease of its performance and the use of whole serum instead of extracted immunoglobulin. Unfortunately, the method lacks the sensitivity and specificity of the stimulation assay; false-negative results usually occur with sera of low stimulating potency, and some positive results are due to the presence of TBAb. The assay can also be performed with cultured cells exposed to IgG in a low-salt medium, a procedure still confined to research laboratories. Results from all procedures are expressed as a TBI index, with positive values starting at 10 to 15% and maximum inhibition being 100%, a level almost never attained by even the most potent TSAb (Fig. 7). TBAb is equally effective in blocking TSH- and TSAb-induced stimulation of cAMP accumulation (Fig. 8A), and the activity is often termed the thyroid stimulation-blocking antibody (TSBAb). When measured in the TBI assay (Fig. 7), the activity is designated TSH binding-inhibiting antibody. The highest titers of TBAb so far described have been found in mothers of infants with transient neonatal hypothyroidism (Fig. 7).

It has been long recognized that TSAb and TBAb may coexist in some patients with either Graves' disease or Hashimoto's thyroiditis. This is reflected in a biphasic dose-response in the stimulation-type assay (Fig. 8B) and a higher

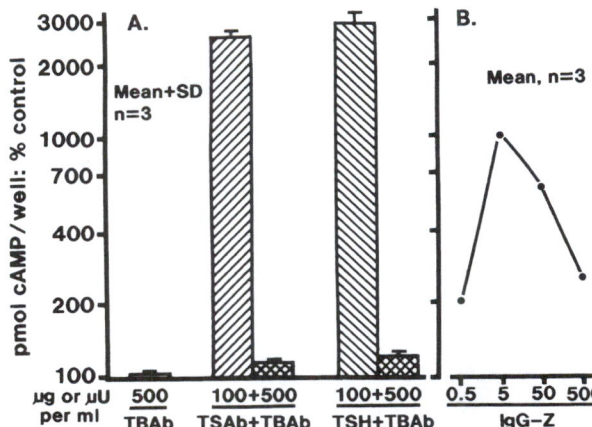

FIGURE 8 Assays with CHO–TSH-R cells in a low-salt medium. (A) Inhibitory effect of TBAb on TSAb- and TSH-induced accumulation of cAMP. (B) Biphasic effect of a patient's IgG (IgG-Z). Cells were incubated for 2 h with the test substances (TRAb as purified IgG) and concentrations indicated, and cAMP in the medium was measured.

inhibition of ^{125}I-TSH binding than would be expected from the TSAb activity alone. Thus, if they are used as an aid in clinical management, results from a single assay and a fixed concentration of TRAb should be interpreted with caution.

Characteristics of TSH-R Antibodies

Despite tremendous advances in the fields of immunology and molecular biology, TRAb have not been obtained in monoclonal form, and they are still defined by their biological activities in in vitro assays. With the use of immunochemical techniques for purification, TSAb was shown to be oligoclonal (and sometimes even monoclonal) in terms of its IgG subclass distribution (exclusively IgG1) and light chaintype association (predominantly λ). Resolution by preparative isoelectric focusing, showing a peak TSAb activity at pH 8.5 to 9, supports the notion of its oligoclonal origin. Limited data for TBAb show less subclass restriction, and an exclusive association with κ light chain was found in a single patient of four tested. Both TRAb are also effective as Fab fragments, suggesting that cross-linking of the receptor is not the basis of their action.

That the stimulating activity might not be the property of a single species of antibody came from the analyses of sera from patients with unusual clinical presentations. Two antibodies, distinct from TSAb, have been characterized by their properties in different assays; one appears to be human TSH-R specific, and the stimulating effect of the other is not inhibitable by TBAb (16). The incidence of these antibodies is unknown, since differing bioactivities cannot be detected in a single stimulation-type assay, a common practice in screening patients' sera. Heterogeneity of TBAb has also been suggested by the finding that some patients' sera block TSH-induced stimulation without affecting the binding (16).

Cloning of the TSH-R has contributed to the understanding of its structure-function relationship and interactions of TRAb and TSH. It is clear that TRAb bind to highly conformational epitopes on the extracellular domain of TSH-R and do not recognize linear sequences (12), a fact reflected in their failure to facilitate cloning of the receptor (22). Part of individual conformational epitopes for TSAbs, TBAb, and TSH obviously overlap. Studies with TSH-R-luteinizing hormone

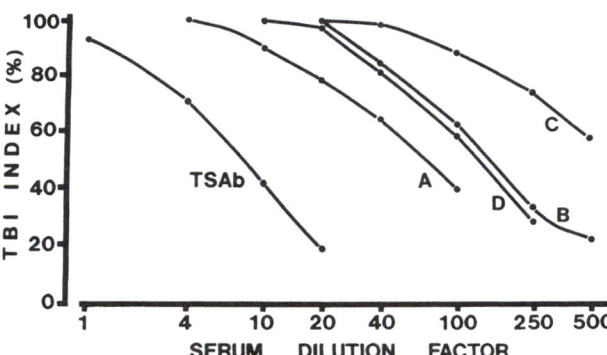

FIGURE 7 TBI assay with a commercial kit (Kronus, Inc., Boise, Idaho). Dilutions were carried out with pooled serum from healthy humans. A, B, C, and D refer to sera from mothers, all on replacement therapy, who had hypothyroid neonates. TSAb was from a mother who was treated with ^{131}I for hyperthyroidism of Graves' disease and subsequently had two hyperthyroid neonates. (Reprinted, with permission of The Endocrine Society, from M. Zakarija, J. M. McKenzie, and M. S. Eidson, Transient neonatal hypothyroidism: characterization of maternal antibodies to the thyrotropin receptor, *J. Clin. Endocrinol. Metab.* **70:**1239–1246, 1990.)

receptor chimeras were able to distinguish two populations of stimulating antibodies (17), and the coexistence of TSAb and TBAb in some hypothyroid patients was confirmed using TSH-R mutants (14). Further characterization of TRAb, especially at the molecular level, will depend on their availability as monoclonal antibodies. So far, only one adequately characterized human monoclonal TSAb-IgG has been reported (19).

The importance of the cAMP cascade in the regulation of thyroid function and growth has recently been reinforced by the discovery of spontaneously occurring mutations in the TSH-R and their consequences (20, 21), thus supporting the notion that the effect of TSAb and TBAb on the thyroid is sufficient to explain the respective clinical presentations. Lack of absolute correlation of TSAb titers with the degree of hyperthyroidism and goiter size could be attributed to modifying influences of various cytokines, elaborated by thyroid-infiltrating lymphocytes. Lymphocytic infiltration of the thyroid in Graves' disease varies widely, from none to that seen in Hashimoto's thyroiditis, and there is evidence for negative correlation between the size of the gland and the degree of infiltration. In addition, some TRAb have been shown to activate phospholipases C and A_2 (13). Another variable probably contributing to the disparity is the coexistence of TBAb in approximately 30% of patients with Graves' disease (16).

Clinical Application of Assays for TSH-R Antibodies

The assays offered by commercial diagnostic laboratories are quite expensive and, in most instances, unnecessary; the usual clinical and biochemical criteria are sufficient for establishing the diagnosis. Circumstances in which the assay of TRAb, as TSAb and/or TBAb, is merited in the clinical management of patients with autoimmune thyroid disease encompass the following situations. Persistence of TSAb at the end of a course of antithyroid drugs predicts the relapse of hyperthyroidism and the need for thyroid ablation (surgical resection or administration of radioactive iodide). In pregnancy complicated by Graves' disease, high titers of TSAb in maternal blood at the end of gestation are predictive of neonatal hyperthyroidism, which may have a deleterious effect on the child's development if not recognized and treated on time. Since ablative treatment, with consequent eu- or hypothyroidism, does not necessarily ensure immunologic remission, i.e., the disappearance of TSAb, the measurement of TSAb in pregnant women so treated is imperative; without the protection of antithyroid drugs, stimulation of the fetal thyroid by TSAb and the ensuing hyperthyroidism can lead to irreversible abnormalities. Screening for a specific TRAb is also necessary in all pregnant women who have had a previous child with neonatal hyper- or hypothyroidism. We stress here that all such women are clinically affected, but the diagnosis does not always match the outcome in the neonate; women with hypothyroidism of Hashimoto's thyroiditis may give birth to a hyperthyroid infant, and those previously treated for Graves' hyperthyroidism and still having TSAb may give birth to a hypothyroid infant. Thus, autoimmune thyroid disease cannot be distinguished solely on the basis of the type of TRAb. Different TRAb can occur any time during the autoimmune process and may coexist in an individual patient, with the more potent antibody responsible for the clinical presentation in the neonate. Postnatal effects are transient, with the duration related to the initial level of TRAb and the time required for catabolism of maternal IgG. Timely, but limited in duration, treatment of affected infants usually leads to an excellent outcome.

The usefulness of TRAb assays will undoubtedly increase in the future. Achieving this increased usefulness will entail full characterization of all TRAb, both currently known and still to be identified, and the development of simpler techniques with high sensitivities and specificities for their detection.

PANCREAS

(This section was written by L. Yu, J. Wang, and G. S. Eisenbarth.)

Introduction

Diabetes mellitus is made up of a heterogeneous group of disorders. Approximately 10% of patients with diabetes mellitus have the immune-mediated form of the disease, now termed type 1A diabetes (American Diabetes Association 2004 [25]). Prior terms for this form of diabetes include juvenile-onset diabetes and insulin-dependent diabetes. In that as many patients develop type 1A diabetes as adults as children, and that at the time of diagnosis many individuals are not dependent upon insulin for survival, the term type 1A has been adopted to reflect disease etiology. A type 1B form of diabetes represents severe loss of insulin secretion on a nonautoimmune basis, but at present a clear example of this form of the disorder is lacking. Type 2 diabetes is characterized by insulin resistance and moderate loss of insulin secretory capacity and makes up the bulk of patients with diabetes. Finally, separate diabetes mellitus categories consist of gestational diabetes and "specific types of diabetes" usually with defined mutations or accompanying pathology (e.g., pancreatic abnormalities, endocrinopathies, or drug induced).

The great majority of non-Hispanic Caucasian (>90%) and approximately 50% of Hispanic and African-American children developing diabetes have the type 1A form of the disease, while between 5 and 15% of adults presenting with diabetes (depending upon the population) have type 1A diabetes. Type 1A diabetes is highly associated with specific HLA class II (DR and DQ) alleles, with both high-risk and protective genotypes present. In particular, DQ8 (DQA1*0301 and DQB1*0302) and DQ2 (DQA1*0501 and DQB1*0201) are present in 90% of Caucasian patients with the disease and 40% of the general population, and DQ6 (DQA1*0102 and DQB1*0602) is present in 20% of the population and 1% of children with type 1A diabetes. The nomenclature and detailed associations of specific HLA alleles and additional genetic polymorphisms with type 1A diabetes can be found at http://www.barbaradaviscenter.org, *Immunology of Diabetes* web textbook, chapter 7. There are no tests that can absolutely exclude a diagnosis of type 1A diabetes, and it is possible for individuals to have evidence of both type 1A (e.g., anti-islet autoantibodies) and type 2 diabetes (e.g., severe insulin resistance). In general, however, the presence of anti-islet autoantibodies measured with highly specific assays (≥99% specificity) in a patient with diabetes is pathognomonic of the disorder, and the presence of anti-islet autoantibodies can be used to predict the disease with various positive predictive values (45) depending on the spectrum of autoantibodies expressed (Fig. 9). Though there is general agreement that T lymphocytes rather than autoantibodies are the primary pathogenic mechanism, at present there is a lack of assays for anti-islet T cells with sufficient specificity and sensitivity to contribute to laboratory diagnosis or disease prediction.

Autoantibodies

Anti-islet autoantibodies are usually present years before clinical onset of type 1A diabetes (45). A decade ago, anti-islet

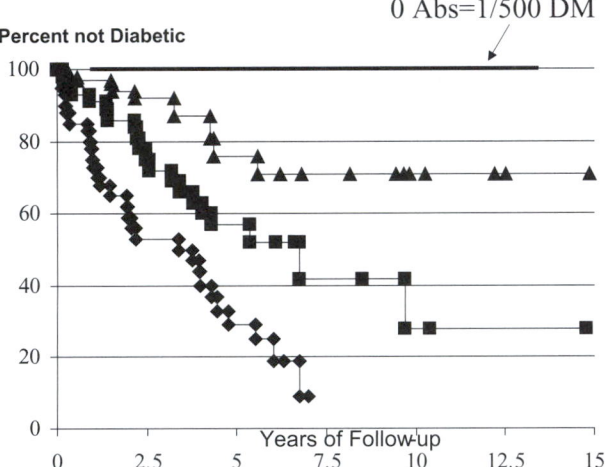

Percent not Diabetic

0 Abs=1/500 DM

Years of Follow-up

FIGURE 9 Progression to overt type 1A diabetes of first-degree relatives of patients with type 1A diabetes (DM) relative to number of anti-islet autoantibodies expressed (autoantibodies to GAD65, ICA512, and insulin). ◆, three antibodies; ■, two antibodies; ▲, one antibody. (From http://www.barabaradaviscenter.org, *Immunology of Diabetes.*)

autoantibody tests were limited to measuring cytoplasmic islet cell autoantibodies (ICA) and insulin autoantibodies (IAA). Currently, recombinant autoantibody assays with biochemically defined autoantigens (Table 1), including insulin, glutamic acid decarboxylase (GAD), ICA512 (IA-2), I-A2β (phogrin), and carboxypeptidase H, are available.

ICA were first discovered in the early 1970s in patients with polyendocrine autoimmunity (29), and antibodies in the sera from these patients reacted with frozen sections of human pancreas. These patients with type 1A diabetes have ICA that frequently persist for decades, while in the majority of patients with type 1A diabetes the ICA slowly disappear. ICA was soon identified in patients with the more common form of type 1A diabetes and was found to be present long before clinical onset of diabetes (36, 37). The Diabetes Prevention Trial—Type 1 (DPT-1) demonstrated that all

TABLE 1 Biochemically characterized autoantigens

Antigen	Sensitivity (%)	Comment
Insulin	49–92	Higher levels in young children
GAD	84	Higher sensitivity with sera from patients with adult-onset type 1A diabetes
ICA512/IA-2	74	Tyrosine phosphatase-like molecule
IA-2β/phogrin	61	Tyrosine phosphatase-like molecule
Carboxypeptidase H	10	Infrequent
GLIMA38	14–38	Not yet sequenced
GM2-1	?	Ganglioside: chromatography assay
ICA69	?	Western blot assay with poor specificity
ICA12	<20	Diabetes relatedness requires further study

anti-islet autoantibodies tested for in the trial, including ICA, GAD autoantibodies (GAA), and ICA512 autoantibodies (ICA512AA), in relatives were relatively stable, with 75 to 85% of all positivity (90 to 95% with high levels) confirmed during follow-up. ICA has been shown to be present in 70 to 80% of newly diagnosed type 1A diabetics and is predictive for the development of diabetes in both relatives of patients with diabetes and the general population. ICA is a heterogeneous mixture of IgG isotype autoantibodies against a variety of islet cell molecules. To date, three autoantigens have been defined that contribute to the ICA positivity, including GAD, insulinoma antigen 2 (IA-2 [ICA512] and a homologous antigen, IA-2β), and glycolipids (26, 28, 31, 38, 42). However, there are likely other autoantibodies still to be identified (Fig. 10). Approximately 5% of ICA-positive individuals without biochemical autoantibodies in the DPT-1 trial progressed to diabetes, indicating that there is another autoantigen(s) playing a role in type 1A diabetes autoimmunity. We believe that the current three major autoantibody assays in general can replace the ICA test for initial screening even though there remains an additional unidentified ICA autoantigen(s) (antigen "X" [Fig. 10]).

The first ICA antigen component to be determined was a 64-kDa protein that was later identified (26) as the enzyme GAD. GAD is present in all human islet cells (e.g., α, β, and δ) and other endocrinological organ tissues like testes, ovary, and neurons, though only pancreatic β cells are destroyed in type 1A diabetes. The GAA of patients with stiff man syndrome had been previously identified and are unusual in that they react with fixed sections of the brain and react with denatured GAD molecules on Western blots and with GAD protein fragments (33). In contrast, most sera from diabetic patients only target GAD protein epitopes dependent on protein conformation and do not bind GAD protein fragments or react with denatured GAD protein. There are two isomers of GAD, GAD65 and GAD67, which are 76% homologous in amino acid sequence. Autoantibodies to GAD65 are predominant over those to GAD67, and the autoantibodies binding to GAD67 in diabetic patients seem to represent antibodies to epitopes shared with GAD65 (35).

The second identified ICA antigen component was IA-2 (or ICA512), a protein tyrosine phosphatase, and its homologous antigen IA-2β (phogrin) (38, 42). The two isomers are most homologous in their antigenic intracellular regions to which essentially all of the autoantibodies are directed. Almost all autoantibodies to IA-2β also react with IA-2, while approximately 10% of diabetic patients have autoantibodies only reacting with IA-2 and not with IA-2β. In addition, two differentially spliced ICA512 (IA-2) mRNAs are expressed in islets, with one form lacking exon 13, which includes the transmembrane region of the molecule (40). In our laboratory, an ICA512 clone (ICA512bdc) was used to develop an autoantibody radioassay. Approximately 10% of patients developing type 1 diabetes have autoantibodies reacting with only one of the two forms of alternatively spliced IA-2 molecules.

To date, insulin is the only known β cell-specific autoantigen of humans (all other islet autoantigens are also produced by human non-β islet cells). IAA were found by Palmer and coworkers (39) in patients with newly diagnosed type 1A diabetes and were soon demonstrated to be present for many years before the clinical onset of disease. IAA is so far the only autoantibody dramatically age dependent in its prevalence and level (34). The levels of IAA inversely correlate with the age of disease onset, and less than half of individuals developing type 1A diabetes after age 15 have detectable

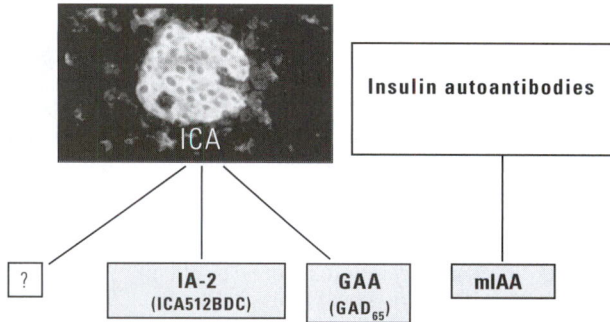

FIGURE 10   The current well-identified anti-islet autoantibody assays. (From http://www.barbaradaviscenter.org, *Immunology of Diabetes*.) Islet autoimmunity is defined as one or more autoantibodies *persistent* for at least 3 to 6 months.

IAA levels. IAA is usually the first autoantibody to appear in young children developing type 1 diabetes (46). For most patients, treatment with exogenous insulin also induces insulin antibodies. The current IAA assay is not able to distinguish between natural IAA and induced insulin antibodies. In the rare insulin autoimmune syndrome (44), also termed Hirata syndrome, patients express high levels of IAA, often with episodes of severe hypoglycemia.

General Assay Methodology

The first useful islet autoantibody assay was the ICA test utilizing indirect IF with frozen sections of human pancreas as a substrate. A standard for ICA was established utilizing a serial dilution of a calibrated serum with assigned JDF (for the Juvenile Diabetes Foundation) units. To date, the ICA test remains cumbersome, and the Immunology of Diabetes Society (IDS) workshops demonstrated that there existed large variation among laboratories in terms of sera called ICA positive.

The current major format for determination of islet autoantibodies uses fluid-phase radioimmunobinding assays,

applied to all three major islet autoantibody tests, including GAA, ICA512AA, and IAA. A semiautomated format is available where labeled antigen is incubated with patient sera; both are placed in 96-well filtration plates, where the immune complex is precipitated with protein A- and/or protein G-coupled Sepharose; free radioactivity is separated by filtration washing; scintillation fluid is added directly to the plates; and counting is performed on multichannel beta counters able to handle the plates (Fig. 11).

ELISAs employing plate-bound antigen are the most common assay formats for basic immunologic research. In multiple diabetes autoantibody workshops, for either human or mouse models, standard ELISA formats lack both sensitivity and specificity compared to the fluid-phase radioassay formats. In the most recent international workshop only a single modified ELISA (for GAA) attained levels of specificity and sensitivity equivalent to those of the radioassays (30).

It is recommended that all laboratories attempting to measure anti-islet autoantibodies take part in Diabetes Antibody Standardization Program (DASP) workshops organized by the IDS and the Centers for Disease Control and Prevention. As demonstrated in multiple workshops, though the majority of laboratories have excellent assays for GAA and ICA512AA, many laboratories have IAA assays with unacceptable sensitivity and specificity when evaluating in blind the DASP panel of 100 control sera and 50 sera from patients with type 1A diabetes of recent onset.

Determination of ICA by Indirect IF

Sample Requirements

Samples are stored at −20°C or below until analyzed. Approximately 200 μl of serum per sample is needed for this assay. Hemolyzed or lipemic blood samples may have artificially low ICA titers and thus should not be used for analysis with this method. In order to obtain high-quality serum and prevent or decrease the possibility of hemolysis, the yellow-top gel serum separator tubes are recommended.

1. Mix ^{125}I-insulin and sera

2. Incubate 72 hours at 4°C

3. Add Protein A/G-Sepharose to reaction mix in a 96-well filtration plate

4. Incubate for 45 min at 4°C

5. Wash each well using the vacuum-operated 96-well plate washer

6. Count radioactivity with 96-well plate beta counter

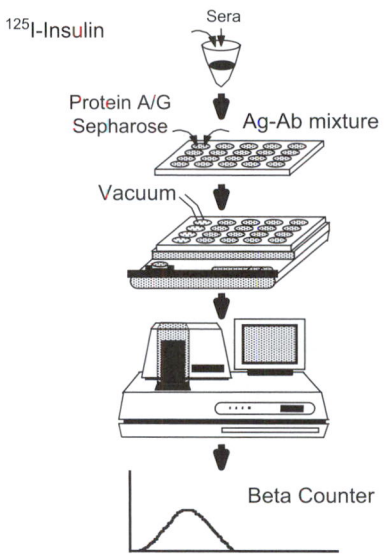

FIGURE 11   General outline of fluid-phase 96-well plate assays for autoantibodies. In this example ^{125}I-insulin is utilized, but the format is identical for GAD65 and ICA512 assays.

Materials, Reagents, and Equipment

Cryostat

Frozen 5-µm sections of human blood group O pancreas

Fluorescein-antibody conjugate [goat anti-human IgG F(ab)₂ fragment-FITC or rabbit fluorescein-conjugated antihuman IgG (Behringwerke AG, Marburg, Germany) or sheep anti-human IgG–FITC conjugate (Sigma, St. Louis, Mo.)]

Fluorescence microscope with epi-illumination 20× objective (Leica, Wetzlar, Germany)

Reciprocal shaker

Principle

We highly recommend human pancreas with blood type O of cadaveric donors taken while the heart is still beating, because the pancreas is very prone to autolysis. Five-millimeter cubes of the pancreas are quickly frozen in isopentane at −70°C, sealed in a freezer-container, and stored at −80°C. Five-micrometer-thick frozen sections are cut with the temperature of cryostat held between −25 and −30°C and then placed onto the glass microscope slides (usually four sections per slide), air dried for 30 min with a fan, and then directly used or stored at −80°C. The freezer-stored slides must be brought to room temperature with air drying in front of a fan for 30 min before use. The slides to be used should be well labeled, and the sections on the same slide need to be isolated from each other with a hydrophobic marker. Serum sample is then applied on each section, and tissue-bound specific autoantibodies from patient's serum will be revealed by an animal (goat, sheep, or rabbit) anti-human IgG–fluorescein conjugate under a fluorescence microscope with epi-illumination.

Procedure

1. In the initial experiment, 50 µl of undiluted serum is applied on each tissue section and incubated for 30 min at room temperature in a moisture chamber.

2. Each slide is rinsed gently with 0.5 M PBS (pH 7.4), with care to not damage or remove each tissue section.

3. The slides are completely submerged in 0.5 M PBS (pH 7.4) and gently washed on a reciprocal shaker for 5 min; this wash step is repeated twice, each time in fresh PBS for 5 min.

4. Both sides of the slides are then quickly dried with a low-lint Kim Wipe, with care to not touch the tissue sections on each slide, and then placed back into the incubation chamber to prevent complete dehydration before the next step.

5. Each section is then covered with 50 µl of diluted (often 1/20 dilution determined empirically) fluorescein-antibody conjugate in PBS (containing 1% bovine serum albumin [BSA]) and incubated for 30 min at room temperature in a moist chamber.

6. The slides are washed as in steps 2 and 3.

7. The slides are quickly dried as in step 4, a slide cover is placed with a glycerol solution (90% glycerol–10% [wt/vol] PBS), and a coverslip is applied and sealed with nail polish.

8. The slide is observed for islet cell-specific fluorescence under a fluorescence microscope fitted with a 20× epi-illumination objective.

9. All samples with detectable ICA are titrated by retesting the serum in serial dilution. The endpoint titer is compared with the 80-JDF unit international standard used by the IDS workshops.

Standardization, Quality Control, and Quality Assurance

1. To determine the appropriate dilution of fluorescein-antibody conjugate, a known negative serum sample, a weakly positive serum sample, and a strongly positive serum sample need to be tested with various dilutions of conjugate; the optimal dilution is the highest dilution that gives the strongest specific islet cell reaction with a lower nonspecific staining.

2. A standardization procedure should be applied for each new lot of pancreas by serially diluting the 80-JDF unit standard in both negative sera and PBS. A five-point curve of standard diluted in negative serum versus standard diluted in PBS should be linear, and JDF units are calculated from this curve by interpolation of patient serum endpoint titer in PBS.

3. Strongly positive, weakly positive, and negative control samples should be included in each assay. A known positive serum sample is recommended for storage in aliquots and testing every 3 months to monitor assay drift. The ICA assay, including quality control samples, should be analyzed with the reader blinded to the sample identity.

Biochemically Defined Autoantibody Radioassay

Sample Requirements

We recommend that the serum be obtained from red top or tiger top (separator) blood collecting tubes and be hemolysis and lipemia free. Only 5 µl of serum is required to measure both GAA and ICA512AA, and 12 µl of serum is required for micro-IAA (mIAA). The method we utilize measures GAA and ICA512AA (IA-2AA) simultaneously.

Materials, Reagents, and Equipment

Human GAD65 cDNA clone

Human ICA512 (IA-2) cDNA clone. The two most utilized clones are IA-2ic (intracytoplasmic IA-2) and ICA512BDC (clone lacking exon 13 [transmembrane] domain of IA-2).

TNT Sp6 coupled in vitro translation kit (Promega)

RNasin RNase inhibitor (Promega)

[³⁵S]methionine (GE Health Care)

[³H]leucine (GE Health Care)

¹²⁵I-insulin (GE Health Care)

Protein A-Sepharose Fast Flow (GE Health Care)

Protein G-Sepharose Fast Flow (GE Health Care)

NAP-5 column (GE Health Care)

48-well PCR plate (Fisher)

96-well filtration plates (Fisher)

Bottle-top 500-ml filter units (Fisher)

TopSeal (Perkin-Elmer)

MicroScint-20 (Perkin-Elmer)

TopCount beta counter (Perkin-Elmer)

Vacuum-operated 96-well plate washer (Millipore)

96-well plate shaker (Wallac-Delfi)

GAA and ICA512AA Assay

General Principle

Labeled GAD65 and ICA512 are produced by in vitro transcription/translation with differential labeling (³H-GAD65 and ³⁵S-ICA512). The patient serum is incubated with the labeled antigens together overnight, and antibody-bound labeled antigens are separated from unbound labeled antigens with protein A-Sepharose precipitation in a 96-well plate. Radioactivity is counted on a 96-well plate beta counter. Emission spectra of ^{35}S and ^{3}H partially overlap and can be corrected, allowing simultaneous measurement of antibodies against the two antigens. Results are expressed as standard World Health Organization (WHO) units as in DASP workshops and are described in detail in the procedure below. Many laboratories are currently still using their own index that adjusts the counts per minute of the test serum for the counts per minute of positive and negative control sera in each assay with the following formula: (cpm of the test serum – cpm of the negative serum)/(cpm of positive serum – cpm of the negative serum), where cpm is counts per minute. A cutoff for positivity above the 99th percentile of normal controls is often utilized.

Procedure

Part I: In vitro transcription/translation to produce labeled GAD65 and ICA512 (IA-2)

IMPORTANT NOTES. All reagents, tubes, and tips must be RNase free. All reagents should be kept on ice while on the bench. An incubation temperature of 30°C is critical for production efficiency. The reticulocyte lysate must be stored at −80°C and thawed rapidly just before use. Each tube can be thawed only twice, after which there will be a significant decrease in its efficiency.

PROCEDURE

1. Follow the kit protocol for one-step in vitro transcription/translation. The total reaction volume can be adjusted (decreased or increased) as needed.
2. Purify the labeled product with the NAP-5 column.
3. Analyze the activity of labeled antigen by trichloroacetic acid precipitation as described in the kit protocol. The labeling efficiency significantly varies with different cDNAs and plasmids.

Part II: Radioassay (2 days)

DAY 1

1. Prepare antigen-buffer solution: With the optimized condition, 20,000 cpm in 50 µl of buffer is usually applied per well. For a 96-well plate with 25% extra volume to ensure enough volume for aliquoting into each well, the total counts per minute is $96 \times 20,000$ cpm $\times 125\%$, i.e., 2.4×10^6 cpm for both ^{3}H-GAD65 and ^{35}S-ICA512; the total volume is 96×50 µl $\times 125\%$, i.e., 6 ml.
2. Prepare the serial dilution of a calibrated standard serum with known WHO unit. The calibrated standard sera with known WHO units in serial dilution are available from the Centers for Disease Control and Prevention and many laboratories. We recommend a standard curve covering a wide range of antibody levels with calibrated standard serum in each assay.
3. Incubation of serum with antigen-buffer: One well per serum sample will be used for incubation and then split into two wells during precipitation with protein A-Sepharose. Add 5 µl of serum and 125 µl of antigen-assay buffer (150 mM NaCl, 20 mM Tris-HCl, 0.1% BSA, and 0.1% sodium azide, pH 7.4) containing both ^{3}H-GAD65 and ^{35}S-ICA512 into a 48-well PCR plate and incubate overnight at 4°C. The standard positive control and negative control serum samples for both GAA and ICA512AA must be included in each

assay, and only one corresponding labeled antigen is added into these control wells, from which the spill rates of ^{3}H and ^{35}S into two windows of the beta counter will be obtained.

4. Preparation of 96-well filtration plates: Coat the plate with BSA by adding 200 µl of assay buffer to each well, put the plate on aluminum foil, and incubate overnight at room temperature.
5. Preparation of protein A-Sepharose: Use only plastic tubes because the protein A sticks to glass. Pull 20 ml of protein A-Sepharose into a 50-ml tube, spin the solution down at 1,500 rpm for 3 min, remove the fluid phase, and resuspend into assay buffer. Repeat this twice and make a final 50% (vol/vol) solution of protein A-Sepharose assay buffer.

DAY 2

1. Remove the assay buffer from the 96-well filtration plate and add 25 µl of well-mixed 50% protein A-Sepharose to each well.
2. Transfer 50 µl from each well of the overnight incubation to two wells on the 96-well filtration plate, and shake the plate on a plate shaker at low speed for 45 min at 4°C.
3. Place the plate on a vacuum plate washer and wash the plate three times with 200 µl of assay buffer per well each time. Then remove the plate, add 100 µl of assay buffer per well, and shake the plate for at least 5 min at 4°C.
4. Wash the plate two more times with 200 µl of assay buffer per well each time, change the plate orientation, and wash the plate another two times.
5. Blot the plate on a paper towel and place the plate under a lamp for around 15 min. After drying, add 30 µl of scintillation liquid (MicroScint-20) to each well, seal the plate with a piece of TopSeal, and count the plate on a TopCount beta counter with window A set at 2.9 to 10 for ^{3}H and window B set at 10 to 256 for ^{35}S.
6. Obtain the counts-per-minute distribution of ^{3}H and ^{35}S in windows A and B from positive control wells in which only one corresponding labeled antigen was added. Correct the spill rate and calculate the ^{3}H and ^{35}S counts per minute for each sample well.
7. Calculate the index with the following formula: (cpm of the test serum – cpm of the negative serum) / (cpm of positive serum – cpm of the negative serum).
8. Calculate WHO units: Using the counts per minute from the serial dilution (seven to nine points) of a calibrated standard serum with known WHO units, plot a chart with $\log_2$ (WHO units) versus counts per minute in Excel as in Fig. 12. With the curve formula, $\log_2$ units can be calculated for each test sample by replacing "x" in the formula with the counts per minute of the test sample and then converting $\log_2$ units into WHO units by anti-$\log_2$ (power 2).

Standardization, Quality Control, and Quality Assurance

1. The laboratory should keep enough volume of the calibrated standard sera and positive and negative control sera for long-term use. Each of these serum samples should be aliquoted and stored at −20°C.
2. All the assays are run in duplicate, with a standard curve for WHO unit calculation and including positive and negative control samples for quality control and for lab index calculation. In our assay, GAA positivity is any value greater than index 0.032 and ICA512AA value greater than 0.049.
3. The results of analysis of negative and positive controls should be monitored to detect drift and evaluate assay

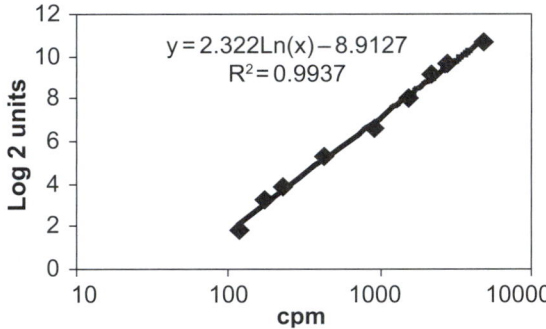

FIGURE 12 Standard curve for calculation of WHO units. The *x* axis shows the counts per minute from the assay after removing the background counts per minute, and the *y* axis shows known $\log_2$ WHO units.

performance. Our positive control range for both GAA and ICA512 is an index of 1.0 (±25%) (0.75 to 1.25). The negative control must be less than the 99th percentile of normal controls for the assay results to be valid (e.g., <0.032 [GAD65Ab] or <0.05 [ICA512] for our assay and index standards).

4. Every positive sample in the first assay is confirmed by retesting that sample in a different assay. If the confirmatory assay result is negative, a third run is performed. We utilize the results of two assays which agree (negative and negative or positive and positive) for the determination of a positive or negative result.

mIAA Assay

General Principle

The mIAA assay is a competitive radioassay. The patient serum is incubated with ^{125}I-insulin with and without cold human insulin overnight, and antibody-bound labeled antigens are separated from unbound labeled antigens with protein A/G-Sepharose precipitation in a 96-well plate. Radioactivity is counted directly on a 96-well plate beta counter for the β emission of ^{125}I. The levels are expressed as index that adjusts the delta counts per minute of the test serum for the delta counts per minute of positive and negative control sera in a particular assay. A WHO unit is not available for IAA at present.

Procedure (2 Days)

Day 1

1. Prepare ^{125}I-insulin-buffer solution with and without cold human insulin: Use 1 ml of 5% BSA in PBS to dissolve the powder of 10 μCi of ^{125}I-insulin as stock solution. We utilize 20,000 cpm in 30 μl of buffer per well. For a 96-well plate with 10% extra to ensure enough volume for aliquoting into each well, the total counts per minute is $96 \times 20,000$ cpm $\times$ 110%, i.e., 2.1×10^6 cpm, which is equal to 160 μl of ^{125}I-insulin stock solution; the total volume is $96 \times 30\,\mu l \times 110\%$, i.e., 3.2 ml, which needs to be divided in half (half with and half without cold human insulin [100 U/ml]) as follows:

1,520 μl of buffer 1	1,392 μl of buffer 1
80 μl of ^{125}I-insulin	80 μl of ^{125}I-insulin
1.6 ml	128 μl of cold insulin
	1.6 ml

2. Incubation of serum with antigen buffer: Four wells per serum sample are used for both competition and noncompetition in duplicate. Add 6 μl of serum and 30 μl of antigen assay buffer (150 mM NaCl, 20 mM Tris-HCl, 1% BSA, and 0.1% sodium azide, pH 7.4) to a 96-well PCR plate, mix well, keep at room temperature for 2 h, and then incubate overnight at 4°C. The index positive control and negative control serum samples must be included in each assay.

3. Preparation of 96-well filtration plates: Coat the plate with BSA by adding 200 μl of assay buffer to each well, put the plate on an aluminum foil sheet, and incubate overnight at room temperature.

4. Preparation of protein A/G-Sepharose: Use only plastic tubes because proteins A and G stick to glass. Pull 20 ml of protein A-Sepharose and 5 ml of protein G-Sepharose into two 50-ml tubes, spin the solution down at 1,500 rpm for 3 min, remove the fluid phase, and resuspend into assay buffer. Repeat this twice and make a final 62.5% (vol/vol) solution for protein A-Sepharose with assay buffer and a 40% (vol/vol) solution for protein G-Sepharose. Mix 4 parts protein A-Sepharose solution with 1 part protein G-Sepharose solution to form a final working solution with 50% (vol/vol) protein A-Sepharose and 8% protein G-Sepharose.

Day 2

1. Remove the assay buffer from the 96-well filtration plate and add 50 μl of well-mixed protein A/G-Sepharose to each well.

2. Transfer 30 μl from each well of the overnight incubation to a corresponding well on the 96-well filtration plate, and shake the plate on a plate shaker at low speed for 45 min at 4°C.

3. Place the plate on a vacuum plate washer and wash the plate three times with 200 μl of washing buffer (150 mM NaCl, 20 mM Tris-HCl, 0.1% BSA, and 0.1% sodium azide, pH 7.4) per well each time. Then remove the plate, add 100 μl of assay buffer per well, and shake the plate for at least 5 min at 4°C.

4. Wash the plate two more times with 200 μl of assay buffer per well each time, change the plate orientation, and wash the plate another two times.

5. Blot the plate on a paper towel and place the plate under a lamp for around 15 min. After drying, add 50 μl of scintillation liquid (MicroScint-20) to each well, seal the plate with a piece of TopSeal, and count the plate on a TopCount beta counter.

6. Calculate the index with the following formula: (Δcpm of test sample − Δcpm of negative control) / (Δcpm of negative control − Δcpm of negative control).

Standardization, Quality Control, and Quality Assurance

1. The laboratory should keep enough volume of the positive and negative control sera for long-term use. Each of these serum samples should be aliquoted and stored at −20°C.

2. All of the assays are run in duplicate and must include positive and negative control samples. In our assay, mIAA positivity is any value greater than index 0.010, the 99th percentile of normal controls.

3. The results of controls should be monitored to detect drift and general assay performance. In addition to the index of positive and negative control samples, a pair of standard positive and negative serum samples were included in each assay in our laboratory. The standard positive serum is at

very low level of mIAA. The acceptable standard low positive control range is an index of 0.02 to 0.08 for our low-positive standard. The negative control must be <0.01 for results of the assay run to be utilized.

4. Every positive sample in the first run is confirmed by retesting that sample in a different assay. If the confirmatory assay comes out negative, a third assay is necessary. The results of two assays which agree (positive and positive or negative and negative) will be the final determination of positivity or negativity.

New Technology

ELISA

For most autoimmune disorders and for basic immunologic research, ELISAs employing plate-bound antigen are popular. Many laboratories and biotech companies have adopted this method for anti-islet autoantibody assays, and different ELISA kits are available. Multiple workshops utilizing sera from patients with type 1 diabetes and multiple mouse strains have demonstrated that standard ELISA formats lack both sensitivity and specificity compared to fluid-phase radioassay formats. For IAA, the ELISA formats were able to detect high-capacity antibodies following insulin immunization (e.g., therapy with subcutaneous injections of human insulin), but not the IAA of prediabetic individuals. To date in international workshops only one ELISA kit for GAA has attained a level of specificity and sensitivity equivalent to those of the radioassay. This assay depends on using a free antibody arm to capture biotinylated GAD (developed by Kronus and published in May of 2003 [30]). In brief, the ELISA plate was coated with GAD65 protein, and 25 μl of test serum was added for incubation with shaking for 1 h at room temperature. The wells were then washed three times with washing buffer, and 100 μl of biotinylated GAD65 was added. After a further 1-h incubation, the plate wells were washed three times and incubated for 20 min with 100 μl of streptavidin peroxidase conjugate. A wash step was then followed by addition of 100 μl of tetramethylbenzidine and, after 20 min, 100 μl of 0.5-mol/liter H_2SO_4 and measurement of absorbance at 405 and 450 nm. This "ELISA" is actually a form of fluid-phase reaction of labeled antigen with bound autoantibody with specificity enhanced by the requirement for each arm of the immunoglobulin to react with antigen.

Epitope Assays

Comparisons of the epitope repertoires of autoantibodies to insulin, GAD65 and ICA512, provide a tool to further analyze type 1 diabetes-related autoantibodies (23, 35, 47). Most sera from type 1 diabetes patients only target GAD65 protein epitopes dependent on protein conformation and do not bind GAD65 protein fragments or react with denatured GAD65 protein with immunoblotting. In contrast, sera from patients with stiff man syndrome have antibodies that bind GAD65 protein fragments consisting of N-terminal, middle, and C-terminal regions. The majority of sera from type 1 diabetes patients target more than two epitopes on ICA512 molecules, while non-disease-related antibodies usually react with only one epitope. For the methodology of these epitope assays, laboratories usually use the same radioimmunoassay format as described above with cloned protein fragments containing the epitope to be utilized or with a chimerical protein (e.g., GAD65/GAD67, which contains epitopes of GAD65 and sequences of non-antibody-reactive GAD67 to retain protein conformation). For IAA epitope

testing, proinsulin, insulin analogs, and insulin molecules from different spices are used as competitive inhibitors in the regular IAA radioassay.

Autoantibody Subclass and Isotype Determination

There were some reports that there is heterogeneity of immunoglobulin subclass antibodies to GAD65 in newly diagnosed type 1A diabetic patients and ICA-positive first-degree relatives who progressed or did not progress to diabetes (32). New-onset diabetics and progressors were found to have a predominance of IgG1, GAA, and ICA, while nonprogressors had predominantly IgG2 and/or IgG4. A recent study on IAA also indicated that heterogeneity of IgG subclass is related to the risk of developing type 1A diabetes (24).

For the methodology of isotype analysis, a modified standard radioimmunoassay format is used. On day 1, prepare reagent and serum mixtures for overnight incubation at 4°C in two separate tubes. In one tube, incubate 2.5 μl of serum with 25 μl of radiolabeled antigen; in the other tube, incubate 5 μl of biotin-labeled anti-IgG subclass monoclonal antibody with 10 μl of streptavidin-Sepharose (BD Pharmingen), with shaking. On day 2, after washing the Sepharose incubation tube three times, mix two incubations together in a 96-well filtration plate and incubate for 1 h at 4°C, with shaking. The rest of the steps for washing and counting are the same as described above.

Interpretation

Analysis of Data

In general it is important to utilize assays for anti-islet autoimmunity that have high specificity, usually defined as a specificity of ≥99%. Even with specificities set at this level, if one is measuring three different anti-islet autoantibodies, 3% of the "normal" population will be found to express one or more of the autoantibodies. Obviously expression of multiple anti-islet autoantibodies is a relatively rare event, though even here for low-risk populations (1/300 children, for instance, in the United States develop type 1 diabetes) there will be some individuals expressing anti-islet autoantibodies who may never progress to overt diabetes. As with all autoantibody tests it is also important to recognize that for low values, particularly for levels just above the cutoff points for defined "positivity," a repeat assay of the same sample (particularly for low-risk populations) may fail to confirm the presence of the autoantibody as often as one-third of the time (27). Repeat analysis of an independent sample is important for assessing risk, as subjects with "transient" islet autoantibodies are at relatively low risk. After the onset of type 1A diabetes a significant subset of patients lose (over decades) their GAD65 and ICA512 anti-islet autoantibodies.

A major caveat is that insulin antibodies appear in most individuals treated with subcutaneous insulin (even human insulin). Thus, after approximately 10 days of insulin therapy, the presence of insulin antibodies (which cannot be distinguished from autoantibodies with current assays) cannot be used to diagnose type 1A diabetes.

Clinical Application

Anti-islet autoantibodies find their primary application in the differential diagnosis of the forms of diabetes and in predicting risk of progression to overt diabetes.

It is clear that adults presenting with diabetes who express anti-islet autoantibodies (in particular GAD65 autoantibodies) more rapidly progress to utilization of insulin compared to typical patients with type 2 diabetes (43). Such adults with "type 1A" diabetes are termed LADA patients (for latent autoimmune diabetes of adults). In a similar manner, a significant number of obese children presenting with diabetes do not have anti-islet autoantibodies and appear to have forms of type 2 diabetes (41), and it is likely that this will become an increasingly common problem. For many endocrinologists, having the diagnosis, for example, of atypical type 1A diabetes (e.g., LADA) leads to the immediate initiation of insulin therapy rather than a trial of oral hypoglycemic agents. For children with presumed type 2 diabetes who lack all anti-islet autoantibodies and have evidence of insulin resistance, there are trials evaluating oral medications such as metformin. In addition, a diagnosis of type 1A diabetes alerts one to the risk of accompanying autoimmune disorders (e.g., thyroid autoimmunity in 1/4, celiac disease in 1/20, and Addison's disease in approximately 1/200). Relatives who are being evaluated for renal donation to a patient with type 1A diabetes may express anti-islet autoantibodies, and knowledge of increased diabetes risk may influence donor considerations. In addition, young children expressing anti-islet autoantibodies should be carefully monitored for metabolic abnormalities (e.g., glucose determination at 3-month intervals), as early diagnosis of diabetes can prevent hospitalization with ketoacidosis.

REFERENCES

CHRONIC THYROIDITIS, ADDISON'S DISEASE, AND PERNICIOUS ANEMIA

1. **Beaune, P., D. Pessayre, P. Dansette, D. Mansuy, and M. Manns.** 1994. Autoantibodies against cytochromes P450: role in human diseases. *Adv. Pharmacol.* **30:**199–245.
2. **Betterle, C., G. Coco, and R. Zanchetta.** 2005. Adrenal cortex autoantibodies in subjects with normal adrenal function. *Best Pract. Res. Clin. Endocrinol. Metab.* **19:**85–99.
3. **Bigazzi, P. E., C. L. Burek, and N. R. Rose.** 1992. Antibodies to tissue-specific, endocrine, gastrointestinal, and surface-receptor antigens, p. 765–774. *In* N. R. Rose, E. Conway de Macario, J. L. Fahey, H. Friedman, and G. M. Penn (ed.), *Manual of Clinical Laboratory Immunology*, 4th ed. American Society for Microbiology, Washington, D.C.
4. **Bresler, H. S., C. L. Burek, W. H. Hoffman, and N. Rose.** 1990. Autoantigenic determinants on human thyroglobulin. II. Determinants recognized by autoantibodies from patients with chronic autoimmune thyroiditis compared to healthy subjects. *Clin. Immunol. Immunopathol.* **54:**76–86.
5. **Burek, C. L., and N. R. Rose.** 1996. Thyroglobulin antibodies, p. 810–815. *In* J. B. Peter and Y. Shoenfeld (ed.), *Autoantibodies.* Elsevier, Amsterdam, The Netherlands.
6. **Czarnocka, B., J. Ruf, M. Ferrand, P. Carayon, and S. Lissitzky.** 1985. Purification of the human thyroid peroxidase and its identification as the microsomal antigen involved in autoimmune thyroid diseases. *FEBS Lett.* **190:**147–152.
7. **Gleeson, P. A., I. R. van Driel, and B. Toh.** 1996. Parietal cell autoantibodies, p. 600–606. *In* J. B. Peter and Y. Shoenfeld (ed.), *Autoantibodies.* Elsevier, Amsterdam, The Netherlands.
8. **Lazarus, J. H.** 1998. Prediction of postpartum thyroiditis. *Eur. J. Endocrinol.* **139:**12–13.
9. **Rapoport, B., and S. M. McLachlan.** 1996. Thyroid peroxidase autoantibodies, p. 816–821. *In* J. B. Peter and Y. Shoenfeld (ed.), *Autoantibodies.* Elsevier, Amsterdam, The Netherlands.
10. **Toh, B. H., and F. Alderuccio.** 2004. Pernicious anaemia. *Autoimmunity* **37:**357–361.
11. **Weetman, A. P.** 1995. Autoimmunity to steroid-producing cells and familial polyendocrine autoimmunity. *Bailliere's Clin. Endocrinol. Metabol.* **9:**157–174.

HYPERTHYROIDISM OF GRAVES' DISEASE AND ANTIBODIES TO THE THYROTROPIN RECEPTOR

12. **Chazenbalk, G. D., F. Latrofa, S. M. McLachlan, and B. Rapoport.** 2004. Thyroid stimulation does not require antibodies with identical epitopes but does involve recognition of a critical conformation at the N terminus of the thyrotropin receptor A-subunit. *J. Clin. Endocrinol. Metab.* **89:**1788–1793.
13. **Di Cerbo, A., R. Di Paola, C. Menzaghi, V. De Filippis, K. Tahara, D. Corda, and L. D. Kohn.** 1999. Graves' immunoglobulins activate phospholipase A2 by recognizing specific epitopes on the thyrotropin receptor. *J. Clin. Endocrinol. Metab.* **84:**3283–3292.
14. **Kosugi, S., T. Ban, T. Akamizu, W. Valente, and L. D. Kohn.** 1993. Use of thyrotropin receptor (TSHR) mutants to detect stimulating TSHR antibodies in hypothyroid patients with idiopathic myxedema, who have blocking TSHR antibodies. *J. Clin. Endocrinol. Metab.* **77:**19–24.
15. **McKenzie, J. M., and M. Zakarija.** 1995. Hyperthyroidism, p. 676–711. *In* L. J. DeGroot et al. (ed.), *Endocrinology*, 3rd ed., vol. 1. The W. B. Saunders Co., Philadelphia, Pa.
16. **McKenzie, J. M., and M. Zakarija.** 1996. Antibodies in autoimmune thyroid disease, p. 416–432. *In* L. E. Braverman and R. D. Utiger (ed.), *Werner and Ingbar's The Thyroid*, 7th ed. J. B. Lippincott Co., Philadelphia, Pa.
17. **Nagayama, Y., and B. Rapoport.** 1992. Thyroid stimulatory autoantibodies in different patients with autoimmune thyroid disease do not all recognize the same components of the human thyrotropin receptor: selective role of receptor amino acids Ser25-Glu30. *J. Clin. Endocrinol. Metab.* **75:**1425–1430.
18. **Rapoport, B., and S. M. McLachlan.** 2001. Thyroid autoimmunity. *J. Clin. Investig.* **108:**1253–1259.
19. **Sanders, J., J. Jeffreys, H. Depraetere, M. Evans, T. Richards, A. Kiddie, K. Brereton, L. D. K. E. Premawardhana, D. Y. Chirgadze, R. Nunez Miguel, T. L. Blundell, J. Furmaniak, and B. Rees Smith.** 2004. Characteristics of a human monoclonal autoantibody to the thyrotropin receptor: sequence structure and function. *Thyroid* **14:**560–570.
20. **Tonacchera, M., P. Agretti, A. Pinchera, V. Resellini, A. Perri, P. Collecchi, P. Vitti, and L. Chiovato.** 2000. Congenital hypothyroidism with impaired thyroid response to thyrotropin (TSH) and absent circulating thyroglobulin: evidence for a new inactivating mutation of the TSH receptor gene. *J. Clin. Endocrinol. Metab.* **85:**1001–1008.
21. **Van Sande, J., J. Parma, M. Tonacchera, S. Swillens, J. Dumont, and G. Vassart.** 1995. Genetic basis of endocrine disease. Somatic and germline mutations of the TSH receptor gene in thyroid disease. *J. Clin. Endocrinol. Metab.* **80:**2577–2585.
22. **Vassart, G., J. Parma, J. Van Sande, and J. E. Dumont.** 1994. The thyrotropin receptor and the regulation of thyrocyte function and growth: update 1994. *Endocrine Rev. Monogr.* **3:**77–80.

PANCREAS

23. **Achenbach, P., K. Koczwara, A. Knopff, H. Naserke, A. G. Ziegler, and E. Bonifacio.** 2004. Mature high-affinity immune responses to (pro)insulin anticipate the autoimmune cascade that leads to type 1 diabetes. *J. Clin. Investig.* **114:**589–597.
24. **Achenbach, P., K. Warncke, J. Reiter, H. E. Naserke, A. J. Williams, P. J. Bingley, E. Bonifacio, and A. G. Ziegler.** 2004. Stratification of type 1 diabetes risk on the

basis of islet autoantibody characteristics. *Diabetes* **53:** 384–392.

25. **American Diabetes Association.** 2004. Diagnosis and classification of diabetes mellitus. *Diabetes Care* **27** (Suppl. 1): S5–S10.

26. **Baekkeskov, S., H. J. Aanstoot, S. Christgau, A. Reetz, M. Solimena, M. Cascalho, F. Folli, H. Richter-Olesen, and P. De Camilli.** 1990. Identification of the 64K autoantigen in insulin-dependent diabetes as the GABA-synthesizing enzyme glutamic acid decarboxylase. *Nature* **347:**151–156.

27. **Barker, J. M., et al.** 2004. Prediction of autoantibody positivity and progression to type 1 diabetes: Diabetes Autoimmunity Study in the Young (DAISY). *J. Clin. Endocrinol. Metab.* **89:**3896–3902.

28. **Bleich, D., M. Polak, S. Chen, K. M. Swiderek, and C. Levy-Marchal.** 1999. Sera from children with type 1 diabetes mellitus react against a new group of antigens composed of lysophospholipids. *Horm. Res.* **52:**86–94.

29. **Bottazzo, G. F., A. Florin-Christensen, and D. Doniach.** 1974. Islet-cell antibodies in diabetes mellitus with autoimmune polyendocrine deficiencies. *Lancet* **ii:**1279–1283.

30. **Brooking, H., R. Ananieva-Jordanova, C. Arnold, M. Amoroso, M. Powell, C. Betterle, R. Zanchetta, J. Furmaniak, and B. R. Smith.** 2003. A sensitive nonisotopic assay for GAD65 autoantibodies. *Clin. Chim. Acta* **331:**55–59.

31. **Colman, P. G., R. C. Nayak, I. L. Campbell, and G. S. Eisenbarth.** 1988. Binding of cytoplasmic islet cell antibodies is blocked by human pancreatic glycolipid extracts. *Diabetes* **37:**645–652.

32. **Couper, J. J., L. C. Harrison, J. J. E. Aldis, P. G. Colman, M. C. Honeyman, and A. Ferrante.** 1998. IgG subclass antibodies to glutamic acid decarboxylase and risk for progression to clinical insulin-dependent diabetes. *Hum. Immunol.* **59:**493–499.

33. **Daw, K., N. Ujihara, M. Atkinson, and A. C. Powers.** 1996. Glutamic acid decarboxylase autoantibodies in stiff-man syndrome and insulin-dependent diabetes mellitus exhibit similarities and differences in epitope recognition. *J. Immunol.* **156:**818–825.

34. **Eisenbarth, G. S., R. Gianani, L. Yu, M. Pietropaolo, C. F. Verge, H. P. Chase, M. J. Redondo, P. Colman, L. Harrison, and R. Jackson.** 1998. Dual-parameter model for prediction of type I diabetes mellitus. *Proc. Assoc. Am. Physicians* **110:**126–135.

35. **Hagopian, W. A., B. Michelsen, A. E. Karlsen, F. Larsen, A. Moody, C. E. Grubin, R. Rowe, J. Petersen, R. McEvoy, and A. Lernmark.** 1993. Autoantibodies in IDDM primarily recognize the 65,000-M(r) rather than the 67,000-M(r) isoform of glutamic acid decarboxylase. *Diabetes* **42:**631–636.

36. **Lendrum, R., G. Walker, and D. R. Gamble.** 1975. Islet-cell antibodies in juvenile diabetes mellitus of recent onset. *Lancet* **i:**880–882.

37. **Maclaren, N., S. Huang, and J. Fogh.** 1975. Antibody to cultured human insulinoma cells in insulin-dependent diabetes. *Lancet* **i:**997–1000.

38. **Notkins, A. L., J. Lu, Q. Li, F. P. Vander Vegt, C. Wasserfall, N. K. Maclaren, and M. S. Lan.** 1996. IA-2 and IA-2 beta are major autoantigens in IDDM and the precursors of the 40 kDa and 37 kDa tryptic fragments. *J. Autoimmun.* **9:**677–682.

39. **Palmer, J. P., C. M. Asplin, P. Clemons, K. Lyen, O. Tatpati, P. K. Raghu, and T. L. Paquette.** 1983. Insulin antibodies in insulin-dependent diabetics before insulin treatment. *Science* **222:**1337–1339.

40. **Park, Y. S., E. Kawasaki, K. Kelemen, L. Yu, M. Schillers, M. Rewers, M. Mizuta, G. S. Eisenbarth, and J. C. Hutton.** 2000. Humoral autoreactivity to an alternatively spliced variant of ICA512/IA-2 in type 1 diabetes. *Diabetologia* **43:**1293–1301.

41. **Pinhas-Hamiel, O., and P. Zeitler.** 1998. Type 2 diabetes in adolescents, no longer rare. *Pediatr. Rev.* **19:**434–435.

42. **Rabin, D. U., S. M. Pleasic, J. A. Shapiro, H. Yoo-Warren, J. Oles, J. M. Hicks, D. E. Goldstein, and P. M. M. Rae.** 1994. Islet cell antigen 512 is a diabetes-specific islet autoantigen related to protein tyrosine phosphatases. *J. Immunol.* **152:**3183–3188.

43. **Turner, R., et al., for the UK Prospective Diabetes Study Group.** 1997. UKPDS 25: autoantibodies to islet-cell cytoplasm and glutamic acid decarboxylase for prediction of insulin requirement in type 2 diabetes. *Lancet* **350:**1288–1293.

44. **Uchigata, Y., S. Kuwata, T. Tsushima, K. Tokunaga, M. Miyamoto, K. Tsuchikawa, Y. Hirata, T. Juji, and Y. Omori.** 1993. Patients with Graves' disease who developed insulin autoimmune syndrome (Hirata disease) possess HLA-Bw62/Cw4/DR4 carrying DRB1*0406. *J. Clin. Endocrinol. Metab.* **77:**249–254.

45. **Verge, C. F., R. Gianani, E. Kawasaki, L. Yu, M. Pietropaolo, R. A. Jackson, H. P. Chase, and G. S. Eisenbarth.** 1996. Prediction of type 1 diabetes in first-degree relatives using a combination of insulin, GAD, and ICA512bdc/IA-2 autoantibodies. *Diabetes* **45:**926–933.

46. **Yu, L., D. T. Robles, N. Abiru, P. Kaur, M. Rewers, K. Kelemen, and G. S. Eisenbarth.** 2000. Early expression of antiinsulin autoantibodies of humans and the NOD mouse: evidence for early determination of subsequent diabetes. *Proc. Natl. Acad. Sci. USA* **97:**1701–1706.

47. **Ziegler, A. G., M. Hummel, M. Schenker, and E. Bonifacio.** 1999. Autoantibody appearance and risk for development of childhood diabetes in offspring of parents with type 1 diabetes. The 2-year analysis of the German BABYDIAB study. *Diabetes* **48:**460–468.

Autoantibodies to Glycolipids in Peripheral Neuropathy

HUGH J. WILLISON

121

Peripheral neuropathies constitute a diverse group of diseases caused by a wide range of genetic, toxic, metabolic, and inflammatory insults to the peripheral nervous system. A considerable proportion of neuropathies are believed to have an autoimmune basis, either as a feature of systemic autoimmune diseases, vasculitides, paraneoplastic or postinfectious syndromes, in association with lymphoproliferative diseases, or as isolated peripheral nerve syndromes. In clinical practice, the cause of sporadic neuropathies is often obscure, resulting in the frequent use of multiple screening tests to aid in diagnosis. Over the last 15 years, there has been a widespread increase in the use of antiganglioside antibody assays as diagnostic tools, based on the recognition from research studies that gangliosides are important autoantigens in many patients with autoimmune peripheral nerve disorders (20).

Early progess in this field stemmed from the discovery that immunoglobulin M (IgM) paraproteins with anti-myelin-associated glycoprotein (anti-MAG) activity present in patients with IgM paraproteinemic neuropathy also reacted with carbohydrate epitopes on a sulfated glucuronic acid-containing glycosphingolipid termed sulfated glucuronyl paragloboside (SGPG) (10). Further studies soon showed that cases of IgM paraproteinemic neuropathy that were anti-MAG or anti-SGPG antibody negative often had antibodies reactive with various other glycolipid and ganglioside antigens. Anti-GM1 ganglioside IgM antibodies were then found in a large proportion of patients with a syndrome termed multifocal motor neuropathy (MMN), thereby catalyzing a vast body of clinical research into the association between anti-GM1 antibodies and other motor nerve syndromes (12). At the same time, interest centered on identifying antiganglioside antibodies in Guillain-Barré syndrome (GBS) and its variant forms, including Miller-Fisher syndrome (MFS) (3, 5), an area of research that remains highly topical.

Both preceding and in parallel with this evolving field of neuropathy research and clinical practice, antiganglioside and antiglycolipid antibodies have also been reported in a vast range of other diseases and syndromes, as well as for persons of normal health (8, 11). Antiglycolipid antibodies are viewed as forming an important part of the natural autoantibody repertoire directed towards microbial carbohydrate structures, which has the potential to be expanded in both specific and nonspecific ways. This may explain their ubiquitous presence in both healthy and diseased patient populations and may account for some of the misleading studies that have claimed disease-specific associations, further confounded by technical difficulties in their measurement. This chapter only addresses their relationship to autoimmune neuropathy, for which diagnostic testing is widespread.

Table 1 displays the main clinical syndromes in which a well-defined antiglycolipid antibody specificity has been identified. In patients with IgM paraproteinemic demyelinating neuropathy, paraproteins with anti-MAG activity also react with carbohydrate epitopes on SGPG and its higher lactosaminyl homologue SGLPG. Another paraproteinemic neuropathy syndrome is a chronic large fiber sensory neuropathy with prominent ataxia (18). The IgM paraprotein reacts with gangliosides bearing NeuNAc(α2-8)NeuNAc-linked disialosyl groups, including, but not limited to, GD3, GD1b, GT1a, GT1b, and GQ1b. The patients may also have cold agglutinin syndrome by virtue of the presence of sialylated glycan epitopes on human red blood cells with which the IgM paraproteins can cross-react. Ophthalmoplegia is also variably present in this syndrome.

In MMN with demyelinating conduction block, antibodies to GM1 ganglioside are present in about half of the cases (9). Patients with MMN and anti-GM1 antibodies are mostly male and have a clinical picture comprising a chronic asymmetric motor syndrome, usually with distal onset in an upper limb. The average age of onset is in the fourth decade and the illness runs an indolent course, with patients usually remaining ambulant and physically independent 10 to 20 years after onset. The electrophysiological examination classically shows focal motor conduction block, and intravenous human immunoglobulin is standard therapy.

A wide variety of antiganglioside and antiglycolipid antibodies have been reported in up to 50% of GBS cases in many series (4, 21). Antibodies against GM1, GD1a, GM1b, and GalNAc-GD1a mark a form of GBS with prominent motor axonal involvement, now called AMAN (acute motor axonal neuropathy). In MFS, an acute self-limiting variant of GBS comprising ataxia, areflexia, and ophthalmoplegia, anti-GQ1b and anti-GT1a IgG antibodies are present in over 90% of cases; the antibodies also react with GD1b and/or GD3 in about half the cases (3, 20).

As research into clinical-serological associations between neuropathy phenotypes and antiglycolipid antibodies

TABLE 1 Clinical syndromes associated with specific antiglycolipid autoantibodies

Clinical syndrome	Antibody specificity	Antibody isotype
Chronic sensorimotor demyelinating neuropathy	MAG, SGPG, SGLPG	IgM (monoclonal)
Chronic ataxic neuropathy	NeuNAc(α2-8)NeuNAc epitopes on GD1b, GD3 GQ1b, GT1b, GT1a, and GD2	IgM (monoclonal)
MMN	Gal(β1-3)GalNAc epitopes on GM1, GA1, and GD1b	IgM
Chronic motor neuropathy	GM2, GalNAc-GM1b, and GalNAc-GD1a	IgM
AMAN	GM1a, GM1b, GD1a, and GalNAc-GD1a	IgG
Demyelinating GBS	GalC, LM1, SGPG, GM1, and GM2	IgG
MFS	GQ1b, GT1a, GD3, and GD1b	IgG

evolves, it is likely that more requests for clinical testing will enter the diagnostic laboratory. The most commonly sought antibodies at present are to GM1 and GQ1b gangliosides.

METHODS

Sample Requirements

Antiganglioside antibodies are best measured in serum, although they can also be estimated in plasma. Cerebrospinal fluid may contain small amounts of antiganglioside antibody (filtered from the systemic circulation), but there is no evidence to indicate any local intrathecal synthesis of antibody, and measurement in cerebrospinal fluid has no advantage over measurement in serum. Serum antiganglioside antibodies are stable for short periods (i.e., days) at standard ambient temperature and can be stored at 4°C for 1 to 2 weeks without adverse effect. Interlaboratory shipping of serum can be conducted at ambient temperature. Repeated freeze-thawing prior to testing should be avoided. In chronic peripheral neuropathy syndromes, antiganglioside antibodies are usually IgM, occurring either as paraproteins (often monoclonal gammopathies of undetermined significance) or as polyclonal antibodies. Measurement can be performed at any stage of the clinical illness. In acute-onset, self-limiting neuropathies such as

GBS, the antiganglioside antibodies are usually IgG but may be IgM or IgA. They are at highest titer at clinical onset and then disappear over ensuing weeks or months and should therefore be sought immediately after clinical presentation, ideally before any therapeutic intervention. Plasma exchange or intravenous immunoglobulin therapy may substantially reduce or mask titers.

Materials and Reagents

Gangliosides are sialic acid-containing glycosphingolipids composed of a long-chain aliphatic amine, ceramide, attached to between one and five hexoses, at least one of which must be sialylated. It is the presence of a sialic acid molecule(s) attached to a galactose residue(s) in the hexose core which defines a glycosphingolipid as a ganglioside. In the human nervous system, the sialic acid is N-acetylneuraminic acid (NeuNAc). Common structures are shown in Table 2. Ganglioside nomenclature is according to that of Svennerholm (6), in which the prefix G refers to ganglio; M, D, T, and Q refer to the number of sialic acid molecules (mono, di, tri, and quad); and the Arabic numerals and lowercase letters refer to the order of migration of the gangliosides on thin-layer chromatograms (TLC).

Although total chemical or enzymatic synthesis of gangliosides is possible in specialized laboratories, most diagnostic laboratories purchase purified gangliosides from commercial

TABLE 2 Examples of clinically relevant ganglioside structures

Name	Carbohydrate sequence
GM1	Gal(β1-3)GalNAc(β1-4)Gal(β1-4)Glc(β1-1) ceramide (α2-3) NeuNAc
GD1a	Gal(β1-3)GalNAc(β1-4)Gal(β1-4)Glc(β1-1) ceramide (α2-3) (α2-3) NeuNAc NeuNAc
GD1b	Gal(β1-3)GalNAc(β1-4)Gal(β1-4)Glc(β1-1) ceramide (α2-3) NeuNAc (α2-8)
GQ1b	Gal(β1-3)GalNAc(β1-4)Gal(β1-4)Glc(β1-1) ceramide (α2-3) (α2-3) NeuNAc NeuNAc (α2-8) (α2-8) NeuNAc NeuNAc

sources or purify them from bovine brain. Chloroform-methanol extraction followed by DEAE-Sephadex chromatography is one of several commonly used procedures (14). Characterization is aided by chemical and enzymatic derivatization, TLC, and more sophisticated techniques such as fast atom bombardment mass spectrometry and high-performance liquid chromatography. The major gangliosides in brain are GM1, GD1a, GD1b, and GT1b, but there are also many minor gangliosides in both brain and peripheral nerve and in other tissues.

Gangliosides can be purchased from a wide variety of commercial sources. Rare gangliosides should be sought by personal requests to relevant investigators. Many preparations are only partially pure; for example, commercial preparations of GT1a and GT1b are often contaminated by significant amounts of GQ1b and vice versa. Care should be taken to control for this in nondiscriminatory immunoassays, such as enzyme-linked immunosorbent assays (ELISAs) or dot blots.

Antiganglioside autoantibodies are referred to by their specificity, either in terms of individual gangliosides (e.g., anti-GM1 IgG antibodies) or in terms of the reactive carbohydrate epitope [e.g., anti-Gal(β1-3)GalNAc IgM antibodies]. When generalizing, it is often more appropriate to use the term antiglycolipid antibodies (as opposed to antiganglioside antibodies), since many neuropathy-associated autoantibodies react with glycolipids which are not strictly gangliosides, such as SGPG, sulfatide, asialo-GM1, and galactocerebroside, as these molecules do not contain sialic acid.

The Current Procedure

Methodology for antibody detection presents difficulties, largely because the physical properties of gangliosides do not lend themselves well to development of uniform assays. Although antiganglioside antibodies can be detected by a variety of different methods, the principal and most commonly used screening method is ELISA (13, 19). A typical ELISA procedure is as follows.

1. Using a standard 96-well ELISA plate selected for high glycolipid binding properties (e.g., Immulon 2; Dynatech), coat each well of rows A, C, E, and G with 200 ng of GM1 or GQ1b in 100 μl of 100% ethanol and each well of rows B, D, F, and H with 100 μl of 100% ethanol alone by evaporation to dryness at room temperature, and then store at least overnight at 4°C. Coated plates are stable at 4°C for up to 2 weeks.

2. Block all 96 wells with 200 μl of phosphate-buffered saline–bovine serum albumin (PBS-BSA) (pH 7.4, 1% BSA) for 2 h at 4°C. Discard PBS-BSA by flicking or automated washing.

3. Prepare serum samples by mixing gently and then centrifuge out any fibrin or particulate debris. Dilute test serum to 1/100 in PBS–0.1% BSA, add in duplicate to ganglioside-coated and uncoated wells, and serially dilute from 1/100 to 1/500, 1/2,500, and 1/12,500.

4. Leave test serum to incubate overnight at 4°C.

5. Wash plate six times in PBS wash buffer cooled to 4°C, by dunking and flicking or using an automated washer.

6. Add 100 μl of peroxidase-conjugated anti-human IgM or IgG, diluted to 1/3,000 (dilution optimized by checkerboard analysis) in PBS–0.1% BSA. Incubate for 2 h at 4°C.

7. Wash plate six times in PBS wash buffer.

8. Develop plate by adding substrate solution comprising one 15-mg o-phenylenediamine tablet in 60 ml of citrate buffer with 20 μl of 30% hydrogen peroxide and letting it stand for 20 min.

9. Stop peroxidase reaction with 50 μl of 3 M H_2SO_4.

10. Read optical densities (ODs) in an automated plate reader at 490 nm.

11. Calculate titers by endpoint dilution analysis as follows.

    a. Subtract blank-well ODs from coated-well ODs to obtain working ODs.

    b. Obtain means of working ODs from duplicate wells.

    c. On semilog paper, plot linear ODs (x axis) against the log test serum dilution (y axis).

    d. Draw a best-fit dilution curve and assign the titer to the point at which the dilution curve crosses the OD at 0.1 unit.

There have been some attempts to recommend standard methodology, although most laboratories have established in-house protocols. In multicenter comparative studies there has been fair agreement on clearly positive or negative cases but variable results with borderline samples (22). Important factors in setting up the ELISA include (i) the choice of ELISA plates, including glycolipid binding properties, batch variations, and storage conditions (checks on individual batches of plates are made by using a positive serum sample and calculating the lowest coefficient of variance over the whole plate while giving an optimal signal); (ii) the temperature at which the assay is performed, including all incubation and washing steps, 4°C being most commonly recommended; (iii) the duration of serum incubation, which should be at least 4 h; and (iv) the presence or absence of Tween 20 as a detergent (gangliosides are soluble in detergent and will therefore be removed from the polystyrene plate). Assay results are usually reported as titers calculated by endpoint analysis.

In addition to ELISA, the TLC overlay technique is widely used (17). TLC overlay involves separating glycolipids on aluminum-backed silica plates in a solvent system and then performing an immunoverlay with serum and labeled antibodies. Although not readily amenable to quantitative titration, TLC overlay has the advantage of allowing unambiguous identification of a particular glycolipid and is thus considered the "gold standard" method. This is especially useful when specific glycolipids are not available in pure form. Dot blots are also widely used, but as with TLC, it is harder to obtain readily quantifiable data. A technically straightforward and rapid agglutination assay has recently been reported (2). Antibodies have been recently described that react with ganglioside complexes (7), and the important role of accessory lipids also needs consideration; however, these issues at present remain outside the scope of a routine diagnostic laboratory.

CONSIDERATIONS

There is no antiganglioside antibody investigation that is absolutely essential for diagnosis of a particular subtype of peripheral neuropathy, since independent investigation, principally electrodiagnostic tests in the context of an appropriate clinical picture and exclusion of other causes, is usually adequate. However, an antiganglioside antibody investigation may be useful (i) to confirm a diagnosis, such as MMN, AMAN, or MFS; (ii) to subclassify an existing diagnosis, such as IgM paraproteinemic neuropathy, into those with anti-NeuAc(α2-8)NeuAc activity or anti-SGPG activity, etc.; and (iii) to exclude or differentiate among several possible diagnoses, such as botulism, brain stem demyelinating disease, and MFS (anti-GQ1b antibody testing), or between MMN and amyotrophic lateral sclerosis (anti-GM1 antibody testing).

INTERPRETATION

A normal range of IgG and IgM titers for each glycolipid antigen must be established within a laboratory since antiglycolipid antibodies form part of the normal autoantibody repertoire and antibodies to some gangliosides may be found at low titer in both normal and disease control sera. The distribution of antiganglioside antibodies in the population does not follow a normal pattern but is skewed, with some control subjects having high antibody levels against some gangliosides (titers of >1/1,000) and most having undetectable levels (titers of <1/100). As a result, defining a clinically meaningful normal range or reference range, even when using logarithmically transformed data, is problematic. In my laboratory we set the upper limit of the normal range as 2 standard deviations above titers obtained using a panel of at least 50 healthy control subjects of all ages and both sexes; for most antiganglioside antibodies this equates with an antibody titer being positive if >1/500 by endpoint dilution analysis (19).

With respect to the sensitivity and specificity of antiganglioside antibodies in particular clinical settings, no clear data are available from large multicenter studies. Some syndromes (e.g., "anti-MAG neuropathy") are to an extent defined by the presence of a particular antiglycolipid antibody. Anti-GQ1b IgG antibodies are a highly sensitive (>90%) and specific (>90%) marker for MFS and related syndromes accompanied by ophthalmoplegia (16). Anti-GM1 IgM antibodies are found in ~50% of cases of MMN (1, 9, 15). Anti-GM1 and anti-GD1a IgG antibodies are very specifically associated with acute motor dominant forms of GBS, including AMAN, occurring in ~50% of cases (4). Anti-MAG antibodies are found in ~50% of cases of IgM paraproteinemic neuropathy, and a proportion of the remainder react with other glycolipid antigens. Anti-GD1b IgM antibodies are highly specific for a rare form of chronic ataxic neuropathy termed CANOMAD, although the sensitivity is unknown.

REFERENCES

1. Adams, D., T. Kuntzer, D. Burger, M. Chofflon, M. R. Magistris, F. Regli, and A. J. Steck. 1991. Predictive value of anti-GM1 ganglioside antibodies in neuromuscular diseases—a study of 180 sera. *J. Neuroimmunol.* **32**:223–230.
2. Alaedini, A., I. Wirguin, and N. Latov. 2001. Ganglioside agglutination immunoassay for rapid detection of autoantibodies in immune-mediated neuropathy. *J. Clin. Lab. Anal.* **15**:96–99.
3. Chiba, A., S. Kusunoki, H. Obata, R. Machinami, and I. Kanazawa. 1993. Serum anti-GQ1b IgG antibody is associated with ophthalmoplegia in Miller Fisher syndrome and Guillain-Barre syndrome: clinical and immunohistochemical studies. *Neurology* **43**:1911–1917.
4. Ho, T. W., H. J. Willison, I. Nachamkin, C. Y. Li, J. Veitch, H. Ung, G. R. Wang, R. C. Liu, D. R. Cornblath, A. K. Asbury, J. W. Griffin, and G. M. McKhann. 1999. Anti-GD1a antibody is associated with axonal but not demyelinating forms of Guillain-Barre syndrome. *Ann. Neurol.* **45**:168–173.
5. Ilyas, A. A., H. J. Willison, R. H. Quarles, F. B. Jungalwala, D. R. Cornblath, B. D. Trapp, D. E. Griffin, J. W. Griffin, and G. M. McKhann. 1988. Serum antibodies to gangliosides in Guillain-Barre syndrome. *Ann. Neurol.* **23**:440–447.
6. IUPAC-IUB Commission on Biochemical Nomenclature (CBN). 1977. The nomenclature of lipids. *Eur. J. Biochem.* **79**:11–21.
7. Kaida, K., D. Morita, M. Kanzaki, K. Kamakura, K. Motoyoshi, M. Hirakawa, and S. Kusunoki. 2004. Ganglioside complexes as new target antigens in Guillain-Barre syndrome. *Ann. Neurol.* **56**:567–571.
8. Kissel, J. T. 1998. Autoantibody testing in the evaluation of peripheral neuropathy. *Semin. Neurol.* **18**:83–94.
9. Kornberg, A. J., A. Pestronk, K. Bieser, T. W. Ho, G. M. McKhann, H. S. Wu, and Z. Jiang. 1994. The clinical correlates of high-titer IgG anti-GM1 antibodies. *Ann. Neurol.* **35**:234–237.
10. Latov, N. 1994. Antibodies to glycoconjugates in neuropathy and motor-neuron disease. *Proc. Brain Res.* **101**:295–303.
11. Mizutamari, R. K., H. Wiegandt, and G. A. Nores. 1994. Characterization of anti-ganglioside antibodies present in normal human plasma. *J. Neuroimmunol.* **50**:215–220.
12. Pestronk, A. 1998. Multifocal motor neuropathy: diagnosis and treatment. *Neurology* **51**:S22–S24.
13. Ravindranath, M. H., R. M. H. Ravindranath, D. L. Morton, and M. C. Graves. 1994. Factors affecting the fine specificity and sensitivity of serum antiganglioside antibodies in ELISA. *J. Immunol. Methods* **169**:257–272.
14. Schnaar, R. L. 1994. Isolation of glycosphingolipids. *Methods Enzymol.* **230**:348–370.
15. Vanschaik, I. N., P. M. M. Bossuyt, A. Brand, and M. Vermeulen. 1995. Diagnostic value of GM1 antibodies in motor-neuron disorders and neuropathies—a metaanalysis. *Neurology* **45**:1570–1577.
16. Willison, H. J., and G. M. O'Hanlon. 1999. The immunopathogenesis of Miller Fisher syndrome. *J. Neuroimmunol.* **100**:3–12.
17. Willison, H. J., G. M. O'Hanlon, G. Paterson, J. Veitch, G. Wilson, M. Roberts, T. Tang, and A. Vincent. 1996. A somatically mutated human antiganglioside IgM antibody that induces experimental neuropathy in mice is encoded by the variable region heavy chain gene, V1-18. *J. Clin. Investig.* **97**:1155–1164.
18. Willison, H. J., C. P. O'Leary, J. Veitch, L. D. Blumhardt, M. Busby, M. Donaghy, P. Fuhr, H. Ford, A. Hahn, S. Renaud, H. A. Katifi, S. Ponsford, M. Reuber, A. Steck, I. Sutton, W. Schady, P. K. Thomas, A. J. Thompson, J. M. Vallat, and J. Winer. 2001. The clinical and laboratory features of chronic sensory ataxic neuropathy with anti-disialosyl IgM antibodies. *Brain* **124**:1968–1977.
19. Willison, H. J., J. Veitch, A. V. Swan, N. Baumann, G. Comi, N. A. Gregson, I. Illa, B. C. Jacobs, J. Zielasek, and R. A. C. Hughes. 1999. Inter-laboratory validation of an ELISA for the determination of serum anti-ganglioside antibodies. *Eur. J. Neurol.* **6**:71–77.
20. Willison, H. J., and N. Yuki. 2002. Peripheral neuropathies and anti-glycolipid antibodies. *Brain* **125**:2591–2625.
21. Yuki, N. 1998. Anti-ganglioside antibody and neuropathy: review of our research. *J. Periph. Nerv. Sys.* **3**:3–18.
22. Zielasek, J., G. Ritter, S. Magi, H. P. Hartung, and K. V. Toyka. 1994. A comparative trial of anti-glycoconjugate antibody assays—IgM antibodies to GM1. *J. Neurol.* **241**:475–480.

Detection of Antimitochondrial Autoantibodies in Primary Biliary Cirrhosis and Liver Kidney Microsomal Antibodies in Autoimmune Hepatitis

PATRICK S. C. LEUNG, MICHAEL P. MANNS, ROSS L. COPPEL, AND M. ERIC GERSHWIN

122

The immunodetection of autoantibodies has been technically difficult because (i) serum autoantibodies from patients usually react to a broad spectrum of antigens, (ii) some of these autoantibodies may have low titers, (iii) the biochemical nature of these autoantigens has been unknown, and (iv) many autoantigens are present at low concentrations and often require sophisticated procedures for their biochemical purification. The development and application of immunohistochemical, biochemical, and molecular biological techniques have redefined approaches for the study of autoimmune diseases, in particular the immunological detection of autoantigens. This is exemplified by two autoimmune diseases of the liver, namely, primary biliary cirrhosis (PBC) and autoimmune hepatitis (AIH). This chapter will focus on the detection of antimitochondrial antibodies in PBC and the detection of liver-kidney microsomal antibodies (LKM antibodies) in AIH.

PBC

PBC is an autoimmune disease of the liver characterized by autoimmunity-mediated destruction of intrahepatic bile ducts with progressive inflammatory scarring and, eventually, liver function failure (23). Immunologically, PBC is characterized by the presence of antimitochondrial autoantibodies (AMA) in the circulation (32) and the infiltration of T cells into the liver (24, 25). AMA can be detected in >95% of patients with the disease (15, 29). These mitochondrial autoantigens were shown to be the E2 subunits of the 2-oxo-acid dehydrogenase complex (14, 59, 62) (Table 1). Subsequently, extensive molecular and immunological studies of PBC, including cloning of mitochondrial autoantigens (16), antigen-specific isotype studies (52, 59), mapping of B- and T-cell epitopes (10, 21, 28, 30, 48, 53, 56, 57), and analyses of human, murine, and baculovirus monoclonal antibodies (5, 12, 13, 28, 51), have provided valuable information and reagents for an understanding of the immunopathogenesis of PBC as well as for the development of accurate and specific diagnostic reagents with recombinant autoantigens (27, 42, 58). Immunohistochemical studies have shown the presence of either pyruvate dehydrogenase complex subunit E2 (PDC-E2) or a cross-reactive molecule in the luminal region of bile duct epithelial cells (BDEC) for PBC, but not in control cells (4, 5, 22, 41, 55). These data, together with recent reports on apoptotic cleavage of PDC-E2 in apoptotic BDEC (39, 40, 44), suggest that antibodies targeting BDEC of the PBC liver may be pathogenic. Recently, immunoglobulin G (IgG) and IgA AMA were detected in saliva and urine from patients with PBC, suggesting that a locally driven mucosal response is involved in PBC (46, 54).

DETECTION OF AMA

AMA can be detected by the following methods: (i) indirect immunofluorescence (IF) (61), (ii) immunoblotting (30), and (iii) enzyme-linked immunosorbent assays (ELISAs) (27, 58).

Immunohistochemical Staining for AMA in PBC Sera by IF

Among the various methods of detection of AMA, IF is by far the most commonly used clinical test for AMA and is performed with HEp-2 cells or tissue sections from mice or rats. A detailed protocol is described below.

1. Prepare smears of HEp-2 cells on clean glass slides and air dry.
2. Fix cells in cold acetone for 10 min at 4°C and air dry.
3. Place each glass slide in phosphate-buffered saline (PBS) for 5 min.
4. Apply diluted patient sera (usually 1:40, 1:80, 1:160, 1:320, and 1:640) onto slides and incubate the slides for 60 min at room temperature.
5. Wash the slides with PBS three times for 3 min each time.
6. Apply diluted fluorescein isothiocyanate (FITC)-conjugated goat anti-human IgG with Evans blue, and incubate the slides for 60 min at room temperature.
7. Wash the slides with PBS three times for 3 min each time.
8. Mount samples with 90% glycerol in PBS.
9. Examine samples under a fluorescence microscope.

HEp-2 slides can also be obtained commercially (e.g., Immunoconcepts, Sacramento, Calif., or Immco Diagnostics, Buffalo, N.Y.). Results of a typical IF test with AMA-positive PBC serum on HEp-2 cells are shown in Fig. 1. Alternatively, rat and mouse kidney sections can also be used for immunohistochemical staining for AMA. However, IF lacks the specificity of identifying specific

TABLE 1 Summary of 2-oxo-acid dehydrogenase mitochondrial antigens in PBC

Antigen	Molecular mass (kDa)[a]	Frequency (%) in PBC patients[b]
PDC-E2	70	>95
Branched-chain 2-oxo-acid dehydrogenase complex E2 subunit (BCOADC-E2)	52	53–55
2-Oxo-glutarate dehydrogenase complex E2 subunit (OGDC-E2)	48	39–88
PDC-E1α	41	41–66
E3BP (protein X)	55	>95

[a]Determined by immunoblotting of beef heart mitochondrial preparations.
[b]Determined from different studies.

antigens. In addition, background levels which are caused by nonspecific binding are common. Therefore, accurate detection of AMA by IF requires serial dilutions of sera (usually 1:40, 1:80, 1:160, 1:320, and 1:640) and also an optimal dilution of FITC-labeled anti-human Ig. The precise optimal dilution of secondary FITC-antibody may also vary from batch to batch. Thorough washing steps and changes of washing solutions are also necessary to reduce the background.

Immunoblotting for Detection of Specific AMA against Mitochondrial Antigens

A total mitochondrial homogenate from mammalian tissues is best suited to testing of AMA by immunoblotting. Briefly, mitochondrial preparations from a bovine heart, rat liver, human placenta, or other tissues are resolved in a sodium dodecyl sulfate (SDS)-polyacrylamide gel, transferred onto nitrocellulose filters, and probed with sera from patients with PBC. AMA reactivity against mitochondrial antigens is usually detected by enzyme-conjugated anti-human Ig and chemiluminescence.

Preparation of Mitochondria from Mammalian Liver

A convenient method for preparing mitochondria is described below.

1. Homogenize rat or mouse liver (15 g) in 30 ml of ice-cold buffer I (0.5 M sorbitol, 0.1 mM EDTA, 50 mM Tris, pH 7.4) and centrifuge the homogenate at $250 \times g$ for 10 min.
2. Filter the supernatant through four layers of cheese-cloth.
3. Spin the supernatant at $250 \times g$ for 10 min at 4°C.
4. Take the supernatant and spin it at $8,000 \times g$ for 10 min at 4°C.
5. Resuspend the pellet in 15 ml of buffer I and spin it again as in step 4.
6. Repeat step 5.
7. Resuspend the pellet in 4 ml of buffer I with 0.05% bovine serum albumin (BSA) and store it in a 1-ml aliquot. Store the sample at −20°C; the final concentration should be about 40 to 60 mg/ml.

Test of AMA Reactivity against Mammalian Mitochondria by Immunoblotting

1. Electrophoretically resolve 20 μg of mitochondrial preparations in an SDS–10% polyacrylamide gel, using a preparative comb (Hoefer Scientific, San Francisco, Calif.). Run molecular weight protein standards in parallel.
2. Stop the gel when the bromophenol blue dye reaches the bottom of the gel and transfer the resolved protein onto a nitrocellulose filter.
3. After the transfer, stain the blot with Ponceau S (Sigma, St. Louis, Mo.) to check for the efficiency of transfer. If the transfer is satisfactory, cut 3-mm strips from the blot with a sharp razor blade.
4. Incubate each strip with 1 ml of diluted PBC serum (1:1,000) for 1 h at room temperature. Run positive control sera and negative control sera in parallel.
5. After incubation, wash each strip with PBS containing 0.05% Tween three times for 10 min each time.

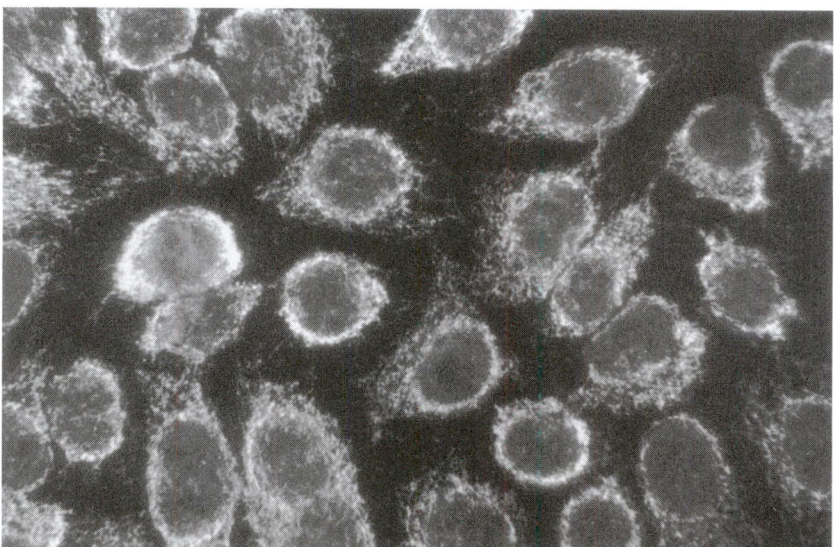

FIGURE 1 Detection of AMA by IF on HEp-2 cells. Note the characteristic mitochondrial staining pattern by PBC sera.

6. Incubate each strip with a predetermined optimal dilution of secondary antibody (e.g., enzyme-conjugated secondary antibodies) and wash as in step 5.

7. Detect signals with a substrate for the enzyme-conjugated secondary antibodies. If horseradish peroxidase-conjugated secondary antibodies are used, the blots can be blocked with milk for 10 min after being washed and the signals can be detected by chemiluminescence on X-ray film. Chemiluminescence kits can be obtained from common vendors such as Pierce.

Figure 2 depicts typical patterns of AMA reactivity against various subunits of the 2-oxo-acid dehydrogenase complex. AMA reactivites are directed against the 70-kDa PDC-E2, 55-kDa E3 binding protein (protein X), 52-kDa branched-chain 2-oxo-acid dehydrogenase complex E2 subunit (BCOADC-E2), 48-kDa 2-oxo-glutarate dehydrogenase complex E2 subunit OGDC-E2, and 41-kDa PDC-E1α proteins. Note that sera from PBC patients do not necessarily react to all five mitochondrial autoantigens and that the pattern of reactivity may vary from patient to patient (29, 31).

Test for AMA Reactivity in PBC Sera by ELISA with Recombinant Autoantigens

Several studies have demonstrated the successful application of recombinant proteins as test antigens for PBC by ELISA (20, 30, 43). An ELISA using recombinant proteins is versatile, specific, and sensitive. In addition, ELISA is also efficient and allows the testing of multiple sera at several serial dilutions simultaneously. cDNAs encoding PDC-E2, BCOADC-E2, OGDC-E2, E3BP, and PDC-E1α have been cloned and expressed in *Escherichia coli* with isopropyl-β-D-thiogalactopyranoside (IPTG)-inducible plasmid vectors. Recombinant proteins can be easily purified from IPTG-induced bacterial cultures as described previously (43). Recently, the use of designer molecules (42) expressing AMA-reactive epitopes has greatly facilitated the testing of multiple sera for AMA. The availability and application of recombinant proteins clearly provide the cleanest and most specific reagents for AMA assays.

A standard procedure is as follows:

1. Dilute recombinant antigen to 5 μg/ml in carbonate buffer, pH 9.6.

2. Coat a 96-well ELISA plate with 100 μl of recombinant antigen from step 1/well. Store the plate at 4°C overnight.

3. Wash the plate three times with 100 μl of PBS containing 0.05% Tween (washing buffer). Shake off the washing buffer between washes.

4. Block the plate with 100 ml of 1% BSA in PBS; incubate the plate at room temperature for 1 h.

5. Add test sera (serial dilutions) in PBS containing 1% BSA and 0.05% Tween; incubate the plate at room temperature for 1 h.

6. Wash the plate as in step 3, and then add 100 μl of a predetermined dilution of secondary antibody, such as horseradish peroxidase-conjugated anti-human Ig. Incubate the plate at room temperature for 1 h.

7. Wash the plate as in step 3. The presence of bound AMA can be determined by adding 100 μl of substrate for horseradish peroxidase (e.g., ABTS [2, 2-azinobis 3-ethylbanzthiazoline sulfonic acid] [Sigma]). Incubate the plate for 10 min at room temperature, and stop the reaction by adding 100 μl of 5% SDS. The intensity of color developed can be measured in an ELISA plate reader at 405 nm.

For ELISA, it is necessary to include a positive serum control, a negative serum control, and a well containing no primary antibody to correct any data or values caused by nonspecific binding of antibodies and background. A test serum is considered positive when the optical density reading is at least two times higher than the normal serum reading and the data are reproducible.

INTERPRETATION OF AMA DATA

Although AMA are highly reliable for the diagnosis of PBC, some limitations and precautions are noted below. Firstly, the high titer of AMA and the sensitivity of the test demand

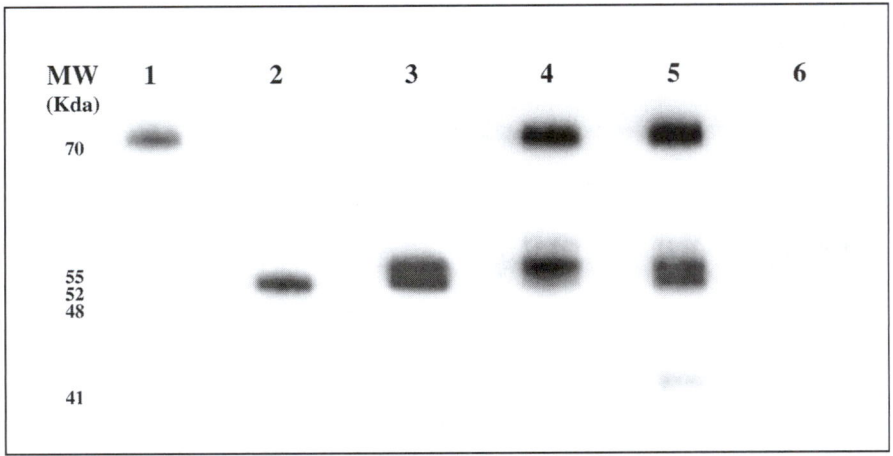

FIGURE 2   Reactivity of PBC sera to bovine heart mitochondria. Bovine heart mitochondria were resolved by SDS-PAGE, transferred to a nitrocellulose filter, and tested for their reactivity with PBC sera (lanes 1 to 5). Note the different patterns of AMA reactivities for various patients with PBC to the 70-kDa PDC-E2, 55-kDa E3 binding protein (protein X), 52-kDa BCOADC-E2, 48-kDa OGDC-E2, and 41-kDa PDC-E1α proteins. Sera from healthy controls do not react to any of these mitochondrial proteins (lane 6).

extreme caution to avoid cross-contamination of sera and false-positive results. Secondly, about 5 to 10% of PBC patients are AMA negative. Other clinical diagnostic features are also critical for a differential diagnosis (Table 2). Thirdly, neither the titer nor the specificity of autoantigens is related to the severity of the disease and therefore cannot be used to monitor the clinical course. Most importantly, positive and negative antibody controls should be included in the assay. Despite these limitations, cloned autoantigens and their recombinant proteins are extremely valuable diagnostic tools for clinicians.

AIH

Chronic hepatitis is a heterogeneous syndrome characterized by clinical, biochemical, and morphological criteria (8). Hepatitis viruses B and C may cause chronic hepatitis. In contrast, AIH, drug-induced hepatitis, and cryptogenic hepatitis are other subgroups of chronic hepatitis that presumably differ etiologically. AIH is a syndrome of unknown etiology. The annual incidence of AIH among Northern Europeans is 1.9 per 100,000. Women are more affected than men, but all ages are susceptible (3). The loss of tolerance against the patient's own liver is regarded as the main pathogenic mechanism. While hitherto poorly defined defects of the immune system are responsible for chronic viral hepatitis, a hyperreaction of the patient's immune system towards autologous

TABLE 2 Clinical characteristics of PBC

Clinical symptoms
  Skin itching or jaundice appears in some cases
  Portal hypertension and ascites or esophageal varices may
    appear
  Osteoporosis according to the insufficiency of vitamin D or
    calcium may occur

Laboratory data
  Presence of AMA
  Elevation of bile duct-associated enzymes (ALP, γ-GTP) in serum
  Elevation of serum bile acid
  Elevation of total cholesterol
  Elevation of serum IgM

Histological parameter
  Chronic nonsuppurative destructive cholangitis (CNSDC) in
    middle-size interlobular or septal bile ducts, vanishing bile
    ducts, and granulomas

Complications
  Skin xanthoma (especially when hypercholesterolemia continues)
  Autoimmune diseases such as Sjögren syndrome, rheumatoid
    arthritis, and chronic thyroiditis also occur

Diagnosis
  The patient is determined to have PBC when one of the following features is recognized.
    1. CNSDC is recognized in a liver specimen, and laboratory
       data are compatible with PBC. In some rare cases, the AMA
       test is negative.
    2. AMA or anti-pyruvate dehydrogenase antibody test is
       positive, and liver histology is compatible with PBC even
       though CNSDC is not recognized.
    3. AMA or anti-pyruvate dehydrogenase antibody test is
       positive and clinical features or present history is compatible
       with PBC even though liver histology is not checked.

TABLE 3 Diagnostic criteria for AIH

Parameter[a]	Score[b]
Hypergammaglobulinemia	+3
Autoantibodies	
ANA, SMA, LKM-1	+3
SLA, ASPRG, LP	+2
AMA	−2
Female sex	+2
AST ALT of <3.0	+2
Complete response to immunosuppression	+2
Anti-HAV IgM, HBsAg, anti-HBc IgM	−3
HCV RNA (PCR)	−2
Other virus infections	−3
Ethanol intake	
Males, <35 g/day; females < 25 g/day	+2
Immunogenetics: HLA-B8-DR3 or -DR4	+1

[a]ASPRG, antibodies against asialoglycoprotein receptor; AST, aspartate aminotransferase; ALT, alanine aminotransferase; HAV, hepatitis A virus; HBsAg, hepatitis B serum antigen; HCV, hepatitis C virus.

[b]If the total value of scores is >15 before or >17 after therapy, then AIH is certain; if the total value of scores is 10 to 15 before or 12 to 17 after therapy, then AIH is probable.

liver tissue is responsible for autoimmune hepatitis (9). Autoantibodies are the hallmarks of the diagnosis of autoimmune hepatitis (Table 3). It is debated whether different patterns of autoantibodies characterize clinically or etiologically distinct subgroups of autoimmune hepatitis (6, 19, 34). For example, antinuclear antibodies (ANA) are very heterogeneous, but their association with autoimmune liver diseases has not been identified, whereas smooth muscle antibodies (SMA) in autoimmune liver diseases are particularly directed against F-actin. Serologically, AIH can be divided into the following three subgroups: antinuclear and smooth muscle antibody positive (ANA/SMA; type 1), liver-kidney microsomal antibody positive (LKM-1; type 2), and soluble liver antigen/liver-pancreas antigen antibody positive (SLA/LP; type 3) (49). However, there are no significant clinical implications resulting from this classification. Recently, significant progress has been achieved in the characterization of microsomal antigens associated with liver diseases (Table 4). Three members of the cytochrome P450 supergene family and two members of the UDP-glucuronosyl-transferases (UGTs) have been identified as hepatocellular autoantigens. These antigens are of particular interest since they characterize subgroups of autoimmune hepatitis and some forms of drug-induced hepatitis and also occur in a small proportion of patients with chronic viral hepatitis C or D (33). Recent data showed that autoantibodies to SLA (anti-SLA) and autoantibodies to a cytoplasmic antigen shared by the liver and pancreas (anti-LP) recognize the same target antigen, which was identified as a non-liver-specific cytosolic UGA-suppressor tRNA-associated protein (60).

LKM antibodies have been defined due to their typical immunofluorescent staining of liver and kidney tissue. LKM-1 antibodies homogeneously stain the whole liver lobule and the proximal renal tubule (47). They react mainly with human cytochrome P450 2D6 (18, 35). LKM-2 antibodies react with cytochrome P450 IIC9 (2), and LM antibodies react with liver-specific cytochrome P450 IA2 (37). LKM-3 antibodies react with a major autoepitope on family 1 UGTs, and some sera react in addition with a minor epitope on family 2 UGTs (45). LKM-1 antibodies are serological markers of

TABLE 4 Heterogeneity of microsomal antigens

Antibody	Size (kDa)	Target antigen	Associated disease
LKM-1	50	Cytochrome P450 2D6	AIH type II (hepatitis C)
LKM-2	50	Cytochrome P450 2C9	Ticrynafen-induced hepatitis
LKM-3	55	Family 1 UGT	Hepatitis D-associated AIH
LM	52	Cytochrome P450 1A2	Dihydralazine-induced hepatitis (AIH), autoimmune polyendocrine syndrome type 1 (APS-1)
Unknown	50	Cytochrome P450 2A6	Autoimmune polyendocrine syndrome type 1, hepatitis C
	57	Disulfide isomerase	Halothane-induced hepatitis
	59	Carboxylesterase	Halothane-induced hepatitis
	59	Unknown	Chronic hepatitis C
	64	Unknown	AIH
	70	Unknown	Chronic hepatitis C

autoimmune hepatitis type 2 (Table 4), a syndrome that frequently starts in childhood. In autoimmune hepatitis, the main epitope is an eight-amino-acid linear epitope that shares sequence homology with the immediate-early protein of herpes simplex virus type 1 (IE 175). LKM-1 antibodies occur in 0 to 7% of patients with hepatitis C; these microsomal antibodies react either with a larger sequence of P450 IIC9, other epitopes on this protein, or conformational epitopes that are not recognized on immunoblots. Furthermore, sera from patients with hepatitis C may react with other microsomal proteins. LKM-2 antibodies did occur in a drug-induced form of hepatitis caused by a diuretic drug called tienilic acid which has only been used in the United States and France. The drug has been withdrawn from the market, and thus these antibodies have only been described in France. LKM-3 antibodies are associated with 5 to 13% of patients with chronic hepatitis D and also occur in some patients with autoimmune hepatitis type 2 (Table 4). In rare cases, they may be the only marker of autoimmune hepatitis (50). LM antibodies occur in a proportion of patients with autoimmune hepatitis type 2 and drug-induced hepatitis caused by dihydralazine. Interestingly, like the case for LKM-1 antibodies, these LKM-3 autoantibodies in autoimmune liver diseases have a higher titer, because the autoepitope is linear and small, than low-titer antibodies to conformational epitopes in viral hepatitis. It is unknown whether LKM antibodies are involved in pathogenesis. It is likely that the antibodies themselves do not mediate tissue destruction, but rather that tissue damage is mediated by liver-infiltrating T lymphocytes, possibly directed against cytochrome P450 molecules.

METHODS OF DETECTION OF LKM ANTIBODIES

LKM autoantibodies can be detected by the following methods: (i) IF (47), (ii) competitive ELISA (17, 36), (iii) immunoblotting with human liver microsomes (1, 26), and (iv) immunoblotting with recombinant antigens (35, 38).

Detection of LKM Autoantibodies in AIH by IF

IF (38, 47) on rat liver and kidney sections is commonly used to detect LKM autoantibodies in patients with autoimmune hepatitis. Patient sera are serially diluted 1:40, 1:80, and 1:160. Additionally, the optimal dilution of the FITC-conjugated secondary antibody must be determined for each batch of

antibody to avoid strong background fluorescence, which makes the evaluation of LKM-positive sera difficult. The method is described in detail below.

1. Prepare frozen sections from rat livers and kidneys on glass slides and air dry.
2. Apply patient sera to slides at the appropriate dilutions and incubate the slides at room temperature for 1 h.
3. Wash the slides three times with PBS.
4. Apply FITC-conjugated goat anti-human IgG and incubate the slides for 30 min at room temperature.
5. Wash the slides three times with PBS.
6. Mount the samples with 90% glycerol in PBS.
7. Evaluate slides under a fluorescence microscope.

There are some similarities between AMA and LKM antibodies, which sometimes causes problems to investigators inexperienced in routine immunofluorescence. While LKM antibodies do not stain distal renal tubules, LM antibodies do not stain the kidney at all, since they react with a liver-specific antigen. For IF, LKM antibodies very strongly stain the whole liver lobule (Fig. 3A), while on kidney tissue, they only stain proximal renal tubules (Fig. 3B). In contrast, AMA stain proximal and distal renal tubules. If the medulla of the kidney is not part of the tissue, LKM antibodies may be misdiagnosed as AMA. Since only two childhood cases of PBC have been reported (7), a positive AMA result for children is almost always due to LKM antibodies. If in IF only the liver stains and no reaction is seen in the kidney, one must suspect LM antibodies, which are directed against the liver-specific cytochrome P450 IA2.

Detection of LKM Autoantibodies by Competitive ELISA

An additional method to detect and further differentiate LKM autoantibodies in patient serum is competitive ELISA. An immunoglobulin fraction of serums, e.g., an LKM-1- or LKM-3-positive serum, is used to coat the plates. At the same time, an aliquot of this immunoglobulin fraction is biotinylated.

Preparation of Microsomes from Rat Liver for ELISA

Microsomes from rat liver tissue isolated by differential centrifugation are used as antigens for the competitive ELISA to test for LKM autoantibodies.

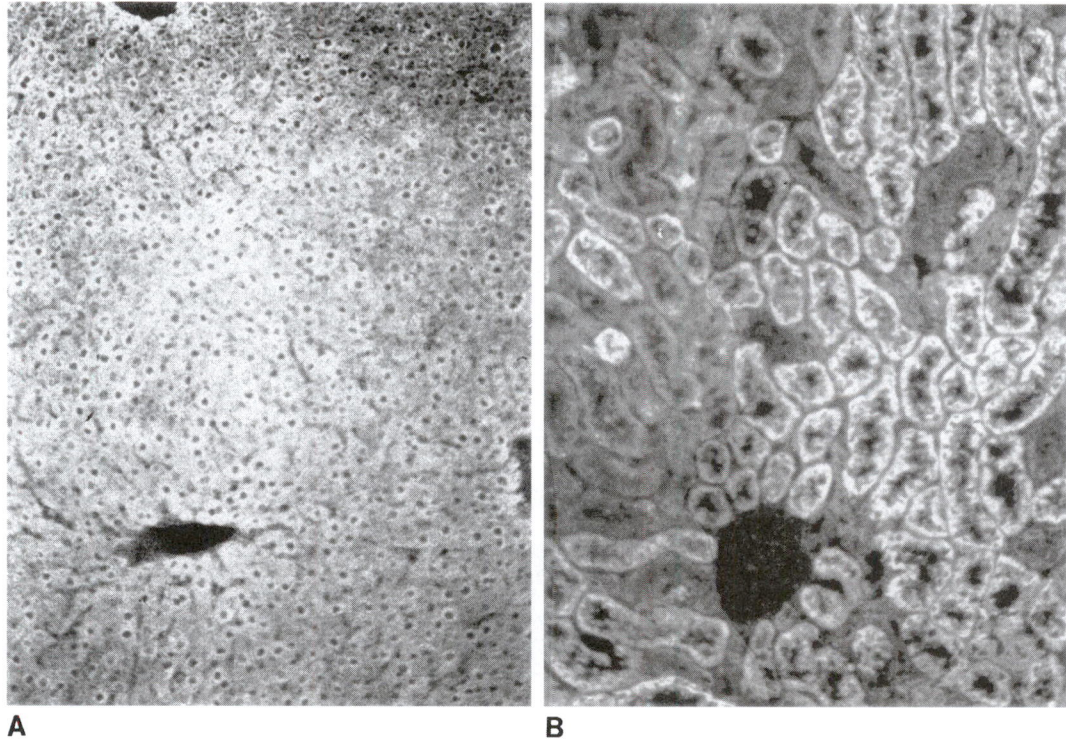

FIGURE 3 Detection of LKM antibodies and AMA by IF on cryostat rat liver and kidney sections. (A) Staining of liver lobule by LKM-1 antibodies. (B) Staining of proximal but not distal renal tubules by LKM-1 antibodies.

Procedure

All steps should be done at 4°C.

1. Remove liver and wash in 0.9% NaCl.
2. Homogenize liver in ice-cold 250 mM sucrose.
3. Centrifuge sample for 10 min at $1,800 \times g$.
4. Centrifuge supernatant for 15 min at $12,000 \times g$.
5. Spin supernatant for 60 min at $200,000 \times g$.
6. Resuspend pellet in a small volume of PBS and determine the protein concentration.

Biotinylation and Preparation of IgG Fraction from Patient Sera for ELISA

An IgG fraction is prepared from LKM-1- or LKM-3-positive patient serum by precipitation with ammonium sulfate. An aliquot of this fraction is biotinylated according to the instructions given by the manufacturer.

Procedure

1. Dilute the IgG fraction of an LKM-positive patient serum to a concentration of 20 mg/ml in PBS.
2. Coat an ELISA plate with 50 μl of the IgG fraction/well.
3. Wash the plate once with PBS containing 0.1% Tween.
4. Block the plate with 200 μl of 1% BSA in PBS/well and incubate it for 24 to 48 h at 4°C.
5. Wash the plate once with PBS-Tween.
6. Dilute liver microsomes to a concentration of 100 μg/ml and place them in an ultrasound water bath for 3 min.

7. Add liver microsomes (50 ml/well) and incubate the plate at room temperature for 60 min.
8. Wash the plate two times with PBS-Tween.
9. Dilute patient sera (1:10) in PBS containing 10 mM EDTA, add 50 ml/well, and incubate the plate for 60 min at room temperature.
10. Wash the plate as in step 8.
11. Dilute biotin-labeled immunoglobulin fraction (1 mg/ml) 1:100 in PBS-BSA, add 50 μl/well, and incubate the plate for 60 min at room temperature.
12. Wash the plate three times with PBS-Tween.
13. Dilute avidin peroxidase appropriately in PBS-BSA, add 50 ml/well, and incubate the plate for 60 min; wash the plate as in step 8.
14. Add ABTS (50 ml/well), wait for the color reaction, add stop buffer (100 mM citric acid, pH 2), and measure the color intensity in an ELISA reader at 450 nm.

Immunoblotting with Human Liver Microsomes to Test for LKM

Procedure

1. Prepare liver microsomes as described for ELISA. Instead of rat liver, use a small piece of human liver tissue.
2. Resolve 1 mg of microsomes in sample buffer by SDS–10% polyacrylamide gel electrophoresis (SDS–10% PAGE). In parallel, run a molecular weight standard.
3. Stop the gel when the bromophenol blue dye reaches the bottom of the gel, and transfer the proteins onto a nitrocellulose filter.

4. Cut the nitrocellulose filter into 3-mm strips, block the strips for 60 min in Tris-buffered saline (TBS)–Tween containing 2% milk powder, and then add patient sera, positive control sera, and negative control sera diluted 1:100. Incubate the strips in 1 ml of diluted sera for 60 min at room temperature.

5. Wash each strip three times with TBS-Tween for 5 min each time.

6. Add 1 ml of an appropriately diluted alkaline phosphatase-conjugated goat anti-human IgG and incubate the strip for 60 min at room temperature.

7. Wash the strip three times and then detect the signal by using a substrate for the enzyme-conjugated second antibody, such as NBT/BCIP (Nitro Blue Tetrazolium/5-bromo-4-chloro-indolyl phosphate).

Interpretation

Characteristic LKM-1 autoantibodies react with a 50-kDa microsomal protein of human liver microsomes, and some sera from patients with autoimmune hepatitis type 2 react with a protein of 64 kDa. LKM-1 antibodies in patients with chronic hepatitis C are more heterogeneous (11). They may react with other microsomal proteins of 59 and 70 kDa. Approximately 50% of sera from patients with hepatitis C do not react with human microsomes in immunoblots since these antibodies react with conformational epitopes.

Immunoblotting with Recombinant Liver Antigens

P450 IIC9 (38) and P450 IA2 (37) cDNAs were expressed in *E. coli*. UGT 1.1 cDNA (45) was expressed in baculovirus.

Procedure

1. Resolve 50 mg of recombinant P450 11D6 or IA2 or 200 mg of UGT 1.1 by SDS–10% PAGE. In parallel, run a molecular weight standard.

2. Stop the gel when the bromophenol blue dye reaches the bottom of the gel, and transfer the proteins onto a nitrocellulose filter.

3. Follow steps 3 to 7 from the previous section.

Interpretation

Since almost all cytochrome P450 enzymes have a molecular mass of about 50 kDa, a precise differentiation of different cytochrome P450 antibodies may only be possible if recombinant antigens are used. The identification of cytochrome P450 IA2 as a hepatocellular antigen resulted from the observation that a serum reacted with a 50-kDa protein but not with the recombinant cytochrome P450 IID6. In immunoblots with human liver microsomes, a distinction between P450 IID6 and P450 IA2 was not possible.

GENERAL REAGENTS

PBS, pH 7.4: Dissolve 32 g of NaCl, 0.8 g of KCl, 4.6 g of Na_2PO_4 (anhydrous), and 0.8 g of KH_2PO_4 (anhydrous) in 4 liters of distilled water. Adjust the pH to 7.2 to 7.4.

TBS-Tween: Dissolve 1.2 g of Tris and 8.7 g of NaCl in 1 liter of distilled water. Adjust the pH to 8.0 and add 500 µl of Tween 20.

3% milk in PBS: Dissolve 3 g of nonfat dry milk in 100 ml of PBS. Adjust the pH to 7.2 to 7.4 by adding a few drops of 2 N NaOH.

Carbonate coating buffer: Dissolve 0.8 g of Na_2CO_3, 1.46 g of $NaHCO_3$, and 0.1 g of NaN_3 in distilled water. Adjust to a pH of 9.6 and a final volume of 500 ml.

5× citrate buffer, pH 5.2: Dissolve 50.0 g of citric acid monohydrate and 7.4 g of Na_2HPO_4 in 150 ml of distilled water. Adjust the pH to 5.2. Adjust the final volume to 200 ml.

ABTS substrate: Prepare 1 mM ABTS solution by adding 55 mg of ABTS to 100 ml of citrate buffer. Add hydrogen peroxide to 0.05% immediately before use.

NBT/BCIP substrate: Mix together 33 µl of NBT and 16.5 µl of BCIP in 5 ml of alkaline phosphatase buffer.

Alkaline phosphatase buffer: Dissolve 12.1 g of Tris and 1.0 g of $MgCl_2$ in 1 liter of distilled water. Adjust the pH to 9.5.

REFERENCES

1. **Alvarez, F., O. Bernard, J. C. Homberg, and G. Kreibich.** 1985. Anti liver kidney microsomal antibody recognizes a 50,000 molecular weight protein of the endoplasmic reticulum. *J. Exp. Med.* **161:**1231–1236.
2. **Beaune, P., P. M. Dansette, D. Mansuy, L. Kiffel, M. Finck, C. Amar, J. P. Leroux, and J. C. Homberg.** 1987. Human antiendoplasmic reticulum autoantibodies appearing in drug-induced hepatitis are directed against a human cytochrome P450 that hydroxylates the drug. *Proc. Natl. Acad. Sci. USA* **84:**551–555.
3. **Boberg, K. M.** 2002. Prevalence and epidemiology of autoimmune hepatitis. *Clin. Liver Dis.* **6:**347–359.
4. **Cha, S., P. S. Leung, R. L. Coppel, J. Van de Water, A. A. Ansari, and M. E. Gershwin.** 1994. Heterogeneity of combinatorial human autoantibodies against PDC-E2 and biliary epithelial cells in patients with primary biliary cirrhosis. *Hepatology* **20:**574–583.
5. **Cha, S., P. S. Leung, M. E. Gershwin, M. P. Fletcher, A. A. Ansari, and R. L. Coppel.** 1993. Combinatorial autoantibodies to dihydrolipoamide acetyltransferase, the major autoantigen of primary biliary cirrhosis. *Proc. Natl. Acad. Sci. USA* **90:**2527–2531.
6. **Czaja, A. J., and M. P. Manns.** 1995. The validity and importance of subtypes in autoimmune hepatitis: a point of view. *Am. J. Gastroenterol.* **90:**1206–1211.
7. **Dahlan, Y., L. Smith, D. Simmonds, L. D. Jewell, I. Wanless, E. J. Heathcote, and V. G. Bain.** 2003. Pediatric-onset primary biliary cirrhosis. *Gastroenterology* **125:**1476–1479.
8. **Desmet, V., M. A. Gerber, J. H. Hoofnagle, M. Manns, and P. Scheuer.** 1994. Classificaton of chronic hepatitis: diagnosis, grading and staging. *Hepatology* **19:**1513–1520.
9. **Diamantis, I., and D. T. Boumpas.** 2004. Autoimmune hepatitis: evolving concepts. *Autoimmun. Rev.* **3:**207–214.
10. **Dubel, L., A. Tanaka, P. S. Leung, J. Van de Water, R. Coppel, T. Roche, C. Johanet, Y. Motokawa, A. Ansari, and M. E. Gershwin.** 1999. Autoepitope mapping and reactivity of autoantibodies to the dihydrolipoamide dehydrogenase-binding protein (E3BP) and the glycine cleavage proteins in primary biliary cirrhosis. *Hepatology* **29:**1013–1018.
11. **Durazzo, M., T. H. Philipp, F. N. van Pelt, B. Luttig, E. Borghesio, G. Michel, E. Schmidt, S. Loges, M. Rizzetto, and M. P. Manns.** 1995. Heterogeneity of microsomal autoantibodies (LKM) in chronic hepatitis C and D virus infection. *Gastroenterology* **108:**455–462.
12. **Fukishima, N., M. Nakamura, M. Matsui, H. Ikematsu, K. Koike, H. Ishibashi, K. Hayashida, and Y. Niho.** 1995.

Establishment and structural analysis of human mAb to the E2 component of the 2-oxoglutarate dehydrogenase complex generated from a patient with primary biliary cirrhosis. *Int. Immunol.* 7:1047–1055.

13. Fukushima, N., G. Nalbandian, J. Van De Water, K. White, A. A. Ansari, P. Leung, T. Kenny, S. G. Kamita, B. D. Hammock, R. L. Coppel, F. Stevenson, H. Ishibashi, and M. E. Gershwin. 2002. Characterization of recombinant monoclonal IgA anti-PDC-E2 autoantibodies derived from patients with PBC. *Hepatology* 36:1383–1392.

14. Fussey, S. P., J. R. Guest, O. F. James, M. F. Bassendine, and S. J. Yeaman. 1988. Identification and analysis of the major M2 autoantigens in primary biliary cirrhosis. *Proc. Natl. Acad. Sci. USA* **85**:8654–8658.

15. Gershwin, M. E., R. L. Coppel, and I. R. Mackay. 1988. Primary biliary cirrhosis and mitochondrial autoantigens—insights from molecular biology. *Hepatology* 8:147–151.

16. Gershwin, M. E., I. R. Mackay, A. Sturgess, and R. L. Coppel. 1987. Identification and specificity of a cDNA encoding the 70 kd mitochondrial antigen recognized in primary biliary cirrhosis. *J. Immunol.* 138:3525–3531.

17. Gruber, R., E. Felber, G. R. Pape, W. Hochtlen-Vollmar, and G. Riethmuller. 1994. Detection of autoantibodies against M2, LKM-1, and SLA in liver diseases by standardized uniform ELISA techniques. *J. Clin. Lab. Anal.* **8**: 284–292.

18. Gueguen, M., A. M. Yamamoto, O. Bernard, and F. Alvarez. 1989. Anti-liver kidney microsome antibody type 1 recognizes human cytochrome P450 db 1. *Biochem. Biophys. Res. Commun.* 159:542–547.

19. Homberg, J. C., N. Abauf, O. Bernard, S. Islam, F. Alvarez, S. H. Khalil, R. Poupon, F. Darnis, V. G. Levy, P. Grippon, et al. 1987. Chronic active hepatitis associated with anti-liver/kidney microsome antibody type I: a second type of "autoimmune hepatitis." *Hepatology* 7:1333.

20. Iwayama, T., P. S. Leung, M. Rowley, S. Munoz, M. Nishioka, T. Nakagawa, E. R. Dickson, R. L. Coppel, I. R. Mackay, and M. E. Gershwin. 1992. Comparative immunoreactive profiles of Japanese and American patients with primary biliary cirrhosis against mitochondrial autoantigens. *Int. Arch. Allergy Immunol.* 99:28–33.

21. Jones, D. E. J., J. M. Palmer, O. F. W. James, S. J. Yeaman, M. F. Bassendine, and A. G. Diamond. 1995. T-cell responses to the components of pyruvate dehydrogenase complex in primary biliary cirrhosis. *Hepatology* 21:995–1002.

22. Joplin, R., L. L. Wallace, G. D. Johnson, J. G. Lindsay, S. J. Yeaman, J. M. Palmer, A. J. Strain, and J. M. Neuberger. 1995. Subcellular localization of pyruvate dehydrogenase dihydrolipoamide acetyltransferase in human intrahepatic biliary epithelial cells. *J. Pathol.* 176:381–390.

23. Kaplan, M. M. 1996. Primary biliary cirrhosis. *N. Engl. J. Med.* 21:1570–1580.

24. Kita, H., Z. X. Lian, J. Van de Water, X. S. He, S. Matsumura, M. Kaplan, V. Luketic, R. L. Coppel, A. A. Ansari, and M. E. Gershwin. 2002. Identification of HLA-A2-restricted CD8(+) cytotoxic T cell responses in primary biliary cirrhosis: T cell activation is augmented by immune complexes cross-presented by dendritic cells. *J. Exp. Med.* 195:113–123.

25. Kita, H., S. Matsumura, X. S. He, A. A. Ansari, Z. X. Lian, J. Van de Water, R. L. Coppel, M. M. Kaplan, and M. E. Gershwin. 2002. Quantitative and functional analysis of PDC-E2-specific autoreactive cytotoxic T lymphocytes in primary biliary cirrhosis. *J. Clin. Investig.* 109: 1231–1240.

26. Kyraitsoulis, A., M. Manns, G. Gerken, A. W. Lohse, W. Ballhausen, K. Reske, Z. Meyer, and K. H.

Buschenfelde. 1987. Distinction between natural and pathological autoantibodies by immunoblotting and densitometric subtraction: liver-kidney-microsomal antibody (LKM) positive sera identity multiple antigens in human liver tissue. *Clin. Exp. Immunol.* **79**:53–60.

27. Leung, P. S., T. Iwayama, T. Prindiville, D. T. Chuang, A. A. Ansari, R. M. Wynn, R. Dickson, R. Coppel, and M. E. Gershwin. 1992. Use of designer recombinant mitochondrial antigens in the diagnosis of primary biliary cirrhosis. *Hepatology* **15**:367–372.

28. Leung, P. S., S. Krams, S. Munoz, C. P. Surh, A. Ansari, T. Kenny, D. L. Robbins, J. Fung, T. E. Starzl, W. Maddrey, R. L. Coppel, and M. E. Gershwin. 1992. Characterization and epitope mapping of human monoclonal antibodies to PDC-E2, the immunodominant autoantigen of primary biliary cirrhosis. *J. Autoimmun.* 5: 703–718.

29. Leung, P. S., J. Van de Water, R. L. Coppel, and M. E. Gershwin. 1991. Molecular characterization of the mitochondrial autoantigens in primary biliary cirrhosis. *Immunol. Res.* 10:518–527.

30. Leung, P. S. C., D. T. Chuang, R. M. Wynn, S. Cha, D. J. Danner, A. Ansari, R. Coppel, and M. E. Gershwin. 1995. Autoantibodies to BCOADC-E2 in patients with primary biliary cirrhosis recognize a conformational epitope. *Hepatology* **22**:505–513.

31. Leung, P. S. C., M. P. Manns, and M. E. Gershwin. 1996. *Inflammatory Hepatobiliary Cirrhosis*, vol. II. Mosby Year Book, Inc., St. Louis, Mo.

32. Mackay, I. R. 1958. Primary biliary cirrhosis showing high titer of autoantibody: report of a case. *N. Engl. J. Med.* **254**:185.

33. Manns, M. 1994. Autoantibodies in chronic hepatitis: diagnostic reagents and scientific tools to study etiology, pathogenesis and cell biology, vol. XII. W.B. Saunders Company, Philadelphia, Pa.

34. Manns, M., G. Gerken, A. Kyriatsoulis, M. Staritz, and K. H. Meyer zum Buschenfelde. 1987. Characterization of a new subgroup of autoimmune chronic active hepatitis by autoantibodies against a soluble liver antigen. *Lancet* i:292.

35. Manns, M., E. F. Johnson, K. J. Griffin, E. M. Tan, and K. F. Sullivan. 1989. Major target antigen of liver and kidney microsomal autoantibodies in idiopathic autoimmune hepatitis in cytochrome P450db1. *J. Clin. Investig.* 83: 1066–1072.

36. Manns, M., K. H. Meyer zum Buschenfelde, J. Slusarczyk, and H. P. Dienes. 1984. Detection of liver-kidney microsomal autoantibodies by radioimmunoassay and their relation to anti-mitochondrial antibodies in inflammatory liver diseases. *Clin. Exp. Immunol.* **57**:600–608.

37. Manns, M. P., K. J. Griffin, L. C. Quattrochi, M. Sacher, H. Thaler, R. H. Tukey, and E. F. Johnson. 1990. Identification of cytochrome p450 IA2 as a human autoantigen. *Arch. Biochem. Biophys.* **280**:229–232.

38. Manns, M. P., and E. F. Johnson. 1991. Identification of human microsomal cytochrome P450 using autoantibodies. *Methods Enzymol.* 206:210–219.

39. Matsumura, S., J. Van De Water, H. Kita, R. L. Coppel, T. Tsuji, K. Yamamoto, A. A. Ansari, and M. E. Gershwin. 2002. Contribution to antimitochondrial antibody production: cleavage of pyruvate dehydrogenase complex-E2 by apoptosis-related proteases. *Hepatology* 35:14–22.

40. Matsumura, S., J. Van De Water, P. Leung, J. A. Odin, K. Yamamoto, G. J. Gores, K. Mostov, A. A. Ansari, R. L. Coppel, Y. Shiratori, and M. E. Gershwin. 2004. Caspase induction by IgA antimitochondrial antibody: IgA-mediated biliary injury in primary biliary cirrhosis. *Hepatology* 39:1415–1422.

41. Migliaccio, C., A. Nishio, J. Van de Water, A. A. Ansari, P. S. Leung, Y. Nakanuma, R. L. Coppel, and M. E. Gershwin. 1998. Monoclonal antibodies to mitochondrial E2 components define autoepitopes in primary biliary cirrhosis. *J. Immunol.* **161:**5157–5163.

42. Moteki, S., P. S. C. Leung, R. L. Coppel, E. R. Dickson, M. M. Kaplan, S. Munoz, and M. E. Gershwin. 1996. Use of designer triple expression hybrid clone for three different lipoyl domains for the detection of anti-mitochondrial antibodies. *Hepatology* **24:**97–103.

43. Moteki, S., P. S. C. Leung, E. R. Dickson, D. H. Van Thiel, C. Galperin, T. Buch, D. Alarcon-Segovia, D. Kershenobich, K. Kawano, R. L. Coppel, S. Matuda, and M. E. Gershwin. 1996. Epitope mapping and reactivity of autoantibodies to the E2 component of 2-oxoglutarate dehydrogenase complex (OGDC-E2) in primary biliary cirrhosis using recombinant OGDC-E2. *Hepatology* **23:**436–444.

44. Odin, J. A., R. C. Huebert, L. Casciola-Rosen, N. F. LaRusso, and A. Rosen. 2001. Bcl-2-dependent oxidation of pyruvate dehydrogenase-E2, a primary biliary cirrhosis autoantigen, during apoptosis. *J. Clin. Investig.* **108:**223–232.

45. Philipp, T., M. Durazzo, C. Trautwein, B. Alex, P. Straub, J. G. Lamb, E. F. Johnson, R. H. Tukey, and M. P. Manns. 1994. Recognition of uridine diphosphate glucuronosyl transferase by LKM-3 antibodies in chronic hepatitis D. *Lancet* **344:**578–581.

46. Reynosa-Paz, S., P. S. C. Leung, J. Van de Water, A. Tanaka, S. Munoz, N. Bass, K. Lindor, P. J. Donald, R. L. Coppel, A. Ansari, and M. E. Gershwin. 2000. Evidence for a local driven mucosal response and the presence of mitochondrial antigens in saliva in primary biliary cirrhosis. *Hepatology* **31:**24–29.

47. Rizzetto, M., G. Swana, and D. Doniaach. 1973. Microsomal antibodies in active chronic hepatitis and other disorders. *Clin. Exp. Immunol.* **15:**331–344.

48. Shimoda, S., M. Nakamura, H. Ishibashi, K. Hayashida, and Y. Niho. 1995. HLA DRB4 0101-restricted immunodominant T cell autoepitope of pyruvate dehydrogenase complex in primary biliary cirrhosis: evidence of molecular mimicry in human autoimmune diseases. *J. Exp. Med.* **181:**1835–1845.

49. Strassburg, C. P., and M. P. Manns. 2002. Autoantibodies and autoantigens in autoimmune hepatitis. *Semin. Liver Dis.* **22:**339–352.

50. Strassburg, C. P., P. Obermayer-Straub, B. Alex, T. Philipp, R. H. Tukey, and M. P. Manns. 1995. Autoepitopes on UDP-lucuronosyltransferase (LKM-3) in autoimmune hepatitis differ from those on hepatitis C. *Gastroenterology* **108:**A1177.

51. Surh, C. D., A. Ahmed-Ansari, and M. E. Gershwin. 1990. Comparative epitope mapping of murine monoclonal and human autoantibodies to human PDH-E2, the major mitochondrial autoantigen of primary biliary cirrhosis. *J. Immunol.* **144:**2647–2652.

52. Surh, C. D., A. E. Cooper, R. L. Coppel, P. Leung, A. Ahmed, R. Dickson, and M. E. Gershwin. 1988. The predominance of IgG3 and IgM isotype antimitochondrial autoantibodies against recombinant fused mitochondrial polypeptide in patients with primary biliary cirrhosis. *Hepatology* **8:**290–295.

53. Surh, C. D., R. Coppel, and M. E. Gershwin. 1990. Structural requirement for autoreactivity on human pyruvate dehydrogenase-E2, the major autoantigen of primary biliary cirrhosis. Implication for a conformational autoepitope. *J. Immunol.* **144:**3367–3374.

54. Tanaka, A., G. Nalbandian, P. S. C. Leung, G. D. Benson, M. Santiago, J. A. Findor, A. D. Branch, R. L. Coppel, A. A. Ansari, and M. E. Gershwin. 2000. Mucosal immunity and primary biliary cirrhosis: presence of antimitochondrial antibodies in urine. *Hepatology* **32:**910–915.

55. Tsuneyama, K., J. Van de Water, P. S. C. Leung, S. Cha, Y. Nakanuma, M. Kaplan, R. De Lellis, R. Coppel, A. Ansari, and M. E. Gershwin. 1995. Abnormal expression of the E2 component of the pyruvate dehydrogenase complex on the luminal surface of biliary epithelium occurs before major histocompatibility complex class II and BB1/B7 expression. *Hepatology* **21:**1031–1037.

56. Tuaillon, N., C. Andre, J. P. Briand, E. Penner, and S. Muller. 1992. A lipoyl synthetic octadecapeptide of dihydrolipoamide acetyltransferase specifically recognized by anti-M2 autoantibodies in primary biliary cirrhosis. *J. Immunol.* **148:**445–450.

57. Van de Water, J., A. Ansari, T. Prindiville, R. L. Coppel, N. Ricalton, B. L. Kotzin, S. Liu, T. E. Roche, S. M. Krams, S. Munoz, et al. 1995. Heterogeneity of autoreactive T cell clones specific for the E2 component of the pyruvate dehydrogenase complex in primary biliary cirrhosis. *J. Exp. Med.* **181:**723–733.

58. Van de Water, J., A. Cooper, C. D. Surh, R. Coppel, D. Danner, A. Ansari, R. Dickson, and M. E. Gershwin. 1989. Detection of autoantibodies to recombinant mitochondrial proteins in patients with primary biliary cirrhosis. *N. Engl. J. Med.* **320:**1377–1380.

59. Van de Water, J., M. E. Gershwin, P. Leung, A. Ansari, and R. L. Coppel. 1988. The autoepitope of the 74-kD mitochondrial autoantigen of primary biliary cirrhosis corresponds to the functional site of dihydrolipoamide acetyltransferase. *J. Exp. Med.* **167:**1791–1799.

60. Volkmann, M., L. Martin, A. Baurle, H. Heid, C. P. Strassburg, C. Trautwein, W. Fiehn, and M. P. Manns. 2001. Soluble liver antigen: isolation of a 35-kd recombinant protein (SLA-p35) specifically recognizing sera from patients with autoimmune hepatitis. *Hepatology* **33:**591–596.

61. Walker, J. G., D. Doniach, I. M. Roitt, and S. Sherlock. 1965. Serological tests in the diagnosis of primary biliary cirrhosis. *Lancet* **39:**827–830.

62. Yeaman, S. J., S. P. Fussey, D. J. Danner, O. F. James, D. J. Mutimer, and M. F. Bassendine. 1988. Primary biliary cirrhosis: identification of two major M2 mitochondrial autoantigens. *Lancet* **i:**1067–1070.

Skin Diseases

CARLOS H. NOUSARI AND GRANT J. ANHALT

123

The dermis and epidermis have a dense network of adhesion proteins and fibrous structural proteins that provide mechanical strength to the skin. A number of these adhesion molecules are known to become targets of autoantibodies, and antigen-antibody interactions in the skin lead to the clinical manifestations of autoimmune bullous skin diseases. Demonstration of the characteristic autoantibodies in the tissue and circulating in the blood is the critical diagnostic feature of numerous such diseases. In most of these diseases, the circulating autoantibodies have also been shown, by passive transfer in animal models, to directly cause the characteristic tissue injury. For each of these diseases, we describe the expected findings in tissue and serum and outline immunochemical tests that may be useful in diagnosis. Additionally, there are some inflammatory skin diseases in which immunologic changes have been identified, but these changes are not essential diagnostic features and causality has not been established. These diseases are discussed in brief.

IIF OF SERUM FOR DIAGNOSIS OF SKIN DISEASES

Technical Aspects

Indirect immunofluorescence (IIF) is a semiquantitative procedure whereby a double immunolabeling is performed to evaluate the presence and titer of circulating autoantibodies (16, 46, 73). Blood is drawn into a tube without anticoagulant, and serum is serially diluted with phosphate-buffered saline (PBS) with 0.05% sodium azide. An initial dilution of 1:10 and doubling dilutions thereafter are usually used. Substrates most commonly used are 6-mm frozen sections of monkey skin and esophagus, human skin, guinea pig lip or esophagus, and murine bladder. All nonhuman substrate sections are available from commercial laboratories. Human skin is usually obtained from neonatal foreskins or discarded surgical specimens. Use of multiple substrates may increase the sensitivity of detection of circulating antibodies (3). The sections are incubated with serum dilutions for 30 min at room temperature and then washed with PBS-azide. Antibodies bound to the substrate are detected by incubation with fluorescein isothiocyanate-labeled hyperimmune goat serum (a source of anti-human class-specific immunoglobulins), followed by two washings with PBS (48, 50). Routinely, anti-human immunoglobulin M(IgM), IgG, and IgA are used.

Salt-Split Skin IIF

The sensitivity and specificity of IIF for basement membrane zone (BMZ) autoantibodies when human skin is used are markedly increased by salt splitting the tissue before use. Normal human skin is trimmed into 4-mm squares, the dermis is shaved as thin as possible, the squares are incubated for 48 to 72 h in 1 M NaCl at 4°C, excess salt is removed by washing in PBS-azide, and then the epidermis is manually separated from the dermis. (Additional details are found in chapter 48 of this volume.) The epithelium is placed on the dermis, and the tissue is frozen and sectioned at 6 μm. The use of this substrate for IIF is crucial for the diagnosis of subepidermal bullous diseases characterized by deposition of immunoreactants along the BMZ, e.g., to differentiate bullous pemphigoid (BP) from epidermolysis bullosa acquisita (EBA) (86) and to identify the anti-epiligrin (laminin 5) mucous membrane pemphigoid (MMP) from other types of MMP (57).

Immunochemical Techniques

Immunochemical detection and definition of the antigenic specificity of serum autoantibodies in bullous diseases constitute a powerful way of defining these diseases but are not yet widely used. Research applications of these tests have been common since the early 1980s and generally employ three techniques: Western immunoblotting using sodium dodecyl sulfate (SDS) extracts of skin, immunoprecipitation using metabolically labeled keratinocyte cultures, and enzyme-linked immunosorbent assay (ELISA) using recombinant antigens. These techniques are applicable in those cases where circulating antibodies are present in reasonably high titers (essentially all cases of pemphigus and approximately up to 85% of cases of subepidermal blistering diseases) and provide precise diagnosis by documenting binding of autoantibodies to skin autoantigens, identified by their characteristic molecular weights. Technical problems that have delayed implementation are as follows. (i) These adhesion molecules are present in small quantities in tissue, are insoluble, and are difficult to extract and prepare in commercial quantities. (ii) Western blotting still requires separation of skin antigens by SDS-polyacrylamide gel electrophoresis immunoblotting with serum and comparison with internal controls. This is very time-consuming and expensive. (iii) In many cases, Western immunoblotting is no more sensitive than IIF in detecting circulating autoantibodies. (iv) Immunoprecipitation requires use of cell cultures, SDS-polyacrylamide gel electrophoresis, and radioactive amino acids, techniques not used in most diagnostic laboratories.

Fortunately, development of ELISA techniques has progressed substantially in recent years. Recombinant proteins that contain the major antigenic epitopes recognized by autoantibodies have been successfully used for pemphigus vulgaris (PV) and pemphigus foliaceus (PF) (desmogleins 3 and 1, respectively) and for the BP 180 antigen (BP antigen 2 [BP Ag2]). The ELISA for desmogleins 1 and 3 and BP 180 is currently available commercially from Medical and Biological Laboratories (Nagoya, Japan; http://www.mbl.co.jp). However, because the technology to produce the protein is intensive, the cost of the plates is quite high, and in some states, the reimbursement for the test falls short of the material costs. A standardized ELISA to detect circulating autoantibodies for paraneoplastic pemphigus (PNP) and EBA is not available yet, but recently, significant progress has been made in this area (15, 20, 28, 75, 80).

SKIN DISEASES IN WHICH IMMUNOLOGIC ABNORMALITIES ARE AN ESSENTIAL COMPONENT OF THE DIAGNOSTIC CRITERIA

Pemphigus

There are four major forms of pemphigus: PV, PF, PNP, and IgA pemphigus. All forms are characterized by a loss of normal epidermal cell-to-cell adhesion (acantholysis) and by the presence of pathogenic autoantibodies reacting against desmosomal adhesion molecules. Pemphigus is a potentially lethal disease; to establish the diagnosis with certainty, the presence of both tissue-bound and circulating autoantibodies must be demonstrated.

PV

Tissue

Direct immunofluorescence (DIF) of perilesional skin shows the characteristic linear deposition of IgG and C3 on the surface of epidermal cells (Fig. 1) (62, 67). Previously, it was thought that the autoantibodies bound a substance in the intercellular spaces between keratinocytes, and the staining pattern was referred to as intercellular space or intercellular substance staining. It is known that this pattern is due to binding of autoantibodies to a transmembrane adhesion molecule of the keratinocyte, desmoglein 3 and 1, but the older terminology is still used. IgG deposition is rather uniform throughout the epithelium, although there may be some preferential staining of the suprabasilar cells, especially in oral biopsy samples. C3 immunostaining is more focal, occurring in areas where acantholysis is evident. The absence of deposition of immunoreactants at the BMZ, in the context of positive cell surface immunostaining, constitutes the hallmark IF features of PV (Fig. 1). False-positive deposition of IgG is not expected but can be seen if the skin biopsy sample is not adequately washed prior to sectioning or if the transport medium is old and has become acidic. False negatives can occur if the biopsy is too distant from lesional tissue. Isolated C3 deposition on the epidermal cell surfaces without concomitant deposition of IgG can be found in impetigo and in some cases of drug-induced pemphigus.

Serologic Studies

IIF should be positive for all patients with active disease, and monkey esophagus is the optimal substrate for detection (3, 31). The expected finding is a linear binding of IgG over the epithelial cell surfaces, producing a chicken wire pattern of fluorescence. There is no binding to the esophageal BMZ (Fig. 2).

Sensitivity and Specificity

The titers of circulating autoantibody show a rough correlation with disease activity, although detection of circulating antibodies can lag behind the development of clinical disease, especially early in the course, and low titers (up to 1:160) may not have a reliable direct correlation to clinical activity (23). Low titers of antiepithelial antibodies, directed at other cell surface proteins such as blood group antigens, have been detected occasionally in patients with skin burns, in penicillin-allergic individuals, in those with dermatophyte infections, and in some healthy subjects, but they are not frequently observed (2, 5, 26, 32).

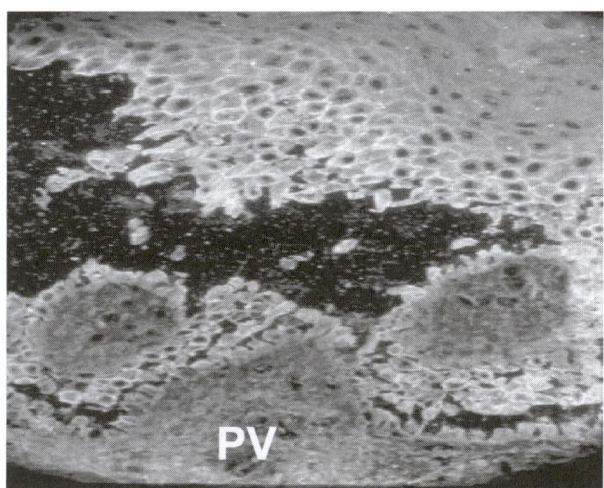 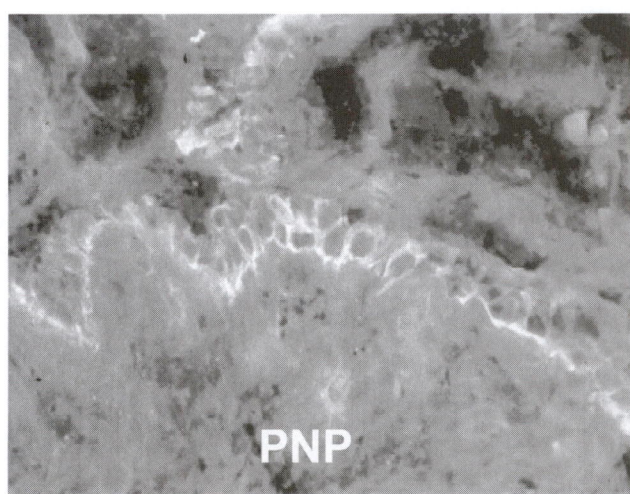

FIGURE 1 (Left) DIF of oral mucosa in PV showing linear IgG deposits on the epithelial cell surfaces; (right) DIF of oral mucosa in PNP showing linear IgG deposits on the epithelial cell surfaces as well as along the BMZ.

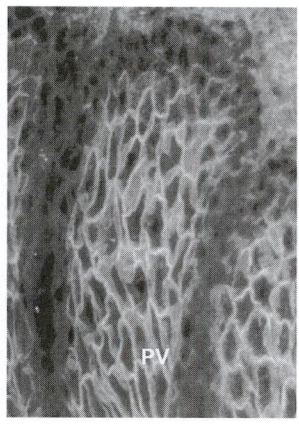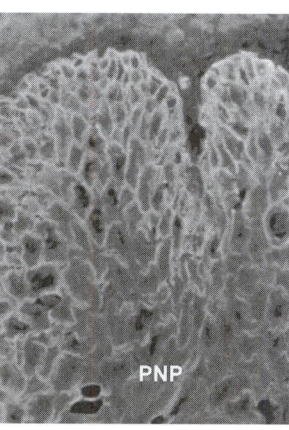

FIGURE 2 (Left) IIF in PV showing the presence of circulating IgG autoantibodies binding the epithelial cell surfaces of monkey esophagus substrate with sparing of BMZ and the basal third of the epithelial stratum; (right) IIF in PNP showing the presence of circulating IgG autoantibodies binding the epithelial cell surfaces as well as the BMZ of monkey esophagus substrate.

Immunochemical Techniques

The epitopes recognized by autoantibodies in PV are largely conformational and usually cannot readily be detected by a denaturing technique such as Western immunoblotting. Immunoprecipitation in the presence of nondenaturing detergents is relatively sensitive and very specific for characterization of these antibodies; however, the technique is expensive and of limited availability and thus is used only in research protocols or for unusual cases. For these reasons, ELISA using the extracellular portion of the desmoglein 3 molecule, produced in a baculovirus expression system, is becoming a useful diagnostic test (45). The sensitivity of the ELISA for PV and PF is approximately 95%, and the specificity approaches 98%, when only samples with very significantly elevated levels of antibody are considered true positives (6). In PV, when only oral epithelium is affected, elevated levels of serum antibodies against desmoglein 3 alone are expected. If patients have both skin and oral lesions, the serum autoantibodies should react with both desmoglein 3 and desmoglein 1 (Table 1) (7).

PF

Four clinical subsets of PF have been identified: idiopathic PF, endemic PF, drug-induced PF (72, 81), and pemphigus erythematosus.

TABLE 1 Antibody profiles in pemphigus variants

Disease	Antibody reactivity
PF	Desmoglein 1
PV (oral lesions only)	Desmoglein 3
PV (oral and skin lesions)	Desmogleins 3 and 1
IgA pemphigus	
	Desmocollins 1, 2, and 3
	Desmogleins 3 and 1
PNP	
	Plakins
	Desmogleins 3 and 1

Tissue
With the exception of pemphigus erythematosus, the pattern of IgG deposition in the epidermis is the same in all subsets of PF and indistinguishable from that observed in PV. In pemphigus erythematosus, there is combined immunoreactant deposition similar to that seen in pemphigus and in lesions of lupus erythematosus (LE); i.e., there is linear IgG on the epidermal cell surfaces as well as granular deposition of immunoreactants along the epidermal BMZ (37, 83). IgA PF, also known as intercellular IgA dermatosis, is a newly described and rare condition characterized by linear deposition of only IgA on the epidermal cell surfaces. The inclusion of this entity as a form of pemphigus is controversial.

Serologic Studies
Patients with PF produce an autoantibody specific for another transmembrane adhesion molecule of stratified squamous epithelium, desmoglein 1. IIF using monkey esophagus as a substrate will detect circulating IgG autoantibodies in more than 90% of patients with PF, and the titer of autoantibody roughly correlates with the clinical disease activity (29). The pattern of binding of PF antibodies is indistinguishable from that of PV.

Sensitivity and Specificity
About 10% of patients have levels of circulating autoantibody that are undetectable when monkey esophagus is used. Guinea pig lip or esophagus appears to be somewhat more sensitive, in that it will identify most of these false-negative sera. Additionally, the IF titer on guinea pig mucosa is usually higher than that measured using monkey esophagus (79). In pemphigus erythematosus, antinuclear antibody activity may also be detected in the serum. In IgA PF, circulating IgA antiepithelial antibodies may be detected, but the incidence is not certain and the antigen specificity is not clear. There is some evidence that IgA autoantibodies may react with two related transmembrane adhesion molecules, desmocollins 1 and 2.

Immunochemical Techniques
As in PV, Western blotting and immunoprecipitation techniques are difficult and expensive and are not routinely performed. The ELISA for desmoglein 1 is also proving very useful. In PF, the expected result is the detection of autoantibodies against desmoglein 1 but not desmoglein 3. With a sensitivity of about 95%, this assay should soon become standard for the diagnosis of PF.

PNP
PNP is associated with underlying lymphoproliferative disease or thymomas and has clinical and immunologic specificities that clearly distinguish it from other forms of pemphigus.

Tissue
DIF of perilesional tissue shows deposition of IgG in the intercellular spaces of the affected skin and mucosal epithelial cells, in a pattern similar to that seen in PV or PF, but the deposition can be faint and/or focal. A distinctive finding is the combined presence of linear complement deposition along the BMZ in addition to the epithelial cell surface binding of IgG (Fig. 1) (11). Frequently, patients have high levels of coexistent autoantibodies against cytoskeletal proteins, producing high background cytoplasmic staining in the epithelium and obscuring specific autoantibody deposition.

Serologic Studies

In most cases of PNP, circulating IgG autoantibodies reactive with the cell surface of monkey esophagus will be detectable by IIF. In most cases, the pattern of binding will be similar to that observed with PV or PF serum antibodies. In a minority of cases, circulating antibodies that additionally bind along the epithelial BMZ are present, but in most cases it is not possible to distinguish PNP from other forms of pemphigus by this technique alone. Patients with PNP have a complex humoral autoimmune response, with serum antibodies known to be specific for proteins of the desmosomes and hemidesmosomes (desmoplakins I and II and the BP Ag1) as well as two keratinocyte proteins, envoplakin and periplakin. The key to differentiation of PNP from other forms of pemphigus by IIF lies in the tissue distribution of these autoantigens. The PV and PF antigens, desmogleins 1 and 3, are produced only by stratified squamous epithelia. Serologic markers for PNP are autoantibodies against plakin proteins, which include desmoplakins I and II, envoplakin, periplakin, and plectin (Table 2) (9). Desmoplakins are expressed in stratified squamous epithelia and in many other epithelia and adhesion structures throughout the body. The finding of autoantibody reactivity that is either (i) restricted solely to stratified squamous epithelia or (ii) reactive with both stratified squamous and other epithelia implies the presence or absence, respectively, of antidesmoplakin autoantibodies. The most commonly used nonstratified squamous epithelium for this purpose is rat or mouse urinary bladder epithelium. By IIF, binding of serum antibodies to the cell surface of only esophagus indicates PV or PF, and binding to both esophagus and urinary bladder epithelium indicates PNP (Fig. 3). With monkey esophagus as a substrate, the fact that the PNP autoantibodies would bind the epithelial cell surfaces consistently and homogeneously throughout the entire epithelial stratum (due to the ubiquitous location of plakin proteins), in conjunction with the BMZ staining, should raise a strong suspicion for PNP (Fig. 2).

Sensitivity and Specificity

The sensitivity and specificity of IIF for PNP using urinary bladder are estimated to be 75 and 83%, respectively (Fig. 3) (44).

Immunochemical

Although IIF procedures are reasonable for diagnostic screening in suspected cases of PNP, up to 25% of cases cannot be diagnosed by IF alone. Definition of the complex antigen specificity of the autoantibodies requires more precise techniques. Almost all patients with PNP have antibodies against desmoglein 3 that can be detected by ELISA, and about two-thirds have antibodies also against desmoglein 1. To properly distinguish PV from PNP, one must show antibodies both against the desmogleins and against the plakin proteins. Immunoprecipitation with ^{14}C-labeled keratinocytes

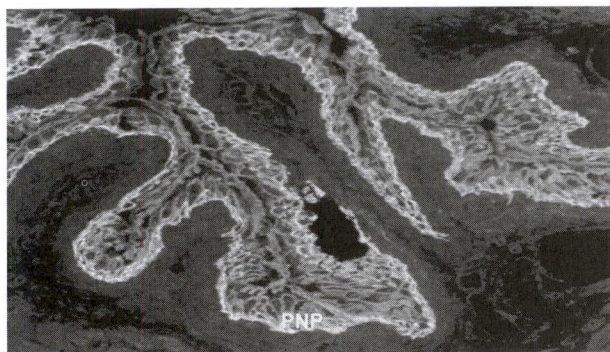

FIGURE 3 IIF in PNP showing the presence of circulating IgG autoantibodies binding the epithelial cell surfaces as well as the BMZ of murine bladder, a plakin-rich substrate.

remains the standard diagnostic method (11) but is available only from laboratories doing research in this field. By immunoblotting for antibodies to the plakin proteins, usually only envoplakin and periplakin antibodies can be detected; however, the demonstration of antibodies against these two plakin proteins in addition to desmoglein autoantibodies is usually confirmatory of the diagnosis. Antidesmoplakin antibodies have recently been detected in some PV patients, namely, children with significant mucosal disease and even in patients with BP. Therefore, strict clinical and immunopathological correlation as well as exclusion of other antiplakin antibodies, e.g., envoplakin and periplakin, by immunoblotting or immunoprecipitation is recommended for these patients.

BP and GP

Both BP and gestational pemphigoid (GP) are characterized by subepidermal cutaneous blisters and by the presence of autoantibodies against hemidesmosomal proteins (8, 66).

Tissue

By DIF, BP is characterized by linear deposition of C3 along the epidermal BMZ in virtually all perilesional specimens and by similar linear deposition of IgG in up to 90% of specimens (59, 65). Occasionally, concomitant but much weaker linear deposition of IgA is observed. Linear deposition of IgM along the BMZ has been reported as a rare and sole DIF finding in BP (43). With direct NaCl-split biopsy specimens (see chapter 48), the linear IgG deposition is found exclusively on the epidermal side (roof) of the induced blister. However, the linear C3 deposition may be observed at both epidermal and dermal locations, even in patients with IgG exclusively on the epidermal side. GP (also known as herpes gestationis) is a form of BP that occurs during pregnancy. Immunologic abnormalities are almost identical, with perilesional skin consistently showing linear deposition of C3 along the BMZ and linear deposition of IgG in 40% of the biopsy specimens (64).

Serologic Studies

Standard IIF using monkey esophagus will detect circulating anti-epidermal BMZ autoantibodies in only about 50% of cases. BP antibody titers do not correlate well with the clinical disease activity (Fig. 2). The detection of these antibodies is increased to about 70% if normal human salt-split skin is used as the substrate. Additionally, the IgG autoantibodies will be localized only on the epidermal side (roof) of the induced blister (Fig. 4) (41), which differentiates the disease

TABLE 2 Plakin proteins

Desmosomal
  Desmoplakin I/II
  Envoplakin
  Periplakin

Hemidesmosomal
  BP 230 (BP Ag1)
  Plectin

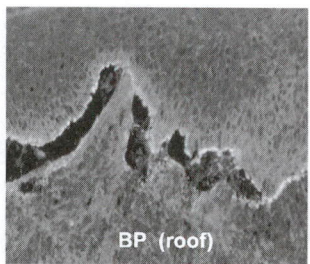 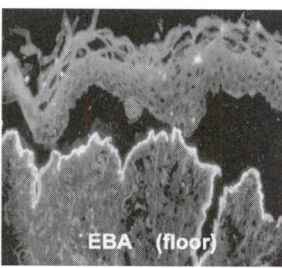

FIGURE 4 (Left) IIF in BP showing the presence of circulating IgG autoantibodies binding the epidermal side (roof) of human salt-split skin; (right) IIF in EBA showing the presence of circulating IgG autoantibodies binding the dermal side (floor) of human salt-split skin.

from EBA and other dermolytic subepidermal blistering diseases with certainty. In GP, low titers of complement-fixing IgG autoantibody, also specific for keratinocyte hemidesmosomal proteins, are present in the serum. This autoantibody was originally called the herpes gestationis factor, before its identity as an immunoglobulin was proven, but the terminology still persists. The autoantibody is generally present in titers too low to be detected by standard IIF techniques, and so a complement immunofixation technique is required to demonstrate its presence. Salt (1 M NaCl)-split normal human skin is sequentially incubated with a 1:10 dilution of heat-inactivated patient serum, fresh normal human serum as a source of complement, and fluorescein isothiocyanate-labeled anti-C3. The anti-C3 detects complement that is activated and bound to the IgG on the roof of the induced blister. This method is positive for the majority of the patients with active disease (49, 51).

Specificity

The finding of anti-BMZ antibodies that bind the epidermal side of split skin is abnormal and is expected to occur only in variants of pemphigoid.

Immunochemical Techniques

In BP and GP, autoantibodies against two distinct proteins of the keratinocyte hemidesmosome are present: (i) a 230-kDa intracellular hemidesmosomal plaque protein called BP Ag1 and (ii) a 180-kDa transmembrane protein of the hemidesmosome called BP Ag2. Antibodies against a small epitope present on the extracellular domain of the BP 180 antigen have been shown by passive transfer into mice to induce blister formation in vivo (58). It is not known whether antibodies against BP Ag1 can cause tissue injury, and so studies on antigen detection have focused on the BP 180 antigen (BP Ag2). Antibodies specific for the BP 180 antigen can be detected by Western blotting and by ELISA, using recombinant proteins representing the immunodominant epitope of BP Ag2 (38). In general, immunoblotting is not more sensitive than IIF on salt-split skin for detection of antibody, but the ELISA technique is much more sensitive and is capable of detecting specific antibody in about 94% of cases of BP and GP (89). The finding of (i) epidermal BMZ localization of in vivo-bound IgG on the epidermal side of salt-split skin by DIF or (ii) circulating IgG on the epidermal side of salt-split skin by IIF is so characteristic of pemphigoid that antigen-specific serologic testing is simply not necessary for diagnosis in most cases.

MMP (Cicatricial Pemphigoid)

MMP is a variant in which lesions occur primarily on mucous membranes and the lesions heal with scarring. MMP is a clinical diagnosis, and the typical clinical, histologic, and immunopathological features can be associated with more than a single antigen-antibody system. The majority of patients with cicatricial pemphigoid have antibody reactivity with the BP antigens; however, a minority have a similar clinical syndrome but with antibodies directed against laminin 5, type VII collagen, hemidesmosomal integrins (17), or other BMZ antigens.

Tissue

DIF findings are similar to those for BP except that coincident weaker linear deposition of IgA along the BMZ is often seen (12, 33, 56). Using IIF of salt-split human skin, the linear deposition of IgG is seen on the epidermal side in most cases, but in a minority, IgG deposition is seen on the floor of the induced blister as in anti-epiligrin MMP or predominantly mucosal EBA (30, 53, 55).

Specificity

The diagnosis cannot be made without showing immunoreactants along the BMZ. There is substantial sampling error, and false-negative DIF is common, occurring in as many as 10% of cases after a single biopsy. If clinical suspicion warrants it, biopsies should be repeated. Also, when perilesional mucosa is biopsied, the epithelium often peels off the lamina propria and can be lost during processing of the tissue.

Serologic Studies

In most cases where lesions are localized to mucosal surfaces, circulating antibodies will not be detectable. In about 15% of cases, IgG anti-BMZ antibodies are present but in low titers.

Immunochemical Techniques

Immunochemical techniques are not possible in most cases because of the absence of circulating autoantibodies. Preliminary studies show that the BP 180 ELISA yields more sera with detectable antibodies, but the level of detection is still low (less than one-third).

DH

Dermatitis herpetiformis (DH) is an extremely pruritic papulovesicular eruption of the skin, associated with the HLA-B8,DQ2 haplotype and an asymptomatic gluten-sensitive enteropathy.

Tissue

DH is diagnosed by the characteristic deposition of granular IgA scattered along the BMZ, with more dense accumulation in the tips of the dermal papillae and along the dermal microfibrils since these IgA deposits have high binding affinity for fibrillin 1 (Fig. 5). These IgA deposits persist even after treatment with dapsone and will decrease only after prolonged observance of a strict gluten-free diet (34).

Serologic Studies

Antiendomysial IgA antibodies, now known to react with tissue transglutaminase, are present in DH patients. They can be detected in most cases by ELISA (78) and in 50 to 80% of cases by IIF binding with the endomysial lining of smooth muscle bundles in the muscularis mucosa of monkey esophagus. These autoantibodies are present in most active cases of DH with gluten-sensitive enteropathy of grades III

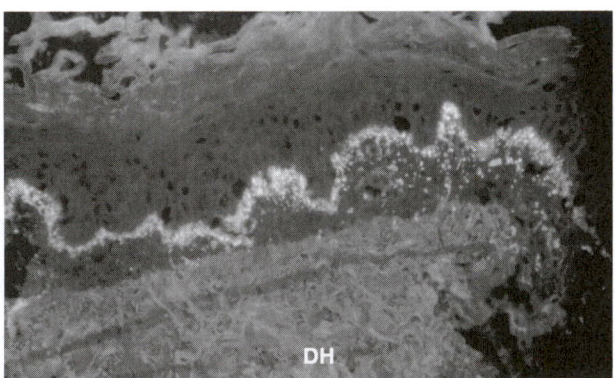

FIGURE 5 DIF of DH showing characteristic granular IgA deposits along the BMZ, with accentuation at the tip of the dermal papillae and microfibrils.

and IV (21). Despite their potential use in monitoring the clinical response to a gluten-free diet, they are not often used in clinical practice.

LABD and CBDC

Linear IgA bullous disease (LABD) and chronic bullous disease of childhood (CBDC) are characterized by pruritic blisters of skin, but disease subsets exist. Most patients have IgA antibodies against a secreted fragment of BP Ag2 and have a blistering cutaneous disease that resembles BP (77, 87). However, up to 20% of LABD patients have a scarring mucosal disease similar to MMP (52), in some cases induced by drugs such as vancomycin (68). Therefore, the diagnosis of LABD or CBDC includes several different conditions that are mediated by a single immunoglobulin isotype.

Tissue

LABD and CBDC are defined by the finding on DIF of linear deposition of IgA along the epidermal BMZ. Other immunoreactants, aside from very weak deposition of C3, are not detected.

Serologic Studies

In LABD and CBCD, circulating IgA anti-BMZ antibodies are detectable in about 50% of patients when human split skin is used (85). In the majority of LABD sera, circulating IgA reacts with the BP 180 antigen on the epidermal side of the induced blister. However, in some cases of both LABD and CBCD, namely, the vancomycin-induced variant, the immunoreactant may be found on the dermal surface, again reflecting the heterogeneity of the disease as currently defined.

EBA and BSLE

The cutaneous immunologic features of EBA and bullous systemic LE (BSLE) are identical: in both syndromes, subepidermal blistering is caused by autoantibodies against type VII collagen. In EBA, the autoantibodies are the sole immunologic abnormality; in BSLE, they arise in a patient with coexistent systemic LE.

Tissue

There is dense linear deposition of IgG and C3 along the epidermal BMZ. The deposition is similar to that observed in pemphigoid but on close inspection may appear thicker and more fibrillar (14, 35). In direct NaCl-split biopsy specimens,

the linear deposition of immunoreactants in EBA and BSLE is characteristically present on the dermal side (floor) of the induced blister (36).

Serologic Studies

Circulating autoantibodies are detectable in about 50% of patients. Salt-split human skin IIF shows linear deposition of IgG only on the floor of the induced blister (86). Western immunoblotting is as sensitive as IIF for detection of these antibodies, and an ELISA has been developed (20); however, both techniques are currently available only from research laboratories. These techniques are useful in that they can distinguish with certainty EBA and BSLE from less common and incompletely characterized bullous diseases that may have similar IF findings (19, 22, 88).

Cutaneous Vasculitides

Tissue

Even though the diagnosis of vasculitis is made on histologic grounds (82), DIF plays a very important role, in some cases a critical, if not sine qua non, role in the classification and workup of cutaneous vasculitides, namely, in the small size types.

In the so-called "cutaneous leukocytoclastic angiitis" (previously known as hypersensitivity vasculitis), rare systemic disease is encountered and thus granular weak IgM with even weaker C3 is commonly found in small dermal vessels. In contrast, in cutaneous vasculitides associated with high titer of rheumatoid factor, such as rheumatoid vasculitis and cryoglobulinemia II, strong granular IgM and C3 is almost the rule on skin DIF examination. In antineutrophil cytoplasmic antibody-mediated cutaneous vasculitides, granular IgG and weaker IgM and C3 constitute a common vascular pattern, whereas in connective tissue disease-associated vasculitides, strong vascular IgG and C3 deposits are characteristically found.

DIF plays a sine qua non role in IgA vasculitis and hypocomplementemic urticarial vasculitis. In IgA vasculitis (Henoch-Schoenlein purpura) in children and adults, granular IgA with or without other weaker immunoreactants is found in eventually all patients from early lesions, in the very superficial postcapillary papillary venules (13). Hypocomplementemic urticarial vasculitis almost always presents as a syndrome that falls into the spectrum of systemic LE; therefore, the DIF vascular pattern is typically characterized by granular IgG deposits along the BMZ and in and around upper dermal vessels (27) (Fig. 6).

Serologic Studies

An assay for detection of circulating IgG or IgA immune complexes can be performed but is of very limited clinical value.

DISEASES IN WHICH IMMUNOLOGIC ABNORMALITIES ARE HELPFUL BUT NOT ESSENTIAL IN DIAGNOSIS

Cutaneous Porphyria

Porphyria cutanea tarda is diagnosed by demonstration of increased urinary excretion of uroporphyrins and coproporphyrins. Because of the presence of subepidermal blisters, DIF is frequently performed; the results demonstrate thick, homogeneous, and linear deposition of IgG, IgA, and weaker C3 both around superficial dermal vessels and along the BMZ. The blood vessels are typically thickened, giving a

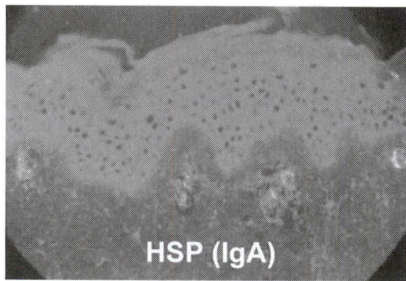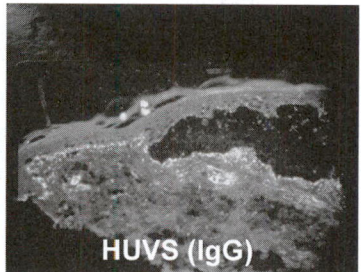

FIGURE 6 (Left) DIF of skin of IgA vasculitis (Henoch-Schoenlein purpura) showing granular IgA deposits in and around superficial papillary dermal vessels; (right) DIF of skin in hypocomplementemic urticarial vasculitis showing granular IgG deposits in and around superficial papillary dermal vessels as well as along the BMZ (lupus band-like).

doughnut-like appearance (24, 61). These IF findings represent not an antigen-antibody reaction but a trapping phenomenon of immunoglobulins to increased and altered glycoproteins in BMZ and blood vessels. Similar IF findings are seen in pseudoporphyria (74), a condition that mimics porphyria cutanea tarda but has no demonstrable abnormality of porphyrin metabolism. Pseudoporphyria is often precipitated by treatment with nonsteroidal anti-inflammatory drugs from the caproic acid group and furosemide, exposure to UVA light in tanning parlors, or hemodialysis (8).

Erythema Multiforme

In early lesions of erythema multiforme, there may be deposition of IgM and C3 in the walls of superficial dermal vessels. The sensitivity and specificity of these findings are still debatable (18).

Cutaneous Lupus

DIF findings in skin can often assist the diagnosis of LE, but one must ascertain whether the biopsy was obtained from lesional or nonlesional skin.

Lesional Skin

In cutaneous lupus, there is granular deposition of IgM and C3, as well as IgG and IgA, along the BMZ of epidermis and adnexal structures (25). This pattern can be seen in lesional specimens from a variety of cutaneous lupus conditions, including discoid LE, systemic LE, subacute cutaneous LE, and lupus profundus (54). A similar pattern is also seen in dermatomyositis and mixed connective tissue disease. However, subtle differences in the DIF pattern often help

lead to a better clinicopathological correlation in the evaluation of cutaneous connective tissue diseases.

In discoid LE, dense granular IgM with weaker other immunoreactants primarily found around adnexal BMZ is quite characteristic (Fig. 7).

Most cases of subacute and anti-Ro cutaneous LE are characterized by granular IgG along the BMZ as well as throughout the lower third of the epidermal stratum, giving a characteristic cytoplasmic "dusting" or fine speckling (84).

The so-called tumid LE, which is characterized by minimal epidermal-dermal junction but periadnexal inflammation, typically presents with immunoreactants deposited around the adnexal rather than the epidermal BMZ.

Systemic LE is characterized by granular IgG and C3 along the epidermal BMZ (Fig. 7). On the other hand, dermatomyositis is characterized by granular C5b-9 and weaker IgG and IgM and C3 (60).

Nonlesional Skin

Biopsy of normal skin to aid in the diagnosis of systemic LE is known as a lupus band test (4, 76). The demonstration of IgG or IgM deposition along the BMZ of normal skin is considered a positive lupus band test and implies but does not directly correlate with (i) the presence of circulating immune complexes, (ii) antibodies against native DNA, (iii) the frequent presence of anti-Sm antibodies, and (iv) a high incidence of lupus nephritis (42, 69). The need for this test is questionable, as there are much more sensitive and specific diagnostic tests to detect the presence of circulating immune complexes and complement activation in lupus.

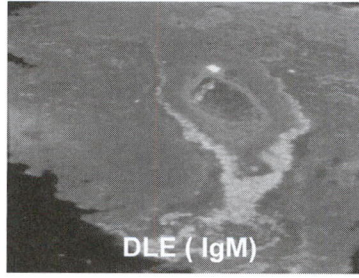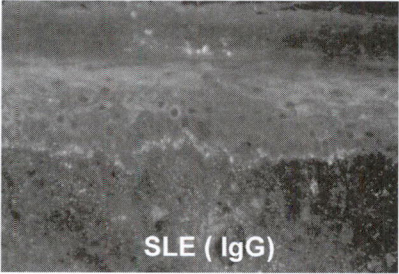

FIGURE 7 (Left) DIF of skin in discoid LE showing dense granular IgM deposits along the follicular (adnexal) BMZ; (right) DIF of skin in systemic LE showing granular IgG deposits along the epidermal BMZ.

Lichen Planus

Tissue

In oral lesions of lichen planus, a distinctive dense linear and shaggy deposition of fibrin along the BMZ extending into the lamina propia is present in most cases. The presence of abundant cytoid bodies scattered along the BMZ is also characteristic (1, 39, 40, 56). In cutaneous lesions, IF findings are less helpful, characteristic fibrin deposition is not detected, and frequently only cytoid bodies are found.

In oral biopsy samples, this pattern of fibrinogen and cytoid bodies often helps differentiate lichen planus from other lichenoid mucositis such as contact allergic mucositis, graft-versus-host disease, oral connective tissue diseases, and lichenoid variant of PNP.

Serologic Studies

There have been reports of circulating antibodies specific for a lichen planus-specific antigen and detectable by IIF (71), but this test has not proven to be useful.

REFERENCES

1. **Abell, E., D. G. Presbury, R. Marks, and D. Ramnarain.** 1975. The diagnostic significance of immunoglobulin and fibrin deposition in lichen planus. *Br. J. Dermatol.* **93:**17–24.
2. **Ablin, R. J., K. Milgrom, K. Kano, F. T. Rapaport, and E. H. Beutner.** 1969. Pemphigus-like antibodies in patients with skin burns. *Vox Sang.* **16:**73–75.
3. **Acosta, E., and L. Ivanyi.** 1982. Comparison of the reactivity of various epithelial substrates for the titration of pemphigus antibodies by indirect immunofluorescence. *Br. J. Dermatol.* **107:**537–541.
4. **Ahmed, A. R., and T. T. Provost.** 1979. Incidence of positive lupus band test using sun-exposed and unexposed skin. *Arch. Dermatol.* **115:**228–229.
5. **Ahmed, A. R., and S. Workman.** 1983. Anti-intercellular substance antibodies: presence in serum samples of 14 patients without pemphigus. *Arch. Dermatol.* **119:**17–21.
6. **Amagai, M., A. Komai, T. Hashimoto, K. Hashimoto, T. Yamada, Y. Kitajima, K. Ohya, H. Iwanami, and T. Nishikawa.** 1999. Usefulness of enzyme-linked immunosorbent assay using recombinant desmogleins 1 and 3 for serodiagnosis of pemphigus. *Br. J. Dermatol.* **140:**351–357.
7. **Amagai, M., K. Tsunoda, D. Zillikens, T. Nagai, and T. Nishikawa.** 1999. The clinical phenotype of pemphigus is defined by the anti-desmoglein autoantibody profile. *J. Am. Acad. Dermatol.* **40:**167–170.
8. **Anderson, K. E.** 1993. Pseudoporphyria versus porphyria cutanea tarda. *J. Pediatr.* **123:**841–842.
9. **Anhalt, G. J.** 1999. Making sense of antigens and antibodies in pemphigus. *J. Am. Acad. Dermatol.* **40:**763–766.
10. **Anhalt, G. J., and L. A. Diaz.** 1981. The dermal-epidermal junction in normal and disease states. *Prog. Dis. Skin* **1:**161–176.
11. **Anhalt, G. J., C. H. Kim, J. R. Stanley, N. J. Korman, D. A. Jabs, M. Kory, H. Izumi, H. Ratrie III, D. Mutasim, L. Ariss-Abdo, and R. S. Labib.** 1990. Paraneoplastic pemphigus: an autoimmune mucocutaneous disease associated with neoplasia. *N. Engl. J. Med.* **323:** 1729–1735.
12. **Anhalt, G. J., and L. H. Morrison.** 1991. Bullous and cicatricial pemphigoid. *J. Autoimmun.* **4:**17–35.
13. **Baart de la Faille-Kuyper, E. M., L. Kater, C. J. Kooiker, and E. J. Dorhout Mees.** 1973. IgA deposits in cutaneous blood vessel walls and mesangium in Henoch-Schoenlein syndrome. *Lancet* **i:**892–893.
14. **Bauer, E. A., Y. H. Kim, D. T. Woodley, J. Vitto, P. Verrando, and J. P. Ortonne.** 1993. Epidermolysis bullosa, p. 257–272. *In* T. T. Provost and W. L. Weston (ed.), *Bullous Diseases.* Mosby, St. Louis, Mo.
15. **Bekou, V., S. Thoma-Uszynski, O. Wendler, W. Uter, S. Schwietzke, T. Hunziker, C. C. Zouboulis, G. Schuler, L. Sorokin, and M. Hertl.** 2005. Detection of laminin 5-specific auto-antibodies in mucous membrane and bullous pemphigoid sera by ELISA. *J. Investig. Dermatol.* **124:** 732–740.
16. **Beutner, E. H., V. Kumar, S. A. Krasny, and T. P. Chorzelski.** 1987. Defined immunofluorescence in immunodermatology, p. 3–40. *In* E. H. Beutner, T. P. Chorzelski, and V. Kumar (ed.), *Immunopathology of the Skin*, 3rd ed. Wiley, New York, N.Y.
17. **Bhol, K. C., J. E. Colon, and A. R. Ahmed.** 2003. Autoantibody in mucous membrane pemphigoid binds to an intracellular epitope on human beta4 integrin and causes basement membrane zone separation in oral mucosa in an organ culture model. *J. Investig. Dermatol.* **120:** 701–702.
18. **Bushkell, L. L., S. E. Mackel, and R. E. Jordon.** 1980. Erythema multiforme: direct immunofluorescence and detection of circulating immune-complexes. *J. Investig. Dermatol.* **74:**372–374.
19. **Chan, L. S., J. D. Fine, R. A. Briggaman, D. T. Woodley, C. Hammerberg, R. J. Drugge, and K. D. Cooper.** 1993. Identification and partial characterization of a novel 105-Dalton lower lamina lucida autoantigen associated with a novel immune-mediated subepidermal blistering disease. *J. Investig. Dermatol.* **101:**262–267.
20. **Chen, M., L. S. Chan, X. Cai, E. A. O'Toole, J. C. Sample, and D. T. Woodley.** 1997. Development of an ELISA for rapid detection of anti-type VII collagen autoantibodies in epidermolysis bullosa acquisita. *J. Investig. Dermatol.* **108:**68–72.
21. **Chorzelski, T. P., E. H. Beutner, J. Sulej, H. Tchorzewska, S. Jablonska, V. Kumar, and A. Kapuscinska.** 1984. IgA-endomysium antibody, a new immunological marker of dermatitis herpetiformis and coeliac disease. *Br. J. Dermatol.* **111:**395–402.
22. **Cotell, S. L., J. C. Lapiere, J. D. Chen, T. Iwasaki, P. A. Krusinski, L. S. Chan, and D. T. Woodley.** 1994. A novel 105-KDa lamina lucida autoantigen: association with bullous pemphigoid. *J. Investig. Dermatol.* **103:**78–83.
23. **Creswell, S. N., M. M. Black, B. Bhogal, and M. V. Skeete.** 1981. Correlation of circulating intercellular antibody titers in pemphigus with disease activity. *Clin. Exp. Dermatol.* **6:**477–483.
24. **Dabski, C., and E. H. Beutner.** 1991. Studies of laminin and type IV collagen in blisters of porphyria cutanea tarda and drug-induced pseudoporphyria. *J. Am. Acad. Dermatol.* **25:**28–32.
25. **Dahl, M. V.** 1983. Usefulness of direct immunofluorescence in patients with lupus erythematosus. *Arch. Dermatol.* **119:**1010–1017.
26. **Dahl, M. V., J. H. McGowen, S. I. Katz, and W. R. Vineyard.** 1974. Pemphigus-like antibodies in sera of patients with thermal burns, gunshot wounds and skin grafts. *Mil. Med.* **139:**196–198.
27. **Davis, M. D., M. S. Daoud, B. Kirby, L. E. Gibson, and R. S. Rogers III.** 1998. Clinicopathologic correlation of hypocomplementemic and normocomplementemic urticarial vasculitis. *J. Am. Acad. Dermatol.* **38**(Part 1):899–905.
28. **Delbaldo, C., M. Chen, A. Friedli, C. Prins, J. Desmeules, J. H. Saurat, D. T. Woodley, and L. Borradori.** 2002. Drug-induced epidermolysis bullosa acquisita with antibodies to type VII collagen. *J. Am. Acad. Dermatol.* **46**(Suppl.):S161–S164.

29. Diaz, L. A., S. A. Sampaio, E. A. Rivitti, C. R. Martin, P. R. Cunha, C. Lombardi, F. A. Almeida, R. M. Castro, M. L. Macca, and C. Lavrado. 1989. Endemic pemphigus foliaceus (fogo selvagem). I. Clinical features and immunopathology. *J. Am. Acad. Dermatol.* **20:**657–669.

30. Domloge-Hultsch, N., G. J. Anhalt, W. R. Gammon, Z. Lazarova, R. Briggaman, M. Welch, D. A. Jabs, C. Huff, and K. B. Yancey. 1994. Antiepiligrin cicatricial pemphigoid: a subepithelial bullous disorder. *Arch. Dermatol.* **130:** 1521–1529.

31. Feibelman, C., G. Stolzner, and T. T. Provost. 1981. Pemphigus vulgaris. Superior sensitivity of monkey esophagus in the determination of pemphigus antibody. *Arch. Dermatol.* **117:**561–562.

32. Fellner, M. J., K. Fukujama, A. Moshell, and M. V. Klaus. 1973. Intercellular antibodies in blood and epidermis: a histochemical study of IgG immunoglobulins in patients with late reactions to penicillins and their comparison with similar antibodies in patients with pemphigus vulgaris. *Br. J. Dermatol.* **89:**115–126.

33. Fine, J. D., G. R. Neises, and S. I. Katz. 1985. Immunofluorescence and immunoelectron microscopic studies in cicatricial pemphigoid. *J. Investig. Dermatol.* **84:**39–43.

34. Fry, L., G. Haffeden, F. Wojnarowska, B. R. Thompson, and P. P. Seah. 1978. IgA and C3 complement in the uninvolved skin in dermatitis herpetiformis after gluten withdrawal. *Br. J. Dermatol.* **99:**31–37.

35. Gammon, W. R., and R. A. Briggaman. 1993. Epidermolysis bullosa acquisita and bullous systemic lupus erythematosus. *Dermatol. Clin.* **11:**535–547.

36. Gammon, W. R., C. Kowaleski, and T. P. Chorzelski. 1990. Direct immunofluorescence studies of sodium chloride-separated skin in the differential diagnosis of bullous pemphigoid and epidermolysis bullosa acquisita. *J. Am. Acad. Dermatol.* **22:**664–670.

37. Gianetti, A. 1974. Immunofluorescence studies in the Senear-Usher syndrome. *Arch. Dermatol. Forsch.* **248:**287.

38. Giudice, G. J., K. C. Wilske, G. J. Anhalt, J. A. Fairley, A. F. Taylor, D. J. Emery, R. G. Hoffman, and L. A. Diaz. 1994. Development of an ELISA to detect anti-BP180 autoantibodies in bullous pemphigoid and herpes gestationis. *J. Investig. Dermatol.* **102:**878–881.

39. Gogate, P., R. Valenzuela, S. Deodhar, W. F. Bergfeld, and M. Yeip. 1980. Globular deposition of immunoglobulins and complement in the papillary dermis: clinical significance. *Am. J. Clin. Pathol.* **73:**512–517.

40. Goldstein, B. H., and S. M. Katz. 1979. Immunofluorescent findings in oral bullous lichen planus. *J. Oral Med.* **34:**8–12.

41. Gomes, M. A., C. Dambuyant, J. Thivolet, and R. Bussy. 1982. Bullous pemphigoid: a correlative study of autoantibodies, circulating immune complexes and dermo-epidermal deposits. *Br. J. Dermatol.* **107:**43–51.

42. Halberg, P., S. Ullman, and F. Jorgensen. 1982. The lupus band test as a measure of disease activity in systemic lupus erythematosus. *Arch. Dermatol.* **118:**572–576.

43. Helm, T. N., and R. Valenzuela. 1992. Continuous dermoepidermal junction IgM detected by direct immunofluorescence: a report of nine cases. *J. Am. Acad. Dermatol.* **26:** 203–206.

44. Helou, J., J. Allbritton, and G. Anhalt. 1995. Accuracy of indirect immunofluorescence testing in the diagnosis of paraneoplastic pemphigus. *J. Am. Acad. Dermatol.* **32:** 441–447.

45. Ishii, K., M. Amagai, R. P. Hall, T. Hashimoto, A. Takayanagi, S. Gamou, N. Shimizu, and T. Nishikawa. 1997. Characterization of autoantibodies in pemphigus using antigen-specific enzyme-linked immunosorbent assays with baculovirus-expressed recombinant desmogleins. *J. Immunol.* **159:**2010–2017.

46. Jablonska, S., T. P. Chorzelski, E. H. Beutner, B. Michel, R. H. Cormane, K. Holubar, S. F. Bean, K. M. Blaszczyk, J. Ploem, and N. K. Sackia. 1975. Cooperative study: uses for immunofluorescence tests of skin and sera. *Arch. Dermatol.* **11:**371–381.

47. Jiao, D., and J. C. Bystryn. 1998. Antibodies to desmoplakin in a patient with pemphigus foliaceus. *J. Eur. Acad. Dermatol. Venereol.* **11:**169–172.

48. Johnson, G. D., R. S. Davidson, K. C. McNamee, G. Russell, D. Goodwin, and E. J. Holborow. 1982. Fading of immunofluorescence during microscopy. A study of the phenomenon and its remedy. *J. Immunol. Methods* **55:** 231–242.

49. Jordon, R. E., K. G. Heine, G. Tappeiner, L. L. Bushkell, and T. T. Provost. 1976. The immunopathology of herpes gestationis. Immunofluorescence studies and characterization of "HG factor." *J. Clin. Investig.* **57:**1426–1433.

50. Kaplan, D. S., and G. L. Picciolo. 1983. IF standardization by quantitative microfluorometry. II. Reduction in fading by reducing agents. *Immunol. Commun.* **12:**107.

51. Katz, S. I., K. C. Hertz, and H. Yaoita. 1976. Herpes gestationis. Immunopathology and characterization of the HG factor. *J. Clin. Investig.* **57:**1434–1444.

52. Kelly, S. E., P. A. Frith, P. R. Millard, F. Wojnarowska, and M. M. Black. 1988. A clinicopathological study of mucosal involvement in linear IgA disease. *Br. J. Dermatol.* **119:**161–170.

53. Kelly, S. E., and F. Wojnarowska. 1988. The use of chemically split tissue in the detection of circulating anti-basement membrane zone antibodies in bullous pemphigoid and cicatricial pemphigoid. *Br. J. Dermatol.* **118:**31–40.

54. Landry, M., and W. M. Sams, Jr. 1973. Systemic lupus erythematosus. Studies of the antibodies bound to skin. *J. Investig. Dermatol.* **52:**1871–1880.

55. Laskaris, G., and A. Angelopoulus. 1981. Cicatricial pemphigoid, direct and indirect immunofluorescent studies. *Oral Surg. Oral Med. Oral Pathol.* **51:**48–54.

56. Laskaris, G., A. Sklavounou, and A. Angelopoulus. 1982. Direct immunofluorescence in oral lichen planus. *Oral Surg.* **53:**483–487.

57. Lazarova, Z., C. Sitaru, D. Zillikens, and K. B. Yancey. 2004. Comparative analysis of methods for detection of anti-laminin 5 autoantibodies in patients with anti-epiligrin cicatricial pemphigoid. *J. Am. Acad. Dermatol.* **51:**886–892.

58. Liu, Z., S. D. Shapiro, S. S. Twining, R. M. Senior, G. J. Giudice, J. A. Fairley, and L. A. Diaz. 2000. A critical role for neutrophil elastase in experimental bullous pemphigoid. *J. Clin. Investig.* **105:**113–123.

59. Logan, R. A., B. Bhogal, A. K. Das, P. M. McKee, and M. M. Black. 1987. Localization of bullous pemphigoid antibody—an indirect immunofluorescence study of 228 cases using a split-skin technique. *Br. J. Dermatol.* **117:** 471–478.

60. Mascaro, J. M., Jr., G. Hausmann, C. Herrero, J. M. Grau, M. C. Cid, J. Palou, and J. M. Mascaro. 1995. Membrane attack complex deposits in cutaneous lesions of dermatomyositis. *Arch. Dermatol.* **131:**1386–1392.

61. Maynard, B., and M. S. Peters. 1992. Histologic and immunofluorescence study of cutaneous porphyrias. *J. Cutan. Pathol.* **19:**40–47.

62. Michel, B., Y. Milner, and K. David. 1973. Preservation of tissue fixed immunoglobulins in skin biopsies of patients with lupus erythematosus and bullous diseases. Preliminary report. *J. Investig. Dermatol.* **59:**449–452.

63. Mimouni, D., D. Foedinger, D. J. Kouba, S. J. Orlow, K. Rappersberger, J. J. Sciubba, O. V. Nikolskaia, B. A. Cohen, G. J. Anhalt, and C. H. Nousari. 2004. Mucosal

dominant pemphigus vulgaris with anti-desmoplakin autoantibodies. *J. Am. Acad. Dermatol.* **51**:62–67.

64. **Morrison, L. H., and G. J. Anhalt.** 1991. Herpes gestationis. *J. Autoimmun.* **4**:37–45.

65. **Mutasim, D. F., G. J. Anhalt, L. A. Diaz, and H. P. Patel.** 1987. Linear immunofluorescence staining of the cutaneous basement membrane zone produced by pemphigoid antibodies: the result of hemidesmosome staining. *J. Am. Acad. Dermatol.* **16**:75–82.

66. **Mutasim, D. F., and L. A. Diaz.** 1991. The use of immunohistochemical techniques in the differentiation of subepidermal bullous diseases. *Am. J. Dermatopathol.* **13**:77–83.

67. **Nisengard, R. J., M. Blaszczyk, T. P. Chorzelski, and E. Beutner.** 1978. Immunofluorescence of biopsy specimens. Comparison of methods of transportation. *Arch. Dermatol.* **114**:1329–1332.

68. **Nousari, H. C., A. Kimyai-Asadi, J. P. Caeiro, and G. J. Anhalt.** 1999. Clinical, demographic and immunohistologic features of vancomycin-induced linear IgA bullous disease. *Medicine* (Baltimore) **78**:1–8.

69. **Ojeda-Duran, S., R. Vargas-Rosendo, and J. Fernandez-Diez.** 1980. Skin immunofluorescence in patients with systemic lupus erythematosus, SLE: relationship between the immunohistochemical pattern and systemic activity. *Arch. Investig. Med.* **11**:215–226.

70. **Okura, M., Y. Tatsuno, M. Sato, S. Hashizume, Y. Kubota, K. Matumura, T. Hashimoto, and M. Mizoguchi.** 1997. Vesicular pemphigoid with antidesmoplakin autoantibodies. *Br. J. Dermatol.* **136**:794–796.

71. **Olsen, R. G., D. du Plessis, C. Barron, E. J. Schulz, and W. Villet.** 1983. Lichen planus dermopathy: demonstration of a lichen planus specific epidermal antigen in affected patients. *J. Clin. Lab. Immunol.* **10**:103–106.

72. **Parfrey, P., M. Clement, M. Vanderburg, and P. Wright.** 1980. Captopril-induced pemphigus. *Br. Med. J.* **281**:194.

73. **Peck, S. M., K. E. Osserman, L. B. Weiner, A. Lefkovits, and R. S. Osserman.** 1968. Studies in bullous diseases. Immunofluorescent serologic tests. *N. Engl. J. Med.* **279**: 951–958.

74. **Poh-Fitzpatrick, M. B.** 1986. Porphyria, pseudoporphyria, pseudopseudoporphyria . . . ? *Arch. Dermatol.* **122**:403–404.

75. **Powell, A. M., Y. Sakuma-Oyama, N. Oyama, S. Albert, B. Bhogal, F. Kaneko, T. Nishikawa, and M. M. Black.** 2005. Usefulness of BP180 NC16a enzyme-linked immunosorbent assay in the serodiagnosis of pemphigoid gestationis and in differentiating between pemphigoid gestationis and pruritic urticarial papules and plaques of pregnancy. *Arch. Dermatol.* **141**:705–710.

76. **Provost, T. T., G. Andres, P. J. Maddison, and M. Reichlin.** 1980. Lupus band test in untreated SLE patients: correlation of immunoglobulin deposition in the skin of the extensor forearm with clinical renal disease and serologic abnormalities. *J. Investig. Dermatol.* **74**:407–412.

77. **Roh, J. Y., C. Yee, Z. Lazarova, R. P. Hall, and K. B. Yancey.** 2000. The 120-kDa soluble ectodomain of type XVII collagen is recognized by autoantibodies in patients with pemphigoid and linear IgA dermatosis. *Br. J. Dermatol.* **143**:104–111.

78. **Rose, D. W., E. B. Brocker, D. Schuppan, and D. Zillikens.** 1999. Circulating autoantibodies to tissue transglutaminase differentiate patients with dermatitis herpetiformis from those with linear IgA disease. *J. Am. Acad. Dermatol.* **41**:957–961.

79. **Sabolinski, M. L., E. H. Beutner, S. Krasny, V. Kumar, J. Huang, T. P. Chorzelski, S. Sampaio, and J. C. Bystryn.** 1987. Substrate specificity of anti-epithelial antibodies of pemphigus vulgaris and pemphigus foliaceus sera in immunofluorescence tests on monkey and guinea pig esophagus sections. *J. Investig. Dermatol.* **88**:545–549.

80. **Sakuma-Oyama, Y., A. M. Powell, N. Oyama, S. Albert, B. S. Bhogal, and M. M. Black.** 2004. Evaluation of a BP180-NC16a enzyme-linked immunosorbent assay in the initial diagnosis of bullous pemphigoid. *Br. J. Dermatol.* **151**:126–131.

81. **Santa-Cruz, D. J., P. G. Prioleau, M. D. Marcus, and J. Vitto.** 1981. Pemphigus-like lesions induced by d-penicillamine. Analysis of clinical, histopathological and immunofluorescence features in 34 cases. *Am. J. Dermatopathol.* **3**:85–92.

82. **Schroeter, A. L., P. W. M. Copeman, R. E. Jordon, W. M. Sams, and R. K. Wilkelmann.** 1971. Immunofluorescence of cutaneous vasculitis associated with systemic disease. *Arch. Dermatol.* **104**:254–259.

83. **Senear, E., and B. Usher.** 1926. An unusual type of pemphigus combining features of lupus erythematosus. *Arch. Dermatol. Syphil.* **13**:761.

84. **Srivastava, M., A. Rencic, G. Diglio, H. Santana, P. Bonitz, R. Watson, E. Ha, G. J. Anhalt, T. T. Provost, and C. H. Nousari.** 2003. Drug-induced, Ro/SSA-positive cutaneous lupus erythematosus. *Arch. Dermatol.* **139**:45–49.

85. **Wojnarowska, F., R. A. Marsden, B. Bhogal, and M. M. Black.** 1988. Chronic bullous disease of childhood, childhood cicatricial pemphigoid, and linear IgA disease of adults: a comparative study demonstrating clinical and immunopathologic overlap. *J. Am. Acad. Dermatol.* **19**: 792–805.

86. **Woodley, D. T.** 1990. Immunofluorescence on salt-split skin for the diagnosis of epidermolysis bullosa acquisita. *Arch. Dermatol.* **126**:229.

87. **Zillikens, D., K. Herzele, M. Georgi, E. Schmidt, I. Chimanovitch, H. Schumann, J. M. Mascaro, L. A. Diaz, L. Bruckner-Tuderman, E. B. Brocker, and G. J. Giudice.** 1999. Autoantibodies in a subgroup of patients with linear IgA disease react with the NC16A domain of BP 180. *J. Investig. Dermatol.* **113**:947–953.

88. **Zillikens, D., Y. Kawahara, A. Ishiko, H. Shimizu, J. Mayer, C. V. Rank, Z. Liu, G. J. Giudice, H. H. Tran, M. P. Marinkovich, E. B. Brocker, and T. Hashimoto.** 1996. A novel subepidermal blistering disease with autoantibodies to a 200-kDa antigen of the basement membrane zone. *J. Investig. Dermatol.* **106**:1333–1338.

89. **Zillikens, D., J. M. Mascaro, P. A. Rose, Z. Liu, S. M. Ewing, F. Caux, R. G. Hoffman, L. A. Diaz, and G. J. Giudice.** 1997. A highly sensitive enzyme-linked immunosorbent assay for the detection of circulating anti-BP180 autoantibodies in patients with bullous pemphigoid. *J. Investig. Dermatol.* **109**:679–683.

Cardiovascular Diseases

J. BRUCE SUNDSTROM, C. LYNNE BUREK, NOEL R. ROSE, AND AFTAB A. ANSARI

124

Cardiovascular diseases comprise a broad spectrum of disorders which cause cardiac dysfunction. Vascular diseases such as hypertension, atherosclerosis, and acute and chronic coronary artery disease, which adversely influence systemic hemodynamics, indirectly cause cardiac dysfunction by causing acute myocardial infarction (AMI) or by promoting heart muscle disease. A standardized classification and definition of heart muscle diseases or cardiomyopathies was most recently established in 1995 by the World Health Organization and International Society and Federation of Cardiology Task Force (24). Cardiomyopathies are classified as hypertropic, restrictive, dilated, arrhythmogenic right ventricular, unclassified, or specific. Specific cardiomyopathies describe heart muscle diseases that have been further defined based in part on their etiologies and their association with specific systemic or cardiac disorders. These include (i) ischemic cardiomyopathy, (ii) valvular cardiomyopathy, (iii) hypertensive cardiomyopathy, (iv) metabolic cardiomyopathy, (v) general system disease, (vi) muscular dystrophies, (vii) neuromuscular disorders, (viii) sensitivity and toxic reactions, (ix) peripartum cardiomyopathy, and (x) inflammatory cardiomyopathy. Inflammatory cardiomyopathy, which is now defined as myocarditis with cardiac dysfunction, is further categorized as idiopathic, autoimmune, or infectious. Multiple factors, including age, genetics, infection, and nutrition, contribute to the morbity and mortality of heart disease. However, this chapter will focus exclusively on the current knowledge of immunologic aspects involved in the etiology and pathogenesis of cardiomyopathies and the application of immunological and molecular techniques for measuring and characterizing relevant biomarkers used in the detection and assessment of myocardial damage and in determining the diagnosis and prognosis of related cardiovascular diseases.

SEROLOGIC DIAGNOSIS AND ASSESSMENT OF AMI

AMI most often results from a lack of sufficient blood supply to the heart, a condition usually associated with acute coronary syndrome (ACS). When emergency room or crisis care patients with ACS present with symptoms of chest pains, a rapid diagnosis and characterization of the extent of AMI are essential for prescribing appropriate treatment, e.g., early intervention with antithrombolytic therapy or angioplasty, to minimize the risk of (further) cardiac injury and death. The ability

to accurately interpret symptoms of chest pains and to be able to distinguish between patients with unstable angina and those with AMI is required so that high-risk patients needing immediate attention and low-risk patients that can be clinically managed by outpatient care can be properly sorted by triage. Serologic measurements of soluble biomarkers released during myocyte necrosis are used in conjunction with electrocardiograms and more sophisticated imaging techniques, e.g., echocardiography and perfusion scintigraphy, to characterize the presence and extent of AMI. Serum biomarkers have a greater advantage of detecting recent myocardial injury, which is not easily distinguishable by cardiac imaging techniques, in patients with clinical evidence of preexisting heart disease.

Serologic monitoring of myocardial injury involves the measurement of levels of serum biomarkers that correlate well with levels of cardiac myocyte injury and necrosis. In ACS, myocardial injury results from insufficient oxygen during episodes of ischemia. Whether the cellular damage is reversible or irreversible usually depends on the duration of ischemia. Myocyte necrosis is an example of irreversible injury that results in the rapid and complete release of cytoplasmic proteins that soon become detectable in the serum. However, under mild ischemic conditions or stress, proportionally smaller amounts of cytoplasmic proteins and macromolecules may be released from cardiac myocytes at levels correlating with reversible myocardial tissue injury. The ideal serum biomarker of myocardial injury would have the following characteristics. (i) It would be heart specific, expressed only in cardiac tissues and not in noncardiac tissues, even during pathological conditions. (ii) It would be highly sensitive, so that clinically significant interpretations could be made at low levels of expression. (iii) The levels of expression would be proportional to the extent of myocardial damage and therefore would provide the ability to discriminate between reversible and irreversible myocardial injury. (iv) It would be able to allow monitoring of reperfusion therapy and an estimation of infarct size and prognosis. (v) The release and decay kinetics would allow rapid diagnosis and the ability to distinguish recent from recurrent myocardial injuries. (vi) It would be rapid, sensitive, quantitative, and cost-effective (23).

Historical Background

The earliest conventional serum biomarkers used to assess AMI were enzymes involved in cellular metabolism, such as aspartate aminotransferase (AST; formerly called ASAT or SGOT) (1). Levels of AST in the serum appeared to correlate with AMI, and biochemical assays that measured their functional enzymatic activity were very sensitive. Nevertheless, assays measuring AST expression lacked cardiac tissue specificity, thus detracting from their clinical relevance for the diagnosis of AMI.

Lactate dehydrogenase (LD), a cellular enzyme involved in the conversion of pyruvate to lactate in glucose metabolism, later replaced AST. Although LD is expressed in almost all tissues, it exists as five different isoenzymes and thus had the advantage of increased specificity and improved clinical efficacy as a biomarker for AMI. The LD isoenzymes have a tetrameric structure made up of different combinations of 34-kDa "M" (muscle) and "H" (heart) subunits with the following structures: LD-1, H_4; LD-2, H_3M_1; LD-3, H_2M_2; LD-4, H_1M_3; and LD-5, M_4. LD is found in many tissues, but the distribution of different isoforms varies among different tissues. Although LD-1 is the major isoform found in the heart, it is also present in other tissues, including the kidneys, brain, red blood cells, stomach, and pancreas. A significant amount of LD-2 is also present in cardiac tissues, but LD-3, LD-4, and LD-5 are only present in trace amounts. Levels of LD-2 in the plasma rise relative to those of LD-1 within 8 to 12 h after AMI, and LD-1/LD-2 ratios have been used to detect and monitor the development of recent cardiac tissue necrosis (28). LD-1/LD-2 ratios of ≤0.76 measured in plasma are consider normal, whereas LD-1/LD-2 ratios of ≤1.0 are considered reasonably specific for AMI. However, increased LD-1/LD-2 ratios in plasma may occur in the absence of AMI in patients with chronic skeletal muscle injury, stomach, kidney, or pancreatic disorders, or significant erythrocyte damage, thus limiting its positive predictive value (23).

Myoglobin is a low-molecular-mass (17.8 kDa) heme-binding protein abundant in both cardiac and skeletal muscle that is rapidly released (1 to 2 h) after AMI, peaks at ~7 h, and returns to normal levels in plasma by 24 h after the onset of symptoms in the absence of renal disease. Myoglobin is one of the earliest expressed plasma markers of myocyte necrosis, and thus the frequent collection of blood samples early after the onset of symptoms is recommended. A doubling of myoglobin levels above the baseline has been considered diagnostic of AMI. However, due to their lack of specificity, myoglobin measurements only have a reported predictive value of 43% and therefore are mainly used in conjunction with measurements of more heart-specific biomarkers (15). Nevertheless, myoglobin does have a high predictive negative value and thus has been used for identifying patients with unstable angina without AMI. Creatine kinase (CK), a cellular enzyme that catalyzes the transfer of high-energy phosphate from ATP to creatine, later replaced LD as the preferred serum biomarker of AMI.

The active CK enzyme is a dimer consisting of "M" (muscle) and "B" (brain) subunits, each with a molecular mass of approximately 41 kDa. Cytosolic CK exists as three isoenzymes; namely, CKBB (CK-1), CKMB (CK-2), and CKMM (CK-3). Although CK is present in most tissues, CKMB constitutes approximately 15 to 30% of CK in myocardial tissue and only 1 to 3% in skeletal muscle tissue (19). Biochemical assays that measure total CK activity in the serum or plasma required that samples be pretreated with reducing agents, e.g., β-mercaptoethanol, to prevent oxidation and a loss of activity. Determination of the levels of the three CK isoenzymes in plasma requires electrophoretic separation in agarose gels which are subsequently overlaid with appropriate substrates. Quantitative measurements of CK isoenzymes are made by densitometry. However, these measurements can be technically complicated by artifacts present in patient serum, e.g.,

bilirubin, drugs, etc. The introduction of monoclonal antibody-based assays that measure the total CKMB mass in either serum or plasma has not only eliminated these concerns but also given significantly greater sensitivity (34). Levels of CKMB in plasma increase by 6 to 10 h after the onset of symptoms, peak around 24 h, and then return to normal by 36 to 72 h. Measurements of levels of CKMB in plasma of ≥7 ng/ml are considered diagnostic of AMI. CKMB has generally been considered a specific biomarker for irreversible myocardial injury; however, the specificity for AMI is not 100%. Vigorous exercise, chronic renal failure, or skeletal myopathies and hypothyroidism can all increase levels of CKMB in plasma. Furthermore, reports of studies of endomyocardial biopsies performed on patients with unstable angina have revealed evidence of micronecrosis in the absence of elevated levels of CKMB in serum (11). Modifications in CKMB measurements have been introduced in efforts to increase the specificity of CKMB measurements for myocardial necrosis. The CKMB index represents the following: (total CKMB/total CK) × 100%. Values of >2.5% (ranging from 2 to 5%) are considered to represent the myocardium-derived MB isoenzyme (19). Measurements in serum of the two CKMB isoforms, CKMB2 (tissue subform) and CKMB1 (plasma-modified subform), have also been used to increase the assay specificity. The two isoforms can be separated and quantitated by high-voltage electrophoresis. A CKMB2/CKMB1 ratio of >1.5 has been used as a threshold for heart-specific tissue necrosis with a sensitivity of >90% (37). Furthermore, CKMB isoform ratios are apparently diagnostic of AMI earlier than those of CKMB mass. Nevertheless, the implementation of testing for new more sensitive and specific biomarkers, such as cardiac troponins, as well as a strategy for utilizing multiple biomarkers of myocyte necrosis, is currently being practiced in select clinical settings for more accurate diagnosis of AMI.

Cardiac troponins (Tns) represent a class of serum biomarkers that are emerging as the new "gold standard" for the diagnosis of AMI due to their greater specificity and sensitivity for myocardial necrosis. The Tns comprise a group of regulatory proteins uniquely located on the thin filament of striated muscle. The Tn complex is composed of the following three subunits: TnT, which serves to attach the Tn complex to tropomyosin; TnI, which regulates actin-myosin interactions by attenuating actinomyosin ATPase; and TnC, which binds calcium (20). Immunoassays for cardiac TnT (cTnT) and cTnI first introduced in the early 1990s have been improved and so extensively implemented in clinical settings that cTn levels are now included in the Joint European Society of Cardiology/American College of Cardiology Committee's consensus definition of MI (3). Heart-specific isoforms exist for TnI (cTnI) and TnT (cTnT) and can be detected in plasma or serum by specific monoclonal antibodies without cross-reactivity with skeletal muscle Tns. Unlike CKMB, cTns are not found in the sera of healthy patients (i.e., in the absence of cardiac tissue injury), thus providing troponin measurement with a superior signal-to-noise ratio and enhancing their usefulness and risk stratification for the evaluation of patient responses to therapy. However, troponins are released relatively slower after myocardial injury and have a longer half-life in serum than CKMB. Thus, despite their superior specificity, troponins are not as effective for the diagnosis of recent AMIs. Therefore, it has been recommended that cTn testing be used in combination with myoglobin testing when patients are admitted within 2 to 6 h and with CKMB mass measurement when they are admitted within 6 to 8 h. Other clinical studies have shown that combined measurements of myoglobin, CKMB, and cTnI at 0, 3, 6, 9 to 12, and 24 h offer the best strategy for therapeutic monitoring and optimal risk stratification of recurring AMI or death within 30 days (33, 49).

Need for Improved Assays for Cardiac Markers of AMI

Cardiovascular disease holds the distinction of having the highest morbidity and mortality rates in the Western world. Approximately 8,000,000 patients are evaluated in hospital chest pain centers for acute cardiovascular disorders in the United States each year, and of these approximately 3,000,000 are classified as having no evidence of AMI (41). The rate of AMI misdiagnosis among these 3,000,000 patients ranges from 1 to 3% (or between 30,000 and 90,000 patients) (35). Thus, there is a critical need for early and accurate diagnosis after the onset of symptoms for risk stratification and optimal patient care and survival from AMI. Toward this objective, a strategy of utilizing rapid point-of-care testing and assays that screen for multiple biomarkers of myocyte necrosis is currently being pursued for faster and more accurate diagnosis of ACS. New immunoassays are being introduced to improve the early diagnosis of AMI and to provide rapid turnaround times and point-of-care results. New testing methods for serum fatty acid binding protein (FABP) provide an example of this evolving trend in serological testing. FABP is an intracellular fatty acid carrier that exhibits release kinetics during AMI similar to those of myoglobin. Due to its relatively low expression in plasma in the absence of myocardial injury, it has been considered to be more sensitive for the detection of AMI. However, the turnaround time for standard capture enzyme-linked immunosorbent assays (ELISAs) for FABP is approximately 45 to 60 min. Microparticle-enhanced turbidimetric assays for plasma FABP have been developed that can now be performed on clinical chemistry analyzers with a turnaround time of 10 min (38). More sensitive capture immunoassays for FABP, utilizing electrochemical immunosensors and an amperometric detection system, have been described and have a performance time of 20 min (38). In addition, biotechnology companies are now offering new multiplexed assays featuring arrays for multiple cardiac markers, including CKMB. Troponin-1, CKMB, and C-reactive protein assays (see below) are also being developed, utilizing chemiluminescent detection systems for enhanced sensitivity (Panomics, Redwood City, Calif.). One

major limitation is that at present, standardization for many of these new testing methods has not yet been established. A list of biomarkers currently used for diagnosis risk stratification for AMI is provided in Table 1.

PATHOGENESIS OF CMI

Serum biomarkers used for clinical diagnosis, monitoring, and risk stratification for AMI are selected because they possess release and decay kinetics that correlate well with sudden necrotic cardiac myocyte death. On the other hand, chronic myocardial injury (CMI) is characterized by a much slower process accompanied by myocyte dropout, which is usually associated with apoptotic processes involved in the pathogenesis of dilated cardiomyopathy (DCM). DCM is a consequence of maladaptive compensatory tissue remodeling responses to reduced cardiac systolic output that evolves in a complex manner in the context of different genetic and environmental backgrounds over sustained but variable periods of time. These remodeling responses are mediated by a variety of endogenous stress-induced proteins, including tumor necrosis factor alpha (TNF-α), interleukin-1 (IL-1), IL-6, endothelin 1, angiotensin II (ANG-II), matrix metalloproteinases (MMPs) (2, 16, 17, 39, 50), transforming growth factor beta (TGF-β) acidic and basic fibroblast growth factors, vascular endothelial growth factor (VEGF), and others (10, 25–27, 51). These stress-induced proteins act directly on both cardiac myocytes, to induce hypertrophy, cytoprotection, or repair, and nonmyocyte cardiac tissues, to increase vascularization and to effect extracellular matrix (ECM) remodeling and fibrosis. Thus, cardiac tissue remodeling results in changes in both myocyte volume and the volume of supporting nonmyocyte cardiac tissues. Regardless of the initial precipitating event, the progression towards heart failure eventually proceeds independently along a common pathway for all forms of DCM. In some cases, DCM is thought to arise subsequent to a low-grade inflammation of cardiac tissue, usually (but not necessarily always) secondary to a viral infection of cardiac tissues by adenovirus or specific strains of coxsackievirus (22). Experimental animal models of postinfectious autoimmune myocarditis (14) or autoimmune myocarditis induced by immunization of mice with heart-specific peptides in the presence of complete Freund adjuvant and in the absence of cardiotropic viral infection (45) all develop

TABLE 1 Serum biomarkers used for diagnosis of AMI

Plasma or serum biomarker	Value (%) at indicated time					
	2–4 h		6–10 h		18–24 h	
	Sensitivity	Specificity	Sensitivity	Specificity	Sensitivity	Specificity
Enzymes						
LD					95	90
CKMB activity	40.7	98.8	97.5	96.2	97.9	96.9
CKMB mass	39.3	98.8	100	90.4	95.7	99.6
CKMB isoforms	46.4	88.9	96.2	90.2	80.9	89.9
Nonstructural proteins						
Myoglobin	90	38.3				
Heart FABP	90	19.2				
Structural and regulatory proteins						
cTns						
cTnT	35.7	98.3	86.5	96.4	78.7	95.7
cTnI	57.5	94.3	92.3	94.6	95.7	93.4
Myosin light chains	75	64.2	78.6	61.1	81.5	52.5

DCM and cardiac-specific autoimmunity. Left ventricular (LV) hypertrophy and dilatation with a reduced ejection fraction are common manifestations in DCM. This is a compensatory response to a chronic volume overload that results from myocyte loss and reduced contractile function. Thus, LV tissue remodeling in response to acute or chronic cardiac tissue injury is a common factor of DCM. Tissue remodeling responses are initiated and directed in part by cellular components of innate immunity resident in cardiac tissues, such as cardiac mast cells and dendritic cells. These responses are focused on both directly reorganizing the cardiovascular architecture by degrading ECM components through MMPs, promoting replacement fibrosis, and developing new ECM and vascular beds and recruiting and directing other components of adaptive immunity to remove damaged and necrotic tissues. During this process of tissue remodeling and repair, certain cryptic cardiac antigens, e.g., myosin, mitochrondrial proteins, heat shock proteins, etc., become exposed to immature dendritic cells, which under the influence of other "danger signals" present during the injury and remodeling process (such as CD40 ligand expressed on activated platelets) undergo maturation and become able to initiate subsequent heart-specific autoimmune responses which may or may not contribute significantly to further cardiac tissue injury. Therefore, the level of cardiac tissue injury required to result in irreversible DCM is determined by three major factors: (i) the extent or severity of the original insult, (ii) the extent or severity of the tissue injury and remodeling response by innate immune components, and (iii) the extent of severity of heart-specific autoimmune responses engendered and directed by reparative innate immune responses. Another variable in the etiology of DCM that may be dependent on these three major factors is the period of time from the original insult required for DCM to develop. Furthermore, the presence of bacterial and viral products capable of signaling through Toll-like receptors on cardiac dendritic cells and mast cells may further contribute to the remodeling and subsequent autoimmune phenomena involved in DCM. As a result, DCM develops along with evidence of heart-specific autoimmune responses in the form of antibodies specific for heart-specific autoantigens.

Increases in the hemodynamic burden and volume overload can also contribute to cardiomyocyte damage and DCM. Several reports from different laboratories indicate that cardiac hypertrophy is associated with signaling through the Gαq subtype of G proteins (GTP-binding proteins) expressed on cardiac myocytes (9, 47). Molecules such as endothelin 1 and ANG-II, which are upregulated in response to increased pulmonary pressure and chronic volume overload, signal through Gαq-mediated pathways, causing a reactivation of embryonic genes such as atrial natriuretic factor (ANF), skeletal α-actin, and β-myosin heavy chain and ultimately resulting in cardiac myocyte hypertrophy. However, excessive hemodynamic stress can lead to myocyte apoptosis instead of hypertrophy, resulting in rapid decompensation and DCM. Reports from studies involving chronic volume overload in experimental murine models of pulmonary hypertension have indicated a role for mast cells in LV remodeling (46). Increases in pulmonary artery blood pressure lead to rapid increases in the number of activated mast cells in the heart. Furthermore, in experimental models of chronic volume overload, cardiac mast cell chymase replaces angiotensin-converting enzyme (ACE) as the major enzyme responsible for producing ANG-II from ANG-I (40). In addition, other mast cell-expressed mediators, such as MMPs, TNF-α, TGF-β, tryptase, prostaglandin E2, VEGF, and others, have also been shown to be involved in processes of cardiac tissue remodeling, including cardiac myocyte apoptosis, proliferation of nonmyocyte

cardiac tissues, fibrosis replacement, and ECM remodeling. Other nonmyocyte cardiac tissues also express mediators that contribute to the process of cardiac tissue remodeling, e.g., endothelial expressed endothelin-1 and reactive oxygen species, which have been associated with cardiomyopathy. Reactive oxygen species also activate mast cells, thus further contributing to chronic tissue remodeling and LV remodeling. Thus, monitoring serum biomarkers that correlate with the dysregulation of pulmonary normotension and compensatory cardiac tissue remodeling is useful in the diagnosis and risk assessment of DCM and congestive heart failure (CHF).

Serologic Monitoring of CMI

During CHF, chronic overstimulation of the renin-angiotensin-aldosterone system leads to increases in blood pressure and electrolyte concentrations and edema, thus inducing compensatory vasodilation and diuretic and natriuretic responses by the natriuretic peptide system (42). A-type natriuretic peptides (ANP) are produced by and released from the atria in response to dilatation. C-type natriuretic peptides (CNP) are produced by cardiovascular endothelial tissues in response to sheer stress. B-type natriuretic peptides (BNP) are released from the ventricles in response to prolonged increases in end-diastolic volume and pressure and thus have emerged as an excellent biomarker for LV dysfunction in DCM. BNP is derived from its high-molecular-weight precursor, pro-BNP (amino acids [aa] 1 to 108), whose expression is genetically regulated and which is not stored preformed in vesicles. The mature form, BNP-32, consists of the 32 C-terminal amino acid residues (aa 77 to 108) of the parent pro-BNP. It has been suggested that elevated levels of amino-terminal pro-BNP (Nt-proBNP) in plasma are better indicators of early cardiac dysfunction that BNP-32 (36). Levels of Nt-proBNP in plasma are determined with a competitive inhibition enzyme immunoassay (EIA). Individual replicate wells contain constant amounts of immobilized antibody specific for Nt-proBNP and of peroxidase-labeled Nt-proBNP (tracer) and variable amounts of unlabeled Nt-proBNP (present in standards or patient plasma). With increasing concentrations of unlabeled peptide, the binding of the competing tracer is proportionally reduced. After an incubation period, the unbound tracer is removed by washing, and a colorimetric peroxidase substrate is added. The amount of (peroxidase enzyme-mediated) color change is inversely proportional to the amount of Nt-proBNP in the sample. Increasing concentrations of serum BNP or Nt-proBNP significantly correlate with decreasing ejection fractions ($P < 0.001$) and with increasing levels of heart failure according to the New York Heart Association classification (36). Currently, the only commercially available clinical ELISAs for BNP that are U.S. Food and Drug Administration approved have a diagnostic sensitivity of 90%, specificity of 76%, positive predictive value of 79%, and negative predictive value of 89% (31). However, new rapid point-of-care tests for Nt-proBNP are likely to also become approved soon for use in clinical immunology laboratories.

Other biomarkers that are associated with CMI fall into three overlapping categories: (i) markers of inflammation, (ii) markers of tissue remodeling, and (iii) markers of vascular endothelial activation. The clinical significance of most, if not all, of the biomarkers listed in Table 2 continues to be defined in research studies involving animal models and in human clinical investigations.

Markers of Tissue Remodeling Associated with CMI

Myocardial tissue remodeling is triggered by LV dysfunction and is associated with cardiomyocyte hypertrophy and

TABLE 2 Serum biomarkers for CMI

Marker
Markers of tissue remodeling
Nt-proBNP
BNP
Annexin V
FAS/APO-1
Endothelin-1
ACE
MMP2
MMP7
MMP9
TGF-β
Fibrinogen
Homocysteine
Markers of inflammation
C-reactive protein
CD40 ligand
IL-6
IL-1
TNF-α
Gamma interferon
Markers of vascular endothelial activation
Soluble intracellular adhesion molecule 1 (sICAM-1)
Soluble vascular cellular adhesion molecule 1 (VCAM-1)
sE-Selectin
sP-Selectin
VEGF
Platelet-derived growth factor
Placental growth factor
NO

death, remodeling of the ECM, and replacement fibrosis. Chronic low but significant levels of myocyte dropout induce structural remodeling of the LV ECM to compensate for the loss of LV function. Increased expression levels of MMPs and cardiac mast cell tryptase in plasma and tissue correlate with evidence of LV remodeling and dysfunction in CHF (21, 44).

Markers of Inflammation Associated with CMI

Levels of IL-6 and certain related cytokines of the IL-6 family, e.g., cardiotrophin-1, in plasma have been shown to increase proportionally with the severity of CHF in both human clinical studies and experimental animal models (6, 43). Although the exact tissue sources of IL-6-related cytokines have not been identified, vascular endothelium and smooth tissues, as well as cardiac tissues, have been implicated. Intracellular signaling on cardiac myocytes is mediated via different multimeric IL-6 family cytokine receptors, which all share a common gp130 transmembrane subunit. The homeostatic regulation of IL-6 expression during CHF is complex and is influenced by a larger network of other cytokines and neurohormones, including TNF-α, ANG-II, epinephrine, and norepinephrine. Indeed, ACE inhibitors or β-blockers have been shown to have a lowering effect on IL-6 expression during CHF (13). IL-6 appears to mediate the detrimental effects of CHF by influencing the hypertrophy and apoptosis of cardiac myocytes (48). TNF-α promotes LV remodeling by altering the ECM. TNF-α mediates such structural modifications through its ability to activate proenzyme forms of MMPs in

myocardial tissues. TNF-α also promotes the activation of vascular endothelium. The expression of TNF-α is triggered by myocardial tissue damage and by inflammation, especially in viral myocarditis.

IL-1 is another cytokine whose expression is interrelated to the cascade of proinflammtory mediators released during CHF. IL-1 causes a negative inotropic effect on LV function by inducing NO expression and by promoting the production and release of IL-18.

Markers of Vascular Endothelial Activation

Inflammation associated with tissue remodeling and the progression towards CHF in DCM also results in increases in serum of the levels of soluble adhesion molecules, e.g., sICAM-1, E-selectin, P-selectin, and VCAM-1, expressed by activated cardiovascular endothelial cells. Although such measurements are not yet approved for clinical monitoring and staging of CHF, recent research reports have shown that levels of sICAM-1 in serum, as measured by capture ELISA, accurately correlated (p < 0.001) with the intramyocardial expression of ICAM-1 in patients with DCM and correlated with the New York Health Association classification of DCM (32). Thus, multiple serum biomarkers of tissue remodeling, inflammation, and endothelial activation have been shown to correlate with the development and progression of DCM (Table 3); however, other, more invasive procedures involving immunohistochemical characterization of endomyocardial biopsies are required for definitive diagnosis and staging of inflammatory cardiomyopathies.

PATHOGENESIS AND IMMUNODIAGNOSIS OF INFLAMMATORY CARDIOMYOPATHIES

Inflammatory cardiomyopathies belong to a class of dilated cardiomyopathies that do not result from the effects of ischemia or increased hemodynamic burden, but rather result from multiple infectious (viral, bacterial, fungal, and parasitic) and noninfectious (drugs, genetics, nutrition, age, idiopathies, etc.) etiologies (Table 3). As mentioned above, inflammatory cardiomyopathy is defined as myocarditis with cardiac dysfunction and includes idiopathic, autoimmune, and infectious myocarditis. In infectious myocarditis, myocyte damage occurs through both the direct and indirect effects of pathogenic agents (30). Certain cardiotropic viruses, e.g., coxsackie B virus (CVB), can cause direct myocyte damage and necrosis. Other viruses, e.g., adenoviruses, may induce apoptosis as a way of escaping immune system recognition. Infectious agents can also cause heart disease indirectly by inducing immunopathological responses that result in myocyte damage. Myocytolysis may occur due to the nonspecific cytotoxic effects of cytokines expressed by infiltrating lymphocytic effector cells, or it can be secondary to hypoxic ischemia due to vasospasms or endothelial dysfunction caused by viral myocarditis (18). Immunity-mediated myocyte damage may also result from the specific cell-mediated cytotoxic actions of T cells and NK cells, or it can be caused by the humoral cytotoxic effects of complement-fixing heart-reactive antibodies produced by epitope mimicry in autoimmune myocarditis (Table 4). Chronic rheumatic heart disease is one of the best examples of the involvement of epitope mimicry in valvular heart disease (12). In rheumatic fever, a sequel to group A streptococcal pharyngitis, antibodies specific for epitopes on the M surface protein cross-react with human tissue antigens. The valvular heart disease is thought to be mediated by antibodies that cross-react with streptococcal sialyl Lewis X oligosaccharide residues and human cardiac selectin.

TABLE 3 Infectious and noninfectious etiologies of inflammatory cardiomyopathy

Category	Disease or organism	Etiology
Infectious		
Viral myocarditis	Enterovirus	Coxsackie B3, B4 virus
	Herpesvirus	Cytomegalovirus, varicella-zoster virus
	Orthomyxovirus	Influenza virus
	Paramyxovirus	Parainfluenza virus
	Parvovirus	
	Retrovirus	Human immunodeficiency virus
	Adenovirus	
	Flavivirus	Hepatitis C virus
	Reovirus	
Bacterial myocarditis	*Streptococcus*	Pyogenese group A
	Staphylococcus	S. *aureus*
	Serratia	S. *marcescens*
	Chlamydia	
	Salmonella	
	Aerococcus	A. *urinae*
	Erlichia	
	Vibrio	V. *cholerae*
Parasitic/protozoal/ spirochetal myocarditis	Chagas' disease	*Trypanosoma cruzi*
		Toxoplasma gondii
	Lyme disease	*Borrelia*
Rickettsial myocarditis	Q fever	
	Rocky Mountain spotted fever	
	Scrub typhus	
Fungal myocarditis	*Cryptococcus*	C. *neoformans*
	Candidiasis	C. *albicans*
	Histoplasmosis	
	Aspergillus	
Noninfectious		
Autoimmune myocarditis	Rheumatic fever	
	Systemic lupus erythematosis	Systemic
	Sjögren's syndrome	
	Dressler's syndrome	Post-MI
	Postpartum cardiomyopathy	
	Kawasaki disese	
	Sarcoidosis	
Drug-induced myocarditis	Cardiotoxic myocarditis	Cocaine 999, catecholamines, doxorubicin
	Hypersensitivity myocarditis	Antibiotics, diuretics, others

Laboratory diagnosis is made after the onset of rheumatic fever by measuring elevated anti-streptolysin O titers. Elevated titers of anti-DNase B, antihyaluronidase, and antistreptozyme are also used to confirm this disease (Table 4).

The same immune responses engendered during the infectious phase of myocarditis may persist after viral clearance and develop into autoimmune postinfectious myocarditis. Such immunopathologies can evolve from a breakdown of tolerance (or from immunologic ignorance) to self antigens due to epitope mimicry, as in chronic rheumatic fever, or from sensitization by sequestered immunogenic self antigens exposed to the host immune system as a result of myocyte necrosis (Table 4). Supporting experimental evidence for the latter scenario comes from murine studies with susceptible (BALB/cA/J, BALB/cA.CA, and BALB/cA.SW) and nonsusceptible (C57B1/10 and C57B1/6) strains infected with cardiotropic CVB3 (8). Results from these studies describe a pathogenic pathway in which infiltrating macrophages or resident cardiac dendritic cells take up and process antigenic host cardiac myosin (released by virally damaged myocytes in susceptible hosts), which is then presented to specific T cells during the inductive phase. Macrophage-derived cytokines, e.g., IL-1β, TNF-α, and IL-12, not only cause further myocyte damage but also support and direct a TH1 type of immune response and the induction of myocyte-specific CD8+ cytotoxic T cells. The significance of the influence of cytokines in the induction of CVB-initiated autoimmune myocarditis is evidenced by the observation that the introduction of recombinant IL-1β or TNF-α into genetically resistant B.10 mice restores the progression from virus infection to autoimmune myocarditis. Primary autoimmune myocarditis can be induced by immunizing susceptible strains with murine cardiac myosin in complete Freund's adjuvant and nonsusceptible strains with the coadministration of IL-1β or TNF-α. In this model, both cellular and humoral immune responses develop, with complement-fixing heart-reactive antibodies recognizing myosin on the surfaces of cardiac myocytes, as well as BCKD and ANT. It has been proposed that cellular and humoral autoimmune responses to cardiac tissues evolve during the chronic activation of Toll-like receptors (TLRs) expressed on

TABLE 4 Autoantibodies detected in inflammatory cardiomyopathies

Antigen specificity	Type of mimicry
Alpha cardiac actin	Enterovirus
HSP-60	Enterovirus
β-Adrenergic receptor	T. cruzi
M2-cholinergic receptor	T. cruzi
Laminin	
Actin	
Myosin	Bacterial, enterovirus
ANT	
Vimentin	
Sarcolemma	Enterovirus
Desmin	
Mitochrondrial antigen	Bacterial, enterovirus
Carnitin	
Laminin	
Myolemma	
Sarcolemma	
DNase B	Bacterial
Hyaluronidase	
Streptosyme	

cardiac dendritic cells primed with cardiac antigens in post-infectious myocarditis (7). Thus, the development of autoimmune myocarditis relies on cooperation between innate and adaptive immunity during prolonged periods of (smoldering) inflammation. Since similar cellular and humoral autoimmune responses are detected in human patients with inflammatory cardiomyopathies, immunosuppression has been considered as a therapy option. However, the results of the recent Myocarditis Treatment Trial showed no significant improvement in LV ejection fraction or mortality after immunosuppressive therapy with either cyclosporin, azathioprine, or prednisolone in patients with Dallas criteria-diagnosed myocarditis (29). Although some controversy still exists regarding the criteria utilized for the diagnosis of myocarditis, it may be that immunosuppressive therapy might be more effective at earlier stages of disease or, indeed, may be more effective for primary autoimmune myocarditis,

whereas when applied to cases of infectious myocarditis, it may inhibit immune clearance of the pathogen. Therefore, what is needed is effective diagnosis and treatment and refined techniques for identifying true etiologies when myocarditis is suspected.

The diagnosis of myocarditis, inflammatory myocarditis, or lymphocytic myocarditis has traditionally been determined by histochemical analysis of endomyocardial biopsies (EMBs) by use of the Dallas criteria in conjunction with evidence of a fourfold increase in antibody titers between acute- and convalescent-phase sera (5). The Dallas criteria, established in 1986 by Aretz (4), define active, borderline, and absent myocarditis as the presence of lymphocytic infiltrates with adjacent myocyte necrosis, the presence of lymphocytic infiltrates without myocyte necrosis, and the absence of infiltrating lymphocytes, respectively. This approach has several limitations. The collection of EMBs is a relatively invasive procedure, with a bias toward select tissues of the heart; furthermore, accurate diagnosis relies on histochemical evidence of a focal lesion, which may be easily missed upon biopsy and which is often only expressed during the acute phase of an active infection, when such biopsies may be difficult to obtain.

Currently, immunohistochemical staining and molecular immunological techniques, e.g., PCR and in situ hybridization, are being applied to EMB to enhance the sensitivity and specificity of this procedure for the diagnosis of myocarditis. Enzyme-conjugated monoclonal antibodies with specificities for lymphocyte CD antigens are used to distinguish different subsets of infiltrating lymphocytes, macrophages, and neutrophils. Molecular assays, e.g., PCR and in situ hybridization, are now being applied to detect specific viral sequences within EMBs. These techniques, which are able in some cases to distinguish between productive and nonproductive infections, are useful for discriminating between active, chronic, and postinfectious cases of myocarditis.

Although the immunohistological characterization of leukocytic infiltrates in EMBs is improving, histological confirmation of myocyte damage has been a greater challenge and a source of interobserver variability in the clinical diagnosis of myocarditis by the Dallas criteria. This difficulty in assessing myocyte damage in EMBs may be one explanation for the low frequency (10%) of Dallas criterion-positive EMBs reported in 1996 in the Myocarditis Treatment Trial, which enrolled over 2,200 patients with reduced ventricular

TABLE 5 Clinical immunological assays for detection and characterization of inflammatory heart disease

Specimen type	Result	Method[a]	Criterion
EMB	Lymphocytic infiltrates	H&E histology	Cellular morphology
	B-cell infiltrates	IHC/IFA	Detection of CD20 surface antigen
	CD4+ T-cell infiltrates	IHC/IFA	Detection of CD3/CD8 surface antigen
	CD8+ T-cell infiltrates	IHC/IFA	Detection of CD3/CD8 surface antigen
	NK cell infiltrates	IHC/IFA	Detection of CD56 surface antigen
	Macrophage infiltrates	IHC/IFA	Detection of CD14/CD68 surface antigen
	Infection with specific virus	IHC/PCR	Detection of virus-specific DNA or RNA
	Necrosis	H&E histology	Cellular morphology
	Apoptosis	Cardiac TUNEL assay	Fragmented DNA
Serum	Heart-reactive antibodies	IFA/EIA	Detection of immunoglobulin G anti-cardiac myosin antibodies
	Cardiac myocyte damage	EIA	Dectection of TnT, TnI, or CKMB
	Cardiac myocyte damage	Anti-myosin scintigraphy	Nuclear imaging with [111]indium–anti-myosin
	Diagnosis of viral myocarditis	ELISA	Fourfold rise in specific immunoglobulin G titer
	Diagnosis of rhematic myocarditis	Anti-streptolysin O test	

[a]H&E, hematoxylin and eosin, IHC, immunohistochemistry; IFA, immunofluorescence assay; ISH, in situ hybridization.

function and no evidence of coronary artery diseases (29). A number of new, currently available histochemical and molecular assays, e.g., annexin binding assays, terminal deoxynucleotidyltransferase dUDP-biotin nick end labeling-based assays, and immunochemical assays for the detection of apoptosis-related caspases, are now being used to identify and discriminate between apoptotic and necrotic cells within EMBs (Table 5).

REFERENCES

1. **Adams, J. E., III, D. R. Abendschein, and A. S. Jaffe.** 1993. Biochemical markers of myocardial injury. Is MB creatine kinase the choice for the 1990s? *Circulation* **88**:750–763.

2. **Altieri, P., C. Brunelli, S. Garibaldi, A. Nicolino, S. Ubaldi, P. Spallarossa, L. Olivotti, P. Rossettin, A. Barsotti, and G. Ghigliotti.** 2003. Metalloproteinases 2 and 9 are increased in plasma of patients with heart failure. *Eur. J. Clin. Investig.* **33**:648–656.

3. **Apple, F. S., H. E. Quist, P. J. Doyle, A. P. Otto, and M. M. Murakami.** 2003. Plasma 99th percentile reference limits for cardiac troponin and creatine kinase MB mass for use with European Society of Cardiology/American College of Cardiology consensus recommendations. *Clin. Chem.* **49**:1331–1336.

4. **Aretz, H. T.** 1987. Myocarditis: the Dallas criteria. *Hum. Pathol.* **18**:619–624.

5. **Aretz, H. T., M. E. Billingham, W. D. Edwards, S. M. Factor, J. T. Fallon, J. J. Fenoglio, Jr., E. G. Olsen, and F. J. Schoen.** 1987. Myocarditis. A histopathologic definition and classification. *Am. J. Cardiovasc. Pathol.* **1**:3–14.

6. **Aukrust, P., T. Ueland, E. Lien, K. Bendtzen, F. Muller, A. K. Andreassen, I. Nordoy, H. Aass, T. Espevik, S. Simonsen, S. S. Froland, and L. Gullestad.** 1999. Cytokine network in congestive heart failure secondary to ischemic or idiopathic dilated cardiomyopathy. *Am. J. Cardiol.* **83**:376–382.

7. **Eriksson, U., R. Ricci, L. Hunziker, M. O. Kurrer, G. Y. Oudit, T. H. Watts, I. Sonderegger, K. Bachmaier, M. Kopf, and J. M. Penninger.** 2003. Dendritic cell-induced autoimmune heart failure requires cooperation between adaptive and innate immunity. *Nat. Med.* **9**:1484–1490.

8. **Fairweather, D., Z. Kaya, G. R. Shellam, C. M. Lawson, and N. R. Rose.** 2001. From infection to autoimmunity. *J. Autoimmun.* **16**:175–186.

9. **Feuerstein, G. Z., and D. Rozanski.** 2000. G proteins and heart failure: is Gαq a novel target for heart failure? *Circ. Res.* **87**:1085–1086.

10. **Flesch, M., A. Hoper, L. Dell'Italia, K. Evans, R. Bond, R. Peshock, A. Diwan, T. A. Brinsa, C. C. Wei, N. Sivasubramanian, F. G. Spinale, and D. L. Mann.** 2003. Activation and functional significance of the renin-angiotensin system in mice with cardiac restricted overexpression of tumor necrosis factor. *Circulation* **108**:598–604.

11. **Gotlieb, A. I., M. R. Freeman, T. A. Salerno, S. V. Lichtenstein, and P. W. Armstrong.** 1991. Ultrastructural studies of unstable angina in living man. *Mod. Pathol.* **4**:75–80.

12. **Guilherme, L., and J. Kalil.** 2002. Rheumatic fever: the T cell response leading to autoimmune aggression in the heart. *Autoimmun. Rev.* **1**:261–266.

13. **Gullestad, L., P. Aukrust, T. Ueland, T. Espevik, G. Yee, R. Vagelos, S. S. Froland, and M. Fowler.** 1999. Effect of high- versus low-dose angiotensin converting enzyme inhibition on cytokine levels in chronic heart failure. *J. Am. Coll. Cardiol.* **34**:2061–2067.

14. **Hill, S. L., and N. R. Rose.** 2001. The transition from viral to autoimmune myocarditis. *Autoimmunity* **34**:169–176.

15. **Hillis, G. S., N. Zhao, P. Taggart, W. C. Dalsey, and A. Mangione.** 1999. Utility of cardiac troponin I, creatine

16. **Inoue, T., T. Kato, K. Takayanagi, T. Uchida, I. Yaguchi, H. Kamishirado, S. Morooka, and N. Yoshimoto.** 2003. Circulating matrix metalloproteinase-1 and -3 in patients with an acute coronary syndrome. *Am. J. Cardiol.* **92**:1461–1464.

17. **Kai, H., H. Ikeda, H. Yasukawa, M. Kai, Y. Seki, F. Kuwahara, T. Ueno, K. Sugi, and T. Imaizumi.** 1998. Peripheral blood levels of matrix metalloproteases-2 and -9 are elevated in patients with acute coronary syndromes. *J. Am. Coll. Cardiol.* **32**:368–372.

18. **Kawai, C.** 1999. From myocarditis to cardiomyopathy: mechanisms of inflammation and cell death: learning from the past for the future. *Circulation* **99**:1091–1100.

19. **Keffer, J. H.** 1996. Myocardial markers of injury. Evolution and insights. *Am. J. Clin. Pathol.* **105**:305–320.

20. **Levin, E. R., D. G. Gardner, and W. K. Samson.** 1998. Natriuretic peptides. *N. Engl. J. Med.* **339**:321–328.

21. **Li, Y. Y., C. F. McTiernan, and A. M. Feldman.** 2000. Interplay of matrix metalloproteinases, tissue inhibitors of metalloproteinases and their regulators in cardiac matrix remodeling. *Cardiovasc. Res.* **46**:214–224.

22. **MacLellan, W. R., and A. J. Lusis.** 2003. Dilated cardiomyopathy: learning to live with yourself. *Nat. Med.* **9**:1455–1456.

23. **Mair, J.** 1997. Progress in myocardial damage detection: new biochemical markers for clinicians. *Crit. Rev. Clin. Lab. Sci.* **34**:1–66.

24. **Maisch, B., I. Portig, A. Ristic, G. Hufnagel, and S. Pankuweit.** 2000. Definition of inflammatory cardiomyopathy (myocarditis): on the way to consensus. A status report. *Herz* **25**:200–209.

25. **Mann, D. L.** 2002. Angiotensin II as an inflammatory mediator: evolving concepts in the role of the renin angiotensin system in the failing heart. *Cardiovasc. Drugs Ther.* **16**:7–9.

26. **Mann, D. L.** 2002. Inflammatory mediators and the failing heart: past, present, and the foreseeable future. *Circ. Res.* **91**:988–998.

27. **Mann, D. L.** 2003. Stress-activated cytokines and the heart: from adaptation to maladaptation. *Annu. Rev. Physiol.* **65**:81–101.

28. **Marshall, T., J. Williams, and K. M. Williams.** 1991. Electrophoresis of serum isoenzymes and proteins following acute myocardial infarction. *J. Chromatogr.* **569**:323–345.

29. **Mason, J. W.** 1996. Immunopathogenesis and treatment of myocarditis: the United States Myocarditis Treatment Trial. *J. Card. Fail.* **2**:S173–S177.

30. **Mason, J. W.** 2003. Myocarditis and dilated cardiomyopathy: an inflammatory link. *Cardiovasc. Res.* **60**:5–10.

31. **McCullough, P. A., R. M. Nowak, J. McCord, J. E. Hollander, H. C. Herrmann, P. G. Steg, P. Duc, A. Westheim, T. Omland, C. W. Knudsen, A. B. Storrow, W. T. Abraham, S. Lamba, A. H. Wu, A. Perez, P. Clopton, P. Krishnaswamy, R. Kazanegra, and A. S. Maisel.** 2002. B-type natriuretic peptide and clinical judgment in emergency diagnosis of heart failure: analysis from Breathing Not Properly (BNP) Multinational Study. *Circulation* **106**:416–422.

32. **Noutsias, M., C. Hohmann, M. Pauschinger, P. L. Schwimmbeck, K. Ostermann, U. Rode, M. H. Yacoub, U. Kuhl, and H. P. Schultheiss.** 2003. sICAM-1 correlates with myocardial ICAM-1 expression in dilated cardiomyopathy. *Int. J. Cardiol.* **91**:153–161.

33. **Panteghini, M., F. S. Apple, R. H. Christenson, F. Dati, J. Mair, and A. H. Wu.** 1999. Proposals from IFCC Committee on Standardization of Markers of Cardiac Damage (C-SMCD): recommendations on use of biochemical markers of cardiac damage in acute coronary syndromes. *Scand. J. Clin. Lab. Investig.* **230**(Suppl.):103–112.

34. Pettersson, T., O. Ohlsson, and N. Tryding. 1992. Increased CKMB (mass concentration) in patients without traditional evidence of acute myocardial infarction. A risk indicator of coronary death. *Eur. Heart J.* **13:**1387–1392.

35. Pope, J. H., T. P. Aufderheide, R. Ruthazer, R. H. Woolard, J. A. Feldman, J. R. Beshansky, J. L. Griffith, and H. P. Selker. 2000. Missed diagnoses of acute cardiac ischemia in the emergency department. *N. Engl. J. Med.* **342:**1163–1170.

36. Prontera, C., M. Emdin, G. C. Zucchelli, A. Ripoli, C. Passino, and A. Clerico. 2003. Natriuretic peptides (NPs): automated electrochemiluminescent immunoassay for N-terminal pro-BNP compared with IRMAs for ANP and BNP in heart failure patients and healthy individuals. *Clin. Chem.* **49:**1552–1554.

37. Puleo, P. R., P. A. Guadagno, R. Roberts, M. V. Scheel, A. J. Marian, D. Churchill, and M. B. Perryman. 1990. Early diagnosis of acute myocardial infarction based on assay for subforms of creatine kinase-MB. *Circulation* **82:**759–764.

38. Robers, M., F. F. Van der Hulst, M. A. Fischer, W. Roos, C. E. Salud, H. G. Eisenwiener, and J. F. Glatz. 1998. Development of a rapid microparticle-enhanced turbidimetric immunoassay for plasma fatty acid-binding protein, an early marker of acute myocardial infarction. *Clin. Chem.* **44:**1564–1567.

39. Schwartzkopff, B., B. Fassbach, B. Pelzer, M. Brehm, and B. E. Strauer. 2002. Elevated serum markers of collagen degradation in patients with mild to moderate dilated cardiomyopathy. *Eur. J. Heart Fail.* **4:**439–444.

40. Stewart, J. A., Jr., C. C. Wei, G. L. Brower, P. E. Rynders, G. H. Hankes, A. R. Dillon, P. A. Lucchesi, J. S. Janicki, and L. J. Dell'Italia. 2003. Cardiac mast cell- and chymase-mediated matrix metalloproteinase activity and left ventricular remodeling in mitral regurgitation in the dog. *J. Mol. Cell. Cardiol.* **35:**311–319.

41. Storrow, A. B., and W. B. Gibler. 2000. Chest pain centers: diagnosis of acute coronary syndromes. *Ann. Emerg. Med.* **35:**449–461.

42. Suzuki, T., T. Yamazaki, and Y. Yazaki. 2001. The role of the natriuretic peptides in the cardiovascular system. *Cardiovasc. Res.* **51:**489–494.

43. Tsutamoto, T., T. Hisanaga, A. Wada, K. Maeda, M. Ohnishi, D. Fukai, N. Mabuchi, M. Sawaki, and M. Kinoshita. 1998. Interleukin-6 spillover in the peripheral circulation increases with the severity of heart failure, and the high plasma level of interleukin-6 is an important prognostic predictor in patients with congestive heart failure. *J. Am. Coll. Cardiol.* **31:**391–398.

44. Upadhya, B., J. L. Kontos, F. Ardeshirpour, J. Pye, W. S. Boucher, T. C. Theoharides, G. J. Dehmer, and E. N. Deliargyris. 2004. Relation of serum levels of mast cell tryptase of left ventricular systolic function, left ventricular volume or congestive heart failure. *J. Card. Fail.* **10:**31–35.

45. Wang, Y., M. Afanasyeva, S. L. Hill, and N. R. Rose. 1999. Characterization of murine autoimmune myocarditis induced by self and foreign cardiac myosin. *Autoimmunity* **31:**151–162.

46. Wei, C. C., P. A. Lucchesi, J. Tallaj, W. E. Bradley, P. C. Powell, and L. J. Dell'Italia. 2003. Cardiac interstitial bradykinin and mast cells modulate pattern of LV remodeling in volume overload in rats. *Am. J. Physiol. Heart. Circ. Physiol.* **285:**H784–H792.

47. Wettschureck, N., H. Rutten, A. Zywietz, D. Gehring, T. M. Wilkie, J. Chen, K. R. Chien, and S. Offermanns. 2001. Absence of pressure overload induced myocardial hypertrophy after conditional inactivation of Galphaq/Galpha11 in cardiomyocytes. *Nat. Med.* **7:**1236–1240.

48. Wollert, K. C., and H. Drexler. 2001. The role of interleukin-6 in the failing heart. *Heart Fail. Rev.* **6:**95–103.

49. Wu, A. H., F. S. Apple, W. B. Gibler, R. L. Jesse, M. M. Warshaw, and R. Valdes, Jr. 1999. National Academy of Clinical Biochemistry Standards of Laboratory Practice: recommendations for the use of cardiac markers in coronary artery diseases. *Clin. Chem.* **45:**1104–1121.

50. Yamazaki, T., J. D. Lee, H. Shimizu, H. Uzui, and T. Ueda. 2004. Circulating matrix metalloproteinase-2 is elevated in patients with congestive heart failure. *Eur. J. Heart Fail.* **6:**41–45.

51. Zolk, O., J. Quattek, U. Seeland, A. El-Armouche, T. Eschenhagen, and M. Bohm. 2002. Activation of the cardiac endothelin system in left ventricular hypertrophy before onset of heart failure in TG(mREN2)27 rats. *Cardiovasc. Res.* **53:**363–371.

Kidney and Lung Disease Mediated by Anti-Glomerular Basement Membrane Antibodies: Detection by Western Blot Analysis

A. BERNARD COLLINS AND ROBERT B. COLVIN

125

Several diseases of the kidney with overlapping histological and clinical features are characterized by a rapid loss of renal function, crescentic glomerulonephritis, and sometimes lung hemorrhage. In affected patients it is crucial to establish the diagnosis as quickly as possible, since early medical treatment can inhibit the rampant downhill course of the disease, which results in permanent renal failure or even death due to lung hemorrhage. The histological examination of renal biopsy specimens typically shows a lesion of crescentic necrotizing glomerulonephritis in all of these diseases. Direct immunofluorescence studies performed on frozen tissue can distinguish these diseases into the following categories: (i) anti-glomerular basement membrane (anti-GBM)-mediated glomerulonephritis (Goodpasture syndrome), (ii) immune complex-mediated glomerulonephritis, and (iii) pauci-immune glomerulonephritis. The last category of diseases includes Wegener's granulomatosis, microscopic polyarteritis nodosa, Churg-Strauss syndrome, and related overlapping forms of these vasculitides (16, 24). Anti-neutrophil cytoplasmic antibodies (ANCA) are almost always detected in this group, and these diseases are currently referred to as ANCA-associated diseases (36a).

Serological assays for the detection of ANCA and anti-GBM autoantibodies are important diagnostic tools in the evaluation of patients with rapidly progressive renal failure and/or pulmonary hemorrhage, providing a rapid noninvasive method for establishing a diagnosis. These tests are sensitive and highly specific and can provide definitive diagnostic information for the effective clinical management of patients with a rapidly progressive course of disease. This chapter describes the detection of circulating anti-GBM antibodies by serological techniques. ANCA assays are described in reference 36a.

Goodpasture syndrome is an autoimmune disease mediated by circulating autoantibodies with specificity to the GBM and alveolar basement membrane. The nephrotoxic activity of these antibodies in the pathogenesis of this disease has been clearly shown (6, 9, 23, 38). The anti-GBM antibodies react with type IV collagen, the major structural component of mammalian basement membranes (35). The protomeric form of type IV collagen is composed of three α chains which are divided into three structural domains: a 7S, or minor collagenous, domain in the N-terminal region; a triple helical, or major collagenous, domain in the middle region; and an NC1, or noncollagenous globular, domain in the C-terminal region (10). The three α chains are assembled into a network with NC1-NC1 and 7S-7S interactions to form a macromolecular superstructure. Most basement membranes in the body contain only the classical α chains, α1(IV) and α2(IV) (17, 34), but specialized basement membranes such as those of the kidney, lung, and eye contain the novel α chains α3(IV) and α4(IV) (10, 11, 13). The α5(IV) chain also has limited distribution in basement membranes of the body. The gene encoding the α5(IV) chain is located on the X chromosome, and mutations of this gene are responsible for approximately 85% of the cases of Alport syndrome (1, 12, 39, 40). Ultrastructurally the GBM of patients with Alport syndrome is abnormal, showing areas of thickening and thinning, scalloping, and laminations. In the normal GBM the α3(IV) and α5(IV) chains are incorporated together, but in the case of patients with Alport syndrome with an X-linked mode of inheritance for the disease, there may be partial or complete loss of the α3(IV) chain as well as the α5(IV) chain. Staining by indirect immunofluorescence for the α3(IV) chain using Goodpasture serum is frequently negative (15, 25, 30). Therefore, there is a risk that patients with Alport syndrome who receive a renal transplant may develop alloantibodies to antigens in the donor GBM. We have detected in the sera of patients with Alport syndrome who develop posttransplant anti-GBM nephritis antibodies that are directed against either the α3(IV) chain (Fig. 1) or the α5 chain (Fig. 2). Similar findings have been reported elsewhere (3, 19). Anti-GBM nephritis in Alport syndrome patients posttransplantation is rare but has been reported (20) to occur in approximately 3 to 4% of male Alport syndrome patients who have undergone transplantation. It usually occurs within the first year following transplantation, with approximately 75% of the transplanted kidneys failing irreversibly within the first few weeks or first few months following transplantation. Posttransplantation anti-GBM nephritis usually recurs in patients receiving subsequent new transplants and usually recurs at an accelerated rate. The length of the interval between retransplantation or the absence of detectable circulating anti-GBM antibodies appears to have no effect on the likelihood of recurrence. The gene for the α6(IV) chain was discovered in 1993 by Zhou et al. (41). Specifically, the reactivity of anti-GBM antibodies has been shown to be directed to the noncollagenous, or NC1, domain of the α3(IV) chain, termed the Goodpasture antigen (13, 35, 36).

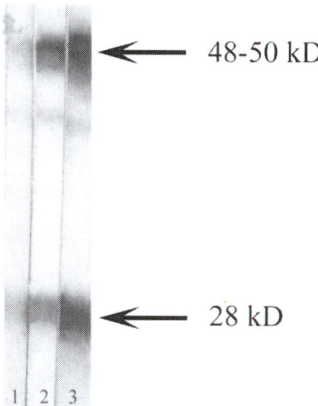

FIGURE 1 Western blot analysis of a serum sample from an Alport syndrome patient who developed posttransplant anti-GBM nephritis (lane 1). The reactivity of the antibody is to the α3(IV) chain, the Goodpasture antigen, at 28 and 48 to 50 kDa. The reactivity is identical to that seen with a monoclonal antibody to the α3(IV) collagen chain (lane 2) and with that of a serum from a patient with renal-biopsy-proven Goodpasture syndrome (lane 3).

All patients with Goodpasture syndrome have autoantibodies that react primarily with the α3 chain of type IV collagen (10, 32, 33); however, lower-titer reactivity to other α chains has been reported (10). The α3(IV) NC1 antibodies recognize a restricted group of epitopes, as demonstrated by the fact that the autoantibodies in the sera of most patients are partially blocked by monoclonal antibodies to the α3(IV) NC1 chain (31). Kalluri et al. in 1991 (18) further localized the Goodpasture epitope to the carboxyl-terminal region of the α3(IV) NC1, encompassing residues 198 to 223, as the primary antibody interaction site. The Goodpasture antigen is released as NC1 hexamers after bacterial collagenase treatment of the GBM (35). The hexamers are composed of the subunits of the NC1 domains of the various α chains

that comprise the two intertwined protomers. When the hexamers are then subjected to sodium dodecyl sulfate-polyacrylamide gel electrophoresis (SDS-PAGE), they further dissociate into monomeric and dimeric subunits, which are used as an antigen in Western blot analysis for detecting reactivity to the Goodpasture antigen (13).

The earliest technique used for the detection of circulating anti-GBM antibodies was indirect immunofluorescence (13, 26, 27). In the assay, normal human kidney frozen tissue sections are incubated with the patient's serum, as well as with positive and negative control sera. Specific bound immunoglobulin to the GBM, usually immunoglobulin G (IgG), is detected by using a fluorescein-labeled antiserum to human IgG or to human immunoglobulins (IgG, IgA, and IgM). Difficulties in interpretation of the assay are related to the nonspecific accumulation of IgG along the GBM in the normal kidney tissue substrate used as a source of GBM, particularly in autopsy tissue. This nonspecific accumulation makes subjective interpretation of positive staining very difficult and results in a high percentage of false positives and negatives. Furthermore, standardization is difficult or impossible since there is a great variability in the reactivity between different kidney specimens.

Wilson in 1974 (37) developed a radioimmunoassay (RIA) for detecting anti-GBM antibodies, using a collagenase digest of the GBM as an antigen. The assay was a double-antibody RIA which incorporated the use of radiolabeled human IgG to assess the adequacy of immunoglobulin precipitation by the second antibody. Quantitation and objectivity were the greatest advantages that the RIA technique offered over the indirect immunofluorescence technique. The disadvantage, however, was that the crude digest of human GBM contained not only the Goodpasture antigen but also other components of the glomerular basement, such as laminin and entactin. Therefore, false-positive binding could arise from antibodies reactive with other basement membrane components; such reactivity has been reported for several glomerular diseases (5).

WESTERN BLOT ANALYSIS

Our laboratory has developed a sensitive and specific assay for the detection of circulating anti-GBM antibodies using Western blot analysis. The assay has the advantage that the exact molecular weight of the antigen recognized by the autoantibody can be determined accurately and compared to the reactivity of a known Goodpasture serum to the α3(IV) chain. The antigen used in the assay is a collagenase digest of isolated human GBM prepared by the enzymatic digestion of the GBM, which releases the NC1 domains of the type IV collagen, including the α3(IV) NC1, the Goodpasture antigen. Separation of the soluble proteins by PAGE followed by transfer to nitrocellulose paper for immunoblotting allows discrimination between antibody reacting to the Goodpasture antigen and those reacting with other components of the GBM.

Isolation of Glomeruli and Preparation of GBM

GBM is prepared from normal human kidneys obtained at autopsy or from nephrectomy specimens in the operating room. Use of autopsy specimens is limited to no more than 10 to 12 h after death, and in the case of surgical specimens, only the normal portion at least 1 to 2 cm distal from any tumor is taken. The kidneys are then stored frozen at −70°C for glomerular isolation.

The tissue is thawed in 0.01 M phosphate-buffered saline (PBS), pH 7.2, containing 10 mM phenylmethylsulfonyl

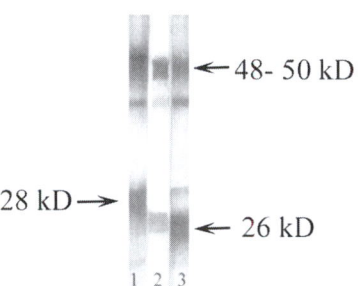

FIGURE 2 Western blot analysis of another serum sample from an Alport syndrome patient who also developed posttransplant anti-GBM nephritis. However, when immunoblotted on the collagenase digest of the human GBM it shows reactivity to a lower-molecular-mass antigen in the monomer region of the NC1 domain, at approximately 26 kDa instead of 28 kDa (lane 3). It shows the same reactivity to a higher-molecular-mass antigen in the dimer region, at approximately 48 to 50 kDa. The reactivity is to α5(IV) chain collagen and is identical to reactivity of a monoclonal antibody to the α5(IV) chain collagen (lane 2). Serum from a patient with renal-biopsy-proven Goodpasture syndrome is in lane 1.

fluoride as a protease inhibitor. All subsequent isolation steps are carried out in the presence of phenylmethylsulfonyl fluoride. The cortical portion of the kidneys is cut away from the medulla and placed in ice-cold PBS. Glomeruli are isolated from the cortical tissue using differential sieving according to the method of Edgington et al. (7), as modified by Gang (8). The glomeruli are washed two or three times with PBS. After the final wash with PBS, the glomeruli are washed twice with distilled water to rupture the cell membranes. To further remove cellular material, the glomeruli are sonicated by pulsation using a W200 P Sonifier cell disrupter (Heat Systems—Ultrasonics, Inc., Plainview, N.Y.) equipped with a microtip at 40% duty cycle. After the initial sonication the preparation is examined using phase microscopy and the sonication step is repeated until only refractile GBM remains. The GBM is dialyzed against distilled water overnight at 4°C, lyophilized, and stored in a desiccator at 4°C.

Enzymatic Digestion of the GBM

The GBM is digested using chromatographically purified collagenase type VII prepared from *Clostridium histolyticum* (Sigma, St. Louis, Mo.). The collagenase preparation is substantially free of nonspecific protease, clostripain, and tryptic activities. Ten milligrams of lyophilized GBM is suspended in 2 ml of 0.1 M Tris-HC1 (pH 7.5) in a 15-ml centrifuge tube with 5 mM $CaCl_2$ added to facilitate digestion. The mixture is sonicated for 30 min in a Bransonic 220 water bath sonicator (Branson Co., Shelton, Conn.). Collagenase type VII (1,000 U/mg of GBM) is added and the GBM is digested at 37°C in a shaking water bath for 48 h according to the method of Wieslander et al. (35). The pH is monitored at 30, 60, and 120 min and adjusted to 7.5 if necessary using 1 N Tris-HC1 or 1 N Trizma base. After digestion, 1 ml of 0.1 M Tris-HC1, pH 7.5, containing 2 mM EDTA is added to chelate free Ca^{2+} and thus quench the reaction. The particulate solution is centrifuged at 1,500 × g for 30 min at 4°C. The clear supernatant is recovered and assayed for protein concentration using the Lowry method (22). The solubilized antigen is then stored frozen at −70°C in 50-µl aliquots.

In initial studies the GBM was subjected to various durations of enzymatic digestion from 24 to 96 h to maximize the degradation of the collagenous portions of the membrane. Protein determinations by the Lowry method were performed, and the results obtained showed that approximately 50 to 60% (wt/wt) of the membrane was solubilized in the first 24 h. The solubilization occurred less rapidly after that, but continued up to 72 to 96 h.

PAGE and Transfer to Nitrocellulose Paper

An aliquot of the soluble antigen preparation obtained from the collagenase digestion of the GBM is thawed, and 200 µg is added to each gel and then separated by SDS-PAGE as described by Laemmli (21) in 12% unreduced gels using a Mighty Small II gel apparatus (Hoefer Scientific, San Francisco, Calif.) at a constant current of 40 mA for 1 h. Included as a marker is a low-molecular-weight standard (Bio-Rad, Richmond, Calif.). After PAGE, the separated proteins are transferred to nitrocellulose paper (Pharmacia Biotech, San Francisco, Calif.) using a TE series Transphor electrophoresis unit (Hoefer Scientific) and a PS 500X DC power supply. The transfer electrophoresis is carried out using a constant current of 200 mA for 1 h with a circulating water cooling system according to the method of Burnette (4). In order to verify and visualize the separated

transferred proteins, the nitrocellulose paper is cut from one side of the paper to include the molecular weight standard and the soluble GBM antigen digest and placed into 0.1% India ink on a slow rotator for 30 to 60 min, followed by a PBS wash. The remainder of the nitrocellulose paper is stored dry between two pieces of Whatman filter paper at room temperature. Storing paper in this manner allows sera to be tested quickly and efficiently. Paper can be stored dry for up to 2 months.

Western Blotting

Upon receiving sera for anti-GBM testing by Western blot analysis, an appropriate piece of the dried nitrocellulose paper is cut for the number of sera to be tested and placed into 5% skim milk buffer for 1 h, with agitation for blocking. After blocking, the nitrocellulose paper is cut into 3- to 4-mm wide strips and placed into the wells of a Mighty Small incubation tray (Hoefer Scientific). The strips are incubated in 1 ml of test serum diluted 1:10 in 0.5% skim milk buffer for a minimum of 1 h. After incubation, the excess serum is aspirated and the strips are washed three times for 5 min each time with 0.5% skim milk buffer and then incubated with 1 ml of biotin-conjugated goat anti-human IgG (heavy and light chains; Vector Labs, Burlingame, Calif.) at 1:250 for 1 h, with agitation. After incubation, excess conjugate is aspirated and the strips are washed with 0.5% skim milk buffer. To detect bound labeled antibody, the strips are incubated in 1 ml of avidin-biotin complex (Vector Labs) for 60 min, the excess reagent is aspirated, and the nitrocellulose strips are washed in the 0.5% skim milk buffer as described above. The last incubation is with 3-amino-9-ethyl carbazole (1 ml per well), a chromogen for horseradish peroxidase. Finally, the strips are washed in distilled water for 5 to 10 min and blotted dry between two pieces of Whatman filter paper, so that the strips can be examined for reactivity to the α3(IV) NC1 (the Goodpasture antigen) or reactivities to other NC1 domains of type IV collagen. The total time for performance of the test is 4 to 5 h.

Background

Western blot analysis for the detection of anti-GBM antibodies was developed in our reference laboratory at Massachusetts General Hospital in 1988, and since then it has been used routinely for analysis of sera referred for screening of anti-GBM antibodies, typically in a setting of rapidly progressive disease with kidney and lung involvement. Since January 2004 approximately 10,000 (9,597) sera have been tested for anti-GBM antibodies. Subsequently we retested by Western blot analysis samples of frozen sera from 1981 to 1988 that had previously been found to be positive by indirect immunofluorescence, enzyme-linked immunosorbent assay (ELISA), or RIA in order to compare sensitivities. We have detected anti-GBM antibodies in the sera of 165 (1.7%) patients from samples sent to our reference laboratory between 1981 and 2003. Virtually all patients with a positive test for anti-GBM antibodies have been found to have clinical or pathological features consistent with anti-GBM disease. In a series of 18 patients with biopsy-proven anti-GBM disease and a positive Western blot, 85 to 90% were positive by indirect immunofluorescence and 100% were positive by RIA or ELISA.

A comprehensive serological workup for patients with a pulmonary renal syndrome should include ANCA testing since, in our experience, the syndrome of lung hemorrhage and glomerulonephritis is most often due to an ANCA-associated disease (28). In 1996, Niles et al. (28) reviewed the medical records of 750 patients that had serum sent to our laboratory for anti-GBM testing from 1981 to 1993.

In this group, 88 patients had evidence of lung hemorrhage and glomerulonephritis and 48 were found to have ANCA, 6 had anti-GBM antibodies, 7 had both, and 27 were negative for both. Furthermore, 30 to 40% of patients with anti-GBM antibodies also have ANCA (2, 14). Studies from our laboratory by Niles et al. in 1991 (29) reported that of 123 patients with rapidly progressive glomerulonephritis who were studied serologically for anti-GBM antibodies and ANCA, 42 had pauci-immune necrotizing glomerulonephritis by light microscopy, 18 had anti-GBM disease, and 63 had other forms of renal disease as diagnosed by renal biopsy. The 63 patients with other forms of glomerulonephritis included those with minimal change, systemic lupus erythematosus, membranoproliferative glomerulonephritis types I and II, membranous glomerulonephritis, IgA nephropathy, Henoch-Schönlein purpura, focal segmental glomerulosclerosis, antitubular basal membrane disease, acute hemolytic-uremic syndrome, mixed cryoglobulinemia, systemic light chain disease, and postinfectious glomerulonephritis. Healthy laboratory personnel were analyzed as controls. Only the sera of the patients with biopsy-proven crescentic and necrotizing glomerulonephritis by light microscopy and positive direct immunofluorescence (diffuse, linear IgG along the GBM) reacted with the specific molecular weight components of the Goodpasture antigen when screened for circulating anti-GBM antibodies by Western blot analysis (Fig. 3). No positivity was detected in the sera of patients with other forms of glomerulonephritis or in the sera of the 917 healthy controls that were also analyzed. Of the 18 patients with anti-GBM antibodies, 8 also had ANCA; 2 were specific for proteinase 3 and 6 were specific for myeloperoxidase. Histologically, there was no clear difference seen between patients with anti-GBM alone and those with both anti-GBM and ANCA.

Our Western blot analysis results showed that only the sera from patients with biopsy-proven anti-GBM reacted with the Goodpasture antigen in the 28-kDa and 48- to 50-kDa regions corresponding to the monomeric and dimeric forms of α3(IV) NC1 (the Goodpasture antigen) as defined by Weislander et al. (35). In approximately 40% of the sera

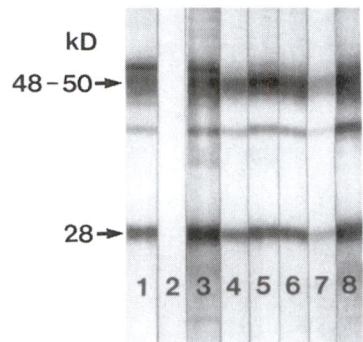

kD
48–50→
28→
1 2 3 4 5 6 7 8

FIGURE 3 Western blot analysis of sera from seven patients with biopsy-proven anti-GBM nephritis (lanes 3 to 8). Note the reduced intensity of the bands in lane 7 compared to lane 8. The serum sample in lane 7 was from the same patient as that in lane 8, but after 11 plasmapheresis exchanges. Positive control serum and normal control serum are in lanes 1 and 2, respectively. The antigen preparation is a collagenase digest of human GBM, which is separated by PAGE and immunoblotted onto nitrocellulose paper. The reactivity seen in the positive sera is to the same two molecular mass regions at 28 and 50 kDa, which represent the α3(IV) NC1 (Goodpasture antigen) in its monomeric and dimeric forms.

analyzed, reactivity to antigens of different molecular weights was detected. Thus, Western blot analysis provides a definitive means of differentiating between the specific reactivity of anti-GBM antibody in the sera of patients with anti-GBM disease and the reactivities of antibodies with other specificities. These other reactivities are probably due to a secondary antibody response to other proteins released from the damaged GBM as a result of the binding of the nephritogenic anti-GBM antibodies to the GBM.

ELISA FOR α3(IV) NC1

Western blot analysis is a sensitive and specific assay for detecting anti-GBM antibodies, but quantitation is needed for the purpose of monitoring disease activity. Therefore, in positive sera the level of anti-GBM antibody is quantitated using an antigen-specific immunoassay (ELISA). A reasonably satisfactory monitoring commercial ELISA kit (SciMedex Corp., Denville, N.J.) uses microtiter strips coated with the monomer of the α3(IV) NC1 subunit. The value, in ELISA units (EU), for each unknown serum is determined from a standard curve constructed from analysis of known positive sera containing assigned values of 5, 20, 80, and 320 EU/ml. A positive serum and a negative serum are also included in each determination. The level of antibody is expressed as EU per milliliter; a value equal to or greater than 15 EU/ml is considered positive, a value equal to 5.1 to 14.9 EU/ml is considered equivocal, and a value equal to or less than 5 EU/ml is considered negative. Differences in sensitivity and specificity were observed when the results of ELISA and Western blot analysis using the same serum were compared. The differences in results were evident for treated patients, particularly when plasmapheresis was part of the treatment regimen. However, the ELISA is clearly less sensitive than Western blotting. Often after treatment, the ELISA will become negative, while the Western blot analysis remains positive. False positives are also a problem in this ELISA; we have obtained positive ELISA results with sera from nine patients with no evidence of anti-GBM disease by biopsy or Western blot analysis. Therefore, the most sensitive and specific current method for detecting circulating anti-GBM antibodies is Western blot analysis. In our laboratory, positive anti-GBM antibody results obtained by ELISA are never reported without confirmation by Western blot analysis. It is also important to note that the antibody "titer" obtained in the ELISA for different patients cannot be used as a measure of the disease severity, since the antibodies may have different affinities and biological activities. The test is most useful for monitoring an individual patient, comparing subsequent samples with the initial sample.

REFERENCES

1. Barker, D. F., S. L. Hostikka, J. Zhou, L. T. Chow, A. R. Oliphant, S. C. Gerken, M. C. Gregory, M. H. Skolnick, C. L. Atkin, and K. Tryggvason. 1990. Identification of mutations in the COL4A5 collagen gene in Alport syndrome. *Science* **248:**1224–1227.
2. Bosch, X., E. Mirapeix, J. Font, X. Borrellas, R. Rodriguez, A. Lopez-Soto, M. Ingelmo, and L. Revert. 1991. Prognostic implication of anti-neutrophil cytoplasmic autoantibodies with myeloperoxidase specificity in anti-glomerular basement membrane disease. *Clin. Nephrol.* **36:**107–113.
3. Brainwood, D., C. Kashtan, M. C. Gubler, and A. N. Turner. 1998. Targets of alloantibodies in Alport anti-glomerular basement membrane disease after renal transplantation. *Kidney Int.* **53:**762–766.

4. **Burnette, W. N.** 1981. "Western blotting": electrophoretic transfer of proteins from sodium dodecyl sulfate-polyacrylamide gels to unmodified nitrocellulose and radiographic detection with antibody and radioiodinated protein A. *Anal. Biochem.* **112:**195–203.

5. **Bygren, P., B. Cederholm, D. Heinegard, and J. Wieslander.** 1989. Non-Goodpasture anti-GBM antibodies in patients with glomerulonephritis. *Nephrol. Dial. Transplant.* **4:**254–261.

6. **Couser, W. G.** 1992. Glomerular disorders, p. 551–568. *In* J. B. Wyngaarden, L. H. Smith, and C. J. Bennett (ed.), *Cecil Textbook of Medicine.* W. B. Saunders, Philadelphia, Pa.

7. **Edgington, T. S., R. J. Glassock, J. I. Watson, and F. J. Dixon.** 1967. Characterization and isolation of specific renal tubular epithelial antigens. *J. Immunol.* **99:**1199–1210.

8. **Gang, N. F.** 1970. A rapid method for the isolation of glomeruli from the human kidney. *Am. J. Clin. Pathol.* **53:**267–269.

9. **Glassock, R. J., A. H. Cohen, S. G. Adler, and H. J. Ward.** 1991. Secondary glomerular diseases, p. 1280–1368. *In* B. M. Brenner and F. C. Rector (ed.), *The Kidney,* 4th ed. W. B. Saunders, Philadelphia. Pa.

10. **Hellmark, T., C. Johansson, and J. Wieslander.** 1994. Characterization of anti-GBM antibodies involved in Goodpasture's syndrome. *Kidney Int.* **46:**823–829.

11. **Hostikka, S. L., R. L. Eddy, M. G. Byers, M. Hoyhtya, T. B. Shows, and K. Tryggvason.** 1990. Identification of a distinct type IV collagen alpha chain with restricted kidney distribution and assignment of its gene to the locus of X chromosome-linked Alport syndrome. *Proc. Natl. Acad. Sci. USA* **87:**1606–1610.

12. **Hudson, B. G., K. Tryggvason, M. Sundaramoorthy, and E. G. Neilson.** 2003. Alport's syndrome, Goodpasture's syndrome, and type IV collagen. *N. Engl. J. Med.* **348:**2543–2556.

13. **Hudson, B. G., J. Wieslander, B. J. Wisdom, Jr., and M. E. Noelken.** 1989. Goodpasture syndrome: molecular architecture and function of basement membrane antigen. *Lab. Investig.* **61:**256–269. (Erratum, **61:**690.)

14. **Jayne, D. R., P. D. Marshall, S. J. Jones, and C. M. Lockwood.** 1990. Autoantibodies to GBM and neutrophil cytoplasm in rapidly progressive glomerulonephritis. *Kidney Int.* **37:**965–970.

15. **Jenis, E. H., J. E. Valeski, and P. L. Calcagno.** 1981. Variability of anti-GBM binding in hereditary nephritis. *Clin. Nephrol.* **15:**111–114.

16. **Jennette, J. C., A. S. Wilkman, and R. J. Falk.** 1989. Anti-neutrophil cytoplasmic autoantibody-associated glomerulonephritis and vasculitis. *Am. J. Pathol.* **135:**921–930.

17. **Johnson, G. D., R. S. Davidson, K. C. McNamee, G. Russell, D. Goodwin, and E. J. Holborow.** 1982. Fading of immunofluorescence during microscopy: a study of the phenomenon and its remedy. *J. Immunol. Methods* **55:**231–242.

18. **Kalluri, R., S. Gunwar, S. T. Reeders, K. C. Morrison, M. Mariyama, K. E. Ebner, M. E. Noelken, and B. G. Hudson.** 1991. Goodpasture syndrome. Localization of the epitope for the autoantibodies to the carboxyl-terminal region of the alpha 3(IV) chain of basement membrane collagen. *J. Biol. Chem.* **266:**24018–24024.

19. **Kalluri, R., M. Weber, K. O. Netzer, M. J. Sun, E. G. Neilson, and B. G. Hudson.** 1994. COL4A5 gene deletion and production of post-transplant anti-alpha 3(IV) collagen alloantibodies in Alport syndrome. *Kidney Int.* **45:**721–726.

20. **Kashtan, C. E., R. J. Butkowski, M. M. Kleppel, M. R. First, and A. F. Michael.** 1990. Posttransplant anti-glomerular basement membrane nephritis in related males with Alport syndrome. *J. Lab. Clin. Med.* **116:**508–515.

21. **Laemmli, U. K.** 1970. Cleavage of structural proteins during the assembly of the head of bacteriophage T4. *Nature* **227:**680–685.

22. **Lowry, O. H., N. J. Rosebrough, A. L. Farr, and R. J. Randall.** 1951. Protein measurement with the Folin phenol reagent. *J. Biol. Chem.* **193:**265–275.

23. **Martinez, J. S., and P. F. Kohler.** 1971. Variant "Goodpasture's syndrome"? The need for immunologic criteria in rapidly progressive glomerulonephritis and hemorrhagic pneumonitis. *Ann. Intern. Med.* **75:**67–76.

24. **McCluskey, R., A. Collins, and J. Niles.** 1995. Kidney, p. 109. *In* R. Colvin, A. Bhan, and R. McCluskey (ed.), *Diagnostic Immunopathology,* 2nd ed. Raven Press, Ltd., New York, N.Y.

25. **McCoy, R. C., H. K. Johnson, W. J. Stone, and C. B. Wilson.** 1982. Absence of nephritogenic GBM antigen(s) in some patients with hereditary nephritis. *Kidney Int.* **21:**642–652.

26. **McPhaul, J. J., Jr., and F. J. Dixon.** 1969. The presence of anti-glomerular basement membrane antibodies in peripheral blood. *J. Immunol.* **103:**1168–1175.

27. **McPhaul, J. J., Jr., and J. D. Mullins.** 1976. Glomerulonephritis mediated by antibody to glomerular basement membrane. Immunological, clinical, and histopathological characteristics. *J. Clin. Investig.* **57:**351–361.

28. **Niles, J. L., E. P. Bottinger, G. R. Saurina, K. J. Kelly, G. Pan, A. B. Collins, and R. T. McCluskey.** 1996. The syndrome of lung hemorrhage and nephritis is usually an ANCA-associated condition. *Arch. Intern. Med.* **156:**440–445.

29. **Niles, J. L., G. L. Pan, A. B. Collins, T. Shannon, S. Skates, R. Fienberg, M. A. Arnaout, and R. T. McCluskey.** 1991. Antigen-specific radioimmunoassays for anti-neutrophil cytoplasmic antibodies in the diagnosis of rapidly progressive glomerulonephritis. *J. Am. Soc. Nephrol.* **2:**27–36.

30. **Olson, D. L., S. K. Anand, B. H. Landing, E. Heuser, C. M. Grushkin, and E. Lieberman.** 1980. Diagnosis of hereditary nephritis by failure of glomeruli to bind anti-glomerular basement membrane antibodies. *J. Pediatr.* **96:**697–699.

31. **Pusey, C. D., A. Dash, M. J. Kershaw, A. Morgan, A. Reilly, A. J. Rees, and C. M. Lockwood.** 1987. A single autoantigen in Goodpasture's syndrome identified by a monoclonal antibody to human glomerular basement membrane. *Lab. Investig.* **56:**23–31.

32. **Saxena, R., P. Bygren, R. Butkowski, and J. Wieslander.** 1989. Specificity of kidney-bound antibodies in Goodpasture's syndrome. *Clin. Exp. Immunol.* **78:**31–36.

33. **Segelmark, M., R. Butkowski, and J. Wieslander.** 1990. Antigen restriction and IgG subclasses among anti-GBM autoantibodies. *Nephrol. Dial. Transplant.* **5:**991–996.

34. **Timpl, R.** 1989. Structure and biological activity of basement membrane proteins. *Eur. J. Biochem.* **180:**487–502.

35. **Wieslander, J., J. F. Barr, R. J. Butkowski, S. J. Edwards, P. Bygren, D. Heinegard, and B. G. Hudson.** 1984. Goodpasture antigen of the glomerular basement membrane: localization to noncollagenous regions of type IV collagen. *Proc. Natl. Acad. Sci. USA* **81:**3838–3842.

36. **Wieslander, J., P. Bygren, and D. Heinegard.** 1984. Isolation of the specific glomerular basement membrane antigen involved in Goodpasture syndrome. *Proc. Natl. Acad. Sci. USA* **81:**1544–1548.

36a.**Wiik, A.** 2002. Antineutrophil cytoplasmic antibodies (ANCAs) and ANCA testing, p. 981–986. *In* N. R. Rose, R. G. Hamilton, and B. Detrick (ed.), *Manual of Clinical Laboratory Immunology,* 6th ed. ASM Press, Washington, D.C.

37. **Wilson, C.** 1980. Radioimmunoassay for anti-glomerular basement membrane antibodies, p. 376–380. *In* N. Rose

and H. Friedman (ed.), *Manual of Clinical Immunology*, 2nd ed. American Society for Microbiology, Washington, D.C.

38. **Wilson, C. B., and F. J. Dixon.** 1973. Anti-glomerular basement membrane antibody-induced glomerulonephritis. *Kidney Int.* **3:**74–89.

39. **Zhou, J., D. F. Barker, S. L. Hostikka, M. C. Gregory, C. L. Atkin, and K. Tryggvason.** 1991. Single base mutation in alpha 5(IV) collagen chain gene converting a conserved cysteine to serine in Alport syndrome. *Genomics* **9:**10–18.

40. **Zhou, J., S. L. Hostikka, L. T. Chow, and K. Tryggvason.** 1991. Characterization of the 3′ half of the human type IV collagen alpha 5 gene that is affected in the Alport syndrome. *Genomics* **9:**1–9.

41. **Zhou, J., T. Mochizuki, H. Smeets, C. Antignac, P. Laurila, A. de Paepe, K. Tryggvason, and S. T. Reeders.** 1993. Deletion of the paired alpha 5(IV) and alpha 6(IV) collagen genes in inherited smooth muscle tumors. *Science* **261:**1167–1169.

Autoimmunity of Testis, Ovary, and Spermatozoa

RICHARD A. BRONSON, JULIA LUBORSKY, AND KENNETH S. K. TUNG

126

Experimental studies indicate that infertility may have an immune basis, resulting from spontaneous or induced autoimmune disease that targets the testis, the ovary, or the spermatozoa (51). In humans, these diseases are represented by granulomatous orchitis, premature ovarian failure (POF), and sperm antibody-associated infertility in male and female subjects (50). Two immunologic mechanisms may be operative. Sperm antibodies can impair spermatozoal motility or viability by complement-dependent cytotoxicity, interfere with spermatozoal transport in the female genital tract, or block the cellular interaction in the fertilization process. Alternatively, antibody- and T-cell-mediated inflammation may result in atrophy of the gonads, associated with loss of germ cells.

In this chapter, we describe spermatozoal antibody-mediated infertility, with emphasis on the methods of sperm antibody detection with respect to the laboratory procedure, clinical indications, and interpretation of results. We describe an emerging assay for detection of antibodies to ovarian antigens. We then briefly discuss the human testicular and ovarian autoimmune diseases and the diagnostic dilemma they present.

SPERM-ASSOCIATED ANTIBODY AS MECHANISM OF MALE AND FEMALE INFERTILITY

When endocrinologic problems or sequelae of genital infection have been excluded, there remain a substantial number of patients with idiopathic infertility. In this subset of patients, spermatozoal antibodies may have an important causal role. Antisperm antibodies also develop in men following vasectomy, and they may account for infertility in some men following vasovasostomy for restoration of fertility (41, 49). Autoantibodies to sperm may also occur in patients with cystic fibrosis and congenital absence of the vas deferens (6, 12, 21).

Normally, spermatozoal antigens do not elicit immune responses in normal males and females. This is because systemic tolerance mechanisms are operative, and seminal plasma contains immunosuppressive molecules that may normally control immunity to spermatozoa. Autoimmunity ensues following stimulation by foreign microbial antigen that mimics gonadal antigen (19), when antigen is presented to T cells in the context of a vasectomy-induced granuloma, or

invoked by endogenous antigen when an immunoregulatory mechanism, such as regulatory T cells, is defective (49, 54).

Most clinical evidence for spermatozoal antibodies in infertility has come from correlative studies. These studies do not define the causal nature of the antibodies in the infertile state. More direct evidence has come from clinical studies in in vitro fertilization (IVF) and embryo transfer programs. In the presence of spermatozoal head-directed antibodies, when nearly all spermatozoa are coated with immunoglobulin (Ig), the fertilization rate has been significantly reduced, according to reports from several IVF programs (8, 9, 28, 39, 44). When serum from women with antisperm antibodies was used in IVF medium, fertilization rates were decreased. Sixty percent of women with unsuccessful pregnancy had sperm head-directed serum antibodies, compared with 6% of women with successful pregnancy (39, 52).

Spermatozoal Antibody Detection Methods

Spermatozoal antibodies may be detected in serum, or they are bound to the ejaculated spermatozoa. Studies comparing methods of sperm antibody detection indicated that antibodies to surface antigens of viable spermatozoa correlate best with infertility, whereas antibodies to internal spermatozoal antigens do not. Tests based on sperm agglutination were quite reproducible but lacked sensitivity (40). In contrast, the immunobead test, the mixed-antiglobin reaction (MAR) test, and the complement sperm immobilization tests are most sensitive. These tests are used most frequently by clinical laboratories and are described below in detail (see also references 3 and 40).

Direct Immunobead Assay

In the direct immunobead method, which detects Ig (presumed antibody) bound to spermatozoa in vivo, ejaculated spermatozoa are reacted with polyacrylamide beads coated with antibody to human Ig (immunobeads) (3, 5, 8). Immunobeads coated with rabbit anti-human IgA, IgG, or IgM (Irving Scientific, Santa Ana, Calif.) in phosphate-buffered saline (PBS) are dispensed in concentrations that optimize spermatozoal contact. This concentration is usually 6 to 7 mg/ml, although the exact concentration should be determined for each lot of immunobeads. Sodium azide is removed from the immunobeads by centrifugation in 4 ml of PBS at $800 \times g$ for 10 min. Immunobeads are then suspended in PBS containing 10 mg of bovine serum albumin fraction V (BSA;

ICN Immunobiologicals) per ml that has been presterilized by passage through a 0.22-μm-pore-size filter unit (Millipore). To avoid bead aggregation, each class of beads is sonicated before initial use for approximately 20 s at continuous pulse and at medium setting. Thereafter, beads can be vortexed to remain in suspension if they are allowed to stand for more than 2 h. Beads should be stored at 4°C. Lyophilized beads appear to be stable for at least a year, while beads reconstituted in buffer have a shelf life of at least 4 to 6 weeks if not contaminated. A convenient approach is to weigh out a small aliquot of dry immunobeads and suspend them in sterile PBS every 2 weeks. Immunobeads contaminated by bacteria or human serum will not bind to spermatozoa coated with antibodies.

To prepare sperm suspension, fresh semen samples (10 to 50 μl), liquefied at room temperature for 45 min postcollection, are added to glass test tubes (12 by 75 mm) and mixed with 4 ml of PBS containing 5 mg of BSA per ml (PBS–0.5% BSA). For samples with low spermatozoal count and those with poor motility and progression, a larger amount of semen is required. After centrifugation at $300 \times g$ for 8 min, the cell pellet is suspended in 500 μl of PBS–0.5% BSA. The spermatozoal suspension is transferred to a 0.5-ml Microfuge tube and centrifuged for 8 s on a Beckman Microfuge E. After the Microfuge procedure has been repeated twice, the spermatozoal pellet is suspended in 80 μl of PBS–0.5% BSA. When necessary, to promote motility in samples with weak spermatozoal motility, 10 to 20 μl of horse serum (Flow Laboratories) is added. Horse serum is prepared by heating the sample at 80°C for 10 min and discarding the coagulum by dislodging it with a Pasteur pipette and centrifuging the sample. Small aliquots of heat-inactived horse serum are kept at −20°C.

To evaluate the reaction between immunobeads and spermatozoa, a 10- to 15-μl volume of the spermatozoal suspension is added to 50 μl of immunobeads in a glass tube (12 by 75 mm). The contents are mixed by gentle pipetting with a mechanical pipetter (Eppendorf); then a drop of the suspension is placed on a glass slide and covered with a coverslip (22 by 22 mm). Slide preparations are examined serially under phase-contrast optics, at ×200 magnification, over a 10- to 15-min interval. At a final cell concentration of 10^6/ml, the spermatozoal suspension yields approximately 10 cells per microscopic field. Results obtained include (i) percent motile spermatozoa with bound immunobeads, (ii) approximate number of immunobeads per cell, and (iii) location of bound immunobeads on the spermatozoa. Immunobeads on the slides are kept in suspension by tapping the coverslip occasionally, and observation should be completed within 10 to 15 min. Observation is made in areas with high concentrations of immunobeads, and replicates of 100 motile spermatozoa are examined. If the duplicates differ by more than 10%, an additional 200 spermatozoa are recorded.

As controls, known positive and negative sera are studied simultaneously based on the indirect immunobead test (see below). Also, the specificity of a positive reaction may be verified by the addition of normal human serum (10 μl) to the reaction mixture. Serum Igs block anti-Ig on the immunobeads and prevent binding of anti-Ig to spermatozoa.

Indirect Immunobead Test

In the indirect immunobead method, antisperm antibodies are first reacted with the biological fluids; the antibodies captured on the spermatozoa are in turn detected by reaction with immunobeads (3, 5, 10).

1. Spermatozoa, preferably from the husband or from a fertile donor known to be free of antisperm antibodies, are obtained by the swim-up method. This is accomplished by overlaying 0.5 ml of PBS–0.5% BSA in a test tube (12 by 75 mm). After incubation at 37°C for 60 min, the spermatozoa in the top 0.4 ml of the pooled PBS–5% BSA layers are carefully collected and counted.

2. Spermatozoa are added to serum samples from the patient and to known positive and negative control sera that have been heated (56°C, 30 min) and diluted appropriately in PBS. The final serum dilutions are 1:10 and 1:100.

3. The sperm-serum mixture is incubated in a water bath at 37°C for 60 min. Following centrifugation at $300 \times g$ for 8 min, the cell pellet is suspended in 400 μl of PBS–5% BSA and transferred to the 500-μl Microfuge tubes.

4. The spermatozoa are washed four times by centrifugation for 8 s in a Beckman Microfuge E. Care must be taken to remove all supernatant from the cell pellets during the washing steps, as residual serum Ig can interfere with the immunobead assay by blocking the anti-Ig sites on the beads.

5. The washed spermatozoa are suspended to an appropriate concentration, mixed with immunobeads, and examined as described for the direct immunobead test.

Comment: The currently available immunobeads are not specifically manufactured for use in clinical laboratories. Although the lot-to-lot variability in sensitivity appears to be low, it is important to compare the results between assays. It should be stressed that serum and microbial contamination of immunobeads will interfere with the sensitivity of the immunobead test.

MAR Test

The MAR test (26), popular in Europe, detects IgG and IgA antisperm antibodies bound in vivo to the plasma membrane of motile spermatozoa. Whereas immunobeads coupled with anti-Ig are able to bind directly to the sperm-bound Ig, in the MAR antiserum, anti-IgG or anti-IgA is added to agglutinate the spermatozoa with Ig-coated, glutaraldehyde-fixed sheep erythrocytes.

1. Prepare Ig-bound sheep erythrocytes as follows. Sheep erythrocytes in Alsever's solution are washed four times by centrifugation at $2,000 \times g$ for 5 min in a total of 20 volumes of phosphate-buffered glucose (PBG; 76 ml of 0.15 M disodium phosphate, 24 ml of 0.15 M monopotassium phosphate, and 100 ml of 5.4% glucose in distilled water, pH 7.2) and after centrifugation are resuspended in PBG as a 20% solution. The erythrocytes are fixed by addition of an equal volume of 0.2% glutaraldehyde dissolved in PBG and incubation with the erythrocyte mixture in a 37°C water bath for 15 min. The erythrocytes, washed five times with 0.85% sodium chloride and resuspended as a 10% solution in 0.85% sodium chloride containing 0.1% sodium azide, are stored at 4°C. The shelf life of fixed cells exceeds 4 years.

To coat erythrocytes with Ig, fixed erythrocytes (5 ml) are washed twice with PBG (pH 7.2) and suspended in 2 ml of PBS. Then 1 ml of purified human IgG or colostral IgA (LN antisera; Behringwerke AG, Marburg, Germany) at 1 mg/ml is added together with 0.5 ml of 1% sodium azide. After thorough mixing, the cells are incubated at 37°C for 16 h on a rotating platform. The cells are washed three times in PBS, resuspended as a 20% solution in 2 ml of 50% glycerol in PBS, and stored at 4°C. The shelf life exceeds 2 years.

2. For the MAR test, the Ig-coated cells are washed three times and resuspended in PBS as a 2% solution. On a slide, 10 μl of the erythrocytes is added to 10 μl of fresh, liquefied semen from the patient or from antibody-negative and antibody-positive individuals. To this mixture is added 10 μl

of undiluted rabbit antiserum IgG to human IgG or IgA. The rabbit antisera are first dialyzed against PBS to remove the preservatives and are kept at −70°C. The cell-antibody mixture is covered with a coverslip and incubated in a moist chamber at 37°C for 15 min for IgG-specific MAR. The cell reaction is examined by phase-contrast microscopy at ×400 magnification. The percentage of motile spermatozoa involved in mixed agglutination with one or more erythrocytes is determined; a result of 10% or greater is considered positive.

Comment: The MAR test detects IgG class antisperm antibody with sensitivity comparable to that of the immunobead assay. In contrast, the MAR test detects IgA class antibody with a sensitivity lower than that of the immunobead test (40). Ig-bound erythrocytes are also not commercially available.

Complement-Dependent Spermatozoal Immobilization Test (25)

1. Test sera and positive and negative control sera are heated at 56°C for 30 min and centrifuged at $1,350 \times g$ for 10 min.
2. Guinea pig sera nontoxic to human spermatozoa with complement activity exceeding 200 50% hemolytic complement units are stored at −80°C until used. An active but nontoxic guinea pig complement source is critical for a successful assay.
3. A fresh sample of ejaculated human semen is liquefied for 20 min at room temperature, counted, and centrifuged at $1,350 \times g$ for 5 min. After being washed once with 10% negative control human serum in normal saline, actively motile spermatozoa are collected by the swim-up method as described earlier. The spermatozoal number is adjusted to 40×10^6/ml.
4. Next, 0.25 ml of test or control serum, 0.025 ml of human spermatozoal suspension, and 0.05 ml of guinea pig serum (containing approximately 10 50% hemolytic complement units) are mixed in a small test tube and incubated in a gently shaking water bath at 32°C for 60 min.
5. To ensure that the guinea pig serum is not toxic to the spermatozoa, an important control is to add guinea pig serum to spermatozoa without test serum. The test is not valid when guinea pig serum is toxic.
6. A drop of spermatozoal mixture is transferred by Pasteur pipette to a clean glass slide and examined immediately, without a coverslip, at ×200 magnification. The percentage of motile spermatozoa among 200 spermatozoa is recorded in triplicate samples. The percentages of motile spermatozoa in the negative control (%C) and test (%T) samples are obtained. The ratio of these percentages is designated the spermatozoal immobilization value. A value of 2 or higher is determined to be positive for antisperm antibodies.

Comment: Complement-dependent immobilization, popular in Japan, is highly specific, with minimal false-positive reactions. However, the test does not detect non-complement-fixing antibodies. The concentration of antibody on the sperm surface also dictates the extent of complement-mediated immobilization (5).

PCT To Assess Function of Antibody-Bound Spermatozoa

Antibodies may interfere with penetration of cervical mucus by spermatozoa and impede the transport of spermatozoa to the ovulated oocyte. Since the postcoital test (PCT) directly examines the interaction between spermatozoa and cervical mucus, it provides a functional assessment of spermatozoal antibodies (4).

Cervical mucus of good quality is best inspected by phase-contrast microscopy for the presence of motile spermatozoa. It should be collected from the endocervical canal, after cleaning the cervix with a dry cotton swab. Its volume should be noted, as well as its clarity and stretchiness (spinnbarkeit) and pH. A low pH (<7) suggests contamination of the specimen with vaginal secretions during its collection. At low magnification, the mucus is surveyed microscopically for distribution of spermatozoa and heterogeneity of spermatozoal density. At high (×400) magnification, the number of viable spermatozoa per high-power field in selected areas is determined. The presence of white blood cells is noted, as this suggests the possibility of local infection and the need to screen for sexually transmitted diseases.

Since the quality of cervical mucus is hostile to spermatozoa during most of the menstrual cycle, the timing of PCT is critical. Cervical mucus obtained within a short time before ovulation is optimal for spermatozoal penetration, and this is the optimum time for PCT. In the past, accurate timing was possible only retrospectively by noting a rise of basal body temperature 1 to 2 days following PCT. Currently, monitoring of urinary luteinizing hormone is used to determine the best time for PCT. Daily monitoring should begin 3 to 4 days before the anticipated ovulation. It should be noted that the sensitivity of commercially available kits to detect luteinizing hormone within urine varies widely. The preovulatory gonadotropin surge may be initiated in approximately two-thirds of women in the morning and one-third in the afternoon. The couple should be advised to have sexual relations on the evening of the day the ovulation predictor test turns positive, and cervical mucus should be assessed the next morning, within 12 h of coitus. There is controversy about what constitutes a normal test (4). The presence of fewer than five motile sperm per high-power field, or restricted motion of sperm within preovulatory cervical mucus of good quality (immobilization or shaking motions), requires further evaluation, including semen analysis and tests for antisperm antibodies. Poor mucus may result from cervicitis, prior in utero exposure to diethylstilbestrol, or cervical cauterization.

Clinical Indications of Antisperm Antibody Tests

Spontaneous Agglutinated Ejaculated Spermatozoa
For the rare patient, the finding of agglutinated spermatozoa in the semen specimens should alert one to the possibility of autoimmunity to spermatozoa.

Abnormal PCT
An important indication of the presence of antisperm antibody is an abnormal PCT, particularly when the semen quality is normal and the cervical mucus, obtained at late follicular phase, is well hydrated and acellular. In this setting, if the number of spermatozoa in the cervical mucus is unexpectedly low or spermatozoa are absent, it is important to rule out the presence of antisperm antibodies.

If the antibodies are bound to the principal piece of spermatozoal tail or to the spermatozoal head, the spermatozoa may exhibit a shaking or "cogwheel" motion, with little forward progression, or they may be completely immobilized after a period of 5 to 6 h following entry into the mucus after coitus. Antibodies confined to the end piece of the spermatozoal tail are not associated with a reduced fertility rate.

Patients with Idiopathic Infertility

While an abnormal PCT is suggestive of the presence of antibodies, a negative result does not preclude antibody testing. Patients with infertility for which there is not an apparent cause, despite rigorous clinical evaluation, are also candidates for antisperm antibody testing.

Prospective Vasovasostomy Patients

Men who have had vasectomy and subsequent sterilization reversal should also be screened for spermatozoal antibodies. However, while the majority of these men have serum antisperm antibodies, only a minority of them have antibody-coated sperm in their ejaculates. In the latter group, impaired fertility has been found. It should be noted that infertility in these patients is not always immune mediated.

Correlation between Antisperm Antibodies Detected by the Immunobead Test and Clinical Status

One in 150 healthy young men screened for antisperm antibodies in a semen donor recruitment program was found to have Ig on more than 20% of the spermatozoa, whereas 7% of men among unselected infertile couples have similar antibodies (4).

A general correlation has been found between the proportion of spermatozoa with bound immunobeads and reduction of motile spermatozoa within postcoital cervical mucus. When 100% of the spermatozoa were coated with antibodies, zero to five spermatozoa were found per high-power field in a well-timed PCT. When less than 50% of spermatozoa were coated with Ig, the number of spermatozoa within cervical mucus was within the normal range.

The presence of spermatozoal antibodies also parallels in a general way the reduction in pregnancy rate. Among 108 infertile couples wherein more than 50% of the husbands' spermatozoa were coated with antibodies, the pregnancy rate was 22%. In contrast, among couples in whom less than 50% of the spermatozoa were coated with antibodies, 44% became pregnant. In a subset of infertile patients in whom the dominant or sole factor leading to infertility was identified as autoimmunity to spermatozoa, the conception rate in couples in whom more than 50% of the spermatozoa were Ig bound was 15%, whereas for the couples in whom less than 50% of the spermatozoa had bound Ig, the conception rate was 60%.

The antigenic locations also have clinical significance. Head-directed antibodies significantly reduced the fertility rate, antibodies to the spermatozoal tail (main piece) had variable effects on fertility, and antibodies to the tip of the spermatozoal tail had no effect (39). Antibodies of the IgG and IgA classes are more predictive of fertility reduction, whereas IgM antibodies are not predictive of infertility. IgM antibodies may be detected within serum but only rarely are detected in the ejaculate, on spermatozoa.

In some infertile patients, antibodies to spermatozoa are detected only in the seminal plasma (23). Since antibodies are not detected in the sera of these patients, the antibodies are likely produced locally. In a group of men suspected of autoimmunity to spermatozoa, for whom matched serum samples and serum samples from women were directly compared, antibodies were found solely in the ejaculate in 15% of the patients, and they were mainly of the IgA class.

At this stage of development, without the benefit of quantitative assay and a "gold standard," the clinical interpretation of antisperm antibody is in part an art. Care must be exercised in distinguishing between a positive result and a clinically significant result based on the immunobead or any antisperm antibody assay. If most spermatozoa are not present within cervical mucus and the majority of the spermatozoa have detectable Ig on their surface, the result of immunobead binding is considered clinically significant. However, apart from the unequivocal cases, direct immunobead binding results should not be interpreted in the absence of clinical correlates. Similarly, serological tests for antisperm antibodies in men, including indirect immunobead binding, are not sufficient by themselves to document the presence of clinically significant autoimmunity to spermatozoa. Finally, a decision on therapy should not be implemented solely on the basis of a serological test, whatever the detection method.

Future Prospects

A useful diagnostic autoantibody assay would be one that recognizes antigens that are responsible for the pathogenesis of the autoimmune process. An important approach in sperm and oocyte antigen identification has benefited from recent contraceptive vaccine research (reviewed in reference 18). Antibodies from infertile couples have been used to identify sperm-specific molecules as potential contraceptive vaccine immunogens. In addition, monoclonal antibodies to sperm and oocytes that inhibit fertility or fertilization in vitro have been generated. These antibodies have identified antigens that are available as recombinant proteins or as peptides representing defined native B-cell epitopes. The antigen function has been verified in some cases by antibody interference during IVF assays, and in others in rodent and primate fertility trials following active immunization. This systematic approach has identified sperm and oocyte antigens that may serve as target antigens in future serological tests.

OVARY-ASSOCIATED ANTIBODY IN DIAGNOSIS OF OVARIAN AUTOIMMUNE DISEASE, POF, AND FEMALE INFERTILITY

The evidence for an autoimmune disease of the ovary includes (i) frequent association with other autoimmune diseases, (ii) lymphocytic infiltration of the ovary, and (iii) association with serum ovarian antibodies (36). Approximately 70% of patients with POF and 70% of women with unexplained infertility had serum antibody to ovarian and/or oocyte antigens. The predictive value of a poor pregnancy outcome after IVF in individuals with autoantibodies was 82% (33).

Ovarian dysfunction is determined by abnormalities in menstrual cycle patterns and measurement of early follicular-phase follicle-stimulating hormone and estradiol. However, endocrine tests do not differentiate between endocrine and autoimmune etiologies for ovarian dysfunction (32, 36). Detection of ovarian autoantibodies supports the diagnosis of ovarian autoimmunity. Autoantibodies are associated with POF and unexplained infertility and are rarely detected in sera of women from a blood bank or other infertility clinics (31). About 1% of women in the United States have POF (35), and 60 to 70% of these may be due to an etiology of ovary autoimmunity (15, 29). From clinical studies, 20% of women with infertility have an unexplained cause, and of the women with unexplained infertility, 50 to 70% have ovarian and/or oocyte antibodies.

In addition, during ovarian hyperstimulation for IVF, about 20% of women do not respond with adequate estradiol production in response to follicle-stimulating hormone stimulation. When this occurs in younger women with ovarian or oocyte antibody, an autoimmune basis is considered (36, 42). In general, women with ovarian autoimmunity have lower success rates during infertility treatment (20, 24, 33). The ovarian antibody test is useful in (i) confirming a diagnosis of autoimmune premature menopause, (ii) potentially predicting the risk for premature menopause, (iii) diagnosing and differentiating an autoimmune etiology from an endocrine etiology in female infertility, and (iv) predicting poor responses to estrogen-induced ovulation and reduced probability of pregnancy following IVF.

Antiovarian and Antioocyte Antibody Immunoassays

Serum antibody of some patients with autoimmune ovarian disease reacts with either oocyte extracts, ovarian extracts, or both. Therefore, independent immunoassays for ovarian antibodies and oocyte antibodies (37) have been developed for clinical diagnosis. The nature of the target oocyte or ovarian antigen has not been determined. For antiovarian antibody, an 85% concordance was noted between results based on human versus rat ovarian antigens, so rat ovarian extract is used in the assay. Human oocytes are obtained as a by-product of IVF treatment for infertility. Positive values are determined by comparison to values for control sera from women of similar age with normal menstrual cycles without clinical evidence of autoimmune disease.

Reagents

Enzyme-linked immunosorbent assay (ELISA) buffer: 10 mM phosphate buffer, 30 mM NaCl, and 1 mM MgCl$_2$, pH 7.4

Wash buffer: 0.05% Triton X-100 in ELISA buffer

Dilution buffer for serum and antibody: Wash buffer plus 1% BSA (A7050; Sigma)

Blocking solution: Wash buffer plus 5% BSA

Alkaline phosphatase (AP) substrate buffer: 24 mM MgCl$_2$, 1 M diethanolamine (pH 9.8) (D8885; Sigma), and AP reagent (1 mg of p-nitrophenylphosphate/ml of AP buffer). AP reagent is not stable and should be prepared immediately before use.

Homogenization buffer: 40 mM Tris-HCl, 5 mM MgSO$_4$, and 0.25 M sucrose, pH 7.4

Comments: For blocking nonspecific reaction, we use BSA preselected for maximum antibody binding but minimal nonspecific binding. The BSA preparations obtained from the manufacturer change over time, and each new batch should be monitored. Quality control water is purchased from Baxter (no. 2F7115) and is used in all buffer preparations and cell washes.

Ovarian Extract Preparation

Rat ovaries are removed from 3-week-old rats 36 to 48 h after they have been stimulated by serum from a pregnant mare and human chorionic gonadotropin (34).

1. Add chilled homogenization buffer, at 1 ml per 80 to 100 mg (wet weight) of tissue (or ~1 rat ovary), to a Dounce homogenizer.
2. Homogenize by hand with 10 to 20 strokes on ice.
3. Centrifugation

    a. Transfer homogenate to a cold 15-ml conical centrifuge tube, bring final volume to 10 ml with homogenization buffer, and centrifuge at 1,000 × g, and 4°C for 10 min.

    b. Transfer supernatant to a 15-ml centrifuge tube and centrifuge at 10,000 × g, 4°C for 30 min.

    c. Discard supernatant and suspend the pellet in homogenization buffer at 1 ml per 100 mg (wet weight) of tissue.

    d. Freeze aliquots on dry ice and store at −70°C.

Oocyte Extract Preparation

The antioocyte assay uses oocytes that failed to fertilize during IVF procedures (37). The oocytes should be intact, and adherent granulosa cells should have been removed. However, it is critical to freeze and store oocytes in the homogenization buffer and to inactivate any enzymes that were used for isolation (14).

1. Collect human oocytes into homogenization buffer and rinse once by centrifugation in a 1.5-ml Microfuge tube in a Microfuge system at 1,000 × g for 0.5 min.
2. Freeze the final pellet, devoid of buffer, in aliquots on dry ice and store at −70°C.
3. Disrupt oocytes by freezing, homogenization, and vigorous mixing.
4. Thaw frozen oocytes (~15 min), and rinse ~100 oocytes by centrifugation in a Microfuge system (~1,000 rpm) for 0.5 min, remove supernatant, and repeat rinse twice in homogenization buffer.
5. Add 0.1 ml of cold Tris buffer (no sucrose) per 20 oocytes and vortex at high speed for 15 to 30 s.
6. Homogenize in a Microfuge tube with a micropestle by hand with 10 to 20 strokes and vortex; repeat until solution appears uniform (repeating three or four times), and use immediately.

Preparation of Antigen-Coated Immunoassay Plates

1. Use high-protein-binding plate (for example, Nunc Maxisorb).
2. Thaw tissue extract just before use and vortex well. Dilute the tissue in ELISA buffer to 2 μg of protein per ml (human) or 1 μg of protein per ml (rat). Vortex well and use immediately. For oocytes, dilute the homogenate with ELISA buffer to ~0.1 ml per oocyte (i.e., 10 oocytes/1 ml).
3. With a multichannel pipette, add 100 /μl of extract to each well; place in a moisture box.
4. Wrap plates individually in Saran Wrap and incubate for 1 h at room temperature.
5. Store in a −70°C freezer for up to 6 months.

ELISA

Day 1

1. Thaw plates in a moisture box for 1 h at room temperature.
2. Discard excess fluid in wells by "flicking" the plate; blot quickly on fresh paper towels.
3. Add 200 μl of blocking buffer to all wells with a multipipette; cover plates and incubate in a moisture box at room temperature for about 1 h and then overnight in a refrigerator.

Day 2

1. Bring plates to room temperature and thaw stored serum.
2. Dilute each serum sample to 1:100 in dilution buffer.
3. Flick excess fluid from plates and wash wells three times with 200 μl of wash buffer.

4. Add test or control sera (100 µl at 1:100) in duplicate.

5. Incubate for 1.5 h at room temperature and then wash three times with wash buffer.

6. During incubation, dilute conjugated second antibody [Sigma; goat anti-human F(ab')$_2$-specific IgG conjugated to AP] in dilution buffer, at an appropriate dilution determined previously (about 1:10,000).

7. Add 100 µl of conjugated second antibody to the wells and incubate at room temperature for 1 h.

8. Wash twice with 200 µl of ELISA buffer (no Triton X-100) and then four times with 200 µl of distilled quality control water.

9. *Immediately* before use add AP reagent to AP substrate buffer at 1 mg/ml. Plates can be "held" in ELISA buffer (no Triton X-100) from step 8, after removal of second antibody, while substrate is being prepared.

10. Develop color reaction by adding 100 µl of AP substrate reagent to each well.

11. Determine absorbance at 405 nm (optical density [OD]) in an ELISA reader. Endpoint readings should be taken at 15, 30, 45, and 60 min (Fig. 1). Data should be determined at the linear portion of the enzyme reaction curve just below the plateau (usually within 30 to 60 min). Alternatively, add appropriate stop solution at 45 to 60 min and determine absorbance.

Comments: A small amount (10 µl each) of second antibody solution and AP substrate should be mixed in a test tube to test for a yellow color reaction prior to the addition of the substrate to the plate. If no color reaction occurs, prepare fresh substrate buffer (check pH) and test again. If a color reaction still fails to occur, test a new antibody-AP conjugate.

Control Sera Included in Each ELISA

Second antibody control: for each plate two wells contain antigen, conjugated second antibody, and reagent only (omit primary serum), to assess nonspecific background, which should be less than 0.10.

Negative controls: Serum from normally cycling women without diagnosed autoimmune disease. Use at least 6 to 8 controls.

Positive control: Serum previously identified to be positive for ovarian or oocyte antibody

Buffer control (optional): for each plate two wells contain antigen, blocking solution, and substrate solution only (no antibodies), to monitor any substrate reaction with tissue enzyme; their absorbance should be <0.1.

Data Analysis

1. Determine the cutoff value for positive results. Calculate (i) the average total OD of the controls and (ii) the standard deviation (SD) of average total OD for controls. The SD of the controls is usually <0.1 unless there is an outlier among the controls. The cutoff value for positive results is the control average plus 2 SDs (95% confidence level, or $P < 0.05$). The coefficient of variation for the assay should be less than 10%.

2. Evaluate assay performance. The second antibody control should be less than 0.1 OD unit below the control mean. If this control is similar to the values of test sera on the plate, then the block might have been omitted (or there is a problem with the BSA in the blocking buffer). In addition, the control mean should be 0.5 to 0.6 OD unit or less, with an SD of <0.1. If the SD for the control mean is large, check if

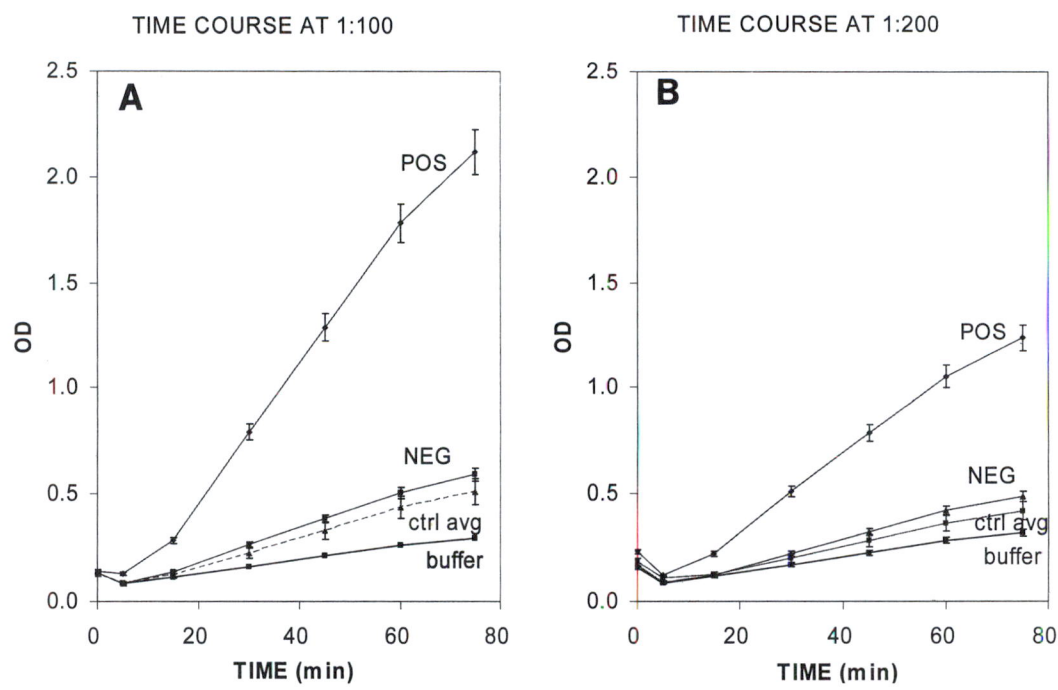

FIGURE 1 Kinetics of enzyme immunoassay reaction for ovarian antibody test. The graph compares the OD (at 405 nm) for the control average (ctrl avg) ($n = 5$) at each time point with the ODs of a positive control sample (POS), a negative sample (NEG), and the background (buffer) for serum dilutions of 1:100 (A) and 1:200 (B).

(i) there are outliers among the control values (with five or more controls, one outlier control can be omitted, as is routine in radioimmunoassay analysis) or (ii) the values of multiple replicates are too far apart (i.e., check individual SDs for replicates). This is usually an operator error, either in plate preparation or assay performance, and the assay will need to be repeated. Positive control values should be at least two times greater than the control mean (preferably three to four times at 1:100). The size of this difference is an indication of the "differentiation power" of the assay. If the positive control is less than 1.5 times over the assay control mean, the assay should be repeated. Consider inadequate antigen, too much antigen, or incorrect serum dilution as a potential source of error.

3. Result interpretation. Calculate the specific signal for all test samples by subtracting the cutoff value from the total average OD for each sample. The result is considered positive if the sample shows a definite signal above the cutoff value. It is considered negative when a specific signal is detected at or below the cutoff value. It is indeterminant when the sample, on repeated testings, yields variable results.

Human Autoimmune Ovarian Disease

Human autoimmune ovarian disease is associated with POF or unexplained infertility (17, 29). POF may occur as an isolated disease or as a component of the autoimmune polyglandular syndromes (APS) in association with adrenal or thyroid autoimmunity. About 20% of APS patients have been reported to have POF (53). The antigen in Addison's disease is CYP21, a member of the P450 steroidogenic enzyme family, and is found at a high rate in Addison's disease and APS associated with Addison's disease (38). Antibodies to P450 enzymes are found in POF associated with APS but rarely in isolated POF (2, 7, 11, 38, 46). Although it is hypothesized that the corresponding ovarian CYP17 homolog is a major antigen in POF, only 10 to 20% of sera from patients with isolated POF had detectable antibody to CYP17 (11, 30). It has been suggested that women with POF and anti-CYP17 or steroid cell autoantibodies are at risk for APS or Addison's disease and should be further evaluated.

Recent studies indicate that APS type 1 is associated with mutations of the autoimmune regulator gene (27, 47); however, an association with isolated POF has not been reported. Several antigens have been suggested as targets of ovarian autoantibodies (1, 16, 17, 22, 29), but information on a major antigen still is needed.

Diagnosis of ovarian autoimmunity depends on the detection of serum autoantibodies to crude preparations of ovarian antigens or to oocyte antigens and the exclusion of an infectious cause for the ovarian inflammation (reviewed in reference 29).

HUMAN AUTOIMMUNE TESTICULAR DISEASE

Male infertility can result from autoimmune disease that affects the testis and its excurrent ducts. Some human testicular diseases have immunopathological features that resemble the testicular changes of autoimmune orchitis of the infertile mink (50). They include (i) granulomatous orchitis of noninfectious basis that presents as enlarged testis (a differential diagnosis of testicular tumor) (43), (ii) aspermatogenesis without orchitis in testis with local immune complexes, and (iii) epididymal granulomas of noninfectious origin (50). Nonspecific orchitis associated with viral infections, such as

mumps virus and human immunodeficiency virus, may also have an autoimmune basis (13).

EXPERIMENTAL AUTOIMMUNE DISEASE OF THE OVARY AND TESTIS

Spontaneous autoimmune orchitis and spontaneous infertility occur in mink, horses, dogs, and rats (51). In contrast, spontaneous autoimmune ovarian disease in experimental animals has not been reported. Experimentally, autoimmune orchitis and oophoritis are induced by immunization with testis and ovarian antigen in adjuvant. In addition, both diseases occur spontaneously in mice thymectomized on day 3 of life (45, 48). Orchitis is associated with T-cell and antibody responses to sperm antigens, whereas oophoritis is associated with responses to oocyte antigens (oocyte cytoplasmic antigens and the zona pellucida) and antigen of steroid-producing cells. In both diseases, antigen-specific $CD4^+$ T cells elicit inflammation of the gonads, and this is followed by atrophy, loss of the germ cells, and appearance of serum autoantibodies. Studies based on the thymectomy model indicate that occurrence of the autoimmune diseases is prevented by a population of regulatory T cells that express the CD25 (interleukin 2 receptor alpha chain) marker, present in normal adult humans or mice.

SUMMARY

Antibody to spermatozoa appears to be responsible for infertility in some men and women with unexplained infertility, particularly in the setting of an abnormal PCT. The popular sperm antibody assays include the immunobead, MAR, and sperm immobilization assays described in this chapter. Regardless of the assay, the result of the antibody test should be interpreted in the context of clinical findings. It is likely that the current efforts to discover sperm antigens relevant to the fertilization process will advance sperm antibody detection assays in the future. Autoimmune testicular disease results in infertility of animals, but its human counterpart has not been unequivocally documented. Human autoimmune ovarian disease is better defined; however, the diagnosis is difficult, further refinement of diagnostic assay is required, and the prevalence of disease remains speculative.

REFERENCES

1. **Arif, S., R. Varela-Calvino, G. S. Conway, and M. Peakman.** 2001. 3 beta hydroxysteroid dehydrogenase autoantibodies in patients with idiopathic premature ovarian failure target N- and C-terminal epitopes. *J. Clin. Endocrinol. Metab.* **86:**5892–5897.
2. **Betterle, C., C. Dalpra, N. Greggio, M. Volpato, and R. Zanchetta.** 2001. Autoimmunity in isolated Addison's disease and in polyglandular autoimmune diseases type 1, 2 and 4. *Ann. Endocrinol.* (Paris) **62:**193–201.
3. **Bronson, R., G. Cooper, T. Hjort, R. Ing, W. R. Jones, S. X. Wang, S. Mathur, H. O. Williamson, P. F. Rust, and H. H. Fudenberg.** 1985. Anti-sperm antibodies, detected by agglutination, immobilization, microcytotoxicity and immunobead-binding assays. *J. Reprod. Immunol.* **8:**279–299.
4. **Bronson, R. A.** 1999. Antisperm antibodies: a critical evaluation and clinical guidelines. *J. Reprod. Immunol.***45:**159–183.
5. **Bronson, R. A., G. W. Cooper, and D. L. Rosenfeld.** 1982. Correlation between regional specificity of antisperm antibodies to the spermatozoan surface and complement-mediated sperm immobilization. *Am. J. Reprod. Immunol.* **2:**222–224.

6. Bronson, R. A., W. J. O'Connor, T. A. Wilson, S. K. Bronson, F. I. Chasalow, and K. Droesch. 1992. Correlation between puberty and the development of autoimmunity to spermatozoa in men with cystic fibrosis. *Fertil. Steril.* **58**:1199–1204.

7. Chen, S., J. Sawicka, C. Betterle, M. Powell, L. Prentice, M. Volpato, S. B. Rees, and J. Furmaniak. 1996. Autoantibodies to steroidogenic enzymes in autoimmune polyglandular syndrome, Addison's disease, and premature ovarian failure. *J. Clin. Endocrinol. Metab.* **81**:1871–1876.

8. Clarke, G. N. 1988. Sperm antibodies and human fertilization. *Am. J. Reprod. Immunol. Microbiol.* **17**:65–71.

9. Clarke, G. N., H. Bourne, and H. W. Baker. 1997. Intracytoplasmic sperm injection for treating infertility associated with sperm autoimmunity. *Fertil. Steril.* **68**:112–117.

10. Clarke, G. N., P. J. Elliott, and C. Smaila. 1985. Detection of sperm antibodies in semen using the immunobead test: a survey of 813 consecutive patients. *Am. J. Reprod. Immunol.* **7**:118–123.

11. Dal Pra, C., S. Chen, J. Furmaniak, B. R. Smith, B. Pedini, A. Moscon, R. Zanchetta, and C. Betterle. 2003. Autoantibodies to steroidogenic enzymes in patients with premature ovarian failure with and without Addison's disease. *Eur. J. Endocrinol.* **148**:565–570.

12. D'Cruz, O. J., G. G. Haas, Jr., R. de La Rocha, and H. Lambert. 1991. Occurrence of serum antisperm antibodies in patients with cystic fibrosis. *Fertil. Steril.* **56**:519–527.

13. Dejucq, N., and B. Jegou. 2001. Viruses in the mammalian male genital tract and their effects on the reproductive system. *Microbiol. Mol. Biol. Rev.* **65**:208–231.

14. Eppig, J. J., and E. E. Telfer. 1993. Isolation and culture of oocytes. *Methods Enzymol.* **225**:77–84.

15. Fenichel, P., C. Sosset, P. Barbarino-Monnier, B. Gobert, S. Hieronimus, M. C. Bene, and M. Harter. 1997. Prevalence, specificity and significance of ovarian antibodies during spontaneous premature ovarian failure. *Hum. Reprod.* **12**:2623–2628.

16. Forges, T., P. Monnier-Barbarino, and G. Faure. 2003. What are the antigenic targets in the ovary? *Gynecol. Obstet. Fertil.* **31**:759–765. (In French.)

17. Forges, T., P. Monnier-Barbarino, G. C. Faure, and M. C. Bene. 2004. Autoimmunity and antigenic targets in ovarian pathology. *Hum. Reprod. Update* **10**:163–175.

18. Frayne, J., and L. Hall. 1999. The potential use of sperm antigens as targets for immunocontraception; past, present and future. *J. Reprod. Immunol.* **43**:1–33.

19. Garza, K. M., and K. S. Tung. 1995. Frequency of molecular mimicry among T cell peptides as the basis for autoimmune disease and autoantibody induction. *J. Immunol.* **155**:5444–5448.

20. Geva, E., G. Fait, L. Lerner-Geva, J. B. Lessing, T. Swartz, I. Wolman, Y. Daniel, and A. Amit. 1999. The possible role of antiovary antibodies in repeated in vitro fertilization failures. *Am. J. Reprod. Immunol.* **42**:292–296.

21. Girgis, S. M., E. M. Ekladious, R. Iskander, R. El Dakhly, and F. N. Girgis. 1982. Sperm antibodies in serum and semen in men with bilateral congenital absence of the vas deferens. *Arch. Androl.* **8**:301–305.

22. Gobert, B., C. Jolivet-Reynaud, P. Dalbon, P. Barbarino-Monnier, G. C. Faure, M. Jolivet, and M. C. Bene. 2001. An immunoreactive peptide of the FSH involved in autoimmune infertility. *Biochem. Biophys. Res. Commun.* **289**:819–824.

23. Hellstrom, W. J., J. W. Overstreet, S. J. Samuels, and E. L. Lewis. 1988. The relationship of circulating antisperm antibodies to sperm surface antibodies in infertile men. *J. Urol.* **140**:1039–1044.

24. Horejsi, J., J. Martinek, D. Novakova, J. Madar, and M. Brandejska. 2000. Autoimmune antiovarian antibodies and their impact on the success of an IVF/ET program. *Ann. N. Y. Acad. Sci.* **900**:351–356.

25. Isojima, S., and K. Koyama. 1989. Techniques for sperm immobilization test. *Arch. Androl.* **23**:185–199.

26. Jager, S., J. Kremer, and T. Slochteren-Draaisma. 1978. A simple method of screening for antisperm antibodies in the human male. Detection of spermatozoal surface IgG with the direct mixed antiglobulin reaction carried out on untreated fresh human semen. *Int. J. Fertil.* **23**:12–21.

27. Kumar, P. G., M. Laloraya, and J. X. She. 2002. Population genetics and functions of the autoimmune regulator (AIRE). *Endocrinol. Metab. Clin. N. Am.* **31**:321–338, vi.

28. Lahteenmaki, A., I. Reima, and O. Hovatta. 1995. Treatment of severe male immunological infertility by intracytoplasmic sperm injection. *Hum. Reprod.* **10**:2824–2828.

29. Luborsky, J. 2002. Ovarian autoimmune disease and ovarian autoantibodies. *J. Womens Health Gender-Based Med.* **11**:585–599.

30. Luborsky, J. 2002. Test for ovarian autoimmunity by detecting autoantibodies to CYP17. U.S. patent 6,458,550.

31. Luborsky, J., B. Llanes, S. Davies, Z. Binor, E. Radwanska, and R. Pong. 1999. Ovarian autoimmunity: greater frequency of autoantibodies in premature menopause and unexplained infertility than in the general population. *Clin. Immunol.* **90**:368–374.

32. Luborsky, J., B. Llanes, R. Roussev, and C. Coulam. 2000. Ovarian antibodies, FSH and inhibin B: independent markers associated with unexplained infertility. *Hum. Reprod.* **15**:1046–1051.

33. Luborsky, J., and R. Pong. 2000. Pregnancy outcome and ovarian antibodies in infertility patients undergoing controlled ovarian hyperstimulation. *Am. J. Reprod. Immunol.* **44**:261–265.

34. Luborsky, J. L., L. J. Dorflinger, K. Wright, and H. R. Behrman. 1984. Prostaglandin F2 alpha inhibits luteinizing hormone (LH)-induced increase in LH receptor binding to isolated rat luteal cells. *Endocrinology* **115**:2210–2216.

35. Luborsky, J. L., P. Meyer, M. F. Sowers, E. B. Gold, and N. Santoro. 2003. Premature menopause in a multi-ethnic population study of the menopause transition. *Hum. Reprod.* **18**:199–206.

36. Luborsky, J. L., P. Thiruppathi, B. Rivnay, R. Roussev, C. Coulam, and E. Radwanska. 2002. Evidence for different aetiologies of low estradiol response to FSH: age-related accelerated luteinization of follicles or presence of ovarian autoantibodies. *Hum. Reprod.* **17**:2641–2649.

37. Luborsky, J. L., I. Visintin, S. Boyers, T. Asari, B. Caldwell, and A. DeCherney. 1990. Ovarian antibodies detected by immobilized antigen immunoassay in patients with premature ovarian failure. *J. Clin. Endocrinol. Metab.* **70**:69–75.

38. Maclaren, N., Q. Y. Chen, A. Kukreja, J. Marker, C. H. Zhang, and Z. S. Sun. 2001. Autoimmune hypogonadism as part of an autoimmune polyglandular syndrome. *J. Soc. Gynecol. Investig.* **8**:S52–S54.

39. Mandelbaum, S. L., M. P. Diamond, and A. H. DeCherney. 1987. Relationship of antisperm antibodies to oocyte fertilization in in vitro fertilization-embryo transfer. *Fertil. Steril.* **47**:644–651.

40. Meinertz, H., and R. Bronson. 1988. Detection of antisperm antibodies on the surface of motile spermatozoa. Comparison of the immunobead binding technique (IBT) and the mixed antiglobulin reaction (MAR). *Am. J. Reprod. Immunol. Microbiol.* **18**:120–123.

41. Meinertz, H., L. Linnet, P. Fogh-Andersen, and T. Hjort. 1990. Antisperm antibodies and fertility after vasovasostomy: a follow-up study of 216 men. *Fertil. Steril.* **54**:315–321.

42. Meyer, W. R., G. Lavy, A. H. DeCherney, I. Visintin, K. Economy, and J. L. Luborsky. 1990. Evidence of gonadal

and gonadotropin antibodies in women with a suboptimal ovarian response to exogenous gonadotropin. *Obstet. Gynecol.* **75:**795–799.

43. **Morgan, A. D.** 1976. Inflammation and infestation of the testis and paratesticular structures, p. 79–138. *In* R. C. B. Pugh (ed.), *Pathology of the Testis.* Blackwell Scientific Publications, Ltd., Oxford, United Kingdom.

44. **Nagy, Z. P., G. Verheyen, J. Liu, H. Joris, C. Janssenswillen, A. Wisanto, P. Devroey, and A. C. Van Steirteghem.** 1995. Results of 55 intracytoplasmic sperm injection cycles in the treatment of male-immunological infertility. *Hum. Reprod.* **10:**1775–1780.

45. **Nishizuka, Y., and T. Sakakura.** 1969. Thymus and reproduction: sex-linked dysgenesia of the gonad after neonatal thymectomy in mice. *Science* **166:**753–755.

46. **Reimand, K., P. Peterson, H. Hyoty, R. Uibo, I. Cooke, A. P. Weetman, and K. J. Krohn.** 2000. 3beta-hydroxysteroid dehydrogenase autoantibodies are rare in premature ovarian failure. *J. Clin. Endocrinol. Metab.* **85:** 2324–2326.

47. **Ruan, Q. G., and J. X. She.** 2004. Autoimmune polyglandular syndrome type 1 and the autoimmune regulator. *Clin. Lab. Med.* **24:**305–317.

48. **Taguchi, O., and Y. Nishizuka.** 1981. Experimental autoimmune orchitis after neonatal thymectomy in the mouse. *Clin. Exp. Immunol.* **46:**425–434.

49. **Tung, K. S.** 1996. Autoimmune diseases of the testis and the ovary, p. 153–170. *In* R. A. Bronson et al. (ed.), *Reproductive Immunology.* Blackwell Science, Inc., Cambridge, United Kingdom.

50. **Tung, K. S., and C. Y. Lu.** 1991. Immunologic basis of reproductive failure, p. 308–333. *In* F. T. Krause, I. Damjanov, and N. Kaurman (ed.), *Pathology of Reproductive Failure.* The Williams & Wilkins Co., Baltimore, Md.

51. **Tung, K. S. K.** 1998. Autoimmune disease of the testis and the ovary, p. 687–704. *In* N. R. Rose and I. R. Mackay (ed.), *The Autoimmune Diseases,* 3rd ed. Academic Press Inc., San Diego, Calif.

52. **Vazquez-Levin, M., P. Kaplan, I. Guzman, L. Grunfeld, G. J. Garrisi, and D. Navot.** 1991. The effect of female anti-sperm antibodies on in vitro fertilization, early embryonic development, and pregnancy outcome. *Fertil. Steril.* **56:** 84–88.

53. **Winqvist, O., G. Gebre-Medhin, J. Gustafsson, E. M. Ritzen, O. Lundkvist, F. A. Karlsson, and O. Kampe.** 1995. Identification of the main gonadal autoantigens in patients with adrenal insufficiency and associated ovarian failure. *J. Clin. Endocrinol. Metab.* **80:**1717–1723.

54. **Witkin, S. S.** 1988. Mechanisms of active suppression of the immune response to spermatozoa. *Am. J. Reprod. Immunol. Microbiol.* **17:**61–64.

Immunologic Testing for Celiac Disease and Inflammatory Bowel Disease

JAMES A. GOEKEN

127

The diagnostic usefulness of serological testing for celiac disease (CD) is well established since the antigens and the immune response involved in its pathogenesis are now known. The importance of serological screening of patients suspected to have CD has been recently emphasized by the 2004 National Institutes of Health (NIH) Consensus Conference on Celiac Disease (http://consensus.nih.gov/cons/118/118celiac.htm). Numerous publications have reported the clinical utility of these tests, encouraging clinicians to utilize them routinely for patient screening and monitoring.

Serological tests for inflammatory bowel diseases (IBDs) (Crohn's disease and ulcerative colitis [UC]) have been relatively recently developed, and although clinical use is growing, controversy about their role in diagnosis and management continues.

CD

CD (also known as celiac sprue or gluten-sensitive enteropathy) was first described in 1888 by Samuel Gee. Typical symptoms include diarrhea, intestinal cramps, frequent stools, flatulence, weight loss, chronic fatigue, and poor growth in children. Signs may include chronic anemia (usually due to iron deficiency), poor dentition, amenorrhea and infertility in adult females, and osteoporosis in adults of both sexes (14, 17, 23). Dietary intolerance was considered a possible etiology of CD soon after its recognition but was not proven until 1953 (10). CD was believed until relatively recently to be a rare disease primarily affecting children, but with the advent of better serological tests and availability of endoscopic biopsy to obtain histological confirmation, increasing numbers of both children and adults been diagnosed with CD. CD is now recognized to be one of the most common inherited diseases in humans, and serological testing has become an indispensable tool for detecting it (13, 15, 22). The latter is true because in addition to its high prevalence, clinical signs and symptoms are varied in both location and intensity. Although the small intestine is the primary organ involved, extraintestinal complaints may predominate, making it possible for physicians to miss the diagnosis without an effective screening test (5, 24).

Population Affected by CD

CD occurs most frequently in Caucasians, Middle Easterners, North Africans, and East Indians but is uncommon in East Asians and Black populations. In Europe and other parts of the world settled by Europeans, the prevalence of symptomatic CD is relatively high. In Europe and the United States, recent population studies indicate a frequency of CD of approximately 0.5 to 1% (13, 15).

CD is a familial disorder linked to two haplotypes of the major histocompatibility locus, HLA-DQ2 and HLA-DQ8. Expression of HLA-DQ2 is found in 90 to 95% of individuals with CD, while HLA-DQ8 is found in 5 to 10%. Other factors, including non-HLA genes and the environment, are also involved, since approximately 30% of the Caucasian population is positive for either HLA-DQ2 or -DQ8 but the majority do not develop CD (30).

Pathogenesis

CD is due to immunologic intolerance to gluten, a protein-carbohydrate complex of wheat, or to similar components of the related grains barley and rye (17, 24). Individuals with CD make an immune response directed at a combinatorial antigen involving gliadin (the ethanol-soluble protein of gluten) and tissue transglutaminase (tTG), a ubiquitous enzyme which uses gliadin as a source of glutamine residues that it adds to tissue proteins (12). The initial response is mediated by T lymphocytes, which infiltrate the small intestinal epithelial cells. Increased numbers of intraepithelial lymphocytes (IEL) are the initial histological evidence of CD (24). Non-antigen-specific T gamma/delta lymphocytes are the first to accumulate, followed by gliadin-specific CD8[+] T alpha/beta lymphocytes. CD4[+] T cells are present in small numbers among the IEL but are the majority of the cells that infiltrate the intestinal submucosa. It is believed that CD4[+] T cells are responsible for most of epithelial cell injury via their secretion of gamma interferon and other cytokines (19).

The destruction of intestinal epithelial cells causes intestinal villi to shorten and atrophy, resulting in loss of absorptive surface and malabsorption leading to the characteristic disease symptoms and signs of diarrhea and weight loss. More than half of affected individuals are asymptomatic or have only extraintestinal manifestations despite typical small intestinal histological abnormalities and positive serological tests associated with CD (5, 17, 23, 31). This condition is known as "silent CD." Even asymptomatic patients are at risk for the long-term complications of untreated CD, including iron deficiency anemia, osteoporosis, and intestinal malignancies (particularly T-cell lymphomas in the small intestine) (23).

Test Methods for CD

AGA

Antigliadin antibody (AGA) was the first serological test used to detect CD and to monitor patient compliance with a gluten-free diet (10, 23). Both immunoglobulin G (IgG) AGA (AGA-G) and IgA AGA (AGA-A) are clinically employed (17, 23). Reported sensitivities for both AGA-A and AGA-G vary from ~60 to 90%, with reports differing as to which has greater sensitivity, although clinicians believe that AGA-G does (17, 23, 28). AGA-G levels become elevated in a variety of intestinal inflammatory processes, and therefore this test lacks high specificity for CD (17, 29). Its chief value is in screening patients with selective IgA deficiency for CD. That condition is found in 1 to 3% of CD patients, in whom it is about 10 times more frequent than in the normal population (4, 7). Reported AGA-A specificity for CD ranges from 74 to 93%, with the majority between 80 and 85% (5, 6, 18, 24, 29).

Enzyme immunoassay (EIA) is the method most commonly used to measure AGA. Gliadin extracts are usually employed as the substrate, but deamidated gliadin has been recently reported to give greater test sensitivity and specificity for CD (1). Commercial EIAs utilizing this substrate are now available.

Anti-R1 Reticulin Antibodies

IgA anti-R1 reticulin antibody was identified in CD in the 1980s and was discovered to be more specific than AGA (Table 1). It is detected by indirect immunofluorescence microscopy (IIFM) on connective tissue fibers surrounding proximal renal tubules and hepatocytes on frozen sections of murine kidney and liver. Only IgA anti-R1 reticulin antibodies are specific for CD. This assay is more difficult to interpret than antiendomysial antibody (AEMA) (discussed below) because antibody to other variants of reticulin can be confused with anti-R1 reticulin (2). This test has proven sensitive and specific in specialized laboratories that frequently perform it; however, AEMA immunofluorescence assay and anti-tTG EIA (discussed below) have proven to be more sensitive and specific. Participants in the NIH Consensus Conference on Celiac Disease did not recommend IgA anti-R1 reticulin antibody testing since it does not add diagnostic sensitivity to that achieved with either AEMA or anti-tTG testing (http://consensus. nih.gov/cons/118/118celiac.htm).

AEMA

AEMA reacts with a cell membrane component of the smooth muscle cell demonstrated to be tissue tTG (discussed

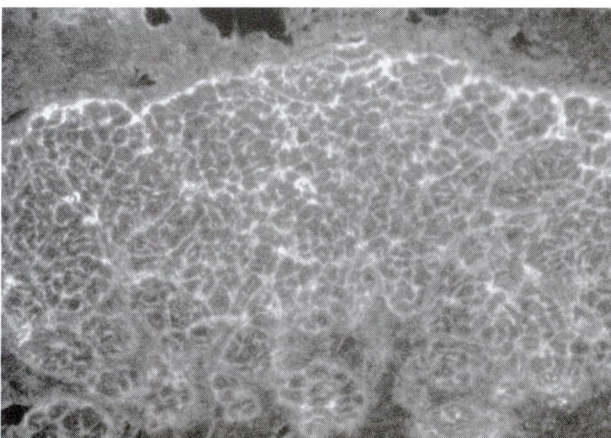

FIGURE 1 Characteristic staining pattern of IgA AEMA on monkey esophagus section as revealed by IIFM.

below). It is detected by indirect IIFM on fresh frozen sections of monkey esophagus or human umbilical cord. On cross-sections of esophagus, AEMA is detected as a grid-like pattern of staining surrounding smooth muscle cells in the muscularis mucosa, vessel walls, and muscularis propria (2) (Fig. 1). AEMA is best demonstrated in the muscularis mucosa. On human umbilical cord sections, AEMA stains the exterior surface of vascular wall smooth muscle cells and cells within Wharton's jelly (23).

Both IgA and IgG class AEMA (AEMA-A and AEMA-G) are clinically useful. AEMA-A is very specific (94 to 100%) for CD in individuals with normal IgA levels (6, 8, 16, 18, 23). The test is also very sensitive, with reports of up to 100% sensitivity published. This high sensitivity is based on the diagnosis of CD by intestinal biopsy showing villous atrophy. Test sensitivity is lower for patients tested very early in the course of their disease before histological evidence of villous atrophy is detectable (although some patients are seropositive when increased IEL are the only abnormality of the small intestinal mucosa) (29). When patients with early CD are added to those with IgA deficiency (see below) and a chronically seronegative group estimated to be 3 to 6% of the total, AEMA-A sensitivity achievable in a clinical laboratory is unlikely to exceed 90% (8, 17). One study comparing AEMA-A testing in six reference laboratories using sera from controls and confirmed CD patients demonstrated sensitivities ranging from 57 to 90%, but with 100% specificity (25). Determination of AEMA-A titer has been used to monitor dietary compliance since titers decrease after patients adopt gluten-free diets and typically fall below detectable limits within 6 months (6, 7).

AEMA-G is useful to detect CD in patients with IgA deficiency (6, 7, 21). Similar to AGA-G, AEMA-G does not disappear after patients go on a gluten-free diet, so the test is not useful to monitor dietary compliance.

AEMA testing requires a fluorescence microscope and experienced laboratory personnel. Monkey esophagus substrate slides are available commercially from several sources or can be prepared in the lab if fresh monkey tissue is available. Tissue from the distal two-thirds of the esophagus should be selected because it contains the necessary smooth muscle. Screening for AEMA-A should be carried out at serum dilutions of no more than 1:5 due to risk of missing significant low-titer AEMA at higher dilutions. In testing for

TABLE 1 Sensitivity and specificity of serological tests for CD[a]

Test name	Method	Sensitivity (%)	Specificity (%)
AGA-A	EIA	63–91	74–93
AGA-G	EIA	63–94	63–76
Anti-R1 reticulin-A	IIFM	~75	90
AEMA-A	IIFM	90–100	94–100
AEMA-G	IIFM	NA	NA
Anti-hutTG-A	EIA	91–100	85–100
Anti-gptTG-A	EIA	76–100	35–100
Anti-hutTG-G	EIA	98[b]	98[b]

[a]Data from references 3, 4, 8, 9, 16, 19, 22, 28, and 33. Abbreviations: NA, not available; hutTG , human tTG; gptTG, guinea pig tTG.

[b]IgA-deficient patients.

AEMA-G, I have found use of monkey-absorbed anti-human IgG conjugates as the secondary antibody superior to nonabsorbed reagents because they reduce the level of background staining caused by cross-reactivity of anti-human antibody with the monkey tissue substrate. A 1:5 screening dilution of serum is satisfactory in AEMA-G testing if monkey-absorbed conjugate is employed.

Anti-tTG Antibody

tTG (EC 2.3.2.13) is a widely distributed calcium-rich enzyme that cross-links gliadin peptides to connective tissue proteins (collagens II, V, and XI; procollagen; fibronectin; etc.) (12). It is highly expressed in areas of tissue damage and healing, where it is thought to strengthen the provisional extracellular matrix. It was identified in 1997 as the autoantigen of CD and the antigenic specificity of AEMA (12). EIA is the method of choice for detecting anti-tTG. The antigen source initially utilized for this test was isolated from guinea pig liver; however, human tTG purified from erythrocytes or produced with recombinant DNA technology is now preferred. Studies comparing guinea pig anti-tTG EIA with human anti-tTG EIA have demonstrated that the human tTG-based tests have greater sensitivity and specificity (3, 33). Human tTG-based test kits are available from multiple commercial sources (33). Sensitivities and specificities reported for human anti-tTG EIAs are up to 100%; however, the issues mentioned above regarding AEMA-A also apply to this test. IgG class anti-tTG (anti-tTG-G) EIA using human antigen has shown greater sensitivity and specificity for CD in IgA-deficient patients than AGA-G (20).

IgA Antiactin Antibody

IgA antiactin antibody, previously considered mainly as a source of interference in IIFM detection of AEMA-A, has been reported to be positively associated with the degree of intestinal mucosal atrophy present in patients with CD (26). EIA is utilized to detect this antibody. Extensive evaluations have not been reported yet, so the value of this assay is not firmly established. IgG antiactin (anti-smooth muscle) antibody is quite common at low titers in healthy individuals, moderate titers in many chronic liver diseases, and high titers in autoimmune hepatitis type 1; it is therefore unlikely to be of use in IgA-deficient CD patients.

Test Selection

The NIH Consensus Conference on Celiac Disease (2004) issued the following statement concerning diagnostic testing (http://consensus.nih.gov/cons/113/118celiac.htm):

> In summary, serological testing is recommended for screening individuals whose clinical signs and symptoms suggest possible celiac disease. Either AEMA-A or ATTG-A may be utilized for initial screening test because of their comparable high sensitivity and specificity. It was felt there was no additional advantage of performing AGA-A, AGA-G or ARA-A due to the lesser sensitivity and specificity of these tests. If AEMA-A or ATTG-A is negative, quantitative IgA should be performed to rule out IgA deficiency. If IgA is absent, test for AGA-G, AEMA-G, or ATTG-G to rule out CD.

Some reports state that an additional 20% of patients proven to have CD on subsequent small bowel biopsy can be serologically identified by performing AGA testing in addition to AEMA and anti-tTG testing at initial screening (11). A significant number of false positives will also be detected if the gliadin extract AGA tests are utilized, however. The clinical advantage of additional testing is not clear since it would lead to significantly increased numbers of small intestinal biopsies to identify relatively few additional patients.

Despite the NIH Celiac Disease Consensus Conference opinion that screening with either AEMA-A or anti-tTG-A is sufficient, there are circumstances in which performance of both assays seems warranted. There have been a number of reports concerning false-positive anti-tTG assays, the majority of which appear to have occurred with guinea pig tTG-based tests (3, 32). One study of patients with congestive heart failure and no evidence of CD found false-positive anti-tTG results with both guinea pig and human tTG-based tests and proved by Western blotting that the patients did have anti-tTG autoantibody (27). Reports have also shown that the specificity of AEMA-A is slightly higher than that of anti-tTG-A, so when patients have positive anti-tTG-A tests but no clinical evidence of CD, it is probably worthwhile to perform confirmatory AEMA-A testing before subjecting the patient to intestinal biopsy (32).

Remarks and Conclusions

Serological screening is useful in selecting patients with suspected CD for endoscopic biopsy, a procedure involving significant risk as well as being invasive and costly.

AEMA-A and anti-tTG-A are the most sensitive and specific tests currently available and are useful in monitoring dietary compliance. AGA-A and AGA-G antibodies are commonly available in clinical laboratories and have been traditionally used for screening but lack the sensitivity and specificity of the two newer tests.

IBD

IBD is a general term for noninfectious, idiopathic chronic inflammation of the intestines. The two major IBDs are Crohn's disease and UC. Although the clinical behavior and pathological features of these diseases differ, many of their symptoms and signs are similar. These include cramping, abdominal pain, intermittent diarrhea (sometimes bloody), nausea, vomiting, and laboratory evidence of inflammation in the form of increased levels of the acute-phase reaction proteins, such as C-reactive protein and fibrinogen (34, 42). Physical examination is rarely able to distinguish Crohn's disease and UC. Invasive radiographic studies, endoscopy, and mucosal biopsy are usually necessary for that purpose. Discussion continues as to whether these are fundamentally different diseases or are opposite ends of a continuum of intestinal inflammatory processes. Evidence for the latter view has been increasing. About 10 to 15% of IBD patients have clinical and histological features of both diseases and are designated as having "indeterminate colitis" (42). Half of these eventually assume the features of either Crohn's disease or UC, while the rest remain diagnostically indeterminate. Treatment of both diseases primarily involves rectal administration of anti-inflammatory drugs (corticosteroids and various nonabsorbable 5-aminosalicylate-based compounds, e.g., sulfasalazine) (42).

UC

UC primarily affects the colon and rectum. The mucosa is infiltrated with neutrophils, and inflammation is symmetrical and continuous. Crypt abscesses form in the deeper parts of the colonic and rectal mucosa, and superficial ulceration is widespread. Patients often have severe bowel cramps and bloody diarrhea. Occasionally, the colon becomes greatly dilated (toxic megacolon) and may rupture, causing peritonitis (34, 42). The clinical course of UC is characterized by remissions and relapses, similar to most autoimmune diseases. After 10 or more years of ulcerative colitis, rapid intestinal epithelial cell turnover leads to a 20- to 30-fold increase in carcinoma of the colon (34, 42). Total colectomy may be prophylactically performed in some UC patients after passage of this length of time or when dysplasia is detected in colonic mucosal cells. Patients with Crohn's colitis have a similar risk of colon carcinoma.

Crohn's Disease

Crohn's disease in the majority of patients predominantly affects the small intestine, although 20 to 30% of patients have colon-limited disease (Crohn's colitis) (42). Inflammation in Crohn's disease is segmental, with affected areas alternating with normal areas in the small intestine. Ulcers and "skip areas" of uninvolved mucosa alternate with diseased segments. The pathology involves deeply penetrating mucosal ulcers extending into the muscularis propria and sometimes through the serosa. Thickening of the involved bowel wall and narrowing of the lumen occur in areas of inflammation. Where the serosa is involved, an adhesion between segments of bowel occurs. Both adhesions and luminal narrowing may lead to bowel obstruction, a major complication of Crohn's disease. Histological features of the disease are mixed acute and chronic inflammation in the involved mucosa and the penetrating ulcers. Noncaseating granulomata are found in the bowel wall in approximately 50% of patients, but are not numerous. Their absence does not rule out Crohn's disease (42).

Treatment of Crohn's disease was formerly limited to anti-inflammatory drugs, rest, and good supportive care. Surgical intervention was not undertaken unless bowel perforation or obstruction occurred because the disease has a marked tendency to recur at bowel segment anastomoses (34, 42). Within the past few years, a new approach to therapy has proven very successful in patients with predominantly small intestinal involvement. Monoclonal antibodies to tumor necrosis factor alpha (TNF-α), a cytokine critical in the inflammatory pathways in Crohn's disease, or TNF-α receptor analogues are able to block TNF-α activity and dramatically reduce inflammation and clinical symptoms (42). Not all patients respond to this therapy, particularly those with Crohn's colitis.

Populations Affected by IBDs

Both Crohn's disease and UC affect men and women in equal numbers. Both diseases have their onset between 15 and 30 years, with a second, smaller peak between 50 and 70 years. The adult incidence of UC is $\sim 6 \times 10^5$ to 12×10^5 and that of CD is $\sim 5 \times 10^5$ to 7×10^5 in the United States and northern Europe (34, 42). Children are also affected but with lower frequency than adults. IBD is most common in industrialized countries of the northern hemisphere; southern Europe, South Africa, and Australia all have a lower incidence of IBD (2×10^5 to 8×10^5 for UC and 0.1×10^5 to 4×10^5 for Crohn's disease) (34, 42). Both forms of IBD have an increased incidence (10- to 15-fold) in immediate relatives of patients with IBD, and family studies have found that 10 to 35% of patients have affected family members (42). Northern Europeans and Ashkenazi Jews have the highest incidence (43). Genetic factors (especially involving components of the immune response) contribute to disease susceptibility, but environmental factors also play a role in pathogenesis, as demonstrated by differences in incidence rates in the northern and southern hemispheres in populations with similar genetic makeup (42).

Testing for IBD

Two serological tests are most often ordered in the workup of patients with suspected IBD. These tests are described below.

ANCA

Anti-neutrophil cytoplasmic antibody (ANCA) is widely used to screen patients for small vessel necrotizing vasculitides (SVV) such as Wegener's granulomatosis, microscopic polyangiitis, and Churg-Strauss syndrome (46, 50). ANCA testing is done by IIFM on ethanol-fixed human neutrophil substrate. Two patterns of ANCA are associated with SVV: C-ANCA and P-ANCA, so named for the area of ethanol-fixed neutrophils stained (cytoplasm or perinuclear zone) (50).

Association of UC with antibodies to neutrophils (so-called "granulocyte-specific ANA") preceded discovery of ANCA in vasculitis patients (40). Antibodies to neutrophil antigens in patients with IBD were rediscovered early in the investigation of ANCA in vasculitis. In most cases, these produce a P-ANCA staining pattern on ethanol-fixed neutrophils (atypical cytoplasmic, mixed atypical cytoplasmic and perinuclear, and, rarely, "typical" C-ANCA patterns may also be found) (Fig. 2). P-ANCA in IBD may be indistinguishable from vasculitis-associated P-ANCA, although staining is generally restricted to the nuclear membrane rather than extending into the nucleus. Variability in reproducibility of the staining pattern due to a variety of factors led the International Group for Consensus on ANCA Testing and Reporting to recommend using the generic term "P-ANCA" for both IBD- and vasculitis-associated variants (45, 46). Since much of the literature concerning ANCA in IBD utilizes the term "atypical P-ANCA" (UC-ANCA, X-ANCA, and antineutrophil nuclear antibody were also used in early references), it is used in this chapter for convenience. In most instances, sera positive for atypical P-ANCA produce no staining or weak, patchy, nongranular cytoplasmic staining of formalin-fixed neutrophils. This is in contrast to myeloperoxidase (MPO)-specific P-ANCA, which usually produces granular cytoplasmic staining (although rare examples fail to stain formalin-fixed neutrophils) (46). Atypical P-ANCA does not have specificity for either anti-MPO or anti-proteinase 3 (anti-PR3), the two major vasculitis-associated specificities most commonly associated with P-ANCA and C-ANCA, respectively (46). The specificity of atypical P-ANCA has not yet been satisfactorily defined; several different specificities have been reported, including bactericidal/permeability-increasing protein, catalase, elastase, α-enolase, histone H1, high-mobility-group proteins (HMG1 and HMG2), lactoferrin, and nuclear membrane proteins (39, 45). Most do not have specificity for neutrophil nuclear membrane, which IIFM staining suggests is important.

Approximately 50 to 70% of UC patients are positive for atypical P-ANCA (36, 37, 39, 41, 44). Atypical P-ANCA is also found in approximately 10 to 30% of Crohn's disease patients, 65 to 80% of primary sclerosing cholangitis (PSC) patients, 90% of autoimmune hepatitis type 1 patients, 90% of Felty syndrome patients, and up to 30% of patients with active rheumatoid arthritis (45). These diseases are probably not all associated with the same autoantibody specificity, but proof awaits identification of the antigen or antigens involved. Atypical P-ANCA may be the same in UC, Crohn's disease, and PSC patients. ANCA-positive Crohn's patients typically have colon-limited rather than the more common small intestinal fibrostenotic disease (49). PSC is associated with coexisting IBD, usually UC (47). In contrast, neither

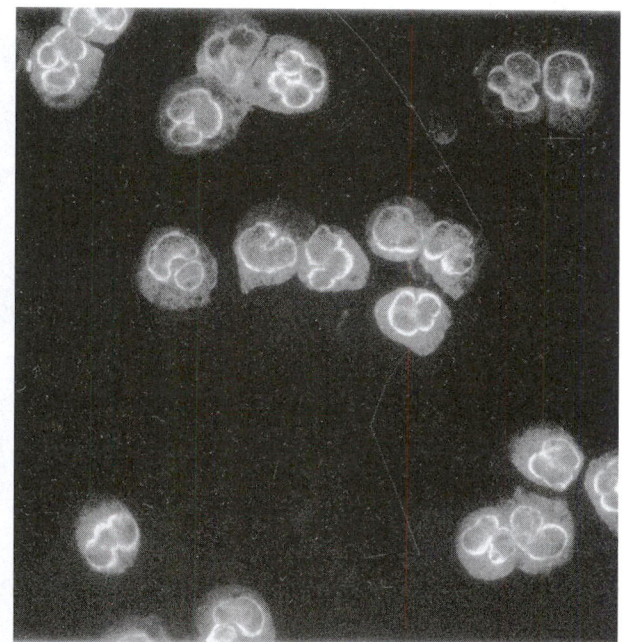

FIGURE 2 Staining pattern of atypical P-ANCA associated with IBD on ethanol-fixed human neutrophils as revealed by IIFM. Contrast with typical P-ANCA in Fig. 2, chapter 118, this volume (12).

patients with autoimmune hepatitis, Felty syndrome, nor rheumatoid arthritis typically have any form of IBD.

Testing Methods for ANCA

The routine procedure for ANCA testing is described by Wiik (50). Commercial substrate slides are readily available and satisfactory. Recommendations concerning interpretation and reporting of ANCA made by an international consensus group included the following points. (i) P-ANCA$^+$ sera should be tested for ANA and by EIA for anti-MPO and anti-PR3 to eliminate false-positive ANCA reports due to ANA and to specifically identify vasculitis-associated ANCAs. (ii) P-ANCA$^+$ sera with negative anti-MPO and anti-PR3 EIA results should be reported as atypical ANCA. (iii) Titration of atypical ANCA in IBD is not necessary, as it has not been demonstrated to have clinical significance (45).

ASCA

Anti-*Saccharomyces cerevisiae* antibody (ASCA) is directed at an oligomannoside of bread and beer yeast (43) and is present in individuals with Crohn's disease more frequently and at higher titers than in patients with UC (35, 37, 38, 41–44, 47–49). Both IgG and IgA class ASCA determinations appear to be useful. IgG ASCA is present in 50 to 80% of patients with Crohn's disease, and IgA ASCA is present in 35 to 50%, compared with 2 to 14% of UC patients and 1 to 7% of healthy controls (35, 37, 38, 41–44, 47–49). Test specificity is higher for Crohn's disease if both IgG and IgA ASCAs are present but test sensitivity of this combination is only 50 to 55%.

EIA is the method used for ASCA testing. Various investigators of ASCA used different preparations of the antigen, ranging from whole-yeast extracts to highly purified *S. cerevisiae* oligomannoside, so reported ASCA sensitivities and specificities are variable. Commercial sources of IgA ASCA

and IgG ASCA reagents are available. Comprehensive comparison studies of various commercial ASCA kits are not yet published.

Remarks and Conclusions

The clinical utility of combined ANCA and ASCA testing for IBD continues to be debated. The combination of these tests may have utility in evaluation of patients with symptoms consistent with IBD. One or more positive tests would provide an argument for performing the invasive procedures (radiographic, endoscopic, and biopsy) necessary for diagnosis.

REFERENCES

CELIAC DISEASE

1. **Aleanzi, M., A. M. Demonte, C. Esper, S. Garcilazo, and M. Waggener.** 2001. Celiac disease antibody recognition against native and selectively deamidated gliadin peptides. *Clin. Chem.* **47:**2023–2028.
2. **Beutner, E., T. P. Chorzelski, and V. Kumar (ed.).** 1987. *Immunopathology of the Skin*, 3rd ed., sections 24–28. Churchill Livingstone, New York, N.Y.
3. **Carroccio, A., G. Vitale, L. Di Prima, N. Chifari, S. Napoli, C. La Russa, G. Gulotta, M. R. Averna, G. Montalto, S. Mansueto, and A. Notarbartolo.** 2002. Comparison of anti-transglutaminase ELISAs and an anti-endomysial antibody assay in the diagnosis of celiac disease: a prospective study. *Clin. Chem.* **48:**1546–1550.
4. **Cataldo, F., V. Marino, G. Botturo, P. Greco, and A. Ventura.** 1997. Celiac disease and selective IgA deficiency. *J. Pediatr.* **131:**306–308.
5. **Catassi, C., I.-M. Rätsch, E. Fabiani, M. Rossini, G. V. Coppa, P. L. Giorgi, F. Bordicchia, and F. Candela.** 2000. Celiac disease in the year 2000: exploring the iceberg. *Lancet* **343:**200–203.
6. **Chorzelski, T. P., J. Sulej, H. Tchorzewska, S. Jablonska, E. H. Beutner, and V. Kumar.** 1983. IgA class endomysium antibodies in dermatitis herpetiformis and coeliac disease. *Ann. N. Y. Acad. Sci.* **420:**325–334.
7. **Collin, P., M. Maki, O. Keyrilainen, O. Hallstrom, T. Reunala, and A. Pasternack.** 1992. Selective IgA deficiency and coeliac disease. *Scand. J. Gastroenterol.* **27:**367–371.
8. **Dahele, A. V., M. C. Aldhous, K. Humphreys, and S. Ghosh.** 2001. Serum IgA tissue transglutaminase antibodies in celiac disease and other gastrointestinal diseases. *Q. J. Med.* **94:**195–205.
9. **Dahlbom, I., M. Olsson, N. K. Forooz, A. G. Sjöholm, L. Truedsson, and T. Hansson.** 2005. Immunoglobulin G (IgG) anti-tissue transglutaminase antibodies used as markers for IgA-deficient celiac disease patients. *Clin. Diagn. Lab. Immunol.* **12:**254–258.
10. **Dicke, W. K., H. A. Weijers, and J. H. Van de Kanmer.** 1953. The presence in wheat of a factor having a deleterious effect in cases of coeliac disease. *Acta Paediatr. Scand.* **42:**34–42.
11. **Dickey, W., D. F. Hughes, and S. A. McMillan.** 2000. Reliance on serum endomysial antibody testing underestimates the true prevalence of coeliac disease by one-fifth. *Scand. J. Gastroenterol.* **35:**181–183.
12. **Dieterich, W., T. Ehnis, M. Bauer, P. Donner, U. Volta, E. O. Riecken, and D. Schuppan.** 1997. Identification of tissue transglutaminase as the autoantigen of celiac disease. *Nat. Med.* **3:**797–801.
13. **Dubé, C., A. Rostom, R. Sy, A. Cranney, N. Saloojee, C. Garritty, M. Sampson, L. Zhang, F. Yazdi, V. Mamaladze, I. Pan, J. Macneil, D. Mack, D. Patel, and D. Moher.** 2005. The prevalence of celiac disease in average-risk and at-risk Western European populations: a systemic review. *Gastroenterology* **128:**S57–S67.

14. **Fasano, A.** 2005. Clinical presentation of celiac disease in the pediatric population. *Gastroenterology* **128:**S68–S73.

15. **Fasano, A., I. Berti, T. Gerarduzzi, T. Not, R. B. Colletti, S. Drago, Y. Elitsur, P. H. R. Green, S. Guandalini, I. D. Hill, M. Pietzak, A. Ventura, M. Thorpe, D. Kryszak, F. Fornaroli, S. S. Wasserman, J. A. Murray, and K. Horvath.** 2003. Prevalence of celiac disease in at-risk and not-at-risk groups in the United States: a large multi-center study. *Arch. Intern. Med.* **163:**286–292.

16. **Feighery, L., C. Collins, C. Feighery, N. Malumud, G. Coughlan, R. Willoughby, and J. Jackson.** 2003. Anti-transglutaminase antibodies and the serological diagnosis of coeliac disease. *Br. J. Biomed. Sci.* **60:**14–18.

17. **Green, P. H. R., K. Rostami, and M. N. Marsh.** 2005. Diagnosis of celiac disease. *Best Pract. Res. Clin. Gastroenterol.* **19:**389–400.

18. **Horvath, K., and I. D. Hill.** 2002. Anti-tissue transglutaminase antibody as the first line screening for celiac disease: good-bye antigliadin tests? *Am. J. Gastroenterol.* **97:**2702–2704.

19. **Koning, F., D. Schuppan, N. Cerf-Bensussan, and L. M. Sollid.** 2005. Pathomechanisms in celiac disease. *Best Pract. Res. Clin. Gastroenterol.* **19:**373–387.

20. **Korponay-Szabo, I. R., I. Dahlbom, K. Laurila, S. Koskinen, N. Woolley, J. Partenen, J. B. Kovacs, M. Maki, and T. Hansson.** 2003. Elevation of IgG antibodies against tissue transglutaminase as a diagnostic tool for coeliac disease in selective IgA deficiency. *Gut* **52:**1567–1571.

21. **Kumar, V., M. Jarzabek-Chorzelska, J. Sulej, K. Karnewska, T. Farrell, and S. Jablonska.** 2002. Celiac disease and immunoglobulin A deficiency: how effective are the serological methods of diagnosis? *Clin. Diagn. Lab. Immunol.* **9:**1295–1300.

22. **Mäki, M., K. Mustalahti, J. Kokkonen, P. Kulmala, M. Haapalahti, T. Karttunen, J. Ilonen, K. Laurila, I. Dahlbom, T. Hansson, P. Höpfl, and M. Knip.** 2003. Prevalence of celiac disease among children in Finland. *N. Engl. J. Med.* **348:**2517–2524.

23. **Marsh, M. N. (ed.).** 1992. *Coeliac Disease,* p. 192–214. Blackwell Scientific, Oxford, United Kingdom.

24. **Marsh, M. N.** 1992. Gluten, major histocompatibility complex and the small intestine. *Gastroenterology* **102:**330–354.

25. **Murray, J. A., A. J. Herlein, F. Mitros, and J. A. Goeken.** 2000. Serologic testing for celiac disease in the United States: results of a multilaboratory comparison study. *Clin. Diagn. Lab. Immunol.* **7:**584–587.

26. **Pedreina, S., E. Sugai, M. Moreno, H. Vazquez, S. Niveloni, E. Smecuol, R. Mazure, Z. Kogan, E. Maurino, and J. C. Bai.** 2005. Significance of smooth muscle/anti-actin autoantibodies in celiac disease. *Acta Gastroenterol. Latinoam.* **35:**83–93.

27. **Peracchi, M., C. Trovato, M. Longhi, M. Gasparin, D. Conte, C. Tarantino, D. Prati, and M. T. Bardella.** 2002. Tissue transglutaminase antibodies in patients with end-stage heart failure. *Am. J. Gastroenterol.* **97:**2850–2854.

28. **Stern, M., and the Working Group on Serologic Screening for Celiac Disease.** 2000. Comparative evaluation of serologic tests for celiac disease: a European initiative towards standardization. *J. Pediatr. Gastroenterol. Nutr.* **31:**513–519.

29. **Tursi, A., G. Brandimarte, and G. M. Giorgetti.** 2003. Prevalence of antitissue transglutaminase antibodies in different degrees of intestinal damage in celiac disease. *J. Clin. Gastroenterol.* **36:**219–221.

30. **van Heel, D. A., K. Hunt, L. Greco, and C. Wijmenga.** 2005. Genetics in coeliac disease. *Best Pract. Res. Clin. Gastroenterol.* **19:**323–339.

31. **Volta, U., A. Granito, L. De Franceschi, N. Petrolini, and F. B. Bianchi.** 2001. Anti-tissue transglutaminase antibodies as predictors of silent celiac disease in patients with hypertransaminasaemia of unknown origin. *Dig. Liver Dis.* **33:**420–425.

32. **Weiss, B., Y. Bujanover, B. Avidan, A. Frandkin, I. Weintraub, and B. Shainberg.** 2004. Positive tissue transglutaminase antibodies with negative endomysial antibodies: low rate of celiac disease. *Isr. Med. Assoc. J.* **6:**9–12.

33. **Wong, R. C. W., R. J. Wilson, R. H. Steele, G. Rodford-Smith, and S. Adelstein.** 2002. A comparison of 13 guinea pig and human anti-tissue transglutaminase antibody ELISA kits. *J. Clin. Pathol.* **55:**488–494.

INFLAMMATORY BOWEL DISEASE

34. **Andres, P. G., and L. S. Friedman.** 1999. Epidemiology and natural course of inflammatory bowel disease. *Gastroenterol. Clin. N. Am.* **28:**255–281.

35. **Glas, J., H.-P. Török, F. Vilsmaier, K.-H. Herbinger, M. Hoelscher, and C. Folaczny.** 2002. Anti-*Saccharomyces cerevisiae* antibodies in patients with inflammatory bowel disease and their first-degree relatives: potential clinical value. *Digestion* **66:**173–177.

36. **Hardarson, S., D. R. Labrecque, F. A. Mitros, G. A. Neil, and J. A. Goeken.** 1993. Anti-neutrophil cytoplasmic antibody (ANCA) in inflammatory bowel and hepatobiliary diseases: high prevalence in ulcerative colitis, primary sclerosing cholangitis and autoimmune hepatitis. *Am. J. Clin. Pathol.* **99:**277–281.

37. **Hoffenberg, E., S. Fidanza, and A. Sauaia.** 1999. Serologic testing for inflammatory bowel disease. *J. Pediatr.* **134:**447–452.

38. **Klebl, F. H., F. Bataille, C. R. Bertea, H. Herfarh, E. Hofstädter, J. Schölmerich, and G. Rogler.** 2003. Association of perinuclear antineutrophil cytoplasmic antibodies and anti-*Saccharomyces cerevisiae* antibodies with Vienna classification subtypes of Crohn's disease. *Inflamm. Bowel Dis.* **9:**302–307.

39. **Mulder, A. H. L., J. Broekroelofs, G. Horst, P. C. Limburg, G. F. Nelis, and C. G. M. Kallenberg.** 1994. Anti-neutrophil cytoplasmic antibodies (ANCA) in inflammatory bowel disease: characterization and clinical correlates. *Clin. Exp. Immunol.* **95:**490–497.

40. **Nielsen, H., A. Wiik, and J. Elmgreen.** 1983. Granulocyte specific antinuclear antibodies in ulcerative colitis. Aid in differential diagnosis of inflammatory bowel disease. *Acta Pathol. Microbiol. Scand. Sect. C* **91:**23–26.

41. **Papadakis, K. A., and S. R. Targan.** 1999. Serologic testing in inflammatory bowel disease: its value in indeterminate colitis. *Curr. Gastroenterol. Rep.* **1:**482–485.

42. **Podolsky, D. K.** 2002. Inflammatory bowel disease. *N. Engl. J. Med.* **347:**417–429.

43. **Quinton, J. F., B. Sendid, D. Reumaux, P. Duthilleul, A. Cortot, B. Grandbastien, G. Charrier, S. R. Targan, J. F. Colombel, and D. Poulain.** 1998. Anti-*Saccharomyces cerevisiae* mannan antibodies combined with antineutrophil cytoplasmic autoantibodies in inflammatory bowel disease: prevalence and diagnostic role. *Gut* **42:**788–791.

44. **Ruemmele, F. M., S. R. Targan, G. Levy, M. Dubinsky, J. Braun, and E. G. Seidman.** 1998. Diagnostic accuracy of serological assays in pediatric inflammatory bowel disease. *Gastroenterology* **115:**822–829.

45. **Savige, J., W. Dimech, M. Fritzler, J. Goeken, E. C. Hagen, D. Jayne, J. C. Jennette, R. McEvoy, W. Pollock, C. Pusey, M. Trevisin, A. Wiik, and R. Wong.** 2003. Addendum to the International Consensus Statement on

Testing and Reporting of Antineutrophil Cytoplasmic Antibodies (ANCA)—quality control guidelines, comments and recommendations for testing in other autoimmune diseases. *Am. J. Clin. Pathol.* **120:**312–318.

46. **Savige, J., D. Gillis, E. Benson, D. Davies, V. Esnault, R. J. Falk, E. C. Hagen, D. Jayne, J. C. Jennette, B. Paspaliaris, W. Pollock, C. Pusey, C. O. Savage, R. Silvestrini, F. van der Woude, J. Wieslander, and A. Wiik.** 1999. International Consensus Statement on Testing and Reporting of Antineutrophil Cytoplasmic Antibodies (ANCA). *Am. J. Clin. Pathol.* **111:**507–513.

47. **Seibold, F., P. Weber, R. Klein, P. A. Berg, and K. H. Weidman.** 1992. Clinical significance of antibodies against neutrophils in patients with inflammatory bowel disease and primary sclerosing cholangitis. *Gut* **37:**657–662.

48. **Stotland, B. R., R. R. Stein, and G. Lichtenstein.** 2000. Advances in inflammatory bowel disease. *Med. Clin. N. Am.* **84:**1107–1124.

49. **Vasiliauskas, E. A., L. Y. Kam, L. C. Karp, J. Gaiennie, H. Yang, and S. R. Targan.** 2000. Marker antibody expression stratifies Crohn's disease into immunologically homogenous subgroups with distinct clinical characteristics. *Gut* **47:**487–496.

50. **Wiik, A.** 2002. Antineutrophil cytoplasmic antibodies (ANCAs) and ANCA testing, p. 981–986. *In* N. R. Rose, R. G. Hamilton, and B. Detrick (ed.), *Manual of Clinical Laboratory Immunology,* 6th ed. ASM Press, Washington, D.C.

Autoimmune Thrombocytopenia

THOMAS S. KICKLER

128

The diagnosis of autoimmune thrombocytopenia is one of exclusion. In patients with a low platelet count and the absence of other hematologic disorders, administration of thrombocytopenia-producing drugs, or splenomegaly, the diagnosis is usually made. Either immunoglobulin G (IgG) or IgM antiplatelet antibodies directed against membrane platelet glycoprotein mediate reticuloendothelial destruction of platelets. This process may be acute and self-limited, as is frequently the case in children. A chronic form of autoimmune thrombocytopenia exists and is the clinical course most often seen in adults. With characterization of the immunopathological features of autoimmune thrombocytopenia, a variety of methods have been developed to measure the antiplatelet autoantibodies that mediate the immune destruction of platelets in this disorder (1, 3, 7).

ACUTE IMMUNE THROMBOCYTOPENIA

Acute immune thrombocytopenia occurs primarily in children, with a peak age of 2 to 6 years. Typically, there is a history of an antecedent viral infection followed by the acute onset of bruising, petechiae, and mucosa bleeding. If thrombocytopenia persists longer than 6 months despite therapy, the child should be considered to have chronic autoimmune thrombocytopenia. The risk of chronicity increases with increased age of the child; otherwise, there are no prognostic features, either clinical or laboratory, that will predict whether a child with acute immune thrombocytopenia will recover spontaneously. Our understanding of the pathogenic mechanisms of acute immune thrombocytopenia is lacking. It appears that viral illnesses are responsible for evoking an immune response and that antibodies to platelets or immune complexes are involved in shortened platelet survival. Increased levels of immunoglobulin found on the platelets of these patients may reflect the deposition of immune complexes that have bound to the platelet Fc receptor. It is also possible that transient production of autoantibodies may be induced by viral infections. There is little evidence to suggest that microbial agents produce some factor that alters the surface of platelets, making them immunogenic (3).

CHRONIC AUTOIMMUNE THROMBOCYTOPENIA

Immunopathological Features

Early observations by Harrington and coworkers showed that thrombocytopenic pregnant women frequently delivered babies with thrombocytopenia (4). This suggested that some plasma factor crossing the placenta mediated the newborn's thrombocytopenia. Plasma infusions from patients with thrombocytopenia were shown to produce thrombocytopenia in healthy volunteers Subsequently, Shulman et al. (16) showed that the degree of thrombocytopenia was dependent on the amount of plasma infused, with splenectomized or corticosteroid-treated subjects being more resistant to the effects of the infused autoimmune thrombocytopenic plasma. The pathogenic factor present in the plasma reacted with normal and autologous platelets and could be isolated and removed from the gamma fraction of plasma by adsorption with platelets. These early studies provided a basic understanding of the pathogenic mechanisms of the factors involved in platelet destruction (16).

The first direct evidence that autoantibodies are present on platelets was the observation that eluates prepared from the platelets of patients with autoimmune thrombocytopenia bind to normal platelets (19). These eluate studies also documented that the major antigenic target for these antibodies was platelet glycoprotein IIB/IIIA. This observation was based on the failure of the eluates to react with platelets from patients who are deficient for platelet glycoprotein IIb/IIIa (Glanzmann thrombasthenia). Subsequent studies using Western blotting (immunoblotting) or immunoprecipitation demonstrated that the autoantigens were principally found on platelet glycoprotein IIIa. Some patients may have autoantibodies that react with one or more platelet glycoproteins, including platelet glycoprotein Ib/IX or Ia/IIa (8, 13, 20).

The distribution of the heavy chain type of autoantibodies present on the platelets, frequently referred to as platelet-associated immunoglobulin, is a follows: 95% of patients have IgG either alone or in combination with IgA or IgM; 5% have IgM alone. A variety of studies have shown a broad range for the IgG subclass distribution that may be found; however, subclass determination has not been shown to have prognostic importance (5).

The autoantibodies found in chronic autoimmune thrombocytopenia may bind to megakaryocytes and possibly impair thrombopoiesis. The binding of antiplatelet antibodies to megakaryocytes was first demonstrated by immunofluorescent studies. Careful isotopic platelet kinetic studies have demonstrated increased platelet turnover associated with normal or decreased thrombopoiesis. Using in vitro culture systems for megakaryocyte colony formation, investigators have shown that antibodies can impair megakaryocyte differentiation and platelet production (3).

Clinical Features

Patients with chronic autoimmune thrombocytopenia typically present with petechiae and mucosa bleeding. Symptoms may be present for months, or some patients may experience more acute manifestations. If bleeding has been significant, anemia may be present. Alternatively, some patients may have concomitant autoimmune hemolytic anemia, which accounts for the assisted anemia. Physical examination is unremarkable except for bleeding manifestations. The peripheral smear shows reduced to absent platelets having

an increased mean platelet volume. The bone marrow is normal (3).

Platelet Autoantibody Detection

A variety of methods to measure antiplatelet antibodies are available (9–12, 14). The earlier assays employing complement fixation or platelet lysis lacked sensitivity and are no longer used. Quantitative measurements based on antiglobulin consumption give falsely high values for platelet-associated immunoglobulin because antiglobulin binds differently to membrane-bound IgG than to the IgG in the solution used to calibrate the standard curve. Assays for total platelet immunoglobulin performed by detergent lysis of platelets and then measurement of the immunoglobulin by radial diffusion or nephelometry were developed before it was realized that a large amount of normal immunoglobulin constituted the platelet alpha granule. These assays should be considered of little clinical importance (2, 15).

Of the available approaches, the platelet glycoprotein capture assays offer the best sensitivity and specificity. There are two types of capture assays, the solid-phase (immunobead) method and the monoclonal antibody-specific immobilization of platelet antigen assay (MAIPA). Figure 1 gives a general description of these assays. Both of these methods are straightforward and can measure both platelet-associated and plasma

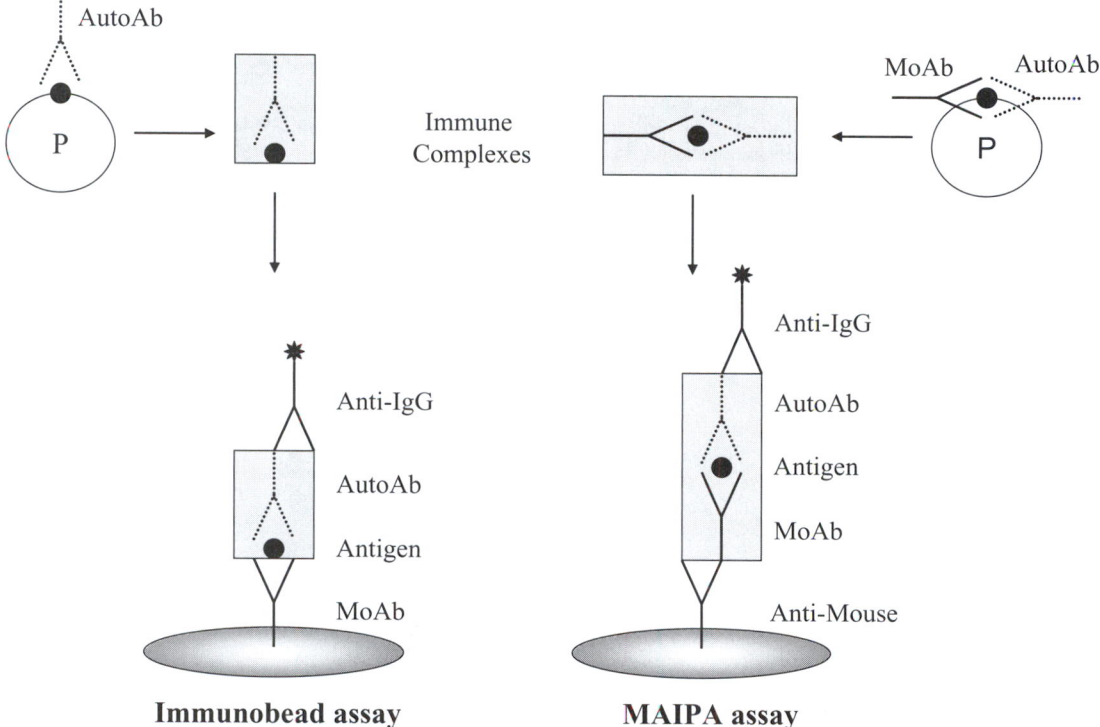

Immunobead assay   **MAIPA assay**

FIGURE 1 Platelet autoantibody assays. In the solid-phase assay, a microtiter well or plastic bead is coated with a monoclonal antibody (MoAB) to a specific platelet glycoprotein, such as GPIIb-IIIa or Ib-IX. Platelets from a patient with idiopathic thrombocytopenia purpura are washed, solubilized with detergent, and added to the coated surface to allow capture by platelet glycoprotein complex and bound autoantibody (AutoAb). The autoantibody is measured using labeled anti-human IgG. The MAIPA is similar, except that the murine monoclonal antiplatelet glycoprotein antibody is added to the autoantibody-sensitized platelets and the immune complex composed of platelet glycoprotein, mouse monoclonal antibody, and human immunoglobulin is captured with an anti-mouse antibody.

antibodies. When platelet-associated antibodies are assayed, approximately 80% of samples will have detectable antibody when a panel of monoclonal antibodies is employed to capture the platelets. The relative sensitivity for serum antibodies is approximately 50% (1, 12–14, 18). The details of performing the MAIPA are given below. Since IgG, IgM, and IgA autoantibodies may be found in autoimmune thrombocytopenia, the labeled antiglobulin used should have specificity for these three classes of immunoglobulin.

Antigen capture assays have advantages over the previously mentioned tests for detecting autoimmune antibodies because interference by nonspecific immunoglobulin is reduced, native conformation of platelet antigens is maintained by using nondenaturing detergents, and determination of target platelet glycoprotein is possible. Tsubakio and coworkers pointed out the importance of monoclonal antibodies being used as a determinant in the detection of platelet autoantibodies (18). They showed that if the monoclonal antibody was directed to epitopes identical or closely adjacent to those to which the autoantibody was directed, no binding would occur. Conversely, they hypothesized that if the epitopes were widely separated, maximum antibody binding would occur. If epitope locations were relatively close, intermediate antibody binding might occur (13). Subsequent investigators have confirmed these observations in the detection of autoantibodies.

Immunoblotting has been utilized as a research tool rather than as a diagnostic test (6, 17). After the platelet membranes are washed and solubilized, the various platelet glycoproteins are separated by sodium dodecyl sulfate-polyacrylamide gel electrophoresis. The platelet proteins are then electrophoretically transferred to nitrocellulose paper. Patient serum is then incubated with the membranes, and a labeled secondary antibody is used to determine the proteins against which the patient's antibody is directed. When this technique is applied, one may find detectable antibody present in normal sera. Since many patients with autoimmune thrombocytopenia may have cytosolic antibodies to platelet glycoprotein, immunoblotting may detect antibodies that have no pathological significance.

TEST PROCEDURE: MAIPA

Reagents

Coating buffer: 1.59 g of Na_2CO_3, 2.93 g of $NaHCO_3$, and 0.2 g of NaN_3. Add distilled H_2O to 1 liter and adjust pH to 9.6.

TBS wash buffer: 3.03 g of Tris, 22 g NaCl, 12.5 ml of Nonidet P-40, 1.25 ml of Tween 20, and 1.25 ml of 1 M $CaCl_2$. Add distilled H_2O to 2.5 liters.

Solubilization buffer: 1.21 g of Tris dissolved in 950 ml of isotonic saline, pH 7.4. Add 5 ml of Nonidet P-40, and add isotonic saline to 1 liter.

Goat anti-mouse IgG (code 115-005-071; Jackson ImmunoResearch). Dilute to 3 µg/ml in coating buffer.

Peroxidase-conjugated goat anti-human IgG (code 109-035-008; Jackson ImmunoResearch). Dilute to 1 in 5,000 to 1 in 30,000 (determined by previous experiment) in TBS wash buffer.

Substrate solution: Dissolve four 3.5-mg tablets of 1,2-phenylenediamine dihydrochloride (OPD·2HCl) (code S 2045; Dako) in 12 ml of distilled water in a foil-covered container. Add 5 µl of 30% H_2O_2 immediately before use.

Stop solution: Add 28 ml of 95 to 97% H_2SO_4 to 972 ml of distilled water.

Warning: Use only freshly prepared reagents.

MAIPA (Microplate Method)

Method

A. Preparation of coated F-well microplate
1. Prepare goat anti-mouse IgG as described above and aliquot 100 µl/well into two flat-well microplates (44204A; Nunc) for duplicate testing.
2. Incubate microplates at 4°C overnight (or at least 2 h at room temperature).
3. Store sealed coated plates for up to 2 weeks at 4°C.
4. Thirty minutes before the plates are required on the day of testing, wash them four times with TBS wash buffer.
5. Leave last wash in wells for 30 min at 4°C to block plates and prevent nonspecific binding at subsequent stages. Decant buffer before use.

B. Preparation of platelets
1. Take blood from group O donors into EDTA or citrate.
2. Centrifuge at 1,800 rpm for 10 min in a benchtop centrifuge.
3. Remove the top three-fourths of the PRP from the top of the tube and transfer to a 10-ml conical centrifuge tube.
4. Add phosphate-buffered saline (PBS)-EDTA buffer to 10 ml and centrifuge at 1,500 × g for approximately 5 min.
5. Decant supernatant, resuspend cells gently in 2 ml of buffer, and repeat step B.4 twice.
6. Resuspend platelets in PBS-EDTA at approximately 200×10^9/liter. Store at 4°C for up to 2 weeks.

C. First incubation
1. For each sample to be tested, aliquot 100 µl of platelet suspension into a U-well microplate and spin at 1,500 × g in a benchtop microplate centrifuge for 3 min. Include two negative controls and one weakly positive control.
2. Decant supernatant and resuspend platelet pellets in 50 µl of test serum or plasma and incubate at 37°C for 30 min.
3. Wash platelets by adding 200 µl of PBS-EDTA to each test and centrifuge at 1,500 × g for 3 min. Resuspend platelet pellet by using a microplate shaker and wash once more.

D. Incubation with monoclonal antibody
1. Resuspend platelet pellets in 40 µl of diluted mouse monoclonal antibody (make sure cells are fully resuspended using a microplate shaker or pipette) and incubate for 30 min at 37°C.
2. Wash platelets three times.

E. Lysis
1. Lyse platelets by resuspending each pellet in 130 µl of solubilization buffer. Resuspend cell pellet using a pipette, *not* the microplate shaker, to avoid carryover. Incubate for 30 min at 4°C.
2. Block the coated F-well microplate; see steps A.4 and A.5 above.
3. Centrifuge microplate at maximum speed in a benchtop centrifuge (approximately 3,000 rpm) for 15 min at room temperature.

4. For each test, aliquot 130 μl of TBS wash buffer into a U-well microplate.
5. Remove 100 μl from each supernatant from step E.3 and dilute in 130 μl of TBS wash buffer from step E.4.

F. Attachment to solid phase
1. Transfer 100 μl of diluted platelet lysate, in duplicate, to a precoated and blocked well microplate; add 100 μl of TBS wash buffer to four to eight precoated wells on each plate (reagent blank). Incubate at 4°C for 90 min or overnight.
2. Wash microplate wells four times with 200 μl of TBS wash buffer.

G. Anti-IgG incubation
1. Add 100 μl of diluted peroxidase-labeled anti-human IgG to each well and incubate at 4°C for 90 min.
2. Wash microplate wells six times with 200 μl of TBS wash buffer. Blot top face of microplate dry between washes by placing on absorbent paper.

H. Color development
1. Add 100 μl of substrate solution to each well and leave plate at room temperature.
2. Stop the reaction by adding 100 μl of 0.5 M H_2SO_4 when a suitable color intensity has developed. Read the absorbance at 490 nm (for dual-wavelength enzyme-linked immunosorbent assay readers, a reference filter between 630 and 650 nm is suitable) within 1 h.

Note: Two-milliliter microcentrifuge tubes can be used instead of U-well microplates, in which case the centrifugation in step E.3 can be increased to >10,000 × g for 20 min at 4°C.

Specimen

Serum or EDTA- or citrate-collected plasma or platelets prepared from EDTA-anticoagulated whole blood are used.

Interpretation

1. Calculate the mean optical density for all controls and samples.
2. The positive cutoff is the mean of the negative control plus three standard deviations.
3. The positive control should be at least three times the optical density of the negative control.

REFERENCES

1. Berchtold, P., and M. Wenger. 1993. Autoantibodies against platelet glycoproteins in autoimmune thrombocytopenic purpura: their clinical significance and response to treatment. *Blood* **81:**1246–1255.
2. George, J. 1990. Platelet immunoglobulin G: its significance for the evaluation of thrombocytopenia and for understanding the origin of alpha granule proteins. *Blood* **76:**859–870.
3. George, J. N., M. A. El-harangue, and G. E. Rasion. 1995. Chronic idiopathic thrombocytopenia purpura. *N. Engl. J. Med.* **331:**1207–1211.
4. Harrington, W. J., V. Minnich, J. W. Hollingsworth, and C. V. Moore. 1951. Demonstration of a thrombocytopenic factor in the blood of patients with thrombocytopenic purpura. *J. Lab. Clin. Med.* **38:**1–10.
5. He, R., D. M. Reid, C. E. Jones, and N. R. Shulman. 1994. Spectrum of Ig classes, specificities and titers of serum antiplatelet glycoproteins in chronic idiopathic thrombocytopenia purpura. *Blood* **83:**1024–1032.
6. Herman, J. H., T. S. Kickler, and P. M. Ness. 1986. The resolution of platelet serologic problems using western blotting. *Tissue Antigens* **28:**257–268.
7. Kickler, T. S. 1994. Platelet immunology, p. 304–315. *In* K. L. Anderson and P. M. Ness (ed.), *Scientific Basis of Transfusion Medicine.* The W. B. Saunders Co., Philadelphia, Pa.
8. Kiefel, V., M. S. Santoso, E. Kaufmann, and C. Mueller Eckhardt. 1991. Autoantibodies against platelet glycoprotein Ib/IX: a frequent finding in autoimmune thrombocytopenic purpura. *Br. J. Haematol.* **79:**256–262.
9. Kiefel, V., M. S. Santoso, M. Weisheit, and C. Mueller Eckhardt. 1987. Monoclonal antibody-specific immobilization of platelet antigens (MAIPA): a new tool for the identification of platelet reactive antibodies. *Blood* **70:**1722–1726.
10. Kim, H. O., S. D. Kennedy, and T. S. Kickler. 1995. Studies using immobilized platelet glycoproteins for detection of platelet alloantibodies. *Am. J. Clin. Pathol.* **104:**258–263.
11. LoBuglio, A. F., W. S. Court, L. Vinocur, G. Maglott, and G. M. Shaw. 1983. Use of a ^{125}I labeled anti-human IgG monoclonal antibody to quantify platelet bound IgG. *N. Engl. J. Med.* **309:**459–463.
12. McMillan, R. 1990. Antigen-specific assays in immune thrombocytopenia. *Transfus. Med. Rev.* **14:**136–143.
13. McMillan, R., P. Tani, and F. Millard. 1987. Platelet associated and plasma antiglycoprotein autoantibodies in chronic ITP. *Blood* **70:**1040–1045.
14. Mueller-Eckhardt, C., and V. Kiefel. 1989. Laboratory methods for the detection of platelet antibodies and identification of antigens, p. 436–453. *In* T. J. Kunicki and J. N. George (ed.), *Platelet Immunobiology.* J. B. Lippincott, Philadelphia, Pa.
15. Rosse, W. F., D. V. Devine, and R. Ware. 1984. Reactions of immunoglobulin G-binding ligands with platelets and platelet-associated immunoglobulin G. *J. Clin. Investig.* **73:**489–496.
16. Shulman, N. R., V. J. Marder, M. C. Hiller, and E. M. Collier. 1964. Platelet and leukocyte isoantigens and their antibodies: serologic, physiologic and clinical studies, p. 222–304. *In Progress in Hematology,* 4th ed. Grune and Stratton, New York, N.Y.
17. Smith, J. W., C. P. M. Hayward, T. E. Warkentin, P. Horsewood, and J. G. Kelton. 1993. Investigation of human platelet alloantigens and glycoproteins using nonradioactive immunoprecipitation. *J. Immunol. Methods* **158:**77–85.
18. Tsubakio, T., P. Tani, V. L. Woods, and R. McMillan. 1987. Autoantibodies against platelet GPIIb/IIIa in chronic ITP react with different epitopes. *Br. J. Haematol.* **67:**345–348.
19. van Leeuwen, E. F., J. T. M. van der Ven, C. P. Engelfriet, and A. E. G. von dem Borne. 1982. Specificity of autoantibodies in autoimmune thrombocytopenia. *Blood* **59:**23–26.
20. Woods, V. L., E. H. Oh, D. Mason, and R. McMillan. 1984. Autoantibodies against the platelet glycoprotein IIb/IIIa complex in patients with chronic ITP. *Blood* **64:**368–375.

Monitoring Autoimmune Reactivity within the Retina

JOHN J. HOOKS, MARIAN S. CHIN, CHI-CHAO CHAN, AND BARBARA DETRICK

129

Immune-mediated vision loss is a rapidly expanding area of research and therapy. This chapter deals with the identification of antiretinal immune reactivity in patients with retinal diseases.

EYE: IMMUNE UNIQUE (PRIVILEGE) SITE

It is important to note that there are at least two major distinctive features of the eye. The first unique characteristic of the eye is easy visibility (17). When examining the eye, one has the remarkable advantage of being able to visualize inflammatory processes, vascular leakage, and cellular damage without using invasive procedures. Moreover, electrophysiological testing is easily performed and readily evaluates the retina's ability to respond to light stimulus. The second extraordinary feature of the eye is its immune status. The immune response that occurs within the eye is different from the systemic immune response, and this unique characteristic has been referred to as immune privilege. Several components contribute to this state. Anatomic features, such as the lack of lymphatic drainage and the presence of a blood-ocular barrier, limit access by the immune system. Additional factors contributing to immune uniqueness include limited expression of the major histocompatibility complex molecules; increased expression of the cell surface molecule CD57, which inhibits complement activation; local production of the immunosuppressive cytokine transforming growth factor β; and constitutive expression of the regulatory molecule FasL. Despite these remarkable features of ocular immunity, inflammatory processes do occur in the eye, and these are frequently referred to as uveitis. Uveitis is the fifth leading cause of vision loss in the world (18). Most ocular inflammatory processes that we recognize have a cellular component associated with them. Here, the severity of the inflammation can be graded by direct visualization of the inflammatory processes. The laboratory can be useful in identifying lymphocyte reactivity to specific retinal antigens and in distinguishing between primary intraocular lymphoma and inflammatory processes. We also know that antibody-mediated pathology can occur. Laboratory assays are designed to detect and characterize antiretinal antibody reactivity.

CLASSIC EXAMPLES OF AUTOIMMUNE DISEASE IN THE RETINA

Retinal autoimmunity exists as a naturally occurring disease in humans and as an experimentally designed animal model system. In humans, sympathetic ophthalmia (SO) is a classic example of a T-cell-mediated disease (4, 5). SO is an ocular inflammatory (autoimmune) disease that occurs after a perforating injury to one eye. The injured eye undergoes a massive lymphocytic granulomatous infiltration. At any time from the first week to several years following the trauma (peak is second week to 3 months), a spontaneous lymphocytic granulomatous infiltration occurs in the noninjured, "sympathizing" eye. Several studies have shown that the infiltrate consists predominantly of T cells. Today, SO is a rare disease; posterior uveitis is more frequently seen and is also associated with lymphocytic infiltrates that can be predominantly of T-cell origin. Within the retina, a number of uveitogenic antigens have been identified and characterized. Two of these, retinal S antigen (arrestin) and interphotoreceptor retinal binding protein (IRBP), have been used to develop a model of T-cell-mediated autoimmune ocular disease which is termed experimental autoimmune uveoretinitis. These retinal proteins are now utilized to monitor human T-cell reactivity to retinal tissue.

RETINOPATHIES ASSOCIATED WITH ANTIRETINAL ANTIBODIES

Human retinopathies associated with the production of antiretinal antibodies can be categorized into three groups: (i) visual paraneoplastic disorders, (ii) infection-associated retinopathies, and (iii) retinal degenerative disorders (Table 1).

Progressive blindness as a remote effect of cancer was first reported in 1976 (19). The two most frequently observed forms of visual paraneoplastic disorders are referred to as cancer-associated retinopathy (CAR) and melanoma-associated retinopathy (MAR). Clinical and experimental observations in CAR and MAR probably provide the best evidence for a pathological role of autoreactive antibodies in human retinopathies. First, affected patients suffer from a retinopathy that is characterized by retinal tissue damage and the presence of antiretinal antibodies. Second, some patients respond to plasma exchange and immunosuppressive therapy. Third, retinal cell damage can be induced by the autoreactive antibodies in vitro, and there is evidence of passive transfer of disease to animals (1, 10).

CAR is most commonly associated with small-cell carcinoma of the lung, but it has also been reported for patients with breast, endometrial, and other cancers (15, 21). In

TABLE 1 Antibody responses directed against retinal antigens in sera from patients with retinal diseases[a]

Retinal disease	Immunologic reactivity	Ag
Visual paraneoplastic disorders		
CAR	Photoreceptor outer segment	Recoverin (23 kDa), retinal enolase, TULP1, and others
MAR	Outer plexiform layer and INL	Bipolar cells
Infection-associated retinopathies		
Toxoplasmosis	Photoreceptor layer	Not known
Onchocerciasis	Neural retina and RPE	Cross-reactivity between *O. vulvulus* Ag (OV39) and RPE Ag (hr44)
Retinal degenerative diseases		
RP	Neural retina	Carbonic anhydrase II (30 kDa) and enolase (45 kDa)
RAR	Photoreceptor outer segment	Recoverin (23 kDa)
ARMD	Photoreceptors	Neurofilaments
Idiopathic retinopathy	Neural retina	Variety of retina Ags: S Ag, IRBP, and LEDGF
Neurologic disease (stiff man syndrome)	Neural retina	GAD

[a]Ag, antigen; RP, retinitis pigmentosa; RAR, recoverin-associated retinopathy; ARMD, age-related macular degeneration.

these patients, antibodies develop with reactivity to the retina, and this response is associated with rod and cone dysfunction. Visual loss occurs over months and may even precede the identification of the malignancy. Using immunofluorescent-antibody (IFA) assays on retinal tissue sections, one can demonstrate that sera from CAR patients react with the photoreceptor outer segments and ganglion cells. Analysis of retinal antigens has revealed that a variety of antigens may be involved in this process. The primary antigens identified are a 23-kDa antigen (recoverin), a retinal enolase (46 kDa), and a group of reactivities with retinal antigens identified as 40-, 43-, and 60-kDa molecules. Although over 15 retinal antigens have been described in the CAR syndrome, the most common antigen linked to CAR is the 23-kDa recoverin, a calcium-binding protein found in both rods and cones.

MAR is a second paraneoplastic syndrome that occurs in patients with melanoma (12, 14). Progressive visual loss develops over months and is frequently associated with metastatic cutaneous melanoma. Again, IFA technology can be used to identify antibody in MAR patient sera that reacts to bipolar cells in the outer nuclear layer and their dendrites in the outer plexiform layer of the retina.

The second group of retinopathies associated with antiretinal antibodies is retinal disorders that are triggered by an infectious agent (9). In humans, onchocerciasis and toxoplasmosis fall into this category. Infection with the nematode parasite *Onchocerca volvulus* can result in severe eye disease, often referred to as river blindness. It is estimated that approximately 18 million people in tropical Africa, the Arabian Peninsula, and Latin America are infected with this organism, and of these approximately 1 million to 2 million are blind or have severe visual impairment. Humans are infected with the helminth larvae by the bite of a black fly of the *Simulium* genus.

Posterior ocular onchocerciasis is characterized by atrophy of the retinal pigment epithelium (RPE), and as lesions advance, subretinal fibrosis occurs. A number of studies indicate that affected patients have antiretinal antibodies in

their sera and vitreous (6). Reactivity was observed in the inner retina and photoreceptor layers by IFA analysis. Characterization of the autoantigens revealed that a recombinant antigen in *O. volvulus* showed immunologic cross-reactivity with a component of the RPE. By Western blot analysis, an antibody to a 22,000-molecular-weight antigen (OV39) of *O. volvulus* recognized a 44,000-molecular-weight component (hr44) of the RPE cell. Although OV39 and hr44 are not homologous, they did show limited amino acid sequence identity. Immunizations of Lewis rats with either OV39 or hr44 induce ocular pathology. These studies indicate that molecular mimicry between *O. vovulus* and human RPE protein may contribute to the retinopathy found in patients with onchocerciasis (2, 13).

Toxoplasmosis, which occurs in over 500 million humans worldwide, is caused by the obligate intracellular parasite *Toxoplasma gondii*. *T. gondii* is also the most frequently identified infectious agent in posterior uveitis, and *Toxoplasma* retinochoroiditis is an important cause of blindness in young adults. Since the 1980s, several reports have documented a high prevalence of antiretinal antibodies in sera from *T. gondii*-infected patients (23). These antibodies are directed against the photoreceptor layer. Moreover, leukocytes from these patients have been shown to proliferate in response to retinal S antigen (16).

The third group of retinopathies associated with antiretinal antibodies is classified as the retinal degenerative disorders. These include retinitis pigmentosa with cystoid macula edema, recoverin-associated retinopathy, age-related macular degeneration, idiopathic retinopathies, and retinopathies associated with autoimmune neurologic diseases. Table 1 identifies serum antibody responses directed against retinal antigens in patients with retinal diseases. These are described in more detail in reference 10. Recently, we have characterized a subgroup of patients with retinal degenerative disease, referred to as a cone rod degeneration, that has reactivity to retinal ganglion and inner nuclear layer (INL) (Chin et al., unpublished data).

LABORATORY MONITORING OF ANTIRETINAL ANTIBODIES

Standard immunohistochemical assays or immunofluorescent assays are used to identify antibody reactivity within the retina. In addition to human retina, rodent (mouse or rat) or monkey eyes are frequently used as the substrate. After enucleation, eyes are immediately placed in OCT and frozen and stored at −70°C. Using a cryostat, whole rodent eye sections can be prepared and placed on SuperFrost slides. When using monkey or human eye tissue as the substrate, the frozen eye must be cut into smaller blocks of tissue before cryosections of the eye are cut. Slides containing the retina are stored at −70°C until used.

Procedure

1. Briefly, the standard procedure consists of fixing and permeabilizing the ocular tissue sections with acetone-methanol (1:1) and rinsing them with phosphate-buffered saline (PBS), pH 7.4. Endogenous peroxidase activity is quenched by incubating the sections in 0.6% H_2O_2 prior to incubating the tissue in a blocking solution. A standard blocking solution is 10% normal goat (NGS) or rabbit (NRS) serum in PBS. Bovine serum albumin, glycine, and/or cold-water fish gelatin can be added to the standard blocking solution if necessary to reduce nonspecific binding by the primary antibody.

2. Serial twofold dilutions of sera (1:40 to 1:640) from patients with retinal degeneration and healthy controls are incubated with the tissue sections either for 1 to 2 h at room temperature or overnight at 4°C.

3. Slides are washed in PBS with 1% NGS or NRS, and a dilution of the secondary antibody (horseradish peroxidase-conjugated anti-human immunoglobulin G) is applied to the tissue for 1 h.

4. Detection of bound immunoglobulin molecules is accomplished using a peroxidase substrate such as 3,3′-diaminobenzidine. Instead of horseradish peroxidase, the secondary antibody may be conjugated to alkaline phosphatase.

However, the peroxidase substrates produce more pronounced precipitates and give sharper localization than alkaline phosphatase substrates.

5. Slides are counterstained, dehydrated, and cleared and coverslips are mounted prior to examining the tissue sections under a microscope.

Interpretation

Studies in our laboratory demonstrate that immunofluorescence or immunocytochemical tests using rodent or monkey tissue and serum from individuals with no history of retinal disease are usually negative or reactive only at low serum dilution. In contrast, high titers of antibody are found in patients with selected retinal degenerative diseases. Sera from 18 healthy individuals demonstrated immunoreactivity to normal mouse ocular tissue in 33% of samples at a 1:40 dilution, in 13% of samples at a 1:80 dilution, and in 3% of samples at a 1:160 dilution, and no reactivity was noted at a dilution of 1:320 or 1:640. In contrast, in selected patients with retinal degenerative disorders we can detect reactivity in serum samples at dilutions of 1:160 to 1:1,280. Because the majority of the serum samples from healthy individuals did not show immunoreactivity to mouse ocular tissues at a dilution of 1:160 and the sera from patients with retinal degenerations were immunoreactive at a dilution of 1:1,280, we have selected 1:160 as the dilution that can discriminate between healthy individuals and patients with retinal degenerative disorders. It is interesting that this is similar to the dilution scheme used to discriminate antinuclear antibody reactivity in patients with systemic lupus erythematosus from positive antinuclear antibody results for healthy individuals (20).

Cellular location can be important to report. At least five patterns of immune reactivity are commonly observed: photoreceptor outer segments, INL, outer nuclear layer, ganglion cells, and RPE cells. In CAR patients, reactivity with the outer segment layer of photoreceptors is frequently seen and is associated with antirecoverin antibodies. In MAR patients, staining is frequently observed with bipolar cells in

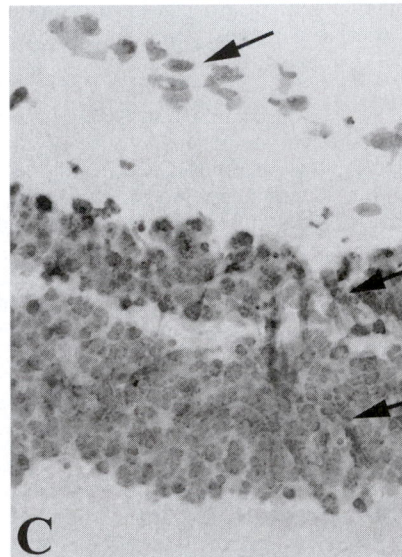

FIGURE 1 Immunohistochemical staining for antiretinal antibodies. Frozen sections of normal mouse retina were incubated with "normal" nonreactive human sera (A) or with sera from patients with retinal degenerative disease (B and C). Note reactivity with photoreceptor outer segments in panel B (arrowhead) or with ganglion cells (upper arrow), INL (middle arrow), and outer nuclear layer (lower arrow) in panel C.

the INL. An example of patterns of immune reactivity in the retina is shown in Fig. 1.

LABORATORY MONITORING OF T-CELL REACTIVITY

Procedure

1. Approximately 10 ml of heparinized or EDTA venous blood is needed for T-cell assays. Peripheral blood leukocytes (PBL) are recovered following Ficoll-Hypaque separation techniques. PBL are resuspended in RPMI medium supplemented with 5% (vol/vol) fetal bovine serum.

2. Determine the number of viable PBL by trypan blue exclusion. Adjust the cell concentration to 2×10^6 ml.

3. Deliver 100 µl of the cell suspension into triplicate wells of a 96-well plate.

4. Add 100 µl of stimulant or control as follows: medium (negative control), phytohemagglutinin or concanavalin A (positive control), and retinal antigen (S antigen or IRBP).

5. Incubate cells at 37°C for 72 h.

6. Assay the response of lymphocytes to stimulation by monitoring cell proliferation or production and release of cytokines. Cell proliferation assay can measure [^{3}H]thymidine incorporation into cellular DNA. Alternatively, one can use enzyme immunoassays (EIAs) to measure the release of gamma interferon or interleukin 2 (IL-2) in the supernatant fluid.

Interpretation

The appropriate incorporation of controls into these assay systems is essential for interpretation. PBL from a healthy individual (known nonresponder) should be used each time the test is performed. In addition, in each test a medium control (negative/baseline) and a T-cell stimulant (phytohemagglutinin, concanavalin A, etc.) must be included. When determining cell proliferation by [^{3}H]thymidine assay, the samples are evaluated by stimulation index (SI). The SI is obtained by dividing the counts per minute for retinal-antigen-treated cells by those for medium-treated cells. An SI of >2.0 is considered positive.

LABORATORY MONITORING OF OCULAR CYTOKINES (IL-6 AND IL-10)

Vitreous biopsies are frequently performed to distinguish between ocular inflammation associated with uveitis and ocular malignancy due to primary intraocular lymphoma (PIOL) or primary central nervous system lymphoma (PCNSL). Cells within the vitreous are collected by cytospin and evaluated by a cytopathologist to identify lymphoma cells. The majority of PIOLs and PCNSLs are diffuse large B-cell lymphomas (7, 11). These tumor cells produce high levels of IL-10, a growth and differentiation factor for B cells. In contrast, the inflammatory cells in uveitis produce high levels of IL-6, a proinflammatory cytokine. We and other investigators have found elevation of vitreal IL-10 with a ratio of IL-10 to IL-6 greater than 1 in PIOL (3, 8, 22, 24). Using this ratio analysis, the sensitivity and specificity of the assay are 75%. Evaluation of IL-10 and IL-6 concentrations in vitreous samples is performed using standard EIA methodology.

SUMMARY AND FUTURE DIRECTIONS

Analysis of immune-mediated vision loss is in its infancy. In patients with established retinal disease, the presence of autoantibodies can help define the nature of the disease and

provide markers to classify the disease and to monitor therapy. Today, laboratory monitoring of antiretinal antibodies is frequently used to assess patients with paraneoplastic syndrome. Laboratory monitoring of T-cell reactivity to retinal antigens is frequently used to assess uveitic patients undergoing immunomodulatory therapies. Finally, laboratory monitoring of ocular cytokines is frequently used to aid in the differential diagnosis of ocular inflammation and ocular malignancy.

Measurement of antiretinal immune reactivity is difficult to perform in the clinical laboratory. Analysis of immunocytochemical or immunofluorescent staining of retina tissue sections requires special training for interpretation. Nevertheless, with the characterization of specific retinal antigens, the future should include the development of standard EIA and Western blot assays to monitor patients with this form of vision loss.

REFERENCES

1. Adamus, G., M. Machnicki, H. Elerding, B. Sugden, Y. S. Blocker, and D. A. Fox. 1998. Antibodies to recoverin induce apoptosis of photoreceptor and bipolar cells in vivo. *J. Autoimmun.* 11:523–533.
2. Braun, G., N. M. McKechnie, and W. Gurr. 1995. Molecular and immunological characterization of hr44, a human ocular component immunologically cross-reactive with antigen Ov39 of Onchocerca volvulus. *J. Exp. Med.* 182:1121–1131.
3. Cassoux, N., H. Merle-Beral, P. Lehoang, C. Herbort, and C. C. Chan. 2001. Interleukin-10 and intraocular-central nervous system lymphoma. *Ophthalmology* 108:426–427.
4. Chan, C. C., and M. Mochizuki. 1999. Sympathetic ophthalmia: an autoimmune ocular inflammatory disease. *Springer Semin. Immunopathol.* 21:125–134.
5. Chan, C. C., R. B. Nussenblatt, L. S. Fujikawa, A. G. Palestine, G. Stevens, Jr., L. M. Parver, M. W. Luckenbach, and T. Kuwabara. 1986. Sympathetic ophthalmia. Immunopathological findings. *Ophthalmology* 93:690–695.
6. Chan, C. C., R. B. Nussenblatt, M. K. Kim, A. G. Palestine, K. Awadzi, and E. A. Ottesen. 1987. Immunopathology of ocular onchocerciasis. 2. Anti-retinal autoantibodies in serum and ocular fluids. *Ophthalmology* 94:439–443.
7. Chan, C. C., and D. J. Wallace. 2004. Intraocular lymphoma: update on diagnosis and management. *Cancer Control* 11:285–295.
8. Chan, C. C., S. M. Whitcup, D. Solomon, and R. B. Nussenblatt. 1995. Interleukin-10 in the vitreous of patients with primary intraocular lymphoma. *Am. J. Ophthalmol.* 120:671–673.
9. Hooks, J. J., B. Detrick, and R. Nussenblatt. 2004. Infections associated with retinal autoimmunity, p. 691–700. *In* Y. Shoenfeld and N. R. Rose (ed.), *Infection and Autoimmunity.* Elsevier, Amsterdam, The Netherlands.
10. Hooks, J. J., M. O. Tso, and B. Detrick. 2001. Retinopathies associated with antiretinal antibodies. *Clin. Diagn. Lab. Immunol.* 8:853–858.
11. Hormigo, A., L. Abrey, M. H. Heinemann, and L. M. DeAngelis. 2004. Ocular presentation of primary central nervous system lymphoma: diagnosis and treatment. *Br. J. Haematol.* 126:202–208.
12. Lei, B., R. A. Bush, A. H. Milam, and P. A. Sieving. 2000. Human melanoma-associated retinopathy (MAR) antibodies alter the retinal ON-response of the monkey ERG in vivo. *Investig. Ophthalmol. Vis. Sci.* 41:262–266.
13. McKechnie, N. M., W. Gurr, and G. Braun. 1997. Immunization with the cross-reactive antigens Ov39 from Onchocerca volvulus and hr44 from human retinal tissue

induces ocular pathology and activates retinal microglia. *J. Infect. Dis.* **176:**1334–1343.

14. **Milam, A. H., J. C. Saari, S. G. Jacobson, W. P. Lubinski, L. G. Feun, and K. R. Alexander.** 1993. Autoantibodies against retinal bipolar cells in cutaneous melanoma-associated retinopathy. *Invest. Ophthalmol. Vis. Sci.* **34:**91–100.

15. **Murphy, M. A., C. E. Thirkill, and W. M. Hart, Jr.** 1997. Paraneoplastic retinopathy: a novel autoantibody reaction associated with small-cell lung carcinoma. *J. Neuroophthalmol.* **17:**77–83.

16. **Nussenblatt, R. B., I. Gery, E. J. Ballintine, and W. B. Wacker.** 1980. Cellular immune responsiveness of uveitis patients to retinal S-antigen. *Am. J. Ophthalmol.* **89:**173–179.

17. **Nussenblatt, R. B., and S. M. Whitcup.** 2003. *Uveitis: Fundamentals and Clinical Practice*, 3rd ed. Mosby, Philadelphia, Pa.

18. **Resnikoff, S., D. Pascolini, D. Etya'ale, I. Kocur, R. Pararajasegaram, G. P. Pokharel, and S. P. Mariotti.** 2004. Global data on visual impairment in the year 2002. *Bull. W. H. O.* **82:**844–851.

19. **Sawyer, R. A., J. B. Selhorst, L. E. Zimmerman, and W. F. Hoyt.** 1976. Blindness caused by photoreceptor degeneration as a remote effect of cancer. *Am. J. Ophthalmol.* **81:**606–613.

20. **Tan, E. M., T. E. Feltkamp, J. S. Smolen, B. Butcher, R. Dawkins, M. J. Fritzler, T. Gordon, J. A. Hardin, J. R. Kalden, R. G. Lahita, R. N. Maini, J. S. McDougal, N. F. Rothfield, R. J. Smeenk, Y. Takasaki, A. Wiik, M. R. Wilson, and J. A. Koziol.** 1997. Range of antinuclear antibodies in "healthy" individuals. *Arthritis Rheum.* **40:**1601–1611.

21. **Thirkill, C. E., P. FitzGerald, R. C. Sergott, A. M. Roth, N. K. Tyler, and J. L. Keltner.** 1989. Cancer-associated retinopathy (CAR syndrome) with antibodies reacting with retinal, optic-nerve, and cancer cells. *N. Engl. J. Med.* **321:**1589–1594.

22. **Whitcup, S. M., V. Stark-Vancs, R. E. Wittes, D. Solomon, M. J. Podgor, R. B. Nussenblatt, and C. C. Chan.** 1997. Association of interleukin 10 in the vitreous and cerebrospinal fluid and primary central nervous system lymphoma. *Arch. Ophthalmol.* **115:**1157–1160.

23. **Whittle, R. M., G. R. Wallace, R. A. Whiston, D. C. Dumonde, and M. R. Stanford.** 1998. Human anti-retinal antibodies in toxoplasma retinochoroiditis. *Br. J. Ophthalmol.* **82:**1017–1021.

24. **Wolf, L. A., G. F. Reed, R. R. Buggage, R. B. Nussenblatt, and C. C. Chan.** 2003. Vitreous cytokine levels. *Ophthalmology* **110:**1671–1672.

CANCER

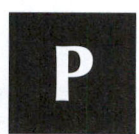

VOLUME EDITOR
ROBERT G. HAMILTON
SECTION EDITOR
MARK RAFFELD

Introduction

As succinctly stated by Winters et al. (chapter 134), "Cancer is a disease of dysregulated protein function and expression. Altered protein networks and signaling pathways drive the malignant phenotype, resulting in cell survival, invasion, and metastasis." The Cancer section in this 7th edition of the *Manual of Molecular and Clinical Laboratory Immunology* contains four chapters that focus on immunologic methods that are useful in detecting and quantifying proven and investigational tumor markers. These markers are mostly proteins that have proven or anticipated use in the diagnosis and management of cancer patients and patients receiving immunologic therapies. Where possible, molecular biology methods are introduced, and the Cancer section concludes with an exciting glimpse into the application of proteonomics in the quest to identify new cancer markers that will lead to enhanced diagnosis and management of oncology patients.

Diagnostic oncology and immunology laboratories all over the world currently measure a number of biomolecules released from tissue into body fluids that are markers of tumor presence and growth. The measurement of these analytes assists oncologists in making more accurate diagnoses and managing their patients with cancer, especially as it relates to monitoring therapy, detecting cancer recurrence, and assessing the patient's prognosis. This has been a challenging area of diagnostic immunology because most tumor markers are not elevated under all cancerous conditions and others are elevated under non-cancer conditions such as benign or nonmalignant disease. Fortunately, the concentrations of select tumor markers are known to correlate with tumor progression and aggressiveness. Rai and Chan overview the design and performance of several well-established tumor marker assays in chapter 131. They discuss the limitations and potential interferences of these assays within the context of three tumor marker examples: prostate-specific antigen (human kallikrein-3), a serine protease of ~33 kDa that is used to screen and monitor prostate cancer; cancer antigen 125, a membrane protein involved in ovarian cancer detection; and carcinoembryonic antigen, an oncofetal glycoprotein of ~200 kDa that is useful in assessment of colon and lung cancer.

Chapter 132 examines immunologic and molecular tumor markers that have been useful in the diagnosis and classification of malignancies of the immune system, namely, lymphomas and, to a lesser extent, non-lymphoid neoplasms that originate from cells involved in antigen presentation and processing. After an historical overview of the development of current classification schemes, Raffeld and Jaffe discuss the use of flow cytometry in quantifying the presence and density of cell surface markers and immunohistochemistry, using paraffin and frozen sections to visualize the immunologic phenotype of cancerous cells within the context of their in situ organization and cellular morphology. The authors highlight advances related to the availability of new monoclonal antibody specificities, molecular biology assays for clonality and molecular cytogenetic analyses involving in situ hybridization, and PCR-based assays for the detection of chromosomal translocations, chromosome copy number, gene copy number, and mRNA expression. Finally, the chapter provides an excellent overview of how these test results are interpreted within the context of the diagnostic algorithm for tumors of the immune system.

Chapter 133 focuses on the selection, performance, and quality control of immunological tests that are used to monitor the vast array of immunologic therapies involving monoclonal antibodies, cytokines, growth factors, activated cells, cellular products, immunotoxins, and immunomodulatory agents. Therapeutic use of these immunomodulating agents is designed to enhance capabilities of the innate and adaptive immune system to control disease. Whiteside overviews the design characteristics for clinical trials involving these biological agents. Selection of the appropriate specimens to assess the humoral and cellular compartments and timing of sample collection need to be tailored so that the specific hypothesis at the basis of the study is appropriately investigated. The chapter then highlights criteria for selecting the appropriate assays for soluble cell products (e.g., immunoglobulins, cytokines, complement components, lymphocyte receptors, enzymes); cell surface phenotypic markers and intracytoplasmic markers with flow cytometry; and assays that assess cell function. Emphasis is placed on the rationale behind systematic selection of the most informative assays, based on the specific hypothesis being tested and the design of appropriate controls to ensure assay quality.

Winters et al. complete the Cancer section by discussing the future of proteomics and immunoproteomics in cancer diagnostics. The proteome encompasses the large complement of expressed proteins some of which are overexpressed in cancerous cells. The goal of proteomics is to identify protein patterns and indicators of posttranslational modifications to proteins (e.g., phosphorylation, glycosylation, cleavage) in biological fluids that reflect abnormal or excessive cellular growth. Surface-enhanced laser-desorption ionization/time-of-flight (SELDI-TOF) mass spectroscopy and artificial-intelligence-based pattern recognition algorithms are combined to assess the complex patterns of the proteome. The chapter tantalizes the reader by introducing new technologies involving high-resolution mass spectrometers, isotope-coded affinity tag methods, and two-dimensional polyacrylamide gel electrophoresis run in tandem with mass spectrometry. Finally, examples of specific applications are presented, such as the identification of major histocompatibility class I and class II molecules that are associated with cancer cells, and the quantification of plasma telomerase, an enzyme detected in approximately 90% of all tumor types that is elevated in malignant cells.

Immunologic Approaches to Tumor Markers: Assays, Applications, and Discovery

ALEX J. RAI AND DANIEL W. CHAN

131

A tumor marker is defined as a molecule, whether protein or nucleic acid, from a tissue or body fluid, that can be used to determine the presence of a tumor (2). The first tumor marker, which was discovered in the 1800s, was used in the treatment of multiple myeloma (3). In recent decades, several additional markers have been identified by immunizing mice with extracts from cancerous cell lines or tumors derived from animals with malignancies. These explanted cells elicit immune responses in the new host, and the resulting antibodies are used to screen new samples. Many of the cancer antigens, e.g., cancer antigen 125 (CA-125), were discovered in this manner.

Today, tumor markers are used daily in diagnostic laboratories all over the world (see Table 1 for Food and Drug Administration-cleared tumor markers). Many clinicians rely on their measurement to monitor patient therapy and to detect cancer recurrence. In this chapter, we review the design, performance, and application of tumor marker assays; interferences; specific tumor markers; and the impact of new technologies on the discovery of novel tumor markers.

CLINICAL PARAMETERS AND CONSIDERATIONS IN THE USE OF TUMOR MARKER ASSAYS

Several terms are used in evaluating the performance of tumor marker assays (8). These include diagnostic sensitivity and specificity, and positive and negative predictive values. The diagnostic sensitivity of an assay reflects the fraction of those subjects with a specific disease that the assay correctly identifies as positive. The diagnostic specificity of an assay reflects the fraction of those subjects without the disease that the assay correctly identifies as negative. The positive predictive value refers to the probability that an individual with a positive test result has the disease. The negative predictive value corresponds to the probability that an individual with a negative result does not have the disease.

There is an inverse relationship between the sensitivity and specificity which is related to the assigned cutoff value that is used for a particular test to segregate diseased populations from those with no disease. In most populations, there is an overlap between the noncancer and cancer groups, since individuals without cancer may exhibit elevated levels of a marker and some individuals with cancer may not show elevations in a particular marker. Hence, the

cutoff value for a particular assay will determine the diagnostic sensitivity and specificity of the test based on the numbers of individuals that are diagnosed with and without disease.

The optimal cutoff value can be selected using a receiver operating characteristic curve, where the sensitivity is plotted against 1-specificity (false-positive rate). This analysis allows for the determination of the accuracy of a test by continuously varying the threshold over the entire range of values (11).

APPLICATIONS OF TUMOR MARKERS

The possible applications for tumor markers include screening, diagnosis, monitoring of therapy, detection of disease recurrence, and determination of prognosis. Each of these applications will be described further along with the ideal characteristics of the tumor markers that are required for each application.

Screening

An ideal screening test would identify those individuals in a population who have disease. However, most of the present tumor marker assays do not exhibit the appropriate sensitivity and specificity to be useful for this purpose. Many tumor markers are not elevated under all cancerous conditions (i.e., corresponding assays are not highly sensitive), and others are elevated under noncancerous conditions such as the presence of benign or nonmalignant disease (i.e., corresponding assays are not highly specific). Thus, the possibility of false-positive and false-negative results exists in the use of such markers for screening. The prevalence of most cancers in the population is low, but with the inappropriate sensitivity and specificity of some tumor marker assays, false-positive results may be generated. False-positive results can induce emotional and psychological distress in addition to an unnecessary and costly medical workup for the patient in question. However, there are limited cases in which screening for cancer within a population is possible, under particular conditions (Table 1).

Diagnosis

Diagnosis is the process by which an individual is investigated for the disease of interest. Most tumor marker assays lack the diagnostic sensitivity and specificity to be useful for

TABLE 1 Food and Drug Administration-approved tumor marker tests

Cancer type	Tumor marker(s)	Applications	Gene ontology classification
Breast	CA 15-3, CA 27.29	Detection of recurrence; monitoring of therapy and disease progression in metastatic disease	Membrane protein fragment
	HER-2/neu	Determination of prognosis; detection of recurrence; monitoring of therapy	Membrane protein (extracellular domain)
Prostate	Free PSA (fPSA), total PSA (tPSA), complexed PSA (cPSA)	Screening and diagnosis; detection of recurrence	Secreted protease
Ovarian	CA-125	Monitoring of therapy; determination of prognosis; detection of recurrence	Membrane protein fragment
Colorectal	CEA	Identification of patients with aggressive disease; determination of prognosis; detection of recurrence; monitoring of response to treatment	Membrane protein fragment
Pancreatic	CA 19-9	Monitoring of disease progress and response to therapy; detection of recurrence	Membrane protein fragment
Liver	Alpha fetoprotein (AFP)	Screening of high-risk populations (in conjunction with ultrasound); detection of residual disease; monitoring of therapy; detection of recurrence	Secreted protein
Bladder	NMP-22 (urine)	Detection of residual disease	Nuclear protein

this purpose. In select cases, tumor markers can be used as an adjunct to other diagnostic modalities in the detection of cancer. Possibilities for increasing the sensitivity and specificity for diagnosis include the use of multiple, instead of single, markers.

Monitoring of Treatment

Treatment monitoring is one of the most important applications of tumor markers in clinical use today. Remission and relapse of disease can be monitored by the fall and rise in concentrations of defined tumor markers. It is important to note that this monitoring should be done with serial samples measured by the same assay. Baseline values for a particular patient should be established, and evaluation of subsequent samples can use this value for comparison. It is important to note that different assays may produce different values. Such differences can be related to the use of antibodies with different specificities or other subtle variations in assay methodologies and instruments. It is also important to note that standardization among different assays may be difficult because of the use of different reagent systems or calibrators.

Concerns related to the diagnostic specificity of an assay also are important when the assay is used for monitoring treatment. Inflammation and/or illness can cause increases in levels of particular tumor markers, and a lack of assay specificity may be mistaken for relapse. Nevertheless, the success of surgery, treatment, and drug therapy has been effectively monitored using tumor marker assays. The rate at which the tumor marker falls or rises also provides important information. Surgical removal of the tumor should result in a dramatic fall of the tumor marker, consistent with its half-life.

In contrast, the rise in a tumor marker may indicate relapse; a steep increase may suggest that treatment is no longer effective and requires modification.

Detection of Recurrence of Disease

Once the patient has been diagnosed with disease, they often undergo surgery to remove the tumor. As the cancer type is already known, the specificity of the tumor marker assay becomes less of a concern. Sensitivity in this case becomes the critical factor since it is important to measure low concentrations of the analyte as an indicator of disease recurrence. The rate of increase can be used to dictate the frequency of testing, and it may influence the therapy that is prescribed.

The assay format and sample requirements make the measurement of tumor markers for the monitoring of disease recurrence a popular choice. The levels of certain circulating tumor markers have been shown to be increased before the appearance of other physical manifestations of tumor recurrence.

Determination of Prognosis

The ability of a particular tumor marker to assist in predicting the outcome of a patient's disease defines its application in determining prognosis. Concentrations of tumor markers are known to correlate with tumor progression and aggressiveness. Thus, high levels of a particular marker at the time of diagnosis may indicate a disease that has progressed rapidly and may be indicative of poor prognosis. Low levels of the same tumor marker indicate that the disease is still in its early stages or confined to a particular organ. More research is needed to better stratify good- and poor-prognosis patients by using levels of tumor markers.

Prediction of Therapeutic Response

Some tumor markers can act as surrogate markers for disease characterization, and thus, they can be used to aid clinicians in determining the most appropriate therapy. Examples include the use of estrogen receptor testing to predict response to chemotherapy and HER2/neu testing to predict response to specific cytotoxic agents.

IMMUNOASSAYS

In the 1950s, Michaelis and Menten and others elaborated on the specificities and kinetics of enzyme-substrate interactions. Clinical laboratorians sought to take advantage of these new findings by using enzymes as the basis for quantitative measurement of analytes. These were the first quantitative assays developed to measure specific molecules. It was later realized that the specificity of the antibody-antigen interaction is greater than that of the enzyme-substrate interaction and, therefore, the antibody-antigen interaction could also be exploited for the selective targeting of analytes.

Immunoassays take advantage of the unique properties of antibodies for the specific targeting of their cognate antigens. The antigen harbors an epitope, which is a region of the molecule recognized by a specific portion of the antibody, a region called the paratope. Antibodies can be employed for specific targeting of analytes in many complex biological matrices, including blood (whole or a portion thereof), urine, and other fluids. For an overview of immunoassays and their practical application, the reader is referred to reference 1 and chapter 3, this volume. Over the last few decades, there have been many improvements and advancements in the field of immunoassays, including developments in monoclonal antibody technology, availability of new solid phases, and the development of new labels for more sensitive detection (9).

TYPES OF IMMUNOASSAYS

Limited-Reagent Versus Excess-Reagent Assays

There are two major formats for immunoassays—limited-reagent and excess-reagent formats. Limited-reagent assays use a fixed amount of antibody that is not present in saturating amounts. This limited amount of antibody is captured in the microwell. Subsequently, the sample is added in the presence of a labeled antigen and a competition is thus established (Fig. 1). The antigens, both that in the sample and the labeled antigen, compete for the limited antibody binding sites. The greater the concentration of analyte in the sample, the fewer labeled molecules will bind and the lower the generated signal. Thus, there is an inverse relationship between the concentration of the antigen in the sample and the signal obtained. These competitive binding assays are particularly useful for smaller analytes which do not have a second epitope that is recognized by an antibody.

In the excess-reagent format, an excess quantity of antibody is used to bind an antigen. The most common version of these assays is the two-site immunometric assay ("sandwich" assay) (Fig. 2). This assay uses two antibodies to capture and detect the antigen. The capture antibody is present in excess and is bound to a solid phase. A sample is added containing the antigen of interest. Subsequently, a second antibody (detection antibody) is added. The latter reagent

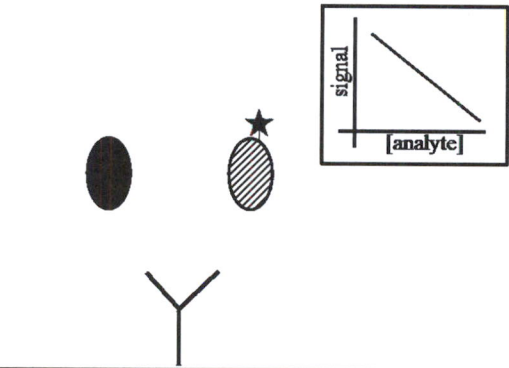

FIGURE 1 Competitive assay format. In this format, a labeled antigen is added in the presence of antigen from the sample. A competition is established, resulting in an inverse relationship between the sample concentration and the assay signal.

binds to a second, noninterfering epitope of the molecule of interest and forms a sandwich. Coupled to this detection antibody is a signal molecule, such as an enzyme, radioisotope, or fluorophore, which aids in detection. Addition of a substrate for the enzyme, or the measurement of radioactivity or fluorescence, is used to obtain a signal. This signal correlates with the level of the analyte of interest and provides accurate quantification. Most tumor marker assays in use today are monoclonal antibody-based noncompetitive immunometric assays.

For noncompetitive immunoassays, there are at least two format types that can be employed. Both are enzyme immunoassays, the first of which employs antibodies from two different species and the second of which uses two different monoclonal antibodies (see Fig. 2). In the first, two different antibodies are selected that target different epitopes on the antigen molecule. To increase the sensitivity of the system, one should select the polyclonal antibody for coating so that the greatest number of molecules present in the sample will be captured in the microwell. Only those that bind to the second detection antibody will be used in quantitation.

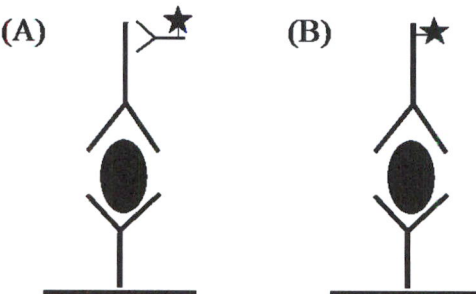

FIGURE 2 Sandwich enzyme-linked immunosorbent assay (ELISA) format. There are two alternatives for this design, as shown in the figure. In panel A, the analyte is sandwiched by the capture and detection antibodies, and a third antibody coupled to a signal molecule is added. An example of this format would be the use of two antibodies from two different species and a third universal reagent. In panel B, the detection antibody is directly coupled to the signal molecule; when it forms the sandwich, it can generate signal for quantification. An example of this format would be a custom antibody coupled to horseradish peroxidase.

In this one-step incubation procedure, the sample and detection antibodies are added simultaneously, resulting in greater sensitivity and a faster turnaround time relative to a two-step procedure. The hook effect may, however, occur when this format is used. In this situation, the concentration of analyte is too high and it results in a reduced signal (see below).

The second assay format uses a two-step procedure in which two different monoclonal antibodies target separate epitopes (Fig. 2B). The coating antibody captures the sample while the labeled detection antibody binds a different epitope of the same molecule.

CONSIDERATIONS FOR TEST DESIGN

In designing a clinical test, one must consider the test's intended use. Present tumor markers are used mostly for monitoring therapy. In this case, precision and a wide dynamic range are the most important performance parameters. In contrast, for assays detecting recurrence, sensitivity is the most important factor. At the core of optimizing each of these parameters is the appropriate selection of antibodies used in assay design.

Antibody Selection

Most tumor markers are present in very low concentrations in serum. Thus, assays are preferred that detect low levels of the specified analyte and that involve low cross-reactivity. These performance parameters are largely dependent on the antibodies used in assay. Ideally, the solid-phase antibody should be of high affinity. In the competitive format, there is only one antibody and it should be of high affinity and specificity.

The antigen that is measured should be the same as the antigen used for antibody production. Proteins are known to be present in many forms throughout the body. Their conformations change during periods of maturation, processing, secretion, and degradation, which can result in fragments that enter the circulation. Heterogeneity of the protein antigen can result in subtle differences that may manifest as altered biochemical characteristics, including the ability or inability to be bound by antibodies.

The specificity of the antigen-antibody interaction, coupled with the exquisite sensitivity of enhanced signal detection methods available today, makes immunoassays the method of choice in laboratory medicine. Quantitative measurements can be made from complex fluids, including serum, plasma, urine, and other body fluids.

INTERFERENCES IN IMMUNOASSAYS

An interference is defined as any condition that can cause a deviation of the measured value of an analyte from its true value (8a). There are a number of interferences which have been described. Most testing errors occur during the analytical phase and are related to bias and imprecision. In general, these can be minimized by good internal quality control procedures. However, there are errors that escape detection using even good quality control procedures. Thus, external proficiency checks are also needed for broader surveillance. There may also be endogenous errors that are caused by problems with the specimens. Some of these occur sporadically while others are specimen dependent. In these cases, clinical suspicion and error detection are facilitated by good communication with clinicians. Examples of interferences include those inherent to samples, cross-reactivity, the presence of antireagent antibodies, the presence of rheumatoid factor, and the high-dose-antigen hook effect (see reference 8a).

Types of Analytical Errors

- Sample interferences, e.g., lipemic specimens. In some cases, specimens from fasting subjects are preferred over lipid-rich specimens. The results obtained from postprandial samples need to be treated with caution, as the excess lipids may interfere with the immunoassay. Other examples of sample interferences include hemolyzed or icterus specimens, which can cause falsely low or high results for particular analytes and assays.

- Cross-reactivity. Errors relating to cross-reactivity can be either positive or negative. These are less likely to occur with the use of monoclonal antibodies than with polyclonal antibodies. The former are directed towards a single epitope, and the latter target multiple epitopes. These errors are also less likely with two-site immunometric assays, which employ two noninterfering epitopes on the same molecule and, hence, confer greater specificity. However, even in the latter case, some analytes, e.g., glycoprotein hormones, are still problematic.

- The presence of antireagent antibodies. Antireagent antibodies bind both the capture and detection antibodies and can form an immune complex. These interfering antibodies produce either a negative or positive result, depending upon the assay design. Nonimmune immunoglobulin G (IgG) can be used to quench this reaction and suppress interference. However, the amount of IgG required will need to be determined empirically. Heterophilic antibodies are produced mostly against animal Igs. The production of some of these antibodies may be iatrogenic (see the example of human anti-mouse antibody interference described below). They have been characterized in individuals such as farm workers that have been exposed to animals, individuals that have a large number of pets, and also individuals that consume large quantities of dairy products. In the last case, there is a transfer of dietary antigens through the gut wall, which elicits an immune response. Some individuals may also experience a similar heterophilic antibody response if they have been recently treated with pharmaceutical or diagnostic remedies derived from animals, e.g., cancer patients that are treated therapeutically with mouse antibodies. Human anti-mouse antibodies can interfere with immunoassays, particularly tumor marker assays. Patients treated with these antibodies harbor antibodies to the animal Igs in their blood, and thus, their sera interfere in laboratory assays that employ mouse antibodies.

- The presence of rheumatoid factor. Rheumatoid disease produces autoantibodies that can bind to the Fc fragment of assay antibodies. These autoantibodies are usually of low affinity and can cause a problem in assays based on turbidimetry, latex particles, and agglutination. Several possibilities for circumventing the interferences exist, including the use of blocking agents, dilution studies, testing for the presence of autoantibodies, the use of other methods to check questionable results, and the use of other samples such as serum or urine to measure and verify the presence of the same analyte.

- The presence of protein complexes. This interference is not abolished by nonimmune serum and is caused by the presence of oligomeric complexes of the target protein. Discrepant results have been anecdotally described in the case of prolactin, specific steroids, and troponin, among others.

- The hook effect. The hook effect occurs when there is an excess of antigen present in the sample. This can occur

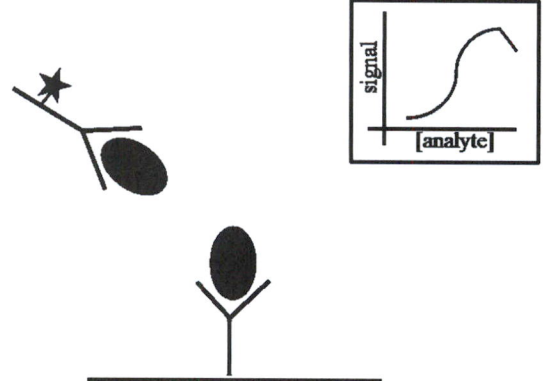

FIGURE 3 Hook effect. Excess analyte results in the binding of both antibodies, but no signal is generated.

with an analyte whose concentration can vary widely, such as a tumor marker. When there is an excess of antigen in the sample, the capture and detection antibodies will both bind to the antigen, but a sandwich will not be formed (Fig. 3). Thus, the signal obtained from such an event will not be proportional to the amount of antigen present but instead will be lower than expected. A true result can be measured by subsequent dilution and reassay of the sample.

Erroneous results are sometimes subtle and may not be questioned. However, they can have serious consequences, and thus it is important to limit immunoassay interferences. To circumvent the issues of interference, there are a number of possible solutions. In the case of heterophilic antibodies, one can use blocking reagents, which are commercially available. Simply preincubating the patient's sample with blocking solution prior to measuring the sample by immunoassay should remove the interference. Another approach is specimen dilution. If a linear response is not observed, then it is likely that there is interference. Another option is to use a different antibody or a different assay (preferably employing a different methodology) to reassay the sample. Depending on the nature of the interfering substance, it may or may not produce a similar result when reassayed.

ILLUSTRATIVE TUMOR MARKERS

Three representative tumor markers will now be discussed: prostate-specific antigen (PSA), a secreted molecule useful in the assessment of prostate cancer; CA-125, a membrane protein involved in ovarian cancer detection; and carcinoembryonic antigen (CEA), an oncofetal antigen which is useful in the assessment of colon and lung cancer.

PSA

PSA, also known as human kallikrein 3 (hK3), is a serine protease of ~33 kDa. It is a member of the hK family, which comprises approximately 15 genes located on chromosome 19 (6). Many of the proteins encoded by this locus are expressed highly in the prostate, including hK2, hK4, and hK15, in addition to PSA. As a secreted protein, PSA undergoes maturation during its progression through the secretory pathway in prostate epithelial cells. It is initially expressed in a "prepro" form in these cells. This prepro protein contains a 17-amino-acid signal sequence which is later removed to form proPSA. This proPSA molecule is inactive

but is targeted for cleavage by hK2, expressed in the prostate lumen ducts. The hK2 protease cleaves PSA and converts it into its mature form of 237 amino acids. It is this mature molecule that is secreted into the serum, where it forms complexes with other circulating proteins.

PSA plays an important role in the treatment of prostate cancer. It is one of the only markers employed for cancer detection. It is also used to monitor therapy and to detect the recurrence of disease. PSA is known to be elevated in the presence of prostate cancer but can also be elevated under benign conditions of this organ, such as benign prostatic hyperplasia and prostatitis. The reference value for normal individuals is <4 ng/ml, whereas levels of >10 ng/ml usually indicate the presence of disease. Levels between 4 and 10 ng/ml correspond to the diagnostic grey zone. At these values, it is difficult to assess cancer presence and it is helpful to assess additional analytes to evaluate the presence of disease, including specific forms of PSA. PSA exhibits significant heterogeneity in serum. While some assays measure total PSA (tPSA), other fractions can be measured. The majority of PSA protein circulates in the serum as a complex with protease inhibitors. The main protease inhibitors include α1-antichymotrypsin, α1-protease inhibitor, and inter-α-trypsin inhibitor. This complexed PSA corresponds to 70 to 90% of tPSA, and the remaining 10 to 30% is unbound and is known as free PSA (fPSA). This fPSA component can be further fractionated into additional forms—proPSA, benign prostatic hyperplasia-associated PSA, and intact PSA. Recent studies using two-dimensional gel electrophoresis suggest that there are additional protein variants in this fraction that are less appreciated (5). It is desirable to have fPSA levels as high as possible, preferably >25%. fPSA values of <10% are usually associated with disease.

CA-125

CA-125 was first identified and characterized with a murine monoclonal antibody raised against an antigen from an ovarian cancer cell line. The antigen is associated with a large glycoprotein of >200 kDa that resides in the plasma membrane. CA-125 is elevated in >80% of nonmucinous epithelial ovarian cell cancers, the most common of which are serous ovarian cancers. In contrast, it is not usually elevated in individuals with nonserous ovarian cancers, including mucinous, endometriod, and clear cell carcinomas. It is widely used for the assessment of ovarian cancer, although it can be elevated in individuals suffering from benign conditions such as inflammatory conditions, pregnancy, menstruation, and endometriosis. Presently, it is widely used in the monitoring of therapy and follow-up in ovarian cancer.

CA-125 levels have been shown to decrease during tumor regression and increase with tumor progression. Once ovarian cancer patients are treated with chemotherapy, a baseline value can be measured and they can be tested periodically by CA-125 measurement. A rise in the level of CA-125 can be used to detect recurrent or metastatic disease, even before clinical signs are evident. The lead time of CA-125 elevation before the clinical progression of disease has been shown to range between 1 and 15 months. However, it is not yet clear whether this lead time translates into improved patient outcomes or a better quality of life for patients.

Recently, the gene which encodes CA-125, *MUC16*, was cloned. It resides on chromosome 19. The encoded polypeptide consists of three domains—the carboxy-terminal, extracellular, and amino-terminal domains. There are a number of commercial assays that measure CA-125. They utilize a limited number of antibodies and target various fragments of the CA-125 molecule. Values of >35 U/ml are considered to be elevated and associated with disease.

CEA

CEA was one of the first tumor markers described. It is a glycoprotein of approximately 200 kDa and belongs to the class of tumor markers that are oncofetal antigens. It is expressed in the fetal and embryonic gut, but its expression usually stops before birth so it is not present in normal, healthy adults.

It has been widely used in the treatment of individuals with colon cancer and lung cancer but may also be present in individuals with pancreatic, breast, and ovarian cancers. It has also been shown to be elevated under nonmalignant conditions including chronic obstructive pulmonary disease, cirrhosis, ulcerative colitis, and Crohn's disease. It is increased in the bloodstreams of smokers relative to those of nonsmokers.

CEA is one of several similar antigens which were first described in the 1960s by Gold and Freedman (4). It was initially thought to be specific to gastrointestinal cancers but was later shown to be more nonspecific. Its applications include determining whether cancer is localized or metastatic (particularly for colon cancer), monitoring cancer treatment, and also checking for recurrence.

There are presently several assays available for CEA, and the reference intervals vary among assays. The reference interval is usually 0 to 3 ng/ml for nonsmokers and 0 to 5 ng/ml for smokers. Levels of >20 ng/ml are highly suggestive of cancer.

RECENT DEVELOPMENTS IN TUMOR MARKER DISCOVERY

Single Markers Versus Multiple Markers

It has become evident during the last ~15 years that single markers will not likely be able to distinguish between diseased and nondiseased groups. Instead, it is more likely that a multimarker panel will be more useful in segregating these populations (10). Much of this situation may be due to the fact that cancer is a heterogeneous disease. There are subtypes of cancers, each characterized by mutations in different genes causing activation and inactivation of different signal transduction pathways and resulting in different phenotypes. Thus, it is appropriate that over the last few years, new technologies with the ability to simultaneously investigate the expression of hundreds of genes or proteins have been developed. These technologies include the use of nucleic acid arrays and protein-based methods and are described in more detail in subsequent paragraphs and in other reports (e.g., reference 7). These techniques will become the new tumor marker assays of the future. The new approaches use the power of multiple markers, whereas the previous methods and assays measured only single entities.

NEW TECHNOLOGIES

cDNA- or Oligonucleotide-Based Arrays

Gene expression analyses have been used for the last 7 to 8 years to identify differences in gene expression levels between two samples. Although differences can be identified, it is important to verify the alteration at the protein level, as proteins are the functional workhorses in the cell. Furthermore, RNA levels and protein levels do not necessarily correlate well. Thus, a protein-based detection method

should be used as an adjunct to confirm alterations that are suspected based on genetic assessments.

Protein-Based Methods: Mass Spectrometry, Gel Electrophoresis, and Antibody Arrays

With regard to protein-based methods for tumor marker discovery, there have been tremendous advancements over the last 10 to 20 years. Most discovery paradigms comprise several steps, including protein separation, bioinformatics analysis, protein identification and characterization, database searching, and verification of alterations. With each of these steps, there have been advancements over the last few years that have enhanced our ability to detect more proteins. Protein separation has been enhanced through the use of newly developed reagents such as improved detergents for greater protein solubility, better reducing agents, improved protocols, and commercially available kits for protein fractionation and improvements in two-dimensional gel technology allowing for greater reproducibility. Taken together, these advances allow us to visualize a greater portion of the proteome than previously possible.

With regard to bioinformatics, there has been great progress. First, there are newly developed algorithms that allow us to analyze large volumes of data from high-throughput experiments. The algorithms employ one of many procedures for the analysis of data. Multiple procedures are available and can be selected for custom applications (10). Nucleotide and protein databases are another aspect of bioinformatics that has contributed greatly to the assessment of the human genome and proteome. The genomes of a number of organisms have been completely sequenced, and gene or protein candidates can now be mapped to cDNA or genes, with the corresponding full-length proteins being identified. The presence of orthologs from different species can also be quickly determined for follow-up studies and for in-depth functional analyses using genetically tractable organisms.

Lastly, protein identification methods have advanced over the last ~15 years. High-resolution instrumentation, e.g., the Pro-TOF mass spectrometer (Perkin Elmer), and new methods, e.g., FTICR-MS (Fourier transform ion-cyclotron resonance-mass spectrometry), allow for the precise measurement of peptides, affording unambiguous identification of peptides after protease digestion.

FUTURE PROSPECTS

The future looks hopeful for the discovery of new tumor markers. With the completion of the sequencing of the human genome, strides are being made in the characterization of the human proteome and there are advancements in high-throughput nucleic acid and protein analysis technologies. It is envisioned that these advancements will help identify new tumor markers with greater capabilities that can be used alone or in combination with other markers or diagnostic modalities with greater accuracy than was previously possible. The increased sensitivity and specificity will result in the development of improved assays for tumor markers. This will provide the laboratorian and clinician with earlier and more accurate information on cancer biomarkers and the prospects of translation into improved patient care.

REFERENCES

1. **Chan, D. W. (ed.).** 1987. *Immunoassay: a Practical Guide.* Academic Press Inc., San Diego, Calif.
2. **Chan, D. W., and M. K. Schwartz.** 2002. Tumor markers: introduction and general principles, p. 9–18. *In* E. P. Diamandis, H. A. Fritsche, H. Lilja, D. W. Chan, and

M. K. Schwartz (ed.), *Tumor Markers: Physiology, Pathobiology, Technology, and Clinical Applications.* AACC Press, Washington, D.C.

3. **Diamandis, E. P.** 2002. Tumor markers: past, present, and future, p. 3–8. *In* E. P. Diamandis, H. A. Fritsche, H. Lilja, D. W. Chan, and M. K. Schwartz (ed.), *Tumor Markers: Physiology, Pathobiology, Technology, and Clinical Applications.* AACC Press, Washington, D.C.

4. **Gold, P., and S. O. Freedman.** 1965. Demonstration of tumor specific antigens in human colonic carcinomata by immunological tolerance and absorption techniques. *J. Exp. Med.* **121:**439–462.

5. **Jung, K., J. Reiche, A. Boehme, C. Stephan, S. A. Loening, D. Schnorr, W. Hoesel, and P. Sinha.** 2004. Analysis of subforms of free prostate-specific antigen in serum by two-dimensional gel electrophoresis: potential to improve diagnosis of prostate cancer. *Clin. Chem.* **50:**2292–2301.

6. **Lilja, H.** 2003. Biology of prostate-specific antigen. *Urology* **62**(Suppl. 5A):27–33.

7. **Rai, A. J., and D. W. Chan.** 2004. Cancer proteomics: serum diagnostics for tumor marker discovery. *Ann. N. Y. Acad. Sci.* **1022:**286–294.

8. **Solberg, H. E.** 2001. Establishment and use of reference values, p. 251–261. *In* C. A. Burtis and E. R. Ashwood (ed.), *Tietz Fundamentals of Clinical Chemistry.* W. B. Saunders, Philadelphia, Pa.

8a. **Sturgeon, C. M.** 2002. Limitations of assay techniques for tumor markers, p. 65–81. *In* E. P. Diamandis, H. A. Fritsche, H. Lilja, D. W. Chan, and M. K. Schwartz (ed.), *Tumor Markers: Physiology, Pathobiology, Technology and Clinical Applications.* AACC Press, Washington, D.C.

9. **Wu, J. T.** 2000. *Quantitative Immunoassay: a Practical Guide for Assay Establishment, Troubleshooting, and Clinical Application.* AACC Press, Washington, D.C.

10. **Zhang, Z.** 2002. Combining multiple markers in clinical diagnostics: a review of methods and issues, p. 133–140. *In* E. P. Diamandis, H. A. Fritsche, H. Lilja, D. W. Chan, and M. K. Schwartz (ed.), *Tumor Markers: Physiology, Pathobiology, Technology, and Clinical Applications.* AACC Press, Washington, D.C.

11. **Zweig, M. H., and G. Campbell.** 1993. Receiver operating characteristic plots: a fundamental tool in clinical medicine. *Clin. Chem.* **39:**561–577.

Malignancies of the Immune System: Use of Immunologic and Molecular Tumor Markers in Classification and Diagnostics

MARK RAFFELD AND ELAINE S. JAFFE

132

Malignancies of the immune system are primarily represented by the malignant lymphomas and a smaller number of non-lymphoid neoplasms that originate from cells involved in antigen presentation and processing. The diagnosis and classification of these tumors have benefited enormously from advances in cellular and molecular immunology, as well as from careful dissection of the molecular genetics of the cancers themselves. Our ability to correctly diagnose tumors of the immune system, which in many instances show little morphological variation, requires the careful application of both immunologic tumor markers and molecular (DNA- or RNA-based) tumor markers. Therefore, malignancies of the immune system not only are interesting models of normal immune cells but also are excellent examples of the variety of molecular and immunologic approaches for assessing cancers.

The classification of the malignant lymphomas and non-lymphoid tumors of immune cells has undergone significant reappraisal over the past 40 years. Early classification systems of malignant lymphomas, such as the Rappaport classification and the Working Formulation, were based on architectural and cytological characteristics of the neoplastic elements (71, 82). However, with increasing knowledge of the complexity of the immune system a more functional approach was sought. The next generation of classification schemes (Kiel, and Lukes and Collins) attempted to integrate immunologic function with morphological parameters, with the premise that each of the lymphomas was an expansion of normal cellular counterparts (34, 65). These classification schemes still relied heavily upon the ability to correlate cytological characteristics of tumor cells with the cytological characteristics of normal counterparts. In practice, this proved to be an extremely difficult endeavor, even for experienced hematopathologists, and it became apparent that a more objective and reproducible classification scheme was needed. The decades from the 1970s through the 1990s saw an explosion of basic information in both cellular and molecular immunology, and in cancer genetics. The application of monoclonal antibodies, developed in the course of studying the normal immune system, provided one powerful approach for establishing objective diagnostic criteria, while the development of molecular testing based on rapid advances in the molecular genetic understanding of these tumors provided a second approach. By incorporating these technologies into the diagnostic armamentarium, it became possible to develop a more objective classification scheme that would take into account the molecular and immunologic characterization of the tumors.

In 1994 the International Lymphoma Study Group, a consortium of hematopathologists from the United States and Europe, met and concluded that a classification system should consist of a list of agreed-upon disease entities defined by multiple parameters, rather than being driven by a single overriding principle, such as clinical outcome (Working Formulation) or cellular differentiation (Kiel). For the first time immunophenotype and molecular genotype were recognized as critical elements in establishing a biologically meaningful classification scheme (39). This breakthrough meeting led to the development of the first modern lymphoma classification system based upon biological principles, the REAL classification, and its successor, the current World Health Organization (WHO) classification (Table 1) (48).

A major premise underlying the current classification systems was that lineage must be the starting point for a lymphoma classification. The application of modern immunologic techniques and concepts has permitted the development of a conceptual framework that may be used to decipher the morphological diversity of these neoplasms and has shown the relationship of lymphoid and mononuclear phagocytic neoplasms to the normal immune and hematopoietic systems. The development of monoclonal antibodies reactive with lymphoid, monocytic, and myeloid subsets can be used in the classification, primary diagnosis, and staging of hematopoietic malignancies and as adjunctive tools for immunotherapy in both in vivo and in vitro settings. In addition, many disease entities, particularly among the B-cell lymphomas, have a highly specific immune profile that can aid greatly in differential diagnosis. Other markers associated with lineage and cellular differentiation help to relate the various lymphoproliferative disorders to distinct stages in the development of the normal immune cells, and they are of particular interest in evaluating lymphoblastic neoplasms and in differentiating germinal-center (GC) from postgerminal-center B-cell neoplasms. Monoclonal antibodies to oncogene or tumor suppressor gene products such as cyclin D1, BCL-2, and p53 have also proved useful in diagnosis and prognostication, and in understanding the pathogenetic mechanisms of lymphomagenesis.

The WHO and REAL classification schemes also recognized the importance of cytogenetic and correlative

TABLE 1 WHO classification of lymphoid neoplasms

B-cell neoplasms
    Precursor B-cell neoplasm
        Precursor B-lymphoblastic leukemia/lymphoma
    Mature (peripheral) B-cell neoplasms
        SLL/CLL
            B-cell prolymphocytic leukemia
            LPL
            Splenic MZL (with or without villous lymphocytes)
            Hairy cell leukemia
            Plasma cell myeloma/plasmacytoma
            Extranodal MZL of MALT type
            Nodal MZL (with or without monocytoid B cells)
            FCL
            MCL
            DLBCL
                Mediastinal large-B-cell lymphoma
                Primary effusion lymphoma
                Intravascular large-B-cell lymphoma
            Burkitt lymphoma/Burkitt cell leukemia

T- and NK-cell neoplasms
    Precursor T-cell neoplasm
        Precursor T-lymphoblastic lymphoma/leukemia
    Mature (peripheral) T-cell and NK-cell neoplasms
        T-cell prolymphocytic leukemia
        T-cell granular lymphocytic leukemia
        Aggressive NK-cell leukemia
        ATL(HTLV-1$^+$)
        Extranodal NK/T-cell lymphoma, nasal type
        Enteropathy-type T-cell lymphoma
        Hepatosplenic T-cell lymphoma
        Subcutaneous panniculitis-like T-cell lymphoma
        Mycosis fungoides/Sézary syndrome
        ALCL, T/null cell, primary cutaneous type
        PTL, not otherwise characterized
        AILT
        ALCL, T/null cell, primary systemic type

molecular genetic abnormalities in contributing to the pathogenesis of particular entities. At the time the REAL classification was proposed, it had become clear that certain lymphoid neoplasms possess recurrent cytogenetic abnormalities involving oncogenes or tumor suppressor genes that play key roles in the pathogenesis of particular tumors. Many of the morphological entities that hematopathologists had long recognized were found to be associated with specific translocations, such as the t(8;14) translocation and its variants that involve the c-MYC gene in Burkitt's lymphoma (20), the t(11;14) translocation that involves the cyclin D1 gene in mantle cell lymphoma (MCL) (114), and the t(14;18) translocation that involves the BCL-2 gene in the vast majority of follicle center lymphomas (104). These associations not only validated the morphological component of the classification scheme but also enabled the further development and refinement of categories of lymphomas that were difficult to separate by morphology alone. The continued molecular dissection of lymphomas has further revealed characteristic cytogenetic and molecular genetic abnormalities in mucosa-associated lymphoid tissue (MALT) lymphomas, in anaplastic large-cell lymphomas (ALCLs), and in plasma cell neoplasms, as well as in many other lymphoma subtypes. The development of molecular technologies, particularly fluorescent in situ hybridization (FISH) and PCR,

has brought molecular diagnostics into the routine clinical laboratory and has enabled molecular genotyping to increasingly become a part of the classification criteria.

MOLECULAR AND IMMUNOLOGIC TESTS UTILIZED IN LYMPHOMA DIAGNOSTICS

Immunologic Approaches

Lymphoid and histiocytic neoplasms can be studied in fluid phase by flow cytometry or in paraffin or frozen sections by immunohistochemistry. Flow cytometry is particularly useful in assessing cell surface markers and has the advantage of being able to provide semiquantitative information regarding antigen density. Furthermore, advances in fluorescent-dye chemistry and in laser technology have made the simultaneous detection of multiple antigens routine (9). The disadvantages of flow cytometry are that in situ tissue organization is lost and the detection of cytoplasmic and nuclear antigens is technically challenging, requiring permeabilization of the cells during specimen processing. In addition, cell suspensions may not be representative of the pathological process due to fibrosis or abundant stromal elements, and specimens must be processed at the time of procurement, necessitating careful planning when obtaining the sample.

In contrast to flow cytometry, immunohistochemical techniques allow one to visualize the immunologic phenotype in the context of the in situ organization and cellular morphology. This approach is useful when one considers that lymphomas are rarely pure populations of neoplastic cells, and that a variety of normal cell types are invariably present. Moreover, in some situations, such as in Hodgkin's disease (HD) and T-cell-rich large-B-cell lymphomas, the neoplastic cells represent a minority of the cells present. Such minor populations of cells may be difficult to study by flow cytometry but can be easily identified by the combination of immunohistochemistry and morphology.

In recent years, an increasing number of mouse monoclonal antibodies have become available for use in paraffin sections, eliminating the need to perform immunohistochemistry on frozen tissue sections (Table 2). The development of these reagents has occurred not by chance, but rather by targeting the antigenic conformations present in fixed tissues (67). Another important advance in immunohistochemistry has been the recent development of rabbit monoclonal antibodies (95). These antibodies generally have a much higher affinity than comparable mouse monoclonal antibodies and have shown great promise for diagnostic applications (89).

Paraffin section immunohistochemistry has also been greatly facilitated by the development of heat-induced antigen retrieval techniques (57, 93). Previous antigen retrieval techniques involving chemicals or proteolytic enzymes had relatively limited success in diagnostic immunohistochemistry, beyond their ability to improve intermediate filament staining. Heat-induced antigen retrieval procedures proved to have broad applicability, allowing for the detection of numerous antigens rendered nonreactive during the fixation and paraffin embedding processes. The advances in antigen retrieval techniques eliminated the need for the specialized processing at the time of surgical removal and made it possible for immunophenotyping to be performed on all diagnostic biopsy specimens. There are excellent reviews of both flow cytometry and immunohistochemistry in chapters 20 and 47 of this manual.

TABLE 2 Antigens detectable in paraffin sections by immunohistochemistry[a]

Antigen (antibody)	Immune cells and/or tumor cells detected
CD20 (L-26)	B cells, L&H cells, RS cells +/−
CD79a (mb-1)	Pre-B cells, B cells, plasma cells
Kappa, lambda	Pre-B cells +/− (cytoplasmic), B cells, plasma cells
CD3	T cells
CD45RO	Memory T cells
CD43	T cells, some B cells, myeloid cells
CD15	Granulocytes, RS cells
CD30	RS cells, ALCL, immunoblasts
MPO	Myeloid cells
CD68	Histiocytes, myeloid cells
TdT	Lymphoblasts
MIB-1/Ki-67	Proliferating cells
Bcl-2	Useful in differential diagnosis of FH vs. FL Negative in GCs, positive in FL and other low-grade lymphomas
CD4, CD8	T-cell subsets
CD5	T cells, CLL, MCL
CD10	FL, follicle center cells, AILT
BCL6	Normal and neoplastic GC cells
IgD	Mantle cells, MCL, SMZL
CD21	FDCs, AILT
CD23	FDCs, CLL
CD1a	LC, cortical thymocytes
TIA-1, perforin, granB	Cytotoxic T cells, NK cells
CD56	NK cells, nasal T/NK-cell lymphoma, γδ TCL
CD57	Cytotoxic T cells, NK cells
LMP-1	RS cells, EBV + cells with latency 2 and 3 phenotypes
EMA	ALCL, plasma cells, L&H cells
Clusterin	ALCL, FDCs, FDC neoplasms
CD-99	Lymphoblastic lymphoma, Ewing's sarcoma
Langerin	LC and related neoplasms
Cyclin D1	MCL, HCL (weak)
ALK	ALCL
MUM-1	Subpopulation of GC B cells and plasma cells
p53	Tumor suppressor gene, accumulates when mutated

[a]Abbreviations: MPO, myeloperoxidase; LMP-1, latent membrane protein; GranB, granzyme B; TCL, T-cell lymphoma; FH, follicular hyperplasia; FL, follicular lymphoma, SMZL, splenic MZL; HCL, hairy cell leukemia.

Molecular Approaches

The molecular tests that are commonly applicable to tumors of immune cells fall into two categories: assays for clonality and molecular cytogenetic assays. Clonality assays are rarely used in nonlymphoid malignancies; however, there are occasions in which they may be useful. The clinically applicable molecular cytogenetic assays include in situ hybridization (ISH) studies and PCR-based assays which are utilized primarily for translocation detection. The principles behind molecular cytogenetic assays are applicable to both lymphoid and nonlymphoid tumors.

Clonality Assays

By far the most common molecular test used in the assessment of hematologic malignancies is clonality testing. Many reactive conditions simulate lymphomas, and it is critical to distinguish between a self-limited benign lymphoid proliferation caused by an immune response to a drug or virus and an uncontrolled neoplastic proliferation. The basis of clonality testing in lymphoid proliferations lies within the unique molecular biology of antigen receptor genes. When progenitor hematopoietic stem cells become committed to either the B- or T-cell lineage, they undergo a structural change in their DNA encoding their respective antigen receptor genes.

This structural change is maintained throughout the life of that cell and is inherited in all daughter cells. Likewise, if a neoplastic event occurs in a lymphoid cell possessing a rearranged antigen receptor gene, all daughter cells will inherit the identical rearrangement, creating a tumor-specific molecular marker. Structural changes of antigen receptor genes have traditionally been evaluated using restriction fragment analysis of genomic DNA followed by Southern blotting (106). In this procedure, DNA is digested by restriction enzymes that cut at known sites in the germ line. The restricted DNA is size fractionated, generally by agarose gel electrophoresis. The fractionated DNA is transferred by Southern blotting to a solid nylon or nitrocellulose matrix, and the position (which is proportional to the size) of the fragment containing the antigen receptor gene of interest is visualized by hybridization with a labeled probe that is directed to the antigen receptor gene. Germ line DNA (i.e., DNA that has not undergone rearrangement) generates a single restriction fragment that reflects the distance between the restriction enzyme sites that encompass the probe sequence. However, DNA that has undergone rearrangement will show an altered restriction fragment, different in size from the germ line fragment, reflecting the structural change that has occurred as a result of the rearrangement.

Although this procedure is capable of accurately assessing nearly 100% of all clonal B- or T-cell neoplasms, it is time-consuming and requires a relatively large amount of DNA (>20 μg) and is therefore not as well suited as PCR techniques for clinical laboratory testing.

Unlike restriction fragment analysis, the basis of PCR assays for clonality lies within differences in the sizes of the *junctional* regions that are formed during V-J or V-D-J segment recombinations. The biological basis of these size differences lies primarily with the activity of terminal deoxynucleotidyltransferase (TdT) and exonuclease activities that add and delete nucleotides in a nontemplated manner, generating junctional regions of various lengths. Physiologically this process plays a major role in creating antibody diversity, in combination with somatic mutation of the antigen receptor genes. The junctional "repertoire" can be analyzed using consensus primers that span the junctions (V and J region primers). In a reactive polyclonal population of B or T cells, the junctional sequences generated by PCR will vary from one cell to the next, generating many different-sized PCR fragments visualized as a ladder of bands on an ethidium-stained acrylamide gel. In lymphomas, all daughter tumor cells bear the identical rearranged antigen receptor gene containing identical junctional sequences. In this case, PCR will generate a single-sized product visible on the ethidium-stained gel. This product is specific for and a signature of the tumor from which it was generated.

PCR can be performed with 100 ng or less of DNA, is rapid, and is extremely easy to perform. For these reasons PCR has become the assay of choice in the clinical laboratory to test for clonality. Detection of the resulting PCR fragments is most frequently performed by gel or capillary electrophoresis. The disadvantage of PCR is that it typically has a much higher false-negativity rate than the genomic Southern blot approach, approximating 20% or more for B-cell clonality and 10% or more for T-cell clonality, depending upon the specific method chosen and the primers used. Recently a large consortium of European laboratories collaborated in a large study designated as BIOMED-II (105). The consortium developed and tested a multiplex system comprised of multiple primer pairs designed to lower the false-negativity rate of the commonly used assays for B- and T-cell clonality. These sets of primers were shown to perform extremely well, approaching detection rates of 100% for both B- and T-cell rearrangements. However, in order to reach this high level of diagnostic sensitivity, more than 31 primers multiplexed in five separate reactions were required for the assessment of immunoglobulin heavy-chain gene (IGH) rearrangements, and 44 primers multiplexed in five separate reactions were required for the assessment of T-cell receptor (TCR) rearrangements. Furthermore, these primer sets were validated primarily for freshly isolated DNA and did not perform as well in paraffin tissue, in which DNA may be partially degraded. Nonetheless, this comprehensive study demonstrates that it is possible to attain high levels of diagnostic sensitivity using PCR assays for clonality. The BIOMED-II primers are available through InVivoScribe Technologies (Carlsbad, Calif.; http://www.invivoscribe.com).

Clonality testing is rarely used in nonlymphoid malignancies, but there are occasions in which it can be useful. Simple PCR-based approaches for the assessment of clonality in nonlymphoid malignancies are the HUMARA (see below) and related assays that exploit X-linked chromosomal inactivation (23). Since the cells comprising a tumor are descendants of a single progenitor cell, the entire population of tumor cells will carry the identical inactivated maternal or paternal X chromosome that was present in the ancestral progenitor. This phenomenon has been known for many years, and the immunologic assessment of the A and B isoforms of the X-linked glucose-6-phosphate dehydrogenase enzyme, with all of its limitations, was the common method for assessing clonality until the development of molecular technologies (72). A molecular genetic feature of X-linked chromosomal inactivation is promoter hypermethylation of genes located on the inactivated chromosome (85). In a monoclonal population of cells, either 100% of the paternal or 100% of the maternal alleles will be hypermethylated, while in a polyclonal population of cells, 50% of the paternal and 50% of the maternal alleles will be hypermethylated, as a result of random X inactivation in the population. The assessment of hypermethylation is performed through the use of methylation-sensitive restriction enzymes, in combination with PCR. Prior to PCR, the DNA of interest is cut using a methylation-sensitive restriction endonuclease. Subsequently, PCR is performed using primers that encompass the promoter region. The methylated alleles remain uncut and generate a PCR product, while the nonmethylated alleles are cut by the restriction enzyme, which prevents the generation of a PCR product. In order to assess whether both maternal and paternal alleles have been amplified, the promoter chosen must also contain a highly polymorphic site that allows one to distinguish between the two alleles. The complete loss of one allele (maternal or paternal) indicates the presence of a clonal population. Because the X-linked human androgen receptor (HUMARA) gene contains a highly polymorphic sequence in proximity to its promoter, this locus has become the target of choice for X-linked clonality assays (55). The HUMARA assay can be performed on DNA extracted from formalin-fixed paraffin-embedded tissue, is relatively simple, and is adaptable to the clinical molecular diagnostics laboratory. As for all assays exploiting X inactivation, the primary disadvantage of the HUMARA assay it that it can be performed only for female patients.

Molecular Cytogenetics

ISH

ISH is a powerful technology that allows in situ visualization of specific chromosomal translocations, chromosome copy number, gene copy number, and mRNA expression. Translocations are assessed through the use of DNA probes that recognize regions of chromosomes involved in translocations. These probes fall into two general categories: so-called break-apart probes, which are generally used singly, and fusion probes, which are used in pairs. Break-apart probes are designed to span a breakpoint region of interest. Therefore, if the targeted chromosome is split by a translocation, three signals will appear, one from the normal nontranslocated chromosome and one from each of the two derivative translocated chromosomes. Break-apart probes can provide information that the targeted region is involved in a translocation; they do not provide information identifying the partner chromosome. Break-apart probes are particularly useful when one does not know one translocation partner, or when multiple partners exist, such as for translocations involving the *bcl*-6 locus on 3q27. Fusion probes, on the other hand, are designed to recognize both chromosomal regions involved in the translocations, so that one can precisely identify both translocation partners. In the case of fusion probes, each member of the differentially labeled probe pair hybridizes with its targeted chromosomal region, generating four signals. In cells containing the targeted translocation, two of the signals from each of the chromosomes involved in the translocation fuse into one and only three signals are seen. In practice, fusion probes are generally labeled in different colors (green and red), so that the fusion signal generally is a mixture of the two different probe colors (yellow). Probes are generally labeled with fluorescent dyes (FISH), but chromogens (CISH) have been used successfully as well for some applications. FISH can be performed on metaphase chromosome spreads, but its greatest success in diagnostic pathology has been its adaptation to interphase nuclei in either frozen or fixed tissues (53). FISH has the highest diagnostic sensitivity of any available test for identifying specific chromosomal translocations and numerical chromosome alterations. However, FISH is labor-intensive and is not available in all diagnostic laboratories due to the high cost of the associated equipment.

FISH overcomes some of the limitations of PCR in the assessment of translocations, since large chromosomal regions can be analyzed, greatly reducing the problem of false negatives due to the focal nature of PCR. As previously mentioned, the disadvantages of FISH are that it is technically challenging when applied to tissue sections, is time-consuming, and requires relatively expensive equipment and an experienced practitioner, preferably a cytogeneticist. Nonetheless, when available, FISH is the method of choice to identify most of the lymphoma-specific translocations. Probes for most of the clinically important translocations are available commercially through Vysis, Inc. (Downers Grove, Ill.).

PCR

PCR of chromosomal breakpoint junctions is also a popular method for identifying translocations because of its rapidity and simplicity. The translocations that occur in lymphoid neoplasms are of two general types, those that result in the deregulation of normal cellular genes without disrupting the coding sequence (type 1) and those that result in the fusion of two normal cellular genes to create a novel chimeric gene product (type 2). The majority of type 1 translocations involve one of the antigen receptor gene loci. These include translocations such as t(8;14) involving the MYC gene on chromosome 8 and the IGH locus on chromosome 14, t(11;14) involving the cyclin D1 locus on chromosome 11 and the IGH locus, and t(14;18) involving the BCL-2 gene and the IGH locus. In all of these cases, the translocations deregulate the target gene by disrupting its regulatory elements or by placing it under the control of elements of the involved antigen receptor gene. A minority of the type 1 translocations do not involve an antigen receptor gene, such as some of the variant translocations involving the BCL-6 gene on chromosome 3q27. Nonetheless, the result is similar in that the target gene's coding sequence is left intact, but its regulatory elements are altered through the substitution of control elements from the various genes on the partnering chromosomes. Whereas the type 1 translocations leave the coding sequences of the potential oncogenes intact, type 2 tranlocations occur between two unrelated genes and result in the creation of a novel mRNA and protein encoded by portions of the two fused genes. Typically both genes are transcription factors and the resulting chimeric proteins display highly aberrant transcriptional activities. Representative of the type 2 translocation is the pre-B-cell acute lymphocytic leukemia (ALL) t(12;21) translocation, which fuses the TEL gene on chromosome 12 to the AML1 gene on chromosome 21.

The molecular detection strategies for the two types of translocations differ in that for the type 1 translocations the targeted template is generally the junctional sequence *within the DNA*, while in the type 2 translocations the primers generally target the junctional sequence *within the message (cDNA)* encoding the novel protein. For both types of translocations, a PCR product will be generated only from the tumor cells bearing the junctional DNA or cDNA sequences created by the translocation, which therefore serves as a tumor-specific marker. Detection is generally carried out by either gel or capillary electrophoresis. Alternatively, PCR and detection may be combined in real-time PCR instruments. These instruments monitor the accumulation of product during the PCR using fluorescent detection technologies (6).

The use of PCR to detect type 1 translocations can be highly effective when the breakpoints on the partnering chromosomes are clustered, as occurs with the t(14;18) translocations in follicle center lymphomas. However, if the breakpoints are instead spread over a larger area, as they are with the t(11;14) translocation in MCLs, this technique will miss many translocations. While DNA-based PCR assays have a very high analytic sensitivity, capable of identifying 1 in 10^6 abnormal cells, these tests have a much lower diagnostic sensitivity than FISH, since each PCR primer set can target only a DNA segment of a few hundred base pairs, while an appropriate FISH probe can identify translocations involving all potential breakpoint regions.

Type 2 translocations occur most frequently in pre-B-cell and B-lymphoblastic lymphoma/leukemias, but they also occur in some of the mature B- and T-cell lymphomas, including ALCL and MALT lymphoma. These are extremely interesting events from the biological point of view, as they create chimeric proteins that have novel oncogenic activities. For diagnostic purposes, the chimeric RNA serves as the tumor-specific PCR product. Reverse transcription (RT)-PCR assays targeting the chimeric RNA sequences generally have a much higher diagnostic sensitivity than those that target the corresponding chromosomal breakpoint regions because in most cases, gene splicing events create junctions precisely between the exons of the fused genes, even when the breakpoint sequences themselves may be spread diffusely throughout intronic sequences. For example, 75% of ALCLs possess a t(2;5) translocation joining the nucleophosmin (NPM) gene on chromosome 5 to the ALCL tyrosine kinase (ALK) gene on chromosome 2. The breakpoints are spread throughout intron 4 of the NPM gene and within a single intron of the ALK gene, which presents difficulties in the design of a simple DNA-based PCR test. However, splicing events in the novel transcript bring exon 4 of the NPM gene into contiguity with a 5′ coding exon of the ALK gene in all cases. This allows the design of a simple RT-PCR assay, using only a single primer pair, that can reliably identify all of the t(2;5) translocation.

Other Molecular Tests Used in Lymphoma Diagnostics

PCR is also used to identify the presence of viruses that are associated with different lymphoma subtypes. Chapters in section J (Viral Diseases) of this manual (e.g., chapter 89) discuss these viral detection assays in more detail. PCR to detect viral DNA can be especially helpful in the diagnosis of human T-cell leukemia virus type 1 (HTLV-1)-associated lymphomas, human herpesvirus 8 (HHV-8)-associated pleural effusion lymphomas, and lymphoproliferations associated with Epstein-Barr virus (EBV), such as EBV posttransplant lymphoproliferative disorders, nasal NK/T-cell lymphoma, angioimmunoblastic T-cell lymphoma (AILT), and Burkitt's lymphoma. However, the identification of a viral product by PCR should be correlated with in situ or morphological studies since the presence of these viruses is not tumor specific. For example, HHV-8 may also be found in Kaposi's sarcoma and Castleman's disease, and EBV may be identified in non-neoplastic immunoproliferative conditions, particularly when immunosuppression is present. Furthermore, it is important to recognize that because of the extremely high sensitivity of PCR-based tests, nonpathological levels of some viruses that are present at low levels, such as EBV, may be detected.

FISH and the related technique CISH are also well suited for identification of mRNA in situ and for identifying viruses such as EBV (4). The advantage of CISH is that it can be assessed using an ordinary light microscope. However, it is limited by the number of chromogens available and by the resolution of the technology. CISH can be used as a secondary technique to assess light-chain exclusion, when exclusion cannot be definitively assessed at the protein level. CISH is commonly used in hematopathology laboratories for the identification of EBV infection and has become an important ancillary test for diagnosing cases of NK/T-cell lymphoma, Burkitt's lymphoma, AILT, and other EBV-associated lymphoproliferative disorders, including posttransplant lymphoproliferative disorders.

cDNA microarray studies have recently been utilized to further the classification of lymphomas (2, 35, 86, 88, 91). Clinically significant subcategories within morphologically homogeneous lymphoma entities, such as diffuse large-B-cell lymphoma (DLBCL) and chronic lymphocytic leukemia (CLL), have been identified through the use of this technology. While cDNA microarrays are not yet ready for clinical diagnostics, it is only a matter of time before this powerful technology evolves into a more user-friendly format and becomes an integral part of the molecular diagnostic laboratory. cDNA microarray technology is discussed in detail in chapters 4 and 5.

INTERPRETATION AND APPLICATION OF IMMUNOLOGIC AND MOLECULAR MARKERS IN THE DIAGNOSIS OF TUMORS OF THE IMMUNE SYSTEM

Precursor Lymphoid Neoplasms

Lymphoblastic malignancies (LBL) are neoplasms of precursor T and B lymphocytes. They may present clinically as either lymphoblastic lymphoma or ALL, and morphologically the T- and B-lineage varieties of LBL are indistinguishable. Virtually 100% of these neoplasms are positive for TdT, which can be detected by immunocytochemical techniques using rabbit antisera or murine monoclonal antibodies directed against it.

Precursor T-cell LBL most often present as lymphoma, usually with a mediastinal mass, with or without bone marrow involvement and a leukemic phase. They usually have an immature T-cell phenotype that correlates with different stages of intrathymic maturation (Fig. 1). The earliest T-cell-associated antigen with some lineage specificity is CD7. However, it is also expressed in rare cases of acute myeloid leukemia, where it may represent evidence of lineage infidelity, often seen in primitive hematopoietic malignancies. CD3, linked to the T-cell antigen receptor, is expressed in the cytoplasm prior to its presence on the surface and thus may not be revealed by immunofluorescence techniques on living cells (77). In this situation a T-cell LBL may be CD3 positive in tissue sections but negative by routine flow cytometry. However, techniques that permeabilize the cell membrane are available to detect cytoplasmic antigens by flow cytometry. It should be noted that the normal thymocytes

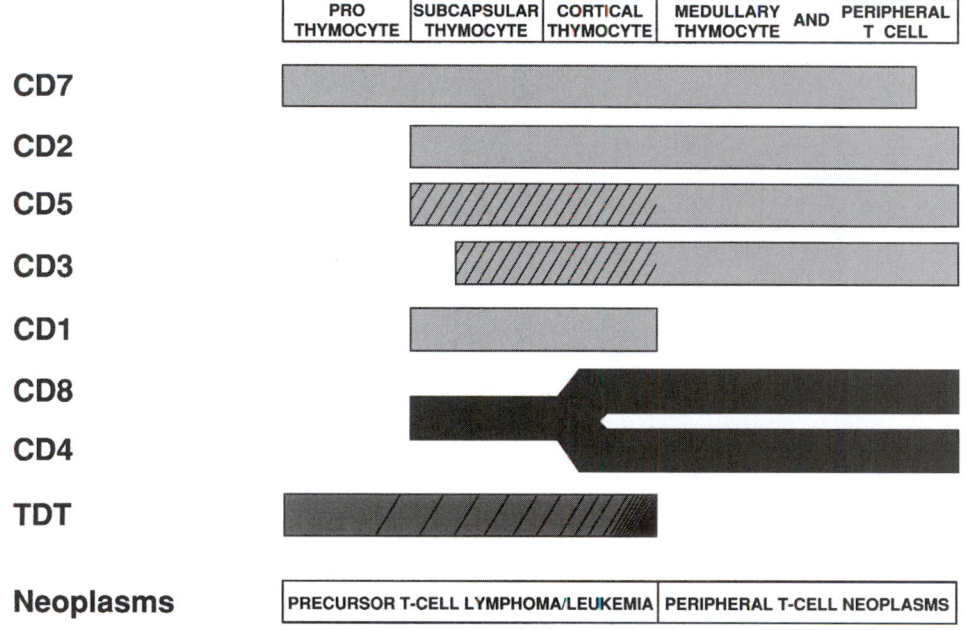

FIGURE 1   Schematic diagram showing stages of T-cell differentiation. Neoplasms can be related to precursor and mature or peripheral T lymphocytes. Antigenic phenotype correlates with maturational stage. Note that CD7 is the earliest T-associated antigen.

encountered in a lymphocyte-rich thymoma would be phenotypically similar to the cells of a T-cell LBL. Immunohistochemical analysis will be necessary to detect the thymic epithelial cells numerous in the former condition.

T-lymphoblastic lymphomas are clonal neoplasms, and most will have TCRβ or TCRγ rearrangements (99). About 20% of T-lymphoblastic lymphomas also have IGH rearrangements, a phenomenon known as lineage infidelity (100). Lineage infidelity is common in early-lineage T- and B-cell neoplasms but is rare in mature B- and T-cell neoplasms. Therefore, when assessing clonality in lymphoblastic lymphomas, antigen receptor rearrangements cannot be used to assign B- or T-cell lineage. Up to 50% of T-lymphoblastic lymphoma/leukemias have recurrent translocations most frequently involving one of the TCR gene loci (Table 3). These can be detected by FISH and in many cases by PCR.

Precursor B-cell LBL present as leukemia more often than as lymphoma. In cases presenting as lymphoma, common clinical manifestations include skin involvement (often of the scalp or face), lytic bone lesions, or lymphadenopathy. The risk of involvement of the central nervous system is less than for pre-T-cell LBL. Although these precursor B-cell tumors do not normally express immunoglobulin, other markers of B-cell lineage, such as CD19 and CD79a, will be present (Fig. 2) (13). These antigens are expressed at the time of IGH rearrangement, usually indicating commitment to the B-cell lineage. In cases of so-called pre-B-cell ALL, the cells contain cytoplasmic μ heavy chains but are still negative for surface immunoglobulin. The CD20 antigen is not acquired until the stage of light-chain gene rearrangement, and it is expressed in approximately 50% of cases (56). Thus, pre-B-cell LBL is often negative for CD20 in paraffin sections.

TABLE 3 Chromosomal translocations, involved genes, and detection methods in B- and T-cell lymphoma/leukemias[a]

Translocation	Genes	Tumor	Translocation type	Primary test(s)
B-lymphoblastic leukemia/lymphoma				
t(12;21)(p13;q22)	TEL-AML1	B-ALL	2	FISH, RT-PCR
t(1;19)(q23;p13)	PBX1-E2A	B-ALL	2	FISH, RT-PCR
t(17;19)(q22;p13)	HLF-E2A	B-ALL	2	FISH, RT-PCR
t(9;22)(q34;q11)	BCR-ABL	B-ALL	2	FISH, RT-PCR
t(4;11)(q21;q23)	MLL-AF4	B-ALL	2	FISH, RT-PCR
t(11;19)(q23;p13.3)	MLL-ENL	B-ALL	2	FISH, RT-PCR
Mature B-cell lymphomas				
t(14;18)(q32;q21)	BCL-2–IGH	FL	1	PCR, FISH
t(11;14)(q13;q32)	CCND1-IGH	MCL, MM	1	PCR[b], RT-PCR[c], FISH
t(4;14)(p16;q32)	FGFR3-IGH	MM	1	FISH
t(6;14)(p16;q32)	IRF4-IGH	MM	1	FISH
t(14;16)(q32;q23)	IGH-MAF	MM	1	FISH
t(8;14)(q24;q32)	MYC-IGH	BL, B-ALL	1	FISH
t(8;22)(q24;q11)	MYC-IGλ	BL, B-ALL	1	FISH
t(2;8)(p12;q24)	MYC-IGκ	BL, B-ALL	1	FISH
t(11;18)(q21;q21)	API2-MLT	MALT	1	FISH, RT-PCR
t(14;18)(q32;q21)	IGH-MLT	MALT	1	FISH
t(1;14)(p22;q32)	BCL-10–IGH	MALT	1	FISH
t(3;14)(q27;q32)	BCL-6–IGH	DLBCL	1	FISH
t(3;v)(p27;v)[d]	BCL-6–MPS[e]	DLBCL	1	FISH
t(9;14)(p13;q32)	PAX5-IGH	LPL	1	FISH
T-lymphoblastic leukemia/lymphoma				
t(1;14)(p32;q11)	TAL1-TCRδ	T-ALL	1	FISH, RT-PCR
t(1;7)(p32;q34)	TAL1-TCRβ	T-ALL	1	FISH, RT-PCR
t(1;7)(p34;q34)	LCK-TCRβ	T-ALL	1	FISH, RT-PCR
t(11;14)(p15;q11)	LMO1-TCRδ	T-ALL	1	FISH, RT-PCR
t(11;14)(p13;q11)	LMO2-TCRδ	T-ALL	1	FISH, RT-PCR
t(7;9)(q34;q32)	TAL2-TCRβ	T-ALL	1	FISH, RT-PCR
t(7;9)(q34;q34)	TAN1-TCRβ	T-ALL	1	FISH, RT-PCR
t(7;11)(q34;p13)	RHOM2-TCRβ	T-ALL	1	FISH, RT-PCR
t(7;19)(q34;p13)	LYL1-TCRβ	T-ALL	1	FISH, RT-PCR
t(7;10)(q34;q24)	TCRβ-HOX11	T-ALL	1	FISH, RT-PCR
t(10;14)(q24;q11)	HOX11-TCRδ	T-ALL	1	FISH, RT-PCR
t(8;14)(q24;q11)	MYC-TCRα/δ	T-ALL	1	FISH, RT-PCR
Mature T-cell lymphomas				
t(2;5)(p23;q35)	ALK-NPM	ALCL	2	FISH, RT-PCR

[a]Abbreviations: B-ALL, pre-B, B-cell ALL; FL, follicular lymphoma; MM, multiple myeloma; BL, Burkitt lymphoma; MALT; MZL lymphoma of MALT type; T-ALL, T-cell lymphoblastic lymphoma/leukemia.
[b]Major cluster region primers identify about 35% of translocations.
[c]RT-PCR to the cyclin D1 mRNA will detect close to 100% of cases.
[d]3q27 partners with various (v) chromosomal partners and loci.
[e]MPS, multiple partner genes.

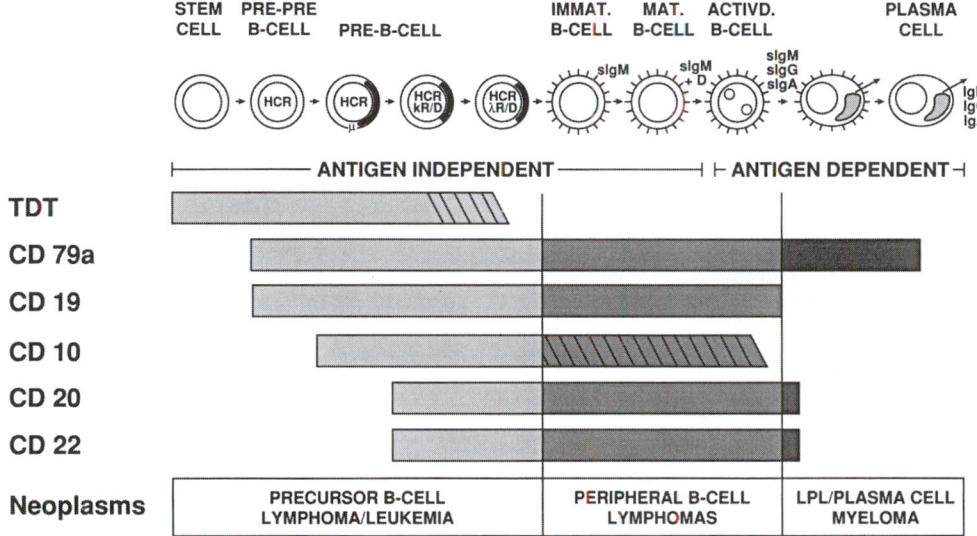

FIGURE 2 Schematic diagram showing stages of B-cell differentiation. Lymphomas can be related to precursor B-cell, mature B-cell, and secretory B-cell (plasma cell) stages of differentiation. Note that CD79a has the broadest range of reactivity, staining precursor, mature, and secretory B cells. Abbreviations: PRE, precursor; IMMAT, immature; MAT, mature; ACTIVD, activated; HCR, heavy-chain gene rearrangement; κ and λ R/D, κ and λ light-chain gene rearrangement/deletion; sIg, surface immunoglobulin; LPL, lymphoplasmacytic lymphoma.

All pre-B-cell and B-cell lymphoblastic lymphomas are clonal neoplasms, and the vast majority have IGH rearrangements. In some cases the IGH rearrangements are incomplete, showing only D-to-J segment joining (101). B-cell lymphoblastic lymphomas have an extremely high frequency of lineage infidelity, with 90% of cases having clonal rearrangements of one or more TCR loci (TCRβ [35%], TCRγ [60%], or TCRδ [55%]) (98). About 30% of cases have characteristic chromosomal translocations (Table 3). A high percentage of these involve two non-antigen receptor genes that can be identified by FISH or by RT-PCR.

Both pre-T-cell and pre-B-cell LBL may be negative for the leukocyte common antigen (CD45). In addition, they both express CD99, the *mic-2* gene product, in a large proportion of cases. This antigen is expressed in Ewing's sarcoma, a nonlymphoid malignancy presenting in children and young adults, often with lytic bone lesions of the distal extremities. Because of potentially overlapping histological and clinical features, an extensive immunohistochemical panel as well as molecular analysis may be required for accurate differential diagnosis (74).

Mature B-Cell Lymphomas

A variety of malignancies composed of small mature B lymphocytes are recognized in the WHO classification. These include small lymphocytic lymphoma (SLL)/CLL, follicular lymphoma (FCL), MCL, extranodal marginal zone lymphoma (MZL) of MALT type, nodal MZL, splenic MZL, and hairy cell leukemia. In most of these neoplasms, the cells are arrested prior to the secretory stage of B-cell development and express pan-B-cell antigens such as CD19, CD20, and CD22. Evidence of plasmacytoid differentiation is most commonly seen in MZL and is a consistent feature of lymphoplasmacytic lymphoma (LPL). Each of the small B-cell malignancies has a characteristic immunophenotypic signature that is highly useful in differential diagnosis (Table 4).

Monoclonal surface immunoglobulin expression is usually readily detected in frozen sections but is generally not evident in paraffin sections. Even in frozen sections, abundant serum

TABLE 4 Differential diagnosis of small B-cell lymphomas[a]

Disease	CD5	CD10	CD23	CD43	Cyclin D1	Immunoglobulin class(es)[b]
FL	−	+	±	−	−	IgM, IgG
MCL	+	−	−	+	+	IgM/IgD
CLL/SLL	+	−	+	+	−	IgM/IgD
LPL	−	−	−	±	−	IgM (c)
MALT	−	−	−	±	−	IgM (c, s)
SMZL	−	−	−	−	−	IgM/IgD
HCL	−	−	−	−	±	IgG

[a]Abbreviations: FL, follicular lymphoma; MALT, MZL of MALT type; SMZL; splenic MZL; HCL, hairy cell leukemia; c, cytoplasmic; s, surface.
[b]Most commonly expressed heavy-chain class.

immunoglobulins in the interstitial space may result in high background staining, which can obscure cellular staining and make interpretation difficult. This problem is frequently observed in tissues from patients with polyclonal hypergammaglobulinemia. In paraffin sections, cytoplasmic immunoglobulin can be detected, but it is usually most evident in cells showing evidence of plasmacytoid differentiation. Positive staining in the perinuclear space is highly reliable and is usually not subject to technical problems.

The ability of the cells to form follicles correlates with the presence of dendritic reticulum cells (DRC), which can be identified in frozen and paraffin sections by using monoclonal antibodies reactive with CD21, CD23, CD35, or clusterin. DRC are numerous in FCL and intimately associated with the neoplastic nodules, even in extranodal locations. Staining for DRC will often enhance a vaguely nodular pattern that is difficult to see in routine histological sections. DRC are rare in SLL but are present with an irregular, vaguely nodular distribution in MCL.

CD5 is very useful in the subclassification of low-grade B-cell lymphomas. This antigen is found on normal T cells but on few normal B cells. Both SLL and MCL are usually positive for CD5, but it is almost never expressed in true FCL. Thus, this antigen is useful in the differential diagnosis of MCL with a vaguely nodular growth pattern versus a true FCL. CD5 is also useful in the differential diagnosis of SLL and MCL with lymphomas of MALT. MALT lymphomas arise in extranodal sites (e.g., lung, gastrointestinal tract, and salivary gland) and are composed of small round and small-cleaved (centrocyte-like) cells, which may resemble the cells of SLL and MCL. MALT lymphomas are usually CD5 negative (29). CD23 is very useful in the differential diagnosis of SLL/CLL and MCL, since SLL/CLL is nearly always CD23 positive and MCL is nearly always CD23 negative (59). The common ALL antigen (cALLa) or CD10 is found much more often in FCL than in the other small B-cell lymphomas (51). For unknown reasons, MCL and hairy cell leukemia both express λ light chain much more frequently than do the other B-cell lymphomas, which usually express κ.

Cytogenetic and molecular genetic studies are also extremely valuable in differential diagnosis, and monoclonal antibodies to oncogene products can be used as surrogate markers in some situations (Table 5). FCL is characterized by the t(14;18) translocation that juxtaposes the *BCL-2* gene with the IGH promoter/enhancer, resulting in BCL-2 overexpression (104). While the translocation results in BCL-2 overexpression, BCL-2 expression, however, is not specific for the translocation, as other low-grade lymphomas express this antiapoptotic protein (32). Thus, while the detection of overexpressed BCL-2 by immunohistochemistry is useful in differentiating follicular lymphoma from follicular hyperplasia, it is not helpful in distinguishing follicular lymphoma from other SLLs. PCR assays targeting the most common breakpoint cluster involved in the t(14;18) translocation can identify up to 65% of cases, while FISH analysis is capable of detecting all cases (42).

The t(11;14) translocation is present in all MCLs (68). This translocation involves the cyclin D1 gene, resulting in the overexpression of the protein, which is not expressed in nonneoplastic lymphoid cells or in other small lymphocytic neoplasms, with the exception of a small percentage of myeloma cases that have t(11;14) and hairy cell leukemias which express very low levels of cyclin D1 (81). The development of new mouse and rabbit monoclonal antibodies to cyclin D1 have greatly improved the detection of these aggressive SLLs, and molecular testing for the translocation is generally not necessary (95). PCR analysis for identification of t(11;14) breakpoint sequences has a relatively low yield unless multiple primer pairs are used, and therefore this method is not widely used. However, RT-PCR targeting the overexpressed cyclin D1 transcripts has been successfully employed in diagnostics (12). This assay exploits the fact that normal lymphocytes and other lymphomas do not express cyclin D1 message, except for a minority of myelomas and hairy cell leukemias at low levels. FISH assays for t(11;14) will identify 100% of cases. Recently cDNA microarray analyses have been performed on cases of MCL (88). While these studies have confirmed the homogeneity of this lymphoma, they have also shown that it is possible to stratify cases and predict survival based upon the expression of a set of genes associated with cellular proliferation.

The t(11;18) translocation involving *API2/MLT (MALT)* genes is the most common recurring cytogenetic abnormality in MALT lymphomas of the gastrointestinal tract and lung, where it is found in about one-third of all cases (8). However, other less common translocations also occur in MALT lymphomas, including the t(14;18) translocation involving the IGH gene and the MLT gene and the t(1;14) translocation involving BCL-10 and IGH (43). The t(14;18) translocation preferentially involves non-gastrointestinal tract MALT lymphomas such as those in the lung and ocular

TABLE 5   Evaluation of oncogenes and tumor suppressor genes by immunohistochemistry and molecular diagnostic techniques[a]

Antigen	Disease association	Genetic abnormality	Applicable genetic test(s)	Immunohisto-chemistry result
BCL-2	Follicular lymphoma	t(14;18)	GS, PCR, FISH[b]	+, nonspecific
Cyclin D1	MCL	t(11;14)	GS, PCR, FISH[b]	+, specific[b]
	Multiple myeloma (15%)	t(11;14)	RT-PCR[b] (cyclin D1)	+, specific[b]
p53	Progressed lymphomas	17q deletion	LOH, SSCP, FISH	+, probable[b,c]
	Aggressive lymphomas	Mutation	Sequencing[c]	Mutation
BCL-6	DLBCL (GCB > ABC)	t(3;14)	GS, FISH[b]	+, nonspecific
	3q26 variants	Mutation		
ALK	ALCL	t(2;5)	GS, RT-PCR, FISH[b]	+, specific[b]
		2p23 variants		

[a]Abbreviations: GS, genomic Southern blot analysis; SSCP, single-strand conformational polymorphism analysis; GCB, germinal center B cell-like; ABC, activated B cell-like.
[b]Method(s) of choice for detection of genetic abnormalities in the clinical molecular diagnostics laboratory.
[c]p53 overexpression is generally correlated with the presence of mutation; however, lack of expression is poorly correlated with lack of mutation. Sequencing is required for definitive proof of mutation.

adnexa, while the t(1;14) translocation tends to be found in advanced-stage MALT lymphoma. It is of interest that these three translocations perturb two genes (BCL-10 and MLT) that are involved in antigen receptor NF-κB activation (43). The most common of these translocations, t(11;18), can be readily assessed using commercially available FISH probes, or by RT-PCR using published primers to the API2 and MLT genes.

CLL lacks a characteristic recurrent translocation but displays other cytogenetic abnormalities, including deletions of 13q14, trisomy 12, and deletions of 11q and 17p, which are both associated with a more aggressive clinical course (25). The 13q14 deletion occurs in a very high percentage of CLL cases and results in the consistent loss of genes encoding micro-RNAs (15). Micro-RNAs are small antisense RNAs encoded in the genome that appear to regulate the translation of critical proteins (16). The micro-RNAs that are deleted at 13q14 are miR15 and miR16, which are regulators of the antiapoptotic BCL-2 protein, implicating the loss of these micro-RNAs in the abnormally high levels of BCL-2 found in CLL (18). FISH analysis tends to underestimate the frequency of micro-RNA loss because a significant number of the deletions at 13q14 are small.

Over the past several years there have been a number of studies that have clearly shown that there are two distinct clinicopathological subtypes of CLL that can be distinguished by the presence or absence of IGH mutation, CD38 expression, and ZAP70 expression (103, 110). Nonmutated CLL tends to be CD38 positive and ZAP70 positive. Patients with nonmutated CLL have a 5-year survival of about 40 months, compared to 120 months for their counterparts with ZAP70-negative mutated CLL. Gene microarray studies have confirmed the presence of these two clinicopathological subgroups (86). At present, either mutational analysis or ZAP70 expression by immunohistochemistry or flow cytometry is recommended to distinguish these two CLL subtypes.

Tumors of fully differentiated B cells synthesize and secrete immunoglobulin, giving rise to monoclonal immunoglobulin spikes that can be detected by serum immunoelectrophoresis. LPL is the histological counterpart of Waldenström macroglobulinemia. In this disease the cell is arrested between the B lymphocyte and the plasma cell. Class switching from immunoglobulin M (IgM) to IgG, IgA, etc., has not yet occurred, and clinically the process resembles a low-grade lymphoma with widespread involvement of lymphoid organs. Although rare patients carry the t(9;14) translocation which juxtaposes the PAX5 gene to the IGH locus, the molecular pathogenesis of these rare tumors is largely unstudied.

Multiple myeloma, which arises from terminally differentiated B cells, may show monoclonal IgG, IgA, IgM, or IgD, in that order of frequency. The cells at this stage of differentiation lose most B-cell markers, such as CD20, CD19, and CD22. However, CD79a is still found (67). All myelomas have clonally rearranged immunoglobulin genes and express monoclonal immunoglobulin, which is mainly cytoplasmic and can be most readily detected in paraffin sections. Of practical significance, it should be noted that normal and neoplastic plasma cells are CD45 (leukocyte common antigen) negative but are positive for epithelial membrane antigen. The pathologist should be alert to these characteristics in the eventual differential diagnosis of anaplastic carcinoma versus multiple myeloma. Multiple myeloma has several characteristic recurrent translocations (Table 3). Interestingly, many of these result in the overexpression of cyclin D, either directly or indirectly, and it has been proposed that overexpression of cyclin D is a common pathogenetic mechanism unifying all of the different translocations (11). FISH is the method of choice for detection of the various translocations.

DLBCL is not a single disease entity but a category that includes both primary aggressive B-cell lymphomas and histologically progressed lymphomas. Because there are as yet no immunophenotypic or morphological features that lead to reliable subclassification of these lymphomas, it was deemed most advisable to retain most morphological variants of DLBCL in a single category, pending further data and delineation of other entities. Notably, some specific entities have been defined, and these include mediastinal or thymic-B-cell lymphoma, primary effusion lymphomas (HHV-8 associated), and intravascular DLBCL (17, 24, 63, 64).

Therefore, it is not unexpected that most cases of DLBCL do not display unique phenotypic profiles but express the mature-B-cell characteristics seen in diverse low-grade B-cell tumors. For example, expression of CD10 usually correlates with the presence of the t(14;18) translocation (27). In some cases, the presence of CD5 indicates that the process arose in the background of a small lymphocytic malignancy (SLL/CLL), so-called Richter's syndrome, although de novo CD5⁺ DLBCLs also exist. p53 is commonly expressed and is often an indication of an acquired *p53* mutation associated with histological progression (90). p53 protein expression also is a poor prognostic marker (113). *BCL-6* is expressed in the majority of DLBCL cases, in many instances indicating a derivation from the germinal center (GC). However, both translocations and mutations of *BCL-6* occur frequently as well. While translocations of *BCL-6* are clearly important pathogenetically, *BCL-6* mutations are a normal physiological event in the GC. Recent data from several laboratories using cDNA microarray studies have begun to identify distinct differences within the DLBCLs (2, 92). Mediastinal B-cell lymphomas have been shown to be quite distinct in their gene expression signature from other DLBCLs and, in fact, have a signature closer to that of HD (92). "Standard" DLBCL has been shown to be composed of at least three different subgroups: a GCB subgroup, simulating the gene expression signature of GC B cells; an activated B cell-like (ABC) subgroup, simulating the signature of activated peripheral B cells; and a third, unclassified subgroup (2, 87). The ABC subgroup has been shown to have a significantly worse prognosis than the GCB subgroup, demonstrating that the subclassification has clinical relevance. Pathologists have been able to extract from these data a small panel of genes, amenable to immuohistochemical study, that have been shown to be effective in dividing the GCB group (BCL-6, CD10) from the ABC group (MUM-1/IRF4) (38).

A morphological variant of DLBCL is so-called T-cell-rich large-B-cell lymphoma. The neoplastic cells comprise less than 5% of the population in the lymph nodes, with most of the infiltrating cells being reactive polyclonal T cells. Staining of paraffin sections with L-26 is especially helpful in the recognition of T-cell-rich large-B-cell lymphoma and will highlight the large tumor cells. Cell suspensions prepared from such lymph nodes usually contain >75% T cells (up to 90% or more) and may be erroneously diagnosed as T-cell lymphomas with flow cytometric techniques. In many of these cases, the neoplastic cells resemble the L&H cells (so-called lymphocytic plus histiocytic variants) of nodular lymphocyte predominant Hodgkin's lymphoma, and a relationship between these entities has been postulated (22). There is as yet no reliable immunohistochemical or molecular test to distinguish these two disease entities, and the diagnosis remains heavily reliant upon clinical-pathological parameters.

Another DLBCL variant that has been clearly separated from the vast majority of DLBCLs is the pleural effusion lymphomas associated with human immunodeficiency virus (HIV) infection. Not only do these B-cell lymphomas have the unusual clinical feature of presenting as an effusion, most often without a solid or leukemic phase, but also they have an unusual immunophenotype and contain HHV-8 (17). These lymphomas have a plasmablast-like B-cell phenotype, but paradoxically generally do not display membrane or cytoplasmic immunoglobulin by immunohistochemistry. However, all cases have rearrangement of their immunoglobulin genes as detected by either genomic Southern blotting or PCR. HHV-8 can be easily demonstrated in the tumor cells by specific antibodies to the ORF76 protein or by PCR of involved fluids (73).

Burkitt's lymphoma is a high-grade malignancy that expresses CD20, CD19, and CD22. Surface immunoglobulin is usually of the IgM class, and the cALL antigen (CD10) is nearly always positive. Burkitt's lymphoma can rarely present as acute leukemia (L3) in the FAB (French-American-British) scheme. This lymphoma is TdT negative, helping to distinguish it from LBL, which is always TdT positive. Burkitt's lymphoma is characterized by translocations involving the MYC gene (54). Translocations involving MYC are best detected by FISH, as the chromosomal breakpoints are not sufficiently clustered to allow simple PCR testing. Burkitt's lymphoma is a highly proliferative tumor, with 100% of the cells in cycle (MIB-1$^+$), and is consistently BCL-2 negative. It is positive for BCL-6, indicating a relationship to the GC.

Mature T-Cell Neoplasms

Neoplasms of mature or peripheral T-cell origin demonstrate marked cytological heterogeneity. However, in contrast to the case with B-cell lymphomas, cytological features are less useful in defining disease entities. While nearly all cases of peripheral T-cell lymphoma (PTL) possess clonal rearrangements of at least one of the TCR genes, these lymphomas do not display consistent immunophenotypic profiles. In addition, the molecular pathogenesis remains to be defined for most of the T-cell lymphomas. Therefore, at present, clinical parameters play a major role in the classification of T-cell lymphomas, as cytological, immunophenotypic, and molecular features are insufficient to define these neoplasms. As a group they tend to be much more aggressive than B-cell lymphomas (70).

PTL, unspecified, is a category somewhat analogous to DLBCL (50). It is felt to be heterogeneous, and probably contains several yet-to-be-recognized entities. PTLs display a wide morphological spectrum, with cells of diverse sizes and appearances. PTL often has an inflammatory background composed of eosinophils, histiocytes, and plasma cells. This polymorphous cellular composition may lead to difficulty in distinction from HD. The presence of cytological

atypia in the background lymphocytes argues against a diagnosis of HD. Immunophenotypic markers are also useful in this differential diagnosis.

Immunophenotypic markers for clonality are not readily available in the T-cell system. Therefore, molecular assays for the assessment of clonality are often extremely helpful. The major subset antigens CD4 and CD8 are not clonal markers analogous to light-chain restriction in the B-cell system. Although most PTLs express only CD4 or CD8, some reactive conditions can also show marked subset restriction, most commonly of the CD4 subset. If a proliferation coexpresses CD4 and CD8 or fails to express either CD4 or CD8, that profile is suggestive of malignancy (75).

Other abnormalities of antigenic phenotype are commonly observed in PTL (Table 6). If a battery of pan-T-cell monoclonal antibodies is used, PTL will often fail to express one or more of the major markers CD7, CD5, CD3, and CD2. The antigen most frequently absent is CD7. However, because this antigen is expressed on only 85% of normal T cells, its absence is not unequivocal evidence of a malignancy. Indeed, some reactive T-cell proliferations will be CD7 negative.

A prominence of postcapillary venules is a feature often noted in PTL. AILT is a specific subtype of PTL characterized by an especially florid proliferation of postcapillary venules (31). The predominant infiltrating cells in AILT are CD4-positive T cells. Interestingly, the tumor cells have recently been shown to express CD10 and CXCR13, suggesting that these tumors originate from a subset of CD10-positive T cells that populate the GCs (7, 37). A prominent inflammatory background is present, including polyclonal plasma cells, histiocytes, and eosinophils. A disordered meshwork of CD21-positive reticulum cells distributed around blood vessels is highly characteristic of this lymphoma type.

Most cases of AILT show clonal TCRβ or TCRγ gene rearrangement. B cells are variable in frequency and in some cases may be numerous. In addition, some B cells positive for EBV are seen in nearly all cases (107). These EBV$^+$ cells may be monoclonal as detected by IGH PCR techniques, and in rare cases the EBV$^+$ B cells may progress to a DLBCL (1). In other rare instances the EBV$^+$ cells may also simulate Hodgkin's lymphoma morphologically and immunophenotypically (79). It is postulated that the expansion of EBV$^+$ B cells is secondary to the underlying immunodeficiency so characteristic of this disease.

Adult T-cell leukemia/lymphoma (ATL) is a unique clinicopathological entity associated with the human retrovirus HTLV-1 (14). The neoplastic cells have a mature T-cell phenotype. They are CD4 positive and strongly express interleukin-2 receptors (CD25). Elevated levels of soluble interleukin-2 receptors may be found in the serum and correlate with disease activity. They have a high proliferative rate with MIB-1, in keeping with the aggressive clinical

TABLE 6 Immunophenotype in the differential diagnosis of nodal PTLs^a

Disease	Immunophenotypic features
AILT	CD10 +, mixed CD4/CD8, proliferation of FDCs (CD21$^+$ cells), EBV$^+$ blasts
PTL, unspecified	CD4 > CD8, Ag loss (CD7, CD5, CD2)
ATLL	CD4$^+$, CD25$^+$, CD7-, CD30$^{+/-}$, CD15$^+$
ALCL	ALK$^+$, CD30$^+$, clusterin $^+$, EMA $^+$, CD25 $^+$, CD4 $^+$, CD3$^{+/-}$
TCRBCL	Large CD20 $^+$ blasts in CD3 $^+$ background
Reactive	Mixed CD4/CD8, intact architecture, variable CD25, CD30; scattered CD20 $^+$

^{a}Abbreviations: Ag, antigen; TCRBCL, T-cell-rich large-B-cell lymphoma.

TABLE 7 Extranodal NK/T-cell lymphomas[a]

Subtype	EBV	CD3	TIA-1	GranB/Per	CD56	TCR Major	TCR Minor
SPTCL	−	+ s	+	+	±	αβ	γδ
EATL	±	+ s	+	+	±	αβ	γδ/NK
Nasal	+	+ c	+	+	+	NK	γδαβ?
Hep/spl	−	+ s	+	−	+	γδ	αβ

[a]Abbreviations: SPTCL, subcutaneous panniculitis-like T-cell lymphoma, EATL, enteropathy-associated T-cell lymphoma; Nasal, nasal NK/T-cell lymphoma; Hep/spl, hepatosplenic T-cell lymphoma; GranB/Per, granzyme B/perforin; s, surface CD3; c, cytoplasmic CD3.

course. In vitro they exhibit suppressor cell function. As with many PTLs, they are CD7 negative. All cases of ATL have clonal TCRβ and TCRγ rearrangements and are associated with clonally integrated HTLV-1 retrovirus. Serologic testing for HTLV-1 as well as the identification of viral genomic sequences by PCR can be of great help in diagnosing this lymphoid neoplasm. However, only a minority of infected patients will develop ATL, and it is important to correlate serologic positivity for HTLV-1 or a positive PCR result with the presence of a clonal T-cell lymphoproliferation. Recurrent translocations are not reported in ATL, but numerical abnormalities and deletions of the long arm of chromosome 6 as assessed by both cytogenetic and loss-of-heterozygosity (LOH) studies are frequent (40).

Extranodal NK/T-cell lymphomas represent a distinctive group and share many histological and immunophenotypic features (49). This observation is in keeping with the close relationship between NK cells and cytotoxic T cells (96). They include intestinal T-cell lymphoma, subcutaneous panniculitis-like T-cell lymphoma, and nasal and extranasal NK/T-cell lymphoma. Most of the extranodal T-cell lymphomas appear to be derived from cytotoxic T cells; they express granzyme B, the cytotoxic granule-associated protein TIA-1 (also known as granule membrane protein GM-17), and perforin (21). CD56, an antigen expressed on NK cells, may also be present, but it is most common in nasal NK/T-cell lymphoma (Table 7). These lymphomas as a group present in and spread to extranodal sites, with infrequent lymph node involvement. They frequently contain extensive necrosis, sometimes associated with angioinvasion. Apoptosis of tumor cells also is prominent, in part related to the cytotoxic features of the neoplastic cells. EBV is universally found in nasal and extranasal NK/T-cell lymphoma and may be seen sporadically in intestinal T-cell lymphoma. EBV is generally absent in subcutaneous panniculitis-like T-cell lymphoma. Hepatosplenic T-cell lymphoma also belongs to this broad group of cytotoxic T-cell lymphomas.

Within the extranodal NK/T-cell lymphomas, there is some variation in lineage, a feature which departs from the general principle that lineage is a defining feature of disease entities. For example, nasal NK/T-cell lymphoma is usually of NK-cell derivation, but in rare cases it may be derived from either γδ or αβ T cells. Similarly, intestinal T-cell lymphoma is usually of αβ T-cell derivation, but a minor proportion of cases are derived from γδ T cells.

Nasal NK/T-cell lymphomas express some T-cell-associated antigens but are probably of NK-cell derivation (46). Necrosis is seen in most cases. The midline nasal area is the most common site of involvement, but the disease can also present itself in other extranodal sites. In other sites it is referred to as nasal-type NK/T-cell lymphoma (46). The

neoplastic cells generally lack T-cell gene rearrangements. The cells are positive for CD2 and CD7 but negative for surface CD3. However, they usually express CD3ε within the cytoplasm, which can be detected in paraffin sections with both polyclonal and monoclonal antibodies. CD56 is present in virtually all cases. The neoplastic cells are EBV positive, and the EBV genome is monoclonal based on terminal-repeat analysis (41). p53 is overexpressed in nearly all cases, but there have been no confirmatory mutational studies (80). There are few classical cytogenetic studies of these lymphomas, and while numerical abnormalities have been reported, no recurrent translocations have been identified (115). LOH studies show a high frequency of chromosomal loss at 6q, 13q, 11q, and 17p (the site of the p53 gene) (94). Recent studies using spectral karyotyping have identified a cryptic translocation involving Xp21 and 8p23 (116). The genes involved have not been identified.

The hepatosplenic T-cell lymphomas are most often derived from immature γδ T cells (19). The cells express the cytotoxic granule-associated protein TIA-1, but they lack expression of the effector proteins, the granzymes and perforin. This feature may explain the lack of tissue necrosis in these tumors. In addition to expressing TCRδ, an indication of a γδ cell receptor, the cells are positive for CD56 and either CD4⁻/CD8⁻ or positive for CD8. CD5 is usually absent as well. This lymphoma, as the name implies, presents with marked hepatosplenomegaly, but occult bone marrow involvement is usually present as well. However, lymph node involvement is absent. This lymphoma is associated with isochromosome 7q and trisomy 8 as consistent cytogenetic abnormalities (3). Interestingly, an identical form of hepatosplenic lymphoma composed of αβ T cells can be encountered in rare cases (62).

A distinctive subtype of T-cell lymphoma is ALCL (10). It can occur at any age but is most common in children and adolescents (26). Although the cells express some T-cell antigens, they usually have a markedly aberrant phenotype, and some cases may appear to be of null cell phenotype (Table 8). However, at the genotypic level, all cases appear to have rearranged TCR genes (30). CD30 is an antigen initially detected on the neoplastic cells in HD. It is found on Reed-Sternberg (RS) cells, a subset of activated T cells, EBV-infected B cells, and in all cases of ALCL. Other characteristic markers include epithelial membrane antigen (EMA) and clusterin (109). The neoplastic cells also exhibit cytotoxic molecules (58).

Histologically, ALCL most often is composed of large, often lobulated, cells that preferentially involve lymph node sinuses, and in the past such lesions were often interpreted as malignant histiocytosis (97). Tissue section immunohistochemistry is very helpful in the diagnosis of this entity because the malignant cells may not be numerous and staining for CD30 highlights their sinusoidal distribution. The

TABLE 8 Differential diagnosis of ALCL and HD[a]

Disease	CD30	CD15	LCA	CD3	TIA-1	EMA	Clusterin	ALK	CD20
ALCL	+	−	+	±	+	+	+	+	−
cHD	+	+	−	−	−	−	−	−	±
NLPHD		−	−	+	−	±	−	−	+
PTL, unspecified	±	−	+	+	±	−	−	−	−
DLBCL	±	−	+	−	−	±	−	−	+

[a]LCA, leukocyte common antigen; cHD, classical HD.

CD30 antigen can be detected in either paraffin or frozen sections.

ALCL was first recognized based on characteristic histological features (sinusoidal invasion) and a distinctive immunophenotype (CD30⁺). However, neither sinusoidal invasion nor CD30 positivity proved to be entirely specific. Subsequently, a characteristic cytogenetic abnormality was identified, the t(2;5) translocation, which led to identification of the genes involved in the most common translocation of ALCL (*NPM/ALK*) and insights into the pathogenesis (69, 83). Generation of monoclonal antibodies to the aberrantly expressed ALK can be used diagnostically and has led to improved definition of the diagnostic entity, with important clinical and prognostic implications (78). Utilizing these biological tools, the ultimate histological spectrum of ALCL is both broader and narrower than originally believed. ALK expression can now be considered a defining feature, as ALK-negative cases of ALCL probably represent different entities (44).

In addition to the classical t(2;5) translocation that is found in about 75% of ALCLs, additional variant translocations occur in the remainder of cases (61). All variant translocations involve the ALK gene on chromosome 2, but a different partner chromosome. Regardless of the partnering gene involved in the translocation, ALK is activated in all cases and is believed to play a central role in ALCL pathogenesis (108). The diagnosis of ALCL can be assisted by RT-PCR, which will identify the 75% of cases with classical NPM/ALK fusion genes, or by FISH, which will detect both classical and variant translocations.

Primary cutaneous ALCL is a different disease and is closely related to lymphomatoid papulosis, a chronic lymphoproliferative disease of the skin (111). These cases do not have a t(2;5) translocation and do not express ALK protein. Notably, although all cases of true ALCL are ALK positive, ALK expression can be detected in other rare entities, such as myofibroblastic tumors, and ALK-positive CD30-negative large-B-cell lymphomas.

HD (Hodgkin's Lymphoma)

HD is an unusual neoplastic disorder because the neoplastic cells represent only a minority of the cells present in the tumor mass. The neoplastic cells, the RS cells and their mononuclear variants, are admixed with normal lymphocytes, histiocytes, eosinophils, neutrophils, and plasma cells. The paucity of RS cells has led to difficulty in their characterization by flow cytometric techniques and has severely impeded the molecular analysis of this neoplasm. The normal lymphocytes within HD are usually identifiable as T cells, predominantly CD4⁺. However, the nature of the malignant cell in HD has taken a long time to unravel.

The tumor cells express CD15, an antigen found in normal granulocytes, histiocytes, and many epithelial cells. They also express the CD30 antigen, first identified on cell lines derived from HD. Leukocyte common antigen (CD45) is frequently absent. The identification of CD20 on at least some of the neoplastic cells led to speculation that HD was B-cell derived (76). Immunohistochemistry to assess light-chain restriction is also usually not helpful for the assessment of clonality, as the amount of immunoglobulin produced is small, the cells tend to stain nonspecifically, and background staining for immunoglobulin tends to be high. Traditional molecular studies of HD generally failed to detect clonal IGH rearrangements because of the low percentage of tumor cells in the population. The diagnostic sensitivity of IGH PCR is about 2 to 3% tumor cells (of total B cells), and frequently the number of clonal RS cells is below this threshold. However, by enriching RS cells through the use of microdissection techniques, several investigators were able to confirm a clonal B-cell origin in virtually all cases (52, 60). In addition, the cells were shown to have somatic mutations of the IGH genes, indicative of a GC stage of differentiation. Similar to the classical forms of HD, the nodular lymphocyte-predominant variant (NLPHD) has also been shown to be of B-cell origin; however, because of its distinctive immunophenotypic and clinicopathological characteristics, NLPHD is now considered to be a separate entity (66). There are no characteristic recurrent translocations of significance known in either classical HD or in NLPHD, and molecular profiling studies have been difficult to perform due to the difficulty in obtaining pure populations of tumor cells.

NONLYMPHOID TUMORS OF THE IMMUNE SYSTEM: "HISTIOCYTIC" DISORDERS

Normal Histiocytic Subsets

The cells of the histiocytic system consist of two major subsets of antigen-presenting cells: dendritic cells and phagocytic cells (45). The follicular DRC are found in follicles and present antigen to B lymphocytes, but they may not be of hematopoietic origin. They are positive for CD21, CD23, CD35, and clusterin but are CD45 negative. The interdigitating dendritic cells (IDC) and Langerhans cells (LC) are bone marrow-derived cells that present antigen to T lymphocytes. LC are found primarily in the skin but also in other organs. IDC are found in lymph nodes and other lymphoid organs. Both LC and IDC are S100 positive. The relationship between these cells is controversial. Both types are CD1a positive, although IDCs show variable expression dependent upon their maturational stage. However, unlike LCs, IDCs do not possess the characteristic Birbeck granule. Fibroblastic reticular cells are involved in transport of cytokines and other mediators (36). In lymph nodes, they ensheathe the postcapillary venules. They are of mesenchymal rather than hematopoietic origin, and they express smooth muscle actin (5).

All of the macrophages of lymph nodes share many enzyme histochemical and immunophenotypic characteristics. They have abundant and diffuse activity for lysosomal enzymes, including acid phosphatase and nonspecific esterase. As stated above, all of these cells can also demonstrate phagocytosis under appropriate conditions. Activity for lysozyme and alpha-1-antitrypsin can be seen in all of the above subtypes but is most prominent in epithelioid histiocytes. Activity for lysozyme decreases abruptly with phagocytosis, presumably because of its loss into lysosomal vacuoles. CD68 is the most useful antigen for detection of macrophages in routine paraffin sections.

A variety of monoclonal antibodies that react with monocytes and macrophages have been derived. Unfortunately, most of these antibodies lack specificity for the mononuclear phagocytic system, and many react with other hematopoietic cells as well: myeloid cells, T cells, or B cells. For example, CD11c is present on monocytes and macrophages, and is weak or absent on normal T and B lymphocytes. However, this antigen is found on the cells of hairy cell leukemia (a B-cell lymphoproliferative disorder) and in some cases of B-cell CLL. Cross-reactivities with T cells are present as well. For example, CD4 is found in normal monocytes and macrophages. CD25, in addition to being found on activated T lymphocytes, is found on normal monocytes and macrophages. CD68, strongly positive on histiocytes, also reacts with granulocytic precursors. The CD14 antigen is present on monocytes and macrophages and probably has the greatest specificity for the macrophage lineage among available reagents.

Proliferative Histiocytic Lesions

Proliferative lesions of antigen-presenting cells are relatively rare (28). The principal proliferative lesion of the dendritic cell system is LC histiocytosis (LCH). Recent studies, using the HUMARA method described above, have shown that the cells of LCH are monoclonal, but the disease usually has a self-limited course, especially in older children and adults (112). It may be fatal in infants. The cells of LCH have the characteristics of LC, including CD1 expression, langerin expression, and Birbeck granules (33). In contrast to normal LC, the cells also express antigens associated with phagocytic histiocytes, such as CD14 and CD11c. While comparative genomic hybridization studies have revealed losses or gains of a variety of chromosomal regions, there are no consistent genetic abnormalities associated with this disease.

Although the cells of LCH may sometimes appear to be cytologically atypical, even with abnormal mitotic figures, histological features are said not to be an important prognostic indicator in this disease. The prognosis is best correlated with the age at presentation and the extent of organ system involvement. Patients under 2 years of age tend to have a poor prognosis, whereas those older than 6 years have an excellent prognosis. Multisystem disease also is a poor prognostic factor.

There are rare tumors described that have a derivation from IDC. These lesions are usually based in lymph nodes and are often associated with an inflammatory background and/or necrosis. There is overlap in histology and phenotype with true histiocytic tumors, and they may have an aggressive clinical course. By contrast, follicular dendritic cell (FDC) sarcomas usually present with localized lymph node involvement. They may recur locally but usually do not disseminate. These neoplasms are also rare. Rare tumors of fibroblastic reticular cell origin also are seen in lymph nodes. The expression of clusterin, CD21 (DRC sarcomas), S100

(IDC tumors), CD1a (IDC tumors), and actin (fibroblastic reticular cell tumors) can be helpful in distinguishing these three stromal neoplasms of lymph nodes (5). There are no specific cytogenetic abnormalities or molecular tests associated with these tumors.

Malignancies of mononuclear phagocytes include acute monocytic leukemia and histiocytic sarcoma. In rare instances, histiocytic sarcomas may be disseminated, fulfilling criteria for what has been termed in the past "malignant histiocytosis." However, most instances of malignant histiocytosis reported previously represent other entities, such as ALCL (45).

Acute monocytic leukemia relates to a bone marrow-derived monoblast. This malignancy arises in the bone marrow compartment, with secondary involvement of the peripheral blood and usually a markedly elevated leukocyte count. In contrast to acute myeloid leukemia, there is a somewhat higher incidence of involvement of non-hematopoietic sites, with frequent involvement of skin and gingiva.

Histiocytic sarcoma represents a malignancy of the mononuclear phagocytic series at the stage of the fixed-tissue histiocyte. Therefore, the lesions in histiocytic sarcoma represent localized, relatively discrete tumefactions. In addition to the reticuloendothelial system, common sites of involvement include skin and bone. Because there are few, if any, markers with absolute specificity for macrophages, the investigator must rigorously exclude other cell lineages with both immunophenotypic and molecular means.

In the absence of special studies, morphological evidence of phagocytosis by the neoplastic cells, most commonly erythrophagocytosis, had been proposed as a criterion for a derivation from mononuclear phagocytes. However, phagocytosis is inconspicuous in most mononuclear phagocytic malignancies. Moreover, it is not a specific finding and has been described for lymphoid, plasmacytic, and even epithelial tumors. Even if phagocytosis is observed, it is virtually always clinically insignificant. The hemophagocytic syndrome is the most common and clinically significant of the proliferative disorders of macrophages. However, it is not a neoplastic process. It is usually seen in association with immunodeficiency or another hematopoietic malignancy (47, 84). This syndrome appears to be pathogenetically related to an excessive production of cytokines and chemokines capable of stimulating mononuclear phagocytes (102). The cells in hemophagocytic syndromes are morphologically and phenotypically activated macrophages.

CONCLUSIONS

Tumors of the immune system are of interest not only because they represent models of normal immune cells but also because they provide excellent examples of how immunologic and molecular tumor markers may be used in clinical diagnosis. Because the lymphomas simulate normal cellular counterparts, it has been possible to develop modern classification schemes that take advantage of and utilize the large panels of antibodies that were primarily developed to study and characterize normal immune cells. The investigation of the molecular genetic abnormalities found in tumors of the immune system, particularly the translocations that occur in lymphoid neoplasms, has resulted in the discovery of oncogenic classes of genes that have been further exploited for the development of diagnostic testing and tumor classification purposes. The assimilation of both immunologic and molecular approaches has been largely responsible for the current biologically based WHO classification scheme.

The example provided by the WHO classification scheme has not gone unnoticed in the study and classification of other cancers. While many of the other tissues in which cancers arise may not be as complex as the immune system, the classification of nonlymphoid tumors has also benefited from advances in the detection of immunologic and molecular genetics of the tumors. One such example has been the refinements that have occurred in the classification and diagnosis of the so-called small cell tumors of childhood, in which both protein and molecular markers have been used to dissect out the origins and provide the tools to accurately classify these morphologically similar tumors. Small blue cell tumors include neuroblastomas, rhabdomyosarcomas, Ewing's sarcomas, and other rare tumors. Each of these is now known to be associated with characteristic cell surface markers and tumor-specific translocations. Thus, the same approaches discussed for the lymphomas can be applied to the investigation and classification of these and other cancers. There is little doubt that the next generation of classification schemes developed for both tumors of the immune system and other types of tumors will continue to benefit from and incorporate information from advances in our understanding of the biology of normal cellular counterparts, as well as from the voluminous data being generated from the ongoing molecular dissection of the tumors themselves.

REFERENCES

1. Abruzzo, L. V., K. Schmidt, L. M. Weiss, E. S. Jaffe, L. J. Medeiros, C. A. Sander, and M. Raffeld. 1993. B-cell lymphoma after angioimmunoblastic lymphadenopathy: a case with oligoclonal gene rearrangements associated with Epstein-Barr virus. *Blood* **82:**241–246.

2. Alizadeh, A. A., M. B. Eisen, R. E. Davis, C. Ma, I. S. Lossos, A. Rosenwald, J. C. Boldrick, H. Sabet, T. Tran, X. Yu, J. I. Powell, L. Yang, G. E. Marti, T. Moore, J. Hudson, Jr., L. Lu, D. B. Lewis, R. Tibshirani, G. Sherlock, W. C. Chan, T. C. Greiner, D. D. Weisenburger, J. O. Armitage, R. Warnke, L. M. Staudt, et al. 2000. Distinct types of diffuse large B-cell lymphoma identified by gene expression profiling. *Nature* **403:**503–511.

3. Alonsozana, E. L., J. Stamberg, D. Kumar, E. S. Jaffe, L. J. Medeiros, C. Frantz, C. A. Schiffer, B. A. O'Connell, S. Kerman, S. A. Stass, and L. V. Abruzzo. 1997. Isochromosome 7q: the primary cytogenetic abnormality in hepatosplenic gamma delta T cell lymphoma. *Leukemia* **11:**1367–1372.

4. Ambinder, R. F., and R. B. Mann. 1994. Detection and characterization of Epstein-Barr virus in clinical specimens. *Am. J. Pathol.* **145:**239–252.

5. Andriko, J. W., E. P. Kaldjian, M. Tsokos, S. L. Abbondanzo, and E. S. Jaffe. 1998. Reticulum cell neoplasms of lymph nodes: a clinicopathologic study of 11 cases with recognition of a new subtype derived from fibroblastic reticular cells. *Am. J. Surg. Pathol.* **22:**1048–1058.

6. Arya, M., I. S. Shergill, M. Williamson, L. Gommersall, N. Arya, and H. R. Patel. 2005. Basic principles of real-time quantitative PCR. *Expert Rev. Mol. Diagn.* **5:**209–219.

7. Attygalle, A., R. Al-Jehani, T. C. Diss, P. Munson, H. Liu, M. Q. Du, P. G. Isaacson, and A. Dogan. 2002. Neoplastic T cells in angioimmunoblastic T-cell lymphoma express CD10. *Blood* **99:**627–633.

8. Baens, M., B. Maes, A. Steyls, K. Geboes, P. Marynen, and C. De Wolf-Peeters. 2000. The product of the t(11;18), an API2-MLT fusion, marks nearly half of gastric MALT type lymphomas without large cell proliferation. *Am. J. Pathol.* **156:**1433–1439.

9. Baumgarth, N., and M. Roederer. 2000. A practical approach to multicolor flow cytometry for immunophenotyping. *J. Immunol. Methods* **243:**77–97.

10. Benharroch, D., Z. Meguerian-Bedoyan, L. Lamant, C. Amin, L. Brugieres, M. J. Terrier-Lacombe, E. Haralambieva, K. Pulford, S. Pileri, S. W. Morris, D. Y. Mason, and G. Delsol. 1998. ALK-positive lymphoma: a single disease with a broad spectrum of morphology. *Blood* **91:**2076–2084.

11. Bergsagel, P. L., W. M. Kuehl, F. Zhan, J. Sawyer, B. Barlogie, and J. Shaughnessy, Jr. 2005. Cyclin D dysregulation: an early and unifying pathogenic event in multiple myeloma. *Blood* **106:**296–303.

12. Bijwaard, K. E., N. S. Aguilera, Y. Monczak, M. Trudel, J. K. Taubenberger, and J. H. Lichy. 2001. Quantitative real-time reverse transcription-PCR assay for cyclin D1 expression: utility in the diagnosis of mantle cell lymphoma. *Clin. Chem.* **47:**195–201.

13. Buccheri, V., B. Mihaljevic, E. Matutes, M. J. Dyer, D. Y. Mason, and D. Catovsky. 1993. mb-1: a new marker for B-lineage lymphoblastic leukemia. *Blood* **82:**853–857.

14. Bunn, P. A., Jr., G. P. Schechter, E. Jaffe, D. Blayney, R. C. Young, M. J. Matthews, W. Blattner, S. Broder, M. Robert-Guroff, and R. C. Gallo. 1983. Clinical course of retrovirus-associated adult T-cell lymphoma in the United States. *N. Engl. J. Med.* **309:**257–264.

15. Calin, G. A., C. D. Dumitru, M. Shimizu, R. Bichi, S. Zupo, E. Noch, H. Aldler, S. Rattan, M. Keating, K. Rai, L. Rassenti, T. Kipps, M. Negrini, F. Bullrich, and C. M. Croce. 2002. Frequent deletions and downregulation of micro-RNA genes miR15 and miR16 at 13q14 in chronic lymphocytic leukemia. *Proc. Natl. Acad. Sci. USA* **99:**15524–15529.

16. Calin, G. A., C. Sevignani, C. D. Dumitru, T. Hyslop, E. Noch, S. Yendamuri, M. Shimizu, S. Rattan, F. Bullrich, M. Negrini, and C. M. Croce. 2004. Human microRNA genes are frequently located at fragile sites and genomic regions involved in cancers. *Proc. Natl. Acad. Sci. USA* **101:**2999–3004.

17. Cesarman, E., Y. Chang, P. S. Moore, J. W. Said, and D. M. Knowles. 1995. Kaposi's sarcoma-associated herpesvirus-like DNA sequences in AIDS-related bodycavity-based lymphomas. *N. Engl. J. Med.* **332:**1186–1191.

18. Cimmino, A., G. A. Calin, M. Fabbri, M. V. Iorio, M. Ferracin, M. Shimizu, S. E. Wojcik, R. I. Aqeilan, S. Zupo, M. Dono, L. Rassenti, H. Alder, S. Volinia, C. G. Liu, T. J. Kipps, M. Negrini, and C. M. Croce. 2005. miR-15 and miR-16 induce apoptosis by targeting BCL2. *Proc. Natl. Acad. Sci. USA* **102:**13944–13949.

19. Cooke, C. B., M. Krenacs, M. Stetler-Stevenson, T. C. Greiner, M. Raffeld, D. W. Kingma, L. Abruzzo, C. Frantz, M. Kaviani, and E. S. Jaffe. 1996. Hepatosplenic gamma/delta T-cell lymphoma: a distinct clinicopathologic entity of cytotoxic gamma/delta T-cell origin. *Blood* **88:**4265–4274.

20. Dalla-Favera, R., M. Bregni, J. Erikson, D. Patterson, R. C. Gallo, and C. M. Croce. 1982. Human c-myc onc gene is located on the region of chromosome 8 that is translocated in Burkitt lymphoma cells. *Proc. Natl. Acad. Sci. USA* **79:**7824–7827.

21. de Bruin, P. C., J. A. Kummer, P. van der Valk, P. van Heerde, P. M. Kluin, R. Willemze, G. J. Ossenkoppele, T. Radaszkiewicz, and C. J. Meijer. 1994. Granzyme B-expressing peripheral T-cell lymphomas: neoplastic equivalents of activated cytotoxic T cells with preference for mucosa-associated lymphoid tissue localization. *Blood* **84:**3785–3791.

22. Delabie, J., E. Vandenberghe, C. Kennes, G. Verhoef, M. Foschini, M. Stul, J. Cassiman, and C. De Wolf-Peeters. 1992. Histiocyte-rich B-cell lymphoma. A distinct clinicopathologic entity possibly related to lymphocyte predominant Hodgkin's disease, paragranuloma subtype. *Am. J. Surg. Pathol.* **16:**37–48.

23. Diaz-Cano, S. J., A. Blanes, and H. J. Wolfe. 2001. PCR techniques for clonality assays. *Diagn. Mol. Pathol.* **10:**24–33.

24. DiGiuseppe, J. A., W. G. Nelson, E. J. Seifter, J. K. Boitnott, and R. B. Mann. 1994. Intravascular lymphomatosis: a clinicopathologic study of 10 cases and assessment of response to chemotherapy. *J. Clin. Oncol.* **12:**2573–2579.

25. Dohner, H., S. Stilgenbauer, K. Dohner, M. Bentz, and P. Lichter. 1999. Chromosome aberrations in B-cell chronic lymphocytic leukemia: reassessment based on molecular cytogenetic analysis. *J. Mol. Med.* **77:**266–281.

26. Falini, B., S. Pileri, P. L. Zinzani, A. Carbone, V. Zagonel, C. Wolf-Peeters, G. Verhoef, F. Menestrina, G. Todeschini, M. Paulli, M. Lazzarino, R. Giardini, A. Aiello, H.-D. Foss, I. Araujo, M. Fizzotti, P.-G. Pelicci, L. Flenghi, M. F. Martelli, and A. Santucci. 1999. ALK+ lymphoma: clinico-pathological findings and outcome. *Blood* **93:**2697–2706.

27. Fang, J. M., W. G. Finn, J. W. Hussong, C. L. Goolsby, A. R. Cubbon, and D. Variakojis. 1999. CD10 antigen expression correlates with the t(14;18)(q32;q21) major breakpoint region in diffuse large B-cell lymphoma. *Mod. Pathol.* **12:**295–300.

28. Favara, B. E., A. C. Feller, M. Pauli, E. S. Jaffe, L. M. Weiss, M. Arico, P. Bucsky, R. M. Egeler, G. Elinder, H. Gadner, M. Gresik, J. I. Henter, S. Imashuku, G. Janka-Schaub, R. Jaffe, S. Ladisch, C. Nezelof, and J. Pritchard. 1997. Contemporary classification of histiocytic disorders. The WHO Committee On Histiocytic/ Reticulum Cell Proliferations. Reclassification Working Group of the Histiocyte Society. *Med. Pediatr. Oncol.* **29:**157–166.

29. Ferry, J. A., W. I. Yang, L. R. Zukerberg, A. C. Wotherspoon, A. Arnold, and N. L. Harris. 1996. CD5+ extranodal marginal zone B-cell (MALT) lymphoma. A low grade neoplasm with a propensity for bone marrow involvement and relapse. *Am. J. Clin. Pathol.* **105:**31–37.

30. Foss, H. D., I. Anagnostopoulos, I. Araujo, C. Assaf, G. Demel, J. A. Kummer, M. Hummel, and H. Stein. 1996. Anaplastic large-cell lymphomas of T-cell and null-cell phenotype express cytotoxic molecules. *Blood* **88:**4005–4011.

31. Frizzera, G., Y. Kaneko, and M. Sakurai. 1989. Angioimmunoblastic lymphadenopathy and related disorders: a retrospective look in search of definitions. *Leukemia* **3:**1–5.

32. Gaulard, P., M. d'Agay, M. Peuchmaur, N. Brousse, C. Gisselbrecht, P. Solal-Celigny, J. Diebold, and D. Mason. 1992. Expression of the bcl-2 gene product in follicular lymphoma. *Am. J. Pathol.* **140:**1089–1095.

33. Geissmann, F., Y. Lepelletier, S. Fraitag, J. Valladeau, C. Bodemer, M. Debre, M. Leborgne, S. Saeland, and N. Brousse. 2001. Differentiation of Langerhans cells in Langerhans cell histiocytosis. *Blood* **97:**1241–1248.

34. Gerard-Marchant, R., I. Hamlin, K. Lennert, F. Rilke, A. Stansfeld, and J. van Unnik. 1974. Classification of non-Hodgkin's lymphomas. *Lancet* **ii:**406–408.

35. Golub, T. R., D. K. Slonim, P. Tamayo, C. Huard, M. Gaasenbeek, J. P. Mesirov, H. Coller, M. L. Loh, J. R. Downing, M. A. Caligiuri, C. D. Bloomfield, and E. S. Lander. 1999. Molecular classification of cancer: class discovery and class prediction by gene expression monitoring. *Science* **286:**531–537.

36. Gretz, J. E., A. O. Anderson, and S. Shaw. 1997. Cords, channels, corridors and conduits: critical architectural elements facilitating cell interactions in the lymph node cortex. *Immunol. Rev.* **156:**11–24.

37. Grogg, K. L., A. D. Attygalle, W. R. Macon, E. D. Remstein, P. J. Kurtin, and A. Dogan. 2005. Angioimmunoblastic T-cell lymphoma: a neoplasm of germinal-center T-helper cells? *Blood* **106:**1501–1502.

38. Hans, C. P., D. D. Weisenburger, T. C. Greiner, R. D. Gascoyne, J. Delabie, G. Ott, H. K. Muller-Hermelink, E. Campo, R. M. Braziel, E. S. Jaffe, Z. Pan, P. Farinha, L. M. Smith, B. Falini, A. H. Banham, A. Rosenwald, L. M. Staudt, J. M. Connors, J. O. Armitage, and W. C. Chan. 2004. Confirmation of the molecular classification of diffuse large B-cell lymphoma by immunohistochemistry using a tissue microarray. *Blood* **103:**275–282.

39. Harris, N. L., E. S. Jaffe, H. Stein, P. M. Banks, J. K. Chan, M. L. Cleary, G. Delsol, C. De Wolf-Peeters, B. Falini, K. C. Gatter, et al. 1994. A revised European-American classification of lymphoid neoplasms: a proposal from the International Lymphoma Study Group. *Blood* **84:**1361–1392.

40. Hatta, Y., Y. Yamada, M. Tomonaga, I. Miyoshi, J. W. Said, and H. P. Koeffler. 1999. Detailed deletion mapping of the long arm of chromosome 6 in adult T-cell leukemia. *Blood* **93:**613–616.

41. Ho, F., G. Srivastava, S. Loke, K. Fu, B. Leung, R. Liang, and D. Choy. 1990. Presence of Epstein-Barr virus DNA in nasal lymphomas of B and T cell type. *Hematol. Oncol.* **8:**271–281.

42. Horsman, D. E., R. D. Gascoyne, R. W. Coupland, A. J. Coldman, and S. A. Adomat. 1995. Comparison of cytogenetic analysis, Southern analysis, and polymerase chain reaction for the detection of t(14; 18) in follicular lymphoma. *Am. J. Clin. Pathol.* **103:**472–478.

43. Isaacson, P. G., and M. Q. Du. 2004. MALT lymphoma: from morphology to molecules. *Nat. Rev. Cancer* **4:**644–653.

44. Jaffe, E. S. 2001. Anaplastic large cell lymphoma: the shifting sands of diagnostic hematopathology. *Mod. Pathol.* **14:**219–228.

45. Jaffe, E. S. 1995. Malignant histiocytosis and true histiocytic lymphomas, p. 560–593. *In* E. S. Jaffe (ed.), *Surgical Pathology of Lymph Nodes and Related Organs*, 2nd ed. W. B. Saunders Co., Philadelphia, Pa.

46. Jaffe, E. S., J. K. C. Chan, I. J. Su, G. Frizzera, S. Mori, A. C. Feller, and F. Ho. 1996. Report of the workshop on nasal and related extranodal angiocentric T/NK cell lymphomas: definitions, differential diagnosis, and epidemiology. *Am. J. Surg. Pathol.* **20:**103–111.

47. Jaffe, E. S., J. Costa, A. S. Fauci, J. Cossman, and M. Tsokos. 1983. Malignant lymphoma and erythrophagocytosis simulating malignant histiocytosis. *Am. J. Med.* **75:**741–749.

48. Jaffe, E. S., N. L. Harris, J. Diebold, and H. K. Muller-Hermelink. 1998. World Health Organization classification of lymphomas: a work in progress. *Ann. Oncol.* **9** (Suppl. 5):S25–S30.

49. Jaffe, E. S., L. Krenacs, S. Kumar, D. W. Kingma, and M. Raffeld. 1999. Extranodal peripheral T-cell and NK-cell neoplasms. *Am. J. Clin. Pathol.* **111**(Suppl. 1):S46–S55.

50. Jaffe, E. S., L. Krenacs, and M. Raffeld. 1997. Classification of T-cell and NK-cell neoplasms based on the REAL classification. *Ann. Oncol.* **8**(Suppl. 2):S17–S24.

51. Jaffe, E. S., M. Raffeld, and L. J. Medeiros. 1993. Histopathologic subtypes of indolent lymphomas: caricatures of the mature B-cell system. *Semin. Oncol.* **20:**3–30.

52. Kanzler, H., R. Kuppers, M. L. Hansmann, and K. Rajewsky. 1996. Hodgkin and Reed-Sternberg cells in Hodgkin's disease represent the outgrowth of a dominant

tumor clone derived from (crippled) germinal center B cells. *J. Exp. Med.* **184:**1495–1505.

53. **Kluin, P. H., and E. Schuuring.** 1997. FISH and related techniques in the diagnosis of lymphoma. *Cancer Surv.* **30:**3–20.

54. **Kluin, P. M., and J. H. van Krieken.** 1991. The molecular biology of B-cell lymphoma: clinicopathologic implications. *Ann. Hematol.* **62:**95–102.

55. **Kopp, P., R. Jaggi, A. Tobler, B. Borisch, M. Oestreicher, L. Sabacan, J. L. Jameson, and M. F. Fey.** 1997. Clonal X-inactivation analysis of human tumours using the human androgen receptor gene (HUMARA) polymorphism: a non-radioactive and semiquantitative strategy applicable to fresh and archival tissue. *Mol. Cell. Probes* **11:**217–228.

56. **Korsmeyer, S. J., A. Arnold, A. Bakhshi, J. V. Ravetch, U. Siebenlist, P. A. Hieter, S. O. Sharrow, T. W. LeBien, J. H. Kersey, D. G. Poplack, P. Leder, and T. A. Waldmann.** 1983. Immunoglobulin gene rearrangement and cell surface antigen expression in acute lymphocytic leukemias of T-cell and B-cell precursor origins. *J. Clin. Investig.* **71:**301–313.

57. **Krenacs, L., T. Krenacs, and M. Raffeld.** 1999. Antigen retrieval for immunohistochemical reactions in routinely processed paraffin sections. *Methods Mol. Biol.* **115:**85–93.

58. **Krenacs, L., A. Wellmann, L. Sorbara, A. W. Himmelmann, E. Bagdi, E. S. Jaffe, and M. Raffeld.** 1997. Cytotoxic cell antigen expression in anaplastic large cell lymphomas of T- and null-cell type and Hodgkin's disease: evidence for distinct cellular origin. *Blood* **89:**980–989.

59. **Kumar, S., G. A. Green, J. Teruya-Feldstein, M. Raffeld, and E. S. Jaffe.** 1996. Use of CD23 (BU38) on paraffin sections in the diagnosis of small lymphocytic lymphoma and mantle cell lymphoma. *Mod. Pathol.* **9:**925–929.

60. **Kuppers, R., K. Rajewsky, M. Zhao, G. Simons, R. Laumann, R. Fischer, and M. Hansmann.** 1994. Hodgkin's disease: Hodgkin and Reed Sternberg cells picked from histological sections show clonal immunoglobulin gene rearrangements and appear to be derived from B cells at various stages of development. *Proc. Natl. Acad. Sci. USA* **91:**1092–1096.

61. **Kutok, J. L., and J. C. Aster.** 2002. Molecular biology of anaplastic lymphoma kinase-positive anaplastic large-cell lymphoma. *J. Clin. Oncol.* **20:**3691–3702.

62. **Lai, R., L. M. Larratt, W. Etches, S. T. Mortimer, L. D. Jewell, L. Dabbagh, and R. W. Coupland.** 2000. Hepatosplenic T-cell lymphoma of alphabeta lineage in a 16-year-old boy presenting with hemolytic anemia and thrombocytopenia. *Am. J. Surg. Pathol.* **24:**459–463.

63. **Lamarre, L., J. Jacobson, A. Aisenberg, and N. Harris.** 1989. Primary large cell lymphoma of the mediastinum. *Am. J. Surg. Pathol.* **13:**730–739.

64. **Lazzarino, M., E. Orlandi, M. Paulli, E. Boveri, E. Morra, E. Brusamolino, S. Kindl, R. Rosso, C. Astori, M. C. Buonanno, et al.** 1993. Primary mediastinal B-cell lymphoma with sclerosis: an aggressive tumor with distinctive clinical and pathologic features. *J. Clin. Oncol.* **11:**2306–2313.

65. **Lukes, R., and R. Collins.** 1974. Immunologic characterization of human malignant lymphomas. *Cancer* **34:**1488–1503.

66. **Mason, D., P. Banks, J. Chan, M. Cleary, G. Delsol, C. de Wolf-Peeters, B. Falini, K. Gatter, T. Grogan, N. Harris, P. Isaacson, E. Jaffe, D. Knowles, H. Muller-Hermelink, S. Pileri, M. Piris, H. Stein, E. Ralfkiaer, and R. Warnke.** 1994. Nodular lymphocyte predominance Hodgkin's disease: a distinct clinico-pathological entity. *Am. J. Surg. Pathol.* **18:**528–530.

67. **Mason, D. Y., J. L. Cordell, M. H. Brown, J. Borst, M. Jones, K. Pulford, E. Jaffe, E. Ralfkiaer, F. Dallenbach, H. Stein, S. Pileri, and K. C. Gatter.** 1995. CD79a: a novel marker for B-cell neoplasms in routinely processed tissue samples. *Blood* **86:**1453–1459.

68. **Medeiros, L. J., J. H. van Krieken, E. S. Jaffe, and M. Raffeld.** 1990. Association of bcl-1 rearrangements with lymphocytic lymphoma of intermediate differentiation. *Blood* **76:**2086–2090.

69. **Morris, S. W., M. N. Kirstein, M. B. Valentine, K. G. Dittmer, D. N. Shapiro, D. L. Saltman, and A. T. Look.** 1994. Fusion of a kinase gene, ALK, to a nucleolar protein gene, NPM, in non-Hodgkin's lymphoma. *Science* **263:**1281–1284.

70. **The Non-Hodgkin's Lymphoma Classification Project.** 1997. A clinical evaluation of the International Lymphoma Study Group classification of non-Hodgkin's lymphoma. *Blood* **89:**3909–3918.

71. **The Non-Hodgkin's Lymphoma Pathologic Classification Project.** 1982. National Cancer Institute sponsored study of classifications of non-Hodgkin's lymphomas: summary and description of a working formulation for clinical usage. *Cancer* **49:**2112–2135.

72. **Nurse, G. T., and T. Jenkins.** 1973. G.-6-P.D. phenotypes and X-chromosome inactivation. *Lancet* **ii:**99–100.

73. **Otsuki, T., S. Kumar, B. Ensoli, D. W. Kingma, T. Yano, M. Stetler-Stevenson, E. S. Jaffe, and M. Raffeld.** 1996. Detection of HHV-8/KSHV DNA sequences in AIDS-associated extranodal lymphoid malignancies. *Leukemia* **10:**1358–1362.

74. **Ozdemirli, M., J. C. Fanburg-Smith, D. P. Hartmann, A. T. Shad, J. M. Lage, I. T. Magrath, N. Azumi, N. L. Harris, J. Cossman, and E. S. Jaffe.** 1998. Precursor B-lymphoblastic lymphoma presenting as a solitary bone tumor and mimicking Ewing's sarcoma: a report of four cases and review of the literature. *Am. J. Surg. Pathol.* **22:**795–804.

75. **Picker, L., L. Weiss, L. Medeiros, G. Wood, and R. Warnke.** 1987. Immunophenotypic criteria for the diagnosis of non-Hodgkin's lymphoma. *Am. J. Pathol.* **128:**181–201.

76. **Pinkus, G. S., and J. W. Said.** 1988. Hodgkin's disease, lymphocyte predominance type, nodular—further evidence for a B cell derivation: L&H variants of Reed-Sternberg cells express L26, a pan B cell marker. *Am. J. Pathol.* **133:**211–217.

77. **Pittaluga, S., M. Uppenkamp, and J. Cossman.** 1987. Development of T3/T cell receptor gene expression in human pre-T neoplasms. *Blood* **69:**1062–1067.

78. **Pulford, K., L. Lamant, S. W. Morris, L. H. Butler, K. M. Wood, D. Stroud, G. Delsol, and D. Y. Mason.** 1997. Detection of anaplastic lymphoma kinase (ALK) and nucleolar protein nucleophosmin (NPM)-ALK proteins in normal and neoplastic cells with the monoclonal antibody ALK1. *Blood* **89:**1394–1404.

79. **Quintanilla-Martinez, L., F. Fend, L. R. Moguel, L. Spilove, M. W. Beaty, D. W. Kingma, M. Raffeld, and E. S. Jaffe.** 1999. Peripheral T-cell lymphoma with Reed-Sternberg-like cells of B-cell phenotype and genotype associated with Epstein-Barr virus infection. *Am. J. Surg. Pathol.* **23:**1233–1240.

80. **Quintanilla-Martinez, L., J. L. Franklin, I. Guerrero, L. Krenacs, K. N. Naresh, C. Rama-Rao, K. Bhatia, M. Raffeld, and I. T. Magrath.** 1999. Histological and immunophenotypic profile of nasal NK/T cell lymphomas from Peru: high prevalence of p53 overexpression. *Hum. Pathol.* **30:**849–855.

81. **Raffeld, M., and E. S. Jaffe.** 1991. bcl-1, t(11;14), and mantle cell derived neoplasms. *Blood* **78:**259–263.

82. **Rappaport, H.** 1966. Tumors of the hematopoietic system. *Atlas of Tumor Pathology.* Armed Forces Institute of Pathology, Washington, D.C.

83. Rimokh, R., J. P. Magaud, F. Berger, J. Samarut, B. Coiffier, D. Germain, and D. Y. Mason. 1989. A translocation involving a specific breakpoint (q35) on chromosome 5 is characteristic of anaplastic large cell lymphoma ('Ki-1 lymphoma'). *Br. J. Haematol.* **71**:31–36.

84. Risdall, R. J., R. W. McKenna, M. E. Nesbit, W. Krivit, H. H. Balfour, Jr., R. L. Simmons, and R. D. Brunning. 1979. Virus-associated hemophagocytic syndrome: a benign histiocytic proliferation distinct from malignant histiocytosis. *Cancer* **44**:993–1002.

85. Robertson, K. D., and P. A. Jones. 1999. Tissue-specific alternative splicing in the human INK4a/ARF cell cycle regulatory locus. *Oncogene* **18**:3810–3820.

86. Rosenwald, A., A. A. Alizadeh, G. Widhopf, R. Simon, R. E. Davis, X. Yu, L. Yang, O. K. Pickeral, L. Z. Rassenti, J. Powell, D. Botstein, J. C. Byrd, M. R. Grever, B. D. Cheson, N. Chiorazzi, W. H. Wilson, T. J. Kipps, P. O. Brown, and L. M. Staudt. 2001. Relation of gene expression phenotype to immunoglobulin mutation genotype in B cell chronic lymphocytic leukemia. *J. Exp. Med.* **194**:1639–1647.

87. Rosenwald, A., G. Wright, W. C. Chan, J. M. Connors, E. Campo, R. I. Fisher, R. D. Gascoyne, H. K. Muller-Hermelink, E. B. Smeland, J. M. Giltnane, E. M. Hurt, H. Zhao, L. Averett, L. Yang, W. H. Wilson, E. S. Jaffe, R. Simon, R. D. Klausner, J. Powell, P. L. Duffey, D. L. Longo, T. C. Greiner, D. D. Weisenburger, W. G. Sanger, B. J. Dave, J. C. Lynch, J. Vose, J. O. Armitage, E. Montserrat, A. Lopez-Guillermo, T. M. Grogan, T. P. Miller, M. LeBlanc, G. Ott, S. Kvaloy, J. Delabie, H. Holte, P. Krajci, T. Stokke, and L. M. Staudt. 2002. The use of molecular profiling to predict survival after chemotherapy for diffuse large-B-cell lymphoma. *N. Engl. J. Med.* **346**:1937–1947.

88. Rosenwald, A., G. Wright, A. Wiestner, W. C. Chan, J. M. Connors, E. Campo, R. D. Gascoyne, T. M. Grogan, H. K. Muller-Hermelink, E. B. Smeland, M. Chiorazzi, J. M. Giltnane, E. M. Hurt, H. Zhao, L. Averett, S. Henrickson, L. Yang, J. Powell, W. H. Wilson, E. S. Jaffe, R. Simon, R. D. Klausner, E. Montserrat, F. Bosch, T. C. Greiner, D. D. Weisenburger, W. G. Sanger, B. J. Dave, J. C. Lynch, J. Vose, J. O. Armitage, R. I. Fisher, T. P. Miller, M. LeBlanc, G. Ott, S. Kvaloy, H. Holte, J. Delabie, and L. M. Staudt. 2003. The proliferation gene expression signature is a quantitative integrator of oncogenic events that predicts survival in mantle cell lymphoma. *Cancer Cell* **3**:185–197.

89. Rossi, S., L. Laurino, A. Furlanetto, S. Chinellato, E. Orvieto, F. Canal, F. Facchetti, and A. P. Dei Tos. 2005. Rabbit monoclonal antibodies: a comparative study between a novel category of immunoreagents and the corresponding mouse monoclonal antibodies. *Am. J. Clin. Pathol.* **124**:295–302.

90. Sander, C. A., T. Yano, H. M. Clark, C. Harris, D. L. Longo, E. S. Jaffe, and M. Raffeld. 1993. p53 mutation is associated with progression in follicular lymphomas. *Blood* **82**:1994–2004.

91. Savage, K. J., and R. D. Gascoyne. 2004. Molecular signatures of lymphoma. *Int. J. Hematol.* **80**:401–409.

92. Savage, K. J., S. Monti, J. L. Kutok, G. Cattoretti, D. Neuberg, L. De Leval, P. Kurtin, P. Dal Cin, C. Ladd, F. Feuerhake, R. C. Aguiar, S. Li, G. Salles, F. Berger, W. Jing, G. S. Pinkus, T. Habermann, R. Dalla-Favera, N. L. Harris, J. C. Aster, T. R. Golub, and M. A. Shipp. 2003. The molecular signature of mediastinal large B-cell lymphoma differs from that of other diffuse large B-cell lymphomas and shares features with classical Hodgkin lymphoma. *Blood* **102**:3871–3879.

93. Shi, S. R., R. J. Cote, and C. R. Taylor. 1997. Antigen retrieval immunohistochemistry: past, present, and future. *J. Histochem. Cytochem.* **45**:327–343.

94. Siu, L. L., K. F. Wong, J. K. Chan, and Y. L. Kwong. 1999. Comparative genomic hybridization analysis of natural killer cell lymphoma/leukemia. Recognition of consistent patterns of genetic alterations. *Am. J. Pathol.* **155**:1419–1425.

95. Spieker-Polet, H., P. Sethupathi, P. C. Yam, and K. L. Knight. 1995. Rabbit monoclonal antibodies: generating a fusion partner to produce rabbit-rabbit hybridomas. *Proc. Natl. Acad. Sci. USA* **92**:9348–9352.

96. Spits, H., B. Blom, A. C. Jaleco, K. Weijer, M. C. Verschuren, J. J. van Dongen, M. H. Heemskerk, and P. C. Res. 1998. Early stages in the development of human T, natural killer and thymic dendritic cells. *Immunol. Rev.* **165**:75–86.

97. Stein, H., D. Mason, J. Gerdes, N. O'Connor, J. Wainscoat, G. Pallesen, K. Gatter, B. Falini, G. Delsol, H. Lemke, R. Schwarting, and K. Lennert. 1985. The expression of the Hodgkin's disease associated antigen Ki-1 in reactive and neoplastic lymphoid tissue: evidence that Reed-Sternberg cells and histiocytic malignancies are derived from activated lymphoid cells. *Blood* **66**:848–858.

98. Szczepanski, T., A. Beishuizen, M. J. Pongers-Willemse, K. Hahlen, E. R. Van Wering, A. J. Wijkhuijs, G. J. Tibbe, M. A. De Bruijn, and J. J. Van Dongen. 1999. Cross-lineage T cell receptor gene rearrangements occur in more than ninety percent of childhood precursor-B acute lymphoblastic leukemias: alternative PCR targets for detection of minimal residual disease. *Leukemia* **13**:196–205.

99. Szczepanski, T., A. W. Langerak, M. J. Willemse, I. L. Wolvers-Tettero, E. R. van Wering, and J. J. van Dongen. 2000. T cell receptor gamma (TCRG) gene rearrangements in T cell acute lymphoblastic leukemia reflect 'end-stage' recombinations: implications for minimal residual disease monitoring. *Leukemia* **14**:1208–1214.

100. Szczepanski, T., M. J. Pongers-Willemse, A. W. Langerak, W. A. Harts, A. J. Wijkhuijs, E. R. van Wering, and J. J. van Dongen. 1999. Ig heavy chain gene rearrangements in T-cell acute lymphoblastic leukemia exhibit predominant DH6-19 and DH7-27 gene usage, can result in complete V-D-J rearrangements, and are rare in T-cell receptor alpha beta lineage. *Blood* **93**:4079–4085.

101. Szczepanski, T., M. J. Willemse, E. R. van Wering, J. F. van Weerden, W. A. Kamps, and J. J. van Dongen. 2001. Precursor-B-ALL with D(H)-J(H) gene rearrangements have an immature immunogenotype with a high frequency of oligoclonality and hyperdiploidy of chromosome 14. *Leukemia* **15**:1415–1423.

102. Teruya-Feldstein, J., J. Setsuda, X. Yao, D. W. Kingma, S. Straus, G. Tosato, and E. S. Jaffe. 1999. MIP-1alpha expression in tissues from patients with hemophagocytic syndrome. *Lab. Investig.* **79**:1583–1590.

103. Tobin, G., and R. Rosenquist. 2005. Prognostic usage of VH gene mutation status and its surrogate markers and the role of antigen selection in chronic lymphocytic leukemia. *Med. Oncol.* **22**:217–228.

104. Tsujimoto, T., J. Cossman, E. S. Jaffe, and C. M. Croce. 1985. Involvement of the bcl-2 gene in human follicular lymphoma. *Science* **288**:1440–1443.

105. van Dongen, J. J., A. W. Langerak, M. Bruggemann, P. A. Evans, M. Hummel, F. L. Lavender, E. Delabesse, F. Davi, E. Schuuring, R. Garcia-Sanz, J. H. van Krieken, J. Droese, D. Gonzalez, C. Bastard, H. E. White, M. Spaargaren, M. Gonzalez, A. Parreira, J. L. Smith, G. J. Morgan, M. Kneba, and E. A. Macintyre. 2003. Design and standardization of PCR primers and protocols for detection of clonal immunoglobulin and T-cell receptor gene recombinations in suspect lymphoproliferations:

report of the BIOMED-2 Concerted Action BMH4-CT98-3936. *Leukemia* **17**:2257–2317.

106. **van Dongen, J. J., and I. L. Wolvers-Tettero.** 1991. Analysis of immunoglobulin and T cell receptor genes. Part II: possibilities and limitations in the diagnosis and management of lymphoproliferative diseases and related disorders. *Clin. Chim. Acta* **198**:93–174.

107. **Weiss, L. M., E. S. Jaffe, X. F. Liu, Y. Y. Chen, D. Shibata, and L. J. Medeiros.** 1992. Detection and localization of Epstein-Barr viral genomes in angioimmunoblastic lymphadenopathy and angioimmunoblastic lymphadenopathy-like lymphoma. *Blood* **79**:1789–1795.

108. **Wellmann, A., T. Otsuki, M. Vogelbruch, H. M. Clark, E. S. Jaffe, and M. Raffeld.** 1995. Analysis of the t(2;5)(p23;q35) translocation by reverse transcription-polymerase chain reaction in CD30+ anaplastic large-cell lymphomas, in other non-Hodgkin's of T-cell phenotype, and in Hodgkin's disease. *Blood* **86**:2321–2328.

109. **Wellmann, A., C. Thieblemont, S. Pittaluga, A. Sakai, E. S. Jaffe, P. Siebert, and M. Raffeld.** 2000. Detection of differentially expressed genes in lymphomas using cDNA arrays: identification of clusterin as a new diagnostic marker for anaplastic large cell lymphomas (ALCL). *Blood* **96**:398–404.

110. **Wiestner, A., A. Rosenwald, T. S. Barry, G. Wright, R. E. Davis, S. E. Henrickson, H. Zhao, R. E. Ibbotson, J. A. Orchard, Z. Davis, M. Stetler-Stevenson, M. Raffeld, D. C. Arthur, G. E. Marti, W. H. Wilson, T. J. Hamblin, D. G. Oscier, and L. M. Staudt.** 2003. ZAP-70 expression identifies a chronic lymphocytic leukemia subtype with unmutated immunoglobulin genes, inferior clinical outcome, and distinct gene expression profile. *Blood* **101**:4944–4951.

111. **Willemze, R., and R. C. Beljaards.** 1993. Spectrum of primary cutaneous CD30 (Ki-1)-positive lymphoproliferative disorders. A proposal for classification and guidelines for management and treatment. *J. Am. Acad. Dermatol.* **28**:973–980.

112. **Willman, C. L., L. Busque, B. B. Griffith, B. E. Favara, K. L. McClain, M. H. Duncan, and D. G. Gilliland.** 1994. Langerhans'-cell histiocytosis (histiocytosis X)—a clonal proliferative disease. *N. Engl. J. Med.* **331**:154–160.

113. **Wilson, W. H., J. Teruya-Feldstein, T. Fest, C. Harris, S. M. Steinberg, E. S. Jaffe, and M. Raffeld.** 1997. Relationship of p53, bcl-2, and tumor proliferation to clinical drug resistance in non-Hodgkin's lymphomas. *Blood* **89**:601–609.

114. **Withers, D. A., R. C. Harvey, J. B. Faust, O. Melnyk, K. Carey, and T. C. Meeker.** 1991. Characterization of a candidate bcl-1 gene. *Mol. Cell. Biol.* **11**:4846–4853.

115. **Wong, K. F., Y. M. Zhang, and J. K. Chan.** 1999. Cytogenetic abnormalities in natural killer cell lymphoma/leukaemia—is there a consistent pattern? *Leuk. Lymphoma* **34**:241–250.

116. **Wong, N., K. F. Wong, J. K. Chan, and P. J. Johnson.** 2000. Chromosomal translocations are common in natural killer-cell lymphoma/leukaemia as shown by spectral karyotyping. *Hum. Pathol.* **31**:771–774.

Monitoring of Immunologic Therapies

THERESA L. WHITESIDE

133

Biologic therapies have gained considerable acceptance in recent years. A broad array of biologic agents have become available for the treatment of inheritable or acquired immunodeficiency, autoimmune diseases, cancer, or persistent infections. Among them, immune system-based therapeutics utilizing antibodies, immune cells, or immunomodulators are now widely available. These agents target the immune system and represent potentially useful alternatives to conventional therapies, and increasingly frequently, they are being used in conjunction with chemotherapy, radiation, surgery, or even behavior-modifying therapies.

Biologic therapies can be categorized as follows: (i) monoclonal antibodies (MAbs), (ii) cytokines, (iii) growth factors, (iv) activated cells, (v) cellular products, (vi) immunotoxins, and (vii) other immunomodulatory agents. The rationale for the therapeutic use of immunomodulating agents is their ability to enhance the capabilities of the innate and/or adaptive immune system to control disease. Because immunotherapies largely remain in the experimental domain, the selection of an immunologic agent for therapy is preceded by extensive in vitro studies and in vivo experiments with animal models of disease designed to define the presumed mechanism(s) of its therapeutic activity. Frequently, however, preclinical studies fail to identify a complete spectrum of biologic activities for a new agent. This reflects the fact that most immune system-based agents are pleiotropic, acting on a variety of cellular targets and components of molecular pathways, so that a precise definition of each activity may not always be possible. Also, their systemic effects might be different from those mediated at the disease site. In general, mechanisms of action defined for immune agents in preclinical studies with animal models of disease often turn out to be quite irrelevant to those operating in vivo in patients with disease. Nevertheless, animal models remain useful for evaluating the toxicity of immunotherapies and their overall effects on the disease process. Ex vivo preclinical studies of the new agent with human mononuclear cells (MNC) are often helpful in providing a rationale for targeting therapy to a particular subset of these cells or for focusing mechanistic studies on a particular cell population.

CLINICAL TRIALS WITH BIOLOGIC AGENTS

Following preclinical evaluations, a therapeutically promising immunologic agent is introduced to the clinic in the form of a phase I protocol. An investigational new drug application is filed with the Food and Drug Administration (FDA). The application includes a clinical protocol. Agency approval is necessary for clinical evaluations of any experimental biologic agent. Following a review of the proposed clinical protocol, preclinical results, and animal safety studies, the FDA will intervene by putting the study on hold if additional information or clarifications are needed. Clinical trials involving gene therapy need approval by the Recombinant Advisory Committee. In addition, institutional approvals from the institutional review board and the biosafety committee have to be obtained prior to opening the trial for patient accrual.

The design of a phase I study is based on the predicted mechanism of action of an immunologic agent, as determined in preclinical experiments. Biologic agents are available as natural or recombinant materials which may have potent immunomodulatory activities. When administered systemically in high doses, they often induce considerable toxicities. However, the maximal tolerated dose (MTD) for a given biologic agent is not necessarily the dose that produces the desired biologic or therapeutic effect. In fact, low doses of biologics might have greater or different therapeutic effects than high doses without accompanying toxicity. This observation suggests that in contrast to the case for pharmacologic or chemotherapeutic agents, which are usually characterized by a linear dose-response curve, biologic agents have a distinctive bell-shaped response curve. The optimal biologic dose (OBD) for each biologic agent is thus likely to be different from the MTD and needs to be defined in phase I/II clinical trials in order to preserve and optimize its therapeutic benefits and limit its toxicity. The developmental strategy for a therapeutic agent involves determination of the mechanism-specific OBD, that is, the dose that optimally activates the postulated mechanism of action with tolerable toxicity. A clinical trial designed to determine the OBD is referred to as phase Ib, in contrast to a phase Ia trial, in which only the clinical toxicity of a new biologic agent is defined as the MTD (12). It is important to remember that the OBD may be different from the MTD for a given biologic agent. In addition, the same agent might have quite disparate OBDs for different immunologic characteristics. Interleukin-2 (IL-2), for example, which is a cytokine currently approved for therapy of renal cell carcinoma and melanoma, has a much lower OBD for the activation of circulating T and natural killer (NK) cells than for supporting the generation of lymphokine-activated killer (LAK) activity (10).

In general, phase Ib trials are intended to measure the pharmacokinetics and biodistribution of a biologic agent, together with selected immunologic parameters which, on the basis of the postulated immune mechanism, are likely to influence the disease process. For example, in a patient with cancer who is treated with IL-2, one postulated mechanism for antitumor effects might be an up-regulation of T-cell and/or NK activity in the peripheral circulation (12). In this case, monitoring of LAK activity in the peripheral blood of this patient during therapy might be expected to serve as a surrogate measure for the therapeutic effects of IL-2, and the dose of IL-2 resulting in the maximal LAK activity or cytolytic T-lymphocyte (CTL) activity with tolerable toxicity would be selected as the OBD. However, it is now known that IL-2, by binding to cells which express the IL-2 receptor (IL-2R), activates $CD4^+$ $CD25^+$ T_{reg} cells, among other cell subsets (19). T_{reg} cells are capable of down-regulating immune responses, including the antitumor activity of effector cells, which is clearly an undesirable situation in a patient being treated for cancer (19). Further, newer data suggest that stimulatory versus inhibitory in vivo effects of IL-2 may be dose dependent. Hence, it seems important to define the OBD for IL-2 which promotes immune activation in a patient with cancer. On the other hand, for subjects with autoimmune diseases, the OBD for IL-2-based therapy might be different, as inhibitory effects are a desired end point. This type of rationale is likely to apply to immune system-based therapy in general, and therefore the goal of establishing the OBD is a critical component of the developmental strategy for biologic agents and their application to various diseases.

In most phase Ib trials performed to date, surrogate immunologic end points are achieved much more easily than clinical responses. During IL-2 therapy for renal cell carcinoma, for example, virtually all patients develop high levels of endogenous LAK activity, while only a fraction of these patients achieve objective antitumor responses (10). In other words, surrogate immunologic end points selected on the basis of preclinical results do not appear to correlate with clinical responses, possibly because these end points seldom reflect the entire spectrum of physiologic mechanisms mediated by a biologic agent. In considering the pleiotropic activities of biologic agents, it appears that no single surrogate end point is likely to correlate with their therapeutic effects and thus with a clinical response. On the other hand, it is possible that a panel of carefully selected monitoring assays might provide a clue about the in vivo effects of an agent. For this reason, the current approaches to monitoring favor multiparameter analyses employing new high-throughput technologies, including genomics and proteomics. The possibilities for multiparameter testing now extend to immunologic monitoring, allowing evaluations of more than one surrogate end point in patients treated with biologic agents to identify those that are clinically meaningful.

In view of the difficulties experienced to date in selecting immunologic end points for monitoring of phase Ib trials, it could be anticipated that a direct measure of the dose of a biologic agent inducing the best therapeutic, e.g., antitumor or antiviral, effects would be preferable to the use of surrogate biomarkers. However, practical and ethical considerations rule out the direct approach of determining the best therapeutic dose. Since antitumor response rates for single biologic agents generally range between 10 and 30%, dose-finding studies would require excessively large numbers of patients and would expose many of them to ineffective doses of the agent tested. For this reason, the goal of phase I trials is to determine the toxicity and to define the promising OBD of a biologic agent, with the caveat that this OBD might relate only to a particular biologic activity of this agent and that it may not relate to its therapeutic activity. In fact, it is not uncommon to see few or even no clinical responses in phase I trials. But having obtained evidence of safety and a lack of toxicity, it is then possible to expand the earlier clinical observations in phase II clinical studies and to begin asking questions about the dose and mechanisms of action of a biologic agent. Ultimately, an agent's therapeutic efficacy has to be determined in large-scale randomized phase III clinical trials in which the placebo arm is compared to the experimental arm. It is encouraging that in recent years several biological therapeutics, including MAbs and cytokines, have reached the stage of being evaluated for efficacy in phase III clinical trials (15).

IMMUNOLOGIC MONITORING OF CLINICAL TRIALS WITH BIOLOGIC AGENTS

The rationale for monitoring immunologic parameters in clinical trials with biologic agents is based on the premise that these agents achieve therapeutic effects as a result of their ability to modify one or more components of the patient's immune system. The expectation is that by serially measuring immune markers, which change relative to the pretherapy baseline level, it might be possible to define the immunologic mechanism responsible for the activity of a biologic agent. In addition, the objective is to determine whether the observed changes in the immunologic phenotype or function correlate with clinical responses, toxicity, resistance to other therapies, or any other phenomena likely to influence the therapeutic outcome.

The first step toward rational immunologic monitoring is the selection of the most informative assays. This selection cannot be arbitrary and has to be based on a specific hypothesis. It is, of course, best to formulate the hypothesis on the basis of preliminary data available to the investigator from personal preclinical experience and from the current literature. The investigator is obliged to use judgment and collective experience to address the likely mechanisms responsible for therapeutic effects. But since most biologic agents have multiple biologic effects, more than one hypothesis of action can be postulated. Which of these hypotheses is ultimately selected for testing depends on the individual insights and preferences of the clinical investigator. However, it is not advisable to test too many hypotheses at once, for fear of making the design of a clinical trial too complex and the accompanying monitoring too extensive. There is no way to guarantee that the hypothesis selected for testing in a clinical trial is correct; hence, the selection of a hypothesis is the most crucial aspect of the trial design and has to be formulated only after a complete review of all preclinical data. As such, a clinical trial is not different from any other hypothesis-driven scientific experiment.

The next step of the scientific process calls for a design of an experimental plan in which the proposed hypothesis can be tested in the most satisfactory fashion. This includes the selection of assays to be performed and the frequency of monitoring. For phase I clinical trials, it is prudent to begin by considering a broad array of immunologic effects because the biologic activity of the evaluated biologic agent may be incompletely understood. It may be advantageous at this stage to consider alternative explanations for its biologic and, possibly, therapeutic effects. Hence, the selected assays should be sensitive rather than specific in order to detect biologic effects when they are induced by therapy. In phase II and III clinical trials, it might be possible to narrow down the selection of immunologic assays to those that were observed to reflect biologic activity or to correlate with clinical responses in previous clinical trials. In place of sensitive screening assays, more specialized specific or confirmatory assays could be introduced at this time to better focus on the mechanisms of activity mediated by the biologic agent. While no well-defined criteria exist for the selection of optimal monitoring assays, a general principle may be defined as follows. The choice of immunologic assays to be used for monitoring of phase I trials has to be based on solid preliminary data derived from relevant animal models of disease as well as in vitro experiments with human cells. In phase II and III clinical trials, the choice of assays to be used has to depend on previous results derived from phase I trials.

STRATEGY FOR IMMUNOLOGIC MONITORING: A PRACTICAL GUIDE

The choice of a strategy for immunologic monitoring of clinical trials with biologic agents is neither simple nor straightforward. No single assay or experimental approach is appropriate for all therapeutic interventions. The selection of the "right" monitoring assays requires familiarity with immunologic assays, judgment, and a considerable understanding of the biologic and therapeutic effects induced by the biologic agent used. Therefore, clinical investigators are obliged to make a number of well-informed and practical decisions, each of which is likely to influence the overall quality of monitoring and, hence, the final results of the trial. To facilitate assay selection and use in monitoring of clinical trials, several practical guidelines are given below, with the proviso that these are neither comprehensive nor applicable to all situations.

The frequency of immunologic assays to be performed is an important component of the trial design. Clearly, it is essential to establish a pretherapy baseline and posttherapy values. Beyond that, the number of time points selected for monitoring during the course of therapy depends on the characteristics of the biologic agent administered. For example, it is well known that cytokines usually have rapid and often dramatic effects on the total number and functions of cells in the circulation or on the levels of other cytokines or soluble cytokine receptors in the serum. Thus, with IL-2 administered as a bolus, rapid lymphopenia followed by a rebound in the number of circulating lymphocytes is observed (20). In contrast, when low intravenous doses of IL-2 are given continuously over a period of time, a gradual rise in the number of circulating $CD3^-$ $CD56^+$ NK cells is observed (5). More recent data suggest that IL-2 delivery may also increase the frequency of T_{reg} cells in the circulation or tissues and promote activation-induced cell death (21). These initial effects of IL-2 are followed by delayed effects due to the induction of secondary cytokines. The well-known result of high-dose IL-2 therapy, i.e., transient hypotension observed 4 to 8 h after IL-2 bolus administration, is induced by the secondary cytokines tumor necrosis factor alpha and IL-1β, which are released in response to IL-2 (18). In clinical trials with cytokines, it is important to measure the pharmacokinetics of the cytokine used for therapy as well as the levels of secondary cytokines in serum, which might be responsible for toxicity of the therapy.

A well-described effect of long-term therapy with biologics is the development of antibodies (Abs) to the administered biologic agent (2). Such antidrug Abs do not arise in every patient treated, and they may not appear until weeks or months into therapy or until multiple courses of the drug are administered. However, their presence in the plasma of individuals treated with the biologic agent is an important factor for the outcome of therapy, because they may either neutralize the drug or contribute to the development of immune complex disease. Therefore, it seems reasonable to monitor for the appearance of such Abs during the course of therapy. This requirement is obviously necessary when therapy with anti-idiotypic Abs is considered, e.g., for some patients with malignancies. Such patients may be treated with an anti-idiotypic Ab (Ab2) which is an internal image of the antigen and can include the production of Ab1 and Ab3, both of which are able to bind the antigen. Since Ab3 is therapeutic and Ab1 may not be, the presence and levels of Ab1 and Ab3 in serum are crucial for the interpretation of immunologic as well as clinical responses (8). Another important consideration is the transient nature of some immune responses. For example, in vaccination protocols for patients with cancer or viral infections, the appearance of antigen-specific effector cells in the circulation may be short-lived after single or even multiple vaccinations. In this case, assays for the detection and frequency of such effector cells have to be performed often and soon after vaccination. With other vaccines, however, the appearance in the peripheral circulation of the effector cells may be delayed, so their frequency will not increase until late into the vaccination regimen. It thus appears that a decision to monitor the immediate versus delayed effects of therapy with any biologic agent has to be made with caution, after considering possible implications of these effects on the interpretation of immunologic and therapeutic results of the trial. The relative complexity and cost of the assay often influence the frequency of monitoring. For this reason, simple, robust assays that can be reliably performed on serially collected, cryopreserved samples are necessary for frequent immunologic monitoring.

A decision to select cellular versus humoral immunologic assays for monitoring is directly related to the mechanism of action proposed for the biologic agent. While it may be difficult to prioritize on the basis of the limited understanding of such mechanisms, the consideration of practical aspects of monitoring can help in reaching a reasonable decision. Limitations in the frequency of phlebotomy or the total blood volume obtained from the patient during treatment are an important consideration. The variability of cell yields, day-to-day assay variability, and problems with the functional activity of cryopreserved effector cells often restrict the use of cellular assays. These assays are more difficult and more costly to perform than serum-based assays. It is advisable to consider serum- or plasma-based (hereafter referred to as serum/plasma) assays first, especially when they can substitute for cellular assays. For example, the levels of cytokines released by activated cells, the enzymatic activity known to be induced by a particular biologic agent (e.g., interferon-induced 2',5'-adenylate synthetase), and the presence of inhibitors or antagonists of biologic agents (e.g., IL-1ra) or products of activated cell subsets (e.g., soluble cytokine receptors, β_2-microglobulin, or neopterin) can be more readily monitored with serum or plasma than with cells.

The only in vivo assay available for measurements of cellular immunity in humans, the skin test for delayed-type hypersensitivity (DTH), is often underutilized or misinterpreted, largely because of difficulties in the recording and interpretation of test results. Yet when performed and read according to the guidelines, a DTH assay remains the best available measure of epitope-specific cell-mediated immunity in patients with immunodeficiencies, particularly when it is combined with a biopsy to confirm the nature of cells infiltrating the skin. Reagents for purified protein derivative, tetanus, *Candida*, and other antigens are commercially available. Other antigens, e.g., tumor-derived purified or synthetic peptides which are not yet commercially available or commercially available viral peptides, can also be used, provided that they have passed the safety requirements. A change in the DTH skin test from unreactive to reactive as a result of biotherapy is a significant result.

Monitoring of numbers or functions of MNC in peripheral blood during therapy often does not adequately reflect immunologic events that take place at the site of disease. Systemic effects of cytokines and certain other biologic agents are generally distinct from their local or locoregional effects, and monitoring of lesions, tissues, or organs involved in a disease is likely to yield more informative data than will the same assays performed with cells or cell subsets obtained from the peripheral blood. The obvious difficulty with this strategy is that blood is more readily available than tissues. Only superficial lesions or sites accessible to repeated biopsies can be monitored. Nevertheless, during a clinical trial, it might be feasible to obtain serial biopsies for in situ studies, and this opportunity should not be overlooked. An alternative possibility is to obtain body fluids (e.g., pleural fluids and ascites), in addition to peripheral blood, to be able to detect longitudinal changes in organ-associated immune cells or their products relative to those in peripheral circulation. This approach is especially recommended when intracavitary therapy with a biologic agent is considered.

Monitoring of immune functions generally requires considerable cell numbers, fairly large volumes of blood or other body fluids, and facilities to process these samples for cell recovery. Vigorous attempts are being made to miniaturize immunologic assays and to perform them with whole blood. Newer, more sensitive technologies, including molecular assessments, flow cytometry, electrochemiluminescence, and more sophisticated single-cell assays, that are generally performed on whole blood greatly facilitate monitoring, decreasing the required blood volume and dispensing with blood processing. The concept of bringing immunologic monitoring to the bedside, with only drops of blood needed for each assay, is slowly beginning to emerge. This approach must wait for further technical advances and for strong correlations to be established between immunologic biomarkers and clinical end points. Meanwhile, it appears that a profile of several immune measures determined in the course of therapy and analyzed using specially created software can provide useful prognostic information (9). These preliminary results are encouraging, and they indicate that immune profiling is likely to be more widely adopted for monitoring in the near future.

In general, a protocol schema specifies the time points for sample collection. These samples must be recovered from the peripheral blood, body fluids, or tissues and either used fresh or preserved for future monitoring. For studies of pharmacokinetics, a special effort has to be made to collect the specimens at the precisely designated time intervals and to process them in accordance with the experimental protocol to avoid degradation, inactivation, or loss of activity. In the planning of immunologic monitoring, not only the timing of

specimen collections but also the nature of anticoagulants needs to be considered. For example, to measure levels of cytokines in body fluids, plasma rather than serum is preferable, since cytokines tend to be trapped in the clot, with subsequently low levels of cytokines measured in the serum (24). While the separation of serum/plasma or MNC from the peripheral blood is a routine laboratory procedure, the recovery and fractionation of cells from tissues or body fluids containing normal or malignant tissue cells are time-consuming and require special expertise and considerable effort (6). The use of individual separated subsets of tissue-infiltrating or blood MNC is not recommended for serial monitoring, mainly because of a need for tissue sampling and large blood volumes. Also, the lack of uniformly acceptable procedures for cell separations and unpredictable yields of cells recovered from tissues hamper the use of cell separation techniques for monitoring. Nevertheless, the advantage of studies performed with highly purified subsets of immune cells obtained from the site of disease is obvious. When it is feasible to obtain a biopsy prior to and after therapy and to recover viable cells for monitoring of cellular functions, or even of cellular phenotypes, investigators are encouraged to incorporate such procedures in a protocol schema.

It is often unclear which immunologic assays can be reliably performed with fresh versus cryopreserved cells. From a practical viewpoint, it would be more convenient to use serially harvested frozen aliquots of serum/plasma or batched cryopreserved immune cells instead of freshly harvested specimens for immunologic monitoring. The ability to reliably cryopreserve immune effector cells for future use in retrospective studies or for batching of serially collected specimens to eliminate the interassay variability is highly desirable. In fact, the only reliable way to determine differences between pretherapy and posttherapy assays is to perform them at the same time. This strategy calls for banking of cryopreserved specimens (batching) and for assays which can be routinely performed with cryopreserved cells. However, certain immunologic assays, especially those that measure cell functions, e.g., cytotoxicity, are best performed with freshly harvested samples. Cryopreservation may introduce artifacts, even when a rate-controlled drop in temperature is implemented. Therefore, each laboratory is obliged to compare fresh and frozen cells to ascertain that a test can be reliably performed with either before attempting to use them for monitoring. Assays which can be reliably performed with frozen cells and batched specimens are the best candidates for monitoring, but in situations that require the use of fresh immune cells, it is essential to determine the interassay variability to be able to distinguish spurious from therapy-induced changes.

Immunologic cellular assays performed with whole blood as opposed to separated MNC are especially useful for serial monitoring. Their advantages include the ability to measure the phenotype and functions of effector cells without separation from other blood cells and plasma. Separation procedures are likely to modulate and alter functions of effector cells. Since phenotypic markers on immune cells are generally assessed in whole blood by flow cytometry, it would seem to be preferable to also monitor functions of these cells in the same way. At the very least, the correlations between the phenotypic and functional immune parameters might improve under these assay conditions. The disadvantage is that whole-blood assays have to be performed with freshly harvested specimens, thus eliminating the possibility of batching serial samples.

Technical advances and new insights into immunologic mechanisms have led to the recent development of new types of immunoassays. As a result, a clinical investigator generally has a choice between phenotypic versus functional, specific versus nonspecific, and direct versus indirect assays. The range of assays currently available for monitoring predicates that careful consideration needs to be given to selection of the optimal assay. Assay validation is expensive and requires special expertise. Monitoring of patients enrolled in clinical trials should only be performed in laboratories with established quality assurance (QA) and quality control (QC) measures which meet the standards for good laboratory practice, as defined by the FDA. It is important for clinical investigators to realize that serial immunologic monitoring of clinical trials is more rigorous and demanding than performing a series of research assays. To monitor trials with credibility, the laboratory has to have methods in place to ensure reliable serial data (see section on QC below).

PHENOTYPIC ASSAYS FOR IMMUNOLOGIC MONITORING

In many trials with biologic agents, a high priority is given to cell surface phenotype assays, which are generally performed with fresh whole-blood specimens or cells separated from the peripheral blood, body fluids, or tissues. Flow cytometry-based assays are now widely and easily accessible and highly accurate. A vast array of labeled MAbs suitable for multicolor and multiparameter flow analyses are commercially available, allowing the measurement of the proportions of various immune cell subsets. Percent changes in these subsets as well as alterations in the activation level of the cells can be readily assessed during immunotherapy. In designing a clinical trial, flow cytometry markers should be judiciously selected. There has been a tendency to indiscriminately include large panels of immunologic markers to monitor changes in the proportions of several MNC subsets induced by therapy. However, phenotypic assays, like all other immunologic assays used for monitoring, should be selected in order to test the hypothesis advanced as part of a clinical trial. Through the skillful selection of marker panels, it is possible to focus on a single population of effector cells or on several phenotypically distinct subsets, on cells expressing activation markers, or on cells that express a particular constellation of adhesion molecules. Various receptors for growth factors and cytokines on the cell surface can further be used to assign the cells to subsets and to relate their phenotypes to the functional potential of these cells. Thus, phenotypic analysis is a powerful tool for monitoring the effects of therapy on immune cells, and the selection of markers to be monitored on T, B, and NK cells and monocytes or granulocytes for shifts induced by therapy and based on the predicted mechanism of action of a tested biologic agent can be informative.

Today, two-color flow cytometry for surface markers on immune cells has been largely replaced by three-color or four-color flow cytometry assays in monitoring of immunotherapies. Improved software for data analysis and a wide application of novel gating strategies have increased acceptance of multiparameter flow cytometry for monitoring. Although complexities associated with the data analysis and interpretation of results are time-consuming, the advantages of multiparameter panels far outweigh their demand for expert execution. A combination of activation markers, growth receptors, cytokine or chemokine binding sites, etc., on distinct and identifiable subsets of MNC provides a powerful tool for monitoring. Whole-blood specimens can be shipped by overnight carriers for flow cytometry analysis

without compromising their quality. If multiparameter analysis is considered desirable but not feasible within one's own institution, it may be advisable to make arrangements with a flow facility specializing in immunologic monitoring. This alternative is strongly recommended for the monitoring of multicenter or cooperative group trials.

Surface phenotypic characteristics of immune cells are often utilized for assessments of absolute numbers of these cells in whole blood. The recent development of single-platform methods, which are performed entirely on a flow cytometer, has significantly improved the assay precision and accuracy. The most popular technique is based on four-color flow cytometry in the presence of counting beads. The identification of lymphocytes by the surface expression of bright CD45 and low side-scatter signals is followed by the quantification of T-cell subsets based on the expression of CD3, CD4, and CD8 and performed in parallel with counting of fluorescent beads. The number of labeled cells per microliter of blood is obtained as follows: number of counted cells × concentration of beads/number of beads counted. In a recent study, we found absolute numbers of CD3$^+$, CD4$^+$, and CD8$^+$ T cells to be significantly decreased in the circulation of patients with head and neck cancer (16). In contrast, the percentages of these cells were not decreased, thus indicating that absolute numbers and not percentages of lymphocyte subsets should be measured in disease. The usually reported cell percentages are misleading because they do not consider a total white blood cell count, which is frequently altered in patients with advanced diseases, particularly after previously administered therapies.

In addition to surface phenotyping, flow cytometry has been widely used to measure intracytoplasmic markers. This method requires cell permeabilization to allow for access of MAbs used for detection to cellular components in the cytosol or cellular compartments. Because this method detects the expression of cytokines, signaling molecules, or enzymes, it has been frequently used as a functional end point in recent clinical trials. Intracytoplasmic proteins, such as granzyme, perforin, antigen-presenting machinery components, caspases, and other enzymes, including cytokines, signal transduction molecules and transcription factors, measured in phenotypically defined cells can provide useful information about the activation state of the individual cells or subsets of cells and about their functional attributes. In performing these assays, use can be made of quantitative flow cytometry, which allows for quantification of the expression level of each protein. By use of a mixture of four types of beads with known fluorescence intensities and unlabeled blank beads, a standard curve is generated which expresses the fluorescence intensities of each bead set in terms of molecular equivalents of soluble fluorochrome (MESF) units for every assay. The mean fluorescence intensity of each unknown sample can be transformed into MESF units by use of this calibration curve. This minimizes day-to-day variability, thus providing a stable and standardized method for use in clinical laboratories. The method has been applied to assessment of the individual antigen-presenting machinery component expression in human dendritic cells (DC) (26) as well as to quantitation of other intracellular molecules such as the T-cell receptor (TCR)-associated ζ chain in human T lymphocytes (26).

Functional attributes of cells, e.g., proliferation and cytotoxicity, can be measured by flow cytometry simply and more efficiently than by familiar radiolabel-based assays, providing not only an estimate of proliferative or lytic activity, respectively, but also the identity of effector cells at the population or single-cell level. By using differently labeled responder and stimulator cells, these methods can be adapted to the quantitation of functional responses in individual cells, cell subsets, or entire populations of cells. For example, the proliferative history of fluorescently labeled cells can be established by determining the number of mitoses experienced by these cells. The principle of the method is that the amount of fluorescent dye taken up by the cell is equally partitioned between daughter cells during mitosis and therefore decreased by half at each cell division. Dyes such as carboxyfluorescein diacetate succinimidyl ester (CFSE) diffuse into a cell and are cleaved by intracellular esterases into compounds that are fluorescent and react with amino groups of intracytoplasmic proteins (11). By combining surface marker staining with CFSE, it is possible to monitor a cell or cell subset through successive mitoses and to determine the number of cell divisions. The use of CFSE allows for quantitative resolution of up to eight cell division cycles (11), and by comparing the number of cells that divided with those that did not divide, a precursor frequency as well as the expansion potential of antigen-specific T cells can be calculated with Cell Quest software.

The frequency of peptide-specific T cells present in mixed lymphocyte populations can be determined based on the use of biotin- or streptavidin-labeled complexes containing the peptide linked to HLA class I molecules (3). These complexes, referred to as tetramers, represent oligomeric complexes of HLA molecules with a peptide, which have an increased avidity for T cells expressing the relevant TCR. When tetramers bind to the TCR on T cells able to recognize the peptide, a strong, easily detectable fluorescent signal is generated that can be measured in a flow cytometer. The specificity of tetramers for peptide-specific T cells, which is considered their greatest asset, cannot be taken for granted, however, as nonspecific binding may occur under unfavorable experimental conditions. Nevertheless, tetramers are currently widely used to monitor changes in the frequency of peptide-specific T cells in lymphocyte populations before and after vaccinations. Tetramer analysis provides the frequency of epitope-specific T cells with a sensitivity of 1/10,000 but gives no information about their function.

Another category of flow cytometry assays that has recently gained wide acceptance is cytokine flow cytometry (CFC) (22). This is another single-cell assay which allows for quantitation of individual cells positive for a cytokine detectable in permeabilized cells by the use of cytokine-specific MAbs. CFC is performed following a brief (4 to 6 h) coincubation of lymphoid cells with an antigen to induce cytokine expression in antigen-responsive cells. CFC has been used to measure the frequency of T cells able to respond to antigens expressed by infectious agents such as cytomegalovirus, Epstein-Barr virus, or human immunodeficiency virus type 1, tumor-associated antigens such as MUC-1, or melanoma differentiation antigens. CFC can provide the phenotype of epitope-specific responder cells and defines the frequency of cells poised to secrete but not yet secreting the cytokine accumulating in the Golgi apparatus. Its sensitivity is perhaps a little better than that of tetramers, and it lends itself well to serial monitoring.

A special advantage of multiparameter flow cytometry for monitoring is the possibility for the use of a combination of tetramers or CFC for a cytokine with differentiation markers characterizing T-lymphocyte subsets. In trials with biologic agents, especially vaccines, which might alter the process of lymphocyte maturation, differentiation or migration from, e.g., the naïve to memory pool or the circulation to target

tissues, the use of such combinations has been found to be informative. Staining of lymphocyte surfaces for markers such as CCR7, CD45RO or CD45RA, CD27, or CD28 and at the same time for tetramer binding or CFC allows determinations of the percentage of naïve, central memory, effector, or terminally differentiated T cells. This type of analysis indicates how a biologic agent modulates the T-cell turnover in the peripheral circulation or changes populations of infiltrating tissue T cells.

Still another type of flow cytometry assays frequently used today provides means for enumerating cells that have initiated apoptosis, i.e., are able to bind annexin V, have an altered mitochondrial membrane potential, express high levels of caspase-3 activity or a high Bax/Bcl2 ratio, show evidence of DNA fragmentation (TUNEL⁺ cells [terminal deoxynucleotidyltransferase-mediated dUTP-biotin nick end labeling-positive cells]), or have decreased or absent expression of the TCR-associated ζ chain (25). In patients with advanced cancer or with chronic, persistent infections, a considerable proportion of circulating T cells are destined to undergo apoptosis, and flow cytometry offers an opportunity to monitor changes in the numbers of these cells before, during, and after immunotherapy. These methods depend on the use of special substrates, chromogens, or MAbs for the detection of proapoptotic or antiapoptotic molecules in the target cell and generally include cell permeabilization as well as a combination of surface and intracellular staining. The availability of reagent kits that are commercially distributed makes measurements of apoptosis relatively simple, with the caveat that freshly harvested cells are required for analyses of annexin binding to cells, as cryopreservation may impair the integrity of cellular membranes.

Multiparameter flow cytometry has greatly expanded opportunities for serial monitoring of therapy-induced changes in immune cells. It has provided means for measuring several molecules at once and for a combination of surface and intracytoplasmic biomarkers. In addition to rare event analysis, including tetramer-based or cytokine-based detection of peptide-specific T cells, flow cytometry has been widely used to quantitate the expression of various cellular components by incorporating calibration beads with different fluorescence intensities. The numerous advantages of flow cytometry have to be counterbalanced by the requirement for special expertise in its performance and data interpretation. The reproducibility of flow cytometry-based assays is strictly governed by the operator's skills of setting the gates and excluding nonspecific events and is therefore open to considerable subjectivity. Aside from gating strategies, which can greatly influence results and thus impose a need for a careful and standardized selection of the most appropriate settings, the interpretation of flow cytometry data in serial monitoring requires stringent controls for interassay variability and a great deal of judgment. While daily calibration solves the problem of instrument variability, other challenges exist. For example, some of the lymphocyte subsets encompass only a small proportion of cells in the gate, and to be able to distinguish shifts induced by therapy from daily assay variability, it may be necessary to acquire a large number of cells for such rare event analyses. Changes in the phenotype of effector cells should be interpreted in conjunction with changes observed in functional assays. Specifically, it is important to consider whether changes in function induced during therapy correlate with changes in the number of effector cells or are due to the augmentation of effector function in a small subset of cells. It is also possible that therapy alters both the number and function of effector cells. During therapy, these changes can be dramatic or subtle, and they can simultaneously occur in several subsets of cells. Analyses of these changes and the establishment of correlations between their magnitude and frequency require special statistical approaches, as discussed below. Since alterations in the proportion or absolute number of effector cells and alterations in function may be mediated by entirely different mechanisms (e.g., increased blood vessel permeability and up-regulation of NK activity during therapy with IL-2, respectively), it should not be expected that phenotypic and functional data will necessarily correlate with clinical responses. More likely, no significant correlations will be detected, even though significant changes in the immune cell number and/or function may be registered during therapy. This should not be interpreted as evidence that the immune system has no impact on the disease but rather as evidence that despite therapy-mediated immunomodulation, the disease process persists, undoubtedly because of the involvement of factors unrelated to immune system activity.

Phenotypic studies of immune cells need not involve flow cytometry. With the broad availability of excellent Abs, the immunohistochemical evaluation of cells in situ is a powerful method for recording therapy-induced changes in the composition or activation state of effector cell subsets. The importance of in situ studies cannot be overemphasized. In a recently completed retrospective study of 132 tumor biopsies obtained from patients with oral carcinoma, we were able to correlate a lack of or low expression of the TCR-associated ζ chain in tumor-infiltrating lymphocytes (TIL) with significantly decreased 5-year survival (17). In a subsequent immunohistologic examination of the number of S100$^+$ DC in the same tumors, both the low number of DC and the

absent or low ζ expression in TIL were found to be independent and highly significant predictors of poor survival for these patients. Thus, these two biologic markers are currently emerging as robust correlates of overall survival, disease-free survival, and time to recurrence for patients with oral carcinoma (17).

FUNCTIONAL ASSAYS FOR IMMUNOLOGIC MONITORING

In Table 1, assays that are currently in use for immunologic monitoring are divided into two broad categories: serum/plasma assays and cellular assays (phenotypic and functional). The rationale for utilizing serum/plasma assays for monitoring instead of more technically demanding and expensive cell-based measurements was discussed above. In the same vein, among cellular assays, flow cytometry is faster, more accessible, and frequently more reproducible than most other assays, particularly those involving radioactive labels. In addition to monitoring changes in levels of serum immunoglobulins or specific antibodies by routinely available rate nephelometry or enzyme-linked immunosorbent assays (ELISAs), a spectrum of other assays can be used to obtain a longitudinal serum profile reflecting changes in one or more cellular products. Generally referred to as proteomics, these assays are discussed below. In some cases, soluble products can serve as activation markers for a particular subset of immune cells, such as neopterin for monocytes or soluble IL-2R α chain (CD25) for T-helper cells. Body fluids can be readily frozen and banked to allow batch processing of the planned assays or for future studies.

TABLE 1 Immunologic assays currently available for monitoring of phase I clinical trails with biologic agents

Assay type and parameter	Sample type
Soluble cellular products	
Immunoglobulin levels	Serum, plasma, body fluids
Cytokine levels and pharmacokinetics (ELISA, multiplex format)	Serum, plasma, body fluids
Cytokine receptors and antagonists	Serum, plasma, body fluids
Other lymphocyte surface receptors (e.g., CD8, CD25, sFas, HLA molecules)	Serum, plasma, body fluids
Ligands (FasL, TRAIL) and growth factors	Serum, plasma, body fluids
Enzymes (e.g., 2',5'-adenylate synthetase and terminal deoxynucleotide transferase)	Serum, plasma, body fluids
Neopterin	Serum, plasma, body fluids
β$_2$-Microglobulin	Serum, plasma, body fluids
Phenotypic markers	
Proportions of cells (antigen specific versus unrestricted)	Whole blood, tissue biopsy, body fluids
Absolute cell numbers	Whole blood, tissue biopsy, body fluids
Cellular subpopulations (e.g., Th1, Th2, effector, memory, or naïve T cells, T$_{reg}$)	Isolated lymphocytes
Single-cell flow cytometry (e.g., CFC, tetramers)	Isolated lymphocytes
Functional assays	
In vivo DTH skin test	Visual inspection or biopsy
Cytotoxicity (ADCC^a, LAK, NK, or T-cell specific)	MNC or subpopulations of MNC
Cytokine production (ELISA, ELISPOT)	MNC or subpopulations of MNC
Proliferation	MNC or subpopulations of MNC
Chemotaxis	MNC or subpopulations of MNC
Signal transduction (ζ chain, Zap-70, NF-κB, other molecules)	MNC or subpopulations of MNC
Superoxide generation	MNC or subpopulations of MNC
Apoptosis assays (annexin V binding, caspase activity, TUNEL)	MNC or subpopulations of MNC

^{a}ADCC, antibody-dependent cellular cytotoxicity.

Monitoring the functions of immune effector cells is considered to be necessary, since their phenotypic characteristics may not adequately convey their functional capabilities. Functional assays are usually performed with peripheral blood MNC and only rarely with effector cells obtained from the site of disease. Thus, functions of "substitute" cells that are easily accessible for monitoring in the circulation are measured instead of those of the effector cells at the sites of disease. This is by far the greatest limitation of monitoring, since systemic effects of biologic agents on immune cells are likely to be different from local or locoregional effects. The surrogate results obtained with peripheral blood lymphocytes should not be expected to closely reflect the biologic activity of the drug on functions of immune cells in situ. Additionally, investigators need to be aware that at any given time point, circulating lymphocytes represent <2% of a total lymphocyte pool, and that the turnover of circulating lymphocytes is responsible for constant changes occurring at the rate determined by the events in the periphery. To overcome these limitations, attempts are being made to study serial tissue biopsies, utilizing immunostaining and/or in situ hybridization or reverse transcription-PCR for cellular proteins and/or mRNA coding for the proteins involved in, e.g., cytotoxicity (perforin, granzymes, and tumor necrosis factor), proliferation (growth factors and cytokines), or signal transduction (the ζ chain and protein tyrosine kinases). The field of genomics has greatly facilitated these studies, providing a new set of tools for rapid screening of gene expression, as discussed below. In some cases, it may be possible to recover a limited number of cells from serial biopsies to perform functional studies. Obviously, these studies are very difficult to perform with human tissues, and they are not practical for the monitoring of many patients at multiple time points. Nevertheless, they are extremely valuable because they allow comparisons to be made between local and systemic effects of a biologic agent on immune effector cells and will eventually justify or discredit the common practice of monitoring alterations in cellular functions in the peripheral blood alone.

Cytotoxicity measurements have occupied a special place in the monitoring of immunotherapies. There is a good rationale for monitoring cytotoxicity in clinical trials with biologics, which often tend to augment this effector function in many different cell types. In oncology protocols, antitumor cytotoxicity, whether mediated by class I major histocompatibility complex (MHC)-restricted autotumor-specific T cells, nonspecific NK cells, monocytes, or antibody-dependent $Fc\gamma R^+$ effector cells, has been extensively monitored. The evidence derived from animal models suggests that tumor growth and the elimination of metastases are mediated, at least in part, by cytotoxic effector cells. In some clinical trials with biologics, autotumor cytotoxicity mediated by tumor antigen-specific T lymphocytes has emerged as the only significant in vitro correlate of clinical responses (1). However, more recent data indicate that tumor regression and metastasis elimination are complex events involving multiple mechanisms and many cellular interactions, only some of which are mediated by immune cells. The process of antitumor cytotoxicity may involve other events in addition to perforin- or granzyme-mediated lysis, as measured in vitro by the release of ^{51}Cr from labeled, sensitive targets. Cellular interactions leading to necrosis, apoptosis, or both and involving activated effector cells of various types, cellular receptors, enzymes, antibodies, cytokines, and other factors may significantly contribute to effector cell-mediated lysis. It is clearly not possible to monitor all of these multiple events in the course of a clinical trial, although assays are available to measure them individually. A great majority of these assays have not yet been used for monitoring, and their value as reliable in vitro correlates of the process of antitumor immune activation in vivo remains to be determined. It is also apparent that a classical cytotoxicity assay measuring only the secretory function of effector cells is not able to adequately reflect the many mechanisms involved in the process of cytotoxicity in vivo. For this reason, the cytotoxicity assay has been largely replaced in monitoring by more informative, simpler, and cheaper single-cell assays based on multiparameter flow cytometry or image analysis and the enumeration of spots reflecting antigen-specific cytokine production by individual cells.

The choice of the type of cytotoxicity assay for monitoring depends on the hypothesis tested and practical considerations of assay availability. For most viral diseases, the presence of virus-specific cytotoxic T cells is necessary for recovery, and at least one goal of immunotherapy in patients with chronic viral infections is to induce the in vivo generation or activation of such virus-specific cytotoxic T cells. Obviously, measurements of virus-specific T-cell-mediated cytotoxicity are advisable in this case, although considerable practical difficulties might be encountered in assembling the components of this demanding assay (as described elsewhere). Similarly, for a cancer patient immunized with a tumor peptide vaccine in order to induce a memory T-cell response directed at the tumor, it might be desirable to monitor for the appearance of tumor-specific cytolytic T cells, under the presumption that they will mediate antitumor effects. Since, however, the number of these cells in the circulation may be small even after reimmunization, in vitro priming followed by enzyme-linked immunospot (ELISPOT) assays to quantitate the responding T cells and/or cytotoxicity assays with the autologous tumor cells as targets would be required. In the assessment of antigen-specific responses, the choice of a specific as well as sensitive assay becomes all important. The currently available data indicate that frequencies of single-epitope-specific T cells in non-antigen-primed circulating lymphocyte populations can be as low as 1 in 10^5 to 1 in 10^6. Considered from this point of view, the standard ^{51}Cr-release cytotoxicity assay does not qualify for monitoring of antigen-specific CTL precursors (CTLp) because of its relatively low sensitivity, which is estimated to be 1 CTL in 1,000. The frequencies reported in the literature for CTLp specific for some of the well-defined human MHC class I-restricted epitopes in the peripheral circulation of patients with cancer are too low to be detected in cytotoxicity assays. Furthermore, cytotoxicity assays measure the activity of the population of cells and provide no information about the frequency of individual tumor-specific T cells without an additional step of limiting dilution analysis. Today, the ELISPOT assay for gamma interferon (IFN-γ)-producing immune cells has largely replaced ^{51}Cr-release assays in monitoring of clinical trials. The ELISPOT assay can be used with cryopreserved MNC and is sufficiently sensitive to detect 1 IFN-γ-secreting T cell among 100,000 plated cells (4). When used with autologous DC pulsed with cell lysates or individual peptides, for example, the assay can detect not only $CD8^+$ but also $CD4^+$ responses, which is important in view of accumulating evidence that $CD4^+$ helper cells play a crucial role in the induction and maintenance of immune responses. The assay does not require labeled, viable cells as targets. Instead, cell lysates, synthetic or natural antigens, or whole cells can be used as stimulators. It can be set up in a variety of formats, allowing for substantial flexibility in the choice of antigen-presenting cells, ratios of responder to stimulator cells, and the use of in vitro sensitization for the expansion of antigen-specific T cells. The ELISPOT assay performed with patients' peripheral blood mononuclear cells without in vitro sensitization measures the frequency of peptide-specific precursor cells able to respond by cytokine production to the cognate peptide. Like all other assays for the detection of antigen- or peptide-specific T cells, it is HLA restricted.

Monitoring of epitope-specific T-cell cytotoxicity in clinical trials is logistically and practically difficult, as it requires prior HLA typing of participants. Often, the nature of antigens necessary for sensitization is unknown, or no appropriate targets are available. Instead, non-MHC-restricted cytotoxicity is measured, and the assay is adjusted to measure lysis mediated by NK cells, activated T cells, NKT cells, monocytes, or granulocytes. The selection of targets (e.g., NK-sensitive K562 versus NK-resistant Daudi cells), length of the assay (4 h for lymphocytes and 18 h for monocytes), and use of targets coated with the target-specific antibody are some of the variables that can be considered. In addition, cytotoxicity is often measured following the in vitro incubation of effectors in the presence of a drug or an activating agent to induce the generation of primed or activated effector cells. A good example is the generation of LAK cells in the presence of IL-2, followed by measurements of cytotoxicity against Daudi cells or other NK-resistant targets (13). LAK activity measured in freshly isolated lymphocytes is a useful measure of the ability of a biologic agent to induce nonspecific cytolytic effector cells in vivo. However, at present, attention has been focused on assays able to measure antigen-specific T-cell responses, largely due to the commonly held conviction that adaptive immune responses are responsible for therapeutic effects.

Assays that measure cytokine levels in serum/plasma or other body fluids have become an important part of monitoring. Both bioassays and immunoassays are available for assessments of cytokine levels (24), but only the latter are practical for the monitoring of clinical trials. Body fluids can be frozen and batched for immunoassays. Currently, multiplex-type assays using antibody-coated colored beads for the capture of multiple cytokines in a small (0.5-ml) sample and laser-type detectors to measure the fluorescence intensity of the individual beads are gaining popularity, replacing conventional ELISA. Like ELISA, mutiplex cytokine assays are antibody based but have the advantage of providing a profile of cytokines in a body fluid at a reasonable cost. Assays for inflammatory cytokines, hematopoietic cytokines, inhibitory cytokines, etc., can be selected to profile cytokines associated with a disease process and to assess changes in this profile following therapy. A number of problems with the assessment of cytokines in sera exist, including the ability of cytokines to bind to and form complexes with serum proteins and the presence of soluble cytokine receptors or antagonists, natural inhibitors, or anticytokine antibodies (24). All of these factors may contribute to difficulties in the interpretation of cytokine profiles, and knowledge of cytokine biology is important for accurate assessments and interpretation of cytokine levels in biologic fluids.

The ability of immune effector cells to produce and release cytokines in response to a biologic agent can be used as a monitoring strategy. This approach calls for incubation of cells alone (spontaneous production) or in the presence of an activating agent (stimulated production) and subsequent quantitation of cytokines in cellular supernatants (24). The assay can be used to measure the immunocompetence of cells by including stimulators such as phytohemagglutinin or lipopolysaccharide or the ability of cells to produce cytokines in response to the stimulator of choice. The assay also allows for the assessment of in vivo activation of cells by measuring spontaneous cytokine release. Once released, cytokines in cellular supernatants can be measured in multiplex-format assays. Cytokine production assays have been reproducibly performed with either fresh or cryopreserved cells (24), allowing for batching of cells or of cellular supernatants. This is a practical advantage of monitoring, as is the possibility of assaying the levels of several cytokines in one supernatant. The assay can also be performed with separated subsets of MNC, permitting the monitoring of cytokine profiles in these cell subsets, and it lends itself especially well to serial monitoring.

The proliferation of immune cells in response to a biologic agent or to mitogens and/or antigens has been in the monitoring repertoire for a long time. It can be used as a measure of immunocompetence following stimulation with an activating agent and can be performed with banked cryopreserved cells or as a whole-blood assay. In newer, modified versions, it can be nonradioactive. Proliferation assays can require very few cells if performed in Terasaki plates. As discussed above, it is also possible to use a flow cytometer to read the assay and to confirm the phenotype of proliferating cells. Proliferation assays can be used in conjunction with measurements of cytokines and cytotoxicity. These assays are informative, practical, and adjustable to fit the specific trial design or circumstances in a monitoring laboratory.

Apoptosis of immune effector cells in the circulation of patients with cancer or persistent infections has been observed and may contribute to the poor immunocompetence associated with these diseases (23). The observation that most T lymphocytes, including the subset responsible for antigen-specific responses, undergo spontaneous apoptosis in patients but not in healthy controls suggests that a rapid turnover of these cells is a characteristic feature of the disease process. Immunotherapy might be able to protect immune cells from apoptosis and prolong their survival. Thus, changes in the proportion of T cells destined to undergo apoptosis during biotherapy might correlate with improved immunologic or clinical responses. For these reasons, apoptosis assays, many of which are flow cytometry based as described above, have assumed an important place in monitoring of clinical trials.

New molecular assays are being introduced for the monitoring of immune cells. In cancer and certain immunodeficiency diseases, abnormalities in signal transduction have been identified, and they appear to be responsible for defective functions of immune cells in these diseases (7). Since it might be possible to correct these abnormalities and thus repair immune functions with immunotherapy, monitoring for the presence and extent of signaling defects is indicated, at least before and after such therapy. The TCR-associated ζ chain is one of the key signaling molecules, and its absence or decreased expression in T cells reflects impaired functions. Since ζ is also a component of FcγRIII, its lower-than-normal expression in NK cells signifies the presence of signaling defects in these effector cells as well. The expression of ζ in MNC is measured by two- or three-color flow cytometry following staining of permeabilized cells with ζ-specific as well as cell surface-specific Abs. Both a lower-than-normal mean fluorescence intensity for ζ and the proportion of MNC with absent ζ expression can be reliably used for quantitative evaluations. The assay can be calibrated against fluorescent beads, with the results expressed in MESF units (see above). As with other immunologic evaluations, pre- and posttherapy comparisons are performed with the same assay, using cryo-preserved cells. The expression of ζ, NF-κB, Zap-70, or other signaling molecules in MNC can also be determined by Western blots or gel mobility shifts, but flow cytometry analyses are quantitative and simpler to use for monitoring. Immunostaining in situ, which allows for assessment of the signaling molecules in T or NK cells accumulating at the site of disease, is a very useful indirect measure of the functional state of these cells. The expression of ζ in TIL is an important biomarker of survival for patients with oral carcinoma, as discussed above, and changes in the mobility of the NF-κB subunits have been related to impaired function of immune cells in renal cell carcinoma. Thus, monitoring for the expression of signaling molecules in immune cells has biologic as well as clinical significance (25).

GENOMICS AND PROTEOMICS IN IMMUNOLOGIC MONITORING

Advances in technology now allow for the simultaneous analysis of different genes in cells or tissues by the use of DNA chips or microarrays. Rapid and cost-effective screening for the expression of multiple genes coding for cytokines, activation markers, components of major signaling pathways, etc., offers a powerful new approach to monitoring of cell activation, differentiation, or proliferation in response to biotherapy. The technology involves mRNA extraction from cells or tissues and its subsequent labeling and hybridization to the microarray. The hybridized products are visualized in a phosphorimager and analyzed with software capable of comparing control with test samples to detect differences in the expression of selected genes. In this way, up-regulation or down-regulation of gene expression in tissues or cells exposed to a biologic agent can be monitored.

Similar to gene arrays, technologies combining two-dimensional polyacrylamide gel electrophoresis with mass spectrometry allow for simultaneous analysis of many hundreds of proteins in body fluids or tissues. It is expected that pathologic changes in tissues or cells are reflected in distinct protein patterns detectable in body fluids or cellular supernatants. Proteomic technologies are able to discriminate between normal and pathologic protein patterns and can be used to map protein changes associated with a disease process. The potential of these technologies for capturing distinct protein patterns that could serve as biomarkers or be correlated with clinical responses or prognoses is being actively explored.

Gene and protein profiling, whether by multiplex immunoassays, microarrays, or proteomic detection methods, may be of special importance in relation to cytokine-based therapies. The clinical use of cytokines for therapy of human diseases has been increasing. Discoveries of new cytokines and their availability as recombinant proteins as well as cytokine gene therapies have facilitated the pharmacologic use of cytokines. Systemic or local therapies with these mediators, which induce one another and amplify cytokine circuits, call for careful monitoring of cytokine levels in relation to clinical end points. Given the dynamic and rapid progress in cytokine assay development, it appears likely that such monitoring will shortly provide a wealth of clinically useful information about cytokine involvement in human disease.

QC IN IMMUNOLOGIC MONITORING

QC of immunologic assays, particularly cellular assays, is difficult, and QC of serial immunologic measures represents a special challenge. To meet the challenge, a well-designed and rigorously maintained QC program is a requirement in a monitoring laboratory. Such a QC program contains several components, including the definition of standard operating procedures, training of personnel, instrument maintenance, reagent control, review of quality, and proficiency testing. Laboratories performing immunologic monitoring for clinical trials are required to implement their own QC programs to ensure that acceptable data are generated. Currently, no model QC programs exist, but monitoring laboratories are encouraged to follow the good-laboratory practice guidelines defined by professional groups such as the College of American Pathologists or the departments of health in some states. No proficiency testing programs are available for most immunologic monitoring assays, except for those designed for flow cytometry or hematology (leukocyte count and differential), and participation in these programs is highly recommended.

An important aspect of serial immunologic monitoring is documenting changes from baseline upon treatment. This is possible only when measurements taken over time are assessed accurately. Thus, each assay selected for monitoring has to be vigorously controlled for intra-assay and interassay variability. Also, the reproducibility of the same assay used for individual patients tested at different times has to be ensured (biologic variability). This requires considerable effort and expense.

The process of QC begins with sample collection and processing, which have to be organized to meet the protocol schema and occur at specified times of the day and, presumably, before the next cycle of therapy. Blood samples for immunologic monitoring need to be routinely harvested in the morning to avoid diurnal variability. The flow of specimens and the recording of the collection and arrival times of samples are important activities in a monitoring laboratory. Although immunologic monitoring assays should be scheduled in advance, times of sample arrival tend to vary. The laboratory is obliged to establish strict guidelines for sample handling and to document problems in accordance with the quality assurance requirements. A precise history of each sample must be maintained. Processing must be uniform and follow standard operating procedures which are available in writing and regularly updated. Frequent checks of reagent quality and equipment performance have to be implemented. The decision to cryopreserve cells or use fresh cells is made prior to the clinical trial and has to be based on preliminary comparative studies using fresh and cryopreserved lots of the same normal MNC, which need to be performed for every assay. This is a crucial decision for monitoring, because the selection of assays that can be batched (i.e., performed at the same time for all cells collected in the course of the trial) will avoid day-to-day variability and considerably decrease the cost of monitoring.

Regardless of whether cryopreserved or fresh samples are used, standardization of all assays has to be performed prior to beginning a clinical trial. The importance of the reproducibility of assays used for longitudinal monitoring cannot be overemphasized. The standardization data are obtained by repeatedly performing the assay with cells obtained from healthy individuals under invariant and previously optimized experimental conditions to establish the mean, median, 80% normal range, and coefficient of variation. The intra-assay variability is also determined. When the standardized assay is ready for monitoring, a set of appropriate controls is selected, and these depend on whether fresh or cryopreserved cells are used. With fresh cells collected at different time points, repeated testing of preserved control samples (e.g., cryopreserved lots of normal MNC with a pre-determined range of reactivity) is necessary to control for day-to-day variability. With fresh cells, it may also be advisable to include fresh control cells obtained from a healthy volunteer. A pool of volunteers repeatedly tested over time can be established for this purpose. A QC program in place will ensure that the values obtained for an individual control sample remain within an acceptable range over time and specify when the assay results are considered out of the normal range. With cryopreserved cells or frozen serum/plasma, it is best to batch and test all serial samples from a patient in one assay. Even in this case, however, it is necessary to control for day-to-day variability to have some assurance that the assay performs equally well for all patients in a protocol. The data obtained from control samples, evaluated in parallel with each patient sample, can help to ensure the validity of the results for a particular day's assay. Whenever universally accepted standards are available (e.g., the World Health Organization standards for cytokines), these should be regularly included in the monitoring of assays. Alternatively, internal controls initially compared with the standards can replace the standards, which are often available in finite quantities, for routine use.

STATISTICAL ANALYSIS OF DATA FROM IMMUNOLOGIC MONITORING

In preparation for final data analysis, the results of immunologic monitoring are "cleaned," i.e., purged of errors made during data entry. We have found it helpful to monitor for such errors at several levels. First, the technologist who performs the test enters the results into the computerized database, after examining the daily controls and finding the assay acceptable. The technologist is least likely to make errors in entering the results of an assay that he or she just performed. Second, prior to the final analysis, a statistician generates summary data sheets, which are screened by the laboratory monitor, often a laboratory supervisor, who is intimately familiar with the assays. All outlier values identified by the computer are checked and verified by the monitor against the laboratory records. Third, all variations from the protocol schema are noted for each patient. It is necessary to confirm that all measurements were made at the time points specified in the original treatment schema. Because of the importance of the timing of samples relative to the treatment, a change in the schedule or dose of therapy or in the sequence of sampling may have profound effects on the results of immunologic monitoring.

The biostatistician performing the analysis of immunologic data should interact closely with the clinical immunologist. The statistician should be consulted with respect to trial design and should be involved in its planning. The statistician's input is vital in determining the number of patients necessary to adequately define an OBD.

Immunologic data are often normalized for analysis with a logarithmic scale. The statistical analysis selected depends on the trial design and hypotheses tested, but since pre- and post-treatment changes are generally measured, the analysis seeks to determine if the changes from baseline are significant. Typically, pretreatment baseline levels are established by computing medians of three pretreatment determinations. Medians are preferable to means, as they are not influenced by extreme data points. Nonparametric tests for differences in posttreatment levels relative to the pretreatment baseline can include tests such as the Wilcoxon signed rank test or analysis of variance with Fisher's protected least-significant-difference

method to determine pairwise differences between two specific time points. Comparisons between treatment groups can be accomplished by multiple regression analysis to permit simultaneous contrasts between groups, using a pooled estimate of the variance for all groups. Dose-response analysis utilizes parametric repeated-measure dose-response models which are fitted to posttreatment data, controlling for between-patient differences by including the pretreatment level as a covariate. Repeated-measure analyses are potentially sensitive to occasional extreme data points, and the use of robust fitting methods, which downweigh the influence of extreme data points, is important. The monitoring data are generally presented as a series of time plots, which are adjusted by subtraction of the estimated contribution of each patient's baseline level, so that the plots depict the relationship that would exist if all patients' baseline values were equal to the overall pretreatment average.

ROLE OF THE CLINICAL IMMUNOLOGIST IN IMMUNOLOGIC MONITORING OF CLINICAL TRIALS

The clinical immunologist should play a major role in the design, execution, and analysis of clinical trials which include immunologic monitoring. Many clinicians fail to consult or include the clinical immunologist in the trial design, expecting only to utilize the technical expertise of such an individual. Equally, many clinicians forget that the interpretation of immunologic data is never straightforward and requires special training and considerable experience. The clinical immunologist is likely to be well aware of the preclinical evidence regarding the biologic agent which is being evaluated and can help design a trial based on the agent's mechanism of action. The clinical immunologist can help not only by formulating a correct and rational hypothesis but also by giving advice regarding how best to test this hypothesis by utilizing the assays at hand. The clinician will be best served by working closely with the laboratory staff when monitoring is ongoing, and close daily interactions between the clinical and laboratory teams are necessary for collecting samples and obtaining meaningful data. It is desirable to have the clinical immunologist oversee the performance of assays and be responsible for the QC program in the monitoring laboratory. Equally important responsibilities of the clinical immunologist are the interpretation of results and data analysis, with the latter being performed in conjunction with the statistician. Ongoing discussion between the principal clinical investigator, the immunologist, and the statistician is necessary for the correct analysis and interpretation of immunologic monitoring data.

Immunologic monitoring of clinical trials has entered a new era. Technical developments and molecular insights into interactions of immune cells have expanded the field of opportunities for capturing and analyzing multiple therapy-induced changes in the phenotype and functions of immune cells. The greatest challenge, i.e., relating these changes to clinical end points, remains, however, and still requires close and effective teamwork between the clinician, the laboratory immunologist, and biostatistical personnel. Contributions from informatics experts are likely to become equally important. Cooperation and insights provided by each team member will facilitate meaningful monitoring, and the benefits of utilizing combined expertise in all aspects of clinical trials with biologic agents or any other trials monitoring immune responses can be considerable.

REFERENCES

1. Aebersold, P. M., C. Hyatt, S. Johnson, K. Hines, L. Korcak, M. Sanders, M. Lotze, S. Topalian, J. Yang, and S. A. Rosenberg. 1991. Lysis of autologous melanoma cells by tumor-infiltrating lymphocytes: association with clinical response. *J. Natl. Cancer Inst.* **83:**932–937.

2. Allegretta, M., M. B. Atkins, R. A. Dempsey, E. C. Bradley, M. W. Konrad, A. Childs, S. N. Wolfe, and J. W. Mier. 1986. The development of anti-interleukin-2 antibodies in patients treated with recombinant human interleukin-2 (IL-2). *J. Clin. Immunol.* **6:**481–490.

3. Altman, J. D., P. A. H. Moss, P. R. Goulder, D. H. Barouch, M. G. McHeyzer-Williams, J. I. Bell, A. J. McMichael, and M. M. Davis. 1996. Phenotypic analysis of antigen-specific T lymphocytes. *Science* **274:**94–96.

4. Asai, T., W. J. Storkus, and T. L. Whiteside. 2000. Evaluation of the modified ELISPOT assay for interferon-γ production in monitoring of cancer patients receiving anti-tumor vaccines. *Clin. Diagn. Lab. Immunol.* **7:**145–154.

5. Caligiuri, M. A., C. Murray, and M. J. Robertson. 1993. Selective modulation of human natural killer cells *in vivo* after prolonged infusion of low dose recombinant interleukin 2. *J. Clin. Investig.* **91:**123–132.

6. Elder, E. M., and T. L. Whiteside. 1992. Processing of tumors for vaccine and/or tumor-infiltrating lymphocytes, p. 817–819. *In* H. Friedman, N. R. Rose, E. C. deMacario, J. L. Fahey, H. Friedman, and G. M. Penn (ed.), *Manual of Clinical Laboratory Immunology*, 4th ed. American Society for Microbiology, Washington, D.C.

7. Elder, M. B., D. Lin, J. Clever, A. C. Chan, T. J. Hope, A. Weiss, and T. G. Parslow. 1994. Human severe combined immunodeficiency due to a defect in ZAP-70, a T cell tyrosine kinase. *Science* **264:**1596–1599.

8. Foon, K. A., W. J. John, M. Chakraborty, R. Das, A. Teitelbaum, J. Garrison, O. Kashala, S. K. Chatterjee, and M. Bhattacharya-Chatterjee. 1999. Clinical and immune responses in resected colon cancer patients treated with anti-idiotype monoclonal antibody vaccine that mimics the carcinoembryonic antigen. *J. Clin. Oncol.* **17:**2889–2895.

9. Friedman, H. 2004. Personal communication.

10. Gambacorti-Passerini, C., J. A. Hank, M. R. Albertini, A. A. Borchert, K. H. Moore, J. H. Schiller, R. Bechhofer, E. C. Borden, B. Storer, and P. M. Sondel. 1993. A pilot phase II trial of continuous-infusion interleukin-2 followed by lymphokine-activated killer cell therapy and bolus-infusion interleukin-2 in renal cancer. *J. Immunother.* **13:**43–48.

11. Givan, A. L., J. L. Fisher, M. Waugh, M. S. Ernstoff, and P. K. Wallace. 1999. A flow cytometric method to estimate the precursor frequencies of cells proliferating in response to specific antigens. *J. Immunol. Methods* **230:**99–112.

12. Hank, J. A., P. C. Kohler, G. Weil-Hillman, N. Rosenthal, K. H. Moore, B. Storer, D. Minkoff, J. Bradshaw, R. Bechhofer, and P. M. Sondel. 1988. *In vivo* induction of the lymphokine-activated killer phenomenon: interleukin 2-dependent human non-major histocompatibility complex-restricted cytotoxicity generated *in vivo* during administration of human recombinant interleukin-2. *Cancer Res.* **48:**1965–1971.

13. Hank, J. A., J. A. Sosman, P. C. Kohler, R. Bechhofer, B. Storer, and P. M. Sondel. 1990. Depressed *in vitro* T cell responses concomitant with augmented interleukin-2 responses by lymphocytes from cancer patients following *in vivo* treatment with interleukin-2. *J. Biol. Response Mod.* **9:**5–19.

14. Herberman, R. B. 1985. Design of clinical trials with biological response modifiers. *Cancer Treat. Rep.* **69:**1161–1164.

15. Ko, B. K., K. Kawano, J. L. Murray, M. L. Disis, C. L. Efferson, H. M. Kuerer, G. E. Peoples, and C. G. Ioannides. 2003. Clinical studies of vaccines targeting breast cancer. *Clin. Cancer Res.* **9:**3222–3234.

16. Kuss, I., B. Hathaway, R. L. Ferris, W. Gooding, and T. L. Whiteside. 2004. Decreased absolute counts of T lymphocyte subsets and their relation to disease in squamous cell carcinoma of the head and neck. *Clin. Cancer Res.* **10:**3755–3762.

17. Reichert, T. E., C. Scheuer, R. Day, W. Wagner, and T. L. Whiteside. 2001. The number of intratumoral dendritic cells and ξ chain expression in T cells as prognostic and survival biomarkers in human oral carcinomas. *Cancer* **91:**2136–2147.

18. Rosenberg, S. A., M. T. Lotze, J. C. Yang, P. M. Aebersold, W. M. Linehan, C. A. Seipp, and D. E. White. 1989. Experience with the use of high-dose interleukin-2 in the treatment of 652 cancer patients. *Ann. Surg.* **210:**474–485.

19. Shevach, E. M. 2004. Fatal attraction: tumors beckon regulatory T cells. *Nat. Med.* **9:**900–901.

20. Sondel, P. M., P. C. Kohler, J. A. Hank, K. H. Moore, N. S. Rosenthal, J. A. Sosman, R. Bechhofer, and B. Storer. 1988. Clinical and immunological effects of recombinant interleukin 2 given by repetitive weekly cycles to patients with cancer. *Cancer Res.* **48:**2561–2567.

21. Van Parijs, L., and A. K. Abbas. 1998. Homeostasis and self-tolerance in the immune system: turning lymphocytes off. *Science* **280:**243–248.

22. Whiteside, T. L. 2000. Monitoring of antigen-specific cytolytic T lymphocytes in cancer patients receiving immunotherapy. *Clin. Diagn. Lab. Immunol.* **7:**327–332.

23. Whiteside, T. L. 2002. Apoptosis of immune cells in the tumor microenvironment and peripheral circulation of patients with cancer: implications for immunotherapy. *Vaccine* **20:**A46–A51.

24. Whiteside, T. L. 2002. Cytokine assays. *Biotechniques* **33:**4–15.

25. Whiteside, T. L. 2004. Down-regulation of ζ chain expression in T cells: a biomarker of prognosis of cancer? *Cancer Immunol. Immunother.* **53:**865–876.

26. Whiteside, T. L., J. Stanson, M. R. Shurin, and S. Ferrone. 2004. Antigen processing machinery (APM) in human dendritic cells: up-regulation by maturation and down-regulation by tumor cells. *J. Immunol.* **173:**1526–1534.

The Future of Cancer Diagnostics:
Proteomics, Immunoproteomics, and Beyond

MARY E. WINTERS, MARK LOWENTHAL, ANDREW L. FELDMAN,
AND LANCE A. LIOTTA

134

Cancer is a disease of dysregulated protein function and expression. Altered protein networks and signaling pathways drive the malignant phenotype, resulting in cell survival, invasion, and metastasis. The large complement of expressed proteins is known collectively as the proteome, and the study of these proteins is known as proteomics. Some potential benefits of advances in proteomics are the abilities to predict who will develop cancer; select optimized, individualized therapy; and monitor how the cancer responds to therapy. Emerging proteomic technologies include identification of diagnostic proteomic patterns in biological fluids, high-throughput protein arrays that immobilize the entire repertoire of proteins from a population of cells, and identification of immunogenic structural features shared and conserved between different antigens, known as immunoproteomics, which could guide development of broadly protective vaccines.

The advent of these technologies has brought the ability to quantitatively measure thousands of proteins, enabling global measurements of protein expression, and the ability to profile the interactions and pathways of these proteins. In addition, these techniques provide data on posttranslational events, such as protein phosphorylation and cleavage, which are not obtainable by gene microarray analysis. Mass spectral analysis of serum proteomic patterns is emerging as an effective method for the early diagnosis of diseases such as ovarian cancer (14). Surface-enhanced laser-desorption ionization–time-of-flight (SELDI-TOF) mass spectrometry rapidly assesses complex protein mixtures in body fluids. Combined with artificial intelligence-based pattern recognition algorithms, this emerging technology can generate highly accurate diagnostic information. Reverse-phase protein microarrays capture the entire repertoire of proteins from a population of cells, enabling the study of changes in protein expression and function before, after, and during treatment. A new paradigm for cancer diagnostics is that the concept of a biomarker for cancer detection and monitoring is not limited to a single protein but can comprise a proteomic pattern of many individual proteins and the changes this pattern undergoes when tissues transform from a normal to a malignant state. The goal is to identify cancer at its earliest stages and to identify people at high risk of developing cancer. Proteomic profiling has emerged as a powerful tool in the large-scale analysis of protein expression, structure, and function, as well as a means to identify proteins and biochemical pathways involved in aberrant biological processes. The techniques are constantly evolving in an effort to provide optimized and validated protocols that will be clinically useful. This chapter will address the issues related to technology development, validation, and quality assurance and discuss trends in future diagnostic strategies.

MS

The importance of mass spectrometry (MS) to the fields of proteomics and cancer diagnostics is undeniable. Mass spectrometers are powerful and versatile analytical instruments with the ability to detect and characterize biomolecular structures on a global scale, both qualitatively and quantitatively. Although the first-generation mass spectrometer was developed by J. J. Thompson in 1897 as no more than a gas phase electron conductor, functional mass spectrometers are in their relative infancy of development. In the early 1950s, Wolfgang Paul envisioned and invented the quadropole mass filter and the quadropole ion trap, designs that continue today to form a basis for mass spectrometer hardware. Over the last decade, design development has been rapid, leading to high-resolution, sensitive instruments. The recent sequencing of the human genome has generated enormous attention in the area of protein and peptide research and has accelerated the mass spectrometer to the forefront of present disease diagnosis and therapeutic monitoring techniques. Although the mass spectrometer can be found in many designs and is used for various functions, nearly all mass spectrometers can be described as the combination of three basic components: the ion source, the mass analyzer, and a detector. Here we describe the importance of the three most popular ionization techniques for MS: matrix-assisted laser desorption ionization (MALDI), SELDI, and electrospray ionization (ESI). In addition, new developments and applications in the field of MS will be discussed.

IONIZATION TECHNIQUES

MALDI-TOF MS

MALDI–time-of-flight (MALDI-TOF) MS is an analytical technique that can measure mass/charge (m/z) ratios of biological compounds with high accuracy and subpicomole sensitivity. Because of its theoretical and technical simplicity and reproducibility, MALDI has become a widespread analytical tool for peptides, proteins, and most other biomolecules (oligonucleotides, carbohydrates, natural products, and lipids). A basic principle of MALDI-MS is the laser-induced ionization of analytes (that are dried onto the surface of a sample plate) by using an efficient and directed energy transfer as a matrix-assisted laser-induced desorption event. Sample preparation is relatively simple and can be adapted for different types of experiments. The analyte is first cocrystallized with a large molar excess of a matrix compound, usually a UV-absorbing weak organic acid. The choice of matrix varies depending upon the physical properties of the analyte, such as molecular weight and chemical composition. Pulse-UV laser radiation of this analyte-matrix mixture results in the vaporization of the matrix, which carries the analyte into a flight tube and eventually to the mass analyzer. In the analyzer, the momentum of the analyte upon a detector plate induces an electron cascade event that allows the quantitative determination of the analyte's m/z (Fig. 1A).

Advantages of using MALDI-MS include the infinite theoretical molecular weight range detection limits of ionized biomolecules, the capacity for direct quantitation of protein m/z values, and the efficient throughput and straightforward laboratory methodology. Investigators may also utilize MALDI-MS for qualitative analysis of enzymatically digested proteins by peptide mass fingerprinting experiments, in which measured peptide masses are compared to information in a theoretically generated database of enzyme-specific cleavage sites. Quantitative techniques, such as isotope-coded affinity tagging (ICAT) (3, 15), stable isotope labeling by amino acids in cell culture (7, 8), and quantitative cysteinyl-peptide enrichment technology (1), allow direct measurement of absolute protein concentrations in complex mixtures as well as the determination of differences between diseased and healthy or before- and after-treatment sample sets. MALDI-MS is also being used for protein profiling directly from sectioned tissue (6). These techniques provide a window into the changes of the cellular proteome in response to disease and provide data sets which may be mined for diagnostic and prognostic information related to the disease state. Disadvantages of MALDI-MS include high intolerances for salts and other species in biological samples, an inability to sequence amino acid structure directly, and the necessity to work with homogeneous samples for peptide mass fingerprinting and isotopic quantitative experiments.

SELDI-TOF MS

SELDI-TOF MS is presently at the forefront of discovery of tumor-associated biomarkers that have potential for development into clinical diagnostic assays. SELDI is a sister technique of MALDI-MS, as both use a laser to desorb and ionize analytes for direct mass determination. The patented protein chip array (Ciphergen Biosystems, Inc.) (21) distinguishes SELDI-TOF MS from other MS-based systems. In contrast to the metal plate used in MALDI-TOF MS for application of the analyte and matrix, SELDI chips provide a variety of surface chemistries for researchers to optimize protein capture and analysis. Each sample is spotted directly onto the chip surface, and the unique affinity capture chemistry binds a subset of the sample proteome. The chip is washed to remove non-covalently bound species, and finally an energy-absorbing molecule solution, which acts like a matrix in MALDI-MS, is spotted on top of the sample. The chip, containing up to eight samples, is inserted into a vacuum chamber, where it is irradiated with a laser. Mass spectra can be analyzed by using complex algorithm-based computer-assisted tools that classify a subset of the spectra by their characteristic patterns of m/z

and relative intensity (Fig. 1B). There are various proprietary chemistries that permit simplification of complex samples ranging from raw serum and other bodily fluids to cell lysates. The choice of binding surfaces includes hydrophobic surfaces for reverse-phase capture, cation and anion exchange surfaces, immobilized metal affinity capture surfaces for metal-binding proteins, and preactivated surfaces for investigation of antibody-antigen, DNA-protein, and receptor-ligand interactions.

The protein chip system (Ciphergen Biosystems, Inc.) detects and accurately calculates the masses of compounds ranging from small molecules and peptides of less than 1,000 Da up to proteins of 500 kDa or more based on a measured TOF to the detector plate. This technology is being applied primarily to the analysis of cancer patient sera to identify distinctive protein patterns that may be characteristic of specific tumor types (19). Patterns that distinguish between cancer patients and normal subjects with remarkable accuracy have been reported for several types of cancer, including breast, ovarian, prostate, and pancreatic cancer.

The proteomic patterns generated by these technologies have broad implications as they represent the sum of many alterations in metabolic and signaling pathways and networks that confer a survival advantage to the cancer cell. Because proteins are the primary functional effectors of these cellular processes, analysis of the proteome offers a snapshot of the state of molecular pathways in vivo. Furthermore, analysis of the proteome allows the detection of functionally relevant posttranslational modifications, such as phosphorylation, and has the potential to provide information not present at the genomic or gene expression level.

ESI MS

ESI MS requires more extensive sample preparation and theoretical expertise than MALDI- or SELDI-MS; however, it is the most powerful MS technique available. ESI MS is a soft ionization technique that produces ions directly from the liquid phase, allowing it to be easily coupled with high-performance liquid chromatography (HPLC) front-end hardware. Hundreds of distinct proteins from a heterogeneous sample can be simultaneously identified by ion fragmentation of proteolytically digested peptides in a single analysis, and homogeneous samples or very simple mixtures can be quantitatively analyzed by isotopic labeling techniques. The dynamic range of protein concentrations present in typical bodily fluids is simplified by prefractionation techniques, including immunochemistry, carrier protein isolation, dissociation, depletion, and multidimensional liquid chromatography. Disadvantages to using an ESI source include low-throughput data analysis, technical intricacy, and high instrumentation cost.

Electrospray mass spectrometers come in many configurations that differ in m/z ranges covered, the mass accuracies, and achievable resolutions. Typical mass spectrometer setups consist of an ionization source (where the liquid phase analytes are ionized into a fine mist and injected into the mass spectrometer), a tandem separation-isolation region coupled to a fragmentation region (these include hybrid configurations of quadrupoles, TOF analyzers, magnetic sectors, and quadrupole ion traps), and a detector (photomultiplier, electron multiplier, and the microchannel plate detectors). ESI is well suited to the analysis of polar molecules ranging from less than 100 Da to more than 1,000,000 Da in molecular mass.

In ESI experiments, samples obtained from polyacrylamide gels or polyvinylidene difluoride membranes or

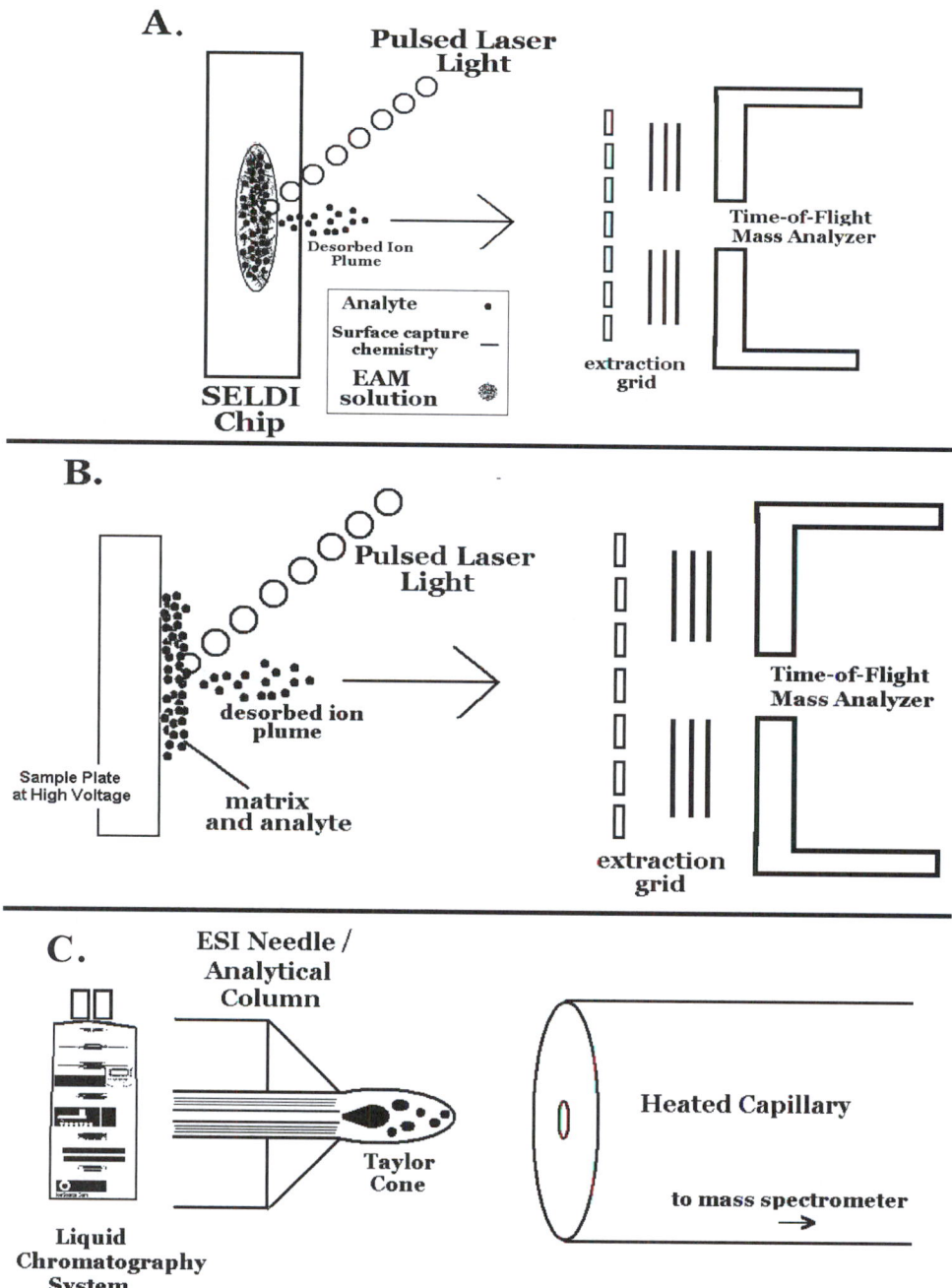

FIGURE 1 Schematic representation of three typical ionization and sample introduction techniques for MS analysis. Following ionization, analyte molecules are accelerated into a mass analyzer and detector of an appropriate instrumental configuration. (A) SELDI utilizes energy-absorbing molecule solution to absorb laser energy and induce ionization of immobilized analyte molecules. The analyte is covalently bound to a chip surface by one of many surface-capture chemistries (e.g., cation-anion exchange or reverse phase). (B) In MALDI, microliter volumes of the analyte and excess matrix can be dissolved in organic solvents and spotted by one of many techniques onto a plate. The matrix (e.g., alpha-cyano-4-hydroxycinnamic acid or sinapic acid) contains a chromophore that absorbs energy from the laser pulse and produces a plasma, resulting in vaporization and ionization of the analyte. Only molecular ions of the analyte molecules are produced, and almost no fragmentation occurs. (C) ESI utilizes a high positive or negative potential at an atmospheric, liquid junction to ionize a sample into the gas phase. This production of ions, called pneumatic nebulization, disperses the emerging solution into a very fine spray of charged droplets. As the solvent evaporates, droplet size decreases while the surface charge increases until, at the Rayleigh limit, Coulomb repulsion overcomes the droplet's surface tension and the droplet explodes. The process continues until each analyte ion is individually charged, often producing multiply charged ions. EAM, energy-absorbing molecule.

directly from solution are digested with a proteolytic enzyme (e.g., trypsin or Lys-C) into peptide fragments prior to injection into an HPLC system. The peptides are bound to solid-phase affinity columns (typically reverse phase or ion exchange) and are eluted (and thus separated in time) from these columns by changing the organic solvent gradient concentration (Fig. 1C). The simplification of peptide heterogeneity over time is essential to the success of a tandem MS (MS-MS) experiment.

Interpretation of data generated by ESI MS relies heavily on computer processing and database searching. Real MS-MS data are compared to theoretically generated fragmentation spectra inferred from a species' genome, and correlation scores are evaluated by the scientist to determine which amino acid sequences suggest unique protein identifications. Advantages of ESI MS include abilities for direct amino acid sequencing, posttranslational modification analysis, quantitative proteomic determination, and the analysis of complex mixtures (1). Disadvantages of using an ESI source include low-throughput data analysis, technical intricacy, and instrumentation cost.

NEW DEVELOPMENTS AND APPLICATIONS

High-Resolution Mass Spectrometers

The most commonly used instrument for MS is the ion trap mass spectrometer, which is reasonably sensitive and has a reputation for being durable, reliable, and easy to use. However, conventional three-dimensional ion traps have limited trap capacity. Newer mass spectrometers have triple quadrupoles of which the last quadrupole can be operated as a conventional quadrupole mass filter, or as a linear ion trap, allowing decoupling of precursor ion isolation and fragmentation from the ion trap itself. This provides more sensitive MS-MS and allows the identification and measurement of low levels of posttranslational modification in a single liquid chromatography–MS-MS run.

Another type of MS is Fourier transform ion cyclotron resonance MS (FTMS), which offers both high resolution and the ability to perform MS-MS experiments. In FTMS, charged particles orbit in the presence of a magnetic field. While the ions are orbiting, a radio frequency signal is used to excite them and the ions produce a detectable image current on the cell in which they are trapped (2, 7). The time-dependent image current can then be Fourier transformed to obtain the component frequencies of the different ions that correspond to their m/z. Combined with ESI and MALDI, FTMS has the potential to become an important research tool offering high accuracy with errors as low as ±0.001%.

Biomarker Amplification by Serum Carrier Protein Binding

Mass spectroscopic analysis of the low-molecular-mass (LMM) range of the serum-plasma proteome is a rapidly emerging frontier for biomarker discovery. Mass spectroscopic analysis of human serum following molecular mass fractionation has demonstrated that the majority of LMM biomarkers exist bound to carrier proteins. Moreover, the pattern of LMM biomarkers bound specifically to albumin has been shown to be distinct from the pattern of those bound to non-albumin carriers. In a recent study (16), prominent SELDI-TOF ionic species (m/z, 6631.7043) previously shown to correlate with the presence of ovarian cancer were amplified by albumin capture. Several insights emerged: (i) accumulation of LMM biomarkers on circulating carrier

proteins greatly amplifies the total concentration of the measurable biomarker in serum and plasma; (ii) the total biomarker concentration in serum and plasma is largely determined by the carrier protein clearance rate, not by the unbound-biomarker clearance rate itself; and (iii) examination of the LMM species bound to a specific carrier protein may reveal important diagnostic information. These findings shift the focus of biomarker detection to the carrier protein and its biomarker content. The value of this technique is that potential biomarkers are amplified to measurable quantities that could be quantified in readily available body fluids such as serum or urine.

ICAT Strategies

ICAT is a quantitative technique that allows direct measurement of absolute protein concentrations in simple mixtures as well as determination of differences between diseased and healthy or before- and after-treatment sample sets. This method relies on the labeling of protein samples from two different sources with two chemically identical reagents that differ only in masses as a result of isotope composition. Differential labeling of samples by mass allows the relative amounts of protein in two samples to be quantified. Protein extract from two different samples is reacted with one of two forms of the ICAT reagent, an isotopically light form in which the linker contains eight hydrogen atoms or a heavy form in which the linker contains eight deuterium atoms. The ICAT reagent reacts with cysteine residues in proteins via a thiol-reactive group and contains a biotin moiety to facilitate purification. Peptides are recovered on the basis of the biotin tag by avidin affinity chromatography and are then analyzed by MS (Fig. 2). The difference in peak heights between heavy and light peptide ions directly correlates with the difference in protein abundances in the cells. Thus, if a protein is present at a threefold higher level in one sample, this will be reflected in a threefold difference in peak heights. Following quantitation of the peptides, they can be fragmented by MS-MS and the amino acid sequence can be obtained. Thus, using this approach, proteins can be identified and their expression levels can be compared in the same analysis. One advantage of this method is the elimination of the two-dimensional (2D) gel for protein separation and quantitation. As a result, an increased amount of sample can be used to elevate levels of low-abundance proteins. Alternatively, the cell lysate can be fractionated prior to reaction with the ICAT reagent. This can allow an increase in levels of low-abundance proteins before analysis. The main disadvantages are that presently this method works only for proteins containing cysteine, even though this includes the majority of proteins. In addition, peptides must contain appropriately spaced protease cleavage sites flanking the cysteine residues. Finally, the ICAT label is large (~500 kDa) and remains with each peptide throughout the analysis. This can make database searching more difficult, especially for small peptides with limited sequences. Sensitivity may also be of concern since tagged peptides derived from low-copy-number proteins are likely to be poorly recovered during the affinity step as a result of nonspecific interactions with avidin-Sepharose. Studies have been performed to optimize the labeling of proteins with the ICAT reagent; therefore, despite these limitations, this approach may have applications for the study of protein expression profiles in cancer and other diseases.

2D PAGE and MS Paradigm

Two-dimensional polyacrylamide gel electrophoresis (2D PAGE) has been used traditionally to separate complex

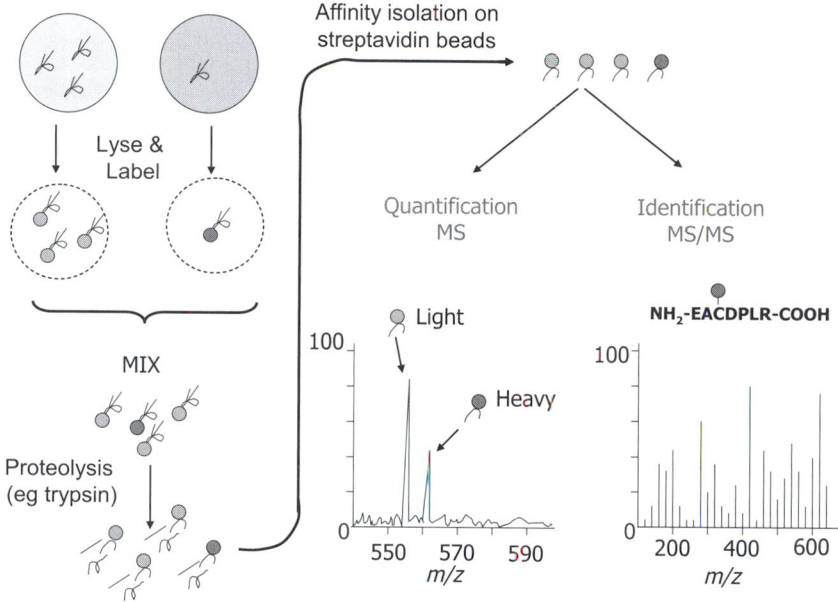

FIGURE 2 ICAT MS-based protein profiling. This method relies on the labeling of protein samples from two different sources with two chemically identical reagents that differ only in masses as a result of isotope composition. Protein extract from two different samples is reacted with one of two forms of the ICAT reagent, an isotopically light form in which the linker contains eight hydrogens or a heavy form in which the linker contains eight deuterium atoms. The ICAT reagent reacts with cysteine residues in proteins via a thiol-reactive group and contains a biotin moiety to facilitate purification. Peptides are recovered on the basis of the biotin tag by avidin affinity chromatography and are then analyzed by MS. Example of a labeled peptide.

mixtures of proteins by both pI (first dimension) and mass (second dimension). Use of 2D gels and MS in tandem is a powerful tool that can highly resolve proteins on a global scale and identify them through querying of DNA and protein databases. This combined technique has the potential for identifying novel as well as known proteins. It also allows the parallel comparison of a number of samples at one time to determine differential protein expression. Miniaturization, automation, and increasing speed of analysis are occurring at both the separation and MS phases. However, separation by 2D PAGE tends to be a time-consuming, labor-intensive technique that is difficult to automate. Also, imperfect separation (and subsequent lack of identification) can occur with basic (pH, >9) proteins, such as hydrophobic or membrane proteins, and high-molecular-mass (>150-kDa) or LMM (<10-kDa) proteins.

TECHNICAL ISSUES

Among the technical issues associated with MS, preanalytical variables may be the most problematic. These include variations due to inconsistent sample collection, handling, and preprocessing procedures. These sources of variations are compounded by biological variables such as unknown subphenotypes among study populations. Preanalytic variation should be eliminated or minimized whenever possible through good experimental design, careful analytic procedures, and quality control protocols. Since collection practices, sample handling, and storage conditions may vary from institution to institution, samples from multiple sites should

be randomly divided into a discovery (training) data set and a validation (testing) data set. Biological variation may be more difficult to account for, especially when a protein profiling experiment is used for de novo discovery. When no prior knowledge exists about the protein the researcher is studying, adequate sample size is hard to define because the complexity of the final model and the peaks included in that model are unknown beforehand.

ANALYTICAL ISSUES

The unified maximum separability analysis algorithm was developed for genomic and proteomic expression data. The rationale behind unified maximum separability analysis is that information about the overall data distribution can be used to prequalify any training sample to be a support vector, i.e., a set containing boundary datum points. After selection of a limited number of protein peaks as candidate biomarkers, more traditional linear modeling techniques may be used. Methods such as logistic regression allow the user to define a relationship between protein peaks as well as evaluate each peak's contribution to the multivariate relationship. To test the robustness of the final model, the full set may be split using a stratified random sampling procedure. Two data sets are constructed from the original data set, and the decision rule derived using one data set is tested for the second data set. Bootstrap analysis may be used if the number of samples collected for the study is too small for a stratified random sampling procedure. Regardless of what technique is employed, verification of analysis results is imperative.

DATA HANDLING

Like the genome project, more sophisticated data mining and learning algorithm software programs will be required to reproducibly and efficiently collect and analyze the information being generated by proteomic technologies. Furthermore, present proteomic projects are generating a wealth of data for a wide range of tissues, and it is critical that results are organized and presented in a form that makes analysis as simple and accessible as possible. To this end, a number of databases have been constructed containing both visual and textual data with extensive links to both protein and nucleic acid databases. The ability to effectively search such databases for the identification of ions from spectral data has become an essential step in the study of proteomes. The ability of analytical techniques used in protein characterization and their associated database query programs to determine identity at the functional group level has been examined for proteins with low levels of homology at the gene-protein sequence level. Such theoretical data manipulations may help predict the utility of data acquired experimentally with non-sequence-dependent software for proteome analysis. Genomes of eight organisms have now been fully sequenced, and the results have been distributed within publicly accessible gene and protein databases. These databases of model organisms have been proposed as a starting point for studies of either the total proteome or the functional proteome (defined as gene product expression under specific environmental or laboratory conditions).

THE FUTURE OF MS

MS is a powerful tool for the detection and characterization of biomolecules. The greatest strength of this technology is its diversity of applications. Selecting the best tool for each application depends on the complexity of the sample, desired throughput times, and the need for sequence determination or mass measurement of an analyte. The laser desorption techniques (MALDI and SELDI) are ideally suited for high-throughput sample analysis of intact proteins. These techniques are relatively simple to perform with minimal training and can be used for global pattern analysis of complex samples. Sequence determination can be performed only with homogeneous samples. SELDI-MS occupies a niche in proteomic research as a technique that can measure m/z "fingerprints" in a specific subproteome. ESI is the most powerful tool for sequencing proteins in complex samples. This technique is well-suited to front-end fractionation, atomic-scale resolution, and subattomole sensitivity (using FTMS). One can envision using ESI for determining posttranslational modification, comparing protein dysregulation levels between samples by using isotopic labeling techniques, or quantitating absolute protein concentrations in complex mixtures. Electrospray devices are found in numerous hardware configurations that differ in operational costs (sensitivity, resolution, speed, and accuracy) and practical costs (technical know-how, instrument size, and monetary considerations).

2D DIGE

In the last few years, improvements in relative protein quantitation have been made using differential gel electrophoresis (DIGE) technology. DIGE labels two protein samples with either Cy3 or Cy5 and then separates these different protein populations on the same 2D PAGE gel. Separation on the same gel eliminates potential errors introduced from overlaying electronic images from two different gels. The stained 2D PAGE gels are converted into fluorescence-specific electronic images and analyzed by algorithms that match and compare protein expression levels from each sample. Zhou et al. utilized 2D DIGE to quantify the differences in protein expression levels between laser capture microdissection (LCM)-procured esophageal carcinoma cells and normal epithelial cells and to define cancer-specific and normal-specific protein markers (23). In addition to confirming down-regulation of annexin I, this study demonstrated up-regulation of tumor rejection antigen (gp96) in esophageal squamous cell cancer.

PROTEIN MICROARRAYS

Techniques

Protein microarrays are presently being utilized in several ways relevant to cancer research: (i) to discover novel ligands or drugs that bind to specific bait molecules on the array, (ii) to conduct multiplexed immunoassays to develop a miniature panel of serum biomarkers or cytokines, and (iii) to profile the activation state of specific members of known signal pathways and protein networks. For categories (i) and (ii), a variety of competing technologies already exist for protein discovery. For category (iii), reverse-phase protein arrays offer a robust new method of quantitatively assessing expression levels and the activation status of proteins (18). Reverse-phase arrays comprise spots containing immobilized analyte molecules. Each spot represents an individual test sample, typically consisting of solubilized proteins extracted either from a tissue section or from a pure population of cells collected by LCM. Each array represents multiple different samples. The reverse-phase array is probed with a single detection molecule, and a single analyte is measured for each spot on the array across multiple samples. This format allows multiple samples to be analyzed under the same experimental conditions for any given analyte. An analyte-specific ligand (e.g., antibody) is applied in the solution phase; bound antibodies are detected by secondary tagging. Signal amplification is critical for achieving the sensitivity required for analysis of low-abundance proteins. A reliable method capitalizes on the catalyzed reporter deposition technology developed for immunohistochemical assays. This technology is based on the enzyme-mediated deposition of biotin-tyramide conjugates at the site of a biotinylated antibody-ligand complex (CSA kit; DakoCytomation, Carpinteria, Calif.) (Fig. 3). Each array is scanned, the spot intensities are analyzed, data are normalized to the total protein level, and a standardized, single value is generated for each sample on the array. This single datum point may then be used for comparison to those of every other spot on the array. Such a data set may be used for generation of protein expression profiles across patient samples and may provide insights into the cellular signaling network for each individual patient.

Analytical Challenges

Protein microarrays pose a significant set of analytical challenges not raised by gene arrays (5, 24). The first challenge is the vast range of analyte concentrations to be detected. Protein concentrations demonstrate a broader dynamic range than mRNA concentrations (by up to a factor of 10^{10}). Furthermore, low-abundance analytes exist in a complex biological mixture containing a vast excess of contaminating proteins. If, for example, the specificity of a detection antibody is 99% but a cross-reacting protein exists in a thousandfold (or greater) excess, then for each analyte

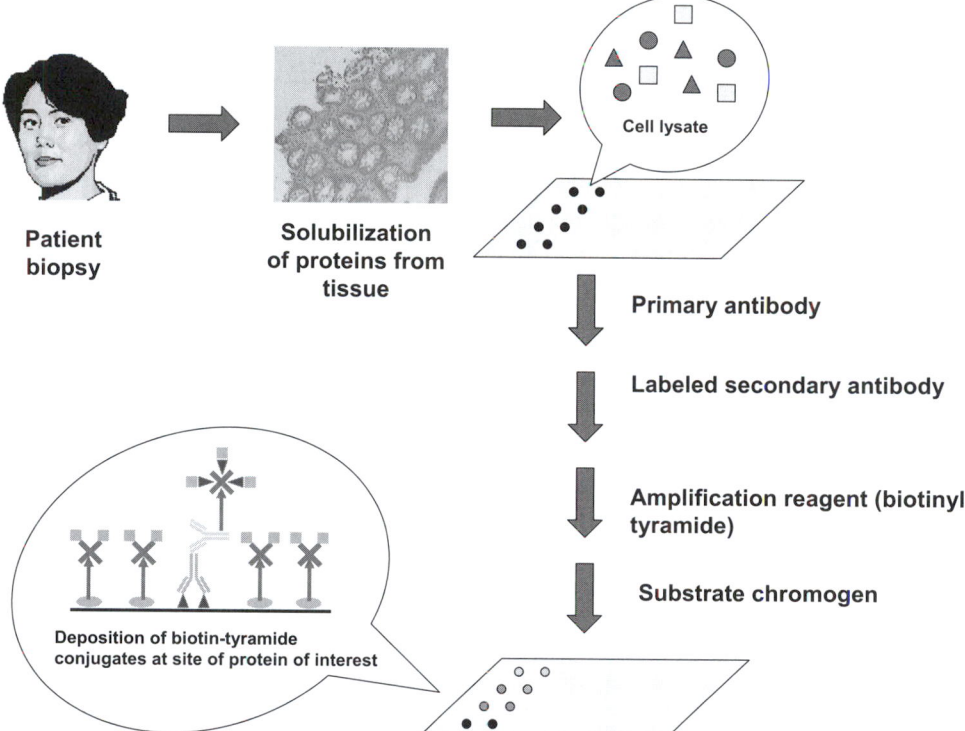

FIGURE 3 Reverse-phase protein microarrays. Nanoliter amounts of tissue lysate are arrayed in dilution curves onto multiple nitrocellulose-coated slides. An analyte-specific ligand (e.g., antibody) is applied in solution phase; bound antibodies are detected by secondary tagging. Signal amplification is a prerequisite for achieving the sensitivity required for analysis of low-abundance proteins. A reliable method capitalizes on the catalyzed reporter deposition technology developed for clinical immunoassays. This technology is based on the enzyme-mediated deposition of biotin-tyramide conjugates at the site of a biotinylated antibody-ligand complex (CSA kit; DakoCytomation). Upon image analysis, the relative proportion of the analyte protein molecules in the total protein can be determined. Each array is scanned, spot intensities are analyzed, data are normalized to the total protein level, and a standardized, single value is generated for each sample on the array. This single datum point may then be used for comparison to those of every other spot on the array. This data set may be used for generation of network profiles across patient samples.

molecule detected, there will be 10 cross-reacting contaminating molecules detected and the signal-to-background ratio will be unacceptable. Another significant challenge for protein microarrays is the requirement for antibodies, or similar detection probes, that are specific for posttranslational modifications representing the activation state of the target protein. Presently, high-quality modification state-specific antibodies are commercially available for only a small percentage of the known proteins involved in signal networks and gene regulation. A significant challenge for cooperative groups, funding agencies, and international consortia is the generation of large, comprehensive libraries of fully characterized specific antibodies, ligands, and probes. A major initiative of the Human Proteome Organization is the production and qualification of antibody libraries that will be made available to the scientific community (9, 22).

Accuracy and precision are paramount for protein microarrays. A small shift in a signaling pathway in the protein circuitry can dramatically affect the ultimate biologic outcome. This issue is critical in pathologic states such as progression of premalignant lesions. Immunohistochemistry (and, by extension, multiplexed tissue arrays) can provide

information about histomorphological and subcellular localization of proteins. However, immunohistochemistry is inherently subjective and semiquantitative at best and may not be adequately sensitive for low-abundance analytes. Variability in the intensities of immunohistochemical staining can result from variation in tissue handling and fixation practices, accessibility of the antigenic epitope based on antigen retrieval procedures, and cellular heterogeneity. In the face of these limitations, the ability to obtain a sensitive, functional proteomic analysis from a sample lysate only a few hundred micrometers in diameter and containing the solubilized cellular material itself is a promising development in cancer research and diagnostics.

Sensitivity Requirements

PCR-like direct amplification methods have not yet been developed for proteins. Consequently, protein microarrays require indirect, and very stringent, amplification chemistries (13, 17, 20). Adequate sensitivity must be achieved (at least in the femtomolar range) with acceptable background. Moreover, the labeling and amplification method must be linear and reproducible to ensure reliable quantitative analysis. Finally, the amplification chemistry must be tolerant of the large dynamic range of the analytes and the complexity of the biologic samples. The biologic sample may naturally contain endogenous biotin, peroxidases, alkaline phosphatases, fluorescent proteins, and immunoglobulins, all of which can substantially reduce the yield or increase the background of the amplification reaction. The high sensitivity of reverse-phase protein arrays is possible in part because the detection probe (e.g., antibody) can be tagged and the signal is amplified independently from the immobilized analyte. Amplification chemistries available take advantage of methods developed for highly sensitive third-generation commercial clinical immunoassays (4, 11). For example, coupling the detection antibody with highly sensitive tyramide-based avidin-biotin signal amplification systems can yield detection sensitivities of fewer than 1,000 to 5,000 molecules/spot. Reverse-phase protein array methodology assesses only one protein per slide but has the advantage that all samples can be analyzed side by side in a single array. This is particularly advantageous for clinical samples for which protein levels across samples can be compared simultaneously under identical conditions on a single slide.

Clinical Samples

The clinical power of protein microarrays can be realized only if the technology can be directly applied to biopsy specimens, tissue cell aspirates, or body fluid samples. In such cases, the input sample for protein microarrays often is small in volume and low in analyte concentration. The total number of cells available for analysis from a core needle biopsy specimen or a cell aspirate may be fewer than 100,000. Moreover, since tissues are highly heterogeneous, the population of target cells may compose a small percentage of the total. Thus, only a few thousand cancer cells may be procurable from a core biopsy specimen. Since many proteins of interest and their phosphorylated counterparts exist in low abundance, the total concentration of analyte proteins in each sample often is low. Consequently, if the analytic method does not have adequate sensitivity, the number of cells required for the assay may not be clinically obtainable.

Sample Preparation

Sample preparation methods are critical in proteomic analysis, as some proteins are insoluble in a heterogeneous mixture of cells. An important advance in sample preparation was the development of LCM. Prior to LCM, "pure" cell populations were obtained from tissues manually. Although manual microdissection can achieve good precision, it is time-consuming and labor-intensive and requires a high degree of manual dexterity. The LCM system allows a one-step procurement of selected cells from a heterogeneous section of tissue. LCM has been used successfully to obtain pure populations of cancer cells from both frozen and paraffin-embedded tissues, stained or unstained, for molecular analysis of macromolecules. LCM is capable of isolating single cells, making it possible to procure pure populations of neoplastic cells from lesions less than 1 mm in diameter without encroachment of adjacent nonneoplastic cells. Using this technique, it has been possible to compare matched samples of normal epithelial cells, stromata, benign cells, preneoplastic cells, and cancer cells.

FUTURE DIAGNOSTIC STRATEGIES

MHC Antigens

Diagnostic strategies based on immunoproteomics exploit the natural response of the human immune system by identifying antigens associated with major histocompatibility complex (MHC) class I and class II molecules that are uniquely associated with cancer cells. These novel diagnostic tools are based on the identification of the following:

- Endogenous antigenic peptides associated with class I and II MHC molecules.
- Autoantibody-reactive proteins identified using serological analysis.
- Membrane proteins on the surfaces of diseased cells that are putative targets for novel monoclonal antibody therapeutics.

New technologies use automated, data-dependent high-throughput MS techniques to sequence all of the peptides extracted from class I and II MHC molecules on a diseased cell. Direct identification of endogenous MHC-associated peptides is very powerful because it identifies multiple shared antigens in the same tumor type from several different patients as well as antigens common to different tumor types. Novel peptide isolation, purification, and MS technologies can determine which MHC-associated peptides and surface-expressed proteins are differentially displayed on normal versus diseased cells by directly comparing the peptides or proteins from the diseased and normal tissues. Differential analysis methodology is also applied to identify autoantigens by screening serum autoantibodies in patients. The MHC-associated antigens can then be compared with information in autoantigen databases to identify diagnostic antigens. This approach, which exploits the presence of tumor-reactive antibodies present in cancer patient serum, identifies antigens that are present at very early stages of disease, before tumors are detectable by other commonly used methods, such as imaging.

Recursive Partitioning of TAAs

The sera of cancer patients contain antibodies which react with a unique group of autologous cellular antigens called tumor-associated antigens (TAAs). The low frequency of positive reactions against any individual antigen has precluded the use of autoantibodies as useful diagnostic markers. However, multiple-antigen arrays may provide accurate and valuable tools for cancer detection and diagnosis. Koziol et al. found that the use of recursive partitioning resulted in the selection of subsets of a panel of seven TAAs which differentiated between tumors and controls, and these subsets were unique to each cancer cohort (12). Recursive partitioning is a multivariate statistical methodology for constructing a decision tree. During the process of decision tree induction, questions must be asked to direct the user down the appropriate path. For instance, if each potential question could have a true or false answer, any particular node would have at most two paths leading from it to the next node(s) in the path. Every possible value of every possible feature within the training set represents a potential split in the decision tree. At each node, the data are split into two independent groups—this is referred to as partitioning. Once there are two new nodes (child nodes) linked to a previous node (the parent node), the process can be repeated for each child node independently by using only the observations present in that child—the recursive step. This initial study was based on seven selected TAAs. Panels of TAAs could be expanded to include other known TAAs such as HER-2/neu, ras, cyclins, and antigens involved in cell-mediated immune reactions, many of which might have concomitant humoral immune responses.

Plasma Telomerase as a Cancer Biomarker

A research group at the University of Maryland is using a telomeric repeat amplification protocol to evaluate the utility of measuring telomerase in body fluids for the diagnosis of malignancy and for use as a monitoring tool during therapy (10). Telomerase, an enzyme detected in approximately 90% of all tumor types, is found in elevated levels in malignant cells. This project is unique because it will assay telomerase levels in body fluids rather than cellular material. Investigators will do the following:

- Use a variety of technologies, including an automated telomeric repeat amplification protocol assay, laser-induced fluorescence detection, quantitative reverse transcription PCR, and other molecular and biochemical techniques, to measure telomerase activity in noncellular fluids for early lung cancer detection.

- Examine a large group of patients with a variety of cancers, including malignancies of the lung, esophagus, and gastrointestinal tract, to evaluate telomerase as a biomarker for early cancer detection.

Combination Strategies for Biomarker Development

The Biomarker Development Laboratory at Moffitt uses a combination of proteomic and DNA-based technologies to evaluate biomarkers for earlier lung cancer detection. The focus of this group is to develop better detection tests for preclinical lung cancer. Some of the biomarkers under investigation include a difucosylated ceramide, lacto-N-fucopentose III, transforming growth factor β receptor type II, SMAD 2, SMAD 4, and SMAD 7. Because the existing technology for early lung cancer detection is not very sensitive, there is a need to improve the sensitivity of detection techniques and develop a screening approach that uses multiple markers. Investigators will do the following:

- Use proteomic and DNA-based strategies in pursuit of the project objectives.

- Evaluate a variety of biomarkers in archived sputum specimens from a cohort of smokers and former smokers. This archive will provide clinical material associated with known subsequent cancer outcome for a case control study of biomarker utility.

- Perform subsequent analyses on a high-throughput screening platform presently under development through a collaborative research and development agreement with an industrial partner.

CONCLUSION

In the dawning age of targeted anticancer therapeutics, the ability to accurately identify the molecular aberrations present within an individual tumor is critical in determining appropriate treatment. For patients, this will mean better management of their disease and better outcomes. Advances in the understanding of cancer biology and the development of powerful proteomic technologies are leading to the identification of many previously unknown abnormalities in preneoplastic cells and cancer cells. This progress has promoted the identification of novel biomarkers and therapeutic agents, leading to important advances in detection, diagnosis, and treatment of human cancers.

REFERENCES

1. Aebersold, R., and M. Mann. 2003. Mass spectrometry-based proteomics. *Nature* 422:198–207.

2. Bergquist, J., M. Palmblad, M. Wetterhall, P. Hakansson, and K. E. Markides. 2002. Peptide mapping of proteins in human body fluids using electrospray ionization Fourier transform ion cyclotron resonance mass spectrometry. *Mass Spectrom. Rev.* 21:2–15.

3. Blagoev, B., I. Kratchmarova, S. E. Ong, M. Nielsen, L. J. Foster, and M. Mann. 2003. A proteomics strategy to elucidate functional protein-protein interactions applied to EGF signaling. *Nat. Biotechnol.* 21:315–318.

4. Bobrow, M. N., K. J. Shaughnessy, and G. J. Litt. 1991. Catalyzed reporter deposition, a novel method of signal amplification. 2. Application to membrane immunoassays. *J. Immunol. Methods* 137:103–112.

5. Celis, J. E. 2003. Clinical proteomics—an emerging discipline in biomedical research. *Mol. Cell. Proteomics* 2:367.

6. Chaurand, P., M. E. Sanders, R. A. Jensen, and R. M. Caprioli. 2004. Proteomics in diagnostic pathology—profiling and imaging proteins directly in tissue sections. *Am. J. Pathol.* 165:1057–1068.

7. Damoc, E., N. Youhnovski, D. Crettaz, J. D. Tissot, and M. Przybylski. 2003. High resolution proteome analysis of cryoglobulins using Fourier transform-ion cyclotron resonance mass spectrometry. *Proteomics* 3:1425–1433.

8. Han, D. K., J. Eng, H. L. Zhou, and R. Aebersold. 2001. Quantitative profiling of differentiation-induced microsomal proteins using isotope-coded affinity tags and mass spectrometry. *Nat. Biotechnol.* 19:946–951.

9. Hanash, S. 2004. HUPO initiatives relevant to clinical proteomics. *Mol. Cell. Proteomics* 3:298–301.

10. Hess, J. L., D. H. Atha, J. F. Xu, and W. E. Highsmith. 2004. Telomerase activity measurement in magnetically captured epithelial cells: comparison of slab-gel and capillary electrophoresis. *Electrophoresis* 25:1852–1859.

11. Hunyady, B., K. Krempels, G. Harta, and E. Mezey. 1996. Immunohistochemical signal amplification by catalyzed reporter deposition and its application in double immunostaining. *J. Histochem. Cytochem.* 44:1353–1362.

12. Koziol, J. A., J. Y. Zhang, C. A. Casiano, X. X. Peng, F. D. Shi, A. C. Feng, E. K. L. Chan, and E. M. Tan. 2003. Recursive partitioning as an approach to selection of immune markers for tumor diagnosis. *Clin. Cancer Res.* 9:5120–5126.

13. Kukar, T., S. Eckenrode, Y. Gu, W. Lian, M. Megginson, J.-X. She, and D. Wu. 2002. Protein microarrays to detect protein-protein interactions using red and green fluorescent proteins. *Anal. Biochem.* 306:50–54.

14. Liotta, L. A., I. Petricoin, F. Emanuel, A. M. Ardekani, B. A. Hitt, P. J. Levine, V. A. Fusaro, S. M. Steinberg, G. B. Mills, and C. Simone. 2003. General keynote: proteomic patterns in sera serve as biomarkers of ovarian cancer. *Gynecol. Oncol.* 88:S25–S28.

15. Liu, T., W. J. Qian, E. F. Strittmatter, D. G. Camp, G. A. Anderson, B. D. Thrall, and R. D. Smith. 2004. High-throughput comparative proteome analysis using a quantitative cysteinyl-peptide enrichment technology. *Anal. Chem.* 76:5345–5353.

16. Mehta, A. I., S. Ross, M. S. Lowenthal, V. Fusaro, D. A. Fishman, E. F. Petricoin, and L. A. Liotta. 2003. Biomarker amplification by serum carrier protein binding. *Dis. Markers* 19:1–10.

17. Morozov, V. N., A. V. Gavryushkin, and A. A. Deev. 2002. Direct detection of isotopically labeled metabolites bound to a protein microarray using a charge-coupled device. *J. Biochem. Biophys. Methods* 51:57–67.

18. Paweletz, C. P., L. Charboneau, V. E. Bichsel, N. L. Simone, T. Chen, J. W. Gillespie, M. R. Emmert-Buck, M. J. Roth, E. F. Petricoin, and L. A. Liotta. 2001. Reverse phase protein microarrays which capture disease progression show activation of pro-survival pathways at the cancer invasion front. *Oncogene* 20:1981–1989.

19. **Petricoin, E. F., and L. A. Liotta.** 2004. SELDI-TOF-based serum proteomic pattern diagnostics for early detection of cancer. *Curr. Opin. Biotechnol.* **15:**24–30.

20. **Schweitzer, B., and S. F. Kingsmore.** 2002. Measuring proteins on microarrays. *Curr. Opin. Biotechnol.* **13:**14–19.

21. **Tang, N., P. Tornatore, and S. R. Weinberger.** 2004. Current developments in SELDI affinity technology. *Mass Spectrom. Rev.* **23:**34–44.

22. **Tyers, M., and M. Mann.** 2003. From genomics to proteomics. *Nature* **422:**193–197.

23. **Zhou, G., H. Li, D. DeCamp, S. Chen, H. Shu, Y. Gong, M. Flaig, J. W. Gillespie, N. Hu, P. R. Taylor, M. R. Emmert-Buck, L. A. Liotta, E. F. Petricoin III, and Y. Zhao.** 2002. 2D differential in-gel electrophoresis for the identification of esophageal scans cell cancer-specific protein markers. *Mol. Cell. Proteomics* **1:**117–123.

24. **Zhu, W., X. N. Wang, Y. M. Ma, M. L. Rao, J. Glimm, and J. S. Kovach.** 2003. Detection of cancer-specific markers amid massive mass spectral data. *Proc. Natl. Acad. Sci. USA* **100:**14666–14671.

TRANSPLANTATION IMMUNOLOGY

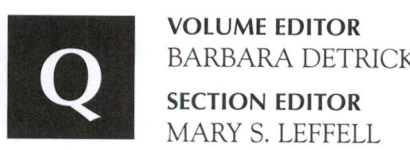

VOLUME EDITOR
BARBARA DETRICK

SECTION EDITOR
MARY S. LEFFELL

Histocompatibility Testing after Fifty Years of Transplantation

MARY S. LEFFELL

135

The year 2004 marks the 50th anniversary of the first successful renal transplant, which was performed by Drs. Murray, Merrill, and Harrison at Peter Bent Brigham Hospital in Boston (18). During the next decade, clinical transplantation was extended to liver, lung, heart, pancreas, and bone marrow transplants (2, 10, 11, 16, 28). Early attempts in human transplantation were limited by the immunosuppressive regimens which comprised primarily steroids, irradiation, and azathioprine. It is generally agreed that major advances in transplantation began with the discovery of cyclosporine (5) and its subsequent introduction in the United States after receiving Food and Drug Administration approval in 1984. Today, second- and third-generation drugs, such as tacrolimus, rapamycin, and mycophenolate mofetil, are continuing to reduce the incidence and severity of allograft rejection while permitting reduced steroid doses with a concomitant reduction in the side effects of immunosuppression. In the United States, 1-year survival rates for renal and renal-pancreatic transplants average 90% and average rates approach or exceed 80% for other solid-organ transplants (24). The development of clinical transplantation has also fostered growth in understanding of the alloimmune response and of the major histocompatibility complex and in histocompatibility assessment. The first recognition that HLA antigens could provoke alloantibodies was in 1952 when Dausset described the antigen "Mac," later to be named HLA-A2 (7). The term HLA was derived from the early studies of leukoagglutinins in the sera of multiparous women or transfused patients, combining the human-1 (Hu-1) and leukocyte antigen (LA) designations of Dausset and Payne et al., respectively (23). Some 30 years later, Bjorkman et al. defined the structural basis for normal and allo-immune antigen recognition with the crystalline structure of HLA-A2 (4). Given the remarkable advances that have occurred during the development of transplantation, it seems fitting that this anniversary was also marked by the initiation of the first collaborative clinical trial to induce human tolerance for transplantation (6).

For much of the past 50 years of transplantation, the primary assay for histocompatibility testing, which can be used both for typing and for alloantibody detection, has been the complement-dependent cytotoxicity test. In 1968, the cytotoxicity assay was miniaturized into "micro-lymphocytotoxicity," which became the standard technique for serologic typing, antibody screening, and crossmatching (19). The "Terasaki" tray was a boon to histocompatibility, not only because it simplified testing, but also because it conserved precious typing sera by requiring only 1 μl per test well. Histocompatibility laboratories no longer rely exclusively on complement-dependent serology, since molecular techniques are available for typing and since solid-phase immunoassays, using solubilized HLA antigens and single recombinant HLA antigens, are providing more sensitive and cost-effective antibody screening and identification. Cytotoxicity still has an important role in histocompatibility laboratories as it remains the standard assay for antibody crossmatches. Today's histocompatibility laboratories, therefore, often utilize multiple techniques and have expanded their testing further to other immunogenetic systems, including the genes encoding cytokines and killer immunoglobulin-like receptors (KIR).

Molecular typing methods and solid-phase immunoassays are enabling histocompatibility laboratories to adapt testing to meet the changing needs of transplant patients. In solid-organ transplantation, the most urgent problem is the shortage of available deceased-donor organs. The number of patients on the national waiting list is over 85,000, with an average of only 20,000 donor organs available annually (29). The donor shortage has placed increased emphasis on attempts to use live donors when possible and on efforts to maximize the longevity of transplanted organs by earlier and better diagnosis of rejection. Ongoing efforts are also aimed at inducing tolerance or graft acceptance such that immunosuppression treatments, particularly steroids, can be safely reduced or withdrawn. More than one-third of renal transplant patients have the additional problem of some degree of prior sensitization to HLA antigens, manifested as circulating anti-HLA antibodies (29). Since the late 1960s, when HLA antibodies were discovered to cause hyperacute rejection of renal allografts, the presence of anti-HLA antibodies at titers sufficient to give a positive cytotoxicity crossmatch has been considered a contraindication for transplantation (14, 22, 30). Clinical protocols using high-dose intravenous immunoglobulin or a combination of intravenous immunoglobulin and plasmapheresis are being used to successfully desensitize and perform transplants on patients who otherwise might have waited years for a compatible deceased-donor organ (12, 31). Similar protocols are also being used for ABO blood group-incompatible organ transplants, and some centers are even finding compatible donors for sensitized patients through paired exchanges of living-donor organs (8). Laboratory support for these innovative clinical protocols is vital and is highly dependent upon the accurate assessment of the levels and specificities of patients' antibodies. Three of the chapters in this section focus on the methods that are being used to monitor and evaluate transplant patients. Reinsmoen and Zeevi discuss approaches to evaluate cellular sensitization that can be employed in steroid withdrawal protocols and post-transplant monitoring for rejection or tolerance. Hartono et al. describe molecular techniques that permit earlier and more-sensitive detection of allograft rejection, and Zachary and colleagues compare the various techniques for defining clinically relevant alloantibodies and illustrate the utility of these assays in clinical desensitization protocols.

The availability of suitable donors is also problematic for many patients who are candidates for bone marrow transplantation or hematopoietic stem cell transplantation (HSCT). The ideal donor for HSCT is an HLA-identical sibling, but at most only 30% of patients have suitable related donors. Efforts to increase the number of available donors have fostered altruistic donor registries, with more than 50 such registries worldwide. One of the largest registries is that of the National Marrow Donor Program (NMDP), which presently lists more than 5 million typed potential marrow and peripheral blood stem cell donors and has more than 30,000 cord blood units (20). The increasing use of registry donors has permitted a recent retrospective analysis of the impact of HLA matching among 1,874 recipients of unrelated-donor HSCT (9). Mismatches at the antigen or low-resolution level, not surprisingly, had greater impact on patient survival and the risk of graft-versus-host disease than did mismatches at the allele level. Importantly, mismatches at HLA-C were found to confer a level of risk similar to those conferred by mismatches at HLA-A, HLA-B, and DRB1; therefore, NMDP recommendations for evaluating unrelated donors now include allele-level typing for HLA-C. The NMDP analysis also highlighted the reduced likelihood of finding "perfect" matches (i.e., those in which the recipient and donor match for both alleles at HLA-A, HLA-B, HLA-C, and DRB1) when typing resolution is increased from the antigen to the allele level. Of the study pairs that were matched for HLA-A, HLA-B, HLA-C, and DRB1 at low resolution, 34% had one or more mismatches as determined by high-resolution typing (9).

In practice, HLA polymorphism reduces the probability of finding perfectly matched unrelated donors unless the candidate has HLA alleles and haplotypes that are relatively common. Consequently, newer HSCT protocols permit certain degrees of HLA mismatching. This includes the use of one-haplotype-matched related donors and one- or two-allele-mismatched unrelated donors. Stem cells from one-haplotype-matched donors can be given as "mini" transplants under protocols that use nonmyeloablative conditioning regimens. Nonmyeloablative conditioning using reduced doses of cytotoxic drugs and other chemotherapy permits transplantation in older patients who cannot tolerate doses for complete ablation (17, 27). Alternative sources of stem cells include cord blood and peripheral blood following mobilization with growth factors (1, 3). Peripheral blood stem cells may be used not only for primary transplantation but also for additional immunotherapy via a secondary infusion to promote the "graft-versus-leukemia" effect (26). Investigations are also under way to determine if mismatching for certain KIR genes can potentiate the anti-cancer effect mediated by natural killer cells (15, 25). These

newer HSCT protocols are requiring additional testing from histocompatibility and cytogenetic laboratories. High-resolution definition of HLA alleles is essential for selection of compatible unrelated donors for HSCT. Evaluation of the degree of donor chimerism is needed in the protocols that result in mixed populations of self- and donor-derived leukocytes in transplant recipients and in assessments to determine when secondary infusions of donor cells may be warranted. For transplants with some degree of HLA mismatching, accurate determination of humoral sensitization is required to assess the risk of engraftment failure due to antibody-mediated rejection. The remaining chapters in this section address these newer issues for bone marrow and stem cell transplantation. The chapter by Hurley and colleagues explains the premises behind the different molecular techniques that can be used to differentiate HLA alleles and how to apply one or more of these methods to achieve the degree of typing resolution required for a given clinical application. Baxter-Lowe discusses the techniques that can be employed to determine both engraftment of donor stem cells and the relative degree of donor-recipient chimerism. Lastly, Tyan and Carrington focus on the polymorphism of the KIR genes and report that defining KIR alleles and haplotypes is applicable not only in HSCT, as KIR genotypes may affect susceptibility to autoimmunity and viral infections (13, 21).

REFERENCES

1. **Barker, J. N., and J. E. Wagner.** 2002. Umbilical cord blood transplantation: current state of the art. *Curr. Opin. Oncol.* **14:**160–164.
2. **Barnard, C. H.** 1967. A human cardiac transplantation interim report of a successful operation performed at Groote Schurr Hospital, Capetown. *S. Afr. Med. J.* **41:** 1271–1274.
3. **Bensinger, W. I., and R. Storb.** 2001. Allogeneic peripheral blood stem cell transplantation. *Rev. Clin. Exp. Hematol.* **5:**67–86.
4. **Bjorkman, P. J., M. A. Saper, B. Samraoui, W. S. Bennett, J. L. Strominger, and D. C. Wiley.** 1987. Structure of the human class I histocompatibility antigen, HLA-A2. *Nature* **329:**506–512.
5. **Borel, J. F., C. Feurer, H. U. Gubler, and H. Stahelin.** 1994. Biological effects of cyclosporin A: a new antilymphocytic agent. *Agents Actions* **43:**179–186. [Reprint of 1976 paper.]
6. **Couzin, J.** 2004. Putting tolerance to the test. *Science* **305:**194–196.
7. **Dausset, J.** 1954. Leuco-agglutinins. IV. Leuco-agglutinins and blood transfusion. *Vox Sang* **4:**190–198.
8. **Delmonico, F. L.** 2004. Exchanging kidneys—advances in living-donor transplantation. *N. Engl. J. Med.* **350:** 1812–1814.
9. **Flomenberg, N., L. Baxter-Lowe, D. Confer, M. Fernandez-Vina, A. Filipovich, M. Horowitz, C. Hurley, C. Kollman, C. Anasetti, H. Noreen, A. Begovich, W. Hildebrand, E. Petersdorf, B. Schmeckpeper, M. Setterholm, E. Trachtenberg, T. Williams, E. Yunis, and D. Weisdorf.** 2004. Impact of HLA class I and class II high-resolution matching on outcomes of unrelated donor bone marrow transplantation: HLA-C mismatching is associated with a strong adverse effect on transplantation outcome. *Blood* **104:**1923–1930.
10. **Hardy, J. D., W. R. Webb, M. L. Dalton, Jr., and G. R. Walker, Jr.** 1963. Lung homotransplantation in man. *JAMA* **186:**1065–1074.

11. **Horowitz, M. M.** 1999. Uses and growth of hematopoietic stem cell transplantation, p. 12–18. *In* E. D. Thomas, K. G. Blume, and S. J. Forman (ed.), *Hematopoietic Cell Transplantation*, 2nd ed. Blackwell Sciences, Malden, Mass.

12. **Jordan, S. C., A. Vo, S. Bunnapradist, M. Toyoda, A. Peng, D. Puliyanda, E. Kamil, and D. Tyan.** 2003. Intravenous immune globulin treatment inhibits crossmatch positivity and allows for successful transplantation of incompatible organs in living-donor and cadaver recipients. *Transplantation* **76**:631–636.

13. **Khakoo, S. I., C. L. Thio, M. P. Martin, C. R. Brooks, X. Gao, J. Astemborski, J. Cheng, J. J. Goedert, D. Vlahov, M. Hilgartner, S. Cox, A. M. Little, G. J. Alexander, M. E. Cramp, S. J. O'Brien, W. M. Rosenberg, D. L. Thomas, and M. Carrington.** 2004. HLA and NK cell inhibitory receptor genes in resolving hepatitis C virus infection. *Science* **305**:872–874.

14. **Kissmeyer-Nielsen, F., S. Olsen, V. P. Peterson, and O. Fjeldborg.** 1966. Hyperacute rejection of kidney allografts associated with pre-existing humoral antibodies against donor cells. *Lancet* **ii**:662–665.

15. **Leung, W., R. Iyengar, V. Turner, P. Lang, P. Bader, P. Conn, D. Niethammer, and R. Handgretinger.** 2004. Determinants of antileukemia effects of allogeneic NK cells. *J. Immunol.* **172**:644–650.

16. **Lillehei, R. C., Y. Idezuki, W. D. Kelly, J. S. Najarian, F. K. Merkel, and F. C. Goetz.** 1969. Transplantation of the intestine and pancreas. *Transplant. Proc.* **1**:230–238.

17. **Maris, M., B. M. Sandmaier, D. G. Maloney, P. A. McSweeney, A. Wollfrey, T. Chauncey, J. Shizuru, D. Niederwieser, K. G. Blume, S. Forman, and R. Storb.** 2001. Non-myeloablative hematopoietic stem cell transplantation. *Transfus. Clin. Biol.* **8**:231–234.

18. **Merrill, J. P., J. E. Murray, J. H. Harrison, and W. R. Guild.** 1956. Successful homotransplantation of the human kidney between identical twins. *JAMA* **160**:277–282.

19. **Mittal, K. K., M. R. Mickey, D. P. Singal, and P. I. Terasaki.** 1968. Serotyping for homotransplantation. 18. Refinement of microdroplet lymphocyte cytotoxicity test. *Transplantation* **6**:913–927.

20. **National Marrow Donor Program.** June 28, 2005, posting date. *About the National Marrow Donor Program.* [Online.] National Marrow Donor Program, Minneapolis, Minn. http://www.marrow.org/NMDP/.

21. **Nelson, G. W., M. P. Martin, D. Gladman, J. Wade, J. Trowsdale, and M. Carrington.** 2004. Cutting edge: heterozygote advantage in autoimmune disease: hierarchy of protection/susceptibility conferred by HLA and killer Ig-like receptor combinations in psoriatic arthritis. *J. Immunol.* **173**:4273–4276.

22. **Patel, R., and P. I. Terasaki.** 1969. Significance of the positive crossmatch test in kidney transplantation. *N. Engl. J. Med.* **280**:735–739.

23. **Payne, R., M. Tripp, J. Wiegle, W. Bodmer, and J. Bodmer.** 1964. A new leukocyte isoantigenic system in man. *Cold Spring Harbor Symp. Quant. Biol.* **29**:285.

24. **Port, F. K., D. M. Dykstra, R. M. Merion, and R. A. Wolfe.** 2004. Organ donation and transplantation trends in the USA, 2003. *Am. J. Transplant.* **4**(Suppl. 9):7–12.

25. **Ruggeri, L., M. Capanni, E. Urbani, K. Perruccio, W. D. Shlomchik, A. Tosti, S. Posati, D. Rogaia, F. Frassoni, F. Aversa, M. F. Martelli, and A. Velardi.** 2002. Effectiveness of donor natural killer cell alloreactivity in mismatched hematopoietic transplants. *Science* **295**:2097–2100.

26. **Slavin, S.** 2001. Immunotherapy of cancer with alloreactive lymphocytes. *Lancet Oncol.* **2**:491–498.

27. **Slavin, S., A. Nagler, M. Y. Shapira, M. Aker, C. Gabriel, and R. Or.** 2002. Treatment of leukemia by alloreactive lymphocytes and nonmyeolablative stem cell transplantation. *J. Clin. Immunol.* **22**:64–69.

28. **Starzl, T. E., C. G. Groth, L. Brettschneider, I. Penn, V. A. Fulginiti, J. B. Moon, H. Blanchard, A. J. Martin, Jr., and K. A. Porter.** 1968. Orthotopic homotransplantation of the human liver. *Ann. Surg.* **168**:392–415.

29. **U.S. Department of Health and Human Services.** 2003. Annual Report of the U.S. Organ Procurement and Transplantation Network and the Scientific Registry of Transplant Recipients: Transplant Data 1993–2002. Department of Health and Human Services, Health Resources and Services Administration, Office of Special Programs, Division of Transplantation, Rockville, Md.; United Network for Organ Sharing, Richmond, Va.; University Renal Research and Education Association, Ann Arbor, Mich.

30. **Williams, G. M., D. M. Hume, R. P. Hudson, Jr., P. J. Morris, K. Kano, and F. Milgrom.** 1968. "Hyperacute" renal-homograft rejection in man. *N. Engl. J. Med.* **279**:611–618.

31. **Zachary, A. A., R. A. Montgomery, L. E. Ratner, M. Samaniego-Picotta, D. Kopchaliiska, and M. S. Leffell.** 2003. Specific and durable elimination of antibody to donor HLA antigens in renal transplant patients. *Transplantation* **76**:1519–25.

Molecular Methods: HLA Alleles

CAROLYN KATOVICH HURLEY, KAI CAO, TING TANG, NORIKO STEINER, ANA M. LAZARO, C. ALAN HOWARD, AND JENNIFER NG

136

INTRODUCTION AND BACKGROUND

A Comparison of HLA Typing Methods

Molecular biology techniques aimed at identification of HLA polymorphism at the gene level have largely replaced HLA typing assays based on identification of HLA proteins (15). Both DNA-based testing and serology are used to evaluate differences found in key HLA protein regions (antigen binding domains) that are known to have significant biologic relevance in modulating the immune system. This evaluation is performed either directly by using human alloantiserum-based assays to define key epitopes within these HLA proteins or by evaluating the sequences of the corresponding DNA regions coding for this portion of the HLA molecule. The advantages of DNA-based testing over the longer-established protein-based assays are summarized in Table 1 and in previous publications (1, 13, 14, 16, 18). Most of the DNA-based assays rely on PCR to amplify the HLA genes and the detection of nucleotide sequence differences among HLA alleles to predict HLA types.

HLA Genes

The HLA genes encode at least six different HLA molecules, HLA-A, -B, and -C (class I molecules) and HLA-DR, -DQ, and -DP (class II molecules). (Note that other HLA genes such as the HLA-G gene are not yet included in HLA typing schemes since their importance in transplantation is not yet known.) The HLA molecules are encoded by the most polymorphic genetic loci known in humans (21). The genes (or loci) encoding one chain of the HLA class I molecules (the heavy chain) and both chains (alpha and beta) of the HLA class II molecules are clustered in one region of human chromosome 6, termed the major histocompatibility complex. The products of the A, B, and C loci associate with the product of the β_2-microglobulin locus to form the class I molecules. The products of alpha (A) and beta (B) loci of DR, DQ, and DP associate with one another to form the class II molecules. For example, the product of the DQB1 locus, the DQ beta chain, associates with the product of the DQA1 locus, the DQ alpha chain, to form a DQ molecule. Other class II A and B gene pairs that may be identified in HLA typing include: DPA1 and DPB1 (specifying a DP molecule), DRA and DRB1 (specifying a DR molecule), DRA and DRB3 (specifying a DR52 molecule), DRA and DRB4 (specifying a DR53 molecule), and DRA and DRB5 (specifying a DR2-like molecule [DR51]).

The numbers that often follow A and B (e.g., DQA1 and DRB3) were added to distinguish these genes from other class II A- and B-like genes in the DNA of the cell. Individuals carry either one or two different functional DRB loci on chromosome 6. Most versions of chromosome 6 found in the population carry the DRB1 locus. Some versions of chromosome 6 also carry a DRB3 or DRB4 or DRB5 locus. Thus, some individuals express two DR molecules encoded by a single copy of chromosome 6 (e.g., carrying DRB1 and DRB5 loci) or, potentially, four DR molecules in all (e.g., encoded by DRB1 and DRB5 loci on one copy of chromosome 6 and by DRB1 and DRB4 on the second copy of chromosome 6).

At the DNA level, the HLA loci have multiple alternate forms (alleles). β_2-Microglobulin is not polymorphic. New alleles are described in reports of the World Health Organization (WHO) HLA nomenclature committee (e.g., reference 11), and a summary appears on a website (http://www.anthonynolan.org.uk/HIG/index.html) (22). The total number of alleles present in the entire human population at each locus differs. For example, more than 360 alleles at the DRB1 locus have been described but only 3 alleles at the DRA locus have been described. Thus, each individual carries a limited set of HLA alleles (e.g., two HLA-A locus alleles, two HLA-B locus alleles, and two HLA-C locus alleles, etc.) while the entire population carries a very diverse and extensive collection of HLA alleles. Because many HLA alleles exist in the population, most outbred individuals carry two different alleles at a locus and are heterozygous. Individuals who carry two identical alleles at a locus are homozygous for that locus. The frequencies of individual alleles vary in different human populations (3).

Within each HLA gene, the polymorphism is clustered into one or two of the approximately six to eight expressed gene segments (exons). In the HLA class I alleles, the majority of the differences among alleles are found in exons 2 and 3; in the HLA class II alleles, the majority of the differences are found in exon 2. DNA-based HLA typing focuses on these polymorphic exons to identify HLA alleles.

HLA Nomenclature

Each HLA allele is designated by the name of the gene followed by an asterisk and a four- to eight-digit number indicating the allele (11; http://www.anthonynolan.org.uk/HIG/index.html). For example, DPB1*010101 is an allele of the

TABLE 1 Comparison of HLA typing methods

Assay parameters	DNA-based molecular assays	Protein-based[a] assays	
		Serology	Cellular assays[b]
Type(s) of assay	SSP, SSOPH, RSCA, SBT, other	Complement-dependent cellular cytotoxicity assay	Mixed lymphocyte culture, primed lymphocyte typing
Sample and quantity	Nucleated cells, e.g., <1 ml of whole blood	Peripheral blood lymphocytes isolated from 5 to 10 ml of blood	Peripheral blood lymphocytes isolated from 10 to 50 ml of blood
Sample limitations	Viable cells not required	Viable cells required; other limitations dependent on patient health, treatment	Viable cells required; other limitations dependent on patient health, treatment
Reagent(s)	Synthetic oligonucleotides	Human alloantisera, some monoclonal antibodies	Lymphocytes or lymphocytes primed in culture
Reagent specificity and resolution	DNA polymorphisms detected based on known alleles; reagents can be developed as new alleles are described; resolution adjustable depending on reagents and techniques used; not known which polymorphisms are relevant for transplantation outcome	Based on sensitization of serum donor; reagent usually reacts with multiple allelic products; difficult to identify reagents for new specificities; reagents derived during sensitization in vivo so may detect biologically relevant differences	Very sensitive to HLA differences; cultured cells may lose specificity; reagents derived during sensitization in vivo so may detect biologically relevant differences
Reagent availability	Unlimited source with defined specificity	Reagents derived from humans so source limited and varied over time	Reagents derived from humans so source limited and varied over time; difficult to generate and maintain cellular reagents
Commercial kit availability	Available	Available	Not available
Time to complete assay[c]	4 h to 3 days depending on the resolution required	1 day	7 to 8 days

[a] Other protein-based assays used in the past but difficult to apply clinically include isoelectric focusing and two-dimensional gel electrophoresis.
[b] Cellular assays are used to identify HLA types and to measure the level of T-cell reactivity to HLA differences between two individuals. Chapter 138, this volume, will cover the latter in more detail.
[c] Single sample.

HLA-DPB1 gene, DQB1*0304 is an allele of the HLA-DQB1 gene, and B*2701 is an allele of the HLA-B gene. The first two numbers in the numerical designation of each allele are based on similarity to other alleles and sometimes on the serologic type of the resultant protein molecule. For example, the HLA-A molecule expressed by the A*02010101 allele bears the A2 serological specificity defining the HLA-A2 molecule (or antigen). The A*0226 allele has a DNA sequence similar to those of alleles specifying molecules bearing the A2 serological specificity; however, the HLA-A molecule specified by A*0226 has not been characterized using serology and so no information is available on its serologic specificity (25). The second example illustrates an allele whose name is based on its similarity to other alleles, in this case, similarity to A*02010101, A*0202, A*0203, and so forth. New alleles which appear significantly different in nucleotide sequence from previously described alleles may receive a unique WHO assignment for the first two digits of their names. Thus, B*8101, whose product was frequently serologically typed as B7, received a unique designation setting it apart from the B*07 allele family (5). The third and fourth digits in an allele designation refer to the order in which the allele was discovered. For example, DRB1*030101 was the first DRB1*03 allele to be discovered and DRB1*030201 was the second.

Some combinations of alleles share the first four digits of a six-digit designation (e.g., DRB1*110101 and DRB1*110102). The digits indicate that the two alleles differ in DNA sequence but that the HLA proteins specified by the two alleles do not differ (i.e., they differ by silent or synonymous substitutions). Some combinations of alleles are identified by eight-digit designations (e.g., DRB4*01030101 and DRB4*01030102). These alleles differ in DNA sequence only outside of their protein-encoding sequences. In some cases, these differences may affect the expression of the alleles. In the case of DRB4*0103102, the allele is not expressed due to a defect in an mRNA splice site. The addition of an "N" indicates the presence of an allele which is not expressed as a normal HLA protein at the cell surface . The N may not always be included but is implied (i.e., DRB4*01030102N = DRB4*01030102). Other letters indicate HLA products that might be secreted (B*44020102S) or expressed at a low level (A*24020102L).

Different HLA alleles defined by DNA typing can specify HLA proteins which are indistinguishable by methods based on protein identification, such as serology (25). For example, an individual carrying the B*070201 allele would be found to have the same serologic type (B7) as an individual carrying the B*0705 allele. Because serologic reagents specific enough to define this subdivision (or "split") are not available, serology cannot distinguish between the two proteins specified by the two alleles B*070201 and B*0705. There are many other examples of alleles defined using DNA typing which cannot be individually identified using protein-based typing methods.

Resolution of Molecular Typing Protocols

Based upon the level of information needed, the DNA-based strategy may focus just on regions of exons 2 and/or 3 that are highly polymorphic or the strategy may also include the evaluation of additional, less common polymorphisms located within rather conserved regions of these exons to obtain a greater level of DNA sequence information (resolution). A multistep approach is often used to identify HLA alleles by DNA-based typing. For this reason, HLA assignments (i.e., types) defined by DNA-based typing may be reported at different levels of resolution: low-resolution (or generic or serologic)-level DNA-based typing produces a result which is similar in appearance and detail to a serologic type. For example, a DNA-defined type, DRB1*04, is the approximate equivalent of the serologic type DR4. At this level of resolution, it is not possible to determine without further testing which of the over fifty DRB1*04 alleles described in the current WHO nomenclature report (e.g., DRB1*0401, DRB1*0402, and DRB1*0403, etc.) is carried by the individual being tested. Intermediate-resolution-level DNA-based typing may narrow down the choices by listing several different possibilities for the type carried by an individual, for example, DRB1*0404 and DRB1*0410. Due to the complexity of the typing system and the frequent need to enter typing information into a database, codes for multiple allele alternatives are sometimes used to express these various possibilities for the types carried by an individual. For example, the possibility DRB1*0404 or DRB1*0410 is expressed as DRB1*04HT in the National Marrow Donor Program database, where HT indicates the 04 or 10 allele combination (codes are listed at http://www.nmdpresearch.org). The letter codes are used to help hematopoietic stem cell transplantation centers identify the most closely matched individuals from a file of more than eight million volunteer donors (9). Additional DNA-based typing is then performed to find the closest match. Allele level resolution DNA-based typing identifies the specific allele carried by an individual (e.g., DRB1*0410).

One caution in interpreting DNA-based typing results is that a type is often defined by a pattern of reactivity of a panel of reagents. DNA sequence differences lying outside of the regions of the gene tested will not be detected (7). Thus, the assignment of a particular type, e.g., DRB1*0410, actually means that the pattern of reagent reactivity is consistent with that particular allele and that only DRB1*0410 is known to exhibit that pattern of reactivity at the time that the typing is carried out. If another allele exists with that same pattern and that second allele has not yet been characterized at the time of the typing, that allele will be missed. In addition, since some typing strategies analyze a mixture of two alleles at a locus, the polymorphisms detected by the typing reagents may be shared by two or more allele combinations. These "ambiguous" combinations are listed on the HLA nomenclature website (http://www.anthonynolan.org.uk/HIG/index.html).

The level of resolution obtained by DNA-typing methods is controlled by the choice of typing protocols. In the widely used sequence-specific priming (SSP) and sequence-specific oligonucleotide probe hybridization (SSOPH) protocols, the level of resolution is controlled by the number of oligonucleotide primers and/or probes used in the assay. This number may depend on the purpose of the typing, the time available for carrying out the typing, the cost of the typing, and the expertise of the laboratory. For example, typing of a cadaveric kidney donor requires results to be obtained in 3 to 6 h. Most DNA-based typing methods can produce a typing result within this time frame; however, the level of resolution obtained in that time will be limited. In the case of solid-organ transplantation, low- to intermediate-resolution assays satisfy the National Organ Procurement and Transplantation Network requirements for antigen level matching.

In the design of an unrelated marrow donor registry, like the one developed by the National Marrow Donor Program, the resolution of donor HLA typing is determined by balancing the need for accurate, cost-effective, high-volume HLA typing in order to provide a sufficiently large registry of HLA types and the desire to provide the maximum HLA information possible to assist a transplant center carrying out a patient search in identifying potentially HLA-matched donors. The low-intermediate level of resolution of HLA typing used for donor recruitment typing effectively allows transplant centers to identify a few potentially matched donors, who may then undergo more-extensive, higher-resolution HLA typing in order to identify the optimally matched unrelated donor for the patient.

It is also important to realize that the decisions made concerning the resolution of the HLA typing of the patient, which will be used to search a registry of unrelated hematopoietic stem cell donors, are also extremely important in the overall outcome of the search process. The results of numerous studies have shown that initially typing the patient at the highest resolution possible creates the best foundation for the search process. The transplant center is thus faced with similar challenges, primarily, the costs of high-resolution typing and the time required to perform this level of typing. Overall, this high-resolution-typing approach will allow an evaluation of the difficulty of the search, will increase the effectiveness of the donor selection process, and finally will allow better matching, which together will result in better transplant outcomes and fewer complications (8).

Correlation of DNA-Based and Serologic Typing

The nomenclature used to assign DNA-based HLA types is based on that used in serology; however, there are many examples in which the assignments applied to an allele and to its product appear to differ from each other. These differences are often the result of the complex nature of serologic testing and the nomenclature system used to assign allele names. A more detailed discussion of this topic has been published previously (25). The National Organ Procurement and Transplantation Network, which is operated under contract by the United Network for Organ Sharing, maintains a list of serology equivalents for molecular types for solid-organ transplantation. The United Network for Organ Sharing list for both alleles and serologic splits can be found at http://www.unos.org/PoliciesandBylaws/policies/ in Policy 3A.

TECHNOLOGY AND INSTRUMENTATION

One common method of DNA-based typing utilizes a panel of sequence-specific oligonucleotide primers in multiple PCRs to define HLA alleles by the presence or absence of amplification. At least one member of each primer pair is designed to bind to a specific polymorphic sequence in the HLA gene being characterized. A second common method of typing utilizes PCR to amplify all alleles at a specific HLA locus. The amplified DNA is denatured and hybridized to a panel of synthetic oligonucleotide probes to identify HLA alleles. This method of typing is termed SSOPH. Comparison of the polymorphic sequences present and absent as detected by the reagents with the sequences of known alleles is used to identify the alleles that might be present (Fig. 1). Still other DNA-based methods in more

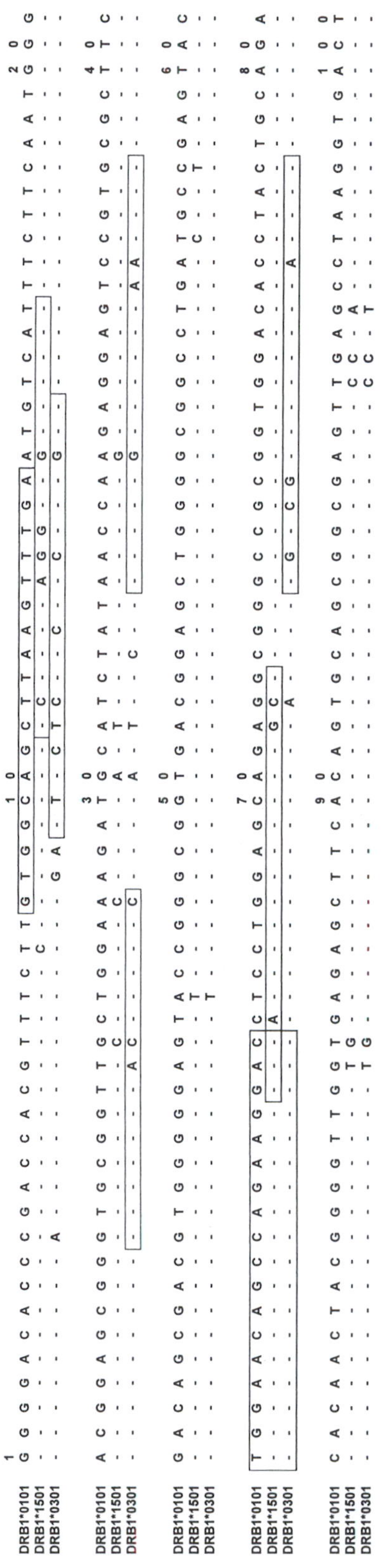

FIGURE 1 DRB1 nucleotide sequences from a few DRB1 alleles. Dashes indicate identity with the sequence of DRB1*0101. The numbers indicate the codons. Only part of the sequence of the DRB1 gene is shown; the polymorphic exon 2 includes codons 5 through 95. Probes identifying polymorphic sequences distinguishing these alleles are boxed.

limited use rely on electrophoresis of DNA strands (heteroduplex analysis, reference strand-mediated conformational analysis [RSCA], and sequence-specific conformational polymorphism) or DNA sequencing (sequence-based typing [SBT]) to identify HLA alleles. The following sections describe the many commercial kits used for DNA preparation and HLA typing and provide a protocol for DNA sequencing. References describing all DNA-based typing methods are found in Tables 2 through 5.

QA AND QC

Extensive guidelines for quality control (QC) and quality assurance (QA) related to all stages of DNA-based HLA testing are described in the American Society for Histocompatibility and Immunogenetics (ASHI) standards for HLA testing (http://www.ashi-hla.org/) and in the ASHI *Laboratory Manual* (10). ASHI, the European Federation for Immunogenetics, and other organizations have standards for DNA-based HLA typing and an accreditation process. Additional ASHI guidelines apply for laboratories performing high-volume (>50,000 tests per year) HLA testing. These include duplicate typing of a subset of the samples tested, use of enhanced sample-tracking mechanisms, and implementation of QC measures for automated procedures and equipment. Proficiency testing samples can be obtained from the College of American Pathologists, the UCLA International Cell Exchange, the Southeast Organ Procurement Foundation, and ASHI.

TEST VALIDATION

HLA typing assays are validated by testing a panel of cells with known HLA alleles. DNA from HLA-characterized reference cells is usually derived from Epstein-Barr virus-transformed B lymphoblastoid cell lines. Such reference cells are available from cell repositories (e.g., the 13th International Histocompatibility Workshop repository [http://www.ihwg.org] and the National Marrow Donor Program [http://www.nmdpresearch.org]). The panel should be large enough to include cells carrying alleles commonly found in the population undergoing routine testing. Typing should also include DNA prepared from sample types (e.g., whole blood) which will be tested in the laboratory. These samples might be tested through parallel testing with a well-established HLA typing laboratory.

COST ASSESSMENT

HLA typing is used primarily to identify histocompatible organ and hematopoietic stem cell donors (6, 20), but it is also used for identification of those at risk for HLA-associated autoimmune diseases (17), for identification of potential responders to peptide-based vaccines (26), and for paternity testing. All of the HLA testing assays described herein require DNA preparation and PCR amplification. The choice of a testing method (i.e., SSP versus SSOPH versus RSCA versus SBT) and selection of a commercial kit will depend on (i) the number of samples to be typed; (ii) the expertise of the laboratory; (iii) the speed, efficiency, cost, and reliability of the method or kit; (iv) the HLA loci to be identified and the resolution required at each locus; and (v) the QA and QC required.

INTERPRETATION

Interpretation of the assays should yield HLA assignments indicating the presence of one or two alleles at a locus for

TABLE 2 References[a] providing primer strategies (SSP) for determining HLA types

HLA-A, -B, and -C

Welsh, K., and M. Bunce. 1999. Molecular typing for the MHC with PCR-SSP. *Rev. Immunogenet.* **1:**157–176.

Bunce, M., C. M. O'Neill, M. C. Barnardo, P. Krausa, M. J. Browning, P. J. Morris, and K. I. Welsh. 1995. Phototyping: comprehensive DNA typing for HLA-A, B, C, DRB1, DRB3, DRB4, DRB5 and DQB1 by PCR with 144 primer mixes utilizing sequence-specific primers (PCR-SSP). *Tissue Antigens* **46:**355–367.

Krausa, P., M. Brywka, D. Savage, K. M. Hui, M. Bunce, J. L. Ngai, D. L. Teo, Y. W. Ong, D. Barouch, C. E. Allsop, et al. 1995. Genetic polymorphism within HLA-A*02: significant allelic variation revealed in different populations. *Tissue Antigens* **45:**223–231.

HLA-DR, -DQ, and -DP

Olerup, O., and H. Zetterquist. 1992. HLA-DR typing by PCR amplification with sequence specific primers (PCR-SSP) in 2 hours: an alternative to serological DR typing in clincial practice including donor-recipient matching in cadaveric transplantations. *Tissue Antigens* **39:**225–235.

Olerup, O., and H. Zetterquist. 1991. HLA-DRB1*01 subtyping by allele-specific PCR amlification: A sensitve, specific and rapid technique. *Tissue Antigens* **37:**197–204.

Zetterquist, H., and O. Olerup. 1992. Identification of the HLA-DRB1*04, -DRB1*07, and -DRB1*09 alleles by PCR amplification with sequence-specific primers (PCR-SSP) in 2 hours. *Hum. Immunol.* **34:**64–74.

Bunce, M., C. J. Taylor, and K. I. Welsh. 1993. Rapid HLA-DQB typing by eight polymerase chain reaction amplifications with sequence-specific primers (PCR-SSP). *Hum. Immunol.* **37:**201–206.

Olerup, O., A. Aldener, and A. Fogdell. 1993. HLA-DQB1 and -DQA1 typing by PCR amplification with sequence-specific primers (PCR-SSP) in 2 hours. *Tissue Antigens* **41:**119–134.

[a]This list is not comprehensive.

each cell. If assays include more than one reagent to define an HLA type, the results must be consistent. Software for data interpretation should be used because of the complexity of the HLA system and should be updated to include the most recently described HLA alleles. The most current and accurate information can be obtained from the HLA nomenclature website (http://www.ebi.ac.uk/imgt/hla/download.html) (22). If a single allele is observed at a locus (i.e., the sample appears to be homozygous for the gene), the amplification results should be reviewed for potential failure to amplify one of the alleles. HLA assignments should be reviewed by an expert to evaluate the frequency of the assigned alleles in the population tested and common associations between alleles at several loci to determine if the result makes sense based on knowledge of the HLA system. All alternative assignments must be listed on the assay report form.

The continuous discovery of new alleles at every HLA locus requires continual updates of the typing strategy and the addition of new reagents or the use of additional assays to achieve the desired resolution. Typing systems may yield ambiguous typing results for certain allele combinations (Fig. 2). In these situations, the typing system does not distinguish among alternative allele combinations; for example, the same DNA sequence of a mixture of two alleles may be interpreted as DRB1*1101, DRB1*1301, or DRB1*1102, and DRB1*1109. In this case, the alternative allele combinations carry the same polymorphisms but the *cis* and *trans* associations of the polymorphic residues differ (i.e., which polymorphisms are located on one copy of chromosome 6 [*cis* association] and which polymorphisms are located on different copies of chromosome 6 [*trans* association]). To resolve this issue, an amplification strategy aimed at amplifying a single allele of the heterozygote for sequencing is required. Alternative typing strategies such as RSCA can also be applied to resolve the typing results to a single combination of two alleles. In some cases, the polymorphism that distinguishes two or more alleles lies outside of the commonly tested exons (e.g., the distinction between A*0101 and A*0104N lies outside of exons 2 and 3, in exon 4). A list of the alleles with these types of differences is provided on the WHO HLA nomenclature website (http://anthonynolan.org/uk/HIG/index.html).

PREPARATION OF DNA

Molecular biology-based HLA typing methods utilize DNA as a starting material. DNA can be prepared from any source of nucleated cells, although whole blood is the usual source of samples. Further isolation of the buffy coat component of blood containing leukocytes and platelets without heme-containing red blood cells yields more DNA at a higher concentration and removes a PCR inhibitor (heme). Protocols for DNA extraction begin with lysis of cells by using detergents and release of DNA from associated proteins. DNA is isolated in one of several ways. DNA can be precipitated from the solution with ethanol, and the dry pellet can be dissolved with sterile water. Alternatively, the DNA can be centrifuged through a solid-phase column that binds the DNA and the DNA is eluted in a subsequent step with a suitable buffer. Another purification protocol involves the addition of solid-phase modified magnetic particles to capture the DNA. The use of magnetic particles allows the use of manual or robotic manipulation based on magnetic separation, filtration, or purification.

Selection of a DNA preparation method or kit should depend on (i) the type of specimen (e.g., whole blood, blood spotted onto filter paper cards, and swabs of epithelial cells) that is regularly processed in the laboratory; (ii) the ability to obtain PCR-amplifiable DNA from the specimen; (iii) the speed, efficiency, and cost of the method; (iv) the number of samples that need to be processed; and (v) the requirement for long-term storage of DNA.

Sample Requirements

Whole blood treated with acid citrate dextrose is the recommended sample. Blood drawn in anticoagulants containing heparin is not recommended since heparin can interfere with the subsequent gene amplification step. Other sample sources include clotted whole blood, buffy coat cells, frozen white blood cell pellets, cryopreserved lymphocytes, lymphoblastoid cell lines, and blood dried on specially treated paper cards. For the latter, IsoCode cards (Schleicher & Schuell Bioscience, Keene, N.H.), FTA cards (Whatman Inc., Clifton, N.J.), Generation capture cards (Gentra

TABLE 3 References[a] providing probe strategies (SSOPH) for determining HLA types

HLA-A, -B, and -C

Oh, S. H., K. Fleischhauer, and S. Y. Yang. 1993. Isoelectric focusing subtypes of HLA-A can be defined by oligonucleotide typing. *Tissue Antigens* **41**:135–142.

Allen, M., L. Liu, and U. Gyllensten. 1994. A comprehensive polymerase chain reaction-oligonucleotide typing system for the HLA class I A locus. *Hum. Immunol.* **40**:25–32.

Bugawan, T. L., R. Apple, and H. A. Erlich. 1994. A method for typing polymorphism at the HLA-A locus using PCR amplification and immobilized oligonucleotide probes. *Tissue Antigens* **44**:137–147.

Cao, K., M. Chopek, and M. A. Fernandez-Vina. 1999. High and intermediate resolution DNA typing systems for Class I HLA-A, -B, -C genes by hybridization with sequence specific oligonucleotide probes (SSOP). *Rev. Immunogenet.* **1**:177–208.

Williams, F., H. Mawhinney, and D. Middleton. 1997. Application of an HLA-B PCR-SSOP typing method to a bone marrow donor registry. *Bone Marrow Transplant.* **19**:205–208.

Kennedy, L. J., K. V. Poulton, P. A. Dyer, W. E. R. Ollier, and W. Thomson. 1995. Definition of HLA-C alleles using sequence-specific oligonucleotide probes (PCR-SSOP). *Tissue Antigens* **46**:187–195.

Levine, J. E., and S. Y. Yang. 1994. SSOP typing of the Tenth International Histocompatibility Workshop reference cell lines for HLA-C alleles. *Tissue Antigens* **44**:174–183.

HLA-DR, -DQ, and -DP

Kimura, A., R. P. Dong, H. Harada, and T. Sasazuki. 1992. DNA typing of HLA class II genes in B-lymphoblastoid cell lines homozygous for HLA. *Tissue Antigens* **40**:5–12.

Gao, X., J. R. Moraes, S. Miller, and P. Stastny. 1991. DNA typing for class II HLA antigens with allele-specific or group-specific amplification. V. Typing for subsets of HLA-DR1 and DR'Br'. *Hum. Immunol.* **30**:147–154.

Moraes, M. E., M. Fernandez-Viña, and P. Stastny. 1991. DNA typing for class II HLA antigens with allele-specific or group-specific amplification. IV. Typing for alleles of the HLA-DR2 group. *Hum. Immunol.* **31**:139–144.

Shaffer, A. L., J. A. Falk-Wade, V. Tortorelli, A. Cigan, C. Carter, K. Hassan, and C. K. Hurley. 1992. HLA-DRw52-associated DRB1 alleles: identification using polymerase chain reaction-amplified DNA, sequence-specific oligonucleotide probes, and a chemiluminescent detection system. *Tissue Antigens* **39**:84–90.

Gao, X., M. Fernandez-Vina, W. Shumway, and P. Stastny. 1990. DNA typing for class II HLA antigens with allele-specific or group-specific amplification: typing for subsets of HLA-DR4. *Hum. Immunol.* **27**:40–50.

Molkentin, J., J. Gorski, and L. A. Baxter-Lowe. 1991. Detection of 14 HLA-DQB1 alleles by oligotyping. *Hum. Immunol.* **31**:114–122.

Bugawan, T., and H. A. Erlich. 1991. Rapid typing of HLA-DQB1 DNA polymorphism using nonradioactive oligonucleotide probes and amplified DNA. *Immunogenetics* **33**:163–170.

Bugawan, T. L., A. B. Begovich, and H. A. Erlich. 1990. Rapid HLA-DPB typing using enzymatically amplified DNA and nonradioactive sequence-specific oligonucleotide probes. *Immunogenetics* **32**:231–241.

Fernandez-Vina, M., M. E. Moraes, and P. Stastny. 1991. DNA typing for class II HLA antigens with allele-specific or group-specific amplification. III. Typing for 24 alleles of HLA-DP. *Hum. Immunol.* **30**:60–68.

[a]This list is not comprehensive.

Systems Inc., Minneapolis, Minn.) or comparable cards are spotted with untreated or anticoagulated blood. The amount of specimen required and the yield depend on the isolation method and kit. In general, 200 μl to 1 ml of whole blood will yield 4 to 12 μg of DNA, and 200 μl of buffy coat will yield about 25 to 50 μg of DNA. Other types of cells, such as epithelial cells isolated with a swab and cells in blood spots on filter paper, can be utilized with modifications to the

TABLE 4 References[a] for alternate methods of DNA-based testing

PCR-restriction fragment length polymorphism

Maeda, M., N. Uryu, N. Murayama, H. Ishii, M. Ota, K. Tsuji, and H. Inoko. 1990. A simple and rapid method for HLA-DP genotyping by digestion of PCR-amplified DNA with allele-specific restriction endonucleases. *Hum. Immunol.* **27**:111–121.

Ota, M., T. Seki, H. Fukushima, K. Tsuji, and H. Inoko. 1992. HLA-DRB1 genotyping by modified PCR-RFLP method combined with group-specific primers. *Tissue Antigens* **39**:187–202.

Sequence-specific conformational polymorphism

Lo, Y. M. D., P. Patel, W. Z. Mehal, K. A Fleming, J. I. Bell, and J. S. Wainscoat. 1992. Analysis of complex genetic systems by ARMS-SSCP: application to HLA genotyping. *Nucleic Acids Res.* **20**:1005–1009.

Hoshino, S., A. Kimura, Y. Fukuda, K. Dohi, and T. Sasazuki. 1992. Polymerase chain reaction-single-strand conformation polymorphism analysis of polymorphism in DPA1 and DPB1 genes: a simple, economical, and rapid method for histocompatibility testing. *Hum. Immunol.* **33**:98–107.

Heteroduplex

Sorrentino, R., I. Cascino, and R. Tosi. 1992. Subgrouping of DR4 alleles by DNA heteroduplex analysis. *Hum. Immunol.* **33**:18–23.

Summers, C., F. Morling, M. Taylor, J. L. Yin, and R. Stevens. 1994. Donor-recipient HLA class I bone marrow transplant matching by multilocus heteroduplex analysis. *Transplantation* **58**:628–629.

Arguello, J. R., and J. A. Madrigal. 1999. HLA typing by reference strand mediated conformation analysis (RSCA). *Rev. Immunogenet.* **1**:209–219.

Turner, D., S. Akpe, J. Brown, C. Brown, A. McWhinnie, A. Madrigal, and C. Navarrete. 2001. HLA-B typing by reference strand mediated conformation analysis using a capillary-based semiautomated genetic analyzer. *Hum. Immunol.* **62**:414–418.

[a]This list is not comprehensive.

TABLE 5 References[a] on direct DNA sequencing (SBT)

Petersdorf, E. W., and J. A. Hansen. 1995. A comprehensive approach for typing the alleles of the HLA-B locus by automated sequencing. *Tissue Antigens* **46**:73–85.

McGinnis, M. D., M. P. Conrad, A. G. M. Bouwens, M. G. J. Tilanus, and M. N. Kronick. 1995. Automated, solid-phase sequencing of DRB region genes using T7 sequencing chemistry and dye-labeled primers. *Tissue Antigens* **46**:173–179.

Versluis, L. F., E. Rozemuller, S. Tonks, S. G. E. Marsh, A. G. M. Bouwens, J. G. Bodmer, and M. G. J. Tilanus. 1993. High-resolution HLA-DPB typing based upon computerized analysis of data obtained by fluorescent sequencing of the amplified polymorphic exon 2. *Hum. Immunol.* **38**:277–283.

Scheltinga, S. A., L. A. Johnston-Dow, C. B. White, A. W. Van der Zwan, J. E. Bakema, E. H. Rozemuller, J. G. Van den Tweel, M. N. Kronick, and M. G. J. Tilanus. 1997. A generic sequencing based typing approach for the identification of HLA-A diversity. *Hum. Immunol.* **57**:120–128.

Versluis, L. F., E. H. Rozemuller, K. Duran, and M. G. Tilanus. 1995. Ambiguous DPB1 allele combinations resolved by direct sequencing of selectively amplified alleles. *Tissue Antigens* **46**:345–349.

[a]This list is not comprehensive.

procedure (10) or with procedures especially designed for the sample type (manufacturers' protocols).

Materials and Reagents

A number of methods and commercial kits are available for the preparation of DNA (Table 6). Reagents required are listed in the manufacturer's protocol for each kit. Water for all protocols is distilled and deionized (ddH$_2$O) unless otherwise specified.

Equipment and Instrumentation

Most of the procedures are carried out in a laminar flow hood. Dedicated pipettors, sterile pipette tips with an aerosol barrier, and sterile tubes or plates are used. Equipment required for all protocols includes a microcentrifuge capable of $12,000 \times g$, a Vortex mixer, an adjustable water bath or heat block that reaches 65 to 70°C, and an ice bucket or benchtop cooler. For work in the laboratory, a suitable lab coat, disposable gloves, and protective goggles should be worn.

DNA Preparation Procedure

All procedures are carried out in a laminar flow hood by using an aseptic technique. Precautions should be taken in

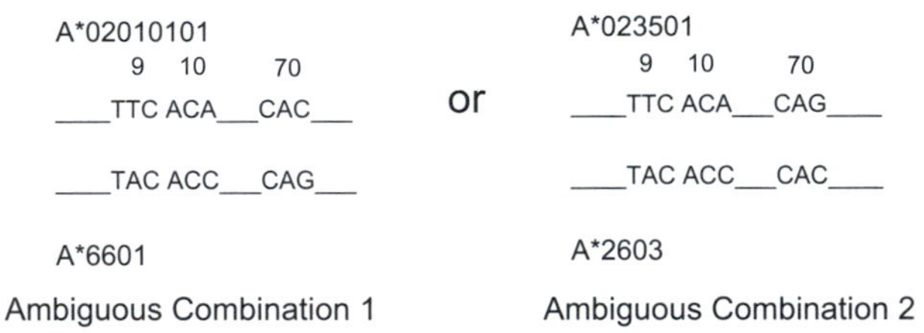

A*02010101
  9 10   70
____TTC ACA___CAC___

____TAC ACC___CAG___

A*6601

Ambiguous Combination 1

or

A*023501
  9 10   70
____TTC ACA___CAG____

____TAC ACC___CAC____

A*2603

Ambiguous Combination 2

FIGURE 2 Example of two heterozygous allele combinations that cannot be distinguished from one another when both HLA-A alleles are characterized as a heterozygous mixture (i.e., ambiguous combinations). Some of the polymorphic nucleotides that distinguish the alleles and their *cis* and *trans* associations are diagrammed in the figure. The heterozygous combination A*02010101 and A*6601 (ambiguous combination 1) cannot be distinguished from the alternative, A*023501 and A*2603 (ambiguous combination 2), unless a single allele is isolated and characterized. Identification of the alleles present relies on the laboratory's ability to link the first polymorphic sequence (located at codons 9-10, TTC ACA) to one of the two alternative second polymorphisms (CAC or CAG at codon 70). If CAC is in *cis* (i.e., found on the same DNA strand) with TTC ACA, then the first ambiguous combination is present.

working with potentially infectious human material. Instructions for each kit are provided by the manufacturer. If purified DNA is to be stored up to 24 h, storage at 2 to 8°C is recommended. For storage for longer than 24 h, the DNA should be dissolved in buffer (10 mM TrisCl, 0.5 mM EDTA [pH 9.0]) and stored in aliquots at −70°C. Since DNA degrades, only the amount of DNA required for the assay should be prepared at any one time. If the Tris-EDTA buffer is not compatible with subsequent applications, DNA may be dissolved in water at pH 7.0. Water with an acid pH may result in DNA degradation.

The work area should be separate from work areas exposed to PCR-amplified DNA. Appropriate precautions must be taken to avoid contamination of samples with previously amplified DNA. The dedication of an isolated work area with a laminar flow hood and dedicated equipment and reagents is recommended. For laboratories doing large-volume testing, a dedicated room with restricted access is recommended.

If whole-blood samples are not processed immediately, it is recommended that they be held at room temperature in the original sterile container. If processing is delayed, it is recommended that the samples be distributed into 0.5- to 1-ml aliquots and frozen at −70°C. Blood samples older than 1 week (stored at 4°C) may produce poor yields and/or poor-quality DNA. Blood can be frozen for at least 1 year to provide a long-term supply of DNA. An advantage of using blood spotted onto cards is the long-term stability of the sample and the ease of storage and shipping. A disadvantage, depending on the type of card, is that the extraction of DNA may be more difficult than that from a fresh blood sample.

Yield is dependent on the white cell count of the sample. For samples with known low counts (<3,000 white blood cells/mm^3), the buffy coat should be isolated. When the sample yields a small cell pellet or a small amount of DNA, amplification may fail due to insufficient DNA. If a cell pellet is brown or green, the PCR failure rate is high, likely due to the contamination with hemoglobin and/or poor proteolytic digestion. If a DNA pellet is isolated, the pellet should not be overdried as it becomes difficult to dissolve. Unbuffered DNA in storage is subject to degradation resulting from low pH as well as from the presence of nucleases. DNA preparation protocols differ in the purity of the prepared DNA and therefore in its stability under long-term storage.

QA and QC

The quality of the DNA is monitored by its ability to be amplified in the PCR as judged by the appearance of an ethidium bromide-stained band of amplified DNA of appropriate size

TABLE 6 Kits for the isolation of DNA

Company, location	Name of kit(s)	Specimen(s) required	Basic process or system
Qiagen, Valencia, Calif.	QIAmp DNA MINI kit	Whole blood, plasma, serum, buffy coat, body fluids, lymphocytes, tissues, swabs, dried blood spots, or cultured cells	Spin column
Pel-Freez Clinical Systems, LLC, Brown Deer, Wis.	DNA isolation kit	Whole blood or buffy coat	DNA precipitation
Gentra, Minneapolis, Minn.	Puregene; GENERATION capture cards	Whole blood or bone marrow; dried blood spots on cards	Elution of DNA or amplification from the immobilized DNA
Eppendorf, Hamburg, Germany	Perfect gDNA blood mini kit	Whole blood or buffy coat	Spin column
Promega, Madison, Wis.	MagneSil blood genomic max yield system	Whole blood or buccal swabs	Paramagnetic particles
	Ready Amp genomic DNA purification system; Wizard SV genomic DNA purification	Whole blood or blood stains; cultured cells or tissues	Resin-based system; spin column
AutoGEN, Holliston, Mass.	AutoGenprep 965 (high-throughput DNA extraction in a 96-well format [automated])	Whole blood	DNA precipitation
Omega, Doraville, Ga.	ENZA blood DNA kit	Whole blood, buffy coat, or specimens on filter paper	HiBind spin column

on an agarose gel. The purity of DNA can also be monitored by taking the ratio of the absorbance at the 260-nm wavelength (measuring primarily DNA) to that at the 280-nm wavelength (measuring protein) by using a spectrophotometer. Values in the range of 1.7 to 1.9 are optimal.

AMPLIFICATION OF HLA GENES

PCR is used to generate a large number of copies of an HLA gene for rapid detection of HLA types. PCR uses sequence-specific primer pairs (a 5' [sense] primer and a 3' [antisense] primer) and *Taq* polymerase to specifically amplify selected segments of DNA. By using two oligonucleotide primers that hybridize to opposite DNA strands and that flank the region of interest in the target DNA, a specific DNA sequence is enzymatically synthesized. If the protocol is followed by further analysis of the amplicon by hybridization, the amplification also serves to reduce nonspecific hybridization of oligonucleotide probes.

Primers are designed to amplify specifically all alleles at a locus or a subset of alleles. For class I typing, primers usually flank the most polymorphic exons, 2 and 3. For class II typing, primers usually flank polymorphic exon 2. The design of primers is based on sequence alignments of the HLA alleles published and available on the Internet (http://www.anthonynolan.org.uk/HIG/index.html) (22). When primers are designed to selectively amplify a group of alleles, the region of polymorphism used to discriminate alleles is positioned at the 3' end of the oligonucleotide primer to eliminate the amplification of mismatched alleles. The length and sequence of the oligonucleotide primer will determine the specificity and hybridization conditions in the PCR. Most HLA typing utilizes oligonucleotide primers that are approximately 21 nucleotides in length.

Genomic DNA is denatured at 94 to 96°C. Synthetic oligonucleotide primers anneal to denatured DNA at temperatures selected to provide specific amplification.

Taq polymerase adds nucleotides onto the primers copying the DNA strands at 72°C. Repetition of the cycle of denaturation, annealing, and extension generates billions of copies of the selected DNA with termini defined by the 5' ends of the primers. DNA can be labeled during amplification when the PCR is conducted using primers which are labeled (e.g., with biotin). Amplified DNA is detected by staining with ethidium bromide following electrophoresis on an agarose gel. Alternatively, the quantification of PCR products can be performed with a fluorescent DNA dye, PicoGreen, that is intercalated into double-stranded DNA but does not bind to single-stranded DNA or RNA.

Sample Requirements

DNA is prepared as described above. Usually, 2 to 10 µl of DNA is required for each 20- to 100-µl PCR mixture (200 to 500 ng of DNA/reaction).

Materials and Reagents

The key materials and reagents needed include PCR tubes or Microamp trays (ISC BioExpress, Kaysville, Utah), PCR buffer, MgCl$_2$, primers, deoxynucleoside triphosphates (dNTPs), and *Taq* polymerase. The PCR buffer often is provided with the enzyme. Commercial HLA typing kits are available which include reagents for amplification of genomic DNA. PicoGreen can be purchased from Molecular Probes, Inc., Eugene, Oreg.

Equipment and Instrumentation

A laminar flow hood or pre-PCR room which is isolated from the post-PCR area, a thermal cycler, a 37°C heat block, a Vortex mixer, and a microcentrifuge are needed.

Amplification Procedure

The amplification reaction mixture is prepared in a laminar flow hood or pre-PCR room by using an aseptic technique. Amplification and gel electrophoresis are carried out in an area separate from the preamplification area.

Briefly, the PCR reaction mix (without genomic DNA) is prepared according to manufacturers' recommendations, the mix is aliquoted into PCR tubes, and then DNA is added into each tube. Alternatively, DNA may be aliquoted into PCR tubes first and then PCR mix added. Precautions should be used when pipetting to avoid contamination. The manufacturer's instructions should be followed if a commercial kit is used. The amplified DNA can be stored at 4°C for a brief period of time. Amplification is detected by gel electrophoresis or by PicoGreen staining (Invitrogen, Carlsbad, Calif., vendor protocol).

The sample identification should be carefully checked to avoid sample switches. When a Microamp tray is used, precautions should be taken to label the tray orientation to avoid sample switches. Care must be taken to avoid contamination of samples and reagents with amplified DNA. Precautions include (i) physical separation of preamplification steps from amplification and postamplification steps, (ii) aliquoting of reagents so that an aliquot will be used up in a single assay, (iii) limitation of the number of PCR cycles used to amplify an HLA gene (<35 cycles), and (iv) use of wipe tests to monitor contamination of laboratory benches and equipment. Care must be taken in handling and storage of the DNA polymerase to avoid loss of activity and to avoid inaccuracies in measurement of the enzyme. Because DNA settles at the bottom of the tube, care must be taken to shake the tube to thoroughly mix the DNA with the enzyme. The PCR mix may evaporate during amplification if the tube is not tightly sealed. Nonspecific amplification or amplification failure may result from suboptimal amplification conditions. These may include an inadequate (in amount or purity) DNA template, incorrect primer concentration, suboptimal magnesium concentration, an annealing temperature that results in nonspecific amplification (temperature is too low) or no amplification (temperature is too high), suboptimal annealing and extension times, inadequate denaturation of the template, or mismatches of the primer to the DNA template. The thermal cycler should be carefully monitored to ensure correct temperature cycling. Oligonucleotides used as primers should be aliquoted into small volumes for storage since multiple freeze-thaw cycles can result in loss of primer specificity.

QA and QC

Controls to monitor and detect contamination with amplified DNA should be included in the assay. These should include tubes which contain all of the PCR reagents except DNA which are carried through the amplification cycles and analyzed by gel electrophoresis or DNA quantification and probe hybridization. Nonspecific amplification can be monitored by the use of reference DNA containing alleles which should be amplified or not amplified by specific primer sets. Equipment, such as thermal cyclers, must be calibrated periodically.

Interpretation

A discrete band of the expected size should be visible under UV light following gel electrophoresis. Additional bands indicate nonspecific amplification. The faster-migrating primers will also stain with ethidium bromide and should not be confused with the amplified DNA. When the PicoGreen method is used, an acceptable reading range should be met for successful amplification and the negative control should be below the preset acceptable reading.

AMPLIFICATION OF HLA GENES FOR HLA TYPING—SSP

In some cases, the goal of the PCR is to define which alleles might be carried by an individual by the presence or absence of amplification (termed SSP) (Table 2). A panel of primer pairs, each amplifying a subset of alleles, is used to narrow down the possible HLA alleles carried by an individual. Many of the concepts are described above under "Amplification of HLA Genes."

Materials and Reagents

A number of commercial kits are available for HLA typing by SSP (Table 7).

QA and QC

Amplification failure is a particular concern in utilizing the SSP typing approach, which requires multiple PCR primer pairs and relies on positive or negative amplification to identify HLA alleles. Each tube should contain a second set of primers which amplify a gene segment that is present in all

TABLE 7 Examples of sequence-specific primer typing kits[a]

Vendor, location	Loci (resolution)	No. of samples
Dynal Biotech Inc., Brown Deer, Wis.	HLA-A, HLA-B, HLA-C, HLA-DR, HLA-DQ (low resolution)	20 tests/kit
Pel-Freez Clinical Systems, LLC, Brown Deer, Wis.	Class I (high resolution), class II (high resolution)	10–12 tests/kit
GenoVision Inc., West Chester, Pa.	HLA-A, HLA-B, HLA-C, HLA-DR, HLA-DQ	12–72 tests/kit
One Lambda Inc., Canoga Park, Calif.	HLA-A, HLA-B, HLA-C, HLA-DR (low and high resolution)	8–40 tests/kit
Bio-Synthesis Inc., Lewisville, Tex.	HLA-A, HLA-B, HLA-C, HLA-DR, HLA-DQ (low and high resolution)	25–48 tests/kit
Biotest Diagnostics Corp., Denville, N.J.	HLA-A, HLA-B, HLA-C, HLA-DR, HLA-DQ (low and high resolution)	12–24 tests/kit

[a]Information on procedures is available from the vendor websites.

DNA samples and that differs in size from the amplified HLA gene segment (19). The primer panel might also contain more than one primer pair to define an HLA type. Each panel of samples to be typed should include positive and negative reference DNA to detect contamination with previously amplified DNA, nonspecific amplification, and human errors. The laboratory should have a set of well-defined reference samples with known HLA alleles to validate the assay and to validate new lots of reagents, especially primers. It is recommended that the reference panel cover most of the polymorphisms that the primers detect.

Cost Assessment

This assay can be used at various levels of resolution depending on the purpose of the testing. SSP is able to obtain allele level resolution, although the number of primers required is large and new alleles might not be detected. SSP is difficult to use for large numbers of samples because of the number of thermocyclers required and the gel electrophoresis step. Use of other protocols besides electrophoresis to monitor amplification will aid in high-volume throughput.

Interpretation

A discrete band of the expected size should be visible under UV light following gel electrophoresis. The positive control band should also be visible, but it may be present in a lower quantity in tubes with positive amplification of HLA due to competition for reagents. Approaches for interpretation of SSP data have been described previously (2).

GEL ELECTROPHORESIS

DNA is negatively charged due to its phosphate composition; thus, amplified DNA will move toward the positively charged pole in an agarose gel matrix. The position of the migration is determined by the size of the DNA fragment; small fragments move faster than large fragments. The double-stranded DNA is visualized by staining with ethidium bromide. The mobility is assessed by using a commercially prepared set of DNA markers to determine the size of the amplicon.

Sample Requirement

3 to 5 μl of amplified PCR product. If large numbers of samples are being typed, only a subset (e.g., 10% of samples) needs to be evaluated by electrophoresis, and this evaluation should include amplified DNA from the positive and negative controls.

Materials and Reagents

Gel loading buffer (6×) made as a sterile solution but not autoclaved: 0.25% (wt/vol) bromophenol blue (Bio-Rad Laboratories, Hercules, Calif.; catalog no. 161-0404), 0.25% (wt/vol) xylene cyanol (Bio-Rad Laboratories; catalog no. 161-0423), and 15% (vol/vol) Ficoll (Sigma-Aldrich Co., St. Louis, Mo.; catalog no. F2637). Filter the buffer through a 0.2-μm-pore-size filter. Store at room temperature.

50× Tris-acetate-EDTA (TAE) gel buffer (autoclaved): 242 g of Tris base, 57.1 ml of glacial acetic acid, and 100 ml of 0.5 M EDTA. Bring the final volume to 1,000 ml with water. Adjust the solution to pH 8.0 with NaOH pellets. For 1× solution, add 10 ml of 50× TAE buffer to 490 ml of ddH$_2$O.

0.5 M EDTA, pH 8.0 (autoclaved and stored at room temperature): For 1,000 ml, dissolve 186.12 g of EDTA (372.24 g/mol) in ddH$_2$O and bring the volume to 700 ml. Adjust the pH to 8.0 with NaOH pellets. EDTA will dissolve when the correct pH has been obtained. Bring the final volume to 1,000 ml with ddH$_2$O.

Ethidium bromide (caution—this hazardous material is a carcinogen): Make as a sterile solution, 5 mg/ml in ddH$_2$O, but do not autoclave. Ethidium bromide can also be purchased as a concentrated solution (10 mg/ml; Bio-Rad Laboratories; catalog no. 161-0433).

Agarose (ultrapure; Gibco BRL, Life Technologies, Gaithersburg, Md.; catalog no. 15510-027)

Molecular weight DNA markers: 1-kb DNA ladder (Gibco BRL; catalog no. 156150-024)

Equipment and Instrumentation

- Heated stirring plate or microwave
- Horizontal agarose gel apparatus
- Power supply
- Short-wave UV box
- Camera

Gel Electrophoresis Procedure

1. Prepare agarose gel: 1.0% (wt/vol) agarose in 1× TAE buffer. Heat to boiling on a hot plate, stirring to dissolve agarose, or in a microwave for 1 to 2 min. When the solution is cool enough to touch, add 5 μl of 5-mg/ml ethidium bromide, swirl to mix, and pour into the gel electrophoresis apparatus. Place the comb (12 to 24 wells) into the gel. The percentage of agarose will be determined by the size of the DNA fragments analyzed (1.2% for analysis of the 300-bp DRB amplicon, 1.0% for the 800-bp class I amplicon). The amount of gel required will be determined by the choice of electrophoresis apparatus. Following solidification of the gel, fill the gel tank with 1× TAE buffer, submerging the gel in ~5 mm of buffer.

2. Add 1 μl of 6× gel loading buffer to 3 to 5 μl of amplified DNA.

3. Load samples and the molecular weight marker into the wells. The marker is diluted according to the manufacturer's instructions prior to loading.

4. Electrophorese the DNA to obtain clear separation of molecular weight ranges. Dye should separate towards the positive pole into two colors. For example, a 300-bp fragment is electrophoresed at 130 V for 30 min.

5. Photograph the gel with the short-wavelength UV-B 280- to 320-nm-wavelength transilluminator.

The dye should not be electrophoresed off the gel. DNA will not separate well with higher voltages or shorter running times. The DNA ladder could be degraded at higher voltage. The solidified gel containing ethidium bromide should be discarded in a solid biohazard waste container.

QA and QC

Markers with known molecular weights are used to measure the size of the DNA.

Cost Assessment

This procedure allows verification of amplification and determination of the size of the amplicon and uses inexpensive reagents. The quantitation of amplified DNA with the PicoGreen double-stranded DNA quantitation reagent (Molecular Probes, Inc.; catalog no. P-7581) can be used in place of gel electrophoresis. The PicoGreen double-stranded DNA quantitation reagent is an ultrasensitive fluorescent nucleic acid stain for double-stranded DNA. The samples are excited at 480 nm, and the fluorescence emission intensity is measured at 520 nm by using a spectrofluorometer or fluorescence microplate reader (e.g., Perkin-Elmer HTS 7000 Plus bioassay fluorescent and absorbance microplate reader; PE Biosystems, Foster City, Calif.). The disadvantage to this technique is that the size of the amplicon and the presence of other DNA fragments are not evaluated; the advantage is the ability to analyze many samples rapidly.

Interpretation

For gel electrophoresis, a single brightly stained band of the correct size shows that the amplification was successful. A fast-moving stained band of unincorporated primers may also be detected. If PicoGreen is used, the sample fluorescence is corrected for background by using a reagent blank and a standard curve generated using reference DNA at various concentrations. The results should be validated locally as the optical density (OD) will vary depending on the size of the PCR product and the efficiency of the primers. Usually, the fluorescence reading for each amplicon must be at least three times the reading for the PCR negative control. The presence of amplification of the primers annealing to themselves is suggested if the fluorescence reading for the negative control is as high as that for the amplicons.

SSOPH

In SSOPH, extracted, amplified, and denatured DNA is hybridized with labeled oligonucleotide probes to identify the HLA type. Oligonucleotide probes are selected to hybridize to specific sequences in HLA alleles (Fig. 1). A panel of probes is used to define alleles or groups of alleles potentially present in the denatured amplified DNA. The design of probes is based on alignment of the HLA allele sequences published and available on the Internet (http://www.anthonynolan. org.uk/HIG/index.html) (22). In probe design, the region of polymorphism is usually positioned in the middle of the oligonucleotide. The length and sequence of the oligonucleotide will determine the specificity and hybridization conditions. Most HLA typing utilizes oligonucleotides that are approximately 18 nucleotides in length. Table 3 lists references for various HLA SSOPH typing strategies.

During hybridization, labeled probe will bind to a specific sequence in the amplified DNA. After several stringent wash steps, DNA that is nonspecifically bound to the probe is removed. Labeled DNA-probe complex is then detected. Probes are labeled so that their binding to denatured amplified DNA can be detected. There are several methods for labeling probes. The label added will depend on the detection system utilized. Probes may be detected by chemiluminescence, chromogenic reactions, fluorescence, or radioactivity. For example, for chemiluminescence detection, terminal transferase adds nucleotides, dATP and dUTP, to the 3' end of the oligonucleotide. The dUTP utilized in the tailing reaction may be coupled to digoxigenin, which is detected with an antibody coupled to alkaline phosphatase. Addition of a substrate, Lumiphos 480 (Tepnel Lifecodes Corp., Stamford, Conn.) or CSPD (Roche Diagnostics, Indianapolis, Ind.), causes the emission of light, which is detected by X-ray film.

A panel of oligonucleotide probes is used to identify HLA alleles. The size of the panel and the specificity of probes will determine the resolution level of the typing (i.e., the ability to distinguish among alleles).

SSOPH Typing Systems

SSOPH HLA typing systems can be divided into two major categories: forward SSOPH and reverse SSOPH. In the forward system, denatured amplified DNA is blotted onto a solid support (e.g., membrane) and then hybridized with labeled oligonucleotide probes, which are in solution. In the reverse typing system, probes are attached to a solid support and hybridized with the labeled amplified DNA solution. For both systems, because the interpretation of the hybridization pattern to determine HLA assignments is very complicated, data analysis requires the help of a software program.

Many SSOPH commercial typing kits are available now. They are well developed and have been used by HLA labs for the past several years. The typing procedures are easy to follow and robust. Laboratories can also design their own probe-based typing systems. This may be cost-effective if they are engaged in large-volume HLA typing. Use of a homemade system will involve probe design, reagent synthesis and labeling, and interpretation software development.

Sample Requirement

DNA amplified by PCR, usually the product of a 100-μl PCR mixture, is sufficient.

Materials and Reagents

Table 8 lists the various kits currently available. Information on primers and probes for SSOPH typing of HLA loci is given in the 13th International Histocompatibility Workshop manual (http://www.ihwg.org/protocols/protocol.htm). An oligonucleotide probe labeling kit for chemiluminescence detection is available with detailed instructions (Roche Diagnostics).

Equipment and Instrumentation

Equipment needs are described in Table 8.

SSOPH Procedure

Information on SSOPH protocols can be downloaded from the kit vendors' websites. The amount of amplified DNA in each sample can be evaluated by agarose gel electrophoresis. It is not necessary to check the quality and quantity of PCR-amplifed DNA from each sample before hybridization. In cases in which a sample fails to produce an interpretable typing result due to absent or poor hybridization, it is better to reamplify the genomic DNA since unsatisfactory typing is most likely caused by failed amplification. The hybridization temperature is very critical for obtaining stringent hybridization, and it must be closely monitored during the operation.

QA and QC

Each panel of samples to be typed should include positive and negative DNA controls to detect contamination with previously amplified DNA, nonspecific probe hybridization, and human errors. In the high-throughput typing lab, it is necessary to add blind random repeats in each sample panel to a level of 1 to 3% to monitor sample mishandling during the entire testing process. The laboratory should have a set of well-defined reference samples with known HLA alleles to test new lots of reagents, especially probes. It is recommended that the reference panel cover most of the polymorphisms that the probes detect. Equipment, such as thermal cyclers, water baths, and detectors, must be calibrated periodically.

TABLE 8 Examples of SSOPH typing kits[a]

Type of SSOPH	Name of kit	Vendor (location)	Loci	Sample size[b]	Major equipment (vendor)	Description
Forward	Lifecodes HLA kit	Tepnel Lifecodes Corp (Stamford, Conn.)	HLA-A, HLA-B, HLA-C, DRB, DQB, DPB	Large	Thermal cycler, shaking water bath, Hydra-96 microdispenser (Art Robbins Instruments, Sunnyvale, Calif.)	PCR-amplified DNA blotted onto membrane; one membrane hybridized with one probe; probe-specific wash temperature may vary; chemiluminescence or colorimetric detection achieved; data reading has no time limit; addition of new probes requires extra membranes and hybridization step.
Reverse	LABType HLA kit	One Lambda (Canoga Park, Calif.)	HLA-A, HLA-B, HLA-C, DRB, DQB	Small, medium, or large	Thermal cycler, centrifuge, Luminex 100 system (Luminex, Austin, Tex.)	Multiplex PCR; probes attached to microspheres (beads); all probes hybridize and are washed at same temperature in one well (up to 100 probes/well); fluorescence detection achieved; data collection by Luminex 100 system can be delayed up to 3 to 7 days; addition of new probes with no extra steps.
	RELI-SSO HLA kit	Dynal Biotech (Brown Deer, Wis.)	HLA-A, HLA-B, HLA-C, DRB, DQB	Small or medium	Thermal cycler, Dynal AutoRELI 48 instrument	Probes bound on membrane strip; probes hybridize and are washed in AutoRELI 48 instrument at same temperature; color detection achieved; data reading has no time limit.
	LifeMatch HLA-SSO kit	Tepnel Lifecodes Corp. (Stamford, Conn.)	HLA-A, HLA-B, HLA-C, DRB	Small, medium, or large	Thermal cycler, Luminex 100 system (Luminex, Austin, Tex.)	Asymmetric PCR; no denaturation step; probes attached on microspheres (beads); all probes hybridize at same temperature in one well (up to 100 probes).
	Inno-LIPA HLA-SSO kit	Innogenetics (Alpharetta, Ga.)	HLA-A, HLA-B, HLA-C, DRB, DQB	Small or medium	Thermal cycler, Auto-LiPA (strip processor)	Probes bound onto membrane strip; probes hybridize and are washed in Auto-LiPA at same temperature; color detection achieved; data reading has no time limit.

[a]Information on procedures is available from the vendor websites.
[b]Sample size: small, 1 to 10 samples per test; medium, 11 to 50 samples per test; large, >50 samples per test.

Cost Assessment

This assay can be used at various levels of resolution, depending on the purpose of the testing. SSOPH is able to reach allele level resolution, although the number of primers and probes required is large and new alleles might not be detected. SSOPH can be used for both small numbers and large numbers of samples.

Interpretation

Kits containing a large number of probes for a single HLA locus or probes designed to link polymorphisms (i.e., to determine whether specific polymorphisms lie within the same allele) will reduce the percentage of results with several alternative HLA assignments and will produce higher-resolution typing data.

RSCA

The method of RSCA relies upon the separation of homo- and hetero-DNA duplexes in a gel matrix (Table 4). PCR is used to amplify a locus or a region of the gene. The strands of the amplification product, containing one or two HLA alleles, are hybridized with a fluorescently labeled reference strand from a known reference HLA allele, forming heteroduplexes. The fluorescent label allows heteroduplexes containing the reference strand to be detected.

The mobility of the labeled heteroduplexes is compared to the mobility of reference homoduplexes after separation by nondenaturing polyacrylamide electrophoresis. The use of laser-based instrumentation (e.g., Prism 310; Applied Biosystems Inc., Foster City, Calif.) and computer software in addition to internal DNA markers for correction of gel-to-gel variability allows discrimination among HLA alleles which may differ by only a single nucleotide within the DNA fragment.

Materials and Reagents
An RSCA kit is available from Pel-Freez Clinical Systems, LLC (Brown Deer, Wis.).

QA and QC
At least two fluorescently labeled DNA references are used to create heteroduplexes with the sample alleles. Fluorescently labeled reference DNA strands flanking the samples are used as markers to measure the mobilities of bands during electrophoresis.

Cost Assessment
RSCA is often useful for resolving typing ambiguities in which determination of the *cis-trans* associations of polymorphic motifs requires an additional typing step. RSCA has been used for high-resolution class I and II typing and matching for bone marrow donor selection.

Interpretation
Sequence differences between the HLA alleles in the sample and the fluorescently labeled reference strands lead to the production of homo- and heteroduplexes following denaturation and cooling. As a particular heteroduplex will migrate different distances relative to homoduplexes, measurement of mobility values allows alleles to be assigned.

DNA SEQUENCING
A final protocol for HLA typing is sequencing of HLA genes (Table 5). Amplification is used to obtain sufficient copies of a specific HLA gene for analysis by DNA sequencing. PCR amplification primers are chosen so that the resultant amplicon contains the genetic information from the polymorphic exons of a single allele or both alleles carried by an individual. For HLA class I genes, the primer sets used in the PCR bracket exon 2 and exon 3, including the intervening intron. For class II genes, the primers flank exon 2. If two alleles are present, their sequences are characterized as a mixture.

DNA synthesis (i.e., the DNA-sequencing reaction) is carried out using a single primer, the four nucleotides (dATP, dTTP, dGTP, and dCTP), and four dideoxynucleotides (dideoxy-dATP [ddATP], ddTTP, ddGTP, and ddCTP) (24). At each position in the sequence, the DNA polymerase has the option of incorporating a normal nucleotide or a dideoxynucleotide. If a normal nucleotide is incorporated, synthesis proceeds. If a dideoxynucleotide is incorporated, synthesis is halted. The result is a mixture containing DNA fragments ending at various positions along the length of the DNA sequence. Following denaturation, the newly synthesized strands are separated by size on a polyacrylamide gel. If the newly synthesized strands are labeled, through labeling of either the primer or the dideoxynucleotides, the strands can be visualized on the gel. The strands terminated by a single dideoxynucleotide are distinguished from the strands terminated by the other three dideoxynucleotides through the use of different fluorescent labels or through analysis of each reaction in a separate lane of the gel. Through this approach, the sequence of nucleotides comprising each HLA allele can be determined. Depending on the length of the region sequenced, two or more sequencing primers are used to obtain sense (forward) and antisense (reverse) sequences of exons 2 and 3 for class I and exon 2 for class II genes (Fig. 3).

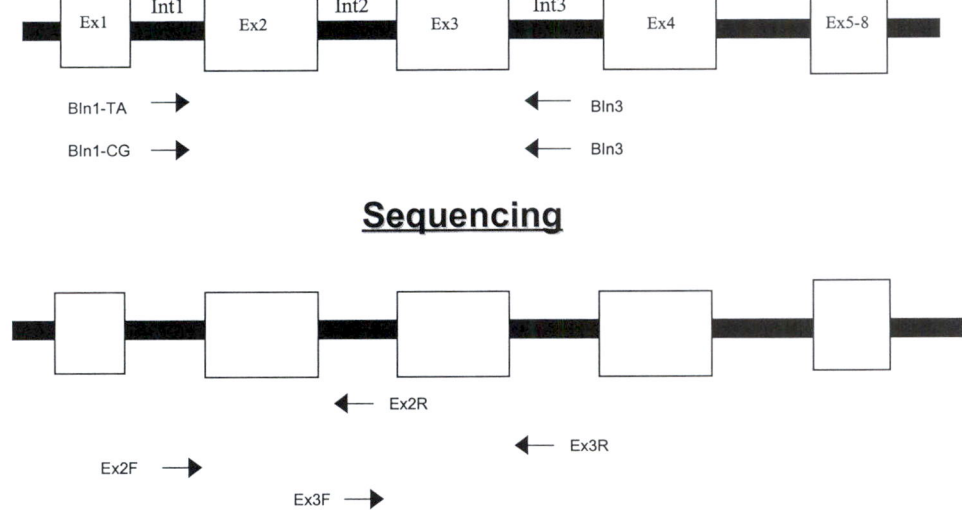

FIGURE 3 Primer locations for sequence-based typing of the HLA-B gene. The locations at which amplification and sequencing primers anneal to the HLA-B gene are indicated by arrows. BIn3 includes both BIn3 and BIn3-AC primers. Ex, exon; Int, intron; F, forward; R, reverse.

Amplification of HLA Class I Genes for Sequencing

The HLA-B gene will be used as an example for amplification of HLA class I genes. PCR amplification primers are chosen so that the resultant amplicon contains the genetic information from the polymorphic exons of a single HLA-B allele or both HLA-B alleles carried by an individual. The primer sets used in the PCR bracket exon 2 and exon 3, including the intervening intron. The two alternative forward (or sense) primers anneal to a polymorphism in the intron before exon 2 (4) which subdivides the HLA-B alleles into two groups. Therefore, approximately half of the time, the two alleles in a heterozygous individual will be individually isolated for subsequent characterization. If the two alleles fall within the same amplification group, their sequences are characterized as a mixture. Two reverse primers are mixed together to achieve amplification of all B locus alleles. The BIn3-AC primer is required to amplify the B*7301 allele, which is not amplified by the BIn3 primer.

Sample Requirement

DNA (200 to 500 ng) previously heated to 95°C for 5 min in a heating block and stored on ice

Materials and Reagents

Automated sequencers and commercial kits for the amplification and sequence analysis of some HLA alleles are available (PE Biosystems; Amersham Pharmacia Biotech, Inc., Piscataway, N.J.; Visible Genetics Inc., Toronto, Ontario, Canada; and Abbott Laboratories, Abbott Park, IL [Atria Genetics Inc., Forensic Analytical Molecular Genetics]).

0.5-ml sterile disposable bubble-top tubes

10× PCR buffer (4): 500 mM Tris-HCl, pH 8.8; 150 mM ammonium sulfate; 500 μM EDTA; 0.1% (wt/vol) Knox gelatin; and 100 mM β-mercaptoethanol. Buffer is made without β-mercaptoethanol, autoclaved, and stored at room temperature. A working solution containing β-mercaptoethanol is made fresh just before use.

dNTP solution: 1.25 mM (each) dNTPs diluted in water and stored at 4°C for no more than 2 weeks. Stock solutions: 100 mM dNTP set (catalog no. 10297-018; Invitrogen, Carlsbad, Calif.)

Platinum *Taq* DNA polymerase at 5 U/μl (Invitrogen; catalog no. 10966-034)

PCR primers for HLA-B: 10 pmol of each sense primer/μl. The antisense primers are dissolved in water at a concentration of 10 pmol/μl, and 4 μl of BIn3 is mixed with 1 μl of BIn3-AC to yield the final antisense mixture.

Sense primers (4):

BIn1-TA, 5′-GGCGGGGGCGCAGGACCTGA-3′

BIn1-CG, 5′-GGCGGGGGCGCAGGACCCGG-3′

Antisense primers:

BIn3, 5′-GGAGSCCATCCCCGSCGACCTAT-3′ (where S is the International Union of Biochemistry code for G and C)

BIn3-AC, 5′-GGAGGCCATCCCGGGCGATCTAT-3′

Dimethyl sulfoxide (catalog no. D-8418; Sigma)

50 mM MgCl₂

Ultrapure reagent-grade water (New England Reagent Laboratory, East Providence, R.I.)

Agarose gel reagents

Equipment and Instrumentation

- Laminar flow hood
- 95°C heating block
- Thermal cycler (GeneAmp PCR system 9600; Perkin-Elmer, Norwalk, Conn.)
- Vortex mixer
- Microcentrifuge
- Agarose gel electrophoresis equipment

Amplification Procedure

In a sterile laminar flow hood:

1. Assemble two PCR mixes for each sample.
   i. To the heat-denatured DNA aliquot, add TA-PCR mix (volume indicated for one sample): 10 μl of PCR buffer (working solution), 10 μl of dimethyl sulfoxide, 2 μl of MgCl₂, 16 μl of diluted dNTP solution, 2 μl of each primer (sense primer BIn1-TA and antisense primer mixture [BIn3–BIn3-AC]), 0.5 μl of *Taq* DNA polymerase, and water to bring volume to 100 μl.
   ii. Assemble the CG-PCR mix as described for the TA-PCR mix but using a different primer set: BIn1-CG and antisense primer mixture.
2. Mix by vortexing and microcentrifuge briefly to bring liquid to the bottom of the tube.
3. Cycle the tubes in a thermal cycler according to the following temperature profile: 96°C for 5 min for one cycle; 96°C for 10 s, 65°C for 30 s, and 72°C for 60 s for five cycles; 96°C for 20 s, 60°C for 30 s, and 72°C for 60 s for 30 cycles; and 72°C for 10 min for one cycle.
4. Analyze an aliquot on an agarose gel. Store the remaining amplified DNA at 4°C.

Interpretation

The identification of amplification products of approximately 1 kb in size on an agarose gel is used to predict the sequencing result. If only one of the two amplifications shows a band upon gel electrophoresis, it is expected that the sequence analysis of the amplified DNA will include one or two alleles. If both amplifications are positive as judged by gel electrophoresis, the sequence analysis of each amplicon should yield a single allele.

Purification of Amplified DNA in Preparation for Nucleotide Sequencing

Amplified DNA is purified to remove any unreacted PCR primers and dNTPs. These components will interfere with the sequencing reaction. The amplified DNA is passed through a microconcentrator with distilled water. DNA is captured on a membrane during centrifugation. The unreacted PCR primers and dNTPs are collected in the waste tube. DNA is then recovered by subsequent centrifugation and denatured.

Sample Requirement

Amplified DNA

Materials and Reagents

Microcon-100 (catalog no. 42413; Amicon, Inc., Beverly, Mass.)

Ultrapure reagent-grade water (New England Reagent Laboratory)

Equipment and Instrumentation

• Fixed-angle microcentrifuge (model no. 5415C; Eppendorf-Netheler-Hinz GmbH, Hamburg, Germany)

Purification Procedure

Details of the purification procedure are provided in the Microcon microconcentrators operating instructions by Amicon, Inc. (publication I-394H).

1. Insert the filtrate cup into one of the Microcon-100 sample reservoirs.

2. Being careful not to touch the filter membrane with the pipette tip, pipette 400 μl of sterile distilled water into the blue concentrator column (filtrate cup).

3. Add the entire PCR mix to 400 μl of water. The total volume of DNA and water should not exceed 500 μl.

4. Place the assembled Microcon unit into the microcentrifuge and centrifuge at 2,000 × g for 8 min.

5. Remove the concentrator assembly from the centrifuge. Separate the filtrate cup from the sample reservoir and remove the spin cap.

6. Carefully place the filtrate cup upside down in a new sample reservoir and centrifuge for an additional 3 min at 2,000 × g.

7. Approximately 2 μl of liquid should be recovered. Bring the volume to 20 to 30 μl with water. The amount of water to be added is estimated by the intensity of the amplified DNA following gel electrophoresis prior to Microcon purification and should yield 30 to 50 ng/μl.

8. Measure the OD at 260 and 280 nm and estimate the amount of DNA (an OD of 1 at 260 nm is equal to 50 μg/ml). The expected yield is 30 to 50 ng/μl after dilution. Ratios of absorbance at 260 nm versus that at 280 nm are about 1.7 to 1.9.

Sometimes Microcon filters are defective and the recovery may be greater than expected. If the yield is more than 20 μl following centrifugation, the mixture should be purified using a second Microcon filter. If the yield is low, the PCR should be repeated.

Nucleotide Sequencing

In the procedure described below, the HLA-B locus PCR product is sequenced by using BigDye terminator cycle sequencing kits with AmpliTaq DNA polymerase, FS (Applied Biosystems). DNA is first denatured at 96°C. Sequencing primers anneal to denatured DNA at 50°C. Four primers are used to obtain sense (forward) and antisense (reverse) sequences of exons 2 and 3 (Fig. 3). DNA polymerase adds nucleotides onto the primers, extending the DNA strands at 60°C until the addition of one of the four dye-labeled terminators ends the extension. Repetition of the cycle of denaturation, annealing, and extension generates billions of copies of the dye-labeled DNA. The DNA fragments obtained using dye terminator chemistry are precipitated with 100% ethanol containing sodium acetate. The supernatant, which contains unincorporated dye terminators, is discarded.

A polyacrylamide gel is formed by the copolymerization of acrylamide and bisacrylamide. The process begins when N, N, N, N-tetramethylethylenediamine (TEMED) reacts with ammonium persulfate (APS), causing linkage of the acrylamide monomers. The polymer chains are randomly cross-linked with bisacrylamide to form the gel matrix. The Long Ranger gel is generated in a similar fashion.

Sample Requirement

The DNA sequencing reaction is performed using 100 ng of purified amplified DNA.

Materials and Reagents

BigDye terminator cycle sequencing kits with AmpliTaq DNA polymerase, FS (Applied Biosystems; catalog no. 4336778 for 5,000 reactions)

Sequencing primers: 5 pmol of each primer. Primers used for HLA-B sequencing include the following:

Exon 2 sense primer, 5′-GCCGGGAGGAGGGTC-3′

Exon 2 antisense primer, 5′-GGATCTCGGACCCG-GAG-3′

Exon 3 sense primer, 5′-GGGGGACGGKGCTGA-CCG-3′ (where K represents G or T)

Exon 3 antisense primer, 5′-AGGCTCCCCACTG-3′

0.2-ml strip PCR tubes (catalog no. T-3013-Y; GeneMate, Kaysville, Utah) or a 0.2 ml-diameter PCR plate (catalog no. 1402-9600; USA Scientific, Inc., Ocala, Fla.)

100% and 70% ethanol

3 M sodium acetate, pH 4.6

Deionized formamide: Mix 10 ml of formamide (catalog no. 0606; Solon, Ohio) with 1 g of Amberlite MB-1 (Sigma; MB-1A). Stir formamide and resin together for 15 to 20 min but no longer than 30 min as the formamide will eventually dissolve the resin. Filter through a 0.2-μm-pore-size filter and store at −20°C.

25 mM EDTA, pH 8.0

Dye: 10 ml of 25 mM EDTA, pH 8.0, and 500 mg of blue dextran

Long Ranger 5% gel and buffer: Long Ranger gel solution (50% stock solution; catalog no. 50611; FMC Bio-Products, Rockland, Maine), APS (American Chemical Society grade; Amresco; catalog no. 0486-100G-APP), TEMED (electrophoresis purity reagent; Amresco; catalog no. 0761-25ML-APP), urea (Invitrogen; catalog no. 15505-035), and 10× Tris-borate-EDTA (TBE) buffer (16.6 g of EDTA, 216 g of Tris, and 110 g of boric acid, with water added to bring the final volume to 2 liters [the pH should be approximately 8.4]), filtered with a 150-ml filter system with 0.22-μm-pore-size nylon (Nalgene; catalog no. 150-0020; Nalge Co., Rochester, N.Y.). Thoroughly mix the follwing ingredients; 18 g of urea, 5 ml of 10× TBE, 5 ml of Long Ranger gel stock solution, and 26 ml of water. Filter the acrylamide solution and degas for 5 min. Prepare 10% APS. Note that APS begins to decompose at once when dissolved in water. The result is loss of activity. For reproducible results, the APS solution should be prepared immediately before each use. Into the degassed acrylamide solution, add the following components gently: 250 μl of 10% APS and 35 μl of TEMED. Gently swirl the solution and pour the gel as indicated in the user manual for the sequencer. Polymerization begins when APS and TEMED are added to the gel solution. Alternatively, use the Long Ranger single pack (catalog no. 50691; Cambrex Bio Science Rockland Inc., Rockland, Maine) and follow the manufacturer's instructions.

1% TBE running buffer made by diluting 10× TBE with water

Equipment and Instrumentation

- Thermal cycler (Perkin-Elmer; model 9600)
- 95°C heating block
- Vortex
- Microcentrifuge with vertical rotor (Eppendorf; model 5403) or tabletop centrifuge with swing plate holder (Sorvall; model RT6000 D)
- Automated DNA sequencer (PE Biosystems; model 377)

Nucleotide Sequencing Procedure

Use an aseptic technique on the lab bench.

1. In 0.2-ml strip tubes or plates, assemble sequencing reaction mixtures (one for each primer) on ice. Add reagents as follows: 50 to 100 ng of purified PCR product (approximately 1 to 2 µl), 1 µl of primer (5 pmol), and 4 µl of terminator ready reaction mix, with water added to bring the total volume to 10 µl. (Alternatively, add reagents as follows: 50 to 100 ng of purified PCR product [approximately 1 to 2 µl], 1 µl of primer [5 pmol], 1 µl of terminator ready reaction mix, and 5 µl of Better Buffer [The Gel Company, San Francisco, Calif.], with water added to bring the total volume to 15 µl.)

2. Place the samples in the thermocycler. Denature DNA at 96°C for 2 min, and then start cycles: 96°C for 10 s, 50°C for 5 s, and 60°C for 3 min for 25 cycles.

3. Store the product at 4°C or ethanol precipitate immediately.

4. Prepare a fresh mix with 1 ml of anhydrous ethanol and 40 µl of 3 M sodium acetate, pH 4.6.

5. To each sequencing reaction mixture, add 25 µl of the ethanol-sodium acetate mix. Vortex to mix.

6. Place tubes or plates in a benchtop vertical microcentrifuge or a tabletop centrifuge with swing plate holders. Centrifuge the tubes or plates for 30 min at 1,500 to 3,000 × g (3,000 rpm; 16- to 17-cm rotor) at room temperature.

7. Immediately invert the tubes or plates onto paper towels. Place the inverted tubes or plates and paper towel in the centrifuge for 1 min at 150 × g (700 rpm; 16- to 17-cm rotor) to remove the remaining supernatant.

8. Add 50 µl of 70% ethanol to the tubes or plates.

9. Centrifuge for 5 min at 1,500 to 3,000 × g.

10. Immediately invert the tubes or plates onto paper towels. Place the inverted tubes or plates and paper towel in the centrifuge for 1 min at 150 × g (700 rpm; 16- to 17-cm rotor) to remove the remaining supernatant.

11. Samples can be stored as dry pellets at −20°C.

12. Prepare the loading buffer by combining deionized formamide and dye in a ratio of 5:1 deionized formamide to EDTA-blue dextran.

13. Resuspend the dried sample in 1.5 to 4 µl of loading buffer, depending on the gel comb size (e.g., for a 96-well comb, use 2 µl) and the intensity of the PCR product prior to sequencing. Vortex and briefly centrifuge the sample to bring liquid to the bottom of the tube.

14. Heat the sample at 95°C for 2 min in a heating block or thermal cycler to denature the DNA. Place the sample on ice until ready to load.

15. Analyze the sample on a 5% Long Ranger gel.

16. Load 0.5 to 2 µl of the preparation into the sequencing gel wells, depending on the size of the lanes and the sequencing chemistry used. The remaining sample can be kept at −20° C for up to 2 weeks.

17. Electrophoresis (1.69 kV; 20 to 30 mA; 5 to 6 h) and analysis should follow guidelines for the automated instrument (ABI PRISM 377-18 DNA sequencer user's manual, part 904210, PE Biosystems, www.pebio.com).

BigDye terminator ready reaction mix contains fluorescent dye and should be kept away from direct sunlight. Suboptimal results as judged by the lack of clearly defined peaks and a high background can be caused by inadequate amounts of the DNA template, poor quality of template, failure to remove contaminants prior to analysis of the sample, and problems with the gel or instrument. Some DNA fragments may have secondary structures which alter their mobility, resulting in incorrect sequence assignment. These anomalies can be identified by comparing to reference HLA sequences and by determining the nucleotide sequences of both coding and noncoding DNA strands. These and other problems are discussed in detail in the PE Biosystems automated DNA sequencing chemistry guide (PE Biosystems).

QA and QC

The conserved region of the HLA gene can serve as a control for the sequencing reaction and electrophoresis. Previously undescribed alleles need to be confirmed from a second independent PCR amplification and sequence reaction. If two alleles are sequenced simultaneously, the positions at which the two alleles differ in nucleotide sequence (i.e., heterozygous peaks) should be reviewed (23). All sequences should be compared to the matched sequence(s) and to the mismatched sequence(s) which most closely resemble the assigned sequence. Criteria for accepting a sequence should include evaluation of the number of uninterpretable positions and signal strength. The use of new lots of reagents should be documented and validated. A record of parameters (run temperature, milliamperes, and volts) for the automated sequencer should be maintained.

Cost Assessment

Sequencing is expensive due to the high cost of the DNA sequencer and the sequencing reagents. It is, however, the best approach to achieve allele level resolution typing of HLA alleles and is the preferred approach for characterization of patients requiring hematopoietic stem cell transplantation and their potential unrelated donors. The laboratory should be prepared to identify and/or design additional PCR or sequencing primers needed to resolve typing of alleles since commercial kits may not provide the resolution needed to obtain allele level resolution.

Interpretation

The sequence of nucleotides is refined using software tools provided with the DNA sequencer. The final sequence is compared to sequences in a database by the software to identify the allele(s) present (12, 23). Positions at which the sequence differs from those of the next most closely related alleles should be reviewed. Allele-specific amplification or sequencing primers may be required to resolve typing of alternative allele combinations (Fig. 2). For example, a sequence result of A*02010101, A*6601, or A*023501, and A*2603 requires the addition of a sequencing primer specific for one of the two alleles in each combination (e.g., annealing to the TTC ACA sequence at codons 9 through 10 which is found in both A*02 alleles). This will allow the laboratory to determine whether the codon 70 polymorphism (CAC) is linked to the TTC ACA sequence at codons 9 and 10 (identifying the allele combination as A*02010101 and A*6601) or not (identifying the allele combination as A*023501 and A*2603). A list of alleles with identical sequences in the commonly sequenced exons is provided on a website (http://www.anthonynolan.org.uk/HIG/index.html). Since no commercial kit includes the reagents required to resolve all ambiguous allele combinations encountered, the laboratory must have the capability to design and validate these primers in-house.

This publication has been supported by funding from the Office of Naval Research (N00014-99-1-0551) to the C. W. Bill Young Marrow Donor Recruitment and Research Program.

The views expressed in this article are those of the authors and do not reflect the official policy or position of the Department of the Navy, the Department of Defense, or the U.S. government.

REFERENCES

1. Bozon, M. V., J. C. Delgado, A. Selvakumar, O. P. Clavijo, M. Salazar, M. Ohashi, S. M. Alosco, J. Russell, N. Yu, B. Dupont, and E. J. Yunis. 1997. Error rate for HLA-B antigen assignment by serology: implications for proficiency testing and utilization of DNA-based typing methods. *Tissue Antigens* **50**:387–394.

2. Bunce, M., M. C. Barnardo, and K. I. Welsh. 1998. The PCR-SSP manager computer program: a tool for maintaining sequence alignments and automatically updating the specificities of PCR-SSP primers and primer mixes. *Tissue Antigens* **52**:158–174.

3. Cao, K., J. Hollenbach, X. Shi, W. Shi, M. Chopek, and M. Fernandez-Vina. 2001. Analysis of the frequencies of HLA-A, B, and C alleles and haplotypes in the five major ethnic groups of the United States reveals high levels of diversity in these loci and contrasting distribution patterns in these populations. *Hum. Immunol.* **62**:1009–1030.

4. Cereb, N., and S. Y. Yang. 1997. Dimorphic primers derived from intron 1 for use in the molecular typing of HLA-B alleles. *Tissue Antigens* **50**:74–76.

5. Ellexson, M. E., G. Z. Zhang, D. Stewart, M. Lau, G. Teresi, P. Terasaki, B. Roe, and W. Hildebrand. 1995. Nucleotide sequence analysis of HLA-B* 1523 and B*8101—dominant α-helical motifs produce complex serologic recognition patterns for the HLA-B"DT" and HLAB "NM5" antigens. *Hum. Immunol.* **44**:103–110.

6. Flomenberg, N., L. A. Baxter-Lowe, D. L. Confer, M. Fernandez-Vina, A. Filipovich, M. Horowitz, C. K. Hurley, C. Kollman, C. Anasetti, H. Noreen, A. Begovich, W. Hildebrand, E. Petersdorf, B. Schmeckpeper, M. Setterholm, E. Trachtenberg, T. Williams, E. J. Yunis, and D. Weisdorf. 2004. Impact of HLA class I and class II high resolution matching on outcomes of unrelated donor bone marrow transplantation: HLA-C mismatching is associated with a strong adverse effect on transplant outcome. *Blood* **104**:1923–1930. [Online.] doi:10.1182/blood-2004-03-0803.

7. Hurley, C. K. 1997. Acquisition and use of DNA-based HLA typing data in bone marrow registries. *Tissue Antigens* **49**:323–328.

8. Hurley, C. K., L. A. Baxter-Lowe, B. Logan, C. Karanes, C. Anasetti, D. Weisdorf, and D. L. Confer. 2003. National Marrow Donor Program HLA-matching guidelines for unrelated marrow transplants. *Biol. Blood Marrow Transplant.* **9**:610–615.

9. Hurley, C. K., M. Setterholm, M. Lau, M. S. Pollack, H. Noreen, A. Howard, M. Fernandez-Vina, D. KuKuruga, C. R. Muller, M. Venance, J. A. Wade, M. Oudshoorn, C. Raffoux, J. Enczmann, P. Wernet, and M. Maiers. 2004. Hematopoietc stem cell donor registry strategies for assigning search determinants and matching relationships. *Bone Marrow Transplant.* **33**:443–450.

10. Kosman, C. 2000. HLA class I and class II DNA extraction methods. *In* A. B. Hahn, G. A. Land, and R. M. Strothman (ed.), *American Society for Histocompatibility and Immunogenetics Laboratory Manual.* American Society for Histocompatibility and Immunogenetics, Lenexa, Kans.

11. Marsh, S. G. E., E. D. Albert, W. F. Bodmer, R. E. Bontrop, B. Dupont, H. A. Erlich, D. E. Geraghty, J. A. Hansen, B. Mach, W. R. Mayr, P. Parham, et al. 2002. Nomenclature for factors of the HLA system, 2002. *Eur. J. Immunogenet.* **29**:463–515.

12. McGinnis, M. D., M. P. Conrad, A. G. M. Bouwens, M. G. J. Tilanus, and M. N. Kronick. 1995. Automated, solid-phase sequencing of DRB region genes using T7 sequencing chemistry and dye-labeled primers. *Tissue Antigens* **46**:173–179.

13. Mickelson, E. M., L. A. Guthrie, R. Etzioni, C. Anasetti, P. J. Martin, and J. A. Hansen. 1994. Role of the mixed lymphocyte culture (MLC) reaction in marrow donor selection: matching for transplants from related haploidentical donors. *Tissue Antigens* **44**:83–92.

14. Mickelson, E. M., G. Longton, C. Anasetti, E. Petersdorf, P. Martin, L. A. Guthrie, and J. A. Hansen. 1996. Evaluation of the mixed lymphocyte culture (MLC) assay as a method for selecting unrelated donors for marrow transplantation. *Tissue Antigens* **47**:27–36.

15. Middleton, D. 1999. History of DNA typing for the human MHC. *Rev. Immunogenet.* **1**:135–156.

16. Mytilineos, J., M. Lempert, S. Scherer, V. Schwarz, and G. Opelz. 1998. Comparison of serological and DNA PCR-SSP typing results for HLA-A and HLA-B in 421 black individuals—a collaborative transplant study report. *Hum. Immunol.* **59**:512–517.

17. Nepom, G. T., and H. Erlich. 1991. MHC class-II molecules and autoimmunity. *Annu. Rev. Immunol.* **9**:493–525.

18. Noreen, H. J., N. Yu, M. Setterholm, M. Ohashi, J. Baisch, R. Endres, M. Fernandez-Vina, U. Heine, S. Hsu, M. Kamoun, Y. Mitsuishi, D. Monos, L. Perlee, S. Rodriguez-Marino, S. Smith, S. Y. Yang, K. Shipp, J. Hegland, and C. K. Hurley. 2001. Validation of DNA-based HLA-A and HLA-B testing of volunteers for a bone marrow registry through parallel testing with serology. *Tissue Antigens* **57**:221–229.

19. Olerup, O., and H. Zetterquist. 1992. HLA-DR typing by PCR amplification with sequence specific primers (PCR-SSP) in 2 hours: an alternative to serological DR typing in clinical practice including donor-recipient matching in cadaveric transplantations. *Tissue Antigens* **39**:225–235.

20. Opelz, G., T. Wujciak, B. Dohler, S. Scherer, and J. Mytilineos. 1999. HLA compatibility and organ transplant survival. *Rev. Immunogenet.* **1**:334–342.

21. Parham, P., and T. Ohta. 1996. Population biology of antigen presentation by MHC class I molecules. *Science* **272**:67–74.

22. Robinson, J., M. J. Waller, P. Parham, J. G. Bodmer, and S. G. E. Marsh. 2001. IMGT/HLA database—a sequence database for the human major histocompatibility complex. *Nucleic Acids Res.* **29**:210–213.

23. Rozemuller, E. H., A. G. M. Bouwens, B. E. J. E. G. Bast, and M. G. J. Tilanus. 1993. Assignment of HLA-DPB alleles by computerized matching based upon sequence data. *Hum. Immunol.* **37**:207–212.

24. Sanger, F., S. Nicklen, and A. Coulson. 1977. DNA sequencing with chain terminating inhibitors. *Proc. Natl. Acad. Sci. USA* **74**:5463–5467.

25. Schreuder, G. M. T., C. K. Hurley, S. G. E. Marsh, M. Lau, M. Maiers, C. Kollman, and H. J. Noreen. 2001. The HLA dictionary 2001: a summary of HLA-A, -B, -C, -DRB1/3/4/5, -DQB1 alleles and their association with serologically defined HLA-A, -B, -C, -DR, and -DQ antigens. *Hum. Immunol.* **62**:826–849.

26. Sidney, J., H. M. Grey, R. T. Kubo, and A. Sette. 1996. Practical, biochemical and evolutionary implications of the discovery of HLA class I supermotifs. *Immunol. Today* **17**:261–266.

Evaluation of the Humoral Response in Transplantation

ANDREA A. ZACHARY, JULIE A. HOUP, RENATO VEGA, KEVIN CHESTERTON, AND DONNA P. LUCAS

137

INTRODUCTION

Relevance of Antibodies in Transplantation

Antibodies of the immunoglobulin G (IgG) class can damage tissues in a variety of ways, including (i) directly through complement activation, (ii) indirectly through the deposition of immune complexes, and (iii) indirectly through the recruitment of cytotoxic or inflammation-inducing cells. Very high levels of antibody result in hyperacute rejection and graft failure, an outcome that can be easily avoided by the performance of a lymphocyte crossmatch test prior to transplantation. However, clear elucidation of the relevance of donor-reactive antibodies of various strengths and specificities and of antibodies that arise after transplantation has been hampered by inadequate technologies and lack of reimbursement for posttransplantation monitoring of antibodies. Nonetheless, a deleterious effect of antibodies specific for mismatched donor HLA antigens has been demonstrated for every type of organ that has been transplanted in sufficient numbers. Further, there is evidence that anti-HLA antibodies are involved in acute and chronic as well as hyperacute rejection of organs (reviewed in reference 26). As the number of composite-tissue and HLA-mismatched bone marrow transplants increases, it is likely that antibodies will be a rejection risk in these transplants as well. In mismatched bone marrow transplants, there is a risk of immunocompetent tissues from sensitized donors producing antibodies to recipient tissues as well as of recipients making anti-donor tissue antibodies. In theory, antibodies specific for any antigen on transplanted tissue should be capable of damaging the transplant. Among those known to be deleterious to transplanted tissue are antibodies specific for antigens of the HLA and ABO systems. More recently, antibodies to MICA antigens encoded by genes in the HLA system have been shown to be involved in graft rejection. The focus of this chapter will be HLA-specific antibodies, and we will use the term donor-specific antibody (DSA) to refer to an antibody(ies) specific for donor HLA.

Among the reasons HLA-specific antibodies are so important are that HLA antigens are present on transplanted tissues (class I [HLA-A, -B, and -C] antigens are expressed on most nucleated cells, and class II [HLA-DR, -DQ, and -DP] expression, although more limited, is likely to be induced at the time of transplant); most transplants involve some degree of HLA mismatch; HLA antigens provoke one of the strongest immune responses; and recipients may become sensitized to HLA antigens prior to transplantation through transfusion, pregnancy, and possibly environmental agents or after transplantation by the graft itself. The risk represented by HLA-specific antibodies is determined by the characteristics of the antibody, including titer, class, specificity, timing, and course (i.e., whether the antibody is increasing or decreasing), and by the relevant characteristics of the tissue, which are the extent and type of antigen expression and the resilience of the tissue to antibody-mediated damage. The level of risk, as measured by the timing and extent of damage to the graft, is directly proportional to the antibody titer. Regarding Ig class, IgG antibodies are established risk factors, the data are ambiguous for IgM antibodies, and there are data suggesting that HLA-specific antibodies of the IgA class are beneficial in transplantation (reviewed in reference 26). It has been clearly demonstrated that antibodies to either HLA class I or HLA class II antigens represent a risk and are capable of producing hyperacute rejection (reviewed in reference 26). However, the level of antigen expression varies among HLA loci. Antigens encoded by the HLA-C, -DRB3 (DR52), and -DRB4 (DR53) and possibly the -DRB5 (DR51) loci are expressed at much lower levels than those encoded by HLA-A, -B, and -DRB1 (5, 12, 21), and there may be a lower risk of rejection associated with their respective antibodies, although there has been at least one case of hyperacute rejection mediated by an antibody specific for a C locus antigen (3). Antibodies that are present at the time of transplantation or that develop after transplantation can damage tissues. In contrast, antibodies that were present only historically appear to represent little risk except in two situations: (i) when the present transplant shares a mismatched antigen with a previous transplant and (ii) when a previous graft was lost to an early immunologic rejection. The courses of antibodies, over time, may be relevant to the level of risk. Antibodies that are increasing in titer or expanding in specificity may represent a recent or ongoing sensitization, which may include newly developing antibodies to donor antigens, and are potentially of greater risk than those that are waning in titer or breadth, which may reflect senescence or an active down-regulation of the immune response and may be more responsive to intervention. Differences among organs and tissues in HLA antigen expression, extent of exposure to antibodies, and impact on function of antibody-mediated damage are well known. However, a variety of factors, such as certain cytokines and hormones which can be released in response to trauma, infection, or certain treatments, can affect antigen expression, which in turn can provoke a humoral response and provide increased target for antibody binding.

Goals and Aims

Despite the danger presented by antibodies to donor HLA, the risk to the transplant can be overcome, in many cases, through appropriate intervention. Thus, the goal in testing for HLA-specific antibody should be to determine the level of risk to the transplanted organ or tissue. This, then, provides an opportunity to determine what treatment, if any, will overcome that risk—i.e., what has to be done to prevent or treat rejection. The risk is present in the form of existing antibody(ies) or an increased probability of making antibody(ies) to donor HLA. The most definitive source of information is the detection and characterization of antibodies both prior to and following transplantation. This includes assessing the antibody characteristics, identified above, that are associated with risk: Ig class, titer, specificity, and trend. However, even routine screening prior to transplantation reveals only a small window in the patient's history and there is a substantial opportunity for undetected sensitization. Therefore, obtaining information about potentially sensitizing events in the patient's history will increase the accuracy of the assessment of risk. This chapter will deal with the technical aspects of obtaining the information necessary to evaluate humoral sensitization to HLA antigens in the transplant patient.

Authors' Note

The minimal testing requirements for compliance with the Clinical Laboratory Improvement Act (1988) can be found in the Code of Federal Regulations, subpart 42, section 493.1278, which can be accessed at http://www.gpoaccess.gov/ cfr/index.html; search for 42CFR493.1278. There has been an ongoing expression of concern by some regarding the expense of testing for humoral sensitization. A review of the literature provides extensive evidence of the benefit of such testing in prolonging graft and patient survival and reducing injurious rejection episodes. More recently, several centers have initiated treatment protocols designed to overcome sensitization, the single largest barrier to transplantation, and antibody testing provides a means to identify the best candidates for these protocols and to monitor treatment efficacy. Given the high cost of treatment for rejection, of reduced graft survival, and of alternative treatment when transplants fail, testing for antibodies is a very cost-effective investment.

METHODS

Creating a Patient Profile

Certain patient information is useful for quantifying the risk of rejection, assessing how aggressive a responder a patient is, and interpreting results of antibody tests. The applicable information is outlined in Table 1. The table is reasonably self-explanatory and merits only a few additional remarks. Information about previous sensitizing events can be used to achieve a gross assessment of how aggressively a patient responds to exposure to HLA. Patients with a previous graft in place have a source of antigen for maintaining sensitization but may have artificially low levels of antibodies because the donor tissue is acting like an immunologic sponge, removing antibodies by adsorption onto the antigens expressed on the tissue or releasing soluble antigens that bind to the antibodies. Samples should be obtained approximately 2 to 4 weeks after a transfusion to optimize detection of a humoral response. Transfusion histories are extremely difficult to obtain, are often inaccurate, and should be

TABLE 1 Patient information

Category	Information needed	Relevance
Diagnosis	Specific disease	Reflects likelihood of presence of autoantibodies
Previous transplants	No. and duration	Degree of immunologic insult; possibility of repeated exposure
	Kind and date of each	Immunogenicity and graft duration
	Current condition[a] of each	Potential source of antigen for maintaining sensitization or absorbing antibody
	HLA type of each	Identity of mismatched antigens
Pregnancies	No.	Potentially sensitizing events
	No. that went to full term	Increased potential for sensitization
	Identity of paternal HLA antigens	Identifies specificity of potentially sensitizing antigens
Transfusions	Occurrence of previous transfusions	Possible sensitization
	Date of most recent	Selection of serum for testing; interpretation of results
Surgeries	Kind and date of each	Possible source of unreported transfusions
Medications administered	Humanized antibodies	Cannot be readily removed
	Therapeutic monoclonal antibodies	Panreactive in lymphocyte-based assays
	Other cytotoxic drugs	May result in nonspecific cell death in lymphocyte-based assays
	Other drugs	Possible interference with assays
Recent immunologically stimulatory events	Infections	May result in lymphocyte-reactive antibodies that are not specific for HLA; may cause a polyclonal activation that results in recurrence or increase of HLA-specific antibodies; may result in cytokine release and increased expression of HLA antigens on donor tissue
	Trauma	
	Hormone therapy	

[a]Whether or not the graft has been removed.

supplemented with information about previous surgeries that might have been occasions for transfusion.

Tests

There are two categories of test used to assess a humoral response, the crossmatch and the antibody screen, the latter of which may be further subdivided into screens that test simply for the presence of antibody and those designed to provide antibody characterization.

Crossmatch Tests

The crossmatch test assesses the presence, in the recipient's serum, of antibody reactive with donor antigens. The most commonly used medium for the antigen is donor lymphocytes, which are readily obtainable and express HLA antigens at high levels, although other cells and tissues have been employed in specialized studies. Recently, efforts have been directed at using solubilized donor antigens as targets in solid-phase immunoassays, the advantages of which are discussed below in "Techniques for Testing Antibodies." In HLA-mismatched transplants that include substantial amounts of immunocompetent tissues, such as transplants of bone marrow and possibly lung and small bowel, a reverse crossmatch test involving donor serum and recipient cells is also appropriate since engrafted tissue from a sensitized donor could produce antibodies reactive with recipient HLA. Another antibody-mediated problem, transfusion-related acute lung injury (TRALI), can occur when transfused blood contains a substantial amount of antibody specific for the transfusion recipient's HLA antigens (10). Although a reverse crossmatch test could identify such situations, it is more efficient and economical to screen plasma units for the presence of HLA-specific antibody.

The advantages of the crossmatch test are that it measures reactivity with donor antigens directly and can be used to track the trend of anti-donor reactivity through serum titration. The disadvantages are that (i) when cellular targets are used, the test does not readily differentiate HLA-specific antibodies from other antibodies that bind to lymphocytes and (ii) donor cells are not always available at the necessary time or in sufficient quantities, although it may be possible to use cells from a surrogate donor, as will be discussed later. New crossmatching methods, solid-phase immunoassays that utilize solubilized donor HLA antigens as targets, may avoid some of the technical problems of lymphocyte-based assays while assessing donor specificity directly. The advantages and disadvantages of the various techniques are discussed further below.

Antibody Screens

An antibody screen is simply a crossmatch or series of crossmatches against individuals selected according to their HLA phenotypes to represent, collectively, most HLA antigens. There are two types of antibody screens, those that utilize a pool of antigens or cells from multiple individuals to determine the presence or absence of antibody and those that utilize a panel of individual phenotypes or antigens to determine the HLA specificities of the antibodies. The antibody screen has multiple advantages. It can be performed at any time prior to or following transplantation and, thus, prevent unnecessary donor testing and/or shipment of organs. It provides information useful in performing and interpreting the results of a crossmatch test, such as which sera represent the array of HLA antibodies that the patient has ever had, which sera might contain interfering antibodies such as

autoantibodies or therapeutic antibodies, what is the most informative crossmatch technique, and whether or not a positive crossmatch result is due to antibodies to the donor HLA antigens. When performed on sequential samples, it provides information about trends in antibody activity. Finally, it provides a means of recognizing when sensitizing events or sample switches might have occurred.

The major disadvantages of the antibody screen are that it neither tests donor cells nor defines antibody directly. That is, most antibody assignments are based on a statistically significant association between the positive reactions of the antibody and the presence of one or more antigens. The development of solid-phase immunoassays using single antigen targets resolves some of that problem, but as will be discussed below, these assays are not a fail-safe method of determining antibody specificity. The high polymorphism of the HLA system mandates the use of panels of 50 to 100 phenotypes to be able to determine HLA specificities reliably. Even then, it is difficult to characterize sera containing multiple antibodies since antibodies to three or four common antigens can render a serum panreactive. Tests using single, purified antigen targets should resolve this problem. However, at present, these reagents are not characterized well enough to provide a stand-alone, definitive method. It should be noted that although using an antibody screening technique that is more sensitive than the crossmatching technique may provide information about levels of DSA too low to be detected in the crossmatch test, using a screening technique that is less sensitive than the crossmatching technique may result in difficulty in interpreting a positive crossmatch result.

Techniques for Testing Antibodies

General Principles

There are two categories of antibody-testing techniques differentiated by type of target: (i) those that utilize cells as targets—namely, cytotoxicity testing and flow cytometry—and (ii) those that utilize soluble HLA molecules bound to a solid matrix. The relevant factors for each type of assay and their advantages and disadvantages are summarized in Tables 2 and 3 and discussed below.

Complement-dependent cytotoxicity tests detect antibodies through a secondary process—cell lysis by a complement which has been activated by antibodies bound to target cells. The test usually consists of a sensitization phase in which target cells and serum are incubated together, followed by the addition of complement and subsequent incubation to allow the complement to be activated by the bound antibody. Microscopic evaluation following the addition of a vital stain permits a gross estimation of the percentage of viable cells (9). The sensitivity of the assay can be modified by altering incubation times and temperatures, performing washes to remove anticomplementary factors, and adding an antiglobulin reagent to enhance complement activation. The test is routinely performed on lymphocytes, which are usually further fractionated into T- and B-lymphocyte populations. Each test uses cells from a single individual.

Cell-based flow cytometry is an indirect assay that measures the binding of antibody to cells through the use of an antiglobulin labeled with a fluorescent marker. The specificity of the antiglobulin reagent permits identification of the Ig class of cell-bound antibodies. Further characterization of the cells can be achieved by gating on cells defined by physical parameters and staining of cells with labeled monoclonal antibodies specific for markers that are unique to certain cell

TABLE 2 Assay characteristics

Factor	Cell-based assays		Solubilized antigen-based assays		
	Cytotoxicity	Flow cytometry	ELISA	Flow cytometry with beads	Luminex
Sensitivity	Low to moderate	High	High	High	High
HLA specificity	Low to moderate	Low to moderate	High	High	High
Isotype detection	Gross; requires serum manipulation	Determined by conjugate specificity	Determined by conjugate specificity	Determined by conjugate specificity	Determined by conjugate specificity
Cost	Low	High	Moderate to high	High	High
Automation	None	Partial	Partial	Partial	Partial
Throughput	Can test multiple sera simultaneously but not rapidly	Limited	High	Limited	Very high

types. Although flow cytometric tests usually employ cells from a single individual, it has been demonstrated that the assay is sufficiently sensitive to detect antibody to cells from one subject in a mixture of cells pooled from up to six different individuals (19).

Solid-phase immunoassays utilize affinity-purified, soluble HLA antigens isolated from culture fluid or human plasma, solubilized from cell membranes, or synthesized via recombination technology. Several test methods are in current use. An enzyme-linked immunosorbent assay (ELISA) uses microtiter or microtest plates with the antigen bound to flat-bottom wells. After the addition of test serum to the wells, the presence of HLA-specific antibody is detected by the addition of an enzyme-conjugated antiglobulin and a chromogenic substrate which results in a color change in wells containing bound HLA-specific antibody. The antigens may be from a single individual or may be pooled from multiple individuals who, collectively, represent all or nearly all HLA antigens, and they may be of a single HLA class or a combination of HLA class I and HLA class II antigens (9, 25). The assay can be read manually, but the use of an auto-

mated reader increases sensitivity and provides finer quantification of the reactions. HLA antigens bound to 5.6-μm-diameter polystyrene beads are employed in two different formats: standard flow cytometry and the Luminex format (4). In standard flow cytometry, a single dye is incorporated into beads in different concentrations to permit differentiation of beads bearing different antigens or antigen combinations. In the Luminex format, two different dyes, each at 10 different dilutions, are incorporated into beads to provide up to 100 different beads differentiated by color. The beads are examined in a specific instrument in which one laser is used to identify the particular bead and another is used to detect the presence of a fluorochrome-conjugated antiglobulin that has bound to the human antibody on the bead. The beads may be coated with pooled class I or class II antigens, antigens from class I or class II phenotypes, or antigens of a single HLA specificity.

Advantages and Disadvantages

Two of the major advantages of the cytotoxicity assay stem from its use for more than three decades: (i) it is usually

TABLE 3 Advantages and disadvantages of different assays

	Cytotoxicity	Flow cytometry	Solid-phase immunoassay
Advantages	No additional training needed Can adjust sensitivity 35 years of experience No special equipment needed Inexpensive; can run multiple dilutions for little additional cost	High sensitivity Can select isotype detected Simultaneous analysis of multiple cell types	High sensitivity Eliminates reactivity of non-HLA-specific antibodies Partial automation possible Readily distinguishes between cI- and cII-specific antibodies
Disadvantages	Extra manipulation required to differentiate between cI- and cII-specific antibodies Need adequate number of viable lymphocytes Does not readily distinguish HLA-specific antibodies from other lymphocyte-reactive antibodies Does not detect extremely low levels of antibody	Requires expensive equipment Cost of reagents Need adequate number of viable lymphocytes Does not readily distinguish HLA-specific antibodies from other lymphocyte-reactive antibodies Software may not interface with existing database	May require additional training Reagents can be expensive May get interference from immune complexes, high levels of IgM, or discoloration of serum Extensive quality control needed No reasonable way to assess levels of various antigens present Software may not interface with existing database

a standard test in laboratories performing histocompatibility tests for transplantation, and (ii) all the test variables, factors affecting the test, and quality control requirements have been well characterized. The test utilizes very small volumes of test materials (1 to 2 μl of serum and 2,000 to 2,500 cells per reaction) and is relatively inexpensive to run. Multiple serum samples can be tested at multiple dilutions, providing information about antibody titers and trends for one or multiple patients. Despite these advantages, however, the test has many shortcomings. It requires an adequate supply of viable lymphocytes, separate testing of T and B lymphocytes, and removal of class I-specific antibodies to identify class II-specific antibodies; depends on the activity of the complement, which is a highly variable and labile reagent; requires adequate amounts of the heterophile antibody found in rabbit serum used routinely as the complement source; is not sufficiently sensitive to detect extremely low levels of antibodies; and, most importantly, does not readily differentiate between HLA-specific and other lymphocyte-binding antibodies. Antibodies that may interfere in the assay include autoantibodies, therapeutic antibodies that react with all or some subsets of lymphocytes, and some anti-Lewis antibodies. Spurious reactions with B lymphocytes have been attributed to anti-viral antibodies. A gross evaluation of the class of antibody reactive in the assay is possible through inactivation of IgM with reducing reagents or heat aggregation. However, neither technique will completely abrogate the reactivity of high levels of IgM.

Cell-based flow cytometry provides a high degree of sensitivity, permits simultaneous analysis of multiple cell types without the need for separation of cells, and facilitates determination of Ig class through the selection of antiglobulin specificity. However, like the cytotoxicity assay, it requires an adequate number of viable cells and does not readily differentiate between HLA-specific and other lymphocyte-binding antibodies that either are of human origin or have been humanized. Further, it requires expensive equipment and specialized training and utilizes expensive reagents.

Solid-phase immunoassays using purified HLA antigens combine a high degree of sensitivity with increased specificity. We have found the sensitivity of ELISA to be comparable to that of cell-based flow cytometry (11, 25) and Luminex tests to be more sensitive. Solid-phase immunoassays readily distinguish between class I- and class II-specific antibodies by using antigens of only one class in a single test. Further, these assays provide a more refined quantification of reactivity with the different phenotypes, which enhances the characterization of antibody specificity. The solid-phase immunoassays have demonstrated an immunity to interference from a variety of non-HLA-specific antibodies, including therapeutic antibodies, including therapeutic antibodies specific for non-HLA lymphocyte surface markers. The high sensitivity of solid-phase immunoassays makes it possible to detect an antibody to a single antigen when a sample is tested against a pool of antigens. This is in contrast to the requirement for performing multiple tests against a variety of individual phenotypes in the cytotoxicity assay or against several sets each composed of a limited number of different phenotypes in the flow cytometric assay. The ability to test against pooled antigens represents a potential for substantial cost savings when sera are tested in batches. Further, beads differentiated by color permit multiple tests to run in a single assay that uses a very small serum volume. These assays have the potential of contributing substantially to our knowledge about the humoral response to HLA antigens and about the immunologic structure of the HLA molecule. However, solid-phase immunoassays are not without

disadvantages. These include a potential need for additional equipment and training, increased reagent cost for some of the assays, and a need for extensive quality control. The high sensitivity of these tests contributes to increased variability and necessitates extensive experience to optimize interpretation and use of the test results. Nonspecific binding of Ig may occur when the test serum contains immune complexes or aggregated Ig, rendering the test invalid. It has been found that high levels of IgM antibodies can affect test results, even when an IgG-specific antiglobulin is used (11). In assays using individual phenotypes, there is no way to ensure that each antigen of the phenotype is present in an adequate quantity. This may be a problem when the antigens are obtained from cell lines that may undergo mutation or viral transformation that affects synthesis of one or more antigens or when natural allele- and locus-specific variability affects antigen expression. There may not be uniform amounts of antigens among different beads that are each coated with HLA molecules of one specificity. HLA molecules may be distorted upon binding to a solid matrix, resulting in the loss of some epitopes or the creation of others. Finally, in any assay with computer-generated results, there is a potential for a problem in interfacing with the laboratory's existing database.

Quality Control

Crossmatch

There are three quality control procedures relevant to the crossmatch test. The objective of the first is to ensure that the cells being tested are from the right individual, which can be achieved by performing HLA typing in parallel to and with the same cells used in the crossmatch test. The objective of the second is to identify reactivity due to non-HLA-specific antibodies. Some of these antibodies, namely, autoantibodies and therapeutic lymphocyte-reactive antibodies, can be detected by performing an autologous crossmatch test. Finally, if one is using the crossmatch test to track the course of an antibody, including as a reference a serum sample that was previously tested by the same technique will provide a measure of variability in sensitivity.

Antibody Screen

Even though a positive control is included in all tests, it usually is not adequate to detect small variations in sensitivity. Such variations could result in a failure to detect antibodies present in levels that are at the border of the test's sensitivity. Inclusion of one or more well-characterized sera diluted to levels near their endpoints of reactivity would provide a means of recognizing this degree of variability.

Cytotoxicity Assay

Information about the cytotoxicity assay and relevant quality control measures is available in two excellent sources (8, 22), and we mention here only a few items particularly important in tests of antibodies.

Frequently, different lymphocyte subsets are used in the cytotoxicity test because of differences in the expression of various antigens. It is helpful to include controls specific for these subsets to estimate the relative purity of the cell preparation and detect contamination with unwanted cell types. These controls are usually monoclonal antibodies specific for a cell surface marker unique to or predominant in a certain cell type and most often are designed to identify T and B lymphocytes and, occasionally, monocytes.

Addition of an antiglobulin reagent is a frequent modification of the cytotoxicity test used for antibody detection. In these cases, it is important to include a control to validate the presence and efficacy of the antiglobulin reagent. This control should be a serum sample that activates complement only in the presence of the antiglobulin reagent.

Most background cell death (i.e., cell death not mediated by HLA-specific antibodies) is detected in the negative control wells. However, there may be occasions, particularly in the crossmatch test, that warrant additional discrimination. In these cases, the question of whether cell death is mediated by antibodies or not can be resolved by running a parallel test using a heat-inactivated (56°C for 30 min) complement.

Solid-Phase Immunoassays

Reagents

There are a number of factors that can contribute to variability among test reagent lots, including (i) changes in any component that affects test sensitivity, (ii) variability in the preparation procedures for one or more individual phenotypes, (iii) contamination of or absence of antigen in one or more wells of an ELISA plate or on one or more beads, (iv) changes in a cell line used as a source of antigens, and (v) manufacturing differences in the solid-phase media used. In turn, these factors can affect the threshold value for a positive test result, the background reactivity associated with an individual phenotype, and the ability of the antigens of an individual phenotype to yield a positive reaction with a specific antibody. Some of this variability can be assessed by testing each lot of reagents with a panel of well-characterized sera that includes sera known to contain HLA-specific antibodies as well as some known to lack such antibodies. In addition, each lot of reagents should be monitored throughout the course of its use to determine if the correct value has been selected as the threshold for a positive reaction and to determine if antigens of any individual phenotype are demonstrating an inordinate number of reactions that are discordant with the assigned antibody specificity (25). Recent reports have shown that normalizing reaction data to the amount of antigen present improves the interpretation of the results. It is likely that this sort of normalization is best conducted by the manufacturer on each lot of reagents rather than by each individual user, providing uniform standardization while minimizing the additional cost.

Tests

Batch tests of sera against pooled antigens provide little or no opportunity for detecting slight variations in test sensitivity or operator error such as sample switching or dilution error. Inclusion of two or more blinded characterized sera serves as a quality control measure of the test system as well as of testing personnel. The sera should vary in strength to provide a meaningful assessment of test sensitivity and should vary from run to run to serve as meaningful unknowns. Background reactivity may be caused by a variety of factors, including high IgM levels and immune complexes, among others. Background reactivity can result in false negatives when it occurs in the negative controls and false positives when it occurs in the test wells or beads. There are commercially available blocking agents designed to reduce nonspecific reactivity. Certain patients, notably those undergoing hemapheresis or plasmapheresis, have reduced background reactivity. In assays that use beads, the wash technique must be appropriate and consistent to avoid variable loss of beads. Of course, standard quality assurance measures, particularly instrument calibration, are essential to ensure consistent and reproducible results. Quality control factors relevant to tests of antibodies are summarized in Table 4.

TEST VALIDATION

The requirements for validation of laboratory assays are described in detail in the federal regulations (see above). Testing for HLA antibodies is confounded by the complexity of the HLA system and the antibody response to HLA antigens and by the lack of reference antibodies. Therefore, test validation can be prolonged and costly. To optimize evaluation of the assays and the clinical utility of the data generated, there should be an ongoing comparison of the

TABLE 4 Quality control factors

Test	Variable	Quality control measure	Purpose
Crossmatching	Cell identity	Serologic typing performed simultaneously with crossmatching	Verify identity of cells used in crossmatch test
	Antibody specificity	Autologous crossmatching	Test for presence of non-HLA-specific antibody
	Titer	Use of reference (previously tested serum)	Account for day-to-day variability
Antibody screening	Test sensitivity	Testing of serum at threshold of reactivity	Test for small variations in assay sensitivity
Cytotoxicity	Cell type	Use of cell-specific antibody	Assess proportion of different cell types in preparation
	Antiglobulin level	Use of antiglobulin-dependent serum	Test efficacy of antiglobulin reagent
	Cause of cell death	Heat inactivation of complement	Abolish antibody-mediated cell death
Solid-phase immunoassays	Presence or absence of nonspecific binding	Use of antigen-free matrix (well or bead)	Measure extent of nonspecific binding
	Phenotype validation	Use of panel of known sera	Test for presence of expected phenotypes
	Threshold for defining positive reaction	Ongoing comparison to results of other assays	Determine if value for positive reaction is correct
	Technical errors	Use of blinded controls	Determine if expected results are obtained

results of various tests—can the crossmatch test and anti-body screen results for a specimen be reconciled? These comparisons reflect the sensitivities and specificities of the various assays. A frequently asked question is how many sera need to be tested for validation of an antibody screen assay. This question is impossible to answer with a specific number because of the thousands of possible combinations of antibodies that can be present in a specimen. The practical answer is that the validation must generate enough data for the user to be able to interpret the test results reliably. Some aspects of an assay's performance may be detectable only after extensive testing. Therefore, evaluation of an assay should continue after sufficient testing has been performed to place the assay into clinical use with confidence.

INTERPRETATION

Antibody Screen

Data Obtained

Five types of data may be obtained from antibody screens: (i) the strength of individual reactions, (iii) Ig isotype, (iii) titer, (iv) percent panel-reactive antibody (PRA), and (v) HLA specificity. Positive reactions of a serum sample with antigens of a variety of phenotypes may vary in strength because of differences among phenotypes in the number of antigens to which the serum contains antibodies; because of normal variability in antigen expression among individuals, cell types, and antigens and within an individual from day to day; and because of differences in the numbers and titers of various antibodies within a serum sample. There are abundant data regarding variability in antigen expression on cells. Class I antigens are expressed at higher levels on B cells than on T cells. Among various loci, HLA-C antigens are expressed at lower levels than are HLA-A and -B locus antigens and antigens encoded by DRB3 and -4 (and possibly -5) loci (DRw52, -53, and -51, respectively) are expressed at approximately 15 to 20% of the level of the DRB1-encoded antigens (DR1 to DR18). In tests of pooled antigens, differences in reaction scores obtained with different serum samples from the same individual reflect differences in the breadths of antibody specificities. Among sera from different individuals, these differences are determined by both the breadth of antibodies and the frequencies of the antigens in the pool. In tests of individual phenotypes, stronger reactions are obtained with phenotypes that are homozygous for a target antigen or that have more than one target antigen. This, in turn, may be useful in verifying antibody specificities. Quantification of the strength of reactivity is more refined in solid-phase immunoassays and flow cytometry than in cytotoxicity testing, and this information may be useful in confirming putative assignments of antibody specificity. Determining the molecular equivalents of soluble fluorochromes (MESFs) for flow cytometric or Luminex results permits comparison of test results from specimen to specimen and day to day. To determine MESFs, a standard calibration curve is created using beads labeled with different known amounts of a fluorochrome. The MESF value for a test serum is then obtained from the standard curve by interpolating the fluorescent channel values of the serum (18).

Ig isotype is most precisely defined in adherence assays that use an isotype-specific antiglobulin. In cytotoxicity

assays, the Ig class may be approximated by heating serum (63°C for 10 min) or by adding reducing reagents to inactivate IgM. However, both methods have limited efficacy. Titer determination is easily achieved by testing serum at multiple dilutions.

The PRA is obtained by using the following equation:

$$\text{PRA} = \frac{\text{number of phenotypes with positive reactions}}{\text{total number of phenotypes tested}} \times 100$$

This statistic is frequently misinterpreted as an indicator of antibody titer, of changes in antibody reactivity in an individual over time, and of the likelihood of a positive crossmatch. PRA may reflect changes in antibody specificities over time but only if the phenotype panel remains constant, and then only when the loss of some antibodies is not compensated for by the addition of others with different specificities. The phenotypes in antibody screening panels are usually selected to optimize identification of antibody specificity and rarely, if ever, reflect the distribution of phenotypes and antigens in the donor population. Thus, PRA is a poor predictor of crossmatch outcome. However, identifying the HLA-specific antibodies in a serum sample permits one to calculate the probability of a positive crossmatch (27). Accurate characterization of the HLA-specific antibodies in a serum sample may provide the most valuable information for transplantation purposes. This information can be used to (i) reduce cold ischemia time by preventing the unnecessary shipment of organs and crossmatch testing of patients incompatible with a specific donor, (ii) avoid incorrectly passing over a sensitized patient by recognizing donors to whom the patient has no antibodies, (iii) determine the clinical relevance of a positive crossmatch by recognizing if the reactivity is due to HLA-specific antibodies or not, and (iv) permit preemptive treatment to avoid antibody-mediated rejection by detecting DSA present at levels too low to be detected in the crossmatch test and/or formed de novo after transplantation.

Phenotype Panel

In tests to determine antibody specificity, the most critical factor is the panel of phenotypes used. There are several goals to consider in establishing a panel, and these goals are often at odds with one another. The HLA antigens, collectively, should include the array of antigens in the donor population and occur in patterns that permit differentiation among antibodies of various specificities. The strong linkage disequilibrium of the HLA system may make it difficult to find a phenotype bearing an antigen without another with which it is frequently associated, such as B8 without A1. This problem is even more pronounced for HLA class II antigens. Also, some antigens are rare and may not be readily available for inclusion in a panel. Fortunately, antibodies to these antigens are also rare and reactivity is usually due to an antibody specific for an epitope shared with another, more common antigen. For example, reactivity with A36 occurs with antibodies specific for A1 and reactivity with B81 is usually mediated by an antibody to an epitope shared with B7. Thus, the absence of a rare antigen from a panel may be accommodated if one is willing to accept an antibody to a common antigen as evidence of sensitization to a rare, cross-reactive antigen.

Sensitized individuals, particularly those sensitized via transplantation, often display broad reactivity. This may be due to either a large number of antibodies to different antigens or a small number of antibodies to epitopes shared among several antigens (7). In either case, precise definition of the antibody specificities may require tests against a large number of phenotypes. Establishing, maintaining, and using such a large panel are usually cost prohibitive. In some cases, information regarding antibody specificity may be obtained from other sources, such as crossmatch tests or special studies, but the possibility that a patient has unrecognized HLA-specific antibodies must always be considered. In these cases, solid-phase immunoassays that use single antigen targets may help resolve questions about critical antibodies.

Solid-phase immunoassays using purified, single HLA molecules as targets are available from more than one supplier; however, precise information about the quantity of each antigen and the extent to which structural conformation may have been compromised is not readily available. Further, when single-antigen reagents are used, the determination of the presence or absence of a particular antibody may rely on only a single reaction. In these cases, a technical failure that involves a key antigen could have serious consequences. Therefore, single-antigen reagents are probably best used as an adjunct to other antibody tests, in particular when other assays do not provide a clear identification of antibody specificities.

Specificity Determination

When a serum sample is tested against a variety of phenotypes, the basis of specificity determination is the association between the occurrence of an antigen and the reactivity of the serum. This can be demonstrated diagrammatically and defined statistically. The association can be shown in either of two ways for the purposes of statistical analysis. The first is a 2×2 table.

		Antigen	
		+	−
Serum	+	a	b	A
	−	c	d	B
		C	D	n

The composition of the 2×2 table is as follows. The concordant reactions, when antigen and serum reactivity are both either present (+) or absent (−), are represented in cells a and d, respectively. The discordant reactions are those in which the serum yields a positive reaction in the absence of the antigen, represented in cell b, and in which the serum yields a negative reaction in the presence of the antigen, represented in cell c. The capital letters A to D represent the marginal totals (e.g., A = a + b), and n is the total sample size (n = A + B = C + D). The values are used in the statistics described below. The 2×2 data can also be presented in a linear display, shown here.

	Serum versus antigen			
Specificity	++	+−	−+	−−
	a	b	c	d

Note that the heading of this display, serum versus antigen, specifies the reaction order. That is, in the third column, "+−" means that the serum is serum positive and the antigen is absent (negative).

A correlation coefficient (r) or chi-squared (χ^2) value can be calculated (2) from these data by using the equations shown below.

$$r = \frac{ad - bc}{\sqrt{ABCD}} \quad \text{or} \quad \chi^2 = \frac{n(ad - bc)^2}{ABCD}$$

The P values for the correlation coefficient are affected by the sample size, and for the chi-squared statistic, they are affected by the degrees of freedom, which are always 1 for a 2×2 table. These values can be found in standard statistical tables (6), and a few are given here.

Statistic	Probability			
	0.05	0.02	0.01	0.001
χ^2	3.841	5.412	6.635	10.827
r (n = 40)	0.304	0.358	0.393	0.490
r (n = 50)	0.273	0.322	0.354	0.443

Either statistic can be used, and the two are algebraically related when an uncorrected chi-squared value is calculated (i.e., $\chi^2 = r^2 n$). The correlation coefficient yields values on a scale of −1 to +1, with +1 and −1 reflecting complete positive and negative associations, respectively, and 0 being the absence of an association. The chi-squared numerical value can range from zero to infinity and varies with different values of n. Thus, the values cannot be compared meaningfully for sera tested against panels of different sizes. Although r values greater than 0.3 are statistically significant for panels in which n is ≥ 40, it is difficult to assign specificities with confidence with correlations below 0.5. In our experience, 95% of assignments have r of ≥ 0.5 and 85% had r of ≥ 0.6. One is more willing to accept correlations with lower values when there are other supportive data. For example, if the titer of an antibody decreases over time, the correlation will diminish with increasing numbers of false negatives. However, the remaining reactivity provides evidence of the antibody's continued presence.

Diagrams showing comparisons of antigen and serum reaction patterns are provided in Fig. 1 to 4. In all the figures, the panel members' phenotypes are shown in the columns, the columns collectively represent the entire panel, and the rows indicate the presence or absence of specific antigens in

phenotype	1	2	3	4	5	6	7	8	9	10	11	12	13	14	15	16	17	18	19	20	21	22	23	24	25	26	27	28	29	30	31	32	33	34	35	36	37	38	39	40	41	42	43	44	45	46	47	48
A2	X				X	X								X											X		X		X														X					
serum 1	X				X	X								X											X		X		X														X					

FIGURE 1 Determination of specificity: serum 1. Reactions and presence of antigen are indicated by X.

phenotype	1	2	3	4	5	6	7	8	9	10	11	12	13	14	15	16	17	18	19	20	21	22	23	24	25	26	27	28	29	30	31	32	33	34	35	36	37	38	39	40	41	42	43	44	45	46	47	48
A9		X								X						X	X	X	X							X					X	X						X						X				X
B35		X	X													X	X														X			X	X									X				
serum 2 vs. A9		X		X				X		X						X	X	X	O							X					X	O		X				X				X		X				O
serum 2 vs. B35		X	O	X				X		X						X	X	X								X					X			X	X	O		X				X		X				

FIGURE 2 Determination of specificity: serum 2, first iteration. Reactions and presence of antigen are indicated by X. Shading of boxes representing serum reactions corresponds to antigen specificity indicated by similar shading. False-positive reactions for assigned specificities are indicated by boldfaced X's. False-negative reactions for assigned specificities are indicated by O.

the phenotypes and the reactivity of test sera with the phenotypes. For economy of space, only specificities being discussed are shown. For example, in Fig. 2, phenotype 1 has neither A9 nor B35, phenotype 2 has both, and phenotype 3 has B35 but not A9. In Fig. 1, it can be seen that the pattern of reactivity of serum 1 with the panel is identical to the pattern of occurrence of the A2 antigen on the panel. The linear display of this association and the 2×2 table are given below.

Serum versus antigen

Specificity	++	+−	−+	−−	r
A2	8	0	0	40	1.0

HLA-A2

		+	−	
Serum 1	+	8	0	8
	−	0	40	40
		8	40	48

There are 8 concordant positives, 40 concordant negatives, and no false positives or false negatives.

Unfortunately, most sera do not yield such unambiguous patterns of reactivity. A more typical example is shown in Fig. 2. We have shown the patterns of the two antigens, A9 and B35, that have the strongest associations with the serum reaction pattern. The 2×2 data and correlations are as follows.

Serum versus antigen

Specificity	++	+−	−+	−−	r
A9	9	4	3	32	0.62
B35	6	7	2	33	0.48

Although both correlations are highly significant statistically, neither is convincing. Both sera have a substantial number of discordant reactions. Since no better correlation was found with a single antigen, the next step is to look for one or more additional antigen patterns that account for the false positives. The high degree of homology among HLA antigens has resulted in sharing of antigenic epitopes among groups of antigens—the so-called cross-reactive groups of antigens, or CREGs. These shared epitopes are also referred to as public determinants, and those unique to a single antigen are referred to as private determinants (15). Antibodies produced in response to sensitization with HLA antigens are often specific for public determinants (16). A9 has been associated with two major CREGs, A2-A9-A28 and A1-A9. Figure 3 shows that neither of these CREGs can account for the serum reactivity. The serum has failed to react with any A1s; A2 accounts for one of the false positives, but the serum missed six other A2s and all three A28s. However, when we examine the B35 CREG (Fig. 4), we see an excellent correlation between the serum reactivity and this group of antigens as shown below.

Serum versus antigen

Specificity	++	+−	−+	−−	r
B35 (6 of 8); 53 (4 of 4); 70 (3 of 3)	12	1	2	33	0.85

Numbers in parentheses indicate the number of positive reactions out of the total number of antigen occurrences.

Note that the correlation coefficient has been calculated for the CREG rather than for each antigen within the CREG. We believe that this provides a more accurate assessment of the serum reactivity.

Reactivity strength in cytotoxicity assays is measured on a discontinuous scale in which the percentages of dead cells are grouped into five categories. There are a large number of

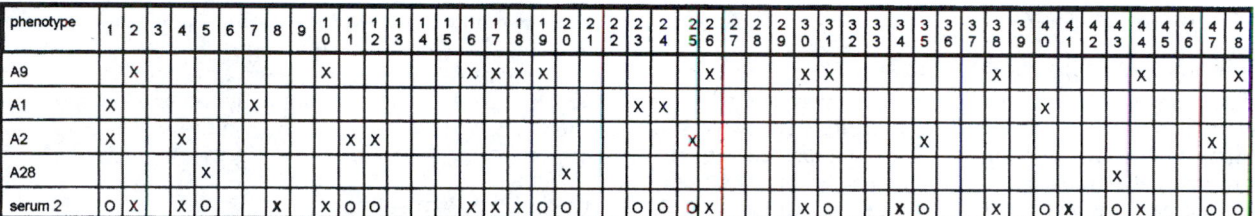

FIGURE 3 Determination of specificity: serum 2, A9 CREGs. Reactions and presence of antigen indicated by X. False-negative reactions for assigned specificities are indicated by boldfaced X's. False-negative reactions for assigned specificities are indicated by O.

phenotype	1	2	3	4	5	6	7	8	9	10	11	12	13	14	15	16	17	18	19	20	21	22	23	24	25	26	27	28	29	30	31	32	33	34	35	36	37	38	39	40	41	42	43	44	45	46	47	48
B35		X	X														X	X												X				X	X									X				
B53					X		X																			X																	X				
B70				X			X																															X										
serum 2		X	O	X			X		X							X	X	X								X			X					X	O			X					X		X			

FIGURE 4 Determination of specificity: serum 2, B35 CREGs. Reactions and presence of antigen are indicated by X. Shading of boxes representing serum reactions corresponds to antigen specificity indicated by similar shading. False-positive reactions for assigned specificities are indicated by bold-faced X's. False-negative reactions for assigned specificities are indicated by O.

variables that can affect the assessed strengths of reactions in a cytotoxicity assay, including day-to-day variability in test conditions and variability among technologists in assessing reaction strengths. Reaction strength is measured on a continuous scale in solid-phase immunoassays, reaction results can be instrument read, and all phenotypes are tested simultaneously. The effect of this is that when the results are listed in descending order of reaction strength, the positively reacting phenotypes are often grouped by target antigen. This facilitates identification of at least some of the antibody specificities. Specificity determination is not an exact science; however, several things can be done to increase the accuracy of the interpretation. We have shown here the value of considering cross-reactivity. Another step is taking into account the phenotype of the person whose serum is being tested, since individuals do not normally make antibodies to their own HLA antigens. Tracking patients' reactivity patterns over time and identifying the phenotypes of the sources of sensitization, particularly transplantation and pregnancy, can provide confirmation of tentative specificity assignments. As noted earlier, the strongest reactions in solid-phase immunoassays are usually with phenotypes that correspond to two or more antigens with which the serum is reactive. For example, for a serum specimen with antibodies to A2 and A9, when the reactions are listed by strength, the phenotypes at the top of the list are likely to be those having both A2 and A9 or homozygous for one or the other, followed by those having A2 but not A9 and then those having A9 without A2. For broadly reactive sera, some specificities can be identified by testing the sera at multiple dilutions since different antibodies in the sera are likely to be present at different titers. In the example given here, the reactions at a 1:8 dilution may be limited to A2-bearing phenotypes and the undiluted serum reacts with all phenotypes having either A2 or A9. Importantly, however, one should avoid the temptation of trying to account for each serum reaction and assign only those specificities that can be assigned with confidence. Additional specialized techniques discussed later in this chapter may be useful in cases in which it may be crucial to confirm the presence or absence of a particular antibody.

Computerized Specificity Analysis

Most computerized analysis programs perform what is referred to as a tail analysis. This is an iterative process in which the pattern of serum reactivity is compared with the patterns of all of the various antigens. The specificity yielding the highest statistical value above a designated threshold is assigned, and then the positive reactions attributable to the assigned specificity are deleted from both the antigen patterns and the serum reaction pattern. The pattern of the remaining reactions is then compared to the abridged set of antigen patterns, and the process is repeated to a designated end point. Unaccounted-for serum reactions are the tail, and the phenotypes of these are then printed out. The problem with this approach is well illustrated in the example of serum 2, shown above. In this case, the A9 specificity would have been assigned, eliminating five of the eight B35 phenotypes, two of five B53s, and one of three B70s, leaving those three antigens with correlation coefficients of 0.30, 0.67, and 0.67, respectively. The most likely computer-assigned specificity would be A9, B53, and B70, with r of 0.80. Clearly, further investigation of this serum would reveal that the presence of antibodies to B35, B53, and B70 is more likely statistically and more logical biologically. Several steps can be taken to overcome this problem, at least in part. CREG patterns could be used for analysis in addition to the antigen patterns. Rather than having accounted-for reactions eliminated, the next most likely specificity could be added and the correlation with the collective specificities could be determined at each step. Finally, one could simply have a list of all the specificities yielding a certain degree of correlation printed out and then direct the computer to analyze for correlations with certain groups of antigens. The problem with any approach is simply that computer programs deal with algorithms, not biology. Thus, computer assignments should not be accepted without manual review of the data.

Crossmatch Test

There are two levels of interpretation to be considered in the crossmatch test: whether or not the test result is positive and what the test result means clinically. Although it is possible to detect cell death and changes in either optical density or fluorescence, the lack of reference reagents has made it impossible to determine what amount of antibody yields what degree of reactivity in any of the assays used. This is further complicated by test variability within and among assays, among laboratories using the same assay, and among treatment protocols and transplantation practices. Therefore, most interpretation is based on clinical outcome. Unfortunately, many of the studies performed to correlate crossmatch results with clinical outcome have not controlled for many of the relevant variables, including (i) timing of acquisition of the serum specimen relative to transplantation, (ii) Ig class of the antibody, (iii) antibody specificity, and (iv) antibody titer. Therefore, the conclusions of these studies are frequently in conflict with one another.

Specialized Procedures

Serum Absorption

Sera containing HLA class I-specific antibodies will react with both T and B cells, confounding the identification of class II-specific antibodies in cell-based assays. When solid-phase immunoassays are not an option for testing for class II-specific antibodies, sera can be absorbed with pooled platelets to remove the class I-specific antibodies. Platelets do not actively synthesize HLA molecules and lose them from their surface over time. Therefore, the age of the platelets will affect their efficacy. The pool should also comprise platelets from a number of individuals sufficient to provide a reasonable assurance that the major HLA specificities are represented (17).

It may be desirable to remove selected HLA-specific antibodies from a serum sample. This can be achieved by absorbing with cells (platelets or lymphocytes) from a single individual. However, the limitations on the number of cells that can be obtained dictates absorbing very small volumes of serum, which in turn increases the risk of introducing a significant dilution factor. An alternative to absorption with cells is absorption with polystyrene beads to which solubilized HLA molecules have been affixed—although this may be cost prohibitive and the HLA molecules may have altered conformational epitopes. Following absorption, control cells must be tested to establish the efficacy of the absorption.

Tests with Selected Cells

Improved characterization of antibody specificity in sera containing multiple antibodies can be achieved by testing such sera against cells selected to have specific, limited antigenic differences from those of the serum donor. Cells can be selected as surrogates for those of a potential or real donor when the donor cells are not available, as frequently occurs with deceased donors. One might select certain types of cells for their particular antigen expression patterns. For example, B cells express both HLA-DR and HLA-DQ antigens. Monocytes express HLA-DR, but only 10% of monocytes express HLA-DQ, providing a means of differentiating antibodies specific for these different sets of class II antigens.

Dealing with Non-HLA-Specific Antibodies

Among the most common interfering antibodies occurring prior to transplantation are autoantibodies. Many of these antibodies are IgM and can be eliminated by heat inactivation or reduction. However, these techniques will not completely abolish reactivity when the antibody is present at high titer, and absorption with autologous cells, more-effective techniques to eliminate IgM such as chromatography and dialysis (1), or tests that use an isotype-specific conjugate may be necessary in order to achieve a meaningful crossmatch. The large IgM molecule may block IgG binding. This can be overcome, in part, by performing the serum-cell incubation at 37°C, a temperature that favors binding of IgG. Autoantibodies of the IgG class are less common but do occur and are much more problematic in tests. The removal of these antibodies requires absorption. Periodically, autoantibodies will be present in a donor otherwise appearing to be healthy. This circumstance is suggested when tests of donor cells persistently yield low background reactivity in the negative controls of cytotoxicity tests despite consistently good pretest viability. When this situation is suspected, it is worthwhile to do a donor autocrossmatch test for confirmation.

Therapeutic antibodies are problematic in cell-based assays. When the antibodies are of nonhuman origin, they can be removed by absorption with magnetic beads coated with a species-specific antiglobulin or the interference can be overcome by performing flow cytometry with antiglobulin reagents that have been absorbed to remove reactivity with all but human Ig. The increasing number of humanized antibodies in use, however, is problematic for cell-based assays.

These antibodies may be reactive in cell-based assays for months after the cessation of treatment. In some cases, the target antigen may be removed from the cell surface, abolishing antibody activity. For example, pronase treatment of B cells removes CD20, the target of rituximab, among other cell surface molecules (24). Pronase-treated cells can then be run in a flow cytometric assay, but the treatment usually renders the cells too fragile for use in a cytotoxicity assay. When the antibody target cannot be removed, absorption with cells bearing the target antigen but lacking donor HLA antigens becomes the only recourse.

APPLICATION

Whom To Test

Three groups of patients are at high risk for an adverse effect of HLA-specific antibodies: organ transplant recipients, patients receiving platelet and/or leukocyte support, and patients receiving HLA-disparate bone marrow transplants. In the case of bone marrow transplants, both the donor and recipient should be tested. A fourth group of patients are those at risk for TRALI (see above). Although this is a serious condition and responsible for more than 10% of transfusion-related fatalities, the incidence is low (<0.5% of all patients transfused) and can be averted by having plasma screened for HLA- and granulocyte-specific antibodies.

When To Test

Conventional wisdom and federal regulations indicate that testing should be performed at regular intervals prior to transplantation and following sensitizing events. Unfortunately, we do not always know about sensitizing events and it is becoming increasingly apparent that we have not identified all possible sensitizing events. Clearly, data from apparently nontransfused patients and evidence of similarities between microbial proteins and HLA antigens indicate that there may be much broader potential for sensitization or reactivation of a humoral response than has been previously appreciated (14). Further, inflammation itself may generate polyclonal B-cell activation that results in the production of HLA-specific antibodies.

It has been suggested that the low rate of sensitization and increasing waiting times dictate testing only when transplantation is imminent. Most data on sensitization are from cytotoxicity testing, and increased use of the more sensitive and specific solid-phase immunoassays indicates that the percentage of patients sensitized may be grossly underestimated (4). Antibody screening can be performed at a low absolute cost and at a cost much lower than that of other components of transplantation. Antibody screening provides information important to selecting patients and sera for and interpreting the results of a crossmatch test and can provide advance notice of the presence of factors, such as autoantibodies, that may adversely affect interpretation of the crossmatch results. Therefore, it would seem that trying to reduce costs by eliminating access to the important information obtained from antibody screening is penny wise and pound foolish.

Special considerations apply to patients being treated in a protocol designed to reduce or eliminate humoral sensitization and will be discussed in a separate section below.

Perhaps one of the greatest and most costly deficiencies of the present standard of practice is the lack of adequate posttransplantation testing, which results from the lack of financial reimbursement for such testing. Three factors argue in favor of such testing: (i) there are now treatment protocols that produce a durable elimination of DSA, (ii) assays presently available are sufficiently sensitive to detect antibodies before a transplanted organ suffers extensive injury, and (iii) prolonging graft survival by avoiding antibody-mediated rejection not only prevents returning a renal transplant patient to costly dialysis but also prevents increasing the number of patients awaiting transplantation.

How To Test

Good management practices dictate applying the minimal number of protocols uniformly to maximize cost saving. Having one or a small number of test protocols does save money in the laboratory, which should mean reduced laboratory charges. However, it is quite possible that this approach extracts a much greater cost in rejection, treatment for rejection, and reduced graft survival. It has been a costly lesson of medicine, learned over and over again, that the shotgun approach cannot be applied to complex issues. Given the complexity of transplantation, it is probably more cost-effective overall to customize testing according to the complexity and emergent nature of the case.

Monitoring for Desensitization Protocols

Patients with HLA-specific antibodies have access to transplantation reduced in proportion to the breadth of their sensitization and, as a group, have poorer graft outcomes. Several treatment protocols have been tried in attempts to achieve long-lasting reduction or elimination of HLA-specific antibodies. Presently, desensitization protocols can be grouped into two general categories: those that utilize high-dose (1 to 2 g/kg of body mass) pooled intravenous Ig (IVIg) and those that use plasmapheresis combined with low-dose (100 mg/kg) cytomegalovirus hyperimmune globulin or IVIg (13, 20, 23). The former is used to eliminate some or all HLA-specific antibodies of patients awaiting transplantation from either a live or deceased donor, the latter is used to down-regulate antibodies specific for a particular donor's HLA, and both are used for rescuing an organ undergoing antibody-mediated rejection. Both types of protocols require accurate identification of the patient's HLA-specific antibodies prior to treatment. The efficacy of the high-dose IVIg protocol can be predicted with in vitro testing (23). The ability of the IVIg reagent to block reactivity of the test serum in vitro correlates with its ability to down-regulate reactivity in vivo. The test must be performed in a fashion that avoids problems associated with the high Ig concentration. After there has been sufficient time after treatment for the serum Ig concentration to return to levels that do not affect testing, the efficacy of the treatment can be assessed with routine crossmatch or antibody screening assays.

The goals of monitoring for the plasmapheresis–low-dose cytomegalovirus hyperimmunoglobulin protocol are to determine the risk of antibody-mediated rejection, monitor treatment efficacy, and generate information that helps guide and fine-tune treatment (13, 20). The pretreatment evaluation of the patient consists of (i) identification of previous, potentially sensitizing events and the response to those events; (ii) creation of an immunologic profile of the present transplant (i.e., the number of current mismatches, the number to which the patient has antibodies, the immunogenicity of the mismatched antigens, and the occurrence of repeat mismatches); and (iii) determination of the specificity and strength of the DSA. The patient's antibodies should have been monitored during the pretransplantation period, and once treatment is started,

serum samples should be obtained before and after each treatment, immediately prior to transplant, and 48 to 72 h after treatment is stopped. The extent of treatment (the number of rounds of plasmapheresis and additional immunosuppressants) needed correlates most strongly with the titer of the DSA. Therefore, a crossmatch test to assess the titer should be performed at a time prior to the initiation of treatment that is sufficient to allow any needed adjustments in the treatment schedule. Once treatment is started, tests should be performed to monitor the course of the DSA. A cost- and time-efficient way to do this is to test all sera in a solid-phase immunoassay that uses pooled target antigens to chart the general trend of the antibodies and to monitor the strength of DSA by performing crossmatch or antibody identification tests on selected sera. Plasmapheresis removes many substances from the plasma, and background reactivity in solid-phase and flow cytometric assays usually decreases during treatment. This should be taken into account when the results of these assays are interpreted. There is a certain amount of day-to-day and technologist-to-technologist variability in the results of complement-dependent cytotoxicity crossmatch tests. This variability can be minimized to a certain extent by having the same technologist perform all crossmatch tests and including in each round of testing a reference serum, which would be a historic serum sample from the patient, with a known titer. Also, normalization of the data through the use of MESFs and other procedures will facilitate a more meaningful interpretation of test results. The data that should be examined are (i) the overall trend of the DSA titer and (ii) the extent of rebound that occurs between treatments. Once the transplant has been performed, a sample should be obtained 48 to 72 h after treatment is completed to check for DSA rebound. Whenever possible, transplant patients should undergo antibody monitoring posttransplantation for a minimum of 3 months and following any potentially sensitizing event.

The Whole Picture: the Assessment of Risk

As the opportunities for reducing antibodies and modulating the immune response improve, it will become increasingly important to produce a body of information that provides an assessment of risk to the transplant. Our increasing understanding of the role of the humoral response in transplantation indicates the need for certain types of information: (i) does the patient have antibodies; (ii) if so, what are the specificities, titers, and Ig classes; (iii) are the antibodies increasing or decreasing in strength or breadth; (iv) has the patient had antibodies in the past; and (v) has the patient experienced potentially sensitizing events. Neither the crossmatch test nor the antibody screen alone can answer these questions—the tests are complementary, and both are needed to get an accurate assessment of the patient's humoral immune status. The antibody screen may reveal very low levels of an antibody, indicating that a very sensitive crossmatching technique, such as flow cytometry, is appropriate or, conversely, may demonstrate that the antibody levels are such that this expensive technique is overkill. Even when both antibody screening and crossmatch tests are performed, it may not be possible to obtain an adequate picture of the patient's humoral immunity. In these cases, specialized techniques may be appropriate. Although the use of such ad hoc procedures will add to costs, in many cases and particularly when the information is applied to clinical care, the investment will be well worth it.

REFERENCES

1. **Andrew, S. M., J. A. Titus, R. Coico, and A. Amin.** 1997. Purification of immunoglobulin M and immunoglobulin D, p. 2.9.1–2.9.8. *In* J. E. Coligan, A. M. Kruisbeek, D. H. Margulies, E. M. Shevach, and W. Strober (ed.), *Current Protocols in Immunology*, vol. 1. John Wiley & Sons, Inc., New York, N.Y.

2. **Barnett, R. N.** 1979. *Clinical Laboratory Statistics*, 2nd ed. Little, Brown and Company, Boston, Mass.

3. **Chapman, J. R., C. J. Taylor, A. Ting, and P. J. Morris.** 1986. Hyperacute rejection of a renal allograft in the presence of anti-HLA-Cw5 antibody. *Transplantation* **42:**91–93.

4. **Earley, M. C., R. F. Vogt, Jr., H. M. Shapiro, F. F. Mandy, K. L. Kellar, R. Bellisario, K. A. Pass, G. E. Marti, C. C. Stewart, and W. H. Hannon.** 2002. Report from a workshop on multianalyte microsphere assays. *Cytometry* **50:**239–242.

5. **Emery, P., B. Mach, and W. Reith.** 1993. The different level of expression of HLA-DRB1 and -DRB3 genes is controlled by conserved isotypic differences in promoter sequence. *Hum. Immunol.* **38:**137–147.

6. **Fisher, R. A., and F. Yates.** 1949. *Statistical Tables for Biological, Agricultural and Medical Research.* Oliver and Boyd, London, England.

7. **Fuller, T. C.** 1991. Monitoring HLA alloimmunization. Analysis of HLA alloantibodies in the serum of prospective transplant recipients, p. 551–570. *In* G. E. Rodey (ed.), *Clinics in Laboratory Medicine*. W. B. Saunders, Philadelphia, Pa.

8. **Hahn, A. B., G. A. Land, and R. M. Strothman.** 2000. *ASHI Laboratory Manual*, 4th ed. ASHI, Lenexa, Kans.

9. **Hopkins, K. A.** 1994. The basic lymphocyte microcytotoxicity test, p. I.B.1.1–I.B.1.13. *In* D. L. Phelan, E. M. Mickelson, H. S. Noreen, T. W. Shroyer, D. M. Cluff, and A. Nikaein (ed.), *ASHI Laboratory Manual*, 3rd ed. ASHI, Lenexa, Kans.

10. **Kleinman, S., T. Caulfield, P. Chan, R. Davenport, J. McFarland, S. McPhedran, M. Meade, D. Morrison, J. Pinsent, P. Robillard, and P. Slinger.** 2004. Toward an understanding of transfusion-related acute lung injury: statement of a consensus panel. *Transfusion* **44:**1774–1789.

11. **Lucas, D. P., M. L. Paparounis, L. Myers, J. M. Hart, and A. A. Zachary.** 1997. Detection of HLA class I-specific antibodies by the QuikScreen enzyme-linked immunosorbent assay. *Clin. Diagn. Lab. Immunol.* **4:**252–257.

12. **McCutcheon, J. A., J. Gumperz, K. D. Smith, C. T. Lutz, and P. Parham.** 1995. Low HLA-C expression at cell surfaces correlates with increased turnover of heavy chain mRNA. *J. Exp. Med.* **181:**2085–2095.

13. **Montgomery, R. A., A. A. Zachary, L. C. Racusen, M. S. Leffell, K. King, J. Burdick, W. R. Maley, and L. E. Ratner.** 2000. Plasmapheresis and intravenous immune globulin provides effective rescue therapy for refractory humoral rejection and allows kidneys to be successfully transplanted into crossmatch positive recipients. *Transplantation* **70:**887–895.

14. **Raybourne, R. B., K. M. Williams, X. K. Cheng, and D. T. Yu.** 1990. Demonstration of shared epitopes between bacterial proteins and HLA class-I proteins using monoclonal antibodies. *Scand. J. Rheumatol. Suppl.* **87:**134–138.

15. **Rodey, G. E., and T. C. Fuller.** 1987. Public epitopes and the antigenic structure of the HLA molecules. *Crit. Rev. Immunol.* **7:**229–267.

16. **Rodey, G. E., J. F. Neylan, J. D. Whelchel, K. W. Revels, and R. A. Bray.** 1994. Epitope specificity of class I alloantibodies. I. Frequency analysis of antibodies to private versus public specificities in potential transplant recipients. *Hum. Immunol.* **39:**272–280.

17. **Rodey, G. E., B. Sturm, and R. H. Aster.** 1973. Cross-reactive HL-A antibodies. Separation of multiple HL-A antibody specificities by platelet absorption and acid elution. *Tissue Antigens* **3:**63–69.

18. **Schwartz, A., E. Fernandez-Repollet, R. Vogt, and J. Gratama.** 1996. Standardizing flow cytometry: construction of a standardized fluorescence calibration plot using matching spectral calibrators. *Cytometry* **26:**22–31.

19. **Shroyer, T. W., M. H. Deierhoi, C. A. Mink, L. R. Cagle, S. L. Hudson, S. D. Rhea, and A. G. Diethelm.** 1995. A rapid flow cytometry assay for HLA antibody detection using a pooled cell panel covering 14 serological crossreacting groups. *Transplantation* **59:**626–630.

20. **Sonnenday, C., L. Ratner, A. Zachary, J. Burdick, M. Samaniego, E. Kraus, D. Warren, and R. Montgomery.** 2002. Preemptive therapy with plasmapheresis/intravenous immunoglobulin allows successful live donor renal transplantation in patients with a positive cross-match. *Transplant. Proc.* **34:**1614–1616.

21. **Stunz, L. L., R. W. Karr, and R. A. Anderson.** 1989. HLA-DRB1 and -DRB4 genes are differentially regulated at the transcriptional level. *J. Immunol.* **143:**3081–3086.

22. **Tardif, G. N., and J. M. MacQueen.** 1993. *SEOPF Tissue Typing Reference Manual*, 3rd ed. SEOPF, Richmond, Va.

23. **Tyan, D. B., V. A. Li, L. A. Czer, A. Trento, and S. C. Jordan.** 1994. Intravenous immunoglobulin suppresssion of HLA alloantibody in highly sensitized transplant candidates and transplantation with a histoincompatible organ. *Transplantation* **57:**553–562.

24. **Vaidya, S., T. Y. Cooper, Y. Avandsalehi, T. Barnes, K. Brooks, P. Hymel, M. Noor, R. Sellers, A. Thomas, D. Stewart, J. Daller, J. C. Fish, K. K. Gugliuzza, and R. A. Bray.** 2001. Improved flow cytometric detection of HLA alloantibodies using pronase: potential implications in renal transplantation. *Transplantation* **71:**422–428.

25. **Zachary, A. A., N. L. Delaney, D. P. Lucas, and M. S. Leffell.** 2001. Characterization of HLA class I-specific antibodies by ELISA using solubilized antigen targets. 1. Evaluation of the GTI QuikID assay and analysis of antibody patterns. *Hum. Immunol.* **62:**228–235.

26. **Zachary, A. A., and J. M. Hart.** 1997. Relevance of antibody screening and crossmatching in solid organ transplantation, p. 477–519. *In* M. S. Leffell, A. D. Donnenberg, and N. R. Rose (ed.), *Handbook of Human Immunology*. CRC Press, Boca Raton, Fla.

27. **Zachary, A. A., and A. G. Steinberg.** 1997. Statistical analysis and applications of HLA population data, p. 132–140. *In* N. R. Rose, E. C. de Macario, J. D. Folds, H. C. Lane, and R. M. Nakamura (ed.), *Manual of Clinical Laboratory Immunology*, 5th ed. ASM Press, Washington, D.C.

Evaluation of the Cellular Immune Response in Transplantation

NANCY L. REINSMOEN AND ADRIANA ZEEVI

138

Solid-organ transplantation has become an increasingly important therapeutic modality for patients with various end-stage diseases. Despite improved immunosuppression protocols, most transplant recipients face a variety of complications. Early posttransplant infection and rejection are the major causes of morbidity and mortality. Drug toxicity, chronic rejection, and malignancies are long-term complications.

Many attempts have been made to develop in vitro procedures that can assess the immunological status of the allograft reliably and accurately. Immunological monitoring could, in theory, differentiate rejection from other forms of dysfunction, such as infection or primary nonfunction. Furthermore, the ideal tool would be able to gauge accurately a patient's response to antirejection therapy and might help prevent overimmunosuppression. Immunological monitoring could also be important in predicting long-term graft outcome and thereby identify which recipients could have their immunosuppression therapy markedly reduced without increasing the risk of acute or chronic rejection.

Although there is no one ideal immunological test that can accomplish all of the above, there are a number of tests that can be used together to assess the immunological status of the transplant recipient. The most informative approach appears to be performing sequential analyses using assays that measure different immune functions.

MLC

Concept

Mixed leukocyte culture (MLC) is perhaps the most widely used of cellular assays. It represents a functional assay of cellular response to stimulatory determinants associated predominantly with HLA class II molecules, including HLA-DR and -DQ and, to a lesser extent, HLA-DP. The first descriptions of this assay as a measurement of cellular immunity (5, 6), together with the development of a one-way method of stimulation, allowed the correlation of proliferative responses between siblings. The conclusion was that a single genetic locus or region, now known as HLA, controlled the MLC reactivity. The recognition of disparate HLA class II molecules and the resulting T-cell activation (as measured by MLC) are thought to represent an in vitro model of the afferent arm of the in vivo allograft reaction.

MLC is an in vitro test of lymphocytes responding to stimulation by disparate HLA class II molecules, which are predominantly expressed on B cells and monocytes of the stimulator cell population. Proliferative reactivity to HLA class I molecules has been reported but plays a minimal role in the overall bulk MLC response. In MLC, stimulator cells have been inactivated, usually by X-irradiation, and can no longer divide. The resulting proliferation of responding cells involves the logarithmic expansion of multiple clones of alloactivated T cells. This expansion can be measured by incorporation of the radioisotope-tritiated thymidine into replicating DNA during the logarithmic phase of cellular expansion, usually on the fifth day of culture. The amount of thymidine incorporated into cellular DNA is then assayed by liquid scintillation spectrophotometry. Exogenous tritiated thymidine added to in vitro cultures is incorporated during DNA replication via the salvage pathway, in which free purine bases are formed by hydrolytic degradation of nucleic acid and nucleotides. Exogenous tritiated thymidine is added to cultures for a period of time that is longer than the S phase of the cell cycle but shorter than the cell cycle itself, usually 18 h.

The degree of reactivity observed correlates with the degree of antigenic disparity between responding and stimulating cells. MLC has been used clinically for donor selection, predominantly for bone marrow transplantation. With the more recent application of DNA-based HLA typing methods, MLC is used less often for donor selection but more often for monitoring of the recipient's posttransplant donor antigen-specific immune status. The difference between posttransplant and pretransplant antidonor MLC responses can be used to define any changes (increases or decreases). Studies have shown that solid-organ recipients who develop a decreased response (i.e., are hyporesponsive) are at low risk for immunological complications, such as late acute rejection episodes and chronic rejection. Hyporeactivity is defined as at least a 60% decrease in reactivity of the posttransplant antidonor response compared with that of the pretransplant antidonor response, assuming the response to third-party cells remains unchanged (33, 34).

Procedure

Sample Requirements

Collection of specimens: Care must be taken throughout the procedure to ensure a sterile specimen. Usually, 20 to 30 ml of sterile heparinized blood is obtained from the blood donor. The specimen may be saved overnight but should be processed within 24 h of the phlebotomy. It should be maintained at room temperature even if it is being shipped by overnight carrier. Poor cell yields may result from temperature conditions that are too cold or too warm.

Materials and Reagents

Lymphocyte separation medium (LSM; Pharmacia Biotechnologies; catalog no. 17084003)

Culture medium: RPMI 1640 with HEPES buffer supplemented with 100 U of penicillin per ml, 100 U of streptomycin (Grand Island Biological; catalog no. 380-2400AJ) per ml, 10 U of preservative-free heparin (Monoparin heparin; Accurate Chemical & Scientific Corp.; catalog no. A6500) per ml, 2 mM L-glutamine, and 10 to 20% pooled human sera

Pooled human sera: sera from 10 to 20 healthy nontransfused male donors, heat inactivated at 56°C for 30 min (see "Pitfalls and Troubleshooting" below for additional specifications)

[³H]thymidine (New England Nuclear; catalog no. NEN-027): specific activity of 6.7 Ci/mM. Commonly used amounts are 0.5 to 1.0 mCi per well.

Hanks balanced salt solution (Grand Island Biological; catalog no. 310-4170PJ)

Equipment and Instrumentation

Radiation source (usually gamma-emitting radiation source); alternatively, mitomycin (Sigma; catalog no. M0503)

Laminar flow hoods (Baker 60; The Baker Co., Sanford, Maine)

Liquid scintillation counter (1205 Betaplate; Pharmacia LKB)

Rate freezer (model 70014; CryoMed)

Liquid nitrogen refrigeration unit (model CAIIIL; CryoMed)

Mechanics and Controls

Mononuclear cells are isolated by centrifugation of peripheral blood diluted 1:2 with Hanks balanced salt solution over LSM. Peripheral blood mononuclear cells (PBMC) are removed from the LSM interface, diluted with Hanks balanced salt solution, and then centrifuged at $500 \times g$ for 10 min. The supernatant is decanted, and the wash steps are repeated two more times. The cells are resuspended in an exact quantity of complete culture medium. A leukocyte count is done, and viability is determined via dye exclusion. The cell suspension is diluted to a final concentration of 5×10^5 PBMC per ml by using the culture medium. Stimulator cells are inactivated either by irradiation at 1,500 to 3,000 rad or by incubation with mitomycin according to the manufacturer's instructions. With a repeating microliter pipette, stimulator and responder cells are added in triplicate to round-bottom microtiter plates (ICN; catalog no. 760-042-05) such that each well receives 100 μl of stimulator cells (5×10^4 PBMC) and 100 μl of responding cells (5×10^4 PBMC).

A complete culture setup includes the following:

1. Allogeneic cultures containing all possible combinations of responder and stimulator cells, including cells from three control cell donors of known HLA phenotypes

2. Autologous cultures containing the responder and stimulator cells from the same cell donor

3. Control wells containing either responder or stimulator cells alone, with an equal volume of complete culture medium

4. Double irradiation control cultures containing stimulator cells from two different cell donors

The cultures are incubated at 37°C in a humidified atmosphere of 5% CO_2 for 5 days, after which 0.5 to 1.0 μCi of tritiated thymidine is added to each well. The cultures are incubated for an additional 18 h. The culture plates can then be harvested immediately or sealed with pressure-sensitive film and placed in the refrigerator until harvesting. A number of different harvesting machines and counting systems are available: the cells can be harvested onto filter disk sheets, or the samples can be counted in vials or cassettes or directly, without the need for scintillation fluid. The manufacturer's instruction manual should describe the appropriate procedures.

Pitfalls and Troubleshooting

1. Drugs: If a patient is taking one of the following drugs, the proliferative response may be compromised: prednisone, Myleran, hydroxyurea, Cytoxan, or L-asparaginase.

2. Serum: One of the most common sources of technical problems in any cellular procedure is a poor serum source. Each individual lot of a serum source or, preferably, each individual serum unit within the lot should be screened for growth support capabilities and possible HLA antibodies. The screen should include a control response to a pool of allogeneic cells to measure maximum response and an autologous control to ensure low backgrounds. If sporadic high backgrounds are observed, an endotoxin test may be advisable.

3. Tritiated thymidine: If low counts per minute are observed, the scintillation counter and the shelf life of tritiated thymidine should be checked. The half-life of the tritium is 12.3 years, but the shelf life of the thymidine is considerably shorter.

4. Frozen cells: Cells to be used as responder cells in the cell cultures can be bulk frozen by a step-down procedure at 4, −30, and −70°C before use. However, viability and cell recovery are better if the cells are rate frozen and stored in the vapor phase of a liquid nitrogen storage unit.

The *American Society for Histocompatibility and Immunogenetics Procedure Manual* (35) is an excellent source of additional information and details on cellular methods.

Interpretation

Results are usually expressed as raw counts per minute of tritiated thymidine incorporation. The data may be reduced to allow for easier interpretation and comparability from one test to another. The two most common forms of data reduction are the stimulation index and the relative response (RR). The stimulation index is a simple ratio of the counts per minute for an experimental MLC combination to the counts per minute for the autologous control. The RR is the ratio of the net counts per minute (after subtraction of the autologous control counts per minute for an allogeneic MLC combination) to the counts per minute for a maximally stimulated or control MLC combination (usually the response to a pool of allogeneic cells), multiplied by 100 to obtain a percentage (35).

MLC VARIATIONS

MTT Method

A nonradioactive alternative to detecting proliferation is a colorimetric (3-4, 5-dimethylthiazol-2-yl)-2.5 diphenyl tetrazolium bromide salt (MTT) reduction assay. This assay detects the activity of a mitochondrial enzyme that is proportional to the number of metabolically active cells present in the culture. The MTT, a yellow aqueous solution, is taken up by the viable cells and reduced in the mitochondria to a purple crystal. After solubilization of these crystals, the reaction is measured with a spectrophotometer. An increase in the measured optical density parallels an increase in mitochondrial enzyme activity, which reflects an increase in the number of cells. This approach can detect increases in an interleukin 2 (IL-2)-sensitive line, CTLL2O. Van Buskirk et al. (47) have demonstrated that colorimetric detection of IL-2 production correlates well with the radioactive detection of T-cell proliferation and can be used interchangeably with the standard MLC.

Multiparameter Flow Cytometry

A second nonradioactive method to detect T-cell activation is a flow cytometry assay (FastImmune assay system; Becton Dickinson). It detects an early activation antigen, CD69, which reaches peak expression within 8 h of stimulation (24). The assay uses a three-color technique to detect CD3-, CD69-, and CD4-positive or CD3-, CD69-, and CD8-positive cells. Advantages are a short activation time (4 h), the absence of radioactivity, avoidance of peripheral blood lymphocyte separation, the ability to identify activated T-cell subsets, a quick turnaround (results can be obtained in hours), simplicity, and high sensitivity (24). This technique may be especially informative when mitogen or antigen stimuli are analyzed; however, analyzing a response to an allogeneic cell stimulus may be more difficult.

RELATED METHODS

T-Cell Precursor Frequency Determination by LDA

The frequency of T-cell precursors is determined by limiting dilution assays (LDA). Limiting numbers of responder cells are cultured with a constant number of stimulator cells and assayed for reactivity (cytotoxicity, proliferation, or cytokine release) against additional stimulator cells. In contrast to MLC, which measures a bulk response, LDA is a quantitative tool. It allows the investigator to estimate the frequency of lymphocytes with a given function and antigen specificity. LDA imply that the lysis is a single-hit process; that is, a single precursor cell will initiate the sequence of events that leads, in the case of cytotoxic precursors, to the eventual lysis of the cell. A frequency can be determined if the lymphocyte population is random; that is, the function of the lymphocyte population is not influenced by the presence of another lymphocyte population. The clear distinction between a response and a lack of that response is imperative. Making this distinction is more difficult in the cytotoxicity assay, where an arbitrary threshold that separates the spontaneous release of ^{51}Cr from the release from the lysed targets is set. The frequency of responding cells is determined by a maximum likelihood estimation by using a computer program (19).

LDA of HTL

Helper T lymphocytes (HTL) are detected by their ability to produce IL-2. The murine IL-2-dependent line CTLL2O is used as the indicator line in this bioassay. Adding CTLL2O cells directly to the micrometer wells is a more sensitive method than removing an aliquot of supernatant and adding it to the CTLL2O cells. Before adding the indicator line, the plates are irradiated to inhibit the responder cells from proliferating and incorporating [^{3}H]thymidine. A low dose of irradiation does not block the continued production of IL-2 by the responding cells. In the absence of IL-2, the CTLL2O cells die rapidly. Therefore, any proliferation detected is due to division of the IL-2-stimulated CTLL2O cells.

Method

LDA can be done on fresh or cryopreserved cells. The cells are prepared as described in the section on the MLC protocol. Limiting numbers of PBMC (2×10^4, 1.0×10^4, 0.5×10^4, 0.25×10^4, 0.125×10^4, 0.0625×10^4, and 0.03125×10^4) are cultured in round-bottom microtiter plates with constant numbers (10×10^4) of irradiated (3,000 rad) stimulator cells. When HLA-identical pairs are tested, increased numbers of cells are often used such that the highest concentration is 4×10^4, 6×10^4, 8×10^4, or 10×10^4 cells per well. Multiple wells per dilution are necessary to ensure an accurate assessment of the frequency. Usually, 24 wells per dilution are set up. The culture medium is the same as that used in the MLC protocol. Control wells consist of 24 wells containing irradiated stimulator cells alone (for calculation of background activity), responder cells in medium alone (negative controls), and responder and stimulator cells set up separately against HLA-mismatched third-party cells (positive controls). The plates are incubated for 64 h at 37°C in a 5% CO_2 environment. The plates are irradiated with 2,500 rad. CTLL2O cells (1×10^3) are added in 25 ml of medium. The plates are incubated for 8 h with 1 mCi of [^{3}H]thymidine in 25 ml per well. Cultures are reincubated for 16 h. Cultures are harvested and counted as outlined in the MLC protocol. The wells are considered positive if [^{3}H]thymidine incorporation is greater than the mean plus 3 standard deviations of results for the 24 control wells. The frequency of responding cells is determined by a maximum likelihood estimation by using a computer program, and the variance is determined by the use of 95% confidence intervals. Regression analysis is used to generate a straight line. Chi-square analysis is used to show that the data obtained are in accordance with single-hit kinetics. A program that does all the necessary calculations for this analysis is listed in reference 19.

Pitfalls and Troubleshooting

The sensitivity of this assay depends on the condition of the IL-2 indicator cells. The proliferation of the CTLL2O line depends on murine or human IL-2 or murine IL-4, without which the cells will die rapidly. The line should be maintained at a concentration of 1×10^4 to 10×10^4 cells per ml in a solution containing RPMI 1640 (with HEPES), 100 U of penicillin/ml, 100 μg of streptomycin/ml, 2 mM L-glutamine, 1% sodium pyruvate (100 mM solution), 1% minimal essential medium amino acids (50×), 0.5% diluted beta mercaptoethanol (diluted 1:57 with phosphate-buffered saline [PBS]), and 10% pooled human serum (PHS) culture medium, supplemented with 500 U of IL-2. Great care should be taken to subculture this line every 2 to 3 days.

LDA of CTL

As mentioned before, the major advantage of the LDA is the ability to quantitate a particular T-cell function in an antigen-specific manner. The LDA for cytotoxic T lymphocytes

(CTL) requires a longer incubation time than that for HTL since the cytotoxic activity must be generated in the presence of growth factors and alloantigen. Thus, the cultures are incubated for 10 days; IL-2 is added on days 3 and 6. The target cells are labeled with ^{51}Cr, which is taken up by the target cells and linked to internal proteins by endogenous enzymes. The unbound ^{51}Cr is washed away. The targets are added to the LDA wells for 4 h. During this time, CTL lyse the targets and ^{51}Cr leaks out of the cell into the culture supernatant. The amount of ^{51}Cr detected in the culture medium is directly related to the number of target cells lysed by the CTL. Although ^{51}Cr does emit gamma rays, it is more efficient to assay for the Auger rays that are also emitted. The Auger rays have an energy level within the same wavelength range as those of tritium and, therefore, can be detected by the conventional scintillation counting method. Frequency determinations are done in a manner similar to that used for the HTL precursor (HTLp) method.

Reagents

Phytohemagglutinin (PHA), 28.75 U/ml (Burroughs Wellcome; catalog no. HA-17)

RPMI 1640

Method

Limiting numbers of PBMC (5×10^4 to 0.125×10^4) are cultured in round-bottom microtiter plates with constant numbers (5×10^4) of irradiated (3,000 rad) stimulator cells. Multiple wells per dilution are necessary to ensure an accurate assessment of the frequency. Usually, 24 wells per dilution are set up. The culture medium is the same as that used for the MLC method. IL-2 and additional culture medium are added on days 3 and 6 so that the final concentration is 5 U/ml. Target cells are prepared on day 7 by using unirradiated stimulator cells from the initial priming combination. The cell concentration is adjusted to 10^6 cells per ml, and 1 ml of the cells is placed with 1 ml of PHA in 4 to 6 wells of a 24-well microtiter plate and incubated at 37°C in a humidified atmosphere of 5% CO_2 for 3 days. On day 10, the cultures are assayed for cytotoxicity (or other functional assays are used) against ^{51}Cr-labeled target cells. PHA-stimulated target cells (2×10^6) are labeled with 0.5 mCi of ^{51}Cr for 1.5 h, washed, and adjusted to a concentration of 2×10^4 cells per ml. One hundred microliters of the medium is replaced in the priming cultures with 100 μl of labeled target cells, and the plates are spun at $100 \times g$ for 5 min and incubated for 4 h. Supernatants are harvested and tested for released ^{51}Cr by using either a gamma counter to detect the gamma rays or a beta counter to detect the Auger rays released. Wells are scored as positive by determining that the reactivity observed is significantly (>3 standard deviations) greater than the control background. Wells containing irradiated stimulator cells incubated without responder cells are used as background controls. As for the HTLp method outlined above, the frequency of cytotoxic cells is determined by a maximum likelihood estimation by using a computer program and the variance is determined by the use of 95% confidence intervals. A regression analysis is used to generate a straight line, and chi-square analysis is used to show that the data obtained are in accordance with single-hit kinetics. A program that does all the necessary calculations for this analysis is listed in reference 20.

Variation

A variation of the target cell labeling procedure for the cytotoxic limiting dilution analysis has been described by Van Besouw et al. (46). In this approach, the T-cell blast target cells are labeled with europium-diethylenetriaminepenta-acetate (Fluka [Buchs, Switzerland] and Sigma Chemicals [St. Louis, Mo.]). The incubation period to measure cytolysis is the same as that previously described. The supernatant (20 μl) is transferred onto a low-background fluorescent 96-well plate (Fluoroimmunoplate; Nunc, Roskilde, Denmark), and 100 μl of enhancement solution (LKB-Wallac, Turku, Finland) is added to each well. Fluorescence of the released europium is measured in a time-resolved fluorometer (Victor 1420 multilabel counter; LKB-Wallac), and results are expressed in counts per second.

Cell Division and Precursor Frequency Analysis Using CFSE

Concept

The ability to determine the division history of specific cell populations proliferating in an immune response is useful in quantifying the phenotype and frequency of the responding cells, as well as functional changes during differentiation of T cells, B cells, and hematopoietic precursor cells. The intracellular fluorescent label carboxyfluorescein diacetate succinimidyl ester (CFSE) can be used to tag the proliferating cells. CFSE is cell permeant and nonfluorescent until cellular esterases cleave carboxyl groups from the molecule, rendering it nonpermeant and fluorescent. The succinimidyl moiety of CFSE covalently attaches to the cytoplasmic amine groups. The covalently bound CFSE is divided equally between the daughter cells, allowing for resolution of up to eight cell division cycles. The CFSE staining in combination with immunophenotyping allows comparison of the kinetics of proliferation in various cell populations. A quantitative assessment of antigen-specific-T-cell proliferation can be made by analysis of the flow cytometric histogram plots. The number of precursors that divided can be extrapolated and summed to determine the number of cells that responded to the antigen. By comparing the number of cells that divided to the number of those that did not divide, a precursor-responder frequency can be determined. The procedure outlined below is for testing human cells. Other references describe procedures for animal models (26, 27, 51).

Procedure

Sample Requirements
The collection requirements are the same as those for the MLC procedure.

Materials and Reagents
The lymphocyte separation medium, culture medium, pooled human sera, and Hanks balanced salt solution are the same as those for the MLC procedure.

CFSE is dissolved in dimethyl sulfoxide to the final concentration determined by the investigator. Aliquots can be stored at $-20°C$ in a desiccator and protected from light for up to 1 year.

Equipment and Instrumentation

- Four-color flow cytometer (FACSCalibur; Becton Dickinson Immunocytometry Systems, San Jose, Calif.) and CellQuest software. Other instrumentation is the same as that for the MLC.

Mechanics and Controls

1. Staining procedure: For best results, the optimal dilution of CFSE in PBS, from a range of 1.25 to 2.5 mM, should be determined. The responder cell population is resuspended in PBS–0.1% bovine serum albumin (BSA) at a concentration of $<1 \times 10^7$ lymphocytes/ml and incubated with CFSE for 5 to 10 min (optimal time will need to be determined) at room temperature. Add an equal volume of pooled human sera and agitate for 1 min to quench the reaction. The cells are then washed three times in PBS and adjusted to the appropriate concentration in the culture medium. Alternatively, RPMI 1640 containing 10% pooled human sera can be used for the last two washes.

2. Culture conditions: As in the MLC, the responder cells are incubated with an equal number of peripheral blood stimulator cells. Epstein-Barr virus (EBV)-transformed lymphoblastoid cell lines (LCL) may be substituted for stimulator cells once the optimal LCL concentration that allows for minimal response to the EBV in seropositive donors is determined. The in vitro culture conditions are the same as those for the MLC, with positive and negative controls. The cell cultures are incubated for an optimal time (4 to 5 days) determined by the investigator. The cells are then harvested, washed, and stained with the appropriate antibodies for immunophenotyping as determined by the investigator (e.g., anti-CD3 [phycoerythrin {PE}] and anti-CD3 [peridinin chlorophyll protein {PerCP}]).

3. Flow cytometry analysis: The flow cytometer is set up for excitation at 488 nm, and the green fluorescence (i.e., CFSE) is collected with a 525-nm-pore-size band-pass filter. The immunophenotyping signals are collected with a 574-nm-pore-size band-pass filter for orange fluorescence (i.e., PE) and a 675-nm-pore-size band-pass filter for red fluorescence (i.e., PerCP and PE-Cy5). Four-color flow cytometry is performed (FACSCalibur), and the cells are analyzed using CellQuest acquisition and analysis software. A gate defining lymphocytes and blasts by forward and side scatter properties is used in all analyses.

Pitfalls and Troubleshooting

As in the MLC, the viability of the cells is crucial. Keeping a small amount of serum protein in the staining step helps to maintain viability. Protein also quenches the CFSE fluorescence; therefore, appropriate protein levels need to be determined by titration. The level of staining must also be determined since too heavy staining can cause problems with viability and compensation during acquisition and analysis.

Approximately eight division cycles can be identified before the autofluorescence obscures the peaks. If clear division peaks are not seen, optimal proliferating conditions may not have been obtained. It is helpful to start by setting parameters and culture conditions assaying a response obtained by stimulating with anti-CD3 or a recall antigen. Once reproducible results are obtained, a response to allogeneic cells can be optimized.

Interpretation

For quantitative assessment of the alloresponse, the number of cells within each CFSE fluorescent peak is determined by analysis of the flow cytometric histogram plots. The number of precursors that divided (P_{div}) is determined by analysis of the number of events comprising the various peaks of daughter cells with identical proliferative histories and extrapolated by dividing by $2n$, where n is the division cycle number. The number of precursors that divided makes up the numerator, and the denominator is the total number of cells (P_{tot}). The P_{div} is relatively straightforward to calculate; however, the P_{tot} determination is more complex and several approaches have been reported. To obtain a precursor frequency, the total number of potentially alloreactive cells, including those plated in culture but not recovered, must be considered as P_{tot}. Alternatively, the number of cells recovered may be considered as P_{tot}. To obtain a responder frequency, the number of cells that were activated but did not proliferate can be considered as P_{tot}. The investigator decides the method for determination of P_{tot}.

EBV-Transformed LCL

Long-term culture of cells can involve either normal cells or transformed cells. Normal B cells can be infected with EBV through the CD21 receptor. EBV-transformed LCL are often simply called LCL. An LCL panel or bank is a valuable source of reference DNA and reference reagents for tissue typing and can be used for cellular studies of epitopes recognized by antibody or T cells. Since the LCL have been transformed, they do not depend on the addition of exogenous lymphokines for their continual growth. These cell lines are easy to grow, but critical attention must be given to the sterility and growth conditions of the lines so that mycoplasma infection does not overtake the cultures.

Mycoplasma is an organism that lacks cell walls and, thus, is not susceptible to many antibiotics, nor is it readily visible by light microscopy. However, the effects of mycoplasma infection are readily evident and severe. *Mycoplasma* contains the thymine kinase enzyme, which interferes with nucleic and amino acid metabolism and subsequently with DNA replication in the contaminated cell culture. The growth rate of infected cells is affected, and they eventually die. Meticulous care must be taken, since mycoplasma infection can easily spread to other cultures in the laboratory. Mycoplasma infection should be suspected in short-term cultures if values for tritiated thymidine incorporation have decreased or are very low.

The single best way to prevent mycoplasma contamination is by using an aseptic culture technique. The cultures must never be allowed to overgrow the culture medium to the point where the medium is yellow. As outlined below, LCL must be checked and split at least every second day. A second common source of mycoplasma contamination is the water bath. When a frozen vial of LCL is thawed in a water bath, the outside of the vial should be wiped with a 2% bleach solution before it is opened. One of the first signs of mycoplasma infection of LCL is a dirty or gritty appearance of the cultures when viewed under the microscope. In addition, LCL generally will not divide at the usual rapid rate. They must be checked regularly for mycoplasma infection.

A variety of methods for mycoplasma detection are available, including Hoechst staining. Biochemical methods include nucleic acid hybridization using DNA probes. Simple kits for mycoplasma detection that rely on DNA hybridization techniques are now available (Gen-Probe; catalog no. 1591). The kit consists of small tritium-labeled DNA probes complementary to known specific sequences of mycoplasma RNA. These probes are added to the supernatant from cell cultures. If *Mycoplasma* is present, the DNA probe will bind to the mycoplasma RNA, forming hybrids that are then detected in a scintillation counter.

Procedure

Generation and Maintenance of LCL

The laminar flow hood must be cleaned daily with a 2% bleach solution, and the filters must be checked routinely.

Incubators must be cleaned monthly, including washing with a 2% bleach solution and autoclaving of all of the racks, and preferably, autoclaved water should be kept in the bottom of the incubator.

1. LCL culture medium: A commonly used medium is RPMI 1640 without HEPES buffer, supplemented with 100 U of penicillin per ml, 100 U of streptomycin per ml, 0.05 mg of gentamicin per ml, 2 mM L-glutamine, and 10% fetal calf serum.

2. EBV supernatant: The supernatant used to transform PBMC can be obtained by the culture of an EBV-shedding line, such as B95-8 cultured in LCL medium. The line is cultured for 2 weeks until the medium is yellow, at which time the culture is centrifuged at $1,500 \times g$ for 10 min and the supernatant is filtered through a 0.4-mm-pore-size filter.

3. CSA: Cyclosporine A (CSA) medium is stored as a stock, 50 mg/ml, at 40°C and is diluted in LCL culture medium to a final concentration of 0.5 μg/ml (also stored at 40°C).

Transformation

PBMC (2×10^6) are suspended in 1 ml of CSA culture medium, 1 ml of EBV supernatant is added, and the mixture is incubated for 21 days. Since the culture is shedding virus during this time, it should be isolated from other cultures. CSA culture medium is added during this period when the culture medium turns yellow. After 21 days, the cultures are removed from CSA culture medium and placed in regular LCL culture medium.

Maintaining LCL

The cultures are inspected for contamination, mycoplasmas, and cell density by using an inverted-phase microscope every other day. The cultures are split by diluting the cells to about 0.2×10^6 cells per ml. The LCL are controlled-rate frozen (usually at 5×10^6 to 10×10^6 LCL per vial) and stored in vapor phase liquid nitrogen.

Graft-Infiltrating Cells—Propagation of Lymphocyte Cultures from Allograft Biopsies

Concept

In solid-organ transplantation, the histological analysis of allograft biopsies remains the "gold standard" for diagnosing rejection (8). Although many cell types have been implicated in rejecting allografts, including B cells, macrophages, neutrophils, and eosinophils, it is generally accepted that CD3$^+$ T lymphocytes initiate allograft rejection (16, 50). Both CD4$^+$ (helper) and CD8$^+$ (cytotoxic) T cells are present in the graft and express IL-2 receptor and HLA-DR antigens, suggesting the presence of activated lymphocytes. The phenotype studies provide little information about the functional characteristics and their alloreactive specificity.

Another approach is to learn about the functional characteristics of graft-infiltrating cells through in vitro propagation in the presence of IL-2 (13, 15, 26, 27, 28, 32, 37, 54). Activation of T cells occurs as a result of recipient allorecognition of donor antigens, which leads to the expression of IL-2 receptors on the activated T cells. The lymphocyte growth assay is straightforward. Biopsy fragments are incubated in tissue culture medium supplemented with 5% human serum and 10 to 30 IU of recombinant IL-2. Lymphocyte growth in cardiac transplant recipients correlates with the histological grade of rejection, and positive growth from histologically negative biopsy fragments is associated with subsequent biopsy-proven rejection

(21, 49). A persistent lack of growth from biopsy fragments is associated with an increase in rejection-free cardiac allograft survival. These studies indicate that in vitro culturing of lymphocytes from endomyocardial biopsy fragments is clinically useful for the early diagnosis of acute cellular rejection. This conclusion may also apply to other organs. For lung transplant recipients, transbronchial biopsy fragments have been cultured to propagate infiltrating alloreactive T cells. Lymphocyte growth is virtually 100% for biopsy fragments with histological diagnosis of acute rejection or active bronchiolitis obliterans, a form of chronic lung rejection, and less than 30% of biopsy fragments with no major abnormalities show growth (29). The presence of activated T cells is indicative of a subsequent rejection episode. Lymphocyte growth from renal transplant biopsy fragments also correlates with acute cellular rejection, and the production of IL-2 by the infiltrating cells is associated with irreversible rejection (22). In liver transplant recipients, more lymphocyte growth is associated with rejection and less growth is seen for patients on OKT3 treatment for rejection (37).

A serious complication of heart transplantation is the development of accelerated graft coronary disease (GCD). Persistent growth from biopsy fragments during the first 3 months post-transplant is associated with a higher risk of GCD. More than 40% of patients whose biopsy fragments persistently grew lymphocytes developed GCD. In contrast, only 6% with non-grower biopsy fragments had subsequent GCD (55).

This section outlines the basic approach used to propagate cells from biopsy fragments. Other approaches, such as the use of donor or allogeneic cells as feeder cells, may be used at the discretion of the investigator. Since the ultimate goal is the early detection of activated cells infiltrating the allograft and not in vitro priming, this section deals with methods that minimize the possibility of priming against the donor antigens in vitro.

Procedure

Sample Requirements

An endomyocardial (or other tissue) biopsy specimen collected in a jar containing sterile physiological saline

Approximately 10 ml of heparinized blood obtained from the patient

Materials and Reagents

LSM Ficoll-Paque (Pharmacia)

500 ml of RPMI 1640 with L-glutamine (GIBCO) plus 12.5 ml of HEPES Buffer Solution 1M (GIBCO) and 2.8 ml of gentamicin reagent solution (10 mg/ml; GIBCO)

Pooled human sera type AB (NormIcera-Plus)—(Gemini Bio-Products)

Recombinant IL-2 (Hoffmann La-Roche)

Equipment and Instrumentation

Laminar flow biological safety cabinet (NuAire, Inc.)

Beckman centrifuge (model TJ-6)

Olympus biological microscope (model BHTU)

Forma Scientific water jacket incubator (model 3154)

Cesium-137 Gammacell irradiator

Test Procedure

Autologous feeder cells are separated from recipient blood by LSM centrifugation (see description of MLC method). The biopsy specimens are placed in a small (35-by-10-mm) sterile petri dish by using a sterile transfer pipette, and with a surgical blade or sterile 20-gauge needles, the biopsy specimens are sectioned into three to four small fragments. Each biopsy fragment is transferred onto a 96-well round- (or flat-) bottom plate that contains 100 μl of IL-2-enriched medium (10 to 30 IU of IL-2 in 5% human serum–RPMI 1640). Autologous feeder cells are irradiated (4,000 rad) and added to each well at a concentration of 0.5×10^6/ml. The biopsy cultures are incubated at 37°C and 5% CO_2. Biopsy cultures are monitored for lymphocyte growth regularly. If the investigator wants to monitor rapid lymphocyte growth as a clinical test for rejection, then the biopsy fragments are incubated in IL-2-enriched medium without autologous feeder cells. This procedure allows the identification of graft-infiltrating cells that emigrate from the tissue to the culture well within 24 to 48 h. In the presence of feeder cells, the earliest report of lymphocyte growth is within 5 to 7 days. Once cell growth is observed, the cultures are split and expanded in culture plates with successively larger wells. The cultures are fed with medium containing IL-2 every other day and with autologous feeder cells once a week. All biopsy-derived cell cultures lacking cell growth are discarded after 3 weeks.

Pitfalls and Troubleshooting

When long-term cultures are required to achieve large numbers of cells, the addition of anti-CD3 monoclonal antibody may help expand the activated population without compromising the specificity. In addition, a cocktail of T-cell growth factors such as IL-2 and IL-4 may enhance the growth of graft-infiltrating cells.

Cytokine Measurements

Concept

The conventional assay of T-cell activation is the measurement of cellular proliferation in response to antigen stimulation. More recently, the determination of the frequency of cytokine-expressing cells has been possible through limiting dilution analysis, intracellular cytokine staining, and the enzyme-linked immunospot (ELISPOT) technique. The CD4 T-helper cells have been subdivided into three categories according to their cytokine secretion profiles: Th1 cells that secrete IL-2, gamma interferon (IFN-γ), and tumor necrosis factor alpha; Th2 cells that secrete IL-4, IL-5, IL-6, and IL-10; and Th0 cells that may secrete IL-2, IL-4, and IFN-γ (12, 29, 30). Many distinct patterns based on differential quantities of expression within the Th1 and Th2 phenotypes and mixtures of these phenotypes (Th0) are associated with graft rejection and acceptance.

ELISPOT Assay

The ELISPOT assay was developed in the laboratories of Peter Heeger, Anna Valujskikh, and Paul Lehmann (17, 36, 44, 45).

Procedure

Sample Requirements

Human peripheral blood collected in three or four green-top Vacutainer tubes with heparin

Antigen (sources are given in parentheses): alloantigen (donor or third-party spleen cells), mitogens (PHA or concanavalin A), or recall antigens (cytomegalovirus or purified protein derivative)

Materials and Reagents

LSM (Isoprep [Robbins Scientific] or Ficoll-Hypaque)

Culture medium: RPMI 1640 containing antibiotics and glutamine with 10% high-quality fetal bovine serum

Blocking solution: PBS–1% BSA—3 g of BSA (Sigma) added to 300 ml of PBS and allowed to sit for 15 min. Filter through a 0.22-mm-pore-size filter and store at 4°C.

PBS-Tween-BSA

Red spots: streptavidin-horseradish peroxidase (Dakoo, Carpenteria, Calif.) diluted 1:2,000 in PBS-Tween-BSA

Buffer for red substrate: 800 ml of 3-amino-g-ethyl carbazole (AEC) added to 24 ml of AEC buffer

AEC buffer (0.1 M sodium acetate buffer, pH 5.0): 0.2 M acetic acid (11.55 ml of glacial acetic acid per liter of distilled water). Add 148 ml of 0.2 M acetic acid to 352 ml of 0.2 M sodium acetate. Bring volume up to 1 liter with distilled water.

AEC: Add 1 g of AEC (ImmunoPure AEC; Pierce; catalog no. 34004) to 100 ml of DMF (N,N-dimethylformamide; Fisher Scientific; catalog no. BP1160-500) using gloves and a mask and working under a fume hood. Wrap the bottle in foil and store at room temperature.

Antibodies from Pharmingen (San Diego, Calif.):

Coating antibody—IFN-γ (clone R46A2) at a final concentration of 2 μg/ml or IL-2 (clone JES6-1A12) at a final concentration of 6 μg/ml

Secondary detection antibodies—IFN-γ (clone XMG1.2 biotin) at a final concentration of 1 μg/ml and IL-2 (clone JES6-5H4 biotin) at a final concentration of 2 μg/ml

ELISPOT plates (Fisher Scientific, Millipore, or Cellular Technologies Ltd. [Cleveland, Ohio]; catalog no. M200-50)

Equipment and Instrumentation

Laminar flow hood

Incubator set a 37°C and 5% CO_2

Immunospot 2 analyzer from Cellular Technologies Ltd.

Test Procedure

Day 1. Mark the ELISPOT plate and add 100 μl of coating antibody/well diluted to the appropriate concentration in PBS. Wrap the plate in plastic and incubate it in a humid environment at 4°C overnight.

Day 2. In a sterile laminar flow hood, discard the coating antibody by shaking the inverted plate. Block the plate with a sterile solution of PBS–1% BSA at 150 μl/well and incubate the plate for 1 h at room temperature. Discard the liquid from the plate and wash the plate three times with sterile PBS. Until the assay, keep the plates with 200 μl of PBS/well at room temperature. Peripheral blood lymphocytes isolated from the whole blood are diluted to a concentration of 3 million per ml and are plated at 100 μl/well. Stimulator cells (irradiated or mitomycin C treated) are counted and resuspended at 3 million per ml, and 100 μl is used in each well. When needed, T-cell-depleted antigen-presenting cells can be used to control the background. Mitogens (PHA) at a final concentration of 2 μg/ml and soluble protein antigens at different concentrations (0.1 to 50 μM) are added to the plates (final volume of 200 μl/well). The plates are incubated for 24 h at 37°C with 5% CO_2.

Day 3. The secondary antibody is diluted in PBS-Tween-BSA. Discard the fluid from the wells and wash the wells three times with PBS. After each wash, remove the liquid by tapping the plate onto clean towels. Wash the plate four times with PBS-Tween. Leave the last wash in the plate and incubate the plate for 5 min at room temperature. Discard the liquid and add 100 μl of the second detecting antibody/well. The plate is wrapped and incubated overnight at 4°C in a humid atmosphere or for 4 to 5 h at room temperature.

Day 4. Discard the second antibody and wash the plate three times with PBS-Tween. Add 100 μl of streptavidin-horseradish peroxidase/well and incubate for 90 min at room temperature. Near the end of incubation, prepare the reagent for spot development (AEC in AEC buffer plus 12 μl of 30% H_2O_2). Wash the plate four times in PBS (200 μl/well), and add 200 μl of substrate to each well. The spots should develop in 15 to 40 min. Stop the reaction before the background color becomes too strong by washing the plate four times with distilled water. Dry the plate and keep it covered because the spots are light sensitive and will fade if exposed to light. The plate can be kept covered in aluminum foil for counting the next day or stored at room temperature for future analysis. When the plate is fully dry, it can be analyzed with a dissecting microscope or with a computer-assisted image analyzer.

Pitfalls and Troubleshooting

The viability of the responder and stimulator cells is very important. Fresh cells are the best; however, frozen specimens can be used if the recovery is sufficient. The sources of fetal calf serum and antibodies are important for the success of the test. Keeping background staining low is crucial, and it is therefore important to stop the reaction in time. Also, the spontaneous release of cytokines from stimulator cells can be diminished by using T-cell-depleted antigen-presenting cells.

Clinical Significance

The ELISPOT assay has a number of advantages over other techniques. The assay is very sensitive and reproducible, and the detection of the secreted molecule occurs directly at the site of the secreting cells. The ELISPOT assay is 100- to 400-fold more sensitive than the enzyme-linked immunosorbent assay performed on culture supernatants. Since this assay can detect antigen-specific cells at the single-cell level, it is more sensitive than intracellular cytokine staining. The analysis is carried out with the help of an automated image analyzer that detects the spots based on predetermined size, shape, and color density characteristics, making the assay very reproducible. The ELISPOT assay may be used to discriminate between in vivo-primed alloreactive cells and naïve T cells. Antigen-primed T cells produce cytokines in less than 24 h after stimulation, but naïve T cells require 3 to 5 days of stimulation in vitro to differentiate into effector cells producing Th1 or Th2 cytokines. Heeger and colleagues have shown that a high frequency of donor-reactive memory T cells producing IFN-γ pretransplant correlates with an increasing risk of posttransplant acute rejection episodes in living related-donor kidney transplant recipients (17).

Intracellular Cytokine Analysis by Two-Color Flow Cytometry

Multiparametric flow cytometry can be used to study cytokine production at the single-cell level. It has the advantage of rapidly measuring the cytokine production by thousands by individual cells and of simultaneously detecting two cytokines in the same cell. Most of the reported studies used PBMC as the starting material (3, 18, 31). In addition, the intracellular cytokine analysis can be performed with whole blood (2, 14, 41). Whole-blood activation preserves the in vivo cellular and biochemical environment. The whole-blood assay is also particularly important to analyze the cytokine production in transplant recipients receiving long-term immunosuppressive drug therapy (2, 48).

Procedure

Sample Requirements

Human peripheral blood collected in two green-top Vacutainer tubes with heparin. In addition, tissue-propagated lymphocytes or cells from bronchoalveolar lavage fluid can be used.

Materials and Reagents

Chemicals for culture and stimulation of cells: phorbol myristate acetate (PMA; Sigma; catalog no. P-8139) and Ca ionophore A23187 (Sigma; catalog no. C7522)

Intracellular transport inhibitor: brefeldin A (Sigma; catalog no. B-7651). Dissolve in 100% dimethyl sulfoxide.

Directly conjugated monoclonal antibodies from Pharmingen: CD8 {mouse anti-human immunoglobulin G(κ) [IgG(κ)] HIT8a}, fluorescein isothiocyanate (FITC) labeled; IL-2 (rat anti-human IgG2a, MQ1-17H12); IFN-γ [mouse anti-human IgG1(κ) 4S.B3]; IL-4 (rat anti-human IgG1, MP4-25D2); and IL-10 (rat anti-human IgG2a, A5-4). All cytokine monoclonal antibodies are PE labeled.

Isotype control antibodies consisting of FITC-conjugated mouse anti-human IgG1(κ) (MOPC-21), PE-conjugated mouse anti-human IgG1 (MOPC-21), and PE-conjugated rat anti-human IgG2a (R23-95), each used at comparable concentrations of the antibody of interest

Staining buffer (fluorescence-activated cell sorter [FACS] medium): Dulbecco's PBS (DPBS) without Mg^{2+} or Ca^{2+}, 1% heat-inactivated fetal calf serum, and 0.1% (wt/vol) sodium azide. Adjust buffer pH to 7.4 to 7.6 filter 0.2 μM, and store at 4°C.

Fixation buffer: 4% (wt/vol) paraformaldehyde. Add paraformaldehyde to DPBS and warm in a 50°C water bath (fume hood) until dissolved (1 to 3 h). Adjust pH to 7.4 to 7.6 and store at 4°C.

Permeabilization buffer: DPBS without Mg^{2+} or Ca^{2+}, 1% heat-inactivated fetal calf serum, 0.1% (wt/vol) sodium azide, and 0.1% (wt/vol) saponin (Sigma; catalog no. S-7900). Adjust pH to 7.4 to 7.6 and filter.

FIX and PERM permeabilization kit (CALTAG Laboratories, Burlingame, Calif.) for whole-blood assay

Ficoll-Hypaque gradient

Human AB serum

"V"-bottom plates (Costar)

Instruments

FACscan flow cytometer (Beckman Coulter, Hialeah, Fla.)

Incubator set at 37°C and 5% CO_2

Test Procedure

Cell culture. PBMC or cells of interest are plated at 50,000 to 350,000 cells in 96-well "V"-bottom plates in a final volume of 100 μl of 5% AB RPMI 1640. Cells are cultured with or without PMA (50 ng/ml) and Ca ionophore (1 μg/ml) and brefeldin A (1.5 μg/ml). Incubate at 37°C in a humidified 5% CO_2 incubator for 4 h for PBMC cultures and for 2 h for bronchoalveolar lavage cells.

Whole blood (1 ml) is stimulated with PMA (50 ng/ml) and Ca ionophore (1 μg/ml) and brefeldin A (1.5 μg/ml). Unstimulated whole blood is cultured with RPMI 1640 alone and brefeldin A. Cell cultures are incubated for 4 h at 37°C in a humidified 5% CO_2 incubator.

Staining Procedure

PBMC cultures.

1. Centrifuge the plate for 5 min at 1,500 rpm (Beckman TJ-6), quickly flick the supernatants, and blot dry the plate.
2. Wash all wells with 150 μl of FACS medium and recentrifuge. Repeat flick, and blot dry.
3. Surface stain with 10 μl of anti-CD8 FITC antibody/well. Place the antibody in the well and gently resuspend cells >8 to 10 times. Wrap the plate it in foil and put it in the refrigerator for at least 20 min.
4. Wash wells with 200 ml of FACS medium and centrifuge for 4 min at 1,500 rpm (Beckman TJ-6).
5. Gently flick out the supernatant and fix cells with 150 μl of 4% paraformaldehyde. Incubate overnight in the refrigerator.
6. Centrifuge plates and blot dry. Add 150 μl of permeabilization buffer to each well.
7. Recentrifuge for 4 min, flick the plate, and repeat once. For the unstained wells, use just 10 μl of permeabilization buffer.
8. Stain with intracellular cytokine antibody for each particular cytokine (10 μl of a 1:10 dilution in permeabilization buffer).
9. Place the plate wrapped in foil at 4°C for 30 min.
10. Wash the plate with 200 μl of FACS medium, and centrifuge for 4 min at 1,500 rpm.
11. Flick the plate, add 200 μl of FACS medium, and transfer cells to labeled flow tubes.

Whole blood.

1. Do the surface marker staining with FITC-labeled anti-CD8 antibody prior to the intracellular staining.
2. Use the FIX and PERM cell kit according to the manufacturer's procedure.
3. Incubate 100 μl of whole-blood culture mixed with 100 μl of reagent A (fixation medium) in a 5-ml Falcon tube for 15 min at room temperature.
4. Wash the cells in PBS.
5. Add 100 μl of reagent B to permeabilize the cells.
6. Add the intracellular cytokine-specific antibody (10 μl), and incubate the mixture in the dark at room temperature for 15 min.

7. Wash the samples once in PBS and once in FACS medium.
8. Resuspend the samples in 200 μl of FACS medium and analyze them on a FACScan cytometer.

Data Analysis

- Typical forward and side scatter gates are set for lymphocytes, and a CD8$^+$ gate is set to exclude any dead or contaminating nonlymphoid cells.
- Ten thousand events per sample are acquired within the specific gate.
- Two-parameter histograms showing cytokine staining are created.
- Quadrant statistics are based on the staining of the negative isotype controls.
- Cytokine production is analyzed by detection of PE staining.
- The number of cells staining for each cytokine is expressed as a percentage of CD8$^-$ and CD8$^+$ cells, and the total number of cells is expressed per million PBMC.

Troubleshooting

Always set aside wells for controls and for unstained cells to use in setting the target cell gates. An appropriate Ig isotype control should be run with each assay. Initial blocking studies with recombinant cytokines should be done to establish antibody specificity. Reagents that block Fc receptors may be used for reducing nonspecific staining (especially when cells other than T cells are stained). After fixation, the plates can be kept overnight at 4°C. This step may also lower nonspecific background staining. The intracellular cytokine antibody should be diluted in permeabilization buffer containing saponin. Titers of antibodies should be determined for each cell type and source of stimulation. Finally, best results will be obtained when samples are run on the flow cytometer within a couple of hours following staining. For additional information on flow cytometry, see chapters 18 and 40, this volume.

Intracellular ATP Synthesis Assay: Immune Cell Function Assay

Recently, a method has been developed to measure the cell-mediated (T-cell, or T-lymphocyte) response directly in whole blood (43, 52, 53). The ImmuKnow assay (Cylex, Inc.) has been used to assess the overall basal immune response and to monitor the efficacy of different immunosuppressive protocols posttransplant (2, 41). This whole-blood assay measures increases in intracellular ATP synthesis by CD4$^+$ cells in response to stimulation with PHA in the presence of immunosuppressive drugs. Most immune cell functions depend directly or indirectly on the production of ATP, and thus, ATP has been used as a marker of lymphocyte activation (1, 4, 9, 10, 11, 39, 42). Reduced ATP levels directly inhibit the cascade of steps required for lymphocyte function, including the transcription of cytokine mRNA, cytokine production, and lymphocyte proliferation. ATP production precedes the appearance of most cytokines measured.

The immune cell function assay measures ATP synthesis which occurs as a result of stimulation with PHA for 15 to 18 h. Whole blood is also incubated in the absence of stimulant to assess basal ATP activity. Anti-CD4 monoclonal antibody-coated magnetic beads are added to immunoselect out CD4$^+$ cells from both the stimulated and nonstimulated wells. After washing of the CD4$^+$ cells on a magnet tray, the cells are lysed to release intracellular ATP. Luminescence reagent (luciferin-luciferase) added to the released ATP produces light according to the following equation:

$$luciferin + ATP + O_2 \xrightarrow[\text{luciferase}]{Mg^{2+}} oxyluciferin + AMP + pyrophosphate + CO_2 + light$$

The amount of light measured by a luminometer is proportional to the concentration of ATP. The concentration of ATP (in nanograms per milliliter) is calculated from a calibration curve and compared to ATP level ranges to assess the cell-mediated immune function of the sample. The ImmuKnow assay has been approved by the Food and Drug Administration and is commercially available.

Procedure: Sample Requirements, Collection, and Handling

Whole blood is collected into a specimen collection tube containing sodium heparin and stored and transported at room temperature. The assay must be set up within 30 h of specimen collection. Blood should be stored and transported at room temperature only (18 to 28°C). It is recommended that a normal control sample be drawn and run with each test sample.

Materials and Reagents

The Food and Drug Administration-approved assay kit ImmunoKnow (catalog no. 4400; Cylex, Inc.) contains the following materials and reagents.

Assay plate and cover: 96-well (12- by 8-well strips) plate coated with an inert substance to prevent nonspecific binding. Store at 2 to 28°C, desiccated in the resealable foil pouch.

Sample diluent: 25 ml. Store at 2 to 8°C.

Stimulant: PHA-L, 12.5 μg/ml. Store at 2 to 8°C.

CD4 Dynabeads (Dynal Biotech A.S.A., Oslo, Norway): magnetic beads coated with mouse monoclonal anti-human CD4, supported in buffered saline with BSA and preservative (6.5 ml). Store at 2 to 8°C.

Wash buffer: buffered saline with BSA (125 ml). Store at 2 to 8°C.

Lysis reagent: hypotonic basic solution with detergent (50 ml). Store at 2 to 8°C.

Calibrator panel: ATP concentrations, 0, 1, 10, 100, and 1,000 ng/ml (0.8 ml each). Store at 2 to 8°C.

Luminescence reagent: luciferin and luciferase in a buffered solution (33 ml). Store frozen upon receipt at −70°C or lower. (If a −70°C or lower-temperature freezer is not available, contact Cylex, Inc., for alternative storage instructions.) Thaw at room temperature (18 to 28°C) only. Mix well after thawing. The reagent may be thawed and refrozen up to four times.

Measurement plate: 96-well (12 8-well strips) black or white opaque plate (two of each plate). Store at 2 to 28°C in the resealable bag.

Reagent and Equipment Requirements

All reagents should be allowed to come to room temperature before use. Luminescence reagent must not be thawed above room temperature (i.e., do not thaw reagent at 37°C). Reagents should be thoroughly mixed immediately before pipetting.

The microtiter plate shaker must provide an adequate mix to fully resuspend settled blood cells following incubation without visible loss of material from the wells (i.e., no visible splashing should be observed on the assay plate cover). Once an appropriate setting is determined, use this setting throughout the assay. A vacuum pump with a strength of 150 to 200 mm Hg is recommended. If a stronger vacuum is used, care should be taken not to aspirate the Dynabeads during wash steps.

Equipment and Instrumentation

Luminometer: The luminometer must be formatted for a 96-well microtiter plate, capable of measuring "glow" luminescence, with a maximum emission of 562 nm, and maintain linearity over a measurement range of 5 decades of light output. A computer with Microsoft Excel version 95, 97, or 2000 is needed to support luminometer function.

Incubator set at 37°C with a 5% CO_2 humidified atmosphere

Magnet tray (Cylex, Inc. [catalog no. 1050]; also available in the Cylex immune cell function assay accessory pack [catalog no. 1004])

Cylex immune cell function assay data analysis software (Cylex, Inc. [catolog no. 1440]; also available in the Cylex immune cell function assay accessory pack [catalog no. 1004])

Vacuum aspiration system (Cylex, Inc. [catalog no. 1040]) or equivalent (also available in the Cylex immune cell function assay accessory pack [catalog no. 1004])

Eight-channel aspiration manifold with tubing connector (Cylex, Inc. [catalog no. 1070]) or equivalent (also available in the Cylex immune cell function assay accessory pack [catalog no. 1004])

Miscellaneous equipment: vacuum source, vacuum apparatus with disposable tubing and receiving flask, microtiter plate shaker, Vortex mixer, adjustable pipettes and tips capable of delivering 25- to 1,000-μl volumes, eight-channel multichannel pipette(s) and tips capable of delivering 50- to 200-μl volumes, reagent reservoirs, 12-by-75-mm tubes, and a timer.

Mechanics and Controls

Assay part 1: cell stimulation. Gently invert each control and patient whole-blood specimen several times to ensure uniform distribution of blood cells. Prepare a 1:4 dilution of each whole-blood specimen using sample diluent (e.g., 500 μl of whole blood plus 1.5 μl of sample diluent). Assemble the assay plate according to the worksheet supplied by the manufacturer by using one eight-well strip for each specimen and 25 μl of sample diluent in the first four wells. Dispense 100 μl of each diluted patient specimen into eight appropriately labeled wells, according to the worksheet. Replace the plate cover and shake the plate on a plate shaker for 30 s. Incubate the covered assay plate cover and shake the plate on a plate shaker for 30 s. Incubate the covered, assay plate in a 37°C and 5% CO_2 incubator for 15 to 18 h.

Assay part 2: CD4 cell selection and ATP release.
Remove the assay plate from the incubator and shake it
on a plate shaker for 3 min. Hand mix by gentle inversion
the CD4 Dynabeads, and dispense 50 µl into each well. The
magnetic beads must be thoroughly suspended to ensure
accurate addition to each well. Cover the plate, shake it on
the plate shaker for 15 s, and incubate it for 30 min at room
temperature (18 to 28°C). Shake the plate for 15 s halfway
through incubation and again at the end of incubation.
Remove the strips from the assay plate and place them onto
the assembled magnet tray. Wait 1 to 2 min for the
Dynabeads to collect on the sides of the wells to isolate CD4
cells from the whole blood. Carefully aspirate whole blood
from each well by using an eight-channel aspiration manifold attached to a vacuum system. Avoid dislodging the
Dynabeads. Wash three times to eliminate residual unbound
cells and interfering substances from the wells. Wash with
200 µl of wash buffer in each well, wait 1 min, and then aspirate. After the last wash step, remove the strip holder from
the magnet base, shake the strips for 1 min on the plate
shaker, and then replace the strip holder on the magnet base.
Wait 1 min, and then aspirate.

Dispense 200 µl of lysis reagent into each well. Remove
the strip holder from the magnet base and shake the strips
on the plate shaker for 5 min. Place the strip holder onto the
magnet base and wait 1 to 2 min.

Assay part 3: ATP measurement. If there will be a delay
of more than 4 h before proceeding to assay part 3, the strips
should be frozen at this time. Remove the strips from the
strip holder and place them in the assay plate frame.
Seal the strips, place the cover on the assay plate, and freeze
at −20°C. Frozen strips are stable for at least 1 month. To
continue, remove the plate from the freezer, allow it to come
to room temperature (18 to 28°C), place the strips in the
strip holder of the magnet tray, and dispense into measurement plates as described below.

The measurement plate should include one strip for each
patient and two strips for the calibrator panel. Using a
multichannel pipette, transfer 50 µl from each well of
the magnet tray to the appropriately labeled wells of the
measurement plate. Change pipette tips for each strip.
Dispense 50 µl of each calibrator into duplicate wells of
the measurement plate according to the worksheet. Using
a multichannel pipette, dispense 150 µl of luminescence
reagent into each well of the measurement plate. Following
the luminometer manufacturer's instructions, read the plate
between 3 and 10 min after addition of the luminescence
reagent.

Calibration
The amount of ATP present in the cell lysate is calculated from an ATP calibration curve generated in each assay
run. Relative light units (RLU) for control and patient samples are obtained from the luminometer and converted into
nanograms of ATP per milliliter based on comparable RLU
signals in the calibrators.

The RLU data from the luminometer are converted and
analyzed using the Cylex immune cell function assay data
analysis software. Luminometer RLU values provided in
Microsoft Excel or tabular formats can be directly copied
and exported into the data analysis software spreadsheet.
ATP calibrator concentrations versus RLU values are plotted on a log-log scale, and linear regression analysis generates a calibration curve. To assess the linearity of the curve,
each calibrator is reanalyzed by plotting RLU values on the

curve and calculating corresponding ATP values. In addition, the correlation coefficient (r^2) of the calibration curve
is calculated.

Calculation of Results
Calculate the ATP concentrations for the control and
patient specimens by using the Cylex immune cell function
assay data analysis software. After RLU values and specimen
identification are entered into the spreadsheet and the calibration curve is generated, the following data are calculated
and displayed in a report: ATP result for each replicate,
average ATP value for replicates, standard deviation for
replicates, and coefficient of variance of replicates. The coefficient of variance for stimulated wells must be <20%. If not,
an analytical method to identify outlier values must be used
and the results must be recalculated. Reported ATP values
must be limited to the defined range of the calibrator panel.
Samples with ATP values above the highest calibrator are
reported as having values of >1,000 ng/ml. Samples with
ATP values below the lowest calibrator are reported as having values of <1 ng/ml.

Pitfalls and Troubleshooting: Limitations
All of the following criteria must be met for the assay run to
be considered valid:

- The ATP result for the nonstimulated control sample
  must be ≤60 ng/ml.
- The ATP result for the stimulated control sample must
  be ≥240 ng/ml.
- The ATP level for the nonstimulated sample must be less
  than the ATP level for the stimulated sample.

If the specimen meets these criteria, proceed with interpretation of the stimulated sample. If the nonstimulated
sample does not meet these criteria, the specimen may have
nonspecific production of ATP and the results are not valid.
A new specimen should be drawn.

The linearity of the calibration curve must be accepted
under the following criteria:

- The calculated value for the 1,000-ng/ml ATP calibrator
  must be 900 to 1,100 ng/ml (refer to the result in the
  "Average" column in Table IV of the data analysis software report).
- The calculated value for the 100-ng/ml ATP calibrator
  must be 85 to 115 ng/ml (refer to the result in the
  "Average" column in Table IV of the data analysis software report).
- The correlation coefficient (r^2) of the ATP calibration
  curve must be ≥0.97.

Interpretation of Results
The assessment of the cellular-mediated immune response
of a specimen is made by comparing the ATP concentration for that specimen to fixed ATP level ranges. The
ATP concentration for each specimen is calculated from
the calibration curve established for the measurement
plate in which the sample was run. Assay standardization is
maintained by running the calibrator and a freshly drawn
specimen from an apparently healthy individual with each
assay run. The cutoffs for the ATP level ranges are 225 and
525 ng/ml (Table 1).

The ATP level ranges for the Cylex immune cell function
assay were established by testing 155 apparently healthy

TABLE 1   Interpretation of PHA-stimulated sample results

ATP level (ng/ml)	Result	Interpretation
≤225	Low immune cell response	The patient's circulating immune cells are showing low response to PHA stimulation
226–524	Moderate immune cell response	The patient's circulating immune cells are showing moderate response to PHA stimulation
≥525	Strong immune cell response	The patient's circulating immune cells are showing strong response to PHA stimulation

adults and 127 transplant recipients with the assay. A cumulative frequency of differences was used to select the ATP levels that give the best balance of results between immunosuppressed and nonimmunosuppressed individuals. Note that this is a qualitative assay, and therefore, the results do not directly quantify the level of immunosuppression. Results of the Cylex immune cell function assay should be used in conjunction with clinical presentation, medical history, and other clinical indicators when establishing the immune status of a patient.

Expected Values

Freshly drawn whole-blood specimens from 155 apparently healthy adults and 127 transplant recipients were evaluated with the Cylex immune cell function assay. The distribution of results of the assay for these populations is summarized in Table 2.

The population of apparently healthy adults consisted of 37 (24%) females, 105 (68%) males, and 13 (8%) individuals of unknown gender, and the age range was 20 to 60 years. The ethnicity of the population was as follows: 59% (91) African-American, 28% (44) Caucasian, and 13% (20) other or unknown. The population of transplant recipients consisted of 55 (43%) females and 72 (57%) males, and the age range was 20 to 64 years. The ethnicity of the population was as follows: 24% (31) African-American, 69% (87) Caucasian, and 7% (9) other or unknown. The organs transplanted included kidneys (59% [75]), livers (34% [43]), pancreases (2% [3]), and multiple organs (5% [6]).

VALIDATION OF NEW CELLULAR ASSAY PROCEDURES

Several of the assays outlined in this chapter are being implemented in the clinical laboratory. A few assays, such as the MLC, have written standards (see the *American Society*

for Histocompatibility and Immunogenetics Procedure Manual [35]); however, most immune assays do not. Every new test must be validated before being implemented for patient testing, either by running parallel testing with another laboratory with a validated test procedure or by running known samples that have been tested by another validated method. Validation of a new test usually also includes an external quality assessment through a proficiency testing program. Although many agencies and associations offer programs for this purpose, none are available for the cellular immune assays outlined in this chapter.

When proficiency testing is not available, alternative validation procedures must be implemented, including split-sample and audit sample procedures. The split-sample procedure evaluates imprecision and testing errors. For external verification of test results, 5 to 10 samples are aliquoted and distributed to one or several other laboratories for parallel testing. Internal split-sample procedures test intertechnologist variation and operator-dependent variation. To test intertechnologist variation, samples are split and run by two different technologists. Audit samples, aliquots of control samples that are stored and analyzed periodically over time, assess the imprecision of the assay but not the accuracy. The standard deviation and coefficient of variation are statistics used to determine acceptable thresholds.

Analysis of Patient and Normal Control Subject Data

Tracking of the daily average of patient data has been used extensively for quality control measures. This technique compares the average of 20 consecutive patient values versus an established patient mean value. Optimal application of this method requires an adequate number of patient values obtained using criteria for exclusion of outlying values likely to be from abnormal subjects. In addition, data from two normal control subjects run with each assay have been used to detect shifts in method performance. Methods to monitor a daily mean or an average for normal control subjects have been applied as quality control measures for a number of clinical tests. For methods with small population variation, 10 to 100 results are required for valid quality control.

Analysis of Data from Validation Procedures

The laboratory should define the limits of acceptability for each validated procedure either by analysis of internal quality control data (e.g., a standard deviation form the mean of ±2 or 3) or by use of data in the literature.

Statistical Evaluation of Split-Sample Data

The laboratories involved in evaluation of split-sample data must agree on the criteria for validation, including the test methods, numbers of tests, criteria for determining agreement, and procedures to resolve discrepancies. The statistical

TABLE 2   Distribution of results of the Cylex immune cell function assay

ATP level (ng/ml)	Immune cell response	No. of transplant recipients with indicated results (n = 127)	No. (%) of apparently healthy adults with indicated results (n = 155)
≤225	Low	51 (40)	9 (6)
226–524	Moderate	66 (52)	102 (66)
≥525	Strong	10 (8)	44 (28)

procedure to determine agreement between laboratories uses a formula to calculate the confidence interval for the difference between two results.

Statistical Evaluation of Patient and Normal Control Data

The result values are placed in rank order. The central 68% of all values are selected, and the mean is calculated. If the distribution of values is normal, the low and high values of the central 68% of all values approximately equal 1 standard deviation below and above the mean. The mean and standard deviation provide measures for comparison with other laboratories, previous data from the same laboratory, and published data.

Proficiency Testing

For every test that is performed, the laboratory must participate in external proficiency testing, when available, to ensure quality of testing. The proficiency test samples must be handled in the same manner as the patient samples; that is, they must be introduced into the laboratory system in the same manner. Testing of the proficiency test samples should be rotated among all technologists who routinely perform the assay in question. The relationship between the results must be defined and evaluated. Corrective action must be initiated if a result is found to be unacceptable when compared to the consensus results. The accuracy for external proficiency testing should be >90%. When no commercial proficiency testing programs are available, parallel testing with another laboratory doing the same test must be done at least every 6 months. In-house proficiency testing should also be performed to assess variability between technologists. This comparison testing should be done at least every 6 months.

Quality Assurance for Cellular Assays

Quality assurance is a comprehensive program to ensure quality results from the initiation of a test through the end of result analysis by conforming to established written policies, monitoring compliance to policies, and documenting corrective actions. Each laboratory must have written policies for the requisition and collection of samples, the volume needed, the type of anticoagulant to be used, labeling, and sample storage and transportation for each test done in the laboratory. The policy must include criteria for sample acceptance or rejection. Each written requisition must match the sample and contain the following information: name of patient, identification number, date and time of sample acquisition, specific testing ordered, and referring facility.

Records of the types of problems encountered in sample acquisition should be kept and monitored for trends. Corrective action should be initiated and documented if problems persist. Compliance with requirements should be 95% or better.

Each laboratory should have a comprehensive procedure manual which details the standard operating procedure for each analysis performed, written in the NCCLS format. The procedure manual should be reviewed yearly by the director and all technical staff and signed and dated by the director prior to implementation. Minor corrections can be handwritten but need to include the date of revision and the director's approval.

Quality Control Procedures for Cellular Programs

The laboratory shall define and document quality control measures for each test performed. These measures must include written policies outlining the criteria for accepting or rejecting results, evaluating reagents for consistent quality, and documenting equipment performance. All quality control problems must be addressed. The corrective actions must be documented in writing and reported in the quality assurance report.

Each procedure description must indicate quality control measures employed and how they are used in the interpretation of the results. Acceptable ranges must be established, and corrective actions must be documented when the controls do not fall within these ranges. Results of the test are not reported if the quality control for the test procedure exceeds the acceptable limit.

Each laboratory shall have a written policy for labeling reagents with the name, date received, date prepared or expiration date, date opened, technologist's initials, and storage conditions. Written procedures for quality control for each reagent prior to use are required. Descriptions of specific quality control procedures should include the appropriate method for testing each reagent, which may include titration, parallel testing, and measure of cell growth support, as well as documentation of acceptable performance. The date the reagent is put into use must also be documented.

Written protocols must be in place for routine equipment performance checks and scheduled preventative maintenance. All maintenance and results must be documented, and such records must be stored. Tolerance limits for each equipment performance check must be established, and compliance must be documented. When acceptable limits are exceeded, corrective action may include a procedure for troubleshooting, criteria for instrument repair, backup procedures or instruments, and a power failure plan.

CLINICAL APPLICATIONS

Currently, cellular assays are used to define donor antigen-specific hyporeactivity, to investigate the function and specificity of graft-infiltrating cells, and to determine T-cell precursor frequencies. The MLC and cell-mediated lympholysis techniques are currently used to investigate the development of donor antigen-specific hyporeactivity posttransplant (34). These assays may be useful for identifying patients who are good candidates for discontinuing or tapering of immunosuppression therapy on the basis of apparent immunoregulation of response to disparate antigens. The development of donor antigen-specific hyporeactivity, as measured by MLC, correlates with improved late solid-organ transplant outcome, as evidenced by fewer late rejection episodes and fewer graft losses (34).

Propagation of T lymphocytes from kidney, heart, and liver allografts demonstrates a strong correlation between long-term T-cell growth and clinical acute cellular rejection (55). The primed lymphocyte test has been used to investigate the specificity of these graft-infiltrating cells. This technique demonstrates functional characteristics of graft-infiltrating cells and provides information on the activation state of the T-cell infiltrate.

Previous studies have suggested a correlation between CTL precursor (CTLp) frequency and the clinical grade of graft-versus-host disease in recipients of bone marrow from unrelated donors (19, 20). Recipients with CTLp frequencies higher than 1:100,000 tended to have more severe graft-versus-host disease than those with lower CTLp frequencies. Schwarer et al. (40) compared helper and cytotoxic anti-recipient T-cell frequencies in recipients who had received unrelated-donor bone marrow. They found that the HTLp and CTLp assays provided similar predictive information for outcome; however, the HTLp method is more rapid and less labor-intensive and, thus, may be more useful for donor selection in unrelated-donor bone marrow transplantation. This approach may be useful in predicting graft-versus-host disease in unrelated-donor bone marrow transplant recipients. More recently, Van Buskirk et al. (47) have described the use of the CTLp assay to identify kidney recipients in whom immunosuppressive therapy can be safely reduced. Their data showed that kidney recipients with low or no frequency of donor-specific CTLp could safely have their immunosuppressive drug load tapered. The frequencies of intracellular IL-2- and IFN-γ-producing cells in normal individuals are similar in whole blood and isolated PBMC. However, in transplant recipients on tacrolimus or CSA, the frequency of IL-2-producing cells may be significantly inhibited in whole blood while little or no inhibition is observed when the cells are isolated prior to the in vitro stimulation (2). In addition, the concentration of tacrolimus in blood does not directly correlate with its inhibitory effect on cytokine production in peripheral T-cell subsets (2). Despite these caveats, monitoring the in vivo efficacy of tacrolimus or CSA in suppressing cytokine production in T-cell subsets may further improve the posttransplant management of transplant recipients. This approach can also identify patients who are less susceptible to tacrolimus- or CSA-mediated inhibition and who therefore may need other immunosuppression (2).

The immune function assay (ImmuKnow; Cylex, Inc.) is a Food and Drug Administration-approved assay currently being implemented as a clinical test at many transplant centers. The assay has been used to directly assess the immune system, individualize immunosuppressive therapy, monitor drug tapering, conduct vaccine trials, monitor the efficacy of different immunosuppressive regimens, and distinguish rejection from infections such as hepatitis C virus infection in transplant recipients. A recent multicenter study evaluated the Cylex ImmuKnow assay for the measurement of immune response in immunosuppressed transplant recipients (23). Most immunosuppressive drugs are currently administered on the basis of weight. However, the baseline levels of immune response in patients awaiting transplant vary enormously and are not a function of body weight. The investigators in this multicenter trial found that the level of tacrolimus as measured by the conventional immunoassay did not correlate with the degree of biological immunosuppression by the PHA-induced ATP levels (23). They observed that following transplant, recipients' responses were statistically distributed among three levels of reactivity (low, intermediate, and high) based on this assay. Further, the effectiveness of the immunosuppressive therapy appears to increase with time posttransplant since the number of recipients in the low-response-level category increased despite lower dosing of the drugs. Zeevi et al. (56) demonstrated that responses to recall antigen, alloantigen, and PHA were measurable by lymphoproliferation assays in immunosuppressed transplant recipients but were apparently suppressed when measured by the ATP assay. In addition, recent studies show that high pretransplant intracellular ATP levels in kidney and lung recipients correlate with an increased risk of early acute rejection episodes (unpublished data). Furthermore, the Cylex assay provides an objective measure of the net state of a patient's immunosuppression while minimizing the drug therapy (57).

CONCLUDING REMARKS

The long-term goals of using the cellular assays described in this chapter are to assess accurately the changing immunological statuses of transplant recipients, to predict long-term graft outcome, and to provide the immune response information needed to individualize immunosuppression therapy. By using methods that measure various immune functions in a serial fashion, an accurate assessment of the recipient's immune status can be obtained. Sequential evaluation of a patient's immune status should be considered in any protocols that incorporate modification of the immunosuppression therapy.

REFERENCES

1. Abbas, A. K., A. H. Lichtman, and J. S. Pober. 2000. *Cellular and Molecular Immunology*, 4th ed. W. B. Saunders Company, Philadelphia, Pa.
2. Ahmed, M., R. Venkataraman, A. Logar, A. S. Rao, B. P. Griffith, R. Keenan, F. S. Dodson, R. Shapiro, J. J. Fung, and A. Zeevi. 2001. Quantitation of immunosuppression by tacrolimus using flow cytometric analysis of interleukin-2 and interferon-γ inhibition in CD8− and CD8+ peripheral blood T cells. *Therapeutic Drug Monitoring* 23:354–362.
3. Anderson, U., G. Hallden, U. Persson, J. Hed, G. Moller, and M. Deley. 1988. Enumeration of IFN-γ producing cells by flow cytometry. *J. Immunol. Methods* 112:139–142.
4. Andreotti, P. E., D. Linder, L. J. Hartman, G. A. Harel, and P. H. Thaker. 1993. *Bioluminescence and Chemiluminescence*, p. 257. John Wiley & Sons, New York, N.Y.
5. Bach, R. H., and K. Hirschhorn. 1964. Lymphocyte interaction: a potential histocompatibility test in vitro. *Science* 143:813–814.
6. Bain, B., M. Vas, and L. Lowenstein. 1964. The development of large immature mononuclear cells in mixed leukocyte cultures. *Blood* 23:108–116.
7. Baker, R. J., M. P. Hernandez-Fuentes, P. A. Brookes, A. N. Chaudhry, H. T. Cook, and R. I. Lechler. 2001. Loss of direct and maintenance of indirect alloresponses in renal allograft recipients: implications for the pathogenesis of chronic allograft nephropathy. *J. Immunol.* 167:7199–7206.
8. Billingham, M. 1979. Diagnosis of cardiac rejection by endomyocardial biopsy. *J. Heart Transplant* 1:25.
9. Buttgereit, F., G. R. Burmester, and M. D. Brand. 2000. Bioenergetics of immune functions: fundamental and therapeutic aspects. *Immunol. Today* 21(4):192–199.
10. Crouch, S. P. M., R. Kozlowski, K. J. Slater, and J. Fletcher. 1993. The use of ATP bioluminescence as a measure of cell proliferation and cytotoxicity. *J. Immunol. Methods.* 160:81–88.
11. Crumpton, M. J., D. Allan, J. Auger, N. M. Green, and V. C. Maino. 1976. p. 85–101. In J. J. Oppenheim and D. L. Rosenstreich (ed.), *Mitogens in Immunobiology*. Academic Press, New York, N.Y.
12. Del Prete, G. F., M. De Carli, M. Ricci, and S. Romagnani. 1991. Helper activity from immunoglobulin synthesis of T helper type 1 (Th1) and Th2 human T cell clones: the help of Th1 clones is limited by their cytolytic capacity. *J. Exp. Med.* 174:809–813.
13. Duquesnoy, R. J., J. D. K. Trager, and A. Zeevi. 1991. Propagation and characterization of lymphocytes from transplant biopsies. *Crit. Rev. Immunol.* 10:455.
14. Ferry, B., P. Antrobus, L. Huzicka, A. Farrell, A. Lane, and H. Chapel. 1997. Intracellular cytokine expression in

whole blood preparations from normals and patients with atopic dermatitis. *Clin. Exp. Immunol.* **110**:410–415.

15. Fung, J. J., A. Zeevi, B. Markus, T. R. Zerbe, and R. J. Duquesnoy. 1986. Dynamics of allospecific T lymphocyte infiltration in vascularized human allografts. *Immunol. Res.* **5**:149.

16. Hancock, W. W. 1984. Analysis of intragraft effector mechanisms associated with human renal allograft rejection: immunohistological studies with monoclonal antibodies. *Immunol. Rev.* **77**:61.

17. Heeger, P. S., N. S. Greenspan, S. Kuhlenschmidt, C. Dejelo, C. Hricik, D. E. Shulak, and J. A. Tary-Lehman. 1999. Pretransplant frequency of donor-specific IFN gamma producing lymphocytes is a manifestation of immunologic memory and correlates with risk of post transplant rejection episodes. *J. Immunol.* **163**:2267–2275.

18. Jung, T., U. Schauer, C. Heusser, C. Neuman, and C. Rieger. 1993. Detection of intracellular cytokines by flow cytometry. *J. Immunol. Methods* **159**:197–207.

19. Kaminski, E., J. Hows, P. Brookes, S. Mackinnon, T. Hughes, O. Avakian, C. Sharrock, J. Goldman, and J. R. Batchelor. 1989. Alloreactive cytotoxic T-cell frequency analysis and HLA matching for bone marrow transplants from HLA matched unrelated donors. *Transplant. Proc.* **21**:2976–2977.

20. Kaminski, E., J. Hows, S. Man, P. Brookes, S. Mackinnon, T. Hughes, O. Avakian, I. M. Goldman, and J. R. Batchelor. 1989. Prediction of graft versus host disease by frequency analysis of cytotoxic T cells after unrelated donor bone marrow transplantation. *Transplantation* **48**:608–613.

21. Kaufman, C. L., A. Zeevi, R. L. Kormos, T. R. Zerbe, R. J. Keenan, B. F. Uretsky, B. P. Griffith, R. L. Hardesty, and R. J. Duquesnoy. 1990. Propagation of infiltrating lymphocytes and graft coronary disease in cardiac transplant recipients. *Hum. Immunol.* **28**:228.

22. Kirk, A. D., M. A. Ibrahim, R. R. Bolinger, and O. Finn. 1992. Renal allograft infiltrating lymphocytes. A prospective analysis of in vitro growth characteristics and clinical relevance. *Transplantation* **53**:329.

23. Kowalski, R., D. Post, M. C. Schneider, J. Britz, J. Thomas, M. Deierhoi, A. Lobashevsky, R. Redfield, E. Schweitzer, A. Heredian, C. Davis, C. Bentlejewski, J. Fung, R. Shapiro, and A. Zeevi. 2003. Immune cell function testing: an adjunct to therapeutic drug monitoring in transplant patient management. *Clin. Transplant.* **17**:77–88.

24. Lopez-Cabrera, M., A. Santis, E. Fernandez-Ruiz, R. Blacher, F. Esch, P. Sanchez-Mareos, and F. Sanchez-Madrid. 1993. Molecular cloning, expression, and chromosomal localization of the human earliest lymphocyte activation antigen AIM/CD69, a new member of the C-type animal lectin superfamily of signal-transmitting receptors. *J. Exp. Med.* **178**:537–547.

25. Lyons, B. 1988. Flow cytometric analysis of cell division by dye dilution, p. 9.11.1–9.11.9. *In* A. Doherty and K. V. Doherty (ed.), *Current Protocols in Cytometry.* John Wiley & Sons, Inc., New York, N.Y.

26. Markus, B. H., A. J. Demetris, S. Saidman, J. J. Fung, A. Zeevi, T. E. Starzl, and R. J. Duquesnoy. 1988. Alloreactive T lymphocytes from liver transplant biopsies: association of HLA specificity with clinicopathological findings. *Clin. Transplant.* **2**:70.

27. Mayer, T. G., A. A. Fuller, T. C. Fuller, A. I. Lazarovits, L. A. Boyle, and J. Kurnick. 1985. Characterization of in vivo-activated allospecific T lymphocytes propagated from human renal allograft biopsies undergoing rejection. *J. Immunol.* **134**:258.

28. Miceli, C., T. S. Barry, and O. J. Finn. 1988. Human allograft derived T-cell lines: donor class I- and class II-directed

cytotoxicity and repertoire stability in sequential biopsies. *Hum. Immunol.* **22**:185–198.

29. Mosmann, T. R., and R. L. Coffman. 1989. Heterogeneity of cytokine secretion patterns and functions of helper T cells. *Adv. Immunol.* **46**:111–147.

30. Mosmann, T. R., and R. L. Coffman. 1989. Th1 and Th2 cells. Different patterns of lymphokine secretion lead to different functional properties. *Annu. Rev. Immunol.* **7**:145–173.

31. Pickler, L. J., M. K. Singh, Z. Zdraveski, J. R. Treer, S. L. Waldrop, P. R. Bergstresser, and V. C. Maino. 1995. Direct demonstration of cytokine synthesis heterogeneity among human memory/effector T cells by flow cytometry. *Blood* **86**:1408–1409.

32. Rabinowich, H., A. Zeevi, S. A. Yousem, I. L. Paradis, J. H. Dauber, R. Kormos, R. Hardesty, B. P. Griffith, and R. J. Duquesnoy. 1991. Alloreactivity of lung biopsy and bronchoalveolar lavage derived lymphocytes from pulmonary transplant patients: correlations with acute rejection and bronchiolitis obliterans. *Clin. Transplant.* **4**:376.

33. Reinsmoen, N. L., D. Kaufman, D. Sutherland, A. J. Matas, J. S. Najarian, and F. H. Bach. 1990. A new in vitro approach to determine acquired tolerance in long-term kidney allograft recipients. *Transplantation* **50**:783–789.

34. Reinsmoen, N. L., and A. J. Matas. 1993. Evidence that improved late renal transplant outcome correlates with the development of in vitro donor antigen-specific hyporeactivity. *Transplantation* **55**:1017–1023.

35. Reinsmoen, N. L., and E. M. Mickelson. 1994. HLA-DW typing, p. II.C.3.1–II.C.3.9. *In* A. Nikaein (ed.), *American Society for Histocompatibility and Immunogenetics Procedure Manual.* American Society for Histocompatibility and Immunogenetics, Lenexa, Kans.

36. Rininsland, F. H., T. Helms, R. J. Asaad, B. O. Boehm, and M. T. Lehmann. 2000. Granzyme B ELISPOT assay for ex vivo measurements of T cell immunity. *J. Immunol. Methods* **240**:143–155.

37. Saidman, S. L., A. J. Demetris, A. Zeevi, and R. J. Duquesnoy. 1990. Propagation of lymphocytes infiltrating human liver allografts: correlation with histologic diagnosis of rejection. *Transplantation* **49**:107–112.

38. Sayegh, M. H., B. Watschinger, and C. B. Carpenter. 1994. Mechanisms of T cell recognition of alloantigen: the role of peptides. *Transplantation* **57**:1295–1302.

39. Schulick, R. D., M. B. Weir, M. W. Miller, D. J. Cohen, B. L. Bermas, and C. M. Shearer. 1993. Longitudinal study of in vitro CD4+ T helper cell function in recently transplanted renal allograft patients undergoing tapering of their immunosuppressive drugs. *Transplantation* **56**:590–596.

40. Schwarer, A. P., Y. Z. Jiang, S. Deacock, P. S. Brookes, A. J. Barrett, J. M. Goldman, J. R. Batchelor, and R. I. Lechler. 1994. Comparison of helper and cytotoxic antirecipient T cell frequencies in unrelated bone marrow transplants. *Transplantation* **58**:1198–1203.

41. Sewell, C. W. A., E. M. North, A. D. B. Webster, and J. Farrant. 1997. Determination of intracellular cytokines by flow cytometry following whole blood culture. *J. Immunol. Methods* **209**:67–74.

42. Shearer, G. M., and M. Clerici. 1994. In vitro analysis of cell-mediated immunity: clinical relevance. *Clin. Chem.* **40/11**:2162–2165.

43. Sottong, P. R., J. A. Rosebrock, and T. R. Kramer. 2000. Measurement of T-lymphocyte responses in whole-blood cultures using newly synthesized DNA and ATP. *Clin. Diagn. Lab. Immunol.* **7**:307–311.

44. Valujskikh, A., and P. S. Heeger. 2000. A closer look at cytokine-secreting T lymphocytes. *Graft* **3**:250–258.

45. Valujskikh, A., and P. S. Heeger. 2001. Enzyme-linked immunosorbent spot (ELISPOT) assay for detection of

alloreactive cytokine-reacting cells—detailed methods. *Graft* **4:**195–201.

46. **Van Besouw, N. M., B. J. Van Der Mast, P. De Kuiper, P. J. H. Smak Gregoor, L. M. B. Vaessen, J. N. M. Ijzermans, T. Van Gelder, and W. Weimar.** 2000. Donor-specific T-cell reactivity identifies kidney transplant patients in whom immunosuppressive therapy can be safely reduced. *Transplantation* **70:**136–143.

47. **Van Buskirk, A. M., P. W. Adams, and C. G. Orosz.** 1995. Nonradioactive alternative to clinical mixed lymphocyte reaction. *Hum. Immunol.* **43:**38–44.

48. **Van Den Berg, A. P., W. N. Twilhaar, W. J. van Son, W. vander Bij, I. J. Klompmaker, M. J. Sloof, T. H. The, and L. H. de Leij.** 1998. Quantitation of immunosuppression by flow cytometric measurement of the capacity of T cells for interleukin 2 production. *Transplantation* **65:**1066–1071.

49. **Weber, T., C. Kaufman, A. Zeevi, T. R. Zerbe, R. J. Hardesty, R. H. Kormos, B. P. Griffith, and R. J. Duquesnoy.** 1989. Lymphocyte growth from cardiac allograft biopsy specimens with no or minimal cellular infiltrates: association with subsequent rejection episode. *J. Heart Transplant.* **8:**233.

50. **Weintraub, D., M. Masek, and M. E. Billingham.** 1985. The lymphocyte subpopulations in cyclosporine treated human heart rejection. *Heart Transplant.* **4:**213.

51. **Wells, A. D., M. C. Walsh, D. Sandaran, and L. A. Turka.** 2000. T cell effector function and anergy avoidance are quantitatively linked to cell division. *J. Immunol.* **165:**2432–2443.

52. **Wier, M.** 1996. Rapid assay of cellular immunity in Q fever. *Abstr. 96th Gen. Meet. Am. Soc. Microbiol. 1996.* American Society for Microbiology, Washington, D.C.

53. **Wier, M. L.** 1998. Methods for measurement of lymphocyte function. U.S. patent 5,773,232.

54. **Zeevi, A., J. Fung, T. R. Zerbe, C. Kaufman, B. S. Rabin, B. P. Griffith, R. L. Hardesty, and R. J. Duquesnoy.** 1986. Allospecificity of activated T cells grown from endomyocardial biopsies from heart transplant patients. *Transplantation* **41:**620–626.

55. **Zeevi, A., C. Kaufman, and R. Duquesnoy.** 1994. Clinical relevance of lymphocyte analysis in cardiac and pulmonary transplantation, p. 181. *In* M. Rose and M. Yacob (ed.), *Immunology of Heart and Lung Transplantation.* Edward Arnold Publishers, London, United Kingdom.

56. **Zeevi, A., C. Bentlejewski, K. Spichty, K. Griffith, K. Abu-Elmagd, N. Hooper, R. Kowalski, and J. Fung.** 2001. Posttransplant immune monitoring-ATP based assay for T cell activation. One Lambda, Inc., Canoga Park, Calif.

57. **Zeevi, A., J. Britz, C. Bentlejewski, D. Guaspari, W. Tong, G. Bond, H. Murase, C. Harris, M. Zak, D. Martin, D. Post, R. Kowalski, and K. Abu Elmagd.** 2005. Monitoring immune function during tacrolimus tapering in small bowel transplant recipients. *Transpl. Immunol.* **15:**17–24.

Molecular Characterization of Rejection in Solid Organ Transplantation

CHOLI HARTONO, DARSHANA DADHANIA, AND MANIKKAM SUTHANTHIRAN

139

Improved knowledge of the alloimmune repertoire, development and clinical application of new therapeutics, advances in surgical techniques, and effective infection prophylaxis have advanced transplantation to the forefront of modern medicine. Nevertheless, diagnostic and therapeutic challenges remain. Herein, we provide an outline of the immune cascade contributing to allograft rejection, emphasize molecular protocols that have been applied to investigate gene expression, and summarize molecular correlates of rejection of human kidney, heart, lung, liver, or pancreatic islet cell allografts.

The immune cascade culminating in allograft rejection is initiated following the physical interaction between the recipient's CD4+ T cells and CD8+ T cells and the antigen-presenting cells of donor origin (the direct pathway of allorecognition) and of recipient origin (the indirect pathway of allorecognition) (35, 92). The allopeptides, displayed on the surface of antigen-presenting cells, impart antigen specificity and provide the "first" signal. A costimulatory signal is obligatory for plenary T-cell activation (69). The activated T cells secrete cytokines such as interleukin 2 (IL-2) and gamma interferon (IFN-γ), and the education and recruitment of cytotoxic CD8+ T cells, antibody-forming B cells, and proinflammatory leukocytes culminate in allograft rejection (91, 92). Major histocompatibility complex (MHC) class I proteins present donor-derived allopeptides to the recipient's CD8+ T cells, whereas the MHC class II molecules present the allopeptides to the recipient's CD4+ T cells. Chemokines and adhesion molecules generate the requisite signals for cell trafficking and transmigration of proinflammatory cells into the allograft (41, 49, 55, 73). Toll-like receptors appear to play an important role not only in eliciting innate immunity but also in the amplification of acquired immunity directed at the allograft (3).

Acute rejection is a risk factor for chronic allograft nephropathy (CAN), and CAN is an established cause for late allograft failure (45). In addition to immunologic factors, nonimmunologic factors such as old donor age, donor death due to cerebrovascular accident, ischemia/reperfusion injury, and toxicity from calcineurin inhibitors contribute to the development of CAN (73), a relentlessly progressive process that is histologically distinguished by fibrosis and obliterative vascular disease.

Compelling evidence supports a dominant role for transforming growth factor β1 (TGF-β1) excess in the pathogenesis of organ fibrosis (14), and CAN is distinguished by overexpression of TGF-β1 (76). In experimental models, epithelial-to-mesenchymal transition (EMT) is a prerequisite for renal interstitial fibrosis (103, 105). The TGF-β1 molecule, normally associated with latency-associated protein, becomes activated by β6 integrin (53, 77). Activated TGF-β1, in turn, downregulates E-cadherin via stimulation of integrin-linked kinase in epithelial cells (44, 105). The downregulation of E-cadherin expression results in the loss of epithelial cell-to-cell contact and paves the way for the epithelial cells to undergo EMT (44).

MOLECULAR TECHNIQUES TO CHARACTERIZE GENE EXPRESSION

The advent of an in vitro assay, PCR, to amplify the nucleic acid sequences has greatly reduced the amount of starting material required for the identification and measurement of mRNAs in biological samples. The current technology not only allows testing of a hypothesis but also facilitates characterization of biological pathways via analysis of a single gene or a large group of genes in clinical samples. The following steps are required for the analysis of gene expression: (i) isolation of RNA (either total RNA or mRNA), (ii) reverse transcription of RNA to cDNA, (iii) amplification of the mRNA of interest, and (iv) detection and quantification of the amplified product.

RT-PCR Assay

Amplification of mRNA is performed using PCR, a technique first utilized for the diagnosis of sickle cell anemia by amplification of the beta globulin gene and restriction site analysis (65). Obtaining high-quality RNA with minimal degradation is a critical step in obtaining an accurate profile of the transcriptome. RNA is unstable and prone to degradation by RNases; precaution should be taken to use RNase-free material. Samples to be processed for RNA isolation should not be left at room temperature for more than 30 min and should be snap frozen in liquid nitrogen and stored in a −80°C freezer. With the use of RNase inhibitors like RNAlater, storage at 4°C for several days is feasible without significant RNA degradation. The starting RNA sample should have an A_{260}/A_{280} ratio of 1.8 to 2.0. RNA degradation and DNA contamination can be assessed by electrophoresis of the sample on a 1% denaturing agarose gel using the Agilent 2100 Bioanalyzer. High-quality RNA samples demonstrate clean 28S and 18S rRNA peaks at a ratio of 1.5 to 2.0 (106). Since cDNA is more stable than RNA, RNA is generally reverse transcribed to cDNA prior to storage. The efficiency of reverse transcription (RT) may vary based on factors such as the presence of inhibitors, starting quantity, and the enzyme used for RT (89). An internal control, such as synthetic cRNA that is similar to the target mRNA but for a small deletion, is useful for monitoring RT efficiency.

Most RNA isolations have some DNA contamination, and the inclusion of DNase in the isolation procedure minimizes contamination. However, the use of DNase is associated with some loss of starting RNA material that may alter the gene expression profile. Furthermore, if the DNase is not properly inactivated prior to RT, there is also a potential for degradation of the cDNA sample.

A typical PCR mixture consists of target cDNA, free nucleotides, oligonucleotides as sense and antisense primers, and thermostable DNA polymerase. The cDNA copies serve as the template for the initial PCR, in which the single-stranded cDNA is converted to a double-stranded DNA. The gene of interest is amplified logarithmically in three sequential steps, denaturation, annealing of the primers, and primer extension, which are repeated with each PCR cycle. The primers are designed to obtain an amplicon of 90 to 150 bp. PCR products are separated by size using either polyacrylamide gel (for 5 to 500 bp) or agarose gel (for 200 bp to 5 kbp) electrophoresis (42). The amount of PCR product can be estimated using the following formula: $X = I(1 + E)^n$, where I is the starting cDNA amount, E is the average efficiency, and n is the number of cycles (65).

Competitive Quantitative PCR Assay

A competitive DNA fragment is constructed which is similar to the cDNA of interest with the exception of either a mutation at a specific enzyme restriction site or insertion of a small intron or sequence of DNA (43, 79). These principles are illustrated in our design and construction of gene-specific DNA competitors for the measurement of mRNAs for the cytotoxic attack molecules granzyme B and perforin and for the cyclophilin B gene, which is a housekeeping gene (Fig. 1).

In the competitive quantitative PCR assay, the cDNA is amplified with different concentrations of the gene-specific DNA competitor. The PCR products are resolved by electrophoresis, stained with ethidium bromide, and scanned by laser densitometry. The concentrations of naturally occurring gene transcripts are quantified by measuring the ratio of the cDNA band to the band of the specific competitor. For accurate calculations, the ratio of the target cDNA to the competitor should be between 0.66 and 1.5 (87).

Kinetic (Real-Time) Quantitative PCR Assay

Real-time quantitative PCR incorporates the use of fluorescent signal that is released in "real-time" linearly with the amplification process. DNA-binding dyes or probes such as TaqMan probes are used to detect and measure the amplified products (29). The guiding principle for the development of the probes is the transfer of fluorescence resonance energy from the reporter dye to the quencher dye because of close physical proximity in the intact probe. When the probe is degraded, the reporter dye is no longer in physical contact

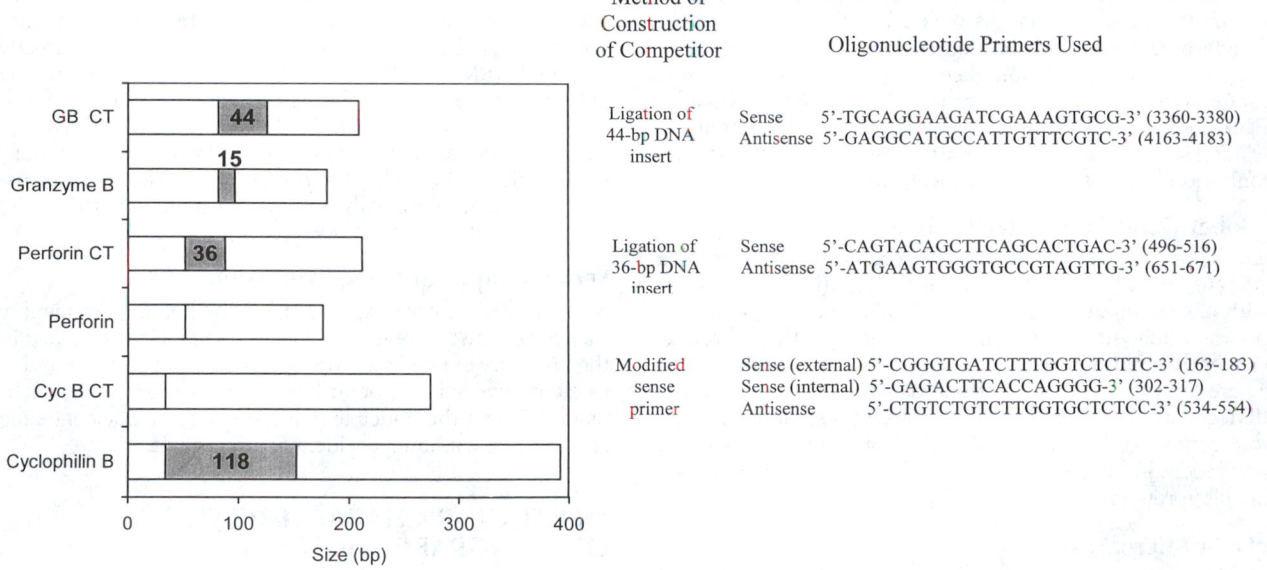

FIGURE 1 Design and construction of DNA competitors. A DNA competitor of granzyme B cDNA was prepared by digestion of the 180-bp naturally occurring product of PCR (GenBank accession no. M28879) with MseI and ligation of the subfragments with a 44-bp DNA insert with appropriate cohesive ends at the 5′ and 3′ ends. A DNA competitor of perforin cDNA was prepared by digestion of the 176-bp naturally occurring product of PCR (GenBank accession no. M28393) with N1aIII and ligation of the subfragments with a 36-bp DNA insert. The 274-bp cDNA competitor of cyclophilin was amplified with the use of a modified sense primer that contains the external sense primer at its 5′ end and a 16-bp subfragment internal sense primer at its 3′ end corresponding to sequences 302 to 317 within the naturally occurring product of PCR (GenBank accession no. M60857). (Reprinted from reference 43 with permission.)

with the quencher dye, which results in the emission of fluorescent signal (29). In real-time TaqMan PCR, the reagent mixture contains the gene-specific probe, sense and antisense primers, unknown cDNA, and DNA *Taq* polymerase. The probe is specific for the mRNA of interest and is designed to be located downstream from one of the primers. As the primer is extended from the 5′ to the 3′ end by *Taq* polymerase, the exonuclease activity of the enzyme degrades the probe and releases the reporter dye from the quencher. This process is repeated with each PCR cycle and as the fluorescent signal increases, an amplification plot of the change in fluorescence against the cycle number is created in real time. An arbitrary threshold is chosen where the fluorescence signal is increasing linearly (usually 10 times the standard deviation of the baseline), and the cycle number at this point is reported as the cycle threshold (CT). The CT value is used to extrapolate the mRNA quantity using a standard curve method or the 2C (delta C [T]) method; in the standard curve method, serial dilutions of known quantities of DNA or amplicons are used (22, 29), and in the comparative CT method, the relative expression compared to a reference sample is calculated after normalizing all of the reference and sample gene expression data to data for a housekeeping gene (29, 48).

The Invader RNA Assay

The Invader RNA assay quantifies the mRNA of interest from the amount of fluorescent signal released from a gene-specific probe. This technique utilizes mRNA without RT, and there is no target amplification (79). The detection limit is 1,000 or more RNA transcripts per cell. The mRNA transcripts themselves are used as the target, and therefore differences in RT efficiencies are not an issue. However, differences in the starting amount of RNA in each reaction can lead to incorrect quantification. This problem is minimized by the use of assays such as biplex Invader RNA assay, in which there is simultaneous detection of two different genes, the target gene and a housekeeping gene, within the same sample (79). Recently, Berggren et al. modified the Invader RNA assay and developed a high-throughput assay for measuring gene expression using matrix-assisted laser desorption ionization–time of flight mass spectrometry (11).

Global Gene Expression Analysis

The steps involved in global gene expression analysis involve (i) synthesis of an expression microarray, (ii) hybridization with labeled unknown cDNA or cRNA, and (iii) quantification and analysis of the signal resulting from the hybridization of the unknown sample to the probes on the microarray. There are two basic types of microarray platforms: an array that consists of gene-specific cDNA probes and an array that consists of synthesized oligonucleotide probes. Marshall and Hodgson have reviewed a number of available microarray platforms (50).

cDNA Microarrays

In cDNA microarrays, gene-specific probes are selected based on biological relevance. In addition, each array contains negative controls (plant or bacterial genes), positive controls (housekeeping genes), and key controls (genes with a known pattern of expression in the system being studied). The cDNAs are generally prepared in bacterial colonies, amplified using PCR, and subsequently purified using nucleic acid isolation procedures. The cDNA elements are arrayed using a robotic system onto a glass slide coated with a DNA binding substrate such as poly-L-lysine or silane (37). The DNA binding substrate is inactivated following the arraying process. The

unknown sample RNA and reference RNA are labeled with different fluorescent markers, such as Cy4 for the unknown sample and Cy5 for the reference sample. The fluorescent markers are linked to one of the nucleotides and incorporated into the samples individually during RT of RNA to cDNA. Unincorporated nucleotides are removed to minimize background noise, and the labeled reference and unknown samples are mixed in a hybridization solution. The mixture is placed on the array and hybridized over 14 to 16 h. The array is then washed and read in a microarray reader.

Oligonucleotide Microarrays

In oligonucleotide arrays, the oligonucleotide probes are synthesized in vitro and subsequently arrayed onto the solid support as in cDNA microarrays, or they can be synthesized in situ as in the Affymetrix GeneChip. The Affymetrix GeneChip system is unique in that multiple oligonucleotides of 20 to 25 nucleotides that are complementary to the different regions of transcript are synthesized in situ for each hybridization unit (37). In addition, the hybridization unit contains a mismatched oligonucleotide probe that differs by one nucleotide for each of the target-specific probes. Hence, a hybridization unit for each gene consists of a series of matched and mismatched probes synthesized in a 24- by 24-μm space.

mRNA is reverse transcribed to cDNA and then transcribed to cRNA using T7 RNA polymerase and biotin-labeled CTP and UTP. The biotinylated cRNA is chemically fragmented into fragments of 35 to 200 bases prior to hybridization. The hybridization cocktail is prepared with the buffer solution, control cRNA, and the biotinylated sample cRNA, which is later placed on the chip for hybridization. After hybridization, the biotinylated cRNA is fluorescently labeled by streptavidin-phycoerythrin. The array is scanned on the Affymetrix GeneChip scanner and analyzed using various software packages. The detection of the transcript is based on the degree of binding to the perfectly matched (PM) and mismatched (MM) probes in the hybridization unit. The software program calculates a discrimination score $[R = (PM - MM)/(PM + MM)]$ that is then adjusted, ranked, and assigned a P value based on nonparametric testing. The determination of whether a transcript is present, marginally present, or absent is based on the P value cutoffs set by the operator.

Serial Analysis of Gene Expression

Serial analysis of gene expression has the potential to identify the entire transcriptome of a biological sample as well as aid in the discovery of new transcripts previously not recognized due to alternative splicing or to low abundance (98). The technique relies on the principle that a site-specific nucleotide tag of 9 to 10 bp can uniquely identify a transcript.

MOLECULAR CHARACTERIZATION OF ALLOGRAFT REJECTION

Molecular Correlates of Acute Rejection of Renal Allografts

Cytotoxic T lymphocytes (CTL) destroy target cells via multiple effector mechanisms. In the granule exocytosis pathway, the cytotoxic attack molecules, perforin and granzyme B, function as molecular executors; in the death receptor pathway, cross-linking of Fas antigen by the Fas ligand results in target cell apoptosis.

Considerable data exist that cytotoxic attack mechanisms contribute to acute rejection of renal allografts. Lipman et al., with the use of RT-PCR assay to measure the levels of expression for granzyme B as well as mRNAs for IL-1β, IL-6, tumor necrosis factor alpha (TNF-α), IL-2, and IL-2 receptor α in 24 core needle renal allograft biopsy samples, demonstrated that acute rejection is associated with a high level of intragraft expression of granzyme B mRNA (46). In this study, the level of expression of other mRNAs examined did not distinguish acute-rejection samples from samples without acute-rejection changes. In a follow-up investigation, Lipman and colleagues utilized competitive quantitative PCR assay to measure transcripts for granzyme B, perforin, and TIA-1 in 35 renal allograft biopsy specimens (10 samples with acute rejection, 6 with chronic rejection, 9 showing both acute and chronic rejection, 9 without any rejection changes, and 1 with cytomegalovirus [CMV] nephritis) and 6 nontransplant biopsy specimens (47). Quantitation of transcript levels showed that the mRNAs for the cytotoxic attack molecules are expressed at significantly higher levels in the acute-rejection samples than in the no-rejection or chronic-rejection samples; also, in the one specimen with CMV nephritis, neither granzyme B nor perforin was detected and TIA-1 mRNA was found at a very low level.

Sharma et al. determined, with the use of RT-PCR assay, intragraft gene expression in 80 renal allograft biopsy specimens obtained from 68 recipients of renal allografts (76). From the 80 biopsies performed to resolve the basis of graft dysfunction, 42 of the samples were classified as acute rejection, 10 as chronic rejection, 11 as both acute and chronic rejection, 10 as cyclosporine (CSA) toxicity, and the remaining 7 as other, using the Banff 97 working classification (61). Measurement of intragraft mRNAs in renal allograft biopsy samples identified heightened expression of transcripts for Fas ligand and granzyme B in samples classified as acute rejection compared to all other diagnostic categories (76).

In M. Suthanthiran's investigation of intragraft expression of cytokine mRNAs in 127 renal allograft biopsy specimens from 107 patients with graft dysfunction, IL-2 mRNA was detected in 10 of 82 acute-rejection samples but in none of the 45 samples without acute rejection (91); IL-10, a cytokine with both anti-inflammatory and proinflammatory activities, was detected in 46 of 82 samples with acute rejection and in 9 of 45 samples without acute rejection (91, 100).

Strehlau et al. applied competitive quantitative PCR assay to measure transcript levels in 60 renal allograft biopsy samples and reported heightened expression of mRNAs for Fas ligand, granzyme B, perforin, IL-7, IL-10, and IL-15 during an episode of acute rejection (90). Data analysis, taking into consideration the levels of expression of granzyme B, perforin, and Fas ligand, showed that acute rejection can be predicted with a sensitivity of 100% and a specificity of 100%. Neither the levels of transcripts for IL-2 nor the levels of mRNAs for IFN-γ and IL-4 were increased in the acute-rejection samples; also, the levels of RANTES (regulated upon activation normal T-cell expressed and secreted) mRNA and IL-8 mRNA were not informative (90).

IL-15, a product of nonlymphoid cells such as macrophages, dendritic cells, and renal tubular cells, promotes the activation, growth, and differentiation of T cells, B cells, and NK cells. Pavlakis et al. investigated intragraft expression of IL-15 and IL-2 mRNA in 45 renal allograft biopsy specimens and reported the detection of IL-15 mRNA in all of the samples and in a heightened fashion in samples classified as acute rejection (60). Intragraft expression of IL-2 mRNA was a rare event; only 3 of the 45 specimens expressed IL-2 mRNAs.

The association between mRNA levels and the Banff rejection grades and the response to antirejection therapy was investigated by Nickel et al. (56). Measurement of levels of mRNAs in 22 renal allograft biopsy samples showed that the levels of mRNAs for perforin, granzyme B, and Fas ligand but not that of Fas are significantly higher in therapy-resistant acute-rejection samples (n = 7) than in therapy-sensitive specimens (n = 8).

Experimental data and emerging literature suggest that the chemokine and chemokine receptor system is a significant participant in the antiallograft response. In the study by Panzer et al. (59), intragraft expression of CXCR3 ligands IP-10 (IFN-γ-inducible protein) and I-TAC were increased 5.2- and 7.2-fold, respectively, in the renal allografts undergoing acute rejection; also, a 5.7-fold increase in the level of expression of RANTES was observed in the rejecting allograft.

Existing data support the idea that acute rejection can be diagnosed with a high degree of accuracy by noninvasive means (34). Vasconcellos and colleagues investigated whether peripheral blood cell mRNA levels predict renal allograft diagnosis (97). Transcripts for Fas ligand, granzyme B, and perforin were measured in 31 paired samples of peripheral blood cells and renal allograft biopsies (11 specimens obtained during an episode of acute rejection and 20 specimens obtained in the absence of acute rejection) from 25 recipients of renal allografts. Coordinate gene expression between peripheral blood cells and allograft biopsy samples was evident, and the levels of any two of the three mRNAs measured were highly informative; the calculated positive and negative predictive values were 100 and 95%, respectively.

The diagnostic utility of peripheral blood cell mRNA levels as predictors of allograft rejection has been extended in a number of studies. Shoker et al. reported that the levels of peripheral blood cell CD40 ligand mRNA are a correlate of the acute-rejection Banff score and the severity of intertubular capillary changes (80). Tan and colleagues, following measurement of peripheral blood cell mRNAs for cytokines in sequential samples obtained from 43 patients (15 with acute rejection and 28 without), concluded that alterations in peripheral blood cell cytokine mRNA levels predict acute rejection as well as responsiveness to antirejection therapy, and that IL-5 and IL-13 mRNA levels increase before and during an episode of acute rejection (93).

Granulysin is expressed by CTL and NK cells and induces mainly caspase-independent cell death. Sarwal and colleagues investigated granulysin expression in peripheral blood cells (n = 61) and in allograft biopsy samples (n = 53) obtained from 97 adult or pediatric recipients (67). Granulysin mRNA levels were higher in peripheral blood cells obtained during an episode of acute rejection or infection. Allograft biopsy samples classified as acute rejection (n = 53) showed mononuclear granulysin staining, and the intensity of staining was higher in steroid-resistant samples (n = 25) than in steroid-sensitive samples (n = 28).

Sabek et al. collected peripheral blood from 27 patients undergoing renal allograft biopsies for graft dysfunction and measured peripheral blood cell levels of mRNA encoding granzyme B, perforin, or HLA-DR with the use of real-time quantitative PCR assay (64). Granzyme B expression was increased during an episode of acute rejection, and its upregulation predicted acute rejection with a 95% specificity. Levels of HLA-DR mRNA were informative as well and predicted acute rejection with an 88% sensitivity (64).

Simon and colleagues examined whether longitudinal monitoring of peripheral blood cell gene expression in the first month of renal transplantation predicts the development of acute rejection (85). In their study of 67 recipients of renal allografts, transcripts for granzyme B and perforin were measured with the use of real-time PCR assay. Renal allograft recipients who developed acute rejection ($n = 17$) had higher levels of granzyme B mRNA and perforin mRNA than those without acute rejection ($n = 50$). Data analysis involving receiver operating characteristic curve analysis demonstrated that gene expression levels are predictive of development of acute rejection and that peripheral blood cell perforin mRNA levels, measured in samples obtained on days 8 to 10 posttransplantation, predicted the occurrence of an episode of acute rejection with a sensitivity of 90% and a specificity of 82%; also, measurement of granzyme B mRNA levels in the samples obtained 8 to 10 days posttransplantation predicted acute rejection with a sensitivity of 87% and a specificity of 72%. In a follow-up investigation of 54 subjects (17 with rejection and 34 without), Simon et al. found that that the positive predictive values and negative predictive values are optimized to 78 to 100% and 82 to 91%, respectively, by taking into consideration the peripheral blood cell perforin and IL-18 mRNA levels together (86).

We and others developed PCR-based protocols for urinary cell mRNA profiling and investigated whether noninvasive diagnosis of acute rejection is feasible by measurement of urinary cell mRNA levels. Li et al. demonstrated that the urinary cell levels of mRNA for perforin and granzyme B are increased in patients with acute rejection compared to those without acute rejection (43). In that single-center study, which included 151 urine specimens from 85 renal allograft recipients, the levels of perforin and granzyme B mRNA, but not those of constitutively expressed cyclophilin B mRNA, were higher in urinary cells from patients with an episode of acute rejection than in those without such an episode. The level (log-transformed mean ± standard error [SE]) of perforin mRNA was 1.4 ± 0.3 fg per μg of total RNA in the patients with an episode of acute rejection (24 samples from 22 patients) and -0.6 ± 0.2 fg per μg of total RNA in the patients without an episode of acute rejection (127 samples from 63 patients) ($P < 0.001$). The levels of granzyme B mRNA were 1.2 ± 0.3 fg per μg of total RNA in the patients with an episode of acute rejection and -0.9 ± 0.2 fg per μg of RNA in the patients without an episode of acute rejection ($P < 0.001$).

The receiver operator characteristic curves, illustrated in Fig. 2, show the fractions of true-positive results (sensitivity) and false-positive results ($1 -$ specificity) for various cutoff levels of perforin mRNA, granzyme B mRNA, and cyclophilin B mRNA. The log-transformed threshold that gave the maximal sensitivity and specificity for perforin mRNA was 0.9 fg per μg of total RNA; at this threshold, the sensitivity and specificity were both 83% ($P < 0.001$). The log-transformed threshold was 0.4 fg per μg of total RNA for granzyme B mRNA; at this threshold, the sensitivity was 79% and the specificity was 77% ($P < 0.001$). The levels of cyclophilin B mRNA were not useful in identifying allografts that would show acute rejection.

In serial studies of urinary cell mRNA profiling, sequential urine samples were obtained from 37 patients during the first 9 days after transplantation. A mixed-level two-way analysis of variance was used to estimate and compare the mean levels of perforin mRNA, granzyme B mRNA, and cyclophilin B mRNA during days 1 through 3, 4 through 6, and 7 through 9 in 8 patients in whom acute rejection developed within 10 days after transplantation and in 29 patients in whom acute rejection did not develop within the first 10 days. The levels of perforin mRNA and granzyme B mRNA, but not those of cyclophilin B mRNA, were higher in urine samples obtained on days 4 through 6 and 7 through 9 from patients in whom acute rejection developed than in samples from those without acute rejection (Fig. 3).

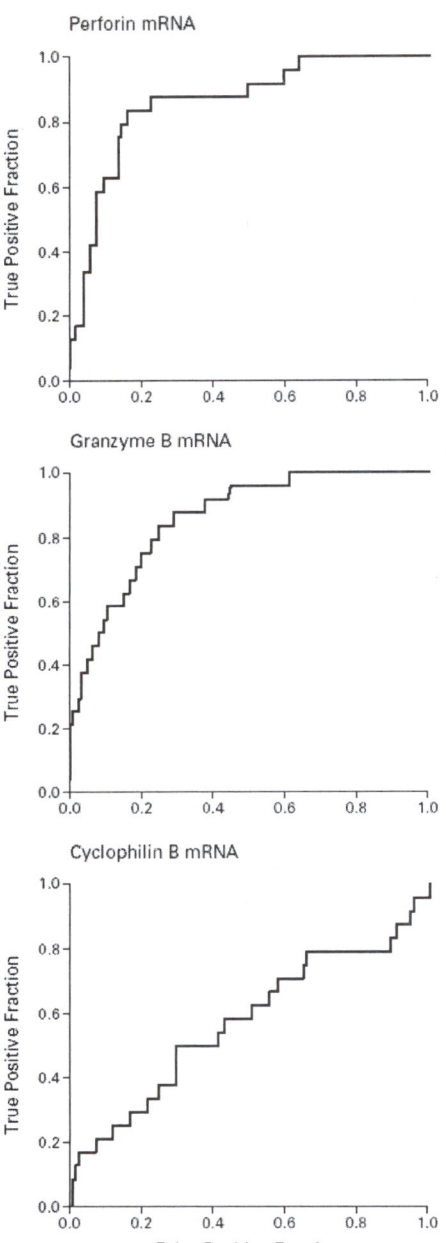

FIGURE 2 Receiver operator characteristic curve of mRNA levels. The fractions of true-positive results (sensitivity) and false-positive results ($1-$specificity) for perforin mRNA levels, granzyme B mRNA levels, and cyclophilin B mRNA levels as markers of acute rejection are shown. The calculated areas under the curve were 0.86 for perforin mRNA levels, 0.86 for granzyme B mRNA levels, and 0.58 for cyclophilin B mRNA levels. A value of 0.5 is no better than expected by chance, and a value of 1.0 reflects a perfect indicator. (Reprinted from reference 43 with permission.)

A key physiological role of chemokines is to mediate the recruitment and activation of host leukocytes to sites of inflammation, including organ transplants undergoing allograft rejection (55, 73). The chemokine IP-10 (CXCL10) and its receptor CXCR3 constitute an important pathway in the rejection of vascularized allografts. We and others measured with the use of real-time quantitative PCR assay the

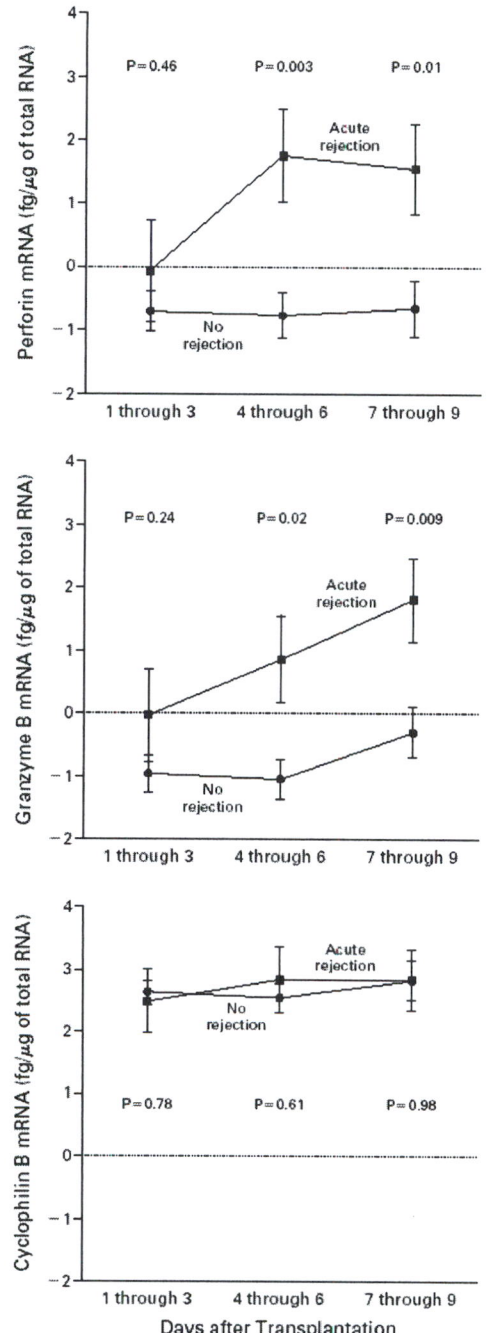

FIGURE 3 Levels (mean ± SE) of perforin mRNA, granzyme B mRNA, and cyclophilin B mRNA in sequential urine samples. The mRNAs were measured in urine samples obtained during the first 9 days after transplantation, using competitive quantitative PCR assay. The levels of perforin mRNA and granzyme B mRNA but not those of cyclophilin B mRNA were higher in the 8 patients in whom acute rejection developed within the first 10 days after transplantation than in the 29 patients in whom acute rejection did not develop within the first 10 days after transplantation. The respective numbers of urine samples obtained from the patients with an episode of acute rejection and those without such an episode were as follows: 6 and 43 on day 1, 2, or 3 after transplantation; 5 and 26 on day 4, 5, or 6; and 6 and 14 on day 7, 8, or 9. Means, SEs, and P values were estimated with use of a mixed-level two-way analysis of variance. In all cases, log-transformed values are shown. (Reprinted from reference 43 with permission.)

levels of IP-10 mRNA and CXCR3 mRNA in 90 urine specimens from 82 kidney transplant recipients with allograft dysfunction (94). Levels of IP-10 and CXCR3 mRNA were significantly higher in the urine of patients with acute rejection than in those with other causes of acute graft dysfunction or with stable function posttransplantation. Receiver operating characteristic curve analysis demonstrated that acute rejection can be predicted by IP-10 levels with a sensitivity of 100% and a specificity of 78% with the use of a cutoff value of 9.11 copies/µg of total RNA, and by CXCR3 levels with a sensitivity of 63% and a specificity of 83% with the use of a cutoff value of 11.59 copies/µg of total RNA (Fig. 4). Also, immunohistologic analysis of transplant biopsy samples showed that IP-10 and CXCR3 are largely absent from grafts with stable function, whereas during acute rejection IP-10 is expressed by renal tubules and infiltrating mononuclear cells, and CXCR3 is expressed by host mononuclear cells, including in areas of tubulitis (94).

CD103 ($\alpha^E\beta_7$-integrin) is displayed on the surface of alloreactive CD8$^+$ cytotoxic T cells and CD103$^+$ cells observed in renal allografts undergoing rejection (31, 63). Because intratubular localization of mononuclear cells is a feature of acute cellular rejection of renal allografts (61), we and others investigated the hypothesis that CD103 mRNA levels in urinary cells predict acute rejection (22). Eighty-nine urine specimens from 79 recipients of renal allografts were collected. RNA was isolated from the urinary cells, and CD103 mRNA levels and levels of a constitutively expressed 18S rRNA were measured with the use of real-time quantitative PCR assay. CD103 mRNA levels, but not 18S rRNA levels, were higher in urinary cells from 30 patients with an episode of acute rejection (32 biopsy samples and 32 urine samples) than in 12 patients with other findings on allograft biopsy (12 biopsy samples and 12 urine samples), 12 patients with biopsy evidence of CAN (12 biopsy samples and 12 urine samples), and 25 patients with stable graft function after renal transplantation (0 biopsy samples and 33 urine samples) ($P = 0.001$, one-way analysis of variance). Acute rejection was predicted with a sensitivity of 59% and a specificity of 75% using a natural log-transformed value of 8.16 CD103 copies/µg as the cutoff ($P = 0.001$).

Serine proteinase inhibitor 9 (PI-9) with a reactive center P1 (Glu)-P1' (Cys) is a natural antagonist of granzyme B and is expressed at high levels in CTL. In view of the role of CTL in acute rejection, we and others investigated the postulate that PI-9 would be hyperexpressed during acute rejection (54). Since PI-9 can protect CTL from its own fatal arsenal and potentially enhance the vitality of CTL, we and others examined whether PI-9 levels correlate with the severity of rejection as well as predict subsequent graft function. Ninety-five urine specimens from 87 renal allograft recipients were obtained. RNA was isolated from the urinary cells, and mRNA encoding PI-9, granzyme B, or perforin and a constitutively expressed 18S rRNA were measured with the use of real-time quantitative PCR assay and the level of expression was correlated with allograft status. The levels of PI-9 ($P = 0.001$), granzyme B ($P < 0.0001$), and perforin mRNAs ($P < 0.0001$), but not the levels of 18S rRNA ($P = 0.54$), were higher in the urinary cells from the 29 patients with a biopsy-confirmed acute rejection than in the 58 recipients without acute rejection. PI-9 levels were significantly higher in patients with type II or higher acute-rejection changes than in those with less than type II changes ($P = 0.01$). Furthermore, PI-9 levels predicted subsequent graft function ($r = 0.43$, $P = 0.01$).

The usefulness of urinary cell mRNA profiling for the noninvasive diagnosis of early acute rejection and delayed acute rejection has been examined by Kotsch et al. (38). Urinary cell

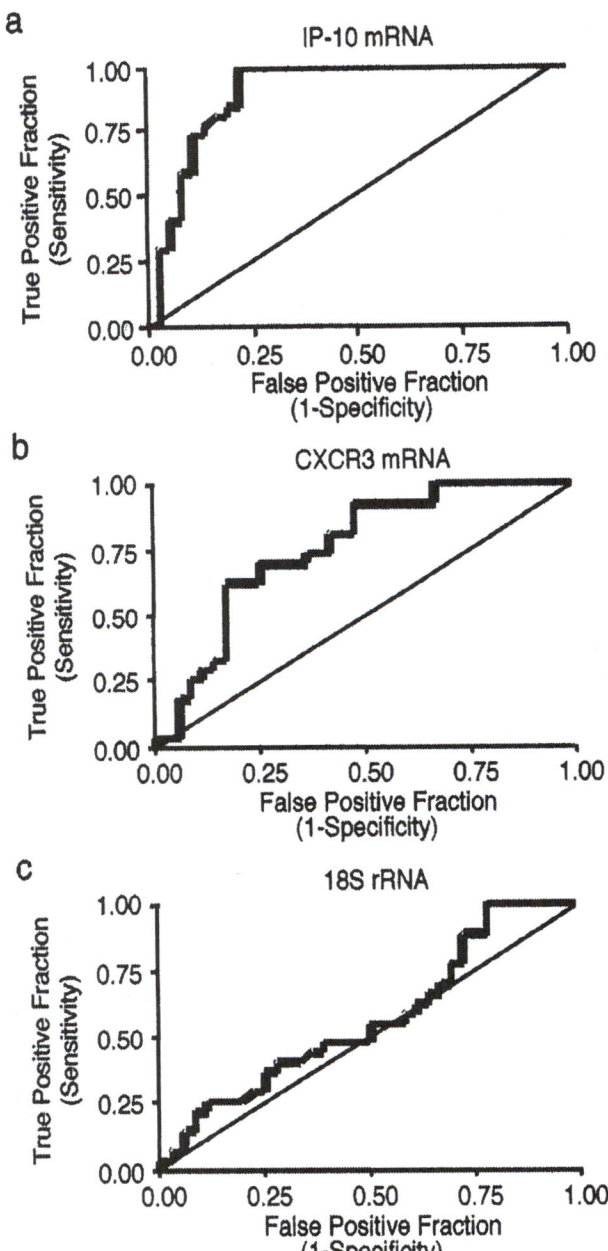

a

IP-10 mRNA

b

CXCR3 mRNA

c

18S rRNA

FIGURE 4 Receiver operating characteristic curve of mRNA and rRNA levels. The fractions of true-positive results and false-positive results for IP-10 mRNA levels, CXCR3 mRNA levels, and 18S rRNA levels as markers of acute rejection are shown. Levels of mRNAs were measured with the use of real-time quantitative PCR assay. The calculated areas under the curve were 0.903 for IP-10 mRNA levels, 0.762 for CXCR3 mRNA levels, and 0.574 for 18S rRNA levels. A value of 0.5 is no better than expected by chance, and a value of 1.0 reflects a perfect indicator. (Reprinted from reference 94 with permission.)

mRNA levels were measured in 221 specimens collected from 26 recipients of renal allografts, and the transcript levels were measured with the use of real-time quantitative PCR assay. An increase in the levels of granulysin mRNA was observed in 11 of 14 acute-rejection episodes. In this investigation, levels of mRNA for granzyme B, perforin, Fas ligand, TNF-α,

RANTES, IL-2, IL-10, IFN-γ, TGF-β1, CD3, and CCR1 were less specific and sensitive in predicting acute rejection than were granulysin mRNA levels (38).

The clinical application of microarray platforms for global mRNA profiling has begun to yield novel insights regarding allograft rejection. Akalin et al. used the first-generation high-density oligonucleotide array composed of 6,800 genes (Affymetrix GeneChip) to investigate gene expression patterns of seven renal allograft biopsy samples with acute rejection and three biopsy samples without acute rejection (2). Compared to the gene expression pattern of the samples without acute rejection, 32 to 219 genes were upregulated in the acute-rejection samples; of these transcripts, only 4 (the HuMig gene, the T-cell receptor active β chain-related gene, the gene for IL-2-stimulated phosphoprotein, and the RING4 gene) were uniformly upregulated in all seven acute-rejection specimens, and 6 additional transcripts (for ISGF-3, C3, nicotinamide N-methyltransferase, MIP-3b, myeloid differentiation protein, and CD18) were upregulated in six of the seven acute-rejection samples. Moreover, upregulation of cytotoxic effector molecules in the acute-rejection biopsies was not observed, and two genes were found to be downregulated (2).

Sarwal et al. used the DNA microarray technology, pioneered at Stanford University, to investigate gene expression patterns of renal allograft biopsy samples from 50 pediatric recipients (66). Exploratory and supervised bioinformatics analyses demonstrated consistent differences in the gene expression profiles of samples classified as acute rejection, drug toxicity, CAN, and normal. Importantly, molecular heterogeneity among histologically indistinguishable acute-rejection samples was evident. Genes that were found to be highly expressed included those that are involved in T-cell activation: those for nuclear factor κB₁, IFN-γ, IL-2, and T-cell receptors. NK cells and macrophage activation were also seen, with high levels of expression of NK cell transcript 4, macrophage receptor, and macrophage matrix metalloproteinase 7. Expression levels of effector molecules such as granzyme A and chemokines such as RANTES were also elevated.

Flechner et al. (26), with the use of oligonucleotide microarrays (Affymetrix HG-U95Av2 gene chip), analyzed 31 human renal biopsy specimens (9 samples from live donor controls [normal], 7 acute-rejection samples, 5 samples from patients with renal dysfunction but no rejection [graft dysfunction], and 10 samples from patients with good transplant function and normal histology [protocol samples]). Peripheral blood lymphocytes (PBLs) that corresponded to acute rejection (7 specimens), protocol biopsies (9 specimens), and graft dysfunction (8 specimens) were also analyzed. Gene expression profiling of allograft biopsy samples showed that 96 genes were upregulated and 619 were downregulated when the acute-rejection gene expression pattern was compared with that of protocol samples, and 44 of the 96 unregulated genes were those implicated in immune and inflammatory functions. Some of the upregulated immune genes in the acute-rejection samples were those for allograft inflammatory factor 1 (AIF-1), CD2 antigen, CD14 antigen, RANTES, the C-X-C motif chemokine receptor 4, granzyme A, endothelial cell growth factor 1 (platelet derived), integrin, IP-30, and IL-10 receptors α and β. Of the 12 immune genes shown to be upregulated during comparison of samples classified as acute rejection to samples from patients with graft dysfunction but without acute-rejection changes, 7 genes corresponded to the genes that were upregulated in the acute-rejection versus stable-function group. The upregulated 7 immune genes were those for IL-10 receptor α, Src-like-adaptor, lymphocyte-specific protein tyrosine kinase, endothelial cell growth factor 1 (platelet derived), AIF-1, integrin, and adipsin. The gene expression pattern of PBLs was found to be different from that of corresponding biopsy samples. Two immune genes, those for β_2-microglobulin and immunoglobulin (Ig) κ constant, were found to be upregulated during comparison of gene expression patterns of PBLs from patients with acute rejection to the PBLs from patients with stable function. The gene expression patterns of PBLs distinguished acute-rejection biopsy samples from stable-function samples but not from biopsy samples from patients with graft dysfunction but without acute rejection.

Molecular Correlates of Chronic Rejection of Renal Allografts

The histologic hallmarks of CAN are interstitial fibrosis and obliterative vasculopathy. We and others have observed high levels of intragraft expression of TGF-β1 mRNA in biopsy samples classified as CAN (76, 91). In mRNA phenotyping studies of 127 renal allograft biopsy samples obtained from 107 recipients of renal allografts, a significant correlation was found between intragraft TGF-β1 mRNA expression and CAN (76). The investigation also showed that neither interstitial fibrosis nor CAN is predicted by intragraft expression of mRNAs for IL-2, IFN-γ, IL-4, IL-10, granzyme B, or perforin.

TGF-β1 is normally associated with latency-associated protein and becomes activated by β6 integrin (53, 77). Sawada et al. have reported heightened expression of β6 integrin in renal allograft biopsy specimens with CAN, whereas β6 integrin was not detected in normal renal allograft biopsy specimens (68). The detection of an endogenous activator of TGF-β1 in biopsy samples classified as CAN may provide a potent mechanism for the downregulation of E-cadherin and EMT.

Intragraft gene expression in transplant nephrectomy specimens has been investigated by Nocera et al. (57). Ten specimens were from patients with CAN, and three were from patients with early (<30 days) graft failure due to intrarenal hemorrhage and vascular thrombosis. Normal renal tissues from kidneys removed for neoplasm served as the control. In biopsy samples classified as Banff CAN grades 2 and 3, genes that were hyperexpressed included those for IL-6, IL-10, IFN-γ, and IL-3. The genes for IL-3 and IL-10 were not expressed in the early graft failure group (57).

Donauer et al., using microarray technology, analyzed renal biopsy specimens from 13 chronically rejected transplant kidneys, 16 normal kidneys, and 12 end-stage polycystic kidneys (23). Compared with normal kidneys and end-stage kidneys from patients with polycystic kidney disease, chronically rejected transplant kidneys displayed higher expression of 21 genes and lower expression of 6 genes. Among the 21 genes that were upregulated, 3 genes were associated with immune response (those for Ig heavy chain, MHC class I, and prostaglandin E receptor EP3 subtype), 2 genes were associated with inflammation (those for complement C1s and KIAA0201), and 3 genes were associated with signaling (those for hepatocyte growth factor activator inhibitor, ceramide glucosyltransferase, and FYN binding protein). The remaining genes that were upregulated represented transcription, protein metabolism, cytoskeleton, and adhesion/extracellular matrix (type IV collagenase). In comparison of gene expression in end-stage renal disease (polycystic kidneys and chronically rejected kidneys) with normal tissues, 11 genes were found to be upregulated whereas 37 genes were downregulated. Among the 11 genes that were upregulated, 8 were associated with immune responses (those for Ig heavy chain, Ig rearranged γ chain, CD53 glycoprotein, secreted cement gland protein, Ig κ chain, SNC73 protein, rearranged Ig heavy chain, and Ig germ line κ chain C18).

Scherer et al. analyzed histologically normal renal allograft biopsy samples obtained at 6 months posttransplantation; one group developed chronic rejection at 12 months and the other did not (70). Allograft gene expression patterns, identified with the use of Affymetrix HG-U95Av2 gene chip, revealed a set of 10 genes that potentially could serve as predictive biomarkers of chronic rejection (70). The differentially expressed genes included those for cytokeratin 15 (KRT15), Hox A7, Hox B7, prolactin receptor, OS9 (APRIL [acidic protein rich in leucines]), G-protein gamma, OBCML (opiate-binding protein-cell adhesion molecular-like), NPRL2 (tumor suppressor), DKFZp5586B1722, and W26469:32f4.

Flechner et al. investigated gene expression patterns of 41 renal allograft biopsy samples obtained from renal graft recipients treated with a regimen of cyclosporine (CSA)-basiliximab mycophenolate mofetil (MMF)-prednisone or sirolimus-MMF-prednisone (27). The biopsies were performed at 2 years posttransplantation and mRNA profiles were determined using high-density oligonucleotide arrays (Affymetrix HG-U95Av2 gene chip). mRNA profiling revealed 379 differentially expressed genes between the two treatment protocols, and 97% of the upregulated genes were observed in the CSA treatment arm. Of the upregulated genes, the top 6 of the 32 functional clusters were composed of genes implicated in transcription, fibrosis/tissue remodeling, immunity/inflammation, intracellular protein transport, signal transduction, and cell growth. In this investigation, biopsy samples classified as CAN were more frequent in the CSA group than in the sirolimus group, and 130 genes were found to be differentially expressed when gene expression patterns of samples with normal histology ($n = 18$) were compared with those of Banff CAN grades 2 and 3 ($n = 9$). The differentially expressed genes included those involved in fibrosis/tissue remodeling and immunity/inflammation.

Molecular Correlates of Acute Rejection of Cardiac Allografts

Endomyocardial biopsy samples obtained during an episode of acute ejection reveal perivascular and interstitial mononuclear cell infiltrates. In severe acute rejection, destruction of myocytes with histologic evidence of necrosis, tissue edema, hemorrhage, and vasculitis is seen (12).

Shulzhenko et al. investigated the expression of mRNAs for CD40 ligand, IFN-γ, and Fas ligand in 39 endomyocardial biopsy samples obtained from 10 adult cardiac allograft recipients within the first 6 months of transplantation and found that the transcripts for CD40 ligand, IFN-γ, and Fas ligand were all expressed at a higher level during an episode of acute rejection than with no rejection (82). Moreover, levels of IFN-γ mRNA were predictive of the development of acute rejection.

The CD27/CD70 costimulatory pathway has been shown to enhance antigen-specific CTL activity via a perforin-dependent pathway (101). Morgun and colleagues investigated with the use of quantitative competitive PCR assay the level of expression of CD27 mRNA in 120 endomyocardial biopsy samples and in 89 peripheral blood mononuclear cell samples collected from 31 recipients of cardiac allografts and reported that the levels of CD27 transcripts were higher in the biopsy samples obtained during acute rejection than with no rejection (52). Interestingly, the CD27 mRNA levels were lower in peripheral blood mononuclear cells collected during acute rejection than during rejection-free periods.

T-cell immune response cDNA 7 (TIRC7) is considered to play a critical role in T-cell signaling. With the use of quantitative competitive PCR assay to measure intragraft and peripheral blood cell TIRC7 mRNA, Shulzhenko et al. found that intragraft expression TIRC7 was increased in endomyocardial biopsy specimens of patients with acute cardiac allograft rejection, whereas the transcript levels were decreased in the peripheral blood cells (83).

CD69 is a human leukocyte membrane protein expressed on T cells, B cells, and NK cells during the early phase of immune activation. Schowengerdt et al., with the use of flow cytometry, investigated CD69 membrane protein expression in peripheral blood T cells collected from pediatric recipients of cardiac allografts and found that CD69 expression is increased in both CD4+ T cells and CD8+ T cells during an episode of acute rejection (72).

The chemokine and chemokine receptor system is a key regulator of immune cell traffic. Melter et al. examined 169 sequential endomyocardial biopsy samples by immunocytochemistry for the expression of CCR1, CCR3, CCR5, or CXCR3 by CD3+ T cells and found a strong association among CD3+ T-cell infiltration, CXCR3 expression, and acute rejection by histology; RT-PCR analysis of 35 endomyocardial biopsy samples showed that eotaxin, lymphotactin, MCP-1, Mig, and SDF-1 (stromal cell-derived factor 1) were present in both normal and rejecting biopsy samples, whereas the CXCR3 ligand IP-10 was exclusively present in samples classified as acute rejection (51).

Fahmy and colleagues measured with the use of real-time quantitative PCR assay levels of mRNAs for chemokines and chemokine receptors in 316 serial and scheduled endomyocardial biopsy specimens from 30 cardiac allograft recipients and reported that the levels of mRNAs for IP-10, Mig, I-TAC, RANTES, CXCR3, and CCR5, but not those of MCP-1 and IL-8, are higher in samples classified as grade 2 or 3 rejection than in samples without rejection (24). In a subsequent study of gene expression patterns of 60 endomyocardial biopsy samples from 24 recipients, Fahmy et al. reported that, despite similar rejection grade by histology, the levels of IP-10, Mig, RANTES, CXCR3, and CCR5 were all higher in samples obtained between 9 and 12 months of transplantation than in samples obtained in the first 3 months of transplantation (25).

The vitronectin receptor integrin αVβ3A participates in multiple aspects of endothelial cell biology, including migration, apoptosis, and T-cell signaling. Yamani et al. investigated the expression of integrin αVβ3, fibronectin receptor α5β1, and tissue factor in endomyocardial biopsy samples and reported positive staining for integrin αVβ3 protein during acute cellular rejection of cardiac allografts but not for α5β1, or tissue factor in lymphocytic aggregates and vascular endothelial cells (102).

As in acute rejection of renal allografts, cardiac allografts undergoing acute rejection are distinguished by intragraft hyperexpression of cytotoxic attack molecules granzyme B, perforin, and Fas ligand. With the use of quantitative competitive PCR assay, Shulzhenko et al. measured levels of mRNA for granzyme B, perforin, and Fas ligand in 29 endomyocardial biopsy samples from 11 cardiac allograft recipients and reported that the levels of mRNAs for granzyme B, perforin, and Fas ligand were all higher in samples showing acute rejection than in those without rejection (84). Also, the levels of any two of the three mRNAs measured were increased in 100% of prerejection biopsy samples, in 92% of rejection samples, and in only 36% of biopsy samples without histologic changes of acute rejection. Upregulation of Fas ligand expression, during an episode of acute rejection, was also found by Oh et al. in their examination of endomyocardial biopsy specimens from 13 consecutive cardiac allograft

recipients (58), and as observed with renal allografts (75), the levels of expression of mRNA for Fas antigen were similar in biopsy samples with and without acute rejection.

Schoels et al. measured peripheral blood cell mRNA levels in 58 peripheral blood cell samples collected from 44 cardiac allograft recipients undergoing endomyocardial biopsies (71). Thirty-nine parameters, including cytokine and chemokine mRNAs, were examined, and data analysis showed that among the 39 mRNAs, peripheral blood mononuclear cell levels of mRNAs for perforin, granzyme B, CD95 ligand, RANTES, CXCR3, ENA 78, and TGF-β1 were significantly higher and the COX2 mRNA level was lower when peripheral blood samples were collected during grade 2 or higher rejection (n = 26) than in samples with no rejection or less than grade 2 rejection (n = 36). Receiver operator characteristic curve analysis showed that rejection of grade 2 or higher can be predicted with a sensitivity of 84% and a specificity of 82% with the use of levels of perforin, CD95 ligand, RANTES, COX2, and SEC7/TIC mRNAs (71).

Vascular endothelial growth factor (VEGF) is a major angiogenesis cytokine and has multiple functional attributes, including proinflammatory activity. Reinders et al. studied the expression of VEGF by immunohistochemistry in 101 endomyocardial biopsy samples from 10 cardiac transplant recipients and reported that whereas VEGF is expressed at a low level in normal endomyocardial biopsy samples, the angiogenic cytokine is induced in specimens with acute rejection and persistent expression is associated with the development of graft vascular disease (62). It was also observed that VEGF expression is associated with graft infiltration by CD3+ T cells and CD68+ monocytes and macrophages.

Molecular Correlates of Chronic Rejection of Cardiac Allografts

Cardiac allograft vasculopathy (CAV) is a form of chronic rejection in which intimal thickening leads to accelerated transplant coronary artery disease. High rejection scores on endomyocardial biopsy samples are an independent predictor of the development CAV (16).

Thrombospondin-1 (TSP-1) is a matrix glycoprotein expressed by smooth muscle cells and endothelial cells in response to vascular injury, platelet-derived growth factor, and basic fibroblast growth factor. TSP-1 stimulates the migration and proliferation of smooth muscle cells. In a study by Zhao et al., quantitative PCR assay was used to measure TSP-1 mRNA levels in endomyocardial biopsy specimens and immunochemistry was used to localize TSP-1 protein expression (108). TSP-1 mRNA levels in cardiac allografts were higher than in normal donor hearts, and cardiac allograft recipients with persistent elevations in TSP-1 mRNA levels in their sequential endomyocardial biopsy samples developed severe CAV (as determined by angiography), whereas those with transient elevations did not develop CAV; TSP-1 protein was localized primarily to cardiac myocytes and neointimal smooth muscle cells.

In a subsequent study, Zhao et al. studied the expression of CXCR3 and its ligands IP-10, I-TAC, and Mig in 133 consecutive endomyocardial biopsy samples from human cardiac allografts and in 11 normal donor hearts (107). mRNAs for IP-10, Mig, and I-TAC were detected only in cardiac allografts and not in normal hearts; sustained elevations of IP-10 and I-TAC were associated with CAV, and both IP-10 and Mig were both increased during acute rejection. CXCR3 was localized to both vascular cells and infiltrating cells, whereas IP-10 and I-TAC were found in vascular cells and Mig was detected primarily in infiltrating macrophages (107).

AIF-1 cDNA was initially cloned in a rat model (Lewis to F344) of chronic rejection, and AIF-1 mRNA and protein were both observed in neutrophils and macrophages infiltrating the cardiac allograft (95). Autieri et al. examined the association between the level of expression of AIF-1 and International Society for Heart and Lung Transplantation (ISHLT) rejection grade and CAV (6). In their study, 157 endomyocardial biopsy specimens from 26 recipients of cardiac allografts were analyzed for AIF-1 mRNA expression with the use of semiquantitative PCR assay. The authors found that the levels of AIF-1 mRNA were a correlate of ISHLT rejection grade and that the levels increase with rejection severity. Also, AIF-1 protein was localized to infiltrating cells in grade 1 specimens, whereas AIF-1 was detected in both infiltrating cells and cardiomyocytes in the biopsy samples showing grade 3 rejections (6).

The transcription factor early growth response factor 1 (Egr-1) participates in multiple immune and inflammatory pathways. Egr-1 is induced in endothelial cells and interacts with the consensus sequence GCGGTGGGCG present in the promoter region of several stress-related genes, including those for intercellular adhesion molecule 1 (ICAM-1), platelet-derived growth factor, TGF-β1, and plasminogen activator inhibitor 1 (PAI-1). Egr-1 induction may play an important role in the proliferation of vascular smooth muscle cells leading to intimal thickening and CAV. Autieri et al. investigated the role of Egr-1 in cardiac allograft rejection by examining 106 endomyocardial biopsy samples from 11 recipients of cardiac allografts (5). Immunohistochemistry and Western blotting were used to investigate Egr-1 expression in coronary arteries from patients with CAV.

Egr-1 protein was not detected in biopsy samples without rejection, and intense nuclear staining was detected in leukocytes and cardiac myocytes from samples with grade 3 rejection. Egr-1 mRNA was detected in 20% (6 of 30), 34% (20 of 58), 22% (2 of 9), and 89% (8 of 9) of the endomyocardial samples classified as ISHLT grades 0, 1, 2, and 3 (5). In this study, Egr-1 hyperexpression was found in the vascular cells of coronary arteries from patients with CAV.

Molecular Correlates of Acute Rejection of Lung Allografts

Acute rejection of lung allografts is distinguished by perivascular mononuclear cell infiltration of venules and arterioles. Various degrees of peribronchiolar mononuclear cell inflammation leading to bronchitis and bronchiolitis are also seen in allograft biopsy specimens (4, 104). Bronchoscopic lung allograft biopsy is the procedure of choice to evaluate acute rejection in lung transplantation.

An immunohistochemical study of 72 transbronchial biopsy specimens from 21 human recipients of lung or heart and lung allografts showed that the CD3+ cells are more abundant in allografts than in controls and that a positive correlation exists between histologic rejection and the number of CD3+, CD8+, CD25+, and CD16+ cells. In this study, the inverted CD4/CD8 ratio was not a correlate of rejection, and the phenotype of the cell infiltration was not predictive of CMV infection (19).

Clement et al. analyzed 31 bronchoalveolar lavage specimens for the level of expression of perforin and granzyme B and reported that their level of expression in alveolar lymphocytes is a correlate of the severity of rejection (17). Immunohistochemical analysis of transbronchial lung biopsy samples from patients with acute lung allograft rejection has shown increased expression of both CD4+ helper and CD8+ cytotoxic T cells and heightened expression of RANTES,

perforin, and Fas ligand during acute rejection (13). Intriguingly, perforin appeared to play a dual role: a cytopathic role contributing to tissue injury as well as a role in the downregulation of antiallograft immunity. Shreeniwas et al. evaluated 52 transbronchial biopsy specimens from 24 recipients of lung allografts and found by immunohistochemical staining that E-selectin expression but not the expression of ICAM-1 is a correlate of acute lung allograft rejection (81). It was also found in this study that endothelial cells displayed a high level of expression of HLA class II proteins even in the absence of acute rejection.

Murine models of acute lung allograft rejection suggest an important role for chemokines CXCL9/CXCR3 and RANTES (8, 10). The participation of the chemoattractant IP-10 and its receptor CXCR3 in lung allograft rejection was explored by Agostini et al. (1). Immunohistochemical examination of transbronchial biopsy specimens showed that acute rejection and obliterative broncholitis were associated with infiltration of cells that express CXCR3. Moreover, the T cells from the bronchoalveolar lavage specimens were positive for CXCR3. In addition to CXCR3, acute rejection was also associated with IP-10-expressing macrophages, and IP-10 levels were high in the bronchoalveolar fluid collected during an episode of acute rejection.

Shi and colleagues investigated with the use of quantitative competitive PCR assay whether the levels of mRNAs encoding IL-15 and granzyme B are diagnostic of acute rejection of lung allografts (78). As found with renal allografts, mRNAs for IL-15 and granzyme B were both expressed at a higher level in bronchoalveolar lavage-derived mononuclear cells from patients with acute lung allograft rejection than in samples from patients with stable lung function. Data analysis involving receiver operator characteristic curve analysis demonstrated that acute rejection can be predicted with a sensitivity of 94% and a specificity of 67% with the use of a cutoff value of 3.1 fg of granzyme B mRNA per μg of RNA.

Gimino et al. used microarray technology (Affymetrix GeneChip) to analyze the gene expression patterns of bronchoalveolar lavage cells of patients with and without acute lung allograft rejection (28). The bronchoalveolar lavage cell counts as well as the differential counts were similar between the two groups. The gene expression profiles, however, were strikingly different. In the acute-rejection group ($n = 7$ patients), 135 genes were upregulated compared to the genes in the no-rejection group ($n = 27$ patients), and the upregulated genes suggested seven biological pathways in the acute-rejection process. The upregulated immune response genes included those for STAT-4, CD28, chemokine (C-C motif) receptor 7, chemokine (C-X-C motif) receptor 3, CTLA-4, granzyme A, perforin 1, IFN-γ, lymphotoxin β, T-cell receptor α locus, T-cell receptor β locus, IL-2-inducible T-cell kinase, CD3ε, human Ig rearranged γ chain, Ig κ chain, and Ig λ locus. Other genes that were found to be significantly changed when specimens with acute rejection versus no rejection were compared included those regulating apoptosis (6 genes) and transcription (5 genes) and genes involved in cell signaling (10 genes).

Molecular Correlates of Chronic Rejection of Lung Allografts

Chronic rejection of lung allografts is a major diagnostic and therapeutic challenge and a significant contributor to morbidity and mortality. It is manifested by the development of bronchiolitis obliterans syndrome (BOS) (36). BOS is not common in the early posttransplantation period, but its incidence progressively rises to involve 60 to 70% of lung transplant recipients within 5 years of transplantation. Histologically, bronchiolitis obliterans is characterized by fibroproliferative growth engulfing airway lumens and obliterating blood vessels. The prognosis is dismal after BOS is diagnosed, with mortality reaching 40% in the 2 years following the diagnosis (4). Acute rejection is the leading cause of BOS (15).

Belperio et al. investigated the role of CXC chemokines Mig, IP-10, and I-TAC in the pathogenesis of bronchiolitis obliterans. With the use of enzyme-linked immunosorbent assay to analyze bronchoalveolar lavage fluid obtained from healthy lung transplant recipients and those who developed BOS, the investigators found that the levels of Mig, IP-10, and I-TAC are all elevated in patients who progress from acute rejection to chronic rejection (9).

Molecular Correlates of Acute Rejection of Liver Allografts

A consensus document, the Banff schema for the grading of liver allograft rejection, has been published (21). Not dissimilar to the histologic criteria used to classify renal allograft rejection, the grading schema for acute liver rejection is based upon the degree and severity of infiltration/inflammation by mononuclear cells of the portal triad, bile duct, and venous endothelium.

Krams et al. investigated intrahepatic expression of granzyme B using semiquantitative RT-PCR (39). Allograft biopsy samples obtained during an episode of acute rejection showed heightened expression of granzyme B mRNA compared to biopsy specimens without rejection, with resolution of rejection, or with only preservation injury.

The levels of expression of granzyme B as well as granzyme A have been examined in fine-needle aspirates of liver allografts, and the levels of both granzymes B and A were significantly higher in the aspirates obtained from grafts undergoing acute rejection than in aspirates from the liver grafts not showing acute rejection, but not higher than in aspirates obtained from patients with CMV infection (40).

Hyperexpression of chemokine receptors CXCR3, CXCR4, and CCR5, at the protein level, has been observed in graft-infiltrating lymphocytes as well as in circulating cells (30). It has been reported that CXCR3 ligands, IP-10, Mig, and I-TAC are all highly expressed on liver allograft endothelium and that the expression of SDF, a ligand for CXCR4, is restricted to biliary epithelium CCR3, and CCR5 is overexpressed in activated Kupffer cells (30).

Bartlett et al. investigated intrahepatic expression of costimulatory molecules CD80, CD86, and CD154 in 44 orthotopic liver allografts, at the levels of mRNA (with the use of semiquantitative RT-PCR) and protein (immunohistochemistry), and observed that intragraft expression of CD80 and CD154, at the protein but not at the mRNA level, is a correlate of acute rejection (7).

Liver allografts undergo acute rejection despite effective suppression of IL-2 expression, suggesting that additional growth factors, such as IL-15, contribute to the rejection process. Support for this hypothesis is provided by the observation of Conti et al. that in situ expression of IL-15 is elevated in patients with acute liver allograft rejection, especially during steroid-resistant rejection, and chronic rejection (18).

High-density microarray analyses, carried out by Sreekumar and colleagues, have begun to yield gene expression patterns that distinguish acute rejection from recurrent hepatitis C virus infection of the liver allograft (88). In their study, liver allograft biopsy samples from patients with acute rejection showed overexpression of genes associated with MHC class I and class II antigens, complement components, T-cell activation, and apoptosis compared to gene expression patterns of recurrent hepatitis C virus infection. Additional genes hyperexpressed during an episode of acute rejection included those for granzyme B, TNF-related apoptosis-inducing ligand, TNF-α-converting enzyme, TNF-α-inducible protein A20, TNF-α, TGF-β1 and insulin-like growth factor 1, transcription factor ISGF-3, IFN-γ-responsive transcription factor, and heat shock protein 70.

Molecular Correlates of Chronic Rejection of Liver Allografts

Compared to that for all other solid organ allografts, the incidence of chronic liver rejection is low; it is reported to be about 5% (20, 99). Also, contrary to the case with other vascularized solid organs, the incidence of chronic liver rejection usually decreases over time. Chronic rejection is typically seen in liver transplant recipients with persistent unresolved acute rejection and can lead to end-stage liver disease within the first year after transplantation.

Vasculopathy of hepatic arteries and terminal venules with loss of bile ducts are the distinguishing histologic features. Patients present with a cholestatic picture with blood tests indicating elevation of γ-glutamyl transpeptidase and alkaline phosphatase.

Van der Leij et al. investigated, with the use of RT-PCR and by immunocytochemistry, the expression of the TGF-β1-induced antiapoptotic factor (TIAF) gene in chronic liver allograft rejection and found that whereas this gene is not expressed in normal liver, its expression is upregulated in liver biopsy specimens with chronic rejection (96).

Molecular Characterization of Acute Rejection of Pancreatic Islet Allografts

Human islet cell transplantation has become a viable clinical therapeutic approach for the treatment of type 1 diabetes (74). The inability to diagnose rejection of islet cell graft prior to the development of hyperglycemia complicates clinical management of the islet graft recipient. Han et al. developed quantitative real-time PCR assays for the measurement of rhesus and cynomolgus monkey mRNAs for perforin, granzyme B, and Fas ligand and investigated whether heightened expression of peripheral blood cell mRNAs for cytotoxic attack molecules precede and/or are diagnostic of islet graft rejection in nonhuman primates (33). Four rhesus monkeys with long-term islet allograft function were studied following discontinuation of anti-CD154 monoclonal antibody therapy; in all four recipients, elevations in the level of expression of mRNAs encoding cytotoxic proteins were observed to precede islet graft rejection, and among the CTL genes, alterations in the levels of granzyme B mRNA were the best predictor of rejection (33).

Han et al. have translated their preclinical observations to the clinic (32). In their study cohort of 13 islet graft recipients with insulin independence, 8 subsequently became insulin dependent. Longitudinal measurement of peripheral blood cell mRNA levels showed that elevations in the levels of mRNAs for perforin, granzyme B, and Fas ligand precede islet graft failure and hyperglycemia. As previously observed by Han and colleagues in the nonhuman primate model (33), alterations in the levels of granzyme B mRNA were the best predictor of islet graft failure. Upregulation of CTL genes was also noted during episodes of infection, but the combination of elevations in CTL transcript levels and cellular sensitization, as identified with the use of mixed leukocyte reaction assay, was observed only in the patients who lost their islet grafts and in not those with infection.

TABLE 1 Noninvasive diagnosis of acute rejection of allografts

Type of allograft	Cell type	Molecular correlate of acute rejection	Reference
Renal	Peripheral blood	Granzyme B↑, perforin↑, Fas ligand↑	97
Renal	Peripheral blood	CD40 ligand ↑	80
Renal	Peripheral blood	IL-5 and IL-13 ↑	93
Renal	Peripheral blood	Granulysin ↑	67
Renal	Urinary	Granzyme B ↑, perforin ↑	43
Renal	Peripheral blood	Granzyme B ↑, HLA-DR ↑	64
Renal	Peripheral blood	Granzyme B ↑, perforin ↑	85
Renal	Urinary	CD103 ↑	22
Renal	Urinary	PI-9 ↑	54
Renal	Peripheral blood	IL-18 ↑	86
Renal	Urinary	IP-10 ↑, CXCR3 ↑	94
Renal	Urinary	Granulysin ↑	38
Heart	Peripheral blood	TIRC 7 ↓	83
Heart	Peripheral blood	CD27 ↓	52
Heart	Peripheral blood	Granzyme B ↑, perforin ↑, CD95 ligand ↑, RANTES ↑, CXCR3 ↑, ENA 78 ↑, COX2 ↓	71
Lung	Bronchoalveolar lavage	Granzyme B ↑, perforin ↑	17
Lung	Bronchoalveolar lavage	CXCR3 ↑, IP-10 ↑	1
Lung	Bronchoalveolar lavage	Granzyme B ↑, IL-15 ↑	78
Islet	Peripheral blood	Granzyme B ↑	32

CONCLUDING REMARKS

We have reviewed data regarding molecular correlates of rejection of human renal, cardiac, lung, liver, and pancreatic islet cell allografts. Nucleic acid-based strategies have proven useful for the detection and quantification of gene expression in the clinic. Recent refinements have paved the way for devising noninvasive molecular diagnostic tests for acute rejection of allografts (Table 1). Global expression profiling with technologies such as microarrays will add to our knowledge and provide further insights into molecular pathways, and several pathways are likely to be responsible for the rejection process. Future challenges will include sorting out the vast genomic data and identifying of critical pathways and targetable nodal points. We envision molecular studies to be of value not only from a diagnostic perspective but also in the development and application of mechanism-based therapeutics. The ultimate objective, personalized medicine for the transplant recipient, is an accomplishable goal.

We are grateful to Linda Stackhouse for her meticulous help in the preparation of the manuscript. The studies from the authors' laboratory were supported in part by awards from the National Institutes of Health (R01 AI 51652 and R01 AI60706). In this focused survey of literature related to molecular correlates of allograft rejection, some of the key and original contributions may not have been cited, and we regret the inadvertent omission.

REFERENCES

1. **Agostini, C., F. Calabrese, F. Rea, M. Facco, A. Tosoni, M. Loy, G. Binotto, M. Valente, L. Trentin, and G. Semenzato.** 2001. CXCR3 and its ligand CXCL10 are expressed by inflammatory cells infiltrating lung allograft and mediate chemotaxis of T cells at sites of rejection. *Am. J. Pathol.* **158:**1703–1711.
2. **Akalin, E., R. C. Hendrix, R. G. Polavarapu, T. C. Pearson, J. F. Neylan, C. P. Larsen, and F. G. Lakkis.** 2001. Gene expression analysis in human renal allograft biopsy samples using high-density oligoarray technology. *Transplantation* **72:**948–953.
3. **Akira, S., and K. Takeda.** 2004. Toll-like receptor signaling. *Nat. Rev. Immunol.* **4:**499–511.
4. **Arcasoy, S. M., and R. M. Kotloff.** 1999. Lung transplantation. *N. Engl. J. Med.* **340:**1081–1091.
5. **Autieri, M. S., E. Keleman, J. P. Gaughan, and H. Eisen.** 2004. Early growth responsive gene (Egr)-1 expression correlates with cardiac allograft rejection. *Transplantation* **78:**107–111.
6. **Autieri, M. V., S. Kelemen, B. A. Thomas, E. D. Feller, B. I. Goldman, and H. J. Eisen.** 2002. Allograft inflammatory factor-1 expression correlates with cardiac rejection and development of cardiac allograft vasculopathy. *Circulation* **106:**2218–2223.
7. **Bartlett, A. S. R., J. L. McCall, R. Ameratunga, M. L. Yeong, E. Gane, and S. R. Munn.** 2003. Analysis of intragraft gene and protein expression of the costimulatory molecules, CD80, CD86 and CD154, in orthotopic liver transplant recipients. *Am. J. Transplant.* **3:**1363–1368.
8. **Belperio, J. A., M. D. Burdick, M. P. Keane, Y. Y. Xue, J. P. Lynch III, B. L. Daugherty, S. L. Kunkel, and R. M. Strieter.** 2000. The role of the CC chemokine, RANTES, in acute lung allograft rejection. *J. Immunol.* **165:**461–472.
9. **Belperio, J. A., M. P. Keane, M. D. Burdick, J. P. Lynch III, Y. Y. Xue, K. Li, D. J. Ross, and R. M. Strieter.** 2002. Critical role for CXCR3 chemokine biology in the pathogenesis of bronchiolitis obliterans syndrome. *J. Immunol.* **169:**1037–1049.
10. **Belperio, J. A., M. P. Keane, M. D. Burdick, J. P. Lynch III, D. A. Zisman, Y. Y. Xue, K. Li, A. Ardehali, D. J. Ross, and R. M. Strieter.** 2003. Role of CXCL9/CXCR3 chemokine biology during pathogenesis of acute lung allograft rejection. *J. Immunol.* **171:**4844–4852.
11. **Berggren, W. T., T. Takova, M. C. Olson, P. S. Eis, R. W. Kwiatkowski, and L. M. Smith.** 2002. Multiplexed gene expression analysis using the invader RNA assay with MALDI-TOF mass spectrometry detection. *Anal. Chem.* **74:**1745–1750.
12. **Billingham, M. E., N. R. B. Cary, M. E. Hammond, J. Kemnitz, C. Marboe, H. A. McCallister, D. C. Snovar, G. L. Winters, and A. Zerbe.** 1990. A working formulation for the standardization of nomenclature in the diagnosis of heart and lung rejection: heart rejection study group. *J. Heart Transplant.* **9:**587–593.

13. Bittmann, I., C. Muller, J. Behr, J. Groetzner, L. Frey, and U. Lohrs. 2004. Fas/FasL and perforin/granzyme pathway in acute rejection and diffuse alveolar damage after allogeneic lung transplantation—a human biopsy study. *Virchows Arch.* **445:**375–381.

14. Border, W. A., and N. A. Noble. 1994. Transforming growth factor β in tissue fibrosis. *N. Engl. J. Med.* **331:**1286–1292.

15. Bowdish, M. E., S. M. Arcasoy, J. S. Wilt, J. V. Conte, R. D. Davis, E. R. Garrity, M. L. Hertz, J. B. Orens, B. R. Rosengard, and M. L. Barr. 2004. Surrogate markers and risk factors for chronic lung allograft dysfunction. *Am. J. Transplant.* **4:**1171–1178.

16. Cafario, A. L. P., F. Tona, A. B. Fortina, A. Angelini, S. Piaserico, A. Gambino, G. Feltrin, A. Ramondo, M. Valente, S. Iliceto, G. Thiene, and G. Gerosa. 2004. Immune and nonimmune predictors of cardiac allograft vasculopathy onset and severity: multivariate risk factor analysis and role of immunosuppression. *Am. J. Transplant.* **4:**962–970.

17. Clement, M. V., S. Legros-Maida, D. Israel-Biet, F. Carnot, A. Soulie, P. Reynaud, J. Guillet, I. Gandjbakch, and M. Sasportes. 1994. Perforin and granzyme B expression is associated with severe acute rejection. Evidence for in situ localization in alveolar lymphocytes of lung-transplanted patients. *Transplantation* **57:**322–326.

18. Conti, F., J. Frappier, S. Dharancy, C. Chereau, D. Houssin, B. Weill, and Y. Calmus. 2003. Interleukin-15 production during liver allograft rejection in humans. *Transplantation* **76:**210–216.

19. de Blic, J., M. Peuchmaur, F. Carnot, C. Danel, M. Deruesne, P. Reynaud, P. Scheinmann, and N. Brousse. 1992. Rejection in lung transplantation—an immunohistochemical study of transbronchial biopsies. *Transplantation* **54:**639–644.

20. Demetris., A., et al. 2000. Update of the International Banff Schema for Liver Allograft Rejection: working recommendations for the histopathologic staging and reporting of chronic rejection. *Hepatology* **31:**792–799.

21. Demetris, A. J., et al. 1997. Banff schema for grading liver allograft rejection: an international consensus document. *Hepatology* **25:**658–663.

22. Ding, R., B. Li, T. Muthukumar, D. Dadhania, M. Medeiros, C. Hartono, D. Serur, S. V. Seshan, V. K. Sharma, S. Kapur, and M. Suthanthiran. 2003. CD103 mRNA levels in urinary cells predict acute rejection of renal allografts. *Transplantation* **75:**1307–1312.

23. Donauer, J., B. Rumberger, M. Klein, D. Faller, J. Wilpert, T. Sparna, G. Schieren, R. Rohrbach, P. Dern, J. Timmer, P. Pisarski, G. Kirste, and G. Walz. 2003. Expression profiling on chronically rejected transplant kidneys. *Transplantation* **76:**539–547.

24. Fahmy, N. M., M. H. Yamani, R. C. Starling, N. B. Ratliff, J. B. Young, P. M. McCarthy, J. Y. Feng, A. C. Novick, and R. L. Fairchild. 2003. Chemokine and chemokine receptor gene expression indicates acute rejection of human cardiac transplants. *Transplantation* **75:**72–79.

25. Fahmy, N. M., M. H. Yamani, R. C. Starling, N. B. Ratliff, J. B. Young, P. M. McCarthy, J. Y. Feng, A. C. Novick, and R. L. Fairchild. 2003. Chemokine and receptor-gene expression during early and late acute rejection episodes in human cardiac allografts. *Transplantation* **75:**2044–2047.

26. Flechner, S. M., S. M. Kurian, S. R. Head, S. M. Sharp, T. C. Whisenant, J. Zhang, J. D. Chismar, S. Horvath, T. Mondala, T. Gilmartin, D. J. Cook, S. A. Kay, J. R. Walker, and D. R. Salomon. 2004. Kidney transplant rejection and tissue injury by gene profiling of biopsies and peripheral blood lymphocytes. *Am. J. Transplant.* **4:**1475–1489.

27. Flechner, S. M., S. M. Kurian, K. Solez, D. J. Cook, J. T. Burke, H. Rollin, J. A. Hammond, T. Whisenant, C. M. Lanigan, S. R. Head, and D. R. Salomon. 2004. *De novo* kidney transplantation without use of calcineurin inhibitors preserves renal structure and function at two years. *Am. J. Transplant.* **4:**1776–1785.

28. Gimino, V. J., J. D. Lande, T. R. Berryman, R. A. King, and M. I. Hertz. 2003. Gene expression profiling of bronchoalveolar lavage cells in acute lung rejection. *Am. J. Respir. Crit. Care Med.* **168:**1237–1242.

29. Giulietti, A., L. Overbergh, D. Valckx, B. Decallonne, R. Bouillon, and C. Mathieu. 2001. An overview of real-time quantitative PCR: applications to quantify cytokine gene expression. *Methods* **25:**386–401.

30. Goddard, S., A. Williams, C. Morland, S. Qin, R. Gladue, S. G. Hubscher, and D. H. Adams. 2001. Differential expression of chemokines and chemokine receptors shapes the inflammatory response in rejecting human liver transplants. *Transplantation* **72:**1957–1967.

31. Hadley, G. 2004. Role of integrin CD103 in promoting destruction of renal allografts by CD8$^+$ T cells. *Am. J. Transplant.* **4:**1026–1032.

32. Han, D., X. Xu, D. Baidal, J. Leith, C. Ricordi, R. Alejandro, and N. S. Kenyon. 2004. Assessment of cytotoxic lymphocyte gene expression in the peripheral blood of human islet allograft recipients. *Diabetes* **53:**2281–2290.

33. Han, D., X. Xu, R. L. Pastori, C. Ricordi, and N. S. Kenyon. 2002. Elevation of cytotoxic lymphocyte gene expression is predictive of islet allograft rejection in nonhuman primates. *Diabetes* **51:**562–566.

34. Hartono, C., D. Dadhania, and M. Suthanthiran. 2004. Noninvasive diagnosis of acute rejection of solid organ transplants. *Front. Biosci.* **9:**145–153.

35. Heeger, P. S. 2003. T-cell allorecognition and transplant rejection: a summary and update. *Am. J. Transplant.* **3:**525–533.

36. Heng, D., L. D. Sharples, K. McNeil, S. Stewart, T. Wreghitt, and J. Wallwork. 1998. Bronchiolitis obliterans syndrome: incidence, natural history, prognosis, and risk factors. *J. Heart Lung Transplant.* **17:**1255–1263.

37. Jordan, B. R. (ed.). 2001. *DNA Microarrays: Gene Expression Applications.* Springer, New York, N.Y.

38. Kotsch, K., M. F. Mashreghi, G. Bold, P. Tretow, J. Beyer, M. Matz, J. Hoerstrup, J. Pratschke, R. C. Ding, M. Suthanthiran, H. D. Volk, and P. Reinke. 2004. Enhanced granulysin mRNA expression in urinary sediment in early and delayed acute renal allograft rejection. *Transplantation* **77:**1866–1875.

39. Krams, S. M., J. C. Villaneuva, M. B. Quinn, and O. M. Martinez. 1995. Expression of the cytotoxic T cell mediator granzyme B during liver allograft rejection. *Transpl. Immunol.* **3:**162–166.

40. Kuijf, M. M. L., J. Kwekkeboom, M. A. Kuijpers, M. Willems, P. E. Zondervan, H. G. M. Niesters, W. C. J. Hop, C. E. Hack, T. Paavonen, K. Hockerstedt, H. W. Tilanus, I. Lautenschlager, and H. J. Metselaar. 2002. Granzyme expression in fine-needle aspirates from liver allografts is increased during acute rejection. *Liver Transplant.* **8:**952–956.

41. Lakkis, F. G., A. Arakelov, B. T. Konieczny, and Y. Inoue. 2000. Immunologic 'ignorance' of vascularized organ transplants in the absence of secondary lymphoid tissue. *Nat. Med.* **6:**686–688.

42. Lantz, P. G., W. Abu al-Soud, R. Knutsson, B. Hahn-Hagerdal, and P. Radstrom. 2000. Biotechnical use of polymerase chain reaction for microbiological analysis of biological samples. *Biotechnol. Annu. Rev.* **5:**87–130.

43. Li, B., C. Hartono, R. Ding, V. K. Sharma, R. Ramaswamy, B. Qian, D. Serur, J. Mouradian, J. E.

Schwartz, and M. Suthanthiran. 2001. Noninvasive diagnosis of renal-allograft rejection by measurement of messenger RNA for perforin and granzyme B in urine. *N. Engl. J. Med.* **344:**947–954.

44. Li, Y., J. Yang, C. Dai, C. Wu, and Y. Liu. 2003. Role for integrin-linked kinase in mediating tubular epithelial to mesenchymal transition and renal interstitial fibrogenesis. *J. Clin. Investig.* **112:**503–516.

45. Libby, P., and J. S. Pober. 2001. Chronic rejection. *Immunity* **14:**387–397.

46. Lipman, M. L., A. C. Stevens, R. C. Bleackley, J. H. Helderman, T. R. McCune, W. E. Harmon, M. E. Shapiro, S. Rosen, and T. B. Strom. 1992. The strong correlation of cytotoxic T lymphocyte-specific serine protease gene transcripts with renal allograft rejection. *Transplantation* **53:**73–79.

47. Lipman, M. L., A. C. Stevens, and T. B. Strom. 1994. Heightened intragraft CTL gene expression in acutely rejecting renal allografts. *J. Immunol.* **152:**5120–5127.

48. Livak, K. J., and T. D. Schmittgen. 2001. Analysis of relative gene expression data using real-time quantitative PCR and the 2(-delta delta C(T)) method. *Methods* **25:**402–408.

49. Luster, A. D. 1998. Chemokines—chemotactic cytokines that mediate inflammation. *N. Engl. J. Med.* **338:**436–445.

50. Marshall, A., and J. Hodgson. 1998. DNA chips—an array of possibilities. *Nat. Biotechnol.* **16:**27–31.

51. Melter, M., A. Exeni, M. E. J. Reinders, J. C. Fang, G. McMahon, P. Ganz, W. H. Hancock, and D. M. Briscoe. 2001. Expression of the chemokine receptor CXCR3 and its ligand IP-10 during human cardiac allograft rejection. *Circulation* **104:**2558–2564.

52. Morgun, A., N. Shulzhenko, G. F. Rampim, A. P. Chinellato, R. V. Z. Diniz, D. R. Almeida, M. M. Souza, M. Franco, and M. Gerbase-DeLima. 2003. Blood and intragraft CD27 gene expression in cardiac transplant recipients. *Clin. Immunol.* **107:**60–64.

53. Munger, J. S., X. Huang, H. Kawakatsu, M. J. D. Griffiths, S .L. Dalton, J. Wu, J. F. Pittet, N. Kaminski, C. Garat, M. A. Matthay, D. B. Rifkin, and D. Sheppard. 1999. The integrin αvβ6 binds and activates latent TGFβ1: a mechanism for regulating pulmonary inflammation and fibrosis. *Cell* **96:**319–328.

54. Muthukumar, T., R. Ding, D. Dadhania, M. Medeiros, B. Li, V. K. Sharma, C. Hartono, D. Serur, S. V. Seshan, H. D. Volk, P. Reinke, S. Kapur, and M. Suthanthiran. 2003. Serine proteinase inhibitor-9, an endogenous blocker of granzyme B/perforin lytic pathway, is hyperexpressed during acute rejection of renal allografts. *Transplantation* **75:**1565–1570.

55. Nelson, P. J., and A. M. Krensky. 2001. Chemokines, chemokine receptors, and allograft rejection. *Immunity* **14:**377–386.

56. Nickel, P., J. Lacha, S. Ode-Hakim, B. Sawitzki, N. Babel, U. Frei, H. D. Volk, and P. Reinke. 2001. Cytotoxic effector molecule gene expression in acute renal allograft rejection: correlation with clinical outcome; histopathology and function of the allograft. *Transplantation* **72:**1158–1160.

57. Nocera, A., A. Tagliamacco, R. De Palma, F. Del Galdo, A. Ferrante, I. Fontana, S. Barocci, F. Ginevri, D. Rolla, J. L. Ravetti, and U. Valente. 2004. Cytokine mRNA expression in chronically rejected human renal allografts. *Clin. Transplant.* **18:**564–570.

58. Oh, S. I., I. W. Kim, H. C. Jung, J. W. Seo, I. H. Chae, H. S. Kim, and B. H. Oh. 2001. Correlation of Fas and Fas ligand expression with rejection status of transplanted heart in human. *Transplantation* **71:**906–909.

59. Panzer, U., R. R. Reinking, O. M. Steinmetz, G. Zahner, U. Sudbeck, S. Fehr, B. Pfalzer, A. Schneider,

F. Thaiss, M. Mack, S. Conrad, H. Huland, U. Helmchen, and R. A. K. Stahl. 2004. CXCR3 and CCR5 positive T-cell recruitment in acute human renal allograft rejection. *Transplantation* **78:**1341–1350.

60. Pavlakis, M., J. Strehlau, M. Lipman, M. Shapiro, W. Maslinski, and T. B. Strom. 1996. Intragraft IL-15 transcripts are increased in human renal allograft rejection. *Transplantation* **62:**543–545.

61. Racusen, L. C., K. Solez, R. B. Colvin, S. M. Bonsib, M. C. Castro, T. Cavallo, B. P. Croker, A. J. Demetris, C. B. Drachenberg, A. B. Fogo, P. Furness, L. W. Gaber, I. W. Gibson, D. Glotz, J. C. Goldberg, J. Grande, P. F. Halloran, H. E. Hansen, B. Hartley, P. J. Hayry, C. M. Hill, E. O. Hoffman, L. G. Hunsicker, A. S. Lindblad, N. Marcussen, M. J. Mihatsch, T. Nadasdy, P. Nikerson, T. S. Olsen, J. C. Papadimitriou, P. S. Randhawa, D. C. Rayner, I. Roberts, S. Rose, D. Rush, L. Salinas-Madrigal, D. R. Salomon, S. Sund, E. Taskinen, K. Trpkov, and Y. Yamaguchi. 1999. The Banff 97 working classification of renal allograft pathology. *Kidney Int.* **55:**713–723.

62. Reinders, M. E., J. C. Fang, W. Wong, P. Ganz, and D. Briscoe. 2003. Expression patterns of vascular endothelial growth factor in human cardiac allografts: association with rejection. *Transplantation* **76:**224–230.

63. Robertson, H., W. K. Wong, D. Talbot, A. D. Burt, and J. A. Kirby. 2001. Tubulitis after renal transplantation: demonstration of an association between CD103+ T cells, transforming growth factor β1 expression and rejection grade. *Transplantation* **71:**306–313.

64. Sabek, O., M. T. Dorak, M. Kotb, A. O. Gaber, and L. Gaber. 2002. Quantitative detection of T-cell activation markers by real-time PCR in renal transplant rejection and correlation with histopathologic evaluation. *Transplantation* **74:**701–707.

65. Saiki, R. K., S. Scharf, F. Faloona, K. B. Mullis, G. T. Horn, H. A. Erlich, and N. Arnheim. 1985. Enzymatic amplification of beta-globin genomic sequences and restriction site analysis for diagnosis of sickle cell anemia. *Science* **230:**1350–1354.

66. Sarwal, M., M. S. Chua, N. Kambham, S. C. Hsieh, T. Satterwhite, M. Masek, and O. Salvatierra, Jr. 2003. Molecular heterogeneity in acute renal allograft rejection identified by DNA microarray profiling. *N. Engl. J. Med.* **349:**125–138.

67. Sarwal, M. M., A. Jani, S. Chang, P. Huie, Z. Wang, O. Salvatierra, Jr., C. Clayberger, R. Sibley, A. M. Krensky, and M. Pavlakis. 2001. Granulysin expression is a marker for acute rejection and steroid resistance in human renal transplantation. *Hum. Immunol.* **62:**21–31.

68. Sawada, T., M. Abe, K. Kai, K. Kubota, S. Fuchinoue, and S. Teraoka. 2004. β6 integrin is up-regulated in chronic renal allograft dysfunction. *Clin. Transplant.* **18:**525–528.

69. Sayegh, M. H., and L. A. Turka. 1998. The role of T-cell costimulatory activation pathways in transplant rejection. *N. Engl. J. Med.* **338:**1813–1821.

70. Scherer, A., A. Krause, J. R. Walker, A. Korn, D. Niese, and F. Raulf. 2003. Early prognosis of the development of renal chronic allograft rejection by gene expression profiling of human protocol biopsies. *Transplantation* **75:**1323–1330.

71. Schoels, M., T. J. Dengler, R. Richter, S. C. Meuer, and T. Giese. 2004. Detection of cardiac allograft rejection by real-time PCR analysis of circulating mononuclear cells. *Clin. Transplant.* **18:**513–517.

72. Schowengerdt, K. O., F. J. Fricker, K. S. Bahjat, and S. T. Kuntz. 2000. Increased expression of the lymphocyte early activation marker CD69 in peripheral blood correlates with histologic evidence of cardiac allograft rejection. *Transplantation* **69:**2102–2107.

73. Segerer, S., Y. Cui, F. Eitner, T. Goodpaster, K. L. Hudkins, M. Mack, J. P. Cartron, Y. Colin, D. Schlondorff, and C. E. Alpers. 2001. Expression of chemokines and chemokine receptors during human renal transplant rejection. *Am. J. Kidney Dis.* **37:** 518–531.

74. Shapiro, A. M. J., J. R. T. Lakey, E. A. Ryan, G. S. Korbutt, E. Toth, G. L. Warnock, N. M. Kneteman, and R. V. Rajotte. 2000. Islet transplantation in seven patients with type 1 diabetes mellitus using a glucocorticoid-free immunosuppressive regimen. *N. Engl. J. Med.* **343:**230–238.

75. Sharma, V. K., R. M. Bologa, B. Li, G.P. Xu, M. Lagman, W. Hiscock, J. Mouradian, J. Wang, D. Serur, V. K. Rao, and M. Suthanthiran. 1996. Molecular executors of cell death—differential intrarenal expression of Fas ligand, Fas, granzyme B, and perforin during acute and/or chronic rejection of human renal allografts. *Transplantation* **62:**1860–1866.

76. Sharma, V. K., R. M. Bologa, G. P. Xu, B. Li, J. Mouradian, J. Wang, D. Serur, V. Rao, and M. Suthanthiran. 1996. Intragraft TGF-beta 1 mRNA: a correlate of interstitial fibrosis and chronic allograft nephropathy. *Kidney Int.* **49:**1297–1303.

77. Sheppard, D., C. Rozzo, L. Starr, V. Quaranta, D. J. Erle, and R. Pytela. 1990. Complete amino acid sequence of a novel integrin β subunit (β6) identified in epithelial cells using the polymerase chain reaction. *J. Biol. Chem.* **265:**11502–11507.

78. Shi, R., J. Yang, A. Jaramillo, N. S. Steward, A. Aloush, E. P. Trulock, G. A. Patterson, M. Suthanthiran, and T. Mohanakumar. 2004. Correlation between interleukin-15 and granzyme B expression and acute lung allograft rejection. *Transpl. Immunol.* **12:**103–108.

79. Shimkets, R. A. 2004. *Gene Expression Profiling: Methods and Protocols.* Humana, Totowa, N.J.

80. Shoker, A., D. George, H. Yang, and M. Baltzan. 2000. Heightened CD40 ligand gene expression in peripheral CD4+ T cells from patients with kidney allograft rejection. *Transplantation* **70:**497–505.

81. Shreeniwas, R., L. L. Schulman, M. Narasimhan, C. C. McGregor, and C. C. Marboe. 1996. Adhesion molecules (E-selectin and ICAM-1) in pulmonary allograft rejection. *Chest* **110:**1143–1149.

82. Shulzhenko, N., A. Morgun, M. Franco, M. M. Souza, D. R. Almeida, R. V. Z. Diniz, A. C. C. Carvalho, A. Pacheco-Silva, and M. Gerbase-DeLima. 2001. Expression of CD40 ligand, interferon-gamma and Fas ligand genes in endomyocardial biopsies of human cardiac allografts: correlation with acute rejection. *Braz. J. Med. Biol. Res.* **34:**779–784.

83. Shulzhenko, N., A. Morgun, G. F. Rampim, M. Franco, D. R. Almeida, R. V. Z. Diniz, A. C. C. Carvalho, and M. Gerbase-DeLima. 2001. Monitoring of intragraft and peripheral blood TIRC7 expression as a diagnostic tool for acute cardiac rejection in humans. *Hum. Immunol.* **62:**342–347.

84. Shulzhenko, N., A. Morgun, X. X. Zheng, R. V. Diniz, D. R. Almeida, N. Ma, T. B. Strom, and M. Gerbase-DeLima. 2001. Intragraft activation of genes encoding cytotoxic T lymphocyte effector molecules precedes the histological evidence of rejection in human cardiac transplantation. *Transplantation* **72:**1705–1708.

85. Simon, T., G. Opelz, M. Wiesel, R. C. Ott, and C. Susal. 2003. Serial peripheral blood perforin and granzyme B gene expression measurements for prediction of acute rejection in kidney graft recipients. *Am. J. Transplant.* **3:**1121–1127.

86. Simon, T., G. Opelz, M. Wiesel, S. Pelzl, R. C. Ott, and C. Susal. 2004. Serial peripheral blood interleukin-18 and perforin gene expression measurements for prediction of acute kidney graft rejection. *Transplantation* **77:**1589–1595.

87. Souaze, F., A. Ntodou-Thome, C. Y. Tran, W. Rostene, and P. Forgez. 1996. Quantitative RT-PCR: limits and accuracy. *BioTechniques* **21:**280–285.

88. Sreekumar, R., D. L. Rasmussen, R. H. Wiesner, and M. R. Charlton. 2002. Differential allograft gene expression in acute cellular rejection and recurrence of hepatitis C after liver transplantation. *Liver Transplant.* **8:**814–821.

89. Stahlberg, A., J. Hakansson, X. Xian, H. Semb, and M. Kubista. 2004. Properties of the reverse transcription reaction in mRNA quantification. *Clin. Chem.* **50:**509–515.

90. Strehlau, J., M. Pavlakis, M. Lipman, M. Shapiro, L. Vasconcellos, W. Harmon, and T. B. Strom. 1997. Quantitative detection of immune activation transcripts as a diagnostic tool in kidney transplantation. *Proc. Natl. Acad. Sci. USA* **94:**695–700.

91. Suthanthiran, M. 1998. Human renal allograft rejection: molecular characterization. *Nephrol. Dial. Transplant.* **13:**(Suppl. 1):21–24.

92. Suthanthiran, M., and T. B. Strom. 1994. Renal transplantation. *N. Engl. J. Med.* **331:**365–376.

93. Tan, L., W. M. Howell, J. L. Smith, and S. A. Sadek. 2001. Sequential monitoring of peripheral T-lymphocyte cytokine gene expression in the early post renal allograft period. *Transplantation* **71:**751–759.

94. Tatapudi, R. R., T. Muthukumar, D. Dadhania, R. Ding, B. Li, V. K. Sharma, E. Lozada-Pastorio, N. Seetharamu, C. Hartono, D. Serur, S. V. Seshan, S. Kapur, W. W. Hancock, and M. Suthanthiran. 2004. Noninvasive detection of renal allograft inflammation by measurements of mRNA for IP-10 and CXCR3 in urine. *Kidney Int.* **65:**2390–2397.

95. Utans, U., R. J. Arceci, Y. Yamashita, and M. E. Russell. 1995. Cloning and characterization of allograft inflammatory factor-1: a novel macrophage factor identified in rat cardiac allografts with chronic rejection. *J. Clin. Investig.* **95:**2954–2962.

96. Van der Leij, J., A. Van den Berg, E. W. J. A. Albrecht, T. Blokzijl, R. Roozendaal, A. S. H. Gouw, K. P. De Jong, C. A. Stegeman, H. Van Goor, N. S. Chang, and S. Poppema. 2003. High expression of TIAF-1 in chronic kidney and liver allograft rejection and in activated T-helper cells. *Transplantation* **75:**2076–2082.

97. Vasconcellos, L. M., A. D. Schachter, X. X. Zheng, L. H. Vasconcellos, M. Shapiro, W. E. Harmon, and T. B. Strom. 1998. Cytotoxic lymphocyte gene expression in peripheral blood leukocytes correlates with rejecting renal allografts. *Transplantation* **66:**562–566.

98. Velculescu, V. E., L. Zhang, B. Vogelstein, and K. W. Kinzler. 1995. Serial analysis of gene expression. *Science* **270:**484–487.

99. Wiesner, R. H., K. P. Batts, and R. A. Krom. 1999. Evolving concepts in the diagnosis, pathogenesis, and treatment of chronic hepatic allograft rejection. *Liver Transpl. Surg.* **5:**388–400.

100. Xu, G. P., V. K. Sharma, B. Li, R. Bologa, Y. Li, J. Mouradian, J. Wang, D. Serur, V. Rao, and K. H. Stenzel. 1995. Intragraft expression of IL-10 messenger RNA: a novel correlate of renal allograft rejection. *Kidney Int.* **48:**1504–1507.

101. Yamada, S., K. Shinozaki, and K. Agematsu. 2002. Involvement of CD27/CD70 interactions in antigen-specific cytotoxic T-lymphocyte (CTL) activity by perforin-mediated cytotoxicity. *Clin. Exp. Immunol.* **130:**424–430.

102. Yamani, M. H., J. Yang, C. S. Masri, N. B. Ratliff, M. Bond, R. C. Starling, P. McCarthy, E. Plow, and J. B. Young. 2002. Acute cellular rejection following human heart transplantation is associated with increased expression of vitronectin receptor (integrin αvβ3). *Am. J. Transplant.* **2:**129–133.

103. Yang, J. W., and Y. H. Liu. 2002. Blockage of tubular epithelial to myofibroblast transition by hepatocyte growth factor prevents renal interstitial fibrosis. *J. Am. Soc. Nephrol.* **13:**96–107.

104. Yousem, S. A., G. J. Berry, P. T. Cagle, D. Chamberlain, A. N. Husain, R. H. Hruban, A. Marchevsky, N. P. Ohori, J. Ritter, S. Stewart, and H. D. Tazelaar. 1996. Revision of the 1990 working formulation for the classification of pulmonary allograft rejection: Lung Rejection Study Group. *J. Heart Lung Transplant.* **15:**1–15.

105. Zeisberg, M., J. I. Hanai, H. Sugimoto, T. Mammoto, D. Charytan, F. Strutz, and R. Kalluri. 2003. BMP-7 counteracts TGF-β1-induced epithelial-to-mesenchymal transition and reverse chronic renal injury. *Nat. Med.* **9:**964–968.

106. Zhang, W., I. Shmulevich, and J. Astola. 2004. *Microarray Quality Control.* John Wiley & Sons, Hoboken, N.J.

107. Zhao, X. M., H. Yenya, G. G. Miller, A. D. Luster, R. N. Mitchell, and P. Libby. 2002. Differential expression of the IFN-γ-inducible CXCR3-binding chemokines, IFN-inducible protein 10, monokine induced by IFN, and IFN-inducible T cell α chemoattractant in human cardiac allografts: association with cardiac allograft vasculopathy and acute rejection. *J. Immunol.* **169:**1556–1560.

108. Zhao, X. M., H. Yenya, G. G. Miller, R. N. Mitchell, and P. Libby. 2001. Association of thrombospondin-1 and cardiac allograft vasculopathy in human cardiac allografts. *Circulation* **103:**525–531.

Human Natural Killer Cell Receptors

DOLLY B. TYAN AND MARY CARRINGTON

140

Natural killer (NK) cells are one of the first lines of defense of the innate immune system. Typically described as large granular lymphocytes and sharing a common progenitor with T cells (24), they function both prior to initiation of the adaptive immune response and when the latter system is subverted, as happens in some viral infections and cancer. They respond early and rapidly after infection by producing gamma interferon from prestored transcripts before T cells in the adaptive immune system have had time to expand and differentiate in response to antigen. Likewise, they express granzymes and perforin and their lytic reactions can be triggered in minutes without requirement of transcription, translation, or proliferation (27, 29). In a mature immune response, they can sense varying levels of HLA class I or other ligands on target cells that the adaptive immune system does not see and perform spontaneous target cell killing of virally infected or transformed cells.

Regulation of NK cytolytic activity is a function of engagement of one or more NK surface receptors that may be activating or inhibitory. Unlike receptors in the adaptive immune system, NK receptors are in germ line configuration and do not rearrange (24). Two of the primary sets of receptors present on human NK cells are called the killer immunoglobulin (Ig)-like receptors (KIR; previously known as the killer inhibitory receptors) and the CD94/NKG2 lectin-like receptors. These sets each correspond to a family of genes with exceptionally interesting features in terms of both their genetics and their signaling. The KIR genes (15 genes and 2 pseudogenes) have enormous genetic diversity generated by a combination of variable gene content, alternative splicing, and allelic polymorphism, and they recognize a limited set of HLA class I molecules or epitopes, whereas the more ancestral CD94/NKG2 genes (four genes plus NKG2D) have less diversity but an intriguing array of unconventional HLA class I-like target ligands. These two receptor gene families and their roles in the immune response are the topic of this chapter. Other NK receptor gene families (e.g., leukocyte Ig-like receptor [LIR] and natural cytotoxicity receptor [NCR] genes) also present on some NK cells (4, 35, 56) will not be discussed here.

KIR GENETICS

The KIR genes occupy about 150 kb of the leukocyte receptor complex located on chromosome 19q13.4 (24) residing in a region comprising several families of leukocyte receptor genes (Fig. 1). They encode type I glycoproteins (extracellular amino terminus) with either two or three external Ig-like loop domains, a stem region, a transmembrane (TM) region, and either a short or a long cytoplasmic tail (CYT). The nomenclature is descriptive: the first three-letter designation indicates the gene family (KIR), the number and letter following (2D or 3D) indicate the number (i.e., two or three) of external Ig-like domains present, the letter following (L or S) indicates the presence of a long or short CYT, and the last digit indicates a gene variant with similar organization but >2% sequence difference (Fig. 2). For example, KIR2DL1 is the first variant in a series of KIR (KIR2DL1, KIR2DL2, etc.) with two external domains (i.e., 2D) and a long CYT (i.e., L). KIR exist as monomers with the exception of KIR3DL, which can also form homodimers (24). KIR are found primarily on NK cells but also on NKT cells (a subset of memory T cells with NK receptors), where they may modulate the adaptive immune response by competition with the T-cell receptor for ligand or by modulation of the response depending on which KIR genes are present (56).

A prototype KIR gene (KIR3DL1) has nine exons, as shown in Fig. 3 (8, 33, 56), and all of the other KIR genes can be derived from it by alternative splicing and subsequent mutation. Most KIR have two external Ig-like domains and are of two types. Type 1 KIR2D genes have functional exons 4 (D1) and 5 (D2), but exon 3 (D0) is a pseudoexon that is shorter by one codon and is spliced out even with the correct splicing sites and the correct reading frame (56). Type 2 KIR2D genes have exons 3 (D0) and 5 (D2) present but have spliced out >2 kb containing the fourth exon (D1). Figure 3 portrays the usual variants, but additional splicing variants also exist that are relatively unique (reviewed in references 54 and 56).

The TM and CYT of the KIR are of paramount importance for the function of NK cells because signaling occurs through these portions of the molecule. In general, KIR with long CYTs are inhibitory and those with short CYTs are activating. The long CYTs contain ITIM motifs [immunoreceptor tyrosine-based inhibitory motifs: sequence, (V/I)XYXX(L/V)] (29, 35, 49) which when phosphorylated become docking sites for the SHP-1 protein tyrosine phosphatase involved in inhibitory signaling (31). KIR with a charged residue (Lys) in the TM and short CYTs are generally activating. The short CYTs lack the ITIM motifs, and the charged TM residues interact with adaptor molecules containing ITAM

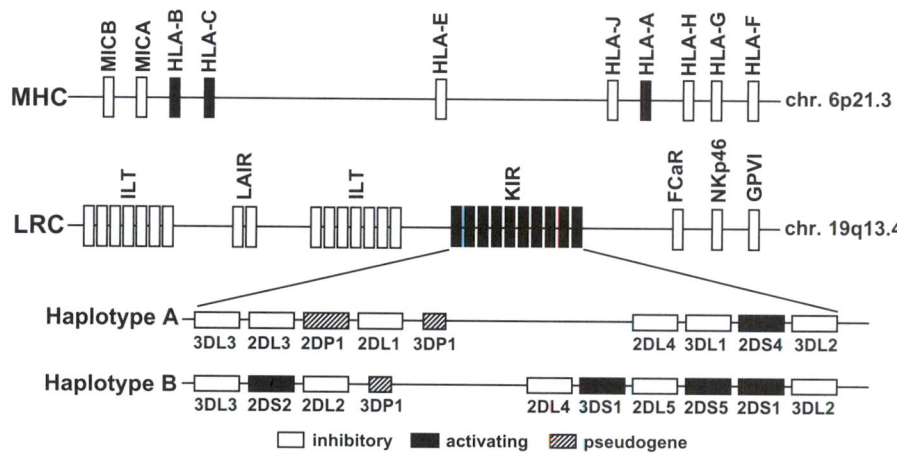

FIGURE 1 HLA class I and KIR gene loci: functionally related gene clusters that exhibit extreme polymorphism. The HLA class I genes map within the MHC at 6p21.3, and the KIR genes map within the leukocyte receptor complex (LRC) at 19q13.4. The KIR gene order is shown for the two distinct KIR haplotypes that have been sequenced in their entirety. Chr., chromosome; ILT, Ig-like transcript; LAIR, leukocyte-associated Ig-like receptor; FCaR, FCα receptor; GPVI, glycoprotein VI.

motifs [immunoreceptor tyrosine-based activation motifs; sequence, $D/EXXYXXL/IX_{(6-8)}YXXL/I$] connecting them to protein tyrosine kinase (PTK) activation pathways (31). KIR2DL4 may be divergent in that it appears to be activating despite its long tail due to the presence of a charged residue (Arg) in the TM domain and a substitution of Cys for Tyr in the CYT ITIM domain (56). KIR CYTs can also have different lengths despite similar exon lengths and sequences due to point substitutions in the exons that lead to premature stop codons (e.g., KIR3DS1) (50). The multiple examples of shortened

CYTs suggest that the generation of activating KIR is evolutionarily important (56). Finally, KIR with similar extracellular domains can have CYTs with opposite signaling motifs that may dictate the ultimate effector function of the NK cell.

In addition to the variations in splicing and CYT composition, most of the KIR genes are known to be polymorphic (56). The polymorphism varies by gene locus and is thought

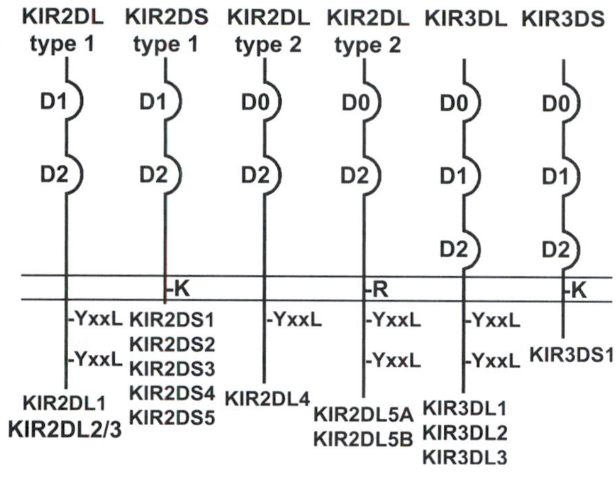

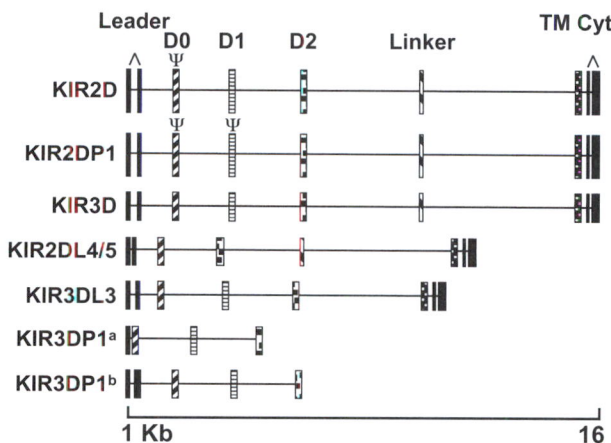

FIGURE 3 Exon-intron structure of the KIR genes. Exons 1 and 2 correspond to the leader (signal) sequence; exons 3 to 5 correspond to the Ig domains D0, D1, and D2, respectively; exons 6 and 7 correspond to the linker and TM regions, respectively; and exons 8 and 9 correspond to the cytoplasmic domain. All exons are design coded. The genes for type 1 two-domain KIR genes, KIR2DL1, KIR2DL2 and -3, and all 2DS genes, have a genomic organization identical to that of the genes encoding KIR molecules with three Ig domains, but exon 3 (encoding D0) of the genes for two-domain KIR is a pseudoexon (ψ). Exon 3 is also a pseudoexon in the KIR2DP1 gene, which also contains a pseudoexon 4. The genes encoding type 2 two-domain KIR, which include KIR2DL4, KIR2DL5A, and KIR2DL5B, are characterized by the absence of exon 4. (This figure was adapted from http://web.ncbi.nlm.nih.gov:2441/books/bookres.fcgi/mo no_003/ch1d1.pdf.)

FIGURE 2 The basis of KIR nomenclature: domain structure of the KIR molecules. KIR genes express molecules with either two or three extracellular Ig-like domains. The cytoplasmic domains of the inhibitory receptors are long and contain ITIM (I/VXYXXL/V) sequences, whereas a charged amino acid residue, which facilitates interaction with the adaptor molecule DAP12/KARAP, is located in the TM of the short-tailed activating receptors. KIR2DL4 contains signature sequences of both activating and inhibitory receptors. (This figure was adapted from http://web.ncbi.nlm.nih.gov:2441/books/bookres.fcgi/mo no_003/ch1d1.pdf.)

to be a result of point mutations and homologous recombination. The full extent of the polymorphism has not yet been established and is just beginning to be understood as new populations are studied. The polymorphic sites lie along the entire length of the gene (as opposed to HLA genes where there are "hot spots" of variability) but frequently occur in the Ig-like loop domains, suggesting that the polymorphisms contribute to the interactions with KIR ligands (56).

One of the most intriguing features of the KIR system is that individuals have haplotypes (genes linked on one chromosome) with variable gene content. Multiple examples of unequal recombination exist within the KIR region (reviewed in reference 56), giving rise to gene duplication or, in some cases (e.g., the KIR3DL1 and KIR3DS1 genes), to genes with the same binding capacities but different signaling potentials where these genes segregate as alleles. The arrangement of KIR loci is given in Fig. 4 (8). There are three framework genes, the KIR3DL3, KIR2DL4, and KIR3DL2 genes, present in most individuals. However, individuals have varying numbers of the remaining genes. In general, there are considered to be two supertypic haplotypes, called A and B. The A haplotypes are missing many of the activating genes and generally have KIR2DS4 as their only activating receptor. The B haplotypes contain more genes and have more activating receptors while retaining

many or all of the inhibitory ones. Variation in the A haplotypes results from allelic polymorphism, whereas that in the B haplotypes results from both allelic diversity and the variable number of genes present. There is a growing array of haplotypes (at least 37) that have been identified as different populations have been studied (Fig. 4). Since all individuals inherit both a paternal and a maternal haplotype, this serves to increase the diversity of KIR genes present in any one individual (e.g., a person may inherit two different B haplotypes or one A and one B haplotype). One of the difficulties in typing individuals for their KIR genes stems from the inability to distinguish homozygosity from hemizygosity for any given gene.

NK cell function in recognizing abnormal cells or those in which there is selective downregulation of HLA class I genes is dependent on the expression of the KIR genes present and the relative numbers of inhibitory versus activating receptors. With minor exceptions in some individuals with promoter polymorphisms, all of the KIR genes present in any given individual are transcribed and would be found in the whole population of their NK cells collectively. However, the number and types of receptors (inhibitory or activating) present on any individual NK cell or clone are variable, and different cells would express only some of the encoded KIR genes. Determining which genes are expressed appears to be a stochastic process but one in

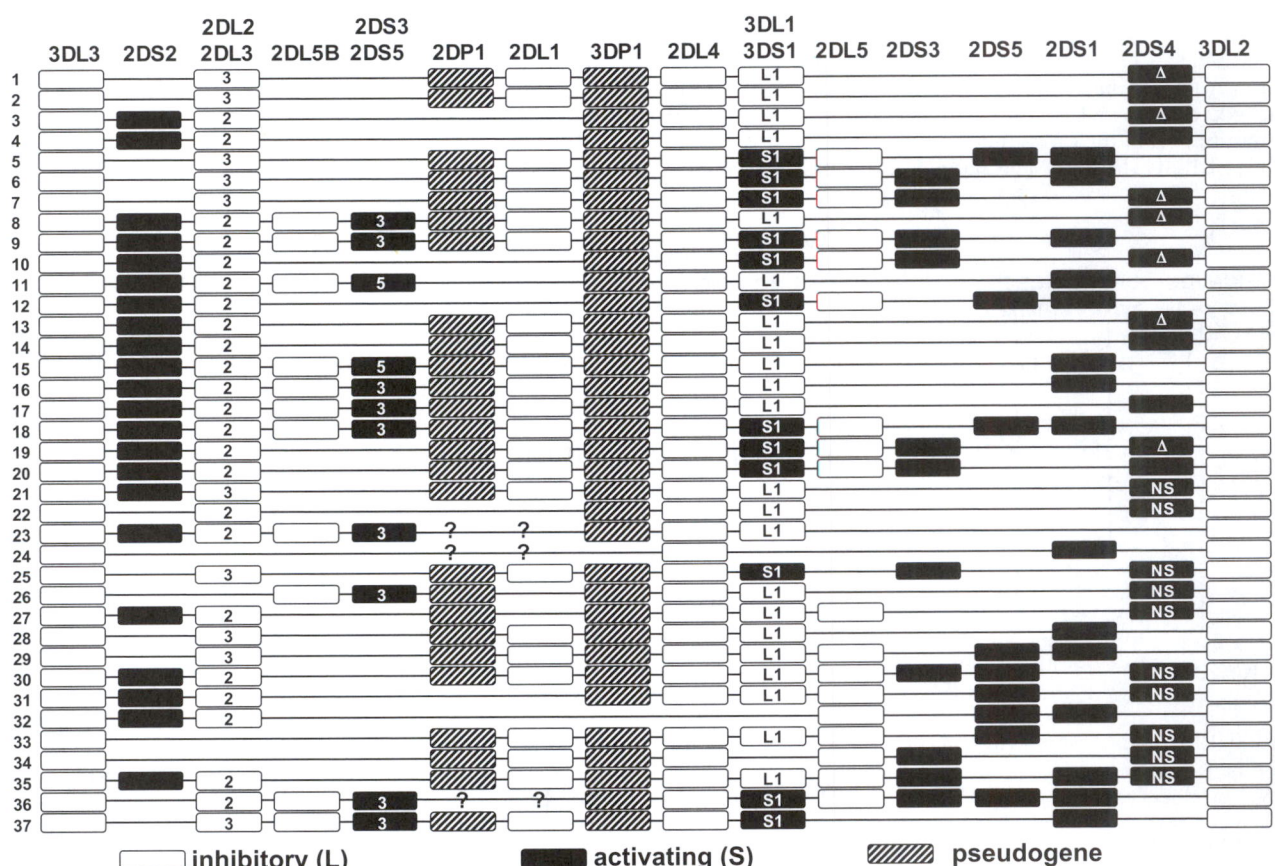

FIGURE 4 KIR haplotypes identified by segregation analysis. Segregation analysis was used to determine the haplotypes shown, many of which are not yet definitive, since it is not always possible to determine gene copy number precisely, even when using family material (14, 19, 46, 52). KIR2DS4 alleles with the 21-bp deletion are indicated by Δ, and those that were not subtyped are marked NS. (This figure was adapted from http://web.ncbi.nlm.nih.gov:2441/books/bookres.fcgi/mono_003/ch1d1.pdf.)

which the expression is stable over time (56). Allelic exclusion may occur in a clonally specific manner but is not a requirement, and both alleles can be expressed on the same NK cell or in the NK cell population as a whole (56). Every NK cell will have at least one inhibitory receptor expressed that recognizes self class I ligands in order to avoid autoimmunity. No additional NK receptor is essential. However, the expression of as many as six additional activating genes has been observed (56). Even given this diversity of receptor expression on individual cells, it is conceivable that one could have a combination of KIR haplotypes and HLA genes that would not yield a single inhibitory pair. Despite the presence of the inhibitory receptor CD94/NKG2A (see below), the resulting diminished inhibitory capability could theoretically lead to autoimmunity and/or pathogenesis. As was mentioned above, the function of the NK cell depends on the array of receptors it expresses and is the sum of the signaling potentials of the activating and inhibiting receptors. Determination of the ultimate effector function of a given NK cell requires that these activating and inhibiting receptors reside on the same cell. Additionally, the stimulating antigen and relevant major histocompatibility complex (MHC) must be present on the same cell to avoid killing of normal bystander cells (28).

Taken together, the variable gene content of haplotypes, the alternative splicing of exons, the allelic polymorphism, and the ethnic distributions contribute to a system with enormous diversity, perhaps beginning to approximate that seen for HLA.

KIR LIGANDS

The ligands for the KIR are the HLA classical class I molecules A, B, and C and the nonclassical class I molecule HLA-G. HLA class II does not appear to be involved (27). The best-known interaction occurs between inhibitory KIR and HLA-C (35, 37, 38). HLA-C has a dimorphism at position 80 (Asn/Lys). KIR2DL1 recognizes C locus molecules with Lys at this position (Cw2, Cw4, Cw5, and Cw6; group C2), whereas KIR2DL2 and KIR2DL3 (products of alleles recognizing the same ligands [36]) recognize those with Asn at this position (Cw1, Cw3, Cw7, and Cw8; group C1). The dichotomy in recognition of the C locus molecules is also dependent on a dimorphism at position 44 in the D1 domain of the KIR2DL proteins, where KIR2DL1 has Met but KIR2DL2 and KIR2DL3 have Lys.

KIR2DS1 (activating) can also recognize C locus molecules with Lys80, but substitution of Lys for Thr at position 70 lowers the affinity compared to that of KIR2DL1 (56). In the case of KIR2DS2, on the other hand, substitution of tyrosine for phenylalanine in one of the loops enhances the affinity for C (Asn80) compared to that of KIR2DL2 (56). In general, high-affinity ligands for the activating genes are unknown, but differences in affinities between inhibitory and activating receptors are key to the ultimate cytolytic signal, or lack thereof, given to the NK cells.

Other KIR genes recognize other class I molecules. KIR3DL1 receptors recognize an epitope on HLA-B molecules that also differs in the region around position 80 (56). This region (positions 77 to 83) gives rise to a peptide dimorphism, known as Bw4 or Bw6, found on all B locus molecules, and each B locus gene has a predictable Bw4 or Bw6 epitope. Because one or the other of these epitopes occurs on every B locus protein, they have very high frequencies in the population. The Bw4 epitope can also be present on some HLA-A locus molecules (e.g., A23, A24, A25, and

A32). KIR3DL1 can distinguish Bw4 from Bw6 and delivers an inhibitory signal when the Bw4 epitope is present on the target cell. While KIR3DL1 appears to be specific to Bw4-positive HLA-B allotypes, KIR3DL2 apparently has a much more restricted set of ligands recognizing HLA-A3 and HLA-A11 (56), although A3 is a moderately high frequency antigen at least in the Caucasian population (3). Lastly, KIR2DL4 recognizes HLA-G (7, 40), which is found preferentially on human extravillous cytotrophoblast (EVT) cells at the maternal-fetal interface. It was originally thought to mediate inhibition of decidual NK cells (56), but as noted above, KIR2DL4 is different from the other KIR with long CYTs and can also be an activating receptor. Other data suggest that the response depends on the activation state of the effector cells (18). In any case, the interaction of HLA-G and KIR2DL4 is likely to be involved in supporting proper maternal-fetal interactions (39, 40). The fact that the KIR2DL4 gene is unique among the KIR genes in being conserved in humans and Old World primates (56) and ubiquitously expressed suggests that its role is important evolutionarily.

CD94/NKG2 RECEPTORS

In addition to the KIR family, another family of receptors belonging to the C-type lectins exists on NK cells. This is the family of CD94/NKG2 receptors (35, 56) encoded by the NK gene complex located on chromosome 12p12.3–p13.1 (24). These receptors are type 2 membrane glycoproteins (intracellular amino terminus), and each subunit has an extracellular C-type lectin domain connected by a stalk region of 25 to 75 residues to the TM and CYT domains. CD94 is the product of a single monomorphic gene, whereas the NKG2 family is a limited family of receptors encoded by the NKG2A gene (and its splice variant the NKG2B gene) and the NKG2C, NKG2E, and NKG2F genes. The NKG2A, -C, -E, and -F molecules have only limited polymorphism but are structurally diverse, suggesting differences in ligands and signaling (24). With the possible exception of the NKG2F gene, which encodes an orphan receptor (21), all of these NKG2 genes encode receptors that are functional only as heterodimers with CD94 (35). CD94 appears to be required for cell surface expression of the NKG2 molecules and may act as a chaperone (24). CD94 can also homodimerize. NKG2A and NKG2B have long CYTs, whereas NKG2C and NKG2E have short CYTs. As with the KIR, those with the long CYTs are inhibitory and those with the short CYTs are activating. There is another gene in the same NK cluster, but only distantly related, called the NKG2D gene (9). Its product does not require CD94, can homodimerize, and is an activating receptor found also on all CD8+ T cells (27). It is relatively nonpolymorphic, and no inhibitory form of it has been detected. Further, cells activated through NKG2D are relatively resistant to inhibition by inhibitory KIR engaged through HLA class I except when inhibitory KIR are present in high abundance or when the ligand is HLA-G (see below) (9). NKG2D has been extensively studied, and its ligand binding has revealed novel mechanisms by which viruses can subvert the immune system to escape killing.

CD94/NKG2 AND NKG2D LIGANDS

Unlike those of the KIR, the CD94/NK2 and NKG2D ligands are generally HLA class Ib molecules (for which there was previously no known function) or atypical class I-like molecules. NKG2A binds the class Ib molecule HLA-E (6).

In contrast to the usual class Ia peptides bound in the groove, HLA-E presents the leader sequence peptides from the other class Ia genes (including the leader from HLA-G) (23). NKG2D, on the other hand, binds to stress-inducible nonclassical HLA class I-like molecules (9). These include the MICA (MHC class I-related chain A) and MICB (9) proteins as well as the UL16 binding proteins (ULBP), also named the retinoic acid-inducible transcript proteins (RAET). These ligands are induced by cellular stress such as heat shock, transformation, and viral or bacterial infection (e.g., UL16 is a protein derived from cytomegalovirus [CMV]) (41). MICA and ULBP are expressed in lipid rafts at the cell surface (12), which may be relevant for signaling. MICA and MICB have the heavy chain of a classical HLA class I molecule but lack beta-2 microglobulin and peptide. The ULBP have only the alpha-1 and -2 domains of a classical HLA class I molecule, lacking both the alpha-3 domain and beta-2 microglobulin, and have glycosylphosphatidylinositol anchors instead of the traditional TM and CYT domains. Levels of these ligands can be modulated both transcriptionally and posttranslationally, and release of soluble forms of MICA or ULBP can contribute to pathogenesis.

PATHOGENESIS

Viruses

Because killing by NK cells is dependent on the strength of signal resulting from the inhibitory-activating receptor competition, pathogenesis can result when either the levels of the signals or the ligands are perturbed. CMV is instructive in this regard but is by no means the only viral type in which NK cells play a putative role. CMV expresses proteins that trap class I heavy chains in the endoplasmic reticulum (US3) or translocate them to the cytosol for degradation (US2, US11). Another (US6) downregulates the expression of HLA class I genes by interfering with peptide transport via TAP (transporter associated with antigen processing) and trapping the class I proteins inside the cell (31, 53). In addition, UL18 produced by CMV mimics an HLA class I molecule and may act as a decoy. CMV also subverts the NKG2D (activating) pathway by producing UL16, a CMV-encoded TM glycoprotein that binds to MICB (but not MICA) and to ULBP. UL16 causes upregulation of ULBP but causes the binding of UL16 to MICB, ULBP1, and ULBP2 to occur inside the endoplasmic reticulum (43, 59). This impedes or prevents the transit of these ligands to the cell surface, thus reducing the surface ligand density necessary to deliver the NKG2D activation signal. Further, in vitro studies have shown that at least one retinoic acid-inducible transcript protein can be secreted from transfected CHO cells (9).

Thus, one could envision a scenario in which the KIR and the CD94/NKG2 inhibitory receptors would have no ligands on a CMV-infected cell and the NK cell would receive an unopposed activating signal. However, if the activating KIR or NKG2D also had no ligand or bound to soluble ligand(s), no cytolysis would ensue, either because the NK cell received no signal at all or because the soluble ligand acted as a decoy away from the infected cell. Additionally, since NKG2D is a coreceptor for CD8$^+$ T cells (9, 48, 56), this arm of the immune system would also not function. Viral replication would then proceed. Clearly, multiple evasion strategies have developed in CMV to subvert both the innate and adaptive immune systems, strategies demonstrated to be highly successful for viral replication and spreading.

KIR genes also have been implicated in viral pathogenesis. Patients infected with hepatitis C virus (HCV) can be subdivided into two basic groups: those who clear the virus and resolve the infection and those who have chronic HCV infection. The affinities of inhibitory KIR2DL proteins for their respective ligands proceed as follows: KIR2DL1 >KIR2DL2>KIR2DL3 (58). Patients who are homozygous for both KIR2DL3 and its cognate HLA-C1 ligands, a receptor-ligand combination that theoretically provides the weakest inhibitory signal, have a significantly better chance of resolving HCV infection than patients who have the KIR2DL1-HLA-C2 or KIR2DL2-HLA-C1 receptor-ligand combinations (20). These data suggest that weak inhibitory receptor-ligand signaling, such as that provided through KIR2DL3-HLA-C1 interactions, may be relatively easily overcome by competing activating signals, resulting in the eliminations of HCV-infected targets. For human immunodeficiency virus (1, 34), individuals with KIR3DS1 in combination with Bw4-positive HLA-B molecules having Ile at position 80 (Bw4-80I) have delayed progression to AIDS when infected with the virus. This delay is dependent on having both KIR3DS1 and Bw4-80I because the presence of one without the other shows no protection. In fact, having two copies of KIR3DS1 in the absence of Bw4-80I is associated with more rapid progression to AIDS. Taken together, these data support an interaction between the products of these genetic determinants in AIDS progression.

Autoimmune Disease

Activating KIR, especially KIR2DS1 and KIR2DS2, have been implicated in autoimmune diseases such as rheumatoid arthritis and psoriatic arthritis (PsA) (36). Since the affinity of the HLA-C group ligand binding is higher for the inhibitory KIR2DL1 and KIR2DL2 and -3 than it is for the activating KIR2DS1 and KIR2DS2, disease appears to ensue when the balance is disrupted. For PsA, it appears that disease susceptibility is a function of the sum of the activating and inhibitory KIR-ligand combinations that are present, where genotypes corresponding with strong activating potential increase the risk of developing disease. Thus, the particular array of KIR present on any given cell will dictate the response of that cell, and the sum of the population of cells will dictate the susceptibility to PsA.

Pregnancy and Recurrent Spontaneous Abortions

Large numbers of NK cells having NKG2A (inhibitory), NKG2C (activating), and a subset of the KIR (e.g., KIR2DL4) are present on maternal NK cells at the fetal-maternal interface with the EVT cells (7, 15). In addition, HLA-C, -E, and -G are expressed on the EVT cells (22), suggesting a balance between activation and inhibition to ensure an appropriate level of fetal trophoblast invasion (in order for proper transfer of essential nutrients and gases from the mother to the fetus) while preventing rejection of the fetal cells. A study of recurrent spontaneous aborters demonstrated that these women have fewer inhibitory KIR (55) than women without pregnancy loss. Along the same lines, HLA-G is the ligand for the inhibitory receptor KIR2DL4. The HLA-G leader sequence can be presented in the context of HLA-E as a ligand for NKG2A. HLA-G has been shown to overcome the signal of the activating receptors and inhibit killing by the NK cells when present in high enough density (32, 39). Further, HLA-G can be present as complexes or in soluble form (15) and either potentially divert the activation of NK cells as described above for

CMV or possibly saturate the inhibitory receptors when present in increased concentrations. HLA-C is the only polymorphic class I molecule expressed by extravillous trophoblast cells, and combinations of maternal KIR on uterine NK cells and fetal HLA-C genotypes expressed on the trophoblast may confer a range of uterine NK cell effects, from relatively strong activation to strong inhibition. Combinations of maternal KIR and fetal HLA-C ligands were tested for their potential effects on the risk of developing preeclampsia. The frequency of possessing two A haplotypes (i.e., those encoding either 0 or 1 expressed activating KIR) was high among preeclamptic mothers relative to that among mothers with healthy pregnancies, specifically when the baby carried at least one HLA-C group 2 allele (17), a receptor-ligand combination that is likely to convey strong inhibitory signals on the uterine NK cells. These data suggest that NK cell activation at the maternal-fetal interface is necessary for maternal and fetal health during pregnancy.

Blood Dyscrasias and Cancer

For lymphoproliferative disease of granular lymphocytes, there is an increase in the number of activating genes with increased production of anti-KIR antibody (13). Pure red-cell aplasia is thought to have an NK cell component in which the inhibitory receptors lack any self ligand and thus destroy autologous $CD34^+$ stem cells via a CD94/NKG2A mechanism (16). These data, together with the situation described earlier, where the NK inhibitory receptors potentially lack any of their ligands, suggest that autoreactive NK cells exist in otherwise healthy individuals.

Many tumors downregulate HLA class I (10). In mice, the upregulation of NKG2D ligands occurring in tumor cells leads to potent rejection of the tumors and conversion to T-cell immunity against the original tumor line (NKG2D ligand negative). In humans, NK cells from colorectal cancer patients lack NKG2D expression due to internalization while soluble MICA is elevated (11). In vitro studies have shown that when soluble MICA is present, NKG2D is internalized within 4 to 24 hours and tumor growth occurs. When soluble MICA is absent from the serum, NKG2D expression is upregulated and the NK cells are tumoricidal, retarding tumor growth in SCID mice. Likewise, MICA-positive leukemia cells are lysed by NKG2D-positive NK cells (45). Leukemia patients, but not healthy donors, were found to have elevated soluble MICA and MICB in their sera, suggesting that the presence of the soluble MIC (shedding) has a regulatory effect on NKG2D either by downregulating it or by acting as a decoy as described above for CMV. The shedding of MIC has also been implicated as instrumental in the progression of prostate cancer (60).

BONE MARROW TRANSPLANTATION

In a landmark paper in 2002 (44), it was shown that donor versus recipient NK alloreactivity could significantly eliminate leukemia relapse and graft rejection and protect acute myelogenous leukemia (AML) patients against graft-versus-host disease (GVHD). The basis for this is as follows: lethally conditioned patients have MHC antigens expressed on their residual cells. MHC differences between donor and recipient can cause failure to engraft due to these residual cells, including mismatches for HLA-C, the ligand for the subset of KIR described above. Conversely, donor cells in the graft, including T cells, can become activated posttransplant by the disparate MHC, setting the stage for GVHD. T cells in the graft are desirable, however, since they both hasten engraftment and enhance the graft-versus-leukemia effect in those surviving any GVHD. The goal of enhancing engraftment and the graft-versus-leukemia effect while reducing or eliminating GVHD (cf. reference 38) has become the holy grail of bone marrow transplantation.

NK cells are among the transplanted donor cells. In a mismatched allogeneic setting, it is possible that the appropriate KIR ligand (class I) might be missing from the recipient cells and trigger NK cell activation and host cell killing. In the study mentioned above, when recipients were stratified according to whether ligand for the donor inhibitory KIR was present or absent, it was found that recipients were totally protected against rejection, GVHD, and AML relapse when the ligands were absent (i.e., transplanted with alloreactive or incompatible NK cells). The probability of event-free survival at 5 years was 60% in the group where the ligands were absent versus 5% in the group where they were present. Multivariate analysis showed that this difference was due strictly to KIR ligand incompatibility in the GVHD direction. This is thought to be due to the killing of the dendritic cells and antigen-presenting cells which predispose to graft failure and GVHD (38). Further studies with mice demonstrated that large numbers of incompatible NK cells do not cause GVHD and that subsequent infusions of alloreactive NK cells into mixed chimeras convert recipients into full donor chimeras. Moreover, infusions of alloreactive NK cells into sublethally conditioned recipients convert them to fully myeloablated status without the need for additional conditioning. The same is not true for patients with acute lymphocytic leukemia (ALL), in whom NK cells are known by in vitro experiments not to be effective (38, 44). Others have had varying levels of success in replicating these findings, but the findings offer an exciting new avenue for improving success in bone marrow transplantation.

SIGNALING

Signaling in NK cells occurs through a variety of receptors, the most well known of which is CD16 (Fc gamma RIII). The following discussion applies only to signaling through the NKG2 and KIR pathways, however, and the reader is referred to the review by Lanier (24) for details of signaling through CD16.

The signaling pathways are dependent upon the family of NK receptor and upon whether the receptor is activating or inhibitory. For the activating receptors (except KIR2DL4 [27]), the KIR associates with the disulfide-linked homodimer DAP12/KARAP (killer cell-activating receptor-associated protein) (25–27, 31, 35, 47). The association occurs due to a Lys in the TM domain of the KIR forming a salt bridge with the ITAM-containing DAP12. When the ligand for the KIR is engaged, tyrosine phosphorylation of the ITAM occurs, causing recruitment of Syk and ZAP70 (tyrosine kinases) through their SH domains, and downstream activation occurs through the Jun N-terminal protein kinase (JNK) and extracellular signal-regulated kinase (ERK) pathways, although the JNK activation may be independent of DAP12. In studies with ULBP activation of NK cells (51), the downstream activation occurred through JNK2, STAT5, ERK, mitogen-activated protein kinase (MAPK), and AKT. The end result was gamma interferon production resulting in CD25 expression, Ca^{2+} influx, increased FasL expression, tyrosine phosphorylation of STAT1, cytokine and chemokine production, degranulation, and cytotoxicity (2, 27, 30). CD94/ NKG2C and CD94/NKG2E also associate through a Lys residue with Asp in the TM segment of DAP12 (25). Antibodies to CD94 have been shown to induce activation of tyrosine kinase and phospholipase C gamma (PLC-γ) and to generate inositol phosphates (24). In contrast, NKG2D associates with DAP10, also through a salt bridge. DAP10 does not have an ITAM but instead has an essential YXXM motif. Activation after ligand binding is through the phosphatidylinositol 3-kinase pathway and involves Vav1 and Rho family GTPases and PLC. The activation is independent of Syk or ZAP70 (5, 27). The YXXM motif is important because it is the binding site for the p85 regulatory subunit of phosphatidylinositol 3-kinase and recruits Grb2 (9).

For the inhibitory genes, ligand binding to the KIR causes tyrosine phosphorylation of the ITIM and the subsequent recruitment of SHP-1 and SHP-2 (tyrosine phosphatases). The latter prevent pp36 binding and inhibit the activation through Vav, PLC-γ, Grb2, Syk, and ZAP70 (24, 26, 27, 29, 35, 42, 54). CD94/NKG2A functions in a similar manner to block signaling. Interestingly, inhibitory KIR which have docking sites for SHP-1 are found in the center of lipid rafts where activation signals accumulate. The rafts increase in size in cytolytic responses and disappear rapidly when the inhibitory response predominates (57).

KIR TYPING

The involvement of KIR genes in viral infections and potentially in bone marrow transplantation suggests that KIR typing may have wider application in the future. For this reason, KIR typing by molecular methods is becoming standardized through an ongoing external quality control program (UCLA Tissue Typing Laboratory, Los Angeles, Calif.). Testing is variably done by sequencing, PCR-sequence-specific priming (PCR-SSP), or PCR-sequence-specific oligonucleotide probing (PCR-SSOP). Because of the high homology among the genes, sequencing can yield erroneous results and should be used only as a means for typing on a restricted level. Individual labs have their own primer-probe sets for assignment of types, but now a commercial kit (KIR Genotyping SSP Priming Kit) is available from Dynal/Pel-Freez (Brown Deer, Wis.) and is in widespread use among those labs performing KIR typing. In general, 16 genes can be defined: the 2DL1, 2DL2, 2DL3, 2DL4, 2DL5, 3DL1, 3DL2, 3DL3, 3DS1, 2DS1, 2DS2, 2DS3, 2DS4, 2DS5, 2DP1, and 3DP1 genes. The kit further distinguishes two alleles each for the 2DL5, 2DS4, and 3DP1 genes. (The DP designation indicates a pseudogene.) This basic typing strategy allows the definition of genes that are present or absent but does not distinguish between homozygotes and hemizygotes at any gene locus. Validation of KIR typing can be done either by using the external quality control program already in place or by requesting DNA from the CEPH (Centre d'Etude du Polymorphisme Humain) families that were tested at the 13th International Histocompatibility Workshop (http://www.ihwc.org). Additional polymorphism is detectable using allele-specific primers (e.g., reference 46), but these primers are not commercially available. It is clear that additional polymorphisms will be discovered, and thus typing for alleles is currently incomplete. Typing for the NKG2 system is not routinely done since the genes appear to be minimally polymorphic and NKG2D is present on all NK cells. Should typing be desirable, monoclonal antibodies are available that detect each of the members of the family.

SUMMARY

NK cells form the first line of immune defense in innate immunity. A complex system of cell surface receptors exists on NK cells. These receptors can be activating or inhibitory and are derived from multiple gene families, including the KIR and the CD94/NKG2 families discussed above. Their ligands are the HLA class I and class I-like molecules. Current data suggest that the effector response of the individual NK cell is determined by competition between the activating and inhibitory receptors and depends on the strength of the overall strongest signal. We are beginning to appreciate the role of NK cells in viral infections, autoimmune disease, cancer, and bone marrow transplantation, and methods to type the KIR genes are now available.

This publication has been funded in whole or in part with federal funds from the National Cancer Institute, National Institutes of Health, under contract no. N01-C0-12400.

REFERENCES

1. **Ahmad, A., and R. Ahmad.** 2003. HIV's evasion of host's NK cell response and novel ways of its countering and boosting anti-HIV immunity. *Curr. HIV Res.* **1:**295–307.
2. **Andre, P., R. Castriconi, N. Espeli, T. Anfossi, T. Juarez, S. Hue, H. Conway, F. Romagne, A. Dondero, M. Nanni, S. Caillat-Zucman, D. H. Raulet, C. Bottino, E. Vivier, A. Moretta, and P. Paul.** 2004. Comparative analysis of human NK cell activation induced by NKG2D and natural cytotoxicity receptors. *Eur. J. Immunol.* **34:**961–971.
3. **Baur, M. P., and J. A. Danilovs.** 1980. Population analysis of HLA-A, B, C, DR, and other genetic markers, p. 958. *In* P. I. Terasaki (ed.), *Histocompatibility Testing 1980.* UCLA Tissue Typing Laboratory, Los Angeles, Calif.
4. **Biassoni, R., C. Cantoni, D. Pende, S. Sivori, S. Parolini, M. Vitale, C. Bottino, and A. Moretta.** 2001. Human natural killer cell receptors and co-receptors. *Immunol. Rev.* **181:**203–214.
5. **Billadeau, D. D., J. L. Upshaw, R. A. Schoon, C. J. Dick, and P. J. Leibson.** 2003. NKG2D-DAP10 triggers human NK cell-mediated killing via a Syk-independent regulatory pathway. *Nat. Immunol.* **4:**557–564.
6. **Braud, V. M., D. S. Allan, C. A. O'Callaghan, K. Soderstrom, A. D'Andrea, G. S. Ogg, S. Lazetic, N. T. Young, J. I. Bell, J. H. Phillips, L. L. Lanier, and A. J. McMichael.** 1998. HLA-E binds to natural killer cell receptors CD94/NKG2A, B and C. *Nature* **391:**795–799.
7. **Cantoni, C., S. Verdiani, M. Falco, A. Pessino, M. Cilli, R. Conte, D. Pende, M. Ponte, M. S. Mikaelsson, L. Moretta, and R. Biassoni.** 1998. p49, a putative HLA class I-specific inhibitory NK receptor belonging to the immunoglobulin superfamily. *Eur. J. Immunol.* **28:**1980–1990.
8. **Carrington, M., and P. Norman.** 2003. *The KIR Gene Cluster.* [Online.] National Library of Medicine, National Center for Biotechnology Information, Bethesda, Md. http://ncbi.nlm.nih.gov/entrez/query.fcgi?db = Books.
9. **Cerwenka, A., and L. L. Lanier.** 2003. NKG2D ligands: unconventional MHC class I-like molecules exploited by viruses and cancer. *Tissue Antigens* **61:**335–343.
10. **Diefenbach, A., and D. H. Raulet.** 2002. The innate immune response to tumors and its role in the induction of T-cell immunity. *Immunol. Rev.* **188:**9–21.
11. **Doubrovina, E. S., M. M. Doubrovin, E. Vider, R. B. Sisson, R. J. O'Reilly, B. Dupont, and Y. M. Vyas.** 2003. Evasion from NK cell immunity by MHC class I chain-related molecules expressing colon adenocarcinoma. *J. Immunol.* **171:**6891–6899.
12. **Eleme, K., S. B. Taner, B. Onfelt, L. M. Collinson, F. E. McCann, N. J. Chalupny, D. Cosman, C. Hopkins, A. I. Magee, and D. M. Davis.** 2004. Cell surface organization of stress-inducible proteins ULBP and MICA that stimulate human NK cells and T cells via NKG2D. *J. Exp. Med.* **199:**1005–1010.

13. Epling-Burnette, P. K., J. S. Painter, P. Chaurasia, F. Bai, S. Wei, J. Y. Djeu, and T. P. Loughran, Jr. 2004. Dysregulated NK receptor expression in patients with lymphoproliferative disease of granular lymphocytes. *Blood* 103:3431–3439.

14. Gomez-Lozano, N., C. M. Gardiner, P. Parham, and C. Vilches. 2002. Some human KIR haplotypes contain two KIR2DL5 genes: KIR2DL5A and KIR2DL5B. *Immunogenetics* 54:314–319.

15. Gonen-Gross, T., R. Gazit, H. Achdout, J. Hanna, S. Mizrahi, G. Markel, V. Horejsi, and O. Mandelboim. 2003. Special organization of the HLA-G protein on the cell surface. *Hum. Immunol.* 64:1011–1016.

16. Grau, R., K. S. Lang, D. Wernet, P. Lang, D. Niethammer, C. M. Pusch, and R. Handgretinger. 2004. Cytotoxic activity of natural killer cells lacking killer-inhibitory receptors for self-HLA class I molecules against autologous hematopoietic stem cells in healthy individuals. *Exp. Mol. Pathol.* 76:90–98.

17. Hiby, S. E., J. J. Walker, K. M. O'Shaughnessy, C. W. Redman, M. Carrington, J. Trowsdale, and A. Moffett. 2004. Combinations of maternal KIR and fetal HLA-C genes influence the risk of preeclampsia and reproductive success. *J. Exp. Med.* 200:957–965.

18. Hofmeister, V., and E. H. Weiss. 2003. HLA-G modulates immune responses by diverse receptor interactions. *Semin. Cancer Biol.* 13:317–323.

19. Hsu, K. C., X. R. Liu, A. Selvakumar, E. Mickelson, R. J. O'Reilly, and B. Dupont. 2002. Killer Ig-like receptor haplotype analysis by gene content: evidence for genomic diversity with a minimum of six basic framework haplotypes, each with multiple subsets. *J. Immunol.* 169:5118–5129.

20. Khakoo, S. I., C. L. Thio, M. P. Martin, C. R. Brooks, X. Gao, J. Astemborski, J. Cheng, J. J. Goedert, D. Vlahov, M. Hilgartner, S. Cox, A.-M. Little, G. J. Alexander, M. E. Cramp, S. J. O'Brien, W. M. C. Rosenberg, D. L. Thomas, and M. Carrington. 2004. HLA and NK cell inhibitory receptor genes in resolving hepatitis C virus infection. *Science* 305:872–874.

21. Kim, D. K., J. Kabat, F. Borrego, T. B. Sanni, C. H. You, and J. E. Coligan. 2004. Human NKG2F is expressed and can associate with DAP12. *Mol. Immunol.* 41:53–62.

22. King, A., S. E. Hiby, L. Gardner, S. Joseph, J. M. Bowen, S. Verma, T. D. Burrows, and Y. W. Loke. 2000. Recognition of trophoblast HLA class I molecules by decidual NK cell receptors—a review. *Placenta* 21(Suppl. A): S81–S85.

23. Lanier, L. L. 1998. Follow the leader: NK cell receptors for classical and nonclassical MHC class I. *Cell* 92:705–707.

24. Lanier, L. L. 1998. NK cell receptors. *Annu. Rev. Immunol.* 16:359–393.

25. Lanier, L. L. 2000. Turning on natural killer cells. *J. Exp. Med.* 191:1259–1262.

26. Lanier, L. L. 2003. Natural killer cell receptor signaling. *Curr. Opin. Immunol.* 15:308–314.

27. Lanier, L. L. 2005. NK cell recognition. *Annu. Rev. Immunol.* 23:225–274.

28. Lanier, L. L., and J. H. Phillips. 1996. Inhibitory MHC class I receptors on NK cells and T cells. *Immunol. Today* 17:86–91.

29. Lanier, L. L., B. Corliss, and J. H. Phillips. 1997. Arousal and inhibition of human NK cells. *Immunol. Rev.* 155:145–154.

30. Liang, S., H. Wei, R. Sun, and Z. Tian. 2003. IFNalpha regulates NK cell cytotoxicity through STAT1 pathway. *Cytokine* 23:190–199.

31. Lopez-Botet, M., A. Angulo, and A. Guma. 2004. Natural killer cell receptors for major histocompatibility complex class I and related molecules in cytomegalovirus infection. *Tissue Antigens* 63:195–203.

32. Mandelboim, O., L. Pazmany, D. M. Davis, M. Vales-Gomez, H. T. Reyburn, B. Rybalov, and J. L. Strominger. 1997. Multiple receptors for HLA-G on human natural killer cells. *Proc. Natl. Acad. Sci. USA* 94:14666–14670.

33. Martin, A. M., E. M. Freitas, C. S. Witt, and F. T. Christiansen. 2000. The genomic organization and evolution of the natural killer immunoglobulin-like receptor (KIR) gene cluster. *Immunogenetics* 51:268–280.

34. Martin, M. P., X. Gao, J. H. Lee, G. W. Nelson, R. Detels, J. J. Goedert, S. Buchbinder, K. Hoots, D. Vlahov, J. Trowsdale, M. Wilson, S. J. O'Brien, and M. Carrington. 2002. Epistatic interaction between KIR3DS1 and HLA-B delays the progression to AIDS. *Nat. Genet.* 31:429–434.

35. Natarajan, K., N. Dimasi, J. Wang, R. A. Mariuzza, and D. H. Margulies. 2002. Structure and function of natural killer cell receptors: multiple molecular solutions to self, nonself discrimination. *Annu. Rev. Immunol.* 20:853–885.

36. Nelson, G. W., M. P. Martin, D. Gladman, J. Wade, J. Trowsdale, and M. Carrington. 2004. Cutting edge: heterozygote advantage in autoimmune disease: hierarchy of protection/susceptibility conferred by HLA and killer Ig-like receptor combinations in psoriatic arthritis. *J. Immunol.* 173:4273–4276.

37. Parham, P. 2004. NK cells lose their inhibition. *Science* 305:786–787.

38. Parham, P., and K. L. McQueen. 2003. Alloreactive killer cells: hindrance and help for haematopoietic transplants. *Nat. Rev. Immunol.* 3:108–122.

39. Pazmany, L., O. Mandelboim, M. Vales-Gomez, D. M. Davis, T. C. Becker, H. T. Reyburn, J. D. Seebach, J. A. Hill, and J. L. Strominger. 1999. Human leucocyte antigen-G and its recognition by natural killer cells. *J. Reprod. Immunol.* 43:127–137.

40. Rajagopalan, S., and E. O. Long. 1999. A human histocompatibility leukocyte antigen (HLA)-G-specific receptor expressed on all natural killer cells. *J. Exp. Med.* 189:1093–1100.

41. Raulet, D. H. 2003. Roles of the NKG2D immunoreceptor and its ligands. *Nat. Rev. Immunol.* 3:781–790.

42. Ravetch, J. V., and L. L. Lanier. 2000. Immune inhibitory receptors. *Science* 290:84–89.

43. Rolle, A., M. Mousavi-Jazi, M. Eriksson, J. Odeberg, C. Soderberg-Naucler, D. Cosman, K. Karre, and C. Cerboni. 2003. Effects of human cytomegalovirus infection on ligands for the activating NKG2D receptor of NK cells: up-regulation of UL16-binding protein (ULBP)1 and ULBP2 is counteracted by the viral UL16 protein. *J. Immunol.* 171:902–908.

44. Ruggeri, L., M. Capanni, E. Urbani, K. Perruccio, W. D. Shlomchik, A. Tosti, S. Posati, D. Rogaia, F. Frassoni, F. Aversa, M. F. Martelli, and A. Velardi. 2002. Effectiveness of donor natural killer cell alloreactivity in mismatched hematopoietics transplants. *Science* 295:2097–2100.

45. Salih, H. R., H. Antropius, F. Gieseke, S. Z. Lutz, L. Kanz, H. G. Rammensee, and A. Steinle. 2003. Functional expression and release of ligands for the activating immunoreceptor NKG2D in leukemia. *Blood* 102:1389–1396.

46. Shilling, H. G., L. A. Guethlein, N. W. Cheng, C. M. Gardiner, R. Rodriguez, D. Tyan, and P. Parham. 2002. Allelic polymorphism synergizes with variable gene content to individualize human KIR genotype. *J. Immunol.* 168: 2307–2315.

47. Snyder, M. R., T. Nakajima, P. J. Leibson, C. M. Weyand, and J. J. Goronzy. 2004. Stimulatory killer Ig-like receptors modulate T cell activation through DAP12-dependent and DAP12-independent mechanisms. *J. Immunol.* 173: 3725–3731.

48. Snyder, M. R., C. M. Weyand, and J. J. Goronzy. 2004. The double life of NK receptors: stimulation or co-stimulation. *Trends Immunol.* 25:25–32.

49. Staub, E., A. Rosenthal, and B. Hinzmann. 2004. Systematic identification of immunoreceptor tyrosine-based inhibitory motifs in the human proteome. *Cell. Signal.* **16**:435–456.

50. Steffens, U., Y. Vyas, B. Dupont, and A. Selvakumar. 1998. Nucleotide and amino acid sequence alignment for human killer cell inhibitory receptors (KIR), 1998. *Tissue Antigens* **51**:398–413.

51. Sutherland, C. L., N. J. Chalupny, and D. Cosman. 2001. The UL16-binding proteins, a novel family of MHC class I-related ligands for NKG2D, activate natural killer cell functions. *Immunol. Rev.* **181**:185–192.

52. Uhrberg, M., P. Parham, and P. Wernet. 2002. Definition of gene content for nine common group B haplotypes of the Caucasoid population: KIR haplotypes contain between seven and eleven KIR genes. *Immunogenetics* **54**:221–229.

53. Ulbrecht, M., V. Hofmeister, G. Yuksekdag, J. W. Ellwart, H. Hengel, F. Momburg, S. Martinozzi, M. Reboul, M. Pla, and E. H. Weiss. 2003. HCMV glycoprotein US6 mediated inhibition of TAP does not affect HLA-E dependent protection of K-562 cells from NK lysis. *Hum. Immunol.* **64**:231–237.

54. Valiante, N. M., K. Lienert, H. G. Shilling, B. J. Smits, and P. Parham. 1997. Killer cell receptors: keeping pace with MHC class I evolution. *Immunol. Rev.* **155**:155–164.

55. Varla-Leftherioti, M., M. Spyropoulou-Vlachou, D. Niokou, T. Keramitsoglou, A. Darlamitsou, C. Tsekoura, M. Papadimitropoulos, V. Lepage, C. Balafoutas, and C. Stavropoulos-Giokas. 2003. Natural killer (NK) cell receptors' repertoire in couples with recurrent spontaneous abortions. *Am. J. Reprod. Immunol.* **49**:183–191.

56. Vilches, C., and P. Parham. 2002. KIR: diverse, rapidly evolving receptors of innate and adaptive immunity. *Annu. Rev. Immunol.* **20**:217–251.

57. Vyas, Y. M., H. Maniar, C. E. Lyddane, M. Sadelain, and B. Dupont. 2004. Ligand binding to inhibitory killer cell Ig-like receptors induces colocalization with Src homology domain 2-containing protein tyrosine phosphatase 1 and interruption of ongoing activation signals. *J. Immunol.* **173**:1571–1578.

58. Winter, C. C., J. E. Gumperz, P. Parham, E. O. Long, and N. Wagtmann. 1998. Direct binding and functional transfer of NK cell inhibitory receptors reveal novel patterns of HLA-C allotype recognition. *J. Immunol.* **161**:571–577.

59. Wu, J., N. J. Chalupny, T. J. Manley, S. R. Riddell, D. Cosman, and T. Spies. 2003. Intracellular retention of the MHC class I-related chain B ligand of NKG2D by the human cytomegalovirus UL16 glycoprotein. *J. Immunol.* **170**:4196–4200.

60. Wu, J. D., L. M. Higgins, A. Steinle, D. Cosman, K. Haugk, and S. R. Plymate. 2004. Prevalent expression of the immunostimulatory MHC class I chain-related molecule is counteracted by shedding in prostate cancer. *J. Clin. Investig.* **114**:560–568.

Detecting Chimerism after Blood and Marrow Transplantation

LEE ANN BAXTER-LOWE

141

In medicine, "chimerism" describes the coexistence of cells that are derived from different zygotes. This term is derived from Chimera, the name of a fire-spitting monster with a lion's head, a goat's body, and a serpent's tail, which is described in Greek mythology. Hematopoietic chimerism has been reported in association with allogeneic transplantation, blood transfusion, and pregnancy (with the condition occurring in mothers and offspring). This chapter discusses fundamental aspects of laboratory assessment of hematopoietic chimerism after blood and marrow transplantation. Clinical indications for chimerism testing in blood and marrow transplantation include posttransplant monitoring of engraftment kinetics and stable mixed chimerism as well as detecting relapse and graft loss. Additional applications include detecting cells engrafted from a third party (e.g., through blood transfusion) and distinguishing monozygotic and dizygotic twins.

Chimerism testing detects the presence of donor cells, preferably providing quantification (e.g., the percentage of donor cells). This objective is accomplished by detecting genetic polymorphism or distinguishing the products of polymorphic genes. Chimerism testing is routinely used after allogeneic blood and marrow transplantation to monitor the status of the allograft and to detect relapse (2, 7, 20). This testing has also become important for guiding certain posttransplant interventions, such as donor lymphocyte infusions. Microchimerism testing, which is usually defined as detecting cells of donor origin when they account for <1% of total cells, is currently used predominantly in research settings. Microchimerism has been reported after solid-organ transplantation (31), blood transfusion (22), and pregnancy (11). The clinical significance of microchimerism remains controversial.

METHODS FOR CHIMERISM TESTING

In the early years of bone marrow transplantation, chimerism testing was primarily limited to use for monitoring donor engraftment. Most donors were HLA-identical siblings, and engraftment of donor cells was often detected using erythrocyte antigens that differed between donor and host. Although flow cytometry and agglutination methods for detecting erythrocyte antigens could detect admixtures of 0.1 to 0.5% for approximately 80% of sibling pairs, transfusions could confound the results and engraftment of other lineages could not be determined (12). Another technique which was used to monitor engraftment was conventional cytogenetic analysis of metaphase chromosomes. Cytogenetic approaches have several limitations, including the lack of an informative marker for many donor-recipient pairs, the necessity for metaphase chromosomes, and substantial labor requirements. For HLA-mismatched donor-recipient pairs, serological HLA typing was also used to monitor engraftment. Limitations included poor sensitivity, qualitative results, and cross-reactivity of reagents, which confounded data interpretation.

In the 1980s, some of the limitations associated with these historical methods were overcome by new methods that detected polymorphism in genomic DNA. One of the earliest of these new methods detected restriction fragment length polymorphism by using gel electrophoresis to separate DNA fragments based upon size and Southern blotting followed by probe hybridization to detect specific fragments (32). There were informative markers for most donor-recipient pairs, but this labor-intensive procedure has since been supplanted by more convenient methods that use DNA amplification.

Another DNA-based method uses in situ hybridization with probes that are specific for sex chromosomes or autosomal markers. This method can be sensitive, specific, and quantitative. For sex-mismatched transplants, fluorescence in situ hybridization is still used today because single cells can be analyzed and counting large numbers of cells allows high precision and sensitivity (30). Methods that detect only Y chromosome markers, inferring that negative cells are of female origin, are subject to errors in overestimation of female cells caused by age- or disease-related loss of the Y chromosome as well as several technical factors that diminish hybridization. These limitations are overcome by procedures that use different chromophores to distinguish probes hybridized to X and Y chromosomes. With the use of both X and Y probes, the false-positive rate for female and male cells is less than 1% (13). This method can be used only for sex-mismatched transplants.

Today, the most widely used methods for chimerism testing detect polymorphic differences in the numbers of tandem repeats of perfect or slightly imperfect sequence motifs in genomic DNA (see Fig. 1). These motifs are generally referred to as variable-number tandem repeat (VNTR) sequences. For a particular VNTR locus, the number of tandemly repeated sequence motifs in each allele shows

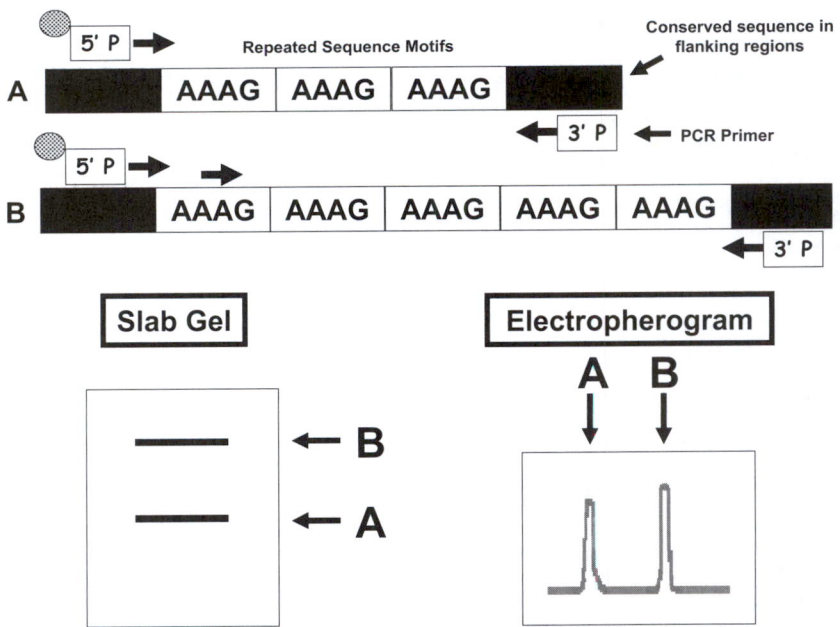

FIGURE 1 STR alleles. Two STR alleles that are distinguished by the numbers of tandem repeats of the sequence motif AAAG are depicted at the top of the figure. The solid black sections represent conserved sequences which are located in the flanking regions of the STR. Oligonucleotides labeled 5′ P and 3′ P anneal to these flanking regions to selectively prime DNA synthesis in the PCR. In this example, the 5′ P primer is labeled with a fluorescent dye molecule. The products of the PCR can be separated using slab gel electrophoresis (bottom left), and the fluorescence is often displayed as an electropherogram (bottom right).

codominant Mendelian inheritance. VNTR loci with sequence motifs of 2 to 8 bp (also called microsatellites) are usually described as short tandem repeats (STR). The acronym VNTR can describe any locus with a repeated sequence motif but is sometimes used to distinguish repeats of long sequence motifs (>8 bp pairs) from STR.

CHIMERISM TESTING USING STR LOCI

In 2005, the predominant methods for chimerism testing involve amplification of STR loci. STR polymorphism is detected using test systems that employ PCR to selectively amplify a target locus (Fig. 1). The assay requires genomic DNA from the test sample and control DNA samples, which can be isolated from any source (e.g., blood, bone marrow, and tissue). PCR primers are designed to specifically anneal to conserved flanking regions of the repeat unit. The PCR products are usually fluorescently labeled and resolved by electrophoresis on capillary or slab gels that can resolve single-nucleotide differences. The size and quantity (i.e., the area under the peak) of each allele are determined and used to calculate the relative proportions of each allele in the test sample.

Most laboratories begin by amplifying a panel of STR loci to determine the sizes of the STR alleles for the host and donor. Alleles that differ between the donor and recipient are referred to as informative alleles. As shown in Fig. 2, there are several possible observations: host and donor alleles are identical (not informative); at least one host and one donor allele is unique (host and donor informative); there is a unique host allele but the donor allele is also present in the host (host informative); or there is a unique donor allele but the host allele is also present in the donor (donor

informative). Thiede et al. compared the frequencies of informative alleles for 27 STR markers in 203 recipients and their HLA-matched related donors (33). Penta E, SE33, D2S1338, and D18S51 were the most frequently informative,

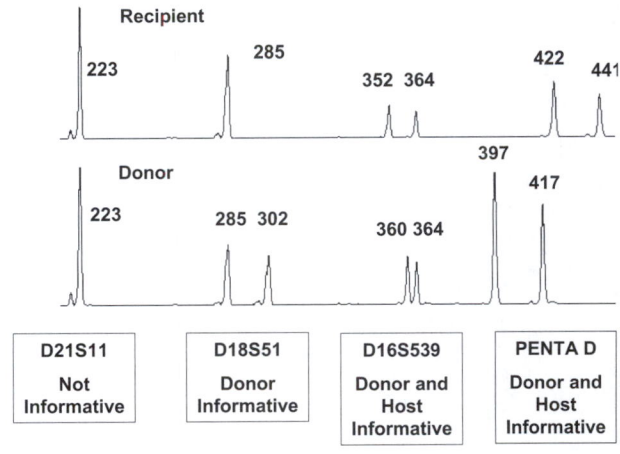

FIGURE 2 Electropherograms for a donor-recipient pair. Electropherograms for multiplex reactions for four loci are shown. For D21S11, the donor and recipient are homozygous for the same allele (223 bp). For D18S51, the recipient is homozygous for an allele with 285 bp. The donor shares this allele and has an additional informative allele (302 bp). For D16S539, the donor and recipient share the 364-bp allele, and there are informative alleles for the donor (360 bp) and recipient (352 bp). For Penta D, there are two informative recipient alleles (422 and 441 bp) and two informative donor alleles (397 and 417 bp).

with each being informative for both the donor and recipient in 25 to 50% of the pairs. The frequency of detecting informative alleles was correlated with the degree of heterozygosity ($r = 0.86$; $P = 0.0001$) but not with the total number of alleles observed for the locus.

For posttransplant specimens, the goal is to estimate the relative proportions of donor and recipient alleles in the sample. These are determined by measuring the areas under the informative peaks for the donor and host. Data from admixtures containing increasing quantities of DNA are shown in Fig. 3. For posttransplant specimens, the results are typically reported as the percentage of donor alleles in the specimen. The percentage of donor alleles (% D) is calculated using the following equation:

$$\% \, D = (D_1 + D_2)/(D_1 + D_2 + H_3 + H_4)$$

where D_1 and D_2 represent the areas under donor-informative peaks 1 and 2 and H_1 and H_2 represent the areas under host-informative peaks 3 and 4. If the host and donor share an allele, the shared allele is eliminated from the equation. Calculations for more complex patterns have been summarized by Nollet et al. (25).

There are two approaches for PCR for posttransplant specimens, (i) multiplex PCR using a panel of primers for many STR loci or (ii) individual PCR using one or two loci that have the most favorable characteristics. Advantages of multiplex test systems include availability of commercial reagents, ease of use, and minimal DNA requirements (25). One drawback of the multiplex approach is that amplification conditions are optimized for the primer mixture rather than a particular locus,

which limits the sensitivity that can be achieved. In addition, inadequate correction for spectral overlap of dyes can increase background variation and sometimes affect quantification of informative alleles (29). An alternative which overcomes some of these limitations is to select one or two loci for posttransplant testing and to perform amplification under conditions that are optimal for each locus (27). Improving the efficiency of the PCR and diminishing background variation are beneficial for achieving maximal sensitivity.

Unfortunately, the area under the peak for each PCR product is not always directly proportional to the quantity of the allele in the genomic DNA template. Factors that contribute to deviations include (i) preferential amplification, (ii) stutter peaks, (iii) artifacts related to spectral overlap, and for slab gels, (iv) artifacts related to lane tracking (27, 29). There are several approaches to overcome these limitations, including (i) determining the mean values for many loci (i.e., multiplex methods), (ii) selecting loci and reaction conditions to minimize these factors, and (iii) using standard curves generated by admixtures of donor and host DNA to adjust for deviations from linearity (25, 27).

Preferential amplification is illustrated in Fig. 2 (for Penta D), where the peak for the smaller allele (397 bp) is approximately 14% larger than expected for equivalent amplification of each donor allele and the peak for the larger allele (417 bp) is 14% smaller than expected. Preferential amplification is influenced by a variety of factors, including the number and the relative size difference of the alleles, amplification efficiency, concentration of reaction components (e.g., DNA, polymerase, and magnesium), and differences in sequence motifs that affect the DNA polymerase (27).

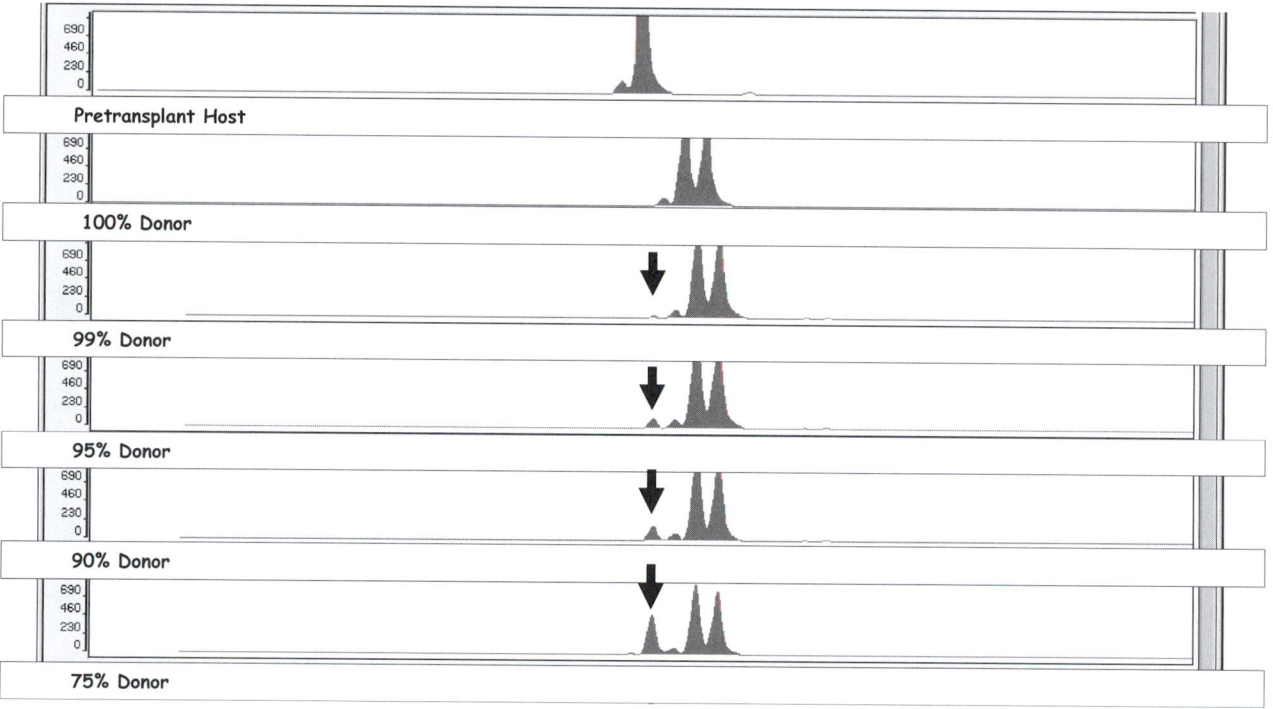

FIGURE 3 Admixtures of control DNA for a donor-recipient pair. The electropherogram for the homozygous recipient is shown in the top panel. The small peak to the immediate left of the main peak is a stutter peak. The panel labeled "100% Donor" shows the alleles from the control DNA from the donor. The small peak to the immediate left of the two large peaks is a stutter peak. Presumably, the stutter peak from the larger of the donor alleles comigrates with the smaller allele. The next panels show the amplification products of admixtures of donor and recipient DNA. Arrows show the host peak in the admixtures.

Preferential amplification can be minimized by selecting loci with informative alleles that have small differences in length.

Stutter peaks can occur during the PCR if the polymerase is dissociated during extension of the new strand of DNA (35). When another polymerase molecule associates with the DNA, loops can form in the template or extending strand which can cause loss or addition of one or more repeat units in the final PCR product. The resulting products, which differ by one or more repeat units, serve as templates during subsequent cycles, creating additional copies of alleles with aberrant lengths. Stutter peaks are also referred to as shadow bands or DNA polymerase slippage products. Examples of stutter peaks are provided in Fig. 3 and 4. Stutter peaks can be included in determining the area for the associated allele. If stutter peaks comigrate with an informative peak, it is necessary to make appropriate adjustments by estimating the contribution of the stutter peak by using admixtures of control DNA or making corrections using a standard curve (27).

MIXED CHIMERISM

There are many situations in which there is coexistence of donor and host hematopoietic cells, and this phenomenon is

referred to as mixed chimerism. In patients with mixed chimerism, the proportion (percentage) of donor cells can change, and this condition is described as increasing mixed chimerism if the percentage of donor cells is increasing or decreasing mixed chimerism if the percentage of donor cells is decreasing. Sometimes there are lineage-specific differences in levels of donor cell engraftment. For example, certain patients with severe combined immunodeficiency (SCID) syndrome have T cells that are of donor origin while all other cells remain of host origin. This situation is referred to as split chimerism.

For patients with mixed chimerism, it is important to understand underlying dynamic processes. Changes in percentages of donor cells may be caused by alterations in engraftment levels for all lineages or in the relative numbers of cells of lineages that have different levels of donor chimerism. Thus, increases in percent donor chimerism do not necessarily indicate improved donor cell engraftment. For example, in a SCID patient with split chimerism, T cells may proliferate during an infection, causing the percentage of donor cells in peripheral blood to increase. This is not an indication of additional donor cell engraftment but rather selective expansion of donor-derived T cells. After the infection subsides and the T cells die, the percentage of donor cells in peripheral blood will decrease.

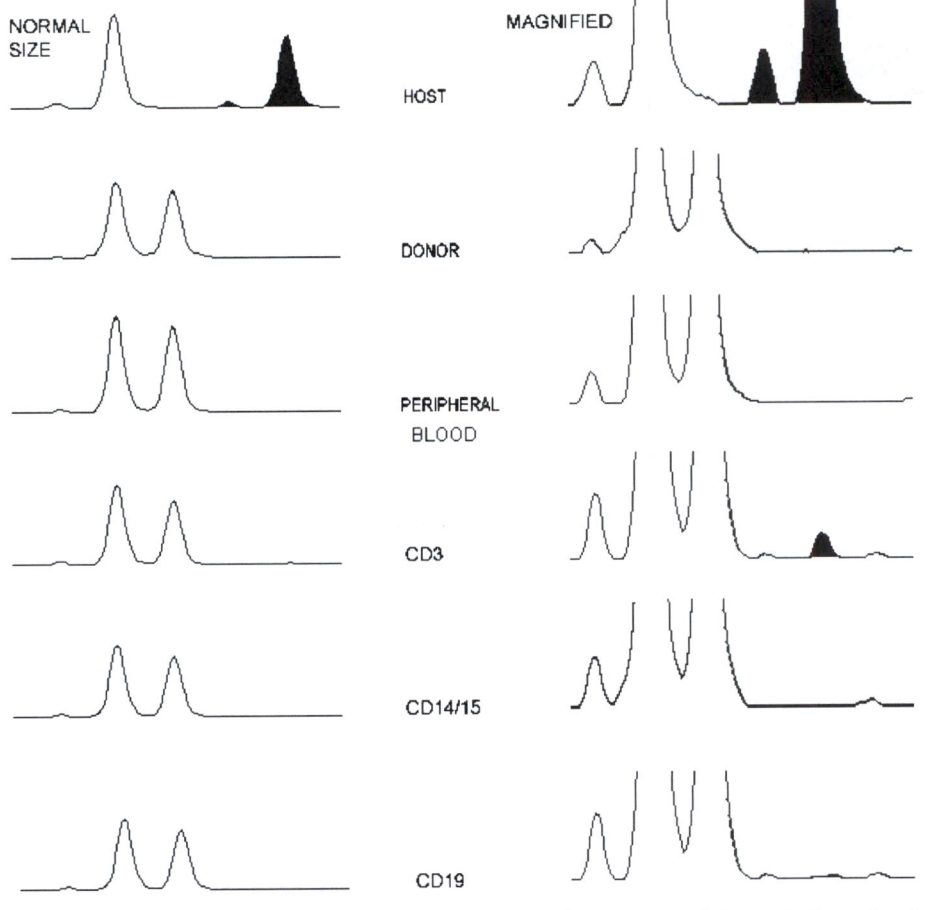

FIGURE 4 Testing of cell subsets to increase sensitivity. The two upper left panels show the electropherograms of the host alleles and donor alleles. The host allele is undetectable in electropherograms for peripheral blood, CD14/15, and CD19 subsets using the standard scale and an expanded scale (right). For the CD3 subset, the host allele is barely detectable in the standard scale but is clearly evident in an expanded scale. Subset analysis not only provides increased sensitivity but also shows the lineage of the autologous cells.

For mixtures of donor and recipient alleles, it is preferable to (i) select loci that have informative alleles for the donor as well as the host, (ii) avoid loci that have alleles with substantial differences in size, because this often results in preferential amplification of the smaller allele, and (iii) avoid loci with informative alleles that comigrate with stutter peaks (± 1 or more core units of the sequence motif) of other alleles. If preferential amplification and/or comigration with stutter peaks occurs, it is possible to correct for deviations from expected rates of amplification by making adjustments according to a standard curve which is determined using admixtures of donor and host DNA (27). Another alternative for diminishing contributions from loci that deviate from normal distribution is to determine the mean percentage of donor cells for many loci.

SENSITIVITY

If only donor alleles are detected in a posttransplant specimen, the condition is described as complete donor chimerism or full donor chimerism. In this situation, the sensitivity of the assay is extremely important because there may be autologous cells in the sample that are present at levels that are below the detection limits of the assay. For example, complete donor chimerism (100% donor cells) may be reported using an assay with 5% sensitivity but a more sensitive technique may detect low levels of residual autologous cells (e.g., a result of 96 to 99% donor cells). Transplant recipients who have become complete donor chimeras can subsequently become mixed chimeras due to proliferation of autologous cells that were previously present at undetectable levels.

If the specimen is predominantly of donor or host origin, sensitivity becomes the most important factor for selecting optimal STR loci. In this situation, the following characteristics are important: (i) preferential amplification of the informative allele(s) for the minority population is advantageous because it improves sensitivity, (ii) low background variation is beneficial because it enhances the ability to detect very small informative peaks, and (iii) separation of peaks allows for avoidance of comigration with stutter peaks, which diminishes sensitivity. With careful selection of loci, sensitivity of at least 0.1% can be achieved with this technique.

Sensitivity can also be increased by testing subsets of cells (2, 24). For example, following allogeneic transplantation, T cells may account for only 10% of peripheral blood leukocytes and 3% of bone marrow cells. If the sensitivity of the method for detecting host cells was 1% and 20% of the T cells were of host origin, 98% of cells in unseparated peripheral blood would be determined to be of donor origin and 100% of those in unseparated bone marrow would be determined to be of donor origin. For isolated T cells, results of chimerism testing would be reported as 80% donor cells for subsets isolated from peripheral blood or bone marrow. If the sensitivity for the informative host allele was 3% rather than 1%, unfractionated peripheral blood would be reported as 100% donor. The usefulness of testing subsets of cells is shown in Fig. 4, in which host cells are detectable only in the T-cell subset. In patients with transplants for hematological malignancies, chimerism testing of a subset of cells that expresses a tumor marker is sometimes used as an indirect test for minimal residual disease.

NEW TECHNIQUES

Real-time PCR assays that detect single-nucleotide polymorphisms (SNPs) have been applied to chimerism testing.

A report on 11 biallelic SNPs described informative alleles for 90% of the donor-recipient pairs and sensitivity of 0.1% (1). One drawback of the real-time PCR techniques is that the coefficient of variation is 30 to 50% (1, 23), in comparison with approximately 5% for STR systems (7, 17, 21, 27). One factor contributing to this variation for real-time PCR is that the cycle threshold for a positive reaction is typically plus or minus one cycle and a difference in one cycle translates into a twofold difference in the number of copies of the target allele. Thus, real-time PCR assays are very useful for applications requiring high levels of sensitivity but are not optimal for quantifying differences in mixed chimerism that are readily detected by STR or in situ hybridization methods. Real-time PCR methods play an important role in detecting microchimerism, because these assays can reach a sensitivity of 1:100,000 cells.

Pyrosequencing, which is a rapid and quantitative sequencing technology, has also been applied to chimerism testing. Hochberg et al. were able to identify at least one informative SNP locus in each of 55 patients with HLA-identical donors by using pyrosequencing to measure donor and recipient alleles for 14 SNPs with high allele frequencies (18). This approach overcomes many of the limitations of STR analysis (e.g., preferential amplification and stutter peaks), and the assays are easier to perform. However, in the current format, sensitivity is inferior to that obtained with STR methods (5%).

CLINICAL INDICATIONS

For blood and marrow transplantation, chimerism analysis has become an important component of posttransplant monitoring. In the peritransplant period, chimerism testing is used to monitor engraftment, rejection, and graft failure. Engraftment kinetics may be important. Rapid engraftment has been associated with increased risk for acute graft-versus-host disease (2, 9). Under certain conditions, persistence of autologous cells of particular lineages (e.g., CD3 and NK cells) has been associated with increased risk for relapse of malignant disease (9). These investigations have provided the foundation for certain treatment interventions, such as donor lymphocyte infusions and modifications in immunosuppressive therapy (5, 6).

For patients receiving transplants for hematological malignancies, detection of persisting or recurrent autologous cells may be an indication of residual disease and/or the presence of normal hematopoietic cells. The risks associated with persistence of residual disease are straightforward. It has been suggested that the persistence of normal autologous cells is also an important risk factor for relapse, because these cells are indicative of tolerance, which may diminish graft-versus-tumor effects (7, 8). Chimerism analysis of subsets of cells can increase the sensitivity for detecting autologous cells and provide an indirect assay to screen for possible recurrent disease. Trends in donor chimerism have also been shown to be important for certain patients. Decreasing donor chimerism in longitudinal specimens has been associated with disease relapse, and patients who have rapid decreases in donor chimerism have the highest risk of relapse (3–6, 10). Reports of these trends have provided the foundation for several clinical trials to prevent disease relapse by using chimerism analysis to prescribe preemptive immunotherapy such as withdrawal of immunosuppression or infusions of donor cells (7). Other investigators have reported correlations by using cells with particular markers (e.g., CD34) or suggested certain thresholds that are associated with relapse (e.g., 75% CD34 cells of donor origin) (28, 34).

There have been many observational studies suggesting that chimerism testing may be useful for prognosis, but contradictory results have created considerable controversy in the field. It is likely that many factors have contributed to apparently discordant observations, including differences in disease, transplant regimens, sampling, and characteristics of chimerism testing (e.g., sensitivity and accuracy). For example, one study reported that mixed chimerism in T cells and NK cells was associated with leukemia relapse in children but not adults (16). Overall, serial and quantitative analysis of chimerism can be useful for identifying patients who are at highest risk for relapse. The frequency of testing is an important factor, because the time between onset of mixed chimerism and relapse can be short for some patients.

Chimerism monitoring can be particularly important for transplant regimens that are associated with delayed or gradual engraftment, such as reduced-intensity conditioning regimens (9, 15). In this setting, measuring the levels of donor chimerism of the peripheral blood cell subset might allow early therapeutic interventions to prevent graft rejection or disease progression.

Transplantation of umbilical cord blood is associated with increased rates of graft failure and delays in engraftment relative to transplantation of cells derived from living donors. One approach that has had early success in overcoming these obstacles is transplantation with multiple cord blood units. For these transplants, chimerism testing must distinguish cells from the host from those from multiple donors. The general principles provided in this chapter apply to this situation, but interpretation of the data can be very complicated due to sharing of alleles. Early reports have suggested that multidonor hematopoietic chimerism gradually evolves into survival of cells derived from a single unit. The importance of engraftment kinetics in this complex setting remains to be determined.

In addition to the indications described above, chimerism testing can be used to test for the presence of third-party cells derived from blood transfusions (14), maternal cell engraftment in immunocompromised children (19), and maternal cell contamination of umbilical cord blood units (26). The STR loci which are used for engraftment testing are also used for identity testing and can be used to distinguish between monozygotic and dizygotic twins.

SUMMARY

The zygotic origin of cells can be determined using a variety of methods. In 2005, the prevalent technique for chimerism testing involves quantification of the products of PCR amplification of highly polymorphic STR loci. These assays have not yet been standardized, and there can be substantial variation in the sensitivity and accuracy. After hematopoietic cell transplantation, chimerism assays are routinely used to monitor donor engraftment and autologous recovery. Analysis of lineage-specific chimerism can improve sensitivity for detecting residual host cells and can be useful for assessing prognostic risks for graft-versus-host disease, rejection, or recurrent malignancy.

I acknowledge and thank Gil Afonso for assistance in preparing the figures.

REFERENCES

1. Alizadeh, M., M. Bernard, B. Danic, C. Dauriac, B. Birebent, C. Lapart, T. Lamy, P. Y. Le Prise, A. Beauplet, D. Bories, G. Semana, and E. Quelvennec. 2002. Quantitative assessment of hematopoietic chimerism after bone marrow transplantation by real-time quantitative polymerase chain reaction. *Blood* **99:**4618–4625.

2. Antin, J. H., R. Childs, A. H. Filipovich, S. Giralt, S. Mackinnon, T. Spitzer, and D. Weisdorf. 2001. Establishment of complete and mixed donor chimerism after allogeneic lymphohematopoietic transplantation: recommendations from a workshop at the 2001 Tandem Meetings of the International Bone Marrow Transplant Registry and the American Society of Blood and Marrow Transplantation. *Biol. Blood Marrow Transplant.* **7:**473–485.

3. Bader, P., W. Holle, T. Klingebiel, R. Handgretinger, N. Benda, P. G. Schlegel, D. Niethammer, and J. Beck. 1997. Mixed hematopoietic chimerism after allogeneic bone marrow transplantation: the impact of quantitative PCR analysis for prediction of relapse and graft rejection in children. *Bone Marrow Transplant.* **19:**697–702.

4. Bader, P., W. Holle, T. Klingebiel, R. Handgretinger, D. Niethammer, and J. Beck. 1996. Quantitative assessment of mixed hematopoietic chimerism by polymerase chain reaction after allogeneic BMT. *Anticancer Res.* **16:**1759–1763.

5. Bader, P., H. Kreyenberg, W. Hoelle, G. Dueckers, R. Handgretinger, P. Lang, B. Kremens, D. Dilloo, K. W. Sykora, M. Schrappe, C. Niemeyer, A. Von Stackelberg, B. Gruhn, G. Henze, J. Greil, D. Niethammer, K. Dietz, J. F. Beck, and T. Klingebiel. 2004. Increasing mixed chimerism is an important prognostic factor for unfavorable outcome in children with acute lymphoblastic leukemia after allogeneic stem-cell transplantation: possible role for pre-emptive immunotherapy? *J. Clin. Oncol.* **22:**1696–1705.

6. Bader, P., H. Kreyenberg, W. Hoelle, G. Dueckers, B. Kremens, D. Dilloo, K. W. Sykora, C. Niemeyer, D. Reinhardt, J. Vormoor, B. Gruhn, P. Lang, J. Greil, R. Handgretinger, D. Niethammer, T. Klingebiel, and J. F. Beck. 2004. Increasing mixed chimerism defines a high-risk group of childhood acute myelogenous leukemia patients after allogeneic stem cell transplantation where pre-emptive immunotherapy may be effective. *Bone Marrow Transplant.* **33:**815–821.

7. Bader, P., D. Niethammer, A. Willasch, H. Kreyenberg, and T. Klingebiel. 2005. How and when should we monitor chimerism after allogeneic stem cell transplantation? *Bone Marrow Transplant.* **35:**107–119.

8. Bader, P., K. Stoll, S. Huber, A. Geiselhart, R. Handgretinger, C. Niemeyer, H. Einsele, P. G. Schlegel, D. Niethammer, J. Beck, and T. Klingebiel. 2000. Characterization of lineage-specific chimerism in patients with acute leukemia and myelodysplastic syndrome after allogeneic stem cell transplantation before and after relapse. *Br. J. Haematol.* **108:**761–768.

9. Baron, F., J. E. Baker, R. Storb, T. A. Gooley, B. M. Sandmaier, M. B. Maris, D. G. Maloney, S. Heimfeld, D. Oparin, E. Zellmer, J. P. Radich, F. C. Grumet, K. G. Blume, T. R. Chauncey, and M. T. Little. 2004. Kinetics of engraftment in patients with hematologic malignancies given allogeneic hematopoietic cell transplantation after nonmyeloablative conditioning. *Blood* **104:**2254–2262.

10. Barrios, M., A. Jimenez-Velasco, J. Roman-Gomez, M. E. Madrigal, J. A. Castillejo, A. Torres, and A. Heiniger. 2003. Chimerism status is a useful predictor of relapse after allogeneic stem cell transplantation for acute leukemia. *Haematologica* **88:**801–810.

11. Bianchi, D. W., G. K. Zickwolf, G. J. Weil, S. Sylvester, and M. A. DeMaria. 1996. Male fetal progenitor cells persist in maternal blood for as long as 27 years postpartum. *Proc. Natl. Acad. Sci. USA* **93:**705–708.

12. Blume, K. G., E. Beutler, K. J. Bross, G. M. Schmidt, W. E. Spruce, and R. L. Teplitz. 1980. Genetic markers in human bone marrow transplantation. *Am. J. Hum. Genet.* **32:**414–419.

13. Dewald, G. W., C. R. Schad, E. R. Christensen, M. E. Law, A. R. Zinsmeister, P. G. Stalboerger, S. M. Jalal, R. C. Ash, and R. B. Jenkins. 1993. Fluorescence in situ hybridization with X and Y chromosome probes for cytogenetic studies on bone marrow cells after opposite sex transplantation. *Bone Marrow Transplant.* **12:**149–154.

14. Drobyski, W., S. Thibodeau, R. L. Truitt, L. A. Baxter-Lowe, J. Gorski, R. Jenkins, J. Gottschall, and R. C. Ash. 1989. Third-party-mediated graft rejection and graft-versus-host disease after T-cell-depleted bone marrow transplantation, as demonstrated by hypervariable DNA probes and HLA-DR polymorphism. *Blood* **74:**2285–2294.

15. Girgis, M., C. Hallemeier, W. Blum, R. Brown, H. S. Lin, H. Khoury, L. T. Goodnough, R. Vij, S. Devine, M. Wehde, S. Postma, A. Oza, J. DiPersio, and D. Adkins. 2004. Chimerism and clinical outcomes of 110 recipients of unrelated donor bone marrow transplants who underwent conditioning with low-dose, single-exposure total body irradiation and cyclophosphamide. *Blood* **105:**3035–3041.

16. Guimond, M., L. Busque, C. Baron, Y. Bonny, R. Belanger, J. Mattioli, C. Perreault, and D. C. Roy. 2000. Relapse after bone marrow transplantation: evidence for distinct immunological mechanisms between adult and paediatric populations. *Br. J. Haematol.* **109:**130–137.

17. Hancock, J. P., N. J. Goulden, A. Oakhill, and C. G. Steward. 2003. Quantitative analysis of chimerism after allogeneic bone marrow transplantation using immunomagnetic selection and fluorescent microsatellite PCR. *Leukemia* **17:**247–251.

18. Hochberg, E. P., D. B. Miklos, D. Neuberg, D. A. Eichner, S. F. McLaughlin, A. Mattes-Ritz, E. P. Alyea, J. H. Antin, R. J. Soiffer, and J. Ritz. 2003. A novel rapid single nucleotide polymorphism (SNP)-based method for assessment of hematopoietic chimerism after allogeneic stem cell transplantation. *Blood* **101:**363–369.

19. Katz, F., S. Malcolm, S. Strobel, A. Finn, G. Morgan, and R. Levinsky. 1990. The use of locus-specific minisatellite probes to check engraftment following allogeneic bone marrow transplantation for severe combined immunodeficiency disease. *Bone Marrow Transplant.* **5:**199–204.

20. Khan, F., A. Agarwal, and S. Agrawal. 2004. Significance of chimerism in hematopoietic stem cell transplantation: new variations on an old theme. *Bone Marrow Transplant.* **34:**1–12.

21. Kreyenberg, H., W. Holle, S. Mohrle, D. Niethammer, and P. Bader. 2003. Quantitative analysis of chimerism after allogeneic stem cell transplantation by PCR amplification of microsatellite markers and capillary electrophoresis with fluorescence detection: the Tuebingen experience. *Leukemia* **17:**237–240.

22. Lee, T. H., T. Paglieroni, H. Ohto, P. V. Holland, and M. P. Busch. 1999. Survival of donor leukocyte subpopulations in immunocompetent transfusion recipients: frequent long-term microchimerism in severe trauma patients. *Blood* **93:**3127–3139.

23. Maas, F., N. Schaap, S. Kolen, A. Zoetbrood, I. Buno, H. Dolstra, T. de Witte, A. Schattenberg, and E. van de Wiel-van Kemenade. 2003. Quantification of donor and recipient hemopoietic cells by real-time PCR of single nucleotide polymorphisms. *Leukemia* **17:**621–629.

24. Matsuda, K., K. Yamauchi, M. Tozuka, T. Suzuki, M. Sugano, E. Hidaka, K. Sano, and T. Katsuyama. 2004. Monitoring of hematopoietic chimerism by short tandem repeats, and the effect of CD selection on its sensitivity. *Clin. Chem.* **50:**2411–2414.

25. Nollet, F., J. Billiet, D. Selleslag, and A. Criel. 2001. Standardization of multiplex fluorescent short tandem repeat analysis for chimerism testing. *Bone Marrow Transplant.* **28:**511–518.

26. Poli, F., S. M. Sirchia, M. Scalamogna, I. Garagiola, L. Crespiatico, L. Pedranzini, L. Lecchi, and G. Sirchia. 1997. Detection of maternal DNA in human cord blood stored for allotransplantation by a highly sensitive chemiluminescent method. *J. Hematother.* **6:**581–585.

27. Scharf, S. J., A. G. Smith, J. A. Hansen, C. McFarland, and H. A. Erlich. 1995. Quantitative determination of bone marrow transplant engraftment using fluorescent polymerase chain reaction primers for human identity markers. *Blood* **85:**1954–1963.

28. Scheffold, C., M. Kroeger, M. Zuehlsdorf, J. Tchinda, G. Silling, G. Bisping, M. Stelljes, T. Buechner, W. E. Berdel, and J. Kienast. 2004. Prediction of relapse of acute myeloid leukemia in allogeneic transplant recipients by marrow CD34+ donor cell chimerism analysis. *Leukemia* **18:**2048–2050.

29. Schraml, E., and T. Lion. 2003. Interference of dye-associated fluorescence signals with quantitative analysis of chimerism by capillary electrophoresis. *Leukemia* **17:**221–223.

30. Shimoni, A., A. Nagler, C. Kaplinsky, M. Reichart, A. Avigdor, I. Hardan, M. Yeshurun, M. Daniely, Y. Zilberstein, N. Amariglio, F. Brok-Simoni, G. Rechavi, and L. Trakhtenbrot. 2002. Chimerism testing and detection of minimal residual disease after allogeneic hematopoietic transplantation using the bioView (Duet) combined morphological and cytogenetical analysis. *Leukemia* **16:**1413–1418, 1419–1422.

31. Starzl, T. E., A. J. Demetris, M. Trucco, H. Ramos, A. Zeevi, W. A. Rudert, M. Kocova, C. Ricordi, S. Ildstad, and N. Murase. 1992. Systemic chimerism in human female recipients of male livers. *Lancet* **340:**876–877.

32. Suttorp, M., N. Schmitz, P. Dreger, J. Schaub, and H. Loffler. 1993. Monitoring of chimerism after allogeneic bone marrow transplantation with unmanipulated marrow by use of DNA polymorphisms. *Leukemia* **7:**679–687.

33. Thiede, C., M. Bornhauser, and G. Ehninger. 2004. Evaluation of STR informativity for chimerism testing—comparative analysis of 27 STR systems in 203 matched related donor recipient pairs. *Leukemia* **18:**248–254.

34. Thiede, C., K. Lutterbeck, U. Oelschlagel, M. Kiehl, C. Steudel, U. Platzbecker, C. Brendel, A. A. Fauser, A. Neubauer, G. Ehninger, and M. Bornhauser. 2002. Detection of relapse by sequential monitoring of chimerism in circulating CD34+ cells. *Ann. Hematol.* **81:**S27–S28.

35. Walsh, P. S., N. J. Fildes, and R. Reynolds. 1996. Sequence analysis and characterization of stutter products at the tetranucleotide repeat locus vWA. *Nucleic Acids Res.* **24:**2807–2812.

LABORATORY MANAGEMENT

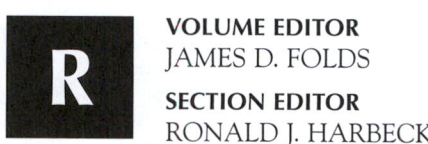

VOLUME EDITOR
JAMES D. FOLDS

SECTION EDITOR
RONALD J. HARBECK

Clinical Immunology Laboratory Accreditation, Licensure, and Credentials

LINDA COOK AND RONALD J. HARBECK

142

It was once possible to perform testing on hospital and clinic patient samples by simply setting up a laboratory and going to work. Many of today's excellent clinical immunology laboratories were spawned in the leading research laboratories across the country as new assays were evaluated and developed by leading researchers and clinicians. Many currently used immunology tests were originally designed, validated, and performed by research technicians, graduate students, or postdoctoral fellows. However, in today's hospital and reference laboratory environment, many government regulations and professional guidelines mandate the education levels of individuals who perform and oversee the testing, recommend test procedures, and define acceptable ordering, result reporting, and billing practices. The U.S. Department of Health and Human Services division of the CMS (formerly the HCFA), which regulates billing practices, has also had a significant impact on the way laboratories must be structured and managed. Today's successful clinical immunology laboratory practitioners must educate themselves about existing guidelines and regulations and keep abreast of the constant changes in order to ensure compliance and professionalism in all areas of the laboratory. This chapter provides a broad overview of the major agencies and regulations which have had an impact on laboratory practices. Laboratory personnel must keep constantly updated by reading appropriate professional articles and reviewing the appropriate Web pages of the responsible agencies and organizations for the latest information.

Various governmental agencies, regulations, organizations, etc., are referred to in this chapter. To assist the reader, a list of abbreviations follows. In addition, an extensive list of websites is provided in Table 1 to help the reader obtain further information regarding specific agencies, regulations, and programs.

Abbreviations. AAAAI, American Academy of Allergy, Asthma and Immunology; **AACC,** American Association of Clinical Chemistry; **ABHI,** American Board of Histocompatibility and Immunogenetics; **AMA,** American Medical Association; **AMLI,** Association of Medical Laboratory Immunologists; **ASCP,** American Society of Clinical Pathologists; **ASHI,** American Society for Histocompatibility and Immunogenetics; **ASM,** American Society for Microbiology; **CAP,** College of American Pathologists; **CDC,** Centers for Disease Control and Prevention; **CLEP,** Clinical Laboratory Evaluation Program; **CLIA,** Clinical

Laboratory Improvement Amendments; **CLSI,** Clinical and Laboratory Standards Institute (formerly National Committee for Clinical Laboratory Standards); **CMS,** Centers for Medicare and Medicaid Services (formerly the Health Care Financing Administration [HCFA]); **CPA,** Clinical Pathology Accreditation Ltd.; **CPT,** Current Procedural Terminology; **DRG,** diagnosis-related group; **FDA,** Food and Drug Administration; **GLP,** good laboratory practice; **HCPCS,** HCFA Common Procedure Coding System; **HMO,** health maintenance organization; **ICD,** International Classification of Diseases; **ISO,** International Organization for Standardization; **JCAHO,** Joint Commission on Accreditation of Healthcare Organizations; **LOINC,** Laboratory Observation Identifier Names and Codes; **OIG,** Office of the Inspector General; **WHO,** World Health Organization.

REGULATORY ISSUES AND AGENCIES OF THE FEDERAL GOVERNMENT

CLIA

In 1965 the federal government enacted Public Law 89-97, which created Medicare and Medicaid under the Social Security Act of 1939. As a result of this law, the Department of Health, Education and Welfare developed standards for clinical laboratories operating in inpatient and outpatient settings. The Department of Health, Education and Welfare appointed JCAHO to set standards and survey the laboratories for accreditation. However, Congress became concerned that significant problems existed in the quality of laboratory testing for Medicare recipients provided by laboratories engaged in interstate commerce. Therefore, in 1967 Congress passed the CLIA (CLIA '67) mandating licensure for laboratories providing testing on more than 100 out-of-state specimens per year in major testing categories such as microbiology, chemistry, serology, and hematology. A letter of exemption could be obtained from the CDC for those laboratories receiving fewer than 100 out-of-state specimens per year.

In 1987 the *Wall Street Journal* published an article which again raised concerns among the public about the quality of laboratory testing, especially cytology (1, 2). This prompted Congress and many state health departments to closely review the operations of the nation's clinical laboratories. This review resulted in Congress passing Public Law 100-578, or the CLIA of 1988 (CLIA '88) (12). In 1992 the final rules for CLIA '88

TABLE 1 Websites of governmental and private agencies setting regulations and guidelines for clinical laboratories

Agency or organization[a]	Website
Federal regulations and guidelines	
Agency for Healthcare Research and Quality	http://www.ahcpr.gov
CAP (Laboratory Accreditation)	http://www.cap.org/apps/cap.portal
Department of Health and Human Services	
CDC	http://www.cdc.gov
CMS	http://www.cms.hhs.gov
CMS lab diagnostic fee schedules (yearly file)	http://www.cms.hhs.gov/suppliers/clinlab
CMS CLIA information	http://www.cms.hhs.gov/clia
FDA	http://www.fda.gov
FDA (waived tests)	http://www.fda.gov/cdrh/clia/cliawaived.html
FDA GLP document 21 Part 58	http://www.access.gpo.gov/nara/cfr
National Institutes of Health	http://www.nih.gov
National Institute of Occupational Safety and Health	http://www.cdc.gov/niosh/homepage.html
OIG (*Federal Register* notices/compliance)	http://www.oig.hhs.gov/authorities/frnotices.html
Environmental Protection Agency	http://epa.gov
Good Laboratory Practices Online	http://www.fda.gov/ora/compliance_ref/bimo/glp/default.htm; http://www2.sjsu.edu/faculty/chem55/55glpout.htm
Medicare, glossary of terms	http://www.medicare.gov/Glossary/Search.asp
Society of Quality Assurance	http://www.sqa.org
State regulations and guidelines	
California Department of Health Services, Division of Laboratory Science, Laboratory Field Services	http://www.dhs.ca.gov/ps/ls/LFSB/default.htm
New York State Clinical Laboratory Evaluation Program	http://www.wadsworth.org/index.html
Oregon	http://www.oregon.gov/DHS/ph/lcqa/docs/all-lab.pdf
Washington State	http://www.doh.wa.gov/hsqa/fsl/LQA_Home.htm
International regulations and guidelines	
External Peer Review Techniques/CASPE Research	http://www.caspe.co.uk/index.html
Institute for Standardization and Documentation in Medical Laboratory	http://www.instand-ev.de
IFCC	http://www.ifcc.org
European Communities Confederation of Clinical Chemistry and Laboratory Medicine	http://www.e-c4.org
ISO	http://www.iso.ch
ISO clinical laboratory testing and in vitro diagnostic test systems	http://www.iso.org/iso/en/CatalogueListPage.CatalogueList?COMMID = 4643&scopelist = PROGRAMME
WHO	http://www.who.int/en
CPA	http://www.cpa-uk.co.uk
Other	
American Association of Blood Banks	http://www.aabb.org
AMA	http://www.ama-assn.org
AMA CPT Coding	http://www.ama-assn.org/ama/pub/category/3113.html
American Osteopathic Association	http://www.aoa-net.org
ASHI	http://www.ashi-hla.org
LAP	http://www.cap.org/apps/docs/laboratory_accreditation/checklists/checklistftp.html
JCAHO	http://www.jcaho.com
CLSI	http://www.nccls.org

[a] See text for abbreviations.

were published (13, 16). CLIA '88 replaced CLIA '67 and the separate Medicare/Medicaid regulations that were in effect up until this time. CLIA '88 required that all facilities performing examinations on materials obtained from the human body for the purpose of providing information for the diagnosis, prevention, or treatment of any disease or impairment of, or the assessment of the health of, human beings were subject to CLIA standards. The sites included in these new regulations were doctors' offices, clinics, health departments, hospitals, and reference laboratories. These requirements mandated additional procedures, reviews, and proficiency testing for all laboratories whether or not they were directly associated with

health care institutions. Laboratories exempt from CLIA '88 include those that are subject to the rules published and enforced by the Veterans Administration and by the Department of Defense (for personnel drug surveillance and enforcement purposes). In addition, laboratories licensed by approved state licensure programs, law enforcement agencies that determine the legal status of individuals, laboratories performing forensic testing, and those performing research testing where the results are not reported for clinical use are also exempt from CLIA '88 regulations.

As part of the CMS's mandates, it is responsible for the administration of the Medicare and Medicaid programs. It is the responsibility of the Division of Outcomes and Improvement within the CMS to ensure that medical laboratories provide quality testing results. This is achieved through a survey and certification program (14). As of August 2005, the Division of Laboratory Services of the CMS reports that 192,533 laboratories are registered, while 104,994 physician office laboratories are registered. Approximately 38,000 labs are authorized to perform high- or moderate-complexity testing. There are 10 regional offices located throughout the United States with at least one laboratory consultant in each office who is a medical technologist.

Many medical laboratories may not be directly affected by the CMS surveys. CMS has granted "deemed" status to several organizations. In other words, the CMS has the authority to establish and oversee a program that allows private, national accreditation organizations to "deem" that a laboratory is in compliance with Medicare requirements. These organizations include the CAP, JCAHO, the American Association of Blood Banks, the American Osteopathic Association, ASHI, and the Commission on Office Laboratory Accreditation. In addition, two states, Washington and New York, are exempt from CLIA regulations since their programs were found to be equal to or exceed Medicare compliance requirements.

CLIA has established four categories of testing,: waived, moderate complexity, provider-performed microscopy, and high complexity. The waived tests are those considered simple laboratory examinations and procedures that pose insignificant risk of producing an erroneous laboratory test result. Laboratories with a certificate of waiver are not subject to inspection for certification. However, it is expected that the laboratory will abide by all quality control measures as specified by the manufacturer of the kits in use. CLIA '88-waived tests include those performed in bacteriology (includes urine catalase, *Helicobacter pylori* test kits, and group A streptococcus antigen detection kits), endocrinology (includes urine human chorionic gonadotropin and ovulation tests by visual color comparison), general chemistry (includes some cholesterol, creatinine, fecal occult blood, fructosamine, gastric occult blood, glucose, microalbumin, and triglyceride tests), hematology (erythrocyte sedimentation rate, hematocrit, hemoglobin, and prothrombin times), toxicology and therapeutic drug monitoring (ethanol and nicotine and/or metabolites such as cotinine), and urinalysis (urine dipsticks). For the immunology laboratory, tests for bladder tumor-associated antigen and antibodies against *H. pylori* and Epstein-Barr virus (infectious mononucleosis) and respiratory syncytial virus have been approved as of August 2005 as waived tests. The FDA maintains a website which contains frequent updates of waived tests (Table 1).

Tests included in the moderately complex category require some basic scientific and technical knowledge of the various analytical phases of the testing. In addition, basic training and experience are required to perform the test. The tests generally are not fully automated and require some monitoring, timing, or simple calculations. Independent technical skill, decision making, or intervention by the analyst may be required. Before the results of a moderately complex test are released, interpretation and judgment by the analyst may be required.

The moderately complex testing category contains one subcategory of provider-performed microscopy. Tests included in this category are procedures which utilize a microscope in which the test specimen is labile or if the test is delayed could compromise the accuracy of the results. They include wet-mount preparations of vaginal, cervical, or skin specimens; KOH preparations; pinworm examinations; fern tests; postcoital examinations of vaginal or cervical mucus; urine sediment examination; nasal smears for eosinophils; fecal leukocyte examination; and examination of semen for the presence or absence of sperm and motility. Tests included in this category must be performed during a patient's visit only by licensed physicians, dentists, or podiatrists or by mid-level practitioners, including nurse practitioners, nurse midwives, and physician assistants.

Highly complex testing involves a manual procedure with multiple steps in the sample or reagent processing or automated procedures requiring significant operator intervention. These tests require specialized scientific and technical knowledge as well as appropriate training and experience in order to perform all phases of the analytical process. Reagents used in these tests may be labile and may require special handling or preparation. The operational steps involved in performing the tests may be complex, requiring manual manipulation and monitoring. A high level of troubleshooting abilities, decision making, intervention, interpretation, and judgment are required. Many tests performed in the clinical immunology laboratory are included in this category.

CLIA '88 has specified the training needed of individuals based on the complexity of the testing. For a laboratory performing moderately complex testing, the directors may include pathologists, M.D.'s, D.O.'s, or Ph.D.'s with appropriate experience and training or individuals with a master's or bachelor's degree in science with appropriate experience and training. For high-complexity laboratories a pathologist, other M.D., or D.O. with 1 year of laboratory training during residency or 2 years' experience directing or supervising high-complexity testing may direct the laboratory. In order for a Ph.D. to direct a high-complexity laboratory, he or she must be certified in one of the laboratory specialties, e.g., by the American Board of Medical Laboratory Immunology, or until September 1994 have had 2 years' laboratory training or experience. At the end of the 2 years the individual must (i) become board certified, (ii) be serving as a laboratory director and qualified on or before 28 February 1992, (iii) be qualified under 14 March 1990 CLIA '67 rules, or (iv) be qualified under state law to direct a laboratory in the state on or before 28 February 1992. Further information regarding the requirements for a laboratory director and updates of requirements can be located at http://www.phppo.cdc.gov/clia/regs/subpart_m.aspx#493.1405.

In addition to the laboratory director, specific qualifications are required for technical supervisors, general supervisors, clinical consultants, and cytotechnologists. The CLIA regulations require that the laboratory employ one or more individuals who are qualified by education and either training or experience to perform the responsibilities of a technical supervisor. For diagnostic immunology the requirements range from board-certified pathologists to individuals with a bachelor's degree in science with 4 years of training in high-complexity testing. For histocompatibility and clinical cytogenetics, individuals must be an M.D., D.O., or Ph.D. with 4 years of training or experience. The CLIA requirements for a general supervisor are an M.D., D.O., or Ph.D., a master's or bachelor's degree in science with 1 year of training or experience in high-complexity testing, or an associate degree in laboratory science or medical laboratory technology and 2 years of training or experience in high-complexity testing. One should refer to the CAP website for additional requirements for education and training for supervisors and testing personnel (http://www.phppo.cdc.gov/clia/regs/toc.aspx).

Reimbursement Issues

Receiving payment for the tests performed in the laboratory has become a very complex issue. Regulations concerning how much will be paid for which tests now rarely match the fee chosen by an individual laboratory. Different billing and reimbursement practices are set by a variety of entities, including private insurance companies, HMOs, the CMS, and a variety of regional carriers who determine local medical review policies. Beginning in 1997 the task of attempting to standardize these policies throughout the country was given to the CMS, a federal agency that is tasked with oversight of the federal program. The CMS created a negotiated rulemaking committee with members consisting of representatives from laboratory organizations, physician groups, and other interested parties. In an ongoing effort, the committee has been tasked to define national reimbursement policies for many lab tests and tries to define through a consensus process policies that reflect good laboratory utilization of testing. National policies are available on the CMS website (http://cms.hhs.gov/coverage). Because of the myriad of reimbursement strategies, each laboratory must establish its own policies and procedures based on information from each of these entities. Because the CMS reimbursement policies have the largest impact on laboratories, a brief review of the most important CMS issues follows. Many other carriers use the CMS policies as guides to set their individual policies. For these reasons, a clear understanding of CMS procedures and guidelines is important. It may also be important for each lab to investigate other agencies and insurance companies when they constitute a significant percentage of the testing population.

Current billing practices for the CMS separate tests into two major types, inpatient and outpatient testing. For inpatient testing, reimbursement is in the form of a single lump payment based on the diagnosis of the patient and any subsequent problems which occur during a hospital stay. The payment system is based on categorization of the patient's disease into a DRG. DRGs consist of 495 groups in 23 major diagnostic categories. The conversion of U.S. hospital billing practices to this billing system occurred in October of 1983 and led to the conversion of hospital laboratories from revenue centers to cost centers. Because hospitals receive the same money for a single patient with a particular disease, the onus is on physicians and laboratory directors to ensure appropriate laboratory utilization by all individuals who order laboratory tests on patients.

Outpatient tests, for which the patient is usually seen in a clinic setting, are being reimbursed per test by Medicare or Medicaid. Payments are subject to a variety of rules and regulations. Many of these issues are dealt with by hospital billing departments, but laboratory directors and managers are responsible for ensuring compliance with the CMS regulations. The most important of these is the selection of the appropriate CPT-4 billing code for each test being performed. Because of the perceived success of the DRG inpatient billing system, a similar system has been designed for outpatient billing. The regulations for outpatient billing have their foundation in the Ambulatory Payment Classification system for coding of procedures and tests. This funding program and associated regulations are administered by the Medicare Outpatient Prospective Payment System, which became functional as of 1 August 2000. The Ambulatory Payment Classification system has 451 groups of outpatient services that must be coded. The Outpatient Prospective Payment Program regulations currently do not include laboratory billing, with the exception of allergy skin testing and some immunopathology testing. This system may in the future be expanded to include all laboratory tests.

Regulations also exist for laboratories which service skilled nursing facilities, kidney dialysis centers (end-stage renal disease regulations), and physicians' office laboratories. In addition to these specialized situations many state governments also have regulations which impact billing practices.

Finally, with the transition of many patients into HMOs, much of the outpatient laboratory services became a capitation system in which the laboratory receives a predetermined amount of money for each covered individual regardless of the number of tests which are done. It is important for individuals responsible for laboratory testing for HMOs to maximize the efficient use of laboratory services and have an accurate idea of test expenses.

Compliance Issues

The OIG within the Department of Health and Human Services is responsible for issuing and monitoring billing regulation for the federal government. The OIG has issued three different regulatory documents which describe the compliance programs for hospital billing departments and clinical laboratories. These can be found on the OIG website under the date of issue; the initial hospital compliance program was issued in 1998 (2/23/98), with supplemental guidelines issued in 2005 (1/27/05); the compliance guidelines for clinical laboratories were issued in 1998 (8/24/98). These documents must be read by individuals responsible for ordering, performing, and billing for laboratory tests so that all laboratory practices are consistent with the regulations. The purpose of these plans is to assist clinical laboratories in developing effective internal controls that will promote adherence to federal and state law, and the program requirement of federal, state, and private health plans (15). The key elements listed in the compliance program should address the following: (i) the development of written standards of conduct that address specific areas of potential fraud, e.g., marketing schemes, CPT coding issues, improper diagnosis coding, and improper claim submissions; (ii) the designation of a chief compliance officer or other appropriate bodies who are charged with the responsibility of operating and monitoring the compliance program and reporting to the chief executive officer and the governing body; (iii) the development and offering of education and training programs to all affected employees; (iv) the maintenance of a process to receive complaints and the adoption of procedures to protect the anonymity of complainants and whistleblowers; (v) the development of a system to respond to allegations of improper and illegal activities and the use of disciplinary action against employees who have violated internal compliance policies or applicable laws or who have engaged in wrongdoing; (vi) the use of audits and/or other evaluation techniques to monitor compliance and ensure a reduction in identified problem areas; and (vii) the investigation and remediation of identified systemic problems and the development of policies addressing the nonemployment or retention of sanctioned individuals.

Each institution and all laboratories must comply with these regulations in order to ensure lack of fraud and abuse in Medicare and Medicaid billing. Immunology laboratories should play a role in the development of laboratory and institutional procedures and policies and ensure that all systems and employees are in compliance with the OIG documents.

Regulations exist which mandate communication between laboratories and the physicians who utilize them. In the OIG compliance documents, the responsibility is placed on the laboratory to inform physicians on a regular basis of the CPT-4 coding and Medicare reimbursement amounts for all tests. This is especially important for tests billed as multiple CPT-4 codes. For example, billing for immunoglobulin quantitations—immunoglobulin G (IgG), IgA, and IgM—could be billed as "3 × 82374, Gammaglobulins, each." The laboratory has the responsibility to inform all patients ordering immunoglobulin quantitations that they are ordering three billable tests in this example. Physician information is also important if "reflex" testing is done. Reflex testing, or the automatic addition of a second test based on the results of the first test, can only be done when the physicians and institution have established the process based on clear medical necessity. All physicians must be aware and agree with any reflex testing strategies being used by the laboratory. This includes all immunofluorescent tests, antinuclear antibodies (ANAs), antimitochondrial antibodies, etc., in which one bill is generated for the initial screen and a second bill is issued for the further analysis of a positive result, e.g., the titration of a positive ANA test.

Another aspect of Medicare and Medicaid billing is that each test must be considered medically necessary. As a part of this determination, each request for laboratory test billing must contain information concerning the diagnosis for the patient. If the test is ordered as part of a panel, all the tests within the panel must also be medically necessary. The diagnostic information for each patient is conveyed using a coding system of diseases termed the ICD-9. ICD-9 was initially published in January of 1979 and is currently the system in use. A federal coordination and maintenance committee meets on a regular basis to examine the ICD-9 code system and adds to or modifies the codes as needed. As this is a federal coding system, it is available in its current form on the CMS website. This disease system is used in both inpatient and outpatient services to code and classify morbidity data for medical records, medical care review, and basic health statistics. The National Center for Health Statistics at the CDC is the WHO collaborating center for North America.

Procedure Coding

In addition to the disease coding, each laboratory test must be coded to indicate the actual test performed. There are over 150 known coding systems that have been developed. The one that is most applicable to U.S. clinical laboratories is the CPT code. CPT coding was developed by the AMA in 1966 and is updated annually (http://www.ama-assn.org). The CPT-4 system has thousands of codes that define a wide variety of medical procedures, including a section for pathology and laboratory medicine. Each test analyte is defined by a five-digit code. Medicare payments have been divided into Part A (the professional component) and Part B (the technical component). Laboratory tests that require significant professional interpretation skills, such as direct skin biopsy immunofluorescent studies or flow cytometry leukemia analysis, can be billed for both a professional and a technical component. The professional component is billed by adding the additional code (-26) modifier onto the five-digit code for the test performed. The reimbursement amount for each technical component (Part B) for each CPT-4 code is published yearly on the CMS website (Table 1) for all CPT-4 codes and for each U.S. state. Part A reimbursements vary widely and should be determined for each local medical carrier. All laboratories should review their CPT-4 coding each

year to ensure the appropriate coding for all laboratory tests. In addition to the CPT-4 coding system, CPT-5 is under development.

Two other coding systems are used, the HCPCS and the LOINC. The HCPCS is referred to as a national code and is approved and maintained jointly by the CMS, the Health Insurance Association, and the Blue Cross and Blue Shield Association. The HCPCS system uses five-position alphanumeric codes for nonphysician procedures and for injectable drugs and their administration. The LOINC was developed by an ad hoc group of clinical pathologists, chemists, and laboratory service vendors. Their goal was to create universal test codes for laboratory tests and procedures.

Advanced Beneficiary Notice

Under Section 1862 (a)(I)(A) of the Medicare Law, Medicare will pay only for services that it determines to be "reasonable and necessary." If the service is not determined to be reasonable and necessary, the beneficiary is not responsible for payment of the service unless prior to the service being rendered, the patient has been notified in writing that Medicare will likely deny payment of the service for his or her specific condition. By signing the advanced beneficiary notice, the patient agrees to assume financial responsibility for the service. The reason given must be specific to the services under consideration. An advance written notice to the beneficiary can protect the provider from liability.

GLP

Clinical laboratories have been increasingly involved in pharmaceutical and diagnostic companies' evaluation of new drugs or diagnostic products. In the 1970s the FDA published regulations governing the conduct of the safety tests on regulated products (GLP regulations, 21 CFR part 58). Compliance with these regulations is intended to ensure the quality and integrity of the safety data prior to the marketing and/or clinical testing of the regulated product. Products that must have evidence of safety include human and animal drugs, human biological products, medical devices, and diagnostic products. The regulations address such issues as the protocol, personnel, facilities, equipment, operations, testing, and controls. The FDA conducts regular inspections and data audits to monitor a laboratory's compliance with GLP requirements. This process is rather detailed and thorough. Before undertaking a GLP project, it is important to consult with a quality assurance professional familiar with GLP regulations. Table 1 lists websites that provide more detailed information on GLP.

ASR

In 1997, the FDA issued a Final Rule regulating analyte-specific reagents (ASR) that are sold for clinical diagnostic applications (Federal Register, 21:8, revised 1 April 2004, 21CFR809.3 and 21CFR809.10). They are defined by the FDA as "antibodies, both polyclonal and monoclonal, specific receptor proteins, ligands, nucleic acid sequences, and similar reagents which, through specific binding or chemical reactions with substances in a specimen, are intended for use in a diagnostic application for identification and quantification of an individual chemical substance or ligand in biological specimens" (6). This rule has made it easier for manufacturers of diagnostic products to develop and market products. The burden of responsibility for the performance of an ASR is on the laboratory. This regulation mandates that each report generated by a laboratory in which an ASR was used must state, "This test was developed and its performance characteristics determined by [*laboratory name*]. It has not been cleared or approved by the U.S. Food and Drug Administration." A laboratory may elect to include additional, clarifying information along with this statement. The CAP has developed some sample statements to go along with the required statement (5). For example, the following statements have been suggested. (i) "The FDA has determined that such clearance or approval is not necessary." (ii) "This test is used for clinical purposes. It should not be regarded as investigational or for research." (iii) "This laboratory is certified under the Clinical Laboratory Improvement Amendments of 1988 (CLIA) as qualified to perform high-complexity clinical testing. Pursuant to the requirements of CLIA, this laboratory has established and verified the test's accuracy and precision." Since the implementation of the ASR regulations, difficulties have surrounded the application of the regulations, so the FDA began a series of hearings beginning in 2005 to improve the process. Revised regulations may be issued in the future to deal with some of these issues.

STATE CERTIFYING PROGRAMS

The CMS has recognized certain states as being exempt from their certifying program. These states can carry out their own laboratory surveillance and issue their own certifications. These states currently include Washington and New York. Prior to 1 January 2000 the laboratories in Oregon were exempt.

Washington State

In 1989 the state legislature passed the Medical Test Site Licensure law, which allowed the state to regulate clinical laboratory testing. In 1993, Washington's program was judged to be equivalent to CLIA and Washington became the first state in the country to be granted deemed status. In 1997 the CMS extended Washington's exempt status under the CLIA program for all laboratories. Washington retains its regulatory activity at the state level, where it claims the process is more accessible and responsive to local needs.

Under the Washington State program, approximately 2,600 test sites are issued licenses or certificates of waiver. Biennial on-site surveys of approximately 600 nonwaived testing sites are conducted. This survey examines quality control and patient records, test performance, test reporting, management policies, and quality assurance programs. Although the state does not offer its own proficiency testing program, testing sites must participate in a program that is approved by the CMS. The state monitors proficiency test results for acceptability.

New York State

In 1996 New York received exempt status under the CLIA program for independent and hospital laboratories. Prior to this New York became the first state, in 1965, to initiate a certification and licensing program for clinical laboratories operating within the state. Since then the program has expanded, and now, through the Clinical Laboratory Evaluation Program (CLEP), it monitors the quality of testing from all clinical laboratories and blood banks within the state of New York as well as all out-of-state facilities that accept clinical specimens obtained from within New York State. In very rare situations, an unusual test can be granted an exception and performed in a lab without a license. CLEP issues permits to over 1,000 laboratories across the nation and 600 patient service centers in New York State.

The three objectives of the CLEP program are "1) to monitor, improve, and broaden the clinical capabilities of participating laboratories and blood banks; 2) to provide guidelines, quality control standards, and procedures to be used by permit-holding clinical facilities; and 3) to expand the clinical and educational background of medical technologists, laboratorians, and other personnel involved in the operation of clinical laboratories through training and remediation programs."

Standards for New York State accreditation can be found at http://www.wadsworth.org/labcert/clep/Survey/standards-menu.htm. To obtain a New York State laboratory permit, the laboratory must complete an application, submit the required fees, designate a laboratory director and assistant directors, if applicable, and obtain certificates of qualification in all permitted categories for which the laboratory has applied. Currently approximately 2,300 certificates of qualification have been issued to individuals to serve as directors or assistant directors of clinical laboratories and blood banks. In addition, the laboratory must successfully participate in two successive New York State proficiency testing events for all applied categories and subcategories and for all analytes for which New York State proficiency testing is offered, submit standard operating procedures and validation data for department review and approval, complete a successful on-site inspection, and submit an acceptable plan of correction for any deficiencies cited during the inspection. An out-of-state laboratory seeking a New York State permit shall pay to the department an on-site survey fee calculated by the department, which shall consist of a transportation expense and a per-diem expense. Details concerning certification of labs and tests and a request form for a nonlicensed exemption can be found at http://www.wadsworth.org/labcert/clep/clep.html.

The specific technical categories and subcategories for tests that relate to a clinical immunology laboratory are listed in Table 2.

California

The California section of Laboratory Field Services (LFS) is responsible for licensing clinical laboratory personnel, including clinical laboratory scientists (formally titled clinical laboratory technologists), bioanalysts, specialty directors, specialty scientists, and cytotechnologists, through an application process and examination. The program also approves training schools for clinical laboratory personnel, including schools that provide instruction in phlebotomy. Finally, the program conducts complaint investigations which may include on-site inspection processes.

California requires all laboratories to participate in proficiency testing programs that have been approved by the California Department of Health Services and the federal government. Currently, proficiency testing is performed three times per year with five specimens to test per analyte.

ACCREDITATION AND LICENSURE OF LABORATORIES

The CLIA regulations issued by the federal government have mandated that all laboratories performing clinical testing must undergo regular inspections by an agency or organization with deemed status, e.g., the CAP, JCAHO, or New York State. These agencies all have detailed requirements which include acceptable education and training for all personnel, content of procedure manuals, documentation of quality control and preventive maintenance procedures, verification of new procedures, ordering and result reporting

TABLE 2 New York State Department of Health technical categories and subcategories[a]

Technical categories and subcategories	Description
Cellular immunology	
Lymphoid function assays (formerly Limited I)	Analysis of lymphocyte functions by in vitro assays, e.g., antigen-induced proliferation, alloantigen-stimulated proliferation, mitogen-stimulated proliferation, cytolytic assays, and cytokine or immunoglobulin production. For determinations of cytokines in serum, plasma, or CSF, refer to "Cytokines" below.
Lymphoid/T-lymphocyte immunophenotyping (formerly Limited IIA and IIB)	Lymphoid immunophenotyping (formerly Limited IIA) is for laboratories that perform tests for any markers in addition to CD3/CD4 and CD3/CD8. T-lymphocyte immunophenotyping (formerly IIB) is for laboratories performing only CD3/CD4 and CD3/CD8 testing.
Nonlymphoid immunophenotyping (formerly Limited III)	Quantification of nonmalignant cells other than lymphocytes, e.g., stem cell analysis, PNH, or LAD
Malignant leukocyte immunophenotyping (formerly Limited IV)	Use of flow cytometry to identify and characterize leukemias or lymphomas in blood and tissue specimens based on cell phenotype, including cell surface and cytoplasmic antigens, with or without ploidy analysis
Diagnostic immunology	Diagnostic services serology subcategories: (i) serological tests for autoantibodies except antibodies to blood cells and spermatozoa; (ii) serological tests for specific markers of infectious diseases or exposure to such diseases, excluding HIV; (iii) tests for nonspecific indicators of infectious diseases or exposure to such diseases; and (iv) IgA, IgE, IgG, IgM, C3, C4, and alpha-1 antitrypsin
	Donor services serology subcategory: for donor banks and laboratories under contract to donor banks that perform any tests on donors of human organs, tissues, and/or blood for transfer, transfusion, or transplantation
HIV	For laboratories performing serological or molecular tests for HIV for diagnostic or prognostic purposes. This category encompasses three subcategories: (i) screening tests only, (ii) general, and (iii) viral identification.
Histocompatibility	Identification of HLA antigens
General	Laboratories performing all phases of histocompatibility testing for organ or tissue transplantation, including MHC class I and class II antigen typing, HLA antibody screening, and, when necessary, cross-matching hold a permit for this category.
HLA typing	This category is for laboratories offering only HLA antigen typing, HLA antibody screening, and/or mixed-lymphocyte cultures. This category would apply to those laboratories performing histocompatibility testing or initial antigen typing for transplant purposes. Laboratories that perform HLA antigen typing for parentage testing only and not as a diagnostic test need only hold a permit in the category of parentage/identity testing only.
Transplant monitoring	This category is for laboratories performing testing for STR to monitor the success of engraftment following the transplantation of hematopoietic progenitor cells (e.g., bone marrow) or other molecular tests to monitor the success of transplant procedures.
Cytokines	This category includes the quantification of cytokines in serum, plasma, or CSF.

[a] Other categories related to a clinical immunology laboratory include fetal defect markers and immunohematology. Abbreviations: CSF, cerebrospinal fluid; PNH, paroxysmal nocturnal hemoglobinuria; LAD, leukocyte adhesion deficiency; MHC, major histocompatibility complex; STR, short tandem repeats.

procedures, and many other details which are necessary for the documentation of appropriate laboratory practice. The requirements by these agencies are equal to or, in most cases, greater than those mandated by CLIA.

LAP

The Laboratory Accreditation Program (LAP) of the CAP has been in existence since 1962 and since that time has developed into the world's largest single voluntary clinical laboratory improvement program. The LAP has been granted deemed status by CMS and is recognized by JCAHO as an equivalent program in JCAHO-accredited institutions. There are currently over 6,000 laboratories accredited by the CAP in the United States and abroad. The focus of the LAP is the use of an educational, peer

review inspection process using teams of laboratory professionals as inspectors. The CAP gives working laboratorians an opportunity to participate in the inspection process. By visiting and inspecting peer laboratories a significant educational component is added to the accreditation process. The CAP selects a team of inspectors of practicing pathologists, laboratory scientists, and medical technologists who are matched to the laboratory's profile as closely as possible. All aspects of the laboratory's operation are evaluated in this process, from sample acquisition to general laboratory management.

The process to become accredited by the CAP begins with the submission of an application. The CAP then forwards to the laboratory checklists for each of the laboratory sections. The checklists are developed and approved by CAP committees and address each laboratory discipline. There are frequent revisions of the checklists to reflect the ever-changing profile of laboratory testing and regulations. It is advisable to check the CAP website (Table 1) to review the current checklists. Since the checklists that are sent to the labs are the checklists that the inspectors use during the on-site visit, the laboratory should review all items and address any deficiencies or problem areas prior to the inspection. The major areas that are covered in the checklist include proficiency testing, quality control and quality improvement (e.g., supervision, procedure manuals, specimen collection and handling, reporting of results, reagents, calibration, controls and standards, instruments, and equipment), personnel, physical facilities, and laboratory safety. Next, the CAP selects an inspection team, and a mutually acceptable date is set for the inspection. However, in 2006, the CAP will conduct unannounced inspections. During the inspection process the inspectors conduct a thorough inspection of each phase of the laboratory's operation using the checklists as guides. After the inspection, the inspectors meet with the laboratory staff for a summation conference to review the findings. The inspectors leave a copy of the final summation report, and the laboratory must correct any deficiencies and provide any requested documents to the CAP. If the deficiencies are corrected to the satisfaction of the CAP, the laboratory is accredited for a 2-year cycle but conducts a self-inspection at the 1-year mark using the most current checklists.

JCAHO

More than 19,000 health care organizations are accredited by JCAHO in the United States and in several foreign countries. JCAHO began evaluating hospital laboratory services in 1979. In 1995 JCAHO's standards were deemed to be certifiable under CLIA '88.

Generally a medical technologist surveyor is assigned to review the laboratory's activities and policies. During the on-site survey, the surveyor will look at administrative, technical, safety, and infection control policies and procedures as well as proficiency testing records. In addition, surveyors will meet with laboratory directors and managers to determine their involvement in the operation of the organization. Specifically, they will be seeking information on the communication between the clinical staff, administrators, and other departments; reviewing in-services; and evaluating the oversight of the laboratory testing and quality assessment and improvement activities. While visiting each laboratory section, the surveyor will review section-specific policies and procedures, infection control and safety practices, preventive maintenance, quality control, and proficiency testing results. The surveyor will also visit patient care areas to assess the processes for testing, specimen collection, and requesting and reporting of results and blood transfusions.

ASHI

ASHI has set standards for histocompatibility testing for many years. The standards include the following areas: general policies, personnel qualifications, quality assurance, HLA antigens, serological typing—HLA class I and II antigens, mixed-leukocyte culture tests, antibody screening, renal transplantation, non-renal organ transplantation, marrow transplantation, platelet and granulocyte transfusion, disease association, parentage testing, nucleic acid analysis, flow cytometry, and enzyme-linked immunosorbent assays. ASHI

maintains these standards and conducts inspections of laboratories for licensing as well as assisting in the certification of technologist and director level individuals (Table 1).

Proficiency Testing

A significant ongoing requirement of all accrediting agencies is the regular performance of testing on blinded samples. Testing should be done in a manner identical to that for patient samples and the results then sent to be compared to those from other laboratories performing testing in a similar manner. Laboratories must show evidence that they are enrolled, participate in a regular proficiency testing process, and regularly review results and make corrections to problems and errors discovered in the process of the testing. In addition, a subset of tests are "regulated analytes" in which a continuing good performance is necessary in order for the laboratory to be able to bill Medicare and Medicaid for these tests. Regulated tests in the immunology laboratory include a number of assays usually performed by nephelometry (IgG, IgA, IgM, IgE, C-reactive protein [CRP], C3, C4, haptoglobin, and alpha-1 antitrypsin) and a few serology tests, including tests for rheumatoid factor, infectious mononucleosis, rubella, and ANA. Any tests performed by laboratories in which proficiency testing is unavailable must be shown to be performing correctly in some other manner. This may include trading samples with other laboratories, regular review of clinical appropriateness, or other strategies.

The CAP is the proficiency test supplier with the largest range of test samples supplied. Details of the surveys available and the analytes contained in each survey are available on the CAP website (Table 1). Many other organizations, including ASHI, the CDC Model Performance Evaluation Program, and certain state programs also supply proficiency materials. A variety of manufacturers of reagents and instruments also produce proficiency testing or quality control materials with which results from labs are compared to each other.

INTERNATIONAL ISSUES AND AGENCIES

While U.S. medical laboratories are required to follow guidelines established by CLIA, laboratories outside of the United States have, in many cases, developed systems for assessment of quality that follow international standards. One such organization is the ISO, headquartered in Geneva, Switzerland. The ISO is a nongovernmental federation of national standards bodies from over 100 countries worldwide. Established in 1947, the mission of the ISO "is to promote the development of standardization and related activities in the world with a view to facilitating the international exchange of goods and services, and to developing cooperation in the spheres of intellectual, scientific, technological and economic activity." During the 1970s and 1980s, with an increase in the global economy, companies found a wide variation in the quality of the goods and services they purchased from sources all over the world. From this the ISO developed internationally accepted standards to ensure product quality. In 1987, the ISO published the ISO 9000 series of international standards and guidelines on quality management and quality assurance. For clinical laboratories, document ISO/TC 212, CD 15189, addresses standardization and guidance in the field of laboratory medicine and in vitro diagnostic test systems. In addition to quality management areas discussed in this document, pre- and postanalytical procedures, analytical performance, laboratory safety, reference systems, and quality assurance are included. Certification by the ISO is a voluntary activity.

In addition to the ISO, other nongovernmental organizations are involved in laboratory quality assurance at the international level (8). These include the International Federation of Clinical Chemistry and Laboratory Medicine (IFCC) and the WHO. The IFCC interacts with several international professional organizations involved in laboratory medicine, including the International Union of Immunological Societies and the World Association of Societies of Pathology and Laboratory Medicine. Among the national organizations are the CLSI (formerly the National Committee for Clinical Laboratory Standards) in the United States and the Institute for Standardization and Documentation in Medical Laboratory in Germany. Regional organizations include the Asian Pacific and Latin American Federation of Clinical Biochemists. In addition to Germany, many other countries in Europe and several clinical

laboratory professional organizations have been actively involved in quality systems and accreditation issues. Among these are the European Communities Confederation of Clinical Chemistry and Laboratory Medicine (7, 10) and External Peer Review Techniques. Further information about the activities of these organizations can be found on their websites (Table 1).

A peer review system for the accreditation of pathology laboratory services in the United Kingdom was inaugurated in 1992. The CPA (Table 1) is associated with the Royal College of Pathologists, the Association of Clinical Pathologists, the Association of Clinical Biochemists, the Institute of Biomedical Science, the Independent Healthcare Association, and the Institute of Health Services Management. The operation functions in a manner similar to that of the CAP in the United States. There are advisory committees that define and review standards, assess applications, recommend inspectors, and advise on decisions after inspection. Survey

TABLE 3 Credentialing agencies and programs[a]

Level	Certifying agency or program	Organization	Education level required	Examination frequency	Website
Director	American Board of Medical Laboratory Immunology	ASM	Ph.D. or M.D. and appropriate experience	Annual	http://www.asm.org
Director	American Board of Medical Microbiology	ASM	Ph.D. or M.D. and appropriate experience	Annual	http://www.asm.org
Director	American Board of Histocompatibility and Immunogenetics	ASHI	Ph.D. or M.D. and appropriate experience	Annual	http://www.ashi-hla.org
Director	American Board of Clinical Chemistry (Immunology)	AACC	Ph.D. and appropriate experience	Annual	http://www.aacc.org
Director	American Board of Clinical Chemistry (Molecular Diagnostics)	AACC	Ph.D. and appropriate experience	Annual	http://www.aacc.org
Director	American Board of Allergy, Asthma and Immunology	AAAAI	M.D. and appropriate experience	Annual	http://www.aaaai.org
Director	CAP (Immunopathology)	ASCP	M.D. and appropriate experience	Biannual	http://www.cap.org
Manager/supervisor	ASCP—Specialist, Immunology	ASCP	B.S. and appropriate experience	Annual	http://www.ascp.org
Manager/supervisor	Clinical Histocompatibility	ABHI	B.S. and appropriate experience	Annual	http://www.ashi-hla.org
Specialist	Flow Cytometry Certificate	ASCP	Appropriate experience	Annual	http://www.ascp.org
Technologist	ASCP—Immunology (only)	ASCP	B.S. and internship	Biannual	http://www.ascp.org
Technologist	ASCP—(General)	ASCP	B.S. and internship	Annual	http://www.ascp.org
Technologist	ASCP—Histology	ASCP	B.S. and internship	Annual	http://www.ascp.org
Technologist	Clinical Histocompatibility	ASHI	B.S. and appropriate experience	Annual	http://www.ashi-hla.org
Specialist	Clinical Histocompatibility	ASHI	B.S. and appropriate experience	Annual	http://www.ashi-hla.org
Technician	ASCP—MLT (General)	ASCP	Associate degree and appropriate experience	Annual	http://www.ascp.org

[a] See text for abbreviations.

teams of voluntary inspectors, each with expertise in the laboratory's specific disciplines, conduct on-site inspections. The inspectors are drawn from practicing pathologists and clinical or biomedical scientists. A recent paper discusses the accreditation process (3).

For a laboratory to become accredited, the process begins with the laboratory assessing itself against the relevant CPA standards, making application, and being subjected to an on-site inspection in order to determine compliance with the standards. After the relevant advisory committee has reviewed the inspectors' assessment, a report is sent back to the laboratory. If there are no problems with the on-site inspection of the laboratory, the board issues a 12-month certificate. If deficiencies are found, accreditation is withheld until the deficiencies have been corrected to the satisfaction of the CPA. When the laboratory has major deficiencies, approval is withheld until the deficiencies have been corrected. In this case reapplication is required. Accreditation is valid for 4 years, with the CPA reserving the right to reinspect at any time without notice. There is a requirement for an annual reregistration and a self-declaration stating continuing compliance with the standards.

CREDENTIALING

A number of organizations are involved in issuing credentials or licenses for individuals who demonstrate technical and management skills in clinical immunology. These programs generally include two components, one which establishes guidelines for training programs and a second which creates and administers the examination process. It is important for all individuals involved in clinical immunology laboratory practice to obtain appropriate certification. These programs encourage professionalism for their members and provide core groups of exceptionally qualified leaders in laboratory immunology. A list of professional societies which provide credentialing programs is shown in Table 3.

LABORATORY STANDARDS

Several professional and voluntary organizations have developed standards for the testing of clinical specimens and provide reagents for the standardization of assays. Among those organizations that have developed procedural standards is the CLSI. The CLSI is a professional volunteer organization that creates standards documents for the testing of clinical samples. A committee of experts develops a document that describes GLP for a test or analyte. After the committee creates a draft, the documents go through three stages, a "proposed" status in which a wide and thorough review takes place, then in some cases a "tentative" stage when the document needs a thorough field evaluation period or when specific data need to be collected, and finally "approved" status when the guideline has achieved wide consensus in the field. Although these are not mandatory guidelines, they are

TABLE 4 Immunology standardization documents available from the CLSI

Document/status [a]	Title
DI02-A2-A	*Immunoprecipitin Analysis: Procedures for Evaluating the Performance of Materials*
DI03-A	*Agglutination Analyses: Antibody Characteristics, Methodology, Limitations, and Clinical Validation*
I/LA20-A	*Quality Assurance for the Indirect Immunofluorescence Test for Autoantibodies to Nuclear Antigen (IFA-ANA)*
I/LA6-A	*Detection and Quantitation of Rubella IgG Antibody: Evaluation and Performance Criteria for Multiple Component Test Products, Specimen Handling, and Use of Test Products in the Clinical Laboratory*
I/LA13-A	*Human Immunodeficiency Virus Type I, Reference Material Specifications*
I/LA15-A	*Apolipoprotein Immunoassays: Development and Recommended Performance Characteristics*
I/LA19-A	*Specifications for Immunological Testing for Infectious Diseases*
I/LA20-A	*Evaluation Methods and Analytical Performance Characteristics of Immunological Assays for Human Immunoglobulin E (IgE) Antibodies of Defined Allergen Specificities*
H42-A	*Clinical Applications of Flow Cytometry: Quality Assurance and Immunophenotyping of Lymphocytes*
H43-A	*Clinical Applications of Flow Cytometry: Immunophenotyping of Leukemic Cells*
H44-A	*Methods for Reticulocyte Counting (Flow Cytometry and Supravital Dyes)*
I/LA21-P	*Clinical Evaluation of Immunoassays*
I/LA1-A2	*Assessing the Quality of Radioimmunoassay Systems (2nd ed.)*
MM2-A	*Immunoglobulin and T Cell Receptor Gene Rearrangement Assays*
MM3-A	*Molecular Diagnostic Methods for Infectious Diseases*
MM4-A	*Quality Assurance for Immunocytochemistry*
MM9-A	*Nucleic Acid Sequencing Methods in Diagnostic Laboratory Medicine*
MM14-A	*Proficiency Testing (External Quality Assessment) for Molecular Methods*
M34-P	*Western Blot Assay for Antibodies to Borrelia burgdorferi*
M29-A	*Protection of Laboratory Workers from Instrument Biohazards and Infectious Disease Transmitted by Blood, Body Fluids, and Tissue*
GP2-A3	*Clinical Laboratory Technical Procedure Manuals*
GP29-A	*Assessment of Laboratory Tests when Proficiency Testing Is Not Available*

[a] A, approved; P, proposed.

TABLE 5 Available standards and reference materials

Standard material	Sponsoring organizations[a]	Analytes available[b]
Reference plasma protein (CRM/BCR 470)	CAP, BRC, IFCC	IgG, IgA, IgM, C3, C4, albumin, alpha-1 antitrypsin, alpha-1-acid glycoprotein, alpha-2 macroglobulin, haptoglobin, transferrin, ceruloplasmin, prealbumin, CRP
Autoantibodies	CLB, NIBSC, CDC	Homogeneous ANA (WHO66/233), anti-dsDNA (Wo/80), smooth muscle antibody (WHO106), RF (WHO1066), CRP (85/506)
WHO reference materials	NIBSC, WHO	RF, ASO, antithyroglobulin, antimicrosomal, TPO, antimitochondrial, anticardiolipin, HIV-1 and HCV RNA, rubella and other infectious disease sera, IgG subclasses, etc.
ANA and ENA[c] sera	AMLI	AF/CDC1 to AF/CDC10; homogeneous, speckled, nucleolar, centromere ANAs; SS-A, SS-B, Sm, U1-RNP, Scl-70, and Jo-1 antibodies
Anti-SS-A/Ro	CAP	Anti-SS-A/Ro (no. C103BG)
Cytokines, interleukins, and growth factors	NCI, NIBSC	Cytokines IFN-α, IFN-β, IFN-γ, IL-1a, IL-1b, IL-2, IL-3, IL-4, IL-5, IL-6, IL-7, IL-8, IL-9, IL-10, LIF, G-CSF, GM-CSF, M-CSF, SCF, TGF-β1, TNF-α, TNF-β, RANTES

[a]Addresses of sponsoring organizations: AMLI, P.O. Box 25, 18500 Barnesville Rd., Barnesville, MD 20838 (http://www.amli.org); BRC, European Community Bureau of References (materials available through NIBSC and IRMM); CAP, 325 Waukegan Rd., Northfield, IL 60093-2759 (http://www.cap.org); CDC, ANA Reference Laboratory, CDC Immunology Branch, Atlanta, GA 30333; CLB, Central Laboratory of The Netherlands, Red Cross Blood Transfusion Service, Plesmanlaan 125, Amsterdam, The Netherlands [phone, 31 (0) 20 512 9222] (http://www.clb.nl); IFCC, http://194.79.144.120/index.html (reagents obtained from IRMM); IRMM, Institute for Reference Materials and Measurements, Retieseweg, B-2440, Geel, Belgium [phone, 132 (0) 14 571 211] (http://www.irmm.jrc.bel); NCI, Craig Reynolds, Biological Response Modifiers Program, NCI-FCRDC, Building 1052, Room 253, Frederick, MD 21702; NIBSC, National Institute of Biological Standards and Controls, Blanche Lane, South Mimms, Potters Bar, Herts, EN6 3QG, United Kingdom (http://www.nibsc.ac.uk); WHO, World Health Organization Immunology Unit, Geneva, Switzerland (http://www.who.org).

[b]dsDNA, double-stranded DNA; RF, rheumatoid factor; ASO, anti-streptolysin O; TPO, thyroid peroxidase; HCV, hepatitis C virus; IFN, interferon; IL, interleukin; LIF, leukemia inhibitory factor; G-CSF, granulocyte colony-stimulating factor; GM-CSF, granulocyte-macrophage colony-stimulating factor; M-CSF, macrophage colony-stimulating factor; TGF, transforming growth factor; TNF, tumor necrosis factor.

[c]ENA, extractable nuclear antigen.

useful documents and in some cases are used as the basis for acceptable performance on inspection checklists for laboratory certification agencies such as the CAP. Table 4 contains a list of available CLSI guidelines for immunology tests. Additional information can be found at the CLSI website (Table 1). Occasionally agencies such as the CDC have published guidelines for the performance of laboratory testing of importance to the clinical immunology laboratory. For example, in 1997 the CDC published guidelines for CD4+-cell determination in persons infected with human immunodeficiency virus (HIV) (4).

The Standards Committee of the AMLI has recently provided an autoantibody reference preparation of 10 sera (http://amli.org/standards.htm). The antibody specificities represented on the panel include double-stranded DNA, SS-A, SS-B, Sm, ribonucleoprotein, Scl-70, centromere, Jo-1, and two negative sera. The Standards Committee has also begun to evaluate and produce other serum panels for detection of cardiolipin, neutrophil cytoplasmic, ribosomal P, thyroid peroxidase, thyroglobulin, tissue transglutaminase, and gliadin autoantibodies. The CDC and the Arthritis Foundation have also described a similar panel of reference sera (11). The IFCC provides serum reference materials for several assays that are performed in the clinical immunology laboratory, including assays for C3, C4, CRP, IgG, IgA, IgM, and prostate-specific antigen (PSA). The Association of the Teaching of Immunology of the French Language Universities maintains a website where reference serum preparations are discussed (http://www.assim.refer.org/serumr~1.htm). In addition, a complete list of national and international reference preparations for the clinical immunology laboratory has recently been published (9). Finally, several companies provide reference serum preparations. For example, Zeus Scientific Company (Raritan, N.J.) provides reference sera for enzyme-linked immunosorbent assay procedures. For further information on available standards and reference materials, see Table 5.

REFERENCES

1. **Bogdanich, W.** 1987. Medical labs, trusted as largely error-free, are far from infallible. *Wall Street Journal*, 2 February 1987, p. 1.
2. **Bogdanich, W.** 1987. The Pap test misses much cervical cancer through labs' errors. *Wall Street Journal*, 2 November 1987, p. 1.
3. **Burnett, D., C. Blair, M. R. Haeney, S. L. Jeffcoate, K. W. M. Scott, and D. L. Williams.** 2002. Clinical pathology accreditation: standards for the medical laboratory. *J. Clin. Pathol.* **55:**729–733.

4. **Centers for Disease Control and Prevention.** 1997. 1997 revised guidelines for performing CD4+ T-cell determinations in persons infected with human immunodeficiency virus (HIV). *Morb. Mortal. Wkly. Rep.* **10:**1–29.

5. **College of American Pathologists.** 1998. "Statline." **14** (20):2–3. 14 October 1998.

6. **Federal Register.** 1997. Medical devices; classification/reclassification; restricted devices; analyte specific reagents. 21 CFR 809. Final rule. *Fed. Regist.* **62:** 62243–62260.

7. **Jansen, R. T., V. Blaton, D. Burnett, W. Huisman, J. M. Querealto, S. Zerah, and B. Allman.** 1997. Essential criteria for quality systems in medical laboratories. *Eur. J. Clin. Chem. Clin. Biochem.* **35:**121–122.

8. **McQueen, M. J.** 1997. Laboratory quality assurance at the international level: the role of nongovernmental organizations. *J. Int. Fed. Clin. Chem.* **9:**144–146.

9. **Nakamura, R. M.** 1998. National and international reference preparations for the clinical diagnostic immunology laboratory, p. 54–63. *In* R. M. Nakamura, C. L. Burek, L. Cook, J. D. Folds, and J. L. Sever (ed.), *Clinical Diagnostic Immunology, Protocols in Quality Assurance and Standardization.* Blackwell Science, Inc., Malden, Mass.

10. **Sanders, G. T., R. T. Jansen, G. Beastall, E. Gurr, D. Kenny, K. P. Kohse, and S. Zerah.** 1999. Recent activities of EC4 in the harmonization of clinical chemistry in the European Union. *Clin. Chem. Lab. Med.* **37:**477–480.

11. **Smolen, J. S., B. Butcher, M. J. Fritzler, T. Gordon, J. Hardin, J. R. Kalden, R. Lahita, R. N. Maini, W. Reeves, M. Reichlin, N. Rothfield, Y. Takasaki, W. J. van Venrooij, and E. M. Tan.** 1997. Reference sera for antinuclear antibodies. II. Further definition of antibody specificities in international antinuclear antibody reference sera by immunofluorescence and western blotting. *Arthritis Rheum.* **40:**413–418.

12. **U.S. Department of Health and Human Services.** 1988. The Clinical Laboratory Improvement Amendments of 1988. Public Law 100–578.

13. **U.S. Department of Health and Human Services.** 1992. Medicare, Medicaid and CLIA programs: regulations implementing the Clinical Laboratory Improvement Amendments of 1988 (CLIA). *Fed. Regist.* **57:**7002–7243.

14. **U.S. Department of Health and Human Services.** 1980. *Survey Procedures and Interpretative Guidelines for Laboratories and Laboratory Services.* HCFA State Operations Manual. Health Care Financing Administration and Food and Drug Administration, Baltimore, Md.

15. **U.S. Department of Health and Human Services, Office of the Inspector General.** 1998. Compliance program guidance for clinical laboratories. *Fed. Regist.* **63:**8987–8998.

16. **Wanamaker, V.** 1999. Health Care Financing Administration/Clinical Laboratory Improvement Amendments of 1988. *Arch. Pathol. Lab. Med.* **123:**478–481.

Author Index

Subject Index

About the Author

ANNA BRADY is Assistant Professor and bibliographer for Irish Studies and Women's Studies at Queens College, City University of New York. She is the compiler of *Union List of Film Periodicals* (Greenwood Press, 1984).

DATE DUE

Demco, Inc. 38-293